D1476300

COLOR PLATES

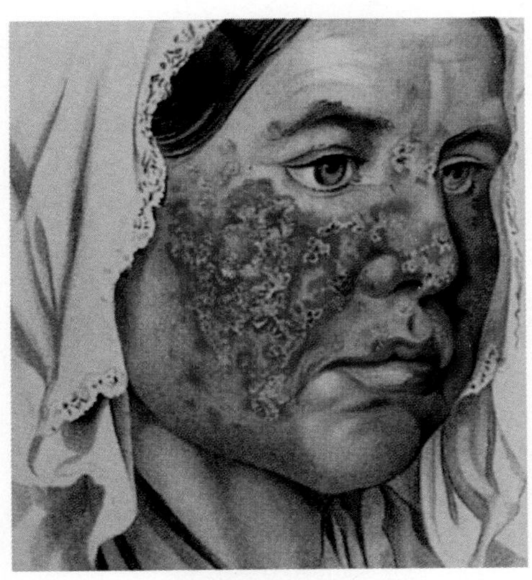

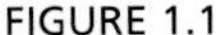

FIGURE 1.1

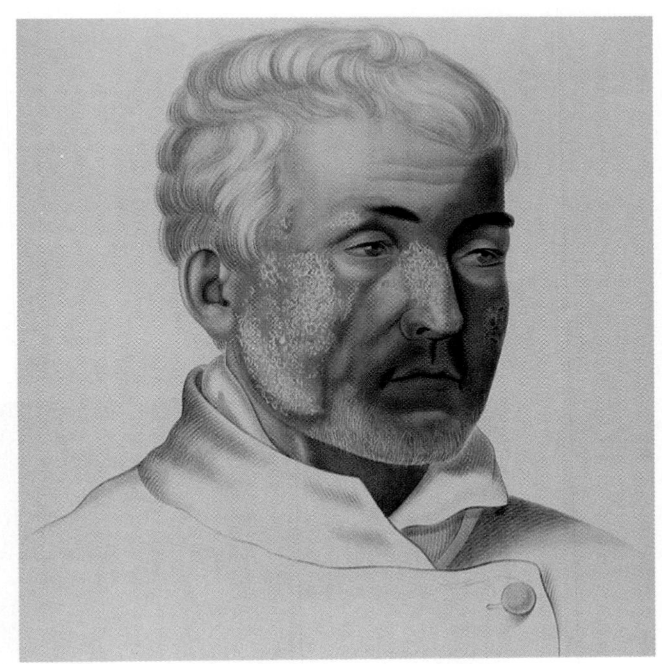

FIGURE 1.2

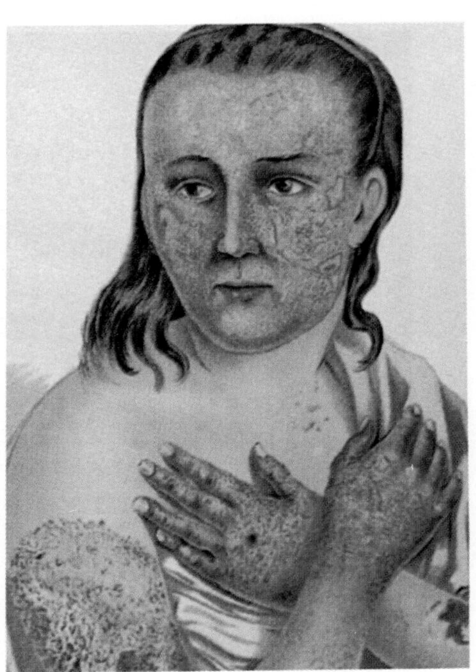

FIGURE 1.3

A 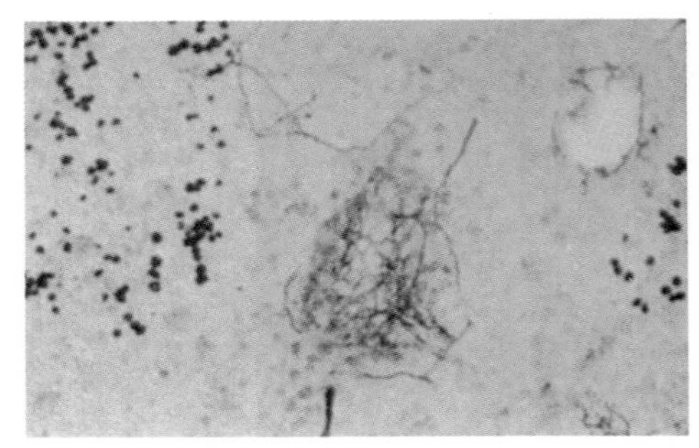 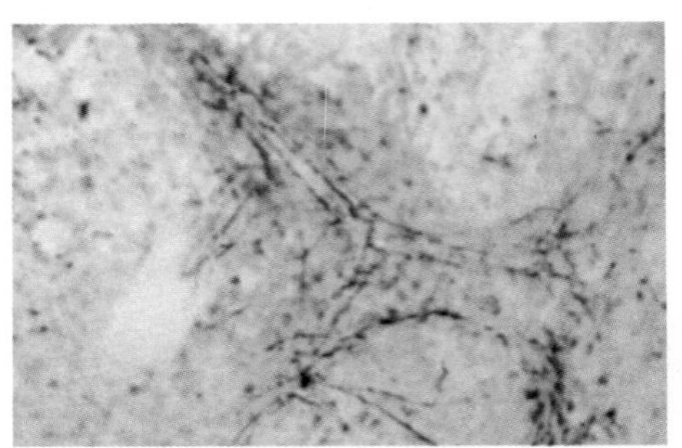 B

FIGURE 17.10

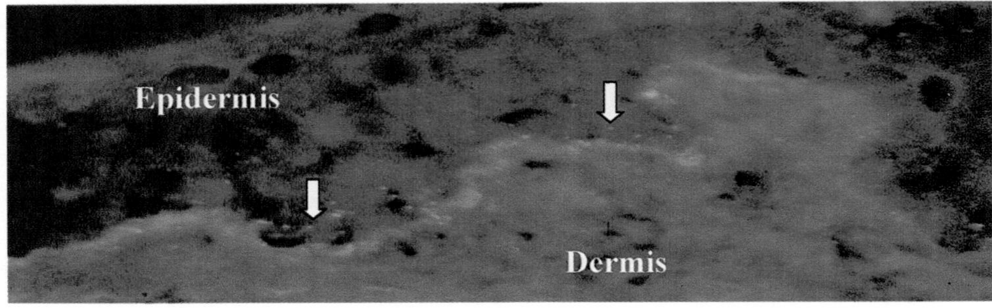

FIGURE 28.4

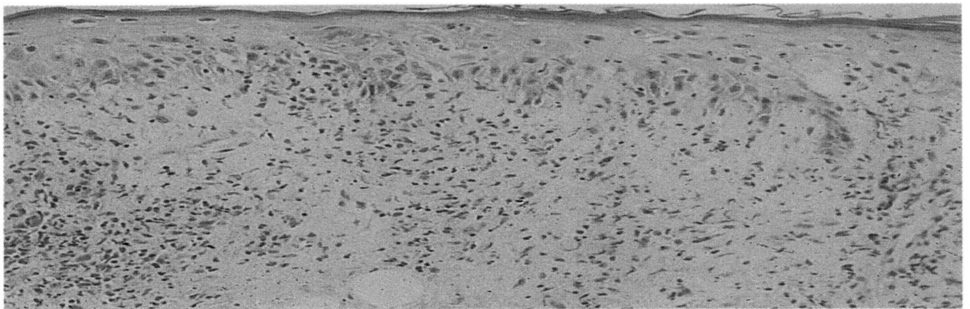

FIGURE 28.5

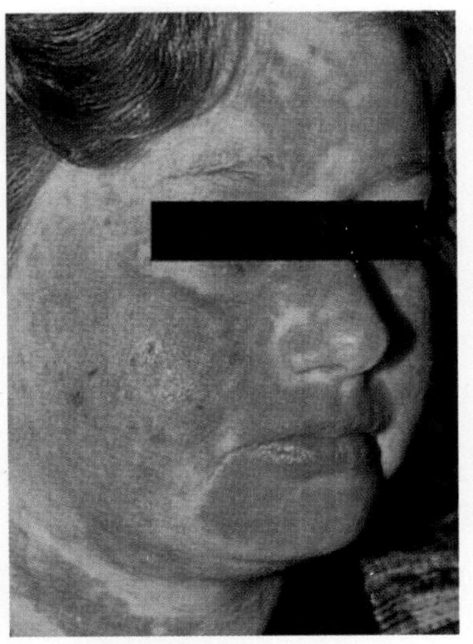

FIGURE 29.1

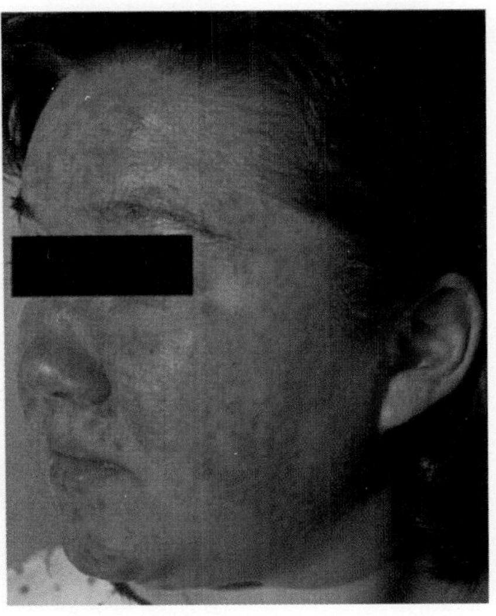

FIGURE 29.2

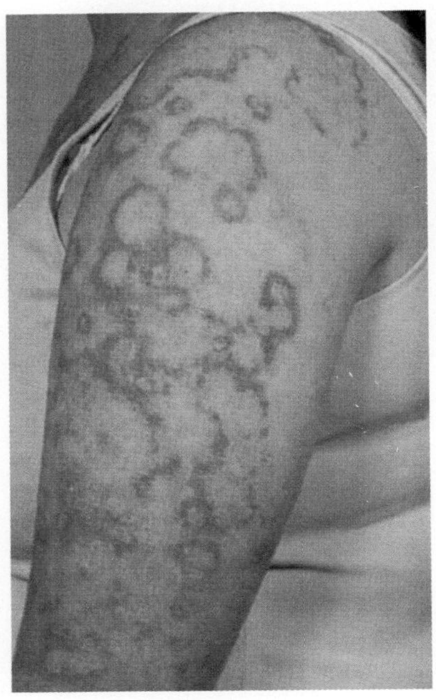

FIGURE 29.7

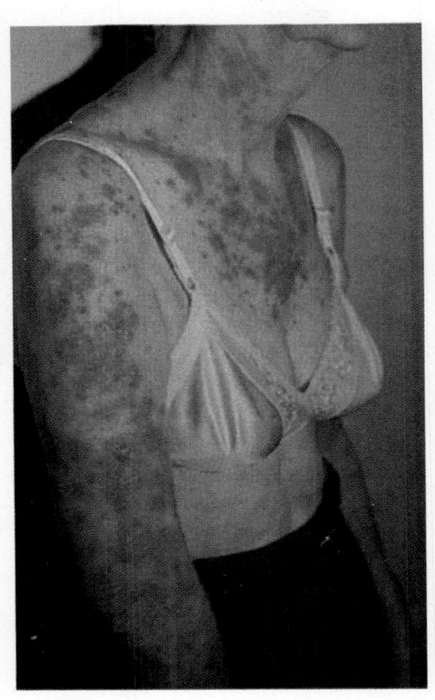

FIGURE 29.8

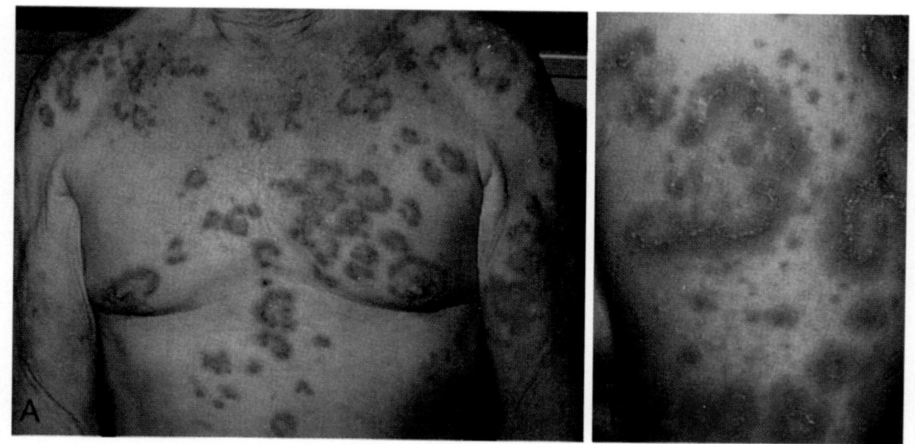

FIGURE 29.12

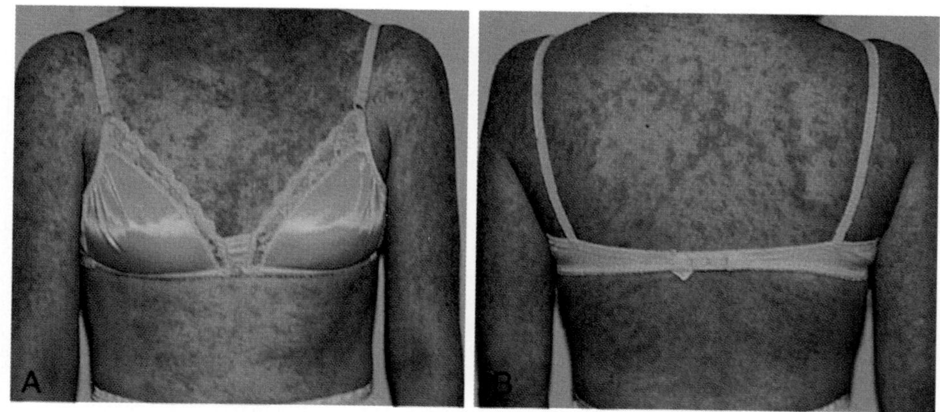

FIGURE 29.13

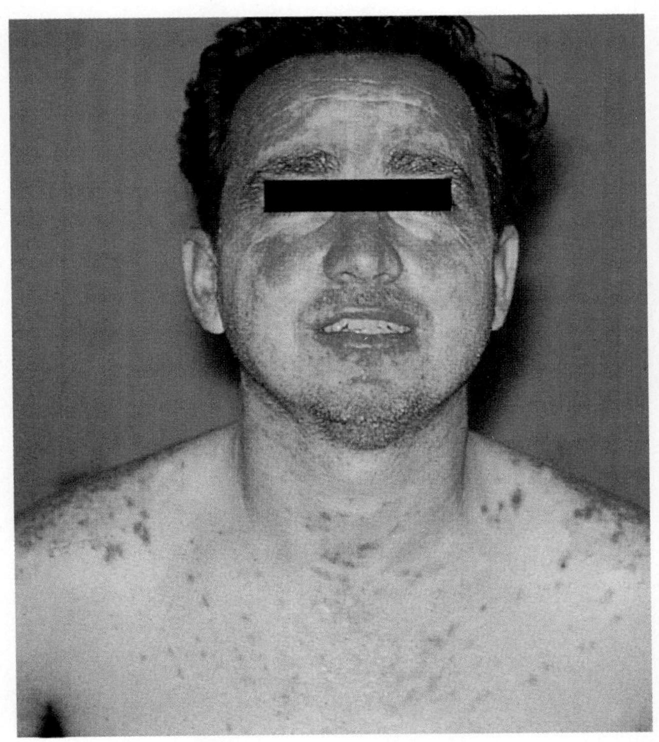

FIGURE 29.15

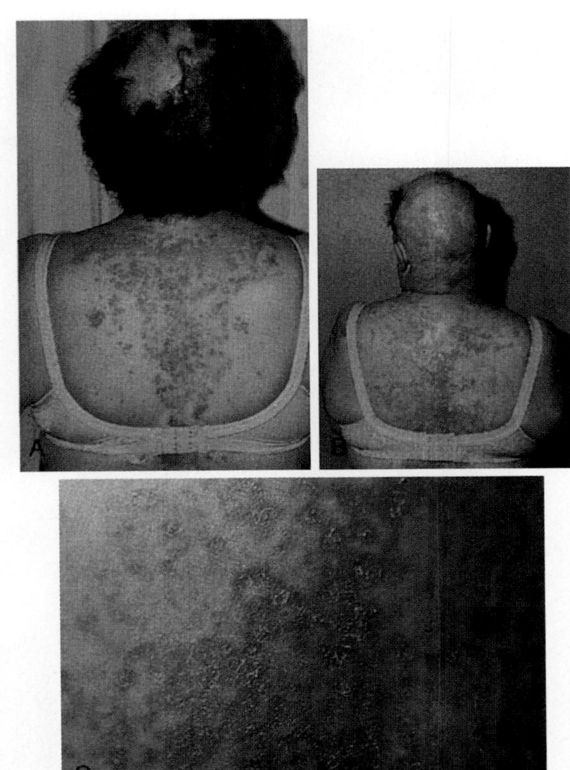

FIGURE 29.16

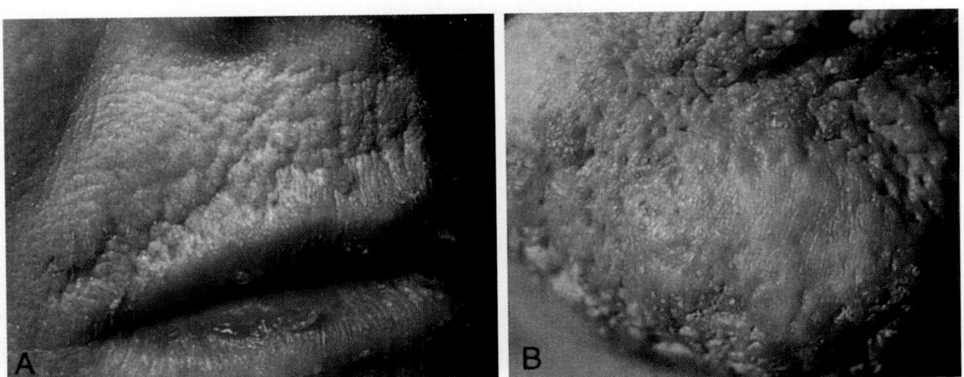

FIGURE 29.23

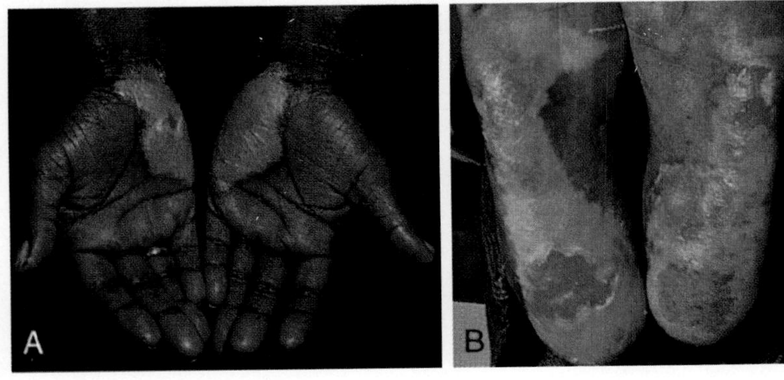

FIGURE 29.28

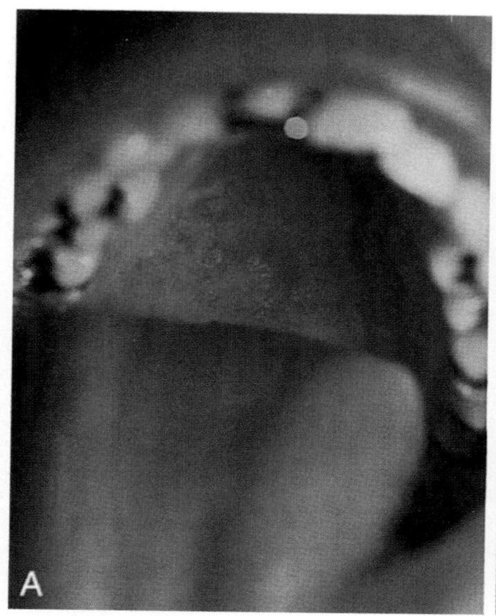

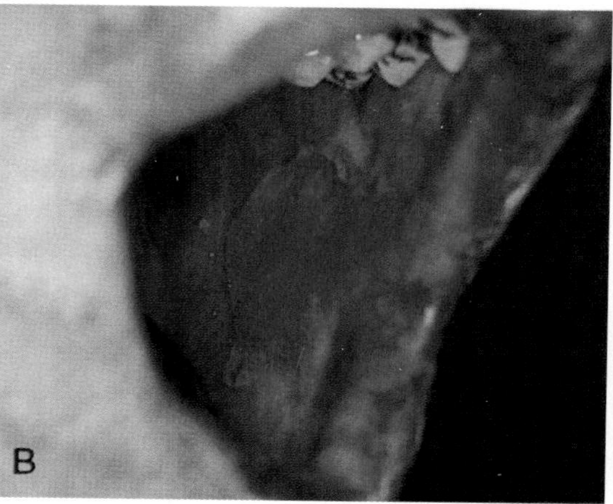

FIGURE 29.34

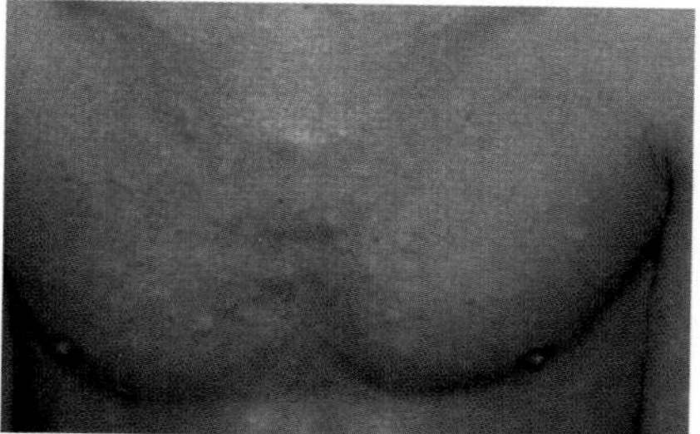

FIGURE 29.44

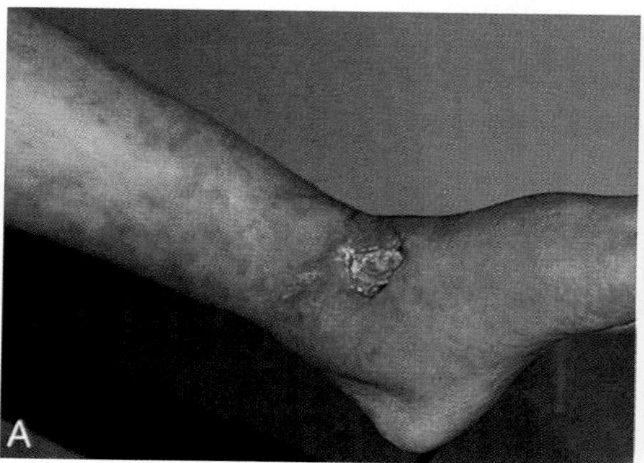

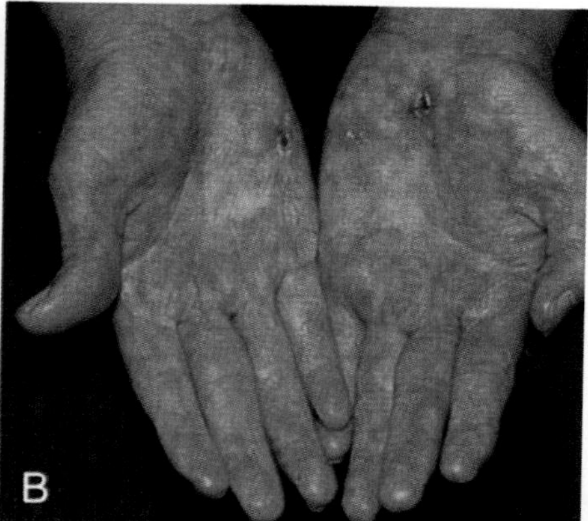

FIGURE 29.45

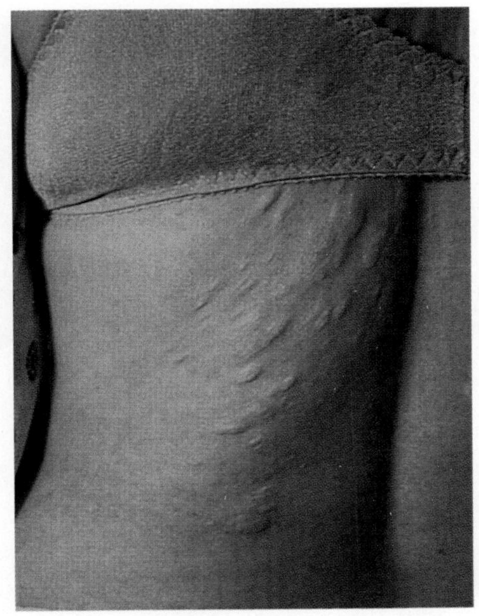

FIGURE 29.46

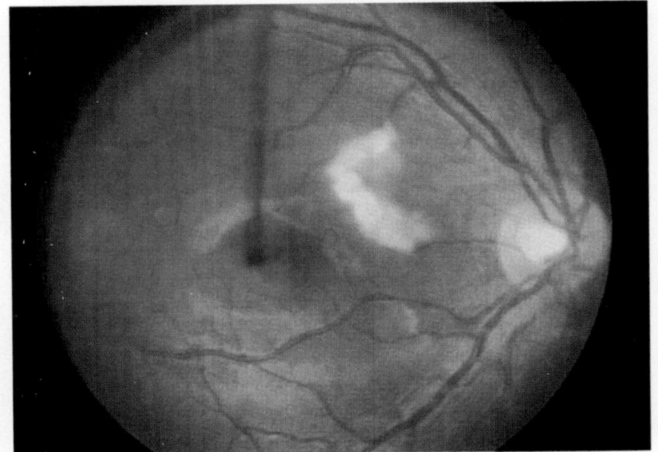

FIGURE 37.3

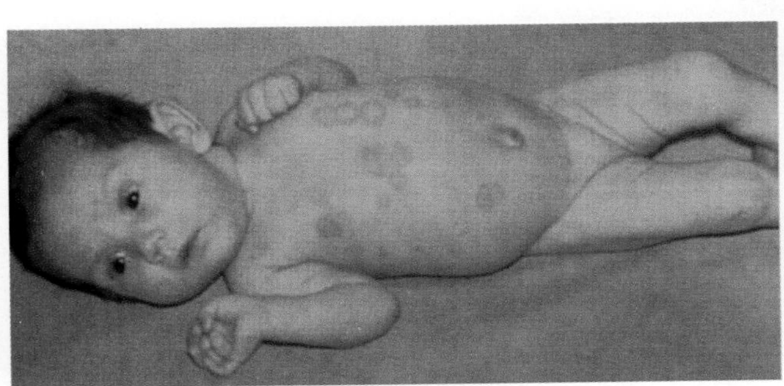

FIGURE 49.1

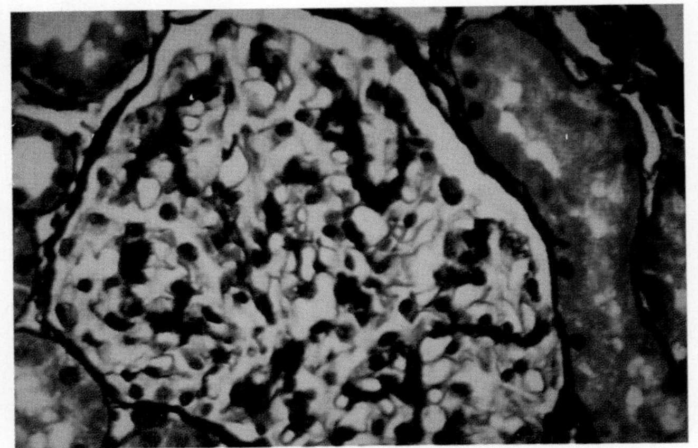

FIGURE 50.1

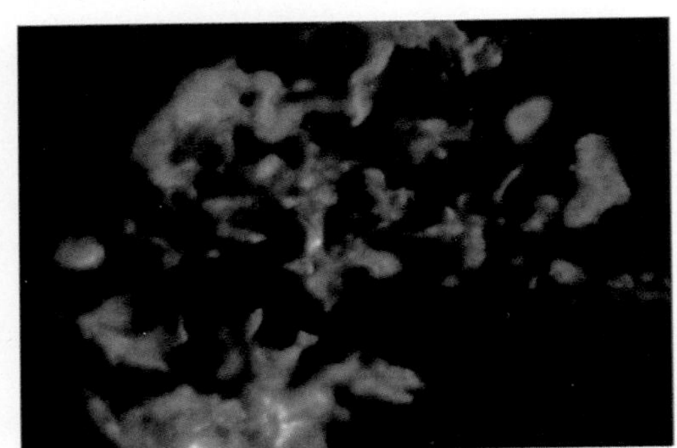

FIGURE 50.2

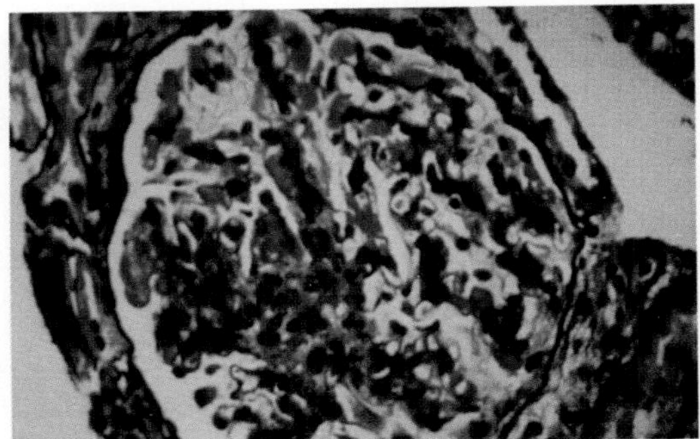

FIGURE 50.4

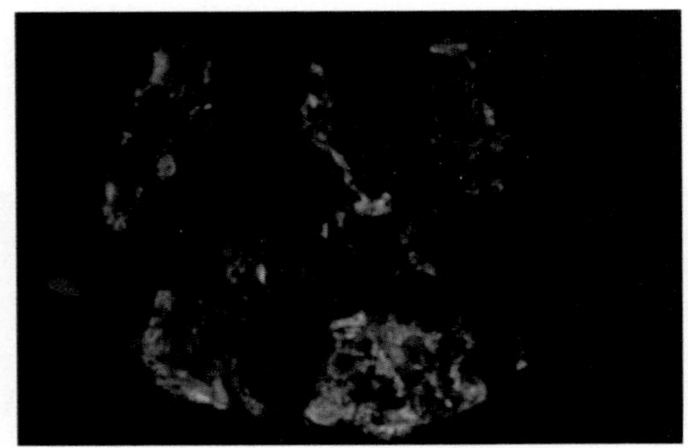

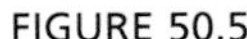

FIGURE 50.5

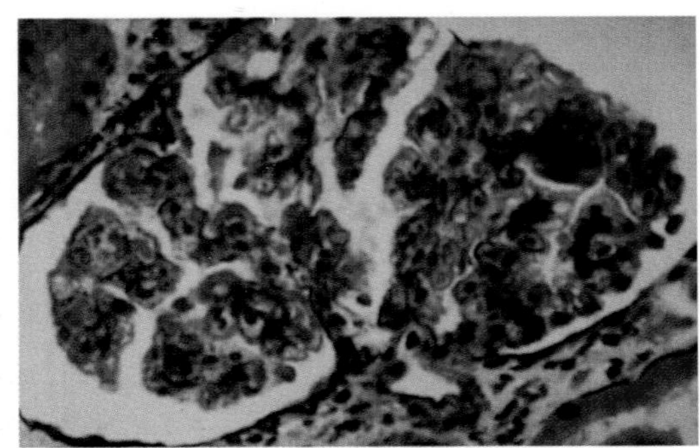

FIGURE 50.7

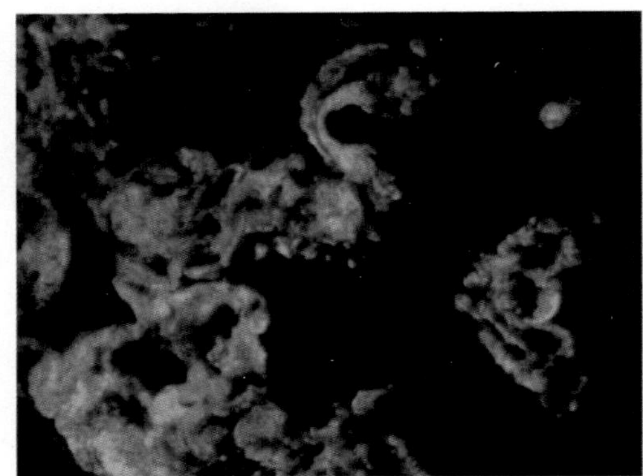

FIGURE 50.8

DUBOIS' LUPUS ERYTHEMATOSUS

SIXTH EDITION

DUBOIS' LUPUS ERYTHEMATOSUS

SIXTH EDITION

Editors

DANIEL J. WALLACE, M.D.

Clinical Professor of Medicine
Cedars-Sinai Medical Center
UCLA School of Medicine
Los Angeles, California

BEVRA HANNAHS HAHN, M.D.

Professor of Medicine
UCLA School of Medicine
Los Angeles, California

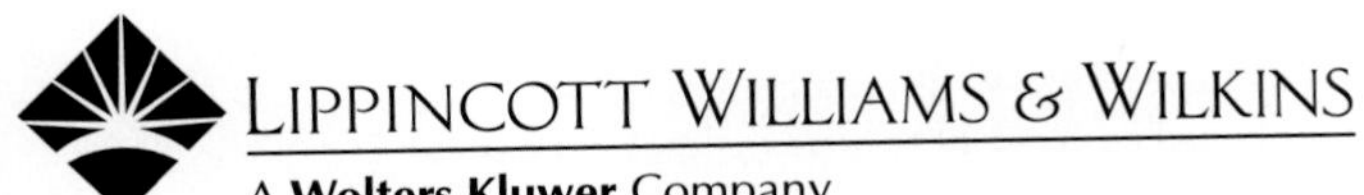

Philadelphia • Baltimore • New York • London
Buenos Aires • Hong Kong • Sydney • Tokyo

Acquisitions Editor: Richard Winters
Developmental Editor: Denise Martin
Production Editor: Robin E. Cook
Manufacturing Manager: Colin Warnock
Cover Designer: Mark Lerner
Compositor: Lippincott Williams & Wilkins Desktop Division
Printer: Maple Press

530 Walnut Street
Philadelphia, PA 19106 USA
LWW.com

Printed in the USA

Library of Congress Cataloging-in-Publication Data
Dubois' lupus erythematosus / editors, Daniel J. Wallace, Bevra Hannahs Hahn. — 6th ed.
p. ; cm.
Includes bibliographical references and index.
ISBN 0-7817-2464-3
1. Systemic lupus erythematosus. 2. Lupus erythematosus. I. Title: Lupus erythematosus. II. Wallace, Daniel J. (Daniel Jeffrey), 1949– III. Hahn, Bevra. IV. Dubois, Edmund L. Lupus erythematosus.
[DNLM: 1. Lupus Erythematosus, Discoid. 2. Lupus Erythematosus, Systemic. WR 152 D8152 2001]
RC924.5.L85 L87 2001
616.7′7—dc21

2001033875

Care has been taken to confirm the accuracy of the information presented and to describe generally accepted practices. However, the authors, editors, and publisher are not responsible for errors or omissions or for any consequences from application of the information in this book and make no warranty, expressed or implied, with respect to the currency, completeness, or accuracy of the contents of the publication. Application of this information in a particular situation remains the professional responsibility of the practitioner.

The authors, editors, and publisher have exerted every effort to ensure that drug selection and dosage set forth in this text are in accordance with current recommendations and practice at the time of publication. However, in view of ongoing research, changes in government regulations, and the constant flow of information relating to drug therapy and drug reactions, the reader is urged to check the package insert for each drug for any change in indications and dosage and for added warnings and precautions. This is particularly important when the recommended agent is a new or infrequently employed drug.

Some drugs and medical devices presented in this publication have Food and Drug Administration (FDA) clearance for limited use in restricted research settings. It is the responsibility of the health care provider to ascertain the FDA status of each drug or device planned for use in their clinical practice.

10 9 8 7 6 5 4 3 2 1

DEDICATION

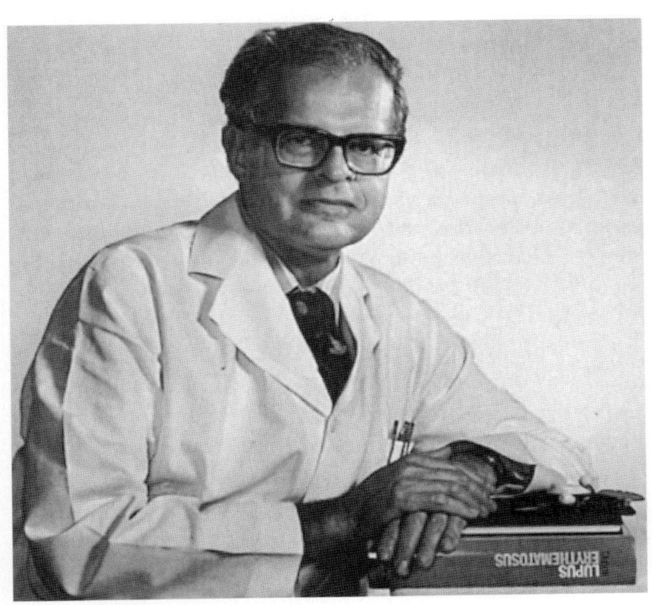

EDMUND LAWRENCE DUBOIS: 1923–1985

Edmund Lawrence Dubois (pronounced "Doo-Boyz") was born on June 28, 1923, to a middle-class Jewish family in Newark, New Jersey. He was the only child of a general surgeon, and his mother worked in the office. Ed, as he was known, graduated from high school in Newark in 1939. He then attended Johns Hopkins University, graduating with a bachelor's degree in 1943. While serving in the Army, he stayed in Baltimore to attend Johns Hopkins Medical School, where he also did his internship under A. McGehee Harvey, the legendary Chief of Service who was a lupus pioneer in his own right. Ed's tendency to know and train under the best and the brightest continued with a residency in medicine at the University of Utah under Max Wintrobe (author of the hematology textbook) and at Parkland Hospital in Dallas under Tinsley Harrison (author of Harrison's medicine textbook). He also completed an autopsy pathology fellowship at Los Angeles County General Hospital in 1948.

Ed decided to stay in Southern California and went into private practice at his father's office in July 1950. In 1951, he met—and, in 1952, married—Nancy Kully, the beautiful daughter of Barney Kully, a local ear, nose, and throat specialist. To keep professionally busy, he volunteered his time at the Los Angeles County General Hospital. The "General," as it was known, was the largest hospital in the United States at the time, with over 3000 beds. Dr. Paul Starr, then Chairman of the Department of Medicine, asked him to start a clinic consisting of eight patients who had a newly diagnosed disorder that was characterized by a positive result on a recently described laboratory test known as the "LE cell prep." Within 10 years, Ed had the largest lupus practice in the world, caring for 500 patients at the General Tuesday morning Lupus Clinic and another 500 patients in his private practice.

By the mid-1980s, more than one-half of the rheumatologists in Southern California could say that Ed Dubois had taught them nearly everything they knew about lupus. His first publications on lupus appeared in the *Journal of the American Medical Association* (four of them!) and the *American Journal of Medicine* (two papers) in 1951 and 1952. They described autoimmune hemolytic anemia as a manifestation of systemic lupus erythematosus (SLE), showed that steroids ameliorate the disease, and described the general clinical and laboratory features of patients who had positive LE cell preps.

As the General became more closely affiliated with the University of Southern California, university resources allowed the establishment of lupus research laboratories. Ed Dubois' keen clinical instincts and his demands for perfection among those who worked with him permitted him to publish seminal works that established him as the first, or among the first, to propose insights that we now take for granted. These include: use of nitrogen mustard for serious SLE (1954); use of Atabrine for cutaneous and mild systemic lupus (1954); high-dose steroid protocol for managing central nervous system disease (1956); analysis of why hydralazine induced LE cells (1957); the first description of avascular necrosis in lupus (1960); the first description of steroid-induced peptic ulcers (1960); the first description of gangrene from lupus vasculitis (1962); anticonvulsant drug-induced lupus (1963); establishment of one of the first NZB/NZW mouse research laboratories in the United States (1963), detailed analysis of an accrued, incredible series of 520 patients with lupus (1964); one of the first probes into familial SLE (1964); use of cyclophosphamide in SLE (1967); the first large series of procainamide-induced lupus (1968); absence of erosions in lupus synovitis (1970); phenothiazine-induced lupus (1972); the first report of lupus with myelofibrosis (1973); the first large analysis of causes of death, containing 212 patients (1974); HLA typing of patients with lupus (1974); ibuprofen for SLE (1975); and the incidence of septic arthritis in lupus (1975).

In 1966, Ed wrote the first edition of his monograph, *Lupus Erythematosus: A Review of the Current Status of Discoid and Systemic Lupus Erythematosus and Their Variants.* Dedicated "to the patients from whom we have learned," this remarkable, largely single-authored textbook was enormously successful and now—with this volume—is in its fifth edition. More than any other publication, this book has shaped how rheumatologists approach and treat this disease. Although he authored 175 papers, abstracts, book chapters, and received numerous international honors while traveling, Ed was most proud of being the founding medical director of The American Lupus Society and President of the Southern California Rheumatism Society.

Ed Dubois was a tireless workaholic. He would rise at 5 am and write for an hour or two before going to work. A humanist of the first order, one-half of his time was spent giving free medical care. Ed was known to be exacting and did not suffer fools easily. Although he seemed to be a man of few words, his gentle kind-heartedness was always evident. Ed's probing intellect was apparent within moments of meeting him, and he was always relaxed, modest, and approachable. Ed could be a wonderful teacher when confronted with a student physician who had an inquiring mind and a capacity to work hard. Although he had well-known Hollywood luminaries as private patients, he was never snobbish or conceited, and he felt much more at home seeing indigent patients at the General's lupus clinic.

More than anything else, Ed Dubois was a private man who was devoted to his family. He was happily married and had four children, all of whom now have successful careers. His first grandchild (of six) was born shortly before he died. He was an expert yachtsman who relaxed best on his boat. (When he was terminally ill, he bought a new boat that he named *Dubious.*) His other consuming passion was photography. Able to be privately tutored by the likes of Ansel Adams, his office was filled with creative and wonderful pictures showing his love of life.

While still a youthful 54 years of age in 1977, Ed complained of low back and knee pain, which turned out to be a compression fracture from multiple myeloma. He privately confided to me that excessive exposure to radiation during his training and in various research laboratories was responsible for this. A fighter to the end, Ed lived with myeloma for 8 years, which must be close to a record. He saw a full schedule of patients 2 weeks before he died, in February 1985, from pneumonia complicated by renal shut-down. I was fortunate to meet Ed Dubois as a medical student at the University of Southern California and as a resident at Cedars-Sinai Medical Center. Among the greatest honors in my life was when he asked me to help in his office part-time in 1977, while I was still a fellow in training, and to edit his book along with him in 1982. I will always value his friendship.

Daniel J. Wallace, MD

Acknowledgment: I gratefully acknowledge the assistance of Mrs. Nancy (Edmund) Dubois in preparing this dedication.

CONTENTS

CONTRIBUTING AUTHORS

Steven B. Abramson, M.D. Professor of Medicine and Pathology, New York University School of Medicine, Chairman, Division of Rheumatology, Hospital for Joint Diseases, New York University Medical Center, New York, New York

Jenny Thorn Allan Publications Director, Lupus Foundation of America, Rockville, Maryland

H. Michael Belmont, M.D. Assistant Professor of Medicine, New York University School of Medicine, and Chief Medical Officer, Hospital for Joint Diseases, New York, New York

Thomas G. Benedek, M.D. Professor of Medicine, Department of Medicine, University of Pittsburgh School of Medicine, Pittsburgh, Pennsylvania

Dimitrios T. Boumpas, M.D. Professor of Medicine and Rheumatology, Medical School, University of Crete, Director, Divisions of Internal Medicine and Rheumatology, University Hospital Heraklion, Greece, Adjunct Professor of Medicine and Rheumatology, Uniformed Services University for the Health Sciences, Bethesda Maryland

Jill P. Buyon, M.D. Professor of Medicine, Department of Rheumatology, New York University School of Medicine, and Vice Chairman, Department of Rheumatology, Hospital for Joint Diseases, New York, New York

Joseph E. Craft, M.D. Professor of Medicine and Immunobiology, Chief, Section of Rheumatology, Yale School of Medicine, and Attending Physician, Department of Internal Medicine, Yale-New Haven Hospital, New Haven, Connecticut

Dr David D'Cruz, M.D., F.R.C.P. Consultant Rheumatologist, The Lupus Research Unit, The Rayne Institute, The Louise Coote Lupus Unit, St. Thomas' Hospital, London, United Kingdom

Betty Diamond, M.D. Professor, Department of Microbiology and Immunology, Division of Rheumatology, Department of Medicine, Albert Einstein College of Medicine, Bronx, New York

Jan Dutz, M.D., F.R.C.P.C. Assistant Professor, Department of Medicine, Vancouver Hospital and Health Sciences Center, University of British Columbia, Vancouver, British Columbia, Canada

Fanny M. Ebling, Adjunct Professor, Department of Medicine, Division of Rheumatology, UCLA School of Medicine, Los Angeles, California

Keith B. Elkon, M.D. Head, Division of Rheumatology, University of Washington, Seattle, Washington

Robert I. Fox, M.D., Ph.D. Member, Allergy and Rheumatology Medical Clinic, Scripps Medical and Research Foundation, Rheumatology Division, Scripps Memorial Hospital, La Jolla, California

Marvin Fritzler, M.D., Ph.D. Professor and Arthritis Society Chair, Department of Medicine, University of Calgary, Calgary, Alberta, Canada

Michael Froncek, M.D. Clinical Assistant Professor, Division of Rheumatology and Immunology, Keck School of Medicine, University of Southern California, Los Angeles, California, and Associate, Orrin M. Troum, M.D., and Associates, Santa Monica, California

Ian P. Giles, M.B.B.S., M.R.C.P. Arthritis Research Campaign Clinical Research Fellow, Department of Medicine, University College London, Clinical Research Fellow, Department of Medicine, Middlesex Hospital, London, United Kingdom

Ellen M. Ginzler, M.D., M.P.H. Professor and Chief of Rheumatology, Department of Medicine, State University of New York Downstate Medical Center, Brooklyn, New York

Dafna D. Gladman, M.D., F.R.C.P.C. Professor, Department of Medicine, University of Toronto, Rheu-matologist and Deputy Director, Centre for Prognosis Studies in The Rheumatic Diseases, Toronto Western Hospital, Toronto, Ontario, Canada

T. Murphy Goodwin, M.D. Associate Professor of Obstetrics and Gynecology, Department of Obstetrics and Gynecology, Chief, Division of Maternal-Fetal Medicine, Keck School of Medicine, University of Southern California, Los Angeles, California

J. Dixon Gray, Ph.D. Assistant Professor of Research Medicine, Division of Rheumatology and Immunology, Keck School of Medicine, University of Southern California, Los Angeles, California

Jennifer M. Grossman, M.D. Clinical Instructor, Division of Rheumatology, Department of Medicine, UCLA School of Medicine, Los Angeles, California

Bevra Hannahs Hahn, M.D. Professor of Medicine, UCLA School of Medicine, Los Angeles, California

David Hallegua, M.D. Clinical Instructor, Division of Rheumatology, Cedars-Sinai Medical Center/UCLA School of Medicine, Los Angeles, California

John B. Harley, M.D., Ph.D. Professor of Medicine, Oklahoma University College of Medicine, Oklahoma University Health Sciences Center, Member and Program Head, Arthritis and Immunology Program, Oklahoma Medical Research Foundation, Oklahoma City, Oklahoma

Evelyn V. Hess, M.D., M.A.C.P., M.A.C.R. Professor of Medicine, Division of Immunology, University of Cincinnati College of Medicine, Cincinnati, Ohio

Marc C. Hochberg, M.D., M.P.H. Head, Division of Rheumatology, Professor, Department of Medicine, University of Maryland Medical School, Baltimore, Maryland

David A. Horwitz, M.D. Professor of Medicine and Immunology, Chief, Division of Rheumatology and Immunology, Keck School of Medicine, University of Southern California, LAC+USC Medical Center, Los Angeles, California

Graham Hughes, M.D. Head, The Lupus Research Unit The Rayne Institute, Consultant Rheumatologist, The Louise Coote Research Unit, St. Thomas' Hospital, London, United Kingdom

Ellen Ignatius, R.N. Vice President of Education and Science Information, Department of Education and Research, Lupus Foundation of America, Rockville, Maryland

Karen Johnson, R.N., M.Ed. Health Educator, Lupus Foundation of America, Rockville, Maryland

David Isenberg, M.D., M.R.C.P. Arthritis Research Campaign's Professor of Rheumatology, Department of Medicine, University College London, Consultant Rheumatologist, Department of Medicine, Middlesex Hospital, London, United Kingdom

Jatinderpal K. Kalsi, Ph.D. Visiting Scholar, UCLA School of Medicine, Los Angeles, California

Kenneth C. Kalunian, M.D. Division of Rheumatology, Department of Medicine, UCLA School of Medicine, Los Angeles, California

Michael Kashgarian, M.D. Professor, Department of Pathology, Yale University School of Medicine, Director, Diagnostic Electron Microscopy and Renal Pathology, Yale-New Haven Hospital, New Haven, Connecticut

Munther A. Khamashta, M.D., M.R.C.P., Ph.D. Senior Lecturer, Lupus Research Unit, The Rayne Institute, St. Thomas Hospital, London, United Kingdom

Kyriakos A. Kirou, M.D. Assistant Professor of Medicine, The Hospital for Special Surgery, Weill Medical College of Cornell University, New York, New York

Rodanthi C. Kitridou, M.D. Professor of Medicine, Department of Medicine/Rheumatology, University of Southern California, Director Clinical Rheumatology, Department of Medicine/Rheumatology, Los Angeles County and USC Medical Center, Los Angeles, California

Lloyd B. Klickstein, M.D., Ph.D. Assistant Professor of Medicine, Department of Medicine, Harvard Medical School, Associate Physican, Division of Rheumatology, Department of Medicine, Brigham and Women's Hospital, Boston, Massachusetts

John H. Klippel, M.D. Medical Director, Arthritis Foundation, Atlanta, Georgia

Hirsh D. Komarow, M.D. Clinical Associate, Genetics Section, Arthritis and Rheumatism Branch, National Institute of Arthritis and Musculoskeletal and Skin Diseases, National Institutes of Health, Bethesda, Maryland

Dwight H. Kono, M.D. Associate Professor, Department of Immunology, The Scripps Research Institute, La Jolla, California

Thomas J. A. Lehman, M.D. Professor, Department of Pediatrics, Cornell University, and Chief, Division of Pediatric Rheumatology, Hospital for Special Surgery, New York, New York

Stamatis-Nick C. Liossis, M.D. Assistant Professor of Medicine, Department of Medicine, Uniformed Services University of the Health Sciences, Bethesda, Maryland

Gale A. McCarty M.D., F.A.C.P., F.A.C.R. Professor of Medicine, Division of Rheumatology/Immunology, University of Virginia, Charlottesville, Virginia

Daniel P. McCauliffe, M.D. Associate Professor of Dermatology, Department of Dermatology, University of North Carolina, Chapel Hill, North Carolina

W. Joseph McCune, M.D. Professor of Internal Medicine, University of Michigan Hospitals, Ann Arbor, Michigan

Paul Michelson, M.D. Chairman, Division of Ophthalmology, Scripps Medical Research Foundation Hospital, La Jolla, California

Patricia Moore, M.D. Professor of Neurology, University of Pittsburgh, Pittsburgh, Pennsylvania

Anne-Barbara Mongey, M.D., D.C.H., M.R.C.P.I. Associate Professor of Medicine, Division of Immunology, University of Cincinnati College of Medicine, Cincinnati, Ohio

Elena Peeva, M.D. Instructor of Medicine, Department of Microbiology and Immunology, Albert Einstein College of Medicine, Bronx, New York

Michelle A. Petri, M.D., M.P.H. Professor, Department of Medicine, Johns Hopkins University School of Medicine, Baltimore, Maryland

Chaim Putterman, M.D. Assistant Professor, Department of Microbiology and Immunology, Director, Arthritis Clinic, Division of Rheumatology, Montefiore Medical Center, Bronx, New York

Francisco P. Quismorio, Jr, M.D. Professor of Medicine and Pathology, Department of Medicine, Kent School of Medicine, University of Southern California, and Vice Chief, Division of Rheumatology, Department of Medicine, Los Angeles County-University of Southern California Medical Center, Los Angeles, California

Morris Reichlin, M.D. Professor of Medicine, Oklahoma University College of Medicine, Oklahoma University Health Sciences Center, Vice President of Research and Scientific Director, Member, Arthritis and Immunology Program, Oklahoma City, Oklahoma

Mona Riskalla, M.D. Fellow, Pediatric Rheumatology, Department of Pediatrics and Communicable Diseases, University of Michigan, Ann Arbor, Ann Arbor, Michigan

Robert L. Rubin, Ph.D. La Jolla Institute for Allergy and Immunology, San Diego, California

Violeta Rus, M.D. Assistant Professor of Medicine, Division of Rheumatology and Clinical Immunology, Department of Medicine, University of Maryland Medical School, University Hospital, Baltimore, Maryland

Jane E. Salmon, M.D. Professor, Weill Medical College of Cornell University, Attending Physician, Department of Medicine, Hospital for Special Surgery, New York, New York

Peter H. Schur, M.D. Professor of Medicine, Department of Medicine, Harvard Medical School, Senior Physician, Department of Medicine/Rheumatology, Brigham and Women's Hospital, Boston, Massachusetts

Howard Shapiro, M.D. Assistant Clinical Professor, Department of Psychiatry, University of Southern California School of Medicine, Attending Staff, Department of Psychiatry, Cedars-Sinai Medical Center, Los Angeles, California

Josef Smolen, M.D. Departments of Rheumatology, Lainz Hospital and General Hospital, University of Vienna, Austria

Richard D. Sontheimer, M.D. John S. Strauss Endowed Chair in Dermatology, Professor and Head, Department of Dermatology, University of Iowa Health Care, Iowa City, Iowa

Esther M. Sternberg, M.D. Director, Integrative Neural-Immune Program, National Institute of Mental Health, National Institues of Health, Bethesda, Maryland

William Stohl, M.D., Ph.D. Division of Rheumatology and Immunology, Keck School of Medicine, University of Southern California, Los Angeles, California

Argyrios N. Theofilopoulos, M.D. Professor, Department of Immunology, The Scripps Research Institute, La Jolla, California

Betty P. Tsao, Ph.D. Department of Medicine/Rheumatology, UCLA School of Medicine, Los Angeles, California

George C. Tsokos, M.D. Professor of Medicine, Director, Division of Immunology and Rheumatology, Department of Medicine, Uniformed Services University of the Health Sciences, Bethesda, Maryland, and Chief, Cellular Injury, Department of Cellular Injury, Walter Reed Army Institute of Research, Silver Spring, Maryland

Murray B. Urowitz, M.D., F.R.C.P.C. Professor of Medicine and Associate Dean of Postgraduate Affairs, University of Toronto, Rheumatologist and Director, Centre for Prognosis Studies in The Rheumatic Diseases, Toronto Western Hospital, Toronto, Ontario, Canada

Sara E. Walker, M.D. M.A.C.P. Professor, Department of Internal Medicine, University of Missouri School of Medicine, MA406G Health Sciences Center, Columbia, Missouri

Daniel J. Wallace, M.D. Clinical Professor of Medicine, Cedars-Sinai Medical Center, UCLA School of Medicine, Los Angeles, California

Michael Weisman, M.D. Professor of Medicine, Department of Rheumatology, UCLA School of Medicine, Director, Division of Rheumatology, Cedars-Sinai Medical Center, Los Angeles, California

Sterling G. West, M.D. Professor, Department of Medicne, University of Colorado Health Sciences Center, Denver, Colorado

Keyvan Yousefi, M.D. Clinical Fellow, Division of Rheumatology, Department of Medicine, Cedars-Sinai Medical Center, Los Angeles, California

PREFACE

The sixth edition of *Dubois' Lupus Erythematosus* continues to highlight important advances in the field. In the last few years, there has been an explosion of newly published information germane to SLE. Basic science and cellular immunology insights relate macrophage dysfunction, cell signaling defects, costimulatory molecules, T cell subsets, proinflammatory mediators (adhesion molecules, nitric oxide, cyclooxygenase), apoptosis, aberrant cytokine production, and tolerance defects to the disorder. Linkage studies, genome scans, and association studies led investigators to describe 20-30 potential lupus susceptibility genes. Ultraviolet light can damage lupus skin, direct cytotoxicity, and promote an inflammatory reaction. Humeral research has explored idiotypic networks, the phylogenetically important antibodies to the nucleosome, the ability of autoantibodies to penetrate living cells, nerve tissue antibodies, and the pathogenicity of catanionic IgG anti-DNA antibodies. Lupologists have formed consortiums to better define lupus-related disorders such as undifferentiated connective tissue disease, update the American College of Rheumatology criteria, develop clinical indices to assess damage and response to therapy, and develop quality of life measures. Clinical trials of cox-2-selective antagonists, hormonal interventions, inhibitors of lipooxygenase and adhesion molecules, newer generation immune suppressives, and at least six biologics targeting specific immune interactions have been studied or are in progress. This represents a quantum leap for lupology, which until recently had not seen any meaningful clinical trials in over 20 years. In the next decade peptide vaccinations, gene transfer therapies, stem cell transplantation and interventions which influence apoptosis will be adapted to help the suffering of lupus patients.

To chronicle these advances and place these in perspective, the 64 sections of *Dubois' Lupus Erythematosus*, 6th ed. have undergone some changes. Twenty-five percent of the chapters have new authors or coauthors. Greater international authorship participation highlights the global fight against lupus. New clinical chapters and sections highlight biologic therapies, disability, cox-2 interventions, clinical trial methodologies, the new classification for lupus, undifferentiated connective tissue disease, and outcomes research. The basic science sections have generally been completely rewritten and updated to reflect the above-mentioned advances in genetics, inflammatory mediator biology, cytokine physiology, cell signaling, tolerance and newly described animal models and autoantibodies. The authors continue to thank their families for their loving support and appreciate the hard work of Richard Winters, Robin Cook, and Denise Martin at Lippincott Williams & Wilkins.

Daniel J. Wallace
Bevra Hannahs Hahn
Los Angeles, CA

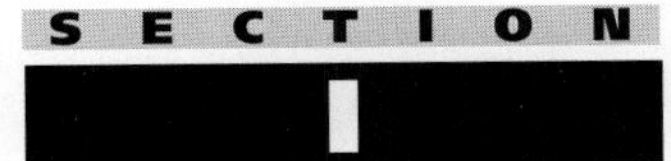

HISTORY

1

HISTORICAL BACKGROUND OF DISCOID AND SYSTEMIC LUPUS ERYTHEMATOSUS

THOMAS G. BENEDEK

THE PRESCIENTIFIC PERIOD

Lupus (wolf) was an ancient Roman family name, and there was a St. Lupus who lived in central France in about 600 A.D. (1). How the name of this large carnivore came to have a disease association is obscure. The earliest known medical use of "lupus" appeared in a 10th century biography of St. Martin, who had lived in 4th century Gaul. The Bishop of Liege was healed at St. Martin's shrine in Tours:

> He was seriously afflicted and almost brought to the point of death by the disease called lupus. . . . The location of the disease . . . was not to be seen, nonetheless, a sort of thin red line remained as a mark of the scar (2).

Toward the end of the 12th century Rogerius Frugardi, a Salernitan surgeon, introduced the term *noli me tangere* (touch me not) to designate a facial ulcer. He also stated, "Sometimes lupus arises in the thighs and the lower legs [and is] distinguished from cancer" (3). This distinction was clarified somewhat by his student, Roland of Parma: "In the early stages it [cancer] is called sclirosis [hardening] or negrosis [blackening]. After it begins to rot it is called cancrena [gangrene ?]; finally it is called carcinoma [cancer]." This progressive lesion also is named according to its location: on the face he used Roger's term, *noli me tangere,* on the trunk, *cingulum* [girdle]. "However, in the lower body, as in the feet, thighs and hips, it is called *lupula* [little she-wolf] and it is incurable . . . in this place" (4).

"Lupus" remained associated with ulcerated lesions of the legs until the 16th century, after which it was considered primarily a facial lesion. Most authors considered it to be a distinctive disease rather than a phase of an evolving ailment, but no one described lupus in sufficient detail for a modern diagnosis to be inferred. Various ailments likely bore the name. Paracelsus (1493–1541) presents an example of the undefined use of the term:

> The art of medicine resides in recognizing the site wherein lies the cure, such as cancer, lupus, gout, plague, fever, hydrops, polyuria, menses, worms, etc. (5).

DIFFERENTIATION FROM TUBERCULOSIS

Discussion of whether this skin disease is merely a manifestation of tuberculosis, which itself was just being defined, began early in the 19th century. According to the dermatologist Thomas Bateman (1778–1821), his mentor, Robert Willan (1757–1812) had defined lupus:

> . . . to comprise, together with the "noli me tangere" affecting the nose and lips, other slow tubercular affections, especially about the face, commonly ending in ragged ulcerations of the cheeks, forehead, eyelids, and lips, and sometimes occurring in other parts of the body, where they gradually destroy the skin and muscular parts to a considerable depth (6).

In 1853 Sir James Paget (1814–1899), calling the lesion a "rodent ulcer," identified *noli me tangere* as a neoplasm (7).

In 1845 Ferdinand von Hebra (1816–1880, Vienna) proposed a classification of skin diseases based on abnormalities of specific components of the skin. Under "hyperactivity of sebaceous glands" he described "seborrhea congestiva," which a few years later was renamed *lupus erythemateux*. Here is his description:

> One sees at the beginning of this illness—mainly on the face, on the cheeks and the nose in a distribution not dissimilar to a butterfly—on an erythematous but not infiltrated base the sebum filled openings of the sebaceous glands as white flat dots (8).

Laurent T. Biett (1761–1840, Paris) may in 1833 have described the same disease as "erytheme centrifuge," but this was first published in 1851 (Fig. 1.1) by his student, Pierre L. Cazenave (1795–1877, Paris):

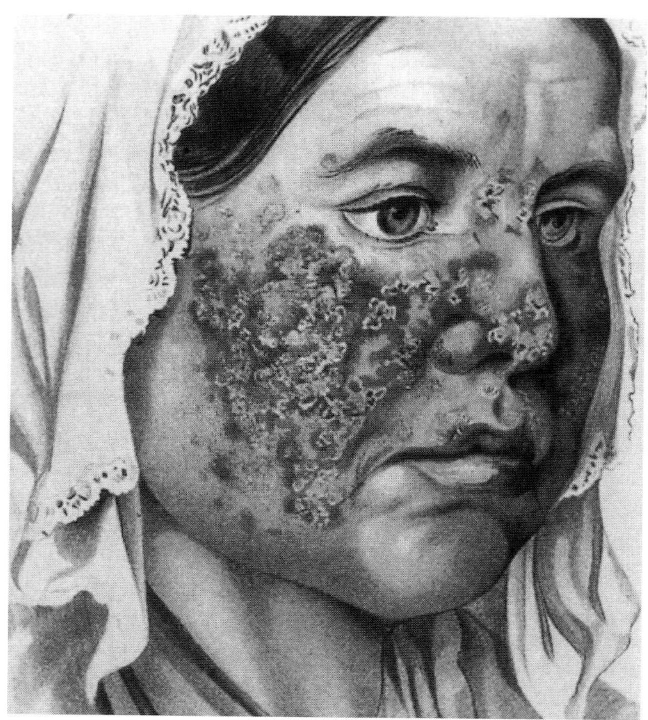

FIGURE 1.1. (See color plate.) Disseminated lupus erythematosus (LE) showing "livid red slightly raised lesions with flat, depressed, paler centers resembling scars; or covered by an adherent thin scale which feels greasy." (From Kaposi M. Neue Beiträge zur Kenntnis des Lupus erythematosus. *Arch Dermatol Syph* 1872;4:36–78.)

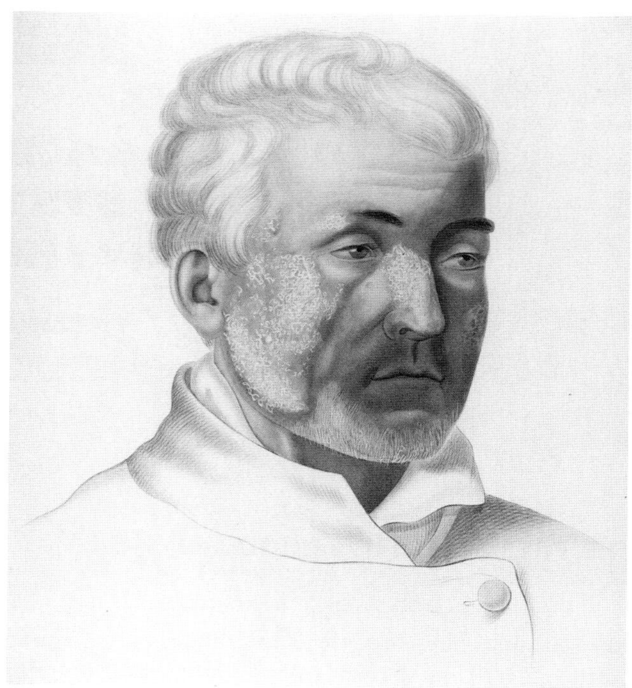

FIGURE 1.2 (See color plate.) The first modern illustration of cutaneous lupus, labeled "Lupus erythemateux," in Cazenave (11) in 1856. (From Wallace DJ, Lyon I. Pierre Cazenave and the first detailed modern description of lupus erythematosus. *Semin Arthritis Rheum* 1999;28:305–313. Reproduced with permission.)

> It is a very rare occurrence, and appears most frequently in young people, especially in females, whose health is otherwise excellent. It attacks the face chiefly. It generally appears in the form of round red patches, slightly elevated, and about the size of a 30 sous piece: these patches generally begin by a small red spot, slightly papular, which gradually increases in circumference, and sometimes spreads over the greater part of the face. The edges of the patches are prominent, and the centre, which retains its natural color, is depressed . . . (9)

At a meeting in 1851 Cazenave also described a case and after giving credit to Biett for having described a variety of lupus as "erytheme centrifuge," introduced the term *lupus erythemateaux* (10).

In the 1856 edition of his textbook Cazenave wrote extensively about lupus erythematosus (LE). He mentions the potential occurrence of "fever and even pain," but his presentation is entirely dermatologic. Cazenave herein is the first to note alopecia as a symptom. He does not mention the "butterfly rash," but states that the eruption "is very common on the face and the nose." He emphasizes that lesions heal with scarring, but do not ulcerate—an important distinction from lupus vulgaris—and states that these patients are not necessarily scrofulous (11) (Fig. 1.2).

The distinction from scrofulous (i.e., tuberculous) was important because lupus was considered a tuberculous disease, "tuberculous" having a different meaning in this prebacteriologic time. According to Erasmus Wilson (1809–1884; 1862, London):

> Destruction, then, we may take as the leading character of lupus. A further inquiry into the nature of lupus is served, however, to show that this destructive disease was preceded by a circumscribed thickening and prominence of the skin, commonly termed a *tubercle*, hence, lupus is considered as a tuberculous affection of the skin. . . . Now, the destructive action implied by the term lupus was, in the first instance, intended to be restricted to that form of tubercle which commonly issues in destructive ulceration, but as cutaneous diseases came to be more carefully observed, it was perceived that there existed a kind of tubercle which did not of a necessity ulcerate, which was chronic and lasting in its nature, and which . . . left behind it a deep pit or a strongly marked cicatrix. . . . This form of cutaneous disease . . . has been distinguished by Cazenave under the name of *lupus erythematosus* (12).

Unfortunately, Wilson then confuses this finding with a syphilitic lesion. However, the fact that the medieval description of "lupus" depended mainly on ulceration makes it likely that the nonulcerative lupus was first recognized in the 1830s.

Moriz (Kohn) Kaposi (1837–1902, Vienna) with his publications of 1869 (13) and especially 1872 called attention to LE. He confirmed Wilson's observation that LE occurs more frequently in women and considered that it also is more likely to be severe in them (14). Kaposi believed that tuberculosis and LE may occur in the same patient, but was convinced that LE is not a manifestation of tuberculosis. He became quite annoyed at the confusion:

> . . . the disease called lupus erythematosus does not have the least in common with lupus vulgaris, and it is not enough to criticise even leading surgeons for confusing these two entirely different processes that have not the least in common, and even less to justify many dermatologic specialists who assume transitional or mixed forms of lupus erythematosus and lupus vulgaris, as has occurred recently (15).

From 1866 to 1871 Kaposi made the diagnosis of LE in 22 patients, while he diagnosed lupus vulgaris (LV) (cutaneous tuberculosis) in 279. He introduced the term "discoid" for lesions that expand from single foci and "discrete and aggregate" for lesions that enlarge by the merger of multiple pinhead size foci (14). Subsequently he altered the latter term to "disseminate and aggregate" (15). Confusion resulted from Kaposi's intention for "disseminate" to refer to cases where the lesions were not limited to the head, while it so happened that systemic symptoms (Fig. 1.3) were observed only in patients with disseminate skin lesions.

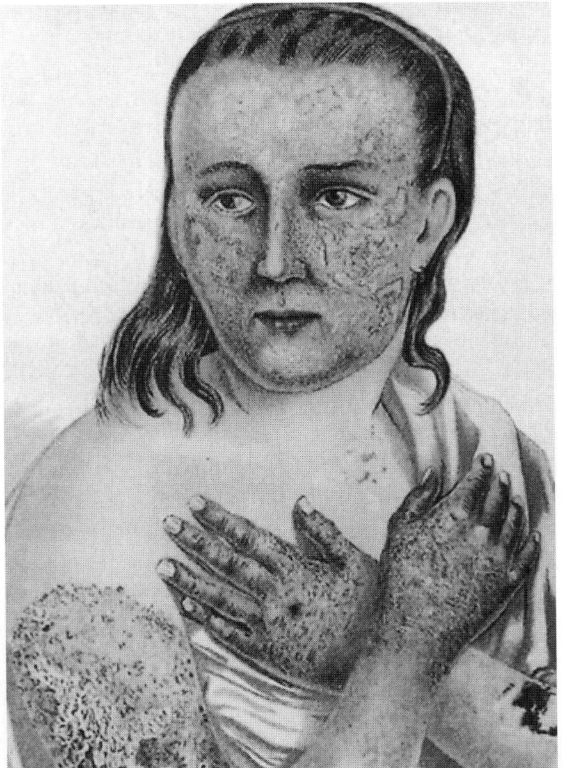

FIGURE 1.3. (See color plate.) Disseminated LE involving scalp, face, trunk, and extremities. (From Kaposi M. Neue Beiträge zur Kenntnis des Lupus erythematosus. *Arch Dermatol Syph* 1872;4: 36–78.)

> Lupus erythematosus may occur and progress with manifestations of a disseminated or universal acute or subacute febrile eruption, and may then frequently involve the entire body with intense local and general symptoms, indeed to endanger and destroy life (14).

Of the 11 cases Kaposi described in 1872, four had pneumonia, three had arthralgias, and three had major adenopathy. Of the three who came to autopsy, two had pneumonia, one of whom also had amyloidosis, and one had tuberculosis. No renal disease was described. He was uncertain whether the relationship between the cutaneous and other findings was more than coincidental. The first American publication on LE, by W. H. Geddings in 1869, described the cutaneous findings of case no. 1 of Kaposi's 1872 publication (16).

Many investigators recognized that the relative prevalence of LE and LV was influenced by socioeconomic factors, LV being particularly associated with poverty. Thus, Jonathan Hutchinson (1828–1913, London) cited Wilson as having seen an equal number of cases of these two diseases among 10,000 dermatologic patients from among the "wealthier classes," and attributed this to referral bias (17). One generation later, H. R. Crocker (1845–1909), another English dermatologist, found LV to be twice as prevalent as LE among 10,000 dermatologic clinic cases (1.27% versus 0.63%), while the opposite was true among 5,000 private patients (0.98% versus 1.80%) (18).

Hutchinson in 1888 made the principal distinctions between the major members of the lupus family (Table 1.1). Hutchinson concluded, "The features which distinguish these two diseases . . . are useful rather for the purposes of clinical diagnosis and arrangement than as implying essential differences. . . . The two are closely allied and . . . are in a general way induced by a similar kind of causative influence. . . . In the lupus family vulgaris and erythematosus stand as brother and sister, having many essential resemblances and many marked but superficial differences." In his descriptions of the symmetry of LE lesions he substituted "the bat's wing form" for Hebra's "butterfly." Six years after the discovery of the tubercle bacillus Hutchinson conceded that no one had detected them in cases of LE, "but

TABLE 1.1. DISTINCTIVE FEATURES OF LUPUS VULGARIS AND LUPUS ERYTHEMATOSUS

Feature	Lupus Vulgaris	Lupus Erythematosus
"Apple jelly" growth	Characteristic	Little or none
Tendency to ulcerate	Yes	No
Symmetrical lesions	No	As a rule
Childhood occurrence	Yes	No
Sex ratio	Almost equal	Far commoner in women
Related to chilblains	No	Yes
Fatal	Very seldom	Sometimes

this, no doubt is only a question of time" (17). Hutchinson was in a shrinking minority of advocates of a direct tuberculous etiology of LE. In view of the inability to recover tubercle bacilli from LE lesions, but with no persuasive alternative etiologic hypothesis, the most acceptable compromise was that LE "is a chronic inflammatory process produced by toxic substances of tuberculous origin" (19). Goeckerman (20) in 1921 analyzed Mayo Clinic data and found tuberculosis equally prevalent among cases of discoid lupus erythematosus (DLE) and those with other dermatoses. In 1933 Keil (New York), in reviewing autopsy reports of cases of systemic LE, found that only 20% showed evidence of active or remote tuberculosis. He also concluded that the occurrence of the two diseases is coincidental and, in view of the prevalence of tuberculosis, not surprising (21).

RECOGNITION OF SYSTEMIC LUPUS ERYTHEMATOSUS

Between 1872 and the first of William Osler's (1849–1919) three long articles describing a disease he initially called "erythema exudativum multiforme" (EEM), a few cases of LE were described in which some extracutaneous symptoms were present (22,23). In 1895 Osler described a disease

> . . . of unknown etiology with polymorphic skin lesions—hyperaemia, oedema, and hemorrhage—arthritis occasionally, and a variable number of visceral manifestations, of which the most important are gastro-intestinal crises, endocarditis, pericarditis, acute nephritis, and hemorrhage from the mucous surfaces. Recurrence is a special feature of the disease, and attacks may come on month after month, or even throughout a long period of years. . . . The attacks may not be characterized by skin manifestations; the visceral symptoms alone may be present, and to the outward view the patient may have no indication whatever of erythema exudativum (24).

The relevance of Osler's contributions to the understanding of LE have been misinterpreted. In 1900 he acknowledged that the cases he was assembling were not uniform: "While I feel that in bringing together a somewhat motley series of cases I may only have contributed to make the 'confusion worse confounded,' on the other hand there is, I think, a positive advantage in recognizing the affinities and the strong points of similarity in affections usually grouped as separate diseases" (25). Therefore, he withdrew the term EEM in favor of the less specific "erythema group." At no time did he use "LE."

In the last paper (1904), Osler summarized his 29 cases, and they differ markedly in gender and age from typical LE: 18 were male and 12 were between the ages of 3 and 12; 19 had purpura and "colic." All had some sort of cutaneous findings. The most frequent extracutaneous symptoms were arthralgia in 17 and "nephritis" in 14. None of the seven fatal cases came to autopsy. Osler made no etiologic hypotheses, but in regard to pathogenesis he stated: "The essential process is a vascular change with exudate, blood, serum, alone or combined" (26).

Osler's three articles drew praise for calling attention to the association of cutaneous and visceral symptoms (27,28). The modern diagnosis of most of these patients undoubtedly would be Schönlein-Henoch purpura, a possibility about which Osler equivocated (25). Harry Keil, a dermatologist in New York, in 1937 became the first to point out that Osler's 29 cases included two descriptions of typical acute (systemic) LE (29,30).

Various modifications of "lupus erythematosus" came to be preferred over Osler's "erythema group." In 1908 Kraus and Bohac (31) in Prague introduced "acute LE" to indicate the presence of both cutaneous and visceral symptoms. "Chronic LE" became a synonym for DLE. "Acute disseminated LE" was used for "cases which start acutely [i.e., with systemic symptoms], assume a disseminated [cutaneous] form and run acutely throughout" (32). That cutaneous lesions are not a prerequisite for a diagnosis of SLE was rediscovered in 1936 (33), and emphasized in 1942 (34). While various authors used cumbersome descriptive terms, "LE" never was discarded. Brunsting (35) in 1952 in Rochester, Minnesota, introduced "disseminated (systemic) LE," and Harvey et al. (36) in 1954 in Baltimore finally popularized the contemporary "systemic lupus erythematosus" (SLE) (Table 1.2).

Once visceral symptoms began to be associated with cutaneous LE, the question of whether they are causally related had to be resolved. Consequently there is a gap between the first description of many findings and the recognition that they are a component of LE. Kaposi had mentioned the occurrence of fever and pneumonia in 1872, but Kraus and Bohac (31) concluded in 1908–1909 from their eight cases that pneumonia may be a component of LE and that fever is not necessarily due to infection.

In 1911 Emanuel Libman (1872–1946, New York) hospitalized a 10-year-old girl who had been ill for 10 weeks with polyarthralgia, followed by precordial pain, dyspnea, and oliguria. "There was an erythematous eruption of butterfly pattern, which resembled acute lupus erythematosus disseminatus." Blood cultures were sterile. Hematuria and a precordial rub developed during a febrile 8-week course. The autopsy revealed "endocarditis of a peculiar type, particularly because of the unusual manner of spread of the endocardial lesions along the posterior wall of the left ventricle," and also glomerulonephritis. This case was first reported in 1924 as the fourth of four cases of nonbacterial valvular and mural endocarditis treated by Libman and autopsied by Benjamin Sacks (37). Cases 1 and 2 had already been reported in 1923 (38). Two of the four had the butterfly facial eruption and three had nephritis. Libman and Sacks pointed out "the similarity of certain of the symptoms to those observed in the erythema group of

TABLE 1.2. FIRST DESCRIPTIONS AS COMPONENTS OF SYSTEMIC LUPUS ERYTHEMATOSUS

Component	Author, Year	Site	Reference
Clinical			
Butterfly rash	von Hebra, 1845	Vienna	8
Panniculitis	Kaposi, 1869	Vienna	13
Arthralgia	Kaposi, 1872		14
Adenopathy	Kaposi, 1872		14
Arthritis	Philippson, 1892	Hamburg	23
Nephritis	Osler, 1895	Baltimore	24
Purpura	Osler, 1895		24
Psychosis	Bowen, 1896	New York	48
Pneumonia	Kraus and Bohac, 1908	Prague	31
Raynaud's phenomenon	MacLeod, 1908	London	46
Photosensitivity	Pulay, 1921	Vienna	118
Endocarditis	Libman & Sacks, 1923	New York	38
Retinopathy	Pillat, 1935	Vienna	55
Peritonitis	Friedberg et al., 1936	New York	33
Encephalopathy	Daly, 1945	Minneapolis	49
Myelopathy	Piper, 1953	Madison, WI	52
Laboratory			
BFP reaction	Reinhart, 1909	Hamburg	65
Leukopenia	Goeckerman, 1923	Rochester, MN	60
Anemia	Keefer and Felty, 1924	Baltimore	59
Hematoxylin bodies	Gross, 1932	New York	117
Thrombocytopenia	Lyon, 1933	Philadelphia	62
"Wire loop" glomeruli	Baehr et al., 1935	New York	44
"Onion skin" splenic lesion	Kaiser, 1942	Baltimore	45
Hypergammaglobulinemia	Coburn & Moore, 1943	Baltimore	69
LE cell	Hargraves, 1948	Rochester, MN	73
Lupus anticoagulant	Conley and Hartman, 1952	Baltimore	151
Antinuclear antibody	Miescher and Fauconnet, 1954	Geneva, Switz.	83

BFP, biologically false positive; LE, lupus erythematosus.

Osler," but declined to make a definite diagnosis of SLE in any case.

Dermatologists, upon reviewing published cases in 1936, came to the confusing conclusion that the "Libman-Sacks syndrome is a subvariety of the Osler erythema group," but probably not LE (39). An internist and a pathologist finally stated unequivocally in 1940 that this form of endocarditis is a manifestation of SLE, irrespective of the presence of characteristic skin lesions (40). Libman-Sacks endocarditis has become a less common pathologic finding since the introduction of corticosteroid therapy—59% of cases of SLE reported during 1924–1951 versus 36% of cases during 1953–1976 (41).

At least two of the patients in whom Osler found signs of nephritis did have LE (26,30). Sequeira and Balean (42) in 1902 in London found proteinuria in five of ten cases of disseminated (cutaneous) LE, of whom the one fatal case had a pathologic diagnosis of nephritis. Similar single cases were published in the next few years. Keith and Rowntree (43) in 1922 in Rochester, Minnesota, pointed out that nephritis is "a common complication of disseminated LE." In a pathologic study of 23 cases of SLE, Baehr et al. (44) in 1935 in New York differentiated a type of nephritis in 13 (56%), which they considered to be peculiar to LE. "The commonest and most characteristic glomerular alteration was a peculiar hyaline thickening of the capillary walls. . . . The thickened wall appears rigid, as if made of heavy wire. We have, therefore, called it the 'wire loop lesion.' . . . It is quite different from the hyaline degeneration seen in glomeruli of arteriosclerotic kidneys or of chronic glomerulonephritis. It apparently represents a toxic degenerative process" (44). Nevertheless, renal failure was not considered a principal cause of death in LE, probably because early death usually resulted from infection. The importance of renal involvement was recognized by Harvey et al., who found that in two thirds of their autopsied cases "SLE alone was responsible for varying degrees of renal damage." They pointed out "the inability to correlate the degree of renal involvement disclosed clinically and the extent of renal damage at postmortem examination" (36).

Libman and Sacks (37), incidentally to their description of the cardiac lesion, also described a splenic abnormality: "The greater part of each malpighian body [lymph follicle] was occupied by a number of arterioles, each of which was surrounded by a broad zone of hyaline-like connective tissue. The arteriolar lumen in each instance was diminished in caliber." Kaiser (45) in 1942 in Baltimore studied this "onion skin" periarterial splenic fibrosis in detail and found it in 83% of cases of SLE, but in only 3% of other diseases. "Its discovery post mortem should at least raise the suspicion of that diagnosis . . . [and] its coincidence with the other well recognized lesions of the connective tissue such as verrucous endocarditis and the 'wire loop' glomerular changes can serve to strengthen the post mortem diagnosis of disseminated lupus erythematosus" (45). Abdominal symptoms were recognized as peritonitis, which tended to be associated with pleurisy, but there were no primarily gastrointestinal findings (33).

In regard to cerebral involvement, Osler considered as "peculiarly obscure" the delirium in one case (no. 1), and in case no. 15 recurrent episodes of hemiplegia and aphasia, which he speculated "were associated with changes in the brain of essentially the same nature which subsequently occurred . . . in the skin. They remind one somewhat of the attacks of recurrent aphasia with paralysis in cases of Raynaud's disease" (24). Whether these patients actually had SLE is equivocal, but this allegation has repeatedly been made. Peripheral Raynaud's phenomenon was associated with SLE by MacLeod (46) in 1908 in London. Until the 1940s abnormalities of cerebral function were generally attributed to fever or uremia. Even though seizures are the most frequent cerebral manifestation of SLE, this symptom was alluded to only incidentally before 1951, when it was also pointed out that seizures may precede diagnosable SLE for years (47). Harvey et al. (36) attributed seizures to SLE in 11% of their patients. According to Bowen (1896), "I have often met with cases of extreme melancholia in the subjects of this disease [LE] and in a number of instances the mind has become really affected" (48). Toxic delirium was described (49), but the range of psychotic manifestations that may occur was not comprehensively reviewed until 1960 (50). Cerebral vasculitis to which the various manifestations might be attributed was described by Jarcho (51) in 1936 in Baltimore and Daly (49) in 1945 in Minneapolis). Paraplegia due to spinal vasculitis was identified in 1953 (52).

Attention to ocular symptoms antedates modern descriptions of cerebral symptoms. Retinal vasculitis was demonstrated pathologically in the 1930s (53,54). The first more extensive investigation (1935, Vienna) concluded that the ophthalmoscopic findings of some cases of DLE and SLE are further evidence of a tuberculous disease (55). Maumenee (56) in 1940 in Baltimore introduced the term "cotton-wool spots" for the retinal lesions as a synonym for the older term "cytoid bodies." However, they "should not be regarded as pathognomonic of acute lupus erythematosus." More recent investigations have shown that cotton-wool spots are ischemic lesions in the retina, while cytoid bodies are microscopic neural lesions; they coexist, but are not identical (57). Prior to 1970 cotton-wool spots were described in about 10% of cases of SLE, but less frequently more recently (58).

The absence of anemia in early descriptions of SLE can be attributed to the rudimentary state of hematologic methods. However, it is surprising that "secondary anemia often with a normal leukocyte count" was not described until 1924 (59). A case with leukopenia was cited by Goeckerman (60) in 1923. However, Rose and Pillsbury (61) in 1939 in Philadelphia were the first to consider this "the principal feature of the blood picture." Purpura had been described by Kaposi (14) and by Osler (24), but the thrombocytopenia with which it occurs was not recognized until the 1930s (62,63). Conversely, the infrequency of purpura among platelet deficient patients was pointed out in 1951 (64).

SEROLOGIC ASPECTS

The Wassermann test for syphilis was devised in 1906 and rapidly gained wide use. It soon was discovered that some, mainly tropical, diseases frequently gave positive results in nonsyphilitic individuals. The first such cases of SLE were reported from Germany in 1909 and 1910 (65,66). The latter author suggested that this result is evidence that LE is *not* a manifestation of tuberculosis, since falsely positive reactions had not been reported in the latter disease. The incidence of biologically false-positive [BFP] reactions has ranged from less than 3% to 44% of cases of LE (67,68). The variation may in part be due to insufficient distinction having been made between DLE and SLE, since BFP rarely occurs in the former. Coburn and Moore (69) in 1943 in New York demonstrated hypergammaglobulinemia in SLE and related the BFP reaction to this. With the discovery of the specific *Treponema pallidum* immobilization (TPI) test for syphilis in 1949, complement fixation tests of the Wassermann type gradually were abandoned (70). Haserick and Long (71) in 1952 found that BFP reactions may precede clinical signs of SLE by years. Testing for BFP reactors was abandoned within a few years after the discovery of the LE cell.

In 1943 Malcolm M. Hargraves, a hematologist at the Mayo Clinic, found "peculiar rather structureless globular bodies taking purple stain" in the marrow aspirate of a child with an undiagnosed disease; 2½ years later he made a similar observation. Symptoms in a third case with this finding, in 1946, suggested that this patient had SLE. Two important observations were made in addition to the association of this unusual cell with the diagnosis of SLE: (a) more of these cells were found when the specimen was not fixed immediately; and (b) two similar cells needed to be differentiated. These findings were first reported in January 1948 (72). The "tart cell" (named after a patient, not the pastry) is not disease specific. Its distinguishing feature "is that the secondary nucleus has retained definite chromatin structure."

> The "LE cell" . . . is the end result . . . either of phagocytosis of free nuclear material . . . or an actual autolysis of one or more lobes of the nucleus. . . . The "LE" cell is practically always a mature neutrophylic polymorphonuclear leukocyte in contradistinction to the "tart" cell which is most often a histiocyte (73).

John R. Haserick at the Cleveland Clinic suggested already in 1948 that "the greatest value of the 'LE' cell lies in its possible presence in suspected cases of acute disseminated lupus erythematosus in which the classic dermatologic manifestations are lacking" (74). Hargraves (75) in 1949 demonstrated LE cells in the buffy coat of centrifuged specimens of peripheral blood of patients in whose marrow LE cells had been detected. Then Haserick did the converse, inducing LE cells by incubating non-LE marrow with serum from LE patients. Thus, LE cells are formed by a factor in the blood of LE patients (76). Then in 1950 he showed that this factor is a gamma globulin (77). In the same year Klemperer et al. in New York discovered "hematoxylin bodies" (78). These appeared to be identical with the phagocytosed substance within LE cells, in various tissues obtained at autopsy of cases of SLE. This strengthened the hypothesis that the LE cell reaction is related to the pathogenesis of the disease (78). LE cells also were demonstrated *in vivo* in the content of artificially raised blisters (79). Peripheral blood replaced bone marrow as the source of LE cells, and of several techniques the one described by Zimmer and Hargraves (80) in 1952 was generally adopted.

Reliance on the LE cell to diagnose SLE began to diminish after a few years. Kievits et al. (81) in 1956 demonstrated LE cells in 16% of cases of rheumatoid arthritis, increasing doubt about the specificity of the reaction, and Rothfield et al. (82) in 1961 showed that LE cells cannot be detected in about a quarter of cases of SLE, proving poor sensitivity. In 1954, investigators in Switzerland had found that isolated cell nuclei can absorb the serum factor that induces LE cell formation. They therefore postulated that the factor is an antibody against a component of the nucleus (83). In 1957 Friou et al. (84) at Yale devised a technique to demonstrate the antibody semiquantitatively by indirect immunofluorescence microscopy. The reactive substance was identified in 1959 as a DNA-histone nucleoprotein (85) and Beck (86) in 1961 in London showed that at least three fluorescent staining patterns could be distinguished. In the next decade, refined laboratory methods permitted the discovery of numerous antibodies, some of which could be correlated clinically with subsets of SLE and other diseases. The discovery of the LE cell had initiated the discipline of immunopathology.

In 1957 three laboratories almost simultaneously demonstrated a factor in the serum of some cases of SLE that reacts specifically with DNA (87,88). Tan et al. (89) in 1966 in New York detected anti-DNA antibodies in SLE sera. Koffler et al. (90) in 1969 in New York found that the detection of native (double-stranded) DNA (dsDNA) is more specific for SLE, but less sensitive than antibody to denatured (single-stranded) DNA. Schur et al. (91) in 1971, using more sensitive techniques, confirmed the specificity of the reaction with dsDNA, but obtained positive reactions in only one half of SLE sera. Tan and Kunkel (92) in 1966 in New York detected a cytoplasmic (RNP) antigen in SLE serum that they designated Sm. It was the first antibody to a nonhistone nuclear antigen and highly specific for SLE, although found in only one third of cases.

The next discoveries about the antibody systems related to SLE were gained from the development of techniques to extract uncomplexed histones from nuclei and recombining them with DNA, free of other components (93). Histones are small basic proteins associated with nucleic acids in cell nuclei. Some extracted recombined antigens, depending on the precise histone structure, can be used to detect antihistone antibodies. The important findings were that antihistone antibodies occur more frequently in drug-induced than in idiopathic SLE, and that lupus-inducing drugs vary in their ability to induce these antibodies, procaine amide doing so most consistently (94,95).

The role of antinuclear antibodies (ANAs) in SLE became uncertain when clinically typical cases in which ANAs could not be detected began to be described (96). These cases comprise fewer than 5% of cases of SLE, and most have antibody reactive against the cytoplasmic RNA antigen Ro (97).

The introduction in 1963 of a convenient pathologic technique complemented the ever-increasing number of serologic tests. The "lupus band test" determines by immunofluorescence microscopy of skin biopsies whether immunoglobulins are deposited at the dermo-epidermal junction (98). In DLE it is positive in lesional but not in uninvolved skin. It also is positive in the "normal" skin of at least half of cases of SLE (99). It has proven not to be a highly specific finding, since it occurs in about 15% of cases of rheumatoid arthritis (100) and in various bullous dermatoses (101).

EPIDEMIOLOGY

In contrast to DLE, until the 1950s SLE was considered a rare disease. At the Johns Hopkins Hospital as of 1936 five cases were found among 7,500 autopsies (50). Twelve cases were diagnosed at the University of Pennsylvania Hospital during 1932 to 1938 (61). The large referral clientele of the Mayo Clinic included 154 cases from 1918(?) through 1937 and 132 cases during 1938 to 1947 (68). At Columbia-Presbyterian Hospital in New York, 44 cases were recognized during 1937 to 1952 (102). SLE was diagnosed in 11 cases at the Los Angeles County Hospital during 1946 to 1949, but in 44 cases during the next 2 years. Dubois (103) attributed the increase to use of the LE cell test and better diagnostic acumen. On the other hand, the incidence of hospitalization for SLE in a Swedish city remained about one per 100,000 in 1938 to 1939 and 1948 to 1949, but increased to 4.8 per 100,000 during 1954 to 1955. These authors considered this increase genuine, although unexplained (104). The first survey of a circumscribed population in which case findings included outpatient records was conducted in New York in 1951 to 1960. SLE was found to have a higher incidence in the African-American than the white population, and the prevalence showed a greater increase than the incidence (105).

Various factors influencing the prevalence and survivorship with SLE were discussed by Merrell and Shulman (106) in 1955 in Baltimore. They also introduced the calculation of survival probability by life table analysis. Of the cases Harvey et al. (36) diagnosed during 1949 to 1953, 52% survived for 4 years. The extent to which the subsequent prolongation of survival should be attributed to the introduction in 1950 (107) of corticosteroid therapy has remained unsettled (108). Certainly, earlier diagnosis and recognition of less severe cases has contributed factitiously to lengthening the mean life expectancy. Urman and Rothfield (109) found that in a series of SLE patients treated principally with corticosteroids during 1957 to 1967, 10-year survival was 63%, while in a similarly treated series during 1968 to 1975 it increased to 84%. Haserick (110) in 1953 recognized that nephropathy benefits less from corticosteroids than do other manifestations. The 10-year survival of the patient cohort begun by Dubois' group (111), which was treated during 1950 to 1971 with multiple agents, was 87%, but only 65% in those with renal involvement.

SLE AND "COLLAGEN DISEASE"

Development of the modern pathogenetic concept of SLE required the rejection of two principles: that of Giovanni B. Morgagni (1682–1771, Padua) who had concluded in 1761 that every disease resides primarily in a certain organ, and that of Paul Ehrlich (1854–1915, Frankfurt) in 1901, who concluded that an organism cannot react against any of its own constituents. The former was first contradicted by the German pathologist, Fritz Klinge (112) (1892–1974), who showed in 1928 to 1934 that the morbid process in rheumatic fever is not limited to the synovium and heart, but affects connective tissue diffusely, and that such a process is also present in rheumatoid arthritis. Klemperer et al. (113) in 1941 in New York, in their study of the pathology of SLE, reported the following:

> The apparent heterogeneous involvement of various organs in this disease had no logic until it became apparent that the widespread lesions were identical in that they were mere local expressions of a morbid process affecting the entire collagenous tissue system. The most prominent of these alterations is fibrinoid degeneration—a descriptive morphologic term [E. Neumann, 1880] (113) indicating certain well-defined optical and tinctorial alterations in the collagenous fibers and ground substance (76).

This is the origin in 1942 of the term *collagen disease*, which initially was limited to SLE and scleroderma (113).

Ehrlich's doctrine was first questioned by Wilhelm Generich (115), a German dermatologist, who in 1921 speculated about the etiology of SLE:

> Lymphocytic [leukocytic ?] ferments are liberated by the disintegration of lymph nodes. They act on the organism as denatured protein and in sufficient quantity cause anaphylaxis. Furthermore, the liberated ferments exert their biologic effect, which seemingly consists of sensitizing the vascular endothelium and destroying certain components of connective tissue cells, especially, predisposed components of the skin and eventually also of all parenchymatous organs, if an abundant accumulation (acute LE) of the ferments develops in the blood.

This hypothesis gained acceptance in the 1940s due to the research of Arnold Rich (1893–1968, Baltimore), who advocated that the primary lesions of SLE affected endothelium and collagen by anaphylaxis (116). The initiator of such hypersensitivity, however, remained obscure. Gross (117) in 1932 in New York had described microscopic "granular hematoxylin-stained bodies" in the hearts of cases of Libman-Sacks endocarditis. In 1950 Klemperer et al. (78) detected these abnormalities "in 32 of 35 cases of this disease, often widely distributed throughout the body." Whether they were (or contained) the pathogen could not be ascertained.

PHOTOSENSITIVITY

The main symptom that the popular press has associated with LE is aggravation of the disease by exposure to bright sunlight. This was first described by a Viennese dermatologist in 1921 in regard to a fair-complected woman on whom DLE developed following intensive sun exposure. After several months, when the lesions had diminished, she received one ultraviolet irradiation to the back. On the next day there was a marked proliferation of lesions in the irradiated area (118). Rasch (119) in 1926 in Copenhagen stated that he had seen many such cases since 1907, with the lesions typically limited to the uncovered skin. He concluded that LE (i.e., SLE) "is very decidedly aggravated by light, in fact caused by it."

Rose and Pillsbury (62) in 1939 in Philadelphia take precedence in the description of exacerbations of SLE following exposure to sun or therapeutic ultraviolet light, and also photosensitivity long preceding the development of recognized symptoms of this disease. Reports of the prevalence of photosensitivity have varied considerably: e.g., 11% of 105 cases (36), 32.7% of 520 cases (120).

DRUG-INDUCED AND AGGRAVATED LUPUS ERYTHEMATOSUS

Sulfonamides (initially sulfanilamide) began to be used to treat DLE in 1938 (121) and a few years later also SLE, with some benefit being described. In 1945 florid SLE developed in a young soldier who was being treated with sulfadiazine for presumed pyelonephritis (122). Gold (123) in 1951 in London hypothesized that the aggravation of LE by sulfonamide treatment, as had recently been reported, is due to the sensitization of patients by prior exposure to these drugs.

Gold compounds also acquired a reputation for exacerbating preexisting SLE. Their use in treating DLE began and ended long before their use in rheumatoid arthritis, the initial rationale also having been the presumed tuberculous etiology of the disease (124). A review in 1927 concluded that "in the treatment of lupus erythematosus we possess a systemic remedy of real efficacy. When one considers how refractory and unresponsive to therapeutic endeavor lupus erythematosus has been, . . . the results now achieved are all the more gratifying" (125). As recently as 1956, a therapeutic comparison of gold sodium thiosulfate and chloroquine, the latter first advocated for DLE in 1954 (126), showed similar efficacy (127).

Despite the lack of any effective treatment for SLE, as of 1937: "The general opinion that this method of treatment [gold] is contraindicated for acute and subacute disseminated lupus erythematosus is well founded on sad experience. . . . The capillaries seem unduly sensitive not only to gold therapy but also to a wide variety of therapeutic agents. . . . This is understandable in the case of therapy with gold preparations, since it affects the structures (capillaries) attacked by lupus erythematosus itself" (128). It still was deemed necessary in 1949 to warn that "gold is especially dangerous in the acute phases and probably should never be used" (129). This danger never was well documented.

Chronologically, the first commonly used drugs that were implicated to possibly induce rather than aggravate SLE were hydralazine (1954) (130), hydantoins (1957) (131), and procainamide (1962) (132). In the case of hydralazine the development of symptoms clearly was related to the chronic use of large doses to control hypertension. The first reported manifestation was arthritis, and additional symptoms more definitely suggestive of SLE developed if hydralazine was not discontinued. Comens and Schroeder (133) in 1956 found that, although LE cells were not found consistently in patients whose symptoms suggested SLE, these cells could also be demonstrated in some asymptomatic patients who were taking hydralazine. A Mayo Clinic study (1965) compared 50 cases of "hydralazine syndrome" with 100 hypertensive patients who were receiving another therapy. The authors concluded from the prehydralazine histories that "antedating manifestations possibly suggesting lupus diathesis" were nearly six times as frequent in the hydralazine cases as in the controls. Hence, this drug probably uncovers an "underlying lupus diathesis" (134).

Diphenylhydantoin and mesantoin were the first, but not the only, anticonvulsants to be related to the induction of SLE (131,135). Since seizures may be an early manifestation of this disease, the possibility that certain drugs "uncover" SLE gained support from these observations.

By far the most unequivocal inducing agent has been the antiarrhythmic drug procainamide. Dubois (136) in 1969 compared 33 well-documented cases against his cohort of 520 cases of idiopathic SLE. This supported the impression that the drug-induced disease tends to exhibit fewer and milder symptoms, particularly lacking gastrointestinal, renal, and neurologic involvement. In a prospective study Blomgren et al. (137) in 1969 in Rochester, New York, showed that ANA developed within 6 months in one half of patients who were placed on procainamide, "making it unlikely that the drug simply unveils a latent predisposition to idiopathic lupus erythematosus."

DIAGNOSTIC CRITERIA

Valid, agreed-upon diagnoses are essential for epidemiologic and therapeutic research. The method for developing disease specific diagnostic criteria was pioneered in 1944 on rheumatic fever (138). When the technique was applied to LE in 1971, the extraordinarily large number of 74 clinical and laboratory items were considered and refined into 14 diagnostic criteria, one of which was the presence of DLE (139). The revision of 1982 placed greater reliance on serologic findings and the number of criteria was reduced to 11. The presence of at least four criteria was required in both schemes. Using the revised set, false-negative diagnoses decreased without a change in the small percentage of false-positive diagnoses (140).

THE RELATIONSHIP OF DLE TO SLE

Agreement with Kaposi's belief that DLE and SLE are expressions of the same disease has waxed and waned. For example, MacLeod (141) in 1913 in London concluded: "Lupus erythematosus of the acute disseminated type has from time to time been found to occur in association with more or less general toxaemia. . . . The circumscribed cases have probably a different etiology from those of the acute disseminated type." Reliance on skin lesions to diagnose SLE was abandoned reluctantly. According to a 1952 textbook, "Diagnosis may be impossible until the appearance of the characteristic rash" (142). Of the pre-1938 cases of SLE diagnosed at the Mayo Clinic, the onset was considered to be with DLE in 47%. This decreased to 17% of those seen in the next decade, perhaps because of greater experience

(68). Keil (128) in 1937 pointed out the *lack* of correlation between the severity of cutaneous and internal manifestations, and considered it probable that the two are variants of the same disorder. However, Baehr et al. (143) still held in 1951 that "disseminate lupus erythematosus bears no relationship whatever . . . to the benign indolent skin lesion known to dermatologists as discoid lupus." Among Dubois' 520 cases of SLE (1950–1963), 10.8% initially had discoid lesions, thrice as many as had a "butterfly rash" (120). According to a more recent multicenter study, 13% of 353 cases of SLE "at some time during the course of their illness" manifested discoid lesions (144). Conversely, none of 120 cases of DLE developed systemic findings during a 5-year follow-up (145). The two opinions were moderated by Burch and Rowell (146) in 1968 in Leeds, England, who theorized that there is a different polygenic predisposition for the development of DLE and SLE: "When a genuine transition from DLE to SLE occurs, the affected patient is genetically predisposed to both diseases." The question remains open.

FOUR SUBSETS OF LUPUS ERYTHEMATOSUS

Antiphospholipid Syndrome

In 1941 Pangborn (147) in Albany, New York, discovered that the substance in the beef heart extract that was used in the complement fixation test for syphilis was a phospholipid. Keil (148) had recently surmised that the "false positive" reactions in cases of SLE are not merely coincidental. However, evidence of a mechanism to explain "biologic false positive [BFP] reactivity did not accrue until 1983, when a sensitive method to test for anti-cardiolipin [antiphospholipid] antibodies was devised" (149).

In 1948 Conley et al. (150) in Baltimore demonstrated an endogenous circulating anticoagulant in nonhemophilic bleeding patients. Four years later two cases of SLE with hemorrhaging attributed to such an anticoagulant were briefly described (151). Lee and Sanders (152) in 1955 in New York found that this substance is not a rarity in SLE, but that it usually does not cause bleeding. This observation was followed in 1963 by the surprising discovery that the anticoagulant may be associated not only with bleeding, but also with thromboses (153). In 1975 spontaneous abortion during the course of SLE was first associated with the lupus anticoagulant (154), and this relationship was subsequently confirmed prospectively (155). In 1988 anticardiolipin antibodies associated with syphilis were differentiated from those related to SLE (156).

Lupus Erythematosus Profundus

"Lupus erythematosus profundus" was coined by Samuel Irgang (157) in 1940 in New York to differentiate from DLE cases with nodular lesions in the deeper portions of the skin, but little epidermal involvement. Such a case had been described by Kaposi (13) in 1869, and this manifestation has been called Kaposi-Irgang syndrome in the dermatologic literature (158). The first American report is attributed to Fordyce (159) in 1924 in New York. Before the 1940s this variant probably was usually misdiagnosed as sarcoid (160). Winkelmann (161) in 1970 suggested that "LE panniculitis" would be a more accurate term, thereby endorsing the pathologic interpretation of Fountain (162) in 1968 in London.

Subacute Cutaneous Lupus Erythematosus

"Subacute cutaneous LE," described by Sontheimer et al. (163) in 1979 in Dallas, appears to be clinically intermediate between DLE and SLE. The lesions may be preceded by those of DLE and coincide with these at some time in about 20% of cases. They differ from discoid lesions in being annular or resembling psoriasis, lacking follicular plugging, and are less likely to heal with scarring. Patients are more frequently light sensitive than those with either DLE or SLE. About half fulfill the diagnostic criteria for SLE. Most cases are ANA-positive, but resemble "ANA-negative SLE" in being anti-Ro positive (163). Occurrence as a drug-induced phenomenon was first described in 1985, associated with hydrochlorothiazide (164).

Neonatal Lupus Erythematosus

The innocuous transplacental transfer of the LE factor (anti-DNA antibody) was demonstrated in 1954 (165). In the same year a case of transient DLE was described in an infant whose mother subsequently developed SLE (166). Since then, neonatal DLE has usually been found to resolve within the first year. In 1957 a woman with SLE delivered a boy who had complete heart block and died on the second day. His myocardium was found to contain hematoxylin bodies (167). By 1977, sufficient cases of neonatal complete heart block had been described that this became recognized as the most characteristic sign of neonatal LE, occurring in about half of these infants (168–170). Second most frequent are cutaneous lesions. SS-A (anti-Ro) antibody was pointed out in 1981 to be the most consistent serologic finding in both neonatal DLE and SLE (171, 172).

HOW DID SLE COME TO BE TRANSFERRED FROM THE REALM OF DERMATOLOGY TO INTERNAL MEDICINE?

With few exceptions, such as the clinical observations of Osler and of Libman, the delineation and treatment of LE remained in the domain of dermatologists until the 1940s.

There are two complementary explanations for this: (a) SLE was recognized by its cutaneous findings and thereby was linked, albeit equivovally, to DLE, a cutaneous disease. SLE was diagnosed much less frequently than DLE and its visceral manifestations were considered secondary to the cutaneous. The 1939 edition of Sutton and Sutton's *Diseases of the Skin* contained 13 pages on DLE and SLE (173), while the 1944 edition of Comroe's *Arthritis and Allied Conditions* had three (174). It only became accepted in the 1940s that SLE may occur without skin lesions (35), one factor that moved the disease toward the internist. (b) A medical specialty, when it is circumscribed by more than the patient's age or gender, results from particular technical and/or therapeutic expertise. Although the beginnings of rheumatology may be placed in the late 1920s, its pioneers had neither technical nor therapeutic superiority over other internists. This changed abruptly with the almost simultaneous discovery of two diagnostic methods: the rheumatoid factor and the LE cell in 1948, and cortisone therapy in 1949, followed in 1950 by the establishment of the Institute of Arthritis and Metabolic Diseases in the National Institutes of Health. The LE cell test increased the diagnosis of SLE, and corticosteroids conveyed not only that these patients could be helped, but that the treatment required specialized knowledge, thereby enhancing the status of rheumatology (175).

Interest in LE has shifted from clinical description to immunologic research, with the still frustrated goal of elucidating the etiology, whether it be single or multiple. The continued intensification of scientific interest is reflect in the listing of articles in the *Index Medicus.* These have been increasing steadily, from eight columns in 1960 to 21 in 1982, 25 in 1987, 31 in 1992, and 47 in 1997!

REFERENCES

1. de Voragnine RJ. *The golden legend.* Ryan G, Ripperger H, trans. New York: Arno Press, 1969:515–516.
2. Smith CD, Cyr M. The history of lupus erythematosus from Hippocrates to Osler. *Rheum Dis Clin North Am* 1988;14:1–19.
3. Neuburger M. *Geschichte der Medizin,* vol 2. Stuttgart: F Enke, 1911:307.
4. Michelson HE. The history of lupus vulgaris. *J Invest Dermatol* 1946;7:261–267.
5. Paracelsus TB. *Bücher und Schriften.* Huser J, ed. 1639. (Reprint: *Von dem Buch der Arznei kompt,* vol 1. Hildesheim: G Olms, 1971:235.)
6. Bateman T. *A practical synopsis of cutaneous diseases.* 1st American edition from the 4th London ed. Philadelphia: Collins & Croft, 1818:305.
7. Paget J. *Lectures on surgical pathology.* Philadelphia: Lindsay & Blakiston, 1854:588–589.
8. Von Hebra F. *Jahresbericht über die Fortschritte der gesammten Medecin in allen Ländern im Jahre,* 1845. Canstatt BF, Eisermann G, eds. Erlangen: F Enke, 1846:226–227.
9. Cazenave A, Schedel HE. *Manual of diseases of the skin,* 2nd American ed. New York: SS & W Wood, 1852:35–36.
10. Wallace DJ, Lyon I. Pierre Cazenave and the first detailed modern description of lupus erythematosus. *Semin Arthritis Rheum* 1999;28:305–313.
11. Cazenave A, Chausit M. Conference 4 June 1951. *Ann Mal de la Peau* 1851;3:297–299. Cited in Holubar K. Terminology and iconography of lupus erythematosus. *Am J Dermatopathol* 1980; 2:239–242.
12. Wilson E. *On diseases of the skin,* 5th American edition from the 5th London ed. Philadelphia: Blanchard & Lea, 1863:315.
13. Kaposi (Kohn) M. Zum Wesen und zur Therapie des Lupus erythematosus. *Arch Dermatol Syph* 1869;1:18–41.
14. Kaposi M. Neue Beiträge zur Kenntnis des Lupus erythematosus. *Arch Dermatol Syph* 1872;4:36–78.
15. Kaposi M. *Pathologie und Therapie der Hautkrankheiten.* Wien: Urban & Schwarzenberg, 1893:714.
16. Geddings WH. On lupus erythematosus. *Am J Med Sci* 1869; 58:58–69.
17. Hutchinson J. Harveian lectures on lupus. *Br Med J* 1888;1: 6–10,58–63,113–118.
18. Crocker HR. *Diseases of the skin,* vol 2, 3rd ed. Philadelphia: P Blakiston, 1897:1402,1404.
19. Hartzell MB. *Diseases of the skin. Their pathology and treatment.* Philadelphia: JB Lippincott, 1917:362.
20. Goeckerman WH. Is lupus erythematosus discoides chronicus due to tuberculosis? *Arch Dermatol Syph* 1921;3:788–801.
21. Keil H. Relationship between lupus erythematosus and tuberculosis. *Arch Dermatol Syph* 1933;28:765–779.
22. Hardaway WA. A case of lupus erythematosus presenting unusual complications. *J Cutan GU Dis* 1889;7:447–450.
23. Philippson L. Ein Fall von Lupus erythematosus disseminatus mit Gelenkaffectionen. *Berl Klin Wochenschr* 1892;29:870–871.
24. Osler W. On the visceral complications of erythema exudativum multiforme. *Am J Med Sci* 1895;110:629–646.
25. Osler W. The visceral lesions of the erythema group. *Br J Dermatol* 1900;12:227–245.
26. Osler W. On the visceral manifestations of the erythema group of skin diseases (third paper). *Trans Assoc Am Phys* 1903;18: 599–624. Also *Am J Med Sci* 1904;127:1–23.
27. Christian HA. Visceral disturbances in patients with cutaneous lesions of the erythema group. *JAMA* 1917;69:125–129.
28. Engman MF, Weiss RS. The "erythema group" of skin diseases. *Arch Dermatol Syph* 1925;12:325–333.
29. Keil H. Conception of lupus erythematosus and its morphologic variants. *Arch Dermatol Syph* 1937;36:729–757.
30. Benedek TG. William Osler and development of the concept of systemic lupus erythematosus. *Semin Arthritis Rheum* 1997;27: 48–56.
31. Kraus A, Bohac C. Bericht über acht Fälle von Lupus erythematosus acutus. *Arch Dermatol Syph* 1908–09;43:117–156.
32. Scholz M. Lupus erythematosus acutus disseminatus hemorrhagicus. Report of a case. *Arch Dermatol Syph* 1922;6: 466–472.
33. Friedberg CK, Gross L, Wallach K. Nonbacterial thrombotic endocarditis associated with prolonged fever, arthritis, inflammation of serous membranes and wide-spread vascular lesions. *Arch Intern Med*1936;58:662–684.
34. Rakov HL, Taylor JS. Acute disseminated lupus erythematosus without cutaneous manifestations and with heretofore undescribed pulmonary lesions. *Arch Intern Med* 1942;70:88–100.
35. Brunsting LA. Disseminated (systemic) lupus erythematosus. *Proc Staff Mayo Clin* 1952;27:410–412.
36. Harvey AM, Shulman LE, Tumulty PA, et al. Systemic lupus erythematosus. Review of the literature and clinical analysis of 138 cases. Medicine 1954;33:291–437.
37. Libman E, Sacks B. A hitherto undescribed form of valvular and mural endocarditis. *Arch Intern Med* 1924;33:701–737.

38. Libman E, Sacks B. A hitherto undescribed form of valvular and mural endocarditis. *Trans Assoc Am Physicians* 1923;38:46–61.
39. Belote GH, Ratner HS. The so-called Libman-Sacks syndrome. Its relation to dermatology. *Arch Dermatol Syph* 1936;33: 642–664.
40. Ginzler AM, Fox TT. Disseminated lupus erythematosus. a cutaneous manifestation of a systemic disease (Libman-Sacks). *Arch Intern Med* 1940;65:26–50.
41. Doherty NE, Siegel RJ. Cardiovascular manifestations of systemic lupus erythematosus. *Am Heart J* 1985;110:1257–1265.
42. Sequeira JH, Balean H. Lupus erythematosus: a clinical study of seventy-one cases. *Br J Dermatol* 1902;14:367–379.
43. Keith NM, Rowntree LG. A study of renal complications of disseminated lupus erythematosus: report of four cases. *Trans Assoc Am Physicians* 1922;37:487–502.
44. Baehr G, Klemperer P, Schifren A. A diffuse disease of the peripheral circulation (usually associated with lupus erythematosus and endocarditis). *Trans Assoc Am Physicians* 1935;50: 139–155.
45. Kaiser IH. The specificity of periarterial fibrosis of the spleen in disseminated lupus erythematosus. *Bull J Hopkins Hosp* 1942; 71:31–42.
46. MacLeod JM. A lecture on lupus erythematosus: its nature and treatment. *Lancet* 1908;2:1271–1275.
47. Russell PW, Haserick JR, Zucker EM. Epilepsy in systemic lupus erythematosus. Effect of cortisone and ACTH. *Arch Intern Med* 1951;88:78–92.
48. Bowen JT. Lupus erythematosus. In: Stedman TL, ed. *Twentieth century practice*, vol 5. New York: W Wood, 1896:691–708.
49. Daly D. Central nervous system in acute disseminate lupus erythematosus. *J Nerv Ment Dis* 1945;102:461–465.
50. Fessel WJ, Solomon GF. Psychosis and systemic lupus erythematosus. A review of the literature and case reports. *Calif Med* 1960;92:266–270.
51. Jarcho S. Lupus erythematosus associated with visceral vascular lesions. *Bull J Hopkins Hosp* 1936;59:262–270.
52. Piper PG. Disseminated lupus erythematosus with involvement of the spinal cord. *JAMA* 1953;153:215–217.
53. Goldstein I, Wexler D. Retinal vascular disease in a case of acute lupus erythematosus disseminatus. *Arch Ophthalmol* 1932;8: 852–857.
54. Semon H, Wolff E. Acute lupus erythematosus with fundus lesions. *Proc R Soc Med* 1933;27:153–157.
55. Pillat A. Über das Vorkommen von Choroiditis bei lupus erythematodes. *Arch Ophthalmol* 1935;133:566–577.
56. Maumenee AE. Retinal lesions in lupus erythematosus. *Am J Ophthalmol* 1940;23:971–981.
57. Lieberman TW. Retinal cotton wool spots and cytoid bodies. *Mt Sinai Hosp J* 1972;39:604–609.
58. Gold DH, Morris DA, Henkind P. Ocular findings in systemic lupus erythematosus. *Br J Ophthalmol* 1972;56:800–804.
59. Keefer CS, Felty AR. Acute disseminated lupus erythematosus. *Bull Johns Hopkins Hosp* 1924;35:294–304.
60. Goeckerman WH. Lupus erythematosus as a systemic disease. *JAMA* 1923;80:542–547.
61. Rose E, Pillsbury DM. Acute disseminated lupus erythematosus—a systemic disease. *Ann Intern Med* 1939;12:951–963.
62. Lyon JM. Acute lupus erythematosus. *Am J Dis Child* 1933;45: 572–583.
63. Templeton HJ. Thrombocytopenia in acute disseminated lupus erythematosus. *Arch Dermatol Syph* 1934;29:700–702.
64. Michael SR, Vural IL, Bassen FA, et al. The hematologic aspects of disseminated (systemic) lupus erythematosus. *Blood* 1951;6: 1059–1072.
65. Reinhart A. Erfahrungen mit der Wassermann-Neisser-Bruckschen Syphilis-reaktion. *Munch Med Wochenschr* 1909;41: 1092–2097.
66. Hauck L. Positiver Ausfall der Wassermann-Neisser-Bruckschen Syphilis-reaktion bei Lupus erythematosus acutus. *Münch Med Wochenschr* 1910;57:17.
67. Rein CR, Kostant GH. Lupus erythematosus. serologic and chemical aspects. *Arch Dermatol Syph* 1950;61:898–903.
68. Montgomery H, McCreight WG. Disseminate lupus erythematosus. *Arch Dermatol Syph* 1949;60:356–372.
69. Coburn AF, Moore DH. The plasma proteins in disseminate lupus erythematosus. *Bull Johns Hopkins Hosp* 1943;73: 196–204.
70. Moore JE, Lutz WB. The natural history of systemic lupus erythematosus. an approach to its study through chronic biologic false positive reactors. *J Chron Dis* 1955;1:297–316.
71. Haserick JR, Long R. Systemic lupus erythematosus preceded by false-positive serologic tests for syphilis. presentation of five cases. *Ann Intern Med* 1952;37:559–565.
72. Hargraves MM. Discovery of the LE cell and its morphology. *Mayo Clin Proc* 1969;44:579–599.
73. Hargraves MM, Richmond H, Morton R. Presentation of two bone marrow elements. the "tart" cell and the "LE" cell. *Proc Staff Mayo Clin* 1948;23:25–28.
74. Haserick JR, Sundberg RD. The bone marrow as a diagnostic aid in acute disseminated lupus erythematosus. *J Invest Dermatol* 1948;11:209–213.
75. Hargraves MM. Production in vitro of the LE cell phenomenon: use of normal bone marrow elements and blood plasma from patients with acute disseminated lupus erythematosus. *Proc Staff Mayo Clin* 1949;24:234–237.
76. Haserick JR, Bortz DW. A new diagnostic test for acute disseminated lupus erythematosus. *Cleve Clin Q* 1949;16: 158–161.
77. Haserick JR. Blood factor in acute disseminated lupus erythematosus. II. Induction of specific antibodies against LE factor. *Blood* 1950;5:718–722.
78. Klemperer P, Gueft B, Lee SL, et al. Cytochemical changes of acute lupus erythematosus. *Arch Pathol* 1950;49:503–515.
79. Watson JB, O'Leary PA, Hargraves MM. Neutrophiles resembling LE cells in artificial blisters. *Arch Dermatol Syph* 1951;63; 328–333.
80. Zimmer FE, Hargraves MM. The effect of blood coagulation on LE cell formation. *Proc Staff Mayo Clin* 1952;27:424–430.
81. Kievits JH, Goslings J, Schuit HR, et al. Rheumatoid arthritis and the positive LE-cell phenomenon. *Ann Rheum Dis* 1956;15: 211–216.
82. Rothfield NF, Phythyon JM, McEwen C, et al. The role of antinuclear reactions in the diagnosis of systemic lupus erythematosus: a study of 53 cases. *Arthritis Rheum* 1961;4:223–239.
83. Miescher P, Fauconnet M. L'absorption du facteur "LE" par des noyaux cellulaires isoles. *Experientia* 1954;10:252–254.
84. Friou, GJ, Finch, SC, Detre KD. Interaction of nuclei and globulin from lupus erythematosus serum demonstrated with fluorescent antibody. *J Immunol* 1958;80:324–329.
85. Holman HR, Deicher HR. The reaction of the LE cell factor with deoxy-ribonucleoprotein of the cell nucleus. *J Clin Invest* 1959;38:2059–2072.
86. Beck JS. Antinuclear antibodies: methods of detection and significance. *Mayo Clin Proc* 1969;44:600–619.
87. Ceppelini R, Polli E, Celada F. A DNA-reacting factor in serum of a patient with lupus erythematosus diffusus. *Proc Soc Exp Biol Med* 1957;96:572–574.
88. Robbins WC, Holman HR, Deicher HR, et al. Complement fixation with cell nuclei and DNA in lupus erythematosus. *Proc Soc Exp Biol Med* 1957;96:575–579.

89. Tan EM, Schur PH, Carr RI, et al. Deoxyribonucleic acid (DNA) and antibodies to DNA in the serum of patients with systemic lupus erythematosus. *J Clin Invest* 1966;45: 1732–1740.
90. Koffler D, Carr RI, Agnello V, et al. Antibodies to polynucleotides: distribution in human serum. *Science* 1969;166: 1648–1649.
91. Schur PH, Stollar D, Steinberg AD, et al. Incidence of antibodies to double-stranded RNA in systemic lupus erythematosus and related diseases. *Arthritis Rheum* 1971;14:342–347.
92. Tan EM, Kunkel HG. Characteristics of a soluble nuclear antigen precipitating with sera of patients with systemic lupus erythematosus. *J Immunol* 1966;96:464–471.
93. Fritzler MJ, Tan EM. Antibodies to histones in drug-induced and idiopathic lupus erythematosus. *J Clin Invest* 1978;62: 560–567.
94. Tan EM, Robinson J, Robitaille P. Studies on antibodies to histones immunofluorescence. *Scand J Immunol* 1976;5:811–817.
95. Portanova JP, Rubin, RL, Joslin FG, et al. Reactivity of anti-histone antibodies induced by procainamide and hydralazine. *Clin Immunol Immunopathol* 1982;25:57–79.
96. Fessel WJ. ANA-negative systemic lupus erythematosus. *Am J Med* 1977;64:80–86.
97. Maddison RJ, Provost TT, Reichlin M. Serological findings with ANA-negative systemic lupus erythematosus. *Medicine* 1981;60:87–94.
98. Burnham TK, Neblett TR, Fine G. The application of the fluorescent antibody technic to the investigation of lupus erythematosus and various dermatoses. *J Invest Dermatol* 1963;41: 451–456.
99. Burnham TK, Fine G. The immunofluorescent "band" test for lupus erythematosus. III. Employing clinically normal skin. *Arch Dermatol* 1971;103:24–32.
100. Ma AS, Soltani K, Bristol LA, et al. Cutaneous immunofluorescence studies in adult rheumatoid arthritis in sun-exposed and non-sun-exposed areas. *Int J Dermatol* 1984;23:269–272.
101. Jablonska S, Beutner EH, Micehl B, et al. Uses for immunofluorescent tests of skin and sera. *Arch Dermatol* 1975;111:371–381.
102. Jessar RA, Lamont-Havers RW, Ragan C. Natural history of lupus erythematosus disseminatus. *Ann Intern Med* 1953;38: 1265–1294.
103. Dubois EL. The effect of the LE cell test on the clinical picture of systemic lupus erythematosus. *Ann Intern Med* 1953;38: 1265–1294.
104. Svanbord A, Solvell L. Incidence of disseminated lupus erythematosus. *JAMA* 1957;165:1126–1128.
105. Siegel M, Reilly EB, Lee SL, et al. Epidemiology of Systemic lupus erythematosus. Time trend and racial differences. *Am J Public Health* 1964;54:33–43.
106. Merrell M, Shulman LE. Determination of Prognosis in chronic disease, illustrated by systemic lupus erythematosus. *J Chron Dis* 1955;1:12–32.
107. Hench PS, Kendall EC, Slocumb CH, et al. Effects of cortisone acetate and pituitary ACTH on rheumatoid arthritis, rheumatic fever and certain other conditions. *Arch Intern Med* 1950;85: 545–666.
108. Albert DA, Hadler NH, Ropes MW. Does corticosteroid therapy affect the survival of patients with systemic lupus erythematosus? *Arthritis Rheum* 1979;22:945–953.
109. Urman JD, Rothfield NF. Corticosteroid treatment in systemic lupus erythematosus. Survival studies. *JAMA* 1977;238: 2272–2276.
110. Haserick JR. Effect of cortisone and corticotropin on prognosis of systemic lupus erythematosus. *Arch Dermatol Syph* 1953;68: 714–725.
111. Wallace DJ, Podell T, Weiner J, et al. Systemic lupus erythematosus—survival patterns. Experience with 609 patients. *JAMA* 1981;245:934–938.
112. Klinge F. Der Rheumatismus; pathologisch-anatomische und experimentell-pathologische Tatsachen. *Ergeb Allg Pathol Pathol Anat* 1933;27:1–355.
113. Klemperer P, Pollack AD, Baehr G. Diffuse collagen disease. Acute disseminated lupus erythematosus and diffuse scleroderma. *JAMA* 1942;119:331–332.
114. Benedek TG. Subcutaneous nodules and the differentiation of rheumatoid arthritis from rheumatic fever. *Semin Arthritis Rheum* 1984;13:305–321.
115. Gennerich W. Über die Ätiologie des Lupus erythematodes. *Arch Dermatol Syph* 1921;135:184–207.
116. Rich AR. Hypersensitivity in disease, with special reference to periarteritis nodosa, rheumatic fever, disseminated lupus erythematosus and rheumatoid arthritis. *Harvey Lect* 1947;42: 106–147.
117. Gross L. The heart in atypical verrucous endocarditis. In: *Contributions to the medical sciences in honor of Dr. Emanuel Libman*, vol 2. New York: International Press, 1932:527–550.
118. Pulay E. Stoffwechselpathologie und Hautkrankheiten. XVII. *Dermatol Wochenschr* 1921;73:1217–1234.
119. Rasch C. Some historical and clinical remarks on the effect of light on the skin and skin diseases. *Proc R Soc Med* 1926;20: 11–30
120. Tuffanelli DL, Dubois EL. Cutaneous manifestations of systemic lupus erythematosus. *Arch Dermatol Syph* 1964;90:377–386.
121. Ingels AE. Lupus erythematosus treated with sulfanilamide. *Arch Dermatol Syph* 1938;37:879–884.
122. Hoffman, BJ. Sensitivity to sulfadiazine resembling acute disseminated lupus erythematosus. *Arch Dermatol Syph* 1945;51: 190–192.
123. Gold S. Role of sulphonamides and penicillin in the pathogenesis of systemic lupus erythematosus. *Lancet* 1951;1:268–272.
124. Ruete A. Ueber den Wert des Aurium-Kalium cyanatum bei der Behandlung des Lupus vulgaris und erythematodes. *Dtsch Med Wochenschr* 1913;39:1727–1729.
125. Schamberg JF, Wright CS. The use of gold and sodium thiosulfate in the treatment of lupus erythematosus. *Arch Dermatol Syph* 1927;15:119–137.
126. Pillsbury DM, Jacobson C. Treatment of chronic discoid lupus erythematosus with chloroquine (Aralen). *JAMA* 1954; 1330–1333.
127. Crissey JT, Murray PF. A comparison of chloroquine and gold in the treatment of lupus erythematosus. *Arch Dermatol Syph* 1956;74:69–72.
128. Keil H. Conception of lupus erythematosus and its morphologic variants. *Arch Dermatol Syph* 1937;36:729–757.
129. Lansbury J. The collaen diseases. In: Hollander JL, ed. *Arthritis and allied conditions*, 4th ed. Philadelphia: Lea & Febiger, 1949: 670.
130. Dustan HP, Taylor RD, Corcoran AC, et al. Rheumatic and febrile syndrome during prolonged hydralazine treatment. *JAMA* 1954;154:23–29.
131. Ruppli H, Vossen R. Nebenwirkung der Hydantoinkörpertherapie unter dem Bilde eines visceralen Lupus erythematosus. *Schweiz Med Wochenschr* 1957;87:1555–1558.
132. Ladd AT. Procainamide-induced lupus erythematosus. *N Engl J Med* 1962;267:1357–1358.
133. Comens P, Schroeder HA. The LE cell as a manifestation of delayed hydralazine intoxication. *JAMA* 1956;160:1134–1136.
134. Alarcon-Segovia D, Worthington JW, Ward E, et al. Lupus diathesis and the hydralazine syndrome. *N Engl J Med* 1965; 272:462–466.

135. Lindqvist T. Lupus erythematosus disseminatus after administration of mesantoin. *Acta Med Scand* 1957;158:131–138.
136. Dubois EL. Procainamide induction of a systemic lupus erythematosus-like syndrome. *Medicine* 1969;48:217–228.
137. Blomgren SE, Condemi JJ, Bignall MC. Antinuclear antibody induced by procainamide. *N Engl J Med* 1969;281:64–66.
138. Jones TD. The diagnosis of rheumatic fever. *JAMA* 1944;126: 481–484.
139. Cohen AS, Reynolds WE, Franklin EC, et al. Preliminary criteria for the classification of systemic lupus erythematosus. *Bull Rheum Dis* 1971;21:643–648.
140. Tan EM, Cohen AS, Fries JF, et al. The 1982 revised criteria for the classification of systemic lupus erythematosus. *Arthritis Rheum* 1982;25:1271–1277.
141. MacLeod JM. Discussion on the nature, varieties, causes, and treatment of lupus erythematosus. *Br Med J* 1913;2:313–319.
142. Traut EF. *Rheumatic diseases. Diagnosis and treatment*. St. Louis: CV Mosby, 1952:613.
143. Baehr G. Disseminated lupus erythematosus. In: Cecil RL, Loeb RF, eds. *A textbook of medicine*, 8th ed. Philadelphia. WB Saunders, 1951:483.
144. Hay EM, Gordon BC, Isenberg DA, et al. The BILAG index. a reliable and valid instrument for measuring clinical disease activity in systemic lupus erythematosus. *Q J Med* 1993;86: 447–458.
145. Beck JS, Rowell NR. Discoid lupus erythematosus. *Q J Med* 1966;35:119–136.
146. Burch PR, Rowell NR. The sex- and age-distribution of chronic discoid lupus erythematosus in four countries. *Acta Derm Venereol* 1968;48:33–46.
147. Pangborn MC. A new serologically active phospholipid from beef heart. *Proc Soc Exp Biol Med* 1941;48:484–486.
148. Keil H. Dermatomyositis and systemic lupus erythematosus. II. Comparative study of essential clinicopathologic features. *Arch Intern Med* 1940;66:339–383.
149. Harris EN, Boey ML, Mackworth-Young CG, et al. Anticardiolipin antibodies: detection by radioimmunoassay and association with thrombosis in systemic lupus erythematosus. *Lancet* 1983;2:1211–1214.
150. Conley CL, Rathbun HK, Morse WI, et al. Circulating anticoagulant as a cause of hemorrhagic diathesis in man. *Bull Johns Hopkins Hosp* 1948;83:288–296.
151. Conley CL, Hartman RC. A hemorrhagic disorder caused by circulating anti-coagulant in patients with disseminated lupus erythematosus. *J Clin Invest* 1952;31:621–622.
152. Lee SL, Sanders M. A disorder of blood coagulation in systemic lupus erythematosus. *J Clin Invest* 1955;34:1814–1822.
153. Bowie EJ, Thompson JH, Pacussi CA, et al. Thrombosis in systemic lupus erythematosus despite circulating anticoagulants. *J Lab Clin Med* 1963;62:416–430.
154. Nilsson IM, Astedt B, Hedner U, et al. Intrauterine death and circulating anticoagulant ("antithromboplastin"). *Acta Med Scand* 1975;197:153–159.
155. Lockshin MD, Druzin ML, Goei S, et al. Antibody to cardiolipin as a predictor of fetal distress or death in pregnant patients with systemic lupus erythematosus. *N Engl J Med* 1985;313:152–156.
156. Harris EN, Gharavi AE, Wasley GD, et al. Use of an enzyme-linked immunoabsorbent assay and of inhibition studies to distinguish between antibodies to cardiolipin from patients with syphilis or autoimmune disorders. *J Infect Dis* 1988;157: 23–31.
157. Irgang S. Lupus erythematosus profundus. *Arch Dermatol Syph* 1940;42:97–108.
158. Arnold HL. Lupus erythematosus profundus (Kaposi-Irgang). *Arch Dermatol Syph* 1948;57:196–203.
159. Fordyce JA. Lupus erythematosus with nodular lesions suggesting sarcoid. *Arch Dermatol Syph* 1925;11:852–853.
160. Arnold HL. Lupus erythematosus profundus. Commentary and report of four more cases. *Arch Dermatol Syph* 1956;73:15–33.
161. Winkelmann RK. Panniculitis and systemic lupus erythematosus. *JAMA* 1970;211:472–475.
162. Fountain RB. Lupus erythematosus profundus. *Br J Dermatol* 1968;80:571–579.
163. Sontheimer RD, Thomas JR, Gilliam JN. Subacute cutaneous lupus erythematosus. A cutaneous marker for a distinct lupus erythematosus subset. *Arch Dermatol* 1979;115:1409–1415.
164. Sontheimer RD. Subacute cutaneous lupus erythematosus: a decade's perspective. *Med Clin North Am* 1989;73:1073–1090.
165. Reed BR, Huff JC, Jones SK, et al. Subacute cutaneous lupus erythematosus associated with hydrochlorothiazide therapy. *Ann Intern Med* 1985;103:49–51.
166. Bridge RG, Foley FE. Placental transmission of the lupus erythematosus factor. *Am J Med Sci* 1954;227:1–8.
167. McCuiston CH, Schoch EP. Possible discoid lupus erythematosus in newborn infant. *Arch Dermatol Syph* 1954;63:782–785.
168. Hogg GR. Congenital acute lupus erythematosus associated with subendocardial fibroelastosis. *Am J Clin Pathol* 1957;28: 648–654.
169. McCue CM, Mantakas ME, Tingelstad JB, et al. Congenital heart block in newborns of mothers with connective tissue disease. *Circulation* 1977;56:82–90.
170. Chamaides L, Truex RC, Vetter V, et al. Association of maternal systemic lupus erythematosus with congenital complete heart block. *N Engl J Med* 1977;297:1204–1207.
171. McCune AB, Weston WL, Lee LA. Maternal and fetal outcome in neonatal lupus erythematosus. *Ann Intern Med* 1987;106: 518–523.
172. Kephart DC, Hood AF, Provost TT. Neonatal lupus erythematosus: new serologic findings. *J Invest Dermatol* 1981;77:331–333.
173. Sutton RL, Sutton RL Jr. *Diseases of the skin*, 10th ed. St. Louis: CV Mosby, 1939:359–372.
174. Comroe BI. *Arthritis and allied conditions*, 3d ed. Philadelphia: Lea & Febiger, 1944:846–848.
175. Benedek TG. A century of American rheumatology. *Ann Intern Med* 1987;106:30.

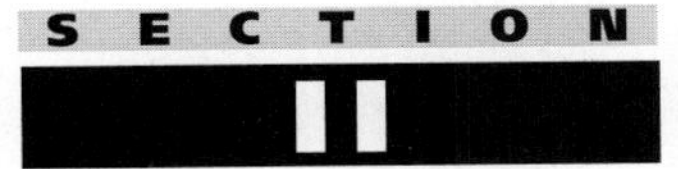

DEFINITION, CLASSIFICATION, AND EPIDEMIOLOGY

2

DEFINITION, CLASSIFICATION, ACTIVITY, AND DAMAGE INDICES

JENNIFER M. GROSSMAN
KENNETH C. KALUNIAN

DEFINITION OF SYSTEMIC LUPUS ERYTHEMATOSUS

Systemic lupus erythematosus (SLE) is a multisystem disease that is caused by tissue damage resulting from antibody and complement-fixing immune complex deposition. There is a wide spectrum of clinical presentations, which are characterized by remissions and exacerbations. The pathogenic immune responses probably result from environmental triggers acting in the setting of certain susceptibility genes. Ultraviolet light and certain drugs are the only known environmental triggers to date.

SLE CLASSIFICATION CRITERIA

In 1971, the American Rheumatism Association (ARA) published preliminary criteria for the classification of SLE. These criteria were developed for clinical trials and population studies rather than for diagnostic purposes (1). The criteria were based on information from 52 rheumatologists in clinics and hospitals in the United States and Canada; each physician provided 74 items of information on five patients in each of the following categories: unequivocal SLE, probable SLE, classic rheumatoid arthritis (RA), and medical patients with nonrheumatic diseases.

Based on computer analysis of the data, 14 manifestations were selected. The ARA committee proposed that a person can be said to have SLE if any four or more of the following manifestations are present, either serially or simultaneously, during any period of observation:

1. Facial erythema (i.e., butterfly rash): Diffuse erythema, flat or raised, over the malar eminence(s) and/or bridge of the nose; may be unilateral.
2. Discoid lupus: Erythematous-raised patches with adherent keratotic scaling and follicular plugging; atrophic scarring may occur in older lesions; may be present anywhere on the body.
3. Raynaud's phenomenon: Requires a two-phase color reaction, by patient's history or physician's observation.
4. Alopecia: Rapid loss of a large amount of scalp hair, by patient's history or physician's observation.
5. Photosensitivity: Unusual skin reaction from exposure to sunlight, by patient's history or physician's observation.
6. Oral or nasopharyngeal ulceration.
7. Arthritis without deformity: One or more peripheral joints involved with any of the following in the absence of deformity: (a) pain on motion, (b) tenderness, (c) effusion or periarticular soft tissue swelling. (Peripheral joints include feet, ankles, knees, hips, shoulders, elbows, wrists, and metacarpophalangeal, proximal interphalangeal, terminal interphalangeal, and temporomandibular joints.)
8. Lupus erythematosus (LE) cells: Two or more classic LE cells seen on one or more occasions, or one cell seen on two or more occasions, using an accepted, published method.
9. Chronic false-positive serologic test for syphilis (STS): Known to be present for at least 6 months and confirmed by *Treponema pallidum* immobilization (TPI) or Reiter's tests.
10. Profuse proteinuria: Greater than 3.5 g/d.
11. Urinary cellular casts: May be red cell, hemoglobin, granular, tubular, or mixed.
12. One or both of the following: (a) pleuritis, good history of pleuritic pain; or rub heard by a physician; or radiographic evidence of both pleural thickening and fluid; and/or (b) pericarditis, documented by electrocardiogram (ECG) or rub.
13. One or both of the following: (a) psychosis, and/or (b) convulsions, by patient's history or physician's observation in the absence of uremia and offending drugs.
14. One or more of the following: (a) hemolytic anemia; (b) leukopenia, white blood cell count of less than 4000/mL on two or more occasions; and/or (c) thrombocytopenia, platelet count less than 100,000/mL.

These criteria were selected because of their high sensitivity and specificity; the committee noted a 90% sensitivity and 99% specificity against RA and a 98% specificity against a miscellany of nonrheumatic diseases (1). In a retrospective pilot study of 500 male veterans with scleroderma, only ten patients satisfied the SLE criteria at the time of diagnosis (1).

These criteria subsequently were tested in other centers; sensitivities varied between 57.2% to 98.0% (2–6). The studies with the lowest sensitivities involved patients who were seen either initially or at only one particular point in time (4); these investigators noted that a higher proportion of their patients eventually demonstrated four or more criteria with time. Lom-Orta et al. (8) studied 31 patients who were thought to have SLE who did not fulfill the ARA criteria; 21 of them fulfilled the criteria within a few years.

Numerous suggestions were made for improvement of the classification criteria, including the inclusion of antinuclear antibody (ANA) and other autoantibodies (9–11) and use of a weighted scoring system in which certain criteria are given more weight than others (12). An ARA subcommittee was created to evaluate these considerations; their study led to the publication of revised criteria in 1982 (13). Thirty potential criteria were studied, including numerous serologic tests and histologic descriptions of skin and kidney, as well as each of the original 1971 criteria. These 30 variables were compared in patients with SLE and matched controls. Eighteen investigators representing major clinics contributed patient report forms; these forms indicated the presence or absence of each variable at the time of examination or any time in the past. Abnormalities that could be attributed to comorbid conditions or concurrent medications were not reported (14). Each investigator was instructed to report data on ten consecutive patients and the next age-, race-, and sex-matched patient with a nontraumatic, nondegenerative, connective tissue disease seen at that clinic. This generated data from 177 patients with SLE and 162 control patients from 18 institutions. Cluster and other multivariate analysis techniques were used in studying the variables; numerous potential criteria sets were analyzed.

The final revised criteria consist of 11 items, compared with 14 in the preliminary criteria; five of the criteria are composites of one or more abnormalities. As in the preliminary data, patients must fulfill four or more criteria; no single criterion is absolutely essential. These criteria are the same as the 1997 revised criteria shown in Table 2.1 with the exception of criterion 10, which according to the revised 1982 criteria read: immunologic disorder (a) positive LE-cell preparation OR (b) anti–double-stranded DNA OR (c) anti-Sm OR (d) biologically false positive (BFP) [false-positive serologic test for syphilis positive for at least 6 months with negative TPI or fluorescein treponema antibody (FTA) test].

TABLE 2.1. THE 1997 REVISED CRITERIA FOR THE CLASSIFICATION OF SYSTEMIC LUPUS ERYTHEMATOSUS (SLE)

Criterion	Definition
1. Malar rash	Fixed malar erythema, flat or raised
2. Discoid rash	Erythematous-raised patches with keratotic scaling and follicular plugging; atrophic scarring may occur in older lesions
3. Photosensitivity	Skin rash as an unusual reaction to sunlight, by patient history or physician observation
4. Oral ulcers	Oral or nasopharyngeal ulcers, usually painless, observed by physician
5. Arthritis	Nonerosive arthritis involving two or more peripheral joints, characterized by tenderness, swelling, or effusion
6. Serositis	a. Pleuritis (convincing history of pleuritic pain or rub heard by physician or evidence of pleural effusion) OR b. Pericarditis (documented by ECG, rub, or evidence of pericardial effusion)
7. Renal disorder	a. Persistent proteinuria (>0.5 g/d or >3+) OR b. Cellular casts of any type
8. Neurologic disorder	a. Seizures (in the absence of other causes) OR b. Psychosis (in the absence of other causes)
9. Hematologic disorder	a. Hemolytic anemia OR b. Leukopenia (<4,000/mL on two or more occasions) OR c. Lymphopenia (<1,500/mL on two or more occasions) OR d. Thrombocytopenia (<100,000/mL in the absence of offending drugs)
10. Immunologic disorder	a. Anti–double-stranded DNA OR b. Anti-Sm OR c. Positive finding of antiphospholipid antibodies based on (1) an abnormal serum level of IgG or IgM anticardioliin antibodies, (2) a positive test result for lupus anticoagulant using a standard method, or (3) a false-positive serologic test for syphilis known to be positive for at least 6 months and confirmed by *Treponema pallidum* immobilization or fluorescent treponemal antibody absorption test
11. Antinuclear antibody	An abnormal titer of antinuclear antibody (ANA) by immunofluorescence or an equivalent assay at any time and in the absence of drugs known to be associated with "drug-induced lupus syndrome."

For identifying patients in clinical studies, a person shall be said to have SLE if any four or more of the 11 criteria are present, either serially or simultaneously, during any interval or observation.
Ig, immunoglobulin.
From Hochberg MG. Updating the American College of Rheumatology revised criteria for the classification of systemic lupus erythematosus (letter). *Arthritis Rheum* 1997;40:1725, with permission.

Skin and kidney biopsies were not used in the final criteria set, because they were infrequently obtained. Raynaud's phenomenon and alopecia were eliminated, because their combined sensitivity/specificity scores were low. Renal criteria were consolidated. In the preliminary criteria set, cellular casts and proteinuria were separate criteria; in the revised set, there is only a single renal criterion, which is satisfied if a patient has cellular casts and/or proteinuria. In addition, the revised criteria reduced the amount of proteinuria that is needed for fulfillment, from greater than 3.5 g/d in the preliminary set to more than 0.5 g/d (or >3+ if quantitation is not performed) in the revised set.

ANA, anti-DNA, and anti-Sm antibodies were included, and the importance of false-positive serology for syphilis and LE-cell preparations was downgraded. ANAs were felt to be the most important addition to the criteria set, because they were positive at some point during the course of disease in 176 of the 177 patients. Despite their nonspecificity (they were present in 51% of the controls studied), the subcommittee felt their almost universal positivity made them a necessary criterion.

Using the patient database on which they were based, the revised criteria were 96% sensitive and specific, compared with 78% and 87%, respectively, for the 1971 criteria (13). The subcommittee further tested the revised criteria against an ARA database of 590 patients with SLE, scleroderma, or dermatomyositis/polymyositis. Using the revised criteria against this database population, sensitivity in patients with SLE was 83%, and specificity against the combined scleroderma and dermatomyositis/polymyositis patients was 89%. Using the preliminary criteria, sensitivity for SLE was only 78% and specificity only 87% (14).

In a subsequent comparison of the relative sensitivities of the 1971 and 1982 criteria, Levin et al. (15) studied 156 patients with SLE at the University of Connecticut (a participating center in devising the revised criteria). Eighty-eight percent met the preliminary criteria, whereas 83% met the revised criteria when arthritis was strictly defined (i.e., nonerosive arthritis). Ninety-one percent met the revised criteria when arthritis was more liberally defined (i.e., nondeforming arthritis). These differences were not statistically significant. Their analysis also noted that of the three serologic tests added in the revised criteria (i.e., ANA, anti-Sm, and anti-DNA antibodies), ANA accounted for the increased sensitivity of the revised criteria. Levin et al. noted that both the preliminary and the revised criteria were inappropriate for diagnostic purposes, in that over 50% of their patients fulfilled neither set of criteria when tested at the time of diagnosis. These patients subsequently fulfilled both sets of criteria at the same rate (77.5% fulfilled preliminary criteria and 78.5% revised criteria 5 years after diagnosis, and 84.5% and 83.0% for preliminary and revised criteria, respectively, at 7 years).

Passas et al. (16) compared specificity of the preliminary and revised criteria in 207 University of Connecticut patients with non-SLE rheumatic diseases that are important in the differential diagnosis of SLE. The specificity was 98% for the preliminary criteria and 99% for the revised criteria. The preliminary and revised criteria also were tested on 285 Japanese patients with SLE and 272 control patients with non-SLE connective tissue diseases (17). The preliminary criteria had a sensitivity of 78% and a specificity of 98%, compared with a sensitivity of 89% and specificity of 96% for the revised criteria. Davis and Stein (18) applied the preliminary and revised criteria to 18 Zimbabwean patients with SLE reported up to 1989; they noted a sensitivity of 83% for the preliminary and 94% for the revised criteria. When serologic criteria were excluded, the sensitivity of the revised criteria was only 78%. They concluded that in many areas of Zimbabwe, where serologic tests are not readily available, the preliminary criteria may be more valuable than the revised criteria in the classification of patients with SLE, because the preliminary criteria rely more on clinical rather than serologic variables. An Iranian study (19) noted an improvement in sensitivity with the revised criteria (90% vs. 81% for the revised and preliminary criteria, respectively) in a study of 135 patients with SLE in Tehran. They noted that this improvement was attributed to the inclusion of ANA, anti-DNA antibodies, and the decrease in the level of proteinuria needed to fulfill the renal criterion.

The patient data set on which the revised criteria were based was reanalyzed by Edworthy et al. (20) using recursive partitioning methodology to develop two classification trees; the intent was to provide a simpler means of classifying patients with SLE. The simple tree requires knowledge of only two variables: immunologic disorder and malar rash. If a patient has an immunologic disorder [defined as the presence of LE cells, a false-positive Venereal Disease Research Laboratory (VDRL) test, anti-DNA antibodies, or anti-Sm antibodies], then the patient meets the classification criteria; if the patient does not fulfill the immunologic criterion but has a malar rash, then the patient is classified as having SLE. A more complex classification tree also was derived that requires the knowledge of six variables, including ANA, anti-DNA antibodies, malar rash, discoid rash, pleurisy, and hypocomplementemia; all of these variables were included in the revised criteria set, except for hypocomplementemia. When applied to the patient data sets used in the development of the 1982 revised criteria, the sensitivity and specificity of the simple classification tree were both 92%. Using the complex tree, they noted a 97% sensitivity, 95% specificity, and 96% accuracy. Antibodies to DNA were found to be the best overall discriminator. These classification trees, however, have not been used clinically in studies of SLE.

Because the presence of antiphospholipid antibodies and the antiphospholipid syndrome was increasingly recognized in SLE patients, the Diagnostic and Therapeutic Criteria Committee of the American College of Rheumatology (ACR) reviewed the 1992 revised criteria for SLE (21). They recommended that the immunologic criteria be modified with the removal of the LE cell preparation and the addition of immunoglobulin G (IgG) or M (IgM) anticardiolipin antibodies or a lupus anticoagulant. The 1997 revised criteria are listed in Table 2.1.

None of the methods for classifying patients with SLE was intended for diagnostic purposes. The findings of Levin et al. (15) underscore the problems that are associated with use of classification criteria for diagnostic purposes. Over 50% of their patients with SLE did not fulfill the criteria at one particular point in time, and while all eventually did, it required 9 to 20 years in some cases. In addition, the sensitivity of these classification criteria for milder cases of SLE is not known. In a study of Swedish patients with SLE, Jonsson et al. (22) noted that the number of criteria in the 1982 revised set fulfilled by their patients was similar to or higher than that in other reported series despite overall mild disease. However, no strict measure of disease activity was applied, and no comparisons of disease activity in other populations were made.

SLE ACTIVITY INDICES

Defining the degree of disease activity is essential in quantitating changes in patients, standardizing differences between patients, and evaluating clinical responses to therapy, especially in therapeutic trials. Although over 60 systems to assess disease activity in SLE exist, agreement on a definition for SLE activity has not been reached (23). Most studies of the usefulness of the various available indices have focused on (a) the British Isles Lupus Assessment Group (BILAG) scale, (b) the Systemic Lupus Erythematosus Disease Activity Index (SLEDAI), (3) the Systemic Lupus Activity Measure (SLAM), and (4) the University of California, San Francisco/Johns Hopkins University Lupus Activity Index (LAI).

The BILAG system, which was developed by clinical investigators from four centers in the United Kingdom and one in the Republic of Ireland, rates the activity of SLE in eight organ systems (24). Scoring in each organ system is based on the principle of intention to treat using the following ratings: A, disease that requires urgent, disease-modifying therapy; B, disease that demands close attention and, perhaps, modification of minor therapy (e.g., addition of such medications as low-dose corticosteroids or hydroxychloroquine) with maintenance, but not institution, of new major modalities (including medications such as high-dose corticosteroids or cytotoxic agents); C, static or inactive disease requiring no or only symptomatic therapy (including pain medications and nonsteroidal antiinflammatory agents); and D, absence of symptoms or laboratory abnormalities. Ratings are made based on the patient's clinical condition within the last month before evaluation. For statistical comparison with other numerically based indices, the following weights have been given to the four categories: A = 9, B = 4, C = 1, and D = 0 (25). Possible scores with this system vary from a minimum of 0 to a maximum of 72.

The SLEDAI was developed at the University of Toronto. Several clinicians rated the importance of 37 variables in defining SLE activity (26). Using the highest-ranking 24 variables, 39 fictitious patients were created, and 14 rheumatologists ordered these patients in terms of disease activity. The implied weights of each variable in contributing to the judgment of activity in the group of fictitious patients were derived from multiple regression analysis. Real patients were then used to compare the instrument with the physician's global assessment of activity, and significant correlations were seen. The index is a one-page form with 24 items. The most recent version is shown in Figure 2.1. Definitions of the items are provided on the form. Items that are present are noted, and scoring is calculated by summing the predetermined weights for the items that are present. Items that are life-threatening have higher weights. Possible scores using this instrument vary from 0 to 105. Manifestations must be present in the 10 days preceding evaluation.

Two modifications of SLEDAI have been proposed: MEX-SLEDAI, and SELENA-SLEDAI. MEX-SLEDAI (27) was developed for use in Third World countries where immunologic and complement assays are costly and/or unavailable. The instrument uses most aspects of SLEDAI with some modifications, but it does not include anti-DNA antibodies or complement descriptors. MEX-SLEDAI also does not include the following SLEDAI clinical descriptors: visual disturbance, lupus headache, and pyuria. MEX-SLEDAI descriptors that are not part of SLEDAI include creatinine increase of greater than 5 mg/dL, hemolysis, peritonitis, fatigue, and lymphopenia. Whereas the proteinuria descriptor in the SLEDAI is defined as greater than 0.5 g per 24 hours of new onset or a recent increase of more than 0.5 g per 24 hours, the proteinuria descriptor of MEX-SLEDAI is new onset of greater than 0.5 g/L on random specimen. MEX-SLEDAI requires that significant proteinuria be new to denote activity, whereas active renal involvement in SLEDAI can be interpreted as significant new proteinuria or a significant increase in existing proteinuria. In a prospective study of 39 patients representing a spectrum of disease activity, five physicians scored disease activity using SLEDAI and MEX-SLEDAI on three consecutive patient visits (27); both instruments demonstrated validity and responsiveness.

SELENA-SLEDAI was adapted from the SLEDAI for use in a multicenter safety study of estrogens in women with SLE; it has been validated through its prospective use in the ongoing study (28). SELENA-SLEDAI differs from SLEDAI in the definitions of some descriptors for clarification and attribution. The definition of the seizure descriptor has been expanded to exclude seizures resulting from past, irreversible central nervous system damage. Scleritis and episcleritis have been added to the definition of the visual disturbance descriptor, and vertigo has been added to the cranial nerve disorder descriptor. The cerebrovascular accident descriptor excludes hypertensive causes in SELENA-SLEDAI. The pleurisy and pericarditis descriptors have been

SLEDAI-2K: DATA COLLECTION SHEET

Study No.: __________ Patient Name: ______________________________ Visit Date: ____ ____ ____
d m yr

(Enter weight in SLEDAI-2K Score column if descriptor is present at the time of the visit or in the preceding 10 days.)

SLEDAI 2K Weight	SCORE	Descriptor	Definition
8	______	Seizure	Recent onset, exclude metabolic, infectious or drug causes.
8	______	Psychosis	Altered ability to function in normal activity due to severe disturbance in the perception of reality. Include hallucinations, incoherence, marked loose associations, impoverished thought content, marked illogical thinking, bizarre, disorganized, or catatonic behavior. Exclude uremia and drug causes
8	______	Organic brain syndrome	Altered mental function with impaired orientation, memory, or other intellectual function, with rapid onset and fluctuating clinical features, inability to sustain attention to environment, plus at least 2 of the following: perceptual disturbance, incoherent speech, insomnia or daytime drowsiness, or increased or decreased psychomotor activity. Exclude metabolic, infectious, or drug causes.
8	______	Visual disturbance	Retinal changes of SLE. Include cytoid bodies, retinal hemorrhages, serous exudate or hemorrhages in the choroid, or optic neuritis. Exclude hypertension, infection, or drug causes.
8	______	Cranial nerve disorder	New onset of sensory or motor neuropathy involving cranial nerves.
8	______	Lupus headache	Severe, persistent headache; may be migrainous, but must be nonresponsive to narcotic analgesia.
8	______	CVA	New onset of cerebrovascular accident(s). Exclude arteriosclerosis.
8	______	Vasculitis	Ulceration, gangrene, tender finger nodules, periungual infarction, splinter hemorrhages, or biopsy or angiogram proof of vasculitis.
4	______	Arthritis	$\geq$ 2 joints with pain and signs of inflammation (i.e., tenderness, swelling or effusion).
4	______	Myositis	Proximal muscle aching/weakness, associated with elevated creatine phosphokinase/aldolase or electromyogram changes or a biopsy showing myositis.
4	______	Urinary casts	Heme-granular or red blood cell casts.
4	______	Hematuria	>5 red blood cells/high power field. Exclude stone, infection or other cause.
4	______	Proteinuria	>0.5 gram/24 hours
4	______	Pyuria	>5 white blood cells/high power field. Exclude infection.
2	______	Rash	Inflammatory type rash.
2	______	Alopecia	Abnormal, patchy or diffuse loss of hair.
2	______	Mucosal ulcers	Oral or nasal ulcerations.
2	______	Pleurisy	Pleuritic chest pain with pleural rub or effusion, or pleural thickening.
2	______	Pericarditis	Pericardial pain with at least 1 of the following: rub, effusion, or electrocardiogram or echocardiogram confirmation.
2	______	Low complement	Decrease in CH50, C3, or C4 below the lower limit of normal for testing laboratory
2	______	Increased DNA binding	Increased DNA binding by Farr assay above normal range for testing laboratory.
1	______	Fever	>38° C. Exclude infectious cause.
1	______	Thrombocytopenia	<100,000 platelets / $x10^9/L$, exclude drug causes.
1	______	Leukopenia	< 3,000 white blood cells / $x10^9/L$, exclude drug causes.

TOTAL SCORE ______

FIGURE 2.1. The Systemic Lupus Erythematosus Disease Activity Index 2K. (From Bombardier C, Gladman DD, Urowitz MB, et al. Derivation of the SLEDAI. A disease activity index for lupus patients. The Committee on Prognosis Studies in SLE. *Arthritis Rheum* 1992;35:630–640, with permission.)

modified as well; rather than defining pleurisy as pleuritic chest pain with pleural rub or effusion or pleural thickening, SELENA-SLEDAI defines this descriptor as classic and severe pleuritic chest pain, pleural rub, effusion, or new pleural thickening with attribution to lupus. Pericarditis is similarly redefined; instead of pericardial pain with rub, effusion, ECG, or echocardiographic confirmation, SELENA-SLEDAI defines this descriptor as classic and severe pericardial pain, rub, effusion, or ECG confirmation. In addition, the proteinuria descriptor in SELENA-SLEDAI simplifies the SLEDAI descriptor. The SELENA-SLEDAI definition of proteinuria is the new onset or recent increase of more than 0.5 g per 24 hour, whereas the SLEDAI definition can be interpreted to include all patients with proteinuria of greater than 0.5 g per 24 hours.

The SLAM, which was developed at Brigham and Women's Hospital (29), lists 33 clinical and laboratory manifestations of SLE, and each manifestation is assessed as either active or inactive. Graded estimates of activity are based on severity of increasing disability, organ destruction, need to follow the patient more closely, or need to consider major treatment change. Possible scores with this instrument vary from 0 to 86. Manifestations must be present in the month before evaluation. This index includes subjective symptoms such as fatigue, myalgias, arthralgias, and abdominal pain felt to be attributable to SLE, and therefore may detect smaller changes in disease activity.

The LAI (30) is a five-part scale. Part one is the physician's global disease activity assessment on a 0- to 3-point visual analogue scale (VAS). Part two is an assessment of four symptoms (i.e., fatigue, rash, arthritis, serositis), each on a 0- to 3-point VAS. Part three scores the activity of four organ systems (i.e., neurologic, renal, pulmonary, hematologic), each on a 0- to 3-point VAS. Part four involves medication, that is, prednisone (1 point for 0 to 15 mg/d, 2 points for 16 to 39 mg/d, 3 points for ≥40 mg/d) and cytotoxic agents (3 points for use of cyclophosphamide, chlorambucil, azathioprine, or methotrexate). Part five scores for three laboratory parameters: (a) proteinuria (0 points for negative or trace, 1 point for 1+, 2 points for 2 to 3+, and 3 points for 4+ on urine dipstick); (b) anti-DNA antibodies (0 to 3 points assigned according to range used in the local laboratory); and (c) C3, C4, or CH50 (0 to 3 points assigned according to range used in the local laboratory). The LAI summary score is the arithmetic mean of the part one score, the mean of the four values in part two, the maximum of the four values in part three, the mean of the two values in part four, and the mean of the three laboratory values. Possible LAI scores range from 0 to 3. Scores reflect the manifestations, laboratory abnormalities, and medications during the 2-week period before scoring.

In a study that did not include the LAI, Liang et al. (23) looked at six indices for their reliability and validity in assessing disease activity in patients with SLE at one center. Twenty-five patients, who were selected to represent a spectrum of disease activity, were independently evaluated by two physicians on two occasions approximately 1 month apart. Validity of the six instruments was demonstrated by significant correlations of scores among the different indices (r = 0.81–0.97). BILAG, SLEDAI, and SLAM demonstrated the best intervisit and interrater reliability.

An international group sponsored by the North Atlantic Treaty Organization (NATO) studied the operational validity, reliability, and sensitivity to change of several indices when used by physicians at different centers (25). This group chose to limit its studies to BILAG, SLEDAI, and SLAM because of the prior work of Liang et al. (23), who did not study LAI. The NATO group (25) initially studied the validity of the three indices when used by physicians from eight different centers to assess the same patients; the indices were tested using data on patients from chart review. Indices were compared to the clinician's judgment of disease activity using a VAS. The three indices correlated significantly with each other and with the VAS ($p \leq .05$ for all correlation coefficients). However, the activity scores for the same patients using different indices varied widely among two of the eight physician scorers. This suggested that the indices are complex and require familiarity for effective use, and that the considerable intra- and interobserver variation may make the indices difficult to correlate in multicenter comparison studies of patient groups or treatment protocols in which different investigators use different indices to assess activity. The group suggested that uniform use of one or two of these indices might improve our ability to compare the results of studies from different centers.

The NATO group next studied the same three indices for their reproducibility and validity in the assessment of patients in an actual clinical setting (31). Seven patients, representing a spectrum of disease activity and disease manifestations, were each examined by four of seven physicians from seven different centers; physicians from the center where the study patients received their care were excluded. Each observer completed the three indices and a VAS of disease activity on each of the examined patients. All the indices significantly correlated with each other, and there was no significant interobserver variation. All three indices detected differences among patients. This study suggests that physicians from different countries and health care systems can evaluate patients reproducibly, regardless of the instruments used and the disease activity of the patients and without significant interobserver variation. Differences in the findings of the two NATO studies may be attributable to the methodologies that were used. The problems with inter- and intraobserver variations seen in the first study may have resulted from difficulties associated with chart abstraction of clinical information, and these problems may not exist when the indices are used in an actual clinical setting.

Petri et al. (32) characterized the validity and reliability of the SLEDAI and LAI using patients from the Johns Hopkins lupus cohort. Validity was assessed by comparing the indices with the physician's global assessment of disease activity; the correlation of M-LAI (LAI modified so as not to contain part one, which assesses the physician's global assessment [PGA]) and SLEDAI with the physician's global assessment was 0.64 and 0.55, respectively. Reliability was tested in six patients who were seen twice, 1 week apart, by nine physicians; the interrater reliability and test-retest reliability was greater for LAI than for SLEDAI. This study demonstrates that the indices can be readily assimilated into routine clinical practice.

To establish the reliability of SLEDAI among less experienced clinicians who were not familiar with it as a tool for patient assessment, Hawker et al. (33) studied the reliability of SLEDAI by having three second-year rheumatology fellows apply the instrument on nine outpatients with SLE; each fellow independently interviewed and examined the patients. SLEDAI distinguished between patients (p = .0009), and physician variability was not statistically significant (p = .27). Inter- and intraobserver agreement was 78.7% and 98.0%, respectively.

DISEASE INDICES AND SENSITIVITY TO CHANGE

The NATO group studied the comparative ability of BILAG, SLEDAI, and SLAM to assess change in disease activity over time (34). Clinical and laboratory features of eight patients with SLE who were seen on three consecutive visits were abstracted and sent to eight physicians at different centers in three separate packages. Order of the patient-visit summaries was randomized, and the three indices were rated in one of six specific sequences. The three indices were significantly correlated (p ≤0.01 for all comparisons); the sequence presented, patient order, and order of index scoring did not significantly contribute to the variation of any of the indices. All three indices detected differences among patients (p ≤.01); differences between visits were detectable with SLEDAI (p = .04) but not with SLAM or BILAG.

Petri et al. (35) have demonstrated that both LAI and SLEDAI are sensitive to change. As part of an ongoing, prospective study, the physician's global assessment of disease activity, LAI, and SLEDAI have been completed at least quarterly for 185 patients with SLE followed by rheumatologists at Johns Hopkins Hospital. Using a definition of disease flare as a change of greater than 1.0 in the physician's global assessment of disease activity (measured on a 0 to 3 scale) from the previous visit or one within the prior 93 days, mean SLEDAI scores increased by 3.0, and mean LAI scores (modified to omit the physician's global assessment) increased by 0.26 at times of flare. These increases in the SLEDAI and LAI scores were found to be significant changes. These findings suggest that both SLEDAI and LAI can detect changes in activity with time, and that they may be useful in following changes of disease activity in the clinic setting.

Fortin and colleagues (36) evaluated 96 patients monthly for 5 months, completing at each visit a SLAM-R, a SLEDAI, a physician's global assessment, and a physician's transition score, which coded a patient as stable, improved, or worse. Using multiple statistically methods, they found that both SLEDAI and SLAM-R were sensitive to change, but that the SLAM-R was consistently more sensitive. Ward and colleagues (37) further evaluated the disease activity indices for sensitivity to change; 23 patients were evaluated prospectively at 2-week intervals for up to 40 weeks. SLEDAI, SLAM, BILAG, LAI, and ECLAM (European Consensus Lupus Activity Measure), as well as a physician's and patient's global assessment, were determined at each visit. Compared to the physician's global assessment, all indices were sensitive to change (r = 0.52 to 0.75). LAI and ECLAM were the most sensitive to change; however, the LAI score incorporates the PGA and thus may be artificially elevated. The SLEDAI was the least sensitive to change. When compared to the patient's global assessment, only SLAM correlated with changes in disease activity and this correlation was weak. Patients in this study had mildly to moderately active lupus, and patients with more severe disease may have correlated better with the disease activity indices. These results are important when considering the design of clinical trials.

The above studies demonstrate that there are numerous indices that are valid, sensitive measures of disease activity in lupus. However, further research is needed to determine the most responsive instrument to maximize the ability to evaluate outcome in clinical trials. Ongoing studies are under way to define response for the purposes of determining whether an intervention is effective. Once a consensus is reached on this definition, these activity indices will be tested for their ability to assess response.

DISEASE FLARE

Petri et al. (35) have defined disease flare as an increase in the LAI part one physician's global assessment of 1.0 or greater. In following 185 patients with SLE at least quarterly over several years, 98 (53%) had at least one flare; the total number of flares was 146. The incidence of flare was 0.65 per each patient-year of follow-up; the median time from the first study visit to flare was 12 months. Flares were frequently characterized by constitutional symptoms, musculoskeletal involvement, cutaneous involvement, and hypocomplementemia. At the time of flare, mean SLEDAI scores increased by 3.0 and mean LAI scores by 0.26. Overall, 44.8% of flares prompted a change in treatment. Patients who experienced flares fulfilled more of the SLE criteria at entry and had been followed for a longer duration after entry into the cohort compared with those who did not have flares. No specific clinical or laboratory variables present at entry were found to predict time to first flare. These data demonstrate that quantification of flare is possible, that flares are frequent in patients with disease of long duration, and that most flares involve minor organ systems.

An alternative means of identifying important changes in lupus activity is the physician's decision to initiate or increase treatment. This is the basis of the BILAG.

TerBorg et al. (38) defined criteria for both major and minor exacerbations based on a Dutch activity index. A patient is considered to have a major exacerbation if one or more criteria for major flare are fulfilled; these include severe manifestations of disease with specific definitions or severe changes in laboratory parameters without improvement after prednisolone therapy at a maximum of 30 mg/d for at least 1 week. Criteria for minor exacerbation include an increase of the activity index by at least two points, with a minimum activity index of three points, with the clinical necessity of beginning a regimen of prednisolone at a dosage of at least 10 mg/d, of increasing the prednisolone dosage by at least 5 mg/d, or of starting an antimalarial or immunosuppressive drug.

Criteria for mild/moderate and severe flare have been developed for use in the SELENA study; these criteria will be prospectively validated as part of that study. Criteria for mild/moderate flare include a change in SLEDAI of 3 points or more, new or worse discoid rash, photosensitivity, lupus profundus, cutaneous vasculitis or bullous lesions, nasopharyngeal ulcers, pleuritis, pericarditis, arthritis, or fever attributable to lupus. Other criteria of mild/moderate flare include a need to increase prednisone, but not to doses greater than 0.5 mg/kg/d, because of lupus activity and an increase in the physician's global assessment of 1.0 to 2.5 (on a 0- to 3-point VAS). Criteria for a severe flare include a change in SLEDAI to greater than 12 points, new or worse central nervous system lupus activity, vasculitis, nephritis, myositis, thrombocytopenia of less than 60,000 per mL, or hemolytic anemia with hemoglobin levels of less than 7 or a decrease in hemoglobin of greater than 3 requiring a doubling of prednisone dosage or the need for prednisone doses of greater than 0.5 mg/kg/d, or hospitalization. Other criteria for severe flare include the institution of cyclophosphamide, azathioprine, methotrexate, or prednisone >0.5 mg/kg/d or hospitalization because of lupus activity, or an increase in the physician's global assessment to a level greater than 2.5 (on a 0- to 3-point VAS).

Abrahamowicz et al. (39) evaluated the relationship between SLAM and SLEDAI scores of 30 paper patients based on actual cases and 38 lupus experts' decision to start therapy. They found that the disease activity as measured by SLAM-R or SLEDAI predicted the institution of steroid or alternative treatments. Using modeling, the authors determined that at least 70% of the physicians would initiate treatment at a score of 10 for both instruments. These indices have their limitations. SLAM-R scores include subjective symptoms that may be difficult to determine attribution to lupus, while SLEDAI does not include many manifestations of SLE. Furthermore, different patients with similar scores had markedly different percentages of physicians who would start therapy. Thus, these instruments can be useful in clinical practice and in clinical trials; however, they cannot replace physician judgment.

Gladman and colleagues (40) compared the SLEDAI score of 230 patients with five visits determined at the time of the visit to the score on a 5-point scale (no activity, mild activity but no change in treatment, mild activity but improvement, persistent activity, and flare with a preset definition) determined by review of the medical record by a nontreating clinician. Based on this analysis, they propose that a flare be defined as an increase in SLEDAI of >3, improvement as a decrease in SLEDAI of >3, persistent active disease as a change in SLEDAI by ±3, and remission as a SLEDAI score of 0.

Measuring response to therapy is another important aspect of monitoring SLE. This aspect of clinical activity is not captured in the current disease activity indices. Validation of a new instrument RIFLE (Responder Index for Lupus Erythematosus) is under way. This instrument, which was developed by members of SLICC (Systemic Lupus International Collaborating Clinics), characterizes numerous manifestations of lupus activity and rates the activity of these manifestations at different points in time as improved or worsened with degrees of change. With this instrument, a patient's response to a therapeutic intervention can be characterized as a complete response, partial response, or nonresponse.

DAMAGE INDEX

To compare patient groups and measure outcome in treatment protocols, the SLICC/ACR Damage Index (DI) for SLE (Fig. 2.2) was developed by the Systemic Lupus International Collaborating Clinics and accepted by the ACR as a valid measure of damage in patients with lupus (41). This instrument measures accumulated organ damage occurring since the onset of SLE. Damage can result from either the disease process, its sequelae, or treatment, because attribution often is difficult in patients with SLE. The index is assessed irrespective of current disease activity, amount, or duration of any therapy and/or disability of the patient.

In developing the index, a list of items considered to reflect damage in SLE was generated through a group process. This group, representing international clinicians who were considered to be experts in lupus, reached a consensus as to which items should be included in an index. Each clinician submitted clinical information on four patients at two points in time (average interval between visits, 5 years). Two patients from each center had active disease and two patients inactive disease; some patients had increased damage with time and others stable damage. Nineteen clinicians completed the index on 42 case scenarios. Analysis of variance revealed that the index could identify changes in damage seen in patients with both active and inactive disease.

The index includes descriptors in 12 organ systems. For the purposes of the SLICC/ACR index, damage is considered only if present for at least 6 months.

Item	Score
Ocular (either eye, by clinical assessment)	
Any cataract ever	1
Retinal change *or* optic atrophy	1
Neuropsychiatric	
Cognitive impairment (e.g., memory deficit, difficulty with calculation, poor concentration, difficulty in spoken or written language, impaired performance level) *or* major psychosis	1
Seizures requiring therapy for 6 months	1
Cerebrovascular accident ever (score 2 if >1)	1 (2)
Cranial or peripheral neuropathy (excluding optic)	1
Transverse myelitis	1
Renal	
Estimated or measured glomerular filtration rate <50%	1
Proteinuria ≥3.5 gm/24 hours	1
or	
End-stage renal disease (regardless of dialysis or transplantation)	3
Pulmonary	
Pulmonary hypertension (right ventricular prominence, or loud P2)	1
Pulmonary fibrosis (physical and radiograph)	1
Shrinking lung (radiograph)	1
Pleural fibrosis (radiograph)	1
Pulmonary infarction (radiograph)	1
Cardiovascular	
Angina *or* coronary artery bypass	1
Myocardial infarction ever (score 2 if >1)	1 (2)
Cardiomyopathy (ventricular dysfunction)	1
Valvular disease (diastolic murmur, or systolic murmur >3/6)	1
Pericarditis for 6 months, *or* pericardiectomy	1
Peripheral vascular	
Claudication for 6 months	1
Minor tissue loss (pulp space)	1
Significant tissue loss ever (e.g., loss of digit or limb) (score 2 if >1 site)	1 (2)
Venous thrombosis with swelling, ulceration, *or* venous stasis	1
Gastrointestinal	
Infarction or resection of bowel below duodenum, spleen, liver, or gall bladder ever, for any cause (score 2 if >1 site)	1 (2)
Mesenteric insufficiency	1
Chronic peritonitis	1
Stricture *or* upper gastrointestinal tract surgery ever	1
Musculoskeletal	
Muscle atrophy or weakness	1
Deforming or erosive arthritis (including reducible deformities, excluding avascular necrosis)	1
Osteoporosis with fracture or vertebral collapse (excluding avascular necrosis)	1
Avascular necrosis (score 2 if >1)	1 (2)
Osteomyelitis	1
Skin	
Scarring chronic alopecia	1
Extensive scarring or panniculum other than scalp and pulp space	1
Skin ulceration (excluding thrombosis) for >6 months	1
Premature gonadal failure	1
Diabetes (regardless of treatment)	1
Malignancy (exclude dysplasia) (score 2 if >1 site)	1 (2)

Damage (nonreversible change, not related to active inflammation) occurring since onset of lupus, ascertained by clinical assessment and present for at least 6 months unless otherwise stated. Repeat episodes must occur at least 6 months apart to score 2. The same lesion cannot be scored twice.

FIGURE 2.2. The Systemic Lupus International Collaborating Clinics/American College of Rheumatology Damage Index for SLE. (From Gladman DD, Ginzler E, Goldsmith C, et al. The development and initial validation of the Systemic Lupus International Collaborating Clinics/American College of Rheumatology Damage Index for systemic lupus erythematosus. *Arthritis Rheum* 1996;39:363–369, with permission.)

The instrument has been demonstrated to have construct validity using clinical data on patients abstracted from chart review (41). The SLICC/ARC DI also was noted to have reliability and validity when used by ten physicians from five countries in the assessment of ten actual patients with SLE representing a spectrum of damage and activity; each of these patients was assessed by six of the ten physicians (42). The SLICC/ACR DI detected differences among patients (p <.001); there was no detectable observer difference (p = .933) and no order effect (p = .261). There was concordance in the

TABLE 2.2. THE MEDICAL OUTCOME SURVEY SHORT-FORM GENERAL HEALTH SURVEY

1. In general, would you say your health is: ________
   1 = Excellent
   2 = Very good
   3 = Good
   4 = Fair
   5 = Poor
2. *Compared to one year ago,* how would you rate your health in general now? ________
   1 = Much better now than one year ago
   2 = Somewhat better now than one year ago
   3 = About the same as one year ago
   4 = Somewhat worse now than one year ago
   5 = Much worse now than one year ago
3. The following items are about activities you might do during a typical day. Does your health now limit you in these activities? If so, how much? 1 = Yes, limited a lot
   2 = Yes, limited a little
   3 = No, not limited at all
   a. *Vigorous activities,* such as running, lifting heavy objects, participating in strenuous sports ________
   b. *Moderate activities,* such as moving a table, pushing a vacuum cleaner, bowling, or playing golf ________
   c. Lifting or carrying groceries ________
   d. Climbing *several* flights of stairs ________
   e. Climbing *one* flight of stairs ________
   f. Bending, kneeling, or stooping ________
   g. Walking *more than one mile* ________
   h. Walking *several blocks* ________
   i. Walking *one block* ________
   j. Bathing or dressing yourself ________
4. During the *past 4 weeks,* have you had any of the following problems with your work or other regular daily activities *as a result of your physical health?* 1 = Yes, 2 = No
   a Cut down on the *amount of time* you spent on work or other activities ________
   b. *Accomplished less* than you would like ________
   c. Were limited in the *kind* of work or other activities ________
   d. Had difficulty performing the work or other activities (for example, it took extra effort) ________
5. During the *past 4 weeks,* have you had any of the following problems with your work or other regular daily activities *as a result of any emotional problems* (such as feeling depressed or anxious) 1 = Yes, 2 = No
   a. Cut down on the *amount of time* you spent of work or other activities ________
   b. *Accomplished less* than you would like ________
   c. Didn't do work or other activities as *carefully* as usual ________
6. During the *past 4 weeks*, to what extent has your physical health or emotional problems interfered with your normal social activities with family, friends, neighbors, or groups? ________
   1 = Not at all
   2 = Slightly
   3 = Moderately
   4 = Quite a bit
   5 = Extremely
7. How much bodily pain have you had during the past 4 weeks? ________
   1 = None
   2 = Very mild
   3 = Mild
   4 = Moderate
   5 = Severe
   6 = Very severe
8. During the *past 4 weeks* how much did pain interfere with your normal work (including both work outside the home and housework)? ________
   1 = Not at all
   2 = A little bit
   3 = Moderately
   4 = Quite a bit
   5 = Extremely
9. These questions are about how you feel and how things have been with you *during the past 4 weeks.* For each question, please give one answer that comes closest to the way you have been feeling.
   1 = All of the time
   2 = Most of the time
   3 = A good bit of the time
   4 = Some of the time
   5 = A little of the time
   6 = None of the time

TABLE 2.2. *(continued)*

How much of the time during the *past 4 weeks*....
- a. Did you feel full of pep? ________
- b. Have you been a very nervous person? ________
- c. Have you felt so down in the dumps that nothing could cheer you up? ________
- d. Have you felt calm and peaceful? ________
- e. Did you have a lot of energy? ________
- f. Have you felt downhearted and blue? ________
- g. Did you feel worn out? ________
- h. Have you been a happy person? ________
- i. Did you feel tired?

10. During the past 4 weeks, how much of the time has your physical health or emotional problems interfered with your social activities (like visiting your friends, relatives, etc.)? ________
    - 1 = All of the time
    - 2 = Most of the time
    - 3 = Some of the time
    - 4 = A little of the time
    - 5 = None of the time

11. How **TRUE** or **FALSE** is each of the following statements for you?
    - 1 = Definitely true
    - 2 = Mostly true
    - 3 = Don't know
    - 4 = Mostly false
    - 5 = Definitely false

- a. I seem to get sick a little easier than other people. ________
- b. I am as healthy as anybody I know. ________
- c. I expect my health to get worse. ________
- d. My health is excellent. ________

From Stewart AL, Hays RD, Ware JE Jr. The MOS short-form general health survey. Reliability and validity in a patient population. *Med Care* 1988;26(7):724–735, with permission.

SLICC/ACR DI among observers despite a wide spectrum of disease activity detected by the SLEDAI. The authors concluded that physicians from different centers are able to reproducibly assess patients with SLE using the SLEDAI to assess disease activity and the SLICC/ACR DI to assess accumulated damage.

In a study of 200 lupus patients from five centers, 61% were noted to have damage within 7 years of disease onset with a mean of 3.8 years (43). Furthermore, in a study of 1,297 patients from eight centers, the SLICC/ACR DI has also been shown to increase over time (44); 99 patients died, and these patients had significantly higher DI early in their illness compared to those patients who had survived (1.56 versus 0.99, $p = .0003$). This index may be useful in clinical practice as a further means of identifying patients with a poor prognosis.

HEALTH STATUS

In addition to disease activity and damage, quality of life is a third important component in the assessment of patients with SLE. Assessment of health status has been shown to be an important independent outcome measure in lupus (45). This was confirmed in a second study where SLEDAI, SLICC/ACR DI, and the SF-20 did not correlate well with each other (46). Fortin and colleagues (47) found that in a cross-sectional analysis, the SLAM-R score correlated with most subscales of the SF-36, but SLEDAI did not. However, longitudinal changes in both disease activity scales did correlate with changes in the SF-36. Sutcliffe and colleagues (48) found that higher disease activity is associated with worse physical and emotional function, pain, and general health. The study also found that patients who were more satisfied with health care and had greater social support had a better general view of their health, suggesting a potential nonpharmacologic intervention to improve health care of lupus patients. The Medical Outcomes Study Short Form 36 (SF-36) (Table 2.2) is an instrument that has been validated and is one of the most commonly used to in lupus (49). The SF-36 was chosen as the health status measure of choice at a SLICC workshop in 1995 (50).

In 1998, OMERACT (Outcome Measures in Rheumatology) IV was held and included a module on SLE (51). The investigators considered 21 domains and concluded that randomized controlled trials and longitudinal observational series should include a minimum of four domains: a measure of disease activity, a measure of health-related quality of life, a measure of damage, and toxicity/adverse events. The institution of these core domains will improve the quality of clinical trials and the efficacy of evaluating new therapies.

REFERENCES

1. Cohen AS, Reynolds WE, Franklin EC, et al. Preliminary criteria for the classification of systemic lupus erythematosus. *Bull Rheum Dis* 1971;21:643–648.
2. Cohen AS, Canoso JJ. Criteria for the classification of systemic lupus erythematosus status 1972 (editorial). *Arthritis Rheum* 1972;15:540–543.
3. Davis P, Atkins B, Josse RG, et al. Criteria for classification of SLE. *Br Med J* 1973;3:90–91.
4. Fries JF, Siegel RC. Testing the preliminary criteria for classification of SLE. *Ann Rheum Dis* 1973;32:171–177.

5. Gibson TP, Dibona GF. Use of the American Rheumatism Association's preliminary criteria for the classification of systemic lupus erythematosus. *Ann Intern Med* 1972;77:754–756.
6. Trimble RB, Townes AS, Robinson H, et al. Preliminary criteria for the classification of systemic lupus erythematosus (SLE). Evaluation in early diagnosed SLE and rheumatoid arthritis. *Arthritis Rheum* 1974;17:184–188.
7. Deleted in page proofs.
8. Lom-Orta H, Alarcon-Segovia D, Diaz-Jouanen E. Systemic lupus erythematosus. Differences between patients who do and who do not fulfill classification criteria at the time of diagnosis. *J Rheumatol* 1980;7:831–837.
9. Canoso JJ, Cohen AS. A review of the use, evaluations, and criticisms of the preliminary criteria for the classification of systemic lupus erythematosus. *Arthritis Rheum* 1979;22:917–921.
10. Deleted in page proofs.
11. Weinstein A, Bordwell B, Stone B, et al. Antibodies to native DNA and serum complement (C3) levels. Application to diagnosis and classification of systemic lupus erythematosus. *Am J Med* 1983;74:206–216.
12. Tan PLJ, Borman GB, Wigley RD. Testing clinical criteria for systemic lupus erythematosus in other connective tissue disorders. *Rheumatol Int* 1981;1:147–149.
13. Tan EM, Cohen AS, Fries JF, et al. Special article: the 1982 revised criteria for the classification of systemic lupus erythematosus. *Arthritis Rheum* 1982;25:1271–1277.
14. Fries JF. Methodology of validation of criteria for systemic lupus erythematosus. *Scand J Rheumatol* 1987;65(suppl):25–30.
15. Levin RE, Weinstein A, Peterson M, et al. A comparison of the sensitivity of the 1971 and 1982 American Rheumatism Association criteria for the classification of systemic lupus erythematosus. *Arthritis Rheum* 1984;27:530–538.
16. Passas CM, Wond RL, Peterson M, et al. A comparison of the specificity of the 1971 and 1982 American Rheumatism Association criteria for the classification of systemic lupus erythematosus. *Arthritis Rheum* 1985;28:620–623.
17. Yokohari R, Tsunematsu T. Application to Japanese patients, of the 1982 American Rheumatism Association revised criteria for the classification of systemic lupus erythematosus. *Arthritis Rheum* 1985;28:693–698.
18. Davis P, Stein M. Evaluation of criteria for the classification of SLE in Zimbabwean patients (letter). *Br J Rheumatol* 1989;28: 546–556.
19. Davatchi F, Chams C, Akbarian M. Evaluation of the 1982 American Rheumatism Association revised criteria for the classification of SLE (letter). *Arthritis Rheum* 1985;28:715.
20. Edworthy SM, Zatarain E, McShane DJ, et al. Analysis of the 1982 ARA lupus criteria data set by recursive partitioning methodology: new insights to the relative merit of individual criteria. *J Rheumatol* 1988;15:1493–1498.
21. Hochberg MC. Updating the American College of Rheumatology Revised Criteria for the Classification of Systemic Lupus Erythematosus (letter). *Arthritis Rheum* 1997;40:1725.
22. Jonsson H, Nived O, Sturfelt G. Outcome in systemic lupus erythematosus: a prospective study of patients from a defined population. *Medicine* 1989;68:141–150.
23. Liang MH, Socher SA, Larson MG, et al. Reliability and validity of six systems for the clinical assessment of disease activity in systemic lupus erythematosus. *Arthritis Rheum* 1989;32: 1107–1118.
24. Symmons DPM, Coopock JS, Bacon PA, et al. Development and assessment of a computerized index of clinical disease activity in systemic lupus erythematosus. *Q J Med* 1988;68:927–937.
25. Kalunian KC, Gladman DD, Bacon PA, et al. Development and assessment of a computerized index of clinical disease activity in systemic lupus erythematosus. Unpublished manuscript.
26. Bombardier C, Gladman DD, Urowitz MB, et al. Derivation of the SLEDAI. A disease activity index for lupus patients. The Committee on Prognosis Studies in SLE. *Arthritis Rheum* 1992; 35:630–640.
27. Guzman J, Cardiel MH, Arce-Salinas A, et al. Measurement of disease activity in systemic lupus erythematosus. Prospective validation of 3 clinical indices. *J Rheumatol* 1992;19:1551–1558.
28. Petri M, Buyon J, Skovron ML, et al. Reliability of SELENA SLEDAI and flares as a clinical trial outcome measure. *Arthritis Rheum* 1998;41:S218.
29. Liang MH, Socher SA, Roberts WN, et al. Measurement of systemic lupus erythematosus activity in clinical research. *Arthritis Rheum* 1988;31:817–825.
30. Petri M, Bochemstedt L, Colman J, et al. Serial assessment of glomerular filtration rate in lupus nephropathy. *Kidney Int* 1988; 34:832–839.
31. Gladman DD, Goldsmith CH, Urowitz MB, et al. Cross-cultural validation and reliability of three disease activity indices in systemic lupus erythematosus. *J Rheumatol* 1992;19: 608–611.
32. Petri M, Hellman D, Hochberg M. Validity and reliability of lupus activity measures in the routine clinic setting. *J Rheumatol* 1992;19:53–59.
33. Hawker G, Gabriel S, Bombardier C, et al. A reliability study of SLEDAI: a disease activity index for systemic lupus erythematosus. *J Rheumatol* 1993;20:657–660.
34. Gladman DD, Goldsmith CH, Urowitz MB, et al. Sensitivity to change of 3 systemic lupus erythematosus disease activity indices: internation validation. *J Rheumatol* 1994;21:1468–1471.
35. Petri M, Genovese M, Engle E, et al. Definition, incidence and clinical description of flare in systemic lupus erythematosus: a prospective cohort study. *Arthritis Rheum* 1991;34:937–944.
36. Fortin PR, Abrahamowicz M, Clarke AE, et al. Do lupus disease activity measures detect clinically important change? *J Rheumatol* 2000;27:1421–1428.
37. Ward MM, Marx AS, Barry NN. Comparison of the validity and sensitivity to change of 5 activity indices in systemic lupus erythematosus. *J Rheumatol* 2000;27:664–670.
38. TerBorg EJ, Horst G, Huymmel EJ, et al. Measurement of increases in anti-double-stranded DNA antibody levels as a predictor of disease exacerbation in systemic lupus erythematosus. *Arthritis Rheum* 1990;33:634–643.
39. Abrahamowicz M, Fortin P, du Berger R, et al. The relationship between disease activity and expert physician's decision to start major treatment in active systemic lupus erythematosus: a decision aid for development of entry criteria for clinical trials. *J Rheumatol* 1998;25:277–284.
40. Gladman DD, Urowitz ME, Kagal A, et al. Accurately describing changes in disease activity in systemic lupus erythematosus. *J Rheumatol* 2000;27:377–379.
41. Gladman DD, Ginzler E, Goldsmith C, et al. The development and initial validation of the Systemic Lupus International Collaborating Clinics/American College of Rheumatology Damage Index for systemic lupus erythematosus. *Arthritis Rheum* 1996; 39:363–369.
42. Gladman D, Urowitz, Goldsmith C, et al. The reliability of the Systemic Lupus International Collaborating Clinics/American College of Rheumatology damage index in patients with systemic lupus erythematosus. *Arthritis Rheum* 1997;40: 809–813.
43. Rivest C, Lew RA, Welsing PMJ, et al. Association between clinical factors, socioeconomic status, and organ damage in recent onset systemic lupus erythematosus. *J Rheumatol* 2000;27: 680–684.
44. Gladman DD, Goldsmith CH, Urowitz MB, et al., for the Systemic Lupus International Collaborating Clinics. The Systemic

Lupus International Collaborating Clinics/American College of Rheumatology (CLICC/ACR) Damage Index for Systemic Lupus Erythematosus International Comparison. *J Rheumatol* 2000;27:373–376.

45. Gladman DD, Urowitz MB, Ong A, et al. Lack of correlation among the 3 outcomes describing SLE: disease activity, damage and quality of life. *Clin Exp Rheumatol* 1996;14:305–308.
46. Hanly JG. Disease activity, cumulative damage and quality of life in systematic (sic) lupus erythematosus: results of a cross-sectional study. *Lupus* 1997;6:243–247.
47. Fortin PR, Abrahamowicz M, Neville C, et al. Impact of disease activity and cumulative damage on the health of lupus patients. *Lupus* 1998;7:101–107.
48. Sutcliffe N, Clarke AE, Levinton C, et al. Associates of health status in patients with systemic lupus erythematosus. *J Rheumatol* 1999;26:2352–2356.
49. Stoll T, Gordon C, Seifert B, et al. Consistency and validity of patient administered assessment of quality of life by the MOS SF-36; its association with disease activity and damage in patients with systemic lupus erythematosus. *J Rheumatol* 1997;24:1608–1614.
50. Gladman D, Urowitz M, Fortin P, et al. Systemic Lupus International Collaborating Clinics conference on assessment of lupus flare and quality of life measures in SLE. *J Rheumatol* 1996;23: 1953–1955.
51. Smolen J, Strand V, Cardiel M, et al. Randomized clinical trials and longitudinal observational studies in systemic lupus erythematosus: consensus on a preliminary core set of outcome domains. *J Rheumatol* 1999;26:504–507.

3

THE ROLE OF ENVIRONMENT IN SYSTEMIC LUPUS ERYTHEMATOSUS AND ASSOCIATED DISORDERS

ANNE-BARBARA MONGEY
EVELYN V. HESS

Systemic lupus erythematosus (SLE) and associated diseases of connective tissue are believed to be immune mediated. The specific etiology of these disorders remains unknown. Genetic factors are believed to play an important role because of the clustering of these diseases among families and within ethnic groups (1–4) as well as reported human leukocyte antigen (HLA) associations (5,6). However, discordance for SLE has been reported for identical twins and for those belonging to the same ethnic group but who live in different parts of the world (7,8). This suggests that the environment plays an important role in providing either a triggering and/or a modifying influence in the development of autoimmune diseases. One of the most popular theories today is that an autoimmune disease develops in a genetically susceptible host who has been exposed to a triggering, probably environmental, agent. Genetic susceptibility may reside in the presence of certain HLA genes and/or genes coding for a variety of enzymes. This latter group of genes would have the ability to determine the duration of exposure of the host to a particular agent that may be important in determining which individuals will go on to develop clinical diseases.

Over the past 50 years, many agents, and drugs in particular, have been associated with the development of lupus-like syndromes (9–11). Observations dating back to 1969 have also implicated certain metals and a variety of chemical, infectious, and dietary agents in the development of autoimmune-like diseases (Table 3.1). This chapter reviews the possible role of environmental agents in the etiopathogenesis of autoimmune diseases, in particular SLE.

CHEMICAL FACTORS (TABLE 3.2)

Aromatic Amines and Hydrazines

Many of the drugs implicated in drug-related lupus (DRL), such as procainamide and hydralazine, are aromatic amines or hydrazines. These drugs are metabolized by means of the acetylation pathway. Studies show that DRL and autoantibody formation are more likely to occur in patients who are genetically slow acetylators (12), suggesting that the free amine or hydrazine moiety is the inciting agent.

Hydrazines

Both naturally occurring hydrazines and aromatic amines are potential inciting agents in the development of lupus. Hydrazine and its derivatives are present in a variety of compounds that are used in agriculture and industry. They have numerous commercial applications as intermediates in the synthesis of plastics, anticorrosives, rubber products, herbicides, pesticides, photographic supplies, preservatives, textiles, dyes, and pharmaceuticals.

Hydrazine occurs naturally in tobacco, tobacco smoke, mushrooms, and penicillium. A case-control study of 282 lupus patients revealed a significant increased risk for SLE among smokers, while there was an inverse association with alcohol and milk intake (13). This was similar to results reported by Benoni et al. (14), who had reported a slight increased risk for smokers. These results are of some interest since it has previously been suggested that smoking has immunosuppressive effects.

Reidenberg et al. (15) reported the development of a lupus-like syndrome in a 25-year-old technician who used hydrazine sulfate intermittently in her work. She developed recurrent episodes of arthralgias, fever, photosensitive rash, and a positive antinuclear antibody (ANA). Avoidance of contact with hydrazine resulted in the remission of symptoms. Subsequently, the patient had recurrences of the symptoms when reexposed to hydrazine or its derivatives, or following ingestion of a tartrazine-containing medication. Of interest, the patient was a slow acetylator.

Tartrazine

Aromatic amines are present in the diet as reduction products of azo food dyes by the intestinal bacteria. Tartrazine or

TABLE 3.1. AGENTS WITH A POTENTIAL ROLE AS TRIGGERS OF LUPUS SYNDROMES AND ASSOCIATED DISORDERS

Chemical factors
Metals
Dietary factors
Radiation
Infectious agents

Food, Drug, and Cosmetic (FD&C) Act yellow no. 5 is an azo dye that is present in thousands of foods and drugs and has been reported to cause asthma, urticaria, angioedema, rhinorrhea, allergic vascular purpura, and peripheral eosinophilia, and to have phototoxic potential. Pereyo (16) described the development of a lupus-like syndrome characterized by photosensitivity, arthralgias, and myalgias following ingestion of tartrazine in a patient who previously had drug-related lupus secondary to procainamide. Subsequently, he reported exacerbations of cutaneous disease in five patients with SLE after they ingested medicines containing tartrazine (17). Another patient developed arthralgias, myalgias, malaise, photosensitivity, and a positive ANA after an oral challenge with tartrazine (17).

Hair Dyes

Aromatic amines are also present in permanent hair coloring solutions and can be absorbed through the scalp (18). Paraphenylenediamine, a hair-dyeing compound, reproduced features consistent with those of connective tissue diseases in experimental animals. Geschickter et al. (19) found that, following repeated daily brushings of *N,N*1-dimethyl *p*-phenylenediamine to the shaved skins of rats, various focal lesions seen in collagen vascular diseases were reproduced histologically. Scleroderma-like lesions were seen in the skin of those animals receiving high doses or those receiving treatment for a very prolonged period. In a case-control study, Hochberg and Kaslow (20) found an increase in the prior use of hair dyes among 74 patients with SLE, but this difference was not statistically significant. In another case-control study, Freni-Titulaer et al. (21) reported a positive association between the use of hair care products and the development of connective tissue diseases. The study included 23 patients with SLE, ten with scleroderma, two with polymyositis, and nine with undifferentiated connective tissue disease. Environmental factors were only considered if the exposure occurred in the 5-year period prior to onset of the disease for patients or in the equivalent period for the controls. In the crude analyses, exposures to hair dyes, hair permanent solutions, and hair spray all showed statistically significant associations; however, using multivariate analyses, only the association with hair dyes remained statistically significant. Petri and Allbritton (22), in a subsequent case-control study of their 218 lupus patients, failed to find a statistically significant association between SLE and exposure to hair permanents or dyes before the diagnosis of SLE or between disease activity and subsequent hair product usage. In a case-control study of 159 patients, Reidenberg et al. (23) failed to find a significant association between SLE and environmental exposure to amines, which included drugs containing aromatic amines (e.g., procainamide and sulfonamides), usage of hair dyes, or a history of cigarette smoking.

In a cohort study Sanchez-Guerrero et al. (24) investigated the possible role of permanent hair dye usage in the development of SLE using data obtained from the Nurses Health study, which is a prospective cohort study containing 106,390 women as participants who have been followed for up to 14 years. The age-adjusted relative risk for development of SLE among users of permanent hair dye was 0.96, which was not significantly different from that of the never-users. In addition, the risk of developing SLE was not related to the duration of use of the hair dye, age at first use, or frequency of uses of these dyes.

Similarly, a more recent study by Hardy et al. (25) did not find a significant association between various hair treatments, including permanent and nonpermanent dyes, bleach, highlights, and lowlights in the development of SLE. These authors evaluated 150 SLE patients by interviewed administered questionnaire and compared the results to 300 controls from the same geographic region. Of interest, a significant negative association was noted between ever having used highlights and SLE; cases used highlights less frequently than the healthy controls. The reason for this is unclear, although it did not appear to be an artifact of analysis since there was not an unusually low number of responses from participants.

Thus, while some smaller studies had suggested an association between hair dye usage and the development of SLE, the more recent larger studies have failed to show an association. Given the failure of these more recent, larger controlled studies to find an association, we do not advise

TABLE 3.2. CHEMICAL FACTORS REPORTED TO BE ASSOCIATED WITH AUTOIMMUNE DISEASE

Aromatic amines and hydrazines
Hydrazines
Tartrazine
Hair dyes
Silica
Vinyl chloride
Organic solvents
Hydrocarbon solvents
Trichloroethylene
Hexachlorobenzene
Dioxins (e.g., TCDD)
Epoxy resins
Silicone

TCDD, 2,3,7,8-tetrachlorodibenzo-*p*-dioxin.

our patients with lupus to refrain from usage of these products.

Other Amines

Scleroderma, characterized by Raynaud's phenomenon, skin induration, and restrictive pulmonary disease, was reported to develop in two patients following exposure to meta-phenylaminediamine (26).

Silica

Occupational exposure to silica dust may cause chronic pulmonary inflammation and has been reported as a possible risk factor for the development of autoimmune diseases including SLE and scleroderma. Crystalline silica or quartz is an abundant mineral found in rock, sand, and soil, and silica is also part of the small particulate fraction of air pollution. Sources of occupational exposure to silica dust include many manufacturing and construction processes such as mining, quarrying and tunneling, stone cutting, dressing, polishing and cleaning monumental masonry, and use of abrasives or abrasive blasting; occupations requiring manufacturing of glass, foundry work, vitreous enameling, and boiler scaling; and occupations involving pottery, porcelain, and lining bricks. In the last 45 years, there have been reports of the development of autoantibodies and connective tissue diseases in workers exposed to silica. It has been suggested that silica may have a potent nonspecific adjuvant effect that may be responsible for the development of autoimmunity in some patients.

Erasmus (27) reported 17 cases of scleroderma among underground gold miners in South Africa who had a predominance of pulmonary features that occurred in more than 50% of their patients. In their experience of more than 150 scleroderma patients, Rodnan et al. (28) found that 43% of their 60 male patients had worked in occupations marked by prolonged and heavy exposure to silica dust. Pulmonary manifestations were more frequent than in other patients with scleroderma. Lippmann et al. (29) reported that 34% of 156 coal miners with pneumoconiosis had ANAs, although only nine had positive rheumatoid factors. There was a geographic association with the presence of ANAs, which occurred most frequently in those areas in which pneumoconiosis was most prevalent. Bailey et al. (30) reported that 2 of 22 silicotic sandblasters in the New Orleans area had positive lupus erythematosus (LE) cells, ANAs, and lupus-like features consisting of arthritis and rash.

Ziskind et al. (31) reported that approximately 10% of sandblasters developed connective tissue disease, including scleroderma, rheumatoid arthritis, and SLE, which were often associated with the accelerated type of silicosis. Cowie (32) reported an annual incidence of scleroderma among black men who were gold miners of 81.8 per million, which was significantly higher than the estimated incidence of approximately 3.4 per million (p <.001) for the general population of black men of a similar age; all had been exposed to silica dust as part of their occupation. Martin et al. (33) reported on six male subjects with scleroderma among a work force of two open-pit iron ore operations who had been exposed to high levels of silica-containing dust. Five cases had diffuse sclerodermatous changes while the sixth case had only sclerodactyly and digital pulp scars.

Jones et al. (34) reported two cases of SLE among 73 silicotic sandblasters. Hatron et al. (35) diagnosed SLE in five coal miners exposed to silica in the area of Lille, France. In addition there have been other reports of associations between silica exposure and SLE with a variable chronologic relationship between the development of SLE and silicosis (36). Bolton et al. (37) reported the development of rapidly progressive renal failure in four patients who had been exposed to silica. Three of these patients had clinical and/or serologic studies that were consistent with SLE. Renal function improved in one patient following treatment with pulse methylprednisolone.

Sanchez-Roman et al. (38) reported a higher than expected number of patients with connective tissue diseases among 50 workers from a factory producing scouring powder with a high silica content. Thirty-two (64%) of these 50 subjects had systemic symptoms; of these, using American Rheumatism Association (ARA) criteria, six were diagnosed with Sjögren's syndrome, five with systemic sclerosis, three with SLE, and five with an overlap syndrome. Thirty-six subjects (72%) had antinuclear and four anti–double-stranded DNA (dsDNA) antibodies.

Steenland and Brown (39), using multiple-cause analysis, reported significant excesses of a number of connective tissue diseases, including SLE, scleroderma, and arthritis, among 3,328 gold miners who had worked underground for at least 1 year between 1940 and 1965 in South Dakota. Koeger et al. (36) evaluated all patients with connective tissue diseases who had been hospitalized between January 1979 and December 1989 for chronic occupational exposure to silica. Twenty-four (3%) of 764 patients with connective tissue diseases were found to have been exposed to silica for a minimum of 3 years, of whom eight patients had scleroderma, five rheumatoid arthritis, four SLE, one discoid lupus, three dermatomyositis, and three other connective tissue diseases. The male predominance, with all five lupus patients being male, most likely reflects the fact that the occupations classically associated with chronic exposure to silica are in heavy industry. The mean duration of exposure to silica prior to the onset of connective tissue disease was 13.6 ± 7 years. ANAs occurred in 75% of patients with connective tissue diseases compared with 36.6% of those with non–silica-associated connective tissue diseases. Wilke et al. (40) reported the development of a lupus-like disease in a 58-year-old caucasian man who had presented with new-onset renal insufficiency. Renal biopsy revealed glomerulosclerosis and chronic interstitial nephritis, and immunofluorescence was positive for granular deposition of C3, fibrin, and immunoglobulin M (IgM) peripherally. Serologic studies revealed a high titer positive ANA of 1 : 2,560 and antibodies to Ro, La, and cardiolipin, antineutrophil cytoplasmic antibodies (p-ANCA), and antimyeloperoxidase antibodies. A skin biopsy revealed leukocytoclastic vasculitis. Brown et al. (41) reported a sixfold excess mortality from a variety of musculoskeletal diseases, consisting of rheumatoid arthritis, SLE, and Sjögren's syndrome, among patients hospitalized for silicosis in Sweden between 1965 and 1983 and in Denmark from 1977 to 1989.

Rosenman et al. (42) reviewed the medical records and questionnaires from 583 individuals with silicosis reported to a state surveillance system for silicosis and determined that there was approximately a 2.5- to 15-fold increase in connective tissue diseases among these individuals. The prevalence of rheumatoid arthritis was 5.2%, scleroderma was 0.2%, and SLE was 0.2% among these patients. Of note, all patients were male. However, there was only one patient with lupus included in this study and he had developed the disease 42 years after his first exposure to silica.

Masson et al. (43) reported the development of SLE in seven patients and subacute cutaneous lupus erythematosus in one patient after exposure to mineral dusts for periods varying from 7 to 33 years. Seven of these patients were male, of whom six were slate miners and one a fine-gravel worker. The eighth patient was a dental laboratory technician who had been exposed to a variety of minerals including silica. All eight patients had lymphocytopenia and ANAs, generally in high titer, and the majority also had arthritis. Other clinical features included pericarditis, pleurisy, malar rash, oral ulcer, Raynaud's phenomenon, and renal involvement. Four patients had antibodies to dsDNA and four antibodies to Ro/SS-A antigen. Rheumatoid factor was present in three patients. The lupus features developed after the signs of silicosis in six of eight patients. This is similar to findings reported by Conrad et al. (44) of 28 definite (four or more ARA criteria) and 15 probable (two to three ARA criteria) cases of SLE among 30,000 uranium miners with a history of heavy (>20 mg respirable particles/m^3) exposure to silica. Clinical features included malar rash, discoid lesions, photosensitivity, oral ulcers, arthritis, serositis, and renal involvement. Contrary to the preceding study, only 57.1% of patients had arthritis. ANAs were present in all 28 patients with definite lupus and 73% of those with probable lupus. In addition, antibodies to dsDNA were found in 38.9% and antibodies to Ro/SSA in 38.9% of patients with definite lupus. In a subsequent study, Conrad et al. (45) reported an increase in the prevalence of the 16/6 idiotype, which is a major cross-reactive idiotype of anti-DNA antibodies that has been reported in SLE and patients treated with procainamide (46), among uranium miners exposed to heavy quartz dust compared with healthy blood donors. The group consisted of miners with definite and probable SLE, those with symptoms suggestive of SLE, and those with medium to high titers of anti-dsDNA antibodies. All the miners with the 16/6 Id idiotype had antibodies to dsDNA. Of interest, after short-term follow-up, two of the miners who were 16/6 Id positive developed progression of their diseases compared with none of the miners who were 16/6 Id negative, suggesting that this idiotype may indicate a higher risk for the development of SLE. Other studies by Conrad et al. (47) reported the presence of antibodies to CENP-B, a centromere specific protein, among miners exposed to quartz dust, and suggested that the presence of these antibodies may indicate an increased risk the development of scleroderma.

Other antibodies including the antineutrophilic cytoplasmic antibodies have also been reported among patients exposed to silica. Wichmann et al. (48) detected antibodies to myeloperoxidase in 14 of 52 patients with a history of occupational exposure to silica at a scouring powder factory for a mean of 7 years. Sixteen of the 52 patients had SLE and 12 systemic sclerosis; in comparison antimyeloperoxidase antibodies were not detected in control groups consisting of six patients with SLE and 15 healthy subjects. These findings would suggest that chronic exposure to silica may induce polyclonal immune activation. Case-control studies have reported association between exposure to silica and the development of ANCA-associated disease (49,50). Satterly et al. (51) reported a significantly higher frequency of exposure to silica among 41 patients with ANCA-associated glomerulonephritis compared with matched controls. In contrast, only 11% of 19 patients with lupus nephritis reported silica exposure compared with 16% of matched controls.

Possible Mechanisms

Experimental studies have indicated that silica has the ability to activate microvascular endothelial cells, peripheral blood mononuclear cells, and dermatofibroblasts, and have suggested that this mechanism may play a role in the development of the scleroderma seen in patients exposed to silica (52). Silica particles are phagocytosed by macrophages, which in turn become activated and release a variety of inflammatory cytokines. Silica has an adjuvant affect on antibody production. It has been postulated that the activation of macrophages may lead to increased antigen processing and acceleration of production of antibodies. It has also been suggested that silica may activate the immune system by release of reactive oxygen species (53). Ueki et al. (54) reported polyclonal activation of human T cells by silica *in vitro* and suggested that silica may act on human lymphocytes as a superantigen. Of interest are previous reports of lymphocyte activation and the induction of polyclonal autoantibody responses by both mercury and gold, suggesting that organic substances may have the ability to act as superantigens.

Silica has been reported to induce apoptosis in macrophages, lymphocytes, and alveolar and granulomatous cells (53). Otsuki et al. (55) reported that messenger RNA (mRNA) expression for soluble Fas was dominantly expressed, as compared with mRNA expression for the membrane form of Fas, in peripheral blood mononuclear cells obtained from 69 patients with silicosis but without evidence of autoimmune diseases. In addition levels of serum soluble Fas were significantly higher in these patients compared with those seen in healthy volunteers and patients with scleroderma. These findings would suggest persistence of autoreactive cells in patients with silicosis as a result of decreased apoptosis, which may in turn lead to the development of autoantibodies and autoimmunity.

It has been suggested that genetic factors may also play a role in the development of autoimmune diseases in patients exposed to silica. Studies by Frank et al. (56) reported a difference in the frequency of the HLA class II and III genes between patients with antitopoisomerase-1 antibodies with idiopathic scleroderma compared with those who had scleroderma and a history of silica exposure. The prevalence of the tumor necrosis factor-α_2 (TNF-α_2) allele was reported to be increased significantly in patients with scleroderma and silicosis and was decreased in patients with idiopathic scleroderma.

One of the confounding factors in determining the association between silica and the development of autoimmune disease is that occupational exposure generally results in exposure to a wide range of other minerals as well, such as iron ore and other metals that may also have adjuvant activity. Since most of the studies have been retrospective, it is difficult to accurately assess the exposure level, although it would appear that the development of autoimmune diseases tends to occur in patients who have very high levels of exposure to silica.

These data suggest the possibility that exposure to silica may predispose to or precipitate the development of SLE and other connective tissue diseases in certain individuals. Controlled prospective studies are needed to confirm this.

Vinyl Chloride

Occupational exposure to vinyl chloride has been associated with the development of scleroderma. Sclerodermatous-like skin lesions have been found among workers involved in the industrial process of polymerizing polyvinyl chloride, which is used in the plastics industry. A small percentage ($\leq 3\%$) of these workers have been reported to develop occupational acro-osteolysis, which is characterized by Raynaud's-like phenomenon involving the hands, sclerodermatous-like changes involving the skin of the hands and forearms, and osteolytic and sclerotic lesions of the bones, especially the extremities and sacroiliac joints. In some cases, synovial thickening of the small joints of the hands was seen (57,58). Cutaneous involvement is characterized by diffuse, waxy thickening of the skin of the digits of the hands, which is most noticeable over the flexor and extensor tendons but also may involve the feet. Unlike scleroderma, the skin appendages continue to function. ANAs and rheumatoid factors are negative. Duration of exposure to the polyvinyl chloride before onset of the disease is variable. The syndrome appears to occur only in workers involved in manual cleaning of the polyvinyl chloride reactor vessels, suggesting that the etiologic agent(s) may be one or more of the incomplete products of polymerization.

Susceptibility to the autoimmune effects of vinyl chloride has been associated with the HLA-DR5 antigen, with disease severity linked to the haplotype A1,B8,DR3, which suggests a genetic influence (59,60). Vinyl chloride may bind to nucleotides. However, more recent data have indicated that its oxidized metabolites, chloroethylene oxide and chloroacetaldehyde, are also highly reactive (61). These metabolites may bind to the sulfhydryl groups present on self proteins and may thus alter their antigenicity or modify their structure, leading to the development of an autoimmune response similar to that seen with mercury.

Avoidance of exposure to the chemical is thought to prevent further progression of the skin disease but has no effect on the further progression of the bony lesions.

Organic Solvents

Solvents are used for cleaning (degreasing) and are constituents of paints, varnish, lacquers, thinners, paint and varnish removers, waxes, floor and shoe polish, inks, adhesives, antifreeze mixtures, motor fuel, pharmaceutical products, and preservatives. They are also used in the manufacture of artificial rubber, leather, plastics, explosives, textiles, formulations for pesticide, fumigants, and other disinfectants. Vapor inhalation is believed to be the most important means by which patients are exposed to these solvents.

A number of polyhalogenated hydrocarbons, which have become ubiquitous in the environment, have been associated with the development of immunotoxicity in experimental animals. Abnormalities in immune function have been reported in humans exposed to polychlorinated biphenyls, which are present in contaminated rice oil, and to polybrominated biphenyls (62,63). Exposure to hydrocarbon solvents has been associated with the development of Goodpasture's syndrome. Beirne and Brennan (64) reported a history of extensive occupational exposure to various industrial solvents, including paint solvents and sprays, jet propulsion fuel, degreasing solvents, and hair sprays, in six of eight patients with anti–glomerular basement membrane antibody-mediated glomerulonephritis. Duration of exposure was a minimum of 1 year in five cases and generally was to a vapor or fine mist form of the solvent in question. Klavis and Drommer (65), who described a patient with Goodpasture's syndrome who became ill after a single, massive exposure to a gasoline-based paint spray, also reported the development of pulmonary hemorrhage and glomerular damage in rats that were chronically exposed to gasoline vapors. It has been suggested that chronic or massive exposure to these chemicals may result in chemical interaction with possible injury to the lung and glomerular basement membranes, which leads to the formation of autoantibodies directed against these membranes in susceptible individuals. In a study of rabbits (66), it was found that intratracheal instillation of minute amounts of gasoline resulted in the binding of anti–basement membrane antibodies to the alveolar basement membrane. This would suggest that the chemical facilitates binding of the antibody to the tissue antigen rather than producing an autoimmune response itself.

Vojdani et al. (67) screened 289 subjects with a history of exposure of at least 10 years' duration to industrial chemicals, resulting from working in computer manufacturing plants, for evidence of immunologic abnormalities. These chemicals included phthalic anhydride, formaldehyde, isocyanate, trimellitic anhydride, and aliphatic and aromatic hydrocarbons. A significantly higher percentage of exposed subjects had immune abnormalities compared to a control group of 120 nonexposed individuals. These abnormalities included evidence of immune dysregulation such as abnormal T-helper: T-suppressor cell ratios, elevated numbers of T and B cells and activated T cells, suppression of lymphocyte blastogenic responses to T- and B-cell mitogens, and a biphasic natural killer (NK)-cell cytotoxic activity. Significant elevation of both IgG and IgM chemical hapten antibodies, in particular those directed against formaldehyde, trimellitic anhydride, phthalic anhydride, and benzene ring, also were found. In addition, significantly elevated levels of IgM rheumatoid factor, ANAs, antibodies to myelin basic protein, and IgM, IgG, and IgA immune complexes were detected in the study group. These were poorly controlled studies and have not been confirmed.

There have been numerous reports of associations of exposure to organic solvents and the development of connective tissue diseases including scleroderma-like illnesses. Many of these have been in the form of case reports that provide weak evidence for an association. Aromatic solvents and chlorinated solvents are the two groups that have been most commonly implicated in the development of scleroderma. Aromatic solvents, especially benzene, has been associated with the development of skin fibrosis (68,69). There have been case reports of exposure to a variety of chemicals including benzene, toluene, and other related substances and the development of scleroderma-like illnesses, although many of these patients lacked the typical sclerodermatous changes or had features that are atypical for scleroderma (70). A sclerodermatous syndrome characterized by skin thickening with involvement of the hands, arms, face, and trunk; myopathy; and esophageal dysfunction was reported in a man following exposure to herbicides consisting of aminotriazole, bromouracil, and diuron with some improvement occurring after corticosteroid therapy. A patient reported by Dunnill and Black (71) had developed a generalized cutaneous sclerosis associated with a myopathy and esophageal involvement 6 months after he had spent 3 months spraying a herbicide containing aminotriazole, bromouracil, and diuron. Beer et al. (72) reported the development of a dermatitis, leukopenia, and ANAs in a father and daughter who had been exposed to an insecticide containing 1,1,1-trichloroethane, propane, S-methoprene, and permethrin after the father had used this insecticide in his trailer home. The father also developed thrombocytopenia, and the daughter antibodies to dsDNA and Smith. Clinical improvement occurred following treatment with steroids. Walder (69) reported the development of scleroderma in 11 patients who had close contact with a variety of solvents including toluene, benzene, white spirits xylene, and dieselene.

Chlorinated Hydrocarbons

Exposure to the chlorinated hydrocarbon, trichloroethylene (TCE), has resulted in the greatest number of reported cases. TCE is a chlorinated ethene that is primarily used as a solvent for removing grease from metal parts. It is also found in a variety of products including adhesives, spot removers, carpet-cleaning fluids, paint removers, and strippers, and has been detected at hazardous waste dump sites. Exposure to TCE can occur through the air as a result of evaporation from degreasing operations or waste disposal sites and ground water contamination through leeching. TCE is closely related to vinyl chloride and has also been reported to be associated with the development of scleroderma, eosinophilic fasciitis, and scleroderma-like illness (73,74). Duration of exposure prior to the development of scleroderma has been reported to range from 2 to 14 years, although one woman developed typical scleroderma with acute swelling of her hands after only 2½ hours of intense exposure to the chemical. Waller et al. (74) reported the development of biopsy-proven fasciitis in two patients following exposure to TCE. One of these patients had been exposed to TCE through ingestion of contaminated well water, and she had noticed improvement in her symptoms following the use of bottled water. Autoantibodies have been detected among patients developing scleroderma-like syndromes following exposure to TCE in contrast to the vinyl chloride–associated sclerodermatous disease. Vinyl chloride is a halogenated ethylene, while TCE is a halogenated aliphatic organic compound that is chemically similar to vinyl chloride. A syndrome similar to that seen with vinyl chloride has been reported in a patient who was exposed to perchloroethylene (tetrachloroethylene), which is another closely related halogenated aliphatic hydrocarbon (75).

A number of immunologic abnormalities including persistent T lymphocytosis, increased CD4/CD8 ratio, and an increased prevalence of autoantibodies was reported among residents of Woburn, Massachusetts, who had been exposed to water contaminated by TCE and, to a lesser extent, tetrachloroethylene, 1,2-*trans*-dichloroethylene, 1,1,-trichloroethane, and chloroform (76).

Kilburn and Warshaw (77) implicated TCE in the development of SLE among residents exposed to contaminated well water. They reported an elevated prevalence of ANAs and lupus-like symptoms among 362 subjects exposed to contaminated well water in the southwest Tucson area and suggested that chemicals such as TCE may induce or promote the development of autoantibodies and autoimmune diseases such as SLE. The study group was compared to a control group of 158 nonexposed individuals, matched for age range and educational level, who were living in southwest Phoenix. The principal contaminants in the well water consisted of TCE but also trichloroethane, inorganic chromium, and other chemicals. Using the 1971 ARA preliminary criteria for SLE, the authors reported that the prevalences of all ten SLE symptoms were greater in the study group than in the control group. Of these arthritis/arthralgias, Raynaud's phenomenon, malar rash, heliotropic skin lesions, and seizure/convulsion reached statistical significance. The frequency of ANAs was also increased in the study group: a fluorescent ANA (FANA) titer of 1 : 160 or greater was seen in 10.7% of the study group compared with 4.7% of the controls. However, the clinical data in this study were obtained only by questionnaires, and matching for ethnicity and socioeconomic groups was not addressed. The authors used the 1971 ARA preliminary criteria for SLE, which included nonspecific features of SLE as well as features such as "heliotrope skin lesions," which are seen with dermatomyositis. In addition, 13 of the 32 subjects with high FANA titers had other predisposing factors: three had rheumatoid arthritis, one a sister with SLE, six had taken methyldopa, and three had taken Dilantin, all of which can be associated with ANAs. Properly controlled studies using 1982 ARA classification criteria and including complete histories and examinations of all subjects are required to test this postulated association (78). Subsequently, a possibly higher than expected prevalence of SLE was reported among Mexican residents of Nogales, Arizona, although this again has yet to be confirmed (79).

Studies in animals have demonstrated inhibition of humoral- and cell-mediated immunity in mice exposed to TCE (80,81). In a subsequent study, the same group reported depression of the humoral immunity in CD1 mice exposed to 1,1,2-trichloroethane, but there was no effect on cell-mediated immunity (82). Studies by Khan et al. (83) suggested that TCE and its metabolite dichloroacetyl chloride (DCAC) could induce and/or accelerate the development of autoimmune responses among female MRL +/+ mice following exposure to TCE and DCAC by intraperitoneal injections. ANAs developed in the majority of the mice exposed to DCAC and all of those exposed to TCE. Anti–single-stranded DNA (ssDNA) antibodies were detected in 50% of the mice exposed to TCE and all of those exposed to DCAC. Anticardiolipin antibodies were detected in the majority of those exposed to DCAC but not to TCE. Antibodies to Sm, histones, and dsDNA were not detected. Of note, these responses were induced at a much lower dose by DCAC compared with TCE, suggesting that this metabolite may be important in the development of autoimmunity. More recently Griffin et al. (84) reported that MRL +/+ mice that had been exposed to TCE in their drinking water for 4 weeks developed a T-helper-1 (Th1)-type immune response characterized by a dose-dependent increase in interferon-γ but without any effect on interleukin-4 (IL-4). Other data reported by this group indicated that the metabolic activation of TCE by cytochrome P-450 2E1 resulted in the production of a reactive metabolite that was suggested to be important in mediating these changes. In contrast, TCE did not produce any effect on the immune systems of the brown Norway (BN) rats (85), suggesting that different immune systems vary in their responses.

Hexachlorobenzene (HCB) is a chemical that has the ability to affect the immune system. (86). In contrast to TCE, exposure to HCB in the diet resulted in the development of an inflammatory infiltration consisting of eosinophils and some mononuclear cells around large- and medium-sized arteries and the large bronchi of BN rats (87). An increase in immunoglobulin levels, which included IgG and particularly IgM, have been reported in workers who have been occupationally exposed to this chemical (88). Accidental exposure to HCB over a 4-year period, from 1955 to 1959 as a result of ingestion of wheat that had been treated with the fungicide HCB, led to the development of porphyria among an estimated 4,000 people (89). A follow-up study of 204 patients reported the persistence of symptoms including arthritis, scarring of the skin, enlargement of the thyroid gland (90). The development of HCB-induced skin lesions in rats correlated with immune parameters including increased levels of IgM to ssDNA, suggesting a possible autoimmune etiology.

Pre- and perinatal exposure to certain chemicals has been reported to affect the development of the immune system in both human and animal studies. Gestational exposure to the organochlorine insecticide chlordane or to the polycyclic aromatic hydrocarbon benzo[*a*]pyrene exposure has been reported to result in apparent lifelong immunosuppression in mice. Long-term depression of both delayed-type hypersensitivity and mixed lymphocyte reactivity was noted in mice exposed to chlordane *in utero*, although similar effects are not seen in adult mice exposed to this chemical (91).

Prenatal exposure to certain halogenated aromatic hydrocarbons, notably dioxins, can lead to severe long-lasting immunosuppression in rodents (92).

The environmental agent 2,3,7,8-tetrachlorodibenzo-*p*-dioxin (TCDD) is a polycyclic halogenated hydrocarbon. It has been reported to produce effects on the fetal thymus, which included inhibition of maturation of the thymocytes and downregulation of expression of thymic major histocompatibility complex class I molecules (93). Exposure of mice predisposed to the development of autoimmune diseases to TCDD *in utero* led to exacerbation of postnatal autoimmunity. It has been suggested that gestational exposure to certain immunotoxins may be important in the expression of autoimmunity in humans. Such exposure may impair the development of self tolerance and may in turn lead to the development of autoimmunity in individuals exposed to TCDD *in utero*.

Exposure of adult SNF_1 male mice to monthly exposures of TCDD in an oil depot accelerated the development of an autoimmune lupus-like nephritis (94). There was a decrease in the proliferative response to concanavalin A (ConA) and in the *in vitro* stimulated production of IgG by cells of animals treated with TCDD. The production of IgG antibodies to ssDNA was produced at the same level, suggesting a shift with expansion of cells producing pathogenic antibodies. Administration of TCDD to mice resulted in impaired generation of cytotoxic T lymphocytes in response to allogeneic cells (95).

Epoxy Resins

There have been a few reports suggesting an association between exposure to epoxy resins and the development of morphea, a variant of scleroderma. Yamakage et al. (96) reported the development of cutaneous sclerosis in six of 233 workers who were exposed to the vapor of epoxy resins while engaged in the polymerization process of epoxy resins at a factory in Japan. Histologic examination revealed changes similar to generalized morphea rather than to systemic scleroderma. Both patients also developed marked muscle weakness. The systemic manifestations and the sclerotic skin changes disappeared within 5 years and no evidence of internal involvement was found (97). Follow-up skin biopsy revealed atrophy of the dermis but restoration of the normal fine collagen bundles. It was suggested that *bis*-(4-amino-3-methyl-cyclohexyl) methane, entering through the lungs in vapor form, was the most likely causative agent. This compound, which is one of the cyclohexylamines, had been applied to the polymerization of epoxy resins as a new type of plasticizer at the time of exposure of these workers. This agent is chemically related to a number of drugs including procainamide, *d*-penicillamine, chlorpromazine, and isoniazid, all of which have been implicated in the development of drug-related lupus.

Epidemiologic Studies

Several epidemiologic studies have sought an association between exposure to solvents and the development of scleroderma. A Swedish study reported that exposure to chemicals was higher than expected among scleroderma patients (98). Subsequently, a French study reported that 56% of 25 males with scleroderma had been exposed to either silica dust or chemicals over a mean duration of 14.5 years as a result of their occupation (99). A later study from Italy reported a significant association between scleroderma and occupational exposure to organic solvents and silica among 21 scleroderma patients compared with controls (100). However, a well-designed control study by Silman and Jones (101) of 56 men with scleroderma failed to show evidence of an association between the disease and exposure to silica. Only two patients were classified as having possible silica exposure. Occupational exposure to epoxy resins, formaldehyde, and vinyl chloride was rarely reported. Occupation analysis suggested that 11% of patients had probable exposure and a further 34% possible exposure to organic solvents. However, case-control analysis did not confirm a significant increase in risk in exposure to organic solvents, although the confidence intervals were wide.

A recent study by Nietert et al. (102) evaluated occupational exposure to solvents as a risk factor for the development of scleroderma. They determined work exposures to solvents using job exposure matrixes that were verified by a blinded industrial expert. Men with scleroderma were reported to be more likely than controls to have a high cumulative intensity score and a high maximum intensity score for any solvent exposure and, in particular, for exposure to TCE. They also reported a significant association of exposure to any solvent with scleroderma among those patients who tested positive for the anti–Scl-70 antibody compared with those who are negative for this antibody. Since the anti–Scl-70 antibody has been associated with certain HLA genotypes, these results suggest that both genetic and environmental factors may play a role in the pathogenesis of scleroderma.

A population-based case-control study of 274 women with scleroderma in Michigan failed to find any association with silicone breast implants (103). This group did report equivocal evidence of risk for other silicone exposures but found no evidence of risk from exposure to silica. This same group reported that exposure to halogenated solvents, trichloroethane and TCE, or to pesticides/herbicides was a significant risk factor for the development of scleroderma based on the results of a case-control study of 274 Michigan women diagnosed with scleroderma (104). This group also conducted a parallel population-based case-control study in Ohio in which 1,989 women who were diagnosed with scleroderma between 1985 and 1992 were evaluated for possible risk factors for the development of scleroderma. Evaluation of this patient group did not reveal any association between scleroderma and silicone-gel breast implants or silica exposure. However, there was a significant association with sculpting and pottery making (105). The scleroderma patients and controls included in both the Michigan and Ohio studies were subsequently evaluated for exposure to solvents by telephone interview. Among occupational activities considered to have a potential for exposure to solvents, professional cleaning and maintenance were both associated with a significant increased risk of scleroderma. In addition, self-reported exposure to paint thinners and removers was significantly associated with an increased risk, while TCE and gasoline exposure were suggestive of an increased risk of scleroderma (106). Another study by the same group reported that exposure to paint thinners and removers was associated with a significant increased risk for undifferentiated connective tissue disease (107).

Koeger et al. (108) suggested that occupational exposure to silicone spray may be a risk factor for the development of connective tissue disease. They conducted a cross-sectional study of 245 patients with a variety of connective tissue diseases of whom 28 were males who had been hospitalized during an 18-month study period. Five male patients were considered to have significant exposure to silicone spray as defined by a daily exposure of 6 to 8 hours for 3 years or longer prior to the onset of connective tissue disease. Of these five patients, two developed SLE, two rheumatoid arthritis, and one mixed connective tissue disease. All five patients had interstitial lung disease based on x-ray and pulmonary function test studies in addition to hypercellularity on bronchoalveolar lavages.

Nietert et al. (109) evaluated the role of exposure to solvents as part of recreational hobbies as a risk factor for the development of systemic sclerosis. Solvent exposure based on hobbies and occupations was determined for 178 patients with systemic sclerosis and 200 controls by interview. Participation in solvent-oriented hobbies was similar for patients with scleroderma and controls; however, the odds of high cumulative solvent oriented hobby exposure was three times greater for those patients with scleroderma who had the anti–Scl-70 antibody compared to patients who were negative, and the odds were 2.5 times higher for the antibody-positive scleroderma patients compared with controls. These results suggest a possible role for exposure to solvents in the development of scleroderma associated with anti–Scl-70 antibodies. This would also indicate that there may be different etiologic pathways for the development of scleroderma.

Silicone

Autoimmune diseases have been reported to occur after the injection or implantation of paraffin or silicone (110,111). Miyoshi et al. (112) first described the development of autoimmune phenomena in humans after inframammary injections of paraffin, which he termed human adjuvant disease. Characteristics of the disease were the development of hypergammaglobulinemia, autoantibody formation (including ANA), and granuloma formation approximately 2 years after the injection of silicone or related substances, with improvement following their removal. Subsequently, Yoshida (113) also included arthralgias, arthritis, adenopathy, elevated erythrocyte sedimentation rate, and positive rheumatoid factor as characteristics. However, not all patients showed clinical improvement following removal of the injected materials. Studies in rats using the type II collagen arthritis model have also suggested that silicone gel, acting as an adjuvant, has the ability to mediate collagen-induced arthritis in dark Agouti rats when it was mixed with bovine collagen II (114). Despite these findings, silicone gel alone did not appear to be arthritogenic. This report of an adjuvant effect was in contrast to previous findings reported by the same group in which silicone gel did not promote the onset of arthritis in Lewis rats.

In 1984, Kumagai et al. (115) reported an association between the injection of either paraffin or silicone and the development of autoimmune-like diseases in 46 patients. Of these, 24 had definite evidence of SLE, mixed connective tissue diseases, rheumatoid arthritis, Sjögren's syndrome, Hashimoto's thyroiditis, or scleroderma. ANAs with antigenic specificities similar to those seen with connective tissue diseases have been detected in patients with silicone breast implants or those who had silicone injections (116). Overall, there have been at least 100 cases of patients developing autoimmune-like diseases up to 25 years after augmentation mammoplasty procedures, some of which have resolved following removal of the implants. However, most of the evidence has been based primarily on case reports, which provide very weak evidence for a causal relationship.

Over a dozen studies have assessed the risk of implants in the development of connective tissue disease, in particular scleroderma. Many of these studies have methodologic flaws and most have failed to confirm an association.

A retrospective cohort study by Gabriel et al. (117) of 749 women who received a breast implant between 1964 and 1991 and who were both age- and sex-matched with 1,498 community controls failed to find a statistically significant association. Similarly, in their case series study, Bridges et al. (118) did not find a significant association. Sanchez-Guerrero et al. (119) analyzed data from 14 years of follow-up on 87,501 women enrolled in the Nurses' Health Study cohort: of these, 516 had a connective tissue disease, and 1,183 had breast implants. Based on these data, they calculated that the age-adjusted relative risk of a connective tissue disease was 0.6 for women with any type of breast implant and 0.3 for women with silicone gel–filled implants compared to women without implants. These results were not significant using 95% confidence intervals.

The study by Hennekens et al. (120) had the highest statistical power for the detection of a potential risk given the large sample size of their study population. They evaluated the possible association of breast implants with the development of connective tissue disease in a retrospective cohort study of 395,543 female health professionals using a questionnaire. A total of 10,830 women reported having breast implants and 11,805 connective tissue diseases. The relative risk of any connective tissue disease among those women reporting breast implants was 1.24 (95% confidence interval of 1.08 to 1.41), which was statistically significant (p = .0015). No statistical significant association was found for rheumatoid arthritis, Sjögren's syndrome, dermatomyositis, polymyositis, scleroderma, or SLE. These results suggest the possibility of a small increased risk for the development of a connective tissue disease among patients with breast implants, but would exclude the presence of a large risk. Of note, the data analyzed were limited to those obtained before 1992 in order to avoid a potential reporting bias as a result of widespread publicity. This study was limited by the fact that the data were self-reported; this may bias the subject to possible overreporting of connective tissue diseases. Clinical verification of the reported connective tissue diseases would need to be performed to confirm the results of this survey and validate the increased risk.

Other studies have also evaluated the risk of implants in the development of connective tissue disease but have not found an association. However, the smaller number of subjects included in these studies would not allow for the detection for relative risks less than 2.0. Hochberg et al. (121) in a multicenter case-control study examined the possible association of augmentation mammoplasty with scleroderma; 837 women with a clinical diagnosis of scleroderma recruited from three university-based tertiary-care scleroderma clinical research centers were compared to 2,507 race matched local controlled women. Eleven (1.31%) of the scleroderma patients reported a history of augmentation mammoplasty prior to the diagnosis of their disease compared with 31 (1.24%) of the controls. No statistically significant association between the augmentation mammoplasty and scleroderma was demonstrated.

In a more recent study, Edworthy et al. (122) evaluated 1,576 women who had undergone breast implantation between 1978 and 1986 for possible connective tissue disease. The women were initially evaluated by an extensive questionnaire and by blood sample, and those with features suggestive of connective tissue disease were subsequently assessed blindly by a rheumatologist. Age- and sex-adjusted prevalence rates for rheumatoid arthritis, SLE, scleroderma, and Sjögren's syndrome among the study group were consistent with those published reports for Caucasian women. Breast implant recipients reported significantly greater frequencies of symptoms and in particular thought problems, numbness in extremities, muscle pain, headache, and hand pain than the controls. However, there was no increase in the postsurgical incident rates for any of the connective tissue diseases compared with the control population. Hence, similarly to other studies, no significant association was noted between silicone gel–filled implants and the development of connective tissue diseases. In addition, serologic analysis did not reveal any significant differences between the breast implant recipients and controls when adjusted for age.

Similar results were reported by Karlson et al. (123), who evaluated 200 randomly selected women who had had silicone breast implants but did not have a history of connective tissue disease and 500 age-matched nonexposed women, of whom 100 had a connective tissue disease, for the presence of a variety of autoantibodies, including ANAs, antibodies to dsDNA, ssDNA, Smith, ribonucleoprotein (RNP), Ro, La, Scl-70, cardiolipin, thyroglobulin, thyroid microsomes and silicone, rheumatoid factor, and immunoglobulins. ANAs were present in 14% of the women with silicone breast implants compared to 20% of healthy controls. There was a higher frequency of anti-ssDNA antibodies at 41% among silicone breast implants compared with 29% for the control group. However, there were no other significant differences in the frequency of antibodies between the two groups. Since anti-ssDNA antibodies are generally considered to have little clinical relevance, the results of these studies would suggest a lack of association between autoimmunity and silicone breast implants.

Taken in combination, the results of the aforementioned epidemiologic studies would rule out a large increase in the risk for the development of connective tissue diseases as a result of silicone breast implantation. Although associations cannot be definitively ruled out as yet, given the relatively low prevalence of some connective tissue diseases (e.g., scleroderma) any association with the more common diseases (e.g., SLE and rheumatoid arthritis) is unlikely.

Other Chemicals and Toxins

Exposure to beryllium, which is used in the ceramic, electronics, aerospace, and nuclear weapons industries, can lead to immune-mediated lung disease in certain individuals. In a controlled study, Richeldi et al. (124) reported an association between the development of chronic beryllium disease (CBD) and HLA-DPB1* 0201 alleles.

In vitro and *in vivo* studies have demonstrated modulation of the immune response by cocaine (125). Cocaine abuse has resulted in the development of clinical features and syndromes that simulate connective tissue diseases such as SLE, vasculitis, and polymyositis (126–129). It is as yet unclear whether cocaine produces its effects through direct toxicity, repeated vascular injury, repeated antigenic stimulation, modulation of the immune system, or a combination of all these.

Colchicine, which is derived from the autumn crocus, has been reported to cause (130) a myopathy that is similar to that seen in patients with polymyositis.

Eosin, which is contained in lipstick and is used in the laboratory for tissue staining, has been reported to cause photosensitivity rashes and contact dermatitis (131). It has the ability to bind strongly to body tissue *in vitro*, and it has been suggested that if the same happened *in vivo*, through application of lipstick, it might act as an immunologic trigger for SLE. Photosensitivity is one recognized feature of lupus, and one could hypothesize that the presence of eosin in lipstick might suggest an explanation for the female predominance seen in this disease. However, no studies have investigated this, so at present it is not necessary to advise patients to refrain from using lipstick.

METALS (TABLE 3.3)

Chronic exposure to certain metals has been reported to induce immune complex mediated kidney disease in both animals and humans (132–134).

Gold

Chronic administration of gold may lead to development of a glomerulopathy and antibody formation. Diffuse granular deposits of IgG, IgM, and complement have been found in glomerular lesions in humans. Silverberg et al. (135) reported gold deposits in the proximal tubules of four patients with gold-induced nephrotic syndrome and of one patient who had a renal biopsy while receiving gold but who did not have proteinuria. The deposits were more marked in the three patients who had received the largest doses of gold; these patients also had deposits in the interstitium, glomerular tufts, and distal tubules. The patient without proteinuria had deposits that were similar in location and extent to those found in patients receiving similar amounts of gold who had developed nephrotic syndrome. The lack of correlation between the dose of gold and proteinuria/nephrotic syndrome would argue against a direct toxic effect and in favor of a hypersensitivity mechanism.

Gold also has an effect on neutrophil, monocyte, and lymphocyte function. The risk of gold-induced proteinuria is increased 32 times in patients who possess HLA-DR2 and -DR3, suggesting a genetic predisposition (136). Administration of gold has been associated with the development of immune complex–mediated nephropathy in animals, the production of antibodies to renal epithelial antigens, and the formation of granular immune deposits consisting of these antibodies and their antigens, in addition to the development of ANAs and antinucleolar antibodies in some murine strains and antilaminin antibodies in BN rats (137,138).

TABLE 3.3. METALS REPORTED TO BE ASSOCIATED WITH AUTOIMMUNE DISEASE

Gold
Cadmium
Mercury
Pristane

Cadmium

Long-term oral exposure to cadmium has been reported to induce a membranous glomerulonephropathy in rats that is thought to be mediated by immune complexes (139) and is similar to that seen in humans. Granular, irregular, dense deposits of IgG were found in most glomeruli. Cadmium also has been reported to induce the formation of ANAs in mice (140), which may be the result of either direct or indirect polyclonal activation of B cells. Development of a marked proliferation of B cells in rats receiving high doses of cadmium that resulted in antibody formation also has been reported (141). Miners and alkaline battery workers are exposed to cadmium in the course of their occupation.

Mercury

Mercury has been found to have the ability to induce autoimmunity both in animals and humans and to both activate and inhibit immune responses. Mercury is a xenobiotic that is widely present in the environment. Its levels are increasing as a result of mining and processing of raw oils as part of various industrial activities and in the discharge of medical and scientific waste products. Mercuric compounds are used in fluorescent lights, batteries, and electronic devices in addition to dental amalgam. At this point it is unclear whether the load levels of mercury present in dental amalgam constitute a significant risk for the development of mercury-induced autoimmunity. Apart from occupational exposure, mercury intake is primarily through ingestion of contaminated food especially fish (142). It may also be present in some dietary supplements and over-the-counter health remedies and is also used as a preservative in some immunoglobulin and vaccine preparations. Medications containing mercury, such as the organomercurial diuretics, mercury-containing laxatives, and the ammoniated mercury in skin ointments that were used to treat psoriasis, have been associated with the development of an autoimmune-mediated nephrotic syndrome (143). Immunofluorescent studies demonstrated the presence of IgG and C3 at the level of the renal glomerular basement membrane in these patients. There has been a decrease in the incidence of these syndromes with the decrease in the use of medications. A slight increase in antibodies to DNA was reported among a cohort of workers who were exposed to mercury vapor (144). Although there have been a few reports of autoimmune disease and ANAs occurring in workers exposed to mercury, occupational exposure to mercury generally does not result in autoimmunity (145,146).

Mercury has been shown to affect the functions of some immune cells, in particular, macrophages, polymorphonuclear leukocytes, and T lymphocytes (147). *In vitro* treatment with mercuric chloride resulted in inhibition of mitogen stimulated proliferation and decreased production of

IL-2 from human T-cells. Similarly, *in vitro* exposure to mercuric chloride appears to inhibit proliferation and immunoglobulin syntheses by human B cells. In contrast, *in vivo* exposure to mercury has been reported to increase T-lymphocyte responses in the BALB/c mice and stimulate the production of IgE and other immunoglobulin isotypes by B lymphocytes in both rats and mice (148).

Mercuric chloride can induce the development of several types of immune complex–mediated glomerulopathies in susceptible strains of rats, and in some cases there was concomitant production of antibodies directed against a nuclear nonhistone chromatin protein (148). Antibodies to self antigens, such as ssDNA, laminin, and collagen II and IV, and to nonself antigens, such as trinitrophenyl and sheep red blood cells, have been described in BN rats treated with mercuric chloride (149). Antilaminin autoantibodies accounted for most of the antiglomerular basement membrane antibodies in the glomerular deposits (150). High titers of antinucleolar antibodies also developed in SJL/N and B10.S (H-2s) mice following mercury administration (151,152). These antinucleolar antibodies were directed against a U3-RNP-associated protein, believed to be fibrillarin, and were very similar to the antibodies found in some patients with scleroderma (152). Some mice also had ANAs, including some directed against histones.

Murine strains appear to vary in their susceptibility to the development of antibody formation and clinical disease. Goter Robinson et al. (137) demonstrated variation in antibody responses to mercuric chloride and found that susceptibility appeared to be determined by the H-2s haplotype. Antibodies directed against nucleolar antigen(s) were induced in Swiss ICR mice by the administration of mercuric chloride (153). However, unlike the BN rat, none of these mice developed true glomerulopathy. This may result from a difference in antigen specificity between the two animal models or from inadequate immune complex formation because of antibody excess. Other strains of mice did develop immune deposits and glomerulonephritis following treatment with mercuric chloride, suggesting a genetic influence.

Animal studies indicated that mercury can induce renal disease that is comparable to an autoimmune glomerulonephropathy, although the autoantigen is as yet unknown. Studies of mice and rats suggest that the autoantigens may be laminin 1, fibrillarin, or nuclear histones. BN, Maxx, and DZB rats develop nephrotic syndrome and antibodies to laminin 1, which is a component of renal glomerular basement membrane and may have a pathogenic role in the development of the disease. Mercury has been reported to induce polyclonal B-cell activation with high levels of IgG1, IgG3, and IgE immunoglobulins, intense autoantibody production against dsDNA, IgG, and collagen, and renal immune complex deposits in (NZBXNZW) F1 mice (154). Mercuric chloride can inhibit the production of interferon-γ in susceptible BN rats and induce the production of IL-4, suggesting a skewing of the Th response toward Th2.

Mercury may also interact with exposed sulfhydrl groups present on endigenous proteins and thus may modify self proteins through mercuric-thiol interactions, resulting in modification of the molecular and antigenic properties of the self protein. This may lead to a T-cell induced B-cell response against these mercury modified proteins, resulting in the development of autoantibodies. Mercury-triggered immune responses may then recognize the native self proteins. Data from Kubicka-Muranyi et al. (155) suggest that mercury may induce antigen presentation of a novel epitope as a result of binding to the nucleolar protein fibrillarin. These authors also reported upregulation of the presentation of unaltered fibrillarin epitopes and stimulation of fibrillarin-specific T-cell clones. Genetic control of this autoimmune response was mapped to the H-2A region of the major histocompatibility complex of susceptible mice.

In a subsequent study, Pollard et al. (156) suggested that overall protein structure was important in dictating interaction with mercury. They had noted that some proteins that were cysteine rich were not modified by mercury but that the cysteines present in the fibrillarin molecule were not disulfide bonded, resulting in exposure of sulfhydryl (SH) groups that could be modified by interaction with mercury. Although mercury-modified fibrillarin generates a T-cell–induced B-cell response, the antibodies that are produced have the ability to recognize unmodified fibrillarin, which may then potentiate the immune response. ANAs, which may react with fibrillarin, can be seen in many patients with scleroderma. It is possible that chemical modification of the exposed cysteines of fibrillarin may be important in the induction of an autoimmune response that leads to the development of scleroderma, although there is little clinical evidence implicating mercury as the culprit. Thus, mercury can elicit a genetically restricted autoantibody response in mice that targets the nucleolar autoantigen fibrillarin. Other *in vitro* studies by Pollard et al. (157) have indicated that modification of fibrillarin by mercuric chloride accompanies cell death; mercury can then elicit a specific protease activity that results in cleavage of fibrillarin, producing novel protein fragments that may be released and act as sources of antigenic determinants for self reactive T cells. Other studies by this group indicated that exposure to mercury may significantly accelerate the onset of systemic autoimmune disease in a strain-dependent manner, suggesting that genetic susceptibility may predispose to mercury-induced exacerbations of autoimmunity (158). Genetic predisposition may be important in the development of xenobiotic-induced autoimmunity in humans as well.

In a small study of 13 patients, Arnett et al. (159) evaluated exposure to mercury as a possible environmental trigger for the development of scleroderma. Since animal studies indicated that exposure to mercury can induce antifibrillarin antibodies, 13 patients with antifibrillarin antibodies of whom 11 had scleroderma were evaluated and compared to 39 scleroderma patients without antifibrillarin antibodies and 32 healthy controls. Exposure to mercury was determined by measuring urinary mercury levels. Urinary mercury levels were significantly elevated in the 13 antifibrillarin-positive patients compared with the two control groups. These values remained significantly elevated even when urinary mercury levels were corrected for urinary creatinine levels. However, the urinary mercury levels, although significantly elevated, remained within what is considered to be the normal unexposed range. Thus, these data are insufficient to either rule out or confirm a possible association between mercury exposure and the development of autoantibodies to fibrillarin and/or scleroderma in humans.

El-Fawal et al. (160) reported that titers of IgG to neurofilaments and myelin basic protein were prevalent in male workers exposed to lead or mercury and that they correlated significantly with levels of blood lead or urinary mercury. IgG antibodies to neuronal cytoskeletal proteins were also noted. IgG titers to these antibodies correlated significantly with subclinical neurologic deficits in these workers. Of note these antibodies were not found in a control group of frozen-food packing plant workers. Autoantibodies to neuronal and glial antigens have also been detected in animals exposed to lead (161), suggesting that lead may play a role in the pathogenesis of autoimmunity.

Possible Mechanisms

Gold and mercury can activate the immune system by directly stimulating immune cells or acting as immunogenes or haptens. Possible mechanisms of action by which heavy metals can alter immune function include the binding to thiol-rich proteins with the formation of disulfide bonds between –SH groups and thiols of self proteins with alteration of the antigenic structure and function of these proteins or exposure of cryptic epitopes, the generation of free radicals, by direct interaction with regulatory factors that modify gene activity, or by direct cytotoxicity resulting in release of intracellular constituents. Heavy metals may also exert effects on the immune system through upregulation of calreticulin at the protein and RNA levels. Calreticulin is a new human rheumatic disease–associated autoantigen that recent evidence has suggested may function as a heat shock/stress response gene. It has been implicated in a number of autoimmune processes including molecular mimicry, epitope spreading, complement inactivation, and stimulation of inflammatory mediators such as production of nitric oxide (162,163). Autoantibodies to calreticulin have been demonstrated in sera from patients with SLE in addition to other rheumatic diseases. Mercuric chloride may bind to the thiol groups present on the antioxidant glutathione, leading to oxidative damage, which may result in the expression of stress proteins that may possibly augment an autoimmune response (164). A single mechanism is unlikely to be responsive for the induction of autoimmunity by metals. Laboratory investigations have indicated that gold and mercury induce autoimmunity in only a few strains of inbred mice and rats, suggesting that immunogenetic and pharmacogenetic factors are required for expression of autoimmune disease induced by metals (165).

Pristane

In contrast to gold and mercury, pristane has been reported to induce a lupus-like syndrome characterized by autoantibody production and glomerulonephritis in some inbred strains of mice. SJL/J mice treated with pristane developed autoantibodies to ribosomal P antigen and immune complex glomerulonephritis. BALB/c mice treated with pristane developed a rheumatoid factor–positive erosive arthritis in addition to immune complex–mediated glomerulonephritis and antibodies to nRNP/Sm, Su, and ssDNA (166). Shaheen et al. (167) reported that both mineral oil and one of its components, pristane, could induce the development of a lupus-like syndrome in nonautoimmune strains of mice by increasing the production of proinflammatory cytokines including IL-6 and IL-12. Intraperitoneal injection of pristane resulted in the production of high levels of antibodies to dsDNA, Sm, and nRNP in addition to other autoantibodies and immune complex–mediated glomerulonephritis in these mice. Immunohistochemical staining revealed phagocytosis of pristane by the macrophages in these mice. Lipopolysaccharide (LPS)-stimulated macrophages obtained from the pristane-treated mice produce significantly more IL-6 and IL-12 than the PBS-treated controls, suggesting that there is a defect in macrophage function caused by exposure to pristane, which in turn may lead to the overproduction of proinflammatory cytokines and the development of autoantibodies and autoimmune disease.

It had been postulated that pristane induces nonspecific activation of the immune system. However, more recent work by Hamilton et al. (168) suggested that the microbial environment may be important in determining the magnitude of the immune response in this inducible lupus model. They reported a marked increase in total IgM and IgG3 2 weeks after interperitoneal pristane injection, which was followed by an increase in IgG1, IgG2a, and IgG2b in conventionally housed mice; in contrast, there was a decrease in the levels of IgG and an increase in IgM levels in mice treated with pristane that were housed in a pathogen-free environment. In addition, there was an increase in the duration of onset and a decrease in the levels of anti-nRNP/Sm and Su autoantibodies in the mice housed in the pathogen-free environment compared with those conventionally housed. These data would suggest that microbial stimulation is important in the development of hypergammaglobulinemia and in autoantibody production in this lupus model. These data would also suggest that multiple environmental factors may influence the development of autoimmune disease in mice and it is likely that this may also be true for development of SLE in humans.

DIETARY FACTORS (TABLE 3.4)

Amino Acids

A lupus-like syndrome has been described in adult female cynomolgus macaques (monkeys) fed semipurified diets containing alfalfa sprouts or seeds (169,170). The syndrome was characterized by the development of ANAs, elevated anti-dsDNA binding, LE cells, hypocomplementemia, antiglobulin-positive anemia, alopecia, dermatitis, and nephrotic syndrome. ANAs were present in high titers with rim, homogeneous, and occasionally speckled patterns of staining. Skin biopsy of one animal revealed deposits along the dermal-epidermal junction that stained with antisera to human IgG, IgA, and C3. Renal biopsy of the same animal revealed a diffuse glomerulonephritis with coarse granular deposits of IgG and C3. Withdrawal of alfalfa seeds from the diet resulted in normalization of hematologic parameters and negative antiglobulin tests in two animals, with recurrence of lupus-like disease following a rechallenge with alfalfa seeds. Addition of L-canavanine, a nonprotein amino acid that occurs in relatively large amounts in alfalfa seeds and sprouts, to the diet of three monkeys that had previously developed this lupus-like syndrome following ingestion of alfalfa resulted in reactivation of the syndrome (170). Not all monkeys exposed to alfalfa seeds or sprouts developed this syndrome, suggesting that L-canavanine induces lupus-like syndrome only in genetically susceptible primates.

The development of ANAs and pancytopenia has been reported in one human following prolonged ingestion of alfalfa seeds (171), and reactivation of SLE was observed in two patients with clinically and serologically quiescent diseases following ingestion of alfalfa tablets (172). Lupus-like symptoms consisting of arthralgias, myalgias, rash, and ANAs developed in four previously healthy individuals after taking 12 to 24 alfalfa tablets per day for 3 weeks to 7 months (173). Patients became asymptomatic after discontinuing the tablets, and ANAs disappeared in two patients.

Because L-canavanine is a competitive analogue of L-arginine, it may interfere with protein synthesis or enzymatic reactions involving L-arginine. *In vitro* studies have revealed dose-related effects of L-canavanine on normal human peripheral blood mononuclear cells, which included diminution of the mitogenic response (174). L-canavanine also was found to stimulate intracytoplasmic immunoglobulin synthesis, autoantibody production, including dsDNA antibodies, and antibody-mediated glomerular damage in both normal and autoimmune mice. It was noted to increase intracytoplasmic immunoglobulin synthesis in some normal human subjects and patients taking alfalfa tablets, suggesting a B-cell effect; however, no significant difference in mitogen responses to L-canavanine was found between these two groups (173). Although no controlled trials definitively implicate alfalfa in the pathogenesis of SLE, the results of the reports discussed here would suggest caution in the use of this and other health-food products in SLE patients.

TABLE 3.4. DIETARY FACTORS WITH POTENTIAL IMMUNOMODULATING EFFECTS

Amino acids
L-Canavanine
Phenylalanine and tyrosine
Herbal medicines
Adulterated rapeseed Oil—TOS
L-Tryptophan—EMS
Lipids
Omega-3 and omega-6 fatty acids
Vitamins and minerals
β-carotene
α-tocopherol acetate
Vitamin C

EMS, eosinophilia-myalgia syndrome.

Other Amino Acids

Restrictions of some amino acids in the diet have been reported to modify the severity of autoimmune disease in mice. Dubois and Strain (175) reported that feeding low-phenylalanine or low-tyrosine diets prevented the development of renal diseases and prolonged the survival of autoimmune-prone (NZBXNZW) F1 (B/W) mice.

Herbal Medicines

There have been reports suggesting that a number of herbal medications may have the ability to modulate the immune system. Kao et al. (176) noted resolution of severe lupus nephritis in a Chinese patient in the United States after she had treated herself with an extract of *Tripterygium wilfordii* hook F (TWH), which is a vine-like Chinese plant with known *in vitro* immunosuppressive properties.

Jordan et al. (177) reported that a Chinese herbal decoction suppressed the phytohemagglutinin (PHA)-stimulated proliferative response of lymphocytes obtained from a child with active steroid-resistant lupus nephritis. This compound decreased the expression of T-cell activation markers and inhibited the pokeweed mitogen–stimulated production of immunoglobulins by peripheral blood mononuclear cells.

In another study, Yu and Stseng (178) reported that substances extracted from a Chinese herbal drug called Fu-ling, using 50% hot ethanol, significantly augmented the secretion of IL-1β and IL-6 six hours after *in vitro* culture with human peripheral blood mononuclear cells. This effect was noted to be dose dependent. In contrast, the Fu-ling extract significantly suppressed the secretion of transforming growth factor-β (TGF-β) *in vitro*. Fu-ling is a widely used Chinese herbal drug and is the scleroderma of *Poria Cocos* (Schw.) Wolf, which grows on the roots of pine trees. It is one of the major ingredients of the drug Bu-Chy, which also contains other ingredients that have been demonstrated to have immunoregulatory effects. This includes Ren-Shen-Yang-Rong-Tang, which can modulate the production of granulocyte-macrophage colony-stimulating factor (GM-CSF) and IL-6 from human peripheral blood mononuclear cells.

In a case report, Kava-Kava, a herbal medicine commonly used to treat anxiety that is derived from the roots of the pepper plant *Piper methysticum*, was suggested to be implicated in the development of dermatomyositis in a 47-year-old white woman (179).

Thus, certain herbal medicines appear to have immunomodulating properties; depending on the agent, they may play a role in the induction/exacerbation or may be useful in the treatment of autoimmune diseases.

Autoimmune-Like Syndromes Induced by Dietary Agents

Toxic Oil Syndrome

In 1981, Tabuenca (180) reported the appearance of a new multisystem syndrome in Spain that seemed to be related to the ingestion of rapeseed oil that had been denatured with aniline and contained acetanilide. Approximately 20,000 people were affected with this syndrome and over 350 died because of it. Following removal of the oil from the market, the incidence of new cases dropped sharply. A marked predominance of females among those with more severe and chronic disease was noted on follow-up. Patients initially presented with fever, generalized malaise, headache, cough, dyspnea, and myalgias (181). A diffuse interstitial alveolar pattern was characteristically seen on chest radiographs and was associated with hypoxia and peripheral eosinophilia. With remission of the initial symptoms, patients developed intense myalgias, severe muscle weakness and atrophy, joint contractures, dysphagia, scleroderma-like cutaneous lesions, alopecia, Raynaud's phenomenon, peripheral neuropathy, sicca syndrome, and occasionally pulmonary arterial hypertension. The skin was indurated and had a shiny, wax-like appearance with changes occurring most commonly in the legs and forearms, beginning both proximally and distally. Most patients also developed flexion contractures and many also had a sicca syndrome and/or dysphagia. Esophageal manometry showed a reduction in primary waves and an increase in tertiary waves. Skin changes reached their maximal extent 5 to 10 months after onset, followed by atrophy and hyperpigmentation. Late in the course of the disease, carpal tunnel syndrome and digital tuft changes were seen. Histologic studies demonstrated vascular lesions, which included partial or total obliteration of the lumen of the affected artrioles, capillaries, and veins, as well as predominant lymphocyte and histiocyte infiltration and obliterative fibrosis of the intima in the late phases of the disease. Deposits of fibrillar mucin and eosinophilic fibrosis that extended into the subcutaneous fat tissue were found in some patients. Many had ANAs whose titers subsequently decreased and became negative in most cases. Histone antibodies were also detected but not anti-DNA or anti-extractable nuclear antibodies (ENA).

In 1993, Alonso-Ruiz et al. (182) reported the results of an 8-year follow-up of 332 patients who had been diagnosed with the toxic oil syndrome. Thirty patients (9%) went into complete clinical remission following the acute phase, while 275 (82.8%) developed late clinical features. At the 8-year follow-up, however, 49.1% of patients were in remission while 47.3% still had symptoms. Organ involvement was documented in 16.6%, although it was considered severe in only 5%. Only 6.8% of patients had evidence of functional limitation. Hence, while the manifestations were severe and disabling during the initial 2-year period, marked improvement was noted in the majority of patients at long-term follow-up. Thus, this so-called toxic oil syndrome had many features of the connective tissue diseases and provides evidence of a supporting role for the induction of collagen vascular diseases by an environmental toxin to which large populations were exposed.

It has been suggested that the primary candidate for the induction of the toxic oil syndrome were the fatty acid esters of oleylanilide and 3 (*N*-phenylamino)-1,2-propanediol. Of interest is the fact that this latter substance is chemically related to 3-(phenylamino) alanine, which is one of the contaminants in case-associated L-tryptophan, which in turn was implicated in the development of the eosinophilic myalgia syndrome. More recently, similar contaminants have been found in melatonin, which is a commonly used over-the-counter product to reduce jet lag (183). High circulating levels of IgE and antibodies to collagen, DNA and muscle have been detected in patients with the toxic oil syndrome. An association with HLA-DR3 and -DR4 haplotypes has also been reported. Although the pathogenesis of this syndrome remains unclear, studies evaluating cytokine mRNA expression in lung tissue from patients with toxic oil syndrome have suggested that although there is activation of both Th1 and Th2 cytokines, the balance may be in favor of the Th2-mediated mechanism (184). Other studies have suggested that an increase in the production of interferon-γ may have activated indothiamine-2,3-deoxygenase, leading to an abnormally rapid metabolism of tryptophan. Bell et al. (185) reported an increase in mRNA levels for interferon-γ, IL-1β, and IL-6 in the splenocytes, and induction of IgE in a murine model for the toxic oil syndrome. It has been hypothesized that treatment with anilide resulted in the breakdown of tolerance, leading to polyclonal B-cell activation.

Tryptophan and Eosinophilia-Myalgia Syndrome

In late 1989, an apparently new clinical entity, which became known as the eosinophilia-myalgia syndrome (EMS), was described by the Centers for Disease Control and Prevention. Case-control studies demonstrated an association between the syndrome and use of L-tryptophan–containing products (186). Similar to the Spanish toxic oil syndrome, EMS reached epidemic proportions early on; following nationwide withdrawal of L-tryptophan–containing products, there was a dramatic decrease in the number of new cases. More than 1,500 cases have been reported thus far, and at least 26 patients have died (187). The syndrome appeared to have a subacute onset (188), although the clinical features, severity of disease, and duration of L-tryptophan exposure before illness were variable. Patients typically presented with fatigue, myalgias, and arthralgias. Many had mild respiratory symptoms and some had an inflammatory pulmonary parenchymal process. A variety of cutaneous lesions were seen that generally resolved spontaneously within a few weeks. Modest transient elevations of hepatic and muscle enzymes were reported (189,190). Muscle biopsies typically revealed perivascular, primarily mononuclear cell, infiltrates in the perimysium and fascia and, less frequently, the endomysium. Peripheral blood eosinophilia, often with absolute eosinophil counts greater than 2,000 cells/mL, was invariably seen. ANAs, most frequently with a speckled staining pattern, were detected, but antibodies to dsDNA and other nuclear and cytoplasmic antigens were absent.

Following the initial acute phase, a chronic phase characterized by a predominance of cutaneous, neurologic, and/or pulmonary involvement developed in a large number of patients (188). Cutaneous involvement, which resembled scleroderma or diffuse fasciitis, was frequently prominent. Although there was sparing of the digits, some developed joint contractures. Skin biopsy typically revealed thickening of the fascia and inflammatory cell infiltration of the deep layers of the dermis with progression to fibrosis in some cases. Some patients subsequently had slow regression of their skin disease. The course and progress of the disease was variable, with rapid resolution following discontinuation of L-tryptophan in some while others had progression of their disease.

The etiopathogenesis of this syndrome has yet to be elucidated. Case-control studies have found a strong association between the ingestion of L-tryptophan and development of the syndrome, but it is unclear whether L-tryptophan itself or a contaminant or impurity is the etiologic factor. L-tryptophan is present in the average protein diet throughout the Western world in amounts equal to or greater than those found in the preparations ingested by some affected patients, and had previously been commonly used in tablet form in the United States without the widespread occurrence of this syndrome. This would argue against the amino acid itself being the inciting factor. It is more likely that, similar to the Spanish toxic oil syndrome, a contaminant is at fault (191) that either incited an inflammatory response or was autosensitizing in a susceptible host either by direct means or through hapten formation. There is evidence to implicate 1,1-ethylidenebis (EBT) as a possible etiologic agent (192). Lewis rats treated with case-associated L-tryptophan or EBT developed significant myofascial thickening compared with controls (192), in addition to pancreatic changes; however, evidence of immune activation was only seen in those animals treated with case-associated L-trytophan. Hence, the exact etiologic agent(s) has yet to be determined.

Lipids

Dietary factors can modify the severity of murine lupus. Studies by Fernandes (193) reported that a decrease in caloric intake with an increase in physical activity can reduce the severity of autoimmune diseases in mice and possibly humans. The autoimmune disease seen in New Zealand black (NZB) mice occurred significantly later and was less severe in those mice fed low-fat diets (194). In addition, lower titers of autoantibodies and increased cellular cytotoxicity after tumor immunization were noted (195). Restriction of caloric intake initiated from the time of weaning led to a significant prolongation of life and alteration of lymphoid cell immune function in lupus-prone [NZB × New Zealand white (NZW)] F1 (B/W) mice (196,197). Histopathologic studies, performed when the mice were 10 months old, revealed advanced renal disease with extensive deposits of immunoglobulin and complement in the glomerular capillaries of the group receiving the high-calorie diet, whereas those receiving the low-calorie diet had little glomerular proliferation, virtually no wire loops or evidence of glomerulosclerosis, and minimal immunoglobulin deposits (197). Antibody titers to native DNA also were significantly lower in the latter group. Restriction of caloric and fat intake was found to inhibit the development of vasculitis and glomerulonephritis in B/W mice, while a high intake of saturated fat in the diet enhanced the development of these lesions (195).

Some reports have suggested that the source of lipid intake may significantly alter the development of autoimmune diseases (193). Fatty acids are of major importance in maintaining cell structure and are key factors in determining the function of membrane-bound enzymes and receptors. In this way they may be important regulators of immune responses. Diets enriched with the polyunsaturated fatty acid eicosapentaenoic acid has been shown to delay the rise of anti-ssDNA and -dsDNA antibody titers, inhibit the development of glomerular disease, and prolong the life of female NZB × NZW/F1 mice (198). A diet using fish oil as the exclusive source of lipid suppressed both autoimmunity and the development of glomerulonephritis in Medical Research Laboratory (MRL)/*lpr* mice (199). Polyunsaturated omega-6 fatty acids derived from vegetable sources, such as corn oil, and monounsaturated animal fat, such as lard, are highly proinflammatory compared to the omega-3 fatty acids found in highly polyunsaturated fat–rich marine oils. A significant increase in the incidence of autoimmune diseases was reported among animals fed a diet containing highly polyunsaturated oils when compared to those receiving the marine oils containing omega-3 fatty acids. Mice fed 20% fish oils lived significantly longer than those fed with 20% corn oils, which would support the proinflammatory nature of the omega-6 lipids (200). These differences were independent of calorie intake. Omega-6 and omega-3 dietary lipids have also been reported to have effects on cytokine production. Lower TGF-β_1 mRNA expression was found in splenocytes from mice fed corn oil compared with those fed fish oils. There was a significant increase in TGF-β_1 mRNA expression in the kidneys of mice corn oil compared with those receiving fish oil suggesting that the dietary lipids may regulate expression of TGF-β_1 in an organ-specific manner (201).

Chandrasekar et al. (202) reported that NZB × NZW (F1) (B/W) mice that were fed fish oils had a greatly reduced amount of proteinuria, serum anti-dsDNA antibodies, improvement in survival, and reduction in renal TGF-β_1 mRNA and protein levels, suggesting that the beneficial effects of fish oil on renal disease in murine models of lupus may be attributed, at least in part, to a reduction in TGF-β_1 expression in the kidneys. More recent data (203) suggests that fish oils may delay the onset of autoimmune renal disease in NZB × NZW mice by suppressing both Th1 and Th2 cytokine production.

Administration of fish oil that contains the omega-3 fatty acids has been shown to suppress the production of IL-1α, IL-1β, IL-2, IL-6, and TNF-α by peripheral blood mononuclear cells from healthy volunteers, and the effect was noted to last up to 10 weeks after discontinuation of the fish oil (204,205). Other studies have shown that omega-3 fatty acids can reduce the activation of macrophages in both animals and humans as shown by a decrease in the expression of class II antigen and the production IL-1 and TNF-α mRNA levels (204,206). Calder et al. (207) reported a reduction in *in vitro* proliferation of lymphocytes by the addition of eicosapentaeonic acid (EPA), which is found in fish oils, or by the addition of serum obtained from volunteers who have been treated with EPA. Dietary supplementation with omega-3 fatty acids to healthy volunteers for 6 to 12 weeks resulted in suppression of mitogen-stimulated lymphocyte proliferation and decreased cytokine production (208,209). In contrast, Kremer et al. (210) reported an enhancement of proliferation of lymphocytes obtained from patients who had received fish oils.

Rossetti et al. (211) reported that administration of gammalinolenic acid (GLA) to volunteers and patients with rheumatoid arthritis and SLE reduced T-cell proliferation when peripheral blood mononuclear cells were stimulated with either PHA or anti-CD3/CD4 monoclonal antibodies. Both GLA and EPA have been reported to suppress the long-term growth of IL-2–dependent lymphocytes isolated from the synovium of patients with rheumatoid arthritis (212). It had been suggested that GLA has the ability to interfere with early events in the signal transduction pathway in human T cells. Fatty acids may have the ability to regulate the activation of both T and B cells and may therefore have the potential to be useful in the treatment of SLE. Gammalinolenic acid and dihomogammalinolenic (DGLA) have been demonstrated to suppress the production of IL-1β and TNF-α in a dose-dependent manner when added to stimulated human peripheral blood mononuclear cells. In addition, the administration of GLA over a period of hours and of months also suppressed the production of IL-1β and TNF-α by stimulated human peripheral blood mononuclear cells (213). Gammalinolenic acid is present in relatively large amounts in seeds of the evening primrose and borage plants and is converted rapidly to DGLA.

The effects of dietary modulation on disease severity in humans have not been well defined. There have been only a few studies and they have had variable results. A 1-year study of fish oil treatment for SLE patients did not show any clinical benefit, although there was a possible reduction in the frequency of active nephritis among the treated patients (214). In another open study, 17 patients with SLE were treated for 1 year with a diet reduced in polyunsaturated fats and enriched in saturated fat (215). There was a significant reduction in the number of patients with active disease and in prednisolone consumption, suggesting a beneficial effect. However, the numbers are too small to draw any definite conclusions, and a placebo effect cannot be ruled out. In a subsequent placebo- (olive oil) controlled study in which fish oils were administered for 34 weeks to lupus patients, there was improvement in the clinical symptoms by patient assessment, although no objective data were reported (216). This was a prospective, double-blind, crossover study to assess the effects of a low-fat, high–margarine-oil (eicosapentaenoic acid was used) diet on the course of disease in 27 patients with active SLE. Of the 17 patients who completed the 34-week study, 14 had either "ideal" or "useful" improvement in their disease while receiving eicosapentaenoic acid, compared with only four of those receiving placebo. Thirteen patients had no change or deterioration in their disease while receiving placebo, compared with only three of those receiving eicosapentaenoic acid. A significant difference ($p < .01$) in outcome was found when the "ideal" and "useful" categories were combined and compared with the "static" and "worse" groups, suggesting a beneficial effect from the margarine oil-supplemented diet.

However, two other studies in which patients were supplemented for 6 months with eicosapentaenoic acid failed to demonstrate any benefit (217). In a double-blind crossover study of 17 patients with SLE supplementation with 10 to 15 capsules of a commercial fish oil, MaxEPA, for 6 months did not demonstrate any detectable benefit (218). Clinical improvement has been reported in patients with rheumatoid arthritis receiving a 12-week supplement of eicosapentaenoic acid (219). It has been suggested that increased consumption of omega-6 or a vegetable source of oils may promote autoimmunity and increase the incidence and severity of autoimmune diseases by increasing the free radical formation through a decrease in the levels of antioxidant enzyme levels (193). This in turn may result in an impairment of immune function through an effect on the production of antiinflammatory cytokines, such as IL-2 and TGF-β. In contrast, omega-3 lipids, obtained from marine oils, in the presence of an antioxidant supplement may exert a beneficial effect on the development of autoimmune diseases in humans, although well-controlled studies evaluating this need to be done.

Thus, although the benefits of administration of fish oil to animals have resulted in a striking decrease in the development and progression of autoimmune diseases, results of human studies have indicated only a modest benefit so far. Because the possible benefits of such dietary changes have yet to be proven in human autoimmune diseases, dietary recommendations should be made on an individual basis, taking into account the general nutritional status of the patient.

Vitamins and Minerals

Single or multiple deficiencies in vitamins and/or minerals may result in impaired immunologic function, which can be restored with correction of the deficiencies (220). Depression of humoral- and cellular-mediated immunity has been reported in vitamin A–deficient animals. Deficiencies in B vitamins also result in the impairment of humoral-mediated responses in animals. Vitamin C has been reported to enhance cellular immunity both *in vivo* and *in vitro* and to promote the motility of neutrophils. Some data suggest that 1,25-dihydroxyvitamin D inhibits activation of T-helper cells. Vitamin E deficiency in animals has been associated with depressed humoral and cellular responses, and one report in humans suggested that supplementation of vitamin E above the recommended daily allowance enhanced cell-mediated immune responsiveness in healthy elderly subjects, partly through lymphocyte stimulation (221).

Damage mediated by free radical oxidative products has been implicated in the pathogenesis of a number of inflammatory diseases, including rheumatoid arthritis and SLE. It has been proposed by Weimann and Weiser (222) that oxidative modification of cellular structures by free radicals that are being continuously produced through normal aerobic metabolism may play a role in the pathogenesis of autoimmune diseases. These authors demonstrated a beneficial effect of supplementation with antioxidants consisting of β-carotene, α-tocopherol acetate, and vitamin C on the development of lupus-like disease in MRL/*lpr* mice. They reported an increase in the survival time of the mice that received the supplementation in addition to decreased lymphoproliferation and IgG levels, including antibodies to dsDNA. Histopathologic studies also indicated improvement in those animals that received the supplementation with antioxidants. In addition these authors reported that rats that normally do not develop autoimmune diseases could be induced to develop serologic changes, which included elevated IgG levels and antibodies to dsDNA, by vitamin E deficiency, although no histopathologic changes were noted in the kidney.

Comstock et al. (223) evaluated the possible role of serum concentrations of antioxidants, α-tocopherol, β-carotene, and retinol in the pathogenesis of rheumatoid arthritis and SLE. It was hypothesized that low antioxidant levels may be a risk factor or marker for these diseases. The study included 21 rheumatoid arthritis and six SLE cases that were compared to controls. Lower serum concentrations of α-tocopherol, β-carotene, and retinol were found in both SLE and rheumatoid arthritis compared with the controls. However, only the difference for β-carotene among rheumatoid patients reached statistical significance. These results suggest the possibility that low antioxidant levels may be important in the pathogenesis of these diseases possibly through inhibition of free radical oxidative damage. It has been suggested that exposure to certain chemicals may result in the development of inflammatory diseases including SLE due to production of reactive oxygen species as a result of activation of the cytochrome P-450 by the chemical agent (224,225).

Deficiences in certain minerals have been associated with impairment in immune responsiveness (220). Iron deficiency has been associated with a high frequency of infections. It results in impairment of neutrophil and lymphocyte function, both of which also are depressed in zinc deficiency. Improvement of immune responsiveness was noted in a group of institutionalized, healthy elderly subjects given zinc supplementation. Other evidence suggests that zinc may directly enhance immune responsiveness. Deficiency of selenium has been associated with an impaired humoral immune response as well.

Thus, a variety of vitamin and/or mineral deficiencies can lead to impaired immunologic function. In addition, some of these nutritional factors appear to have the ability to enhance immune responsiveness, which theoretically could be important in the pathogenesis of autoimmune diseases.

RADIATION

Exposure to sunlight is a well-established environmental factor in the induction and exacerbation of both cutaneous and systemic lupus erythematosus. Artificial ultraviolet (UV) radiation has been associated with exacerbations of SLE (226), and experimental reproduction of cutaneous lupus lesions by exposure to UV radiation has been reported in both animals and humans (227,228). An increase in mortality and acceleration of autoimmunity has been reported in BXSB mice exposed to UV light (229). UV-A radiation can induce the formation of ANAs in mice (230) and increase the susceptibility to DNA damage in murine lupus (231). UV irradiation of DNA can phototransform the molecule and render it immunogenic (UV-DNA). Lupus skin lesions were induced in mice by first immunizing them with UV-DNA to induce high titers of antibody and then irradiating them with UV light (228). Mouse Ig and complement were seen in the dermal-epidermal areas and in the nuclei of peridermal cells in areas of irradiated skin similar to that seen in SLE.

Furukawa et al. (232) demonstrated augmentation of extranuclear antigen expression on keratinocyte cell surfaces following UV irradiation that was dose, UV-B light, and glycosylation dependent and involved expression of SSA/Ro, SSB/La, and Ul-RNP antigens. Binding of autoantibodies to SSA and SSB antigens expressed on keratinocytes in the skin may provide the immunologic trigger for the development of cutaneous lupus. Of interest is the report of a controlled study by McGrath et al (233), who found that long-term exposure to low-dose UV-A light prolonged the survival of NZB × NZW mice. Those mice who received UV-A irradiation combined with depilation had significantly augmented *in vitro* cellular immunologic function and decreased levels of antibodies to DNA compared with the group that received neither treatment, suggesting a possible immune-modulating effect. The apparent discrepancy between these results and those of other studies may reflect administration of smaller doses of UV-A light.

Cutaneous lesions tend to occur in the sun-exposed areas of patients with lupus and often are associated with exposure to UV light. In one study of 128 patients with lupus (227), exposure to either UV-A or UV-B light induced cutaneous lesions consistent with lupus in 64% of patients with subacute cutaneous lupus erythematosus, 42% of patients with discoid lupus erythematosus, and 25% of those with SLE. Photosensitivity to fluorescent light has been reported in a patient with lupus (234) and fluorescent light has been reported to have the ability to activate *cis*-urocanic acid, a potent immunologic mediator present in the epidermis (235). Photochemotherapy with long-wave UV light and oral 8-methoxypsoralen [psoralen plus UV-A (PUVA)] has been associated with the development of lupus and sclerodermatous-like syndromes in some patients with psoriasis, although a causal relationship has not been proven. In one report, a patient with psoriasis developed pancytopenia, antibodies to dsDNA and SSA/Ro, hypocomplementemia, and cutaneous lesions consistent with subacute cutaneous lupus erythematosus while receiving PUVA treatment. There was complete resolution of cutaneous lesions and improvement of the hematologic abnormalities following discontinuation of PUVA therapy (236). Eyanson et al. (237) reported the development of SLE in a 23-year-old woman with psoriasis during PUVA treatment that was characterized by rash, alopecia, nephritis, seizures, coma, high-titer ANAs, and hypocomplementemia. Bjellerup et al. (238) reported the occurrence of ANAs in 7 of 34 patients (21%) with severe psoriasis receiving PUVA therapy compared with 3 (6%) of 50 patients before PUVA treatment. ANA titers were low and antibodies to dsDNA were not detected. In a sequential study of 99 patients receiving PUVA therapy, 31 developed a positive ANA (239), but none developed systemic disease. However, Stern et al. (240), as part of a prospective study of 1,023 patients who were treated with PUVA, failed to detect a significant increase in the incidence of ANAs in these patients over a 2-year period. In addition, Levin et al. (241) found no association between ANAs and PUVA treatment in their 2-year study of 22 patients. Thus, the relationship remains equivocal.

A number of studies have demonstrated a reduction in lymphocyte function following exposure of normal individuals to sunlight or UV lamps. It has been suggested that UV radiation especially in the intermediate- to short-wave range (at rather low doses) may alter subcellular kinetics in cell activation and may in this way modify the immune response (242).

INFECTIOUS AGENTS

Data published in the last few years have provided support for the role of infection and, in particular, viral agents in the etiology of SLE (Table 3.5).

TABLE 3.5. INFECTIOUS AGENTS WITH A POSSIBLE ETIOPATHOGENIC ROLE IN SLE AND OTHER ASSOCIATED DISORDERS

Viruses
Epstein-Barr virus
Cytomegalovirus
Type C oncornaviruses
Human endogenous retroviruses
Human parvovirus B19
Bacteria
Streptococcal cell wall
Freund's adjuvant
Bacterial lipopolysaccharide

Viruses

Viruses have been proposed as possible triggering factors for autoimmune diseases. There are reports of virus-like intracellular inclusions in vascular walls, circulating leukocytes and glomerular endothelial cytoplasm of patients with lupus, and virus-like extracellular particles within the glomerular membranes (243–245). These inclusions resemble filamentous forms of myxoviruses and reoviruses, and they have been associated with disease activity. However, they have also been seen in patients with idiopathic membranous nephropathy, infectious mononucleosis, neoplasia, and acquired immunodeficiency syndrome (AIDS), suggesting that they are not specific for SLE. Rich et al. (246) found that interferon-α endogenous to patients with SLE induced inclusions in the human B lymphoblastoid cell line Daudi, and suggested that the same might occur *in vivo*; an association with disease activity also was noted. Persistent, high endogenous levels of interferon-α have been reported in patients with SLE and patients with AIDS; hence, lupus inclusions may only be a marker of elevated interferon-α and thus of disease activity. A role for a viral agent in the pathogenesis of SLE has also been proposed by Plotz (247), who suggested that the autoantibodies found in lupus patients are antiidiotype antibodies to antiviral antibodies. However, this mechanism would not explain the polyclonal B-cell activation seen in SLE.

Significant elevations of antibody titers to a number of viruses, such as measles; rubella; parainfluenza types 1, 2, and 3; reovirus type 2; mumps; and Epstein-Barr virus (EBV), have been reported in patients with SLE (248–250). They may represent nonspecific activation of B lymphocytes; however, no correlation has been found between virus antibody titers and IgG levels with disease activity. Evans et al. (251) reported significantly elevated antibody titers to EBV among patients with SLE compared with controls. The ratio of patient to control titers was 6.1421, which was highly significant. Dror et al. (252) reported the case of a 14-year-old girl who presented concurrently with acute onset of SLE and clinical and laboratory findings consistent with acute EBV infection. Serologic studies and the detection of specific EBV antigens on histopathologic examination of renal biopsy confirmed the acute EBV infection. More recently, James et al. (253) reported an association between EBV infection and SLE, and suggested that this virus may be important in the pathogenesis of lupus. Because of the high prevalence of EBV infection among adults, they chose to evaluate only young lupus patients. IgG antibodies to EBV viral capsid antigen was detected in 116 of 117 (99%) of their lupus patients who were between 4 and 19 years old compared with 107 of 153 (70%) of the controls. Significant cross-reactivity with the spliceosome as an etiology for this difference was ruled out by absorption studies. A subset of lupus patients was further evaluated for the presence of EBV DNA in the peripheral blood mononuclear cells. All 32 patients had EBV DNA in their lymphocytes compared with only 23 of 32 matched controls. No significant difference was found in the seroconversation rates for IgG antibodies to four other herpes virus—cytomegalovirus, herpes types 1 and 2, and the varicella zoster virus—between patients and controls. These data suggest that EBV infection may be important in the pathogenesis of lupus, although a causal relationship has not been established.

Animal studies have indicated that immunization with a peptide derived from the amino acid sequence Sm B/B′ can induce a lupus-like autoimmunity in rabbits (254). Similarly, immunization with a closely related sequence found in the Epstein-Barr nuclear antigen-1 (EBNA-1) can also induce a lupus-like autoimmune disease. Marchini et al. (255) reported that 38 of their patients with SLE had antibodies to the EBNA-1 35 to 38 sequence, which is highly homologous to the 95 to 119 region of SmD; antibodies to the SmD 95 to 119 peptide were detected in 32 of the patients with SLE who were studied. Although anti–EBNA-1 antibodies also were detected in patients with EBV-related diseases and healthy individuals, only those antibodies from patients with SLE demonstrated similar affinity for the viral peptide and the SmD sequence peptide, suggesting cross-reactivity of antiviral antibodies with an autoantigen.

In a follow-up study, James et al. (256) suggested that the immune response to EBNA-1 is different among lupus patients compared with normal controls. They evaluated the relative quantity of antibodies generated against a variety of fragments of EBNA-1 using sera from 20 lupus patients and 20 EBV-infected controls and noted a stronger average binding to the N-terminal fragment and the C-terminal fragment for sera from lupus patients compared with matched controls. Further studies using overlapping octapeptides suggest a fine specificity between the reactivities of the sera obtained from lupus patients compared with EBV-positive matched normal controls. These data suggest that the two groups mount different immune responses to EBNA-1, which may be of importance in the pathogenesis of lupus.

Incaprera et al. (257) reported that 50% of their lupus patients and all the patients with acute infectious mononucleosis but none of the healthy individuals with a past history of EBV infection had IgG antibodies to a 20 amino acid peptide derived from the virus-encoded nuclear antigen of EBV virus (EBNA-2). Further analysis revealed a high degree of homology between this peptide and the C-terminal domain of the SmD1 ribonucleoprotein, which is a target of autoantibodies among 25% to 40% of patients with lupus. These data suggest that antibodies elicited by the EBNA-2 antigen may cross-react with the spliceosome and may play a role in the development of autoantibodies in SLE patients. In addition these authors demonstrated the presence of EBV type 1 DNA, using polymerase chain reaction (PCR) analysis, in the oropharyngeal secretions in 8 of 15 SLE patients. The virus was also isolated from six of the eight DNA-positive specimens, suggesting that there is persistent EBV infection in a certain number of SLE patients, which may be of pathogenic importance.

An increased immune response to EBV early antigens has been reported among patients with a variety of rheumatic diseases including rheumatoid arthritis, SLE, and Sjögren's syndrome (258). It was suggested that these results indicate the presence of reactivated virus among these patients.

Several studies have looked for a possible association between EBV and Sjögren's syndrome, and they have had varied results (259–264). Results indicated an apparent increase in EBV load in the salivary glands of patients with primary Sjögren's syndrome. However, EBV has also been found in the tissues of many apparently healthy individuals, and as yet there is insufficient evidence to definitively implicate this virus in the etiopathogenesis of Sjögren's syndrome.

Other studies have suggested that cytomegalovirus (CMV) may be important in the pathogenesis of SLE. Rider et al. (265) reported that 88 of 97 (90.7%) serum samples obtained from patients with SLE were seropositive for the human CMV compared with only 32 of 50 (64%) patients with rheumatoid arthritis and 42 of 97 (43.3%) of normal controls. The difference in prevalence of the human CMV virus between lupus patients and normal controls was significant. In contrast, 78 (80.4%) of lupus patients, 40 (80%) of rheumatoid arthritis patients, and 57 (58.8%) of normal controls were seropositive for the herpes simplex virus-1. CMV infection has also been implicated in disease exacerbations of two patients with lupus (266).

Type C oncornaviruses have been implicated in the pathogenesis of glomerulonephritis in NZB mice (267,268), and immunochemical studies have shown evidence of type C RNA virus expression in tissues from patients with SLE (269,270). However, further studies have failed to confirm these findings (271).

Human endogenous retroviruses have also been implicated as etiologic factors in autoimmune disease (272). Antibodies that are reactive with human retroviral proteins have been found in patients with a variety of connective tissue diseases, including SLE (273). Reports have suggested a pathogenic role for gene products of human endogenous retroviruses in lupus nephritis. Krieg et al. (274) reported an association between murine lupus and expression of an endogenous retroviral transcript. Indirect evidence suggesting a role of human endogenous retroviruses in the development of lupus has been provided by Hishikawa T et al. (275). They reported the presence of antibodies to a recombinant p30 gag protein derived from a clone of the human endogenous retrovirus among 48.3% of SLE patients, 35% of Sjögren's syndrome patients, and 33.3% of mixed connective tissue disease (MCTD) patients but in no healthy subjects. In another study, Bengtsson et al. (276) reported an increase in the frequencies of antiretroviral antibodies against two peptides derived from the *env* gene of the type C–like class of human endogenous retroviruses and against two peptides derived from the gag region of human T lymphotropic virus type 1–related endogenous sequence among patients with SLE. Longitudinal evaluation of one patient over a period of 12 years indicated that the concentrations of certain antiretroviral antibodies varied according to the lupus disease activity.

Human endogenous retrovirus-3 has also been suggested to play a pathogenic role in the development of congenital heart block (277). Elevated levels of antibodies to endogenous retrovirus-3 were reported among normal pregnant women and in patients with Sjögren's syndrome and SLE. However, levels of these antibodies were significantly higher among the mothers with babies with congenital heart block compared to normal sera. Antibodies in the sera of three of the mothers with babies with congenital heart block demonstrated binding to sections of fetal cardiac tissue. These authors also reported high levels of expression of endogenous retrovirus-3 in fetal heart, with a peak expression occurring between 11 and 17 weeks of gestation, and suggested that this retrovirus may play a role in the development of congenital heart block.

Human retrovirus-5 (HRV-5) infection has been proposed as another possible etiologic factor in the development of autoimmune disease. Early reports indicated the presence of HRV-5 RNA in the tissues obtained from patients with autoimmune diseases and normal salivary glands (278). However, subsequent work by the same group using PCR analysis to detect proviral DNA failed to support an association between this virus and Sjögren's syndrome (279). In a more recent study, using nested PCR analysis, HRV-5 proviral DNA was detected in 53% of synovial samples obtained from patients with rheumatoid arthritis, reactive arthritis, osteoarthritis, and psoriatic arthritis and in the blood samples of 11 (16%) of 69 SLE patients but in none of the synovial samples obtained from normal individuals (280).

Antibodies to retroviral gag proteins have been reported in patients with SLE. Talal et al. (281) reported the presence of antibodies to the p24 gag protein of HIV-1 in 22 of 61 patients with lupus using Western blotting. Twenty of these patients (91%) also expressed an immunodominant idiotype (Id 4B4), which previously had been demonstrated on a human anti-Sm monoclonal antibody called 4B4. Sm antigen partially inhibited antibody binding of p24 gag, which suggests cross-reactivity between the two antigens. The Sm antigen contains a region of amino acid sequence that is homologous to one contained in the p24 gag protein and that reacts with autoantibodies bearing the 4B4 idiotype (282). Antibodies reacting with human T-lymphotropic-1 (HTLV-1) or human immunodeficiency virus-1 (HIV-1) core proteins, most frequently p55 and p24, or with the HIV-1 Nej protein were detected in 64% of 22 patients with SLE and 63% of eight patients with discoid lupus erythematosus and associated with recurrent infections and widespread acral discoid skin lesions. However, others (283) have failed to detect antibodies to the p24 gag protein among patients with SLE. These patients may be positive for HIV by enzyme-linked immunosorbent assay, but this can be distinguished from true infection by Western blot analysis (284).

Gul et al. (285) detected antibodies to HIV-1 using an enzyme immunoassay in 12 (27%) of 44 Turkish patients with SLE. Immunoblot analysis demonstrated antibodies primarily to retroviral gag proteins in 23 (52%) of the patients with the most frequent reactivity directed against the p18 gag protein. Despite previous reports, antibodies to the p24 antigen were found in only two patients.

Serum antibodies to HIV-1 proteins also have been described in patients with primary Sjögren's syndrome (286). Antibodies to HIV p24 core protein antigen has been reported in about one third of patients with either Sjögren's syndrome or SLE who did not have any evidence of exposure to or infection with HIV itself (287). Further studies by this group, using peptides representing fragments of the p24 core protein, revealed that there were characteristic epitope-specific profiles for Sjögren's syndrome and SLE patients. They also suggest that the specificity of these reactivities were indicative of a specific pattern of a nonrandom cross-reactivity between HIV type 1 p24 and autoimmune sera, which may be partially specific for the individual diseases. A possible association between the HTLV-1 infection and Sjögren's syndrome was suggested by Nakamura et al. (288). They reported a high prevalence of Sjögren's syndrome among patients with HTLV-1 associated myelopathy.

In animal studies, transgenic mice containing the HTLV-1 tax gene have been shown to develop an exocrinopathy that histologically resembles Sjögren's syndrome (289). HTLV-1 has been associated with some connective tissue diseases. Detection of HTLV-1 proviral DNA and its gene expression in synovial cells in a special type of inflammatory arthritis (290) has been reported. Danao et al. (291), however, have shown that some of the descriptions of antibodies to HTLV-1 among patients with SLE most likely represent artifactual reaction with cellular components in the antigenic extract.

In other studies, Query and Keene (292) cloned a 68-kd U1-RNP protein that they found contained a region of amino acid sequence that was homologous with a p30 gag sequence of several mammalian C-type viruses. This homologous region was cross-reactive with the retroviral p30 gag antigen. Rabbits have been induced to produce anti-RNP antibodies by immunization with the p30 gag protein.

These data suggest that exposure to certain retroviruses leads to an immune response that, through molecular mimicry, may result in the production of autoantibodies that are cross-reactive with a variety of nuclear proteins.

Blomberg et al. (293) provided some further circumstantial evidence of a role for retroviruses. They found an increased frequency of antibodies that were cross-reactive with baboon endogenous retrovirus and murine leukemia virus among 72 patients with SLE compared with 88 controls. The former antibodies correlated with the presence of anti-RNP and anti-Sm antibodies. An increase in reactivity with some retroviral env and gag synthetic peptides also was noted in the patients with SLE. However, although a variety of antiretroviral antibodies, some of which cross-react with nuclear proteins, have been reported in patients with SLE and other autoimmune diseases, attempts to isolate infectious retroviruses from such patients generally have been unsuccessful. Also, SLE rarely occurs and ANAs infrequently are found in patients with AIDS, although the sex ratio may be important here (294).

Other data suggesting an etiologic role for retroviruses in SLE come from reports of the incorporation of a 5.3-kilobase (kb) ETn retrotransposition sequence into the second intron of the *Fas* gene, resulting in low expression of the normal Fas protein in MRL/*lpr* mice. It is believed that this genetic defect thus leads to a failure of apoptosis and, hence, development of a lymphoproliferative and lupus-like disease in these mice (295).

Human parvovirus B19 has been suggested as a triggering agent for SLE since acute parvovirus infection may present with lupus-like features. Nesher et al. (296) reported that striking similarities exist between SLE and human parvovirus B19 (HPV-B19) infection; they noted that most of their patients with parvovirus infection presented with rash, arthropathy, myalgia, fever, and a positive ANA. Various cytopenias, hypocomplementemia, and anti-DNA antibodies have also been described. However, a recent study by Bengtsson et al. (297) failed to detect a difference in the prevalence of IgG parvovirus antibodies between a group of 99 lupus patients and 99 age- and sex-matched healthy controls.

Immunization

There have been some reports of patients developing lupus following immunization (298–300). SLE has been reported to occur most frequently after immunization for hepatitis B, but it has also been reported following administration of typhoid/paratyphoid, anthrax, tetanus, and a combination of vaccines (301). However, no prospective studies have evaluated this possible association.

Results of animal studies have indicated that immunization of rats and mice with proteins or oligopeptides that are lupus autoantigens may lead to the development of immune response to other SLE-associated autoantigens in addition to the immunogen (254). Some of these animals have developed a lupus-like disease as well. Animal studies reported by Gharavi and Pierangeli (302) demonstrated that antiphospholipid antibodies and anti-β_2-GPI antibodies with properties similar to those found in patients with the antiphospholipid antibody syndrome could be induced by immunization of mice with phospholipid-binding viral peptides. Based on these results it was suggested that exposure to viral or bacterial products may induce the production of antiphospholipid antibodies in humans.

Studies by Saraux et al. (303) evaluated the relative contributions of genetic and environmental factors to the production of anticardiolipin antibodies among 32 SLE patients and their family members. Anticardiolipin antibodies were restricted to certain families, which included spouses. There was a significant correlation between titers of IgG anticardiolipin antibodies in lupus patients and their spouses, suggesting that environmental factors, possibly infectious agents, are important.

Possible Mechanisms

A number of pathogenic mechanisms have been proposed by which retroviruses might induce the development of autoimmune disease. These include upregulation of proinflammatory cytokines by specific viral proteins, leading to stimulation of the immune system and molecular mimicry between retroviral core proteins and RNP antigens as suggested by the similarity between peptides derived from EBV and the spliceosome. The molecular mimicry hypothesis would also be supported by work of Haaheim et al. (304), who evaluated the epitope recognition pattern of La autoantibodies in sera obtained from 14 patients with Sjögren's syndrome and six lupus patients using 18 different decapeptides obtained from the human La autoantigen. The linear epitopes that were most frequently recognized by these sera demonstrated sequence similarities with proteins from a range of ubiquitous human viruses and, in particular, the herpes virus group.

Bacteria

Chronic polyarthritis has been induced in animals by injecting cell walls from certain bacteria, such as streptococci and Freund's complete adjuvant, that consist of a dispersion of dried, heat-killed tubercle bacilli in mineral oil with or without an emulsifying agent (305,306). The polyarthritis resembles human rheumatoid arthritis. In addition to the articular features, nodular skin lesions, weight loss, malaise, uveitis, iritis, dermatitis, urethritis, and alopecia also may be present. Although the exact pathogenetic mechanism remains unknown, a delayed hypersensitivity to constituents of the bacterial cell wall most likely is responsible; whether a similar event is responsible for the induction of rheumatoid arthritis in humans remains unclear. Bacterial products may play a role in the pathogenesis of lupus nephritis. Cavallo and Granholm (307) noted enhanced polyclonal B-cell activation, elevated levels of anti-DNA antibodies, and development of a diffuse proliferative glomerulonephritis in the NZB/W mice who received bacterial lipopolysaccharide. The potential significance of this in relation to human disease has yet to be determined.

The work of Pisetsky (308) has shown that bacterial DNA is a potent immune stimulant that can induce a wide range of both specific and nonspecific immune responses. These observations have led to a new model for induction of anti-DNA antibodies in SLE. It is possible that bacterial DNA could serve as a molecular mimic since it has sites that are present on both self and foreign DNA. Studies in mice have shown that injection of bacterial DNA can elicit various cross-reactive autoantibodies in NZB/NZW mice, suggesting a possible adjuvant property of bacterial DNA (309). It is possible that some such mechanism could account for the flares in human SLE in relation to infections.

Thus, a large body of circumstantial evidence exists to strengthen the clinical observations that infections may be associated with the onset and flare-ups of SLE.

MECHANISMS

While SLE is believed to be immunologically mediated, the exact etiopathogenic mechanisms remain unknown. SLE likely develops as a result of a genetically controlled immune response following exposure to certain trigger factor(s). These agents may produce their effects in a variety of ways (Table 3.6):

1. The agent, which normally elicits an antigen-specific immune response, may induce polyclonal B-cell activation in certain individuals, resulting in autoantibody production.
2. Agents may mediate their effects by means of direct toxic effects on immune or other cells, leading to impairment of immune responses and/or cytotoxicity, resulting in release of intracellular constituents with consequent induction of autoantibodies.
3. Cross-reactivity may occur through molecular mimicry because of structural similarities between the agent(s)

TABLE 3.6. POSSIBLE MECHANISMS FOR INDUCTION OF AUTOIMMUNITY BY ENVIRONMENTAL AGENT(S)

Polyclonal B-cell activation
Direct cytotoxicity
Molecular mimicry
Modulation of immune response through alternation of composition of cellular membranes
Direct interaction with factors that regulate gene activity
Alteration of antigenic structure and/or function
Generation of free radicals

and cellular constituent(s) or through the sharing of molecular epitopes by the agent, such as a microbe, and the host.

4. Modulation of the immune response may occur through dietary factors, resulting in amelioration or acceleration of the disease. The effects of fatty acids may be mediated through alterations in the composition of cellular membranes, especially those of lymphocytes.
5. Agents may directly interact with regulatory factors that modify gene activity. Impairment of T-cell DNA methylation by environmental agents has been demonstrated and may result in the emergence of autoreactive T cells and autoimmunity (310). Certain pharmacologic agents, such as procainamide and hydralazine, can inhibit T-cell DNA methylation. Adoptive transfer of murine T cells that are made autoreactive with DNA methylation inhibitors resulted in development of a lupus-like disease in otherwise healthy syngeneic recipients.
6. Agent may bind to self proteins with alteration of the antigenic structure and function of these proteins or exposure of cryptic epitopes leading to the induction of an autoimmune response.
7. Agents may induce the generation of free radicals that induce an inflammatory response.

SUMMARY

Despite intensive research, the etiology and pathogenesis of SLE and other diseases of connective tissue remain to be elucidated. Many environmental agents have the ability to induce autoimmune disease in both humans and animals, but they probably require certain conditions, such as genetic predisposition, to do so (311) (Table 3.6). Pharmacogenetic studies have shown that the activity of various enzymes systems is genetically determined. Some of these genetic differences are believed to be important in determining which individuals are likely to develop toxic effects from drugs and other agents; certain phenotypes have been reported to be associated with a variety of diseases, including some connective tissue diseases (312).

Pharmacogenetic differences may explain the variability in disease susceptibility. Metabolic rates play a role in determining duration of exposure to chemical and pharmacologic agents that may be important in inducing immune dysregulation. One possible mechanism is that only individuals with certain pharmacogenetic phenotypes will develop autoimmune diseases when exposed to potential triggering environmental agents. Given the numerous reports linking environmental agents to the development of autoimmunelike diseases, it clearly is essential to take a complete occupational and environmental history, including the use of drugs and other agents, such as herbal medicines, when evaluating patients with these diseases.

A major problem in the identification and definition of possible environmentally associated rheumatic disorders has been the traditional reliance on comparisons of disease incidence or prevalence in exposed and unexposed cohorts. This has not been ideal for some multifactorial disorders when there may be only small populations for study. It became clear, then, that for identification, description, and more precise definition of an environmentally associated rheumatic disease such as SLE, more was needed. The Environmental Diseases Study Group of the American College of Rheumatology has suggested a more orderly, staged process based on current paradigms in toxicology, epidemiology, and epistemology (313). The group's publication outlines the four stages for identification and definition of such disorders:

Stage 1: Proposing the association. Case reports or case series, defined by certain conditions, suggest the possible association of a clinical disorder with an environmental exposure.

Stage 2: Testing the association. Epidemiologic, clinical, and laboratory studies test the hypothesis that the exposure is associated with the disorder.

Stage 3: Defining the disorder. If the approaches in stage 2 support an association, classification and other criteria are developed.

Stage 4: Refining the disorder. An ongoing reassessment and revision of classification and other criteria are performed in light of additional clinical and laboratory information.

It is hoped that these strategies will be useful in increasing our understanding and detection of environmental agents that may be involved in the pathogenesis of autoimmune diseases.

REFERENCES

1. Hart HH, Grigor RR, Caughey DE. Ethnic difference in the prevalence of systemic lupus erythematosus. *Ann Rheum Dis* 1983;42:529–532.
2. Kaslow RA, Masi AT. Age, sex, and race effects on mortality from systemic lupus erythematosus in the United States. *Arthritis Rheum* 1978;32:493–497.
3. Morton RO, Gershwin ME, Brady C, et al. The incidence of systemic lupus erythematosus in North American Indians. *J Rheumatol* 1976;3:186–190.
4. Serdula MK, Rhoads GG. Frequency of systemic lupus erythematosus in different ethnic groups in Hawaii. *Arthritis Rheum* 1979;22:328–333.
5. Fielder AH, Walport MJ, Batchelor JR, et al. Family study of the major histocompatibility complex in patients with systemic lupus erythematosus: importance of null alleles of C4A and C4B in determining disease susceptibility. *Br Med J (Clin Res)* 1983; 286:425–428.
6. Howard PF, Hochberg MC, Bias WB, et al. Relationship between C4 null genes, HLA-D region antigens and genetic susceptibility to systemic lupus erythematosus in Caucasians and black Americans. *Am J Med* 1986;81:187–193.

7. Nai-Zheng C. Rheumatic diseases in China. *J Rheumatol* 1983; 10(suppl 10):4144.
8. Fessel WJ. Systemic lupus erythematosus in the community. Incidence, prevalence, outcome, and first symptoms; the high prevalence in black women. *Arch Intern Med* 1974;134: 1027–1035.
9. Morrow JD, Schroeder HA, Perry HM Jr. Studies on the control of hypertension by Hyphex. II. Toxic reactions and side effects. *Circulation* 1953;8:829–839.
10. Ladd AT. Procainamide-induced lupus erythematosus. *N Engl J Med* 1962;267:1357–1358.
11. Mongey A-B, Adams LE, Donovan-Brand RJ, et al. Serological evaluation of patients receiving procainamide. *Arthritis Rheum* 1992;35:219–222.
12. Adams LE, Mongey A-B. Role of genetic factors in drug-related autoimmunity. *Lupus* 1994;3:443–449.
13. Nagata C, Fujita S, Iwata H, et al. Systemic lupus erythematosus: a case-control epidemiologic study in Japan. *Int J Dermatol* 1995;34:333–337.
14. Benoni C, Nilsson A, Nived O. Smoking and inflammatory bowel disease comparison with systemic lupus erythematosus a case control study. *Scand J Gastroenterol* 1990;25:751–755.
15. Reidenberg MM, Durant PJ, Harris RA, et al. Lupus erythematosus-like disease due to hydrazine. *Am J Med* 1983;75:365–370.
16. Pereyo N. Tartrazine and drug-induced lupus. *Schock Lett* 1980; 30:1.
17. Pereyo N. Tartrazine, hydrazine, amino compounds and systemic lupus erythematosus. *Science-Ciencia* 1987;14:31–35.
18. Reidenberg MM. The chemical induction of systemic lupus erythematosus and lupus-like illnesses. *Arthritis Rheum* 1981; 24:1004–1008.
19. Geschickter CF, Athanasiadou PA, O'Malley WE. The role of mucinolysis in collagen disease. *Am J Clin Pathol* 1958;30: 93–111.
20. Hochberg MC, Kaslow RA. Risk factors for the development of systemic lupus erythematosus: a case-control study. *Clin Res* 1983;31:732A(abst).
21. Freni-Titulaer LWJ, Kelley DB, Grow AG, et al. Connective tissue disease in southeastern Georgia: a case control study of etiologic factors. *Am J Epidemiol* 1989;130:404–409.
22. Petri M, Allbritton J. Hair product use in systemic lupus erythematosusa case controlled study. *Arthritis Rheum* 1992;35: 625–629.
23. Reidenberg MM, Drayer DE, Lorenzo B, et al. Acetylation phenotypes and environmental chemical exposure of people with idiopathic systemic lupus erythematosus. *Arthritis Rheum* 1993; 36:971–973.
24. Sanchez-Guerrero J, Karlson EW, Colditz GA, et al. Hair dye use and the risk of developing systemic lupus erythematosus. *Arthritis Rheum* 1996;39:657–662.
25. Hardy CJ, Palmer BP, Muir KR, et al. Systemic lupus erythematosus (SLE) and hair treatment: a large community based case-control study. *Lupus* 1999;8:541–544.
26. Owens GR and Medsger TA. Systemic sclerosis secondary to occupational exposure. *Am J Med* 1988;85:114–116.
27. Erasmus LD. Scleroderma in gold-miners on the Witwatersrand with particular reference to pulmonary manifestations. *S Afr J Clin Lab* 1957;3:209–231.
28. Rodnan GP, Benedek TG, Medsger TA Jr, et al. The association of progressive systemic sclerosis (scleroderma) with coal miners' pneumoconiosis and other forms of silicosis. *Ann Intern Med* 1967;66:323–334.
29. Lippmann, M., Eckert, HL, Hahon, N, et al. Circulating antinuclear and rheumatoid factors in coal miners. A prevalence study in Pennsylvania and West Virginia. *Ann Intern Med* 1973; 79:807–811.
30. Bailey, WC, Brown, M, Buechner HA, et al. Silico-mycobacterial disease in sandblasters. *Am Rev Respir Dis* 1974;110: 115–125.
31. Ziskind M, Jones RN, Weill H. Silicosis. *Am Rev Respir Dis* 1976; 113:643–665
32. Cowie RL. Silica-dust-exposed mine workers with scleroderma (systemic sclerosis). *Chest* 1987;92:260–262.
33. Martin JR, Griffin M, Moore E, et al. Systemic sclerosis (scleroderma) in two iron ore mines. *Occup Med* 1999;49(3): 161–169.
34. Jones RN, Turner-Warwick M, Ziskind M, et al. Autoimmune diseases and autoantibodies in silicosis. *Am Rev Respir Dis* 1975; 112:105(abst).
35. Hatron PY, Plouvier B, Francois M, et al. Association lupus erythemateux et silicose. *Rev Med Interne* 1982;3:245–246.
36. Koeger, A-C, Lang, T, Alcaix, D, et al. Silica-associated connective tissue disease, a study of 24 cases. *Medicine* 1995;74: 221–237.
37. Bolton WK, Suratt PM, Sturgill BC. Rapidly progressive silicon cephropathy. *Am J Med* 1981;71:823–828.
38. Sanchez-Roman J, Wichmann I, Salaberri J, et al. Multiple clinical and biological autoimmune manifestations in 50 workers after occupational exposure to silica. *Ann Rheum Dis* 1993;52: 534–538.
39. Steenland, K and Brown, D. Mortality study of gold miners exposed to silica and nonasbestiform amphibole minerals: an update with 14 more years of follow-up. *Am J Ind Med* 1995; 27:217–229.
40. Wilke RA, Salisbury S, Abdel-Rahman E, et al. Lupus-like autoimmune disease associated with silicosis. *Nephrol Dial Transplant* 1996;11:1835–1838.
41. Brown LM, Gridley G, Olsen JH, et al. Cancer risk and mortality patterns among silicotic men in Sweden and Denmark. *J Occup Environ Med* 1997;39:633–638.
42. Rosenman KD, Moore-Fuller M, Reilly MJ. Connective tissue disease and silicosis. *Am J Ind Med* 1999;35:375–381.
43. Masson C, Audran M, Pascaretti C, et al. Silica-associated systemic erythematosus lupus or mineral dust lupus? *Lupus* 1997; 6:1–3.
44. Conrad K, Mehlhorn J, Luthke K, et al. Systemic lupus erythematosus after heavy exposure to quartz dust in uranium mines: clinical and serological characteristics. *Lupus* 1996;5:62–69.
45. Conrad K, Levy Y, Blank M, et al. The pathogenic 16/6 idiotype in patients with silica associated systemic lupus erythematosus (SLE) and uranium miners with increased risk for development of SLE. *J Rheumatol* 1998;24:660–666.
46. Shoenfeld Y, Vilner Y, Resheft, et al. Increased presence of common systemic lupus erythematosus anti-DNA idiotypes (16/6 Id, 32/15 Id) is induced by procainamide. *J Clin Immunol* 1987;7:410–417.
47. Conrad K, Stahnke G, Liedvogel B, et al. Anti-CENP-B response in sera of uranium miners exposed to quartz dust and patients with possible development of systemic sclerosis (scleroderma). *J Rheumatol* 1995;22:1286–1294.
48. Wichmann I, Sanchez-Roman J, Morales J, et al. Antimyeloperoxidase antibodies in individuals with occupational exposure to silica. *Ann Rheum Dis* 1996;55:205–207.
49. Gregorini G, Ferioli A, Donato F, et al. Association between silica exposure and necrotizing crescentic glomerulonephritis with p-ANCA and anti-MPO antibodies: a hospital-based case-control study. *Adv Exp Med Biol* 1993;336:435–440.
50. Nuyts GD, Vlem EV, Vos AD, et al. Wegener's granulomatosis is associated with exposure to silicon compounds: a case-control study. *Nephrol Dial Transplant* 1995;10:1162–1165.
51. Satterly KK, Hogan SL, Nachman, et al. ANCA-associated diseases with renal involvment (ANCA-GN) but not lupus nephri-

tis (LN) are associated with silica exposure. *Clin Exp Immunol* 1998;11:25(abst).

52. Haustein U-F and Anderegg U. Silica induced scleroderma—clinical and experimental aspects. *J Rheumatol* 1998;25: 1917–1926.
53. Parks CG, Conrad K, Cooper GS. Occupational exposure to crystalline silica and autoimmune disease. *Environ Health Perspect* 1999;107(suppl 5):793–802.
54. Ueki A, Yamaguchi M, Ueki H, et al. Polyclonal human T-cell activation by silicate in vitro. *Immunology* 1994;82:332–335.
55. Otsuki T, Sakaguchi H, Tomokuni A, et al. Soluble fas mRNA is dominantly expressed in cases with silicosis. *Immunology* 1998;94:258–262.
56. Frank KH, Fussel M, Conrad K, et al J. Different distribution of HLA class II and tumor necrosis factor alleles (TNF-308.2, TNF alpha 2 microsatellite) in anti-topoisomerase I responders amongst scleroderma patients with and without exposure to quartz/metal dust. *Arthritis Rheum* 1998;41:1306–1311.
57. Dodson VN, Dinman BD, Whitehouse WM, et al. Occupational acroosteolysis. *Arch Environ Health* 1971;22:83–91.
58. Markowitz SS, McDonald CJ, Fethiere W, et al. Occupational acroosteolysis. *Arch Dermatol* 1971;106:219–233.
59. Black CM, Perira S, McWhirter A, et al. Genetic susceptibility to scleroderma-like syndrome in symptomatic and asymptomatic workers exposed to vinyl chloride. *J Rheumatol* 1986;13: 1059–1062.
60. Yoshida S, Gershwin ME. Autoimmunity in selected environmental factors of disease induction. *Semin Arthritis Rheum* 1993;22:399–419.
61. Chiang SY, Swenberg JA, Weisman WH, et al. Mutagenicity of vinyl chloride and its reactive metabolites, chloroethylene oxide and chloroacetaldehyde, in a metabolically competent human B-lymphoblastoid line. *Carcinogenesis* 1997;18:31–36.
62. Chang KJ, Hsieh KH, Lee TP, et al. Immunologic evaluation of patients with PCB poisoning: determination of lymphocyte subpopulations. *Toxicol Appl Pharmacol* 1981;61:58–63.
63. Bekesi JG, Roboz JP, Solomon S, et al. Persistent immune dysfunction in Michigan dairy farm residents exposed to polybrominated biphenyls. In: Hadden JW, Chedid L, Dukor P, et al., eds. *Advances in immunopharmacology*, vol 2. New York: Pergamon Press, 1983:33–39.
64. Beirne GJ, Brennan JT. Glomerulonephritis associated with hydrocarbon solvents. *Arch Environ Health* 1972;25:365–369.
65. Klavis G, Drommer W. Goodpasture's syndrome and effect of benzene. *Arch Toxicol* 1970;26:40–50.
66. Yamamoto T, Wilson CB. Binding of anti-basement membrane antibody to alveolar basement membrane after intratracheal gasoline instillation in rabbits. *Am J Pathol* 1987;126:497–505.
67. Vojdani A, Choneum M, Brautbar N. Immune alteration associated with exposure to toxic chemicals. *Toxicol Ind Health* 1992;8:239–254.
68. Czirjak L, Szegedi G: Benzene exposure in systemic sclerosis (SSC). *N Engl J Med* 1987;107:118.
69. Walder BK. Do solvents cause scleroderma? *Int J Dermatol* 1983;22:157–158.
70. Steen VD. Occupational scleroderma. *Curr Opin Rheumatol* 1999;11:490–494.
71. Dunnill MGS, Black CM. Sclerodermatous syndrome after occupational exposure to herbicides—response to systemic steroids. *Clin Exp Dermatol* 1994;19:518–520.
72. Beer KR, Lorincz AL, Medenica MM, et al. Insecticide-induced lupus erythematosus. *Int J Dermatol* 1994;33:860–862.
73. Lockey JE, Kelly CR, Cannon GW, et al. Progressive systemic sclerosis associated with exposure to trichlororethylene. *Gen Occup Med* 1985;29:493–496.
74. Waller PA, Clauw D, Cupps T, et al. Fasciitis (not scleroderma) following prolonged exposure to an organic solvent (tricholoroethylene). *J Rheumatol* 1994;21:1567–1570.
75. Sparrow GA. A connective tissue disorder similar to vinyl chloride disease in a patient exposed to perchloroethylene. *Clin Exp Dermatol* 1977;2:17–22.
76. Byers VS, Levin AS, Ozonoff DM, et al. Association between clinical symptoms and lymphocyte abnormalities in a population with chronic domestic exposure to industrial solvent-contaminated domestic water supply and a high incidence of leukaemia. *Cancer Immunol Immunother* 1988;27:77–81.
77. Kilburn KH, Warshaw RH. Prevalence of symptoms of systemic lupus erythematosus (SLE) and of fluorescent antinuclear antibodies associated with chronic exposure to trichloroethylene and other chemicals in well water. *Environ Res* 1992;57:1–9.
78. Wallace DJ, Quismorio FP Jr. The elusive search for geographic clusters of systemic lupus erythematosus: a critical review. *Arthritis Rheum* 1995;38:1564–1567.
79. Walsh BT, Reed M, Emerson J, et al. A large cluster of systemic lupus erythematosus individuals in a Mexican-American border town in Arizona. *Arthritis Rheum* 1993;36:S145(abst).
80. Tucker AN, Sanders VM, Barnes DW, et al. Toxicology of trichloroethylene in the mouse. *Toxicol Appl Pharmacol* 1982; 62:351–357.
81. Sanders VM, Tucker AN, White Jr. KL, et al. Humoral and cell-mediated immune status in mice exposed to trichloroethylene in the drinking water. *Toxicol Appl Pharmacol* 1982;62: 358–368.
82. Sanders VM, White Jr. KL, Shopp Jr. GM, et al. Humoral and cell-mediated immune status of mice exposed to 1,1,2-trichloroethane. *Drug Chem Toxicol* 1985;8(5):357–372
83. Khan MF, Kaphalia BS, Prabhakar BS, et al. Trichloroethene-induced autoimmune response in female MRL +/+ mice. *Toxicol Appl Pharmacol* 1995;134:155–160.
84. Griffin JM, Gilbert KM, Pumford NR. Cytochrome P450 activation of trichloroethylene initiates a Th_1 T-cell response in MRL +/+ mice. National Institute of Environmental Health Sciences, Linking Environmental Agents and Autoimmune Diseases, September 1–3, 1998, NIEHS Research Triangle Park, NC. Abstract presented at the Environmental meeting.
85. White KL Jr, Booker CD, Llewellyn CG. Experimental studies of environmental exposures and systemic lupus erythematosus. National Institute of Environmental Health Sciences, Linking Environmental Agents and Autoimmune Diseases, September 1–3, 1998, NIEHS Research Triangle Park, NC. Abstract presented at the Environmental meeting.
86. Schielen P, Schoo W, Tekstra J, et al. Autoimmune effects of hexachlorobenzene in the rat. *Toxicol Appl Pharmacol* 1993;122: 233–243.
87. Michielsen CPPC, Muis A, Vos JG, et al. Ingestion of the environmental pollutant hexachlorobenzene (HCB) causes eosinophilic inflammation and airways hyperreactivity in the Brown Norway rat. National Institute of Environmental Health Sciences, Linking Environmental Agents and Autoimmune Diseases, September 1–3, 1998, NIEHS Research Triangle Park, NC. Abstract presented at the Environmental meeting
88. Queiroz ML, Bincoletto C, Perlingeiro RC, et al. Immunoglobulin levels in workers exposed to hexachlorobenzene. *Hum Exp Toxicol* 1998;17:172–175.
89. Vos JG: Hexachlorobenzene and Autoimmune Disease. National Institute of Environmental Health Sciences, Linking Environmental Agents and Autoimmune Diseases, September 1–3, 1998, NIEHS Research Triangle Park, NC. Abstract presented at the Environmental meeting.
90. Cripps DJ, Peters HA, Gocmen A, et al. Porphyria turcica. Twenty years after hexachlorobezene intoxication. *Br J Dermatol* 1984;111(10):413–422.

91. Holladay SD. Prenatal immunotoxicant exposure and postnatal autoimmune disease. *Environ Health Perspect* 1999;107(5): 687–691.
92. Fine JS, Gasiewicz TA, Silverstone AE. Lymphocyte stem cell alterations following perinatal exposure to 2,3,7,8-tetrachlorodibenzo-p-dioxin. *Mol Pharmacol* 1989;35:18–25.
93. Holladay S. Development vs. Adult Exposure to Environmental Agents and Autoimmune Disease. National Institute of Environmental Health Sciences, Linking Environmental Agents and Autoimmune Diseases, September 1–3, 1998, NIEHS Research Triangle Park, NC. Abstract presented at the Environmental meeting
94. Silverstone AE, Gavalchin J, Shanley P, et al. TCDD potentiates a lupus-like autoimmune nephritis in male NZB × SWR (SNF_1) mice. National Institute of Environmental Health Sciences, Linking Environmental Agents and Autoimmune Diseases, September 1–3, 1998, NIEHS Research Triangle Park, NC. Abstract presented at the Environmental meeting.
95. Clark DA, Sweeney G, Safe S, et al. Cellular and genetic basis for suppression of cytotoxic T-cell generation by haloaromatic hydrocarbons. *Immunopharmacology* 1983;6:143–153.
96. Yamakage A, Ishikawa H, Saito Y, et al. Occupational scleroderma-like disorder occurring in men engaged in the polymerization of epoxy resins. *Dermatologica* 1980;161:33–44.
97. Ishikawa O, Warita S, Tamura A, et al. Occupational scleroderma. A 17-year follow-up study. *Br J Dermatol* 1995;133: 786–789.
98. Swerdrup B: Do workers in the manufacturing industry run an increased risk of getting scleroderma? *Int J Dermatol* 1984;23: 629.
99. Gabay C, Kahn MF. Male-type scleroderma: the role of occupational exposure. *Schweiz Med Wochenschr* 1992;14:1746–1752.
100. Bovenzi M, Barbone F, Betta A, et al. Scleroderma and occupational exposure. *Scand J Work Environ Health* 1995;21: 289–292.
101. Silman AJ, Jones S. What is the contribution of occupational environmental factors to the occurrence of scleroderma in men? *Ann Rheum Dis* 1992;51:1322–1324.
102. Nietert PJ, Sutherland SE, Silver RM, et al. Is occupational organic solvent exposure a risk factor for scleroderma? *Arthritis Rheum* 1998;41(6):1111–1118.
103. Burns CJ, Laing TJ, Gillespie BW, et al. The epidemiology of scleroderma among women: assessment of risk from exposure to silicone and silica. *J Rheumatol* 1996;23(11):1904–1911.
104. Laing T, Gillespie B, Burns C, et al. Risk factors for scleroderma among Michigan women. *Arthritis Rheum* 1995;38:S341.
105. Lacey Jr. JV, Laing TJ, Gillespie BW, et al. Epidemiology of scleroderma among women: assessment of risk from exposure to silicone and silica. *J Rheumatol* 1997;24:1854–1855.
106. Lacey Jr. JV, Garabrant DH, Gillespie BW, et al. Self-reported exposure to solvents in women with systemic sclerosis (SSc). *Arthritis Rheum* 1997;40:S201.
107. Lacey Jr. JV, Garabrant DH, Gillespie BW, et al. Self-reported exposure to solvents in women with undifferentiated connective tissue disease (UCTD). *Arthritis Rheum* 1997;40:S201.
108. Koeger AC, Rozenberg S, Chaibi P, et al. Connective tissue disease associated with silicone alveolitis due to silicone-spray. A prospective series. *Arthritis Rheum* 1995;38:S342(abst).
109. Nietert PJ, Sutherland SE, Silver RM, et al. Solvent oriented hobbies and the risk of systemic sclerosis. *J Rheumatol* 1999;26: 2369–2372.
110. Kaiser W, Biesenbach G, Stuby U, et al. Human adjuvant disease: remission of silicone induced autoimmune disease after explanation of breast augmentation. *Ann Rheum Dis* 1990;49: 937–938.
111. Sergott TJ, Limoli JP, Baldwin CM Jr, et al. Human adjuvant disease, possible autoimmune disease after silicone implantation: a review of the literature case studies, and speculation for the future. *Plast Reconstruct Surg* 1986;78:104–114.
112. Miyoshi K, Miyamura T, Kobayashi Y, et al. Hypergammaglobulinemia by prolonged adjuvanticity in man. Disorders developed after augmentation mammoplasty. *Jpn Med J* 1964;2122: 9–14.
113. Yoshida K. Post mammaplasty disorder as an adjuvant disease of man. *Shikoku Igaku Zasshi* 1973;29:318–332.
114. Naim JO, Ippolito KML, Lanzafame RJ, et al. Induction of type II collagen arthritis in the DA rat using silicone gels and oils as adjuvant. *J Autoimmunity* 1995;8:751–761.
115. Kumagai Y, Shiokawa Y, Medsger TA Jr, et al. Clinical spectrum of connective tissue disease after cosmetic surgery. *Arthritis Rheum* 1984;27:1–12.
116. Press RI, Peebles CL, Kumagai Y, et al. Antinuclear antibodies in women with silicone breast implants. *Lancet* 1992;340: 1304–1307.
117. Gabriel SE, O'Fallon WM, Kurland LT, et al. Risk of connective tissue diseases and other disorders after breast implantation. *N Engl J Med* 1994;330:1697–1702.
118. Bridges AJ, Conley C, Wang G, et al. A clinical and immunologic evaluation of women with silicone breast implants and symptoms of rheumatoid disease. *Ann Intern Med* 1993;118: 929–936.
119. Sanchez-Guerrero J, Colditz GA, Karlson EW, et al. Silicone breast implants and the risk of connective-tissue diseases and symptoms. *N Engl J Med* 1995;332:1666–1670.
120. Hennekens CH, Lee I-M, Cook NR, et al. Self-reported breast implants and connective-tissue disease in female health professionals. *JAMA* 1996;275:616–621.
121. Hochberg MC, Perlmutter DL, Medsger TA Jr, et al. Lack of association between augmentation mammoplasty and systemic sclerosis (scleroderma). *Arthritis Rheum* 1996;39:125–131.
122. Edworthy SM, Martin L, Barr SG, et al. A clinical study of the relationship between silicone breast implants and connective tissue disease. *J Rheumatol* 1996;25:254–260
123. Karlson EW, Hankinson SE, Liang MH, et al. Association of silicone breast implants with immunologic abnormalities: a prospective study. *Am J Med* 1999;106:11–19.
124. Richeldi L, Sorrentino R, Saltini C. HLA-DPB1 glutamate 69: a genetic marker of beryllium disease. *Science* 1993;262: 242–244.
125. Watzl B, Watson RR. Immunomodulation by cocainea neuroendocrine mediated response. *Life Sci* 1990;46:1319–1329.
126. Lie JT. Medical complications of cocaine and other illicit drug abuse simulating rheumatic disease. *J Rheumatol* 1990;17: 736–737.
127. Zamora-Quezada JC, Dinerman H, Stadecker MJ, et al. Muscle and skin infarction after free-basing cocaine (crack). *Ann Intern Med* 1988;108:564–566.
128. Mody CK, Miller BL, McIntyre HB, et al. Neurologic complications of cocaine abuse. *Neurology* 1988;38:1189–1193.
129. Orser B. Thrombocytopenia and cocaine abuse. *Anesthesiology* 1991;74:195–196.
130. Kunci RW, Duncan G, Watson D, et al. Colchicine myopathy and neuropathy. *N Engl J Med* 1987;316:1562–1568.
131. Burry JN. Lipstick and lupus erythematosus. *N Engl J Med* 1969;281:620–621.
132. Bigazzi PE. Autoimmunity and heavy metals. *Lupus* 1994;3: 449–453.
133. Druet P, Bernard A, Hirsch F, et al. Immunologically mediated glomerulonephritis induced by heavy metals. *Arch Toxicol* 1982; 50:187–194.
134. Harrison DJ, Thomson D, McDonald MK. Membranous glomerulonephritis. *J Clin Pathol* 1986;39:167–171.

135. Silverberg DS, Kidd EG, Shnitka TK, et al. Gold nephropathy. A clinical and pathologic study. *Arthritis Rheum* 1970;13: 812–825.
136. Wooley PH, Griffin J, Panayi GS, et al. HLA DR antigens and toxic reaction to sodium thiomalate and d-penicillamine in patients with rheumatoid arthritis. *N Engl J Med* 1980;303: 300–302.
137. Goter Robinson CJ, Balazs T, Egorov IK. Mercuric chloride-, gold sodium thiomalate-, and d-Penicillamine-induced antinuclear antibodies in mice. *Toxicol Appl Pharmacol* 1986;86: 159–169.
138. Schumann D, Kubicka-Muranyi M, Mirtschewa J, et al. Adverse immune reactions to gold. I. Chronic treatment with an Au (I) drug sensitizes mouse T cells not to Au (I), but to Au (III) and induces autoantibody formation. *J Immunol* 1990; 145:2132–2139.
139. Joshi BC, Dwivedi C, Powell A, et al. Immune complex nephritis in rats induced by long-term oral exposure to cadmium. *J Comp Pathol* 1981;91:11–15.
140. Ohsawa M, Takahashi K, Otsuka F. Induction of anti-nuclear antibodies in mice orally exposed to cadmium at low concentrations. *Clin Exp Immunol* 1988;73:98–102.
141. Powell AL, Joshi B, Dwivedi C, et al. Immunopathological changes in cadmium treated rats. *Vet Pathol* 1979;16:116–118.
142. Bernier J, Brousseau P, Krzystyniak K, et al. Immunotoxicity of heavy metals in relation to great lakes. *Environ Health Perspect* 1995;103(suppl 9):23–34.
143. Lindqvist KJ, Makene WJ, Shaba JD, et al. Immunofluorescence and electron microscopic studies of kidney biopsies from patients with nephrotic syndrome, possibly induced by skin lightening creams containing mercury. *E Afr Med J* 1974;51: 168–169.
144. Cardnas A, Roels HR, Bernard AM, et al. Markers of early renal changes induced by industrial pollutants: application to workers exposed to mercury vapor. *Br J Ind Med* 1999;50:17–27.
145. Schrallhammer-Benkler K, Ring J, Przybilla B, et al. Acute mercury intoxication with lichenoid drug eruption followed by mercury contact allergy and development of antinuclear antibodies. *Acta Derm Venereol (Stockh)* 1992;72:294–296.
146. Roger J, Zilikens D, Burg G, et al. Systemic autoimmune disease in a patient with long standing exposure to mercury. *Eur J Dermatol* 1992;2:168–170.
147. Weening JJ, Hoedemaeker PHJ, Bakker WW. Immunoregulation and anti-nuclear antibodies in mercury-induced glomerulopathy in the rat. *Clin Exp Immunol* 1981;45:64–71.
148. Bigazzi PE. Metals and kidney autoimmunity. *Environ Health Perspect* 1999;107(suppl 5):753–765.
149. Goldman M, Druet P, Gleichmann E. Th2 cells in systemic autoimmunity: insights from allogeneic diseases and chemically-induced autoimmunity. *Immunol Today* 1991;12: 223–271.
150. Guery JC, Druet E, Glotz D, et al. Specificity and cross reactive idiotypes of antiglomerular basement membrane autoantibodies in HgCl2-induced autoimmune glomerulonephritis. *Eur J Immunol* 1990;20:93–100.
151. Hultman P, Enestrom S, Pollard KM, et al. Anti-fibrillarin autoantibodies in mercury-treated mice. *Clin Exp Immunol* 1989;78:470–472.
152. Reuter R, Tessaro G, Vohr HW, et al. Mercuric chloride induces autoantibodies against U3 small ribonucleoprotein in susceptible mice. *Proc Natl Acad Sci USA* 1989;86:237–241.
153. Goter Robinson CJ, Abraham AA, Balazs T. Induction of antinuclear antibodies by mercuric chloride in mice. *Clin Exp Immunol* 1984;58:300–306.
154. Al-Balaghi S, Moller E, Moller G, et al. Mercury induces polyclonal B-cell activation, autoantibody production and renal immune complex deposits in young (NZBXNZW) F1 hybrids. *Eur J Immunol* 1996;26:1519–1526
155. Kubicka-Muranyi M, Griem P, Lubben B, et al. Mercuric chloride induced autoimmunity in mice involves up regulated presentation by spleen cells of altered and unaltered nucleolar cell antigen. *Int Arch Allergy Immunol* 1995;108:1–10.
156. Pollard KM, Lee DK, Casiano CA, et al. Do autoimmunity-inducing xenobiotic mercury interacts with the autoantigen fibrillarin and modifies its molecular and antigenic properties. *J Immunol* 1997;158:3521–3528.
157. Pollard KM, Kono DH, Pearson DL, et al. Autoimmunity induced by xenobiotics. *Mol Exp Med* 1998–1999;267–269.
158. Pollard KM, Pearson DL, Hultman P, et al. Xenobiotic-induced acceleration of Systemic Autoimmune Disease. National Institute of Environmental Health Sciences, Linking Environmental Agents and Autoimmune Diseases, September 1–3, 1998, NIEHS Research Triangle Park, NC. Abstract presented at the Environmental meeting
159. Arnett RC, Fritzler MJ, Ahn, C, et al. Urinary mercury levels in patients with autoantibodies to U3–RNP (fibrillarin). *J Rheumatol* 2000;27:405–410.
160. El-Fawal HAN, DeFeo A, Shamy MY. Neuorimmunotoxicology:A marriage whose time has come. National Institute of Environmental Health Sciences, Linking Environmental Agents and Autoimmune Diseases, September 1–3, 1998, NIEHS Research Triangle Park, NC. Abstract presented at the Environmental meeting
161. DeFeo A, El-Fawal HAN. Serum with autoantibodies to nervous system antigens blocks neuromuscular activity. National Institute of Environmental Health Sciences, Linking Environmental Agents and Autoimmune Diseases, September 1–3, 1998, NIEHS Research Triangle Park, NC. Abstract presented at the Environmental meeting
162. Eggleton P, Llewellyn DH. Pathophysiological roles of calreticulin in autoimmune disease. *Scand J Immunol* 1999;49: 466–473.
163. Nguyen TO, Capra JD, Sontheimer RD. Calreticulin is transcriptionally up regulated by heat shock, calcium and heavy metals. *Mol Immunol* 1996;33:379–386.
164. Naganuma A, Anderson ME, Meister A. Cellular glutathione as a determinant of sensitivity to mercuric chloride toxicity. *Biochem Pharmacol* 1990;40:693–697.
165. Bigazzi PE. Mercury. In: Zelikoff J, Thomas P, eds. *Immunotoxocology of environmental and occupational metals.* London: Taylor and Francis, 1998:131–161.
166. Satoh M, Hamilton KJ, Ajmani AK, et al. Autoantibodies to ribosomal P antigens with immune complex glomerular nephritis in SJL mice treated with pristane. *J Immunol* 1996;157: 3200–3206.
167. Shaheen V, Satoh M, Richards HB, et al. Role of macrophages in the induction of lupus by an environmental agent. National Institute of Environmental Health Sciences, Linking Environmental Agents and Autoimmune Diseases, September 1–3, 1998, NIEHS Research Triangle Park, NC. Abstract presented at the Environmental meeting.
168. Hamilton KJ, Satoh M, Swartz J, et al. Influence of microbial stimulation on hypergammaglobulinemia and autoantibody production in pristane-induced lupus. *Clin Immunol Immunopathol* 1998;86:271–279.
169. Bardana EJ Jr, Manilow MR, Houghton DC, et al. Diet-induced systemic lupus erythematosus (SLE) in primates. *Am J Kidney Dis* 1982;l:345–352.
170. Manilow MR, Bardana EJ Jr, Pirokský B, et al. Systemic lupus erythematosus-like syndrome in monkeys fed alfalfa sprouts: role of a nonprotein amino acid. *Science* 1982;216: 415–417.

171. Manilow MR, Bardana EJ Jr, Goodnight SH. Pancytopenia during ingestion of alfalfa seeds (letter). *Lancet* 1981;1:615.
172. Roberts JL, Hayashi JA. Exacerbation of SLE associated with alfalfa ingestion (letter). *N Engl J Med* 1983:308:1361.
173. Prete P. The mechanism of action of l-canavanine in inducing autoimmune phenomena. *Arthritis Rheum* 1985;28: 1198–2000.
174. Alcocer-Varela J, Iglesias A, Llorente L, et al. Effects of l-canavanine on T cells may explain the induction of systemic lupus erythematosus by alfalfa. *Arthritis Rheum* 1985;28:52–57.
175. Dubois EL, Strain L. Effect of diet on survival and nephropathy of NZB NZW hybrid mice. *Biochem Med* 1973;7:336–342.
176. Kao NL, Richmond GW, Moy JN. Resolution of severe lupus nephritis associated with *Tripterygium wilfordii* hook F ingestion. *Arthritis Rheum* 1993;36:1751–1752.
177. Jordan SC, Yap H-K, Lee B-W, et al. Characterization of the immunosuppressive properties of a Chinese herbal decoction (CH) used in the treatment of lupus nephritis. *J Invest Med* 1996;44:142A.
178. Yu S-J, Stseng J. Fu-ling, a Chinese herbal drug, modulates cytokine secretion by human peripheral blood monocytes. *Int J Immunopharmocol* 1996;18:37–44.
179. Guro-Razuman S, Anand P, Hu G, et al. Dermatomyositis-like illness following kava-kava ingestion. *J Clin Rheumatol* 1999;5: 342–345.
180. Tabuenca JM. Toxic-allergic syndrome caused by ingestion of rapeseed oil denatured with aniline. *Lancet* 1981;2:567–568.
181. Alonso-Ruiz A, Zea-Mendoza AC, Salazar-Vallinas JM, et al. Toxic oil syndrome: a syndrome with features overlapping those of various forms of scleroderma. *Semin Arthritis Rheum* 1986; 15:200–212.
182. Alonso-Ruiz, Calabozo M, Perez-Ruiz F, et al. Toxic oil syndrome. A long term follow up of a cohort of 332 patients. *Medicine* 1993;72:285–295.
183. Gershwin ME. Evidence for the role of environmental agents in the initiation or progression of autoimmune conditions. National Institute of Environmental Health Sciences, Linking Environmental Agents and Autoimmune Diseases, September 1–3, 1998, NIEHS Research Triangle Park, NC. Abstract presented at the Environmental meeting.
184. DelPozo V, De Andraes B, Gallardo S, et al. Cytokine mRNA expression among tissue from toxic oil syndrome patients: a Th2 immunological mechanism. *Toxicology* 1997;118:61–70.
185. Bell SA, Hobbs MV, Rubin RL. Isotype-restricted hyperimmunity in a murine model of toxic oil syndrome. *J Immunol* 1992; 148:3369–3376.
186. Edison M, Philen RM, Sewell CM, et al. L-Tryptophan and eosinophilic-myalgia syndrome in New Mexico. *Lancet* 1990; 335:645–648.
187. Hertzman PA, Falk H, Kilbourne EM, et al. The eosinophilia myalgia syndrome: the Los Alamos Conference. *J Rheumatol* 1991;18:867–873.
188. Kilbourne EM, Swygert LA, Philen RM, et al. Interim guidance on the eosinophilia-myalgia syndrome. *Ann Intern Med* 1990; 112:85–86.
189. Varga J, Heiman-Patterson TD, Emery DL, et al. Clinical spectrum of the systemic manifestations of the eosinophilia-myalgia syndrome. *Semin Arthritis Rheum* 1990;19:313–328.
190. Martin RW, Duffy J, Engel AG, et al. The clinical spectrum of the eosinophilia-myalgia syndrome associated with l-tryptophan ingestion. Clinical features in 20 patients and aspects of pathophysiology. *Ann Intern Med* 1990;113:124–134.
191. Belongia EA, Hedberg CW, Gleich GJ, et al. An investigation of the cause of the eosinophilia-myalgia syndrome associated with tryptophan use. *N Engl J Med* 1990;323:357–365.
192. Love LA, Radar JI, Crofford LJ, et al. Pathological and immunological effects of ingesting l-tryptophan and 1,1-ethylidenebis (l-tryptophan) in Lewis rats. *J Clin Invest* 1993;91: 804–811.
193. Fernandes G. Dietary lipids and risk of autoimmunity. *Clin Immunol Immunopathol* 1994;72:193–197.
194. Fernandes G, Yunis EJ, Smith J, et al. Dietary influence on breeding behavior, hemolytic anemia and longevity in NZB mice. *Proc Soc Exp Biol Med* 1972;139:1189– 1196.
195. Fernandes G, Yunis EJ, Jose DG, et al. Dietary influence on antinuclear antibodies and cell-mediated immunity in NZB mice. *Int Arch Allergy* 1973;44:770–782.
196. Fernandes G, Alonso DR, Tanaka T, et al. Influence of diet on vascular lesions in autoimmune-prone B/W mice. *Proc Natl Acad Sci USA* 1983;80:874–877.
197. Fernandes G, Friend P, Yunis EJ, et al. Influence of dietary restriction on immunologic function and renal disease in (NZB X NZW) F1 mice. *Proc Natl Acad Sci USA* 1978;75: 1500–1504.
198. Prickett JD, Robinson DR, Steinberg AD. Effects of dietary enrichment with eicosapentaenoic acid upon autoimmune nephritis in female NZB × NZW/F1 mice. *Arthritis Rheum* 1983;26:133–139.
199. Kelley VE, Ferreti A, Izui S, et al. A fish oil diet rich in eicosapentaenoic acid reduces cyclooxygenase metabolites, and suppresses lupus in MRL/lpr mice. *J Immunol* 1985;134: 1914–1919.
200. Prickett JD, Robinson DR, Steinberg AD. Dietary enrichment with the polyunsaturated fatty-acid eicosapaentoic acid acid prevents proteinuria and prolongs survivial in NZB × NZW F1 mice. *J Clin Invest* 1981;68:556.
201. Fernandes G, Chandrasekar B, Venkatraman JT, et al. Increased transforming growth factor and decrease oncogene expression by omega-3 fatty-acids in the spleen delays the onset of autoimmune disease in B/W mice. *J Immunol* 1994;152:5979–5987.
202. Chandrasekar B, Troyer DA, Venkatraman JT, et al. Dietary omega-3 lipids delay the onset and progression of autoimmune lupus nephritis by inhibiting transforming growth factor β mRNA and protein expression. *J Autoimmunity* 1995;8: 381–393.
203. Jolly CA, Fernandes G. Diet modulates Th-1 and Th-2 cytokine production in the peripheral blood of lupus-prone mice. *J Clin Immunol* 1999;19:172–178.
204. Endres S, Ghorbani R, Kelley VE, et al. The effect of dietary supplementation with n-3 PUFA on the synthesis of interleukin-1 and tumor necrosis factor by mononuclear cells. *N Engl J Med* 1989;320:265–271.
205. Meydani SN, Lithtenstin AH, Cornwall S, et al. Immunological effects of national cholesterol education panel step-2 diets with and without fish-derived n-3 fatty acid in Richmond. *J Clin Invest* 1993;92:105–113.
206. Huang SC, Misfeldt ML, Fritsch KL. Dietary fat influences ia antigen expression and immune cell populations in the murine, peritoneum and spleen. *J Nutr* 1992;122:1219–1231.
207. Calder PC, Bevan SJ, Newsholme EA. The inhibition of T-lymphocyte proliferation by fatty acids is via eicosanoid-independent mechanism. *Immunology* 1992;75:108–115.
208. Meydani SN, Endres S, Woods MM, et al. Oral (n-3) fatty acid supplementation suppresses cytokine production and lymphocyte proliferation: comparison between young and older women. *J Nutr* 1991;121:547–555.
209. Endres S, Meydani SN, Ghorbani S, et al. Dietary supplementation with n-3 fatty acids suppresses interleukin-2 production and mononuclear cell proliferation. *J Leukoc Biol* 1993;54: 599–603.
210. Kremer JM, Laurence DL, Jubiz W, et al. Dietary fish oil and olive oil supplementation in patients with rheumatoid arthritis:

clinical and immunological effects. *Arthritis Rheum* 1990;33: 810–820.

211. Rossetti RG, DeLuca P, Seiler CM, et al. Modification of human lymphocyte and monocyte function by gammalinolenic acid (GLA), and unsaturated fatty acid: Studied in vitro and in vivo. *Arthritis Rheum* 1997;40:4187(abst).
212. DeMarco DM, Santoli D, Zurier RB. Effects of fatty acids on proliferation and activation of human snow wheel compartment lymphocytes. *J Leukoc Biol* 1994;56:612–616.
213. Rossetti RG, Seiler CM, DeLuca P, et al. Oral administration of unsaturated fatty acids: effects on human peripheral blood T lymphocyte proliferation. *J Leukoc Biol* 1997;62:438–443.
214. Moore GF, Yarboro C, Sebring N, et al. Eicosapentaenoic acid in the treatment of systemic lupus erythematosus. *Arthritis Rheum* 1987;30:533(abst).
215. Thorner A, Walldius G, Nillson E, et al. Beneficial effects of reduced intake of polyunsaturated fatty acids in the diet for one year in patients with systemic lupus erythematosus (letter). *Ann Rheum Dis* 1990;49:134.
216. Walton AJE, Snaith ML, Locniskar M, et al. Dietary fish oil and the severity of symptoms in patients with systemic lupus erythematosus. *Ann Rheum Dis* 1991;50:463–466.
217. Krieg AM. Environmental and infectious factors. In: Steinberg AD, moderator. Systemic lupus erythematosus. *Ann Intern Med* 1991;115:548–559.
218. Westberg G, Tarkowski A. Effect of MaxEPA in patients with SLE. A double-blind, crossover study. *Scand J Rheumatol* 1990; 19:137–143.
219. Kremer JM, Bigauoette J, Michalek AV, et al. Effects of manipulation of dietary fatty acids on clinical manifestations of rheumatoid arthritis. *Lancet* 1985;1:184–187.
220. Delafuente JC. Nutrients and immune responses. *Rheum Dis Clin North Am* 1991;17:203–212.
221. Meydani SN, Barklund MP, Liu S, et al. Vitamin E supplementation enhances cell-mediated immunity in healthy elderly subjects. *Am J Clin Nutr* 1990;52:557–563.
222. Weimann BJ, Weiser H. Effects of antioxidant vitamins C, E, and β-carotene on immune functions in MRL/lpr mice and rats. *Ann NY Acad Sci* 1997;669:390–392
223. Comstock GW, Burke AE, Hoffman SC, et al. Serum concentrations of α tocopherol, β carotene, and retinol preceding the diagnosis of rheumatoid arthritis and systemic lupus erythematosus. *Ann Rheum Dis* 1997;56:323–325.
224. Parke DV, Parke AL: Chemical-induced inflammation and inflammatory diseases. *Int J Occ Med Environ* 1996;9(3): 211–217.
225. Parke DV, Sapota A: Chemical toxicity and reactive oxygen species. *Int J Occ Med Environ* 1996;9(4):331–340.
226. Stern RS, Docken W. An exacerbation of SLE after visiting a tanning salon. *JAMA* 1986;255:3120.
227. Lehman P, Holzle E, Kind P, et al. Experimental reproduction of skin lesions in lupus erythematosus by UVA and UVB radiation. *J Am Acad Dermatol* 1990;22:181–187.
228. Natali PG, Tan EM. Experimental skin lesions in mice resembling systemic lupus erythematosus. *Arthritis Rheum* 1973;16: 579–589.
229. Ansel JC, Mountz J, Steinberg AD, et al. Effects of UV radiation on autoimmune strains of mice: increased mortality and accelerated autoimmunity in BXSB male mice. *J Invest Dermatol* 1985;85:181–186.
230. Bruze M, Forsgren A, Ljunggren B. Antinuclear antibodies in mice induced by long wave ultraviolet radiation (UVA). *Acta Derm Venereol (Stockh)* 1985;65:25–33.
231. Golan DT, Borel Y. Increased photosensitivity to near-ultraviolet light in murine SLE. *J Immunol* 1984;132:705–710.
232. Furukawa F, Kashihara-Sawami M, Lyons MB, et al. Binding of antibodies to the extractable nuclear antigens SS;n-A;n/Ro and SS-B/La is induced on the surface of human keratinocytes by ultraviolet light (UVL): implications for the pathogenesis of photosensitive cutaneous lupus. *J Invest Dermatol* 1990;94: 77–85.
233. McGrath H Jr, Bak E, Michalski JP. Ultraviolet-A light prolongs survival and improves immune function in (New Zealand black × New Zealand white) F1, hybrid mice. *Arthritis Rheum* 1987; 30:557–561.
234. Martin L, Chalmers IM. Photosensitivity to fluorescent light in a patient with systemic lupus erythematosus. *J Rheumatol* 1983; 10:811–812.
235. McGrath H, Bell JM, Haycock JW. Fluorescent light activates the immunomodulator cisurocanic acid in vitro: implications for patients with systemic lupus erythematosus. *Ann Rheum Dis* 1994;53:396–399.
236. Dowdy MJ, Nigra TP, Barth WF. Subacute cutaneous lupus erythematosus during PUVA therapy for psoriasis: case report and review of the literature. *Arthritis Rheum* 1989;32:343–346.
237. Eyanson S, Greist MC, Brandt KD, et al. Systemic lupus erythematosus: association with psoralen-ultraviolet-A treatment of psoriasis. *Arch Dermatol* 1979;115:54–56.
238. Bjellerup M, Bruze M, Forsgren A, et al. Antinuclear antibodies during PUVA therapy. *Acta Derm Venereol (Stockh)* 1979;59: 73–75.
239. Kubba R, Steck WD, Clough JD. Antinuclear antibodies and PUVA photochemotherapy. *Arch Dermatol* 1981;117:474–477.
240. Stern RS, Morison WL, Thibodeau LA, et al. Antinuclear antibodies and oral methoxsalen photochemotherapy (PUVA) for psoriasis. *Arch Dermatol* 1979;115:1320–1324.
241. Levin DL, Roenigk HH, Caro WA, et al. Histologic, immunofluorescent and antinuclear antibody findings in PUVA-treated patients. *J Am Acad Dermatol* 1982;6:328–333.
242. Deeg HJ. Ultraviolet irradiation in transplantation biology. *Transplantation* 1988;45:845–851.
243. Fresco R. Virus-like particles in systemic lupus erythematosus. *N Engl J Med* 1970;283:1231–1233.
244. Grausz H, Earley LE, Stephens BG, et al. Diagnostic import of virus-like particles in the glomerular endothelium of patients with systemic lupus erythematosus. *N Engl J Med* 1970;283:506–511.
245. Gyorkey F, Min K-W, Sincovics JG, et al. Systemic lupus erythematosus and myxovirus (letter). *N Engl J Med* 1969;280: 333.
246. Rich SA, Owens TR, Anzola C, et al. Induction of lupus inclusions by sera from patients with systemic lupus erythematosus. *Arthritis Rheum* 1986;29:501–507.
247. Plotz PH. Autoantibodies are antiidiotype antibodies to antiviral antibodies. *Lancet* 1987;ii:824–826.
248. Hollinger FB, Sharp JT, Lidsky MD, et al. Antibodies to viral antigens in systemic lupus erythematosus. *Arthritis Rheum* 1971;14:1–11.
249. Philips PE, Christian CL. Myxovirus antibody increases in human connective tissue disease. *Science* 1970;168:982–984.
250. Rothfield NF, Evans AS, Niederman JC. Clinical and laboratory aspects of raised virus antibody titers in systemic lupus erythematosus. *Ann Rheum Dis* 1973;32:238–246.
251. Evans AS, Rothfield NF Niederman NF. Raised antibody titers to EB Virus and systemic lupus erythematosus. *Lancet* 1971;1: 167–168.
252. Dror Y, Blachar Y, Cohen P, et al. Systemic lupus erythematosus associated with acute Epstein-Barr virus infection. *Am J Kidney Dis* 1988;32:825–828.
253. James JA, Kaufman KM, Farris AD, et al. An increased prevalence of Epstein-Barr virus infection in young patients suggests a possible etiology for systemic lupus erythematosus. *J Clin Invest* 100:3019–3026, 1997.

254. James JA, Gross RH, Scofield R, et al. PPGMRPP immunization generates anti-Sm humoral autoimmunity and induces systemic lupus erythematosus in rabbits. *J Exp Med* 1995;181: 453–461.
255. Marchini B, Dolcher MP, Sabbatini A, et al. Immune response to different sequences of the EBNA-I molecule in Epstein-Barr virus related disorders and in autoimmune diseases. *J Autoimmunity* 1994;7:179–191.
256. James JA, Kaufman KM, Harley JB. Immune response differences between systemic lupus erythematosus patients and normal controls in their immune response to Epstein Barr virus nuclear antigen. National Institute of Environmental Health Sciences, Linking Environmental Agents and Autoimmune Diseases, September 1–3, 1998, NIEHS Research Triangle Park, NC. Abstract presented at the Environmental meeting.
257. Incaprera M, Rindi L, Bazzichi A, et al. Potential role of the Epstein-Barr virus in systemic lupus erythematosus autoimmunity. *Clin Exp Rheumatol* 1998;16:289–294.
258. Newkirk MM, Shiroky JB, Johnson N, et al. Rheumatic disease patients, prone to Sjogren's syndrome and/or lymphoma, mount an antibody response to BHRF1, the Epstein-Barr viral homologue of BCL-2. *Br J Rheumatol* 1996;35:1075–1081.
259. Fox RI, Pearson G, Vaughan JH. Detection of Epstein-Barr virus associated antigens and DNA in salivary gland biopsies from patients with Sjogren's syndrome. *J Immunol* 1986;137: 3162–3168.
260. Saito I, Servenius B, Compton T, et al. Detection of Epstein-Barr virus DNA by polymerase chain reaction in blood and tissue biopsies from patients with Sjogren's syndrome. *J Exp Med* 1989;169:2191–2198.
261. Mariette X, Gozlan J, Clerc D, et al. Detection of Epstein-Barr virus DNA by in situ hybridization and polymerase chain reaction in salivary gland biopsy specimens from patients with Sjogren's syndrome. *Am J Med* 1991;90:286–294.
262. Schuurman HJ, Schemmann MH, de Weger RA, et al. Epstein Barr virus in the sublabial salivary gland in Sjogren's syndrome. *Am J Clin Pathol* 1989;91:461–463.
263. Venables PJ, Teo CG, Baboonian C, et al. Persistence of Epstein-Barr virus in salivary gland biopsies from healthy individuals and patients with Sjogren's syndrome. *Clin Exp Immunol* 1989;75:359–364.
264. Venables PJ, Baboonian C, Horsfall AC, et al. The response to Epstein-Barr virus infection in Sjogren's syndrome. *J Autoimmunity* 1989;2:439–448.
265. Rider JR, Ollier WE, Lock RJ, et al. Human cytomegalovirus infection and systemic lupus erythematosus. *Clin Exp Rheumatol* 1997;15:405–409.
266. Hayashi T, Lee S, Ogasawara H, et al. Exacerbation of systemic lupus erythematosus related to cytomegalovirus infection. *Lupus* 1998;7:561–564.
267. Levy JA, Pincus T. Demonstration of biological activity of a murine leukemia virus of New Zealand black mice. *Science* 1970;170:326–327.
268. Mellors RC, Aoki T, Huebner FJ. Further implications of murine leukemia-like virus in the disorders of NZB mice. *J Exp Med* 1969;129:1045–1061.
269. Mellors RC, Mellors JW. Antigen related to mammalian type C RNA viral p30 proteins is located in renal glomeruli in human systemic lupus erythematosus. *Proc Natl Acad Sci USA* 1976;73: 233–237.
270. Panem S, Ordonez NG, Kirsten WH, et al. Type-C virus expression in systemic lupus erythematosus. *N Engl J Med* 1976;295:470–475.
271. Hicks JT, Aulakh GS, McGrath PP, et al. Search for Epstein-Barr and type C oncornaviruses in systemic lupus erythematosus. *Arthritis Rheum* 1979;22:845–857.
272. Urnovitz HB, Murphy WH. Human endogenous retroviruses: nature, occurrence, and clinical implications in human disease (see comments). *Clin Microbiol Rev* 1996;9:72–99.
273. Ranki A, Kurki P, Riepponen S, et al. Antibodies to retroviral proteins in autoimmune connective tissue disease. *Arthritis Rheum* 1992;35:1483–1487.
274. Krieg AM, Khan AS, Steinberg AD. Expression of an endogenous retroviral transcript is associated with murine lupus. *Arthritis Rheum* 1989;32:322–329.
275. Hishikawa T, Ogasawara H, Kaneko H, et al. Detection of antibodies to a recombinant gag protein derived from human endogenous retrovirus clone 4-1 in autoimmune diseases. *Viral Immunol* 1997;10:137–147.
276. Bengtsson A, Blomberg J, Nived O, et al. Selective antibody reactivity with peptides from human endogenous retroviruses and nonviral poly (amino acids) in patients with systemic lupus erythematosus. *Arthritis Rheum* 1996;39:1654–1663.
277. Li JM, Fan WS, Horsfall AC, et al. The expression of human endogenous retrovirus-3 in fetal cardiac tissue and antibodies in congenital heart block. *Clin Exp Immunol* 1996;104: 388–393.
278. Griffiths DJ, Venables PJ, Weiss RA, et al. A novel exogenous retrovirus sequence identified in humans. *J Virol* 1997;71: 2866–2872.
279. Rigby SP, Griffiths DJ, Weiss RA, et al. Human retrovirus-5 proviral DNA is rarely detected in salivary gland biopsy tissues from patients with Sjogren's syndrome. *Arthritis Rheum* 1997; 40:2016–2021.
280. Griffiths DJ, Cooke SP, Herve C, et al. Detection of human retrovirus 5 in patients with arthritis and systemic lupus erythematosus. *Arthritis Rheum* 1999;42:448–454.
281. Talal N, Garry RF, Schur PH, et al. A conserved idiotype and antibodies to retroviral proteins in systemic lupus erythematosus. *J Clin Invest* 1990;85:1866–1871.
282. Krieg AM, Gourley MF, Perl A. Endogenous retroviruses: potential etiologic agents in autoimmunity. *FASEB J* 1992;6: 2537–2544.
283. Herrmann M, Baur A, Nebel-Schickel H, et al. Antibodies against p24 of HIV-1 in patients with systemic lupus erythematosus. *Viral Immunol* 1992;5:229–231.
284. DeVita VT Jr, Hellman S, Rosenberg SA. *Serologic tests for HIV infection in AIDS-etiology diagnosis, treatment and prevention*, 3rd ed. Philadelphia: JB Lippincott, 1992:141–155.
285. Gul A, Inanc M, Yilmaz G, et al. Antibodies reactive with HIV-1 antigens in systemic lupus erythematosus. *Lupus* 1996;5: 120–122.
286. Talal N, Dauphinee MJ, Dang H, et al. Detection of serum antibodies to retroviral proteins in patients with primary Sjogren's syndrome (autoimmune exocrinopathy). *Arthritis Rheum* 1990;33:774–781.
287. Deas JE, Liu LG, Thompson JJ, et al. Reactivity of sera from systemic lupus erythematosus and Sjogren's syndrome patients with peptides derived from human immunodeficiency virus p24 capsid antigen. *Clin Diagn Lab Immunol* 1998;5:181–185.
288. Nakamura H, Kawakami A, Tominaga M, et al. Relationship between Sjogren's syndrome and human T-lymphotropic virus type 1 infection: follow-up study of 83 patients. *J Lab Clin Med* 2000;135:139–144.
289. Green JE, Hinrichs SH, Vogel J, et al. Exocrinopathy resembling Sjogren's syndrome in HTLV-I tax transgenic mice. *Nature* 1989;341:72–74.
290. Kitajima I, Yamamoto K, Sato K, et al. Detection of human T cell lymphotropic virus type I proviral DNA and its gene expression in synovial cells in chronic inflammatory arthropathy. *J Clin Invest* 1991;88:1315–1322.
291. Danao T, Reghetti G, Yen-Lieberman B, et al. Antibodies to the

human T lymphocytotropic type I in systemic lupus erythematosus. *Clin Exp Rheum* 1991;9:55–58.

292. Query CC, Keene JD. A human autoimmune protein associated with U1-RNA contains a region of homology that is cross-reactive with retroviral p30 gag antigen. *Cell* 1987;51:211–220.
293. Blomberg J, Nived O, Pipkorn R, et al. Increased antiretroviral antibody reactivity in sera from a defined population of patients with systemic lupus erythematosus. Correlation with autoantibodies and clinical manifestations. *Arthritis Rheum* 1994;37:57–66.
294. Solinger AM, Adams LE, Friedman-Kien AE, et al. Acquired immune deficiency syndrome (AIDS) and autoimmunity-mutually exclusive entities? *J Clin Immunol* 1988;8:32–42.
295. Watanabe-Fukunaga R, Brannan CI, Copeland NG, et al. Lymphoproliferation disorder in mice explained by defects in Fas antigens that mediates apoptosis. *Nature* 1992;356:314–317.
296. Nesher G, Osborn TG, Moore TL. Parvovirus infection mimicking systemic lupus erythematosus. *Semin Arthritis Rheum* 1995;24:297–303.
297. Bengtsson A, Widell A, Elmstahl S, et al. No serological indications that systemic lupus erythematosus is linked with exposure to human parvovirus B19. *Ann Rheum Dis* 2000;59:64–66.
298. Finielz P, Lam-Kam-Sang LF, Guiserix J. Systemic lupus erythematosus and thrombocytopenic purpura in two members of the same family following hepatitis B vaccine (letter). *Nephrol Dial Transplant* 1998;13:2420–2421.
299. Scofield RH, James JA. Immunization as a model for systemic lupus erythematosus. *Semin Arthritis Rheum* 1999;29:140–147.
300. Older SA, Battafarano DF, Enzenauer RJ, et al. Can immunization precipitate connective tissue disease? Report of five cases of systemic lupus erythematosus and review of the literature. *Semin Arthritis Rheum* 1999;29:131–139.
301. Shoenfeld Y, Aharon-Maor A, Sherer Y. Vaccination as an additional player in the mosaic of autoimmunity. *Clin Exp Rheumatol* 2000;18:181–184.
302. Gharavi AE, Pierangeli SS. Origin of antiphospholipid antibodies: induction of aPL by viral peptides. *Lupus* 1998;7(suppl 2):S52–S54.
303. Saraux A, Jouquan J, Goff PL, et al. Environmental factors may modulate antiphospholipid antibody production in family members of patients with systemic lupus erythematosus. *Arthritis Rheum* 1999;42:1062–1065.
304. Haaheim LR, Halse AK, Kvakestad R, et al. Serum antibodies from patients with primary Sjogren's syndrome and systemic lupus erythematosus recognize multiple epitopes on the La(SS-B) autoantigen resembling viral protein sequences. *Scand J Immunol* 1996;43:115–121.
305. Koga T, Pearson CM, Narita T, et al. Polyarthritis induced in the rat with cell walls from several bacteria and two streptomyces species. *Proc Soc Exp Biol Med* 1973;143:824–827.
306. Pearson CM. Development of arthritis, periarthritis, periostitis in rats given adjuvants. *Proc Soc Exp Biol Med* 1956;91:95–101.
307. Cavallo T, Granholm NA. Bacterial lipopolysaccharide transforms mesengial into proliferative lupus nephritis without interfering with processing of pathogenic immune complexes in NZB/W mice. *Am J Pathol* 1990;137:971–978.
308. Pisetsky DS. The role of bacterial DNA in host defense and autoimmunity. The Syllabus, American College of Rheumatology, November 1999.
309. Gilkeson GS, Pippen AMM, Pisetsky DS. Induction of cross reactive anti-ds-DNAantibodies in pre-autoimmune NZB/NZW mice by immunization with bacterial DNA. *J Immunol* 1995;95:1398–1402.
310. Yung RL, Richardson BC. Role of T cell DNA methylation in lupus syndromes. *Lupus* 1994;3:487–491.
311. Hess EV. Drug and environmental lupus syndromes. *Br J Rheumatol* 1995;34:597–601.
312. Waring RH, Emery P. The genetic basis of responses to drugs—a rheumatological perspective. *Br J Rheumatol* 1993;32:181–188.
313. Miller FW, Hess EV, Clauw D, et al. Approaches for identifying and defining environmentally associated rheumatic disorders. *Arthritis Rheum* 2000;43:243–249.

4

THE EPIDEMIOLOGY OF SYSTEMIC LUPUS ERYTHEMATOSUS

VIOLETA RUS
MARC C. HOCHBERG

Epidemiology can be defined as the study of the frequency and distribution of disease and the determinants (i.e., factors) associated with disease occurrence and outcome in populations. Epidemiologists design and conduct four major types of studies to evaluate chronic disease: (a) descriptive studies to estimate the incidence and prevalence of and the mortality from disease in relation to characteristics of person, place, and time; (b) observational studies, either retrospective or prospective in design, to derive inferences about etiologic factors associated with the occurrence of disease; (c) observational cohort studies to determine the course and prognosis of patients with a disease; and (d) experimental studies to evaluate preventive or therapeutic measures.

Epidemiologic studies of systemic lupus erythematosus (SLE) have focused on (a) development and validation of criteria for disease classification; (b) estimation of morbidity and mortality rates in different populations at different times; (c) determination of etiologic factors, both host and environmental; (d) estimation of prognosis and survival of patients; and (e) evaluation of treatments in randomized controlled trials. This chapter reviews major findings in the epidemiology of SLE in the first four areas: disease classification, morbidity and mortality rates, etiologic factors, and prognosis and survival. The reader is referred to Chapters 3 and 6 for detailed discussion of the mechanisms underlying the association of genetic and environmental factors, respectively, with SLE.

CLASSIFICATION CRITERIA

In 1971, the American Rheumatism Association (ARA) published preliminary criteria for the classification of SLE (1). At present, the American College of Rheumatology (ACR) 1982 revised criteria for the classification of SLE (2), as modified in 1997 (3), are used for case definition (Table 4.1). The original 1982 data set was reanalyzed by Edworthy et al. (4) using recursive partitioning to generate two classification trees in an attempt to identify simpler and more explicit rules to classify patients with SLE. The resulting simple classification tree requires knowledge of only two variables: immunologic disorder and malar rash. A more complex tree requires knowledge of six variables, including serum complement levels, which is not included within the 1982 revised criteria. The sensitivity, specificity, and accuracy were 96% for the 1982 revised criteria and 92% for the simple classification tree (Table 4.1). Perez-Gutthann et al. (5) compared the sensitivity of the 1982 revised criteria in the traditional format and both classification trees in 198 patients from the Johns Hopkins Lupus Cohort. The revised criteria were significantly more sensitive than the simple classification tree, correctly identifying 184 (93%) compared with 168 (85%) cases, respectively ($p = .016$); the full classification tree correctly identified 186 cases (94%). Thus, these data support the use of the 1982 revised criteria in the traditional format to classify patients with SLE.

Other groups have examined the relative value of an individual criterion in selected patient populations using receiver operating characteristic curves (6) and Bayesian theory (7,8); however, the use of weighted criterion scores has not proven to be more reliable in epidemiologic studies.

Recently, the Diagnostic and Therapeutic Criteria Committee of ACR has updated the 1982 criteria (3). Within criterion 10, item (a), the positive LE cell test, was deleted and item (d) was changed to the positive test for antiphospholipid antibodies including 1) an abnormal serum level of immunoglobulin G (IgG) or M (IgM) anticardiolipin antibodies, 2) a positive test for lupus anticoagulant using a standard method, or 3) a false-positive serologic test for syphilis known to be positive for at least 6 months and confirmed by *Treponema pallidum* immobilization or fluorescent treponemal antibody adsorption test. The updated version was more sensitive (78% vs. 72%), but slightly less specific (88% vs. 91%) than the 1982 criteria in a cohort of 346 patients with connective tissue disease (9).

TABLE 4.1. 1982 REVISED CRITERIA FOR SYSTEMIC LUPUS ERYTHEMATOSUS

	Sensitivity	Specificity	Accuracy[a]
1. Malar rash	57	96	76
2. Discoid rash	18	99	57
3. Photosensitivity	43	96	68
4. Oral ulcers	27	96	60
5. Nonerosive arthritis	86	37	63
6. Pleuritis or pericarditis	56	86	70
7. Renal disorder	51	94	71
8. Seizures or psychosis	20	98	57
9. Hematologic disorder	59	89	73
10. Immunologic disorder	85	93	88
11. Positive antinuclear antibody	99	49	77
>4 criteria	96	96	96
Simple classification tree	92	92	92
Full classification tree	97	95	96

[a]Accuracy is defined as the average of sensitivity and specificity. For definitions of individual criterion items, see Tan et al. (2)
Data from Tan et al. (2) and Edworthy et al. (4).

None of the methods for classifying patients with SLE was designed for diagnostic purposes. These criteria should be used mainly for the purpose of classifying patients in clinical, epidemiologic, and pathogenetic studies of SLE. Assuring homogeneity of the case population is ideal for epidemiologic studies that address etiology or risk factors. However, classification criteria lack sensitivity for recognizing milder cases of SLE, which becomes a limitation for descriptive studies of morbidity and observational studies of prognosis, because subjects with a multisystem disease that is consistent with SLE will not be included if they fail to fulfill the criteria. Data from the Rochester study suggest that the prevalence of suspected SLE is comparable to that of definite SLE: 64 versus 54 per 100,000 in white females and 33 versus 40 per 100,000 overall, respectively (10). For understanding the social burden of the disease and guiding health care and research policy, all patients should be included.

Criteria for classifying the subsets of neuropsychiatric SLE were developed by the Ad Hoc Neuropsychiatric Lupus Workshop Group in 1990 (11). An ad hoc multidisciplinary committee developed standard nomenclature as well as detailed diagnostic and exclusion criteria for 19 neuropsychiatric syndromes in 1997. A detailed discussion of these subsets is included in Chapter 35.

MORBIDITY DATA

Prevalence

The overall prevalence of SLE in the continental United States and Hawaii has been reported to range between 14.6 and 122 cases per 100,000 persons (Table 4.2). Studies have varied over time and place and used different methods of case ascertainment (10,12–18). The studies conducted in San Francisco, California, and Rochester, Minnesota, used both inpatient and outpatient records for case identification and published criteria for case validation; the major differences were the sampling frame (members of the Kaiser Foundation Health Plan and resi-

TABLE 4.2. PREVALENCE OF SLE BY SEX/RACE GROUP IN THE UNITED STATES[a]

Authors	Location	Year	WM	WF	BM	BF	Overall
Siegel and Lee (15)	New York	1965	3	17	3	56	14.6
Fessel (13)	San Francisco	1973	7	71	53	283	50.8
Michet et al. (10)	Rochester, MN	1980	19	54	ND	ND	40.0
Maskarinec and Katz (17)	Hawaii	1989	ND	ND	ND	ND	41.8

[a]Rates per 100,000 persons.
BF, black females; BM, black males; ND, no data; WF, white females; WM, white males.

dents of Olmsted County, respectively) and racial composition of the populations (81% and 99% white, respectively). The sex- and race-specific prevalence estimates for white males and females, however, are comparable, because the 95% confidence intervals (CIs) for these ratios overlap. Estimates of the overall prevalence in whites were 44 and 40 per 100,000, respectively (Table 4.2). The most current estimate in blacks is that from the San Francisco study, but it is based on only 19 patients, 16 of whom were women. Thus, the confidence intervals are wide, limiting the reliability of this estimate.

Applying the rates obtained from the San Francisco study to the 1990 U.S. population, the National Arthritis Data Workgroup estimated that 239,000 cases of suspected or definite SLE were present in the United States: 4,000 white males, 31,000 black males, 163,000 black females, and 41,000 white females (19). Because of limited data on other racial and ethnic groups, no estimates for Hispanics and Asians were attempted. Both of these groups have a higher reported prevalence of SLE than whites (vide infra). In a meta-analysis based on 16 population-based prevalence studies from Europe and North America, Jacobson et al. (20) estimated the weighted mean prevalence rate of SLE at 23.8/100,000. By applying these rates to the 1996 U.S. census data, the authors estimated that a total of 63,052 persons are afflicted with the disease.

Two studies based on self-reported, physician-diagnosed SLE in the United States using data from telephone screening (12,18) suggested that the prevalence of SLE might be much higher. In one study, the prevalence of SLE by unsubstantiated claim was 1 in 177 (18). The prevalence reported by Hochberg et al. (12) after validating the diagnosis of SLE by medical record review was 124 per 100,000. This increased prevalence was confirmed in the most recent study from Rochester, Minnesota, that reported age- and sex–adjusted prevalence rates as of January 1, 1993 to be of 1.22 in 1000 (16).

International studies to estimate the prevalence of SLE have been conducted in Sweden (21,22), Finland (23), Iceland (24,25), New Zealand (26,27), Malaysia (28), England and Wales (29–32), China (33,34), Japan (35,36), the Caribbean island of Curacao (37), and Northern Ireland (38) (Table 4.3). Of the studies conducted in countries with predominantly white populations, prevalence estimates varied from a low of 12.5 per 100,000 females in England (32) to a high of 39 per 100,000 of both sexes combined in Sweden (22). This variability may result from differences in methodology of case ascertainment, including use of general practice diagnostic registries (32), hospital discharge records (23,27,35), outpatient clinic records, surveys of physicians, or combinations thereof (22,25,29–31), as well as from differences in host and environmental factors among different populations. In comparing studies using similar methodologies for case identification and validation, the prevalence of SLE is almost identical. Studies from the United States and Sweden that used hospital records for case identification reported similar prevalence rates of about 40 per 100,000 (10,22), while studies from the United Kingdom using multiple case-finding methods found consistently lower prevalence rates of about 25 per 100,000 (29–31). The lowest rate at 12 per 100,000 was determined through use of general practice diagnostic registries (32). However, true geographic differences in the prevalence of SLE among whites cannot be excluded and may result from differences in genetic and other host or environmental factors (39).

Incidence

The average annual incidence of SLE in the continental United States has been estimated in several studies; inci-

TABLE 4.3. PREVALENCE OF SLE: SELECTED INTERNATIONAL STUDIES

Study	Country	Year	Cases (*n*)	Rate[a]
Meddings and Grennan (27)	New Zealand	1980	16	15
Nived et al. (21)	Sweden	1982	61	39
Helve (23)	Finland	1978	1,323	28
Hochberg (32)	England	1982	20	12[b]
Nakae et al. (35)	Japan	1984	NS	21
Gudmundsson and Steinsson (25)	Iceland	1990	86	36
Samanta et al. (29)	England	1992	50	26
Nossent (37)	Curacao	1992	69	48
Hopkinson et al. (30)	England	1993	137	25
Anstey et al. (51)	Australia	1993	22	52
Johnson et al. (31)	England	1995	242	28
Gourley et al. (38)	N. Ireland	1993	467	254

[a]Rate per 100,000; both sexes combined.
[b]Females only; as no cases identified among males.
NS, not stated.

TABLE 4.4. INCIDENCE OF SLE BY SEX/RACE GROUP IN THE UNITED STATES[a]

Study	Location	Date	WM	WF	BM	BF	Overall
Siegel and Lee (15)	New York	1956–65	0.3	2.5	1.1	8.1	2.0
Fessel (13)	San Francisco	1965–73	ND	ND	ND	ND	7.6
Michet et al. (10)	Rochester, MN	1950–79	0.9	2.5	ND	ND	1.8
		1970–79	0.8	3.4	ND	ND	2.2
Hochberg (40)	Baltimore, MD	1970–77	0.4	3.9	2.5	11.4	4.6
McCarty et al. (41)	Pittsburgh, PA	1985–90	0.4	3.5	0.7	9.2	2.4
Uramoto et al. (16)	Rochester, MN	1950–79	ND	ND	ND	ND	1.51
		1980–92	ND	ND	ND	ND	5.56

[a]Incidence rates per 100,000 persons per year.
BF, black females; BM, black males; ND, no data; WF, white females; WM, white males.

dence rates vary from 1.8 to 7.6 cases per 100,000 persons per year (10,13–16,40,41) (Table 4.4). International studies from Iceland (25), Sweden (21,31,42), the United Kingdom (30,31), Japan (36), and the Caribbean island of Curacao (37) reported incidence rates for SLE of similar magnitude (Table 4.5).

Despite using different methods for case ascertainment, average annual incidence rates of SLE from 1985 to 1990 in Allegheny County, Pennsylvania (41), are quite similar to those reported in Baltimore during an earlier period (40). Of particular interest are the differences in incidence reported by Kurland et al. (14), Michet et al. (10) and Uramoto et al. (16) for the same population using the identical medical record retrieval system. Michet et al. attributed these differences to changes in diagnostic classification. Nonetheless, a temporal trend in incidence among whites can be inferred from the Rochester data. Rates nearly tripled from 1.5 in the 1950–1979 cohort to 5.56 per 100,000 in the 1980–1992 cohort (16). Possible explanations for the increase in incidence is improved recognition of mild disease, increased exposure to hormones such as oral contraceptives and estrogen replacement therapy, and greater exposure to ultraviolet light because of depletion in the ozone layer.

Effects of Age and Sex on Morbidity Rates

The variability in prevalence and incidence rates in different published studies may be explained in part by the effect of age, gender, and race. Overall, prevalence and incidence rates are higher in females compared to males, and higher in African Americans, Afro-Caribbeans, and Asians than in Caucasian populations.

In white females, age-specific incidence rates have varied among studies, and peak incidence rates per 100,000 per year occurred in the 15- to 44-year age group (15), the 20- to 39-year age group (41), the 25- to 44-year age group (10), the 35- to 54-year age group (40), the 45- to 64-year age group (22), the 50- to 74-year age group (25), the 50- to 59-year age group (30), and among those aged 18 and 19 years (31). Median age at diagnosis for white females in these studies ranged from 37 to 50 years, emphasizing that SLE is not necessarily a disease of young women.

Age-specific incidence rates in white males are difficult to interpret because of the small numbers of cases. In those studies with adequate data, peak rates occurred in the 50- to 59-year age group (30) and in those aged 65 and older (10,15). The later onset of SLE in white males

TABLE 4.5. INCIDENCE OF SLE: SELECTED INTERNATIONAL STUDIES

Study	Country	Date	Cases (*n*)	W	M	Overall[a]
Nived et al. (21)	Sweden	1982	61	7.6	2.0	4.8
Jonsson et al. (42)	Sweden	1986	39	—	—	4.0
Iseki et al. (36)	Japan	1984	566	5.3	0.6	3.0
Gudmundsson and Steinsson (25)	Iceland	1990	76	5.8	0.8	3.3
Nossent (37)	Curacao	1992	94	7.9	1.1	4.6
Hopkinson et al. (30)	England	1993	23	6.1	1.3	3.7
Johnson et al. (31)	England	1995	33	6.8	0.5	3.8

[a]Rate per 100,000; both sexes combined.

compared with white females was also noted in the Baltimore study (40) and the Leicester, United Kingdom, study (29).

Age-specific incidence rates in black females were greatest in the 15- to 44-year age group in New York City (15), the 20- to 39-year age group in Pittsburgh (41), and the 25- to 34-year age group in Baltimore (40) and Birmingham, United Kingdom (31), exceeding 20 per 100,000 per year. Age-specific rates in black males can be reliably estimated only from the Baltimore study and reached a peak in the 45- to 64-year age group of 5 per 100,000 per year (40). Among Afro-Caribbeans on the island of Curacao, peak age-specific incidence rates occurred in the 45- to 64-year age group in women and among those aged 65 and older in men (37).

Age-specific prevalence rates for females in the United States are best estimated by the data of Fessel (13): approximately 1 and 4 per 1,000 for white and black women aged 15 to 64 years, respectively. The prevalence of SLE among white women in southern Sweden, 99 per 100,000, is similar to that among white women in the United States (21). Age-standardized prevalence among white women in Iceland was slightly lower, at 62 per 100, 000 (25), while that among white women in the United Kingdom was markedly less, at 32 per 100,000 (29) and 36 per 100,000 (31).

Clinical studies have consistently demonstrated a female predominance approaching 90% of SLE cases. This excess is especially noteworthy in the 15- to 64-year age group, wherein ratios of age- and sex-specific incidence rates show a six- to tenfold female excess in whites and blacks. No such excess was noted in the 14 and younger or the 65 and older age groups in New York City (15), Rochester, Minnesota (10), Sweden (21), or Nottingham, UK (30). A fourfold greater incidence rate in females age 65 and older than in males was found among whites but not blacks in Baltimore (40). These age-related differences in the ratio of sex-specific incidence rates have been thought to relate to hormonal changes that occur during puberty and the child-bearing years.

Effect of Race on Morbidity Rates

The relative increased frequency of SLE in people of African origin was examined by Symmons (43) and more recently by Bae et al. (44). A greater incidence and prevalence of SLE has consistently been found in blacks than in U.S. whites (13,15,40,41). Studies in both New York City (15) and San Francisco (13) found a three- to fourfold greater prevalence in black females aged 15 to 64 than in white females (Table 4.2), and studies in Baltimore and Pittsburgh found a threefold greater age-adjusted average annual incidence rate in black females compared with white females (40,41) (Table 4.4). A study in Birmingham, England, found higher age-adjusted incidence and prevalence rates in Afro-Caribbeans than in whites (31). Age-adjusted incidence rates were 25.8 and 4.3 per 100,000 for Afro-Caribbeans and whites, respectively, and age-adjusted prevalence rates were 112 and 21 per 100,000 for Afro-Caribbeans and whites, respectively. Despite the apparent predilection for women of African origin in Northern Europe, North America, and the Caribbean, the frequency of SLE in West African countries where most of their ancestors originated, as estimated from case reports and small series, is low (44). This "prevalence gradient" may be related to genetic and environmental factors as well as gene-environment interactions (44,45).

In a number of studies, the age distribution of incident cases differed significantly, with a younger median age and earlier peak incidence rates in women of African origin. Mean age in Afro-Caribbean females was 34.5 years, compared with 41 years in white females, and the peak incidence rate was in the 30- to 39-year age group compared with the 40- to 49-year age group, respectively (31). These results are almost identical to those from a study in Baltimore, wherein the mean age of black females with SLE was 35.5 years, compared with 41.7 years for white females (40), and those from a study in Pittsburgh, wherein the mean age of black females was 35.2 years, compared with 39.8 years for white females (41). The mean age at diagnosis was 31 years, with a peak age at diagnosis in the 21- to 30-year age group, in 93 Afro-Caribbean patients from Jamaica; no comparison with white patients was available (46). On the island of Curacao, the mean age at diagnosis was 34 years, with a peak age at diagnosis in the 45- to 64-year age group, in 94 Afro-Caribbean patients; again, no comparison with whites was available (37).

Conflicting data exist regarding excess prevalence of SLE among Asians compared with whites (26,29–31,33–35, 47–49). In Hawaii, compared to Caucasians, the prevalence odds ratio (OR) was 1.3 for Japanese, 1.5 for Filipinos, 2.4 for Chinese, and 0.8 in Hawaiians (17). An earlier study performed by Serdula and Rhoads (47) from 1970 through 1975 reports an estimated age-adjusted prevalence of 5.8 per 100,000 in whites, compared with 17.0 per 100,000 among Asians (Chinese, Filipino, and Japanese). Age-adjusted prevalence rates of SLE in Auckland, New Zealand, were 14.6 and 50.6 per 100,000 in whites and Polynesians, respectively (26). Three studies from the United Kingdom (29–31) found higher age-adjusted incidence and prevalence rates of SLE in Asians (Indian, Pakistani, Bangladeshi) than in whites. In Leicester, England, the age-adjusted prevalence of SLE was 64.0 per 100,000 in Asians, compared with 26.1 per 100,000 in whites (29). In Birmingham, England, the age-adjusted incidence and prevalence rates of SLE in Asians were 20.7 and 46.7 per 100,000 compared with 4.3 and 20.7 per 100,000 in whites, respectively (31). Of interest, neither incidence nor prevalence rates differed by country of birth among Asians in this study.

Casting doubt on real differences between Asians, specifically Chinese, and whites are the findings of Fessel (13) and Nai-Zheng (33,34). In the San Francisco study, the prevalence of SLE was not increased among Chinese compared with whites (13). Data from China based on population surveys suggest a prevalence of SLE between 40 and 70 per 100, 000 (34). Finally, a survey in Taiwan identified only one case of SLE among 1,836 residents and no cases among 2,000 female students (48). Thus, population-based data in three countries fail to support an excess prevalence of SLE among Chinese compared with Caucasians. Prevalence data from Japan also fail to support the observations in Hawaii of an excess prevalence in Japanese compared with whites (35).

No published data exist about incidence rates in Hispanic Americans, but an ongoing study is comparing genetic, clinical, and outcome features in Hispanics, African Americans, and Caucasians (50).

The incidence and prevalence of SLE estimated in an Australian Aboriginal population in the Top End Northern Territory (51) were 11 per 100,000 per year and 52 per 100,000, respectively. The authors suggested these rates were higher than those for Australian whites; however, estimates for the European population in Australia are not available.

An excess incidence and prevalence of SLE among Native American Indians compared with whites was suggested by three studies (52–54). This excess was isolated to only 3 of 75 American Indian tribes (52); a single Pacific Northwest Indian population, the Nootka (53); and three different Indian groups, the Tlingit, Haida, and Tsimshian, living in coastal southeast Alaska (54). Of interest, the prevalence of SLE among Alaskan Inuits is not increased over that which would be expected (55,56). These isolated observations could represent chance findings; on the other hand, inbreeding and/or environmental factors may explain this clustering. Further studies of American Indian populations could identify additional clusters with excess morbidity from SLE in an effort to test hypotheses regarding risk factors.

MORTALITY DATA

Mortality attributed to SLE in the continental United States has been estimated from community-based (15) as well as national data (58,61,62,67) (Table 4.6). Lopez-Acuna et al. (61) identified all deaths attributed to both discoid and systemic lupus erythematosus from National Center for Health Statistics (NCHS) data tapes for the period 1968 to 1978. A total of 11,156 deaths were identified, 2, 568 (23.0%) of which were attributed to discoid lupus and 8,588 (77.0%) to SLE. There were no differences in the distribution of deaths from discoid lupus and SLE by sex/race, region, or year; therefore, the authors combined results for their analysis. There were a total of 6,452 deaths in white females, 2,573 in black females, 1,760 in white males, and 371 in black males, with average age-adjusted mortality rates of 6.0, 17.6, 1.8, and 3.0 per 1 million persons per year, respectively (Table 4.6). Age-specific average annual mortality rates showed a unimodal distribution for all sex/race groups, with maximum rates occurring in the 45- to 54-year age group for blacks and the 65- to 74-year age group for whites (Fig. 4.1).

Kaslow (62) analyzed a subset of these mortality records and examined deaths attributed to SLE alone from 1968 through 1976 in the 12 states with 88% of U.S. residents of Asian descent. Mortality rates were threefold greater among blacks and twofold greater among Asians compared with whites—8.4, 6.8, and 2.8 per 1 million person-years, respectively. Age- and sex-adjusted mortality rates for Chinese, Japanese, and Filipinos were 7.5, 6.8, and 5.1 per 1 million persons-years, respectively. Age- and sex-adjusted race-specific mortality rates in Hawaii were greatest among Filipinos and higher in the combined Asian group than for the U.S. mainland population, confirming previous observations (47). A study from Hawaii reported that mortality rates were three times higher in non-Caucasian than Cau-

TABLE 4.6. CAUSE-SPECIFIC MORTALITY FROM SLE BY SEX/RACE GROUP IN THE UNITED STATES[a]

Study	Years	WM	WF	BM	BF
Cobb (67)	1959–61	1.1	4.0	1.8	10.6
Siegel and Lee (15)	1956–65	1.6	6.6	4.4	20.0
Kaslow and Masi (59)	1972–76	1.5	5.2	2.2	14.8
Gordon et al. (58)	1972–76	1.2	4.5	1.9	13.1
Lopez-Acuna et al. (61)[b]	1968–78	1.8	6.0	3.0	17.6

[a]Rates per 1 million persons per year.
[b]Includes deaths attributed to both discoid lupus erythematosus and SLE.
BF, black females; BM, black males; WF, white females; WM, white males.

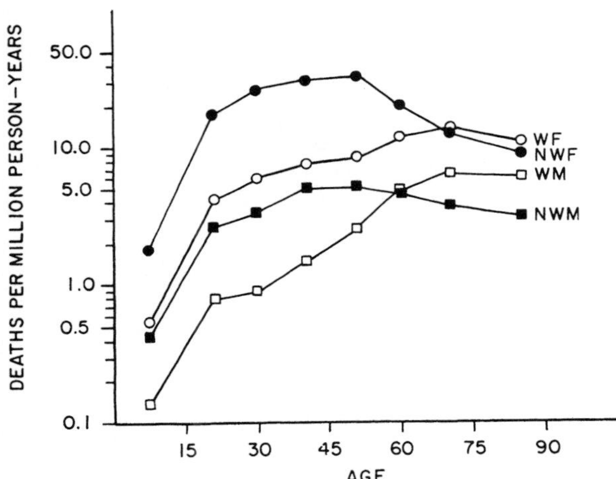

FIGURE 4.1. Average annual age-specific mortality rates attributed to lupus erythematosus by sex/race group in the United States, 1968 to 1978. (White males □, white females ○, black males ■, black females ●).

casians in 1985–1989 (17). It is unclear whether the differences in mortality rates between Asians and whites mirror true differences in incidence rates as seen with blacks (vide supra).

Siegel and Lee (15) noted greater mortality and morbidity from SLE among Puerto Ricans compared with whites in New York City. Lopez-Acuna et al. (63) analyzed mortality from SLE in Puerto Rico from 1970 through 1977 as well as a subset of the NCHS data set for five western and southwestern states with the highest proportion of Hispanics: Arizona, California, Colorado, New Mexico, and Texas. A total of 92 deaths from SLE occurred in Puerto Rico; the average age-adjusted mortality rates of 7.5 and 2.0 deaths per 1 million person-years in females and males, respectively, were not significantly different from those noted among U.S. whites over this period. A correlation between the proportion of Spanish-heritage population and county-specific mortality rates from SLE was noted for females but not males in these five states; the implications of this finding may reflect both ethnic/racial and socioeconomic factors. Cause-specific mortality data from Latin American countries have not been reported.

Data on nationwide mortality from SLE have been reported from Finland (23), Iceland (25), England and Wales (64), and the island of Curacao (37). Average mortality rates were 4.7, 2.5, and 17.0 per 1 million person-years in Finland, England and Wales, and Curacao, respectively. Patterns of age-specific mortality rates in Finland as well as England and Wales were similar to those in U.S. whites. The fourfold greater age-adjusted mortality among English females compared with males is similar to that seen in the United States as well. Patterns of age-specific mortality rates in Curacao were similar to those in blacks, with a peak mortality rate in the 45- to 64-year age group and a fourfold greater mortality in women than in men (37).

Temporal trends in mortality rates have been examined in the United States (58,61) and in England and Wales (64). In the United States, there was a significant decline in age-adjusted annual mortality rates between 1968 and 1978 for all sex/race groups (61) (Fig. 4.2). A significant temporal decline in age-adjusted annual mortality rates from SLE also was observed among females in England and Wales from 1974 to 1983 but not among males, probably because of the small numbers of deaths from SLE among males (64). A similar decline in mortality was observed in the Toronto Cohort, where estimated risk for death was compared for patients entered in the cohort between 1970–1977, 1978–1986, and 1987–1994 (65). The standardized mortality ratios declined from 10.1 in the first group to 3.3 in the last group. The same decline was observed for the first two groups followed over the next time period. The decline in mortality rates observed in these developed countries is probably due to improved survival in patients with SLE, as reflected by (a) a temporal increase in the mean age at death from SLE in the United States between 1968 and 1978 (61) (Fig. 4.3), and (b) 10-year cumulative survival rates approaching or exceeding 90% in some studies (66) (vide infra).

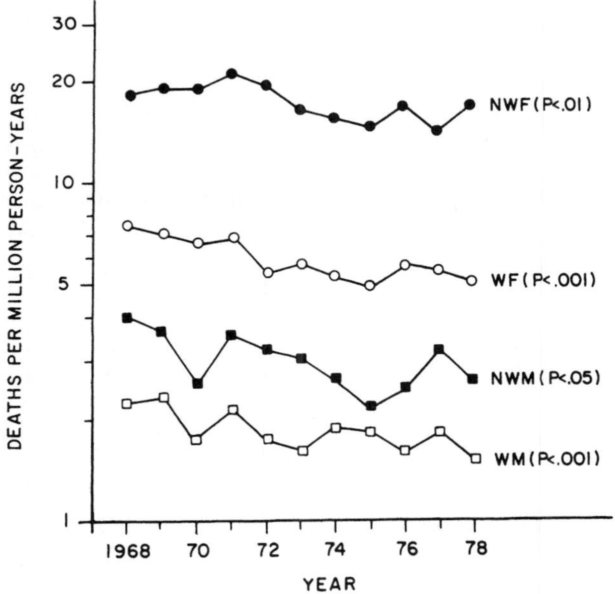

FIGURE 4.2. Trends in age-adjusted annual mortality rates from lupus erythematosus by sex/race group in the United States, 1968 to 1978. (White males □, white females ○, black males ■, black females ●).

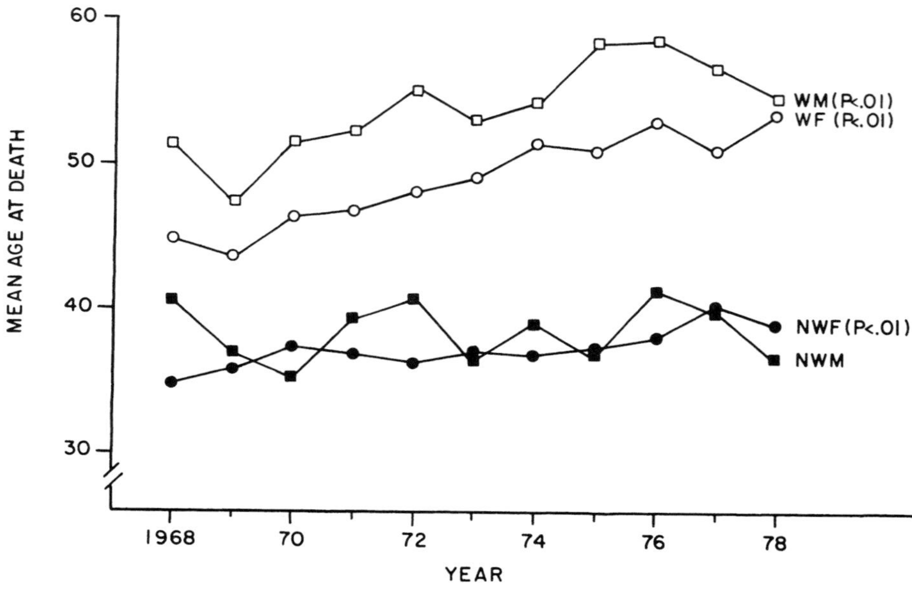

FIGURE 4.3. Trends in mean age at death from lupus erythematosus by sex/race group in the United States, 1968 to 1978. (White males □, white females ○, black males ■, black females ●).

PROGNOSIS AND SURVIVAL

Longitudinal observational studies of patients with SLE to estimate prognosis with respect to survival have been conducted for over four decades (Table 4.7). The first such study found a 51% cumulative survival rate at 4 years after diagnosis (68), while current studies in developed countries suggest that the 10-year cumulative survival rate approaches or exceeds 90% and the 20-year cumulative survival rate approaches 70% (16,65,69,70). The improved survival in patients with SLE may have resulted from advances in medical therapy in general, more judicious use of lupus-specific therapy, earlier diagnosis, and inclusion of milder cases in more recent studies. In developing countries like India and among black Caribbean patients, poorer survival has been recorded (71–73). This section highlights host and disease factors that are associated with decreased survival and the causes of death in

TABLE 4.7. CUMULATIVE SURVIVAL RATES IN SLE: 1954 TO 1995

Study	Center	Year	5 Years	10 Years	15 Years
Merrill and Shulman (68)	Baltimore	1954	51	—	—
Kellum and Haserick (75)	Cleveland	1964	69	54	—
Estes and Christian (76)	New York	1971	77	60	—
Feinglass et al. (77)	Baltimore	1976	94	82	—
Hochberg et al. (78)	Baltimore	1981	97	90	—
Wallace et al. (79)	Los Angeles	1981	88	79	—
Ginzler et al. (80)	Multicenter	1982	88	71	—
Rubin et al. (81)	Toronto	1985	88	—	—
Stafford-Brady et al. (82)	Toronto	1988	84	75	—
Swaak et al. (83)	Netherlands	1989	94	87	—
Jonsson et al. (22)	Sweden	1989	95	—	—
Reveille et al. (84)	Birmingham	1990	90	87	—
Gripenberg and Helve (85)	Finland	1991	—	91	—
Pistiner et al. (103)	Los Angeles	1991	97	93	—
Ward et al. (69)	Durham	1993	82	71	63
Abu-Shakra et al. (86)	Toronto	1993	93	85	—
Nossent (72)	Curacao	1993	56	—	—
Massardo (88)	Chile	1994	92	77	66
Tucker et al. (89)	London	1995	93	85	79

patients with SLE as well as measures of morbidity among long-term survivors. Reviews of prognostic studies in SLE have been published elsewhere (66,74).

Factors Associated with Survival

A number of demographic features such as gender, age at onset, race, and socioeconomic status may be predictive for mortality in patients with SLE. Although cause-specific mortality rates from SLE increase with advancing age, studies of age at diagnosis as an independent predictor of survival have been conflicting. Several studies suggested that a higher age at presentation was a risk factor for death (69,80, 84,86). However, in a study comparing adult- and childhood-onset SLE patient populations, no significant differences in the 1- to 5-year mortality were demonstrated (89). In contrast, Wallace et al. (79) found that an earlier age at diagnosis of SLE was detrimental to survival. The effect of gender on mortality has been controversial (36,90–93). However, in general, once differences in age distribution between male and female patients with SLE are considered, gender is not a significant predictor of survival.

Race, on the other hand, does appear to be a significant predictor of survival, with blacks having a worse prognosis than U.S. whites (80,84,94), and Asians living in England having a worse prognosis than English whites (95). In addition, Asian Indian, black Caribbean, and Chilean patients with SLE all appear to have a worse prognosis than either North American or European whites (72,88,96).

Ginzler et al. (80) noted a worse prognosis for blacks compared with whites in the Multicenter Lupus Survival Study. When they entered the study, blacks had more severe disease than whites, as reflected by a higher mean number of ARA criteria, higher mean serum creatinine level, lower mean hematocrit, and greater frequency of central nervous system involvement. Blacks also were more likely to have public rather than private medical insurance. When these confounding variables were considered in a multivariate model, however, black race was no longer a significant predictor of decreased survival. Reveille et al. (84) studied survival among 389 patients with SLE seen at the University of Alabama at Birmingham between 1975 and 1984. They also found that black patients had a worse prognosis than whites, even after adjustment in multivariate analysis for the source of medical insurance. Of interest was their finding of a higher frequency of renal involvement in black compared with white patients. Black patients have been found to have a greater frequency of renal disease in other studies (97,98), one of which attributed this in part to a higher frequency of hypertension and poor compliance with medical care (98).

Studenski et al. (94) studied the survival of 411 patients with SLE seen at the Duke University Medical Center between 1969 and 1984. Nonwhite race and public funding of medical care both were significantly associated with decreased survival, even after adjustment in a multivariate model. Ward et al. (69) extended these observations to a median duration of observation of 11 years in the same cohort of patients. Old age, male sex, black race, lack of private medical insurance, and low household income were associated with decreased survival in univariate analysis, but only age, sex, and socioeconomic indicators remained associated in multivariate analysis. When analysis was limited to lupus-related mortality, only lower household income remained an independent predictor of survival. Recently, the same author (99) compared the rate of in-hospital mortality in almost 10,000 patients and reported a lower mortality risk in patients admitted at hospitals with more than 50 urgent or emergency SLE admissions per year compared to patients admitted at hospitals with less experience in caring for SLE (OR = .34, 95% CI 0.19–0.58).

Regarding the clinical and laboratory features of SLE, renal disease, as measured by either serum creatinine or qualitative urine protein excretion, is by far the most important predictor of poor outcome (79,80,84,86,88,100–103). In an analysis of 51 deaths occurring among 310 patients with SLE with 1,234 patient-years of follow-up, patients with systolic blood pressure of 145 mm Hg or greater, especially in combination with a serum urea nitrogen level of 40 mg/dL or greater, had the worst prognosis (71). In patients with lupus nephritis, those with diffuse proliferative nephritis on biopsy have the worst prognosis compared with other World Health Organization classes (101,102). Among those with diffuse proliferative glomerulonephritis, chronic changes involving the glomerulus and interstitium suggest a poorer prognosis (102,104,105). In one study of an inception cohort of 87 patients with lupus nephritis, those with evidence of either severe disease or renal damage at presentation, marked by a serum creatinine level of 1.5 mg/dL or greater, 24-hour urine protein of 2.6 g or greater, or concomitant hypertension, had a worse prognosis (106). In another study of 123 patients with lupus who underwent renal biopsy between 1970 and 1984, the 18 patients with serum creatinine greater than 120 mol/L had a worse prognosis; among the 105 patients with normal serum creatinine levels, those with either proliferative or chronic lesions on biopsy had a worse prognosis (102). The role of chronic lesions on biopsy as a poor prognostic marker was confirmed in a study of 116 patients with lupus nephritis from the Netherlands (104). Central nervous system involvement has also been associated with decreased survival (76, 80,83,107), although not to the same degree as renal involvement, and not in all cohorts in which it was studied (77). Sibley et al. (108) suggested that central nervous system involvement was a poor prognostic factor only in patients with active disease in other organs.

Lung involvement including pleuritis, lupus pneumonitis, pulmonary hemorrhage, and pulmonary hypertension was found to be a predictive factor for mortality (86). When using the Systemic Lupus International Collaborative Clinics/American College of Rheumatology (SLICC/ACR) Damage Index, the mean pulmonary damage score at 1 year significantly predicted death at 10 years after diagnosis (109).

Greater overall disease activity, as measured by the Systemic Lupus Erythematosus Disease Activity Index (SLEDAI) at the time of first visit to a lupus clinic, was shown to be an independent predictor of worse survival in a published study of a cohort of Canadian patients (86). The SLICC/ACR Damage Index was not independently associated with poorer survival in a study on 90 Afro-Caribbean patients (110), but predicted poor outcome defined as death in an international study (111).

Laboratory markers of SLE, particularly antibodies to native DNA, Sm, and other nuclear antigens, although useful in diagnosis, are not independent predictors of outcome (81,102,103,112,113). Two studies, however, have found decreased survival in patients with positive tests for antiphospholipid antibodies (114,115). Anemia was found to be an independent predictor of poor survival in one study even after adjustment for the presence of renal disease (80). Thrombocytopenia has been also found to be an independent predictor of survival in several studies (84,86,88, 103,116).

Causes of Death

Fatalities among patients with SLE are primarily attributable to active disease such as renal and central nervous system involvement and systemic vasculitis, followed by infections and thromboses (69,72,103,112,117–120). The infections may be bacterial and involve multiple organisms, often occurring in the setting of active SLE, or opportunistic, occurring in patients receiving high-dose steroids and cytotoxic therapy (118,119,121,122). Comorbid conditions and other complications of therapy account for the remainder of deaths.

During the past decade, increasing attention has been directed toward a potentially preventable cause of mortality: corticosteroid-associated coronary artery disease (81,112, 123,124). Indeed, in one study the incidence of myocardial infarction was ninefold higher than in the control population (22), while another found that women with lupus in the 35- to 44-year age group were over 50 times more likely to have a myocardial infarction than were women of similar age in the Framingham Offspring Study (125). In a study of 229 patients with SLE, Petri et al. (126) identified 19 patients with coronary artery disease and examined factors associated with this outcome. Univariate analysis identified male gender, older age at diagnosis, longer duration of SLE, longer duration of prednisone therapy, history of hypertension, hypercholesterolemia, and obesity as predictors of coronary artery disease in these subjects. In multivariate analysis, age at diagnosis, duration of prednisone therapy, use of antihypertensive therapy, hypercholesterolemia, and obesity were all independently associated with increased risk. Another study of 64 patients from England confirmed the role of hyperlipidemia as a risk factor for the development of cardiovascular disease (127), while a third study of 75 patients from Sweden confirmed the association of corticosteroid therapy with cardiovascular disease (128). Rahman et al. (129) showed that SLE patients with a cardiac event have fewer traditional risk factors than non-SLE patients with premature atherosclerosis; therefore, variables independent of traditional risk factors contribute to the development of coronary artery disease in SLE. Thus, efforts in patient management should be directed not only at keeping corticosteroid doses as low as possible with use of hydroxychloroquine and other steroid-sparing agents, but also at preventing and aggressively treating known risk factors for coronary artery disease, including hypercholesterolemia, obesity, hypertension, and diabetes, and at counseling against smoking and a sedentary lifestyle (113,114).

An increased risk of malignancy in patients with SLE was shown in some but not all studies. Compared with age- and sex-specific cancer incidence rates from the Finnish Cancer Registry, the relative risk of developing cancer in 205 patients with SLE was 2.6; the relative risk exceeded 40.0 for non-Hodgkin's lymphoma (130). The standardized incidence ratio (SIR) for all malignancies in 616 women with SLE from Cook County, Illinois, was 2.0 (131), while among 219 female patients residents of Allegheny County, Pennsylvania, was only 1.4 (132). Further multicenter, longitudinal cohort studies are needed to determine if there is an increased incidence of malignancy in patients with SLE and if factors such as immunosuppressive therapy are related to the development of cancer in these patients.

MORBIDITY OUTCOMES

In the face of improving survival among patients with SLE, attention over the past decade has been directed increasingly toward outcome measures other than survival. It has been suggested that three aspects of the disease are necessary to describe prognosis in SLE: disease activity, accumulated damage, and health status/quality of life (133).

Measurement of disease activity using validated quantitative indices has been recommended as both an outcome and an independent variable (134). A number of reliable indices have been developed for use in clinical research (115,135–139). These indices have been validated (138, 140–143) and shown to be sensitive to change over time (144); this area is reviewed in Chapter 2.

Gladman and Urowitz (145) reviewed disease-related morbidity outcomes, including renal failure, atherosclerosis and coronary artery disease, avascular necrosis of bone, and cognitive neuropsychologic dysfunction, and Urowitz (124) suggested the use of a damage index for clinical epidemiologic studies. SLICC, in conjunction with the ACR, has developed and validated the SLICC/ACR Damage Index for use in clinical studies of SLE (146,147). This index summarizes damage across 12 organ systems and describes accumulated organ damage since the onset of SLE. The index has been proven to be reliable (148) and valid (109).

In addition to the description of disease activity and damage in patients with SLE, several investigators have studied physical disability and psychosocial adjustment as health status outcomes in patients with SLE (133, 149–153). Hochberg et al. (149,150) as well as others (154, 155) have studied physical disability, measured with the Health Assessment Questionnaire, and psychosocial adjustment as health status outcomes in patients with SLE. These studies have demonstrated significant interrelationships between physical disability, psychosocial adjustment, coping mechanisms, and self-efficacy behaviors; patients with greater levels of physical disability had worse psychosocial adjustment and poorer coping mechanisms and self-efficacy behaviors. In addition, sociodemographic factors, including lower formal educational level, and selected clinical features, including arthritis and fatigue, were associated with greater degrees of physical disability and worse psychosocial adjustment.

Finally, several groups have examined perceived quality of life as a health status outcome in patients with SLE (156, 157). These studies support the clinical observations that morbidity outcomes in SLE are multidimensional (158). Indeed, the preliminary core set for outcome in SLE adopted at the OMERACT IV meeting includes disease activity, health-related quality of life, damage, and toxicity/adverse events (159).

ETIOLOGIC FACTORS

Epidemiologic studies of etiologic factors in SLE have focused on three broad areas: (a) endocrine-metabolic factors, (b) environmental factors, and (c) genetic factors.

Endocrine-Metabolic Factors

The strongest risk factor for the development of SLE is female gender. In a review of five series of juvenile-onset and seven series of adult-onset SLE, totaling 317 and 1, 177 cases, respectively, Masi and Kaslow (160) showed that the sex ratio at age of onset or diagnosis rises with puberty from 2 : 1 to approximately 6 : 1, peaks in young adulthood at 8 : 1, and then declines with female menopause in the sixth decade of life (Table 4.8). The authors felt these data indicated that study of sex-related factors offered a clue to the pathogenesis of SLE. Studies in the New Zealand black/white (NZB/W) F1 hybrid mouse, a murine model of SLE, support a role for female hormones in the modulation of autoantibody production, development of renal disease, and death (161). Indeed, Lahita as well as others have reported abnormalities in the metabolism of estrogens and androgens in both males and females with SLE (162,163).

TABLE 4.8. FEMALE-TO-MALE SEX RATIO AT AGE OF ONSET OR DIAGNOSIS IN SLE

Age of Onset (y)	Female (*n*)	Male (*n*)	F:M Ratio
0–9	39	19	2.0
10–19	220	39	5.6
20–29	369	49	7.5
30–39	298	37	8.0
40–49	183	35	5.2
50–59	98	25	3.9
60+	58	25	2.3
Total	1,265	229	5.5

Adapted from Masi AT, Kaslow RA. Sex effects in systemic lupus erythematosus: a clue to pathogenesis. *Arthritis Rheum* 1978;21: 480–484.

Two case-control studies have investigated the role of clinically recognizable endocrine factors in the etiology of SLE. Grimes et al. (164) found no association of age at menarche, parity, history of infertility, fetal wastage, or oral contraceptive usage with SLE. Hysterectomy appeared to be protective, with a crude odds ratio of 0.55; however, after adjustment for age, the odds ratio was 0.73 (95% CI 0.4–1.5) (164). Simultaneous adjustment for age and race was not performed. A history of endometriosis was more common in women with SLE, but the odds ratio did not significantly differ from unity.

Hochberg and Kaslow (165) found no significant differences between cases and controls in age at menarche, age at first intercourse, and proportion with irregular menses, history of infertility, or usage of oral contraceptives. History of pregnancy ending in miscarriage was associated with SLE (OR = 2.7, 95% CI 1.4–5.2), as was being pregnant on one or more occasions without having a live birth (OR = 17.3, p = .006). Fetal-maternal microchimerism resulting from passage of the fetal cells in maternal circulation during pregnancy has not been found to be a risk factor for the development of SLE (166).

Sanchez-Guerrero et al. (167) used the Nurses' Health Study as a prospective cohort to study the role of the use of oral contraceptives in the development of SLE, and found that past use of oral contraceptives was associated with a slightly increased risk of developing SLE (relative risk of 1.4, 95% CI 1.1–3.3). The oral contraceptives used by this cohort in 1960 to 1970 contained higher estrogen doses than the oral contraceptives used currently. In two case-control studies, oral contraceptives use prior to diagnosis was not associated with an increased risk for lupus (164, 168). Overall the current data do not definitely support an association between the use of oral contraceptives and an increased risk for SLE. In a subset of nurses who were postmenopausal at entry into the cohort, Sanchez-Guerrero et al. (169) analyzed the relation between postmenopausal hormone use and development of SLE. An increase in the risk for SLE of 2.1 (95% CI 1.1–4.0) for ever-users, 2.5 (95% CI 1.2–5.0) for current users, and 1.8 (95% CI 0.8–4.1) for past users was observed. The risk was proportionally related to the duration of use of postmenopausal hormones (test for trend, $p = .011$). The role of hormonal manipulation on disease activity is also an active area of investigation (170). Large prospective double-blind placebo-controlled studies such as the Safety in Estrogens in Lupus Erythematosus-National Assessment (SELENA) trial should provide the basis for definitive recommendations.

Environmental Factors

Historically, SLE has been considered to probably have a viral etiology (171,172). Despite several decades of investigation, however, no firm documentation of a definite viral etiology has been identified. Some studies have focused on human retroviruses, especially human T-lymphotropic virus type 1 (HTLV-1) and human immunodeficiency virus (HIV). Most studies have failed to demonstrate an association between antibodies to HTLV-1 and SLE (173–176). Talal et al. (177) found a higher incidence of antibodies to HIV, but this finding was not confirmed in other populations (178).

Antibodies to specific viruses have been shown to cross-react with autoantigens such as vesicular stomatitis virus with Ro (179) and Epstein-Barr virus with Sm antigen (180). Hardgrave et al. (179) found that a greater proportion of patients with SLE than controls had antibodies against the viral proteins of vesicular stomatitis virus. Also, in SLE patients the antibodies displayed a different binding pattern that included the internal viral matrix and nucleocapsid proteins.

Blomberg et al. (181) examined the frequency of antibodies cross-reactive with purified C-type retrovirus particles and with synthetic retroviral peptides in patients with SLE and population controls; they found that a greater proportion of patients with SLE reacted with viral proteins, including whole baboon endogenous virus and murine leukemia virus, and that reactivity with whole baboon endogenous virus correlated with the presence of antibodies to U1 ribonucleoproteins.

James and colleagues (180) have reported a higher rate of seroconversion to Epstein-Barr virus in young patients with SLE compared with controls (OR = 49.9, 95% CI 9.3–10.25) and Rider et al. (182) reported an increased prevalence for cytomegalovirus (CMV) in SLE patients compared with normal controls (OR = 14.53, 95% CI 6.39–33.04). In both studies, no difference was found in the seroconversion rates against other herpes viruses. However, in a case-control study by Strom et al. (168), the occurrence of herpes zoster before the diagnosis of SLE was associated with a risk of developing SLE (age-, sex-, and race-adjusted OR = 6.4, 95% CI 1.4–28.0). The implications for a viral etiology of SLE, however, are unclear.

The presence of a transmissible agent, presumably viral, was hypothesized to explain the co-occurrence of human and canine SLE in the same household (183). One study found no association of dog ownership with SLE (165) and another study found no excess cases of SLE or asymptomatic subjects with anti-DNA antibodies among household contacts of index dogs (184). In one study, fewer than half of the dogs owned by patients with SLE had abnormal serum protein electrophoresis and elevated titers of anti-DNA antibodies compared with none of the control dogs (185). However, the control dogs, owned by pharmaceutical companies, were housed in special environments, and were not comparable to the pets owned by the patients.

The most likely noninfectious environmental factors with an etiologic role in SLE are chemicals. The syndrome of drug-induced lupus, most commonly reported with hydralazine, procainamide, and isoniazid (186), and environmental lupus syndromes (187) provide models to study the possible effects of chemicals, especially aromatic amines (188). In one initial case-control study, Freni-Titulaer et al. (189) found an association between use of hair dyes and connective tissue diseases, including SLE (OR = 7.2, 95% CI 1.9–26.9), but two subsequent case-control studies (190,191) and one cohort study (192) failed to demonstrate an association between the use of hair products and the development of SLE.

Reidenberg (188) hypothesized that slow acetylation was a risk factor for the development of SLE as an explanation for drug-induced lupus and the possible association of exposure to aromatic amines with SLE. Several studies, however, failed to confirm an independent association of slow acetylation with SLE (57,60,190). Thus, data from controlled epidemiologic studies fail to support a role for environmental factors in the etiology of idiopathic SLE.

Several epidemiologic studies have examined the association between SLE and silica dust exposure. A high SLE prevalence of 93 per 100,000 found in male uranium workers (193), a higher than expected number of SLE and SLE overlap syndrome cases among workers at a silica-containing scouring powder plant (194), and a significantly increased number of hospitalizations for treatment of SLE among silicotic men [relative risk (RR) = 23.8, 95% CI 11.9–86.3] (195) suggest that workers occupationally exposed to silica have a higher probability of developing clinical manifestations of SLE. Other putative environmental or occupational triggers and the mechanisms underlying their possible association with SLE have been recently reviewed (196).

Four case-control and four cohort studies have examined the association between breast implants and connective tissue diseases including SLE (197–204). In a recent meta-analysis of these studies, Janowsky et al. (206) found a summary, unadjusted OR of 0.63 (95% CI 0.44–0.86). When the data were reanalyzed after limiting the analysis to five studies that provided an adjusted estimate, the adjusted relative risk for SLE was 1.01; hence, silicon-breast implants do not appear to be associated with a risk for SLE (206).

Dietary factors including antioxidants were explored by Comstock et al. (207) in a nested case-control study of six SLE patients and 24 controls. Although the number of cases was too small to allow definite conclusions, the levels of α-tocopherol, β-carotene, and retinol measured in serum that was collected more than 2 years prior to the onset of disease were 13% to 20% lower in SLE patients compared to controls. As dietary factors are potentially modifiable risk factors, future epidemiologic studies should investigate their possible association with SLE.

Genetic Factors

The application of genetic epidemiology to SLE has generated strong evidence for a hereditary predisposition to this disorder. These data have been reviewed elsewhere (205, 208) and are discussed in detail in Chapter 6.

Familial aggregation of SLE has been demonstrated in two studies (209,210). Hochberg et al. (209) studied the occurrence of SLE among first-degree relatives of 77 patients with SLE and age-, sex-, and race-matched controls without a history of rheumatic disease. Eight (10.4%) of the SLE probands had one or more first-degree relatives with SLE, compared with only 1 (1.3%) of the controls (RR = 8, p = .03). SLE occurred in 9 (1.67%) of 541 first-degree relatives of SLE probands but in only 1 (0.19%) of 540 first-degree relatives of controls (RR = 9, p = .01). Of the nine affected first-degree relatives of SLE probands, seven were female and two male, while the only affected control first-degree relative was female. The prevalence of SLE in female first-degree relatives was 2.64 per 100 for patients versus 0.40 per 100 for controls (RR = 6.8, p = .04).

Lawrence et al. (210) studied 41 consecutive patients with SLE, identified from hospital registers, who had 147 available first-degree relatives aged 15 and older, of whom 128 were fully evaluated with examinations and serologic studies. Control relatives were selected from family surveys of probands with osteoarthritis, psoriasis, and colitis. Definite SLE was found in 5 (3.9%) of the first-degree relatives of SLE probands, compared with only 1 (0.8%) of the 128 matched first-degree relatives of controls (p = .001).

Twin studies have demonstrated a concordance rate among monozygotic twins ranging between 24% and 69%, compared to the 2% to 9% concordance rate among dizygotic twins, providing further support for a genetic contribution to the mechanism of familial aggregation of SLE (211–214). Block et al. (211) found a concordance for clinical SLE in 4 (57%) of the seven monozygotic pairs and in none of the three dizygous pairs. Of the 12 monozygotic pairs in the literature, concordance for SLE was documented in seven (58%). A more recent study based on self-reported diagnoses of persons listed in a nationwide, chronic disease twin registry in the United States found a lower rate of concordance in monozygous twin pairs (212). Of 45 same-sex monozygous twin pairs, 11 (24%) reported concordance for SLE, compared with only 1 (3%) of 38 same-sex dizygous twin pairs. In a study from Finland, only one of nine monozygotic twin pairs was definitely concordant for SLE, while two additional monozygotic twin pairs probably were concordant for SLE (i.e., the co-twin fulfilled only three of the ACR classification criteria). None of ten dizygotic twin pairs were concordant for SLE in yet another study (213). Grennan et al. (214) found that 25% of monozygotic twins were concordant for SLE, while none of the 18 human leukocyte antigen (HLA) identical, same-sex siblings of SLE probands had definite SLE, suggesting that most of the genetic predisposition to SLE may be attributed to genes outside the HLA region (214). Arnett and Shulman (215) noted a striking concordance for clinical and laboratory features of SLE in monozygotic twin pairs compared with nontwin sib pairs. The concordance of autoantibody profiles in monozygotic twin pairs was confirmed by Reichlin et al. (216). These observations also support a genetic influence on disease expression in SLE.

Two separate analyses support a polygenic mode for inheritance of SLE. Using Block's data on concordance for SLE in monozygotic twin pairs, Winchester and Nunez-Roldan (217) calculated that a multigenic hypothesis with either three or four dominant alleles best explained the familial inheritance of SLE. Lawrence et al. (210) determined that a pattern of polygenic inheritance with only moderate heritability best fit their family data. Advances in quantitative methods of segregation analysis, however, have allowed the study of single-gene effects in other conditions thought to have a polygenic mode of inheritance.

Segregation or pedigree analysis has been applied to SLE to determine the mode of mendelian inheritance in multicase families. Arnett et al. (218) studied 19 multicase SLE families with 232 relatives, of whom 24 had SLE, 27 other autoimmune diseases, and 47 serologic abnormalities including high-titer antinuclear antibodies, antibody to single-stranded DNA, or a false-positive test for syphilis. They postulated a single, genetically determined autoimmune trait and applied segregation analysis to the family data. The results were consistent with a mendelian dominant inheritance pattern with a gene frequency of 0.06 and 91% penetrance. The expression of autoimmunity was modified by gender and age at the time of study, but not by HLA-DR phenotype. Further studies by this group estimated the population frequency of the autoimmune gene as 0.10, with penetrance of 92% in females and 49% in males (219). Linkage of this autoimmune gene to other genetic markers was also studied by Arnett's group (219), but they failed to demonstrate linkage with any HLA phenotype, immunoglobulin allotype, or 21 other polymorphic genetic markers. More recently, genome screens for human SLE by linkage analysis have indicated candidate genes on chromosome 1 and several other chromosomal regions (220–222).

Other genetic factors identified in SLE to date, including HLA genes, genes involved in immune complex clearance, genes implicated in tolerance, and regulation of inflammation, are reviewed in detail in Chapter 6.

SUMMARY

Descriptive epidemiologic studies of SLE have been conducted worldwide; the most extensive data are available for the United Kingdom, Scandinavia (especially Sweden), and the United States. In the United States, blacks have threefold higher incidence and prevalence rates of SLE, as well as cause-specific mortality rates, compared with whites, while in England, Asian Indians and Afro-Caribbeans have higher incidence and prevalence rates than whites. The reasons for this excess, however, remain unknown. Analytic and genetic epidemiologic studies suggest a multifactorial etiology of SLE, and results support a polygenic mode of inheritance, including important roles for a theoretic, autosomal-dominant autoimmune gene and female sex hormones. Although a viral etiology remains attractive, there is little direct evidence to support such a hypothesis. Similarly, epidemiologic studies provide little if any support for the role of environmental factors, including chemical exposures, as risk factors for idiopathic SLE. Finally, observational epidemiologic studies have demonstrated an increasingly favorable prognosis for patients with SLE, allowing the identification of potentially preventable causes of death and a better understanding of long-term morbidity and impact on overall health status.

REFERENCES

1. Cohen AS, Reynolds WE, Franklin EC, et al. Preliminary criteria for the classification of systemic lupus erythematosus. *Bull Rheum Dis* 1971;21:643–648.
2. Tan EM, Cohen AS, Fries JF, et al. The 1982 revised criteria for the classification of systemic lupus erythematosus. *Arthritis Rheum* 1982;25:1271–1277.
3. Hochberg MC. Updating the American College of Rheumatology revised criteria for the classification of systemic lupus erythematosus [letter] [see comments]. *Arthritis Rheum* 1997;40: 1725.
4. Edworthy SM, Zatarain E, McShane DJ, et al. Analysis of the 1982 ARA lupus criteria data set by recursive partitioning methodology: new insights into the relative merit of individual criteria [see comments]. *J Rheumatol* 1988;15:1493–1498.
5. Perez-Gutthann S, Petri M, Hochberg MC. Comparison of different methods of classifying patients with systemic lupus erythematosus. *J Rheumatol* 1991;18:1176–1179.
6. Manu P. Receiver operating characteristic curves of the Revised Criteria for the Classification of Systemic Lupus Erythematosus [letter]. *Arthritis Rheum* 1983;26:1054–1055.
7. Clough JD, Elrazak M, Calabrese LH, et al. Weighted criteria for the diagnosis of systemic lupus erythematosus. *Arch Intern Med* 1984;144:281–285.
8. Somogyi L, Cikes N, Marusic M. Evaluation of criteria contributions for the classification of systemic lupus erythematosus. *Scand J Rheumatol* 1993;22:58–62.
9. Gilboe IM, Husby G. Application of the 1982 revised criteria for the classification of systemic lupus erythematosus on a cohort of 346 Norwegian patients with connective tissue disease. *Scand J Rheumatol* 1999;28:81–87.
10. Michet CJ Jr, McKenna CH, Elveback LR, et al. Epidemiology of systemic lupus erythematosus and other connective tissue diseases in Rochester, Minnesota, 1950 through 1979. *Mayo Clin Proc* 1985;60:105–113.
11. Singer J, Denburg JA. Diagnostic criteria for neuropsychiatric systemic lupus erythematosus: the results of a consensus meeting. The Ad Hoc Neuropsychiatric Lupus Workshop Group. *J Rheumatol* 1990;17:1397–1402.
12. Hochberg MC, Perlmutter DL, Medsger TA, et al. Prevalence of self-reported physician-diagnosed systemic lupus erythematosus in the USA. *Lupus* 1995;4:454–456.
13. Fessel WJ. Systemic lupus erythematosus in the community. Incidence, prevalence, outcome, and first symptoms; the high prevalence in black women. *Arch Intern Med* 1974;134:1027–1035.
14. Kurland LT, Hauser WA, Ferguson RH, et al. Epidemiologic features of diffuse connective tissue disorders in Rochester, Minn., 1951 through 1967, with special reference to systemic lupus erythematosus. *Mayo Clin Proc* 1969;44:649–663.
15. Siegel M, Lee SL. The epidemiology of systemic lupus erythematosus. *Semin Arthritis Rheum* 1973;3:1–54.
16. Uramoto KM, Michet CJ Jr, Thumboo J, et al. Trends in the incidence and mortality of systemic lupus erythematosus, 1950–1992 [see comments]. *Arthritis Rheum* 1999;42:46–50.
17. Maskarinec G, Katz AR. Prevalence of systemic lupus erythematosus in Hawaii: is there a difference between ethnic groups? *Hawaii Med J* 1995;54:406–409.
18. Lahita RG. Special report: adjusted lupus prevalence. Results of a marketing study by the Lupus Foundation of America. *Lupus* 1995;4:450–453.
19. Lawrence RC, Helmick CG, Arnett FC, et al. Estimates of the prevalence of arthritis and selected musculoskeletal disorders in the United States [see comments]. *Arthritis Rheum* 1998;41: 778–799.
20. Jacobson DL, Gange SJ, Rose NR, et al. Epidemiology and estimated population burden of selected autoimmune diseases in the United States. *Clin Immunol Immunopathol* 1997;84: 223–243.
21. Nived O, Sturfelt G, Wollheim F. Systemic lupus erythematosus in an adult population in southern Sweden: incidence, prevalence and validity of ARA revised classification criteria. *Br J Rheumatol* 1985;24:147–154.
22. Jonsson H, Nived O, Sturfelt G. Outcome in systemic lupus erythematosus: a prospective study of patients from a defined population. *Medicine (Baltimore)* 1989;68:141–150.
23. Helve T. Prevalence and mortality rates of systemic lupus erythematosus and causes of death in SLE patients in Finland. *Scand J Rheumatol* 1985;14:43–46.
24. Teitsson I, Thorsteinsson J. Systemic lupus erythematosus in Iceland. *Iceland Med J* 1978;64(suppl):116.
25. Gudmundsson S, Steinsson K. Systemic lupus erythematosus in Iceland 1975 through 1984. A nationwide epidemiological study in an unselected population. *J Rheumatol* 1990;17: 1162–1167.

26. Hart HH, Grigor RR, Caughey DE. Ethnic difference in the prevalence of systemic lupus erythematosus. *Ann Rheum Dis* 1983;42:529–532.
27. Meddings J, Grennan DM. The prevalence of systemic lupus erythematosus (SLE) in Dunedin. *NZ Med J* 1980;91:205–206.
28. Frank AO. Apparent predisposition to systemic lupus erythematosus in Chinese patients in West Malaysia. *Ann Rheum Dis* 1980;39:266–269.
29. Samanta A, Roy S, Feehally J, et al. The prevalence of diagnosed systemic lupus erythematosus in whites and Indian Asian immigrants in Leicester city, UK. *Br J Rheumatol* 1992;31:679–682.
30. Hopkinson ND, Doherty M, Powell RJ. The prevalence and incidence of systemic lupus erythematosus in Nottingham, UK, 1989–1990. *Br J Rheumatol* 1993;32:110–115.
31. Johnson AE, Gordon C, Palmer RG, et al. The prevalence and incidence of systemic lupus erythematosus in Birmingham, England. Relationship to ethnicity and country of birth. *Arthritis Rheum* 1995;38:551–558.
32. Hochberg MC. Prevalence of systemic lupus erythematosus in England and Wales, 1981–2. *Ann Rheum Dis* 1987;46: 664–666.
33. Nai-Zheng C. Rheumatic diseases in China. *J Rheumatol* 1983; 10(suppl 10):41–44.
34. Nai-Zheng Z. Epidemiology of systemic lupus erythematosus (SLE) in China. In: *Proceedings of the Second International Conference on Systemic Lupus Erythematosus.* Tokyo: Professional Postgraduate Services, Int., 1989:29–31.
35. Nakae K, Furusawa F, Kasukawa R. A nationwide epidemiological survey on diffuse collagen diseases: estimation of prevalence rates in Japan. In: Kasukawa R, Missouri GC, eds. *Mixed connective tissue disease and antinuclear antibodies.* Amsterdam: Elsevier, 1987:9–20.
36. Iseki K, Miyasato F, Oura T, et al. An epidemiologic analysis of end-stage lupus nephritis. *Am J Kidney Dis* 1994;23:547–554.
37. Nossent JC. Systemic lupus erythematosus on the Caribbean island of Curacao: an epidemiological investigation. *Ann Rheum Dis* 1992;51:1197–1201.
38. Gourley IS, Patterson CC, Bell AL. The prevalence of systemic lupus erythematosus in Northern Ireland. *Lupus* 1997;6: 399–403.
39. Hopkinson N. Epidemiology of systemic lupus erythematosus. *Ann Rheum Dis* 1992;51:1292–1294.
40. Hochberg MC. The incidence of systemic lupus erythematosus in Baltimore, Maryland, 1970–1977. *Arthritis Rheum* 1985;28: 80–86.
41. McCarty DJ, Manzi S, Medsger TA Jr, et al. Incidence of systemic lupus erythematosus. Race and gender differences. *Arthritis Rheum* 1995;38:1260–1270.
42. Jonsson H, Nived O, Sturfelt G, et al. Estimating the incidence of systemic lupus erythematosus in a defined population using multiple sources of retrieval [see comments]. *Br J Rheumatol* 1990;29:185–188.
43. Symmons DP. Frequency of lupus in people of African origin. *Lupus* 1995;4:176–178.
44. Bae SC, Fraser P, Liang MH. The epidemiology of systemic lupus erythematosus in populations of African ancestry: a critical review of the "prevalence gradient hypothesis" [see comments]. *Arthritis Rheum* 1998;41:2091–2099.
45. Polednak AP. Connective tissue responses in blacks in relation to disease: further observations. *Am J Phys Anthropol* 1987;74: 357–371.
46. Wilson WA, Hughes GR. Rheumatic disease in Jamaica. *Ann Rheum Dis* 1979;38:320–325.
47. Serdula MK, Rhoads GG. Frequency of systemic lupus erythematosus in different ethnic groups in Hawaii. *Arthritis Rheum* 1979;22:328–333.
48. Chou CT, Lee FT, Schumacher HR. Modification of a screening technique to evaluate systemic lupus erythematosus in a Chinese population in Taiwan. *J Rheumatol* 1986;13: 806–809.
49. Catalano MA, Hoffmeier M. Frequency of systemic lupus erythematosus in different ethnic groups of Hawaii. *Arthritis Rheum* 1989;22:328–333(abst).
50. Reveille JD, Moulds JM, Ahn C, et al. Systemic lupus erythematosus in three ethnic groups: I. The effects of HLA class II, C4, and CR1 alleles, socioeconomic factors, and ethnicity at disease onset. LUMINA Study Group. Lupus in minority populations, nature versus nurture. *Arthritis Rheum* 1998;41: 1161–1172.
51. Anstey NM, Bastian I, Dunckley H, et al. Systemic lupus erythematosus in Australian aborigines: high prevalence, morbidity and mortality. *Aust NZ J Med* 1993;23:646–651.
52. Morton RO, Gershwin ME, Brady C, et al. The incidence of systemic lupus erythematosus in North American Indians. *J Rheumatol* 1976;3:186–190.
53. Atkins C, Reuffel L, Roddy J, et al. Rheumatic disease in the Nuu-Chah-Nulth native Indians of the Pacific Northwest. *J Rheumatol* 1988;15:684–690.
54. Boyer GS, Templin DW, Lanier AP. Rheumatic diseases in Alaskan Indians of the southeast coast: high prevalence of rheumatoid arthritis and systemic lupus erythematosus. *J Rheumatol* 1991;18:1477–1484.
55. Boyer GS, Lanier AP. Spondyloarthropathy and rheumatoid arthritis in Alaskan Yupik Eskimos. *J Rheumatol* 1990;17:489–496.
56. Boyer GS, Lanier AP, Templin DW. Prevalence rates of spondyloarthropathies, rheumatoid arthritis, and other rheumatic disorders in an Alaskan Inupiat Eskimo population. *J Rheumatol* 1988;15:678–683.
57. Baer AN, Woosley RL, Pincus T. Further evidence for the lack of association between acetylator phenotype and systemic lupus erythematosus. *Arthritis Rheum* 1986;29:508–514.
58. Gordon MF, Stolley PD, Schinnar R. Trends in recent systemic lupus erythematosus mortality rates. *Arthritis Rheum* 1981;24: 762–769.
59. Kaslow RA, Masi AT. Age, sex, and race effects on mortality from systemic lupus erythematosus in the United States. *Arthritis Rheum* 1978;21:473–479.
60. Ong ML, Mant TG, Veerapen K, et al. The lack of relationship between acetylator phenotype and idiopathic systemic lupus erythematosus in a South-east Asian population: a study of Indians, Malays and Malaysian Chinese. *Br J Rheumatol* 1990; 29:462–464.
61. Lopez-Acuna D, Hochberg MC, Gittelsson AM. Mortality from discoid and systemic lupus erythematosus in the United States, 1968–1978. *Arthritis Rheum* 1982;25(suppl):S80(abst).
62. Kaslow RA. High rate of death caused by systemic lupus erythematosus among U. S. residents of Asian descent. *Arthritis Rheum* 1982;25:414–418.
63. Lopez-Acuna D, Hochberg MC, Gittelson AM. Do persons of Spanish-heritage have an increased mortality from systemic lupus erythematosus compared to other Caucasians? *Arthritis Rheum* 1982;25(suppl):S67(abst).
64. Hochberg MC. Mortality from systemic lupus erythematosus in England and Wales, 1974–1983. *Br J Rheumatol* 1987;26: 47–441.
65. Urowitz MB, Gladman DD, Abu-Shakra M, et al. Mortality studies in systemic lupus erythematosus. Results from a single center. III. Improved survival over 24 years. *J Rheumatol* 1997; 24:1061–1065.
66. Roubenoff K, Hochberg MC. Systemic lupus erythematosus. In: Bellamy N, ed. *Prognosis in the rheumatic diseases.* Lancaster: Kluwer Academic, 1991:193–212.

67. Cobb S. *The frequency of the rheumatic diseases.* Cambridge, MA: Harvard University Press, 1971:99.
68. Merrill M, Shulman LE. Determination of prognosis in chronic disease, illustrated by systemic lupus erythematosus. *J Chron Dis* 1955;1:12–32.
69. Ward MM, Pyun E, Studenski S. Long-term survival in systemic lupus erythematosus. Patient characteristics associated with poorer outcomes. *Arthritis Rheum* 1995;38:274–283.
70. Kiss E, Regeczy N, Szegedi G. Systemic lupus erythematosus survival in Hungary. Results from a single centre. *Clin Exp Rheumatol* 1999;17:171–177.
71. Seleznick MJ, Fries JF. Variables associated with decreased survival in systemic lupus erythematosus. *Semin Arthritis Rheum* 1991;21:73–80.
72. Nossent JC. Course and prognostic value of Systemic Lupus Erythematosus Disease Activity Index in black Caribbean patients. *Semin Arthritis Rheum* 1993;23:16–21.
73. Malaviya AN, Chandrasekaran AN, Kumar A, et al. Systemic lupus erythematosus in India [published erratum appears in *Lupus* 1998;7(5):370]. *Lupus* 1997;6:690–700.
74. Klippel JH. Systemic lupus erythematosus: demographics, prognosis, and outcome. *J Rheumatol* 1997;48(suppl):6771.
75. Kellum RE, Haserick JR. Systemic lupus erythematosus. A statistical evaluation of mortality based on a consecutive series of 229 patients. *Arch Intern Med* 1964;113:200–207.
76. Estes D, Christian CL. The natural history of systemic lupus erythematosus by prospective analysis. *Medicine (Baltimore)* 1971;50:85–95.
77. Feinglass EJ, Arnett FC, Dorsch CA, et al. Neuropsychiatric manifestations of systemic lupus erythematosus: diagnosis, clinical spectrum, and relationship to other features of the disease. *Medicine (Baltimore)* 1976;55:323–339.
78. Hochberg MC, Dorsch CA, Feinglass EJ, et al. Survivorship in systemic lupus erythematosus: effect of antibody to extractable nuclear antigen. *Arthritis Rheum* 1981;24:54–59.
79. Wallace DJ, Podell T, Weiner J, et al. Systemic lupus erythematosus—survival patterns. Experience with 609 patients. *JAMA* 1981;245:934–938.
80. Ginzler EM, Diamond HS, Weiner M, et al. A multicenter study of outcome in systemic lupus erythematosus. I. Entry variables as predictors of prognosis. *Arthritis Rheum* 1982;25: 601–611.
81. Rubin LA, Urowitz MB, Gladman DD. Mortality in systemic lupus erythematosus: the bimodal pattern revisited. *Q J Med* 1985;55:87–98.
82. Stafford-Brady FJ, Urowitz MB, Gladman DD, et al. Lupus retinopathy. Patterns, associations, and prognosis [see comments]. *Arthritis Rheum* 1988;31:1105–1110.
83. Swaak AJ, Nossent JC, Bronsveld W, et al. Systemic lupus erythematosus. I. Outcome and survival: Dutch experience with 110 patients studied prospectively. *Ann Rheum Dis* 1989;48: 447–454.
84. Reveille JD, Bartolucci A, Alarcon GS. Prognosis in systemic lupus erythematosus. Negative impact of increasing age at onset, black race, and thrombocytopenia, as well as causes of death. *Arthritis Rheum* 1990;33:37–48.
85. Gripenberg M, Helve T. Outcome of systemic lupus erythematosus. A study of 66 patients over 7 years with special reference to the predictive value of anti-DNA antibody determinations. *Scand J Rheumatol* 1991;20:104–109.
86. Abu-Shakra M, Urowitz MB, Gladman DD, et al. Mortality studies in systemic lupus erythematosus. Results from a single center. II. Predictor variables for mortality. *J Rheumatol* 1995; 22:1265–1270.
87. Jouhikainen T, Stephansson E, Leirisalo-Repo M. Lupus anticoagulant as a prognostic marker in systemic lupus erythematosus. *Br J Rheumatol* 1993;32:568–573.
88. Massardo L, Martinez ME, Jacobelli S, et al. Survival of Chilean patients with systemic lupus erythematosus. *Semin Arthritis Rheum* 1994;24:1–11.
89. Tucker LB, Menon S, Schaller JG, et al. Adult- and childhood-onset systemic lupus erythematosus: a comparison of onset, clinical features, serology, and outcome [see comments]. *Br J Rheumatol* 1995;34:866–872.
90. Miller MH, Urowitz MB, Gladman DD, et al. Systemic lupus erythematosus in males. *Medicine (Baltimore)* 1983;62: 327–334.
91. Kaufman LD, Gomez-Reino JJ, Heinicke MH, et al. Male lupus: retrospective analysis of the clinical and laboratory features of 52 patients, with a review of the literature. *Semin Arthritis Rheum* 1989;18:189–197.
92. Inman RD, Jovanovic L, Markenson JA, et al. Systemic lupus erythematosus in men. Genetic and endocrine features. *Arch Intern Med* 1982;142:1813–1815.
93. Folomeev M, Alekberova Z. Survival pattern of 120 males with systemic lupus erythematosus [see comments]. *J Rheumatol* 1990;17:856–859.
94. Studenski S, Allen NB, Caldwell DS, et al. Survival in systemic lupus erythematosus. A multivariate analysis of demographic factors. *Arthritis Rheum* 1987;30:1326–1332.
95. Samanta A, Feehally J, Roy S, et al. High prevalence of systemic disease and mortality in Asian subjects with systemic lupus erythematosus. *Ann Rheum Dis* 1991;50:490–492.
96. Kumar A, Malaviya AN, Singh RR, et al. Survival in patients with systemic lupus erythematosus in India. *Rheumatol Int* 1992;12:107–109.
97. Hochberg MC, Boyd RE, Ahearn JM, et al. Systemic lupus erythematosus: a review of clinico-laboratory features and immunogenetic markers in 150 patients with emphasis on demographic subsets. *Medicine (Baltimore)* 1985;64: 285–295.
98. Petri M, Perez-Gutthann S, Longenecker JC, et al. Morbidity of systemic lupus erythematosus: role of race and socioeconomic status. *Am J Med* 1991;91:345–353.
99. Ward MM. Hospital experience and mortality in patients with systemic lupus erythematosus. *Arthritis Rheum* 1999;42: 891–898.
100. Esdaile JM, Levinton C, Federgreen W, et al. The clinical and renal biopsy predictors of long-term outcome in lupus nephritis: a study of 87 patients and review of the literature. *Q J Med* 1989;72:779–833.
101. McLaughlin J, Gladman DD, Urowitz MB, et al. Kidney biopsy in systemic lupus erythematosus. II. Survival analyses according to biopsy results. *Arthritis Rheum* 1991;34: 1268–1273.
102. McLaughlin JR, Bombardier C, Farewell VT, et al. Kidney biopsy in systemic lupus erythematosus. III. Survival analysis controlling for clinical and laboratory variables. *Arthritis Rheum* 1994;37:559–567.
103. Pistiner M, Wallace DJ, Nessim S, et al. Lupus erythematosus in the 1980s: a survey of 570 patients. *Semin Arthritis Rheum* 1991;21:55–64.
104. Nossent HC, Henzen-Logmans SC, Vroom TM, et al. Contribution of renal biopsy data in predicting outcome in lupus nephritis. Analysis of 116 patients. *Arthritis Rheum* 1990;33: 970–977.
105. Austin HA, Muenz LR, Joyce KM, et al. Prognostic factors in lupus nephritis. Contribution of renal histologic data. *Am J Med* 1983;75:382–391.
106. Goulet JR, MacKenzie T, Levinton C, et al. The long-term

prognosis of lupus nephritis: the impact of disease activity. *J Rheumatol* 1993;20:59–65.
107. Ward MM, Pyun E, Studenski S. Long-term survival in systemic lupus erythematosus. Patient characteristics associated with poorer outcomes. *Arthritis Rheum* 1995;38:274–283.
108. Sibley JT, Olszynski WP, Decoteau WE, et al. The incidence and prognosis of central nervous system disease in systemic lupus erythematosus. *J Rheumatol* 1992;19:47–52.
109. Stoll T, Seifert B, Isenberg DA. SLICC/ACR Damage Index is valid, and renal and pulmonary organ scores are predictors of severe outcome in patients with systemic lupus erythematosus. *Br J Rheumatol* 1996;35:248–254.
110. Nossent JC. SLICC/ACR Damage Index in Afro-Caribbean patients with systemic lupus erythematosus: changes in and relationship to disease activity, corticosteroid therapy, and prognosis. *J Rheumatol* 1998;25:654–659.
111. Gladman DD, Goldsmith CH, Urowitz MB, et al. The Systemic Lupus International Collaborating Clinics/American College of Rheumatology (SLICC/ACR) Damage Index for Systemic Lupus Erythematosus International Comparison. *J Rheumatol* 2000;27:373–376.
112. Urowitz MB, Bookman AA, Koehler BE, et al. The bimodal mortality pattern of systemic lupus erythematosus. *Am J Med* 1976;60:221–225.
113. Petri M, Spence D, Bone LR, et al. Coronary artery disease risk factors in the Johns Hopkins Lupus Cohort: prevalence, recognition by patients, and preventive practices. *Medicine (Baltimore)* 1992;71:291–302.
114. Petri M, Lakatta C, Magder L, et al. Effect of prednisone and hydroxychloroquine on coronary artery disease risk factors in systemic lupus erythematosus: a longitudinal data analysis. *Am J Med* 1994;96:254–259.
115. Petri M, Hellmann D, Hochberg M. Validity and reliability of lupus activity measures in the routine clinic setting. *J Rheumatol* 1992;19:53–59.
116. Nossent JC, Swaak AJ. Prevalence and significance of haematological abnormalities in patients with systemic lupus erythematosus. *Q J Med* 1991;80:605–612.
117. Rosner S, Ginzler EM, Diamond HS, et al. A multicenter study of outcome in systemic lupus erythematosus. II. Causes of death. *Arthritis Rheum* 1982;25:612–617.
118. Duffy KN, Duffy CM, Gladman DD. Infection and disease activity in systemic lupus erythematosus: a review of hospitalized patients. *J Rheumatol* 1991;18:1180–1184.
119. Abu-Shakra M, Urowitz MB, Gladman DD, et al. Mortality studies in systemic lupus erythematosus. Results from a single center. I. Causes of death. *J Rheumatol* 1995;22:1259–1264.
120. Cervera R, Khamashta MA, Font J, et al. Morbidity and mortality in systemic lupus erythematosus during a 5-year period. A multicenter prospective study of 1,000 patients. European Working Party on Systemic Lupus Erythematosus. *Medicine (Baltimore)* 1999;78:167–175.
121. Hellmann DB, Petri M, Whiting-O'Keefe Q. Fatal infections in systemic lupus erythematosus: the role of opportunistic organisms. *Medicine (Baltimore)* 1987;66:341–348.
122. Nived O, Sturfelt G, Wollheim F. Systemic lupus erythematosus and infection: a controlled and prospective study including an epidemiological group. *Q J Med* 1985;55:271–287.
123. Ward MM. Premature morbidity from cardiovascular and cerebrovascular diseases in women with systemic lupus erythematosus. *Arthritis Rheum* 1999;42:338–346.
124. Urowitz MB. Late mortality and morbidity. In: *Proceedings of the Second International Conference on Systemic Lupus Erythematosus.* Professional Postgraduate Services, Int., Tokyo: 1989: 190–193.
125. Manzi S, Meilahn EN, Rairie JE, et al. Age-specific incidence rates of myocardial infarction and angina in women with systemic lupus erythematosus: comparison with the Framingham Study. *Am J Epidemiol* 1997;145:408–415.
126. Petri M, Perez-Gutthann S, Spence D, et al. Risk factors for coronary artery disease in patients with systemic lupus erythematosus. *Am J Med* 1992;93:513–519.
127. MacGregor AJ, Dhillon VB, Binder A, et al. Fasting lipids and anticardiolipin antibodies as risk factors for vascular disease in systemic lupus erythematosus. *Ann Rheum Dis* 1992;51: 152–155.
128. Sturfelt G, Eskilsson J, Nived O, et al. Cardiovascular disease in systemic lupus erythematosus. A study of 75 patients form a defined population. *Medicine (Baltimore)* 1992;71:216–223.
129. Rahman P, Urowitz MB, Gladman DD, et al. Contribution of traditional risk factors to coronary artery disease in patients with systemic lupus erythematosus. *J Rheumatol* 1999;26: 2363–2368.
130. Pettersson T, Pukkala E, Teppo L, et al. Increased risk of cancer in patients with systemic lupus erythematosus. *Ann Rheum Dis* 1992;51:437–439.
131. Ramsey-Goldman R, Mattai SA, Schilling E, et al. Increased risk of malignancy in patients with systemic lupus erythematosus. *J Invest Med* 1998;46:217–222.
132. Sweeney DM, Manzi S, Janosky J, et al. Risk of malignancy in women with systemic lupus erythematosus. *J Rheumatol* 1995; 22:1478–1482.
133. Gladman D, Urowitz M, Fortin P, et al. Systemic Lupus International Collaborating Clinics conference on assessment of lupus flare and quality of life measures in SLE. Systemic Lupus International Collaborating Clinics Group. *J Rheumatol* 1996; 23:1953–1955.
134. Liang MH, Socher SA, Roberts WN, et al. Measurement of systemic lupus erythematosus activity in clinical research. *Arthritis Rheum* 1988;31:817–825.
135. Liang MH, Socher SA, Larson MG, et al. Reliability and validity of six systems for the clinical assessment of disease activity in systemic lupus erythematosus. *Arthritis Rheum* 1989;32: 1107–1118.
136. Bombardier C, Gladman DD, Urowitz MB, et al. Derivation of the SLEDAI. A disease activity index for lupus patients. The Committee on Prognosis Studies in SLE. *Arthritis Rheum* 1992; 35:630–640.
137. Symmons DP, Coppock JS, Bacon PA, et al. Development and assessment of a computerized index of clinical disease activity in systemic lupus erythematosus. Members of the British Isles Lupus Assessment Group (BILAG). *Q J Med* 1988;69:927–937.
138. Guzman J, Cardiel MH, Arce-Salinas A, et al. Measurement of disease activity in systemic lupus erythematosus. Prospective validation of 3 clinical indices. *J Rheumatol* 1992;19: 1551–1558.
139. Vitali C, Bencivelli W, Isenberg DA, et al. Disease activity in systemic lupus erythematosus: report of the Consensus Study Group of the European Workshop for Rheumatology Research. II. Identification of the variables indicative of disease activity and their use in the development of an activity score. The European Consensus Study Group for Disease Activity in SLE. *Clin Exp Rheumatol* 1992;10:541–547.
140. Hawker G, Gabriel S, Bombardier C, et al. A reliability study of SLEDAI: a disease activity index for systemic lupus erythematosus [published erratum appears in *J Rheumatol* 1993;20(6): 1091]. *J Rheumatol* 1993;20:657–660.
141. Gladman DD, Goldsmith CH, Urowitz MB, et al. Cross-cultural validation and reliability of 3 disease activity indices in systemic lupus erythematosus. *J Rheumatol* 1992;19:608–611.

142. Bencivelli W, Vitali C, Isenberg DA, et al. Disease activity in systemic lupus erythematosus: report of the Consensus Study Group of the European Workshop for Rheumatology Research. III. Development of a computerised clinical chart and its application to the comparison of different indices of disease activity. The European Consensus Study Group for Disease Activity in SLE. *Clin Exp Rheumatol* 1992;10:549–554.
143. Hay EM, Bacon PA, Gordon C, et al. The BILAG index: a reliable and valid instrument for measuring clinical disease activity in systemic lupus erythematosus. *Q J Med* 1993;86:447–458.
144. Gladman DD, Goldsmith CH, Urowitz MB, et al. Sensitivity to change of 3 Systemic Lupus Erythematosus Disease Activity Indices: international validation. *J Rheumatol* 1994;21: 1468–1471.
145. Gladman DD, Urowitz MB. Morbidity in systemic lupus erythematosus. *J Rheumatol* 1987;14(suppl 13):223–226.
146. Gladman D, Ginzler E, Goldsmith C, et al. Systemic lupus international collaborative clinics: development of a damage index in systemic lupus erythematosus. *J Rheumatol* 1992;19: 1820–1821.
147. Gladman D, Ginzler E, Goldsmith C, et al. The development and initial validation of the Systemic Lupus International Collaborating Clinics/American College of Rheumatology damage index for systemic lupus erythematosus [see comments]. *Arthritis Rheum* 1996;39:363–369.
148. Gladman DD, Urowitz MB, Goldsmith CH, et al. The reliability of the Systemic Lupus International Collaborating Clinics/American College of Rheumatology Damage Index in patients with systemic lupus erythematosus. *Arthritis Rheum* 1997;40:809–813.
149. Hochberg MC, Sutton JD. Physical disability and psychosocial dysfunction in systemic lupus erythematosus. *J Rheumatol* 1988;15:959–964.
150. Engle EW, Callahan LF, Pincus T, et al. Learned helplessness in systemic lupus erythematosus: analysis using the Rheumatology Attitudes Index. *Arthritis Rheum* 1990;33:281–286.
151. Gladman DD, Urowitz MB, Ong A, et al. A comparison of five health status instruments in patients with systemic lupus erythematosus (SLE). *Lupus* 1996;5:190–195.
152. Stoll T, Gordon C, Seifert B, et al. Consistency and validity of patient administered assessment of quality of life by the MOS SF-36; its association with disease activity and damage in patients with systemic lupus erythematosus. *J Rheumatol* 1997; 24:1608–1614.
153. Petri M, Barr SG, Zonana-Nach A, et al. Measures of disease activity, damage, and health status: the Hopkins Lupus Cohort experience. *J Rheumatol* 1999;26:502–503.
154. Callahan LF, Pincus T. Associations between clinical status questionnaire scores and formal education level in persons with systemic lupus erythematosus. *Arthritis Rheum* 1990;33:407–411.
155. Ward MM, Lotstein DS, Bush TM, et al. Psychosocial correlates of morbidity in women with systemic lupus erythematosus. *J Rheumatol* 1999;26:2153–2158.
156. Burckhardt CS, Archenholtz B, Bjelle A. Measuring the quality of life of women with rheumatoid arthritis or systemic lupus erythematosus: a Swedish version of the Quality of Life Scale (QOLS). *Scand J Rheumatol* 1992;21:190–195.
157. Gordon C, Clarke AE. Quality of life and economic evaluation in SLE clinical trials. *Lupus* 1999;8:645–654.
158. Hochberg MC. Outcome measures in perspective: systemic lupus erythematosus. In: Strand V, ed. *Proceedings: early decisions in DMARD Development III biologic agents in autoimmune disease.* Atlanta: Arthritis Foundation, 1994:147–153.
159. Smolen JS, Strand V, Cardiel M, et al. Randomized clinical trials and longitudinal observational studies in systemic lupus erythematosus: consensus on a preliminary core set of outcome domains. *J Rheumatol* 1999;26:504–507.
160. Masi AT, Kaslow RA. Sex effects in systemic lupus erythematosus: a clue to pathogenesis. *Arthritis Rheum* 1978;21:480–484.
161. Roubinian JR, Talal N, Greenspan JS, et al. Effect of castration and sex hormone treatment on survival, anti-nucleic acid antibodies, and glomerulonephritis in NZB/NZW F1 mice. *J Exp Med* 1978;147:1568–1583.
162. Jungers P, Nahoul K, Pelissier C, et al. Low plasma androgens in women with active or quiescent systemic lupus erythematosus. *Arthritis Rheum* 1982;25:454–457.
163. Lahita RG. The connective tissue diseases and the overall influence of gender. *Int J Fertil Menopausal Stud* 1996;41:156–165.
164. Grimes DA, LeBolt SA, Grimes KR, et al. Systemic lupus erythematosus and reproductive function: a case-control study. *Am J Obstet Gynecol* 1985;153:179–186.
165. Hochberg MC, Kaslow RA. Risk factors for the development of systemic lupus erythematosus: a case control study. *Clin Res* 1983;153:179–186(abst).
166. Rus V, Luzina IG, Atamas SP, et al. Is micro-engraftment of fetal cells a risk factor for the development of systemic lupus erythematosus? *Arthritis Rheum* 1999;42:9S:A1438.
167. Sanchez-Guerrero J, Karlson EW, Liang MH, et al. Past use of oral contraceptives and the risk of developing systemic lupus erythematosus. *Arthritis Rheum* 1997;40:804–808.
168. Strom BL, Reidenberg MM, West S, et al. Shingles, allergies, family medical history, oral contraceptives, and other potential risk factors for systemic lupus erythematosus. *Am J Epidemiol* 1994;140:632–642.
169. Sanchez-Guerrero J, Liang MH, Karlson EW, et al. Postmenopausal estrogen therapy and the risk for developing systemic lupus erythematosus [see comments]. *Ann Intern Med* 1995;122:430–433.
170. Petri M, Robinson C. Oral contraceptives and systemic lupus erythematosus. *Arthritis Rheum* 1997;40:797–803.
171. Pincus T. Studies regarding a possible function for viruses in the pathogenesis of systemic lupus erythematosus. *Arthritis Rheum* 1982;25:847–856.
172. Phillips PE. The potential role of microbial agents in the pathogenesis of systemic lupus erythematosus. *J Rheumatol* 1981;8: 344–347.
173. Boumpas DT, Popovic M, Mann DL, et al. Type C retroviruses of the human T cell leukemia family are not evident in patients with systemic lupus erythematosus. *Arthritis Rheum* 1986;29: 185–188.
174. Koike T, Kagami M, Takabayashi K, et al. Antibodies to human T cell leukemia virus are absent in patients with systemic lupus erythematosus. *Arthritis Rheum* 1985;28:481–484.
175. McDougal JS, Kennedy MS, Kalyanaraman VS, et al. Failure to demonstrate (cross-reacting) antibodies to human T lymphotropic viruses in patients with rheumatic diseases. *Arthritis Rheum* 1985;28:1170–1174.
176. Murphy EL Jr, De Ceulaer K, Williams W, et al. Lack of relation between human T-lymphotropic virus type I infection and systemic lupus erythematosus in Jamaica, West Indies. *J Acquir Immune Defic Syndr* 1988;1:18–22.
177. Talal N, Flescher E, Dang H. Are endogenous retroviruses involved in human autoimmune disease? *J Autoimmun* 1992; 5(suppl A):61–66.
178. Kalden JR, Gay S. Retroviruses and autoimmune rheumatic diseases. *Clin Exp Immunol* 1994;98:1–5.
179. Hardgrave KL, Neas BR, Scofield RH, et al. Antibodies to vesicular stomatitis virus proteins in patients with systemic lupus erythematosus and in normal subjects. *Arthritis Rheum* 1993;36:962–970.
180. James JA, Kaufman KM, Farris AD, et al. An increased prevalence of Epstein-Barr virus infection in young patients suggests a possible etiology for systemic lupus erythematosus. *J Clin Invest* 1997;100:3019–3026.

181. Blomberg J, Nived O, Pipkorn R, et al. Increased antiretroviral antibody reactivity in sera from a defined population of patients with systemic lupus erythematosus. Correlation with autoantibodies and clinical manifestations. *Arthritis Rheum* 1994;37: 57–66.
182. Rider JR, Ollier WE, Lock RJ, et al. Human cytomegalovirus infection and systemic lupus erythematosus. *Clin Exp Rheumatol* 1997;15:405–409.
183. Beaucher WN, Garman RH, Condemi JJ. Familial lupus erythematosus. Antibodies to DNA in household dogs. *N Engl J Med* 1977;296:982–984.
184. Reinertsen JL, Kaslow RA, Klippel JH, et al. An epidemiologic study of households exposed to canine systemic lupus erythematosus. *Arthritis Rheum* 1980;23:564–568.
185. Jones DR, Hopkinson ND, Powell RJ. Autoantibodies in pet dogs owned by patients with systemic lupus erythematosus [see comments]. *Lancet* 1992;339:1378–1380.
186. Yung RL, Richardson BC. Drug-induced lupus. *Rheum Dis Clin North Am* 1994;20:61–86.
187. Hess EV. Environmental lupus syndromes [editorial]. *Br J Rheumatol* 1995;34:597–599.
188. Reidenberg MM. Aromatic amines and the pathogenesis of lupus erythematosus. *Am J Med* 1983;75:1037–1042.
189. Freni-Titulaer LW, Kelley DB, Grow AG, et al. Connective tissue disease in southeastern Georgia: a case-control study of etiologic factors. *Am J Epidemiol* 1989;130:404–409.
190. Reidenberg MM, Drayer DE, Lorenzo B, et al. Acetylation phenotypes and environmental chemical exposure of people with idiopathic systemic lupus erythematosus. *Arthritis Rheum* 1993; 36:971–973.
191. Petri M, Allbritton J. Hair product use in systemic lupus erythematosus. A case-control study. *Arthritis Rheum* 1992;35: 625–629.
192. Sanchez-Guerrero J, Karlson EW, Colditz GA, et al. Hair dye use and the risk of developing systemic lupus erythematosus. *Arthritis Rheum* 1996;39:657–662.
193. Conrad K, Mehlhorn J, Luthke K, et al. Systemic lupus erythematosus after heavy exposure to quartz dust in uranium mines: clinical and serological characteristics. *Lupus* 1996;5:62–69.
194. Sanchez-Roman J, Wichmann I, Salaberri J, et al. Multiple clinical and biological autoimmune manifestations in 50 workers after occupational exposure to silica [see comments]. *Ann Rheum Dis* 1993;52:534–538.
195. Brown LM, Gridley G, Olsen JH, et al. Cancer risk and mortality patterns among silicotic men in Sweden and Denmark. *J Occup Environ Med* 1997;39:633–638.
196. Cooper GS, Dooley MA, Treadwell EL, et al. Hormonal, environmental, and infectious risk factors for developing systemic lupus erythematosus. *Arthritis Rheum* 1998;41:1714–1724.
197. Goldman JA, Greenblatt J, Joines R, et al. Breast implants, rheumatoid arthritis, and connective tissue diseases in a clinical practice. *J Clin Epidemiol* 1995;48:571–582.
198. Hennekens CH, Lee IM, Cook NR, et al. Self-reported breast implants and connective-tissue diseases in female health professionals. A retrospective cohort study [see comments] [published erratum appears in *JAMA* 1998;279(3):198]. *JAMA* 1996;275: 616–621.
199. Strom BL, Reidenberg MM, Freundlich B, et al. Breast silicone implants and risk of systemic lupus erythematosus. *J Clin Epidemiol* 1994;47:1211–1214.
200. Edworthy SM, Martin L, Barr SG, et al. A clinical study of the relationship between silicone breast implants and connective tissue disease [see comments]. *J Rheumatol* 1998;25: 254–260.
201. Friis S, Mellemkjaer L, McLaughlin JK, et al. Connective tissue disease and other rheumatic conditions following breast implants in Denmark [see comments]. *Ann Plast Surg* 1997;39:1–8.
202. Nyren O, Yin L, Josefsson S, et al. Risk of connective tissue disease and related disorders among women with breast implants: a nation-wide retrospective cohort study in Sweden [see comments]. *BMJ* 1998;316:417–422.
203. Sanchez-Guerrero J, Colditz GA, Karlson EW, et al. Silicone breast implants and the risk of connective-tissue diseases and symptoms [see comments]. *N Engl J Med* 1995;332:1666–1670.
204. Teel WB. *A population-based case-control study of risk factors for connective tissue diseases.* Ph.D. dissertation. Seattle: University of Washington, 1997.
205. Hochberg MC. Genetic epidemiology of systemic lupus erythematosus. In: *Proceedings of the Second International Conference on Systemic Lupus Erythematosus.* Tokyo: Professional Postgraduate Services, Int., 1989:9–19.
206. Janowsky EC, Kupper LL, Hulka BS. Meta-analyses of the relation between silicone breast implants and the risk of connective-tissue diseases. *N Engl J Med* 2000;342:781–790.
207. Comstock GW, Burke AE, Hoffman, SG, et al. Serum concentrations of alpha tocopheral, beta carotene and retinal preceding the diagnosis of rheumatoid arthritis and systemic lupus erythematosus. *Ann Rheum Dis* 1997; 56:323–325.
208. Hochberg MC. The application of genetic epidemiology to systemic lupus erythematosus. *J Rheumatol* 1987;14:867–869.
209. Hochberg MC, Florsheim F, Scott J, et al. Familial aggregation of systemic lupus erythematosus. *Am J Epidemiol* 1985;122: 526–527(abst).
210. Lawrence JS, Martins CL, Drake GL. A family survey of lupus erythematosus. 1. Heritability. *J Rheumatol* 1987;14:913–921.
211. Block SR, Winfield JB, Lockshin MD, et al. Studies of twins with systemic lupus erythematosus. A review of the literature and presentation of 12 additional sets. *Am J Med* 1975;59: 533–552.
212. Deapen D, Escalante A, Weinrib L, et al. A revised estimate of twin concordance in systemic lupus erythematosus [see comments]. *Arthritis Rheum* 1992;35:311–318.
213. Jarvinen P, Kaprio J, Makitalo R, et al. Systemic lupus erythematosus and related systemic diseases in a nationwide twin cohort: an increased prevalence of disease in MZ twins and concordance of disease features. *J Intern Med* 1992;231:67–72.
214. Grennan DM, Parfitt A, Manolios N, et al. Family and twin studies in systemic lupus erythematosus. *Dis Markers* 1997;13: 93–98.
215. Arnett FC, Shulman LE. Studies in familial systemic lupus erythematosus. *Medicine (Baltimore)* 1976;55:313–322.
216. Reichlin M, Harley JB, Lockshin MD. Serologic studies of monozygotic twins with systemic lupus erythematosus. *Arthritis Rheum* 1992;35:457–464.
217. Winchester RJ, Nunez-Roldan A. Some genetic aspects of systemic lupus erythematosus. *Arthritis Rheum* 1982;25: 833–837.
218. Arnett FC, Reveille JD, Wilson RW, et al. Systemic lupus erythematosus: current state of the genetic hypothesis. Semin *Arthritis Rheum* 1984;14:24–35.
219. Bias WB, Reveille JD, Beaty TH, et al. Evidence that autoimmunity in man is a Mendelian dominant trait. *Am J Hum Genet* 1986;39:584–602.
220. Moser KL, Neas BR, Salmon JE, et al. Genome scan of human systemic lupus erythematosus: evidence for linkage on chromosome 1q in African-American pedigrees. *Proc Natl Acad Sci USA* 1998;95:14869–14874.
221. Tsao BP, Cantor RM, Kalunian KC, et al. Evidence for linkage of a candidate chromosome 1 region to human systemic lupus erythematosus. *J Clin Invest* 1997;99:725–731.
222. Gaffney PM, Ortmann WA, Selby SA, et al. Genome screening in human systemic lupus erythematosus: results from a second Minnesota cohort and combined analyses of 187 sib-pair families. *Am J Hum Genet* 2000;66:547–556.

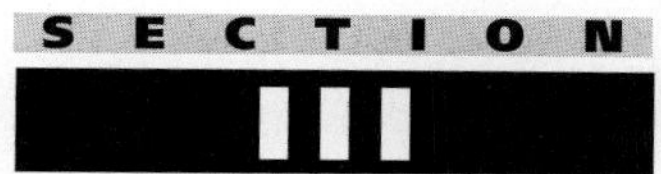

PATHOGENESIS

5

AN OVERVIEW OF THE PATHOGENESIS OF SYSTEMIC LUPUS ERYTHEMATOSUS

BEVRA HANNAHS HAHN

In systemic lupus erythematosus (SLE), tissue damage is mediated by autoantibodies, immune complexes, T cells, cytokines, chemokines, and other proinflammatory molecules such as activated oxygen radicals and products of activated complement. Individuals who develop the disease have two major characteristics: (a) they can make pathogenic subsets of autoantibodies (autoAbs), immune complexes (ICs), and T cells; and (b) they cannot regulate production and clearance of autoAbs, ICs, and activated T cells properly.

Why do these abnormal responses occur? A simple overview of the pathogenesis of SLE is shown in Fig. 5.1, and a more complex illustration of the web of interactions required to develop the disease is shown in Fig. 5.2. Disease pathogenesis has been reviewed by others (1–3) and is discussed in detail throughout this book. As shown in Fig. 5.1, it is likely that multiple susceptibility genes and environmental agents interact to begin and then perpetuate the activation of T and B lymphocytes that leads to the production of pathogenic autoAbs and ICs. Direct infiltration of target tissues by T cells and monocytes/macrophages also plays a role in disease. Although healthy individuals can make autoAbs that react with most (probably all) of the antigens (Ags) that are hallmarks of SLE, patients with the disease are more susceptible to damage from autoAbs and ICs. This may result from the ability to make subsets that are particularly harmful and/or the inability to appropriately regulate hyperactivated B and helper T cells and their products, in which case the sheer quantities of autoAbs and ICs as well as the prolonged exposure of tissue to them permits tissue damage.

The structural characteristics and physiologic properties of many pathogenic autoAb and IC subsets are known, but whether differences between SLE and healthy individuals are quantitative or qualitative is not yet clear. Virtually every regulatory network that influences antibody and IC production and metabolism is abnormal in both mice and humans with SLE. Thus, disease pathogenesis may depend on abnormalities of immunoregulation. At the heart of this problem are hyperactivated B- and T-helper cells, and at the head of the problem is the susceptibility genome of individuals who are at risk to develop SLE. I visualize this disease as originating in the genome of each individual and coming to clinical importance as multiple interacting factors, at some point in time, permit sustained production of the harmful products of the immune response (autoAbs, ICs, and T cells) that initiate tissue damage.

The portions of this book that deal with disease pathogenesis explore in detail most of the factors that play important roles in disease susceptibility, induction, or perpetuation (Fig. 5.2). Each of those chapters is extensively referenced. This chapter briefly summarizes the current state of knowledge regarding these factors and the questions that must be answered if we are to move forward to prevention and more effective therapies.

WORLDWIDE DISTRIBUTION

Systemic lupus erythematosus is found virtually everywhere, implying that most ethnic groups are susceptible. Therefore, there must be genes in common, or combinations of different genes, that produce similar immune dysregulation, or there must be environmental agents that are ubiquitous. On the other hand, there are some fascinating ethnic/environmental differences. For example, SLE is relatively common in United States and Caribbean blacks, but it is unusual among blacks indigenous to the African continent. Is this difference accounted for by the addition of genes from nonblack races in the Americas, or are there environmental stimuli present in one region that are absent in the other? Compared with whites in North America, blacks have not only an increased prevalence of SLE but also higher mortality. This could result from differences in socioeconomic status (as in other diseases, lower socioeconomic groups have worse outcomes), environmental exposures, or modifying genes. For example, genetic predisposi-

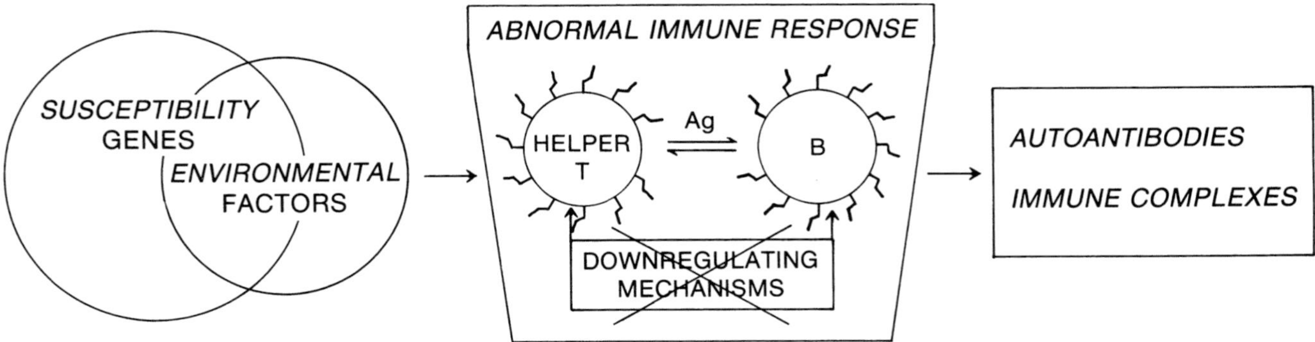

FIGURE 5.1. An overview of the pathogenesis of SLE. Interactions between susceptibility genes and environmental factors lead to abnormal immune responses. Those responses consist of hyperactive T-cell help for hyperactive B cells, with both polyclonal activation and specific antigenic stimulation of both types of cell. Downregulating mechanisms that shut off such hyperactive responses in normal individuals are impaired in patients with SLE. The result of the abnormal immune response is production of autoantibodies (autoAbs), some of which form immune complexes (ICs). Pathogenic subsets of the autoAb and the IC deposit in or on tissues and initiate the damage that is characteristic of SLE.

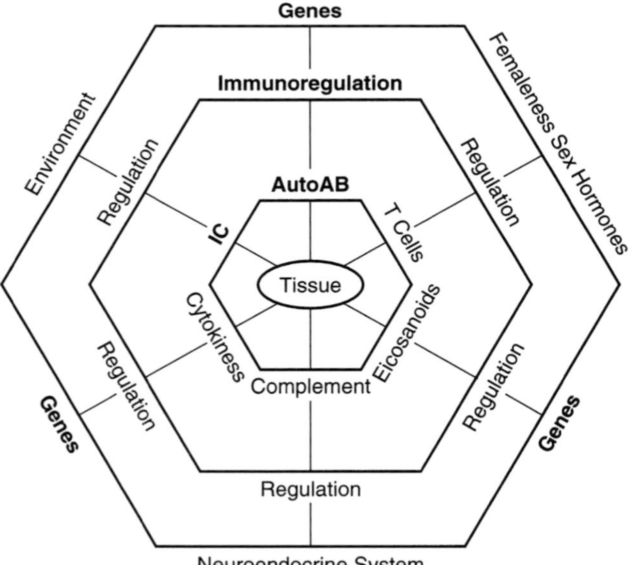

FIGURE 5.2. Some of the complex interactions that must occur to result in the clinical syndromes of SLE. At the center is target tissue, which is subjected to damage by autoAbs, ICs, T cells, cytokines, and eicosanoids. Critical for permitting sustained production of pathogenic autoAbs, IC, and T cells are multiple defects in immunoregulation. The root causes of all these abnormalities are genetic predisposition modified by environmental stimuli, sex hormones, and the neuroendocrine system.

tion to hypertension in many U.S. blacks surely would increase the morbidity and mortality of individuals with lupus nephritis. Thus, in each population, numerous genetic, social, economic, and environmental factors influence disease.

GENETIC SUSCEPTIBILITY

Since the previous edition of this book, published in 1997, a large amount of new information about genes and gene regions that predispose to SLE is available. At the time of the current writing, it seems likely that most of the genes predisposing to SLE are normal; that is, an individual inherits an unlucky combination of normal genetic polymorphisms, each of which permits a little immune overresponse and/or a bit of regulatory underresponse, or the presentation of high quantities of target antigens in certain tissues, the combination of which is just enough to permit SLE to evolve after some environmental stimulus provokes an immune response that contains anti-self elements. There is good evidence for this hypothesis in the genetics of murine lupus (4,5). Adding to the genome of normal mice selected gene segments that predispose to SLE in a lupus strain has shown that more than one segment is required to produce clinical disease, and that each has a different activity. For example a gene segment designated Sle1 breaks tolerance to nucleosomes, Sle2 provides B-cell hyperactivity, and Sle3 provides T-cell hyperactivity. Interestingly, in these experiments (5) the murine parental strain that donated Sle1, 2, and 3 is healthy, and thus must have regulatory epistatic genes that protect it from disease. The gene region containing at least one of these has been defined; adding that epistatic gene, Sle1-s, to the normal genome along with Sle1 and Sle3 protects the mouse partially from clinical nephritis. This interaction of multiple normal genes is likely to mirror the picture in most humans with SLE.

In humans, several genes have been identified that predispose to SLE. Those most widely agreed upon are listed in Table 5.1 and have been reviewed (6).

Many different genes contribute to susceptibility. In a small proportion of patients (6–8), a single gene may be responsible. Almost all individuals who are homozygous for deficiencies of C1q, an early component of complement, develop SLE. About half of individuals with homozygous deficiencies of C2 develop lupus-like diseases, and complete or partial deficiencies of C4 predispose to disease, but in a minority of individuals. Complete deficiency of C1q is uncommon, C2 deficiencies account for <5% of patients with SLE, and C4 partial deficiencies are common. For the other 95% of patients with SLE, multiple genes are required. It has been intriguing to speculate on how C1q is so potent: What does its product do that is so protective from SLE? Several possibilities have been suggested: (a) It is important enough in clearing of immune complexes that its absence cannot be completely substituted by alternate pathways. (b) It binds to apoptotic blebs and is probably critical to clearing apoptotic cells (which provide autoantigens to the immune system). (c) Its absence permits sustained infection, which keeps triggering autoimmune responses.

Genes of the human leukocyte antigen (HLA) complex [major histocompatibility complex (MHC) in mice] clearly play a role in susceptibility to SLE. The class II and III regions are particularly important. Class II genes, especially DR and DQ, influence the autoAb repertoire, the ability of T and B cells to recognize particular peptides and antigens, the age of disease onset, and some clinical subsets of disease. HLA-DR2 and -DR3 increase relative risk for SLE about threefold. They tend to occur in different populations and to be associated with different clinical subsets. HLA-DR2 in some studies is associated with early onset of disease with nephritis, and HLA-DR3 with later onset and dermatitis, Sjögren's syndrome, and less nephritis. However, there are many exceptions to these "rules." The MHC portion of the genome shapes the autoAb repertoire, and the autoAb repertoire determines clinical subsets. For example, anti-Ro–linked syndromes, such as neonatal lupus and subacute cutaneous lupus, may occur primarily in individuals with DQ1 and DQ2 linked with appropriate HLA-B and DR haplotypes. We have already discussed the MHC class III genes C2 and C4; this region also contains the gene encoding tumor necrosis factor-α (TNF-α). In some ethnic groups, the polymorphism of TNF-α associated with SLE

TABLE 5.1. EXAMPLES OF GENES THAT INCREASE SUSCEPTIBILITY TO SYSTEMIC LUPUS ERYTHEMATOSUS (SLE) IN HUMANS

In the MHC region on chromosome 6:
- C2, C4: Individuals with deficiencies in these complement components have increased risk for SLE (they are less rare than C1q deficiencies, but many individuals with deficiencies of C2 and C4 do not develop SLE)
- DR2, DR3: Each predisposes to SLE, usually in different clinical subsets (e.g., nephritis more likely with DR2, dermatitis and Sjögren's more likely with DR3); vary in different ethnic groups
- TNF-α polymorphisms: In some ethnic groups; may not be independent risk factor from extended haplotype containing allele that encodes synthesis of low quantities of TNF-α

In non-MHC regions:
- C1q: The majority of individuals with homozygous deficiency of C1q (which is rare) have SLE (C1q is cleaved when activated by immune complexes; it also binds to apoptotic blebs and probably participates in clearing of apoptotic cells; its absence may also predispose to infection)
- Region on chromosome 1; 1q41–42 (PARP is possible; agreement on the susceptibility gene in this region has not been reached)
- Fc-γ RIIA and RIIIA (determines binding, phagocytosis, and ultimate disposal of immune complexes containing IgG2 for RIIA and IgG1 and IgG3 for RIIIA; particularly predisposing to lupus nephritis in African-American, European Caucasian, and some South Korean populations)
- IL-10 and Bcl polymorphisms inherited together (particularly in Hispanic Americans)
- Polymorphisms in a region near IL-6
- Several regions on chromosomes other than chromosome 1 found in genome scanning from multiple centers (genes not yet defined)
- Polymorphism of mannose-binding protein

Ig, immunoglobulin; IL, interleukin; MHC, major histocompatibility complex; PARP, poly(ADP-ribose) polymerase; TNF, tumor necrosis factor.

correlates with low synthesis of the molecule. Whether this is an independent risk factor or merely part of an extended haplotype that predisposes to SLE has been debated. It does raise the interesting issue of whether administration of TNFα inhibitors might be detrimental in some patients who have those haplotypes.

Genes outside the HLA region also clearly predispose to SLE. Most human genome scans as well as studies of candidate gene regions have shown that at least two regions on chromosome 1 increase susceptibility to the disease. These include 1q23 and 1q41–43. Within the first region are the genes that encode two Fc receptors: FcγRIIA and FcγRIIIA (6,9). In several ethnic groups, including African Americans, European Caucasians, and some South Koreans, certain polymorphisms of one or both predispose to lupus nephritis. The characteristics of the lupus-predisposing polymorphisms are that the molecule they encode binds the Fc of immunoglobulin (Ig) weakly, and/or phagocytoses it poorly. FcγRIIA binds IgG2, and RIIIA binds IgG1 and IgG3. Since most pathogenic autoantibodies, such as nephritogenic anti-C1q, contain at least one of these subsets, failure to clear complexes containing those antibodies would clearly be detrimental (9). The gene or genes within the 1q41 region may include polyadenosine diphosphate (ADP)-ribose] polymerase (PARP) or a gene located quite near it (6). Other genes that have been confirmed as increasing susceptibility to SLE in more than one cohort include the following polymorphisms: one encoding interleukin-10 (IL-10), with risk especially increased when associated with one encoding *bcl-2* (in Hispanic Americans) (10), one in a region near the gene encoding IL-6, and one encoding mannose-binding protein. It is encouraging that several different investigative groups studying different cohorts have frequently identified some of the same genes or gene regions in these cohorts. This suggests that our opportunity to understand many of the genetic influences on SLE will be fulfilled over the next few years.

Finally, we must consider the possibility that genetic control of antigen expression in target tissues is crucial to development of SLE. Infusion of autoantibodies into certain strains of mice causes disease (hemolysis or nephritis, for example), whereas other strains are resistant. Could this relate to differences in quality or quantity of target antigens in the different strains? In a recent example, a polymorphism in the β_2-glycoprotein I (gpI) gene identifies which persons with antibodies to β_2-gpI will experience clotting episodes (among Asians but not other ethnic groups) (11).

ENVIRONMENTAL TRIGGERS

Ultraviolet (UV) light, especially UVB, flares SLE in most patients with the disease. It is unclear whether exposure to UV light can initiate the illness, but onset after a sunburn is not unusual. There is good evidence that exposure of skin to UV light alters the location and chemistry of DNA as well as the availability of Ro and RNP antigens. For example, when keratinocytes are exposed to UV light, apoptosis is induced, and as part of that process nucleosomal and Ro antigens move to the cell surface. If a person has anti-DNA or anti-Ro, or T cells that recognize peptides from either antigen, then antibody- or T-cell–mediated inflammation can occur, resulting in lupus dermatitis. Additional mechanisms must be involved in some patients who have rash but do not have either of these autoAb sets (12).

Although there has been substantial effort to identify other factors, none has been convincingly demonstrated in more than one study. Ingestion of alfalfa sprouts and exposure to hair dye, lipstick, and organic compounds such as trichloroethylene all have been suspect, but none has been confirmed at the time of this writing. Ingestion of medications such as procainamide, phenothiazines, isoniazid, and hydralazine can induce lupus-like syndromes in a small proportion of exposed individuals, but these syndromes usually differ clinically from spontaneous SLE and subside after the offending drug is withdrawn. It is likely that understanding susceptibility to drug-induced lupus will provide important clues to the pathogenesis of spontaneous disease.

Finally, there has been continuing interest in the possibility that infectious agents might initiate or flare SLE. Mechanisms might include molecular mimicry between the external Ag and a self-Ag, epitope spreading (an initial Ag-specific response over time spreads to include T and B cells with related but not identical specificities, eventually including cells that recognize self-Ag), nonspecific activation of T and B cells in a host that cannot downregulate those responses, or damage caused to tissue by the infection resulting in release of altered, more immunogenic self-Ag. Although there has been little agreement between investigative groups on what infections can potentially cause SLE, there has been recent interest in Epstein-Barr virus (EBV) (13) and the related herpes virus cytomegalovirus (CMV). Time will tell whether these ubiquitous viruses, or other infectious agents, play a role in SLE.

THE SOURCE OF AUTOANTIGENS IN SLE

Recently there has been renewed interest in the source of autoantigens that stimulate the autoAb characteristic of SLE (Table 5.2). The process of activation-induced cell death, a programmed cell death known as "apoptosis," is probably a major source of autoantigens (14,15). As mentioned above, a cell undergoing apoptosis develops surface blebs resulting from Ag moving from cytoplasm into cell membrane. In this position near the surface of cells, the Ag can activate immune response. Many of the autoAg characteristic of SLE can be found in these blebs, including nucleosomes, Ro, and U1 RNP. Furthermore, in cells that have been activated, the antigenic "heads" of phospholipid mol-

TABLE 5.2. SOURCE OF ANTIGENS THAT STIMULATE AUTOANTIBODIES

Apoptotic cells: surface blebs contain nucleosome, Ro, U1 RNP, phospholipids
Activated cells: molecules move from cytoplasm to cell membrane where they can be recognized by the immune system: in activated cells the phospholipids flip direction so that antigenic portions are exposed toward the outer surface of the membrane
Proteins modified during process of apoptosis: for example, different antibodies can arise to 70-kd U1 RNP-associated protein recognizing either unmodified or phosphorylated protein.
Infectious agents: by processes of (a) molecular mimicry (i.e., autoantibodies against the organism cross-react with similar self molecules); (b) epitope spreading (i.e., the immune response is initially directed toward a protein or lipid specific for the infecting organism, but as the immune response matures and involves increasing numbers of T and B cells the number of antigens recognized expands until self is included); (c) nonspecific activation of T and B lymphocytes; or (d) presentation of self antigens from damage to tissues resulting from cytokine/chemokine release during infection

ecules flip from inward to outward orientation—again offering an opportunity to be recognized by the immune system. In platelets that are activated, cytosolic Ags move to the surface where autoAbs can bind them and cause the thrombocytopenia of SLE. Intracellular molecules are modified structurally during cell activation and apoptosis, and such modifications may render the proteins antigenic. In lymphocytes, DNA is also modified during apoptosis, with changes in methylation and increased content of deoxycytosine-deoxyguanine (16)—changes known to render DNA more immunogenic than unmodified mammalian DNA. Finally, interactions between apoptotic cells and antibodies against them activate bystander monocytes/macrophages with release of cytokines such as TNF-α and interferon-α (IFN-α) (17–19). But, since all of us have cells undergoing apoptosis continually, why does this process become pathogenic in persons predisposed to SLE? The answer may be simply a matter of increases in quantity and duration of apoptotic cells and apoptotic bodies. There is substantial evidence that lymphocytes from people with SLE undergo increased levels of apoptosis upon stimulation (14,15), and that clearance of apoptotic materials is impaired in lupus patients (20).

Other sources of autoAg could be provided by infectious agents, as discussed in the preceding section.

THE IMPORTANCE OF FEMALE GENDER AND SEX HORMONES

In every human adult population, females with SLE greatly outnumber males with the disease. Furthermore, the sex difference is most prominent during the female reproductive years. In New Zealand black/white (NZB/NZW) F1 mice, disease can be strongly influenced by manipulating sex hormones. Castrating females and/or providing androgens or antiestrogens protects from disease, whereas castrating males and providing estrogens accelerates and worsens SLE. In contrast, BXSB mice (in which the disease occurs in males because of an accelerating factor on the Y chromosome) develop disease that is influenced little by the sex-hormone status of the animal. Thus, it seems that the importance of female gender in disease susceptibility depends, at least in part, on genetic background, yet in human populations, female predilection is universally striking.

The metabolism of sex hormones is abnormal in some patients with SLE. Men and women with the disease metabolize testosterone more rapidly than normal, and estrogenic metabolites of estradiol persist longer in women with the disease. In many mammals, females have a more vigorous antibody response to immunization than do males, and female gender may be one more factor in the web of SLE that contributes to T- and B-cell hyperactivity. There is recent evidence that estradiol prevents tolerance of some autoreactive B cells (21), thus setting the stage for release of autoAb, which can mature into pathogenic subsets. A major breakthrough in understanding the role of female gender in SLE would advance our understanding of pathogenesis tremendously.

THE ROLE OF THE NEUROENDOCRINE SYSTEM IN SLE

There are additional hormonal/cytokine factors that contribute to the pathogenesis of SLE. Best documented are the observations that some patients have hyperprolactinemia and others have inappropriate levels of antidiuretic hormone. These findings suggest abnormalities in hypothalamic and/or pituitary function. Hyperprolactinemia also occurs in some of the murine lupus strains. In addition, there is accumulating evidence that cortisol output in response to stress stimuli may be abnormal in animals predisposed to autoimmune disorders and in humans with fibrositis. These individuals probably have difficulty suppressing inflammatory responses. Such abnormalities are likely to occur in human lupus, and they may play important roles in some disease manifestations, such as fibrositis and arthritis.

B- AND T-CELL HYPERACTIVITY

Multiple regulatory abnormalities have been described in murine and human SLE, and there is a huge body of work in this area (reviewed in refs. 3 and 22–24). The overriding abnormalities are hyperactivity in B and T lymphocytes (Fig. 5.1). As a result, T-cell–dependent autoAbs are made in high quantity, and subsets of those autoAbs and the ICs they form with Ag mediate tissue damage. Possible mechanisms for T- and B-cell hyperactivity are listed in Table 5.3.

A major factor accounting for sustained activation of T and B cells in patients with SLE may be the persistence of antigens presented by poorly cleared and increased quantities of apoptotic cells, as discussed above. In addition, the autoAbs themselves provide peptides that activate T-cell help, which keeps driving production of the same autoAbs (22,23). Thus, B cells serve as antigen-presenting cells (APCs) offering up peptides from their own molecules as well as those from inciting antigens to responding T cells. Although the major role of B cells has previously been considered as precursors for cells synthesizing pathogenic autoAb, they also serve as APCs. In Medical Research Laboratory (MRL)-Fas/*lpr* lupus mice with B cells altered so that they cannot release Ig, interstitial nephritis and vasculitis still occur (22). Presumably these manifestations are caused primarily by T cells activated by the B cells serving as APCs. It is no surprise that treatment of lupus mice with soluble receptors (TACI) that prevent binding of B cell surface receptors by Blys released by monocytes, and subsequent cell activation, prevent disease (25). Epitope spreading is also a major stimulus sustaining T- and B-cell activation. In this process, a strictly antigen-specific response begins in B and T cells, but expands as additional closely related but not identical T and B cells are recruited into the response. Eventually, some of those recently recruited cells recognize self Ag, related in some way to the original stimulating non-self Ag.

Another mechanism accounting for increased T- and B-lymphocyte functions may be increased expression of activation molecules on cell surfaces (23). Activated APCs and B cells, particularly in the presence of high levels of IFN-γ or IL-4, express high quantities of HLA class II receptors, which in turn can present increased quantities of peptides to activate T-helper $CD4^+CD8^-$ cells. Similar high expression of MHC class I surface molecules should present peptides to regulatory T cells, but in SLE, these $CD4^-CD8^+$ cells can supply help rather than suppression. Similarly, high expression of IL-2R on T cells primes them for stimulation by circulating IL-2. In this manner, B- and T-cell activation can cycle repeatedly. Lymphocytes from patients with SLE also express elevated levels of surface CD40L, making them easy targets for engagement by CD40 and activation of second signaling, which can result in cell activation and synthesis of Ig.

The possibility that T and B lymphocytes in individuals with SLE possess a genetically encoded, intrinsic mechanism for cell activation that is hyperactive following surface-induced signaling is particularly appealing (27). Thus, alterations in intra- or extracellular calcium flux or phosphatidylinositol 4,5-biphosphate (PIP_2) hydrolysis, or activation of calmodulin-dependent tyrosine kinases and phosphatases or of diacylglycerol-activated protein kinase C (PKC), with abnormal phosphorylation of multiple substrates along the intracellular activation cascade, could upregulate the synthesis of products of cell activation such

TABLE 5.3. MECHANISMS FOR B- AND T-CELL HYPERACTIVITY IN SLE

Sustained presence of autoantigens: related to increased apoptosis in lymphocytes, impaired clearance of apoptotic bodies, and self antigens provided continually by tissue damage
Epitope spreading in both B- and T-cell populations: a single antigen initiates a response, but in the absence of appropriate control mechanisms, the immune response continues to mature, to engage more T and B cells with specificities somewhat related to the initiating antigen, until both T and B cells are activated by multiple antigens, many of which are self
Increased expression of surface molecules participating in cell activation (e.g., CD40L) in both B and T cells
Autoantibodies activating T cells help to continue their production by providing T-cell–activating peptides from their own molecules
Increased intracellular responses to activating signals (e.g., elevated release of intracellular calcium), in both B and T cells
Skewing of multiple subsets of T cells ($CD4^+CD8^-$, $CD4^-CD8^+$, $CD4^-CD8^-$, possibly CD1-restricted T cells, with both alpha/beta and gamma/delta TCR) toward T cells help autoantibody production
Abnormalities in cytokine production: defective production of IL-2 required to develop regulatory T cells, defective production of TGF-β to mediate suppression, overproduction of IL-6 and IL-10 to promote B-cell maturation and Ig secretion
Defective regulatory mechanisms

Ig, immunoglobulin; IL, interleukin; TCR, T-cell reactivity; TGF, transforming growth factor.

as cytokines or immunoglobulins. To date, a defect in the 3′,5′-cyclic adenosine monophosphate (cAMP)-dependent phosphorylation of proteins mediated by membrane-associated protein kinase A (PKA) has been identified in T cells from patients with SLE, probably because a subunit of PKA translocates to the nucleus aberrantly (27). In addition, some patients with SLE, particularly in Japan, have mutations in T-cell receptor zeta chain, which may interfere with the phosphorylation of zeta that begins T-cell activation.

It is also possible that APCs in individuals with SLE process Ag differently from APCs in individuals without SLE. Thus, peptides that are particularly likely to activate T cells are generated. Such a process also could differ quantitatively, rather than qualitatively, in patients with SLE. Alternatively, self Ag and autoAb may contain peptide sequences that are unique to the disease. In that case, APCs would be normal, but the peptides generated from Ag breakdown would be particularly stimulatory.

A large body of work has been done in murine lupus searching for abnormalities of tolerance in B- and T-cell compartments of individuals with lupus. Tolerance is complex, with several different mechanisms available for the animal to eliminate or inactivate T and B cells that are strongly autoreactive. That tolerance can occur in one compartment [e.g., T-helper-1 (Th1) cells] but not another (e.g., Th2 cells) in the same animal adds confusion to interpreting data that depend on suppressed T-cell proliferation as a readout for tolerance. Early work showed that it is difficult to suppress antibody responses in lupus mice after tolerization and immunization with protein Ag. More recent work in transgenic mice suggests that subtle defects in B-cell deletion, anergy, and allelic exclusion all occur in mice predisposed to SLE, and these defects are more prominent as the animals age. The mechanisms that account for these defects, however, are yet to be delineated.

One of the important mysteries in SLE is the fact that T cells with multiple surface phenotypes mediate help for autoAb production—both in human and murine lupus (3). Help is provided by the classic $CD4^+CD8^-$ cell, but also by $CD4^-CD8^+$ (the traditional "suppressor" T cell) and $CD4^-CD8^-$ double negative cells with either α/β or γ/δ T-cell receptors (TCRs). What abnormalities underlie this skewing of cells toward help? The answer to this question will unveil important information about pathogenesis.

Perhaps the hyperactivity of T and B cells depends largely on abnormalities of lymphocytes. In mice with SLE, IL-2 production falls as mice age and disease begins, and in most strains large quantities of IFN-γ and IL-4 or IL-6 are found. These cytokines drive production of the complement-fixing autoAbs that dominate in murine SLE—IgG2a, IgG2b, and Ig1 antinucleosome, anti-DNA, anti-C1q, and others. In human SLE, cytokine patterns are less predictable. In some patients disease activity is associated with drops in lymphocyte production of IL-2, and in most IL-6 levels are high. There is probably considerably more variability in the human cytokine pattern than in mice, given the larger array of participating genes. One of the most interesting recent observations regarding lymphocytes in human SLE is their general inability to make transforming growth factor-β (TGF-β) (29). If some regulatory T cells require TGF-β to mediate their effects, absence of that cytokine might account for sustained T- and B-cell hyperactivity.

As implied by the cytokine data, there is renewed interest in identifying defects in regulatory T cells in patients with SLE (24). Normal mice have regulatory T cells that protect them from autoreactive cells and prevent autoimmunity. Similar cells exist in humans. If we could find ways to activate them, a new therapeutic strategy might result.

THE IMPORTANCE OF AUTOANTIBODIES

The structure of autoAb is likely to be important to disease pathogenesis. There is considerable evidence that antibodies to DNA that can bind structures present in basement membranes or other constituents of tissue such as glomeruli are pathogenic (30,31). Thus, anti-DNA, which also bind nucleosomes, laminin, collagen type IV, or heparan sulfate, are likely to induce nephritis. Ag-binding ability depends on the structure of the antibody. Although no unique germline information is required to produce a pathogenic autoAb, there are probably important point mutations that account for the pathogenicity of some immunoglobulin molecules. Many SLE autoAbs may be disease markers and not direct pathogens, but anti-DNA, antiphospholipid, antineuronal, anti-Ro, antierythrocyte, antilymphocyte, and antiplatelet antibodies are likely to participate directly in tissue damage. Therefore, it is important to identify the forces that drive somatic mutation of autoAbs.

An additional caveat regarding the importance of autoAbs in SLE is the recent observation that autoAbs are processed into peptides that activate T-cell help for additional autoAb production, discussed above.

Another possible factor in B- and T-cell hyperactivity could be composition of the target tissues in individuals with SLE. For example, strains of mice subject to autoimmune myocarditis present different cardiac Ag than do resistant mice. To date, there is no evidence that individuals with SLE have a different composition of glomerular basement membrane, synovium, or neural tissue, but data regarding genetic differences in β_2-gpI that relate to whether anti–β_2-gpI can cause clotting (11) may be a start in this direction.

DEFECTIVE IMMUNE REGULATION IN SLE

With the background of the preceding section regarding T- and B-cell hyperactivity, it is useful to mention again the multiple abnormalities of immune regulation that have been found in mice and humans with SLE. These are enumerated in Table 5.4.

Both humans and mice with SLE exhibit defective clearance of ICs, both particulate and soluble. The defects are complex and discussed elsewhere in this volume. The role of Fcγ receptors and of CR1 receptors in clearing immune complexes has become prominent because of observations that either alleles of the FcR that do not bind IgG well predispose to SLE, and/or consumption or mutations in CR1 alleles also increase risk for this disease. Thus, multiple abnormalities can contribute to the persistence of harmful ICs in individuals who are predisposed to SLE.

Antibody normally serves as a negative feedback to production of more antibody by at least two mechanisms: (a) co–cross-linking of B-cell receptors with Fc receptors, and (b) induction of antiidiotypic networks. On a single B cell, Ig receptors bind Ag, while Fc receptors bind Ig in an Ag/Ab complex. In the absence of second signal molecules (CD40, BLys), this cross-linking of B-cell surface Ig and FcR constitutes a downregulating signal that can lead to apoptosis. This process is apparently not fully operational in many patients with SLE. The abnormality could result from defective FcR, defective cell signaling, or the presence of second signal molecules on cell surfaces that program the cell for activation rather than death (Table 5.4). On the other hand, inactivating B cells by cross-linking receptors and FcR is the basis of recently successful experimental treatments of patients with LJP394 (reviewed in ref. 31). If patients have anti-DNA that strongly binds the nucleotides in the LJP394 tetramer, the B cells make less anti-DNA, and numbers of renal flares are decreased.

Antiidiotypic networks fail to suppress idiotype-bearing antibodies in the normal fashion (reviewed in ref. 32). Several investigators have shown that antiidiotypes against public idiotypes on circulating Ig are suppressed in patients with active SLE, only to return during periods of disease remission. The regulatory abnormalities that account for this are unknown. Murine lupus can be worsened or suppressed by manipulation of the idiotypes on autoAbs; therefore, understanding these networks better could lead to useful clinical interventions. Idiotype/antiidiotype networks are discussed in detail in Chapter 15.

TABLE 5.4. DEFECTIVE REGULATORY MECHANISMS IN SLE

Clearance of apoptotic cells and apoptotic bodies
Clearance of immune complexes: may relate in part to alleles of gamma RIIA and RIIIA that do not bind/phagocytose IgG1, IgG2, and IgG3 well; may also relate to inherited or acquired low expression of CR1 receptors
Cytokine/chemokine networks: favor continued autoantibody production and continuing tissue damage that provides new antigens; includes adhesion molecules that keep pathogenic cells in regions of damage and activation molecules on endothelial cells
Idiotypic networks: idiotypes of pathogenic autoantibodies are normally downregulated by antiidiotypes
Generation of regulatory T cells: may relate to defective production of IL-2 and TGF-β

Humans and mice with SLE are clearly not tolerant to self. In normal individuals, T and B cells that have high affinity for self are eliminated by various tolerance mechanisms. It is likely that multiple abnormalities permit autoreactive cells to survive in greater-than-normal numbers in SLE. These could include defects in apoptosis, increased activation of second signal surface molecules on T and B cells that favor cell activation rather than cell death, and quantitative increases in activated B-cell or helper T-cell populations.

Much work has been done to understand the defects in T and natural killer cell regulation that contribute to SLE (29). This body of research is described in detail in Chapters 9 and 10. It is likely that in healthy individuals, most autoimmune responses evoke a T-cell response designed to downregulate that response. In the autoimmune model experimental allergic encephalomyelitis (EAE), immunization with myelin basic protein induces disease mediated by Ag-specific T cells. Disease remission occurs when regulatory $CD4^{+}CD8^{-}$ T cells arise that recognize the TCR of disease-inducing T cells. It is possible that a similar process accounts for spontaneous remissions or improvement in disease among patients with SLE. Some years ago, several investigators demonstrated defective T-cell suppression of autoAb production in animal models of SLE. Interest in this phenomenon has revived, and it is clear that normal mice and humans have T cell repertoires designed to suppress autoreactive T and B cells (24). Where are the downregulating cells in patients with active lupus? Are the TCRs of patients with SLE nonimmunogenic? Do the regulatory T cells secrete cytokines that make them helpers instead of suppressors? Are there basic, genetically controlled defects in the ability to make active forms of the suppressive cytokine TGF-β? The answers to these and similar questions should provide major clues to the pathogenesis of SLE.

THE MEDIATORS OF TISSUE DAMAGE

Several chapters in this book deal with substances that contribute to tissue damage in SLE. AutoAbs are the hallmark of this disease. Although virtually all autoAbs can be made by normal individuals, subsets of some Abs are directly pathogenic. This has been shown for anti-DNA (some subsets cause nephritis when transferred to normal mice), antiphospholipid (some cause clotting and/or fetal loss when transferred to mice), antilymphocyte (some impair T-cell functions), antierythrocyte (some cause hemolysis on transfer to animals), and antiplatelet antibodies. Each of these antibodies is considered in detail in chapters dedicated to them. Antibodies that are not directly pathogenic can bind to tissue by virtue of charge or via ICs. Whether the autoAbs of SLE are structurally different from autoAbs made by normal individuals is still a point of interest.

It is likely that T cells mediate at least some tissue lesions of SLE. For example, the bulk of evidence suggests that polymyositis is mediated by T cells that are cytotoxic for muscle; the polymyositis of SLE is probably no exception. Patients with dermatitis mediated by anti-Ro(SSA) often do not have Ig deposition at the dermal-epidermal junction. Many experts suspect that Ro-specific T cells account for much of the tissue damage in those rashes. Interstitial nephritis and vasculitis are predominantly T cell lesions (22). As mentioned earlier, the dramatic skewing of T cells toward subsets that produce help for autoAb synthesis is a dramatic feature of SLE. In murine SLE, elimination or inactivation of T cells with antibodies targeted toward CD4 or second signal molecules such as B7-1/B7-2 or CD40 ligand is quite effective in preventing or reversing autoAb production and clinical manifestations of SLE.

As with other inflammatory processes, the pathogenesis of SLE cannot be confined to B- and T-cell dysfunction. Activation of complement pathways clearly is essential for many disease manifestations. The influx of monocyte/macrophages and neutrophils into damaged tissue releases scores of molecules that enhance tissue damage as well as begin repair. Endothelial cells are activated in glomeruli and blood vessels; this must be crucial to the pathogenesis of ischemic lesions in some instances. Furthermore, the continuing long-term attack on endothelial cells by IC must contribute to the arteriosclerotic disease that becomes so important in patients after one or two decades of SLE. The activation of chemokines, upregulation of adhesion molecules, upregulation of molecules on lymphocytes that mediate second signals, and release of toxic oxygen radicals by infiltrating inflammatory cells all play important roles in tissue damage (33). Each of these nonlymphoid cells, the relevant chemokines and cytokines, and other products of inflammation are discussed elsewhere in this volume.

SUMMARY

Systemic lupus erythematosus is a very complex disease. It consists of several syndromes that share enough in common to justify grouping them under the heading SLE. What will we know about pathogenesis in the next decade? There will be multiple additional genes identified that predispose individuals to the disease: some will be shared across ethnic groups, some will be syntenic in murine and human lupus, and some will be unique to given families, ethnic groups, or clinical subsets of the disease. We will learn what the genes do, and how those activities are influenced by environment, sex hormonal status, and neuroendocrine factors. The genes will encode multiple factors that influence the immune response—mostly permitting T- and B-cell hyperactivity and impairing the normal downregulating responses. The lessons learned not only will improve our understanding of SLE but lead to new, more specific therapies and a broader understanding of normal immune and inflammatory responses.

REFERENCES

1. Boumpas DT, Austin HA III, Fessler BJ, et al. Systemic lupus erythematosus: emerging concepts. Part 1: renal, neuropsychiatric, cardiovascular, pulmonary and hematologic disease. *Ann Intern Med* 1995;122:940–950.
2. Boumpas DT, Fessler BJ, Austin HA III, et al. Systemic lupus erythematosus: emerging concepts. Part 2: dermatologic and joint disease, the antiphospholipid antibody syndrome, pregnancy and hormonal therapy, morbidity and mortality and pathogenesis. *Ann Intern Med* 1995;123:42–53.
3. Mohan C, Datta SK. Lupus: key pathogenic mechanisms and contributing factors. *Clin Immunol Immunopathol* 1995;77: 209–220.
4. Kono DH, Theofilopoulos AN. Genetic studies in systemic autoimmunity and aging. *Immunologic Res* 2000;21:111–22.
5. Mohan C, Morel L, Yang P, et al. Genetic dissection of lupus pathogenesis: a recipe for nephrophilic autoantibodies. *J Clin Invest* 1999;103:1685–1695.
6. Tsao BP, Cantor RM, Kalunian KC, et al. The genetic basis of systemic lupus erythematosus. *Proc Assoc Am Physicians* 1998; 110:113–117.
7. Walport MJ, Davies KA, Botto M. C1q and systemic lupus erythematosus. *Immunobiology* 1998;199:265–285.
8. Taylor PR, Carugati A Fadok VA, et al. A hierarchical role for classical pathway complement proteins in the clearance of apoptotic cells in vivo. *J Exp Med* 2000;192:359–366.
9. Haseley LA, Wisnieski JJ, Denburg MR, et al. Antibodies to C1q in systemic lupus erythematosus: characteristics and relation to Fc gamma RIIA alleles. *Kidney Int* 1997;52:1375–1380.
10. Mehrian R, Quismorio FP Jr, Strassmann G, et al. Synergistic effect between IL-10 and bcl-2 genotypes in determining susceptibility to systemic lupus erythematosus. *Arthritis Rheum* 1998; 41:596–602.
11. Hirose N, Williams R, Alberts AR, et al. A role for the polymorphism at position 247 of the beta2-glycoprotein I gene in the generation of anti-beta2-glycoprotein I antibodies in the antiphospholipid syndrome. *Arthritis Rheum* 1999;42: 1655–1661.
12. Sontheimer RD. Photoimmunology of lupus erythematosus and dermatomyositis: a speculative review. *Photochem Photobiol* 1996; 63:583–594.
13. James JA, Kaufman KM, Farris AD, et al. An increased prevalence of Epstein-Barr virus infection in young patients suggests a possible etiology for systemic lupus erythematosus. *J Clin Invest* 1997;100:3019–3026.
14. Andrade F, Cascioloa-Rosen L, Rosen A. Apoptosis in systemic lupus erythematosus. Clinical implications. *Rheum Dis Clin North Am* 2000;26:215–227.
15. Levine JS, Koh JS, The role of apoptosis in autoimmunity: immunogen, antigen and accelerant. *Semin Nephrology* 1999;19: 34–47.
16. Huck S, Deveaud E, Namane A, et al. Abnormal DNA methylation and deoxycytosine-deoxyguanine content in nucleosomes from lymphocytes undergoing apoptosis. *FASEB J* 1999;3: 1415–1422.

17. Manfredi AA, Rovere P, Galati G, et al. Apoptotic cell clearance in systemic lupus erythematosus. I. Opsonization by antiphospholipid antibodies. *Arthritis Rheum* 1998;41:205–214.
18. Bave U, Alm GV, Ronnblom L. The combination of apoptotic U937 cells and lupus IgG is a potent IFN-alpha inducer. *J Immunol* 2000;165:3519–3526.
19. Pittoni V, Ravirajan CT, Donohoe S, et al. Human monoclonal anti-phospholipid antibodies selectively bind to membrane phospholipid and beta2-glycoprotein I (beta2-GPI) on apoptotic cells. *Clin Exp Immunol* 2000;199:533–543.
20. Herrmann M, Voll RE, Zoller OM, et al. Impaired phagocytosis of apoptotic cell material by monocyte-derived macrophages from patients with systemic lupus erythematosus. *Arthritis Rheum* 1998;41:1241–1250.
21. Bynoe MS, Grimaldi CM, Diamond B. Estrogen up-regulates Bcl-2 and blocks tolerance induction of naïve B cells. *Proc Natl Acad Sci USA* 2000;97:2703–2708.
22. Chan OT, Madaio MP, Shlomchik MJ. The central and multiple roles of B cells in lupus pathogenesis. *Immunol Rev* 1999;169: 107–121.
23. Singh RR, Hahn BH. Reciprocal T-B determinant spreading develops spontaneously in murine lupus: implications for pathogenesis. *Immunol Rev* 1998;164:201–208.
24. Shevack EM. Regulatory T cells in autoimmunity. *Annu Rev Immunol* 2000;18:423–449.
25. Gross JA, Johnston J, Mudri S, et al. TACI and BCMA are receptors for a TNF homologue implicated in B-cell autoimmune disease. *Nature* 2000;404:995–999.
26. Kammer GM. High prevalence of T cell type I protein kinase A deficiency in systemic lupus erythematosus. *Arthritis Rheum* 1999;42:1458–1465.
27. Mishra N, Khan IU, Tsokos GC, et al. Association of deficient type II protein kinase A activity with aberrant nuclear translocation of the RII beta subunit in systemic lupus erythematosus T lymphocytes. *J Immunol* 2000;165:2830–2840.
28. Tsuzaka K, Takeuchi T, Onoda N, et al. Mutations in T cell receptor zeta chain mRNA of peripheral T cells from systemic lupus erythematosus patients. *J Autoimmun* 1998;11:381–5.
29. Ohtsuka K, Gray JC, Quismorio FP Jr, et al. Cytokine-mediated downregulation of B cell activity in SLE: effects of interleukin-2 and transforming growth factor-beta. *Lupus* 1999;8: 95–102.
30. Madaio MP. The role of autoantibodies in the pathogenesis of lupus nephritis. *Semin Nephrol* 1999;19:48–56.
31. Hahn BH. Antibodies to DNA. *N Engl J Med* 1998;338: 1359–1368.
32. Sherer Y, Shoenfeld Y. Idiotypic network dysregulation: a common etiopathogenesis of diverse autoimmune diseases. *Appl Biochem Biotechnol* 2000;83:155–162.
33. Sfikakis PP, Mavrikakis M. Adhesion and lymphocyte costimulatory molecules in systemic rheumatic diseases. *Clin Rheumatol* 1999;18:317–327.

6

THE GENETICS OF HUMAN LUPUS

BETTY P. TSAO

The importance of genetic influences on systemic lupus erythematosus (SLE) has been recognized through cumulative genetic epidemiology studies. Early genetic studies were primarily focused on genes located within the major histocompatibility complex (MHC). Subsequent studies have emphasized the participation of both MHC genes and non-MHC genes in the pathogenesis of SLE. Many population-based studies have shown associations between the disease and alleles of immunologically relevant genes, including certain MHC loci, deficiencies of complement components, Fcγ receptors, and cytokines. Complementary to association studies of candidate genes, linkage analysis is another tool that tests whether a particular chromosomal region is likely to harbor a gene conferring a disease phenotype by testing whether genetic markers and a disease phenotype show correlated transmission within pedigrees. Using the identified murine SLE susceptibility loci as a guide, a targeted search of the homologous human chromosome 1 region has yielded evidence for linkage of 1q41-42 to SLE. Most recently, five genome-scans for susceptibility loci in human SLE have been reported. These linkage results have shown that no single locus is shared in all collections of SLE-multicase families. In addition, multiple genes are necessary to predispose to disease susceptibility, and may vary depending on ethnic and genetic heterogeneity. Encouragingly, cumulative studies have colocalized several linked regions that are likely to contain SLE susceptibility genes. All these studies are reviewed in this chapter, focusing on those that have been published since the last edition.

GENETIC EPIDEMIOLOGY STUDIES

Familial Aggregation of SLE

The prevalence of lupus in the United States population is approximately 1 in 2,000, but it varies among racial and ethnic groups (e.g., more prevalent in Hispanics and African-Americans) (1) (see Chapter 4). In contrast, a familial prevalence of 10% to 12% has been documented using surveys of several hundreds of SLE patients who reported having at least one first-degree relative with the disease (2,3). Using a case-control design of 77 SLE patients and 77 controls (matched for age, gender, and race), Hochberg (4) also reported significant familial aggregation of SLE and that 10% of the SLE probands have at least one first-degree relative affected with disease compared to only 1% in the controls. The prevalence of SLE in female first-degree relatives was estimated to be 2.64 per 100 SLE patients and 0.4 per 100 normal controls. A subsequent study that examined the first-degree relatives of patients affected with SLE, discoid lupus erythematosus (LE), or other rheumatic diseases found definite SLE in 3.9% of relatives of the SLE probands, 2.6% of the relatives of discoid LE patients, and 0.3% of the disease control relatives (5). Taken together, familial aggregation of SLE has been consistently observed in multiple studies, which can be caused by genetic factors, environmental factors, or both.

Twin Studies

Twin studies can offer clues to distinguish between genetic and environmental influences in the pathogenesis of a disease. Because twins usually share the same environment, concordance of disease in monozygotic twins and discordance in dizygotic twins imply genetic contribution to disease susceptibility. The concordance rate in monozygotic twins (24% to 58%) is approximately ten times the rate in dizygotic twins or in siblings (2% to 5%) (6,7). The deviation from 100% concordance in monozygotic twins indicates non-germline factors also are required for the development of disease, which may include environmental triggers, the diverse repertoire of immunoglobulin genes and T-cell receptor genes, the inactivation of X chromosome, or genetic imprinting (8). In the largest twin study in SLE thus far, the 24% concordance rate in 45 monozygotic versus 2% in 62 dizygotic twins (7) is similar to those found in type 1 diabetes, multiple sclerosis, and rheumatoid arthritis (8,9).

Sibling Recurrence Risk

The risk for siblings of SLE patients to develop disease [λ_s, sibling recurrence risk (10); 2% in sibs versus 1/1,000 to 1/2,000 in the U.S. population] can be 20 to 40 times higher than that of the general population. The value of λs has been used to assess evidence for sibling familial clustering of a disease. The λs of at least 20 in SLE is in the range of that observed in other autoimmune diseases, for example, 8 in rheumatoid arthritis, 15 in type 1 diabetes, 20 in multiple sclerosis, and 54 in ankylosing spondilitis (9).

In summary, the importance of genetic influences on SLE has been consistently supported by studies of populations, twin concordance rates, and aggregation of disease in families. In addition, the existence of multiple inbred strains of mice that spontaneously develop lupus-like disease further lends support for a genetic basis for SLE (reviewed in Chapter 7). What were these genes that increase risk for SLE? Many investigators have addressed this question. These studies are reviewed next.

GENETIC STUDIES IN SLE

Genetic Terms and Methods for Genetic Studies

The term *complex trait* refers to the lack of direct correlation between a phenotype and a genotype (11). For example, SLE is a complex trait that does not exhibit classic mendelian recessive or dominant inheritance attributable to a single gene locus. The complexity can arise either because the same genotype can result in different phenotypes (modified by effects of environment, stochastic events, or interactions with other genes) or different genotypes can result in the same phenotype. Since the disease definition is dependent on fulfillment of 4 of the 11 American College of Rheumatology (ACR) criteria (12,13), SLE represents an array of heterogeneous phenotypes and thus further increases its complexity.

Genetic dissection of complex traits has been approached by two main methods: association and linkage (11). Historically, association studies that use the case-control design have been commonly used to compare unrelated affected and unaffected individuals from a given population. An allele A of a candidate gene is associated with the disease of interest if it is present at a significantly higher frequency in affected patients than unaffected controls. This method is suitable to detect genes with small effect because it is relatively easier to recruit large numbers of unrelated subjects than families with particular family structures. This study design needs to carefully match the subjects and the controls with respect to the age, gender, genetic background, and environmental exposure to avoid false-positive assertions caused by unanticipated differences between the two groups. Positive association suggests that the tested allele (or a polymorphism in linkage disequilibrium with it) is a risk factor for the development of disease. Negative results of the polymorphism of a candidate gene do not rule out the possibility that other polymorphisms of the test gene may still predispose to disease susceptibility.

The availability of large numbers of mapped DNA markers throughout the whole genome has facilitated linkage analysis. The commonly used markers are called microsatellites, which are di-, tri-, or tetranucleotide repeats varying greatly among individuals in size. Linkage analysis use families with multiple affected members to assess co-segregation of the test maker allele with a phenotype of interest. A model can be proposed to explain the inheritance pattern of phenotypes and genotypes observed in pedigrees (11). Alternatively, in the absence of a known mode of inheritance of the trait, an allele-sharing method can be used because affected relatives should show excess allele sharing of the test marker if it is near the gene conferring the phenotype. Both methods have pros and cons. The model-based approach tends to be more powerful than model-free methods (11,14–16). However, a misspecification of the mode of inheritance generally results in an overestimation of the recombination fraction that may be misleading (15,17). The application of genetic linkage in complex diseases usually lead to the identification of large genomic intervals of 10 to 20 centimorgan (cM) that are likely to contain disease susceptibility genes.

Once an approximate estimate of the location of the trait gene is identified, one can make use of linkage disequilibrium for a more accurate location. Linkage disequilibrium occurs when certain alleles of two physically closely located genes (or DNA markers) appear to be jointly transmitted more frequently than expected from their respective frequency. Thus, marker loci near a susceptibility gene are often observed to be in linkage disequilibrium with the disease, resulting in significant differences in the relative frequencies of marker alleles among affected individuals from those in the general population. Although population-based association studies are powerful, the family-based association design, for example, the transmission disequilibrium test (TDT) (18), has the advantage of avoiding population stratification that may cause spurious associations (11). The TDT method on families uses the preferential transmission of the test allele(s) from heterozygous parents to affected children as evidence for association between the test allele and the disease (18). As the result of linkage disequilibrium, a particular combination of alleles at a set of closely linked loci, termed a haplotype, tends to be transmitted as a block from generation to generation. Genome-wide linkage disequilibrium mapping has been proposed as a powerful approach for detecting subtle genetic effects underlying common human diseases (19,20). Improved techniques in the near future for high-throughput identification and genotyping densely mapped polymorphisms will make this approach feasible. Regardless of the adopted approach, a functional contribution of the tested allele in the pathogenesis of the disease needs to be demonstrated to provide evidence for a susceptibility gene.

The MHC Region

The MHC [also referred as human leukocyte antigen (HLA)] region at chromosome 6p21.31 contains 224 identified loci within 3.6 million base pairs (bp) (Fig. 6.1). It is the most gene-dense region of the human genome that has been completely sequenced thus far (21). Historically, the MHC region is known to specify histocompatibility genes and can be subdivided into class II (centromeric), class III, and class I (telomeric) regions. The class I and II molecules are the most polymorphic human proteins known to date. Since these molecules shape the immune repertoire of an individual, the extreme polymorphism is thought to evolve in response to infectious pathogens. Perhaps it is the reason why the MHC is associated with more diseases than any other region of the human genome, and is linked to most, if not all, autoimmune disorders (21,22).

The MHC class I region contains the HLA-A, B, C, E, F, G, H, and J loci (Fig. 6.1) (21,23,24). Each individual expresses at least three different class I proteins encoded by HLA-A, B, and C in combination with a nonpolymorphic protein—β_2-microglobulin. The gene for β_2-microglobulin, although it encodes a part of the MHC class I molecule, is located on chromosome 15. The MHC class I A, B, and C molecules are expressed on all nucleated cells and most highly in hematopoietic cells. They are highly polymorphic; the numbers of HLA-A, B, and C alleles that have been identified in various populations continue to increase. The additional genes in the class I region, E, F, G, H, and J loci, are class I–like genes encoding class IB molecules. Class IB molecules may function in innate immunity mediating recognition by natural killer (NK) cells.

As shown in Fig. 6.1, the MHC class II region includes the genes for the α and β chains of the antigen-presenting class II MHC-molecules HLA-DR, DP, and DQ, the genes encoding the DMα and DMβ chains, and the genes encoding the α and β chains of the DO molecule (encoded by DNα and DOβ) (21,23). In addition, the large multifunctional protease (LMP)-2 and -7 genes encoding proteosome subunits (necessary for generating peptide fragments from endogenous proteins to bind class I molecules), and the transporters associated with antigen processing (TAP)-1 and -2 genes (jointly encoding a TAP heterodimer to transport peptide from the cytosol to the endoplasmic reticulum) are also in the class II region. The DM molecules act as a chaperon and catalyze peptide binding to class II DR, DP, and DQ molecules, while DO molecules serve as a negative regulator of DM. The class II molecules are also highly polymorphic. There are 239 DRβ alleles, 20 DQα, 35 DQβ, 12 DPα, and 80 DPβ alleles found mainly in Caucasian populations with the exception of a single DRα allele (23). The true polymorphic nature of these molecules awaits detailed studies worldwide. An individual can use DR, DP, or DQ molecules to present peptide antigens to T cells that are recognized by T-cell receptors

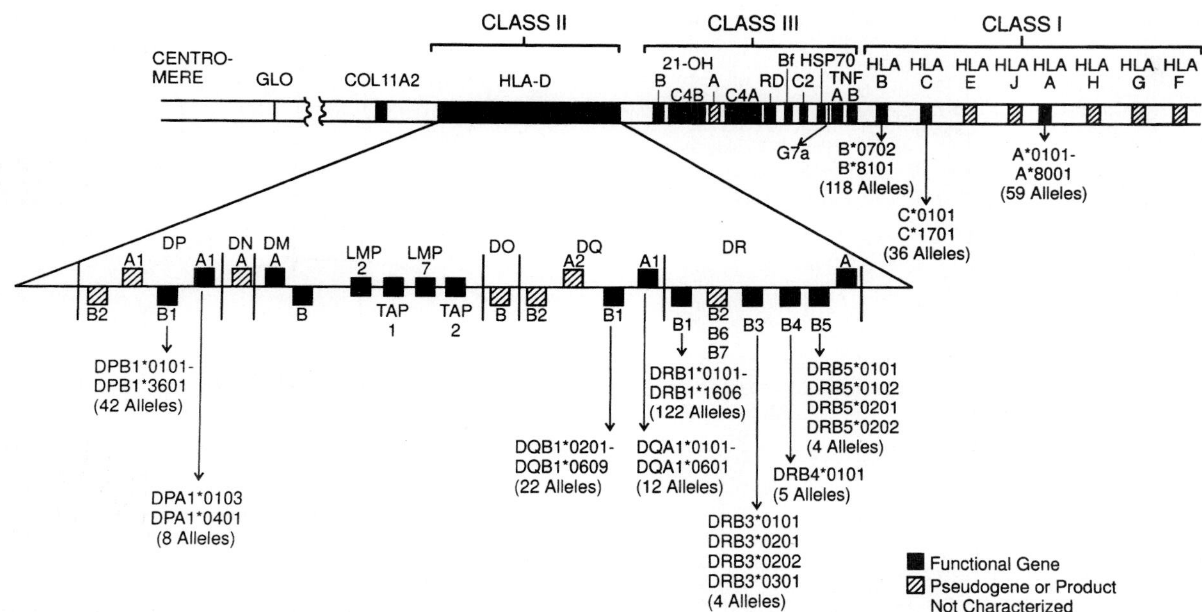

FIGURE 6.1. Schematic of the human major histocompatibility complex (MHC) or human leukocyte antigen (HLA) region located on the short arm of chromosome 6. The multiple genes and their order are shown. The area between HLA-A and DP spans approximately 3.6×10^6 base pairs of DNA and represents a distance of approximately 2 centimorgans (cM) (i.e., map or recombinational units). (Adapted from Reveille JD. The molecular genetics of systemic lupus erythematosus and Sjögren's syndrome. *Curr Opin Rheumatol* 1992;4:644–656, with permission.)

(TCRs) initiating immune responses (Fig. 6.2). These MHC class II molecules are glycosylated heterodimer membrane proteins normally expressed in a subset of hematopoietic cells and thymic stromal cells. Upon exposure to inflammatory cytokine interferon-γ, other cell types can be induced to express class II molecules.

It is worth noting that there is no wild type for class I and II molecules. Particular alleles of these antigen-presenting molecules that have been associated with autoimmune diseases are also commonly found in a normal, unaffected population (21). The presence of multiple class I and II loci allows a broad spectrum of peptides that can be presented to T cells of an individual. A diagram of the trimolecular complex (MHC class II–peptide antigen T-cell receptor) is presented in Fig. 6.3. Allelic variation of these molecules appears to be restricted to the amino-terminal domains (α1 and α2 domains of class I molecules and β1 domain of class II molecules) at positions that line the peptide-binding cleft or at exposed surfaces of the outer domain of the molecule (23). In addition, most individuals are heterozygotes expressing different alleles inherited from both parents at class I and II loci. The large number of different alleles of these antigen-presenting molecules also allows a diverse immune response to a pathogen in any population. The distribution of allelic frequency of class I and II molecules varies among ethnic groups, and may show regional differences as well. This frequency variation and linkage disequilibrium of the MHC region give rise to various extended haplotypes frequently observed among separate populations.

The MHC class III region contain genes encode the complement component C4 (*C4A* and *C4B* genes), C2 and factor B (*Bf* gene), cytokine tumor necrosis factor-α (TNF-α) (*TNFA* gene), and lymphotoxins (*LTA* and *LTB* genes), and heat-shock protein (HSP)-70 (Fig. 6.1). Physically near the two *C4* genes is the gene encoding 21-hydoxylase, an enzyme involved in steroid synthesis. Within the class III region C4A and C4B are the most polymorphic genes

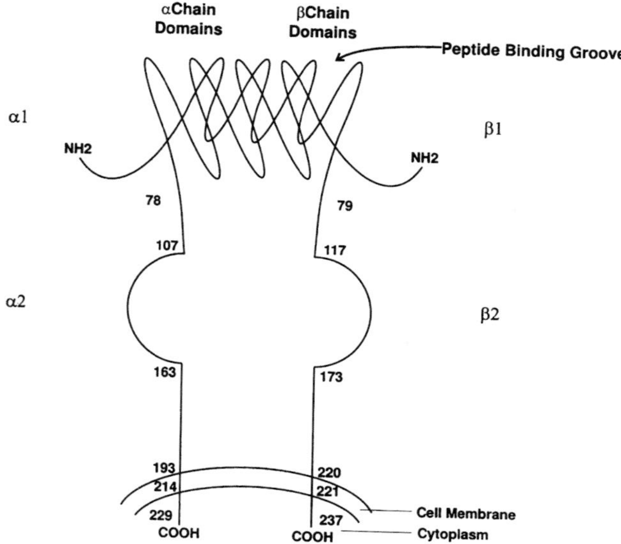

FIGURE 6.2. Schematic of an MHC class II heterodimer composed of α and β chains. The amino (NH2) terminus is the most external domain, while the carboxy (COOH) terminus is intracytoplasmic. There are two external domains on each of the α and β chains, with the most outermost containing the polymorphic amino acid sequences.

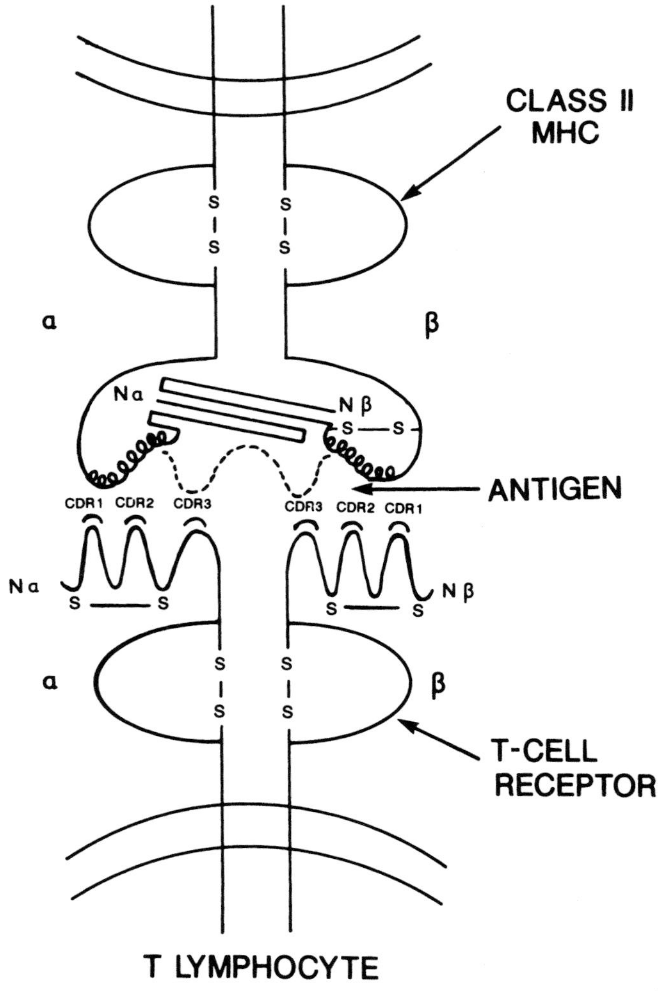

FIGURE 6.3. Schematic representation of the trimolecular HLA class II molecule-peptide-TCR complex. Processed antigen (*curved dotted line*) is presented by the HLA class II *αβ* heterodimer (*top*) to the TCE *αβ* heterodimer (*bottom*). The first two complmentarity-determining regions (CDR1 and CDR2, indicated by the *double loop*) interact with the *α* helix of the HLA class II heterodimer containing the third hypervariable amino acid segment of the outermost (first) domains and forming the wall of the antigen-presenation cleft. The putative contact points for antigen include CDR3 on the TCR and, in the floor of the antigen-presentation cleft of the HLA class II heterodimer (in *β*-pleated configuration), the first and second hypervariable amino acid segments of the outermost domains. (From Reveille JD, Arnett FC. Immunogenetics of systemic autoimmune diseases. In: Reichlin M, Bigazzi P, eds. Systemic autoimmunity. New York: Marcel Dekker, 1992:97–140.)

including at least 14 C4A and 17 C4B alleles (25,26). Frequent deletions and gene duplication events of the *C4* genes further contribute to their genetic polymorphism (27–29).

GENETIC ASSOCIATION OF MHC ALLELES WITH SLE

MHC Class II Molecules and SLE

Approximately 30 years ago, positive association between HLA-B8 and SLE was reported (30–32). Later studies showed weak or no association between SLE and class I molecules, but very consistent association with HLA-DR2 and DR3 in many populations (33–35). The more recent DNA typing has subdivided the previous DR2 and DR3 specificity into continuously increasing numbers of DRB1 alleles. Case-control studies have demonstrated the association between SLE and HLA-DR3 (or HLA-*DRB1*0301*; one of the allele from the previous DR3 specificity) in many Caucasian populations including American Caucasians, Australians, British Caucasians, Spaniards, Italians, Germans, and Scandinanvians (36–47). The association of SLE susceptibility and DR2 (or HLA-*DRB1*1501*; one of the allele from the previous DR2 specificity) has also been shown in studies of Caucasians from the United States, Australia, United Kingdom, and Germany, as well as Asians from Japan, China, Korea, and Singapore (39,41,48–56). There are reports showing no association between SLE susceptibility and DR3 or DR2, which include studies of Bulgarians, Greeks, Indians, and Chinese in Taiwan (57–60). Taken into account the heterogeneous manifestations of SLE including various autoantibodies, the confirmed association of DR2 and DR3 with SLE is an important and remarkable finding. The estimated relative risk of either DR2 or DR3 for the development of SLE is approximately two- to three fold in Caucasians.

In Mexican Americans (who have ancestry of Mexicans, European Caucasians, and Native Americans), HLA-*DRB1*0301*(DR3) (61) and *DRB1*08* (DR8) (45) have been associated with SLE. African Americans are known to have varying degrees of African, European Caucasian, and Native American ancestry. Several studies of African Americans yielded weak and varying associations of DR alleles (none, DR2, DR3, or DR7) with SLE (45,62–68). In genetic studies of Mexican Americans and African-Americans, it is especially challenging to match ethnic ancestry of the cases and controls. The lack of consistency of the observed association might be derived from the unmatched SLE cases and normal controls (11).

MHC Class II Alleles and Autoantibodies

MHC class II alleles may be more strongly associated with autoantibody subsets than with the disease status of SLE because of their pivotal role in T-cell–dependent antibody responses. A few examples of genetic association between class II alleles and specific autoantibodies are described next.

Anti-Ro (SSA) and Anti-La (SSB)

These antibodies are frequently present in patients affected with either SLE or Sjögren's syndrome. These antibodies were initially associated with HLA-DR3 (48,69–71) or DR2 in Caucasians. Hochberg et al. (64) showed that the presence of both anti-Ro and anti-La together with DR3 occurred frequently in SLE patients with older age of disease onset, while anti-Ro in the absence of anti-La and DR2 were present in patients with younger age of disease onset. Subsequently, antibodies to Ro and La seem to be most significantly associated with the HLA-DQ alleles in linkage disequilibrium with DR2, DR3 and other MHC haplotypes (72–74). Molecularly, they are commonly the HLA-DQA alleles with glutamine at position 34 and DQB alleles with leucine at position 26 (75,76). The anti-Ro response has been resolved into antibodies to 52-kd and 60-kd Ro/SSA molecules. The response to the 52-kd Ro protein has been associated with HLA-DR3 and *DRB1*0301, DQA1*0501*, and *DQB1*0201* (77,78).

Antiphospholipid Antibodies

These antibodies [anticardiolipin (aCL) antibodies and lupus anticoagulant (LAC)] are frequently found in patients affected with primary antiphospholipid syndrome (APS) and a subset of SLE patients. Clinically, they are associated with both venous and arterial thrombosis and recurrent fetal loss. An increased frequency of class II alleles HLA-DR7, DR4, and DRw53 (*DRB4*0101*) were reported in studies of primary APS (79–81) and supported by studies of patients affected with SLE or with secondary APS (82–86). The *DRB1*0402* allele (one of the alleles of DR4 specificity) was highly represented in both aCL and anti-β_2-glycoprotein I (β_2-gpI)-positive patients from a large cohort of European SLE patients (86). A sharing of HLA-DR4 haplotype in affected members was noted in two families multiplex for SLE and manifestations of APS (87,88). However, a study of seven families in which 30 of the 101 family members met criteria for APS failed to show linkage of HLA with APS (89). Segregation studies of these families suggested an autosomal-dominant (or codominant) inheritance of the disease.

A subset of aCLs bind to β_2-gpI, a phospholipid-binding plasma protein. In a combined cohort of patients with primary APS, SLE, or another connective tissue disease, anti–β_2-gpI autoantibodies were found to be associated with HLA-*DQB1*0302* carried on DR4 haplotypes and DRB4*0101 in Mexican Americans, and with HLA-DR6 (DR13) haplotype *DRB1*1302-DQB1*0604/5* in blacks, but not with HLA-DR7 in any of the studied Caucasians, Mexican Americans, and African Americans (90). When analyzed as a combined multiethnic cohort, HLA-

*DQB1*0302*, and the combined *DQB1*0301, *0302,* and **0303* alleles showed the most powerful association with anti–β_2-gpI (90). β_2-gpI is a member of the complement control protein (CCP) superfamily. Genetic variations of the 5th CCP domain of β_2-gpI (at amino acid positions 247, 306, and 316) that may affect its binding to phospholipids have been suggested to influence the generation of anti–β_2-gpI antibodies in APS patients (90–94). A correlation between the valine/leucine polymorphism at position 247 and the production of anti–β_2-gpI in primary APS patients was observed in British Caucasians (92), and was subsequently supported by studies of Asian patients with APS (especially as a major risk factor in those V/V homozygotes) but not of American Caucasians and African-Americans (93). Kamboh et al. (95) reported that polymorphisms at codons 306 and 316 had a gene-dosage effect on plasma concentrations of β_2-gpI, and the Trp to Ser at codon 316 protected against the production of anti–β_2-gpI in American Caucasian SLE patients (95). The protective association of this polymorphism was not supported by studies of SLE and APS patients from the Netherlands (96) and the United States (94). Instead, Gushiken et al. (94) suggested that Ser316 polymorphism may be an independent risk factor for thrombosis in patients with SLE.

Anti-Sm and RNP Antibodies

Anti-Sm antibodies are highly specific for SLE including the binding specificity to U1, U2, U4, U5, and U6 small nuclear ribonucleoproteins (snRNPs). These autoantibodies are present frequently in African-American SLE patients(97). Anti-RNPs often occur with anti-Sm in SLE patients, or in the absence of anti-Sm in patients with mixed connective tissue diseases (MCTDs). Many class II alleles have been implicated in association with anti-Sm or anti-RNP including HLA-DR4 in Caucasians (70,98) and Asians (99) and DR2 in Caucasians (98) and blacks (100), as well as HLA-DQB1*0302 in Caucasians (99) or in Mexican Americans (61).

Anti–Double-Stranded DNA (dsDNA) Antibodies

These antibodies may contribute to the development of glomerulonephritis. This antibody response has been associated with HLA-DR3 (101), DR2 (48,102), and DR7 (103). The antibodies' respective linked HLA-DQ alleles may also responsible for the observed associations.

In summary, the MHC associations with many autoantibodies including anti-dsDNA, antiphospholipid, anti-RNP, and Sm are very complex and inconclusive at present. Other MHC class II genes including DP, DM, Tap1, and Tap2 alleles have either no or weak and inconsistent associations with SLE.

Complement Component C2 and C4

The complement component genes within the class III region include C2, C4A, C4B, and factor B. They are closely linked and usually inherited as a single group termed a complotype. Hereditary C2 deficiency in Caucasians is located on an HLA-A25, B18, DR2 *(DRB1*1501), DQB1*0602* haplo-

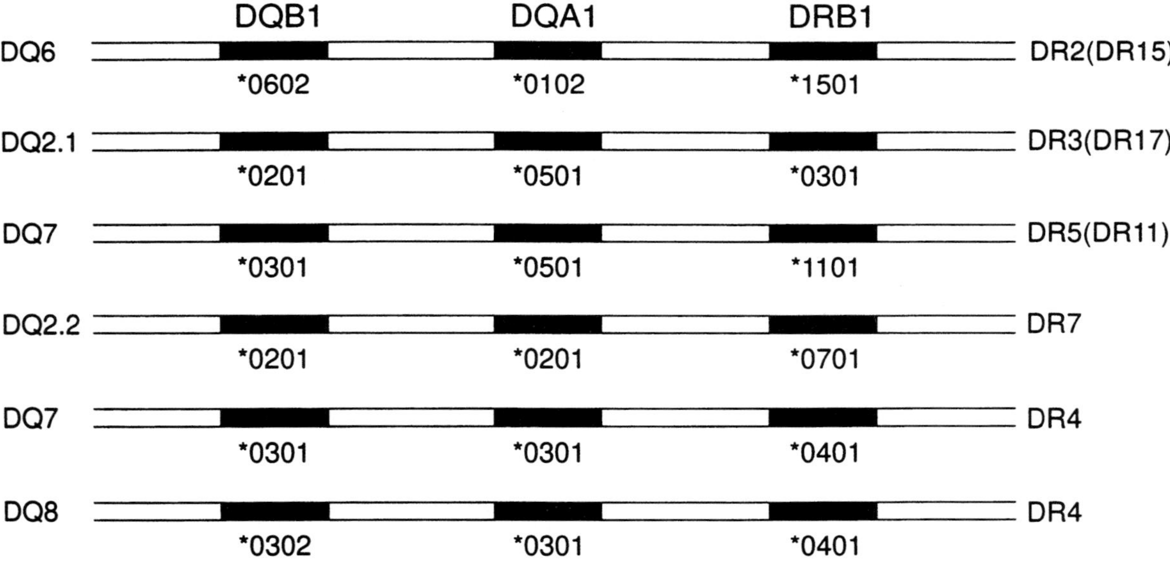

FIGURE 6.4. Several representative haplotypes of HLA-DQA1 and DQB1 alleles; the World Health Organization (WHO) allelic designations are given under each (*darkened areas*). To the *left* are the HLA specificities encoded by the HLA-DQB1 alleles. Note that different HLA-DQA1 alleles may accompany the same HLA-DQB1 allele (i.e., DQ2.1 vs. DQ2.2 and DQ7). To the *right* are the usual DR alleles, which are in linkage disequilibrium with these DQ allelic combinations.

type (104,105). This deficiency is the result of a 28-bp deletion leading to a splicing defect of the C2 transcript (106). Heterozygous deficiency is common in Caucasian populations (approximately 1% to 2%), and is increased among SLE patients in several studies (105,107,108), but not in another report (109). Homozygous C2 deficiency is present in approximately 1 in 10,000 Caucasians, and about 30% of them develop SLE or lupus-like disease (110,111). These patients frequently have anti-Ro (but not anti-La) autoantibodies (112,113). In summary, C2 deficiency may represent an infrequent risk factor for SLE in Caucasian patients (105), but not in Asians (57) or African Americans (108).

Plasma C4 is the protein product of two C4A genes and two C4B genes. Although double homozygous deficiency of C4 (producing no C4) is rare, approximately 70% of these individuals develop SLE or lupus-like disease (114–121). More commonly, individuals have homozygous null alleles at either C4A or C4B locus, often with reduced levels of serum C4. Functional differences between C4A and C4B have been demonstrated. Many Caucasian populations studied revealed an association of C4A deficiency with SLE in which *C4A*QO* (the null allele of C4) allele frequencies are 0.25 to 0.41 in patients versus 0.10 to 0.23 in controls (41,122–127). The *C4A*QO* is most often caused by the deletion of the C4A and 21-OHA genes on the HLA-*B8, Cw7, DR3, C4A*QO, C4B1* haplotype, a common MHC haplotype in Caucasians (126,128–130). Because the frequency of DR3 is also increased in patients, and because the C4A null allele is not increased in DR3-negative patients (41,131), it is difficult to determine the relative contribution of separate loci within the extended MHC haplotype. Studies of Asians in whom C4A null alleles are within other MHC haplotypes (Fig. 6.4) have supported that the lack of C4A protein may predispose to SLE. In summary, cumulative data have shown consistent associations of *C4A*QO* with SLE. However, other genes within the MHC haplotypes harboring null alleles also may contribute to disease susceptibility.

Tumor Necrosis Factor

In addition to complement components C2 and C4 loci, within the MHC class III region the loci for tumor necrosis factor (TNF) encoding TNF-α, TNF-β, and lymphotoxin-β have also been implicated in SLE susceptibility. Polymorphisms of the *TNFA* gene, which is located within the MHC class III region, have been associated with SLE. Reduced levels of TNF-α production associated with genetic polymorphisms at or near the *TNFA* gene were observed in one lupus-prone mouse model and in DR2 positive SLE patients (132–134). Compared to the DR3 positive SLE patients, DR2 positive patients were also associated with increased incidence of lupus nephritis (132). In mice, recombinant TNF-α replacement could delay in the development of lupus nephritis (133,134). In humans, treatment with a monoclonal antibody to TNF-α (Remicade; Centocor, Malvern, PA) in rheumatoid arthritis patients occasionally induced anti-dsDNA antibody and a self-limiting clinical lupus syndrome (135). These findings suggest that (a) reduced levels of TNF-α may predispose to SLE, and (b) polymorphisms of the *TNFA* gene may influence its level of production.

In recent years, polymorphisms in the promoter region of the human *TNFA* gene have been studied extensively in association with many autoimmune diseases (reviewed in ref. 136). Among them, −308A *TNFA* has been a major focus of these studies for its association with SLE either independently or as a part of an extended MHC haplotype HLA-*A1-B8-DRB1*0301-DQ2* (137) in Caucasians (138–140), Asians (57), and African Americans (141). The −308A *TNFA* allele has been shown to confer higher transcriptional activity than the −308G *TNFA* allele (142). However, neither the disease association nor the enhanced activity has been consistently demonstrated in other similar studies (136,142). Therefore, additional studies are needed to help clarify the role of genetic polymorphisms of the *TNFA* in susceptibility to SLE.

MHC Haplotypes and SLE

Figure 6.4 depicts MHC haplotypes associated with SLE. The early finding of the association of B8 with SLE is likely attributable to B8-DR3 (*DRB*0301* according to the new nomenclature) extended haplotype, which contains a complement C4A null allele (*C4A*QO), DQA*0501*, and *DQB1*0201* (127,128). This haplotype is fairly common in Caucasian populations at a frequency of approximately 25%, and is associated with multiple autoimmune disorders (22,143). The other DR3-containing extended haplotype—HLA-*B18-C4B*QO-DRB1*0301-DQA1*0501-DQB1*0201*—frequently found in Southern European and Mexican/Mexican Americans has also been associated with SLE (40,61). The DR2-containing SLE-associated haplotype—*HLA-B7-DRB5*0101-DRB1*1501-DQA1*0102-DQB1*0602*—is frequently found in Western Europeans, Africans (*DRB1*1503*), and Asians (50–53, 55–57,144–149). In Asians, C4A null phenotypes appear to have different genetic deletions from those frequently found in Caucasians (52,55,149). Various studies have used different ethnic populations to investigate the role of C4A null in SLE. Because of the tight linkage disequilibrium of the MHC region, it has been difficult to determine whether a single locus or multiple independent loci mediate the observed association of extended haplotypes.

In summary, the MHC region is likely to contain multiple genes influencing susceptibility to lupus via separate pathways. The impact of these genes appears to be quite variable among the studied groups using the current approaches. It is generally agreed that determination of the relative contribution of each implicated locus within the MHC is a very difficult but important task for the next decade.

TABLE 6.1. GENES ASSOCIATED WITH SYSTEMIC LUPUS ERYTHEMATOSUS (SLE)

Names	Gene Symbols	Chromosomal Locations
Complement component C1q	*C1q*	1p36
Tumor necrosis receptor 2	*TNFR2*	1p36
T-cell receptor-ζ	*TCRZ*	1q23
IgG Fc receptor IIIb	*FCGR3B*	1q23
IgG Fc receptor IIIa	*FCGR3A*	1q23
IgG Fc receptor IIa (CD32)	*FCGR2a*	1q24
Interleukin-10	*IL10*	1q32
Complement receptor 1	*CR1*	1q32
Poly(ADP-ribose) polymerase	*PARP*	1q42
Immunoglobulin κ locus	*IGK*	2p12
MHC class II genes	*DRB, DQA*	6p21
MHC class III genes	*C2, C4, TNF*	6p21
Interleukin-6	*IL6*	7p21-p15
T-cell receptor γ locus	*TCRG*	7p15-14
T-cell receptor β locus	*TCRB*	7q35
Mannose-binding lectin	*MBL*	10q11
T-cell receptor α locus	*TCRA*	14q11.2
T-cell receptor δ locus	*TCRD*	14q11.2
Ig heavy chain locus (V,D,J,C)	*IGH*	14q32-33
Interleukin-4 receptor	*IL4R*	16p11-12
Interferon-α receptor 1	*IFNAR1*	21q22.11
Interferon-α receptor 2	*IFNAR2*	21q22.11
Ig λ locus	*IGL*	22q11

MHC, major histocompatibility complex.
Ig, immunoglobulin.

GENETIC ASSOCIATION OF NON-MHC LOCI WITH SLE

Genome scans for mapping susceptibility loci in both murine models and human lupus have clearly demonstrated that both genes within the MHC complex and many other non-MHC genomic loci all contribute to risk for the development of SLE (143) (see Chapter 7, and linkage studies described in this chapter). Many genes encoding molecules with relevant immunologic functions have been associated with SLE (Table 6.1). The following subsections summarize the association studies of candidate genes and their chromosomal locations (to facilitate correlation to the mapped SLE susceptibility loci by linkage analyses).

C1q (Mapped at 1p36)

Three genes (*a*, *b*, and *c* genes) encode the first component of the complement system. Homozygous deficiency in any of the three *C1q* genes is almost invariably associated with SLE (150). This is a powerful disease susceptibility gene since >90% identified individuals with this deficiency developed SLE. However, homologous *C1q* deficiency is extremely rare in the population (approximately 40 cases in the world reported thus far). Despite various ethnic and genetic backgrounds, these patients develop disease at a young age without a female predominance. They share a nearly invariant feature of severe photosensitive skin rash, often with high titers of anti-Ro autoantibodies (112,151).

To understand how the absence of *C1q* can predispose to SLE, *C1q*-deficient mice were established (152). A significant portion developed glomerulonephritis with immune deposits in certain genetic backgrounds but not in others. These data are consistent with genetic interactions, suggesting that either a single susceptibility gene (*C1q*) is necessary but not sufficient for expression of murine SLE, or genetic modifiers are present in resistant strains to suppress phenotypes mediated by *C1q*. Interestingly, significantly higher numbers of glomerular apoptotic bodies were observed in *C1q*-deficient mice independent of their disease status, but not in wild-type mice (152). These *in vivo* findings are consistent with the previous *in vitro* data showing direct binding of *C1q* to apoptotic blebs on ultraviolet (UV)-irradiated keratinocytes in the absence of antibody (153). These investigators postulate that *C1q* plays a role in the maintenance of immunologic tolerance by clearing apoptotic cells, thus preventing the autoimmune response to autoantigen-containing apoptotic blebs (152).

The combined data of both humans and mice have provided compelling evidence that homozygous deficiency of *C1q* is a clear genetic risk for the development of SLE. In addition, the murine study provides a mechanism for how this genetic deficiency can play a role in the disease pathogenesis. However, the low frequency of this genetic defect makes it a rare genetic risk for SLE.

TNFR2 (1p36)

The p75 tumor necrosis factor receptor (*TNFR2*), the larger of the two membrane receptors that bind to either TNF-α or TNF-β, mediates effector functions in different cell types. *TNFR2* may be particularly important in T cells for being the major TNF receptor on circulating T cells and the major known mediator for autoregulatory apoptosis of CD8$^+$ T cells (154). Since *TNFA* is a strong candidate gene for SLE susceptibility, molecules participating in the TNF-mediated pathway are also likely to influence the pathogenesis of SLE.

TNFR2 has been considered as a candidate gene within the murine susceptibility loci [the New Zealand black (NZB)-derived *Nba-1*, *Imh-1*, and *Mott-1* loci) for SLE (155–157). The autoimmune phenotypes linked to these loci include fatal glomerulonephritis, immunoglobulin M (IgM) hypergammaglobulinemia, and formation of aberrant plasma cells (Mott cells). *TNFR2* is located on the distal end of mouse chromosome 4, a region homologous to the short arm of human chromosome 1 (1p36) where tentative linkage to human SLE has been reported in two independent genome scans (158,159). A single nucleotide polymorphism (SNP) of *TNFR2* results in arginine instead of methionine at position 196 of exon 6, which was associated with SLE in Japanese (160) but not in a Spanish or British population (161). Whether this amino acid difference has functional significance is yet to be determined. No association between SLE and a *TNFR2* intronic microsatellite was found in a recent Italian case-control study (162). Thus, current evidence for association between SLE and polymorphisms of *TNFR2* is weak and inconsistent. Further studies will help clarify whether genetic variants of *TNFR2* are risk factors for lupus.

FcγRIIa, FcγRIIIa, and FcγRIIIb (1q23-24)

These receptors are a family of molecules that bind to the Fc portion of IgG molecules. Each Fc receptor recognizes one or a few closely related IgG isotypes, and is expressed on the cell membrane of different leukocytes (23,163). Both FcγRII and FcγRIII have low affinity that bind to polymeric IgG present in immune complexes. Upon binding, they mediate internalization of immune complexes, antibody-mediated cytotoxicity, and the release of cytokines, thus connecting humoral and cellular immune responses. Because impaired clearance and subsequent tissue deposition of immune complexes are believed to play an important role in the pathogenesis of SLE, genetically determined polymorphisms that affect optimal functioning of FcγRII and FcγRIII molecules have been the focus of studies described below.

FcγRIIa (CD32) molecules are expressed on cell membranes of monocytes, macrophages, neutrophils, and platelets (23). FcγRIIa is capable of binding to all IgG isotypes, but it is the major receptor for the IgG2 subclass (23,163). Two codominantly expressed alleles are present in multiple studied ethnic groups that encode either the histidine [H] or the arginine [R] residue at codon 131 due to a single nucleotide polymorphism (SNP) in genomic DNA (164,165). *FcγRIIa-R131* binds less efficiently to IgG2 than *FcγRIIa-H131* allele, resulting in potentially delayed clearance of immune complexes. The R131 allele and R131 homozygotes were significantly overrepresented in lupus nephritis patients of Dutch Caucasians (164). Supporting this report, lupus nephritis patients had significant underrepresentation of *FcγRIIa-H131* homozygosity in African Americans (165). This skewed distribution of FcγRIIa alleles was further confirmed in Korean lupus nephritis patients and SLE patients as a whole (166). Taken together, these three studies suggest that the *FcγRIIa-R131* allele increases the risk for lupus nephritis (164–166). However, this conclusion has not been supported in many similar studies in American, British, Italian, Dutch, or German Caucasians, Afro-Caribbeans, Chinese, or Koreans (152,162,165, 168–179,276). Despite the lack of association in German Caucasians, SLE patients homozygous for the *FcγRIIa-R131* allele had higher frequencies of proteinuria, hemolytic anemia, hypocomplementemia, and an earlier age of onset of SLE (276). There was a strong trend toward skewing of FcγRIIa in Dutch SLE patients, and in a subset of 13 SLE patients, homozygous *R/R* patients showed significantly slower clearance of *in vivo* clearance of IgG-coated erythrocytes than *H/R* and *H/H* patients (170). These data are consistent with the interpretation that the *FcγRIIa-R131* allele can be either a weak risk factor or a disease modifier for certain clinical manifestations. Two independent studies have also supported the view that *FcγRIIa-R131* may not be a genetic risk for the development of SLE, but may be a risk factor for lupus nephritis, especially in SLE patients positive for IgG2 antibodies to *C1q* (277,278). These investigators postulated that IgG2 autoantibodies to *C1q* might be particularly nephritogenic in lupus patients with *R131/R131* genotypes because of poor efficiency in clearing IgG2 containing immune complexes.

FcγRIIIa (CD16) is expressed on cell surfaces of NK cells, monocytes, and macrophages. It binds to both IgG1 and IgG3 subclasses (23,163). A common polymorphism of T to G substitution at position 559 results in an amino acid substitution of phenylalanine (F) to valine (V) (at amino acid 176 counting in the leader sequence or at amino acid 158 of the mature sequence) (167). Normal individuals homozygous for *V/V* bind IgG1 and IgG3 more efficiently than those with *F/F* genotypes (167). Wu et al. (167) showed a strong association between the low-affinity allele and SLE in an ethnically diverse population, and especially an underrepresentation of homozygous *V/V* in lupus nephritis patients. This skewed allele distribution of *FcγRIIIa-158V/F* in SLE patients was further supported by studies of Caucasians (168) and Koreans (169), but not by similar studies of Dutch Caucasian (170) and African Americans (171). Seligman et al. (172) have recently demonstrated an association between the low-affinity *FcγRIIIa-158F* allele and risk of lupus nephritis among Caucasians but not among non-Caucasians (172). In contrast, the low-affinity *FcγRIIa-131R* allele was not associated with lupus nephritis in the examined Caucasians, Hispanics, African-Americans, and Asian/Pacific Islanders (172).

FcγRIIa and FcγRIIIa are transmembrane proteins. In contrast, FcγRIIIb is attached to cell membrane by a phosphatidylinositol anchor. FcγRIIIa and FcγRIIIb both bind to IgG1 and IgG3 but are expressed in different cell types, the former mainly in NK cells and macrophages and the latter in neutrophils. Earlier reports of a few SLE patients with rare alleles deficient in surface expression of FcγRIIIb suggested its possible involvement in the development of SLE (173,174). In addition, two common variants of FcγRIIIb gene, *NA1* and *NA2* alleles, were identified with differences in four amino acids (175). Functionally, individuals homozygous for *NA2* have lower capacity to mediate phagocytosis than *NA1* homozygotes. Hatta et al. (176) have reported that individuals with *FcγRIIIB-NA2/NA2* are at risk for lupus nephritis in a Japanese population. Of interest, in this study genetic association between alleles of FcγRIIa, FcγRIIIa, or FcγRIIIb and SLE were simultaneously compared. Only the *FcγRIIIB-NA2* but not the *FcγRIIA-R131* or *FcγRIIIA-158F* was a risk factor for SLE. However, a similar study of Dutch Caucasians found the *NA1* allele was at a significantly higher frequency among lupus nephritis patients than nonnephritis patients (170). Another study conducted in a combined American and

Dutch Caucasian cohort, however, found a significant association of the *FcγRIIIA-158F* allele with SLE, but not the *FcγRIIA-R131* or *FcγRIIIB-NA2* allele (168).

The overall emerging theme from cumulating data is that the low-affinity allele of FcγRII or FcγRIII may be a risk factor for SLE or lupus nephritis, presumably because of less efficiency in binding and clearing of immune complexes. The relative importance of these receptors in the pathogenesis of disease may vary among populations depending on IgG isotypes of pathogenic autoantibodies. This growing body of genetic studies of Fcγ receptors has shown how difficult it is to reach consensus in establishing a role of the tested candidate gene in pathogenesis of a multifactorial, complex disease such as SLE. Inconsistent findings may be best explained by disease heterogeneity and by genetic admixture. Since neither plays a role in inbred murine models, mice deficient in the common γ subunit that knock out the expression of FcγRI and FcγRIII were established to study the importance of Fcγ receptors in glomerulonephritis. These *FcγR*-deficient mice are protected from the development of glomerulonephritis despite deposition of pathogenic autoantibodies and immune complexes in kidneys, suggesting that Fcγ receptors are necessary for autoantibody-mediated renal injury (177,178).

TCRZ (1q23)

Decreased expression of TCR-ζ chain in studies of the TCR/CD3-mediated signaling was observed in the majority of SLE patients, and this defect is independent of disease activity, medication, or clinical manifestations (179). Each of the TCR-ζ chain or the CD3-γ, -δ, or -ε chain contains one or more immunoreceptor tyrosine-based activation motifs (ITAMs). They associate noncovalently with the antigen-binding TCR α/β (or γ/δ) chains to mediate signal transduction in T lymphocytes. A critical early event in the signal transduction pathway of TCR activation is phosphorylation of ITAM and its subsequent dephosphorylation. Given the known T cell defects in SLE patients and the pivotal role of the ζ chain in T-cell activation, several studies focused on this gene as a candidate susceptibility gene for SLE. The absence of exon 7 [encoding the guanosine triphosphate/guanosine diphosphate (GTP/GDP) binding site proximal to the third ITAM] of TCR-ζ messenger RNA (mRNA) was observed in two Japanese SLE patients (180). Subsequently, frequent mutations in the cloned polymerase chain reaction (PCR) products of TCR-ζ mRNA were demonstrated in six of eight Japanese SLE patients, but not in two systemic sclerosis patients and two normal controls (181). However, no unique mutations in TCR-ζ mRNA were found in a study using direct sequencing of PCR products derived from Caucasian, African American, Hispanic, Chinese, or Japanese SLE patients living in North America (182). Instead, novel single-nucleotide polymorphisms of the ζ chain gene were shared similarly among normal and SLE patients (182). These investigators suggest that polymorphisms of TCR-ζ chain gene are unlikely to play an important role in genetic susceptibility to SLE. It appears that the discrepancy in mutations of TCR-ζ mRNA of the reported SLE patients may be attributed to how mutations are detected. Mutations in the cloned PCR products but not in PCR products from the total amplified ζ mRNA suggest that these mutations are present somatically in a small proportion of mRNA without corresponding alterations in genomic DNA. This interpretation is consistent with recent findings that peripheral B and T cells derived from SLE patients contain abnormal mRNA transcripts (183,184).

Interleukin-10 (IL-10) (1q32)

IL-10 is an excellent candidate gene for SLE susceptibility because (a) increased IL-10 production promotes B-cell hyperactivity and autoantibody production (185), (b) the frequency of IL-10 secreting cells is elevated in peripheral blood samples of sporadic cases of SLE (186), and (c) studies of SLE patients and their relatives suggest genetic influences on IL-10 production (187,188). Llorente et al. (187) showed that both SLE patients and their relatives from 13 Mexican extended pedigrees had higher levels of spontaneous release of IL-10 and mRNA than normal controls. Grondal et al. (188) subsequently confirmed this finding in Caucasians; both SLE patients and their relatives from an extended Icelandic pedigree had higher numbers of IL-10 secreting cells than healthy controls. The increased production of IL-10 in SLE patients appears to be constitutive and not affected by disease activity or treatment. In addition, environmental factors may impact on IL-10 production; spouses of SLE patients had significantly higher number of IL-10 producing cells compared to controls.

The molecular mechanisms that cause increased IL-10 production among SLE patients have been actively explored. Levels of IL-10 secretion have been correlated with specific haplotypes containing either two microsatellite markers or three single nucleotide polymorphisms within the *IL-10* promoter (189–191). Association between these *IL-10* promoter polymorphisms and SLE has been reported in case-control studies of two Caucasian (162,189) and one Mexican American (192) but not in similar studies of another Caucasian (193) or one Asian (194) population(s). Mehrian et al. (192) also reported synergistic effect between *IL-10* and *bcl-2* genotypes in susceptibility to SLE (192). To our knowledge, this finding has not been replicated in another cohort. In the two negative association studies with SLE, there was significant association with renal disease in lupus patients (193,194). Thus, it appears to be a very consistent finding that polymorphisms of the *IL-10* promoter region increase risk for either SLE or lupus nephritis; however, the molecular basis for this observation awaits further elucidation. Recently, novel polymorphisms in the *IL-10* promoter region have been identified (279), which may help elucidate the interindividual variability of IL-10 quantitative production and the molecular basis of *IL-10* in the genetic susceptibility to SLE.

CR1 (1q32)

Complement receptor 1 (CR1) is the binding receptor for complement component C3b and C4b expressed on the cell membrane of erythrocytes, granulocytes, all B and some T lymphocytes, monocytes, glomerular podocytes, and follicular dendritic cells (23). Functionally, it is important in effective removal of circulating immune complexes that have fixed complements. Excessive amounts of immune complexes in SLE may be caused by dysregulated overproduction of autoantibodies or impaired clearance of immune complexes. Wilson et al. (196) quantified the C3b receptors on erythrocytes from 38 SLE patients, 14 of their spouses, and 47 relatives as well as from 113 normal subjects, and concluded that the decreased number of C3b receptors frequently observed in lupus patients was inherited in an autosomal-codominant manner. Subsequently, a *HindIII* restriction enzyme restriction fragment length polymorphism (RFLP) (7.4- or 6.9-kb fragment) that correlated with the number of CR1 receptors on erythrocytes further supported the genetic basis of decreased CR1 receptors observed in SLE patients (195,197–199). However, the correlation between *HindIII RFLP* and SLE susceptibility was not found in nine SLE multicase Mexican families (200) or in an Indian case-control study (201). Kumar et al. (201) observed that while the numbers of CR1 remained stable in consecutive patients among controls, they varied significantly in lupus patients, correlating with serum levels of C3d, circulating immune complexes, and the severity of the disease (201). Thus, low levels of CR1 expression in erythrocytes among lupus patients may be an acquired defect.

CR1 exhibits allelic size variants that has different numbers of C3b-binding sites (195,198,202–204). Because this molecular weight polymorphism may affect clearance of immune complexes, several studies investigated whether the smallest allele (the *CR1-C* allele with the lowest C3b binding site) was associated with SLE susceptibility. An association between SLE and the C allele was suggested in one large SLE multiplex pedigree (202), but not in case-control studies of a French (205), Hispanic, African American, or American Caucasian populations (45,206). The *CR1* size polymorphism appears unlikely to a risk factor to the development of SLE.

PARP (1q41-42)

Poly (ADP-ribose) polymerase (PARP) is a zinc-finger DNA-binding protein that is involved in DNA repair and apoptosis (207). The potential involvement of PARP in SLE was previously suggested by its subnormal levels of activity and of mRNA in SLE patients, and by its intermediate levels in unaffected relatives of SLE patients (208–210). Autoantibodies that bind to the two zinc-finger motifs of PARP are frequently found in patients with autoimmune rheumatic and bowel diseases (211). These autoantibodies do not significantly affect PARP enzyme activity, but efficiently prevent caspase-3–mediated PARP cleavage during apoptosis and prolong cell survival, which can cause failure to eliminate autoimmune cells and sustain autoimmune stimulation (212). Recently, genetic polymorphisms of the *PARP* gene were tested for association with SLE because the gene is located within the genomic interval linked to human SLE in several independent studies (158,213–216).

Tsao et al. (216,261) originally linked a 15-cM region on chromosome 1q41-q42 with susceptibility to SLE, and subsequently narrowed this region approximately 5 cM. Three positional candidate genes within the narrowed region were tested for an association with SLE using the TDT (18), which tests whether alleles of the test candidate gene are preferentially transmitted from heterozygous parents to the oldest affected offspring in each nuclear family, thus avoiding the potential spurious association caused by the population admixture in the case-control study. Of the three tested candidate genes, only *PARP* alleles showed an overall skewed transmission to affected offspring using a multiethnic cohort containing 124 families (216). A particular *PARP* allele (85-bp allele) appeared to be preferentially transmitted to affected offspring but not to unaffected offspring. Tsao et al. concluded that *PARP* might be the susceptibility gene within the chromosome 1q41-q42 region, or might be close to it.

Subsequently, case-control studies in French and German Caucasians found no significant association of the 85-bp *PARP* allele with SLE (217,218). In addition, no association of the 85-bp *PARP* allele with SLE susceptibility was observed using the TDT analysis of three multiethnic cohorts comprised of 187 sib pair families, 126 multiplex families, and 119 simplex families (219). A case-control study of *PARP* alleles in African Americans found a significant difference between the *PARP* allele frequencies in SLE patients and controls, and a significant deviation from Hardy-Weinberg equilibrium (HWE) in SLE genotypes, but not in controls (220). Departure from HWE at a marker locus can provide evidence for linkage disequilibrium between the marker and susceptibility locus, and for heterogeneity of disease susceptibility (221,222). Considering this growing body of studies, it appears that the studied *PARP* polymorphism is not a risk factor for SLE (223), but may be in linkage disequilibrium with the SLE susceptibility locus within the 1q41-q42 region (220). An additional positional candidate gene, *HRES-1*, has been recently suggested (224). HRES-1 is an endogenous retrovirus related to human T-lymphotropic virus. Many SLE patients have autoantibodies to the HRES-1 encoded nuclear protein (225). Further studies will help identify the gene variant that increases risk for SLE within the 1q41-q42 region linked to lupus susceptibility.

IL-6 (7p21-p15)

Interleukin-6 is an important B-cell growth and differentiation factor. Polymorphisms of the 3′ flanking region of IL-6 have been shown to be associated with SLE in Caucasians and African-Americans, which may enhance the stability of IL-6 mRNA, thus contributing to elevated levels of IL-6 in SLE patients (226–228). The SLE-associated polymorphisms are short adenine and thymine (AT)-rich minisatellite alleles that were found exclusively in SLE patients (13% among the studied Caucasian and 9% among African Americans). To our knowledge, this finding has not been replicated in independent studies.

Mannose-Binding Lectin (10q11)

Mannose-binding lectin (MBL) binds mannose on surfaces of bacteria or viruses, initiates a pathway for opsonization of pathogens, and activates complement components by MBL-associated proteases. MBL deficiency results in low levels of circulating MBL, impaired opsonization of microorganisms, and frequent infections, which occurs in 5% to 10% of the general population (229). MBL is very similar to *C1q* in three-dimensional structure. The well-known association of complement deficiencies and SLE has prompted genetic studies of *MBL* in SLE patients. Case-control studies in Caucasians, African Americans, and southern Chinese have found polymorphisms in the promoter region and exon 1, which correlate with lower levels of MBL that are significantly more frequent in SLE patients than in controls (230–232). Recently, Garred et al. (233) reported that homozygosity of *MBL* variant alleles could explain the increased risk for infections in a small subset of Danish SLE patients. It is generally agreed that MBL variant alleles represent a minor risk factor for developing SLE.

Interleukin-4 Receptor (IL-4R; 16p11-12) and Interferon-α Receptors (IFN-AR; 21q22)

Cytokine profiles of SLE patients have been a subject of great interest (see Chapter 10). Because IL-4 and IL-4 receptor (IL-4R)-mediated signaling pathway is important for the commitment of the T-helper-2 (Th2) phenotype, functional polymorphisms of these two genes may predispose susceptibility to autoimmune diseases. A recent study of 50 Japanese SLE patients and 100 Japanese controls showed significant association of SLE with the *IL-4Rα* chain gene polymorphisms (codons 50 and 551) but not with the IL-4 gene promoter polymorphism (234). One of the important cytokines that the Th1 cell type produces is IFN-γ. Genetic associations between SLE susceptibility and variants of IFN-γ receptor 1 and 2 genes were recently reported in a Japanese population (235,236). These findings await confirmation in other populations.

T-Cell Receptor Genes

The most common TCR is the αβ TCR present on the majority of T cells. Other T cells bear the γδ TCRs. The *TCR α* and *δ* chain genes reside on human chromosome 14, while the *TCR β* and *γ* chain genes map to human chromosome 7. Within a *TCR* gene locus, the DNA rearrangement process brings together one variable gene segment (one diversity gene segment), one joining gene segment, and one constant gene segment to encode gene products. A diverse TCR repertoire can present various processed peptides to MHC class I/II molecules to mount immune responses. A number of studies examining *TCR* RFLP in SLE patients have yielded weak and inconsistent results. Tebib et al. (237) reported an association between the constant region of the *TCR α* chain and SLE in American Caucasians but not in Mexicans. Huang et al. (238) did not support this observation in a study of North American Caucasians (14 SLE multiplex families as well as 41 cases and 88 controls). Dunckley et al. (239) found no association between *TCR* (*α*, *β*, and *γ*) RFLP and SLE or MHC class II molecules. Frank et al. (240) reported an association of *TCR β* RFLP with anti-Ro (SSA) antibodies but not with SLE. No linkage of *TCR α*, *β*, and *γ* chain genes to SLE was observed in five multiplex Caucasian families (241). The family studies had fairly small sample sizes and might lack power to detect linkage. Data available thus far fail to support the contribution of *TCR* gene variants to risk for SLE.

Immunoglobulin Heavy and Light Chain Genes

Earlier association studies of the immunoglobulin heavy chain locus (map to chromosome 14) and Ig heavy chain Gm allotypes as well as the kappa light chain gene (chromosome 2) and kappa light chain (km) allotypes yielded conflicting results. An association of Gm phenotype to SLE was observed in American and Australian Caucasians (242,243), Japanese (244), African Americans (245), but not in Hungarians or central Europeans (246,247). An association between Km phenotype and SLE was reported in North American Caucasians (248) but not in central Europeans (247). Kumar et al. (249) found a significant association of a Ig heavy chain constant region polymorphism with SLE in unrelated Mexicans and Mexican SLE multiplex families but not in SLE patients from the United States. No association between the lambda light chain polymorphism and SLE was observed by Blasini et al. (250). Since the Gm/Km allotypes or Ig RFLP can detect only limited polymorphism present within the vast variation of immunoglobulin gene loci, these studies do not rule out the possibility that immunoglobulin gene variants can confer genetic risk for SLE.

The expression of a particular V gene and receptor editing may regulate the production of autoantibodies (251). Olee et al. (252) reported the deletion of the *Humhv3005* gene (likely to encode heavy chains of rheumatoid factors) in 25% of the studied rheumatoid arthritis and SLE patients and 2% of the normal controls. A subsequent study from the same group concluded the deletion of this V gene contributed a weak genetic risk for SLE (238).

GENETIC LINKAGE OF GENOMIC LOCI TO HUMAN SLE

Linkage analysis studies families containing multiple relatives affected with the same disease. The rationale is that DNA markers located near a susceptibility gene will be transmitted together with the disease gene in affected members of each family because they are likely to share the same susceptibility gene allele at a particular disease locus (11). A genome scan typically uses a panel of genetic markers spaced 10 to 20 cM (1 cM equals about 1 million base pairs of DNA) apart to cover the whole genome for mapping susceptibility loci. The large number of the studied markers (approximately 350 microsatellite markers) markedly increases the likelihood of false-positive linkage results, thus the need to replicate and confirm linkage in independent samples (253). However, it is not a trivial task to determine whether a given study has replicated the previous linkage results of complex human diseases. The statistical evidence required for confirmation and the acceptable variation in mapped positions have not reached a consensus among experts (223,253–255).

As shown in Table 6.2, five independent genome scans for mapping loci containing SLE susceptibility genes have been conducted in the last three years (158,159,213, 214,258). A comparison of these reports of genetic linkage to SLE susceptibility clearly shows that (a) multiple genes predispose to SLE, (b) no single locus appears to be shared in all studied SLE multiplex families, (c) 16 loci identified in two or more independent scans are putative susceptibility loci (Table 6.3), and (d) 11 loci listed in Table 6.4 may also contain susceptibility loci. Because these 11 loci were identified only in a single scan, we used more stringent criteria of a lod >2 or nonparametric linkage (NPL) >2.5 than the criteria used for agreement of loci in two or more scans (lod >1 or NPL >1.5 and intermarker distance of 25 cM or less). Thus these 27 loci identified by linkage analyses are likely to contain SLE susceptibility genes. Because the statistical evidence for linkage at many loci is rather weak, it is important to distinguish true susceptibility loci from false positives.

The differences in mapped loci among studies may be attributed to many factors, including genetic heterogeneity, disease heterogeneity, power differences to detect linkage, stochastic fluctuation of allele frequencies in samples (especially if the sample size is small), and the method employed for linkage analyses (11,253–255). As shown in Table 6.2, there is a large variation among studied samples in size, ethnic composition, and family structure. Gaffney et al. (158,213) studied affected sib-pair families including 105 families in cohort 1 and 82 families in cohort 2, that were composed of approximately 80% Caucasian. Shai et al. (159) studied 80 multiplex families (predominantly sib-pair families) composed of 43 Mexican American and 37 Caucasian families (159). Both Gaffney et al. and Shai et al. performed model-free multipoint linkage analyses using the GENEHUNTER program (257). Moser et al. (214) used mainly model-based two-point linkage analysis to study 94 extended pedigrees consisting of 55 Caucasian and 31 African American families (214). Linqvist et al. (258) also used model-based two-point linkage analysis to study six

TABLE 6.2. COMPARISONS OF COHORTS STUDIED IN GENOME SCANS FOR MAPPING SLE SUSCEPTIBILITY LOCI

Study Design	UMN[a] 1 Sibpairs	UMN 2 Sibpairs	UMN Combined Sibpairs	OMRF[b] Extended Pedigrees	USC[c] Extended Pedigrees	Uppsala[d] Extended Pedigrees	
No. of families	105	82	187	94	80	8	11
% Caucasian	80	78	79	58	46	(Icelandic)	(Swedish)
% Hispanic	8	6	7	nd	54	0	0
% Afr.-Amer.	5	15	10	33	0	0	0
% Asian	3	0	2	nd	0	0	0
% Other	4	1	2	nd	0	0	0
No. of SLE patients	220	179	399	220	188	16	28
No. of unaffecteds	155	101	256	311	246	80	26
Total subjects	375	280	655	531	434	96	54
References	158	213	213	214	159	256,258	258

[a]A study conducted at University of Minnesota (UMN).
[b]A study conducted at Oklahoma Medical Research Foundation (OMRF).
[c]A study conducted at University of Southern California (USC).
[d]A study conducted at University of Uppsala.

TABLE 6.3. PROPOSED HUMAN SLE SUSCEPTIBILITY LOCI IDENTIFIED IN TWO OR MORE LINKAGE ANALYSES OF MULTIPLEX FAMILIES

Locus	UMN 1 (158)	UMN 2 (213)	UMN Combined (213)	OMRF (214)	OMRF (263)	USC (159)	UCLA[a] (261)	UCLA[a] (216)	Uppsala[b] (258)	Interval (cM)[*,c]
1p36	+[f]	+				+				24
1q23-24				+		+				1
1q31				+					+	6
1q41-42	+		+	+[d]	+[e]	+	+	+		10
2q32-35		+		+						17
3q11	+			+						10
4p16-15			+	+						0
4q28-31	+	+		+						16
6p11-22	+		+			+			+	14
14q21-23	+					+				21
16q12-13	+					+				2
18q21						+			+	10
19q13				+					+	0
20p12-13	+					+				7
20q11-13	+			+		+				4
21q21				+					+	10

*Intervals were defined as lod >1.0 or NPL >1.5 and intermarker distance ≤25 cM.
[a]Targeted genomic scan of chromosome 1q only.
[b]Positive linkage observed in either six extended Icelandic pedigrees or 11 Swedish pedigrees, but not in the combined sample.
[c]Marker locations were derived from maps available at the Genetics Location Database, University of Southampton.
[d]Observed in 31 African-American pedigrees.
[e]Observed in 51 European American pedigrees.
[f]Markers within the genomic interval yielding lod >1.0 or NPL >1.5 and intermarker distance ≤25 cM.

Icelandic extended pedigrees and 11 Swedish multiplex pedigrees.

Despite all of these confounding factors, promising agreement in 16 loci has been found in these studies as summarized in Table 6.3. This table and the criteria used (lod >1 or NPL >1.5 and intermarker distance ≤25 cM) were adapted from Gaffney et al. (213) and expanded to incorporate the recent publication by Linqvist et al. (258). Among these loci, 1q23-24, 1q41-42, 6p11-22, and 16 q12-13 appear most promising with positive linkage results in three independent data sets.

Linkage at 1q23 with a lod score of 3.37 in African Americans was described by Moser et al. (214). This region is syntenic to linkage in murine models of SLE, and contains several Fcγ receptor polymorphisms that have been associated with human SLE. Further support for linkage of this

TABLE 6.4. DISPARATE LOCI IDENTIFIED IN A SINGLE INDEPENDENT COHORT THAT HAD LOD >2.0 OR NPL >2.5

Loci	UMN 2 (213)	UMN Combined (213)	OMRF (214)	USC (159)	Uppsala (258)
1q44				+[a]	
2p15		+			
2q37					+
6q26-27			+		
7p22	+				
7q21	+				
7q36	+				
10p13	+				
11q25			+		
12p12-11			+		
13q32			+		

[a]Markers within the genomic interval yielding lod >2.0 or NPL >2.5.

region to SLE has been described in the extended pedigrees (259) as well as by two independent studies (159,260).

Tsao et al. (261) originally linked the 1q41-42 region with susceptibility to SLE by conducting a targeted genome scan of a candidate genomic interval syntenic to the established murine susceptibility loci (the overlapping *Sle1/Nba2/Lbw7* loci mapped to the distal end of mouse chromosome 1; reviewed in ref. 143). A 15-cM region of 1q41-42 showed evidence for linkage to SLE using a multiethnic cohort of families containing 52 sib pairs affected with SLE (approximately 50% Caucasians, 28% Asians, and 22% African Americans). These results support the hypothesis that the same genes may predispose to lupus susceptibility in both mice and humans. Subsequently, using an enlarged sample containing 78 affected sib pairs, a multipoint linkage analysis of this region yielded a peak of lod score of 3.3 and narrowed the region of interest to approximately 5 cM (216). Linkage of this region to SLE was supported by a lod score of 1.33 in the UM combined cohort of 187 sib-pair families (213), and by highly significant p values in the OMRF cohort (215,262). Risch (223) raised the issue of variation in mapped positions among these studies. The distance of 10 cM or less is well within the range that can be expected in mapping complex human diseases with pedigree materials available (254). Data thus far strongly support a susceptibility gene within this region.

Both 6p11-22 and 16q12-13 had a lod >3.6 in the combined Gaffney cohort of 187 SLE sib-pair families, the largest sample analyzed thus far (213). Using the guidelines proposed by Lander and Kruglyak (253), a lod ≥3.6 is considered to indicate significant linkage. The interval 6p11-22 contains the MHC region where many genes important to the immune system reside. Although Shai et al. (159) supported linkage at these loci, their respective p values did not reach .01, a threshold put forth by Lander and Kruglyak (253) for confirmed linkage. Lindqvist et al. (258) supported linkage of the MHC region to SLE in the Swedish but not Icelandic pedigrees. Tsao et al. (260) supported linkage of 16q13 to SLE in a recent preliminary report.

Most recently, a novel linkage of 4p16-15.2 to SLE was identified (p = .0003 and lod = 3.84) using 126 pedigrees from OMRF and confirmed (lod = 1.5) using the UM cohort (263). In addition, an epistatic interaction between 4p16-15.2 and 5p15 in American Caucasians (p = .038) was noted in the OMRF cohort. This study utilized multiple statistical tools and suggested the application of a single linkage method to a given data set may fail to detect important linkage.

Of interest, three of these regions (1q42, 11p15, 16q13) identified in linkage analysis using SLE families have also been implicated in other human autoimmune diseases. The genomic segment of 1q42 has been linked to type 1 diabetes mellitus using a combined genome scan data containing 679 affected sib pairs (264). Gaffney et al. (158), who linked the genomic segment of 11p to SLE, noted that this region was also linked with asthma, multiple sclerosis, and type 1 diabetes. Similarly, the chromosome 16q13 region was linked to SLE, Crohn's disease, Blau syndrome, psoriasis, type 1 diabetes, and asthma (265–272). These findings support the hypothesis that common susceptibility genes may predispose to clinically distinct autoimmune diseases (158,273,274). However, the linked intervals usually are rather large and may contain hundreds of genes. Thus, it is highly likely that different genes within the shared regions contribute to separate autoimmune diseases. Recently, the identification of a shared genetic variant of IL-2 contributing to risk for two separate autoimmune diseases supports this hypothesis. Independent genetic studies of the murine models for type 1 diabetes and multiple sclerosis identified a common genomic interval linked to both autoimmune diseases. Subsequent studies showed that the two susceptible strains of both autoimmune diseases shared the identical genetic variant of the IL-2 gene within the shared genomic interval, but the resistant strains had a different variant (275). Because of the important physiologic role of IL-2 in these two diseases, the investigators suggested that the genetic variant shared in susceptible strains is a risk factor for both autoimmune diseases. Whether any of the 1q42, 11p15, and 16q13 regions contains a shared genetic variant predisposing to lupus and other autoimmune diseases awaits further studies.

SUMMARY

This chapter clearly illustrates an important role of genetic contributions to susceptibility of SLE as well as the complexity of such genetic effects. Both MHC and non-MHC genes predispose to SLE similarly to other autoimmune diseases. Many studies during the past quarter of a century showed consistent associations of MHC class II and III genes with SLE in various populations. The search for non-MHC genes including mapping susceptibility loci in genome-wide screens has been actively pursued more recently. The presence of susceptibility genes within several chromosomal regions linked to SLE has been confirmed. The recently completed draft sequence of the human genome provides tremendous information that will greatly facilitate mapping and the eventual identification of susceptibility genes. The identification of these genes will almost certainly provide new insights into the genetic mechanisms that are disrupted in susceptible individuals, and may lead to novel therapeutic targets for disease intervention.

REFERENCES

1. Kotzin BL. Systemic lupus erythematosus. *Cell* 1996;85: 303–306.
2. Buckman KJ, Moore SK, Ebbin AJ, et al. Familial systemic lupus erythematosus. *Arch Intern Med* 1978;138(11): 1674–1676.

3. Pistiner M, Wallace DJ, Nessim S, Lupus erythematosus in the 1980s: a survey of 570 patients. *Semin Arthritis Rheum* 1991; 21(1):55–64.
4. Hochberg MC. The application of genetic epidemiology to systemic lupus erythematosus. *J Rheumatol* 1987;14(5):867–869.
5. Lawrence JS, Martins CL, Drake GL. A family survey of lupus erythematosus. 1. Heritability. *J Rheumatol* 1987;14(5): 913–921.
6. Block SR, Winfield JB, Lockshin MD, et al. Studies of twins with SLE. A review of the literature and presentation of 12 additional sets. *Am J Med* 1979;59:533–552.
7. Deapen D, Escalante A, Weinrib L, et al. A revised estimate of twin concordance in SLE. *Arthritis Rheum* 1992;35:311.
8. Gregersen PK. Discordance for autoimmunity in monozygotic twins. Are "identical" twins really identical? *Arthritis Rheum* 1993;36(9):1185–1192.
9. Vyse TJ, Todd JA. Genetic analysis of autoimmune disease. *Cell* 1996;85:311–318.
10. Risch N. Assessing the role of HLA-linked and unlinked determinants of disease. *Am J Hum Genet* 1987;40:1–14.
11. Lander ES, Schork NJ. Genetic dissection of complex traits. *Science* 1994;265:2037–2048.
12. Hochberg MC. Updating the American College of Rheumatology revised criteria for the classification of systemic lupus erythematosus. *Arthritis Rheum* 1997;40(9):1725–1734.
13. Tan EM, Cohen AS, Fires JF, et al. Special article: the 1982 revised criteria for the classification of SLE. *Arthritis Rheum* 1982;25:1271–1277.
14. Abreu PC, Greenberg DA, Hodge SE. Direct power comparisons between simple LOD scores and NPL scores for linkage analysis in complex diseases. *Am J Hum Genet* 1999;65(3): 847–857.
15. Clerget-Darpoux F, Bonaiti-Pellie C, Hochez J. Effects of misspecifying genetic parameters in lod score analysis. *Biometrics* 1986;42(2):393–399.
16. Hodge SE, Abreu PC, Greenberg DA. Magnitude of type I error when single-locus linkage analysis is maximized over models: a simulation study. *Am J Hum Genet* 1997;60(1):217–227.
17. Ott J. Complex traits on the map. *Nature* 1996;379(6568): 772–773.
18. Spielman RS, McGinnis RE, Ewens WJ. Transmission test for linkage disequilibrium: the insulin gene region and insulin-dependent diabetes mellitus (IDDM). *Am J Hum Genet* 1993; 52:506–516.
19. Kruglyak L. Prospects for whole-genome linkage disequilibrium mapping of common disease genes. *Nat Genet* 1999;22(2): 139–144.
20. Risch N, Merikangas K. The future of genetic studies of complex human diseases. *Science* 1996;273:1516–1517.
21. Beck S, Trowsdale J. The human major histocompatibility complex: lessons from the DNA sequence. In: Lander ES, Page DC, Lifton R, eds. *Annual review of genomics and human genetics.* Palo Alto: Annual Reviews, 2000:117–137.
22. Price P, Witt C, Allcock R, et al. The genetic basis for the association of the 8.1 ancestral haplotype (A1, B8, DR3). with multiple immunopathological diseases. *Immunol Rev* 1999;167: 257–274.
23. Janeway CA, Travers P, Walport M, et al. *ImmunoBiology: the immune system in health and disease*, 4th ed. London: Current Biology, 1999.
24. MHC Sequencing Consortium. Complete sequence and gene map of a human major histocompatibility complex. *Nature* 1999;401:921–923.
25. Mauff G, Brenden M, Braun-Stilwell M. Relative electrophoretic migration distances for the classification of C4 allotypes. *Complement Inflamm* 1990;7(4–6):277–281.
26. Mauff G, Alper CA, Dawkins R, et al. C4 nomenclature statement (1990). *Complement Inflamm* 1990;7(4–6):261–268.
27. Tokunaga K, Saueracker G, Kay PH, et al. Extensive deletions and insertions in different MHC supratypes detected by pusled field gel electrophoresis. *J Exp Med* 1988;168(3): 933–940.
28. Campbell RD, Law SK, Reid KB, et al. Structure, organization, and regulation of the complement genes. *Annu Rev Immunol* 1988;6:161–195.
29. Yu CY. Molecular genetics of the human MHC complement gene cluster. *Exp Clin Immunogenet* 1998;15(4):213–230.
30. Goldberg MA, Arnett FC, Bias WB, Shulman LE. Histocompatibility antigens in systemic lupus erythematosus. *Arthritis Rheum* 1976;19(2):129–132.
31. Grumet FC, Coukell A, Bodmer JG, et al. Histocompatibility (HL-A) antigens associated with systemic lupus erythematosus. A possible genetic predisposition to disease. *N Engl J Med* 1971; 285(4):193–196.
32. Waters H, Konrad P, Walford RL. The distribution of HL-A histocompatibility factors and genes in patients with systemic lupus erythematosus. *Tissue Antigens* 1971;1(2):68–73.
33. Nies KM, Brown JC, Dubois EL, et al. Histocompatibility (HL-A) antigens and lymphocytotoxic antibodies in systemic lupus erythematosus (SLE). *Arthritis Rheum* 1974;17(4):397-402.
34. Gibofsky A, Winchester RJ, Patarroyo M, et al. Disease associations of the Ia-like human alloantigens. Contrasting patterns in rheumatoid arthritis and systemic lupus erythematosus. *J Exp Med* 1978;148(6):1728–1732.
35. Reinertsen JL, Klippel JH, Johnson AH, et al. B-lymphocyte alloantigens associated with systemic lupus erythematosus. *N Engl J Med* 1978;299(10):515–518.
36. Black CM, Welsh KI, Fielder A, et al. HLA antigens and Bf allotypes in SLE: evidence for the association being with specific haplotypes. *Tissue Antigens* 1982;19(2):115–120.
37. Celada A, Barras C, Benzonana G, et al. Increased frequency of HLA-DRw3 in systemic lupus erythematosus. *Tissue Antigens* 1980;15(3):283–288.
38. Cowland JB, Andersen V, Halberg P, et al. DNA polymorphism of HLA class II genes in systemic lupus erythematosus. *Tissue Antigens* 1994;43(1):34–37.
39. Dunckley H, Gatenby PA, Serjeantson SW. DNA typing of HLA-DR antigens in SLE. *Immunogenetics* 1986;24:158–162.
40. Gomez-Reino JJ, Martinez-Laso J, Vicario JL, et al. Immunogenetics of systemic lupus erythematosus in Spanish patients: differential HLA markers. *Immunobiology* 1991;182(5): 465–471.
41. Hartung K, Baur MP, Coldewey R, et al. Major histocompatibility complex haplotypes and complement C4 alleles in systemic lupus erythematosus. Results of a multicenter study. *J Clin Invest* 1992;90(4):1346–1351.
42. Lulli P, Sebastiani GD, Trabace S, et al. HLA antigens in Italian patients with systemic lupus erythematosus: evidence for the association of DQw2 with the autoantibody response to extractable nuclear antigens. *Clin Exp Rheumatol* 1991;9(5): 475–479.
43. Reinharz D, Tiercy JM, Mach B, et al. Absence of DRw15/3 and of DRw15/7 heterozygotes in Caucasian patients with systemic lupus erythematosus [see comments]. *Tissue Antigens* 1991;37(1):10–15.
44. Reveille JD, Anderson KL, Schrohenloher RE, et al. Restriction fragment length polymorphism analysis of HLA-DR, DQ, DP and C4 alleles in Caucasians with SLE. *J Rheumatol* 1991;18: 14–18.
45. Reveille JD, Moulds JM, Ahn C, et al. Systemic lupus erythematosus in three ethnic groups: I. The effects of HLA class II,

C4, and CR1 alleles, socioeconomic factors, and ethnicity at disease onset. LUMINA Study Group. Lupus in minority populations, nature versus nurture. *Arthritis Rheum* 1998;41(7): 1161–1172.
46. Ruuska P, Hameenkorpi R, Forsberg S, et al. Differences in HLA antigens between patients with mixed connective tissue disease and systemic lupus erythematosus. *Ann Rheum Dis* 1992;51(1):52–55.
47. Skarsvag S, Hansen KE, Holst A, et al. Distribution of HLA class II alleles among Scandinavian patients with systemic lupus erythematosus (SLE): an increased risk of SLE among non[DRB1*03,DQA1*0501,DQB1*0201] class II homozygotes? *Tissue Antigens* 1992;40(3):128–133.
48. Ahearn JM, Provost TT, Dorsch CA, et al. Interrelationships of HLA-DR, MB, and MT phenotypes, autoantibody expression, and clinical features in systemic lupus erythematosus. *Arthritis Rheum* 1982;25(9):1031–1040.
49. So AK, Fielder AH, Warner CA, et al. DNA polymorphisms of MHC class II and class III genes in SLE. *Tissue Antigens* 1990; 35:144–147.
50. Hashimoto H, Tsuda H, Matsumoto T, et al. HLA antigens associated with systemic lupus erythematosus in Japan. *J Rheumatol* 1985;12(5):919–923.
51. Hirose S, Ogawa S, Nishimura H, et al. Association of HLA-DR2/DR4 heterozygosity with systemic lupus erythematosus in Japanese patients. *J Rheumatol* 1988;15(10):1489–1492.
52. Doherty DG, Ireland R, Demaine AG, et al. Major histocompatibility complex genes and susceptibility to systemic lupus erythematosus in southern Chinese. *Arthritis Rheum* 1992; 35(6):641–646.
53. Savage DA, Ng SC, Howe HS, et al. HLA and TAP associations in Chinese systemic lupus erythematosus patients. *Tissue Antigens* 1995;46(3 pt 1):213–216.
54. Dong RP, Kimura A, Hashimoto H, et al. Difference in HLA-linked genetic background between mixed connective tissue disease and systemic lupus erythematosus. *Tissue Antigens* 1993; 41(1):20–25.
55. Hong GH, Kim HY, Takeuchi F, et al. Association of complement C4 and HLA-DR alleles with systemic lupus erythematosus in Koreans. *J Rheumatol* 1994;21(3):442–447.
56. Hawkins BR, Wong KL, Wong RW, et al. Strong association between the major histocompatibility complex and systemic lupus erythematosus in southern Chinese. *J Rheumatol* 1987; 14(6):1128–1131.
57. Lu L-Y, Ding W-Z, Fici D, et al. Molecular analysis of major histocompatibility complex allelic associations with systemic lupus erythematosus in Taiwan. *Arthritis Rheum* 1997;40(6): 1138–1145.
58. Marintchev LM, Naumova EJ, Rashkov RK, et al. HLA class II alleles and autoantibodies in Bulgarians with systemic lupus erythematosus. *Tissue Antigens* 1995;46(5):422–425.
59. Mehra NK, Pande I, Taneja V, et al. Major histocompatibility complex genes and susceptibility to systemic lupus erythematosus in northern India. *Lupus* 1993;2(5):313–314.
60. Reveille JD, Arnett FC, Olsen ML, et al. HLA-class II alleles and C4 null genes in Greeks with systemic lupus erythematosus. *Tissue Antigens* 1995;46(5):417–421.
61. Reveille JD, Moulds JM, Arnett FC. Major histocompatibility complex class II and C4 alleles in Mexican Americans with systemic lupus erythematosus. *Tissue Antigens* 1995;45(2): 91–97.
62. Alarif LI, Ruppert GB, Wilson R Jr, et al. HLA-DR antigens in Blacks with rheumatoid arthritis and systemic lupus erythematosus. *J Rheumatol* 1983;10(2):297–300.
63. Gladman DD, Terasaki PI, Park MS, et al. Increased frequency of HLA-DRw2 in SLE. *Lancet* 1972;2:902–905.
64. Hochberg MC, Boyd RE, Ahearn JM, et al. SLE: a review of clinico-laboratory features and immunogenetic markers in 150 patients with emphasis on demographic subsets. *Medicine* 1985; 64:285–295.
65. Kachru RB, Sequeira W, Mittal KK, A significant increase of HLA-DR3 and DR2 in systemic lupus erythematosus among blacks. *J Rheumatol* 1984;11(4):471–474.
66. Wilson WA, Scopelitis E, Michalski JP. Association of HLA-DR7 with both antibody to SSA(Ro) and disease susceptibility in blacks with systemic lupus erythematosus. *J Rheumatol* 1984; 11(5):653–657.
67. Barron KS, Silverman ED, Gonzales J, et al. Clinical, serologic, and immunogenetic studies in childhood-onset systemic lupus erythematosus. *Arthritis Rheum* 1993;36(3):348–354.
68. Reveille JC, Schronhenloher RE, Acton RT, et al. DNA analysis of HLA-DR and DQ genes in American Blacks with SLE. *Arthritis Rheum* 1989;32:1243–1251.
69. Bell DA, Maddison PJ. Serologic subsets in systemic lupus erythematosus: an examination of autoantibodies in relationship to clinical features of disease and HLA antigens. *Arthritis Rheum* 1980;23(11):1268–1273.
70. Smolen JS, Klippel JH, Penner E, et al. HLA-DR antigens in systemic lupus erythematosus: association with specificity of autoantibody responses to nuclear antigens. *Ann Rheum Dis* 1987;46(6):457–462.
71. Hartung K, Ehrfeld H, Lakomek HJ, et al. The genetic basis of Ro and La antibody formation in systemic lupus erythematosus. Results of a multicenter study. The SLE Study Group. *Rheumatol Int* 1992;11(6):243–249.
72. Fujisaku A, Frank MB, Neas B, et al. HLA-DQ gene complementation and other histocompatibility relationships in man with the anti-Ro/SSA autoantibody response of systemic lupus erythematosus. *J Clin Invest* 1990;86(2):606–611.
73. Hamilton RG, Harley JB, Bias WB, et al. Two Ro (SS-A) autoantibody responses in systemic lupus erythematosus. Correlation of HLA-DR/DQ specificities with quantitative expression of Ro (SS-A) autoantibody. *Arthritis Rheum* 1988;31(4): 496–505.
74. Harley JB, Reichlin M, Arnett FC, et al. Gene interaction at HLA-DQ enhances autoantibody production in primary Sjogren's syndrome. *Science* 1986;232(4754):1145–1147.
75. Reveille JD, Macleod MJ, Whittington K, et al. Specific amino acid residues in the second hypervariable region of HLA-DQA1 and DQB1 chain genes promote the Ro (SS-A)/La (SS-B) autoantibody responses. *J Immunol* 1991;146(11): 3871–3876.
76. Scofield RH, Harley JB. Association of anti-Ro/SS-A autoantibodies with glutamine in position 34 of DQA1 and leucine in position 26 of DQB1. *Arthritis Rheum* 1994;37(6):961–962.
77. Buyon JP, Slade SG, Reveille JD, et al. Autoantibody responses to the "native" 52-kDa SS-A/Ro protein in neonatal lupus syndromes, systemic lupus erythematosus, and Sjogren's syndrome. *J Immunol* 1994;152(7):3675–3684.
78. Ehrfeld H, Hartung K, Renz M, et al. MHC associations of autoantibodies against recombinant Ro and La proteins in systemic lupus erythematosus. Results of a multicenter study. SLE Study Group. *Rheumatol Int* 1992;12(5):169–173.
79. Asherson RA, Doherty DG, Vergani D, et al. Major histocompatibility complex associations with primary antiphospholipid syndrome. *Arthritis Rheum* 1992;35(1):124–125.
80. Trabace S, Nicotra M, Cappellacci S, et al. HLA-DR and DQ antigens and anticardiolipin antibodies in women with recurrent spontaneous abortions. *Am J Reprod Immunol* 1991;26(4): 147–149.
81. Goldstein R, Moulds JM, Smith CD, et al. MHC studies of the primary antiphospholipid antibody syndrome and of antiphos-

pholipid antibodies in systemic lupus erythematosus. *J Rheumatol* 1996;23(7):1173–1179.

82. Granados J, Vargas-Alarcon G, Drenkard C, et al. Relationship of anticardiolipin antibodies and antiphospholipid syndrome to HLA-DR7 in Mexican patients with systemic lupus erythematosus (SLE). *Lupus* 1997;6(1):57–62.
83. McHugh NJ, Maddison PJ. HLA-DR antigens and anticardiolipin antibodies in patients with systemic lupus erythematosus [letter;comment]. *Arthritis Rheum* 1989;32(12):1623–1624.
84. Savi M, Ferraccioli GF, Neri TM, et al. HLA-DR antigens and anticardiolipin antibodies in northern Italian systemic lupus erythematosus patients [see comments]. *Arthritis Rheum* 1988; 31(12):1568–1570.
85. Hartung K, Coldewey R, Corvetta A, et al. MHC gene products and anticardiolipin antibodies in systemic lupus erythematosus results of a multicenter study. SLE Study Group. *Autoimmunity* 1992;13(2):95–99.
86. Galeazzi M, Sebastiani GD, Tincani A, et al. HLA class II alleles associations of anticardiolipin and anti-beta2GPI antibodies in a large series of European patients with systemic lupus erythematosus. *Lupus* 2000;9(1):47–55.
87. Dagenais P, Urowitz MB, Gladman DD, et al. A family study of the antiphospholipid syndrome associated with other autoimmune diseases. *J Rheumatol* 1992;19(9):1393–1396.
88. May KP, West SG, Moulds J, et al. Different manifestations of the antiphospholipid antibody syndrome in a family with systemic lupus erythematosus. *Arthritis Rheum* 1993;36(4): 528–533.
89. Goel N, Ortel TL, Bali D, et al. Familial antiphospholipid antibody syndrome: criteria for disease and evidence for autosomal dominant inheritance. *Arthritis Rheum* 1999;42(2): 318–327.
90. Arnett FC, Thiagarajan P, Ahn C, et al. Associations of anti-beta2-glycoprotein I autoantibodies with HLA class II alleles in three ethnic groups. *Arthritis Rheum* 1999;42(2):268–274.
91. Kamboh MI, Mehdi H. Genetics of apolipoprotein H (beta2-glycoprotein I) and anionic phospholipid binding. Lupus 1998; 7(suppl 2):S10–S13.
92. Atsumi T, Tsutsumi A, Amengual O, et al. Correlation between beta2-glycoprotein I valine/leucine247 polymorphism and anti-beta2-glycoprotein I antibodies in patients with primary antiphospholipid syndrome. *Rheumatol (Oxf)* 1999;38(8): 721–723.
93. Hirose N, Williams R, Alberts AR, et al. A role for the polymorphism at position 247 of the beta2-glycoprotein I gene in the generation of anti-beta2-glycoprotein I antibodies in the antiphospholipid syndrome. *Arthritis Rheum* 1999;42(8): 1655–1661.
94. Gushiken FC, Arnett FC, Ahn C, et al. Polymorphism of beta2-glycoprotein I at codons 306 and 316 in patients with systemic lupus erythematosus and antiphospholipid syndrome. *Arthritis Rheum* 1999;42(6):1189–1193.
95. Kamboh MI, Manzi S, Mehdi H, et al. Genetic variation in apolipoprotein H (beta2-glycoprotein I) affects the occurrence of antiphospholipid antibodies and apolipoprotein H concentrations in systemic lupus erythematosus. *Lupus* 1999;8(9): 742–750.
96. Horbach DA, van Oort E, Lisman T, et al. Beta2-glycoprotein I is proteolytically cleaved in vivo upon activation of fibrinolysis. Thromb Haemost 1999;81(1):87–95.
97. Arnett FC, Hamilton RG, Reveille JD, et al. Genetic studies of Ro (SS-A) and La (SS-B) autoantibodies in families with systemic lupus erythematosus and primary Sjogren's syndrome. *Arthritis Rheum* 1989;32(4):413–419.
98. Kaneoka H, Hsu KC, Takeda Y, et al. Molecular genetic analysis of HLA-DR and HLA-DQ genes among anti-U1-70-kd autoantibody positive connective tissue disease patients. *Arthritis Rheum* 1992;35(1):83–94.
99. Kuwana M, Okano Y, Kaburaki J, et al. Major histocompatibility complex class II gene associations with anti-U1 small nuclear ribonucleoprotein antibody. Relationship to immunoreactivity with individual constituent proteins. *Arthritis Rheum* 1995; 38(3):396–405.
100. Olsen ML, Arnett FC, Reveille JD. Contrasting molecular patterns of MHC class II alleles associated with the anti-Sm and anti-RNP precipitin autoantibodies in systemic lupus erythematosus. *Arthritis Rheum* 1993;36(1):94–104.
101. Griffing WL, Moore SB, Luthra HS, et al. Associations of antibodies to native DNA with HLA-DRw3. A possible major histocompatibility complex-linked human immune response gene. *J Exp Med* 1980;152(2 pt 2):319s-325s.
102. Alvarellos A, Ahearn JM, Provost TT, et al. Relationships of HLA-DR and MT antigens to autoantibody expression in systemic lupus erythematosus [letter]. *Arthritis Rheum* 1983; 26(12):1533–1535.
103. Schur PH. Associations between SLE and the MHC complex: clinical and immunological considerations. *Clin Immunol Immunopathol* 1982;24:263–275.
104. Awdeh ZL, Raum DD, Glass D, et al. Complement-human histocompatibility antigen haplotypes in C2 deficiency. *J Clin Invest* 1981;67(2):581–583.
105. Araujo MN, Silva NP, Andrade LE, et al. C2 deficiency in blood donors and lupus patients: prevalence, clinical characteristics and HLA-associations in the Brazilian population. *Lupus* 1997;6(5):462–466.
106. Johnson CA, Densen P, Hurford RK Jr, et al. Type I human complement C2 deficiency. A 28-base pair gene deletion causes skipping of exon 6 during RNA splicing. *J Biol Chem* 1993; 268(3):2268.
107. Glass D, Raum D, Gibson D, et al. Inherited deficiency of the second component of complement. Rheumatic disease associations. *J Clin Invest* 1976;58(4):853–861.
108. Sullivan KE, Petri MA, Schmeckpeper BJ, et al. Prevalence of a mutation causing C2 deficiency in systemic lupus erythematosus. *J Rheumatol* 1994;21(6):1128–1133.
109. Pickering MC, Walport MJ. Links between complement abnormalities and systemic lupus erythematosus. *Rheumatol (Oxf)* 2000;39(2):133–141.
110. Walport MJ. Inherited complement deficiency—clues to the physiological activity of complement in vivo. *Q J Med* 1993; 86(6):355–358.
111. Walport MJ. The Roche Rheumatology Prize Lecture. Complement deficiency and disease. *Br J Rheumatol* 1993;32(4): 269–273.
112. Meyer O, Hauptmann G, Tappeiner G, et al. Genetic deficiency of C4, C2 or *C1q* and lupus syndromes. Association with anti-Ro (SS-A) antibodies. *Clin Exp Immunol* 1985;62(3): 678–684.
113. Provost TT, Arnett FC, Reichlin M. Homozygous C2 deficiency, lupus erythematosus, and anti-Ro (SSA) antibodies. *Arthritis Rheum* 1983;26(10):1279–1282.
114. Ballow M, McLean RH, Einarson M, et al. Hereditary C4 deficiency—genetic studies and linkage to HLA. *Transplant Proc* 1979;11(4):1710–1712.
115. Hauptmann G, Grosshans E, Heid E. Lupus erythematosus syndrome and complete deficiency of the fourth component of complement. *Boll Ist Sieroter Milan* 1974;53(1):suppl.
116. Kjellman M, Laurell AB, Low B, et al. Homozygous deficiency of C4 in a child with a lupus erythematosus syndrome. *Clin Genet* 1982;22(6):331–339.
117. Mascart-Lemone F, Hauptmann G, Goetz J, et al. Genetic deficiency of C4 presenting with recurrent infections and a SLE-

like disease. Genetic and immunologic studies. *Am J Med* 1983; 75(2):295–304.

118. Schaller JG, Gilliland BG, Ochs HD, et al. Severe systemic lupus erythematosus with nephritis in a boy with deficiency of the fourth component of complement. *Arthritis Rheum* 1977; 20(8):1519–1525.
119. Tappeiner G, Hintner H, Scholz S, et al. Systemic lupus erythematosus in hereditary deficiency of the fourth component of complement. *J Am Acad Dermatol* 1982;7(1):66–79.
120. Tappeiner G. Disease states in genetic complement deficiencies. *Int J Dermatol* 1982;21(4):175–191.
121. Urowitz MB, Gladman DD, Minta JO. Systemic lupus erythematosus in a patient with C4 deficiency. *J Rheumatol* 1981;8(5): 741–746.
122. Christiansen FT, Zhang WJ, Griffiths M, et al. Major histocompatibility complex (MHC) complement deficiency, ancestral haplotypes and systemic lupus erythematosus (SLE): C4 deficiency explains some but not all of the influence of the MHC. *J Rheumatol* 1991;18(9):1350–1358.
123. Davies EJ, Rigsby R, Stiller CR, et al. HLA-DQ, DR and complement C4 variants in SLE. *Br J Rheumatol* 1993;32(1): 870–875.
124. Dunckley H, Gatenby PA, Hawkins B, et al. Deficiency of C4A is a genetic determinant of systemic lupus erythematosus in three ethnic groups. *J Immunogenet* 1987;14(4–5): 209–218.
125. Fielder AH, Walport MJ, Batchelor JR, et al. Family study of the major histocompatibility complex in patients with systemic lupus erythematosus: importance of null alleles of C4A and C4B in determining disease susceptibility. *Br Med J (Clin Res Ed)* 1983;286(6363):425–428.
126. Kemp ME, Atkinson JP, Skanes VM, et al. Deletion of C4A genes in patients with systemic lupus erythematosus. *Arthritis Rheum* 1987;30(9):1015–1022.
127. Schur PH, Marcus-Bagley D, Awdeh Z, et al. The effect of ethnicity on major histocompatibility complex complement allotypes and extended haplotypes in patients with systemic lupus erythematosus. *Arthritis Rheum* 1990;33(7):985–992.
128. Carroll MC, Palsdottir A, Belt KT, et al. Deletion of complement C4 and steroid 21-hydroxylase genes in the HLA class III region. *EMBO J* 1985;4(10):2547–2552.
129. Goldstein R, Arnett FC, McLean RH, et al. Molecular heterogeneity of complement component C4 "null" and 21-hydroxylase genes in systemic lupus erythematosus. *Arthritis Rheum* 1988;31:736–744.
130. Hartung K, Fontana A, Klar M, et al. Association of class I, II, and III MHC gene products with systemic lupus erythematosus. Results of a Central European multicenter study. *Rheumatol Int* 1989;9(1):13–18.
131. Batchelor JR, Fielder AH, Walport MJ, et al. Family study of the major histocompatibility complex in HLA DR3 negative patients with systemic lupus erythematosus. *Clin Exp Immunol* 1987;70(2):364–371.
132. Jacob CO, Fronek Z, Lewis GD, et al. Heritable major histocompatibility complex class II-associated differences in production of tumor necrosis factor : relevance to genetic predisposition to systemic lupus erythematosus. *Proc Natl Acad Sci USA* 1990;87:1233–1237.
133. Jacob CO, McDevitt HO. Tumour necrosis factor- in murine autoimmune lupus nephritis. *Nature* 1988;331:356–358.
134. Jacob CO, Lee SK, Strassmann G. Mutational analysis of TNF-alpha gene reveals a regulatory role for the 3′-untranslated region in the genetic predisposition to lupus-like autoimmune disease. *J Immunol* 1996;156(8):3043–3050.
135. Charles PJ, Smeenk RJ, De Jong J, et al. Assessment of antibodies to double-stranded DNA induced in rheumatoid arthritis patients following treatment with infliximab, a monoclonal antibody to tumor necrosis factor alpha: findings in open-label and randomized placebo-controlled trials [In Process Citation]. *Arthritis Rheum* 2000;43(11):2383–2390.
136. Bidwell J, Keen L, Gallagher G, et al. Review: Cytokine gene polymorphism in human disease: on-line databases. *Genes Immunity* 1999;1:3–19.
137. Wilson AG, de Vries N, Pociot F, et al. An allelic polymorphism within the human tumor necrosis factor alpha promoter region is strongly associated with HLA A1, B8, and DR3 alleles. *J Exp Med* 1993;177(2):557–560.
138. Rood MJ, van Krugten MV, Zanelli E, et al. TNF-308A and HLA-DR3 alleles contribute independently to susceptibility to systemic lupus erythematosus. *Arthritis Rheum* 2000;43(1): 129–134.
139. Rudwaleit M, Tikly M, Khamashta M, et al. Interethnic differences in the association of tumor necrosis factor promoter polymorphisms with systemic lupus erythematosus. *J Rheumatol* 1996;23(10):1725–1728.
140. Wilson AG, Gordon C, di Giovine FS, et al. A genetic association between systemic lupus erythematosus and tumour necrosis factor-alpha. *Eur J Immunol* 1994;24:191–195.
141. Sullivan KE, Wooten C, Schmeckpeper BJ, et al. A promoter polymorphism of tumor necrosis factor a associated with systemic lupus erythematosus in African-Americans. *Arthritis Rheum* 1997;40(12):2207–2211.
142. Wilson AG, Symons JA, McDowell TL, et al. Effects of a polymorphism in the human tumor necrosis factor alpha promoter on transcriptional activation. *Proc Natl Acad Sci USA* 1997; 94(7):3195–3199.
143. Vyse TJ, Kotzin BL. Genetic susceptibility to systemic lupus erythematosus. *Annu Rev Immunol* 1998;16:261–292.
144. Dupont B. *Immunobiology of HLA, Vol II: Immunogenetics and histocompatibility.* New York: Springer-Verlag, 1989.
145. Awdeh ZL, Raum D, Yunis EJ, et al. Extended HLA/complement allele haplotypes: evidence for T/t-like complex in man. *Proc Natl Acad Sci USA* 1983;80(1):259–263.
146. Baur MP, Danilovs JA. Population analysis of HLA-A,B,C,DR and other genetic markers. In: Terasaki PI, ed. *Histocompatibility testing 1980.* Los Angeles: UCLA Press, 1980:955–958.
147. Hurley CK, Ziff BL, Silver J, et al. Polymorphism of the HLA-DR1 haplotype in American blacks. Identification of a DR1 beta-chain determinant recognized in the mixed lymphocyte reaction. *J Immunol* 1988;140(11):4019–4023.
148. Hurley CK, Gregersen PK, Gorski J, et al. The DR3(w18), DQw4 haplotype differs from DR3(w17),DQw2 haplotypes at multiple class II loci. *Hum Immunol* 1989;25(1):37–50.
149. Yamada H, Watanabe A, Mimori A, et al. Lack of gene deletion for complement C4A deficiency in Japanese patients with systemic lupus erythematosus. *J Rheumatol* 1990;17(8):1054–1057.
150. Morgan BP, Walport MJ. Complement deficiency and disease. *Immunol Today* 1991;12(9):301–306.
151. Navratil JS, Korb LC, Ahearn JM. Systemic lupus erythematosus and complement deficiency: clues to a novel role for the classical complement pathway in the maintenance of immune tolerance. *Immunopharmacology* 1999;42(1–3):47–52.
152. Botto M, Dell'Agnola C, Bygrave AE, et al. Homozygous *C1q* deficiency causes glomerulonephritis associated with multiple apoptotic bodies. *Nat Genet* 1998;19:56–59.
153. Korb LC, Ahearn JM. Cutting Edge. *C1q* binds directly and specifically to surface blebs of apoptotic huiman keratinocytes: complement deficiency and systemic lupus erythematosus revisited. *J Immunol* 1997;158:4525–4528.
154. Zheng L, Fisher G, Miller RE, et al. Induction of apoptosis in mature T cells by tumour necrosis factor. *Nature* 1995; 377(6547):348–351.

155. Drake CG, Babcock SK, Palmer E, et al. Genetic analysis of the NZB contribution to lupus-like autoimmune disease in (NZB × NZW)F1 mice. *Proc Natl Acad Sci USA* 1994;91(9):4062–4066.
156. Hirose S, Tsurui H, Nishimura H, et al. Mapping of a gene for hypergammaglobulinemia to the distal region on chromosome 4 in NZB mice and its contribution to systemic lupus erythematosus in (NZB × NZW)F1 mice. *Int Immunol* 1994;6(12): 1857–1864.
157. Jiang Y, Hirose S, Hamano Y, et al. Mapping of a gene for the increased susceptibility of B1 cells to Mott cell formation in murine autoimmune disease. *J Immunol* 1997;158(2):992–997.
158. Gaffney PM, Kearns GM, Shark KB, et al. A genome-wide search for susceptibility genes in human systemic lupus erythematosus sib-pair families. *Proc Natl Acad Sci USA* 1998;95(25): 14875–14879.
159. Shai R, Quismorio FP Jr, Li L, et al. Genome-wide screen for systemic lupus erythematosus susceptibility genes in multiplex families. *Hum Mol Genet* 1999;8(4):639–644.
160. Komata T, Tsuchiya N, Matsushita M, et al. Association of tumor necrosis factor receptor 2 (*TNFR2*) polymorphism with susceptibility to systemic lupus erythematosus. *Tissue Antigens* 1999;53(6):527–533.
161. Al Ansari AS, Ollier WE, Villarreal J, et al. Tumor necrosis factor receptor II (TNFRII) exon 6 polymorphism in systemic lupus erythematosus. *Tissue Antigens* 2000;55(1):97–99.
162. D'Alfonso S, Rampi M, Bocchio D, et al. Systemic lupus erythematosus candidate genes in the Italian population: evidence for a significant association with interleukin-10. *Arthritis Rheum* 2000;43(1):120–128.
163. Ravetch JV, Clynes RA. Divergent roles for Fc receptors and complement in vivo. *Annu Rev Immunol* 1998;16:421–432.
164. Duits AJ, Bootsma H, Derksen RHWM, et al. Skewed distribution of IgG Fc receptor IIa (CD32. polymorphism is associated with renal disease in systemic lupus erythematosus patients. *Arthritis Rheum* 1995;39:1832–1836.
165. Salmon JE, Millard S, Schachter LA, et al. Fc gamma RIIA alleles are heritable risk factors for lupus nephritis in African Americans. *J Clin Invest* 1996;97(5):1348–1354.
166. Song YW, Han CW, Kang SW, et al. Abnormal distribution of Fc gamma receptor type IIa polymorphisms in Korean patients with systemic lupus erythematosus. *Arthritis Rheum* 1998; 41(3):421–426.
167. Wu J, Edberg JC, Redecha PB, et al. A novel polymorphism of FcRIIIa (CD16. alters receptor function and predisposes to autoimmune disease. *J Clin Invest* 1997;100(5):1059–1070.
168. Koene HR, Kleijer M, Swaak AJ, et al. The Fc gammaRIIIA-158F allele is a risk factor for systemic lupus erythematosus. *Arthritis Rheum* 1998;41(10):1813–1818.
169. Salmon JE, Ng S, Yoo DH, et al. Altered distribution of Fcgamma receptor IIIA alleles in a cohort of Korean patients with lupus nephritis. *Arthritis Rheum* 1999;42(4):818–819.
170. Dijstelbloem HM, Bijl M, Fijnheer R, et al. Fcgamma receptor polymorphisms in systemic lupus erythematosus: association with disease and in vivo clearance of immune complexes [In Process Citation]. *Arthritis Rheum* 2000;43(12):2793–2800.
171. Oh M, Petri MA, Kim NA, et al. Frequency of the Fc gamma RIIIA-158F allele in African American patients with systemic lupus erythematosus. *J Rheumatol* 1999;26(7):1486–1489.
172. Seligman VASC, Lum R, Inda SE, et al. The FcRIIIA-158F allele is a major risk factor for the development of lupus nepjritis among Caucasians but not non-Caucasians. *Arthritis Rheum* 2001;44(3):618–625.
173. Clark MR, Liu L, Clarkson SB, et al. An abnormality of the gene that encodes neutrophil Fc receptor III in a patient with systemic lupus erythematosus. *J Clin Invest* 1990;86(1): 341–346.
174. Enenkel B, Jung D, Frey J. Molecular basis of IgG Fc receptor III defect in a patient with systemic lupus erythematosus. *Eur J Immunol* 1991;21(3):659–663.
175. Salmon JE, Edberg JC, Kimberly RP. Fc gamma receptor III on human neutrophils. Allelic variants have functionally distinct capacities. *J Clin Invest* 1990;85(4):1287–1295.
176. Hatta Y, Tsuchiya N, Ohashi J, et al. Association of Fc gamma Receptor III B polymorphism with SLE. *Genes Immunity* 1999; 1:53–60.
177. Clynes R, Dumitru C, Ravetch JV. Uncoupling of immune complex formation and kidney damage in autoimmune glomerulonephritis. *Science* 1998;279:1052–1054.
178. Park SY, Ueda S, Ohno H, et al. Resistance of Fc receptor- deficient mice to fatal glomerulonephritis. *J Clin Invest* 1998; 102(6):1229–1238.
179. Liossis S-NC, Ding XZ, Dennis GJ, et al. Altered pattern of TCR/CD3-mediated protein-tyrosyl phosphorylation in T cells from patients with systemic lupus erythematosus. *J Clin Invest* 1998;101:1448–1457.
180. Takeuchi T, Tsuzaka K, Pang M, et al. TCR zeta chain lacking exon 7 in two patients with systemic lupus erythematosus. *Int Immunol* 1998;10(7):911–921.
181. Tsuzaka K, Takeuchi T, Onoda N, et al. Mutations in T cell receptor zeta chain mRNA of peripheral T cells from systemic lupus erythematosus patients. *J Autoimmun* 1998;11(5): 381–385.
182. Wu J, Edberg JC, Gibson AW, et al. Single-nucleotide polymorphisms of T cell receptor zeta chain in patients with systemic lupus erythematosus. *Arthritis Rheum* 1999;42(12): 2601–2605.
183. Dorner T, Heimbacher C, Farner NL, et al. Enhanced mutational activity of Vkappa gene rearrangements in systemic lupus erythematosus. *Clin Immunol* 1999;92(2):188–196.
184. Nambiar MP, Enyedy EJ, Warke VG, et al. Polymorphisms/mutations of TCR-zeta-chain promoter and 3' untranslated region and Selective Expression of TCR zeta-chain with an alternatively spliced 3' untranslated region in patients with systemic lupus erythematosus. *J Autoimmun* 2001;16:133–142.
185. Llorente L, Zou W, Levy Y, et al. Role of interleukin 10 in the B lymphocyte hyperactivity and autoantibody production of human systemic lupus erythematosus. *J Exp Med* 1995;181(3): 839–844.
186. Hagiwara E, Gourley MF, Lee S, et al. Disease severity in patients with systemic lupus erythematosus correlates with an increased ratio of interleukin-10: interferon-gamma- secreting cells in the peripheral blood. *Arthritis Rheum* 1996;39(3): 379–385.
187. Llorente L, Richaud-Patin Y, Couderc J, et al. Dysregulation of interleukin-10 production in relatives of patients with systemic lupus erythematosus. *Arthritis Rheum* 1997;40(8):1429–1435.
188. Grondal G, Kristjansdottir H, Gunnlaugsdottir B, et al. Increased number of interleukin-10–producing cells in systemic lupus erythematosus patients and their first-degree relatives and spouses in Icelandic multicase families. *Arthritis Rheum* 1999; 42(8):1649–1654.
189. Eskdale J, Wordsworth P, Bowman S, et al. Association between polymorphisms at the human IL-10 locus and systemic lupus erythematosus [published erratum appears in *Tissue Antigens* 1997;50(6):699]. *Tissue Antigens* 1997;49(6):635–639.
190. Eskdale J, Gallagher G, Verweij CL, et al. Interleukin 10 secretion in relation to human IL-10 locus haplotypes. *Proc Natl Acad Sci USA* 1998;95(16):9465–9470.
191. Turner DM, Williams DM, Sankaran D, et al. An investigation of polymorphism in the interleukin-10 gene promoter. *Eur J Immunogenet* 1997;24(1):1–8.

192. Mehrian R, Quismorio FPJ, Strassmann, et al. Synergistic effect between IL-10 and bcl-2 genotypes in determining susceptibility to SLE. *Arthritis Rheum* 1998;41:596–602.
193. Lazarus M, Hajeer AH, Turner D, et al. Genetic variation in the interleukin 10 gene promoter and systemic lupus erythematosus [see comments]. *J Rheumatol* 1997;24(12):2314–2317.
194. Mok CC, Lanchbury JS, Chan DW, et al. Interleukin-10 promoter polymorphisms in Southern Chinese patients with systemic lupus erythematosus [see comments]. *Arthritis Rheum* 1998;41(6):1090–1095.
195. Vik DP, Wong WW. Structure of the gene for the F allele of complement receptor type 1 and sequence of the coding region unique to the S allele. *J Immunol* 1993;151(11):6214–6224.
196. Wilson JG, Wong WW, Schur PH, et al. Mode of inheritance of decreased C3b receptors on erythrocytes of patients with systemic lupus erythematosus. *N Engl J Med* 1982;307(16): 981–986.
197. Wilson JG, Murphy EE, Wong WW, et al. Identification of a restriction fragment length polymorphism by a CR1 cDNA that correlates with the number of CR1 on erythrocytes. *J Exp Med* 1986;164(1):50–59.
198. Wong WW, Kennedy CA, Bonaccio ET, et al. Analysis of multiple restriction fragment length polymorphisms of the gene for the human complement receptor type I. Duplication of genomic sequences occurs in association with a high molecular mass receptor allotype. *J Exp Med* 1986;164(5):1531–1546.
199. Wilson JG, Ratnoff WD, Schur PH, et al. Decreased expression of the C3b/C4b receptor (CR1) and the C3d receptor (CR2) on B lymphocytes and of CR1 on neutrophils of patients with systemic lupus erythematosus. *Arthritis Rheum* 1986;29(6): 739–747.
200. Tebib JG, Martinez C, Granados J, et al. The frequency of complement receptor type 1 (CR1. gene polymorphisms in nine families with multiple cases of systemic lupus erythematosus. *Arthritis Rheum* 1989;32(11):1465–1469.
201. Kumar A, Kumar A, Sinha S, et al. Hind III genomic polymorphism of the C3b receptor (CR1) in patients with SLE: low erythrocyte CR1 expression is an acquired phenomenon. *Immunol Cell Biol* 1995;73(5):457–462.
202. Van Dyne S, Holers VM, Lublin DM, et al. The polymorphism of the C3b/C4b receptor in the normal population and in patients with systemic lupus erythematosus. *Clin Exp Immunol* 1987;68(3):570–579.
203. Wong WW, Cahill JM, Rosen MD, et al. Structure of the human CR1 gene. Molecular basis of the structural and quantitative polymorphisms and identification of a new CR1-like allele. *J Exp Med* 1989;169(3):847–863.
204. Wong WW, Farrell SA. Proposed structure of the F′ allotype of human CR1. Loss of a C3b binding site may be associated with altered function. *J Immunol* 1991;146(2):656–662.
205. Cornillet P, Gredy P, Pennaforte JL, et al. Increased frequency of the long (S) allotype of CR1 (the C3b/C4b receptor, CD35) in patients with systemic lupus erythematosus. *Clin Exp Immunol* 1992;89(1):22–25.
206. Moulds JM, Reveille JD, Arnett FC. Structural polymorphisms of complement receptor 1 (CR1) in systemic lupus erythematosus (SLE) patients and normal controls of three ethnic groups. *Clin Exp Immunol* 1996;105(2):302–305.
207. Oliver FJ, Menissier-de Murcia J, de Murcia G. Poly(ADP-ribose) polymerase in the cellular response to DNA damage, apoptosis, and disease. *Am J Hum Genet* 1999;64(5): 1282–1288.
208. Haug BL, Lee JS, Sibley JT. Altered poly-(ADP-ribose) metabolism in family members of patients with systemic lupus erythematosus. *J Rheumatol* 1994;21:851–856.
209. Lee JS, Haug BL, Sibley JT. Decreased mRNA levels coding for poly(ADP-ribose) polymerase in lymphocytes of patients with SLE. *Lupus* 1994;3(2):113–116.
210. Sibley JT, Haug BL, Lee JS. Altered metabolism of poly(ADP-ribose) in the peripheral blood lymphocytes of patients with systemic lupus erythematosus. *Arthritis Rheum* 1989;32(8): 1045–1049.
211. Decker P, Briand JP, de Murcia G, et al. Zinc is an essential cofactor for recognition of the DNA binding domain of poly(ADP-ribose) polymerase by antibodies in autoimmune rheumatic and bowel diseases. *Arthritis Rheum* 1998;41(5): 918–926.
212. Decker P, Isenberg D, Muller S. Inhibition of caspase-3-mediated poly(ADP-ribose) polymerase (PARP) apoptotic cleavage by human PARP autoantibodies and effect on cells undergoing apoptosis. *J Biol Chem* 2000;275(12):9043–9046.
213. Gaffney PM, Ortmann WA, Selby SA, et al. Genome screening in human systemic lupus erythematosus: results from a second Minnesota cohort and combined analyses of 187 sib-pair families. *Am J Hum Genet* 2000;66(2):547–556.
214. Moser KL, Neas BR, Salmon JE, et al. Genome scan of human systemic lupus erythematosus: evidence for linkage on chromosome 1q in African-American pedigrees. *Proc Natl Acad Sci USA*1998;95(25):14869–14874.
215. Moser KL, Gray-McGuire C, Kelly J, et al. Confirmation of genetic linkage between human systemic lupus erythematosus and chromosome 1q41. *Arthritis Rheum* 1999;42(9): 1902–1907.
216. Tsao BP, Cantor RM, Grossman JM, et al. PARP alleles within the linked chromosomal region are associated with systemic lupus erythematosus. *J Clin Invest* 1999;103(8):1135–1140.
217. Delrieu O, Michel M, Frances C, et al. Poly(ADP-ribose) polymerase alleles in French Caucasians are associated neither with lupus nor with primary antiphospholipid syndrome. GRAID Research Group. Group for Research on Auto-Immune Disorders [see comments]. *Arthritis Rheum* 1999; 42(10):2194–2197.
218. Boorboor P, Drescher BE, Hartung K, et al. Poly(ADP-ribose) polymerase polymorphisms are not a genetic risk factor for systemic lupus erythematosus in German Caucasians [letter] [In Process Citation]. *J Rheumatol* 2000;27(8):2061.
219. Criswell LA, Moser KL, Gaffney PM, et al. PARP alleles and SLE: failure to confirm association with disease susceptibility [letter;comment] [see comments]. *J Clin Invest* 2000;105(11): 1501–1502.
220. Tan FK, Reveille JD, Arnett FC, et al. Poly(ADP)-ribose polymerase and susceptibility to systemic lupus erythematosus and primary antiphospholipid syndrome: comment on the article by Delrieu et al [letter]. *Arthritis Rheum* 2000;43(6):1421–1423.
221. Feder JN, Gnirke A, Thomas W, et al. A novel MHC class I-like gene is mutated in patients with hereditary haemochromatosis [see comments]. *Nat Genet* 1996;13(4):399–408.
222. Nielsen DM, Ehm MG, Weir BS. Detecting marker-disease association by testing for Hardy-Weinberg disequilibrium at a marker locus. *Am J Hum Genet* 1998;63(5):1531–1540.
223. Risch N. Searching for genes in complex diseases: lessons from systemic lupus erythematosus [comment]. *J Clin Invest* 2000; 105(11):1503–1506.
224. Magistrelli C, Samoilova E, Agarwal RK, et al. Polymorphic genotypes of the HRES-1 human endogenous retrovirus locus correlate with systemic lupus erythematosus and autoreactivity. *Immunogenetics* 1999;49(10):829–834.
225. Perl A, Colombo E, Dai H, et al. Antibody reactivity to the HRES-1 endogenous retroviral element identifies a subset of patients with systemic lupus erythematosus and overlap syndromes. Correlation with antinuclear antibodies and HLA class II alleles. *Arthritis Rheum* 1995;38(11):1660–1671.

226. Linker-Israeli M, Deans RJ, Wallace DJ, et al. Elevated levels of endogenous IL-6: a putative role in pathogenesis. *J Immunol* 1991;147(1):117–123.
227. Linker-Israeli M, Wallace DJ, Prehn J, et al. A greater variability in the 3′ flanking region of the IL-6 gene in patients with systemic lupus erythematosus (SLE). *Autoimmunity* 1996;23:199–209.
228. Linker-Israeli M, Wallace DJ, Prehn J, et al. Association of IL-6 gene alleles with systemic lupus erythematosus (SLE) and with elevated IL-6 expression. *Genes Immunity* 1999;1:45–52.
229. Turner MW. Deficiency of mannan binding protein—a new complement deficiency syndrome. *Clin Exp Immunol* 1991; 86(suppl 1):53–56.
230. Davies EJ, Snowden N, Hillarby MC, et al. Mannose-binding protein gene polymorphism in systemic lupus erythematosus. *Arthritis Rheum* 1995;38(1):110–114.
231. Ip WK, Chan SY, Lau CS, et al. Association of systemic lupus erythematosus with promoter polymorphisms of the mannose-binding lectin gene. *Arthritis Rheum* 1998;41(9):1663–1668.
232. Sullivan KE, Wooten C, Goldman D, et al. Mannose-binding protein genetic polymorphisms in black patients with systemic lupus erythematosus. *Arthritis Rheum* 1996;39(12):2046–2051.
233. Garred P, Madsen HO, Halberg P, et al. Mannose-binding lectin polymorphisms and susceptibility to infection in systemic lupus erythematosus. *Arthritis Rheum* 1999;42(10):2145–2152.
234. Kanemitsu S, Takabayashi A, Sasaki Y, et al. Association of interleukin-4 receptor and interleukin-4 promoter gene polymorphisms with systemic lupus erythematosus. *Arthritis Rheum* 1999;42(6):1298–1300.
235. Nakashima H, Inoue H, Akahoshi M, et al. The combination of polymorphisms within interferon-gamma receptor 1 and receptor 2 associated with the risk of systemic lupus erythematosus. *FEBS Lett* 1999;453(1–2):187–190.
236. Tanaka Y, Nakashima H, Hisano C, et al. Association of the interferon-gamma receptor variant (Val14Met) with systemic lupus erythematosus. *Immunogenetics* 1999;49(4):266–271.
237. Tebib JG, Alcocer-Varela J, Alarcon-Segovia D, et al. Association between a T cell receptor restriction fragment length polymorphism and systemic lupus erythematosus. *J Clin Invest* 1990;86(6):1961–1967.
238. Huang DF, Siminovitch KA, Liu XY, et al. Population and family studies of three disease-related polymorphic genes in systemic lupus erythematosus. *J Clin Invest* 1995;95(4): 1766–1772.
239. Dunckley H, Gatenby PA, Serjeantson SW. T-cell receptor and HLA class II RFLPs in systemic lupus erythematosus. *Immunogenetics* 1988;27(5):393–395.
240. Frank MB, McArthur R, Harley JB, et al. Anti-Ro(SSA) autoantibodies are associated with T cell receptor beta genes in systemic lupus erythematosus patients. *J Clin Invest* 1990;85(1):33–39.
241. Wong DW, Bentwich Z, Martinez-Tarquino C, et al. Nonlinkage of the T cell receptor alpha, beta, and gamma genes to systemic lupus erythematosus in multiplex families. *Arthritis Rheum* 1988;31(11):1371–1376.
242. Whittingham S, Mathews JD, Schanfield MS, et al. HLA and Gm genes in systemic lupus erythematosus. *Tissue Antigens* 1983;21(1):50–57.
243. Schur PH, Pandey JP, Fedrick JA. Gm allotypes in white patients with systemic lupus erythematosus. *Arthritis Rheum* 1985;28(7):828–830.
244. Nakao Y, Matsumoto H, Miyazaki T, et al. IgG heavy chain allotypes (Gm) in autoimmune diseases. *Clin Exp Immunol* 1980;42(1):20–26.
245. Fedrick JA, Pandey JP, Chen Z, et al. Gm allotypes in black patients with systemic lupus erythematosus. *Arthritis Rheum* 1985;28(7):828–830.
246. Stenszky V, Kozma L, Szegedi G, et al. Interplay of immunoglobulin G heavy chain markers (Gm) and HLA in predisposing to systemic lupus nephritis. *J Immunogenet* 1986; 13(1):11–17.
247. Hartung K, Coldewey R, Rother E, et al. Immunoglobulin allotypes in systemic lupus erythematosus—results of a central European multicenter study. SLE Study Group. *Exp Clin Immunogenet* 1991;8(1):11–15.
248. Hoffman RW, Sharp GC, Irvin WS, et al. Association of immunoglobulin Km and Gm allotypes with specific antinuclear antibodies and disease susceptibility among connective tissue disease patients. *Arthritis Rheum* 1991;34(4):453–458.
249. Kumar A, Martinez-Tarquino C, Maria-Forte A, et al. Immunoglobulin heavy chain constant-region gene polymorphism in systemic lupus erythematosus. *Arthritis Rheum* 1991; 34(12):1553–1556.
250. Blasini AM, Delgado MB, Valdivieso C, et al. Restriction fragment length polymorphisms of constant region genes of immunoglobulin lambda chains in Venezuelan patients with systemic lupus erythematosus. *Lupus* 1996;5(4):300–302.
251. Suzuki N, Harada T, Mihara S, et al. Characterization of a germline Vk gene encoding cationic anti-DNA antibody and role of receptor editing for development of the autoantibody in patients with systemic lupus erythematosus. *J Clin Invest* 1996; 98(8):1843–1850.
252. Olee T, Yang PM, Siminovitch KA, et al. Molecular basis of an autoantibody-associated restriction fragment length polymorphism that confers susceptibility to autoimmune diseases. *J Clin Invest* 1991;88(1):193–203.
253. Lander ES, Kruglyak L. Genetic dissection of complex traits: guidelines for interpreting and reporting linkage results. *Nat Genet* 1995;11:241–247.
254. Roberts SB, MacLean CJ, Neale MC, et al. Replication of linkage studies of complex traits: an examination of variation in location estimates. *Am J Hum Genet* 1999;65(3):876–884.
255. Xu J, Wiesch DG, Taylor EW, et al. Evaluation of replication studies, combined data analysis, and analytical methods in complex diseases. *Genet Epidemiol* 1999;17(suppl 1):S773–S778.
256. Lindquist A-K, Steinsson K, Kristjansdottir H, et al. Complete genome scan on Icelandic multicase families with systemic lupus erythematosus. Cancun, Mexico, 5th Internat'l Conf. on SLE. *Lupus* 1998;7(suppl 1):11.
257. Kruglyak L, Lander ES. Parametric and nonparametric linkage analysis: a unified multipoint approach. *Am J Hum Genet* 1996; 58:1347–1363.
258. Lindqvist AK, Steinsson K, Johanneson B, et al. A susceptibility locus for human systemic lupus erythematosus (hSLE1) on chromosome 2q. *J Autoimmun* 2000;14(2):169–178.
259. Harley JB, Gray-McGuire C, Kelly J, et al. Seven established linkages to human systemic lupus erythematosus. *Arthritis Rheum* 2000;43(9):S279.
260. Tsao BP, Grossman JM, Arnett FC, et al. Investigation of SLE-linked regions identified by genome scans: support for 1q24, 16q13, and 20p12. *Arthritis Rheum* 2000;43(9):S278.
261. Tsao BP, Cantor RM, Kalunian KC, et al. Evidence for linkage of a candidate chromosome 1 region to human systemic lupus erythematosus. *J Clin Invest* 1997;99(4):725–731.
262. Harley JB, Gray-McGuire C, Kelly J, et al. Seven established linkages to human systemic lupus erythematosus. *Arthritis Rheum* 2001;43(9):S279.
263. Gray-McGuire C, Moser KL, Gaffney PM, et al. Genome scan of human systemic lupus erythematosus by regression modeling: evidence of linkage and epistasis at 4p16-15.2. *Am J Hum Genet* 2000;67(6):1460–1469.
264. Concannon P, Gogolin-Ewens KJ, Hinds DA, et al. A second-generation screen of the human genome for susceptibility to

insulin-dependent diabetes mellitus. *Nat Genet* 1998;19(3): 292–296.

265. Curran ME, Lau KF, Hampe J, et al. Genetic analysis of inflammatory bowel disease in a large European cohort supports linkage to chromosomes 12 and 16. *Gastroenterology* 1998;115(5): 1066–1071.
266. Daniels SE, Bhattacharrya S, James A, et al. A genome-wide search for quantitative trait loci underlying asthma. *Nature* 1996;383(6597):247–250.
267. Davies JL, Kawaguchi Y, Bennett ST, et al. A genome-wide search for human type 1 diabetes susceptibility genes. *Nature* 1994;371(6493):130–136.
268. Hampe J, Schreiber S, Shaw SH, et al. A genomewide analysis provides evidence for novel linkages in inflammatory bowel disease in a large European cohort. *Am J Hum Genet* 1999;64(3): 808–816.
269. Hugot JP, Laurent-Puig P, Gower-Rousseau C, et al. Mapping of a susceptibility locus for Crohn's disease on chromosome 16. *Nature* 1996;379(6568):821–823.
270. Mirza MM, Lee J, Teare D, et al. Evidence of linkage of the inflammatory bowel disease susceptibility locus on chromosome 16 (IBD1) to ulcerative colitis. *J Med Genet* 1998;35(3):218–221.
271. Nair RP, Henseler T, Jenisch S, et al. Evidence for two psoriasis susceptibility loci (HLA and 17q) and two novel candidate regions (16q and 20p) by genome-wide scan. *Hum Mol Genet* 1997;6(8):1349–1356.
272. Tromp G, Kuivaniemi H, Raphael S, et al. Genetic linkage of familial granulomatous inflammatory arthritis, skin rash, and uveitis to chromosome 16. *Am J Hum Genet* 1996;59(5): 1097–1107.
273. Becker KG, Simon RM, Bailey-Wilson JE, et al. Clustering of non-major histocompatibility complex susceptibility candidate loci in human autoimmune diseases. *Proc Natl Acad Sci USA* 1998;95(17):9979–9984.
274. Bias WB, Reveille JD, Beaty TH, et al. Evidence that autoimmunity in man is a Mendelian dominant trait. *Am J Hum Genet* 1986;39(5):584–602.
275. Encinas JA, Wicker LS, Peterson LB, et al. QTL influencing autoimmune diabetes and encephalomyelitis map to a 0.15– cM region containing Il2 [letter]. *Nat Genet* 1999;21(2):158–160.
276. Manger K, Repp R, Spriewald BM, et al. Fcγ receptor IIa polymorphism in Caucasian patients with systemic lupus erythematosus: association with clinical symptoms. *Arthritis Rheum* 1998;41:1181–1189.
277. Haseley LA, Wisnieski JJ, Denburg, MR, et al. Antibodies to Clq in systemic lupus erythematosus: characteristics and relation to Fc gamma RIIA alleles. *Kidney Int* 1997;52:1375–1380.
278. Norsworthy P, Theodoridis E, Botto M, et al. Overrepresentation of the Fcgamma receptor type IIA R131/R131 genotype in caucasoid systemic lupus erythematosus patients with autoantibodies to Clq and glomerulonephritis. *Arthritis Rheum* 1999;42:1828–1832.
279. Gibson AW, Edberg JC, Wu J, et al. Novel single nucleotide polymorphisms in the distal il-10 promoter affect il-10 production and enhance the risk of systemic lupus erythematosus. *J Immunol* 2001;166:3915–3922.

7

THE GENETICS OF MURINE SYSTEMIC LUPUS ERYTHEMATOSUS

DWIGHT H. KONO
ARGYRIOS N. THEOFILOPOULOS

Although the etiology of systemic lupus erythematosus (SLE) is multifactorial, genetic susceptibility appears to be an important and possibly essential component. Thus, elucidation of the processes leading to disease induction and maintenance will likely require knowledge of the key genetic alterations and their contributions. Deciphering the genetics of lupus, however, has proven to be a formidable task, in large part because of the size of the human genome and the complexity of polygenic inheritance in heterogeneous human populations. Studies of inbred strains of mice that, spontaneously or by induction, develop SLE-like systemic autoimmunity have provided an excellent opportunity to examine genetic susceptibility and genes vital to the development of lupus in well-defined experimental model systems. Mouse models are particularly useful in dissecting polygenic traits because of homogeneous genetic backgrounds, standardized environmental conditions, and the ability to obtain sufficient numbers for genetic mapping and for accurate phenotype determination. Furthermore, the mouse genome is well characterized and its gene composition is sufficiently similar to the human genome to allow comparative analysis. Mice are also the premier mammalian species for genetic manipulation and importantly, their immune system is nearly identical to humans and as well defined, making it possible to study in considerable detail the immunologic alterations associated with different genetic backgrounds.

SPONTANEOUS AND INDUCED MOUSE MODELS OF SLE

Mouse models of systemic autoimmunity used in genetic studies encompass monogenic, polygenic, spontaneous, and induced diseases (Table 7.1). Descriptions of the major strains can be found in Chapter 18. Most genetic studies have focused on the spontaneous models, particularly the New Zealand black (NZB), New Zealand white (NZW), Medical Research Laboratory (MRL)-*Fas^{lpr}* (lymphoproliferative), and BXSB strains. Autoimmunity in these mice is polygenically inherited, although both the MRL- *Fas^{lpr}* and BXSB strains have single genes (*Fas^{lpr}* and *Yaa*, respectively) that exhibit mendelian inheritance and contribute to a large proportion of the total variance. A number of recombinant inbred lines, derived from crosses of lupus-prone and nonautoimmune strains [recombinant inbred (RI) lines in Table 7.1], have also been generated. These lines develop a spectrum of phenotypes indicating polygenic inheritance of traits; however, the relatively small number of substrains have precluded more detailed analysis. One of these RI lines, NZM/Aeg2410, derived from the NZB and NZW strains, however, has been useful for studying recessive susceptibility genes (see below). Two long-lived (*-ll*) sublines derived from the BXSB and MRL-*Fas^{lpr}* strains have also been described (1,2). Both have less severe disease than the original parental strain from which they spontaneously arose, and may be caused by single mutations. Studies of the MRL-*Fas^{lpr}*-ll substrain revealed decreases in interferon-γ (IFN-γ), as well as immunoglobulins IgG2a and IgG3 subclasses, suggesting that a reduction in pathogenic T-helper-1 (Th1)-type responses may play a role in disease resistance (3).

Genetic predisposition is also important for the induced mouse models, particularly mercury-induced autoimmunity (HgIA). Exposure of susceptible strains to mercury results in a constellation of immunopathologic manifestations including lymphoproliferation, hypergammaglobulinemia, autoantibodies, and immune complexes (4,5). Although most strains develop lymphoid hyperplasia and elevated IgG levels, autoantibody and immune complex deposits are dependent on H-2 haplotype and other background genes (6,7). Notably, the antinucleolar antibody response, which is mainly directed against fibrillarin (8) [a specificity also observed in scleroderma (9)], requires the

TABLE 7.1. SPONTANEOUS AND INDUCED MOUSE MODELS OF LUPUS

Spontaneous disease models
NZ and related strains
NZB
NZW
(NZB × NZW)F_1 (BWF_1)
(NZB × SWR)F_1
(NZB × NZW) recombinant inbred (RI) lines "NZM/Aeg" lines (275)
(NZB × SM) RI lines "(NXSM)RI"
(NZB × C58) RI lines "(NX8)RI"
MRL (*Fas*^{lpr} and wild-type) and related strains
MRL-*Fas*^{lpr}. *ll* (long-lived substrain) (2)
MRL-*Fas*^{lpr}, *Yaa* (146)
SCG/Kj-*Fas*^{lpr} (BXSB × MRL-*lpr*)RI (276)
BXSB and related strains
BXSB-*ll* (long-lived substrain) (1)
(NZW × BXSB)F_1
(NZB × BXSB)F_1
(SJL × SWR)F_1 (277)
Palmerston North (278)
Motheaten strains (131–133)
Induced disease models
Heavy metal–induced autoimmunity (4)
Drug-induced lupus (279)
Pristane-induced (280)
Antiidiotypic (281)
Graft-versus-host disease

MRL, Medical Research Laboratory; NZB, New Zealand black mouse; NZW, New Zealand white mouse; SCG, spontaneous crescentic glomerulonephritis-forming mouse/kinjoh; SJL, Swiss Jim Lambert.

I-A^s haplotype (7). Among the various backgrounds examined, the DBA/2 strain is the most resistant (6), and strains susceptible to spontaneous lupus appear to be more sensitive to mercury exposure (10).

More recently, transgenic or gene knockout manipulations of nonautoimmune background strains have generated new autoimmune mouse models with manifestations similar to spontaneous SLE (see later section). Finally, interval-specific congenic strains have been generated that contain introgressed genomic regions encompassing susceptibility loci defined in genome-wide mapping studies. Such substrains are being used to define component phenotypes and to precisely map the location of susceptibility alleles. Insights gained from novel substrains of mice based on new information and technologies will undoubtedly continue to fuel the constant evolution and advancement of this field.

SPECIFIC "LUPUS" PREDISPOSING GENES

Spontaneous variants or mutations leading to accelerated autoantibody production or other lupus-like manifestations in mice have been documented for the major histocompatibility complex (MHC) class II genes, Fas, Fas ligand (Fasl) and hematopoietic cell phosphatase (Hcph or SHP-1) (Table 7.2). The Y accelerator of autoimmunity and lymphoproliferation (*Yaa*) gene, which is responsible for the male predisposition to lupus in BXSB mice, is known to be located on the Y chromosome, but the identity of the gene is not known. Defects or polymorphisms in other immune-related genes have been postulated to predispose to lupus, but their roles have not been firmly established. These genes include the T-cell receptor (*Tcr*) (11–16), immunoglobulin (*Ig*) (17–19) and tumor necrosis factor (TNF) (*Tnf*) (20–23), FcγRIIB1 (24), and CD22 (25).

MHC Class II Genes

Predisposition to systemic autoimmunity is strongly linked to specific MHC (H-2 in mice) haplotypes in certain lupus backgrounds, particularly the BXSB (26) and BWF_1 mice (27,28). For the BXSB strain, H-2^b is the lupus-predisposing haplotype (26,29), whereas the heterozygous H-$2^{d/z}$ is associated with the greatest susceptibility in BWF_1 hybrids (reviewed in ref. 30). Although certain MHC haplotypes can promote susceptibility, additional predisposing genes are required for the development of SLE since autoimmunity does not develop when the predisposing MHC haplotypes are on normal backgrounds or crosses (30,31). For example, (NZB×NZW)F1 mice (H-$2^{d/z}$) are highly susceptible to lupus, whereas F1 hybrids between NZB and PL/J or B10.PL (H-2^u, which is identical to H-2^z in the antigen-binding domains), or BALB/c mice congenic for H-2^z, are not susceptible (32–34). Other examples are the BXSB.*ll*

TABLE 7.2. SPONTANEOUS MUTATIONS ASSOCIATED WITH LUPUS-LIKE MANIFESTATIONS

Name	Gene	Chr	cM	Susceptible Allele	Alteration	Major Autoimmune-Manifestations
Fas ligand	*Fasl*	1	85.0	*gld* (generalized lymphoproliferative disease)	T→C, 847 nt. (Phe→Leu)	Lymphoproliferation, DN T cells, auto-Abs, GN
SHP-1, PTP-1C, hemopoietic cell phosphatase	*Hcph*	6	60.2	*me* (motheaten)	C deletion, 228 nt. aberrant RNA splicing	Auto-Abs (both *me* and *me^v* mutations)
				me^v (viable motheaten)	T→A 1,076 nt. disrupts splice donor site	
MHC	*H-2*	17	18.6	Depends on background strain	H-2$^{d/z}$ (BWF$_1$), H-2^b (BXSB), H-2^{bm12} (NZB), others	Enhanced autoimmunity, including auto-Ab, GN, lymphoproliferation (depending on MHC and background)
Fas, APO-1, CD95	*Fas*	19	23.0	*lpr* (lymphoproliferation)	ETn insertion with aberrant RNA splicing	Lymphoproliferation, expansion of DN T cell subset, auto-Abs, GN, arthritis depending on background (both *lpr* and *lpr^{cg}* mutations)
				lpr^{cg} (lymphoproliferation complementing *gld*)	T→A, 786 nt. (Ile→Asn) disrupts binding of Fas to Fasl	
Y accelerated autoimmunity and lymphoproliferation	*Yaa*	Y	ND		ND	Accelerated autoimmunity, enhanced Ab responses to foreign and self antigens

Chr, chromosome; GN, glomerulonephritis; MHC, major histocompatibility complex; ND, not determined; PTP, protein tyrosine phosphatase.
Chromosomal locations are based on the Mouse Genome Database, The Jackson Laboratory (*http://www.informatics.jax.org*). See text for references

and MRL-*Fas^{lpr}*.ll substrains that have identical H-2 haplotypes, but are much less susceptible to disease because of possibly single mutations in non-MHC genes (1–3).

The actual gene (or genes) within the MHC complex that promotes lupus susceptibility still remains to be determined. The polymorphic class II genes are strong candidates based on findings in H-2 congenic mice and their central roles in both repertoire shaping and antigen recognition (26,35,36). NZB mice congenic for H-2^{bm12}, but not the closely related H-2^b, develop accelerated disease despite the fact that these haplotypes are apparently similar except for the I-A molecule. This seems to implicate three amino acids in the I-Aβ chain at positions 67, 70, and 71 since the H-2^{bm12} and H-2^b sequences differ by these residues in the MHC peptide-binding groove. Strong linkage with lupus disease in NZ background mice is also observed with the hemizygous H-2^z haplotype in combination with either the d, b, or v haplotypes (27,28,37–39). It has been proposed that in this instance, autoimmune-promoting MHC class II specificities are created by transcomplementation of the different α and β chains with formation of novel hybrid molecules (40,41). The finding that other heterozygous H-2^z haplotypes including H-2$^{v/z}$ (39) and H-2$^{b/z}$ (37,38) also increase susceptibility makes it less likely that novel class II hybrid molecules are responsible. Another possibility is that the two different H-2 haplotypes may regulate the production of different sets of nephritogenic autoantibodies (42). In this case, heterozygous H-2$^{d/z}$ haplotype mice would produce both sets of pathogenic antibodies resulting in greater susceptibility to nephritis. Recent studies attempted to directly implicate class II molecules by expressing I-A^z or I-E^z transgenes in the NZB × C57BL/6 background; however, no increased susceptibility was found in mice expressing either of these transgenes (43,44). Although the inference is that the class II molecules are not responsible, it is also possible that the transgene did not adequately recapitulate the expression patterns required to promote autoimmunity, since it is known that slight changes in class II expression result in substantial effects on disease susceptibility, e.g., homozygous versus heterozygous expression (45) or the presence or absence of I-E (46). In this regard, transgenic mice would not have the same levels of class II molecules as wild-type mice since they would have normal levels of class II in addition to the transgene.

Other studies have sought to explain why H-2^d (I-E$^+$) congenic BXSB mice [normally H-2^b (I-E$^-$)] do not develop lupus (36,46,47). Lack of susceptibility was not from I-E–dependent, endogenous superantigen-induced modifications of the TCRVβ (BV) repertoire imposed by H-2^d, because H-$2^{b/d}$ haplotype mice are susceptible to disease despite similar deletion of the appropriate BV-bearing T cells (26). Interestingly, BXSB mice expressing a high copy number (~50) of an I-$E\alpha^d$ transgene with ~20-fold higher $E\alpha^d$ messenger RNA (mRNA) levels than H-$2^{b/d}$ mice were found to be resistant to the development of autoimmunity, similarly to H-2^d BXSB mice (46). Protection by the I-Eα transgene has also been reported for I-E^+ haplotype lupus backgrounds (48,49). It is postulated that this resistance is due to competitive inhibition of autoantigenic peptide binding to I-A^b by a large excess of transgenic I-Eα peptide. However, this does not fully explain the lack of susceptibility of H-2^d BXSB mice that have normal copy number of I-$E\alpha^d$. Nonetheless, these findings suggest a novel mechanism, whereby excess production of MHC-binding peptide from I-Eα, or perhaps other proteins, may alter antigen presentation and possibly disease susceptibility. Whether the mechanism is due to inhibition of autoantigen presentation or to repertoire shaping during central thymic selection or in the peripheral immune system is not known.

Other potential genes within the H-2 complex include a polymorphic NZW TNF-α gene that appears to promote lupus in the BWF_1 hybrid (20,21) and a recessive NZW locus (*Sles1*) that appears to suppress the development of autoimmunity in NZW mice (50). However, the relationship of *Sles1* to the known class II and TNF-α polymorphisms in the NZW strain has yet to be determined. The NZW TNF-α polymorphism, which is also found in several nonautoimmune mouse strains, results in lower TNF-α levels presumably because of a regulatory-affecting mutation in the 3′ UT region of the gene (21,51). However, it has yet to be established whether this specific mutation is responsible for disease susceptibility. Nevertheless, the potential importance of TNF-α in lupus is supported by the recent finding that heterozygous deficiency of TNF-α in (NZB × TNFko)F1 hybrids leads to enhanced autoimmunity with accelerated antinuclear autoantibodies (ANAs), hyperproliferating B cells, and immune complex–mediated renal disease (52). Similarly, reduction in TNF-mediated signaling by gene knockout of *Tnfr1* resulted in accelerated lymphadenopathy and autoimmune disease in MRL-*Fas^lpr^* mice (53).

Fas and Fas Ligand

Fas (APO-1 or CD95) is a 306-amino acid, 45-kd, cell surface membrane protein related to the TNF receptor superfamily of type I membrane glycoproteins. Fas is expressed on actively proliferating cells in the thymus, liver, ovary heart, skin, and gut epithelium with particularly high levels on $CD4^+CD8^+$ thymocytes, activated T and B cells, and some neoplastic cells (54,55). Following binding to its ligand, Fas transduces signals leading, in most instances, to apoptotic cell death (56,57). The ligand for Fas, FasL, is a 40-kd type II transmembrane glycoprotein belonging to the TNF ligand family of proteins. It is expressed almost exclusively on T-cell lineages, primarily upon activation (58) and in certain immunologically sequestered sites such as the testis, eye, and placenta (58–61). In these areas, FasL may contribute to maintenance of immune privilege by inducing Fas-mediated apoptosis in invading inflammatory cells, reducing inflammatory responses (62), and in the case of the retina, may also control the growth of new vision-damaging subretinal blood vessels (63). Further details on Fas/FasL induced apoptosis can be found in Chapter 8.

Two spontaneous loss-of-function mutations in Fas (Fas^{lpr} and $Fas^{lpr\text{-}cg}$) and one in FasL ($Fasl^{gld}$) result in similar autoimmune manifestations (Table 7.2). The Fas^{lpr} defect is caused by an early retroviral transposon (ETn) insertion within the second intron between exons 2 and 3, which causes aberrant RNA splicing, a frame shift, and premature termination of the mRNA at the long terminal repeat region of the ETn (64–68). Low levels (~10%) of wild-type Fas mRNA and surface protein, however, are detectable (66–70), and recombinant *Fas* knockout mice, but not *lpr* mice, develop liver hyperplasia in addition to lymphoproliferation (71). The $Fas^{lpr\text{-}cg}$ stands for *lpr* complementing *gld* (72), and the *gld* for generalized lymphoproliferative disease (73). The $Fas^{lpr\text{-}cg}$ mutation is caused by a single point mutation (T→A at nucleotide 786; isoleucine→asparagine; this residue is valine in humans) within the intracytoplasmic domain of Fas that modifies an amino acid in the so-called death domain essential for signal transduction (65). Finally, the $Fasl^{gld}$ allele is a point mutation in the carboxy-terminal extracellular domain (T→C at nucleotide 847, phenylalanine→leucine) of FasL on chromosome 1, which abolishes the binding of Fas to the FasL (74–76).

Mice homozygous for these mutations have accumulation of $CD4^-CD8^-$ (double negative, DN), $B220^+$, $TCR\alpha\beta^+$ T cells, and the induction or acceleration of systemic autoimmunity (30,77). Both severity of the autoimmune disease and degree of lymphoproliferation, however, depend on other background genes (30). Fas^{lpr} does not complement $Fasl^{gld}$, whereas the $Fas^{lpr\text{-}cg}$ allele, as suggested by its name, can complement both the Fas^{lpr} allele and to a slightly lesser degree, the $Fasl^{gld}$ allele. Furthermore, in contrast to the recessive Fas^{lpr} mutation, autoimmunity and lymphoproliferation is observed in heterozygous MRL-$Fas^{lpr\text{-}cg}/+$ mice, although less severe and without the characteristic expansion of DN T cells (78). In humans, defects in Fas have been identified as a cause of the rare autoimmune lymphoproliferative syndrome [ALPS or Canale-Smith syndrome] (79–81). This syndrome has also been described with loss-of-function mutations in caspase 10, a cysteine protease involved in the downstream apoptosis-promoting pathway of Fas (82). The majority of SLE patients, however, do not appear to have deficiencies or mutations in *Fas* or *Fasl* (83–86).

Because of the important role that Fas/FasL plays in apoptosis, defects in clonal deletion of T and B cells have been sought to explain the *lpr* phenotype. Clearly a T-cell defect is evident by the accumulation of DN *lpr* cells. Most studies, however, have found no defects in central thymic deletion in Fas-deficient mice to exogenous and endogenous superantigens (87–90) and conventional class I and II presented antigens (91–93). In contrast, abnormalities in the receptor-mediated apoptosis of mature T cells (90,91,94,95) along with the early expansion of a distinct BV8.3/BD1.1/BJ1.1 T-cell receptor in $CD4^+$ cells from MRL-*Fas*^{lpr}, but not MRL-+/+ (96), have implicated defective peripheral T-cell deletion as a possible mechanism contributing to autoimmunity. Thus, Fas/FasL interactions are important for activation-induced cell death (AICD) (97,98). AICD is initiated by antigen receptor engagement, which upregulates Fas and induces FasL in T cells, primarily in $CD8^+$ cells and the Th0 and Th1 $CD4^+$ subsets. Subsequent binding of Fas and FasL, which also can occur cell-autonomously (97,99), leads to RNA-dependent apoptosis (97,99–101). Fas-mediated killing is essential for $CD4^+$ Th1 T-cell–mediated cytotoxicity and is one of at least two cytotoxic T lymphocyte (CTL) pathways for $CD8^+$ T cells (102–106). The Fas-dependent CTL pathway, however, in contrast to the perforin-dependent CTL pathway, cannot kill pathogen-infected targets (107), suggesting that Fas/FasL functions primarily in maintaining cell homeostasis, i.e., killing expanded clones that have outlived their immunologic function.

Evidence from the TCR BV repertoire of DN $B220^+$ T cells (89,96), DN cell cytolytic activity and positive perforin expression (108), anti-CD8 treatment, and targeted gene knockouts of MHC class I (β_2-microglobulin) (109–112), CD8 (113), or CD4 (113) indicate that the majority of DN cells are derived from $CD8^+$ T cells. DN *lpr* cells are likely activated peripheral T cells that fail to undergo AICD, a finding consistent with their activated phenotype, which includes $CD44^{hi}$, expression, and phosphorylation of $p57^{fyn}$, constitutive tyrosine phosphorylation of Vav, and high expression of FasL in both *gld* and *lpr*mice (114,115). The elevated constitutive expression of FasL has been postulated to cause the unidirectional *lpr*-associated wasting syndrome (i.e., graft-versus-host disease–like abnormality) observed when *lpr* bone marrow is adoptively transferred to wild-type recipients (114,116–118).

An important role for T cells in *lpr* disease was suggested by reversal of both lymphoaccumulation and autoimmunity in MRL-*Fas*^{lpr} mice expressing a wild-type Fas transgene under the control of the CD2 promoter (119). However, the significance of this became less certain when subsequent studies of nonautoimmune mice expressing the same CD2-Fas transgene revealed a lack of thymic atrophy and other T-cell characteristics normally associated with aging (120), thereby indicating alteration of normal T-cell development. Subsequently, more specific transgenic expression of Fas in T cells (lck promoter), but not B cells, was found to block lymphoproliferation, but not autoimmunity. This suggests that Fas expression in B cells may be a critical factor (121).

This is supported by other studies, which have clearly implicated B cells in the development of *lpr*-mediated autoimmunity. Mixed bone marrow chimera studies have demonstrated that autoantibodies are produced from Fas-defective, but not wild-type donor, B cells (122). B cells from *lpr* and *gld* mice exhibit resistance to spontaneous apoptosis *in vitro* (123). Double-transgenic mice expressing the antibody to hen egg-white lysozyme (HEL) and either membrane-bound or soluble HEL were used to study the fate of autoreactive B cells in Fas-deficient *lpr* mice (124). Elimination of self-reactive *lpr* B cells recognizing membrane-bound HEL and functional inactivation of B cells to soluble HEL appeared to occur normally; however, an age-related breakdown of tolerance to soluble HEL was observed, suggesting a defect in the censoring of autoreactive B cells. Further studies have indicated that anergic B cells normally are eliminated by $CD4^+$ T cells through the Fas/FasL pathway, but without Fas killing, B cells are triggered to proliferate (125,126). Consistent with this are the findings that anti–double-stranded DNA (dsDNA) B cells in Fas-deficient mice are not developmentally arrested and excluded from splenic follicles as in nonautoimmune mice, but migrate into the follicles (127), and that there are abnormal increases in IgG2a- and rheumatoid factor (RF)–secreting B cells in the T-rich zones of the periarteriolar lymphoid sheath (PALS) (128). Fas/FasL-mediated apoptosis also may further contribute to B-cell homeostasis by eliminating bystander B cells that are activated by CD40L alone (129).

Protein Tyrosine Phosphatase and Motheaten Mice

SHP-1 is a protein tyrosine phosphatase (PTP) ubiquitously expressed in hematopoietic lineage cells. Two recessive spontaneous mutations, motheaten (me) and motheaten viable (me^v), result in similar severe developmental and functional abnormalities of multiple hematopoietic cells lineages, leading to mortality of *me* and *me*^{v} mice at around 3 and 9 weeks of age, respectively (130). Motheaten mice are immunodeficient, but paradoxically develop features of systemic autoimmunity such as hypergammaglobulinemia, antinuclear antibodies, and immune complex deposits in multiple tissues (131). The hypergammaglobulinemia is produced by an expanded population of atypical plasmacytoid cells and a reduced B-cell population composed primarily of $CD5^+$ B1 cells. The T-cell compartment is normal at birth, but by 4 weeks of age there is involution, absent lymphoid follicles, impaired CTLs, and reduced responses to both mitogens and alloantigens. Other hematopoietic alterations include defective natural killer cell differentiation and function, increased erythroid precursors, and enormous expansions of monocytes/macrophages and neutrophil populations. The term *motheaten* refers to a characteristic skin pattern of patchy inflammation and alopecia caused by large subcutaneous and dermal accumulations of neutrophils that rupture and scar.

SHP-1 consists of an N-terminal catalytic domain and two in tandem SH2 (src homology 2) domains that are important for its function. The *me* mutation is a single cytidine residue deletion at position 228 within the N-terminal SH2 domain that converts the normal sequence to a donor splice-site consensus sequence. This results in aberrant splicing and deletion of the 101-base pair (bp) portion of exon downstream from the newly created splice site. The me^{v} mutation disrupts a normal GT 5′ splice donor site (GT→GA, residue 1076), which also leads to aberrant splicing, this time within the SHP-1 catalytic domain, 15 bp upstream of the normal splice site (132,133). SHP-1 activity in the *me* mutant is absent, whereas a profound reduction is found in the me^{v} mutant (134), findings consistent with the greater severity of disease in *me* mice.

SHP-1 is normally recruited by negative regulatory molecules that contain immunoreceptor tyrosine-based inhibitory motifs (ITIMs) (135), such as CD22, FcγRIIB, and CD72, to specific sites where it then inhibits molecular complexes that require tyrosine phosphorylation for activation, such as the B-cell receptor (BCR) and T-cell receptor (TCR). Loss of this essential inhibitory function in *me* mice appears responsible for the exuberant activation and expansion of hematopoietic cell populations and the resulting disease manifestations. Although *me* mice have increased immunoglobulin levels and autoantibodies, the major clinical sequelae that lead to early mortality are not observed in spontaneous SLE, and are not mediated by autoantibodies or T and B lymphocytes (132,133,136–138). Autoantibody production may be caused by the inability of CD22 and possibly FcγRIIB to negatively regulate the B-cell antigen receptor when SHP-1 is absent (139).

Yaa Gene

BXSB mice have a marked male predilection for systemic autoimmunity in contrast to the female predominance in humans and other susceptible mouse strains. This striking sexual dichotomy is due not to hormonal factors but to a gene on the Y chromosome, designated *Yaa* (140–142). Since conventional genetic mapping approaches are not possible for the nonrecombining Y chromosome, *Yaa* has yet to be cloned. Nevertheless there is some information about its contribution to systemic autoimmunity.

Transfer of the *Yaa* gene (Y-chromosome) to nonautoimmune and autoimmune strains has demonstrated that it contributes additively to lupus, but is dependent on other background genes. Nonautoimmune strains, such as CBA/J or C57BL/6, are largely unaffected by the *Yaa* gene, whereas all lupus-susceptible strains examined, including the BXSB, NZB, NZW, and MRL-Fas^{lpr}, have accelerated disease that generally maintains the clinical characteristics of the background strain (30,143–145). Mice with mild lupus appear affected more by the *Yaa* gene than are strains with already accelerated disease (26). This selective augmentation by *Yaa* contrasts with the induction of generalized autoimmunity by the *lpr* and *gld* mutations (145) and suggests different mechanisms are involved. This is further supported by the findings that *lpr* and *Yaa* congenic mice with identical backgrounds have different phenotypes (30) and that the *lpr* and *Yaa* mutations are additive (146). Interestingly, DBA/1.*Yaa* (consomic for the BXSB Y-chromosome) were less susceptible to collagen-induced arthritis (CIA) than were wild-type DBA/1 mice, suggesting that *Yaa* plays different roles in CIA and lupus (147).

Regarding the mechanisms responsible for the *Yaa* phenotype, double bone-marrow chimera experiments using a mixture of Yaa^{+} and Yaa^{-} cells of different IgH allotypes revealed selective production of anti-DNA antibody and hypergammaglobulinemia by Yaa^{+} B cells (148). The antibody-promoting effect of the *Yaa* gene is applicable not only to self antigens but to foreign antigens as well (149), and analogous to the effects in lupus mice, enhancement was observed mainly for antigens eliciting low T-cell–dependent antibody responses and not for those eliciting high antibody responses (149). Accordingly, the *Yaa* gene was postulated to increase the expression of an "intercellular adhesion molecule" on B cells, which promotes low-avidity, T- helper–B-cell interactions (142). Thus, nontolerant T-helper cells that normally are quiescent in Yaa^{-} animals because of insufficient antigen presentation become activated in Yaa^{+} animals. Other mechanisms that increase antigen presentation, intracellular signaling, and co-receptor molecule expression can also be postulated, and elucidation undoubtedly will require identification of the molecular defect.

Similar types of mixed bone marrow chimera experiments with Yaa^{+} and Yaa^{-} T cells that differ by Thy-1 allotypes revealed that autoimmunity was mediated with similar efficiency regardless of whether Yaa^{+} cells were present or eliminated by anti–Thy-1 antibodies (49). This suggests that the *Yaa* defect does not require expression in T cells. That B cells, but not T cells, from Yaa^{+} mice have enhanced proliferative responses compared with cells from Yaa^{-} mice is also consistent with this possibility (150).

LUPUS-LIKE MANIFESTATIONS IN GENE KNOCKOUT AND TRANSGENIC MICE

Genetic manipulation of nonautoimmune background strains has helped define not only the role of specific genes in the immune system, but also possible mechanisms of sys-

TABLE 7.3. GENES ASSOCIATED WITH LUPUS-LIKE MANIFESTATIONS IN KNOCKOUT AND TRANSGENIC NORMAL BACKGROUND MICE

Name	Gene	Chr	cM	Major Autoimmune Manifestations	Ref.
Knockouts					
CTLA-4	*Cd152*	1	30.1	Multiorgan lymphoproliferative disease, myocarditis, pancreatitis	181–183
CD45 (protein tyrosine phosphatase, receptor type C)	*Ptprc*	1	74.0	Lymphoproliferation, anti-dsDNA, splenomegaly, GN	202
Serum amyloid P component	*Sap*	1	94.2	Antichromatin Ab, GN, female predominance	222
IL-2Rα	*Il2ra*	2	6.4	Lymphoproliferation, hyper-IgG, auto-Ab, anti-RBC Ab	191
IL-2	*Il2*	3	19.2	Lymphoproliferation, hyper-IgG, auto-Ab, anti-RBC Ab	190
lyn	*Lyn*	4	0.0	Enhanced B-cell activation, splenomegaly, hyper-IgM, auto-Ab, GN	151,152
C1q	*C1qa*	4	66.1	Auto-Ab, GN	219,282
	C1qb	4	66.1		
	C1qc	4	66.1		
TGF-β_1	*Tgfb1*	7	6.5	Multiorgan lymphocytic and monocytic infiltrates	205
CD22	*Cd22*	7	9.0	Enhanced B cell activation, auto-Ab	153,283
Zfp-36 (tristetraprolin)	*Zfp36*	7	10.2	Complex systemic disease: cachexia, dermatitis, arthritis	232,234,284
IL-2Rβ	*Il2rb*	15	43.3	Lymphoproliferation, hyper-IgG, auto-Ab, anti-RBC Ab	192
Dnase1	*Dnase1*	16	1.7	ANA, immune complex GN	252
p21 cyclin-dependent Kinase inhibitor 1A	*Cdkn1a*	17	15.23	Antichromatin Ab, GN, female predominance	250
Complement component 4	*C4*	17	18.8	Impaired immune complex clearance, ANA, GN, female predominance	221
Pten (+/– mice)	*Pten*	19	24.5	Lymphadenopathy, auto-Ab, GN, decreased survival, female predominance	247
Aiolos (zinc finger protein, subfamily 1A, 3)	*Znfn1a3*	ND	ND	Activated B cells, increased IgG, auto-Ab	171
Bim (Bcl2 interacting mediator of cell death)	*Bim*	ND	ND	Lymphoid/myeloid cell accumulation, auto-Ab, GN, vasculitis	211
Cbl-b	ND	ND	ND	Multiorgan lymphoid infiltrates, anti-dsDNA Ab	243
PD-1 (programmed cell death 1)	*Pdcd1*	hu2	q37.3	Proliferative arthritis, GN, glomerular IgG3 deposits	199
Transgenics					
FLIP (retrovirus-mediated expression)	*Cflar*	1	30.1	Hyper-IgG, auto-Abs, GN	218
Bcl-2 (B cell promotor)	*Bcl2*	1	59.8	Lymphoid hyperplasia, hyper-IgG, auto-Ab, GN	212
CD19	*Cd19*	7	59.0	Increased B-cell activation, B1 cell population, IgG, auto-Ab	157
Fli-1 (class I promotor)	*Fli1*	9	16.0	Lymphoid hyperplasia, auto-Ab, GN	249
IFN-γ (keratin promotor)	*Ifng*	10	67.0	Auto-Ab, GN, female predominance	224
IL-4 (class I promotor)	*Il4*	11	29.0	Hyper-IgG1/E, auto-Ab, GN	225
BAFF (α_1-antitrypsin or β-actin promotor)	*Tnfsf13b*	ND	ND	Auto-Ab (RF, CIC, dsDNA Ab), GN	179,180

Genes are listed by chromosomal locations. Gene names and chromosomal locations are from the Mouse Genome Database (Jackson Laboratories).
ANA, antinuclear antibody; CTLA, cytotoxic T-lymphocyte associated; Ig, immunoglobulin; ND, not determined; TGF, transforming growth factor

temic autoimmunity (Table 7.3). The number and diversity of genes that have resulted in phenotypes resembling lupus after manipulation is remarkable, considering the total number of genes examined, and suggests a potentially large pool of abnormalities that could lead to lupus-like disease. The systemic autoimmunity produced by these mutations, however, is sometimes only vaguely similar to spontaneous lupus, and often there are additional unique findings not observed in SLE. Thus, the relevance of many of these genes to spontaneous SLE remains to be determined. Manifestations of lupus have been observed following manipulation of genes affecting B- and T-lymphocyte activation, comple-

TABLE 7.4. MECHANISMS FOR INDUCTION OF SYSTEMIC AUTOIMMUNITY

Enhanced B-cell activation[a]
Lyn, CD22 or SHP-1 knockout
FcγRII knockout
Aiolos knockout
CD19 transgenic
Tnfsf13b (BAFF, BlyS, TALL-1, or THANK) transgenic
Enhanced T-cell activation
CTLA-4 knockout
IL-2 or IL-2R knockout
CD45 E613R knock-in mutation (B cells as well)
PD-1 knockout (probably B cells as well)
TGF-β deficiency (knockout/dominant negative)
Defective apoptosis
Fas or FasL mutations (lpr and gld mice, ALPS in humans; also caspace 10)
Bim knockout (not related to Fas)
Bcl-2 transgenic
Flip transgenic
Complement and related genes
C1q knockout
C4 knockout
SAP knockout
Cytokine-mediated activation
IL-4 transgenic
IFN-γ transgenic
TTP (Zfp-36) deficiency (excessive TNF-α)
TNF-α transgenic
Defective signal transduction
Cb1-b knockout (increased activation of T cells, possibly B cells)
$Pten^{+/-}$ knockout (defective Fas from increased PIP-3 elevating Akt levels)
Fli-1 transgenic
Unopposed cell cycling
$p21^{cip1/waf1}$ knockout (cyclin kinase inhibitor, primarily T cells)
Other mechanisms
Dnase1 knockout

[a]Genes are categorized according to the most likely or predominant mechanism.
IFN, interferon; IL, interleukin; SAP, serum amyloid P component; TNF, tumor necrosis factor; TTP, tristetraprolin

ment, cytokines, apoptosis, signal transduction, and the cell cycle (Tables 7.3 and 7.4).

Genes Related to B-Cell Activation

The fate of B cells following antigen receptor (BCR) engagement is a complex process that involves direct or indirect interaction of the BCR with numerous molecules that can promote or inhibit cell activation. Among these are several tyrosine kinases (lyn, fyn, Btk, Blk, Syk), phosphatases (CD45, SHP-1, SHP-2, and SHIP), and accessory molecules (CD19, CD22, FcRγIIB). Genetic manipulation of many of these B-cell regulatory molecules has resulted in mice with features similar to lupus, e.g., gene knockouts of lyn (151,152) or CD22 (153–155), and spontaneous mutations of SHP-1 in motheaten mice (see above) (132,133).

Lyn is a nonreceptor scr-related tyrosine kinase involved in negative regulation of BCR signaling. Although lyn also plays a role in positive signaling, this function appears largely redundant since deficiency of lyn leads to hypersensitivity to BCR-mediated triggering. Mice with homozygous deletions of lyn have increased activation and higher turnover rates of B cells, splenomegaly, elevated IgM levels, autoantibodies, and glomerulonephritis (GN). Homozygous deficiency of CD22, a B-cell–specific cell surface sialoadhesin that specifically binds to asialoglycoproteins, results in a similar picture with hyperresponsiveness to BCR signaling, expansion of the peritoneal B1 cell population, and autoantibodies. Similarities between the lyn and CD22 knockouts stem from the fact that the inhibitory action of CD22 requires the recruitment and phosphorylation of lyn, which then, in turn, recruits SHP-1, bringing it in proximity to the BCR where it can dephosphorylate the BCR and downregulate the response. Heterozygous deletions of CD22, lyn, and SHP-1 were shown to have additive effects on B-cell abnormalities consistent with the notion that they are limiting elements to a common pathway (156).

CD19 along with CD21 and Tapa-1 (CD81) on B cells form the functional cell surface receptor complex for C3 fragments, which enhances BCR signal transduction and is crucial for B-cell development and tolerance. Mice overexpressing a CD19 transgene develop hyperresponsive B cells to BCR cross-linking, marked expansion of the B1 cell population, hypergammaglobulinemia, and autoantibodies (157). Furthermore, expression of the CD19 transgene in anti–hen egg lysozyme Ig (HEL-Ig)/soluble HEL double transgenic mice led to the appearance of anti-HEL antibodies, suggesting that a defect in anergy to certain soluble antigens might be the underlying mechanism (158).

The FcγRIIb on B cells also inhibits B-cell antigen receptor signaling (159), primarily by recruiting, through its intracytoplasmic immunoreceptor tyrosine-based inhibitory motif, the inositol phosphatase SHIP rather than the phosphotyrosine phosphatase SHP-1 (160,161). Gene knockout of FcγRII amplifies humoral and anaphylactic responses (162) and promotes the development of lupus-like disease (163), as well as type II collagen-induced arthritis (164) and type IV collagen-induced Goodpasture's syndrome (165). Interestingly, two deletions in the promoter region of FcγRIIb in NZB mice have been identified, which is associated with lower levels of FcγRII expression in germinal centers and hypergammaglobulinemia (24). This polymorphism maps to NZB loci on chromosome 1 linked to autoantibody production (*Lbw7* and *nba2*, see below and Table 7.4); however, whether this is the actual allele remains to be determined. Overall, these studies suggest that enhancement of BCR signaling, as shown by overexpression of CD19 and knockouts of CD22, lyn, SHP-1, or FcγRII, may be a potential pathogenic mechanism for lupus.

Aiolos is a zinc finger DNA-binding protein that shares a common GGGA core sequence binding motif with the closely homologous nuclear factor Ikaros (166). It is highly expressed in mature B cells and, to a lesser extent, in developing bone marrow B cells and thymocytes. In the nucleus, aiolos is mainly localized to the 2 MD chromatin remodeling complex that also contains Ikaros, the Mi-2 adenosine triphosphatase (ATPase), histone deacetylases, and other components of the nucleosome remodeling histone deacetylase (NURD) complex (166–169). These findings suggest that Ikaros family members regulate gene expression during lymphocyte development by recruiting certain histone deacetylase complexes to specific promoters (170). Mice with homozygous deletions of the aiolos gene develop defects primarily in the B-cell compartment, with hyperresponsiveness to BCR and CD40 stimulation, increased number of conventional B cells but a marked reduction in B1 cells, increased proportion of B cells with activated phenotype, hypergammaglobulinemia (particularly of IgE and IgG1), a threefold reduction in IgM, and positive ANAs in about half of animals by 16 weeks of age (171). Detected T-cell abnormalities were limited to only a slight increase in proliferative capacity of thymocytes and mature T cells. Thus, deficiency of aiolos appears to facilitate B-cell entry into cell cycle, maturation to germinal center lymphocytes, and a breakdown of B-cell tolerance.

Tnfsf13b (also called BAFF, BlyS, TALL-1, THANK, or zTNF4) is a newly identified member of the TNF ligand superfamily expressed primarily on cells of myeloid origin, such as monocytes and dendritic cells (172–175). Both the transmembrane protein and a secreted homotrimeric form, released by cleavage at a furin canonical motif in the stalk region, are active in the co-stimulation of B cells, the main cell type known to express its receptor. Two TNF family members, TACI and BCMA, have been identified as the receptors for Tnfsf13b (176). Tnfsf13b promotes peripheral B-cell survival, particularly the transitional type 2B cells, a subset of splenic immature B cells that are considered targets for negative selection (177,178). Overexpression of *Tnfsf13b* in the liver (α_1-antitrypsin promoter with the APO E enhancer) (179) or in multiple tissues (β-actin promoter) (180) resulted in a similar picture, consisting of elevated numbers of B cells and, to a lesser extent, T cells, as well as increases in activated bcl-2–expressing mature B cells, memory/effector phenotype T cells, and syndecan-1-positive plasma cells. B cells from transgenic mice survived longer in culture than those from wild-type controls. Furthermore, transgenic mice developed a lupus-like disease characterized by elevated levels of all immunoglobulin subclasses, rheumatoid factor, anti-DNA antibodies, circulating immune complexes and kidney immunoglobulin deposits with proteinuria and elevated blood urea nitrogen. Importantly, elevations in *Tnfsf13b* was also recently shown in both BWF_1 and MRL-*Fas*^{lpr} mice, and treatment of BWF_1 mice with a soluble TACI-Ig fusion protein, which blocks *Tnfsf13b* function, inhibited proteinuria, and prolonged survival (176).

Genes Related to T-Cell Activation

Systemic autoimmunity also develops after knockout deletion of certain genes that primarily effect T-cell function (Table 7.4). Cytotoxic T-lymphocyte antigen-4 (CTLA-4), a surface glycoprotein expressed exclusively on T cells, acts as an inhibitor of the CD28-B7.1/B7.2 co-stimulatory pathway in part by binding with higher affinity to B7.1 and B7.2. Consequently, mice with homozygous deletion of CTLA-4 develop a multiorgan lymphoproliferative disease associated with increased frequency of activated B and T cells, hypergammaglobulinemia, and early mortality at 3 to 4 weeks of age with severe myocarditis and pancreatitis (181–183). The abnormal T-cell expansion and disease manifestations are not due to alteration in thymocyte development (184), but to a failure to maintain homeostasis of activated peripheral T cells, primarily the CD4$^+$ subset (185,186). The precise mechanism through which this occurs has yet to be determined (187).

Gene knockouts of interleukin-2 (IL-2) (188–190) or either of its high (IL-2Rα) (191) or low (IL-2Rβ) (192) affinity receptors result in a similar syndrome consisting of late immunosuppression with defective antibody and CTL responses, but also lymphoproliferation, expansion of memory/effector phenotype T cells, polyclonal hypergammaglobulinemia, autoantibodies, and immune-mediated hemolytic anemia. Inflammatory bowel disease similar to human ulcerative colitis occurs in mice lacking IL-2 (193) or IL-2Rα (191), but not IL-2β (192). Autoantibody production depends on the expanded CD4$^+$ T cells (192) and CD40/CD40L interaction (188). The accumulation of T lymphocytes appears to be due to resistance of IL-2–deficient T cells to activation-induced cell death, at least partly from decreased Fas-mediated apoptosis (194). Other studies of mice maintained under germ-free conditions demonstrated that colitis, but not other autoimmune manifestations, requires exposure to environmental pathogens (195).

PD-1 is a 55-kd ITIM-containing transmembrane cell surface glycoprotein expressed on activated T and B lymphocytes and monocytic cells that appears to play an important nonredundant role in maintaining the homeostasis of lymphocytes and myeloid cells following their activation (196). Engagement of PD-1 by its ligand, PD-L1, has been shown to inhibit TCR-mediated lymphocyte proliferation and cytokine secretion (197); however, it is anticipated to act on a wider range of cell types as evident by gene knockout studies. Mice deficient for PD-1 develop moderate hyperplasia of lymphoid and myeloid cells, increases in several Ig isotypes (particularly IgG3), enhanced responses to IgM cross-linking, and alterations in peritoneal B1 cells (198). Older (14-month-old) C57BL/6-PD-1$^{-/-}$ mice spontaneously develop GN and proliferative arthritis, but not elevated anti-dsDNA antibodies or rheumatoid factor (199). Further acceleration of GN and arthritis occurs when the PD-1 deletion is combined with the *Fas*^{lpr} mutation. Interestingly, manifestations appear highly dependent on background genes. For example, in contrast to the findings in the C57BL/6 strain, BALB/c mice-PD-$1^{-/-}$ mice reportedly develop lethal pancreatitis with massive thrombosis. Thus PD-1 deficiency may accelerate background predisposition to autoimmunity similar to the *Fas^lpr^* and *Yaa* mutations.

CD45 is a receptor protein tyrosine phosphatase expressed on all nucleated hematopoietic lineages, where it is required for antigen receptor signal transduction and functions to promote cell activation. Homodimerization of CD45 inhibits phosphatase activity by symmetrical interactions, wherein the catalytic site of one molecule is blocked by a structural wedge from the other (200,201). Replacement of the glutamine at residue 613 by an arginine (E613R) destroys the inhibitory capacity of the wedge, and knock-in mice with this mutation were generated to examine the significance of dimerization (202). Although mice appeared normal at 4 weeks, they subsequently developed progressive lymphadenopathy and splenomegaly, increased number of activated T and B cells, anti-dsDNA autoantibodies, immune-complex GN, and early mortality. Autoimmunity was dominantly transmitted.

TGF-β1 gene knockout mice rapidly develop massive necrotizing lymphocytic and monocytic infiltrates in multiple organs soon after birth, and succumb by around 3 weeks of age (203,204). Serum IgG autoantibodies to nuclear antigens as well as Ig glomerular deposits are detected, but appear to play a minor role in overall disease severity (205). Although deficiencies of either class II or class I (β2m) molecules combined with transforming growth factor (TGF)-$\beta_1^{-/-}$ reduced both tissue inflammation and autoimmunity, implicating both $CD4^+$ and $CD8^+$ T cells in these processes; in both instances there was only partial improvement in survival because of the remaining lethal myeloproliferative abnormalities (206,207). Direct inhibition of TGF-β_1 in T cells by a dominant negative TGF-β receptor type II transgene under the control of a modified CD4 promoter specific for $CD4^+$ and $CD8^+$ T cells resulted in sickness, wasting, and diarrhea at around 3 to 4 months of age, monocytic infiltrates in multiple tissues, enlarged peripheral lymphoid organs, increased percentage of memory/effector phenotype T cells, hypergammaglobulinemia, autoantibodies and glomerular immune complex deposits (208). Thus, TGF-β is crucial for maintenance of T-cell homeostasis and suppression of autoimmunity.

Apoptosis Genes

Bim is a proapoptotic ligand of the Bcl-2 family that shares homology with other members in only the short (nine amino acid) BH3 motif (209). Through this domain, Bim binds to antiapoptotic Bcl-2 molecules and blocks their function. Bim is largely bound to the cytoplasmic dynein light chain LC8 that, under normal circumstances, is sequestered in the microtubule-associated dynein motor complex (210). Certain apoptotic signals release LC8, allowing LC8 together with Bim to translocate to Bcl-2 and inhibit its function. Homozygous knockout of Bim resulted in an incompletely penetrant embryonic lethal phenotype apparently for nonimmunologic reasons. In the surviving offspring, however, alterations in the homeostasis of multiple hematopoietic cell lineages developed (211). As anticipated, Bim-deficient B and T lymphocytes were resistant to certain apoptosis-promoting signals, but not to FasL. The knockout mice were found to have lymphoid hyperplasia with increases in naive T and B cells, altered thymocyte subset composition, and increases in granulocytes and monocytes in the peripheral blood. With age, these mice developed systemic autoimmunity manifested by progressive lymphadenopathy and splenomegaly; dramatic expansion of plasma cells; hyper-IgM, -IgG, and -IgA; antinuclear antibodies; immune complex GN; and vasculitis with a 55% survival at 1 year.

Similarly, transgenic expression of the *bcl-2* gene in B cells under the immunoglobulin enhancer resulted in lymphoid hyperplasia, hypergammaglobulinemia, high titers of antinuclear antibodies, and immune complex GN (212). Studies thus far have suggested that the constitutive *bcl-2* expression may promote autoimmunity by blocking apoptosis of autoantibody-producing B cells that normally arise spontaneously in germinal centers during the primary response to foreign antigens (213–215).

Finally, FLIP (gene name *Cflar*, for caspase 8 and FADD-like apoptosis regulator, and also called I-FLICE, CASH, Casper, CLARP, FLAME, and MRIT) is a death-effector domain-containing protein similar in structure to the apoptosis-promoting CASP8 (FLICE), but devoid of a caspase domain. In contrast to FLICE, FLIP inhibits death receptor-induced apoptosis by blocking the recruitment and activation of CASP8 (216,217). Transplantation of bone marrow cells retrovirally transfected with FLIP resulted in the resistance of B and T cells to activation-induced cell death, expansion of these cell populations, and in 4- to 6-month-old animals the development of hypergammaglobulinemia, anti-dsDNA autoantibodies, and glomerular immunoglobulin deposits with histologic evidence of GN characterized by glomerular sclerosis and thickening of mesangium and basement membranes (218). Despite the fact that FLIP blocks Fas signaling of activation-induced cell death, there were no accumulations of $B220^+$ or $CD4^-CD8^-$ DN T cells or activated T cells. This suggests that Fas and/or FLIP may affect other nonoverlapping pathways.

Complement Genes

Deficiencies of early complement components (C1q-s, C2, or C4) have long been know to predispose to SLE, indicating an important regulatory role for the complement pathway in suppressing autoimmunity. Although inadequate clearance of immune complexes was postulated to be the most likely mechanism, this did not fully explain the loss of tolerance to nuclear antigens. Gene knockout mice for C1q and C4 were therefore generated to address this issue. Homozygous C1q-deficient mice recapitulated the human disorder with the development of mild, but typical, features of lupus, including autoantibodies and a 25% incidence of immune complex GN (219). A large number of apoptotic bodies were discovered in the glomeruli of these mice, suggesting that C1q plays an essential role in the clearance of apoptotic bodies. In the case of C4 deficiency, accelerated lupus-like disease has been reported in both *Fas*^{lpr} (220) and normal background mice (221) (Table 7.3). Using a HEL Ig transgenic model, B cells from C4-deficient mice were shown to have a tolerance defect to soluble HEL (220). Thus, it was hypothesized that early complement components may be vital for maintaining self tolerance by virtue of their role in presenting tolerizing antigens to B cells. Clearance of immune complexes is also impaired in C4 knockout mice by a mechanism that is independent of CR1/CR2 complement receptors (221).

A similar mechanism was also proposed to explain the unexpected development of lupus-like autoimmunity in mice with homozygous deficiency of serum amyloid P (SAP) component, a highly conserved plasma protein originally named for its presence in amyloid deposits (222,223). Manifestations included a female predominance; autoantibodies to chromatin and its components, but not to other nuclear, tissue, or organ antigens; immune complex GN; and low incidence of mortality. In contrast to C1q deficiency, no accumulation of apoptotic bodies was detected in glomeruli. SAP binds to DNA and chromatin, and can displace H1-histones, thereby increasing solubility and reducing the rate of degradation and clearance of chromatin (222). It was hypothesized that SAP functions to promote self-tolerance to chromatin and its subunits by preventing immunogenic antigen-processing and/or by tolerizing chromatin reactive lymphocytes.

Cytokine Ligand and Receptor Genes

Under certain circumstances, systemic autoimmunity also develops in mice transgenic for the major Th1 and Th2 cytokines, IFN-γ and IL-4, respectively. Expression of IFN-γ in the suprabasal layer of the epidermis under the control of the involucrin promoter resulted in not only a severe inflammatory skin disorder, but also the generation of autoantibodies to dsDNA and histone, and an immune complex proliferative GN, particularly in females (224). This suggests that presentation of nuclear antigen by skin Langerhans cells and perhaps keratinocytes may be sufficient for the production of ANAs, and provides a possible explanation for the ultraviolet (UV) sensitivity of SLE patients. Similarly, C3H mice transgenic for the IL-4 gene under the control of the MHC class I promoter also developed systemic autoimmunity characterized by elevated MHC class II molecules and CD23, enhanced responses to polyclonal stimuli *in vitro*, increased levels of IgG1 and IgE, anemia, ANAs, and immune complex GN (225). These manifestations were likely due to direct IL-4–induced polyclonal activation of B cells, since CD4^{+} T cells were not required and there was no evidence of inefficient negative selection of B cells. The role of IL-4 in promoting lupus, however, is more complicated since autoimmunity was not observed in other transgenics expressing IL-4 on B cells or T cells (226–229), and in a spontaneous model of lupus expression of an IL-4 transgene did not exacerbate disease, but was protective (230). This would imply that a number of factors, such as the level and site of IL-4 production, and background genetic susceptibility, can modify the effects of IL-4 on systemic autoimmunity.

Tristetraprolin (TTP or Zfp-36) is a widely expressed zinc-binding protein initially thought to function as a transcription factor, particularly in lymphoid tissues, where high levels are found (231). Mice with homozygous knockout of TTP develop a complex syndrome consisting of cachexia, patchy alopecia, dermatitis, conjunctivitis, erosive arthritis, myeloid hyperplasia, glomerular mesangial thickening, and ANAs (232). These manifestations are mainly caused by excessive TNF-α production by macrophages and are reversed almost entirely by treatment with anti–TNF-α antibody (232,233). Thus, TTP must function as a nonredundant negative regulator of TNF-α. The mechanism was later discovered to be due to the binding of TTP to an AU-rich element contained in the TNF-α mRNA, which destabilizes the mRNA (234). In contrast to the autoimmune-promoting effects of elevated levels of TNF-α, physiologic amounts may, under certain circumstances, play a role in suppressing systemic autoimmunity. In studies of TNFR1 (p55) knockout mice, nonautoimmune mice did not develop defects in apoptosis or autoimmunity (235,236), yet the same knockout in the lupus-prone C57BL/6-*Fas*^{lpr} mice resulted in accelerated lymphoproliferation and autoimmune disease (53). Since TNF can induce death of activated peripheral T cells (93), these findings might be attributable to TNF compensating for the lack of Fas in *Fas*^{lpr} mice.

Cell Signaling Genes

Cbl-b is member of the cbl family of adapter proteins that predominantly function to inhibit receptor and nonreceptor tyrosine kinases (237,238). Two members, cbl-b and cbl, share a complex structure consisting of an amino-terminal phosphotyrosine-binding (PTB) domain, a C3HC4 RING finger, a proline-rich region capable of binding proteins with SH3 domains, several phosphotyrosine residues for binding SH2 domains, a ubiquitin recognition sequence, and, at the carboxy-terminal, a putative leucine zipper. Recently, a smaller third member (cbl-c or cbl-3) has been identified that contains the PTB, RING finger and a truncated proline-rich region, but is missing the rest of the carboxy portion (239,240). Cbl-b proteins appear to function as a negative regulator by inhibition of receptor clustering and raft aggregation in cell membranes (241). Cbl-b is expressed in normal and malignant mammary epithelial cells, a variety of normal tissues, and in hematopoietic tissues and cell lines. In accordance with their negative regulatory role, T cells from mice homozygous for the cbl-b gene knockout exhibit enhanced proliferation to antigen receptor signaling and do not require CD28 co-stimulation for IL-2 production or generation of T-dependent antibodies (242,243). Significantly, enhanced basal and activated levels of Vav, a guanine exchange factor for Rac-1/Rho/CDC42, was the only alteration in TCR signaling identified in these knockout mice. This was consistent with the previous findings that cbl-b binds to Vav and, when overexpressed, inhibits Vav stimulation of the c-Jun terminal kinase (244). Cbl-$b^{-/-}$ mice exhibit increased susceptibility to autoimmunity, both to experimental autoimmune encephalomyelitis (242) and to a spontaneous generalized autoimmune disease (243). The latter consisted of multiorgan lymphoaccumulation of polyclonal activated B and T cells with parenchymal damage, increased plasma cells, and antibodies to dsDNA by 6 months of age. Curiously, spontaneous autoimmunity occurred in only one (243) of the two Cbl-b knockout studies, suggesting that background strain, environment or other factors are important.

Phosphate and tensin homologue (PTEN) is a protein/lipid phosphatase initially identified as a tumor suppressor gene on chromosome 10q23, which is associated with a wide range of human malignancies (245,246). Germline mutations of PTEN also cause three autosomal-dominant disorders: Cowden disease, Lhermitte-Duclos syndrome, and Bannayan-Zonana syndrome. Homozygous knockouts of PTEN are embryonic lethal, but heterozygous mice develop an autoimmune disorder characterized by severe polyclonal lymphadenopathy, diffuse inflammatory cell infiltrates of most organs, hypergammaglobulinemia, anti-DNA antibodies, immune complex GN, and decreased survival (247). Females were more severely affected, with survivals of less than 12 months compared with over 15 months in males. Defective Fas-mediated activation-induced cell death of T and B lymphocytes was observed in PTEN-deficient mice due to impaired Fas signaling associated with increases in the survival factor Akt. It was therefore postulated that uninhibited increases in phosphatidylinositol (3,4,5-triphosphate (PIP_3), the major substrate for PTEN (248), leads to the recruitment and activation of Akt, and possibly other factors, which then inhibits Fas-mediated killing (247). PTEN-deficient mice, however, in contrast to *Fas*^{lpr} mice, did not have increases in either B220$^+$ or CD4$^-$CD8$^-$ DN T-cell populations, and furthermore, PTEN heterozygous knockouts had more severe disease than nonautoimmune background Fas-deficient mice. Thus, the development of autoimmunity in PTEN-deficient mice cannot be completely accounted for by Fas deficiency.

In another study, aberrant expression of a transgenic *ets* family proto-oncogene, Fli-1, under the control of the MHC class I promoter, resulted in a constellation of lupus-like manifestations that included lymphoid hyperplasia, hypergammaglobulinemia, elevated ANAs, and severe immune complex GN (249). Fli-$1^{-/-}$ B cells were hyperresponsive to a variety of stimuli, showed resistance to activation-induced cell death, and had prolonged survival compared to nontransgenic B cells. Although these findings suggest an important regulatory function for Fli-1 in B-cell response and homeostasis, a more limited role was indicated by the finding that immunologic defects in Fli-1 knockout mice were confined to a mild generalized thymic hypocellularity.

Cell Cycle–Related Genes

Gene knockout of the cyclin inhibitor p21$^{cip1/waf1}$ in mixed background C57BL/6 × 129/Sv also resulted in the development of systemic autoimmunity characterized by lymphoid hyperplasia, elevated IgG1, IgG antinuclear antibodies, GN, and early mortality (250). *In vitro* T-cell proliferation was enhanced in these mice, and there was an accumulation of effector/memory phenotype (CD44^{high}) CD4$^+$ T cells, although levels of other activation/effector/memory cell markers, such CD25, CD62L, CD69, and CD45RB, were similar to those in wild-type mice. An increased proportion of splenic B cells also expressed an activated (HSA^{low}, IgG^{low}) phenotype. Interestingly, females had more severe disease than males, similar to human SLE. Based on these findings, it was suggested that p21 negatively regulates T-cell proliferation following long-term stimulation, as is presumably the situation for autoantigen-reactive CD4$^+$ T cells. In sharp contrast, other studies in lupus-prone BXSB mice found an increase in p21 and other cyclin inhibitors in the expanded memory/effector CD4$^+$ T cells that are predominantly arrested in G1 (251). This led to just the opposite hypothesis, that the accumulating CD4$^+$ T cells, following successive rounds of division, become unable to enter into cell cycle and are resistant to apoptosis because of the buildup of cyclin inhibitors, a state similar to replicative senescence. Although no longer cycling, such cells may nonetheless secrete cytokines and activate B cells. Overall, it may be that both insufficient and excessive p21 may predispose to lupus by two independent mechanisms. Further studies will be needed to determine the precise role of p21 in spontaneous SLE.

Other Genes

Dnase1 is a 32- to 38-kd protein that is the major nuclease present in the blood, urine, and secretions. Interestingly, knockout of the Dnase1 gene in nonautoimmune background mice was recently reported to increase the incidence of SLE manifestations, including positive ANAs, anti-DNA antibodies, and immune complex GN (252). Although this suggests that accumulation of self DNA may trigger loss of tolerance and lupus, the precise mechanism is not known and other possibilities such as reduced degradation of exogenous nonmethylated CpG-rich DNA from pathogens might also play a role. This observation is somewhat unexpected since mammalian DNA alone is a poor immunogen for generating anti-DNA antibodies, and cell transfer studies in mice have suggested that genetic susceptibility for lupus is expressed in bone marrow–derived cells (30). Nevertheless, reduced Dnase1 activity, as observed in sera of lupus patients (252), may contribute to overall SLE susceptibility.

LUPUS SUSCEPTIBILITY LOCI

Current approaches to identifying genes predisposing to quantitative traits generally entail four main steps. First, mapping of traits is performed by genome-wide scans using evenly distributed markers spanning the chromosomes. Next, interval-specific congenic strains are generated that contain a generous portion of an introgressed genomic fragment to confirm the mapping studies and to identify the major intermediate phenotypes. A relatively large region is generally taken to assure that the specific gene or genes are indeed present within the interval. Third, panels of congenics with crossovers or smaller intervals are generated to finely map the location of the susceptibility gene or genes. This may be performed in one or two stages, i.e., localization first to ~5-centimorgan (cM) sized fragments and then to <1-cM sized fragments (253). The final step requires cloning, sequencing, and identifying of the genes within the fragment. Candidate genes are then selected based on expression, structure, function, or other characteristics for screening the parental strains for polymorphisms. The bulk of the work in this final step is the physical cloning and sequencing of the entire interval, which will be expedited by the forthcoming complete sequence of the mouse genome.

Over the past few years several groups have embarked on delineating lupus-related loci using genome-wide scans. Such searches involving a variety of crosses have revealed multiple quantitative and binary trait loci as summarized in Table 7.5. Thus far, at least 45 named loci distributed over 17 of the 19 autosomal chromosomes have been reported to be linked with one or more lupus traits. These and additional unnamed loci are listed by chromosome and chromosomal location (distance in centimorgans from the centromere) in Table 7.2. Some of these loci, identified by different groups, appear to be identical, whereas others appear to represent unique loci. Overall, the data suggest that susceptibility to spontaneous lupus in these strains is not due to the presence of a large number of common predisposing loci, but rather to different specific sets of a few major loci.

Loci Identified in Crosses of NZB and NZW Mice

The NZB and NZW strains have been the most extensively studied of the lupus-prone strains. Genome-wide scans of intercrosses, backcrosses, and crosses to normal background strains have resulted in the identification of loci contributing to one or more lupus-related traits on 15 of the 19 autosomal chromosomes (Table 7.2). Importantly, non-MHC loci that appear confirmed in more than one cross, include *Sle1* (NZW derived) and *Lbw7/Nba2* (NZB derived) on chromosome 1, *Lbw2/Sle2/nba1/Imh1/Mott* (NZB derived) on chromosome 4, *Lbw5/Sle3* (NZW derived) on chromosome 7, *Lbw8* (NZB derived) on proximal chromosome 8, and *nwa1* (NZW derived) on chromosome 16. The mapping studies indicate that inheritance of lupus traits is multiplicative, dependent on the number and specific combination of susceptibility loci (epistasis) and suggests that different sets of loci contributed to different traits, i.e., lymphoid hyperplasia, autoantibody production, GN, and mortality (50,254–256). Furthermore, at least one of the autoimmune-predisposing loci, *baa1* (chromosome 9), was from the normal BALB/c background (257), implying that either disease-predisposing alleles may be present in nonautoimmune strains or that susceptible strains may have alleles that suppress autoimmunity (50).

The roles of *Sle1*, *Sle2*, and *Sle3* in lupus pathogenesis have been further defined using interval-specific congenic C57BL/6 (B6) mice, which contain introgressed genomic fragments of chromosomes 1, 4, and 7, respectively, from the NZB/NZW-derived recombinant inbred strain NZM/Aeg2410 (258,259). *Sle1* congenic mice (B6.NZMc1) developed elevated IgG ANAs (particularly targeting H2A/H2B/DNA subnucleosomes), but no GN (260). Adoptive cotransfer of bone marrow from B6.NZMc1 and wild-type B6 mice revealed that autoantibodies were mainly produced by B6.NZMc1 B cells, thus implying that *Sle1* is functionally expressed in B cells (261). B6.NZMc4 congenic mice exhibited generalized B-cell hyperactivity, expansions of B1 cells, and elevated levels of polyclonal IgM, but no increases in IgG ANAs or GN (262). It was hypothesized that the expanded B1 cell population, which expressed higher levels of co-stimulatory molecules such as B7, might promote autoimmunity by facilitating the presentation of self antigens to T cells (263). B6.NZMc7 congenic mice developed elevated, but low, levels of ANAs and a low incidence of GN. A marked increase in activated T

TABLE 7.5. LOCI PREDISPOSING TO LUPUS-RELATED TRAITS IN SPONTANEOUS DISEASE MODELS

Name	Chr	cM	Marker	Cross	Major Associations	Parental Allele	Reference
Bxs4	1	7.7	D1Mit3	B10 × (B10 × BXSB)F_1	LN	BXSB	273
Bxs1	1	32.8	D1Mit5	BXSB × (B10 × BXSB)F_1	GN/ANA/spleen	BXSB	272
Bxs2	1	63.1	D1Mit12	BXSB × (B10 × BXSB)F_1	GN/ANA/spleen	BXSB	272
Sle1	1	87.9	D1Mit15	(NZM × B6) × NZM	GN	NZM (NZW)	38
				(NZM × B6)F_2	dsDNA/GN/spleen		266
Lbw7	1	92.3	D1Mit36	BWF2	Chr/spleen	NZB	254
Nba2	1	92.3	D1Mit111	(B × SM) × W	GN	NZB	39
		92.3	D1Mit148	(B × SM) × W/(B6.H2^z × B) × B	ANA/gp70/GN		285
		94.2	Crp/Sap	((B6.H2^z & Ba.H2^z) × B)F_1 × B	GN		286
Bxs3	1	100.0	D1Mit403	BXSB × (B10 × BXSB)F_1	dsDNA	BXSB	272
Sles2	3	35.2	D3Mit137	(B6.NZMc1 × NZW)F_1 × NZW	dsDNA/GN (resistance)	NZW	50
Bxs5	3	39.7	D3Mit40	B10 × (B10 × BXSB)F_1	ANA/IgG3	BXSB	273
Lprm2	3	64.1	D3Mit14	(MRL-lpr × C3H-lpr)BC & F_2	Vasculitis (resistance)	MRL	268,287
Arvm2	4	19.8	D4Mit89	(MRL-lpr × C3H-lpr)BC & F_2	Vasculitis	MRL	287
Lprm1	4	32.5	D4Mit82	MRL-lpr × (MRL-lpr × C3H-lpr)F_1	Vasculitis	MRL	268
Acla2	4	40.0	D4Mit79	NZW × (NZW × BXSB)F_1	CL	BXSB	274
Sle2	4	44.5	D4Mit9	(NZM × B6) × NZM	GN	NZM	38
Spm1	4	45.9	D4Mit58	(B6 × NZB)F_1 × NZB	Spleen	NZB	288
Lbw2	4	55.6	D4Nds2	BWF2	Mortality/GN/spleen	NZB	254
Sles2	4	57.6	D4Mit12	(B6.NZMc1 × NZW)F_1 × NZW	dsDNA/GN (resistance)	NZW	50
Arvm2	4	57.6	D4Mit147	(MRL-lpr × C3H-lpr)BC & F_2	Vasculitis	MRL	287
Asm2	4	65.0	D4Mit199	MRL-lpr × (MRL-lpr × C3H-lpr)F_1	Sialadenitis	MRL female	270
nba1	4	65.7	Epb4.1[a]	BWF1 × W	GN	NZB	289
Lmb1	4	69.8	D4Mit12	(B6-lpr × MRL-lpr)F_2	Lprn/dsDNA	B6	267
Imh1/Mott	4	69/69.8	D4Mit66/48	BWF1 × W	hyper IgM/GN/dsDNA	NZB	290,291
Sle6	5	20.0	D5Mit4	(B6.NZMc1 × NZW)F_1 × NZW	GN	NZW	50
Lmb2	5	41.0	D5Mit356	(B6-lpr × MRL-lpr)F_2	Lprn/dsDNA	MRL	267
Lprm4	5	54.0	D5Mit23	MRL-lpr × (MRL-lpr × C3H-lpr)F_1	Spleen	MRL	268
Lbw3	5	84.0	D5Mit101	BWF2	Mortality	NZW	254
Lbw4	6	64.0	D6Mit25	BWF2	Mortality	NZB	254
Sle5	7	0.5	D7Mit178	(NZM × B6)F_2	dsDNA	NZM (NZW)	266
Lrdm1	7	6.0	Pou2f2	(MRL-lpr × CAST)F_1 × MRL-lpr	GN	MRL	269
Sle3	7	16.0	D7Mit25	(NZM × B6)F_2	GN	NZM (NZW)	266
Lbw5	7	23.0	D7Nds5	BWF2	Mortality	NZW	254
Lmb3	7	27.0	D7Mit211	(B6-lpr × MRL-lpr)F_2	Lprn/dsDNA	MRL	267
Sle3	7	28.0	p	(NZM × B6) × NZM	GN	NZM (NZW)	38
Aem2	7	28.4	D7Mit30	(B6 × NZB)F_1 × NZB	RBC	NZB	288
Myo1	7	69.0	D7Mit14	NZW × (NZW × BXSB)F_1	MI	BXSB	274
Pbat2	8	11	D8Mit96	NZW × (NZW × BXSB)F_1	Platelet	BXSB	274
baa1	9	28.0	D9Mit22	(W × Ba)F_1 × W	IgM ssDNA/IgM histone	Balb/c	257
Asm1	10	38/40	D10Mit115/259	MRL-lpr × (MRL-lpr × C3H-lpr)F_1	Sialadenitis	MRL	270
Aem3	10	41.5	D10Mit42	(B6 × NZB)F_1 × NZB	RBC	NZB	288
Lmb4	10	51.0	D10Mit11	(B6-lpr × MRL-lpr)F_2	Lprn/GN	MRL	267
Lbw8	11	28.0	IL4	BWF_2	chr	NZB	254
Lrdm2	12	27.0	D12Nyu3	(MRL-lpr × CAST)F_1 × MRL-lpr	GN	MRL	269
Yaa1	13	35.0	D13Mit250	B6 × (W × B6-Yaa)F_1	gp70	NZW	292
Myo2	14	39.0	D14Mit68	NZW × (NZW × BXSB)F_1	MI	BXSB	274
Lprm3	14	44.0	D14Mit195	MRL-lpr × (MRL-lpr × C3H-lpr)F_1	GN (resistance)	MRL	268
Lprm5	16	21.0	D16Mit3	MRL-lpr × (MRL-lpr × C3H-lpr)F_1	dsDNA	MRL	268
nwa1	16	38.0	D16Mit5	(W × Ba)F_1 × W	Histone	NZW	257
nwa1	16	38.0	D16Mit5	(B × W)F_1 × W	GN/dsDNA	NZW	293
Acla1	17	18.2	D17Mit16	NZW × (NZW × BXSB)F_1	CL	NZW/BXSB	274
Sles1	17	18.8	H2/D17Mit34	(B6.NZMc1 × NZW)F_1 × NZW	GN/dsDNA (resistance)	NZW	50
Pbat1	17	18.9	D17Nds2	NZW × (NZW × BXSB)F_1	Platelet	NZW/BXSB	274
Lbw6	18	47.0	D18Mit8	BWF_2	Mortality/GN	NZW	254
nwa2	19	41.0	D19Mit11	(W × Ba)F_1 × W	ssDNA	NZW	257

Table includes only named loci with linkages $p < .01$ or loci >1.9. Loci are listed by their approximate chromosomal locations based on the marker with the highest association. Chr, chromosome. cM distances are based on the Mouse Genome Database. Abbreviations for mouse strains (Cross column): B = NZB, B6 = C57BL/6, B10 = C57BL/10, Ba = Balb/c, CAST = CAST/Ei, lpr = *Fas*^{lpr}, NZM = NZM/Aeg2410, W = NZW, (MRL-lpr × C3H-lpr)BC and F_2 = both MRL-lpr × (MRL-lpr × C3H-lpr)F_1 and (MRL-lpr × C3H-lpr)F_2 crosses. Original phenotypes that mapped to loci are shown: chr, antichromatin autoantibody; CL, anticardiolipin autoantibody; dsDNA, anti-dsDNA autoantibody; GN, glomerulonephritis; gp70, gp70 immune complexes; histone, antihistone autoantibody; LN, lymphadenopathy; Lprn, lymphoproliferation; MI, myocardial infarct; platelet, antiplatelet auto-Ab and thrombocytopenia; RBC, antiRBC auto-Ab; spleen, splenomegaly. Autoantibodies are IgG unless otherwise specified.
[a]Formerly named *elp-1*

cells, elevated CD4/CD8 ratios, and resistance to activation-induced cell death were observed, suggesting that *Sle3* may promote generalized T-cell activation (264). Bicongenic B6.NZMc1/7 mice developed severe GN associated with elevated IgG ANAs to multiple chromatin components, expanded B- and T-cell populations, and splenomegaly (265). Although the precise mechanisms have yet to be defined, based on these initial findings, a simple additive model was initially proposed wherein lupus develops in NZM/Aeg2410 mice from distinct gene alterations that cause loss of tolerance to nucleosome components (*Sle1*), a B-cell defect (Sle2), and a T-cell defect (*Sle3*) (256). However, more recent studies involving crosses of these congenic mice have demonstrated a more complex inheritance of lupus traits (50,266).

Loci Identified in MRL-*Fas^{lpr}* Crosses

Although the *Fas^{lpr}* mutation promotes loss of tolerance and autoimmunity, the type of manifestations and severity of lupus-like disease is highly dependent on background susceptibility genes. This has led several groups to define lupus-related quantitative trait loci (QTL) in crosses of MRL-*Fas^{lpr}* mice, a strain that develops particularly severe spontaneous accelerated systemic autoimmunity (Table 7.2). QTL for one or more lupus traits have been identified on 13 of the 19 autosomal chromosomes. The large number of loci may be attributable, in part, to the different traits assessed, such as sialadenitis, GN, and vasculitis, which are most likely caused by overlapping, but distinct, sets of susceptibility genes, and to the fact that crosses involved different strains. Nevertheless, several loci on chromosomes 5 (*Lmb2*, *Lprm4*), 7 (Lmb3, *Ldrm1*) and 10 (*Lmb4*, Asm1) had overlapping intervals and may be identical (267–270). Interestingly, another locus, *Lmb1* (chromosome 4), which mapped to the nonautoimmune B6 background, had an additive effect on lymphoproliferation equal to the other *Lmb* QTL (267). This demonstrates that so-called nonautoimmune mice can harbor bona fide susceptibility genes, but presumably the number and combination of such genes are insufficient for disease induction. Such genes undoubtedly account for the background effects observed when using different strain combinations to map QTLs.

Loci Identified in BXSB Crosses

BXSB males develop severe accelerated lupus largely due to the presence of the *Yaa* gene (271); however, other background genes are clearly important since significant autoimmune responses are not observed in consomic nonautoimmune background CBA/J.BXSB-Y (143) or B6.BXSB-Y (144). Genome-wide searches have identified non-MHC loci encompassing 6 chromosomes in backcrosses to C57BL/10 (B10) and NZW strains (Table 7.2). Interestingly, genome-wide scans of reciprocal backcrosses of BXSB to B10 mice revealed five QTLs, four of which were located on chromosome 1 (272,273). In contrast, none of the non-MHC BXSB loci identified in NZW×(NZW×BXSB)F1 backcrosses overlapped with these loci (274). Further studies will be needed to determine the significance of these observations.

Summary of the Lupus Susceptibility Loci

Overall, from these mapping studies involving a variety of crosses of four different lupus-prone background strains, a number of generalizations can be surmised. Each strain appears to contain a few major susceptibility loci; however, there is minimal overlap of susceptibility genes among the various lupus-predisposed strains, indicating the potential for a large pool of susceptibility genes. Predisposition to the different traits appears to be governed by different sets of genes, some of which are common to several traits. The genetic contributions are in general additive, but can depend substantially on specific combinations (epistasis). This suggests the presence of common mechanisms or pathways, and raises the possibility that intervention directed toward such loci might have a strong therapeutic impact. Finally, the fact that interval-specific congenic strains manifest highly penetrant component phenotypes clearly opens the way for ultimately cloning the underlying genes.

CONCLUSION

The progress from only a handful of genetic alterations known to cause loss of tolerance and lupus-like manifestations 8 years ago, when Fas mutations were identified as the cause of the *lpr* phenotype, to now, when over 30 specific genes and over 40 loci have been identified, illustrates clearly the enormous strides made in the study of mouse models of SLE. Common immunopathologic mechanisms, such as altered regulation of antigen-receptor signaling, defective apoptosis, and ineffective complement-mediated clearance of antigen, appear to be emerging, which future studies using genetic manipulation of additional immunologically relevant genes should bring into sharper focus. The feasibility of cloning quantitative lupus traits in mouse models appears no longer to be an issue, and the eventual identification of predisposing mutations should help reveal major etiologic factors. Ultimately, definition of the genetics of systemic autoimmunity should provide a rational basis for assessing susceptibility and for devising therapeutic interventions.

ACKNOWLEDGMENTS

This is publication number 13866-IMM from the Department of Immunology, the Scripps Research Institute, 10550 N. Torrey Pines Road, La Jolla, CA 92037. This work was supported in part by National Institutes of Health grants AR42242, ES08666, AR93555, and AR31203.

REFERENCES

1. Kofler R, McConahey PJ, Duchosal MA, et al. An autosomal recessive gene that delays expression of lupus in BXSB mice. *J Immunol* 1991;146:1375–1379.
2. Fossati L, Takahashi S, Merino R, et al. An MRL/MpJ-lpr/lpr substrain with a limited expansion of lpr double-negative T cells and a reduced autoimmune syndrome. *Int Immunol* 1993;5: 525–532.
3. Takahashi S, Fossati L, Iwamoto I, et al. Imbalance towards Th1 predominance is associated with acceleration of lupus-like autoimmune syndrome in MRL mice. *J Clin Invest* 1996;97: 1597–1604.
4. Pollard KM, Hultman P. Effects of mercury on the immune system. *Met Ions Biol Sys* 1997;14:421–440.
5. Bigazzi PE. Metals and kidney autoimmunity. *Environ Health Perspect* 1999;107:753–765.
6. Hultman P, Bell LJ, Enestrom S, et al. Murine susceptibility to mercury. I. Autoantibody profiles and systemic immune deposits in inbred, congenic, and intra-H-2 recombinant strains. *Clin Immunol Immunopathol* 1992;65:98–109.
7. Hultman P, Bell LJ, Enestrom S, et al. Murine susceptibility to mercury. II. Autoantibody profiles and renal immune deposits in hybrid, backcross, and H-2d congenic mice. *Clin Immunol Immunopathol* 1993;68:9–20.
8. Hultman P, Enestrom S, Pollard KM, et al. Anti-fibrillarin autoantibodies in mercury-treated mice. *Clin Exp Immunol* 1989;78:470–477.
9. Ochs RL, Lischwe MA, Spohn WH, et al. Fibrillarin: a new protein of the nucleolus identified by autoimmune sera. *Biol Cell* 1985;54:123–133.
10. Pollard KM, Pearson DL, Hultman P, et al. Lupus prone mice as models to study xenobiotic-induced acceleration of systemic autoimmunity. *Environ Health Perspect* 1999;107(suppl 5): 729–735.
11. Kotzin BL, Barr VL, Palmer E. A large deletion within the T-cell receptor beta-chain gene complex in New Zealand White mice. *Science* 1985;229:167–171.
12. Noonan DJ, McConahey PJ, Cardenas GJ. Correlations of autoimmunity with H-2 and T cell receptor beta chain genotypes in (NZB × NZW) F2 mice. *Eur J Immunol* 1990;20: 1105–1110.
13. Woodland DL, Kotzin BL, Palmer E. Functional consequences of a T cell receptor D·2 and J·2 gene segment deletion. *J Immunol* 1990;144:379–385.
14. Ghatak S, Sainis K, Owen FL, et al. T-cell-receptor b- and I-A b-chain genes of normal SWR mice are linked with the development of lupus nephritis in NZB × SWR crosses. *Proc Natl Acad Sci USA* 1987;84:6850–6853.
15. Hirose S, Tokushige K, Kinoshita K, et al. Contribution of the gene linked to the T cell receptor β chain gene complex of NZW mice to the autoimmunity of (NZB × NZW)F1 mice. *Eur J Immunol* 1991;21:823–826.
16. Kumar V, Sercarz E. Holes in the T cell repertoire to myelin basic protein owing to the absence of the D beta 2–J beta 2 gene cluster: implications for T cell receptor recognition and autoimmunity. *J Exp Med* 1994;179:1637–1643.
17. Bailey NC, Bona A, Dikman S, et al. Correlation between the occurrence of lupus nephritis, anti-erythrocyte autoantibodies and V kappa haplotype in NZB × 129/J and NZB × SM/J recombinant inbred murine strains. *Eur J Immunol* 1991;21: 959–965.
18. Halpern MD, Fisher CL, Cohen PL, et al. Influence of the Ig H chain locus on autoantibody production in autoimmune mice. *J Immunol* 1992;149:3735–3740.
19. Halpern MD, Craven SY, Cohen PL, et al. Regulation of anti-Sm autoantibodies by the immunoglobulin heavy chain locus. *J Immunol* 1993;151:7268–7272.
20. Fujimura T, Hirose S, Jiang Y, et al. Dissection of the effects of tumor necrosis factor-alpha and class II gene polymorphisms within the MHC on murine systemic lupus erythematosus (SLE). *Int Immunol* 1998;10:1467–1472.
21. Jacob CO, Lee SK, Strassmann G. Mutational analysis of TNF-alpha gene reveals a regulatory role for the 3′-untranslated region in the genetic predisposition to lupus-like autoimmune disease. *J Immunol* 1996;156:3043–3050.
22. Bazzoni F, Beutler B. Comparative expression of TNF-alpha alleles from normal and autoimmune-prone MHC haplotypes. *J Inflamm* 1995;45:106–114.
23. Richter G, Qin ZH, Diamantstein T, et al. Analysis of restriction fragment length polymorphism in lymphokine genes of normal and autoimmune mice. *J Exp Med* 1989;170: 1439–1443.
24. Jiang Y, Hirose S, Sanokawa-Akakura R, et al. Genetically determined aberrant down-regulation of FcgammaRIIB1 in germinal center B cells associated with hyper-IgG and IgG autoantibodies in murine systemic lupus erythematosus. *Int Immunol* 1999;11:1685–1691.
25. Mary C, Laporte C, Parzy D, et al. Dysregulated expression of the Cd22 gene as a result of a short interspersed nucleotide element insertion in Cd22a lupus-prone mice. *J Immunol* 2000; 165:2987–2996.
26. Merino R, Fossati L, Lacour M, et al. H-2-linked control of the Yaa gene-induced acceleration of lupus- like autoimmune disease in BXSB mice. *Eur J Immunol* 1992;22:295–299.
27. Hirose S, Nagasawa R, Sekikawa I, et al. Enhancing effect of H-2 linked NZW genes on the autoimmune traits of (NZB × NZW)F1 mice. *J Exp Med* 1983;158:228–233.
28. Kotzin BL, Palmer E. The contribution of NZW genes to lupus-like disease in (NZB × NZW)F1 mice. *J Exp Med* 1987; 165:1237–1251.
29. Theofilopoulos AN. Murine models of SLE. In: Lahita RG. *Systemic lupus erythematosus*, 2nd ed. San Deigo: Academic Press, 1992;2:121–194.
30. Theofilopoulos AN, Dixon FJ. Murine models of systemic lupus erythematosus. *Adv Immunol* 1985;37:269–390.
31. Theofilopoulos AN, Kono DH. Murine lupus models: gene-specific and genome-wide studies. In: Lahita RG, ed. *Systemic lupus erythematosus*, 3rd ed. San Diego: Academic Press, 1999:145–181.
32. Theofilopoulos AN. Immunologic genes in mouse lupus models. In: Bona CA, Siminovitch KA, Zanetti M, et al., eds. *The molecular pathology of autoimmune diseases*. New York: Harwood Academic, 1993:281–316.
33. Ogawa S, Nishimura H, Awaji M, et al. Nucleotide sequence analysis of MHC class II genes in autoimmune disease-prone (NZB×NZW)F1 mice. *Immunogenetics* 1990;32:295–299.
34. Schiffenbauer J, Wegrzyn L, Croker BP. Background genes mediate the development of autoimmunity in (NZB × PL/J)F1 or (NZB × BIO.PL)F1 mice. *Clin Immunol Immunopathol* 1992;62:227–234.
35. Chiang B, Bearer E, Ansari A, et al. The BM12 mutation and autoantibodies to dsDNA in NZB.H-2bm12 mice. *J Immunol* 1990;145:94–101.
36. Iwamoto M, Ibnou-Zekri N, Araki K, et al. Prevention of murine lupus by an I-E alpha chain transgene: protective role of I-E alpha chain-derived peptides with a high affinity to I-A^b molecules. *Eur J Immunol* 1996;26:307–314.
37. Kawano H, Abe M, Zhang D, et al. Heterozygosity of the major histocompatibility complex controls the autoimmune disease in (NZW × BXSB)F1 mice. *Clin Immunol Immunopathol* 1992; 65:308–314.

38. Morel L, Rudofsky UH, Longmate JA, et al. Polygenic control of susceptibility to murine systemic lupus erythematosus. *Immunity* 1994;1:219–229.
39. Drake CG, Rozzo SJ, Hirschfeld HF, et al. Analysis of the New Zealand black contribution to lupus-like renal disease. Multiple genes that operate in a threshold manner. *J Immunol* 1995; 154:2441–2447.
40. Gotoh Y, Takashima H, Noguchi K, et al. Mixed haplotype A beta z/A alpha d class II molecule in (NZB × NZW)F1 mice detected by T cell clones. *J Immunol* 1993;150:4777–4787.
41. Nygard NR, McCarthy DM, Schiffenbauer J, et al. Mixed haplotypes and autoimmunity. *Immunol Today* 1993;14:53–56.
42. Vyse TJ, Halterman RK, Rozzo SJ, et al. Control of separate pathogenic autoantibody responses marks MHC gene contributions to murine lupus. *Proc Natl Acad Sci USA* 1999;96: 8098–8103.
43. Vyse TJ, Rozzo SJ, Drake CG, et al. Contributions of Ea(z) and Eb(z) MHC genes to lupus susceptibility in New Zealand mice. *J Immunol* 1998;160:2757–2766.
44. Rozzo SJ, Vyse TJ, David CS, et al. Analysis of MHC class II genes in the susceptibility to lupus in New Zealand mice. *J Immunol* 1999;162:2623–2630.
45. Ibnou-Zekri N, Vyse TJ, Rozzo SJ, et al. MHC-linked control of murine SLE. *Curr Top Microbiol Immunol* 1999;246: 275–280.
46. Merino R, Iwamoto M, Fossati L, et al. Prevention of systemic lupus erythematosus in autoimmune BXSB mice by a transgene encoding I-E alpha chain. *J Exp Med* 1993;178:1189–1197.
47. Ibnou-Zekri N, Iwamoto M, Fossati L, et al. Role of the major histocompatibility complex class II Ea gene in lupus susceptibility in mice. *Proc Natl Acad Sci USA* 1997;94:14654–14659.
48. Ibnou-Zekri N, Iwamoto M, Gershwin ME, et al. Protection of murine lupus by the Ead transgene is MHC haplotype-dependent. *J Immunol* 2000;164:505–511.
49. Fossati L, Sobel ES, Iwamoto M, et al. The Yaa gene-mediated acceleration of murine lupus: *Yaa*$^-$ T cells from non-autoimmune mice collaborate with Yaa$^+$ B cells to produce lupus autoantibodies in vivo. *Eur J Immunol* 1995;25:3412–3417.
50. Morel L, Tian XH, Croker BP, et al. Epistatic modifiers of autoimmunity in a murine model of lupus nephritis. *Immunity* 1999;11:131–139.
51. Jacob CO, McDevitt HO. Tumour necrosis factor-alpha in murine autoimmune "lupus" nephritis. *Nature* 1988;331:356–358.
52. Kontoyiannis D, Kollias G. Accelerated autoimmunity and lupus nephritis in NZB mice with an engineered heterozygous deficiency in tumor necrosis factor. *Eur J Immunol* 2000;30: 2038–2047.
53. Zhou T, Edwards CK, Yang P, et al. Greatly accelerated lymphadenopathy and autoimmune disease in lpr mice lacking tumor necrosis factor receptor I. *J Immunol* 1996;156:2661–2665.
54. Watanabe-Fukunaga R, Brannan CI, Itoh N, et al. The cDNA structure, expression, and chromosomal assignment of the mouse Fas antigen. *J Immunol* 1992;148:1274–1279.
55. Drappa J, Brot N, Elkon KB. The Fas protein is expressed at high levels on CD4+CD8+ thymocytes and activated mature lymphocytes in normal mice but not in the lupus-prone strain, MRL lpr/lpr. *Proc Natl Acad Sci USA* 1993;90: 10340–10344.
56. Alderson MR, Armitage RJ, Maraskovsky E, et al. Fas transduces activation signals in normal human T lymphocytes. *J Exp Med* 1993;178:2231–2235.
57. Lynch DH, Ramsdell F, Alderson MR. Fas and FasL in the homeostatic regulation of immune responses. *Immunol Today* 1995;16:569–574.
58. Suda T, Okazaki T, Naito Y, et al. Expression of the Fas ligand in cells of T cell lineage. *J Immunol* 1995;154:3806–3813.
59. Bellgrau D, Gold D, Selawry H, et al. A role for CD95 ligand in preventing graft rejection. *Nature* 1995;377:630–632.
60. Griffin TS, Brunner T, Fletcher SM, et al. Fas ligand-induced apoptosis as a mechanism of immune privilege. *Science* 1995; 270:1189–1192.
61. Hunt JS, Vassmer D, Ferguson TA, et al. Fas ligand is positioned in mouse uterus and placenta to prevent trafficking of activated leukocytes between the mother and the conceptus. *J Immunol* 1997;158:4122–4128.
62. Gao Y, Herndon JM, Zhang H, et al. Antiinflammatory effects of CD95 ligand (FasL)-induced apoptosis. *J Exp Med* 1998; 188:887–896.
63. Kaplan HJ, Leibole MA, Tezel T, et al. Fas ligand (CD95 ligand) controls angiogenesis beneath the retina. *Nat Med* 1999; 5:292–297.
64. Oehm A, Behrmann I, Falk W, et al. Purification and molecular cloning of the APO-1 cell surface antigen, a member of the tumor necrosis factor/nerve growth factor receptor superfamily. Sequence identity with the Fas antigen. *J Biol Chem* 1992; 267:10709–10715.
65. Watanabe-Fukunaga R, Brannan CI, Copeland NG, et al. Lymphoproliferative disorder in mice explained by defects in Fas antigen that mediates apoptosis. *Nature* 1992;356:314–317.
66. Adachi M, Watanabe-Fukunaga R, Nagata S. Aberrant transcription caused by the insertion of an early transposable element in an intron of the Fas antigen gene of lpr mice. *Proc Natl Acad Sci USA* 1993;90:1756–1760.
67. Chu JL, Drappa J, Parnassa A, et al. The defect in Fas mRNA expression in MRL/lpr mice is associated with insertion of the retrotransposon, ETn. *J Exp Med* 1993;178:723–730.
68. Wu J, Zhou T, He J, et al. Autoimmune disease in mice due to integration of an endogenous retrovirus in an apoptosis gene. *J Exp Med* 1993;178:461–468.
69. Mariani SM, Matiba B, Armandola EA, et al. The APO-1/Fas (CD95) receptor is expressed in homozygous MRL/lpr mice. *Eur J Immunol* 1994;24:3119–3123.
70. Booker JK, Reap EA, Cohen PL. Expression and function of Fas on cells damaged by gamma-irradiation in B6 and B6/lpr mice. *J Immunol* 1998;161:4536–4541.
71. Adachi M, Suematsu S, Kondo T, et al. Targeted mutation in the Fas gene causes hyperplasia of peripheral lymphoid organs and liver. *Nat Genet* 1995;11:294–300.
72. Matsuzawa A, Moriyama T, Kaneko T. A new allele of the *lpr* locus, lpr^{cg}, that complements the *gld* gene in induction of lymphadenopathy in the mouse. *J Exp Med* 1990;171:519–531.
73. Roths JB, Murphy ED, Eicher EM. A new mutation, *gld*, that produces lymphoproliferation and autoimmunity in C3H/HeJ mice. *J Exp Med* 1984;159:1–20.
74. Lynch DH, Watson ML, Alderson MR, et al. The mouse Fas-ligand gene is mutated in gld mice and is part of a TNF family gene cluster. *Immunity* 1994;1:131–136.
75. Takahashi T, Tanaka M, Brannan CI, et al. Generalized lymphoproliferative disease in mice, caused by a point mutation in the Fas ligand. *Cell* 1994;76:969–976.
76. Hahne M, Peitsch MC, Irmier M, et al. Characterization of the non-functional Fas ligand of gld mice. *Int Immunol* 1995;7: 1381–1386.
77. Murphy ED, Roths JB. Autoimmunity and lymphoproliferation: induction by mutant gene lpr and acceleration by a male associated factor in BXSB mice. In: Rose NL, Bigazzi PE, Warner NL, eds. *Genetic control of autoimmune disease*. Amsterdam: Elsevier, 1979:207–220.
78. Ogata Y, Kimura M, Shimada K, et al. Distinctive expression of lpr^{cg} in the heterozygous state on different genetic backgrounds. *Cell Immunol* 1993;148:91–102.
79. Rieux-Laucat F, Le Deist F, Hivroz C, et al. Mutations in Fas

associated with human lymphoproliferative syndrome and autoimmunity. *Science* 1995;268:1347–1349.

80. Fisher GH, Rosenberg FJ, Straus SE, et al. Dominant interfering Fas gene mutations impair apoptosis in a human autoimmune lymphoproliferative syndrome. *Cell* 1995;81:935–946.
81. Drappa J, Vaishnaw AK, Sullivan KE, et al. Fas gene mutations in the Canale-Smith syndrome, an inherited lymphoproliferative disorder associated with autoimmunity. *N Engl J Med* 1996;335:1643–1649.
82. Wang J, Zheng L, Lobito A, et al. Inherited human Caspase 10 mutations underlie defective lymphocyte and dendritic cell apoptosis in autoimmune lymphoproliferative syndrome type II. *Cell* 1999;98:47–58.
83. Mysler E, Bini P, Drappa J, et al. The apoptosis-1/Fas protein in human systemic lupus erythematosus. *J Clin Invest* 1994;93: 1029–1034.
84. Wu J, Wilson J, He J, et al. Fas ligand mutation in a patient with systemic lupus erythematosus and lymphoproliferative disease. *J Clin Invest* 1996;98:1077–1113.
85. Kojima T, Horiuchi T, Nishizaka H, et al. Analysis of fas ligand gene mutation in patients with systemic lupus erythematosus. *Arthritis Rheum* 2000;43:135–139.
86. McNally J, Yoo DH, Drappa J, et al. Fas ligand expression and function in systemic lupus erythematosus. *J Immunol* 1997; 159:4628–4636.
87. Singer PA, Balderas RS, McEvilly RJ, et al. Tolerance-related V beta clonal deletions in normal CD4–8–, TCR- alpha/beta + and abnormal lpr and gld cell populations. *J Exp Med* 1989; 170:1869–1877.
88. Zhou T, Bluethmann H, Zhang J, et al. Defective maintenance of T cell tolerance to a superantigen in MRL-lpr/lpr mice. *J Exp Med* 1992;176:1063–1072.
89. Herron LR, Eisenberg RA, Roper E, et al. Selection of the T cell receptor repertoire in Lpr mice. *J Immunol* 1993;151:3450–3459.
90. Mogil RJ, Radvanyi L, Gonzalez-Quintial R, et al. Fas (CD95) participates in peripheral T cell deletion and associated apoptosis *in vivo*. *Int Immunol* 1995;7:1451–1458.
91. Singer GG, Abbas AK. The fas antigen is involved in peripheral but not thymic deletion of T lymphocytes in T cell receptor transgenic mice. *Immunity* 1994;1:365–371.
92. Sidman CL, Marshall JD, von Boehmer H. Transgenic T cell receptor interactions in the lymphoproliferative and autoimmune syndromes of lpr and gld mutant mice. *Eur J Immunol* 1995;22:499–504.
93. Sytwu HK, Liblau RS, McDevitt HO. The roles of Fas/APO-1 (CD95) and TNF in antigen-induced programmed cell death in T cell receptor transgenic mice. *Immunity* 1996;5:17–30.
94. Bossu P, Singer GG, Andres P, et al. Mature CD4+ T lymphocytes from MRL/lpr mice are resistant to receptor-mediated tolerance and apoptosis. *J Immunol* 1993;151:7233–7239.
95. Russell JH, Rush B, Weaver C, et al. Mature T cells of autoimmune lpr/lpr mice have a defect in antigen-stimulated suicide. *Proc Natl Acad Sci USA* 1993;90:4409–4413.
96. Musette P, Pannetier C, Gachelin G, et al. The expansion of a CD4+ T cell population bearing a distinctive beta chain in MRL lpr/lpr mice suggests a role for the fas protein in peripheral T cell selection. *Eur J Immunol* 1994;24:2761–2766.
97. Dhein J, Walczak H, Baumler C, et al. Autocrine T-cell suicide mediated by APO-1/(Fas/CD95). *Nature* 1995;373:438–441.
98. Podack ER. Execution and suicide: cytotoxic lymphocytes enforce Draconian laws through separate molecular pathways. *Curr Opin Immunol* 1995;7:11–16.
99. Brunner T, Mogil RJ, LaFace D, et al. Cell-autonomous Fas (CD95)/Fas-ligand interaction mediates activation-induced apoptosis in T-cell hybridomas. *Nature* 1995;373:441–444.
100. Ju ST, Panka DJ, Cui H, et al. Fas(CD95)/FasL interactions required for programmed cell death after T-cell activation. *Nature* 1995;373:444–448.
101. Yang Y, Mercep M, Ware CF, et al. Fas and activation-induced Fas ligand mediate apoptosis of T cell hybridomas: inhibition of Fas ligand expression by retinoic acid and glucocorticoids. *J Exp Med* 1995;181:1673–1682.
102. Ju ST, Cui H, Panka DJ, et al. Participation of target Fas protein in apoptosis pathway induced by CD4+ Th1 and CD8+ cytotoxic T cells. *Proc Natl Acad Sci USA* 1994;91:4185–4189.
103. Lowin B, Hahne M, Mattmann C, et al. Cytolytic T-cell cytotoxicity is mediated through perforin and Fas lytic pathways. *Nature* 1994;370:650–652.
104. Hanabuchi S, Koyanagi M, Kawasaki A, et al. Fas and its ligand in a general mechanism of T-cell-mediated cytotoxicity. *Proc Natl Acad Sci USA* 1994;91:4930–4934.
105. Berke G. The CTL's kiss of death. *Cell* 1995;81:9–12.
106. Kagi D, Vignaux F, Ledermann B, et al. Fas and perforin pathways as major mechanisms of T cell-mediated cytotoxicity. *Science* 1994;265:528–530.
107. Walsh CM, Matloubian M, Liu CC, et al. Immune function in mice lacking the perforin gene. *Proc Natl Acad Sci USA* 1994; 91:10854–10858.
108. Hammond DM, Nagarkatti PS, Gote LR, et al. Double-negative T cells from MRL-lpr/lpr mice mediate cytolytic activity when triggered through adhesion molecules and constitutively express perforin gene. *J Exp Med* 1993;178:2225–2230.
109. Mixter PF, Russell JQ, Durie FH, et al. Decreased CD4–CD8– TCR-alpha beta + cells in lpr/lpr mice lacking beta 2-microglobulin. *J Immunol* 1995;154:2063–2074.
110. Ohteki T, Iwamoto M, Izui S, et al. Reduced development of CD4–8–B220+ T cells but normal autoantibody production in lpr/lpr mice lacking major histocompatibility complex class I molecules. *Eur J Immunol* 1995;25:37–41.
111. Giese T, Davidson WF. In CD8+ T cell-deficient lpr/lpr mice, CD4+B220+ and CD4+B220– T cells replace B220+ double-negative T cells as the predominant populations in enlarged lymph nodes. *J Immunol* 1995;154:4986–4995.
112. Maldonado MA, Eisenberg RA, Roper E, et al. Greatly reduced lymphoproliferation in lpr mice lacking major histocompatibility complex class I. *J Exp Med* 1995;181:641–648.
113. Koh DR, Ho A, Rahemtulla A, et al. Murine lupus in MRL/lpr mice lacking CD4 or CD8 T cells. *Eur J Immunol* 1995;25: 2558–2562.
114. Watanabe D, Suda T, Hashimoto H, et al. Constitutive activation of the Fas ligand gene in mouse lymphoproliferative disorders. *EMBO J* 1995;14:12–18.
115. Mimura T, Minota S, Nojima Y, et al. Constitutive tyrosine phosphorylation of the vav proto-oncogene product in MRL/Mp-lpr/lpr mice. *J Immunol* 1997;158:2977–2983.
116. Chu JL, Ramos P, Rosendorff A, et al. Massive upregulation of the Fas ligand in lpr and gld mice: implications for Fas regulation and the graft-versus-host disease-like wasting syndrome. *J Exp Med* 1995;181:393–398.
117. Theofilopoulos AN, Balderas RS, Gozes Y, et al. Association of the lpr gene with a graft-versus-host-like disease. *J Exp Med* 1985;162:1–18.
118. Via CS, Nguyen P, Shustov A, et al. A major role for the Fas pathway in acute graft-versus-host disease. *J Immunol* 1996; 157:5387–5393.
119. Wu J, Zhou T, Zhang J, et al. Correction of accelerated autoimmune disease by early replacement of the mutated lpr gene with the normal Fas apoptosis gene in the T cells of transgenic MRL-lpr/lpr mice. *Proc Natl Acad Sci USA* 1994;91:2344–2348.
120. Zhou T, Edwards CK, Mountz JD. Prevention of age-related T cell apoptosis defect in CD2–fas– transgenic mice. *J Exp Med* 1995;182:129–137.

121. Fukuyama H, Adachi M, Suematsu S, et al. Transgenic expression of Fas in T cells blocks lymphoproliferation but not autoimmune disease in MRL-lpr mice. *J Immunol* 1998;160: 3805–3811.
122. Sobel ES, Katagiri T, Katagiri K, et al. An intrinsic B cell defect is required for the production of autoantibodies in the lpr model of murine systemic autoimmunity. *J Exp Med* 1991; 173:1441–1449.
123. Reap EA, Leslie D, Abrahams M, et al. Apoptosis abnormalities of splenic lymphocytes in autoimmune lpr and gld mice. *J Immunol* 1995;154:936–943.
124. Rathmell JC, Goodnow CC. Effects of the lpr mutation on elimination and inactivation of self-reactive B cells. *J Immunol* 1994;153:2831–2842.
125. Rathmell JC, Townsend SE, Xu JC, et al. Expansion or elimination of B cells in vivo: dual roles for CD40– and Fas (CD95)-ligands modulated by the B cell antigen receptor. *Cell* 1996; 87:319–329.
126. Rathmell JC, Cooke MP, Ho WY, et al. CD95 (Fas)-dependent elimination of self-reactive B cells upon interaction with CD4+ T cells. *Nature* 1995;376:181–183.
127. Mandik-Nayak L, Seo SJ, Sokol C, et al. MRL-lpr/lpr mice exhibit a defect in maintaining developmental arrest and follicular exclusion of anti-double-stranded DNA B cells. *J Exp Med* 1999;189:1799–814.
128. Jacobson BA, Panka DJ, Nguyen KA, et al. Anatomy of autoantibody production: dominant localization of antibody-producing cells to T cell zones in Fas-deficient mice. *Immunity* 1995; 3:509–519.
129. Rothstein TL, Wang JK, Panka DJ, et al. Protection against Fas-dependent Th1-mediated apoptosis by antigen receptor engagement in B cells. *Nature* 1995;374:163–165.
130. Green MC, Shultz LD. Motheaten, an immunodeficient mutant of the mouse. *J Hered* 1975;66:250–258.
131. Bignon JS, Siminovitch KA. Identification of PTP1C mutation as the genetic defect in motheaten and viable motheaten mice: a step toward defining the roles of protein tyrosine phosphatases in the regulation of hemopoietic cell differentiation and function. *Clin Immunol Immunopathol* 1994;73: 168–179.
132. Shultz LD, Schweitzer PA, Rajan TV, et al. Mutations at the murine motheaten locus are within the hematopoietic cell protein-tyrosine phosphatase (Hcph) gene. *Cell* 1993;73:1445–1454.
133. Tsui HW, Siminovitch KA, deSouza L, et al. Motheaten and *viable motheaten* mice have mutations in the haematopoietic cell phosphatase gene. *Nat Genet* 1993;4:124–129.
134. Kozlowski M, Mlinaric RI, Feng GH, et al. Expression and catalytic activity of the tyrosine phosphatase PTP1C is severely impaired in motheaten and viable motheaten mice. *J Exp Med* 1993;178:2157–2163.
135. Thomas ML. Of ITAMs and ITIMs:turning on and off the B cell antigen receptor. *J Exp Med* 1995;181:1953–1956.
136. Van Zant G, Shultz LD. Hematologic abnormalities of the immunodeficient mouse mutant, viable motheaten (*me*^{v}). *Exp Hematol* 1989;17:81–87.
137. Scribner CL, Hansen CT, Klinman DM, et al. The interaction of the xid and me genes. *J Immunol* 1987;138:3611–3617.
138. Yu CC, Tsui HW, Ngan BY, et al. B and T cells are not required for the viable motheaten phenotype. *J Exp Med* 1996;183: 371–380.
139. Doody GM, Justement LB, Delibrias CC, et al. A role in B cell activation for CD22 and the protein tyrosine phosphatase SHP. *Science* 1995;269:242–244.
140. Murphy ED, Roths JB. A Y chromosome associated factor in strain BXSB producing accelerated autoimmunity and lymphoproliferation. *Arthritis Rheum* 1979;22:1188–1194.
141. Eisenberg RA, Izui S, McConahey PJ, et al. Male determined accelerated autoimmune disease in BXSB mice: transfer by bone marrow and spleen cells. *J Immunol* 1980;125:1032–1036.
142. Izui S, Iwamoto M, Fossati L, et al. The Yaa gene model of systemic lupus erythematosus. *Immunol Rev* 1995;144:137–156.
143. Hudgins CC, Steinberg RT, Klinman DM, et al. Studies of consomic mice bearing the Y chromosome of the BXSB mouse. *J Immunol* 1985;134:3849–3854.
144. Izui S, Higaki M, Morrow D, et al. The Y chromosome from autoimmune BXSB/MpJ mice induces a lupus-like syndrome in (NZW × C57BL/6)F1 male mice, but not in C57BL/6 male mice. *Eur J Immunol* 1988;18:911–915.
145. Merino R, Shibata T, de Kossodo S, et al. Differential effect of the autoimmune Yaa and lpr genes on the acceleration of lupus-like syndrome in MRL/MpJ mice. *Eur J Immunol* 1989;19: 2131–2137.
146. Suzuka H, Yoshifusa H, Nakamura Y, et al. Morphological analysis of autoimmune disease in MRL-lpr,Yaa male mice with rapidly progressive systemic lupus erythematosus. *Autoimmunity* 1993;14:275–282.
147. Jansson L, Holmdahl R. The Y chromosome-linked "autoimmune accelerating" yaa gene suppresses collagen-induced arthritis. *Eur J Immunol* 1994;24:1213–1217.
148. Merino R, Fossati L, Lacour M, et al. Selective autoantibody production by Yaa $^{+}$ B cells in autoimmune Yaa^{+}-Yaa^{-} bone marrow chimeric mice. *J Exp Med* 1991;174:1023–1029.
149. Fossati L, Iwamoto M, Merino R, et al. Selective enhancing effect of the Yaa gene on immune responses against self and foreign antigens. *Eur J Immunol* 1995;25:166–173.
150. DesJardin LE, Butfiloski EJ, Sobel ES, et al. Hyperproliferation of BXSB B cells is linked to the Yaa allele. *Clin Immunol Immunopathol* 1996;81:145–152.
151. Nishizumi H, Taniuchi I, Yamanashi Y, et al. Impaired proliferation of peripheral B cells and indication of autoimmune disease in lyn-deficient mice. *Immunity* 1995;3:549–560.
152. Hibbs ML, Tarlinton DM, Armes J, et al. Multiple defects in the immune system of *Lyn*-deficient mice, culminating in autoimmune disease. *Cell* 1995;83:301–311.
153. O'Keefe TL, Williams GT, Davies SL, et al. Hyperresponsive B cells in CD22-deficient mice. *Science* 1996;274:798–801.
154. Otipoby KL, Andersson KB, Draves KE, et al. CD22 regulates thymus-independent responses and the lifespan of B cells. *Nature* 1996;384:634–637.
155. Sato S, Miller AS, Inaoki M, et al. CD22 is both a positive and negative regulator of B lymphocyte antigen receptor signal transduction: altered signaling in CD22 deficient mice. *Immunity* 1996;5:551–562.
156. Cornall RJ, Cyster JG, Hibbs ML, et al. Polygenic autoimmune traits: Lyn, CD22, and SHP-1 are limiting elements of a biochemical pathway regulating BCR signaling and selection. *Immunity* 1998;8:497–508.
157. Tedder TF, Inaoki M, Sato S. The CD19-CD21 complex regulates signal transduction thresholds governing humoral immunity and autoimmunity. *Immunity* 1997;6:107–118.
158. Inaoki M, Sato S, Weintraub BC, et al. CD19-regulated signaling thresholds control peripheral tolerance and autoantibody production in B lymphocytes. *J Exp Med* 1997;186:1923–1931.
159. Coggeshall KM. Inhibitory signaling by B cell Fc gamma RIIb. *Curr Opin Immunol* 1998;10:306–312.
160. Ono M, Okada H, Bolland S, et al. Deletion of SHIP or SHP-1 reveals two distinct pathways for inhibitory signaling. *Cell* 1997;90:293–301.
161. Nadler MJS, Chen B, Anderson JS, et al. Protein-tyrosine phosphatase SHP-1 is dispensable for Fc gammaRIIB-mediated inhibition of B cell antigen receptor activation. *J Biol Chem* 1997;272:20038–20043.

162. Takai T, Ono M, Hikida M, et al. Augmented humoral and anaphylactic responses in FcgRII-deficient mice. *Nature* 1996; 379:346–349.
163. Bolland S, Ravetch JV. Spontaneous autoimmune disease in Fc(gamma)RIIB-deficient mice results from strain-specific epistasis. *Immunity* 2000;13:277–285.
164. Yuasa T, Kubo S, Yoshino T, et al. Deletion of fc gamma receptor IIB renders H-2(b) mice susceptible to collagen-induced arthritis. *J Exp Med* 1999;189:187–194.
165. Nakamura A, Yuasa T, Ujike A, et al. Fcg Receptor IIB-deficient mice develop Goodpasture's Syndrome upon immunization with type IV collagen: a novel murine model for autoimmune glomerular basement membrane disease. *J Exp Med* 2000;191: 899–906.
166. Morgan B, Sun L, Avitahl N, et al. Aiolos, a lymphoid restricted transcription factor that interacts with Ikaros to regulate lymphocyte differentiation. *EMBO J* 1997;16:2004–2013.
167. Xue Y, Wong J, Moreno GT, et al. NURD, a novel complex with both ATP-dependent chromatin-remodeling and histone deacetylase activities. *Mol Cell* 1998;2:851–861.
168. Zhang Y, Ng HH, Erdjument-Bromage H, et al. Analysis of the NuRD subunits reveals a histone deacetylase core complex and a connection with DNA methylation. *Genes Dev* 1999;13: 1924–1935.
169. Knoepfler PS, Eisenman RN. Sin meets NuRD and other tails of repression. *Cell* 1999;99:447–450.
170. Koipally J, Renold A, Kim J, et al. Repression by Ikaros and Aiolos is mediated through histone deacetylase complexes. *EMBO J* 1999;18:3090–3100.
171. Wang JH, Avitahl N, Cariappa A, et al. Aiolos regulates B cell activation and maturation to effector state. *Immunity* 1998;9: 543–553.
172. Moore PA, Belvedere O, Orr A, et al. BLyS: member of the tumor necrosis factor family and B lymphocyte stimulator. *Science* 1999;285:260–263.
173. Schneider P, MacKay F, Steiner V, et al. BAFF, a novel ligand of the tumor necrosis factor family, stimulates B cell growth. *J Exp Med* 1999;189:1747–1756.
174. Shu HB, Hu WH, Johnson H. TALL-1 is a novel member of the TNF family that is down-regulated by mitogens. *J Leukoc Biol* 1999;65:680–683.
175. Mukhopadhyay A, Ni J, Zhai Y, et al. Identification and characterization of a novel cytokine, THANK, a TNF homologue that activates apoptosis, nuclear factor-kappaB, and c-Jun NH2-terminal kinase. *J Biol Chem* 1999;274:15978–15981.
176. Gross JA, Johnston J, Mudri S, et al. TACI and BCMA are receptors for a TNF homologue implicated in B-cell autoimmune disease. *Nature* 2000;404:995–999.
177. Batten M, Groom J, Cachero TG, et al. BAFF mediates survival of peripheral immature B lymphocytes. *J Exp Med* 2000;192: 1453–1466.
178. Thompson JS, Schneider P, Kalled SL, et al. BAFF binds to the tumor necrosis factor receptor-like molecule B cell maturation antigen and is important for maintaining the peripheral B cell population. *J Exp Med* 2000;192:129–135.
179. Mackay F, Woodcock SA, Lawton P, et al. Mice transgenic for BAFF develop lymphocytic disorders along with autoimmune manifestations. *J Exp Med* 1999;190:1697–1710.
180. Khare SD, Sarosi I, Xia XZ, et al. Severe B cell hyperplasia and autoimmune disease in TALL-1 transgenic mice. *Proc Natl Acad Sci USA* 2000;97:3370–3375.
181. Waterhouse P, Penninger JM, Timms E, et al. Lymphoproliferative disorders with early lethality in mice deficient in Ctla-4. *Science* 1995;270:985–988.
182. Tivol EA, Borriello F, Schweitzer AN, et al. Loss of CTLA-4 leads to massive lymphoproliferation and fatal multiorgan tissue destruction, revealing a critical negative regulatory role of CTLA-4. *Immunity* 1995;3:541–547.
183. Tivol EA, Boyd SD, McKeon S, et al. CTLA4Ig prevents lymphoproliferation and fatal multiorgan tissue destruction in CTLA-4–deficient mice. *J Immunol* 1997;158:5091–5094.
184. Chambers CA, Cado D, Truong T, et al. Thymocyte development is normal in CTLA-4–deficient mice. *Proc Natl Acad Sci USA* 1997;94:9296–9301.
185. Chambers CA, Sullivan TJ, Allison JP. Lymphoproliferation in CTLA-4–deficient mice is mediated by costimulation-dependent activation of CD4+ T cells. *Immunity* 1997;7:885–895.
186. Chambers CA, Kuhns MS, Allison JP. Cytotoxic T lymphocyte antigen-4 (CTLA-4) regulates primary and secondary peptide-specific CD4(+) T cell responses. *Proc Natl Acad Sci USA* 1999; 96:8603–8608.
187. Bachmann MF, Kohler G, Ecabert B, et al. Cutting edge: lymphoproliferative disease in the absence of CTLA-4 is not T cell autonomous. *J Immunol* 1999;163:1128–1131.
188. Schorle H, Holtschke T, Hunig T, et al. Development and function of T cells in mice rendered interleukin-2 deficient by gene targeting. *Nature* 1991;352:621–624.
189. Kundig TM, Schorle H, Bachmann MF, et al. Immune responses in interleukin-2–deficient mice. *Science* 1993;262: 1059–1061.
190. Sadlack B, Lohler J, Schorle H, et al. Generalized autoimmune disease in interleukin-2–deficient mice is triggered by an uncontrolled activation and proliferation of CD4+ T cells. *Eur J Immunol* 1995;25:3053–3059.
191. Willerford DM, Chen J, Ferry JA, et al. Interleukin-2 receptor alpha chain regulates the size and content of the peripheral lymphoid compartment. *Immunity* 1995;3:521–530.
192. Suzuki H, Kundig TM, Furlonger C, et al. Deregulated T cell activation and autoimmunity in mice lacking interleukin-2 receptor. *Science* 1995;268:1472–1476.
193. Sadlack B, Merz H, Schorle H, et al. Ulcerative colitis-like disease in mice with a disrupted interleukin-2 gene. *Cell* 1993;75: 253–261.
194. Van Parijs L, Biuckians A, Ibragimov A, et al. Functional responses and apoptosis of CD25 (IL-2R alpha)-deficient T cells expressing a transgenic antigen receptor. *J Immunol* 1997; 158:3738–3745.
195. Contractor NV, Bassiri H, Reya T, et al. Lymphoid hyperplasia, autoimmunity, and compromised intestinal intraepithelial lymphocyte development in colitis-free gnotobiotic IL-2–deficient mice. *J Immunol* 1998;160:385–394.
196. Ishida Y, Agata Y, Shibahara K, et al. Induced expression of PD-1, a novel member of the immunoglobulin gene superfamily, upon programmed cell death. *EMBO J* 1992;11:3887–3895.
197. Freeman GJ, Long AJ, Iwai Y, et al. Engagement of the PD-1 immunoinhibitory receptor by a novel B7 family member leads to negative regulation of lymphocyte activation. *J Exp Med* 2000;192:1027–1034.
198. Nishimura H, Minato N, Nakano T, et al. Immunological studies on PD-1 deficient mice: implication of PD-1 as a negative regulator for B cell responses. *Int Immunol* 1998;10: 1563–1572.
199. Nishimura H, Nose M, Hiai H, et al. Development of lupus-like autoimmune diseases by disruption of the PD-1 gene encoding an ITIM motif-carrying immunoreceptor. *Immunity* 1999;11:141–151.
200. Desai DM, Sap J, Schlessinger J, et al. Ligand-mediated negative regulation of a chimeric transmembrane receptor tyrosine phosphatase. *Cell* 1993;73:541–554.
201. Bilwes AM, den Hertog J, Hunter T, et al. Structural basis for inhibition of receptor protein-tyrosine phosphatase-alpha by dimerization. *Nature* 1996;382:555–559.

202. Majeti R, Xu Z, Parslow TG, et al. An inactivating point mutation in the inhibitory wedge of CD45 causes lymphoproliferation and autoimmunity. *Cell* 2000;103:1059–1070.
203. Shull MM, Ormsby I, Kier AB, et al. Targeted disruption of the mouse transforming growth factor-β1 gene results in multifocal inflammatory disease. *Nature* 1992;359:693–699.
204. Kulkarni AB, Karlsson S. Transforming growth factor-beta 1 knockout mice. A mutation in one cytokine gene causes a dramatic inflammatory disease. *Am J Pathol* 1993;143:3–9.
205. Dang H, Geiser AG, Letterio JJ, et al. SLE-like autoantibodies and Sjögren's syndrome-like lymphoproliferation in TGF-β knockout mice. *J Immunol* 1995;155:3205–3212.
206. Letterio JJ, Geiser AG, Kulkarni AB, et al. Autoimmunity associated with TGF-beta1–deficiency in mice is dependent on MHC class II antigen expression. *J Clin Invest* 1996;98:2109–2119.
207. Kobayashi S, Yoshida K, Ward JM, et al. Beta 2-microglobulin-deficient background ameliorates lethal phenotype of the TGF-beta 1 null mouse. *J Immunol* 1999;163:4013–4019.
208. Gorelik L, Flavell RA. Abrogation of TGFbeta signaling in T cells leads to spontaneous T cell differentiation and autoimmune disease. *Immunity* 2000;12:171–181.
209. O'Connor L, Strasser A, O'Reilly LA, et al. Bim: a novel member of the Bcl-2 family that promotes apoptosis. *EMBO J* 1998; 17:384–395.
210. Puthalakath H, Huang DC, O'Reilly LA, et al. The proapoptotic activity of the Bcl-2 family member Bim is regulated by interaction with the dynein motor complex. *Mol Cell* 1999;3: 287–296.
211. Bouillet P, Metcalf D, Huang DC, et al. Proapoptotic Bcl-2 relative Bim required for certain apoptotic responses, leukocyte homeostasis, and to preclude autoimmunity. *Science* 1999;286: 1735–1738.
212. Strasser A, Whittingham S, Vaux DL, et al. Enforced bcl-2 expression in B-lymphoid cells prolongs antibody responses and elicits autoimmune disease. *Proc Natl Acad Sci USA* 1991;88: 8661–8665.
213. Ray SK, Putterman C, Diamond B. Pathogenic autoantibodies are routinely generated during the response to foreign antigen: a paradigm for autoimmune disease. *Proc Natl Acad Sci USA* 1996;93:2019–2024.
214. Kuo P, Bynoe M, Diamond B. Crossreactive B cells are present during a primary but not secondary response in BALB/c mice expressing a bcl-2 transgene. *Mol Immunol* 1999;36:471–479.
215. Mandik-Nayak L, Nayak S, Sokol C, et al. The origin of antinuclear antibodies in bcl-2 transgenic mice. *Int Immunol* 2000; 12:353–364.
216. Irmler M, Thome M, Hahne M, et al. Inhibition of death receptor signals by cellular FLIP. *Nature* 1997;388:190–195.
217. Tschopp J, Irmler M, Thome M. Inhibition of fas death signals by FLIPs. *Curr Opin Immunol* 1998;10:552–558.
218. Van Parijs L, Refaeli Y, Abbas AK, et al. Autoimmunity as a consequence of retrovirus-mediated expression of C-FLIP in lymphocytes. *Immunity* 1999;11:763–770.
219. Botto M, Dell'Agnola C, Bygrave AE, et al. Homozygous C1q deficiency causes glomerulonephritis associated with multiple apoptotic bodies. *Nat Genet* 1998;19:56–59.
220. Prodeus AP, Goerg S, Shen LM, et al. A critical role for complement in maintenance of self-tolerance. *Immunity* 1998;9: 721–731.
221. Chen Z, Koralov SB, Kelsoe G. Complement C4 inhibits systemic autoimmunity through a mechanism independent of complement receptors CR1 and CR2. *J Exp Med* 2000;192: 1339–1352.
222. Bickerstaff MC, Botto M, Hutchinson WL, et al. Serum amyloid P component controls chromatin degradation and prevents antinuclear autoimmunity. *Nat Med* 1999;5:694–697.
223. Paul E, Carroll MC. SAP-less chromatin triggers systemic lupus erythematosus. *Nat Med* 1999;5:607–608.
224. Seery JP, Carroll JM, Cattell V, et al. Antinuclear autoantibodies and lupus nephritis in transgenic mice expressing interferon gamma in the epidermis. *J Exp Med* 1997;186:1451–1459.
225. Erb KJ, Ruger B, von Brevern M, et al. Constitutive expression of interleukin (IL)-4 in vivo causes autoimmune-type disorders in mice. *J Exp Med* 1997;185:329–339.
226. Muller W, Kuhn R, Rajewsky K. Major histocompatibility complex class II hyperexpression on B cells in interleukin 4–transgenic mice does not lead to B cell proliferation and hypergammaglobulinemia. *Eur J Immunol* 1991;21:921–925.
227. Burstein HJ, Tepper RI, Leder P, et al. Humoral immune functions in IL-4 transgenic mice. *J Immunol* 1991;147:2950–2956.
228. Tepper RI, Levinson DA, Stanger BZ, et al. IL-4 induces allergic-like inflammatory disease and alters T cell development in transgenic mice. *Cell* 1990;62:457–467.
229. Lewis DB, Yu CC, Forbush KA, et al. Interleukin 4 expressed in situ selectively alters thymocyte development. *J Exp Med* 1991;173:89–100.
230. Santiago M, Fossati L, Jacquiet C, et al. Interleukin-4 protects against a genetically linked lupus-like autoimmune syndrome. *J Exp Med* 1997;185:65–70.
231. Worthington MT, Amann BT, Nathans D, et al. Metal binding properties and secondary structure of the zinc-binding domain of Nup475. *Proc Natl Acad Sci USA* 1996;93:13754–13759.
232. Taylor GA, Carballo E, Lee DM, et al. A pathogenetic role for TNF alpha in the syndrome of cachexia, arthritis, and autoimmunity resulting from tristetraprolin (TTP) deficiency. *Immunity* 1996;4:445–454.
233. Carballo E, Gilkeson GS, Blackshear PJ. Bone marrow transplantation reproduces the tristetraprolin-deficiency syndrome in recombination activating gene-2 (–/–) mice. Evidence that monocyte/macrophage progenitors may be responsible for TNFalpha overproduction. *J Clin Invest* 1997;100:986–995.
234. Carballo E, Lai WS, Blackshear PJ. Feedback inhibition of macrophage tumor necrosis factor-alpha production by tristetraprolin. *Science* 1998;281:1001–1005.
235. Rothe J, Lesslauer W, Lotscher H, et al. Mice lacking the tumour necrosis factor receptor 1 are resistant to TNF-mediated toxicity but highly susceptible to infection by *Listeria monocytogenes. Nature* 1993;364:798–802.
236. Pfeffer K, Matsuyama T, Kundig TM, et al. Mice deficient for the 55 kd tumor necrosis factor receptor are resistant to endotoxic shock, yet succumb to *L. monocytogenes* infection. *Cell* 1993;73:457–467.
237. Lupher ML, Jr., Rao N, Eck MJ, et al. The Cbl protooncoprotein: a negative regulator of immune receptor signal transduction. *Immunol Today* 1999;20:375–382.
238. Keane MM, Rivero-Lezcano OM, Mitchell JA, et al. Cloning and characterization of cbl-b: a SH3 binding protein with homology to the c-cbl proto-oncogene. *Oncogene* 1995;10: 2367–2377.
239. Keane MM, Ettenberg SA, Nau MM, et al. cbl-3: a new mammalian cbl family protein. *Oncogene* 1999;18:3365–3375.
240. Kim M, Tezuka T, Suziki Y, et al. Molecular cloning and characterization of a novel cbl-family gene, cbl-c. *Gene* 1999;239: 145–154.
241. Krawczyk C, Bachmaier K, Sasaki T, et al. Cbl-b is a negative regulator of receptor clustering and raft aggregation in T cells. *Immunity* 2000;13:463–473.
242. Chiang YJ, Kole HK, Brown K, et al. Cbl-b regulates the CD28 dependence of T-cell activation. *Nature* 2000;403:216–220.
243. Bachmaier K, Krawczyk C, Kozieradzki I, et al. Negative regulation of lymphocyte activation and autoimmunity by the molecular adaptor Cbl-b. *Nature* 2000;403:211–216.

244. Bustelo XR, Crespo P, Lopez-Barahona M, et al. Cbl-b, a member of the Sli-1/c-Cbl protein family, inhibits Vav-mediated c-Jun N-terminal kinase activation. *Oncogene* 1997;15:2511–2520.
245. Cantley LC, Neel BG. New insights into tumor suppression: PTEN suppresses tumor formation by restraining the phosphoinositide 3–kinase/AKT pathway. *Proc Natl Acad Sci USA* 1999; 96:4240–4245.
246. Di Cristofano A, Pandolfi PP. The multiple roles of PTEN in tumor suppression. *Cell* 2000;100:387–390.
247. Di Cristofano A, Kotsi P, Peng YF, et al. Impaired Fas response and autoimmunity in Pten+/– mice. *Science* 1999;285:2122–2125.
248. Maehama T, Dixon JE. The tumor suppressor, PTEN/MMAC1, dephosphorylates the lipid second messenger, phosphatidylinositol 3,4,5–trisphosphate. *J Biol Chem* 1998;273:13375–13378.
249. Zhang L, Eddy A, Teng YT, et al. An immunological renal disease in transgenic mice that overexpress Fli-1, a member of the ets family of transcription factor genes. *Mol Cell Biol* 1995; 15:6961–6970.
250. Balomenos D, Martin-Caballero J, Garcia MI, et al. The cell cycle inhibitor p21 controls T-cell proliferation and sex-linked lupus development. *Nat Med* 2000;6:171–176.
251. Sabzevari H, Propp S, Kono DH, et al. G1 arrest and high expression of cyclin kinase and apoptosis inhibitors in accumulated activated/memory phenotype CD4+ cells of older lupus mice. *Eur J Immunol* 1997;27:1901–1910.
252. Napirei M, Karsunky H, Zevnik B, et al. Features of systemic lupus erythematosus in Dnase1-deficient mice. *Nat Genet* 2000; 25:177–181.
253. Darvasi A. Experimental strategies for the genetic dissection of complex traits in animal models. *Nat Genet* 1998;18:19–24.
254. Kono DH, Burlingame RW, Owens DG, et al. Lupus susceptibility loci in New Zealand mice. *Proc Natl Acad Sci USA* 1994; 91:10168–10172.
255. Vyse TJ, Kotzin BL. Genetic susceptibility to systemic lupus erythematosus. *Annu Rev Immunol* 1998;16:261–292.
256. Morel L, Wakeland EK. Susceptibility to lupus nephritis in the NZB/W model system. *Curr Opin Immunol* 1998;10:718–725.
257. Vyse TJ, Morel L, Tanner FJ, et al. Backcross analysis of genes linked to autoantibody production in New Zealand White mice. *J Immunol* 1996;157:2719–2727.
258. Morel L, Mohan C, Yu Y, et al. Functional dissection of systemic lupus erythematosus using congenic mouse strains. *J Immunol* 1997;158:6019–6028.
259. Morel L, Yu Y, Blenman KR, et al. Production of congenic mouse strains carrying genomic intervals containing SLE-susceptibility genes derived from the SLE-prone NZM2410 strain. *Mamm Genome* 1996;7:335–339.
260. Mohan C, Alas E, Morel L, et al. Genetic dissection of SLE pathogenesis. Sle1 on murine chromosome 1 leads to a selective loss of tolerance to H2A/H2B/DNA subnucleosomes. *J Clin Invest* 1998;101:1362–1372.
261. Sobel ES, Mohan C, Morel L, et al. Genetic dissection of SLE pathogenesis: adoptive transfer of Sle1 mediates the loss of tolerance by bone marrow-derived B cells. *J Immunol* 1999;162: 2415–2421.
262. Mohan C, Morel L, Yang P, et al. Genetic dissection of systemic lupus erythematosus pathogenesis: Sle2 on murine chromosome 4 leads to B cell hyperactivity. *J Immunol* 1997;159: 454–465.
263. Mohan C, Morel L, Yang P, et al. Accumulation of splenic B1a cells with potent antigen-presenting capability in NZM2410 lupus-prone mice. *Arthritis Rheum* 1998;41:1652–1662.
264. Mohan C, Yu Y, Morel L, et al. Genetic dissection of Sle pathogenesis: Sle3 on murine chromosome 7 impacts T cell activation, differentiation, and cell death. *J Immunol* 1999;162: 6492–6502.
265. Mohan C, Morel L, Yang P, et al. Genetic dissection of lupus pathogenesis: a recipe for nephrophilic autoantibodies. *J Clin Invest* 1999;103:1685–1695.
266. Morel L, Mohan C, Yu Y, et al. Multiplex inheritance of component phenotypes in a murine model of lupus. *Mamm Genome* 1999;10:176–181.
267. Vidal S, Kono DH, Theofilopoulos AN. Loci predisposing to autoimmunity in MRL- *Fas*^{lpr} and C57BL/6-Fas^{lpr} mice. *J Clin Invest* 1998;101:696–702.
268. Wang Y, Nose M, Kamoto T, et al. Host modifier genes affect mouse autoimmunity induced by the lpr gene. *Am J Pathol* 1997;151:1791–1798.
269. Watson ML, Rao JK, Gilkeson GS, et al. Genetic analysis of MRL-lpr mice: relationship of the Fas apoptosis gene to disease manifestations and renal disease-modifying loci. *J Exp Med* 1992;176:1645–1656.
270. Nishihara M, Terada M, Kamogawa J, et al. Genetic basis of autoimmune sialadenitis in MRL/lpr lupus-prone mice: additive and hierarchical properties of polygenic inheritance. *Arthritis Rheum* 1999;42:2616–2623.
271. Izui S, Merino R, Fossati L, et al. The role of the Yaa gene in lupus syndrome. *Intern Rev Immunol* 1994;11:211–230.
272. Hogarth MB, Slingsby JH, Allen PJ, et al. Multiple lupus susceptibility loci map to chromosome 1 in BXSB mice. *J Immunol* 1998;161:2753–2761.
273. Haywood ME, Hogarth MB, Slingsby JH, et al. Identification of intervals on chromosomes 1, 3, and 13 linked to the development of lupus in BXSB mice. *Arthritis Rheum* 2000;43:349–355.
274. Ida A, Hirose S, Hamano Y, et al. Multigenic control of lupus-associated antiphospholipid syndrome in a model of (NZW × BXSB) F1 mice. *Eur J Immunol* 1998;28:2694–2703.
275. Rudofsky UH, Evans BD, Balaban SL, et al. Differences in expression of lupus nephritis in New Zealand mixed H-2z homozygous inbred strains of mice derived from New Zealand black and New Zealand white mice. Origins and initial characterization. *Lab Invest* 1993;68:419–426.
276. Kinjoh K, Kyogoku M, Good RA. Genetic selection for crescent formation yields mouse strain with rapidly progressive glomerulonephritis and small vessel vasculitis. *Proc Natl Acad Sci USA* 1993;90:3413–3417.
277. Vidal S, Gelpi C, Rodriguez-Sanchez JL. (SWR x SJL)F1 mice: a new model of lupus-like disease. *J Exp Med* 1994;179:1429–1435.
278. Walker SE, Gray RH, Fulton M, et al. Palmerston North mice, a new animal model of systemic lupus erythematosus. *J Lab Clin Med* 1978;92:932–45.
279. Rubin RL. Etiology and mechanisms of drug-induced lupus. *Curr Opin Rheumatol* 1999;11:357–363.
280. Satoh M, Kumar A, Kanwar YS, et al. Anti-nuclear antibody production and immune-complex glomerulonephritis in BALB/c mice treated with pristane. *Proc Natl Acad Sci USA* 1995;92:10934–10938.
281. Mendlovic S, Fricke BH, Shoenfeld Y, et al. The genetic regulation of the induction of experimental SLE. *Immunology* 1990; 69:228–236.
282. Walport MJ, Davies KA, Botto M. C1q and systemic lupus erythematosus. *Immunobiology* 1998;199:265–285.
283. O'Keefe TL, Williams GT, Batista FD, et al. Deficiency in CD22, a B cell-specific inhibitory receptor, is sufficient to predispose to development of high affinity autoantibodies. *J Exp Med* 1999;189:1307–1313.
284. Lai WS, Carballo E, Strum JR, et al. Evidence that tristetraprolin binds to AU-rich elements and promotes the deadenylation and destabilization of tumor necrosis factor alpha mRNA. *Mol Cell Biol* 1999;19:4311–4323.
285. Vyse TJ, Rozzo SJ, Drake CG, et al. Control of multiple autoantibodies linked with a lupus nephritis susceptibility

locus in New Zealand black mice. *J Immunol* 1997; 158:5566–5574.

286. Rozzo SJ, Vyse TJ, Drake CG, et al. Effect of genetic background on the contribution of New Zealand black loci to autoimmune lupus nephritis. *Proc Natl Acad Sci USA* 1996; 93:15164–15168.
287. Qu W, Miyazaki T, Terada M, et al. Genetic dissection of vasculitis in MRL/lpr lupus mice: a novel susceptibility locus involving the $CD72^c$ allele. *Eur J Immunol* 2000;30: 2027–2037.
288. Ochiai K, Ozaki S, Tanino A, et al. Genetic regulation of anti-erythrocyte autoantibodies and splenomegaly in autoimmune hemolytic anemia-prone New Zealand black mice. *Int Immunol* 2000;12:1–8.
289. Drake CG, Babcock SK, Palmer E, et al. Genetic analysis of the NZB contribution to lupus-like autoimmune disease in (NZB × NZW)F1 mice. *Proc Natl Acad Sci USA* 1994;91:4062–4066.
290. Hirose S, Tsurui H, Nishimura H, et al. Mapping of a gene for hypergammaglobulinemia to the distal region on chromosome 4 in NZB mice and its contribution to systemic lupus erythematosus in (NZB × NZW)F1 mice. *Int Immunol* 1994;6: 1857–1864.
291. Jiang Y, Hirose S, Hamano Y, et al. Mapping of a gene for the increased susceptibility of B1 cells to Mott cell formation in murine autoimmune disease. *J Immunol* 1997;158:992–997.
292. Santiago ML, Mary C, Parzy D, et al. Linkage of a major quantitative trait locus to Yaa gene-induced lupus- like nephritis in (NZW × C57BL/6)F1 mice. *Eur J Immunol* 1998;28:4257–4267.
293. Vyse TJ, Drake CG, Rozzo SJ, et al. Genetic linkage of IgG autoantibody production in relation to lupus nephritis in New Zealand hybrid mice. *J Clin Invest* 1996;98:1762–1772.

8

APOPTOSIS

KEITH B. ELKON

MORPHOLOGY AND TISSUE RESPONSE

Necrosis is the familiar form of cell death that rapidly occurs following the exposure of cells to ischemic or toxic insults. During necrosis, the cell membrane becomes permeable, resulting in irreversible swelling and rupture of the cell (Fig. 8.1). The cellular nucleic acids and proteins are released into the tissues, usually resulting in inflammation at the site. Apoptosis is the form of cell death seen during normal physiologic processes, such as embryogenesis and metamorphosis, as well as in certain pathologic situations, such as cancers. The term was first applied to the morphologic appearance of these cells as depicted by electron microscopy (1). In contrast to necrotic cells, apoptotic cells are shrunken, have condensed nuclei, and undergo dissolution by blebbing (Fig. 8.1). The resulting apoptotic bodies are phagocytosed by surrounding cells and rapidly degraded in lysozymes.

An important difference between programmed (i.e., apoptotic) and accidental/toxic (i.e., necrotic) death is that programmed cell death results in the ordered fragmentation of the cell. Because apoptosis occurs through complex biochemical pathways, death of the cell is slow (6 to 48 hours). *In vivo*, however, removal of apoptotic fragments is so rapid at sites of normal cell turnover that apoptotic cells are rarely seen. In these circumstances, phagocytosis of apoptotic bodies by neighboring cells and/or professional phagocytes does not cause activation of the engulfing cell; therefore, an inflammatory response does not ensue.

Although necrosis and apoptosis are described as entirely distinct, this is not necessarily the case. Many stimuli can induce either apoptosis or necrosis depending on the dose

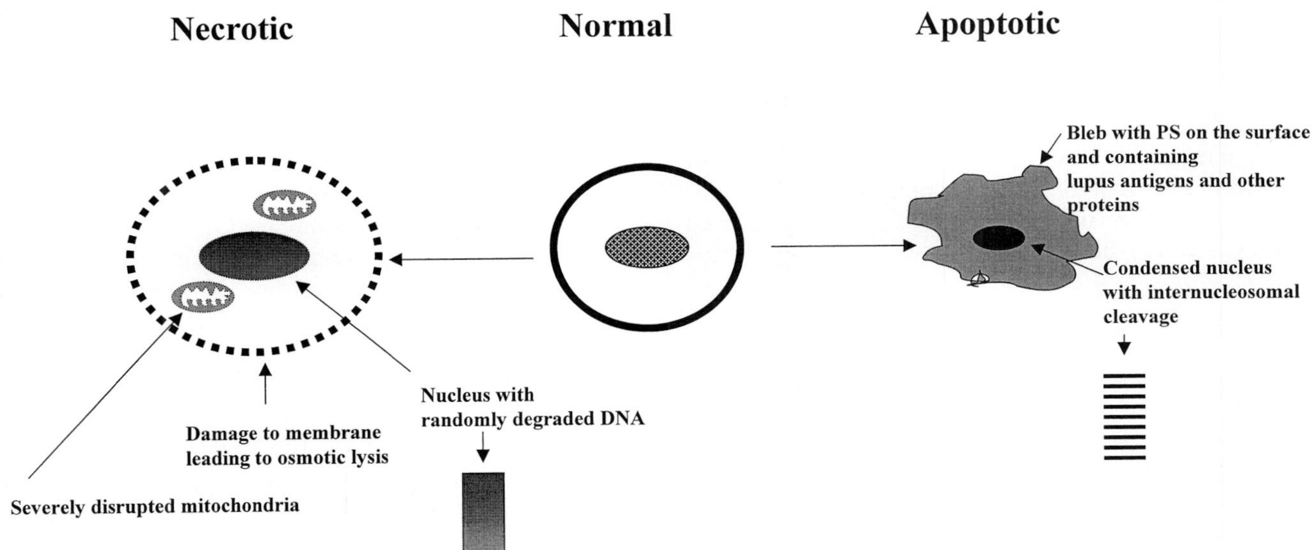

FIGURE 8.1. Morphology of cell death: schematic depiction of necrosis and apoptosis. The necrotic cells are swollen with severely disrupted cell surface and mitochondrial membranes. In contrast, apoptotic cells are shrunken, express blebs on the surface, and the DNA is cleaved into discrete nucleosomal fragments. The ordered appearance of these fragments as a "ladder" on agarose gels can clearly be distinguished from the "smear" of randomly degraded DNA that occurs during necrosis.

or duration of exposure (2,3). For example, cells immediately adjacent to an infarct are necrosed, whereas those further away show apoptotic changes. Also, apoptosis can be induced by pathogens, and in this case inflammation will ensue. For example, bacteria such as *Shigella flexneri* induce apoptosis of macrophages, which, through the activation of caspase-1 [interleukin-1 (IL-1) converting enzyme (ICE)], cause an inflammatory response (4).

THE BIOCHEMISTRY OF APOPTOSIS

Although the morphologic descriptions of apoptosis were reported more than 30 years ago (1), the complex biochemical pathways that are responsible for its regulation have only begun to be dissected over the last decade. Progress in the field has been so rapid that apoptotic pathways can only be summarized in this chapter, and readers are referred to two series of reviews in *Science* August 28, 1998, and *Nature* October 12, 2000, for additional details. Similarly, space limitations preclude most primary references but recent reviews on subtopics are indicated.

Understanding the basic biochemical pathways in mammalian cells has been considerably enhanced by genetic studies of apoptosis in the nematode *Caenorhabditis elegans* (5). Fourteen genes that regulate apoptosis during development of *C. elegans* were identified and named CED 1 to 14 (cell death abnormal). Ced-3 and Ced-4 are proteases that promote cell death, whereas Ced-9 is a protein that promotes cell survival. It is thought that most of the remaining Ced proteins are required for engulfment of apoptotic cells.

The cell death process can be divided into a number of stages (Fig. 8.2): inductive stimulus, signal transduction, activation of caspases (cysteine-containing proteases with a substrate specificity for peptidyl sequences with a P1 aspartate residue), activation of nuclease(s) with nuclear condensation, redistribution of the cellular contents into apoptotic bodies, and removal of the dying cells. Since the nature of the inductive stimulus dictates the initial biochemical pathways engaged, the "stress" and "death receptor" induced pathways are described separately.

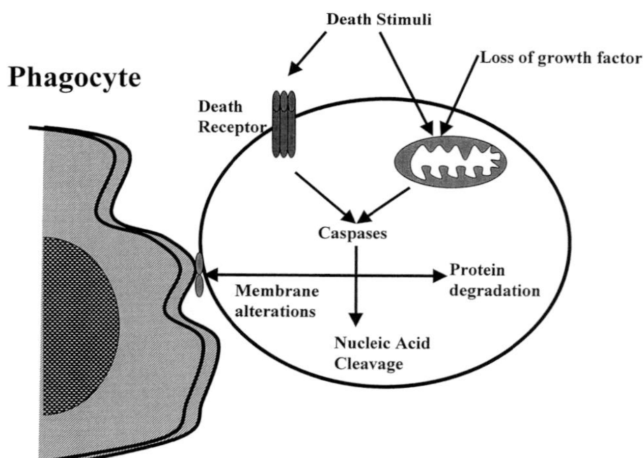

FIGURE 8.2. Outline of the main events in apoptosis. Death of the cells is either actively induced through a death receptor on the surface of the cell, through loss of growth factors, or through stress stimuli that induce apoptosis via the mitochondrial pathway. These events activate caspases, which in turn selectively cleave substrates (including other caspases). The major consequences of caspase cleavage are alterations to the cell surface membrane, disassembly of the cytoskeleton and nuclear membrane, and activation of nucleases. The apoptotic program is not complete until the corpses are removed by phagocytes that recognize signals on the apoptotic cells. Each of these events is described in more detail in the text and illustrated in subsequent figures.

Stress Induced Apoptosis

Exposure of cells to many chemical (e.g., corticosteroids, alkylating agents, topoisomerase inhibitors) or physical (ultraviolet light, gamma irradiation) insults induces damage to protein, DNA, and lipids that trigger repair and stress responses. In addition, cytokine withdrawal and intense signaling through the lymphocyte antigen receptor at certain stages of differentiation also trigger the intrinsic cell death pathway that is executed by the mitochondria. Mitochondria are cytoplasmic organelles that contain their own 16-kilobase (kb) genome encased by inner and outer membranes with cytochrome *c* lodged in between. Mitochondria help to maintain the redox potential and provide energy to the cell through the generation of adenosine triphosphate (ATP) by oxidative phosphorylation. These biochemical pathways create an electrochemical gradient ($\Delta\Psi$) that is positive and acidic on the outside and alkaline on the inner side of the mitochondrial membrane. Spanning the membranes, a protein permeability transition (PT) pore comprising the adenine nuclear translocator (ANT), the voltage dependent anion channel (VDAC), and cyclophillin D regulates mitochondrial membrane potential (6). In some cases, severe reduction in energy reserves may lead to disruption of the outer mitochondrial membrane (7).

Cell stresses converge on the mitochondria and result in the release of cytochrome *c* from the intermitochondrial space into the cytosol (Fig. 8.3A). In the cytosol, cytochrome *c*, together with the cofactors Apaf-1 and ATP or dATP, promotes the cleavage of pro-caspase 9 into its active form (8). Multimers containing these proteins and cofactors assemble to form the apoptosome (see below). Caspase 9 acts on effector caspases such as caspase 3, resulting in the caspase cascade that leads to the cleavage and inactivation of a wide variety of substrates within the cell. Cytochrome *c* is not the only proapoptotic protein released by the mitochondria. Recently a caspase-independent apoptosis-inducing factor (AIF) as well as a protein called smac/diablo have been characterized. As discussed below, Smac/diablo is absolutely required in some cell types for the

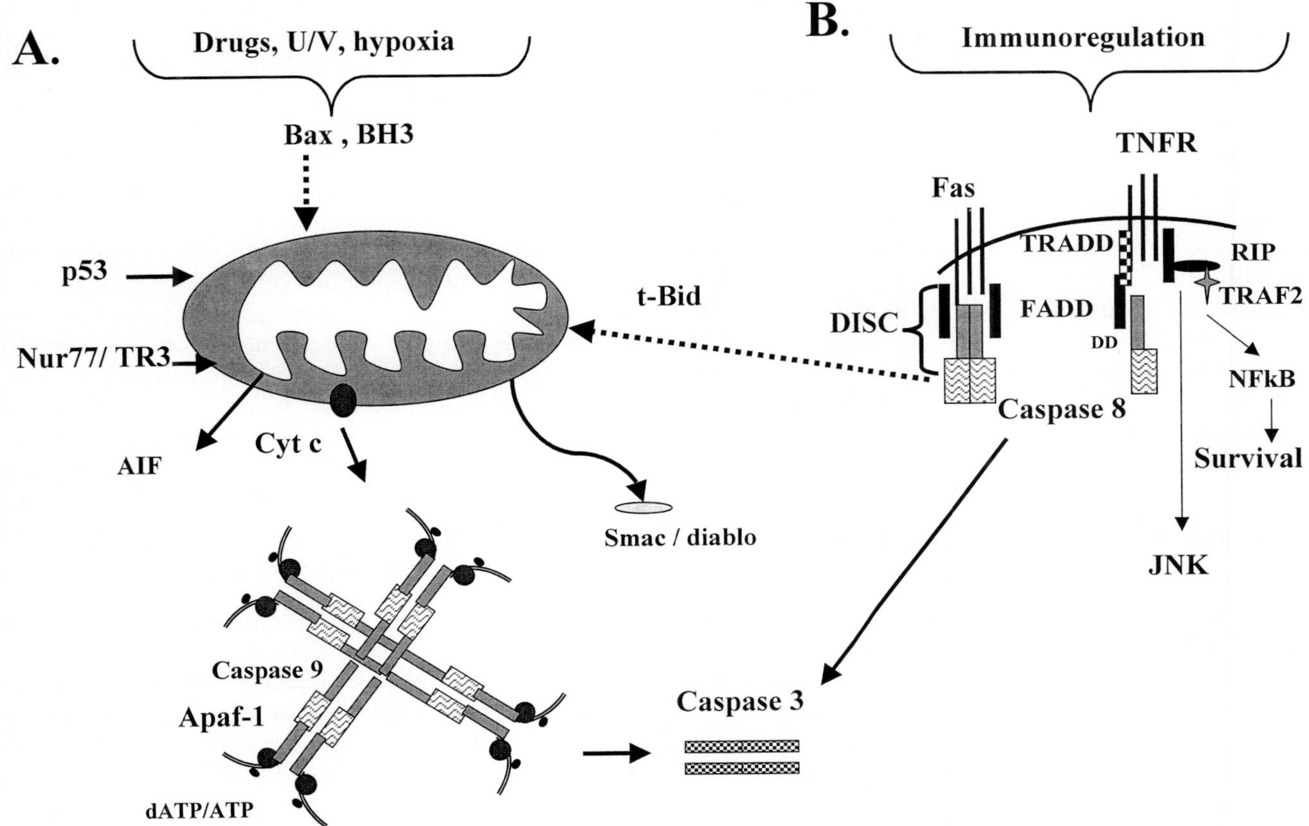

FIGURE 8.3. The biochemistry of apoptosis. **A:** Stress-induced apoptosis. Cells that are injured, for example by hypoxia, ultraviolet (UV) irradiation, or drugs, activate a variety of stress responses that impinge on the mitochondria. The net result is the release of proapoptotic factors that include cytochrome *c*, apoptosis-inducing factor (AIF), and smac/DIABLO. In the cytoplasm, cytochrome *c* and adenosine triphosphate (ATP) or dATP bind to Apaf-1, which in turn binds to caspase 9 to form a multiprotein complex called the apoptosome. Processing of caspase 9 into an active tetramer results in the cleavage of the effector caspase, caspase 3, which may also be found in the apoptosome. **B:** Death receptor–mediated apoptosis. Death receptors are preassembled as trimers on the surface of cells. When engaged by ligand, they are clustered and recruit the adapter molecules (FADD and TRADD for Fas and TNFR1, respectively). Binding of FADD to the Fas death domain (DD) leads to the recruitment and autocatalytic cleavage of caspase 8. The active caspase 8 tetramer cleaves pro-caspase 3, leading to the caspase cascade required for apoptosis. In some cell types, minimal activation of caspase 8 is sufficient to cleave the antiapoptotic Bcl-2 family member Bid. The truncated Bid protein (t-Bid) promotes the release of cytochrome *c* either by directly inserting into the membrane or by forming a complex with Bax. The TNFR1/TRADD complex can also recruit FADD and initiate apoptosis as for Fas. However, in most cells, TNFR causes cell activation and promotes survival, through recruitment of TRAF2, RIP (a kinase), and activation of NF-κB.

induction of apoptosis by inactivating the inhibitors of apoptosis (IAPs) that bind to caspase 3, thus releasing caspase 3 from inhibition.

How are stress responses linked to the mitochondria? There are many routes to death from within and much controversy regarding the sequence of events (9). A few pertinent examples will be given. During the deletion of thymocytes by high-affinity interaction with self antigen (negative selection), signaling through the Jun kinase (JNK, also known as stress activated protein kinase, SAPK) pathway leads to activation of the Nur 77 family of transcription factors (reviewed in ref. 10). Nur 77, also called TR3, has recently been shown translocate from the nucleus to the mitochondria and may directly induce the release of proapoptotic factors. Similarly, JNK activation has been implicated in many other forms of cellular stress (osmotic, redox, radiation) that induce the release of mitochondrial cytochrome *c*, although the precise pathways remain to be determined.

Genotoxic cell injury has dire consequences for the cell in terms of the potential for mutagenesis and neoplastic transformation. Cells have therefore evolved sophisticated DNA repair mechanisms as well as a default suicide pathway when damaged DNA cannot be repaired. This type of stress response is orchestrated by the p53 family of proteins (reviewed in ref. 11). P53 is a transcription factor that upregulates the expression of p21 (Cip1/waf1) which, in turn, induces a cell cycle arrest. If the DNA damage is severe, the cell initiates suicide, in part by upregulation of a proapoptotic Bcl-2 family protein, Bax (see below). Additional biochemical pathways leading to apoptosis remain to be fully clarified.

Death Receptor–Induced Apoptosis

Of particular importance to the immune system are receptors and ligands belonging to the tumor necrosis factor (TNF) superfamily (TNFSF) (reviewed in ref. 12). This family now comprises about 20 members, six of which [Fas, TNFR I, DR-3 (TRAMP/wsl/APO-3), DR-4 (TRAIL), DR-5, and DR-6] are death receptors characterized by the presence of a homologous stretch of ~80 amino acids in the cytoplasmic signal transducing portion of the molecule called the death domain. In addition, three decoy receptors have been identified, two (DcR1 and DcR2) that bind and inhibit their ligand, TRAIL, and one (DcR3) that binds Fas ligand. These decoy receptors presumably modulate cytotoxic function of the ligands but the biologic contexts remain to be defined. The two best characterized receptor-mediated death pathways, Fas and TNF-α, will briefly be described, although it should be noted that many other members of this family (CD30, CD40, and BLyS/TALL-1/BAFF/THANK/zTNF4) regulate survival in cells of the immune system.

Fas (APO-1/CD95) is a 48-kd cell surface glycoprotein receptor that is expressed at high levels in the thymus and on activated T cells, B cells, and macrophages; it also is expressed in nonlymphoid organs such as the liver, heart, skin, and cells within the gastrointestinal tract. The FasL (ligand) is predominantly expressed on activated T cells of the $CD4^+$ T-helper-1 (Th1) and CD8 subtypes. Like TNF, the receptor does not appear to be required for negative selection of high-affinity cells in the thymus. Whether Fas/TNF plays any role in thymic selection remains to be determined, but most studies indicate that Fas-mediated apoptosis is required for termination of the immune response in the peripheral immune response (discussed later).

Ligation of either Fas or TNFR by the corresponding ligand induces receptor clustering and recruitment of intracellular adapter molecules leading to the formation of a death-inducing signaling complex (DISC) (Fig.8.3B). Initially, aggregation of Fas induces recruitment of the adapter protein FADD/MORT1 to the death domain of Fas. FADD has two structural domains: a C-terminal death domain, which mediates Fas binding, and an N-terminal death effector domain (DED). The FADD DED allows recruitment of pro-caspase 8 and pro-caspase 10b via DED–DED interactions. Pro-caspases 8 and 10b have a bipartite structure comprising a DED and an enzymatic caspase domain, the latter linking Fas aggregation with the execution phase of apoptosis. The apposition of pro-caspases 8 and 10b to the activated Fas complex, leads to autocatalytic cleavage (13) and conversion of the proenzymes to activated proteases, which are released and able to initiate a proteolytic cascade leading to programmed cell death. In some cell lines, caspase 8 cleavage also results in cleavage of the proapoptotic molecule Bid to form the truncated t-Bid. T-Bid inserts into the mitochondria, thereby releasing cytochrome *c* and amplifying the caspase cascade [type II pathway (14)] (Fig. 8.3).

TNF-α is a cytokine produced by macrophages, T cells, and other cell types both within and outside of the immune system. TNF-α can be membrane bound or can be cleaved from the surface by the metalloproteinase, TNF converting enzyme (TACE). TNF-α binds to two structurally distinct receptors, type I (p55) and type II (p75) with similar high affinities. Both receptors are ubiquitously expressed, although type II receptors are highly inducible. The most important function of TNF appears to be activation of the innate and adaptive immune system in response to infection. This pathway is transmitted through TRADD, TRAF-2, and NFκB (Fig. 8.3.B). TNF-α was so named for its ability to induce death in a number of tumors and tumor cell lines. TNF-α can also kill certain T-cell subsets by activation induced cell death (AICD), similar to Fas (12). In these cells, TNF signals death through FADD and caspase 8 with the resulting recruitment of downstream caspases similar to Fas (Fig. 8.3B). How can a cytokine signal opposite cell fates? The life or death decision cannot simply be correlated with engagement of type I or II receptors. The response, to a large extent, is made at the level of the target cell (hardwiring, previous signals received, state of activation). At the level of the inducer, membrane TNF-α (expressed predominantly on T cells) predominantly mediates apoptosis, whereas soluble TNF may mediate either activation or death.

EXECUTION OF APOPTOSIS: COMMON DOWNSTREAM PATHWAYS OF STRESS AND RECEPTOR MEDIATED APOPTOSIS

During execution of apoptosis, cells detach from their matrix (if adherent), begin to form blebs, and condense. These key alterations are orchestrated mainly by caspases, but other proteases such as calpains are also implicated in this phase of apoptosis. Processing of intracellular substrates inactivates the cell and prepares it for engulfment. Here, the pathways whereby upstream caspase activation leads to execution of apoptosis will briefly be described.

The upstream caspases 9, 8, and 10 discussed above, have large prodomains that interact with regulatory/adapter proteins such as Apaf-1 for caspase 9 and FADD for caspases 8 and 10. Presumably, clustering of these complexes allows for autocatalytic cleavage of the large and small subdomains to form the active tetramers. As in many biologic processes, catalytic cleavage is enhanced by the assembly of a large (700-kd) multiprotein complex called the "apoptosome" (Fig. 8.3A). The Apaf-1 apoptosome contains caspases 9, 3, and 7, and is biologically active (15).

Effector caspases such as 3, 6, and 7 have small prodomains and are cleaved into their active forms by the upstream caspases. The effector caspases are necessary for the execution of apoptosis. They cleave specific substrates such as the structural proteins fodrin, gelsolin, and lamins, key intracellular enzymes involved in DNA repair [e.g., poly–adenosine diphosphate (ADP) ribose polymerase, DNA-PK]. These changes facilitate inactivation of synthetic functions of the cell, dissolution of the nuclear membrane, and the packaging of cellular proteins into apoptotic blebs on the cell surface. Release, blebbing, and condensation are associated with actin rearrangement, actin-myosin II contraction, and actin dissolution, respectively (reviewed in ref. 16).

One of the earliest changes observed is the translocation of charged phospholipids such as phosphatidylserine (PS) to the outer surface of the cell membrane. This alteration is associated with downregulation of the amino phospholipid translocase that normally maintains phospholipid asymmetry and with activation of a nonspecific lipid scramblase (17). Phosphatidylserine is a ligand for a receptor that promotes phagocytosis of apoptotic cells and can be detected on the cell surface through calcium-dependent binding to annexin V (18). This alteration is of special interest in relation to antiphospholipid antibodies that bind to negatively charged phospholipids (see below).

In addition, caspases cleave regulatory proteins such as Bcl family members and the inhibitor of caspase-activated Dnase (ICAD, also called DFF45). Cleavage of ICAD leads to the release of active CAD, which in turn enters the nucleus and cleaves nucleosomes at the linker region yielding the characteristic "DNA ladder" (Fig. 8.1). DNA fragmentation results in free 3-OH groups, which can be detected within the nuclei in tissue sections using biotinylated dNTPs. It should be noted that not all caspases are involved in the execution of apoptosis. Caspases 1, 4, 5, 11, 12, and 13 are, most likely, involved in inflammation. The best understood example in this context is caspase 1, the enzyme that cleaves IL-1 into its active form (19).

Since caspases play a critical role in apoptosis, some additional points should be mentioned. Caspases can be divided into functional subgroups based on their substrate specificities (20). Group I (caspases 1, 4, and 5) that are potently inhibited by the serpin, CrmA; group II (caspases 2, 3, and 7) are specific for DExD; and group III (caspases 6, 8, 9, and 10) that are specific for I/V/LExD, a sequence that is also contained at the junctions of the caspase subunits themselves. Significantly, granzyme B produced by cytotoxic T cells has a similar substrate specificity to group III caspases and is also capable of inducing apoptosis through this pathway. Identification of the substrate specificity of caspases has led to a number of practical applications including the ability to quantify activity using fluorogenic tetrapeptide substrates and to the inhibition of proteolytic activity with noncleavable cell-permeable tetrapeptide analogues.

The penultimate step in apoptosis is redistribution of nuclear and cytosolic contents into apoptotic blebs. As discussed earlier, this process is greatly facilitated by proteolysis of the cell matrix proteins. Disposal of dying cells is considered below.

SURVIVAL SIGNALS AND REGULATION OF APOPTOSIS

As mentioned above, most cells within the immune system die by default, but specific signals can prolong survival in order to recruit cells into the immune response. Survival signals include low-affinity binding by lymphocyte antigen receptors, growth factor/cytokine (e.g., IL-4, IL-7) receptors, and ligation of co-stimulatory receptors (CD28 on T cells, CD40 and BlyS on B cells) (21). Many of the survival pathways activate protein kinase C (PKC) (22). Engagement of antigen and co-stimulatory receptors on mature T cells lead to PI3-kinase activation. PI3-kinase promotes the phosphorylation of protein kinase B/Akt (phospho-Akt), a potent antiapoptotic enzyme (23). Phospho-Akt promotes cell survival through a number of pathways, some of which are cell type specific. These pathways include inhibition of synthesis or function of the proapoptotic proteins Bad, caspase 9 and Fas ligand, and facilitation of the activity of I kappa B kinase (IKK) α leading to increased activity of nuclear factor NF-κB, a known antiapoptotic transcription factor (Fig. 8.3B).

Among the most important regulators of survival are more than 15 proteins belonging to the Bcl family (reviewed in ref. 24). Mammalian Bcl-2 homologues are Bcl-XL, Bcl-w, Mcl-1, A1, and the virus homologues are BHRF1, LMW5-HL, ORF16, KS-Bcl-2, and E1B-19K. Proapoptotic members of this family include Bax, Bak, Bok, Bik, Blk, Hrk, BNIP3, Bim, Bad, and Bid. How do Bcls regulate apoptosis? One level of regulation is conferred by binding interactions (homo- or heterodimerization) between members, effected largely by their BH1, 2, and 3 domains (25). Although the outcomes vary for each specific pair, homodimerization of Bcl-2 or Bax potentiates their anti- or proapoptotic function, respectively, whereas heterodimers may potentiate or abrogate function of one member of the pair. Bcls such as Bcl-2 and Bcl-XL may also bind to Apaf-1 and prevent it from activating caspase 9, analogous to the regulation of CED-4 by CED-9 in *C. elegans*.

Bcls regulation of cell death is closely connected to mitochondrial function (reviewed in ref. 25). The physical association of Bcl-2 family proteins with the outer mitochondrial membrane, as well as the close structural similarity between the BH1 and 2 domains, and bacterial pore forming proteins such as colicins (26) allow them to regulate ion fluxes or the transfer of small molecules from the PT pore in the outer membrane. *In vitro* models suggest that Bax and Bak promote opening of the VDAC allowing the release of cytochrome *c* (and presumably smac/diablo) into the cytosol, whereas Bcl-2 binds directly to VDAC and closes it (27). Regulation of the release of the caspase independent AIF from the mitochondria is incompletely defined (28).

Caspase Inhibitors

As mentioned above, Bcl-2 and other antiapoptotic members of this family may bind to caspase 9/Apaf-1, inhibiting activity. At the level of death receptors, a protein called FLIP inhibits Fas-mediated apoptosis (Fig. 8.4). Flice inhibitory protein (FLIP) has high sequence homology to caspase 8 but lacks the active site cysteine required for proteolytic activity. When FLIP is recruited to the DISC, it prevents caspase 8 recruitment and therefore inhibits caspase activation.

Intracellular IAPs are a separate family of antiapoptotic proteins that are highly conserved through evolution. The

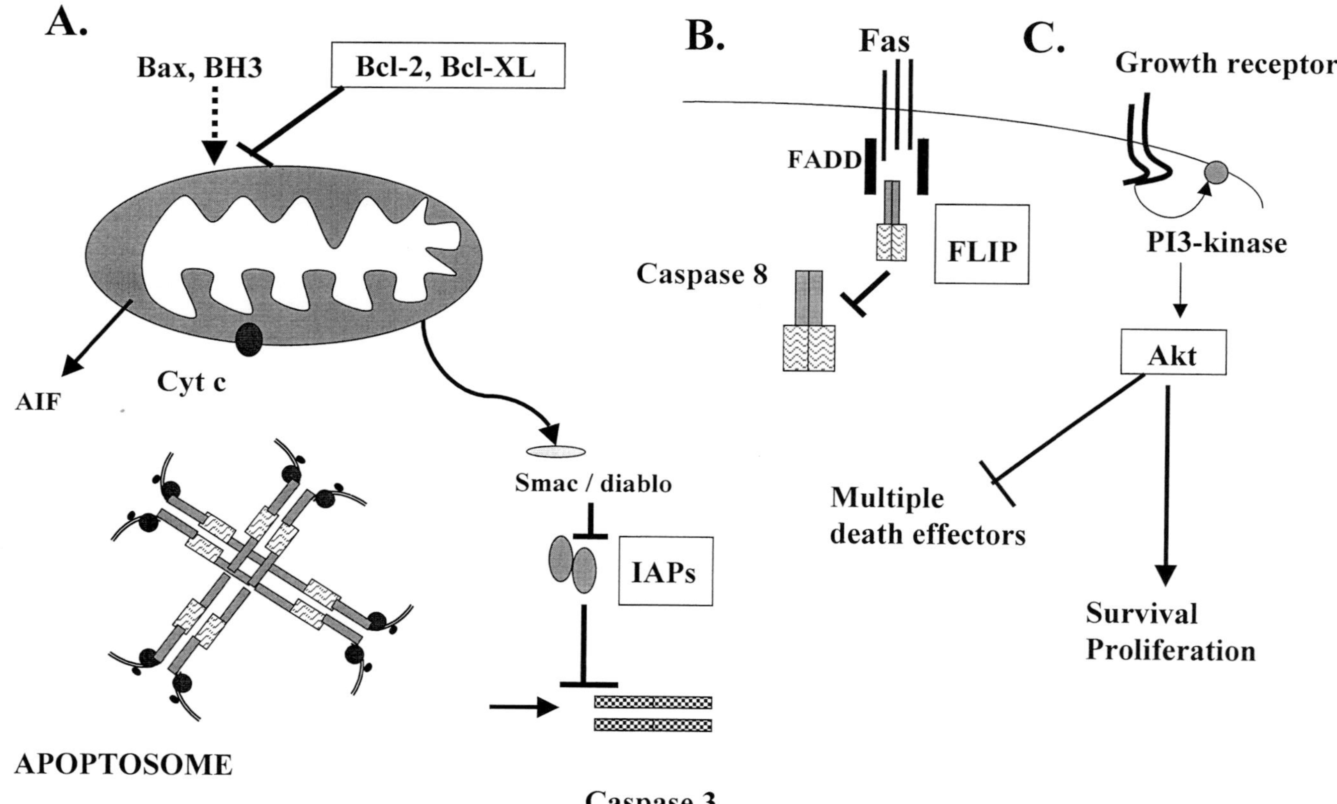

FIGURE 8.4. Apoptosis inhibitors. Both the mitochondrial and receptor-mediated apoptotic pathways are subject to regulation by cellular apoptosis inhibitors indicated by a frame (see text for virus homologues). In the mitochondrial pathway (**A**), Bcl-2 and Bcl-XL inhibit apoptosis by dimerizing with proapoptotic Bcl family members such as Bax, by interacting with mitochondrial membranes (most likely conductance channels), and possibly by inhibiting productive apaf-1/caspase 9 interactions. Inhibitors of apoptosis (IAPs) block caspase 3 activation, which can be attenuated by the release of mitochondrial protein smac/DIABLO. In the Fas death receptor pathway (**B**), activation is inhibited by the protein FLIP. **C:** Growth receptors induce phosphorylation of Akt (PKB) through PI3-kinase. Akt inhibits apoptosis through multiple pathways including phosphorylation of caspase 9, inactivation of Bad, and inhibition of Fas ligand transcription.

neuronal IAP [neuronal apoptosis inhibitory protein (NAIP)] was discovered through the association of NAIP mutations in patients with the severe form of spinal muscular atrophy. Additional members of the family (e.g. c-IAP-1, 2, X-IAP, and survivin) have subsequently been identified. Recent studies suggest that the major mechanism of action of IAPs is inhibition of effector caspases and that the protein Smac/diablo acts to release this inhibition (29,30) (Fig. 8.4).

Mammalian DNA viruses synthesize proteins that inhibit cell death, including a Bcl-2 homologue, BHRF (Epstein-Barr virus), and the E1B 19-kd protein (adenovirus). Herpes viruses also produce a protein called v-FLIP that competes for binding to FADD, similar to c-FLIP described above. The insect virus baculovirus produces at least two inhibitors of apoptosis: p35, which inhibits proteolysis by caspase 1; and IAP, which is thought to act upstream of the proteolytic pathway. CrmA, a cowpox virus product, also attenuates apoptosis through caspase inhibition.

DISPOSAL OF APOPTOTIC CELLS AND IMPLICATIONS FOR IMMUNITY

A number of different ligands and receptors have been implicated in the recognition and phagocytosis of apoptotic cells by macrophages *in vitro* (Fig. 8.5)(reviewed in ref. 31). These include integrin receptors αvβ5 or αvβ3, CD36, which shares the αvβ3/CD36/ thrombospondin recognition mechanism, class A and B scavenger receptors, the ATP-binding cassette transporter ABC1, and CD14. In addition, a receptor that binds to phosphatidylserine (PS) has recently been cloned (32). This receptor was reported to have high expression in the heart, skeletal muscle, and kidney, but only low to moderate expression in spleen and thymus (32). Recent studies have also suggested an important role for serum opsonins such as complement and acute phase proteins in the phagocytosis of dying cells in the peripheral immune system (33,34). The relevance of serum opsonins in relation to autoantibody selection and the pathogenesis of SLE is discussed below.

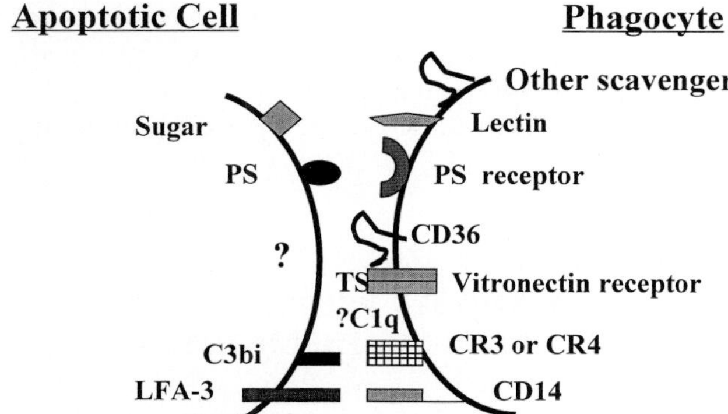

FIGURE 8.5. Receptors and ligands implicated in recognition and/or phagocytosis of apoptotic cells. Signals such as phosphatidylserine (PS) and certain sugars are exposed on the cell as it undergoes apoptosis. Other serum-derived ligands [complement components, thrombospondin (TS)] act as opsonins. Phagocytosis of apoptotic cells induces antiinflammatory cytokines such as transforming growth factor-β (TGF-β).

APOPTOSIS AND ITS RELEVANCE TO NORMAL IMMUNE FUNCTION

More than 10^9 lymphocytes are produced in bone marrow each day. In addition, large numbers of lymphocytes are clonally expanded in the periphery following contact with antigens. To maintain the size of the lymphoid pool, an equivalent rate of cell death must occur. Each mature cell type within the immune system has a normal life span. For neutrophils the average life span is ~1 day, and for lymphocytes a few weeks. However, pressures to develop immune tolerance and immunologic memory require that the life span for clonal populations of lymphocytes vary from less than a day (high-affinity autoreactive cells) to many years (memory cells). This remarkable variation is influenced first and foremost by engagement of the lymphocyte antigen receptor, and secondly by multiple additional signals, some of which promote cell survival and others that induce or enable the apoptotic program (see above).

In addition to the maintenance of homeostasis in relation to the number of cells, apoptosis is crucial for the induction and preservation of immunologic tolerance. The basic principles that determine the initial fate of lymphocytes are that self-reactive cells commit suicide, useless lymphocytes die, and cells recruited into an immune response by foreign antigens in the context of co-stimulation initiate a survival pathway. However, as discussed later, even this latter group of cells will need to be eliminated to maintain immunologic homeostasis and avoid autoimmunity. A more complete discussion of tolerance is given elsewhere (35).

The Central Lymphoid Organs (Thymus and Bone Marrow)

Lymphocytes are poised to die at all stages of maturation. Immature cells die when their antigen receptors fail to undergo productive rearrangement. In cells that have undergone productive rearrangement and express antigen receptors on the cell surface, cells are signaled to die when these receptors bind with high affinity to antigens (i.e., negative selection). To be saved from a default death pathway, immature T cells (i.e., thymocytes) require low-affinity binding to self–major histocompatibility complex

(MHC) through their antigen receptor (i.e., positive selection) to survive. These cells then seed into the periphery.

There are many parallels between the maturation of T cells in the thymus and B cells in the bone marrow. Large numbers of pro-B cells die due to faulty rearrangement of the genes encoding components of the B-cell receptor (BCR), μ heavy chain and κ or λ light chain. Like $CD4^+$/$CD8^+$ thymocytes, B cells that have reached the maturational stage of "early B cells," immunoglobulin M (IgM^+) and IgD^-, are very sensitive to apoptosis when engaged by high-density cross-linking of their antigen receptor. Unlike thymocytes, however, early B cells that react with high affinity to self antigen have a chance to avoid death by expressing a different light chain on the cell surface—"receptor editing." Whereas B cells were thought to lack any element for positive selection, experimental evidence is accumulating that B cells may also be rescued from death by interaction with self antigen (36).

The Peripheral Immune System (Spleen, Lymph Nodes, Mucosa)

As mentioned earlier, most of the newly emergent lymphocytes circulate for days or weeks. Here, potentially autoreactive lymphocytes become activated and may undergo apoptosis or anergy (functional inactivation) on their first encounter with antigen in the periphery. Cells that do not encounter antigen most likely die by a different cell death program.

Following activation by foreign microorganisms, lymphocytes become fully armed and express and/or secrete cytotoxic molecules and proinflammatory cytokines. To avoid unnecessary tissue damage, it is imperative that, once the initiating organism is destroyed, the activated lymphocytes are also removed. In addition, since co-stimulatory molecules are upregulated during inflammation and most of the antigens presented by the MHC are self peptides (37), a significant opportunity for self reactivity occurs at this time. Persistence of activated lymphocytes in the presence of highly expressed co-stimulatory molecules on antigen-presenting cells allows the activated cells to cross-react with or, in the case of B cells, somatically mutate toward self specificity. The critical role of apoptosis in the maintenance of peripheral tolerance is illustrated by systemic autoimmunity that develops in humans and mice with Fas and Fas ligand mutations (see below).

Apoptosis of activated cells (activation-induced cell death, AICD) occurs by two phenomena: (a) cytokine withdrawal, leading to apoptosis by the intrinsic pathway; and (b) active death induction through death receptors (see above)(38). At least two death receptors are implicated in apoptosis of activated peripheral lymphocytes, Fas, and TNF-α, although TRAIL may play a role when induced by cytokines such as type 1 interferons (39). Fas ligand is expressed on activated CD8, CD4 T cells of the Th1 subset and natural killer (NK) cells. These cells therefore can kill themselves as well as activated Th2 $CD4^+$ T cells, B cells, and macrophages. The role of TNF-α is less well established, especially since TNF-α–deficient mice do not develop autoimmunity. Nevertheless, both *in vivo* and *in vitro* experiments suggest that TNF-α plays a role in AICD of subsets of T cells.

Downmodulation of the immune responses does not only occur by apoptosis; the T-cell surface molecule CTLA-4 also turns off activated T cells (reviewed in ref. 40). CTLA-4 is normally expressed at very low levels on resting T cells but is markedly upregulated following activation. CTLA-4 binds to the same co-stimulatory molecules on antigen-presenting cells, B7.1 and B7.2, that CD28 does, but, because of its much higher affinity of binding, outcompetes CD28. By reducing engagement of CD28, and by transducing inhibitory signals to the activated T cells, CTLA-4 helps to terminate an immune response. The importance of CTLA-4 in downregulating immune responses is illustrated by the massive inflammation and lymphocytic infiltration of organs in mice deficient for this molecule (40).

Disposal of Apoptotic Cells and Tolerance

In view of the vast numbers of apoptotic cells phagocytosed in the thymus and bone marrow, it is reasonable to assume that the endogenous cellular material is degraded and presented to lymphocytes. This would ensure that lymphocytes with high affinity for self antigens are eliminated. However, low-affinity positively selected self-reactive lymphocytes seed to the periphery. Here, these cells also encounter antigen-presenting cells that have engulfed dying cells. How is self reactivity avoided? A key element is the innate immune response of macrophages to the phagocytosis of apoptotic cells. Avoidance of an immune response to self is ensured by the production of antiinflammatory molecules such as transforming growth factor-β_1 (TGF-β_1) and prostaglandin E_2 (PGE_2) (41).

APOPTOSIS AND ITS RELEVANCE TO SYSTEMIC LUPUS ERYTHEMATOSUS

Considering the pivotal roles that apoptosis plays in tolerance induction and maintenance, as well as the huge burden of self antigens that must be disposed of by this process, it is not surprising that abnormalities in these pathways can result in systemic autoimmunity. The specific genes involved are listed in Table 8.1 and the mechanisms briefly discussed below.

TABLE 8.1. SPONTANEOUS AND GENETICALLY ENGINEERED MUTATIONS THAT AFFECT APOPTOSIS AND PREDISPOSE TO LUPUS-LIKE DISEASE[a]

Defective Apoptosis	Defective Clearance (?)
Fas, Fas ligand	C1q, C2, C4
Bcl-2 Tg	SAP/CRP
Bim	sIgM
? IL-2, IL-2R	DNAse 1
PTEN +/–	
? BlyS/TALL Tg	

[a]Mutations lead to underexpression of the protein product except for Tg (transgenic) mice that overexpress the relevant gene product. In the case of PTEN, heterozygotes (+/–) express the disease. See text for discussion of the mechanisms proposed. ? indicates that the mechanism remains uncertain.
CRP, c reactive protein; IL, interleukin; SAP, serum amyloid protein; Tg, transgenic.

Defects in the Induction or Regulation of Apoptosis

Three independent autosomal recessive mutations of the Fas receptor or its ligand have arisen in three different mouse strains, all of which develop massive lymphadenopathy and lupus-like autoimmunity (42). The molecular mechanisms responsible for these mutations have been characterized, and all result in impaired Fas-mediated apoptosis. It is interesting to note the highly variable expression of lupus in terms of severity, organ involvement, and autoantibody production in these strains as well as other normal strains onto which the lpr mutation has been crossed (43). This variability stresses the importance of background genes as modifiers of the clinical phenotype. Humans with Fas, Fas ligand, or caspase 10 mutations also develop a lupus-like disease although very few develop four American College of Rheumatology (ACR) criteria for the disease (44). The disease in humans is characterized by lymphadenopathy, splenomegaly, and autoimmune cytopenias with variable expression of rash, neuropathy, or nephritis (45,46).

Manipulations of genes in the Bcl-2 family [overexpression of the antiapoptotic protein Bcl-2 (47), knockout of the proapoptotic protein Bim (48)] have led to lupus-like diseases in mice. Although some studies have reported higher expression of Bcl-2 in T cells from patients with systemic lupus erythematosus (SLE), a consistent association has not been observed in all studies. PTEN +/– (heterozygous) mice also develop lupus and die from glomerulonephritis (49). PTEN deficiency leads to increased activation of Akt with its attendant promotion of survival pathways (see above), as well as reduced sensitivity to Fas-mediated apoptosis. Overexpression of the TNF family member BlyS in transgenic mice leads to a lupus-like disease (50,51) due to co-stimulation and inhibition of apoptosis of B cells.

Deficiencies of IL-2 (52) as well as the IL-2α and β receptors (53,54) cause lupus-like diseases in mice. At least part of the mechanism responsible is that IL-2 is required for reducing the expression of FLIP, the protein that competes for caspase 8 binding to death receptors (Fig. 8.4B). Although inappropriately low IL-2 and IL-2R expression have long been known to exist in human SLE, it is unclear whether these abnormalities are primary or secondary and whether they contribute to disease pathogenesis.

In summary, these findings demonstrate that mutations in apoptosis-inducing molecules or overexpression of molecules that promote lymphocyte survival may result in a lupus-like syndrome. How does this occur? Autoimmunity could arise when potentially autoreactive cells emerging from the thymus are activated by self antigens but fail to be deleted. When lymphocytes are stimulated by foreign antigen but fail to die through AICD, they also have an increased opportunity to cross-react with self antigens in the periphery. This is a significant problem for B cells, which would have the opportunity to mutate their antigen receptor toward higher-affinity binding for self antigens in germinal centers. Finally, since antigen-presenting cells present self peptides on MHC class I or class II (through cross-priming), defective apoptosis of antigen-presenting cells promotes the availability of self peptides to be seen by low-affinity self-reactive lymphocytes (55).

Defective Handling of Dying Cells

Accumulating evidence supports the notion that the products of dying cells are immunogenic in SLE. This evidence includes the prominent B- and T-cell immune reactivity toward antigens that are expressed on, or are products of, apoptotic cells such as nucleosomes and negatively charged phospholipids (56,57). Furthermore, UV irradiation of keratinocytes caused a redistribution of lupus autoantigens such that small surface apoptotic blebs contain RNA, ribosomes, and Ro/SSA, and larger blebs contain DNA and Ro/SSA, La/SSB, and small nuclear ribonucleoproteins (snRNPs) (58). Exactly how this redistribution causes immunization is unclear, but it has been suggested that protein autoantigens are modified by caspases or granzymes such that they become immunogenic (59). These findings are of interest since UV light is a known inducer of flares of SLE and may cause a greater degree of exposure of antigens in SLE keratinocytes compared with normal controls (60). Despite these provocative observations, the evidence that autoantibodies are induced by apoptotic cells or their fragments remains indirect.

As discussed above, phagocytosis of apoptotic cells is not a neutral process but actively induces immunosuppression. In contrast, phagocytosis of necrotic cells frequently results in a proinflammatory response. It follows that if apoptotic cells are not rapidly cleared, they may undergo postapoptotic necrosis, which in turn induces the expression of cytokines such as TNF-α (41,61). How could this situation arise? In theory, if apoptosis overwhelmed the clearance capacity of macrophages or if macrophage clearance was defective, an abnormal immune response to self could arise. Some evidence in support of enhanced apoptotic rates and defective clearance has been reported in human SLE (62,63).

As shown in Table 8.1, in four different knockout mice the lupus-like phenotype might be caused by impaired clearance of dying cells. In C1q-deficient mice, increased numbers of apoptotic cells were observed in the kidneys (64). Taken together with the evidence that apoptotic cells bind (65) and activate (34) complement and that complement opsonizes apoptotic cells for phagocytosis *in vitro* (34), early complement deficiencies may predispose to SLE through impaired clearance of dying cells. Similarly, the human homologue of SAP, CRP, was recently shown to opsonize apoptotic cells for clearance by macrophages (33), and SAP-deficient mice also have an abnormal clearance of chromatin (66). The lupus-like disease associated with DNAse 1 deficiency has been attributed to lack of timely clearance of DNA from dying cells (67), and at least one explanation for the tendency for secretory IgM deficiency to cause a lupus-like disease (68,69) is impaired clearance of self antigens by natural antibodies.

In summary, circumstantial evidence as well as direct experimentation through genetic manipulation of mice and *in vitro* experiments support the idea that autoantigen specificity and possibly the immunogenicity of self antigens can be explained by defective handling or processing of dying cells.

SUMMARY

Studies over the last decade have provided fundamental insights into biochemical pathways that regulate cell death and the mechanisms whereby dying cells are removed. Through spontaneous and engineered mutations, the importance of these pathways for immune homeostasis and the avoidance of autoimmunity have become abundantly clear. Although only a very small number of humans with SLE or SLE-like diseases have been shown to have defined mutations in apoptotic pathways, it is quite possible that previously established links between SLE and deficiencies in early complement pathways are attributable to defective clearance of apoptotic cells. Further studies in this field should be enlightening.

REFERENCES

1. Kerr J, Wyllie A, Currie A. Apoptosis: a basic biological phenomenon with wide-ranging implications in tissue kinetics. *Br J Cancer* 1972;26:239–257.
2. Bonfoco E, Krainc D, Ankarcrona M, et al. Apoptosis and necrosis: two distinct events induced, respectively, by mild and intense insults with N-methyl-D-aspartate or nitric oxide/superoxide in cortical cell cultures. *Proc Natl Acad Sci USA* 1995;92(16): 7162–7166.
3. Leist M, Single B, Castoldi AF, et al. Intracellular adenosine triphosphate (ATP) concentration: a switch in the decision between apoptosis and necrosis. *J Exp Med* 1997;185:1481–1486.
4. Sansonetti PJ, Phalipon A, Arondel J, et al. Caspase-1 activation of IL-1beta and IL-18 are essential for *Shigella flexneri*-induced inflammation. *Immunity* 2000;12(5):581–590.
5. Horvitz H, Shaham S, Hengartner M. The genetics of programmed cell death in the nematode *Caenorhabditis elegans. Cold Spring Harbor Symp Quant Biol* 1994;59:377–385.
6. Kroemer G, Zamzami N, Susin SA. Mitochondrial control of apoptosis. [Review] [71 refs]. *Immunol Today* 1997;18(1):44–51.
7. Vander Heiden MG, Chandel NS, Schumacker PT, et al. Bcl-xL prevents cell death following growth factor withdrawal by facilitating mitochondrial ATP/ADP exchange. *Mol Cell* 1999;3(2): 159–167.
8. Zou H, Henzel W, Liu Z, et al. Apaf-1, a human protein homologous to C. elegans CED-4, participates in cytochrome c-dependent activation of caspase 3. *Cell* 1997;90:405–413.
9. Brenner C, Kroemer G. Apoptosis. Mitochondria—the death signal integrators [comment]. *Science* 2000;289(5482): 1150–1151.
10. Amsen D, Kruisbeek AM. Thymocyte selection: not by TCR alone. *Immunol Rev* 1998;165:209–229.
11. Levine AJ. P53, the cellular gatekeeper for growth and division. *Cell* 1997;88:323–331.
12. Wallach D, Varfolomeev EE, Malinin NL, et al. Tumor necrosis factor receptor and Fas signaling mechanisms. *Annu Rev Immunol* 1999;17:331–367.
13. Muzio M, Chinnaiyan A, Kischkel F, et al. FLICE, a novel FADD-homologous ICE/CED-3-like protease, is recruited to the CD95 (Fas/APO-1) death-inducing signaling complex. *Cell* 1996;85:817–827.
14. Scaffidi C, Fulda S, Srinivasan A, et al. Two CD95 (APO-1/Fas) signaling pathways. *EMBO J* 1998;17:1675–1687.
15. Cain K, Bratton SB, Langlais C, et al. Apaf-1 oligomerizes into biologically active approximately 700-kDa and inactive approximately 1.4-MDa apoptosome complexes. *J Biol Chem* 2000; 275(9):6067–6070.
16. Mills JC, Stone NL, Pittman RN. Extranuclear apoptosis. The role of the cytoplasm in the execution phase. *J Cell Biol* 1999;146(4):703–708.
17. Verhoven B, Schlegel RA, Williamson P. Mechanisms of phosphatidylserine exposure, a phagocyte recognition signal, on apoptotic T lymphocytes. *J Exp Med* 1995;182:1597–1601.
18. Vermes I, Haanen C, Steffens-Nakken H, et al. A novel assay for apoptosis: flow cytometric detection of phosphatidylserine expression on early apoptotic cells using fluorescein- labeled annexin V. *J Immunol Methods* 1995;184:39–51.
19. Yuan J, Shaham S, Ledoux S, et al. The *C. elegans* cell death gene ced-3 encodes a protein similar to mammalian interleukin-1-converting enzyme. *Cell* 1993;75:641–652.
20. Garcia-Calvo M, Peterson EP, Leiting B, et al. Inhibition of human caspases by peptide-based and macrophage inhibitors. J Biol Chem 1998;273:32608–32613.
21. Do RK, Hatada E, Lee H, et al. Attenuation of apoptosis underlies B lymphocyte stimulator enhancement of humoral immune response [In Process Citation]. *J Exp Med* 2000;192(7):953–964.
22. Perandones CE, Illera VA, Peckham D, et al. Regulation of apoptosis in vitro in mature murine spleen T cells. *J Immunol* 1993; 151:3521–3529.
23. Downward J. Mechanisms and consequences of activation of protein kinase B/Akt. *Curr Opin Cell Biol* 1998;10:262–267.

24. Adams JM, Cory S. The Bcl-s protein family: arbiters of cell survival. *Science* 1998;281:1322–1326.
25. Gross A, McDonnell JM, Korsmeyer SJ. BCL-2 family members and the mitochondria in apoptosis. *Genes Dev* 1999;13(15): 1899–1911.
26. Muchmore SW, Sattler M, Liang H, et al. X-ray and NMR structure of human Bcl-xL, an inhibitor of programmed cell death. Nature 1996;381(6580):335–341.
27. Shimizu S, Narita M, Tsujimoto Y. Bcl-2 family proteins regulate the release of apoptogenic cytochrome-c by the mitochondrial channel VDAC. *Nature* 1999;399:483–487.
28. Susin SA, Lorenzo HK, Zamzami N, et al. Molecular characterization of mitochondrial apoptosis-inducing factor. *Nature* 1999; 397:441–446.
29. Du C, Fang M, Li Y, et al. Smac, a mitochondrial protein that promotes cytochrome c-dependent caspase activation by eliminating IAP inhibition. *Cell* 2000;102(1):33–42.
30. Verhagen AM, Ekert PG, Pakusch M, et al. Identification of DIABLO, a mammalian protein that promotes apoptosis by binding to and antagonizing IAP proteins. *Cell* 2000;102(1): 43–53.
31. Gregory CD. CD14-dependent clearance of apoptotic cells: relevance to the immune system. *Curr Opin Immunol* 2000;12: 27–34.
32. Fadok VA, Bratton DL, Rose DM, et al. A receptor for phosphatidylserine-specific clearance of apoptotic cells [see comments]. *Nature* 2000;405(6782):85–90.
33. Gershov D, Kim S, Brot N, et al. C-Reactive Protein Binds to Apoptotic Cells, Protects the cells from assembly of the terminal complement components, and sustains an antiinflammatory innate immune response. Implications for systemic autoimmunity. *J Exp Med* 2000;192(9):1353–1364.
34. Mevorach D, Mascarenhas J, Gershov DA, et al. Complement-dependent clearance of apoptotic cells by human macrophages. *J Exp Med* 1998;188:2313–2320.
35. Elkon K. Clinical immunology. In: Rich RR, Kotzin B, Shearer W, et al., eds. *Clinical immunology*, 2nd ed. London: Harcourt International, *in press*.
36. Hayakawa K, Asano M, Shinton SA, et al. Positive selection of natural autoreactive B cells. *Science* 1999;285:113–116.
37. Chicz RM, Urban RG, Lane WS, et al. Predominant naturally processed peptides bound to HLA-DR1 are derived from MHC-related molecules and are heterogeneous in size. *Nature* 1992; 358:764–768.
38. Van Parijs L, Abbas AK. Homeostasis and self tolerance in the immune system: turning lymphocytes off. *Science* 1998;280: 243–248.
39. Kayagaki N, Yamaguchi N, Nakayama M, et al. Type I interferons (IFNs) regulate tumor necrosis factor-related apoptosis-inducing ligand (TRAIL) expression on human T cells: A novel mechanism for the anti-tumor effects of type I IFNs. *J Exp Med* 1999;189:1451–1460.
40. Oosterwegel MA, Greenwald RJ, Mandelbrot DA, et al. CTLA-4 and T cell activation. *Curr Opin Immunol* 1999;11:294–300.
41. Fadok VA, Bratton DL, Konowal A, et al. Macrophages that have ingested apoptotic cells in vitro inhibit proinflammatory cytokine production through autocrine/paracrine mechanisms involving TGF-beta, PGE2, and PAF. *J Clin Invest* 1998;101: 890–898.
42. Nagata S. Apoptosis by death factor. *Cell* 1997;88:355–365.
43. Cohen PL, Eisenberg RA. lpr and gld: single gene models of systemic autoimmunity and lymphoproliferative disease. *Annu Rev Immunol* 1991;9:243–269.
44. Vaishnaw AK, Toubi E, Ohsako S, et al. Both quantitative and qualitative apoptotic defects are associated with the clinical spectrum of disease, including systemic lupus erythematosus in humans with Fas (APO-1/CD95) mutations. *Arthritis Rheum* 1999;42:1833–1842.
45. Martin DA, Zheng L, Siegel RM, et al. Defective CD95/APO-1/Fas signal complex formation in the human autoimmune lymphoproliferative syndrome, type Ia [In Process Citation]. *Proc Natl Acad Sci USA* 1999;96(8):4552–4557.
46. Vaishnaw AK, Orlinick JR, Chu JL, et al. Molecular basis for the apoptotic defects in patients with CD95 (Fas/Apo-1) mutations. *J Clin Invest* 1999;103:355–363.
47. Strasser A, Whittingham S, Vaux DL, et al. Enforced Bcl-2 expression in B-lymphoid cells prolongs antibody responses and elicits autoimmune disease. *Proc Natl Acad Sci USA* 1991;88: 8661–8665.
48. Bouillet P, Metcalf D, Huang DCS, et al. Preapoptotic Bcl-2 relative Bim required for certain apoptotic responses, leukocyte homeostasis, and to preclude autoimmunity. *Science* 1999;286: 1735–1738.
49. Di Cristofano A, Kotsi P, Peng YP, et al. Impaired Fas response and autoimmunity in Pten (+/–) mice. *Science* 1999;285:2122–2125.
50. Khare SD, Sarosi I, Xia XZ, et al. 2000. Severe B cell hyperplasia and autoimmune disease in TALL-1 transgenic mice. *Proc Natl Acad Sci USA* 2000;97(7):3370–3375.
51. Mackay F, Woodcock SA, Lawton P, et al. Mice transgenic for BAFF develop lymphocytic disorders along with autoimmune manifestations. *J Exp Med* 1999;190(11):1697–1710.
52. Sadlack B, Lohler J, Schorle H, et al. Generalized autoimmune disease in interleukin-2-deficient mice is triggered by an uncontrolled activation and proliferation of CD4+ T cells. *Eur J Immunol* 1995;25:3053–3059.
53. Suzuki H, Kundig TM, Furlonger C, et al. Deregulated T cell activation and autoimmunity in mice lacking interleukin-2 receptor. *Science* 1995;268:1472–1476.
54. Willerford DM, Chen J, Ferry JA, et al. Interleukin-2 receptor à chain regulates the size and content of the peripheral lymphoid compartment. *Immunity* 1995;3:521–530.
55. Ashany D, Song X, Lacy E, et al. Lymphocytes delete activated macrophages through the Fas/APO-1 pathway. *Proc Natl Acad Sci USA* 1995;92:11225–11229.
56. Mohan C, Adams S, Stanik V, et al. Nucleosome: a major immunogen for pathogenic autoantibody-inducing T cells of lupus. *J Exp Med* 1993;177:1367–1381.
57. Price BE, Rauch J, Shia MA, et al. Antiphospholipid autoantibodies bind to apoptotic, but not viable, thymocytes in a beta2-glycoprotein I-dependent manner. *J Immunol* 1996;157: 2201–2208.
58. Casciola-Rosen LA, Anhalt G, Rosen A. Autoantigens targeted in systemic lupus erythematosus are clustered in two populations of surface structures on apoptotic keratinocytes. *J Exp Med* 1994; 179:1317–1330.
59. Rosen A, Casciola-Rosen L. Autoantigens as substrates for apoptotic proteases: implications for the pathogenesis of systemic autoimmune disease. *Cell Death Differ* 1999;6:6–12.
60. Golan TD, Elkon KB, Gharavi AE, et al. Enhanced membrane binding of autoantibodies to cultured keratinocytes of SLE patients after UVB/UVA irradiation. *J Clin Invest* 1992;90: 1067–1076.
61. Stern M, Savill J, Haslett C. Human monocyte derived macrophage phagocytosis of senescent eosinophils undergoing apoptosis. *Am J Pathol* 1996;149:911–921.
62. Emlen W, Niebur J-A, Kadera R. Accelerated in vitro apoptosis of lymphocytes from patients with systemic lupus erythematosus. *J Immunol* 1994;152:3685–3692.
63. Manfredi AA, Rovere P, Galati G, et al. Apoptotic cell clearance in systemic lupus erythematosus. *Arthritis Rheum* 1998;41: 205–214.
64. Botto M, Dell'Agnola C, Bygrave AE, et al. Homozygous C1q

deficiency causes glomerulonephritis associated with multiple apoptotic bodies. *Nat Genet* 1998;19:56–59.
65. Korb LC, Ahearn JM. C1q binds directly and specifically to surface blebs of apoptotic human keratinocytes. *J Immunol* 1997; 158:4525–4528.
66. Bickerstaff MCM, Botto M, Hutchinson WL, et al. Serum amyloid P component controls chromatin degradation and prevents antinuclear autoimmunity. *Nat Med* 1999;5:694–697.
67. Napirei M, Karsunky H, Zevnik B, et al. Features of systemic lupus erythematosus in Dnase1-deficient mice [see comments]. *Nat Genet* 2000;25(2):177–181.
68. Boes M, Schmidt T, Linkemann K, et al. Accelerated development of IgG autoantibodies and autoimmune disease in the absence of secreted IgM. *Proc Natl Acad Sci USA* 2000;97(3): 1184–1189.
69. Ehrenstein MR, Cook HT, Neuberger MS. Deficiency in serum immunoglobulin (Ig)M predisposes to development of IgG autoantibodies. *J Exp Med* 2000;191(7):1253–1258.

9

T LYMPHOCYTES, NATURAL KILLER CELLS, AND IMMUNE REGULATION

DAVID A. HORWITZ
WILLIAM STOHL
J. DIXON GRAY

SLE IS A T-CELL–DEPENDENT DISEASE

Systemic lupus erythematosus (SLE) is a systemic disease that is characterized by generalized autoimmunity. Unlike organ-specific autoimmune diseases such as insulin-dependent diabetes mellitus or myasthenia gravis, SLE is characterized by autoantibodies against nuclear, cytoplasmic, and cell surface molecules that transcend organ-specific boundaries. It is the inflammatory responses triggered by local formation and/or deposition of antigen-antibody immune complexes that are responsible for the clinical manifestations of vasculitis and multiorgan system disease.

The production of pathogenic autoantibodies in SLE is T-cell dependent (1–6). In murine models of SLE, depletion of $CD4^+$ T cells blocks disease onset (7), and athymic mice do not develop SLE (8,9). In humans, the effects of human immunodeficiency virus (HIV) infection on $CD4^+$ lymphocytes may ameliorate SLE activity and spur remission (10).

Although numerous abnormalities of T-cell function have been described in this autoimmune disease, investigators have failed to find a common abnormality expressed by all patients. There is no evidence that autoantigen-specific T cells in SLE patients reflect a defect in the generation of the T-cell repertoire. Instead, the T-cell response to self antigens reflects a breakdown of tolerance to these structures.

It is now appreciated that T-cell recognition of foreign and self antigens is similar, and self reactivity to histocompatibility molecules is not only physiologic but also indispensable to the generation of normal immune responses. Moreover, since a T-cell receptor can recognize multiple peptide antigens, one might ask how a limited number of highly cross-reactive T cells can respond to the large number of foreign peptides and yet remain tolerant, or nonresponsive, to self peptides? In fact, thymic deletion of T cells that are capable of reacting against certain self peptides is incomplete, and autoreactive T cells capable of initiating SLE exist in healthy individuals (11). From this information, one might expect that SLE should be a common disorder in the general population instead of occurring only rarely.

With the realization that every individual harbors T cells that could potentially induce autoimmune disease (12), it becomes necessary to understand the mechanisms that initiate and sustain nonresponsiveness or tolerance. Just as autoreactive T cells are not completely eliminated during ontogeny, B cells that have the potential to make autoantibodies are also not completely deleted (13). In SLE, B cells spontaneously producing antibodies are increased (14,15). Immunoglobulin M (IgM) autoantibodies with anti-DNA or anti-IgG (i.e., rheumatoid factor) specificities may arise through nonspecific (i.e., T-cell–independent) stimulation of B cells. Because they are of the IgM class, these autoantibodies generally are not pathogenic. However, following the breakdown of tolerance in SLE, normally quiescent T cells become activated (16,17). These T cells provide the necessary help for IgM-producing B cells to undergo class switching and secrete pathogenic IgG anti-DNA (18,19). As discussed later, many discrete and seemingly disparate T-cell abnormalities may lead to this same common end result. Moreover, ineffective attempts by the immune system to downregulate the ongoing autoimmunity may lead to a variety of secondary T-cell abnormalities.

To make this complex topic more understandable to the nonimmunologist, this chapter provides background information on the general properties of T cells and their two principal responses to antigen, summarizes the properties of natural killer (NK) cells, reviews T cell and NK cell abnormalities in SLE, and presents a current view of the role of T cells in the induction and perpetuation of SLE. Two caveats are offered at the outset. First, the present concepts of immune dysregulation in SLE largely have been largely derived from studies involving murine models of SLE. The great advantages of murine models are that *in vivo* studies can be undertaken so the lymphoid organs, where autoimmunity is generated and sustained, can be studied directly. In contrast, most of the information concerning human SLE has been derived from the study of blood lymphocytes, and one cannot absolutely guarantee that the *ex vivo* properties of blood lymphocytes precisely reflect those events occurring in lymphoid organs *in vivo*. Second, while human SLE typically is a disease of exacerbations and remissions even in the absence of immunosuppression medications, animal models generally have a progressive course. Dynamic regulatory mechanisms, therefore, are especially important in human SLE. Confusing the picture further is the heterogeneity of SLE syndromes and the differences in patient populations studied by individual investigators. Nonetheless, in general, studies of blood lymphocytes in human SLE have complemented those in murine lupus and shed considerable light on the immune dysfunctions underlying SLE.

T LYMPHOCYTES AND NATURAL KILLER CELLS IN HEALTHY INDIVIDUALS

General Properties of T Cells

T cells are thymus-derived lymphocytes that develop effector or regulatory functions depending on how they are stimulated. The properties of the various T-cell populations are summarized in Table 9.1. Unlike B cells, T cells are unable to bind antigen directly; rather, they recognize antigen complexed to major histocompatibility complex (MHC) molecules. $CD4^+$ T cells recognize peptides complexed to MHC class II [human leukocyte antigen (HLA)-DR, -DP, -DQ]. $CD4^+$ cells typically recognize microbial peptides after phagocytosis and processing by professional antigen-presenting cells (APCs). $CD8^+$ cells recognize peptides complexed to MHC class I (HLA-A, -B, -C). These cells generally recognize peptide fragments of newly synthesized intracellular proteins, and therefore can eliminate virus-infected cells. The T-cell antigen receptor (TCR) expressed on the T-cell surface consists of a two-chain, $\alpha\beta$ heterodimer that is noncovalently complexed to the signal-transducing CD3 structure. Although $CD4^+$ cells usually provide B-cell help and $CD8^+$ cells become killer cells (20), each of these populations can develop the opposite function (21,22). These cells are positively selected by self histocompatibility antigens in the thymus, and following release they recirculate continuously between blood and peripheral lymph nodes.

T cells are called naive or virgin when they leave the thymus. Because of the low avidity of their TCR for antigen, naive T cells can be activated only in the presence of professional APCs under optimal conditions. Once they are activated, however, cell surface adhesion molecule expres-

TABLE 9.1. HUMAN T AND NATURAL KILLER (NK) CELL POPULATIONS

Population	TCR Structure	Comment
$CD4^+$	$\alpha\beta$ chains	Recognize peptide antigens complexed to self MHC class II structures (HLA-DR, -DP, -DQ)
$CD8^+$	$\alpha\beta$ chains	Recognize peptide antigens complexed to self MHC class I structures (HLA-A, -B, -C)
$CD4^+$ $CD25^+$	$\alpha\beta$ chains	Minor population that first appears in the thymus in the postnatal period; very potent regulatory effects that include the constant inhibition of potentially pathogenic autoreactive T cells
Gamma delta; generally $CD3^+$ $CD4^-$, $CD8^-$ (double negative)	Restricted expression of $\gamma\delta$ chains	Minor population in blood, abundant in intestine; directly recognizes phosphorylated and stress-induced proteins; important immunoregulatory functions
NKT, express CD3 and NK markers (i.e., CD56); generally $CD4^-$, $CD8^-$ (double negative)	Restricted expression of $\alpha\beta$ chains	Minor population in blood, but present in skin and mucosal tissues such as intestine, liver, lungs; recognize CD1, glycolipid antigens
Natural killer (NK) $CD3^-$, $CD4^-$, $CD8^{+/-}$ $CD56^+$, $CD16^+$, $CD11b^+$	Germline	Found in blood, spleen, and mucosal tissues including female reproductive organs; rare in peripheral lymph nodes; produce immunoregulatory cytokines that include IFN-γ or TGF-β

HLA, human leukocyte antigen; IFN, interferon; MHC, major histocompatibility complex; TCR, T-cell receptor; TGF, transforming growth factor.

sion is upregulated, and these "memory" cells can be restimulated by antigen under much less stringent conditions (23–26). Such CD4$^+$ cells respond well to soluble antigens and support B-cell differentiation. Corresponding memory CD8$^+$ cells, which are the precursors of antigen-specific killer cells, also are generated (27,28). Naive and memory T cells can be identified by reciprocal expression of CD45 isoforms on their cell surfaces. (CD45 is a membrane tyrosine phosphatase that has a vital role in signal transduction.) Naive T cells display the high molecular weight CD45RA isoform, and memory T cells express the low molecular weight CD45RO isoform (23–27).

The distinction between naive and memory T cells is especially important in the development of autoimmunity, because potentially harmful autoreactive T cells are in the immature, naive state. Because of clonal anergy or T-cell suppression, these cells will be maintained in the resting state. Once tolerance is broken and these autoreactive T lymphocytes become memory cells, autoimmunity would be easily sustained.

Properties of NKT cells and NK Cells

Conventional CD4$^+$ and CD8$^+$ T cells also need to be distinguished from other CD3$^+$ T cells that generally do not express CD4 or CD8, which are also called "double-negative" cells. These cells often express NK cell markers and have been called NKT cells (29,30). These cells are derived from either the thymus or the liver from a common precursor of T cells and NK cells. Unlike conventional cells that respond to peptide antigens, NKT cells respond to glycolipid antigens in the context of "nonclassical" MHC antigens such as CD1. Two thirds of double negative T cells express TCRs that are composed of αβ and one third express γδ chains. While rare in peripheral lymphoid tissue, double-negative T cells are abundant in mucosal tissues and have potent immunoregulatory effects (31).

Narural killer (NK) cells comprise a lymphocyte population that clearly is distinct from T and B cells (31). NK cells were named for their ability to lyse particular tumor target cells in the absence of any obvious activating stimulus (32–34), and they can also kill certain cells that are infected by intracellular organisms (35). Although NK cells share CD2 in common with T cells (36,37), they also recognize classical class I HLA molecules by killer cell inhibitory receptors (KIRs). NK cells bind the nonclassical class I molecule, HLA-E, to a heterodimer receptor formed by the association of CD94 with various members of the NKG2 proteins. Monoclonal antibodies to CD11b, CD16, and CD56 react predominantly with NK cells (38–41). Both CD11b and CD56 identify virtually identical lymphocyte populations (42). An important feature that distinguishes NK cells from T and B cells is their ability to respond directly to interleukin-2 (IL-2) and interferon-γ (IFN-γ) (43,44). Resting T and B cells generally require a first signal to respond to these cytokines.

NK cells can spontaneously lyse certain tumor target cells and can kill IgG-coated cells by a mechanism called antibody-dependent cellular cytotoxicity (ADCC). In addition to their cytotoxic properties, NK cells can enhance or suppress antibody production (45–47). IL-2–activated NK cells express CD40 ligand (48) and can induce resting B cells to become antibody-producing cells (47). Depending on the subset and the way they are stimulated, NK cells can produce IFN-γ, tumor necrosis factor-α (TNF-α), IL-10, or transforming growth factor-β (TGF-β) (49). When NK cells are added to CD4$^+$ cells and B cells, they enhance antibody production. However, when CD8$^+$ cells are also present, IgG production is markedly inhibited. The interaction of activated NK cells and CD8$^+$ cells results in NK release of active TGF-β, and this cytokine induces CD8$^+$ T cells to suppress antibody production. NK cells can constitutively produce active TGF-β and are the principal immediate lymphocyte source of this cytokine (Fig. 9.1).

MECHANISMS INVOLVED IN TOLERANCE INDUCTION AND MAINTENANCE

The properties of the various mechanisms are summarized in Table 9.2.

Clonal Deletion

During ontogeny, pluripotent stem cells migrate to the thymus and become thymocytes, which potentially are capable of differentiating into mature T cells. However, only a small percentage of thymocytes actually survive intrathymic development and fully mature into immunocompetent T cells. This is the result of two processes, termed positive and negative selection. Positive selection refers to those events through which only those T cells that recognize self MHC are allowed to survive (50). These T cells recognizing self MHC class II or class I molecules become CD4$^+$ or CD8$^+$ cells, respectively. Through a sequence of events called negative selection, these T cells migrate to the thymic medulla, where those T cells that bind strongly to self peptide MHC complexes presented by stromal cells are eliminated (50). In this manner, only T cells that are capable of recognizing self MHC molecules reach the periphery, but those T cells with exceptionally avid autoreactivity (i.e., potential autoaggressive T cells) are physically deleted from the T-cell repertoire.

Clonal Anergy and Activation-Induced Cell Death

Because thymic stromal cells lack many important tissue-specific autoantigens, clonal deletion of potential autoaggressive T cells in the thymus is incomplete. Studies with

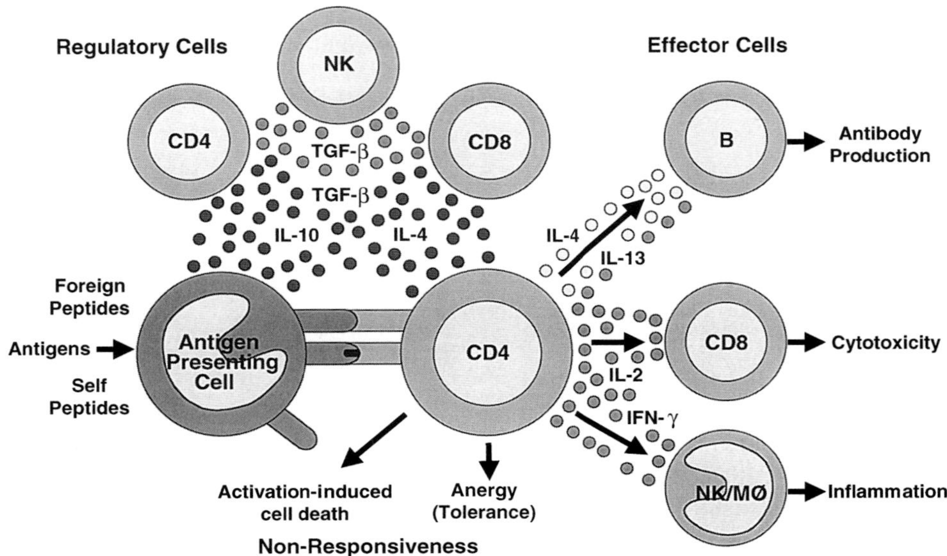

FIGURE 9.1. Development of immunity, autoimmunity, or tolerance. T cells respond to antigen by either becoming activated or anergic (nonresponsive). Upon presentation of foreign peptides, CD4+ T cells become activated and produce cytokines that provide help for antibody production or the induction of cell-mediated immunity. By contrast, self antigens generally induce anergy. Autoimmune diseases such as systemic lupus erythematosus (SLE) develop when tolerance is broken and self-reactive T cells become activated. Activation requires a second, co-stimulatory signal in addition to antigen recognition. Regulatory T cells maintain tolerance to self antigens by blocking co-stimulatory signals. CD4+ and CD8+ regulatory cells inhibit other T cells by producing immunosuppressive cytokines. Besides its immunosuppressive effects, transforming growth factor-β (TGF-β) co-stimulates activated CD4+ and CD8+ T cells to become regulatory cells. Natural killer (NK) cells can serve as an immediate source of the active form of TGF-β. Self tolerance is also maintained by activation-induced apoptosis. This is a feedback regulatory mechanism that serves to maintain the total numbers of T cells relatively constant.

TABLE 9.2. MECHANISMS INVOLVED IN TOLERANCE INDUCTION AND MAINTENANCE

Mechanism	Site	Comment
Clonal deletion	Thymus and periphery	Not all potentially autoaggressive T cells are deleted from the repertoire; in the periphery these cells are deleted by activation induced cell death.
Clonal anergy	Thymus and periphery	T cells that recognize self peptides (signal 1) without the required co-stimulatory signal (signal 2) become nonresponsive; clonal anergy is reversible
Regulatory cells	Periphery	Several subsets, which include CD4+, CD8+, and NKT cells; prevent autoimmunity by blocking critical co-stimulatory signals for T-cell activation
Clonal ignorance	Periphery	Immunologically dormant, self-reactive T cells Infectious agents bearing antigens cross reactive with self can activate these T cells Regulatory cells normally prevent the activation of these T cells

NKT, natural killer T cells.

transgenic mice have revealed that some potentially autoaggressive T cells do physically exist, but they are rendered anergic (i.e., immunologically nonresponsive) (11,51) in the periphery. T cells require at least two signals to proliferate or develop effector function: specific antigen (signal 1), and a critical co-stimulatory signal (signal 2). If T cells bind antigen in the absence of proper co-stimulatory signals, they have two possible outcomes. First, they may undergo a series of events that prevents them from becoming activated by antigen at a later time (52); this is called clonal anergy. Alternatively, they may proliferate briefly but then undergo apoptosis; this is called activation-induced cell death (53). Because anergic cells physically persist, this nonresponsiveness can be reversed by certain cytokines, such as IL-2 (54). Thus, bystander autoreactive, anergic T cells may be converted into fully competent, autoaggressive T cells that are capable of promoting an autoimmune response if, by chance, these anergic cells come in close proximity to other cells producing IL-2 in response to some unrelated foreign antigen.

Clonal Ignorance

T cells with low-affinity receptors for organ-specific self antigens (i.e., thyroid, pancreatic islet cell) may escape both clonal deletion and clonal anergy. Transgenic mouse models of autoimmune disease have revealed the existence of competent T cells that are specific for self peptides and that under normal physiologic conditions fail to react with these self peptides. Following a microbial infection, however, these cells can possibly become activated and initiate autoimmunity (55).

Regulatory T Cells

Professional regulatory T cells comprise a third mechanism to control the activation of potentially autoaggressive T cells and maintain tolerance to self antigens. During the past few years considerable progress has been made in identifying regulatory T cell subsets and learning how to induce T cells to develop regulatory activity. While formerly most attention was given to $CD8^+$ suppressor T cells, it is now clear that subsets of $CD4^+$ cells also develop marked downregulatory activity. In addition to conventional $CD4^+$ and $CD8^+$ T cells, the thymus produces potent regulatory T cells that appear during the early neonatal period (56). Some are $CD4^+$ cells that also express IL-2 receptor α chains (CD25) (57), and others also express NK cell markers (58). These T-cell subsets have critical protective regulatory effects since neonatal thymectomy leads to a generalized multiorgan autoimmune disease (56,57). Thus, autoreactive T cells previously believed to be "ignorant" are continuously held in check by small numbers of naturally occurring regulatory T cells.

Other $CD4^+$ cells that produce TGF-β and IL-10 have been called Th3 cells. These T cells prevent autoimmune disease in mice and probably have a similar role in humans. They can be generated by oral administration of antigen. In addition to well-described immunosuppressive effects, TGF-β co-stimulates immature T cells to become regulatory cells. $CD8^+$ T cells activated in the presence of TGF-β suppress antibody production (49), and peripheral $CD4^+$ cells activated in the presence of this cytokine develop the phenotype and suppressive effects of the thymus-derived $CD25^+$ regulatory subset (59). The need for TGF-β in the development of regulatory T cells is shown in Fig. 9.1. IL-10 also has a role in the induction of regulatory T cells. $CD4^+$ cells repeatedly stimulated with IL-10 become anergic and develop strong suppressive activity (60).

Another mechanism to block tissue injury caused by activated Th1 cells is by "immune deviation." By slightly altering the antigen or the way it is presented, Th2 rather than Th1 cells are activated, and these cells produce anti-inflammatory cytokines. In this case, Th2 lymphocytes act like regulatory T cells.

Development of Immunity, Autoimmunity, or Tolerance

Antigen recognition by peripheral T cells can have two very different outcomes. The first is activation and differentiation to become effector cells. The second is to become anergic or nonresponsive to further stimulation. These two pathways are shown in Fig. 9.1. Whether T cells become activated or anergic following interaction with the APCs is determined by many factors, which include the peptide fragment presented by MHC molecules, the duration of antigen exposure, the strength of co-stimulation, and the cytokine milieu.

T cells are activated by foreign antigens. Immunogenic peptides are presented to T cells by professional APCs such as macrophages or dendritic cells. The interaction of T cells with these APCs results in the co-stimulatory signals needed for activation. These include ligation of CD28 on the T-cell surface by CD80 (B7.1) or CD86 (B7.2) expressed by the APCs (61,62). Other pairs of co-stimulatory molecules include CD2 with CD58 (LFA-3) or CD59, CD40 ligand (CD154) with CD40, and CD11a [lymphocyte function-associated antigen-1 (LFA-1)] with CD54 [intercellular adhesion molecule-1 (ICAM-1)]. Cytokines such as IL-2, IL-4, IL-12, and TNF-α can provide co-stimulatory signals to antigen-activated T cells.

By contrast, T cells are rendered tolerant or anergic by self antigens. In this case, T-cell binding of a self peptide is not accompanied by an activating co-stimulatory signal. Regulatory $CD4^+$ $CD25^+$ T cells can block co-stimulatory signals. Anergic $CD4^+$ T cells cannot produce IL-2, and anergic $CD8^+$ T cells cannot develop IL-2 receptors (57).

Regulatory T cells also express CD152 (CTLA-4), which, like CD28, also binds CD80 and CD86, but transduces strongly inhibitory signals.

ANTIGEN RECOGNITION BY T CELLS IN SLE

Tolerance Induction

Studies of mouse models of SLE suggest that T-cell tolerance induction is intact. Clonal deletion of self-reactive T cells is normal in two models of SLE (63–66). Deletion of T cells stimulated with superantigen is also intact (65). Since New Zealand black/white (NZB/W) F1 mice are resistant to tolerance induction following administration of soluble antigens (67), the development of peripheral clonal anergy may be abnormal. In a recent study, however, T-cell tolerance induction in B/W mice carrying a transgene encoding beef insulin was completely normal (68). In human SLE, short-term T-cell lines were resistant to anergy induction. This resistance was associated with increased expression of CD40L and persistent activation of one particular mitogen-activated protein kinase, extracellular signal-regulated kinase (ERK) (69) (Table 9.3).

Antigen Specificities of Autoreactive T Cells

Although SLE is characterized by anti-DNA antibodies, native mammalian DNA is a poor immunogen. Even purified denatured DNA that is complexed to an immunogenic carrier protein does not induce antibodies to native DNA (70,71). Bacterial DNA, however, can induce anti–double-stranded DNA (dsDNA) antibodies in nonimmune mice (72), and DNA-protein complexes can trigger pathogenic anti-DNA antibodies in SLE. DNA that is bound to histone or complexed to other proteins is in fact a common target of autoantibodies in SLE (73,74). Anti-DNA antibodies that are similar to those detected in human SLE have been raised in nonautoimmune mice immunized with a human DNA-protein complex that is present at high levels in the circulation of patients with SLE (75).

It has become evident that nucleosomes are the principal immunogen for autoantibodies that cause lupus nephritis (70,76–78) (Table 9.3). Conformational epitopes on native chromatin and the (H2A-H2B)2-DNA subnucleosome induce specific antibodies, which then spread in a stepwise manner to include IgG antihistone and antinative DNA antibodies (5,77), which may be complement fixing. Nucleosomes typically express cationic residues that bind to complementary-charged domains of TCRs that are expressed by autoreactive T cells (78,79). Thus, the epitopes that T cells recognize are peptide fragments of the proteins that are complexed with DNA or histones in nucleosomes.

The critical peptide epitopes from the core histones of the nucleosome particle that stimulate autoreactive helper T cells in human SLE have been identified. $CD4^+$ T cells from lupus patients recognize peptides from histone regions H2B, H4, and H3. At least two peptides from the H2A and H4 were recurrently recognized by autoreactive T cells from different lupus patients (80). Since lupus T-helper cells do not respond to free histones, the immunogenic peptides are generally not processed and presented by APCs. To identify these "cryptic" peptides, 154 peptides spanning the entire length of core histone were tested. The peptides that stimulate human helper cells overlapped with the major epitopes for the T-helper cells that induce anti-DNA antibodies in lupus-prone mice (80).

T-Cell Lines and Clones

Unlike most peptide antigens, the nucleosomal epitopes do not obey the rule of MHC-restriction. Nucleosomal epitopes can be presented and recognized in the context of diverse MHC alleles. As stated above, the immunogenic peptides and the lupus TCRs bear reciprocally charged residues that result in high-affinity interactions between the α chain of lupus TCRs and the APCs. Approximately half of cloned human lupus T helper cells responded to nucleosomal antigens that contained cationic residues (78). The CDR3 loops of TCR α chains contained a recurrent motif of anionic residues, whereas the TCR β chains contained both anionic and cationic residues in their CDR3, suggesting that these pathogenic clones probably recognize autoantigens with epitopes of mixed charges (79).

Cytokines produced by autoreactive SLE T-helper cell lines or clones stimulated with immunogenic histone peptides have been identified. Some peptides preferentially induced a strong Th1 (IFN-γ) response, while others favored Th2 (IL-10 and/or IL-4) production (80). Another group found that most autoreactive Th clones secreted IL-

TABLE 9.3. ANTIGEN RECOGNITION IN SYSTEMIC LUPUS ERYTHEMATOSUS (SLE)

- Defect in tolerance induction associated with increased expression of CD40L
- Core histones in nucleosomes are the principal immunogens for anti-DNA autoantibodies that cause lupus nephritis
- Peptides from pathogenic anti-DNA autoantibodies can stimulate autoreactive T-helper cells
- T-helper cells for autoantibody production are derived from $CD4^+$ and NKT$\alpha\beta$ and $\gamma\delta$ $CD4^-$ $CD8^-$ (double negative) T cells

2, IFN-γ, and IL-4, whereas some produced predominantly IL-2 and IFN-γ (81). Notwithstanding the characteristic B-cell hyperactivity and impaired cell-mediated immunity in SLE, these studies indicate that it is an oversimplification to consider SLE as a Th2 cytokine disease.

Nonnucleosomal peptides can also stimulate the autoreactive lupus T cells that provide help for pathogenic anti-DNA antibodies. Several peptides immunogenic for T cells derived from the VH region of a pathogenic anti-DNA antibody have been identified. Immunization of NZB/W F1 mice with either of three specific VH peptides increased anti-DNA levels, accelerated nephritis, and decreased survival. T cells that are immunized with these peptides produced either a Th1 or Th2 profile of cytokines, but adoptive transfer of either of these T cells accelerated disease (82).

These immunogenic, VH region peptides can stimulate autoreactive T cells to provide help for a variety of B cells displaying a cross-reactive version of the original immunogen, a form of determinant spreading. This reciprocal T-B-cell stimulation spreads until large cohorts of T and B cells have expanded (82). Presumably, similar spreading occurs in human SLE.

Human T-cell clones generated from the peripheral blood mononuclear cells (PBMCs) of patients with SLE or mixed connective tissue disease (MCTD) were found to react against uridine-rich, RNA-small nuclear ribonucleoprotein (snRNP) antigen. Similar clones, however, were produced from MHC genotype-matched normal controls. These were oligoclonal CD4$^+$ memory cells (83). A proliferative response to a ribosomal P fusion protein has been reported (84), notwithstanding the impaired response of SLE T cells to soluble antigens.

Another approach to identify previously activated autoreactive T cells in SLE has been to take advantage of the increased mutation rate of cells that have undergone frequent cell division *in vivo*. The frequency of these mutant T cells increases with the degree of immunologic stimulation, as reflected by the overall magnitude of disease, the number of flares, and the presence of photosensitive skin rash. Mutations were found in CD4$^+$, CD8$^+$, and the minor CD3$^+$ CD4$^-$ CD8$^-$ populations. When these T cells were cloned, a substantial number were able to provide help for autologous B cells to produce anti–single-stranded DNA (ssDNA) (85,86).

As discussed, T-cell recognition of and response to both foreign and self antigens is determined by the class I and II MHC gene products of the host. T-cell cytokine production and subsequent helper activity, therefore, is influenced by the expression of MHC alleles on APCs. For example, expression of HLA-DR3 is associated with decreased production of IL-1 and IL-2 (87); expression of HLA-DR2 and DQw1 correlates with elevated anti-dsDNA autoantibody titers, decreased production of TNF-α *in vitro*, and lupus nephritis (88); and expression of both HLA-DR3 and DQw2 correlates with detectable anti-Ro/SSA and anti-La/SSB antibodies (89,90).

Drugs also can induce lupus syndromes by causing DNA damage and releasing altered nucleosomes (77) in addition to inhibiting DNA methylation (91–93). Studies of apoptotic keratinocytes have revealed blebs containing nucleosomes and spliceosomes, which bear most of the predominant SLE autoantigens (94,95). These structures are subject to oxidative modification. Following phagocytosis and processing by APCs, the altered epitopes may be rendered strongly immunogenic for nontolerant CD4$^+$ T cells.

T CELLS AND NK CELLS IN SLE

Percentage and Absolute Numbers of T-Cell Subsets

Decreased numbers of T, B, and NK cells are a common manifestation of active SLE (96–101). Most patients with active SLE have total lymphocyte counts of less than 1,000 cells/mm^3. Because of the relative decrease of lymphocytes in SLE in comparison to monocytes, the percentage of CD3$^+$ T cells often is decreased in mononuclear cell preparations. The apparent percentage of T cells may be further decreased by the contamination of immature granulocytes that copurify with mononuclear cells in patients with active disease.

Within the context of T-cell lymphopenia, certain T-cell subsets may be affected more than others in SLE. Early reports indicated a relative decrease in CD8$^+$ cells in SLE (102,103). One group indicated that patients with sicca syndrome, central nervous system (CNS) disease, lung disease, and muscle disease exhibit increased CD4/CD8 ratios (104). Other studies have indicated that the relative percentage of CD8$^+$ cells is either normal or increased, and that CD4$^+$ cells often are decreased in active SLE (105,106). In such cases, the decrease in CD4$^+$ cells results in an abnormally low CD4/CD8 ratio, a finding that frequently is observed in patients with severe lupus nephritis (104,107). Corticosteroid therapy preferentially decreases CD4$^+$ cells and thus decreases the CD4/CD8 ratio (105). Decreased CD4$^+$ cells correlate with antilymphocyte antibodies (ALAs) that are specifically reactive against this T-cell subset (108,109), and a strong relationship exists between high titers of ALAs, lymphopenia, and disease activity (96,109,110). Within the CD4$^+$ and CD8$^+$ T-cell subsets, CD28$^+$ cells are decreased in SLE (111,112).

In addition to alterations in the number or percentage of CD4$^+$ cells, an association between SLE and expression of a genetically determined variant of the CD4$^+$ molecule in Jamaican blacks has been described (113,114). Whether expression of this variant CD4 molecule truly predisposes certain individuals to develop SLE or simply acts as a marker for some other SLE-predisposing factor remains unknown at present.

NK Cells

Both the percentage and the absolute numbers of NK cells generally are decreased in patients with active SLE. The percentages of $CD16^+$ cells are decreased (115–118), and the percentages of $CD3^-CD11b^+$ lymphocytes also are decreased (117). In patients with inactive SLE, values for NK cells usually are normal. In comparison to normal donors, patients with SLE have decreased NK cytotoxic activity; the decrease tends to be more pronounced in more active patients (119–124). Decreased NK activity may be explained by decreased percentages of NK cells. However, since the numbers of lymphocytes binding NK-sensitive targets are comparable between normal donors and patients with SLE (121), it is more likely that NK cells in patients with active SLE have an impaired capacity to lyse target cells. Antibody-dependent cellular cytotoxicity mediated by CD16 is also decreased in SLE (125–128).

The mechanism(s) responsible for decreased cytotoxic activity of NK cells in SLE are unknown. Serum factors such as immune complexes or ALAs could possibly account for this defect, at least in part. Serum from lupus patients can contain high levels of both immune complexes and ALAs. Immune complexes have been shown to suppress or decrease NK cytotoxic activity (120,124,129). Several groups have reported that incubation with serum from patients with SLE followed by treatment with complement greatly decreased NK cytotoxic activity (119,123,124). The inability of serum alone to decrease NK activity suggests that immune complexes were not involved. Whether the ALAs are specific for NK cells is unknown. One study demonstrated that serum from patients with SLE plus complement did kill a substantial number of NK cells (123). In this study, preincubation of the serum with T lymphocytes removed the cytotoxic activity, suggesting that the antibodies were not NK cell specific. However, another study described the presence of autoantibodies that were specific for CD16 (130). There are ALAs in SLE that react with a variety of cell surface structures, some of which may have the potential to react with NK cells specifically or to prevent mediation of full functional activity.

As stated above, the combination of NK cells and $CD8^+$ cells suppresses T-cell–dependent antibody production in healthy individuals. In SLE, however, the effect is the opposite. NK cells and $CD8^+$ cells added separately together enhance IgG production (131). This is probably because of defective production of TGF-β by NK cells in SLE (132).

The significance of the NK cells' role in the suppression of antibody production has been demonstrated in several murine models of SLE. With certain strain combinations, the injection of parental spleen cells into F1 hybrid mice can result in the development of a lupus-like disease with autoantibody production. An inverse correlation was found between the levels of anti-dsDNA antibody and both the number and function of NK cells (133). The significance of this observation was shown by the reduction of autoimmunity through procedures that elevate NK activity and the exacerbation of symptoms by depleting the animals of NK cells. Similarly, it has been reported that development of autoimmunity in C56BL/6 *lpr* mice correlated with the disappearance of NK cells (134). In a more recent study of C57BL/6 *lpr* mice, the onset of autoimmunity correlated with the disappearance of a distinct population of cells that expressed the phenotype of NK cells but that also expressed TCRs (135). Taken together, these studies suggest that NK cells have an important role in the regulation of antibody production *in vivo*.

$CD4^-$ $CD8^-$ (Double-Negative) and NKT Cells

In addition to almost all $CD4^+$ and $CD8^+$ T cells, which are restricted to protein MHC class I and II molecules (see above), a small percentage of T cells recognize glycolipid determinants in association with CD1. These cells express the NK cell markers such as CD56 or NKR-P1 and are called NKT cells. Most but not all of these cells lack CD4 and CD8 and have been called double-negative (DN) cells. Increased percentages of DN T cells have been reported in SLE. Moreover, cloning these cells revealed that some αβ and γδ cells could provide help for autoantibody production (3,19). These observations have been confirmed and extended. Two groups reported an increase in the DN subset in Caucasian and Japanese populations (136,137), although another could not find a significant increase in Chinese patients with SLE. One group reported an increase in the γδ subset (138).

As the case for NKT cells, SLE DN T-cell clones are restricted by CD1c (137,137a). The DN T cells were stimulated by CD1c on B cells and could provide help for IgG production. Whereas in healthy subjects they produced only IFN-γ, in SLE they produced both IFN-γ and IL-4. Interestingly, in active SLE, they produced high levels of IFN-γ. Another group reported that DN T cells in SLE produced IL-4 (138a).

Besides helper activity, certain subsets of DN or NKT cells possess potent suppressive effects. A small subset that bears an invariant Vα24JαQ TCR is one example. These T cells are decreased in the affected sibling of identical twins discordant for autoimmune diabetes, and marked changes in gene expression have been reported in T-cell clones from these twin pairs (139). There is one report of decreased Vα24JαQ-positive T cells in a Japanese SLE population (140). Decreased percentages of the NKT γδ subset also been reported with an inverse correlation with disease activity (141). γδ T cells have been proposed to have an important role in mediating self tolerance (141a). Thus, although NK T cells are present in only small numbers, different subsets may have important effects in the pathogenesis of SLE.

Naive and Memory T Lymphocyte Subsets

CD4+ T cells with the naive phenotype (i.e., CD45RA+) were reported to be decreased in SLE (142–144). Because serum from patients with SLE contain autoantibodies against CD45RA, it was suggested that this subset was deleted (145,146). However, decreased CD45RA+ cells and a proportionate increase in CD45RO+ cells could reflect T-cell activation *in vivo* with the expected increase in the activated state. Alternately, this shift and the characteristic lymphopenia of lupus could reflect impaired generation and export of naive T cells by the thymus.

T-Cell Apoptosis

Since it was reported that lymphocytes isolated from patients with SLE undergo spontaneous apoptosis in culture at a faster rate than lymphocytes from normal or rheumatoid arthritis control subjects do (147), there has been considerable interest in this area. Most reports confirm increased apoptosis (148–152), with one exception (153). Although one group correlated increased apoptosis with disease activity (147), this was not confirmed in another study (150). Increased T-cell apoptosis does not appear to be specific for SLE, but occurs in other vasculitides (148,149,152). In addition to T cells undergoing cell death, there is also evidence of increased apoptosis of monocytes and neutrophils in SLE (153–155). Thus, increased apoptosis provides further evidence of increased activation of several hematopoietic cell types. Investigators have measured a panel of gene activation-induced gene products in SLE patients and did not find a difference with normal controls (152). However, this group and others have reported that levels of Bcl-2 are increased in SLE T cells and B cells (152,156–160). Bcl-2 is a proto-oncogene protein that protects cells from apoptosis. Enforced expression of Bcl-2 leads to enhanced cell survival and growth (161–163). Mice transgenic for Bcl-2 under the control of an Ig μ chain enhancer not only develop elevated numbers of B cells and serum Ig levels but also spontaneously develop autoantibodies and immune-complex glomerulonephritis (164). Thus, elevated expression of Bcl-2 in freshly isolated SLE peripheral blood lymphocytes could reflect the impaired demise of cells involved in the development of clinical autoimmunity. On the basis of these data, it has been proposed that the reason for the higher values of apoptotic cells in SLE is not because of increased numbers of cells undergoing cell death, but rather because of decreased clearance by phagocytic cells (165). Monocytes have been reported to protect T cells from undergoing apoptosis (166). There are several reasons, therefore, why one or more monocyte defects in SLE could contribute to increased percentages of apoptotic T cells.

Since certain strains of mice with defects in T-cell expression of Fas or Fas ligand develop a SLE-like disease, there has been a considerable interest in Fas expression in SLE. Fas-mediated cytotoxicity represents a major pathway leading to cell death (167–170) and is an important mechanism in peripheral tolerance. Mice that are homozygous for either *lpr*, a mutation in the Fas gene (171), or *gld*, a point mutation resulting in defective or absent Fas ligand expression (172–175), develop generalized lymphadenopathy in association with lupus-like features (176). These mice have impaired deletion of self-reactive B cells and expansion of autoreactive T cells (66,177). Conversely, Medical Research Laboratory (MRL)-*lpr*/*lpr* mice that are transgenic for the intact *Fas* gene under the control of a T-cell–specific CD2 promoter and enhancer do not develop the lymphadenopathy, glomerulonephritis, or clinical autoimmunity that their nontransgenic littermates do (178). Although Fas expression is not decreased in human SLE and actually may be increased (179,180), the potential ramifications of the observations in murine *lpr* and *gld* mice for human disease have been highlighted by an association in humans between Fas mutations and clinical autoimmunity and/or lymphadenopathy (181–183). Moreover, soluble Fas protein, which can inhibit apoptosis of stimulated cells under appropriate conditions, has been reported to be elevated in the serum of many patients with SLE (184,185), although this finding has been challenged (186,187).

Fas ligand (CD95L or CD178) expression by T cells plays an important role in triggering CD95-based apoptosis of CD95+ target cells. CD95-based cell death represents an essential regulatory pathway for activated T cells and, under certain circumstances, for activated B cells as well (188–197). Unfortunately, CD95 ligand surface expression is difficult to detect presumably due to its rapid cleavage from the cell surface by endogenous metalloproteinases. As a consequence, CD95 ligand has been usually measured at the messenger RNA (mRNA) level, an approach that may not accurately reflect surface CD95 ligand expression. One group reported that CD95 ligand surface expression by *in vitro*–activated SLE T cells is increased (198), raising the possibility that elevated CD95 ligand expression contributes to the increased *ex vivo* apoptosis of SLE lymphocytes and the *in vivo* lymphopenia (199–201). Regulation and kinetics of CD95 ligand expression are topics of intense active research, and we anticipate that important insights will be garnered during the next few years regarding the role of CD95 ligand dysregulation in SLE.

ABNORMALITIES OF T CELL FUNCTION IN SLE

In the early 1970s, workers from several laboratories reported that patients with active SLE responded poorly to intradermal injected skin-test antigens (202–205). This observation was followed by numerous reports of impaired T-cell proliferative responses to mitogens, to soluble antigens, and to MHC class II antigens on both allogeneic or autologous APCs. Generation of antigen-specific, cytolytic T cells also was found to be decreased. A partial summary of T-cell functional defects is presented in Table 9.4.

TABLE 9.4. T LYMPHOCYTE FUNCTIONAL ACTIVITIES *IN VITRO*

Function	Activity
Proliferation	
Mitogenic lectins	Decreased or normal
Anti-CD3	Decreased or normal[a]
Anti-CD2	Decreased
Soluble antigens	Decreased
Allogeneic mixed lymphocyte reaction	Decreased
Autologous mixed lymphocyte reaction	Markedly decreased
Response to IL-2	Decreased or normal
Helper cell activity	
Nonspecific	Decreased or normal
Antigen specific	Decreased
Suppressor cell activity	
ConA induced	Decreased or normal
Antigen specific	Decreased
Spontaneous inhibitors of IL-2 production	Increased
Cytotoxic cell activity	
In response to allogeneic or xenogeneic antigens	Decreased
In response to hapten-modified antigens	Increased
In response to anti-CD3	Decreased
In response to IL-2	Decreased

[a]When isolated T cells are used instead of peripheral blood mononuclear cells (PBMCs), the response to αCD3 is normal or increased.
ConA, concanavalin A; IL-2, interleukin-2.

Decreased T-Cell Proliferation to Mitogens and Antigens and Mechanisms to Explain This Effect

Decreased proliferative responses of SLE blood leukocytes or mononuclear cells to mitogenic lectins [i.e., phytohemagglutinin (PHA), concanavalin A (ConA), and pokeweed mitogen] and soluble antigens have been reported by many workers (112,205–214). Similarly, T-cell responsiveness to both allogeneic and autologous lymphocytes is also decreased in SLE (215–219). However, some groups have reported normal T-cell proliferation in response to various activating agents (220–224).

The lack of uniformity of the findings of various investigators can be explained by differences in patient populations, disease activity, cell-preparation procedures, or culture conditions. The explanations for these T-cell defects can be grouped into three major categories. First, there is considerable evidence in SLE of T-cell activation *in vivo*. T cells subjected to constant stimulation become refractory to further stimulation. The second category includes various specific functional defects. Inherent defects in T-cell signaling need to be differentiated from defects in the interactions of T cells with APCs. Third, humoral factors such as autoantibodies or certain cytokines could be responsible for poorly responsive T cells. Each of these categories will be reviewed.

Increased Spontaneous T-Cell Activation In Vivo

Blood lymphocytes isolated from patients with active SLE exhibit numerous signs of activation *in vivo* (Table 9.5).

TABLE 9.5. EVIDENCE OF *IN VIVO* T-CELL ACTIVATION IN SUBJECTS WITH ACTIVE SLE

Increased expression of proliferating cell nuclear antigen in unstimulated T cells
High levels of circulating early apoptotic blood mononuclear cells
Increased levels of mRNA transcripts for interleukin-2 and c-rel (NF-kappa B) in unstimulated T cells
Increased cell surface expression in unstimulated T cells of MHC class II (HLA-DR, -DP) structures, Fas, Fas ligand, CTLA-4, and a modest increase in interleukin-2 receptors
Increased serum levels of soluble interleukin-2 receptors, tumor necrosis factor-α receptors (p55 and p75), soluble Fas, and soluble CD40L
Increased frequency of circulating T cells bearing somatic mutations as evidence of previous cell divisions

CTLA, cytotoxic T-lymphocyte associated; HLA, human leukocyte antigen; MHC, major histocompatibility complex; mRNA, messenger RNA; NF, nuclear factor.

Increased numbers of circulating T cells from these patients express proliferating cell nuclear antigen (i.e., cyclin) (225) and are proliferating spontaneously (226). Increased numbers of T cells have undergone somatic mutation (227,228), or are undergoing apoptosis (147–150). There is increased T-cell expression of MHC class II molecules (229–231), expression of IL-2 and *c-rel* [nuclear factor(NF)-κB] mRNA (232,233), release of soluble IL-2 receptors (234–238), TNF receptors (239–243), and CD40 ligand (244) into the serum (Table 9.5). Polyclonal T-cell activation is an integral component of murine SLE (245).

Defects in Expression of Co-Stimulatory and Effector Surface Molecules

While mitogens bind the TCR and accessory molecules, anti-CD3 binds only to the CD3/TCR. Although CD3/TCR-mediated proliferation of purified T cells in SLE ranges from normal to enhanced (222–224), accessory cell-dependent, CD3/TCR-mediated proliferation in unfractionated PBMC cultures is often abnormally low in SLE (214,217,246). This suggests that T-cell–accessory-cell interactions in SLE may be impaired. Several pairs of receptor/co-receptor pairs on T cells and accessory cells that are crucial to T-cell co-stimulation have been identified, including CD2/CD58 (LFA-3), CD11a (LFA-1)/CD54 (ICAM-1), and CD28 or CD152 (CTLA-4)/CD80 (B7-1) or CD86 (B7-2). Blockade with specific monoclonal antibody (mAb) or soluble fusion proteins of the receptor/co-receptor interactions can inhibit T-cell proliferation, T-cell–dependent B-cell differentiation, and/or induction of T-cell cytolytic activity (247–255).

Of note, expression of CD11a and CD54 is increased in SLE (91,256), and increased T cell CD11a expression has been associated with development of autoreactivity (91). On the other hand, expression of CD80 and CD86 following activation is decreased in SLE (256–258). CD80-delivered signals to SLE T cells do result in normal enhancement in anti-CD3–induced T-cell proliferation (259), but the role of CD86-delivered signals in SLE remains to be determined.

The proliferative response to anti-CD2 also is depressed (112,260). As was the case for anti-CD3, an accessory cell defect was documented in the majority of patients, because the defect disappeared following depletion of these cells. Most important, the addition of anti-CD28 also reversed the defect (112). Others have found that the co-stimulatory effect of anti-CD28 markedly enhanced the capacity of patients with active SLE lymphocytes to produce IL-2. (111). This defective proliferative response to anti-CD2 in SLE may be important, because signaling through this pathway selectively triggers the TGF-β–dependent suppressor-cell pathway (261).

Other T-cell surface antigens that are upregulated during the course of an immune response that play vital roles in T-cell helper function and T-cell cytolytic function are CD40 ligand (CD154) and CD95 (Fas) ligand, respectively. The interaction between CD40L and CD40 on the surface of B cells has many effects on B cells, which include a differentiation signal, rescuing them from apoptosis, or priming them for cell death (262—268). CD40L is transiently expressed by CD4$^+$ T cells soon after activation and is quickly downregulated, especially in the presence of B cells (269,270). This tight regulation of CD40 ligand expression presumably protects the host against induction of indiscriminate polyclonal B-cell differentiation by activated T-helper cells. CD40L is, in fact, hyperexpressed by both CD4$^+$ and CD8$^+$ T cells in SLE (271,272), and biologically active circulating soluble CD40L is increased in SLE (273). Clinical trials with an anti-CD40L monoclonal antibody have begun, which should help ascertain the role of dysregulated CD40L expression in the characteristic polyclonal hypergammaglobulinemia and elevated circulating autoantibody titers of SLE.

Defects in T-Cell Signaling Pathways

Intuitively, T-cell effector function is the culmination of an ordered sequence of specific intracellular biochemical processes. Subtle alterations in these processes may lead to loss of effector function or change in effector function. Several laboratories have demonstrated normal to enhanced CD3/T-cell antigen receptor (TCR)-mediated proliferation of purified T cells in SLE (222–224), whereas CD3/TCR-mediated generation of T-cell cytolytic activity in SLE is subnormal (103,274,275). This dissociation of normal T-cell proliferation from subnormal T-cell cytolytic activity in SLE strongly suggests that multiple chains of intracellular biochemical processes coexist in parallel. SLE T cells, upon activation, may trigger one chain of intracellular events, leading to a normal response for a certain T-cell parameter but may also trigger another chain of intracellular events leading to an abnormal response for a different T-cell parameter.

Physiologic activation of T cells begins with binding of ligand to the surface CD3/TCR complex. In SLE, T-cell expression of the TCR chain is impaired in a large percentage of patients (276–278) (Table 9.6). Mutations of the chain have been proposed to explain this finding (277). However, this defect could also be the consequence of prolonged T-cell activation since recovery of expression has been observed when the cells are rested (278). Given the reduced expression of this vital CD3/TCR component, it is not surprising that many CD3/TCR-triggered events in SLE are abnormal.

Although it may be naive to believe that a few biochemicals generated intracellularly can completely control T-cell fate, it is well established that certain such biochemicals (intracellular second messengers) are indeed crucial to ultimate T-cell responses. Binding of ligand to T-cell surface

TABLE 9.6. DEFECTS OF SIGNAL TRANSDUCTION IN SLE T LYMPHOCYTES

Abnormal intracellular free calcium concentrations
Decreased expression of CD3/T cell receptor ζ chain
Decreased expression of protein kinase C
Decreased activity of protein tyrosine phosphatase activity of CD45
Decreased protein kinase A type I and type II isoenzyme activity
Decreased levels of the p65-RelA subunit of the NF-κB nuclear transcription factor
Increased binding of the transcriptional inhibitor pCREM (cyclic AMP response element modifier) to the IL-2 promotor
Defective phosphorylation of Cbl, an adaptor protein that negatively regulates transmembrane signaling, which correlates with increased expression of CD40 ligand and resistance to tolerance induction

Cyclic AMP, 3′,5′-cyclic adenosine monophosphate.

CD3/TCR triggers a sequence of events leading to phospholipase C activation with hydrolysis of phosphatidylinositol-1,4-bisphosphate (PIP_2) to diacylglycerol (DAG) and inositol 1,4,5-trisphosphate (1,4,5-IP_3) (279). DAG is the physiologic activator of protein kinase C (PKC) (280), whereas 1,4,5-IP_3 promotes calcium mobilization from internal stores and, in T cells, may promote calcium influx across the plasma membrane as well (281). In addition to the role of PIP_2 hydrolysis in generating intracellular DAG, a major portion of intracellular DAG generation (leading to PKC activation) may also arise via hydrolysis of phosphatidylcholine (PC) (282,283).

Changes in intracellular free calcium concentration play a key role in T-cell activation. Elevations in intracellular free calcium levels through mobilization of intracellular stores may not generate the same functional consequences to the cell as elevations of intracellular free calcium through influx of extracellular calcium (284). Influx of exogenous calcium is critical, since depletion of extracellular calcium with chelating agents or pharmacologic blockade of calcium channels profoundly inhibits lymphocyte activation (285,286), and calcium chelators may affect gene expression and production of vital lymphokines such as IL-2 (287). In SLE, impaired calcium responses to PHA and anti-CD3 mAb in T-cell–enriched populations have been reported (288,289), as has increased calcium responses to anti-CD3 mAb (290). The reasons for the disparate results remain unclear at present.

Other early activation-associated biochemical events include activation of several protein tyrosine kinases such as $p56^{lck}$ and $p59^{fyn}$, activation of PKC, and generation of 3′,5′-cyclic adenosine monophosphate (cAMP). Activation of PKC is absolutely essential for IL-2 production (291), and inhibition of PKC activity correlates well with inhibition of T-cell proliferation (292). On the other hand, increased intracellular levels of cAMP correlate with inhibition of IL-2 production by, and proliferation of, T cells, presumably by activating protein kinase A (PKA) (293).

NF-κB activation is crucial to expression of many genes, and CD3/TCR-mediated activation of NK-κB is abnormal in T cells from patients with SLE but not in T cell from patients with rheumatoid arthritis (RA) (294). In addition, PKC activity in response to phorbol ester may be somewhat lower in SLE T cells than in normal T cells (295). Protein tyrosine phosphatase activity of surface CD45, vital to regeneration of substrates for activation-associated tyrosine kinases, is modestly reduced in SLE (296,297). Generation of intracellular cAMP levels in response to multiple different stimuli is impaired in SLE PBMC and T-cell–enriched populations (298,299), and PKA activity is abnormal in T cells from active SLE patients in comparison to T cells from either normal donors or patients with RA or Sjögren's syndrome (300). More recently, deficiencies in PKA type I and type II isozyme activities have each been described in SLE (301–303). Since PKA generally negatively affects membrane-based signaling events, impaired PKA activity in SLE may, at least in part, be responsible for some of those CD3/TCR-triggered events that are exaggerated in SLE. However, PKA-I-catalyzed protein phosphorylation also promotes growth and proliferation (304). In fact, transient transfection of SLE T cells with a plasmid vector carrying a construct for Riβ partially restored IL-2 production by activated T cells (305). Deficient PKA-I isozyme activity may contribute to the pathogenesis of SLE by hindering effective signal transduction and impairing T-cell effector functions (306).

Two important abnormalities of T-cell activation in SLE have recently been characterized. Increased binding of pCREM (phosphorylated cAMP response element modifier) to the IL-2 promoter may explain decreased IL-2 production. CREM is a transcriptional inhibitor of IL-2 gene activation (307). Increased levels of CREM bound to the IL-2 promoter was found in unstimulated T cells from patients with inactive disease. Second, a defect involving Cbl, an adapter protein that negatively regulates transmembrane immune signaling, may contribute to resistance in tolerance induction in SLE. Defective phosphorylation of Cbl correlated with persistent hyperexpression of CD40 ligand and resistance to anergy induced by immobilized anti-CD3 (69).

Serum Inhibitors of T-Cell Function

Factors extrinsic to the cells such as autoantibodies or nonantibody serum components can inhibit the T-cell proliferative response. SLE sera inhibit lymphocyte proliferation in response to mitogenic lectins (210,308–310), soluble antigens (311), and allogeneic (312–314) as well as autologous MHC antigens (213,315–317). These sera also block the generation of cytotoxic T cells (274) and interfere with antigen presentation by macrophages (318). Much of this inhibitory capacity can be ascribed to IgM and IgG antibodies, which react with various lymphocyte cell surface molecules. SLE ALAs react with activated lymphocytes more strongly than resting lymphocytes (311,319,320). IgG ALAs inhibit suppressor cell generation and activity (321–323). In addition, IgG ALAs inhibit mitogen- and mixed lymphocyte reaction (MLR)-induced proliferation (308,309,312,313,316,320,321) and preferentially inhibit the T-cell response to soluble antigens (311).

Although initially reported only to react with T-suppressor cells (321–323), ALAs react with both $CD4^+$ and $CD8^+$ cells (324,325) and may react preferentially with $CD4^+$ cells (326). Such autoantibodies may result in altered CD4/CD8 ratios, leading to altered immune function. In addition, IgM autoantibodies that are reactive with the membrane tyrosine phosphatase CD45 molecule have been described in SLE (327,328). These antibodies preferentially react with the high molecular weight CD45RA isoform that is expressed on naive T cells (23). Such autoantibodies may interfere with T-cell signal transduction. Autoantibodies against the MHC class I associated β_2-microglobulin (329) and MHC class II molecules (316) also have been described. Such autoantibodies could inhibit T-cell function by blocking cell-to-cell interactions.

In addition to ALAs, which were described in the 1980s, it was reported more recently that hyperactive B cells secrete TGF-β complexed to IgG, and these complexes inhibit macrophage and neutrophil function (330,331). Increased levels of IgG-TGF-β complexes have been found in lupus sera (331) and can explain, at least in part, some of the inhibitory effects of lupus sera on T-cell function.

Altered Cytokine Homeostasis

One consequence of active SLE, and a product of continuous immune stimulation, is elevated IL-10 production (332,333). IL-10 inhibits T-cell function by blocking the effects of APCs and T-cell function. Among the cytokines that are downregulated by IL-10 are IL-2, TNF-α, and IFN-γ (334–337). Each of these cytokines has been considered to have an important role in the generation of cytotoxic T cells and those that downregulate antibody production. This issue is discussed in detail in Chapter 10.

Overview of Explanations for Impaired T-Cell Proliferation

Each of the mechanisms discussed contributes to the impaired T-cell proliferative response in SLE. T-cell activation *in vivo*, an integral component of active disease, and the humoral inhibitory factors that are a consequence of disease activity probably play significant roles. In studies where T-cell reactivity in SLE under standard conditions and the effect of serum inhibitors was studied simultaneously, T-cell responsiveness to several mitogenic lectins was only mildly reduced in comparison with healthy controls. Serum from patients with active disease, however, markedly inhibited responsiveness (206,207,309). Although there is no consensus that decreased T-cell proliferation correlates with disease activity, in general T-cell defects in SLE are less severe when the disease is inactive.

Substantial progress has been made in characterizing several apparently inherited molecular defects of T-cell activation in SLE. These include defects in PKA (301–303,305,306), in the p65-RelA subunit of NF-κB (294), and in CREM expression (307). These inherent T-cell defects and the abnormalities in the expression of co-stimulatory and effector surface molecules described above contribute to abnormalities of T-cell function described below. However, each of the inherent T-cell defects cannot by itself account for the proliferative defect, since accessory cell-independent T-cell proliferation in response to anti-CD3 is normal.

T-Cell Cytolytic Activity

The importance of intact generation of T-cell cytolytic activity has long been appreciated by viral and tumor immunologists who have recognized the central role of cytotoxic T lymphocytes (CTLs) in ridding the host of infectious viruses and of incipient tumors. Although abnormalities in T-cell–dependent or T-cell–mediated cytolytic activity have been reported in SLE, including impaired pokeweed mitogen (PWM)-induced cytotoxicity (338), impaired generation of cytotoxic T cells against allogeneic or xenogeneic targets (274,339), and impaired anti-CD3–driven cytolytic activity (224,275), the relevance of these abnormalities to *in vivo* pathophysiology remained enigmatic.

However, there is also increasing evidence from both mice and humans that defects in generation of CTL responses (resulting in decreased target cell death and prolonged target cell survival) may be important not only in impaired clearance of unwanted pathogens and/or neoplasms but also in promoting autoimmunity in general and SLE in specific.

In a graft-versus-host (GVH) murine model, inoculation of (C57BL/6 [B6] × DBA/2 [DBA])F1 (B6D2F1) mice with T cells from one parental strain (B6) triggers an "immunosuppressive" disease (B6 GVH) without clinical autoimmune features, whereas inoculation of B6D2F1 recipients with T cells from the other parental strain (DBA) triggers an "immunostimulatory" disease (DBA GVH) with clinical features resembling SLE (340). This dramatic difference in clinical outcome occurs despite the fact that in either case the infused parental $CD4^+$ T-helper cells become polyclonally activated in response to foreign class II MHC antigens on the host cells. That is, the critical determinant of clinical outcome in this model is not based on differential activation of $CD4^+$ (helper) T cells.

Rather, the critical feature lies in the $CD8^+$ T-cell population. Of great importance, the number of anti-B6D2F1 CTL precursor cells (CTLp) is markedly lower in DBA T cells than in B6 T cells, and elimination of B6 $CD8^+$ T cells (presumably containing the relevant CTLp) prior to inoculation of the B6D2F1 recipients or administering perforin-deficient B6 T cells also results in "immunostimulatory" disease (340,341). These findings suggest that the development of an SLE-like illness requires not just the presence of polyclonally activated $CD4^+$ T cells (with presumed helper activity for autoantibody production) but also requires the absence of polyclonally activated $CD8^+$ CTLp that can effect "full" cytolytic function. Older studies of murine chronic GVH reactions also support this notion (342,343).

SLE patients, never having received foreign tissues, do not experience GVH reactions per se. Nevertheless, polyclonal T-cell activation leading to autoreactivity and help for autoantibody production could arise following exposure to environmental infectious agents. A compelling argument for the role of microbial superantigens (SAgs) (which, like anti-CD3 mAbs, activate T cells via surface CD3/TCR) in the triggering of polyclonal T-cell helper activity resulting in SLE has been offered (344). SAg can promote T-cell–dependent B-cell differentiation (345,346) as well as regulate antibody production, at least in part, by a mechanism involving $CD4^+$ and $CD8^+$ T-cell–mediated SAg-dependent killing of B-cell targets via a CD95-based pathway (347–349). Moreover, as has been documented for HIV (350) but likely also the case for other viruses, T cells, following their infection with certain viruses and incorporation of the viral genomes, can become potent unrestricted helpers for Ig production. In either of these two scenarios, T cells, under *in vivo* physiologic conditions, would be activated through antigen-independent processes, for which antigen-independent activation of T cells by anti-CD3 mAbs should be an excellent model. Thus, the observed *in vitro* defect in anti-CD3–driven CTL activity in SLE (224,275), which is caused by both non–T-cell and T-cell defects (351), may reflect *in vivo* defects in generating polyclonal CTL activity, resulting in dysregulated polyclonal T-cell helper activity and predisposing to the development of SLE. Indeed, the CTL defect in SLE is independent of disease activity and of immunosuppressive medications (275). Moreover, in monozygotic twins discordant for SLE, the defect is often detectable in the clinically healthy co-twins (352), suggesting that the CTL defect in SLE truly antedates onset of clinical disease.

The mechanisms responsible for impaired CTL activity in SLE are not well understood. The defect appears to be independent of Fas, TNF-α, TNF-β, and adenosine triphosphate (ATP), but is dependent on extracellular calcium and associated with low levels of perforin (353). Twin studies have revealed evidence of non–T cells contributing to impaired CTL activity. In five of seven monozygotic twin pairs studied, the addition of non–T cells from the SLE twin to T cells of the healthy co-twin appreciably diminished cytolytic responses (351).

T-Helper Cell Activity in SLE

T-helper cell activity *in vitro* induced by PWM is either decreased (15,354) or normal (355,356). T-helper cell activity induced by specific antigens is decreased in SLE. Unlike normal lymphocytes, SLE cells that are immunized *in vitro* with trinitrophenyl polyacrylamide beads were unable to generate antigen-specific, antibody-forming cells. SLE B cells responded when cocultured with normal T cells, but SLE T cells were unable to provide help for normal B cells (357). The ability of SLE T cells to support B-cell colony formation also is defective in SLE (358). Again, the failure of SLE T cells to respond normally to mitogens or antigens may be explained by the fact that *in vivo* activated T cells respond poorly to subsequent *in vitro* stimulation. Alternatively, aberrant regulatory cells that are generated by chronic antigenic stimulation *in vivo* may inhibit T-cell activation *in vitro* (359). Importantly, the T-cell helper defect in SLE may not prevent the development of essential memory responses. Although primary antibody responses may be depressed, secondary responses are normal (360,361).

Regulatory T-Cell Activity

In addition to cytotoxic T cells that can downregulate antibody production, professional regulatory T cells formerly called suppressor T cells have this function. In the past, numerous investigators reported a defect of this T-cell function in SLE (321,362–374). Formerly, suppressor activity was generated *in vitro* by culturing mononuclear cells with ConA, and the effects of these activated T cells on other lymphocytes were determined. While the biologic significance of ConA suppressor cells was questioned, evidence for functionally significant regulatory T cells has been accumulating for many years. In SLE, one group analyzed DNA-induced antibody synthesis in a pair of identical twins who were discordant for SLE; only B cells from the SLE co-twin could produce anti-DNA antibodies. Addition of the SLE co-twin's T cells to her own B cells promoted anti-DNA antibody production induced by calf thymus DNA. On the other hand, T cells from the unaffected co-twin did not promote anti-DNA antibody synthesis unless $CD8^+$ cells were depleted. This finding suggested that the healthy co-twin had anti-DNA specific T-helper cells, but that they were kept nonfunctional by $CD8^+$ suppressor cells (18). The more recent finding that autoreactive T cells are continuously held in check by regulatory $CD4^+$ $CD25^+$ regulatory T cells has been comprehensively reviewed (57). These studies and the recent description of both $CD4^+$ and $CD8^+$ T cells that produce inhibitory cytokines such as TGF-β has revitalized interest in suppressor T cells.

Although the combination of $CD8^+$ cells and NK cells inhibits IgG synthesis in healthy subjects, this is not the case in SLE. The addition of NK cells and $CD8^+$ cells separately or together enhances IgG production (131). This is because in SLE the cross-talk between $CD8^+$ and NK cells does not induce the latter to produce the active form of TGF-β. This cytokine serves as a critical co-stimulatory factor for the generation of regulatory $CD8^+$ T cells (49,375, 376). Importantly, constitutive production of active TGF-β by NK cells is decreased in SLE (132). Mitogen-induced production of both the latent form and active TGF-β is also decreased in SLE. The former is decreased only in patients with active disease, but decreased production of active TGF-β does not correlate with disease activity (377). Mitogen-stimulated lymphocyte production of active TGF-β is also much less in patients with SLE than in those with rheumatoid arthritis. Thus, lymphocytes from patients with SLE have a decreased capacity to secrete the latent form TGF-β and a decreased ability to convert the latent precursor to its active form.

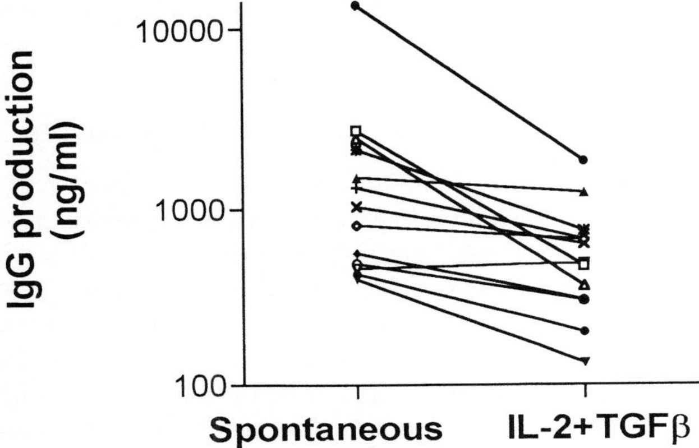

FIGURE 9.2. Cytokine-mediated suppression of spontaneous B-cell activity in SLE. Unstimulated peripheral blood mononuclear cells from patients with active SLE were cultured with the indicated cytokines for 72 hours, washed, and cultured for an additional 7 days. The combination of interleukin-2 (IL-2) and TGF-β inhibited immunoglobulin G (IgG) production, especially in those with very high values. IgG synthesis in healthy controls was generally less than 0.5 μg/mL. (From Ohtsuka K, Gray JD, Quismorio FP Jr, et al. Cytokine mediated down-regulation of B cell activity in SLE: effects of interleukin 2 and transforming growth factor beta. *Lupus* 1999;8:95–102.)

IL-2 and TGF-β are needed to induce $CD8^+$ T cells to become suppressor cells, and production of both of these cytokines is decreased in SLE. Studies using these cytokines to restore T-cell suppressive activity in human SLE have been encouraging. Briefly exposing blood mononuclear cells from patients with active SLE to IL-2 and TGF-β markedly reduced polyclonal IgG and antinucleoprotein antibody production (Fig. 9.2). $CD8^+$ T cells needed to be present for these inhibitory effects (378). These studies suggest that T cells from SLE patients retain the potential to downregulate antibody production and can regain this function with proper cytokine conditioning.

THE ROLE OF T CELLS IN THE INITIATION OF SLE

A proposed sequence of events leading to SLE is outlined in Table 9.7.

Genetic Factors

Genetic factors predispose certain individuals to develop SLE. In mouse lupus, chromosomal loci have been identified that affect T-cell activation, differentiation, and cell death (379). Genes shape the T-cell repertoire and regulate the antigens that are presented to T cells. In human SLE, a genome-wide scan has revealed linkage with SLE susceptibility in at least nine chromosomal loci (380). One of these sites is in the MHC region on chromosome 6. Others have reported separate loci that encode Bcl-2 and IL-10 that act synergistically to increase susceptibility (381). Individuals with inherited deficiencies of early complement components have an increased susceptibility to SLE. C1, C4, and C2 are needed to clear immune complexes and apoptotic cells from the circulation (382). Patients with lupus who possess HLA-DR2/DQw1 have low TNF-α production and increased susceptibility to develop nephritis within the first 5 years after diagnosis (88).

As stated earlier, $CD8^+$ lymphocytes have an impaired ability to become killer cells in SLE (224,275). Indeed, the CTL defect in SLE is independent both of disease activity and of immunosuppressive medications (275). Moreover, as discussed, in monozygotic twins who are discordant for SLE, the defect often is detectable in the clinically healthy co-twins (352), raising the possibility that the CTL defect in SLE may be inherited. These individuals may have an increased risk of developing SLE if they are exposed to one or more inciting environmental factors.

The genes encoding many IgM anti-IgG and low-affinity, cross-reactive nuclear autoantibodies are transcribed directly from the germline and are highly conserved in phylogeny. It has been proposed that the role of B cells with surface IgM anti-IgG may be to capture immune complexes bearing infectious agents, thus serving as APCs for T cells

TABLE 9.7. INITIATION OF SYSTEMIC LUPUS ERYTHEMATOSUS

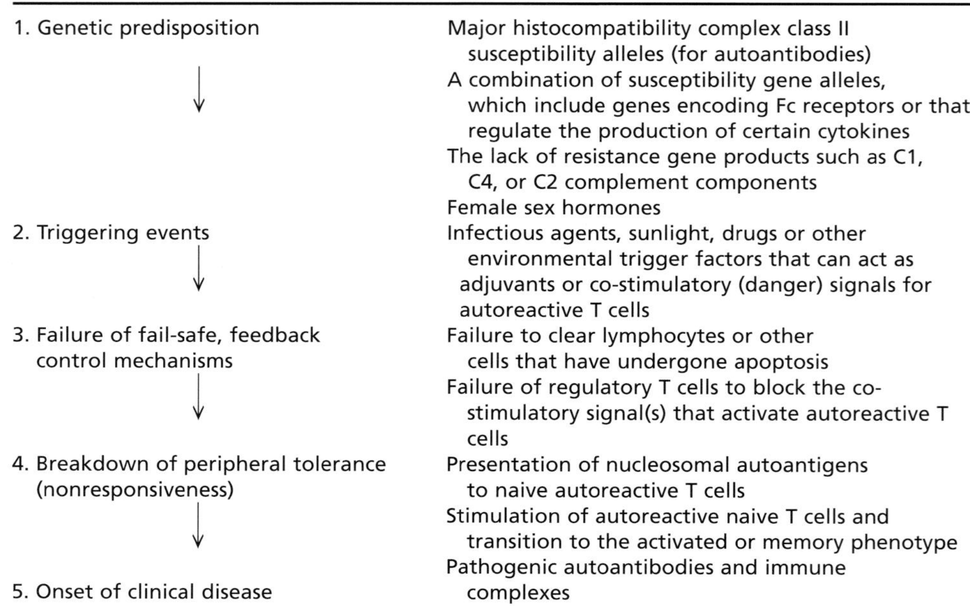

1. Genetic predisposition ↓	Major histocompatibility complex class II susceptibility alleles (for autoantibodies) A combination of susceptibility gene alleles, which include genes encoding Fc receptors or that regulate the production of certain cytokines The lack of resistance gene products such as C1, C4, or C2 complement components Female sex hormones
2. Triggering events ↓	Infectious agents, sunlight, drugs or other environmental trigger factors that can act as adjuvants or co-stimulatory (danger) signals for autoreactive T cells
3. Failure of fail-safe, feedback control mechanisms ↓	Failure to clear lymphocytes or other cells that have undergone apoptosis Failure of regulatory T cells to block the co-stimulatory signal(s) that activate autoreactive T cells
4. Breakdown of peripheral tolerance (nonresponsiveness) ↓	Presentation of nucleosomal autoantigens to naive autoreactive T cells Stimulation of autoreactive naive T cells and transition to the activated or memory phenotype
5. Onset of clinical disease	Pathogenic autoantibodies and immune complexes

(383). These autoantigen-specific B cells do not generally produce autoantibodies. In normal individuals who are exposed to intense immunologic stimulation, these cells may transiently produce IgM autoantibodies. In individuals who develop SLE, however, T-cell help induces a switch to IgG-autoantibody–producing cells.

Inciting Factors

The ultraviolet (UV) radiation from sunlight can generate the autoantigens that precipitate SLE. UV-A and UV-B in sunlight induce keratinocytes to undergo apoptosis and generate reactive oxygen species that alter nucleosomal DNA, Ro, La, and small nuclear ribonucleoproteins. These altered structures appear as blebs on the cell surface of apoptotic cells where they can serve as autoantigens (94,384,385). Evidence was reviewed earlier indicating increased numbers of activated T cells in patients with SLE and these cells are also the source of nuclear autoantigens. Activated cells are more susceptible than resting cells to the induction of apoptosis (387,388). Thus, because of apoptosis of various cells and decreased clearance of the fragmented nuclei, plasma nucleosome levels may be increased in SLE patients (386) and various epitopes are recognized by self-reactive T cells.

Infectious agents can act as the trigger factors to induce polyclonal B-cell activation and autoimmunity. A compelling argument for microbial superantigens has been offered in triggering polyclonal T-cell helper activity, which may result in SLE (344). Microbial superantigens, like anti-CD3 monoclonal antibodies, activate T cells via surface CD3/TCR. Certain bacteria such as staphylococci, streptococci, and mycoplasmas bear structures called superantigens that simultaneously bind to specific structures on the variable (V) region of the TCR chain and to the class II MHC molecules of antigen-presenting B cells. Therefore, these structures bring $CD4^+$ cells into close contact with B cells. Such bridging of T and B cells by microbial superantigens can induce polyclonal IgM and IgG formation. Moreover, specific autoantibodies may be produced if there also is concurrent cross-linking of the B-cell receptor by autoantigen (344).

Failure of Feedback Control Mechanisms

Since cell death from apoptosis is a noninflammatory event and bacterial superantigens challenge the immune system of everyone, T cells must have internal feedback regulators to control their activation. These include the negative regulatory cell surface molecules CD30 and PD-1 (389,390). Deletion of PD-1, a transmembrane protein containing an ITIM (immunoreceptor tyrosine-based inhibitory motif) in normal mice results in a lupus-like syndrome (390). Similarly, deletion of the cell cycle regulator p21 leads to a lupus syndrome in normal female mice (391).

In addition to these internal circuits, there are decreased numbers and/or functional regulatory T cells in SLE. As stated above, IL-2 and the active form of TGF-β are needed for the generation of both $CD8^+$ and $CD4^+$ regulatory T cells (49,59), and production of these cytokines is decreased in SLE (see Chapter 10). Dysfunctional $CD8^+$ killer cells also contribute to the pathogenesis of SLE. The lupus-like syndrome resulting from chronic graft versus host disease in mice is a particularly illustrative example of the importance of $CD8^+$ T cells (340) and is supported by older studies of murine chronic GVH reactions as well (342,343,392,393). NKT cells also have important positive and negative regulatory effects in SLE, and the abnormalities in these cells described above may be significant (135–138,140,141).

Without functional suppressor cells, the adjuvant effect of microbial infections might permit naive autoreactive anergic or ignorant (see above) T cells to undergo clonal expansion and become memory T cells. In fact, T cells that provide specific help for anti-DNA antibody production in SLE display the memory phenotype (19). Because memory cells have a low threshold for activation, subsequent exposure to nucleoprotein antigens along with the appropriate co-stimulatory factors can precipitate the onset of autoimmune disease.

Breakdown of Peripheral Tolerance

Disruption of normal immunologic homeostasis provides the opportunity for the activation of autoreactive T cells. Decreased clearance of apoptotic cells, the persistence of infectious agents, and certain drugs are examples of conditions that can lead to breakdown of immune tolerance. In addition to decreased clearance, increased enriched guanine plus cytosine (GC)-containing DNA fragments are found in the sera of SLE patients (394). In SLE, abnormal DNA methylation of GC-rich regions in apoptotic nucleosomes further increases the immunogenicity of these autoantigens (395).

Since the host defense to combat infectious agents is decreased in SLE (396), the adjuvant-like effects of the organisms persisting in the inflammatory exudate enhance the potential of APCs to alter self proteins or increase the chance of foreign proteins cross-reactive with self to trigger bystander autoreactive T cells. In SLE, decreased macrophage phagocytosis (397), decreased levels of the chromatin-binding C-reactive protein (CRP), snRNPs, some histones, and membrane phospholipids (398), and decreased levels of the early complement components (399,400) result in persistent high concentrations of potentially pathogenic autoantigens. Treatment of NZB/W F1 mice with CRP decreases autoantibody formation and increases survival (401).

Certain drugs can also cause lupus-like syndromes. Some drugs are capable of converting anergic, autoreactive T cells to immunocompetent ones through a mechanism involving DNA methylation. Inhibitors of DNA methylation induce gene expression, and it has been reported that drugs such as procainamide and hydralazine induce self-reactivity in cloned T-cell lines by this mechanism (91–93).

Persistent T-cell activation and/or polyclonal B-cell activation and impaired regulation of antibody production (discussed later) set the stage for the breakdown of T-cell tolerance and generalized autoimmunity. Because B cells that are reactive to self nuclear and certain cytoplasmic antigens are not fully deleted, these cells are prime candidates for being the cells responsible for the breakdown of self tolerance. Considerable evidence has been accumulated indicating that B cells have an important, if not critical role, as APCs in autoimmune diseases, including SLE (402–406).

The charge and repetitive structure of SLE autoantigens cross-link immunoglobulin receptors on nondeleted, self-reactive B cells. For example, B cells can bind DNA, which then endocytose the DNA-DNA-binding protein complex. B cells then process this complex and present the relevant peptides to T cells. This reaction normally would result in T-cell anergy, because resting B cells cannot provide the required co-stimulatory signals that are needed for activation. Activated B cells, however, can deliver this co-stimulatory signal and trigger certain T cells to become fully responsive to self antigens. Alternatively, activated T cells can induce resting B cells to become responsive. This is the case in graft versus host disease, where activated donor $CD4^+$ cells can provide this second signal to permit B-cell activation and trigger autoantibody production (340,392, 393). Either of these situations therefore permits the development of expanded clones of autoreactive T cells and memory B cells that are capable of making specific autoantibodies. As stated, once memory cells have been generated, the opportunity for further autoantibody production is substantially increased.

Thus, the loss of tolerance to certain nuclear and cytoplasmic antigens occurs through a combination of genetic and environmental factors that include immunogenic concentrations of pathogenic autoantigens, defects in regulatory and killer T cells, and intrinsic B-cell defects described in Chapter 11. Autoantigen-specific T cells emerge that have the ability to provide B-cell help for a panoply of autoantibodies. Although the initial self antigen that is recognized may be very specific, the phenomenon of epitope spreading with presentation of cryptic peptides by B cells broadens the original response. Recruitment of other non-tolerant self-reactive T cells broadens the response even further and leads to generalized autoimmunity. Ultimately, B cells produce IgG pathogenic, complement fixing, autoantibodies that induce lupus nephritis and autoantibodies that are responsible for the other lupus syndromes.

T CELLS IN THE PERPETUATION OF SLE

Pathologic Regulatory Circuits

The response of nontolerant autoreactive T cells to nucleosomal antigens, along with pathologic regulatory circuits that sustain this reactivity, result in the perpetuation of SLE (Table 9.8). Both cell surface structures and cytokines are involved in these regulatory circuits. As stated earlier, CD40L is upregulated in SLE and persistent ligation of

TABLE 9.8. PERPETUATION OF SLE

Constant presence of immunogenic concentrations of nucleosomal autoantigens
Continuous stimulation of clonally expanded, autoreactive T and B memory cells
Production of cytokines such as IL-10 that sustain B-cell activity, but inhibit T-cell function
Failure of feedback regulatory networks to shut down autoreactive lymphocytes and restore normal homeostasis

CD40 with CD40L may result in chronic T-cell help for antibody and autoantibody production (136,271). The interaction between CD40 expressed by B cells and CD40L expressed by activated T cells is a critical signal for B-cell differentiation (262,263). A brief treatment of lupus mice with a monoclonal antibody against CD40 ligand greatly decreased the onset of lupus nephritis (407). As stated above, hyperexpression of CD40L is associated with a defect in anergy induction (69). Interestingly, $CD8^+$ T suppressor cells directly inhibit the CD40 signaling pathway (408), and the activity of these cells is decreased in SLE.

Sustained, high levels of IL-10, discussed in the following chapter, directly sustain B-cell proliferation and differentiation. Moreover, IL-10 downregulates IL-2, TNF-α, and TGF-β (132,334–336), cytokines that are needed for feedback regulation of B-cell activity. TNF-α has a protective effect in lupus mice (409), and the treatment of rheumatoid arthritis with a monoclonal antibody that antagonizes TNF-α leads to the appearance of anti-DNA antibodies in approximately 10% of the patients (410). As we have reviewed, both IL-2 and TGF-β are needed for the generation of regulatory T cells, and insufficient amounts of these cytokines probably explain why $CD8^+$ cells support rather than suppress B-cell activity in SLE (49).

Restoring Normal Homeostasis

One would predict that restoration of normal immune function would correlate with disease remission. In fact, remissions with reconstitution of T-cell function have been observed in patients who are treated with oral cyclophosphamide. In these patients, clinical improvement, disappearance of anti-DNA antibodies, normalization of complement, and disappearance of the sequelae of chronic inflammation were followed by the normalization of T-cell proliferation in SLE (411). One case was described in which clinical remission correlated with the normalization of IL-2 production, normalization of serum IL-2-receptor levels, and increase in $CD8^+$ DR^+ memory cells (412). More recently, an early study with the use of anti–IL-10 in human SLE resulted in a decrease in disease activity and improvement in some measures of immune function (413). Resetting the immune system of SLE patients with high-dose cyclophosphamide followed by autologous stem cell transplantation has resulted in complete clinical remission and normalization of the T-cell phenotype and repertoire (414). Based on the current, rapid progress in clarifying the circuits that are involved in normal and pathologic immune regulation, innovative strategies to manage SLE can be developed that allow normal homeostatic mechanisms to be reestablished.

REFERENCES

1. Datta SK, Patel H, Berry B. Induction of a cationic shift in IgG anti-DNA antibodies: role of helper T cells with classical and novel phenotypes in three models of lupus nephritis. *J Exp Med* 1987;165:1252–1268.
2. Santoro TJ, Portanova JP, Kotzin BL. The contribution of L3T4 T cells to lymphoproliferation and autoantibody production in MRL*lpr/lpr* mice. *J Exp Med* 1988;167:713–721.
3. Rajagopalan S, Zordan, Tsokos GC, et al. Pathogenic anti-DNA autoantibody-inducing T helper cell lines from patients with lupus nephritis: isolation of $CD4^-$ $CD8^-$ T helper cell lines that express the gamma-delta T cell antigen receptor. *Proc Natl Acad Sci USA* 1990;87:7020–7024.
4. Diamond B, Katz JB, Aranow C, et al. The role of somatic mutation in the pathogenic anti-DNA response. *Annu Rev Immunol* 1992;10:731–777.
5. Burlingame RW, Rubin RL, Balderas RS, et al. Genesis and evolution of anti-chromatin antibodies in murine lupus implicates immunization with self antigen. *J Clin Invest* 1993;91:1687–1696.
6. Radic MZ, Weigert M. Genetic and structural evidence for antigen selection of anti-DNA antibodies. *Annu Rev Immunol* 1994;12:487–520.
7. Wofsy D, Seaman WE. Reversal of advanced murine lupus in NZB/NZW F1 mice by treatment with monoclonal antibody to L3T4. *J Immunol* 1987;138:3247–3253.
8. Mihara M, Ohsugi Y, Saito K, et al. Immunologic abnormality in NZB/NZW F1 mice. Thymus-independent occurrence of B cell abnormality and requirement for T cells in the development of autoimmune disease, as evidenced by an analysis of the athymic nude individuals. *J Immunol* 1988;141:85–90.
9. Shoenfeld Y, Mozes E. Pathogenic idiotypes in autoimmunity: lessons from new experimental models of SLE. *FASEB J* 1990; 4:2646–2651.
10. Molina JF, Citera G, Rosler D, et al. Coexistence of human immunodeficiency virus infection and systemic lupus erythematosus. *J Rheumatol* 1995;22:347–345.
11. Burkley LC, Lo D, Flavell RA. Tolerance in transgenic mice expressing major histocompatibility molecules extrathymically on pancreatic cells. *Science* 1990;248:1364–1368.
12. Miller JF, Flavell RA. T-cell tolerance and autoimmunity in transgenic models of central and peripheral tolerance. *Curr Opin Immunol* 1994;6(6):892–899.
13. Goodnow CC, Adelstein S, Basten A. The need for central and peripheral tolerance in the B cell repertoire. *Science* 1990;248: 1373–1379.
14. Budman DR, Merchant EB, Steinberg AD, et al. Increased spontaneous activity of antibody-forming cells in the peripheral

blood of patients with active SLE. *Arthritis Rheum* 1977;20: 829–833.

15. Ginsburg WW, Finkelman FD, Lipsky PE. Circulating and pokeweed mitogen-induced immunoglobulin-secreting cells in systemic lupus erythematosus. *Clin Exp Immunol* 1979;35: 76–88.
16. O'Dell JR, Bizar-Scheebaum A, Kotzin BL. In vitro anti-histone antibody production by peripheral blood cells from patients with SLE. *Clin Immunol Immunopathol* 1988;47: 343–353.
17. Gharavi AE, Chu JL, Elkon KB. Autoantibodies to intracellular proteins in humans SLE are not due to random polyclonal B cell activation. *Arthritis Rheum* 1988;31:1337–1345.
18. Takeuchi T, Abe T, Koide J, et al. Cellular mechanism of DNA-specific antibody synthesis by lymphocytes from systemic lupus erythematosus patients. *Arthritis Rheum* 1984;27:766–773.
19. Shivakumar S, Tsokos GC, Datta SK. T cell receptor alpha/beta expressing double negative(CD4–/CD8–) and $CD4^+$ T helper cells in human augment the production of pathogenic anti-DNA autoantibodies associated with lupus nephritis. *J Immunol* 1989;143:103–112.
20. 22. Chess L, MacDermott P, Schlossman SF. Immunologic functions of isolated human lymphocyte populations. *J Immunol* 1985;1113–1121.
21. Karpus WJ, Swanborg RH. $CD4^+$ suppressor cells inhibit the function of effector cells of experimental autoimmune encephalomyelitis through a mechanism involving transforming growth factor-beta. *J Immunol* 1991;146:1163–1168.
22. Takahashi T, Gray JD, Horwitz DA. Human $CD8^+$ lymphocytes stimulated in the absence of $CD4^+$ cells enhance IgG production by antibody-secreting B cells. *Clin Immunol Immunopathol* 1991;58:352–365
23. Akbar AN, Terry L, Timms A, et al. Loss of CD45R and gain of UCHL1 is a feature of primed T cells. *J Immunol* 1988;140: 2171–2178.
24. Beverley P. Immunological memory in T cells. *Curr Opin Immunol* 1991;3:355–360.
25. Byrne JA, Butler JL, Cooper MD. Differential activation requirements for virgin and memory T cells. *J Immunol* 1988; 141:3249–3257.
26. Clement LT, Yamashita N, Martin AM. The functionally distinct subpopulations of human $CD4^+$ helper/inducer T lymphocytes defined by anti-CD45R antibodies derive sequentially from a differentiation pathway that is regulated by activation-dependent post-thymic differentiation. *J Immunol* 1988;141: 1464–1470.
27. Merkenschlager M, Beverley PC. Evidence for differential expression of CD45 isoforms for memory dependent and independent cytotoxic responses: human CD8 memory CTL precursors selectively express CD45RO (UCHL1). *Int Immunol* 1989;1:450–457.
28. Yamashita N, Clement LT. Phenotypic characterization of the post-thymic differentiation of human alloantigen-specific $CD8^+$ cytotoxic T lymphocytes. *J Immunol* 1989;143: 1518–1523.
29. Lanier LL, Chang C, Spits H, et al. Expression of cytoplasmic CD3 epsilon proteins in activated human adult natural killer (NK) cells and CD3 gamma, delta, epsilon complexes in fetal NK cells. Implications for the relationship of NK and T lymphocytes. *J Immunol* 1992;149(6):1876–1880.
30. Exley M, Porcelli S, Furman M, et al. CD161 (NKR-P1A) co-stimulation of CD1d-dependent activation of human T cells expressing invariant V alpha 24 J alpha Q T cell receptor alpha chains. *J Exp Med* 1998;188(5):867–876.
31. Seaman WE. Natural killer cells and natural killer T cells. *Arthritis Rheum* 2000;43(6):1204–1217.
32. Jondal M, Pross H. Surface markers on human B and T lymphocytes. VI. Cytotoxicity against cell lines as a functional marker for lymphocyte subpopulations. *Int J Cancer* 1975;15: 596–605.
33. Takasugi M, Mickey MR, Terasaki PI. Reactivity of lymphocytes from normal persons on cultured tumor cells. *Cancer Res* 1973;33:2898–2902.
34. West WH, Cannon GD, Kay HD, et al. Natural cytotoxic reactivity of human lymphocytes against a myeloid cell line: characterization of the effector cells. *J Immunol* 1977;118: 355–361.
35. Biron CA, Byron KS, Sullivan JL. Susceptibility to viral infections in an individual with a complete lack of natural killer cells. *Nat Immun Cell Growth Regul* 1988;7:47–49.
36. Griffin JD, Hercend T, Beveridge R, et al. Characterization of an antigen expressed by human natural killer cells. *J Immunol* 1983;130:2947–2951.
37. Zarling JM, Clouse JA, Biddison WE, et al. Phenotypes of human natural killer cells populations detected with monoclonal antibodies. *J Immunol* 1981;127:2575–2580.
38. Hercend T, Griffin Bensussan A, Schmidt RE, et al. Generation of monoconal antibodies to a human natural killer clone. Characterization of two natural killer-associated antigens, NKH1A and NKH2, expressed on a subset of large granular lymphocytes. *J Clin Invest* 1985;75:932–943.
39. Kay HD, Horwitz DA. Evidence by reactivity with hybridoma antibodies for a probable myeloid origin of peripheral blood cells active in natural cytotoxicity and antibody-dependent cell-mediated cytotoxicity. *J Clin Invest* 1980;66:847–851.
40. Lanier LL, Cwirla S, Yu G, et al. Membrane anchoring of a human IgG Fc receptor (CD16) determined by a single amino acid. *Science* 1989;246:1611–1613.
41. Perussia B, Starr S, Abraham S, et al. Human natural killer cells analyzed by B73.1, a monoclonal antibody blocking Fc receptor functions. I. Characterization of the lymphocyte subset reactive with B73.1. *J Immunol* 1983;130:2133–2141.
42. w3.pmWerfer T, Witter W, Gotze O. CD11b and CD11c antigens are rapidly increased in human natural killer cells upon activation. *J Immunol* 1991;147:2423–2427.
43. Domzig W, Stadler BM, Herberman RB. Interleukin 2 dependence on human natural killer cell activity. *J Immunol* 1983;130:1970–1973.
44. Trinchieri G, Santoli D. Antiviral activity induced by culturing lymphocytes with tumor-derived or virus-transferred cells. Enhancement of human natural killer cell activity by interferon and inhibition of susceptibility of target cells to lysis. *J Exp Med* 1978;147:1314–1333.
45. Tilden AB, Abo T, Balch CM. Suppressor cell function of human granular lymphocytes identified by the HNK-1 (Leu 7) monoclonal antibody. *J Immunol* 1983;130:1171–1175.
46. Abo W, Gray JD, Bakke AC, et al. Studies on human blood lymphocytes with iC3b (type 3) complement receptors. II.Characterization of subsets which regulate pokeweed mitogen-induced lymphocyte proliferation and immunoglobulin synthesis. *Clin Exp Immunol* 1987;67(3):544–555.
47. Gray JD, Horwitz DA. Activated human NK cells can stimulate resting B cells to secrete immunoglobulin. *J Immunol* 1995; 154(11):5656–5664.
48. Carbone E, Ruggiero G, Terrazzano G, et al. A new mechanism of NK cell cytotoxicity activation: the CD40-CD40 ligand interaction. *J Exp Med* 1997;185(12):2053–2060.
49. Horwitz DA, Gray JD, Ohtsuka K. Role of NK cells and TGF-beta in the regulation of T-cell-dependent antibody production in health and autoimmune disease. *Microbes Infect* 1999;1: 1305–11.
50. Blackman M, Kappler J, Marrack P. The role of the T cell recep-

tor in positive and negative selection of developing T cells. *Science* 1990;248:1335–1341.

51. Burkly Rathmell JC, Goodnow CC. Effects of the lpr mutation in elimination and inactivation of self-reactive B cells. *J Immunol* 1994;153:2831–2842.
52. Schwartz RH. A cell culture model for T lymphocyte clonal anergy. *Science* 1990;248:1349–1356.
53. Green DR, Scott DW. Activation-induced apoptosis in lymphocytes. *Curr Opin Immunol* 1994;6:476–487.
54. Norton SD, Hovinen DE, Jenkins MK. IL-2 secretion and T cell clonal anergy are induced by distinct biochemical pathways. *J Immunol* 1991;146:1125–1129.
55. Ohashi PS, Oehen S, Buerki K, et al. Ablation of tolerance and induction of diabetes by virus infection in viral antigen transgenic mice. *Cell* 1991;65:305–317.
56. Seddon B, Mason D. The third function of the thymus. *Immunol Today* 2000;21:95.
57. Shevach EA. Regulatory T cells in autoimmunity. *Annu Rev Immunol* 2000;18:423.
58. Hammond K, Cain W, van Driel I, et al. Three day neonatal thymectomy selectively depletes NK1.1$^+$ T cells. *Int Immunol* 1998;10(10):1491–499.
59. Yamagiwa S, Gray JD, Horwitz DA. A Role for TGF-β in the generation of human CD4$^+$ CD25$^+$ regulatory cells from naive peripheral blood T cells. *J Immunol* 2001; in press.
60. Groux H, O'Garra A, Bigler M, et al. A CD4$^+$ T-cell subset inhibits antigen-specific T-cell responses and prevents colitis. *Nature* 1997;389(6652):737–742.
61. Freeman GJ, Borriello F, Hodes RJ, et al. Murine B7-2, an alternative CT-A4 counter-receptor that costimulates T cell proliferation and interleukin 2 production. *J Exp Med* 1993;178: 2185–2192.
62. Harding FA, Allison JP. CD28-B7 interactions allow the induction of CD8$^+$ cytotoxic T lymphocytes in the absence of exogenous help. *J Exp Med* 1993;177:1791–1796.
63. Fatenejad S, Peng SL, Disorbo O, et al. Central T cell tolerance in lupus-prone mice: influence of autoimmune background and the lpr mutation. *J Immunol* 1998;161(11):6427–6432.
64. Kotzin BL, Kappler JW, Marrack PC, et al. T cell tolerance to self antigens in New Zealand hybrid mice with lupus-like disease. *J Immunol* 1989;143(1):89–94.
65. Scott DE, Kisch WJ, Steinberg AD. Studies of T cell deletion and T cell anergy following in vivo administration of SEB to normal and lupus-prone mice. *J Immunol* 1993;150:664–672.
66. Roark JH, Kuntz CL, Nguyen CA, et al. Breakdown of B cell tolerance in a mouse model of systemic lupus erythematosus. *J Exp Med* 1995;181:1157–1167.
67. Laskin CA, Taurog JD, Smathers PA, et al. Studies of defective tolerance in murine lupus. *J Immunol* 1981;127(5):1743–1747.
68. Wither J, Vukusic B. T-cell tolerance induction is normal in the (NZB × NZW)F1 murine model of systemic lupus erythematosus. *Immunology* 2000;99(3):345–351.
69. Yi Y, McNerney M, Datta SK. Regulatory defects in cbl and mitogen-activated protein kinase (extracellular signal-related kinase) pathways cause persistent hyperexpression of CD40 ligand in human lupus T cells. *J Immunol* 2000;165(11): 6627–6634.
70. Monestier M, Kotzin BL. Antibodies to histones in systemic lupus erythematosus and drug-induced lupus syndromes. *Clin Rheum Dis* 1992;18:415–436.
71. Amoura Z, Chabre H, Koutouzov S, et al. Nucleosome restricted antibodies are detected before anti-dsDNA in the sera of MRL-Mp lpr/lpr and +/+ mice and are present in the kidney eluates of lupus mice with proteinuria. *Arthritis Rheum* 1994; 37:1684–1688.
72. Gilkeson GS, Grudier JP, Karounos DG, et al. Induction of anti-double stranded DNA antibodies in normal mice by immunization with bacterial DNA. *J Immunol* 1989;142: 1482–1486.
73. Jacob L, Lety MA, Louvard D, et al. Binding of a monoclonal anti-DNA autoantibody to identical protein(s) present at the surface of several human cell types involved in lupus pathogenesis. *J Clin Invest* 1985;75:315–317.
74. Jacob L, Viard JP, Allenet B, et al. A monoclonal anti-double-stranded DNA autoantibody binds to a 94-kDa cell-surface protein on various cell types via nucleosomes or a DNA-histone complex. *Proc Natl Acad Sci USA* 1989;86:4669–4673.
75. Rieber M, Urbina C, Rieber MS. DNA on membrane receptors: a target for monoclonal anti-DNA antibody induced by a nucleoprotein shed in systemic lupus erythematosus. *Biochem Biophys Res Commun* 1989;159:1441–1447.
76. Datta SK. Production of pathogenic antibodies: cognate interactions between autoimmune T and B cells. *Lupus* 1998;7(9): 591–596.
77. Burlingame RW, Boey ML, Starkebaum G, et al. The central role of chromatin in autoimmune responses to histones and DNA in systemic lupus erythematosus. *J Clin Invest* 1994;94: 184–192.
78. Mohan C, Adams S, Stanik V, et al. Nucleosome: a major immunogen for pathogenic autoantibody-inducing T cells of lupus. *J Exp Med* 1993;177:1367–1381.
79. Mao C, Osman GE, Adams S, et al. T cell receptor alpha-chain repertoire of pathogenic autoantibody-inducing T cells in lupus mice. *J Immunol* 1994;152:1462–1470.
80. Lu L, Kaliyaperumal A, Boumpas DT, et al. Major peptide autoepitopes for nucleosome-specific T cells of human lupus. *J Clin Invest* 1999;104(3):345–355.
81. Voll RE, Roth EA, Girkontaite I, et al. Histone-specific Th0 and Th1 clones derived from systemic lupus erythematosus patients induce double-stranded DNA antibody production. *Arthritis Rheum* 1997;40(12):2162–2171.
82. Singh RR, Kumar V, Ebling FM, et al. T cell determinants from autoantibodies to DNA can upregulate autoimmunity in murine systemic lupus erythematosus. *J Exp Med* 1995;181: 2017–2027.
83. Hoffman RW, Takeda Y, Sharp GC, et al. Human T cell clones reactive against U-small nuclear ribonucleoprotein autoantigens from connective tissue disease patients and health individuals. *J Immunol* 1993;151:6460–6469.
84. Crow MK, DelGiudice-Asch G, Zehetbauer JB, et al. Autoantigen-specific T cell proliferation induced by the ribosomal P2 protein in patients with systemic lupus erythematosus. *J Clin Invest* 1994;94:345–352.
85. Dawisha SM, Gmelig-Meyling F, Steinberg AD. Assessment of clinical parameters associated with increased frequency of mutant T cells in patients with systemic lupus erythematosus. *Arthritis Rheum* 1994;37:270–277.
86. Theocharis S, Sfikakis PP, Lipnick RN, et al. Characterization of in vivo mutated T cell clones from patients with systemic lupus erythematosus. *Clin Immunol Immunopathol* 1995;74: 135–142.
87. Hashimoto S, Michalsky JP, Berman MA, et al. Mechanism of a lymphocyte abnormality associates with HLA-B8/DR3: role of interleukin-1. *Clin Exp Immunol* 1990;79:227–232.
88. Jacob CO, Fronek Z, Lewis GD, et al. Heritable major histocompatibility complex class II-associated differences in production of tumor necrosis factor: relevance to genetic predisposition to systemic lupus erythematosus. *Proc Natl Acad Sci USA* 1990;87:1233–1237.
89. Alexander EL, McNicholl J, Watson RM, et al. The immunogenetic relationship between anti-Ro(SS-A)/La(SS-B) antibody positive Sjogren's/lupus erythematosus overlap syndrome and

the neonatal lupus syndrome. *J Invest Dermatol* 1989;93: 751–756.

90. Arnett FC, Bias WB, Reveille JD. Genetic studies in Sjogren's syndrome and systemic lupus erythematosus. *J Autoimmun* 1989;2:403–413.
91. Richardson BC, Strahler JR, Pivirotto TS, et al. Phenotypic and functional similarities between 5-azacytidine-treated T cells and a T cell subset in patients with active systemic lupus erythematosus. *Arthritis Rheum* 1992;35:647–662.
92. Cornacchia E, Golbus J, Maybaum J, et al. Hydralazine and procainamide inhibit T cell DNA methylation and induce autoreactivity. *J Immunol* 1988;140:2197–2200.
93. Richardson BC, Liebling MR, Hudson JL. $CD4^+$ cells treated with DNA methylation inhibitors induce autologous B cell differentiation. *Clin Immunol Immunopathol* 1990;55:368–381.
94. Casciola-Rosen LA, Anhalt G, Rosen A. Autoantigens targeted in systemic lupus erythematosus are clustered in two populations of surface structures on apoptotic keratinocytes. *J Exp Med* 1994;179:1317–1330.
95. Chung JH, Kwon OS, Eun HC, et al. Apoptosis in the pathogenesis of cutaneous lupus erythematosus. *Am J Dermatopathol* 1998;20(3):233–241
96. Glinski W, Gershwin ME, Steinberg AD. Fractionation of cells on a discontinuous Ficoll gradient. Study of subpopulations of human T cells using anti-T cell antibodies from patients with systemic lupus erythematosus. *J Clin Invest* 1976;57:604–614.
97. Horwitz DA, Juul-Nielsen K. Human blood L, lymphocytes in patients with active systemic lupus erythematosus, rheumatoid arthritis, and scleroderma. *Clin Exp Immunol* 1977;30: 370–378.
98. Messner RP, Kindstrom FD, Williams JR Jr. Peripheral blood lymphocyte cell surface markers during the course of systemic lupus erythematosus. *J Clin Invest* 1973;52:3046–3056.
99. Moretta LM, Mingari MC, Webb SR, et al. Imbalances in T cell subpopulations associated with immunodeficiency and autoimmune syndromes. *Eur J Immunol* 1984;7:696–700.
100. Rivero SJ, Diaz-Jouanen E, Alarcon-Segovia D. Lymphopenia in systemic lupus erythematosus. *Arthritis Rheum* 1978;21: 295–305.
101. Rivero SJ, Llorente L, Diaz-Jouanen E, et al. T-lymphocyte subpopulation in untreated systemic lupus erythematosus. Variations with disease activity. *Arthritis Rheum* 1977;20: 1169–1173.
102. Morimoto C, Reinherz EL, Schlossman SF, et al. Alteration in T cell subsets in active systemic lupus erythematosus. *J Clin Invest* 1980;66:1171–1174.
103. Tsokos GC, Balow JE. Phenotypes of T lymphocytes in systemic lupus erythematosus: decreased cytotoxic/suppressor subpopulation is associated with deficient allogenic cytotoxic responses rather than with concanavalin A-induced suppressor cells. *Clin Immunol Immunopathol* 1983;26:267–276.
104. Smolen JS, Chused TM, Leiserson WM, et al. Heterogeneity of immunoregulatory T-cell subsets in systemic lupus erythematosus. *Am J Med* 1982;72:783–790.
105. Bakke AC, Kirkland PA, Kitridou RC, et al. T lymphocyte subsets in systemic lupus erythematosus. *Arthritis Rheum* 1983;26: 745–750.
106. McInerney MF, Clough JD, Senitzer D, et al. Two distinct subsets of patients with systemic lupus erythematosus. *Clin Immunol Immunopathol* 1988;49:116–132.
107. Fornasieri A, Sinico R, Fiorini G, et al. T-lymphocyte subsets in primary and secondary glomerulonephritis. *Proc Eur Dial Transplant Assoc* 1983;19:635–641.
108. Yamada A, Winfield JB. Inhibition of soluble antigen-induced T cell proliferation by warm-reactive antibodies to activated T cells in systemic lupus erythematosus. *J Clin Invest* 1984;74: 1948–1960.
109. Butler WT, Sharp JT, Rossen RD, et al. Relationship of the clinical course of systemic lupus erythematosus to the presence of circulating lymphocytotoxic antibodies. *Arthritis Rheum* 1972; 15:231–238.
110. Winfield JB, Winchester RJ, Kunkel HG. Association of cold-reactive anti-lymphocyte antibodies with lymphopenia in systemic lupus erythematosus. *Arthritis Rheum* 1975;18:587–594.
111. Alvarado C, Alcocer-Varela J, Llorente L, et al. Effect of CD28 antibody on T cells from patients with systemic lupus erythematosus. *J Autoimmun* 1994;7:763–773.
112. Horwitz DA, Tang FL, Stimmler MM, et al. Decreased T cell response to anti-CD2 in systemic lupus erythematosus and reversal by anti-CD28: evidence for impaired T cell-accessory cell interaction. *Arthritis Rheum* 1997;40:822–833.
113. Stohl W, Crow MK, Kunkel HG. Systemic lupus erythematosus with deficiency of the T4 epitope on T helper/inducer cells. *N Engl J Med* 1985;312:1671–1678.
114. Stohl W, Singer JZ. Correlation between systemic lupus erythematosus and T4 epitope phenotype. *Arthritis Rheum* 1987;30: 1412–1415.
115. Alarcon-Segovia D, Ruiz-Arguelles A. Decreased circulating thymus-derived cells with receptors for the Fc portion of immunoglobulin G in systemic lupus erythematosus. *J Clin Invest* 1978;62:1390–1394.
116. Fauci AS, Steinberg AD, Haynes BF, et al. Immunoregulatory aberrations in systemic lupus erythematosus. *J Immunol* 1978; 121:1473–1479.
117. Gray JD, Lash A, Baake AC, et al. Studies on human blood lymphocytes with iC3b (type 3) complement receptors: III. Abnormalities in patients with active systemic lupus erythematosus. *Clin Exp Immunol* 1987;67:556– 564.
118. Struyf NJ, Snoeck HW, Bridts CH, et al. Natural killer cell activity in Sjogren's syndrome and systemic lupus erythematosus: stimulation with interferons and interleukin 2 and correlation with immune complexes. *Ann Rheum Dis* 1990;49: 690–693.
119. Goto M, Tanimoto K, Horiuchi Y. Natural cell mediated cytotoxicity in systemic lupus erythematosus. Suppression by anti-lymphocyte antibody. *Arthritis Rheum* 1980;23:1274–1281.
120. Hoffman T. Natural killer function in systemic lupus erythematosus. *Arthritis Rheum* 1980;23:30–35.
121. Katz P, Zaytoun AM, Lee JH Jr, et al. Abnormal natural killer cell activity in systemic lupus erythematosus: an intrinsic defect in the lytic event. *J Immunol* 1982;129:1966–1971.
122. Oshimi K, Sumiya M, Gonda N, et al. Natural killer cell activity in untreated systemic lupus erythematosus. *Ann Rheum Dis* 1982;41:417–420.
123. Rook AH, Tsokos GC, Quinnan GV Jr, et al. Cytotoxic antibodies to natural killer cells in systemic lupus erythematosus. *Clin Immunol Immunopathol* 1982;24:179–185.
124. Silverman SL, Cathcart ES. Natural killing in systemic lupus erythematosus: inhibitory effects of serum. *Clin Immunol Immunopathol* 1980;17:219–226.
125. Diaz-Jouanen E, Bankhurst AD, Williams RC. Antibody-mediated lymphocytotoxicity in rheumatoid arthritis and systemic lupus erythematosus. *Arthritis Rheum* 1976;19:133–141.
126. Feldmann J, Becker MJ, Moutsopoulos H, et al. Antibody dependent cell-mediated cytotoxicity in selected autoimmune diseases. *J Clin Invest* 1976;58:173–179.
127. Scheinberg MA, Cathcart ES. Antibody-dependent direct cytotoxicity of human lymphocytes. I. Studies on peripheral blood lymphocytes and sera of patients with systemic lupus erythematosus. *Clin Exp Immunol* 1976;24:317–322.
128. Schneider J, Chin W, Friou GJ, et al. Reduced antibody-depen-

dent cell-mediated cytotoxicity in systemic lupus erythematosus. *Clin Exp Immunol* 1975;20:187–192.

129. Perussia B, Acuto O, Terhorst C, et al. Human natural killer cells analyzed by B73.1, a monoclonal antibody blocking FcR functions. II. Studies of B73.1 antibody-antigen interaction on the lymphocyte membrane. *J Immunol* 1983;130:2142–2148.
130. Sipos A, Csortos C, Sipka S, et al. The antigen/receptor specificity of antigranulocyte antibodies in patient with SLE. *Immunol Lett* 1988;19:329–334.
131. Linker-Israeli M, Quismorio FP, Jr, Horwitz DA. CD8+ lymphocytes from patients with systemic lupus erythematosus sustain rather than suppress spontaneous polyclonal IgG production and synergize with CD4+ cells to support autoantibody synthesis. *Arthritis Rheum* 1990;33:1216–1225.
132. Ohtsuka K, Gray JD, Stimmler MM, et al. Decreased production of TGF-β by lymphocytes from patients with systemic lupus erythematosus. *J Immunol* 1998;60:2539–2545.
133. Harada M, Lin T, Kurosawa S, et al. Natural killer cells inhibit the development of autoantibody production in (C57BL/6 × DBA/2)F1 hybrid mice injected with DBA/2 spleen cells. *Cell Immunol* 1995;161:42–49.
134. Pan LZ, Dauphinee MJ, Ansar Ahmed S, et al. Altered natural killer and natural cytotoxic cellular activities in lpr mice. *Scand J Immunol* 1986:23:415–423.
135. Takeda K, Dennert G. The development of autoimmunity in C57BL/6 lpr mice correlates with the disappearance of natural killer type 1positive cells: evidence for their suppressive action on bone marrow stem cell proliferation, B cell immunoglobulin secretion, and autoimmune symptoms. *J Exp Med* 1993;177: 155–164.
136. Devi BS, Van Noordin S, Krausz T, et al. Peripheral blood lymphocytes in SLE—hyperexpression of CD154 on T and B lymphocytes and increased number of double negative T cells. *J Autoimmun* 1998;11(5):471–475.
137. Sieling PA, Porcelli SA, Duong BT, et al. Human double-negative T cells in systemic lupus erythematosus provide help for IgG and are restricted by CD1c. *J Immunol* 2000;165(9): 5338–5344.
137a. Liu MF, Li JS, Weng TH, Lei HY. Double-negative (CD4– CD8–) TCRalphabeta+ cells in patients with systemic lupus erythematosus. *Scand J Rheumatol* 1998;27:130–134.
138. Gerli R, Agea E, Bertotto A, et al. Analysis of T cells bearing different isotypic forms of the gamma/delta T cell receptor in patients with systemic autoimmune diseases. *J Rheumatol* 1991; 18:1504–1510.
138a. Funauchi M, Yu H, Sugiyama M, et al. Increased interleukin-4 production by NK T cells in systemic lupus erythematosus. *Clin Immunol* 1999;92:197–202.
139. Wilson SB, Kent SC, Horton HF, et al. Multiple differences in gene expression in regulatory Valpha 24Jalpha Q T cells from identical twins discordant for type I diabetes. *Proc Natl Acad Sci USA* 2000;97(13):7411–7416.
140. Oishi Y, Iwamoto I. [Role of TCR V alpha 24 J alpha Q+ T cells in autoimmune diseases]. *Nippon Rinsho* 1997;55(6): 1425–1430.
141. Riccieri V, Spadaro A, Parisi G, et al. Down-regulation of natural killer cells and of gamma/delta T cells in systemic lupus erythematosus. Does it correlate to autoimmunity and to laboratory indices of disease activity? *Lupus* 2000;9(5):333–337.
141a. Hanninen A, Harrison LC. Gamma delta T cells as mediators of mucosal tolerance: the autoimmune diabetes model. *Immunol Rev* 2000;173:109–119.
142. Morimoto C, Steinberg AD, Letvin NL, et al. A defect of immunoregulatory T cell subsets in systemic lupus erythematosus patients demonstrated with anti-2H4 antibody. *J Clin Invest* 1987;79:762–768.
143. Raziuddin S, Nur MA, Al Wabel AA. Selective loss of the CD4+ inducers of suppressor T cell subsets (2H4+) in active systemic lupus erythematosus. *J Rheumatol* 1991;16:1315–1319.
144. Sato K, Miyasaka N, Yamaoka K, et al. Quantitative defect of CD4+2H4+ cells in systemic lupus. *Arthritis Rheum* 1987;30: 1407–1411.
145. Mimura T, Fernsten P, Jarjour W, et al. Autoantibodies specific for different isoforms of CD45 in systemic lupus erythematosus. *J Exp Med* 1990;172:653–656.
146. Tanaka S, Matsuyama T, Steinberg AD, et al. Antilymphocyte antibodies against CD4+2H4+ cell populations in patients with systemic lupus erythematosus. *Arthritis Rheum* 1989;32: 398–405.
147. Emlen W, Niebur J, Kadera R. Accelerated in vitro apoptosis of lymphocytes from patients with systemic lupus erythematosus. *J Immunol* 1994;152:3685–3692.
148. Georgescu L, Vakkalanka RK, Elkon KB, et al. Interleukin-10 promotes activation-induced cell death of SLE lymphocytes mediated by Fas ligand. *J Clin Invest* 1997;100(10):2622–2633.
149. Courtney PA, Crockard AD, Williamson K, et al. Lymphocyte apoptosis in systemic lupus erythematosus: relationships with Fas expression, serum soluble Fas and disease activity. *Lupus* 1999;8(7):508–513.
150. Perniok A, Wedekind F, Herrmann M, et al. High levels of circulating early apoptic peripheral blood mononuclear cells in systemic lupus erythematosus. *Lupus* 1998;7(2):113–118.
151. Hernandez-Fuentes MP, Reyes E, Prieto A, et al. Defective proliferative response of T lymphocytes from patients with inactive systemic lupus erythematosus. *J Rheumatol* 1999;26(7): 1518–1526.
152. Lorenz HM, Grunke M, Hieronymus T, et al. In vitro apoptosis and expression of apoptosis-related molecules in lymphocytes from patients with systemic lupus erythematosus and other autoimmune diseases. *Arthritis Rheum* 1997;40:306–317.
153. Caricchio R, Cohen PL. Spontaneous and induced apoptosis in systemic lupus erythematosus: multiple assays fail to reveal consistent abnormalities. *Cell Immunol* 1999;198(1):54–60.
154. Richardson BC, Yung RL, Johnson KJ, et al. Monocyte apoptosis in patients with active lupus. *Arthritis Rheum* 1996;39(8): 1432–1434.
155. Courtney PA, Crockard AD, Williamson K, et al. Increased apoptotic peripheral blood neutrophils in systemic lupus erythematosus: relations with disease activity, antibodies to double stranded DNA, and neutropenia. *Ann Rheum Dis* 1999;58(5): 309–314.
156. Miret C, Font J, Molina R, et al. Bcl-2 oncogene (B cell lymphoma/leukemia-2) levels correlate with systemic lupus erythematosus disease activity. *Anticancer Res* 1999;19(4B):3073–3076.
157. Alvarado-de la Barrera C, Alcocer-Varela J, Richaud-Patin Y, et al. Differential oncogene and TNF-alpha mRNA expression in bone marrow cells from systemic lupus erythematosus patients. *Scand J Immunol* 1998;48(5):551–556.
158. Aringer M, Wintersberger W, Steiner CW, et al. High levels of bcl-2 protein in circulating T lymphocytes, but not B lymphocytes, of patients with systemic lupus erythematosus. *Arthritis Rheum* 1994;37(10):1423–1430.
159. Gatenby PA, Irvine M. The bcl-2 proto-oncogene is overexpressed in systemic lupus erythematosus. *J Autoimmun* 1994; 7(5):623–631.
160. Ohsako S, Hara M, Harigai M, et al. Expression and function of Fas antigen and bcl-2 in human systemic lupus erythematosus lymphocytes. *Clin Immunol Immunopathol* 1994;73: 109–114.
161. Vaux DL, Cory S, Adams JM. *Bcl-2* gene promotes haemopoietic cell survival and cooperates with *c-myc* to immortalize pre-B cells. *Nature* 1988;335:440–442.

162. Nunez G, Seto M, Seremetis S, et al. Growth- and tumor-promoting effects of deregulated *BCL2* in human B-lymphoblastoid cells. *Proc Natl Acad Sci USA* 1989;86:4589–4593.
163. Tsujimoto Y. Overexpression of the human BCL-2 gene product results in growth enhancement of Epstein-Barr virus-immortalized B cells. *Proc Natl Acad Sci USA* 1989;86:1958–1962.
164. Strasser A, Whittingham S, Vaux DL, et al. Enforced BCL2 expression in B-lymphoid cells prolongs antibody responses and elicits autoimmune disease. *Proc Natl Acad Sci USA* 1991;88:8661–8665.
165. Kalden JR. Defective phagocytosis of apoptotic cells: possible explanation for the induction of autoantibodies in SLE. *Lupus* 1997;6(3):326–327.
166. Sakata K, Sakata A, Kong L, et al. Monocyte rescue of human T cells from apoptosis is CD40/CD154 dependent. Scand *J Immunol* 1999;50(5):479–484.
167. Kgi D, Vignaux F, Ledermann B, et al. Fas and perforin pathways as major mechanisms of T cell-mediated cytotoxicity. *Science* 1994;265:528–530.
168. Lowin B, Hahne M, Mattmann C, et al. Cytolytic T-cell cytotoxicity is mediated through perforin and Fas lytic pathways. *Nature* 1994;370:650–652.
169. Walsh CM, Matloubian M, Liu C-C, et al. Immune function in mice lacking the perforin gene. *Proc Natl Acad Sci USA* 1994;91:10854–10858.
170. Kojima H, Shinohara N, Hanaoka S, et al. Two distinct pathways of specific killing revealed by perforin mutant cytotoxic T lymphocytes. *Immunity* 1994;1:357–364.
171. Watanabe-Fukunaga R, Brannan CI, Copeland NG, et al. Lymphoproliferation disorder in mice explained by defects in Fas antigen that mediates apoptosis. *Nature* 1992;356:314–317.
172. Lynch DH, Watson ML, Alderson MR, et al. The mouse Fas-ligand gene is mutated in gld mice and is part of a TNF family gene cluster. *Immunity* 1994;1:131–136.
173. Takahashi T, Tanaka M, Brannan CI, et al. Generalized lymphoproliferative disease in mice, caused by a point mutation in the Fas ligand. *Cell* 1994;76:969–976.
174. Ramsdell F, Seaman MS, Miller RE, et al. gld/gld Mice are unable to express a functional ligand for Fas. *Eur J Immunol* 1994;24:928–933.
175. Cohen PL, Eisenberg RA. Lpr and gld: single gene models of systemic autoimmunity and lymphoproliferative disease. *Annu Rev Immunol* 1991;9:243–269.
176. Reap EA, Leslie D, Abrahams M, et al. Apoptosis abnormalities of splenic lymphocytes in autoimmune lpr and gld mice. *J Immunol* 1995;154:936–943.
177. Roark JH, Kuntz CL, Nguyen CA, et al. Breakdown of B cell tolerance in a mouse model of systemic lupus erythematosus. *J Exp Med* 1995;181:1157–1167.
178. Wu J, Zhou T, Zhang J, et al. Correction of accelerated autoimmune disease by early replacement of the mutated lpr gene with the normal Fas apoptosis gene in the T cells of transgenic MRL-lpr/lpr mice. *Proc Natl Acad Sci USA* 1994;91:2344–2348.
179. Mysler E, Bini P, Drappa J, et al. The apoptosis-1/Fas protein in human systemic lupus erythematosus. *J Clin Invest* 1994;93:1029–1034.
180. Amasaki Y, Kobayashi S, Takeda T, et al. Up-regulated expression of Fas antigen (CD95) by peripheral naive and memory T cell subsets in patients with systemic lupus erythematosus (SLE): a possible mechanism for lymphopenia. *Clin Exp Immunol* 1995;99:245–250.
181. Lenardo M, Chan KM, Hornung F, et al. Mature T lymphocyte apoptosis—immune regulation in a dynamic and unpredictable antigenic environment. *Annu Rev Immunol* 1999;17:221–253.
182. Rieux-Laucat F, Le Deist F, Hivroz C, et al. Mutations in Fas associated with human lymphoproliferative syndrome and autoimmunity. *Science* 1995;268:1347–1349.
183. Fisher GH, Rosenberg FJ, Straus SE, et al. Dominant interfering Fas gene mutations impair apoptosis in a human autoimmune lymphoproliferative syndrome. *Cell* 1995;81:935–946.
184. Cheng J, Zhou T, Liu C, et al. Protection from Fas-mediated apoptosis by a soluble form of the Fas molecule. *Science* 1994;263:1759–1762.
185. Bijl M, van Lopik T, Limburg PC, et al. Do elevated levels of serum-soluble fas contribute to the persistence of activated lymphocytes in systemic lupus erythematosus? *J Autoimmun* 1998;11(5):457–463.
186. Knipping E, Krammer PH, Onel KB, et al. Levels of soluble Fas/APO-1/CD95 in systemic lupus erythematosus and juvenile rheumatoid arthritis. *Arthritis Rheum* 1995;38:1735–1737.
187. Goel N, Ulrich DT, St. Clair EW, et al. Lack of correlation between serum soluble Fas/APO-1 levels and autoimmune disease. *Arthritis Rheum* 1995;38:1738–1743.
188. Garrone P, Neidhardt E-M, Garcia E, et al. Fas ligation induces apoptosis of CD40-activated human B lymphocytes. *J Exp Med* 1995;182:1265–1273.
189. Schattner EJ, Elkon KB, Yoo D-H, et al. CD40 ligation induces Apo-1/Fas expression on human B lymphocytes and facilitates apoptosis through the Apo-1/Fas pathway. *J Exp Med* 1995;182:1557–1565.
190. Yellin MJ, Sippel K, Inghirami G, et al. CD40 molecules induce down-modulation and endocytosis of T cell surface T cell-B cell activating molecule/CD40-L: potential role in regulating helper effector function. *J Immunol* 1994;152:598–608.
191. Ranheim EA, Kipps TJ. Activated T cells induce expression of B7/BB1 on normal or leukemic B cells through a CD40-dependent signal. *J Exp Med* 1993;177:925–935.
192. Suda T, Takahashi T, Golstein P, et al. Molecular cloning and expression of the Fas ligand, a novel member of the tumor necrosis factor family. *Cell* 1993;75:1169–1178.
193. Ramsdell F, Seaman MS, Miller RE, et al. Differential ability of Th1 and Th2 T cells to express Fas ligand and to undergo activation-induced cell death. *Int Immunol* 1994;6:1545–1553.
194. Stalder T, Hahn S, Erb P. Fas antigen is the major target molecule for $CD4^+$ T cell-mediated cytotoxicity. *J Immunol* 1994;152:1127–1133.
195. Hanabuchi S, Koyanagi M, Kawasaki A, et al. Fas and its ligand in a general mechanism of T-cell-mediated cytotoxicity. *Proc Natl Acad Sci USA* 1994; 91:4930–4934.
196. Vignaux F, Golstein P. Fas-based lymphocyte-mediated cytotoxicity against syngeneic activated lymphocytes: a regulatory pathway? *Eur J Immunol* 1994;24:923–927.
197. Alderson MR, Tough TW, Davis-Smith T, et al. Fas ligand mediates activation-induced cell death in human T lymphocytes. *J Exp Med* 1995;181:71–77.
198. Brunner T, Mogil RJ, LaFace D, et al. Cell-autonomous Fas (CD95)/Fas-ligand interaction mediates activation-induced apoptosis in T-cell hybridomas. *Nature* 1995;373:441–444.
199. Dhein J, Walczak H, Bumier C, et al. Autocrine T-cell suicide mediated by APO-1/(Fas/CD95). *Nature* 1995;373:438–441.
200. Ju S-T, Panka DJ, Cui H, et al. Fas(CD95)/FasL interactions required for programmed cell death after T-cell activation. *Nature* 1995;373:444–448.
201. Rothstein TL, Wang JKM, Panka DJ, et al. Protection against Fas-dependent Th1-mediated apoptosis by antigen receptor engagement in B cells. *Nature* 1995;374:163–165.
202. Abe T, Homma M. Immunological reactivity in patients with systemic lupus erythematosus. Humoral antibody and cellular immune responses. *Acta Rheumatol Scand* 1971;17(1):35–46.
203. Horwitz DA. Impaired delayed hypersensitivity in systemic lupus erythematosus. *Arthritis Rheum* 1972;15(4):353–359.

204. Hahn BH, Bagby MK, Osterland CK. Abnormalities of delayed hypersensitivity in systemic lupus erythematosus. *Am J Med* 1973;55:25–31.
205. Paty JG Jr, Sienknecht CW, Townes AS, et al. Impaired cell-mediated immunity in systemic lupus erythematosus (SLE). A controlled study of 23 untreated patients. *Am J Med* 1975;59:769–779.
206. Horwitz DA, Garrett MA. Lymphocyte reactivity to mitogens in subjects with systemic lupus erythematosus, rheumatoid arthritis and scleroderma. *Clin Exp Immunol* 1977;27:92–99.
207. Horwitz DA, Garrett MA, Craig AH. Serum effects of mitogenic reactivity in subjects with systemic lupus erythematosus, rheumatoid arthritis and scleroderma. Technical considerations and lack of correlation with anti-lymphocyte antibodies. *Clin Exp Immunol* 1977;27:100–110.
208. Rosenthal CJ, Franklin EC. Depression of cellular-mediated mediated immunity in systemic lupus erythematosus. Relation to disease activity. *Arthritis Rheum* 1975;18:207–217.
209. Markenson JA, Lockshin MD, Fuzesi L, et al. Suppressor monocytes in patients with systemic lupus erythematosus. Evidence of suppressor activity associated with a cell-free soluble product of monocytes. *J Lab Clin Med* 1980;95:40–48.
210. Bell DA. Cell-mediated immunity in systemic lupus erythematosus: observations on in vitro cell-mediated immune responses in relationship to number of potentially reactive T cells, disease activity, and treatment. *Clin Immunol Immunopathol* 1978;9:301–317.
211. Malave I, Cuadra C. Impaired function of peripheral lymphocytes in systemic lupus erythematosus. *Intern Arch Allergy Appl Immunol (NY)* 1977;55:412–419.
212. Patrucco R, Rothfield NF, Hirschhorn K. The response of cultured lymphocytes from patients with systemic lupus erythematosus to DNA. *Arthritis Rheum* 1967;10:32–37.
213. Sucia-Foca N, Buda JA, Thiem T, et al. Impaired responsiveness of lymphocytes in patients with systemic lupus erythematosus. *Clin Exp Immunol* 1974;18:295–303.
214. Gottlieb AB, Lahita RG, Chiorazzi N, et al. Immune function in systemic lupus erythematosus. Impairment of in vitro T-cell proliferation and in vivo antibody response to exogenous antigen. *J Clin Invest* 1979;63:885–892.
215. Takada S, Ueda Y, Suzuki N, et al. Abnormalities in autologous mixed lymphocyte reaction-activated immunologic processes in systemic lupus erythematosus and their possible correction by interleukin 2. *Eur J Immunol* 1985;15:262–267.
216. Kumagai S, Steinberg AD, Green I. Immune responses to hapten-modified self and their regulation in normal individuals and patients with systemic lupus erythematosus. *J Immunol* 1981; 127:1643–1658.
217. Kuntz MM, Innes JB, Weksler ME. The cellular basis of the impaired autologous mixed lymphocyte reaction in patients with systemic lupus erythematosus. *J Clin Invest* 1979;63:151–153.
218. Sakane T, Steinberg AD, Arnett FC, et al. Studies of immune functions of patients with systemic lupus erythematosus. III. Characterization of lymphocyte subpopulations responsible for defective autologous mixed lymphocyte reactions. *Arthritis Rheum* 1979;22:770–776.
219. Sakane T, Steinberg AD, Green I. Failure of autologous mixed lymphocyte reactions between T and non-T cells in patients with systemic lupus erythematosus. *Proc Natl Acad Sci USA* 1978;75:3464–3468.
220. Utsinger PD, Yount WJ. Phytohemagglutinin response to systemic lupus erythematosus. Reconstitution experiments using highly purified lymphocyte subpopulations and monocytes. *J Clin Invest* 1977;60:626–638.
221. Goldman JA, Litwin A, Adams LE, et al. Cellular immunity to nuclear antigens in systemic lupus erythematosus. *J Clin Invest* 1972;51:2669–2677.
222. Martorell J, Font J, Rojo I, et al. Responsiveness of systemic lupus erythematosus T cells to signals provided through LCA T200 (CD45) and T1 (CD5) antigens. *Clin Exp Immunol* 1989;78:172–176.
223. Stekman IL, Blasini AM, Leon-Ponte M, et al. Enhanced CD3-mediated T lymphocyte proliferation in patients with systemic lupus erythematosus. *Arthritis Rheum* 1991;34:459–467.
224. Stohl W. Impaired generation of polyclonal T cell-mediated cytolytic activity despite normal polyclonal T cell proliferation in systemic lupus erythematosus. *Clin Immunol Immunopathol* 1992;63:163–172.
225. Murashima A, Takasaki Y, Ohgaki M, et al. Activated peripheral blood mononuclear cells detected by murine monoclonal antibodies to proliferating cell nuclear antigen in active lupus patients. *J Clin Immunol* 1990;10:28–37.
226. Horwitz DA, Stastny P, Ziff M. Circulating deoxyribonucleic acid-synthesizing mononuclear leukocytes. I. Increased numbers of proliferating mononuclear leukocytes in inflammatory disease. *J Lab Clin Med* 1970;76:391–402.
227. Dawisha SM, Gmelig-Meyling F, Steinberg AD. Assessment of clinical parameters associated with increased frequency of mutant T cells in patients with systemic lupus erythematosus. *Arthritis Rheum* 1994;37:270–277.
228. Theocharis S, Sfikakis PP, Lipnick RN, et al. Characterization of in vivo mutated T cell clones from patients with systemic lupus erythematosus. *Clin Immunol Immunopathol* 1995;74:135–142.
229. Raziuddin S, Nur MA, Al Wabel AA. Increased circulating HLA-DR+ CD4+ T cells in systemic lupus erythematosus: alterations associated with prednisolone therapy. *Scand J Immunol* 1990;31:139–145.
230. Tsuchiya N, Mitamura T, Goto M, et al. 2-Dimensional flow cytometric analysis of peripheral blood T lymphocytes from patients with systemic lupus erythematosus: preferential expression of HLA-DR antigen on the surface of Leu 2a+ cells. *J Rheumatol* 1988;15:946–951.
231. Hishikawa T, Tokano Y, Sekigawa I, et al. HLA-DP+T cells and deficient interleukin-2 production in patients with systemic lupus erythematosus. *Clin Immunol Immunopathol* 1990;55:285–296.
232. Horwitz DA, Wang H, Gray JD. Cytokine gene profile in circulating blood mononuclear cells from patients with systemic lupus erythematosus: increased interleukin-2 but not interleukin 4 mRNA. *Lupus* 1994;3:423–428.
233. Burgos P, Metz C, Bull P, et al. Increased expression of c-rel, from the NF-kappaB/Rel family, in T cells from patients with systemic lupus erythematosus. *J Rheumatol* 2000;27:116–127.
234. Campen DH, Horwitz DA, Quismorio FP Jr, et al. Serum levels of interleukin-2 receptor and activity of rheumatic disease characterized by immune system activation. *Arthritis Rheum* 1988;31:1358–1364.
235. Manoussakis MN, Papadopoulos GK, Drosos AA, et al. Soluble interleukin 2 receptor molecules in the serum of patients with autoimmune diseases. *Clin Immunol Immunopathol* 1989;50:321–332.
236. ter Borg EJ, Horst G, Limburg PC, et al. Changes in plasma levels of interleukin 2 receptor in relation to disease exacerbations and levels of anti-dsDNA and complement in systemic lupus erythematosus. *Clin Exp Immunol* 1990;82:21–26.
237. Samsonov MY, Tilz GP, Egorova O, et al. Serum soluble markers of immune activation and disease activity in systemic lupus erythematosus. *Lupus* 1995;4:29–32.
238. Spronk PE, ter Borg EJ, Huitema MG, et al. Changes in levels of soluble T-cell activation markers, sIL-2R, sCD4 and sCD8,

in relation to disease exacerbations in patients with systemic lupus erythematosus: a prospective study. *Ann Rheum Dis* 1994; 53:235–239.

239. Heilig B, Fiehn C, Brockhaus M, et al. Evaluation of soluble tumor necrosis factor (TNF) receptors and TNF receptor antibodies in patients with systemic lupus erythematosus, progressive systemic sclerosis, and mixed connective tissue disease. *J Clin Immunol* 1993;13:321–328.
240. Aderka D, Wysenbeek A, Engelmann H, et al. Correlation between serum levels of soluble tumor necrosis factor receptor and disease activity in systemic lupus erythematosus. *Arthritis Rheum* 1993;36:1111–1120.
241. Davas EM, Tsirogianni A, Kappou I, et al. Serum IL-6, TNFalpha, p55 srTNFalpha, p75srTNFalpha, srIL-2alpha levels and disease activity in systemic lupus erythematosus. *Clin Rheumatol* 1999;18(1):17–22.
242. Gabay C, Cakir N, Moral F, et al. Circulating levels of tumor necrosis factor soluble receptors in systemic lupus erythematosus are significantly higher than in other rheumatic diseases and correlate with disease activity. *J Rheumatol* 1997;24(2): 303–330.
243. Studnicka-Benke A, Steiner G, Petera P, et al. Tumour necrosis factor alpha and its soluble receptors parallel clinical disease and autoimmune activity in systemic lupus erythematosus. *Br J Rheumatol* 1996;35(11):1067–1074.
244. Kato K, Santana-Sahagun E, Rassenti LZ, et al. The soluble CD40 ligand sCD154 in systemic lupus erythematosus. *J Clin Invest* 1999;104:947–955.
245. Rozzo SJ, Drake CG, Chiang BL, et al. Evidence for polyclonal T cell activation in murine models of systemic lupus erythematosus. *J Immunol* 1994;153:1340–1351.
246. Kaneoka H, Morito F, Yamaguchi M. Low responsiveness to the anti Leu 4 antibody by T cells from patients with active systemic lupus erythematosus. *J Clin Lab Immunol* 1989;28: 15–26.
247. Bierer BE, Barbosa J, Herrmann S, et al. Interaction of CD2 with its ligand, LFA-3, in human T cell proliferation. *J Immunol* 1988;140:3358–3363.
248. Emilie D, Wallon C, Galanaud P, et al. Role of the LFA3-CD2 interaction in human specific B cell differentiation. *J Immunol* 1988;141:1912–1918.
249. Damle NK, Linsley PS, Ledbetter JA. Direct helper T cell-induced B cell differentiation involves interaction between T cell antigen CD28 and B cell activation B7. Eur *J Immunol* 1991;21:1277–1282.
250. Dohlsten M, Hedlund G, Lando PA, et al. Role of the adhesion molecule ICAM-1 (CD54) in staphylococcal enterotoxin-mediated cytotoxicity. *Eur J Immunol* 1991;21:131–135.
251. Linsley PS, Brady W, Urnes M, et al. CTLA-4 is a second receptor for the B cell activation antigen B7. *J Exp Med* 1991;174: 561–569.
252. Tohma S, Hirohata S, Lipsky PE. The role of CD11a/CD18-CD54 interactions in human T cell-dependent B cell activation. *J Immunol*1991;146:492–499.
253. Tohma S, Lipsky PE. Analysis of the mechanisms of T cell-dependent polyclonal activation of human B cells: induction of human B cell responses by fixed activated T cells. *J Immunol* 1991;146:2544–2552.
254. Azuma M, Cayabyab M, Buck D, et al. CD28 interaction with B7 costimulates primary allogeneic proliferative responses and cytotoxicity mediated by small, resting T lymphocytes. *J Exp Med* 1992;175:353–360.
255. Azuma M, Cayabyab M, Phillips JH, et al. Requirements for CD28-dependent T cell-mediated cytotoxicity. *J Immunol* 1993;150:2091–2101.
256. Takeuchi T, Amano K, Sekine H, et al. Upregulated expression and function of integrin adhesive receptors in systemic lupus erythematosus patients with vasculitis. *J Clin Invest* 1993;92: 3008–3016.
257. Tsokos GC, Kovacs B, Sfikakis PP, et al. Defective antigen-presenting cell function in patients with systemic lupus erythematosus: role of the B7-1 (CD80) costimulatory molecule. *Arthritis Rheum* 1996;39:600–609.
258. García-Cózar FJ, Molina IJ, Cuadrado MJ, et al. Defective B7 expression on antigen-presenting cells underlying T cell activation abnormalities in systemic lupus erythematosus (SLE) patients. *Clin Exp Immunol* 1996;104:72–79.
259. Sfikakis PP, Oglesby R, Sfikakis P, et al. B7/BB1 provides an important costimulatory signal for CD3-mediated T lymphocyte proliferation in patients with systemic lupus erythematosus (SLE). *Clin Exp Immunol* 1994;96:8–14.
260. Fox, D, Millard JA, Treisman J, et al. Defective CD2 pathway T cell activation in systemic lupus erythematosus. *Arthritis Rheum* 1991;34:561–571.
261. Gray JD, Hirokawa M, Ohtsuka K, et al. Generation of an inhibitory circuit involving CD8$^+$ T cells, interleukin 2, and NK cell-derived TGF-: Contrasting effects of anti-CD2 and anti-CD3. *J Immunol* 1998;160:22–48.
262. Lederman S, Yellin MJ, Krichevsky A, et al. Identification of a novel surface protein on activated CD4$^+$ T cells that induces contact-dependent B cell differentiation (help). *J Exp Med* 1992;175:1091–1101.
263. Noelle RJ, Roy M, Shepherd DM, et al. A 39-kDa protein on activated helper T cells binds CD40 and transduces the signal for cognate activation of B cells. *Proc Natl Acad Sci USA* 1992; 89:6550–6554.
264. Holder MJ, Wang H, Milner AE, et al. Suppression of apoptosis in normal and neoplastic human B lymphocytes by CD40 ligand is independent of Bcl-2 induction. *Eur J Immunol* 1993; 23:2368–2371.
265. Tsubata T, Wu J, Honjo T. B-cell apoptosis induced by antigen receptor crosslinking is blocked by a T-cell signal through CD40. *Nature* 1993;364:645–648.
266. Lederman S, Yellin MJ, Cleary AM, et al. T-BAM/CD40–L on helper T lymphocytes augments lymphokine-induced B cell Ig isotype switch recombination and rescues B cells from programmed cell death. *J Immunol* 1994;152:2163–2171.
267. Garrone P, Neidhardt E-M, Garcia E, Galibert L, et al. Fas ligation induces apoptosis of CD40–activated human B lymphocytes. *J Exp Med* 1995;182:1265–1273.
268. Schattner EJ, Elkon KB, Yoo D-H, et al. CD40 ligation induces Apo-1/Fas expression on human B lymphocytes and facilitates apoptosis through the Apo-1/Fas pathway. *J Exp Med* 1995; 182:1557–1565.
269. Yellin MJ, Sippel K, Inghirami G, et al. CD40 molecules induce down-modulation and endocytosis of T cell surface T cell-B cell activating molecule/CD40-L: potential role in regulating helper effector function. *J Immunol* 1994;152:598–608.
270. Ranheim EA, Kipps TJ. Activated T cells induce expression of B7/BB1 on normal or leukemic B cells through a CD40-dependent signal. *J Exp Med* 1993;177:925–935.
271. Desai-Mehta A, Lu L, Ramsey-Goldman R, et al. Hyperexpression of CD40 ligand by B and T cells in human lupus and its role in pathogenic autoantibody production. *J Clin Invest* 1996; 97:2063–2073.
272. Koshy M, Berger D, Crow MK. Increased expression of CD40 ligand on systemic lupus erythematosus lymphocytes. *J Clin Invest* 1996;98:826–837.
273. Vakkalanka RK, Woo C, Kirou KA, et al. Elevated levels and functional capacity of soluble CD40 ligand in systemic lupus erythematosus. *Arthritis Rheum* 1999;42:871–881.
274. Charpentier B, Carnaud C, Bach JF. Selective depression of the

xenogeneic cell-mediated lympholysis in systemic lupus erythematosus. *J Clin Invest* 1979;64:351–360.
275. Stohl W. Impaired polyclonal T cell cytolytic activity: a possible risk factor for systemic lupus erythematosus. *Arthritis Rheum* 1995;38:506–516.
276. Liossis SN, Ding XZ, Dennis GJ, et al. Altered pattern of TCR/CD3-mediated protein-tyrosyl phosphorylation in T cells from patients with systemic lupus erythematosus: deficient expression of the T cell receptor zeta chain. *J Clin Invest* 1998; 101:1448–1457.
277. Takeuchi T, Tsuzaka K, Pang M, et al. TCR chain lacking exon 7 in two patients with systemic lupus erythematosus. *Int Immunol* 1998;10:911–921.
278. Brundula V, Rivas LJ, Blasini AM, et al. Diminished levels of T cell receptor chain in peripheral blood T lymphocytes from patients with systemic lupus erythematosus. *Arthritis Rheum* 1999;42:1908–1916.
279. Stewart SJ, Prpic V, Powers FS, et al. Perturbation of the human T-cell antigen receptor-T3 complex leads to the production of inositol tetrakisphosphate: evidence for conversion from inositol trisphosphate. *Proc Natl Acad Sci USA* 1986;83:6098–6102.
280. Nishizuka Y. The role of protein kinase C in cell surface signal transduction and tumour promotion. *Nature* 1984;308: 693–698.
281. Gardner P. Calcium and T lymphocyte activation. *Cell* 1989;59: 15–20.
282. Bocckino SB, Blackmore PF, Wilson PB, et al. Phosphatidate accumulation in hormone-treated hepatocytes via a phospholipase D mechanism. *J Biol Chem* 1987;262:15309–15315.
283. Rosoff PM, Savage N, Dinarello CA. Interleukin-1 stimulates diacylglycerol production in T lymphocytes by a novel mechanism. *Cell* 1988;54:73–81.
284. Gelfand EW, Cheung RK, Mills GB, et al. Uptake of extracellular Ca^{2+} and not recruitment from internal stores is essential for T lymphocyte proliferation. *Eur J Immunol* 1988;18: 917–922.
285. Stohl W, Kaplan MS, Gonatas NK. A quantitative assay for experimental allergic encephalomyelitis in the rat based on permeability of spinal cords to ^{125}I-human-globulin. *J Immunol* 1979;122:920–925.
286. Arai H, Gordon D, Nabel EG, et al. Gene transfer of Fas ligand induces tumor regression *in vivo*. *Proc Natl Acad Sci USA* 1997;94:13862–13867.
287. Gardner P, Alcover A, Kuno M, et al. Triggering of T-lymphocytes via either T3-Ti or T11 surface structures opens a voltage-insensitive plasma membrane calcium-permeable channel: requirement for interleukin-2 gene function. *J Biol Chem* 1989;264:1068–1076.
288. Sierakowski S, Kucharz EJ, Lightfoot RW, et al. Impaired T-cell activation in patients with systemic lupus erythematosus. *J Clin Immunol* 1989;9:469–476.
289. Portales-Perez D, Gonzalez-Amaro R, Abud-Mendoza C, et al. Abnormalities in CD69 expression, cytosolic pH and Ca2+ during activation of lymphocytes from patients with systemic lupus erythematosus. *Lupus* 1997;6:48–56.
290. Vassilopoulos D, Kovacs B, Tsokos GC. TCR/CD3 complex-mediated signal transduction pathway in T cells and T cell lines from patients with systemic lupus erythematosus. *J Immunol* 1995;155:2269–2281.
291. Truneh A, Albert F, Golstein P, et al. Early steps of lymphocyte activation bypassed by synergy between calcium ionophores and phorbol ester. *Nature* 1985;313:318–320.
292. Nel AE, Bouic P, Lattanze GR, et al. Reaction of T lymphocytes with anti-T3 induces translocation of C-kinase activity to the membrane and specific substrate phosphorylation. *J Immunol* 1987;138:3519–3524.
293. Averill LE, Stein RL, Kammer GM. Control of human T-lymphocyte interleukin-2 production by a cAMP-dependent pathway. *Cell Immunol* 1988;115:88–99.
294. Wong HK, Kammer GM, Dennis G, et al. Abnormal NF-B activity in T lymphocytes from patients with systemic lupus erythematosus is associated with decreased p65-RelA protein expression. *J Immunol* 1999;163:1682–1689.
295. Tada Y, Nagasawa K, Yamauchi Y, et al. A defect in the protein kinase C system in T cells from patients with systemic lupus erythematosus. *Clin Immunol Immunopathol* 1991;60: 220–231.
296. Takeuchi T, Pang M, Amano K, et al. Reduced protein tyrosine phosphatase (PTPase) activity of CD45 on peripheral blood lymphocytes in patients with systemic lupus erythematosus (SLE). *Clin Exp Immunol* 1997;109:20–26.
297. Blasini AM, Alonzo E, Chacon R, et al. Abnormal pattern of tyrosine phosphorylation in unstimulated peripheral blood T lymphocytes from patients with systemic lupus erythematosus. *Lupus* 1998;7:515–523.
298. Mandler R, Birch RE, Polmar SH, et al. Abnormal adenosine-induced immunosuppression and cAMP metabolism in T lymphocytes of patients with systemic lupus erythematosus. *Proc Natl Acad Sci USA* 1982;79:7542–7546.
299. Phi NC, Takáts A, Binh VH, et al. Cyclic AMP level of lymphocytes in patients with systemic lupus erythematosus and its relation to disease activity. *Immunol Lett* 1989;23:61–64.
300. Hasler P, Schultz LA, Kammer GM. Defective cAMP-dependent phosphorylation of intact T lymphocytes in active systemic lupus erythematosus. *Proc Natl Acad Sci USA* 1990;87: 1978–1982.
301. Kammer GM, Khan IU, Malemud CJ. Deficient type I protein kinase A isozyme activity in systemic lupus erythematosus T lymphocytes. *J Clin Invest* 1994;94:422–430.
302. Laxminarayana D, Khan IU, Mishra N, et al. Diminished levels of protein kinase A RIα and RIβ transcripts and proteins in systemic lupus erythematosus T lymphocytes. *J Immunol* 1999; 162:5639–5648.
303. Mishra N, Khan IU, Tsokos GC, et al. Association of deficient type II protein kinase A activity with aberrant nuclear translocation of the RIIβ subunit in systemic lupus erythematosus T lymphocytes. *J Immunol* 2000;165:2830–2840.
304. Cho-Chung YS, Pepe S, Clair T, et al. cAMP-dependent protein kinase: role in normal and malignant growth. *Crit Rev Oncol Hematol* 1995;21:33–61.
305. Khan IU, Kammer GM. Pre-translational block of protein kinase A Riβ synthesis in lupus T cells. *FASEB J* 2000; 14:A1206.
306. Laxminarayana D, Kammer GM. mRNA mutations of type I protein kinase A regulatory subunit alpha in T lymphocytes of a subject with systemic lupus erythematosus. *Int Immunol* 2000;12:1521–1529.
307. Solomou EE, Juang Y-T, Gourley M, et al. Molecular basis of deficient IL-2 production in T cells from patients with SLE: cAMP responsive element modulator (CREM) binds to the −180 site of the IL-2 promoter instead of cAMP responsive element binding protein (CREB). *Arthritis Rheum* 2000;43:S38.
308. Horwitz DA. Mechanisms producing decreased mitogenic reactivity in patients with systemic lupus erythematosus and other rheumatic diseases in mitogens. In: Oppenheim JJ, Rosenstreich DL, eds. *Mitogens and immunobiology*. New York: Academic Press, 1976:625–638.
309. Horwitz DA, Cousar JB. A relationship between impaired cellular immunity, humoral suppression of lymphocytes function and severity of systemic lupus erythematosus. *Am J Med* 1975; 58:829–835.
310. Horwitz DA, Garrett MA, Craig AH. Serum effects on mito-

genic reactivity in subjects with systemic lupus erythematosus, rheumatoid arthritis and scleroderma. *Clin Exp Immunol* 1977; 27:100–110.

311. Yamada A, Winfield JB. Inhibition of soluble antigen-induced T cell proliferation by warm-reactive antibodies to activated T cells in systemic lupus erythematosus. *J Clin Invest* 1984;74: 1948–1960.
312. Wernet P, Kunkel HG. Antibodies to a specific surface antigen on T cells in human sera inhibiting mixed leukocyte culture reactions. *J Exp Med* 1973;138:1021–1026.
313. Williams RC Jr, Lies RB, Messner RP. Inhibition of mixed leukocyte culture responses by serum and gamma globulin fractions from certain patients with connective tissue disorders. *Arthritis Rheum* 1973;16:597–605.
314. Suciu-Foca N, Herter FP, Buda JA, et al. Comparison of lymphocyte reactivity in patients with cancer, systemic lupus erythematosus and renal allografts. *Oncology* 1975;31(3–4): 125–132.
315. Hahn BH, Pletcher LS, Muniain M, et al. Suppression of the normal autologous mixed lymphocyte reaction by sera from patients with systemic lupus erythematosus. *Arthritis Rheum* 1982;25:381–389.
316. Okudaira K, Searles RP, Goodwin JS, et al. Antibodies in the sera of patients with systemic lupus erythematosus that block the binding of monoclonal anti-Ia to Ia-positive targets also inhibit the autologous mixed lymphocyte response. *J Immunol* 1982;129:582–586.
317. Stephens HAF, Fitzharris P, Knight RA, et al. Inhibition of proliferative and suppressor responses in the autologous mixed lymphocyte reaction by serum from patients with systemic lupus erythematosus. *Ann Rheum Dis* 1982;41:495–501.
318. Brozek CM, Hoffman CL, Savage SM, et al. Systemic lupus erythematosus sera inhibit antigen presentation by macrophages to T cells. *Clin Immunol Immunopathol* 1988;46:299–313.
319. Cohen PL, Litvin DA, Winfield JB. Association between endogenously activated T cells and immunoglobulin-secreting B cells in patients with active systemic lupus erythematosus. *Arthritis Rheum* 1982;25:168–173.
320. Litvin DA, Cohen PL, Winfield JB. Characterization of warm-reactive IgG anti-lymphocyte antibodies in systemic lupus erythematosus. Relative specificity for mitogen-activated T cells and their soluble products. *J Immunol* 1983;130:181–186
321. Sagawa A, Abdou NI. Suppressor-cell antibody in systemic lupus erythematosus. Possible mechanism for suppressor-cell dysfunction. *J Clin Invest* 1979;63:536–539.
322. Morimoto C, Abe T, Toguchi T, et al. Studies of anti-lymphocyte antibody in patients with active SLE. *Scand J Immunol* 1979;10:213–221.
323. Sakane T, Steinberg AD, Reeves JP, et al. Studies of immune functions of patients with systemic lupus erythematosus. 4. T-cell subsets and antibodies to T-cell subsets. *J Clin Invest* 1979; 64:1260–1269.
324. Morimoto C, Reinherz EL, Distaso JA, et al. Relationship between systemic lupus erythematosus T cell subsets, anti-T cell antibodies and T cell functions. *J Clin Invest* 1984;73;689–700.
325. Yamada A, Shaw M, Winfield JB. Surface antigen specificity of cold-reactive IgM antilymphocyte antibodies in systemic lupus erythematosus. *Arthritis Rheum* 1985;28:44–51.
326. Yamada A, Cohen PL, Winfield JB. Subset specificity of antilymphocyte antibodies in systemic lupus erythematosus. Preferential reactivity with cells bearing the T4 and autologous erythrocyte receptor phenotypes. *Arthritis Rheum* 1985;28:262–270.
327. Tanaka S, Matsuyama T, Steinberg AD, et al. Antilymphocyte antibodies against $CD4^{+}$2H4+ cell populations in patients with systemic lupus erythematosus. *Arthritis Rheum* 1989;32: 398–405.
328. Gorla R, Airo P, Franceschini F, et al. Decreased number of peripheral blood $CD4^{+}$ $CD29^{+}$ lymphocytes and increased spontaneous production of anti-DNA antibodies in patients with systemic lupus erythematosus. *J Rheumatol* 1990;17: 1048–1053.
329. Messner RP, De Horatius RJ, Ferrone S. Lymphocytotoxic antibodies in systemic lupus erythematosus patients and their relatives. Reactivity with the HLA antigenic molecular complex. *Arthritis Rheum* 1980;23:265–272.
330. Stach RM, Rowley DA. A first or dominant immunization. II. Induced immunoglobulin carries transforming growth factor beta and suppresses cytolytic T cell responses to unrelated alloantigens. *J Exp Med* 1993;78:841–852.
331. Caver TE, O'Sullivan FX, Gold LI, et al. Intracellular demonstration of active TGFbeta1 in B cells and plasma cells of autoimmune mice. IgG-bound TGFbeta1 suppresses neutrophil function and host defense against Staphylococcus aureus infection. *J Clin Invest* 1996;98(11):2496–2506.
332. Llorente L, Richaud-Patin Y, Wijdenes J, et al. Spontaneous production of interleukin-10 by B lymphocytes and monocytes in systemic lupus erythematosus. *Eur Cytokine Network* 1993;4: 421–427.
333. Houssiau FA, Lefebvre C, Vanden Berghe M, et al. Serum interleukin 10 titers in systemic lupus erythematosus reflect disease activity. *Lupus* 1995;4:393–395.
334. Mosmann TR. Properties and functions of interleukin-10. *Adv Immunol* 1994;56:1–26.
335. de Waal Malefyt R, Yssel H, De Vries JE. Direct effect of IL-10 on subsets of human $CD4^{+}$ T cell clones and resting T cells. Specific inhibition of IL-2 production and proliferation. *J Immunol* 1993;150:4754–4765.
336. Ding L, Shevach EM. IL-10 inhibits mitogen-induced T cell proliferation by selectively inhibiting macrophage costimulatory function. *J Immunol* 1992;148:3133–3139.
337. Sagawa K, Mochizuki M, Sugita S, et al. Suppression by IL-10 and IL-4 of cytokine production induced by two-way autologous mixed lymphocyte reaction. *Cytokine* 1996;8:501–506.
338. Warrington RJ, Rutherford WJ. Normal mitogen-induced suppression of the interleukin-6 (IL-6) response and its deficiency in systemic lupus erythematosus. *J Clin Immunol* 1990;10:52–60.
339. Tsokos GC, Smith PL, Christian BC, et al. Interleukin-2 restores the depressed allogeneic cell-mediated lympholysis and natural killer cell activity in patients with systemic lupus erythematosus. *Clin Immunol Immunopathol* 1985;34:379–386.
340. Via CS, Sharrow SO, Shearer GM. Role of cytotoxic T lymphocytes in the prevention of lupus-like disease occurring in a murine model of graft-vs-host disease. *J Immunol* 1987;139: 1840–1849.
341. Shustov A, Luzina I, Nguyen P, et al. Role of perforin in controlling B-cell hyperactivity and humoral autoimmunity. *J Clin Invest* 2000;106:R39–R47.
342. Rolink AG, Gleichmann E. Allosuppressor- and allohelper-T cells in acute and chronic graft-vs.-host (GVH) disease. III. Different Lyt subsets of donor T cells induce different pathological syndromes. *J Exp Med* 1983;158:546–558.
343. Pals ST, Gleichmann H, Gleichmann E. Allosuppressor and allohelper T cells in acute and chronic graft-vs.-host disease. V. F_1 mice with secondary chronic GVHD contain F_1-reactive allohelper but no allosuppressor T cells. *J Exp Med* 1984;159: 508– 523.
344. Friedman SM, Posnett DN, Tumang JR, et al. A potential role for microbial superantigens in the pathogenesis of systemic autoimmune disease. *Arthritis Rheum* 1991;34:468–480.
345. Stohl W, Elliott JE, Linsley PS. Human T cell-dependent B cell differentiation induced by staphylococcal superantigens. *J Immunol* 1994;153:117–127.

346. Crow MK, Zagon G, Chu Z, et al. Human B cell differentiation induced by microbial superantigens: unselected peripheral blood lymphocytes secrete polyclonal immunoglobulin in response to *Mycoplasma arthritidis* mitogen. *Autoimmunity* 1992;14:23–32.
347. Stohl W, Elliott JE. Differential human T cell-dependent B cell differentiation induced by staphylococcal superantigens (SAg): regulatory role for SAg-dependent B cell cytolysis. *J Immunol* 1995;155:1838–1850.
348. Stohl W, Elliott JE, Lynch DH, et al. CD95 (Fas)-based, superantigen-dependent, CD4+ T cell-mediated down-regulation of human in vitro immunoglobulin responses. *J Immunol* 1998; 160:5231–5238.
349. Stohl W, Lynch DH, Starling GC, et al. Superantigen-driven, CD8+ T cell-mediated down-regulation: CD95 (Fas)-dependent down-regulation of human Ig responses despite CD95-independent killing of activated B cells. *J Immunol* 1998;161: 3292–3298
350. Macchia D, Parronchi P, Piccinni M-P, et al. In vitro infection with HIV enables human CD4+ T cell clones to induce noncognate contact-dependent polyclonal B cell activation. *J Immunol* 1991;146:3413–3418.
351. Stohl W, Hamilton AS, Deapen DM, et al. Impaired cytotoxic T lymphocyte activity in systemic lupus erythematosus following *in vitro* polyclonal T cell stimulation: a contributory role for non-T cells. *Lupus* 1999;8:293–299.
352. Stohl W, Elliott JE, Hamilton AS, et al. Impaired recovery and cytolytic function of CD56+ T and non-T cells in systemic lupus erythematosus following in vitro polyclonal T cell stimulation: studies in unselected patients and monozygotic disease-discordant twins. *Arthritis Rheum* 1996;39:1840–1851.
353. Stohl W, Elliott JE, Li L, et al. Impaired nonrestricted cytolytic activity in systemic lupus erythematosus: involvement of a pathway independent of Fas, tumor necrosis factor, and extracellular ATP that is associated with little detectable perforin. *Arthritis Rheum* 1997;40(6):1130–1137.
354. Tan P, Pang G, Wilson JD. Immunoglobulin production in vitro by peripheral blood lymphocytes in systemic lupus erythematosus: helper T cell defect and B cell hyperreactivity. *Clin Exp Immunol* 1981;44:548–554.
355. Fauci AS, Moutsopoulos HM. Polyclonally triggered B cells in the peripheral blood and bone marrow of normal individuals and in patients with systemic lupus erythematosus and Sjogren's syndrome. *Arthritis Rheum* 1981;24:577–583.
356. Nies KM, Stevens RH, Louie JS. Normal T cell regulation of IgG synthesis in systemic lupus erythematosus. *J Clin Lab Immunol* 1980;4:69–75.
357. Delfraissy JF, Second P, Galanaud P, et al. Depressed primary in vitro antibody response in untreated systemic lupus erythematosus. *J Clin Invest* 1980;11:141–142.
358. Kumagai S, Sredni B, House S, et al. Defective regulation of B lymphocyte colony formation in patients with systemic lupus erythematosus. *J Immunol* 1982;128:258–262.
359. Linker-Israeli M, Baake AC, Quismorio FP Jr, et al. Correlation of interleukin-2 production in patients with systemic lupus erythematosus by removal of spontaneously activated suppressor cells. *J Clin Invest* 1985;75:762–768.
360. Brodman R, Gilfillan, Glass D, et al. Influenza response in systemic lupus erythematosus. *Ann Intern Med* 1978;88:735–740.
361. Louie JS, Nies KM Shoji KT, et al. Clinical and antibody responses after influenza immunization in systemic lupus erythematosus. *Ann Intern Med* 1978;88:790–792.
362. Abdou NI, Sagawa A, Passual E, et al. Suppressor T cell abnormality in idiopathic systemic lupus erythematosus. *Clin Immunol Immunopathol* 1976;6:192–199.
363. Bresnihan B, Jasin HE. Suppressor function of peripheral blood mononuclear cells in normal individuals and in patients with systemic lupus erythematosus. *J Clin Invest* 1977;59:106–116.
364. Horowitz S, Borcherding H, Moothy AV, et al. Induction of suppressor T cells in systemic lupus erythematosus by thymosin and cultured thymic epithelium. *Science* 1977;197:999–1001.
365. Morimoto C. Loss of suppressor T lymphocyte function in patients with systemic lupus erythematosus. *Clin Exp Immunol* 1978;32:125–133.
366. Sakane T, Steinberg AD, Green I. Studies of immune functions of patients with systemic lupus erythematosus. I. Dysfunction of suppressor T cell activity related to impaired generation of, rather than response to, suppressor cells. *Arthritis Rheum* 1978; 21:657–664.
367. Kaufman DV, Bostwick E. Defective suppressor T cell activity in systemic lupus erythematosus. *Clin Immunol Immunopathol* 1979;13:9–18.
368. Morimoto C, Abe T, Homma M. Altered function of suppressor T lymphocytes in patients with active systemic lupus erythematosus. *Clin Immunol Immunopathol* 1979;13:161–170.
369. Newman B, Blank R, Lomnitzer R, et al. Lack of suppressor activity in systemic lupus erythematosus. *Clin Immunol Immunopathol* 1979;13:187–193.
370. Ilfeld DN, Krakauer RS. Suppression of immunoglobulin synthesis of systemic lupus erythematosus patients by concanavalin A activated normal human spleen cell supernatants. *Clin Immunol Immunopathol* 1980;17:196–202.
371. Gladman D, Keystone E, Urowitz M, et al. Impaired antigen specific suppressor cell activity in patients with systemic lupus erythematosus. *Clin Exp Immunol* 1980;40:77–82.
372. Alarcon-Segovia D, Palacios R. Differences in immunoregulatory T cell circuits between diphenylhydantoin related and spontaneously occurring SLE. *Arthritis Rheum* 1981;24:1086–1092.
373. Coovadia HM, Mackay IR, d'Aspice AJF. Suppressor cells assayed by three different methods in patients with chronic active hepatitis and systemic lupus erythematosus. *Clin Immunol Immunopathol* 1981;18:268–275.
374. Tsokos GC, Magrath IT, Balow JE. Epstein Barr virus induces normal B cell responses but defective T cell responses in patients with systemic lupus erythematosus. *J Immunol* 1983;131: 1797–1801.
375. Gray JD, Hirokawa M, Horwitz DA. The role of transforming growth factor beta in the generation of suppression: an interaction between CD8;pl T cells and NK cells. *J Exp Med* 1994; 180:1937–1942.
376. Gray JD, Hirokawa M, Ohtsuka K, et al. Generation of an inhibitory circuit involving CD8+ T cells, IL-2 and NK cell derived TGF: contrasting effects of anti-CD2 and anti-CD3. *J Immunol* 1998;160:2248–2254.
377. Ohtstuka K, Gray JD, Stimmler MM, et al. Defects in lymphocyte production of transforming growth factor-β1 do not correlate with disease activity or severity. *Lupus* 1999;8:90–94.
378. Ohtsuka K, Gray JD, Quismorio FP Jr, et al. Cytokine mediated down-regulation of B cell activity in SLE: effects of interleukin 2 and transforming growth factor beta. *Lupus* 1999;8:95–102.
379. Mohan C, Yu Y, Morel L, et al. Genetic dissection of Sle pathogenesis: Sle3 on murine chromosome 7 impacts T cell activation, differentiation, and cell death. *J Immunol* 1999;162(11): 6492–6502.
380. Gray-McGuire C, Moser KL, Gaffney PM, et al. Genome scan of human systemic lupus erythematosus by regression modeling: evidence of linkage and epistasis at 4p16-15.2. *Am J Hum Genet* 2000;67(6):1460–1469.
381. Mehrian R, Quismorio FP Jr, Strassmann G, et al. Synergistic effect between IL-10 and bcl-2 genotypes in determining susceptibility to systemic lupus erythematosus. *Arthritis Rheum* 1998;41(4):596–602.

382. Taylor PR, Carugati A, Fadok VA, et al. A hierarchical role for classical pathway complement proteins in the clearance of apoptotic cells in vivo. *J Exp Med* 2000;192(3):359–366.
383. Carson DA, Chen PP, Kipps TJ. New roles for rheumatoid factor. *J Clin Invest* 1991;87:379–383.
384. Lawley W, Doherty A, Denniss S, et al. Rapid lupus autoantigen relocalization and reactive oxygen species accumulation following ultraviolet irradiation of human keratinocytes. *Rheumatology (Oxf)* 2000;39(3):253–261.
385. Pablos JL, Santiago B, Galindo M, et al. Keratinocyte apoptosis and p53 expression in cutaneous lupus and dermatomyositis. *J Pathol* 1999;188(1):63–68.
386. Amoura Z, Piette JC, Chabre H, et al. Circulating plasma levels of nucleosomes in patients with systemic lupus erythematosus: correlation with serum antinucleosome antibody titers and absence of clear association with disease activity. *Arthritis Rheum* 1997;40:2217–2225.
387. Owen-Schaub LB, Yonehara S, Crump WL III, et al. DNA fragmentation and cell death is selectively triggered in activated human lymphocytes by Fas antigen engagement. *Cell Immunol* 1992;140:197–205.
388. Nishioka WK, Welsh RM. Susceptibility to cytotoxic T lymphocyte-induced apoptosis is a function of the proliferative status of the target. *J Exp Med* 1994;179:769–774.
389. Kurts C, Carbone FR, Krummel MF, et al. Signalling through CD30 protects against autoimmune diabetes mediated by CD8 T cells. *Nature* 1999;398(6725):341–344.
390. Nishimura H, Nose M, Hiai H, et al. Development of lupus-like autoimmune diseases by disruption of the PD-1 gene encoding an ITIM motif-carrying immunoreceptor. *Immunity* 1999;11(2):141–151.
391. Balomenos D, Martin-Caballero J, Garcia MI, et al. The cell cycle inhibitor p21 controls T-cell proliferation and sex-linked lupus development. *Nat Med* 2000;6(2):171–176.
392. Gleichmann E, Pals ST, Rolink AG, et al. Graft-versus-host reactions: clues to the etiopathology of a spectrum of immunological diseases. *Immunol Today* 1984;5:324–332.
393. Gleichmann E, Van Elven EH, Van der Veen JP. A systemic lupus erythematosus (SLE)-like disease in mice induced by abnormal T-B cell cooperation. Preferential formation of autoantibodies characteristic of SLE. *Eur J Immunol* 1982;12: 152–159.
394. Huck S, Deveaud E, Namane A, et al. Abnormal DNA methylation and deoxycytosine-deoxyguanine content in nucleosomes from lymphocytes undergoing apoptosis. *FASEB J* 1999;13: 1415–1422.
395. Sato Y, Miyata M, Sato Y, et al. CpG motif-containing DNA fragments from sera of patients with systemic lupus erythematosus proliferate mononuclear cells in vitro. *J Rheumatol* 1999;26:294–301.
396. Hellmann DB, Petri M, Whiting-O'Keefe Q. Fatal infections in systemic lupus erythematosus: the role of opportunistic organisms. *Medicine (Baltimore)* 1987;66:341–348.
397. Frank MM, Hamburger MI, Lawley TJ, et al. Defective reticuloendothelial system Fc-receptor function in systemic lupus erythematosus. *N Engl J Med* 1979;300:518–523.
398. Robey FA, Jones KD, Steinberg AD. C-reactive protein mediates the solubilization of nuclear DNA by complement in vitro. *J Exp Med* 1985;161:1344–1356.
399. Pickering MC, Botto M, Taylor PR, et al. Systemic lupus erythematosus, complement deficiency, and apoptosis. *Adv Immunol* 2000;76:227–324.
400. Taylor PR, Carugati A, Fadok VA, et al. A hierarchical role for classical pathway complement proteins in the clearance of apoptotic cells in vivo. *J Exp Med* 2000;192(3):359–366.
401. Du Clos TW, Zlock LT, Hicks PS, et al. Decreased autoantibody levels and enhanced survival of (NZB×NZW) F1 mice treated with C-reactive protein. *Clin Immunol Immunopathol* 1994;70:22–27.
402. Bartnes K, Hannestad K. Engagement of the B lymphocyte antigen receptor induces presentation of intrinsic immunoglobulin peptides on major histocompatibility complex class II molecules. *Eur J Immunol* 1997;27(5):1124–1130.
403. Roth R, Nakamura T, Mamula MJ. B7 costimulation and autoantigen specificity enable B cells to activate autoreactive T cells. *J Immunol* 1996;157(7):2924–2931.
404. Chan OT, Madaio MP, Shlomchik MJ. The central and multiple roles of B cells in lupus pathogenesis. *Immunol Rev* 1999; 169:107–121.
405. Serreze DV, Fleming SA, Chapman HD, et al. B lymphocytes are critical antigen-presenting cells for the initiation of T cell-mediated autoimmune diabetes in nonobese diabetic mice. *J Immunol* 1998;161(8):3912–3918.
406. Falcone M, Lee J, Patstone G, et al. B lymphocytes are crucial antigen-presenting cells in the pathogenic autoimmune response to GAD65 antigen in nonobese diabetic mice. *J Immunol* 1998;161(3):1163–1168.
407. Mohan C, Shi Y, Laman JD, et al. Interaction between CD40 and its ligand gp39 in the development of murine lupus nephritis. *J Immunol* 1995;154:1470–1480.
408. Liu Z, Tugulea S, Cortesini R, et al. Inhibition of CD40 signaling pathway in antigen presenting cells by T suppressor cells. *Hum Immunol* 1999;60:568–574.
409. Jacob CO, McDevitt HO. Tumour necrosis factor-alpha in murine autoimmune "lupus" nephritis. *Nature* 1988;331 (6154):356–358.
410. Charles PJ, Smeenk RJ, De Jong J, et al. Assessment of antibodies to double-stranded DNA induced in rheumatoid arthritis patients following treatment with infliximab, a monoclonal antibody to tumor necrosis factor alpha: findings in open-label and randomized placebo-controlled trials. *Arthritis Rheum* 2000;43(11):2383–2390.
411. Horwitz DA. Selective depletion of B lymphocytes with cyclophosphamide in patients with rheumatoid arthritis and systemic lupus erythematosus: guidelines for dosage. *Arthritis Rheum* 1974;17:363–374.
412. Dau PC, Callahan J, Parker R, et al. Immunologic effects of plasmapheresis synchronized with pulse cyclophosphamide in systemic lupus erythematosus (case report). *J Rheumatol* 1991; 18:270–276.
413. Llorente L, Richaud-Patin Y, Garcia-Padilla C, et al. Clinical and biologic effects of anti-interleukin-10 monoclonal antibody administration in systemic lupus erythematosus. *Arthritis Rheum* 2000;43:1790–1800.
414. Traynor AE, Schroeder J, Rosa RM, et al. Treatment of severe systemic lupus erythematosus with high-dose chemotherapy and haemopoietic stem-cell transplantation: a phase I study. Lancet 2000;356:701–707.

10

CYTOKINES IN THE PATHOGENESIS OF SYSTEMIC LUPUS ERYTHEMATOSUS

MICHAEL J. FRONCEK
DAVID A. HORWITZ

Systemic lupus erythematosus (SLE) is a multiorgan autoimmune disease characterized by a breakdown of self-tolerance, resulting in autoantibodies against nuclear, cytoplasmic, and cell surface antigens. Although the precise mechanism for the breakdown of self tolerance is not known, patients with active disease have demonstrable abnormalities in immune regulation. B-cell hyperactivity with polyclonal B-cell activation and consequent autoantibody formation is a prominent feature of SLE. Cellular immunity is also altered, with impairments in T cell and natural killer (NK) cell functions that lead to impaired host defenses (see Chapter 9). Alterations in cytokine production and cytokine networks strongly contribute to tolerance defects, B-cell hyperactivity, and impaired cellular immunity in SLE (1).

Cytokines are low molecular weight proteins that control the growth and differentiation of the cells of the immune system. They are produced and secreted by activated cells and act at very low concentrations in the range of endocrine hormones and neurotransmitters. Unlike hormones, which operate a long distance from secretion, cytokines generally act locally on cells within the immediate vicinity. Unlike neurotransmitters, which also have local effects, cytokines are not preformed but are synthesized following antigenic stimulation. These low molecular weight molecules tightly regulate the immune systems' complex feedback networks.

The role of cytokines in the pathogenesis of SLE has received strong attention, both as a framework for understanding the disease as well as a source of new therapeutic targets. This chapter discusses the properties of cytokines in general and groups them according to their principal effects on T-cell function, reviews the data on the production of these cytokines in human SLE, and reviews the data in a model proposed to reflect our current understanding of cytokine involvement in the pathogenesis of SLE.

GENERAL PROPERTIES OF CYTOKINES

Cytokines are secreted as simple polypeptides or low molecular weight glycoproteins [except for transforming growth factor-β (TGF-β)]. Many form higher molecular weight oligomers and one [interleukin-12 (IL-12)] is a heterodimer. Constitutive production of cytokines is usually low or absent, but production can be increased dramatically by various inducing stimuli acting at either the transcriptional or translational levels. Such induced cytokine production is usually transient unless the stimulus is maintained, and the distance over which the cytokine produced exerts its effect is generally short, that is, of an autocrine or paracrine nature.

Cytokines are both pleiotropic and redundant. While each cytokine has multiple functions, any one can be mediated by more than one cytokine and at least some of the effects of each are directed against cells of the hematopoietic lineage. They can be classified into distinct families based on similarities in their molecular structures, which correlate to some degree with functional relatedness. A detailed discussion of cytokine families is beyond the scope of this chapter, and the reader is referred to other resources for further information (2). When grouped by structural homology, some cytokine families include molecules with distinct and sometimes antagonistic effects on cell function. For the purpose of understanding their role in autoimmune phenomena, a useful grouping of cytokines is by their functional consequences, i.e., promotion of cell-mediated or humoral immunity.

Cytokines generally exert their effects by binding high-affinity ($\sim 10^{-11}$ M) receptors expressed at low numbers (~100 to 1,000) on different cell types. These receptors are generally not expressed constitutively but, like cytokines, appear following activation. Most cytokine actions can be attributed to an altered pattern of gene expression in the target cells. These changes are generally mediated by coupling between the cell surface receptor and intracellular protein kinases, which phosphorylate and activate cytokine-specific transcription factors. The combinatorial nature of this mechanism accounts for the overlapping yet distinct activities of different cytokines in the same structural family.

Because they have such potent effects, their action is highly regulated to avoid harmful effects of overdose. The production of cytokines and their receptors is generally transient, ranging from a few hours to a few days. Their function is also closely regulated by circulating cytokine inhibitors, which are often truncated forms of the extracellular domains of specific cytokine receptors. Production of a specific cytokine is closely followed by the production of respective soluble inhibitor(s). Cytokines such as IL-2, IL-4, IL-6, and tumor necrosis factor-α (TNF-α) are found in serum complexed to soluble receptors so that the levels of cytokines found in serum may not correlate with biologic activity or the amount produced.

SLE and the Th1/Th2 Paradigm

In 1986, Mosmann et al. (3) showed that mouse $CD4^+$ T-cell clones could be classified into distinct subsets according to their cytokine production pattern (3). Clones that produced IL-2 and interferon-γ (IFN-γ) were designated T-helper-1 (Th1) and those that produced IL-4 and IL-5 were designated Th2. Immature T cells, called ThO cells, produce a wide range of cytokines, and these cells differentiate to become Th1 or Th2 cells. Subsequently, with the discovery of other cytokines, Th1 cells were also found to respond to IL-12, and Th2 cells were found to additionally produce IL-6, IL-9, IL-10, and IL-13. These distinct cytokine profiles have functional significance. Th1 cytokines favor T-cell–mediated cellular immunity and cytotoxicity, delayed-type hypersensitivity, and monocyte activation with consequent production of proinflammatory cytokines (Table 10.1) Th2 cytokines favor B-cell–mediated humoral immunity, immunoglobulin E (IgE) class switching (IL-4), eosinophil activation (IL-5), and monocyte deactivation with resulting decrease in proinflammatory cytokine production. Moreover, IL-4 and IL-10 inhibit Th1 cytokine production and, correspondingly, IFN-γ inhibits Th2 cytokine production. Thus, cytokines such as IFN-γ and IL-4 are able to polarize cytokine production toward either the Th1 or Th2 profiles where the predominant response would be cell-mediated immunity or antibody production. Since there is a striking imbalance between these two arms of the immune response in SLE, one would predict Th2 cytokine polarization in this disease. This is the case in certain mouse models of SLE.

Although SLE has features consistent with Th2-type cytokine predominance, it would be an oversimplification to consider SLE as simply a disorder of excess T-cell production of Th2 cytokines for several reasons. The generalization that Th1 cytokines promote cell-mediated immunity and that Th2 cytokines support antibody production is not strictly true because of considerable overlap in cytokine activities. Both IFN-γ, a Th1 cytokine, and IL-4, a Th2 cytokine, play important roles in different aspects of the humoral response. Whereas IL-4 is important in B-cell differentiation, especially in IgM to IgG or IgE class switching, IFN-γ is required for the production of the complement fixing IgG antibodies. Complement fixing IgG anti-DNA antibodies are especially pathogenic in lupus nephritis. The timing of cytokine production is also important. In animal models of experimentally induced SLE, it has been reported that Th1-type cytokines predominate at the time of initiation of the disease, whereas Th2 cytokines are more prominent in later phases of disease (4). Finally, certain nucleosomal histone peptides that trigger autoreactive T cells in SLE preferentially induce Th1 cytokines, while others induce Th2 cytokines (5).

Another problem with the original Th1/Th2 classification is that non-T cells are the principal source of IL-12 and IL-10, two cytokines that have major roles in polarizing T-cell cytokine production. IL-12, which clearly plays the major role promoting Th1 cytokine production, is not produced by T cells, but rather by macrophages. A useful classification of cytokines, therefore, is to group them by their primary biologic activities without reference to their cellular source. Th1-like cytokines are those whose primary function is to promote cell-mediated immunity, such as IL-12, IL-2, IFN-γ, and TNF-β (lymphotoxin). Th2-like cytokines include IL-10, IL-4, IL-5, IL-6, and IL-13. This classification is imperfect, as some cytokines affect both compartments of the immune response. TNF-α has been considered a proinflammatory cytokine, but its effects are complex. This cytokine can also stimulate B-cell proliferation and differentiation (6) and possibly has a major role in the generation and effector activities of regulatory T cells (see below). IL-1 and TGF-β do not fit well into the type 1 or Th2-like grouping, and will be considered separately.

Th1-Like Cytokines in SLE

Interleukin-2

IL-2 delivers activation, growth, and differentiation signals to T, B, and NK cells, and thereby plays a central role in the development and propagation of immune responses. IL-2 also has an important role in the mechanisms that terminate immune responses, which include activation-induced cell death and suppressor T cells. $CD4^+$ lymphocytes are the principal producers of IL-2. $CD8^+$ cells, in general, are poor producers of IL-2 in response to mitogenic or antigenic stimulation, but they can generate substantial amounts of this cytokine in response to phorbol esters (7,8). $CD3^+CD4^-CD8^-$ cells also produce IL-2 when stimulated by mitogens,

TABLE 10.1. MAJOR CYTOKINES INVOLVED IN HUMORAL AND CELLULAR IMMUNITY IN SYSTEMIC LUPUS ERYTHEMATOSUS (SLE)

Cytokine	Cellular Source	Major Activities	Findings in SLE
Th1-like cytokines			
Interleukin-2	T cells	Activation of T and B cells Induction of killer and regulatory T cells	Production *in vivo* in response to autoreactive helper T cells may be increased Production *in vitro* in response to antigens and mitogens is decreased
Interferon-γ	T cells and NK cells	Induction of macrophage and killer T cell activity Co-stimulates B cells to produce complement fixing IgG antibodies	Production *in vitro* by mitogen-stimulated blood T cells is decreased
Interleukin-12	Dendritic cells and macrophages, also produced by B cells	Crucial role in host defense against intracellular pathogens Upregulates IFN-γ production and differentiation Promotes Th1 cell differentiation	Production is decreased in SLE Inverse correlation with IL-10 levels
Th2-like cytokines			
Interleukin-4	T cells and basophils	Promotes Th2 cell differentiation, B cell activation and Ig-class switching	No convincing evidence of increased production by CD4+ T cells in human SLE
Interleukin-10	Macrophages, T cells, and B cells	Stimulates B-cell growth and differentiation Decreases macrophage activation and cytokine production Can induce T-cell anergy	Constitutive production is greatly increased Contributes to B-cell activity and impaired cell-mediated immunity Enhances Fas-mediated T-cell apoptosis
Interleukin-6	Macrophages, Th2 cells, and B cells	Enhances induction of IL-4 producing T cells and supports terminal B-cell differentiation	Production is increased
Interleukin-5	T cells, NK cells, mast cells, eosinophils	Differentiation of eosinophils	Increased mRNA in SLE skin lesions
Other cytokines			
Interleukin-1	Macrophages and B cells	Activation of T cells and macrophages Proinflammatory	Spontaneous release is increased Stimulated production is decreased
TNF-α	Macrophages, T cells, NK, and B cells	Proinflammatory, and supports B cell differentiation Promotes adhesion molecule expression and migration of leukocytes to inflammatory sites Also contributes to regulatory T cell differentiation	Serum levels increased, complexed to TNF receptors Production *in vitro* generally decreased Complex effects *in vivo,* can accelerate or delay autoimmunity in mouse models depending on dose and timing
TGF-β	Macrophages, NK, T cells, and B cells	Broad immunosuppressive effects Produced as latent complex, must be converted to active form Co-stimulates the generation of regulatory T cells	Lymphocyte production of the active form of TGF-β is decreased in patients with active and inactive disease Low levels contribute to the impaired generation of regulatory T cells

IFN, interferon; Ig, immunoglobulin; NK, natural killer; TGF, transforming growth factor; TNF, tumor necrosis factor.

but to a lesser degree than $CD4^+$ cells (9). Co-stimulation through CD28 synergizes with T-cell receptor (TCR) signaling at the level of the IL-2 promoter and increases IL-2 messenger RNA (mRNA) stabilization. This signal promotes T-cell activation and prevents anergy induction. As the immune response proceeds, IL-2R expression diminishes, resulting in both a decline in IL-2 synthesis and a decrease in the number of high-affinity receptors, thus providing for termination of the normal T-cell immune response.

The IL-2 receptor is assembled from three components. The IL-2R α chain (p55, CD25) by itself is of low affinity, and may be expressed in soluble form, but in combination with the β and γ chains forms a high-affinity receptor site for IL-2 binding. The γ subunit (p64) is the so-called common γ chain also utilized by IL-4, IL-7, IL-13, and IL-15. The intermediate affinity β-subunit is also utilized by IL-15. Signal transduction is mediated by the complex of the β and γ receptor chains by the phosphorylation of JAK1 and JAK3, resulting in the activation of multiple signaling molecules, including signal transducers and activators of transcription (STATs) 1, 3, 5α, and 5β, phosphatidylinositol-3 (PI_3)-kinase, and mitogen-activated protein (MAP) kinase.

IL-2 production and responsiveness in SLE has been well studied with increasing evidence that this cytokine has an important role in pathogenesis. Several lines of evidence suggest that at least some T cells may be producing this cytokine *in vivo*. First, increased levels of IL-2 in the serum of SLE patients has been reported (10), and these levels correlate with clinical activity (11). Second, increased IL-2 production by SLE peripheral blood mononuclear cells (PBMCs) cultured at low cell densities has been documented (12). Third, IL-2 mRNA transcripts can be detected in unstimulated PBMCs only from patients with SLE, but not from healthy controls or patients with tuberculosis (13). Fourth, anti–IL-2 antibodies markedly decreased spontaneous Ig production by SLE B cells (13). Thus, it is not unlikely that some stimulated autoreactive T cells produce IL-2 *in vivo*.

Most studies of IL-2 production *in vitro*, however, have indicated that T cells from patients with SLE secrete lower amounts of IL-2 in response to mitogenic or antigenic stimulation than do those from healthy controls, although there is considerable heterogeneity within the groups studied (14–25). Defective IL-2 production has not been confirmed by all groups (26). This variability could be explained on the basis of differences in the clinical manifestations of SLE, disease activity, effects of treatment, the stimulus used to activate T cells, and by differences in the numbers and functional capacity of the responding cells. In general, decreased IL-2 activity is found in patients with active as well as patients with inactive SLE (17) and in relatives of these patients (27). Hagiwara and colleagues (28) have shown that the peripheral blood of lupus patients contains significantly fewer IL-2–secreting cells than that of healthy control subjects. Another study quantifying IL-2–producing lymphocytes following mitogen stimulation revealed a decrease that correlated with disease activity (29). Via and co-workers (25) have demonstrated heterogeneity in the ability of T cells from lupus patients to produce IL-2 following antigenic stimulation. The heterogeneity observed may be explained, in part, by variations in the production of IL-2 during the disease course, which has been observed in animal models (30–33).

Several mechanisms have been proposed to account for impaired IL-2 production. Defective IL-2 production may be a manifestation of an intrinsic T-cell defect. Horwitz and Garrett (34) showed in 1977 that PBMCs from patients with SLE proliferate less than those from controls when stimulated with mitogens (34). Tada and colleagues (35) have described an intrinsic defect in the protein kinase C system in SLE patients. A number of investigators were able to bypass this defect and attain normal IL-2 production by adding another activating agent to a phorbol ester such as phorbol myristate acetate (PMA) (20,36,37). Neither PMA alone, nor combinations of other stimuli such as phytohemagglutinin antigen (PHA), IL-1α, concanavalin A (ConA), or ionomycin are able to overcome the IL-2 secretion defect in human SLE-derived lymphocytes.

Decreased production of 3′,5′-cyclic adenosine monophosphate (cAMP) by lymphocytes from SLE patients was proposed to explain defective IL-2 production, and this defect did not correlate with disease activity (38). Kammer's group (39) has accumulated considerable evidence for deficient type I and type II protein kinase A activity in SLE. Recent analysis of the PKA-1 defect has revealed a pretranslational block in the RIβ subunit in SLE (40).

A second mechanism that can result in decreased IL-2 production in some individuals with SLE is decreased co-stimulation by antigen-presenting cells (25). Decreased expression of B7 on antigen-presenting cells as well as decreased expression of CD28 on T cells has been reported (41). Bypassing the need for co-stimulatory molecules by anti-CD28 can enhance IL-2 production (42,43).

A third causal mechanism is the "exhaustion" hypothesis. If T cells or PBMCs from normal subjects are stimulated with mitogens for 4 days, they acquire an IL-2 production defect that resembles that of lupus T cells. Indeed, resting SLE PBMCs for 2 or 3 days before stimulating these cells with PHA plus phorbol ester normalized IL-2 production (18). Others reported the decreased IL-2 production correlated with increased surface expression of the major histocompatibility complex (MHC) class II marker, human leukocyte antigen (HLA)-DP. After culturing SLE lymphocytes, decreased numbers of HLA-DP^+ cells correlated with increased IL-2 production (44). In a more recent study of mitogen-induced production of other Th1-like cytokines in SLE, resting SLE T cells for 48 hours was unable to correct the observed defects (45).

Factors external to the IL-2–producing T cells comprise a fourth causal mechanism to explain impaired production of this cytokine. Removal of radiosensitive $CD8^+$ cells normalized IL-2 production in SLE (46). These lymphocytes produced a soluble factor that had inhibitory activity. Recently, one group reported that $CD8^+$ T cells in SLE secrete increased amounts of IL-4 and IL-10 (47). The production of these cytokines by $CD8^+$ T cells could explain the inhibition of IL-2 production.

A fifth mechanism involves inhibitory factors in serum. Antibodies in SLE serum have been described that inhibit IL-2 production by normal cells (48). On the other hand, the levels of IL-2 inhibiting activity normally present in human serum is decreased in SLE (49,50). It was previously reported that the serum from patients with active SLE had strong inhibitory activity on the mitogenic reactivity of T cells and that this inhibitory activity was in the IgG fraction (51,52). It has been reported that strongly activated B cells can produce TGF-β complexed to IgG, and there are some data that these complexes are increased in SLE serum (53).

This IgG–TGF-β complex could explain some of the T-cell defects described in SLE, which include the production of IL-2 and other Th1 cytokines by activated T cells.

Besides production of IL-2, the lymphocyte response to this cytokine is also decreased in SLE (16,54,55,56). This is due to decreased expression of IL-2 receptors following mitogenic stimulation. This defect appears to correlate with disease activity. In a longitudinal study, the decreased proliferative response to IL-2 normalized within 6 months after therapy, but 18 months were needed for the expression of high-affinity IL-2 receptors to become normal (29).

Although freshly isolated T cells from patients with active SLE may have increased IL-2R α-chain expression, the β chain is not increased (56). Moreover, in response to mitogenic stimulation, there is less upregulation of both the α and β chains (54,56,57), predominantly in CD4+ T cells (21,57). This abnormality may reflect decreased generation *ex vivo* in SLE of the recently described CD4+ CD25+ regulatory T-cell subset (58).

Decreased IL-2-receptor expression also may reflect a regulatory defect. The precursor frequencies of IL-2–responsive cells increase after resting them for 24 hours before mitogenic stimulation (22). The addition of IL-2 or IFN to SLE lymphocytes partially corrects the defect (59–61). Of interest, although T cells are hyporesponsive, B cells in SLE show increased responsiveness to IL-2 (62).

In addition, high serum levels of soluble IL-2 receptor (sIL-2R) have been documented in patients with active disease (63–66). T-cell activation is known to trigger release of p55 sIL-2R, and despite its low affinity, sIL-2R can neutralize IL-2 effects *in vitro*. Thus, the increased levels of circulating sIL-2R could complex with newly released IL-2 and block the ability of T cells to respond to this cytokine.

It is possible to resolve the apparently conflicting observations that suggest increased IL-2 production by at least some SLE T cells *in vivo*, but impaired production and response to this cytokine *in vitro*. The spontaneous production of IL-2 by circulating T cells of patients with active SLE could be due to autoreactive T cells responding to nuclear autoantigens *in vivo*. This pathologic immune response triggers feedback regulatory mechanisms that result in an unsuccessful attempt by CD8+ cells and other regulatory T cells to terminate this autoimmune response. The inhibitory cytokines produced by these ineffective regulatory cells explain the impaired responsiveness of SLE T cells to mitogens and antigens *in vitro* (See below).

Interferon-γ

Interferon-γ is a 20- to 25-kd glycoprotein produced and secreted by T and NK cells as a homodimer in response to a variety of stimuli, both in a polyclonal and in an antigen-specific, clonally restricted manner. It is produced by CD8+ cells from infected individuals in response to *in vitro* stimulation with viral antigens (67). IFN-γ is also produced by virus-specific, MHC class II restricted CD4+ Th1 cells during infection. IFN-γ preferentially inhibits the proliferation of Th2 cells, and its presence during an immune response results in the preferential expansion of Th1 cells (68).

The IFN-γ receptor consists of a 90-kd a chain (also known as IFN-γ RI) that binds the IFN-γ homodimer, and an associated β chain (also known as IFN-γ RII) is required for biologic activity, e.g., induction of MHC class II (69–73). A single IFN-γ homodimer binds two receptor α chains that do not physically interact with each other (74). Receptor binding results in activation of the intracellular tyrosine kinases JAK1 and JAK2, which in turn phosphorylate STAT1, causing its dimerization and translocation to the nucleus. STAT1 dimers act as transcription factors capable of binding and activating gamma activation site (GAS) promoter elements present in IFN-γ inducible genes.

One of the major activities of IFN-γ is its ability to induce class II MHC expression on T cells, B cells, and antigen-presenting cells. IFN-γ can potentiate many of the actions of IL-12 and can also sensitize antigen-presenting cells to produce heightened levels of this cytokine in response to stimuli. IFN-γ also functions in the innate immune system by promoting increased macrophage killing in response to intracellular microbes and parasites. As stated above, IFN-γ induces class switching of IgM to IgG complement-fixing antibodies, and autoantibodies that have this property can be pathogenic.

There is evidence that IFN-γ has a pathogenic role in organ damage in SLE. Certain nucleosomal histone peptides stimulate autoreactive T cells to produce IFN-γ in lupus mice (5). Administration of IFN-γ greatly accelerates the development of lupus nephritis (75). Interferons may exacerbate and even precipitate human SLE, as has been reported in mice. Administration of IFN-γ to a patient with presumed rheumatoid arthritis induced an exacerbation of SLE (78,80). Administration of IFN-α, a related molecule, to patients with hematologic malignancies has also led to the appearance of autoantibodies and even clinical SLE (76,77). Moreover, IFN-α has also been implicated as a pathogenetic factor in lupus central nervous system (CNS) disease, in that a strong correlation has been reported between IFN-α levels in the cerebrospinal fluid (CSF) and lupus CNS disease (127).

Alterations in the production of IFN-γ in SLE are similar to IL-2. There is evidence of increased serum levels, but levels secreted by mitogen-stimulated cells are decreased in human SLE. One group reported increased serum levels in patients with active disease (81), although others found no difference in patients with early disease (82). Another group found no relationship between serum levels and disease activity, but instead a correlation of IFN-γ levels with those of TNF-α and IL-6, whose levels did parallel disease activity (83).

Several groups have reported decreased production of IFN-γ by mitogen-stimulated PBMCs in SLE (84–87), and the peripheral blood of SLE patients with active disease contains fewer IFN-γ–secreting cells than that of healthy control subjects (28). Yet another group has demonstrated no difference in either basal or mitogen-stimulated IFN-γ production between SLE patients and controls, but instead noted a correlation between IFN-γ levels and SLE disease activity as measured by the Systemic Lupus Activity Measure (SLAM) index (88).

Levels of IFN-γ may be critical at different stages of SLE. High levels at the onset could increase MHC class II gene expression, an effect that may be important in breaking tolerance to self antigens. Also, this cytokine would facilitate the production of pathogenic complement-fixing autoantibodies. Later in the disease, decreased levels of IFN-γ would allow high levels of Th2 cytokines that would enhance B-cell activity. One way of demonstrating this connection would be to show a genetic relationship between specific alleles of genes encoding IFN-γ or its receptor and the development of SLE, similar to what has been observed in mice.

Recently, polymorphisms have been identified within the genes for the two chains of the IFN-γ receptor associated with the risk of developing SLE. There is a higher frequency of the Val14Met polymorphism, located in the C-terminal signal peptide portion of IFN-γR1, in SLE patients than in healthy controls (89). In persons with this polymorphism, there is increased induction of HLA-DR antigen expression on B cells and a shift toward the Th2 phenotype in T cells as indicated by intracellular cytokine staining. Such a shift toward a Th2 response could theoretically increase the carrier's susceptibility to lupus. Further investigation showed that the greatest risk for development of SLE was in individuals who were both heterozygous for the Val14Met polymorphism and homozygous for Gln64 in the other chain of the γ receptor (90). These data imply that there is some link between the IFN-γ receptor structure—and by inference, function—and the development of SLE. *In vitro* studies of these mutant receptors may provide further clues.

Interleukin-12

IL-12 is a heterodimeric cytokine composed of p35 and p40 subunits. It is produced mainly by monocytes, macrophages, neutrophils, and dendritic cells, and to a lesser extent by B cells. Its receptor is a dimeric complex of β1 and β2 chains, so designated because of their homology to the gp130 molecule, shared by other cytokine receptors. Both chains are inducible on naive and memory $CD4^+$ T-cell clones within 48 hours of activation, and are further upregulated by stimulation through CD28. IL-2 can augment IL-12Rβ1 chain expression (91). Conversely, treatment of T cells with IL-10 or TGF-β blocks induction of the high-affinity IL-12 receptor by inhibiting the expression of the IL-12Rβ2 chain (92,93). Functional signaling via the IL-12R results in phosphorylation of $p56^{lck}$, the Janus kinases Tyk2 and Jak2, and the transcription activators STAT3 and STAT4.

IL-12, alone or in combination with IL-2, promotes the expansion and survival of activated T and NK cells and can modulate the cytotoxic activity of cytotoxic T lymphocytes (CTLs) and NK cells. It is required for $CD5^+$ B-cell activation *in vitro* (94), which may be associated with SLE development. IL-12 has been implicated in the pathogenesis of Th1-mediated autoimmune disease, such as experimental autoimmune encephalomyelitis (95).

Tokano and colleagues (96) reported elevated serum levels of IL-12 in SLE patients compared with normal controls, although there was a wide variability, with some patients having normal levels. The patients with high IL-12 levels also tended to have high levels of IFN-γ. They seem to have composed a subset because the majority of patients were reported to have elevations of Th2 cytokines. However, the relevance of serum cytokine levels to SLE pathogenesis is not clear. Interestingly, all the patients in their series with pulmonary involvement had elevated IL-12 levels, although the number of cases was small.

In contrast, most groups have found an impairment in IL-12 production in SLE. Horwitz and co-workers (45) have shown that even early in the course of SLE that monocyte production of IL-12 is decreased. Liu and Jones (97,98) also showed that IL-12 production by SLE PBMCs was significantly impaired, and that this impairment was due to monocyte function, not number. Furthermore, neutralizing antibody to IL-10 enhanced IL-12 production, but did not restore it to normal levels. The authors also found a correlation between low IL-12 production and active SLE as measured by Systemic Lupus Erythematosus Disease Activity Index (SLEDAI) scores. IFN-γ was able to restore IL-12 production level to normal, but clearly is not able to overcome the inhibition caused by high IL-10 levels. In their series, plasma IL-10 levels correlated negatively with IL-12 production by PBMCs *in vitro*. IL-12 production correlated negatively with anti–double-stranded DNA (dsDNA) antibody level and positively with IFN-γ levels (97,98).

The addition of IL-12 to SLE PBMCs can reduce B-cell activity *in vitro*. Houssiau et al. (99) reported that spontaneous polyclonal IgG production and anti-dsDNA-secreting cells were dramatically reduced by addition of IL-12. This appeared to be a direct effect of IL-12 and not due to upregulation of IFN-γ or downregulation of IL-10. Thus, decreased IL-12 production in SLE may possibly contribute to the imbalance between humoral and cellular immunity in this disease.

Th2-Like Cytokines in SLE

Interleukin-4

IL-4 regulates early T-cell activation events and can promote the production of Th2-like cytokines. The major sources of IL-4 are Th2 cells and CD4$^+$ NKT cells. In B cells IL-4 stimulates proliferation and is responsible for the switching of IgM to IgG1 and IgE. In contrast, IL-4 downregulates the proinflammatory and certain Th2-like cytokines in monocytes. It upregulates MHC class II and FcεRII expression. IL-4 shares, as part of its receptor complex, the common γ chain of the IL-2 receptor.

Although IL-4 production in many mouse models of lupus is increased and likely contributes to the pathogenesis of the disease, the role of IL-4 in human SLE is unclear. One might expect IL-4 levels to be elevated, but this has not been a consistent observation among different investigators. Dueymes and colleagues (100) have reported elevated serum IL-4 levels in some lupus patients. Elevated mRNA levels for IL-4 in PBMCs from lupus patients have also been shown (101). In particular, T cells expressing IL-4 appear to be of the NK phenotype, that is CD4$^-$ CD8$^-$ CD57$^+$ (102). Renal biopsies of SLE patients with active nephritis have been found to contain CD4$^+$ T cells expressing IL-4, which might suggest that overexpression is associated with glomerulonephritis (103). In contrast, Furusu and colleagues (104) have found a negative correlation between IL-4 and IL-4R expression levels and the degree of glomerular injury in lupus nephritis.

The current consensus is that IL-4 production in SLE is not increased. Horwitz and colleagues (13) found that IL-4 mRNA transcripts detected by semiquantitative polymerase chain reaction (PCR) were not increased in freshly prepared lymphocytes from their SLE patients. Moreover, in their study, mitogen-induced IL-4 levels were normal and serum IL-4 levels were not increased. Other groups have found that both spontaneous and induced IL-4 production by SLE PBMCs was comparable to or lower than that of controls (105,106). One group has shown an inverse relationship between IL-4 and IL-10 in SLE patients compared to controls, with increased IL-10 mRNA levels elevated in the presence of a simultaneous decrease in IL-4 and IL-13 (107). However, only IL-10 mRNA levels correlated with disease activity as measured by SLEDAI.

Recently, polymorphisms in the IL-4 promoter and IL-4 receptor genes have been associated with the development of SLE (108). The role of IL-4 in the pathogenesis of SLE may be related to its effect on other cytokines, rather than a direct effect. It has been reported that *in vitro* neutralization of endogenous IL-4 enhances spontaneous IgG production by SLE PBMCs, partly due to upregulated IL-6 production (109), while addition of exogenous IL-4 downregulated IL-6 production (110).

Interleukin-5

This cytokine has not been investigated thoroughly in human SLE. Of interest, NK cells can produce this cytokine (111), and it has been reported that NK cells also have the capacity to induce resting B cells to become immunoglobulin-secreting cells (112). Stein and colleagues (113) have shown elevated IL-5 mRNA levels in cutaneous lupus erythematosus (LE) lesions compared to control skin, implying a role for Th2 cells in the development of skin disease in SLE.

Interleukin-6

IL-6 is a pleiotropic cytokine that shares proinflammatory effects with IL-1β and TNF-α, as well as regulating the immune response by providing important positive and negative control signals to activated T and B cells. There is considerable evidence that IL-6 supports B-cell hyperreactivity in SLE. Cultured SLE PBMCs spontaneously release increased amounts of this cytokine (114), and increased levels are detectable in both resting and stimulated whole blood cultures (115). Increased numbers of IL-6–secreting cells have been documented in SLE, with analysis of single cells revealing macrophages as the principal source (28).

Increased serum IL-6 levels have also been demonstrated in SLE patients with active disease when compared to patients whose disease is inactive or healthy controls (116). Others have found a correlation between IL-6 levels and disease activity (117,118). Activity has also been shown to correlate with increased levels of other members of the IL-6 family, including leukemia inhibitory factor (LIF), oncostatin M (OSM), and ciliary neurotrophic factor (CNTF) (119). Ultraviolet A (UVA) irradiation induces transcription of IL-6 (and TNF-α) in human keratinocytes and dermal fibroblasts (120,121). UVA also induces blood mononuclear cells from patients with SLE to produce IL-6 (122). There is increased renal expression of IL-6 in SLE nephritis (123).

However, some groups have not been able to document a correlation between *in vitro* levels of IL-6 and immunoglobulin production (124), and at least one group has shown a lack of correlation between IL-6 levels and disease exacerbation in a retrospective study (125). Two groups have reported increased CSF levels of IL-6 in active CNS SLE (126,127).

In addition to SLE, high serum IL-6 concentrations are found in a variety of conditions, including rheumatoid arthritis, bacterial infections, burns, and alcoholic cirrhosis (128). In these diseases, IL-6 stimulates the liver to produce the acute-phase reactant C-reactive protein (CRP), which is often used clinically as a surrogate marker for IL-6 levels.

This protein, however, usually is not increased in active SLE, and in fact there is a lack of correlation between several key cytokines (IL-6, IL-10, TNF-α, and IFN-γ) and several acute-phase proteins (CRP, α_1-acid-glycoprotein (AGP), α_1-antichymotrypsin (ACT), suggesting their independence from cytokine regulation in SLE (129).

Increased IL-6 production in SLE could also be a consequence of autoimmunity, rather than a precipitant. The principal nuclear autoantigens are derived from free nucleosomes that are the product of cells undergoing apoptosis. It has been reported that exposure of SLE PBMCs to UV light induces keratinocytes in the skin to undergo apoptosis (130). Others have reported that nucleosomes induce the spleen of lupus mice to produce IL-6 (131), and in humans one group has reported that exposure of lupus PBMCs to UV light induces IL-6 production (122). Because apoptotic cells generally are phagocytosed by macrophages, it is not inconceivable that following exposure to sunlight, IL-6 could be produced by macrophages as a consequence of the phagocytosis of nucleosomal autoantigens. These cells also could process these autoantigens for presentation to autoreactive T cells. Autoreactive T-cell clones have been shown to provide help for polyclonal antibody production in part through the production of IL-6 (132).

There is also an intrinsic abnormality in lupus B cells in their response to IL-6. Although low-density B cells from healthy subjects did not respond to IL-6, low-density B cells from patients with active SLE directly differentiated into immunoglobulin-secreting cells without an additional costimulatory signal (133). While freshly isolated B cells from normal individuals do not spontaneously express IL-6 receptors, freshly isolated B cells from patients with SLE do express these receptors, which explains their responsiveness to IL-6 (134,135).

Interleukin-10

IL-10 is a potent stimulator of B-cell proliferation and differentiation and as such would be expected to play an important role in producing the B-cell hyperactivity that characterizes SLE. This cytokine also has other properties that contribute to immune dysregulation in SLE. IL-10 attenuates macrophage activation, cytokine production, and antigen presentation. Macrophage MHC class II expression is decreased, and production of IL-1, IL-6, and TNF-α is usually decreased (136). These indirectly inhibit T-cell function. IL-10 can also induce $CD4^+$ T cells to become anergic and has both inhibitory and stimulatory effects on $CD8^+$ T cells (137,138).

Both functional and genetic and studies suggest a strong pathogenetic link between IL-10 and human SLE. Feedback inhibition of TNF-α by IL-10 is important since the repeated administration of anti–IL-10 to B/W F1 mice delayed the onset of SLE, and this could be attributed to an increase in TNF-α levels (139). Twin studies and family studies have suggested that IL-10 production is genetically determined. Approximately 75% of the variation in IL-10 production can be explained on this basis (140). When at least two members of a family develop SLE, IL-10 production is increased in the relatives. This increase is not observed, however, if only one family member is affected (141). IL-10 production appears to be controlled at the transcriptional level (142), and microsatellite studies have suggested associations with certain alleles (143). In a study of a Mexican-American cohort, positive associations with SLE were found with alleles for IL-10 and Bcl-2, and these gene effects were synergistic. This was especially significant since the Bcl-2 and IL-10 genes reside on different chromosomes. The synergism, therefore, could not be attributed to linkage disequilibrium (144).

Llorente and colleagues (145,146) originally showed that human lupus peripheral blood B cells and monocytes, but not T cells, spontaneously produce large amounts of IL-10 mRNA and protein *in vitro* compared to PBMCs from controls, and this finding has been replicated by others (45). Serum IL-10 levels in SLE patients are elevated compared to controls, and, more importantly, correlate positively with disease activity by SLEDAI and anti-DNA antibody titers and negatively with C3 levels (28,98,147). Disease severity in lupus has been shown to correlate with an elevated ratio of IL-10 to IFN-γ secreting cells (28). In addition to monocytes, B cells, $CD4^+$ $CD45RO^+$ "memory" T cells, and even $CD8^+$ cells produce IL-10 in SLE patients (47,148,149). Llorente et al. (149) have shown that the spontaneous *in vitro* immunoglobulin production by PBMCs from SLE patients was strongly increased by IL-10, but only weakly by IL-6. Furthermore, production was not significantly affected by the addition of anti–IL-6 antibody, but was decreased by an anti–IL-10 monoclonal antibody.

The antagonistic properties of IL-10 on antigen-presenting cell functions have recently been shown to be important in the impaired cellular immune response in SLE (150). Serum IL-10 concentrations were higher in patients whose lymphocytes were "poor-responders" to recall or alloantigens, and addition of anti–IL-10 blocking antibody significantly increased their proliferative response. Furthermore, supernatants from SLE PBMCs could inhibit the normal allogeneic response between healthy controls and downregulate IL-12 p35 and p40 gene expression. An inverse relationship between IL-10 and IL-12 production has been noted by other investigators (151,152).

While IL-10 normally inhibits monocyte IL-6 production (151), this is not the case in SLE. The presence of increased spontaneous IL-10 production from cultures of B cells or monocytes from SLE patients who also have high IL-6 levels implies a defect in responsiveness to IL-10–mediated feedback (153). In SLE, therefore, there may be an intrinsic defect in IL-10–induced suppression of cytokine synthesis. Such a defect could account for the concomitant elevations of IL-10 and IL-6 seen in this disease and the correlation found between the two cytokine levels (129,154). This may be a key factor in perpetuating the polyclonal B-cell activation that characterizes SLE.

Finally, besides inhibiting T-cell activation, IL-10 may also promote activation-induced apoptosis. There is evidence for increased Fas-mediated activation-induced apoptosis in SLE, at least *in vitro*. Neutralization of IL-10 markedly reduced this phenomenon (155).

Other Cytokines

Interleukin-1

IL-1 has multiple biologic activities and is a regulator of the host response to infection and injury. The IL-1 family consists of three distinct, but structurally related molecules: IL-1α, IL-1β, and IL-1 receptor antagonistic (IL-1ra). The latter is the only known naturally occurring cytokine antagonist. IL-1ra acts as a competitive inhibitory of IL-1α and IL-1β by binding to receptors without transducing a signal. The binding of IgG to Fc receptors on monocytes triggers IL-1ra release (156).

In the 1980s increased spontaneous release of IL-1 from SLE monocytes was reported by several groups (157–159) with one exception (160). In one study, increased release of IL-1α and -1β correlated with serum antibodies to ribonucleoprotein (158). Spontaneous release of IL-1β was not observed in a recent study (161). In addition to monocytes, B cells can produce IL-1 as well as IL-6. It has been reported that IL-1 and IL-6 produced by SLE B cells sustain B-cell activity in an autocrine fashion (157,159,162), although others have reported that T-cell help is essential (163–166).

In contrast to increased spontaneous release of IL-1, the ability of monocytes or adherent cells to produce detectable IL-1 after stimulation is decreased in most patients with active disease (167–171). Decreased *in vitro* IL-1 production in SLE could be reversed by indomethacin, a finding suggesting that prostaglandins might be responsible for decreased IL-1 production (172). Increased prostaglandin production by SLE monocytes has indeed been reported in SLE (170,173), but there has been no recent progress in this area.

Two studies of IL-1ra production in SLE have been completed. One group reported decreased Fcγ receptor-mediated production of IL-1ra in patients with active, but not inactive SLE (161). Another group reported low levels of IL-1ra in patients with lupus nephritis (174).

Tumor Necrosis Factor

Although TNF-α is usually considered to be a proinflammatory, this cytokine has multiple functional properties. TNF-α can accelerate murine SLE or protect these mice from developing the disease. Both human SLE and mouse models of this disease show a strong association with specific alleles of MHC gene products. Stimulated blood mononuclear cells from patients with SLE or healthy individuals who are DQw1 or DR2 positive produce lower amounts of TNF-α than DR3 or DR4 positive subjects. Furthermore the MHC II alleles DR2, Dqw-1, and DR3 are strongly associated with SLE (175). It has been suggested that the true association is with the TNF-α since this gene is located in MHC class III region close by HLA-DR on the same chromosome. Polymorphisms associated with TNF-α production have been described. One group found an association independent of MHC II alleles (176), but the association reported by the other was MHC-linked (177). Another group reported an association of several TNF microsatellite alleles with SLE, but these were linked to the extended HLA-DRB1*0301 haplotype (178). One group reported a TNF receptor II polymorphism in Japanese SLE patients (179), but genetic linkage with this marker was not confirmed in SLE populations in Spain or the United Kingdom (180). Decreased TNF-β production in Korean patients homozygous for a specific TNF allele are strongly predisposed to develop SLE (181).

Several groups including our own have reported that *in vitro* production of TNF by mitogen-stimulated PBMCs is decreased in human SLE (45,169,182,183). This is controversial, however, since others have reported high levels of TNF mRNA (101) and increased TNF-α production *in vitro* (184). Another group found that serum levels of TNF-α were normal, but soluble TNF receptors were increased and the levels correlated with disease activity (185).

Whether TNF-α accelerates or prevents the development of autoimmune disease depends on the maturation state of the immune system. This phenomenon is best exemplified in the nonobese diabetic (NOD) mice, which spontaneously develop diabetes mellitus. Different workers at the same institution have made transgenic NOD mice that express TNF-α solely in islet cells. In one model these mice were protected from developing diabetes. Potentially pathogenic self-reactive T cells capable of triggering this disease were rendered nonfunctional. Moreover, the adoptive transfer of their T cells to athymic mice failed to produce diabetes, unlike the T cells of their nontransgenic littermates (186).

The generation of additional transgenic NOD mice that also expressed TNF-α only in islet cells had a different outcome (187). This time the progression of diabetes was greatly accelerated. Analysis of these two models revealed that in mice with rapid disease progression, TNF-α was expressed in the early neonatal period and resulted in accelerated islet antigen presentation to the self-reactive T cells. In the first model, expression of TNF-α in islet cells was delayed and, in this instance, the effects of this cytokine on immune cells resulted in a protective response.

These observations resemble the effects of TNF-α administered to New Zealand black (NZB) × New Zealand white (NZW) F1 mice. Administration of TNF-α to 4-month-old mice just before they begin to develop SLE delays the onset of lupus nephritis (18,188). Administration of TNF-α to younger B/W F1 mice, however, accelerated lupus nephritis instead (190). Dosage effects were also noted. High-dose, but not low-dose, TNF-α accelerated disease.

There are at least two explanations for the protective effects of TNF-α in SLE. Repeated administration of this cytokine leads to T-cell hyporesponsiveness (191). Recent unpublished studies from our laboratory suggest that this cytokine plays a critical role in generating the suppressive effects of human CD8+ regulatory T cells. Antagonism of TNF-α with a neutralizing antibody completely abolished the suppressive effects of these cells on antibody production. We have shown that the combination of IL-2 and TNF-α markedly enhance the production of the active form of TGF-β (192), and we believe that both of these cytokines strongly contribute to the suppressive effects of CD8+ regulatory T cells.

Transforming Growth Factor-β

TGF-βs are a multifunctional family of cytokines important in tissue repair, inflammation, and immunoregulation (193,194). Suppressive effects on the immune system are well described (195). Lymphocytes and monocytes produce the β1 isoform of this cytokine. TGF-β is unlike most other cytokines in that the protein released is biologically inactive and unable to bind to specific receptors (196). The latent complex is cleaved extracellularly to release active cytokine, as discussed below. Thus, the conversion of latent to active TGF-β is the critical step that determines the biologic effects of this cytokine. In addition to its immunosuppressive effects, TGF-β has positive effects on the growth and development of T cells. It upregulates its own production. T cells activated in the presence of TGF-β produce increased amounts of this cytokine (197).

Besides its immunosuppressive effects, there is increasing evidence that TGF-β also co-stimulates activated naive T cells to become regulatory T cells rather than Th1 or Th2 effector cells. CD8+ T cells activated in the presence of IL-2 and TGF-β develop the capacity to inhibit IgG production (198,199). Recently, Yamagiwa and co-workers (200) have documented that a subset of naive CD4+ T cells activated in the presence of TGF-β develop the capacity to prevent CD8+ T cells from responding to alloantigens. Less than one regulatory T cell per 100 T cells was needed for the demonstration of this effect. The phenotypic properties of the potent regulatory T cells were identical to the naturally occurring thymic-derived CD4+ CD25+ regulatory T cells described by others.

The finding that TGF-β apparently has a critical role in the development of regulatory T cells is especially relevant in SLE. Ohtsuka and co-workers (192) recently reported decreased production of both the active and latent forms of lymphocyte-derived TGF-β in SLE. Decreased production of total TGF-β, but not active TGF-β, was related to disease activity (202). Studies of cytokine regulation of TGF-β revealed that IL-2 and TNF-α increased the production of active TGF-β, whereas IL-10 had the opposite effect. Antagonism of IL-10 with a neutralizing antibody significantly increased the level of active TGF-β. SLE peripheral blood lymphocytes now produced levels of active TGF-β that would enable CD8+ cells to develop inhibitory activity (193). Evidence was obtained that the addition of IL-2 and TGF-β to CD8+ cells in SLE could markedly alter the regulatory effects of these cells. While untreated CD8+ cells enhanced IgG production, these cells developed significant inhibitory effects after activation in the presence of these cytokines (201).

It is important to emphasize that TGF-β is present in considerable quantities in serum. However, it is present in its latent form. Plasmin is the principal protease that converts the latent form of TGF-β produced by hematopoietic cells to its active form. Although there are scanty data on the conversion of latent to active TGF-β in SLE, it was reported previously that levels of plasmin activator in SLE serum are decreased and levels of plasmin activator inhibitor are increased (203). Thus, there are several reasons why the production of active TGF-β is decreased in SLE. The lack of IL-2 and TNF-α, increased amounts of IL-10, and decreased protease activity would all contribute to a cytokine defect that would block the generation of regulatory T cells.

Preliminary evidence was obtained that the addition of IL-2 and TGF-β to the blood mononuclear cells of patients with active SLE could downregulate both polyclonal IgG and antinuclear antibody production. PBMCs from 12 patients with active SLE were exposed to IL-2 with or without TGF-β for 3 days, washed, and cultured for 7 more days. This procedure markedly reduced both polyclonal IgG and autoantibody production. The inhibition was IL-2 dependent. In some cases IL-2 only was sufficient, but anti–TGF-β blocked this effect (201). These results provided additional evidence for the importance of IL-2 in the generation of active TGF-β. The finding that antagonism of IL-10 in SLE could increase lymphocyte-derived active TGF-β and that cytokines may be able to restore regulatory T-cell activity are encouraging observations. The potential exists to correct pathogenic immunoregulatory defects *in vivo*.

Although adequate levels of TGF-β in lymphoid tissues are required for immunoregulation, similar levels elsewhere can have deleterious consequences. TGF-β in the kidney can accelerate lupus nephritis (204–206). Interestingly, plasma cells can secrete TGF-β complexed to IgG, and phagocytosis of these complexes by neutrophils or macrophages has immunosuppressive effects (53,207). Serum from patients with active SLE has marked suppressive activity on T-cell function (51), and the suppressive activity was found in the IgG fraction (52). It is possible, therefore, that TGF-β in serum contributes to the many defects of immune function reported in SLE, including an impaired capacity of these patients to resist infection (208).

CYTOKINES AND THE IMBALANCE OF HUMORAL AND CELLULAR IMMUNITY IN SLE

A review of the current literature has revealed evidence strongly suggesting that some T cells from subjects with SLE produce Th1 cytokines such as IL-2 and IFN-γ *in vivo* as well as Th2 cytokines. Most studies also indicate decreased production of Th1 cytokines *in vitro*. These are not necessarily conflicting observations. Spontaneous production of IL-2 by circulating T cells of patients with active SLE could reflect autoreactive T cells responding to nuclear autoantigens *in vivo*. Certain nucleosomal histone peptides stimulate autoreactive T cells to produce IFN-γ in lupus mice (5). It is important to emphasize that feedback control mechanisms, which include cytokines, normally block the reactivity of these autoreactive T cells in healthy subjects. In SLE these homeostatic mechanisms have been altered, and cytokines instead of downregulating autoreactive cells sustain autoimmunity.

In healthy subjects, IL-10 and TGF-β are the principal cytokines responsible for feedback regulation of antibody production and cytotoxic T-cell activity following antigen stimulation (Fig. 10.1). TGF-β directly inhibits B-cell activity and also downregulates IL-10 production (193). Sustained production of Th2-like cytokines in SLE, therefore, could be the consequence of impaired production of active TGF-β. Without the attenuating effects of TGF-β, IL-10 and IL-6 sustain B-cell hyperactivity. In addition, the inhibitory effects of IL-10 on Th1 cytokine production could account for decreased levels of protective antibody following primary immunizations (209–212).

We have indicated the importance of the balance between TNF-α and IL-10 in SLE and that the disproportionally higher levels of IL-10 in this disease has pathogenic significance. As stated above, repeated administration of anti–IL-10 to NZB/W F1 mice delays the onset of SLE and increases survival. Interestingly, feeding NZB/W F1 mice long-chain omega-3 fatty acids also delays onset of autoimmune disease in these mice, and one of the principal effects of this diet was to reverse defects in cytokine production in these mice. Production of TGF-β and IL-2 by mitogen-stimulated splenocytes increased, and correspondingly, production of IL-4 decreased (213). In another study, long-chain omega 3 fatty acids decreased IL-10 and IL-6 levels in lupus mice (214).

High levels of IL-10 also contribute to impaired cellular immunity in SLE. In response to antigen-stimulation, production of the Th1-like cytokines IL-12, IL-2, and IFN-γ is

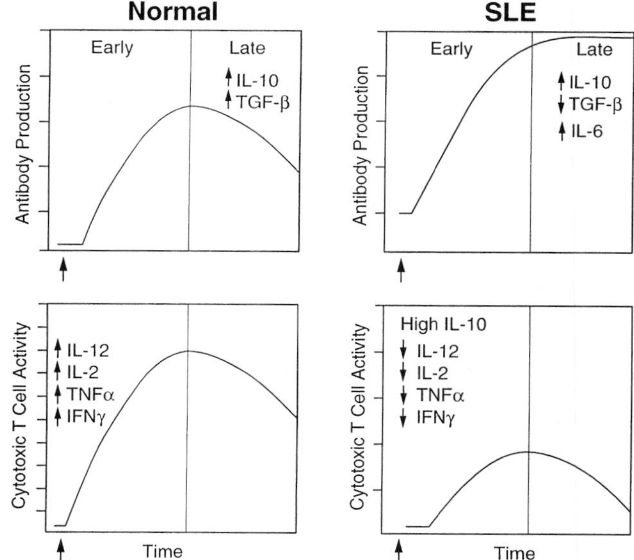

FIGURE 10.1. Abnormal cytokine feedback regulation of humoral and cellular immunity in systemic lupus erythematosus (SLE). In response to antigen stimulation, production of Th1 and Th2 cytokines is followed by production of interleukin-10 (IL-10) and transforming growth factor-β (TGF-β), which act as feedback regulators and inhibit antibody production and the number of cytotoxic T cells. TGF-β also downregulates IL-10 production, but lymphocyte production of active TGF-β is impaired in SLE. Levels of the Th2 cytokines IL-6 and IL-10 remain high and sustain B-cell hyperactivity. High levels of IL-10 also inhibit production of the Th1-like cytokines needed for the generation of cytotoxic T cells. The imbalance between IL-10 and TGF-β production results in B-cell hyperactivity and impaired cytotoxic T lymphocyte (CTL) activity in SLE.

decreased, as is production of TNF-α. The lack of appropriate amounts of these cytokines could account for an inadequate T-cell response to microbial agents and impaired host defense. As indicated above, blockade of IL-10 in SLE significantly increased the T-cell response of these patients to recall antigens and alloantigens. Llorente and co-workers (215) gave a single dose of murine anti–IL-10 to patients with SLE. Improvement in disease activity was noted as well as an increased in the T-cell proliferation *in vitro*. This is an important first step in showing the restoration of the balance between the production of Th1-like and Th2-like cytokines in SLE is likely to result in significant clinical improvement, if not remission.

REFERENCES

1. Horwitz DA, Jacob CO. The cytokine network in the pathogenesis of systemic lupus erythematosus and possible therapeutic implications. *Springer Semin Immunopathol* 1994;16:181–200.
2. Vilcek J. The cytokines: an overview. In: Thompson A, ed. *The cytokine handbook*, 3rd ed. San Diego: Academic Press, 1998:1–20.

3. Mosmann TR, Cherwinski H, Bond MW, et al. Two types of murine helper T cell clone. I. Definition according to profiles of activities and secreted proteins. *J Immunol* 1986;136: 2348–2357.
4. Segal R, Bermas BL, Dayan M, et al. Kinetics of cytokine production in experimental systemic lupus erythematosus: involvement of t helper cell 1/ T helper cell 2—type cytokines in disease. *J Immunol* 1997;158:3009–3016.
5. Lu L, Kaliyaperumal A, Boumpas DT, et al. Major peptide autoepitopes for nucleosome-specific T cells of human lupus. *J Clin Invest* 1999;104:345–55.
6. Jelinek DF, Lipsky PE. Enhancement of human B cell proliferation and differentiation by tumor necrosis factor-alpha and interleukin 1. *J Immunol* 1987;139(9):2970–2976.
7. Luger TA, Smolen JS, Chused TM, et al. Human lymphocytes with either OKT4 or OKT8 phenotype produce interleukin 2 in culture. *J Clin Invest* 1982;70:470–473.
8. Meuer SC, Hussey RE, Penta AC, et al. Cellular origin of interleukin 2 (IL 2) in man: evidence for stimulus-restricted IL 2 production by T4+ and T8+ T lymphocytes. *J Immunol* 1982; 129:1076–1079.
9. Bender A, Kabelitz D. CD4–CD8– human T cells: phenotypic heterogeneity and activation requirements of freshly isolated "double negative" T cells. *Cell Immunol* 1988;128:542–554.
10. Fukushima T, Kobayashi K, Kasama T, et al. Inhibition of interleukin-2 by serum in healthy individuals and in patients with autoimmune disease. *Int Arch Allergy Appl Immunol* 1987;84: 135–141.
11. Huang YP, Perrin LH, Miescher PA, et al. Correlation of T and B cell activities in vitro and serum IL-2 levels in systemic lupus erythematosus. *J Immunol* 1988;141:827–833.
12. Warrington RJ. Interleukin-2 abnormalities in systemic lupus erythematosus and rheumatoid arthritis. A role for overproduction of interleukin-2 in human autoimmunity? *J Rheumatol* 1988;15:616–620.
13. Horwitz DA, Wang H, Gray JD. Cytokine gene profile in circulating blood mononuclear cells from patients with systemic lupus erythematosus: increased interleukin-2 but not interleukin-4 mRNA. *Lupus* 1994;3:423–428.
14. Sierakowski S, Kucharz EJ, Lightfoot RW, et al. Impaired T-cell activation in patients with systemic lupus erythematosus. *J Clin Immunol* 1989;9:469–476.
15. Crispin JC, Alcocer-Varela J. Interleukin-2 and systemic lupus erythematosus—fifteen years later. *Lupus* 1998;7:214–222.
16. Alcocer-Varela, J, Alarcon-Segovia, D. Decreased production of and response to interleukin-2 by cultured lymphocytes from patients with systemic lupus erythematosus. *J Clin Invest* 1982; 69:1388–1392.
17. Linker-Israeli M, Bakke AC, Kitridou RC, et al. Defective production of interleukin 1 and interleukin 2 in patients with systemic lupus erythematosus (SLE). *J Immunol* 1983;130: 2651–2655.
18. Huang YP, Miescher PA, Zubler RH. The interleukin 2 secretion defect in vitro in systemic lupus erythematosus is reversible in rested cultured T cells. *J Immunol* 1986;137:3515–3520.
19. Miyasaka Y, Nakamura T, Russell IJ, et al. Interleukin-2 deficiencies in rheumatoid arthritis and systemic lupus erythematosus. *Clin Immunol Immunopathol* 1984;31:109–117.
20. Murakawa Y, Sakane T. Deficient phytohemagglutinin-induced interleukin-2 activity in patients with inactive systemic lupus erythematosus is correctable by the addition of phorbol myristate acetate. *Arthritis Rheum* 1988;31:826–833.
21. Murakawa Y, Takada S, Ueda Y, et al. Characterization of T lymphocyte subpopulations responsible for deficient interleukin 2 activity in patients with systemic lupus erythematosus. *J Immunol* 1985;134:187–195.
22. Warrington RJ, Sauder PJ, Homik J, et al. Reversible interleukin-2 response defects in systemic lupus erythematosus. *Clin Exp Immunol* 1989;77:163–167.
23. De Faucal P, Godard A, Peyrat MA, et al. Impaired IL-2 production by lymphocytes of patients with systemic lupus erythematosus. *Ann Immunol* 1984;135:161–168.
24. Takada S, Ueda Y, Suzuki N, et al. Abnormalities in autologous mixed lymphocyte reaction-activated immunologic processes in systemic lupus erythematosus and their possible correction by interleukin 2. *Eur J Immunol* 1985;15:262–267.
25. Via CS, Tsokos GC, Bermas B, et al. T cell-antigen presenting cell interactions in human systemic lupus erythematosus. Evidence for heterogeneous expression of multiple defects. *J Immunol* 1993;151:3914–3922.
26. Draeger AM, Swaak AJ, van den Brink HG, et al. T cell function in systemic lupus erythematosus: normal production of and responsiveness to interleukin 2. *Clin Exp Immunol* 1986; 64(1):80–87.
27. Sakane T, Murakawa Y, Nhoboru S, et al. Familial occurrence of impaired interleukin-2 activity and increased peripheral blood B cells actively secreting immunoglobulins in systemic lupus erythematosus. *Am J Med* 1989;86:385–390.
28. Hagiwara E, Gourley MF, Lee S, et al. Disease severity in patients with systemic lupus erythematosus correlates with an increased ratio of interleukin-10: interferon-g-secreting cells in the peripheral blood. *Arthritis Rheum*1996;39:379–385.
29. Alcocer-Varela J, Alarcon-Segovia D. Longitudinal study on the production of and cellular response to interleukin-2 in patients with systemic lupus erythematosus. *Rheumatol Int* 1995;15: 57–63.
30. Bermas BL, Petri M, Goldman D, et al. T helper cell dysfunction in systemic lupus erythematosus (SLE): relation to disease activity. *J Clin Immunol* 1994;14(3):169–177.
31. Via CS. Kinetics of T cell activation in acute and chronic forms of murine graft-versus-host disease. *J Immunol* 1991;146(8): 2603–2609.
32. Rus V, Svetic A, Nguyen P, et al. Kinetics of Th1 and Th2 cytokine production during the early course of acute and chronic murine graft-versus-host disease. Regulatory role of donor CD8+ T cells. *J Immunol* 1995;155:2396–2406.
33. Segal R, Bermas BL, Dayan M, et al. Kinetics of cytokine production in experimental systemic lupus erythematosus: involvement of T helper cell 1/T helper cell 2–type cytokines in disease. *J Immunol* 1997;158(6):3009–3016.
34. Horwitz DA, Garrett MA. Lymphocyte reactivity to mitogens in subjects with systemic lupus erythematosus, rheumatoid arthritis and scleroderma. *Clin Exp Immunol* 1977;27:92–99.
35. Tada Y, Nagasawa K, Yamauchi Y, et al. A defect in the protein kinase C system in T cells from patients with systemic lupus erythematosus. *Clin Immunol Immunopathol* 1991;60(2): 220–231.
36. Linker-Israeli M, Quismorio FP Jr, Horwitz DA. Further characterization of interleukin-2 production by lymphocytes of patients with systemic lupus erythematosus. *J Rheumatol* 1988; 15(8):1216–1222.
37. Sierakowski S, Kucharz EJ. Phorbol myristate acetate (PMA) reverses inhibition of interleukin-2 production by T lymphocytes of patients with systemic lupus erythematosus. *Med Interne* 1988;26(1):67–73.
38. Phi NC, Takats A, Binh VH, et al. Cyclic AMP level of lymphocytes in patients with systemic lupus erythematosus and its relation to disease activity. *Immunol Lett* 1989;23(1):61–64.
39. Mishra N, Khan IU, Tsokos GC, et al. Association of deficient type II protein kinase A activity with aberrant nuclear translocation of the RII beta subunit in systemic lupus erythematosus T lymphocytes. *J Immunol* 2000;165(5):2830–2840.

40. Kammer GM. High prevalence of T cell type I protein kinase A deficiency in systemic lupus erythematosus. *Arthritis Rheum* 1999;42(7):1458–1465.
41. Tsokos GC, Kovacs B, Sfikakis PP, et al. Defective antigen-presenting cell function in patients with systemic lupus erythematosus. *Arthritis Rheum.* 1996;39(4):600–609.
42. Alvarado C, Alcocer-Varela J, Llorente L, et al. Effect of CD28 antibody on T cells from patients with systemic lupus erythematosus. *J Autoimmun* 1994;7:763–773.
43. Horwitz DA, Tang FL, Stimmler MM, et al. Decreased T cell response to anti-CD2 in systemic lupus erythematosus and reversal by anti-CD28: evidence for impaired T cell-accessory cell interaction. *Arthritis Rheum* 1997;40(5):822–833.
44. Hishikawa T, Tokano Y, Sekigawa I, et al. HLA-DP+ T cells and deficient interleukin-2 production in patients with systemic lupus erythematosus. *Clin Immunol Immunopathol* 1990;55: 285–296.
45. Horwitz DA, Gray JD, Behrendsen SC, et al. Decreased production of interleukin-12 and other Th1–type cytokines in patients with recent-onset systemic lupus erythematosus. *Arthritis Rheum* 1998;41:838–844.
46. Linker-Israeli M, Baake AC, Quismorio FP Jr, et al. Correlation of interleukin-2 production in patients with systemic lupus erythematosus by removal of spontaneously activated suppressor cells. *J Clin Invest* 1985;75:762–768.
47. Reuss-Borst MA, Geyer A, Berner B. Cytokine-producing T cells in systemic lupus erythematosus: comment on the article by Akahoshi et al. *Arthritis Rheum* 2000;43(3):711–712.
48. Miyagi J, Minato N, Sumiya M, et al. Two types of antibodies inhibiting interleukin-2 production by normal lymphocytes in patients with systemic lupus erythematosus. *Arthritis Rheum* 1989;32:1356–1364.
49. Fukushima T, Kobayashi K, Kasama T, et al. Inhibition of interleukin-2 by serum in healthy individuals and in patients with autoimmune disease. *Int Arch Allergy Appl Immunol* 1987;84: 135–141.
50. Kucharz EJ, Sierakowski S, Goodwin JS. Decreased activity of interleukin-2 inhibitor in plasma of patients with systemic lupus erythematosus. *Clin Rheumatol* 1988;7:87-90.
51. Horwitz DA, Cousar JB. A relationship between impaired cellular immunity, humoral suppression of lymphocyte function, and severity of systemic lupus erythematosus. *Am J Med* 1975; 58:829–835.
52. Horwitz DA. Mechanisms producing decreased mitogenic reactivity in patients with systemic lupus erythematosus and other rheumatic diseases. In: Oppenheim JJ, Ronsenstreich DL, eds. *Mitogens in immunobiology.* New York: Academic Press, 1976: 625–637.
53. Caver TE, O'Sullivan FX, Gold LI, et al. Intracellular demonstration of active TGFbeta1 in B cells and plasma cells of autoimmune mice. IgG-bound TGFbeta1 suppresses neutrophil function and host defense against Staphylococcus aureus infection. *J Clin Invest* 1996;98(11):2496–2506.
54. Ishida H, Kumagai S, Unehara H, et al. Impaired expression of high affinity interleukin 2 receptor on activated lymphocytes from patients with systemic lupus erythematosus. *J Immunol* 1987;139:1070–1074.
55. Jira M, Strejcek J, Zavadil Z, et al. Interleukin-2 activated cells from peripheral blood of patients with systemic lupus erythematosus. *Z Rheumatol* 1990;49:30–33.
56. Tanaka T, Saiki O, Negoro S, et al. Decreased expression of interleukin-2 binding molecules (p70/75) in T cells from patients with systemic lupus erythematosus. *Arthritis Rheum* 1989;32:552–559.
57. Saiki O, Tanaka T, Kishimoto S. Defective expression of p70/75 interleukin-2 receptor in T cells from patients with systemic lupus erythematosus: a possible defect in the process of increased intracellular calcium leading to p70/p75 expression. *J Rheumatol* 1990;17:1303–1307.
58. Shevach EM. Regulatory T cells in autoimmunity. *Annu Rev Immunol* 2000;18:423–449.
59. Takada S, Ueda Y, Suzuki N, et al. Abnormalities in autologous mixed lymphocyte reaction-activated immunologic processes in systemic lupus erythematosus and their possible correction by interleukin 2. *Eur J Immunol* 1985;15:262–267.
60. Tsokos GC, Smith PL, Christian CB, et al. Interleukin-2 restores to depressed allogeneic cell-mediated lympholysis and natural killer cell activity in patients with systemic lupus erythematosus. *Clin Immunol Immunopathol* 1985;34:379–386.
61. Volk HD, Diamantstein T. IL-2 normalizes defective suppressor T cell function of patients with systemic lupus erythematosus in vitro. *Clin Exp Immunol* 1986;66:525–531.
62. Wigfall DR, Sakai RS, Wallace DJ, et al. Interleukin-2 receptor expression in peripheral blood lymphocytes from systemic lupus erythematosus patients: relationship to clinical activity. *Clin Immunol Immunopathol* 1988;47:354–362.
63. Semenzato G, Bambara LM, Biasi D, et al. Increased serum levels of soluble interleukin-2 receptor in patients with systemic lupus erythematosus and rheumatoid arthritis. *J Clin Immunol* 1988;8(6):447–452.
64. Campen DH, Horwitz DA, Quismorio FP Jr, et al. Serum levels of interleukin-2 receptor and activity of rheumatic diseases characterized by immune system activation. *Arthritis Rheum* 1988;31(11):1358–1364.
65. Manoussakis MN, Papadopoulos GK, Drosos AA, et al. Soluble interleukin 2 receptor molecules in the serum of patients with autoimmune diseases. *Clin Immunol Immunopathol* 1989;50(3): 321–332.
66. Ward MM, Dooley MA, Christenson VD, et al. The relationship between soluble interleukin 2 receptor levels and anti-double stranded DNA antibody levels in patients with systemic lupus erythematosus. *J Rheumatol* 1991;18(2):235–240.
67. Celis E, Miller RW, Wiktor TJ, et al. Isolation and characterization of human T cell lines and clones reactive to rabies virus: antigen specificity and production of interferon-gamma. *J Immunol* 1986;136(2):692–697.
68. Gajewski TF, Fitch FW. Anti-proliferative effect of IFN-gamma in immune regulation. I. IFN-gamma inhibits the proliferation of Th2 but not Th1 murine helper T lymphocyte clones. *J Immunol* 1988;140:4245–4252.
69. Farrar MA, Fernandez-Luna J, Schreiber RD. Identification of two regions within the cytoplasmic domain of the human interferon- receptor required for function. *J Biol Chem* 1991;266: 19626–19635.
70. Soh J, Donnely RJ, Kotenko S, et al. Identification and sequence of an accessory factor required for activation of the human interferon γ receptor. *Cell* 1994;76:793–802.
71. Hibino Y, Mariano TM, Kumar CS, et al. Expression and reconstitution of a biologically active mouse interferon gamma receptor in hamster cells: chromosomal location of an accessory factor. *J Biol Chem* 1991;266:6948–6951.
72. Hibino Y, Kumar CS, Mariano TM, et al. Chimeric interferon-gamma receptors demonstrate that an accessory factor required for activity interacts with the extracellular domain. *J Biol Chem* 1992;267:3741–3749.
73. Kalina U, Ozmen L, Di Padova K, et al. The human gamma interferon receptor accessory factor encoded by chromosome 21 transduces the signal for the induction of 2′,5′-oligoadenylate-synthetase, resistance to virus cytopathic effect, and major histocompatibility complex class I antigens. *J Virol* 1993;67: 1702–1706.
74. Walter MR, Windsor WT, Nagabhushan TL, et al. Crystal

structure of a complex between interferon-gamma and its soluble high-affinity receptor. *Nature* 1995;376:230–235.
75. Jacob CO, van der Meide PH, McDevitt HO. In vivo treatment of (NZB × NZW)F1 lupus-like nephritis with monoclonal antibody to gamma interferon. *J Exp Med* 1987;166(3): 798–803.
76. Schilling PJ, Kurzrock R, Kantarjian H, et al. Development of systemic lupus erythematosus after interferon therapy for chronic myelogenous leukemia. *Cancer* 1991;68:1536–1537.
77. Shiozawa S, Kuroki Y, Kim M, et al. Alpha-interferon in lupus psychosis (abstract). *Arthritis Rheum* 1991;34(suppl):S51.
78. Graninger WB, Hassfeld WB, Pesau BB, et al. Induction of systemic lupus erythematosus by interferon-gamma in a patient with rheumatoid arthritis. *J Rheumatol* 1991;18:1621–1622.
79. Deleted in page proofs.
80. Machold KP, Smolen JS. Interferon-gamma induced exacerbation of systemic lupus erythematosus. *J Rheumatol* 1990;17: 831–832.
81. Al-JAnadi M, Al-Balla S, Al-Dalaan A, et al. Cytokine profile in systemic lupus erythematosus, rheumatoid arthritis, and other rheumatic diseases. *J Clin Immunol* 1993;13:58–67.
82. Ishida H, Yanagida H. Clinical evaluation of serum cytokines from patients with collagen diseases (Japanese). *Jpn J Clin Pathol* 1999;47:327–334.
83. Robak E, Sysa-Jedrzejewska A, Dziankowska B, et al. Association of interferon gamma, tumor necrosis alpha and interleukin 6 serum levels with systemic lupus erythematosus activity. *Arch Immunol Ther Exp* 1998;46:375–380.
84. Tsokos GC, Bounpas DT, Smith PL, et al. Deficient g- interferon production in patients with systemic lupus erythematosus. *Arthritis Rheum* 1986;29:1210–1215.
85. Sibbitt WL Jr, Likar L, Spellman CW, et al. Impaired natural killer cell function in systemic lupus erythematosus: relationship to interleukin-2 production. *Arthritis Rheum* 1983;26: 1316–1320.
86. Tsokos GC, Rook AH, Djeu JY, et al. Natural killer cells and interferon responses in patients with systemic lupus erythematosus. *Clin Exp Immunol* 1982;5:239–245.
87. Stolzenburg T, Binz H, Fontana A, et al. Impaired mitogen-induced interferon-gamma production in rheumatoid arthritis and related diseases. *Scand J Immunol* 1988;27:73–81.
88. Viallard JF, Pellegrin JL, Ranchin V, et al. Th1 (IL-2, interferon-gamma (IFN-gamma)) and Th2 (IL-10, IL-4) cytokine production by peripheral blood mononuclear cells (PBMC) from patients with systemic lupus erythematosus (SLE). *Clin Exp Immunol* 1999;115:189–195.
89. Tanaka Y, Nakashima H, Hisano C, et al. Association of the interferon-gamma receptor variant (Val14Met) with systemic lupus erythematosus. *Immunogenetics* 1999;49:266–271.
90. Nakashima H, Inoue H, Akahoshi M, et al. The combination of polymorphisms within interferon-gamma receptor 1 and receptor 2 associated with the risk of systemic lupus erythematosus. *FEBS Lett* 1999;453:187–190.
91. Naume B, Gately M, Espevik T. A comparative study of IL-12 (cytotoxic lymphocyte maturation factor)–, IL-2–, and IL-7–induced effects on immunomagnetically purified CD56+ NK cells. *J Immunol* 1992;148(8):2429–2436.
92. Pardoux C, Asselin-Paturel C, Chehimi J, et al. Functional interaction between TGF-beta and IL-12 in human primary allogeneic cytotoxicity and proliferative response. *J Immunol* 1997;158(1):136–143.
93. Wu C, Warrier RR, Wang X, et al. Regulation of interleukin- 12 receptor beta1 chain expression and interleukin-12 binding by human peripheral blood mononuclear cells. *Eur J Immunol* 1997;27:147–154.
94. Jones BM. Effect of 12 neutralizing anti-cytokine antibodies on in vitro activation of B-cells. Interleukin-12 is required by B1a but not B2 cells. *Scand J Immunol* 1996;43:64–72.
95. Leonard JP, Waldburger KE, Goldman SJ. Prevention of experimental autoimmune encephalomyelitis by antibodies against interleukin 12. *J Exp Med* 1995;181:381–386.
96. Tokano Y, Morimoto S, Kaneko H, et al. Levels of IL-12 in the sera of patients with systemic lupus erythematosus (SLE)-relation to Th1- and Th2-derived cytokines. *Clin Exp Immunol* 1999;116:169–173.
97. Liu TF, Jones BM. Impaired production of IL-12 in systemic lupus erythematosus. I. Excessive production of IL-10 suppresses production of IL-12 by monocytes. *Cytokine* 1998; 10(2):140–147.
98. Liu TF, Jones BM. Impaired production of IL-12 in system lupus erythematosus. II: IL-12 production in vitro is correlated negatively with serum IL-10, positively with serum IFN-gamma and negatively with disease activity in SLE. *Cytokine* 1998; 10(2):148–153.
99. Houssiau FA, Mascart-Lemone F, Stevens M, et al. IL-12 inhibits in vitro immunoglobulin production by human lupus peripheral blood mononuclear cells (PBMC). *Clin Exp Immunol* 1997;108(2):375–380.
100. Dueymes M, Barrier J, Besancenot JF, et al. Relationship of interleukin-4 to isotypic distribution of anti-double-stranded DNA antibodies in systemic lupus erythematosus. *Int Arch Allergy Immunol* 1993;101:408–415.
101. Richaud-Patin Y, Alcocer-Varela J, Llorente L. High levels of Th2 cytokine gene expression in systemic lupus erythematosus. *Rev Invest Clin* 1995;47:267–276.
102. Funauchi M, Yu H, Sugiyama M, et al. Increased interleukin-4 production by NK T cells in systemic lupus erythematosus. *Clin Immunol* 1999;92(2):197–202.
103. Okada H, Konishi K, Nakazato Y, et al. IL-4 expression in mesangial proliferative glomerulonephritis. *Am J Kidney Dis* 1994;23:242–246.
104. Furusu A, Miyazaki M, Koji T, et al. Involvement of IL-4 in human glomerulonephritis: an in situ hybridization study of IL-4 mRNA and IL-4 receptor mRNA. *J Am Soc Nephrol* 1997;8: 730–741.
105. Tan PL, Blumenstein M, Yeoman S, et al. B cell lymphokines in human systemic lupus erythematosus. *Ann Rheum Dis* 1989; 48(11):941–945.
106. Linker-Israeli M. Cytokine abnormalities in human lupus. *Clin Immunol Immunopathol* 1992;63:10–12.
107. Rus V, Luzina, IL, Atamas S, et al. Simultaneous elevation of IL-10 and depression of IL-4 and IL-13 mRNA in lupus (SLE) patients. *Arthritis Rheum* 1999;42:5310.
108. Kanemitsu S, Takabayashi A, Sasaki Y, et al. Association of interleukin-4 receptor and interleukin-4 promoter gene polymorphisms with systemic lupus erythematosus. *Arthritis Rheum* 1999;42:1298–1300.
109. Linker-Israeli M, Deans RJ, Wallace DJ, et al. Elevated levels of endogenous IL-6 in systemic lupus erythematosus. A putative role in pathogenesis. *J Immunol* 1991;147:117–123.
110. Linker-Israeli M, Honda M, Nand R, et al. Exogenous IL-10 and IL-4 down-regulate IL-6 production by SLE-derived PBMC. *Clin Immunol* 1999;91:6–16.
111. Warren HS, Kinnear BF, Phillips JH, et al. Production of IL-5 by human NK cells and regulation of IL-5 secretion by IL-4, IL-10, and IL-12. *J Immunol* 1995;154(10):5144–5152.
112. Gray JD, Horwitz DA. Activated human natural killer cells can stimulate resting B lymphocytes to secrete immunoglobulin. *J Immunol* 1995;154:5656–5664.
113. Stein LF, Saed GM, Fivenson DP. T-cell cytokine network in cutaneous lupus erythematosus. *J Am Acad Dermatol* 1997;36(2 pt 1):191–196.

114. Klashman DJ, Martin RA, Martinez-Maza O, et al. In vitro regulation of B cell differentiation by interleukin-6 and soluble CD23 in systemic lupus erythematosus B cell subpopulations and antigen-induced normal B cells. *Arthritis Rheum* 1991;34: 276–286.
115. Viallard JF, Taupin JL, Miossec V, et al. Analysis of interleukin-6, interleukin-10 and leukemia inhibitory factor (LIF) production by peripheral blood cells from patients identifies LIF as a potential marker of disease activity. *Eur Cytokine Netw* 1999;10: 17–24.
116. Davas EM, Tsirogianni A, Kappou I, et al. Serum IL-6, TNFalpha, p55 srTNFalpha, p75srTNFalpha, srIL-2alpha levels and disease activity in systemic lupus erythematosus. *Clin Rheumatol* 1999;18(1):17–22.
117. Spronk PE, Ter Borg EJ, Limburg PC, et al. Plasma concentration of IL-6 in systemic lupus erythematosus: an indicator of disease activity? *Clin Exp Immunol* 1992;90:106–110.
118. Robak T, Gladalska A, Stepien H, et al. Serum levels of interleukin-6 type cytokines and soluble interleukin-6 receptor in patients with rheumatoid arthritis. *Mediators Inflamm* 1998; 7(5):347–353.
119. Rovensky J, Jurankova E, Rauova L, et al. Relationship between endocrine, immune, and clinical variables in patients with systemic lupus erythematosus. *J Rheumatol* 1997;24(12):2330–2334.
120. Avalos-Diaz E, Alvarado-Flores E, Herrera-Esparza R. UV-A irradiation induces transcription of IL-6 and TNF alpha genes in human keratinocytes and dermal fibroblasts. *Rev Rhum (Engl Ed)* 1999;66(1):13–19.
121. Kirnbauer R, Kock A, Neuner P, et al. Regulation of epidermal cell interleukin-6 production by UV light and corticosteroids. *J Invest Dermatol* 1991;96(4):484–489.
122. Pelton BK, Hylton W, Denman AM. Activation of IL-6 production by UV irradiation of blood mononuclear cells from patients with systemic lupus erythematosus. *Clin Exp Immunol* 1992;89(2):251–254.
123. Herrera-Esparza R, Barbosa-Cisneros O, Villalobos-Hurtado R, et al. Renal expression of IL-6 and TNFalpha genes in lupus nephritis. *Lupus* 1998;7(3):154–158.
124. Hashimoto C. Studies on synthesis of interleukin-6 and gammaglobulin in peipheral blood mononuclear cells of patients with systemic lupus erythematosus. *Tohoku J Exp Med* 1990; 162:323–335.
125. Swaak AJG, van Rooyen A, Aarden LA. Interleukin-6 (IL-6) and acute phase proteins in the disease course of patients with systemic lupus erythematosus. *Rheumatol Int* 1989;8:263–268.
126. Jara LJ, Irigoyen L, Ortiz MJ, et al. Prolactin and interleukin-6 in neuropsychiatric lupus erythematosus. *Clin Rheumatol* 1998; 17(2):110–114.
127. Hirohata S, Miyamoto T. Elevated levels of interleukin-6 cerebrospinal fluid from patients with systemic lupus erythematosus and central nervous system involvement. *Arthritis Rheum* 1990; 33:644–649.
128. Kroemer G, Martinez AC. Cytokines and autoimmune disease. *Clin Immunol Immunopathol* 1991;61:275–295.
129. Lacki JK, Leszczynski P, Kelemen J, et al. Cytokine concentration in serum of systemic lupus erythematosus patients: the effect on acute phase response. *J Med* 1997;28:99–107.
130. Casciola-Rosen LA, Anhalt G, Rosen A. Autoantigens targeted in systemic lupus erythematosus are clustered in two populations of surface structures on apoptotic keratinocytes. *J Exp Med* 1994;179:1317–1330.
131. Hefeneider SH, Brown LE, McCoy SL, et al. Immunization of BALB/c mice with a monoclonal anti-DNA antibody induces an anti-idiotypic antibody reactive with a cell-surface DNA binding protein. *Autoimmunity* 1993;15:187–194.
132. Takeno M, Nagafuchi H, Kaneko S, et al. Autoreactive T cell clones from patients with systemic lupus erythematosus support polyclonal autoantibody production. *J Immunol* 1997;158(7): 3529–3538.
133. Kitani A, Hara M, Hirose T, et al. Heterogeneity of B cell responsiveness to interleukin 4, interleukin 6, and low molecular weight B cell growth factor in discrete stages of B cell activation in patients with systemic lupus erythematosus. *Clin Exp Immunol* 1989;77:31–36.
134. Kitani A, Hara M, Hirose T, et al. Autostimulatory effects of IL-6 on excessive B cell differentiation in patients with systemic lupus erythematosus: analysis of IL-6 production and IL-6R expression. *Clin Exp Immunol* 1992;88:75–83.
135. Nagafuchi H, Suzuki N, Mizushima Y, et al. Constitutive expression of IL-6 receptors and their role in the excessive B cell function in patients with systemic lupus erythematosus. *J Immunol* 1993;151:6525–6534.
136. Moore KW, O'Garra A, de Waal Malefyt R, et al. Interleukin-10. *Annu Rev Immunol* 1993;11:165–190.
137. Groux H, Bigler M, de Vries JE, et al. Inhibitory and stimulatory effects of IL-10 on human CD8+ T cells. *J Immunol* 1998;160(7):3188–3193.
138. Groux H, Bigler M, de Vries JE, et al. Interleukin-10 induces a long-term antigen-specific anergic state in human CD4+ T cells. *J Exp Med* 1996;184(1):19–29.
139. Ishida H, Muchamuel T, Sakaguchi S, et al. Continuous administration of anti-interleukin 10 antibodies delays onset of autoimmunity in NZB/W F1 mice. *J Exp Med* 1994;179: 305–310.
140. Westendorp RG, Langermans JA, Huizinga TW, et al. Genetic influence on cytokine production and fatal meningococcal disease. *Lancet* 1997;349(9046):170–173. [Published erratum *Lancet* 1977;349:656.]
141. Llorente L, Richaud-Patin Y, Couderc J, et al. Dysregulation of interleukin-10 production in relatives of patients with systemic lupus erythematosus. *Arthritis Rheum* 1997;40(8):1429–1435.
142. Bienvenu J, Doche C, Gutowski MC, et al. Production of proinflammatory cytokines and cytokines involved in the TH1/TH2 balance is modulated by pentoxifylline. *J Cardiovasc Pharmacol* 1995;25(suppl 2):S80–84.
143. Eskdale J, Wordsworth P, Bowman S, et al. Association between polymorphisms at the human IL-10 locus and systemic lupus erythematosus. *Tissue Antigens* 1997;49(6):635–639.
144. Mehrian R, Quismorio FP Jr, Strassmann G, et al. Synergistic effect between IL-10 and bcl-2 genotypes in determining susceptibility to systemic lupus erythematosus. *Arthritis Rheum* 1998;41(4):596–602.
145. Llorente L, Richaud-Patin Y, Wijdenes J, et al. Spontaneous production of interleukin-10 by B lymphocytes and monocytes in systemic lupus erythematosus. *Eur Cytokine Netw* 1993; 4(6):421–427.
146. Llorente L, Richaud-Patin Y, Fior R, et al. In vivo production of interleukin-10 by non-T cells in rheumatoid arthritis, Sjogren's syndrome, and systemic lupus erythematosus. *Arthritis Rheum* 1994;11:1647–1655.
147. Houssiau FA, Lefebvre C, Berghe MV, et al. Serum interleukin 10 titres in systemic lupus erythematosus reflect disease activity. *Lupus* 1995;4:393–395.
148. Al-Janadi M., Al-Dalaan A, Al-Balla S, et al. Interleukin-10 (IL-10) secretion in systemic lupus erythematosus and rheumatoid arthritis: IL-10–dependent CD4+CD45RO+ Tcel-B cell antibody synthesis. *J Clin Immunol* 1996;16:198–207.
149. Llorente L, Zou W, Levy Y, et al. Role of interleukin 10 in the B lymphocyte hyperactivity and autoantibody production of human systemic lupus erythematosus. *J Exp Med* 1995;181(3): 839–844.
150. Lauwerys BR, Renauld J-C, Houssiau FA. Interleukin-10

blockade corrects in vitro impaired allogeneic immune responses of SLE patients. *Arthritis Rheum* 1999;42:9(abst).
151. de Waal Malefyt R, Abrams J, Bennett B, et al. Interleukin 10(IL-10) inhibits cytokine synthesis by human monocytes: an autoregulatory role of IL-10 produced by monocytes. *J Exp Med* 1991;174(5):1209–1220.
152. Takenaka H, Maruo S, Yamamoto N, et al. Regulation of T cell-dependent and -independent IL-12 production by the three Th2-type cytokines IL-10, IL-6, and IL-4. *J Leukoc Biol* 1997; 61(1):80–87.
153. Mongan AE, Ramdahin S, Warrington RJ. Interleukin-10 response abnormalities in systemic lupus erythematosus. *Scand J Immunol* 1997;46:406–412.
154. Lacki JK, Samborski W, Mackiewicz SH. Interleukin-10 and interleukin-6 in lupus erythematosus and rheumatoid arthritis, correlations with acute phase proteins. *Clin Rheumatol* 1997;16: 275–278.
155. Georgescu L, Vakkalanka RK, Elkon KB, et al. Interleukin-10 promotes activation-induced cell death of SLE lymphocytes mediated by Fas ligand. *J Clin Invest* 1997;100(10):2622–2633.
156. Arend WP, Joslin FG, Massoni RJ. Effects of immune complexes on production by human monocytes of interleukin 1 or an interleukin 1 inhibitor. *J Immunol* 1985;134:3868–3875.
157. Tanaka Y, Saito K, Shirakawa F, et al. Production of B cell-stimulating factors by B cells in patients with systemic lupus erythematosus. *J Immunol* 1988;141:3043–3049.
158. Aotsuka S, Nakamura K, Nakano T, et al. Production of intracellular and extracellular interleukin-1 alpha and interleukin-1 beta by peripheral blood monocytes from patients with connective tissue diseases. *Ann Rheum Dis* 1991;50:27–31.
159. Jandl RC, George JL, Silberstein DS, et al. The effect of adherent cell-derived factors on immunoglobulin and anti-DNA synthesis in systemic lupus erythematosus. *Clin Immunol Immunopathol* 1987;42:344–359.
160. Hirose T. Spontaneous production of interleukin-1 and B cell stimulating factors by B cells from patients with systemic lupus erythematosus. *Ryumachi* 1989;29:277–283.
161. Andersen LS, Petersen J, Svenson M, et al. Production of IL-1beta, IL-1 receptor antagonist and IL-10 by mononuclear cells from patients with SLE. *Autoimmunity* 1999;30(4):235–242.
162. Pelton BK, Speckmaier M, Hylton W, et al. Cytokine-independent progression of immunoglobulin production in vitro by B lymphocytes from patients with systemic lupus erythematosus. *Clin Exp Immunol* 1991;83:274–279.
163. Morris SC, Cheek RL, Cohen PL, et al. Autoantibodies in chronic graft versus host result from cognate T-B interactions. *J Exp Med* 1990;171:503–517.
164. Takeuchi T, Abe T, Koide J, et al. Cellular mechanism of DNA-specific antibody synthesis by lymphocytes from systemic lupus erythematosus patients. *Arthritis Rheum* 1984;27:766–773.
165. Linker-Israeli M, Quismorio FP, Jr, Horwitz DA. CD8;pl lymphocytes from patients with systemic lupus erythematosus sustain rather than suppress spontaneous polyclonal IgG production and synergize with CD4+ cells to support autoantibody synthesis. *Arthritis Rheum* 1990;33:1216–1225.
166. Cohen PL, Litvin DA, Winfield JB. Association between endogenously activated T cells and immunoglobulin-secreting B cells in patients with active systemic lupus erythematosus. *Arthritis Rheum* 1982;25:168–173.
167. Sierakowski S, Kucharz EJ, Lightfoot RW Jr, et al. Interleukin-1 production by monocytes from patients with systemic lupus erythematosus. *Clin Rheum* 1987;6:403–407.
168. Alcocer-Varela J, Laffon A, Alarcon-Segovia D. Defective monocyte production of, and T lymphocyte response to, interleukin-1 in the peripheral blood of patients with systemic lupus erythematosus. *Clin Exp Immunol* 1983;55:125–132.
169. Muzes G, Vien CV, Gonzalez-Cabello R, et al. Defective production of interleukin-1 and tumor necrosis factor alpha by stimulated monocytes from patients with systemic lupus erythematosus. *Acta Med Hung* 1989;46:245–252.
170. Takei M, Kang H, Tomura K, et al. Aberration of monokine production and monocyte subset in patients with systemic lupus erythematosus. *J Clin Lab Immunol* 1987;22:169–173.
171. Whicher JT, Gilbert AM, Westacott C, et al. Defective production of leucocytic endogenous mediator (interleukin 1) by peripheral blood leucocytes of patients with systemic sclerosis, systemic lupus erythematosus, rheumatoid arthritis and mixed connective tissue disease. *Clin Exp Immunol* 1986;65:80–89.
172. Horwitz DA, Linker-Israeli M, Gray JD. Lymphocyte and lymphokine abnormalities in patients with systemic lupus erythematosus. *EOS J Immunol Immunopharm* 1987;7:43–52.
173. Markenson JA, Lockshin MD, Fuzesi L, et al. Suppressor monocytes in patients with systemic lupus erythematosus. Evidence of suppressor activity associated with a cell-free soluble product of monocytes. *J Lab Clin Med* 1980;95:40–48.
174. Sturfelt G, Roux-Lombard P, Wollheim FA, et al. Low levels of interleukin-1 receptor antagonist coincide with kidney involvement in systemic lupus erythematosus. *Br J Rheumatol* 1997; 36(12):1283–1299.
175. Jacob CO, Fronek Z, Lewis GD, et al. Heritable major histocompatibility complex class II-associated differences in production of tumor necrosis factor: relevance to genetic predisposition to systemic lupus erythematosus. *Proc Natl Acad Sci USA* 1990;87:1233–1237.
176. Sullivan KE, Wooten C, Schmeckpeper BJ, et al. A promoter polymorphism of tumor necrosis factor alpha associated with systemic lupus erythematosus in African-Americans. *Arthritis Rheum* 1997;40:2207–2011.
177. Rudwaleit M, Tikly M, Khamashta M, et al. Interethnic differences in the association of tumor necrosis factor promoter polymorphisms with systemic lupus erythematosus. *J Rheumatol* 1996;23(10):1725–1728.
178. Hajeer AH, Worthington J, Davies EJ, et al. TNF microsatellite a2, b3 and d2 alleles are associated with systemic lupus erythematosus. *Tissue Antigens* 1997;49(3 pt 1):222–227.
179. Komata T, Tsuchiya N, Matsushita M, et al. Association of tumor necrosis factor receptor 2 (TNFR2) polymorphism with susceptibility to systemic lupus erythematosus. *Tissue Antigens* 1999;53(6):527–533.
180. Al-Ansari AS, Ollier WE, Villarreal J, et al. Tumor necrosis factor receptor II (TNFRII) exon 6 polymorphism in systemic lupus erythematosus. *Tissue Antigens* 2000;55(1):97–99.
181. Lee SH, Park SH, Min JK, et al. Decreased tumour necrosis factor-beta production in TNFB*2 homozygote: an important predisposing factor of lupus nephritis in Koreans. *Lupus* 1997;6(7): 603–609.
182. Mitamura K, Kang H, Tomita Y, et al. Impaired tumour necrosis factor-alpha (TNF-alpha) production and abnormal B cell response to TNF-alpha in patients with systemic lupus erythematosus (SLE). *Clin Exp Immunol* 1991;85:386–391.
183. Malave I, Searles RP, Montano J, et al. Production of tumor necrosis factor/cachectin by peripheral blood mononuclear cells in patients with systemic lupus erythematosus. *Int Arch Allergy Appl Immunol* 1989;89:355–361.
184. Jones BM, Liu T, Wong RW. Reduced in vitro production of interferon-gamma, interleukin-4 and interleukin-12 and increased production of interleukin-6, interleukin-10 and tumour necrosis factor-alpha in systemic lupus erythematosus. Weak correlations of cytokine production with disease activity. *Autoimmunity* 1999;31(2):117–124.
185. Gabay C, Cakir N, Moral F, et al. Circulating levels of tumor necrosis factor soluble receptors in systemic lupus erythemato-

sus are significantly higher than in other rheumatic diseases and correlate with disease activity. *J Rheumatol* 1997;24(2): 303–308.

186. Grewal IS, Grewal KD, Wong FS, et al. Local expression of transgene encoded TNF alpha in islets prevents autoimmune diabetes in nonobese diabetic (NOD) mice by preventing the development of auto-reactive islet-specific T cells. *J Exp Med* 1996;184(5):1963–1974.
187. Green EA, Eynon EE, Flavell RA. Local expression of TNFalpha in neonatal NOD mice promotes diabetes by enhancing presentation of islet antigens. *Immunity* 1998;9(5):733–743.
188. Jacob CO, McDevitt HO. Tumour necrosis factor-alpha in murine autoimmune "lupus" nephritis. *Nature* 1988;331 (6154):356–358.
189. Gordon C, Ranges GE, Greenspan JS, et al. Chronic therapy with recombinant tumor necrosis factor-alpha in autoimmune NZB/NZW F1 mice. *Clin Immunol Immunopathol* 1989;52(3): 421–434.
190. Brennan DC, Yui MA, Wuthrich RP, et al. Tumor necrosis factor and IL-1 in New Zealand Black/White mice. Enhanced gene expression and acceleration of renal injury. *J Immunol* 1989;143(11):3470–3475.
191. Cope AP, Liblau RS, Yang XD, et al. Chronic tumor necrosis factor alters T cell responses by attenuating T cell receptor signaling. *J Exp Med* 1997;185(9):1573–1584.
192. Ohtsuka K, Gray JD, Stimmler MM, et al. Decreased production of TGF-beta by lymphocytes from patients with systemic lupus erythematosus. *J Immunol* 1998;160(5):2539–2545.
193. Border WA, Ruoslahti E. Transforming growth factor- in disease: The dark side of tissue repair. *J Clin Invest* 1992;90:1–7.
194. Wahl SM, Orenstein JM, Shen W. TGF-beta influences the life and death decisions of T lymphocytes. *Cytokine Growth Factor Rev* 2000;11(1–2):71–79.
195. Letterio JJ, Roberts AB. Regulation of immune responses by TGF-beta. *Annu Rev Immunol* 1998;16:137–161.
196. Sporn MB, Roberts AB, Wakefield LM, et al. Some recent advances in the chemistry and biology of TGF-β. *J Cell Biol* 1987;105:1039–1045.
197. Seder RA, Marth T, Sieve MC, et al. Factors involved in the differentiation of TGF-beta-producing cells from naive CD4+ T cells: IL-4 and IFN-gamma have opposing effects, while TGF-beta positively regulates its own production. *J Immunol* 1998; 60:5719–5728.
198. Gray JD, Hirokawa M, Horwitz DA. The role of transforming growth factor beta in the generation of suppression: an interaction between CD8+ T and NK cells. *J Exp Med* 1994;180 (5):1937–1942.
199. Gray JD, Hirokawa M, Ohtsuka K, et al. Generation of an inhibitory circuit involving CD8+ T cells, IL-2, and NK cell-derived TGF-beta: contrasting effects of anti-CD2 and anti-CD3. *J Immunol* 1998;160(5):2248–2254.
200. Yamagiwa S, Gray JD, Horwitz DA. A Role for TGF-β in the generation of human CD4+ CD25+ regulatory cells from naive peripheral blood T cells. *J Immunology* 2001. In press.
201. Ohtsuka K, Gray JD, Quismorio FP Jr, et al. Cytokine-mediated down-regulation of B cell activity in SLE: effects of interleukin-2 and transforming growth factor-beta. *Lupus* 1999;8 (2):95–102.
202. Ohtsuka K, Gray JD, Stimmler MM, et al. The relationship between defects in lymphocyte production of transforming growth factor-beta1 in systemic lupus erythematosus and disease activity or severity. *Lupus* 1999;8(2):90–94.
203. Glas-Greenwalt P, Kant KS, Dosekun A, et al. Ancrod: normalization of fibrinolytic enzyme abnormalities in patients with systemic lupus erythematosus and lupus nephritis. *J Lab Clin Med* 1985;105(1):99–107.
204. Grande JP. Mechanisms of progression of renal damage in lupus nephritis: pathogenesis of renal scarring. *Lupus* 1998;7(9): 604–610.
205. Yamamoto T, Watanabe T, Ikegaya N, et al. Expression of types I, II, and III TGF-beta receptors in human glomerulonephritis. *J Am Soc Nephrol* 1998;9(12):2253–2261.
206. Yamamoto K, Loskutoff DJ. Expression of transforming growth factor-beta and tumor necrosis factor-alpha in the plasma and tissues of mice with lupus nephritis. *Lab Invest* 2000;80(10): 1561–1570.
207. Stach RM, Rowley DA. A first or dominant immunization. II. Induced immunoglobulin carries transforming growth factor beta and suppresses cytolytic T cell responses to unrelated alloantigens. *J Exp Med* 1993;78:841–852.
208. Hellmann DB, Petri M, Whiting-O'Keefe Q. Fatal infections in systemic lupus erythematosus: the role of opportunistic organisms. *Medicine (Baltimore)* 1987;66(5):341–348.
209. Mitchell DM, Fitzharris P, Knight RA, et al. Kinetics of specific anti-influenza antibody production by cultured lymphocytes from patients with systemic lupus erythematosus following influenza immunization. *Clin Exp Immunol* 1982;49(2):290–296.
210. Brodman R, Gilfillan R, Glass D, et al. Influenzal vaccine response in systemic lupus erythematosus. *Ann Intern Med* 1978;88(6):735–740.
211. Louie JS, Nies KM, Shoji KT, et al. Clinical and antibody responses after influenza immunization in systemic lupus erythematosus. *Ann Intern Med* 1978;88(6):790–792.
212. Jarrett MP, Schiffman G, Barland P, et al. Impaired response to pneumococcal vaccine in systemic lupus erythematosus. *Arthritis Rheum* 1980;23(11):1287–1293.
213. Fernandes G, Bysani C, Venkatraman JT, et al. Increased TGF-beta and decreased oncogene expression by omega-3 fatty acids in the spleen delays onset of autoimmune disease in B/W mice. *J Immunol* 1994;152(12):5979–5987.
214. Venkatraman JT, Chu WC. Effects of dietary omega-3 and omega-6 lipids and vitamin E on serum cytokines, lipid mediators and anti-DNA antibodies in a mouse model for rheumatoid arthritis. *J Am Coll Nutr* 1999;18(6):602–613.
215. Llorente L, Richaud-Patin Y, Garcia-Padilla C, et al. Clinical and biologic effects of anti-interleukin-10 monoclonal antibody administration in systemic lupus erythematosus. *Arthritis Rheum* 2000;43(8):1790–1800.

11

B-CELL ABNORMALITIES IN SYSTEMIC LUPUS ERYTHEMATOSUS

STAMATIS-NICK C. LIOSSIS
GEORGE C. TSOKOS

B-lymphocyte overactivity represents the hallmark of immune cell dysregulation in systemic lupus erythematosus (SLE). Overactive B lymphocytes produce a spectrum of autoantibodies (autoAbs) against soluble and cellular constituents. While all cellular constituents represent potential targets of the lupus autoAb response, the most characteristic, as well as the most common, autoAbs in SLE are those targeting the macromolecular complexes of the cell nucleus, the antinuclear antibodies (ANAs). While the spectrum of autoAb specificity in SLE seems unrestricted, only a small number have been shown to contribute convincingly to disease-related tissue injury. The latter are best represented by the anti–blood cell antibodies that activate complement and cause cytopenias and the cationic anti–double-stranded DNA (dsDNA) autoAbs that are thought to contribute to the expression of nephritis (1,2). The presence of some autoAbs correlates with clinical subsets of the disease and is used in disease diagnosis. The majority of the autoAbs have not been assigned a pathogenic role and may represent innocent bystanders. Besides patients with SLE and patients with a variety of autoimmune and nonautoimmune diseases, normal individuals have autoAbs in their sera, albeit transiently and in low concentrations (3).

The small number of B cells in the peripheral blood has been the main limiting factor in the study of their function and their role in the pathophysiology of SLE. This chapter reviews pertinent human data and presents findings from the study of B cells in different murine lupus models.

AUTOREACTIVE B CELLS

Older theories portrayed the view that normally autoreactive B cells do not exist because their presence would provoke overt autoimmunity, and they are therefore eliminated during the maturation process. Nevertheless, it is currently well established that such B cells do exist in the normal person. Moreover, while the naturally autoreactive B-cell pool was initially thought to be rather small, novel studies have presented evidence that this is an underestimation. B cells often respond to autoantigens for which they have such small affinities that they cannot be detected with the use of older, conventional assays (4).

Under normal conditions or in disease states ranging from viral infections to malignancy, normal, autoreactive B cells produce a variety of natural autoAbs that do not cause autoimmune disease or tissue damage. Natural autoAbs usually belong to the immunoglobulin M (IgM) isotype, and do not undergo isotype switching and affinity maturation. They are poly- and cross-reactive with auto- and alloantigens, their appearance may be helpful for the host in order to efficiently eliminate an invader, and natural autoAbs usually appear in the circulation for a short time due to tight regulatory mechanisms imposed on their existence. The above characteristics are in sharp contrast with the autoAb response in SLE, where isotype switching and affinity maturation occur, their presence is not helpful for the host since they can cause tissue damage, their production is continuous, and their presence is long-lived, indicating that regulatory mechanisms governing their appearance and/or elimination are profoundly defective.

Autoreactive antibodies arise from autoreactive B cells, but the mechanisms involved in the preservation of autoreactive B cells are unclear. One view favors that immature B cells having autoreactive potential are eliminated by negative selection so the mature B-cell population contains a few or no autoreactive cells. Escaping the negative selection processes may thus represent a mechanism for nonelimination of immature autoreactive B cells. The generation of the hen-egg lysozyme (HEL) transgenic mouse model improved our understanding on the preservation of autoreactive B cells and the appearance of autoimmunity. Data derived from the study of this model indicate that all B cells inherently exhibit a certain level of autoreactivity. Thus, it may be dangerous for the host to eliminate too many developing immature B cells that bear autoimmune potential because it may restrict severely the repertoire that is necessary for development of normal immune response. It may be equally dangerous to eliminate too few, because this may cause overt autoimmunity. Such a dynamic equilibrium between immunity and autoimmunity is maintained at the stage of the preimmune B cell and is driven by specific selection processes. These selection functions include the strength of B-cell antigen receptor (BCR)-generated intracellular signals (the stronger the BCR-initiated signal, the more likely the rapid elimination of the preimmune B cell) and the interclonal competition. In the presence of a normal B-cell repertoire, the autoantigen weakly binding B cells cannot compete for entry into the follicles of the lymph nodes and spleen in order to receive cell-survival signals. The nonautoimmune B cells are arithmetically superior, and they enter and occupy the follicles rather easily. The follicle-excluded B cells deprived of important survival signals die. When the B-cell repertoire becomes compromised, the autoantigen-binding B cells face less competition, so they eventually enter the follicles, receive survival signals, and become long-lived cells (5–10). The increased occurrence of autoimmunity in conditions of immunodeficiency is in agreement with this theory (11,12).

In contrast to the circulating T-cell pool, B cells in patients with SLE are not arithmetically decreased. Instead, they display increased rates of proliferation, and spontaneously secrete increased amounts of immunoglobulin (13–16). These immunoglobulins are natural antibodies, natural autoAbs, and autoAbs reactive with nuclear, cytoplasmic, and cell-membrane self antigens. The number of cells spontaneously releasing immunoglobulin correlates rather accurately with disease activity (17,18). Polyclonal hypergammaglobulinemia represents a common finding in SLE patients, but correlation with disease activity is less impressive (16). Polyclonal hypergammaglobulinemia is also commonly found in healthy relatives of patients with SLE (19). Nevertheless, challenging SLE peripheral B cells with polyclonal activators or antigens *in vitro* results in substantially decreased amounts of specific Ab production compared to the responses of B cells obtained from normal individuals (20,21).

B-CELL SUBPOPULATIONS

An interesting subpopulation of B cells, known as B-1, has been implicated in the pathogenesis of lupus. B-1 cells are phenotypically distinguished from the other, conventional B cells (B-2 cells), because they bear the T-cell surface marker CD5 in humans (Ly-1 in mice). It is known that B-1 cells represent the majority of B cells during fetal life, and that despite the fact that they are found at high percentages in cavities such as the peritoneum, their numbers in the circulation progressively decrease following birth until they become no more than 20% of the circulating B-cell pool in the adult. B-1 cells have interesting and distinct properties. They represent a B-cell subpopulation that is self-reconstituting and long-lived. They produce highly cross-reactive and low-affinity autoAbs that usually belong to the IgM class (22,23).

It seems that B-1 cells are involved in the pathophysiology of some human and murine autoimmune diseases. Several pieces of evidence implicate them in the pathophysiology of Sjögren's syndrome and rheumatoid arthritis because they produce IgM rheumatoid factor (24,25). B-1 cells are expanded in certain murine lupus-prone models where they have been reported to contribute significantly to the production of important autoAbs. While this may be the case for murine autoimmunity models such as the New Zealand black (NZB), the (NZB×NZW) F1, and the motheaten mouse, where B-1 cells produce antierythrocyte and anti-DNA antibodies, it is not the case for other experimental animal lupus models (23,26,27). In other murine lupus models B-1 cells are not expanded in the circulation, nor does their induced expansion in nonautoimmunity prone mouse strains correlate with the development of autoimmune features (26,28).

It is not clear whether B-1 cells have any prominent pathogenic contribution in human lupus. First, the number of B-1 cells in patients with SLE is not increased, compared to normal individuals, and second, it was reported that in patients with SLE both B-1 and B-2 cells contribute to the production of pathogenic autoAbs such as anti-dsDNA (29). The characteristics of the antibodies produced by the B-1 cell subpopulation (usually IgM class, low affinity for the antigen, and high cross-reactivity) lie closer to the characteristics encountered in the natural autoAbs and are in contrast to those encountered in SLE autoimmunity.

THE ABNORMAL IMMUNOREGULATORY ENVIRONMENT

The features of the autoAbs (isotype switching and affinity maturation) indicate that the lupus autoAb response is a T-cell dependent, (auto)antigen-driven immune process. In fact, there is little doubt regarding the influence of T cells in the function of the lupus B cell. Is it the T-cell compartment responsible for the immune hallmark of the disease, namely the B-cell hyperreactivity? If this is correct, then B cells should be under either decreased T-cell–mediated suppression, or under excessive, unopposed T-cell–derived help. In the past it was considered that autoreactive B cells in SLE are not properly controlled by suppressor T cells (30–32). On the contrary, there is evidence that supports the position that increased T-cell help is responsible for the increased production of antibodies and autoAbs in SLE. Apart from $CD4^+$ helper T cells, other T-cell subpopulations have been reported to provide help to SLE B cells to produce pathogenic autoAbs such as $CD8^+$, or $CD3^+CD4^-CD8^-TCR\alpha\beta^+$, or $CD3^+CD4^-CD8^-TCR\gamma\delta^+$ cells (33–35) (see Chapter 9).

The above studies conclude that B-cell overactivity and the production of autoAbs are due to factors exogenous to the B cell and lie within the T-cell compartment. While the previously mentioned data clearly document the contribution of the T-cell compartment to the production of autoAbs, there are novel functional as well as genetic studies challenging the view that this is an entirely T-cell–dependent process. Studies of murine and human lupus have produced direct or indirect evidence that B cells in SLE are not innocent bystanders but that their contribution to disease initiation and perpetuation may be more central.

FUNCTIONAL STUDIES SUGGESTING THAT B CELLS IN SLE ARE INTRINSICALLY DERANGED

Lately, a number of studies have concluded that the B cell in lupus may contribute in a T-cell–independent manner to the production of autoAbs. These studies have shown the following:

1. Contrary to earlier beliefs, the immunologic tolerance of B cells can be violated rather easily *in vitro* under conditions that could be readily reproduced *in vivo* (36). B-cell tolerance can be broken during viral infections, during immunizations, and upon stimulation with polyclonal activators (37–42). Polyclonally triggered B cells are found in the circulation of patients with SLE and Sjögren's syndrome (43,44). In addition, chronic polyclonal B-cell stimulation may lead to autoimmunity in mice (45). Nevertheless, polyclonal activation is not considered as the principal cause of the production of autoAbs (46). Bretscher and Cohn (47) have proposed the two-signal hypothesis suggesting that contact with (self) antigen, in the absence of T-cell–derived help, tolerizes B cells. Initial B-cell contact with a self antigen and T-cell–derived help at the same time result in B-cell tolerance breakdown (48,49). Nevertheless, experimental data supporting that this rule can be violated and that B-cell tolerance can be broken without the support of T-cell–mediated help were recently published (50).
2. Lupus-prone murine strains genetically manipulated do not have $\alpha\beta^+$ (or $CD4^+$) T cells but were still able to produce significant amounts of pathogenic IgG autoantibodies (51). Medical Research Laboratory/lymphoproliferative (MRL/*lpr*) mice congenitally deficient in $TCR\alpha\beta$ T cells develop autoimmunity characterized by hypergammaglobulinemia, autoAbs to native DNA and to small nuclear ribonucleoproteins, and manifest immune-complex mediated nephritis (52).
3. When pre–B cells obtained from the embryonic liver of (NZB×NZW) F1 mice were transferred to mice with severe combined immunodeficiency (SCID), they were able to produce anti-dsDNA autoAbs and to sustain a lupus-like disease (53). These data are in contrast with previous studies reporting that the transfer of autoreactive B cells into nonautoimmune animals caused the production of relatively small amounts of autoAb (54). In contrast, transfer of normal B cells into autoimmunity-prone recipients was associated with autoantibody production within a month from the transfer (55,56).

The former studies underscore that B cells of lupus-prone experimental animals are able to produce autoAbs and to cause lupus-like disease even in host environments where they receive no $CD4^+$-mediated T-cell help. This ability is preserved in the absence of $\alpha\beta^+$ T cells and even in the total absence of T cells, and hence in the total absence of either T-cell–mediated increased help or decreased suppression. But is it the presence of B cells that is causally related to the development of disease, or the presence of autoAbs that results from B-cell overactivity? Lupus-prone MRL/*lpr* mice that were genetically manipulated to express B cells bearing surface Ig (sIg) BCR but unable to secrete any antibody were studied. These mice developed autoimmunity characterized by nephritis with cellular infiltrates, indicating that autoimmune B cells, rather than the production of autoAb and formed immune-complexes, are important in the expression of the disease (57). The absolute dependence of the expression of SLE on either direct or indirect interactions of B cells with either hyperactive or autoreactive T cells is therefore questionable under certain experimental conditions.

THE LUPUS B CELL IS AN EFFICIENT (AUTO)ANTIGEN-PRESENTING CELL

Investigators taking into account the particularly efficient antigen-presenting capacity of the B cell have produced data indicating that the B cell in lupus represents the central pathogenic cell that triggers other immune cells toward hyperactivity. Studies in the MRL/*lpr* lupus murine model have shown that when these mice undergo genetic manipulation to eliminate B cells, they fail to produce autoAbs and deposit immune-complexes in tissues. These animals do not have circulating activated T cells that appear in the MRL/*lpr* animals and inflamed tissues with infiltrating T cells. While the vast majority of the circulating T cells in the unmanipulated animal have a particular activated/memory phenotype, the vast majority of the T cells in the manipulated animals are naive T cells. It is thus proposed that the abnormal B cells of the MRL/*lpr*/*lpr* model are not only responsible for the production of pathogenic autoAbs, but also mediate activation of T cells (58–60). More specifically, this T-cell activating function of B cells has been shown for CD8$^+$ T cells in the MRL/*lpr* mouse (61). In the above models the presence or the absence of B cell was the one and only determinant of the appearance, or not, of the autoimmune murine syndrome. In the absence of B cells these autoimmune mice had neither activated T cells nor lupus. It is thus possible that under certain circumstances, lupus B cells are not restricted to the production of autoAbs only, but also mediate abnormal T-cell activation.

A potential downside of these studies is that they stem from the MRL/*lpr/lpr* model. The *lpr/lpr* genotype is responsible for the deficiency of the apoptosis-mediator CD95 (Fas/Apo-1) (62). However, apart from sporadic cases, a Fas defect is not apparent in human SLE (63,64). It may be thus questionable the extent to which data from this mouse apply to the human disease. Recently, restoration of the function of the Fas molecule in the MRL/*lpr* murine strain corrected some apoptosis-related abnormalities such as lymphoaccumulation, but did not alter significantly their autoimmune features, thus increasing the likelihood of applicability of such data to the human disease (65). In addition, in the MRL/*lpr* mouse, similarly to human disease, B-1 cells do not contribute to the production of autoAbs (66). Furthermore, in the Fas-replenished mice bearing the MRL background, B cells were again required for the induction of lupus-like nephritis, suggesting that the autoreactive B cells are essential for the development of systemic autoimmunity in a murine model that is independent of Fas-mediated apoptosis (67).

GENETIC STUDIES

The description of functional aberrations in lupus B cells indicating a potentially intrinsic defect suggest that such a defect(s) may reflect the product of genetic alteration(s). Only recently the first three large-scale genetic studies on multiplex lupus families were reported using microsatellite genome-wide searches (68–70). Studies of the genetic composition of lupus-prone mice began several years ago. Three independent research groups analyzing the whole genome of the (NZB×NZW) F1 mouse mapped genetic loci that contribute to development of murine lupus (71–73). It is currently thought that these disease-predisposing genetic loci work in an additive manner; the more disease-predisposing loci an animal inherits, the higher the likelihood it will develop the full-blown lupus-like illness. It is interesting that all three groups reached similar conclusions when mapping disease-susceptibility loci (74,75).

One lupus-prone strain analyzed was the NZM2410 mouse. This is a recently produced substrain of the (NZB×NZW) F1 strain characterized by a highly penetrant and early-onset lupus-like illness. In the NZM2410 model, disease-susceptibility maps to four genetic intervals named Sle1, Sle2, Sle3, and H2 (76). The other two groups similarly mapped disease susceptibility loci; one lupus-related genetic locus called nba-1 by one group and the one called Lbw-2/Sbw-2 by others were identified as the locus with a particularly eminent pathogenetic contribution (71,73). Nba-1, Lbw-2/Sbw-2, as well as Sle2 map in a 9-centimorgan (cM)–spanning region of murine chromosome 4, possibly within the context of a single gene. The investigators studying the NZM2410 mouse managed to express each one of the disease-susceptibility genetic loci in the context of a lupus-resistant background, in order to study the relative contribution of each one of them in the development of the disease. Such crossing experiments produced a new strain expressing Sle2 only that developed a clinical picture characterized by hypergammaglobulinemia and IgM-class autoAbs, which could be attributed to dysfunction of the B-cell compartment only. Nevertheless, mice expressing Sle2 only or other disease-susceptibility genetic loci did not develop full-blown lupus. Such experiments suggest that Sle2 may represent a "lupus B-cell overactivity genetic locus" (77). In addition, the presence of Sle2 but not of Sle1, Sle3, and H2, is crucial for the expansion of B-1 cells seen in the NZM2410 mouse. Such B-1 cells are functionally efficient antigen-presenting cells (78).

Equally interesting are the data stemming from the novel murine models expressing the isolated disease-susceptibility locus Sle1. Sle1 maps on murine chromosome 1 and is associated with the production of antihistone autoAbs in lupus mice. Histones are well-known T-cell–dependent (auto)antigens and the production of antihistone autoAbs is a well-characterized T-cell–dependent (auto)immune-response. Sle1 expressed isolated in a lupus-resistant background was associated with the production of IgG anti-H2A/H2B/DNA autoAbs. This type of autoimmunity was not associated with epitope spreading, and was not characterized by generalized autoimmune defects. While it was initially hypothesized that Sle1 may represent a "lupus T-cell gene," the investigators hypothesized that Sle1 is expressed in murine lupus B cells only, pointing to another "lupus B-cell gene." In fact, using adoptive bone marrow transfer and mixed chimeric experimental models, the same group disclosed that Sle1 mediates loss of tolerance to chromatin in B and T cells and that Sle1 is functionally expressed in the B lymphocyte (79,80). Isolated expression of the genetic interval Sle3 that maps on chromosome 7 was associated with low-grade polyclonal T- and B-cell activation and mildly penetrant glomerulonephritis (81). However, the simultaneous presence of Sle1 and Sle3 was associated with an aggressive autoimmune phenotype, particularly in female mice. Sle1 and Sle3 bicongenic mice developed splenomegaly, significantly expanded B cells and CD4$^+$ T cells with activated phenotypes, widespread humoral autoimmunity including pathogenic autoAbs, and a highly penetrant glomerulonephritis (82).

Based on their elegant studies, the Wakeland group (83) proposed an epistatic model for the development of autoimmunity, where a combination of multiple defects in the genome allow for the expression of autoimmune aberrations culminating up to the expression of lupus-like disease. To complicate things further, the same group identified autoimmunity-suppressing modifiers. One of these, assigned Sles1, was shown to specifically suppress the autoimmune features that should ensue due to the presence of the Sle1, but not the Sle2 or Sle3, locus. It is thus the presence of autoimmunity-promoting and/or the absence or loss of autoimmunity-suppressing genetic elements that integrates into the development of overt autoimmunity in experimental models.

DERANGED CYTOKINE ENVIRONMENT

It was recently reported that the production of and the response to cytokines such as interleukin-6 (IL-6) and IL-10 is abnormally increased in SLE B cells. Both IL-6 and IL-10 are B-cell stimulatory cytokines, while IL-10 also inhibits type-1 cytokine responses (84,85). Patients with active SLE have elevated serum levels of IL-6 (86,87), increased numbers of IL-6 secreting cells (88), and increased IL-6 messenger RNA (mRNA) content in their peripheral blood mononuclear cells (89). B cells from patients with SLE express constitutively cell-surface IL-6 receptors, but normal B cells do not (90). IL-6 generates an *in vitro* increase in the lupus B-cell output of IgG and an increase of IgG anti-DNA autoAbs, and the addition of anti–IL-6 mAb inhibits the IL-6 induced effects (86,90). The autocrine action of IL-6 has been shown clearly in B cells from (NZB×NZW) F1 and from MRL/*lpr* mice (91–93).

Similarly to IL-6, patients with SLE have elevated serum levels of IL-10 (94), increased numbers of IL-10 secreting cells (88), and increased IL-10 mRNA content in their peripheral blood mononuclear cells (89). IL-10 overproduction was shown to have functional significance since an anti–IL-10 mAb used in that study suppressed the *in vitro* production of autoAbs from B cells obtained from patients with SLE, but recombinant human IL-10 promoted it (95). In support of the above is that continuous administration of anti–IL-10 mAb delays the onset of autoimmunity in (NZB×NZW) F1 mice (96). It could be proposed that increased production of IL-10 may represent a product (rather than a cause) of a hyperproliferating B-cell population. Because the degree of B-cell proliferation correlates with disease activity and the overproduction of IL-10 was disease activity-independent, these data point to a putative intrinsic B-cell defect in SLE. In agreement with this hypothesis are reports that increased production of IL-10 is found in B cells from relatives of SLE patients. The mRNA of IL-10 was found in lupus B cells but was undetectable in control B cells. The B-cell subpopulation that contains and releases increased amounts of IL-10, not only in patients with SLE but also in their first- and second-degree relatives, is incompletely characterized (97).

PHENOTYPIC CHANGES OF THE LUPUS B CELL

Desai-Mehta et al. (98) described for the first time the appearance of a co-stimulatory molecule, CD40 ligand (CD40L, CD154) on the surface membrane of lupus B cells, a marker considered to be characteristic of activated T cells. This finding was disease-specific. In the peripheral blood of patients with active SLE, the number of CD40L$^+$ B cells was 20.5-fold greater than in healthy donors. In patients with inactive SLE the numbers of CD40L$^+$ B cells were comparable to those in the controls. Nevertheless, activation-induced CD40L expression on the surface of lupus B cells was 17-fold greater than the baseline levels, compared to a 7.6-fold increase recorded in control subjects. CD40L was actively synthesized within the lupus B cell as supported by data of CD40L mRNA detection in lupus B cells.

CD40L expressed on the surface of lupus B cells retains full functional properties. The addition of a neutralizing anti-CD40L mAb in *in vitro* cell-culture settings decreased the cationic anti-dsDNA production. Because not only T cells but also B cells from SLE patients express functional CD40L on their cell surface, and because both kinds of lymphocytes express CD40, a bidirectional cognate stimulatory loop may function between lupus T and B cells (99). Moreover, it was reported that CD40L expressed on the surface of B cells co-stimulates other B cells as well (100).

In addition to CD40L, CD80 and CD86 are aberrantly expressed on the surface of lupus B cells. Fresh, small, resting, peripheral B cells but also large, activated B cells from patients with SLE were studied for the expression of CD80 and CD86. While CD80 expression was only slightly increased on the surface of large, activated lupus B cells, the expression of CD86 showed a 2.5- and 7-fold increase on the surface of activated and resting lupus B cells, respectively, when compared to B cells obtained from patients with allergic disorders (101). While only patients in remission were studied, and the functional integrity of the co-stimulatory molecules was not assessed, this study provides evidence that B cells from patients with SLE overexpress molecules that belong to the B7 family of co-stimulatory molecules. Expression of B7-family molecules has been shown to be a prerequisite for the disruption of immune tolerance to self antigen (102).

ABERRANT B-CELL ANTIGEN RECEPTOR SIGNAL TRANSDUCTION

The studies discussed above present evidence supporting the view that B cells from patients with SLE have functional as well as phenotypic abnormalities that are at least in part independent of the activity of the underlying disease. It is thus possible that such aberrations represent intrinsic lupus B-cell defects. It is also possible that the heterogeneous defects described above may have a common underlying central biochemical abnormality. Crucial aspects of lymphocyte function, such as activation, proliferation, cytokine production, effector functions, and apoptosis, are determined by the signaling biochemical pathway initiated following ligation of the surface antigen receptor (103–109). Physiologically, the ligand for BCR is the relevant antigen, and for the autoreactive B cell it is the autoantigen. We now know that the biochemical cascade triggered in the B cell following the interaction between BCR and antigen can be closely mimicked by anti-BCR antibodies (Fig 11.1).

We have addressed the question of possible antigen-receptor–mediated signaling aberrations in B cells of lupus patients using anti-Ig antibodies (110). Stimulation of circulating B cells from patients with SLE through their sIgM BCR produced significantly higher fluxes of free intracytoplasmic Ca^{2+} when compared to similarly induced responses of B cells from patients with other systemic rheumatic diseases, or to the responses obtained from normal B cells. This phenomenon was not limited to signaling through the sIgM BCR, but was also observed when the sIgD BCR was used for triggering the signaling process. The elevated Ca^{2+} responses were contributed significantly from the intracellular calcium stores. Nevertheless, the production of inositol 1,4,5-trisphosphate (the principal mediator of free calcium release from the intracellular compartment) was only slightly elevated, raising the possibility of either a hypersensitive Ca^{2+} release machinery or of dominant inositol trisphosphate–independent pathway(s) of Ca^{2+} release. To date, the pathway(s) has been incompletely characterized (111,112).

The earliest known BCR-mediated signaling event is the activation of protein tyrosine kinases, which results in tyrosyl phosphorylation of cellular proteins (113–115). The tyrosyl phosphorylation reaction has numerous substrates; only a few such substrates have been identified. In lupus B cells, the overall level of sIgM-initiated protein tyrosyl phosphorylation was significantly enhanced and correlated with the augmented BCR-mediated free calcium responses. More specifically, at least four cellular proteins with molecular sizes between 36 and 64 kd were significantly hyperphosphorylated in anti-IgM–treated lupus B cells compared to the response of B cells from normal controls (110). The aberrant BCR-mediated signaling process was not associated with disease activity, treatment status, or specific clinical manifestations. Moreover, enhanced tyrosyl protein phosphorylation was disease-specific, implying a possible intrinsic lupus B-cell defect, which may have pathogenic impact. Furthermore, the increased Ca^{2+} responses could represent a biochemical and molecular basis for the enhanced expression of CD40L on the surface of lupus B cells upon stimulation. It has been previously reported that CD40L upregulation on the cell surface is predominantly NFAT-, and hence Ca^{2+}-, dependent (116). Moreover, strikingly similar abnormalities of antigen-receptor signaling have previously been reported from the study of fresh T cells, T-cell lines, and autoantigen-specific T cells from patients with SLE (117,118), pointing to a potentially unifying Ag-receptor–mediated signaling defect(s) in lupus lymphocytes. It

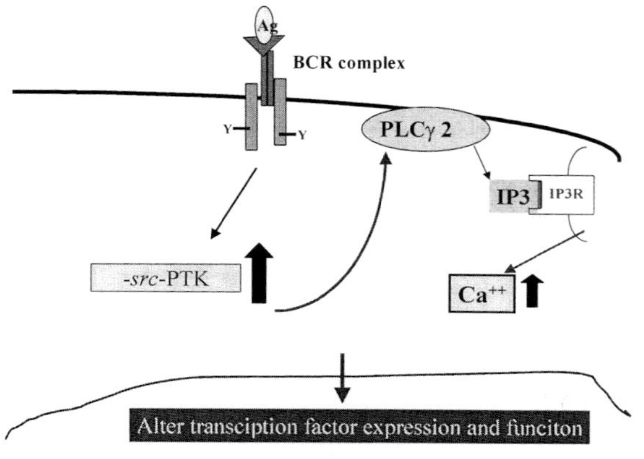

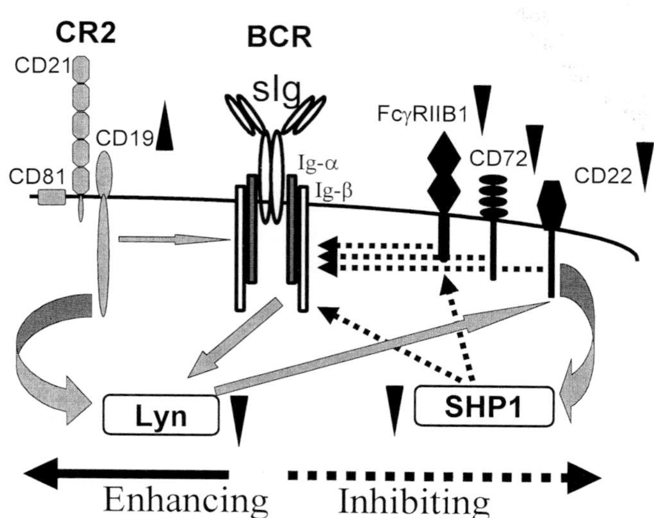

FIGURE 11.1. B-cell signaling regulatory molecules and abnormalities leading to B-cell overactivity and lupus-like autoimmunity. **A:** B-cell receptor (BCR)-initiated activating signals. Occupancy of the BCR by antigenic peptide initiates a biochemical signal that activates nonreceptor tyrosine kinases. Tyrosine phosphorylation of phospholipase Cγ2 (PLC-γ2) hydrolyzes inositol bisphosphate to inositol trisphosphate (IP3) and diacylglyceride. IP3 binds to IP3 receptor (IP3R) and stimulates the rapid release of and subsequent rise in intracellular calcium. Intracellular calcium is a second messenger molecule that is required for activation of molecules such as calcineurin, protein kinase C isozymes, and calmodulin kinases. In lupus B cells engagement of the BCR leads to increased protein tyrosine phosphorylation of various cytoplasmic proteins. **B:** BCR-initiated signaling is tightly controlled by additional membrane receptor-generated signals that either enhance or decrease the initial stimulatory sIg-triggered events. Signaling enhancers (CR2) and/or inhibitors (FcγRIIB1, CD22, CD5, CD72) participate in the regulation of BCR-initiated events. Theoretically, CD72 can bind CD5 present on the surface membrane of the same cell or on the surface of T cells. In the cytoplasm, tyrosine kinase Lyn and tyrosine phosphatase SHP-1 form tight regulatory and interlocking feedback loops. An increase of substrate activity *(solid gray arrows)* and a decrease in activity (*broken black arrows*) are shown. BCR-initiated signaling in SLE B cells is increased. Changes in either membrane or cytoplasmic signaling mediators (*arrowheads*) generated in genetically manipulated animals have been well correlated with the development of B-cell overactivity and/or autoimmunity.

has been proposed that the signaling abnormalities encountered in SLE lymphocytes may provide a biochemical and molecular background for such diverse abnormalities as lymphocyte activation, anergy, and cell death (119).

It is interesting that abnormalities similar to the human lupus BCR-initiated signaling abnormalities were encountered in a study of experimental animal lupus. Feuerstein et al. (120) induced systemic lupus-like autoimmunity through the development of graft-versus-host disease in a background of double-transgenic sIg/sHEL murine tolerance model. Induction of autoimmunity correlated with phenotypical as well as with signal-transduction changes of B cells similar to those in the human disease. B-cell surface expression of CD21 [part of the complement receptor 2 (CR2) complex] was significantly decreased in the autoimmune state. In addition, changes in the BCR-mediated protein tyrosyl phosphorylation pattern in B cells developed following the induction of autoimmunity. In the autoimmune but not in the tolerant state, two substrates with apparent molecular masses of 78 and 60 kd were hyperphosphorylated following BCR cross-linking. The similarity of BCR-induced signaling in patients with SLE and in this particular autoimmunity model underscores the potentially central pathogenic role of aberrantly functioning B cells in both conditions (Fig 11.1A).

ESTROGENS AND THE LUPUS B LYMPHOCYTE

Estrogens are indisputably involved in the pathogenesis of SLE in humans as well as in murine models. Hormonal manipulations dramatically alter the expression of SLE in lupus-prone mice, and women of child-bearing age are afflicted more commonly than men. Estrogens are steroid hormones that exert their effects via binding to their cytoplasmic receptors and following that to estrogen responsive elements (EREs) found in the context of promoters of distinct genes. Nevertheless, the mechanisms involved in the contribution of estrogens to the pathogenesis of SLE are unknown.

It was reported that estrogens upregulate calcineurin expression in T cells from patients with SLE, but this issue has not been addressed for the lupus B cell; nevertheless, similarly to T cells, B cells also possess estrogen receptors (121). These data suggest that estrogens may modulate antigen receptor-mediated cell signaling, since this pathway is deranged in lupus T as well as B cells (see above), and calcineurin represents a major target enzyme of this signaling pathway (122). A recent study showed that estrogens, estradiol in particular, can break B-cell tolerance and cause a lupus-like disease in a previously nonautoimmune mouse that transgenically expresses the heavy chain of a pathogenic anti-DNA autoAb (123). Estradiol induced high titers of anti-DNA autoAb and glomerulonephritis. This was the result of nondeletion or anergization of naive autoreactive B cells that normally should be tolerized. Estradiol-induced autoimmunity in the above murine model was associated with increased expression of the antiapoptotic molecule Bcl-2 by such autoreactive B cells.

ABNORMALITIES OF BCR-SIGNALING REGULATORY MOLECULES

When B cells encounter antigen, other B-cell surface molecules are also engaged, and some of them provide regulatory control over the intensity, the duration, and the fate of the biochemical signal generated by the interaction of BCR with the antigen. Engagement of signaling regulatory molecules triggers separate intracytoplasmic biochemical cascades; the net sum of these signals may result in an increased, an attenuated, or a qualitatively different BCR-initiated signal outcome (124) (Fig. 11.1B).

Complement Receptors on Lupus B Cells

The most important signal-augmenting B-cell surface molecule is the complement receptor type 2 (CR2). This is better perceived as a hetero-oligomeric complex (the CR2 complex) contributed by the molecules CD21 (CR2), CD19 (the signaling molecule of the complex), and CD81. Physiologically, CR2 binds iC3b, C3dg, or C3d. The cytoplasmic signal produced when B-cell antigens are presented to the BCR bound with the aforementioned complement fractions is the sum of co–cross-linking BCR and CR2 and is several orders of magnitude higher when compared to the signal produced by the same antigens via the BCR alone (reviewed in ref. 125).

It was reported that the expression of both CR2 and CR1 is decreased on the surface of B cells from patients with SLE. Because this defect was also present in healthy relatives of patients with SLE, it was proposed that it may be a genetically determined alteration (126). Decreased expression of B-cell surface complement receptors is also seen on MRL/*lpr* B cells during the development of autoimmunity (127). On the contrary, according to a more recent study and to our own experience, it was found that decreased CR2 expression levels correlate well with increased disease activity (128).

CR2 also represents the B-cell surface receptor for Epstein-Barr virus (EBV). An epidemiologic study disclosed that young patients with recent-onset SLE have indexes of EBV infection more commonly than their healthy counterparts (99% vs. 70%) (129). A previous *in vitro* study reported that in circulating lymphocytes, EBV infection of lupus B cells cannot be contained by lupus T cells (130). Moreover, EBV causes hyperactivation of B cells in SLE and decreases their apoptotic death because it induces overexpression of the antiapoptotic molecule bcl-2 in the cytoplasm (131).

CR2 deficiency on the surface of lupus B cells does not help in explaining the pathophysiology of the overactive lupus B cell. Nevertheless, a novel concept on CR2 (and CR1) function supported by experimental data proposes that complement receptor-mediated signaling maintains B-cell immune tolerance to self antigens (132). This view may provide a molecular background for understanding how lupus B cells, expressing low amounts of membrane complement receptors (due to genetic or acquired defects), display deranged immune self-recognition. A hypothesis was formulated that complement participates in the early stages of B-cell–negative selection. According to this proposal, circulating natural autoantibodies identify highly conserved self antigens and activate the classic pathway of complement. Such complexes bind to the BCR and complement receptors of autoreactive immature B cells arising daily in the bone marrow; this process represents an efficient means to get rid of these highly autoreactive B cells. In the case of early complement factor (or complement receptor) deficiencies, autoreactive immature B cells are not efficiently removed, and lupus-like autoimmunity develops (133). Finally, complement activation products can trigger B-cell signaling events. The membrane-attack complex (C5b-9) found in the serum at sublytic concentrations may induce activation of the B-cell kinases Ras, Raf-1, and extracellular signal-regulated kinase (ERK)-1 in a B-cell line via a mechanism involving G proteins (134). Circulating sublytic C5b-9 complex concentrations are reportedly increased in the serum of patients with SLE (135).

B-CELL SURFACE RECEPTORS THAT PROVIDE NEGATIVE REGULATION

There are several different B-cell surface signaling inhibitory receptors (136). Among them, the functions of CD5, CD22, and FcγRIIB1 are better understood. The ligand for CD5 was shown to be CD72 (137). The role of $CD5^+$ B cells in SLE and in experimental animal lupus is discussed above. The role of co-receptor CD22 was incompletely understood until a study that used CD22-knockout mice clearly disclosed that CD22 is a signaling inhibitory molecule. Young CD22-knockout mice displayed autoimmunity, increased BCR-initiated cytoplasmic calcium responses, hypergammaglobulinemia, and circulating IgM autoAbs (138). Adult CD22-knockout mice displayed glomerulonephritis, circulating IgG anti-dsDNA, and anticardiolipin autoAbs (139). This is a particularly interesting model of systemic lupus-like autoimmunity, because it is monogenic, and because a B-cell molecular defect created an autoAb response that included isotype switching and affinity maturation of the (auto)antibody, characters very reminiscent of a T-cell–dependent immune response. Nevertheless, CD22 expression on the surface of B cells from patients with either active or inactive SLE is similar to that of normal controls (140).

A B-cell surface inhibitory receptor with a role that is well appreciated is the one for the Fc fraction of IgG type IIB1 (FcγRIIB1, CD32). When antigen bound to IgG is presented to the BCR, then BCR and FcγRIIB1 are co–cross-linked. The net signal is of smaller magnitude than the signal generated by antigen alone (141,142). The cytoplasmic free Ca^{2+} response is of shorter duration and the B-cell response is incomplete, not resulting in full B-cell activation and proliferation. Previous studies have reported that the system of receptors for the Fc fraction of IgG overall is malfunctioning in SLE, resulting perhaps in the production of excess antibodies and the accumulation of immune complexes (143). Genetically manipulated mice having B-cell surface FcγRIIB1 deficiency manifested hypergammaglobulinemia (144). In NZB as well as in (NZB×NZW) F1 mice, the B-cell surface expression of FcγRIIB1 was recently reported to be decreased in follicular germinal center B cells of adult (autoimmune) mice, but not in the circulating B-cell pool. Moreover, young (not autoimmune) mice of these strains produced the same effect when exposed to foreign antigens, suggesting that FcγRIIB1 downregulation is an acquired phenotype. The NZB allele for FcγRIIB1 was found to have two deletion sites that included transcription factor-binding sites, thus increasing the likelihood that such deletions have a functional impact (145). This defect correlated with IgG hypergammaglobulinemia. Nevertheless, the expression and function of the specific FcγRIIB1, the only Fc receptor found on the surface of B cell, has not been evaluated in patients with SLE.

The co-receptors CD22 and FcγRIIB1 bear a signaling inhibitory domain in their cytoplasmic tail called ITIM (immunoreceptor tyrosine-based inhibitory motif) (146–148). ITIM becomes functional when the tyrosyl residues lying in its context become phosphorylated under the influence of protein tyrosine kinases (149). Tyrosyl phosphorylated ITIMs become the docking and activating sites for the SH2-domain containing protein tyrosine phosphatases, particularly SHP-1 and SHIP (150–152). It is interesting that SHP-1 is absent or dysfunctional in another autoimmunity model, the motheaten or the viable motheaten mouse, respectively (153).

The phosphorylation of ITIM tyrosyl residues is accomplished by protein tyrosine kinases. The ITIM lying in the cytoplasmic tail of the FcγRIIB1 and CD22 co-receptor undergoes tyrosyl phosphorylation by the *src*-family kinase *lyn* (154). In the absence of *lyn*, the CD22-initiated signaling inhibitory pathway is not triggered, despite adequate amounts of B-cell surface CD22 expression (155). Until recently, *lyn* was considered as an integral part of the BCR-initiated B-cell activation machinery (156,157). Yet, knockout experimental models disclosed that *lyn* is redundant in its stimulatory mediator role. In $lyn^{-/-}$ animals immature B cells developed normally but mature B cells were decreased. Rather unexpectedly it was shown that BCR-initiated signaling events were not only propagated but in fact they were enhanced. The $lyn^{-/-}$ mice develop autoimmunity with features quite reminiscent of lupus; they have hypergammaglobulinemia and increased sensitivity to IL-4, and they develop autoAbs and glomerulonephritis (158–161).

Lyn is crucial for the phosphorylation of CD22 and FcγRIIB1, and phosphorylation of CD22 and FcγRIIB1 are crucial for the activation of SHP-1 and SHIP, respectively. Based on recent experimental animal studies, it appears that *lyn*, CD22, and SHP-1 are present in limiting quantities in B cells. A reduction in the quantity of each of the above mediators promotes a state of B-cell hyperreactivity that eventually correlates with the development of autoimmunity (162).

Furthermore, it also appears that the signaling inhibitory co-receptor CD22 and the signaling enhancer CD19 molecule (part of the CR2-complex) are interrelated and form a regulatory feedback loop that tunes BCR-initiated signaling (163). CD19-deficient B cells are hyporesponsive, but B cells expressing even slightly increased CD19 levels are hyperresponsive and develop autoimmunity (164,165). CD19 amplifies *src*-family protein tyrosine kinase activity and has been shown to allow for optimal CD22 function (166). Similarly, CD22 expression negatively regulates CD19-mediated functions. There are several pieces of experimental data suggesting that CD19 amplifies the activity of *lyn* that in turn phosphorylates CD22. CD22 ITIM phosphorylation recruits SHP-1 that negatively regulates the activity of CD19 by tyrosyl dephosphorylating it (163). A study recently investigated the expression of CD22 and *lyn* in B cells from SLE patients (167). Preliminary data disclose that while CD22 expression is comparable to control B cells, the content *lyn* in lupus B cells is significantly decreased in two thirds of patients with SLE (168). Although the function of the CD22/*lyn* signaling inhibitor was not addressed, it is likely that decreased *lyn* in SLE B cells contributes to B-cell overactivity by deficiently regulating the BCR-initiating response.

SUMMARY

An overview of the main B-cell abnormalities in SLE in given in Table 11.1. The single most characteristic abnormality of immune cells encountered in both patients with SLE and in animal lupus models is B-cell overactivity. The pathogenic contribution of factors exogenous to the B cell itself, be it an aberrantly functioning T-cell compartment or the local cytokine environment, is well established. Recent data support a more central pathogenic role for the lupus B cell itself. It is revealed that lupus-like autoimmunity can ensue with either minimal or no contribution from T cells. Genetic as well as functional studies support a role for the lupus B cell as an independent contributor to the appearance of the disease, apart from the well-known contribution of potentially harmful autoAb production. Studies unraveling the biochemistry of lupus B-cell function reveal that there are disease-specific signal transduction aberrations that may represent a common background for other disturbed effector functions. The contribution of signal transduction regulators is appreciated using well-characterized genetically manipulated experimental models. Improving our understanding of the lupus B-cell physiology and pathophysiology

TABLE 11.1. ESTABLISHED B-CELL ABNORMALITIES IN HUMAN/MURINE SYSTEMIC LUPUS ERYTHEMATOSUS (SLE)

B-cell function
Increased numbers of spontaneously activated B cells secreting IgG, IgA, and IgM
Decreased responsiveness *in vitro* to mitogens and antigens
$CD5^+$ B cells produce autoantibodies
Phenotypic changes
Increased expression of CD40 ligand
Increased CD86 expression
Decreased CD21 (CR2) expression
B-cell receptor–initiated cell signaling
Increased free intracytoplasmic calcium response
Increased cytosolic protein tyrosine phosphorylation
Decreased protein kinase lyn content
Cytokines
Increased IL-6 production
Increased IL-10 production
Centrality of B cells in development of lupus
Infections and polyclonal B-cell activators break B-cell tolerance
T-cell–deficient MRL/*lpr* mice develop autoimmunity
B-cell–deficient MRL/*lpr* mice do not develop autoimmunity
B cells from BXW F1 mice >SCID mice cause autoimmunity
B-cell genetics and lupus
Family members of SLE patients have B-cell overactivity
B-cell overactivity loci have been identified in congenic lupus mice

Ig, immunoglobulin; IL, interleukin; MRL, Medical Research Laboratory; SCID, severe combined immunodeficiency disease.

will ultimately improve our understanding of the disease and may provide us with useful tools to deal with SLE more rationally.

REFERENCES

1. Hahn BH. Antibodies to DNA. *N Engl J Med* 1998;338:1359–1368.
2. Raz E, Brezis M, Rosenmann E, et al. Anti-DNA antibodies bind directly to renal antigens and induce kidney dysfunction in the isolated perfused rat kidney. *J Immunol* 1989;142:3076–3082.
3. Guilbert B, Dighiero G, Avrameas S. Naturally occurring antibodies against nine common antigens in human sera. *J Immunol* 1982;128:2779–2787.
4. Lang J, Jackson M, Teyton L, et al. B cells are exquisitively sensitive to central tolerance and receptor editing induced by ultralow affinity, membrane-bound antigen. *J Exp Med* 1996;184:1685–1698.
5. Cyster JG, Hartley SB, Goodnow CC. Competition for follicular niches excludes self-reactive cells from the recirculating B-cell repertoire. *Nature* 1994;371:389–395.
6. Cyster JG, Goodnow CC. Antigen-induced exclusion from follicles and anergy are separate and complementary processes that influence peripheral B cell fate. *Immunity* 1995;3:691–701.
7. Healy JI, Dolmetsch RE, Timmerman LA, et al. Different nuclear signals are activated by the B cell receptor during positive versus negative signaling. *Immunity* 1997;6:419–428.
8. Schmidt KN, Hsu CW, Griffin CT, et al. Spontaneous follicular exclusion of SHP1-deficient B cells is conditional on the presence of competitor wild-type B cells. *J Exp Med* 1998;187:929–937.
9. Schmidt KN, Cyster JG. Follicular exclusion and rapid elimination of hen egg lysozyme autoantigen-binding B cells are dependent on competitor B cells, but not on T cells. *J Immunol* 1999;162:284–291.
10. Cyster JG. Signaling thresholds and interclonal competition in preimmune B-cell selection. *Immunol Rev* 1997;156:87–101.
11. Sherer Y, Shoenfeld Y. Autoimmune diseases and autoimmunity post-bone marrow transplantation. *Bone Marrow Transplant* 1998;22:873–881.
12. Calligaris-Cappio F. Relationship between autoimmunity and immunodeficiency in CLL. *Hematol Cell Ther* 1997;39:S13–16.
13. Ginsburg WW, Finkelman FD, Lipsky PE. Circulating and pokeweed-mitogen-induced immunoglobulin-secreting cells in systemic lupus erythematosus. *Clin Exp Immunol* 1979;35:76–88.
14. Blaese RM, Grayson J, Steinberg AD. Increased immunoglobulin-secreting cells in the blood of patients with active systemic lupus erythematosus. *Am J Med* 1980;69:345–350.
15. Becher TM, Lizzio EF, Mercant LP, et al. Increased multiclonal antibody-forming cell activation in the peripheral blood of patients with SLE. *Int Arch Allergy Appl Immunol* 1981;66:293–298.
16. Quismorio FP, Friou GJ. Serological factors in SLE and their pathogenetic significance. *CRC Crit Rev Clin Lab Sci* 1970;1:639–715.
17. Tsokos GC, Balow JE. Spontaneous and pokeweed mitogen-induced plaque-forming cells in systemic lupus erythematosus. *Clin Immunol Immunopathol* 1981;21:172–183.
18. Balow JE, Tsokos GC. T and B lymphocyte function in patients with lupus nephritis: correlation with renal pathology. *Clin Nephrol* 1984;21:93–101.
19. Clark J, Bourne T, Salaman MR, et al. B lymphocyte hyperactivity in families of patients with systemic lupus erythematosus. *J Autoimmun* 1996;9:59–65.
20. Gottlieb AB, Lahita RG, Chiorazzi N, et al. Immune functions in systemic lupus erythematosus: impairment of in vitro T-cell proliferation and in vivo antibody response to exogenous antigen. *J Clin Invest* 1979;63:885–892.
21. Kallenberg CG, Limburg PC, Van Slochteren C. The T helper B cell activity in SLE: depressed in vivo humoral immune response to a primary antigen (hemocyanin) and decreased in vitro spontaneous Ig synthesis. *Clin Exp Immunol* 1983;53:371–378.
22. Casali P, Notkins AL. 1989. CD5+ B lymphocytes, polyreactive antibodies and the human B-cell repertoire. *Immunol Today* 1989;10:364–368.
23. Hayakawa K, Hardy RR, Parks DR, et al. The Ly-1 B cell subpopulation in normal, immunodefective, and autoimmune mice. *J Exp Med* 1983;157:202–218.
24. Hardy RR, Hayakawa K, Shimizu M, et al. Rheumatoid-factor secretion from human Leu-1 B cells. *Science* 1987;236:81–83.
25. Youinou P, Mackenzie L, Le Masson G, et al. CD5 expressing B lymphocytes in the blood and salivary glands of patients with primary Sjogren's syndrome. *J Autoimmun* 1988;1:188–194.
26. Wofsy D, Chiang NY. Proliferation of Ly-1 B cells in autoimmune NZB and (NZB × NZW)F1 mice. *Eur J Immunol* 1987;17:809–814.
27. Sidman CL, Shultz LD, Hardy RR, et al. Production of immunoglobulin isotypes by Ly-1+ B cells in viable motheaten and normal mice. *Science* 1986;232:1423–1425.
28. Hera A, Marcos MAR, Toribio ML, et al. Development of Ly-1 B cells in immunodeficient CBA/n mice. *J Exp Med* 1987;166:804–809.
29. Suzuki N, Sakane T, Engleman EG. Anti-DNA antibody production by CD5+ and CD5− B cells in patients with systemic lupus erythematosus. *J Clin Invest* 1990;85:238–247.
30. Abdou NI, Sagawa A, Passual E, et al. Suppressor T cell abnormality in idiopathic SLE. *Clin Immunol Immunopathol* 1976;6:192–199.
31. Bresnihan B, Jasin HE. Suppressor function of peripheral blood mononuclear cells in normal individuals and in patients with systemic lupus erythematosus. *J Clin Invest* 1977;59:106–116.
32. Fauci AS, Steinberg AD, Haynes BF, et al. Immunoregulatory aberrations in systemic lupus erythematosus. *J Immunol* 1978;121:1473–1479.
33. Linker-Israeli M, Quismorio FP Jr, Horwitz DA. CD8+ lymphocytes from patients with systemic lupus erythematosus sustain, rather than suppress, spontaneous polyclonal IgG production and synergize with CD4+ cells to support autoantibody synthesis. *Arthritis Rheum* 1990;33:1216–1225.
34. Shivakumar S, Tsokos GC, Datta SK. T cell receptor alpha/beta expressing double-negative ($CD4^-/CD8^-$) and $CD4^+$ T helper cells in humans augment the production of pathogenic anti-DNA autoantibodies associated with lupus nephritis. *J Immunol* 1989;143:103–112.
35. Rajagopalan S, Zordan T, Tsokos GC, et al. Pathogenic anti-DNA autoantibody-inducing T helper cell lines from patients with active lupus nephritis: isolation of $CD4^-8^-$ T helper cell lines that express the gamma/delta T cell antigen receptor. *Proc Natl Acad Sci USA* 1990;87:7020–7024.
36. Dong X, Hamilton KJ, Satoh M, et al. Initiation of autoimmunity to the p53 tumor suppressor protein by complexes of p53 and SV40 large T antigen. *J Exp Med* 1994;179:1243–1252.
37. Ohashi PS, Oehen S, Buerki K, et al. Ablation of "tolerance" and induction of diabetes by virus infection in viral antigen transgenic mice. *Cell* 1991;65:305–317.
38. Caton AJ, Swartzentruber JR, Kuhl AL, et al. Activation and

negative selection of functionally distinct subsets of antibody-secreting cells by influenza hemagglutinin as a viral and a neo-self antigen. *J Exp Med* 1996;183:13–26.
39. Fritz RB, Chou CH, McFarlin DE. Relapsing murine experimental allergic encephalomyelitis induced by myelin basic protein. *J Immunol* 1983;130:1024–1026.
40. Akkaraju S, Canaan K, Goodnow CC. Self-reactive B cells are not eliminated or inactivated by autoantigen expressed on thyroid epithelial cells. *J Exp Med* 1997;186:2005–2012.
41. McHeyzer-Williams MG, Nossal GJ. Clonal analysis of autoantibody producing cell precursors in the preimmune B cell repertoire. *J Immunol* 1988;141:4118–4123.
42. Rocken M, Urban JF, Shevach EM. Infection breaks T-cell tolerance. *Nature* 1992;359:79–82.
43. Fauci AS, Moutsopoulos HM. Polyclonally triggered B cells in the peripheral blood and bone marrow of normal individuals and in patients with SLE and Sjögrens syndrome. *Arthritis Rheum* 1979;24:577–583.
44. Klinman DM. Polyclonal B cell activation in lupus-prone mice precedes and predicts the development of autoimmune disease. *J Clin Invest* 1990;86:1249–1254.
45. Hang L, Slack JH, Amundson C, et al. Induction of murine autoimmune disease by chronic polyclonal B cell activation. *J Exp Med* 1983;157:874–883.
46. Gharavi AE, Chu EL, Elkon KB. Autoantibodies to intracellular proteins in human SLE are not due to random polyclonal B cell activation. *Arthritis Rheum* 1988;31:1337–1345.
47. Bretscher P, Cohn M. A theory of self-nonself discrimination. *Science* 1970;169:1042–1044.
48. Cooke MP, Heath AW, Shokat KM, et al. Immunoglobulin signal transduction guides the specificity of B cell-T cell interaction and is blocked in tolerant self-reactive B cells. *J Exp Med* 1994;179:425–438.
49. Fulcher DA, Lyons AB, Korn SL, et al. The fate of self-reactive B cells depends primarily on the degree of antigen-receptor engagement and availability of T cell help. *J Exp Med* 1996; 183:2313–2328.
50. Kouskoff V, Lacaud G, Nemazee D. T cell-independent rescue of B lymphocytes from peripheral immune tolerance. *Science* 2000;287:2501–2503.
51. Wen L, Roberts S, Wong FS, et al. Immunoglobulin synthesis and generalized autoimmunity in mice congenitally deficient in alpha beta (+) T cells. *Nature* 1994;369:654–658.
52. Peng SL, Madaio MP, Hughes DP, et al. Murine lupus in the absence of alpha beta T cells. *J Immunol* 1996;156:4041–4049.
53. Reininger L, Radaszkiewitz T, Kosco M, et al. Development of autoimmune disease in SCID mice populated with long-term in vitro proliferating (NZB × NZW) F1 pre-B cells. *J Exp Med* 1992;176:1343–1353.
54. Klinman DM, Steiberg AD. Proliferation of anti-DNA producing B cells in a non-autoimmune environment. *J Immunol* 1986;137:69–75.
55. Klinman DM, Steiberg AD. Similar in vivo expansion of B cells from normal DBA/2 and autoimmune NZB in mice in xid recipients. *J Immunol* 1987;139:2284–2289.
56. Klinman DM, Ishigatsubo Y, Steinberg AD. Pathogenesis of generalized autoimmunity: in vivo studies of the interaction between B cells and their internal milieu. *Cell Immunol* 1988; 17:360–368.
57. Chan OT, Hannum LG, Haberman AM, et al. A novel mouse with B cells but lacking serum antibody reveals an antibody-independent role for B cells in murine lupus. *J Exp Med* 1999; 189:1639–1648.
58. Shlomchik MJ, Madaio MP, Ni D, et al. The role of B cells in lpr/lpr-induced autoimmunity. *J Exp Med* 1994;180: 1295–1306.
59. Chan O, Shlomchik MJ. A new role for B cells in systemic autoimmunity: B cells promote spontaneous T cell activation in MRL-lpr/lpr mice. *J Immunol* 1998;160:51–59.
60. Chan O, Madaio MP, Shlomchik MJ. The roles of B cells in MRL/lpr murine lupus. *Ann NY Acad Sci* 1997;815:75–87.
61. Chan OT, Shlomchik MJ. Cutting edge: B cells promaote CD8+ T cell activation in MRL-Fas(lpr) mice independently of MHC class I antigen presentation. *J Immunol* 2000;164: 1658–1662.
62. Watanabe-Fukunaga R, Brannan CI, Copeland NG, et al. Lymphoproliferative disorder in mice explained by defects in Fas antigen that mediates apoptosis. *Nature* 1992;356:314–317.
63. Mysler E, Bini P, Drappa J, et al. The apoptosis-1/Fas protein in human systemic lupus erythematosus. *J Clin Invest* 1994;93: 1029–1034.
64. Vaishnaw AK, Toubi E, Ohsako S, et al. The spectrum of apoptotic defects and clinical manifestations, including systemic lupus erythematosus, in humans with CD95 (Fas/Apo-1) mutations. *Arthritis Rheum* 1999;42:1833–1842.
65. Fukuyama H, Adachi M, Suematsu S, et al. Transgenic expression of Fas in T cells blocks lymphoproliferation but not autoimmune disease in MRL-lpr mice. *J Immunol* 1998;160: 3805–3811.
66. Reap EA, Sobel ES, Cohen PL, et al. Conventional B cells, not B-1 cells, are responsible for producing autoantibodies in lpr mice. *J Exp Med* 1993;177:69–78.
67. Chan OT, Madaio MP, Shlomchik MJ. B cells are required for lupus nephritis in the polygenic, Fas-intact MRL model of systemic autoimmunity. *J Immunol* 1999;163:3592–3596.
68. Tsao BP, Cantor RM, Kalunian KC, et al. Evidence for linkage of a candidate chromosome 1 region to systemic lupus erythematosus (SLE). *J Clin Invest* 1997;99:725–731.
69. Moser LK, Neas BR, Salmon JE, et al. Genome scan of human systemic lupus erythematosus: Evidence for linkage on chromosome 1q in African-American pedigrees. *Proc Natl Acad Sci USA* 1999;95:14869–14874.
70. Gaffney PM, Kearns GM, Shark KB, et al. A genome-wide search for susceptibility genes in human systemic lupus erythematosus sib-pair families. *Proc Natl Acad Sci USA* 1999;95: 14875–14879.
71. Drake CG, Babcock SK, Palmer E, et al. Genetic analysis of the NZB contribution to lupus-like renal disease: multiple genes that operate in a threshold manner. *Proc Natl Acad Sci USA* 1994;91:4062–4066.
72. Morel L, Rudofsky UH, Longmate JA, et al. Polygenic control of susceptibility to murine systemic lupus erythematosus. *Immunity* 1994;1:219–229.
73. Kono DH, Burlingame RS, Owens D, et al. Lupus susceptibility loci in New Zealand mice. *Proc Natl Acad Sci USA* 1994; 91:10168–10172.
74. Theofilopoulos AN. Murine models of lupus. In: Lahita RG, ed. *Systemic lupus erythematosus.* New York: Churchill-Livingstone, 1992:121–194.
75. Theofilopoulos AN. The basis of autoimmunity: part II. Genetic predisposition. *Immunol Today* 1995;16:150–159.
76. Morel L, Mohan C, Yu Y, et al. Functional dissection of systemic lupus erythematosus using congenic mouse strains. *J Immunol* 1997;158:6019–6028.
77. Mohan C, Morel L, Yang P, et al. Genetic dissection of systemic lupus erythematosus pathogenesis: Sle2 on murine chromosome 4 leads to B cell hyperactivity. *J Immunol* 1997;159: 454–465.
78. Mohan C, Morel L, Yang P, et al. Accumulation of splenic B1a cells with potent antigen-presenting capability in NZM2410 lupus-prone mice. *Arthritis Rheum* 1998;41:1652–1662.
79. Mohan C, Alas E, Morel L, et al. Genetic dissection of systemic

lupus erythematosus pathogenesis: Sle1 on murine chromosome 1 leads to selective loss of tolerance to H2A/H2B/DNA subnucleosomes. *J Clin Invest* 1998;101:1362–1372.
80. Sobel ES, Mohan C, Morel L, et al. Genetic dissection of SLE pathogenesis: adoptive transfer of Sle1 mediates the loss of tolerance by bone marrow B cells. *J Immunol* 1999;162: 2415–2421.
81. Mohan C, Yu Y, Morel L, et al. Genetic dissection of SLE pathogenesis: Sle3 on murine chromosome 7 impacts T cell activation, differentiation, and cell death. *J Immunol* 1999;162: 6492–6502.
82. Mohan C, Morel L, Yang P, et al. Genetic dissection of lupus pathogenesis: a recipe for nephrophilic autoantibodies. *J Clin Invest* 1999;103:1685–1695.
83. Morel L, Tian XH, Croker BP, et al. Epistatic modifiers of autoimmunity in a murine model of lupus nephritis. *Immunity* 1999;11:131–139.
84. Fitch FW, Lanki DW, Gajewski TF. T-cell mediated immune regulation. In: Paul WE, ed. *Fundamental immunology*. New York: Raven Press, 1993:733–761.
85. Durum SK, Oppenheim JJ, Proinflammatory cytokines and immunity. In: Paul WE, ed. *Fundamental immunology*. New York: Raven Press, 1993:801–835.
86. Linker-Israeli M, Deans RJ, Wallace DJ, et al. Elevated levels of endogenous IL-6 in systemic lupus erythematosus: a putative role in pathogenesis. *J Immunol* 1991;147:117–123.
87. Spronk PE, Ter Borg EJ, Limburg PC, et al. Plasma concentration of IL-6 in systemic lupus erythematosus, an indicator of disease activity? *Clin Exp Immunol* 1992;90:106–110.
88. Hagiwara E, Gourley MF, Lee S, et al. Disease severity in patients with systemic lupus erythematosus correlates with an increased ratio of interleukin 10: interferon-γ-secreting cells in the peripheral blood. *Arthritis Rheum* 1996;39:379–385.
89. Richaud-Patin Y, Alcocer-Varela J, Llorente L. High levels of TH2 cytokine gene expression in systemic lupus erythematosus. *Rev Invest Clin* 1995;47:267–276.
90. Nagafuchi H, Suzuki N, Mizushima Y, et al. Constitutive expression of IL-6 receptor and their role in the excessive B cell function in patients with systemic lupus erythematosus. *J Immunol* 1993;151:6525–6534.
91. Finck BK, Chan B, Wofsy D. Interleukin 6 promotes murine lupus in NZB/NZW F1 mice. *J Clin Invest* 1994;94:585–591.
92. Tang B, Matsuda T, Akira S, et al. Age-associated increase in interleukin-6 in MRL/lpr mice. *Int Immunol* 1991;3:273–278.
93. Alarcon-Riquelme ME, Moller G, Fernandez C. Macrophage depletion decreases IgG anti-DNA in cultures from (NZB × NZW) F1 spleen cells by eliminating the main source of IL-6. *Clin Exp Immunol* 1993;91:220–225.
94. Houssiau FA, Lefebvre C, Van den Berghe M, et al. Serum interleukin 10 titers in systemic lupus erythematosus reflect disease activity. *Lupus* 1995;4:393–395.
95. Llorente L, Zou W, Levy Y, et al. Role of interleukin 10 in B cell overactivity and autoantibody production of human systemic lupus erythematosus. *J Exp Med* 1995;181:839–844.
96. Ishida H, Muchamuel T, Sakaguchi S, et al. Continuous administration of anti-interleukin-10 antibodies delays onset of autoimmunity in NZB/NZW F1 mice. *J Exp Med* 1994;179:305–310.
97. Llorente L, Richaud-Patin Y, Couderc J, et al. Dysregulation of IL-10 production in relatives of patients with systemic lupus erythematosus. *Arthritis Rheum* 1997;40:1429–1435.
98. Desai-Mehta A, Lu L, Ramsey-Goldman R, et al. Hyperexpression of CD40 ligand by B and T cells in human lupus and its role in pathogenic autoantibody production. *J Clin Invest* 1996; 97:2063–2073.
99. Datta SK, Kalled SL. CD40-CD40L interaction in autoimmune disease. *Arthritis Rheum* 1997;40:1735–1745.
100. Grammer AC, Bergman MC, Miura Y, et al. The CD40L expressed by human B cells costimulates B cell responses. *J Immunol* 1995;154:4996–5010.
101. Folzenlogen D, Hofer MF, Leung DYM, et al. Analysis of CD80 and CD86 expression on peripheral blood B lymphocytes reveals increased expression of CD86 in lupus patients. *Clin Immunol Immunopathol* 1997;83:199–204.
102. Roth R, Nakamura T, Mamula MJ. B7 costimulation and autoantigen-specificity enables B cells to activate T cells. *J Immunol* 1996;157:2924–2931.
103. Reth M, Hombach J, Wienands J, et al. The B cell antigen receptor complex. *Immunol Today* 1991;12:196–201.
104. Reth M. Antigen receptors on B lymphocytes. *Annu Rev Immunol* 1992;10:97–121.
105. Cambier JC, Pleiman CM, Clark MR. Signal transduction by the B cell receptor and its coreceptors. *Annu Rev Immunol* 1994; 12:457–486.
106. Weiss A, Littman DR. Signal transduction by lymphocyte antigen receptors. *Cell* 1994;76:263–274.
107. Cambier JC, Campbell KS. Membrane immunoglobulin and its accomplices-new lessons from an old receptor. *FASEB J* 1992;6:3207–3217.
108. Pleiman CM, D'Ambrosio D, Cambier JC. The B-cell antigen receptor complex: structure and signal transduction. *Immunol Today* 1994;15:393–399.
109. DeFranco AL. The complexity of signaling pathways activated by the BCR. *Curr Opin Immunol* 1997;9:296–308.
110. Liossis SNC, Kovacs B, Dennis GJ, et al. B cells from patients with systemic lupus erythematosus display abnormal antigen-receptor mediated early signal transduction events. *J Clin Invest* 1996;98:2549–2557.
111. Niklinska BB, Yamada H, O'Shea JJ, et al. Tyrosine kinase regulated and inositol phosphate independent Ca2+ elevation and mobilization in T cells. *J Biol Chem* 1992;267:7154–7159.
112. Takata M, Sabe H, Hata A, et al. Tyrosine kinases Lyn and Syk regulate B cell receptor-coupled Ca++ mobilization through distinct pathways. *EMBO J* 1994;13:1341–1349.
113. Gold MR, Matsuchi L, Kelly RB, et al. Tyrosine phosphorylation of components of the B-cell antigen receptors following receptor crosslinking. *Proc Natl Acad Sci USA* 1991;88: 3436–3440.
114. Gold MR, Law DA, DeFranco AL. Stimulation of protein tyrosine phosphorylation by the B lymphocyte antigen receptor. *Nature* 1990;345:810–813.
115. Burkhardt AL, Brunswick M, Bolen JB, et al. Anti-immunoglobulin stimulation of B lymphocytes activates src-related protein tyrosine kinases. *Proc Natl Acad Sci USA* 1991; 7410–7414.
116. Nusslein HG, Frosch KH, Woith W, et al. Increase of intracellular Ca is the essential signal for the expression of CD40L. *Eur J Immunol* 1996;26:840–850.
117. Vassilopoulos D, Kovacs B, Tsokos GC. TCR/CD3 complex-mediated signal transduction pathway in T cells and T cell lines from patients with systemic lupus erythematosus. *J Immunol* 1995;155:2269–2281.
118. Liossis SNC, Hoffman RW, Tsokos GC. Abnormal early TCR/CD3-mediated signaling events of a snRNP-autoreactive lupus T-cell clone. *Clin Immunol Immunopathol* 1998;88: 305–310.
119. Tsokos GC, Liossis SNC. Immune cell signalling in lupus: activation, anergy and death. *Immunol Today* 1999;20:119–124.
120. Feuerstein N, Chen F, Madaio M, et al. Induction of autoimmunity in a transgenic model of B cell receptor peripheral tolerance: changes in coreceptors and B cell receptor-induced tyrosine-phosphoproteins. *J Immunol* 1999;163:5287–5297.
121. Rider V, Foster RT, Evans M, et al. Gender differences in

autoimmune diseases: estrogen increases calcineurin expression in systemic lupus erythematosus [see comments]. *Clin Immunol Immunopathol* 1998;89:171–180.

122. Kammer GM, Tsokos GC. Emerging concepts of the molecular basis for estrogen effects on T lymphocytes in systemic lupus erythematosus. *Clin Immunol Immunopathol* 1998;89: 192–195.
123. Bynoe MS, Grimaldi CM, Diamond B. Estrogen up-regulates Bcl-2 and blocks tolerance induction of naïve B cells. *Proc Natl Acad Sci USA* 2000;97:2703–2708.
124. O'Rourke L, Tooze R, Fearon DT. Co-receptors of B lymphocytes. *Curr Opin Immunol* 1997;9:324–329.
125. Tolnay M, Tsokos GC. Complement receptor 2 in the regulation of the immune response. *Clin Immunol Immunopathol* 1998;88:123–132.
126. Wilson JG, Ratnoff WD, Schur PH, et al. Decreased expression of the C3b/C4b receptor (CR1) and the C3d receptor (CR2) on B lymphocytes and of CR1 on neutrophils of patients with systemic lupus erythematosus. *Arthritis Rheum* 1986;29: 739–747.
127. Takahashi K, Kozono Y, Waldschmidt TJ, et al. Mouse complement receptors type 1 (CR1; CD35) and type 2 (CR2; CD21): expression on normal B cell subpopulations and decreased levels during the development of autoimmunity in MRL/lpr mice. *J Immunol* 1997;159:1557–1569.
128. Marquart HV, Svendsen A, Rasmussen JM, et al. Complement receptor expression and activation of the complement cascade on B lymphocytes from patients with systemic lupus erythematosus (SLE). *Clin Exp Immunol* 1995;101:60–65.
129. James JA, Kaufman KM, Farris AD, et al. An increased prevalence of Epstein-Barr virus infection in young patients suggests a possible etiology for systemic lupus erythematosus. *J Clin Invest* 1997;100:3019–3026.
130. Tsokos GC, Magrath IT, Balow JE. Epstein-Barr virus induces normal B cell responses but defective suppressor T cell responses in patients with systemic lupus erythematosus. *J Immunol* 1983; 131:1797–1801.
131. Gatenby PA, Irvine M. The bcl-2 protooncogene is overexpressed in systemic lupus erythematosus. *J Autoimmun* 1994; 7:623–631.
132. Prodeus AP, Goerg S, Shen LM, et al. A critical role for complement in maintenance of self-tolerance. *Immunity* 1998;9: 721–731.
133. Gommerman JL, Carroll MC. Negative selection of B lymphocytes: a novel role for innate immunity. *Immunol Rev* 2000;173: 120–130.
134. Niculescu F, Rus H, van Biesen T, et al. Activation of Ras and mitogen-activated protein kinase pathway by terminal complement complexes is G protein dependent. *J Immunol* 1997; 158:4405–4412.
135. Manzi S, Rairie JE, Carpenter AB, et al. Sensitivity and specificity of plasma and urine complement split products as indicators of lupus disease activity. *Arthritis Rheum* 1996;39: 1178–1188.
136. Cambier JC. Inhibitory receptors abound? *Proc Natl Acad Sci USA* 1997;94:5993–5995.
137. Van de Velde H, von Hoegen I, Luo W, et al. The B-cell surface protein CD72/Lyb-2 is the ligand of CD5. *Nature* 1991;351: 662–665.
138. O'Keefe TL, Williams GT, Davies SL, et al. Hyperresponsive B cells in CD22-deficient mice. *Science* 1996;274:798–801.
139. O'Keefe TL, Williams GT, Batista FD, et al. Deficiency of CD22, a B cell-specific inhibitory receptor, is sufficient to predispose to development of high affinity autoantibodies. *J Exp Med* 1999;189:1307–1313.
140. Liossis SNC, Dimopoulos MA, Sfikakis PP. Expression of the B cell inhibitory molecule CD22 in patients with systemic lupus erythematosus. *Arthritis Rheum* 1999;42:S55.
141. Wilson HA, Greenblatt D, Taylor CW, et al. The B lymphocyte calcium response to anti-Ig is diminished by membrane immunoglobulin crosslinkage to the Fcγ receptor. *J Immunol* 1987;138:1712–1718.
142. Bijsterbosch MK, Klaus GGB. Crosslinking of surface immunoglobulins and Fc receptors on B lymphocytes inhibits stimulation of inositol phosphate breakdown via the antigen receptors. *J Exp Med* 1985;162:1825–1827.
143. Frank MM, Hamburger MI, Lawley TJ, et al. Defective reticuloendothelial system Fc-receptor function in systemic lupus erythematosus. *N Engl J Med* 1993;300:518–523.
144. Takai T, Ono M, Hikida M, et al. Augmented humoral and anaphylactic responses in FcγRII-deficient mice. *Nature* 1996; 379:346–349.
145. Jiang Y, Hirose S, Sanokawa-Akakura R, et al. Genetically determined aberrant down-regulation of FcgammaRIIB1 in germinal center B cells associated with hyper-IgG and IgG autoantibodies in murine systemic lupus erythematosus. *Int Immunol* 1999;11:1685–1691.
146. Muta T, Kurosaki T, Misulovin Z, et al. A 13-amino-acid motif in the cytoplasmic domain of FcγRIIB modulates B-cell receptor signalling. *Nature* 1994;368:70–73.
147. Daeron M. Fc receptor biology. *Annu Rev Immunol* 1997;15: 203–234.
148. Tedder TF, Tuscano J, Sato S, et al. CD22, a B lymphocyte-specific adhesion molecule that regulates antigen receptor signaling. *Annu Rev Immunol* 1997;15:481–504.
149. Schulte RJ, Campbell MA, Fischer WH, et al. Tyrosine phosphorylation of CD22 during B cell activation. *Science* 1992; 258:1001–1004.
150. D'Ambrosio D, Hippen KL, Minskoff SA, et al. Recruitment and activation of PTP1C in negative regulation of antigen receptor signaling by Fc gamma RIIB1. *Science* 1995;268: 293–297.
151. Campbell MA, Klinman NR. Phosphotyrosine-dependent association between CD22 and protein tyrosine phosphatase 1C. *Eur J Immunol* 1995;25:1573–1579.
152. Ono M, Bolland S, Tempst P, et al. Role of the inositol phosphatase SHIP in negative regulation of the immune system by the receptor FcγRIIB. *Nature* 1996;383:263–266.
153. Kozlowski M, Mlinaric-Rascan I, Feng GS, et al. Expression and catalytic activity of the tyrosine phosphatase PTP1C is severely impaired in motheaten and viable motheaten mice. *J Exp Med* 1993;178:2157–2163.
154. Nishizumi H, Horikawa K, Mlinaric-Rascan I, et al. A double-edged kinase Lyn: a positive and negative regulator for antigen receptor-mediated signals. *J Exp Med* 1998;187:1343–1348.
155. Smith KGC, Tarlinton DM, Doody GM, et al. Inhibition of the B cell by CD22: a requirement for Lyn. *J Exp Med* 1998; 187:807–811.
156. Yamanashi Y, Kakiuchi T, Mizuguchi J, et al. Association of B cell antigen receptor with protein tyrosine kinase Lyn. *Science* 1991;251:192–194.
157. Yamanashi Y, Fukui Y, Wongsasant B, et al. Activation of Src-like protein-tyrosine kinase Lyn and its association with phosphatidylinositol 3-kinase upon B-cell antigen receptor-mediated signaling. *Proc Natl Acad Sci USA* 1992;89:1118–1122.
158. Wang J, Koizumi T, Watanabe T. Altered antigen receptor signaling and impaired Fas-mediated apoptosis of B cells in Lyn-deficient mice. *J Exp Med* 1996;184:831–838.
159. Chan VW, Meng F, Soriano P, et al. Characterization of the B lymphocyte populations in Lyn-deficient mice and the role of Lyn in signaling initiation and down-regulation. *Immunity* 1997;7:69–81.

160. Nishizumi H, Taniuchi I, Yamanashi Y, et al. Impaired proliferation of peripheral B cells and indication of autoimmune disease in lyn-deficient mice. *Immunity* 1995;3:549–560.
161. Hibbs ML, Tarlinton DM, Armes J, et al. Multiple defects in the immune system of Lyn-deficient mice, culminating in autoimmune disease. *Cell* 1995;83:301–311.
162. Cornall RJ, Cyster JG, Hibbs ML, et al. Polygenic autoimmune traits: Lyn, CD22 and SHP-1 are limiting elements of a biochemical pathway regulating BCR signaling and selection. *Immunity* 1998;8:497–508.
163. Fujimoto M, Bradney AP, Poe JC, et al. Modulation of B lymphocyte antigen receptor signal transduction by a CD19/CD22 regulatory loop. *Immunity* 1999;11:191–200.
164. Engel P, Zhou LJ, Ord DC, et al. Abnormal B lymphocyte development, activation and differentiation in mice that lack or overexpress the CD19 signal transduction molecule. *Immunity* 1995;3:39–50.
165. Sato S, Ono N, Steeber DA, et al. CD19 regulates B lymphocyte signaling thresholds critical for the development of B-1 lineage cells and autoimmunity. *J Immunol* 1996;157:4371–4378.
166. Sato S, Jansen PJ, Tedder TF. CD19 and CD22 reciprocally regulate Vav tyrosine phosphorylation during B lymphocyte signaling. *Proc Natl Acad Sci USA* 1997;94:13158–13162.
167. Liossis SNC, Mavrikakis M, Dimopoulos MA, et al. Expression of B cell signaling regulatory molecules in patients with systemic lupus erythematosus. *Arthritis Rheum* 1999;42:S309.
168. Liossis SNC, Solomou EE, Dimopoulos MA, et al. B-cell kinase lyn deficiency in patients with systemic lupus erythematosus. *J Invest Med* 2001;49:157–165.

12

ABNORMALITIES IN IMMUNE COMPLEX CLEARANCE AND Fcγ RECEPTOR FUNCTION

JANE E. SALMON

Systemic lupus erythematosus (SLE), the prototype human disease mediated by immune complexes, is characterized by circulating antigen/antibody complexes that may be removed by the mononuclear phagocyte system or deposited in tissues. The fate of circulating immune complexes depends on the lattice of the immune complexes (i.e., number of antigens and antibody molecules in a given complex), the nature of the antigen and antibodies composing the immune complexes, and the status of the mononuclear phagocyte system. The efficiency of mononuclear phagocyte system immune complex clearance depends on the function of Fcγ receptors, receptors recognizing the Fc region of immunoglobulin, and the complement receptors. In SLE, inadequate clearance results in tissue immune complex deposition, detected by immunofluorescence and electron microscopy, that initiates release of inflammatory mediators and influx of inflammatory cells. If sustained, this leads to tissue damage with resultant, clinically apparent disease, such as glomerulonephritis. Through *in vivo* and *in vitro* studies of patients with SLE, there clearly is both FcγR-dependent and complement-dependent mononuclear phagocyte dysfunction in SLE that has inherited and acquired components. This chapter reviews the role of the mononuclear phagocyte system in immune complex clearance, describes abnormalities in the mononuclear phagocyte function in SLE, and discusses mononuclear phagocyte system Fcγ receptor dysfunction as a mechanism for abnormal immune complex clearance in SLE.

THE ROLE OF THE MONONUCLEAR PHAGOCYTE SYSTEM IN THE CLEARANCE OF IMMUNE COMPLEXES

Early studies of the blood clearance of bacteria in mice, rabbits, and guinea pigs demonstrated that the mononuclear phagocyte system (previously known as the reticuloendothelial system) performed this function for opsonized particles. Infused bacteria were internalized by hepatic and splenic phagocytes (1). The rate of clearance of bacteria from the blood and the site of their clearance depended on the level of antibodies to the bacteria in the serum of the animal. Rapidly cleared, well-opsonized bacteria were principally phagocytosed in the liver, while the more slowly cleared, less efficiently internalized bacteria (and presumably less opsonized) were removed by splenic phagocytes. These observations are remarkable for their similarity to the models of immune complex clearance in animals and humans that are described later.

The role of the mononuclear phagocyte system in the clearance of soluble immune complexes infused into the circulation has been defined in several experimental animal models. In mice and rabbits a major proportion of infused immune complexes formed with rabbit antibodies is taken up by the liver, indicating that the mononuclear phagocyte system serves an important role as a site for complex removal (2,3). This system may be saturated with increasing amounts of infused immune complexes, resulting in glomerular deposition of immune complexes (4). These early studies suggested that modulation of mononuclear phagocyte system function regulates the localization of immune complexes.

Several lines of evidence support this model and demonstrate that defective mononuclear phagocyte system clearance of immune complexes may be important in the development of immune complex diseases, especially glomerulonephritis. Increased glomerular deposition of immune complexes is found when the clearance rates of infused immune complexes are decreased by blockade of the mononuclear phagocyte system with colloidal carbon (5), by cortisone treatment (6), or by reduction and alkylation of antibodies (7,8). In mouse strains with intrinsically lower clearance rates, there is a high degree of immune complex glomerular deposition (9); in contrast, decreased deposition of immune complexes in the kidney is found when mononuclear phagocyte system clearance is enhanced by pretreatment with *Corynebacterium parvum* (10) or zymosan (11).

While impaired immune complex clearance leads to increased tissue deposition, the absence of activating FcγR on phagocytes prevents an inflammatory response at the sites of immune complex deposition. Mice with targeted deletions of stimulatory FcγR are protected from fatal antigen-antibody Arthus reactions and immune complex–mediated glomerulonephritis. In contrast, mice lacking inhibitory FcγR have exaggerated responses to immune complexes (12–14).

Animal models of endogenous immune complex deposition also support the relationship between depressed mononuclear phagocyte system clearance and the genesis of glomerulonephritis. In chronic serum sickness, there is decreased clearance of aggregated albumin (15) and aggregated human immunoglobulin G (IgG) (16). Decreased clearance of heat-aggregated IgG in murine nephritis (associated with lymphocytic choriomeningitis virus infection) (17) and of polyvinyl pyrrolidine in New Zealand black/white (NZB/W) mice (18) has been observed, although some studies of endogenous immune complex-mediated disease have not found dysfunction of the mononuclear phagocyte system. Studies of NZB/W nephritis (19) and Heyman nephritis (20) have concluded that mononuclear phagocyte system function is either normal or supranormal. These results are not in conflict, however; rather, they highlight the importance of the mononuclear phagocyte system probe, the site of clearance, and the timing of the study in relation to the genesis of disease (discussed later).

The principle to be derived from these animal models of immune complex disease, whether from infused immune complexes or endogenous disease, is that immune complex deposition is influenced by the efficiency of mononuclear phagocyte system clearance. Specifically, impairment of mononuclear phagocyte system clearance is associated with tissue deposition of immune complexes and the potential for local organ damage.

MECHANISMS OF IMMUNE COMPLEX CLEARANCE

A number of factors govern the physical characteristics of immune complexes and, hence their biologic properties (Table 12.1). These include the nature of the antibody in the complex, the nature of the antigen, and the antigen-antibody interaction. Antigen and antibodies in the circulation may rapidly form immune complexes, but the immunochemical properties of these circulating immune complexes determine their ultimate fate, either removal by the mononuclear phagocyte system or deposition in tissues. The potential of immune complexes to interact with FcγRs, to fix complement, and to react with complement receptors influences their rate of clearance. Immune complexes without complement will be cleared primarily by FcγRs on fixed tissue macrophages. Complexes that are opsonized with sufficient complement may bind to the receptor for C3b on circulating erythrocytes and subsequently be removed by FcγRs and complement receptors. Thus, two classes of receptors, the FcγRs on phagocytes and the complement receptors on both erythrocytes and phagocytes, participate in the clearance of immune complexes (Fig. 12.1).

TABLE 12.1. FACTORS INFLUENCING THE CHARACTERISTICS OF IMMUNE COMPLEXES

Antigen
Availability
Valence, size
Epitope density and distribution
Tissue tropism/charge
Antibody
Quantity
Class, subclass
Capacity to fix complement
Binding avidity
Charge and distribution
Antigen-antibody interaction
Molar ratio

Complement Mechanisms: Immune Adherence and Erythrocyte CR1 System

Complement component 3 and the receptor for C3b on erythrocytes are important in processing and transporting large immune complexes (21) (see Chapter 13). Incorporation of complement components, C3b in particular, modifies the solubility of large immune complexes (22,23) and mediates the binding of immune complexes to human and other primate erythrocytes. Although both the liver and spleen are the major sites of immune complex uptake, erythrocytes in primates (21,24) and platelets in rodents (25,26) are important in clearing/processing immune complexes from the circulation. It has long been known that large complement-opsonized immune complexes bind to human erythrocytes (27). Termed immune adherence, this reaction has been shown to participate in the handling of nascent circulating immune complexes in primates (28).

Human erythrocytes express complement receptor type 1 (CR1), which permits binding of complement-fixing immune complexes. CR1 on erythrocytes can be conceptualized as having three main functions, which are not mutually exclusive: buffering, transporting, and processing (Fig. 12.1). The role of immune complex buffer has been suggested because erythrocyte-bound immune complexes are unavailable for tissue deposition, whereas nonbound complexes can deposit in the tissues. Bound immune complexes are transported to the liver or spleen where fixed tissue phagocyte FcγRs and complement receptors strip the immune complexes from the erythrocytes, which then return to the circulation to continue this process, thus per-

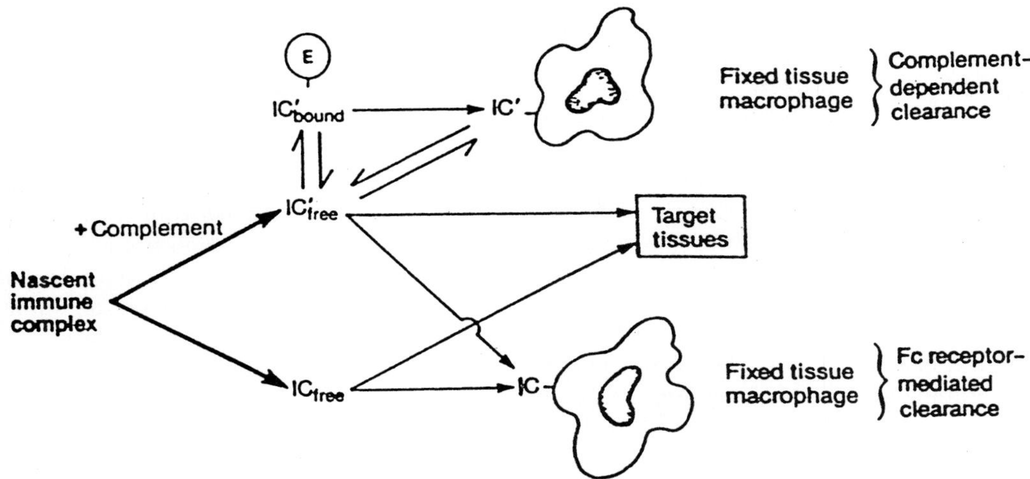

FIGURE 12.1. Framework for immune complex handling. Nascent immune complexes (ICs) that fix complement efficiently are rapidly bound by erythrocytes (E). ICs containing complement may cycle between E-bound and unbound; they usually are rapidly taken up in the liver. Unbound complexes also may deposit in the tissues, and with impaired complement-dependent uptake, they may be taken up by Fc receptor-dependent mechanisms. ICs that do not bind complement are either taken up by Fc receptor-dependent mechanisms or deposited in tissues. (From Kimberly RP. Immune complexes in rheumatic diseases. In: Pisetsky DS, Snyderman R, eds. *Immunology of the rheumatic diseases. Rheum Dis Clin North Am* 1987;13:583–596, with permission.)

forming the transporting function. Finally, CR1 promotes degradation of captured C3b on immune complexes, thereby modifying their subsequent handling.

The human CR1 (the complement receptor for C3b/C4b and, to a lesser degree, iC3b) is a single-chain, intrinsic membrane glycoprotein expressed on several different cells, including erythrocytes, granulocytes, monocytes, and macrophages (see Chapter 13). There are four codominantly expressed alleles of CR1, with molecular weights of 220,000, 250,000, 190,000, and 280,000 d (29–32). This structural polymorphism reflects differences in the number of long homologous repeat units comprising the receptors (33). Inherited and acquired differences in the numeric expression of CR1 on erythrocytes also have been described and associated with SLE (34–38). Two alleles with codominant expression determine erythrocyte CR1 number in healthy individuals (37,39). Although the CR1 number expressed on erythrocytes is low compared with that on leukocytes, approximately 90% of the total circulating CR1 is on erythrocytes, because there are far more erythrocytes than leukocytes in the circulation (40,41).

The binding of immune complexes to CR1 occurs rapidly *in vivo*, and it represents multivalent binding between multiple C3b molecules on the complex and clusters of CR1 on erythrocytes (28,42–45). *In vivo* studies have demonstrated that immune complexes preferentially bind to circulating erythrocytes that express multiple CR1 clusters, and that the capacity of each erythrocyte for binding correlates with the density of cell surface CR1. Because CR1 on erythrocytes tends to cluster more than that on resting neutrophils, most immune complexes that are bound to circulating cells are bound to erythrocytes (22,24,40,41,46–50). A reduction in the number of functional CR1 limits the capacity of erythrocytes to transport and buffer immune complexes, and *in vivo* studies have demonstrated that repeated administration of antigens in immunized humans and primates with immune complex formation results in a decrease in erythrocyte CR1 levels (46,51). Studies with primates have suggested that circulating immune complexes that are not bound to erythrocytes are more easily trapped in the microvasculature and can be recovered in the lungs and kidneys (50,52). Taken together, these findings have obvious implications for immune complex–mediated diseases.

The efficiency of immune complex binding to erythrocytes via CR1 relates to the nature of the immune complex, particularly the ability to activate complement and capture C3b, the spatial organization of the captured C3b, and the final size of the complex (53). Several models have been used to analyze the characteristics of immune complexes interacting with the erythrocyte CR1 system, including DNA/human anti-DNA, bovine serum albumin (BSA)/anti-BSA, tetanus toxoid/human antitetanus toxoid, and hepatitis B surface antigen/human antihepatitis B surface antigen (24,28,48,50,54). In each system, large immune complexes bind to erythrocytes better than do small immune complexes. The antigen and antibody also influence this reaction, because the capacity to fix complement varies with antibody class and certain antigens alone may capture C3b. Erythrocyte CR1 immune complex binding is avid but reversible, and the rate of dissociation also varies according to the particular immune complex, which dictates the nature of C3b capture (43,55).

The erythrocyte CR1 system also may have a second physiologic function: providing a processing mechanism for immune complexes (56). In addition to being a carrier for opsonized immune complexes, CR1 has a potent inhibitory function in the complement cascade, which may enhance clearance. It participates in the inactivation of C3b and may alter the size of complexes, thus affecting their subsequent handling. Specifically, CR1 is a cofactor for factor I in the cleavage of C3b to iC3b and then to C3dg (57,58). Therefore, the binding of immune complexes containing C3b to erythrocyte CR1 facilitates proteolytic cleavage of the C3b to iC3b and C3dg, which do not bind to CR1. This reaction is the basis for the degradation of complement on immune complexes with their subsequent release from the receptor (59), and its rate varies with the physicochemical properties of the individual complexes (55). If the immune complex can again activate complement and bind C3b, it can rebind to CR1 (60). Although repeated cycles of binding and release are likely, these immune complexes are not constantly bound to erythrocytes and thus are available for either deposition or (enhanced) removal by the mononuclear phagocyte system. The fraction of immune complexes in whole blood that is erythrocyte bound depends on several dynamic processes: complement fixation and C3b capture, erythrocyte binding, and C3b degradation and immune complex release.

Fc Receptor Mechanisms

Immune complexes are removed from the circulation by the mononuclear phagocyte system of the liver and spleen through engagement of FcγRs and complement receptors. The interaction of immune complexes with the phagocyte involves a qualitatively different process than that with erythrocytes (47). The relative contribution of each receptor system depends on the immunochemical properties of the complex. The liver, which is much larger than the spleen, is the principal site for the uptake of immune complexes (52,61,62); however, immune complexes that escape clearance by hepatic macrophages, which may be smaller and of lower valence, are taken up by the spleen (61). The role of FcγRs in immune complex clearance of both soluble and particulate immune complexes is shown by studies wherein blockade of FcγRs by an infusion of aggregated IgG into the portal venous system (40) or of antibodies against FcγRs (47) suppresses uptake of these immune complexes (Fig. 12.2). Supporting the pivotal role of FcγRs in handling certain immune complexes, studies of complement depletion show no effect on the efficiency of uptake of immune complexes by the liver or spleen and actually show an acceleration in the rate of removal of complexes from the circulation, presumably resulting from trapping in the microvasculature (50).

FcγRs appear to play a key role in the transfer and retention of immune complexes by mononuclear phagocytes. Studies of DNA/anti-DNA complexes that are bound to radiolabeled erythrocytes and injected into chimpanzees show that while immune complexes are removed by the

ABNORMALITIES IN IMMUNE COMPLEX CLEARANCE AND Fc RECEPTOR FUNCTION

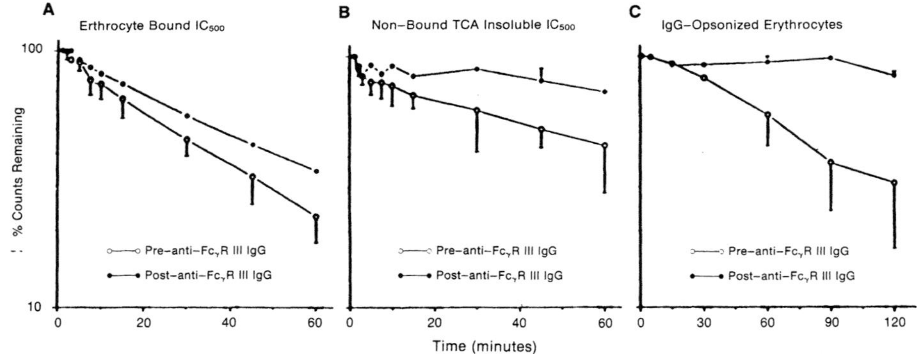

FIGURE 12.2. Effect of anti-FcγRIII monoclonal antibody (MAb) on the handling of soluble immune complex (IC). The effects of anti-FcγRIII MAb infusions on the handling of several different radiolabeled model IC probes in chimpanzees are presented with data expressed as the percentage counts remaining relative to the counts infused. **A:** Following intravenous infusion of soluble radiolabeled IC, clearance of erythrocyte (E)-bound IC was measured and found to be slowed by treatment with anti-FcγRIII MAb IgG. **B:** After intravenous infusion of soluble IC, clearance of non–E-bound IC was slowed more by anti-FcγRIII MAb IgG. **C:** Clearance of IgG-opsonized E was most markedly slowed by anti-FcγRIII infusions. (From Kimberly RP, Edberg JC, Merriam LT, et al. In vivo handling of soluble complement fixing Ab/dsDNA immune complexes in chimpanzees. *J Clin Invest* 1989;84:962–970, with permission.)

mononuclear phagocyte system, the erythrocytes are not sequestered; rather, they are stripped of immune complexes and promptly recirculated (24). Although the mechanism of this stripping is not well defined, the involvement of complement proteases has been implicated (63). In this model of immune complex clearance, infusion of erythrocyte-bound DNA/anti-DNA complexes after treatment with anti-FcγR monoclonal antibody results in a significant amount of non-erythrocyte-bound circulating immune complexes, documenting the participation of FcγRs in the retention of immune complexes by phagocytes (Fig. 12.2B) (47).

In addition to stripping erythrocyte-bound complexes, FcγRs as well as CR3/CR4 are responsible for the clearance of those complexes that are unable to bind to erythrocyte CR1 because of inadequate C3b capture or degradation of C3b. This interpretation is supported by experiments in primates that were treated with anti-FcγR monoclonal antibodies and showed impaired clearance of infused immune complexes, which was most pronounced in the fraction of complexes that did not bind to erythrocytes (47). It has been shown that immune adherence is not a prerequisite for the efficient handling of immune complexes by the mononuclear phagocyte system (51), but immune complexes that do not fix complement or that fix complement poorly cannot be cleared if FcγR function is impaired (Fig. 12.1).

ABNORMAL IMMUNE COMPLEX CLEARANCE IN SLE

Human Models of Immune Complex Clearance

Probes that have been used to assess the efficiency of immune complex clearance in humans are (a) autologous erythrocytes sensitized with IgG antibodies that are directed against the D antigen of the Rh system, (b) preformed immune complexes or aggregated IgG, and (c) antigen infused into passively immunized subjects. Because each of these probes has distinct immunochemical properties, they interact differently with the complement and FcγR systems, as expected. Thus, the results of *in vivo* studies comparing immune clearance in patients with SLE and in healthy individuals vary depending on the probe used.

Analysis of the Clearance of IgG-Sensitized Autologous Erythrocytes

The technique introduced by Frank et al. (64) to measure mononuclear phagocyte system function employs autologous ^{51}Cr-radiolabeled erythrocytes that are sensitized with IgG anti-(Rh)D antibodies and injected into study subjects, and clearance or removal of these cells from the circulation is determined by serial bleeding. External surface counting of sensitized radiolabeled erythrocytes shows initial rapid sequestration in the liver, followed by splenic accumulation of most of the injected cells. The semilogarithmic plot of mean data for the clearance of sensitized cells in normal control subjects is curvilinear, with a rapid initial loss of radiolabeled cells followed by a slower, sustained loss of radioactivity (Fig. 12.3) (65–67).

Although originally conceptualized as a measure of FcγR capacity, kinetic analysis of *in vivo* clearance studies and *in vitro* studies with IgG anti-(Rh)D–coated erythrocytes suggests that complement also plays a role in clearance of this probe. Further support comes from studies of C4-deficient patients, who show delayed clearance relative to healthy individuals (68). A proposed model to describe the series of steps in handling of IgG anti-(Rh)D–sensitized erythrocytes is as follows: Circulating cells initially sequestered by a complement-dependent process are deactivated and released back into the circulation or are phagocytosed. Released cells are sequestered and phagocytosed by an FcγR-mediated process. Circulating cells also may be directly sequestered and phagocytosed by FcγRs (66–68).

The role of complement in the clearance of anti-(Rh)D–sensitized erythrocytes is a function of the level of antibody sensitization (69). Erythrocytes that are prepared with a low density of surface anti-(Rh)D are cleared primarily by splenic FcγRs, while at higher-density sensitizations, hepatic complement receptor-mediated clearance becomes increasingly important. This observation is highlighted in studies of splenectomized patients, which show that the clearance of erythrocytes sensitized with low levels of anti-(Rh)D antibody is more markedly prolonged than that of more

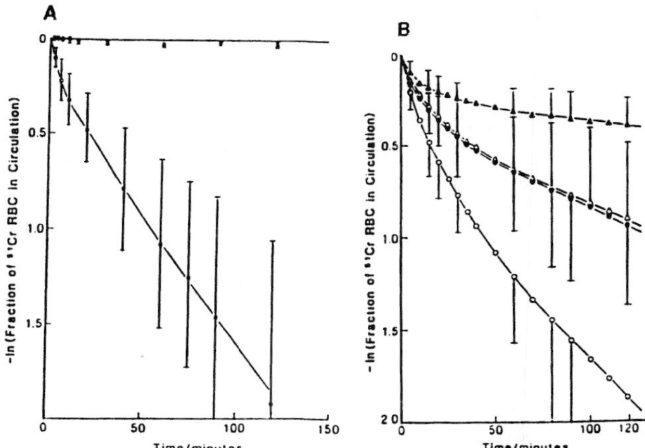

FIGURE 12.3. A: Survival of 51Cr-labeled autologous erythrocytes in normal controls. Data are shown for unsensitized erythrocytes in six normal controls (*upper curve*) and anti-Rh(D)–sensitized erythrocytes in 49 normal controls (*lower curve*). **B:** Survival of 51Cr-labeled autologous anti-Rh(D)–sensitized erythrocytes in 32 patients with SLE: comparison between disease active subgroups. ○-○ inactive/nonrenal (*n* = 5); ●-● active/nonrenal (*n* = 7); •-• active/nonrenal (*n* = 12); ▲-▲, active/renal (*n* = 8). (From Kimberly RP, Meryhew NL, Runquist OA. Mononuclear phagocyte function in SLE. I. Bipartite Fc- and complement-dependent dysfunction. *J Immunol* 1986;137:91–96, with permission.

densely opsonized erythrocytes, which fix complement and may be cleared by hepatic C3b receptors. Because the density of opsonization determines the relative contribution of FcγRs and complement mechanisms in clearance, the results of *in vivo* clearance studies in patients with SLE must be interpreted in the context of the sensitization of the probe.

In Vivo Studies of IgG-Sensitized Autologous Erythrocytes in SLE

Abnormal mononuclear phagocyte system function in patients with SLE has been demonstrated in several studies performed with IgG anti-(Rh)D–sensitized erythrocytes (64,70–73). Clearance half-times for radiolabeled autologous IgG-sensitized erythrocytes were prolonged in these patients compared with normal individuals and were longer in patients with renal disease than in those without renal disease (Figs. 12.3 and 12.4). In these studies, the prolongation of clearance half-time of erythrocytes (low-density sensitization) was attributed to impaired splenic FcγR function. At this low level of sensitization, hepatic complement-mediated clearance is negligible, and the rate of clearance indeed reflects the efficiency and capacity of FcγRs. The abnormality in clearance is receptor specific, because clearance of heat-damaged erythrocytes and aggregated albumin was not prolonged in these patients with SLE (64,74).

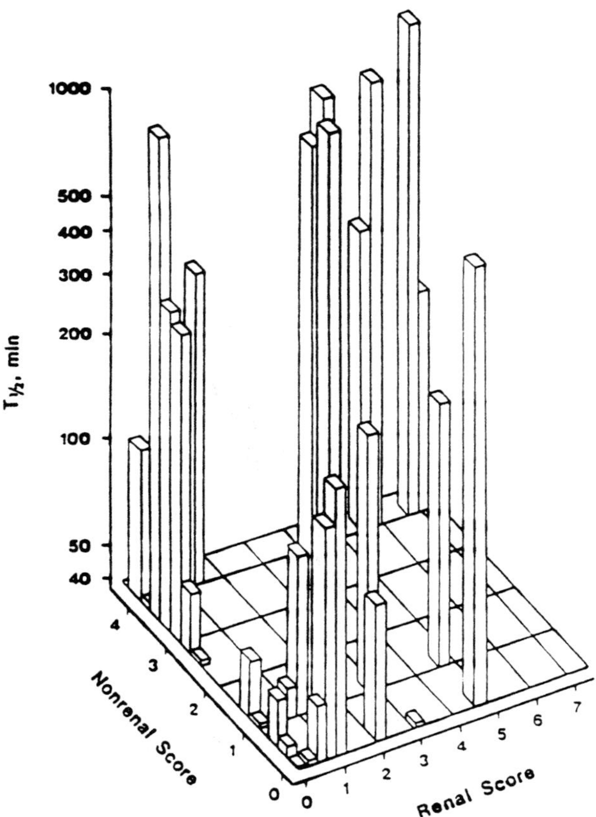

FIGURE 12.4. Relationship of clinical activity and FcγR-mediated mononuclear phagocyte system dysfunction. Clinical activity was assessed in terms of both renal and nonrenal manifestations. Longer (taller) clearance half-time values represent greater degrees of dysfunction. Patients with active renal and nonrenal disease showed the greatest degree of FcγR-mediated clearance impairment. (From Kimberly RP, Salmon JE, Edberg JC, et al. The role of Fc receptors in mononuclear phagocyte system function. *Clin Exp Rheum* 1989;7(suppl):S130–S138, with permission.)

In a contrasting study, clearance of more heavily sensitized erythrocytes in patients with SLE was similar to that of normal controls (75). At this higher level of sensitization, clearance half-times are primarily a measure of hepatic complement receptor function rather than splenic FcγR function (69). Because complement-dependent clearance often is normal in patients with SLE but without renal involvement (discussed later), the overall clearance of heavy opsonized erythrocytes may be normal despite marked FcγR dysfunction.

When clinical activity in patients with SLE was assessed, there was a significant but independent association between impaired FcγR clearance and the level of both renal and nonrenal disease activity (72). Increased activity along either parameter was associated with more impaired clearance. As shown in Fig. 12.4, patients with active renal and nonrenal disease are most likely to have the highest degree of clearance dysfunction. Longitudinal studies in patients with SLE showed that mononuclear phagocyte system function changed concordantly with changes in clinical status, indicating that clearance dysfunction is dynamic and closely related to disease activity (70,71).

Semilogarithmic plots of the mean data for clearance in patients with SLE, grouped according to disease activity and the presence or absence of renal involvement, show differences in slope and duration of the initial, rapid loss of radiolabeled cells from the circulation (predominantly complement-dependent clearance) and in the slope of the slow, sustained clearance reaction (predominantly FcγR-mediated clearance) (Fig. 12.3B). Rate constants governing the FcγR- and complement-dependent steps of the clearance process were derived from kinetic analysis of these curvilinear clearance data. Rate constants were evaluated for four steps: (a) complement-dependent sequestration, (b) C3b deactivation and release, (c) complement-mediated phagocytosis, and (d) FcγR-mediated sequestration and phagocytosis. Such analysis of the studies of patients with SLE grouped by disease activity revealed both FcγR- and complement-dependent dysfunction (67). Impaired FcγR function was evident in all patients except those with neither renal involvement nor any other manifestation of activity. Complement-mediated phagocytic dysfunction was seen only in patients with renal disease. These data suggest that altered complement-mediated phagocytosis in combination with abnormal FcγR-mediated phagocytosis by fixed tissue macrophages contributes to the pathogenesis of lupus nephritis.

In hypocomplementemic patients with SLE, examination of clearance rate constants revealed a good correlation between disease activity and FcγR-mediated clearance function (68). With decreased complement levels, there may be deficient complement opsonization of complexes, impaired binding and processing by erythrocytes, and reduced clearance by hepatic complement receptors. Such circulating immune complexes with little or no complement must be cleared by FcγRs. While rapid hepatic complement-dependent clearance appears to be the first line of defense against immune complex deposition, FcγR-mediated clearance becomes pivotal when this mechanism fails. In disease processes that are associated with hypocomplementemia, tissue immune complex deposition and increased disease activity occur when there is a concomitant defect in FcγR clearance. Similarly to human SLE, studies in four murine models of lupus demonstrated an early progressive defect in FcγR-mediated clearance of IgG-sensitized erythrocytes, whereas the efficiency of complement-mediated clearance varied among the murine strains (76). The consistent finding of impaired FcγR-specific clearance in patients with active SLE emphasizes the potential importance of the mechanism for immune complex disease.

Given the role of immune complex deposition in the pathogenesis of SLE, circulating immune complex levels in patients were measured by a series of different assay systems (i.e., C1q binding, staphylococcal protein A binding assay, Raji cell assay) at the time of *in vivo* erythrocyte clearance in many studies. There was a relationship between the levels of immune complexes and FcγR dysfunction in some, but not all, groups of patients with SLE (84,91,95). The lack of direct correlation between mononuclear phagocyte system function and immune complex level in all studies is not surprising, however, given the complexity of immune complex handling and the range of variables determining net complex levels (70,72).

Although partly acquired and related to disease activity, the FcγR mononuclear phagocyte dysfunction also may have a genetic component. Normal individuals with a human leukocyte antigen (HLA) haplotype containing either DR2 or DR3, which are some gene products found with increased frequency in SLE populations (see Chapter 6), are more likely to have an abnormally prolonged FcγR-mediated clearance of IgG-sensitized erythrocytes than their normal counterparts without these haplotypes (77,78). While the magnitude of the FcγR dysfunction is substantially larger in patients with SLE and has a large dynamic component associated with disease activity (64,70,72), individuals with an immunogenetically associated decrease in FcγR function might be more susceptible to the secondary FcγR abnormalities associated with SLE. Allelic polymorphisms of FcγR also are potential inherited factors influencing immune complex clearance (discussed later). Thus, basal genetically determined mononuclear phagocyte clearance in normal individuals may contribute to the predisposition and pathogenesis of SLE.

Analysis of Clearance of Infused Soluble Immune Complexes

As another measure of mononuclear phagocyte system function, the clearance of preformed, large, soluble, complement-fixing immune complexes has been studied in humans. Radiolabeled tetanus toxoid/antitetanus toxoid, hepatitis B surface antigen/antibody, or aggregated human IgG are infused, and then sequential blood samples are obtained and analyzed for whole blood and erythrocyte-bound radioactivity to monitor clearance (48,54,79). Clearance of these preformed immune complexes (free or erythrocyte bound) from the circulation of humans has been shown to involve the activation of complement with capture of C3b, binding to erythrocyte CR1 receptors, uptake by complement, and FcγR tissue mononuclear phagocytes as described earlier. Factors that cause the erythrocyte transport system to fail, such as hypocomplementemia or CR1 deficiency, are associated with an initially more rapid disappearance of immune complexes, presumably caused by trapping in capillary beds outside the mononuclear phagocyte system. For example, clearance of injected hepatitis B surface antigen/antibody complexes in patients with essential mixed cryoglobulinemia is accelerated compared with that in normal subjects, presumably because of immune complex deposition in tissues outside the liver and spleen as a result of impaired immune adherence. The basis for defective erythrocyte transport and buffering of complexes in these patients appears to be a result of complement depletion and monoclonal rheumatoid factor inhibition of immune complex opsonization and binding (54).

Because the relevance of these large, preformed complexes (40S) to human SLE is not entirely clear, studies of the clearance of smaller (19S) complexes formed *in vivo* have been performed. Patients with ovarian cancer were infused with murine antitumor antibodies followed by human antimurine IgG (46). In this model, complexes were cleared rapidly by the liver, although the role of erythrocyte CR1 was unclear. *In vivo* immune complex formation was associated with systemic complement activation, reduction in erythrocyte CR1, and increased erythrocyte C3 and C4 (similar to the findings in SLE described later), which could predispose to less efficient handling of further complexes.

Given the different kinds of information obtained from each of these *in vivo* probes, examination of multiple models of immune complex clearance is necessary to define the mechanisms of immune complex deposition in SLE.

In Vivo Studies of Infused Soluble Immune Complexes in SLE

In vivo studies of infused soluble immune complexes complement the sensitized erythrocyte model of clearance and demonstrate multifactorial mononuclear phagocyte dysfunction. Abnormalities in erythrocyte CR1 system, the early buffer for circulating immune complexes, are described in patients with SLE, and for these models it is important to recognize that such patients tend to have an acquired, decreased numeric expression of CR1 on erythrocytes that correlates with disease activity (80,81) and may result from repeated immune complex/erythrocyte CR1 interactions (48,51). There also is evidence of an inherited deficiency of CR1 in some patients (36,38).

Diminished CR1 resulting in impaired immune adherence is one of the mechanisms for abnormal clearance of infused soluble complexes in SLE. For example, patients with SLE who were infused with radiolabeled aggregated human IgG showed decreased binding of the probe to erythrocytes and a more rapid initial distribution phase compared with that in normal controls (62,78). Similarly, complement-mediated binding of tetanus toxoid/antitetanus toxoid immune complexes to erythrocytes was decreased in SLE, and this correlated with erythrocyte CR1 number (48). With these model immune complexes, a rapid first phase of elimination was noted in patients with low complement, low CR1, and low immune adherence, which was ascribed to inappropriate tissue deposition of complexes (49).

The second, slower elimination phase of infused aggregated IgG also is abnormal in SLE, presumably because of impaired splenic uptake as well as generalized mononuclear phagocyte dysfunction. Whereas studies in normal individuals show preferential hepatic uptake of aggregated IgG, and those who are splenectomized show hepatic compensation for splenic loss with normal elimination half-times, patients with SLE have both minimal splenic uptake and prolonged clearance half-times (62,78,82). Studies of the infusion of large, soluble immune complexes (hepatitis B surface antigen/antibody) in patients with SLE reveal both impairment of hepatic clearance and retention of complexes as well as impairment of splenic clearance and retention of complexes (83). With this probe, the dysfunction is related to hypocomplementemia and decreased number of erythrocyte CR1 receptors. Similarly, in a patient with hereditary homozygous C2 deficiency, treatment with fresh frozen plasma to normalize classic pathway complement activity normalized the binding of hepatitis B surface antigen/antibody complexes to erythrocytes and corrected defects in splenic clearance and retention (84). Regardless of the mechanism, however, abnormalities in both splenic and hepatic clearance function allow for a spillover of complexes beyond the mononuclear phagocyte system in SLE.

Blockade of FcγRs by elevated levels of IgG interferes with this key mechanism for the elimination of soluble circulating immune complexes (85,86). That serum concentrations of IgG are an important factor predicting the rate of aggregated IgG clearance in SLE (78) emphasizes the importance of FcγR mechanisms in this model and supports the conclusions derived from the sensitized erythrocyte model of immune complex clearance. Specifically, FcγR-mediated clearance efficiency is crucial in SLE because of the defects in complement-dependent function.

BIOLOGY OF HUMAN Fcγ RECEPTORS

With evidence of both the genetic and acquired components of FcγR-mediated clearance defect, further information about FcγR structure and function should enhance our understanding of immune complex handling and provide novel therapeutic options. Human FcγR structure is much more varied than simply being one type of receptor for IgG, as assumed in many of the early studies cited in this chapter. Recent, dramatic growth in our knowledge of FcγRs has revealed extreme diversity accompanied by great complexity. The nomenclature for FcγR follows that proposed by Ravetch and Kinet (87): uppercase letters refer to genes, and lower case letters refer to proteins (i.e., gene products).

Structure and Distribution

FcγRs are an essential receptor system that is engaged by immune complexes as they trigger internalization, release of inflammatory mediators, cytokines, and degranulation. In contrast to complement receptors, FcγR recognize ligand in its native form. In humans, there are three distinct but closely related classes of FcγR—FcγRI (CD64), FcγRII (CD32), and FcγRIII (CD16)—that are identified by immunochemical and physicochemical properties, cellular distribution, and complementary DNA (cDNA) sequences (88–92). There are eight FcγR genes, each of which may lead to unique protein products. Extensive structural diversity among FcγR family members leads to differences in binding capacity, distinct signal transduction pathways, and cell-specific expression patterns (Fig. 12.5). This chapter considers structure-function relationships in the context of each receptor family and provides a framework for understanding how FcγR may contribute to susceptibility, pathogenesis, and therapeutic intervention in SLE.

FcγRs on the surface of hematopoietic cells are often expressed as stimulatory and inhibitory pairs. Given the protean and potent reactivity initiated by stimulatory FcγR, cell activation must be modulated to respond appropriately to variations in environmental stimuli. Studies have suggested that inhibitory FcγRs, which modulate thresholds for activation and terminate stimulating signals, are a key element in the regulation of effector function (13,14). When coaggregated with stimulatory receptors on the cell surface, inhibitory FcγRs can abolish cellular signaling, whereas when self-aggregated, they do not trigger effector functions. Inhibitory FcγRs play a central role in afferent and efferent immune responses as negative regulators of both antibody production and immune complex–triggered activation.

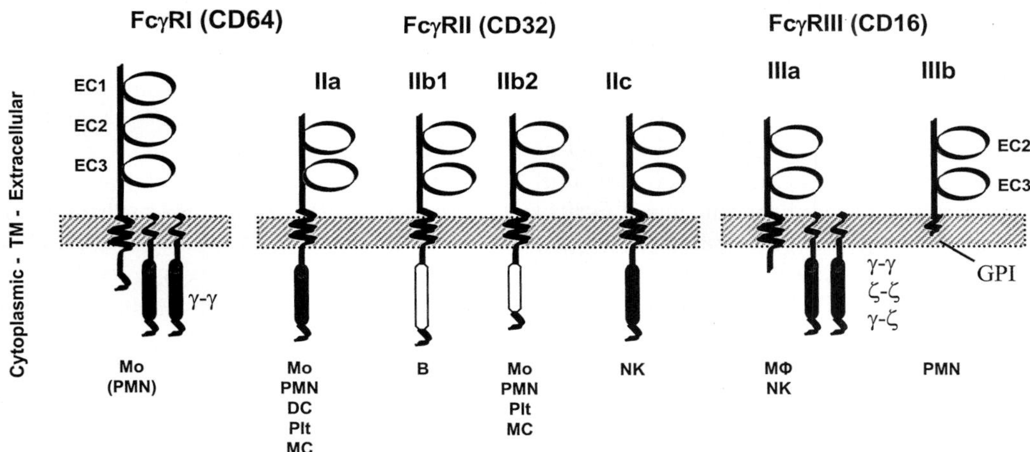

FIGURE 12.5. Schematic representation of the human Fcγreceptor family members. FcγR α-chains contain two or three disulfide-linked immunoglobulin-like extracellular domains (ellipses) that mediate binding to IgG. All FcγRs, except the glycosyl phosphatidylinositol-anchored FcγRIIIb, have a transmembrane region (TM), some of which can interact with accessory chains to yield a multichain signaling complex. The cytoplasmic domains of FcγR or their associated subunits are responsible for signal transduction. FcγRIIIb is the only FcγR that lacks a cytoplasmic tail. FcγRI and FcγRIIIa are multichain receptors that associate with immunoreceptor tyrosine activation motif (ITAM)-containing γ- or ζ-chain dimers (*black cylinders*) to mediate positive signaling. FcγRIIa and FcγRIIc are single-chain stimulatory receptors containing ITAM motifs in their cytoplasmic tails. FcγRIIb (isoforms FcγRIIb1 and FcγRIIb2) are single-chain inhibitory receptors containing immunoreceptor tyrosine inhibitory motif (ITIM) in their cytoplasmic tails (*white cylinders*). The cellular distribution FcγR is listed below each receptor: monocytes (Mo), macrophages (Mφ), dendritic cells (DC), mast cells (MC), B lymphocytes (B), platelets (pLT), natural killer cells (NK), and polymorphonuclear leukocytes (PMN). (Adapted from Salmon JE, Pricop L. Human receptors for immunoglobulin G: Key elements in the pathogenesis of rheumatic disease. *Arthritis Rheum* 2001;44:739–750, with permission.)

FcγRs belong to the immunoglobulin supergene family and are encoded for by multiple genes, which have been mapped to the long arm of chromosome 1q21-23 (93–95). Within the three FcγR families, the presence of multiple distinct genes (arising from gene reduplication) and alternative splicing variants leads to a variety of receptor isoforms that are most strikingly different in transmembrane and intracellular regions, whereas they share similar but not identical extracellular domains (Fig. 12.5).

FcγRs capable of triggering cellular activation possess intracellular activation motifs, termed immunoreceptor tyrosine-based activation motifs (ITAMs), similar to those of B-cell receptors and T-cell receptors (96,97). Inhibitory FcγRs have extracellular domains that are homologous to their activating counterparts, but their cytoplasmic domains contain an immunoreceptor tyrosine-based inhibitory motif (ITIM). Stimulatory FcγRs are typically multichain receptors composed of a ligand-binding α subunit, which confers ligand specificity and affinity, and associated signaling subunits with ITAMs in the cytoplasmic domains (Fig. 12.5). FcγR α chains are transmembrane molecules that share the structural motif of two or three extracellular immunoglobulin-like domains, but vary in their affinity for IgG and in their preferences for binding different IgG subclasses (IgG1, IgG2, IgG3, and IgG4). There are also allelic variations in the ligand-binding region of specific FcγRs that influence the ability to bind certain IgG subclasses and alter the responses of phagocytes to IgG-opsonized antigens (98–100). The transmembrane domains of the α subunits contain a basic residue to mediate the physical interaction with associated signaling chains required for efficient expression and signal transduction. The two multichain FcγR isoforms are termed FcγRI, a high-affinity receptor for IgG that binds monomeric IgG, and FcγRIIIa, an intermediate-affinity receptor, that binds only multivalent IgG. Homodimeric γ-chains are transducing modules for FcγRI and FcγRIIIa (Fig.12.5). Heterodimers of ζ-chains and γ-chains or ζ-ζ-chain homodimers can also transduce signals through FcγRIIIa in human natural killer (NK) cells. The other isoform, FcγRIIIb, has neither an ITAM nor a transmembrane domain, but is maintained in the plasma membrane outer leaflet by a glycosyl phosphatidylinositol anchor (Fig. 12.5). In addition to multichain receptors, there are two other types of activating FcγR and one inhibitory receptor with two different splice variants. FcγRIIa and FcγRIIc are single-chain receptors that include an extracellular ligand-binding domain and ITAM in the cytoplasmic domain. Inhibitory FcγRs, FcγRIIb1 and FcγRIIb2, are single-chain receptors with extracellular domains highly homologous to their activating counterparts and cytoplasmic domains with ITIMs (Fig. 12.5) (101).

FcγRI (CD64) is distinguished by its relatively high affinity for IgG (102). It is the only FcγR that is capable of binding monomeric IgG; other FcγRs require multivalent ligands. In contrast to the low-affinity FcγRII and FcγRIII, which have only two immunoglobulin-like domains homologous to the first two extracellular domains of FcγRI, FcγRI has three extracellular immunoglobulin-like domains, the last of which is postulated to confer high affinity (103–105) (Fig. 12.5). FcγRI is encoded for by at least three different genes, thus suggesting the possibility of the expression of different isoforms. Only FcγRIa has been detected on the cell surface. FcγRIa, a heavily glycosylated 72-kd protein, associated with homodimers of the γ-subunit of the high-affinity receptor for IgE (106) (Fig. 12.5). FcγRIa is present on monocytes, macrophages, and dendritic cells (107). Monocyte expression of FcγRI is markedly enhanced by interferon-γ (IFN-γ) (108,109), though neutrophils that do not constitutively express FcγRI can be induced to express this receptor by IFN-γ and granulocyte colony-stimulating factor (G-CSF) (110,111).

The FcγRII (CD32) family contains 40-kd receptors with low affinity for IgG, interacting only with IgG in complexes. They are the most widely expressed FcγR, and this family has the greatest range of structural heterogeneity. FcγRII family members are present on nearly all cells that bear FcγRs, including most leukocytes and platelets (112–114). Density of expression varies with cell type but generally is higher than that for FcγRI (115). The structural heterogeneity of FcγRII has a complex genetic basis with at least three genes (FcγRIIA, FcγRIIB, and FcγRIIC) and alternative splicing, resulting in the expression of six different isoforms (89–92,116) (Fig. 12.5). The three genes are nearly identical in their extracellular and transmembrane domains but differ in their cytoplasmic domains. The divergence in cytoplasmic tails determines the effector functions that are mediated by each isoform. FcγRIIA, FcγRIIB, and FcγRIIC represent single-protein gene products (α-chains) that are competent for ligand binding (extracellular domain) and signal transduction (cytoplasmic domain incorporating structural motifs essential for signaling). This contrasts with the other FcγRs that assemble in multimolecular signaling complexes (Fig. 12.5). Among the FcγRII family members there are receptors activating and inhibiting receptors, which differ mainly in the signaling motif in the cytoplasmic domain. FcγRIIA and FcγRIIC are contain ITAMs (discussed later). FcγRIIA and FcγRIIC are preferentially expressed on cells of myeloid lineage, monocytes, neutrophils, platelets, and dendritic cells. FcγRIIC has been identified on NK cells (117).

FcγRIIB is the only FcγR gene encoding for an inhibitory receptor. It encodes for single-chain low-affinity receptors with extracellular domains highly homologous to FcγRIIA and FcγRIIC, but with cytoplasmic domains containing an ITIM (101) (Fig. 12.5). Alternative splicing generates two isoforms, FcγRIIb1 and FcγRIIb2, which differ only in their intracytoplasmic regions (116). FcγRIIb1 contains an insertion of 19 amino acids that significantly alters receptor function. FcγRIIb is widely expressed on hematopoietic cells: FcγRIIb1 on B lymphocytes and FcγRIIb2 on myeloid cells. Neither isoform can trigger cell activation. Instead, both isoforms of FcγRIIb, when coaggregated with ITAM-bearing receptors, are negative regulators of activation. In addition, FcγRIIb2 participates in endocytosis of multivalent ligands by phagocytes and antigen-presenting cells while the intracytoplasmic insertion in FcγRIIb1 inhibits internalization (118). FcγRIIb can modulate cell activation by stimulatory FcγR, as well as responses triggered by the B-cell receptor (BCR), the T-cell receptor (TCR), and Fc receptors for IgE (119). However, to inhibit cell activation, FcγRIIb must be coaggregated with ITAM-expressing receptors by a multivalent ligand, and cell activation must be triggered by the receptors that are coaggregated with FcγRIIb (120). For example, FcγRIIb coaggregation with FcγRIIa by IgG-opsonized particles blocks phagocytosis, and FcγRIIb co-ligation to BCR by antibody-antigen complexes inhibits B-cell proliferation and antibody production (121,122). Thus, FcγRIIb-mediated negative regulation of ITAM-dependent cell activation endows IgG-containing immune complexes with the capacity to regulate B cells and inflammatory cells. The balance between stimulatory and inhibitory input determines cellular response.

In addition to different isoforms, there are two allelic forms of FcγRIIA (R131 and H131), resulting in further polymorphism in this receptor class. The FcγRIIA alleles differ functionally because of a single base difference that encodes for the amino acid position 131 in the second extracellular domain (arginine and histidine, respectively). These alleles are expressed codominantly on neutrophils, monocytes, and platelets and have differing IgG subclass-binding specificities (discussed later) (90,98,99).

The FcγRIII (CD16) family of low-affinity receptors for IgG contains two members, each of which is encoded for by different but highly homologous genes (FcγRIIIA and FcγRIIIB), and each is selectively expressed in specific cell types (90,91,123). FcγRIIIa is the most abundant class of FcγR on macrophages and thus is a key receptor of the mononuclear phagocyte system. It is present at high density on Kupffer cells in the liver and on macrophages in the spleen, both important areas for immune complex clearance binding and internalization. In addition, it has been described on a subpopulation of monocytes (124) and on mesangial cells (125). One source of diversity between isoforms of FcγRIIIa is differences in glycosylation, which may account for the variations in receptor affinity noted for NK versus macrophage forms of FcγRIIIa and for FcγRIIIa versus FcγRIIIb (126). FcγRIIIa associates with members of a family of signal transduction molecules that bear ITAMs within their cytoplasmic domains (Fig. 12.5) (127). These molecules also are used by FcγR1 and the high-affinity receptor for IgE. These accessory molecules form disulfide-linked dimeric complexes (homo- or heterodimers) that noncovalently associate with the transmembrane region of FcγRIIIa to enable cell surface expression and signal transduction. FcγRIIIa also has the capacity to associate with the β-subunit of the high-affinity IgE receptor (128).

FcγRIIIb is the most densely expressed FcγR on neutrophils and therefore is the most abundant FcγR in the circulation. The major difference between the two subclasses of FcγRIII is that FcγRIIIa, which is the form expressed on macrophages and NK cells, is a conventional transmembrane protein, whereas FcγRIIIb, which is the form expressed exclusively on neutrophils, is anchored to the outer membrane leaflet by a glycosyl phosphatidylinositol moiety (129,130) (Fig. 12.5). Further diversity in FcγRIII structure is provided by an allotypic variation in FcγRIIIb. The two recognized allelic forms of the glycosyl phosphatidylinositol-anchored neutrophil isoform of FcγRIIIb, termed NA1 and NA2, differ by several amino acids and N-linked glycosylation sites (131,132). The alleles are inherited in a classic mendelian manner and are expressed in a codominant fashion. In addition to different isoforms, there are two allelic forms of FcγRIIIA (F176 and V176), which differ in one amino acid at position 176 in the extracellular domain (phenylalanine or valine, respectively) (100,133,134). These alleles differ in binding capacity for IgG1 and IgG3 (discussed later).

Another potentially important form of FcγR in the context of immune complex handling is circulating soluble receptor. Normal sera contain soluble FcγRII and FcγRIII (135,136). These soluble FcγRs lack transmembrane domains and presumably derive from alternative splicing or release from circulating leukocytes (135–137). The physiologic significance of these circulating IgG-binding proteins is not yet clear, but a proposed biologic function of plasma FcγRs is to suppress IgG production by B cells (138). The role of plasma FcγRs in immune complex clearance is open to speculation. Certainly, they may influence the clearance of immune complexes by blocking the ligand-binding site for FcγRs and thereby inhibiting both FcγR-mediated clearance and FcγR-triggered inflammation at sites of tissue deposition. Immune complex binding of plasma FcγR also has the potential to affect clearance by changing the size of the complexes, altering their solubility, modifying their capacity to activate complement and capture C3b, and shifting binding from macrophage FcγRs to complement receptors.

Ligands

Ligand specificity for FcγRs is relative rather than absolute, and it depends on the valency or degree of opsonization of the study probe. Table 12.2 shows the binding specificity of human FcγRs for human IgG subclasses. The IgG subclass of the antibody in immune complexes and the valence of the complex influence the efficiency of the interaction with FcγRs (139). Further, a single immune complex may bind simultaneously to different classes of FcγR. FcγRI, the high-affinity receptor and the only FcγR capable of univalent binding of IgG (174,175), and FcγRII and FcγRIIIb, which are lower-affinity FcγRs, preferentially bind IgG1 and IgG3. There is differential binding affinity for allelic variants of FcγRIIIa (100). While the affinity of FcγRIIIa-expressed macrophages and NK cells is higher than that of FcγRIIIb on neutrophils, the pattern of specificity for subclasses is similar for all FcγR (126). For all three classes of FcγR, IgG2 is the ligand with lowest affinity (Table 12.2), although studies have shown efficient binding to IgG2 by the H131 allele of FcγRIIa (discussed later) (98,99,140).

In addition to classic IgG-FcγR interactions, FcγR may bind ligands through lectin-carbohydrate interactions. The internalization of nonopsonized *Escherichia coli* bearing mannose-binding lectin requires neutrophil FcγRIIIb, which has high mannose oligosaccharides (141). Monocyte FcγRs also participate in lectin-carbohydrate interactions (142). These observations suggest that nonclassic engagement of FcγRs through lectin-carbohydrate interaction, perhaps by antigens in complexes, can affect clearance by phagocytes. In addition, recent studies have shown that FcγRI and FcγRIIa are critical receptors for C-reactive protein (CRP), and that FcγRIIa is the main receptor on human phagocytes for CRP, which raises the possibility that FcγRs are important for the clearance of nucleosomes bound to CRP, which may also be influenced by allelic polymorphisms (143–145).

TABLE 12.2. FcR AFFINITY AND IgG SUBCLASS SPECIFICITY

	MW (kd)	Genes	Affinity for IgG (Ka)	IgG Specificity
FcRI	72	FcRI	10^8–10^9 M^{-1}	1,3>4>>2
FcRII	40–50	FcRIIA-R131	<10^7 M^{-1}	1,3>>2,4
		FcRIIA-H131	<10^7 M^{-1}	1,3,2>>>4
		FcRIIB, C	<10^7 M^{-1}	1,3>>2,4
FcRIII	60–70	FcRIIIA	10^7 M^{-1}	1,3>>>2,4
	50–80	FcRIIIB	<10^7 M^{-1}	1,3>>2,4

Ig, immunoglobulin; MW, molecular weight.

FcγR Signal Transduction

Effector cell activation is initiated when FcγRs are clustered at the cell surface by multivalent antigen-antibody complexes. Monovalent ligand binding is insufficient to generate a signal. Signal transduction by FcγR following aggregation involves a number of early cellular biochemical changes that lead to cellular activation. Like many other immune system receptors, such as the TCR and BCR, FcγR initiates tyrosine phosphorylation as a critical early signaling event (96,97). Stimulatory FcγRs have no intrinsic enzymatic activity, but are associated with membrane anchored src family kinases. The presence of two YxxL motifs separated by seven variable residues in the signaling subunit (γ-chain) of activating FcγRI and FcγRIIIa, or 12 residues in the case of FcγRIIa and FcγRIIc, is necessary for docking the protein tyrosine kinase syk and for initiation of positive signaling. Tyrosine kinases phosphorylate many intracellular substrates, including phospholipid kinases, phospholipases, adapter molecules, and cytoskeletal proteins. Activation of phospholipase C and phosphatidylinositol-3 (PI_3) kinase by syk leads to the production of phosphoinositol messengers and a sustained increase in cytoplasmic Ca^{2+} (146). Recruitment of the adapter protein shc allows signals triggered by FcγR to reach the nucleus via the ras pathway, leading to phosphorylation of mitogen-activated protein (MAP) kinase, activation of transcription factors, and induction of gene expression (147).

FcγRIIb isoforms are important negative regulators of ITAM-dependent activation and establish the threshold for effector cell activation. Inert when self-aggregated, inhibitory FcγRIIb abolishes cellular signals when co-ligated with stimulatory receptors. The ITIM motif (V/IxYxxL), contained in a 13-amino acid sequence present in the intracytoplasmic domain of both FcγRIIb1 and FcγRIIb2, is essential for the negative regulatory properties of FcγRIIb and other inhibitory receptors (reviewed in refs. 148–150). Like ITAMs, ITIMs are phosphorylated by protein tyrosine kinases and then recruit SH2-containing cytoplasmic molecules. Inhibitory function requires the recruitment of phosphatases to the phosphorylated ITIM. Although the protein tyrosine phosphatases SHP-1 and SHP-2 bind to FcγRIIb-phosphorylated ITIM motifs, the inositol polyphosphate 5′-phosphatase SHIP has been shown to be preferentially recruited to FcγRIIb and appears to play the predominant role in FcγRIIb-mediated inhibition by preventing Ca^{2+} influx (151–153).

Since most cells express more than one FcγR isoform, it is likely that antigen-antibody complexes coaggregate more than one type of receptor. Coclustering of stimulatory FcγR represents a mechanism where different FcγR cooperate to amplify signals and produce more efficient activation of effector cells. FcγR that act synergistically transphosphorylate each other, leading to activation of tyrosine kinases and downstream substrates and initiation of $[Ca^{2+}]_i$ transients, with subsequent cytoskeletal changes and transcriptional activation. In contrast, the regulation of ITAM-dependent cell activation by inhibitory FcγR is a mechanism for negative cooperation. Coclustering of inhibitory FcγRIIb with ITAM-bearing FcγR prevents the influx of extracellular Ca^{2+} and attenuates effector cell activation (148,149). By providing activated protein tyrosine kinases to phosphorylate the ITIM of FcγRIIb, stimulatory FcγRs play a role in their own inhibition. In cells that express both stimulatory and inhibitory receptors for IgG, the relative levels of these two types of receptors determine the state of cell activation after interaction with immune complexes.

FcγR-Mediated Effector Functions

The multivalent interaction of phagocytes with immune complexes leads to internalization of the complex, generation of reactive oxygen intermediates, and release of inflammatory mediators, including prostaglandins, leukotrienes, hydrolytic enzymes, and cytokines [e.g., IFN-γ, interleukin-6 (IL-6), tumor necrosis factor-α (TNF-α), and so on] (154–158). The role of individual isoforms of FcγRs in initiating these effector functions has been investigated in experiments using anti-FcγR monoclonal antibodies, cell lines with limited expression of FcγRs, and transfectants. There is significant overlap among the biologic activities mediated by each family of FcγR, and the relative contribution of each receptor family depends on the nature of the ligand, the state of phagocyte activation, and the effector function being assessed.

Binding and internalization are the most important effector functions for immune complex clearance. Experiments using erythrocytes coated with Fab fragments of anti-FcγR monoclonal antibodies show that in cultured human monocytes (a model system for fixed-tissue macrophages), FcγRI, FcγRIIa, and FcγRIIIa mediate phagocytosis (159). FcγRI is a key receptor on monocytes involved in the binding of IgG anti-(Rh)D–sensitized erythrocytes and small complexes *in vitro* (160). A role for FcγRIIIa is evident from studies showing that blockade of FcγRIII by infusion of anti-FcγRIII monoclonal antibody in humans and nonhuman primates inhibits clearance of IgG anti-D–sensitized erythrocytes as well as clearance of soluble and erythrocyte-bound DNA/anti-DNA immune complexes, but to a lesser extent (Fig. 12.2) (47,161,162). Studies revealing an altered distribution of the allelic variants of FcγRIIa and FcγIIIa in patients with lupus nephritis compared to control subjects without SLE highlight the importance of these receptors as inherited risk factors in the pathogenesis of SLE, presumably related to altered immune complex handling associated with the genotypes (discussed later). Taken together, these studies underscore the crucial role of each FcγR family in particulate and soluble immune complex handling by mononuclear phagocytes.

On neutrophils, while FcγRIIa mediates phagocytosis, the capacity of FcγRIIIb to independently mediate internalization is minimal (159,163,164). Although FcγRIIIb, the glycosyl phosphatidylinositol-anchored molecule, independently generates intracellular signals and initiates several other effector functions, it is conceptualized by some as a trap for circulating immune complexes that focuses IgG ligand for more efficient recognition by other FcγR species on neutrophils (202,211). Recent studies suggest a far more significant role for FcγRIIIb in triggering neutrophil responses—as a potentiator of other receptors on the cell. Cross-linking of FcγRIIIb enhances the amount of FcγRIIa-specific internalization, and co-ligation of FcγRII and FcγRIIIb results in a synergistic phagocytic response: internalization that is greater than the sum of the FcγRII and FcγRIIIb (164–166). This synergistic capacity of FcγRIIIb also enables complement receptor-mediated phagocytosis.

Regarding the intact phagocyte, the mechanisms triggering individual receptor-mediated function as well as engagement of multiple families of receptors in an interactive framework must be considered. In this context, studies of the ligation of individual receptor species (discussed earlier) demonstrate the functional potential of a given receptor. Alternatively, engagement of two receptors may lead to quantitatively, and perhaps qualitatively, distinct cell functions in relation to the engagement of either receptor alone. With engagement of mononuclear phagocyte FcγRs by immune complex, there are both heterotypic and homotypic receptor clusters, resulting in intracellular interactions between the signals that are generated by each receptor family. In monocytes, FcγRI and FcγRIIa cooperate in triggering activation, presumably by heterotypic clustering. In neutrophils, FcγRIIIb acts synergistically with FcγRIIa to mediate phagocytosis (165,166). Coaggregation of activating FcγR with inhibitory FcγRIIb alters the threshold and magnitude of effector functions. Interactions between FcγRs and other leukocyte receptors modulate FcγR-initiated functions; for example, engagement of complement receptor type 3 enhances FcγR-mediated phagocytosis by monocytes. In the interaction of immune complexes with leukocytes, effector function capacity is a consequence of positive and negative cooperation among FcγR families and between FcγRs and other receptors, all of which may be simultaneously engaged.

Cytokines elaborated during an immune response alter FcγR expression and functional capacity. For example, IFN-γ and G-CSF upregulate FcγRI on monocytes and induce its expression on polymorphonuclear cells (PMNs), whereas IL-4 inhibits the expression of all ITAM-bearing FcγR (167–169). Granulocyte-macrophage CSF (GM-CSF) specifically increases FcγRIIa, and transforming growth factor-β (TGF-β) increases FcγRIIIa (169). In contrast to their effects on stimulatory receptors, IFN-γ decreases and IL-4 increases the expression of the inhibitory receptor, FcγRIIb2 on human monocytes (170). It has been proposed that FcγRIIb functions to modulate inflammatory response by establishing the threshold of immune complex-stimulated activation of macrophages. That IFN-γ [a prototypic T-helper-1 (Th1) cytokine] and IL-4 (a prototypic Th2 cytokine) differentially regulate the expression of FcγR isoforms with opposite functions provides a mechanism for regulation of activating and inhibitory signals delivered by FcγRs on phagocytes. Cytokines released within an inflammatory milieu thus act in an autocrine and paracrine manner to modulate effector cell function.

Inherited Differences in FcγRs

Mechanisms for the diversity of FcγR within an individual were discussed earlier. Inherited or acquired differences in FcγR structure, expression, or function provide the basis for differences in FcγR function between individuals, and these differences may contribute to disease susceptibility and pathogenesis. Heritable differences include gene deletions, promoter polymorphisms, and allelic forms. Individuals with the rare deficiency of FcγRIa1 are free of clinical disease, circulating immune complexes, and increased susceptibility to infection (171). The initial report of FcγRIIIb deficiency in a patient with SLE focused attention of the genetics of FcγR and immune complex disease (172). Defects in the expression of FcγRIIIb as a consequence of alterations at the genomic level have been identified in multiple unrelated individuals completely lacking FcγRIIIB alleles (173–175), but they have no consistent clinical pattern of increased infections or immune complex-mediated diseases (176). Although a second report of SLE in FcγRIIIb deficiency raises the possibility that this receptor functions in immune complex handling, perhaps as a carrier for circulating complexes, more extensive population and family studies are required (177).

The concept that the balance of stimulatory and inhibitory FcγR is a determinant of the susceptibility to and severity of immune complex–induced inflammatory disease has been validated by data from murine models (12–14). Recent descriptions of deletions in the promoter region of FcγRIIB in all major autoimmune-prone mice strains have underscored these findings. These deletions are associated with a reduction in the expression and function of the inhibitory FcγRIIb on macrophages and activated B cells, defects that would be expected to promote autoimmunity (178–180). As yet, there have been no reports of deficiency of inhibitory FcγRIIb function in antibody-mediated human disease. However, it is possible that differences in the relative expression of ITAM- and ITIM-containing FcγR influence an individual's risk of developing autoimmune disease.

Genetically determined alterations in FcγR structure provide a basis for inherited predisposition to disease. Allelic variants of human FcγR profoundly influence phagocyte biologic activity. Single amino acid substitutions within the extracellular domains of some stimulatory FcγR alter the capacity of these receptors to bind IgG and have been associated with risk for and phenotype of autoimmune and infectious disease (Fig. 12.6). Allelic polymorphisms have been identified in three FcγR family members: FcγRIIa, FcγRIIIa, and FcγRIIIb. Inherited variants of FcγR have differential binding avidity for different IgG subclasses.

FcγRIIa, expressed on mononuclear phagocytes, neutrophils, and platelets, has two codominantly expressed alleles, H131 and R131, which differ at amino acid position 131 in the extracellular domain (histidine and arginine, respectively), an area that strongly influences ligand binding (Fig. 12.6). The allelic variants differ substantially in their ability to bind human IgG2 (98,99,118,181). FcγRIIa-H131 is the high-binding allele and R131 is low binding, while heterozygotes have intermediate function. Because IgG2 is a poor activator of the classic complement pathway, FcγRIIa-H131 is essential for handling IgG2 immune complexes. Even with model immune complexes containing IgG2 in combination with other IgG subclasses, there is differential handling in PMNs from homozygous individuals related to host FcγRIIa genotype (11). The genotype distribution of FcγRIIA in Caucasian and African-American populations is approximately 25% homozygous for H131, 50% heterozygous, and 25% homozygous for R131. Among Asians the frequency of the R131 allele is much lower, and less than 10% of the population is homozygous for R131 (reviewed in ref. 182).

FcγRIIa has substantial clinical importance for host defense against infection with encapsulated bacteria known to elicit IgG2 responses, such as *Neisseria meningitidis, Hemophilus influenzae,* and *Streptococcus pneumoniae* (183–185). There is an increased frequency of homozygosity for FcγRIIa-R131 among otherwise healthy children who suffer from recurrent respiratory tract infections or fulminant meningococcal sepsis. FcγRIIa-R131 has also been shown to be a risk factor for invasive pneumococcal infection in patients with systemic lupus erythematosus (186). Like IgG2, CRP binds to several encapsulated bacteria. The recent report of a reciprocal relationship between the binding affinities of IgG2 and CRP for FcγRIIa suggests a mechanism for partial protection from invasive infection in individuals homozygous for FcγRIIa-R131 (144). That FcγRIIa is the main receptor for CRP raises the possibility that handling of nucleosomes bound to CRP may also be influenced by allelic polymorphisms (145).

FcγRIIIa, expressed on mononuclear phagocytes and NK cells, also displays codominantly expressed biallelic variants, F176 and V176, which differ in one amino acid at position 176 in the extracellular domain (phenylalanine or valine, respectively) (100,187,188) (Fig. 12.6). FcγRIIIa alleles differ in IgG1 and IgG3 binding; V176 homozygotes bind IgG1 and IgG3 more avidly than F176. These differences in IgG binding have implications for antibody-mediated immune surveillance [antibody-dependent cell-mediated cytotoxicity (ADCC)] and antibody-mediated host defense against pathogens and autoimmune disease. The

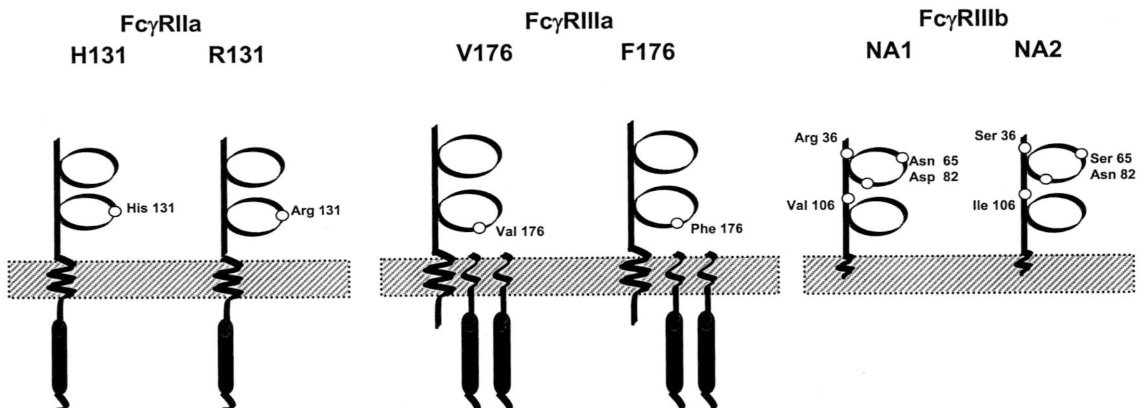

FIGURE 12.6. Allelic variants of human FcγR. **Left:** The FcγRIIa polymorphism is a consequence of an arginine (R131) to histidine (H131) substitution at amino acid position 131 in the extracellular domain, which causes differences in binding affinity for human IgG2 and C-reactive protein (CRP). **Middle:** The FcγRIIIa polymorphism is the consequence of a valine (V176) to phenylalanine (F176) substitution at position 176, leading to changes in binding affinity for human IgG1 and IgG3. **Right:** The NA1 and NA2 polymorphism of FcγRIIIb reflects four amino acid substitutions with consequent differences in N-linked glycosylation sites and quantitative differences in phagocytic function.(Adapted from Salmon JE, Pricop L. Human receptors for immunoglobulin G: key elements in the pathogenesis of rheumatic disease. *Arthritis Rheum* 2001;44:739–750, with permission.)

distribution of genotypes of FcγRIIIA in disease-free Caucasian and African-American populations has been reported to be 40% to 50% homozygous F176, and 40% to 50% heterozygous and 8% to 18% homozygous V176 (182).

Two common allelic variants of FcγRIIIb, a receptor exclusively expressed on neutrophils, have been characterized and shown to alter neutrophil function. The allotypes, known as neutrophil antigen (NA)1 and NA2, were identified as a consequence of their involvement in blood transfusion reactions and alloimmune neutropenias. They differ by five nucleotides, which results in a substitution of four amino acids in the membrane-distant first extracellular domain (132) (Fig. 12.6). Although binding of IgG does not seem to be affected, the NA1 and NA2 allelic forms do have different levels of quantitative function (99,166,189,190). Neutrophils obtained from NA1 homozygous donors have a more robust FcγR-mediated phagocytic response as compared to cells from NA2 donors, despite equivalent receptor density (189,190). Functional differences between the NA1 and NA2 alleles appear to have clinical significance. Homozygous NA1 individuals may be more resistant to bacterial infection, especially when FcγRIIa cannot be effectively engaged, as suggested by the finding of increased *N. meningitidis* infection among hosts with complement component 6 or 8 deficiency who are homozygous for FcγRIIIb-NA2 and FcγRIIa-R131 (191).

Studies of the allelic polymorphisms of FcγR demonstrate functional consequences of subtle structural differences, and these models suggest the potential impact of the rich structural diversity in FcγRs on immune complex handling.

ABNORMALITIES IN Fc RECEPTORS IN SLE

FcγR saturation by circulating immune complexes with decreased receptor availability was initially proposed as a potential mechanism for defective FcγR-mediated clearance (64). The complexity of FcγR structure was not appreciated at the time of these studies, however. Support for this hypothesis was derived from *in vitro* induction of loss of surface FcγRs in monocytes by culture with immune complexes (192,193) and *in vivo* production of mononuclear phagocyte blockade by infusion of immune complexes (4). Even so, several different studies of blood monocytes from patients with SLE demonstrated an increase rather than the predicted decrease in FcγR binding (194–196). In experiments quantitating the binding of monomeric IgG, oligomeric IgG, and IgG-sensitized erythrocytes to monocytes, there was an increase in the levels of binding in patients with SLE compared with the levels in controls. The observed increase in FcγR binding correlated with SLE disease activity in some studies and thus was highest in the population most likely to have the greatest abnormality in FcγR-mediated clearance (194). In other studies, FcγR binding directly correlated with levels of immune complexes (197). Whether the increased binding capacity is specific to one class of FcγR or generalized is not known. The basis for the observed increase in patients with SLE is speculative, but this increase may result from exposure to cytokines and cellular activation (142,197,198).

Despite enhanced binding of FcγR ligand *in vitro*, FcγR-mediated phagocytosis of IgG-sensitized erythrocytes was markedly impaired in monocytes derived from patients with SLE (196) (Fig. 12.7). The defect in phagocytosis *in vitro* was most profound in those patients with the most significantly impaired *in vivo* mononuclear phagocyte system clearance. These observations, along with those from other studies demonstrating a correlation between *in vivo* clearance and *in vitro* FcγR phagocytosis, support the role of defective phagocytosis as an important component of altered FcγR-mediated clearance (77,86). The dissociation of FcγR-mediated binding and FcγR-mediated internalization suggests relative receptor-effector uncoupling. Because the probes used in these studies could not discriminate among the FcγR expressed on monocytes, the contribution of a given class (or classes) of FcγR to this dysfunction is not yet known.

The net FcγR-mediated phagocytic capacity in SLE is a result of at least two factors. The first is inherited, such as that associated with associated with allelic polymorphisms of FcγR or with HLA-DR2 or -DR3; the second is disease acquired and may be related to disease activity. Disease-free individuals with an HLA haplotype containing DR2 or DR3 (both of which are associated with SLE) have decreased FcγR-mediated phagocytosis by blood monocytes, which may contribute to their impaired clearance of IgG-sensitized erythrocytes and their genetic predisposition

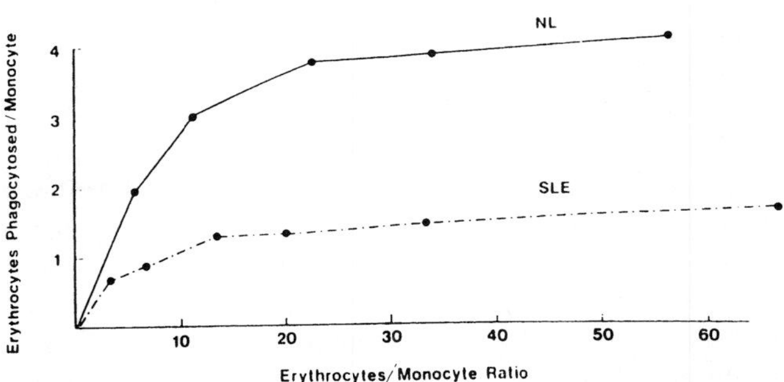

FIGURE 12.7. *In vitro* phagocytosis of ^{51}Cr-labeled IgG-sensitized erythrocytes (EAs) by monocytes from normal volunteers (● – ●) and patients with SLE (● – • – ●) was measured at various ratios of erythrocytes to monocytes. Phagocytic capacity was dependent on the ratio of erythrocytes to monocytes in the incubation mixture. At all ratios, the patients with SLE had lower FcγR-mediated internalization). (From Salmon JE, Kimberly RP, Gibofsky A, et al. Defective mononuclear phagocyte function in systemic lupus erythematosus: dissociation of Fc receptor-ligand binding and internalization. *J Immunol* 1984;133:2525–2531, with permission.)

to SLE (77,196,199). The decrease in FcγR capacity is less profound than that observed in patients with SLE who have similar HLA haplotypes.

A second mechanism for inherited differences in FcγR-mediated mononuclear phagocyte function is allelic polymorphisms of FcγR. It has been hypothesized that low-binding FcγR alleles are susceptibility factors for SLE. Association studies indicate that FcγRIIa-R131 and FcγRIIIa-F176 alleles are highly enriched in some groups of patients with SLE (200–205). In the initial studies with African Americans, a group with a high prevalence and severity of SLE, an association between FcγRIIA alleles and lupus nephritis was described (200). There was an increased frequency of FcγRIIA-R131 gene in the patients with SLE and a corresponding decrease in FcγRIIa-H131, the only human FcγR with the ability to efficiently recognize human IgG2 in black patients with lupus (Fig. 12.6). The skewing in FcγRIIA gene distribution was most marked in the nephritis group as compared with control subjects without SLE. The H131/H131 genotype was uncommon among patients with nephritis, suggesting that FcγRIIA-H131 plays a protective role in the homozygous state, an idea that is supported by *in vitro* experiments showing that the FcγRIIa-R131 gene product is characterized by deficient IgG2 handling in both homozygotes and heterozygotes. Thus, it appears that FcγRIIa-R131/R131 homozygotes and R131/H131 heterozygotes, which have the potential for less-efficient immune complex clearance, are at a greater risk for immune complex deposition. Similar results are been observed in for FcγRIIIA. There is a strong association of low-binding F176/F176 genotype (Fig. 12.6) with SLE, especially nephritis, and a corresponding underrepresentation of the homozygous high-binding V176/V176 genotype (100). As a consequence of these studies, FcγR were considered the first non–major histocompatibility complex (MHC) genes associated with SLE. Indeed, there is now evidence from a genome-wide scan of linkage of the region of the FcγR gene cluster on chromosome 1 with SLE (206).

Although homozygosity for low-binding alleles at either the FcγRIIA or the FcγRIIIA locus can lead to impaired binding of immune complexes, an association between low-binding alleles of FcγR and lupus, and especially lupus nephritis, has not been demonstrated in all ethnic groups studied (100,200,207–209). Nonetheless, meta-analysis (comprising more than 1,000 patients) of studies seeking to establish a relationship between SLE and FcγR variants clearly shows that FcγRIIa-R131 is associated with SLE, especially in African Americans, and that FcγRIIIa-F176 is associated with SLE in Caucasians and in other groups (182). Even within ethnic groups where associations have been demonstrated, there have been conflicting results. Such lack of uniformity has been ascribed to population admixture, lack of appropriate internal controls, differences in disease phenotype, and the confounding influence of other inherited susceptibility factors.

An alternative explanation for these inconsistencies is that the role of specific loci varies with the qualitative nature of the immune response. Differences in the IgG subclass of pathogenic autoantibodies have a profound effect on the relative importance of FcγR alleles in disease. For example, in the presence of anti-C1q antibodies, which correlate with severe renal disease and are largely of the IgG2 subclass, FcγRIIA genes appear to play a crucial role in determining disease severity (210,211). Two studies have found that FcγRIIa-R131 alleles were associated with renal disease among Caucasian lupus patients with anti-C1q antibodies, whereas analysis of the population as a whole revealed no significant difference in the frequencies of FcγRIIa-R131 and -H131 alleles compared with controls (210,211). Indeed, IgG2 is a predominant IgG subclass found in glomeruli of patients with proliferative nephritis. Thus, with precisely defined phenotypes, FcγRIIa variants have been identified as disease modifiers, in this example, conferring inherited risk for nephritis.

The finding that other autoantibodies associated with nephritis, specifically anti–double-stranded DNA (dsDNA) and antinucleosome antibodies, are predominantly IgG1 and IgG3 supports the importance of FcγRIIIA variants as disease modifying genes (212,213). For both FcγRIIa and FcγRIIIa, optimal handling of pathogenic immune complexes is provided only in the homozygous state for high-binding alleles; heterozygotes at either locus have intermediate-binding capacity. Low affinity for IgG2-containing immune complexes by FcγRIIa-R131 and for IgG1 and IgG3 by FcγRIIIa-F176 results in impaired removal of circulating immune complexes, increased tissue deposition, and accelerated organ damage. An alternative explanation for the association of FcγRIIA and FcγRIIIA with lupus is that these genes are in linkage disequilbrium with other candidate proteins. The fact that IgG2 and IgG3 subclasses are present in immune deposits of proliferative glomerulonephritis, however, supports a role for both FcγR genes in conferring risk for SLE and the possibility that these receptors act additively in the pathogenesis of disease (214–216).

The relative importance of interactions between alleles and the potential role of linkage disequilibrium between two FcγR genes within the same cluster on chromosome 1q21-23 is not yet established. However, in a cohort of Hispanic patients with a high prevalence of lupus nephritis there was selection for haplotypes containing both FcγRIIa-R131 and FcγRIIIa-F176 (217). Given that the distance between any of the low-affinity FcγR genes is less than 300 kilobase (kb), linkage disequilibrium of haplotypes might be expected (94,95). Subtle variations in genes controlling immune function, which may have little or no effect in the general population, can assume greater significance in individuals with autoimmune diatheses. The physiology of FcγR alleles provides a new framework within which the interplay between humoral immune response and host genotype may be defined and heritable risk factors for disease susceptibility and disease severity may be identified.

In addition to FcγR dysfunction, there is impaired phagocytosis of other probes in SLE monocytes. Internalization of apoptotic cells is decreased in SLE, which may promote autoimmunity (218). In addition, reduced uptake of nonopsonized particles and complement-opsonized particles has been clearly demonstrated in SLE monocytes (195,219). Thus, as predicted by the *in vivo* clearance studies, there are bipartite defects in internalization by SLE monocytes, dysfunction of FcγRs, and complement mechanisms (67,68).

Collectively, *in vivo* clearance data and *in vitro* monocyte data indicate that FcγRs play a central role in immune complex handling. Regarding conditions with decreased complement-dependent immune complex uptake by fixed tissue macrophages, such as hypocomplementemia or deficiency in erythrocyte CR1 receptors, both of which are seen in SLE, it has been proposed that FcγR-mediated clearance mechanisms can handle both complement- and noncomplement-fixing complexes. In contrast, even in the face of intact complement mechanisms, immune complexes that do not fix complement, or that fix complement poorly (e.g., such as IgG2 containing complexes), are cleared less efficiently if there is abnormal FcγR-mediated function (Fig. 12.1). In this context, the observations that normal subjects with DR2 and DR3 handle an erythrocyte-bound FcγR ligand probe less efficiently and that allelic variants of FcγR have distinct functional capacities provide a compelling argument that certain individuals may be at higher risk for the development of immune complex disease. In contrast to the complement system, the defect in FcγR function in SLE is not associated with decreased receptor number or saturation, but rather with a dissociation of receptor-ligand binding and internalization superimposed on possible inherited differences in FcγR function (194–196).

STRATEGIES FOR MODULATING FcγR-MEDIATED IMMUNE COMPLEX CLEARANCE

The emerging picture of the extensive structural diversity of human FcγRs, the importance of FcγRs in immune complex clearance, and the evidence of FcγR dysfunction in SLE present the opportunity for novel treatment strategies.

A variety of cytokines can regulate total receptor expression, modulate relative isoform predominance, and modulate receptor function (115). For example, *in vivo* and *in vitro* studies have shown that IFN-γ and G-CSF upregulate FcγRI expression (108,115,220,221), and that TGF-β, IFN-γ, and M-CSF upregulate FcγRIIIa on monocytes (169,222), while IL-4 and IL-13 downregulate expression of all three classes of stimulatory FcγRs (186,223). In contrast, IL-4 increases the expression of FcγRIIb2 on monocytes (170). The identification and utilization of cytokines that increase the ratio of expression of inhibitory and stimulatory FcγR represents a new approach for the treatment of autoimmune diseases. Similarly, targeted pharmacologic manipulation of protein kinases or phosphatases may yield effective treatments.

Steroid hormones also have major effects on FcγR expression and function. Estrogens augment and progesterones inhibit (224,225), but steroid effects may vary with the level of activation of the mononuclear system (226). For example, glucocorticoids enhance the IFN-γ–induced augmentation of monocyte FcγR function, whereas alone they are inhibitory for normal donors (228–232). Interestingly, for monocytes from patients with SLE, which may be primed *in vivo* with IFN-γ (227,233,234), glucocorticoids enhance function. Patients with active SLE who are treated with high-dose intravenous pulse methylprednisolone have improved clearance of IgG-sensitized autologous erythrocytes, enhanced monocyte FcγR expression and phagocytosis, and decreased levels of circulating immune complexes (198). These data raise the possibility that pharmacologic therapies can act synergistically with endogenous cytokines to achieve the desired outcome.

Endogenous and pharmacologic agents also modify FcγR function either directly or as consequence of interacting with cytokines to alter net FcγR function (198,235). Released at sites of tissue injury, adenosine interacts with two classes of cell surface receptors on macrophages. Occupancy of high-affinity adenosine A1 receptors enhances FcγR-mediated internalization, whereas ligation of low-affinity adenosine A2 receptor is inhibitory (236). The rapid and potent modulation of FcγR-mediated function suggests that adenosine is an important local regulator of the inflammatory response, and that receptor-specific adenosine analogues may provide novel therapies for immune complex disease.

Soluble FcγRs may be novel antiinflammatory agents. Circulating forms of FcγRII and FcγRIII are present in normal individuals (135,136). In animal models, infusion of soluble FcγR inhibits immune complex–mediated activation of phagocytes by blocking access to FcγR on effector cells (237). Circulating FcγRs have also been shown to suppress IgG production by B cells and may therefore be immunosuppressive (238). With the development of soluble TNF receptors and soluble complement receptors as therapeutic modalities, one can envision the use of soluble FcγRs to block antibody-mediated tissue injury (239,240). The unique properties of different FcγRs—affinity and IgG subclass preference—could be exploited to target specific pathogenic antibodies with specific soluble FcγR variants.

With our increasing recognition of the role of FcγRs in the pathophysiology of SLE and such a range of receptor-modulating agents, successful therapeutic intervention will be feasible and form the basis of further advances in the treatment of SLE.

REFERENCES

1. Benacerraf B, Sebestyen MM, Schlossman S. A quantitative study of the kinetics of blood clearance of P32-labelled *Escherichia coli* and staphylococci by the reticuloendothelial system. *J Exp Med* 1959;10:27–46.
2. Arend WP, Mannik M. Studies on antigen antibody complexes. II. Quantitation of tissue uptake of soluble complexes in normal and complement-depleted rabbits. *J Immunol* 1971;107:63–75.
3. Mannik M, Arend WP, Hall AP, et al. Studies on antigen-antibody complexes. I. Elimination of soluble complexes from rabbit circulation. *J Exp Med* 1971;133:713–739.
4. Haakenstad AO, Mannik M. Saturation of the reticuloendothelial system with soluble immune complexes. *J Immunol* 1974;112:1939–1948.
5. Ford PM. The effect of manipulation of reticuloendothelial system activity on glomerular deposition of aggregated protein and immune complexes in two different strains of mice. *Br J Exp Pathol* 1975;56:523–529.
6. Haakenstad AO, Case JB, Mannik M. Effect of cortisone on the disappearance kinetics and tissue localization of soluble immune complexes. *J Immunol* 1975;114:1153–1160.
7. Haakenstad AO, Mannik M. The disappearance kinetics of soluble immune complexes prepared with reduced and alkylated antibodies and with intact antibodies in mice. *Lab Invest* 1976; 35:283–292.
8. Haakenstad AO, Striker GE, Mannik M. The glomerular deposition of soluble immune complexes prepared with reduced and alkylated antibodies and with intact antibodies in mice. *Lab Invest* 1976;35:293–301.
9. Ford PM. Glomerular localization of aggregated protein in mice: effect of strain differences in relationship to systemic macrophage function. *Br J Exp Pathol* 1976;56:307–313.
10. Barcelli U, Rademacher R, Ooi YM, et al. Modification of glomerular immune complexes deposition in mice by activation of the reticuloendothelial system. *J Clin Invest* 1981;67:20–27.
11. Raij L, Sibley RK, Keane WF. Mononuclear phagocyte stimulation. Protective role from glomerular immune complex deposition. *J Lab Clin Med* 1981;98:558–567.
12. Ravtech JV, Clynes RA. Divergent roles for Fc receptors and complement in vivo. *Annu Rev Immunol* 1998;16:421–32.
13. Takai T, Ono M, Hikida M, et al. Augmented humoral and anaphylactic responses in FcγRII-deficient mice. *Nature* 1996; 379:346–349.
14. Clynes R, Maizes JS, Guinamard R, et al. Modulation of immune complex-induced inflammation in vivo by the coordinate expression of activation and inhibitory Fc receptors. *J Exp Med* 1999;189:179–186.
15. Wilson CB, Dixon FJ. Quantitation of acute and chronic serum sickness in the rabbit. *J Exp Med* 1975;134(suppl):7S–18S.
16. Wardle EN. Reticuloendothelial clearance studies in the course of horse serum induced nephritis. *Br J Exp Pathol* 1974;55:149–152.
17. Hoffsten PE, Swerdlin A, Bartell M, et al. Reticuloendothelial and mesangial function in murine immune complex glomerulonephritis. *Kidney Int* 1979;15:144–159.
18. Morgan AG, Steward MW. Macrophage clearance function and immune complex disease in New Zealand black/white F1 hybrid mice. *Clin Exp Immunol* 1976;26:133–136.
19. O'Regan S. The clearance of preformed immune complexes in rats with Heymann's nephritis. *Clin Exp Immunol* 1979;37:432–435.
20. Finbloom DS, Plotz PH. Studies of reticuloendothelial function in the mouse with model immune complexes. II. Serum clearance, tissue uptake, and reticuloendothelial saturation in NZB/W mice. *J Immunol* 1979;123:1600–1603.
21. Hebert L. The clearance of immune complexes from the circulation of man and other primates. *Am J Kidney Dis* 1991;17: 352–361.
22. Schifferli JA, Bartolotti SR, Peters DK. Inhibition of immune precipitation by complement. *Clin Exp Immunol* 1980;1: 387–394.
23. Schifferli JA, Steiger G, Hauptmann G, et al. Formation of soluble immune complexes by complement in sera of patients with various hypocomplementemic states. Difference between inhibition of immune precipitation and solubilization. *J Clin Invest* 1985;74:2127–2133.
24. Cornacoff JB, Hebert LA, Smead WL, et al. Primate erythrocyte-immune complex-clearing mechanism. *J Clin Invest* 1983; 71:236–247.
25. Manthei U, Nickells MW, Barnes SH, et al. Identification of a C3b/iC3b binding protein of rabbit platelets and leukocytes. A CR1-like candidate for the immune adherence receptor. *J Immunol* 1988;140:1228–1235.
26. Taylor RP, Kujala G, Wilson K, et al. In vivo and in vitro studies of the binding of antibody/dsDNA immune complexes to rabbit and guinea pig platelets. *J Immunol* 1985;134: 2550–2558.
27. Nelson DS. Immune adherence. *Adv Immunol* 1963;3: 131–180.
28. Edberg JC, Kujala GA, Taylor RP. Rapid immune adherence reactivity of nascent, soluble antibody/DNA immune complexes in the circulation. *J Immunol* 1987;139:1240–1244.
29. Dykman TR, Cole JL, Iida K, et al. Polymorphism of the human erythrocyte C3b/C4b receptor. *Proc Natl Acad Sci USA* 1983;80:1698–1702.
30. Dykman TR, Hatch JA, Atkinson JP. Polymorphism of the human C3b/C4b receptors: identification of third allele and analysis of receptor phenotypes in families and patients with systemic lupus. *J Exp Med* 1989;159:691–703.
31. Holers VM, Seya T, Brown E, et al. Structural and functional studies on the human C3b/C4b receptor (CR1) purified by affinity chromatography using a monoclonal antibody. *Complement* 1986;3:63–78.
32. Wong WW, Wilson JG, Fearon DT. Genetic regulation of a structural polymorphism of human C3b receptor. *J Clin Invest* 1983;72:685–693.
33. Klickstein LB, Wong WW, Smith JA, et al. Human C3b/C4b receptor: demonstration of long homologous repeating domains that are composed of the short consensus repeats characteristic of C3/C4 binding proteins. *J Exp Med* 1987;165:1095–1112.
34. Walport MJ, Ross GD, Mackworth-Young C, et al. Family studies of erythrocyte complement type 1 levels: reduced levels in patients with SLE are acquired, not inherited. *Clin Exp Immunol* 1985;59:547–554.
35. Wilson JG, Fearon DT. Altered expression of complement receptors as a pathogenic factor in systemic lupus erythematosus. *Arthritis Rheum* 1984;27:1321–1328.
36. Wilson JG, Murphy EE, Wong WW, et al. Identification of a restriction fragment length polymorphism by a CR1 cDNA that correlates with the number on erythrocytes. *J Exp Med* 1986;164:50–59.
37. Wilson JG, Wong WW, Murphy EE, et al. Deficiency of the C3b/C4b receptor (CR1) of erythrocytes in systemic lupus erythematosus: analysis of the stability of the defect and of a restriction fragment length polymorphism of the CR1 gene. *J Immunol* 1987;138:2706–2710.
38. Wilson JG, Wong WW, Schur PH, et al. Mode of inheritance of decreased C3b receptors on erythrocytes of patients with systemic lupus erythematosus. *N Engl J Med* 1982;307:981–986.
39. Moldenhauer F, David J, Felder AHL, et al. Inherited deficiency of erythrocyte complement receptor type 1 does not cause sus-

ceptibility to systemic lupus erythematosus. *Arthritis Rheum* 1988;30:961–966.
40. Hebert LA, Cosio FG. The erythrocyte-immune complex-glomerulonephritis connection in man. *Kidney Int* 1987;31: 877–885.
41. Schifferli JA, Ng YC, Peters DK. The role of complement and its receptor in the elimination of immune complexes. *N Engl J Med* 1986;315:488–495.
42. Chevalier J, Kazatchkine MD. Distribution in clusters of complement receptor type one (CR1) on human erythrocytes. *J Immunol* 1989;142:2031–2036.
43. Edberg JC, Wright E, Taylor RP. Quantitative analyses of the binding of soluble complement-fixing antibody/dsDNA immune complexes to CR1 on human red blood cells. *J Immunol* 1987;139:3739–3747.
44. Horgan C, Taylor RP. Studies on the kinetics of binding of complement-fixing dsdna/anti-DNA immune complexes to the red blood cells of normal individuals and patients with systemic lupus erythematosus. *Arthritis Rheum* 1984;27:320–329.
45. Paccaud J-P, Carpentier J-L, Schifferli JA. Direct evidence for the clustered nature of complement receptors type I on the erythrocyte membrane. *J Immunol* 1988;141:3889–3894.
46. Davies KA, Hird V, Stewart S, et al. A study of in vivo immune complex formation and clearance in man. *J Immunol* 1990; 144:4613–4620.
47. Kimberly RP, Edberg JC, Merriam LT, et al. In vivo handling of soluble complement fixing Ab/dsDNA immune complexes in chimpanzees. *J Clin Invest* 1989;84:962–970.
48. Schifferli JA, Ng YC, Estreicher J, et al. The clearance of tetanus toxoid/anti-tetanus toxoid immune complexes from the circulation of humans. Complement- and erythrocyte complement receptor 1-dependent mechanisms. *J Immunol* 1988;140: 899–904.
49. Schifferli JA, Ng YC, Paccaud J-P, et al. The role of hypocomplementaemia and low erythrocyte complement receptor type 1 numbers in determining abnormal immune complex clearance in humans. *Clin Exp Immunol* 1989;75:329–335.
50. Waxman FJ, Hebert LA, Cornacoff JB, et al. Complement depletion accelerates the clearance of immune complexes from the circulation of primates. *J Clin Invest* 1984;74:1329–1340.
51. Hebert LA, Cosio FG, Birmingham DJ, et al. Experimental immune complex-mediated glomerulonephritis in the nonhuman primate. *Kidney Int* 1991;39:44–56.
52. Waxman FJ, Hebert LA, Cosio FG, et al. Differential binding of immunoglobulin A and immunoglobulin G1 immune complexes to primate erythrocytes in vivo: immunoglobulin A immune complexes bind less well to erythrocytes and are preferentially deposited in glomeruli. *J Clin Invest* 1986;77:82–89.
53. Edberg JC, Tosic CL, Wright E, et al. Quantitative analysis of the relationship between C3 consumption, C3b capture, and immune adherence of complement fixing antibody/DNA complexes. *J Immunol* 1988;141:4258–4265.
54. Madi N, Steiger G, Estreicher J, et al. Defective immune adherence and elimination of hepatitis B surface antigen/antibody complexes in patients with mixed essential cryoglobulinemia type II. *J Immunol* 1991;147:495–502.
55. Horgan C, Burge J, Crawford L, et al. The kinetics of dsDNA/anti-DNA immune complex formation, binding by red blood cells, and release into serum: effect of DNA m.w. and conditions of antibody excess. *J Immunol* 1984;133: 2079–2084.
56. Medof ME. Complement-dependent maintenance of immune complex solubility. In: Rother K, Till GO, eds. *The complement system*. Berlin: Springer-Verlag, 1988:418–443.
57. Medof ME, Iida K, Mold C, et al. Unique role of the complement receptor CR1 in the degradation of C3b associated with immune complexes. *J Exp Med* 1982;156:1739–1754.
58. Ross GD, Lambris JD, Cain JA, et al. Generation of three different fragments of bound C3 with purified factor I or serum: requirement of factor H vs CR1 cofactor activity. *J Immunol* 1982;129:2051–2060.
59. Davis AE, Harrison RA, Lachmann PJ. Physiologic inactivation of fluid phase C3b: isolation and structural analysis of C3c, C3dg, and C3g. *J Immunol* 1984;132:1960–1966.
60. Medof ME, Lam T, Prince GM, et al. Requirement for human red cells in inactivation of C3b in immune complexes and enhancement of binding to spleen cells. *J Immunol* 1983; 130:1336–1340.
61. Hosea SW, Brown EJ, Hamburger MI, et al. Opsonic requirements for intravascular clearance after splenectomy. *N Engl J Med* 1981;304:245–250.
62. Lobatto S, Daha MR, Breedveld FC, et al. Abnormal clearance of soluble aggregates of human immunoglobulin G in patients with systemic lupus erythematosus. *Clin Exp Immunol* 1988; 72:55–59.
63. Medof ME, Prince GM, Mold C. Release of soluble immune complexes from immune adherence receptors on human erythrocytes is mediated by C3b inactivator independently of B1H and is accompanied by generation of C3c. *Proc Natl Acad Sci USA* 1982;79:5047–5051.
64. Frank MM, Hamburger MI, Lawley TJ, et al. Defective reticuloendothelial system Fc-receptor function in systemic lupus erythematosus. *N Engl J Med* 1979;300:518–523.
65. Schreiber AD, Frank MM. The role of antibody and complement in the immune clearance and destruction of erythrocytes. I. In vivo effects of IgG and IgM complement fixing sites. *J Clin Invest* 1972;51:575–582.
66. Meryhew N, Runquist OA. A kinetic analysis of immune-mediated clearance of erythrocytes. *J Immunol* 1981;126: 2443–2449.
67. Kimberly RP, Meryhew NL, Runquist OA. Mononuclear phagocyte function in SLE. I. Bipartite Fc- and complement-dependent dysfunction. *J Immunol* 1986;137:91–96.
68. Meryhew NL, Kimberly RP, Messner RP, et al. Mononuclear phagocyte system in SLE. II. A kinetic model of immune complex handling in systemic lupus erythematosus. *J Immunol* 1986;137:97–102.
69. Meryhew NL, Messner RP, Wasiluk KR, et al. Assessment of mononuclear phagocyte system function by clearance of anti-D sensitized erythrocytes: the role of complement. *J Lab Clin Med* 1985;105:277–281.
70. Kimberly RP, Parris TM, Inman RD, et al. Dynamics of mononuclear phagocyte system Fc receptor function in systemic lupus erythematosus. Relation to disease activity and circulating immune complexes. *Clin Exp Immunol* 1983;51: 261–268.
71. Hamburger MI, Lawley TJ, Kimberly RP, et al. A serial study of splenic reticuloendothelial system Fc receptor functional activity in systemic lupus erythematosus. *Arthritis Rheum* 1982;25; 48–54.
72. Parris TM, Kimberly RP, Inman RD, et al. Defective Fc receptor-mediated function of the mononuclear phagocyte system in lupus nephritis. *Ann Intern Med* 1982;97:526–532.
73. Van der Woude FJ, Van der Giessen M, Kallenberg GM, et al. Reticuloendothelial Fc receptor function in SLE patients. I. Primary HLA linked defect or acquired dysfunction secondary to disease activity. *Clin Exp Immunol* 1984;55:473–480.
74. Elkon KB, Sewell JR, Ryan PF, et al. Splenic function in nonrenal systemic lupus erythematosus. *Am J Med* 1980;69:80–82.
75. Kabbash L, Esdaile J, Shenker S, et al. Reticuloendothelial sys-

tem Fc receptor function in systemic lupus erythematosus. *J Rheumatol* 1982;9:374–379.
76. Meryhew NL, Shaver C, Messner RP, et al. Mononuclear phagocyte system dysfunction in murine SLE: abnormal clearance kinetics precedes clinical disease. *J Lab Clin Med* 1991; 117:181–193.
77. Kimberly RP, Gibofsky A, Salmon JE, et al. Impaired Fc-mediated mononuclear phagocyte system clearance in HLA-DR2 and MT1-positive healthy young adults. *J Exp Med* 1983;157: 1698–1703.
78. Lawley TJ. Immune complexes and reticuloendothelial system function in human disease. *J Invest Dermatol* 1980;74:339–343.
79. Halma C, Breedveld FC, Daha MR, et al. Elimination of soluble 123I-labeled aggregates of IgG in patients with systemic lupus erythematosus. Effect of serum IgG and number of erythrocyte complement receptor type 1. *Arthritis Rheum* 1991; 34:442–452.
80. Ross GD, Yount WJ, Walport MJ, et al. Disease-associated loss of erythrocyte complement receptors (CR1, C3b receptors) in patients with systemic lupus erythematosus and other diseases involving autoantibodies and/or complement activation. *J Immunol* 1985;135:2005–2014.
81. Walport MJ, Lachmann PJ. Erythrocyte complement receptor type 1, immune complexes, and the rheumatic diseases. *Arthritis Rheum* 1988;31:153–158.
82. Halma C, Daha MR, van Furth R, et al. Elimination of soluble 123I-labeled aggregates of IgG in humans: the effects of splenectomy. *Clin Exp Immunol* 1989;77:62–66.
83. Davies KA, Peters AM, Beynon HL, et al. Immune complex processing in patients with systemic lupus erythematosus. In vivo imaging and clearance studies. *J Clin Invest* 1992;90: 2075–2083.
84. Davies KA, Erlendsson K, Beynon HL, et al. Splenic uptake of immune complexes in man is complement-dependent. *J Immunol* 1993;151:3866–3873.
85. Kelton JG, Singer J, Rodger C, et al. The concentration of IgG in the serum is a major determinant of Fc-dependent reticuloendothelial function. *Blood* 1985;66:490–495.
86. Kimberly RP, Salmon JE, Bussel JB, et al. Modulation of mononuclear phagocyte function by intravenous gamma-globulin. *J Immunol* 1984;132:745–750.
87. Ravetch JV, Kinet JP. Fc receptors. *Annu Rev Immunol* 1991;9: 457–492.
88. Heijen IA, van de Winkel JG. Human IgG Fc receptors. *Int Rev Immunol* 1997;16:29–55.
89. Hulett MD, Hogarth PM. Molecular basis of Fc receptor function. *Adv Immunol* 1994;57:1–127.
90. Salmon JE, Pricop L. Human receptors for immunoglobulin G: Key elements in the pathogenesis of rheumatic disease. *Arthritis Rheum* 2001;44:739–750.
91. Kimberly RP, Salmon JE, Edberg JC. Receptors for immunoglobulin G. Molecular diversity and implications for disease. *Arthritis Rheum* 1995;38:306–314.
92. Daeron M. Fc receptor biology. *Annu Rev Immunol* 1997;15: 203–234.
93. Grundy HO, Peltz G, Moore KW, et al. The polymorphic Fc receptor II gene maps to human chromosome 1q. *Immunogenetics* 1989;29:331–339.
94. Qiu WQ, de Bruin D, Brownstein BH, et al. Organization of the human and mouse low affinity Fc R genes: evidence for duplication and recombination. *Science* 1990;248:732–735.
95. Peltz GA, Grundy HO, Lebo RV, et al. Human FcγRIII: cloning, expression, and identification of the chromosomal locus of two Fc receptors for IgG. *Proc Natl Acad Sci USA* 1989;86:1013–1017.
96. Reth M. Antigen receptor tail clue [letter]. *Nature* 1989;338: 383–384.
97. Cambier JC. Antigen and Fc receptor signaling. The awesome power of the immunoreceptor tyrosine-based activation motif (ITAM). *J Immunol* 1995;155:3281–3285.
98. Warmerdam PA, van de Winkel JG, Vlug A, et al. A single amino acid in the second Ig-like domain of the human Fcγ receptor II is critical for human IgG2 binding. *J Immunol* 1991; 147:1338–1343.
99. Salmon JE, Edberg JC, Brogle NL, et al. Allelic polymorphisms of human Fcγ receptor IIA and Fcγ receptor IIIB. Independent mechanisms for differences in human phagocyte function. *J Clin Invest* 1992;89:1274–1281.
100. Wu J, Edberg JC, Redecha PB, et al. A novel polymorphism of FcγRIIIa (CD16) alters receptor function and predisposes to autoimmune disease. *J Clin Invest* 1997;100:1059–1070.
101. Muta T, Kurosaki T, Misulovin Z, et al. A 13-amino-acid motif in the cytoplasmic domain of FcγRIIB modulates B-cell receptor signalling. *Nature* 1994;368:70–73.
102. Anderson CL. Isolation of the receptor for IgG from a human monocyte cell line (U937) and from human peripheral blood monocytes. *J Exp Med* 1982;156:1794–1806.
103. Allen JM, Seed B. Isolation and expression of functional high affinity Fc receptor cDNAs. *Science* 1989;243:378–380.
104. Van de Winkel JGJ, Ernst LK, Anderson CL, et al. Gene organization of the human high affinity receptor for IgG, FcRI (CD64): characterization and evidence for a second gene. *J Biol Chem* 1991;266:13449–13455.
105. Ernst LK, van de Winkel JGJ, Chiu I-M, et al. Three genes for the human high affinity Fc receptor for IgG (FcR1) encode four distinct transcription products. *J Biol Chem* 1992;267: 15692–15700.
106. Ernst LK, Duchemin A-M, Anderson CL. Association of the high affinity receptor for IgG (FcγRI) with the γ-subunit of the IgE receptor. *Proc Natl Acad Sci USA* 1993;90:6023–6027.
107. Fanger NA, Voigtlaender D, Lui C, et al. Characterization of expression, cytokine regulation, and effector function of the high affinity IgG receptor FcγRI (CD64) expressed on human dendritic cells. *J Immunol* 1997;158:3090–3098.
108. Guyre PM, Morganelli PM, Miller R. Recombinant immune interferon increases immunoglobulin G Fc receptors on cultured human mononuclear phagocytes. *J Clin Invest* 1983;72: 393–397.
109. Perussia B, Dayton ET, Lazarus R, et al. Immune interferon induces the receptor for monomeric IgG1 on human monocytic and myeloid cells. *J Exp Med* 1983;158:1092–1113.
110. Shen L, Guyre PM, Fanger MW. Polymorphonuclear leukocyte function triggered through the high affinity Fc receptor for monomeric IgG. *J Immunol* 1987;139:534–538.
111. Buckle A, Hoss N. The effect of IFN- and colony-stimulating factors on the expression of neutrophil cell membrane receptors. *J Immunol* 1989;143:2295–2301.
112. Looney RJ, Abraham GN, Anderson CL. Human monocytes and U937 cells bear two distinct Fc receptors for IgG. *J Immunol* 1986;136:1641–1647.
113. Looney RJ, Anderson CL, Ryan DH, et al. Structural polymorphism of the human platelet Fc receptor. *J Immunol* 1988;141: 2680–2683.
114. Looney RJ, Ryan DH, Takahashi K, et al. Identification of a second class of IgG Fc receptors on human neutrophils: a 40 kD molecule also found on eosinophils. *J Exp Med* 1986;163: 826–836.
115. Fanger MW, Shen L, Graziano RF, et al. Cytotoxicity mediated by human Fc receptors for IgG. *Immunol Today* 1989;10:92–99.
116. Brooks DG, Qiu WQ, Luster AD, et al. Structure and expression of a human IgG FcRII (CD32): functional heterogeneity is encoded by the alternatively spliced products of multiple genes. *J Exp Med* 1989;170:1369–1386.

117. Metes D, Ernst LK, Chambers WH, et al. Expression of functional CD32 molecules on human NK cells is determined by an allelic polymorphism of the FcγRIIC gene. *Blood* 1998;91: 2369–2380.
118. Van Den Herik-Oudijk IE, Westerdaal NA, Henriquez NV, et al. Functional analysis of human FcγRII (CD32) isoforms expressed in B lymphocytes. *J Immunol* 1994;152:574–585.
119. Daeron M, Latour S, Malbec O, et al. The same tyrosine-based inhibition motif, in the intracytoplasmic domain of FcγRIIB, regulates negatively BCR-, TCR-, and FcR-dependent cell activation. *Immunity* 1995;3:635–646.
120. Daeron M, Malbec O, Latour S, et al. Regulation of high-affinity IgE receptor-mediated mast cell activation by murine low-affinity IgG receptors. *J Clin Invest* 1995;95:577–585.
121. Hunter S, Indik ZK, Kim MK, et al. Inhibition of Fcγ receptor-mediated phagocytosis by a nonphagocytic Fcγ receptor. *Blood* 1998;91:1762–1768.
122. Phillips NE, Parker DC. Cross-linking of B lymphocyte Fcγ receptors and membrane immunoglobulin inhibits anti-immunoglobulin-induced blastogenesis. *J Immunol* 1984;132:627–632.
123. Kurosaki T, Ravetch JV. A single amino acid in the glycosyl phosphatidylinositol attachment domain determines the membrane topology of FcRIII. *Nature* 1989;342:805–807.
124. Passlick B, Flieger D, Siegler-Heitbrock HWL. Identification and characterization of a novel monocyte subpopulation in human peripheral blood. *Blood* 1989;74:2527–2534.
125. Santiago A, Satriano J, DeCandido S, et al. Specific Fc receptor on cultured rat mesangial cells. *J Immunol* 1989;143:2575–2582.
126. Edberg JC, Barinsky M, Redecha PB, et al. FcRIII expressed on cultured monocytes is a N-glycosylated transmembrane protein distinct from FcRIII expressed on natural killer cells. *J Immunol* 1990;144:4729–4734.
127. Anderson P, Caligiuri M, O'Brien C, et al. Fc receptor type III (CD16) is included in the NK receptor complex expressed by human natural killer cells. *Proc Natl Acad Sci USA* 1990;87: 2274–2278.
128. Kurosaki T, Gander I, Wirthmueller U, et al. The β subunit of FceRI is associated with FcγRIII on mast cells. *J Exp Med* 1992; 175:447–451.
129. Ravetch JV, Perussia B. Alternative membrane forms of FcRIII (CD16) on human NK cells and neutrophils: cell-type specific expression of two genes which differ in single nucleotide substitutions. *J Exp Med* 1989;170:481–497.
130. Selvaraj P, Rosse WF, Silber R, et al. The major Fc receptor in blood has a phosphatidylinositol anchor and deficient in paroxysmal nocturnal haemoglobinuria. *Nature* 1988;333:565–567.
131. Huizinga TWJ, Kleijer M, Tetteroo PAT, et al. Biallelic neutrophil NA-antigen system is associated with a polymorphism on the phosphoinositol-linked Fc receptor III (CD16). *Blood* 1990;75:213–217.
132. Ory PA, Goldstein IM, Kwoh EE, et al. Characterization of polymorphic forms of FcRIII on human neutrophils. *J Clin Invest* 1989;83:1676–1681.
133. de Haas M, Koene HR, Kleijer M, et al. A triallelic Fcγ receptor type IIIA polymorphism influences the binding of human IgG by NK cell FcγRIIIa. *J Immunol* 1996;156:3948–3955.
134. Koene HR, Kleijer M, Algra J, et al. FcγRIIIa-158V/F polymorphism influences the binding of IgG by natural killer cell FcγRIIIa, independently of the FcγRIIIa-48L/R/H phenotype. Blood 1997;90:1109–1114.
135. Huizinga TWJ, De Haas M, Kleijer M, et al. Soluble Fc receptor III in human plasma originates from release by neutrophils. *J Clin Invest* 1990;86:416–423.
136. de Haas M, Kleijer M, Minchinton RM, et al. Soluble FcγRIIIa is present in plasma and is derived from natural killer cells. *J Immunol* 1994;152:900–907.
137. Rappaport EF, Cassel DL, McKenzie SE, et al. A soluble form of the human Fc receptor FcγRIIA: cloning, transcript analysis and detection. Exp Hematol 1993;21:689–696.
138. Bich-Yhuy LT, Samarut C, Brochier J, et al. Suppression of the late stages of mitogen-induced human B-cell differentiation by Fc receptors released from polymorphonuclear neutrophils. *J Immunol* 1981;127:1299–1403.
139. Jeffries R. Structure/function relationships of IgG subclasses. In: Shakib F, ed. *The human IgG subclasses: molecular analysis of structure, function, and regulation.* Oxford: Pergamon Press, 1990:93–108.
140. Parren P, Warmerdam PAM, Boeiji LCM, et al. On the interaction of IgG subclasses with the low affinity FcRIIA (CD32) on human monocytes, neutrophils and platelets. Analysis of a functional polymorphism to human IgG2. *J Clin Invest* 1992;90: 1537–1546.
141. Salmon JE, Kapur S, Kimberly RP. Opsonin-independent ligation of Fcγ receptors. The 3G8-bearing receptors on neutrophils mediate the phagocytosis of concanavalin-A treated erythrocytes and non-opsonized Escherichia coli. *J Exp Med* 1987;166:1798–1813.
142. Salmon JE, Kimberly RP. Phagocytosis of concanavalin A-treated erythrocytes is mediated by the Fcγ receptor. *J Immunol* 1986;137:456–462.
143. Marnell LL, Mold C, Volzer MA, et al. C-reactive protein binds to FcγRI in transfected COS cells. *J Immunol* 1995;155: 2185–2193.
144. Bharadwaj D, Stein MP, Volzer M, et al. The major receptor for C-reactive protein on leukocytes is Fcγ receptor II. *J Exp Med* 1999;190:585–590.
145. Stein MP, Edberg JC, Kimberly RP, et al. C-reactive protein binding to FcγRIIa on human monocytes and neutrophils is allele-specific. *J Clin Invest* 2000;105:369–376.
146. Lowry MB, Duchemin AM, Coggeshall KM, et al. Chimeric receptors composed of phosphoinositide 3-kinase domains and Fcγ receptor ligand-binding domains mediate phagocytosis in COS fibroblasts. *J Biol Chem* 1998;273:24513–24520.
147. Karimi K, Lennartz MR. Mitogen-activated protein kinase is activated during IgG-mediated phagocytosis, but is not required for target ingestion. *Inflammation* 1998;22:67–82.
148. Bolland S, Ravetch JV. Inhibitory pathways triggered by ITIM-containing receptors. *Adv Immunol* 1999;72:149–177.
149. Malbec O, Fridman WH, Daeron M. Negative regulation of hematopoietic cell activation and proliferation by FcγRIIB. *Curr Top Microbiol Immunol* 1999;244:13–27.
150. Coggeshall KM. Negative signaling in health and disease. *Immunol Res* 1999;19:47–64.
151. Ono M, Bolland S, Tempst P, et al. Role of the inositol phosphatase SHIP in negative regulation of the immune system by the receptor FcγRIIB. *Nature* 1996;383:263–266.
152. Bolland S, Pearse RN, Kurosaki T, et al. SHIP modulates immune receptor responses by regulating membrane association of Btk. *Immunity* 1998;8:509–516.
153. Chacko GW, Tridandapani S, Damen JE, et al. Negative signaling in B lymphocytes induces tyrosine phosphorylation of the 145-kDa inositol polyphosphate 5-phosphatase, SHIP. *J Immunol* 1996;157:2234–2238.
154. Anegon I, Cuturi MC, Trinchieri G, et al. Interaction of Fc receptor (CD16) ligands induces transcription of interleukin 2 receptor (CD25) and lymphokine genes and expression of their products in human natural killer cells. *J Exp Med* 1988;167: 452–472.
155. Cardella CJ, Davies P, Allison AC. Immune complexes induce selective release of lysosomal hydrolyses from macrophages. *Nature* 1974;247:46–48.
156. Debets JMH, van de Winkel JGJ, Ceuppens JL, et al. Cross-

linking of both FcRI and FcRII induces secretion of tumor necrosis factor by human monocytes, requiring high affinity Fc-FcR interactions. *J Immunol* 1990;144:1304–1310.
157. Krutmann J, Kirnbauer R, Kock A, et al. Cross-linking Fc receptors on monocytes triggers IL-6 production. *J Immunol* 1990;145:1337–1342.
158. Rouzer CA, Scott WA, Kempe J, et al. Prostaglandin synthesis by macrophages requires a specific receptor-ligand interaction. *Proc Natl Acad Sci USA* 1980;77:4279–4282.
159. Anderson CL, Shen L, Eicher DM, et al. Phagocytes mediated by three distinct Fc receptor classes on human leukocytes. *J Exp Med* 1990;171:1333–1345.
160. Gomez F, Chien P, King M, et al. Monocyte Fc receptor recognition of cell-bound and aggregated IgG. *Blood* 1989;74: 1058–1065.
161. Clarkson SB, Bussel JB, Kimberly RP, et al. Treatment of refractory immune thrombocytopenic purpura with an anti-Fcγ receptor antibody. *N Engl J Med* 1986;314:1236–1239.
162. Clarkson SB, Kimberly RP, Valinsky JE, et al. Blockade of clearance of immune complexes by an anti-Fcγ receptor monoclonal antibody *J Exp Med* 1986;164:473–489.
163. Edberg JC, Kimberly RP. Receptor-specific probes for the study of Fc receptor specific function. *J Immunol Methods* 1992;148:179–187.
164. Edberg JC, Kimberly RP. Modulation of Fc and complement receptor function by the glycosyl-phosphatidylinositol-anchored form of FcRIII. *J Immunol* 1994;152:5826–5835.
165. Salmon JE, Brogle NL, Edberg JE, et al. Fc receptor III induces actin polymerization in human neutrophils and primes phagocytosis mediated by Fc receptor II. *J Immunol* 1991;146: 997–1004.
166. Salmon JE, Millard SS, Brogle NL, et al. Fc receptor IIIb enhances Fc receptor IIa function in an oxidant-dependent and allele-sensitive. *J Clin Invest* 1995;95:2877–2885.
167. Pan LY, Mendel DB, Zurlo J, et al. Regulation of the steady state level of FcγRI mRNA by IFN-γ and dexamethasone in human monocytes, neutrophils, and U-937 cells. *J Immunol* 1990;145:267–275.
168. te Velde AA, Huijbens RJ, de Vries JE, et al. IL-4 decreases FcγR membrane expression and FcγR-mediated cytotoxic activity of human monocytes. *J Immunol* 1990;144:3046–3051.
169. Welch GR, Wong HL, Wahl SM. Selective induction of FcγRIII on human monocytes by transforming growth factor-beta. *J Immunol* 1990;144:3444–3448.
170. Pricop L, Redecha P, Teillaud J-L, et al. Differential modulation of stimulatory and inhibitory Fcγ receptors on human monocytes by TH1 and TH2 cytokines. *J Immmunol* 2001;166:531–537.
171. Ceuppens JL, Baroja ML, Van Vaeck F, et al. A defect in the membrane expression of high affinity 72 kD Fc receptors on phagocytic cells in four healthy subjects. *J Clin Invest* 1988;82: 571–578.
172. Clark MR, Lui L, Clarkson SB, et al. An abnormality of the gene that encodes neutrophil Fc receptor III in a patient with systemic lupus erythematosus. *J Clin Invest* 1990;86:341–346.
173. Huizinga TWJ, Kuijpers RWAM, Kleijer M, et al. Maternal genomic neutrophil FcRIII deficiency leading to neonatal isoimmune neutropenia. *Blood* 1990;76:1927–1932.
174. Stroncek D, Skubitz KM, Plachta LB, S et al. Alloimmune neonatal neutropenia due to an antibody to the neutrophil Fc receptor III with maternal deficiency of CD16 antigen. *Blood* 1991;77:1572–1580.
175. Fromont P, Bettaieb A, Skouri H, et al. Frequency of the polymorphonuclear neutrophil FcRIII deficiency in the French population and its involvement in the development of neonatal alloimmune neutropenia. *Blood* 1992;79:2131–2134.
176. Cartron J, Celton JL, Gane P, et al. Iso-immune neonatal neutropenia due to an anti-Fc receptor III (CD16) antibody. *Eur J Pediatr* 1992;151:438–441.
177. Enenkel B, Jung D, Frey J. Molecular basis of IgG Fc receptor III defect in a patient with systemic lupus erythematosus. *Eur J Immunol* 1991;21:659–663.
178. Luan JJ, Monteiro RC, Sautes C, et al. Defective FcγRII gene expression in macrophages of NOD mice: genetic linkage with up-regulation of IgG1 and IgG2b in serum. *J Immunol* 1996;157:4707–4716.
179. Pritchard NR, Cutler AJ, Uribe S, et al. Autoimmune-prone mice share a promoter haplotype associated with reduced expression and function of the Fc receptor FcγRII. *Curr Biol* 2000;10:227–230.
180. Jiang Y, Hirose S, Abe M, et al. Polymorphisms in IgG Fc receptor IIB regulatory regions associated with autoimmune susceptibility. *Immunogenetics* 2000;51:429–435.
181. Clark MR, Stuart SG, Kimberly RP, et al. A single amino acid distinguishes the high-responder from the low-responder form of Fc receptor II on human monocytes. *Eur J Immunol* 1991; 21:1911–1916.
182. Lehrnbecher T, Foster CB, Zhu S, et al. Variant genotypes of the low-affinity Fcγ receptors in two control populations and a review of low-affinity Fcγ receptor polymorphisms in control and disease populations. *Blood* 1999;94:4220–4232.
183. Sanders LA, van de Winkel JG, Rijkers GT, et al. Fcγ receptor IIa (CD32) heterogeneity in patients with recurrent bacterial respiratory tract infections. *J Infect Dis* 1994;170: 854–861.
184. Bredius RG, Derkx BH, Fijen CA, et al. Fcγ receptor IIa (CD32) polymorphism in fulminant meningococcal septic shock in children. *J Infect Dis* 1994;170:848–853.
185. Platonov AE, Shipulin GA, Vershinina IV, et al. Association of human FcγRIIa (CD32) polymorphism with susceptibility to and severity of meningococcal disease. *Clin Infect Dis* 1998;27: 746–750.
186. Yee AM, Ng SC, Sobel RE, et al. FcγRIIA polymorphism as a risk factor for invasive pneumococcal infections in systemic lupus erythematosus. *Arthritis Rheum* 1997;40:1180–1182.
187. de Haas M, Koene HR, Kleijer M, et al. A triallelic Fcγreceptor type IIIA polymorphism influences the binding of human IgG by NK cell FcγRIIIa. *J Immunol* 1996;156: 3948–3955.
188. Koene HR, Kleijer M, Algra J, et al. FcγRIIIa-158V/F polymorphism influences the binding of IgG by natural killer cell FcγRIIIa, independently of the FcγRIIIa-48L/R/H phenotype. *Blood* 1997;90:1109–1114.
189. Salmon JE, Edberg JC, Kimberly RP. Fcγ receptor III on human neutrophils. Allelic variants have functionally distinct capacities. *J Clin Invest* 1990;85:1287–1295.
190. Bredius RG, Fijen CA, De Haas M, et al. Role of neutrophil FcγRIIa (CD32) and FcγRIIIb (CD16) polymorphic forms in phagocytosis of human IgG1- and IgG3-opsonized bacteria and erythrocytes. *Immunology* 1994;83:624–630.
191. Platonov AE, Kuijper EJ, Vershinina IV, et al. Meningococcal disease and polymorphism of FcγRIIa (CD32) in late complement component-deficient individuals. *Clin Exp Immunol* 1998;111:97–101.
192. Mellman IS, Plutner H, Steinman RM, et al. Internalization and degradation of macrophage Fc receptors during receptor-mediated phagocytosis. *J Cell Biol* 1983;96:887–895.
193. Michl J, Unkeless JC, Pieczonka MM, et al. Modulation of Fc receptors of mononuclear phagocytes by immobilized antigen-antibody complexes. *J Exp Med* 1983;157:1746–1757.
194. Fries LF, Mullin WW, Cho KR, et al. Monocyte receptors for the Fc portion of IgG are increased in systemic lupus erythematosus. *J Immunol* 1984;132:695–700.

195. Kavai M, Lukacs K, Sonkloly I, et al. Circulating immune complexes and monocyte Fc receptor function in autoimmune diseases. *Ann Rheum Dis* 1979;38:79–83.
196. Salmon JE, Kimberly RP, Gibofsky A, et al. Defective mononuclear phagocyte function in systemic lupus erythematosus: dissociation of Fc receptor-ligand binding and internalization. *J Immunol* 1984;133:2525–2531.
197. Kavai M, Zsindely A, Sonkloly I, et al. Signals of monocyte activation in patients with SLE. *Clin Exp Immunol* 1983;51: 255–260.
198. Salmon JE, Kapur S, Meryhew NL, et al. High-dose, pulse intravenous methylprednisolone enhances Fc receptor-mediated mononuclear phagocyte function in systemic lupus erythematosus. *Arthritis Rheum* 1989;32:717–725.
199. Salmon JE, Kimberly RP, Gibofsky A, et al. Altered phagocytosis by monocytes from HLA-DR2 and DR3-positive healthy adults is Fc receptor-specific. *J Immunol* 1986;136: 3625–3632.
200. Salmon JE, Millard S, Schachter LA, et al. Fcγ RIIA alleles are heritable risk factors for lupus nephritis in African Americans. *J Clin Invest* 1996;97:1348–1354.
201. Duits AJ, Bootsma H, Derksen RHWM, et al. Skewed distribution of IgG Fc receptor IIa (CD32) polymorphism is associated with renal disease in SLE patients. *Arthritis Rheum* 1996; 38:1832–1836.
202. Salmon JE, Ng S, Yoo DH, et al. Altered distribution of Fcγ receptor IIIA alleles in a cohort of Korean patients with lupus nephritis. *Arthritis Rheum* 1999;42:818–819.
203. Koene HR, Kleijer M, Swaak AJ, et al. The FcγRIIIA-158F allele is a risk factor for systemic lupus erythematosus. *Arthritis Rheum* 1998;41:1813–1818.
204. Manger K, Repp R, Spriewald BM, et al. Fcγ receptor IIa polymorphism in Caucasian patients with systemic lupus erythematosus: association with clinical symptoms. *Arthritis Rheum* 1998;41:1181–1189.
205. Song YW, Han CW, Kang SW, et al. Abnormal distribution of Fcγ receptor type IIa polymorphisms in Korean patients with systemic lupus erythematosus. *Arthritis Rheum* 1998;41: 421–426.
206. Moser KL, Neas BR, Salmon JE, et al. Genome scan of human systemic lupus erythematosus: evidence for linkage on chromosome 1q in African-American pedigrees. *Proc Natl Acad Sci USA* 1998;95:14869–14674.
207. Botto M, Theodoridis E, Thompson EM, et al. FcγRIIa polymorphism in systemic lupus erythematosus (SLE): no association with disease. *Clin Exp Immunol* 1996;104:264–268.
208. Smyth LJ, Snowden N, Carthy D, et al. FcγRIIa polymorphism in systemic lupus erythematosus. *Ann Rheum Dis* 1997;56: 744–746.
209. Oh M, Petri MA, Kim NA, et al. Frequency of the FcγRIIIA-158F allele in African American patients with systemic lupus erythematosus. *J Rheumatol* 1999;26:1486–1489.
210. Haseley LA, Wisnieski JJ, Denburg MR, et al. Antibodies to C1q in systemic lupus erythematosus: characteristics and relation to FcγRIIA alleles. *Kidney Int* 1997;52:1375–1380.
211. Norsworthy P, Theodoridis E, Botto M, et al. Overrepresentation of the Fcγ receptor type IIA R131/R131 genotype in caucasoid systemic lupus erythematosus patients with autoantibodies to C1q and glomerulonephritis. *Arthritis Rheum* 1999;42: 1828–1832.
212. Amoura Z, Koutouzov S, Chabre H, et al. Presence of antinucleosome autoantibodies in a restricted set of connective tissue diseases: antinucleosome antibodies of the IgG3 subclass are markers of renal pathogenicity in systemic lupus erythematosus. *Arthritis Rheum* 2000;43:76–84.
213. Zouali M, Jefferis R, Eyquem A. IgG subclass distribution of autoantibodies to DNA and to nuclear ribonucleoproteins in autoimmune diseases. *Immunology* 1984;51:595–600.
214. Lewis EJ, Busch GJ, Schur PH. Gamma G globulin subgroup composition of the glomerular deposits in human renal diseases. *J Clin Invest* 1970;49:1103–1113.
215. Imai H, Hamai K, Komatsuda A, et al. IgG subclasses in patients with membranoproliferative glomerulonephritis, membranous nephropathy, and lupus nephritis. *Kidney Int* 1997;51: 270–276.
216. Zuniga R, Markowitz, D'Agati V, et al. IgG subclass glomerular deposition and its relationship to FcγRIIA alleles in lupus. *Arthritis Rheum* 1999;42:S174.
217. Zuniga R, Ng S, Reveille JD, et al. Independent contribution to the risk of nephritis by allelic variants of FcγRIIa and FcγRIIIa in Hispanic patients with systemic lupus erythematosus. *Arthritis Rheum* 2001;44:361–367.
218. Herrmann M, Voll RE, Zoller OM, et al. Impaired phagocytosis of apoptotic cell material by monocytes-derived macrophages from patients with systemic lupus erythematosus. *Arthritis Rheum* 1998;41:1241–1250.
219. Hurst NP, Nuki G, Wallington T. Evidence for intrinsic cellular defects of complement' receptor-mediated monocyte phagocytosis in patients with systemic lupus erythematosus (SLE). *Clin Exp Immunol* 1984;55:303–312.
220. Guyre PM, Campbell AS, Kniffin W, et al. Monocytes and polymorphonuclear neutrophils of patients with streptococcal pharyngitis express increased numbers of type I IgG Fc receptors. *J Clin Invest* 1990;86:1892–1896.
221. Valerius T, Repp R, de Wit TP, et al. Involvement of the high affinity receptor for IgG (FcγRI;CD64) in enhanced tumor cell cytotoxicity for neutrophils during granulocyte colony-stimulating factor therapy. *Blood* 1993;82:931–939.
222. Allen JB, Wong HL, Guyre PM, et al. Association of circulating receptor FcRIII-positive monocytes in AIDS patients with elevated levels of transforming growth factor-β. *J Clin Invest* 1991; 87:1773–1779.
223. de Waal Malefyt R, Figdor CG, de Vries JE. Effects of interleukin 4 on monocyte functions: comparison to interleukin 13. *Res Immunol* 1993;144:629–633.
224. Friedman D, Nettl F, Schreiber AD. Effect of estradiol and steroid analogues on the clearance of immunoglobulin G-coated erythrocytes. *J Clin Invest* 1985;75:162–167.
225. Schreiber AD, Nettl FM, Sanders MC, et al. Effect of endogenous and synthetic sex steroids on the clearance of antibody-coated cells. *J Immunol* 1988;141:2959–2966.
226. Warren MK, Vogel SN. Opposing effects of glucocorticoids on interferon—induced murine macrophage Fc receptor and Ia antigen expression. *J Immunol* 1985;134:2462–2469.
227. Hook JJ, Moutsopoulos HM, Geis SA, et al. Immune interferons in the circulation of patients with autoimmune disease. *N Engl J Med* 1979;310:5–8.
228. Atkinson JP, Frank MM. Complement-independent clearance of IgG-sensitized erythrocytes: inhibition of cortisone. *Blood* 1974;44:629–637.
229. Atkinson JP, Schrieber AD, Frank MM. Effects of glucocorticoids and splenectomy on the immune clearance and destruction of erythrocytes. *J Clin Invest* 1973;52:1509–1517.
230. Crabtree GR, Munck A, Smith KA. Glucocorticoids inhibit expression of Fc receptors of the human granulocyte cell line HL-60. *Nature* 1979;279:338–339.
231. Fries LF, Brickman CM, Frank MM. Monocyte receptors for the Fc portion of IgG increases in number in autoimmune hemolytic anemic and other hemolytic states and are decreased by glucocorticoid therapy. *J Immunol* 1983;131: 1240–1245.
232. Hoyoux C, Foidart J, Rigo P, et al. Effects of methylpred-

nisolone on Fc receptor function of human reticuloendothelial system in vivo. *Eur J Clin Invest* 1984;14:60–66.

233. Preble OT, Black RJ, Friedman RM, et al. Systemic lupus erythematosus: presence in human serum of the unusual acid labile leukocyte interferon. *Science* 1982;216:429–431.
234. Preble OT, Rothko K, Klippel JH, et al. Interferon-induced 2–5 adenylate synthetase in vivo and interferon production by lymphocytes from systemic lupus erythematosus patients with and without circulating interferon. *J Exp Med* 1983;157:2140–2146.
235. Girand MT, Hjaltadottir S, Fejes-Toth AN, et al. Glucocorticoids enhance the gamma-interferon augmentation of human monocyte immunoglobulin G Fc receptor expression. *J Immunol* 1987;138:3235–3241.
236. Salmon JE, Cronstein BN. Fc receptor-mediated functions in neutrophils are modulated by adenosine receptor occupancy. A1 receptors are stimulatory and A2 receptors are inhibitory. *J Immunol* 1990;145:2235–2240.
237. Ierino FL, Powell MS, McKenzie IF, et al. Recombinant soluble human FcγRII: production, characterization, and inhibition of the Arthus reaction. *J Exp Med* 1993;178:1617–1628.
238. Galon J, Paulet P, Galinha A, et al. Soluble Fcγ receptors: interaction with ligands and biological consequences. *Int Rev Immunol* 1997;16:87–111.
239. Moreland LW, Schiff MH, Baumgartner SW, et al. Etanercept therapy in rheumatoid arthritis. A randomized, controlled trial. *Ann Intern Med* 1999;130:478–486.
240. Weisman HF, Bartow T, Leppo MK, et al. Soluble human complement receptor type 1: in vivo inhibitor of complement suppressing post-ischemic myocardial inflammation and necrosis. *Science* 1990;249:146–151.

13

COMPLEMENT AND SYSTEMIC LUPUS ERYTHEMATOSUS

PETER H. SCHUR
LLOYD KLICKSTEIN

There is considerable evidence that much of the pathology in patients with systemic lupus erythematosus (SLE) can be attributed to immune complexes (1,2) and, thereby, complement activation (2,271). These immune complexes may either form in the circulation and later deposit in tissues or form *in situ*. Immune complexes may cause tissue inflammation directly or through activation of the complement system. Complement activation causes the release of various mediators, promotes cell interaction, and ultimately results in inflammation. Evaluation of the complement system, which can serve as an indirect measure of the presence of immune complexes, often correlates with clinical aspects of SLE. Monitoring blood levels of complement may be useful in adjusting therapy for the patient.

THE COMPLEMENT SYSTEM

The complement system consists of a group of plasma proteins and cellular receptors that interact sequentially to protect the host from microorganisms and also to facilitate clearance of immune complexes. Complement may also affect other systems of inflammation (3–14). Some of these activities occur on cell surfaces, some on the surfaces of immune complexes, and some in various body fluids.

The complement system (Fig. 13.1) consists of four pathways. The first two are the classic and the alternative (or properdin) pathways, and these two pathways enter into the terminal (or membrane) attack pathway. The classic complement pathway involves complement components C1, C4, and C2. In the fourth, or lectin pathway, mannan-binding lectin (MBL) and its associated serine proteases MASP-1 and MASP-2 substitute for C1. Human immune complexes containing immunoglobulin M (IgM) and/or the IgG subclasses IgG1, IgG2, or IgG3 will bind the C1q portion of C1. Such binding leads to the sequential activation of C1r and C1s; cleavage of C2 and C4 into C2a, C2b, C4a, C4c, and C4d; and the eventual cleavage of C3 by C3 convertase (i.e., the complex C4b2a) into C3a and C3b. There are natural controls or modulators for activation of this system. C1 inhibitor (C1INH), C4b-binding protein (C4bp), and factor I (C3b inactivator; obC3bINA;cb, KAF) prevent complement activation in the fluid phase. Decay acceleration factor (DAF) and membrane cofactor protein (MCP) inhibit classic pathway activation on host cell surfaces.

Cleavage of C3 also can come about through an alternative pathway: the properdin system. This phylogenetically older system can be activated by some immunoglobulins, including aggregated IgA and possibly IgE, as well as polysaccharides, including bacterial endotoxin and foreign surfaces. The pathway involves a number of proteins, including properdin, factor B, factor D, and C3, that interact to create another C3 convertase (C3bBb), which cleaves C3. Interaction of both pathways leads to cleavage of the third component into C3a and C3b, and by various enzymes into even smaller fragments: C3c, C3d, C3dg, C4dk, C3e, and C3g (some of which may still have biologic properties). The larger fragment, C3b, can interact further with components of the properdin system, causing a positive feedback cycle and resulting in further activation and cleavage of C3.

An inactivator of C3b (C3bINA) (factor I) in concert with beta IH (factor H) can block the hemolytic potential of C3b by cleaving it into two inactive fragments: (a) C3d, which remains bound to the antigenantibody complex; and (b) C3c, which is released into the fluid. Properdin or C3 nephritic factor (C3NEF) stabilizes the inherently labile C3 convertases and thus facilitates progression of the system.

The terminal pathway begins at C3. Cleavage of C3b by C3 convertase may lead to formation of either (C3b)2Bb or C46362a, the alternative or classic C5 convertases, respectively. The C5 convertases lead to sequential cleavage or activation of C5, C6, C7, and C9. Deposition of the multimolecular complex consisting of C5 through C9 on a cell membrane leads to the formation of cell membrane defects

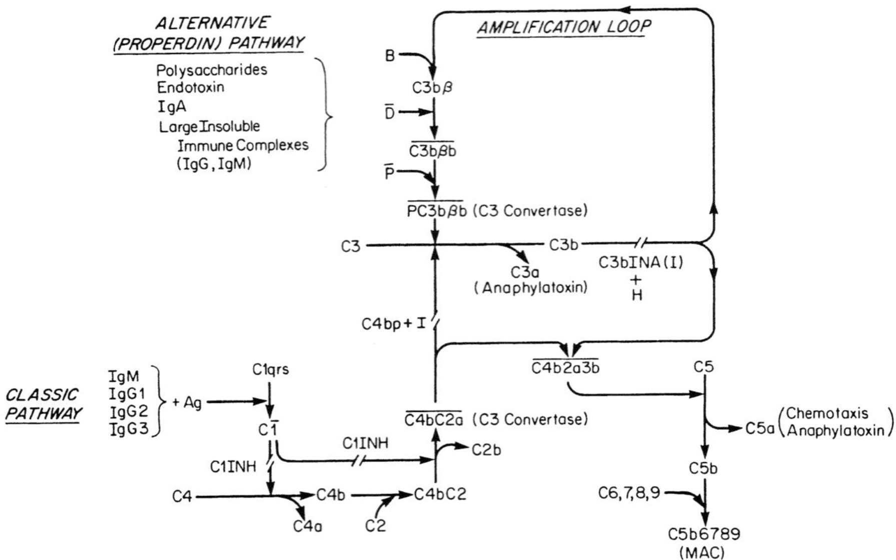

FIGURE 13.1. The complement cascade.

that cause increased permeability and release of intracellular contents, such as hemoglobin. Release of hemoglobin thus provides a means for assaying the overall function of the complement system in the common hemolytic assays used *in vitro*. The terminal pathway is regulated by the inherent instability of the nascent C5b-7 complex and by CD59, which binds C8 in membrane-associated C5b-8 and prevents pore formation and assembly of C9. Inherited deficiency of CD59 leads to a hemolytic illness with the same phenotype as paroxysmal nocturnal hemoglobinuria (275).

Many cells have receptors for complement components or fragments, including C1q, C3a, C3b, C3d, C3bi, C3e, and C5a (3,5,6,15). Receptor CR1 reacts with C3b, iC3b, C4b, C1q, and MBL; CR2 reacts with iC3b, C3dg, and C3d; and CR3 reacts with iC3b. There are specific G-protein–coupled receptors for C3a and C5a that are widely expressed (276). CR1 on erythrocytes has an important role in clearing immune complexes, while complement receptors on other cells participate in enhancing phagocytosis, augmenting antibody-dependent cellular cytotoxicity, and in chemotaxis, leukocyte respiratory bursts, secretion, and B-cell proliferation.

Immunobiologic Aspects of the Complement System

A number of biologic functions have been ascribed to various complement components. C1, C4, and C2 are involved in viral neutralization. The cleavage products C3a and C5a have anaphylatoxic properties and release histamine from mast cells. In addition, C5a also is chemotactic for monocytes and polymorphonuclear leukocytes. Both C3a and C5a have been implicated in the regulation of the humoral immune response (13–15,276).

The presence of C3b on antigen-antibody complexes helps bind these to specific receptors on erythrocytes, B lymphocytes, monocytes, or polymorphonuclear leukocytes, and it promotes clearance and subsequent phagocytosis of these complement complexes. Immune complexes coated with C3b may bind to platelets, causing release of vasoactive amines and resulting in inflammatory reactions. These biologic activities of C3b can be modified by factor I processing C3b to iC3b. Complement activation by immune complexes is also important for limiting the size of the complexes and for promoting their solubility.

Measurement of Complement

The complement system can be assessed by (a) measurement of total hemolytic complement activity (CH_{50}); (b) immunochemical or hemolytic measurement of individual components; (c) measurements of complement fragments, activation-dependent neoepitopes, and complexes that arise from complement activation; and (d) determination of complement metabolism. The total hemolytic complement level (CH_{50}) represents the sum of all components of the system. By adding diluted serum to antibody-sensitized sheep erythrocytes and quantitating the amount of released hemoglobin, one can measure this level in units that represent the reciprocal of that dilution of serum that causes 50% of cells to lyse (i.e., CH_{50}). A CH_{100} represents that dilution of serum that lyses 100% of sensitized cells; this measurement is not nearly as accurate as a CH_{50}, which reflects actual hemolysis in a more linear fashion than CH_{100} (16–18).

Separate complement components generally are measured by immunochemical means: radial immunodiffusion, electroimmunodiffusion, or nephelometry. However, such determinations yield no information about the functional biologic integrity or hemolytic potential of the components being measured. Such functional tests of complement components are rarely employed because of their difficulty in routine clinical assays.

When measuring CH_{50} or components, it is important to remember that some components are thermolabile. Serum stored at room temperature, even for a few days, is adequate for immunochemical measurement of individual components as proteins (as, for instance, by immunodiffusion). However, it is essential to store samples [preferably ethylenediaminetetraacetic acid (EDTA) plasma] as soon as possible at −70°C when measurement of the hemolytic levels of individual components is desired. The CH_{50} will remain relatively stable for a few hours at room temperature or overnight at −20°C; however, samples are best stored at −70°C as soon as possible. Heating for 30 minutes at 56°C also is known to inactivate complement components and decrease/abolish CH_{50} activity.

These assays give but a glimpse of the dynamic state of the complement system. Serial values may be helpful in assessing this dynamic state: falling values suggest more catabolism (e.g., via immune complex fixation) than synthesis is taking place, while rising levels suggest more synthesis than catabolism is taking place.

Measurement of both the native components and the activation products of individual components is a way of assessing the catabolic state of the complement system without necessarily doing serial measurements. The activation products in EDTA plasma generally are measured by enxyme-linked immunosorbent assay (ELISA) using monoclonal antibodies. However, the levels of complement activation factors also can be affected by binding to complement (fragment) receptors, degradation by serum proteases, and renal and hepatic clearance (17).

Complement metabolism is a better way of assessing the dynamic state (i.e., synthesis and catabolism) of individual complement components (19). However, these studies rarely are performed because of the great difficulty both in isolating hemolytically and biologically active purified components and in maintaining their activity after radiolabeling. The liver is the primary source of synthesis of complement components, with the notable exception of C1q, which is probably produced primarily by macrophages (20).

Complement Abnormalities

Understanding the role of complement in disease requires analysis of the whole system (i.e., CH_{50} levels and levels of individual components) (21). For instance, a depressed CH_{50} level could be the result of inherited depletion of a single component and/or acquired depletion of multiple components through immune and nonimmune processes. Further, static measurements of serum CH_{50} levels or of individual complement components should be confirmed whenever possible by serial studies to estimate the metabolism of these proteins. Because most disorders of the complement system affect either the classic or the alternative pathway, we recommend a serum hemolytic CH_{50} and immunochemical analysis of C1q, C4, C3, and factor B proteins for routine blood analysis. Late or terminal components rarely are affected unless C3 is affected as well; measurement of C5 protein has been useful in this regard. Generally, a decrease in CH_{50} activity corresponds well with a decrease in C1q, C4, C2, and C3 component levels, and vice versa. When, on the other hand, CH_{50} levels do not correlate with levels of these components, one should consider abnormalities of another component, serum-handling problems, or nonimmune abnormalities (e.g., malnutrition) (22).

Inherited Defects of Complement

Four types of inherited complement abnormalities are most readily recognized: (a) homozygous deficiency, (b) heterozygous deficiency, (c) dysfunctional proteins, and (d) allotypy (i.e., electrophoretically defined alleles). Certain allotypes also are expressed as null genes (i.e., the gene is present but the protein is not), resulting in either hetero- or homozygous deficiency. Molecular biologic techniques, including restriction fragment length polymorphism (RFLP), have revealed more heterogeneity and abnormalities among complement genes than were recognized by immunochemical techniques (7,8,11,13,14,21,23–30).

Persons who are homozygous deficient in a complement component generally show virtually no CH_{50} activity and are missing one component (assessed hemolytically or immunochemically); levels of all other components are normal. Those who are heterozygous deficient in a component, in particular C1, C4, C2, or C3, have approximately one-half the normal levels of that component and approximately one-half the normal CH_{50} levels; levels of all other components are normal (16) (Table 13.1). The inherited nature of the defect can be confirmed by family studies demonstrating homozygous and/or heterozygous defects in other family members. Inheritance of most complement abnormalities and complete deficiencies is autosomal recessive; however, C1 inhibitor deficiency is autosomal dominant and properdin deficiency is x-linked. In most studies performed in white populations, the frequency of complement deficiencies is approximately the same among males and females. Many of the cases of recurrent neisserial infection in patients with terminal complement deficiencies have occurred in blacks (25).

The frequency of homozygous complement deficiencies in the general population is probably low. To determine this frequency, 10,000 English blood-bank donors were screened for CH_{50} levels. Only one person was found to

TABLE 13.1. COMPLEMENT PROFILES IN HEREDITARY AND ACQUIRED DEFICIENCIES IN SYSTEMIC LUPUS ERYTHEMATOSUS (SLE)

Condition	CH_{50} (μ/mL)	C1q (mg/dL)	C4 (mg/dL)	C2 (mg/dL)	C3 (mg/dL)
Normal	150–250	35–56	26–83	1.6–3.9	91–198
Homozygous C2 deficiency	0	35–56	26–83	0	91–198
Heterozygous C2 deficiency	100–150	35–56	26–83	1.0–1.5	91–198
Homozygous C4 deficiency	0	35–56	0	1.6–3.9	91–198
Heterozygous C4 deficiency	100–150	35–56	10–25	1.6–3.9	91–198
SLE					
Arthritis	100–150	18–34	10–25	1.6–3.9	91–150
Vasculitis	50–100	5–25	5–15	1.0–1.5	80–120
Glomerulonephritis	25–125	10–30	5–20	1.0–1.5	70–75
Nephrotic syndrome[a]	100–150	18–34	26–83	1.6–3.9	91–198

[a]Any nephrotic syndrome
CH_{50}, complement activity.

have a homozygous deficiency of a complement component, C2 (31). In a study of 146,000 Japanese blood-bank donors, 16 late-acting deficiencies were found: two cases of C5, four of C6, six of C7, and four of C8 deficiency, all without any deficiencies of early complement components. Twelve individuals were asymptomatic (32). These observations suggest that complement deficiencies may differ by race, and that disease associations with early complement component deficiencies do not represent ascertainment bias. One can estimate the frequency of homozygous deficiency in a population by determining the frequency of the (more common) heterozygous deficiency.

To determine whether an association between a particular complement deficiency and some clinical entity exists, it is important to determine whether the observed association is a real phenomenon or the result of an ascertainment bias. This becomes relevant when one recognizes that physicians tend to order complement levels primarily in patients with immune, rheumatic, renal, and infectious disorders. It also is important to remember that deficiency of a particular component may not be associated with any disease. The first case of homozygous complement deficiency (C2) was described in an immunologist who donated his blood to a colleague for a complement-fixing experiment that did not work (33)! Nevertheless, approximately two thirds of individuals with homozygous deficiency of the classic pathway suffer from immune/rheumatic disorders such as SLE, glomerulonephritis, anaphylactic purpura/vasculitis, and related disorders (Table 13.2) (7,8,11,13,14,26–29). The strongest associations are between SLE and C1q, C2, and C4 deficiency. Terminal component deficiencies are significantly associated with recurrent pyogenic infection, particularly that caused by *Neisseria* sp. 20 (25) (Table 13.2). However, infections also are noted among individuals with classic component deficiencies, and immune/rheumatic diseases are found in individuals with terminal component deficiencies. It is not clear whether these associations are greater than would be expected by chance alone.

C1

At least 23 pedigrees of C1 (i.e., C1q, C1r, and/or C1s subunit) deficiencies have been described (25,34–37,239–241, 243,248,252,253,270). The clinical profile of many of these families reveals lupus erythematosus or a lupus-like disease, glomerulonephritis, and skin lesions. Many of the children have had infections, and many of the siblings died young of either infections or lupus-like diseases. Heterozy-

TABLE 13.2. COMPLEMENT COMPONENT DEFICIENCIES

Component	Clinical Associations[a]
Classical pathway	
C1q	SLE, GN
C1r	SLE, GN, infection
C1r and C1s	Infection, SLE
C4	SLE, infection, GN
C2	SLE, infection, various immune disorders, normality
Alternative pathway	
C3	Infection, GN
P	Infection
D	Infection
Effector (terminal) pathway	
C5	Infection (*Neisseria*)
C6	Infection (*Neisseria*)
C7	Infection (*Neisseria*), GN
C8	Infection (*Neisseria*), normality, xeroderma
C9	Normality, infection (*Neisseria*)
Control proteins	
C1INH	Hereditary angioedema, SLE
I	Infection
H	Normality, hemolytic uremic syndrome
Complement receptors	
CR1	SLE

[a]Only the more common associations are given.
GN, glomerulonephritis; C1INH, C1 inhibitor.

gotes within families are difficult to identify. C1q deficiency is a very strong disease susceptibility gene for lupus. More than 90% of those individuals have SLE or a lupus-like disease. Of 23 families with C1q deficiency, six are from Turkey (241,270). Four Turkish families had C to T mutation in exon II of the *C1qA* gene. In other families, single base mutations, deletions, and/or transitions led to either termination (stop) codons, frame shift, or amino acid exchanges (251,270). The strong association between C1q deficiency and SLE suggests that functional C1q protects against SLE. Studies in humans (263) and mice (250,252) show that C1q binds apoptotic keratinocytes and that C1q knockout mice develop glomerulonephritis characterized by multiple apoptotic cell bodies and immune deposits (250,252). These observations suggest that C1q deficiency causes autoimmunity by an impaired clearance of apoptotic cells (250,252) as well as by an impaired clearance of immune complexes (270). It should be also noted that clearance of apoptotic cells appears to be impaired in patients with SLE. Monocyte-derived macrophages from patients with SLE exhibit impaired phagocytosis of apoptotic cells (252a). C1s deficiency was shown to be due to a 4–base pair (bp) deletion at nucleotides 1087 to 1090 (TTTG), creating a stop codon (TGA) at position 94 downstream on exon 10 (253).

C4

Less than 1 in 10,000 whites (in Boston) are homozygous C4 deficient (38). Homozygous C4 deficiency has been recognized in many families (25,39–45), and lupus (or lupus-like) erythematosus disease is found in most of them.

Analysis of C4 is more complicated, because it consists of two isotypic forms, C4A and C4B. At least 13 C4A alleles and 16 C4B alleles as well as a null allele at each locus are presently known (46). Null alleles are ascertained by both electrophoresis (i.e., allotyping) and family studies to confirm the null state, a necessary test to prove that the apparent C4A or C4B null state is not acquired, as may happen in SLE because of immune complex binding and activation. Further, there is no good relationship between C4A or C4B null states and serum C4 levels (47,48), and most patients with SLE have low C4 levels (16). C4A null probably is the most common inherited complement deficiency occurring in varying frequency within different normal populations (e.g., Japanese, 6.7%; blacks, 7.1–22.1%; English, 28.4%; French, 13.2%; Germans, 8.7%) (49,50). The frequency of homozygous C4A deficiency in normal whites (in Boston) is 3% and for C4B 2% (37). An increased frequency (50–80%) of C4A protein deficiency has been noted in studies of American, English, Australian, French, Swedish, and Spanish white patients (40,41, 51–62), black patients (40,53,63,64), and Chinese Korean and Japanese patients with SLE (65–68), but not in our study in Boston (69) or in French (70,71), French Canadian (72), Central European (39), or other Japanese patients with SLE (73). However, when our Boston patients were categorized into two groups based on their European ancestry (i.e., English/Irish vs. other), there was an increased frequency of C4AQ0, human leukocyte antigen (HLA)-DR3, and the complotype SC01 in patients of English/Irish descent as compared to ethnically matched controls (69). The increase in C4AQ0 (and DR3) could be accounted for by their being part of the extended haplotype (HLA-B8;SC01;DR3) (69). Most of the other early observations of increased C4AQ0 were indeed in patients of English/Irish descent with SLE in whom an association with DR3 also was noted. Other studies of patients with SLE have reported an increase of the C4A protein null allele without an increase in DR3. Most of these studies have not confirmed the inheritance of the C4A null state by family studies. An increased frequency of C4B null alleles in SLE has been noted only in France and Spain (254,255).

RFLP analysis of individuals with C4A null allele (C4AQ0/C4AQ0Q0) and DR3 using the restriction enzyme HindIII and a 5-kilobase (kb) C4 complementary DNA (cDNA) probe has revealed loss of a 15-kb restriction fragment and appearance of an 8.5-kb fragment (62,74, 75,76). However, in non-DR3 individuals, C4A gene deletion failed to account for the C4A protein deficiency (56,67,75,76). Further analysis of the C4d region of the C4A gene by polymerase chain reaction and RFLP using the N1a IV enzyme revealed that homoexpression of C4B at both loci also was not responsible for C4A deficiency in non-DR3 individuals (75). However, some non-DR3 individuals have a 2-bp insertion in exon 29, which leads to a premature stop codon and C4A protein deficiency (246).

Patients with genetic deficiency of C4 tend to have antibodies to Ro (77), although this association, or association with other clinical features, has not been noted by others (39–41,59). Patients with homozygous C4A deficiency tend to have milder disease, are less likely to have renal disease, and tend to have less C3 decreases (256). There is an increased frequency of the C4A null allele in patients with hydralazine-induced SLE (78) and of C4A null and C4B null in procainamide-induced lupus erythematosus (LE) (79). C4A null does not appear to predispose to neonatal LE (80).

In summary, the role of C4AQ0 is not entirely clear. C4AQ0 undoubtedly contributes to the pathogenesis of SLE. Some ethnic groups express it as part of an extended haplotype and thereby are at increased risk for developing SLE. However, C4AQ0 is not a necessary risk factor for lupus in all ethnic groups (81).

C2

Deficiency of complement component C2 is the second most common genetic complement deficiency in whites; 1% to 2.2% of individuals are heterozygous deficient, and approximately 1 in 10,000 have homozygous deficiency (31,82,258). The C2 deficiency gene frequency is 0.007 to 0.01 in North American whites and Swedes (83,84). C2 deficiency was not found in U.S. blacks (85). Homozygous C2 deficiency has been recognized in over 60 families, while heterozygous deficiency has been found in many more (82,83,85,86). It is inherited as autosomal recessive.

About 30% of the homozygous C2-deficient individuals have SLE or lupus-like disease (272). Most homozygous C2-deficient patients with SLE have relatively mild disease, with mostly skin and joint manifestations; renal disease is uncommon (87). One patient developed severe lupus nephritis after a transfusion, which suggests that lack of C2 prevented immune complex–mediated glomerulonephritis (88). Many patients had either absent or low-titer antinuclear antibodies (ANAs), and this often made it difficult to diagnose lupus (82); however, most had anti-Ro antibodies (82a). The frequency of C2 heterozygous deficiency was increased among patients with SLE and patients with juvenile rheumatoid arthritis, but not in patients with rheumatoid arthritis—6% to 6.6%, 3%, and 1%, respectively; the frequency is 1% to 2.2% in normals (82,258). Others, however, have found no increase of heterozygous C2 deficiency in SLE (271). Clinically, there was no difference between SLE patients with or without heterozygous C2 deficiency, except for the aforementioned tendency toward low ANA titers (81) and a high frequency of antibodies to Ro (64,77). Infections do not appear to be a major problem for most C2-deficient families (87).

C2 deficiency is found in strong linkage disequilibrium with HLA-A10, B18, DR2, C4A4, C4B2, and BFS (89,258). C2 deficiency is caused by a splicing defect resulting from a 28-bp genomic deletion, leading to excision of a 134-bp exon, and predicted premature termination of the C2 translation product (90).

C3–9

SLE occasionally has been noted in association with C3, C5, C6, C7, C8, and C9 deficiency (25,91–93). C5 deficiency also has been noted in a patient with discoid LE (94), C3 deficiency in a patient with subcutaneous lupus erythematosus (SCLE) (95), C3 dysfunction in a patient with SLE-like syndrome (96), and C7 and C4B deficiency in a patient with SLE (97). However, these deficiencies usually are associated with infections (25). LE occasionally also has been noted in individuals with C1INH deficiency associated with hereditary angioedema (25,98.99).

Mannan-Binding Lectin Gene

A dysfunctional allele of the MBL gene has been associated with SLE in a Spanish population (264), a Danish population (274), and a Chinese population (277). Particular MBL alleles also predispose to infection (274).

CR1 and CR2

Deficiency of the erythrocyte receptor for C3b (CR1) also has been described in patients with LE. Whether this deficiency is acquired or inherited, or both, in patients with SLE and normal individuals has become an area of some controversy. Using functional studies and later immunoassays, investigators in Japan concluded that erythrocyte CR1 deficiency is inherited in patients with SLE (100,101). Subsequently, using immunoassays, investigators in New York City (102), Japan (103), United States (104), Denmark (105), Italy (106), and Norway (107) demonstrated low levels in patients with SLE that correlated with disease activity.

In our own studies, we have demonstrated, using both polyclonal monospecific antisera and monoclonal antibodies to the C3b receptor, that a significant number of relatives of probands (of both patients and normals) had reduced levels of CR1, and that three phenotypes could be identified, having high, intermediate, and low levels of CR1 (108). Family studies indicated that the levels were inherited in an autosomal-codominant manner (109). Molecular studies including RFLP demonstrated further the genetic basis for CR1 levels (109). However, subsequent studies from Great Britain, North Carolina, Australia, France, Argentina, and Greece suggested that CR1 levels were under genetic influence, but that the low levels seen in patients with SLE were primarily acquired, and generally reflected disease activity (110–119).

Normal erythrocytes transfused into patients with SLE lost 60% of CR1 within 5 days (120). In a study of normal individuals and hypertensive patients who developed hydralazine-induced SLE, low erythrocyte CR1 levels were noted in some relatives. However, in the patients, low CR1 levels were inversely correlated with circulating immune complex levels and thought to be acquired defects (121). Erythrocyte CR1 levels increased after patients with SLE were treated with erythropoietin (122), and nephritis in patients with active SLE may improve, too (278).

How to reconcile these differences of acquired versus inherited abnormalities of erythrocyte CR1 levels in patients with SLE is not clear (114,123). However, ethnic analysis of our Boston patients suggests that while the C4A null patients tend to have an Anglo-Saxon heritage, the patients with erythrocyte CR1 deficiency mostly have a non–Anglo-Saxon heritage (124). However, in more recent studies of Mexicans with lupus, there was no association of the RFLP (associated with low erythrocyte CR1 number) and SLE (125), further substantiating the hypothesis that genetic associations with SLE usually have an ethnic basis.

In summary, both inherited (probably ethnically defined) and acquired factors contribute to low erythrocyte CR1 levels in SLE (111).

CR1 and CR2 deficiencies on SLE B lymphocytes (126,127) and CR1 deficiencies on SLE neutrophils have been noted (126,128,129). Some of these deficiencies may be familial (126). Low levels of lymphocyte CR3 also have been observed in active SLE (130–132).

POSSIBLE MECHANISMS OF INHERITED COMPLEMENT DEFICIENCY DISEASE ASSOCIATIONS

What is the role of these inherited complement component deficiencies in predisposing to disease? The association of deficiency of either C3, C5, C6, C7, C8, or C3b inactivator with repeated infections is easiest to understand in light of the importance of these complement components in chemotaxis and phagocytosis. The nature of the association between inherited complement component deficiencies, particularly the early components, and SLE, however, is not as clear (133,134).

These early components, including C1q, C4 (especially C4A), and C2, do play a role in immune complex solubilization, clearance of immune complexes, generation of immunoregulatory factors, clearance of apoptotic cells, and viral neutralization (135–141,270). Porter (142) speculated that relatively inefficient particular C4 alleles in individuals may predispose to SLE, and Briggs et al. (143) observed that C4A null patients with SLE tended to have low C4d levels. However, while C4 null individuals have deficient C4-dependent function, they have normal C3 convertase activity, which suggests a normal ability to activate C3 and all biologic functions associated with that (144). Carroll (273) has also suggested that complement deficiency may lead to abnormal binding of nuclear antigens to complement receptors on bone marrow cells. B lymphocytes bearing receptors for these autoantigens would then not be tolerant for these autoantigens, not be eliminated, and would then, in the presence of T cells, be activated and produce autoantibodies. The association of immune disease with heterozygous C2 and C4 deficiency, where there is adequate complement to participate in the usual complement-dependent reactions, suggests that the complement deficiency primarily represents a genetic rather than a biologic marker, and that the association between complement deficiency and SLE results from some other factor(s).

The genes for C4 and C2 (and factor B) are on the short arm of the sixth chromosome between HLA-B and HLA-DR. The linkage of C4A and C2 null genes with HLA-DR3 and DR2, respectively, provides a clue to another possible interrelationship, that is, that these null alleles are part of an extended haplotype (e.g., A1,B8,DR3,C4AQ0) that predisposes to SLE rather than the C4AQ0 allele itself (39,69,81). There is now increasing evidence that immune response genes may be closely linked to those of HLA. Further, a number of studies have shown an increased frequency of either HLA-DR3 and DR2 in certain patients with SLE (81). Therefore, the HLA-linked complement deficiencies also may be linked to immune response genes that may express themselves as immunologically mediated disease. In a sense, C2 and C4 may be only a marker gene for a subset of patients with SLE. On the other hand, C4A deficiency also may not be associated with HLA-DR3 or other HLA. In these instances, the C4A deficiency may indeed contribute to SLE directly. The strong association of C1q deficiency in predisposing to lupus-like disease suggests a direct functional role for complete complement component deficiency rather than through some gene in linkage dysequilibrium of some immune response gene with the MHC complex.

SLE also has been reported with deficiencies of other complement components (C5, C6, C7, C8, C9, C1INH). However, the frequency of association is so low that ascertainment bias, or chance, probably accounts for it.

The mechanism whereby deficiency of C3b receptors (CR1) on erythrocytes predisposes to SLE is not clear, but that these proteins are important in immune complex clearance mechanisms provides a rationale for their association (123). These receptors promote immune complex clearance by binding immune complexes with the red blood cell surface and bringing them to the reticuloendothelial system, where the immune complexes are stripped from the erythrocyte (145). The erythrocytes of patients with SLE bind immune complexes of DNA–anti-DNA less well than in normals, probably because of the low number of CR1 receptors (146,147). Thus, the low number of C3b receptors may result in increased levels of pathogenic immune complexes in the circulation of patients with SLE.

The recent finding that MBL, C1q, C4b, and C3b all bind CR1 and the recognition that homozygous deficiencies of MBL, C1q, C2, and C4 predispose to SLE have led to the hypothesis that abnormal intravascular clearance of apoptotic cell fragments may contribute to the development of SLE (279). As noted above, erythrocyte CR1 normally serves as the carrier for complement opsonized complexes and cell fragments, which are delivered to phagocytic cells in the liver or spleen. C2 deficiency has the lowest disease association among C1, C4, and C2 deficiencies. C2 deficiency would prevent C3b formation via the classic or lectin pathways, but would still allow C1q and C4b opsonization of immune complexes and cells, which may be adequate to mediate clearance via erythrocyte CR1. C4 deficiency would prevent C4b and C3b opsonization, but C1q would still be present and could mediate binding of complexes and cell fragments to CR1 on erythrocytes. C1q deficiency, in which over 90% of affected patients develop severe lupus-like illness, would not permit any classic pathway opsonization. Thus the severity of complement deficiency-associated autoimmune disease parallels the order of the classic activation sequence.

In addition to genetic reasons, acquired C1q, C2, C4, and C3b receptor deficiencies may themselves magnify clinical expression of disease. In summary, complement deficiency, such as C1q, C4A, C2, and CR1, can contribute to predisposition directly and also by their linkage to immune response genes.

Acquired Serum Complement Abnormalities

Vaughan et al. (148) were among the first to show that serum complement levels are decreased in patients with SLE. Subsequently, many studies have demonstrated the association of low CH_{50}, C1q, C4, C2, C3, and/or C1INH levels with clinical activity (149–161,270,271), although some studies have not observed this association (162–166,266). Patients with active LE also tended to have elevated plasma levels of complement activation products, including C1s:C1INH (167), C4a (156,168,169), C4d (170–172,268), C3a (156,173,174), C3d (170–172,175), iC3b neoantigen (176), C3a/C3 (156), C3bP (167), C3dg (157), C3b(Bb)P (245), C4BP (177), Ba (158,178), Bb (158,169,268), C5a (174), and the terminal complement complex (TCC) C5b-9 (158,167,169,173,179–181,245). One study showed no association between clinical activity and elevated levels of Bb (182); another study showed no association between clinical activity and low levels of factor B (173); a third study showed no association with low levels of C1rs-C1INH (245). Patients with SLE and renal disease tend to have lower mean levels of CH_{50}, C1q, C4, and C3 than those without renal disease (149–151,153,154) and higher levels of the TCC (183). Patients with active SLE tend to have elevated levels of the complement regulatory protein sCD46 (MCP) (249). Patients with diffuse proliferative nephritis tend to have abnormal levels of complement regulatory proteins, including decreased levels of CR1 on erythrocytes, and increased levels of DAF and CD59 on the glomerular basement membrane (244).

As noted, static measurements, and even serial measurement, of complement may not accurately reflect the metabolism of complement in the individual with SLE. Metabolic studies are the key, but they are infrequently done because of the difficulty in isolating biologically active complement components. In the few studies that have been performed, patients with SLE and active disease generally had increased catabolism and increased synthesis of C3 and C4 (19,20,184–186) and C9 (269), even though serum levels of C3 and C4 were normal or decreased. Several patients had low synthetic rates of certain complement components (184).

The complement component profile in patients with active lupus nephritis differs somewhat from that seen in other forms of glomerulonephritis. In SLE, there usually are marked depressions of C1q and C4 and less substantial depressions of C3. While there may be early depressions of C1q and C4 in patients with acute poststreptococcal glomerulonephritis, this disease, as well as chronic membranoproliferative glomerulonephritis, is characterized by marked depressions of C3 (187).

Associations have been noted between low levels of individual components and various facets of SLE (Table 13.3). Low factor B levels were found to be one of the best (complement) indicators of active nephritis. Patients with active vasculitis and/or cryoglobulinemia have especially low C1q and C4 levels, and a normal C3 level suggests the absence of active renal disease. These studies demonstrate the qualitative and quantitative differences in the complement system of patients with SLE, depending on the presence of active nephritis and/or active extrarenal disease. Patients with both renal and extrarenal manifestations tend to have the lowest levels; patients with extrarenal manifestations alone generally have the most minor abnormalities. Some patients (10) may have minor depressions of complement components without apparent clinical activity (165); this is especially true for C4.

Serial measurements of complement parameters have demonstrated that complement levels often increase coincidentally with clinical improvement and decrease with exacerbation (150). We (150) and others (153,267) have noted low C4 levels before exacerbation in patients who developed extrarenal manifestations, who developed active nephritis alone, and virtually all patients who developed active nephritis and active extrarenal manifestations. The most significant fall in C4, CH_{50}, and C1q occurred early in exacerbation, whereas C3 continued to decline during the height of clinical illness. We and others also have observed exacerbations associated or even preceded by falls in CH_{50} levels and/or rises in anti–double stranded DNA (dsDNA) antibody levels (149,267). Normal C3 and anti-DNA levels usually are associated with inactive disease and carry a good prognosis (150).

We and others also have observed an inverse relationship between C1q-binding immune complex levels and CH_{50}, C1q, C4, and C3 levels (150). Patients with low complement levels, low titers of anti-DNA antibodies, and low lev-

TABLE 13.3. ASSOCIATIONS WITH LOW SERUM LEVELS OF COMPLEMENT COMPONENTS

C1q	C4	C3	Factor B
Azotemia	Anti-NP	Anti-DNA	Azotemia
Casts	Casts	Casts	Casts
High ANAs		Leukopenia	Pyuria
			Hematuria
			Anemia

Other Associations

C1q	C4
Cryoglobulins	Arthritis
Vasculitis	Rashes
Immune complexes	Nephritis

Anti-NP, antibodies to nucleoprotein; ANAs, antinuclear antibodies.

els of immune complexes may not have active disease (150,165).

Normal women who are pregnant tend to have elevated levels of CH_{50} (158) and of C3 and C4d (188), but normal (158,189) or low C4 (188) and elevated C3a levels (158,189). Patients with active SLE who are pregnant tend to have somewhat decreased levels of CH_{50}, C3, and C4 (158,189–193) and elevated levels of Ba, C3a, C4d, C5b-9, especially CH_{50}/C5a (158,189), whereas patients with preeclampsia (but not LE) have normal levels of CH_{50}, C3, and C4 (158,189,190) but may have minimally elevated levels of Ba, C3a, C4d, and C5b-9 (158,189). Pregnant patients with SLE and hypocomplementemia tend to do worse, and are more likely to have intrauterine growth retardation (IUGR) than those with normal complement levels (247). Patients with primary habitual abortion and high serum levels of anticardiolipin antibodies had low (presumably acquired) C4 levels (194).

Immunologic tests have been used as a guide to therapy for patients with SLE. Lange et al. (195) administered steroid therapy to 15 patients with lupus nephritis based on the degree of hypocomplementemia and hypergammaglobulinemia. They observed normalization of gamma globulin, anti-DNA levels, and CH_{50} by 21 months. Appel et al. (196), in a prospective study of 25 patients, guided immunosuppressive therapy by changes in CH_{50} and antibody to dsDNA. The 5-year follow-up suggested that normalization of complement resulted in a trend toward stabilization of renal histology, creatinine clearance, and serum creatinine at a lower final mean dose of prednisone (197).

In summary, an isolated value of any one serologic parameter may assist in diagnosis but is not of any great therapeutic consequence. Clinical exacerbations may be predicted by serial monitoring of either C4, CH_{50}, C1q-binding assay, C3, or anti-DNA antibodies (Table 13.4). Different serologic profiles exist for different types of clinical exacerbation. Combinations of serologic tests appear to be more useful in predicting exacerbations and in guiding therapy, and this view is shared by others (150,151,198). In our hands, CH_{50}, C4, and C3, have appeared to be the most helpful.

TABLE 13.4. ABILITY OF IMMUNE TESTS TO PREDICT CLINICAL EXACERBATIONS IN SLE

CH_{50}	C3	Anti-DNA	Immune Complexes	Clinical Evidence
↓↓	↓	↑↑	Slight ↑	None necessarily
↓↓	↓↓	↑↑↑	↑↑↑	Active nephritis
↓	↓ (but normal)	↑↑↑	Slight ↑	Active extrarenal
↓↓↓	↓↓↓	↑	↑↑↑	Active nephritis and extrarenal

Other Studies on SLE Serum

Atkinson et al. (199) described two patients with SLE and low CH_{50} levels, low levels of complement components measured by hemolytic assay, but normal levels of complement components measured as proteins (i.e., antigenically). Plasma had normal complement levels, as did serum incubated at 37°C. These sera could be shown to activate complement *in vitro* at 5°C. These observations reemphasize that not all patients with low complement have active SLE: some may have genetic deficiencies, while others have complement activation *in vitro* but not *in vivo*.

A minority of patients with SLE and isolated hemolytic anemia and/or idiopathic thrombocytopenic purpura may have mildly depressed CH_{50} levels. A group of acutely ill, hospitalized patients with SLE and hypoxemia, unassociated with lung disease, were noted to have elevated C3a levels (200). Complement activation was associated with abnormal expression of adhesion molecules on endothelial cells, resulting in leuko-occlusive (i.e., lung) vasculopathy (201).

Complement levels tend to be inversely related to cryoglobulin concentration (202,203). These mixed cryoglobulins, which are considered to be cold-precipitable immune complexes, may consist of IgG, IgM, Clq, C4, and/or C3 (203,204). Some cryoglobulins fix complement *in vitro*, resulting in falsely low hemolytic (e.g., CH_{50}) but not antigen (i.e., C3, C4 protein) measurements.

Patients with drug-induced, LE-like syndromes generally have normal complement levels (205). However, hydralazine and isoniazid, both of which have been implicated in drug-induced LE, inhibit the binding of C4 to an *in vitro* activating system (206), and patients with hydralazine-induced lupus tend to have (inherited) low erythrocyte CR1 levels, thereby perhaps reducing their ability to efficiently clear immune complexes (121). One can speculate that this has a genetic basis, recognizing that drug-induced LE often is associated with DR4 and that certain C4 alleles are associated with DR4. Thus, complement may be directly or indirectly involved in this entity.

Although Davis and Bollet (207) observed an inverse correlation between low complement levels and the presence of rheumatoid factors in patients with lupus nephritis, others have not been able to confirm this observation.

Antibodies to complement components have been observed, including in patients with SLE (208–211). Antibodies to C1q may cause false-positive (C1q binding) assay results for immune complexes (208). The presence of anti-C1q antibodies correlated with activity (242,270), renal disease (209,216,262,270), active renal disease (259), proliferative nephritis (257,261,265), and (even preceded nephritis) in one study (209) but not another (242). Antibodies to C1q did not affect complement activation (214), and were associated with low complement levels (216,218,242,260,270). Antibodies to C1q were deposited and concentrated in the renal glomeruli of patients with proliferative glomerulonephritis (261). Anti-C1q was primarily of the IgG2 subclass (210,212). However, in children anti-C1q was not correlated with glomerulonephritis (260).

Immunoconglutinins (anti-C3b) have been noted in SLE, but they are not associated with clinical activity (219). Nephritic factor, which is an IgG antibody to neoantigen determinants of the alternative C3 convertase (C3b.Bb), has now been observed in six patients with SLE (220,271). This antibody stabilizes the convertase and leads to an acquired state of complement deficiency by a consumptive process.

Anticardiolipin antibodies correlated inversely with low levels of erythrocyte CR1 levels (221). Anticardiolipin antibodies correlated directly with low levels of C4 (222) and activation of complement (223,224) (see Chapter 27).

Complement in the Cerebrospinal Fluid of Patients with SLE

Complement levels have been measured in the cerebrospinal fluid (CSF) of patients with SLE. Because of the low protein levels in this fluid, it is impossible to do CH_{50} levels; however, individual components have been measured.

Petz et al. (225) noted that CSF hemolytic C4 levels were low in patients with SLE and central nervous system (CNS) involvement, while normal levels were found in those patients with SLE but without CNS involvement. The authors commented on the rapid (7.5/d) decay of C4 in spinal fluids from normal individuals, even when stored at −50°C, and thus reported on samples that were stored for 7 days or less.

Hadler et al. (226) found normal levels of CSF hemolytic C4 in both normal individuals and patients with SLE both with and without CNS involvement. However, when serial C4 levels were determined on patients who went from active CNS involvement into remission, it was apparent that C4 levels went from a low-normal value to either normal or high-normal levels, suggesting that serial C4 levels might be of value in evaluating patients with definite or questionable CNS involvement in SLE. Hadler et al.'s study also suggests that these assays must be done within a few hours after spinal tap, because nearly all hemolytic activity was lost within 24 hours after routine storage of CSF from patients with SLE and CNS involvement, while C4 in other CSF specimens decayed less rapidly. Hadler et al. also concluded that serum C4 values were not helpful in evaluating their four patients with SLE and active CNS involvement.

More recently, activated terminal complement component C5b-9 has been found in the CSF of patients with SLE and active CNS disease (181).

In summary, there is complement activation in the CSF of patients with SLE. However, practical methods to measure these phenomena are not currently available.

Complement in Tissue SLE

Further evidence for the participation of complement in SLE has been the detection of complement components in inflamed tissue, particularly in the same locations as immunoglobulins and antigens. Complement components detected in renal lesions included C1q, C1s, C4, C2, C3, C5, C6, C9, TCC, properdin, and factor B (187,227–231, 268) as well as increased levels of the regulatory complement components DAF and CD59 (244) but decreased levels of intact podocyte CR1 receptors (268). However, C4 and factor B were seen infrequently, despite the fact that serum levels of these components were often low in patients with nephritis. There was no apparent difference in the components deposited in patients with predominantly membranous or proliferative nephritis (231).

Similar complement components, including C5b-9, have been found at the dermal-epidermal junction of patients with skin lesions (229,230,232–237). The presence of C4 at this site is highly suggestive of SLE.

Complement activation products, including C3d, also have been found in the urine of patients with SLE, especially those with nephritis (238,268).

SUMMARY

SLE is characterized by a host of immune abnormalities. It is not clear to date which of these are primary and which are secondary, but the observation of a number of genetic defects suggests that some are primary. Multiple genetic defects may then lead to abnormal immune responses to common pathogens, antigens, or even autoantigens. Because of this abnormal immune response, immune complexes form, with resultant complement fixation and activation. These immune complexes interacting with cells and complement initiate an inflammatory response. One also can speculate that this inflammatory response represents a normal response to an abnormal event or is also abnormal in the patient with SLE. The ultimate result is tissue inflammation nand often damage. While therapy at present is aimed at controlling these secondary inflammatory phenomena mediated by immune complexes and complement, therapy ultimately may be more successful after the primary defects are corrected.

REFERENCES

1. Gatenby PA. The role of complement in the aetiopathogenesis of systemic lupus erythematosus. *Autoimmunity* 1991;11:61–66.
2. Porcel JM, Vergani D. Complement and lupus: old concepts and new directions. *Lupus* 1992;1:343–349.
3. Frank MM. Complement in the pathophysiology of human disease. *N Engl J Med* 1987;316:1525–1530.

4. Muller-Eberhard HJ. The membrane attack complex of complement. *Annu Rev Immunol* 1986;4:503–528.
5. Ochs HD, Wedgwood RJ, Heller SR, et al. Complement, membrane glycoproteins, and complement receptors: their role in regulation of the immune response. *Clin Immunol Immunopathol* 1986;40:94–104.
6. Schifferli JA, Ng YC, Peters DK. The role of complement and its receptor in the elimination of immune complexes. *N Engl J Med* 1986;315:488–495.
7. Colten HR, Rosen FS. Complement deficiencies. *Annu Rev Immunol* 1992;10:809–834.
8. Davies KA. Complement. *Baillieres Clin Haematol* 1991;4: 927–955.
9. Lim HW. The complement system. Activation, modulation, and clinical relevance. *Dermatol Clin* 1990;8:608–618.
10. Morgan BP. Clinical complementology: recent progress and future trends. *Eur J Clin Invest* 1994;24:219–228.
11. Bartholomet WR, Shanahan TC. Complement components and receptors: deficiencies and disease associations. *Immunol Ser* 1990;52:33–51.
12. Boackle R. The complement system. *Immunol Ser* 1993;58: 135–159.
13. McLean RH. Complement and glomerulonephritis: an update. *Pediatr Nephrol* 1993;7:226–232.
14. Moulds JM, Krych M, Holers VM, et al. Genetics of the complement system and rheumatic diseases. *Rheum Dis Clin North Am* 1992;18:893–914.
15. Krych M, Atkinson JP, Holers VM. Complement receptors. *Curr Opin Immunol* 1992;4:8–13.
16. Schur PH. Complement testing in the diagnosis of immune and autoimmune disease. *Am J Clin Pathol* 1977;68:647–659.
17. Oppermann M, Hopken U, Gotze O. Assessment of complement activation in vivo. *Immunopharmacology* 1992;24: 119–134.
18. Porcel JM, Peakman M, Senaldi G, et al. Methods for assessing complement activation in the clinical immunology laboratory. *J Immunol Methods* 1993;157:1–9.
19. Ruddy S, Carpenter CB, Chin KW, et al. Human complement metabolism: an analysis of 144 studies. *Medicine* 1975;54: 165–178.
20. Colten HR. Biosynthesis of complement. *Adv Immunol* 1976;22:67–118.
21. Frank MM. Detection of complement in relation to disease. *J Allergy Clin Immunol* 1992:89:641–648.
22. Herbert LA, Cosio, Neff JC. Diagnostic significance of hypocomplementemia. *Kidney Int* 1991;39:811–821.
23. Walport MJ. Inherited complement deficiency clues to the physiological activity of complement in vivo. *Q J Med* 1993;86:355–358.
24. Campbell RD, Carroll MC, Porter RR. The molecular genetics of components of complement. *Adv Immunol* 1986;38: 203–244.
25. Ross SC, Densen P. Complement deficiency states and infection: epidemiology, pathogenesis and consequences of Neisserial and other infections in an immune deficiency. *Medicine* 1984;63:243–273.
26. Schur PH. Inherited complement component abnormalities. *Annu Rev Med* 1986:37;333–346.
27. Sjoholm AG. Inherited complement deficiency states and disease. *Complement Inflamm* 1991;8:341–346.
28. Kolble K, Reid KB. Genetic deficiencies of the complement system and association with disease early components. *Int Rev Immunol* 1993;10:17–36.
29. Davies KA, Schifferli JA, Walport MJ. Complement deficiency and immune complex disease. *Springer Semin Immunopathol* 1994;15:397–416.
30. Lokki ML, Colten HR. Genetic deficiencies of complement. *Ann Med* 1995;27:451–459.
31. Stratton F, cited by Lachman PJ. Genetic deficiencies of the complement system. *Boll 1st Sieroter Milan* 1974;53(suppl 1): 195–207.
32. Inai S, Akagaki Y, Moriyama T, et al. Inherited deficiencies of the late-acting complement components other than C9 found among healthy blood donors. *Int Arch Allergy Appl Immunol* 1989;90:274–279.
33. Silverstein AM. Essential hypocomplementemia: report of a case. *Blood* 1960;16:1338–1341.
34. Kirschfink M, Petry F, Khirwadkar K, et al. Complete functional C1q deficiency associated with systemic lupus erythematosus (SLE). *Clin Exp Immunol* 1993;94:267–272.
35. Bowness P, Davies KA, Norsworthy PJ, et al. Hereditary C1q deficiency and systemic lupus erythematosus. *Q J Med* 1994;87: 455–464.
36. Chevailler A, Drouet C, Ponard D, et al. Non-coordinated biosynthesis of early complement components in a deficiency of complement proteins C1r and C1s. *Scand J Immunol* 1994;40: 383–388.
37. Suzuki Y, Ogura Y, Otsubo O, et al. Selective deficiency of C1s associated with a systemic lupus erythematosus-like syndrome. Report of a case. *Arthritis Rheum* 1992;35:576–579.
38. Marcus-Bagley D, Alper CA. Personal communication, 1995.
39. Hartung K, Baur MP, Coldewey R, et al. Major histocompatibility complex haplotypes and complement C4 alleles in systemic lupus erythematosus. Results of a multicenter study. *J Clin Invest* 1992;90:1346–1351.
40. Petri M, Watson R, Winkelstein JA, et al. Clinical expression of systemic lupus erythematosus in patients with C4A deficiency. *Medicine* 1993;72:236–244.
41. Sturfelt G, Truedsson L, Johansen P, et al. Homozygous C4A deficiency in systemic lupus erythematosus: analysis of patients from a defined population. *Clin Genet* 1990;38: 427–433.
42. Lhotta K, Thoenes W, Glatzi J, et al. Hereditary complement deficiency of the fourth component of complement: effects on the kidney. *Clin Nephrol* 1993;39:117–124.
43. Nordin Fredrickson G, Truedsson L, Trudsson L, et al. DNA analysis in a MHC heterozygous patient with complete C4 deficiency homozygosity for C4 gene deletion and C4 pseudogene. *Exp Clin Immunogenet* 1991;8:29–37.
44. Komine M, Matsuyama T, Nojima Y, et al. Systemic lupus erythematosus with hereditary deficiency of the fourth component of complement. *Int J Dermatol* 1992;31:653–656.
45. Fremeaux-Bacchi V, Uring-Lambert B, Weiss L, et al. Complete inherited deficiency of the fourth complement component in a child with systemic lupus erythematosus and his disease-free brother in a north African family. *J Clin Immunol* 1994; 14:273–279.
46. Mauff G, Alper CA, Dawkins R, et al. C4 nomenclature statement (1190). *Complement Inflamm* 1990;7:261–268.
47. Briggs DC, Senaldi G, Isenberg DA, et al. Influence of C4 null alleles on C4 activation in systemic lupus erythematosus. *Ann Rheum Dis* 1991;50:251–254.
48. Moulds JM, Warner NB, Arnett FC. Complement component C4A and C4B levels in systemic lupus erythematosus: quantitation in relation to C4 null status and disease activity. *J Rheumatol* 1993;20:433–437.
49. Baur MP, Danilovs JA. Population analysis of HLA-A,B,C,DR and other genetic markers. In: Terasaki P, ed. *Histocompatibility testing 1980*. Los Angeles: UCLA Tissue Typing Laboratory, 1981:955–975.
50. Baur MP, Neugebauer M, Deppe H, et al. Population analysis on the basis of deducted haplotypes from random families. In:

Albert ED, Bauer MP, Mayr WR, eds. *Histocompatibility testing 1984*. New York: Springer-Verlag, 1984:333–341.

51. Dawkins RL, Christiansen FT, Kay PH, et al. Disease associations with complotypes, supratypes, and haplotypes. *Immunol Rev* 1983;70:5–22.
52. Fielder AH, Walport MJ, Batchelor JR, et al. Family study of the major histocompatibility complex in patients with systemic lupus erythematosus: importance of null alleles of C4A and C4B in determining disease susceptibility. *Br Med J* 1983; 286:425–428.
53. Howard PF, Hochberg MC, Bias WB, et al. Relationship between C4 null genes, HLA-D region antigens and genetic susceptibility to systemic lupus erythematosus in Caucasians and black Americans. *Am J Med* 1986;81:187–193.
54. Davies EJ, Steers G, Ollier WE, et al. Relative contributions of HLA-DQA and complement C4A loci in determining susceptibility to systemic lupus erythematosus. *Br J Rheumatol* 1995; 34:221–225.
55. Ang DF, Siminovitch KA, Liu XY, et al. Population and family studies of three disease-related polymorphic genes in systemic lupus erythematosus. *J Clin Invest* 1995;95:1766–1772.
56. Fran Q, Uring-Lambert B, Weill B, et al. Complement component C4 deficiencies and gene alterations in patients with systemic lupus erythematosus. *Eur J Immunogenet* 1993;20:11–21.
57. De Juan D, Martin-Villa JM, Gomez-Reino JJ, et al. Differential contribution of C4 and HLA-DQ genes to systemic lupus erythematosus susceptibility. *Hum Genet* 1993;91:579–584.
58. Christiansen FT, Zhang WJ, Griffiths M, et al. Major histocompatibility complex (MHC) complement deficiency, ancestral haplotypes and systemic lupus erythematosus (SLE): C4 deficiency explains some but not all of the influence of the MHC. *J Rheumatol* 1991;18:1350–1358.
59. Reveille JD, Anderson KL, Schrohenloher RE, et al. Restriction fragment length polymorphism analysis of HLA-DR, DQ, DP and C4 alleles in Caucasians with systemic lupus erythematosus. *J Rheumatol* 1991;18:14–18.
60. Stephansson EA, Koskimies S, Lokki ML. HLA antigens and complement C4 allotypes inpatients with chronic biologically false positive (CBFP) seroreactions for syphilis: a follow-up study of SLE patients and CBFP reactors. *Lupus* 1993;2:77–81.
61. So AK, Fielder AH, Warner CA, et al. DNA polymorphism of major histocompatibility complex class II and class III genes in systemic lupus erythematosus. *Tissue Antigens* 1990;35:144–147.
62. Kemp ME, Atkinson JP, Skanes VM, et al. Deletion of C4A genes in patients with systemic lupus erythematosus. *Arthritis Rheum* 1987;30:1015–1022.
63. O'Regan S. The clearance of preformed immune complexes in rats with Heymann's nephritis. *Clin Exp Immunol* 1979;37: 432–435.
64. Wilson WA, Perez MC, Aramantis PE. Partial C4A deficiency is associated with susceptibility to systemic lupus erythematosus in black Americans. *Arthritis Rheum* 1988;31:1171–1175.
65. Dunckley H, Gatenby PA, Hawkins B, et al. Deficiency of C4A is a genetic determinant of systemic lupus erythematosus in three ethnic groups. *J Immunogenet* 1987;14:209–218.
66. Hawkins BR, Wong KL, Wong RW, et al. Strong associations between the major histocompatibility complex and systemic lupus erythematosus in southern Chinese. *J Rheumatol* 1987; 14:1128–1131.
67. Doherty DG, Ireland R, Demaine AG, et al. Major histocompatibility complex genes and susceptibility to systemic lupus erythematosus in southern Chinese. *Arthritis Rheum* 1992; 35:641–646.
68. Hong GH, Kim HY, Takeuchi F, et al. Association of complement C4 and HLA-DR alleles with systemic lupus erythematosus in Koreans. *J Rheumatol* 1994;21:442–447.
69. Schur PH, Marcus-Bagley D, Awdeh Z, et al. The effect of ethnicity on major histocompatibility complex complement allotypes and extended haplotypes in patients with systemic lupus erythematosus. *Arthritis Rheum* 1990;33:985–992.
70. Gougerot A, Stopopa-Lyonnet D, Poirer JC, et al. HLA markers and complotypes: risk factors in SLE. *Ann Dermatol Venerol* 1987;113:329–334.
71. Clemenceau S, Castellano F, Montes de Oca M, et al. C4 null alleles in childhood onset systeic lupus erythematosus. Is there any relationship with renal disease? *Pediatr Nephrol* 1990;4: 207–212.
72. Goldstein R, Sengar DPS. Comparative study of the major histocompatibility complex in French-Canadian Caucasians and non-French-Canadian Caucasians with systemic lupus erythematosus. *Arthritis Rheum* 1993;36:1121–1127.
73. Yamada M, Watanabe A, Minori A, et al. Lack of gene deletion for complement C4A deficiency in Japanese patients with systemic lupus erythematosus. *J Rheumatol* 1990;17:1054–1057.
74. Goldstein R, Arnett FC, McLean RH, et al. Molecular heterogeneity of complement component C4-null and 21-hydroxylase genes in systemic lupus erythematosus. *Arthritis Rheum* 1988;31:736–744.
75. Kumar A, Kumar P, Schur PH. DR3 and non-DR3 associated complement component C4A deficiency in systemic lupus erythematosus. *Clin Immunol Immunopathol* 1991;60:55–64.
76. Goldstein R, Moulds JM, Sengar DP. A rare complement component C4 restriction fragment length polymorphism in two families with systemic lupus erythematosus. *J Rheumatol* 1991; 18:345–348.
77. Meyer O, Hauptmann G, Tappeiner G, et al. Genetic deficiency of C4, C2 or C1q and lupus syndromes. Association with anti-Ro (SSA) antibodies. *Clin Exp Immunol* 1985;62:678–684.
78. Spiers C, Fielder AHL, Chapel H, et al. Complement system protein C4 and susceptibility to hydralazine-induced systemic lupus erythematosus. *Lancet* 1989;1:922–924.
79. Adams LE, Balakrishnan K, Roberts SM, et al. Genetic, immunologic and biotransformation studies of patients on procainamide. *Lupus* 1993;2:89–98.
80. Watson RM, Scheel JN, Petri M, et al. Neonatal lupus erythematosus syndrome: analysis of C4 allotypes and C4 genes on 18 families. *Medicine* 1992;71:84–95.
81. Schur PH. Genetics of systemic lupus erythematosus. *Lupus* 1995;4:425–437.
82. Glass D, Raum D, Gibson D, et al. Inherited deficiency of the second component of complement. Rheumatic disease associations. *J Clin Invest* 1976;58:853–861.

82a. Provost TT, Arnett FC, Reichlin M. Homozygous C2 deficiency, lupus erythematosus, and anti-Ro (SSA) antibodies. *Arthritis Rheum* 1983;26:1279–1282.

83. Sullivan KE, Petri MA, Schmeckpeper BJ, et al. Prevalence of a mutation causing C2 deficiency in systemic lupus erythematosus. *J Rheumatol* 1994;21:1128–1133.
84. Truedsson L, Sturfelt G, Nived O. Prevalence of the type 1 complement C2 deficiency gene in Swedish systemic lupus erythematosus patients. *Lupus* 1993;2:325–327.
85. Bittleman DB, Maves KK, Bertolatus JA, et al. Recurrent infections, pericarditis and renal disease in a patient with total C2 deficiency and decreased NK cell function consistent with acute rheumatic fever and systemic lupus erythematosus. *Ann Rheum Dis* 1994;53:280–281.
86. Borradori L, Gueissaz F, Frenk E, et al. Systemic lupus erythematosus associated with homozygous C2 deficiency. Apropos of a case report and literature review. *Schweiz Med Wochenschr* 1991;121:418–423.
87. Agnello V. Complement deficiency states. *Medicine* 1978;57: 1–24.

88. Roberts JL, Schwartz MM, Lewis EJ. Hereditary C2 deficiency and systemic lupus erythematosus associated with severe glomerulonephritis. *Clin Exp Immunol* 1978;31:328–338.
89. Awdeh ZL, Raum DD, Glass D, et al. Complement-HLA haplotypes in C2 deficiency. *J Clin Invest* 1981;67:581–583.
90. Johnson CA, Densen P, Hurford RK, et al. Type I human complement C2 deficiency: a 28 base pair gene deletion causes skipping of exon 6 during RNA splicing. *J Biol Chem* 1993;267: 9347–9353.
91. Kawai T, Katoh K, Narita M, et al. Deficiency of the 9th component of complement (C9) in a patient with systemic lupus erythematosus. *J Rheumatol* 1989;16:542–543.
92. Tedesco F, Silvani CM, Agelli M, et al. A lupus like syndrome in a patient with deficiency of the sixth component complement. *Arthritis Rheum* 1981;24:1438–1440.
93. Nilsson B, Nilsson UR, Karlsson-Parra A, et al. Constitution of the alternative pathway of complement by plasma infusions given to a patient with an SLE-like syndrome associated with a hereditary C3 dysfunction. *Ann Rheum Dis* 1994;53: 691–694.
94. Asghar SS, Venneker GT, van Meegen M, et al. Hereditary deficiency of C5 in association with discoid lupus erythematosus. *J Am Acad Dermatol* 1991;24:376–378.
95. van Hess CL, Boom BW, Vermeer BJ, et al. Subacute cutaneous lupus erythematosus in a patient with inherited deficiency of the third component of complement. *Arch Dermatol* 1992;128: 700–701.
96. Nilsson UR, Nilsson B, Storm KE, et al. Hereditary dysfunction of the third component of complement associated with a systemic lupus erythematosus-like syndrome and meningococcal meningitis. *Arthritis Rheum* 1992;35:580–586.
97. Segurado OG, Arnaiz-Villena AA, Iglesias-Casarrubios P, et al. Combined total deficiency of C7 and C48 with systemic lupus erythematosus (SLE). *Clin Exp Immunol* 1992;87:410–414.
98. Duhra P, Holmes J, Porter DI. Discoid lupus erythematosus associated with hereditary angioneurotic oedema. *Br J Dermatol* 1990;123:241–244.
99. Perkins W, Stables GI, Lever RS. Protein S deficiency in lupus erythematosus secondary to hereditary angio-oedema. *Br J Dermatol* 1994;130:381–384.
100. Minota S, Terai C, Nojima Y, et al. Low C3b receptor reactivity on erythrocytes from patients with systemic lupus erythematosus detected by immune adherence hemagglutination and radioimmunoassays with monoclonal antibody. *Arthritis Rheum* 1984;27:1329–1335.
101. Miyakawa Y, Yamada A, Kosaka K, et al. Defective immune adherence (C3b) receptor on erythrocytes from patients with systemic lupus erythematosus. *Lancet* 1981;2:493–497.
102. Iida K, Mornaghi R, Nussenzweig V. Complement receptor (CR1) deficiency in erythrocytes from patients with systemic lupus erythematosus. *J Exp Med* 1982;155:1427–1438.
103. Satch H, Yokota E, Tokiyama K, et al. Distribution of the HindIII restriction fragment length polymorphism among patients with systemic lupus erythematosus with different concentrations of CR1. *Ann Rheum Dis* 1991;50:765–768.
104. Tausk F, Harpster E, Gigli I. The expression of C3b receptors in the differentiation of discoid lupus erythematosus and systemic lupus erythematosus. *Arthritis Rheum* 1990;33:888–892.
105. Jepsen HH, Moller Rasmussen J, Teisner B, et al. Immune complex binding to erythrocyte-CR1 (CD 35), CR1 expression and levels of erythrocyte-fixed C3 fragments in SLE outpatients. *APMIS* 1990;98:637–644.
106. Corvetta A, Pomponio G, Bencivenga R, et al. Low number of complement C3b/C4b receptors (CR1) on erythrocytes from patients with essential mixed cryoglobulinemia, systemic lupus erythematosus and rheumatoid arthritis: relationship with disease activity, anticardiolipin antibodies, complement activation and therapy. *J Rheumatol* 1991;18:1021–1025.
107. Iversen BM, Vedeler CA, Matre R, et al. CR1 activity on erythrocytes and renal glomeruli in patients with renal disorders. *Nephrol Dial Transplant* 1993;8:1211–1214.
108. Wilson JG, Wong WW, Schur PH, et al. Mode of inheritance of decreased C3b receptors on erythrocytes of patients with systemic lupus erythematosus. *N Engl J Med* 1982;307:981–986.
109. Wilson JG, Wong WW, Murphy EE, et al. Deficiency of the C3b/C4b receptor (CR1) of erythrocytes in systemic lupus erythematosus: analysis of the stability of the defect and of a restriction fragment length polymorphism of the CR1 gene. *J Immunol* 1987;138:2706–2710.
110. Walport MJ, Ross GD, Mackworth-Young C, et al. Family studies of erythrocyte complement type 1 levels: reduced levels in patients with SLE are acquired, not inherited. *Clin Exp Immunol* 1985;59:547–554.
111. Ross GD, Yount WJ, Walport MJ, et al. Disease-associated loss of erythrocyte complement receptors (CR1, C3b receptors) in patients with systemic lupus erythematosus and other diseases involving autoantibodies and/or complement activation. *J Immunol* 1985;135:2205–2214.
112. Moldenhauer F, David J, Felder AHL, et al. Inherited deficiency of erythrocyte complement receptor type 1 does not cause susceptibility to systemic lupus erythematosus. *Arthritis Rheum* 1988;30:961–966.
113. Jouvin MH, Wilson JG, Bourgeois P, et al. Decreased expression of C3b receptor (CR1) on erythrocytes of patients with SLE contrasts with its normal expression in other systemic diseases and does not correlate with the occurrence or severity of SLE nephritis. *Complement* 1986;3:88–96.
114. Wilson JG, Andriopoulos NA, Fearon DT. CR1 and the cell membranes that bind C3 and C4. A basic and clinical review. *Immunol Res* 1987;6:192–209.
115. Uko G, Dawkins RL, Kay P, et al. CR1 deficiency in SLE: acquired or genetic? *Clin Exp Immunol* 1985;62:329–336.
116. Holme E, Fyfe A, Zoma A, et al. Decreased C3b receptors (CR1) on erythrocytes from patients with systemic lupus erythematosus. *Clin Exp Immunol* 1986;63:41–48.
117. Cornillet P, Gredy P, Pennaforte JL, et al. Increased frequency of the long (S) allotype of CR1 (the C3b/C4b receptor, CD35) in patients with systemic lupus erythematosus. *Clin Exp Immunol* 1992;89:22–25.
118. Cohen JH, Lutz HU, Pennaforte JL, et al. Peripheral catabolism of CR1 (the C3b receptor, D35) on erythrocytes from healthy individuals and patients with systemic lupus erythematosus (SLE). *Clin Exp Immunol* 1992;87:422–428.
119. Said PB, Sarano J, Manni JA, et al. Erythrocyte CR1 receptor reactivity in patients with systemic lupus erythematosus. *Medicina* 1990;50:21–24.
120. Walport M, Ng YC, Lachmann PJ. Erythrocytes transfused into patients with SLE and haemolytic anaemia lose complement receptor type 1 from their cell surface. *Clin Exp Immunol* 1987; 69:501–507.
121. Mitchell JA, Batchelor JR, Chapel H, et al. Erythrocyte complement receptor type 1 (CR1) expression and circulating immune complex (CIC) levels in hydralazine-induced SLE. *Clin Exp Immunol* 1987;68:446–456.
122. Hebert LA, Birmingham DJ, Dillon JJ, et al. Erythropoietin therapy in humans increases erythrocyte expression of complement receptor type 1 (CD35). *J Am Soc Nephrol* 1994;4: 1786–1791.
123. Wilson JG, Fearon DT. Altered expression of complement receptors as a pathogenic factor in systemic lupus erythematosus. *Arthritis Rheum* 1984;27:1321–1328.
124. Schur PH. Caucasian ethnic variation and the evaluation of

genetic, clinical and immunological factors in patients with SLE (abstract). *Clin Res* 1988;36:537A.
125. Tebib JG, Martinez C, Granados J, et al. The frequency of complement receptor type 1 (CR1) gene polymorphisms in nine families with multiple cases of systemic lupus erythematosus. *Arthritis Rheum* 1989;32:1465–1468.
126. Wilson JG, Ratnoff WD, Schur PH, et al. Decreased expression of the C3b/C4b receptor (CR1) and the C3d receptor (CR2) on B lymphocytes and of CR1 on neutrophils of patients with systemic lupus erythematosus. *Arthritis Rheum* 1986;29: 739–747.
127. Marquart HV, Svendsen A, Rasmussen JM, et al. Complement receptor expression and activation of the complement cascade on B lymphocytes from patients with systemic lupus erythematosus (SLE). *Clin Exp Immunol* 1995;101:60–65.
128. Yoshida K, Yukiyama Y, Miyamoto T. Quantification of the complement receptor function on polymorphonuclear leukocytes: its significance in patients with systemic lupus erythematosus. *J Rheumatol* 1987;14:490–496.
129. Yu CL, Tsai CY, Chiu CC, et al. Defective expression of neutrophil C3b receptors and impaired lymphocyte Na(+)-K(+)-ATPase activity in patients with systemic lupus erythematosus. *Proc Natl Sci Counc Repub China* 1991;15:178–185.
130. Gray JD, Lash A, Baake AC, et al. Studies on human blood lymphocytes with iC3b (type 3) complement receptors: III. Abnormalities in patients with active systemic lupus erythematosus. *Clin Exp Immunol* 1987;67:556–564.
131. Witte T, Dumoulin FL, Gessner JE, et al. Defect of a complement receptor 3 epitope in a patient with systemic lupus erythematosus. *J Clin Invest* 1993;92:1181–1187.
132. Mitte T, Gessner JE, Gotze O, et al. Complement receptor 3 deficiency in systemic lupus erythematosus. *Immun Infekt* 1992; 20:60–61.
133. Gatenby PA. The role of complement in the aetiopathogenesis of systemic lupus erythematosus. *Autoimmunity* 1991;11: 61–66.
134. Lachmann PJ. Complement deficiency and the pathogenesis of autoimmune immune complex disease. *Chem Immunol* 1990; 49:245–263.
135. Fearon DT. Complement as a mediator of inflammation. *Clin Immunol Allergy* 1981;1:225–242.
136. Fearon DT, Wong WW. Complement ligand-receptor interactions that mediate biological responses. *Annu Rev Immunol* 1983;1:243–271.
137. Frank MM, Atkinson JP. Complement in clinical medicine. *DM* 1975;Jan:154.
138. Mayer MM. Complement, past and present. *Harvey Lett* 1978; 72:139–193.
139. McDonald E, Jarrett MP, Schiffman G, et al. Persistence of pneumococcal antibodies after immunization in patients with systemic lupus erythematosus. *J Rheumatol* 1984;11:306–308.
140. Meryhew NL, Kimberly RP, Messner RP, et al. Mononuclear phagocyte system in SLE. II. A kinetic model of immune complex handling in systemic lupus erythematosus. *J Immunol* 1986;137:97–102.
141. Sturfelt G, Nived O, Sjoholm AG. Kinetic analysis of immune complex solubilization: complement function in relation to disease activity in SLE. *Clin Exp Rheumatol* 1992; 10:241–247.
142. Porter RR. Complement polymorphism, the major histocompatibility complex and associated disease: a speculation. *Mol Biol Med* 1983;1:161–167.
143. Briggs DC, Senaldi G, Isenberg DA, et al. Influence of C4 null alleles on C4 activation in systemic lupus erythematosus. *Ann Rheum Dis* 1991;50:251–254.
144. Welch TR, Beischel L, Berry A, et al. The effect of null Cr alleles on complement function. *Clin Immunol Immunopathol* 1985;34:316–325.
145. Cornacoff JB, Hebert LA, Smead WL, et al. Primate erythrocyte-immune complex-clearing mechanism. *J Clin Invest* 1983; 71:236–247.
146. Horgan C, Taylor RP. Studies on the kinetics of binding of complement-fixing dsDNA/anti-DNA immune complexes to the red blood cells of normal individuals and patients with systemic lupus erythematosus. *Arthritis Rheum* 1984;27:320–329.
147. Taylor RP, Horgan C, Buschbacher R, et al. Decreased complement mediated binding of antibody/3H-dsDNA immune complexes to the red blood cells of patients with systemic lupus erythematosus, rheumatoid arthritis, and hematologic malignancies. *Arthritis Rheum* 1983;26:736–744.
148. Vaughan JH, Bayles TB, Savour CB. The response of serum gammaglobulin level and complement titer to adrenocorticotrophic hormone therapy in lupus erythematosus disseminatus. *J Lab Clin Med* 1961;37:698–702.
149. Schur PH, Sandson J. Immunologic factors and clinical activity in systemic lupus erythematosus. *N Engl J Med* 1968;278: 533–538.
150. Lloyd W, Schur PH. Immune complexes, complement, and anti-DNA in exacerbations of systemic lupus erythematosus (SLE). *Medicine* 1981;60:208–217.
151. Swaak AJG, Gorenwold J, Bronsveld W. Predictive value of complement profiles and anti-dsDNA in systemic lupus erythematosus. *Ann Rheum Dis* 1986;45:359–366.
152. Ricker DM, Hebert LA, Rohde R, et al. Serum C3 levels are diagnostically more sensitive and specific for systemic lupus erythematosus activity than are serum C4 levels. The Lupus Nephritis Collaborative Study Group. *Am J Kidney Dis* 1991; 18:678–685.
153. Ling CK, Hsieh KH. A long-term immunological study of childhood onset systemic lupus erythematosus. *Ann Rheum Dis* 1992;51:45–51.
154. Houssian FA, D'Crue D, Vienna J, et al. Lupus nephritis: the significance of serological tests at the time of biopsy. *Clin Exp Rheumatol* 1991;9:345–349.
155. Zonana-Nacach A, Salar M, Sanchez ML, et al. Measurement of clinical activity of systemic lupus erythematosus and laboratory abnormalities: a 12-month prospective study. *J Rheumatol* 1995;22:45–49.
156. Milis L, Timmermans V, Morris CA, et al. The value of complement measurements in the assessment of lupus activity. *Aust NZ J Med* 1992;22:338–344.
157. Lim KL, Jones AC, Brown NS, et al. Urine neopterin as a parameter of disease activity in patients with systemic lupus erythematosus: comparison with serum sIL-2R and antibodies to dsDNA, erythrocyte sedimentation rate, and plasma C3, C4, and C3 degradation products. *Ann Rheum Dis* 1993;52: 429–435.
158. Buyon JP, Tamerius J, Ordorica S, et al. Activation of the alternative complement pathway accompanies disease flares in systemic lupus erythematosus during pregnancy. *Arthritis Rheum* 1992;35:55–61.
159. Nakamura S, Yoshinari M, Saku Y, et al. Acquired C1 inhibitor deficiency associated with systemic lupus erythematosus affecting the central nervous system. *Ann Rheum Dis* 1991;50: 713–716.
160. Jazwinska EC, Gatenby PA, Dunckley H, et al. C1 inhibitor functional deficiency in systemic lupus erythematosus (SLE). *Clin Exp Immunol* 1993;92:268–273.
161. Honisky S, Intrator L, Wechsler J, et al. Acquired C1 inhibitor deficiency revealing systemic lupus erythematosus. *Dermatology* 1993;186:261–263.
162. Abrass CK, Nies KM, Louie JS, et al. Correlation and predic-

tive accuracy of circulating immune complexes with disease activity in systemic lupus erythematosus. *Arthritis Rheum* 1980;23:273–282.

163. Cairns SA, London A, Mallick NP. The value of three immune complex assays in the management of systemic lupus erythematosus: an assessment of immune complex levels, size and immunochemical properties in relation to disease activity and manifestations. *Clin Exp Immunol* 1980;40:273–282.
164. Cameron JS, Lessof MH, Ogg CS, et al. Disease activity in the nephritis of systemic lupus erythematosus in relation to serum complement concentrations. DNA-binding capacity and precipitating anti-DNA antibody. *Clin Exp Immunol* 1976;25: 418–427.
165. Valentijn RM, Overhagen HV, Hazevoet HM, et al. The value of complement and immune complex determinations in monitoring disease activity in patients with systemic lupus erythematosus. *Arthritis Rheum* 1985;28:904–913.
166. LeBlanc BA, Gladman DD, Urowitz MB. Serologically activity clinically quiescent systemic lupus erythematosus predictors of clinical flares. *J Rheumatol* 1994;21:2239–2241.
167. Auda G, Holme ER, Davidson JE, et al. Measurement of complement activation products in patients with chronic rheumatic diseases. *Rheumatol Int* 1990;10:185–189.
168. Wild G, Watkins J, Ward AM, et al. C4a anaphylatoxin levels as an indicator of disease activity in systemic lupus erythematosus. *Clin Exp Immunol* 1990;80:167–170.
169. Falk RJ, Dalmasso AP, Kim Y, et al. Radioimmunoassay of the attack complex of complement in serum from patients with systemic lupus erythematosus. *N Engl J Med* 1985;315: 1584–1589.
170. Kerr LD, Adelsberg BR, Spiera H. Complement activation in systemic lupus erythematosus: a marker of inflammation. *J Rheumatol* 1986;13:313–319.
171. Senaldi G, Ireland R, Bellingham AJ, et al. IgM reduction in systemic lupus erythematosus (letter). *Arthritis Rheum* 1988; 31:12–13.
172. Sturfelt G, Johnson U, Sjoholm AG. Sequential studies of complement activation in systemic lupus erythematosus. *Scand J Rheumatol* 1985;14:184–196.
173. Porcel JM, Ordi J, Castro-Salomo A, et al. The value of complement activation products in the assessment of systemic lupus erythematosus flares. *Clin Immunol Immunopathol* 1995;74: 283–288.
174. Belmont HM, Hopkins P, Edelson HS, et al. Complement activation during systemic lupus erythematosus. C3a and C5a anaphylatoxins circulate during exacerbations of disease. *Arthritis Rheum* 1986;29:1085–1089.
175. Rother E, Lang B, Coldewey R, et al. Complement split product C3d as an indicator of disease activity in systemic lupus erythematosus. *Clin Rheumatol* 1993;12:31–35.
176. Negoro N, Okamura M, Takeda T, et al. The clinical significance of iC3b neoantigen expression in plasma from patients with systemic lupus erythematosus. *Arthritis Rheum* 1989;32: 1233–1242.
177. Barnum SR, Dahlback B. C4b-binding protein, a regulatory component of the classical pathway of complement, is an acute-phase protein and is elevated in systemic lupus erythematosus. *Complement Inflamm* 1990;7:71–77.
178. Kajdaosy-Balla A, Doe EM, Bagasra O. Activation of factor B of the alternative pathway of complement. Assessment by rocket immunoelectrophoresis. *Am J Clin Pathol* 1987;88:66–73.
179. Garwryl MA, Chudwin DS, Longlois PF, et al. The terminal complement complex, C5b-9, a marker of disease activity in patients with systemic lupus erythematosus. *Arthritis Rheum* 1988;31:188–195.
180. Hagiwara M, Katayose K, Kan R, et al. The feature of epileptic seizures in systemic lupus erythematosus. *Jpn J Psychiatry Neurol* 1987;41:533–534.
181. Sanders ME, Alexander EL, Koski CL, et al. Detection of activated terminal complement (C5b-9) in cerebrospinal fluid from patients with central nervous system involvement of primary Sjogren's syndrome or systemic lupus erythematosus. *J Immunol* 1987;138:2095–2099.
182. Clough JD, Chang RK. Effectiveness of testing for anti-DNA and the complement components iC3b, Bb, and C4 in the assessment of activity of systemic lupus erythematosus. *J Clin Lab Anal* 1990;4:268–273.
183. Horigome I, Seino J, Sudo K, et al. Terminal complement complex in plasma from patients with systemic lupus erythematosus and other glomerular disease. *Clin Exp Immunol* 1987;70: 417–424.
184. Alper CA, Rosen FS. Studies of the in vivo behavior of human C3 in normal subjects and patients. *J Clin Invest* 1967;46: 2021–2034.
185. Sliwinski AJ, Zvaifler NJ. Decreased synthesis of the third component in hypo-complementemic systemic lupus erythematosus. *Clin Exp Immunol* 1972;11:21–29.
186. Tsukamoto H, Ueda A, Nagasawa K, et al. Increased production of the third component of complement (C3) by monocytes from patients with systemic lupus erythematosus. *Clin Exp Immunol* 1990;82:257–261.
187. Lewis E, Lachin J. Primary outcomes in the controlled trial of plasmapheresis therapy in severe lupus nephritis. *Kidney Int* 1987;31:208.
188. Hopkinson ND, Powell RJ. Classical complement activation induced by pregnancy: implications for management of connective tissue disease. *J Clin Pathol* 1992;45:66–67.
189. Ramson SB, Buyon JP. Activation of the complement pathway: comparison of normal pregnancy, preeclampsia, and systemic lupus erythematosus during pregnancy. *Am J Reprod Immunol* 1992;28:183–187.
190. Buyon JP, Cronstein BN, Morris M, et al. Serum complement values (C3 and C4) do differentiate between systemic lupus activity and preeclampsia. *Am J Med* 1986;81:194–200.
191. Lockshin MD, Harpel PC, Druzin ML, et al. Lupus pregnancy. II. Unusual pattern of hypocomplementemia and thrombocytopenia in the pregnant patient. *Arthritis Rheum* 1985;28: 58–66.
192. Shibata S, Sasaki T, Hirabayashi Y, et al. Risk factors in the pregnancy of patients with systemic lupus erythematosus: association of hypocomplementaemia with poor prognosis. *Ann Rheum Dis* 1992;51:619–623.
193. Rubbert A, Pirner K, Wildt L, et al. Pregnancy course and complications in patients with systemic lupus erythematosus. *Am J Reprod Immunol* 1992;28:205–207.
194. Unander AM, Norberg R, Hahn L, et al. Anticardiolipin antibodies and complement in ninety-nine women with habitual abortion. *Am J Obstet Gynecol* 1987;156:114–119.
195. Lange K, Ores R, Strauss W, et al. Steroid therapy of systemic lupus erythematosus based on immunologic considerations. *Arthritis Rheum* 1965;8:244.
196. Appel AE, Sablay LB, Golden RA, et al. The effect of normalization of serum complement and anti-DNA antibody on the course of lupus nephritis: a two-year prospective study. *Am J Med* 1978;64:274–283.
197. Jarrett MP, Sablay LB, Walter L, et al. The effect of continuous normalization of serum hemolytic complement on the course of lupus nephritis. A five year prospect study. *Am J Med* 1981; 70:1067–1072.
198. Morrow WJW, Isenberg DA, Todd-Pokropek A, et al. Useful laboratory measurements in the management of systemic lupus erythematosus. *Q J Med* 1982;51:125–138.

199. Atkinson JP, Gorman JC, Curd J, et al. Cold dependent activation of complement in discrepancy between clinical and laboratory parameters. *Arthritis Rheum* 1981;24:592–601.
200. Abramson SB, Dabro J, Eberle MA, et al. Acute reversible hypoxemia in systemic lupus erythematosus. *Ann Intern Med* 1991;114:941–947.
201. Belmont HM, Buyon J, Giorno R, et al. Up-regulation of endothelial cell adhesion molecules characterizes disease activity in systemic lupus erythematosus. The Shwartzman phenomenon revisited. *Arthritis Rheum* 1994;37:376–383.
202. Gough W, Lightfoot RW, Christian CL. Cryoglobulins and complement in immune complex disease (abstract). *Arthritis Rheum* 1974;17:497.
203. Stastny P, Ziff M. Cold-insoluble complexes and complement levels in SLE. *N Engl J Med* 1969;280:1376–1381.
204. Schur PH. Human gamma G subclasses. *Prog Clin Immunol* 1972;1:71–104.
205. Blomgren SE, Condemi JJ, Bignall MC. Antinuclear antibody induced by procainamide. A prospective study. *N Engl J Med* 1969;281:64–66.
206. Sim E, Gill EW, Sim RB. Drugs that induce systemic lupus erythematosus inhibit complement component C4. *Lancet* 1984; 25(1):422–424.
207. Davis JS, Bollet AJ. Complement levels, rheumatoid factor and renal disease in SLE (abstract). *Arthritis Rheum* 1966;9: 499–500.
208. Antes U, Heniz H-P, Loos M. Evidence for the presence of autoantibodies to the collagen-like portion of C1q in SLE. *Arthritis Rheum* 1988;31:457–464.
209. Siegert CE, Daha MR, Tseng CM, et al. Predictive value of IgG autoantibodies against C1q for nephritis in systemic lupus erythematosus. *Ann Rheum Dis* 1993;52:851–856.
210. Wisnieski JJ, Jones SM. Comparison of autoantibodies to the collagen-like region of C1q in hypocomplementemic urticarial vasculitis syndrome and systemic lupus erythematosus. *J Immunol* 1992;148:1396–1403.
211. Siegert CE, Breedveld FC, Daha MR. Autoantibodies against C1q in systemic lupus erythematosus. *Behring Inst Mitt* 1993; 93:279–286.
212. Prada AE, Strife CF. IgG subclass restriction of autoantibody to solid-phase C1q in membranoproliferative and lupus glomerulonephritis. *Clin Immunol Immunopathol* 1993;63:84–88.
213. Siegert CE, Saha MR, Swaak AJ, et al. The relationship between serum titers of autoantibodies to C1q and age in the general population and in patients with systemic lupus erythematosus. *Clin Immunol Immunopathol* 1993;67:204–209.
214. Siegert CE, Daha MR, Lobatto S, et al. IgG autoantibodies to C1q do not detectably influence complement activation in vivo and in vitro in systemic lupus erythematosus. *Immunol Res* 1992;11:91–97.
215. Cook AD, Rowley MJ, Wines BD, et al. Antibodies to the collagen-like region of C1q and type II collagen are independent non-cross-reactive populations in systemic lupus erythematosus and rheumatoid arthritis. *J Autoimmun* 1994;7:369–378.
216. Siegert C, Daha M, Westedt ML, et al. IgG autoantibodies against C1q are correlated with nephritis, hypocomplementemia, and dsDNA antibodies in systemic lupus erythematosus. *J Rheumatol* 1991;18:230–234.
217. Wisnieski JJ, Jones SM. IgG autoantibody to the collagen-like region of C1q in hypocomplementemic urticarial vasculitis syndrome, systemic lupus erythematosus, and 6 other musculoskeletal or rheumatic diseases. *J Rheumatol* 1992;19:884–888.
218. Antes U, Heinz HP, Hartung K, et al. Autoantibodies against the complement component C1q in systemic lupus erythematosus. *Klin Wochenschr* 1990;68:1066–1070.
219. Nilsson B, Ekdahl KN, Sjoholm A, et al. Detection and characterization of immunoconglutinins in patients with systemic lupus erythematosus (SLE): serial analysis in relation to disease course. *Clin Exp Immunol* 1992;90:251–255.
220. Walport MJ, Davies KA, Botto M, et al. C3 nephritic factor and SLE: report of four cases and review of the literature. *Q J Med* 1994;87:609–615.
221. Hammond A, Rudge AC, Loizou S, et al. Reduced numbers of complement receptors type 1 on erythrocytes are associated with increased levels of anticardiolipin antibodies. Findings in patients with systemic lupus erythematosus and the antiphospholipid syndrome. *Arthritis Rheum* 1989;32:259–264.
222. Hazeltine M, Rauch J, Danoff D, et al. Antiphospholipid antibodies in systemic lupus erythematosus: evidence of an association with positive Coombs' and hypocomplementemia. *J Rheumatol* 1988;15:80–86.
223. Norberg R, Nived O, Sturfelt G, et al. Anticardiolipin and complement activation: relation to clinical symptoms. *J Rheumatol* 1987;18:149–153.
224. Davis WD, Brey RL. Antiphospholipid antibodies and complement activation in patients with cerebral ischemia. *Clin Exp Rheumatol* 1992;10:455–460.
225. Petz LD, Sharp GC, Cooper NR, et al. Serum and cerebral spinal fluid complement and serum autoantibodies in systemic lupus erythematosus. *Medicine* 1971;50:259–275.
226. Hadler NM, Gerwin RD, Frank MM, et al. The fourth component of complement in the cerebrospinal fluid in SLE. *Arthritis Rheum* 1973;16:507–521.
227. Cochrane CG, Koffler D. Immune complex disease in experimental animals and man. *Adv Immunol* 1973;16:185–253.
228. Koffler D, Bieseker G. Immunopathogenesis of tissue injury. In: Schur PH, ed. *The clinical management of systemic lupus erythematosus*. New York: Grune & Stratton, 1983:29–47.
229. Rothfield N, Ross HA, Minta JO, et al. Glomerular and dermal deposition of properdin in systemic lupus erythematosus. *N Engl J Med* 1972;287:681–685.
230. Schur PH. Complement in lupus. *Clin Rheum Dis* 1975;1: 519–543.
231. Verroust PJ, Wilson CB, Cooper NR, et al. Glomerular complement components in human glomerulonephritis. *J Clin Invest* 1974;53:77–84.
232. Gilliam JN, Cheatum DE, Hurd ER, et al. Immunoglobulin in clinically uninvolved skin in systemic lupus erythematosus: association with renal disease. *J Clin Invest* 1974;43: 1434–1440.
233. Provost TT, Tomasi TB Jr. Evidence for complement activation via the alternative pathway in skin diseases, herpes gestationis, systemic lupus erythematosus, and bullous pemphigoid. *J Clin Invest* 1973;52:1779–1787.
234. Tan EM, Kunkel HG. An immunofluorescent study of the skin lesions in systemic lupus erythematosus. *Arthritis Rheum* 1966; 9:37–46.
235. Helm KF, Peters MS. Deposition of membrane attack complex in cutaneous lesions of lupus erythematosus. *J Am Acad Dermatol* 1993;28:687–691.
236. French LE, Polla LL, Tschopp J, et al. Membrane attack complex (MAC) deposits in skin are not always accompanied by S-protein and clusterin. *J Invest Dermatol* 1992;98:758–763.
237. Takematsu H, Tagami H. Complement fragment C4d and Bb levels in inflammatory skin diseases (e.g., SLE, atopic dermatitis, erythroderma and pustulosis palmaris et plantaris) for assessment of complement activation. *Tohoku J Exp Med* 1991;163: 263–268.
238. Kelly RH, Carpenter AB, Sudol KS, et al. Complement C3 fragments in urine: detection in systemic lupus erythematosus patients by western blotting. *Appl Theor Electrophor* 1993;3:265–269.
239. Stone NM, Williams, A, Wilkinson JD, et al. Systemic lupus erythematosus with C1q deficiency. *Br J Dermatol* 2000;142: 521–524.

240. Topaloglu R, Bakkaloglu A, Slingsby JH, et al. Survey of Turkish systemic lupus erythematosus patients for a particular mutation of C1q deficiency. *Clin Exp Rheum* 2000;18:75–77.
241. Berkel AI, Birben E, Oner C, et al. Molecular, genetic and epidemiologic studies on selective complete C1q deficiency in Turkey. *Immunobiology* 2000;201:347–355.
242. Kumar A, Gupta R, Varghese T, et al. Anti-C1q antibody as a marker of disease activity in systemic lupus erythematosus. *Indian J Med Res* 1999;110:190–193.
243. Slingsby JH, Norsworthy P, Pearce G, et al. Homozygous hereditary C1q deficiency and systemic lupus erythematosus. *Arthritis Rheum* 1996;39:663–670.
244. Arora M, Arora R, Tiwari SC, et al. Expression of complement regulatory proteins in diffuse proliferative glomerulonephritis. *Lupus* 2000;9:127–131.
245. Nagy G, Brozik M, Varga L, et al. Usefulness of detection of complement activation products in evaluating SLE activity. *Lupus* 2000;9:19–25.
246. Sullivan KE, Kim NA, Goldman D, et al. C4A deficiency due to a 2 bp insertion is increased in patients with systemic lupus erythematosus. *J Rheumatol* 1999;26:2144–2147.
247. Kobayashi N, Yamada H, Kishida T, et al. Hypocomplementemia correlates with intrauterine growth retardation in systemic lupus erythematosus. *Am J Reprod Immunol* 1999;42:153–159.
248. Navratil JS, Korb LC, Ahearn JM. Systemic lupus erythematosus and complement deficiency: clues to a novel role for the classical complement pathway in the maintenance of immune tolerance. *Immunopharmacology* 1999;42:47–52.
249. Kawano M, Seva T, Koni I, et al. Elevated serum levels of soluble membrane cofactor protein (CD46, MCP) in patients with systemic lupus erythematosus. *Clin Exp Immunol* 1999;116:542–546.
250. Botto M. C1q knock-out mice for the study of complement deficiency in autoimmune disease. *Exp Clin Immunogenet* 1998;15:231–234.
251. Petry F. Molecular basis of hereditary C1q deficiency. *Immunobiology* 1998;199:286–294.
252. Walport MJ, Davies KA, Botto M. C1q and systemic lupus erythematosus. *Immunobiology* 1998;199:265–285.
252a. Herrmann M, Voll RE, Zoller OM, et al. Impaired phagocytosis of apoptotic cell material by monocyte-derived macrophages from patients with systemic lupus erythematosus. *Arthritis Rheum* 1998;41:1241–1250.
253. Inoue N, Saito T, Masuda R, et al. Selective complement C1s deficiency caused by homozygous four-base deletion in the C1s gene. *Hum Genet* 1998;103:415–418.
254. Naves M, Hajeer AH, The LS, et al. Complement C4B null allele status confers risk for systemic lupus erythematosus in a Spanish population. *Eur J Immunogenet* 1998:317–320.
255. Fan Q, Uring-Lambert B, Weill B, et al. Complement component C4 deficiencies and gene alterations in patients with systemic lupus erythematosus. *Eur J Immunogenet* 1993; 20:11–21.
256. Welch TR, Brickman C, Bishof N, et al. The phenotype of SLE associated with complete deficiency of complement isotype C4A. *J Clin Immunol* 1998;18:48–51.
257. Hasely LA, Wisnieski JJ, Denburg MR, et al. Antibodies to C1q in systemic lupus erythematosus: characteristics and relation to Fc gamma RIIA alleles. *Kidney Int* 1997;52:1375–1380.
258. Arujo MN, Silva NP, Andrade LE, et al. C2 deficiency in blood donors and lupus patients: prevalence, clinical characteristics and HLA-associations in the Brazilian population. *Lupus* 1997;6:462–466.
259. Trendelenberg M, Marfurt J, Gerber I, et al. Lack of occurrence of severe lupus nephritis among anti-C1q autoantibody-negative patients. *Arthritis Rheum* 1999;42:187–188.
260. Ravelli A, Wisnieski JJ, Ramenghi B, et al. IgG autoantibodies to complement C1q in pediatric-onset systemic lupus erythematosus. *Clin Exp Rheumatol* 1997;15:215–219.
261. Mannik M, Wener MH. Deposition of antibodies to the collagen-like region of C1q in renal glomeruli of patients with proliferative lupus glomerulonephritis. *Arthritis Rheum* 1997;40:1504–1511.
262. Sjoholm AG, Martensson U, Sturfelt G. Serial analysis of autoantibody responses to the collagen-like region of C1q, collagen type II, and double stranded DNA in patients with systemic lupus erythematosus. *J Rheumatol* 1997;24:871–878.
263. Korb LC, Ahearn JM. C1q binds directly and specifically to surface blebs of apoptotic human keratinocytes: complement deficiency and systemic lupus erythematosus revisited. *J Immunol* 1997;158:4525–4528.
264. Davies EJ, The LS, Ordi-Ros J, et al. A dysfunctional allele of the mannose binding protein gene associates with systemic lupus erythematosus in a Spanish population. *J Rheumatol* 1997;24:485–488.
265. Gunnarsson I, Ronnelid J, Huang YH, et al. Association between ongoing anti-C1q antibody in peripheral blood and proliferative nephritis in patients with active systemic lupus erythematosus. *Br J Rheumatol* 1997;36:32–37.
266. Esdaile JM, Joseph L, Abrahamowicz M, et al. Routine immunologic tests in systemic lupus erythematosus: is there a need for more studies? *J Rheumatol* 1996;23:1891–1896.
267. Sullivan KE, Wisnieski JJ, Winkelstein JA, et al. Serum complement determinations in patients with quiescent systemic lupus erythematosus. *J Rheumatol* 1996;23:2063–2067.
268. Manzi S, Rairie JE, Carpenter AB, et al. Sensitivity and specificity of plasma and urine complement split products as indicators of lupus disease activity. *Arthritis Rheum* 1996;39:1178–1188.
269. Greenstein JD, Peake PW, Charlesworth JA. The metabolism of C9 in normal subjects and in patients with autoimmune disease. *Clin Exp Immunol* 1996; 104:160–166.
270. Pickering MC, Botto M, Taylor PR, et al. Systemic lupus erythematosus, complement deficiency, and apoptosis. *Adv Immunol* 2000;76:227–324
271. Pickering MC, Walport MJ. Links between complement abnormalities and systemic lupus erythematosus. *Rheumatology* 2000;39:133–141.
272. Figueroa JE, Densen P. Infectious disease associated with complement deficiencies. *Clin Microbiol Rev* 1991:4:359–395.
273. Carroll M. The role of complement and complement receptors in induction and regulation of immunity. *Annu Rev Immunol* 1998;16:545–568.
274. Garred P, Madsen HO, Halberg P, et al. Mannose-binding lectin polymorphisms and susceptibility to infection in systemic lupus erythematosus. *Arthritis Rheum* 1999;42:2145–2152.
275. Yamashina M, Ueda E, Kinoshita T, et al. Inherited complete deficiency of 20-kilodalton homologous restriction factor (CD59) as a cause of paroxysmal nocturnal hemoglobinuria. *N Engl J Med* 1990;323:1184–1189.
276. Hollman TJ, Haviland DL, Kildsgaard J, et al. Cloning, expression, sequence determination and chromosomal localization of the mouse complement C3a anaphylatoxin gene. *Mol Immunol* 1998;35:137–148.
277. Ip WK, Chan SY, Lau CS, et al. Association of systemic lupus erythematosus with promoter polymorphisms of the mannose-binding lectin gene. *Arthritis Rheum* 1998;41:1663–1668.
278. Kiss E, Kavai M, Csipo I, et al. Recombinant human erythropoietin modulates erythrocyte complement receptor type 1 functional activity in patients with lupus nephritis. *Clin Nephrol* 1998;49:364–369.
279. Klickstein LB, Barbashov SF, Liu T, et al. Complement receptor type 1 (CR1, CD35) is a receptor for C1q. *Immunity* 1997;7:345–355.

14

MECHANISMS OF ACUTE INFLAMMATION AND VASCULAR INJURY IN SYSTEMIC LUPUS ERYTHEMATOSUS

H. MICHAEL BELMONT
STEVEN B. ABRAMSON

Inflammation in systemic lupus erythematosus (SLE) is mediated by a complex interaction of the cellular and humoral components of the immune system. In contrast to the host immune response to infection that begins with a known inflammatory trigger, the etiologies of connective tissue diseases such as SLE remain undefined. In the absence of known etiologies, treatment strategies rely on the dissection of inflammatory processes into component parts while keeping in mind the complex interaction of these components. This chapter reviews inflammatory mediators released from cells—neutrophils, monocytes, and platelets—as well as humoral activators of these cells, such as chemoattractants, complement components, and immune complexes. A particular focus is placed on the pathogenic mechanisms by which inflammatory cells and mediators provoke vascular injury in SLE. Additionally, since endothelial injury and subsequent alteration of endothelial adhesiveness and permeability to leukocytes and platelets are principal mechanisms of both the inflammatory states that characterize exacerbated SLE as well as atherosclerosis, we discuss the relationship between atherosclerosis and autoimmunity.

THE ROLE OF CIRCULATING PHAGOCYTIC CELLS AND PLATELETS IN IMMUNE INJURY

The activation of phagocytic cells and platelets in response to chemoattractants, immune complexes, and other stimuli provokes the release of inflammatory mediators that account for diverse manifestations of inflammation in autoimmune disease (Table 14.1). The major effector cells and their functions are discussed in the following sections.

NEUTROPHILS

Neutrophils, together with monocyte/macrophages, are the body's "professional phagocytes." While in the circulation neutrophils are maintained in a resting state, with their wide array of cytoxic mediators either stored in cytoplasmic granules or separated into plasma membrane and cytosolic compartments. Activation of the cell may be triggered by the engagement of particles, such as invading microorganisms, or in the case of autoimmune disease, in response to soluble stimuli that engage specific cell surface receptors.

Directed Migration or Chemotaxis

In inflammation, the initial step of neutrophil activation requires movement toward a target. Such directed migration, or chemotaxis, occurs along a chemical gradient originating at the target. Welldescribed "chemoattractants" include bacterial products such as formulated peptides, and activated complement components, such as C5a. These chemoattractants interact with specific surface receptors that have seven hydrophobic transmembrane domains (1). Ligand/receptor interactions lead to conformational changes of the receptor that allow it to interact with, and activate, heterotrimeric G [guanosine triphosphate (GTP)-binding] proteins. Activation of G proteins results in the generation of an intracellular signal that triggers chemotaxis and related functional responses.

The activation of ligand/receptor complexes not only is capable of initiating chemotaxis, but also can trigger other cellular responses, as described below.

Phagocytosis

Following directed migration along a chemoattractant gradient, phagocytosis is initiated by the attachment or bind-

TABLE 14.1. PROINFLAMMATORY MEDIATORS RELEASED BY NEUTROPHILS, MACROPHAGES, AND PLATELETS

- Secretory products produced by neutrophils and macrophages
  - Reactive oxygen intermediates (e.g., superoxide anion)
  - Proteolytic enzymes
  - Reactive nitrogen intermediates (e.g., nitric oxide)
  - Bioactive lipids
    - Cyclooxygenase products: prostaglandin E_2 (PGE_2), prostaglandin F_{2a}, prostacyclin, thromboxane
  - Lipooxygenase products: monohydroxyeicosatetraenoic acids, dihydroxyeicosatetraenoic acids, leukotrienes B_4, C, D and E[a]
  - Platelet-activating factors
    - (1 O-alkyl-2-acetyl-*sn*-glyceryl-3-phosphorylcholine)
  - Chemokines (e.g., interleukin-8)
- Secretory products produced by macrophages
  - Polypeptide hormones
    - Interleukin 1α and 1β (collectively, IL-1)
    - Tumor necrosis factor-α (cachectin, TNF)
    - Interferon-α
    - Interferon-α (confirmation needed)
    - Platelet-derived growth factor(s)
    - Transforming growth factor-β
    - β-endorphin
  - Complement (C) components
    - Classic path: C1, C4, C2, C3, C5
    - Alternative path: factor B, factor D, properdin
  - Coagulation factors
    - Intrinsic path: IX, X, V, prothrombin
    - Extrinsic path: VII
    - Surface activities: tissue factor, prothrombinase
    - Prothrombolytic activity: plasminogen activator inhibitors, plasmin inhibitors
- Secretory products produced by platelet
  - Plasminogen
  - α_2-plasmin inhibitor
  - Platelet-derived growth factor
  - Platelet factor IV
  - Transforming growth factors α and β
  - Serotonin
  - Adenosine diphosphate
  - Thromboxane A_2
  - 12-hydroxytetraenoic acid

[a]Not produced by neutrophils

ing of target particles to the neutrophil surface. Attachment is followed by enclosure of the particle within a plasma membrane pouch. Upon closure this pouch becomes a vacuole in the cytoplasm, termed a phagosome. In most instances, soon after particle ingestion, primary or secondary lysosomes fuse with the phagosome, which are then termed phagolysosomes. Fusion of the respective membranes permits entry of lysosomal contents into the phagosome and the shielded enzymatic degradation of ingested material, an important aspect of the scavenging function of both neutrophils and macrophages. Thus, phagocytosis can deliver a microbial prey to a sequestered compartment in which the noxious action of host cytotoxins (e.g., degradative enzymes) can be confined.

Macrophages and neutrophils "recognize" certain serumderived molecules when these molecules coat particles to be phagocytosed. These molecules, antibodies and/or complement components, (originally called opsonins, from the Greek "to prepare food for") bind to bacteria, cells, or other surfaces and increase the efficiency of phagocytosis. It is important to emphasize that the phagocytes recognize antibody and/or complement-coated particles because they have surface receptors for immunoglobulin and for the C3 fragments C3b and iC3b. Using this strategy, phagocytes can consume a wide variety of different particles, since the stimulus to phagocytosis depends not on the characteristics of the organism, but rather on recognition of the two major opsonins by specific cell surface receptors.

Although designed primarily to ingest invading microorganisms, macrophages and neutrophils can be triggered by opsonins to release cytotoxic products in the absence of phagocytosis. This occurs in autoimmune disease where antibodies activate the complement system and where soluble immune complexes with covalently bound (i)C3b can engage neutrophil Fc and complement receptors. While the host has multiple inhibitory proteins in extracellular biologic fluids that inactivate released products, such protective mechanisms can be overcome with resultant tissue injury as observed in necrotizing vasculitis, arthritis, and glomerulonephritis (2).

Release of Toxic Proteolytic Enzymes

Neutrophils contain two morphologically distinct granules (specific and azurophilic) that contain proteases, which under normal circumstances are sequestered within the granule and the phagolysosome, presenting no threat to the host. However the extracellular release of granule contents may promote inflammation and damage at tissue sites. Phagocytosis is not necessary for neutrophil degranulation, which may be provoked by soluble stimuli (e.g., C5a, interleukin-8). Degranulation is augmented when neutrophils encounter stimuli deposited on a surface: lysosomal release unfolds by a process of reverse endocytosis, or what has been called "frustrated phagocytosis." This exuberant release of lysosomal enzymes from neutrophils may be relevant to the pathogenesis of tissue injury in diseases characterized by the deposition of immune complexes on cell surfaces or on such extracellular surfaces as vascular basement membranes or articular cartilage (3).

In glomerulonephritis, neutrophil-derived proteases can be demonstrated in urine and are involved in the degradation of the extracellular matrix proteins of the glomerular basement membrane (GBM) and mesangium. The principal proteases that promote GBM degradation appear to be serine proteases, elastase, and cathepsin G, as well as neutrophil collagenase (4). In addition to proteases, neutrophils also release cationic proteins with bactericidal activity, such as lysozyme, bactericidal/permeability increasing factor

(BPI), and the defensins, which increase glomerular permeability by neutralizing the anionic components of the GBM.

Production of Toxic Oxygen Radicals

When phagocytic leukocytes are activated, molecular oxygen consumption by the leukocyte is increased. The majority of this oxygen is transformed directly into superoxide anion radicals. Oxygen-derived free radicals are significant mediators of inflammation causing tissue injury and irreversible modification of macromolecules (5). Superoxide anion is produced by the addition of an extra electron to molecular oxygen by a multiprotein complex that requires membrane-bound cytochrome b_{558} and key cytosolic proteins (including a *ras*-related low molecular weight GTP-binding protein). The multiprotein complex, known as the reduced nicotinamide adenine dinucleotide phosphate (NADPH) oxidase, is assembled at the plasma membrane in response to cell activation. The NADPH oxidase transfers electrons from NADPH to oxygen, forming free radical derivatives of oxygen that are highly reactive, particularly with proteins containing Fe-S centers, lipids, and DNA, and are therefore broadly cytotoxic. Stimulated neutrophils also produce hydrogen peroxide, hydroxyl radicals, and possibly, singlet oxygen.

Some of the most toxic oxygen metabolites produced by neutrophils are generated by the myeloperoxidase (MPO)-hydrogen peroxidehalide system. MPO is a highly cationic enzyme present in the azurophilic granules that catalyzes the reaction of hydrogen peroxide with a halide such as chloride to form hypohalous acids (e.g., hypochlorous acid). These products are capable of killing a variety of microorganisms as well as mammalian cells. There is evidence that the MPOhydrogen peroxide-halide system plays a significant role in phagocyte-mediated injury in glomerulonephritis (4).

MACROPHAGES

Macrophages as Secretory Cells in Inflammation

Macrophages/monocytes play an important role in immune-mediated tissue injury particularly in nephritis (6). These cells express the three major classes of Fc receptors as well as β1, β2, and β3 integrins, which facilitate phagocytosis of opsonized particles, intercellular adhesion, and adhesion to extracellular matrix proteins. Monocytes are recruited into tissues from the circulation in response to chemotactic factors [e.g., C5a, interleukin-8 (IL-8), transforming growth factor-β (TGF-β), fragments of collagen and fibronectin] produced at inflammatory sites. Recruitment requires the expression of adhesion molecules on activated vascular endothelium [e.g., intercellular adhesion molecule-1 (ICAM-1), vascular cell adhesion molecule (VCAM-1)], which are recognized by counterligands of the circulating monocyte (e.g., lymphocyte function associated antigen 1 [LFA-1] and very late antigen 1 [VLA-1], respectively). When monocytes emigrate into tissues they can be transformed into activated macrophages following exposure to cytokines such as interferon-γ (IFN-γ), IL-1, and tumor necrosis factor (TNF). Macrophage activation results in an increase in cell size, increased synthesis of proteolytic enzymes, and the secretion of a variety of inflammatory products.

Release of Inflammatory Mediators and Proteases

Macrophages secrete up to 100 substances, ranging from free radicals, such as superoxide anion, to large macromolecules, such as fibronectin (5). Some products are secreted in response to inflammatory stimuli, while others are constitutively released. For example, plasminogen activator, which converts plasminogen to plasmin, is secreted at low levels by monocytes or nonstimulated macrophages, and is augmented by inflammatory stimuli. Plasmin not only degrades fibrin, but also activates complement components C1 and C3. Activated macrophages produce plasminogen activator in two forms: a soluble form released into the extracellular medium and a cellassociated form. Collagenase is another neutral protease constitutively secreted at low levels by non-activated macrophages; stimulation with IL-1 and toxin augments secretion. In such chronic inflammatory sites as the rheumatoid synovium, collagen may be partially degraded by macrophagesecreted collagenases. Lysozyme, a cationic protein that hydrolyses the glucose linkages in bacterial cell walls, is also a macrophage secretory product. It has also been detected in human osteoarthritic cartilage where it is believed to be secreted by activated chondrocytes.

When stimulated by exposure to immune complexes, endotoxin, IL-1, or C3bcoated particles, macrophages and monocytes exhibit a procoagulant activity (7). The procoagulant products include tissue factor (identified as a receptor for factor VII), factor X activator, prothrombin activator, and vitamin (K-dependent clotting factors II, VII, IX, and X. Monocytes in rheumatic disease patients display a higher procoagulantproducing activity than normal, likely a result of exposure to cytokines and cleavage products of complement. Increased procoagulant activity may contribute to fibrin deposition at sites of inflammation and has been implicated in the formation of crescent formation in glomerulonephritis. Whether such increased macrophage procoagulant activity observed in these conditions also promotes a systemic "hypercoagulable" state in SLE remains unknown.

Production of Cytokines

Macrophages also secrete a variety of polypeptide hormones that regulate immune function and inflammation as well as wound healing and repair (8). Macrophages, for example, produce three cytokines, IL1-α, IL1-β, and TNF-α, which not only have overlapping functions, but also are capable of inducing each others' release by macrophages themselves (5). Macrophages also produce the cytokine neutrophilactivating peptide1/IL-8, which is a potent neutrophil chemoattractant. The production of IL-8, induced by IL1-α, IL1-β, and TNF-α has been described in a variety of tissues, including alveolar macrophages, renal mesangial cells, and psoriatic skin lesions (9). IL-8 is now known to be a member of a family of macrophage inflammatory proteins (MIPs) or chemokines.

The chemokines form a superfamily of small molecular mass proteins that consists of greater than 30 cloned members. These proteins were originally classified based on their structural and restricted functional similarities (10,11). Two families of chemokines are distinguished depending on the arrangement of the first two of four conserved cysteines, which are either separated by one amino acid (CXC chemokines) or adjacent (CC chemokines). IL-8 and the other CXC chemokines act preferentially on neutrophils, while the CC chemokines (MCP-1, MCP-2, MCP-3, RANTES, MIP1-α, and MIP-1β) act on monocytes, but not neutrophils, and have additional activities toward basophil and eosinophil granulocytes, and T lymphocytes. Several chemokine receptors have been identified, all of which belong to the seventransmembranedomain type and are coupled to G proteins. The discovery of chemokines has provided the basis for the understanding of leukocyte recruitment and activation in inflammation and other disturbances of tissue homeostasis.

Nitric Oxide as a Modulator of Inflammation

Macrophages are also among the cellular sources of reactive nitrogen intermediates such as nitric oxide (NO). NO, although originally identified as a product of endothelial cells, which accounts for "endothelium-derived relaxation factor" activity, is now appreciated to be a highly reactive molecule with diverse biologic functions. The exposure of macrophages to cytokines (e.g., IL1-B, IFN-γ) markedly increases NO production. Activities of NO that may be important in the inflammatory response include vasodilation and its capacity to react with superoxide anion to form toxic peroxynitrite compounds. Consistent with a proinflammatory role in SLE, the inhibition of NO synthesis has been demonstrated to reduce the severity of glomerulonephritis in Medical Research Laboratory lymphoproliferative (MRL/*lpr*) mice (12). In human arthritis the production of NO by both synovial macrophages and articular chondrocytes has been demonstrated in both rheumatoid and osteoarthritis (1,13). NO, constitutively produced by vascular endothelium, may exert antiinflammatory properties (14). For example, NO inhibits neutrophil and platelet aggregation, inhibits the adhesion of neutrophils to endothelial cells, inhibits neutrophil oxidant production, and thereby may serve as a "Teflon coat" for blood vessel walls against cellular injury (15). Thus, the role of NO in inflammation is complex. The pro or antiinflammatory properties will depend on (a) whether NO is constitutive (and therefore physiologic) or induced (usually pathologic), (b) the potential for the formation of toxic derivatives such as peroxynitrite, and (c) the adaptive responses of target cells.

PLATELETS

Platelets as Inflammatory Cells

Platelets, derived from marrow megakaryocytes, are involved in hemostasis, wound healing, and cellular responses to injury (16,17). In addition to its important hemostatic function, the platelet may also act as an inflammatory effector cell. In primitive organisms, a single cell type served both leukocyte and platelet functions. In higher organisms, platelets have retained some properties of inflammatory cells. For example platelets (a) display chemotaxis to a variety of stimuli including platelet-activating factor (PAF) and collagen fragments, (b) can endocytose immune complexes via Fc receptors, (c) release inflammatory mediators upon activation and aggregation, (d) are activated by phlogistic agents (such as complement activation products), (e) play a role in animal models of inflammatory disease, and (f) have been identified in localization and activation at tissue injury sites in human inflammatory diseases. Platelet activation at sites of tissue injury is achieved by such hemostatic factors as thrombin, adenosine diphosphate, arachidonate derivates, and exposed subendothelial collagen. There is evidence of platelet activation in immunologically mediated diseases such as asthma, cold urticaria, scleroderma, and SLE (18–20).

Upon exposure to subendothelial matrix proteins, platelets undergo three reactions: adhesion and shape change, secretion of granular contents, and aggregation. Normal adhesion to extracellular matrix proteins requires von Willebrand factor (vWF), which binds to the platelet surface glycoprotein gpIb and serves as a molecular bridge between platelets and subendothelial collagen. Following adhesion, platelets release granular contents that promote clotting and platelet aggregation. During this process, activated platelets release a variety of both protein and lipid-derived mediators with inflammatory potential, and factors with chemotactic, proliferative, thrombogenic, and proteolytic activity. Stimuli that activate platelet adhesion and degranulation also trigger the release of arachidonic acid from the membrane. This initiates the synthesis of thromboxane A_2 (TxA_2) and 12-hydroxytetraenoic acid (12HETE). TxA_2 promotes platelet aggregation and vasoconstriction; 12HETE activates neutrophils and macrophages.

Products released from platelets, which may promote local inflammation, are classified according to their intracellular granule of origin. Dense granules release adenosine diphosphate (ADP), which activates platelet fibrinogen binding sites of the $\gamma 3$ integrin gpIIb/IIIa, and serotonin, a potent vasoconstrictor. α-Granule components include platelet factor 4 and β-thromboglobulin, which have been reported to activate both mononuclear and polymorphonuclear leukocytes. α-Granules are also the source of platelet-derived growth factor (PDGF), which stimulates proliferation of smooth muscle cells and fibroblasts; thrombospondin, which promotes neutrophil adherence to blood vessel walls; factor VIII (vWF); factor V; fibrinogen; and fibronectin.

Platelets express two surface adhesion-promoting molecules: First, gpIIb/IIIa (activated by ADP) binds fibrinogen, fibronectin, vitronectin, and vWF (21). Second, P-selectin (GMP140, PADGEM), a member of the selectin family of adhesion molecules, is a membrane glycoprotein located in the α granules of platelets and Weibel-Palade bodies of endothelium. When these cells are activated by agents such as thrombin, P-selectin is rapidly translocated to the plasma membrane where it functions as a receptor for neutrophils and monocytes. Expression of P-selectin on activated platelets may therefore facilitate recruitment of neutrophils and monocytes to sites of thrombosis or inflammation (22).

Platelets in Glomerulonephritis

Platelets have been identified in the glomeruli of patients with SLE nephritis where they are believed to play a particularly important role (23). Urinary thromboxane levels are elevated in patients with active lupus nephritis, a finding that has several implications: first, it is a sign of abnormal platelet aggregation in the microvasculature with the potential for thrombosis and endothelial injury; second, the vasoconstrictive properties of TxA_2 would be expected to decrease glomerular filtration rate (GFR) and renal blood flow (RBF); and third, the release of growth factors and other mediators by activated platelets could aggravate the proliferative glomerular lesion. Studies of the administration of specific TxA_2 antagonists have shown promise in the improvement of both GFR and RBF in SLE nephritis (24).

Platelet activation in lupus glomerulonephritis has been attributed to a variety of substances, including immune complexes, activated complement components (including C3a and the membrane attack complex, C5b-9), PAF, and vasopressin. In addition, neutrophils may also be able to activate platelets via the release of oxidants and proteases. Platelets may aggravate immune injury in glomerulonephritis via several mechanisms, which include (a) promoting thrombosis; (b) reducing GFR through the production of thromboxane and other vasoactive substances; and (c) releasing products that activate macrophages, neutrophils, and glomerular mesangial cells (4).

THE ROLE OF RECEPTORS FOR COMPLEMENT AND IMMUNE COMPLEXES IN INFLAMMATION

Complement Receptors

The first event in an inflammatory process that begins with chemotaxis requires the margination, attachment, and egress of activated neutrophils from the circulation. As noted above, phagocytic cells express receptors for the complement fragment C3b (receptor designated CR1) and its inactivated cleavage product iC3b (receptor designated CR3, or CD11b/CD18) (25). On the surface of phagocytes, both CR1 and CD11b/CD18 play important roles in the clearance of particles, such as opsonized bacteria, to which C3b or iC3b are bound. This clearance mechanism is also essential for the removal of immune complexes containing C3b and iC3b (26). In addition to its role as a receptor for iC3b, CD11b/CD18 is the major neutrophil adhesion molecule responsible for the capacity of the neutrophil to adhere to vascular endothelium and to other neutrophils (27). CD11b/CD18 is a member of a family of surface glycoproteins known as β_2-integrins, which are heterodimers consisting of a common β subunit (CD18) and distinct α subunits (CD11a, CD11b, CD11c). In the neutrophil the most important β_2-integrin appears to be CD11b/CD18 (CD11B/CD18), required for normal phagocytosis, aggregation, adhesion, and chemotaxis. ICAM1, expressed on resting and activated endothelial cells, has been identified as a ligand for the CD18 integrins (28). Interaction between CD18 and ICAM-1 modulates both the adhesion of neutrophils to vascular endothelium and their egress to the extravascular space. The initial rolling of activated neutrophils on endothelium, a prerequisite for CD18-dependent adhesion under conditions of flow, is mediated by a separate molecular interaction—that between the selectins, E-selectin and P-selectin, on the endothelial cell and a carbohydrate ligand, sialyl-Lex, on the neutrophil (22,23,29). In addition, the neutrophil expresses L-selectin on its surface, which also promotes rolling, and is shed from the plasma membrane upon cell activation. The redundancy with regard to selectin function may in part be explained by the different kinetics of their participation in the events of intracellular adhesion: L-selectin is shed within seconds of neutrophil activation; P-selectin is stored in the Weibel-Palade bodies in endothelial cells and expressed on the surface within minutes following exposure of the cells to acute stimuli, such as thrombin; and E-selectin is upregulated over several hours following cytokine exposure in a process that requires transcription and translation of new protein.

Important therapeutic strategies have evolved from the recent recognition that the ability of toxic mediators released by activated neutrophils to injure vascular endothelium is dependent on their capacity to adhere to the target cell. Experimental models of immune complex–mediated lung injury, ischemiareperfusion injury, and adjuvant arthritis can each be ameliorated by strategies that utilize blocking antibodies to CD18, ICAM-1 or selectins in order to prevent neutrophilendothelial cell attachment. It is likely that these antiadhesion strategies will lead to novel clinical interventions.

Fc Receptors

Autoimmune disorders are characterized by the production of autoantibodies of a wide range of specificities. Immunoglobulin M (IgM) and multimeric IgG can trigger complement-mediated endorgan damage by binding to tissuespecific antigens via their antigen-binding sites. Insoluble immune complexes, however, precipitate in tissues and provoke significant destruction by direct activation of inflammatory cells. By activating cells at the site of deposition, these immune aggregates can provoke release of proteolytic enzymes and toxic oxygen metabolites along endothelial basement membranes. Neutrophils, monocytes/macrophages, platelets, B lymphocytes, and natural killer cells all express receptors for immune complexes (30). These receptors primarily bind aggregated IgG, although receptors for IgE, most commonly expressed on mast cells, are found at a low level on these cells. There are three types of receptors for multimeric IgG that bind these complexes via their Fc fragments; hence, these receptors are termed FcRI, II, and III.

Three families of receptors for the Fc region of IgG, FcγR have been identified: FcγRI, II, and III. Within each of these families distinct genes and alternative splicing variants create a variety of receptor isoforms with distinct functional capacities (31). Fc receptor interactions have been reported. For example, the crosslinking of FCγRIIIb, which leads to neutrophil degranulation and oxidant production, in turn amplifies FCγRII-mediated phagocytosis (32).

In addition, FcγR polymorphisms affect phagocytic function and may therefore contribute to disease susceptibility factors in the development of autoimmunity (33).

Immune complexes trigger neutrophil activation by the generation of similar intracellular messengers to those provoked by treatment with chemoattractants. Engagement of FcR provokes rises in inositol phosphates, cytosolic Ca^{2+} (34), diacylglycerol (35,36), and phosphatidic acid. In addition, immune complexes activate membranebound guanosine triphosphatases (GTPases) as well as cytosolic tyrosine kinases in inflammatory cells (37–39). However, immune complex activation of inflammatory cells utilizes enzymatic pathways of signal transduction that are distinct from those triggered by chemoattractants. The generation of these second messengers by immune complexes differ kinetically and in sensitivity to inhibitors (pertussis toxin, gonococcal Por protein) from those triggered by chemoattractants (35,36,40–42).

Because of the multiple classes of FcR expressed on individual cell types, it has been difficult to dissect the role of the various receptors in cell activation (although platelets, possessing only FcRII are an exception). By means of monoclonal antibodies (mAbs) generated against FcRII (mAb IV.3) or FcRIII (mAb 3G8) that block binding of immune complexes to the respective receptor on neutrophils (35,40), it has been demonstrated that ligation of the unblocked FcR can still provoke lysosomal enzyme release from neutrophils. Similar effects have been shown for other neutrophil functions, such as actin polymerization (43), phagocytosis (44), and superoxide anion generation (45). However, the maximal cellular response to immune complexes is a synergistic one, requiring engagement of both FcRII and III. One would infer from these data that the engagement of either receptor activates a distinct signal transduction mechanism, sufficient in itself for cell activation but capable of "priming" the other. Clear evidence for this has been demonstrated with regard to calcium fluxes; engagement of FcRII can provoke early and sustained increments in Ca^{2+}, whereas FcRIII activation triggers a more transient release of Ca^{2+} (46,47). Whether either receptor can provoke influx of extracellular Ca^{2+} is not yet clear (47,48).

THE ACTIVATION OF PHAGOCYTES AND PLATELETS IN THE DEVELOPMENT OF VASCULAR INJURY IN SLE

Systemic lupus erythematosus is the autoimmune disease that best exemplifies the consequences of the systemic generation of humoral inflammatory mediators and the activation of the cellular constituents of inflammation as outlined above. Immune complex formation, episodic complement activation, the recruitment of stimulated leukocytes and platelets into tissues, and endothelial cell activation produce vascular injury during SLE exacerbations. Vascular disease in SLE can be classified into two broad categories: inflammatory and thrombotic. The former may be associated with local deposition of immune complexes or result from leukocyte-endothelial cell interactions in the absence of immune complex deposition, and the latter is almost invariably associated with circulating antiphospholipid antibodies (Table 14.2).

INFLAMMATORY VASCULAR DISEASE

In most instances inflammatory vascular disease in SLE involves complement activation in the presence or absence of immune complexes, as described below.

The Complement System

The complement system is composed of at least 20 plasma proteins that participate in a variety of host defense and

TABLE 14.2. PATHOLOGIC AND CLINICAL SPECTRUM OF VASCULAR INJURY IN SYSTEMIC LUPUS ERYTHEMATOSUS (SLE)

Pathology	Pathogenesis	Clinical Phenomenon
Capillaritis[a] Vasculitis[a]	Immune complex deposition Activation of complement, neutrophils, and endothelium Modeled by Arthus lesion	[b]Glomerulonephritis, pulmonary alveolar hemorrhage [c]Cutaneous purpura, polyarteritis nodosa-like systemic and cerebral vasculitis
Leukothrombosis	Intravascular activation of complement, neutrophils, and vascular endothelium Absence of local immune complex deposition Modeled by Shwartzman lesion	Widespread vascular injury, hypoxia, cerebral dysfunction, SIRS
Thrombosis	Antibodies to anionic phospholipid-protein complexes interact with endothelial cells, platelets, or coagulation factors Modeled by APS	Arterial and venous thrombosis, fetal wastage, thrombocytopenia, pulmonary hypertension
	Disseminated intravascular platelet aggregation	TTP
Atherosclerosis	Activated endothelium, increased endothelial cell adhesion molecules, increased tissue factor, decreased 27-hydroxylase	MI, CVA

[a]Capillaritis or microvascular angiitis and lupus vasculitis share a similar pathogenesis but are associated with different clinical phenomena, designated here as [b] and [c].
APS, antiphospholipid syndrome; CVA, cerebrovascular accident; MI, myocardial infarction; SIRS, systemic inflammatory response syndrome; TTP, thrombotic thrombocytopenic purpura.

immunologic reactions. Each complement component is cleaved via a limited proteolytic reaction that proceeds by either the classic or alternative pathway. The alternative pathway is more primitive and may be activated by contact with a variety of substances including polysaccharides (such as endotoxin) found in the cell walls of microorganisms. The activation of the classic pathway by immune complexes requires binding of the first complement component, C1, to sites on the Fc portions of immunoglobulins, particularly of the IgG1, IgG3, and IgM isotypes.

Activation of C3

Activation of the third component of complement is central to both the classic and alternative pathways. C3 is cleaved by convertases to two active products, C3a and C3b. C3a, released into the fluid phase, provokes the release of histamine from mast cells and basophils, causes smooth muscle contraction, and induces platelet aggregation. C3b has two functions: C3b is part of the C5 convertase that continues the complement cascade; C3b is also the major opsonin of the complement system. It binds to immune complexes and to a variety of activators such as microbial organisms. The binding of C3b to these particles facilitates the attachment of the particle to the C3b receptor on cells, complement receptor 1 (CR1), which is present on erythrocytes, neutrophils, monocytes, B lymphocytes, and glomerular podocytes. CR1 on phagocytes potentiates phagocytosis. CR1 on erythrocytes, which accounts for approximately 90% of CR1 in blood, facilitates the clearance of immune complexes from the circulation by transporting erythrocyte-bound complexes to the liver and spleen for removal.

Activation of C5

In addition to its role as an opsonin, C3b also forms part of the C5 convertase that leads to the generation of C5a and C5b. C5a, like C3a, is an anaphylotoxin, capable of activating basophils and mast cells. C5a is also among the most potent biologic chemoattractants for neutrophils, as will be discussed below. C5b, which will attach to the surface of cells and microorganisms, is the first component in the assembly of the membrane attack complex, C5b-9.

Membrane Attack Complex

The membrane attack complex (MAC), or the terminal complement assembly of C5b-9, has long been known to produce lysis of bacteria. However, assembly of MAC on homologous leukocytes is not a cytotoxic event. After insertion of MAC into a leukocyte membrane, the cell sheds a small membrane vesicle containing the MAC complex. What is less appreciated is that insertion of MAC into the cell membrane triggers cell activation before it is shed (49,50). MAC acts as an ionophore, provoking increases in cytosolic calcium and consequently triggering cell functions (reviewed in ref. 51). These functions include generation of toxic oxygen products as well as activation of both the cyclooxygenase (platelets, monocyte/macrophages, synoviocytes) and lipoxygenase pathways of arachidonate metabolism. Furthermore, the deposition of MAC increases the surface expression of Pselectin on the endothelial cell surface, promoting adhesion to circulating neutrophils (52). *In vivo* evidence that vascular endothelium represents a site of C5b9 deposition has been demonstrated in immune vasculitis (47,53,54) and infarcted myocardium (55).

Immune Complex Deposition-Dependent Vascular Inflammation

Vasculitis in SLE is most commonly due to the local deposition of immune complexes, particularly those containing antibodies to DNA (anti-DNA), in blood vessel walls (56, 57). This lesion is best modeled by the Arthus reaction and experimental serum sickness. Maurice Arthus reported in 1903 that the repeated cutaneous injection of horse serum into a group of rabbits produced inflammatory reactions characterized by intense polymorphonuclear leukocyte infiltration, hemorrhage, and sometimes necrosis (58). It is now known that this reaction is due the formation of antigenantibody complexes in the vicinity of blood vessel walls, complement activation, and the generation of anaphylatoxins (e.g., C4a, C3a, C5a) and chemotaxins (C5a) (59,60). The resulting infiltration of vessel walls by polymorphonuclear leukocytes leads histologically to leukocytoclastic vasculitis and the release of lysosomal enzymes and oxygen radicals to tissue injury (57).

Modifications of the classic active Arthus reaction include immunization by intravenous rather than cutaneous injection of the antigen as well as the local passive Arthus reaction (e.g., simultaneous cutaneous injection of antigen and antibody), direct passive Arthus reaction (e.g., passive transfer of preformed antibody by the intravenous injection of serum from another immunized rabbit), and the reverse passive Arthus reaction (e.g., antibody injected cutaneously and antigen injected intravenously) (61). The necessary elements of these reactions have been examined and require antigen, precipitating antibody, intact complement pathway, and neutrophils (62). One study suggests that the inflammatory response to immune complexes also requires cell-bound Fc receptors with subsequent amplification by cellular mediators and complement (63).

Immune complex disease in SLE can also be modeled by the acute experimental serum sickness or the glomerulonephritis that accompanies chronic serum sickness. In the acute serum sickness model, the injection of antigen is followed by an immune response, with the generation of antibody and clearance of the antigen by the cells of the reticuloendothelial system. However, during the period of accelerated decay of the antigen the presence of circulating immune complexes produces inflammatory injury involving arteries, glomeruli, and joints (64). Chronic serum sickness requires usually at least 5 weeks of repeated injection of intravenous antigen. The resulting periods of antigen excess leads to circulating immune complexes and glomerulonephritis histologically similar to that observed in patients with SLE (Fig. 14.1) (65).

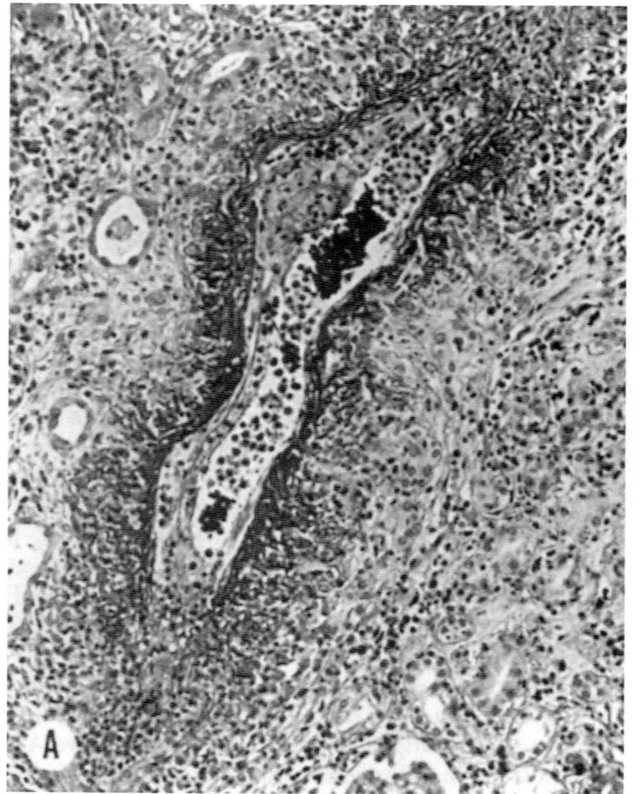

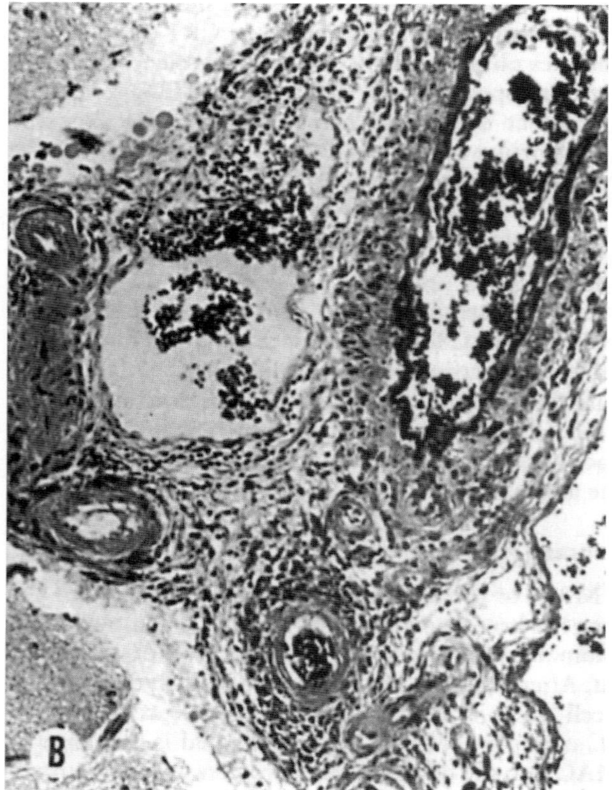

FIGURE 14.1. A: Polyarteritis-type lupus vasculitis with fibrinoid necrosis in the kidney of a patient with systemic lupus erythematosus (SLE). **B:** Polyarteritis-type lupus vasculitis with fibrinoid necrosis in the brain of a patient with SLE. (H&E, ×160.)

A major consequence of immune complex deposition in SLE is the activation of complement. The consumption of complement components and their deposition in tissue is reflected by a decrease in serum levels of C3 and C4 in most patients with active disease (66). However, since the synthesis of both C3 and C4 increases during periods of disease activity, the serum levels of these proteins may be normal despite accelerated consumption (67). Conversely, chronically depressed levels of individual complement components, due to decreased synthesis, hereditary deficiencies, or increased extravascular distribution of complement proteins, has been reported in SLE (68). The decreased serum complement levels in these patients may lead to the mistaken conclusion that excessive complement activation is ongoing. To define more precisely the role of complement activation with respect to clinical disease activity of SLE, circulating levels of complement degradation products during periods of active and inactive disease have been measured (69—74). Levels of plasma C3a, Ba, and the serum complement attack complex, SC5b-9, were each shown to be more sensitive indicators of disease activity than either total C3 or C4 level (69—72,74). Elevations of plasma C3a levels may precede other serologic or clinical evidence of an impending disease flare (74).

The pathologic consequences of immune complex deposition in SLE include both a microvascular angiitis (e.g., glomerulonephritis or pulmonary capillaritis with or without pulmonary hemorrhage) and necrotizing vasculitis (e.g., cutaneous purpura, polyarteritis nodosa—like systemic, cerebral).

Immune Complex "Independent" Vascular Injury

Some patients with SLE have small vessel disease and inflammatory vasculopathy in the absence of local immune complex deposition, particularly those patients with central nervous system (CNS) involvement (71,75,76). Several lines of investigation now suggest yet another mechanism for this complementmediated vascular injury in SLE, one not dependent on immune complex deposition (77—82). This mechanism is best modeled experimentally by the Shwartzman phenomenon. The local Shwartzman lesion requires a preparatory intradermal injection of endotoxin, which is followed in 4 to 18 hours by the intravenous injection of endotoxin (83,84). This results in the intravascular activation of complement triggering the release of anaphylatoxins such as C3a and C5a into the circulation (85). The split products attract and activate inflammatory cells, such as neutrophils and platelets, causing them to aggregate, to adhere to vascular endothelium, to occlude small vessels, and to release toxic mediators. Activation of complement thus leads to an occlusive vasculopathy that may also result in widespread ischemic injury (85).

The Shwartzman phenomenon was originally described as a model of meningicoccal sepsis but it is now recognized that cytokines such as IL-1 and TNF-α can substitute for endotoxin (Fig. 14.2) (86). Such agents stimulate the upregulation on the endothelial cell surface of ICAM1 and E-selectin, which are the counterreceptors for the neutrophil adhesion molecule CD11b/CD18 and Sialyl-Lewis X, respectively (87). It had long been established that complement activation in plasma stimulates circulating neutrophils to produce the local Shwartzman lesion, but it has been recognized that the preparatory phase represents a time of ICAM-1 and E-selectin upregulation (84). The importance of this local endothelial cell activation is supported by the capacity of antibodies to ICAM-1 and E-selectin administered intravenously to prevent the development of the experimental lesion (84).

The episodic, uncontrolled activation of complement proteins is a characteristic feature of SLE. Disease exacerbations are typically accompanied by decreases in total C3 and C4 values in association with elevations in plasma of the

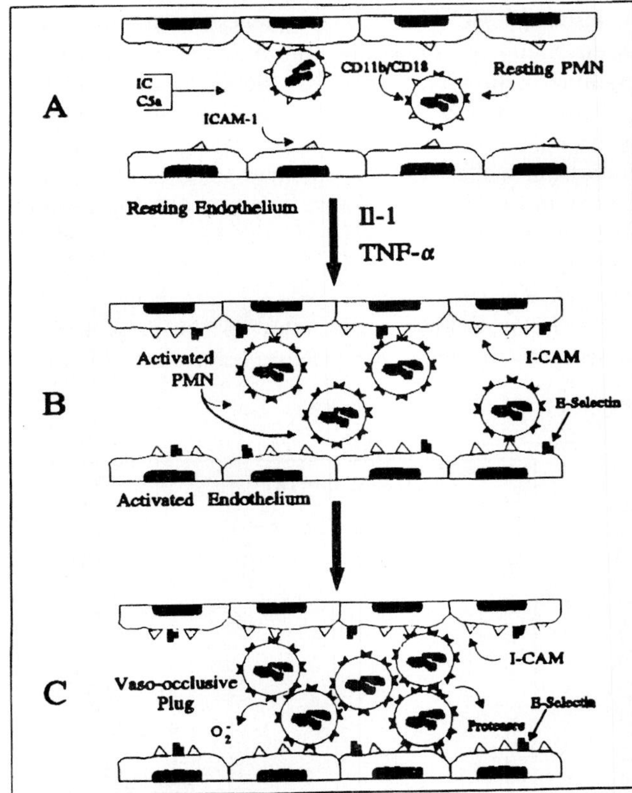

FIGURE 14.2. Schematic presentation of the Shwartzman phenomenon. **A:** Stimulation of polymorphonuclear leukocytes (PMNs) via engagement of C5a or Fc receptors leads to activation of CD11b/CD18, promoting homotypic and heterotypic aggregation. IC, immune complexes. **B:** Endothelial cell activation by cytokines, such as interleukin-1 (IL-1) and tumor necrosis factor-α (TNF-α), leads to upregulation of constitutive intercellular adhesion molecule-1 (ICAM-1) and induces the expression of E-selectin. **C:** The cooccurrence of PMN and endothelial cell activation results in leukothrombosis and vasoocclusive plugs.

biologically active complement split products, C3a desArg and C5a desArg (71,72,88,89). During periods of disease flare, circulating neutrophils are activated to increase their adhesiveness to vascular endothelium, as indicated by the upregulation of the surface $\beta_2$integrin CD11b/CD18 (complement receptor 3) (27,90). One study demonstrated that the surface expression of three distinct endothelial cell adhesion molecules, E-selectin, VCAM-1, and ICAM-1, is also upregulated in patients with SLE (Fig. 14.3) (76). Endothelial cell activation was most marked in patients with disease exacerbations characterized by significant elevations of plasma C3a desArg, and the activation reversed with improvement in disease activity (76). In these studies, endothelial cell adhesion molecule upregulation was observed in otherwise histologically normal skin and was notable for the absence of local immune complex deposition (76). These data suggest that excessive complement activation in association with primed endothelial cells can induce neutrophilendothelial cell adhesion and predispose to leuko-occlusive vasculopathy during SLE disease flares. This pathogenic mechanism may be of particular relevance to vascular beds, which lack the fenestrations that permit the trapping of circulating immune complexes. Such an example is the CNS, where the blood—brain barrier can prevent the access of circulating immune complexes to the perivascular tissues. But in the setting of widespread endothelial cell activation, exuberant systemic complement activation can promote diffuse microvascular injury in the absence of immune complex deposition and produce the most common pathologic finding of CNS lupus, microinfarction (Fig. 14.4) (88,91—94).

Similar pathologic events may also be present in the mesenteric circulation and produce features of SLE enteritis (75) or produce pulmonary leukosequestration and acute, reversible hypoxemia during disease exacerbations (95).

The systemic inflammatory response syndrome (SIRS) is a reaction characterized by widespread inflammation primarily affecting vascular endothelium (96). The same cascade of mediators involved in the Shwartzman phenomenon has been invoked in SIRS (97,98). The main endogenous mediators of SIRS include TNF-α and IL-1 (97). A prominent role for PAF, vasodilator prostaglandins, complement activation, and upregulation of adhesion molecules on leukocytes and endothelial cells has also been identified (97). A consequence of SIRS is multiorgan failure or dysfunction syndrome (MOF or MODS, respectively) with manifestations that include catecholamine unresponsive hypotension, decreased myocardial contractility, cerebral dysfunction, and adult respiratory distress syndrome (ARDS) (96). Interestingly, mAbs directed against the leukocyte integrin CD18 can ameliorate the lung injury in experimental models of SIRS (99).

It is now recognized that SIRS may arise both from sepsis and noninfectious causes, such as immune-mediated organ injury (96). Serious exacerbations of SLE can produce a syndrome that is indistinguishable from SIRS and can be accompanied by MOF. Therefore, the Shwartzman phenomenon may serve as a model for both SIRS and the multiorgan dysfunction that can accompany acute lupus crisis.

Inflammatory vasculopathy independent of immune complex deposition may also occur as a result of antineutrophil cytoplasmic antibodies (ANCAs) or lymphocyte responses. A pathogenic role for ANCAs in vasculitis has been suggested by the demonstration of activation of poly-

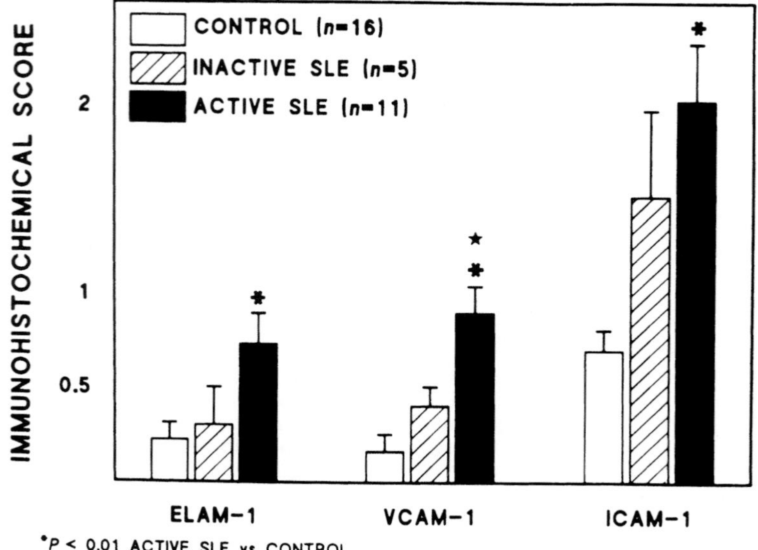

FIGURE 14.3. Systemic lupus erythematous (SLE) disease exacerbation is accompanied by endothelial cell upregulation of three adhesion molecules: Eselectin (ELAM-1), vascular cell adhesion molecule-1 (VCAM-1), and intercellular adhesion molecule-1 (ICAM-1). The mean expression of all three adhesion molecules is significantly greater in patients with active SLE versus healthy controls as well as patients with inactive SLE.

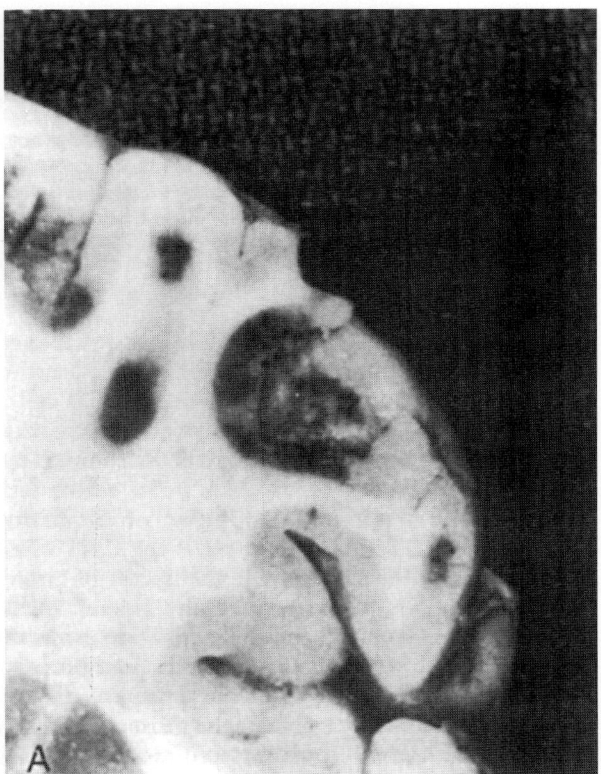

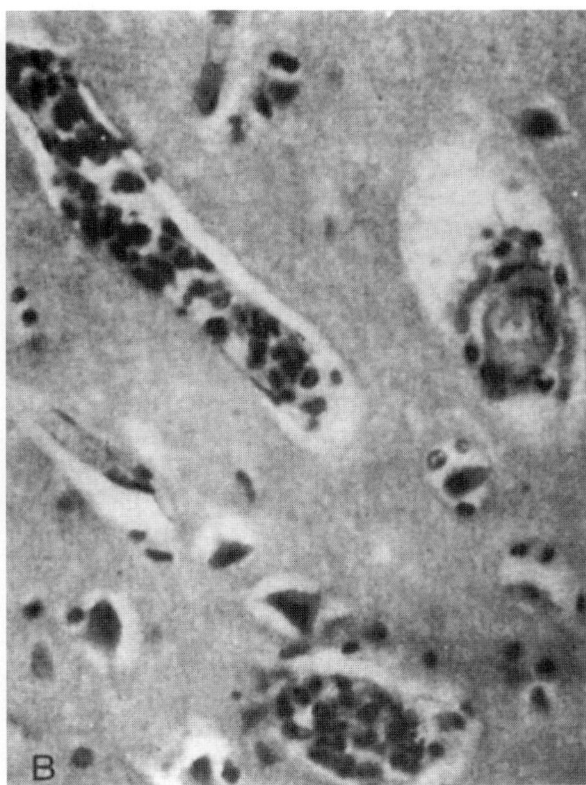

FIGURE 14.4. Specimen of brain obtained postmortem from a patient with fatal exacerbation of neuropsychiatric lupus without antiphospholipid antibodies. **A:** The frontal lobe reveals multiple small cortical infarcts. **B:** High magnification reveals leukothrombosis, with occlusion of small blood vessels by leukocyte aggregates, as well as acute ischemic changes of the neurons. (Photo courtesy of Dr. Nelson Torre, Buffalo, NY.)

morphonuclear leukocytes and enhanced adhesion to endothelial cells by antibodies to proteinase-3 or myeloperoxidase (100). Lymphocytes directly reacting to antigen may release cytokines that result in tissue damage and a mononuclear inflammatory diseases (101). These mechanisms of vascular injury are more typical, however, of Wegener's granulomatosis and Sjögren's syndrome, respectively, than of SLE.

THROMBOTIC NONINFLAMMATORY VASCULAR DISEASE

Antiphospholipid Antibody Syndrome

The presence of antibodies to negatively charged phospholipids is associated with recurrent arterial and venous thrombosis, thrombocytopenia, and fetal wastage (102,103). Antiphospholipid antibody syndrome (APS) requires the demonstration of an antiphospholipid antibody [e.g., biologic false-positive Venereal Disease Research Laboratory (VDRL) test, lupus anticoagulant, anticardiolipin antibodies] and thrombotic phenomena. It is known that the presence in serum of this family of autoantibodies, perhaps operating through cofactors (e.g., β_2-glycoprotein-1 or prothrombin) can generate a thrombotic diathesis (104—108). The mechanism for this hypercoagulable state has not yet been fully understood, although it appears to involve interactions between the antibodies to anionic phospholipidprotein complexes and antigen targets on platelets (109,110), endothelial cells (111—114), or components of the coagulation cascade (115,116). Experimental evidence suggests that increased platelet aggregation, altered endothelial cell function (e.g., decreased prostacyclin or increased thrombomodulin production), or disturbed function of clotting factors (e.g., decreased protein C activation by thrombomodulin, decreased protein S function, as well as decreased prekallikrein and fibrinolytic activity) may explain the predisposition to thrombosis. The role of cytokines in the primary APS or in APS secondary to SLE requires clarification (117). Evidence that antiphospholipid antibodies can activate endothelial cells and increase expression of adhesion molecules suggests another mechanism for the thrombophilia (118).

Thrombotic Thrombocytopenia Purpura

SLE exacerbations are infrequently accompanied by secondary thrombotic thrombocytopenia purpura (TTP) with complete or incomplete features of the clinical pentad: fever, microangiopathic hemolytic anemia, thrombocytopenia, renal disease, and neurologic dysfunction (119). In the absence of antiphospholipid antibodies, the characteristic pathology of TTP, eosinophilic hyaline microthrombi, has been identified in patients with SLE. Large multimers of vWF capable of mediating disseminated intravascular platelet aggregation have been demonstrated in patients with chronic, relapsing TTP as well as SLE (120,121). A consequence of the endothelial cell activation or injury observed in SLE may be the release of vWF multimers or other mediators of platelet aggregation capable of initiating a TTP-like illness (122).

ENDOTHELIAL CELL DYSFUNCTION AND SLE

Systemic lupus erythematosus is increasingly a chronic illness, with rapidly fatal cases now rare and most patients experiencing a long-term disorder with frequent exacerbations and remissions. Therefore, chronic morbidity and late mortality are of greater importance. Abu-Shakra et al. have reported their observations of mortality within the Toronto lupus cohort and described a bimodal distribution of death (122a) Early (within the first year) deaths were most often attributed to active lupus and infection, while late deaths were secondary to atherosclerotic heart disease. Myocardial infarction (MI) accounted for 45% of all deaths. Other studies also document fatal MI in SLE populations but at a significantly lower and constant rate of 3% to 5% of total deaths. In addition to cohort studies of mortality associated with myocardial involvement, the increased prevalence of coronary artery disease in SLE has been documented by case reports and autopsy studies. In 1975, Bulkley and Roberts performed autopsies in 36 SLE patients (33 female and mean age of 32 years). Four (11%) experienced MI, while eight (22%) had greater than 50% narrowing in at least one coronary artery. A second autopsy series of 22 patients age 16 to 37 years demonstrated ten (45%) had coronary artery narrowing that exceeded 75%. The Baltimore lupus cohort reported an 8.3% prevalence of cardiovascular events (MI, sudden cardiac death, and angina) in 229 patients (122b). Aranow and Ginzler from the State University of New York (SUNY) Health Science Center in Brooklyn retrospectively studied 200 patients and found coronary artery disease (CAD) in 30 (15%), MI in 13 (7%), and angina in 24 (12%) (122c). Age-specific incidence rates of MI and angina were compared between 498 women with SLE from the University of Pittsburgh Medical Center and 2,208 female controls. Between the ages of 35 and 44 women with lupus were 50 times more likely than controls to experience MI (122d).

Although coronary artery vasculitis has been described in SLE, it is rare, and the accelerated CAD that is characteristic of SLE is typically otherwise indistinguishable from atherosclerosis that occurs outside the setting of lupus. The pathogenesis of the observed precocious atherosclerosis in SLE includes clustering of traditional risk factors, adverse effects of treatment (e.g., corticosteroids, cyclophosphamide, etc.), and vasculopathy that accompanies disease activity (e.g., hypercoagulable state of secondary antiphospholipid syndrome and neutrophilendothelial cell interactions). Endothelial cell injury and dysfunction with subsequent alteration of endothelial adhesiveness and permeability to leukocytes and platelets are principal mechanisms of both the atherosclerosis and the inflammatory state that characterizes SLE.

Endothelial cells line the lumen of all blood vessels and form the interface between the blood and peripheral tissues. Traditionally, the role of endothelial cells was considered to be that of a gatekeeper. Passive deposition of cholesterol and its metabolites in the artery wall has been thought to be the key step in the pathophysiology of atherosclerosis. In recent years, however, attention has shifted to the role of primary vascular injury. Although many factors cause atherosclerosis, it has become clear now that endothelial cell perturbation and inflammation at the site of vascular injury plays an essential role in the initiation and progression of atherosclerotic disease.

In response to a diverse array of stimuli, activated endothelial cells exhibit a proinflammatory phenotype by upregulation of adhesion molecules on their surface, leading to sequential steps in rolling, firm adhesion, and transmigration of leukocytes and monocytes to the site of injury. Formation and accumulation of foam cells in turn promote neointimal proliferation and thinning of endothelium, which result in dysfunction of the endothelial cells, interaction with the platelets, and stimulation of smooth muscle proliferation, leading to fibrous plaque and thrombus formation (123,124).

The central role of endothelial cell—leukocyte interaction as an early response in the pathogenesis of atherosclerosis was demonstrated by experiments on the C57BL/6 mice model with homozygous mutations for the *ICAM-1* gene. This mutation, resulting in a deficiency of endothelial cell ICAM-1 expression, is associated with a protective role on the development of atherosclerosis in this animal model (125,126). Additionally, SLE, a disease characterized by widespread vascular injury, has a high prevalence of premature atherosclerosis and represents an interesting model to study endothelial perturbation. A summary of the factors altering endothelial cell behavior and specific endothelial responses to these stimuli is given in Table 14.3.

TABLE 14.3. REVIEWED FACTORS STIMULATING ENDOTHELIAL CELLS AND ENDOTHELIAL CELLS' PHENOTYPIC RESPONSES THAT PLAY AN IMPORTANT ROLE IN THE PATHOGENESIS OF ATHEROSCLEROSIS AND INFLAMMATORY VASCULOPATHY

Stimuli	Response
Nonimmunologic	Vascular tone
Mechanical forces: (transmural pressure, tension, hear stress) hypercholesterolemia, oxidized LDL, lysophosphatidylcholine	NO
	Prostacyclin
	Endothelin-1
	Prothrombotic
Immunologic	Tissue factor
Cytokines	vWF
TNF-α	thrombomodulin
IL-1	
IFN-γ	
Activated complement products	Proadhesive
C3a,C3b,C5a,MAC	ICAM-1
Autoantibodies	VCAM-1
aCL	E-selectin
AECA	
Anti-oxLDL	
Anti-dsDNA	
CD40/CD40L interaction	
C1q receptors occupancy	

aCL, anti-cardiolipin; AECA, antiendothelial cell antibody; dsDNA, double-stranded DNA; ICAM, intercellular adhesion molecule; IFN, interferon; IL, interleukin; LDL, low-density lipoprotein; oxLDL, oxidized LDL; NO, nitric oxide; VCAM, vascular cell adhesion molecule; vWF, von Willebrand factor.

Endothelial Phenotype

Endothelium plays a fundamental role in various physiologic functions, including vasoregulation, hemostasis, inflammation, and adhesion biology. What determines the actual difference between the chronic lesion in atherosclerosis and the acute and subacute lesions of inflammatory vasculopathy? An understanding of the details of endothelial perturbation in response to stimuli may provide the explanation. Irrespective of the nature of the stimuli (immunogenic or direct mechanical forces), the endothelium responds by upregulating adhesion molecules and recruiting leukocytes, shifting the phenotype to procoagulant by expressing tissue factor (TF) or vWF, and/or altering vascular tone.

Prothrombotic Phenotype

By shifting the phenotype to procoagulant in response to stimulation, endothelial cells have a direct role in the mechanism of thrombosis, whether this is at a site of atherosclerotic plaque formation or focal vascular inflammation, or in circumstances characterized by diffuse endothelial activation, such as in SLE, catastrophic antiphospholipid syndrome (CAPS), or SIRS (127,128).

Von Willebrand factor (vWF) is a macromolecular protein complex that plays a pivotal role in hemostasis. It functions as a carrier protein for plasma factor VIII, and mediates platelet adhesion to other platelets and to collagen exposed by damaged endothelium. Vascular endothelium is the major source of plasma vWF under physiologic and pathologic conditions. vWF is stored and released from endothelial cell secretory granules, along with its propeptide vWF:AgII. Elevated plasma vWF was found in diabetes and other vasculopathies. Its level and the level of propeptide can serve as a marker of endothelial activation (129). A group from Canada (130) demonstrated decreased peripheral dermal staining for endothelial vWF in SIRS patients, as well as in healthy volunteers after TNF-α injection. This was associated with significantly greater plasma vWF levels, indicating degranulation in response to cytokine stimulation that predisposes to formation of platelet microthrombi, lodging in small capillaries, causing areas of local tissue ischemia.

Cultured endothelial cells *in vitro* express TF in response to a great variety of stimuli (131). The data *in vivo* are controversial; one group found an absence of expression of TF by endothelium overlying atherosclerotic plaques by *in situ* hybridization (132), but a later study reported endothelial expression of TF by using histochemical assessment (133). Solovey et al. (134) demonstrated expression of TF by endothelial cells of sickle cell anemia patients during the acute vasooclusive episode, supported by concurrence between TF antigen and messenger RNA (mRNA) expression.

Proadhesive Phenotype

Adhesion of leukocytes to vascular endothelium is one of the earliest events in acute immunogenic and nonimmunogenic inflammation (123). The initial surface expression of adhesion molecules is the common endothelial response not only to a variety of atherogenic stimuli, but also to complement-mediated vascular injury in SLE (immune complex mediated, as well as immune complex independent).

Many cells, including endothelial cells (ECs), constitutively express ICAM-1, and its expression is upregulated by IL-1 or TNF-α. VCAM-1 is mainly present on ECs activated by IL-1, TNF-α, IFN-γ, or IL-4 (135). ECs activated by IL-1, TNF-α, or thrombin transiently express E-selectin, thereby mediating endothelial adhesion of neutrophils or memory lymphocytes (136). Expression of these molecules promotes formation of vaso-occlusive plaques, by interaction of endothelium with activated neutrophils, displaying upregulation of β_2-integrin CD11b/CD18. The importance of this interaction was demonstrated in a model of vascular injury underlying thrombotic stroke (137). Investigators used neutrophildepleted or ICAM-1—deficient mice and demonstrated resistance of this model to focal cerebral ischemia and reperfusion injury provoked by experimental intraluminal occlusion of the cerebral artery. Elkon's group (138) demonstrated in MRL/MpJ-FAS *lpr* mice that ICAM-1 deficiency results in a striking improvement in survival. Data from several groups analyzing the level of various adhesion molecules in SLE further support the notion that endothelial cells play a central role in systemic inflammatory response by exhibiting their adhesive properties. Immunohistologic examination of non–sun-exposed skin from SLE patients showed upregulation of the surface expression of all three adhesion molecules—E-selectin, ICAM-1, and VCAM-1—in patients with active SLE and with otherwise histologically normal skin with no evidence of local immune complex deposition (76). Elevation of soluble adhesion molecules (E-selectin, sICAM-1, sVCAM-1) also has been reported in active SLE (139). A group from France (135) demonstrated increased level of sVCAM-1 in patients with primary antiphospholipid syndrome (APLS), SLE-related APLS, or SLE, compared to healthy controls or thrombosis controls.

Stimuli that Activate Endothelial Cells

Factors that alter the functional status of endothelium can be divided into two major categories: nonimmunologic, such as direct mechanical forces, vasoactive mediators, and products of oxidation; and immunologic, such as cytokines, complement, and autoantibodies.

Nonimmunologic

The endothelium experiences three primary mechanical forces: transmural pressure, tension, and shear stress. Sprague et al. (140) have demonstrated flow-mediated modulation of endothelial activation markers, and Nagel et al. (141) reported upregulation of ICAM expression in cultured human vascular cells in response to shear stress.

Recent studies have supported the view that hypercholesterolemia and oxidative stress are important inducers of atheroma formation. One of the actions of oxidized low-density lipoprotein (oxLDL) is to induce endothelial dysfunction (142). Erl et al. (143) demonstrated activation of endothelial cells by oxLDL via distinct endothelial ligands, promoting adhesion of monocytes. It is speculated that one of the mechanisms is a disruption of signal transduction (144). Other mechanisms may be related to the lysophosphatidylcholine (LPC) moiety, one of the active components of oxLDL particles that induces superoxide endothelial cytotoxic effect via peroxinitrite production (144,145). Moreover, LPC is a major factor in the antigenicity of oxLDL (146,147). Antibodies against oxLDL were demonstrated both in normal, healthy individuals and in atherosclerotic plaques and were found to correlate with atherosclerosis progression (147). The level of oxLDL antibodies has been correlated with titers for anti-cardiolipin (aCL) in SLE patients (145,148). Several groups (48,149) have demonstrated crossreactivity of aPL and oxLDL underlying the link in development of atherosclerosis and immunologic process.

Immunologic

Cytokines are important mediators of endothelial cell activation. Specifically, TNF-α, IL-1, and macrophage colony-stimulating factor increase binding of LDL to endothelium and increase transcription of the LDL gene (142). TNF-α, IFN-γ, and IL-1 stimulate adhesion molecule expression on endothelial cells, and few studies have reported increased levels of these cytokines in the circulation during vasculitis (150). The Shwartzman phenomenon, originally described as a model of endotoxemia, currently is being used as a model of the widespread vasculopathy of SLE. It is recognized now that cytokines such as IL-1 and TNF-α are the preparatory signals of the inflammatory process (76,127). These proinflammatory cytokines are capable of promoting atherosclerosis by stimulating the adhesive properties of endothelial cells. Accumulation of TNF-α (151) and IL-1 (152) was demonstrated in atherosclerotic plaques of coronary arteries. It is also important to note that while endothelial cells are activated by cytokines, they also can produce IL-1, IL-6, IL-8 and TNF-α while stimulated (150,153). These cytokines can act as autocoids to upregulate adhesion molecule expression. Kaplanski et al. (136) demonstrated induction of IL-8 production in a time- and dose-dependent fashion by thrombin-activated HUVEC; this effect was inhibited by the specific thrombin inhibitor hirudin.

Complement activation that can be either immune complex dependent or independent plays an essential role in the mechanism of endothelial injury. This can explain the development of widespread vascular injury in SLE, an example of immunemediated systemic inflammatory response, even without evidence of immune complex deposition in the tissue. Several products of the activated complement system (C3b, iC3b, and C5a) are known to activate endothelial cells *in vitro*. More recently, Saadi and others (154) demonstrated that interaction of complement with endothelial cells and the assembly of MAC leads to expression of Pselectin and activation of a protease that cleaves and releases heparan sulfate proteoglycan from the EC surface, and induces upregulation of TF and cyclooxygenase-2 (COX-2). They concluded that activation of porcine aortic and microvascular ECs on MAC exposure involves the intermediate step of IL1 release. By using ECs transgenic for human decayaccelerating factor that inhibits complement convertase, these authors demonstrated that complement is required for endothelial activation. The presence of sCR1 prevented activation of aortic as well as microvascular ECs (155).

Granular deposits of immunoglobulin and complement components were found within atherosclerotic lesions

(156), suggesting that complementdependent endothelial activation could play a role in pathogenesis of atherosclerosis.

Antibodies against endothelial cells and cardiolipin were found in a subset of patients with the clinical and angiographic diagnosis of severe premature atherosclerotic peripheral disease (157). Recent research demonstrated that antibodies might contribute to the derangement of functional status of the endothelial cells, rather than simply displaying cell cytotoxicity. It has been reported that both polyclonal as well as monoclonal antiendothelial cell antibodies (AECAs) induce EC activation *in vitro*. AECAs have been shown to mediate release of vWF, arachidonic acid metabolites, and ET-1 from endothelial cells, and to induce a proinflammatory and procoagulant phenotype of EC. A statistically significant increase in expression of endothelial ICAM-1, VCAM-1, and E-selectin was demonstrated on human umbilical vein ECs pretreated with AECA-positive sera from a scleroderma patient compared to cells pretreated with AECA-negative sera (158). Neutralizing antibodies to IL-1, but not antibodies to TNF, substantially inhibited or blocked this activation, providing further evidence for the autocrine actions of IL-1. Del Papa et al. (159) found that AECA IgG from Wegener's granulomatosis patients upregulates the expression of E-selectin, ICAM-1, and VCAM-1 and induces the secretion of IL-1, IL-6, IL-8, and MCP-1. Almost identical results were obtained from analysis of AECA-positive sera from Takayasu arteritis patients (160). Another proposed mechanism is that binding of AECAs makes negatively charged phospholipids accessible to antiphospholipid antibodies (161), thereby further enhancing the activation of EC.

Cross-reactivity between anti–double-stranded DNA (dsDNA) antibodies, cardiolipins, and AECAs has been observed in earlier studies (162,163). By using immunofluorescent staining, Simantov et al. (164) were the first to demonstrate expression of cell adhesion molecules, including E-selectin, VCAM-1, and ICAM-1 by ECs incubated with purified IgG from patients with high titers of anticardiolipin antibodies, even in the absence of clinical or serologic evidence of SLE. They also established that this mechanism is $\beta_2$glycoprotein dependent.

A direct stimulatory effect of anti-dsDNA antibodies on endothelium, as indicated by the release of vWF, may have a pathogenic role on expression of adhesion molecules (165,166). These data can provide a link between SLE and premature atherosclerosis.

The interaction between CD40 and CD40L is another immune-mediated interaction common to both SLE and atherosclerosis that leads to upregulation of adhesion molecules on endothelial cells (146). CD40 is a type 1 member of the TNF receptor superfamily of proteins, and is present on a wide variety of cells, including vascular endothelial cells. Ligation of this receptor on endothelial cells is known to increase expression of inflammatory adhesion molecules. Slupsky and others (167) demonstrated that platelets express the ligand of CD40 within seconds of exposure to agonist, and interact with endothelial cells to participate directly in the induction of an inflammatory response. The same authors also showed that activated platelets induce TF expression on endothelial cells in a CD40/CD40L-dependent manner. Moreover, CD40 ligation on ECs downregulates the expression of thrombomodulin and adhesion molecules, further implicating the procoagulant and proinflammatory phenotype of ECs (168). In a genetically modified murine model with hypercholesterolemia, blocking antibodies to CD40 reduced atherosclerotic lesion formation (169).

In SLE C1q immune complexes may be a source of arterial injury initiating atherogenesis. Lozada et al. (170) showed that immune complexes stimulate endothelial cells to express adhesion molecules E-selectin, ICAM, and VCAM in the presence of a heat-labile complement component C1q. C1q depletion from serum or C1q protein synthesis inhibition on the surface of ECs blocked the expression of adhesive proteins. Moreover, Reiss et al. (171) were able to demonstrate that occupancy of C1q receptors on ECs by immune complexes downregulated mRNA for sterol 27-hydroxylase, the enzyme that mediates peripheral cholesterol metabolism, interfering with the capacity of endothelium to convert cholesterol to antiatherogenic metabolites and therefore enhancing atherogenesis.

In summary, we have described factors leading to endothelial perturbation and overlapping features of endothelial response in autoimmune disorders and atherosclerosis. The conversion of the endothelial phenotype to an adhesive and prothrombotic state and interaction of inflammatory mediators with cholesterol metabolism driven by multiple immunologic and nonimmunologic stimuli are the core of the pathophysiologic link between mechanisms of inflammatory vasculopathy, thrombosis, and atherosclerosis.

THE ROLE OF ACTIVATED ENDOTHELIUM IN SLE

There is a unifying hypothesis to account for the diverse, episodic, and variably distributed (e.g., widespread versus organ restricted; skin, kidney, or CNS, etc.) nature of SLE vascular lesions. Inflammatory lesions would require either circulating immune complexes (e.g., DNA/anti-DNA) or significant complement activation of neutrophils, while thrombotic lesions would require antiphospholipid antibodies. An additional biologic factor, however, is required to explain the waxing and waning nature of disease exacerbations and the limitation of lesions to one or few vascular beds. Immune complexes, activated neutrophils, or antiphospholipid antibodies may be necessary but likely are not sufficient to explain vascular pathology in SLE. Since they may be present in the absence of disease activity and can travel throughout the general circulation, they are incapable of explaining the relapsing and focal nature of vascular injury.

New information regarding the activation of ECs may provide the missing feature. The specificity of vascular injury in SLE may depend on the endogenous capacity of vascular endothelium to respond to stimuli. ECs when activated can express E-selectin, increased ICAM-1, and an inducible form of nitric oxide synthase (iNOS) (76,87). However, there is a restriction to this EC capacity; for example, the upregulation of EC adhesion molecules is limited to postcapillary venules (172). It is therefore possible that the episodic and focal nature of vascular pathology in SLE is dependent on the presence or absence as well as nature of EC activation. EC permissiveness for immune complex deposition or *in situ* formation can result in vasculitis. Activation of EC adhesion molecules by cytokines, immune complexes, complement components, antiendothelial cell antibodies, or antiphospholipid antibodies can result in leukothrombosis if there is simultaneous activation of neutrophils and complement (118). Abnormal iNOS synthesis may also have a role in permitting neutrophilEC interaction and the Shwartzman-like lesion. Additionally, EC activation may lead to the expression of membrane-associated coagulation proteins that are the target of antiphospholipid antibodies.

Additional evidence that activated endothelium contributes to the vasculopathy of exacerbated SLE is the finding that disease flare is accompanied by abnormal levels of circulating endothelial cells (CECs). CEC levels are significantly higher in active SLE patients compared to healthy controls and correlate positively with plasma C3a elevations (173). Furthermore, CECs from patients with active SLE express an activated phenotype, staining for tyrosine. Elevated levels of CEC in active SLE represents a marker for endothelial injury and suggests these cells may further potentiate vascular injury by the production of inflammatory and prothombotic mediators and by engaging in heterotypic aggregation with neutrophil and platelets. In prior studies, the potential for CECs to participate in microinfarction was suggested by studies reported in sickle cell anemia (174) and acute MI (175). In conclusion, the detection of activated CECs in patients with SLE, particularly with higher Systemic Lupus Erythematosus Disease Activity Index (SLEDAI) scores, provides evidence for widespread endothelial injury. Studies are ongoing to determine whether the presence of CECs predicts or is the result of postcapillary vascular damage and microinfarction leading to organ dysfunction or even premature atherosclerosis.

Vascular injury in SLE may require immune complex formation, complement activation, or antiphospholipid antibody production, but we propose that the EC response is responsible for the clinical character of a disease exacerbation by determining the timing and organ distribution of vascular pathology, which includes vasculitis, leukothrombosis, thrombosis, and atherosclerosis.

REFERENCES

1. Snyderman R, Uhing RJ. Chemoattractant stimulus response coupling. In: Goldstein IM, Snyderman R, eds. *Inflammation: basic principles and clinical correlates.* New York: Raven Press, 1992:421–439.
2. Kitsis EA, Weissmann G. The role of the neutrophil in rheumatoid arthritis. *Clin Orthop Rel Res* 1991;265:63–72.
3. Weissmann G, Korchak HM, Perez HD, et al. *Neutrophils as secretory organs.* Boston: PSG, 1981.
4. Johnson RJ, Lovett D, Lehrer RI, et al. Role of oxidants and proteases in glomerular injury. *Kidney Int* 1994;45:352–359.
5. Nathan CF. Secretory products of macrophages. *J Clin Invest* 1987;79:319–326.
6. NikolicPaterson DJ, Lan HY, Hill PA, et al. Macrophages in renal injury. *Kidney Int* 1994;45:S79–S82.
7. Wharram BL, Fitting K, Kunkel SL, et al. Tissue factor expression in endothelial cell/monocyte cocultures stimulated by lipopolysaccharide and/or aggregated IgG. Mechanisms of cell-cell communication. *J Immunol* 1991;146:1437–1445.
8. Schultz G, Rotater DS. EGF and TGF-alpha in wound healing and repair. *J Cell Biol* 1991;45:346–352.
9. Kusner DJ, Luebbers EL, Nowinski RJ, et al. Cytokine and LPS-induced synthesis of interleukin-8 from human mesangial cells. *Kidney Int* 1991;39:1240–1248.
10. Baggiolini M, Loetscher P, Moser B. Interleukin-8 and the chemokine family. *Int J Immunopharmacol* 1995;17:103–108.
11. Schall TJ, Bacon KB. Chemokines, leukocyte trafficking and inflammation. *Curr Opin Immunol* 1994;6:865–873.
12. Weinberg JB, Granger DL, Pisetsky DS, et al. The role of nitric oxide in the pathogenesis of spontaneous murine autoimmune disease: increased nitric oxide production and nitric oxide synthase expression in MRL-1pr Mice, and reduction of spontaneous glomerulonephritis and arthritis by orally administered NG-monomethylarginine. *J Exp Med* 1994;179:651–660.
13. Sakurai H, Kohsaka H, Liu MF, et al. Nitric oxide production and inducible nitric oxide synthase expression in inflammatory arthritides. *J Clin Invest* 1996;96:2357–2363.
14. Clancy RM, Abramson SB. Nitric oxide: a novel mediator of inflammation. *Proc Soc Exp Biol Med* 1995;21093–101.
15. Clancy RM, Leszczynska-Piziak J, Abramson SB. Nitric oxide, an endothelial cell relaxation factor, inhibits neutrophil superoxide anion production via a direct action on the NADPH oxidase. *J Clin Invest* 1992;90:1116–1121.
16. Weksler BB. Platelets. In: Gallin JI, Goldstein M, Snyderman R, eds. *Inflammation. Basic principles and clinical correlates.* New York: Raven Press, 1988:543–557.
17. Skaer RJ. Platelet degranulation. In: Gordon JL, ed. *Platelets in biology and pathology*, vol 2. Amsterdam: Elsevier/NorthHolland, 1981:321–348.
18. Krauer KA. Platelet activation during antigen-induced airway reactions in asthmatic subjects. *N Engl J Med* 1981;304: 1404–1406.
19. Grandel KE, Farr RS, Wanderer AA, et al. Association of platelet activating factor with primary acquired cold urticaria. *N Engl J Med* 1985;313:405–409.
20. Ginsberg MH. Role of platelets in inflammation and rheumatic disease. *Adv Inflamm Res* 1986;2:53–71.
21. Pytela R, Pierschbacher M, Ginsberg M, et al. Platelet membrane glycoprotein IIb/IIIa: member of a family of Arg-Gly-Asp-specific adhesion receptors. *Science* 1986;231:1559–1562.

22. McEver RP, Roder P. Selectins: novel receptors that mediate leukocyte adhesion during inflammation. *Thromb Haemost* 1991;65:223–228.
23. Johnson RJ. Platelets in inflammatory glomerular injury. *Semin Nephrol* 1991;11:276–284.
24. Pierucci A, Simonetti BM, Pecci G. Improvement in renal function with selective thromboxane antagonism in lupus nephritis. *N Engl J Med* 1989;320:421–425.
25. Ross GD, Medof ME. Membrane complement receptors specific for bound fragments of C3. *Adv Immunol* 1985;37: 217–267.
26. Schifferli JA, Ng YC, Peters DK. The role of complement and its receptor in the elimination of immune complexes. *N Engl J Med* 1986;315:488–495.
27. Philips MR, Abramson SB, Weissmann G. Neutrophil adhesion and autoimmune vascular injury. *Clin Aspects Autoimmun* 1989; 3:6–15.
28. Yong K, Khwaja A. Leukocyte cellular adhesion molecules. *Blood Rev* 1990;4:211–225.
29. Lawrence MB, Springer TA. Leukocytes role on a selection of physiologic flow rates: distinction from and prerequisite for adhesion through integrins. *Cell* 1991;65:859–873.
30. Ravetch JV, Kinet J-P. Fc receptors. *Annu Rev Immunol* 1991; 9:457–492.
31. van de Winkel J, Capel P. Human IgG Fc receptor heterogeneity: molecular aspects, clinical implications. *Immunol Today* 1993;14:215–221.
32. Salmon JE, Millard SS, Brogle NL, et al. Fcγ receptor IIIb enhances Fcγ receptor IIa function in an oxidant-dependent and allelesensitive manner. *J Clin Invest* 1995;95:2877–2885.
33. Salmon JE, Edberg JC, Brogle NL, et al. Allelic polymorphisms of human Fc receptor IIA and Fcγ receptor IIIB: independent mechanisms for differences in human phagocyte function. *J Clin Invest* 1992;89:1274–1281.
34. Kimberly RP, Ahlstrom JW, Click ME, et al. The glycosyl phosphatidylinositol-linked FcγRIIIPMN mediates transmembrane signaling events distinct from FcRII. *J Exp Med* 1990;171: 1239–1255.
35. Reibman J, Haines KA, Gude D, et al. Differences in signal transduction between two Fc receptors and receptors for the chemoattractant fMLP in neutrophils: effects of colchicine on pertussis toxin sensitivity and diacylglycerol formation. *J Immunol* 1991;146:988–996.
36. Haines KA, Weissmann G. Protein I of N. gonorrhoeae shows that phosphatidate from phosphatidylcholine via phospholipase C is an intracellular messenger in neutrophil activation by chemoattractants. In: Samuelsson B, Paoletti R, Ramwell PW, et al. , eds. *Advances in prostaglandin, thromboxane and leukotriene research*. New York: Raven Press, 1990:545–552.
37. Blackburn WD Jr, Heck LW. Neutrophil activation by surface bound IgG is via a pertussis toxin insensitive G protein. *Biochem Biophys Res Commun* 1989;164:983–989.
38. Huang MM, Indik Z, Brass LF, et al. Activation of Fc (gamma) RII induces tyrosine phosphorylation of multiple proteins including Fc (gamma) RII. *J Biol Chem* 1992;267:5467–5473.
39. Rubinstein E, Urso I, Boucheix C, et al. Platelet activation by cross-linking HLA class I molecules and Fc receptor. *Blood* 1992;79:2901–2908.
40. Walker BAM, Hagenlocker BE, Stubbs EB Jr, et al. Signal transduction events and Fc R engagement in human neutrophils stimulated with immune complexes. *J Immunol* 1991;146:735–741.
41. Feister AJ, Browder B, Willis HE, et al. Pertussis toxin inhibits human neutrophil responses mediated by the 42-kilodalton IgG Fc receptor. *J Immunol* 1988;141:228–233.
42. Brennan PJ, Zigmond SH, Schreiber AD, et al. Binding of IgG containing immune complexes to a human neutrophil Fc(gamma)RII and Fc(gamma)RIII induces actin polymerization by a pertussis toxin-insensitive transduction pathway. *J Immunol* 1991;146:4282–4288.
43. Salmon JE, Brogle NL, Edberg JC, et al. Fcγ receptor III induces actin polymerization in human neutrophils and primes phagocytosis mediated by Fcγ receptor II. *J Immunol* 1991;146: 997–1004.
44. Rosales C, Brown EJ. Two mechanisms for IgG Fc-receptor-mediated phagocytosis by human neutrophils. *J Immunol* 1991; 146:3937–3944.
45. Brunkhorst BA, Strohmeier G, Lazzari K, et al. Differential roles of Fc(gamma)RII and Fc(gamma)RIII in immune complex stimulation of human neutrophils. *J Biol Chem* 1992;267: 20659–20666.
46. Stadler J, Harbrecht BG, DiSilvio M, et al. Endogenous nitric oxide inhibits the synthesis of cyclooxygenase products and interleukin6 by rat Kupffer cells. *J Leukoc Biol* 1993;
47. Biesecker G, Katz S, Koffler D. Renal localization of the membrane attack complex in systemic lupus erythematosus nephritis. *J Exp Med* 1981;154:1779–1794.
48. Bulkley BH, Roberts WC. The heart in systemic lupus erythematosus and the changes induced in it by corticosteroid therapy. *Am J Med* 1975;58:243–264.
49. Stein JM, Luzio JP. Membrane sorting during vesicle shedding from neutrophils during sublytic complement attack. *Biochem Soc Trans* 1989;16:1082–1083.
50. Morgan BP, Dankert JR, Esser AF. Recovery of human neutrophils from complement attack: Removal of the membrane attack complex by endocytosis and exocytosis. *J Immunol* 1987; 138:246–253.
51. Morgan BP. Complement membrane attack on nucleated cells: resistance, recovery and nonlethal effects. *Biochem J* 1989;264: 1–14.
52. Hattori R, Hamilton KK, McEver RP, et al. Complement proteins C5b9 induce secretion of high molecular weight multimers of endothelial von Willebrand Factor and translocation of granule membrane. *J Biol Chem* 1989;264:9053–9060.
53. Biesecker G, Lavin L, Zisking M, et al. Cutaneous localization of the membrane attack complex in discoid and systemic lupus erythematosus. *N Engl J Med* 1982;306:264–270.
54. Kissel JT, Mendell JR, Rammohan KW. Microvascular deposition of complement membrane attack complex in dermatomyositis. *N Engl J Med* 1986;314:329–334.
55. Schafer H, Mathey D, Hugo F, et al. Deposition of the terminal C5b-9 complement complex in infarcted areas of human myocardium. *J Immunol* 1986;137:1945–1949.
56. Koeffler P, Schur P, Kunkel H. Immunological studies concerning the nephritis of systemic lupus erythematosus. *J Exp Med* 1967;126:607–624.
57. Fauci TY, Haynes BF, Katz P. The spectrum of vasculitis. *Ann Intern Med* 1978;89:660–676.
58. Arthus M. Injections repetees de serum de cheval chez la lapin. *Soc Biol* 1903.
59. Ishizaka K. 1963. Progress in allergy. In: Kallos P, Waksman BH, eds. *Gamma globulin and molecular mechanisms in hypersensitivity reactions*, vol 7. New York: S. Karger, 1963:32–106.
60. Frank MM, Ellman L, Green I, et al. Site of deposition of C3 in Arthus reactions of C4 deficient guinea pigs. *J Immunol* 1973;110:1447–11451.
61. Lawley TJ, Frank MM. Immune complexes and immune complex diseases. In: Parker CW, ed. *Clinical immunology*. Philadelphia: WB Saunders, 1980:143.
62. Cochrane CG. The Arthus reaction. In: Zweifach BW, Grant L, McCluskey RT, eds. *The inflammatory process*. New York: Academic Press, 1965:613–648.
63. Sylvestre DL, Ravetch JV. Fc receptors initiate the Arthus reac-

tion: redefining the inflammatory cascade. *Science* 1994;265: 1095–1098.
64. Dixon FJ, Feldman JD, Vazquez JJ. Experimental glomerulonephritis. The pathogenesis of a laboratory model resembling the spectrum of human glomerulonephritis. *J Exp Med* 1961; 113:899–920.
65. Cochrane CG, Koffler D. 1973. Immune complex disease in experimental animals and man. In: Dixon FJ, Kunkel HG, eds. *Advances in immunology*. New York: Academic Press, 1973: 185–264.
66. Ruddy S, Carpenter CB, Chin KW, et al. Human complement metabolism: an analysis of 144 studies. *Medicine (Baltimore)* 1975;54:165–178.
67. Charlesworth JA, Williams DG, Sherington E, et al. Metabolic studies of the third component of complement and the glycine rich glycoprotein in patients with hypocomplementemia. *J Clin Invest* 1974;53:1578–1587.
68. Sliwinski AJ, Zvaifler NJ. 1972. Decreased synthesis of the third component (C3) in hypocomplemententemic systemic lupus erythematosus. *Clin Exp Immunol* 1972;11:21–29.
69. Kerr L, Adelsberg BR, Schulman P, et al. Factor B activation products in patients with systemic lupus erythematosus: a marker of severe disease activity. *Arthritis Rheum* 1989;32: 1406–1413.
70. Falk RJ, Dalmasso AP, Kim Y, et al. Radioimmunoassay of the attack complex of complement in serum from patients with systemic lupus erythematosus. *N Engl J Med* 1985;312:1594–1599.
71. Belmont HM, Hopkins P, Edelson HS, et al. Complement Activation during systemic lupus erythematosus. C3a and C5a anaphylatoxins circulate during exacerbations of disease. *Arthritis Rheum* 1986;29:1085–1089.
72. Buyon J, Tamerius J, Belmont HM, et al. Assessment of disease activity and impending flare in patients with systemic lupus erythematosus: comparison of the use of complement split products and conventional measurements of complement. *Arthritis Rheum* 1992;35:1028–1037.
73. Buyon J, Tamerius J, Ordica S, et al. Activation of the alternative complement pathway accompanies disease flares in systemic lupus erythematosus during pregnancy. *Arthritis Rheum* 1992;3 5:55–61.
74. Hopkins PT, Belmont HM, Buyon J, et al. Increased levels of plasma anaphylatoxins in systemic lupus erythematosus predict flares of the disease and may elicit vascular injury in lupus cerebritis. *Arthritis Rheum* 1988;31:632–641.
75. Hopkins P, Belmont M, Buyon J, et al. Increased plasma anaphylotoxins in systemic lupus erythematosus predict flares of the disease and may elicit the adult cerebral distress syndrome. *Arthritis Rheum* 1988;31:632–641.
76. Belmont HM, Buyon J, Giorno R, et al. Upregulation of endothelial cell adhesion molecules characterizes disease activity in systemic lupus erythematosus: the Shwartzman phenomenon revisited. *Arthritis Rheum* 1994;37:376–383.
77. Jacob HS, Craddock PR, Hammerschmidt DE, et al. Complementinduced granulocyte aggregation: an unsuspected mechanism of disease. *N Engl J Med* 1980;302:789–794.
78. Hammerschmidt DE, Weaver LJ, Hudson LD, et al. Association of complement activation and elevated plasma-C5a with adult respiratory distress syndrome. *Lancet* 1980;1:947–949.
79. Hakim R, Breillatt J, Lazarus M, et al. Complement activation and hypersensitivity reactions to hemodialysis membranes. *N Engl J Med* 1984;311:878–882.
80. Craddock P, Fehr J, Dalmasso A, et al. Hemodialysis leukopenia. *J Clin Invest* 1977;59:879–888.
81. Chenoweth DE, Cooper SW, Hugh TE, et al. Complement activation during cardiopulmonary bypass. *N Engl J Med* 1981; 304:497–505.
82. Perez HD, Horn JK, Ong R, et al. Complement (C5)-derived chemotactic activity in serum from patients with pancreatitis. *J Lab Clin Med* 1983;101:123–129.
83. Shwartzman G. *Phenomenon of local tissue reactivity*. New York: Paul Hoeber, 1937.
84. Argenbright L, Barton R. Interactions of leukocyte integrins with intercellular adhesion molecule 1 in the production of inflammatory vascular injury in vivo. The Shwartzman phenomenon revisited. *J Clin Invest* 1992;89:259–273.
85. Abramson SB, Weissmann G. Complement split products and the pathogenesis of SLE. *Hosp Pract* 1988;23(12):45–55.
86. Pohlman TM, Stanness KA, Beatty PG, et al. An endothelial cell surface factor(s) induced in vitro by lipopolysaccharide, interleukin 1, and tumor necrosis factor-alpha increases neutrophil adherence by a CDw18-dependent mechanism. *J Immunol* 1986;136:4548–4553.
87. Pober JS, Gimbrone M, Lapierre D, et al. Overlapping patterns of activation of human endothelial cells by interleukin-1, tumor necrosis factor and immune interferon. *J Immunol* 1986;137: 1893–1896.
88. Fletcher MP, Seligmann BE, Gallin JI. Correlation of human neutrophil secretion, chemoattractant receptor mobilization and enhanced functional capacity. *J Immunol* 1982;128:941.
89. Schur PH, Sandson J. Immunologic factors and clinical activity in systemic lupus erythematosus. *N Engl J Med* 1968;278: 533–538.
90. Buyon JP, Shadick N, Berkman R, et al. Surface expression of gp165/95, the complement receptor CR3, as a marker of disease activity in systemic lupus erythematosus. *Clin Immunol Immunopathol* 1988;46:141–149.
91. Johnson RT, Richardson EP. The neurological manifestations of systemic lupus erythematosus: a clinical pathological study of 24 cases and a review of the literature. *Medicine (Baltimore)* 1968;47:337–369.
92. Ellis SG, Verity MA. Central nervous system involvement in systemic lupus erythematosus: a review of the neuropathologic findings in 57 cases, 1955–1977. *Semin Arthritis Rheum* 1979; 8:212–233.
93. Hammad A, Tsukada Y, Torre N. Cerebral occlusive vasculopathy in systemic lupus erythematosus and speculation on the part played by complement. *Ann Rheum Dis* 1992;51:550–552.
94. Devinsky O, Petito CK, Alonso DR. Clinical and neuropathological findings in systemic lupus erythematosus: The role of vasculitis heart emboli and thrombotic thrombocytopenic purpura. *Ann Neurol* 1988;23:380.
95. Abramson SB, Dobro J, Eberle MA, et al. The syndrome of acute reversible hypoxemia of systemic lupus erythematosus. *Ann Intern Med* 1991;114:941–947.
96. Bone RC. Why new definitions of sepsis and organ failure are needed. *Am J Med* 1993;95:348.
97. Nogare D. Septic shock. *Am J Med Sci* 1991;302:50–65.
98. Waage A, Brandtzaeg P, Espevik T, et al. Current understanding of the pathogenesis of gram-negative shock. *Infect Dis Clin North Am* 1991;5:781–789.
99. Walsh CJ, Carey PD, Bechard DE, et al. AntiCD 18 antibody attenuates neutropenia and alveolar capillary-membrane injury during gram-negative sepsis. *Surgery* 1991;110:205–211.
100. Tomer Y, Gilburd B, Blank M, et al. Characterization of biologically active antineutrophil cytoplasmic antibodies induced in mice. Pathogenetic role in experimental vasculitis. *Arthritis Rheum* 1995;38:1375–1381.
101. Alexander EL. Immunopathologic mechanisms of inflammatory vascular disease in primary Sjogren's syndrome—a model. *Scand J Rheumatol* 1986;61:280–285.
102. Hughes GR, Khamashta MA. The antiphospholipid syndrome. *J R Coll Phys Lond* 1994;28:301–304.
103. OrdiRos J, PerezPeman P, Monasterio J. Clinical and therapeutic aspects associated to phospholipid binding antibodies (lupus

anticoagulant and anticardiolipin antibodies). *Haemostasis* 1994;24:165–174.
104. Bevers EM, Galli M. Cofactors involved in the antiphospholipid syndrome. *Lupus* 1992;1:51–53.
105. Ozawa N, Makino T, Matsubayashi H, et al. beta 2-GPIdependent and independent binding of anticardiolipin antibodies in patients with recurrent spontaneous abortions. *J Clin Lab Anal* 1994;8:255–259.
106. Aron AL, Gharavi AE, Shoenfeld Y. Mechanisms of action of antiphospholipid antibodies in the antiphospholipid syndrome. *Int Arch Allerg Immunol* 1995;106:8–12.
107. Pierangeli SS, Harris EN. Antiphospholipid antibodies in an in vivo thrombosis model in mice. *Lupus* 1994;3:247–251.
108. Triplett DA. Antiphospholipid antibodies: proposed mechanisms of action. *Am J Reprod Immunol* 1992;28:211–215.
109. Wiener HM, Vardinon N, Yust I. Platelet antibody binding and spontaneous aggregation in 21 lupus anticoagulant patients. *Vox Sang* 1991;61:111–121.
110. Vazquez-Mellado J, Llorente L, Richaud-Patin Y, et al. Exposure of anionic phospholipids upon platelet activation permits binding of beta 2 glycoprotein I and through it that of IgG antiphospholipid antibodies. Studies in platelets from patients with antiphospholipid syndrome and normal subjects. *J Autoimmun* 1994;7:335–348.
111. Lindsey NJ, Hendeson FI, Malia R, et al. Inhibition of prostacyclin release by endothelial binding anticardiolipin antibodies in thrombosisprone patients with systemic lupus erythematosus and the antiphospholipid syndrome. *Br J Rheumatol* 1994;33:20–26.
112. Westerman EM, Miles JM, Backonja M, et al. Neuropathologic findings in multiinfarct dementia associated with anticardiolipin antibody. Evidence for endothelial injury as the primary event. *Arthritis Rheum* 1992;35:1038–1041.
113. McCraw KR, DeMichele A, Samuels P, et al. Detection of endothelial cell-reactive immunoglobulin in patients with antiphospholipid antibodies. *Br J Haematol* 1991;79:595–605.
114. Silver RK, Adler L, Hickman AR, et al. Anticardiolipin antibodypositive serum enhances endothelial cell platelet-activating factor production. *Am J Obstet Gynecol* 1991;165:1748–1752.
115. Freyssinet JM, TotiOrfanoudakis F, Ravanat C, et al. The catalytic role of anionic phospholipids in the activation of protein C by factor Xa and expression of its anticoagulant function in human plasma. *Blood Coagul Fibrin* 1991;2:691–698.
116. Joseph J, Scopelitis E. Seronegative antiphospholipid syndrome associated with plasminogen activator inhibitor. *Lupus* 1994;3: 201–203.
117. Ahmed K, Vianna J, Khamashta M, et al. IL2, IL6, and TNF levels in primary antiphospholipid antibody syndrome (letter). *Clin Exp Rheumatol* 1992;10:503.
118. Simantov R, LaSala JM, Lo SK, et al. Activation of cultured vascular endothelial cells by antiphospholipid antibodies. *J Clin Invest* 1996;96:2211–2219.
119. Stricker RB, Davis JA, Gershow J, et al. Thrombotic thrombocytopenic purpura complicating systemic lupus erythematosus. Case report and literature review from the plasmapheresis era. *J Rheumatol* 1992;19:1469–1473.
120. Cockerell CJ, Lewis JE. Systemic lupus erythematosus-like illness associated with syndrome of abnormally large von Willebrand's factor multimers. *South Med J* 1993;86:951–953.
121. Moake JL, Rudy CK, Troll JH, et al. Unusually large plasma factor VIII: von Willebrand factor multimers in chronic relapsing thrombotic thrombocytopenic purpura. *N Engl J Med* 1982;303:1432–1435.
122. Takahashi H, Hanano M, Wada K, et al. Circulating thrombomodulin in thrombotic thrombocytopenic purpura. *Am J Hematol* 1991;38:174–177.
122a. Abu-Shakra M, Urowitz MB, Gladman DD, et al. Mortality studies in systemic lupus erythematosus. Results from a single center. II. Predictor variables for mortality. *J Rheumatol* 1995; 22:1265–1270.
122b. Bulkley BH, Roberts WC. The heart in systemic lupus erythematosus and the changes induced in it by corticosteroid therapy. A study of 36 necropsy patients. *Am J Med* 1975;58:243–264.
122c. Aranow C, Ginzler EM. Epidemiology of cardiovascular disease in systemic lupus erythematosus. *Lupus* 2000;9:166–169.
122d. Manzi S, Selzer F, Sutton-Tyrrell K, et al. Prevalence and risk factors of carotid plaque in women with systemic lupus erythematosus. *Arthritis Rheum* 1999;42:51–60.
123. Price DT, Loscalzo J. Cellular adhesion molecules and atherogenesis. *Am J Med* 1999;107:85–97.
124. Vogel RA. Cholesterol lowering and endothelial function. *Am J Med* 1999;107:479–487.
125. Nageh MF, Sandberg ET, Marotti KR, et al. Deficiency of inflammatory cell adhesion molecules protects against atherosclerosis in mice. *Atheroscler Thromb Vasc Biol* 1997;7:1517–1520.
126. Walker G, Lanheinrich AC, Dennhauser E, et al. 3-Deazaadenosine prevents adhesion molecule expression and atherosclerotic lesion formation in the aortas of c57BL/6J mice. *Atheroscler Thromb Vasc Biol* 1999;19(11):2673–2679.
127. Belmont HM, Abramson SB, Lie JT. Pathology and pathogenesis of vascular injury in systemic lupus erythematosus: interactions of inflammatory cells and activated endothelium. *Arthritis Rheum* 1996;39:9–22.
128. Belmont HM, Abramson SB. Systemic inflammatory response syndrome, systemic lupus erythematosus and thrombosis. In: Asherson R, Cervera R, Tripplet DA, et al., eds. *Vascular manifestations of systemic autoimmune diseases.* Chicago: CRC Press, 2001:147–159.
129. Vischer UM, Emeis JJ, Bilo HJ, et al. von Willebrand factor as a plasma marker of endothelial activation in diabetes: improved reliability with parallel determination of the vWf propeptide. *Thromb Haemost* 1998;80:1002–1007.
130. McGill SN, Ahmed NA, Cristou NV. Increased plasma von Willebrand factor in the systemic inflammmatory response syndrome is derived from generalized endothelial cell activation. *Crit Care Med* 1998;26:296–300.
131. Edgington TS, Mackman N, Brand K, et al. The structural biology of expression and function of tissue factor. *Thromb Haemost* 1991;66:67–79.
132. Wilcox JN, Smith KM, Schwartz SM, et al. Localization of tissue factor in the normal vesselwall and in the atherosclerotic plaque. *Proc Natl Acad Sci USA* 1989;86:2839–2843.
133. Thiruvikraman SV, Gudha A, Roboz J, et al. In situ localization of tissue factor in human atherosclerotic plaques by binding of digoxigenin-labeled factors VIIa and X. *Lab Invest* 1996;75: 451–461.
134. Solovey A, Gui L, Key NS, et al. Tissue factor expression by endothelial cells in sickle cell anemia. *J Clin Invest* 1998;101: 899–1904.
135. Kaplanski G, Cacoub P, Farnarier C, et al. Increased soluble vascular adhesion molecule1 concentrations in patients with primary or systemic lupus erythematosus-related antiphospholipid syndrome. *Arthritis Rheum* 2000;43(1):55–64.
136. Kaplanski G, Fabrigoule M, Boulay V, et al. Thrombin induces endothelial type II activation in vitro: IL-1 and TNF-alpha-independent IL-8 secretion and E-selectin expression. *J Immunol* 1997;158:5435–5441.
137. Connolly ES Jr, Winfree CJ, Springer TA, et al. Cerebral protection in homozygous null ICAM1 mice after middle artery occlusion: role of neutrophil adhesion in the pathogenesis of stroke. *J Clin Invest* 1996;97:209–216.
138. Bullard DC, King PD, Hicks MJ, et al. Intercellular adhesion molecule-1 deficiency protects MRL/MpJ-Fas 1pr mice from early lethality. *J Immunol* 1997;159:2058–2067.
139. Nyberg F, Acevedo F, Stephanson E. Different patterns of solu-

ble adhesion molecules in systemic and cutaneous lupus erythematosus. *J Immunol* 1997;65:230–235.
140. Sprague EA, Cayatte AJ, Shwartz CJ. Flow mediated modulation of selected biologic and molecular determinants related to vascular endothelial activation. *J Vasc Surg* 1992;15:919–921.
141. Nagel T, Resnick N, Atkinson WJ, et al. Shear stress selectively upregulates intracellular adhesion molecule-1 expression in cultured human vascular endothelial cells. *J Clin Invest* 1994;94: 885–891.
142. Russell R. Atherosclerosis: an inflammatory disease. *N Engl J Med* 1999;340:115–123.
143. Erl W, Weber PC, Weber C. Monocytic cell adhesion to endothelial cells stimulated by oxidized low density lipoprotein is mediated by distinct endothelial ligands. *Atherosclerosis* 1998;136:297–303.
144. Crossman DC. More problems with endothelium. *Q J Med* 1997;90:157–160.
145. Wu R, Huang YH, Elinder LS. Lysophosphatydylcholine is involved in the antigenicity of oxidized LDL. *Atheroscler Thromb Vasc Biol* 1998;18:626–630.
146. Manzi S, Chester M, Wasko M. inflammation-mediated rheumatic diseases and atherosclerosis. *Ann Rheum Dis* 2000; 50:321–325.
147. Bergmark C, Wu R, de Faire U, et al. Patients with early onset peripheral vascular disease have increased levels of antibodies against oxidized LDL. *Atheroscler Thromb Vasc Biol* 1995;15: 441–445.
148. Vaarala O, Alfthan G, Jauhhiainen M, et al. Crossreaction between antibodies to oxidized lowdensity lipoprotein and to cardiolipin in systemic lupus erythematosus. *Lancet* 1993;341: 923–925.
149. Horkko S, Miller E, Dudl E, et al. Antiphospholipid antibodies are directed against epitopes of oxidized phospholipids: recognition of cardiolipin by monoclonal antibodies to epitopes of oxidized low density lipoprotein. *J Clin Invest* 1996;98:815–825.
150. Warner SJ. Interleukin 1 induces interleukin 1. II. Recombinant human interleukin 1 induces interleukin 1 production by adult human vascular endothelial cells. *J Immunol* 1987;139: 1911–1917.
151. Galea J, Armstrong J, Gadson P, et al. Interleukin-1 beta in coronary arteries of patients with ischemic heart disease. *Atheroscler Thromb Vasc Biol* 1996;16:1000–1006.
152. Barath P, Fishbein MC, Cao J, et al. Detection and localization of tumor necrosis factor in human atheroma. *Am J Cardiol* 1990;65:297–301.
153. Carvalho D, Caroline COS, Isenberg D, et al. IgG antiendothelial cell autoantibodies from patients with systemic lupus erythematosus or systemic vasculitis stimulate the release of two endothelial cell derived mediators which enhance adhesion molecule expression and leukocyte adhesion in an autocrine manner. *Arthritis Rheum* 1999;42:631–639.
154. Saadi S, Holzknecht RA, Patte CP, et al. Complement-mediated regulation of tissue factor activity in endothelium. *J Exp Med* 1995;182:1807–1814.
155. Saadi RA, Holzknecht CP, Patte CP, et al. Endothelial cell activation by poreforming structures: pivotal role for interleukin-1. *Circulation* 2000;101:1867–1873.
156. Bruce IN, Gladman DD, Urowitz MB. Premature atherosclerosis in systemic lupus erythematosus. *Rheum Dis Clin North Am* 2000;26(2):257–278.
157. Nityanand S, Bergmark C, deFaure U, et al. Antibodies against endothelial cells and cardiolipin in young patients with peripheral atherosclerotic disease. *J Intern Med* 1995;238(S):437.
158. Carvalho D, Savage C, Black CM, et al. IgG antiendothelial cell autoantibodies from scleroderman patients induce leukocyte adhesion to human vascular endothelial cells in vitro: induction of adhesion molecule expression and involvement of endothelium-derived cytokines. *J Clin Invest* 1996;97:111–119.
159. Del Papa N, Guidali L, Sironi M, et al. Antiendothelial cell IgG antibodies from patients with Wegener's granulomatosis bind to human endothelial cells I vitro and induce adhesion molecule expression and cytokine secretion. *Arthritis Rheum* 1996;39: 758–767.
160. Blank M, Krause I, Goldkorn T, et al. Monoclonal antiendothelial cell antibodies from a patient with Takayasu arteritis activate endothelial cells from large vessels. *Arthritis Rheum* 1999;42:1421–1432.
161. Bordon A, Dueymes M, Levy Y, et al. Antiendothelial cell antibody binding makes negatively charges phospholipids accessible to antiphospholipid antibodies. *Arthritis Rheum* 1998;41: 1738–1747.
162. Koike T, Tamioka H, Kumagai A. Antibodies cross-reactive with DNA and cardiolipin in patients with systemic lupus erythematosus. *Clin Exp Immunol* 1983;59:449–456.
163. Hassealaar P, Deksen RHWM, Blokzijl L, et al. Crossreactivity of antibodies directed against cardiolipin, DNA, endothelial cells and blood platelets. *Thromb Haemost* 1990;63:169–173.
164. Simantov R, LaSala JM, Lo SK, et al. Activation of cultured endothelial cells by antiphospholipid antibodies. *J Clin Invest* 1995;96:2211–2219.
165. Lai KN, Leung JCK, Lai KB, et al. Increased release of von Willebrand factor antigen from endothelial cells by anti DNA autoantibodies. *Ann Rheum Dis* 1996;55:57–62.
166. Chan TM, Yu PM, Tsang KL, et al. Endothelial cell binding by human polyclonal antiDNA antibodies: relationship to disease activity and endothelial functional alterations. *Clin Exp Immunol* 1995;100:506–513.
167. Slupsky JR, Kalba M, Willuweit A, et al. Activated platelets induce tissue factor expression on human umbilical vein endothelial cells by ligation of CD40. *Thromb Haemost* 1998; 80:1008–1014.
168. Karnmann K, Hughes CD, Schechner J, et al. CD40 on human endothelial cells: inducibility by cytokines and functional regulation of adhesion molecule expression. *Proc Natl Acad Sci USA* 1995;92:4342–4346.
169. Mach F, Schonbeck U, Sukhova GK, et al. Reduction of atherosclerosis in mice by inhibition of CD40 signaling. *Nature* 1998;394:200–203.
170. Lozada C, Levin RI, Huie M, et al. Identification of C1q as the heat-labile serum cofactor required for immune complexes to stimulate endothelial expression of the adhesion molecules Eselectin and intercellular and vascular cell adhesion molecules. *Proc Natl Acad Sci USA* 1995;92:8378–8382.
171. Reiss AB, Mahotra S, Javitt NB, et al. Occupancy of C1q receptors on endothelial cells by immune complexes downregulates mRNA for stero127-hydroxylase, the major mediator of extrahepatic cholesterol metabolism. *Arthritis Rheum* 1998;41(9) S:S79.
172. Paulson JC. *Selectin/carbohydrate-mediated adhesion of leukocytes, adhesion: its role in inflammatory disease.* New York: WH Freeman, 1992.
173. Clancy R, Marder G, Martin V, et al. Circulating activated endothelial cells in SLE: Further evidence for diffused vasculopathy. *Arthritis Rheum* 2001; *in press.*
174. Solovey A, Lin Y, Brown P, et al. Circulating activated endothelial cells in sickle cell anemia. *N Engl J Med* 1997;337:1584–1590.
175. Mutin M, Canavy I, Blann A, et al. Direct evidence of endothelial injury in acute myocardial infarction and unstable angina by demonstration of circulating endothelial cells. *Blood* 1999;93: 2951–2958.

15

IDIOTYPES AND IDIOTYPE NETWORKS

BEVRA HANNAHS HAHN
FANNY M. EBLING
JATINDERPAL K. KALSI

HISTORY

In 1963, Oudin and Michel (1) proposed the concept of idiotypes (Ids) and antiidiotypes (anti-Ids) when describing rabbit antibodies that induce antibodies against themselves. In the same year, Kunkel et al. (2) described Ids on human antibodies. In 1974, Jerne (3) suggested that Ids and anti-Ids participate in self-regulatory immune networks. Since then, many investigators have established the importance of Ids in normal immune regulation and in experimental manipulation of cell function and immune responses.

DEFINITIONS

Terms used in defining Ids and idiotypic networks are listed in Table 15.1. Idiotopes are antigenic regions located in the variable regions of immunoglobulin (Ig) molecules or T-cell antigen receptors (TCRs). Single Ig molecules can express several different idiotopes; the series of idiotopes is referred to as the idiotype for that molecule. Because the exact structural basis of most idiotopes is unknown, the term *idiotype* is widely used to describe the entire antigenic region on Igs or TCRs. An antibody produced in response to antigen (Ag) expresses Id and is called Ab1 to define its place in the Id immune network.

Ids are divided into two general classes: private and public. Private Ids are expressed on Igs or TCRs that expand from a single parent clone. Therefore, private Ids define antibodies or T cells that are clonal and relatively specific for a single stimulating Ag. In contrast, public Ids (also called cross-reactive Ids) are expressed on Igs and TCRs deriving from different parental cells. Therefore, Igs and TCRs displaying public Ids bind several different Ags and are likely to appear in many different individuals of the same species. Further, public Ids may be found on antibodies in individuals of different species. For example, public Ids on anti-DNA antibodies derived from certain mouse strains are found on anti-DNA and other Igs in humans (4,5).

Because idiotypes are antigenic, they stimulate production of anti-Id antibodies, which are referred to as Ab2. Ab2 molecules are divided into at least two subtypes, depending on whether they mimic Ag (6). Ab2α binds Ab1 but otherwise shares no properties of the initial stimulating Ag. Ab2β

TABLE 15.1. DEFINITIONS

1. *Idiotype.* A region on the variable portion of an immunoglobulin molecule or T-cell antigen receptor that is antigenic. When present on an antibody molecule, the antibody may be referred to as Ab1.
2. *Idiotype (Id).* A series of idiotopes on the same molecule.
3. *Private idiotype.* An Id expressed only on the products of a single B- or T-cell clone. Antibodies and T cells bearing private Ids will be specific for only one antigen (Ag).
4. *Public idiotype.* An Id expressed on different B- and T-cell clones that interrelates them. Antibodies and T cells bearing public Ids are in sum able to recognize multiple different Ags. These also are referred to as cross-reactive or shared Ids.
5. *Antiidiotype.* An antibody directed against the idiotope on immunoglobulin, B-cell surface, or T-cell antigen receptor. This antibody may be referred to as Ab2.
6. *Anti-Id type 1.* Also called Ab2α, this Ab2 binds to Ab1 but does not otherwise behave like antigen (Ag).
7. *Anti-Id type 2.* Also called Ab2β, also called homobody, internal image anti-Id, or epibody. This Ab2 binds Ab1 and behaves in additional ways like Ag. For example, it can bind to receptors for Ag and by so doing can trigger cell activation.
8. *Anti–Anti-Id.* An antibody against Ab2. It also may be referred to as Ab3. Some Ab3 molecules share structural similarities to and behave like Ab1; for example, they may bind the Ag to which the original Ab1 is directed.
9. *Epitope.* The region of an antigen bound by Ab1.
10. *Paratope.* The region of an antibody or T-cell receptor bound by anti-Id.
11. *Connectivity.* The property of one Id network influencing the development of another. For example, the Ids on mature immune responses develop in sequence to different Ids, expressed on Ig in fetal mice.
12. *Parallel sets.* A network of Ab1-Ab2-Ab3 that is interactive.
13. *Network antigen.* An Ab2 that can react either with Ag or with Ab1 and therefore can regulate the entire Ag-Ab1-Ab2-Ab3 Id network.

binds Ab1 and behaves in other ways like Ag, and it can stimulate production of more Ab1 and bind to receptors that ordinarily bind Ag. This property was first noted in insulin systems (7). Some Ab2 against antiinsulin Ab1 could bind the insulin receptor on cell surfaces and actually trigger glucose metabolism by those cells. Ab2β anti-Ids are also called internal image anti-Ids, as suggested by Nisonoff and Lamoyi (8), implying that they share structural similarities with Ag. Some authors refer to them as epibodies or homobodies. Another class of Ab2 is Ab2γ, which contains antiidiotypes that are antigen inhibitable because of steric hindrance with the antigen combining site (9). Ab2β has been extensively used to generate internal images of infectious pathogens (10–19), tumor antigens (20–24), and more recently as mimics of self antigen, for example human interferon (IFN), which has antiviral activity (25). Because Ab2 molecules themselves express Ids, they also stimulate production of anti-anti-Ids (Ab3).

Within the variable region of each Ab1 is a region that binds the epitope of the stimulating Ag. The region on Ab1 that binds Ab2 is called a paratope. If the paratope- and epitope-binding regions of the Ab1 molecule overlap or are located close to each other, binding of either (by epitope of Ag or paratope of Ab2) may inhibit binding of the opposite molecule.

IDIOTYPE NETWORKS

Idiotype networks are complex, and three features are particularly important. First, members of the network regulate each other, thus serving to control immune responses. Second, the network links immune responses to self with immune responses to the external environment. Third, the network links the fetal and newborn repertoires to the adult immune response.

Antigen-Antibody Idiotype Networks

There are at least two major concepts of Id networks. The most widely held view, suggested originally by Jerne (3) and later expanded by him and others (6–9,26–29), is illustrated in Fig. 15.1. This concept is based on information suggesting that convex epitopes on Ags are bound by

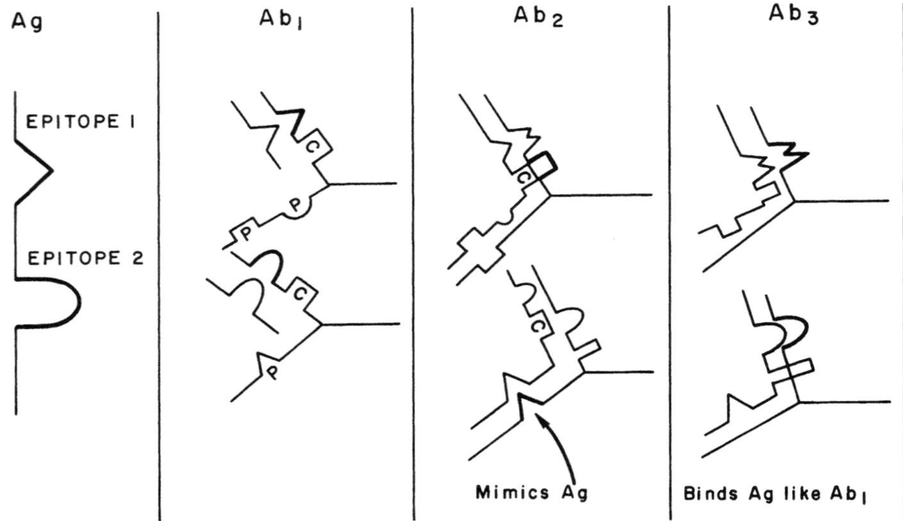

FIGURE 15.1. The antibody Id network. In the first panel, an antigen (Ag) with two epitopes is shown. In the second panel, two antibodies (Ab1) against the antigen are shown: the top Ab1 recognizes epitope 1, and the bottom Ab1 recognizes epitope 2. Each Ab1 has an idiotope specific to that clone, a private Id (p). Both Ab1s contain an identical sequence or conformational idiotope, designated as a cross-reactive (C) or public Id. Thus, the private Ids identify distinct clonal antibody specific for one Ag, and the public Ids identify related families of antibody that derive from different clones and can recognize different epitopes. In the third panel, two anti-Id antibodies (Ab2) have been induced by Ab1. The upper Ab2 is an alpha type; it binds Ab1 but does not mimic Ag. The lower Ab2 is a beta type; it contains a sequence that mimics an epitope on the original Ag and can behave like Ag (bind receptors for Ag, stimulate Ab1, and so on). It is called Ab2β, internal image anti-Id, or an epibody. In the fourth panel, two antibodies (Ab3) induced by Ab2 are shown. The upper Ab3 binds only Ab2. The lower Ab3 has a sequence or conformation that mimics a sequence/conformation in Ab1; it can bind Ag. Some, but not all, members of the network have the capacity to regulate other members.

concave regions in the Ag-binding groove of Ig molecules, as suggested by x-ray crystallographic studies of an Ag-antibody complex (30). Similarly, convex regions on Ab1 molecules are bound by concave regions in the binding groove of Ab2; the same process permits binding of Ab3 to Ab2.

This Id network regulates itself in at least two ways, as shown in Fig. 15.1. First, as discussed earlier, some Ab2 molecules behave like Ag; they stimulate Ab1 production, bind Ag receptors, and can probably trigger cell activation under certain conditions. As illustrated, these Ab2 internal image anti-Ids have sequences or conformations highly similar to those on Ag. This property of anti-Id serving as surrogate Ag has been used to isolate and characterize receptors (7) and to stimulate production of neutralizing Ab1, thus using Ab2 as a vaccine (8,27). Second, some Ab3 molecules have properties of Ab1, in that they can bind the original Ag and are sometimes referred to as Ab1′. An elegant demonstration of the entire network, from Ag to Ab3, has been reported in a study using the O-specific polysaccharide side chain of *Pseudomonas aeruginosa* as Ag to raise Ab1 and Ab3 in mice; both Ab1 and Ab3 were opsonizing, protective antibodies that prevented lethal infection (10). Structural mimicry between Ag and Ab2 has been reported in the GAT system (31); an amino acid motif in GAT was present in Ab2 and recognized by Ab3.

Although experimental results in many Id-anti-Id systems fit the Jerne hypothesis, numerous exceptions have occurred. For example, some Ab2 molecules can serve as surrogate Ags even though their binding to Ab1 is not Ag inhibitable, suggesting that they are not internal image anti-Ids. Such observations have led to another hypothesis of Ag Id-anti-Id interactions, reviewed by Kohler et al. (32). This hypothesis suggests that interactions between Ag, Ab1, Ab2, and so on can occur via side chains/conformations outside the Ag-binding groove of Ig. Some Ab2αs are able to broaden the epitope specificity of the immune response (33). This may be particularly important in situations where a very narrow range of antigenic specificities is recognized by the immune system, for example as in HIV infection. The mechanisms whereby this expansion of response occurs are not clear, but it has been suggested either that Ab2α may bind to both Ab1 and the antigen, thus stabilizing the complex, or that there is formation of a metatope, where new epitopes are revealed through conformational changes that result from the formation of the immune complex (33,34). Both hypotheses regarding Id interactions may be correct, and they may occur simultaneously.

The importance of Id networks in systemic lupus erythematosus (SLE) has been suggested by several investigators who have demonstrated Ab1 and Ab2 in murine or human SLE; some have detected Ab3 (35–43). In several studies, internal image Ab2 has been shown to bind multiple autoAgs and Ab3 to bind Ab1.

T Cells in Idiotype Networks

The preceding discussion addressed Ag induction of circulating Ab1, Ab2, and Ab3. Naturally, B lymphocytes secreting the Abs express the same Ids on their surface Ig. In addition, T lymphocytes are involved in Id-anti-Id networks. Several experiments have shown that Ab2 can bind to and, in some cases, activate T cells (44,45). Figure 15.2 illustrates the mechanisms by which B and T-helper (Th) cells interact to activate each other and to upregulate production of Igs bearing certain Ids. Concepts of T-cell activation require interaction between antigenic peptides presented by the major histocompatibility complex (MHC) to the TCR of T cells. $CD4^+$ T cells recognize Ag presented by MHC class II; $CD8^+$ T cells recognize Ag presented by MHC class I. Such Ag presentation can be provided by B cells, which can process either surface or cytoplasmic Ig into peptides and present them in surface class I or II molecules (46–52). Thus, idiopeptides are presented to TCRs. Activation of a Th cell by this method is shown in Fig. 15.2. Ig can probably stimulate both B and T cells; in the reovirus system, a B-cell epitope has been defined in the CDR2 region of the Ig light chain and a T-cell epitope in the CDR2 of the heavy

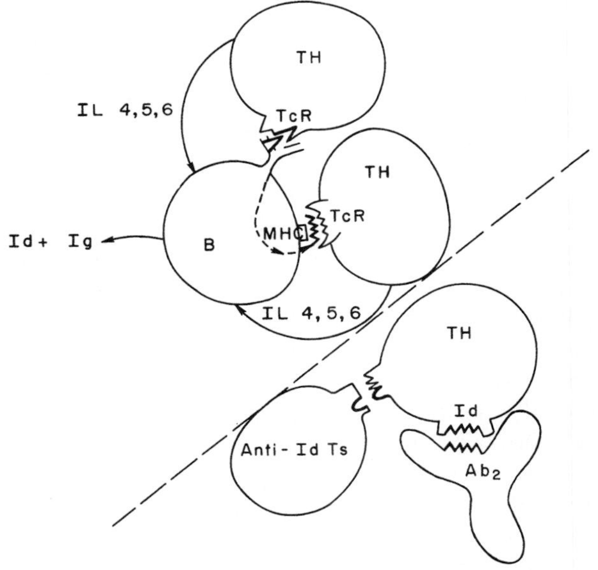

FIGURE 15.2. The T/B-cell Id network. In the upper area, T-helper (Th) cells that augment autoantibody production are shown. They are idiotypic Th cells. The upper Th cell has a T-cell receptor (TCR) that recognizes an Id on the surface Ig of an Id^+ B cell; the lower Th cell has a TCR that recognizes an idiopeptide processed by the B cell from its surface Ig and presented by a major histocompatibility complex (MHC) class II molecule. Both Id Th cells secrete B-cell stimulatory factors (IL-4, -5, and -6) that upregulate production of the Id^+ antibody. In the lower area, the Id Th cell recognizes the idiotope on an Ab2 in one region of its TCR; another region of TCR has induced an anti-Id suppressor T cell (Ts), which can suppress the Id Th cell. Thus, both B and T cells participate in cellular and humoral regulatory networks governed by idiotypes.

chain (53,54). Interestingly, in a murine anti-DNA antibody V88, T- and B-cell epitopes were co-located within the same region of the variable region of the heavy chain of immunoglobulin (VH) (55). There is also evidence that idiotypes may interact directly with TCR (56) and thus activate T cells in a non-MHC restricted fashion.

Activation of Id-recognizing Th cells is probably necessary for full-scale production of Id-bearing antibodies, as shown in Fig. 15.2. Activation of Th cells releases B-cell growth and differentiation lymphokines, which in combination with cell-cell contact results in B-cell production of Ab1, Ab2, and so on (52,57).

TCRs can serve as immunogens for developing the Ab1/Ab2/Ab3 network as well as a regulatory T network, as shown again in Fig. 15.2. For example, immunization of B10.D2 mice with an anti-Id made against the Id on the TCR of a Th clone specific for Sendai virus was effective in producing virus-specific neutralizing antibody, delayed-type hypersensitivity, cytotoxic T cells, and protection against infection (57). Id-recognizing Th cells may be distinct individual cells, or the recognition of Id may be a property of cells that also can recognize Ag epitopes. In several murine antibody systems, including anti-PC and anti-(T,G)A-L, there is collaboration between Th cells that recognize the Ag and the Id or anti-Id. However, Th cells that specifically enrich Id^+ antibodies have been detected (48,58).

T-cell participation in Id networks is not confined to cells with helper function. Manipulation of the Id network can produce T cells that participate in delayed-type hypersensitivity, suppress Ab1 responses, kill cells expressing surface Ag or Ab2, and suppress proliferation of cells expressing the target Ids on their TCRs (57–61). In a recent pilot clinical trial in multiple sclerosis (MS) patients, antiidiotyic $CD8^+$ T cells were induced following vaccination of patients with irradiated autologous myelin basic protein (MBP)-reactive T-cell clones (62). Idiotypic T cells lines were generated from the immunized patients and those reactive against the CDR3 region of the TCR of immunizing MBP-specific clones (63) were able to target and kill autologous MBP-reactive T cells *in vitro*.

Id-reactive T cells have been identified in both lupus-prone and normal mice (52,55,64–70). In the SNF1 model of SLE, $CD4^+$ Id-T cells increase before disease onset ($CD8^+$ do not), and some $CD4^+$Id-T clones from those mice help production of anti-DNA by syngeneic B cells (71,72). Further, disease can be accelerated by adoptive transfer of $CD4^+$ Id $LNF1^+$ T-cell clones in SNF1 mice (65). Similarly, $CD4^+$ T-cell clones from BALB/c mice immunized with monoclonal antibody (mAb) expressing the 16/6 Id proliferated to that Id and induced autoantibodies and nephritis on transfer to naive BALB/c mice (70).

The levels of Id reactive T cells may also vary with disease activity. In patients with myeloma, such T cells are present in early disease but are reduced in later, more advanced stages of cancer (73). Similar reduction in levels of anti-Id T cells have been observed in nonobese diabetic (NOD) mice with progressing disease (74).

THE STRUCTURAL BASIS OF IDIOTYPES

Apart from a few very well-studied Id systems, for example anti-arsonate CR1A (75–78) and the T15Id (79–81) associated with the antiphosphocholine response, the structural basis of most Ids has eluded definition. This is partly related to the tools used to define the Id. Classically, most Ids have been defined serologically, using polyclonal antiidiotypic reagents, which has led to problems of reproducibility inherent with such reagents. For many Ids definition has rested solely on whether it is linear (on H or L chain) or conformational (i.e., needs both H and L chain for expression). Delineation of the exact amino acid residues/sequences defining the Id (or their location) has been possible in only a few systems. Some examples are listed below. Within the heavy chain, two amino acids and/carbohydrate have been defined in the CDR-2 region of the heavy chain (CDR-H2) for antibodies to dextran (82), and D-regions are involved in Id expression in anti-p-arsonate (75–78) and antigalactan antibodies (83). Id 4B4 found on the Ig of some patients with SLE or Sjögren's syndrome (84), Id BH1 on human anticardiolipin antibody (85), and Id cross-reactive idiotype (CRI-EM) described in scleroderma (86) are all associated with the heavy chain. For 16/6Id described in lupus (87,88), and related Ids V-88 (89) and WRI-176β (90), sequences in the FRH2/CDR-H2 (91), CDR-H2/FR-H3 (55,92), and CDR-H2 (93,94) are reported to carry major idiotopes. Id 9G4, which is expressed by cold agglutinins (95), and by a population of immunoglobulins in SLE (96), is located within the CDR-H1 at positions 23 to 25 as the sequence AVY (95). The trytophan at position 7 in the FR-H1 of 9G4 Id^+ heavy chain also contributes to Id expression (97).

Ids associated with the light chain are described in anti-streptococcal group A carbohydrate antibodies (98). In lupus autoantibodies the B3Id is located in the CDR-L1 (99); similarly 8.12Id expression is associated with amino acid residues Tyr32 and Asn 33 in CDR-L1 (100,101). Id H3 described on anticardiolipin antibodies (102) is also associated with the light chain. Other Ids are conformational. Examples can be found in monoclonal cold agglutinins (103), antithyroglobulin antibodies (104), and Id T15 (79).

Although analysis of the V-region amino acid sequences of Id^+ and Id^- Igs has greatly facilitated the identification of such residues, mutational evidence confirming their contribution to Id expression has been reported in a very small number of cases (95,97,101).

An alternative approach to identifying idiotypic determinants has been to use epitope mapping (or pepscan) techniques (105). This method has been used for mapping both B- and T-cell idiotopes and has been employed in studies of Id systems in SLE (55,64,91,94), myeloma (106), and an antithyroglobulin antibody (107). Overlapping peptides of known sequences of VH and/or VL of Id$^+$ Ig are tested against antiidiotypic sera or T cells to determine the sequences of idiotopes contributing to Id expression. In studies of murine and human anti-DNA antibodies expressing public Ids (WRI-176β, V88, and B3Ids) a large number of B-cell idiotopes were identified using sera from lupus-prone mice and patients with SLE (92,94). The idiotopes were located in both the framework regions as well as in the CDRS. Computer models (108,109) of the Id$^+$ anti-DNA antibodies revealed that several of the immunodominant sequences identified were located on the surface of the antibody combining site and were therefore accessible, and that others may become accessible upon binding to antigen (108). In addition, the pepscan method detected noncontiguous epitopes, which in the three-dimensional (3D) binding site structure were situated in close proximity (108; Kalsi, unpublished data). Although individual anti-idiotypic profiles varied, antibody responses to certain sequences were observed more frequently, suggesting that these components may be involved in a regulatory network (92; Kalsi, unpublished data).

Descriptions of TCR-related idiotopes are limited, as they require the generation of T-cell clones known to participate in idiotypic interactions and a determination of what component of the TCR is responsible for Id expression. However, idiotopes located on the TCR CDR3 regions have been identified in murine models of experimental allergic encephalomyelitis (EAE) (110) and in NOD mice (74). In a recent study of patients with MS, a T-cell idiotope was defined in the CDR3 of MBP-reactive TCR (63). This latter idiotope was shown to elicit the generation of CD8$^+$ Id-specific cytolytic cells. Several investigations, however, have concentrated on identifying idiotopes on Id$^+$ Igs that have the capacity to activate T cells. The earliest such study was reported by Ebling et al (64). Using T-cell proliferation assays, three major sites (p34, p58, and p84) on the VH of nephritogenic murine mAb A6.1 were identified. These idiotopes were reported to modulate disease in young lupus-prone mice. In the murine anti-DNA antibody V88, the immunodominant T-cell idiotope was located in the CDR2-FR3 region of the H chain (55). This region also carries at its carboxyl end a major B-cell epitope. Gavalchin and Staines (111) report on two sequences from the CDR2 and CDR2/FR3 region of the heavy chain of an anti-DNA IdLNF1 + mAb 540, which also carry T-cell idiotopes in SNF1 mice. In B-cell lymphoma the CDR1 of the VH contained an idiotope able to elicit CD4$^+$ T-helper cells and release of IFN-γ (112).

The definitive proof of the contribution of residues to Id expression (or indeed antigen binding) would derive from studies employing nuclear magnetic resonance or x-ray crystallographic analysis. Very few Ids have been investigated in this manner. To our knowledge there are currently four known crystal structures of idiotype and antiidiotype interaction (113–116). Mainly these have been generated to determine how closely antiidiotypic antibodies may mimic antigen (116) or not (113,114,117). In a crystal structure (resolution 1.9 Å) of an antilysozyme Fv fragment and the corresponding antiidiotypic Ab E5.2, Fields et al. (116) reported that essentially the same molecular interactions were observable between the Id and anti-Id as were seen between the antibody and the antigen hen-egg lysozyme (HEL). Thus, mimicry involves similar binding characteristics and is not necessarily a result of exact replication of the antigen. In a more recent study, the structure of the Fab fragment of a mouse anti-anti-idiotypic antibody was solved (118). Fab fragments existed in the crystal as dimers and were found to be self complementary. It is suggested that this may be a means of neutralizing an ongoing idiotypic cascade, and, furthermore, interacting antibodies downstream in the idiotypic cascade may be rendered increasingly similar and self reactive. This is an interesting postulate since it has been found that some autoantibodies may in fact be anti-idiotypic for immunoglobulins (119,120).

Very recently, the first description of a crystal structure of an scFv fragment of clonotypic TCR KB5-C20 and its monoclonal anti-clonotypic antibody Désiré-1 at a resolution of 2.6 Å has been presented (121). The anticlonotypic antibody has an unusual mode of binding to the TCR, which is in marked contrast to those defined in earlier antibody Id-anti-idiotype crystal structures. It is arranged almost perpendicular to the antigen combining site and connects with discontinuous regions of the TCR Vα and Vβ. Furthermore, while the anti-clonotypic antibody does not mimic the antigen to which the original TCR is directed, it is able to activate KB5-C20 TCR-bearing T cells.

The composition of an idiotype clearly has a number of components, and the structural feature of the Id which predominants may well depend on the techniques and the tools used in its elucidation. Alongside the structural definition of an Id or a major idiotope there should also be consideration of whether the amino acid residues or sequence being defined as the "structural" idiotope is going to be equivalent in terms of the functional role of the idiotype. For example, when T-cell responses to sequences corresponding to the CDR1 and CDR3 regions of a 16/6+ mAb were examined in normal mice, the predominant response in Balb/c mice was to the CDR1 fragment and in SJL and C3H.SW mice to the CDR3 sequence (122). Thus, depending on the strain and therefore the genetic background of the individual, the structural correlate of the major T-cell idiotope may be different. Furthermore, since epitope mapping studies show that a number of epitopes within the variable region are "idiotypic," it is possible that different idiotopes from the same Ig V region have different effects on the immune response. Clearly, more structure-function studies of idiotypic determinants is required.

IDIOTYPIC REGULATORY CIRCUITS

Some Ids are regulatory, in that they can be suppressed or upregulated by other members of the circuit and in turn can regulate the other members. Early information regarding regulation suggested that anti-Ids served to suppress expression of their complementary Ids on antibodies to specific Ags (123,124). On the other hand, some anti-Ids can upregulate target Ids, even to the extent of activating silent B-cell clones that normally do not express their Id-bearing Ig. For example, BALB/c mice usually do not express the A48Id on their anti-fructosan Abs. However, administration of any of the following can force expression of that Id: (a) A48Id at birth, (b) polyclonal or monoclonal anti-Ids at birth, or (c) keyhole limpet hemacyanian (KLH)-linked polyclonal anti-Id in adults (125). In some systems, certain Ids or anti-Ids are either enhancers or suppressors of Id expression, whereas other Id-bearing mAbs do not regulate the circuit. Furthermore, the nature of the anti-Id (e.g., Ab2β or γ vs Abα) may determine the ability to regulate idiotypic expression (43).

In many experiments with Ids and anti-Ids, the dose and timing of administration are critical to the results. In general, administration of small quantities of Ids or anti-Ids upregulates Id expression, whereas administration of large quantities suppresses Id expression. For example, as shown in Fig. 15.3, immunization of young New Zealand black/white (NZB/NZW) F1 (BW) mice with small quantities (200 ng) of anti-IdX (a public Id on anti-DNA in BW mice) in Freund's adjuvant resulted in accelerated appearance of two autoantibodies: IdX⁺ anti-DNA, and IdX⁺ antihistone (35). In contrast, as shown in Fig. 15.4, repeated administration of large doses of anti-IdX (100 μg every 2 weeks) to adult BW mice suppressed IdX⁺ Ig, anti-DNA, and the lupus-like nephritis associated with anti-DNA in this mouse strain (36,37,126). Thus, the same mAb anti-Id could be used to either enhance or suppress the Id-bearing Ig.

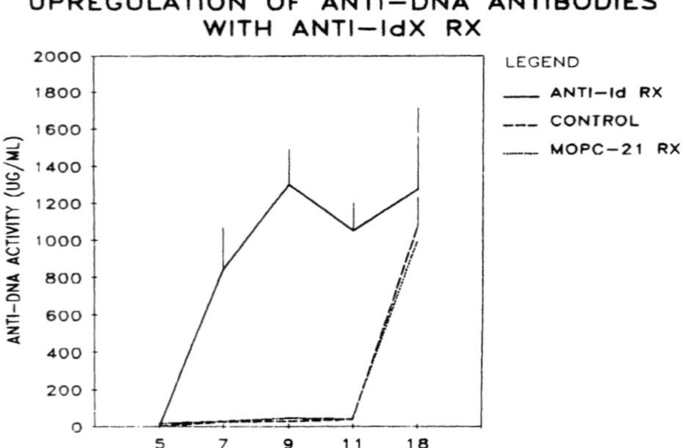

FIGURE 15.3. Upregulation of Id⁺ antibodies to DNA by administration of anti-Id antibodies in New Zealand black/white (NZB/NZW) F1 mice. This is an example of an upregulating Id network. Small doses (200 ng) of a monoclonal anti-IdX (made by immunization with an IdX⁺ antibody to DNA) were injected into young BW mice, and the appearance of anti-DNA in their sera was compared to that of littermates injected with the carrier or with an Id-negative monoclonal antibody (mAb) (MOPC-21). Injections were made at 4 weeks of age. Anti-Id–treated mice developed high titers of antibody to DNA by 7 weeks of age. In the control groups, anti-DNA appeared at 11 weeks (when the mice ordinarily begin to develop antibody); 95 of the anti-DNA in anti-Id–treated mice expressed IdX. The same mice also made IdX⁺ antihistone antibodies at an earlier age than controls. Thus, the anti-Id activated an Id⁺ autoantibody network that resulted in production of different autoantibodies expressing the same cross-reactive, public Id. (These experiments were performed by Karen Dunn, MD.)

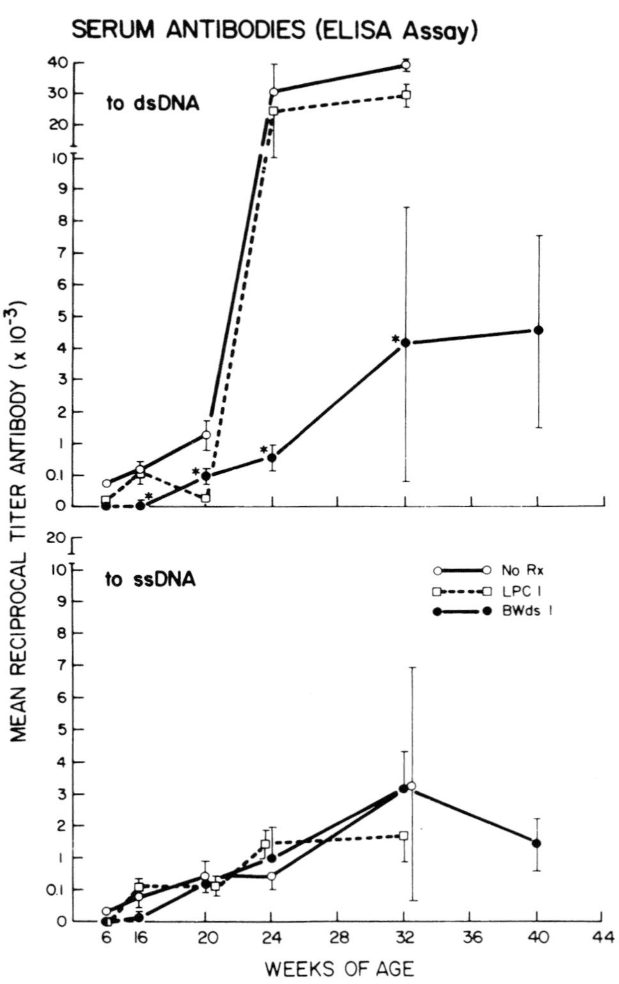

FIGURE 15.4. Downregulation of autoantibody responses by anti-Id antibodies. The idiotypic system is being studied in these experiments and those shown in Fig. 15.3. In this case, high doses of monoclonal IdX (100 μg fortnights), which induce anti-IdX, were given repeatedly to NZB/NZW F1 females beginning at 20 weeks of age. Antibodies to double-stranded DNA (dsDNA) (**upper panel**) were significantly suppressed in IdX-treated mice (*solid line, closed circles*) compared with two control groups (*open symbols*). This is an example of an anti-Id induced by Id downregulating an autoantibody. In contrast, antibodies to single-stranded DNA (ssDNA) were not affected (**lower panel**). (From ref. 126, with permission.)

Id-recognizing T cells also can be used to alter immune responses. For example, infusion of T cells that have been sensitized to Ids of CD4+ T cells that recognize alloAgs results in suppression of the ability of Th cells to proliferate to those Ags and prolongs allograft survival (59).

Although regulatory properties of public Ids can be used to alter *in vivo* immune responses, the Id network in some systems (e.g., B-cell malignancies) escapes from such regulation (36,37,127,128). One mechanism of escape is somatic mutation of the Id so that it no longer is recognized by anti-Id (128). Because mutation of Ig molecules is common in B cells, whereas it is yet to be demonstrated in the TCR of T cells, this escape mechanism probably applies only to Ids on Ig. In NZB/NZW mice treated with anti-Ids, escape of Id+ antibodies from suppression occurs without evidence of mutation of the Ig (126); this might represent a change in Id-directed T-cell help (e.g., a shift from Th1 to Th2 cytokine patterns).

ROLE OF IDIOTYPES IN MATURATION OF THE IMMUNE RESPONSE

In adults, the normal B-cell repertoire probably depends on establishment of essential Id networks during fetal life. Studies of B-cell hybridomas obtained from fetal and 1- to 2-week-old normal BALB/c mice have defined early antibody responses in the pre- and early immune states (129,130). Two properties are clear: (a) many early Ig molecules bind to self Ags, including V regions of Ig; and (b) this preimmune, natural autoantibody network is highly connected via idiotypy.

Many antibodies produced during the first week of gestation bear Ids that are not positively selected later. In contrast, responses to a similar Ag in the neonatal or 1- to 3-week-old mouse carry different Ids, and those Ids are positively selected for expansion, even in adult life. This Id switch probably is independent of environmental stimuli. In fetal antibody responses to dextran or phosphocholine (the first Ag from *Enterobacter cloacae* and the second from pneumococcus), the entire network of Ag, Ab1, Ab2, and Ab3 can be found. Further, a single Ab2 can react with Ab1 from different B cells (i.e., with both anti-PC and antidextran Ab1). Such Ab2 molecules are regulatory (130); they can either suppress the fetal Id+ Ig or enhance the more mature public Ids characteristic of 2- to 3-week-old mice, depending on the mAb Ab2 and the timing of administration. The interplay of the different Ab2 molecules in suppressing or enhancing fetal or mature Ids is an example of connectivity, and it suggests that the original Ab1 responses in the fetus express determinants that activate the Id network and are critical for determining the idiotypic profiles of the adult immune response.

Vakil and Kearney (130) have referred to the early multispecific B cell as a superorganizer, influencing many generations of B cells that follow. This early network can be influenced by administration of Id+ antibodies that do not bind the initiating Ag, so the network is at least partly independent of Ag and can operate via recognition of Id alone. Any interference with the newborn network (by administration of Ag, Ab1, Ab2, or Ab3) results in impairment of normal antibody responses in adult life, especially if a highly public Id is involved (131). It is interesting that the Id F-423 found in fetal Medical Research Laboratory lymphoproliferative (MRL/*lpr*) mice occurs on anti–single-stranded DNA (ssDNA) and also appears in adult MRL/*lpr* and NZB/NZW F1 mice. Administration of IdF-423 accelerates lupus in young MRL/*lpr* mice and of anti-Id F-423 delays disease onset (132). Similarly, Id D23 on natural autoantibodies of normal mice can be found in the glomerular lesions of NZB/NZW F1 mice with lupus nephritis (133). Thus, some public Ids associated with pathogenic autoantibody repertoires are present in fetal or early postnatal life; SLE might result from their dysregulation.

USE OF IDIOTYPIC NETWORKS TO PREVENT INFECTIOUS DISEASES

There has been interest in using the Id network to raise protective B- and T-cell responses to infectious agents (8,10,27,45,11–19,134–138). There are at least three situations in which this approach has advantages over standard immunizations with attenuated, killed, or carrier-linked infectious agents. First, some organisms are so highly infectious that a batch that is not adequately killed or attenuated can produce disease. This is of special concern for organisms with a high mutation rate that allow new, virulent forms to emerge that escape immune surveillance (e.g., HIV). Second, patients who are immunosuppressed are not only poor responders to standard attenuated vaccines (e.g., vaccinia), but may be subject to infection by them. Third, neonates and infants are unable to make good immune response to T-independent Ags (e.g., polysaccharides in cell walls of enteric bacteria). Finally, anti-Id vaccines would be useful in infectious diseases for which there currently are no effective immunizations (e.g., rabies, certain gram-negative bacteria, hepatitis C, HIV).

The use of Id networks to protect against infectious disease relies mainly on immunizations with or induction of Ab2 (anti-Ids). Ab2 molecules that bear the internal image of the Ag then induce Ab1, Ab3, and/or cytotoxic T cells that are Ag specific. (These concepts were discussed earlier.) For bacterial infections, opsonizing antibody responses are probably adequate to prevent infection; for viral infections, both neutralizing antibodies and cytotoxic T cells are desirable. Id or anti-Id vaccines effectively protect animal models from infection with trypanosomes, some viruses (hepatitis B, reovirus encephalitis, Sendai, Venezuelan equine encephalitis virus), and certain bacteria (pneumococcus,

Escherichia coli, capsular polysaccharide of *Neisseria meningitidis* C, O-polysaccharide of *P. aeruginosa*) (10,45,11–19, 135,136). Some Id-anti-Id vaccines activate only Id-based antibody circuits, others only T cells, and still others the entire antibody/T-cell Id network (12,15,45).

The idiotype approach to vaccination may prove to be useful; however, in one series of experiments, immunization with Ab2 increased susceptibility of mice to infection with herpes simplex (139). Such a result is predictable based on the Id regulatory circuits discussed earlier.

To date, no studies in which infection has been prevented in humans by vaccinations with Id, anti-Id, or Id-peptides have been published, although such immunizations have been shown to influence production of desirable antibodies for some infections. There is particular interest in manipulating an Id network in HIV disease, because a public Id is expressed on some human neutralizing antibodies to the gp120 polypeptides of some HIV isolates (137,138). This public Id is expressed in approximately 70% of HIV-1 infected humans and macaques and is recognized by mAb 1F7 (140). Mab 1F7 is not an anti-Id antibody which mimics the antigen (141). It is an example of Ab2α and is reported to broaden the HIV neutralization response. This is particularly important since the virus elicits a very narrow antibody response and the immune system of the affected individual is unable to develop immunity to the emergent variants. An Ab2 (mAb 13 B8.2), which is an antigen mimic of the CDR3-homologous CD4/D1 region thought to be involved in gp120 binding, has also been used in HIV infection (142). This has recently been employed as an immunogen in a phase II randomized trial of 158 patients with early-stage HIV. The antibody was well tolerated and produced an increase in neutralization and anti-HIV gp120 titers.

Several investigators have demonstrated that the maternal idiotypic network has a potent influence in shaping the developing repertoire of the fetus/neonate (130,143–145). It has been suggested that to prevent serious infectious diseases of early childhood, immunizations of the mother be utilized to effect immunity in the offspring (145,146). Aside from passive immunity there is said to be "immunologic imprinting" by maternal idiotypic networks, which provides molecular information about the external environment and presumably skews development toward those idiotypic networks that would be most useful in dealing with local pathogens (143,144). There are a number of examples in the literature reporting the strong association of certain Ids with particular antimicrobial responses (147–149). Furthermore, maternal immunization is reported to alter the kinetics and the quality of the response in successive generations (145,150). For example, the F1 generation of mice immunized with respiratory syncytial virus exhibited characteristics of a secondary immune response when challenged with the original immunogen (150). One report (146) has demonstrated the use of engineered Ab2 fragments mimicking the capsular antigen of group B streptococcus for providing immunity transferable to offspring. Thus far, however, anti-Id vaccines remain an interesting but unproven approach to the prevention of infectious diseases in humans.

IDIOTYPES ON MONOCLONAL PARAPROTEINS AND MALIGNANT CELLS

Monoclonal paraproteins and malignant cells possess idiotypes.

Idiotypes on Paraproteins

The initial studies defining Ids in humans were performed on monoclonal paraproteins. Rheumatoid factor (RF) activity is common among paraproteins from unrelated individuals. Further, many RF$^+$ paraproteins express one of a few public Ids, suggesting that genes capable of encoding them are frequent in unrelated humans. Germline information that codes for those Ids has been identified (151–159). An Id designated Wa by Kunkel et al. (157) is present on 60% of IgM-RF cryoglobulins; a second Id designated Po is expressed on an additional 10%. A common Id on human IgM paraproteins was designated 17.109 by Carson et al. (153). Both Wa$^+$ and 17.109$^+$ RF use restricted VH, VL, and J segments (153–156,158,159). One human germline V gene encodes the 17.109 Id; that gene is designated VkRF, Vk325, or humkv325 (153,154). Most monoclonal RFs using VkRF also use an H chain derived from the VH1 germline gene region designated hv1263 or 783 VH (155,159). Most are synthesized by CD5$^+$ B cells. The VL and VH rearranged genes encoding these RFs vary from germline by 2 to 11 amino acids; therefore, it is possible that closely related but different V gene families are used. Other Ids have been defined using murine monoclonal antibodies that recognize VH1-, VH3-, and VH4-associated CRIs (160). In summary, human paraproteins with RF activity are oligoclonal and use highly restricted germline gene material from both VH and V regions.

One would predict from such data that the mono- or oligoclonal RF products of lymphoproliferative malignancies would display idiotypic restriction, and that is the case. Most express the public Ids 17.109, PSL2, or PSL3 (153). Approximately 20% of neoplastic CD5$^+$ B cells from patients with chronic lymphocytic leukemia express Ig on their surfaces derived from the VkRF gene (156).

In contrast to the situation with monoclonal RFs, the anti–gamma globulins that appear during infections or in autoimmune diseases are polyclonal. The VkRF and VH1 genes are found on a minority of those RFs.

In two studies of IgG M components Williams et al. (161,162) report that 31.3% of 134 samples tested positive for at least one of 16/6, F4, 3I, and 8.12 Ids described in lupus. Several expressed two Ids (16/6 and F4 or 16/6 and 3I), and one sample was positive for three Ids (16/6, F4, and 3I). Several of these M components also bound DNA or $F(ab')_2$. It is common for monoclonal autoantibodies to express public idiotypes. In one group of patients with monoclonal gammopathies, 23% of the proteins had autoantibody activity and among those a few exhibited the public Id PR4 (163).

Idiotypes on Tumors

One of the most active areas of research in idiotypic vaccination is that of cancer therapy. Any malignant cell that expresses an Ig or TCR molecule on its surface should be able to elicit anti-Id responses. Because some Ab2 molecules either contain internal image of Ags or can recognize other sequences/conformations neighboring the Ag-binding site, some tumor-associated surface antigens also might react with anti-Ids. Idiotypic manipulations have been attempted in a variety of tumors. These include human B-cell lymphomas and leukemias, murine B-cell lymphomas, human T-cell leukemias, murine and human breast cancers, melanoma, and colorectal carcinoma.

One of the earliest uses of Id therapy in tumors involved antiidiotypic antibodies. A series of studies (reviewed in ref. 164) spanning 12 years and involving 45 patients demonstrated the use of antiidiotypic antibodies [used alone, with IFN-α, with chlorambucil, or with interleukin-2 (IL-2)] in the treatment of B-cell lymphoma. Levy and colleagues (164) found that most of the patients responded to the therapy (66% overall and 18% complete response) and in six patients (13%) complete remission was observed, which at the time of reporting for five of these six patients was of 4 to 10 years' duration. More recent investigations of these patients in remission showed that the tumor had not been eliminated but became dormant (164). One of the problems with tumors is that the treated Id may mutate and render the therapy invalid. Furthermore, cellular immunity is likely more effective against Id-negative tumors. One approach to overcoming this and generating a broader, polyclonal response is through active immunization of the individual with the Id, producing both humoral and cellular responses. In B-cell lymphoma immunization with Id-KLH conjugate in an immunologic adjuvant resulted in Id-specific responses in 49% of the patients, with 85% of the responders exhibiting antibody responses, while cellular proliferation was observed in 35% (165). The antiidiotypic responses were maintained for several months. The median duration of freedom from disease progression and overall survival was significantly enhanced in Id-responders compared to patients who were nonresponders (165). Two patients who had residual disease at the time of vaccination and generated antiidiotypic responses underwent complete tumor regression, and one of these patients remained in remission for nearly 8 years. In a related study (166) of 16 non-Hodgkin's lymphoma patients, immunization with autologous Id enhanced cytolytic activity in eight of the 11 patients and correlated with disease-free or stable minimal disease, in contrast to nonresponders whose disease progressed. In attempts to improve cellular responses Id-cytokine [granulocyte-macrophage colony-stimulating factor (GM-CSF), IL-2, IL-4] fusion proteins have been used (167–170). GM-CSF is highly effective (171) and is best used in combination with Id-KLH conjugate rather than complexed to it (169,172). Induction of both CD4 and $CD8^+$ cells is reported (170).

Recently, more targeted regimens have evolved. These are centered on improving antigen presentation to T cells, thereby enhancing antitumor activity. Antigen is processed and presented to the T cell in the context of MHC on the surface of an antigen-presenting cell (APC). Provided other second signal molecules are also present, lymphocyte activation takes place. Dendritic cells are highly potent APCs (173,174). A clearer understanding of the characteristics of these cells has allowed their generation from peripheral blood (175,176). Cells thus obtained can be loaded with antigen (Id) *in vitro* prior to inoculation in the individual being treated, thus providing a means of directly targeting the cells most likely to help generate effective immunity, namely the T cells. The use of dendritic cells has been reported in both experimental (177–180) and clinical settings (181–185). Although these cells enhance cellular immunity, some authors voice concerns about the possibility of generating tolerance to the pathogenic Id (186). Monocytes have also been utilized as APCs (182,187), though one group reports that the cytokine profiles differ in the ensuing immune response when compared to dendritic cells (182). Along the same lines one group has recently used the co-stimulatory molecule cytotoxic T-lymphocyte antigen-4 (CTLA-4) conjugated to Id as a means of directly targeting T-cell immunity (188). Ids as a single-chain Fv fragment or DNA encoding the Id have also been used as vaccines to generate antitumor activity (189,190). Studies in murine models of B-cell lymphoma show that the incorporation of constant regions of Ig into the DNA vaccine may enhance antitumor activity (191).

In most cases immunization of the affected individual is carried out to produce immunity. In one study, however, immunization of the donor with the Id was used prior to transplantation of bone marrow to the recipient who was subsequently reported to exhibit antitumor responses (192).

A number of clinical trials are currently under way where antiidiotypic antibody mimics of the offending antigens have been used. In colorectal cancer, two studies—one that employed anti-Id vaccination before and after surgery (21) and one that used vaccine following resection (20)—have reported variable success. The latter study showed lymphocytic infiltration of the resected colon and extravasation of natural killer (NK) cells to the site. In one of these studies (20) the highest success rate was observed in patients who expressed permissive haplotypes for the presentation of the antigen being utilized. Anti-Id antibody vaccine TriAb was used to treat 11 patients with breast cancer (193). Nine of 11 patients showed an Ab3 response after a median of 10 doses, and eight of 11 had a modest T-cell response. At 24 months four patients were alive without evidence of disease progression; these were patients who made a good T-cell response. Mutated p53 is expressed on epithelial cells of a variety of tumors. Ruiz et al. (190) showed that an anti-idiotypic mimic of the mutated antigen may be used to generate antitumor responses in mice. This may offer a more generalized approach to target cancers.

Although idiotypic manipulation of the immune system in cancer holds promise it is becoming clear that these are mostly effective in individuals with minimal disease or low tumor load. Also, it is also evident that optimization of vaccine design, and delivery and timing of vaccination are required.

IDIOTYPES, AUTOIMMUNITY, AND SLE

The Role of Idiotypes in Autoimmunity

Id networks play a central role in autoimmune diseases such as SLE. First, most autoantibodies are characterized by public as well as private Ids; therefore, a limited number of networks regulate a substantial proportion of the autoantibody repertoire (89,194–205). A partial list of autoantibodies containing subsets expressing public Ids is presented in Table 15.2. Second, the Id on any Ab1 that arises may induce internal image Ab2 (epibodies, homobodies), and these internal image anti-Ids can then behave as Ags, thus inducing other Ab1 molecules that react with multiple self-Ags. For example, rabbits immunized with human polyclonal anti-DNA or with monoclonal anti-DNA derived from MRL/*lpr* mice developed autoantibodies that reacted with DNA, cardiolipin, SmRNP, and glomerular extract. All these reactivities were contained in the rabbit anti-Id against the immunizing Ig (38). In fact, some investigators suggest that most autoantibodies are anti-Id responses to antiviral or other protective Ab1 or indeed other autoantibodies (41,119,206,207). Zhang and Reichlin (119) report that some antibodies to Ro and La function as antiidiotypic to anti–double-stranded DNA (dsDNA) antibodies and serve to downregulate them. Antibodies able to bind both dsDNA and F(ab′)2 or idiopeptides have also been reported (55,120,208). In susceptible strains of normal mice, certain Id$^+$ monoclonal anti-DNAs (16/6 and LNF1 for example) or anti-Ids (anti-Id 16/6), when used as immunogens, probably induce a full repertoire of Id network B and T cells, resulting in the appearance of multiple autoantibodies and nephritis (39,40,42,70–72). Only mice that develop anti-Id responses to Ab1 develop SLE-like disease. [It should be noted that one group of investigators could not repeat the work with Id 16/6 (209).] Third, Id networks are probably defective in patients with active SLE. Anti-Ids are detected in the serum during disease remission but are decreased during periods of disease activity (210–212). In fact, both anti-Ids and Id$^+$ Ig can be found in human SLE glomerular deposits and may contribute to nephritis (212–214). The Id network therefore is one of several immunoregulatory abnormalities that contribute to SLE.

Restoration of Id circuitry to normal might suppress active disease, and anti-Ids have been effective in suppressing autoantibody production by murine B cells *in vivo* (4,37–39,42,132,215–217), human B cells *in vitro* (210), and in patients treated with intravenous immunoglobulin (IVIg) (218). Mechanisms by which Ids might participate in the pathogenesis of SLE are reviewed in Table 15.3.

Idiotypes in SLE

Because SLE is considered to be the prototype systemic autoimmune disease, the Id-anti-Id profiles as well as the structure of its most characteristic autoantibody, anti-DNA, have been studied by many investigators (4,5,35–38,42,84, 87–89,100,109,132,133,196–204,210–212,215–217,219 –257). Although most normal subjects, both human and murine, can make anti-DNA bearing public Ids, and although anti-DNA is part of polyreactive neonatal antibodies, most SLE patients have a different anti-DNA repertoire. For example, when MRL/*lpr* mice are immunized with Ars-KLH, the anti-Ars response is idiotypically dis-

TABLE 15.2. PUBLIC IDS ON HUMAN AUTOANTIBODIES

Autoantibody	Ids	References
Anti-DNA	GN2, GN1, X, 16/6, 32/15, PR4, 3I, 8.12, H130, A52, TOF, O-81, NE1, 3E10, D5-M, D5-R, B3, WRI-176β, RT-72	5,36,38–42,70,72,87–90,99,100,219–221,132,133,195–206, 214–217,223–231,243,248,253,265–267,317–320
Rheumatoid factor	Wa, Po, 17.109, PR4, PSL2, RQ	151–159,296–301
Antithyroglobulin	62	286
Anticardiolipin	H3, RT84, 1BH1	85,102,316
Antiacetylcholine receptor	See references	288,289
Antimyelin basic protein	See references	290
Anticollagen	See references	294,295
Anti-Sm	Y2, 4B4	292,293

TABLE 15.3. MECHANISMS BY WHICH IDIOPATHIC NETWORKS PARTICIPATE IN THE PATHOGENESIS OF SLE

1. Many autoantibodies express public Ids. These Ids may be targets of upregulation, thus keeping the levels of the autoantibodies high.
2. Some public Ids on Ab1 induce anti-Ids (Ab2) that bear internal image of Ags. Those Ab2 molecules in turn induce Ab1 molecules that react with multiple self-Ags. Thus, Id+ anti-DNA can induce Id+ anti-Sm, Id+ anticardiolipin, and so on.
3. Certain public Ids are markers of autoantibodies enriched in pathogenic subsets.
4. Idiotypic regulation is skewed toward upregulation of undesirable autoantibodies during periods of disease activity. Restoration of normal Id circuitry might abrogate disease.

tinct from the Ids of most MRL/*lpr* autoantibodies (258). In contrast, humans immunized with pneumovax produce anti-PC antibodies bearing Ids typical of anti-DNA in SLE; however, the Id$^+$ Ig does not bind DNA (253). In general, anti-DNA in healthy individuals is composed largely of IgM with low affinity for ssDNA. In contrast, anti-DNA in mice or humans with active SLE is largely IgG with high affinity for both ssDNA and dsDNA. In fact, IgG anti-dsDNA is relatively specific for SLE.

Several laboratories have defined public Ids on anti-DNA antibodies originating either in human or murine systems (Table 15.4). Many such Ids, especially those occurring near the epitope-binding regions of the Ig molecule, occur in both murine and human SLE. Further, they are found in humans with virtually all known connective tissue diseases (most frequently in Sjögren's syndrome), in first-degree relatives, and in small proportions of healthy individuals (197,223,227,259). Two groups (260,261) have studied Ids in family members of patients with SLE and have found no enrichment in family members or household contacts compared with healthy controls. However, in one study RT-84Id expression was similar in patients and their relatives and also occurred more frequently in spouses than in normal healthy controls (259).

Thus, several lines of evidence suggest that many of the public Ids that characterize autoantibodies in SLE are derived from highly conserved germline genes with little or no mutation. That evidence includes the following: (a) presence of the same Id in unrelated people with or without SLE (223,259–261), (b) presence of the same Id in mice and humans with SLE (5,38,201,225,226), (c) presence of the same Ids in fetal repertoires and natural autoantibodies as on anti-DNA of mature mice with SLE (132,133,236, 260), (d) presence of the same idiotypes on different antibodies to self and to nonself (194,204,237,239,242,244, 251), (e) ability to induce autoantibodies in normal mice by administering Id from human autoantibodies (42), and (f) inability to correlate the presence or quantity of a nephritogenic Id with MHC class II genes that predispose to nephritis (262). In keeping with this idea that public Ids are constructed from commonly available Ig sequences or conformations, few lupus Ids are confined to anti-DNA; in fact, in healthy individuals the Ids may be found (but rarely on anti-DNA). The 16/6 lupus anti-DNA Id has been found on antibodies to cardiolipin, platelets, cytoskeleton, lymphocytes, brain gangliosides, and mycobacteria (227). With a few exceptions, such as 16/6 and 9G4, serum levels of the lupus Ids do not correlate well with disease activity, nor do they accurately predict clinical characteristics of a patient (96,197).

Sequencing of several Id-bearing anti-DNAs from humans and mice has shown that some are derived from the germline with minimal mutation, whereas others have undergone somatic mutation (see Chapters 18 and 21). These two populations could represent those cases arising from polyclonal activation and those responding to specific antigenic stimulation. Not all anti-DNAs are pathogens; only certain subsets can induce disease directly, especially immune glomerulonephritis (224,256). As discussed elsewhere this may be related to the charge, fine specificity, or overall shape of the antigen combining site (263). In studies on antibodies expressing both anti-DNA and anti-F(ab')$_2$ activity, Voss's group (264) showed that the IgG activity was directed toward the hinge region, and suggested that this property may be particularly relevant to immune complex formation and therefore nephritis. Descriptions of unconventional sites within the V regions of some antibodies include the presence of a nucleotide-binding site (265), which may delineate a pathogen in SLE and warrants further investigation.

There is substantial evidence that certain Ids are enriched in pathogenic autoantibody subsets. For example, we found that IdGN2 dominates the Ig in glomeruli of renal biopsy specimens from almost all patients with proliferative histologic forms of lupus nephritis (226); IdGN2 accounted for 28% to 50% of the anti-DNA deposited in glomeruli of patients with diffuse proliferative glomerulonephritis. Other investigators have searched for Id$^+$ Ig in tissue lesions of mice or humans with active SLE. Ids 16/6, 32/15, 3I, GN2, O-81, RT-72, RT-84, B3, 33C.9, and D5-M have been found in glomerular Ig deposits and/or at the dermal-epidermal junction in patients with SLE (196,201, 202,213,214,226,227,266) (Table 15.4). It is likely that each of these Ids is enriched in pathogenic antibody subsets. This also is true in animal models of SLE. In NZB × Swiss Webster F1 mice, lupus nephritis is associated with glomerular deposition of IgG anti-DNA, which is highly enriched in a family of Ids designated IdLN (202). In nephritic NZB/NZW mice, 50% of the glomerular Ig contains IdGN2 and IdGN1$^+$ antibodies. In addition, administration of some (but not all) IdGN2$^+$ monoclonal IgG2 anti-DNA to normal BALB/c mice produces Id$^+$ Ig

TABLE 15.4. PUBLIC IDIOTYPES IN PATIENTS WITH SLE

Id	Source	In Tissue	Location	Special Features	Percent of SLE Patients with Id in Serum	Percent of Normals with Id in Serum	References
GN2	Glomerular	++ (G)	H chain	Dominant Id in glomeruli of pts with DPGN	67	13	197,226
X	mAb aDNA BW mouse	0	?	Dominant Id on serum IgG of BW mice; anti-Id suppresses disease in mice	42	0	196,197
16/6	mAb aDNA	++ (G, S)	H chain germline VH26 or VH4	Immunization of normal mice may induce autoantibody and SLE-like disease	25–28	7	39,40,87,88, 195,223, 225,317
3I	Polyclonal aDNA, SLE patient sera	+ (G)	κ L chain	^{3}I+ aDNA enriched in cationic IgG	50	7	197,229,243
8.12	Polyclonal aDNA, SLE patient sera	+ (G)	λ L chain $V_{\lambda}II$	May be specific for SLE	50	5	98,100,219,220
0–81	mAb a-ssDNA SLE patient	++ (G)	?	Enriched in pts with GN; occurs in BW mice	72 (with GN) 19 (without GN)	0	205,215,254a
NE-1	mAb a-dsDNA	++ (G)	?	Enriched in pts with GN; occurs on a-dsDNA	33 (with GN) 6 (without GN)	0	215,254a
B3	mAb IgG anti-dsDNA, SLE patient sera	+ in vivo ANA	λ L chain	Associated with arthritis in SLE patients	20	0	99
F4	Polyclonal aDNA, SLE patient sera	?	H chain	Expressed only on IgG; enriched in cationic Ig	35	?	243,318
H3	Human mAb from SLE PBC	?	λ L chain	Found on aPL; may be specific for SLE	?	?	303a
RT84	Human mAb from SLE PBC	?	?	Found on aPL and aDNA	19	42	316
3E10	mAb aDNA, MRL/*lpr* mouse	?	Conformational	Found in sera of patients with SLE and GN	75 (without GN)	25 (without GN)	266
KIM4.6.3	mAb IgM anti-ssDNA from normal human tonsil	?	L chain	Id from normal on aDNA in SLE patients	90	24	197,200
134	mAb aDNA, SLE patient sera	?	?	On SLE Ig in serum	42	0	197,319
AM	Polyclonal aDNA in SLE patient sera	?	Conformational	On SLE Ig in serum	25	13	197,320
BEG-2	mAb aDNA, human fetal liver	?	L chain	Fetal antibody Id found on aDNA in SLE patients	8	7	197,321
8EY	mAb aDNA, patients with leprosy	?	?	Id from antibody of patient with infection occurs on aDNA of SLE patients	25	0	197,322
A52	mAb aDNA BW mouse	?	Conformational	Id from BW mice found on human aDNA in SLE patients	>50	?	5
Y2	mAb aSm MRL/*lpr* mouse	?	?	Id from MRL/*lpr* mouse found on aDNA in SLE patients	41	6	292,323
4B4	mAb aSm human	?	H chain	Cross-reacts with Sm and p24 gag protein of HIV-1	52	?	84,293
D5-R	mAb IgG aDNA, human SLE	0 (G)	L chain	Found only on IgG	20–30	5	266
D5-M	mAb aDNA	++ (G)	Conformational	Found only on IgG	20–30	7	266
A24	mAb from normal human cord blood	?	H chain	Newborn has Id/aId network found in aDNA network in adults with SLE	?	?	315

GN, glomerulonephritis; aDNA, anti-DNA; aPL, anti-phospholipid; dsDNA, double-stranded DNA; IgG, immunoglobulin G; mAb, monoclonal antibody; MRL/*lpr*, Medical Research Laboratory lymphoproliferative mice; ssDNA, single-stranded DNA.

deposits in their glomeruli as well as clinical nephritis (230,256). In contrast, monoclonal IgG2 anti-DNA bearing another public Id, IdX, does not induce nephritis in normal mice. Ids D23, 3E10, and 4B1 also have been found in glomeruli of mice with lupus (133,267,268).

As with Ids on antibodies to external Ag, the structural basis of Ids on autoantibodies is known for only a few mAbs. Clearly, the assembly of autoantibodies does not require any special genetic information. They can be constructed from normal germline DNA, with or without somatic mutation; they can be assembled from different VH and VL gene families, although there may be some bias toward use of certain families; and they can resemble antibodies to external Ag (230,232–255,262). Expression of public Ids can depend on amino acid sequences on the H or L chains, or both, or may be conformational (77,82–84,87, 88,98,103,104,219–221). Finally, the structural characteristics of an antibody that make it pathogenic, perhaps related in part to Id expression, are poorly understood; they may determine features such as cross-reactivity, charge, and avidity. (See Chapter 21 for a more complete discussion of the characteristics of pathogenic anti-DNA.)

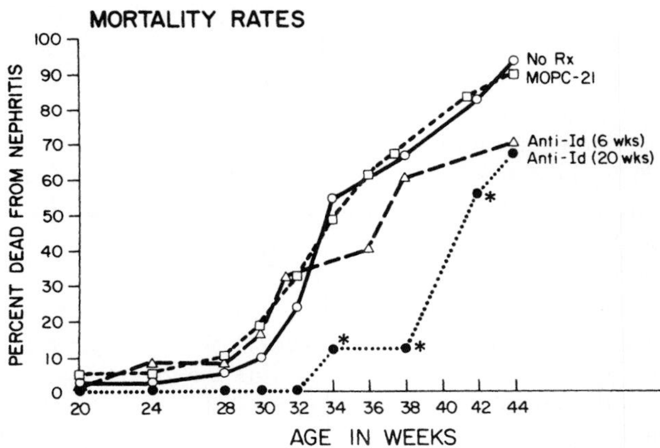

FIGURE 15.5. Suppression of clinical nephritis in NZB/NZW mice by administration of anti-Id antibody. In these experiments, NZB/NZW F1 females were treated once every 2 weeks with injections of a monoclonal anti-IdX or an Id-negative mAb (MOPC-21). Some littermates were untreated. Mice treated with anti-IdX (*dotted line with solid circles*) lived approximately 10 weeks longer than other groups. Their production of anti-dsDNA and IdX$^+$ IgG was suppressed during that period but escaped from control. The appearance of IgG anti-DNA in serum was followed within a few weeks by lethal nephritis. Thus, anti-Id therapy was successful, but only as long as the Id network was sensitive to it. (From ref. 36, with permission.)

Manipulation of Clinical Disease in Mouse Models of SLE by Altering the Idiotypic Network

Id networks have been manipulated by several investigators through administering Ids or anti-Ids in attempts to alter disease in the NZB/NZW, MRL/*lpr*, and SNF1 mouse models of SLE. In some experiments, autoantibody production was suppressed, nephritis was delayed, and survival was prolonged (36,126,132,215–217). In our laboratories, IdGN2, commonly found on glomerular Ig in human lupus DPGN and in nephritic NZB/NZW mice, was downregulated in NZB/NZW mice by administration of a closely related anti-Id (36) (Fig. 15.5). Serum levels of IdGN2 were initially suppressed but escaped from control, and mice died of nephritis with deposits of IdGN2$^+$ and IdGN1$^+$ Ig in their glomeruli. Their lives were prolonged a mean of 10 weeks compared to controls treated with an irrelevant murine mAb. There was no evidence of emergence of mutated or unrecognized Ids in the mice with escape nephritis. It may be that the ability of certain Ids to escape from suppression is a feature that partially explains their enrichment in pathogenic antibody subsets. In a recent study where NOD mice were immunized with 16/6Id, it was reported that instead of developing insulin-dependent diabetes mellitus (IDDM) the animals developed SLE (269). Thus, in susceptible animals, autoimmunity does not go away but simply reemerges under another guise.

Although much work has focused on attempts to suppress the expression of pathogenic Ids in murine lupus, experiments with the 16/6 Id-anti-Id system have shown that lupus and antiphospholipid antibody syndrome can be induced in normal mice by manipulating this Id network (39,40,42,70). Immunization of some normal mice (BALB/c, C3H.SW, AKR, and SJL, but not C57BL/6 or C3H/He) with Ids or anti-Ids resulted in development of circulating Ids and anti-Ids, multiple autoantibodies (including anti-DNA, anti-Sm, and anticardiolipin), leukopenia, and nephritis. The susceptibility of strains to the induction of disease did not seem to correlate with MHC or Ig allotype genes, but it did correlate with the ability to make immune responses within the Id network. That is, susceptible strains immunized with Id or anti-Id responded by producing high-titer anti-Id or Id, respectively; resistant strains did not. This ability depends on characteristics of bone marrow cells, because BALB/c mice chimeric for C57Bl/6 bone marrow are resistant to induction of SLE by Id or anti-Id immunization (270). Clearly, activation of certain Id networks can induce pathogenic reactivity to self.

Recent work on manipulating the idiotypic networks has centered on the use of idiopeptides derived from the V regions of disease-associated autoantibodies. The peptides used have either been selected from the CDRs of the Id$^+$ Ig or chosen through epitope mapping studies that have shown these to be immunodominant for T- or B-cell responses (52,55,64–68,271–274). Since idiotypes are able to enhance or suppress the autoimmune response, it is possible that analyzing the effects different components of the Id have on the autoimmune response may assist in determining what aspects of the idiotypic structure are responsible for stimulation or suppression. In this way motifs pertinent to the reestablishment of regulatory Id networks may be defined. For example, peptides containing the motif KFKGK can stimulate T-cell responses in BW F1 (64) and SNF1 mice (65). The studies thus far have demonstrated the following: Immunizations of normal healthy mice with VH peptides from the murine monoclonal anti-DNA antibody V88 and 16/6Id$^+$ mAb produced symptoms of SLE (66,273). In lupus-prone mice, immunization with idiopeptides of A6.1 VH, IdLNF1 p62-73, 16/6Id, and V88 64-80 accelerated the disease process and reduced survival time (52,65,66,273). In contrast, when a CDR3 peptide was used from a D23Id$^+$ murine monoclonal, immunization was found to have protective effects; up to 50% of lupus-prone mice exhibited prolonged survival times (274). Under high-dose tolerizing regimens, idiopeptides may also be used to tolerize premorbid lupus-prone mice and delay disease onset (66,275). Furthermore, different idiopeptides derived from the same VH may stimulate the production of different cytokine profiles (Th1 vs. Th2) (52). Anti-idiopeptide antibodies are generated in both spontaneous and induced models of SLE, which not only react with the immunizing peptide and the native Id carrying Mab, but may also have specificity for DNA (55,208). This has suggested that the anti-DNA response may arise as part of another response simply through sharing of idiotypic determinants. The other response may be to an external antigen.

Idiotypes in the Treatment of Human SLE

A number of studies have shown that clinical improvement in SLE patients correlates with the presence of circulating antibodies able to interact with Ig variable regions (276–278). As discussed in Chapters 53 and 59, there is interest in treating selected patients with SLE using intravenous gamma globulin (IVIs). These preparations are generated from pools of serum from up to 35,000 normal individuals (277). It has been demonstrated that they carry anti-F(ab′)$_2$ activity, some of which is directed against Ids 8.12, 3I, F4, 4B4, and 16/6, that is characteristic of SLE autoantibodies, and many authors have suggested that these anti-Ids account for improvement in clinical disease (278,279).

Harata et al. (205) reported that affinity columns containing two anti-Ids (D1E2 and 1F5) coupled to sepharose were able to remove 25% to 92% of the anti-DNA antibody repertoire from sera of patients with SLE and could also remove Id$^+$ T cells. In a more recent study of five patients with lupus nephritis, Silvestris et al. (218) compared the effects of using anti-Id (F4 and 8.12) IgG (preparation EL-11) purified from IVIg versus the whole IVIg. In the two SLE patients treated with EL-11 intravenously, a significant improvement compared to the other three patients was noted. There was a rapid reduction of anti-DNA serum antibody and less proteinuria. In a larger study of 20 SLE patients, Levy et al. (280) also report decreases in disease activity and autoantibody production. Immunomodulatory effects of IVIg in experimental models of antiphospholipid antibody syndrome (APS) have been shown and in patients with recurrent abortions treatment with IVIg resulted in successful pregnancies (reviewed in ref. 281). In patients with recurrent abortions treated with IVIg therapy, successful pregnancies have resulted (reviewed in ref. 281). Since M-components express Ids associated with SLE, it has been suggested that they may be used as source material for purification of large amounts of antiidiotypic material for clinical use (282). IVIg have been used to treat a variety of diseases and is thought to operate via a number of mechanisms, excellently reviewed elsewhere (283).

Idiotypic vaccination with murine anti-dsDNA antibody (3E10) of patients with inactive SLE and stable nephritis has recently been tested in a phase I clinical trial (284). Five of the nine subjects developed anti-idiotypic responses to the murine antibody. In a follow-up lasting 2 years, disease exacerbations did not occur. This treatment is therefore considered safe.

Idiotypes in Other Autoimmune Disorders

Antibodies to thyroglobulin (anti-TG) may play a role in autoimmune thyroiditis; many such Ab1 molecules express public Ids. Zanetti et al. (285,286) have shown that mature anti-TG obtained in mice after immunization can bear the same Id as a natural Ab1 in unstimulated neonates. Both mAbs used unmutated germline genes in their VH regions. The public Id62 on murine anti-TG is regulatory and can be used as an immunogen to induce T cells that suppress formation of Ab1; Ab2 can induce the appearance of Ab1 in naive mice or rats.

In autoimmune thyroid disease there also exists a very interesting subset of autoantibodies. These have dual specificity for thyroglobulin and thyroperoxidase (TPO) and are referred to as TGPO autoantibodies. TPO binds to a cross-species idiotope on the variable region of the TG antibody. Using long-term immunization of normal mice with a monoclonal TGPO antibody, antibodies that were similar to the immunogen, i.e., had dual specificity, were generated. Duthoit et al. (287) suggest that the Id of TPGO antibodies is unique because it contains not only the major epitopes of TG but also paratopes of the antibody directed against the major epitopes of TPO. They refer to these epitopes as "intertopes." Clearly such antibodies may play a role in perpetuating the autoimmune response.

Antibodies to the acetylcholine receptor (AcR) of muscle probably cause the autoimmune disease myasthenia gravis in humans and in experimental murine models. Several public Ids have been found on anti-AcR and on non-AcR Ab1 molecules in patients with myasthenia; some are regulatory (288). One study identified Ab2 before or at the onset of disease, followed by the appearance of Ab1 (Id) as clinical symptoms appeared or worsened (289).

In experimental allergic encephalomyelitis, neurologic disease resulting in weakness, paralysis, and death in susceptible murine and rat strains probably is caused exclusively by T cells, although antibodies are produced. Anti-Id Ig or anti-Id T cells made by immunization with effector T cells can prevent disease induced by Ag (myelin basic protein) in certain strains (290). In fact, immunization with peptides derived from the TCR of disease-causing cells can induce a $CD4^+$ regulatory anti-Id T-cell network that causes disease remission (291).

Antibodies to Sm Ag (anti-Sm) are relatively specific for SLE in patients; they also are found in MRL/*lpr* mice. Like anti-DNA, some populations express public Ids (292). A public Id (Y2) defined on a murine mAb anti-Sm was found in 41% of patients with SLE, 27% of their relatives, and 6% of normal individuals. Y2 is found on both anti-Sm and nonanti-Sm in MRL/*lpr* mice, as well as in sera of some normal mouse strains. These observations are similar to those for anti-DNA. Talal et al. (293) reported that a public Id, 4B4, on a monoclonal human anti-Sm is found in sera of patients with SLE who also have antibodies to the p24 gag protein of HIV-1. This brings to mind the possibility that anti-4B4 (anti-Id) may have induced Ab1 molecules that react with a wide variety of self and nonself Ags or, conversely, that antiviral antibodies are the Ids (207).

Antibodies to type II collagen (anti-CII) are produced by mice and rats susceptible to collagen-induced arthritis, which is considered by some experts to be a model for human rheumatoid arthritis. There is evidence that these antibodies can be important in inducing and perpetuating disease, but it also is clear that some T cells can induce joint destruction independent of the antibody response. Twenty to twenty-five percent of anti-CII in DBA/1 mice immunized with bovine CII bear a public Id. That particular Id can be regulated by Ag, but Ab1 molecules that express it are apparently not involved in disease induction as their suppression does not alter disease (294). In contrast, administration of a different anti-Id to rats at the time of immunization with CII suppressed anti-CII and disease; however, the Ab2 was not effective if given 7 days after immunization (295). Interestingly, the effective anti-Id protocol was not associated with suppression of delayed-type hypersensitivity to CII, so the anti-Id may have had a greater effect on Ab2 formation than on the cellular component of the disease.

In human rheumatoid arthritis (RA), several public Ids have been described. Patients with RA usually have polyclonal RFs, with only a small proportion expressing the public Ids characteristic of monoclonal RFs. The polyclonal RF repertoire contains both private and public Ids. Ids defined in other autoantibody systems, such as PR4 on anti-DNA and the H3 Id on anticardiolipin, are increased in patients with RA (296). Some public Ids predominate in the sera of patients with RF-positive disease; others can be found in similar proportions to patients with seropositive or seronegative RA and in hidden RF (i.e., contained in immune complexes and not detected as free populations) (297–301). No public Ids have been defined that are disease specific (as for the other human diseases discussed).

Antibodies to anticardiolipin, associated with hypercoagulable states in some individuals with or without SLE, also bear public Ids (302,303). Harmer et al. (85) described BH1, an idiotype that is expressed on an IgM human monoclonal anticardiolipin antibody that closely resembles the binding characteristics of serum antiphospholipid antibodies of patients with APS. Id expression appears to be highly restricted to patients with APS with eight of nine subjects tested exhibiting raised levels of Id in their serum compared to none of the 15 patients with RA and one of nine SLE patients (304). However, the numbers of patients investigated are extremely small, and confirmation of restriction to APS is required in larger test populations.

One group has described Id CRI-EM (86), a cross-reactive idiotype that is found on autoantibodies and other Igs in patients with scleroderma. Its expression was not observed in normal healthy control sera (n = 40) nor in sera or purified Ig from patients with SLE (n = 17).

Engineered Idiotypes and DNA Vaccines

Recent technologic advances in molecular biology and protein engineering mean that antibody combining sites and therefore idiotypes can be custom built. This can be achieved in a number of ways. First, it is possible to generate single-chain Fv (scFv) fragments that essentially represent the antigen combining site. These consist of the variable region of the heavy chain and the variable region of the light chain joined together with short flexible segment referred to as the linker. They are produced by using the genes that encode for the VH and VL regions, respectively. The scFv is expressed in bacteria and more recently on the surface of filamentous phage (305,306). Clearly, the antigen combining site can be modified genetically to generate a product with a higher affinity or different specificity, or can even be used to express antigenic determinants that may not be naturally located within the combining site (307,308). All this is possible because first, the structure of the antibody-binding site is well conserved and most of the changes that occur in the combining site happen within the CDRs, especially in the CDR3. Second, specific amino acid sequences can be introduced into the CDRs of the V region without altering the overall shape of the combining site. This process is known as CDR grafting. Since B cells are able to process and present their Ig variable regions (46), these "antigenized" Igs (309) can thus be used to elicit highly specific, what are essentially "anti-Id," responses to infectious agents, for example. Zaghouani et al. (308) have used this approach to produce antibodies to a principal neutralizing determinant derived from the V_3 loop of the HIV-1 envelope protein. Earlier reports demonstrated induction of responses to influenza virus (307) and to malaria (310). Xiong et al. (310) demonstrated that as well as CDR-H3, which is the usually site for grafting, CDR-H2 could also be utilized. Furthermore, the introduction of a T-cell epitope into the latter loop enhanced the B-cell response for the malaria antigen that was expressed in the CDR-H3 of the same variable region. This suggests that idiotypic determinants within the variable region may themselves modulate the "anti-idiotypic" response to other determinants within the same site. ScFv can be used as the classic Ab2 antigen mimic. It can also be altered from the wild type to generate a desirable antibody response (307). Features of anti-DNA binding have also been investigated using scFv technology (311). Recombinant antibodies also feature in investigations and treatment of tumors. CDR grafting in fact has been used in a number of cases to produce humanized antibodies so as to minimize the effects of using murine antibodies directed against tumor antigens (312).

A more recent development is the use of DNA vaccines (313,314). Here the DNA encoding for the VH and VL regions itself can be used as an immunogen. The vaccine essentially consists of the genetic material cloned into a bacterial plasmid that is designed to allow expression in eukaryotic cells. The vaccine also contains CpG motifs that can enhance the immune response. The functional protein (Ab2 mimic or Id) when expressed by the vaccinated individual can then elicit immune responses to the antigen, be this infectious agent or tumor antigen. The vaccine can be made effective by conjugating it another component, for example the fragment C of *Clostridium tetani* (313). Clinical trials with these vaccines are currently under way in human follicular lymphoma (313).

Engineered Ids have not been used in SLE as far as we are aware. However, it is tempting to speculate that public Ids that have been described in lupus, may be engineered and used to purify anti-Id reagents for therapy or be used as inoculi singly or linked in a fusion protein with selected cytokines to re-equilibrate dysregulated idiotypic networks.

REFERENCES

1. Oudin J, Michel M. Une nouvelle forme d'allotypic des globulines du serum de lapin apparemment liee a la fonction et a la specificite anticorps. *CR Hebd Seance Acad Sci Ser D, Sci Natur Paris* 1963;257:805–807.
2. Kunkel HG, Mannik M, Williams RC. Individual antigenic specificity of isolated antibodies. *Science* 1963;140:1218–1220.
3. Jerne NK. Towards a network theory of the immune system. *Ann Immunol (Paris)* 1974;125:373–389.
4. Ebling FM, Ando DG, Panosian-Sahakian N, et al. Idiotypic spreading promotes the production of pathogenic autoantibodies. *J Autoimmun* 1988;1:47–61.
5. Eilat DR, Rischel R, Zlotnick A. A central anti-DNA idiotype in human and murine systemic lupus erythematosus. *Eur J Immunol* 1985;15:368–372.
6. Jerne NK, Roland J, Cazenave P-A. Recurrent idiotypes and internal images. *EMBO J* 1982;1:243–246.
7. Sege K, Peterson PA. Use of anti-idiotypic antibodies as cell-surface receptor probes. *Proc Natl Acad Sci USA* 1978; 75:2443–2446.
8. Nisonoff A, Lamoyi E. Implications of the presence of an internal image of the antigen in anti-idiotypic antibodies: possible application to vaccine production. *Clin Immunol Immunopathol* 1989;21:397–402.
9. Dalgleish AG, Kennedy RC. Anti-idiotypic antibodies as immunogens: idiotype-based vaccines [published erratum appears in *Vaccine* 1988;6(4):381]. *Vaccine* 1988;6:215–220.
10. Schreiber JR, Patawaran M, Tosi M, et al. Anti-idiotype-induced, lipopolysaccharide-specific antibody response to *Pseudomona aeruginosa*. *J Immunol* 1990;144:1023–1038.
11. Francotte M, Urbain J. Induction of anti-tobacco mosaic virus antibodies in mice by rabbit anti-idiotypic antibodies. *J Exp Med* 1984;160:1485–1490.
12. Gaulton GN, Greene MI. Anti-idiotypic antibodies of reovirus as biochemical and immunological mimics. *Int Rev Immunol* 1986;1:79–90.
13. Kennedy RC, Melnick JL, Dreesman GR. Antibody to hepatitis B virus induced by injecting antibodies to the idiotype. *Science* 1984;223:930–933.
14. McNamara MK, Ward RE, Kohler H. Monoclonal idiotope vaccine against *Streptococcus* pneumonia infection. *Science* 1984;226:1325–1329.
15. Reagan KJ, Wunner WH, Wiktor TJ, et al. Anti-idiotypic antibodies induce neutralizing antibodies to rabies virus glycoprotein. *J Virol* 1984;48:660–667.
16. Sacks DL, Esser KM, Sher A. Immunization of mice against African trypanosomiasis using anti-idiotypic antibodies. *J Exp Med* 1982;155:1108–1112.
17. Westerink MAJ, Campagnari AA, Wirth MA, et al. Development and characterization of an anti-idiotype antibody to the capsular polysaccharide of *Neisseria* meningitis serogroup C. *Infect Immunol* 1988;56:1120–1125.
18. Thanavala YM, Roitt IM. Monoclonal anti-idiotypic antibodies as surrogates for hepatitis B surface antigen. *Int Rev Immunol* 1986;1:27–36.
19. Pride MW, Shi H, Anchin JM, et al. Molecular mimicry of hepatitis B surface antigen by an anti-idiotype-derived synthetic peptide. *Proc Natl Acad Sci USA* 1992;89:11900–11904.
20. Durrant LG, Maxwell-Armstrong C, Buckley D, et al. A neoadjuvant clinical trial in colorectal cancer patients of the human anti-idiotypic antibody 105AD7, which mimics CD55.*Clin Cancer Res* 2000;6:422–430.
21. Foon KA, John WJ, Chakraborty M, et al. Clinical and immune responses in resected colon cancer patients treated with anti-idiotype monoclonal antibody vaccine that mimics the carcinoembryonic antigen. *J Clin Oncol* 1999;17:2889–2895.
22. Tripathi PK, Qin H, Bhattacharya-Chatterjee M, et al. Construction and characterization of a chimeric fusion protein consisting of an anti-idiotype antibody mimicking a breast cancer-associated antigen and the cytokine GM-CSF. *Hybridoma* 1999; 18:18193–18202.
23. Saito H, Taniguchi M, Fukasawa, T, et al. Establishment of internal-image anti-idiotype monoclonal antibodies to a human antibody to lung cancer.*Cancer Immunol Immunother* 1997; 44:83–87.
24. Foon KA, Lutzky J, Baral RN, et al. Clinical and immune responses in advanced melanoma patients immunized with an anti-idiotype antibody mimicking disialoganglioside GD2. *J Clin Oncol* 2000;18:376–384.
25. Depraetere H, Depla E, Haelewyn J, et al. An anti-idiotypic antibody with an internal image of human interferon-gamma and human interferon-gamma-like antiviral activity. *Eur J Biochem* 2000;267:2260–2267.

26. Jerne NK. The generative grammar of the immune system. *Science* 1985;229:1057–1059.
27. Kennedy RC, Dreesman GR. Anti-idiotypic antibodies as idiotope vaccines that induce immunity against infectious agents. *Int Rev Immunol* 1986;1:67–82.
28. Rodkey LS. Autoregulation of immune responses via idiotype network interactions. *Microbiol Rev* 1980;44:631–636.
29. Urbain J, Wuilmart C, Cazenave PA. Idiotypic regulation in immune networks. *Contemp Top Mol Immunol* 1981;8: 113–117.
30. Amit AG, Mariziuzza RA, Phillips SEV, et al. Three-dimensional structure of an antigen-antibody complex at 2.8A resolution. *Science* 1986;233:747–751.
31. Mazza G, Ollier P, Comme G, et al. A structural basis for the internal image in the idiotypic network: antibodies against synthetic Ab2-D regions cross-react with the original antigen. *Ann Immunol* 1985;136:259–268.
32. Kohler H, Kieber-Emmons T, Srinivasan S, et al. Revised immune network concepts. *Clin Immunol Immunopathol* 1989; 52:104–111.
33. Denisova GF, Zerwanitzer M, Denisov DA, et al. Expansion of epitope cross-reactivity by anti-idiotype modulation of the primary humoral response. *Mol Immunol* 2000;37:53–58.
34. Denisova G, Zwickel J, Gershoni JM. Binding of HIV-1 gp120 to an anti-V3 loop antibody reveals novel antigen-induced epitopes. *FASEB J* 1995;9:127–132.
35. Hahn BH, Ando DG, Dunn K, et al. Idiotype regulatory networks promote autoantibody formation. *J Rheumatol* 1987;14 (suppl 13):143–148.
36. Hahn BH, Ebling FM. Suppression of murine lupus nephritis by administration of an anti-idiotypic antibody to anti-DNA. *J Immunol* 1984;132:187–190.
37. Hahn BH, Ebling FM, Panosian-Sahakian N, et al. Idiotype selection is an immunoregulatory mechanism which contributes to the pathogenesis of systemic lupus erythematosus. *J Autoimmun* 1989;1:673–681.
38. Puccetti A, Migliorini P, Sabbaga J, et al. Human and murine anti-DNA antibodies induce the production of anti-idiotypic antibodies with autoantigen-binding properties (epibodies) through immune-network interactions. *J Immunol* 1990;145: 4229–4237.
39. Mendlovic S, Brocke S, Shoenfeld Y, et al. Induction of a systemic lupus erythematosus-like disease in mice by a common human anti-DNA idiotype. *Proc Natl Acad Sci USA* 1988;85: 2260–2264.
40. Mendlovic S, Fricke H, Shoenfeld Y, et al. The role of anti-idiotypic antibodies in the induction of experimental systemic lupus erythematosus in mice. *Eur J Immunol* 1989;19:729–734.
41. Margaritte C, Gilbert D, Brard F, et al. Structural characterization of an (NZB×NZW)F1 mouse-derived IgM monoclonal antibody that binds through V region-dependent interactions to murine IgG anti-DNA antibodies. *J Autoimmun* 1994;7: 711–725.
42. Shoenfeld Y. Idiotypic induction of autoimmunity: a new aspect of the idiotypic network (review). *FASEB J* 1994;8: 1296–1301.
43. Uner AH, Tatum AH, Knupp CJ, et al. Characteristics of auto anti-idiotypic antibodies reactive with antibodies expressing the pathogenic idiotype, IdLNF1 in the (NZB × SWR)F1 model for lupus nephritis and its parental strains. *J Autoimmun* 1998; 11:233–240.
44. Binz H, Wigzell H. Shared idiotypic determinants on B and T lymphocytes reactive against the same antigenic determinant. I. Demonstration of similar or identical idiotypes on IgG molecules and T-cell receptors with specificity for the same alloantigen. *J Exp Med* 1975;142:197–203.
45. Eichmann K, Rajewsky K. Production of T and B cell immunity by anti-idiotypic antibodies. *Eur J Immunol* 1975;5: 661–665.
46. Weiss S, Bogen B. B-lymphoma cells process and present their endogenous immunoglobulin to major histocompatibility complex-restricted T cells. *Proc Natl Acad Sci USA* 1989;86: 282–285.
47. Bogen B, Weiss S. Processing and presentation of idiotypes to MHC-restricted T cells. *Int Rev Immunol* 1993;10:337–355.
48. Dunn EB, Bottomly K. T15-specific helper T cells: analysis of idiotype specificity by competitive inhibition analysis. *Eur J Immunol* 1985;15:728–733.
49. Cerny J, Smith JS, Webb C, et al. Properties of anti-idiotypic T cell lines propagated with syngeneic B lymphocytes. I. T cells bind intact idiotypes and discriminate between the somatic idiotypic variants in a manner similar to the anti-idiotypic antibodies. *J Immunol* 1988;141:3718–3723.
50. Bikoff EK, Eckhardt LA. Presentation of IgG2a antigens to class II-restricted T cell by stable transfected B lymphoma cells. *Eur J Immunol* 1989;19:1903–1909.
51. Rudensky AY, Preston-Hurlburt P, Hong S-C, et al. Sequence analysis of peptides bound to MHC class II molecules. *Nature (Lond)* 1991;353:622–647.
52. Singh RR, Kumar V, Ebling FM, et al. T cell determinants from autoantibodies to DNA can upregulate autoimmunity in murine systemic lupus erythematosus. *J Exp Med* 1995;181: 2017–2027.
53. Bruck C, Co MS, Slaoui M, et al. Nucleic acid sequence of an internal image bearing monoclonal anti-idiotype and its comparison to the sequence of the external antigen. *Proc Natl Acad Sci USA* 1986;83:6578–6582.
54. Williams WV, Guy HR, Rubin DH, et al. Sequences of the cell-attachment sites of reovirus type 3 and its anti-idiotypic/anti-receptor antibody: modeling of their three-dimensional structures. *Proc Natl Acad Sci USA* 1988;85:6488–6492.
55. Ward FJ, Khan N, Wolger LJ, et al. Immunogenic properties of an anti-DNA antibody-derived peptide, 88H.64–80: location of a dominant idiotope defined by T and B cells. *J Autoimmun* 1998;11:439–447.
56. Osterborg A, Masucci M, Bergenbrant S, et al. Generation of T cell clones binding F(ab′)2 fragments of the idiotypic immunoglobulin in patients with monoclonal gammopathy. *Cancer Immunol Immunother* 1991;34:157–62.
57. Ertl HCJ, Skinner MA, Finberg RW. Induction of anti-viral immunity by an anti-idiotypic antibody directed to a Sendai virus specific T helper cell clone. *Int Rev Immunol* 1986;1: 41–50.
58. Kawahara DJ, Miller A, Sercarz EE. The induction of helper and suppressor cells with secondary anti-hen egg-white lysozyme B hybridoma cells in the absence of antigen. *Eur J Immunol* 1987;17:1101–1107.
59. Batchelor JR, Lombardi G, Lechler RI. Speculations on the specificity of suppression. *Immunol Today* 1989;10:37–40.
60. Dohi Y, Nisonoff A. Suppression of idiotype and generation of suppressor T cells with idiotype-conjugated thymocytes. *J Exp Med* 1979;150:909–912.
61. Dohi Y, Yamada K, Ohno N, et al. Naturally occurring cytotoxic T lymphocyte precursors with specificity for an Ig idiotype. *J Immunol* 1988;141:3804–3809.
62. Zang YC, Hong J, Tejada-Simon MV, et al. Th2 immune regulation by T cell vaccination in patients with multiple sclerosis. *Eur J Immunol* 2000;30:908–913.
63. Zang YC, Hong J, Rivera VM, et al. Preferential recognition of TCR hypervariable regions by human anti-idiotypic T cells induced by T cell vaccination. *J Immunol* 2000;164: 4011–4017.

64. Ebling FM, Tsao BP, Singh RR, et al. A peptide derived from an autoantibody can stimulate T cells in the (NZB x NZW)F1 mouse model of systemic lupus erythematosus. *Arthritis Rheum* 1993;36:355–364.
65. Gavalchin J, Staines NA. T and B cell recognition of idiotypes of anti-DNA autoantibodies. *Lupus* 1997;6:337–343.
66. Waisman A, Ruiz PJ, Israeli E, et al. Modulation of murine systemic lupus erythematosus with peptides based on complementarity determining regions of a pathogenic anti-DNA monoclonal antibody. *Proc Natl Acad Sci USA* 1997;94:4620–4625.
67. Brosh N, Eilat E, Zinger H, et al. Characterization and role in experimental systemic lupus erythematosus of T-cell lines specific to peptides based on complementarity-determining region-1 and complementarity-determining region-3 of a pathogenic anti-DNA monoclonal antibody. *Immunology* 2000;99:257–265.
68. Brosh N, Dayan M, Fridkin M, et al. A peptide based on the CDR3 of an anti-DNA antibody of experimental SLE origin is also a dominant T-cell epitope in (NZB×NZW)F1 lupus-prone mice. *Immunol Lett* 2000;72:61–68.
69. Fricke H, Mendlovic S, Blank M, et al. Idiotype specific T-cell lines inducing experimental systemic lupus erythematosus in mice. *Immunology* 1991;73:421–427.
70. Blank M, Mendlovic S, Mozes E, et al. Induction of systemic lupus erythematosus in naive mice with T-cell lines specific for human anti-DNA antibody SA-1 (16/6 Id+) and for mouse tuberculosis antibody TB/68 (16/6 Id+). *Clin Immunol Immunopathol* 1991;60:471–483.
71. Knupp CJ, Uner AH, Korthas C, et al. Characterization of IdLNF1-specific T cell clones from the (NZB×SWR)F1 murine model for systemic lupus erythematosus. *Clin Immunol Immunopathol* 1993;68:273–282.
72. Knupp CJ, Uner AHJ, Tatum AH, et al. The onset of nephritis in the (NZB×SWR)F1 murine model for systemic lupus erythematosus correlates with an increase in the ratio of CD4 to CD8 T lymphocytes specific for the nephritogenic idiotype (IdLNF1). *Clin Immunol Immunopathol* 1992;65:167–175.
73. Osterborg A, Henriksson L, Mellstedt H. Idiotypic immunity (natural and vaccine-induced) in early stage multiple myeloma. *Acta Oncol* 2000;39:797–800.
74. Elias D, Tikochinski Y, Frankel G, et al. Regulation of NOD mouse autoimmune diabetes by T cells that recognize a TCR CDR3 peptide. *Int Immunol* 1999;11:957–966.
75. Meek K, Jeske D, Slaoui M, et al. Complete amino acid sequence of heavy chain variable region derived from two monoclonal anti-p-azophenyl arsenate antibodies of BALB/c mice expressing the major cross-reactive idiotype of the A/J strain. *J Exp Med* 1984;160:1070–1075.
76. Capra JD, Slaughter C, Milner ECB, et al. The cross-reactive idiotype of A-strain mice: serological and structural analysis. *Immunol Today* 1982;3:332–335.
77. Smith JA, Margolies MN. Complete amino acid sequences of the heavy and light chain variable regions from two A/J mouse antigen non-binding monoclonal antibodies bearing the predominant p-azophenylarsonate idiotype. *Biochemistry* 1987;26: 604–608.
78. Hasemann CA, Capra JD. Mutational analysis of the cross-reactive idiotype of the A strain mouse. *J Immunol* 1991;147(9): 3170–3179.
79. Desaymard C, Giusti AM, Scharff MD. Rat anti-T15 monoclonal antibodies with specificity for VH- and VH-VL epitopes. *Mol Immunol* 1984;21:961–967.
80. Strickland FM, Gleason JT, Cerny J. Serologic and molecular characterization of the T15 idiotype—I. Topologic mapping of idiotopes on TEPC15. *Mol Immunol* 1987;24:631–635.
81. Strickland FM, Gleason JT, Cerny J. Serologic and molecular characterization of the T15 idiotype—II. Structural basis of independent idiotope expression on phosphorylcholine-specific monoclonal antibodies. *Mol Immunol* 1987;24:637–646.
82. Clevinger B, Schilling J, Hood L, et al. Structural correlates of crossreactive and individual idiotypic determinants on murine antibodies to a (1-3)dextran. *J Exp Med* 1980;151:1059–1064.
83. Rudikoff S. Structural correlates of idiotypes expressed on galactan-binding antibodies. In: Greene MI, Nisonoff A, eds. *The biology of idiotypes*. New York: Plenum Press, 1984:15.
84. DeKeyser F, Takei M, Dang H, et al. Characterization of a cross-reactive idiotype on two human autoantibodies associated with systemic autoimmune disease. *Clin Immunol Immunopathol* 1993;69:155–160.
85. Harmer IJ, Loizou S, Thompson KM, et al. A human monoclonal antiphospholipid antibody that is representative of serum antibodies and is germline encoded [see comments]. *Arthritis Rheum* 1995;38:1068–1076.
86. Vázquez-Abad D, Tian L, Zanetti M, et al. A cross-reactive idiotype in scleroderma. *Clin Exp Immunol* 1997;108:420–427.
87. Chen PP, Liu M-F, Sinha S, et al. A 16/6 idiotype-positive anti-DNA antibody is encoded by a conserved VH gene with no somatic mutation. *Arthritis Rheum* 1988;31:1429–1433.
88. Waisman A, Shoenfeld Y, Blank M, et al. The pathogenic human monoclonal anti-DNA that induces experimental systemic lupus erythematosus in mice is encoded by a VH4 gene segment. *Int Immunol* 1995;7:689–696.
89. Staines NA, Ravirajan CT, Morgan A, et al. Expression and relationships of seven public idiotypes of DNA binding autoantibodies on monoclonal antibodies and serum immunoglobulins. *Lupus* 1993;2:25–33.
90. Blanco F, Longhurst C, Watts R, et al. Identification and characterisation of anew human DNA reactive monoclonal antibody and a common idiotype, WRI 176 Id β. *Lupus* 1994;3:15–24.
91. Staines NA, Ward FJ, Denbury AN, et al. Primary sequence and location of the idiotopes of V-88, a DNA-binding monoclonal autoantibody, determined by idiotope scanning with synthetic peptides on pins. *Immunology* 1993;78:371–378.
92. Ward FJ, Knies JE, Cunningham C, et al. Natural antibodies that react with V-region peptide epitopes of DNA-binding antibodies are made by mice with systemic lupus erythematosus as disease develops. *Immunology* 1997;92(3):354–361.
93. Young F, Tucker L, Rubinstein T, et al. Molecular analysis of a germline-encoded idiotypic marker of pathogenic human lupus autoantibodies. *J Immunol* 1990;145:2545–2553.
94. Kalsi J, Ward FJ, Loghurst C, et al. The presence of naturally occurring anti-16/6Id antibodies in SLE sera. *Br J Rheumatol* 1994;suppl 33:40(abst).
95. Potter KN, Li Y, Pascual V, et al. Molecular characterization of a cross-reactive idiotope on human immunoglobulins utilizing the VH4-21 gene segment. *J Exp Med* 1993;178:1419–1428.
96. Isenberg DA, McClure C, Farewell V, et al. Correlation of 9G4 idiotope with disease activity in patients with systemic lupus erythematosus. *Ann Rheum Dis* 1998;57:566–570.
97. Mockridge CI, Chapman CJ, Spellerberg MB, et al. Use of phage surface expression to analyze regions of human V4-34(VH4-21)-encoded IgG autoantibody required for recognition of DNA: no involvement of the 9G4 idiotope. *J Immunol* 1996;157:2449–2454.
98. Nahm MH, Clevinger BL, Davie JM. Monoclonal antibodies to streptococcal group A carbohydrate. I. A dominant idiotypic determinant is located on Vk. *J Immunol* 1982;129:1513–1522.
99. Ehrenstein MR, Longhurst CM, Latchman DS, et al. Serological and genetic characterization of a human monoclonal immunoglobulin G anti-DNA idiotype. *J Clin Invest* 1994;93 (4):1787–1797.
100. Paul E, Iliev AA, Livneh A, et al. The anti-DNA-associated idio-

type 8.12 is encoded by the V lambda II gene family and maps to the vicinity of L chain CDR1. *J Immunol* 1992;149: 3588–3595.

101. Irigoyen M, Kowal C, Young ACM, et al. Molecular mapping of the 8.12 SLE-associated idiotype specificity at the single amino acid level. *Mol Immunol* 1996;33:1255–1265.
102. Hohmann A, Cairns E, Brisco M, et al. Immunoglobulin gene sequence analysis of anti-cardiolipin and anti-cardiolipin idiotype (H3) human monoclonal antibodies. *Autoimmunity* 1995; 22:49–58.
103. Kobzik L, Brown MC, Cooper AG. Demonstration of an idiotypic antigen on a monoclonal cold agglutinin and on its isolated heavy and light chains. *Proc Natl Acad Sci USA* 1976;73: 1702–1705.
104. Zanetti M, Rogers J. Independent expression of a regulatory idiotype on heavy and light chain: further immunochemical analysis with anti-heavy and anti-light chain antibodies. *J Immunol* 1987;139:720–725.
105. Geysen HM, Rodda SJ, Mason TJ, et al. Strategies for epitope analysis using peptide synthesis. *J Immunol Methods* 1987;102: 259–274.
106. Fagerberg J, Yi Q, Gigliotti D, et al. T-cell epitope mapping of the idiotypic monoclonal IgG heavy and light chains in multiple myeloma. *Int J Cancer* 1999;80:671–680.
107. Laune D, Molina F, Mani J-C, et al. Dissection of an antibody paratope into peptides discloses the idiotype recognised by the cognate anti-idiotypic antibody. *J Immunol Methods* 2000;239;63–73.
108. Hobby P, Ward FJ, Denbury AN, et al. Molecular modeling of an anti-DNA autoantibody (V-88) and mapping of its V region epitopes recognized by heterologous and autoimmune antibodies. *J Immunol* 1998;161:2944–2952.
109. Kalsi JK, Martin AC, Hirabayashi Y, et al. Functional and modelling studies of the binding of human monoclonal anti-DNA antibodies to DNA. *Mol Immunol* 1996;33:471–483.
110. Yamamura T, Geng TC, Kozovska MF, et al. An alpha-chain TCR CDR3 peptide can enhance EAE induced by myelin basic protein or proteolipid protein. *J Neurosci Res* 1996;45:706–713.
111. Gavalchin J, Staines NA. T and B cell recognition of anti-DNA autoantibodies. *Lupus* 1997;6:337–343.
112. Wen Y-J, Lim SH. Different properties of T cell epitopes within complementarity-determining regions 1 and 2 of idiotypic VH in B-lymphoma. *Scand J Immunol* 1999;50:296–301.
113. Bentley GA, Boulot G, Riottot MM, et al. Three-dimensional structure of an idiotope-anti-idiotope complex. *Nature* 1990; 348(6298):254–257.
114. Evans SV, Rose DRTo R, Young NM, et al. Exploring the mimcry of polysaccharide antigens by anti-idiotypic antibodies. *J Mol Biol* 1994;241:691.
115. Ban N, Escobar C, Garcia R, et al. Crystal structure of an idiotype-anti-idiotype Fab complex. *Proc Natl Acad Sci USA* 1994; 91:1604–1608.
116. Fields BA, Goldbaum FA, Ysern X, et al. Molecular basis of antigen mimicry by an anti-idiotope. *Nature* 1995;374(6524):739–742.
117. Young NM, Gidney MAJ, Gudmundson B-ME, et al. Molecular analysis for the lack of mimcry of Brucella polysaccharide antigens by Ab2γ antibodies. *Mol Immunol* 1999;36:339–347.
118. Ban N, Day J, Wang X, et al. Crystal structure of an anti-anti-idiotype shows it to be self-complementary. *J Mol Biol* 1996; 255:617–627.
119. Zhang W, Reichlin M. Some autoantibodies to Ro/SS-A and La/SS-B are antiidiotypes to anti-double-stranded DNA. *Arthritis Rheum* 1996;39:522–531.
120. Williams RC Jr, Malone CC, Cimbalnik K, et al. Cross reactivity of human IgG anti-F(ab′)2 antibody with DNA and other nuclear antigens. *Arthritis Rheum* 1997;40:109–123.
121. Mazza G, Housset D, Piras C, et al. Structural features of the interaction between an anti-clonotypic antibody and its cognate T-cell antigen receptor. *J Mol Biol* 1999;287:773–780.
122. Waisman A, Ruiz PJ, Israeli E, et al. Modulation of murine systemic lupus erythematosus with peptides based on complementarity determining regions of a pathogenic anti-DNA monoclonal antibody. *Proc Natl Acad Sci USA* 1997;94:4620–4625.
123. Pawlak L, Hart D, Nisonoff A. Requirements for prolonged suppression of an idiotypic specificity in adult mice. *J Exp Med* 1973;137:1442–1448.
124. Weiler I, Weiler C, Sprenger R, et al. Idiotype suppression by maternal influences. *Eur J Immunol* 1977;7:531–535.
125. Victor-Kobrin C, Barak ZT, Bonilla FA, et al. A molecular and structural analysis of the VH and VK regions of monoclonal antibodies bearing the A48 regulatory idiotype. *J Immunol* 1990;144:614–619.
126. Hahn BH, Ebling FM. Suppression of murine lupus nephritis by administration of a syngeneic monoclonal antibody to DNA. *J Clin Invest* 1983;71:1728–1736.
127. Bogen B. Peripheral T cell tolerance as a tumor escape mechanism: deletion of CD4+ T cells specific for a monoclonal immunoglobulin idiotype secreted by a plasmacytoma *Eur J Immunol* 1996;26:2671–2679.
128. Levy R, Levy S, Cleary ML, et al. Somatic mutations in human B cell tumors. *Immunol Rev* 1987;96:43–50.
129. Holmberg D, Forsgren S, Forni L, et al. Idiotype determinant of natural IgM antibodies that resemble self Ia antigens. *Proc Natl Acad Sci USA* 1984;81:3175–3179.
130. Vakil M, Kearney JF. Regulatory influences of neonatal multispecific antibodies on the developing B cell repertoire. *Int Rev Immunol* 1988;3:117–131.
131. Bernabe RR, Coutinho A, Cazenave PA, et al. Suppression of "recurrent" idiotype results in profound alterations of the whole B cell compartment. *Proc Natl Acad Sci USA* 1981;78: 6416–6420.
132. Ravirajan CT, Staines NA. Involvement in lupus disease of idiotypes Id.F-423 and Id.IV-228 defined, respectively, upon foetal and adult MRL/Mp-lpr/lpr DNA-binding monoclonal autoantibodies. *Immunology* 1991;74:342–347.
133. Hentati B, Ternynck T, Avrameas S, et al. Comparison of natural antibodies to autoantibodies arising during lupus in (NZB×NZW)F1 mice. *J Autoimmun* 1991;4:341–356.
134. Melnick JL. Virus vaccines: principles and prospects. *Bull WHO* 1989;67:105–115.
135. Mathews JH, Roehrig JT, Trent DW. Role of complement and the Fc portion of immunoglobulin G in immunity to Venezuelan equine encephalomyelitis virus infection with glycoprotein-specific monoclonal antibodies. *J Virol* 1985;55: 594–600.
136. Stein KE, Soderstrom T. Neonatal administration of idiotype or antiidiotype primes for protection against Escherichia coli K13 infection in mice. *J Exp Med* 1984;160:1011–1016.
137. Wang QL, Wang HT, Blalock E, et al. Identification of an idiotypic peptide recognized by autoantibodies in human immunodeficiency virus-1-infected individuals. *J Clin Invest* 1995;96: 775–780.
138. Boudet F, Theze J, Zouali M. Anti-idiotypic antibodies to the third variable domain of gp120 induce an anti-HIV-1 antibody response in mice. *Virology* 1994;200:176–188.
139. Kennedy RC, Adler-Stortz C, Burns JW, et al. Anti-idiotype modulation of herpes simplex virus infection leading to increased pathogenicity. *J Virol* 1984;50:951–958.
140. Grant M, Smaill F, Muller S, et al. The anti-idiotypic antibody 1F7 selectively inhibits cytotoxic T cells activated in HIV-1 infection. *Immunol Cell Biol* 2000;78(1):20–27.
141. Müller S, Margolin DH, Nara PL, et al. Stimulation of HIV-

1–neutralizing antibodies in simian HIV-IIIB-infected macaques. *Proc Natl Acad Sci USA* 1998;95:276–281.

142. Schedel I, Sutor G-C, Hunsmann G, et al. Phase II study of anti-CD4 idiotype vaccination in HIV positive volunteers. *Vaccine* 1999;17:1837–1845.
143. Lemke H, Lange H. Is there a maternally induced immunological imprinting phase à la Konrad Lorenz? *Scand J Immunol* 1999;50:348–354.
144. Anderson RW. On the maternal transmission of immunity: a "molecular attention" hypothesis. *Biosystems* 1995;34:87–105.
145. Montesano MA, Colley DG, Eloi-Santos S, et al. Neonatal idiotypic exposure alters subsequent cytokine, pathology, and survival patterns in experimental *Schistosoma mansoni* infections. *J Exp Med* 1999;189:637–645.
146. Magliani W, Polonelli L, Conti S, et al. Neonatal mouse immunity against group B streptococcal infection by maternal vaccination with recombinant anti-idiotypes [see comments]. *Nat Med* 1998;4:705–709.
147. Briles DE, Forman C, Hudak S, et al. The effects of idiotype on the ability of IgG1 anti-phosphorylcholine antibodies to protect mice from fatal infection with *Streptococcus pneumoniae. Eur J Immunol* 1984;14:1027–1030.
148. Nussbaum G, Anandasabapathy S, Mukerjee J, et al. Molecular and idiotypic analyses of the antibody response to *Cryptococcus neoformans* gluronoxylomannan-protein conjugate vaccine in autoimmune and nonautoimmune mice. *Infect Immun* 1999; 67:4469–4476.
149. Hougs L, Juul L, Svejgaard, et al. Structural requirements of the major protective antibody to *Haemophilus influenzae* type b. *Infect Immun* 1999;67:2503–2514.
150. Okamoto Y, Tsutsumi H, Kumar NS, et al. Effect of breast feeding on the development of anti-idiotype antibody response to F glycoprotein of respiratory syncytial virus in infant mice after post-partum maternal immunisation. *J Immunol* 1989;142: 2507–2512.
151. Andrews DW, Capra JD. Complete amino acid sequence of variable domains from two monoclonal human anti-gamma globulins of the Wa cross-idiotypic group: suggestion that the J segments are involved in the structural correlate of the idiotype. *Proc Natl Acad Sci USA* 1981;78:3799–3803.
152. Bentley DL. Most kappa immunoglobulin mRNA in human lymphocytes is homologous to a small family of germ-line V genes. *Nature* 1984;307:77–81.
153. Carson DA, Chen PP, Kipps TJ, et al. Idiotypic and genetic studies of human rheumatoid factors. *Arthritis Rheum* 1987;30: 1321–1327.
154. Chen PP, Albrandt K, Radoux V, et al. Genetic basis for the cross-reactive idiotypes on the light chains of human IgM anti-IgG autoantibodies. *Proc Natl Acad Sci USA* 1986;83: 8318–8322.
155. Chen PP, Liu MG, Glass CA, et al. Characterization of two immunoglobulin VH genes that are homologous to human rheumatoid factors. *Arthritis Rheum* 1989;32:72–78.
156. Goni F, Chen PP, Pons-Estel B, et al. Sequence similarities and cross-idiotypic specificity of L chains among human monoclonal IgMk with anti-gammaglobulin activity. *J Immunol* 1985;135:4073–4078.
157. Kunkel HG, Agnello V, Joslin FG, et al. Cross-idiotypic specificity among monoclonal IgM proteins with anti-gammaglobulin activity. *J Exp Med* 1973;137:331–338.
158. Kunkel HG, Winchester RJ, Joslin FG. Similarities in the light chains of anti-gamma-globulins showing close idiotypic specificities. *J Exp Med* 1974;139:120–128.
159. Newkirk MM, Mageed RA, Jefferis R, et al. Complete amino acid sequences of variable regions of two human IgM rheumatoid factors, BOR and KAS of the Wa idiotypic family, reveal restricted use of heavy and light chain variable and joining region gene segments. *J Exp Med* 1987;166:550–561.
160. Mageed RA, Borretzen M, Moyes SP, et al. Rheumatoid factor autoantibodies in health and disease. *Ann N Y Acad Sci* 1997; 815:296–311.
161. Williams RC Jr, Malone CC, Silvestris F, et al. Benign monoclonal gammopathy with IgG anti-DNA, anti-Sm and anti-F(ab′)2 activity. *Clin Exp Rheumatol* 1997;15(1):33–38.
162. Williams RC Jr, Malone CC, Silvestris F. Cationic myeloma M-components frequently show cross-reacting anti-DNA, Anti-F(ab′)2 and anti-nucleosome specificities. *Scand J Rheumatol* 1997;26(2):79–87.
163. Watts RA, Williams W, Le Page S, et al. Analysis of autoantibody reactivity and common idiotype PR4 expression of myeloma proteins. *J Autoimmun* 1989;2:689–700.
164. Davis TA, Maloney DG, Czerwinski DK, et al. Anti-idiotype antibodies can induce long-term complete remissions in non-Hodgkin's lymphoma without eradicating the malignant clone. *Blood* 1998;92:1184–1190.
165. Hsu FJ, Caspar CB, Czerwinski D, et al. Tumor-specific idiotype vaccines in the treatment of patients with B-cell lymphoma-long term results of a clinical trial. *Blood* 1997;89:3129–3135.
166. Nelson EL, Li X, Hsu FJ, et al. Tumor-specific cytotoxic T lymphocyte response after idiotypic vaccination for B-cell, non-Hodgkin's lymphoma. *Blood* 1996;88:580–589.
167. Chen TT, Tao MH, Levy R. Idiotype-cytokine fusion proteins as cancer vaccines. Relative efficacy of IL-2, IL-4 and granulocyte-macrophage colony-stimulating factor. *J Immunol* 1994;153:4775–4787.
168. Levitsky HI, Montegomery J, Ahmadzadeh M, et al. Immunization with granulocyte-macrophage colony-stimulating factor-transduced, but not B7-1-transduced, lymphoma cells primes idiotype-specific T cells and generates antitumor immunity. *J Immunol* 1996;156:3858–3865.
169. Kwak LW, Young HA, Pennington RW, et al. Vaccination with syngeneic, lymphoma-derived immunoglobulin idiotype combined with granulocyte/macrophage colony-stimulating factor primes mice for a protective T-cell response. *Proc Natl Acad Sci USA* 1996;93:10972–10977.
170. Osterborg A, Yi Q, Henriksson L, et al. Idiotypic immunization combined with granulocyte-macrophage colony-stimulating factor in myeloma patients induced type 1, major histocompatibility complex-restricted, CD8- and CD4-specific T cell responses. *Blood* 1998;91:2459–2466.
171. Mellstedt H, Osterborg A. Active idiotype vaccination in multiple myeloma. GM-CSF may be an important adjuvant. *Pathol Biol* 1999;47:211–215.
172. Chen TT, Levy R. Induction of autoantibody responses to GM-CSF by hyperimmunization with an Id-GM-CSF fusion protein. *J Immunol* 1995;154:3105–3117.
173. Hajek R, Butch AW. Dendritic cell biology and the application of dendritic cells to the immunotherapy of multiple myeloma. *Med Oncol* 2000;17:2–15.
174. Titzer S, Christensen O, Manzke O, et al. Vaccination of multiple myeloma patients with idiotype-pulsed dendritic cells: immunological and clinical aspects. *Br J Haematol* 2000;108: 805–816.
175. Caux C, Dezutter DC, Scmitt D, et al. GM-CSF and TNF-alpha cooperate in the generation of dendritic langerhans cells. *Nature* 1992;360:2548–261.
176. Fisch P, Kohler G, Garbe A, et al. Generation of antigen-presenting cells for soluble protein antigens ex-vivo from peripheral blood $CD34^+$ cells hematopoietic progenitor cells in cancer patients. *Eur J Immunol* 1996;26:595.

177. Timmerman JM, Levy R. Linkage of foreign carrier protein to a self-tumor antigen enhances the immunogenicity of a pulsed dendritic cell vaccine. *J Immunol* 2000;164:4797–4803.
178. Serody JS, Collins EJ, Tisch RM, et al. T cell activity after dendritic cell vaccination is dependent on both the type of antigen and the mode of delivery. *J Immunol* 2000;164:4961–4967.
179. Heimberger AB, Crotty LE, Archer GE, et al. Bone marrow-derived dendritic cells pulsed with tumor homogenate induce immunity against syngeneic intracerebral glioma. *J Neuroimmunol* 2000;103:16–25.
180. Nair SK, Snyder D, Rouse BT, et al. Regression of tumors in mice vaccinated with professional antigen-presenting cells pulsed with tumor extracts. *Int J Cancer* 1997;70:706–715.
181. Reichardt VL, Okada CY, Liso A, et al. Idiotypic vaccination using dendritic cells after autologous peripheral stem cell transplantation for multiple myeloma-a feasibility study. *Blood* 1999;93:2411–2419.
182. Dabadghao S, Bergenbrandt S, Anton D, et al. Anti-idiotypic T cell activation in multiple myeloma induced by M-component fragments presented by dendritic cells. *Br J Haematol*1998;100: 647–654.
183. Santin AD, Hermonat PL, Ravaggi A, et al. Development and therapeutic effect of adoptively transferred T cells primed by tumor lysate-pulsed autologous dendritic cells in a patient with metastatic endometrial cancer. *Gynecol Obstet Invest* 2000;49: 194–203.
184. Lim SH, Bailey-Wood R. Idiotypic protein-pulsed dendritic cell vaccination in multiple myeloma. *Int J Cancer* 1999;83:215–222.
185. Mackensen A, Herbst B, Chen JL, et al. Phase I study in melanoma patients of a vaccine with peptide-pulsed dendritic cells generated in vitro from CD34(+) hematopoietic progenitor cells. *Int J Cancer* 2000;86:385–392.
186. Bodey B, Bodey B Jr, Siegel SE, et al. Failure of cancer vaccines: the significant limitations of this approach to immunotherapy. *Anticancer Res* 2000;20:2665–2676.
187. Ratta M, Curti A, Fogli M, et al. Efficient presentation of tumor to autologous T cells by CD83+ dendritic cells derived from highly purified circulating CD14+ monocytes in multiple myeloma patients. *Exp Hematol* 2000;28:931–940.
188. Huang TH, Wu PY, Lee CN, et al. Enhanced antitumor immunity by fusion of CTLA-4 to a self tumor antigen. *Blood* 2000;96:3663–3670.
189. Tripathi PK, Qin H, Deng S, et al. Antigen mimicry by an anti-idiotypic antibody single chain variable fragment. *Mol Immunol* 1998;35:853–863.
190. Ruiz PJ, Wolkowicz R, Waisman A, et al. Idiotypic immunization induces immunity to mutated p53 and tumor rejection [see comments]. *Nat Med* 1998;4(6):710–712.
191. Syrengelas AD, Chen TT, Levy R. DNA immunization induces protective immunity against B-cell lymphoma. *Nat Med* 1996;2:1038–1041.
192. Kwak LW, Taub DD, Duffey PL, et al. Transfer of myeloma idiotype-specific immunity from an actively immunised marrow donor. *Lancet* 1995;345:1016–1020.
193. Reece DE, Foon KA, Bhattacharya-Chatterjee M, et al. Use of the anti-idiotype vaccine TriAb after autologous stem cell transplantation in patients with metastatic breast cancer. *Bone Marrow Transplant* 2000;26:729–735.
194. McCormack JM, Crossley CA, Ayoub EM, et al. Poststreptococcal anti-myosin antibody idiotype associated with systemic lupus erythematosus and Sjogren's syndrome. *J Infect Dis* 1993; 168:915–921.
195. Stewart AK, Huang C, Stollar BD, et al. High-frequency representation of a single VH gene in the expressed human B cell repertoire *J Exp Med* 1993;177:409–418.
196. Hahn BH, Ebling FM. Idiotypic restriction in murine lupus: high frequency of three public idiotypes on serum IgG in nephritic NZB/NZW F1 mice. *J Immunol* 1987;138: 2110–2118.
197. Isenberg DA, Williams W, Axford J, et al. Comparison of 17 DNA antibody idiotypes in patients with autoimmune diseases, healthy relatives and spouses and normal controls results of an international study from 10 laboratories. *J Autoimmun* 1990;3: 393–414.
198. Marion TN, Lawton AR, Kearney JF, et al. Anti-DNA autoantibody in (NZB/NZW) F1 mice are clonally heterogeneous but the majority share a common idiotype. *J Immunol* 1982;128: 668.
199. Rauch J, Murphy E, Roths JB, et al. A high frequency idiotype marker of anti-DNA autoantibodies in MRL-lpr/lpr mice. *J Immunol* 1982;129:236–241.
200. Cairns E, Massicotte H, Bell DA. Expression in systemic lupus erythematosus of an idiotype common to DNA-binding and nonbinding monoclonal antibodies produced by normal human lymphoid cells. *J Clin Invest* 1989;83:11009.
201. Watts RA, Ravirajan CT, Wilkinson LS, et al. Detection of human and murine common idiotypes of DNA antibodies in tissues and sera of patients with autoimmune diseases. *Clin Exp Immunol* 1991;83:267–273.
202. Gavalchin J, Seder RA, Datta SK. The NZB × SWR model of lupus nephritis. I. Cross-reactive idiotypes of monoclonal anti-DNA antibodies in relation to antigenic specificity, charge and allotype. Identification of inter-connected idiotype families inherited from the normal SWR and the autoimmune NZB parents. *J Immunol* 1986;138:128–137.
203. Dersimonian H, McAdam PWJ, Mackworth-Young C, et al. The recurrent expression of variable region segments in human IgM anti-DNA autoantibodies. *J Immunol* 1989;142:4027–4032.
204. Monestier M, Manheimer-Lory A, Bellon B, et al. Shared idiotypes and restricted immunoglobulin variable region heavy chain genes characterize murine autoantibodies of various specificities. *J Clin Invest* 1986;78:753–759.
205. Harata N, Sasaki T, Shibata S, et al. Selective absorption of anti-DNA antibodies and their idiotype-positive cells in vitro using an anti-idiotypic antibody-affinity column: possible application to plasma exchange. *J Clin Apheresis* 1991;6:34–39.
206. Brohnstein IB, Shuster AM, Gololobov GV, et al. DNA-specific antiidiotypic antibodies in the sera of patients with autoimmune diseases. *FEBS Lett* 1992:314:259–264.
207. Plotz PH. Autoantibodies are antiidiotype antibodies to antiviral antibodies. *Lancet* 1987;2:824–826.
208. Eivazova ER, McDonnell JM, Sutton BJ, et al. Cross-reactivity of antiidiotypic antibodies with DNA in systemic lupus erythematosus. *Arthritis Rheum* 2000;43:429–439.
209. Isenberg DA, Katz D, LePage S, et al. Independent analysis of the 16/6 idiotype lupus model. A role for an environmental factor? *J Immunol* 1991;147:4172–4177.
210. Abdou NI, Wall H, Lindsley HB, et al. Network theory in autoimmunity. In vitro suppression of serum anti-DNA antibody binding to DNA by anti-idiotypic antibody in SLE. *J Clin Invest* 1981;67:1297–1304.
211. Suenaga R, Evans M, Abdou NI. Idiotypic and immunochemical differences of anti-DNA antibodies of a lupus patients during active and inactive disease. *Clin Immunol Immunopathol* 1991;61:320–331.
212. Williams RC Jr, Malone CC, Huffman GR, et al. Active systemic lupus erythematosus is associated with depletion of the natural generic anti-idiotype (anti-F(ab)2) system. *J Rheumatol* 1995;22:1075–1085.
213. Ehrenstein MR, Katz DR, Griffiths MH, et al. Human IgG

anti-DNA antibodies deposit in kidneys and induce proteinuria in SCID mice. *Kidney Int* 1995;48:705–711.
214. Kalsi JK, Ravirajan CT, Wiloch-Winska H, et al. Analysis of three new idiotypes on human monoclonal autoantibodies. *Lupus* 1995;4:375–389.
215. Harata N, Sasaki T, Osaki H, et al. Therapeutic treatment of New Zealand mouse disease by a limited number of anti-idiotypic antibodies conjugated with neocarzinostatin. *J Clin Invest* 1990;86:769–786.
216. Uner AH, Knupp CJ, Tatum AH, et al. Treatment with antibody reactive with the nephritogenic idiotype, IdLNF1, suppresses its production and leads to prolonged survival of (NZB×SWR)F1 mice. *J Autoimmun* 1994;7:27–44.
217. Blank M, Manosroi J, Tomer Y, et al. Suppression of experimental systemic lupus erythematosus (SLE) with specific anti-idiotypic antibody-saporin conjugate. *Clin Exp Immunol* 1994; 98:434–441.
218. Silvestris F, D'Amore O, Cafforio P, et al. Intravenous immune globulin therapy of lupus nephritis: use of pathogenic anti-DNA-reactive IgG. *Clin Exp Immunol* 1996;104(suppl 1): 91–97.
219. Livneh A, Halpern A, Perkins D, et al. A monoclonal antibody to a cross-reactive idiotype on cationic human anti-DNA antibodies expressing lambda light chains: a new reagent to identify a potentially differential pathogenic subset. *J Immunol* 1987; 138:123.
220. Paul E, Diamond B. Characterization of two human anti-DNA antibodies bearing the pathogenic idiotype 8.12. *Autoimmunity* 1993;16:13–21.
221. Irigoyen M, Manheimer-Lory A, Gaynor B, et al. Molecular analysis of the human immunoglobulin V lambda II gene family. *J Clin Invest* 1994;94:532–538.
222. Panosian-Sahakian N, Klotz JL, Ebling F, et al. Diversity of Ig V gene segments found in anti-DNA autoantibodies from a single (NZB × NZW)F1 mouse. *J Immunol* 1989;142: 4500–4506.
223. Datta SK, Naparstek Y, Schwartz RS. In vitro production of an anti-DNA idiotype by lymphocytes of normal subjects and patients with systemic lupus erythematosus. *Clin Immunol Immunopathol* 1986;38:302.
224. Ebling FM, Hahn BH. Pathogenic subsets of antibodies to DNA. *Int Rev Immunol* 1989;5:79–95.
225. Isenberg DA, Shoenfeld Y, Madaio MP, et al. Anti-DNA antibody idiotypes in systemic lupus erythematosus. *Lancet* 1984;2: 417–422.
226. Kalunian KC, Panosian-Sahakian N, Ebling FM, et al. Idiotypic characteristics of immunoglobulins associated with human systemic lupus erythematosus. Studies of antibodies deposited in glomeruli of humans. *Arthritis Rheum* 1989;32:513–522.
227. Shoenfeld R, Isenberg DA. DNA antibody idiotypes:a review of their genetic, clinical and immunopathological features (review). *Semin Arthritis Rheum* 1987;16:215–252.
228. Shoenfeld Y, Isenberg DA, Rauch J, et al. Idiotypic cross-reactions of monoclonal human lupus autoantibodies. *J Exp Med* 1983;158:718–730.
229. Solomon G, Schiffenbauer J, Keiser HD, et al. Use of monoclonal antibodies to identify shared idiotypes on human antibodies to native DNA from patients with systemic lupus erythematosus. *Proc Natl Acad Sci USA* 1983;80:850–854.
230. Tsao BP, Ebling FM, Roman C, et al. Structural characteristics of the variable regions of immunoglobulin genes encoding a pathogenic autoantibody in murine lupus. *J Clin Invest* 1990; 85:530–540.
231. Zouali M, Eyquem A. Idiotypic restriction in human autoantibodies in DNA in systemic lupus erythematosus. *Immunol Lett* 1984;7:187–193.
232. Bona CA. V genes encoding autoantibodies: molecular and phenotypic characteristics. *Annu Rev Immunol* 1988;6: 327–358.
233. Cairns E, Kwong PC, Misener V, et al. Analysis of variable region genes encoding a human anti-DNA antibody of normal origin. Implications for the molecular basis of human autoimmune responses. *J Immunol* 1989;143:685–691.
234. Shlomchik MJ, Aucoin AH, Pisetsky DS, et al. Structure and function of anti-DNA autoantibodies derived from a single autoimmune mouse. *Proc Natl Acad Sci USA* 1987;84: 9150–9154.
235. Trepicchio W Jr, Barrett KJ. Eleven MRL-pr/1pr anti-DNA autoantibodies are encoded by genes from four Vh gene families. A potentially biased usage of Vh genes. *J Immunol* 1987; 138:2323–2331.
236. Trepicchio W Jr, Maruya A, Barrett KJ. The heavy chain genes of a lupus anti-DNA autoantibody are encoded in the germ line of a nonautoimmune strain of mouse and conserved in strains of mice polymorphic for this gene locus. *J Immunol* 1987;139: 3139–3145.
237. Kofler R, Noonan DJ, Levy DE, et al. Genetic elements used for a murine lupus anti-DNA autoantibody are closely related to those for antibodies to exogenous antigens. *J Exp Med* 1985; 161:805–815.
238. Chastagner P, Demaison C, Theze J, et al. Clonotypic dominance and variable gene elements of pathogenic anti-DNA autoantibodies from a single patient with lupus. *Scand J Immunol* 1994;39:165–178.
239. Diamond B, Scharff MD. Somatic mutation of the T15 heavy chain gives rise to an antibody with autoantibody specificity. *Proc Natl Acad Sci USA* 1984;81:5841–5844.
240. O'Keefe TL, Bandyopadhyay S, Datta SK, et al. V region sequences of an idiotypically connected family of pathogenic anti-DNA autoantibodies. *J Immunol* 1990;144:4275–4283.
241. van Es J, Gmelig Meyling FHJ, van de Akker WRM, et al. Somatic mutations in the variable regions of a human IgG anti-ds DNA autoantibody suggest a role for antigen in the induction of systemic lupus erythematosus. *J Exp Med* 1991;173: 461–470.
242. Behar SM, Scharff MD. Somatic diversification of the S107(T15) VH11 germ-line gene that encodes the heavy-chain variable region of antibodies to double-stranded DNA in (NZB × NZW)F1 mice. *Proc Natl Acad Sci USA* 1988;85:3970–3974.
243. Davidson A, Manheimer-Lory A, Aranow C, et al. Molecular characterization of a somatically mutated anti-DNA antibody bearing two systemic lupus erythematosus-related idiotypes. *J Clin Invest* 1990;85:1401–1409.
244. Guisti AM, Chien NC, Zack DJ, et al. Somatic diversification of S107 from an anti-phosphocholine to an anti-DNA autoantibody is due to a single base change in its heavy chain variable region. *Proc Natl Acad Sci USA* 1987;84:2926–2930.
245. Shlomchik M, Mascelli M, Shan H, et al. Anti-DNA antibodies from autoimmune mice arise by clonal expansion and somatic mutation. *J Exp Med* 1990;171:265–292.
246. Shlomchik MJ, Aucoin AH, Pisetsky DS, et al. Structure and function of anti-DNA autoantibodies derived from a single autoimmune mouse. *Proc Natl Acad Sci USA* 1987;84:9150–9154.
247. Behar SM, Lustgarte KL, Corbe S, et al. Characterization of somatically mutated S107 Vh11-encoded anti;n-DNA autoantibodies derived from autoimmune (NZBxNZW)F1 mice. *J Exp Med* 1991;173:731–736.
248. Behar SM, Corbet S, Diamond B, et al. The molecular origin of anti-DNA antibodies. *Int Rev Immunol* 1989;5:23–35.
249. Taki S, Hirose S, Kinoshita K, et al. Somatically mutated IgG anti-DNA antibody clonally related to germ-line encoded IgM anti-DNA antibody. *Eur J Immunol* 1992;22:987–992.

250. Eilat D. The role of germline gene expression and somatic mutation in the generation of autoantibodies to DNA. *Mol Immunol* 1990;27:203–207.
251. Eilat D, Webster DM, Rees AR. V region sequences of anti-DNA and anti-RNA autoantibodies from NZB/NZW F1 mice. *J Immunol* 1988;141:1745–1753.
252. Kofler R, Dixon FJ, Theofilopoulos AN. The genetic origin of autoantibodies (review). *Immunol Today* 1987;80: 375–380.
253. Grayzel A, Solomon A, Aranow C, et al. Antibodies elicited by pneumococcal antigens bear an anti-DNA associated idiotype. *J Clin Invest* 1991;87:8420–846.
254. Marion TN, Bothwell AL, Briles DE, et al. IgG anti-DNA antibodies within an individual autoimmune mouse are the products of clonal selection. *J Immunol* 1989;142:4269–4274.
254a. Muryoi T, Sasaki T, Hatakeyama A, et al. Clonotypes of anti-DNA antibodies expressing specific idiotypes in immune complexes of patients with active lupus nephritis. *J Immunol* 1990;15;144:3856–3861.
255. Marion TN, Tillman DM, Joy N. Interclonal and intraclonal diversity among anti-DNA antibodies from an (NZB×NZW) F1 mouse. *J Immunol* 1990;145:2322–2332.
256. Ohnishi K, Ebling FM, Mitchell B, et al. Comparison of pathogenic and non-pathogenic murine antibodies to DNA: antigen binding and structural characteristics. *Int Immunol* 1994;6: 817–830.
257. Kumar S, Kalsi,J, Ravirajan CT, et al. Molecular Cloning and Expression of the Fabs of Human Autoantibodies in *Escherichia coli*. Determination of the heavy or light chain contribution to the anti-DNA/-cardiolipin activity of the Fab. *J Biol Chem* 2000;275:35129–35136.
258. Very DL Jr, Panka DJ, Weissman D, et al. Lack of connectivity between the induced and autoimmune repertoires of lpr/lpr mice. *Immunology* 1993;80:518–526.
259. Youinou P, Isenberg DA, Kalsi JK, et al. Interplay of four idiotypes and interaction with autoantibodies in lupus patients, their relatives and their spouses *J Autoimmun* 1996;9:767–775.
260. Livneh A, Gazit E, Diamond B. The preferential expression of the anti-DNA associated 8/12 idiotype in lupus is not genetically controlled. *Autoimmunity* 1994;18:16.
261. Shoenfeld Y, Slor H, Shafrir S, et al. Diversity and pattern of inheritance of autoantibodies in families with multiple cases of systemic lupus erythematosus. *Ann Rheum Dis* 1992;51:611–618.
262. Ebling FM, Kalunian KC, Fronek Z, et al. Idiotypic characteristics of immunoglobulins associated with human systemic lupus erythematosus. Association of high serum levels of IdGN2 with nephritis but not with HLA Class II genes predisposing to nephritis. *Arthritis Rheum* 1990;33:978–984.
263. Kalsi J, Ravirajan CT, Rahman A, et al. Structure-function analysis and the molecular origins of anti-DNA antibodies in systemic lupus erythematosus. In: *Expert reviews in molecular medicine*. Cambridge: Cambridge University Press, 1999. *http://www-ermm.cbcu.cam.ac.uk*.
264. Workman CJ, Pfund WP, Voss EW Jr. Two dual-specific (anti-IgG and anti-dsDNA) monoclonal autoantibodies derived from the NZB/NZW F1 recognize an epitope in the hinge region. *J Protein Chem* 1998;17:599–606.
265. Kohler H, Paul S. Superantibody activities: new players in innate and adaptive immune responses. *Immunol Today* 1998;19:221–227.
266. Ehrenstein MR, Hartley B, Wilkinson LS, et al. Comparison of a monoclonal and polyclonal anti-idiotype against a human IgG anti-DNA antibody. *J Autoimmun* 1994;7:349–367.
267. Weisbart RH, Noritake DT, Wong AL, et al. A conserved anti-DNA antibody idiotype associated with nephritis in murine and human systemic lupus erythematosus. *J Immunol* 1990; 144:2653–2658.
268. Gilbert D, Brard F, Margaritte C, et al. An idiotype D23-bearing polyspecific, murine anti-DNA monoclonal antibody forms glomerular immune deposits. Pathogenic role of natural autoantibodies? *Mol Immunol* 1995;32:477–486.
269. Krause I, Tomer Y, Elias D, et al. Inhibition of diabetes in NOD mice by idiotypic induction of SLE. *J Autoimmun* 1999;13: 49–55.
270. Levite M, Zinger H, Mozes E, et al. Systemic lupus erythematosus-related autoantibody production in mice is determined by bone marrow-derived cells. *Bone Marrow Transplant* 1993; 12:179–183.
271. Singh RR, Hahn BH, Sercarz EE. Neonatal peptide exposure can prime T cells and, upon subsequent immunization, induce their immune deviation: implications for antibody vs. T cell-mediated autoimmunity [see comments]. *J Exp Med* 1996;183 (4):1613–1621.
272. Singh RR, Hahn BH, Tsao BP, et al. Evidence for multiple mechanisms of polyclonal T cell activation in murine lupus. *J Clin Invest* 1998;102:1841–1849.
273. Howe CA, Hartley B, Williams DG, et al. Active immunization with anti-DNA autoantibody idiopeptide 88H.64–80 is nephritogenic in (NZB × NZW)F1 and Balb/c mice. *Biochem Soc Trans* 1997;25:316S.
274. Jouanne C, Avrameas S, Payelle-Brogard B. A peptide derived from a polyreactive monoclonal anti-DNA natural antibody can modulate lupus development in (NZB × NZW) F1 mice. Immunology 1999;96:333–339.
275. Singh RR, Ebling FM, Sercarz EE, et al. Immune tolerance to autoantibody-derived peptides delays development of autoimmunity in murine lupus. *J Clin Invest* 1995;96(6): 2990–2996.
276. Abdou NI, Wall H, Lindsley HB, et al. Suppression of serum anti-DNA antibody binding by anti-idiotypy antibody. *J Clin Invest* 1981;67:1297–1302.
277. Williams RC Jr, Malone CC, Huffman GR, et al. Active systemic lupus erythematosus is associated with depletion of the natural generic anti-idiotypic (anti(Fab′)2) system. *J Rheumatol* 1995;22:1075–1085.
278. Silvestris R, Cafforio P, Dammacco F. Pathogenic anti-DNA idiotype-reactive IgG in intravenous immunoglobulin preparations. *Clin Exp Immunol* 1994;97:19–25.
279. Evans M, Abdou NI. In vitro modulation of anti-DNA secreting peripheral blood mononuclear cells of lupus patients by anti-idiotypic antibody of pooled human intravenous immune globulin. *Lupus* 1993;2:371–375.
280. Levy Y, Sherer Y, Ahmed A, et al. A study of 20 SLE patients with intravenous immunoglobulin—clinical and serologic response. *Lupus* 1999;8:705–712.
281. Sherer Y, Levy Y, Shoenfeld Y. Intravenous immunoglobulin therapy of antiphospholipid syndrome. *Rheumatology* 2000;39:421–426.
282. Williams RC Jr, Malone CC, Fry G, et al. Affinity columns containing anti-DNA Id+ human myeloma proteins adsorb human epibodies from intravenous gamma globulin. *Arthritis Rheum* 1997;40:683–693.
283. Rhoades CJ, Williams MA, Kelsey SM, et al. Monocyte-macrophage system as targets for immunomodulation by intravenous immunoglobulin. *Blood Rev* 2000;14;14–30.
284. Spertini F, Leimgruber A, Morel B, et al. Idiotypic vaccination with a murine anti-dsDNA antibody: phase I study in patients with nonactive systemic lupus erythematosus with nephritis. *J Rheumatol* 1999;26:2602–2608.
285. Zanetti M, Glotz D, Rogers J. Perturbation of the autoimmune network. II. Immunization with isologous idiotype induces auto-anti-idiotypic antibodies and suppresses the autoantibody response elicited by antigen: a serologic and cellular analysis. *J Immunol* 1986;137:31–40.

286. Zanetti M, Rogers J, Katz DH. Induction of autoantibodies to thyroglobulin by anti-idiotypic antibodies. *J Immunol* 1984;133:240.
287. Duthoit C, Estienne V, Durand-Gorde JM, et al. Thyroglobulin monoclonal antibody cross-reacting with thyroperoxidase induces in syngeneic mice anti-idiotypic monoclonal antibodies with dual autoantigen binding properties. The intertope hypothesis. *Eur J Immunol* 1999;29:1626–1634.
288. Zweiman B. Theoretical mechanisms by which immunoglobulin therapy might benefit myasthenia gravis. *Clin Immunol Immunopathol* 1989;53:S83.
289. Lefkert AK. Anti-acetylcholine receptor antibody related idiotypes in myasthenia gravis. *J Autoimmunol* 1988;1:63.
290. Owhashi M, Heber-Katz E. Protection from experimental allergic encephalomyelitis conferred by a monoclonal antibody directed against a shared idiotype on rat T cell receptors specific for myelin basic protein. *J Exp Med* 1988;168:2153–2164.
291. Kumar V, Sercarz EE. The involvement of T cell receptor peptide-specific regulatory CD4+ T cells in recovery from antigen-induced autoimmune disease. *J Exp Med* 1993;178:909–916.
292. Pisetsky DS, Semper KF, Eisenberg RA. Idiotypic analysis of a monoclonal anti-Sm antibody. II. Strain distribution of a common idiotypic determinant and its relationship to anti-Sm expression. *J Immunol* 1984;133:2085.
293. Talal N, Garry RF, Schur PH, et al. A conserved idiotype and antibodies to retroviral proteins in systemic lupus erythematosus. *J Clin Invest* 1990;85:1866–1871.
294. Nagler-Anderson C, van-Vollenhove RF, Gurish MF, et al. A cross-reactive idiotype on anti-collagen antibodies in collagen-induced arthritis: identification and relevance to disease. *Cell Immunol* 1988;113:447.
295. Arita C, Kaibara N, Jingushi S, et al. Suppression of collagen arthritis in rats by heterologous anti-idiotypic antisera against anticollagen antibodies. *Clin Immunol Immunopathol* 1987;43:374.
296. Youinou P, Williams W, LeGoff P, et al. Serological abnormalities, including common idiotype PR4, in families with rheumatoid arthritis. *Ann Rheum Dis* 1989;48:898.
297. Bonagura VR, Wedgwood JF, Agostino N, et al. Seronegative rheumatoid arthritis, rheumatoid factor cross reactive idiotype expression, hidden rheumatoid factors. *Ann Rheum Dis* 1989;48:488.
298. Hancock WK, Barnett EV. Demonstration of anti-idiotypic antibodies directed against IgM rheumatoid factor in the serum of rheumatoid arthritis patients. *Clin Exp Immunol* 1989;75:25.
299. Ilowite NT, Wedgwood JF, Bonagura VR. Expression of the major rheumatoid factor cross-reactive idiotype in juvenile rheumatoid arthritis. *Arthritis Rheum* 1989;32:265.
300. Moore TL, Osborn TG, Dorner RW. Cross-reactive antiidiotypic antibodies against human rheumatoid factors from patients with juvenile rheumatoid arthritis. *Arthritis Rheum* 1989;32:699.
301. Ruiz-Arguelles A, Presno-Bernal M. Demonstration of a cross-reactive idiotype (IdRQ) in rheumatoid factors from patients with rheumatoid arthritis but not in rheumatoid factors from healthy, aged subjects. *Arthritis Rheum* 1989;32:134.
302. Krause I, Cohen J, Blank M, et al. Distribution of two common idiotypes of anticardiolipin antibodies in sera of patients with primary antiphospholipid syndrome, systemic lupus erythematosus and monoclonal gammopathies. *Lupus* 1992;1:363–368.
303. Hohmann A, Comacchio R, Boswarva V, et al. The He antiphospholipid idiotype is found in patients with systemic lupus erythematosus (SLE) but not in patients with syphilis. *Clin Exp Immunol* 1991;86:207–211.

303a. Hohmann A, Cains E, Brisco M, et al. Immunoglobulin gene sequence analysis of anti-cardiolipin and anti-cardiolipin idiotype (H3) human monoclonal antibodies. *Autoimmunity* 1995;22:49–58.
304. Mason AN, Harmer IJ, Mageed RA, et al. The BH1 idiotype defines a population of anticardiolipin antibodies closely associated with the antiphospholipid syndrome. *Lupus* 1999;8(3):234–239.
305. Winter G, Griffiths AD, Hawkins RE, et al. Making antibodies by phage display technology. *Annu Rev Immunol* 1994;12:433–455.
306. Chames P, Baty D. Antibody engineering and its applications in tumor targeting and intracellular immunization. *Fems Microbiol Lett* 2000;189:1–8.
307. Bona C, Brumaneau TD, Zaghouani H. Immunogenicity of microbial peptides grafted in self immunoglobulins. *Cell Mol Biol* 1994;40(suppl 1):21–30.
308. Zaghouani H, Anderson SA, Sperber KE, et al. Induction of antibodies to the human immunodeficiency virus type 1 by immunization of baboons with immunoglobulin molecules carrying the principal neutralizing determinant of the envelope protein. *Proc Natl Acad Sci USA* 1995;92:631–635.
309. Zanetti M. Antigenized antibodies. *Nature* 1992;355:476–477.
310. Xiong S, Gerloni M, Zanetti M. Engineering vaccines with heterologous B and T cell epitopes using immunoglobulin genes [see comments]. *Nature Biotech* 1997;15:882–886.
311. Stollar BD. Molecular analysis of anti-DNA antibodies. *FASEB J* 1994;8:337–342.
312. Holliger P, Bohlen H. Engineering antibodies for the clinic. *Cancer Metastasis Rev* 1999;18:411–419.
313. Stevenson, FK. DNA vaccines against cancer: from genes to therapy. *Ann Oncol* 1999;10:1413–1418.
314. Gurunathan S, Wu CY, Freidag BL, et al. DNA vaccines: a key for inducing long-term cellular immunity. *Curr Opin Immunol* 2000;12:442–447.
315. Warrington RJ, Wong SK, Ramdahin S, et al. Normal human cord blood B cells can produce high affinity IgG antibodies to dsDNA that are recognized by cord blood-derived anti-idiotypic antibodies. *Scand J Immunol* 1995;42:397–406.
316. Ravirajan CT, Harmer I, McNally T, et al. Phospholipid binding specificities and idiotype expression of hybridoma derived monoclonal autoantibodies from splenic cells of patients with systemic lupus erythematosus. *Ann Rheum Dis* 1995;54:471–476.
317. Shoenfeld Y, Isenberg DA, Rauch J, et al. Idiotypic cross-reactions of monoclonal human lupus autoantibodies. *J Exp Med* 1983;158:718–730.
318. Davidson A, Smith A, Katz J, et al. A cross-reactive idiotype on anti-DNA antibodies defines a heavy chain determinant present almost exclusively on IgG antibodies. *J Immunol* 1989;143:174–180.
319. Rauch J, Massicotte H, Tannenbaum H. Specific and shared idiotypes found on hybridoma anti-DNA autoantibodies derived from rheumatoid arthritis and systemic lupus erythematosus patients. *J Immunol* 1985;135:2385–2392.
320. Harkiss GD, Hendrie F, Nuki G. Cross-reactive idiotypes in anti-DNA antibodies of systemic lupus erythematosus patients. *Clin Immunol Immunopathol* 1986;39:421–430.
321. Watts R, Ravirajan CT, Staines NA, et al. A human fetal monoclonal DNA-binding antibody shares idiotypes with fetal and adult murine monoclonal DNA-binding antibodies. *Immunology* 1990;69:348–354.
322. Mackworth-Young CG, Sabbaga J, Schwartz RS. Idiotypic

markers of polyclonal B cell activation: public idiotypes shared by monoclonal antibodies derived from patients with systemic lupus erythematosus and leprosy. *J Clin Invest* 1987;79:572–581.

323. Dang H, Takei M, Isenberg D, Shoenfeld Y, et al. Expression of an interspecies idiotype in sera of SLE patients and their first-degree relatives. *Clin Exp Immunol* 1988;71:445–451.

16

THE IMPORTANCE OF SEX HORMONES IN SYSTEMIC LUPUS ERYTHEMATOSUS

SARA E. WALKER

Hormones and the immune system interact through a number of pathways (1,2). Understanding the interdependence of these systems is important in order to appreciate the pathogenesis of autoimmune disease. This chapter discusses the influence of gonads on the thymus and vice versa, as well as the effects of estrogens and androgens in autoimmune disease. It is now apparent that pituitary and hypothalamic hormones that are associated with reproduction and lactation can also direct immune responses and influence expression of autoimmunity. Identification of the stimulating and suppressive properties of specific gonadal, pituitary, and hypothalamic hormones affords the opportunity to design effective and relatively nontoxic treatments for systemic lupus erythematosus (SLE) and related diseases.

GONADAL HORMONES

Immune System–Reproductive System Interactions

The interdependence of the thymus, the pituitary-gonadal axis, and ovaries has been demonstrated in female rodents. A number of thymic peptides have been identified, including thymosin-α_1, thymosin-β_4, thymopoietin, thymulin, and thymic humoral factor-γ_2. These factors regulate T-cell maturation but are also able to influence pituitary and hypothalamic structure and function and act as neurotransmitters. In turn, production of thymulin in the thymic epithelium is controlled by the pituitary hormones prolactin and growth hormone (3).

The thymus is required for normal development and function of ovaries. Congenitally athymic nude mice have small ovaries and premature ovarian failure (4) as well as reduced concentrations of circulating luteinizing hormone (LH), follicle-stimulating hormone (FSH), estrone, and testosterone (5). Neonatal thymectomy results in sterility and ovarian dysgenesis in rodents. B6A mice, thymectomized at 3 days of age, responded with diminished ovarian weight, loss of oocytes, and absent corporea lutea. Circulating antibodies to oocytes were identified, and the ovaries were infiltrated with lymphocytes (6). Neonatal thymectomy also resulted in low levels of FSH, LH, growth hormone, and prolactin (6). A preferential decrease in $CD4^+$ lymphocytes occurred after neonatal thymectomy, and reproductive dysfunction was prevented by injecting $CD4^+$ lymphocytes (7) or by implanting a normal thymus (8).

The thymus is sensitive to gonadal hormones in rodents, and high doses of estradiol or testosterone deplete lymphocytes in the thymic cortex (9). Physiologic doses of estrogen stimulate the thymus. It has been proposed that this stimulation is mediated through the influences of gonadal hormones on thymic factors, such as thymulin, that are secreted by the thymic epithelium. This contention was supported by finding receptors for thymic hormones and for sex hormones colocalized on thymic epithelial cells (10), and by the discovery that estrogen stimulated thymulin secretion (11). Erbach and Bahr (12) found that replacement estradiol increased antibody formation in ovariectomized female rats. Estradiol was effective as long as the rats had an intact thymus or were treated with thymosin factor 5. Mice were "rescued" from thymectomy-induced ovarian dysgenesis if they were treated with estradiol-17β before the thymus was removed. In contrast, injections of 20 μg of estradiol-17β on 4 consecutive days following thymectomy did not prevent involution of the ovaries (13).

Effects of Estrogen in Murine Models of Lupus

Sex hormones play an important role in determining the severity of disease in hybrid New Zealand mice. The F_1 New Zealand black (NZB) × New Zealand white (NZW) hybrid, designated NZB × NZW, spontaneously develops antibodies directed against double-stranded DNA (anti-dsDNA) and immune complex–mediated glomerulonephritis (14). The females have considerably more immunoglobulin G (IgG) anti-DNA antibodies compared to males. Reports from colonies in different parts of the world have verified that disease in NZB × NZW females starts earlier and progresses more rapidly compared to males. At 5 to 6 months of age, there is a switch from IgG plus IgM autoantibodies in females to primarily IgG autoantibodies. This switch occurs 3 months later in males (15). Female NZB × NZW mice die of renal failure at 10 to 12 months of age, and males die at the age of 14 to 16 months (14). Of interest, these hybrid mice have concentrations of serum estradiol and testosterone that are comparable to mice that do not develop autoimmune disease (16,17). Furthermore, the females do not have abnormalities of estrogen metabolism that would alter 2-hydroxylated or 16-hydroxylated products (18).

Treatment with either synthetic estrogen or naturally occurring estradiol-17β accelerates disease in NZB × NZW mice. Mestranol, a synthetic estrogen used in oral contraceptives, induced positive tests for fluorescent antinuclear antibodies in male NZB × NZW mice after 6 weeks of treatment (19). Roubinian et al. (15,20) and Steinberg et al. (21) implanted castrated NZB × NZW mice with crystalline implants that contained high doses (6 to 7 mg) of estradiol-17β. In mice of both sexes, autoantibody levels were stimulated and the recipients of implanted estradiol died prematurely compared with untreated castrates and intact animals (15,20–23).

These early studies clearly linked estrogen with the phenotypic expression of severe autoimmune disease in the NZB × NZW model. It was therefore an unexpected finding that surgical oophorectomy did not reduce severity of lupus in NZB × NZW females (15). In addition, parturition did not lead to immediate postpartum flares of autoimmune disease in NZB × NZW females. Female NZB × NZW mice bred to NZB × NZW males delivered two litters of pups when the dams were 10 and 16 weeks of age, and the pups were removed within 24 hours of whelping. Two weeks after these females whelped, there was no stimulation of anti-dsDNA, serum immunoglobulins, albuminuria, or blood urea nitrogen compared to virgin control females (24). In NZB × NZW females that whelped multiple litters, severity of glomerulonephritis and longevity did not differ from control virgin NZB × NZW females (25).

The experiments of Roubinian et al. (15,20) and Steinberg et al. (21) were repeated (25), and it was found that the traditional high doses of implanted estradiol resulted in extremely high concentrations of circulating estradiol and fatal estrogen toxicity in female NZB × NZW mice. Toxic wasting, bladder distention, endometriosis, and pituitary adenomas were observed in NZB × NZW females that had been implanted with 5 mg or 6 mg of estradiol-17β (23, 26–28). Dosing regimes were developed that more closely mimicked natural levels of estrogen in mice. Brick et al. (16) implanted NZB × NZW mice with 1.5 to 2.0 mg of estradiol-17β, and this dose increased antibody responses in NZB × NZW mice. Carlsten and Tarkowski (29) used biweekly injections of estradiol benzoate, 3.2 μg, to reproduce physiologic levels of estrogen. This treatment accelerated renal disease and shortened longevity in first-generation offspring of NZB × NZW hybrids backcrossed to NZB that had inherited the $H2^d/H2^z$ genotype.

Other models of SLE have been investigated for responses to estrogenic hormones. The MRL/MpJ-*lpr/lpr* (MRL-*lpr*) mouse, which has a defect in the *Fas* gene and impaired thymic apoptosis, develops lymphoproliferation, sialoadenitis, vasculitis, glomerulonephritis, inflammatory arthritis, and antibodies to nuclear antigens. Longevity is not influenced strongly by sex in MRL-*lpr* mice (14). Physiologic doses of estradiol actually suppressed postpartum flares of arthritis in MRL-*lpr* mice (30). Physiologic estradiol stimulated anti-DNA, but short-term treatment did not affect longevity significantly in castrated MRL-*lpr* males (16). Higher doses of estradiol did influence the course of disease. Male castrates that received continuous long-term treatment with a dose of estradiol that exceeded physiologic doses developed enlarged lymph nodes and accelerated glomerular disease and died prematurely (31). MRL-*lpr* females injected with complete Freund's adjuvant, followed by 14 daily injections of high-dose estradiol (0.4 mg/kg/day), responded with proteinuria and early mortality (30). In contrast, the selective estrogen receptor modulator LY139478, an analogue of raloxifene, significantly increased survival in MRL-*lpr* females compared to mice that received either 17α-ethinylestradiol or inert vehicle (32).

Of interest, estrogen stimulates expression of autoimmune disease in mice that were thought traditionally to be "not autoimmune." Aged C57BL/6 mice spontaneously develop anti-DNA antibodies as well as inflammatory changes in multiple organs (33,34). Treatment with estrogen implants stimulated increased anti-DNA titers (34). Long-term exposure to high-dose estradiol implants in C57BL/6 mice resulted in increased plasma cell numbers and increased numbers of spleen and bone marrow cells that secreted IgG and IgM (35). Gender influences the SLE models developed by Wakeland's group (36,37), in which specific lupus susceptibility genes were introduced into C57BL/6 mice by congenic matings. The *Sle 3* gene, which controls glomerulonephritis, had higher penetrance in females than in males (36). B6.NZMc1/c7 mice, which had both the *Sle 1* and *Sle 3* susceptibility loci, had splenomegaly, expanded populations of activated B cells and $CD4^+$ T cells, anti-dsDNA, and glomerulonephritis. Disease was more severe in females compared to males, and it was proposed that the difference in disease severity was due to the stimulating effects of female hormones (37).

Lupus that is induced by manipulating nonautoimmune strains is stimulated by treating the mice with estrogen before inducing the autoimmune disease. Female C57Bl/10 × DBA/2 F1 mice that have been injected with DBA/2 lymphocytes are highly susceptible to chronic graft-versus-host disease. When the lymphocyte recipients were treated with estradiol-17β before induction of the graft-versus-host reaction, there was increased production of multiple autoantibodies, including anti-dsDNA (38). BALB/c mice that are immunized with the 16/6 Id idiotype of human anti-dsDNA will develop anti-DNA antibodies. BALB/c mice of both sexes were implanted with capsules containing 2 to 3 mg of estradiol-17β. Three months later, they were immunized with the idiotype. They developed high titers of antibodies to dsDNA and a number of other autoantigens (39). Treatment of the idiotype-injected mice with either tamoxifen or antiestradiol antibody resulted in decreased severity of proteinuria and protection from deposition of immune complexes in renal glomeruli (40).

Effects of Testosterone in Murine Models of Lupus

In contrast to estradiol, androgenic hormones are protective in NZB × NZW mice. In female NZB × NZW mice, subcutaneous implantation of Silastic capsules containing testosterone or 5-dihydrotestosterone suppressed SLE and prolonged life spans (23). It was not necessary for the females to be castrated in order to benefit from exogenous androgens, and androgen treatment was effective even if it began after the onset of clinical disease (23,41,42). Autoimmune disease in NZB × NZW females is responsive to relatively low doses of androgens. In fact, the low levels of testosterone that are found normally in female mice afford some protection from autoimmune disease. Long-term treatment with flutamide, a specific blocker of androgen receptors, resulted in accelerated mortality in NZB × NZW females (17). The weakly androgenic, naturally occurring steroid dehydroepiandrosterone (DHEA), given as DHEA sulfate, delayed the onset of anti-DNA and prolonged longevity in NZB × NZW females when treatment was started at 2 months of age. In contrast, there was no response if treatment was started at the age of 6 months (43). Treatment of NZB × NZW mice with DHEAS ameliorated imbalances in several cytokines that are associated with progression of autoimmune disease in this model. Circulating levels of interleukin(IL)-10 (IL-10) and IL-6, which are expected to increase with disease onset and exacerbation, were suppressed by DHEAS (43,44).

In NZB × NZW males, the course of disease was accelerated by castration. Surgical removal of the testicles before puberty was followed by early production of anti-DNA antibodies, early switch from 19S to 7S autoantibodies, and early death (41). Early castration was more effective than late castration, and castration of males at the age of 3 months had little effect on anti-DNA antibodies (45).

The rapidly progressive autoimmune disease in MRL-*lpr* mice does not display marked differences between genders, and high-dose estradiol therapy is required to accelerate disease progression. High doses of androgens are effective in suppressing MRL-*lpr* autoimmunity. Suppression of systemic autoimmune disease in males has been achieved with 6 to 8 mg of testosterone, or with 12 mg of 5-dihydrotestosterone, implanted at 2 to 4 weeks of age (46,47). Lacrimal glands of female MRL-*lpr* mice are infiltrated with periductal and perivascular collections of lymphocytes, which disrupt acinar tissue. The involvement of lacrimal glands in MRL-*lpr* females is significantly greater compared to MRL-*lpr* males. Implantation of high-dose pellets that contained 10 or 25 mg of testosterone resulted in dramatic reversal of the inflammatory lesions (48,49).

Immunologic Imprinting of the Fetus

Exposure of the fetal mouse to altered concentrations of gonadal hormones *in utero* can stimulate autoimmune responses in nonautoimmune mice. In the C57BL/6 mouse, treating the dam with estrogen at 14 to 16 days of gestation resulted in offspring that had sialoadenitis and enhanced immune responses, with increased plaque forming cell responses to bromelain-treated erythrocytes (50,51). Immunologic imprinting by gonadal hormones *in utero* can also affect the expression of autoimmunity in NZB × NZW mice. Production of steroid hormones is regulated differently in the maternal-fetal unit that is composed of the NZB dam and NZB × NZW F1 hybrid fetuses, compared with mice that do not spontaneously develop autoimmune disease. Male NZB × NZW fetuses have unexpectedly high levels of serum estradiol, and males have abnormally low concentrations of testicular and placental testosterone (52). The effects of testosterone on the fetus in late gestation were evaluated by treating NZB dams with Silastic implants containing testosterone on days 13 to 18 of gestation. Male NZB × NZW offspring of these dams that had been exposed to increased levels of testosterone while *in utero* had extended life spans compared to male NZB × NZW controls (53).

Mechanisms of Estrogen and Androgen Actions in Murine Lupus

Estrogen influences immune responses through mechanisms that are not limited to one set of immunologically active cells. Exogenous estrogen stimulates production of the T-helper-1 (Th1) cytokine, interferon-γ (IFN-γ) (54), and has the capacity to enhance production of Th2 cytokines (55). Stimulation of these cytokines could explain the effects of estrogenic hormones in murine models of SLE. Expression of IFN-γ transcripts was very high in unstimulated T cells from female NZB × NZW mice (56,57). Furthermore, NZB × NZW females had high expression of IL-6 genes in unfractionated, unstimulated spleen cells (57). Another survey of NZB × NZW females found limited secretion of Th1 cytokines, but unfractionated spleen cells produced high levels of IL-3, IL-4, IL-5, and IL-10 (58).

In addition to its widespread effects on the immune system, estrogen is capable of stimulating immune responses in both nonautoimmune mice and the New Zealand F1 hybrid. Treatment with estrogen, for periods of either 2 or 4 weeks, decreased T-suppressor cell activity in C57BL/6 mice as well as in autoimmune NZB × NZW mice (59). Stimulation was not limited to T cells, or to cells that produced antibodies directed against a specific antigen. CD5+ B cells, which spontaneously produce polyreactive IgM autoantibodies (49), were increased in nonautoimmune mice and in young NZB × NZW mice that were treated with estradiol-17β (60,61).

The widespread immunostimulatory effects of estrogen may result from the hormone's ability to foster abrogation of B-cell tolerance. Autoimmune-susceptible R4A-γ2b BALB/c mice have been made transgenic for the γ2b heavy chain of a nephritogenic anti-DNA antibody. These mice were treated with estradiol-17β implants that were designed to produce constant high serum concentrations of estradiol. Treatment resulted in blockage of tolerance in a population of bone marrow–derived B cells that was capable of producing high-affinity anti-DNA. The proto-oncogene *Bcl-2*, which protects from apoptosis, was increased in splenic B cells of mice that were treated with estradiol (62).

In MRL-*lpr* mice, estrogen appears to have opposing effects on different sets of cells: T-cells are suppressed, and B-cells are stimulated. Estradiol treatment suppressed cutaneous delayed-type hypersensitivity, but serum immunoglobulin concentrations and anti-DNA antibodies were stimulated (31).

Testosterone clearly suppresses autoimmune disease in NZB × NZW mice of both sexes. Earlier studies of the mechanism of androgenic suppression suggested that effects were limited to T cells. Testosterone increased T-suppressor-cell activity (63), and did not affect CD5+ B cells (64) or responses to a thymic-dependent antigen (16) in the NZB × NZW model. More recently, detailed studies of nonautoimmune C57BL/6 mice have demonstrated that surgical removal of the testes is followed by profound changes in B cells and T cells. This reordering of the immune system could explain some aspects of acceleration of autoimmune disease in NZB × NZW male castrates. Surgical castration of male C57BL/6 mice at 6 weeks of age was followed by thymic hypertrophy, splenic enlargement due to expansion of B cells, and decreased numbers of splenic T cells. Spleen cells had increased production of IL-2 and IFN-γ, and antithyroglobulin antibodies and rheumatoid factor production increased (65). B220+ B cells expanded in the bone marrow following castration of C57BL/6 males. However, three subcutaneous injections of testosterone cypionate, 1 mg, or dihydrotestosterone, 0.2 or 0.4 mg, reversed this effect (66).

Experimental Hormone Therapy for Murine Lupus

The observation that estrogen stimulated disease in autoimmune mice led to attempts to control lupus activity with antiestrogens. The aromatase inhibitor 4-hydroxyandrostenedione inhibits estrogen biosynthesis. Treatment of female NZB × NZW mice from 11.5 to 15 weeks of age reduced thymus weights and appeared to retard glomerular inflammation (67). A classic estrogen receptor blocker was highly effective in treating lupus in NZB × NZW females. Tamoxifen, 22 mg/kg body weight, was injected at 2-week intervals and the mice were sacrificed after 5 months of treatment. Beneficial results of treatment were decreased percentages of B cells and CD5+ B cells, decreased serum tumor necrosis factor (TNF) receptor molecules, and decreased immune complex deposition in the kidney (68).

Androgens are beneficial in murine models, and testosterone and 5-dihydrotestosterone produced favorable responses in NZB × NZW (23,41,42) and MRL-*lpr* mice (46–48). Female NZB × NZW mice benefited from long-term intraperitoneal injections of DHEA, 100 μg twice a week, if the injections were started at 2 months of age (before the expected appearance of overt disease). Anti-dsDNA was suppressed and mean longevity was prolonged, so that 71% of treated mice were alive at 41 weeks of age compared to 22% of control mice. DHEA treatment that was started at 6 months of age, after the expected appearance of autoimmune disease, was not effective (43). NZB × NZW females and castrated males also responded favorably to injections of nandrolone decanoate, an androgen with attenuated virilizing properties. Proteinuria and anti-DNA were suppressed, and treatment was effective even if it was begun after disease onset (69,70). The 19-nor-testosterone derivatives norethindrone and norgestrel are progestogens that are used commonly as contraceptives. Each compound was implanted separately in 6-week-old and 24-week-old NZB × NZW females in relatively small doses that were calibrated to suppress reproduction (71). Both progestogens suppressed anti-DNA antibodies, and mice that were implanted with norgestrel at the age of 24 weeks had prolongation of life spans (72).

Sexual Difference in Incidence of SLE in Humans

Hormonal and nonhormonal factors that predispose to the increased incidence of SLE in women have been the subject of several reviews (73–76). Human SLE clearly has a predilection for females of child-bearing age (77) and may appear or exacerbate when serum concentrations of reproductive hormones are elevated and when hormones are undergoing rapid change. In the era before corticosteroids were used to treat SLE, improvement was noted after some women reached menopause, had surgical removal of the uterus and ovaries, or were treated with testosterone. Irradiation of the ovaries, however, did not change the course of disease (78). Signs and symptoms of active lupus have been reported to increase in the 2-week period before onset of the menstrual period (79).

The theory that SLE activity is influenced by reproductive hormones is supported by the finding that disease flares are increased during pregnancy in women with SLE (80–83). The possibility that pregnancy activates lupus has been debated (84). Nevertheless, pregnant SLE patients at the Hopkins Lupus Pregnancy Center had a rate of lupus flares that was significantly higher compared to the same patients after delivery and nonpregnant SLE patients (83). Increased flares during pregnancy have also been observed at the St. Thomas' Lupus Pregnancy Clinic (85). Th1 cytokines, including IL-2, IFN-γ, and TNF-β, are deleterious during pregnancy and may lead to fetal demise. It has therefore been proposed that a shift away from Th1 responses and toward predominant Th2 responses occurs during normal pregnancy and is important in maintaining the intact fetal-maternal unit (86). Are reproductive hormones involved in this shift? Estrogen has the potential to stimulate both Th1 and Th2 responses (54,55). It is of interest to speculate that estrogen in high concentrations, or estrogen acting in concert with other reproductive hormones, can stimulate increased Th2 cytokines. This response would be desirable during a normal pregnancy. In the patient with SLE, excessive Th2 responses could cause increased production of antibodies and lead to activation of disease (87).

Responses of Peripheral Blood Mononuclear Cells to Estrogen in SLE

Peripheral blood mononuclear cells (PBMCs) from patients with SLE have abnormal responses to estrogen stimulation. *In vitro* apoptosis was decreased when lupus patients' PBMCs were cultured with estrogen, a response that could permit abnormal cells to survive and perpetuate autoimmune responses (88). Culturing lupus PBMCs with estradiol-17β enhanced production of IgG anti-dsDNA antibodies. Adding estradiol and exogenous IL-10 to the cultures increased antibody production in the SLE patients' B cells (89).

Estrogen Receptors

Variations in estrogen receptors have been identified in patients with lupus. Normal individuals were found to have both wild-type receptors and an isoform that lacks exon V. In contrast, SLE patients had either the wild type or the truncated form of the receptor. It was suggested that the presence of mutated or differentially spliced forms of estrogen receptor accounted for abnormal responses to estrogen in SLE (90). Calcineurin is an enzyme that participates in T-cell signal transduction and has the potential to promote activation of IL-2 and other cytokine genes. Calcineurin may serve as a link between estrogen and the immune system in lupus. It has been shown that calcineurin messenger RNA (mRNA) expression is increased in response to estradiol in cultured T cells from SLE patients. This effect was independent of medications used to treat SLE (91).

Oral Contraceptives and Postmenopausal Estrogen Replacement

The importance of estrogens in stimulating flares in patients with preexisting SLE was established in the 1960s and 1970s, when oral contraceptives commonly contained high doses of synthetic estrogens. Pimstone (92) and Chapel and Burns (93) reported flares of lupus in patients taking combination pills that contained 50 μg ethinyl estradiol and 100 μg mestranol, respectively.

Other reports documented the initial appearance of autoantibodies and overt SLE in women taking high-estrogen oral contraceptives (94–96). In contrast, other investigators have reported that rheumatic symptoms did not develop in patients taking oral contraceptives (97,98). The current use of small doses of synthetic estrogens in oral contraceptives probably accounts for the apparent decrease in lupus-like side effects. In patients in metropolitan Philadelphia, oral contraceptives were not associated with the appearance of SLE in patients who were diagnosed between 1985 and 1987 (99). However, Sanchez-Guerrero et al. (100) described a prospective cohort study of women in the Nurses' Health Study who were followed every 2 years between 1976 and 1990. When women who had used oral contraceptives were compared with those who never used oral contraceptives, the relative risk for developing SLE, applying a stringent case definition of SLE, was 1.9. It was concluded that past use of oral contraceptives was associated with a small absolute risk for developing SLE.

Postmenopausal estrogen replacement has been associated with flares of SLE. A case has been reported in which a patient with lupus had remission when she became menopausal at 38 years of age. The disease recurred when she was treated with estrogen for osteoporosis at 64 years of age (101). In contrast, two studies of relatively small groups of SLE patients were reassuring. There were no lupus flares associated with conventional hormone replacement (102,103).

It has been suggested that women taking postmenopausal estrogen replacement could be at increased risk to develop SLE. The Nurses' Health Study showed that women who had taken hormone replacement had an increased risk of *de novo* SLE, and the risk was related to duration of therapy (104). In a case-control study, women who used postmenopausal estrogens for 2 years or longer were at risk to develop both discoid lupus and SLE (105).

Abnormal Sex Hormone Levels in SLE

Gonadal hormones are abnormal in SLE. In women with SLE, levels of circulating 16-hydroxyestrone and estriol were increased significantly compared with normal women. The 16-metabolites are potent estrogens that have the potential to stimulate lupus through sustained estrogenic activity (106,107). Women with lupus also have low plasma androgens. Very low levels of circulating androgens have been described in women with active SLE (108). This abnormality could result from increased testosterone oxidation at C-17 or increased tissue aromatase activity (109–111).

Sex hormones have been studied extensively in men with SLE. Imbalances in estrogens and androgens have been reported that could contribute to increased susceptibility to active disease. Estradiol levels were reported to be increased (112,113), normal (114), or low (115) in male patients with SLE. Males with lupus had elevated serum 16-hydroxyestrone (106,110) and estrone (115) concentrations. Some men with SLE have a state of functional hypoandrogenism, with low levels of plasma testosterone (114,115) and elevated LH (116).

PROLACTIN

Prolactin, a peptide hormone secreted in the anterior pituitary, has the potential to stimulate the immune system and has been implicated as a factor that can activate SLE (117). Prolactin is also produced in sites outside the pituitary, including the brain and lymphocytes (118). Prolactin is a cytokine. It has comparable structural motifs, is synthesized in multiple sites including lymphocytes, and has similar receptor structures and signal transduction pathways. Prolactin receptors are distributed throughout the immune system (119) and are included in a novel receptor family that includes receptors for IL-2β, IL-3, IL-4, and IL-6 (120). Prolactin can influence the immune system through the thymus (121), by inducing IL-2 receptors on lymphocytes (122), and by acting as a growth factor for lymphocytes.

Lymphocytes synthesize and release a biologically active form of prolactin (123) that is employed by the cells as an autocrine and paracrine growth factor. It is possible that treatment with corticosteroids affects lymphocyte production of prolactin. Dexamethasone reduces circulating prolactin concentrations and inhibits gene expression of both pituitary prolactin and lymphocyte prolactin (119).

In rodents, prolactin affects the immune system at almost every level and influences T cells, B cells, macrophages, and natural killer cells (124,125). Prolactin is important in maintaining normal immune function and sustaining life. Rats that were deprived completely of prolactin by hypophysectomy and injections of antiprolactin antibody became anergic and anemic and died within 8 weeks. Replacement injections of either prolactin or growth hormone stimulated expression of the c-*myc* growth-promoting gene and reversed involution of the spleen and thymus (126).

High levels of circulating prolactin stimulate immune responses. Hyperprolactinemia that was created in mice by either implanting syngeneic pituitary glands or injecting exogenous prolactin increased primary humoral antibody responses (127), and low levels of prolactin in cysteamine-treated mice were associated with thymic atrophy and immune suppression (128).

Th1 cytokines are involved in initiating autoimmunity, and Th2 cytokines contribute to production of antibodies by B cells. The transcription factor gene, interferon regulatory factor-1 (IRF-1), which is exquisitely sensitive to prolactin, is an important regulator of T cell and B cell differentiation and maturation. IRF-1 is required for Th1 immune responses. Prolactin, which stimulates IRF-1, has the potential to regulate expression of Th1 cytokines such as IFN-γ and IL-15 (125). The potential of IRF-1 to promote autoimmunity was demonstrated when type II collagen-induced arthritis was induced in mice that were either IRF-1 deficient (–/–) or IRF-1 positive (+/–). Disease was reduced in the IRF-1 –/– mice compared to the +/– mice (129).

Estrogen is a potent stimulus for production of pituitary prolactin in rodents, and estrogen stimulates autoimmunity in the NZB × NZW lupus model. Female NZB × NZW mice treated with either ethinyl estradiol or estradiol-17β developed pituitary adenomas and serum prolactin levels that were up to 91 times greater than controls (26). This secondary elevation of prolactin could contribute to the apparent stimulation of autoimmune disease that has been attributed to estrogen.

Hyperprolactinemia in NZB × NZW mice resulted in premature death from autoimmune renal disease. Female NZB × NZW mice were made chronically hyperprolactinemic by grafts of two syngeneic pituitary glands and developed premature glomerulonephritis and early mortality. In contrast, mice treated with the prolactin-lowering drug bromocriptine had delayed appearance of antibodies to dsDNA and significantly prolonged life spans (130). Neidhart (131) treated mature NZB × NZW females from the age of 36 weeks with a dose of bromocriptine (5 mg/kg/day) that suppressed serum prolactin to undetectable levels. After 12 weeks of treatment, autoantibodies were not suppressed in mice that received bromocriptine, but bromocriptine did suppress the occurrence of proteinuria. No mice treated with bromocriptine had histologic evidence of glomerulonephritis, but glomerulonephritis was found in 70% of the control animals.

The effects of very high levels of prolactin were examined in a group of NZB × NZW females that had four transplanted pituitary glands. Twelve weeks after the pituitary glands were implanted, 80% of recipient mice had antibodies to dsDNA and hypergammaglobulinemia (132). Male NZB × NZW mice, which develop an indolent form of SLE, responded to hyperprolactinemia with accelerated disease (124). Another study determined that naturally occurring hyperprolactinemia was detrimental in parous NZB × NZW mice after whelping and suckling two litters, or after experiencing prolonged pseudopregnancy (133). Elbourne et al. (134) found that NZB × NZW mice with high circulating estrogen and high serum prolactin had accelerated albuminuria and premature appearance of antibodies to DNA (75% positive at 16 weeks of age). In contrast, autoimmune disease was retarded in females with high estrogen levels that were treated with bromocriptine. These mice had delayed appearance of albuminuria and antibodies to DNA (10% positive at 16 weeks of age).

Disease-associated autoantibodies have been detected in hyperprolactinemic individuals who did not have clinically apparent autoimmune diseases. Women with prolactinomas had antimicrosomal antibodies and antithyroglobulin, each occurring in 21% of subjects. Antithyroglobulin antibodies were found in 19% of hyperprolactinemic men (135). In another survey of 33 women, 82% of whom had pituitary adenomas, antibodies to at least one autoantigen were detected in 76% and eight subjects had seven or more different autoantibodies. The most common antibody targets were single-stranded DNA (ssDNA) and dsDNA, Sm, pyruvate dehydrogenase, and SSA/Ro. The subjects did not have clinical evidence of autoimmune disease (136). Anticardiolipin antibodies were found in 22% of hyperprolactinemic women and men (137).

Many surveys have shown that hyperprolactinemia is increased in SLE patients. Prolactin concentrations above the norm were found in 12% of serum samples that were submitted for antinuclear antibody testing. High prolactin was most common in women 50 years of age or younger who were diagnosed with SLE and in women over the age of 50 who had antibodies to both SSA/Ro and SSB/La. The expected incidence of hyperprolactinemia was 1.3% (138).

Eight men with SLE had serum prolactin above the mean (139), and five pregnant SLE patients had prolactin values that were greater than expected during gestation (140). In eight additional groups, 15.9% to 40% of patients with SLE had hyperprolactinemia (141–148). In other surveys, prolactin was not elevated in SLE. Ostendorf et al. (149) found that 2% of women with SLE had elevated serum prolactin, and Munoz et al. (150) reported low levels of prolactin in women with SLE during the luteal phase.

Prolactin is not consistently elevated in patients with active lupus. Five reports described positive associations between hyperprolactinemia and clinical or serologic evidence of active SLE (140,141,143,146,150). Miranda et al. (151) classified 26 SLE patients as having mild, moderate, or severely active lupus glomerulonephritis. Those with severe renal disease activity had mean serum prolactin (24.7 ng/mL) that significantly exceeded the mean value of 18.6 ng/mL in patients with mild renal disease activity. In four series, serum prolactin concentrations were not related to activity of lupus disease (142,144,145,147).

Why is serum prolactin elevated in some patients with SLE? Some lupus patients have prolactinomas (152) and others have secondary hyperprolactinemia caused by drugs, hypothyroidism, or renal insufficiency (138,148). Lymphocytes from SLE patients actively secrete prolactin (153), but it is not known if measurable prolactin of lymphocyte origin circulates in these individuals. Antiprolactin antibodies have been identified in SLE patients with idiopathic hyperprolactinemia. The relationship between the antibodies and elevated prolactin has not been explained fully. It is possible that antiprolactin activity interferes with attachment of prolactin to receptors, so that a "false low" level of prolactin is presented to the pituitary, and feedback mechanisms involved in regulation of prolactin secretion are disrupted (148). It is also possible that delayed clearance of prolactin-IgG complexes explains increased serum levels of prolactin in SLE patients with anti-prolactin antibodies (154). The association between inactive SLE and low levels of circulating homovanillic acid suggests that impaired dopamine turnover and altered dopaminergic tone results in hyperprolactinemia (155). Circulating cytokines that cross the blood–brain barrier in SLE may also stimulate the anterior pituitary to release excessive prolactin (124).

Suppression of circulating prolactin with bromocriptine has been reported to control symptoms in patients with SLE (156–158). Seven lupus patients with mild to moderately active disease, six of whom had normal prolactin concentrations before treatment, responded to bromocriptine. After 6 months, bromocriptine was stopped and five patients became hyperprolactinemic. All seven patients had increased lupus disease activity in the 5 months after treatment was discontinued (156). The double-blind study of Alvarez-Nemegyei et al. (157) showed the potential for daily treatment with a fixed dose of bromocriptine (2.5 mg/day) to reduce lupus flares. In a more recent study, patients with active but not life-threatening SLE were randomized to receive either bromocriptine, in a dose designed to suppress serum prolactin to a concentration <1 ng/mL, or hydroxychloroquine, 6 mg/kg. Treatment continued for 1 year. In 11 patients who received bromocriptine, the SLE Activity Measure (SLAM) (7) decreased from 14.0 ± 1.1 (mean ± standard error of the mean) at entry to 7.5 ± 0.8 (p <.05) after 1 year of treatment. In 13 SLE patients who received hydroxychloroquine, the mean SLAM score decreased from 13.4 ± 1.3 at entry to 9.0 ± 1.4 (p <.001) posttreatment. Prednisone doses, the numbers of patients who started and stopped prednisone, and numbers of patients who left the study were similar in both treatment groups (158).

GONADOTROPIN-RELEASING HORMONE

The potential importance of FSH and LH in modulating immune responses and disease activity in SLE was confirmed by the immune-stimulating affects of gonadotropin-releasing hormone (GnRH), which is also known as luteinizing hormone–releasing hormone. GnRH regulates the release of LH and FSH and has the potential to affect the immune system and to modulate disease activity in SLE (117). GnRH receptor mRNA is expressed in lymphocytes.

In rodents, GnRH stimulates expression of the IL-2 receptor, proliferation of T cells and B cells, IFN-γ, and serum IgG. GnRH receptor mRNA is expressed in human, rat, and murine immune cells, and binding studies have confirmed the presence of the receptor in whole spleens and thymuses of rats and mice. In the SWR×NZB F1 hybrid model of SLE, treatment with GnRH antagonists ameliorated autoantibody levels and renal disease and increased survival. Improvement did not depend on changes in gonadal hormones, and was not altered in males and females, gonadectomized mice, or in mice treated with estradiol (159–164).

REFERENCES

1. Grossman CJ. Regulation of the immune system by sex steroids. *Endocr Rev* 1984;5:435–455.
2. Besedovsky HO, del Rey A. Immune-neuro-endocrine interactions: facts and hypotheses. *Endocr Rev* 1996;17:64–102.
3. Dardenne M. Role of thymic peptides as transmitters between the neuroendocrine and immune systems. *Ann Med* 1999;31 (suppl 2):34–39.
4. Lintern-Moore S, Pantelouris EM. Ovarian development in athymic nude mice. I. The size and composition of the follicle population. *Mech Ageing Dev* 1975;4:385–390.
5. Rebar RW, Morandini IC, Erickson GF, et al. The hormonal basis of reproductive defects in athymic mice: diminished gonadotropin concentrations in prepubertal females. *Endocrinology* 1981;108:120–126.
6. Kosiewicz MM, Michael SD. Neonatal thymectomy affects follicle populations before the onset of autoimmune oophoritis in B6A mice. *J Reprod Fertil* 1990;88:427–440.
7. Smith H, Sakamoto Y, Kasai K, et al. Effector and regulatory cells in autoimmune oophoritis elicited by neonatal thymectomy. *J Immunol* 1991;147:2928–2933.
8. Sakakura T, Nishizuka Y. Thymic control mechanism in ovarian development: reconstitution of ovarian dysgenesis in thymectomized mice by replacement with thymic and other lymphoid tissues. *Endocrinology* 1972;90:431–437.
9. Sobhon P, Jirasattham C. Effect of sex hormones on the thymus and lymphoid tissue of ovariectomized rats. *Acta Anat* 1974; 89:211–225.
10. Seiki K, Sakabe K. Sex hormones and the thymus in relation to thymocyte proliferation and maturation. *Arch Histol Cytol (Niigata)* 1997;60:29–38.
11. Savino W, Bartoccioni E, Homo-Delarche F, et al. Thymic hormone containing cells. IX. Steroids in vitro modulate thymulin secretion by human and murine thymic epithelial cells. *J Steroid Biochem* 1988;30:479–484.
12. Erbach GT, Bahr JM. Enhancement of in vivo humoral immunity by estrogen: permissive effect of a thymic factor. *Endocrinology* 1991;128:1352–1358.
13. Chapman JC, Griffin WJ, Vassalo MF, et al. The ovarian dysgenesis normally induced by neonatal thymectomy is prevented by the prior administration of estrogen. *Am J Reprod Immunol* 1995;34:195–199.
14. Andrews BS, Eisenberg RA, Theofilopoulos AN, et al. Spontaneous murine lupus-like syndromes. Clinical and immunopathological manifestations in several strains. *J Exp Med* 1978; 148:1198–1215.
15. Roubinian J, Talal N, Siiteri PK, et al. Sex hormone modulation of autoimmunity in NZB/NZW mice. *Arthritis Rheum* 1979; 22:1162–1169.
16. Brick JE, Wilson DA, Walker SE. Hormonal modulation of responses to thymus-independent and thymus-dependent antigens in autoimmune NZB/W mice. *J Immunol* 1985;134: 3693–3698.
17. Walker SE, Besch-Williford CL, Keisler DH. Accelerated deaths from systemic lupus erythematosus in NZB × NZW F1 mice treated with the testosterone-blocking drug flutamide. *J Lab Clin Med* 1994;124:401–407.
18. Baer AN, Green FA. Estrogen metabolism in the (New Zealand black × New Zealand white) F1 murine model of systemic lupus erythematosus. *Arthritis Rheum* 1990;33:107–112.
19. Walker SE, Bole GG Jr. Influence of natural and synthetic estrogens on the course of autoimmune disease in the NZB/NZW mouse. *Arthritis Rheum* 1973;16:231–239.
20. Roubinian JR, Talal N, Greenspan JS, et al. Effect of castration and sex hormone treatment on survival, anti-nucleic acid antibodies, and glomerulonephritis in NZB/NZW F1 mice. *J Exp Med* 1978;147:1568–1583.
21. Steinberg AD, Melez KA, Raveche ES, et al. Approach to the study of the role of sex hormones in autoimmunity. *Arthritis Rheum* 1979;22:1170–1176.
22. Siiteri PK, Jones LA, Roubinian J, et al. Sex steroid and the immune system. I. Sex difference in autoimmune disease in NZB/NZW hybrid mice. *J Steroid Biochem* 1980;12:425–432.
23. Melez KA, Reeves JP, Steinberg AD. Modification of murine lupus by sex hormones. *Ann Immunol (Paris)* 1978;129C: 707–714.
24. McMurray RW, Keisler D, Izui S, et al. Effects of parturition, suckling and pseudopregnancy on variables of disease activity in the B/W mouse model of systemic lupus erythematosus. *J Rheumatol* 1993;20:1143–1151.
25. Castor R, Walker SE. The course of autoimmune disease in parous NZB/NZW mice. *J Comp Pathol* 1977;87:35–42.
26. Walker SE, McMurray RW, Besch-Williford CL, et al. Premature death with bladder outlet obstruction and hyperprolactinemia in New Zealand black × New Zealand white mice treated with ethinyl estradiol and 17 beta-estradiol. *Arthritis Rheum* 1992;35;1387–1392.
27. Carlsten H, Holmdahl R, Tarkowski A, et al. Oestradiol- and testosterone-mediated effects on the immune system in normal and autoimmune mice are genetically linked and inherited as dominant traits. *Immunology* 1989;68:209–214.
28. Verheul HA, Verveld M, Hoefakker S, et al. Effects of ethinylestradiol on the course of spontaneous autoimmune disease in NZB/W and NOD mice. *Immunopharmacol Immunotoxicol* 1995;17:163–180.
29. Carlsten H, Tarkowski A. Histocompatibility complex gene products and exposure to oestrogen: two independent disease accelerating factors in murine lupus. *Scand J Immunol* 1993; 83:341–347.
30. Ratkay LG, Zhang D, Tonzetich J, et al. Evaluation of a model for post-partum arthritis and the role of oestrogen in prevention of MRL/*lpr* associated rheumatic conditions. *Clin Exp Immunol* 1994;98:52–59.
31. Carlsten H, Tarkowski A, Holmdahl R. Oestrogen is a potent disease accelerator in SLE-prone MRL lpr/lpr mice. *Clin Exp Immunol* 1990;80:467–473.
32. Apelgren LD, Bailey DL, Fouts RL, et al. The effect of a selective estrogen receptor modulator on the progression of spontaneous autoimmune disease in MRL *lpr/lpr* mice. *Cell Immunol* 1996;173:55–63.
33. Hayashi Y, Utsuyama M, Kurashima C, et al. Spontaneous development of organ-specific autoimmune lesions in aged C57BL/6 mice. *Clin Exp Immunol* 1989;78:120–126.
34. Verthelyi D, Ansar Ahmed S. 17-beta estradiol, but not 5-alpha-dihydrotestosterone, augments antibodies to double-

stranded deoxyribonucleic acid in nonautoimmune C57BL/6J mice. *Endocrinology* 1994;135:2615–2622.
35. Verthelyi DI, Ansar Ahmed S. Estrogen increases the number of plasma cells and enhances their autoantibody production in nonautoimmune C57BL/6 mice. *Cell Immunol* 1998;189: 125–134.
36. Morel L, Mohan C, Yu Y, et al. Multiplex inheritance of component phenotypes in a murine model of lupus. *Mamm Genome* 1999;10:176–181.
37. Mohan C, Morel L, Yang P, et al. Genetic dissection of lupus pathogenesis: a recipe for nephrophilic autoantibodies. *J Clin Invest* 1999;103:1685–1695.
38. Van Griensven M, Bergijk EC, Baelde JJ, et al. Differential effects of sex hormones on autoantibody production and proteinuria in chronic graft-versus-host disease-induced experimental lupus nephritis. *Clin Exp Immunol* 1997;107:254–260.
39. Blank M, Mendlovic S, Fricke H, et al. Sex hormone involvement in the induction of experimental systemic lupus erythematosus by a pathogenic anti-DNA idiotype in naive mice. *J Rheumatol* 1990;17:311–317.
40. Dayan M, Zinger H, Kalush F, et al. The beneficial effects of treatment with tamoxifen and anti-oestradiol antibody on experimental systemic lupus erythematosus are associated with cytokine modulations. *Immunology* 1997;90:101–108.
41. Roubinian JR, Papoian R, Talal N. Androgenic hormones modulate autoantibody responses and improve survival in murine lupus. *J Clin Invest* 1977;59:1066–1070.
42. Michalski JP, McCombs CC, Roubinian JR, et al. Effect of androgen therapy on survival and suppressor cell activity in aged NZB/NZW F1 hybrid mice. *Clin Exp Immunol* 1983;52: 229–233.
43. Norton SD, Harrison LL, Yowell R, et al. Administration of dehydroepiandrosterone sulfate retards onset but not progression of autoimmune disease in NZB/W mice. *Autoimmunity* 1997;26;161–171.
44. Yang BC, Lui CW, Chen YC, et al. Exogenous dehydroepiandrosterone modified the expression of T helper-related cytokines in NZB/NZW F1 mice. *Immunol Invest* 1998;27: 291–302.
45. Melez KA, Deleargyros N, Bellanti JA, et al. Effect of partial testosterone replacement or thymosin on anti-DNA in castrated (NZB × NZW) F1 males. *Clin Immunol Immunopathol* 1987; 42:319–327.
46. Shear HL, Wofsy D, Talal N. Effects of castration and sex hormones on immune clearance and autoimmune disease in MRL/Mp-lpr/lpr and MRL/Mp-+/+ mice. *Clin Immunol Immunopathol* 1983;26:361–369.
47. Steinberg AD, Roths JB, Murphy ED, et al. Effects of thymectomy or androgen administration upon the autoimmune disease of MRL/Mp-lpr/lpr mice. *J Immunol* 1980;125:871–873.
48. Ariga H, Edwards J, Sullivan DA. Androgen control of autoimmune expression in lacrimal glands of MRL/Mp-lpr/lpr mice. *Clin Immunol Immunopathol* 1989;53:499–508.
49. Toda I, Sullivan BD, Rocha EM, et al. Impact of gender on exocrine gland inflammation in mouse models of Sjogren's syndrome. *Exp Eye Res* 1999;69:355–366.
50. Ansar Ahmed S, Aufdemorte TB, Chen J-R, et al. Estrogen induces the development of autoantibodies and promotes salivary gland lymphoid infiltrates in normal mice. *J Autoimmun* 1989;2:543–552.
51. Talal N, Dauphinee M, Ansar Ahmed S. CD5 B cells in autoimmunity. *Ann NY Acad Sci* 1992;651:551–556.
52. Keisler LW, vom Saal FS, Keisler DH, et al. Aberrant hormone balance in fetal autoimmune NZB/W mice following prenatal exposure to testosterone excess or the androgen blocker flutamide. *Biol Reprod* 1995;53:1190–1197.
53. Keisler LW, vom Saal FS, Keisler DH, et al. Hormonal manipulation of the prenatal environment alters reproductive morphology and increases longevity in autoimmune NZB/W mice. *Biol Reprod* 1991;44:707–716.
54. Sarvetnick N, Fox HS. Interferon-gamma and the sexual dimorphism of autoimmunity. *Mol Biol Med* 1990;7:323–331.
55. Wilder RL, Elenkov IJ. Hormonal regulation of tumor necrosis factor-alpha, interleukin-12 and interleukin-10 production by activated macrophages. A disease-modifying mechanism in rheumatoid arthritis and systemic lupus erythematosus? *Ann NY Acad Sci* 1999;876:14–31.
56. Sato MN, Minoprio P, Avrameas S, et al. Defects in the regulation of anti-DNA antibody production in aged lupus-prone (NZB × NZW) F1 mice: analysis of T-cell lymphokine synthesis. *Immunology* 1995;85:26–32.
57. McMurray RW, Hoffman RW, Nelson W, et al. Cytokine mRNA expression in the B/W mouse model of systemic lupus erythematosus—analyses of strain, gender, and age effects. *Clin Immunol Immunopathol* 1997;84:260–268.
58. Lin LC, Chen YC, Chou CC, et al. Dysregulation of T helper cell cytokines in autoimmune prone NZB × NZW F1 mice. *Scand J Immunol* 1995;42:466–472.
59. Ansar Ahmed S, Dauphinee MJ, Talal N. Effects of short-term administration of sex hormones in normal and autoimmune mice. *J Immunol* 1985;134:204–210.
60. Ansar Ahmed S, Dauphinee MJ, Montoya AI, et al. Estrogen induces normal murine CD5+B cells to produce autoantibodies. *J Immunol* 1989;142:2647–2653.
61. Talal N, Ansar Ahmed SA. Sex hormones, CD5+ (Ly1+) B-cells, and autoimmune diseases. *Isr J Med Sci* 1988;24:725–728.
62. Bynoe MS, Grimaldi CM, Diamond B. Estrogen up-regulates Bcl-2 and blocks tolerance induction of naive B cells. *Proc Natl Acad Sci USA* 2000;97:2703–2708.
63. Ansar Ahmed S, Dauphinee MJ, Talal N. Effects of short-term administration of sex hormones on normal and autoimmune mice. *J Immunol* 1985;134:204–210.
64. Hayakawa K, Hardy RR, Parks DR, et al. The Ly-1 B cell subpopulation in normal, immunodefective and autoimmune mice. *J Exp Med* 1983;157:202–218.
65. Viselli SM, Stanziale S, Shults K, et al. Castration alters peripheral immune function in normal male mice. *Immunology* 1995; 84:337–342.
66. Viselli SM Reese KR, Fan J, et al. Androgens alter B cell development in normal male mice. *Cell Immunol* 1997;182:99–104.
67. Greenstein BD, Dhaher YY, Bridges E de F, et al. Effects of an aromatase inhibitor on thymus and kidney and on oestrogen receptors in female MRL/MP-lpr/lpr mice. *Lupus* 1993;2: 221–225.
68. Wu WM, Lin BF, Su YC, et al. Tamoxifen decreases renal inflammation and alleviates disease severity in autoimmune NZB/W F1 mice. *Scand J Immunol* 2000;52:393–400.
69. Schuurs AHWM, Verheul HAM. Sex hormones and autoimmune disease. *Br J Rheumatol* 1989;28(suppl 1):59–61.
70. Verheul HAM, Deckers GHJ, Schuurs AHWM. Effects of nandrolone decanoate or testosterone decanoate on murine lupus: further evidence for a dissociation of autoimmunosuppressive and endocrine effects. *Immunopharmacology* 1986;11:93–99.
71. Keisler LW, Walker SE. Suppression of reproductive function in autoimmune NZB/W mice: effective doses of four contraceptive steroids. *Am J Reprod Immunol Microbiol* 1987;14: 115–121.
72. Keisler LW, Kier AB, Walker SE. Effects of prolonged administration of the 19-nor-testosterone derivatives norethindrone and norgestrel to female NZB/W mice: comparison with medroxyprogesterone and ethinyl estradiol. *Autoimmunity* 1991;9:21–32.

73. Isenberg DA. Systemic lupus erythematosus: Immunopathogenesis and the card game analogy. *J Rheumatol* 1997;24(suppl 48):62–66.
74. Cooper GS, Dooley MA, Treadwell EL, et al. Hormonal, environmental, and infectious risk factors for developing systemic lupus erythematosus. *Arthritis Rheum* 1998;41:1714–1724.
75. Lahita RG. The role of sex hormones in systemic lupus erythematosus. *Curr Opin Rheumatol* 1999;11:352–356.
76. Lockshin MD, Gabriel S, Zakeri Z, et al. Gender, biology and human disease: report of a conference. *Lupus* 1999;8:335–338.
77. McCarty DJ, Manzi S, Medsger TA Jr, et al. Incidence of systemic lupus erythematosus. Race and gender differences. *Arthritis Rheum* 1995;38:1260–1270.
78. Rose E, Pillsbury DM. Lupus erythematosus (erythematodes) and ovarian function: observations on a possible relationship, with report of 6 cases. *Ann Intern Med* 1944;21:1022–1034.
79. Steinberg AD, Steinberg BJ. Lupus disease activity associated with menstrual cycle. *J Rheumatol* 1985;12:816–817.
80. Mund A, Simson J, Rothfield N. Effect of pregnancy on course of systemic lupus erythematosus. *JAMA* 1963;183:917–920.
81. Jungers P, Dougados M, Pelissier C, et al. Lupus nephropathy and pregnancy: report of 104 cases in 36 patients. *Arch Intern Med* 1982;142:771–776.
82. Nossent HC, Swaak TJC. Systemic lupus erythematosus: VI. Analysis of the interrelationship with pregnancy. *J Rheumatol* 1990;17:771–776.
83. Petri M, Howard D, Repke J. Frequency of lupus flare in pregnancy. The Hopkins Lupus Pregnancy Center experience. *Arthritis Rheum* 1991;34:1538–1545.
84. Lockshin MD. Pregnancy does not cause systemic lupus erythematosus to worsen. *Arthritis Rheum* 1989;32:665–670.
85. Khamashta MA, Ruiz-Irastorza G, Hughes GRV. Systemic lupus erythematosus flares during pregnancy. *Rheum Dis Clin North Am* 1997;23:15–30.
86. Wegmann TG, Lin H, Guilbert L, et al. Bidirectional cytokine interactions in the maternal-fetal relationship: is successful pregnancy a TH2 phenomenon? *Immunol Today* 1993;14:353–356.
87. Ostensen M. Sex hormones and pregnancy in rheumatoid arthritis and systemic lupus erythematosus. *Ann NY Acad Sci* 1999;876:131–143.
88. Evans MJ, MacLaughlin S, Marvin RD, et al. Estrogen decreases *in vitro* apoptosis of peripheral blood mononuclear cells from women with normal menstrual cycles and decreases TNF-alpha production in SLE but not in normal cultures. *Clin Immunol Immunopathol* 1997;82:258–262.
89. Kanda N, Tsuchida T, Tamaki K. Estrogen enhancement of anti-double-stranded DNA antibody and immunoglobulin G production in peripheral blood mononuclear cells form patients with systemic lupus erythematosus. *Arthritis Rheum* 1999; 42:328–337.
90. Wilson KB, Evans M, Abdou NI. Presence of a variant form of the estrogen receptor in peripheral blood mononuclear cells from normal individuals and lupus patients. *J Reprod Immunol* 1996;31:199–208.
91. Rider V, Foster RT, Evans ME, et al. Gender differences in autoimmune diseases: estrogen increases calcineurin expression in systemic lupus erythematosus. *Clin Immunol Immunopathol* 1998;89:171–180.
92. Pimstone B. Systemic lupus erythematosus exacerbated by oral contraceptives. *S Afr J Obstet Gynecol* 1966;4:62–63.
93. Chapel TA, Burns RE. Oral contraceptives and exacerbation of lupus erythematosus. *Am J Obstet Gynecol* 1971;110:366–369.
94. Kay DR, Bole GG Jr, Ledger WJ. Antinuclear antibodies, rheumatoid factor, and C-reactive protein in the serum of normal women using oral contraceptives. *Arthritis Rheum* 1971;14: 239–248.
95. Schleicher EM. LE cells after oral contraceptives. *Lancet* 1968;1:821–822.
96. Garovich M, Agudelo C, Pisko E. Oral contraceptives and systemic lupus erythematosus. *Arthritis Rheum* 1980;23: 1396–1398.
97. McKenna CH, Weiman KC, Shulman LE. Oral contraceptives, rheumatic disease, and autoantibodies. *Arthritis Rheum* 1969;12:313–314(abst).
98. Tarzy BJ, Garcia CR, Wallach EE, et al. Rheumatic disease, abnormal serology, and oral contraceptives. *Lancet* 1972;2: 501–503.
99. Strom BL, Reidenberg MM, West S, et al. Shingles, allergies, family medical history, oral contraceptives, and other potential risk factors for systemic lupus erythematosus. *Am J Epidemiol* 1994;140;632–642.
100. Sanchez-Guerrero J, Karlson EW, Liang MH, et al. Past use of oral contraceptives and the risk of developing systemic lupus erythematosus. *Arthritis Rheum* 1997;40:804–808.
101. Barrett C, Neylon N, Snaith ML. Oestrogen-induced systemic lupus erythematosus. *Br J Rheumatol* 1986;25:300–301.
102. Arden NK, Lloyd ME, Spector TD, et al. Safety of hormone replacement therapy (HRT) in systemic lupus erythematosus (SLE). *Lupus* 1994;3:11–13.
103. Kreidstein SH, Urowitz MB, Gladmann DD, et al. Hormone replacement therapy in SLE. *Arthritis Rheum* 1995;38:S221 (abst).
104. Sanchez-Guerrero J, Liang MH, Karlson EW,et al. Postmenopausal estrogen therapy and the risk for developing systemic lupus erythematosus. *Ann Intern Med* 1995;122: 430–433.
105. Meier CR, Sturkenboom MCJM, Cohen AS, et al. Postmenopausal estrogen replacement therapy and the risk of developing systemic lupus erythematosus or discoid lupus. *J Rheumatol* 1998;25:1515–1519.
106. Lahita RG, Bradlow HL, Kunkel HG, et al. Alterations of estrogen metabolism in systemic lupus erythematosus. *Arthritis Rheum* 1979;22;1195–1198.
107. Lahita RG, Bradlow HL, Kunkel HG, et al. Increased 16–hydroxylation of estradiol in systemic lupus erythematosus. *J Clin Endocrinol Metab* 1981;53:174–178.
108. Jungers P, Nahoul K, Pelissier C, et al. Low plasma androgens in women with active or quiescent systemic lupus erythematosus. *Arthritis Rheum* 1982;25:454–457.
109. Lahita RG, Bradlow HL, Ginzler E, et al. Low plasma androgens in women with systemic lupus erythematosus. *Arthritis Rheum* 1987;30:241–248.
110. Lahita RG, Bradlow HL, Fishman J, et al. Abnormal estrogen and androgen metabolism in the human with systemic lupus erythematosus. *Am J Kidney Dis* 1982;2(suppl):206–211.
111. Folomeev M, Dougados M, Beaune J, et al. Plasma sex hormones and aromatase activity in tissues of patients with systemic lupus erythematosus. *Lupus* 1992;1:191–195.
112. Inman RD, Jovanovic L, Markenson JA, et al. Systemic lupus erythematosus in men. Genetic and endocrine features. *Arch Intern Med* 1982;142:1813–1815.
113. Miller MH, Urowitz MB, Gladman DD, et al. Systemic lupus erythematosus in males. *Medicine* 1983;62:327–334.
114. Mackworth-Young CG, Parke AL, Morely KD, et al. Sex hormones in male patients with systemic lupus erythematosus: a comparison with other disease groups. *Eur J Rheumatol Inflamm* 1983;6:228–232.
115. Lavalle C, Loyo E, Paniagua R, et al. A correlation study between prolactin and androgens in male patients with systemic lupus erythematosus. *J Rheumatol* 1987;14:268–272.
116. Sequeira JF, Keser G, Greenstein B, et al. Systemic lupus erythematosus: sex hormones in male patients. *Lupus* 1993;2:315–317.

117. Walker SE, Jacobson JD. Roles of prolactin and gonadotropin-releasing hormone in rheumatic diseases. *Rheum Dis Clin North Am* 2000;26:713–736.
118. Ben-Jonathan N, Mershon JL, Allen DL, et al. Extra pituitary prolactin: Distribution, regulation, functions, and clinical aspects. *Endocr Rev* 1996;17:639–669.
119. Weigent DA. Immunoregulatory properties of growth hormone and prolactin. *Pharm Ther* 1996;69:237–257.
120. Thoreau E, Petridou B, Kelly PA, et al. Structural symmetry of the extracellular domain of the cytokine/growth hormone/prolactin receptor family and interferon receptors revealed by hydrophobic cluster analysis. *FEBS Lett* 1991;282:26–31.
121. Dardenne M, Savino W, Gagnerault M-C, et al. Neuroendocrine control of thymic hormonal production. I. Prolactin stimulates *in vivo* and *in vitro* the production of thymulin by human and murine thymic epithelial cells. *Endocrinology* 1989; 125:3–12.
122. Mukherjee P, Mastro AM, Hymer WC. Prolactin induction of interleukin-2 receptors on rat splenic lymphocytes. *Endocrinology* 1990;126:88–94.
123. Montgomery DW, Shen GK, Ulrich ED, et al. Human thymocytes express a prolactin-like messenger ribonucleic acid and synthesize bioactive prolactin-like protein. *Endocrinology* 1992; 131:3019–3026.
124. Walker SE, McMurray RW, Houri JM, et al. Effects of prolactin in stimulating disease activity in systemic lupus erythematosus. *Proc NY Acad Sci* 1998;840:762–772.
125. Yu-Lee, L-Y. Molecular actions of prolactin in the immune system. *Proc Soc Exp Biol Med* 1997;215:35–52.
126. Berczi I, Nagy E, de Toledo SM, et al. Pituitary hormones regulate c-myc and DNA synthesis in lymphoid tissue. *J Immunol* 1991;146:2201–2206.
127. Cross RJ, Campbell JL, Roszman TL. Potentiation of antibody responsiveness after the transplantation of a syngeneic pituitary gland. *J Neuroimmunol* 1989;25:29–35.
128. Bryant, HU, Holaday, JW, Bernton, EW. Cysteamine produces dose-related bidirectional immunomodulatory effects in mice. *J Pharmacol Exp Ther* 1989;249:424–429.
129. Tada Y, Ho A, Matsuyama T, et al. Reduced incidence and severity of antigen-induced autoimmune diseases in mice lacking interferon regulatory factor-1. *J Exp Med* 1997;185: 231–238.
130. McMurray R, Keisler D, Kanuckel K, et al. Prolactin influences autoimmune disease activity in the female B/W mouse. *J Immunol* 1991;147:3780–3787.
131. Neidhart M. Bromocriptine has little direct effect on murine lymphocytes, the immunomodulatory effect being mediated by the suppression of prolactin secretion. *Biomed Pharmacother* 1997;51:118–125.
132. Walker SE, Allen SH, McMurray RW. Prolactin and autoimmune disease. *Trends Endocrinol Metab* 1993;4:147–151.
133. McMurray RW, Keisler D, Izui S, et al. Effects of parturition, suckling and pseudopregnancy on variables of disease activity in the B/W mouse model of systemic lupus erythematosus. *J Rheumatol* 1993;20:1143–1151.
134. Elbourne KB, Keisler D, McMurray RW. Differential effects of estrogen and prolactin on autoimmune disease in the NZB/NZW F1 mouse model of systemic lupus erythematosus. *Lupus* 1998;7:420–427.
135. Pontiroli AE, Falsetti L, Bottazzo G. Clinical, endocrine, roentgenographic, and immune characterization of hyperprolactinemic women. *Int J Fertil* 1987;32:81–85.
136. Buskila D, Berezin M, Gur H, et al. Autoantibody profile in the sera of women with hyperprolactinemia. *J Autoimmun* 1995; 8:415–424.
137. Toubi E, Gabriel D, Golan TD. High association between hyperprolactinemia and anticardiolipin antibodies (letter). *J Rheumatol* 1997;24:1451.
138. Allen SH, Sharp GC, Wang G, et al. Prolactin levels and antinuclear antibody profiles in women tested for connective tissue disease. *Lupus* 1996;5:37–41.
139. Lavalle C, Loyo E, Paniagua R, et al. Correlation study between prolactin and androgens in male patients with systemic lupus erythematosus. *J Rheumatol* 1987;14:268–272.
140. Jara-Quezada L, Graef A, Lavalle C. Prolactin and gonadal hormones during pregnancy in systemic lupus erythematosus. *J Rheumatol* 1991;18:349–353.
141. Jara LJ, Gomez-Sanchez C, Silveira LH, et al. Hyperprolactinemia in systemic lupus erythematosus: Association with disease activity. *Am J Med Sci* 1992;303:222–226.
142. Pauzner R, Urowitz MB, Gladman DD, et al. Prolactin in systemic lupus erythematosus. *J Rheumatol* 1994;21:2064–2067.
143. Neidhart M. Elevated serum prolactin or elevated prolactin/cortisol ratio are associated with autoimmune processes in systemic lupus erythematosus and other connective tissue diseases. *J Rheumatol* 1996;23:476–481.
144. Buskila D, Lorber M, Neumann L, et al. No correlation between prolactin levels and clinical activity in patients with systemic lupus erythematosus. *J Rheumatol* 1996;23:629–632.
145. Huang C-M, Chou C-T. Hyperprolactinemia in systemic lupus erythematosus. *Chin Med J (Taipei)* 1997;59:37–41.
146. Rovensky J, Jurankova E, Rauova L, et al. Relationship between endocrine, immune, and clinical variables in patients with systemic lupus erythematosus. *J Rheumatol* 1997;24:2330–2334.
147. Jimena P, Aguirre MA, Lopez-Curbelo A, et al. Prolactin levels in patients with systemic lupus erythematosus: a case controlled study. *Lupus* 1998;7:383–386.
148. Leanos A, Pascoe D, Fraga A, et al. Anti-prolactin autoantibodies in systemic lupus erythematosus patients with associated hyperprolactinemia. *Lupus* 1998;7:398–403.
149. Ostendorf B, Fischer R, Santen R, et al. Hyperprolactinemia in systemic lupus erythematosus. *Scand J Rheumatol* 1996;25: 97–102.
150. Munoz JA, Gil A, Lopez-Dupla JM, et al. Sex hormones in chronic systemic lupus erythematosus. Correlation with clinical and biological parameters. *Ann Med Intern* 1994;145:459–463.
151. Miranda JM, Prieto RE, Paniagua R, et al. Clinical significance of serum and urine prolactin levels in lupus glomerulonephritis. *Lupus* 1998;7:387–391.
152. McMurray RW, Allen SH, Braun AL, et al. Longstanding hyperprolactinemia associated with systemic lupus erythematosus: possible hormonal stimulation of an autoimmune disease. *J Rheumatol* 1994;21:843–850.
153. Gutierrez MA, Molina JF, Jara LJ, et al. Prolactin and systemic lupus erythematosus: prolactin secretion by SLE lymphocytes and proliferative (autocrine) activity. *Lupus* 1995;4:348–352.
154. Leanos-Miranda A, Chavez-Rueda A, Blanco-Favela F. Biologic activity and plasma clearance of prolactin-IgG complex in patients with systemic lupus erythematosus. *Arthritis Rheum* 2001;44:866–875.
155. Ferreira C, Paes M, Gouveia A, et al. Plasma homovanillic acid and prolactin in systemic lupus erythematosus. *Lupus* 1998;7: 392–397.
156. McMurray RW, Weidensaul D, Allen SH, et al. Efficacy of bromocriptine in an open label therapeutic trial for systemic lupus erythematosus. *J Rheumatol* 1995;22:2084–2091.
157. Alvarez-Nemegyei J, Cobarrubias-Cobos A, Escalante-Triay F, et al. Bromocriptine in systemic lupus erythematosus: a double-blind, randomized, placebo-controlled study. *Lupus* 1998;7: 414–419.
158. Walker SE, Reddy GH, Miller D, et al. Treatment of active systemic lupus erythematosus (SLE) with the prolactin (PRL) low-

ering drug, bromocriptine (BC): comparison with hydroxychloroquine (HC) in a randomized, blinded one-year study. *Arthritis Rheum* 1999;42:S282(abst).

159. Batticane N, Morale MC, Gallo F, et al. Luteinizing hormone-releasing hormone signaling at the lymphocyte involves stimulation of interleukin-2 receptor expression. *Endocrinology* 1991; 129:277–286.
160. Grasso G, Massai L, De Leo V, et al. The effect of LHRH and TRH on human interferon-γ production in vivo and in vitro. *Life Sci* 1998;62:2005–2014.
161. Jacobson JD, Ansari MA, Kinealy M, et al. Gender specific exacerbation of murine lupus by gonadotropin-releasing hormone: potential role of Gα9/11. *Endocrinology* 1999;140: 3429–3437.
162. Marchetti B, Guarcelo V, Morale MC, et al. Luteinizing hormone-releasing hormone (LHRH)agonist restoration of age-associated decline of thymus weight, thymic LHRH receptors, and thymocyte proliferative capacity. *Endocrinology* 1989;125: 1037–1045.
163. Morale MC, Batticane N, Bartoloni G, et al. Blockade of central and peripheral luteinizing hormone-releasing hormone (LHRH) receptors in neonatal rats with a potent LHRH-antagonist inhibits the morphofunctional development of the thymus and maturation of the cell-mediated and humoral immune responses. *Endocrinology* 1991;128:1073–1085.
164. Jacobson JD, Crofford LJ, Sun L, et al. Cyclical expression of GnRH and GnRH receptor mRNA in lymphoid organs. *Neuroendocrinology* 1998;67:117–125.

17

NEUROENDOCRINE IMMUNE INTERACTIONS: PRINCIPLES AND RELEVANCE TO SYSTEMIC LUPUS ERYTHEMATOSUS

ESTHER M. STERNBERG
HIRSH D. KOMAROW

GENERAL PRINCIPLES

A large body of animal and human studies provides evidence of communication between the immune system and the central nervous system (CNS), and of the importance of this communication in susceptibility to inflammatory disease (1–3). This chapter outlines the general principles of this communication, its hormonal and neuronal components, and the physiologic role that it plays in autoimmune/inflammatory disease; defines the afferent and efferent limbs of the communication in more detail; and provides evidence from animal and human studies that these mechanisms are operative in systemic lupus erythematosus (SLE).

The immune system and the CNS are the body's initial interface with the constant environmental perturbations that threaten the organism's homeostasis. These two systems are designed to recognize environmental perturbations and respond to them to re-establish homeostasis. Each system recognizes different kinds of foreign stimuli—chemical, antigenic, or infectious in the case of the immune system, and psychological or physical in the case of the CNS—but they use many of the same transducing systems to translate perturbing signals into stabilizing responses.

These transducing systems can be hormonal or neuronal. Thus, the cytokines of the immune system not only signal other immune cells, but also act as hormones to stimulate the CNS centers that control the stress response. In turn, the hormones of the stress response not only affect neuroendocrine glands, but also suppress and modulate the immune and inflammatory response (Fig. 17.1). The immune system can also signal the CNS via neuronal pathways, such as the vagus nerve, and the CNS can signal the immune system via sympathetic and peripheral neuronal pathways.

These multiple levels of communication between the immune system and the CNS represent an important physiologic mechanism for modulation of the intensity of immune and inflammatory responses, control of susceptibility, and resistance to inflammatory disease. Interruptions of this communication at any point and through any mechanism lead to enhanced susceptibility to or severity of inflammatory/autoimmune disease. Conversely, reconstitution of the communication reduces inflammatory disease. Thus, the degree of inflammation in response to a foreign stimulus depends not only on the nature of the stimulus, its potency, dose, route, and duration of exposure, but also on the intensity of the modulating neuroendocrine and neuronal responses (Fig. 17.2) This principle has important implications for understanding the effects of pharmacologic agents or stress on inflammatory disease. Drugs not primarily designed to affect inflammatory disease severity might alter its course, if they alter the communication between the immune system and the CNS. Similarly, these data provide a rationale and a potential mechanism for anecdotal evidence that "stress" can affect or precipitate autoimmune/inflammatory disease, since the hormones of the stress response that are activated by stress have a profound impact on immune/inflammatory responses.

DEFINITION OF THE NEUROENDOCRINE STRESS RESPONSE

The central anatomic component of the neuroendocrine stress response, the hypothalamus (Fig. 17.3) is located at the base of the brain adjacent to the third ventricle. It responds to a variety of incoming stimuli by synthesizing and secreting the neuropeptide corticotropin-releasing hormone (CRH)

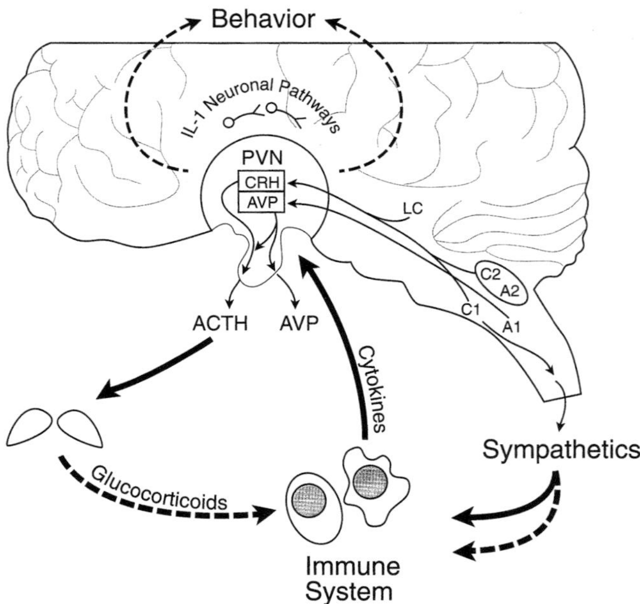

FIGURE 17.1. Schematic of the communication between the immune system and the central nervous system (CNS). Peripheral cytokines stimulate the hypothalamus to release corticotropin-releasing hormone (CRH) and the pituitary gland to release adrenocorticotropin (ACTH). Hypothalamic CRH stimulates ACTH release from the anterior pituitary, and arginine vasopressin (AVP) can act as a co-stimulator to ACTH release. In contrast, AVP released from the posterior pituitary plays a role in salt and water balance. Pituitary ACTH stimulates the adrenal glands to release glucocorticoids, which suppress inflammation, completing this counterregulatory feedback loop between the immune system and the CNS. Neural communications between the hypothalamus, the locus ceruleus, and brainstem noradrenergic nuclei (C1 and A1) stimulate the sympathetic nervous system, which also modulates local inflammation. Cytokines within the brain play a different role than peripheral cytokines, may activate the acute-phase response, and may play a role in neuronal cell death and survival. Cytokines and CRH also induce characteristic behavioral patterns.

(4) (Fig. 17.4). CRH secreted into the rich hypophyseal portal blood supply stimulates the anterior pituitary gland to secrete adrenocorticotropin (ACTH), which in turn stimulates the adrenal glands to secrete corticosteroids (5).

Hypothalamic CRH secretion is held under tight regulatory control by several positive and negative neurotransmitter systems. The noradrenergic, serotonergic, and dopaminergic systems all upregulate CRH, while the opiates γ-aminobutyric acid (GABA) and benzodiazepine as well as glucocorticoid feedback suppress hypothalamic CRH (6,7).

In addition to its neuroendocrine effects via the pituitary, CRH also acts centrally within the brain as a neuropeptide, to induce a characteristic set of behaviors characterized by cautious avoidance, vigilance, enhanced attention, and suppression of vegetative functions such as feeding and reproduction (8). Together this constellation of behaviors is known as the classic "fight or flight" response. Many of these effects are mediated through hypothalamic and extrahypothalamic CRH and through interactions of

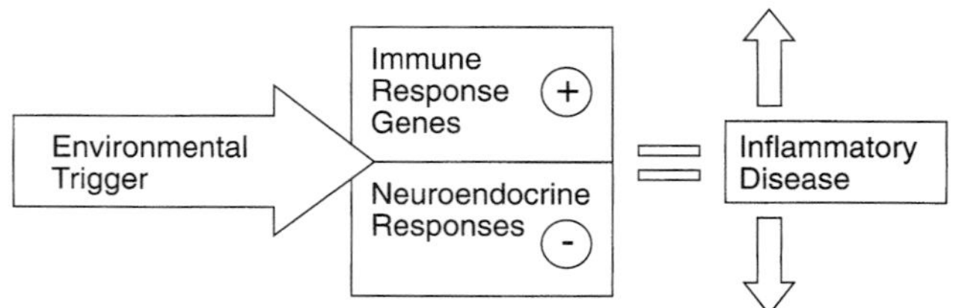

FIGURE 17.2. The degree of inflammation depends on a balance between the characteristics of the proinflammatory environmental stimulus, the host's immune/inflammatory responses, and modulating neuroendocrine responses. (Adapted from Sternberg and Wilder. The role of the hypothalmic-pituitary-adrenal axis in an experimental model of arthritis. *Prog Neuro Endocrin Immunology* 1989;2, with permission.)

these centers with other neurotransmitter systems, such as the brainstem noradrenergic system and the sympathetic nervous system (9–11).

The hypothalamic CRH system communicates with the major noradrenergic pathways also activated during the stress response, via anatomic connections between the hypothalamus and the noradrenergic centers in the brainstem (12) (Fig. 17.3). In turn, the brainstem noradrenergic system sends signals to the periphery via the sympathetic nerves. Through such connections, the physiologic components of the stress response, such as increased heart rate, muscle tone, and sweating, are coordinated with behavioral responses, to form the generalized stress response. Recent studies indicate that the modulation of immune responses

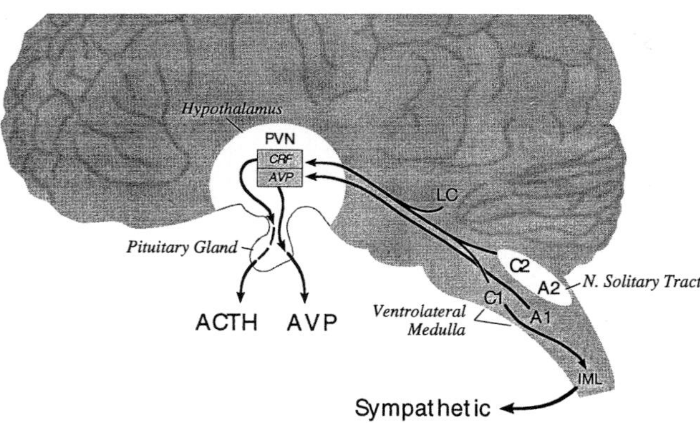

FIGURE 17.3. Anatomic cross-section of brain, including the hypothalamus, pituitary, and brain stem. Corticotropin-releasing factor (CRF), also called CRH, is synthesized in the paraventricular nucleus (PVN) of the hypothalamus, where AVP also is synthesized. These two neuropeptides, released into the vascular system of the median eminence, synergize to stimulate secretion of ACTH from the anterior pituitary gland. AVP from the magnocellular region of the hypothalamus also is secreted from nerve terminals that end in the posterior pituitary gland. Brainstem noradrenergic regions, including the locus ceruleus (LC) and the C1 and C2 and A1 and A2 neurons in the ventrolateral medulla, communicate with the hypothalamic CRH system and the peripheral sympathetic system. The nucleus of the solitary tract [also called nucleus tractus solitarius (NTS)] is a central switching area for the vagus nerve. IML, intermediolateral cell column. (Courtesy of Paul Sawchenko, Salk Institute, San Diego, CA.)

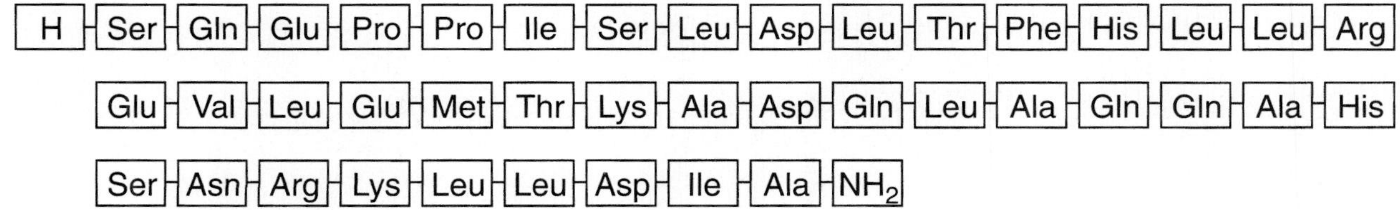

FIGURE 17.4. Peptide structure of CRH. (Adapted from Vale W, Spiess J, Rivier C, et al. Characterization of a 41-residue ovine hypothalamic peptide that stimulates secretion of corticotropin and beta-endorphin. *Science* 1981;213(4514):1394–1397, with permission.)

by both the sympathetic and neuroendocrine systems is also an important physiologic component of the stress response (10,13,14).

AFFERENT LIMB STIMULATION OF THE CNS BY SIGNALS FROM THE IMMUNE SYSTEM

Hormonal Signaling of the Brain by Immune Signals: Routes of Communication

The first suggestion that immune signals could stimulate the brain came from animal experiments (15), which showed that after intraperitoneal injection of bacterial lipopolysaccharide (LPS), interleukin-1 (IL-1) could be detected in brain tissue. The next series of experiments (16–19), which further delineated this signaling between the immune system and the brain, showed that IL-1 itself could directly activate the hypothalamic-pituitary-adrenal (HPA) axis cascade of hormones by direct stimulation of the hypothalamus and pituitary. IL-1 directly stimulates secretion of ACTH from cultured pituitary cells, induces CRH messenger RNA (mRNA) expression in the paraventricular nucleus of the hypothalamus, and induces CRH secretion from explanted hypothalamic tissue in culture (20). Subsequent studies have shown that many cytokines stimulate the hypothalamic pituitary adrenal axis, including IL-6, tumor necrosis factor (TNF), IL-2, interferon-α, and more recently IL-10 (21–29). Other studies suggest that interferon-α may inhibit hypothalamic release via an opiate mechanism (30).

Although there is some debate regarding the mechanisms by which cytokines from the peripheral immune system can stimulate the brain, access probably occurs through several routes (31–38). Cytokines may be actively carried from the blood to the brain across the blood–brain barrier, or may also cross passively at certain anatomically leaky points in the blood–brain barrier, such as the organum vasculosum lamina terminalis (OVLT) or the median eminence (Fig. 17.3). This route may be more prevalent during inflammation or illness, when the blood–brain barrier is more permeable (39). Such conditions are particularly likely to occur in an illness such as SLE in which inflammation may involve the CNS.

However, it is not necessary for cytokines to cross into the brain to exert their effects. Cytokines can be expressed in endothelial cells lining cerebral blood vessels (40,41) (Fig. 17.5) and can stimulate second messenger release in surrounding brain tissue, thus stimulating neurons in these areas. It is likely that some cytokine effects, such as fever, are indirectly mediated through second messengers, such as prostaglandins and nitric oxide (42). The fact that these effects of IL-1 are blocked by prostaglandin antagonists, such as acetyl salicylic acid (ASA) and other non-steroidal anti-inflammatory drugs (NSAIDs), provides evidence for the existence of this mechanism.

Finally, peripheral cytokines can signal the brain, via direct neuronal routes. Studies show that intraperitoneal cytokines can activate specific CNS regions via the vagus nerve (38). The brainstem nucleus of the tractus solitarius (NTS) is the first brain region that exhibits electrical and biochemical activity after intraperitoneal injection of IL-1 (Fig. 17.3). Such NTS activity is prevented by cutting the vagus nerve. Vagotomy has also been shown to block the induction of IL-1β (43). Thus, signaling via peripheral nerves could constitute the most rapid mechanism by which cytokines activate the brain, on the order of milliseconds, and may be an important mechanism for IL-1–induced increases in plasma corticosteroids and hypothalamic norepinephrine depletion (44). Intravenous IL-1β has also been shown to activate efferent activity of branches of the vagal nerve that innervate the thymus (45). Thus, through activation of the vagus, peripheral IL-1 has the potential to simultaneously modulate thymic and hypothalamic function.

Expression of Cytokines Within the CNS

In addition to acting as signals between immune cells and as signals from peripheral immune cells to the brain, cytokines are also expressed within the CNS (46,47). Such CNS cytokines are produced by neurons as well as non-neuronal cells, including cerebral vascular endothelial cells, astrocytes, and glia. Oligodendrocytes, astrocytes, and microglia

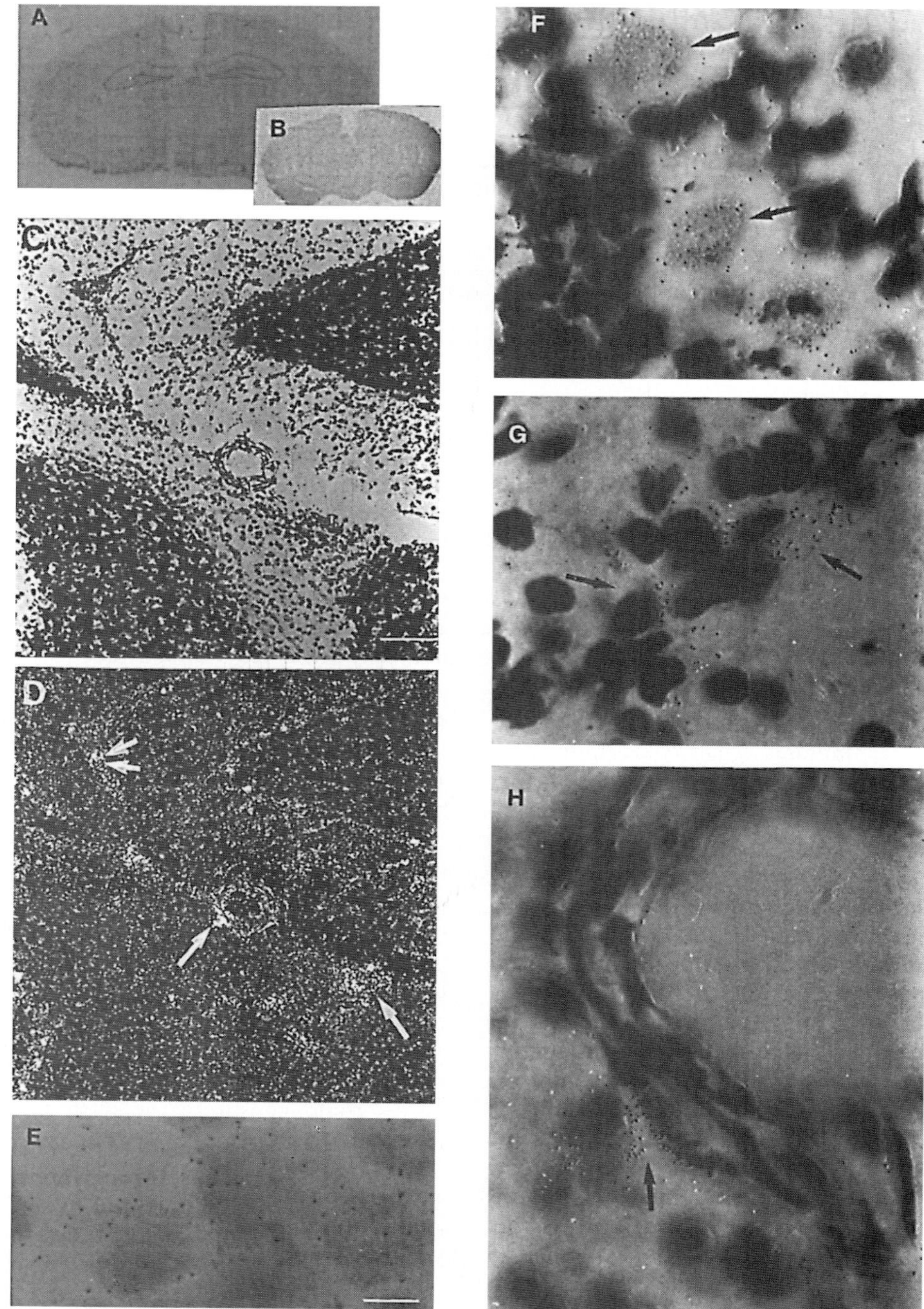

FIGURE 17.5. IL-1 receptor and IL-1 receptor antagonist (IL-1ra) messenger RNA (mRNA) expression in cerebral blood vessels, and *in situ* hybridization of IL-1 receptor type I (IL-1RI) mRNA in rat brain. **A:** Film autoradiograph of IL-1RI mRNA hybridization in hippocampus. **B:** Control for *in situ* hybridization using excess cold probe. **C:** Bright-field photomicrograph of several blood vessels in brain parenchyma. **D:** Dark-field photomicrograph of the same area as in **C**, with localization of IL-1RI mRNA on small blood vessels. **E:** Bright-field photomicrograph of IL-1RI mRNA hybridization in CA-1 neurons of hippocampus. **F:** Bright-field photomicrograph of IL-1RI mRNA hybridization in Purkinje cells of the cerebellar cortex. Note that deposits of silver grains (*black dots*) representing IL-1RI mRNA are concentrated on Purkinje cells bodies. **G:** Bright-field photomicrograph of IL-1RI mRNA hybridization over the endothelial cells of a postcapillary venule. **H:** Bright-field photomicrograph of IL-1RI mRNA hybridization in the perivascular area of an arteriole in brain parenchyma. (**C**, bar = 200 μm; **E**, bar = 20 μm. *Arrows* indicate the localization of IL-1RI mRNA. (From Wong M, Licinio J. Localization of interleukin-1 type I receptor mRNA in rat brain. *Neuroimmunomodulation* 1994;1:110–115, with permission.)

are supporting cells of the CNS; neurons are functional elements of the CNS that transmit neuronal impulses and synthesize and secrete neurotransmitters and neuropeptides. Oligodendrites and astrocytes are derived from neural ectoderm, while microglia are CNS macrophages that are derived from bone marrow. The glial elements produce growth factors, including cytokines, which are important in neuronal cell growth, differentiation, survival, and cell death. Neuronal peptides, which are synthesized in neuronal cell bodies, are transported to neuronal axon terminals, where both peptides and neurotransmitters are stored in vesicles. On stimulation and depolarization, these products are released into the synapse.

Cytokines can be expressed or induced in CNS resident cells (Table 17.1) (48), and can also be expressed in inflammatory cells in inflamed cerebral tissue. This latter situation might be likely to occur in diseases such as SLE, in which CNS inflammation occurs. In addition to cytokines themselves, the entire molecular machinery that allows these molecules to be functional is also found within the brain. The best defined of these systems is the IL-1 system, in which all components have been identified in the brain. These include both types of IL-1 (i.e., IL-1α and β), both types of receptor for IL-1 (i.e., types I and II), the enzyme that activates IL-1β [i.e., IL-1 converting enzyme (ICE)], and the endogenous IL-1 receptor antagonist (IL-1ra), a molecule that blocks the effects of IL-1 (40,49,50).

The CNS cytokine systems serve a different physiologic role than the stimulation of the brain by cytokines produced by peripheral immune cells. Thus, central cytokines appear to play an integral role in modulating nerve cell death and survival (48,51), while peripheral cytokine signals to the CNS have a primarily neuroendocrine function. *In vitro* studies show that IL-1 is toxic to mature neurons in tissue culture, but prevents the naturally occurring neuronal cell death that occurs in immature neurons (52). Evidence that this growth and death effect of cytokines on neuronal tissue is relevant to whole organisms comes from studies in animals and humans. Neurotoxicity results when cytokines are overexpressed in the brain in transgenic mice, in which cytokine genes are targeted to astroglial cells through a promoter specific for astroglia, glial fibrillary acidic protein (53). Such mice develop neuropathology and related neurologic manifestations in areas in which the cytokines are overexpressed. Thus, mice in which IL-6 is targeted to the CNS develop astrogliosis, inflammation, and angiogenesis in areas of the brain including the cerebellum. Clinical manifestations in these mice include paralysis, seizures, and ataxia. Transgenic mice that chronically express IL-6 in brain astrocytes show deficits in avoidance learning (54). However, not all the effects of immune cells and mediators involve neurotoxicity. In certain conditions, as in nerve trauma, antigen-specific T cells have been shown to play a role in neuronal repair, and this immune activation in the CNS can be neuroprotective (55).

In human disease in which cerebral tissue is invaded by inflammatory cells, molecular techniques that allow visualization of gene expression *in situ* show overexpression of cytokines in regions of neurodegeneration. In brain tissue from patients dying with AIDS dementia, overexpression of certain cytokines, including IL-1 and TNF, has been demonstrated, concentrated in areas around the invading giant cells (56). This suggests that some of the neurologic features of AIDS may result from neurotoxicity of cytokines (46,57,58). Furthermore, it suggests the possibility that in other inflammatory diseases characterized by CNS involve-

TABLE 17.1. CYTOKINES EXPRESSED WITHIN GLIAL AND NEURONAL CELLULAR ELEMENTS IN THE CNS

Cytokine	Neuron	Astrocytes	Oligodendrocytes	Microglia
IL-1	+?/R?	+/R	+?/R	+
IL-2	+?/R?		R	R
IL-3	+?/R?	+/R	R	R
IL-4		R	R	R?
IL-5		+		+
IL-6	+?/R	+/R		+/R
IL-7		R?	R	R?
IL-8		+		
TNF-α	R	+/R	R	+/R
IFN-γ		+?/R		R
TGF-β_1		+/R	+/R	+/R
GM-CSF	R	+/R	R	R
M-CSF		R	R	+/R

GM-CSF, granulocyte-macrophage colony-stimulating factor; M-CSF, macrophage colony-stimulating factor; R, presence of receptor; +, production of cytokine; ?, suspected but not definite; IFN, interferon; IL, interleukin; TGF, transforming growth factor; TNF, tumor necrosis factor.
From Sei Y, Vitkovic L, Yokoyama MM. Cytokines in the central nervous system: regulatory roles in neuronal function, cell death and repair. *Neuroimmunomodulation* 1995;2(3):121–133, with permission.

ment, such as SLE, some of the neuropathology and neurologic features might also be caused by cytokine overexpression from inflammatory cells as well (59,60).

IL-1 may also act in concert with other neuropeptides in regulating neuronal cell death and survival. For example, CRH and IL-1 are both induced in neurons during ischemia. Neuronal damage is diminished by the administration of antiserum against CRH and is enhanced by the administration of IL-1ra antisera (61). These data suggest that IL-1ra and CRH play reciprocal roles as neuroprotective and neurodegenerative agents during ischemia. Similarly, IL-1 and TNF-α act synergistically to mediate neurotoxicity through the induction of nitrous oxide by astrocytes (62).

Behavioral Effects of Cytokines on the CNS

One characteristic set of behaviors induced by cytokines is termed sickness behavior (63–65). This is characterized by loss of appetite, decreased mobility, increased somnolence, and fever. Some of these behavioral and functional effects (e.g., fever) are mediated secondarily through prostaglandin; others are initially activated via the vagus nerve (66).

EFFERENT LIMB MODULATION OF IMMUNE AND INFLAMMATORY RESPONSES BY THE NEUROENDOCRINE SYSTEM

Glucocorticoid Modulation of the Immune System

If the stimulation of the CNS by peripheral cytokines is viewed as the afferent limb of the neuroimmune communication, the final end point of the efferent limb of this communication is the glucocorticoid effect of the immune response. Glucocorticoids modulate immune cell function by acting through classic glucocorticoid receptors present on immune cells. The molecular structure and mechanism of action of glucocorticoid receptors is described below. The overall functional effect of glucocorticoids on the immune response, described below, depends on the type, dose, and temporal sequence of glucocorticoid exposure in relation to antigenic or proinflammatory challenge.

Molecular Mechanism of Glucocorticoid Action

Glucocorticoid receptors are members of a hormone receptor superfamily and are structurally related. Hormone receptor members of this superfamily include the glucocorticoid receptor (i.e., binds corticosterone), the mineralocorticoid receptor (i.e., binds corticosterone and aldosterone), and androgen, estrogen, progesterone, thyroid hormone, and retinoic acid receptors. All members of the superfamily act by binding to a soluble cytosolic receptor that is made up of three functional regions: (a) a C-terminal hormone binding region, (b) a DNA binding region, and (c) an N-terminal immunogenic region that is involved in transactivation (Fig. 17.6) (67,68). The unbound receptor is folded and inactive, bound to a 90,000-Da heat shock protein (hsp90) (69,70) (Fig. 17.7A). When the hormonal ligand binds to the receptor, hsp90 is displaced, resulting in a conformational change in the receptor that allows the active ligand-receptor complex to displace to the nucleus and bind either as a homodimer or heterodimer to hormone receptor-binding elements (HREs) on DNA. The hormone-receptor complex acts directly on DNA as a transcription factor, and can either suppress or stimulate DNA gene transcription. Specificity of action is conferred by the hormone-binding site.

The glucocorticoid or type II receptor (GR) binds corticosterone with a lower affinity than the mineralocorticoid or type I receptor (MR). The GR therefore tends to respond to the higher levels of glucocorticoids secreted during stress (i.e., stress levels), while the MR responds to basal or nonstress levels (71–73). While GRs generally bind to glucocorticoid receptor DNA binding elements (GREs) (74,75) as homodimers, several studies indicate that it is possible for GRs and MRs to form heterodimers (76–78). In addition to binding to simple response elements on DNA, hormone-receptor complexes can bind to composite response elements consisting of an HRE and an activator protein-1 (AP1) binding site that binds heterodimers of the protooncogene products c-*Fos* and c-*Jun* or c-*Jun* homodimers (74,79–81). Recent studies indicate that the GR dimers bind to many co-regulatory protein complexes in the course of DNA binding and transcription activation (Fig. 17.7B) (68). These different mechanisms of binding to DNA response elements confer additional specificity of action to the glucocorticoid and mineralocorticoid receptors.

Further specificity of action of these two receptor types is conferred by tissue distribution of the receptors. The primary glucocorticoid receptor in immune cells is the GR, consistent with the physiologic role of glucocorticoid regulation of the immune system by stress levels of these hormones (82–87). An additional level of specificity is conferred by the tissue distribution of the corticosterone-metabolizing enzyme 11β-hydroxysteroid (HDS), which metabolizes corticosterone but not aldosterone. Thus, where this enzyme is present (e.g., kidney), the primary ligand available for binding to the MR is aldosterone rather than corticosterone. Where the enzyme is not present (e.g., brain), the primary ligand for the MR is corticosterone (74). Recent studies have identified subtypes I and II of this enzyme. 11β-HDS type I acts as a reductase *in vivo*, maintaining glucocorticoid levels in target tissues like liver and adipose tissue, whereas 11β-HDS type II protects the MR from occupation and thereby glucocorticoid excess (88,89). The MR in the brain plays a role in regulation of basal HPA function, such as circadian rhythm.

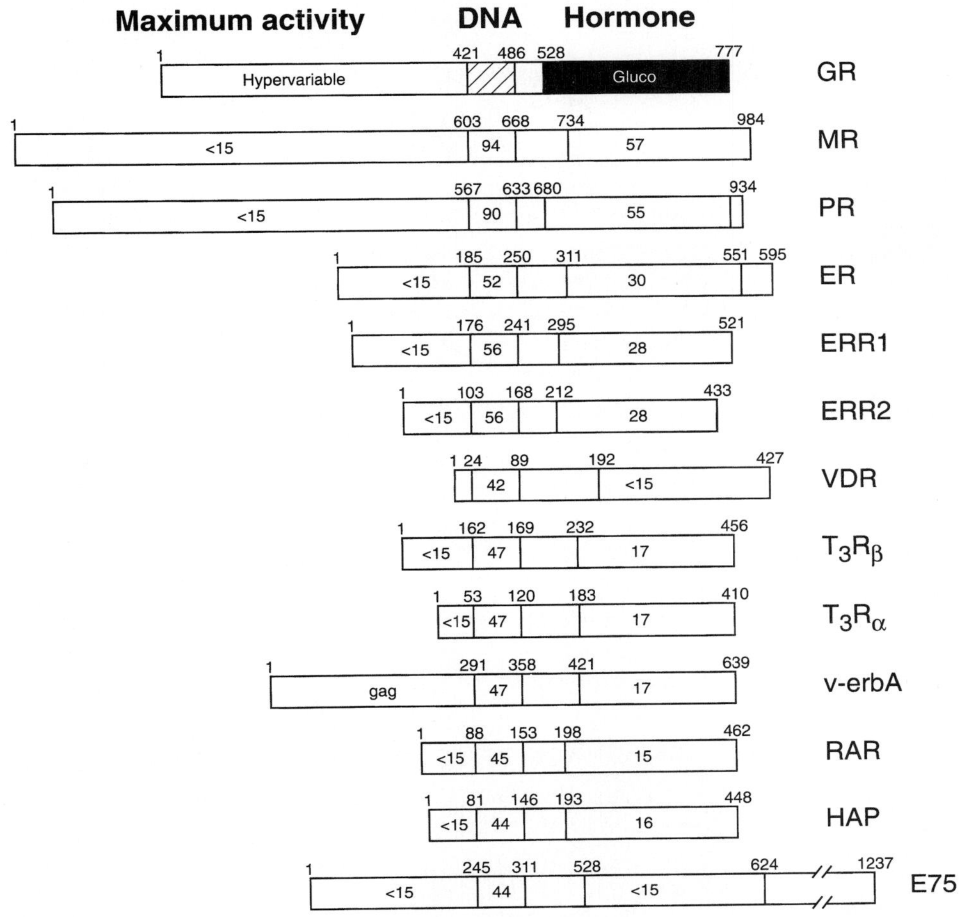

FIGURE 17.6. Schematic structure of the glucocorticoid receptor and related members of the glucocorticoid receptor superfamily, showing hypervariable, DNA-binding and hormone-binding regions. ER, estrogen receptor; ERR1, estrogen receptor type I; ERR2, estrogen receptor type II; PR, progesterone receptor; RAR, retinoic acid receptor; VDR, vitamin D receptor. (Adapted from Evans (67) with permission.)

Glucocorticoid Effects on Immune Responses

The hormones at the final effector end point of the HPA axis, the glucocorticoids, have potent anti-inflammatory and immunosuppressive effects. This overall immunosuppression is attained through suppression of many stimulatory components of the immune cascade and stimulation of some immunosuppressive or anti-inflammatory elements. However, in addition to this suppressive role, glucocorticoids can also stimulate some aspects of the immune or inflammatory response, depending on dose and timing of exposure. Thus, although overall they are immunosuppressive, in this sense glucocorticoids may be viewed as modulators of the immune response (84,90–92).

Glucocorticoids have profound effects on the immune/inflammatory response at the whole organ, cellular, and molecular levels. Exposure to stress levels of glucocorticoids results in rapid involution of the thymus, possibly as a result of glucocorticoid-induced thymocyte apoptosis, or programmed cell death through activation of the glucocorticoid receptor (93–95). Glucocorticoids also cause redistribution of circulating white blood cells (96), with neutrophilic leukocytosis, eosinopenia, monocytopenia, and altered ratios of T-lymphocyte subtypes, resulting in decreased peripheral blood CD4 and increased CD8 cells. At the same time as this peripheral redistribution occurs, there is decreased infiltration of neutrophils and monocytes into tissues.

Glucocorticoids exert greater and more consistent suppressive effects on cell-mediated than on humoral immune function (90). Glucocorticoids have been shown to cause a shift from a T helper-1 (Th1) to a Th2 pattern of cytokines responses, which support humoral immunity and enhanced antibody responses (97–100), while Th1 responses that support cellular immunity are suppressed. In a disease such as SLE, which is characterized by excess or inappropriate

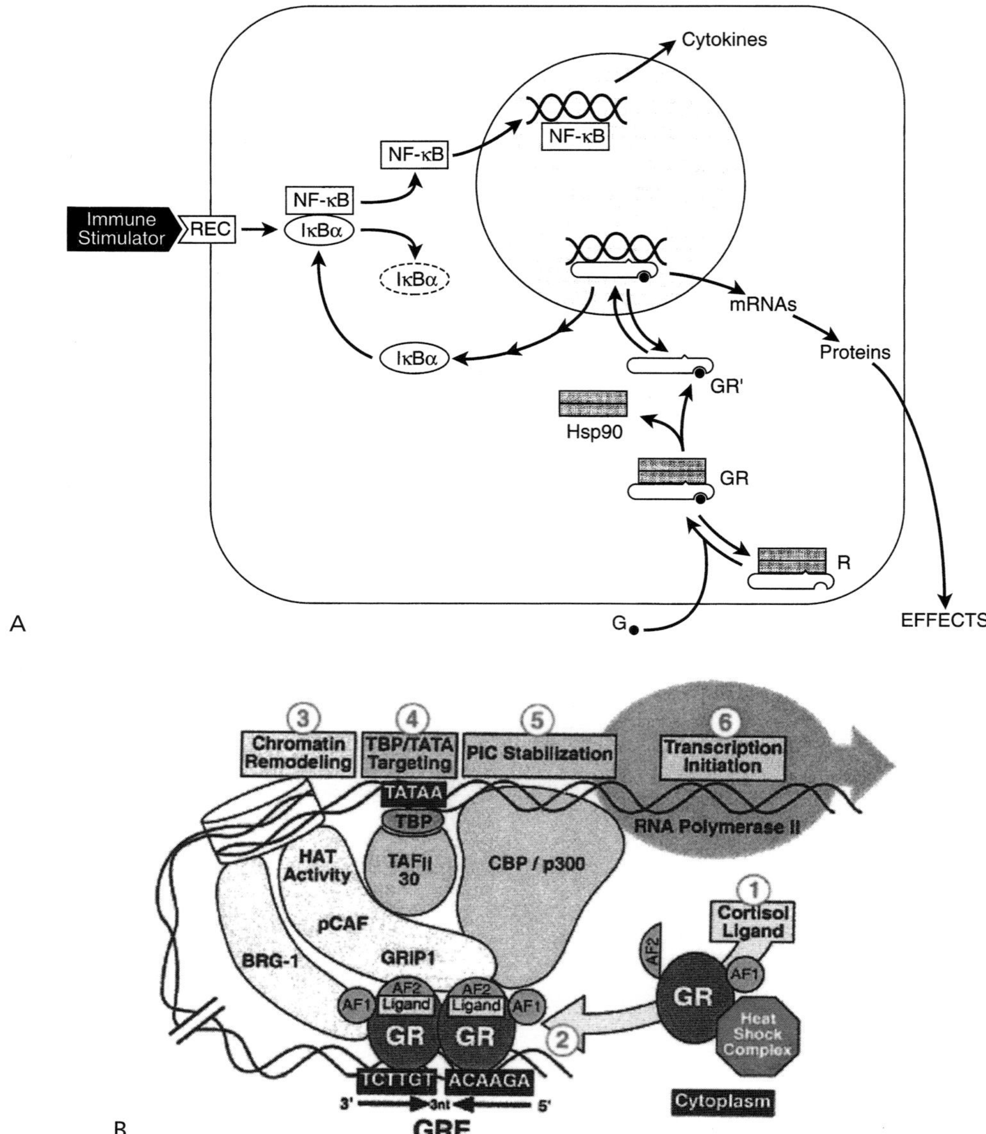

FIGURE 17.7. A: Schematic of glucocorticoid receptor binding and translocation to nucleus, and the modulating role of nuclear transcription factors NF-κB on glucocorticoid effects modified. The glucocorticoid (G) binds to the cytosolic glucocorticoid hormone receptor (GR), displacing heat shock protein 90 (hsp90). The activated hormone receptor complex (GRpr) displaces to the nucleus (GRprn), where it binds to DNA at sites called glucocorticoid response elements (GREs), and induces or decreases mRNAs and proteins encoded by the gene to which it has bound. An additional mechanism by which glucocorticoids regulate immune responses at the genomic level is via stimulation of a production of a protein, IκBa, which binds to NF-κB. In the absence of glucocorticoids, binding of immune stimulators [e.g., tumor necrosis factor (TNF)] to their membrane receptors (REC) leads to destruction of IκBa, allowing NJ-κB to translocate to the nucleus, bind to DNA, and induce transcription of cytokines and other genes. Glucocorticoid stimulation of IκBa production blocks this route of gene transcription. **B:** More detailed schematic showing multiple co-regulatory complexes participating in GR-DNA interactions. Upon binding to cortisol (1), GR dissociates from the cytoplasmic complex, translocates to the nucleus and forms a homodimer on its palindromic GRE (2). Triggered by a ligand-mediated change in GR conformation, the AF1 and AF2 domains then synergize to promote a series of events (3–6) involving the recruitment of co-regulatory complexes. GR, glucocorticoid receptor; GRE, glucocorticoid-responsive element; AF1, activation function 1; AF2, activation function 2. (**A:** Adapted from Munck et al. (55), and Marx J. News and views. *Science* 1995;270:232–233, with permission. **B:** Adapted from Whitfield GK, Jurutka PW, Haussler CA, et al. Steroid hormone receptors: evolution, ligands, and molecular basis of biologic function. *J Cell Biochem* 1999;32–33(suppl):110–122, with permission).

antibody production, it is important to delineate whether glucocorticoids may contribute to or exacerbate this shift.

In functional assays, a large body of data shows that glucocorticoids suppress mitogen- and antigen-stimulated T-cell proliferation (96,101). In contrast, some studies indicate that corticosterone in rats can enhance lymphocyte proliferation, depending on the conditions of culture (102). While the physiologic relevance of these *in vitro* studies is not known, this dual suppressing or enhancing effect of glucocorticoids on lymphocyte proliferation underlines their potential physiologic role as immunomodulators rather than pure immunosuppressors.

Glucocorticoids have been shown to suppress not only differentiation and maturation but also the function of mature effector T-cell subtypes, such as cytolytic and T-helper cells. *In vitro* studies indicate that the degree to which these functions are suppressed is dose dependent and culture-condition dependent. Glucocorticoids also suppress natural killer cell function both *in vitro* and *in vivo* in animals and humans. The suppressive effects of glucocorticoids on B-cell proliferation are variable, depending on the stimulus to proliferation and dose of glucocorticoids used. In general, B-cell proliferation is less consistently suppressed than T-cell proliferation. At the same time, glucocorticoids consistently enhance production of all classes of immunoglobulins. Thus, while the overall effects of glucocorticoids on immune/inflammatory responses at the cellular level are immunosuppressive, some components are enhanced, depending on specific conditions. The relatively greater sensitivity to suppression by glucocorticoids of components of cellular versus humoral immunity tends to shift the immune response from a cellular to a humoral pattern (90).

At the molecular level, glucocorticoids downregulate expression of class II major histocompatibility complex (MHC) antigen expression, thus reducing recognition and binding of antigen. They also inhibit production of proinflammatory molecules and immune mediators (90), including complement components, arachidonic acid products, histamine, bradykinins, and cytokines. At the same time as many of these immunostimulatory/pro-inflammatory molecules are suppressed, their intrinsic suppressors may be enhanced. An example of this balance occurs in the complement system, where glucocorticoids suppress C3 while inducing the complement suppressor factor H. Glucocorticoids suppress production of most postinflammatory cytokines (91,103), but stimulate some antiinflammatory cytokines as well (Fig. 17.8). Thus, IL-1, IL-6, IL-2, interferon-γ, TNF, IL-3, and granulocyte-macrophage colony-stimulating factor are depressed, while IL-4 and IL-10 are increased (98,100). This pattern of a shift from IL-2 to IL-4 production is consistent with the humoral, antibody, and B-cell supportive effects of glucocorticoids, and their tendency to shift the immune response from a Th1 to a Th2 pattern (97,99). In addition, while the glucocorticoids sup-

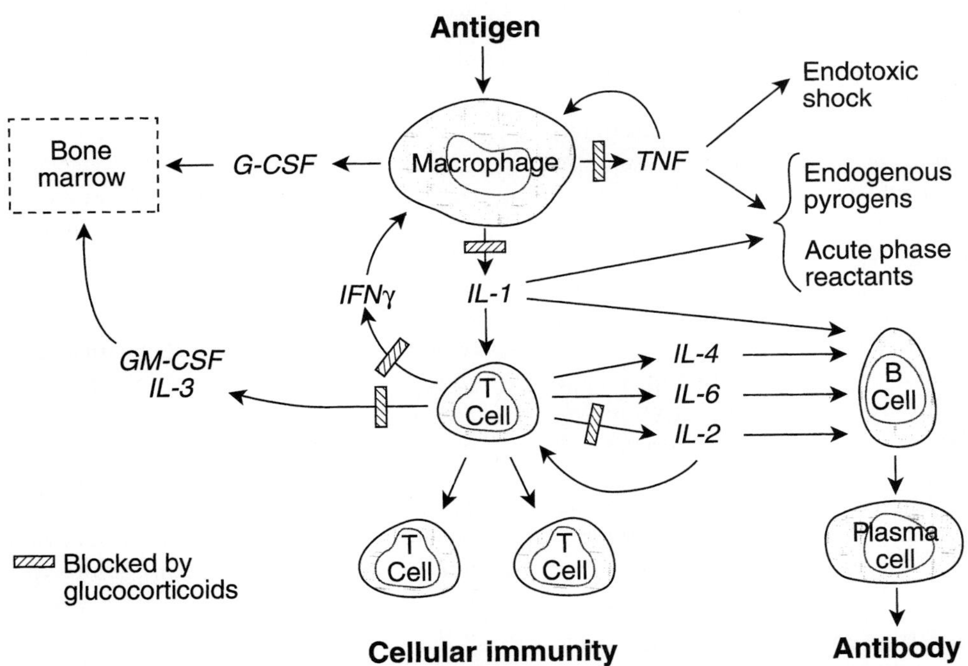

FIGURE 17.8. Glucocorticoid effects on immune responses. *Hatched bars* indicate effects blocks by glucocorticoids. CSF, colony-stimulating factor; GM-CSF, granulocyte-macrophage colony-stimulating factor. (Adapted from Munck et al. (69), with permission.)

press IL-1 production, they also enhance the expression of IL-1β receptor (104). This apparent opposing effect of glucocorticoids actually is consistent with their immunosuppressive role, since it is the type II decoy IL-1 receptor that is induced by glucocorticoids (105,106). Thus, while suppressing IL-1 production, glucocorticoids simultaneously induce expression of the non–signal transducing receptor for IL-1, potentially further reducing the availability of active IL-1.

Glucocorticoids can also regulate the immune response by inducing apoptosis in proliferating lymphocytes (94, 107). Glucocorticoids modulate apoptosis by their effects on T-cell homeostasis, which is regulated in part by crosstalk between glucocorticoid receptor activation triggering apoptosis and effects on the T-cell receptor inhibiting it (95). There is evidence to suggest that such glucocorticoid-regulated apoptosis could take place within the thymus, through induction of an intrathymic glucocorticoid system, since the enzymatic machinery for glucocorticoid synthesis is present within the thymus (108). Indeed, it has been shown that thymic epithelial cells produce glucocorticoids locally, production of which may play a role in positive and negative thymic selection. Based on a model called "mutual antagonism," glucocorticoids can turn up or down the perceived intensity of T-cell receptor (TCR) signaling. Positive selection of T cells in the thymus occurs when there is balance between glucocorticoid signaling and TCR avidity for self antigen/MHC. For positive selection to occur at higher levels of glucocorticoids, a higher TCR avidity is necessary; otherwise, negative selection occurs. On the other hand, lower levels of glucocorticoids enhance TCR signaling efficacy, causing apoptosis to cells that would normally have been positively selected (Fig. 17.9) (95,109–111).

Timing and dose of exposure to glucocorticoids in relation to antigenic or mitogenic exposure also results in variable effects (101), and could explain the variable effects in the whole-organism response to antigenic challenge with its own burst of glucocorticoids. In such situations, a sluggish HPA response to inflammation may be as deleterious in suppressing inflammation as insufficient quantities of glucocorticoid released. In addition, timing of a glucocorticoid pulse may also result in specific deletion of clones of antigen-specific lymphocytes, because proliferating lymphocytes appear to be more susceptible to glucocorticoid-induced apoptosis. Thus, the relatively nonspecific effects of glucocorticoids in suppressing immune responses may take on a specific character if the timing of exposure is appropriate.

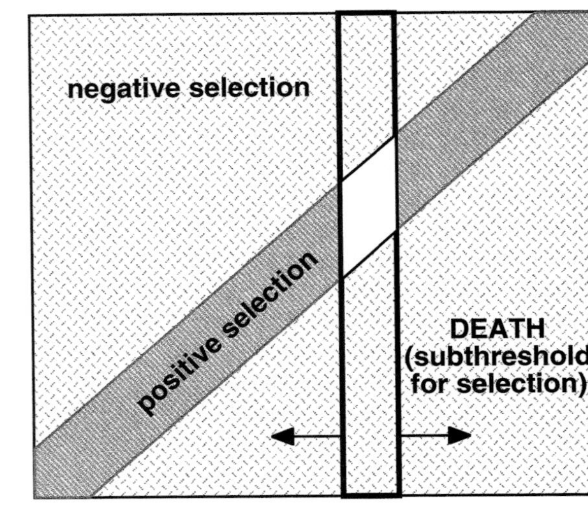

FIGURE 17.9. A model for the influence of T-cell receptor (TCR) avidity and glucocorticoid (GC) responsiveness on TCR selection. At physiologic levels of GCs, thymocytes either die in the thymus due to negative selection or expression of a receptor with subthreshold avidity for self–major histocompatibility complex (MHC) (*hatched area*), or are positively selected (*white area within window*). Diminution of GC signaling shifts the window of selection to the left and results in enhanced efficacy of TCR signaling, causing the apoptosis of thymocytes that would normally be positively selected, and positive selection of a subset of thymocytes whose avidity for self antigen/MHC would have been insufficient in the presence of GC. Similarly, elevated GC responsiveness may shift the window to the right, further suppressing TCR-mediated signals and rescuing a subset of cells with higher avidity for self antigen/MHC that would normally be deleted. (From Vacchio MS, Ashwell JD. Glucocorticoids and thymocyte development. *Semin Immunol* 2000;12(5):475–485, with permission.)

Sympathetic and Peripheral Nervous System Effects on Inflammation and the Immune System

Many immune organs, including spleen, thymus, and lymph nodes, are richly innervated by sympathetic nerves (112) (Fig. 17.10). A number of studies indicate that this neuroanatomic connection plays an important physiologic role in inflammatory responses. Interruptions of such sympathetic innervation alter peripheral immune responses. Immune organs are also innervated by peripheral nerves carrying neuropeptides, such as substance P (SP), which also plays a role in peripheral inflammation.

Evidence that the sympathetic nervous system affects the volume exudation component of peripheral inflammation is provided by sympathetic ablation studies using 6-OH dopamine (6-OHDA) (113), by studies using sympathetic ganglionic blockers such as chlorisondamine (114), or by studies using noradrenergic antagonists and agonists (115). The neuropeptide SP also plays a role in the severity of arthritis (116,117) and in the cellular component of inflammation (118). Substance P, probably released in retrograde fashion from sensory nerve endings, acts as a chemoattractant and stimulator of cellular proliferation and cytokine production, and plays a role in the early arteriolar changes in inflammation (119).

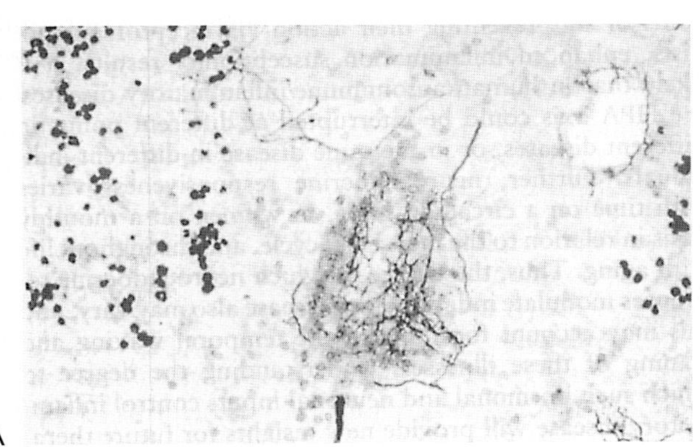
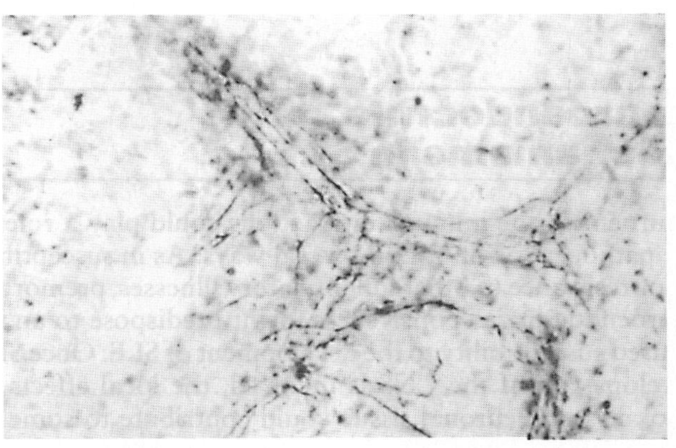

FIGURE 17.10. (See Color Plate 1.) Immunocytochemical-stained sections. **A:** Immunocytochemical staining for tyrosine hydroxylase (TH)-positive (noradrenergic) nerve fibers (*black*) surrounded by T lymphocytes (OX-19–positive cells) in the periarteriolar lymphatic sheath of a F344/N rat (×50). (Courtesy of Suzanne Felten.) **B:** Rat spleen stained for TH-positive nerve fibers (*black*) and OX-19–positive T lymphocytes (*brown*). The TH-positive nerve fibers densely innervate the central arteriole of the white pump (×185). (From Felten SY, Felten DL. Innervation of lymphoid tissue. In: Ader R, Felten DL, Cohen N, eds. *Psychoneuroimmunology*, 2nd ed. San Diego: Academic Press, 1991:27–61, with permission.)

Noradrenergic (NA) and SP denervation studies have shown differential effects on inflammation depending on the location of denervation. Thus, denervation of noradrenergic fibers of lymph nodes (120) is associated with exacerbation of inflammation, while systemic sympathectomy or denervation of joints is associated with decreased severity of inflammation (116,121). Treatment of neonatal rats with 6-OHDA, which interrupts both central and peripheral NA systems, is associated with exacerbation of experimental allergic encephalomyelitis (EAE) (122). Pharmacologic studies show decreased inflammation in experimental arthritis with beta-blockade (123) and decreased severity of EAE with β-adrenergic agonists (122). Both local capsaicin denervation of lymph nodes and systemic capsaicin treatment is associated with diminished peripheral inflammation (116,117,120).

In summary, the effects of interruption or reconstitution of the sympathetic system on inflammation differ, depending on the site of interruption—whether local (in joints), at the draining lymph node, peripheral, or central. Studies have shown that surgical interruption of sympathetic innervation to the spleen is associated with decreased splenic immune cell function (124,125). Similar dying back of noradrenergic splenic innervation during aging may explain some of the deficits of aging (126). Treatment of animals with deprenyl, a monoamine oxidase (MAO) inhibitor, is associated with regrowth of noradrenergic splenic innervation and partial reconstitution of immune function (127,128). These studies suggest that thorough delineation of neural-immune interactions at the immune organ regional level will open new avenues for treatment of immune deficiencies such as those seen in aging.

PHYSIOLOGIC ROLE OF NEUROIMMUNE COMMUNICATION

A multilevel infrastructure exists to allow anatomic, molecular, and functional communications between the immune and nervous systems (1–3,103). Animal studies in which these communications are interrupted on a genetic, pharmacologic, or surgical basis provide evidence that this interaction plays an important role in regulating susceptibility to and severity of inflammatory and autoimmune diseases. Examples in which susceptibility to inflammatory disease is associated with a blunted HPA axis exist in mammalian and avian species. Lewis and Fischer rats are a genetic model for relative inflammatory susceptibility and resistance related to HPA-axis responsiveness in mammalian species (20,129). The obese-strain chicken, which develops spontaneous thyroiditis, and its thyroiditis-resistant counterpart also exhibit relative HPA-axis hypo- and hyperresponsiveness (2).

Lewis rats are highly susceptible to a variety of autoimmune/inflammatory diseases, the patterns of which are related to the nature of the antigen or the proinflammatory stimulus to which they are exposed. Their overall susceptibility to inflammatory disease, however, is related to their profoundly blunted HPA-axis responsiveness. In turn, this results from blunted hypothalamic CRH production and secretion in response to a wide range of proinflammatory and stressful stimuli. Histocompatible Fischer rats exhibit a potent HPA-axis response to these same stimuli in conjunction with relative inflammatory disease resistance compared with that of Lewis rats (Fig. 17.11).

Interruption of the HPA axis in Fischer rats, and in other relatively inflammatory disease resistant strains, renders

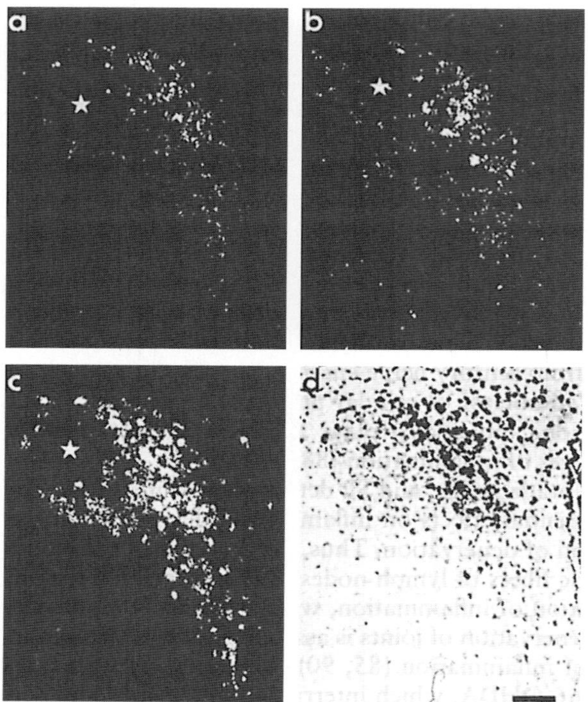

FIGURE 17.11. CRH mRNA expression, by *in situ* hybridization, in the paraventricular nucleus of the hypothalamus of Lewis (LEW)/N and F344/N rats. Photomicrographs of paraventricular nucleus sections labeled *in situ* with CRH oligonucleotide probe. Darkfield photomicrographs (**A–C**) show an increase in CRH mRNA expression in F344/N, but not LEW/N, rats after intraperitoneal streptococcal cell wall (SCW) injection. **A:** F344/N rats at time 0. **B:** LEW;n/N rats 8 hours after injection. **C:** F344/N rats 8 hours after injection. **D:** toluidine staining in same section as **C.** (From Sternberg EM, Young WSd, Bernardini R, et al. A central nervous system defect in biosynthesis of corticotropin-releasing hormone is associated with susceptibility to streptococcal cell wall-induced arthritis in Lewis rats. *Proc Natl Acad Sci USA* 1989; 86(12):4771–4775, with permission.)

these rats highly susceptible to the lethal effects of inflammation, peripherally or centrally. This concept has been shown in such disparate disease models as streptococcal cell wall–induced arthritis (129) and EAE-induced myelin basic protein (130), and in the lethal effects of salmonella (131). Interruptions of the HPA axis in these models have been accomplished surgically, through adrenalectomy or hypophysectomy (i.e., pituitary excision), or pharmacologically with the glucocorticoid receptor antagonist RU-486. Conversely, reconstitution of the HPA axis reverses inflammatory disease susceptibility in inflammatory susceptible strains. Such reconstitution has been accomplished pharmacologically through low-dose physiologic replacement of glucocorticoids in inflammatory susceptible strains (129, 130), as well as surgically by intracerebroventricular transplantation of hypothalamic tissue from inflammatory resistant into inflammatory susceptible strains (132).

Together, these studies underline the biologic principle that neuroendocrine responsiveness plays an important modulating role in susceptibility and resistance to inflammatory and autoimmune disease. When the feedback suppression of the immune system by the antiinflammatory/immunosuppressive effects of the glucocorticoids is interrupted either by blocking production of glucocorticoids or preventing their action via receptor antagonists, enhanced inflammatory susceptibility results. Nonetheless, as in all complex autoimmune inflammatory diseases, many genes contribute to overall disease susceptibility, in addition to neuroendocrine stress-related factors. Thus it has been shown that over 20 different regions on 15 different chromosomes contribute to inflammatory arthritis susceptibility in rats (133–136). While some of these linkage regions contain genes known to regulate both the stress response and inflammation (137), none has yet been associated with disease susceptibilty in a causal manner.

BLUNTED NEUROENDOCRINE STRESS RESPONSE IN HUMAN AUTOIMMUNE/INFLAMMATORY AND ALLERGIC DISEASES

Although the evidence is most clear-cut in animal studies, human studies also provide evidence that such neuroimmune interactions play a role in inflammatory/autoimmune disease. It is reasonable to predict that in human autoimmune/inflammatory diseases, the HPA axis could be interrupted at different points in different diseases or in the same disease in different individuals. Furthermore, variations in neuroendocrine responsiveness with time, on a circadian basis, in women on a monthly basis in relation to the menstrual cycle, and throughout life with aging could be associated with fluctuations of disease activity. Thus, the degree to which neuroendocrine responses modulate inflammatory disease may also vary, and may account for some of the temporal waxing and waning of these illnesses. Studies in rheumatoid arthritis (138), Sjögren's syndrome (139,140), SLE (141,142), fibromyalgia (143,144), chronic fatigue syndrome (145,146), allergic asthma (147,148), and dermatitis (149) have all shown an association of these illnesses with a blunted HPA-axis response to hormonal or psychological stimuli. Understanding the degree to which such hormonal and neuronal inputs control inflammatory disease will provide new insights into future therapeutic approaches for these illnesses.

NEUROENDOCRINE MECHANISMS IN SLE

Neuroendocrine immune interactions could play a role in the pathogenesis of SLE in several ways. As in susceptibility or resistance to other inflammatory illnesses, premorbid neuroendocrine responsiveness might predispose to increased susceptibility to development of SLE. Once SLE develops, and if the CNS is involved, the local effects of cytokines on neuronal tissue could contribute to some of the specific neuropathologic or neuropsychiatric features of SLE. At the effector end point of the axis, differences in glucocorticoid receptor number or sensitivity could play a role in pathogenesis of SLE as well as in the clinical response to treatment with steroids. In addition, regardless of the premorbid reactivity of the HPA axis, chronic inflammation itself could alter HPA-axis responses. Studies supporting these possibilities in animal models and in humans, although still sparse, do suggest that a variety of neuroimmune mechanisms may be relevant to many features in the pathogenesis of SLE.

CNS Cytokines in Animal Models

The classic animal models for SLE are New Zealand black/white (NZB/NZW) F1 mice and Medical Research Laboratory (MRL) mice. These strains of mice develop spontaneous autoimmune disease with many characteristic features seen in human SLE, including renal disease, vasculitis, and antinuclear antibody production. Neuroendocrine responses and CNS expression of cytokine components have been examined in both these strains.

Studies indicate that NZB and (NZB/NZW)F1 mice exhibit a profound deficiency of IL-1 receptor expression in the dentate gyrus of the hippocampus (10% of controls) (150,151) (Fig. 17.12), while MRL mice show no difference in CNS expression of this receptor compared to control nondisease strains. Although this deficiency is present before the mice develop clinical disease, it is not clear what role it plays in the pathogenesis of the syndrome. Differences in expression of the receptor for this cytokine in two strains that develop lupus-like disease could be interpreted to indicate that the defect is unrelated to the pathogenesis of the disease, or that different molecular mechanisms could lead to the same final disease outcome. Further studies in this area are required to determine which of these interpretations is correct.

CNS Cytokines in Human SLE

Two clinical aspects of CNS lupus, vasculitis and neuropsychiatric manifestations, could be related in part to the presence of cytokines in the CNS released from inflammatory cells. Elevated cytokines have been detected in cerebrospinal fluid (CSF) in patients with CNS lupus. In one study, IL-6 was increased during clinical exacerbations of CNS lupus, and fell to control levels in association with clinical improvements after treatment with methylprednisolone (152). Clinical symptoms in these patients included seizures, organic brain syndrome, nonorganic psychosis, chorea, and focal lesions. In a similar study in lupus psychosis, CSF interferon-α (153) increased and returned to baseline corresponding with clinical exacerbations and remissions. In both studies the CSF cytokines were higher than plasma levels, suggesting a CNS source for the cytokines. Furthermore, cytokines were not elevated in patients with seizures from other causes. Although the elevations in CSF cytokines could be viewed as simply a marker for the presence of inflammation, it is noteworthy that in animal models such as transgenic mice in which IL-6 is specifically overexpressed in brain, clinical features such as focal lesions and seizures are seen. This suggests that the elevations in IL-6 measured in human SLE CSF could be playing a pathogenic role in development of some of the neuropathologic features of CNS lupus (154–156).

Evidence of Glucocorticoid Resistance in SLE

In contrast to patients with other autoimmune diseases such as rheumatoid arthritis, patients with SLE often require large doses of glucocorticoids before an effect is seen. Furthermore, even during treatment with large doses of steroids, SLE patients are less likely to develop cushingoid features. This anecdotal clinical evidence suggests that SLE patients may display some degree of glucocorticoid tissue resistance (157,158). The contribution of the glucocorticoid receptor to potential glucocorticoid resistance has been explored in some studies examining the binding number and affinity characteristics of the GR in lupus. The findings of these studies are suggestive and need further investigation.

In a study of SLE patients who had not received steroid treatment within the previous 6 months, the glucocorticoid receptor numbers in peripheral blood mononuclear cells were significantly higher than in controls (159). There was no correlation with disease activity nor was there a difference in affinity of the GR in these patients. In another study, no difference in GR number was found between patients and controls; however, patients on low-dose glucocorticoid treatment were not excluded from this study (160). Because exogenous treatment with glucocorticoids resets the responsiveness of the HPA axis, the GR numbers measured in glucocorticoid-treated patients may reflect treatment rather than intrinsic factors. Thus, the discrepancy between these studies could be related to the differences in exogenous glucocorticoid exposure in these patients, and points out the inherent difficulty in studying GR binding in such patients (161).

Effects of Stress in SLE

Until recently, studies of the effects of stress on physical illness, including autoimmune diseases such as SLE, were viewed with skepticism, related in part to the inherent difficulty in accurately defining and quantitating stressful stimuli and response outcomes. However, recent advances in defining and quantitating not only stressors but also neuroendocrine transducing signals, disease outcomes, and molecular components of the immune/inflammatory response

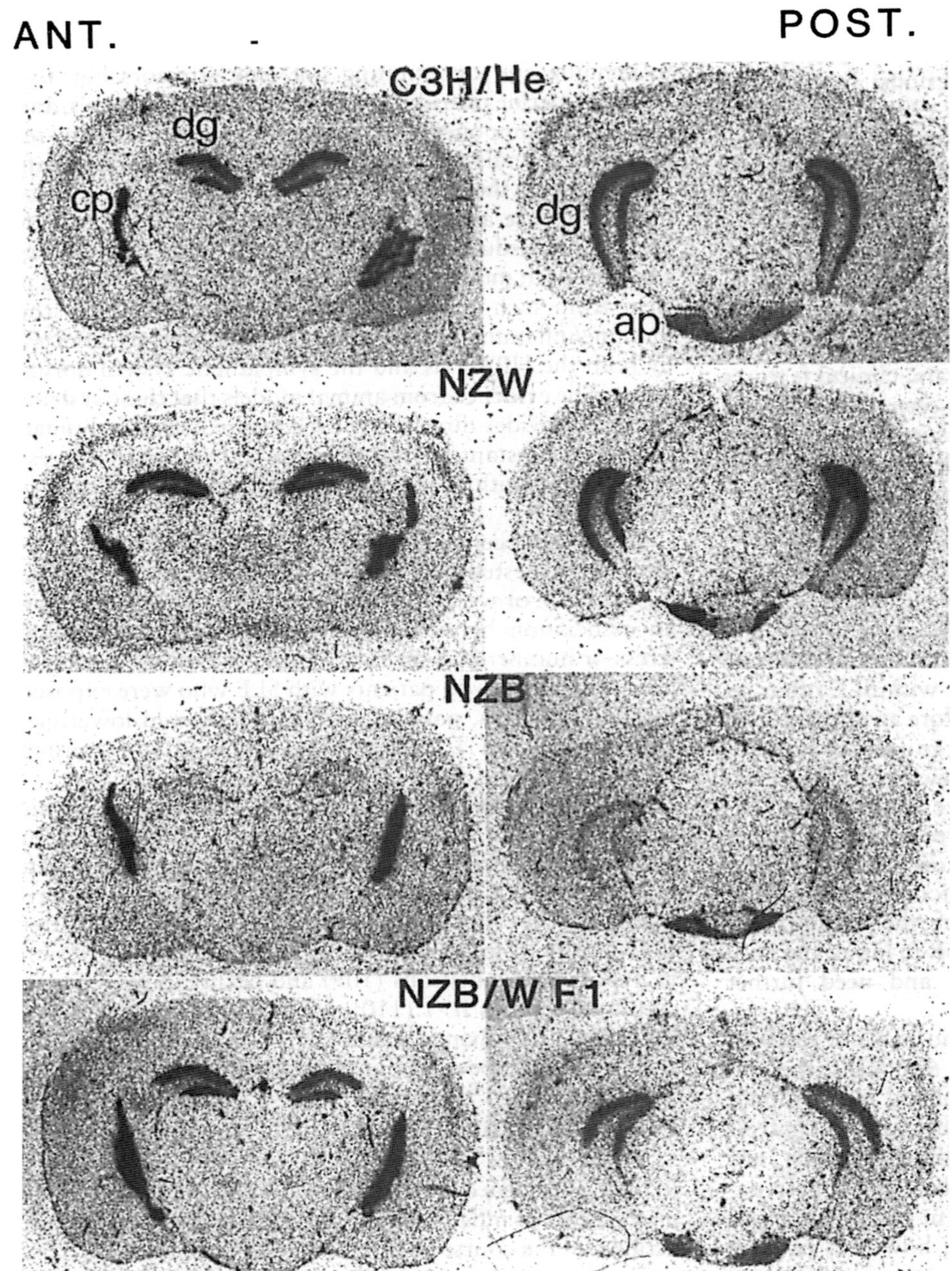

FIGURE 17.12. Autoradiographic localization of interleukin-1 (IL-1) receptor by ^{125}IL-1α-radiolabeled binding in sections from anterior (ANT) and posterior (POST) parts of the brain of 7-month-old female C3H/He, NZW, NZB, and NZB/W F1 mice. *Black areas* indicate IL-1 binding to receptor. Quantitation of expression shows that NZB mice have a profound deficit of IL-1 receptor in the dentate gyrus (dg) of the hippocampus (10% of controls), while NZB/W show a 50% deficit in this area. Other structures, including choroid plexus (cp) and anterior pituitary (ap), show equivalent binding in these strains. (From Jafarian Tehrani et al. (150), with permission.)

in animals and humans have allowed more accurate assessment of the effects of stress on autoimmune/inflammatory disease, and the mechanisms by which such effects are transduced. While most such studies have been carried out in models of infectious disease (162–164), it is clear from such studies that different components of the immune/inflammatory response to pathogens are affected by both the HPA axis and sympathetic system during stress. The evidence from animal models that these systems interact provides direction for future design of human studies to substantiate old or anecdotal claims that stress is associated with exacerbation or precipitation of disease in SLE.

A number of studies have suggested that emotional stress might trigger the onset of SLE or worsen its course

(165–167). Two studies have shown an association between flares of disease and emotional stress or number and severity of daily stressors. In one interventional study in SLE patients exposed to acoustic stress, lupus patients showed lower elevations in B and T lymphocytes compared to normals.

Chronic inflammation itself can be viewed as a chronic stressor that can alter HPA axis responses. The effects of chronic inflammation include hypercortisolism and a shift from primarily CRH control of the stress response to primarily arginine vasopressin (AVP) control (168,169). The latter shift results from a switch from CRH to AVP expression in hypothalamic neurons (170), and occurs in response to cytokines such as IL-1 (171). Multiple sclerosis is one human disease involving chronic CNS inflammation in which such a shift has been demonstrated (169).

Potential Drug Interactions

In light of the evidence for the multiple levels of neuroimmune interactions in inflammatory disease, potential drug interactions on the course of disease should be considered, particularly when instituting therapy with neuropsychiatric agents that may alter HPA-axis function. The effects of such drugs on peripheral inflammatory/immune responses may not always be predictable. For example, imipramine decreases hypothalamic CRH mRNA expression during long-term treatment in rats (172), while it decreases peripheral inflammatory responses (173). This illustrates the importance of directly testing the effects of psychotropic agents in immune/inflammatory disease models, in order to better inform clinical judgments as to the potential effects on course of disease when such agents are used in autoimmune disease, such as SLE.

SUMMARY

It is apparent that neuroendocrine-immune interactions play an important role in the pathogenesis of many features of SLE at multiple levels, within and outside the CNS, at the molecular and whole organ level. This chapter has focused on two aspects of neuroendocrine interactions with the immune system—hypothalamic-pituitary-adrenal and sympathetic immune interactions—as well as on cytokines within the CNS. There are many additional hormonal systems that play an important role in modulating immune function, including the female sex hormones estrogen and progesterone, and prolactin. All these hormones play an important role in the pathogenesis of SLE, and are reviewed elsewhere in this text.

REFERENCES

1. Sternberg EM, Chrousos GP, Wilder RL, et al. The stress response and the regulation of inflammatory disease. *Ann Intern Med* 1992;117(10):854–866.
2. Wick G, Hu Y, Schwarz S, et al. Immunoendocrine communication via the hypothalamo-pituitary-adrenal axis in autoimmune diseases. *Endocr Rev* 1993;14(5):539–563.
3. Bellinger DL, Felten SY, Felten DL. Neural-immune interactions: neurotransmitter signalling of cells of the immune system. In: Tasman A, Riba MB, eds. *Review of psychiatry*. Washington, DC: American Psychiatric Press, 1992:127–144.
4. Vale W, Spiess J, Rivier C, et al. Characterization of a 41-residue ovine hypothalamic peptide that stimulates secretion of corticotropin and beta-endorphin. *Science* 1981;213(4514): 1394–1397.
5. Chrousos GP, Gold PW. The concepts of stress and stress system disorders. *JAMA* 1992;267(9):1244–1252.
6. Calogero AE, Gallucci WT, Gold PW, et al. Multiple feedback regulatory loops upon rat hypothalamic corticotropin-releasing hormone secretion. Potential clinical implications. *J Clin Invest* 1988;82(3):767–774.
7. Imaki T, Nahan J, Rivier C, et al. Differential regulation of corticotropin-releasing factor mRNA in rat brain regions by glucocorticoids and stress. *J Neurosci* 1991;11(3):585–599.
8. Sutton RE, Koob GF, LeMoal M, et al. Corticotropin-releasing factor produces behavioural activation in rats. *Nature* 1982;297: 331–333.
9. Valentino RJ, Foote SL, Aston-Jones G. Corticotropin-releasing hormone activates noradrenergic neurons of the locus coeruleus. *Brain Res* 1983;270:363–367.
10. Irwin M, Hauger R, Brown M. Central corticotropin-releasing hormone activates the sympathetic nervous system and reduces immune function: increased responsivity of the aged rat. *Endocrinology* 1992;131(3):1047–1053.
11. Jansen ASP, Nguyen XV, Karpitskiy V, et al. Central command neurons of the sympathetic nervous system: basis of the fight-or-flight response. *Science* 1995;270:644–646.
12. Cunningham EJ, Bohn MC, Sawchenko PE. Organization of adrenergic inputs to the paraventricular and supraoptic nuclei of the hypothalamus in the rat. *J Comp Neurol* 1990;292(4): 651–667.
13. Madden KS, Felten SY, Felten DL, et al. Sympathetic nervous system modulation of the immune system. II. Induction of lymphocyte proliferation and migration in vivo by chemical sympathectomy. *J Neuroimmunol* 1994;49(1–2):67–75.
14. Madden KS, Moynihan JA, Brenner GJ, et al. Sympathetic nervous system modulation of the immune system. III. Alterations in T and B cell proliferation and differentiation in vitro following chemical sympathectomy. *J Neuroimmunol* 1994;49(1–2): 77–87.
15. Fontana A, Weber E, Dayer JM. Synthesis of interleukin 1/endogenous pyrogen in the brain of endotoxin-treated mice: a step in fever induction. *J Immunol* 1984;133: 1696–1698.
16. Besedovsky HO, Rey dA, Sorkin E, et al. Immunoregulatory feedback between interleukin-1 and glucocorticoid hormones. *Science* 1986;233:652–654.
17. Berkenbosch F, Oers vJ, Rey dA, et al. Corticotropin-releasing factor-producing neurons in the rat activated by interleukin-1. *Science* 1987;238:524–536.
18. Bernton EW, Beach JE, Holaday JW, et al. Release of multiple hormones by a direct action of interleukin-1 on pituitary cells. *Science* 1987;238:519–521.
19. Sapolsky R, Rivier C, Yamamoto G, et al. Interleukin-1 stimulates the secretion of hypothalamic corticotropin releasing factor. *Science* 1987;238:522–524.
20. Sternberg EM, Young WSd, Bernardini R, et al. A central nervous system defect in biosynthesis of corticotropin-releasing hormone is associated with susceptibility to streptococcal cell wall-induced arthritis in Lewis rats. *Proc Natl Acad Sci USA* 1989;86(12):4771–4775.

21. Arimura A, Takaki A, Komaki G. Interactions between cytokines and the hypothalamic-pituitary-adrenal axis during stress. *Ann NY Acad Sci* 1994;739(270):270–281.
22. Fukata J, Usui T, Naitoh Y, et al. Effects of recombinant human interleukin-1a, -1b, 2 and 6 on ACTH synthesis and release in the mouse pituitary tumour cell line atT-20. *J Endocrinol* 1988; 122:33–39.
23. Jones TH, Kennedy RL. Cytokines and hypothalamic-pituitary function. *Cytokine* 1993;5(6):531–538.
24. Mastorakos G, Chrousos GP, Weber JS. Recombinant interleukin-6 activates the hypothalamic-pituitary-adrenal axis in humans. *J Clin Endocrinol Metab* 1993;77(6):1690–1694.
25. McCann SM, Lyson K, Karanth S, et al. Role of cytokines in the endocrine system. *Ann NY Acad Sci* 1994;741(50):50–63.
26. Raber J, Koob GF, Bloom FE. Interleukin-2 (IL-2) induces corticotropin-releasing factor (CRF) release from the amygdala and involves a nitric oxide-mediated signaling: comparison with the hypothalamic response. *J Pharmacol Exp Ther* 1995;272(2): 815–824.
27. Rivier C. Effect of peripheral and central cytokines on the hypothalamic-pituitary-adrenal axis of the rat. *Ann NY Acad Sci* 1993;697(97):97–105.
28. Spangelo BL, Gorospe WC. Role of the cytokines in the neuroendocrine-immune system axis. *Front Neuroendocrinol* 1995; 16(1):1–22.
29. Spath SE, Born J, Schrezenmeier H, et al. Interleukin-6 stimulates the hypothalamus-pituitary-adrenocortical axis in man. *J Clin Endocrinol Metab* 1994;79(4):1212–1214.
30. Saphier D. Neuroendocrine effects of interferon-alpha in the rat. *Adv Exp Med Biol* 1995;373(209):209–218.
31. Banks WA, Kastin AJ, Durham DA. Bidirectional transport of interleukin-1 alpha across the blood-brain barrier. *Brain Res Bull* 1989;23:433–437.
32. Banks WA, Kastin AJ, Ehrensing CA. Blood-borne interleukin-1 alpha is transported across the endothelial blood-spinal cord barrier of mice. *J Physiol (Lond)* 1994;479(pt 2):257–264.
33. Banks WA, Kastin AJ, Gutierrez EG. Interleukin-1 alpha in blood has direct access to cortical brain cells. *Neurosci Lett* 1993; 163(1):41–44.
34. Banks WA, Kastin AJ, Gutierrez EG. Penetration of interleukin-6 across the murine blood-brain barrier. *Neurosci Lett* 1994;179(1–2):53–56.
35. Banks WA, Ortiz L, Plotkin SR, et al. Human interleukin (IL) 1a, murine IL-1a and murine IL-1b are transported from blood to brain in the mouse by a shared saturable mechanism. *J Pharmacol Exp Ther* 1991;259:988–1007.
36. Gutierrez EG, Banks WA, Kastin AJ. Murine tumor necrosis factor alpha is transported from blood to brain in the mouse. *J Neuroimmunol* 1993;47(2):169–176.
37. Waguespack PJ, Banks WA, Kastin AJ. Interleukin-2 does not cross the blood-brain barrier by a saturable transport system. *Brain Res Bull* 1994;34(2):103–109.
38. Watkins LR, Maier SF, Goehler LE. Cytokine-to-brain communication: a review and analysis of alternative mechanisms. *Life Sci* 1995;57(11):1011–1026.
39. Wright JL, Merchant RE. Blood-brain barrier changes following intracerebral injection of human recombinant tumor necrosis factor-alpha in the rat. *J Neurooncol* 1994;20(1):17–25.
40. Wong M, Bongiorno PB, Gold PW, et al. Localization of interleukin-1 beta converting enzyme mRNA in rat brain vasculature: evidence that the genes encoding the interleukin-1 system are constitutively expressed in brain blood vessels. *Neuroimmunomodulation* 1995;2:141–148.
41. Wong M, Licinio J. Localization of interleukin-1 type I receptor mRNA in rat brain. *Neuroimmunomodulation* 1994;1: 110–115.
42. Turnbull AV, Lee S, Rivier C. Mechanisms of hypothalamic-pituitary-adrenal axis stimulation by immune signals in the adult rat. *Ann NY Acad Sci* 1998;840:434–443.
43. Laye S, Bluthe RM, Kent S, et al. Subdiaphragmatic vagotomy blocks induction of IL-1 beta mRNA in mice brain in response to peripheral LPS. *Am J Physiol* 1995;268(5 pt 2):R1327–1331.
44. Fleshner M, Goehler LE, Hermann J, et al. Interleukin-1 beta induced corticosterone elevation and hypothalamic NE depletion is vagally mediated. *Brain Res Bull* 1995;37(6):605–610.
45. Niijima A, Hori T, Katafuchi T, et al. The effect of interleukin-1 beta on the efferent activity of the vagus nerve to the thymus. *J Auton Nerv Syst* 1995;54(2):137–144.
46. Benveniste EN. Cytokine actions in the central nervous system. *Cytokine Growth Factor Rev* 1998;9(3–4):259–275.
47. Hopkins SJ, Rothwell NJ. Cytokines and the nervous system. I: Expression and recognition. *Trends Neurosci* 1995;18(2):83–88.
48. Sei Y, Vitkovic L, Yokoyama MM. Cytokines in the central nervous system: regulatory roles in neuronal function, cell death and repair. *Neuroimmunomodulation* 1995;2(3):121–133.
49. Breder CD, Dinarello CA, Saper CB. Interleukin-1 immunoreactive innervation of the human hypothalamus. *Science* 1988; 240:321–324.
50. Licinio J, Wong ML, Gold PW. Localization of interleukin-1 receptor antagonist mRNA in rat brain. *Endocrinology* 1991; 129(1):562–564.
51. Brenneman D, Schultzberg M, Bartfai T, et al. Cytokine regulation of neuronal cell survival. *J Neurochem* 1992;58:454–460.
52. Brenneman DE, Page SW, Schultzberg M, et al. A decomposition product of a contaminant implicated in L-tryptophan eosinophilia myalgia syndrome affects spinal cord neuronal cell death and survival through stereospecific, maturation and partly interleukin-1-dependent mechanisms. *J Pharmacol Exp Ther* 1993;266(2):1029–1035.
53. Campbell IL. Neuropathogenic actions of cytokines assessed in transgenic mice. *Int J Dev Neurosci* 1995;13(3–4):275–284.
54. Heyser CJ, Masliah E, Samimi A, et al. Progressive decline in avoidance learning paralleled by inflammatory neurodegeneration in transgenic mice expressing interleukin 6 in the brain. *Proc Natl Acad Sci USA* 1997;94(4):1500–1505.
55. Moalem G, Leibowitz-Amit R, Yoles E, et al. Autoimmune T cells protect neurons from secondary degeneration after central nervous system axotomy. *Nat Med* 1999;5(1):49–55.
56. Vitkovic L, Chatham JJ, da Cunha A. Distinct expression of three cytokines by IL-1–stimulated astrocytes in vitro in AIDS brain. *Brain Behav Immun* 1995;9:378–388.
57. Ensoli F, Fiorelli V, DeCristofaro M, et al. Inflammatory cytokines and HIV-1-associated neurodegeneration: oncostatin-M produced by mononuclear cells from HIV-1-infected individuals induces apoptosis of primary neurons. *J Immunol* 1999; 162(10):6268–6277.
58. McGeer PL, McGeer EG. Glial cell reactions in neurodegenerative diseases: pathophysiology and therapeutic interventions. *Alzheimer Dis Assoc Disord* 1998;12(suppl 2):S1–6.
59. Georgescu L, Mevorach D, Arnett FC, et al. Anti-P antibodies and neuropsychiatric lupus erythematosus. *Ann NY Acad Sci* 1997;823:263–269.
60. Jara LJ, Irigoyen L, Ortiz MJ, et al. Prolactin and interleukin-6 in neuropsychiatric lupus erythematosus. *Clin Rheumatol* 1998; 17(2):110–114.
61. Wong M, Loddick SA, Bongiorno PB, et al. Focal cerebral ischemia induces CRH mRNA in rat cerebral cortex and amygdala. *NeuroReport* 1995;6:1785–1788.
62. Chao CC, Hu S, Ehrlich L, et al. Interleukin-1 and tumor necrosis factor-alpha synergistically mediate neurotoxicity: involvement of nitric oxide and of N-methyl-D-aspartate receptors. *Brain Behav Immun* 1995;9(4):355–365.

63. Bluthe RM, Walter V, Parnet P, et al. Lipopolysaccharide induces sickness behaviour in rats by a vagal mediated mechanism. *C R Acad Sci* 1994;317(6):499–503.
64. Dantzer R, Bluthe RM, Gheusi G, et al. Molecular basis of sickness behavior. *Ann NY Acad Sci* 1998;856:132–138.
65. Dantzer R, Bluthe RM, Laye S, et al. Cytokines and sickness behavior. *Ann NY Acad Sci* 1998;840:586–590.
66. Elmquist JK, Scammell TE, Saper CB. Mechanisms of CNS response to systemic immune challenge: the febrile response. *Trends Neurosci* 1997;20(12):565–570.
67. Evans RM. The steroid and thyroid hormone receptor superfamily. *Science* 1988;240:889–895.
68. Whitfield GK, Jurutka PW, Haussler CA, et al. Steroid hormone receptors: evolution, ligands, and molecular basis of biologic function. *J Cell Biochem* 1999;32–33(suppl):110–122.
69. Munck A, Mendel DB, Smith LI, et al. Glucocorticoid receptors and actions. *Am Rev Respir Dis* 1990;141:S2–S10.
70. Wissink S, van Heerde EC, vand der Burg B, et al. A dual mechanism mediates repression of NF-kappaB activity by glucocorticoids. *Mol Endocrinol* 1998;12(3):355–363.
71. De Kloet ER. Brain corticosteroid receptor balance and homeostatic control. *Front Neuroendocrinol* 1991;12(2):95–164.
72. de Kloet ER. Stress in the brain. *Eur J Pharmacol* 2000; 405(1–3):187–198.
73. De Kloet ER, Vreugdenhil E, Oitzl MS, et al. Brain corticosteroid receptor balance in health and disease. *Endocr Rev* 1998; 19(3):269–301.
74. Funder JW. Mineralocorticoids, glucocorticoids, receptors and response elements. *Science* 1993;259:1132–1133.
75. Funder JW. Glucocorticoid and mineralocorticoid receptors: biology and clinical relevance. *Annu Rev Med* 1997;48:231–240.
76. Liu W, Wang J, Sauter NK, et al. Steroid receptor heterodimerization demonstrated in vitro and in vivo. *Proc Natl Acad Sci USA* 1995;92(26):12480–12484.
77. Trapp T, Holsboer F. Heterodimerization between mineralocorticoid and glucocorticoid receptors increases the functional diversity of corticosteroid action. *Trends Pharmacol Sci* 1996; 17(4):145–149.
78. Trapp T, Rupprecht R, Castren M, et al. Heterodimerization between mineralocorticoid and glucocorticoid receptor: a new principle of glucocorticoid action in the CNS. *Neuron* 1994; 13:1457–1462.
79. Malkoski SP, Dorin RI. Composite glucocorticoid regulation at a functionally defined negative glucocorticoid response element of the human corticotropin-releasing hormone gene. *Mol Endocrinol* 1999;13(10):1629–1644.
80. Pearce D, Matsui W, Miner JN, et al. Glucocorticoid receptor transcriptional activity determined by spacing of receptor and nonreceptor DNA sites. *J Biol Chem* 1998;273(46): 30081–30085.
81. Pearce D, Yamamoto KR. Mineralocorticoid and glucocorticoid receptor activities distinguished by nonreceptor factors at a composite response element. *Science* 1993;259:1161–1165.
82. Cole MA, Kim PJ, Kalman BA, et al. Dexamethasone suppression of corticosteroid secretion: evaluation of the site of action by receptor measures and functional studies. *Psychoneuroendocrinology* 2000;25(2):151–167.
83. Deak T, Nguyen KT, Cotter CS, et al. Long-term changes in mineralocorticoid and glucocorticoid receptor occupancy following exposure to an acute stressor. *Brain Res* 1999;847(2): 211–220.
84. Derijk R, Sternberg EM. Corticosteroid action and neuroendocrine-immune interactions. *Ann NY Acad Sci* 1994;746: 33–41; discussion 64–67.
85. Dhabhar FS, McEwen BS, Spencer RL. Stress response, adrenal steroid receptor levels and corticosteroid-binding globulin levels—a comparison between Sprague-Dawley, Fischer 344 and Lewis rats. *Brain Res* 1993;616:89–98.
86. Linthorst AC, Flachskamm C, Barden N, et al. Glucocorticoid receptor impairment alters CNS responses to a psychological stressor: an in vivo microdialysis study in transgenic mice. *Eur J Neurosci* 2000;12(1):283–291.
87. Sternberg EM, Smith CC, Omeljaniuk RJ, et al. Differential type 1 (mineralocorticoid) and type 2 (glucocorticoid) receptor expression in Lewis and Fischer rats. *Neuroimmunomodulation* 1994;1:66–73.
88. Diaz R, Brown RW, Seckl JR. Distinct ontogeny of glucocorticoid and mineralocorticoid receptor and 11beta-hydroxysteroid dehydrogenase types I and II mRNAs in the fetal rat brain suggest a complex control of glucocorticoid actions. *J Neurosci* 1998;18(7):2570–2580.
89. Krozowski Z. The 11beta-hydroxysteroid dehydrogenases: functions and physiological effects. *Mol Cell Endocrinol* 1999; 151(1–2):121–127.
90. DeRijk R, Berkenbosch F. Suppressive and permissive actions of glucocorticoids: a way to control innate immunity and to facilitate specificity of adaptive immunity. In: Grossman CJ, ed. *Bilateral communication between the endocrine and immune systems*. New York: Springer-Verlag, 1994:73–95.
91. Munck A, Guyre PM. Glucocorticoids and immune function. In: Ader R, Felten DL, Cohen N, eds. *Psychoneuroimmunology*. San Diego: Academic Press, 1991:447–474.
92. Elenkov IJ, Webster EL, Torpy DJ, et al. Stress, corticotropin-releasing hormone, glucocorticoids, and the immune/inflammatory response: acute and chronic effects. *Ann NY Acad Sci* 1999;876:1–11; discussion 11–13.
93. Cohen JJ. Programmed cell death and apoptosis in lymphocyte development and function. *Chest* 1993;103(2 suppl):99–101.
94. Evans SR, Cidlowski JA. Regulation of apoptosis by steroid hormones. *J Steroid Biochem Mol Biol* 1995;53(1–6):1–8.
95. Jamieson CA, Yamamoto KR. Crosstalk pathway for inhibition of glucocorticoid-induced apoptosis by T cell receptor signaling. *Proc Natl Acad Sci USA* 2000;97(13):7319–7324.
96. Cupps TR, Fauci AS. Corticosteroid-mediated immunoregulation in man. *Immunol Rev* 1982;65:133–155.
97. Brinkmann V, Kristofic C. Regulation by corticosteroids of Th1 and Th2 cytokine production in human CD4+ effector T cells generated from CD45RO– and CD45RO+ subsets. *J Immunol* 1995;155:3322–3328.
98. Daynes RA, Araneo BA. Contrasting effects of glucocorticoids on the capacity of T cells to produce the growth factors interleukin 2 and interleukin 4. *Eur J Immunol* 1989;19:2319–2325.
99. Snijdewint FGM, Kapsenberg ML, Wauben-Penris PJJ, et al. Corticosteroids class-dependently inhibit in vitro Th1- and Th2-type cytokine production. *Immunopharmacology* 1995;29: 93–101.
100. Elenkov IJ, Chrousos GP. Stress Hormones, Th1/Th2 patterns, pro/anti-inflammatory cytokines and susceptibility to disease. *Trends Endocrinol Metab* 1999;10(9):359–368.
101. Sternberg EM, Parker CW. Immunopharmacologic aspects of lymphocyte regulation. In: Marchalonis JJ, ed. *Lymphocyte structure and function*. New York: Marcel Dekker, 1988:1–53.
102. Wiegers GJ, Reul JMHM, Holsboer F, et al. Enhancement of rat splenic lymphocyte mitogenesis after short-term pre-exposure to corticosteroids in vitro. *Endocrinology* 1994;135:2351–2357.
103. Reichlin S. Neuroendocrine-immune interactions. *N Engl J Med* 1993;329(17):1246–1253.
104. Akahoshi T, Oppenheim JJ, Matsushima K. Induction of high affinity interleukin-1 receptor on human peripheral blood lymphocytes by glucocorticoid hormones. *J Exp Med* 1988; 167:924–936.
105. Colotta F, Dower SK, Sims JE, et al. The type II "decoy" recep-

tor: a novel regulatory pathway for interleukin 1. *Immunol Today* 1994;15(12):562–566.

106. Colotta F, Mantovani A. Induction of the interleukin-1 decoy receptor by glucocorticoids [letter; comment]. *Trends Pharmacol Sci* 1994;15(5):138–139.
107. Cohen JJ. Lymphocyte death induced by glucocorticoids. In: Schleimer RP, Claman HN, Oronsky A, eds. *Anti-inflammatory steroid action: basic and clinical aspects.* San Diego: Academic Press, 1989:111–127.
108. King LB, Vacchio MS, Dixon K, et al. A targeted glucocorticoid receptor antisense transgene increases thymocyte apoptosis and alters thymocyte development. *Immunity* 1995;3(5):647–656.
109. Ashwell JD, Lu FW, Vacchio MS. Glucocorticoids in T cell development and function. *Annu Rev Immunol* 2000;18: 309–345.
110. Vacchio MS, Ashwell JD. Glucocorticoids and thymocyte development [in process citation]. *Semin Immunol* 2000;12(5): 475–485.
111. Vacchio MS, Lee JY, Ashwell JD. Thymus-derived glucocorticoids set the thresholds for thymocyte selection by inhibiting TCR-mediated thymocyte activation. *J Immunol* 1999;163(3): 1327–1333.
112. Felten SY, Felten DL. Innervation of lymphoid tissue. In: Ader R, Felten DL, Cohen N, eds. *Psychoneuroimmunology*, 2nd ed. San Diego: Academic Press, 1991:27–61.
113. Green PG, Luo J, Heller PH, Levine JD. Further substantiation of a significant role for the sympathetic nervous system in inflammation. *Neuroscience* 1993;55(4):1037–1043.
114. Sundar SK, Cierpial MA, Kilts C, et al. Brain IL-1 induced immunosuppression occurs through activation of both pituitary-adrenal axis and sympathetic nervous system by corticotropin-releasing factor. *J Neurosci* 1990;10:3701–3706.
115. Green PG, Luo J, Heller P, et al. Modulation of bradykinin-induced plasma extravasation in the rat knee joint by sympathetic co-transmitters. *Neuroscience* 1993;52(2):451–458.
116. Helme RD, Andrews PV. The effect of nerve lesions on the inflammatory response to injury. *J Neuroscience Res* 1985;13: 453–459.
117. Levine JD, Clark R, Devor M, et al. Intraneuronal substance P contributes to the severity of experimental arthritis. *Science* 1984;226:547–549.
118. Weinstock JV. Neuropeptides and the regulation of granulomatous inflammation. *Clin Immunol Immunopathol* 1992;64(1): 17–22.
119. Pothoulakis C, Castagliuolo I, LaMont JT, et al. CP-96,345, a substance P antagonist, inhibits rat intestinal responses to *Clostridium difficile* toxin A but not cholera toxin. *Proc Natl Acad Sci USA* 1994;91(3):947–951.
120. Felten DL, Felten SY, Bellinger DL, et al. Noradrenergic and peptididergic innervation of secondary lymphoid organs: role in experimental rheumatoid arthritis. *Eur J Clin Invest* 1992; 22(suppl 1):37–41.
121. Levine JD, Dardick SJ, Roizen MF, et al. Contribution of sensory afferents and sympathetic efferents to joint injury in experimental arthritis. *J Neurosci* 1986;6:3423–3429.
122. Chelmicka-Schorr E, Kwasniewski MN, Thomas BE, et al. The b-adrenergic agonist isoproterenol suppresses experimental allergic encephalomyelitis in Lewis rats. *J Neuroimmunol* 1989; 25:203–207.
123. Levine JD, Coderre TJ, Helms C, et al. B2-adrenergic mechanisms in experimental arthritis. *Proc Natl Acad Sci USA* 1988; 85:4553–4556.
124. Madden KS, Bellinger DL, Felten SY, et al. Alterations in sympathetic innervation of thymus and spleen in aged mice. *Mech Ageing Dev* 1997;94(1–3):165–175.
125. Madden KS, Stevens SY, Felten DL, et al. Alterations in T lymphocyte activity following chemical sympathectomy in young and old Fischer 344 rats. *J Neuroimmunol* 2000;103(2): 131–145.
126. Madden KS, Thyagarajan S, Felten DL. Alterations in sympathetic noradrenergic innervation in lymphoid organs with age. *Ann NY Acad Sci* 1998;840:262–268.
127. ThyagaRajan S, Felten SY, Felten DL. Restoration of sympathetic noradrenergic nerve fibers in the spleen by low doses of L-deprenyl treatment in young sympathectomized and old Fischer 344 rats. *J Neuroimmunol* 1998;81(1–2):144–157.
128. ThyagaRajan S, Madden KS, Kalvass JC, et al. L-deprenyl-induced increase in IL-2 and NK cell activity accompanies restoration of noradrenergic nerve fibers in the spleens of old F344 rats. *J Neuroimmunol* 1998;92(1–2):9–21.
129. Sternberg EM, Hill JM, Chrousos GP, et al. Inflammatory mediator-induced hypothalamic-pituitary-adrenal axis activation is defective in streptococcal cell wall arthritis-susceptible Lewis rats. *Proc Natl Acad Sci USA* 1989;86(7):2374–2378.
130. Mason D, MacPhee I, Antoini F. The role of the neuroendocrine system in determining genetic susceptibility to experimental allergic encephalomyelitis in the rat. *Immunology* 1990; 70:1–5.
131. Edwards CKI, Yunger LM, Lorence RM, et al. The pituitary gland is required for protection against lethal effects of *Salmonella typhimurium. Proc Natl Acad Sci USA* 1991;88(6):2274–2277.
132. Misiewicz B, Poltorak M, Raybourne RB, et al. Intracerebroventricular transplantation of embryonic neuronal tissue from inflammatory resistant into inflammatory susceptible rats suppresses specific components of inflammation. *Exp Neurol* 1997;146(2):305–314.
133. Furuya T, Salstrom JL, McCall-Vining S, et al. Genetic dissection of a rat model for rheumatoid arthritis: significant gender influences on autosomal modifier loci [in process citation]. *Hum Mol Genet* 2000;9(15):2241–2250.
134. Dracheva SV, Remmers EF, Chen S, et al. An integrated genetic linkage map with 1,137 markers constructed from five F2 crosses of autoimmune disease-prone and -resistant inbred rat strains. *Genomics* 2000;63(2):202–226.
135. Wilder RL, Griffiths MM, Remmers EF, et al. Localization in rats of genetic loci regulating susceptibility to experimental erosive arthritis and related autoimmune diseases. *Transplant Proc* 1999;31(3):1585–1588.
136. Listwak S, Barrientos RM, Koike G, et al. Identification of a novel inflammation-protective locus in the Fischer rat. *Mamm Genome* 1999;10(4):362–365.
137. Jafarian-Tehrani M, Listwak S, Barrientos RM, et al. Exclusion of angiotensin I-converting enzyme as a candidate gene involved in exudative inflammatory resistance in F344/N rats. *Mol Med* 2000;6(4):319–331.
138. Harbuz MS, Windle RJ, Jessop DS, et al. Differential effects of psychological and immunological challenge on the hypothalamo-pituitary-adrenal axis function in adjuvant-induced arthritis. *Ann NY Acad Sci* 1999;876:43–52.
139. Johnson EO, Vlachoyiannopoulos PG, Skopouli FN, et al. Hypofunction of the stress axis in Sjogren's syndrome. *J Rheumatol* 1998;25(8):1508–1514.
140. Johnson EO, Skopouli FN, Moutsopoulos HM. Neuroendocrine manifestations in Sjogren's syndrome [in process citation]. *Rheum Dis Clin North Am* 2000;26(4):927–949.
141. Shanks N, Moore PM, Perks P, et al. Alterations in hypothalamic-pituitary-adrenal function correlated with the onset of murine SLE in MRL +/+ and lpr/lpr mice. *Brain Behav Immun* 1999;13(4):348–360.
142. Wilder RL. Hormones and autoimmunity: animal models of arthritis. *Baillieres Clin Rheumatol* 1996;10(2):259–271.
143. Neeck G, Crofford LJ. Neuroendocrine perturbations in

fibromyalgia and chronic fatigue syndrome [in process citation]. *Rheum Dis Clin North Am* 2000;26(4):989–1002.
144. Crofford LJ. Neuroendocrine abnormalities in fibromyalgia and related disorders. *Am J Med Sci* 1998;315(6):359–366.
145. Crofford LJ. The hypothalamic-pituitary-adrenal stress axis in fibromyalgia and chronic fatigue syndrome. *Z Rheumatol* 1998; 57(suppl 2):67–71.
146. Demitrack MA, Crofford LJ. Evidence for and pathophysiologic implications of hypothalamic-pituitary-adrenal axis dysregulation in fibromyalgia and chronic fatigue syndrome. *Ann NY Acad Sci* 1998;840:684–697.
147. Hurwitz EL, Morgenstern H. Cross-sectional associations of asthma, hay fever, and other allergies with major depression and low-back pain among adults aged 20–39 years in the United States. *Am J Epidemiol* 1999;150(10):1107–1116.
148. Webster EL, Torpy DJ, Elenkov IJ, et al. Corticotropin-releasing hormone and inflammation. *Ann NY Acad Sci* 1998;840: 21–32.
149. Buske-Kirschbaum A, Jobst S, Hellhammer DH. Altered reactivity of the hypothalamus-pituitary-adrenal axis in patients with atopic dermatitis: pathologic factor or symptom? *Ann NY Acad Sci* 1998;840:747–754.
150. Jafarian Tehrani M, Hu Y, Marquette C, et al. Interleukin-1 receptor deficiency in brains from NZB and (NZB/NZW)F1 autoimmune mice. *J Neuroimmunol* 1994;53:91–99.
151. Jafarian-Tehrani M, Gabellec MM, Adyel FZ, et al. Interleukin-1 receptor deficiency in the hippocampal formation of (NZB × NZW)F2 mice: genetic and molecular studies relating to autoimmunity. *J Neuroimmunol* 1998;84(1):30–39.
152. Hirohata S, Miyamoto T. Elevated levels of interleukin-6 in cerebrospinal fluid from patients with systemic lupus erythematosus and central nervous system involvement. *Arthritis Rheum* 1990;33(5):644–649.
153. Shiozawa S, Kuroki Y, Kim M, et al. Interferon-alpha in lupus psychosis. *Arthritis Rheum* 1992;35(4):417–422.
154. Gilad R, Lampl Y, Eshel Y, et al. Cerebrospinal fluid soluble interleukin-2 receptor in cerebral lupus. *Br J Rheumatol* 1997; 36(2):190–193.
155. Kelley KW, Hutchison K, French R, et al. Central interleukin-1 receptors as mediators of sickness. *Ann NY Acad Sci* 1997; 823:234–246.
156. Zietz B, Reber T, Oertel M, et al. Altered function of the hypothalamic stress axes in patients with moderately active systemic lupus erythematosus. II. Dissociation between androstenedione, cortisol, or dehydroepiandrosterone and interleukin 6 or tumor necrosis factor. *J Rheumatol* 2000;27(4):911–918.
157. Diaz-Borjon A, Richaud-Patin Y, Alvarado de la Barrera C, et al. Multidrug resistance-1 (MDR-1) in rheumatic autoimmune disorders. Part II: increased P-glycoprotein activity in lymphocytes from systemic lupus erythematosus patients might affect steroid requirements for disease control. *Joint Bone Spine* 2000; 67(1):40–48.
158. Greenstein B. Steroid resistance: implications for lupus [editorial]. *Lupus* 1994;3(3):143.
159. Gladman DD, Urowitz MB, Doris F, et al. Glucocorticoid receptors in systemic lupus erythematosus. *J Rheumatol* 1991; 18:681–684.
160. Tanaka H, Akama H, Ichikawa Y, et al. Glucocorticoid receptor in patients with lupus nephritis: relationship between receptor levels in mononuclear leukocytes and effect of glucocorticoid therapy. *J Rheumatol* 1992;19:878–883.
161. Sanden S, Tripmacher R, Weltrich R, et al. Glucocorticoid dose dependent downregulation of glucocorticoid receptors in patients with rheumatic diseases. *J Rheumatol* 2000;27(5): 1265–1270.
162. Brown DH, Sheridan J, Pearl D, et al. Regulation of mycobacterial growth by the hypothalamus-pituitary-adrenal axis: differential responses of *Mycobacterium bovis* BCG-resistant and -susceptible mice. *Infect Immun* 1993;61(11):4793–4800.
163. Hermann G, Tovar CA, Beck FM, et al. Restraint stress differentially affects the pathogenesis of an experimental influenza viral infection in three inbred strains of mice. *J Neuroimmunol* 1993;47(1):83–94.
164. Sheridan JF, Feng NG, Bonneau RH, et al. Restraint stress differentially affects anti-viral cellular and humoral immune responses in mice. *J Neuroimmunol* 1991;31:245–255.
165. Da Costa D, Dobkin PL, Pinard L, et al. The role of stress in functional disability among women with systemic lupus erythematosus: a prospective study. *Arthritis Care Res* 1999;12(2): 112–119.
166. Pawlak CR, Jacobs R, Mikeska E, et al. Patients with systemic lupus erythematosus differ from healthy controls in their immunological response to acute psychological stress. *Brain Behav Immun* 1999;13(4):287–302.
167. Wallace DJ. Does stress or trauma cause or aggravate rheumatic disease? *Baillieres Clin Rheumatol* 1994;8(1):149–159.
168. Lightman SL, Harbuz MS. Expression of corticotropin-releasing factor mRNA in response to stress. *Ciba Found Symp* 1993; 172(173):173–187.
169. Michelson D, Stone L, Galliven E, et al. Multiple sclerosis is associated with alterations in hypothalamic-pituitary-adrenal axis function. *J Clin Endocrinol Metab* 1994;79(3):848–853.
170. Whitnall MH, Anderson KA, Lane CA, et al. Decreased vasopressin content in parvocellular CRH neurosecretory system of Lewis rats. *Neuroreport* 1994;5(13):1635–1637.
171. Schmidt ED, Janszen AW, Wouterlood FG, et al. Interleukin-1-induced long-lasting changes in hypothalamic corticotropin-releasing hormone (CRH)—neurons and hyperresponsiveness of the hypothalamus-pituitary-adrenal axis. *J Neurosci* 1995; 15(11):7417–7426.
172. Brady LS, Whitfield HJJ, Fox RJ, et al. Long-term antidepressant administration alters corticotropin-releasing hormone, tyrosine hydroxylase and mineralocorticoid receptor gene expression in rat brain. Therapeutic implications. *J Clin Invest* 1991;87(3): 831–837.
173. Michelson D, Misiewicz-Poltorak B, Raybourne RB, et al. Imipramine reduces the local inflammatory response to carrageenin. *Agents Actions* 1994;42(1–2):25–28.

18

ANIMAL MODELS OF SYSTEMIC LUPUS ERYTHEMATOSUS

BEVRA HANNAHS HAHN

Since the derivation of the autoimmune New Zealand black (NZB)/B1 mouse in 1959 (1), there has been great interest in several mouse models of spontaneous systemic lupus erythematosus (SLE)-like disease. In addition, recent experiments have shown that eliminating single selected genes can lead to lupus-like disease in normal mice. Studies in all of these animals have shown that genetic factors govern the development of autoimmunity. Multiple genes are involved, however, and some probably are influenced by environmental and hormonal factors. Each model differs from the others in genetic, immunologic, and clinical manifestations of autoimmunity. Information from studies of these animals has contributed to understanding human disease; further, studies of efficacy of therapeutic interventions in spontaneous murine SLE have formed the basis for similar interventions in human disease. Spontaneous SLE also occurs in dogs, and drug- or diet-induced SLE has been reported in cats and monkeys. Investigations are most extensive in mice, so most of this chapter is devoted to murine SLE.

The most widely studied murine models of SLE are described here. These include the New Zealand, Medical Research Laboratory (MRL), BXSB, and Palmerston North strains. In addition, the single gene mutations associated with lupus-like disease in mice are also discussed. Table 18.1 provides an overview of abnormalities in strains with polygenic spontaneous disease.

CLINICAL DISEASE, AUTOANTIBODIES, IMMUNOLOGIC ABNORMALITIES, AND GENETICS IN SPONTANEOUS POLYGENIC MURINE SLE

Numerous murine models of spontaneous SLE have been studied. This section reviews the principal characteristics of the most extensively studied strains.

New Zealand Mice

NZB/Bl (NZB) Mice

The New Zealand Bielschowsky black (NZB/Bl) mouse was bred by Bielschowsky, who was mating mice by coat color to derive cancer-susceptible strains. In 1959, she reported that NZB mice died early from autoimmune hemolytic anemia (1). Shortly thereafter, her colleagues described a hybrid between NZB and unrelated strains including the New Zealand white (NZW) that were characterized by early death in females from nephritis associated with lupus erythematosus (LE) cells, thus providing the first animal models of SLE (2,3).

The characteristics of NZB mice are shown in Tables 18.1 and 18.2. They also are discussed in several review articles (4–8).

Clinical Characteristics and Autoantibodies

NZB mice are characterized by hyperactive B cells, which are present in fetal life, that produce primarily immunoglobulin M (IgM) antibodies to thymocytes, erythrocytes, single-stranded DNA (ssDNA), and the gp70 glycoprotein of murine leukemia virus (5–12). The first antibody to appear in serum is natural thymocytotoxic antibody (NTA) (13,14); by 3 months of age, 100% of mice have this antibody. NTAs are cytotoxic for all thymocytes, 50% to 60% of thoracic duct and peripheral blood lymphocytes (both $CD4^+$ and $CD8^+$ populations), 50% of lymph node cells, 33% of spleen cells, and 5% of bone marrow cells. These figures are similar to the reactivity of anti–Thy-l sera that recognize all T cells. The antigens that are recognized by NTA are varied. Some NTAs react with cell surface molecules on B lymphocytes, granulocytes, and bone marrow myeloid cells; others react with a 55-kd molecule on most T cells. Other reported reactivities include an 88-kd glycoprotein, which is thought to be a T-cell differentiation antigen, and surface molecules of 33- and 30-kd sizes (8,15–17).

TABLE 18.1. MAJOR CHARACTERISTICS OF MURINE STRAINS DEVELOPING SYSTEMIC LUPUS ERYTHEMATOSUS (SLE)

Strain	Coat Color	H-2 Locus	Mls-1 Locus	Age for 50% Mortality (mo)	Sex Dominance	Cause of Death	Autoantibodies
NZB/Bl	Black	d/d	a	16.0	M/F	Hemolytic anemic	NTA, Anti-RBC, Anti-gp70
NZB/NZW F_1 (BW)	Brown	d/z	a/b	8.5	F	GN	IgG anti-DNA
NZB/SWR F_1 (SNF_1)	Brown	d/q	a/a	6.0	F	GN	IgG anti-DNA
MRL-*lpr/lpr* (MRL/l)	White	k/k	b	6.0	M/F	GN	CIC, Anti-DNA, RF, Anti-Sm
BXSB	Brown	b/b	b	5.0	M	GN	IgG anti-DNA

CIC, circulating immune complexes; F, female; M, male; RF, rheumatoid factors; NZB, New Zealand black mice; NZW, New Zealand white mice; MRL-*lpr,* Medical Research Laboratory lymphoproliferative mice.

TABLE 18.2. CHARACTERISTICS OF NZB/BI MICE

A. Clinical
  1. Females live a mean of 431 days, males 467 days
  2. Death usually is caused by autoimmune hemolytic anemia
  3. Fifty-percent mortality by 15 to 17 months of age

B. Histologic
  1. Glomerulonephritis with immunoglobulin and C3 deposits
  2. Marked thymic atrophy
  3. Mild lymphoid hyperplasia

C. Autoantibodies
  1. IgM NTA
  2. IgM and IgG antierythrocyte
  3. IgM anti-ssDNA
  4. Anti-gp70
  5. ANAs by late life
  6. Modest elevations of circulating immune complexes

D. Immune abnormalities
  1. B cells are unusually mature, hyperactivated, and secrete immunoglobulin spontaneously from a very early age (in fetus and in newborn mice); this abnormality is required for autoimmune disease in NZB mice and in hybrids mated with NZB mice
  2. Numbers of B-1 ($CD5^+$) B cells in spleen and peritoneum are increased; these cells make primarily IgM autoantibodies; however, their elimination by introduction of the *xid* gene protects from SLE
  3. B cells resist tolerance to T-independent antigens
  4. Older mice develop aneuploidy in B-1 B cells
  5. Thymic epithelium is atrophic by 1 month of age; this is a striking abnormality in NZB mice
  6. Antithymocyte antibodies react with immune T cells and may inactivate/delete precursors of suppressor T populations
  7. T cells are required for maximal autoantibody formation
  8. A unique form of retroviral gp70 antigen is secreted, and high quantities are found in serum
  9. Clearance of immune complexes by Fc-mediated mechanisms is defective

E. Genetics
  1. Multiple dominant, codominant, and recessive genes participate in the immune abnormalities
  2. One set of genes controls the constellation of polyclonal B-cell activation, expression of gp70, and antithymocyte antibodies; another set of genes controls B-cell tolerance defects, antibodies to gp70, anti-ssDNA, and anti-RBCs; the gene sets segregate independently; neither of these sets is dependent on H-2
  3. The disease is linked to MHC
  4. Analysis of the NZ genome by microsatellites suggests that NZB donates two to five genes located on different chromosomes, some transmitted in a dominant and others in a recessive fashion, to lupus in mice with NZ backgrounds

ANA, antinuclear antibody; IgM, immunoglobulin M; MHC, major histocompatibility complex; ssDNA, single-stranded DNA.

The primary clinical problem in NZB mice is hemolytic anemia, which is fatal in most at between 15 and 18 months of age (1,5,8). There is mild disease acceleration in females, with death occurring approximately 1 month earlier than in males. IgM and IgG antibodies to erythrocytes cause the hemolysis (18–20) and can be directed against erythrocyte surface antigens that are exposed by treating the red blood cell (RBC) with bromelein, against erythrocyte membrane protein band 3 (21–23), or against spectrin (24). Early in life, the antierythrocyte antibodies are polyreactive; later, they become more specific for band 3 or spectrin, suggesting antigenic stimulation (24). Anti-RBC appears in the serum by 3 months of age and is found in 100% of mice by 12 to 15 months. Clinical hemolysis begins 1 to 5 months after the antibodies appear. Severe anemia occurs in 56% to 87% of females and 77% of males (25). The expected sequelae of hemolysis occur (i.e., erythrocyte sequestration and extramedullary hematopoiesis in liver and spleen, splenomegaly, hepatomegaly, and deposits of hemosiderin in multiple tissues).

Clinical glomerulonephritis (GN) may be observed in some NZB mice, but it is mild compared with the nephritis of other lupus murine models, probably because, in contrast to the IgG anti–double-stranded DNA (anti-dsDNA) that arise in the other strains, the IgM anti-ssDNA that dominates the NZB response does not contain many nephritogenic subsets of anti-DNA. However, histologic changes of glomerulonephritis, nephrotic syndrome, and renal insufficiency occur in some mice late in their life span, especially in virgin females (26,27). The incidence of antinuclear antibodies (ANAs) in NZB mice is variable. ANAs are not regularly present in high titers as they are in other lupus-prone strains, but approximately 80% of mice are positive by 9 months of age (5). Some NZB mice exhibit learning disabilities (28), which probably relate both to the cortical ectopias that occur in approximately 40% (possibly similar to the lesions in human dyslexia) and to the autoimmune process. Autoantibodies to Purkinje cells of the cerebellum have been found (29), and the numbers of interleukin-1 (IL-1) receptors that are expressed in the dentate gyrus are much lower than in normal mice (30).

Abnormalities of Stem Cells and B Cells

NZB mice are remarkable for inherent abnormalities in their B cells that probably originate in bone marrow stem cells. In comparison to normal mice, there are increased numbers of IgM-secreting cells and increased synthesis of IgM by individual B cells, which are characteristics that may be controlled by different genes (4,31–33). This hyperactivation of B cells begins quite early and is detectable in fetal liver. The IgM hypergammaglobulinemia of NZB mice may depend on gene(s) in a region on chromosome 4 that is 70 to 90 centimorgan (cM) distal to the centromere (34). Putative bone marrow pre–B cells exhibit increased growth both *in vitro* (35) and *in vivo* (36); this property is lost after 10 months of age (37). The mature B cells are committed to secretion of Ig, particularly IgM. They are resistant to normal control mechanisms involving engagement of the B-cell receptor (BCR). Normally, if the BCR is bound, B cells cannot respond to lipopolysaccharide (LPS) stimulation by secreting Ig; NZB B cells in this situation secrete IgM, probably because of abnormal downstream signaling events. Regulation of B-cell activation is not completely askew, however; binding of major histocompatibility complex (MHC) class II interrupts signaling by LPS in a normal fashion (38).

Another B-cell abnormality that is highly characteristic of NZB mice is the appearance of aneuploidy in B cells, primarily in $CD5^+$ (also designated Ly-1 or B-1) B cells, as the mice age. Hyperdiploid B-1 B cells with additional chromosomes 10, 15, 17, and X are common (39,40). Lymphoid malignancies are more common in NZB than in other murine lupus strains, varying in different colonies between 1% and 20% (13,40–42); they may be a model of B-cell chronic lymphocytic leukemia (40). Malignant B-1 B cells secrete large quantities of IL-10, which can skew T-cell repertoires away from T-helper-1 (Th1) and toward Th2 phenotypes (43). In young NZB mice, numbers of nonmalignant B-1 B cells are increased in the spleen and peritoneum (4,44,45); these cells make IgM autoantibodies to RBCs, thymocytes, and ssDNA (4,44–46). B-2 ($CD5^-$) B cells are more likely to be the source for IgG autoantibodies (47,48). Elimination of B-1 B cells by introducing the X-linked recessive gene, *Xid*(32), or by lysing the cells with water in the peritoneal cavity (where these cells are renewed) reduces antibodies to RBC and hemolytic anemia (49), thus demonstrating the importance of B-1 cells to NZB disease.

Abnormalities of Thymus and T Cells

Abnormalities of the thymus also are characteristic of NZB mice, and T cells interact with hyperactive B cells to further increase autoimmune responses. NZB mice exhibit dramatic involution of thymic tissue; thymic epithelium is atrophied and immunologically defective by 1 month of age (before the appearance of NTA), with epithelial cell degeneration, accumulation of TdT^+ large immature T cells in the subcapsular region of the cortex, cortical atrophy, and increased lymphoid and plasma cell infiltrates in the medulla (5,17,50–53). NZB thymic epithelial cells are functionally defective compared with cells from normal mice, having low expression of surface Ia molecules, low secretion of IL-1, high secretion of prostaglandin E^2 (PGE^2) and PGE^3, and diminished ability to educate nonthymic cells to express Thy-l (51–55).

As in the B-cell compartment, NZB bone marrow contains increased prothymocyte activity, and these prothymoctes have an increased growth advantage when they are transferred to histocompatible recipients (56). T cells probably play a major role in disease, because MHC class II is an important predisposing factor for autoimmunity. The hybrid combination of NZB d/d and NZW z/z or SWR q/q to make d/z or d/q MHC molecules predisposes hybrids to GN that is mediated by IgG anti-dsDNA (57–64), which are antibodies that NZB mice do not make. NZB mice that are congenic for H-2b (NZB.H-2b) have less disease than the wild-type NZB.H-2d. However, introduction of a mutated I-A chain (bm12) converts this animal (i.e., H-2Bbm12) to a phenotype that is similar to the BW hybrid, with high-titer IgG anti-dsDNA and severe clinical GN (65–68). MHC class II likely plays a role in disease by shaping the repertoires of $CD4^+$ T cells. In fact, $CD4^+$ cells that proliferate in response to the RBC membrane protein band 3 and to spectrin (i.e., the major RBC antigens that are recognized by antierythrocyte Ab) have been isolated from NZB spleens (21). The importance of T cells to autoantibody formation also is indicated by experiments in which anti-CD4 nondepleting antibody was administered to NZB mice: antierythrocyte antibodies were significantly decreased, although anemia was not prevented (69,70).

Genetics

NZB mice have a gene(s) located on chromosome 1 (Nba2) linked with elevated serum levels of antibodies to dsDNA, chromatin, histone, and gp7O as well as hypergammaglobulinemia. There are contributions from the MHC region (H-2d/d) that enhance the Nba2 influence on autoantibody formation and nephritis (72,73), and from a region on chromosome 4 that predispose NZB/NZW F1 mice to nephritis (GN) (34,72,73). Studies of backcrosses between (NZB × SM/J) F1 and NZW mice, and of (NZB×NZW) F2 intercross mice, have suggested that NZB genes on chromosomes 1, 4, 7, 10, 13, and 19, in various combinations, contribute to GN (57,73).

Summary

In NZB mice, the combination of inherent B-cell hyperactivity and thymic loss probably results in the abnormal shaping of T- and B-cell repertoires. NZB mice are characterized by a fatal hemolytic anemia that is induced by antierythrocyte antibodies. Other autoantibodies in their repertoire include predominantly IgM NTA, anti-ssDNA, and anti-gp70. Their dominant immunologic abnormalities are hyperactivated B cells from fetal life onward, early degeneration of thymic epithelium, and increased numbers of $CD5^+$ (B-1) B cells that develop aneuploidy with age. These manifestations are controlled by multiple different genes. Sex differences are not marked, but disease is slightly accelerated in females.

New Zealand White Mice (NZW)

This strain is of great interest because it is clinically healthy but provides many genes that predispose to SLE in hybrids with other lupus-prone strains (8,34,57–64,74–83). Therefore, the NZW genome must contain controlling or repressor or epistatic genes that protect from SLE, and those controlling genes must be powerful enough to allow the animal to appear normal.

Clinical Characteristics and Autoantibodies

The NZW mouse has a slightly shortened life span and develops largely nonpathogenic autoantibodies, some of which are only intermittently detectable. The autoantibody pattern is characterized primarily by IgG antibodies to ssDNA and histones (76,84).

Genetics

Two groups of genes are clearly important in predisposing hybrid mice of an NZW parent to lupus and nephritis: (a) the MHC class II gene z, and (b) several non-MHC genes.

Inheritance of the MHC class II z genes from NZW (I-Ez, I-Az, also referred to as I-Eu and I-Au) predisposes hybrid mice to nephritis (76,85–87). H-2d/z mice, compared to H-2 d/d mice, have a higher incidence of nephritis; the d/z haplotype increases the risk for nephritis 30-fold (86). These MHC II genes are important in class switching of various autoantibodies from IgM to IgG (76). H-2d/z predisposes to antibodies to ssDNA, dsDNA, chromatin, and histones, but not to gp-70 (85,86). Because the MHC region is closely linked to the gene encoding tumor necrosis factor-α (TNF-α) in the same gene region, and low production of that cytokine is a dominant genetic feature of NZW mice (88), it has been somewhat difficult to sort out the role of each gene. Fujimura and colleagues (87) made three different H-2 congenic mice of BW bearing distinct haplotypes at class II and TNF-α regions (H-2d/z:A(d/u)E(d/u)TNF-α(d/z), H2(d/u):A(d/u)E(d/u)TNF-α(d/d), and H-2(d/d):A(d/d)E(d/d)TNF-α(d/d); studies of nephritis in each group showed that both the NZW MHC class II and the unique TNF-α allele are important predisposing genes.

Genome scanning has shown regions in several NZW chromosomes outside MHC that increase susceptibility to SLE. These include chromosomes 1, 11, 16, and 19 (which are linked to IgG autoantibody production), with a selective linkage of a region on chromosome 14 with IgG antihistone Ab (76). In addition, chromosomal regions from NZW parents labeled Sle1, Sle2, and Sle3, have been linked with disease susceptibility in NZM2410 mice (products of matings of NZB/NZW F1 brother/sisters with categorization and further mating of various offspring according to severity of nephritis) and congenics of these mice and the normal strain C57B1/6J (reviewed in ref. 74; see also refs. 75–83). Sle1 is located in the distal portion of chromosome 1 and promotes breaking of tolerance to chromatin, with mice developing IgM antichromatin (79,81), which sets the stage for production of IgG anti-dsDNA if other permissive genes are present. Sle2 is located on chromosome 4 and promotes B-cell hyperactivity (78). Sle3 is located on chromosome 7 and promotes T-cell hyperactivity (82). If normal mice are made homozygous for Sle1 or Sle3, few develop clinical nephritis. However, if they are made to express either one or two copies of both Sle1 and Sle2, some 85% develop severe nephritis (74,91). This illustrates the point that more than one susceptibility gene is required to develop clinical SLE. Another gene, probably located in or near the NZW MHC region, labeled Sle1-s (for "Sle1-suppressor"), when expressed in a normal strain along with Sle1 and Sle3, reduces the incidence of severe nephritis approximately 50% (74,91). Therefore, NZW mice appear healthy because their genome contains not only SLE susceptibility genes but also genes that protect from SLE, and the latter dominate in this strain. However, hybrids of NZW in which the other parent also contributes powerful susceptibility genes develop severe SLE. At the time of this writing, the gene(s) within these chromosomal regions have not been identified.

Identifiable single genes other than MHC/TNF-α, Sle1, Sle2, Sle3, and Sle1-s have been proposed as important to SLE susceptibility in NZW mice (93). The p8.6 gene, encoded upstream of the mouse TCRVa1 gene, contains regions that are consensus motifs for SH2 and SH3 binding motifs known to activate phosphorylation of some molecules. A gene mutation present in NZW (and BXSB) mice is associated with dysregulation in signaling through the BCR or T-cell receptor (TCR), which could play a role in the hyperactive responses or these cells in hybrid mice (89). In addition, one of two murine Rt6 genes is deleted in NZW mice (90). Rt6 is a T-cell–restricted GPI-anchored membrane protein, a member of the family of mono[adenosine diphosphate(ADP)-ribosyl]transferases, also known as PARP. These enzymes are activated by apoptosis and play a role in DNA repair.

A portion of the TCR, encompassing Db2-Jb2, is deleted in NZW mice (92). That deletion probably is not important in predisposing BW mice to lupus. Although one genetic backcross study showed lupus-like disease segregating with the abnormal TCRs (62), studies by other groups have not confirmed the importance of this deletion (63).

(NZB/NZW) F1 Mice (BW)

The BW hybrid cross between NZB and New Zealand white (NZW) mice is considered by many to be the murine model that most closely resembles human SLE. The disease is more severe and earlier in females, with high titers of IgG anti-dsDNA, anti-chromatin, ANA, and LE cells occurring in virtually all females; death results from immune glomerulonephritis (5,27,71) (Tables 18.1 and 18.3).

Both NZB and NZW parents contribute genetically to the immune abnormalities that cause disease, as discussed in the preceding sections. The B-cell hyperactivity that is characteristic of the NZB is inherited by the BW, with abnormally high secretion of immunoglobulin being detectable by 1 month of age (6–9). However, the T-cell dependence of the response is more striking than in the NZB parent and probably is responsible for the isotype shift from IgM anti-DNA to IgG anti-DNA that precedes clinical disease (94,95). The ability to make this shift depends in part on genes located on chromosome 1 from the NZB (*Nba2*) parent and gene(s) on chromosome 4 (Sle2) and possibly 7 (*Sle3*) from the NZW (*Sle1*) parent.

Clinical Characteristics and Autoantibodies

The large quantities of IgG antibodies that bind both dsDNA and ssDNA, and are widely designated as anti-dsDNA, are striking and can be abrogated by removal of $CD4^+$ (formerly called $L3T4^+$) T cells (58,96). IgG antibodies to dsDNA clearly contain subsets that cause nephritis. Transfer of certain monoclonal BW IgG2 anti-dsDNA antibodies to normal BALB/c mice induces nephritis in the recipients (97,98). Infusion of anti-DNA into rodent kidneys induces proteinuria (99), and normal mice secreting BW IgG anti-dsDNA encoded by transgenes develop GN (100,101). (Characteristics of pathogenic subsets of anti-DNA are discussed in detail in Chapter 21.)

Anti-DNA and immune complexes containing gp70 and anti-gp70s are the most important autoantibodies made by BW mice that contribute to nephritis (102,103). ANAs are detectable in most females by 2 to 3 months of age; they include antibodies that bind subnucleosomes, nucleosomes, chromatin, dsDNA, ssDNA, dsRNA, transfer RNA (tRNA), polynucleotides, and histones (95–103). IgM anti-DNAs arise in females between 3 and 5 months of age; by 5 to 7 months, IgG anti-DNAs appear (5,94,95). The IgG2a and 2b subclasses are most frequent, which is important because these subclasses fix complement well. The IgM to IgG switch and the dominance of IgG2a and 2b thereafter occur in BW females responding not only to DNA but also to other thymic-independent and -dependent antigens (104). Shortly after the switch to IgG, IgG and complement deposit in the mesangia of BW glomeruli, spreading later to capillary loops and interstitial tubular regions (5). Proteinuria appears between 5 and 7 months; azotemia followed by death occurs at 6 to 12 months of age. Approximately half of the females are dead by 8 months and 90% at 12 months (5,7,98). With regard to immune complexes containing gp70, that antigen is an endogenous retroviral glycoprotein produced by hepatic cells that is found in all mouse strains. However, lupus-prone mice [MRL-Fas(*lpr*), BXSB, NZB, NZW, NZB/NZW F1] all have high serum levels. It is likely that past integrations of murine leukemia viruses into the mouse genome account for production of gp70. DNA/anti-DNA complexes are difficult to detect in mouse sera, whereas gp70/anti-gp7O complexes are found more frequently than free antibody to gp70. It may be that many antibodies to DNA cause nephritis by direct attachment to planted or cross-reactive glomerular and tubular antigens, whereas passive trapping of gp70/anti-gp70 immune complexes is important in inducing nephritis. Ability to make high titer anti-gp70 correlates weakly with the ability to make high quantities of immune complexes. NZB chromosome regions Nba2 (on chromosome 1) and H2 (on chromosome 17) are linked to high levels of gp70/anti-gp70 immune complex production, as they are linked to high

TABLE 18.3. CHARACTERISTICS OF NZB/NZW F_1 MICE

A. Clinical
  1. Females live a mean of 280 days, males 439 days
  2. Death usually is caused by immune glomerulonephritis
  3. Fifty-percent mortality by 8 months in females and 15 months in males

B. Histologic
  1. Glomerulonephritis with proliferative changes in mesangial and endothelial cells of glomeruli, capillary basement membrane thickening, and chronic obliterative changes; mononuclear cell infiltrates in interstitium
  2. Glomerular immune deposits of IgG (predominantly IgG2a) and C3; similar deposits in tubular basement membrane and interstitium
  3. Thymic cortical atrophy by 6 months of age
  4. Myocardial infarcts with hyaline thickening of small arteries
  5. Mild lymph node hyperplasia and splenomegaly

C. Autoantibodies
  1 IgG anti-dsDNA (also binds ssDNA), enriched in IgG2a and 2b
  2. ANA and LE cells in all
  3. IgG antibodies bind chromatin, nucleosomes, and phospholipids
  3. Antithymocyte in most females and some males
  4. Renal eluates contain IgG anti-dsDNA concentrated 25 to 30 times greater than in serum; IgG2a isotype usually is dominant
  5. Modest elevations of circulating immune complexes; these include gp70–anti-gp70
  6. Low serum complement levels by 6 months of age in females

D. Immune abnormalities
  1. Polyclonal B-cell activation
  2. B cells are resistant to tolerance to some antigens
  3. Strict dependence on T-cell help for formation of pathogenic IgG anti-DNA, $CD4^+CD8^-$ and $CD4^-CD8^-$ α/β TCR cells, as well as $CD4^-CD8^-$ γ/Δ TCR cells, can provide help
  4. IgG repertoire becomes restricted with age to certain public Ids; there is some restriction of B-cell clonality in the IgG anti-DNA response
  5. Thymic epithelial atrophy by 6 months of age; medullary hyperplasia; effect of thymectomy on disease varies
  6. Clearance of immune complexes by Fc- and complement-mediated mechanisms is defective
  7. Disease and autoantibody production is sensitive to sex hormone influences

E. Genetics
  1. The expression of high-titer IgG anti-dsDNA requires heterozygosity at MHC, namely $H\text{-}2^{d/z}$
  2. Additional complementary non–H-2-linked genes are required from both NZB and NZW parents to permit full expression of the IgG anti-DNA response; by microsatellite analysis of DNA, there are approximately 10 genes on as many chromosomes, with multiple genes required for early mortality, glomerulonephritis, antichromatin, and splenomegaly; this suggests a multigenic inheritance, with certain groupings predisposing more strongly than others to disease, rather than a simple additive model
  3. The large deletion in the β chain of the TCR of the NZW parent probably does not predispose to disease

dsDNA, double-stranded DNA; TCR, T-cell receptor.

titers of IgG anti-DNA. In contrast, the ability to make high levels of gp70 antigen is linked to regions on chromosomes 4 and 13 (103).

Antibodies eluted from glomeruli are composed predominantly of IgG anti-DNA; 50% of the total IgG is anti-DNA according to some reports (105,106). In colonies in our laboratory, anti-DNA accounts for as much as 85% of the total glomerular IgG (107). IgG2a is the dominant isotype in glomerular deposits, suggesting a role for Th1 cells, because production of IgG2a is dependent on interferon-γ (IFN-γ). Other antigens and antibodies have been reported in glomerular eluates, including gp70, antihistones, anti-C1q, and anti-RNA polymerase (108–110). The high serum levels of IgG anti-DNA occur at about the same time as hypocomplementemia, and levels of circulating immune complexes are elevated (5).

Histologic changes in kidneys include chronic obliterative changes in glomeruli, mesangial and peripheral proliferative changes, capillary membrane thickening, glomerular sclerosis, tubular atrophy, infiltration by mononuclear lymphocytes and monocyte/macrophages, and vasculopathy (primarily degenerative, occasionally inflammatory) (5,27) (Fig. 18.1). In addition, messenger RNA (mRNA) encoding several molecules that contribute to proliferation and inflammation is increased in the kidneys of BW mice with GN; those molecules include platelet-derived growth factor (PDGF), MHC class II, insulin-like growth factor-1 (IGF-1), IFN-γ, and basic fibroblast growth factor (bFGF) (111–114). Other autoantibodies also occur in BW mice. Antibodies to erythrocytes are found in 35% to 78% of BW females, but they rarely cause hemolytic anemia (7). Approximately 50% develop NTAs by 6 months of age. Because the genes governing NTA, anti-DNA, and antierythrocyte antibodies probably segregate separately (6,8,72–83,88–91,93, 115–118), New Zealand mouse strains have been bred that have high-titer NTAs but no autoimmune disease. However, NTAs may serve as an accelerator of the disease process that occurs in mice with IgG anti-DNA, because NTAs may alter T-cell function. Both IgM and IgG antiphospholipid antibodies have been detected and obtained as monoclonal antibodies from BW mice (119). Some have anticardiolipin activity and others lupus anticoagulant properties.

IgG1 antibodies have been eluted from the neurons of BW mice (120); it is not known whether they cross-react extensively with lymphocytes, as do some human lupus antineuronal antibodies. Antibodies to histones, ubiquitin, chromatin, and fibrillarin have been reported, as have cryoglobulins (121–123). Some antibodies to DNA, chromatin, and nucleosomes can bind to and/or penetrate living cells; some of these subsets make glomerular cells proliferate and could impair cellular production of protein (124–128).

The lymphoproliferative features of NZB mice occur in BW hybrids, which exhibit mild lymphadenopathy and splenomegaly (5,7). Lymphoid neoplasia is far less common in BW than in NZB mice. Some investigators have reported

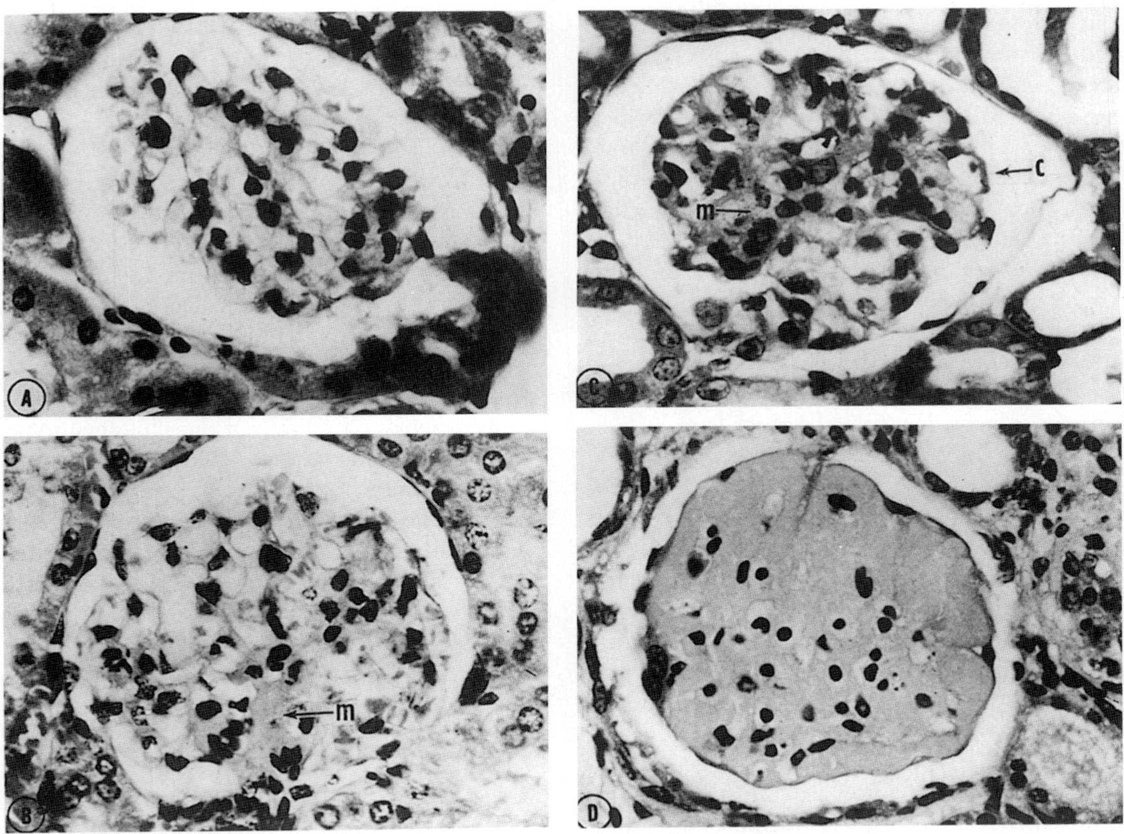

FIGURE 18.1. Glomerulonephritis in New Zealand mice. Each sample is from a kidney section of NZW mice. **A:** Normal mouse glomerulus. **B:** Mesangial proliferation and thickening (m). **C:** Proliferative glomerulonephritis with thickened glomerular capillaries (c). **D:** End-stage glomerulopathy; the glomerulus is obliterated.

a relatively high incidence of thymoma, from 1% to 5% (129), but that has been rare in our colonies unless mice are treated with cytotoxic agents (130). Extrarenal lesions occur in BW mice, including lymphocytic infiltration of salivary glands, mild inflammation around bile ducts in the liver, pancarditis, vasculitis [less common than in MRL-Fas(*lpr*) and BXSB mice], myocardial infarcts, and deposits of DNA and anti-DNA in the dermoepidermal junction of skin and in the choroid plexus (5,131,132).

Sex Hormone Influences on Lupus in BW Mice

The femaleness of spontaneous BW disease has been studied extensively. Most BW males develop ANAs, including antibodies to DNA, but they are predominantly IgM. The IgM to IgG switch occurs relatively late in life, usually after 12 months. Histologic evidence of nephritis can be found in males, and most die of slowly progressive chronic nephritis by 15 to 20 months of age (5,7).

The BW mouse is particularly sensitive to the effect of sex hormones on disease. In general, androgens are protective and suppress the expression of autoantibodies and disease, and estrogens are permissive. Male BW mice (and other hybrids of NZB) develop high titers of IgG autoantibodies as early in life as do females if the males are castrated (6). Males that are castrated and/or treated with estrogens or testosterone antagonists assume a female pattern: early IgM-to-IgG switch of anti-DNA antibodies and early, fatal nephritis (133–135). Females that are treated with castration and androgens, or with antiestrogens, have prolonged survival, with suppression of IgG anti-DNA and nephritis (136–139). In old females, androgens can suppress disease without altering the elevated levels of IgG anti-DNA. Addition of exogenous estrogens cause early death in females, but this may result largely from toxic effects rather than from enhancement of immune responses (135). Hyperprolactinemia occurs in some women with SLE. In BW mice, SLE is accelerated in pseudopregnant females in which cyclical increases of prolactin occur, and administration of prolactin to BW mice accelerates disease, while bromocriptin suppresses it (140–142). Manipulations of BW mice that produce both high levels of estrogen and high levels of prolactin shorten survival about 8 weeks (142).

The effects of sex hormones on immune responses are complex and poorly understood. There are receptors for estrogens, progestogens, and prolactin on lymphocytes (140). The administration of estradiol *in vivo* dramatically suppresses natural killer (NK) cell function, and NK cells downregulate activated B cells (143). In addition, normal mice transgenic for a murine IgG antibody to DNA show defective B-cell tolerance if they are treated with exogenous estradiol (144). Such mice fail to delete B cells producing anti-DNA from unmutated germline genes. In addition to their effects on sex tissues and lymphocytes, sex hormones may regulate the expression of certain genes.

Abnormalities of Stem Cells and B Cells

BW mice exhibit the hyperactivated B-cell phenotype of their NZB parent, except that defects appear later in life. BW mice have abnormally elevated secretion of IgM by 1 month of age. Stem cells of the pre-B lineage can partially transfer disease: severe combined immunodeficiency disease (SCID) mice (a mutant strain that lacks most T cells) that are inoculated with BW bone marrow pre–B cells develop autoantibodies (including IgG anti-dsDNA), and approximately 25% develop clinical nephritis (145). These studies suggest that both B and T cells are required for the full expression of BW disease. The B-cell repertoire that expresses anti-DNA is somewhat restricted. Public idiotypes (Ids) that are expressed on total serum IgG become increasingly restricted as the mice age (146). Although many different V genes can be used to assemble antibodies that bind DNA (147), most BW monoclonal antibody anti-DNA belong to one of approximately 12 families (148–151). This type of restriction is seen in normal, antigen-driven antibody responses.

Abnormalities of Thymus and T Cells

The degeneration of thymic epithelial cells that is characteristic of NZB mice occurs in BW mice, but at 6 months of age in contrast to 1 month of age in the NZB parent (8). Responses to thymectomy have been variable; there are reports of thymectomy failing to alter disease or even accelerating it (51). Full-blown BW lupus depends on the presence of $CD4^+$ helper T cells; T-cell lines from nephritic mice can accelerate disease in naive young syngeneic mice (152,153). Elimination or inactivation of $CD4^+$ T cells prevents the onset of disease and can even partially reverse established nephritis (96,154). As BW mice age, the numbers of $CD4^+$ T cells increase fivefold, and these cells are polyclonal (155). T cells from nephritic BW mice can drive B cells from young normal mice to make pathogenic autoantibodies (152,153), whereas B cells from old mice will not secrete anti-DNA when they are cocultured with T cells from premorbid young normal mice (152,156).

Pathogenic T cells must receive second signals after TCRs are engaged to develop into activated effectors of disease. Interruption of second signals with blockade of the CD28/CTLA4 T-cell surface molecule's interactions with CD80/CD86 (B7-1/B7-2) on antigen-presenting cells (APCs) prevents disease. Experiments showing this include the administration of cytotoxic T-lymphocyte antigen-4 (CTLA-4)–Ig, which binds B7.1 and B7.2, thus preventing interaction with CD28 (157), and the administration of antibodies to CD80 and CD86 (158). In addition, blocking second signals that activate B cells (CD40 interacting with CD40 ligand) by administration of antibody to CD40L prolongs survival in BW and other New Zealand-background lupus mice (159,160). Blocking both CD28/B7 and CD40/CD40L interactions is probably more effective than blocking either one alone (161).

Because $CD4^+$ T cells of the Th1 phenotype (secreting IL-2 and IFN-γ) generally support cell-mediated reactions, whereas $CD4^+$ cells of the Th2 phenotype (secreting IL-4, IL-5, and IL-6) give help to B cells for antibody production, there has been great interest in the possibility that a skewing toward Th2 plays a major role in the SLE of BW mice. Such skewing has been suggested by the well-known fact that T cells from BW mice secrete less and less IL-2 as the mice age, with a diminution in IL-2 receptors on T-cell surfaces (7,156,162). One study (162) showed a concomitant decline in IL-2 and IFN-γ, with an increase in IL-4 secretion by 6 to 8 months of age that would support a shift to Th2. Another study, however, showed a decrease in IL-2 and IL-4 and an increase in IFN-γ as mice aged (156). In our colonies, dramatic increases in plasma levels of IFN-γ and IL-4 occur at the time high quantities of IgG anti-DNA appear. Because the dominant isotype that is eluted from glomerular lesions is IgG2a, which depends on IFN-γ for its synthesis, Th1 cells (or Th0 that secrete IFN-γ) are important in inducing disease. In addition, our laboratory has accelerated disease in young BW mice by the transfer of either Th1 or Th2 cell lines, implying that both subsets play important pathogenic roles. IL-6, which is secreted by Th2 cells and B cells, potentiates autoantibody formation (163). Administration of IL-6 accelerates disease, and antibodies to IL-6 delay it (164). IL-10, which is made predominantly by monocyte/macrophages, also is important, is increased in SLE, and shifts repertoires from Th1 toward Th2, probably by suppressing IL-6. Thus, administration of anti–IL-10 delays disease in BW mice (165).

Transforming growth factor-β (TGF-β) can mediate suppression, which is critical to controlling SLE-like immune responses; IL-1 and TNF-α are both proinflammatory and may be abnormally elevated in BW lupus (166,167). Monocyte/macrophages are primary sources of IL-1; production of that cytokine is reduced in BW and other murine lupus strains (166,168). The role of TNF-α has been debated for several years. NZW mice have an unusual gene that may encode abnormally low levels of TNF-α, and short-term administration of TNF-α to BW mice delays disease (169). However, mRNA for TNF-α is increased in the glomerular tissue of BW mice (167), and chronic administration of the cytokine worsens disease (170,171).

The Role of Defective Regulatory Cells in BW Lupus

Finally, the possibility that regulatory cells that ordinarily suppress activated T and/or B cells are defective or missing from BW repertoires should be considered. CD8$^+$ T cells behave abnormally because they usually are cytotoxic or suppressive. In BW mice, CD8$^+$ T cells are reduced in numbers and possibly in suppressor activity; infusing them can suppress murine lupus (172). B-1 (CD5$^+$) B cells also may downregulate autoantibody production under normal circumstances; these cells, derived from normal CBA/J bone marrow and transferred with BW marrow into chimeric mice, can suppress disease (173). In contrast, mixtures of BW and CBA/N bone marrow (CBA/N carries the *xid* gene, which eliminates B-1 B cells) transfer ordinary BW lupus to recipients (173). Monocytes/macrophages, which are defective in IL-1 production in BW mice, also may serve as downregulators in normal circumstances; it is not clear that they serve this function in the BW model.

Genetic Predisposition

Genetic predisposition is discussed fully in Chapter 7 and was reviewed briefly in the preceding sections on NZB and NZW mice. In BW mice, genetic contributions to disease are provided by both NZB and NZW parents, including MHC genes (heterozygosity for H-2 d/z predisposes to nephritis) and multiple non-MHC genes on at least eight different chromosomes (34,57–65,72–79,82,83,85–93).

Summary

BW mice develop fatal glomerulonephritis, mediated primarily by IgG antibodies to dsDNA and immune complexes of gp70 and anti-gp70, that both occurs earlier and is more severe in females and can be modulated by sex hormones. Multiple genes inherited from both NZB and NZW parents, both MHC and non-MHC, are required for the development of high-titer IgG anti-dsDNA and clinical nephritis. Abnormalities in both T- and B-cell compartments are required for the disease to be fully manifest.

(SWR × NZB) F1 (SNF1) Mice

The SNF1 mouse is a model of lupus nephritis that is produced by mating the normal SWR mouse with the autoimmune NZB mouse (174-179); it does not matter which parent is female and which is male (Table 18.4). In contrast to NZW mice, SWR mice are completely healthy, with normal life spans, low levels of serum gp70, and no evidence of autoimmune disease (174,175). Their B cells can produce Igs bearing the same public Ids that dominate serum Igs in MRL-Fas(*lpr*) mice (179–181).

Clinical Characteristics and Autoantibodies

SNF1 mice are similar to BW mice. Females are dead by 10 to 12 months of age (50% mortality at 6 months) from an immune glomerulonephritis that is mediated primarily by IgG2b antibodies to dsDNA (176,178). This model has been of particular interest because of the oligoclonality of the IgG anti-DNA that is deposited in glomeruli (177,179). Activated B cells of NZB mice make anti-DNAs that are predominantly IgM, bind ssDNA rather than dsDNA, and are anionic in charge (178). In contrast, B cells of SNF1 mice make predominantly IgG2b anti-dsDNA that is cationic (178,179). Cationic charge probably is important in initiating nephritis, because cationic antibodies (or antigens or immune complexes) can bind to polyanions in glomerular basement membranes. IgG in glomerular eluates from BW mice also is enriched in cationic subpopulations (102,107), and it is those populations that bind directly to glomeruli when they are infused into old BW mice (182).

The presumed pathogens, IgG2b cationic anti-dsDNA, also are restricted in Id expression. The IgG in the glomeruli of SNF1 mice can be grouped into two families of Ids (177,179). The first, Id564, is composed entirely of cationic IgG, and most members bear the Igh allotype of the SWR parent. The second Id cluster, Id512, contains immunoglobulin of anionic, neutral, and cationic charge; the allotypes expressed are both SWR and NZB derived. Id564 is unique to SNF1 mice and is not found in either parent. This Id restriction is similar to that reported by our group in BW mice, where only two public Ids (IdGN1 and IdGN2) dominate the glomerular immunoglobulin deposits (146).

Sequence data show that the expression of Id564 depends on the VH region of the immunoglobulin molecule; Id564$^+$ monoclonal antibodies are closely related structurally and

TABLE 18.4. CHARACTERISTICS OF NZB × SWR F$_1$ (SNF$_1$) MICE

A. Clinical
   1. Mean survival in females is 297 days; mean survival in males is 531 days
   2. Females die from immune glomerulonephritis between 5 and 13 months of age

B. Histologic
   1. Glomerulonephritis with proliferative and obliterative lesions

C. Autoantibodies
   1. IgG anti-dsDNA is made by all females
   2. Anti-dsDNA is dominated by IgG2b cationic populations with restricted idiotypes
   3. ANAs in all females

D. Immune abnormalities
   1. B cells are hyperactivated
   2. The development of nephritis depends on the presence of T-cell help for production of IgG anti-DNA
   3. Cationic IgG anti-dsDNA may use the allotype of either the NZB or healthy SWR parent
   4. Anti-dsDNA deposited in glomeruli cluster into two main groups defined by their Ids
   5. CD4$^+$CD8$^-$ and CD4$^-$CD8$^-$ T cells can provide help for the synthesis of cationic IgG anti-dsDNA

E. Genetics
   1. Probably similar to BW mice

probably derive from a germline gene that is unique to the SNF1 mouse (180). One family of Ids, designated as IdLNF$^+$, has been used to track reciprocal T- and B-cell functions that are connected by idiotypy. SNF1 mice also make antihistone antibodies, which are characterized by some clonal restriction and by somatic mutations, as are most autoantibodies in the mouse models (183).

Abnormalities of Stem Cells and B Cells

It is assumed that SNF1 mice inherit hyperactivated B cells from their NZB parent, but there are few data on the subject. The interesting features of this model include the demonstration that a nephritogenic anti-DNA subset can be constructed from the allotype of a normal parent given the appropriate additional genetic background. Idiotypic connectivity between B and T cells also has been particularly well described in this model (184–186). IdLNF$^+$ immunoglobulin does not contain much antibody to DNA, but nephritis and early death correlate with high serum levels of IdLNF$^+$ immunoglobulin and glomerular deposits of the Id, thus illustrating the role of non–DNA-binding immunoglobulin in the glomerular disease. Suppression of IdLNF$^+$ immunoglobulin by the administration of a specific anti-Id does not downregulate serum levels of IgG anti-DNA, but nephritis is delayed and survival prolonged (186).

Abnormalities of T Cells

Studies suggest that the T-cell abnormalities of BW mice are reiterated in the SNF1 model. B cells from SNF1 spleens (or BW spleens) secrete IgG anti-dsDNA (including cationic subsets) only when they are stimulated by T cells in culture (187,188). Those T cells may bear the classic CD4$^+$CDB$^-$ phenotype of helper T cells, or they may be CD4$^-$CD8$^-$ (187).

As mice age, their CD4$^+$, IdLNF$^+$-specific repertoire expands greatly. There is little TCR restriction in the expanding CD4$^+$ cells. Transfer of a few T-cell clones that are specific for the Id increased the Id$^+$ immunoglobulin production in young SNF1 mice (184,185).

Genetics

As in the BW mouse, genes contributed from both parents are necessary for disease in the SNF1. Some genes clearly are linked to H-2. However, one study suggests that nephritis also is influenced by the TCR-β chain (which contains a large deletion similar to the NZW) as well as by the I-A-chain genes of the SWR parent (188).

Summary

The SNF1 mouse is another example of female-dominant, T-cell–dependent lupus nephritis in a hybrid mouse with an NZB background. The nature of the antibodies that deposit in glomeruli has been particularly well studied and is somewhat oligoclonal, thus providing important information about the characteristics and genetic control of pathogenic subsets of autoantibodies.

New Zealand Mixed (NZM) Mice

In 1993, Rudofsky et al. (61) reported a new strain of mice with SLE. They performed selective inbreeding of the progeny of one cross between NZB and NZW mice, selecting for severity of nephritis and coat colors. They derived 27 strains and studied 12, determining homozygosity for NZB and NZW polymorphic gene markers at H-2, Hc (i.e., a polymorphism for C4 on chromosome 2), and coat-color loci on chromosomes 2, 4, and 7. Most NZM strains have IgG anti-dsDNA antibodies. Some strains develop early-onset nephritis in males and others in females similar to the BW F1, and some strains had little nephritis. These initial studies showed that there is not a strict requirement for H-2d/z heterozygosity to develop nephritis.

Subsequently, selected NZM strains were used to study the segregation of genes with manifestations of lupus. For example, the NZM/Aeg2410 line (i.e., more rapid and severe GN than in BW) was backcrossed to normal C57B1 mice for interval mapping of susceptibility loci (189). Three chromosomal intervals containing strong recessive alleles predisposing to GN were found on chromosomes 1, 4, and 7. All of these are contributed by the NZW parent: they have been designated *Sle1*, *Sle2*, and *Sle3*. Studies in single and double congenic mice have shown that *Sle1* allows a mouse to break tolerance to chromatin, *Sle2* permits B-cell hyperactivity, and *Sle3* permits T-cell (and some B-cell) hyperactivity. Normal C57Bl/6J mice expressing *Sle1* or *Sle3* do not develop nephritis, but C57 mice expressing both chromosome regions develop nephritis. See the discussion of genetics of NZW mice above, and Chapter 7 for a more detailed discussion. In SNF1 mice, heterozygosity at H-2 correlates strongly with GN; the MHC alleles seemed to confer susceptibility independently and were additive (189). Subsequent studies in other strains have identified similar regions of chromosomes that contribute to GN, but as more and smaller segments of the mouse genome have been analyzed, the inheritance pattern has looked more like polygenic gene combinations without a strictly additive pattern of inheritance (see Chapter 7). At the time of this writing, the genes in chromosome regions designated *Sle1*, *Sle2*, and *Sle3* have not been identified.

B cells in this strain are abnormal (like the NZB and BW) in that ligation of the BCR does not modulate LPS signals in a normal way (38).

MRL/Mp (MRL+/+) and MRL-Fas(*lpr*) Mice

The MRL-Fas(*lpr*) strain and the congenic MRL/Mp (MRL/+/+) (also called MRL/n) were developed by Murphy and Roths in 1976 (190). They were derived from LG/J mice crossed with AKR/J, C3HDi, and C57B1/6. By the 12th generation of inbreeding, the MRL-Fas(*lpr*) which is characterized by marked lymphadenopathy and splenomegaly, large quantities of antibodies to DNA, antibodies to Sm, and lethal immune nephritis, was derived. Lacking the *lpr* gene, MRL/+/+ mice share over 95% of the genetic material of the MRL-Fas(*lpr*) (7). The *lpr* (i.e., lymphoproliferation) trait occurred as a spontaneous mutation in a single autosomal recessive gene; the mutation results in a defective Fas molecule (191–195). Interactions of Fas and Fas ligand (FasL) are required for the initiation of apoptosis in activated B and T lymphocytes under normal immunoregulatory conditions (196). Therefore, mice that are homozygous for the *lpr* mutation (i.e., Fas (*lpr*), formerly designated *lpr/lpr*) develop massive lymphoproliferation, large quantities of IgG autoantibodies, and autoimmune disease (197–199). Features of this strain are listed in Table 18.5.

TABLE 18.5. CHARACTERISTICS OF MRL/*lpr* MICE

A. Clinical
   1. Massive lymphadenopathy with expansion of $CD4^+$ and $Thy1^+$, $B220^+$, $CD4^-$, $CD8^-$, TCR $\alpha\beta^+$ (double negative or DNT) cells
   2. Early death in males and females (50% mortality at 6 months)
   3. Congenic strain MRL/++ lacks *lpr;* 50% mortality at 17 months
   4. Deaths usually result from immune glomerulonephritis
   5. Approximately one-half develop acute necrotizing polyarteritis
   6. In some colonies, approximately 25% develop destructive polyarthritis

B. Histologic
   1. Subacute proliferation of mesangial and endothelial cells, occasional glomerular crescents, basement membrane thickening; deposits of immunoglobulin and C3 in glomeruli, especially in capillary walls; marked mononuclear cell infiltrate in interstitium
   2. Acute polyarteritis of coronary and renal arteries
   3. Proliferative synovitis, pannus formation, and destruction of articular cartilage—usually detected microscopically, not grossly
   4. Thymic atrophy
   5. Massive hyperplasia of all lymphoid organs, sometimes with hemorrhage and cystic necrosis

C. Autoantibodies
   1. Monoclonal paraproteins in approximately 40%; IgG3 cryoglobulins are common
   2. Most marked elevations of serum IgG, IgM, and immune complexes of all murine SLE models
   3. ANAs at highest levels of all murine SLE models
   4. IgG and IgM anti-dsDNA and anti-ssDNA
   5. Anti-Sm in 10% of females and 35% of males
   6. IgM and IgG rheumatoid factors in 65%; some IgG–IgG complexes
   7. gp70–anti-gp70 complexes
   8. IgM and IgG antibodies to DNA, snRNP particles, and phospholipid often are cross-reactive, suggesting that any of the antigens can activate the entire repertoire
   9. Hypocomplementemia

D. Immune abnormalities
   1. Lymphoid hyperplasia primarily results from expansion of unusual $CD3^+$, $CD4^-$, $CD8^-$, $B220^+$, α/β^+ T cells; they probably derive from activated $CD8^+$ cells that fail to undergo apoptosis
   2. Appearance of these T cells and of early disease is strictly dependent on the *lpr* gene and also is thymus dependent; thymectomy prevents disease
   3. High numbers of hyperactivated B cells appear just before onset of clinical disease
   4. Autoantibodies, nephritis, arthritis, and CNS disease are prevented by elimination of $CD4^+$ cells; lymphoproliferation is not
   5. Lymphoproliferation is prevented by elimination of $CD8^+$ cells; autoantibodies, nephritis, and arthritis are not affected
   6. Defective Fc-mediated phagocytosis and clearance of immune complexes
   7. Monocytes/macrophages are abnormal, with low expression of IL-1β and defective function

E. Genetics
   1. Accelerated disease is produced by a single autosomal recessive gene, *lpr;* this mutation encodes a defective Fas molecule, so that very low levels of Fas are expressed on cell surfaces; engagement between Fas and FasL is infrequent, making Fas-mediated apoptosis defective; Fas/FasL interaction delivers a major signal for deleting activated T cells by apoptosis; mice homozygous for *lpr* develop lymphoproliferation on most backgrounds, but clinical autoimmune disease primarily appears in permissive backgrounds, such as MRL/++ and NZB
   2. The congenic MRL/++ has a B-cell repertoire that makes anti-DNA, anti-Sm, and rheumatoid factors; these autoantibodies probably are controlled by multiple genes, as in the NZB

Clinical Characteristics and Autoantibodies

MRL/+/+ mice are abnormal and develop late-life lupus. They make anti-DNA, anti-Sm, and rheumatoid factors, but serum levels are lower than those of MRL-Fas(*lpr*) mice. Male and female MRL/+/+ are similarly affected; most develop clinical nephritis with advancing age and are dead by 24 months (5,7,190).

In MRL-Fas(*lpr*) mice, the quantities of antibodies that are provided by the MRL/+/+ background are greatly amplified by T-cell help delivered by the $CD4^+$ cells expanded by lymphoproliferation (200–210), probably resulting from delayed/defective apoptosis due to the abnormal Fas gene. The most numerous cells that pack lymph nodes and spleen are not $CD4^+$; they bear the surface phenotype $CD3^+$, $CD4^-$,$CD8^-$, and $B220^+$. They bear α/β TCRs and therefore are part of the T-cell lineage. Presumably in normal mice the double negative cells are rapidly eliminated by apoptosis, and they accumulate in MRL-Fas(*lpr*) mice because of defects in this process. These mice die at 3 to 7 months of age.

Both male and female MRL-Fas(*lpr*) *lpr* mice develop high serum levels of immunoglobulins, monoclonal paraproteins, ANAs, and immune complexes (the highest of all murine lupus strains) (5,7). They make IgM and IgG anti-ssDNA and anti-dsDNA, and they die from immune nephritis at a young age (90% dead by 9 months of age). Other autoantibodies in their repertoire include IgG antibodies that bind chromatin, histone, nucleosomes, nucleobindin (i.e., a DNA-binding protein), cardiolipin, erythrocyte surfaces, thyroglobulin, lymphocyte surfaces, Sm, Ul snRNP, Ro, La, Ku, Su, proteoglycans on endothelial cell membranes, neurons, ribosomal P, RNA polymerase I, C1q, and heat shock proteins (208–229). In addition, they have gp70/anti-gp7O immune complexes (103). A substantial portion of MRL-Fas(*lpr*) mice develop IgG3 cryoglobulins, some containing rheumatoid factor activity (123,230,231). Many of these antibodies are closely related; that is, many antibodies to Sm, La, C1q, and nucleobindin also bind DNA. Anti-DNA, anti-Sm, and anti-La frequently use highly similar VH genes. The following features are found in MRL-Fas(*lpr*) and never, or rarely, in NZB mice and their hybrids: (a) massive lymphoproliferation, (b) inflammatory erosive polyarthritis (usually detected microscopically rather than grossly), (c) IgM rheumatoid factors, (d) severe necrotizing arteritis, and (e) antibodies to snRNP particles (5,7,190,209,221–225,232–234). In addition to the development of fatal nephritis, most MRL-Fas(*lpr*) mice develop lymphocytic infiltration of salivary glands, pancreas, peripheral muscles and nerves, uvea, and thyroid (235–239). In fact, they develop clinical thyroiditis with hypothyroidism, abnormal electrical transmission in muscles and nerves (suggesting clinical polymyositis and polyneuritis), learning disabilities, sensorineural hearing loss, and band keratopathy (237–241).

In females, anti-DNA is detectable in the circulation by 6 to 8 weeks of age, proteinuria begins at 1 to 3 months, and death associated with azotemia occurs at 3 to 6 months (5,7). Males lag behind females by approximately 1 month. IgG2a antibodies to DNA deposit in glomeruli, as do IgG1 and IgG3. The IgG3 cryoglobulins may be associated with either wire-loop, membranous-type lesions or with focal proliferative glomerular disease (123,230,231). The IgG anti-DNA repertoire is dominated by a public Id.H130 (181). Such dominance is reminiscent of the nephritis of BW and SNF1 mice. As for BW mice, there is some evidence that the first stimulating autoantigen is DNA linked to protein, such as chromatin or nucleosomes (226,227). After these antibodies mutate specificities for other autoantigens could develop (e.g., ssDNA, dsDNA, phospholipid, Sm, La, and so on) (218,221,222). Antibodies to small nuclear ribonucleoprotein (snRNP) antigens, such as Sm, Ro, and La, occur in the MRL-Fas(*lpr*) and MRL/+/+ lupus-prone strains (5,7,219–222,228), and not in New Zealand strains. However, antibodies to snRNP have been found in the Palmerston North lupus-prone strain, discussed below (242). In MRL mice, antibodies to snRNP antigens are found in approximately 25% of animals. The reasons why some MRL-Fas(*lpr*) mice express anti-Sm and others do not is unclear; there are no demonstrable genetic or environmental factors that account for these differences (243). There may be a role for antibody specificities, however. The D epitope of Sm may contain helper epitopes that permit antibody expression, and the B epitope may contain suppressor epitopes (219). Antigen specificity for components of the polypeptides/nRNP complex is similar to the specificities of human anti-Sm. The anti-Sm response is dominated by public Ids (e.g., Y2), which can be found on human anti-Sm and on other human and murine autoantibodies (244,245). The ability to make anti-Sm does not correlate with clinical nephritis.

Histologic examination of the kidneys shows proliferation of mesangial and endothelial cells in glomeruli, occasional crescent formation, and basement membrane thickening, as well as interstitial infiltration by lymphocytes. IgG, C3, and anti-DNA are deposited in glomeruli; the presence of gp70 is variable and less constant than in NZB and related strains (246). Antibodies to RNA polymerase I also may contribute to nephritis (211). Renal failure is the primary cause of death.

Polyarthritis occurs in some MRL-Fas(*lpr*) mice with a prevalence between 15% and 25% (5,7,232,233). Years ago, these mice were reported to develop swelling in the hind feet and lower legs; today, most studies are done examining histology rather than observing gross evidence of inflammation (233). By 14 weeks of age, there is synovial cell proliferation with early subchondral bone destruction and marginal erosions. Cartilage is intact in this early lesion, and the synovial stroma is devoid of inflammatory cells. By 19 weeks of age, there is destruction of cartilage and subchondral bone that is associated with proliferating synovial lining cells and pannus formation. Mild inflammation occurs in synovial stroma but is remote from areas of cartilage damage. Focal arteriolitis can occur. By 25 weeks of age, the inflammatory response in synovium is more marked, but proliferating synovial lining cells continue to be present. In addition, joint destruction has progressed to the development of periarticular fibrous scar tissue and new bone formation. The animals have rheumatoid factors and antibodies to collagen type 11 (5,7,232). There also is a correlation between the presence of IgM rheumatoid factor and arthritis. The rheumatoid factors in MRL-Fas(*lpr*) mice differ from those in MRL/+/+ and C57Bl6-*lpr*/*lpr* in that they are more likely to bind IgG2a than to bind other IgG isotypes (231,234). All of these features raise the possibility that MRL-Fas(*lpr*) mice are a model of spontaneous, genetically controlled arthritis, albeit arthritis that is relatively subtle. It is particularly fascinating that the initial destructive lesions are formed by proliferating synovium without inflammatory cells.

Acute necrotizing arteritis, primarily of coronary and renal arteries, is found in over half of MRL-Fas(*lpr*) males and females (5,7). Many have myocardial infarctions, but these seem to be more related histologically to small vessel vasculopathy than to inflammation of medium-sized arteries. The degenerative vascular disease consists of periodic acid-Schiff–positive eosinophilic deposits in the intima and media of small vessels without inflammation. Ig, C3, and occasionally gp70 can be found in the walls of medium and small arteries, venules, and arterioles.

T Cells, B Cells, Stem Cells, and the Thymus

Lymphoproliferation is the hallmark of MRL-Fas(*lpr*) mice. In both males and females, lymphadenopathy begins by 3 months of age (5,7). Nodes can reach 100 times their normal size and may develop hemorrhage and necrosis. Lymphoid malignancies are rare. Normal mouse strains onto which the Fas (*lpr*) gene is engrafted yield homozygotes with lymphoproliferation. Most of these develop anti-DNA, and varying proportions develop nephritis [not as universal or severe as in MRL-Fas(*lpr*) mice] (7,201). Therefore, the *lpr* gene encoding a defective Fas molecule with resultant diminished apoptosis creates a T-lymphocyte population in which highly autoreactive cells are not eliminated in a normal fashion. Other T cells, and probably B cells as well, also proliferate in the absence of some of the usual control mechanisms.

The development of lymphoproliferation may depend on $CD8^+$ cells, which are precursors of the double negative (DN) cells, or some DN cells may be a separate autoreactive lineage that is usually deleted in mice with normal tolerance mechanisms. MRL-Fas(*lpr*) mice that are treated with antibodies to CD8 or genetically engineered to fail to express CD8 or MHC class I molecules do not develop lymphoproliferation (247–249). The unusual $CD3^+$, $B220^+$, $CD4^-$, CD8, TCR-α/β cell that is so greatly expanded may derive from activated $CD8^+$ T cells that do not undergo the usual apoptosis following activation (196,199,250). On the other hand, the DN cell may be an independent lineage capable of certain functions. On *in vivo* transfer to chimeric mice, MRL DN cells did not develop into single positive cells (although the experiment did not strictly rule out the possibility) and their survival was short-lived (251). In other experiments (primarily *in vitro*), activation of DN cells caused them to express perforin and become cytolytic (252). However, the high levels of TGF-β in serum of MRL-Fas(*lpr*) mice after immunization might suppress the cytolytic capacity of the DN cells *in vivo* (253). The DN T cells also may play a role in nephritis; this is the best evidence that they are active *in vivo*. Some T cells cloned from kidney infiltrates have the DN surface phenotype and are autoreactive and kidney-specific, proliferating to renal tubular epithelial and mesangial cells (254,255). When activated *in vitro*, they induce MHC class II and intracellular adhesion molecules (ICAM-1) on cultured tubular epithelial cells; the cytokines encoded by mRNA in the T-cell clones include IL-4, TNF-α, and IFN-γ. Tubular epithelial cells may play an important role in MRL nephritis, because they can process antigen and act as APCs (256).

The autoantibodies, vasculitis, arthritis, and Ig-induced nephritis of MRL-Fas(*lpr*) mice depend largely on $CD4^+$ cells. Studies of mice (a) after the administration of antibodies to CD4, (b) in which MHC class II is knocked out (thus preventing development of $CD4^+$ T cells), or (c) that lack CD4 molecules show that these disease features do not develop (203,247,248,257,258). The presence of the *lpr* gene causes marked expansion of $CD4^+$ cells at the same time that the DN population is increasing. In fact, T-cell help for syngeneic B cells is more marked in MRL-Fas(*lpr*) than in NZB or BXSB mice (7). T cells probably are not entirely incapable of undergoing apoptosis; the protein kinase C–dependent pathway for apoptosis is intact (259). The genes that are used to assemble the TCRs on MRL-Fas(*lpr*) cells are diverse (204). There may be some restriction in clonality at the onset of disease; TCR-β-V8 families were abundant in lymphoid or salivary glands in some studies (260). As disease progresses, however, multiple different clones are involved (204,261). T cells in the periphery have other abnormal features. The ability of MRL-Fas(*lpr*) T cells to cap, proliferate, and express IL-2 surface receptors and to secrete IL-2 after antigenic or mitogenic stimulation is impaired (206,262). This may result from deficient signaling via the phosphoinositide pathway (263). There is increased tyrosine phosphorylation of p561ck in splenic T cells of MRL-Fas(*lpr*) mice with increased levels of intracellular polyamines (264). In lymph nodes, quantities of mRNA encoding IL-6, IL-10, and IFN-γ are increased (265), suggesting the participation of both Th1 and Th2 cells in disease. Cytokine gene therapy has been studied (266), and monthly intramuscular injection of cDNA expression vectors encoding for TGF-β or IL-2 altered MRL-Fas(*lpr*) disease. TGF-β prolonged survival, decreased autoantibodies and total IgG, and suppressed histologic damage to kidneys. IL-2 decreased survival and increased autoantibody and IgG production.

The Fas-defective T cells of MRL-Fas(*lpr*) mice can be destructive in non-*lpr* backgrounds. When T cells are transferred to MRL/+/+ or SCID mice, graft-versus-host wasting disease occurs, probably because there is little Fas on the donor T cells to engage FasL on hepatocytes and other cells in the recipients. Therefore, the donor T cells, when activated, do not enter apoptosis but survive and mediate perforin-induced cytotoxicity of the target recipient organs (267–269).

There is debate regarding the role of B cells in the pathogenesis of MRL-Fas(*lpr*) lupus. The hyperactivation of B cells and abnormalities of pre-B stem cells that clearly are present in NZB mice, their hybrids, and BXSB mice are far less dramatic in the MRL background. However, MRL-Fas(*lpr*) B cells that are isolated from T cells are hyperactivated (270). They hyperrespond to stimulation with LPS or IL-1 (271–273), display increased quantities of IL-6 receptors on their surfaces (274), and do not undergo anergy or receptor editing (two mechanisms of B-cell tolerance) as efficiently as B cells in normal mice (275). Perhaps all of these qualities reflect the importance of normal Fas/FasL interactions in B cells, or the influence of the large populations of helper T cells to which the B cells are exposed. There is restricted B-cell clonality to several autoantigens, such as rheumatoid factor that binds IgG2a, but this is similar to the situation in both BW and normal mice making antibody responses after stimulation by specific antigens (276). In MRL-Fas(*lpr*) mice the contribution of the MRL background apparently provides B cells with appropriate antibody repertoires to cause autoimmunity.

Stem cells in these mice may be less abnormal than stem cells in other SLE mouse models. One group has reported significant delay in disease onset after syngeneic bone marrow transplantation (277). MRL-Fas(*lpr*) mice underwent immunoablation with high-dose cyclophosphamide and then received syngeneic bone marrow that was depleted of Thy1.2 cells. Mean survival was 350 days, compared with 197 days in untreated controls, and lymphadenopathy did not develop. This is a curious finding, because all background genes, as well as the *lpr* gene, would be transferred with the marrow. It suggests that removing T cells can reset the thermostat for autoimmunity, and many weeks are required for disease to begin again.

The thymus is structurally abnormal in MRL-Fas(*lpr*) mice, as it is in all strains that develop spontaneous SLE (278). Thymic cortical atrophy is severe and medullary hyperplasia common, as in NZB and BW mice (50,51). The numbers of epithelial cells in the subcapsular and medullary regions are decreased, and there are cortical holes in which no epithelial cells can be seen. Total cortical thymocytes are decreased in number. Levels of DN cells are high, while levels of single-positive cells are low, thus suggesting the inability of activated DN cells to undergo apoptosis. Studies with superantigens have suggested that early intrathymic deletion of autoreactive T cells is normal in MRL-Fas(*lpr*) mice (279, 280), but that this may be impaired at older ages (281,282). Both thymic and peripheral deletion mechanisms for T cells likely are affected profoundly by the defect in apoptosis, which eliminates highly autoreactive activated T cells from the repertoire (196–199,281,282). In fact, SLE in MRL-Fas(*lpr*) mice may be more thymus dependent than in other strains. Thymectomy of newborn MRL-Fas(*lpr*) mice prevents development of lymphoproliferation and autoimmune disease (6,7,283), and MRL-Fas(*lpr*) thymus engrafted into MRL/+/+ mice causes lymphoproliferation and early death from autoimmune nephritis (7).

Abnormal cell functions also extend to populations other than lymphocytes. Neutrophils from MRL-Fas(*lpr*) (but not MRL/+/+) mice have a marked defect in Fc-receptor–mediated phagocytosis, which develops at the time of onset of autoimmune disease; this may result from elevated levels of TGF-β in the serum. Their ability to access areas of inflammation also may be impaired (284). Macrophages make abnormally small quantities of IL-1 (285,286), and immune complexes are not cleared as efficiently as in normal mice (287).

Genetics

The role of the *lpr* gene (and of the defective Fas molecule it encodes) as a disease accelerator is fairly well understood. The *lpr* allele on chromosome 19 is a mutation in the Fas gene resulting from an early retroviral transposon insertion in the intron between exons 2 and 3, which results in abnormal RNA splicing with a frame shift and premature termination of the mRNA (191–195). Mice that are homozygous for *lpr* express very small amounts of Fas on their cell surfaces. Normal mice express high levels of Fas on activated T and B lymphocytes and on $CD4^+CD8^+$ thymocytes, and lower levels on proliferating cells in the thymus, gut, skin, heart, liver, and ovary. Fas in concert with the FasL transduces signals, which usually results in stimulation via activation of protein tyrosine kinase, which phosphorylates a nuclear RNA-binding protein TIA-1, a ceramide-mediated apoptosis pathway, IL-1–converting enzyme (ICE), cysteine proteases, and protein tyrosine phosphatase 1C gene (PTP1c) to promote apoptosis. On the other hand, Fas/FasL interactions can activate the Abl kinase to inhibit apoptosis (288–298).

Presumably, mice that are homozygous for *lpr* are unable to delete highly autoreactive T (and possibly B) cells in the periphery, which accounts in part for their high production of multiple autoantibodies. Activation-induced cell death has been shown to depend in part on Fas/FasL interactions in $CD8^+$, Th0, and Th1 $CD4^+$ T cells, and B cells (299–301).

Lpr B cells resist apoptosis (302). Fas/FasL also is essential for killing by $CD4^+$ Th1 cells and is one of two pathways that are used by $CD8^+$ cytotoxic lymphocytes (303,304). Anergic autoreactive B cells are normally eliminated by $CD4^+$ T cells; in the absence of normal Fas/FasL interactions, the B cells are activated rather than killed (305). The genetic defect in Fas also accounts for the accumulation of $B220^+$, $CD4^-CD8^-$, and TCR^+ T cells that cause the massive lymphadenopathy associated with *lpr/lpr*. MHC class II knockout MRL-Fas(*lpr*) mice that lack $CD4^+$ cells do not develop SLE despite massive lymphadenopathy (257). MRL-Fas(*lpr*) mice that are transgenic for the gene encoding normal Fas molecules do not exhibit the acceleration of disease characteristic of the wild strain (306). The introduction of Fas(*lpr*) into any mouse strain results in lymphadenopathy of various degrees and production of autoantibodies; only strains that are genetically susceptible to SLE develop high-titer autoantibodies and full-blown clinical autoimmune disease.

MRL+/+ background genes are essential for the development of full-blown SLE. As in NZB and NZB hybrid mice, backcross studies have shown that the abilities to secrete large quantities of immunoglobulin and to make several different autoantibodies segregate independently of each other. More recent analysis of the MRL-Fas(*lpr*) mouse genome by microsatellite methods has identified two regions that associate with nephritis, one on chromosome 7, and one on chromosome 12. Interestingly, no linkage was found with the region on chromosome 17 that encodes the MHC (192). This is different from other murine models of spontaneous SLE. Genome scanning of MRL-Fas(*lpr*) and C57B1/6-Fas (*lpr*) mice (307) showed that lymphadenopathy and splenomegaly are linked to regions on chromosomes 4, 5, 7, and 10, designated *Lmb* l–4. *Lmb* l, 2, and 3 were also linked to anti-DNA but not nephritis; in contrast, *Lmb4* was linked to nephritis. *Lmb 1* was derived from the C57B1 background; *Lmb* 2, 3, and 4 were from MRL. These loci appeared to be additive. At the time of this writing, the single gene(s) within these chromosomal regions have not been identified.

Summary

MRL-Fas(*lpr*) mice are particularly interesting as a model of the accelerating factor for autoimmunity that can be provided by a single gene being added to a susceptible host. The massive lymphoproliferation that is associated with the autosomal-recessive *lpr* gene almost surely results from defective apoptosis. The resultant expansion in $CD4^+$ T cells drives predisposed MRL B cells to make the largest array of autoantibodies that occurs in murine lupus. The production of pathogenic autoantibodies and the presence of cytolytic DN and of $CD4^+$ T cells in target organs such as kidneys and salivary glands result in accelerated autoimmunity and early death from lupus-like nephritis. Some MRL-Fas(*lpr*) mice develop destructive polyarthritis, which often is associated with IgM rheumatoid factors. MRL mice are the only strains that spontaneously make anti-Sm. They also develop vasculitis, which can be severe.

BXSB Mice

The BXSB strain was developed by Murphy and Roths (308,309). BXSB is a recombinant inbred (RI) strain; RI mice are derived by brother/sister matings within each generation, usually extending for 12 to 20 generations. The RI technique is used to produce strains with high frequencies of homozygosity at many loci to see the expression of recessive genes. The initial mating was between a C57BI/6 female and a satin beige (SB/Le male), hence the designation BXSB.

The unique features of BXSB mice are that disease is much worse in males than in females, and the disease-accelerating gene that is responsible for this difference is located on the Y chromosome. The gene is called *Yaa*, for Y chromosome autoimmunity accelerator. The female BXSB gets late-life lupus; therefore, additional genes contribute to disease, as in all other models of spontaneous lupus studied to date (Table 18.6).

Clinical Manifestations and Autoantibodies

BXSB mice make an autoantibody repertoire that includes IgG antibodies to ssDNA and dsDNA, chromatin, C1q, ANA, and antibodies that are directed against brain cells (5,7,310,311). In addition, a small proportion make anti-erythrocyte, NTA, monoclonal paraproteins, and gp70anti-gp70 immune complexes (5,7). By an early age (3 months), they have elevated levels of circulating immune complexes and hypocomplementemia (5). Serum levels of C4 diminish as clinical disease appears (312).

Death is caused by immune glomerulonephritis (5,7, 311). Histologically, the disease is more exudative than in other mouse models. That is, there are neutrophils invading glomeruli along with IgG and C3 deposition, proliferative changes in mesangia and endothelial cells, and basement membrane thickening (5). The progression from nephritis to death is rapid, with 50% of males dead by 5 months of age (5,7,311,312).

T Cells, B Cells, Stem Cells, and the Thymus

Lymphoproliferation occurs in BXSB mice; it is more marked than in BW but less dramatic than in MRL-Fas(*lpr*) (5,7). In contrast to MRL-Fas(*lpr*) mice, the hyperplastic nodes contain predominantly B cells (6,7), and for some time it was thought that B-cell defects were the primary abnormality in BXSB mice. As in the other models, B cells are hyperactivated, higher portions are mature (expressing IgD and IgM on their surfaces), higher proportions display CD40L on their surface, and secretion of IgG and IgM is increased (6,7,313,314). The B cells are resistant to toler-

TABLE 18.6. CHARACTERISTICS OF BXSB MICE

A. Clinical
   1. Males die early of lupus (50% mortality at 5 months; 90% at 8 months)
   2. Females have late-onset lupus (50% mortality at 15 months; 90% at 24 months)
   3. Major cause of death is immune glomerulonephritis
B. Histologic
   1. Males show severe acute to subacute glomerulonephritis, with proliferation and exudation of neutrophils into glomeruli
   2. In males, IgG and C3 deposit in mesangium and glomerular capillary walls by 3 months of age; deposits in tubular basement membranes and interstitium also occur
   3. Lymph node hyperplasia (10–20 times normal size) in males
   4. Myocardial infarcts in 25%, without arteritis
   5. Thymic cortical atrophy with medullary hyperplasia; thymic epithelial cells contain crystalline inclusions
C. Autoantibodies
   1. All males develop ANAs and IgG anti-dsDNA and anti-ssDNA
   2. Less than one-half of males develop monoclonal paraproteins, antierythrocyte antibodies, gp70–anti-gp70, and thymocytotoxic antibodies
   3. Hypocomplementemia in males by 3 months of age; low C4 levels
   4. Elevated levels of circulating immune complexes
   5. Defective monocyte/macrophages
D. Immune abnormalities
   1. B cell is the most frequent cell in hyperplastic lymph nodes
   2. B-cell hyperactivation and advanced maturity
   3. B cells are resistant to tolerance with some antigens
   4. Male bone marrow transferred to female BXSB mice produces accelerated disease; female marrow confers late lupus when transferred to males; mature male B cells do not accelerate disease; abnormality is contained in marrow stem cells
   5. Monocytosis occurs
   6. Elimination of $CD4^+$ T cells diminishes anti-DNA, monocytosis, nephritis, and mortality
   7. Disease is not influenced substantially by thymectomy
   8. Disease is not influenced substantially by sex hormone therapies and/or castration
   9. Defective Fc-mediated immune complex clearance
E. Genetics
   1. A single gene that accelerates disease, *Yaa,* is present on the Y chromosome; it has not been cloned
   2. Additional genes that behave as X-linked recessives confer susceptibility to disease; they may account for late-life SLE in females

ance with human gamma globulin; the resistance is a property of the B cell itself and does not reflect abnormalities in APCs or T cells (315). Studies in Yaa+Yaa– double bone marrow chimeric mice show that Yaa– T cells can activate Yaa+ B cells to make autoantibodies (or increased antibodies to foreign antigens), but Yaa+ T cells cannot drive Yaa– B cells to make autoantibodies (316,317). This probably indicates that Yaa+ B cells present antigen to T cells and the two cells cross-activate each other. However, BXSB T cells play an important role in disease (318,319) by providing help for autoantibody formation. As mice age, they develop the typical T-cell defects of SLE mice (i.e., abnormally low proliferative responses to antigens/mitogens, reduced production of IL-2). Elimination of $CD4^+$ T cells (but not $CD8^+$) suppresses autoantibodies, monocytosis, and nephritis (319). Production of mixed chimerics in BXSB mice created by lethal irradiation followed by transfer of bone marrow from nonautoimmune BALB/c mice plus congenic marrow depleted of T cells prolongs survival, prevents nephritis, and restores normal primary immune responses (which are abnormal in mice receiving only allogeneic cells). Depletion of BXSB T cells is essential to the success of this approach (320). In sum, it is clear that T cells are required for development of full-blown disease. Disease is delayed by the prevention of second signal-mediated T-cell activation after administration of CTLA41g (321). As BXSB males age, their T cells acquire a memory phenotype and secrete lymphokines that are characteristic of both Th1 and Th2 cells (322,323). Recent experiments showed that BXSB disease is not altered in mice deficient in IL-4 (324).

The thymus shows cortical atrophy and defects similar to those in other SLE strains (278,325). Crystalline structures have been described in the thymic epithelial cells of BXSB males; they are thought to represent abnormal storage of thymic hormones (326). Apoptosis of thymic cells is delayed in all SLE strains studied, including BXSB. Thymectomy has accelerated disease in some studies and has not altered it in others (6,327). The effects are not as consistent and dramatic as the protection from disease that is conferred by thymectomy in MRL-Fas(*lpr*) mice (6,7,283).

An additional feature of BXSB mice is monocytosis. By 2 weeks of age, BXSB males have increased numbers of monocyte colony-forming units in spleen and lymph nodes (328). Further, the monocytes/macrophages are abnormal; they make unusually large quantities of procoagulants, which might contribute to the rapid damage of glomeruli that characterizes lupus in this strain (329).

Studies of lymph nodes show dramatic increases in mRNA for IL-1, with some increase in IL-10 and TGF-β, all of which probably come from monocytes. IFN-γ also is increased, suggesting simultaneous increase in monocyte/macrophage and T-cell activity (265).

There is good evidence that a stem cell abnormality is crucial to the development of disease in BXSB mice (7,330), because male BXSB bone marrow can transfer disease and normal marrow grafted into male BXSB mice can prevent disease (7,330–332). This stem cell defect may lead to a single abnormality that affects both B and T cells, or there may be multiple genes influencing multiple responses leading to hyperactivity in each type of lymphocyte and in monocytes.

Manipulations such as castration and androgen therapy do not dramatically alter outcome (6,7,333), in contrast to mice with New Zealand backgrounds.

Genetics

Multiple genes predispose to SLE in BXSB mice, as in the other models. There is an inherent tendency toward autoimmune disease in BXSB mice of both sexes; that tendency is dramatically accelerated by the introduction of the *Yaa* gene on the Y chromosome. This accounts for the earlier, more severe disease in males. If normal mice are generated that bear the *Sle1* gene from NZW mice (a gene associated with ability to break tolerance to nucleosomes) and the *Yaa* gene, fatal autoimmune nephritis occurs (74). The *Yaa* gene alone is not sufficient to permit the development of autoimmunity: MHC and other genes play important roles (334–336). The *Yaa* gene has not been sequenced at the time of this writing. Mice of the H-2b haplotype (BXSB is H-2b) do not express MHC class II I-E molecules; introduction of the I-E α chain into BXSB males permits the mice to display I-E on cell surfaces and prevents disease (337–339). This effect is controlled by MHC and occurs only in mouse strains with "permissive" MHC such as H-2b (340). The I-A molecule in the transgenic mice contains peptides from I-E, and it is possible that those peptides prevent the presentation of other peptides that induce and sustain pathogenic autoantibody production (340). Susceptibility to autoimmunity is transmitted as an autosomal dominant trait in some F1 hybrids that are derived from BXSB (334–336), and in others susceptibility behaves as if it were controlled by autosomal-recessive genes (7).

Results of genome scans of backcrosses between BXSB and B10 mice have been published (341,342). Three to four regions on chromosome 1 and a region on chromosome 3 are linked to nephritis. One publication reports linkage with a region on chromosome 13, the other with regions on chromosomes 4 and 10. The regions on 1 that are telomeric have been linked to SLE in other strains; the other regions may be unique to BXSB.

Summary

In summary, BXSB mice are unique in that lupus nephritis is more severe and occurs earlier in males than in females; this is from the accelerating effect of a single gene, *Yaa*, which is located on the Y chromosome. Disease develops rapidly in BXSB males, with 50% dead of immune glomerulonephritis by 5 months of age.

B cells, T cells, and monocytes all have abnormal functions, most of which suggest hyperactivation. The autoantibody repertoire is directed primarily against nucleosomal and DNA antigens. Multiple genes participate, some of which are shared in other lupus mouse strains and some of which are probably unique to the BXSB background.

The (NZW × BXSB)F1 Model of Antiphospholipid Syndrome and Coronary Artery Disease

Disease Characteristics and Autoantibodies

Male hybrid (NZW × BXSB)F1 mice have been particularly interesting as models of autoimmunity linked to accelerated degenerative coronary artery disease, a combination seen in some patients with SLE. In these mice, 50% of the males are dead by 24 weeks of age, usually with extensive myocardial infarction, with occlusive disease and intimal thickening in small coronary arteries but not extramyocardial coronary arteries. These mice also develop high serum levels of anti-DNA and immune complexes, with antibodies against both platelets and phospholipids. Some monoclonal anticardiolipin antibodies also bind platelets and DNA, similar to some antibodies from BW mice. Most of the antiphospholipids bind 2-glycoprotein I; such subsets may be more likely to be associated with clotting than subsets without that characteristic (343). The males also develop glomerulonephritis, hypertension, leukocytosis, gastrointestinal vasculitis, and thrombocytopenia (343,344).

Abnormalities in Stem Cells, T Cells, and B Cells

All these cells are abnormal, as in BXSB parents. Serum levels of IFN-γ and IL-10 increase as mice age. Treatment with antibodies to CD4 delays disease, whereas treatment with antibodies to CD8 accelerates it (345). Lethal irradiation of (NZW × BXSB)F1 mice followed by transfer of bone marrow from normal C57B1 mice prevents nephritis, coronary artery disease, and thrombocytopenia, suggesting that all of these manifestations result from immune and inflammatory processes (345). On the other hand, treatment with the calcium channel blocker ticlodipine prolongs survival and lowers the prevalence of myocardial infarction without affecting nephritis (347). Similarly, treatment with nifedipine lowers blood pressure and prolongs survival, protects partially from coronary artery stenosis and myocardial infarction, and reduces the amount of histologic nephritis (348). Therefore, the final expression of disease has immune, inflammatory, and degenerative components.

Genetics

One genome scan has shown linkage between various disease features and different chromosomal regions. Antibodies to cardiolipin, platelet-binding antibodies, thrombocytopenia, and myocardial infarction were each controlled by independently segregating dominant alleles. Regions on chromosomes 4 and 17 are linked to anticardiolipin, on chromosomes 8 and 17 to antiplatelet antibodies and thrombocytopenia, and on chromosomes 7 and 14 to myocardial infarction (349). This suggests that there is not a simple direct association between antiphospholipid and myocardial infarct or thrombocytopenia; the antibodies and disease expression have complex genetic requirements.

Gld/Gld Mice with Absence of Fas Ligand

In 1984, Roths et al. (350) reported a spontaneous autosomal-recessive mutation that occurred in the inbred mouse strain C3H/HeJ, which they called gld (for generalized lymphoproliferative disorder). It now is known that the mutation is a single base change in the C-terminal extracellular domain of the FasL molecule, which is encoded on mouse chromosome 6 (351–353); functional FasL molecules are not generated. FasL is expressed on cell surfaces, but the mutation interferes with its ability to bind Fas. Therefore, apoptosis does not proceed normally, highly autoreactive T and B cells persist instead of dying, and SLE results.

FasL plays a major role in apoptosis. Clinically, C3H/gld/gld mice of both sexes develop lymphadenopathy and splenomegaly by 13 weeks of age. Lymphoid organs contain increased numbers of B, T, and double negative lymphocytes. The $B220^+$, $CD4^-$, $CD8^-$, TCR^+ T cell that expands so dramatically in MRL-Fas(*lpr*) mice probably is identical to the major expanded population in gld/gld mice, since both strains have major defects in apoptosis mediated by Fas/FasL interactions. Recent evidence suggests that these DN cells require MHC class I expression for expansion, and contain populations with high avidity for self antigens such as endogenous retroviral superantigens; such a dangerous population is deleted in normal mice (354). C3H/Gld/gld mice have a shortened life span compared with wild-type C3H/HeJ, with male C3H/gld/gld mice living a mean of 396 days and females 368 days, compared with 688 days in females that are not homozygous for gld. Lymphoid cells and macrophages infiltrate the interstitium of lungs extensively, but other organs rarely are involved. Vasculitis does not occur. Most of these mice do not develop histologic lupus nephritis, although all mice older than 22 weeks have immunoglobulin deposits in glomeruli (primarily confined to the mesangium). By that age, serum levels of gamma globulin are approximately five times normal; this increase occurs in all isotypes but is most dramatic in IgA and IgG2b. ANAs begin to appear at 8 weeks of age, and all C3H/gld/gld mice are positive by 16 weeks. By 20 weeks, all have antibodies to thymocytes and antibodies to dsDNA (350,355). The primary cause of early mortality probably is the pulmonary disease. In C3H/gld/gld and BALB/gld/gld mice that live to 1 year of age, B-cell malignancies are common (usually $CD5^+$ malignant plasmacytoid lymphomas) (356). As in other lupus models, genetic backgrounds in addition to the single point mutation determine the extent of disease: B6/gld/gld mice have milder disease than C3H/gld/gld.

The gld mutation has greatly increased our understanding of the importance of Fas/FasL interactions and of apoptosis in maintaining normal immune homeostasis. For example, lethally irradiated mice reconstituted with stem cells from Fas-deficient MRL/*lpr* mice develop chronic graft-versus-host disease (GVHD), but stem cells deficient in both Fas and FasL do not produce GVHD, showing that FasL is an important effector in this syndrome. Interestingly, these double-deficient T cells can induce normal B cells to produce autoantibodies (357) In pristane-induced murine lupus, lpr and gld mutations affect some autoantibody production but not others, suggesting that autoantibodies differ in their dependence on Fas and FasL expression by T cells (358). B6/gld/gld mice can clear cytomegalovirus after infection, but they cannot downregulate the resultant inflammatory responses (359). Nonobese diabetic (NOD) mice spontaneously develop autoimmune diabetes resulting from immune destruction of pancreatic β cells. NOD/gld/gld mice are protected from disease, showing the dependence of the process on FasL-mediated apoptosis (360) The Fas and FasL mutations are discussed later in this chapter and in detail in Chapter 7. Interestingly, lupus-like disease in C3H/gld/gld mice also requires TNF-α: mice deficient in that cytokine or treated with antibodies to TNF-α have milder disease (361). C3H/gld/gld disease can be prevented by lethal irradiation followed by reconstitution with a mixture of normal and gld bone marrow, as long as the normal marrow is not depleted of $Thy1^+$ cells, suggesting that T cells expressing FasL can correct the gld defect; $CD8^+$ $FasL^+$ cells are primarily responsible for suppression of lymphoproliferation (362).

In summary, autoiminune-permissive strains with defective production of FasL develop lymphoproliferation, autoantibodies, and infiltration of organs with lymphocytes that cannot be deleted normally. Their disease has similarities to human SLE, as does disease associated with production of a defective Fas molecule in *lpr*-bearing strains.

Palmerston North Mice (PN)

PN mice are descendants of albino mice that were purchased from a pet shop in 1948 and raised at the Palmerston North Hospital in New Zealand. Inbreeding began in 1964, with animals being selected for ANA positivity. Autoantibodies and nephritis were characterized by Walker et al. (363) in 1978.

Clinical Characteristics and Autoantibodies

Fifty-percent survivals are 11 months for females and 15 months for males. The mice develop two main pathologic lesions: (a) necrotizing vasculitis of small and medium arteries; and (b) proliferative glomerulonephritis with fibrinoid necrosis, crescent formation, and glomerular deposits of IgG and C3. Arteritis occurs in spleen, thymus, kidneys, ovaries, and lungs, with sparing of the aorta. Lymph nodes are hyperplastic in some mice, and malignant lymphoma occurs. Thymic cortical atrophy occurs late (at approximately 11 months).

Anti-DNA and ANAs may be present at birth in some PN mice, and both increase with age until most animals are positive. By 1 month of age, all female PN mice have IgM anti-dsDNA and ssDNA, and the majority also produce IgM antibodies to cardiolipin. By 3 months of age, approximately 90% have IgG anti-ssDNa and -dsDNA. By 6 to 12 months, all females have IgG antibodies to cardiolipin and other phospholipids and the majority have IgG antibodies to erythrocytes (363). LE cells have been reported. As the mice age, the proliferative responses of their T cells tends to diminish, as in other lupus strains (364).

The most remarkable finding in PN mice is vasculitis. A recent report detailed the types of cells and cytokines in perivascular and vascular infiltrates. Perivasculitis dominated in arteries and veins in kidney, liver, brain, and lung; vasculitis dominated in veins and venules. The infiltrates were composed mainly of an unusual cell type with T-cell and B-cell markers mostly $CD4^+$. The predominant cytokines in lesions were IL-4, IL-6, and IL-10 with little to no IL-2, IFN-γ, TGF-β, or TNF-α. Therefore, these T-cell populations are mostly Th2 with little participation of monocytes/macrophages at the time the lesions are full-blown (365).

In summary, the PN mouse is a model of spontaneous autoantibodies, including antibodies to phospholipid, with impressive vasculitis and glomerulonephritis. The genetics are not yet well understood.

INDUCTION OF LUPUS IN NORMAL MOUSE STRAINS

In the previously discussed models of spontaneous SLE, multiple genetic factors likely provide the major if not the only important risk factors. Mutations in Fas (Fas-lpr) and FasL (gld) accelerate autoimmunity in these susceptible strains. However, there are several examples of the induction of SLE-like disease in mice that are otherwise healthy, with genetic backgrounds that do not predispose to autoimmunity. These include (a) induction of chronic GVHD; (b) alteration of expression of single molecules (either upregulation via transgene insertion or deletion in knockout mice); (c) transfer of pathogenic autoantibodies or the B cells that secrete them; (d) forced expression of pathogenic autoantibodies via the introduction of transgenes; (e) activation of idiotypic networks that result in the production of pathogenic autoantibodies; and (f) inoculations of DNA, DNA/protein, other autoreactive proteins or oligopeptides, or pristane. In most of these models, some strains of mice are more susceptible than others, again suggesting that most if not all murine genetic backgrounds contain genes that permit autoimmunity.

Chronic GVHD

GVHD is produced in mice by injecting lymphocytes from a parent into an F1 hybrid differing at one MHC locus from that parent. It is caused by T cells recognizing foreign MHC antigens (366). Acute GVHD is runting disease with failure to thrive, diarrhea, wasting, and early death (367). T cells that are defective in Fas expression (caused by the *lpr* gene) can cause acute GVHD in recipients with identical MHC class II molecules, because they do not undergo apoptosis after activation (368). Acute GVHD is not lupus-like. If lymphocytes are injected after the recipient F1 animal has reached at least 6 weeks of age and if certain H-2 gene interactions occur between parent and F1, chronic GVHD results. Chronic GVHD resembles SLE (366,367, 369–372). Several IgG autoantibodies are made, including anti-dsDNA, anti-ssDNA, and antihistone (366,369,372). In some combinations, fatal lupus-like nephritis mediated by the IgG anti-DNA occurs.

$CD4^+$ effector cells provided by the donor are required for induction of chronic GVHD (366,367); they must be activated by appropriate MHC class II gene products on the surface of the recipient cells (370,371). One combination that results in fatal nephritis of chronic GVHD is H-2d donor lymphocytes into an H-2b recipient (371,372). In contrast, most recipient H2k haplotypes are resistant. The development of clinical nephritis and of autoantibodies can be separated. Many parental hybrid combinations result in the ability of the recipient to make high-titer IgG anti-DNA, but class II genes I-A and I-E (equivalent to human HLA class II DR and DQ) must contain a susceptible haplotype, such as b, for severe nephritis to result (372). Animals without nephritis confine renal deposits of IgG to mesangial regions of glomeruli; animals with nephritis have IgG deposits along the capillary loops (372).

This model provides an excellent example of lupus nephritis resulting from interactions between $CD4^+$ T-helper cells, $CD8^+$ cytotoxic/suppressor cells, and APCs of a host that differs from the donor at MHC. Disease is initiated by donor $CD4^+$ cells activated by host APC to secrete IL-4, and B-cell stimulation with autoantibody production begins. Ability of the host to mount $CD8^+$ cells that kill the B cells determines whether acute or chronic GVHD will occur. Both acute and chronic GVHD may begin as a Th2 cytokine-mediated B-cell stimulation; transition to acute GVHD depends on the education in the host thymus of donor-derived pro-T and pre-T cells to develop into double-positive cells and ultimately $CD8^+$ T cells that terminate the B-cell hyperactivity by eliminating activated B cells (both perforin-mediated cytotoxicity and Fas/FasL killing occur). Activation of $CD8^+$ T is promoted by IFN-γ secretion by donor $CD4^+$ T cells. If thymic education does not occur, IL-4 secretion continues and B cells are not downregulated; sustained autoantibody production and lupus-like chronic GVHD result (373–376). Mice with severe chronic GVHD usually have high levels of IgE and IgG1 in their serum, confirming the important role of Th2 cells in disease. Antibodies to IL-4, or infusion of soluble IL-4 receptor, prevents or suppresses disease (377).

Genetic Alteration of Expression of Single Molecules: Increased Expression in Transgenic Mice

See Chapter 7 for a detailed discussion of genes in murine lupus. Studies in which single genes are overexpressed in transgenic mice, or single genes are deleted in knockout mice, have all suggested that strategies that permit extended lifetimes for autoreactive lymphocytes or for autoantigens promote the development of SLE-like disease in normal mice. For example, overexpression of bcl-2 (which protects cells from apoptotic death) in normal mice transgenic for that molecule causes them to develop mild autoimmunity (378). Bcl-2 transgenic C57B1/6-*lpr* mice have lymphadenopathy but no abnormal autoantibodies (379). In C57B1/6-*lpr* mice transgenic for Pim-l (a cytoplasmic serine/threonine protein kinase that also inhibits apoptosis), lymphoproliferation resulting from the accumulation of $B220^+$ T cells also occurs (380). A molecule that stimulates the growth of B lymphocytes, which is variously named BlyS (B lymphocyte stimulator), BAFF (B cell activating factor belonging to the TNF-α family), THANK (TNF-α homologue that activates apoptosis, nuclear factor [NFI]-xB, c-Jun NH2-terminal kinase), TALL-1 (TNF-α and apoptosis ligand-related leukocyte-expressed ligand 1), and zTNF4, can induce autoimmunity when overexpressed. BLyS is a monocyte-specific TNF-α family cytokine that is a potent co-stimulator with antiimmunoglobulin M *in vitro* and with CD40L *in vivo* for B-cell proliferation. BLyS enhances the humoral responses to T-cell–independent and T-cell–dependent antigens by protecting antigen-activated B cells from apoptosis (381–383).

Genetic Alteration of Expression of Single Molecules: Deleted Molecules in Knockout Mice

Two general categories of single gene deletion have led to generation of lupus-like disease in otherwise healthy mice: (a) removal of genes that downregulate accumulation and/or activation of B or T lymphocytes; and (b) deletion of genes that regulate normal degradation and clearing of DNA, immune complexes, or apoptotic cells and bodies. In the first category, normal mice with deletion of Lyn have a marked increase in IgM-secreting B cells and develop high levels of immune complexes and anti-DNA, along with a glomerulonephritis similar to SLE (384,385). Lyn is a Src protein tyrosine kinase associated with the B-cell receptor (BCR) that participates in an inhibitory signal after BCR activation; Lyn phosphorylates the BCR co-receptor CD22, a process that recruits the tyrosine phosphatase SHP-1 to the BCR/CD22 complex and controls B-cell activation. In the absence of Lyn, B cells exhibit spontaneous hyperreactivity, which doubtless contributes to their lupus-like phenotype (386). Motheaten mice (so called because of patchy alopecia) have spontaneous deletion of a single residue in the N-terminal SH2 domain of the protein tyrosine phosphatase 1C gene (PTP1c). PTP1c activity is absent, which may remove an inhibitory signal for the activation of Lyn and Syk, with resultant B-cell hyperactivation. IgM levels are high, B-1 B cells are abnormally activated, and high-titer ANAs develop, with immune complex deposition in many tissues (387,388). On the T-cell side, deletion of PD-1, an immunoglobulin superfamily member bearing an immunoreceptor tyrosine-based inhibitory motif (ITIM) that affects primarily $CD4^-CD8^-$ thymocytes also results in lupus-like disease (389). Similarly, expression of the cell-cycle regulator p21 prevents accumulation of $CD4^+$ memory cells; deletion of that molecule in normal mice results in loss of tolerance for nuclear antigens. Interestingly, female mice with a p21 deletion are particularly prone to develop SLE; they develop IgG antibodies to dsDNA, lymphadenopathy, Ig-mediated glomerulonephritis, and shortened survival (390).

In the second category—gene deletions that influence clearing of DNA, nucleosomes, apoptotic cells, and apoptotic bodies—several single gene deletions have produced lupus-like phenotypes in normal mice. Humans with homozygous deletions of C1q have a very high prevalence of SLE. Similarly, among mice in which the C1q gene was deleted, approximately half developed high-titer ANAs and 25% had clinical nephritis by the age of 8 months; glomeruli showed unusually abundant deposits of apoptotic bodies (391). C1q probably plays a role in clearance of immune complexes, of apoptotic cells, and of apoptotic bodies (392). Serum amyloid P component (SAP) binds to DNA and chromatin, displaces H-1 histones, and solublizes native long chromatin. SAP also binds to apoptotic cells (surface blebs contain chromatin) and to nuclear debris following cell necrosis. It is probably important in the disposal of these materials. Mice with deletions in the SAP gene developed autoantibodies, including anti-DNA, and severe glomerulonephritis (393). Mice deficient in DNAse1 also developed ANA, Ig deposition in glomeruli, and clinical nephritis (394).

In summary, these single gene knockout mice show that one alteration permitting B- or T-cell hyperactivation, or interfering with the elimination of DNA/nucleosomes or apoptotic and necrotic cells that provide stimulatory nucleosomes and other self antigens, is powerful enough to produce lupus-like phenotypes in mice that otherwise are resistant to clinical autoimmunity.

Lupus Induced by Direct Transfer of Pathogenic Autoantibodies or B Cells that Secrete Those Antibodies

See Chapter 21 for a detailed discussion of this topic. Briefly, our laboratory demonstrated that transfer of B-cell hybridomas secreting pathogenic IgG anti-dsDNA to normal BALB/c mice resulted in the development of SLE, with circulating IgG anti-dsDNA and immune complexes and severe Ig-mediated glomerulonephritis (97,98). In some cases, mice were injected repeatedly with purified IgG rather than with hybridoma cells, with the same results. Injections of the immunoglobulin into C57B1/6 mice did not produce any disease, suggesting that background susceptibility genes, perhaps influencing the composition of the kidney, must be present for this approach to induce disease. SCID mice that were populated with BW pre–B cells developed SLE with the expected secretion of autoantibodies by their adopted B cells (145). Similarly, some human monoclonal antibody anti-DNA inoculated into SCID mice deposited in glomeruli and induced proteinuria (395).

Lupus in Mice Transgenic for Pathogenic Autoantibodies

Transient lupus nephritis developed in normal mice that were transgenic for an IgG2b anti-dsDNA derived from a nephritic BW female (100). The gene construct permitted only small quantities of the transgenic IgG2b to be expressed on B-cell surfaces, thus bypassing early tolerance mechanisms. Therefore, the transgenic mice secreted IgG2b anti-dsDNA for several weeks and, during that time, developed proteinuria. Later, B-cell receptor editing occurred, with resultant elimination of the ability of the immunoglobulin to bind DNA; the proteinuria disappeared and the mice lived a normal life span. Mice carrying transgenes encoding anti-DNA from MRL-Fas(*lpr*) mice have also been generated and studied for B-cell tolerance. In MRL-Fas(*lpr*) mice, anti-dsDNA B cells undergo receptor editing, while anti-ssDNA B cells are functionally silenced (396). In the lupus mice compared to normal BALB/c mice, developmental arrest and accumulation at the T-B interface of splenic follicles does not occur; in the presence of the Fas/*lpr* mutation anti-dsDNA, B cells are found in the follicle, along with CD4 T cells, so that T-B interactions continue to drive clinical autoimmunity (275,397). To summarize, if normal mice express the transgene-encoded immunoglobulin on B-cell surfaces, the cells are developmentally arrested, deleted, anergized, or receptor edited; cells do not reach T-B interaction sites in lymphoid organs, and secretion of the anti-DNA is short-lived if it occurs at all. If the transgenic mouse has an *lpr* background, these mechanisms of tolerance degrade over time, pathogenic B cells reach follicles where they can interact with T cells, and ANAs encoded by the transgene are secreted with steadily increasing titers. In another model using mice transgenic for the R4A-γ2b heavy chain of an anti-DNA monoclonal antibody (mAb) (which can combine with multiple light chains to made a DNA-binding Ig), nonautoimmune hosts display a high-affinity population that is anergic, another high-affinity population that is deleted, and a third population that produced germline-encoded antibodies with low affinity for dsDNA that escaped normal regulation (398). Perhaps these low-affinity cells that normally escape regulation undergo activation and receive T-cell help in mice predisposed to SLE and thus become pathogenic anti-DNA–secreting B cells.

Lupus Following Activation of Id/Anti-Id Networks

The role of Id/anti-Id networks in SLE is discussed in detail in Chapter 15. Immunization with an Id induces anti-Id; immunization with an anti-Id induces anti-anti-Id and/or Id. This principle has been used to study murine models of SLE and of antiphospholipid syndrome. After immunization of BALB/c or other susceptible strains (again, C57B1/6 is resistant) with Id 16/6 (i.e., a frequently occurring Id in patients with SLE) or anti-Id 16/6, a full Id/anti-Id network appeared in the mice along with autoantibodies to DNA, to phospholipids, and to snRNP particles. The mice developed leukopenia, elevated sedimentation rates, and immunoglobulin deposits in glomeruli (399–401). Normal mice that were immunized with a monoclonal antiphospholipid IgM with lupus anticoagulant activity also developed an Id/anti-Id network, along with thrombocytopenia, lupus anticoagulant, and fetal loss (402,403). These models also have been used to test multiple therapeutic interventions (404–409). Both $CD4^+$ and $CD8^+$ cells may be necessary for the development of full-blown disease (408,410). It should be noted that C57B1/6 mice are not completely protected from SLE; when mated with a substrain of NZM/Aeg, some hybrids develop severe immune complex GN (61).

Lupus Induced by Immunization with DNA, DNA/Proteins, RNA/Proteins or Oligopeptides, or Injections of Pristane

There has been great debate regarding the nature of the inciting antigens in SLE. Most investigators agree that DNA/protein and RNA/protein molecules and particles likely are the true immunogens in mice or humans who are predisposed to SLE. In general, naked mammalian DNA is a weak immunogen and does not induce SLE in normal mice unless it is bound to a protein (66,411,412). In contrast, bacterial DNA used to immunize normal mice can induce IgG antibodies to DNA (almost exclusively to ssDNA rather than dsDNA), and some animals develop immune complex nephritis (413). Whether this DNA acquires protein after immunization is unknown. Mammalian DNA used as an immunogen also can induce IgG anti-DNA and nephritis in normal mice if it is bound to protein. Thus, immunization with nucleobindin, which probably combines with nucleosomes that are released from the thymus and other tissues, can induce anti-DNA in normals (213), as can DNA that is combined with a fusion protein (411). Nucleosomes are particles in which DNA is wrapped around histones; they likely are direct immunogens that induce many of the autoantibodies characteristics of SLE.

Immunization of rabbits, mice, and baboons with protein or oligopeptide autoantigens (from Sm B/51, Ro 60-kd peptides, and La/SS-B) have induced epitope spreading, antinuclear antibodies, and proteinuria in a proportion of animals (414–417). However, one group of investigators found more limited epitope spreading in rabbits and mice after immunization with a peptide of Sm B/B′, less ANA production, and no clinical disease (418). This may reflect differences in environmental stimuli to which animals are exposed in different laboratories.

Chronic inflammation may induce autoantibodies in susceptible mice. Satoh et al. (419) injected pristane into the peritoneal cavities of BALB/c mice. Approximately half of these mice developed IgM anti-ssDNA, IgM antihistone, IgG anti-Sm, and IgG anti-Su. IgM, IgG, and C3 were found in glomeruli, predominantly in mesangial areas. This is excellent evidence that inflammatory stimuli can provoke autoantibody production; whether that leads to disease, however, probably depends on concurrent immune responses and genetic susceptibility.

A Brief Overview of the Pathogenesis Of Murine Lupus

Chapter 5 summarizes current concepts regarding the pathogenesis of SLE. Here, the information from murine lupus is briefly synthesized (Table 18.7).

Murine lupus may result almost entirely from genetic predisposition (almost always involving multiple genes in certain pathogenic combinations), from environmental stimuli, or both. It is likely that a susceptible genetic background is always required, because no single environmental trigger that accounts for disease induction or flare in all patients has been identified. However, the relative importance of genes and environmental triggers may vary.

TABLE 18.7. PATHOGENESIS OF AUTOIMMUNITY IN MURINE MODELS OF SLE

A. Genetic susceptibility
    1. MHC genes (NZ and BXSB)
    2. Multiple genes on different chromosomes, not linked to MHC
    3. Single accelerating genes: *lpr, Yaa, me*
B. Immune abnormalities
    1. Excessive T-cell help by $CD4^+$ and $CD4^-CD8^-$ cells
    2. Excessive B-cell activation, partially independent of T cells
    3. Defects in bone marrow stem cells (NZ and BXSB mice)
    4. Abnormal architecture and function of the thymus, with marked cortical atrophy
    5. Defective immune complex clearance
C. Production of autoantibodies
    1. Antibodies against DNA/protein and RNA/protein antigens
    2. Antibodies against cell surface molecules
    3. Antibodies against phospholipids
D. Infiltration of target organs by T cells capable of damaging the organ
E. Environmental factors influencing disease
    1. Diet
    2. Sex hormone status
    3. Infections
    4. Neuroendocrine system

Examples of Spontaneous and Induced Mouse Models of SLE Illustrate These Points

In mice, multiple genes are required for the development of spontaneous SLE. Addition of accelerator genes to these backgrounds makes the disease appear earlier, such as Fas1pr gld and Yaa, each of which is discussed above. In most if not all strains MHC class II genes are critical, probably because they shape the $CD4^+$ T-cell responses that drive abnormal B cells, which already are prone to secrete large quantities of IgM and autoantibodies. Microsatellite analysis of DNA in the mouse genome has shown that multiple genes on different chromosomes are required for development of all SLE manifestations that are known to develop in NZ hybrids. There may be at least two or three genes that influence each manifestation (e.g., anti-DNA, early mortality, glomerulonephritis, and so on). In most strains, there is a region on the telmeric portion of chromosome 1 that contains at least one gene that significantly increases susceptibility; a syntenic region on human chromosome 1 has been associated with SLE in several human populations. In total, there may be ten or more genes in each strain that in combination cause all of the manifestations that are associated with murine lupus, with some providing a higher proportion of susceptibility than others. (These concepts are discussed in detail in Chapter 7.)

In addition, there are several single genes that can be knocked in or knocked out of the genome of normal mice that result in lupus-like clinical disease. Most of them alter B- or T-cell survival and/or affect apoptosis.

The Role of Stem Cells, Thymus Cells, B Cells, and T Cells in Murine Lupus

Most investigators think that abnormalities occur in B and T cells of NZB, NZ hybrids, and BXSB mice. Therefore, a defect (or, more likely, multiple defects) in stem cells may underlie the disease. Transfer of bone marrow cells likely to be stem cells from NZ and BXSB mice have transferred the ability to make autoantibodies and develop disease to otherwise normal recipients (36,119,320,331,332). There is evidence that activation of both T and B cells is abnormal in that cells are too sensitive to stimulation, not eliminated properly after activation, or both. If there are one or a few abnormalities in cell activation that characterize any one strain, however, they have eluded detection thus far.

Thymic architecture is abnormal in all mice with spontaneous SLE (3,50–52,278,325). Basically, cortical atrophy occurs in all, and medullary hyperplasia may be seen. The function of thymic epithelial cells is abnormal. There must be profound effects on positive and negative selection of T-cell repertoires in these thymuses, but again, a basic functional defect that is common to all lupus mice remains to be identified. Thymectomy prevents development of disease in MRL-Fas(*lpr*) mice, but probably not in NZ strains or BXSB mice.

B cells are abnormal in NZ and BSXB mice. They are easily activated and increase in numbers over time (8,12,31–38, 43–49,145,173,176,270,272,273,275,317). The IgM antibodies they make spontaneously probably are the origin of the pathogenic IgG autoantibodies that mediate tissue damage. All that it takes is the addition of T-cell help, and the disease becomes florid. B cells from MRL mice also may be abnormal, although the evidence for this is weaker than in the other strains. After all, the MRL-Fas(*lpr*) mouse makes far more autoantibodies than any other strain, both in terms of antigens that are recognized and total quantities of each antibody. Does this simply mean that any B cell has the capacity to make all of the autoantibodies that are characteristic of SLE? Or does the MRL B cell have characteristics that allow it to recognize a greater number of self antigens?

Finally, the T cell is required for full-blown SLE to develop in all strains with spontaneous disease. Any genes that allow its activation to be upregulated or prevent its removal predispose to the disease. In all of the strains tested, depletion or inactivation of $CD4^+$ cells is a very effective intervention to prevent the appearance of disease and even to at least partially reverse established lupus (69,70,96,154, 157,158,203,247,257,258,319,322). Recent studies have shown that murine lupus can be prevented by interrupting T- and B-cell activation at the level of second signals. After TCR engagement by MHC/peptide, second signals through CD40-CD40 ligand (gp39), through CD28/CTLA4B7-1/B7-2 ligands, or through BlyS-TACI/BCMA are required for the production of cytokines by T cells and of immunoglobulin by B cells. Interruption of these second signals by the administration of antibodies or soluble receptors that prevent ligand interactions, or by knocking out one of the ligands, prevents development of high-titer IgG anti-dsDNA and of nephritis (157,158,321,381,382).

Role of Monocytes/Macrophages and Neutrophils in Murine Lupus

Monocytosis and increased cytokine production by monocytes/macrophages are features of the full-blown autoimmune syndrome in BXSB and MRL-Fas(*lpr*) mice (265, 285,286,315,328). Monocytes/macrophages probably play important roles in disease. The glomeruli of MRL-Fas(*lpr*) mice are infiltrated with monocytes/macrophages (420). Expression of IL-1 and thromboxane (which is induced by IL-1), and of TNF-α, are greatly increased in the glomeruli of MRL-Fas(*lpr*) mice (167,420,421). Kupffer cells from the livers of MRL-Fas(*lpr*) mice also secrete high levels of TNF-α (422). Monocytes/macrophages from BXSB mice also release increased quantities of procoagulants (315). The combined effects of these cytokines would contribute to glomerular damage and accelerate disease.

Defects in Clearance of Immune Complexes

As in humans with SLE, the clearance of circulating immune complexes, and of cells coated with antibodies, may be abnormal in murine lupus. The Fc-mediated clearance of radiolabeled, Ig-sensitized RBCs is delayed in NZB, BW, MRL-Fas(*lpr*), and BXSB mice by the time they reach 6 months of age. Complement receptor-mediated clearance was delayed in MRL-Fas(*lpr*) mice but not in the other strains (280,423). Clearance of heat-aggregated IgG is reduced in old MRL-Fas(*lpr*) mice, but not old MRL/+/+, BXSB, or BW mice (424).

Abnormalities in Target Organs

It is possible that certain mouse strains are susceptible to SLE in part because the organs that are exposed to immunoglobulin and T cells are predisposed to injury. For example, renal tubular cells in MRL-Fas(*lpr*) mice probably process antigens (likely to be self) and act as APCs that activate T cells to induce injury (255,256). Mesangial cells from these mice also proliferate more vigorously than mesangial cells from nonlupus mice when exposed to growth factors (425).

The Role of Environmental Factors

The microenvironment is important in some strains, especially with relation to sex hormones. In all murine lupus strains except BXSB, disease occurs earlier in females than in males (5). In NZB and MRL-Fas(*lpr*) mice, the difference in disease onset is only 1 to 2 months. In BW and SNF1 mice, the difference is several months, and the female predominance in these two strains is striking. Disease in BW mice can be dramatically altered by sex hormone manipulation, with estrogens accelerating disease and androgens delaying it (133–144).

Regarding exogenous stimuli, there is evidence that infections can accelerate murine lupus (103,155,271). This probably results from the formation of additional immune complexes that can add to the immunoglobulin deposits in glomeruli and blood vessels. Polyclonal activation by *in vivo* administration of LPS (similar to the effects of endotoxin) also can accelerate disease in MRL-Fas(*lpr*) mice (271); however, these effects are probably minor. Lupus in mice is almost entirely a genetic disease.

Abnormalities of Immune Regulation

All of the abnormalities in murine lupus, whether spontaneous or induced, likely depend on abnormal regulation to persist and cause disease. In some induced models, regulation simply is overwhelmed by providing huge quantities of pathogenic autoantibodies or by making most B cells express a pathogenic antibody that is encoded by a transgene. In other induced models, regulation is dysregulated by activating undesirable idiotypic circuits. The *Faslpr* gene is an excellent example of a single gene that alters the normal regulation of apoptosis, with catastrophic results for the MRL mouse destined for mild, late-in-life lupus. Some regulatory mechanisms, including B-cell tolerance, are influenced by sex hormones in some genetic backgrounds; in those mice, disease can be profoundly influenced by the manipulation of hormones. The complex interactions that are required to regulate autoimmune responses will continue to be identified in the future.

Summary

Multiple abnormalities are required for a mouse to develop lupus-like disease. These include disturbances in the function of hematopoietic stem cells, B lymphocytes, T lymphocytes, and phagocytic cells. In spontaneous SLE, the abnormalities are determined primarily by genetic influences; most require multiple genes, which are provided by both parents of a susceptible strain. Three accelerating genes, *lpr*, *gld*, and *Yaa*, are not sufficient to cause disease unless they are engrafted onto a host that is genetically susceptible to autoimmunity. The most important results of the abnormalities are production of pathogenic subsets of autoantibodies and immune complexes, which depend on both abnormal B-cell repertoires and unopposed T-cell help. Environmental factors may accentuate these abnormalities but are of minor importance.

THERAPEUTIC INTERVENTIONS IN MURINE LUPUS

A major advantage of each mouse model of SLE is its availability for studies of therapeutic interventions. These interventions are strategies to (a) provide general immunosuppression, (b) eliminate or inactivate helper T cells, (c) inactivate pathogenic B cells, (d) activate suppressor networks, (e) replace stem cells, (f) alter generation of eicosanoids, (g) alter immunoregulation via sex hormones, and (h) alter tissue damage in target organs. Interventions are summarized in Table 18.8.

All successful interventions are most effective when they are introduced before the development of full-blown clinical lupus. The most interesting ones also are effective in mice with established disease, especially those who have advanced to proteinuria.

Strategies that Are Widely Immunosuppressive

Cytotoxic and immunosuppressive drugs that are standard in the management of SLE in patients have been studied in murine models of lupus. These include glucocorticoids, azathioprine, cyclophosphamide, methotrexate, cyclosporine, and newer cytotoxics such as mycophenolate mofetil, rapamycin, and others not yet available for human therapy (e.g., 15-deoxyspergualin and dimethylthiourea), and total lymphoid irradiation. Glucocorticoids suppress hemolysis and prolong life in NZB mice (426). In BW mice, murine chronic GVHD, and MRL-Fas(*lpr*) mice, immunosuppressive agents suppress IgG anti-dsDNA, proteinuria, glomerular immunoglobulin deposits, and nephritis, with resultant prolonged survival (114,426–455). They are effective even in animals with established nephritis although better when introduced before clinical disease appears. The effects on survival of strategies from comparable studies are shown in Fig. 18.2.

Azathioprine as a single agent does not prolong survival in NZB, BW, or chronic GVHD mice. Added to glucocorticoids and/or cyclophosphamide, however, the combination is more effective than any single drug alone (429,430,432).

As a single drug intervention, cyclophosphamide is superior to glucocorticoids or azathioprine in suppressing nephritis and IgG autoantibodies, and it prolongs life in NZB, BW, and chronic GVHD mice (130,429,433–439). It is equally effective whether given daily or intermittently (Fig. 18.3). In combination with glucocorticoid, it suppresses disease in MRL-Fas(*lpr*) mice (433); combinations

TABLE 18.8. THERAPEUTIC INTERVENTIONS IN MURINE LUPUS

Intervention	Strains Studied	Effects
Immunosuppressive drugs		
1. Glucocorticoids	NZB, BW, MRL/*lpr*, BXSB, chronic GVH	Prolong survival Suppress GN Suppress autoantibodies Suppress T abnormalities
2. Cyclophosphamide	Same as 1	Same as 1
3. Azathioprine	BW, chronic GVHD	Not effective as single drug; effective in combination
4. Combinations 1–3	BW	More effective than one drug alone
5. 15-Deoxyspergualin	MRL/*lpr*, BXSB	Suppresses B activity Suppresses lymphoproliferation Suppresses CIC, anti-DNA Suppresses GN
6. Cyclosporin A	MRL/*lpr*, BXSB, BW	Suppresses lymphoproliferation No suppression of anti-DNA, CIC Suppresses GN, arthritis Prolongs survival
7. FK506	MRL/*lpr*	Prolongs survival Suppresses lymphoproliferation Suppresses anti-DNA Suppresses nephritis
Immunosuppressive antibodies and other strategies		
1. Anti-L3T4	BW, MRL/*lpr*, BXSB	Prolongs survival in pre-dz and post-dz mice Depletes or inactivates L3T4$^+$ T, suppresses accumulation of CD8$^+$ T, B, and monocytes in lymphoid organs and kidneys Suppresses anti-DNA Suppresses GN
2. Antiidiotypes	BW, MRL/*lpr*	Prolong survival Suppress anti-DNA Suppress GN
3. Anti-Ia	BW	Anti-IA^z-prolongs survival Suppresses anti-DNA Suppresses GN Anti-IA^d less effective
5. Anti-Ly-2	BW	No effect on survival, autoantibodies, nephritis Depletes Ly-2+ T cells
6. Total nodal irradiation	BW	Prolongs survival No suppression of anti-DNA Suppresses GN Reduction of T-cell help for months, suppression for weeks
Nutritional interventions		
1. Calorie reduction	NZB, BW, MRL/*lpr*, BXSB	Prolongs survival Suppresses lymphoproliferation Suppresses CIC Suppresses nephritis
2. Fat-restricted diet	BW	Same as 1
3. Omega-3 fatty acid–enriched diets (includes fish oil, eicosopentanoic acid)	BW, MRL/*lpr*	Prolong survival Suppress lymphoproliferation Suppress anti-DNA, CIC Suppress nephritis Suppress vasculitis
4. Omega-9 and -6 fatty acid–enriched diets	BW, MRL/*lpr*	Reduce survival Enhance oncogene expression Enhance lymphoproliferation
5. Casein-free diet	BW	Prolongs survival Suppresses anti-DNA Suppresses nephritis
6. Alfalfa sprouts/L-canavanine-enriched diet	NZB, BW	Decrease survival Increase IgG anti-DNA Increase IgG synthesis

continued

TABLE 18.8. (*continued*)

Intervention	Strains Studied	Effects
Sex hormone therapies		
1. Estrogens, castration	BW, MRL/*lpr,* BXSB	Accelerate male dz Increase IgG anti-DNA Increase nephritis Decrease survival Dramatic in BW, modest effects in MRL/*lpr,* no effect in BXSB males
2. Androgens plus castration or antiestrogens	BW, MRL/*lpr*	Suppress female dz Prolong survival Delay IgG anti-DNA Delay nephritis Dramatic in BW, modest effects in MRL/*lpr* females
Gene therapies		
1. Introduction of *xid* NZB, BW gene	NZB, BW	Deletes Ly-1⁺ B cells Decreases IgM synthesis Suppresses autoantibodies Prolongs survival Suppresses nephritis, hemolysis
2. Introduction of nu/nu genes	BW	Deletes T cells Prolongs survival Decreases IgG anti-DNA Suppresses nephritis Decreases lymphoproliferation
3. Administration of TNF-α	BW	Prolongs survival Inhibits T and NK function No suppression of anti-DNA Delays nephritis
Miscellaneous interventions		
1. Prostaglandin E	BW	Prolongs survival Suppresses nephritis
2. UVA light exposure	BW	Prolongs survival Reduces lymphoproliferation Suppresses anti-DNA

CIC, circulating immune complex; dz, disease.

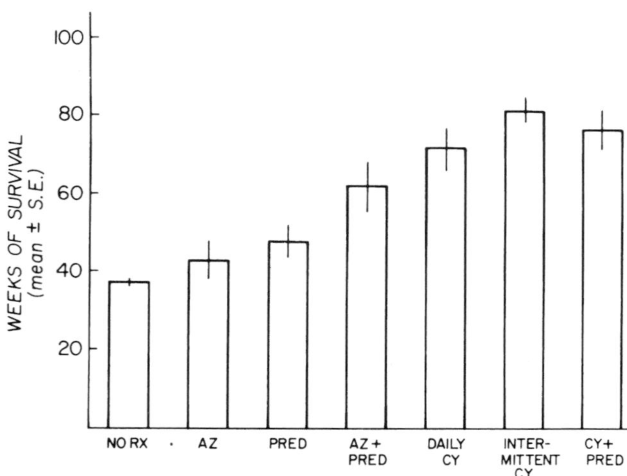

FIGURE 18.2. Survival in (NZBx N2W) F1 female mice treated from 6 weeks of age with daily oral doses of azathioprine (AZ), prednisolone (Pred), cyclophosphamide (Cy), or combination therapies. Bars indicate mean weeks of survival; vertical lines are 1 SEM. Survival was significantly better in Pred vs. No Rx, AZ plus Pred vs. AZ alone, Pred alone, or no RX, and best in all groups receiving Cy, whether daily or intermittent. (See Hahn et al., ref. 130.)

of cyclophosphamide and another immunosuppressive drug such as glucocorticoid or FK506 are more effective than either drug alone (433,441). Administration of cyclophosphamide in any regimen is associated with substantial increases in malignancies, and in some colonies azathioprine also has this effect (130,432,438). Any combination therapy that includes cyclophosphamide suppresses lupus nephritis effectively (433).

Methotrexate delayed the appearance of proteinuria and prolonged survival (without decreasing anti-DNA) in BW and MRL-Fas(*lpr*)mice, but it did not affect disease in NZW × BXSB F1 males (440). A different antifolate, MXX-68, was as effective as methotrexate in delaying nephritis in MRL-Fas(*lpr*) mice (442).

The effects of cyclosporin A (Cy-A) in MRL-Fas(*lpr*), BXSB, and NZB mice also have been studied. Cy-A is highly effective in suppressing lymphoproliferation; the DN T cells that are associated with Fas/*lpr* do not expand (443–446). Cy-A in high doses can suppress the synthesis of anti-DNA *in vitro* (446). However, B-cell hyperactivation with production of high levels of Ig, circulating immune complexes, rheumatoid factors, and anti-DNA was not suppressed when the drug was given *in vivo* (444,445). The effects on nephri-

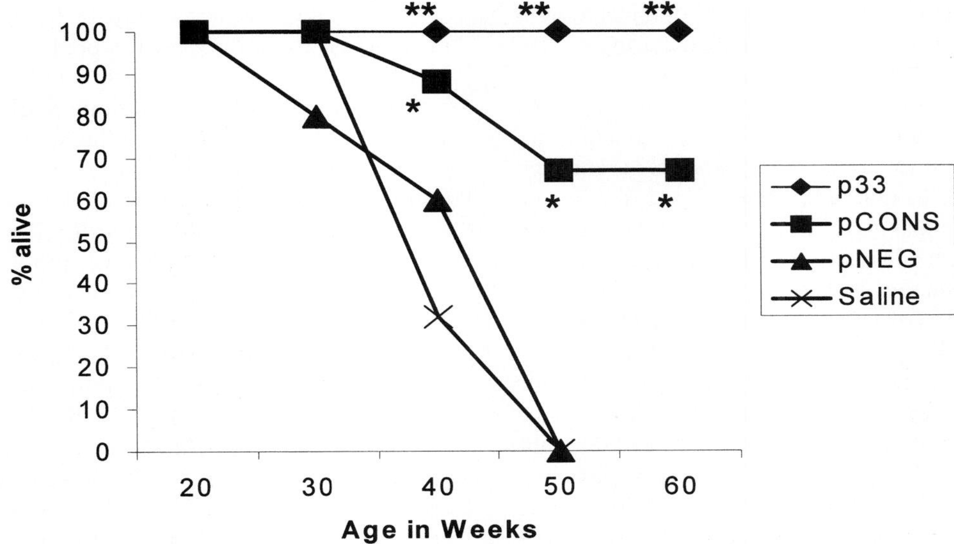

FIGURE 18.3. Effect of immune tolerance to peptides from autoantibody molecules on survival in (NZB/NZW) F1 mice. BW females were treated from the age of 12 weeks with saline (-x-), a negative control peptide that binds major histocompatibility complex (MHC) class II I-Ed but does not cause T-cell activation (pNEG: -Δ-), a wild Ig peptide stimulatory for BW T cells, (p33: -◇-), or a synthetic peptide based on T-cell stimulatory Ig sequences (pCONSENSUS or pCONS: -□-) until 60 weeks of age. Peptides were administered as tolerogens, high doses intravenously once a month. Each group contains 5 to 15 mice. Note that all mice in the saline and pNEG groups were dead by 50 weeks of age, whereas 70% to 100% of mice tolerized with peptides that are stimulatory for T cells were still alive. Survival was significantly longer in the effectively treated groups, $p < .01$ to .05 in the p33 group compared to saline and pNEG by chi square test, $p < .05$ comparing pCONS to saline. Autoantibodies and cytokine increases in interferon-γ (IFN-γ) and interleukin-4 (IL-4) were all significantly delayed in the tolerized groups. These mice mounted normal T- and B-cell responses to immunization with HEL, an external foreign antigen. This illustrates a new approach to achieving specific immune suppression of undesirable autoantibodies.

tis were variable. One group reported no suppression of nephritis and no improvement in survival for either MRL-Fas(*lpr*) or BXSB mice (444), whereas others reported reduction of nephritis and prolonged survival (445). Apparently, renal damage can be suppressed without diminishing B-cell activation and autoantibody synthesis, suggesting that autoantibodies alone may be necessary, but not sufficient, for the development of lethal lupus nephritis. FK506 was given to young MRL-Fas(*lpr*) mice; it prevented lymphoproliferation and nephritis and also reduced titers of anti-dsDNA (447); in another study FK506 was more effective in combination with cyclophosphamide (441).

A recently developed cytotoxic drug, 15-deoxyspergualin, suppresses immune complex formation, anti-DNA, nephritis, and lymphoproliferation in MRL-Fas(*lpr*) and male BXSB mice (448,449). It has been administered primarily to mice before onset of florid disease. It was also effective in treating the immune thrombocytopenia characteristic of (NZW × BXSB)F_1 mice (450). Another newer cytotoxic drug, dimethylthiourea, has been used to treat BW mice (451). When given before disease onset, it is effective at preventing nephritis.

Mycophenolate mofetil has been studied in BW and MRL-Fas(*lpr*) mice. In both strains development of nephritis was suppressed (and in most levels of autoantibodies and total numbers of lymphocytes were also suppressed). In comparison to cyclophosphamide, the numbers of cells infiltrating renal tissue was less with cyclophosphamide (452–455).

Administration of paclitaxel to BW females resulted in significantly prolonged survival, reduced levels of anti-DNA, and delayed onset of nephritis (456).

Several Asian herbal preparations act as general immunosuppressants. Some of these have been effective in suppressing various manifestations of lupus in MRL-Fas(*lpr*) mice (457,458).

Total nodal irradiation has been studied in murine as well as human SLE (439,459–463). Irradiation of BW or MRL-Fas(*lpr*) mice, even after clinical disease is established, results in prolonged survival and markedly diminished nephritis, which is associated with decreased serum levels of anti-DNA. In MRL-Fas(*lpr*) mice, lymphoproliferation is reduced (461,463). Both suppressing and enhancing cell circuits are suppressed for a few weeks after therapy is stopped, but helper circuits return to supernormal, with increased antibody production and proliferation to antigens and mitogens. However, the mice are protected from recurrent high levels of ANA production and from disease for several months after this help appears, despite the fact that suppressive circuits cannot be demonstrated. In one study comparing total node irradiation to cyclophosphamide therapy in BW mice, irradiation was superior in prolonging life, because the incidence of malignant tumors was lower (462).

In summary, immunosuppressive regimens that include glucocorticoids and/or cyclophosphamide, or total nodal irradiation, are impressive in their ability to reverse established nephritis at least partially. The other approaches, such as interfering with synthesis of IL-2, are either more effective when done before clinical organ damage appears or have not been adequately studied in established disease.

Strategies that Deplete or Inactivate T Cells

Because CD4$^+$ helper T cells amplify autoantibody production and are required for the development of full-blown SLE in all SLE mouse models that have been studied to date, elimination or inactivation of those cells is highly effective in preventing disease, and even in partially reversing it once clinical nephritis is manifest. Administration of antibodies to CD4 prolongs survival, suppresses IgG anti-dsDNA and other autoantibodies, and suppresses nephritis and lymphoproliferation in NZ-derived, MRL-Fas(*lpr*), and BXSB mice, and even in normal mice that have been induced to express antiphospholipid antibodies (69,70,96, 154,203,247,258,319,408). Anti-CD4 prolongs survival in BW mice with established nephritis (154). Long-term benefits require continual, repeated treatments throughout the lifetime of the mouse. Apparently, CD4$^+$ cells are not entirely eliminated, or their numbers are repopulated (even in the absence of a thymus), so that autoantibodies and disease eventually appear if the treatment is stopped (464).

The monoclonal antibody used in all of these studies is a rat antimouse L3T4 (CD4); it has the advantage of inducing tolerance to itself in the recipient by preventing antibody responses that require T-cell help (96,465,466). In earlier studies using antibodies against lymphocytes or thymocytes or Thy-1$^+$ cells (CD2$^+$ in humans), results were often obscured by the development of inactivating antibodies and of serum sickness nephritis caused by the immune response to the antilymphocyte globulin (467–470). The rat anti-L3T4 monoclonal antibody is cytotoxic to helper T cells and deletes them from the repertoire. The F(ab)2 fragment of the monoclonal antibody is not cytotoxic, because it cannot fix complement, but it inactivates L3T4$^+$ T cells and is as effective as the whole antibody molecule in preventing the development of anti-DNA and nephritis in BW mice (465). In addition to the predictable effects of anti-L3T4 on diminishing T-cell help and autoantibody formation, non-L3T4$^+$ cells that infiltrate renal and lymphoid tissue as lupus evolves also are influenced. CD8$^+$ T cells and B220$^+$ B cells, as well as CD4$^+$ T cells, are all diminished (466). This suggests a central role for CD4$^+$ T cells in the evolution of activated CD8$^+$ and B cells.

In contrast to the benefit of anti-CD4 in (NZW × BXSB)F1 mice, administration of anti-CD8 worsened disease (345).

Anti-CD4 therapy of MRL-Fas(*lpr*) mice is particularly interesting, because the lymphoproliferative component of their disease is dominated by B220$^+$ CD4CD8$^-$ TCR α/β cells. However, the autoantibodies, arthritis, nephritis, and central nervous system (CNS) disease depend on CD4$^+$ cells (247). Treatment of MRL-Fas(*lpr*) with a combination of anti-CD4 and anti-CD8 abrogates most disease manifestations. However, treatment with anti-CD4 alone suppresses autoantibodies, proteinuria, histologic nephritis, arthritis, and CNS disease, but does not affect lymphocytic proliferation and actually worsens lacrimal gland destruction (247,258,471). Nonmitogenic anti-CD3 also reduces mortality and adenopathy in MRL-Fas(*lpr*) mice (606). The BW mouse has a predictable response, because its disease depends primarily on CD4$^+$ cells: administration of anti-CD8 to tolerized BW mice depleted CD8$^+$ cells but did not influence autoantibody titers, nephritis, or survival (472). Although anti-CD4 therapy is remarkably effective in murine lupus, its use in the human disease has produced disappointing results. Perhaps by the time a patient is diagnosed, desirable immune regulation has developed and is dependent in part on CD4$^+$ cells, so eliminating T-cell help also eliminates T-cell regulation.

BW mice also have been bred with nude mice to produce BW.nu/nu offspring. Nu/nu homozygotes are athymic and develop T-cell repertoires that are small in number and uneducated in the thymus. Without T-cell help, BW-nu/nu mice have prolonged survival that is associated with decreased levels of IgG anti-DNA and little development of nephritis or lymphoproliferation (473,474). However, the animals are not completely disease-free and develop some autoantibodies.

To disable activated CD4$^+$ T cells rather than all CD4$^+$ cells, there has been recent interest in interfering with second signals. T cells receiving only one signal (binding of their TCR) usually undergo activation only if they receive second signals via CD28/CTLA-4 interacting with B7-1 and B7-2 (CD80 and CD86), or CD40 interacting with gp39 (CD40L). Several groups have investigated the effect of disabling B7-1 and/or B7-2. Antibodies to B7-1 plus B7-2 (or to gp39) interrupt signaling, as does soluble CTLA-4–Ig, which binds B7-1 and B7-2 so they cannot interact with CD28 and deliver a second signal. Such treatments are effective in delaying disease in BW and BXSB mice (157,

158,475). Gene deletion of B7.1 worsened nephritis in MRL-Fas(*lpr*) mice, whereas deletion of B7.2 reduced kidney pathology: disabling both molecules by treatment with antibodies to both B7.1 and B7.2 suppressed disease (476). In BW mice, one dose of adenovirus containing CTLA-4–Ig reduced numbers of activated T cells and affected disease as long as the protein was present. B cells requiring T-cell help were impaired, although there was no effect on intrinsic B-cell abnormalities (477). Blockade of CD28-B7 interactions with soluble CTLA-4–Ig fusion protein has been beneficial in other, nonlupus animal models of autoimmunity. For example, gene therapy with adenovirus containing CTLA-4–Ig prevented induction of collagen-induced arthritis (478).

Impairment of CD40/gp39(CD40L) interactions has also been studied in murine lupus. BW mice treated with anti-CD40L had reduced anti-DNA levels, reduced proteinuria, and prolonged survival (159). Treatment with anti-CD40L also prolonged survival in SNF1 mice even if started after nephritis was clinically evident (160). One group reported that better clinical results are obtained in BW mice by blocking both CD28/B7 interactions using CTLA-4–Ig, and CD40/gp39 interactions using anti-gp39. In fact 10 months after a 2-week course of both therapies, 70% of mice were alive compared to 0% to 18% of mice treated with only one of the agents (161). It is likely that combination therapy will be more useful in human disease as well, since there are several routes to B-cell production of autoantibodies.

Finally, inhibition of MHC class II (thus blocking the first signal to $CD4^+$ T cells) has been effective in treating murine lupus. One group studied the efficacy of antibodies to I-A in murine lupus (479). NZB/NZW F1 mice express I-A and I-E MHC class II molecules with two alleles, d and z. Administration of antibodies directed against Az suppressed production of anti-DNA and development of nephritis in BW mice. Anti-I-Ad was somewhat immunosuppressive, but less effective than anti-I-Az. Knockout of MHC class II in MRL-Fas(*lpr*) mice prevented the development of autoantibodies and nephritis, but not of lymphoproliferation (257). A safer strategy to block MHC-peptide activation of TCR is to provide tolerizing peptides in MHC class II molecules, which is discussed below. A report of methimazole treatment benefiting BW mice speculated that the effectiveness depended on downregulation of MHC class I molecules by the drug (480), suggesting that class I activation of $CD8^+$ cells is also important in development of full-blown murine lupus.

Strategies that Prevent B-Cell Activation

Many interventions that interrupt B-cell development or activation also prevent murine SLE. Introduction of the *Xid* gene into NZB or BW backgrounds results in the inability to synthesize normal levels of IgM and near-deletion of B-1 B cells. In that setting, NZB.*xid* and BW.*xid* mice do not develop their characteristic early life, severe lupus (32,481, 482). They are not disease free, however; a few animals develop autoantibodies and nephritis late in life (481). *Xid* is a mutated nonreceptor tyrosine kinase (BTK); the kinase promotes activation of NF-κB via activation of the B-cell receptor, resulting in IgM production (483,484). The hyperactivity of SLE B cells is prevented by *Xid*. In addition, normal B cells may serve a regulatory function that is defective in lupus B cells. Transfer of MHC-matched normal B cells (but not *Xid* B cells) into nonirradiated BW mice decreases serum IgG autoantibody levels, delays proteinuria, and prolongs life (485). Direct inhibition of NF-κB by administration of a p50 antisense nucleotide inhibited NF-κB expression, reduced total IgM and IgG synthesis, and reduced antibodies to dsDNA by 90% (486).

If the IgD or IgM molecules on a B-cell surface are ligated, that cell cannot undergo class switch to produce IgG. When MRL-Fas(*lpr*) mice were treated with multivalent anti-IgD that was conjugated to dextran, development of glomerulonephritis was delayed and survival prolonged (487). Interestingly, removing a major antigen, DNA, that delivers first signals to B-cell receptors in mice with lupus was not effective. DNAse treatment of BW mice reduced numbers of anti-DNA–secreting B cells for one month but did not alter cytokine production, glomerulonephritis, or survival (488).

Manipulation of the idiotypic network by administration of Id or anti-Id can have profound effects on the immune system, and those effects can result in either upregulation or downregulation of autoantibodies. Administration of carefully chosen Ids or anti-Ids in proper doses at the correct time can suppress Id^+ anti-dsDNA and delay the onset of nephritis in BW mice (489–493), MRL-Fas(*lpr*), and SNF1 mice (494,495). Treatment with anti-Ids conjugated to cytotoxic compounds such as neocarzinostatin also is effective in suppressing autoantibodies and nephritis in BW mice, particularly if multiple anti-Ids are included in the regimen (492,493). Anti-Ids also can suppress *in vitro* synthesis of autoantibodies by human B cells (496). There are limitations to Id/anti-Id therapies, however. Some anti-Ids upregulate autoantibodies (497), and variations in dose and time of administration to lupus mice can profoundly influence whether immune responses are enhanced or suppressed. Some anti-Ids do not affect antibody synthesis (498). Beneficial responses can be short-lived, abrogated either by the escape of pathogen-enriched Ids from suppression or by the emergence of pathogenic autoantibodies bearing different Ids (489,491). Finally, pathogenic autoantibodies can express different Ids, so that suppression of multiple public (and possibly some private) Ids may be required for prolonged efficacy. The efficacy of anti-Id therapy in mouse SLE is established. A recent safety study in nine patients with SLE suggested that anti-Id can be induced by immunizations with a selected idiotype (3E10) without adverse effects (499). Treatment of SLE with intravenous gamma globulin may benefit individuals with SLE by suppressing certain Ids, depending on the anti-Ids in each preparation (500). Mice with induced antiphospholipid syndromes have benefited from the administration of intravenous gamma globulin (404).

Interruption of the B-cell growth cytokine IL-4 by administration of soluble IL-4 receptor suppresses autoantibody production in murine lupus (377).

MRL-Fas(*lpr*) B cells respond to IL-1 by secreting Ig, and the level of IL-1 mRNA is elevated in the kidneys of MRL mice with nephritis. Infusion of human recombinant IL-1 receptor antagonist into mice with nephritis suppressed circulating IL-1 but did not change the disease (501). Perhaps earlier treatment would be more effective.

Recently, a new member of the TNF-α family has been described that is a co-receptor for second-signal B-cell activation following BCR ligation. That molecule, BlyS (also called BAFF, TALL-1, and zTNF4) is secreted by monocytes and binds its receptors TACI and BCMA on B cells (383,502–504).

Induction of Tolerance in T and B Cells

There are several mechanisms of immune tolerance: ignorance, anergy, deletion, and receptor editing. One can induce tolerance in T or B lymphocytes in lupus mice by inhibiting the first activating signal (i.e., binding the TCR or BCR with the peptide or antigen it recognizes), by inducing apoptosis in autoreactive cells by anergizing cells via prevention of second signal activations through CD28, CD40 or TACI/BCMA, or by inducing regulatory cells. Induction of tolerance to autoantigens in either helper T or B cells in individuals with SLE would abrogate production of pathogenic antibodies. Several laboratories have developed strategies to tolerize mice with lupus to DNA and related antigens (505–510). Mice so treated have significant delays in the appearance of autoantibodies and nephritis. For example, intrathymic inoculation of Hl-stripped chromatin into BXSB males significantly reduced T-cell proliferation to nucleosomal antigens, and production of IgG antichromatin, anti-dsDNA, and anti-ssDNA, for 8 to 10 weeks (509).

Recently there has been success in both human and murine SLE in tolerizing B cells to a molecule containing short nucleotides displayed on a tetrameric scaffold—a compound called LJP 394 (510,511). BXSB mice treated with this tolerogen have delayed appearance of IgG anti-dsDNA and nephritis, as well as significantly prolonged survival. In patients with SLE who have antibodies to DNA that bind LJP394 with high avidity, there is good clinical response to repeated intravenous injections of LJP394. Quantities of anti-DNA drop significantly, and there are fewer flares of renal disease compared to a placebo-treated control group (608). Another strategy for cross-linking B cells to inactivate them is to administer DNA/anti-DNA soluble immune complexes. That has been effective in improving survival of MRL-Fas(*lpr*) mice (513).

In BW mice, repeated tolerization with monthly intravenous doses of a synthetic peptide based on T helper determinants in the VH region of murine antibodies to DNA, or of combined wild immunoglobulin-derived peptides, produced dramatic delays in nephritis and prolonged survival (512,514,515). Results of one series of experiments are shown in Fig. 18.3. Similarly, tolerization to helper-T-cell–activating peptides from the histone moieties of nucleosomes reduces autoantibody formation and delays Ig deposition in glomeruli in (SWR × NZB)F1 mice (516). In all these studies, peptides that are both T-cell and B-cell epitopes, and induce tolerance to first signals in both T and B cells, were the most effective in delaying clinical disease. One group has reported that repeated oral administration of low doses of whole kidney extract reduced IgG1 and IgG3 anti-dsDNA antibody levels, reduced numbers of inflammatory cells and expression of IL-4 and Il-10 in kidney tissue (while increasing expression of IL-1, IFN-γ, and TNF-α), and prolonged survival (517).

Strategies that Activate Suppressor Networks

Most experts suspect that one of the defects in murine and human SLE is an absence of normal suppressive immunoregulatory networks. Regulatory T cells develop in both thymus and periphery in normal mice; they can be $CD4^+$, $CD8^+$, or double negative; some secrete TGF-β, others IL-10, and still others apparently suppress effector cells without secreting those inhibitory cytokines (518). Vaccination of mice with disease-inducing T cells, or with certain peptides, can activate suppressive networks, with at least some of the regulatory cells ($CD4^+$) recognizing the TCR of the disease-upregulating T cells. De Alboran et al. (519) inoculated young MRL-Fas(*lpr*) mice with irradiated cells from the diseased lymph nodes of older MRL-Fas(*lpr*) mice; peripheral T cells were obtained that protected against disease in adoptive transfer experiments. Normal B cells may also serve a regulatory function; transfer of MHC-matched normal B cells into nonirradiated BW mice decreased serum IgG autoantibody levels, delayed proteinuria, and prolonged life (485). It is likely that attempts to induce regulatory networks in SLE will be successful in the near future.

Therapeutic Strategies Employing Cytokines

Manipulation of cytokines that affect T cells, B cells, or target tissue alters murine lupus. The role of IL-2 in murine lupus is unclear. T cells from virtually all SLE mice develop defects in the production of IL-2 and the presentation of IL-2 receptors on their surfaces. Some experts think that deviation from Th1 (i.e., IL-2–producing) to Th2 (i.e., IL-4–, -5–, and -6–producing) phenotypes promotes autoantibody production. Therefore, one might think that providing IL-2 to increase Th1 cell function would be beneficial; however, there is substantial evidence to the contrary. Gene therapy that provides IL-2 monthly, so that serum levels are elevated, worsens SLE in MRL-Fas(*lpr*) mice (266), and treatment with drugs that inhibit IL-2, such as cyclosporine and FK506, are beneficial (discussed earlier). Rapamycin has some effects that are similar to those of Cy-A and FK506—it prolongs life and reduces lymphoproliferation and nephritis in MRL-Fas(*lpr*) mice (520).

Studies of cytokine mRNA in BW and MRL-Fas(*lpr*) mice with established clinical lupus suggest that both Th1 and Th2 subsets are activated. In BW mice, the largest population of pathogenic anti-DNA are IgG2a, an isotype that depends on IFN-γ (from Th1 cells) for its synthesis. There are high levels of mRNA for both IFN-γ (i.e., a Thl cytokine) and IL-10 (i.e., a promoter of Th2-cell development) in lymphoid tissues. Inhibition of IL-10 by continuous administration of anti–IL-10 significantly delays the onset of lupus in BW mice (165), probably by interfering with the generation of IL-6 (i.e., a B-cell growth factor), because simultaneous administration of anti–IL-6 abrogates the benefit of anti–IL-10 and administration of IL-6 worsens disease (164). In addition to increases in Th1 and Th2 cytokines in lupus mice, proinflammatory cytokines, including IL-1 and TNF-α, that are derived primarily from monocyte/macrophages are increased (265). IFN-γ is a cytokine of central importance in several strains of murine lupus. Administration of this cytokine worsens murine SLE in BW mice; administration of antibodies to IFN-γ or of soluble IFN-γ receptors to BW mice before disease begins significantly prolongs survival and diminishes immunoglobulin deposition and lymphocytic infiltration of kidneys (521). In MRL-Fas(*lpr*) mice, antibodies to IFN-γ do not alter disease (522), but lowering serum levels of IFN-γ with IFN-γR/Fc molecules was effective (523). Gene therapy of MRL-Fas(*lpr*) mice with intramuscular injections of plasmids containing complementary DNA (cDNA) encoding IFN-γR/Fc molecules resulted in reduced serum levels of IFN-γ, and reduced levels of autoantibodies, lymphoid hyperplasia, and glomerulonephritis, with prolonged survival. Treatment after mice had established nephritis was also effective (523). Genetic deletion of IFN-γ receptor significantly delays nephritis in BW mice, although the mice developed lethal lymphomas at 1 year of age (524).

Other cytokines have been studied as therapeutic agents in murine lupus. The response of MRL-Fas(*lpr*) mice to granulocyte colony-stimulating factor (G-CSF) was complex: chronic administration of low doses accelerated nephritis, whereas high doses prolonged survival and prevented inflammation in glomeruli even in the presence of Ig deposits (525). Inhibition of IL-4 in mice transgenic for IL-4 prevented the glomerulosclerosis that occurs in those transgenics (526). Another strategy for changing regulation is to provide large quantities of cytokines. Gene therapy in which cytokines in vectors were injected intramuscularly into MRL-Fas(*lpr*) mice once a month showed that IL-2 accelerated disease, whereas TGF-β suppressed it (266). The effects of TGF-β are complex and vary between suppressing and enhancing inflammatory responses; it generally is suppressive. TNF-α plays a major role in inflammation and immune responses (171). BW mice produce abnormally low quantities of TNF-α, which is a defect that correlates with an unusual restriction fragment length polymorphism in the TNF-α gene (169,527). Initial studies reported that administration of normal recombinant TNF-α delayed the development of nephritis (169). The ability of the recombinant molecule to suppress established nephritis and prolong survival in BW mice was shown, but the benefit was lost after a few months. Another study reported that low doses of TNF-α accelerated nephritis (170). Treatment of normal mice with TNF-α reduced the ability of monocytes to support lymphocyte proliferative responses to mitogens, and it inhibited both T-cell cytotoxicity and NK cell activity (171). Such effects, if they occur in autoimmune mice, should confer substantial benefit, but the therapeutic efficacy of TNF-α administration has been disappointing.

In summary, inhibition of IFN-γ, IL-4, IL-6, and IL-10 has been reported to delay or suppress disease in various models of murine lupus, as discussed earlier (164,165, 377,521).

Bindarit is a propanoic acid derivative that inhibits the chemokine monocyte chemotactic protein-1 (MCP-1) as well as TNF-α production by activated monocytes and macrophages. Treatment of BW mice with bindarit did not reduce autoantibody titers but delayed proteinuria and prolonged survival, even better than did treatment with cyclophosphamide (528,529).

Strategies to Replace Stem Cells

An important question in SLE is whether replacement of bone marrow stem cells with allogeneic cells from MHC-compatible normal mice (331), or with syngeneic cells that have been depleted of T cells (277), will prevent (or at least delay) disease. Immunoablated MRL-Fas(*lpr*) mice receiving bone marrow from MRL+/+ or other H-2–matched strains developed mild rather than the usual marked lymphoproliferation; survival was prolonged (530). Interestingly, immunoablation with radiation or high-dose cyclophosphamide followed by transfer of T-cell–depleted syngeneic MRL-Fas(*lpr*) marrow also prolonged survival (277). In BW mice, transfer of bone marrow–derived pre–B cells from normal donors also suppressed autoantibody production (173). Such stem cells can even be provided from human cord blood (531). Bone marrow stem cell transfer also has benefited BXSB mice (532). These data provided background for the recent studies of immunoablation followed by autologous stem cell transplantation in patients with SLE, several of whom had impressive improvement (533).

Strategies to Alter Generation of Eiconasoids: The Role of Diet

Because inflammation in murine SLE is mediated by multiple molecules, including products of arachadonic acid (AA) metabolism, there has been interest in deviating the products of AA toward less proinflammatory metabolites than the leukotrienes and thromboxanes. This can be done by giving PGE or analogues, or by altering diets. The administration of PGs to BW mice influences their SLE. Repeated injections of PGE_1 suppress nephritis and prolong survival (534–536). Two days of treating MRL-Fas(*lpr*) mice with a PGE analogue, misoprostol, reduced renal cortical IL-1 mRNA levels but not leukotrienes (537).

Dietary factors have a major influence on murine lupus. Calorie reduction alone, to approximately 40% of the usual laboratory mouse dietary intake, significantly prolongs survival and suppresses lymphoproliferation, autoantibody production, increases in Thl and Th2 cytokine production, and nephritis in NZB, BW, MRL-Fas(*lpr*), and BXSB mice (538–543). Restriction of dietary fat seems to be more important than restriction of protein. Diets that are rich in unsaturated fats and in omega-3 fatty acids, such as fish oil, flaxseed, menhaden oil, and eicosapentanoic acid, are associated with improved survival and markedly less lymphoproliferation, autoantibody production, nephritis, and vasculitis in NZB, BW, and MRL-Fas(*lpr*) mice (538,540,544–554). In contrast, diets that are enriched in saturated fats and in omega-9 and omega-6 fatty acids are associated with reduced survival, enhanced oncogene expression, and severe lymphoproliferation (538,540,544, 551,555).

The most likely explanation for the profound effects of diet in murine lupus relate to the conversion of dietary fats to various AA metabolites (i.e., PGs and leukotrienes). Presumably, the omega-3 fatty acids are precursors of molecules that are less inflammatory and/or immunostimulatory than the products of omega-9 and omega-6 fatty acids. Omega-3–rich diets lower the production of leukotriene B_4 and tetraene peptidoleukotrienes by peritoneal macrophages, presumably reducing inflammation (554). In addition, they increase antioxidant enzyme gene expression and decrease tissue levels of proinflammatory cytokines such as IL-6 and TNF-α (541,555).

Dietary factors that are unrelated to lipids also influence murine lupus. BW mice that are raised on a casein-free diet have diminished anti-DNA and nephritis and improved survival (607). The mechanism of this effect is not known. Alfalfa seeds fed to cynomolgus macaque monkeys were associated with the development of autoimmune hemolytic anemia and ANA (556). When the seeds were autoclaved before administration, however, the disease did not occur (557). Several investigators have attributed this phenomenon to the presence of L-canavanine, which is a nonprotein amino acid, in alfalfa. L-Canavanine is immunostimulatory and increases the proliferation of lymphocytes to mitogens and antigens (558,559). The importance of this finding in human SLE, however, is unknown.

Strategies that Manipulate Sex Hormones

The influence of sex hormones on murine lupus is highly variable, depending on the strain. Hybrid mice that are derived from NZ backgrounds, especially BW mice, are exquisitely sensitive to the effects of sex hormones. Females are protected from severe early life lupus by castration plus androgenic hormone, or by antiestrogens (133,136–139, 560). Estrogens worsen their disease, probably through toxic effects as well as immunostimulation (135). Males develop early-onset severe SLE rather than their usual late-onset disease if they are castrated and treated with estrogenic hormones or antiandrogens (133,138,139). Whether this relates to the modification of immune responses by sex hormone receptors in immune cells or to modification of gene expression is unclear. In contrast, male BXSB mice develop rapid-onset, early-life lupus whether or not they are castrated or receive sex hormones (139). MRL-Fas(*lpr*) mice are intermediate between BW and BXSB; that is, estrogenic hormones tend to worsen and androgenic hormones to suppress disease manifestations, but the effects are less dramatic than in BW mice (139). In fact, the effects of estrogen in MRL-Fas(*lpr*) mice are to worsen renal disease but to lessen vasculitis and sialadenitis (561). This could result from the simultaneous stimulation of antibody responses and suppression of T-cell– and NK-cell–mediated immunity (143), but the effects of sex hormones are doubtless more complicated than that. Studies in normal mice transgenic for Ig genes that encode anti-DNA show that estrogen affects B-cell tolerance and permits survival of autoreactive B cells (144). Administration of tamoxifen to MRL-Fas(*lpr*) mice and to BW mice reduces renal damage and prolongs survival (562). Prolactin administration worsens lupus in BW mice, whereas bromocriptine suppresses it (140–142,563). Studies in this interesting area are likely to expand in the next few years.

Strategies that Protect Target Organs from Damage After Immunoglobulin Deposition

Protecting tissue from damage induced by deposition of immunoglobulins, rather than altering immunoglobulin production, is another strategy for treating lupus. For example, administration of NG-monomethyl-l-arginine, which suppresses nitric oxide production, reduces the severity of arthritis and nephritis in MRL-Fas(*lpr*) mice (564). High quantities of inducible nitrous oxide synthetase (iNOS) are expressed in kidneys of MRL-Fas(*lpr*) mice after nephritis begins; administration of linomide significantly decreases iNOS mRNA levels and prevents development of nephritis (565). Similarly, administration of aminoguanidine reduced glomerular expression of both iNOS and TGF-β mRNA in BW mice: this effect was associated with less glomerulosclerosis (566). Antibody MEL-14, which blocks the homing of lymphocytes to lymph nodes, suppressed adenopathy in MRL-Fas(*lpr*) mice; it did not alter autoantibody production (567). Combined treatment with antibodies to LFA-1α and ICAM-1 reduced Ig and C3 deposition in glomeruli and prolonged survival in mice treated after induction of chronic GVHD (568). Inhibition of thromboxane A and endothelin receptors reduces histologic renal damage, hypertension, and proteinuria in BW mice (569,570). Administration of antibodies to ICAM-1 protected MRL-Fas(*lpr*) mice from skin vasculitis and behavioral abnormalities that occurred in the controls (571). Administration of heparin or a heparinoid prevented binding of nucleosome/antinucleosome immune complexes to glomerular basement membrane of BALB/c mice and delayed proteinuria and histologic glomerular damage in MRL-Fas(*lpr*) mice for several weeks (572). Another method to prevent damage is to inhibit development of activated terminal components of complement proteins. Administration of a monoclonal antibody specific for the C5 component of complement blocks cleavage of C5 and generation of C5a and C5b-9. Continuous therapy with anti-C5 for 6 months reduced nephritis and increased survival in BW mice (573). Finally, deposition of immune complexes in glomeruli can be prevented by administration of a soluble peptide selected from a peptide display library for reaction with a mouse monoclonal pathogenic anti-DNA (but not with nonpathogenic monoclonals) (574).

Miscellaneous Interventions

Several additional strategies that affect murine lupus should be noted. Exposure of BW mice to ultraviolet (UV)A light, especially if the mice are shaved to maximize the exposure, was associated with prolonged survival, reduced lymphoproliferation, and suppression of anti-DNA antibodies (575). In contrast, exposure of BXSB mice to UV light that included UVA and UVB, and was reproduced with UVB alone, exacerbated disease (576).

Disease in MRL-Fas(*lpr*) mice has been successfully suppressed by the administration of cholera toxin (577) and of a platelet activating-receptor antagonist (578). Administration of a single dose of thalidomide to NZB, MRL/n, and MRL-Fas(*lpr*) mice reduced the production of IgM and/or IgG, probably by reducing the numbers of $CD5^+$ B cells (579). Treatment of BW mice with lithium chloride prolonged survival through unknown mechanisms (580). The value of these strategies (and of others not mentioned here) will depend on whether these findings can be confirmed and the role of these compounds in altering disease elucidated.

Lupus in Animals Other than Mice

Spontaneous lupus-like disease has been reported in dogs, cats, rats, rabbits, guinea pigs, pigs, monkeys, hamsters, and Aleutian minks (581–588,590,591,593,594). The largest body of literature addresses SLE in dogs. In that animal, the disease can be sporadic or familial.

A colony of dogs particularly susceptible to SLE was created by breeding a male and female German shepherd, each of which had SLE. As healthy sires were introduced to mate with F1 and F2 generations, the disease prevalence declined (586,587). There is a genetic association with MHC, as in mice and in humans (reviewed in ref. 589). The DLA-A7 MHC class I gene confers a relative risk of approximately 12 for SLE whether it is found in sporadic or familial disease; DLA-Al and B5 are negatively correlated with disease (588). Dogs can develop clinical manifestations similar to those in humans, as follows: polyarthritis in 91%, membranous and proliferative forms of glomerulonephritis in 65%, and mucocutaneous lesions in 60%. Other infrequent manifestations include hemolytic anemia, thrombocytopenia, and clotting (587,590–596). Bullous, discoid, and systemic type skin lesions can occur. The predominant autoantibodies, occurring in more than 90% of dogs with SLE, are ANAs and antibodies directed against individual histones. Antibodies against ssDNA, dsDNA, Ro/SSA, Sm, RNP, lymphocytes, and platelets are found, but in less than 30% (584,591,595–599). The H130 Id that is characteristic of anti-DNA from MRL-Fas(*lpr*) mice has been found on anti-DNA in dogs (600). Effective interventions include glucocorticoids, levamisole, apheresis, and tetracyclines. Most dogs respond.

Because of concern that SLE may be transmitted by viruses, studies have been done to determine whether SLE in humans is more common among owners of dogs with SLE. A study of 83 members of 23 households with 19 dogs that had high-titer ANAs showed no excess in the number of cases of human SLE (601).

SLE in cats usually is a spontaneous disease. However, there has been interest in a series of experiments in which the administration of propylthiouracil to cats induces autoantibodies and autoimmune hemolytic anemia (602).

SLE in monkeys can be induced by feeding macaques alfalfa seeds, probably because of the immunostimulatory properties of the L-canavanine nonprotein amino acid that the seeds contain (556–559).

Attempts have been made to induce SLE in animals by transferring plasma from patients with SLE. Histologic evidence of glomerulonephritis was produced by repeated infusions of human plasma containing LE factors into healthy dogs in one set of experiments (603) but not in another (604). Similar experiments were unsuccessful in guinea pigs.

Efforts to induce lupus-like disease in various animals by administering lupus-inducing drugs have been largely unsuccessful. Hydralazine and procainamide have been given to dogs, guinea pigs, swine, and rats, but with little evidence of autoimmune responses (605). On the other hand, immunization of rabbits, mice, and baboons with protein or oligopeptide autoantigens (from Sm B/B′, Ro 60-kd peptides, and La/SS-B) have induced epitope spreading, antinuclear antibodies and proteinuria in a proportion of animals (414–418). This may reflect differences in environmental stimuli to which animals are exposed in different laboratories.

Finally, dogs have been studied for evidence of vertical transmission of infectious agents that cause SLE. In breeding studies performed by Lewis and Schwartz (585), the incidence of positive LE-cell tests in inbred backcrosses and outcross matings was not consistent with any conventional mechanisms of inheritance. The investigators concluded that the results could be explained by vertical transmission of an infectious agent in a genetically susceptible individual. Cell-free filtrates of tissues from seropositive dogs also have been injected into newborn mice (585), and these mice developed ANAs and, in some cases, lymphomas. Passage of cells or filtrates from the tumors to normal newborn puppies resulted in ANA production or positive LE-cell tests. C-type RNA viruses were identified in the tumors. In cats, autoimmunity is highly associated with the feline leukemia virus (582). It may be that autoimmune disease similar to human SLE is more closely linked to viral infections in dogs and cats than in humans.

REFERENCES

1. Bielschowsky M, Helyer BJ, Howie JB. Spontaneous haemolytic anaemia in mice of the NZB/B1 strain. *Proc Univ Otago Med Sch (NZ)* 1959;37:9–11.
2. Helyer BJ, Howie JB. Positive lupus erythematosus tests in a cross-bred strain of mice NZB/B1-NZY/B1. *Proc Univ Otago Med Sch (NZ)* 1961;39:3–4.
3. Helyer BJ, Howie JB. The thymus and autoimmune disease. *Lancet* 1963;2:1026–1029.
4. Wofsy D, Chiang NY. Proliferation of Ly-1 B cells in autoimmune NZB and (NZB × NZW)F1 mice. *Eur J Immunol* 1987; 17(6):809–814.
5. Andrews BS, Eisenberg RA, Theofilopoulos AN, et al. Spontaneous murine lupus-like syndromes. Clinical and immunopathological manifestations in several strains. *J Exp Med* 1978; 148(5):1198–1215.
6. Steinberg AD, Huston DP, Taurog JD, et al. The cellular and genetic basis of murine lupus. *Immunol Rev* 1981;55:121–154.
7. Theofilopoulos AN, Dixon FJ. Etiopathogenesis of murine SLE. *Immunol Rev* 1981;55:179–216.
8. Yoshida S, Castles JJ, Gershwin ME. The pathogenesis of autoimmunity in New Zealand mice. *Semin Arthritis Rheum* 1990;19(4):224–242.
9. DeHeer DH, Edginton TS. Cellular events associated with the immunogenesis of anti-erythrocyte autoantibody responses of NZB mice. *Transplant Rev* 1976;31:116–155.
10. DeHeer DH, Edgington TS. Evidence for a B lymphocyte defect underlying the anti-X anti-erythrocyte autoantibody response of NZB mice. *J Immunol* 1977;118(5):1858–1863.
11. Morton JI, Siegel BV. Transplantation of autoimmune potential. I. Development of antinuclear antibodies in H-2 histocompatible recipients of bone marrow from New Zealand Black mice. *Proc Natl Acad Sci USA* 1974;71(6):2162–2165.
12. Manny N, Datta SK, Schwartz RS. Synthesis of IgM by cells of NZB and SWR mice and their crosses. *J Immunol* 1979;122(4): 1220–1227.
13. Milich DR, Gershwin ME. The pathogenesis of autoimmunity in New Zealand mice. *Semin Arthritis Rheum* 1980;10(2): 111–147.
14. Shirai T, Mellors RC. Natural thymocytotoxic autoantibody and reactive antigen in New Zealand black and other mice. *Proc Natl Acad Sci USA* 1971;68(7):1412–1415.
15. Bray KR, Gershwin ME, Ahmed A, et al. Tissue localization and biochemical characteristics of a new thymic antigen recognized by a monoclonal thymocytotoxic autoantibody from New Zealand black mice. *J Immunol* 1985;134(6):4001–4008.
16. Bray KR, Gershwin ME, Chused T, et al. Characteristics of a spontaneous monoclonal thymocytotoxic antibody from New Zealand Black mice: recognition of a specific NTA determinant. *J Immunol* 1984;133(3):1318–1324.
17. Ohgaki M, Ueda G, Shiota J, et al. Two distinct monoclonal natural thymocytotoxic autoantibodies from New Zealand black mouse. *Clin Immunol Immunopathol* 1989;53(3):475–487.
18. Meryhew NL, Handwerger BS, Messner RP. Monoclonal antibody-induced murine hemolytic anemia. *J Lab Clin Med* 1984; 104(4):591–601.
19. De Heer DH, Edgington TS. Clonal heterogeneity of the anti-erythrocyte autoantibody responses of NZB mice. *J Immunol* 1974;113(4):1184–1189.
20. Holborow EJ, Barnes RD, Tuffrey M. A new red-cell autoantibody in NZB mice. *Nature* 1965;207(997):601–604.
21. Perry FE, Barker RN, Mazza G, et al. Autoreactive T cell specificity in autoimmune hemolytic anemia of the NZB mouse. *Eur J Immunol* 1996;26(1):136–141.
22. Caulfield MJ, Stanko D. A pathogenic monoclonal antibody, G8, is characteristic of antierythrocyte autoantibodies from Coombs'-positive NZB mice. *J Immunol* 1992;148(7):2068–2073.
23. Barker RN, Sa Oliveira GG, Elson CJ, et al. Pathogenic autoantibodies in the NZB mouse are specific for erythrocyte band 3 protein. *Eur J Immunol* 1993;23(7):1723–1726.
24. Hentati B, Payelle-Brogard B, Jouanne C, et al. Natural autoantibodies are involved in the haemolytic anaemia of NZB mice. *J Autoimmun* 1994;7(4):425–439.
25. Howie JB, Helyer BJ. The immunology and pathology of NZB mice. *Adv Immunol* 1968;9:215–266.
26. Bielschowsky M, D'Ath EF. The kidneys of NZB-B1, NZO-B1, NZC-B1 and NZY-B1 mice. *J Pathol* 1971;103(2):97–105.
27. Hicks JD, Burnet FM. Renal lesions in the "auto-immune" mouse strains NZB and F1 NZB×NZW. *J Pathol Bacteriol* 1966;91(2):467–476.
28. Schrott LM, Denenberg VH, Sherman GF, et al. Environmental enrichment, neocortical ectopias, and behavior in the autoimmune NZB mouse. *Brain Res Dev Brain Res* 1992;67(1): 85–93.
29. Harbeck RJ, Hoffman AA, Hoffman SA, et al. A naturally occurring antibody in New Zealand mice cytotoxic to dissociated cerebellar cells. *Clin Exp Immunol* 1978;31(2):313–320.
30. Tehrani MJ, Hu Y, Marquette C, et al. Interleukin-1 receptor deficiency in brains from NZB and (NZB/NZW)F1 autoimmune mice. *J Neuroimmunol* 1994;53(1):91–99.
31. Moutsopoulos HM, Boehm-Truitt M, Kassan SS, et al. Demonstration of activation of B lymphocytes in New Zealand black mice at birth by an immunoradiometric assay for murine IgM. *J Immunol* 1977;119(5):1639–1644.
32. Taurog JD, Moutsopoulos HM, Rosenberg YJ, et al. CBA/N X-

linked B-cell defect prevents NZB B-cell hyperactivity in F1 mice. *J Exp Med* 1979;150(1):31–43.
33. Theofilopoulos AN, Shawler DL, Eisenberg RA, et al. Splenic immunoglobulin-secreting cells and their regulation in autoimmune mice. *J Exp Med* 1980;151(2):446–466.
34. Hirose S, Tsurui H, Nishimura H, et al. Mapping of a gene for hypergammaglobulinemia to the distal region on chromosome 4 in NZB mice and its contribution to systemic lupus erythematosus in (NZB × NZW)F1 mice. *Int Immunol* 1994;6(12): 1857–1864.
35. Schwieterman WD, Wood GM, Scott DE, et al. Studies of bone marrow progenitor cells in lupus-prone mice. I. NZB marrow cells demonstrate increased growth in Whitlock-Witte culture and increased splenic colony-forming unit activity in the Thy-1-, lineage- population. *J Immunol* 1992;148(8):2405–2410.
36. Schwieterman WD, Manoussakis M, Klinman DM, et al. Studies of marrow progenitor abnormalities in lupus-prone mice. II. Further studies of NZB Thy 1(neg)Lin(neg) bone marrow cells. *Clin Immunol Immunopathol* 1994;72(1):114–120.
37. Merchant MS, Garvy BA, Riley RL. B220-bone marrow progenito cells from New Zealand black autoimmune mice exhibit an age-associated decline in Pre-B and B-cell generation. *Blood* 1995;85(7):1850–1857.
38. Anderson CC, Cairns E, Rudofsky UH, et al. Defective antigen-receptor-mediated regulation of immunoglobulin production in B cells from autoimmune strains of mice. *Cell Immunol* 1995;164(1):141–149.
39. Raveche ES, Lalor P, Stall A, et al. In vivo effects of hyperdiploid Ly-1+ B cells of NZB origin. *J Immunol* 1988;141(12): 4133–4139.
40. Marti GE, Metcalf RA, Raveche E. The natural history of a lymphoproliferative disorder in aged NZB mice. *Curr Top Microbiol Immunol* 1995;194:117–126.
41. Holmes MC, Burnet FM. The natural history of autoimmune disease in NZB mice. A comparison with the pattern of human autoimmune manifestations. *Ann Intern Med* 1963;59: 265–276.
42. Denman AM, Denman EJ. Proliferative activity in the lymphatic tissues of germ-free New Zealand black mice. *Int J Cancer* 1970;6(1):108–122.
43. Raveche ES, Phillips J, Mahboudi F, et al. Regulatory aspects of clonally expanded B-1 (CD5+ B) cells. *Int J Clin Lab Res* 1992; 22(4):220–234.
44. Hayakawa K, Hardy RR, Herzenberg LA. Peritoneal Ly-1 B cells: genetic control, autoantibody production, increased lambda light chain expression. *Eur J Immunol* 1986;16(4): 450–456.
45. Hayakawa K, Hardy RR, Parks DR, et al. The "Ly-1 B" cell subpopulation in normal immunodefective, and autoimmune mice. *J Exp Med* 1983;157(1):202–218.
46. Hayakawa K, Hardy RR, Honda M, et al. Ly-1 B cells: functionally distinct lymphocytes that secrete IgM autoantibodies. *Proc Natl Acad Sci USA* 1984;81(8):2494–2498.
47. Conger JD, Pike BL, Nossal GJ. Clonal analysis of the anti-DNA repertoire of murine B lymphocytes. *Proc Natl Acad Sci USA* 1987;84(9):2931–2935.
48. Manohar V, Brown E, Leiserson WM, et al. Expression of Lyt-1 by a subset of B lymphocytes. *J Immunol* 1982;129(2):532–538.
49. Murakami M, Yoshioka H, Shirai T, et al. Prevention of autoimmune symptoms in autoimmune-prone mice by elimination of B-1 cells. *Int Immunol* 1995;7(5):877–882.
50. Vries MD, Hijmans W. Pathological changes of thymic epithelial cells and autoimmune disease in NZB, NZW and (NZB × NZW)F1 mice. *Immunology* 1967;12(2):179–196.
51. Gershwin ME, Ikeda RM, Kruse WL, et al. Age-dependent loss in New Zealand mice of morphological and functional characteristics of thymic epithelial cells. *J Immunol* 1978;120(3): 971–979.
52. Whittum J, Goldschneider I, Greiner D, et al. Developmental abnormalities of terminal deoxynucleotidyl transferase positive bone marrow cells and thymocytes in New Zealand mice: effects of prostaglandin E1. *J Immunol* 1985;135(1):272–280.
53. Minoda M, Horiuchi A. The function of thymic reticuloepithelial cells in New Zealand mice. *Thymus* 1983;5(5–6): 363–374.
54. Minoda M, Horiuchi A. The effects of macrophages on interleukin 2 production in thymocytes of New Zealand black mice. *J Clin Lab Immunol* 1987;22(1):29–34.
55. Minoda M, Senda S, Horiuchi A. The relationship between the defect in the syngeneic mixed lymphocyte reaction and thymic abnormality in New Zealand mice. *J Clin Lab Immunol* 1987;23(2):101–108.
56. Hayes SM, Greiner DL. Evidence for elevated prothymocyte activity in the bone marrow of New Zealand Black (NZB) mice. Elevated prothymocyte activity in NZB mice. *Thymus* 1992; 19(3):157–172.
57. Kono DH, Burlingame RW, Owens DG, et al. Lupus susceptibility loci in New Zealand mice. *Proc Natl Acad Sci USA* 1994;91(21):10168–10172.
58. Tokushima M, Koarada S, Hirose S, et al. In vivo induction of IgG anti-DNA antibody by autoreactive mixed haplotype A beta z/A alpha d MHC class II molecule-specific CD4+ T-cell clones. *Immunology* 1994;83(2):221–226.
59. Song YW, Tsao BP, Hahn BH. Contribution of major histocompatibility complex (MHC) to upregulation of anti-DNA antibody in transgenic mice. *J Autoimmun* 1993;6(1):1–9.
60. Nygard NR, McCarthy DM, Schiffenbauer J, et al. Mixed haplotypes and autoimmunity. *Immunol Today* 1993;14(2):53–56.
61. Rudofsky UH, Evans BD, Balaban SL, et al. Differences in expression of lupus nephritis in New Zealand mixed H-2z homozygous inbred strains of mice derived from New Zealand black and New Zealand white mice. Origins and initial characterization. *Lab Invest* 1993;68(4):419–426.
62. Hirose S, Kinoshita K, Nozawa S, et al. Effects of major histocompatibility complex on autoimmune disease of H-2-congenic New Zealand mice. *Int Immunol* 1990;2(11):1091–1095.
63. Kotzin BL, Palmer E. The contribution of NZW genes to lupus-like disease in (NZB × NZW)F1 mice. *J Exp Med* 1987; 165(5):1237–1251.
64. Schiffenbauer J, McCarthy DM, Nygard NR, et al. A unique sequence of the NZW I-E beta chain and its possible contribution to autoimmunity in the (NZB × NZW)F1 mouse. *J Exp Med* 1989;170(3):971–984.
65. Chiang BL, Bearer E, Ansari A, et al. The BM12 mutation and autoantibodies to dsDNA in NZB.H-2bm12 mice. *J Immunol* 1990;145(1):94–101.
66. Hardin JA. The lupus autoantigens and the pathogenesis of systemic lupus erythematosus. *Arthritis Rheum* 1986;29(4): 457–460.
67. Watanabe Y, Yoshida SH, Ansari AA, et al. The contribution of H-2bm12 and non H-2 background genes on murine lupus in NZB.H-2bm12/b mice. *J Autoimmun* 1994;7(2):153–164.
68. Naiki M, Yoshida SH, Ansari AA, et al. Activation of autoreactive T-cell clones from NZB.H-2bm12 mice. *J Autoimmun* 1994;7(3):275–290.
69. Oliveira GG, Hutchings PR, Lydyard PM. Anti-CD4 treatment of NZB mice prevents the development of erythrocyte autoantibodies but hastens the appearance of anaemia. *Immunol Lett* 1994;39(2):153–156.
70. Oliveira GG, Hutchings PR, Roitt IM, et al. Production of erythrocyte autoantibodies in NZB mice is inhibited by CD4 antibodies. *Clin Exp Immunol* 1994;96(2):297–302.

71. Dubois EL, Horowitz RE, Demopoulos HB, et al. NZB/NZW mice as a model of systemic lupus erythematosus. *JAMA* 1966; 195(4):285–289.
72. Vyse TJ, Rozzo SJ, Drake CG, et al. Control of multiple autoantibodies linked with a lupus nephritis susceptibility locus in New Zealand black mice. *J Immunol* 1997;158(11): 5566–5574.
73. Drake CG, Babcock SK, Palmer E, et al. Genetic analysis of the NZB contribution to lupus-like autoimmune disease in (NZB × NZW)F1 mice. *Proc Natl Acad Sci USA* 1994;91(9): 4062–4066.
74. Morel L, Croker BP, Blenman KR, et al. Genetic reconstitution of systemic lupus erythematosus immunopathology with polycongenic murine strains. *Proc Natl Acad Sci USA* 2000;97(12): 6670–6675.
75. Morel L, Yu Y, Blenman KR, et al. Production of congenic mouse strains carrying genomic intervals containing SLE-susceptibility genes derived from the SLE-prone NZM2410 strain. *Mamm Genome* 1996;7(5):335–339.
76. Vyse TJ, Morel L, Tanner FJ, et al. Backcross analysis of genes linked to autoantibody production in New Zealand White mice. *J Immunol* 1996;157(6):2719–2727.
77. Morel L, Mohan C, Yu Y, et al. Functional dissection of systemic lupus erythematosus using congenic mouse strains. *J Immunol* 1997;158(12):6019–6028.
78. Mohan C, Morel L, Yang P, et al. Genetic dissection of systemic lupus erythematosus pathogenesis: Sle2 on murine chromosome 4 leads to B cell hyperactivity. *J Immunol* 1997;159(1): 454–465.
79. Mohan C, Alas E, Morel L, et al. Genetic dissection of SLE pathogenesis. Sle1 on murine chromosome 1 leads to a selective loss of tolerance to H2A/H2B/DNA subnucleosomes. *J Clin Invest* 1998;101(6):1362–1372.
80. Mohan C, Morel L, Yang P, et al. Accumulation of splenic B1a cells with potent antigen-presenting capability in NZM2410 lupus-prone mice. *Arthritis Rheum* 1998;41(9):1652–1662.
81. Sobel ES, Mohan C, Morel L, et al. Genetic dissection of SLE pathogenesis: adoptive transfer of Sle1 mediates the loss of tolerance by bone marrow-derived B cells. *J Immunol* 1999; 162(4):2415–2421.
82. Mohan C, Yu Y, Morel L, et al. Genetic dissection of Sle pathogenesis: Sle3 on murine chromosome 7 impacts T cell activation, differentiation, and cell death. *J Immunol* 1999;162(11): 6492–6502.
83. Mohan C, Morel L, Yang P, et al. Genetic dissection of lupus pathogenesis: a recipe for nephrophilic autoantibodies. *J Clin Invest* 1999;103(12):1685–1695.
84. Hahn BH, Shulman LE. Autoantibodies and nephritis in the white strain (NZW) of New Zealand mice. *Arthritis Rheum* 1969;12:355–364.
85. Rozzo SJ, Vyse TJ, David CS, et al. Analysis of MHC Class II genes in the susceptibility to lupus in New Zealand mice. *J Immunol* 1999;162(2):623–630.
86. Vyse TR, Halterman RK, Rozzo SJ, et al. Control of separate pathogenic autoantibody responses marks MHC gene contributions to murine lupus. *Proc Natl Acad Sci USA* 1999;96: 8098–8103.
87. Fujimura T, Hirose S, Jiang Y, et al. Dissection of the effects of tumor necrosis factor-alpha and class II gene polymorphisms within the MHC on murine systemic lupus erythematosus (SLE). *Int Immunol* 1998;10:1467–1472.
88. Jacob CO, Lee SK, Strassmann G. Mutational analysis of the TNF-alpha gene reveals a regulatory role for the 3′-untranslated region in the genetic predisposition to lupus-like autoimmune disease. *J Immunol* 1996;156:3053–3050.
89. Maeda T, Webb DR, Chen J, et al. Deletion of signaling molecule genes resembling the cytoplasmic domain of Igbeta in autoimmune-prone mice. *Int Immunol* 1998;10:815–821.
90. Koch-Nolte F, Klein J, Hollmann C, et al. Defects in the structure and expression of the genes for the T cell marker Rt6 in NZW and (NZB×NZW)F1 mice. *Int Immunol* 1995;7: 883–890.
91. Morel L, Tian XH, Croker BP, et al. Epistatic modifiers of autoimmunity in a murine model of lupus nephritis. *Immunity* 1999;11(2):131–139.
92. Noonan DJ, Kofler R, Singer PA, et al. Delineation of a defect in T cell receptor beta genes of NZW mice predisposed to autoimmunity. *J Exp Med* 1986;163(3):644–653.
93. Babcock SK, Appel VB, Schiff M, et al. Genetic analysis of the imperfect association of H-2 haplotype with lupus-like autoimmune disease. *Proc Natl Acad Sci USA* 1989;86(19): 7552–7555.
94. Steward MW, Hay FC. Changes in immunoglobulin class and subclass of anti-DNA antibodies with increasing age in N/ZBW F1 hybrid mice. *Clin Exp Immunol* 1976;126(2):363–370.
95. Papoian R, Pillarisetty R, Talal N. Immunological regulation of spontaneous antibodies to DNA and RNA. II. Sequential switch from IgM to IgG in NZB/NZW F1 mice. *Immunology* 1977;32(1):75–79.
96. Wofsy D, Seaman WE. Successful treatment of autoimmunity in NZB/NZW F1 mice with monoclonal antibody to L3T4. *J Exp Med* 1985;161(2):378–391.
97. Tsao BP, Ebling FM, Roman C, et al. Structural characteristics of the variable regions of immunoglobulin genes encoding a pathogenic autoantibody in murine lupus. *J Clin Invest* 1990; 85(2):530–540.
98. Ohnishi K, Ebling FM, Mitchell B, et al. Comparison of pathogenic and non-pathogenic murine antibodies to DNA: antigen binding and structural characteristics. *Int Immunol* 1994;6(6): 817–830.
99. Raz E, Brezis M, Rosenmann E, et al. Anti-DNA antibodies bind directly to renal antigens and induce kidney dysfunction in the isolated perfused rat kidney. *J Immunol* 1989;142(9): 3076–3082.
100. Tsao BP, Ohnishi K, Cheroutre H, et al. Failed self-tolerance and autoimmunity in IgG anti-DNA transgenic mice. *J Immunol* 1992;149(1):350–358.
101. Tsao BP, Hahn BH. Ig-transgenic mice as models for studying the regulation and role of anti-DNA antibodies in murine lupus. *Immunomethods* 1992;1:185–190.
102. Ebling FM, Hahn BH. Pathogenic subsets of antibodies to DNA. *Int Rev Immunol* 1989;5(1):79–95.
103. Tucker RM, Vyse TJ, Rozzo S, et al. Genetic control of glycoprotein 70 autoantigen production and its influence on immune complex levels and nephritis in murine lupus. *J Immunol* 2000; 165(3):1665–1672.
104. Park CL, Balderas RS, Fieser TM, et al. Isotypic profiles and other fine characteristics of immune responses to exogenous thymus-dependent and -independent antigens by mice with lupus syndromes. *J Immunol* 1983;130(5):2161–2167.
105. Dixon FJ, Oldstone MB, Tonietti G. Pathogenesis of immune complex glomerulonephritis of New Zealand mice. *J Exp Med* 1971;134(suppl 3):71s.
106. Lambert PH, Dixon FJ. Pathogenesis of the glomerulonephritis of NZB/W mice. *J Exp Med* 1968;127(3):507–522.
107. Ebling F, Hahn BH. Restricted subpopulations of DNA antibodies in kidneys of mice with systemic lupus. Comparison of antibodies in serum and renal eluates. *Arthritis Rheum* 1980; 23(4):392–403.
108. Schmiedeke T, Stoeckl F, Muller S, et al. Glomerular immune deposits in murine lupus models may contain histones. *Clin Exp Immunol* 1992;90(3):453–458.

109. Cavallo T, Graves K, Granholm NA, et al. Association of glycoprotein gp70 with progression or attenuation of murine lupus nephritis. *J Clin Lab Immunol* 1985;18(2):63–67.
110. Stetler DA, Cavallo T. Anti-RNA polymerase I antibodies: potential role in the induction and progression of murine lupus nephritis. *J Immunol* 1987;138(7):2119–2123.
111. Nakamura T, Ebihara I, Nagaoka I, et al. Renal platelet-derived growth factor gene expression in NZB/W F1 mice with lupus and ddY mice with IgA nephropathy. *Clin Immunol Immunopathol* 1992;63(2):173–181.
112. Nakamura T, Ebihara I, Tomino Y, et al. Effect of a specific endothelin A receptor antagonist on murine lupus nephritis. *Kidney Int* 1995;47(2):481–489.
113. Ozmen L, Roman D, Fountoulakis M, et al. Experimental therapy of systemic lupus erythematosus: the treatment of NZB/W mice with mouse soluble interferon-gamma receptor inhibits the onset of glomerulonephritis. *Eur J Immunol* 1995;25(1):6–12.
114. Nakamura T, Ebihara I, Nagaoka I, et al. Effect of methylprednisolone on transforming growth factor-beta, insulin-like growth factor-I, and basic fibroblast growth factor gene expression in the kidneys of NZB/W F1 mice. *Renal Physiol Biochem* 1993;16(3):105–116.
115. Maruyama N, Furukawa F, Nakai Y, et al. Genetic studies of autoimmunity in New Zealand mice. IV. Contribution of NZB and NZW genes to the spontaneous occurrence of retroviral gp70 immune complexes in (NZB × NZW)F1 hybrid and the correlation to renal disease. *J Immunol* 1983;130(2):740–746.
116. Datta SK, Owen FL, Womack JE, et al. Analysis of recombinant inbred lines derived from "autoimmune" (NZB) and "high leukemia" (C58) strains: independent multigenic systems control B cell hyperactivity, retrovirus expression, and autoimmunity. *J Immunol* 1982;129(4):1539–1544.
117. Miller ML, Raveche ES, Laskin CA, et al. Genetic studies in NZB mice. VI. Association of autoimmune traits in recombinant inbred lines. *J Immunol* 1984;133(3):1325–1331.
118. Raveche ES, Novotny EA, Hansen CT, et al. Genetic studies of NZB mice. V. Recombinant inbred lines demonstrate that separate genes control autoimmune phenotype. *J Exp Med* 1981; 153:1187–1197.
119. Adachi Y, Inaba M, Amoh Y, et al. Effect of bone marrow transplantation on antiphospholipid antibody syndrome in murine lupus mice. *Immunobiology* 1995;192(3–4):218–230.
120. Moore PM. Evidence for bound antineuronal antibodies in brains of NZB/W mice. *J Neuroimmunol* 1992;38(1–2):147–154.
121. Takeuchi K, Turley SJ, Tan EM, et al. Analysis of the autoantibody response to fibrillarin in human disease and murine models of autoimmunity. *J Immunol* 1995;154:961–971.
122. Elouaai F, Lule J, Benoist H, et al. Autoimmunity to histones, ubiquitin, and ubiquitinated histone H2A in NZB × NZW and MRL-lpr/lpr mice. Anti-histone antibodies are concentrated in glomerular eluates of lupus mice. *Nephrol Dial Transplant* 1994;9(4):362–366.
123. Lemoine R, Berney T, Shibata T, et al. Induction of "wire-loop" lesions by murine monoclonal IgG3 cryoglobulins. *Kidney Int* 1992;41(1):65–72.
124. Okudaira K, Yoshizawa H, Williams RC Jr. Monoclonal murine anti-DNA antibody interacts with living mononuclear cells. *Arthritis Rheum* 1987;30(6):669–678.
125. Vlahakos D, Foster MH, Ucci AA, et al. Murine monoclonal anti-DNA antibodies penetrate cells, bind to nuclei, and induce glomerular proliferation and proteinuria in vivo. *J Am Soc Nephrol* 1992;2(8):1345–1354.
126. Koren E, Koscec M, Wolfson-Reichlin M, et al. Murine and human antibodies to native DNA that cross-react with the A and D SnRNP polypeptides cause direct injury of cultured kidney cells. *J Immunol* 1995;154(9):4857–4864.
127. Yanase K, Smith RM, Cizman B, et al. A subgroup of murine monoclonal anti-deoxyribonucleic acid antibodies traverse the cytoplasm and enter the nucleus in a time-and temperature-dependent manner. *Lab Invest* 1994;71(1):52–60.
128. Reichlin M. Cellular dysfunction induced by penetration of autoantibodies into living cells: cellular damage and dysfunction mediated by antibodies to dsDNA and ribosomal P proteins. *J Autoimmun* 1998;11(5):557–561.
129. Talal N, Steinberg AD. The pathogenesis of autoimmunity in New Zealand black mice. *Curr Top Microbiol Immunol* 1974; 64(0):79–103.
130. Hahn BH, Knotts L, Ng M, et al. Influence of cyclophosphamide and other immunosuppressive drugs on immune disorders and neoplasia in NZB/NZW mice. *Arthritis Rheum* 1975;18(2):145–152.
131. Chandrasekar B, McGuff HS, Aufdermorte TB, et al. Effects of calorie restriction on transforming growth factor beta 1 and proinflammatory cytokines in murine Sjogren's syndrome. *Clin Immunol Immunopathol* 1995;76(3 pt 1):291–296.
132. Jabs DA, Prendergast RA. Murine models of Sjogren's syndrome. *Adv Exp Med Biol* 1994;350:623–630.
133. Roubinian J, Talal N, Siiteri PK, et al. Sex hormone modulation of autoimmunity in NZB/NZW mice. *Arthritis Rheum* 1979; 22(11):1162–1169.
134. Verheul HA, Verveld M, Hoefakker S, et al. Effects of ethinylestradiol on the course of spontaneous autoimmune disease in NZB/W and NOD mice. *Immunopharmacol Immunotoxicol* 1995;17(1):163–180.
135. Walker SE, Besch-Williford CL, Keisler DH. Accelerated deaths from systemic lupus erythematosus in NZB×NZW F1 mice treated with the testosterone-blocking drug flutamide. *J Lab Clin Med* 1994;124:401–407.
136. Duvic M, Steinberg AD, Klassen LW. Effect of the anti-estrogen, Nafoxidine, on NZB/W autoimmune disease. *Arthritis Rheum* 1978;21(4):414–417.
137. Roubinian JR, Talal N, Greenspan JS, et al. Delayed androgen treatment prolongs survival in murine lupus. *J Clin Invest* 1979; 63(5):902–911.
138. Roubinian JR, Talal N, Greenspan JS, et al. Effect of castration and sex hormone treatment on survival, anti- nucleic acid antibodies, and glomerulonephritis in NZB/NZW F1 mice. *J Exp Med* 1978;147(6):1568–1583.
139. Steinberg AD, Melez KA, Raveche ES, et al. Approach to the study of the role of sex hormones in autoimmunity. *Arthritis Rheum* 1979;22(11):1170–1176.
140. Walker SE, Allen SH, Hoffman RW, et al. Prolactin: a stimulator of disease activity in systemic lupus erythematosus. *Lupus* 1995;4(1):3–9.
141. McMurray R, Keisler D, Izui S, et al. Hyperprolactinemia in male NZB/NZW (B/W) F1 mice: accelerated autoimmune disease with normal circulating testosterone. *Clin Immunol Immunopathol* 1994;71(3):338–343.
142. Elbourne KB, Keisler D, McMurray RW. Differential effects of estrogen and prolactin on autoimmune disease in the NZB/NZW F1 mouse model of systemic lupus erythematosus [see comments]. *Lupus* 1998;7(6):420–427.
143. Nilsson N, Carlsten H. Estrogen induces suppression of natural killer cell cytotoxicity and augmentation of polyclonal B cell activation. *Cell Immunol* 1994;158(1):131–139.
144. Bynoe MS, Grimaldi CM, Diamond B. Estrogen up-regulates Bcl-2 and blocks tolerance induction of naive B cells. *Proc Natl Acad Sci USA* 2000;97(6):2703–2708.
145. Reininger L, Radaszkiewicz T, Kosco M, et al. Development of autoimmune disease in SCID mice populated with long-term "in vitro" proliferating (NZB × NZW)F1 pre-B cells. *J Exp Med* 1992;176(5):1343–1353.

146. Hahn BH, Ebling FM. Idiotype restriction in murine lupus; high frequency of three public idiotypes on serum IgG in nephritic NZB/NZW F1 mice. *J Immunol* 1987;138(7):2110–2118.
147. Panosian-Sahakian N, Klotz JL, Ebling F, et al. Diversity of Ig V gene segments found in anti-DNA autoantibodies from a single (NZB × NZW)F1 mouse. *J Immunol* 1989;142(12):4500–4506.
148. Marion TN, Bothwell AL, Briles DE, et al. IgG anti-DNA autoantibodies within an individual autoimmune mouse are the products of clonal selection [see comments]. *J Immunol* 1989; 142(12):4269–4274.
149. Shlomchik M, Mascelli M, Shan H, et al. Anti-DNA antibodies from autoimmune mice arise by clonal expansion and somatic mutation. *J Exp Med* 1990;171(1):265–292.
150. Marion TN, Tillman DM, Jou NT. Interclonal and intraclonal diversity among anti-DNA antibodies from an (NZB × NZW)F1 mouse. *J Immunol* 1990;145(7):2322–2332.
151. Tillman DM, Jou NT, Hill RJ, et al. Both IgM and IgG anti-DNA antibodies are the products of clonally selective B cell stimulation in (NZB × NZW)F1 mice. *J Exp Med* 1992; 176(3):761–779.
152. Ando DG, Sercarz EE, Hahn BH. Mechanisms of T and B cell collaboration in the in vitro production of anti-DNA antibodies in the NZB/NZW F1 murine SLE model. *J Immunol* 1987;138(10):3185–3190.
153. Singh RR, Kumar V, Ebling FM, et al. T cell determinants from autoantibodies to DNA can upregulate autoimmunity in murine systemic lupus erythematosus. *J Exp Med* 1995;181(6): 2017–2027.
154. Wofsy D, Seaman WE. Reversal of advanced murine lupus in NZB/NZW F1 mice by treatment with monoclonal antibody to L3T4. *J Immunol* 1987;138(10):3247–3253.
155. Rozzo SJ, Drake CG, Chiang BL, et al. Evidence for polyclonal T cell activation in murine models of systemic lupus erythematosus. *J Immunol* 1994;153(3):1340–1351.
156. Sato MN, Minoprio P, Avrameas S, et al. Defects in the regulation of anti-DNA antibody production in aged lupus- prone (NZB × NZW)F1 mice: analysis of T-cell lymphokine synthesis. *Immunology* 1995;85(1):26–32.
157. Finck BK, Linsley PS, Wofsy D. Treatment of murine lupus with CTLA4Ig. *Science* 1994;265(5176):1225–1227.
158. Nakajima A, Azuma M, Kodera S, et al. Preferential dependence of autoantibody production in murine lupus on CD86 costimulatory molecule. *Eur J Immunol* 1995;25(11):3060–3069.
159. Early GS, Zhao W, Burns CM. Anti-CD40 ligand antibody treatment prevents the development of lupus- like nephritis in a subset of New Zealand black × New Zealand white mice. Response correlates with the absence of an anti-antibody response. *J Immunol* 1996;157(7):3159–3164.
160. Kalled SL, Cutler AH, Datta SK, et al. Anti-CD40 ligand antibody treatment of SNF1 mice with established nephritis: preservation of kidney function. *J Immunol* 1998;160(5):2158–2165.
161. Daikh DI, Finck BK, Linsley PS, et al. Long-term inhibition of murine lupus by brief simultaneous blockade of the B7/CD28 and CD40/gp39 costimulation pathways. *J Immunol* 1997; 159(7):3104–3108.
162. Lin LC, Chen YC, Chou CC, et al. Dysregulation of T helper cell cytokines in autoimmune prone NZB × NZW F1 mice. *Scand J Immunol* 1995;42(4):466–472.
163. Kanno K, Okada T, Abe M, et al. Differential sensitivity to interleukins of CD5+ and CD5– anti-DNA antibody-producing B cells in murine lupus. *Autoimmunity* 1993;14(3):205–214.
164. Finck BK, Chan B, Wofsy D. Interleukin 6 promotes murine lupus in NZB/NZW F1 mice. *J Clin Invest* 1994;94(2):585–591.
165. Ishida H, Muchamuel T, Sakaguchi S, et al. Continuous administration of anti-interleukin 10 antibodies delays onset of autoimmunity in NZB/W F1 mice. *J Exp Med* 1994; 179(1):305–310.
166. Hartwell DW, Fenton MJ, Levine JS, et al. Aberrant cytokine regulation in macrophages from young autoimmune-prone mice: evidence that the intrinsic defect in MRL macrophage IL-1 expression is transcriptionally controlled. *Mol Immunol* 1995; 32(10):743–751.
167. Brennan DC, Yui MA, Wuthrich RP, et al. Tumor necrosis factor and IL-1 in New Zealand black/white mice. Enhanced gene expression and acceleration of renal injury. *J Immunol* 1989; 143(11):3470–3475.
168. Hartwell D, Levine J, Fenton M, et al. Cytokine dysregulation and the initiation of systemic autoimmunity. *Immunol Lett* 1994;43(1–2):15–21.
169. Jacob CO, McDevitt HO. Tumour necrosis factor-alpha in murine autoimmune "lupus" nephritis. *Nature* 1988;331(6154): 356–358.
170. Gordon C, Ranges GE, Greenspan JS, et al. Chronic therapy with recombinant tumor necrosis factor-alpha in autoimmune NZB/NZW F1 mice. *Clin Immunol Immunopathol* 1989;52(3): 421–434.
171. Gordon C, Wofsy D. Effects of recombinant murine tumor necrosis factor-alpha on immune function. *J Immunol* 1990; 144(5):1753–1758.
172. Ito S, Ueno M, Nishi S, et al. Suppression of spontaneous murine lupus by inducing graft-versus-host reaction with CD8+ cells. *Clin Exp Immunol* 1992;90:260–265.
173. Shao DZ, Yamada S, Hirayama F, et al. Modulation of B-cell abnormalities in lupus-prone (NZB × NZW)F1 mice by normal bone marrow-derived B-lineage cells. *Immunology* 1995; 85(1):16–25.
174. Datta SK, Manny N, Andrzejewski C, et al. Genetic studies of autoimmunity and retrovirus expression in crosses of New Zealand black mice I. Xenotropic virus. *J Exp Med* 1978; 147(3):854–871.
175. Datta SK, McConahey PJ, Manny N, et al. Genetic studies of autoimmunity and retrovirus expression in crosses of New Zealand black mice. II. The viral envelope glycoprotein gp70. *J Exp Med* 1978;147(3):872–881.
176. Eastcott JW, Schwartz RS, Datta SK. Genetic analysis of the inheritance of B cell hyperactivity in relation to the development of autoantibodies and glomerulonephritis in NZB × SWR crosses. *J Immunol* 1983;131(5):2232–2239.
177. Gavalchin J, Datta SK. The NZB X SWR model of lupus nephritis. II. Autoantibodies deposited in renal lesions show a distinctive and restricted idiotypic diversity. *J Immunol* 1987; 138(1):138–148.
178. Gavalchin J, Nicklas JA, Eastcott JW, et al. Lupus prone (SWR × NZB)F1 mice produce potentially nephritogenic autoantibodies inherited from the normal SWR parent. *J Immunol* 1985;134(2):885–894.
179. Gavalchin J, Seder RA, Datta SK. The NZB X SWR model of lupus nephritis. I. Cross-reactive idiotypes of monoclonal anti-DNA antibodies in relation to antigenic specificity, charge, and allotype. Identification of interconnected idiotype families inherited from the normal SWR and the autoimmune NZB parents. *J Immunol* 1987;138(1):128–137.
180. O'Keefe TL, Bandyopadhyay S, Datta SK, et al. V region sequences of an idiotypically connected family of pathogenic anti-DNA autoantibodies. *J Immunol* 1990;144(11):4275–4283.
181. Rauch J, Murphy E, Roths JB, et al. A high frequency idiotypic marker of anti-DNA autoantibodies in MRL-lpr/lpr mice. *J Immunol* 1982;129(1):236–241.
182. Dang H, Harbeck RJ. The in vivo and in vitro glomerular deposition of isolated anti-double-stranded-DNA antibodies

in NZB/W mice. *Clin Immunol Immunopathol* 1984; 30(2):265–278.

183. Portanova JP, Creadon G, Zhang X, et al. An early post-mutational selection event directs expansion of autoreactive B cells in murine lupus. *Mol Immunol* 1995;32(2):117–135.
184. Knupp CJ, Uner AH, Korthas C, et al. Characterization of IdLNF1-specific T cell clones from the (NZB × SWR)F1 murine model for systemic lupus erythematosus. *Clin Immunol Immunopathol* 1993;68(3):273–282.
185. Knupp CJ, Uner AH, Tatum AH, et al. IdLNF1-specific T cell clones accelerate the production of IdLNF1 + IgG and nephritis in SNF1 mice. *J Autoimmun* 1995;8(3):367–380.
186. Uner AH, Knupp CJ, Tatum AH, et al. Treatment with antibody reactive with the nephritogenic idiotype, IdLNF1, suppresses its production and leads to prolonged survival of (NZB × SWR)F1 mice. *J Autoimmun* 1994;7(1):27–44.
187. Datta SK, Patel H, Berry D. Induction of a cationic shift in IgG anti-DNA autoantibodies. Role of T helper cells with classical and novel phenotypes in three murine models of lupus nephritis. *J Exp Med* 1987;165(5):1252–1268.
188. Ghatak S, Sainis K, Owens FL, et al. T-cell-receptor beta and I-A-chain genes of normal SWR mice are linked with the development of lupus nephritis in NZB × SWR crosses. *Proc Natl Acad Sci USA* 1987;84:6850–6853.
189. Morel L, Rudofsky UH, Longmate JA, et al. Polygenic control of susceptibility to murine systemic lupus erythematosus. *Immunity* 1994;1(3):219–229.
190. Murphy ED, Roths JB. A single gene for massive lymphoproliferation with immune complex disease in a new mouse strain MRL. In: *Proceedings of the 16th International Congress in Hematology*. Amsterdam: Excerpta Medica, 1976.
191. Watanabe-Fukunaga R, Brannan CI, Copeland NG, et al. Lymphoproliferation disorder in mice explained by defects in Fas antigen that mediates apoptosis. *Nature* 1992;356(6367): 314–317.
192. Watson ML, Rao JK, Gilkeson GS, et al. Genetic analysis of MRL-lpr mice: relationship of the Fas apoptosis gene to disease manifestations and renal disease-modifying loci. *J Exp Med* 1992;176(6):1645–1656.
193. Wu J, Zhou T, He J, et al. Autoimmune disease in mice due to integration of an endogenous retrovirus in an apoptosis gene. *J Exp Med* 1993;178(2):461–468.
194. Chu JL, Drappa J, Parnassa A, et al. The defect in Fas mRNA expression in MRL/lpr mice is associated with insertion of the retrotransposon, ETn. *J Exp Med* 1993;178(2):723–730.
195. Adachi M, Watanabe-Fukunaga R, Nagata S. Aberrant transcription caused by the insertion of an early transposable element in an intron of the Fas antigen gene of lpr mice. *Proc Natl Acad Sci USA* 1993;90(5):1756–1760.
196. Nagata S, Golstein P. The Fas death factor. *Science* 1995; 267(5203):1449–1456.
197. Drappa J, Brot N, Elkon KB. The Fas protein is expressed at high levels on CD4+CD8+ thymocytes and activated mature lymphocytes in normal mice but not in the lupus-prone strain, MRL lpr/lpr. *Proc Natl Acad Sci USA* 1993;90(21):10340–10344.
198. Lynch DH, Ramsdell F, Alderson MR. Fas and FasL in the homeostatic regulation of immune responses. *Immunol Today* 1995;16(12):569–574.
199. Mountz JD, Bluethmann H, Zhou T, et al. Defective clonal deletion and anergy induction in TCR transgenic lpr/lpr mice. *Semin Immunol* 1994;6(1):27–37.
200. Morse HC III, Davidson WF, Yetter RA, et al. Abnormalities induced by the mutant gene lpr: expansion of a unique lymphocyte subset. *J Immunol* 1982;129(6):2612–2615.
201. Izui S, Kelley VE, Masuda K, et al. Induction of various autoantibodies by mutant gene lpr in several strains of mice. *J Immunol* 1984;133(1):227–233.
202. Katagiri T, Cohen PL, Eisenberg RA. The lpr gene causes an intrinsic T cell abnormality that is required for hyperproliferation. *J Exp Med* 1988;167(3):741–751.
203. Jabs DA, Burek CL, Hu Q, et al. Anti-CD4 monoclonal antibody therapy suppresses autoimmune disease in MRL/Mp-lpr/lpr mice. *Cell Immunol* 1992;141(2):496–507.
204. Singer PA, McEvilly RJ, Noonan DJ, et al. Clonal diversity and T-cell receptor beta-chain variable gene expression in enlarged lymph nodes of MRL-lpr/lpr lupus mice. *Proc Natl Acad Sci USA* 1986;83(18):7018–7022.
205. Singer PA, Theofilopoulos AN. Novel origin of lpr and gld cells and possible implications in autoimmunity. *J Autoimmun* 1990;3(2):123–135.
206. Altman A, Theofilopoulos AN, Weiner R, et al. Analysis of T cell function in autoimmune murine strains. Defects in production and responsiveness to interleukin 2. *J Exp Med* 1981; 154(3):791–808.
207. Cohen PL, Rapoport R, Eisenberg RA. Characterization of functional T-cell lines derived from MRL mice. *Clin Immunol Immunopathol* 1986;40(3):485–496.
208. Fisher CL, Shores EW, Eisenberg RA, et al. Cellular interactions for the in vitro production of anti-chromatin autoantibodies in MRL/Mp-lpr/lpr mice. *Clin Immunol Immunopathol* 1989; 50(2):231–240.
209. Shores EW, Eisenberg RA, Cohen PL. T-B collaboration in the in vitro anti-Sm autoantibody response of MRL/Mp-lpr/lpr mice. *J Immunol* 1988;140(9):2977–2982.
210. Santoro TJ, Portanova JP, Kotzin BL. The contribution of L3T4+ T cells to lymphoproliferation and autoantibody production in MRL-lpr/lpr mice. *J Exp Med* 1988;167(5): 1713–1718.
211. Stetler DA, Sipes DE, Jacob ST. Anti-RNA polymerase I antibodies in sera of MRL lpr/lpr and MRL +/+ autoimmune mice. Correlation of antibody production with delayed onset of lupus-like disease in MRL +/+ mice. *J Exp Med* 1985;162(6): 1760–1770.
212. Kanai Y, Miura K, Uehara T, et al. Natural occurrence of Nuc in the sera of autoimmune-prone MRL/lpr mice. *Biochem Biophys Res Commun* 1993;196(2):729–736.
213. Kanai Y, Takeda O, Kanai Y, et al. Novel autoimmune phenomena induced in vivo by a new DNA binding protein Nuc: a study on MRL/n mice. *Immunol Lett* 1993;39(1):83–89.
214. Kita Y, Sumida T, Ichikawa K, et al. V gene analysis of anticardiolipin antibodies from MRL-lpr/lpr mice. *J Immunol* 1993; 151(2):849–856.
215. Treadwell EL, Cohen P, Williams D, et al. MRL mice produce anti-Su autoantibody, a specificity associated with systemic lupus erythematosus. *J Immunol* 1993;150(2):695–699.
216. Wang J, Chou CH, Blankson J, et al. Murine monoclonal antibodies specific for conserved and non-conserved antigenic determinants of the human and murine Ku autoantigens. *Mol Biol Rep* 1993;18(1):15–28.
217. Uwatoko S, Mannik M, Oppliger IR, et al. C1q-binding immunoglobulin G in MRL/l mice consists of immune complexes containing antibodies to DNA. *Clin Immunol Immunopathol* 1995;75(2):140–146.
218. Bloom DD, St. Clair EW, Pisetsky DS, et al. The anti-La response of a single MRL/Mp-lpr/lpr mouse: specificity for DNA and VH gene usage. *Eur J Immunol* 1994;24(6):1332–1338.
219. James JA, Mamula MJ, Harley JB. Sequential autoantigenic determinants of the small nuclear ribonucleoprotein Sm D shared by human lupus autoantibodies and MRL lpr/lpr antibodies. *Clin Exp Immunol* 1994;98(3):419–426.

220. Fatenejad S, Brooks W, Schwartz A, et al. Pattern of anti-small nuclear ribonucleoprotein antibodies in MRL/Mp- lpr/lpr mice suggests that the intact U1 snRNP particle is their autoimmunogenic target. *J Immunol* 1994;152(11):5523–5531.
221. Bloom DD, Davignon JL, Cohen PL, et al. Overlap of the anti-Sm and anti-DNA responses of MRL/Mp-lpr/lpr mice. *J Immunol* 1993;150(4):1579–1590.
222. Retter MW, Eisenberg RA, Cohen PL, et al. Sm and DNA binding by dual reactive B cells requires distinct VH, V kappa, and VH CDR3 structures. *J Immunol* 1995;155(4):2248–2257.
223. Bernstein KA, Valerio RD, Lefkowith JB. Glomerular binding activity in MRL lpr serum consists of antibodies that bind to a DNA/histone/type IV collagen complex. *J Immunol* 1995; 154(5):2424–2433.
224. Faulds G, Conroy S, Madaio M, et al. Increased levels of antibodies to heat shock proteins with increasing age in Mrl/Mp-lpr/lpr mice [see comments]. *Br J Rheumatol* 1995;34(7):610–615.
225. Dimitriu-Bona A, Matic M, Ding W, et al. Cytotoxicity to endothelial cells by sera from aged MRL/lpr/lpr mice is associated with autoimmunity to cell surface heparan sulfate. *Clin Immunol Immunopathol* 1995;76(3 pt 1):234–240.
226. Amoura Z, Chabre H, Koutouzov S, et al. Nucleosome-restricted antibodies are detected before anti-dsDNA and/or antihistone antibodies in serum of MRL-Mp lpr/lpr and +/+ mice, and are present in kidney eluates of lupus mice with proteinuria. *Arthritis Rheum* 1994;37(11):1684–1688.
227. Burlingame RW, Rubin RL, Balderas RS, et al. Genesis and evolution of antichromatin autoantibodies in murine lupus implicates T-dependent immunization with self antigen. *J Clin Invest* 1993;91(4):1687–1696.
228. Wahren M, Skarstein K, Blange I, et al. MRL/lpr mice produce anti-Ro 52,000 MW antibodies: detection, analysis of specificity and site of production. *Immunology* 1994;83(1):9–15.
229. Moore PM, Joshi I, Ghanekar SA. Affinity isolation of neuron-reactive antibodies in MRL/lpr mice. *J Neurosci Res* 1994; 39(2):140–147.
230. Panka DJ, Salant DJ, Jacobson BA, et al. The effect of VH residues 6 and 23 on IgG3 cryoprecipitation and glomerular deposition. *Eur J Immunol* 1995;25(1):279–284.
231. Berney T, Fulpius T, Shibata T, et al. Selective pathogenicity of murine rheumatoid factors of the cryoprecipitable IgG3 subclass. *Int Immunol* 1992;4(1):93–99.
232. Hang L, Theofilopoulos AN, Dixon FJ. A spontaneous rheumatoid arthritis-like disease in MRL/l mice. *J Exp Med* 1982;155(6):1690–1701.
233. O'Sullivan FX, Fassbender HG, Gay S, et al. Etiopathogenesis of the rheumatoid arthritis-like disease in MRL/l mice. I. The histomorphologic basis of joint destruction. *Arthritis Rheum* 1985;28(5):529–536.
234. Aguado MT, Balderas RS, Rubin RL, et al. Specificity and molecular characteristics of monoclonal IgM rheumatoid factors from arthritic and non-arthritic mice. *J Immunol* 1987;139(4): 1080–1087.
235. O'Sullivan FX, Vogelweid CM, Besch-Williford CL, et al. Differential effects of CD4+ T cell depletion on inflammatory central nervous system disease, arthritis and sialadenitis in MRL/lpr mice. *J Autoimmun* 1995;8(2):163–175.
236. Kanno H, Nose M, Itoh J, et al. Spontaneous development of pancreatitis in the MRL/Mp strain of mice in autoimmune mechanism. *Clin Exp Immunol* 1992;89(1):68–73.
237. Green LM, LaBue M, Lazarus JP, et al. Characterization of autoimmune thyroiditis in MRL-lpr/lpr mice. *Lupus* 1995; 4(3):187–196.
238. Brey RL, Cote S, Barohn R, et al. Model for the neuromuscular complications of systemic lupus erythematosus. *Lupus* 1995; 4(3):209–212.
239. Hoffman RW, Yang HK, Waggie KS, et al. Band keratopathy in MRL/l and MRL/n mice. *Arthritis Rheum* 1983;26(5): 645–652.
240. Hess DC, Taormina M, Thompson J, et al. Cognitive and neurologic deficits in the MRL/lpr mouse: a clinicopathologic study. *J Rheumatol* 1993;20(4):610–617.
241. Kusakari C, Hozawa K, Koike S, et al. MRL/MP-lpr/lpr mouse as a model of immune-induced sensorineural hearing loss. *Ann Otol Rhinol Laryngol Suppl* 1992;157:82–86.
242. Handwerger BS, Storrer CE, Wasson CS, et al. Further characterization of the autoantibody response of Palmerston North mice. *J Clin Immunol* 1999;19(1):45–57.
243. Eisenberg RA, Craven SY, Fisher CL, et al. The genetics of autoantibody production in MRL/lpr lupus mice. *Clin Exp Rheumatol* 1989;7(suppl 3):S35–S40.
244. Pisetsky DS, Semper KF, Eisenberg RA. Idiotypic analysis of a monoclonal anti-Sm antibody. II. Strain distribution of a common idiotypic determinant and its relationship to anti-Sm expression. *J Immunol* 1984;133(4):2085–2089.
245. Dang H, Takei M, Isenberg D, et al. Expression of an interspecies idiotype in sera of SLE patients and their first-degree relatives. *Clin Exp Immunol* 1988;71(3):445–450.
246. Andrews J, Hang L, Theofilopoulos AN, et al. Lack of relationship between serum gp70 levels and the severity of systemic lupus erythematosus in MRL/l mice. *J Exp Med* 1986;163(2): 458–462.
247. Merino R, Fossati L, Iwamoto M, et al. Effect of long-term anti-CD4 or anti-CD8 treatment on the development of lpr CD4– CD8– double negative T cells and of the autoimmune syndrome in MRL-lpr/lpr mice. *J Autoimmun* 1995;8(1):33–45.
248. Koh DR, Ho A, Rahemtulla A, et al. Murine lupus in MRL/lpr mice lacking CD4 or CD8 T cells. *Eur J Immunol* 1995;25(9): 2558–2562.
249. Ohteki T, Iwamoto M, Izui S, et al. Reduced development of CD4–8–B220+ T cells but normal autoantibody production in lpr/lpr mice lacking major histocompatibility complex class I molecules. *Eur J Immunol* 1995;25(1):37–41.
250. Mixter PF, Russell JQ, Budd RC. Delayed kinetics of T lymphocyte anergy and deletion in lpr mice. *J Autoimmun* 1994; 7(6):697–710.
251. Sobel ES, Kakkanaiah VN, Rapoport RG, et al. The abnormal lpr double-negative T cell fails to proliferate in vivo. *Clin Immunol Immunopathol* 1995;74(2):177–184.
252. Hammond DM, Nagarkatti PS, Gote LR, et al. Double-negative T cells from MRL-lpr/lpr mice mediate cytolytic activity when triggered through adhesion molecules and constitutively express perforin gene. *J Exp Med* 1993;178(6):2225–2230.
253. Rowley DA, Becken ET, Stach RM. Autoantibodies produced spontaneously by young 1pr mice carry transforming growth factor beta and suppress cytotoxic T lymphocyte responses. *J Exp Med* 1995;181(5):1875–1880.
254. Diaz GC, Jevnikar AM, Brennan DC, et al. Autoreactive kidney-infiltrating T-cell clones in murine lupus nephritis. *Kidney Int* 1992;42(4):851–859.
255. Diaz-Gallo C, Kelley VR. Self-regulation of autoreactive kidney-infiltrating T cells in MRL-lpr nephritis. *Kidney Int* 1993; 44(4):692–699.
256. Kelley VR, Singer GG. The antigen presentation function of renal tubular epithelial cells. *Exp Nephrol* 1993;1(2):102–111.
257. Jevnikar AM, Grusby MJ, Glimcher LH. Prevention of nephritis in major histocompatibility complex class II- deficient MRL-lpr mice. *J Exp Med* 1994;179(4):1137–1143.
258. Gilkeson GS, Spurney R, Coffman TM, et al. Effect of anti-CD4 antibody treatment on inflammatory arthritis in MRL- lpr/lpr mice. *Clin Immunol Immunopathol* 1992;64(2):166–172.
259. Ohkusu K, Isobe K, Hidaka H, et al. Elucidation of the protein

kinase C-dependent apoptosis pathway in distinct subsets of T lymphocytes in MRL-lpr/lpr mice. *Eur J Immunol* 1995;25(11): 3180–3186.

260. Hayashi Y, Hamano H, Haneji N, et al. Biased T cell receptor V beta gene usage during specific stages of the development of autoimmune sialadenitis in the MRL/lpr mouse model of Sjogren's syndrome. *Arthritis Rheum* 1995;38(8):1077–1084.
261. de Alboran IM, Gonzalo JA, Kroemer G, et al. Attenuation of autoimmune disease and lymphocyte accumulation in MRL/lpr mice by treatment with anti-V beta 8 antibodies. *Eur J Immunol* 1992;22(8):2153–2158.
262. Davignon JL, Cohen PL, Eisenberg RA. Rapid T cell receptor modulation accompanies lack of in vitro mitogenic responsiveness of double negative T cells to anti-CD3 monoclonal antibody in MRL/Mp-lpr mice. *J Immunol* 1988;141(6):1848–1854.
263. Scholz W, Isakov N, Mally MI, et al. Lpr T cell hyporesponsiveness to mitogens linked to deficient receptor- stimulated phosphoinositide hydrolysis. *J Biol Chem* 1988;263(8):3626–3631.
264. Thomas TJ, Gunnia UB, Seibold JR, et al. Defective signal-transduction pathways in T-cells from autoimmune MRL-lpr/lpr mice are associated with increased polyamine concentrations. *Biochem J* 1995;311 (Pt 1):175–182.
265. Prud'Homme GJ, Kono DH, Theofilopoulos AN. Quantitative polymerase chain reaction analysis reveals marked overexpression of interleukin-1 beta, interleukin-1 and interferon-gamma mRNA in the lymph nodes of lupus-prone mice. *Mol Immunol* 1995;32(7):495–503.
266. Raz E, Dudler J, Lotz M, et al. Modulation of disease activity in murine systemic lupus erythematosus by cytokine gene delivery. *Lupus* 1995;4(4):286–292.
267. Hosaka N, Nagata N, Nakagawa T, et al. Analyses of lpr-GVHD by adoptive transfer experiments using MRL/lpr-Thy-1.1 congenic mice. *Autoimmunity* 1994;17(3):217–224.
268. Hosaka N, Nagata N, Miyashima S, et al. Attenuation of lpr-graft-versus-host disease (GVHD) in MRL/lpr spleen cell-injected SCID mice by in vivo treatment with anti-V beta 8.1,2 monoclonal antibody. *Clin Exp Immunol* 1994;96(3):500–507.
269. Ashany D, Hines JJ, Gharavi AE, et al. MRL/lpr—>severe combined immunodeficiency mouse allografts produce autoantibodies, acute graft-versus-host disease or a wasting syndrome depending on the source of cells. *Clin Exp Immunol* 1992; 90(3):466–475.
270. Sobel ES, Katagiri T, Katagiri K, et al. An intrinsic B cell defect is required for the production of autoantibodies in the lpr model of murine systemic autoimmunity. *J Exp Med* 1991; 173(6):1441–1449.
271. Cavallo T, Granholm NA. Lipopolysaccharide from gram-negative bacteria enhances polyclonal B cell activation and exacerbates nephritis in MRL/lpr mice. *Clin Exp Immunol* 1990; 82(3):515–521.
272. Klinman DM, Eisenberg RA, Steinberg AD. Development of the autoimmune B cell repertoire in MRL-lpr/lpr mice. *J Immunol* 1990;144(2):506–511.
273. Lebedeva TV, Singh AK. Increased responsiveness of B. cells in the murine MRL/lpr model of lupus nephritis to interleukin-1 beta. *J Am Soc Nephrol* 1995;5(7):1530–1534.
274. Kobayashi I, Matsuda T, Saito T, et al. Abnormal distribution of IL-6 receptor in aged MRL/lpr mice: elevated expression on B cells and absence on CD4+ cells. *Int Immunol* 1992; 4(12):1407–1412.
275. Roark JH, Kuntz CL, Nguyen KA, et al. Breakdown of B cell tolerance in a mouse model of systemic lupus erythematosus. *J Exp Med* 1995;181(3):1157–1167.
276. Shan H, Shlomchik MJ, Marshak-Rothstein A, et al. The mechanism of autoantibody production in an autoimmune MRL/lpr mouse. *J Immunol* 1994;153(11):5104–5120.
277. Karussis DM, Vourka-Karussis U, Lehmann D, et al. Immunomodulation of autoimmunity in MRL/lpr mice with syngeneic bone marrow transplantation (SBMT). *Clin Exp Immunol* 1995;100(1):111–117.
278. Takeoka Y, Yoshida SH, Van de WJ, et al. Thymic microenvironmental abnormalities in MRL/MP-lpr/lpr, BXSB/MpJ Yaa and C3H HeJ-gld/gld mice. *J Autoimmun* 1995;8(2):145–161.
279. Kotzin BL, Herron LR, Babcock SK, et al. Self-reactive T cells in murine lupus: analysis of genetic contributions and development of self-tolerance. *Clin Immunol Immunopathol* 1989;53(2 pt 2):S35–S46.
280. Singer PA, Balderas RS, McEvilly RJ, et al. Tolerance-related V beta clonal deletions in normal CD4–8–, TCR- alpha/beta + and abnormal lpr and gld cell populations. *J Exp Med* 1989; 170(6):1869–1877.
281. Papiernik M, Pontoux C, Golstein P. Non-exclusive Fas control and age dependence of viral superantigen- induced clonal deletion in lupus-prone mice. *Eur J Immunol* 1995;25(6): 1517–1523.
282. Zhou T, Bluethmann H, Zhang J, et al. Defective maintenance of T cell tolerance to a superantigen in MRL-lpr/lpr mice. *J Exp Med* 1992;176(4):1063–1072.
283. Steinberg AD, Roths JB, Murphy ED, et al. Effects of thymectomy or androgen administration upon the autoimmune disease of MRL/Mp-lpr/lpr mice. *J Immunol* 1980;125(2):871–873.
284. Gresham HD, Ray CJ, O'Sullivan FX. Defective neutrophil function in the autoimmune mouse strain MRL/lpr. Potential role of transforming growth factor-beta. *J Immunol* 1991; 146(11):3911–3921.
285. Levine JS, Pugh BJ, Hartwell D, et al. Interleukin-1 dysregulation is an intrinsic defect in macrophages from MRL autoimmune-prone mice. *Eur J Immunol* 1993;23(11):2951–2958.
286. Hartwell DW, Fenton MJ, Levine JS, et al. Aberrant cytokine regulation in macrophages from young autoimmune-prone mice: evidence that the intrinsic defect in MRL macrophage IL-1 expression is transcriptionally controlled. *Mol Immunol* 1995; 32(10):743–751.
287. Field M, Brennan FM, Melsom RD, et al. MRL mice show an age-related impairment of IgG aggregate removal from the circulation. *Clin Exp Immunol* 1985;61(1):195–202.
288. Eischen CM, Dick CJ, Leibson PJ. Tyrosine kinase activation provides an early and requisite signal for Fas-induced apoptosis. *J Immunol* 1994;153(5):1947–1954.
289. Tian Q, Taupin J, Elledge S, et al. Fas-activated serine/threonine kinase (FAST) phosphorylates TIA-1 during Fas-mediated apoptosis. *J Exp Med* 1995;182(3):865–874.
290. Cifone MG, De Maria R, Roncaioli P, et al. Apoptotic signaling through CD95 (Fas/Apo-1) activates an acidic sphingomyelinase. *J Exp Med* 1994;180(4):1547–1552.
291. Gulbins E, Bissonnette R, Mahboubi A, et al. FAS-induced apoptosis is mediated via a ceramide-initiated RAS signaling pathway. *Immunity* 1995;2(4):341–351.
292. Tekpper CG, Jayadev S, Liu B, et al. Role for ceramide as an endogenous mediator of Fas-induced cytotoxicity. *Proc Natl Acad Sci USA* 92, 8443–8447. 1995.
293. Los M, Van de CM, Penning LC, et al. Requirement of an ICE/CED-3 protease for Fas/APO-1-mediated apoptosis. *Nature* 1995;375(6526):81–83.
294. Enari M, Hug H, Nagata S. Involvement of an ICE-like protease in Fas-mediated apoptosis. *Nature* 1995;375(6526):78–81.
295. Tewari M, Dixit VM. Fas- and tumor necrosis factor-induced apoptosis is inhibited by the poxvirus crmA gene product. *J Biol Chem* 1995;270(7):3255–3260.
296. Kuida K, Lippke JA, Ku G, et al. Altered cytokine export and apoptosis in mice deficient in interleukin-1 beta converting enzyme. *Science* 1995;267(5206):2000–2003.

297. Su X, Zhou T, Wang Z, et al. Defective expression of hematopoietic cell protein tyrosine phosphatase (HCP) in lymphoid cells blocks Fas-mediated apoptosis. *Immunity* 1995;2(4): 353–362.
298. McGahahn AJ, Nishioka WK, Marin SJ, et al. Regulation of the Fas apoptotic cell death pathway by Abl. *J Biol Chem* 1995; 270:22625–22631.
299. Dhein J, Walczak H, Baumler C, et al. Autocrine T-cell suicide mediated by APO-1/(Fas/CD95). *Nature* 1995;373(6513): 438–441.
300. Musette P, Pannetier C, Gachelin G, et al. The expansion of a CD4+ T cell population bearing a distinctive beta chain in MRL lpr/lpr mice suggests a role for the fas protein in peripheral T cell selection. *Eur J Immunol* 1994;24(11):2761–2766.
301. Ju ST, Panka DJ, Cui H, et al. Fas(CD95)/FasL interactions required for programmed cell death after T- cell activation [see comments]. *Nature* 1995;373(6513):444–448.
302. Reap EA, Leslie D, Abrahams M, et al. Apoptosis abnormalities of splenic lymphocytes in autoimmune lpr and gld mice. *J Immunol* 1995;154(2):936–943.
303. Ju ST, Cui H, Panka DJ, et al. Participation of target Fas protein in apoptosis pathway induced by CD4+ Th1 and CD8+ cytotoxic T cells. *Proc Natl Acad Sci USA* 1994;91(10): 4185–4189.
304. Berke G. The CTL's kiss of death. *Cell* 1995;81(1):9–12.
305. Rathmell JC, Cooke MP, Ho WY, et al. CD95 (Fas)-dependent elimination of self-reactive B cells upon interaction with CD4+ T cells. *Nature* 1995;376(6536):181–184.
306. Wu J, Zhou T, Zhang J, et al. Correction of accelerated autoimmune disease by early replacement of the mutated lpr gene with the normal Fas apoptosis gene in the T cells of transgenic MRL-lpr/lpr mice. *Proc Natl Acad Sci USA* 1994;91(6):2344–2348.
307. Vidal S, Kono DH, Theofilopoulos AN. Loci predisposing to autoimmunity in MRL-Fas(lpr) and C57BL/6-Faslpr mice. *J Clin Invest* 1998;101(3):696–702.
308. Murphy ED, Roths JB. New inbred strains. *Mouse News Lett* 1978;58:51–65.
309. Murphy ED, Roths JB. A Y chromosome associated factor in strain BXSB producing accelerated autoimmunity and lymphoproliferation. *Arthritis Rheum* 1979;22(11):1188–1194.
310. Hoffman SA, Arbogast DN, Ford PM, et al. Brain-reactive autoantibody levels in the sera of ageing autoimmune mice. *Clin Exp Immunol* 1987;70(1):74–83.
311. Makin M, Fumiwara M, Watanabe H. Studies on the mechanisms of the development of lupus nephritis in BXSB mic. I. Analyses of immunological abnormalities at the onset preiod. *J Clin Lab Immunol* 1987;22:127–131.
312. Garlepp MJ, Hart DA, Fritzler MJ. Regulation of plasma complement C4 and factor b levels in murine systemic lupus erythematosus. *J Clin Lab Immunol* 1989;28(3):137–141.
313. Blossom S, Chu EB, Weigle WO, et al. CD40 ligand expressed on B cells in the BXSB mouse model of systemic lupus erythematosus. *J Immunol* 1997;159(9):4580–4586.
314. Blossom S, Gilbert KM. Antibody production in autoimmune BXSB mice. I. CD40L-expressing B cells need fewer signals for polyclonal antibody synthesis. *Clin Exp Immunol* 1999;118(1): 147–153.
315. Garnier JL, Merino R, Kimoto M, et al. Resistance to tolerance induction to human gammaglobulin (HGG) in autoimmune BXSB/MpJ mice: functional analysis of antigen-presenting cells and HGG-specific T helper cells. *Clin Exp Immunol* 1988; 73(2):283–288.
316. Fossati L, Iwamoto M, Merino R, et al. Selective enhancing effect of the Yaa gene on immune responses against self and foreign antigens. *Eur J Immunol* 1995;25(1):166–173.
317. Fossati L, Sobel ES, Iwamoto M, et al. The Yaa gene-mediated acceleration of murine lupus: Yaa- T cells from non-autoimmune mice collaborate with Yaa+ B cells to produce lupus autoantibodies in vivo. *Eur J Immunol* 1995;25(12):3412–3417.
318. Dumont FJ, Habbersett RC. Alterations of the T-cell population in BXSB mice: early imbalance of 9F3-defined Lyt-2+ subsets occurs in the males with rapid onset lupic syndrome. *Cell Immunol* 1986;101(1):39–50.
319. Wofsy D. Administration of monoclonal anti-T cell antibodies retards murine lupus in BXSB mice. *J Immunol* 1986;136(12): 4554–4560.
320. Wang B, Yamamoto Y, El Badri NS, et al. Effective treatment of autoimmune disease and progressive renal disease by mixed bone-marrow transplantation that establishes a stable mixed chimerism in BXSB recipient mice. *Proc Natl Acad Sci USA* 1999;96(6):3012–3016.
321. Chu EB, Hobbs MV, Wilson CB, et al. Intervention of CD4+ cell subset shifts and autoimmunity in the BXSB mouse by murine CTLA4Ig. *J Immunol* 1996;156(3):1262–1268.
322. Chu EB, Hobbs MV, Ernst DN, et al. In vivo tolerance induction and associated cytokine production by subsets of murine CD4+ T cells. *J Immunol* 1995;154(10):4909–4914.
323. Chu EB, Ernst DN, Hobbs MV, et al. Maturational changes in CD4+ cell subsets and lymphokine production in BXSB mice. *J Immunol* 1994;152(8):4129–4138.
324. Kono DH, Balomenos D, Park MS, et al. Development of lupus in BXSB mice is independent of IL-4. *J Immunol* 2000; 164(1):38–42.
325. Takeoka Y, Taguchi N, Shultz L, et al. Apoptosis and the thymic microenvironment in murine lupus. *J Autoimmun* 1999;13(3): 325–334.
326. Dardenne M, Savino W, Nabarra B, et al. Male BXSB mice develop a thymic hormonal dysfunction with presence of intraepithelial crystalline inclusions. *Clin Immunol Immunopathol* 1989; 52(3):392–405.
327. Smith HR, Chused TM, Smathers PA, et al. Evidence for thymic regulation of autoimmunity in BXSB mice: acceleration of disease by neonatal thymectomy. *J Immunol* 1983;130(3): 1200–1204.
328. Vieten G, Grams B, Muller M, et al. Examination of the mononuclear phagocyte system in lupus-prone male BXSB mice. *J Leukoc Biol* 1996;59(3):325–332.
329. Cole EH, Sweet J, Levy GA. Expression of macrophage procoagulant activity in murine systemic lupus erythematosus. *J Clin Invest* 1986;78(4):887–893.
330. Scribner CL, Steinberg AD. The role of splenic colony-forming units in autoimmune disease. *Clin Immunol Immunopathol* 1988;49(1):133–142.
331. Ikehara S, Nakamura T, Sekita K, et al. Treatment of systemic and organ-specific autoimmune disease in mice by allogeneic bone marrow transplantation. *Prog Clin Biol Res* 1987;229: 131–146.
332. Eisenberg RA, Izui S, McConahey PJ, et al. Male determined accelerated autoimmune disease in BXSB mice: transfer by bone marrow and spleen cells. *J Immunol* 1980;125(3):1032–1036.
333. Eisenberg RA, Dixon FJ. Effect of castration on male-determined acceleration of autoimmune disease in BXSB mice. *J Immunol* 1980;125(5):1959–1961.
334. Merino R, Fossati L, Lacour M, et al. H-2-linked control of the Yaa gene-induced acceleration of lupus-like autoimmune disease in BXSB mice. *Eur J Immunol* 1992;22(2):295–299.
335. Kawano H, Abe M, Zhang D, et al. Heterozygosity of the major histocompatibility complex controls the autoimmune disease in (NZW × BXSB) F1 mice. *Clin Immunol Immunopathol* 1992; 65(3):308–314.
336. Izui S, Iwamoto M, Fossati L, et al. The Yaa gene model of systemic lupus erythematosus. *Immunol Rev* 1995;144:137–156.

337. Merino R, Iwamoto M, Fossati L, et al. Prevention of systemic lupus erythematosus in autoimmune BXSB mice by a transgene encoding I-E alpha chain. *J Exp Med* 1993;178(4):1189–1197.
338. Iwamoto M, Ibnou-Zekri N, Araki K, et al. Prevention of murine lupus by an I-E alpha chain transgene: protective role of I-E alpha chain-derived peptides with a high affinity to I-Ab molecules. *Eur J Immunol* 1996;26(2):307–314.
339. Ibnou-Zekri N, Iwamoto M, Fossati L, et al. Role of the major histocompatibility complex class II Ea gene in lupus susceptibility in mice. *Proc Natl Acad Sci USA* 1997;94(26): 14654–14659.
340. Ibnou-Zekri N, Iwamoto M, Gershwin ME, et al. Protection of murine lupus by the Ead transgene is MHC haplotype- dependent. *J Immunol* 2000;164(1):505–511.
341. Hogarth MB, Slingsby JH, Allen PJ, et al. Multiple lupus susceptibility loci map to chromosome 1 in BXSB mice. *J Immunol* 1998;161(6):2753–2761.
342. Haywood ME, Hogarth MB, Slingsby JH, et al. Identification of intervals on chromosomes 1, 3, and 13 linked to the development of lupus in BXSB mice. *Arthritis Rheum* 2000;43(2): 349–355.
343. Hashimoto Y, Kawamura M, Ichikawa K, et al. Anticardiolipin antibodies in NZW × BXSB F1 mice. A model of antiphospholipid syndrome. *J Immunol* 1992;149(3):1063–1068.
344. Mizutani H, Engelman RW, Kinjoh K, et al. Gastrointestinal vasculitis in autoimmune-prone (NZW × BXSB)F1 mice: association with anticardiolipin autoantibodies. *Proc Soc Exp Biol Med* 1995;209(3):279–285.
345. Adachi Y, Inaba M, Sugihara A, et al. Effects of administration of monoclonal antibodies (anti-CD4 or anti-CD8) on the development of autoimmune diseases in (NZW × BXSB)F1 mice. *Immunobiology* 1998;198(4):451–464.
346. Good RA. Progress toward production of immunologic tolerance with no or minimal toxic immunosuppression for prevention of immunodeficiency and autoimmune diseases. *World J Surg* 2000;24(7):797–810.
347. Suzuka H, Fujiwara H, Tanaka M, et al. Antithrombotic effect of ticlopidine on occlusive thrombi of small coronary arteries in (NZW×BXSB)F1 male mice with myocardial infarction and systemic lupus erythematosus. *J Cardiovasc Pharmacol* 1995; 25(1):9–13.
348. Tanaka M, Fujiwara H, Shibata Y, et al. Effects of chronic oral administration of nifedipine and diltiazem on occlusive thrombus of small coronary arteries in (NZW × BXSB)F1 male mice. *Cardiovasc Res* 1992;26(6):586–592.
349. Ida A, Hirose S, Hamano Y, et al. Multigenic control of lupus-associated antiphospholipid syndrome in a model of (NZW × BXSB) F1 mice. *Eur J Immunol* 1998;28(9):2694–2703.
350. Roths JB, Murphy ED, Eicher EM. A new mutation, gld, that produces lymphoproliferation and autoimmunity in C3H/HeJ mice. *J Exp Med* 1984;159(1):1–20.
351. Takahashi T, Tanaka M, Brannan CI, et al. Generalized lymphoproliferative disease in mice, caused by a point mutation in the Fas ligand. *Cell* 1994;76(6):969–976.
352. Lynch DH, Watson ML, Alderson MR, et al. The mouse Fas-ligand gene is mutated in gld mice and is part of a TNFALPHA family gene cluster. *Immunity* 1994;1(2):131–136.
353. Hahne M, Peitsch MC, Irmler M, et al. Characterization of the non-functional Fas ligand of gld mice. *Int Immunol* 1995;7(9): 1381–1386.
354. Mixter PF, Russell JQ, Morrissette GJ, et al. A model for the origin of TCR-alphabeta+ CD4–CD8– B220+ cells based on high affinity TCR signals. *J Immunol* 1999;162(10):5747–5756.
355. Bhandoola A, Yui K, Siegel RM, et al. Gld and lpr mice: single gene mutant models for failed self tolerance. *Int Rev Immunol* 1994;11(3):231–244.
356. Davidson WF, Giese T, Fredrickson TN. Spontaneous development of plasmacytoid tumors in mice with defective Fas-Fas ligand interactions. *J Exp Med* 1998;187(11):1825–1838.
357. Zhu B, Beaudette BC, Rifkin IR, et al. Double mutant MRL-lpr/lpr-gld/gld cells fail to trigger lpr-graft-versus-host disease in syngeneic wild-type recipient mice, but can induce wild-type B cells to make autoantibody. *Eur J Immunol* 2000;30(6): 1778–1784.
358. Satoh M, Weintraub JP, Yoshida H, et al. Fas and Fas ligand mutations inhibit autoantibody production in pristane-induced lupus. *J Immunol* 2000;165(2):1036–1043.
359. Zhang HG, Fleck M, Kern ER, et al. Antigen presenting cells expressing Fas ligand down-modulate chronic inflammatory disease in Fas ligand-deficient mice. *J Clin Invest* 2000;105(6): 813–821.
360. Su X, Hu Q, Kristan JM, et al. Significant role for Fas in the pathogenesis of autoimmune diabetes. *J Immunol* 2000;164(5): 2523–2532.
361. Korner H, Cretney E, Wilhelm P, et al. Tumor necrosis factor sustains the generalized lymphoproliferative disorder (gld) phenotype [published erratum appears in *J Exp Med* 2000;191(8): following 1948]. *J Exp Med* 2000;191(1):89–96.
362. Maldonado MA, MacDonald GC, Kakkanaiah VN, et al. Differential control of autoantibodies and lymphoproliferation by Fas ligand expression on CD4+ and CD8+ T cells in vivo. *J Immunol* 1999;163(6):3138–3142.
363. Walker SE, Gray RH, Fulton M, et al. Palmerston North mice, a new animal model of systemic lupus erythematosus. *J Lab Clin Med* 1978;92:932–945.
364. Walker SE, Hewett JE. Responses to T-cell and B-cell mitogens in autoimmune Palmerston North and NZB/NZW mice. *Clin Immunol Immunopathol* 1984;30(3):469–478.
365. Luzina IG, Knitzer RH, Atamas SP, et al. Vasculitis in the Palmerston North mouse model of lupus: phenotype and cytokine production profile of infiltrating cells. *Arthritis Rheum* 1999;42(3):561–568.
366. Van Elven EG, Van Der Veen FM, Rolink AG, et al. Diseases caused by reactions of T lymphocytes against incompatible structures of the major histocompatibility complex. V. high titers of IgG autoantibodies to double-stranded DNA. *J Immunol* 1983;127:2435–2458.
367. Rolink AG, Pals ST, Gleichmann E. Allosuppressor and allohelper T cells in acute and chronic graft-vs.- host disease. II. F1 recipients carrying mutations at H-2K and/or I-A. *J Exp Med* 1983;157(2):755–771.
368. Chu JL, Ramos P, Rosendorff A, et al. Massive upregulation of the Fas ligand in lpr and gld mice: implications for Fas regulation and the graft-versus-host disease-like wasting syndrome. *J Exp Med* 1995;181(1):393–398.
369. Gleichmann E, Van Elven EH, Van der Veen JP. A systemic lupus erythematosus (SLE)-like disease in mice induced by abnormal T-B cell cooperation. Preferential formation of autoantibodies characteristic of SLE. *Eur J Immunol* 1982; 12(2):152–159.
370. Gleichmann H, Gleichmann E, Andre-Schwartz J, et al. Chronic allogeneic disease. 3. Genetic requirements for the induction of glomerulonephritis. *J Exp Med* 1972;135(3): 516–532.
371. Kimura M, Rappard-van der Veen FM, Gleichmann E. Requirement of H-2-subregion differences for graft-versus-host autoimmunity in mice: superiority of the differences at class-II H-2 antigens (I-A/I-E). *Clin Exp Immunol* 1986;65(3):542–552.
372. Portanova JP, Ebling FM, Hammond WS, et al. Allogeneic MHC antigen requirements for lupus-like autoantibody production and nephritis in murine graft-vs-host disease. *J Immunol* 1988;141(10):3370–3376.

373. Rus V, Svetic A, Nguyen P, et al. Kinetics of Th1 and Th2 cytokine production during the early course of acute and chronic murine graft-versus-host disease. Regulatory role of donor CD8+ T cells. *J Immunol* 1995;155(5):2396–2406.
374. Shustov A, Nguyen P, Finkelman F, et al. Differential expression of Fas and Fas ligand in acute and chronic graft-versus-host disease: up-regulation of Fas and Fas ligand requires CD8+ T cell activation and IFN-gamma production. *J Immunol* 1998;161(6):2848–2855.
375. Krenger W, Rossi S, Piali L, et al. Thymic atrophy in murine acute graft-versus-host disease is effected by impaired cell cycle progression of host pro-T and pre-T cells. *Blood* 2000;96(1): 347–354.
376. Shustov A, Luzina I, Nguyen P, et al. Role of perforin in controlling B-cell hyperactivity and humoral autoimmunity [see comments]. *J Clin Invest* 2000;106(6):R39–R47.
377. Schorlemmer HU, Dickneite G, Kanzy EJ, et al. Modulation of the immunoglobulin dysregulation in GvH- and SLE-like diseases by the murine IL-4 receptor (IL-4-R). *Inflamm Res* 1995;44(suppl 2):S194–S196.
378. Strasser A, Whittingham S, Vaux DL, et al. Enforced BCL2 expression in B-lymphoid cells prolongs antibody responses and elicits autoimmune disease. *Proc Natl Acad Sci USA* 1991; 88(19):8661–8665.
379. Reap EA, Felix NJ, Wolthusen PA, et al. bcl-2 transgenic Lpr mice show profound enhancement of lymphadenopathy. *J Immunol* 1995;155(11):5455–5462.
380. Moroy T, Grzeschiczek A, Petzold S, et al. Expression of a Pim-1 transgene accelerates lymphoproliferation and inhibits apoptosis in lpr/lpr mice. *Proc Natl Acad Sci USA* 1993;90(22): 10734–10738.
381. Marsters SA, Yan M, Pitti RM, et al. Interaction of the TNFalpha homologues BLyS and APRIL with the TNFalpha receptor homologues BCMA and TACI. *Curr Biol* 2000;10(13): 785–788.
382. Laabi Y, Strasser A. Immunology. Lymphocyte survival—ignorance is BLys. *Science* 2000;289(5481):883–884.
383. Lhare SD, Sarosi I, Xia XZ, et al. Severe B cell hyperplasia and autoimmune disease in TALL-1 transgenic mice. *Proc Natl Acad Sci USA* 2000;97(7):3370–3375.
384. Hibbs ML, Tarlinton DM, Armes J, et al. Multiple defects in the immune system of Lyn-deficient mice, culminating in autoimmune disease. *Cell* 1995;83(2):301–311.
385. Nishizumi H, Taniuchi I, Yamanashi Y, et al. Impaired proliferation of peripheral B cells and indication of autoimmune disease in lyn-deficient mice. *Immunity* 1995;3(5):549–560.
386. Cornall RJ, Cyster JG, Hibbs ML, et al. Polygenic autoimmune traits: Lyn, CD22, and SHP-1 are limiting elements of a biochemical pathway regulating BCR signaling and selection. *Immunity* 1998;8(4):497–508.
387. Shultz LD, Schweitzer PA, Rajan TV, et al. Mutations at the murine motheaten locus are within the hematopoietic cell protein-tyrosine phosphatase (Hcph) gene. *Cell* 1993;73(7): 1445–1454.
388. Tsui HW, Siminivitch KA, de Souza L, et al. Motheaten and viable motheaten mice have mutations in the haematopoietic cell phosphatase gene. *Nat Genet* 1995;4:124–129.
389. Nishimura H, Honjo T, Minato N. Facilitation of beta selection and modification of positive selection in the thymus of PD-1-deficient mice. *J Exp Med* 2000;191(5):891–898.
390. Balomenos D, Martin-Caballero J, Garcia MI, et al. The cell cycle inhibitor p21 controls T-cell proliferation and sex- linked lupus development. *Nat Med* 2000;6(2):171–176.
391. Walport MJ, Davies KA, Botto M. C1q and systemic lupus erythematosus. *Immunobiology* 1998;199(2):265–285.
392. Taylor PR, Carugati A, Fadok VA, et al. A hierarchical role for classical pathway complement proteins in the clearance of apoptotic cells in vivo. *J Exp Med* 2000;192(3):359–366.
393. Bickerstaff MC, Botto M, Hutchinson WL, et al. Serum amyloid P component controls chromatin degradation and prevents antinuclear autoimmunity [see comments]. *Nat Med* 1999; 5(6):694–697.
394. Napirei M, Karsunky H, Zevnik B, et al. Features of systemic lupus erythematosus in Dnase1-deficient mice [see comments]. *Nat Genet* 2000;25(2):177–181.
395. Ehrenstein MR, Katz DR, Griffiths MH, et al. Human IgG anti-DNA antibodies deposit in kidneys and induce proteinuria in SCID mice. *Kidney Int* 1995;48(3):705–711.
396. Xu H, Li H, Suri-Payer E, et al. Regulation of anti-DNA B cells in recombination-activating gene-deficient mice. *J Exp Med* 1998;188(7):1247–1254.
397. Mandik-Nayak L, Seo SJ, Sokol C, et al. MRL-lpr/lpr mice exhibit a defect in maintaining developmental arrest and follicular exclusion of anti-double-stranded DNA B cells. *J Exp Med* 1999;189(11):1799–1814.
398. Bynoe MS, Spatz L, Diamond B. Characterization of anti-DNA B cells that escape negative selection. *Eur J Immunol* 1999; 29(4):1304–1313.
399. Mendlovic S, Brocke S, Shoenfeld Y, et al. Induction of a systemic lupus erythematosus-like disease in mice by a common human anti-DNA idiotype. *Proc Natl Acad Sci USA* 1988; 85(7):2260–2264.
400. Mendlovic S, Fricke H, Shoenfeld Y, et al. The role of anti-idiotypic antibodies in the induction of experimental systemic lupus erythematosus in mice. *Eur J Immunol* 1989;19(4):729–734.
401. Shoenfeld Y. Idiotypic induction of autoimmunity: a new aspect of the idiotypic network. *FASEB J* 1994;8(15):1296–1301.
402. Bakimer R, Fishman P, Blank M, et al. Induction of primary antiphospholipid syndrome in mice by immunization with a human monoclonal anticardiolipin antibody (H-3). *J Clin Invest* 1992;89(5):1558–1563.
403. Sthoeger ZM, Tartakovsky B, Bentwich Z, et al. Monoclonal anticardiolipin antibodies derived from mice with experimental lupus erythematosus: characterization and the induction of a secondary antiphospholipid syndrome. *J Clin Immunol* 1993; 13(2):127–138.
404. Krause I, Blank M, Kopolovic J, et al. Abrogation of experimental systemic lupus erythematosus and primary antiphospholipid syndrome with intravenous gamma globulin. *J Rheumatol* 1995;22(6):1068–1074.
405. Blank M, Tomer Y, Slavin S, et al. Induction of tolerance to experimental anti-phospholipid syndrome (APS) by syngeneic bone marrow cell transplantation. *Scand J Immunol* 1995;42(2): 226–234.
406. Blank M, Krause I, Buskila D, et al. Bromocriptine immunomodulation of experimental SLE and primary antiphospholipid syndrome via induction of nonspecific T suppressor cells. *Cell Immunol* 1995;162(1):114–122.
407. Shoenfeld Y, Blank M. Effect of long-acting thromboxane receptor antagonist (BMS 180,291) on experimental antiphospholipid syndrome. *Lupus* 1994;3(5):397–400.
408. Tomer Y, Blank M, Shoenfeld Y. Suppression of experimental antiphospholipid syndrome and systemic lupus erythematosus in mice by anti-CD4 monoclonal antibodies. *Arthritis Rheum* 1994;37(8):1236–1244.
409. Levite M, Zinger H, Zisman E, et al. Beneficial effects of bone marrow transplantation on the serological manifestations and kidney pathology of experimental systemic lupus erythematosus. *Cell Immunol* 1995;162(1):138–145.
410. Mozes E, Kohn LD, Hakim F, et al. Resistance of MHC class I-deficient mice to experimental systemic lupus erythematosus. *Science* 1993;261(5117):91–93.

411. Desai DD, Krishnan MR, Swindle JT, et al. Antigen-specific induction of antibodies against native mammalian DNA in nonautoimmune mice. *J Immunol* 1993;151(3):1614–1626.
412. Reeves WH, Satoh M, Wang J, et al. Systemic lupus erythematosus. Antibodies to DNA, DNA-binding proteins, and histones. *Rheum Dis Clin North Am* 1994;20(1):1–28.
413. Gilkeson GS, Grudier JP, Karounos DG, et al. Induction of anti-double stranded DNA antibodies in normal mice by immunization with bacterial DNA. *J Immunol* 1989;142(5): 1482–1486.
414. Scofield RH, Kaufman KM, Baber U, et al. Immunization of mice with human 60-kd Ro peptides results in epitope spreading if the peptides are highly homologous between human and mouse. *Arthritis Rheum* 1999;42(5):1017–1024.
415. Farris AD, Brown L, Reynolds P, et al. Induction of autoimmunity by multivalent immunodominant and subdominant T cell determinants of La (SS-B). *J Immunol* 1999;162(5):3079–3087.
416. Arbuckle MR, Gross T, Scofield RH, et al. Lupus humoral autoimmunity induced in a primate model by short peptide immunization. *J Invest Med* 1998;46(2):58–65.
417. Scofield RH, Henry WE, Kurien BT, et al. Immunization with short peptides from the sequence of the systemic lupus erythematosus-associated 60-kDa Ro autoantigen results in anti-Ro ribonucleoprotein autoimmunity. *J Immunol* 1996;156(10): 4059–4066.
418. Mason LJ, Timothy LM, Isenberg DA, et al. Immunization with a peptide of Sm B/B′ results in limited epitope spreading but not autoimmune disease. *J Immunol* 1999;162(9):5099–5105.
419. Satoh M, Kumar A, Kanwar YS, et al. Anti-nuclear antibody production and immune-complex glomerulonephritis in BALB/c mice treated with pristane. *Proc Natl Acad Sci USA* 1995; 92(24):10934–10938.
420. Boswell JM, Yui MA, Endres S, et al. Novel and enhanced IL-1 gene expression in autoimmune mice with lupus. *J Immunol* 1988;141(1):118–124.
421. Kelley VE, Sneve S, Musinski S. Increased renal thromboxane production in murine lupus nephritis. *J Clin Invest* 1986;77(1): 252–259.
422. Magilavy DB, Rothstein JL. Spontaneous production of tumor necrosis factor alpha by Kupffer cells of MRL/lpr mice. *J Exp Med* 1988;168(2):789–794.
423. Meryhew NL, Shaver C, Messner RP, et al. Mononuclear phagocyte system dysfunction in murine SLE: abnormal clearance kinetics precede clinical disease. *J Lab Clin Med* 1991; 117(3):181–193.
424. Mullins WW Jr, Plotz PH, Schrieber L. Soluble immune complexes in lupus mice: clearance from blood and estimation of formation rates. *Clin Immunol Immunopathol* 1987;42(3): 375–385.
425. Bloom RD, Florquin S, Singer GG, et al. Colony stimulating factor-1 in the induction of lupus nephritis. *Kidney Int* 1993; 43(5):1000–1009.
426. Casey TP, Howie JB. Autoimmune haemolytic anaemia in NZB/B1 mice treated with the corticosteroid drug betamethasone. *Blood* 1965;43:1000–1009.
427. Appleby P, Webber DG, Bowen JG. Murine chronic graft-versus-host disease as a model of systemic lupus erythematosus: effect of immunosuppressive drugs on disease development. *Clin Exp Immunol* 1989;78(3):449–453.
428. Casey TP. Systemic lupus erythematosus in NZB × NZW hybrid mice treated with the corticosteroid drug betamethasone. *J Lab Clin Med* 1968;71(3):390–399.
429. Gelfand MC, Steinberg AD. Therapeutic studies in NZB-W mice. II. Relative efficacy of azathioprine, cyclophosphamide and methylprednisolone. *Arthritis Rheum* 1972;15(3):247–252.
430. Hahn BH, Bagby MK, Hamilton TR, et al. Comparison of therapeutic and immunosuppressive effects of azathioprine, prednisolone and combined therapy in NZP/NZW mice. *Arthritis Rheum* 1973;16(2):163–170.
431. Jevnikar AM, Singer GG, Brennan DC, et al. Dexamethasone prevents autoimmune nephritis and reduces renal expression of Ia but not costimulatory signals. *Am J Pathol* 1992;141(3): 743–751.
432. Casey TP. Azathioprine (Imuran) administration and the development of malignant lymphomas in NZB mice. *Clin Exp Immunol* 1968;3(4):305–312.
433. Kiberd BA, Young ID. Modulation of glomerular structure and function in murine lupus nephritis by methylprednisolone and cyclophosphamide [see comments]. *J Lab Clin Med* 1994; 124(4):496–506.
434. Archer RL, Cunningham AC, Moore PF, et al. Effects of dazmegrel, piroxicam and cyclophosphamide on the NZB/W model of SLE. *Agents Actions* 1989;27(3–4):369–374.
435. Casey TP. Immunosuppression by cyclophosphamide in NZB X NZW mice with lupus nephritis. *Blood* 1968;32(3):436–444.
436. Horowitz RE, Dubois EL, Weiner J, et al. Cyclophosphamide treatment of mouse systemic lupus erythematosus. *Lab Invest* 1969;21(3):199–206.
437. Russell PJ, Hicks JD, Burnet FM. Cyclophosphamide treatment of kidney disease in (NZB × NZW) F1 mice. *Lancet* 1966;1(7450):1280–1284.
438. Walker SE, Bole GG. Augmented incidence of neoplasia in female New Zealand black-New Zealand white NZB/NZW mice treated with long-term cyclophosphamide. *J Lab Clin Med* 178, 978–979. 1971.
439. Waer M, Van Damme B, Leenaerts P, et al. Treatment of murine lupus nephritis with cyclophosphamide or total lymphoid irradiation. *Kidney Int* 1988;34(5):678–682.
440. Mihara M, Katsume A, Takeda Y. Effect of methotrexate treatment on the onset of autoimmune kidney disease in lupus mice. *Chem Pharm Bull (Tokyo)* 1992;40(8):2177–2181.
441. Woo J, Wright TM, Lemster B, et al. Combined effects of FK506 (tacrolimus) and cyclophosphamide on atypical B220+ T cells, cytokine gene expression and disease activity in MRL/MpJ- lpr/lpr mice. *Clin Exp Immunol* 1995;100(1): 118–125.
442. Mihara M, Takagi N, Urakawa K, et al. A novel antifolate, MX-68, inhibits the development of autoimmune disease in MRL/lpr mice. *Int Arch Allergy Immunol* 1997;113(4):454–459.
443. Halloran PF, Urmson J, Ramassar V, et al. Increased class I and class II MHC products and mRNA in kidneys of MRL- lpr/lpr mice during autoimmune nephritis and inhibition by cyclosporine. *J Immunol* 1988;141(7):2303–2312.
444. Berden JH, Faaber P, Assmann KJ, et al. Effects of cyclosporin A on autoimmune disease in MRL/1 and BXSB mice. *Scand J Immunol* 1986;24(4):405–411.
445. Mountz JD, Smith HR, Wilder RL, et al. CS-A therapy in MRL-lpr/lpr mice: amelioration of immunopathology despite autoantibody production. *J Immunol* 1987;138(1):157–163.
446. Pisetsky DS. Inhibition of in vitro NZB antibody responses by cyclosporine. *Clin Exp Immunol* 1988;71(1):155–158.
447. Yamamoto K, Mori A, Nakahama T, et al. Experimental treatment of autoimmune MRL-lpr/lpr mice with immunosuppressive compound FK506. *Immunology* 1990;69(2):222–227.
448. Ito S, Ueno M, Arakawa M, et al. Therapeutic effect of 15-deoxyspergualin on the progression of lupus nephritis in MRL mice. I. Immunopathological analyses. *Clin Exp Immunol* 81, 446–453. 1990.
449. Makino M, Fujiwara M, Aoyagi T, et al. Immunosuppressive activities of deoxyspergualin. I. Effect of the long- term administration of the drug on the development of murine lupus. *Immunopharmacology* 1987;14(2):107–113.

450. Nemoto K, Mae T, Saiga K, et al. Autoimmune-prone (NZW × BXSB)F1 (W/BF1) mice escape severe thrombocytopenia after treatment with deoxyspergualin, an immunosuppressant. *Br J Haematol* 1995;91(3):691–696.
451. Hiyashi T, Kameyama Y, Shirachi T. Long-term treatment with dimethylthiourea inhibits the development of autoimmune disease in NZB×NZW F1 mice. *J Comp Pathol* 1995;112:423–428.
452. Van Bruggen MC, Walgreen B, Rijke TP, et al. Attenuation of murine lupus nephritis by mycophenolate mofetil. *J Am Soc Nephrol* 1998;9(8):1407–1415.
453. McMurray RW, Elbourne KB, Lagoo A, et al. Mycophenolate mofetil suppresses autoimmunity and mortality in the female NZB × NZW F1 mouse model of systemic lupus erythematosus. *J Rheumatol* 1998;25(12):2364–2370.
454. Jonsson CA, Erlandsson M, Svensson L, et al. Mycophenolate mofetil ameliorates perivascular T lymphocyte inflammation and reduces the double-negative T cell population in SLE-prone MRLlpr/lpr mice. *Cell Immunol* 1999;197(2):136–144.
455. Jonsson CA, Svensson L, Carlsten H. Beneficial effect of the inosine monophosphate dehydrogenase inhibitor mycophenolate mofetil on survival and severity of glomerulonephritis in systemic lupus erythematosus (SLE)-prone MRLlpr/lpr mice. *Clin Exp Immunol* 1999;116(3):534–541.
456. Song YW, Kim HA, Baek HJ, et al. Paclitaxel reduces anti-dsDNA antibody titer and BUN, prolonging survival in murine lupus. *Int J Immunopharmacol* 1998;20(11):669–677.
457. Kanauchi H, Imamura S, Takigawa M, et al. Evaluation of the Japanese-Chinese herbal medicine, kampo, for the treatment of lupus dermatoses in autoimmune prone MRL/Mp-lpr/lpr mice. *J Dermatol* 1994;21(12):935–939.
458. Zhou NN, Nakai S, Kawakita T, et al. Combined treatment of autoimmune MRL/MP-lpr/lpr mice with a herbal medicine, Ren-shen-yang-rong-tang (Japanese name: Ninjin-youei-to) plus suboptimal dosage of prednisolone. *Int J Immunopharmacol* 1994;16(10):845–854.
459. Kotzin BL, Arndt R, Okada S, et al. Treatment of NZB/NZW mice with total lymphoid irradiation: long-lasting suppression of disease without generalized immune suppression. *J Immunol* 1986;136(9):3259–3265.
460. Kotzin BL, Strober S. Reversal of nzb/nzw disease with total lymphoid irradiation. *J Exp Med* 1979;150(2):371–378.
461. Moscovitch M, Rosenmann E, Neeman Z, et al. Successful treatment of autoimmune manifestations in MRL/l and MRL/n mice using total lymphoid irradiation (TLI). *Exp Mol Pathol* 1983;38(1):33–47.
462. Slavin S. Successful treatment of autoimmune disease in (NZB/NZW)F1 female mice by using fractionated total lymphoid irradiation. *Proc Natl Acad Sci USA* 1979;76(10): 5274–5276.
463. Theofilopoulos AN, Balderas R, Shawler DL, et al. Inhibition of T cells proliferation and SLE-like syndrome of MRL/1 mice by whole body or total lymphoid irradiation. *J Immunol* 1980;125(5):2137–2142.
464. Connolly K, Roubinian JR, Wofsy D. Development of murine lupus in CD4-depleted NZB/NZW mice. Sustained inhibition of residual CD4+ T cells is required to suppress autoimmunity. *J Immunol* 1992;149(9):3083–3088.
465. Carteron NL, Schimenti CL, Wofsy D. Treatment of murine lupus with F(ab')2 fragments of monoclonal antibody to L3T4. Suppression of autoimmunity does not depend on T helper cell depletion. *J Immunol* 1989;142(5):1470–1475.
466. Carteron NL, Wofsy D, Schimenti C, et al. F(ab')2 anti-CD4 and intact anti-CD4 monoclonal antibodies inhibit the accumulation of CD4+ T cells, CD8+ T cells, and B cells in the kidneys of lupus-prone NZB/NZW mice. *Clin Immunol Immunopathol* 1990;56(3):373–383.
467. Denman AM, Russell AS, Denman EJ. Renal disease in (NZB × NZW)F1 hybrid mice treated with anti- lymphocytic antibody. *Clin Exp Immunol* 1970;6(3):325–335.
468. Denman AM, Russell AS, Loewi G, et al. Immunopathology of New Zealand Black mice treated with antilymphocyte globulin. *Immunology* 1971;20(6):973–1000.
469. Hahn BH, Mehta J, Knotts LL, et al. The effect of altered lymphocyte function on the immunologic disorders of NZB/NZW mice. Response to anti-thymocyte globulin. *Clin Immunol Immunopathol* 1977;8(2):225–237.
470. Wofsy D, Ledbetter JA, Hendler PL, et al. Treatment of murine lupus with monoclonal anti-T cell antibody. *J Immunol* 1985;134(2):852–857.
471. O'Sullivan FX, Vogelweid CM, Besch-Williford CL, et al. Differential effects of CD4+ T cell depletion on inflammatory central nervous system disease, arthritis and sialadenitis in MRL/lpr mice. *J Autoimmun* 1995;8(2):163–175.
472. Wofsy D. The role of Lyt-2+ T cells in the regulation of autoimmunity in murine lupus. *J Autoimmun* 1988;1(2):207–217.
473. Gershwin ME, Castles JJ, Saito W, et al. Studies of congenitally immunologically mutant New Zealand mice. VII: the ontogeny of thymic abnormalities and reconstitution of nude NZB/W mice. *J Immunol* 1982;129(5):2150–2155.
474. Mihara M, Ohsugi Y, Saito K, et al. Immunologic abnormality in NZB/NZW F1 mice. Thymus-independent occurrence of B cell abnormality and requirement for T cells in the development of autoimmune disease, as evidenced by an analysis of the athymic nude individuals. *J Immunol* 1988;141(1):85–90.
475. Chu EB, Hobbs MV, Wilson CB, et al. Intervention of CD4+ cell subset shifts and autoimmunity in the BXSB mouse by murine CTLA4Ig. *J Immunol* 1996;156(3):1262–1268.
476. Liang B, Gee RJ, Kashgarian MJ, et al. B7 costimulation in the development of lupus: autoimmunity arises either in the absence of B7.1/B7.2 or in the presence of anti-b7.1/B7.2 blocking antibodies. *J Immunol* 1999;163(4):2322–2329.
477. Mihara M, Tan I, Chuzhin Y, et al. CTLA4Ig inhibits T cell-dependent B-cell maturation in murine systemic lupus erythematosus. *J Clin Invest* 2000;106(1):91–101.
478. Quattrocchi E, Dallman MJ, Feldmann M. Adenovirus-mediated gene transfer of CTLA-4Ig fusion protein in the suppression of experimental autoimmune arthritis. *Arthritis Rheum* 2000;43(8):1688–1697.
479. Adelman NE, Watling DL, McDevitt HO. Treatment of (NZB × NZW)F1 disease with anti-I-A monoclonal antibodies. *J Exp Med* 1983;158(4):1350–1355.
480. Mozes E, Zinger H, Kohn LD, et al. Spontaneous autoimmune disease in (NZB × NZW)F1 mice is ameliorated by treatment with methimazole. *J Clin Immunol* 1998;18(2):106–113.
481. Ohsugi Y, Gershwin ME, Ahmed A, et al. Studies of congenitally immunologic mutant New Zealand mice. VI. Spontaneous and induced autoantibodies to red cells and DNA occur in New Zealand X-linked immunodeficient (Xid) mice without phenotypic alternations of the Xid gene or generalized polyclonal B cell activation. *J Immunol* 1982;128(5):2220–2227.
482. Klinman DM, Steinberg AD. Similar in vivo expansion of B cells from normal DBA/2 and autoimmune NZB mice in xid recipients. *J Immunol* 1987;139(7):2284–2289.
483. Li T, Tsukada S, Satterthwaite A, et al. Activation of Bruton's tyrosine kinase (BTK) by a point mutation in its pleckstrin homology (PH) domain. *Immunity* 1995;2(5):451–460.
484. Bajpai UD, Zhang K, Teutsch M, et al. Bruton's tyrosine kinase links the B cell receptor to nuclear factor kappaB activation. *J Exp Med* 2000;191(10):1735–1744.
485. Ono S, Shao D, Yamada S, et al. A novel function of B lymphocytes from normal mice to suppress autoimmunity in (NZB × NZW)F1 mice. *Immunology* 2000;100(1):99–109.

486. Khaled AR, Soares LS, Butfiloski EJ, et al. Inhibition of p50 (NKkappaB1) subunit of NF-kappaB by phosphorothioate-modified antisense oligodeoxynucleotides reduces NF-kappaB expression and immunoglobulin synthesis in murine B cells. *Clin Immunol Immunopathol* 1997;83:254–263.
487. Shirai A, Aoki I, Otani M, et al. Treatment with dextran-conjugated anti-IgD delays the development of autoimmunity in MRL-lpr/lpr mice. *J Immunol* 1994;153(4):1889–1894.
488. Verthelyi D, Dybdal N, Elias KA, et al. DNAse treatment does not improve the survival of lupus prone (NZB × NZW)F1 mice. *Lupus* 1998;7(4):223–230.
489. Ebling FM, Ando DG, Panosian-Sahakian N, et al. Idiotypic spreading promotes the production of pathogenic autoantibodies. *J Autoimmun* 1988;1(1):47–61.
490. Hahn BH, Ebling FM. Suppression of NZB/NZW murine nephritis by administration of a syngeneic monoclonal antibody to DNA. Possible role of anti-idiotypic antibodies. *J Clin Invest* 1983;71(6):1728–1736.
491. Hahn BH, Ebling FM. Suppression of murine lupus nephritis by administration of an anti- idiotypic antibody to anti-DNA. *J Immunol* 1984;132(1):187–190.
492. Sasaki T, Muryoi T, Takai O, et al. Selective elimination of anti-DNA antibody-producing cells by antiidiotypic antibody conjugated with neocarzinostatin. *J Clin Invest* 1986;77(4): 1382–1386.
493. Harata N, Sasaki T, Osaki H, et al. Therapeutic treatment of New Zealand mouse disease by a limited number of anti-idiotypic antibodies conjugated with neocarzinostatin. *J Clin Invest* 1990;86(3):769–776.
494. Mahana W, Guilbert B, Avrameas S. Suppression of anti-DNA antibody production in MRL mice by treatment with anti-idiotypic antibodies. *Clin Exp Immunol* 1987;70(3):538–545.
495. Uner AH, Knupp CJ, Tatum AH, et al. Treatment with antibody reactive with the nephritogenic idiotype, IdLNF1, suppresses its production and leads to prolonged survival of (NZB × SWR)F1 mice. *J Autoimmun* 1994;7(1):27–44.
496. Sasaki T, Tamate E, Muryoi T, et al. In vitro manipulation of human anti-DNA antibody production by anti- idiotypic antibodies conjugated with neocarzinostatin. *J Immunol* 1989; 142(4):1159–1165.
497. Teitelbaum D, Rauch J, Stollar BD, et al. In vivo effects of antibodies against a high frequency idiotype of anti- DNA antibodies in MRL mice. *J Immunol* 1984;132(3):1282–1285.
498. Morland C, Michael J, Adu D, et al. Anti-idiotype and immunosuppressant treatment of murine lupus. *Clin Exp Immunol* 1991;83(1):126–132.
499. Spertini F, Leimgruber A, Morel B, et al. Idiotypic vaccination with a murine anti-dsDNA antibody: phase I study in patients with nonactive systemic lupus erythematosus with nephritis. *J Rheumatol* 1999;26(12):2602–2608.
500. Williams RC Jr, Malone CC, Fry G, et al. Affinity columns containing anti-DNA Id+ human myueloma proteins adsorb human epibodies from intravenous gamma globulin. *Arthritis Rheum* 1997;40:683–693.
501. Kiberd BA, Stadnyk AW. Established murine lupus nephritis does not respond to exogenous interleukin-1 receptor antagonist; a role for the endogenous molecule? Immunopharmacology 1995;30(2):131–137.
502. Do RKG, Hatada E, Lee H, et al. Attenuation of apoptosis underlies B lymphocyte stimulator enhancement of humoral immune response. *J Exp Med* 2000;192:953–964.
503. Mackay F, Woodcock SA, Lawton P, et al. Mice transgenic for BAFF develop lymphocytic disorders along with autoimmune manifestations. *J Exp Med* 1999;190(11):1697–1710.
504. Gross JA, Johnston J, Mudri S, et al. TACI and BCMA are receptors for a TNFALPHA homologue implicated in B-cell autoimmune disease [see comments]. *Nature* 2000;404(6781): 995–999.
505. Borel Y, Lewis RM, Stollar BD. Prevention of murine lupus nephritis by carrier-dependent induction of immunologic tolerance to denatured DNA. *Science* 1973;182(107):76–78.
506. Parker LP, Hahn BH, Osterland CK. Modification of NZB/NZW F1 autoimmune disease by development of tolerance to DNA. *J Immunol* 1974;113:292–297.
507. Eshhar Z, Benacerraf B, Katz DH. Induction of tolerance to nucleic acid determinants by administration of a complex of nucleoside D-glutamic acid and D-lysine (D-GL). *J Immunol* 1975;114(2 pt 2):872–876.
508. Borel Y, Lewis RM, Andre-Schwartz J, et al. Treatment of lupus nephritis in adult (NZB + NZW)F1 mice by cortisone-facilitated tolerance to nucleic acid antigens. *J Clin Invest* 1978; 61(2):276–286.
509. Duncan SR, Rubin RL, Burlingame RW, et al. Intrathymic injection of polynucleosomes delays autoantibody production in BXSB mice. *Clin Immunol Immunopathol* 1996;79(2):171–181.
510. Weisman MH, Bluestein HG, Berner CM, et al. Reduction in circulating dsDNA antibody titer after administration of LJP 394. *J Rheumatol* 1997;24(2):314–318.
511. Coutts SM, Plunkett ML, Iverson GM, et al. Pharmacological intervention in antibody mediated disease. *Lupus* 1996;5(2): 158–159.
512. Hahn BH, Ebling FM. Immune tolerance to the artificial peptide pCONSENSUS (pCONS) delays murine lupus by multiple mechanisms, including induction of regulatory cells. *Arthritis Rheum* 2000;43:S93.
513. Burny W, Lebrun P, Cosyns JP, et al. Treatment with dsDNA-anti-dsDNA antibody complexes extends survival, decreases anti-dsDNA antibody production and reduces severity of nephritis in MRLlpr mice. *Lupus* 1997;6(1):4–17.
514. Singh RR, Ebling FM, Sercarz EE, et al. Immune tolerance to autoantibody-derived peptides delays development of autoimmunity in murine lupus. *J Clin Invest* 1995;96(6):2990–2996.
515. Hahn BH, Singh RR, Wong WK, et al. Treatment with a consensus peptide based on amino acid sequences in autoantibodies prevents T cell activation by autoantigens and delays disease onset in murine lupus. *Arthritis Rheum* 2001;44:432–441.
516. Kaliyaperumal A, Michaels MA, Datta SK. Antigen-specific therapy of murine lupus nephritis using nucleosomal peptides: tolerance spreading impairs pathogenic function of autoimmune T and B cells. *J Immunol* 1999;162(10):5775–5783.
517. Ofosu-Appiah W, Sfeir G, Viti D, et al. Suppression of systemic lupus erythematosus disease in mice by oral administration of kidney extract. *J Autoimmun* 1999;13(4):405–414.
518. Shevach EM. Regulatory T cells in autoimmunity. *Annu Rev Immunol* 2000;18:423–449.
519. de Alboran IM, Gutierrez JC, Gonzalo JA, et al. lpr T cells vaccinate against lupus in MRL/lpr mice. *Eur J Immunol* 1992; 22(4):1089–1093.
520. Warner LM, Adams LM, Sehgal SN. Rapamycin prolongs survival and arrests pathophysiologic changes in murine systemic lupus erythematosus. *Arthritis Rheum* 1994;37(2):289–297.
521. Ozmen L, Roman D, Fountoulakis M, et al. Experimental therapy of systemic lupus erythematosus: the treatment of NZB/W mice with mouse soluble interferon-gamma receptor inhibits the onset of glomerulonephritis. *Eur J Immunol* 1995;25(1):6–12.
522. Nicoletti F, Meroni P, Di Marco R, et al. In vivo treatment with a monoclonal antibody to interferon-gamma neither affects the survival nor the incidence of lupus-nephritis in the MRL/lpr-lpr mouse. *Immunopharmacology* 1992;24(1):11–16.
523. Lawson BR, Prud'Homme GJ, Chang Y, et al. Treatment of murine lupus with cDNA encoding IFNGAMMA-gammaR/Fc. *J Clin Invest* 2000;106(2):207–215.

524. Haas C, Ryffel B, Le Hir M. IFN-gamma receptor deletion prevents autoantibody production and glomerulonephritis in lupus-prone (NZB × NZW)F1 mice. *J Immunol* 1998;160(8):3713–3718.
525. Zavala F, Masson A, Hadaya K, et al. Granulocyte-colony stimulating factor treatment of lupus autoimmune disease in MRL-lpr/lpr mice. *J Immunol* 1999;163(9):5125–5132.
526. Ruger BM, Erb KJ, He Y, et al. Interleukin-4 transgenic mice develop glomerulosclerosis independent of immunoglobulin deposition. *Eur J Immunol* 2000;30(9):2698–2703.
527. Bazzoni F, Beutler B. Comparative expression of TNF-alpha alleles from normal and autoimmune- prone MHC haplotypes. *J Inflamm* 1995;45(2):106–114.
528. Sironi M, Guglielmotti A, Polentarutti N, et al. A small synthetic molecule capable of preferentially inhibiting the production of the CC chemokine monocyte chemotactic protein-1. *Eur Cytokine Netw* 1999;10(3):437–442.
529. Guglielmotti A, Aquilini L, D'Onofrio E, et al. Bindarit prolongs survival and reduces renal damage in NZB/W lupus mice. *Clin Exp Rheumatol* 1998;16(2):149–154.
530. Ishida T, Inaba M, Hisha H, et al. Requirement of donor-derived stromal cells in the bone marrow for successful allogeneic bone marrow transplantation. Complete prevention of recurrence of autoimmune diseases in MRL/MP-lpr/lpr mice by transplantation of bone marrow plus bones (stromal cells) from the same donor. *J Immunol* 1994;152(6):3119–3127.
531. Ende N, Czarneski J, Raveche E. Effect of human cord blood transfer on survival and disease activity in MRL-lpr/lpr mice. *Clin Immunol Immunopathol* 1995;75(2):190–195.
532. Himeno K, Good RA. Marrow transplantation from tolerant donors to treat and prevent autoimmune diseases in BXSB mice. *Proc Natl Acad Sci USA* 1988;85(7):2235–2239.
533. Traynor AE, Schroeder J, Rosa RM, et al. Treatment of severe systemic lupus erythematosus with high-dose chemotherapy and haemopoietic stem-cell transplantation: a phase I study. *Lancet* 2000;356(9231):701–707.
534. Zurier RB, Damjanov I, Sayadoff DM, et al. Prostaglandin E1 treatment of NZB/NZW F1 hybrid mice. II. Prevention of glomerulonephritis. *Arthritis Rheum* 1977;20(8):1449–1456.
535. Zurier RB, Sayadoff DM, Torrey AB, et al. Prostaglandin E treatment of NZB/NZW mice. I. Prolonged survival of female mice. *Arthritis Rheum* 1977;20(2):723–728.
536. Yoshikawa T, Suzuki H, Sugiyama E, et al. Effects of prostaglandin E1 on the production of IgM and IgG class anti-dsDNA antibodies in NZB/W F1 mice. *J Rheumatol* 1993; 20(10):1701–1706.
537. Fan PY, Ruiz P, Pisetsky DS, et al. The effects of short-term treatment with the prostaglandin E1 (PGE1) analog misoprostol on inflammatory mediator production in murine lupus nephritis. *Clin Immunol Immunopathol* 1995;75(2):125–130.
538. Fernandes G, Venkatraman J, Khare A, et al. Modulation of gene expression in autoimmune disease and aging by food restriction and dietary lipids. *Proc Soc Exp Biol Med* 1990; 193(1):16–22.
539. Hurd ER, Johnston JM, Okita JR, et al. Prevention of glomerulonephritis and prolonged survival in New Zealand Black/New Zealand White F1 hybrid mice fed an essential fatty acid- deficient diet. *J Clin Invest* 1981;67(2):476–485.
540. Johnson BC, Gajjar A, Kubo C, et al. Calories versus protein in onset of renal disease in NZB × NZW mice. *Proc Natl Acad Sci USA* 1986;83(15):5659–5662.
541. Chandrasekar B, McGuff HS, Aufdermorte TB, et al. Effects of calorie restriction on transforming growth factor beta 1 and proinflammatory cytokines in murine Sjogren's syndrome. *Clin Immunol Immunopathol* 1995;76(3 Pt 1):291–296.
542. Kubo C, Johnson BC, Day NK, et al. Effects of calorie restriction on immunologic functions and development of autoimmune disease in NZB mice. *Proc Soc Exp Biol Med* 1992;201(2): 192–199.
543. Jolly CA, Fernandes G. Diet modulates Th-1 and Th-2 cytokine production in the peripheral blood of lupus-prone mice. J Clin Immunol 1999;19(3):172–178.
544. Alexander NJ, Smythe NL, Jokinen MP. The type of dietary fat affects the severity of autoimmune disease in NZB/NZW mice. *Am J Pathol* 1987;127(1):106–121.
545. Godfrey DG, Stimson WH, Watson J, et al. Effects of dietary supplementation on autoimmunity in the MRL/lpr mouse: a preliminary investigation. *Ann Rheum Dis* 1986;45(12):1019–1024.
546. Morrow WJ, Ohashi Y, Hall J, et al. Dietary fat and immune function. I. Antibody responses, lymphocyte and accessory cell function in (NZB × NZW)F1 mice. *J Immunol* 1985;135(6): 3857–3863.
547. Yamura W, Hattori S, Morrow WJ, et al. Dietary fat and immune function. II. Effects on immune complex nephritis in (NZB X NZW)F1 mice. *J Immunol* 1985;135:3864–3868.
548. Prickett JD, Robinson DR, Steinberg AD. Dietary enrichment with the polyunsaturated fatty acid eicosapentaenoic acid prevents proteinuria and prolongs survival in NZB × NZW F1 mice. *J Clin Invest* 1981;68(2):556–559.
549. Robinson DR, Prickett JD, Polisson R, et al. The protective effect of dietary fish oil on murine lupus. *Prostaglandins* 1985; 30(1):51–75.
550. Watson J, Godfrey D, Stimson WH, et al. The therapeutic effects of dietary fatty acid supplementation in the autoimmune disease of the MRL-mp-lpr/lpr mouse. *Int J Immunopharmacol* 1988;10(4):467–471.
551. Westberg G, Tarkowsky A, Svalender C. Effect of eicosapentaenoic acid rich menhaden oil and Max EPA on the autoimmune disease of MRL/l mice. *Int Arch Allergy Appl Immunol* 1988;88:454–461.
552. Clark WF, Parbtani A. Omega-3 fatty acid supplementation in clinical and experimental lupus nephritis. *Am J Kidney Dis* 1994;23(5):644–647.
553. Hall AV, Parbtani A, Clark WF, et al. Abrogation of MRL/lpr lupus nephritis by dietary flaxseed. *Am J Kidney Dis* 1993; 22(2):326–332.
554. Spurney RF, Ruiz P, Albrightson CR, et al. Fish oil feeding modulates leukotriene production in murine lupus nephritis. *Prostaglandins* 1994;48(5):331–348.
555. Chandrasekar B, Fernandes G. Decreased pro-inflammatory cytokines and increased antioxidant enzyme gene expression by omega-3 lipids in murine lupus nephritis. *Biochem Biophys Res Commun* 1994;200(2):893–898.
556. Malinow MR, Bardana EJ Jr, Pirofsky B, et al. Systemic lupus erythematosus-like syndrome in monkeys fed alfalfa sprouts: role of a nonprotein amino acid. Science 1982;216(4544): 415–417.
557. Malinow MR, McLaughlin P, Bardana EJ Jr, et al. Elimination of toxicity from diets containing alfalfa seeds. *Food Chem Toxicol* 1984;22(7):583–587.
558. Alcocer-Varela J, Iglesias A, Llorente L, et al. Effects of L-canavanine on T cells may explain the induction of systemic lupus erythematosus by alfalfa. *Arthritis Rheum* 1985;28(1):52–57.
559. Prete PE. Effects of L-canavanine on immune function in normal and autoimmune mice: disordered B-cell function by a dietary amino acid in the immunoregulation of autoimmune disease. *Can J Physiol Pharmacol* 1985;63(7):843–854.
560. Matsanuga A, Miller BC, Cottam GL. Dehydroisoandrosterone prevention of autoimmune disease in NZB/W F1 mice; lack of an effect on associated immunological abnormalities. *Biochim Biophys Acta* 1989;992:265–271.
561. Carlsten H, Nilsson N, Jonsson R, et al. Estrogen accelerates

immune complex glomerulonephritis but ameliorates T cell-mediated vasculitis and sialadenitis in autoimmune MRL lpr/lpr mice. *Cell Immunol* 1992;144(1):190–202.
562. Wu WM, Lin BF, Su YC, et al. Tamoxifen decreases renal inflammation and alleviates disease severity in autoimmune NZB/W F1 mice. *Scand J Immunol* 2000;52(4):393–400.
563. Walker SE, McMurray RW, Houri JM, et al. Effects of prolactin in stimulating disease activity in systemic lupus erythematosus. *Ann NY Acad Sci* 1998;840:762–772.
564. Weinberg JB, Granger DL, Pisetsky DS, et al. The role of nitric oxide in the pathogenesis of spontaneous murine autoimmune disease: increased nitric oxide production and nitric oxide synthase expression in MRL-lpr/lpr mice, and reduction of spontaneous glomerulonephritis and arthritis by orally administered NG-monomethyl-L- arginine. *J Exp Med* 1994;179(2):651–660.
565. Hortelano S, Diaz-Guerra MJ, Gonzalez-Garcia A, et al. Linomide administration to mice attenuates the induction of nitric oxide synthase elicited by lipopolysaccharide-activated macrophages and prevents nephritis in MRL/Mp-lpr/lpr mice. *J Immunol* 1997;158(3):1402–1408.
566. Yang CW, Yu CC, Ko YC, et al. Aminoguanidine reduces glomerular inducible nitric oxide synthase (iNOS) and transforming growth factor-beta 1 (TGF-beta1) mRNA expression and diminishes glomerulosclerosis in NZB/W F1 mice. *Clin Exp Immunol* 1998;113(2):258–264.
567. Mountz JD, Gause WC, Finkelman FD, et al. Prevention of lymphadenopathy in MRL-lpr/lpr mice by blocking peripheral lymph node homing with Mel-14 in vivo. *J Immunol* 1988; 140(9):2943–2949.
568. Koostra CJ, Van Der Giezen DM, Van Krieken JH, et al. Effective treatment of experimental lupus nephritis by combined administration of anti-CD11 and anti-CD54 antibodies. *Clin Exp Immunol* 2000;108:324–332.
569. Matsuo Y, Takagawa I, Koshida H, et al. Antiproteinuric effect of a thromboxane receptor antagonist, S-1452, on rat diabetic nephropathy and murine lupus nephritis. *Pharmacology* 1995; 50(1):1–8.
570. Nakamura T, Ebihara I, Tomino Y, et al. Effect of a specific endothelin A receptor antagonist on murine lupus nephritis. *Kidney Int* 1995;47(2):481–489.
571. Brey RL, Amato AA, Kagan-Hallet K, et al. Anti-intercellular adhesion molecule-1 (ICAM-1) antibody treatment prevents central and peripheral nervous system disease in autoimmune-prone mice. *Lupus* 1997;6(8):645–651.
572. Van Bruggen MC, Walgreen B, Fijke TP, et al. Heparin and heparinoids prevent the binding of immune complexes containing nucleosomal antigens to the GBM and delay nephritis in MRL/lpr mice. *Kidney Int* 1996;50:1555–1564.
573. Wang Y, Hu Q, Madri JA, et al. Amelioration of lupus-like autoimmune disease in NZB/WF1 mice after treatment with a blocking monoclonal antibody specific for complement component C5. *Proc Natl Acad Sci USA* 1996;93(16):8563–8568.
574. Gaynor B, Putterman C, Valadon P, et al. Peptide inhibition of glomerular deposition of an anti-DNA antibody. *Proc Natl Acad Sci USA* 1997;94(5):1955–1960.
575. McGrath H Jr, Bak E, Michalski JP. Ultraviolet-A light prolongs survival and improves immune function in (New Zealand black × New Zealand white)F1 hybrid mice. *Arthritis Rheum* 1987; 30(5):557–561.
576. Ansel JC, Mountz J, Steinberg AD, et al. Effects of UV radiation on autoimmune strains of mice: increased mortality and accelerated autoimmunity in BXSB male mice. *J Invest Dermatol* 1985;85(3):181–186.
577. Fan JL, Himeno K, Tsuru S, et al. Treatment of autoimmune MRL/Mp-lpr/lpr mice with cholera toxin. *Clin Exp Immunol* 1987;70(1):94–101.
578. Baldi E, Emancipator SN, Hassan MO, et al. Platelet activating factor receptor blockade ameliorates murine systemic lupus erythematosus. *Kidney Int* 1990;38(6):1030–1038.
579. Vilanova M, Ribeiro A, Carneiro J, et al. The effects of thalidomide treatment on autoimmune-prone NZB and MRL mice are consistent with stimulation of the central immune system. *Scand J Immunol* 1994;40(5):543–548.
580. Hart DA, Done SJ, Benediktsson H, et al. Partial characterization of the enhanced survival of female NZB/W mice treated with lithium chloride. *Int J Immunopharmacol* 1994;16(10):825–833.
581. Akhanzarova VD, Vaso'eva EG. Aleutian mink disease as an experimental model of systemic lupus erythematosus. *Vopr Revmatizma* 1981;1:46–56. 1981.
582. Halliwell RE. Autoimmune diseases in domestic animals. *J Am Vet Med Assoc* 1982;181(10):1088–1096.
583. Shanley KJ. Lupus erythematosus in small animals. *Clin Dermatol* 1985;3(3):131–138.
584. Welin HE, Hansson H, Karlsson-Parra A, et al. Autoantibody profiles in canine ANA-positive sera investigated by immunoblot and ELISA. *Vet Immunol Immunopathol* 1998;61(2–4):157–170.
585. Lewis RM, Andre-Schwartz J, Hirsch MC, et al. The transmissibility of canine systemic lupus erythematosus (SLE). *J Clin Invest* 1974;51:57A.
586. Lewis RM, Schwartz RS. Canine systemic lupus erythematosus. Genetic analysis of an established breeding colony. *J Exp Med* 1971;134(2):417–438.
587. Monier JC, Fournel C, Lapras M, et al. Systemic lupus erythematosus in a colony of dogs. *Am J Vet Res* 1988;49(1):46–51.
588. Teichner M, Krumbacher K, Doxiadis I, et al. Systemic lupus erythematosus in dogs: association to the major histocompatibility complex class I antigen DLA-A7. *Clin Immunol Immunopathol* 1990;55(2):255–262.
589. Wagner JL, Burnett RC, Storb R. Organization of the canine major histocompatibility complex: current perspectives. *J Hered* 1999;90(1):35–38.
590. Center SA, Smith CA, Wilkinson E, et al. Clinicopathologic, renal immunofluorescent, and light microscopic features of glomerulonephritis in the dog: 41 cases (1975–1985). *J Am Vet Med Assoc* 1987;190(1):81–90.
591. Costa O, Fournel C, Lotchouang E, et al. Specificities of antinuclear antibodies detected in dogs with systemic lupus erythematosus. *Vet Immunol Immunopathol* 1984;7(3–4):369–382.
592. Halla JT, Volanakis JE, Schrohenloher RE. Circulating immune complexes in mixed connective tissue disease. *Arthritis Rheum* 1979;22(5):484–489.
593. Fournel C, Chabanne L, Caux C, et al. Canine systemic lupus erythematosus. I: a study of 75 cases. *Lupus* 1992;1(3):133–139.
594. Stone MS, Johnstone IB, Brooks M, et al. Lupus-type "anticoagulant" in a dog with hemolysis and thrombosis. *J Vet Intern Med* 1994;8(1):57–61.
595. Taylor RP, Kujala G, Wilson K, et al. In vivo and in vitro studies of the binding of antibody/dsDNA immune complexes to rabbit and guinea pig platelets. *J Immunol* 1985;134(4):2550–2558.
596. Brinet A, Fournel C, Faure JR, et al. Anti-histone antibodies (ELISA and immunoblot) in canine lupus erythematosus. *Clin Exp Immunol* 1988;74(1):105–109.
597. Kristensen AT, Weiss DJ, Klausner JS, et al. Detection of antiplatelet antibody with a platelet immunofluorescence assay. *J Vet Intern Med* 1994;8(1):36–39.
598. Monesteir M, Novick KE, Karam ET, et al. Autoantibodies to histone, DNA and nucleosome antigens in canine systemic lupus erythematosus. *Clin Exp Immunol* 1995;99:37–41.
599. White SD, Rosychuk RA, Schur PH. Investigation of antibodies to extractable nuclear antigens in dogs. *Am J Vet Res* 1992;53(6):1019–1021.
600. Zouali M, Migliorini P, Mackworth-Young CG, et al. Nucleic

acid-binding specificity and idiotypic expression of canine anti-DNA antibodies. *Eur J Immunol* 1988;18(6):923–927.
601. Reinertsen JL, Kaslow RA, Klippel JH, et al. An epidemiologic study of households exposed to canine systemic lupus erythematosus. *Arthritis Rheum* 1980;23(5):564–568.
602. Aucoin DP, Rubin RL, Peterson ME, et al. Dose-dependent induction of anti-native DNA antibodies in cats by propylthiouracil. *Arthritis Rheum* 1988;31(5):688–692.
603. Clifford GO, McClure J, Conway M, et al. Renal lesions in dogs produced by plasma from patients with systemic lupus erythematosus. *J Lab Clin Med* 1961;58:807–814.
604. Bencze G, Tiboldi T, Lakatos L. Experiments on pathogenetic role of L.E. factor in dogs and guinea pigs. *Acta Rheum Scand* 1963;9:209–215.
605. Dubois EL, Katz YJ, Freeman V, et al. Chronic toxicity studies of hydralazine in dogs. *J Lab Clin Med* 1957;50:119–124.
606. Henrickson M, Giannini EH, Hirsh R. Reduction of mortality and lymphodenopathy in MRL-lpr mice treated with nonmitogenic anti-CD3 monoclonal antibody. *Arthritis Rheum* 1994; 37:587–594.
607. Carr R, Forsyth S, Sadi D. Abnormal responses to ingested substances in murine SLE: apparent effect of a casein-free diet on the development of SLE in N2B/W mice. *J Rheumatol* 1987; 14(suppl B):158–165.
608. Alarcon-Segovia D, Tumlin J, Furie R, et al. SLE trial shows fewer renal flares in LJP 394-treated patients with high-affinity antibodies to LJP 394:90-05 trial results. *Arthritis Rheum* 2000;1231 (abstract).

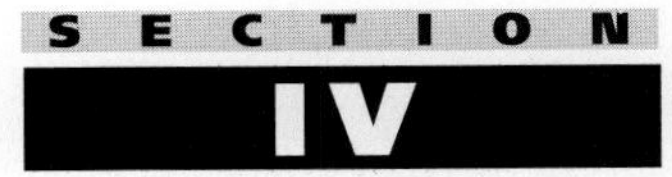

AUTOANTIBODIES

19

THE STRUCTURE AND DERIVATION OF ANTIBODIES AND AUTOANTIBODIES

ELENA PEEVA
BETTY DIAMOND
CHAIM PUTTERMAN

The humoral immune response protects an organism from environmental pathogens by producing antibodies (immunoglobulins) that mediate the destruction or inactivation of microbial organisms and their toxins. To perform this function, the immune system generates antibodies to a diverse and changing array of foreign antigens, yet it must do so without generating pathogenic antibodies to self.

The production of high-affinity antibodies that bind to self-determinants is a prominent feature of systemic lupus erythematosus (SLE) (1). Some autoantibodies in SLE are markers for disease [anti-Sm/ribonucleoprotein (RNP), antinuclear antibody], while others are thought to play a role in pathogenesis and tissue damage (anti-DNA, anticardiolipin, anti-Ro) (2–6).

There have been extensive investigations of autoantibodies in SLE, and these studies have addressed a number of specific questions:

1. Do polymorphisms of immunoglobulin variable region genes contribute to disease susceptibility?
2. Do B cells producing autoantibodies arise from an antigen-triggered and -selected response? If so, are these triggering and selecting antigens self or foreign?
3. Are particular B-cell lineages or differentiation pathways responsible for autoantibody production?
4. What are the characteristics of pathogenic autoantibodies, and how do they mediate pathology?
5. What defects in immune regulation permit the sustained expression of pathogenic autoantibodies?

This chapter discusses autoantibody structure, assembly, and regulation. Based on new advances in our knowledge of autoantibody structure and regulation, novel potential therapeutic strategies are also briefly addressed.

STRUCTURE OF THE ANTIBODY MOLECULE

Antibodies are glycoproteins produced by B lymphocytes in both membrane-bound and secreted forms. They are composed of two heavy chains and two light chains. In general, the two heavy chains are linked by disulfide bonds and each heavy chain is linked to a light chain by a disulfide bond. The intact molecule has two functional regions: a constant region that determines its effector functions, and a variable region that is involved in antigen binding and is unique to a given B-cell clone (7) (Fig. 19.1). The light chains appear to contribute solely to antigen binding and are not known to mediate any other antibody function. In contrast, the heavy chains possess a constant region that determines the isotype [i.e., class: immunoglobulin M (IgM), IgD, IgG, IgA, or IgE] (Fig. 19.2) of the antibody molecule. IgM is the first isotype produced by a B cell and the first to appear in the serum response to a newly encountered antigen. IgM antibodies normally polymerize into pentamers known as macroglobulin, thus conferring higher functional binding strength, or avidity. A 15-kd glycoprotein called the J chain is covalently associated with the pentameric IgM, and mediates the polymerization process (8,9). IgM antibodies can activate complement via the classic pathway and therefore cause lysis of cells expressing target antigens. Under the appropriate conditions, B cells producing IgM can switch to the production of the other isotypes. IgG is the predominant isotype of the secondary (also called memory) immune response. In humans, the IgG isotype is divided into four subclasses, IgG1, IgG2, IgG3, and IgG4, all of which possess different functional attributes. IgG1 is the most abundant in the serum. Antinuclear antibodies in SLE are mainly of IgG1 and IgG3 subclasses (10). In addition to activating complement, IgG antibodies can promote Fc-receptor–mediated phagocytosis of antigen-antibody complexes. High concentrations of antigen-IgG complexes can downregulate an immune response by cross-linking membrane immunoglobulin and FcRII receptors on antigen-specific B cells. This may be an important mechanism for turning off antibody production after all the available antigen is bound to antibody. The IgA constant region allows antibody translocation across epithelial cells into mucosal sites such as saliva, lung, intestine, and the genitourinary

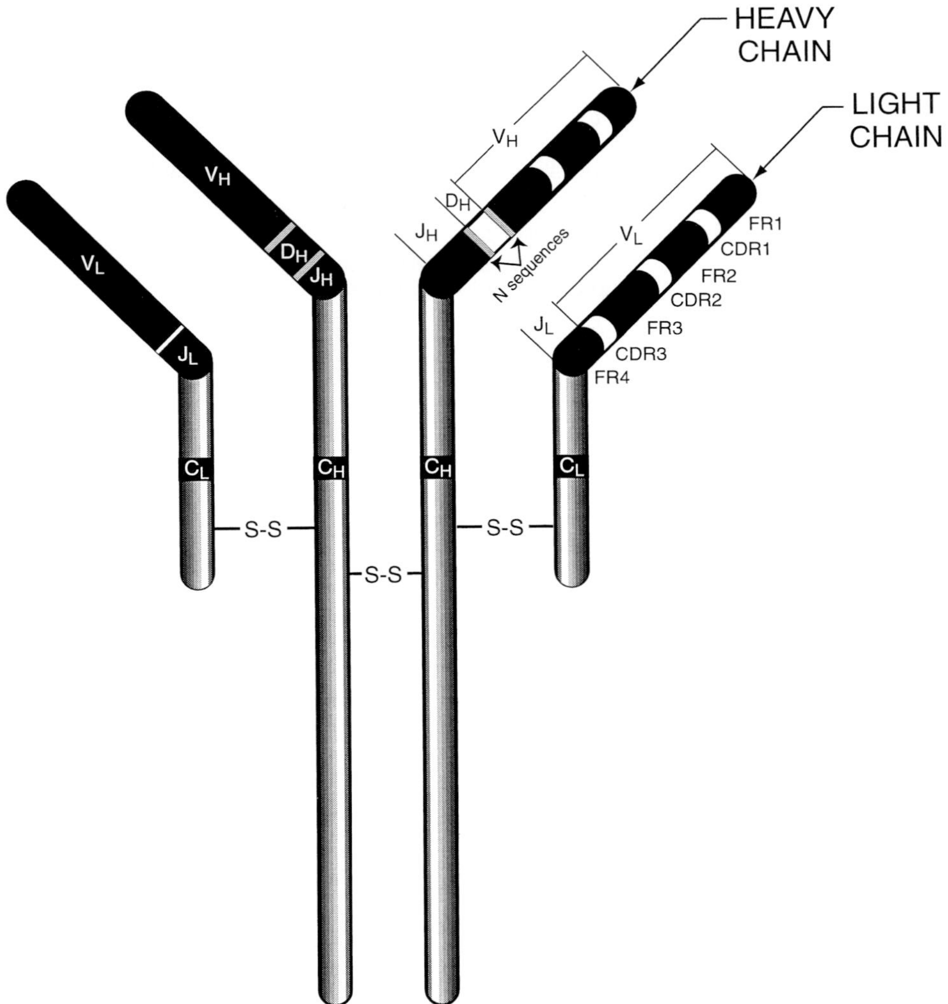

FIGURE 19.1. A prototypic antibody molecule. C, constant region; CDR, complementary-determining region; D, diversity region; FW, framework region; J, joining region; V, variable region.

tract; IgA antibodies can be found as monomers in serum and as dimers in the mucous secretions. The J chain, implicated in IgM polymerization, is not required for IgA dimerization, but does have a role in maintaining IgA dimer stability and is essential for transport of IgA by the hepatic polymeric Ig receptor (11). IgE antibodies can trigger mast cells and eosinophils, which are important cellular mediators of the immune response to extracellular parasites and allergic reactions.

Every complete antibody has two identical antigen-binding sites, each of which is composed of the variable regions of one heavy and one light chain. When the variable regions from both light and heavy chain pair, the hypervariable segments or complementarity determining regions (CDRs) come together and generate a unique antigen-binding site (Fig. 19.1). The antigen-binding site is divided into the highly polymorphic CDRs, and the more conserved framework regions (FRs). The CDRs contain the contact amino

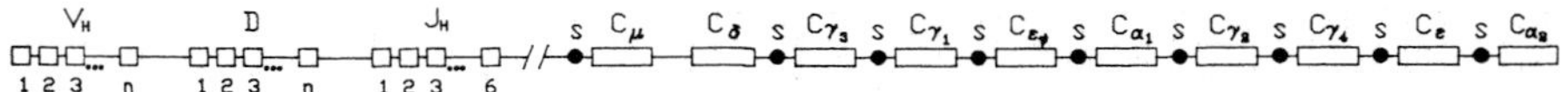

FIGURE 19.2. The heavy-chain immunoglobulin gene locus on chromosome 14. C, constant region; D, diversity gene locus; J, joining gene locus; S, switch region; V, variable gene locus.

acids for antigen binding and thus contribute more than the FRs to antigenic specificity. There are three different CDRs in both the heavy and light chain, and the most variable portion of the antibody molecule is the CDR3 (12,13). There are four FRs. X-ray crystallographic studies have shown that the amino acids of the CDRs are arranged in flexible loops, while the FRs have more rigid structure that maintain the spatial orientation of the antigen-binding pocket (14).

Antibody molecules are Y-shaped structures that can be cleaved into functionally distinct fragments by proteases like papain and pepsin (15,16). Limited digestion with papain cleaves the antibody into three fragments: two identical Fab (fragment antigen binding) fragments and an Fc (fragment crystallizable) fragment. The Fab fragment consists of the entire light chain and the heavy chain variable region with the CH1 domain. It contains the antigen-binding site, which is formed by the variable regions of the light and heavy chain at the tip of each Fab fragment. The Fc fragment is composed of the two carboxy-terminal domains from the heavy chains, the hinge region and CH2 and CH3, and interacts with soluble and cell membrane bound effector molecules. The Fc fragment does not have antigen-binding activity. The Fab portions are linked to the Fc fragment at the hinge region, which allows independent movement of the two Fabs (17). Another protease, pepsin, cleaves the antibody molecule on the carboxy-terminal side of the heavy chain disulfide bridges producing several small fragments and an $F(ab)_2$ fragment, that contains both Fabs linked to each other with an intact hinge region. $F(ab)_2$ cannot be obtained from IgG2 by pepsin. However, lysyl endopeptidase digestion will generate $F(ab)_2$ from IgG2 (18). Based on the fact that the $F(ab)_2$ fragment has the same avidity for antigen as the intact antibody, but does not possess any effector functions, this cleavage product may have therapeutic applications.

The variable region of an antibody may itself serve as an antigen, called an idiotype. Antiidiotypes are antibodies that bind to specific determinants in the CDRs or FRs of other antibodies (19,20) (see Chapter 15). Antibodies that share the same idiotype presumably have a high degree of structural homology and may be encoded by related variable region genes (21). Idiotypes have been postulated to be important in the regulation of the immune response because they can be recognized by both T and B cells (22–25) (see Chapter 15). Antiidiotypic antibodies may therefore be useful reagents for tolerizing pathogenic autoantibody-producing B cells (see below).

ANTIBODY ASSEMBLY

The immunoglobulin light and heavy chain variable region genes are formed by a process of rearrangement of distinct gene segments, separated in the genome in all cells except B lymphocytes. In B cells these genes are rearranged by a process called somatic recombination. During this process, V (variable), D (diversity), and J (joining) segments are brought together to form a heavy chain variable region gene, and V and J segments to form a light chain variable region gene (26–31).

In humans, heavy chain V, D, and J gene segments each come from gene clusters that are tandemly arrayed on chromosome 14 (31,32) (Fig. 19.2). The 50 to 100 functional heavy chain V segment genes are divided into seven families, which share 80% homology by DNA sequence primarily in FRs (33–36). V gene family members are interspersed randomly along the V locus. There are approximately 30 functional D gene segments and six known J gene segments for the human immunoglobulin heavy chain (36).

Each V, D, and J gene segment is flanked by conserved heptamer/nonamer consensus sequences that are crucial for the rearrangement process. The conserved heptamer is always most proximal to the coding sequence, followed by a 12– or 23–base pair (bp) spacer sequence, and then by the conserved nanomer. The length of the spacer corresponds to either one or two turns of the DNA double helix, which allows the heptamer and nanomer to be brought together on one side of the DNA helix and enables them to interact with the proteins that catalyze the recombination process. The heptamer-spacer-nanomer sequence is known as recombination signal sequence (RSS)(37).

Assembly of the complete heavy chain gene begins with the joining of a D segment from the D cluster to a J segment in the J cluster, mediated by DNA cleavage and deletion of the intervening DNA. In a similar manner, a V gene segment is next rearranged to the DJ unit to form a complete VDJ variable region (26,35). This process of variable region recombination is very elaborate and requires a complex of enzymes called V(D)J recombinase (38). Most of these enzymes are also necessary for the maintenance of double-stranded DNA (dsDNA) and are present in all cells. However, for the first cleavage step, specialized enzyme products of the recombination activating-genes RAG-1 and RAG-2 are required (39). The proteins encoded by these genes are active in the early stages of lymphoid development. Signals from both stromal cells and the cytokines interleukin-3 (IL-3), IL-6, and IL-7 are necessary for induction of RAG genes in lymphoid progenitors (40). RAGs bind to the nanomer sequence and initiate VDJ recombination by generating dsDNA breaks at the end of the RSS. Joining of the coding segments is mediated by several enzymes involved in repair of dsDNA breaks: Ku 70, Ku 80, DNA-PKs, XRCC4, ligase, and Mre 11 (41). Members of the high-mobility group family of proteins HMG1 and HMG2 (42) also play a significant role in the formation and stabilization of the precleavage and postcleavage synaptic complex (43,44).

Antibody diversification can be generated by the addition of P and N nucleotides at the VD and DJ junctions. If the single-stranded DNA (ssDNA) that is present after the break can form a hairpin loop, the resulting double-stranded (palindromic, P) sequences are added at the junction. Alternatively, N-nucleotides or non–template-encoded nucleotides, are randomly inserted at the VD and DJ junctions by the enzyme terminal deoxynucleotidyl transferase (TdT) (45). Such N sequences are common in antibodies of the adult immunoglobulin repertoire but are less frequent early in the ontogeny of the B-cell repertoire (46). These random modifications create unique junctions and increase the diversity of the antibody repertoire. Because VDJ joining is imprecise and includes P and N sequences, CDRs of variable length and sequence are generated.

After generation of a functional heavy chain, the light chain gene segments can rearrange from either of two loci, κ or λ. No functional difference has been demonstrated between antibodies that utilize κ or λ light chains. The ratio of the two types of light chains varies in different species. For example, in mice the κ/λ ratio is 20:1 while in humans it is 3:2. The light chain variable region is composed of only two gene segments: V and J. Genes for the V and J segments of κ light chains are located on chromosome 2. The κ locus contains approximately 40 functional V gene segments, which are grouped into seven families, and five J segments (47–51). The λ light chain locus is on chromosome 22, and contains at least seven V gene families, with up to 70 members (52–56). As with the heavy chain, V and J elements of the light chain loci also rearrange by recombination at heptamer/nonamer consensus sites. Only rarely are N sequences inserted at the VJ junction of the light chain (57).

RAG gene expression is high in pro–B and pre–B cells. Once a heavy chain rearrangement successfully occurs, the heavy chain associates with a nonpolymorphic light chain, termed surrogate light chain. The appearance of an Ig heavy chain with surrogate light chain on the cell surface of large pre–B cells coincides with inactivation of the RAG-2 protein. Degradation of both RAG-1 and RAG-2 messenger RNA (mRNA) occurs and there is no further heavy chain rearrangement. Later, RAG-1 and RAG-2 are again expressed and light chain gene rearrangement takes place. When a complete Ig molecule is expressed at the cell surface, RAG expression ceases (58).

The importance of the V(D)J recombination process has been demonstrated in animal studies as well as in some hereditary immune disorders. Mutations that abolish V(D)J recombination cause an early block in lymphoid development resulting in severe combined immune deficiency (SCID) with a complete lack of circulating B and T lymphocytes. Mice missing either RAG-1 or RAG-2 are unable to rearrange immunoglobulin genes or T-cell receptor genes (59). In humans, a loss or marked reduction of V(D)J recombination activity can cause T-B-SCID (60,61) or B-SCID phenotype (62). Mutations that impair but do not completely abolish the function of RAG-1 or 2 in humans result in Omenn syndrome, a form of combined immune deficiency characterized by lack of B cells and oligoclonal, activated T lymphocytes with a skewed T-helper-2 (Th2) profile (63). It is clear, however, from studies of immunodeficient mouse strains that additional gene products also are needed for successful rearrangement to occur. Defects in any of the components of the dsDNA break repair machinery such as Ku70, Ku 80, DNA PKs, DNA ligase IV, and XRCC4 lead to an immunodeficient phenotype with increased radiation sensitivity as a common feature (64).

While the rearranged heavy chain VDJ segment is initially associated with an IgM constant region gene, it can undergo a second kind of gene rearrangement during the secondary response to associate with the other downstream constant region genes (65–67) (Fig. 19.2). Switch sequences located upstream of each constant region gene mediate heavy chain class switching (68).

Although all somatic cells are endowed with two of each chromosome, only one rearranged heavy chain gene and one rearranged light chain gene normally are expressed by a B cell. This phenomenon is known as allelic exclusion. A productive rearrangement on one chromosome inhibits assembly of variable region genes on another chromosome. Rearrangement of the first chromosome often is unproductive because of DNA reading frame shifts or because nonfunctional variable region gene segments called pseudogenes are used. If rearrangement on the first chromosome cannot lead to the formation of a functional polypeptide chain, then the immunoglobulin genes on the other chromosome are allowed to rearrange.

While the heavy chain has a single locus of V, D, and J segments on each chromosome, the light chain has two. The κ locus is the first set of light chain gene segments to rearrange. If these rearrangements are nonproductive on both chromosomes, however, then the V and J segments of the λ locus rearrange to produce an intact light chain (69,70). Thus, while the heavy chain has two loci from which to form a functional gene, the light chain may rearrange at four loci. It has recently been demonstrated that additional rearrangements can occur in B cells already expressing an intact antibody molecule if that antibody has a forbidden autospecificity. These additional rearrangements, which are termed receptor editing, are important in allowing B cells to regulate autoreactivity.

Immune tolerance mediated by receptor editing occurs frequently in developing B cells (71). High-affinity receptor binding to self antigen induces new V(D)J recombination (72) and replacement of the gene encoding self-reactive receptor by a gene encoding a nonautoreactive receptor (73,74). There is some debate about whether Ig gene rearrangement can occur also in mature B cells or only in immature B cells (75). RAG protein expression in germinal centers, as well as after immunization (76,77) has suggested that antibody genes may undergo modification not only in developing but also in mature B cells (77–79). Although the regulation and function of secondary rearrangements of

TABLE 19.1. MECHANISMS OF ANTIBODY DIVERSITY

Combinatorial diversity of V, D, and J gene segments for heavy-chain variable region and V and J gene segments for light-chain variable region
Junctional diversity of rearranged heavy- and light-chain variable regions
  N-terminal addition
  Imprecise joining
Random association of heavy and light chains
Somatic point mutation

Ig genes in mature B cells is not completely elucidated, it seems that in peripheral lymphocytes recombination is not random but represents an antigen-regulated process (74).

GENERATION OF ANTIBODY DIVERSITY

The immune system has several mechanisms to ensure a large antibody repertoire. Before exposure to antigen, B-cell diversity results from (a) combinations of V, D, and J gene segments and V and J segments into heavy and light chain genes, respectively; (b) junctional diversity produced by N or P sequence insertion and/or imprecise joining of gene segments; and (c) the random pairing of heavy and light chains. These three mechanisms are consequences of the process of recombination used to create complete Ig variable regions. The fourth mechanism, called somatic mutation, occurs later on rearranged DNA. This mechanism introduces point mutations into rearranged variable region genes (Table 19.1). These mechanisms are potentially capable of producing a repertoire of 10^{11} different antibodies (80).

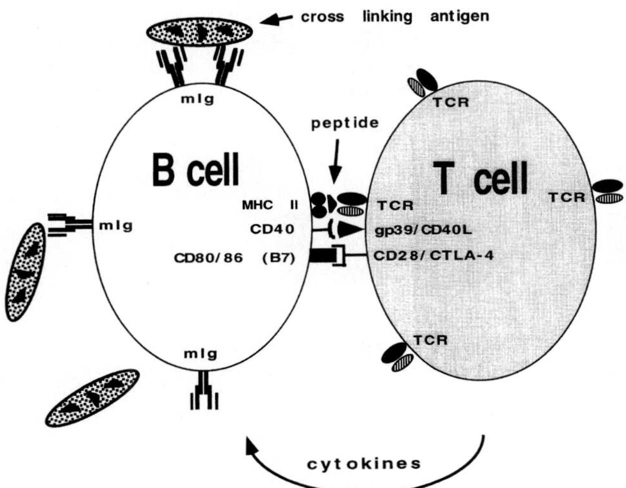

FIGURE 19.3. B-cell–T-cell cognate interactions. MHC II, class II major histocompatibility complex; mIg, membrane immunoglobulin; TCR, T-cell receptor.

Cross-linking of surface immunoglobulin on the B cell by a multivalent antigen is the first in a series of critical steps that eventually can lead to B-cell activation and antibody production. Following cross-linking of membrane immunoglobulin, the antigen-antibody complexes are internalized, and the antigen is cleaved and processed in the cell. Peptide fragments of protein antigen bound to the major histocompatibility complex (MHC) class II molecules are then expressed on the cell surface, where they can be recognized by antigen-specific helper T cells (Fig. 19.3). These T cells provide the co-stimulation and cytokines that are necessary for full B-cell activation.

On initial exposure to an antigen, naive B cells recognizing the antigen enter secondary lymphoid organs such as the spleen or lymph nodes, where they proliferate and begin to secrete IgM. The antibodies of this primary immune response generally are polyreactive and display low affinity to a multitude of antigens, even to antigens without obvious structural homology (Table 19.2). The amplification of antigen-specific B cells occurs in specific regions of the lymphoid tissue called germinal centers. Somatic mutation (discussed later), selection of high-avidity B-cell clones, heavy chain isotype switching, and further differentiation to plasma and memory B cells are thought to occur here.

Recent studies using mice with targeted disruptions of particular genes have shown that in addition to a cognate interaction between the T-cell receptor and an MHC class II molecule, at least two other pairs of B-cell–T-cell contacts are necessary for germinal center formation and function (Fig. 19.3). The first interaction is between the B7-like family (CD80, CD86) of molecules on the B cell and the CD28-like family (CD28, CTLA-4) of co-receptors on the T cell. This is thought to prime the T cell to promote B-cell activation and differentiation (81). The second important interaction is between the CD40 receptor on the B cell and CD40 ligand (CD40L, gp39) expressed on activated CD4 T cells. Activation of the CD40 receptor is thought to be necessary for induction of isotype switching and formation of germinal centers (82,83). Defective CD40 ligand on T cells in humans and mice causes X-linked hyper-IgM syndrome,

TABLE 19.2. DISTINGUISHING FEATURES OF THE NAIVE AND ANTIGEN-ACTIVATED ANTIBODY REPERTOIRE

Feature	Naive	Antigen Activated
Isotype	Primarily IgM	Primarily IgG
Specificity	Polyreactive	Monospecific
Affinity	Low affinity	High affinity
Sequence	Germline gene encoded	Somatically mutated (high R:S ratio)
Titer	Low titer	High titer

Ig, immunoglobulin.

which is characterized by a defect in isotype switching and severe humoral immunodeficiency, leading to increased susceptibility to infections with extracellular bacteria (84). Since the proliferation of autoreactive B cells in SLE is T-cell dependent, there are new therapeutic approaches based on the inhibition of B-cell–T-cell interactions by blockade of the co-stimulatory signals mentioned above.

After the primary immune response runs its course, the germinal center involutes and IgM secretion falls. Reexposure to the antigen and activated T cells, however, can activate memory B cells to initiate the secondary immune response. The secondary serum response is characterized by rapidly produced high titers of IgG antibodies that have greater specificity and increased affinity for antigen through somatic mutation (85–87). Anti-dsDNA antibodies, which are the most well-characterized pathogenic autoantibodies to date, possess all the features of secondary response antibodies (88–91) (Table 19.2) (see Chapter 21).

Somatic point mutations are single nucleotide substitutions that can occur throughout the heavy and light chain variable region genes (92–94) and represent a site-specific, differentiation stage–specific, and lineage-specific phenomenon (95). Somatic mutation takes place in dividing centroblasts, whose rearranged Ig variable region genes undergo a mutation rate of 1 bp per 10^3/cell divisions compared to 1 bp per 10^{10}/cell divisions in all other somatic cells. The DNA mismatch repair system has been implicated in Ig gene mutation because it functions generally to correct point mutations in DNA. A genetic deficiency in a component of the mismatch repair system, PMS2, has been shown to enhance the rate of mutation, suggesting that the DNA mismatch repair system may be altered in hypermutating B cells (96). Similarly, mice deficient in Msh6, a component of the mismatch repair system, have altered nucleotide targeting for mutations (97). Because somatic mutation occurs concurrent with heavy chain class switching, although by a different mechanism, mutation is more common in IgG than in IgM antibodies.

Genealogies of B cells with serial mutations in their immunoglobulin gene sequences demonstrate how point mutations can lead to antibodies with altered affinity for antigen (98–101) (Fig. 19.4). While B cells producing anti-

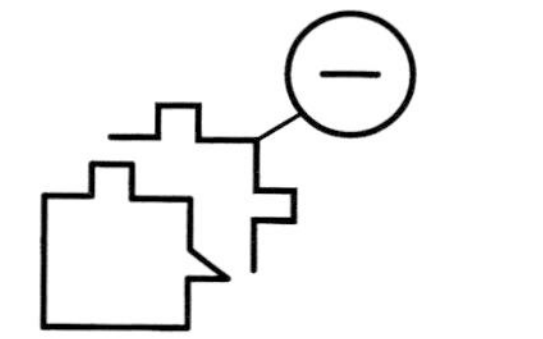

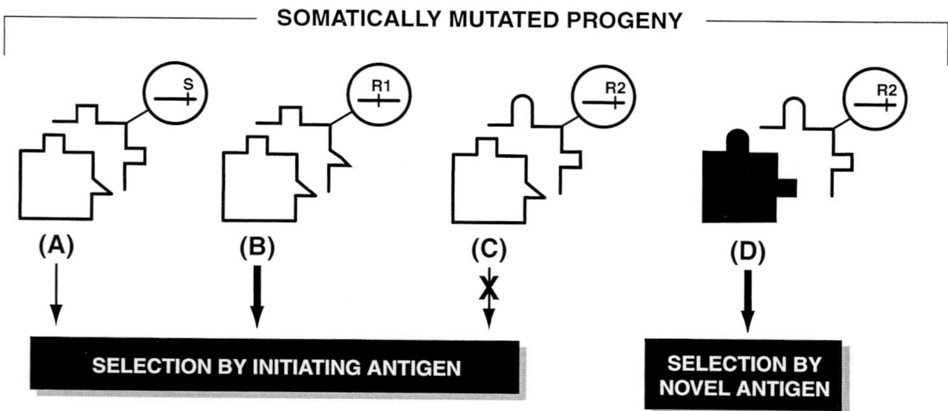

FIGURE 19.4. B-cell genealogy. The progenitor B cell depicted at the top expresses an antibody that is encoded by germline immunoglobulin genes and has a low affinity for antigen. When antigen and T-cell factors trigger B-cell proliferation, class switching, and somatic mutation, numerous B-cell progeny are possible. Three examples are schematized here. **A:** A B cell with a silent (S) point mutation. This nucleotide substitution does not encode a new amino acid. Therefore, the antibody molecule is unaffected, and affinity for antigen does not change. **B:** A B cell whose point mutation encodes an amino acid replacement (R), leading to increased affinity for antigen. This mutated antibody exemplifies affinity maturation. **C:** A B cell with a replacement mutation that alters antigenic specificity. This antibody can no longer bind to the initial triggering antigen. **D:** The same antibody as in **C**, despite no longer being able to bind to the initial triggering antigen, can acquire specificity for a novel (perhaps self) antigen.

bodies with decreased affinity appear within the germinal center, progression of these cells to the plasma or memory cell compartment will be rare, as they are not amplified further in the immune response. In contrast, B cells producing antibodies of higher affinity will continue to be amplified. Ig V gene somatic hypermutation is an important process in the generation of high-affinity antibodies, and a suboptimal frequency of Ig V gene mutation leads to common variable immunodeficiency (CVID) (102). Mutated antibodies also can acquire novel antigenic specificities. In one *in vitro* system, a single amino acid change in a protective antipneumococcal antibody results in reduced binding to pneumococci and a newly acquired affinity for dsDNA (103). Evidence suggests that antibodies to foreign antigen also can acquire autospecificity *in vivo* through somatic point mutation (104,105).

Because a given amino acid can be encoded by more than one DNA triplet, not every point mutation causes an amino acid substitution that can change antibody affinity for an antigen. It is possible to indirectly analyze antigen selection during the course of the germinal center response by calculating the ratio of replacement (R) to silent (S) mutations in rearranged antibody genes (i.e., mutations that lead to amino acid changes vs. those that do not). Purely random point mutations within a DNA sequence containing equal numbers of each possible codon would result in a predicted random R:S ratio of approximately 3:1 (106,107). The random R:S ratio for a particular DNA sequence, however, might be lower or higher than this depending on the actual codon usage (108,109).

In an antigen-selected response, one might expect a higher than random R:S ratio, because B cells containing mutations leading to higher affinity for antigen would be favored to proliferate. Further, antigen selection would predict a higher frequency of R mutations in the CDRs, because these regions include the contact amino acids for antigen binding. This type of analysis has been performed to assess whether certain autoantibodies arise from antigen-selected responses (88–90). There are two concerns, however, with this analysis. First, the assumption of purely random mutation is incorrect; recent studies have shown that bias for particular kinds of mutations occurs and that hot spots of mutation exist (110). Second, while antibodies with a higher-than-random R:S ratio probably are part of an antigen-selected repertoire, the converse clearly is not true: a single amino acid substitution is capable of conferring a tenfold increase in affinity (111,112). Thus, antigen selection may occur in the absence of a high R:S ratio.

B-1 B CELLS AND NATURAL AUTOANTIBODIES IN SLE

B-1 cells (also CD5 or Ly-1) represent a distinct population of B cells (113,114). B-1 cells are the only subset of B lymphocytes that constitutively express the pan–T-cell surface antigen CD5. The significance of this marker has not yet been elucidated. Data showing that CD5 is implicated in the maintenance of tolerance in anergic B cells (115), along with data demonstrating that CD5 mediates negative regulation of B-cell receptor (BCR) signaling in B-1 cells (116), support the hypothesis that the expression of CD5 may help inhibit autoimmune responses.

At present, it is not clear whether the B-1 population is a separate lineage or merely an alternate differentiation pathway of conventional (i.e., B-2) B cells. B-1 cells are unique among mature B lymphocytes in that they appear to be a self-replenishing population, as shown by adoptive transfer experiments in mice (117). Although rare in the spleen and lymph nodes, B-1 cells comprise approximately 10% to 40% of B cells found in the peritoneum. Being a major source of natural autoantibodies (118–120), the B-1 lineage is of particular interest to those studying autoimmunity. Elevated numbers of B-1 cells are present in the autoimmune New Zealand black (NZB) mouse strain (117), and prevention of the autoimmune symptoms has been reported with their elimination (121). B-1 cell expansion is found in some patients with rheumatoid arthritis and Sjögren's syndrome (122), but an association with SLE is weaker (123,124).

Much controversy exists over the physiologic function of the B-1 lymphocytes. B-1 cells generally express germline-encoded, polyreactive IgM antibodies with limited V gene segment usage (117–119). Adoptive transfer experiments have shown that B-1 cells are poor at forming germinal centers (125), which are characteristic of a T-dependent B-cell response and are thought to be necessary for antigen selection and class switching; however, class-switched, somatically mutated B-1 antibodies that appear to show evidence of antigen selection have been isolated from humans (126).

Low titers of low-affinity autoantibodies are part of the normal B-cell repertoire (127–130). They are not unique to any autoimmune disease, nor is there any evidence that they are pathogenic. These natural autoantibodies resemble the antibodies of a primary immune response in that they are mainly IgM and polyreactive, and bind to a wide variety of both autoantigens and foreign antigens that often have no apparent structural homology (131–133). Sequence analysis shows that they are mainly encoded by germline (i.e., unmutated) genes (134–138), although numerous exceptions exist (139). Analysis of the variable regions of natural autoantibodies suggests that they may contain more flexible hydrophilic amino acid residues in their CDRs than somatically mutated, affinity-matured antibodies, as well as longer CDRs (139), which may explain their polyreactivity.

There are some indications that the B cells producing natural antibodies may be clonally related to pathogenic B cells. Idiotypic analyses of natural anti-DNA antibodies from normal individuals and of potentially pathogenic anti-DNA antibodies from patients with SLE demonstrate that cross-reactive idiotypes are present in both populations (140,141). Some investigators have speculated that natural autoantibodies are the precursors to pathogenic autoantibodies (142,143), but more data suggest that the two classes of autoantibodies arise from distinct B-cell populations and that the SLE autoantibodies arise by the somatic mutation of genes that encode protective antibodies (91,144–149). The autoantibodies of SLE distinctly differ from natural autoantibodies. SLE autoantibodies are, in general, IgG antibodies that possess high affinity for antigen and are often extremely cross-reactive (150); for example, anti-DNA antibodies also may bind other phosphate-rich antigens such as cardiolipin and phospholipid (151–153).

PATHOGENIC AUTOANTIBODIES

Indirect evidence for the pathogenicity of several autoantibodies present in SLE includes their association with clinical manifestations in SLE and their presence in affected tissue. For example, antiphospholipid antibodies are associated with fetal wastage and thrombosis (154,155). Anti-Ro antibodies are associated with neonatal SLE and the development of cardiac conduction abnormalities during fetal development (156).

In recent years there is increasing evidence to directly support the pathogenic potential of several lupus-associated autoantibodies. A transgenic mouse expressing the heavy and light chain of the secreted form of an anti-DNA antibody has been shown to develop glomerulonephritis, thereby confirming that anti-DNA antibodies cause renal disease (157). Support for the pathogenic role of anti-DNA antibodies in nephritis can also be found in recent autoimmune disease models displaying high titers of anti-DNA antibodies together with immunoglobulin deposition in the kidney and histologic nephritis (158–161). Perfusion of monoclonal mouse and polyclonal human IgG anti-DNA antibodies through isolated rat kidney induces significant proteinuria and decreased clearance of inulin (162). Addition of plasma as a source of complement markedly increases proteinuria, while preincubation of the antibodies with DNA abolishes binding to renal tissue (162). It is still unknown, however, whether pathogenic anti-DNA antibodies form immune complexes with antigen *in-situ*, or if the antibodies bind to a target antigen that is actually some component of glomerular tissue and/or tubular components. A decrease in binding of anti-DNA antibodies to glomerular elements with DNAse treatment in some experimental models (163) but not in others (164) suggests that both models pertain; some anti-DNA antibodies directly cross-react with glomerular antigens, while other anti-DNA antibodies may bind via a DNA-containing bridge. A number of investigators have administered monoclonal anti-DNA antibodies to nonautoimmune mice, either intraperitoneally in the form of ascites-producing hybridomas or intravenously as purified immunoglobulins (165,166). In these models, it is possible to demonstrate that anti-DNA antibodies differ with respect to pathogenicity (166,167), with some antibodies depositing in the kidney and others not. Moreover, those antibodies that deposit in the kidney may differ with respect to the localization of deposition (166,168).

Recent studies have elegantly demonstrated the arrhythmogenic potential of anti-Ro antibodies. Affinity-purified anti-Ro antibodies from lupus mothers of babies with congenital heart block inhibit calcium currents and induce complete heart block in an *ex vivo* perfused human fetal heart system (169). Immunization of female BALB/c mice with recombinant La and Ro particles leads to first-degree atrioventricular block in 6% to 20% of pups born to immunized mothers, and rarely to advanced conduction defects in offspring of mice immunized with 52-kd Ro (170). Finally, passive transfer of purified human IgG containing anti-Ro and anti-La antibodies to pregnant BALB/c mice results in bradycardia and first-degree atrioventricular block (171).

Experimental evidence has also become available to support the close epidemiologic association between antiphospholipid antibodies and thrombosis. Following experimental induction of vascular injury in mice, injection of affinity-purified immunoglobulin from patients with antiphospholipid syndrome results in a significant increase in thrombus size and a delay in disappearance of the thrombus (172). Injecting human monoclonal anticardiolipin antibodies into pregnant BALB/c mice results in fetal resorption, and a significant decrease in placental and fetal weight (173). Similar results have been obtained by passive transfer of monoclonal murine and polyclonal human anticardiolipin antibodies (174).

Looking at the epidemiologic and experimental data in combination, it seems clear that the importance of several lupus-associated autoantibodies lies not only in their diagnostic significance as markers for the disease, but also in a pathogenic role in tissue damage in affected target organs in SLE. Treating disease with the end point of lowering the titer of specific autoantibodies then becomes a therapeutic goal with a clear pathophysiologic rationale.

Heavy-chain isotype appears to be important in determining the pathogenicity of autoantibodies. For example, marked differences in the severity of induced hemolysis exist among IgG isotype switch variants of an antierythrocytic antibody, related to the capacity of the different isotypes to bind to Fc receptors (175). In murine lupus, the switch from serum IgM anti-DNA activity to IgG anti-DNA activity heralds the onset of renal disease (176). Similarly, human IgG antibodies present in the immune complex deposits within kidneys of patients with SLE appear to trigger mesangial cell proliferation and subsequent tissue damage to a greater extent than IgM antibodies, perhaps because mesangial cells or infiltrating mononuclear cells have Fc receptors for IgG (177). The importance of isotype for anticardiolipin antibodies is intriguing (2); several groups have noted that IgG antiphospholipid and β_2-glycoprotein antibodies correlate better with clinical thrombosis than other isotypes do (see Chapter 25). Nevertheless, pathogenicity has been shown also for the IgM and IgA isotypes (172). IgM and IgA anticardiolipin antibodies also correlate with specific disease phenotypes. For example, IgM antiphospholipid antibodies are associated with hemolytic anemia (178). As a rule, however, heavy-chain class switching to IgG may increase the pathogenicity of lupus antibodies. Other characteristics of autoantibodies that are thought to promote pathogenicity are high avidity for the self antigen, charge, expression of particular idiotypic determinants, and fine specificity (166).

It was formerly widely believed that antibodies could not penetrate live cells, and that nuclear staining of sectioned tissues was an artifact of tissue preparation. There is now evidence that some anti-DNA and antiribosomal P autoantibodies bind to the cell surface, transverse the cytoplasm, and reach the nucleus. Furthermore, there are data to demonstrate a pathogenic effect from cellular penetration by autoantibodies (179–181). While antigen translocation to the cell membrane may explain the accessibility of intranuclear antigens to interaction with autoantibodies (182,183), the capability to penetrate live cells and interact with cytoplasmic or nuclear components may be an additional pathogenic characteristic of some autoantibodies.

While this chapter discusses aspects of autoantibody production, it is possible that autoantibody-mediated tissue damage requires not just the presence of autoantibodies but also the display of a specific antigen in the target organ (184). Differential display of antigen at the level of the target organ may contribute to genetic susceptibility to autoimmune disease. Evidence for such a hypothesis comes, in part, from a murine model of autoimmune myocarditis, where differential susceptibility to antimyosin antibody-induced disease in different mouse strains is dependent on differences in the composition of cardiac extracellular matrix (185). Similarly, in a rat model for tubular nephritis, antibody-mediated disease depends on genetically determined antigen display in the renal tubules (186).

GENETIC AND MOLECULAR ANALYSIS OF ANTI-DNA ANTIBODIES

Genetic analyses of anti-DNA antibodies in both human and murine lupus have provided important information regarding the production of autoantibodies. There is currently no evidence that a distinct set of disease-associated, autoreactive V region genes, present only in individuals with a familial susceptibility to autoimmunity, is used to encode the autoantibodies of autoimmune disease. It is also clear that no particular immunoglobulin V region genes are absolutely required for the production of autoantibodies. Immunoglobulin genes that are present in a nonautoimmune animal clearly are capable of forming pathogenic autoantibodies. The offspring of a nonautoimmune SWR mouse and an NZB mouse (SNF1 mice) spontaneously produce autoantibodies (187), and a large percentage of the anti-DNA antibodies deposited in the kidneys of (NZB × SWR) F1 mice are encoded by genes derived from the nonautoimmune SWR parent (187). In fact, both idiotypic and molecular studies show that the V region genes used to produce autoantibodies in lupus are also used in a protective antibody response in nonautoimmune individuals (188,189). Autoantibodies bear cross-reactive idiotypes that also are present on the antibodies that are made in response to foreign antigens, and V region genes used to encode autoantibodies also encode antibodies to foreign antigen (190–193). Indeed, a number of autoantibodies cross-react with foreign antigens, demonstrating that the same V region gene segments can be used in both protective and potentially pathogenic responses (194–196). These cross-reactive antibodies are capable of binding to bacterial antigen with high affinity, but they also possess specificity for a self antigen. Patients with *Klebsiella* infections and individuals vaccinated with pneumococcal polysaccharide develop antibacterial antibodies expressing anti-DNA cross-reactive idiotypes (188,197). *In vivo*, cross-reactive antibodies with specificity both to pneumococcus and to dsDNA were shown in mice to be protective against an otherwise lethal bacterial infection, yet they also can deposit in the kidney and cause glomerular damage (198). It is possible that cross-reactive antibodies are routinely generated during the course of the normal immune response in the nonautoimmune individual. Ordinarily, however, autoreactive B cells expressing a self specificity are actively downregulated and contribute little to the expressed antibody repertoire.

Although there is no evidence that specific genes encode only autoantibodies, there are data to suggest that autoantibodies are encoded by a somewhat restricted number of immunoglobulin V region genes (199–201). In murine lupus, extensive analyses of anti-DNA–producing B cells show that 15 to 20 heavy-chain V region genes encode most anti-DNA antibodies (202–205). Studying an autoantibody associated J558 gene, investigators (201) found a dramatic increase in frequency of use of heavy chains encoded by this particular gene in autoimmune as compared to normal mice, while nonautoimmune mice immunized with an immunogenic DNA/DNA-binding peptide complex displayed intermediate usage. This supports the concept that differences in V gene usage that may be seen between autoimmune and nonautoimmune mice are quantitative, rather than reflecting a true qualitative difference. While molecular studies of human antibodies are more limited, idiotypic analyses also suggest restricted V gene usage. This is important if antiidiotypes are to play a role in therapeutic strategies. Nevertheless, the anti-DNA response is no more restricted than are many responses to foreign antigen. Furthermore, the restricted V region gene usage does not appear to be skewed toward particular gene families.

Analysis of restriction fragment length polymorphisms, which is a tool used to identify the similarities and differences among particular genes in a population, has been used to examine whether distinct polymorphisms associate with SLE (206–208). A deletion of a specific heavy-chain V gene, *hv-3*, was reported to be more frequent in individuals with SLE or rheumatoid arthritis (209,210). A specific germline Vκ gene, *A30*, was found to increase the cationicity (and therefore the pathogenicity) of human anti-DNA antibodies. A defective *A30* gene was found in eight of nine lupus patients without nephritis, while this gene was normal in all nine lupus patients with nephritis (211). Polymorphism at the *Vκ* gene locus may then contribute to susceptibility to lupus nephritis. While this is not a universal finding, these studies suggest that genetic polymorphisms in immunoglobulin genes may make some contribution to the generation of autoantibodies and expression of human lupus.

Somatic mutation is a possible mechanism by which protective, antiforeign antibodies evolve into pathogenic autoantibodies (Fig. 19.4) (212,213). The characteristics and mechanics of somatic mutation in SLE are therefore of interest. Examining ten human antibodies positive for a specific, lupus-associated idiotype (F4), Manheimer-Lory et al. (214) found no change in the frequency of somatic mutations or the distributions of such mutations in CDRs. While the normal process of somatic mutation is generally random, there is some bias for mutation at specific sequence motifs, termed mutational "hot spots." Surprisingly, F4$^+$ antibodies displayed abnormal somatic mutation as shown by a decrease in hot-spot targeting. As mice transgenic for the antiapoptotic gene *bcl-2* also display this same decreased targeting of mutations to hot spots (215), the decreased targeting in F4$^+$ antibodies derived from lupus patients may reflect an abnormal state of B-cell activation rather than defective machinery for somatic mutation. Studies have been performed (216) on the mutational process in the Vk gene repertoire in individual B cells from a single lupus patient. The frequency of mutations was increased in both productive and unproductive Vκ rearrangements, with evidence of increased targeting to mutational hot spots in framework regions, consistent with altered selection. A single study in mice found essentially no differences in somatic mutation between B cells of an autoreactive and normal strain (217). Abnormal somatic mutation may be due to important alterations in B-cell activation in SLE; however, conflicting data prevent drawing firm conclusions as yet.

AUTOANTIBODY INDUCTION

For the most part, autoantibodies that are present in SLE do not exist in an unstimulated B-cell repertoire. Rather, autoantibodies in SLE usually reflect the process of somatic mutation and apparently are made by B cells following exposure to antigen and T cells. For some autoantibodies, mutation of the germline sequences clearly is crucial in generating the autoantigenic specificity (218). These antibodies have a high R:S ratio, primarily in CDRs; however, the pitfalls of R:S ratio calculations have been discussed and should be considered in the analysis of anti-DNA antibodies (110,111). There also are lupus autoantibodies that have a high R:S ratio in framework regions (219). As these framework region mutations are less likely to alter antigenic specificity, it is tempting to speculate that they instead may facilitate escape from a putative regulatory mechanism. High-affinity anti-dsDNA antibodies also can be encoded by germline genes (220), but these rarely are found in disease.

There are various hypotheses regarding the nature of the eliciting antigen or antigens in SLE (Table 19.3). Several lines of evidence support the role of foreign, microbial antigens in the generation of autoantibodies (221). Lupus-prone strains of mice carrying the xid mutation, which impairs production of the antipolysaccharide antibodies that are required for antibacterial immunity, develop much lower titers of anti-DNA antibodies and decreased renal disease (222). Similarly, autoimmune-prone NZB mice raised in a germ-free environment produce reduced titers of anti-DNA antibodies and show delayed onset of autoimmune manifestations (223). Recently, it has been shown that raising lupus-prone lymphoproliferative (MRL/*lpr/lpr*) mice in a germ-free environment and feeding them a filtered, antigen-free diet significantly decreased the severity of renal disease (224). Evidence that an anti-pneumococcal antibody can spontaneously mutate to become an anti-DNA antibody in an *in vitro* system (103), as well as in response to immunization with a pneumococcal antigen *in vivo* (104), also supports a close structural relationship between the autoantibody response and a protective antibacterial response. Finally, to further demonstrate the close relationship between a protective antibacterial and autoantibody response in lupus, Kowal et al. (225) generated a combinatorial immunoglobulin expression

TABLE 19.3. ANTIGENIC TRIGGERS FOR ANTI-dsDNA ANTIBODIES

Foreign antigen
- Molecular mimics
- Bacterial DNA
- Complexes of DNA and DNA-binding proteins (Fus-1 DNA, T-antigen DNA)

Self-antigen
- RNP autoepitopes
- Histone peptides
- Peptides derived from anti-dsDNA antibodies
- Cryptic autoepitopes (sequestered autoantigens, altered processing/presentation)

Idiotypic network (antiidiotypic antibody = autoantigen)

dsDNA, double-stranded DNA; RNP, ribonucleoprotein.

library on phage from splenocytes of a lupus patient immunized with pneumococcal polysaccharide. Four of eight (50%) of the monovalent Fab fragments selected for expression of a SLE associated idiotype bound both pneumococcal polysaccharide and dsDNA, indicating that a significant portion of the human antipneumococcal response in SLE is cross-reactive with self antigen.

Molecular mimicry as well as somatic mutation might be important mechanisms by which exposure to foreign, bacterial antigen can elicit autoantibodies. Molecular mimicry refers to a sufficient structural homology between foreign and self antigen that allows both antigens to be recognized by a single, cross-reactive B cell. The best-known example for this mechanism in induction of autoimmunity is rheumatic fever, in which the antibodies arising in the antistreptococcal response cross-react with cardiac myosin, leading to antibody deposition in cardiac muscle and carditis. A molecular mimic can induce an autoantibody response by activating cross-reactive B cells specific for both foreign and self antigen. These B cells receive T-cell help for autoantibody production from T cells activated by microbial proteins. In support of a possible role of molecular mimicry in inducing anti-DNA antibodies is the rise in autoantibodies seen even in nonautoimmune hosts following infection (226). Furthermore, nonautoimmune individuals vaccinated with pneumococcal polysaccharide generate antipneumococcal antibodies idiotypically related to anti-DNA antibodies (188). Infection does not usually lead to self-perpetuating autoimmunity, as the T-cell help available for cross-reactive B cells dissipates following the clearing of the infectious agent. Failure to resolve the autoimmune process induced by a molecular mimic may be due to a defect in reinduction of tolerance or persistence of the foreign antigen. Some possible causes for a lack of return to a tolerant state include activation of T cells by antigenic epitopes to which T-cell tolerance had never been established (cryptic epitopes) (227), upregulation of co-stimulatory molecules, the presence of immunomodulatory cytokines, and abnormally enhanced intracellular signaling.

Peptide antigens that structurally mimic DNA can also elicit an autoantibody response (228,229). Screening a phage peptide display library with a pathogenic IgG2b anti-dsDNA antibody, it was possible to identify the D/E W D/E Y S/G consensus motif that is recognized by the antibody (229). DWEYS inhibits the binding of the antibody to dsDNA as well as antibody binding to glomeruli *in vivo*. Immunization of nonautoimmune BALB/c mice with a multimeric peptide containing the consensus motif induces significant serum titers of IgG anti-dsDNA antibodies, as well as antihistone, anti-Sm/RNP, and anticardiolipin antibodies. Monoclonal antibodies from peptide-immunized BALB/c mice resemble anti-dsDNA antibodies present in spontaneous murine lupus, including similar VH and VL gene usage, and generation of arginines in heavy chain CDR3 regions (230).

There is some evidence to suggest that nucleic acids can induce anti-dsDNA antibodies (see also below the discussion of a possible role of disturbed apoptosis in breaking B-cell tolerance). While investigators have long known that mammalian dsDNA is not immunogenic, recent studies have focused on bacterial DNA as a potential trigger for induction of anti-dsDNA antibodies. Bacterial DNA contains unmethylated CpG motifs, which may be an important adjuvant in the immune system (231). Preautoimmune lupus-prone mice immunized with bacterial DNA produce antibodies that not only bind to the immunizing antigen, but are also cross-reactive with mammalian DNA (232). However, the response of nonautoimmune mice to bacterial DNA was non–cross-reactive, indicating that bacterial DNA alone is not sufficient to induce anti-dsDNA antibodies in a non–lupus-prone host.

Another possible model for induction of anti-DNA antibodies is by a hapten-carrier–like mechanism, in which T cells recognize epitopes of a protein carrier associated with DNA and provide help for autoreactive B cells specific for hapten (DNA). Novel peptide determinants of the protein component of the complex may then be presented by DNA-specific B cells to recruit autoreactive T cells, and further perpetuate the autoimmune state. Immunization of nonautoimmune animals with DNA together with DNA-binding proteins such as DNAse I (233), Fus 1 (derived from *Trypanosoma cruzi*) (234), and the polyomavirus transcription factor T antigen (235) results in the generation of anti-dsDNA antibodies with structural similarity to anti-dsDNA antibodies present in spontaneous murine lupus.

Because antiidiotypic antibodies can function like antigen to induce an antibody response, some investigators have emphasized a potential role for antiidiotype in activating autoantibody production. For example, the Ku antigen is a DNA-binding protein (236). Studies of anti-DNA and anti-Ku antibodies suggest that the anti-Ku antibodies are antiidiotypic to anti-DNA antibodies (237). Several studies have found that mice immunized with an anti-DNA antibody and mice immunized with an antiidiotypic antibody to an anti-DNA antibody each develop autoantibodies (238,239). This has also been shown for other autoantigen-autoantibody systems important in lupus, such as anticardiolipin antibodies (240). Interestingly, immunization with antibodies recognizing a DNA-binding protein (anti-p53 antibodies) can generate anti-DNA antibodies (241). While such studies suggest that the idiotypic network may contribute to the production of autoantibodies, others have suggested that antiidiotypes function to induce or maintain clinical remissions (242).

Autoantibody responses to anatomically associated antigens are often simultaneously present in established SLE (Ro/La, Sm/RNP). Yet with longitudinal studies begun early on in the disease course, it is possible to demonstrate that a particular response may be initially limited to a particular peptide epitope, followed by intramolecular (other epitopes in the same polypeptide) and intermolecular (epitopes in distinct, but structurally linked molecules) spread of the response (243). This process is termed epitope spreading, and is the result of processing by antigen-presenting cells (including B cells) of the multimolecular complex, and presentation of novel epitopes to nontolerized T cells. The initial target for epitope spreading may be a molecular mimic derived from a microorganism, or a self antigen. Recent data have suggested that apoptosis can generate novel nuclear autoantigen fragments (244) that may become accessible to interaction with antibody molecules by translocation to the cell surface (183,245). Neoepitopes of particular antigens generated by specific forms of apoptosis might also explain defined autoantibody profiles that are associated with SLE.

The potential role for epitope spreading in diversification of the autoantibody response in SLE has been clearly demonstrated for spliceosome autoimmunity. James and Harley (247) identified two B/B′ octapeptides that were early targets of an anti-Sm response in lupus patients. Rabbits (246) and some inbred mouse strains (247) immunized with one of these octapeptides, PPPGMRPP, develop over time an immune response against other regions of Sm B/B′ and Sm D. Furthermore, in some animals antinuclear antibodies and anti-dsDNA antibodies arose. B-cell epitope spreading has also been demonstrated in the Ro/La autoantigen system (248).

Investigators have (249) identified pathogenic T cells in SNF1 lupus-prone mice that were pathogenic *in vivo*, and accelerated the development of an immune deposit glomerulonephritis in preautoimmune mice. About 50% of these pathogenic T-cell clones were found to respond to nucleosomal antigens, specifically histone peptides. Stimulating these T-cell clones with the histone peptides leads to increased anti-DNA antibody secretion in a coculture system, and peptide immunization induces severe glomerulonephritis (250). Other investigators have focused on the immunogenicity of peptides derived from the VH regions of anti-DNA antibodies themselves (251,252). They (251) reported that three such 12-mer peptides induce a class II restricted proliferation of unprimed T cells from preautoimmune NZB × New Zealand white (NZW) F1 mice. Immunization with one peptide, or transfer of a T-cell line reactive with this peptide, increased the titer of anti-dsDNA antibodies and the severity of the nephritis in NZB × NZW F1 mice. Further support for a possible role of self peptide in induction of anti-dsDNA antibodies can be found in studies showing that tolerization with self peptides can downregulate anti-dsDNA antibody production and nephritis in murine lupus (252–254).

B-CELL TOLERANCE

Several transgenic mouse models have recently been described in which immunoglobulin V regions encoding anti-DNA or other autoantibodies have been introduced into the germline. The importance of these models is multifold: (a) they afford perhaps the best direct evidence that certain anti-DNA antibodies are pathogenic, (b) they have contributed significantly to understanding the tolerizing mechanisms that regulate anti-DNA–producing cells and the defects that allow escape of these cells, and (c) they provide a model in which to test novel therapies designed to block tissue injury or inactivate pathogenic B cells.

B cells expressing autoreactive immunoglobulin receptors arise in all hosts at times of B-cell receptor diversification, both during formation of the naive B-cell repertoire and again during the germinal center response. Regulation of these autoreactive receptors is through inactivation or deletion (255) (Table 19.4). These mechanisms appear to operate when membrane immunoglobulins are cross-linked by antigen in the absence of T-cell help. Whether anergy or deletion occurs depends in part on the extent of membrane immunoglobulin cross-linking (256). Normally, the serum of nonautoimmune mice does not contain high-affinity IgG autoantibodies, illustrating that the normal immune system can efficiently regulate autoantibody-producing B cells. Initial studies of anti-DNA transgenic nonautoimmune mice showed that anti-DNA antibodies are eliminated from the immune repertoire through functional inactivation (i.e., anergy) or deletion (257,258). In lupus-prone mice, there appears to be a defect in some aspect of regulation, allowing the autoreactive B cells to survive and contribute to the expressed antibody repertoire. A more recent study demonstrated that "ignorance" is an additional possible fate of DNA-binding B cells (259). Bynoe et al. (259) isolated low-affinity, DNA-binding B cells from a nonautoimmune mouse transgenic for an anti-DNA heavy chain. These B cells were in a resting state and produced germline-encoded, nonpathogenic antibodies. These cells may be a potential source of pathogenic autoantibodies; they may be recruited into an ongoing immune response, and then become high-affinity (and pathogenic) antibodies via somatic mutation.

Recent studies of mice that are transgenic for autoantibody genes have illuminated an additional mechanism used in maintaining self tolerance. A second immunoglobulin rearrangement may occur, so that the transgenic heavy chain is paired with an endogenous light chain to generate a VH-VL combination that is no longer autoreactive (260). Termed receptor editing, this phenomenon may be another mechanism allowing B cells to maintain tolerance (261). There also is evidence that receptor editing may occur in the heavy-chain locus (262).

TABLE 19.4. MECHANISMS OF B-CELL TOLERANCE

Clonal anergy
Clonal deletion
Clonal ignorance
Receptor editing

Recent transgenic studies have bred anti-DNA transgenes onto autoimmune genetic backgrounds to better understand the differential regulation of the anti-dsDNA specificity in lupus-prone mice (263). An additional innovation has been the application of "knock-in" technology (in which the immunoglobulin transgene is inserted into its proper genetic locus), which provides a more physiologic system in that somatic mutation and isotype switching of the inserted V region may occur (264–266). No one single defect could be identified in tolerance mechanisms (deletion, anergy, receptor editing) to account for the selective expansion of anti-DNA specific B cells in lupus mice. In fact, it has been reported that autoimmune MRL/*lpr*/*lpr* mice can efficiently delete B lymphocytes with a transgenic autoreactive receptor (267).

It is important to understand that the various thresholds for tolerance induction in autoreactive B cells (deletion, anergy, indifference) are not static, but rather may be dynamically altered by immune modulators such as cytokines, hormones, or co-stimulatory molecules. Studies of transgenic and knockout mice, engineered to overexpress or be deficient in molecules of interest, have begun to unravel genes and pathways involved in B-cell regulation and in B-cell tolerance.

The B-cell receptor (BCR) is a complex of surface immunoglobulin with the accessory molecules Igα and Igβ. Following receptor cross-linking by binding of antigen to the BCR, a complex cascade of signaling molecules becomes involved in transducing the signal from the BCR to eventually result in B-cell activation and proliferation, or anergy and death. The potential involvement of enhanced signaling or decreases in negative regulatory signals as possible contributors to autoimmunity is discussed below (Table 19.5).

The finding that expression of a lupus-like syndrome in MRL/*lpr*/*lpr* and C3H *gld*/*gld* mice is due to a single defect in the apoptosis genes Fas and Fas ligand, respectively (268–270), has generated a large amount of interest in examining the role of dysregulated apoptosis in human autoimmunity (Table 19.5). Alterations in Fas and Fas ligand have been described in patients with systemic lupus, with some studies describing a correlation with manifestations of disease and clinical activity (271–275). Interestingly, humans with a variety of defects in the Fas receptor have been described, some of which manifest as significant lymphadenopathy (Canale-Smith syndrome) reminiscent of the lymphoproliferative phenotype of *lpr* mice with defective Fas (276). While only a single lupus patient has been described with a Fas receptor defect, Fas mutations are clearly associated with dysregulated lymphocytes and even rarely defective apoptosis (277).

TABLE 19.5. SINGLE GENE DEFECTS CAUSING AUTOIMMUNITY

Molecules involved in apoptosis
lpr deficiency
gld deficiency
bcl-2 overexpression
Serum amyloid protein deficiency
DNAse I deficiency
C1q deficiency
Signaling molecules
CD19 overexpression
CD22 deficiency
Lyn deficiency
SHP-1 deficiency

Other apoptosis genes have also been implicated in induction of autoimmunity. Transgenic mice overexpressing *bcl-2* have long-lived lymphocytes and enhanced immune responses to immunization, and spontaneously develop antinuclear antigens and immune complex glomerulonephritis (278). Enforced *bcl-2* expression allows recovery of cross-reactive anti-dsDNA, antipneumococcal antibodies from the primary response of nonautoimmune hosts immunized with a pneumococcal cell wall antigen (279). Furthermore, normally anergized or deleted autoreactive anti-DNA B cells could be recovered from mice transgenic both for *bcl-2* and an anti-dsDNA heavy chain (280). Recently it has been shown that estrogen can modify the expressed B-cell repertoire in mice transgenic for an anti-DNA heavy chain, and facilitate the recovery of high-affinity B cells (281). Estrogen may be upregulating *bcl-2*, thus interfering with tolerance induction.

Another possible link between apoptosis and autoimmunity can be found in studies showing that altered clearance of apoptotic particles and persistence of nuclear material in the circulation may induce anti-DNA antibodies. It was shown that immunizing nonautoimmune mice intravenously with syngeneic apoptotic cells induces antinuclear antibodies with specificity for cardiolipin and ssDNA (282). Furthermore, these mice also develop renal immunoglobulin deposition. Recent studies demonstrate a role for complement receptors in clearing of apoptotic cells from the circulation, thus perhaps explaining the apparent paradox that humans with a deficiency in early complement components are more susceptible to SLE. Serum markedly enhances the uptake of apoptotic cells by phagocytes; components of both classic and alternative pathways of complement are responsible for the enhanced uptake (283). Phosphatidylserine on the apoptotic cell surface may activate complement, coating apoptotic cells with C3bi, which facilitates apoptotic cell uptake by macrophage complement receptors (283). Clearance of apoptotic cells via complement receptors may be important in maintaining self tolerance to nuclear antigens. Deficiency in complement receptors CD21/CD35 or complement protein C4 in Fas-deficient mice (284) and C1q deficiency in normal mice (160) accelerates or induces lupus-like features.

Serum amyloid P may also play a role in handling of chromatin from apoptotic cells. Serum amyloid P knockout mice spontaneously develop antinuclear antibodies and severe glomerulonephritis, and display increased anti-DNA antibody levels in response to chromatin immunization (285). A similar lupus phenotype occurs in mice with a targeted deletion in DNAse 1, an enzyme that may be important in degrading DNA generated by apoptosis. Interestingly, patients with SLE had significantly lower serum levels of DNAse 1 when compared to controls with nephritis from other causes (161).

In mice, the complete phenotypic expression of autoimmunity caused by the *lpr* defect (286) or the *bcl-2* transgene (287) is highly dependent on the genetic background. We discussed above several autoimmune disease models, in which defects in apoptosis or in clearing of apoptotic cells lead to antinuclear autoimmunity and glomerulonephritis. It seems reasonable to speculate that Fas, Fas ligand, *bcl-2*, and other genes and regulators of apoptosis, in combination with additional as yet unidentified genes, may be sufficient to induce many of the phenotypic features of systemic lupus in humans.

Abnormalities in signaling pathways can alter regulatory thresholds for B-cell tolerance. The BCR is associated with several molecules that comprise the B-cell co-receptor complex. CD19 is part of the co-receptor complex, and plays a role in regulating signaling thresholds that modulate B-cell activation and autoimmunity (288). CD19 overexpression leads to B-cell hyperresponsiveness and breakdown of peripheral tolerance, as manifested by increased levels of anti-DNA antibodies and rheumatoid factor in mice transgenic for CD19 (289). C22 is a B-cell surface glycoprotein that becomes rapidly phosphorylated following BCR cross-linking. CD22 is a negative signaling regulator, as shown by hyperresponsiveness to receptor signaling in mice deficient for the molecule (290). CD22 knockout mice display a heightened immune response, increased numbers of B-1 B cells, and serum autoantibodies (291). Associated with CD22 are Lyn and SHP-1. Targeted deletion of the genes encoding either of these molecules leads to autoimmune manifestations (292–294). The effects of alterations of these signaling molecules on regulation of tolerance and autoimmunity are evident in mice; however, a definite role for altered signaling in the autoimmune diathesis in patients with lupus is speculative at this time.

THERAPEUTIC INTERVENTIONS

Classic therapeutic interventions in SLE are characterized by their lack of specificity for B cells making particular pathogenic antibodies. Besides the desired decrease in autoantibody production by B cells, these therapies also cause a more generalized immune suppression, with potentially devastating consequences. In recent years, there have been several new and intriguing developments in the treatment of SLE (Table 19.6). Important advances in the molecular biology of B lymphocytes and their regulation have increased our understanding of the immunologic mechanisms that mediate B-cell tolerance and offer new opportunities and novel targets for therapeutic manipulation. Furthermore, antigen-specific therapies may increase the selectivity of the intervention, offering efficacy while potentially decreasing unwanted side effects.

TABLE 19.6. THERAPEUTIC INTERVENTIONS IN SLE

Non–antigen-specific therapies
Classic immunosuppressives (corticosteroids, cytotoxics)
Rapamycin
Mycophenolic acid
Inhibition of co-stimulation (anti-CD40 ligand, CTLA-4–Ig)
Stem cell transplantation
Hormonal manipulation
Antigen-specific therapies
LJP 394 (tetrameric oligonucleotides)
Peptide-based
Immunoglobulin V region–derived peptides
Histone peptides
Peptide mimotopes of dsDNA

CTLA, cytotoxic T-lymphocyte antigen.

Non–Antigen-Specific Therapies: Interfering With Cognate Interactions

Antiself antibodies in SLE clearly arise from T-cell–dependent responses. Among the important accessory molecules in the B-cell–T-cell interaction, CD40 ligand (gp39) is expressed on activated T cells and binds to antigen-specific B cells to transduce a second signal for B-cell proliferation and differentiation (Fig. 19.3). A short treatment of young SNF1 lupus-prone mice with a monoclonal antibody to CD40 ligand markedly delays and reduces the incidence of lupus nephritis for long after the antibody had been cleared (295). Furthermore, treatment of older SNF1 mice with established nephritis reduces the severity of nephritis and prolongs survival (296). Similarly, treating NZB × NZW F1 mice with anti-CD40 ligand leads to decreased anti-dsDNA antibody titers, less renal disease, and most importantly improved survival compared to the control group (297). Inhibition of other co-stimulatory molecules was also found to be beneficial in lupus. Selective inhibition of the interaction of co-stimulatory molecules B7-CD28 by cytotoxic T-lymphocyte antigen-4 (CTLA-4)–Ig (a recombinant fusion molecule between CTLA-4 and the Fc portion of an immunoglobulin molecule) blocks autoantibody production and prolongs life in NZB × NZW F1 mice, even when given late in the course of disease (298,299). Moreover, simultaneous blockade of B7/CD28 and CD40/CD40 ligand with a short course of CTLA-4–Ig and anti-CD40 ligand was significantly more effective than either intervention alone (300). Clinical trials are now under way to study treatment with anti-CD40 ligand and CTLA-4–Ig in human lupus.

Non–Antigen-Specific Therapies: Mycophenolate And Rapamycin

Mycophenolate mofetil inhibits inosine monophosphate dehydrogenase, an enzyme important in the *de novo* synthesis of guanine nucleotides. Inhibition of this metabolic pathway inhibits B- and T-cell proliferation, and results in immunosuppression (301). While mycophenolate mofetil acts as a cytotoxic agent by inhibiting cell division, this effect is relatively selective, and limited to lymphocytes. In MRL/*lpr/lpr* (302) and NZB × NZW F1 (303) murine lupus models, mycophenolate mofetil improves renal disease, decreases serum anti-dsDNA antibody levels, and significantly prolongs survival. In a recent small pilot study in human lupus, mycophenolate mofetil had some beneficial effects in patients with moderate to severe lupus activity (304).

Rapamycin is a novel immunosuppressive macrolide drug, which inhibits lymphocyte proliferation. Rapamycin binds to a protein kinase important in regulating cell cycle progression (305). In MRL/*lpr/lpr* mice, treatment with rapamycin significantly reduces serologic as well as pathologic manifestation of the autoimmune disease (306). Treatment of NZB × NZW F1 mice with early nephritis (5 months of age) with a brief course of anti-B7 antibodies in combination with an 8-week course of rapamycin increases survival at 10 months to 100% versus only 40% in the nontreated mice (307).

Antigen-Based Therapies

There are two possible ways by which antigen conjugates can theoretically improve the course of disease in lupus. First, antigen conjugates may specifically block pathogenic autoantibodies from binding to their target antigen and initiating the inflammatory cascade. Second, antigen conjugates may downregulate antigen-specific B cells and induce specific B-cell tolerance by providing "signal 1" through the antigen receptor without "signal 2" (co-stimulation). One such conjugate, polyethylene-glycol with tetrameric oligonucleotides, was given to BXSB male lupus-prone mice (308). Treatment decreased the number of anti-dsDNA–producing cells, decreased proteinuria, and significantly increased survival. A small, initial study in humans found no major adverse effects, with some decrease in the serum anti-dsDNA titers (309). A much larger phase II/III trial is currently in progress.

A putative role for peptides in induction of anti-DNA antibodies was discussed above; these small antigens may also be suited for therapeutic use. Intravenous treatment of preautoimmune SNF1 mice with nucleosomal peptides postponed the onset of nephritis, while chronic treatment of older mice with established disease improved survival (253). Peptides derived from anti-dsDNA antibodies have been shown to activate autoreactive T cells that provide help for the production of autoantibodies (see above). Treating NZB × NZW F1 mice with several T-cell peptide epitopes derived from an anti-dsDNA antibody induces T-cell tolerance to the peptides, and results in significantly improved renal disease and prolonged mean survival (254). Similarly, neonatal mice treated with CDR-based peptides acquire resistance to subsequent induction of autoimmunity (252).

The recent technology of displaying random peptides in phage permits the identification of peptides that function as surrogate antigens to autoantibodies. The selected peptide does not necessarily have to be the actual sequence that is recognized by pathogenic antibody (although it can be). Studies have demonstrated that peptides can be identified by screening phage peptide display libraries with pathogenic anti-dsDNA antibodies (228,229), and that these peptides may inhibit the deposition of antibody in renal glomeruli *in vivo* (229). Whether peptide dsDNA mimotopes will be useful in inhibiting polyclonal antibody deposition and/or directly tolerizing pathogenic B cells in lupus mouse models is currently under investigation.

SUMMARY

Sequences of many anti-dsDNA antibodies have been analyzed to see how they differ from those of V regions that characterize the human and murine antibody response to foreign antigens. As expected from idiotypic studies in SLE, certain V region genes or families are used preferentially in the anti-DNA response. However, observations of restricted gene usage do not differ in principle from those made in the response of nonautoimmune animals to foreign antigen, in which a small number of V regions dominate the response to any particular antigen. No particular gene family is absolutely necessary for the production of autoantibodies; nonetheless, investigation is continuing into genetic polymorphisms in the Ig locus that are associated with human lupus. It appears that all individuals are capable of generating pathogenic autoantibodies. In autoimmune individuals, however, autoantibodies that have developed high affinity for autoantigen through somatic mutation are present in the expressed B-cell repertoire. At this time this appears to primarily reflect a defect in the mechanisms of self tolerance rather than an abnormality in V-gene repertoire, the process of gene rearrangement, or the process of somatic mutation. While a defect in central tolerance permitting exodus of autoreactive B cells from the bone marrow (perhaps through lack of proper receptor editing or through aberrant signaling) is possible in lupus, it is equally possible that the defect is in peripheral tolerance (in the regulation of B cells maturing in the germinal centers).

The autoantibody response in SLE has the characteristics of an antigen-selected response. Cognate B-T cell interactions are crucial to the maturation of pathogenic anti-dsDNA antibodies, which are primarily IgG, mono- or oligo-specific, and have high affinity for the antigen (dsDNA). Together with the higher-than-random R:S ratio in the CDRs of many anti-dsDNA antibodies, this suggests that the anti-DNA response is both driven and selected by an antigen. Pathogenic, IgG anti-dsDNA antibodies in SLE seem to arise from the conventional B-cell lineage, possibly through somatic mutation of genes encoding protective antibodies. Nevertheless, there is some speculation that natural autoantibodies, perhaps from the B-1 lineage, also could be precursors for anti-DNA antibodies.

While it is likely that more than one immunologic defect can result in the clinical syndrome collectively known as SLE, important advances in understanding different aspects of disease pathogenesis has led to the development of new potential therapeutic modalities. Integration of inhibition of co-stimulation or antigen-specific therapies into the routine management of patients with systemic lupus does not seem to be that far off in the future.

REFERENCES

1. Tan EM. Autoantibodies to nuclear antigens (ANA): their immunobiology and medicine. *Adv Immunol* 1982;33: 167–240.
2. Gharavi AE, Harris EN, Lockshin MD, et al. IgG subclass and light chain distribution of anticardiolipin and anti-DNA antibodies in systemic lupus erythematosus. *Ann Rheum Dis* 1988; 47:286–290.
3. Bootsma H, Spronk PE, Ter Borg EJ, et al. The predictive value of fluctuations in IgM and IgG class anti-dsDNA antibodies for relapses in SLE. A prospective long term observation. *Ann Rheum Dis* 1997;56:661–666.
4. Koffler D. Immunopathogenesis of systemic lupus erythematosus. *Annu Rev Med* 1974;25:149–164.
5. Tan EM, Chan EKL, Sullivan KF, et al. Short analytical review: diagnostically specific immune markers and clues toward the understanding of systemic autoimmunity. *Clin Immunol Immunopathol* 1988;47:121–141.
6. Winfield JB, Faiferman I, Koffler D. Avidity of anti-DNA antibodies in serum and IgG glomerular eluates from patients with systemic lupus erythematosus. Association of high avidity antinative DNA antibody with glomerulonephritis. *J Clin Invest* 1977;59:90–96.
7. Spiegelberg HL. Biological activities of immunoglobulins of different classes and subclasses. *Adv Immunol* 1974;19: 259–294.
8. Niles MJ, Matsuuchi L, Koshland ME. Polymer IgM assembly and secretion in lymphoid and non-lymphoid cell-lines—evidence that J chain is required for pentamer IgM synthesis. *Proc Natl Acad Sci USA* 1995;92:2884–2888.
9. Sorensen V, Rasmussen IB, Sundvold V, et al. Structural requirements for incorporation of J chain into human IgM and IgA. *Int Immunol* 2000;12:19–27.
10. Maddison PJ. Autoantibodies in SLE. Disease associations. *Adv Exp Med Biol* 1999;455:141–145.
11. Hendrikson BA, Conner DA, Ladd DJ, et al. Altered hepatic transport of IgA in mice lacking the J chain. *J Exp Med* 1995; 182:1905–1115.
12. Kabat EA, Wu TT. Attempts to locate complementarity determining residues in the variable positions of light and heavy chains. *Ann NY Acad Sci* 1971;190:382–393.
13. Poljak RJ, Anzel LM, Avey HP, et al. Three dimensional structure of the Fab fragment of a human immunoglobulin at 2.8 A. *Proc Natl Acad Sci USA* 1973;70:3305–3310.
14. Padlan EA. Anatomy of the antibody molecule. *Mol Immunol* 1994;31:169–217.
15. Porter RR. The hydrolysis of rabbit g-globulin and antibodies with crystalline papain. *Biochem J* 1959;73:119–126.
16. Nisonoff A, Wissler FC, Lipman LN, et al. Separation of univalent fragments from the bivalent rabbit antibody molecule by reduction of disulfide bonds. *Arch Biophys,* 1960;89:230–244
17. Gerstein M, Lesk AM, Chothia C. Structural mechanisms for domain movements in proteins. *Biochem* 1994;33:6739–6749.
18. Yamaguchi Y, Kim H, Kato K, et al. Proteolytic fragmentation with high specificity of mouse IgG-mapping of proteolytic cleavage sites in the hinge region. *J Immunol Methods* 1995; 181:259–267.
19. Capra JD, Kehoe JM, Winchester RJ, et al. Structure-function relationship among anti-gamma globulin antibodies. *Ann NY Acad Sci* 1971;190:371–381.
20. Oudin J, Cazenave PA. Similar idiotypic specificities in immunoglobulin fractions with different antibody functions or even without detectable antibody function. *Proc Natl Acad Sci USA* 1971;68:2616–2620.
21. Schiff C, Milili M, Hue I, et al. Genetic basis for expression of the idiotypic network. One unique Ig VH germ line gene accounts for the major family of Ab1 and Ab3 (Ab1) antibodies of the GAT system. *J Exp Med* 1986;163:573–587.
22. Bottomly K. All idiotypes are equal, but some are more equal than others. *Immunol Rev* 1984;79:45–61.
23. Jerne NK. Towards a network theory of the immune system. *Ann Immunol (Paris)* 1974;125:373–389.
24. Rajewsky K, Takemori T. Genetics, expression and function of idiotypes. *Annu Rev Immunol* 1983;1:569–603.
25. Urbain J, Wuilmart C. Some thoughts on idiotypic networks and immunoregulation. *Immunol Today* 1982;3:88–93.
26. Tonegawa S. Somatic generation of immune diversity. *Scand J Immunol* 1993;38:305–317.
27. Waldmann TA. The arrangement of Ig and T cell receptor genes in human lymphoproliferative disorders. *Adv Immunol* 1987; 40:247–321.
28. Early P, Huang H, Davis M, et al. An immunoglobulin heavy chain variable region is generated from three segments of DNA: VH, D, and JH. *Cell* 1980;19:981–992.
29. Kurosawa Y, Tonegawa S. Organization, structure and assembly of immunoglobulin heavy chain diversity DNA segments. *J Exp Med* 1982;155:201–218.
30. Sakano H, Maki R, Kurosawa Y, et al. Two types of somatic recombination are necessary for the generation of complete immunoglobulin heavy chain genes. *Nature* 1980;286: 676–683.
31. Kodaira M, Kinashi T, Umemura I, et al. Organization and evolution of variable region genes of the human immunoglobulin heavy chain. *J Mol Biol* 1986;190:529–541.
32. Walter MA, Sorti V, Hofker MH, et al. The physical organization of the human immunoglobulin heavy chain gene complex. *EMBO J* 1990;9:3303–3313.
33. Berman J, Mellis S, Pollack R, et al. Content and organization of the human Ig VH locus: definition of this new VH families and linkage to the Ig CH locus. *EMBO J* 1988;7:727–738.
34. Pascual V, Capra JD. Human immunoglobulin heavy chain variable region genes: organization, polymorphism, and expression. *Adv Immunol* 1991;49:1–74.
35. Honjo T, Habu S. Origin of immune diversity: genetic variation and selection. *Annu Rev Biochem* 1985;54:803–830.
36. Cook GP, Tomlinson IM. The human immunoglobulin VH repertoire. *Immunol Today* 1995;16:37–42.

37. Lieber M. Immunoglobulin diversity-rearranging by cutting and repairing. *Curr Biol* 1996;6:134–136
38. Lewis SM. The mechanism of V(D)J joining: lessons from molecular, immunological and comparative analysis.*Adv Immunol* 1994;56:27–150
39. Schatz DG, Oettinger MA, Baltimore D. The V(D)J recombination activating gene, RAG-1. *Cell* 1989;59:1035–1048.
40. Muraguchi A, Tagoh H, Kitagawa T, et al. Stromal cells and cytokines in the induction of RAG expression in human lymphoid progenitor cell. *Leuk Lymph* 1998;30:73–85.
41. Paull TT, Gellert M. The 3' to 5 exonuclease activity of Mre 11 facilitates repair of DNA ds breaks. *Mol Cell* 1998:1:969–979.
42. van Gent DC, Hiom K, Paull TT, et al. Stimulation of V(D)J cleavege by high mobility group proteins. *EMBO J* 1997;16: 2665–2670.
43. Jeggo PA, Taccioli GE, Jackson SP. Menage a trois: double strand break repair, V(D)J recombination and DNA-PK. *Bioessays* 1995;17:949–957.
44. Weaver DT. What to do at an end: DNA double strand break repair. *Trends Genet* 1995;11:388–392.
45. Desiderio S. Insertion of N regions into heavy chain genes is correlated with expression of terminal deoxytransferase in B cells. *Nature* 1984;311:752–755.
46. Feeney AJ. Lack of N regions in fetal and neonatal mouse immunoglobulin V-D-J junctional sequences. *J Exp Med* 1990; 172:1377–1390.
47. Jaenichen HR, Pech M, Lindenmaier W, et al. Composite human VK genes and a model of their evolution. *Nucleic Acids Res* 1984;12:5249–5263.
48. Klobeck HG, Meindl A, Combriato G, et al. Human immunoglobulin kappa light chain genes of subgroups II and III. *Nucleic Acids Res* 1985;13:6499–6514.
49. Klobeck HG, Bornkamm GW, Cabriato G, et al. Subgroup IV of human immunoglobulin K light chains is encoded by a single germline gene. *Nucleic Acids Res* 1985;13:6515–6530.
50. Meindl A, Klobeck HG, Ohnheiser R, et al. The V kappa gene repertoire in the human germ line. *Eur J Immunol* 1990;20:1855–1863.
51. Schable KF, Zachau HG. The variable genes of the human immunoglobulin kappa locus. *Biol Chem* 1993;374: 1001–1022.
52. Chuchana P, Blancher A, Brockly F, et al. Definition of the human immunoglobulin variable lambda (IGLV) gene subgroup. *Eur J Immunol* 1990;20:1317–1325.
53. Solomon A, Weiss DT. Serologically defined V region subgroups of human lambda light chains. *J Immunol* 1987;139: 824–830.
54. Lai E, Wilson RK, Hood LE. Physical maps of the mouse and the human immunoglobulin-like loci. *Adv Immunol* 1989;46: 1–59.
55. Chang LY, Yen CP, Besl L, et al. Identification and characterization of a functional human Ig V lambda VI germline gene. *Mol Immunol* 1994;31:531–536.
56. Frippiat JP, Lefranc MP. Genomic organization of 34 kb of the human immunoglobulin lambda locus (IGLV): restriction map and sequences of new V lambda III genes. *Mol Immunol* 1994;31:657–670.
57. Heller M, Owens JO, Mushinski JF, et al. Amino acids at the site of VKJK recombination not encoded by germline sequences. *J Exp Med* 1987;166:637–646.
58. Grawunder U, Leu TMJ, Schatz DG, et al. Down-regulation of RAG1 and RAG2 gene expression in pre-B cells after functional Ig heavy chain rearrangement. *Immunity* 1995;3:601–608.
59. Chen J, Shinkai Y, Young F, et al. Probing immune functions in RAG-deficient mice. *Curr Opin Immunol* 1994;6:313–319.
60. Abe T, Tsunge I, Kamachi Y, et al. Evidence for defects in V(D)J rearrangement in patients with SCID. *J Immunol* 1994;152: 1039–1048.
61. Schwarz K, Gauss GH, Ludwig L, et al. RAG mutations in human B cell negative SCID. *Science* 1996;274:497–499.
62. Schwartz K, Hansen-Hagge TE, Knobloch C, et al. Severe combined immunodeficiency (SCID) in man: B cell-negative (B–) SCID patients exhibit an irregular recombination pattern at the Jh locus. *J Exp Med* 1991;174:1039–1048.
63. Villa A, Santagata S, Bozzi F, et al. Omenn syndrome: a disorder of RAG 1 and RAG2 genes. *J Clin Immunol* 1999;19: 87–97.
64. Notarangelo LD, Villa A, Schwarz K. RAG and RAG defects. *Curr Opin Immunol* 1999;11:435–442.
65. Gritzmacher C. Molecular aspects of heavy chain class switching. *Crit Rev Immunol* 1989;9:173–200.
66. Matsuoka M, Yoshida K, Maeda T, et al. Switch circular DNA formed in cytokine-treated mouse splenocytes: evidence for intramolecular DNA deletion in immunoglobulin class switching. *Cell* 1990;62:135–142.
67. Shimuzu A, Honjo T. Immunoglobulin class switching. *Cell* 1984;36:801–803.
68. Davis MM, Kim SK, Hood LE. DNA sequences mediating class switching in immunoglobulins. *Science* 1980;209: 1360–1365.
69. Heiter P, Korsmeyer SJ, Waldmann TA, et al. Human immunoglobulin kappa light chain genes are deleted or rearranged in lambda producing B cells. *Nature* 1981;290: 368–372.
70. Korsmeyer SJ. A hierarchy of immunoglobulin gene rearrangements in human leukemic pre B-cells. *Proc Natl Acad Sci USA* 1981;78:7096–7100.
71. Retter MW, Namazee D. Receptor editing occurs frequently during normal B cell development. *J Exp Med* 1998;188: 1231–1238.
72. Melamed D, Benschop RJ, Cambier JC, et al. Developmental regulation of B lymphocyte immune tolerance compartmentalizes clonal selection from receptor selection. *Cell* 1998;92: 173–182.
73. Chen C, Park EL, Weigert M. Editing disease-associated autoantibodies. *Immunity* 1997; 6:97–105.
74. Nussenzweig MC. Immune receptor editing: revise and select. *Cell* 1998;95:875–878.
75. Ghia P, Gratwohl A, Singer E, et al. Immature B cells from human and mouse bone marrow can change their surface light chain expression. *Eur J Immunol* 1995;25:3108–3114.
76. Hikida M, Mori M, Takai T, et al. Reexpression of RAG-1 and RAG-2 in activated mature B cells. *Science* 1996;274: 2092–2094
77. Han S, Dillon SR, Zheng B, et al. V(D)J recombinase activity in a subset of germinal center B lymphocytes. *Science* 1997;278: 301–305
78. Papavasiliou F, Casellas R, Suh H, et al. V(D)J recombination in mature B cells: a mechanism for altering antibody responses. *Science* 1997;278:298–301.
79. Hikida M, Nakayama Y, Yamashita Y, et al. Expression of recombination activating genes in germinal center B cells: involvement of interleukin 7 (IL-7) and IL-7 receptor. *J Exp Med* 1998;188:365–372.
80. Berek C, Griffiths GM, Milstein C. Molecular events during maturation of the immune responses to oxazolone. *Nature* 1985;316:412–518.
81. Clark EA, Ledbetter JA. How B and T cells talk to each other. *Nature* 1994;367:425–428.
82. Noelle RJ, Ledbetter JA, Aruffo A. CD40 and its ligand, an essential ligand-receptor pair for thymus-dependent B cell activation. *Immunol Today* 1992;13:431–433.

83. Allen RC, Armitage RJ, Conley ME, et al. CD40 ligand gene defects responsible for X-linked hyper-IgM syndrome. *Science* 1993;259:990–993.
84. DiSanto JP, Bonnefoy JY, Gauchat JF, et al. CD40 ligand mutations in X-linked immunodeficiency with hyper-IgM. *Nature* 1993;361:541–543.
85. Berek C, Milstein C. Mutational drift and repertoire shift in the maturation of the immune response. *Immunol Rev* 1987;96: 23–42.
86. Manser T, Wysocki LJ, Margolies MN, et al. Evolution of antibody variable region structure during the immune response. *Immunol Rev* 1987;96:141–162.
87. Ikematsu H, Harindranath N, Notkins AL, et al. Clonal analysis of a human antibody response II: sequences of the VH genes of human monoclonal IgM, IgG and IgA to rabies virus reveal preferential utilization of the VH III segments and somatic hypermutation. *J Immunol* 1993;150:1325–1337.
88. Radic MZ, Weigert M. Genetic and structural evidence for antigen selection of anti-DNA antibodies. *Annu Rev Immunol* 1994;12:487–520.
89. van Es J, Gmelig Meyling FHJ, van de Akker WRM, et al. Somatic mutations in the variable regions of a human IgG anti-ds DNA autoantibody suggest a role for antigen in the induction of systemic lupus erythematosus. *J Exp Med* 1991;173:461–470.
90. Marion TN, Tillman DM, Jou NT, et al. Selection of immunoglobulin variable regions in autoimmunity to DNA. *Immunol Rev* 1992;128:123–149.
91. Diamond B, Katz JB, Paul E, et al. The role of somatic mutation in the pathogenic anti-DNA response. *Annu Rev Immunol* 1992;10:731–757.
92. Clarke SH, Huppi K, Ruezinsky D, et al. Inter- and intraclonal diversity in the antibody response to influenza hemagglutinin. *J Exp Med* 1985;161:687–704.
93. Clarke SH, Rudikoff S. Evidence for gene conversion among immunoglobulin heavy chain variable region genes. *J Exp Med* 1984;159:773–782.
94. Reynaud C, Anquez V, Dahan A, et al. A single rearrangement event generates most of the chicken immunoglobulin light chain diversity. *Cell* 1985;40:283–291.
95. Wabl M, Steinberg C. Affinity maturation and class switching. *Curr Opin Immunol* 1996;8:89–92.
96. Cascalho M, Wong J, Steinberg C, et al. Mismatch repair coopted by hypermutation. *Science* 1998; 279:1207–1210.
97. Wiesendanger M, Kneitz B, Edelmann W, et al. Somatic hypermutation in Muts homologue (MSH)3-, MSH6-, and MSH3/MSH6-deficient mice reveals a role for the MSH2-MSH6 heterodimer in modulating the base substitution pattern. *J Exp Med* 2000;191:579–584.
98. French DL, Laskov R, Scharff MD. The role of somatic hypermutation in the generation of antibody diversity. *Science* 1989; 244:1152–1157.
99. Griffiths GM, Berek C, Kaartinen M, et al. Somatic mutation and the maturation of immune response to 2-phenyl oxazolone. *Nature* 1984;312:271–275.
100. Kim S, Davis M, Sinn E, et al. Antibody diversity: somatic hypermutation of rearranged VH genes. *Cell* 1981;27:573–581.
101. Sablitzky F, Wildner G, Rajewsky K. Somatic mutation and clonal expansion of B cells in an antigen-driven immune response. *EMBO J* 1985;4:345–350.
102. Levy Y, Gupta N, Le Deist F, et al. Defect in Ig V gene somatic hypermutation in common variable immuno-deficiency syndrome. *Proc Natl Acad Sci USA* 1998;95:131:35–40.
103. Diamond B, Scharff MD. Somatic mutation of the T15 heavy chain gives rise to an antibody with autoantibody specificity. *Proc Natl Acad Sci USA* 1984;81:5841–5844.
104. Ray SK, Putterman C, Diamond B. Pathogenic antibodies are routinely generated during the response to foreign antigen: a paradigm for autoimmune disease. *Proc Natl Acad Sci USA* 1996;93:2019–2024.
105. Hande S, Notidis E, Manser T. Bcl-2 obstructs negative selection of autoreactive, hypermutated antibody V regions during memory B cell development. *Immunity* 1998;8:189–198.
106. Shlomchik MJ, Nemazee D, Sato VL, et al. Variable region sequences of murine IgM anti-IgG monoclonal autoantibodies (rheumatoid factors). A structural explanation of the high frequency IgM anti-IgG B cells. *J Exp Med* 1986;164:407–427.
107. Jukes TH, King JL. Evolutionary nucleotide replacements in DNA. *Nature* 1979;281:605–606.
108. Chang B, Casali P. The CDR1 sequences of a major proportion of human germline Ig VH genes are inherently susceptible to amino acid replacement. *Immunol Today* 1995;15:367–373.
109. Reynaud CA, Garcia C, Hein WR, et al. Hypermutation generating the sheep immunoglobulin repertoire is an antigen-independent process. *Cell* 1995;80:115–125.
110. Betz AG, Neuberger MS, Milstein C. Discriminating intrinsic and antigen-selected mutational hotspots in immunoglobulin V genes. *Immunol Today* 1993;14:405–411.
111. Berek C, Milstein C. The dynamic nature of the antibody repertoire. *Immunol Rev* 1988;105:5–26.
112. Sharon J, Gefter ML, Wysocki LJ, et al. Recurrent somatic mutation in mouse antibodies to p-azophenylarsenate increase affinity to hapten. *J Immunol* 1989;142:596–601.
113. Herzenberg LA, Stall AM, Lalor PA, et al. The Ly-1 B cell lineage. *Immunol Rev* 1986;93:81–102.
114. Hardy RR, Carmack CE, Li YS, et al. Distinctive developmental origins and specificities of murine CD5+ B cells. *Immunol Rev* 1994;137:91–118.
115. Hippen KL, Tze LE, Behrens T. CD5 maintains tolerance in anergic B cells. *J Exp Med* 2000;191:883–889.
116. Bikah G, Carey J, Ciallella JR, et al. CD5-mediated negative regulation of antigen receptor-induced growth signals in B-1 B cells. *Science* 1996;274:1906–1909.
117. Hardy RR, Hayakawa K. CD5 B cells, a fetal B cell lineage. *Adv Immunol* 1994;55:297–339.
118. Kasaian MT, Casali P. Autoimmunity-prone B-1 (CD5 B) cells, natural antibodies and self recognition. *Autoimmunity* 1993;15: 315–329.
119. Hayakawa K, Hardy RR, Honda M, et al. Ly-1 B cells: functionally distinct lymphocytes that secrete IgM antibodies. *Proc Natl Acad Sci USA* 1984;81:2494–2498.
120. Conger JD, Sage HJ, Corley RB. Correlation of antibody multireactivity with variable region primary structure among murine anti-erythrocyte autoantibodies. *Eur J Immunol* 1992; 22:783–790.
121. Murakami M, Yoshioka H, Shirai T, et al. Prevention of autoimmune symptoms in autoimmune-prone mice by elimination of B-1 cells. *Int Immunol* 1995;7:877–882.
122. Casali P, Burastero SE, Balow JE, et al. High affinity antibodies to ssDNA are produced by CD5– B cells in SLE patients. *J Immunol* 1989;143:3476–3483.
123. Casali P, Notkins AL. Probing the human B cell repertoire with EBV: polyreactive antibodies and CD5+ B lymphocytes. *Annu Rev Immunol* 1989;7:513–535.
124. Suzuki N, Sakane T, Engleman EG. Anti-DNA antibody production by CD5+ and CD5– B cells of patients with SLE. *J Clin Invest* 1990;85:238–247.
125. Linton PJ, Lo D, Lai L, et al. Among naive precursor cell subpopulations only progenitors of memory B cells originate germinal centers. *Eur J Immunol* 1992;22:1293–1297.
126. Mantovani L, Wilder RL. Human rheumatoid B-1a (CD5+) cells make somatically hypermutated high affinity IgM rheumatoid factors. *J Immunol* 1993;151:473–488.

127. Lacroix-Desmazes S, Kaveri SV, Mouthon L, et al. Self-reactive antibodies (natural autoantibodies) in healthy individuals. *J Immunol Methods* 1998;216;117–37.
128. Dighiero G, Lymberi P, Holmberg D, et al. High frequency of natural autoantibodies in normal newborn mice. *J Immunol* 1985;134:765–771.
129. Cairns E, Block J, Bell DA. Anti-DNA antibody producing hybridomas of normal lymphoid cell origin. *J Clin Invest* 1984; 74:880–887.
130. Guilbert B, Dighiero G, Avrameas S. Naturally occurring antibodies against nine common antigens in human sera: I. detection, isolation, and characterization. *J Immunol* 1982;128: 2779–2787.
131. Andrzejewski C Jr, Rauch J, Lafer F, et al. Antigen-binding diversity and idiotypic cross-reaction, among hybridoma autoantibodies to DNA. *J Immunol* 1981;126:226–231.
132. Bell DA, Cairns E, Cikalo K, et al. Anti-nucleic acid autoantibody responses of normal human origin: antigen specificity and idiotypic characteristics compared to patients with systemic lupus erythematosus and patients with monoclonal IgM. *J Rheumatol* 1987;14:127–131.
133. Ternynck T, Avrameas S. Murine natural monoclonal autoantibodies. A study of their polyspecificities and their affinities. *Immunol Rev* 1986;94:99–112.
134. Baccala R, Quang TV, Gilbert M, et al. Two murine natural polyreactive autoantibodies are encoded by non-mutated germline genes. *Proc Natl Acad Sci USA* 1989;86:4624–4628.
135. Davidson A, Manheimer-Lory A, Aranow C, et al. Molecular characterization of a somatically mutated anti-DNA antibody bearing two systemic lupus erythematosus-related idiotypes. *J Clin Invest* 1990;85:1401–1409.
136. Hoch S, Schwaber J. Identification and sequence of the VH gene elements encoding a human anti-DNA antibody. *J Immunol* 1987;139:1689–1693.
137. Manser T, Gefter ML. The molecular evolution of the immune response: idiotype specific suppression indicates that B cells express germ-line-encoded V genes prior to antigenic stimulation. *Eur J Immunol* 1986;16:1439–1444.
138. Sanz I, Casali P, Thomas JW, et al. Nucleotide sequences of eight human natural autoantibody VH regions reveals apparent restricted use of VH families. *J Immunol* 1989;142:4054–4061.
139. Avrameas S, Ternynck T. The natural autoantibodies system: between hypotheses and facts. *Mol Immunol* 1993;30: 1133–1142.
140. Halpern R, Davidson A, Lazo A, et al. Familial systemic lupus erythematosus. Presence of a cross-reactive idiotype in healthy family members. *J Clin Invest* 1985;76:731–736.
141. Isenberg DA, Shoenfeld Y, Walport M, et al. Detection of cross-reactive anti-DNA antibody idiotypes in the serum of systemic lupus erythematosus patients and of their relatives. *Arthritis Rheum* 1985;28:999–1007.
142. Dersimonian H, Schwartz RS, Barrett KJ, et al. Relationship of human variable region heavy chain germ-line genes to genes encoding anti-DNA autoantibodies. *J Immunol* 1987;139: 2496–2501.
143. Naparstek Y, Andre-Schwartz J, Manser T, et al. A single VH germline gene segment of normal A/J mice encodes autoantibodies characteristic of systemic lupus erythematosus. *J Exp Med* 1986;164:614–626.
144. Marion TN, Bothwell AL, Briles DE, et al. IgG anti-DNA autoantibodies within an individual autoimmune mouse are the products of clonal selection. *J Immunol* 1989;142:4269–4274.
145. Marion TN, Tillman DM, Jou N. Interclonal and intraclonal diversity among anti-DNA antibodies from an NZB x NZWF1 mouse. *J Immunol* 1990;145:2322–2332.
146. O'Keefe TL, Bandyopadhyay S, Datta SK, et al. V region sequences of an idiotypically connected family of pathogenic anti-DNA autoantibodies. *J Immunol* 1990;144:4275–4283.
147. Shlomchik M, Mascelli M, Shan H, et al. Anti-DNA antibodies from autoimmune mice arise by clonal expansion and somatic mutation. *J Exp Med* 1990;71:265–292.
148. Shlomchik MJ, Aucoin AH, Pisetsky DS, et al. Structure and function of anti-DNA autoantibodies derived from a single autoimmune mouse. *Proc Natl Acad Sci USA* 1987;84: 9150–9154.
149. Shlomchik MJ, Marshak-Rothstein A, Wolfowicz CB, et al. The role of clonal selection and somatic mutation in autoimmunity. *Nature* 1987;328:805–811.
150. Valesini G, Tincani A, Harris EN, et al. Use of monoclonal antibodies to identify shared idiotypes on anti-cardiolipin and anti-DNA antibodies in human sera. *Clin Exp Immunol* 1987;70:18–25.
151. Jacob L, Tron F, Bach JF, et al. A monoclonal anti-DNA antibody also binds cell surface proteins. *Proc Natl Acad Sci USA* 1984;81:3843–3845.
152. Lafer EM, Rauch J, Andrzejewski C Jr, et al. Polyspecific monoclonal lupus autoantibodies reactive with both polynucleotides and phospholipids. *J Exp Med* 1981;153:897–909.
153. Rauch J, Murphy E, Roths JB, et al. A high frequency idiotype marker of anti-DNA autoantibodies in MRL-lpr/lpr mice. *J Immunol* 1982;129:236–241.
154. Sammartino LR, Gharavi AE, Lockshin MD. Antiphospholipid antibody syndrome: immunologic and clinical aspects. *Semin Arthritis Rheum* 1990;20:81–96.
155. Bick RL, Baker WF. Antiphospholipid syndrome and thrombosis. *Semin Thromb Hemost* 1999;25:333–50.
156. Harley JB, Scofield RH, Reichlin M. Anti-Ro in Sjogren's syndrome and systemic lupus erythematosus. *Rheum Dis Clin North Am* 1992;18:337–358.
157. Tsao BP, Ohnishi K, Cheroutre H, et al. Failed self-tolerance and autoimmunity in IgG anti-DNA transgenic mice. *J Immunol* 1992;149:350–358.
158. Ehrenstein MR, Cook HT, Neuberger MS. Deficiency in serum immunoglobulin (Ig)M predisposes to development of IgG autoantibodies. *J Exp Med* 2000;191:1253–1257.
159. Mackay F, Woodcock SA, Lawton P, et al. Mice transgenic for BAFF develop lymphocytic disorders along with autoimmune manifestations. *J Exp Med* 1999;190:1697–1710.
160. Botto M, Dell'Agnola C, Bygrave AE, et al. Homozygous C1q deficiency causes glomerulonephritis associated with multiple apoptotic bodies. *Nat Genet* 1998;19:56–59.
161. Napirei M, Karsunky H, Zevnik B, et al. Features of systemic lupus erythematosus in Dnase1-deficient mice. *Nat Genet* 2000; 25:177–181.
162. Raz E, Brezis M, Rosenmann E, et al. Anti-DNA antibodies bind directly to renal antigens and induce kidney dysfunction in the isolated perfused rat kidney. *J Immunol* 1989;142: 3076–3082.
163. Bernstein K, Bolshoun D, Gilkeson G, et al. Detection of glomerular-binding immune elements in murine lupus using a tissue-based ELISA. *Clin Exp Immunol* 1993;91:449–455.
164. Madiao MP, Carlson J, Cataldo J, et al. Murine monoclonal anti-DNA antibodies bind directly to glomerular antigens and form immune deposits. *J Immunol* 1987;138:2883–2889.
165. Vlahakos DV, Foster MH, Adams S, et al. Anti-DNA antibodies form immune deposits at distinct glomerular and vascular sites. *Kidney Int* 1992;41:1690–1700.
166. Ohnishi K, Ebling FM, Mitchell B, et al. Comparison of pathogenic and non-pathogenic murine antibodies to DNA: antigen binding and structural characteristics. *Int Immunol* 1994;6: 817–830.
167. Putterman C, Limpanasithikul W, Edelman M, et al. The dou-

ble-edged sword of the immune response: Mutational analysis of an anti-pneumococcal, anti-DNA antibody. *J Clin Invest* 1996;97:2251–2259.
168. Katz MS, Foster MH, Madaio MP. Independently derived murine glomerular immune deposit forming anti-DNA antibodies are encoded by near identical VH gene sequences. *J Clin Invest* 1993;91:402–408.
169. Boutjdir M, Chen L, Zhang ZH, et al. Arrhythmogenicity of IgG and anti-52-kD SSA/Ro affinity purified antibodies from mothers of children with congenital heart block. *Circ Res* 1997; 80:354–362.
170. Miranda-Carus ME, Boutjdir M, Tseng CE, et al. Induction of antibodies reactive with SSA/Ro-SSB/LA and development of congenital heart block in a murine model. *J Immunol* 1998; 161:5886–5892.
171. Mazel JA, El-Sherif N, Buyon J, et al. Electrocardiographic abnormalities in a murine model injected with IgG from mothers of children with congenital heart block. *Circulation* 1999; 99:1914–1918.
172. Pierangeli SS, Liu XW, Barker JH, et al. Induction of thrombosis in a mouse model by IgG, IgM, and IgA immunoglobulins from patients with anti-phospholipid syndrome. *Thromb Hemost* 1995;74:1361–1367.
173. Ikematsu W, Luan FL, La Rosa L, et al. Human anti-cardiolipin monoclonal autoantibodies cause placental necrosis and fetal loss in BALB/c mice. *Arthritis Rheum* 1999;41:1026–1039.
174. Piona A, La Rosa L, Tincani A, et al. Placental thrombosis and fetal loss after passive transfer of mouse lupus monoclonal or human polyclonal anti-cardiolipin antibodies in pregnant naïve BALB/c mice. *Scand J Immunol* 1995;41:427–432.
175. Fossati-Jimack L, Ioan-Facsinay A, Reininger L, et al. Markedly different pathogenicity of four immunoglobulin G isotype-switch variants of an antierythrocyte autoantibody is based on their capacity to interact *in-vivo* with the low-affinity Fc-gamma receptor III. *J Exp Med* 2000;191:1293–1302.
176. Papoian R, Pillarisetty R, Talal N. Immunological regulation of spontaneous antibodies to DNA and RNA. II. Sequential switch from IgM to IgG in NZB/NZW F1 mice. *Immunology* 1977;32:7579.
177. Neuwirth R, Singhal P, Diamond B, et al. Evidence for immunoglobulin Fc receptor-mediated prostaglandin E2 and platelet-activating factor formation by cultured rat mesangial cells. *J Clin Invest* 1988;82:936944.
178. Lopez-Soto A, Cervera R, Font J, et al. Isotype distribution and clinical significance of antibodies to cardiolipin, phosphatidic acid, phosphatidylinositol and phosphatidylserine in SLE: prospective analysis of a series of 92 patients. *Clin Exp Rheum* 1997;15:143–149.
179. Vlahakos D, Foster MH, Ucci AA, et al. Murine monoclonal anti-DNA antibodies penetrate cells, bind to nuclei, and induce glomerular proliferation and proteinuria *in-vivo*. *J Am Soc Nephrol* 1992;2:1345–1354.
180. Yanase K, Smith RM, Puccetti A, et al. Receptor-mediated cellular entry of nuclear localizing anti-DNA antibodies via myosin 1. *J Clin Invest* 1997;100:25–31.
181. Kosec M, Koren E, Wolfson-Reichlin M, et al. Autoantibodies to ribosomal P proteins penetrate into live hepatocytes and cause cellular dysfunction in culture. *J Immunol* 1997;159: 2033–2041.
182. Miranda ME, Tseng CE, Rashbaum W, et al. Accessibility of SSA/Ro and SSB/La antigens to maternal autoantibodies in apoptotic human fetal cardiac myocytes. *J Immunol* 1998;161: 5061–5069.
183. Casciola-Rosen LA, Anhalt G, Rosen A. Autoantigens targeted in systemic lupus erythematosus are clustered in two populations of surface structures on apoptotic keratinocytes. *J Exp Med* 1994;179:1317–1330.
184. Tadmor B, Putterman C, Naparstek Y. Embryonal germ-layer antigens: a target for autoimmunity? *Lancet* 1992;339: 975–978.
185. Liao L, Sindhwani R, Rojkind M, et al. Antibody-mediated autoimmune myocarditis depends on genetically determined target organ sensitivity. *J Exp Med* 1995;181:1123–1131.
186. Crary GS, Katz A, Fish AJ, et al. Role of a basement membrane glycoprotein in anti-tubular basement membrane nephritis. *Kidney Int* 1993;43:140–146.
187. Gavalchin J, Nicklas JA, Eastcott JW, et al. Lupus-prone (SWR × NZB) F1 mice produce potentially nephritogenic autoantibodies inherited from the normal SWR parent. *J Immunol* 1985;134:885–894.
188. Grayzel A, Solomon A, Aranow C, et al. Antibodies elicited by pneumococcal antigens bear an anti-DNA associated idiotype. *J Clin Invest* 1991;87:842–846.
189. Shoenfeld Y, Vilner Y, Coates ARM, et al. Monoclonal anti-tuberculosis antibodies react with DNA and monoclonal anti-DNA antibodies react with Mycobacterium tuberculosis. *Clin Exp Immunol* 1986;66:255–261.
190. Kofler R, Noonan DJ, Levy DE, et al. Genetic elements used for a murine lupus anti-DNA autoantibody are closely related to those for antibodies to exogenous antigens. *J Exp Med* 1985;161:805–815.
191. Mackworth-Young CG, Sabbaga J, Schwartz RS, et al. Idiotypic markers of polyclonal B cell activation: public idiotypes shared by monoclonal antibodies derived from patients with systemic lupus erythematosus and leprosy. *J Clin Invest* 1987;79: 572–581.
192. Monestier M, Bonin B, Migliorini P, et al. Autoantibodies of various specificities encoded by genes from the VHJ558 family bind to foreign antigens and share idiotypes of antibodies specific for self and foreign antigens. *J Exp Med* 1987;166: 1109–1124.
193. Naparstek Y, Duggan D, Schattner A, et al. Immunochemical similarities between monoclonal anti-bacterial Waldenstrom's macroglobulins and monoclonal anti-DNA lupus autoantibodies. *J Exp Med* 1985;161:1525–1538.
194. Carroll P, Stafford D, Schwartz RS, et al. Murine monoclonal anti-DNA autoantibodies bind to endogenous bacteria. *J Immunol* 1985;135:1086–1090.
195. Kabat EA, Nickerson KG, Liao J, et al. A human monoclonal macroglobulin with specificity for alpha C-28 linked poly-N-acetyl neuraminic acid, the capsular polysaccharide of group B meningococci and Escherichia coli K1, which cross reacts with polynucleotides and denatured DNA. *J Exp Med* 1986;164: 642–654.
196. Query CC, Keene JD. A human autoimmune protein associated with U1 RNA contains a region of homology that is cross-reactive with retroviral p30 gag antigen. *Cell* 1987;51:211–220.
197. El-Roeiy A, Sela O, Isenberg DA, et al. The sera of patients with Klebsiella infections contain a common anti-DNA idiotype (16/6) Id and anti-polynucleotide activity. *Clin Exp Immunol* 1987;67:507–515.
198. Limpanasithikul W, Ray S, Diamond B. Cross-reactive antibodies have both protective and pathogenic potential. *J Immunol* 1995;155:967–973.
199. Sanz I, Capra JD. The genetic origin of human autoantibodies. *J Immunol* 1988;140:3283–3285.
200. Trepicchio W Jr, Barrett KJ. Eleven MRL-lpr/lpr anti-DNA autoantibodies are encoded by genes from four VH gene families. A potentially biased usage of VH genes. *J Immunol* 1987; 138:2323–2331.

201. Ash-Lerner A, Ginsberg-Strauss M, Pewzner-Jung Y, et al. Expression of an anti-DNA associated Vh gene in immunized and autoimmune mice. *J Immunol* 1997;159:1508–1519.
202. Radic MZ, Weigert M. Origins of anti-DNA antibodies and their implications for B-cell tolerance. *Ann NY Acad Sci* 1995;764:384–396.
203. Marion TN, Tillman DM, Jou N. Interclonal and intraclonal diversity among anti-DNA antibodies from an NZB x NZWF1 mouse. *J Immunol* 1990;145:2322–2332.
204. Eilat D, Webster DM, Rees AR. V region sequences of anti-DNA and anti-RNA autoantibodies from NZB/NZW F1 mice. *J Immunol* 1988;141:1745–1753.
205. Yaoita Y, Takahashi M, Azuma C, et al. Biased expression of variable region gene families of the immunoglobulin heavy chain in autoimmune-prone mice. *J Biochem* 1988;104:337–343.
206. Sanz I, Kelly P, Williams C, et al. The smaller human VH gene families display remarkably little polymorphism. *EMBO J* 1989;8:3741–3748.
207. Souroujon MC, Rubinstein DB, Schwartz RS, et al. Polymorphisms in human H chain V region genes from the VHIII gene family. *J Immunol* 1989;143:706–711.
208. Zouali M, Madaio MP, Canoso RT, et al. Restriction fragment length polymorphism analysis of the V kappa locus in human lupus. *Eur J Immunol* 1989;19:1757–1760.
209. Olee T, Yang PM, Siminovitch KA, et al. Molecular basis of an autoantibody-associated restriction-length polymorphism that confers susceptibility to autoimmune diseases. *J Clin Invest* 1991;88:193–203.
210. Huang DF, Siminovitch KA, Liu XY, et al. Population and family studies of three disease-related polymorphic genes in systemic lupus erythematosus. *J Clin Invest* 1995;95:1766–1772.
211. Suzuki N, Harada T, Mihara S, et al. Characterization of a germline Vk gene encoding cationic anti-DNA antibody and role of receptor editing for development of the autoantibody in patients with SLE. *J Clin Invest* 1996;98:1843–1850.
212. Davidson A, Manheimer-Lory A, Aranow C, et al. Possible mechanisms of autoantibody production. *Biomed Pharmacother* 1989;43:563–570.
213. Rhaman MA, Isenberg DA. Autoantibodies in systemic lupus erythematosus. *Curr Opin Rheum* 1994;6:468–473.
214. Manheimer-Lory AJ, Zandman-Goddard G, Davidson A, et al. Lupus-specific antibodies reveal an altered pattern of somatic mutation. *J Clin Invest* 1997;100:2538–2546.
215. Kuo P, Alban A, Gebhard D, et al. overexpression of bcl-2 alters usage of mutational hot spots in germinal center B cells. *Mol Immunol* 1997;34:1011–1018.
216. Droner T, Heimbacher C, Farner NL, et al. Enhanced mutation activity of V kappa gene rearrangements in systemic lupus erythematosus. *Clin Immunol* 1999;92:188–196.
217. Smith DS, Creadon G, Jena PK, et al. Di- and trinucleotide target preferences of somatic mutagenesis in normal and autoreactive B cells. *J Immunol* 1996;156:2642–2652.
218. van Es J, Gmelig Meyling FHJ, van de Akker WRM, et al. Somatic mutations in the variable regions of a human IgG anti-ds DNA autoantibody suggest a role for antigen in the induction of systemic lupus erythematosus. *J Exp Med* 1991;173:461–470.
219. Behar SM, Scharff MD. Somatic diversification of the S107(T15) VH11 germ-line gene that encodes the heavy-chain variable region of antibodies to double-stranded DNA in NZB x NZWF1 mice. *Proc Natl Acad Sci USA* 1988;85:3970–3974.
220. Shefner R, Kleiner G, Turken A, et al. A novel class of anti-DNA antibodies identified in BALB/c mice. *J Exp Med* 1991;173:287–296.
221. Kuo P, Kowal C, Tadmor B, et al. Microbial antigens can elicit autoantibody production. A potential pathway to autoimmune disease. *Ann NY Acad Sci* 1997;815:230–236.
222. Steinberg B, Smathers P, Frederiksen K, et al. Ability of the xid gene to prevent autoimmunity in (NZB×NZW) F1 mice during the course of their natural history, after polyclonal stimulation, or following immunization with DNA. *J Clin Invest* 1982;70:587–597.
223. Unni KK, Holley KE, McDuffie FC, et al. Comparative study of NZB mice under germ-free and conventional conditions. *J Rheumatol* 1975;2:36–44.
224. Maldanado MA, Kakknaiah V, MacDonald GC, et al. The role of environmental antigens in the spontaneous development of autoimmunity in MRL-lpr mice. *J Immunol* 1999;162:6322–6330
225. Kowal C, Weinstein A, Diamond B. Molecular mimicry between bacterial and self-antigen in a patient with systemic lupus erythematosus. *Eur J Immunol* 1999;29:1901–1911.
226. Argov S, Jaffe CL, Krupp M, et al. Autoantibody production by patients infected with Leishmania. *Clin Exp Immunol* 1989;76:190–197.
227. Moudgil KD, Sercarz EE. The T cell repertoire against cryptic self determinants and involvement in autoimmunity and cancer. *Clin Immunol Immunopathol* 1994;73:283–289.
228. Sibille P, Ternynck T, Nato F, et al. Mimotopes of polyreactive anti-DNA antibodies using phage-display peptide libraries. *Eur J Immunol* 1997;27:1221–1228.
229. Gaynor B, Putterman C, Valadon P, et al. Peptide inhibition of glomerular deposition of an anti-DNA antibody. *Proc Natl Acad Sci USA* 1997;94:1955–1960.
230. Putterman C, Diamond B. Immunization with a peptide dsDNA surrogate induces autoantibody production and kidney immunoglobulin deposition. *J Exp Med* 1998;188:29–38.
231. Pistesky DS. The immunologic properties of DNA. *J Immunol* 1996;156:421–423.
232. Gilkeson GS, Pippen AMM, Pistesky DS. Induction of cross-reactive anti-dsDNA antibodies in pre-autoimmune NZB/NZW mice by immmunization with bacterial DNA. *J Clin Invest* 1995;95:1398–1402.
233. Marchini B, Puccetti A, Dolcher MP, et al. Induction of anti-DNA antibodies in non autoimmune mice by immunization with a DNA-DNAase I complex. *Clin Exp Rheumatol* 1995;13:7–10.
234. Desai DD, Krishnan MR, Swindle JT, et al. Antigen-specific induction of antibodies against native mammalian DNA in non-autoimmune mice. *J Immunol* 1993;151:1614–1626.
235. Rekvig OP, Moens U, Sundsford A, et al. Experimental expression in mice and spontaneous expression in human SLE of polyomavirus T-antigen. *J Clin Invest* 1997;99:2045–2054.
236. Mimori T, Hardin JA. Mechanisms of interaction between Ku protein and DNA. *J Biol Chem* 1986;261:10375–10379.
237. Reeves WH, Chiorazzi N. Interaction between anti-DNA and anti-DNA binding protein autoantibodies in cryoglobulins from sera of patients with systemic lupus erythematosus. *J Exp Med* 1986;164:1029–1042.
238. Mendlovic S, Brocke S, Shoenfeld Y, et al. Induction of a systemic lupus erythematosus-like disease in mice by a common human anti-DNA idiotype. *Proc Natl Acad Sci USA* 1988;85:2260–2264.
239. Mendlovic S, Fricke H, Shoenfeld Y, et al. The role of anti-idiotypic antibodies in the induction of experimental systemic lupus erythematosus in mice. *Eur J Immunol* 1989;19:729–734.
240. Bakimer R, Fishman P, Blank M, et al. Induction of primary anti-phospholipid syndrome in mice by immunization with a human monoclonal anti-cardiolipin antibody (H-3). *J Clin Invest* 1992;89:1558–1663.

241. Erez-Alon N, Herkel J, Wolkowicz R, et al. Immunity to p53 induced by an idiotypic network of anti-p53 antibodies: generation of sequence specific anti-DNA antibodies and protection from tumor metastasis. *Cancer Res* 1998;58:5447–5452.
242. Abdou N, Wall H, Lindsley B, et al. Network theory in autoimmunity: *in-vitro* suppression of serum anti-DNA binding to DNA by antiidiotypic antibody to anti-DNA. *J Clin Invest* 1981;67:1297–1304.
243. Harley JB, James JA. Autoepitopes in lupus. *J Lab Clin Med* 1995;126:509–516.
244. Casciola-Rosen L, Andrade F, Ulanet D, et al. Cleavage by granzyme B is strongly predictive of autoantigen status: implications for initiation of autoimmunity. *J Exp Med* 1999;190: 815–826.
245. Golan TD, Elkon KB, Gharavi AE, et al. Enhanced membrane binding of autoantibodies to cultured keratinocytes of systemic lupus erythematosus patients after ultraviolet B/ultraviolet A irradiation. *J Clin Invest* 1992;90:1067–1076.
246. James JA, Gross T, Scofield RH, et al. Immunoglobulin epitope spreading and autoimmune disease after peptide immunization: Sm B/B′ derived PPPGMRPP and PPPGIRGP induce spliceosome autoimmunity. *J Exp Med* 1995;181:453–461.
247. James JA, Harley JB. A model of peptide-induced lupus autoimmune B cell epitope spreading is strain specific and is not H-2 restricted in mice. *J Immunol* 1998;160:502–508.
248. Reynolds P, Gordon TP, Purcell AW, et al. Hierarchial self-tolerance to T cells determinants within the ubiquitous nuclear self-antigen La (SS-B) permits induction of systemic autoimmunity in normal mice. *J Exp Med* 1996;184:1857–1870.
249. Mohan C, Shi Y, Laman JD, et al. Nucleosome: a major immunogen for the pathogenic autoantibody-inducing T cells of lupus. *J Exp Med* 1993;177:1367–1381.
250. Kaliyaperumal A, Mohan C, Wu W, et al. Nucleosomal peptide epitopes for nephritis-inducing T helper cells of murine lupus. *J Exp Med* 1996;183:2459–2469.
251. Singh RR, Kumar V, Ebling FM, et al. T cell determinants from autoantibodies to DNA can upregulate autoimmunity in murine systemic lupus erythematosus. *J Exp Med* 1995;181: 2017–2027.
252. Waisman A, Ruiz PJ, Israeli E, et al. Modulation of murine systemic lupus erythematosus with peptides based on complementarity determining region of a pathogenic anti-DNA monoclonal antibody. *Proc Natl Acad Sci USA* 1997;94:4620–4625
253. Kaliyaperumal A, Michaels MA, Datta SK. Antigen-specific therapy of murine lupus nephritis using nucleosomal peptides: tolerance spreading impairs pathogenic function of autoimmune T and B cells. *J Immunol* 1999;162:5775–5783
254. Singh RR, Ebling FM, Sercarz EE, et al. Immune tolerance to autoantibody-derived peptides delays development of autoimmunity in murine lupus. *J Clin Invest* 1995;96:2990–2996
255. Goodnow CC. Transgenic mice and analysis of B cell tolerance. *Annu Rev Immunol* 1992;10:489–518.
256. Hartley SB, Crosbie J, Brink R, et al. Elimination from peripheral lymphoid tissues of self-reactive B lymphocytes recognizing membrane-bound antigens. *Nature* 1991;353:765–769.
257. Offen D, Spatz L, Escowitz H, et al. Induction of tolerance to an IgG autoantibody. *Proc Natl Acad Sci USA* 1992;89: 8332–8336.
258. Tsao BP, Chow A, Cheroutre H, et al. B cells are anergic in transgenic mice that express IgM anti-DNA antibodies. *Eur J Immunol* 1993;23:2332–2339.
259. Bynoe MS, Spatz L, Diamond B. Characterization of anti-DNA B cells that escape negative selection. *Eur J Immunol* 1999;29: 1304–1313.
260. Radic MZ, Erikson J, Litwin S, et al. B lymphocytes may escape tolerance by revising their antigen receptors. *J Exp Med* 1993;177:1165–1173.
261. Gay D, Saunders T, Camper S, et al. Receptor editing: an approach by autoreactive B cells to escape tolerance. *J Exp Med* 1993;177:999–1008.
262. Chen C, Radic MZ, Erikson J, et al. Deletion and editing of B cells that express antibodies to DNA. *J Immunol* 1994;152: 1970–1982.
263. Spatz L, Saenko V, Iliev A, et al. Light chain usage in anti-double stranded DNA B cell subsets: Role in cell fate determination. *J Exp Med* 1997;185:1317–1326.
264. Pewzner-Jung Y, Friedmann D, Sonoda E, et al. B cell deletion, anergy, and receptor editing in "knock in" mice targeted with a germline-encoded or somatically mutated anti-DNA heavy chain. *J Immunol* 1998;161:4634–4645.
265. Friedmann D, Yachimovich N, Mostoslavsky G, et al. Production of high affinity autoantibodies in autoimmune NZB/ NZW F1 mice targeted with an anti-DNA heavy chain. *J Immunol* 1999;162:4406–4416.
266. Brard F, Shannon M, Prak EL, et al. Somatic mutation and light chain rearrangements in anti-single stranded DNA transgenic MRL/lpr mice. *J Exp Med* 1999;190:691–704.
267. Kench JA, Russel DM, Nemazee D. Efficient peripheral clonal elimination of B lymphocytes in MRL/lpr mice bearing autoantibody transgenes. *J Exp Med* 1998;108:909–917.
268. Watanabe-Fukunaga R, Brannan CI, Copeland NG, et al. Lymphoproliferation disorder in mice explained by defects in Fas antigen that mediates apoptosis. *Nature* 1992;356:314–317.
269. Chu JL, Drappa J, Parnassa A, et al. The defect in Fas mRNA expression in MRL/lpr mice is associated with insertion of the retrotransposon, ETn. *J Exp Med* 1993;178:723–730.
270. Takahashi T, Tanaka M, Brannan CI, et al. Generalized lymphoproliferative disease in mice, caused by a point mutation in the Fas ligand. *Cell* 1994;76:969–976.
271. Susuki N, Ichino M, Mihara S, et al. Inhibition of Fas/Fas ligand mediated apoptotic cell death of lymphocytes *in-vitro* by circulating anti-Fas ligand autoantibodies in patients with SLE. *Arthritis Rheum* 1998;41:344–353.
272. Courtney PA, Crokard AD, Williamson K, et al. Lymphocyte apoptosis in systemic lupus erythematosus: relationships with Fas expression, serum soluble Fas, and disease activity. *Lupus* 1999;8:508–513.
273. Van Lopik T, Bijl M, Hart M, et al. Patients with SLE with high plasma levels of sFAS risk relapse. *J Rheumatol* 1999;26:60–67.
274. McNally J, Yoo DH, Drappa J, et al. Fas ligand expression and function in SLE. *J Immunol* 1997;159:4628–4636.
275. Nozawa K, Kayagaki N, Tokano Y, et al. Soluble Fas (APO-1, CD95) and soluble Fas ligand in rheumatic diseases. *Arthritis Rheum* 1997;40:1126–1129.
276. Vaishnaw AK, Toubi E, Ohsako S, et al. The spectrum of apoptotic defects and clinical manifestation, including SLE, in humans with CD95 (Fas/APO-1) mutations. *Arthritis Rheum* 1999;42:1833–1842.
277. Drappa J, Vaishnaw AK, Sullivan KE, et al. Fas gene mutation in the Canale-Smith syndrome, an inherited lymphoproliferative disorder associated with autoimmunity. *N Engl J Med* 1996;335:1643–1649.
278. Strasser A, Whittingham S, Vaux DL, et al. Enforced bcl-2 expression in B-lymphoid cells prolongs antibody responses and elicits autoimmune disease. *Proc Natl Acad Sci USA* 1991;88: 8661–8665.
279. Kuo P, Bynoe M, Diamond B. Crossreactive B cells are present during a primary but not secondary response in BALB/c mice expressing a bcl-2 transgene. *Mol Immunol* 1999;36:471–479.
280. Kuo P, Bynoe MS, Wang C, et al. Bcl-2 leads to expression of

anti-DNA B cells but no nephritis: a model for a clinical subset. *Eur J Immunol* 1999;29:3168–3178.

281. Bynoe MS, Grimaldi CM, Diamond B. Estrogen up-regulates bcl-2 and blocks tolerance induction of naïve B cells. *Proc Natl Acad Sci USA* 2000;97:2703–2708.
282. Mevorach D, Zhou JL, Song X, et al. Systemic exposure to irradiated apoptotic cells induces autoantibody production. *J Exp Med* 1998;188:387–392.
283. Mevorach D, Mascarenhas JO, Gershov D, et al. Complement-dependent clearance of apoptotic cells by human macrophages. *J Exp Med* 1998;188:2313–2320.
284. Prodeus AP, Goerg S, Shen LM, et al. A critical role for complement in maintenance of self-tolerance. *Immunity* 1998;9: 721–731.
285. Bickerstaff MC, Botto M, Hutchinson WL, et al. Serum amyloid P component controls chromatin degradation and prevents anti-nuclear autoimmunity. *Nat Med* 1999;5:694–697.
286. Kelly VE, Masuda K, Yoshida H, et al. Induction of various autoantibodies by mutant gene lpr in several strains of mice. *J Immunol* 1984;133:227–233.
287. Strasser A, Harris AW, Cory S. The role of bcl-2 in lymphoid differentiation and neoplastic transformation. *Curr Opin Microbiol Immunol* 1992;182:299–302.
288. Sato S, Ono N, Steeber DA, et al. CD19 regulates B lymphocyte signaling thresholds critical for the development of B-1 lineage cells and autoimmunity. *J Immunol* 1996;157:4371–4378.
289. Inaoki M, Sato S, Weintraub BC, et al. CD19-regulated signaling thresholds control peripheral tolerance and autoantibody production in B lymphocytes. *J Exp Med* 1997;186: 1923–1931.
290. Okeefe TL, Williams GT, Davies SL, et al. Hyperresponsive B cells in CD22-deficient mice. *Science* 1996;274:798–801.
291. O'Keefe TL, Williams GT, Batista FD, et al. Deficiency in CD22, a B cell-specific inhibitory receptor, is sufficient to predispose to development of high affinity autoantibodies. *J Exp Med* 1999;189:1307–1313.
292. Chan VW, Meng F, Soriano P, et al. Characterization of the B lymphocyte populations in Lyn-deficient mice and the role of Lyn in signal initiation and down-regulation. *Immunity* 1997;7: 69–81.
293. Westhoff CM, Whittier A, Kathol S, et al. DNA-binding antibodies from viable motheaten mutant mice: implications for B cell tolerance. *J Immunol* 1997;159:3024–3033.
294. Cornall RJ, Cyster JG, Hibbs ML, et al. Polygenic autoimmune traits: Lyn, CD22, and SHP-1 are limiting elements of a biochemical pathway regulating BCR signaling and selection. *Immunity* 1998;8:497–508.
295. Mohan C, Shi Y, Laman JD, et al. Interaction between CD40 and its ligand gp39 in the development of murine lupus nephritis. *J Immunol* 1995;154:1470–1480.
296. Kalled SL, Cutler AH, Datta SK, et al. Anti-CD40 ligand antibody treatment of SNF1 mice with established nephritis: preservation of kidney function. *J Immunol* 1998;160:2158–2165.
297. Early GS, Zhao W, Burns CM. Anti-CD40 ligand antibody treatment prevents the development of lupus-like nephritis in a subset of NZB x NZW mice. *J Immunol* 1996;157:3159–3164
298. Finck BK, Linsley PS, Wofsy D. Treatment of murine lupus with CTL4Ig. *Science* 1994;265:1225–1227.
299. Mihara M, Tan I, Chuzin Y, et al. CTLA4Ig inhibits T cell-dependent B-cell maturation in murine SLE. *J Clin Invest* 2000; 106:91–101.
300. Daikh DI, Finck BK, Linsley PS, et al. Long-term inhibition of murine lupus by brief simultaneous blockade of B7/CD28 and CD40/gp39 costimulation pathways. *J Immunol* 1997;159: 3104–3108
301. Sievers TM, Rossi SJ, Ghobrial RM, et al. Mycophenolate mofetil. *Pharmacotherapy* 1997;17:1178–1197.
302. Jonsson CA, Svensson L, Carlsten H. Beneficial effects of the inosine monophosphate dehydrogenase inhibitor mycophenolate mofetil on survival and severity of glomerulonephritis in SLE-prone MRL lpr/lpr mice. *Clin Exp Immunol* 1999;116: 534–541.
303. McMurray RW, Elbounre KB, Lagoo A, et al. Mycophenolate mofetil suppresses autoimmunity and mortality in the female NZB x NZW F1 model of systemic lupus erythematosus. *J Rheumatol* 1998;25:2364–2370.
304. Gaubitz M, Schorat A, Schotte H, et al. Mycophenolate mofetil for the treatment of systemic lupus erythematosus: an open pilot trial. *Lupus* 1999; 8:731–736.
305. Abraham RT. Mammalian target of rapamycin: immunosuppressive drugs uncover a novel pathway of cytokine receptor signaling. *Curr Opin Immunol* 1998;10:330–336.
306. Warner LM, Adams LM, Sehgal SN. Rapamycin prolongs survival and arrests pathophysiologic changes in murine systemic lupus erythematosus. *Arthritis Rheum* 1994;37:289–297.
307. Collins MJ, Nagle SL, Goldman SJ, et al. Prolonged inhibition of murine lupus by short term therapy with anti-B7 antibodies and rapamycin during onset of disease. *FASEB J* 2000;14: A1207(abst).
308. Jones DS, Hachmann JP, Osgood SA, et al. Conjugates of double stranded oligonucleotides with polyethylene glycol and keyhole limpet hemocyanin: a model for treating systemic lupus erythematosus. *Bioconjugate Chem* 1994;5:390–399.
309. Weisman MH, Blustein HG, Berner CM, et al. Reduction in circulating dsDNA antibody titer after administration of LJP 394. *J Rheumatol* 1997;24:314–318.

20

ANTINUCLEAR ANTIBODIES: AN OVERVIEW

IAN GILES
DAVID ISENBERG

The antinuclear antibody (ANA) test is often used as a means to determine whether an individual presenting with joint problems has an autoimmune rheumatic disease (ARD) such as systemic lupus erythematosus (SLE) or a related disorder. A positive ANA is thus a serologic indicator of autoimmune disease, although further immunologic investigations coupled with clinical findings are required to make a specific diagnosis. Although initially identified on immunofluorescence microscopy (IFM), more than 30 nuclear antigen-antibody specificities have been identified using more sophisticated techniques, e.g., immunoblotting in patients with SLE and various ARDs (1), reflecting the heterogeneity of the various nuclear targets. However, given the vast number of targets available within the cell (around 2,000), the diversity of autoantibodies produced is actually rather restricted. Distinct autoantibody profiles may provide a specific diagnosis.

The lupus erythematosus (LE) cell phenomenon, of phagocytosis of leukocytes exposed to lupus patients serum, described by Hargreaves et al. (2) in 1948, was the first serologic marker used in the diagnosis of SLE and has now been replaced by ANA testing. For the past 40 years, ANA has been detected by IFM initially on rodent tissue sections (3–5) and more recently using human cell lines (6), which are capable of greater pattern recognition because of the larger size of individual cells and more discrete fluorescence of subcellular organelles while displaying species specificity.

Crucial to the interpretation of the ANA test is the recognition that the main patterns of staining on IFM are rarely specific or diagnostic of any individual autoantibody or disease; an exception to this is the centromere pattern seen with antikinetochore antibodies in limited cutaneous scleroderma. The presence and pattern of staining of ANA is indicative of the presence of an autoantibody, which should be verified with more specific tests (see below) and considered in the clinical context to deduce if the diagnosis of SLE or another autoimmune or separate disease should be considered.

This chapter summarizes the history of ANA testing; discusses choice of substrate, interpretation of IFM with links to target antigens and their clinical relevance, and more specific diagnostic tests; and offers a practical guide to interpretation. The aim is to provide an understanding of the strengths and limitations of ANA determination, its sensitivity and specificity, and above all the importance of a positive ANA result in deciding if the patient has SLE or an autoimmune disease at all.

HISTORY

The initial description of the LE cell test (2) constituted one of the first laboratory abnormalities found to be associated with SLE. Haserick et al. (7) in 1950 then demonstrated that the LE factor is a component of the gamma globulin fraction of serum proteins, while Miescher and Fauconnet (8) in 1954 reported that incubation of sera from lupus patients with a suspension of cell nuclei eliminated the capacity to induce the LE phenomenon. Thus the LE test was the first ANA reactivity ever described, and has been shown to be directed against histone H1 as the major monomeric proteinaceous antigen (9).

Friou and colleagues (3) in 1957 and 1958 first described and partially characterized the phenomenon by which serum from patients with SLE would bind to nuclear antigens in fresh frozen tissue from humans and a range of vertebrate animals. Using fluorochrome labeled antisera, it was shown that the component binding the nucleus was in fact antibody from the patient (3,10). These findings were subsequently confirmed by others (4,5) and clearly demonstrate that an autoimmune pathology was underlying the disease. These findings heralded a new era of research into SLE, and since 1971 it has been one of the 11 American College of Rheumatology (ACR) classification criteria (6,11).

CHOICE OF SUBSTRATE

During the past 40 years a variety of substrates have been used to identify the presence of a positive ANA. In the initial studies rodent tissues of varying types, e.g., mouse kidney, rat liver, were popularized. More recently human cell lines, especially epithelial cells (HEp-2) derived from a human laryngeal carcinoma (12,13), have been widely adopted. The advantages of the HEp-2 cells are that both nuclei and nucleoli are large, which enables a wide range of staining patterns to be recognized on IFM. The cell lines can be cultured in the research laboratory or are available from commercial companies on slides. Analysis of the pattern, intensity, and even presence of immunofluorescence is very time-consuming, requiring careful interpretation by a trained technician or pathologist, which may still give rise to a wide variability between different laboratories experienced in performing ANA tests (14).

More recently, attempts at improved standardization of ANA testing have been introduced using commercially developed enzyme-linked immunosorbent assays (ELISA). There are several different assays available; some coat the ELISA plate with extracts of entire nuclei, while others use only specific antigens. However, the results of these different assays vary significantly from each other, and in some cases from ANA measured by IFM when tested on the same serum. Those ELISAs with the highest sensitivity for the detection of SLE (in patients known to have the disease) have the highest false-positive rate, while those tests with a low false-positive rate have a low sensitivity for the detection of lupus in the same patients (15).

A further disadvantage of the different ELISA kits that use specific antigens is that they cannot detect as yet unknown cellular antigens. In ELISA kits that utilize whole nuclear extracts to coat the plate, it is difficult to monitor the binding of different antigens to the polystyrene plates. Thus, IFM is likely to remain the test of choice using HEp2 cells for some time.

PATTERNS OF IMMUNOFLUORESCENCE AND LINKS TO TARGET ANTIGEN

Demonstration of a positive ANA is merely the start of the journey. Given that the cell nucleus contains DNA, RNA, proteins, and enzymes together with some special structures, e.g., the nucleolus, major attempts have been made in the past 40 years to define more precisely the antigenic targets of a serum that give a positive immunofluorescence pattern.

Six main patterns of IFM on HEp2 cells are recognized, one of which is directed against constituents of the cytoplasm (Table 20.1); not all of these patterns occur commonly in SLE patients. The pattern of staining often reflects the predominant antibody present in the serum. A homogeneous pattern corresponds with antibodies binding to double-stranded DNA (dsDNA) (16) and/or histones (17,18), both of which are described in detail below. The peripheral (rim) pattern has been reported with antibodies to integral glycoproteins of (a) the inner nuclear membrane—lamin B (homogeneous rim pattern) in SLE (19); (b) the nuclear pore complex, glycoprotein (gp)210 (punctate rim pattern) in patients with myositis (20); (c) primary

TABLE 20.1. PATTERNS OF IMMUNOFLUORESCENCE MICROSCOPY (IFM) ON TISSUE CULTURE STAINING

Pattern on IFM	Linked Antigen Specificities	Related Disease
Nuclear		
Homogeneous	Chromatin, histone, dsDNA	SLE, DIL
	Ku	PM-Scl-SLE
Rim enhanced	Lamins, nuclear pore complex	SLE
Speckled		
Coarse	Sm, U1-RNP	SLE
Fine	Ro, La	SS, SCLE, CHB, NL
Distinct	Anti-p80 coilin, anti-p95	PBC
Nucleolar		
Speckles	Scl 70, RNA polymerase 1	Scl
Homogeneous	PM-Scl	Scl
	Ku	PM-Scl-SLE
Clumpy	U3-RNP	Scl
Centromere	Kinetochore	Scl
Different patterns of staining	PCNA	SLE
Cytoplasmic	Ribosomal P protein	SLE

SCLE, subacute cutaneous lupus; CHB, congenital heart block; PBC, primary biliary cirrhosis; DIL, drug-induced lupus; PM-Scl-SLE, polymyositis-scleroderma-SLE overlap; PCNA, proliferating-cell nuclear antigen; RNP, ribonucleoprotein.

biliary cirrhosis (21,22); and (d) chronic active hepatitis (23). The antibodies to lamin B found in the sera of patients with lupus may explain the peripheral rim pattern described in previous reports, which was thought to be due to antibodies to DNA (24). A speckled pattern is commonly found in patients with SLE, indicating binding to a variety of nonhistone, small ribonucleoprotein (RNP) particles including Sm (25), Ro, La, and U1RNP (26). The precise function of these particles is unknown but they may play a role in the processing of messenger RNA. Antibodies to Sm are virtually diagnostic of SLE and are found in 30% of black lupus patients and 5% of Caucasians, frequently in conjunction with anti-U1RNP antibodies. Anti-La antibodies are particularly associated with SLE and Sjögren's syndrome (SS), frequently in conjunction with anti-Ro antibodies (16); lupus patients with anti-La antibodies are less likely to have renal disease (27). Anti-Ro antibodies without anti-La are also detected in subacute cutaneous lupus (SCLE), lupus of homozygous C2 and C4 deficiencies, and neonatal lupus syndrome (28). Some examples of these common patterns of IFM in lupus patients are shown in Fig. 20.1.

Different patterns of cytoplasmic staining exist and are indicative of the distinct target antigens involved. Antibodies directed against components of the cytoskeleton are identified more frequently in ARD but are not specific to lupus (29,30). Approximately 20% of SLE sera display a fine speckled pattern on IFM, which has been identified as antibodies to ribosomal P protein (31,32). The anti-P antibodies have been reported to correlate with neuropsychiatric manifestations (33) and severe depression (34) in SLE; however, these associations were not evident in many published series, and this proposed link remains controversial (35).

The finely granular cytoplasmic fluorescence seen with antiribosomal P antibodies is also seen with autoantibodies to antigens involved in translation and protein synthesis, the aminoacyl-tRNA synthetases—anti-Jo-1 (36), anti-PL-7 (37), anti-PL-12 (38); antibodies to signal recognition particle (39); and anti-KJ (40). The pattern of staining typical of anti-Jo-1 antibodies is demonstrated in Fig. 20.2A. These autoantibodies have not yet been described in lupus, being virtually confined to patients with autoimmune myositis, especially those with accompanying interstitial lung disease (41).

Patterns of IFM rarely seen in SLE sera are the centromere and nucleolar, the presence of which should alert the physician to an alternative diagnosis. Nucleolar patterns are mostly displayed in sera from scleroderma (Scl) patients or overlap syndromes. Antitopoisomerase I antibodies, originally described as anti-Scl-70 (42), are found in approximately 25% of Scl patients and identify the diffuse cutaneous subgroup (DcScl) with systemic involvement. Anticentromere antibodies (ACAs) targeted against the kinetochore are more prevalent, 52% to 82% in Scl patients with local cutaneous disease (43,44). These IFM patterns are illustrated in Fig. 20.3.

Rarely, a homogeneous nuclear and nucleolar IFM pattern is caused by antibodies directed against anti-Ku, which were first described in Japanese polymyositis (PM)-Scl overlap patients (45). Initially there was some confusion with another precipitating antibody system, the anti-Ki, because

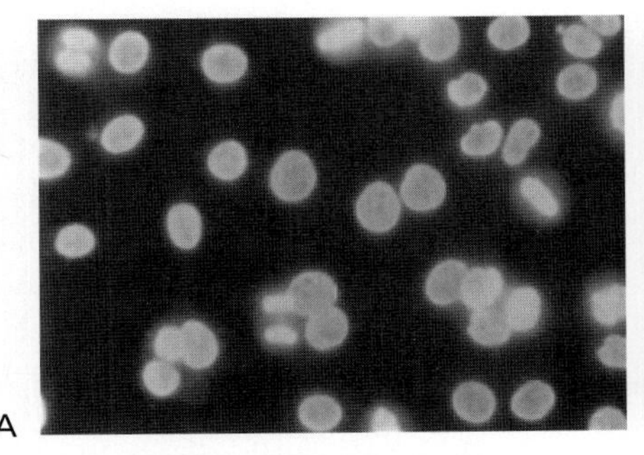

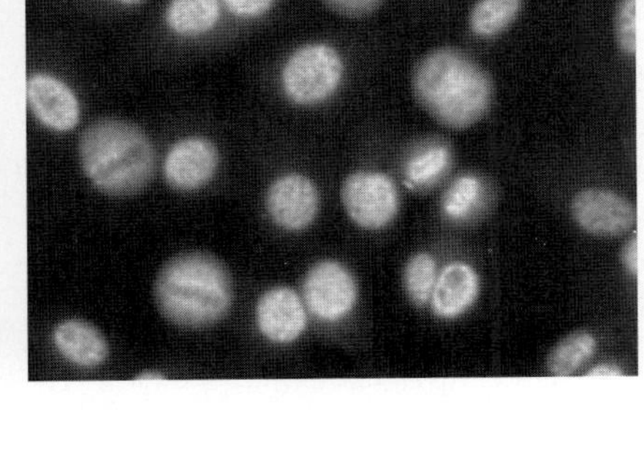

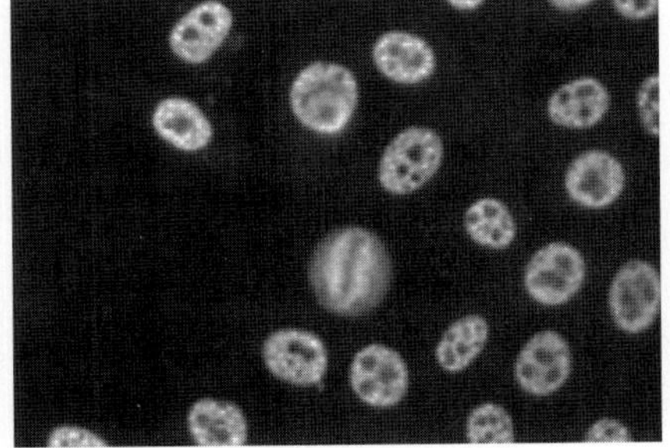

FIGURE 20. 1. Patterns of immunofluorescence microscopy (IFM) upon HEp-2 cells commonly seen in patients with SLE. **A:** Homogeneous staining characteristic of antibodies to double-stranded DNA (dsDNA). **B:** Coarse speckled staining typical of anti-U1RNP/Sm antibodies. **C:** Fine speckled staining characteristic of antibodies to Ro/La antigens.

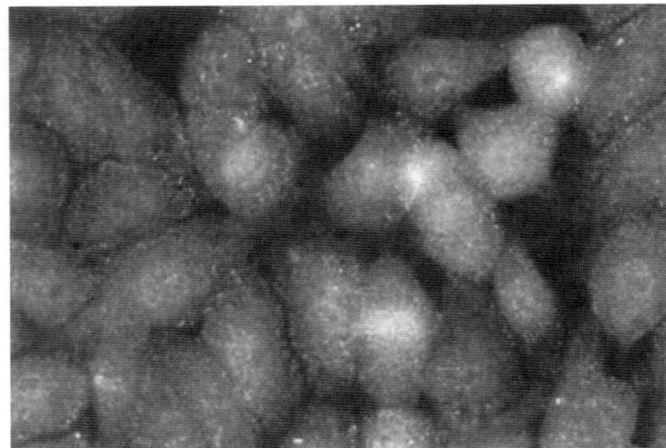

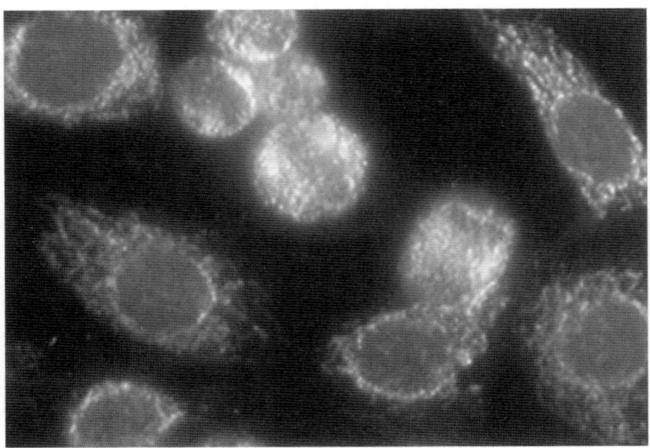

A B

FIGURE 20.2. A: The fine speckled pattern of cytoplasmic IFM, characteristic of antibodies against the aminoacyl t-RNA synthetases. **B:** In contrast, the reticular, lacy cytoplasmic staining characteristic of antibodies to mitochondria typically seen in patients with primary biliary cirrhosis. The substrate in both cases was HEp-2 cells.

of the serum used as prototype in the laboratories (16,46). The Ku antigen consists of two proteins of 66 and 86 kd, which bind tightly to DNA (47,48). Anti-Ku antibodies are found in 55% of Japanese PM-Scl patients (45), 1% to 19% of SLE-PM-Scl patients, and 1% to 14% of Scl patients in North America (41,49).

Anti-Ki antibodies described in 1981 (50) are probably identical to the sicca-lupus (SL) system identified in the same year (51) and found in 7% to 10% of unselected SLE sera by immunodiffusion studies (52). The antibodies recognize a 32-kd nonhistone nuclear antigen and display speckled nuclear patterns on IFM. Subsequent detection of anti-Ki antibodies by ELISA using rabbit thymus extract as substrate revealed frequencies of 19% and a fluctuation of the antibodies with disease activity in the sera from lupus patients (53). Further studies with recombinant Ki antigen on ELISA testing found a frequency of 21% of anti-Ki antibodies and an association with central nervous system (CNS) involvement in SLE patients (54). Despite these reported findings anti-Ki antibodies are not specific for SLE being found in sera of many other patients with ARD.

A rare but specific polymorphonuclear pattern corresponding to different phases of the cell cycle is detected in 3% of SLE sera (16) and is caused by antibodies to proliferating cell nuclear antigen (PCNA, previously called cyclin), an antigen involved in cell cycle regulation. Peak expression of PCNA has been shown to occur immediately before full DNA synthesis, hence its name (55,56). These antibodies are rarely found in other diseases.

Antibodies to RA-33, an antigen contained in nuclear extracts, were initially described in sera from patients with rheumatoid arthritis, but there was no correlation with the presence, absence, or pattern of ANA staining on IFM (57). Subsequently, RA-33 antibodies have been shown to be identical to the A2 protein of the heterogeneous RNP complex (58). It is now recognized that RA-33 antibodies identify a subset of SLE patients who have an erosive arthropathy (59).

CLINICAL INTERPRETATION

In high titers, such as dilutions exceeding 1:320, in an appropriate clinical setting, such as a young woman presenting with a malar rash, polyarthralgia, and leucopenia, the ANA test and interpretation of its significance are straightforward. For every positive ANA result in a case of SLE, however, many more will arise because of drug therapy, old age, chronic infection, chronic liver disease, and other ARD. Very rare cases of ANA-negative lupus are reported (see below), and a positive ANA may be found in healthy individuals and asymptomatic first-degree relatives of lupus patients (60,61).

In healthy individuals of ages 20 to 60 years, ANA determined by IFM on HEp2 cells has been shown to be positive at an increasing frequency with decreasing ANA titer; thus, 3.3% of putatively normal individuals are ANA positive at 1:320 dilution, and up to 31.7% of the same population at 1:40 dilution (14). There is a steady rise in the prevalence of numerous autoantibodies with increasing age such that 10% to 37% of healthy elderly individuals (older than 70 years of age) have a positive ANA albeit of generally low positive titer (62,63).

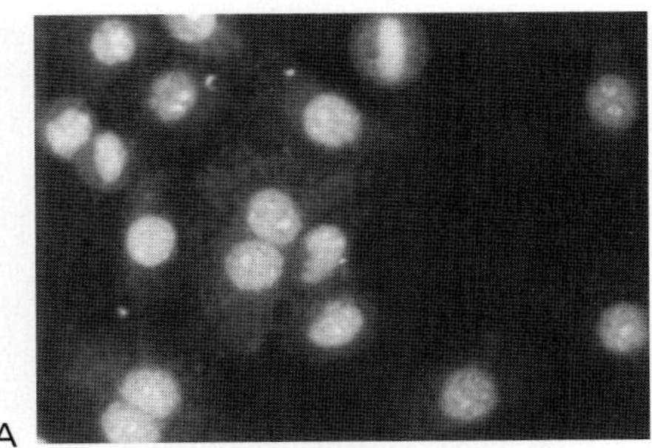

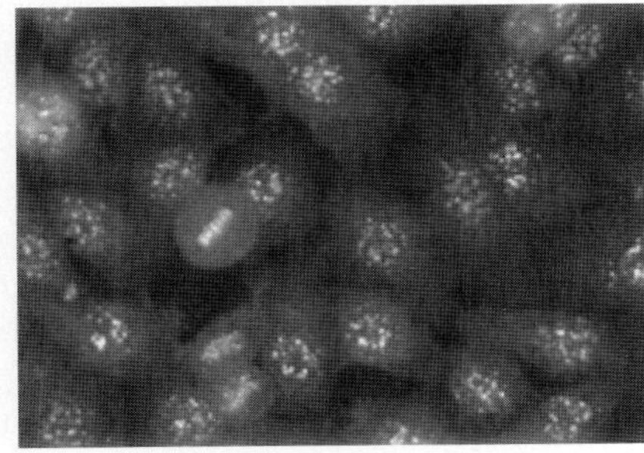

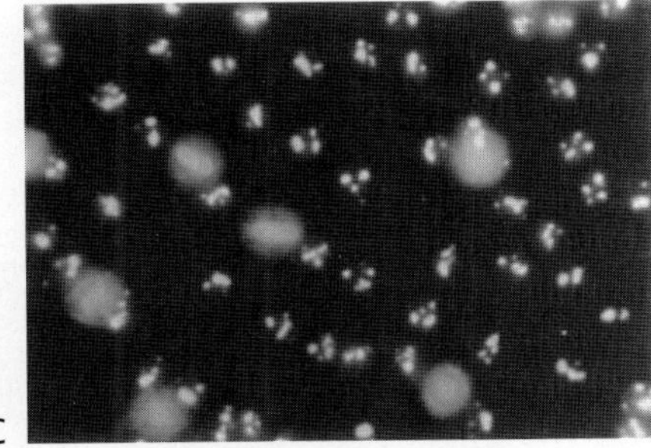

FIGURE 20.3. Immunofluorescence patterns on HEp-2 cells rarely seen in SLE. **A:** Fine granular staining characteristic of anti–Scl-70 antibodies. **B:** The diffuse speckled nuclear pattern of typical antibodies against the centromere in metaphase. **C:** Clumpy nucleolar fluorescence characteristic of antifibrillarin U3RNP antibodies.

A positive ANA has been found in most systemic ARD to varying degrees; however, it occurs with the highest frequency and titer in SLE (Table 20.2). The absolute level of the titer itself does not carry any prognostic significance; however, higher titers are more likely to be significant in making a diagnosis of disease.

Thus the presence and staining pattern of a positive ANA alone is not sufficient to determine the presence of lupus or any ARD. Detection of specific autoantibodies is required by more specific tests, and even then not all autoantibodies can recognize a specific disorder (64). Consideration of autoantibody profiles, however, increases diagnostic predictive value without loss of specificity or sensitivity, for example, in identifying SLE (by the presence of antibodies to dsDNA and/or Sm) from other ARD, such as SS (associated with anti-Ro and/or anti-La) or Scl (ACA and/or Scl 70 antibodies) (65). The same autoantibody profiles have been tested in SLE patients and have been found to identify disease subsets, for example, lupus patients with antibodies to dsDNA and/or Sm had a significant increase in malar rash, hypocomplementaemia, and renal and haematologic involvement, while patients with anti-Ro and/or anti-La antibodies had a worse lupus rash and photosensitivity (66). Therefore, more diagnostic and prognostic power is conferred when autoantibody profiles are considered as a whole in each patient.

A wide variety of drugs can induce a positive ANA and/or symptoms of lupus [drug-induced lupus (DIL)]. Common drugs that do this are hydralazine, procainamide, isoniazid, minocycline, and chlorpromazine, with many others implicated. The homogeneous staining pattern seen on IFM with such drugs is caused by antibodies to histones targeted primarily against the H2A-H2B-DNA complex (67–69) or H2A-H2B alone (70). Antihistone antibodies are also found in 30% to 80% of idiopathic SLE sera directed mainly against H1 and H2B (71), H3 (52), and the H2A-H2B complex (18). The presence of these antibodies is not associated with any particular clinical manifestations in SLE but has been correlated with disease activity (72).

TABLE 20.2. POSITIVE ANTINUCLEAR ANTIBODY (ANA) TESTS IN VARIOUS CONDITIONS USING HEP-2 CELLS AS SUBSTRATE

SLE	Other ARD		Other Disease		Normal Population
98%	Scl	95%	Chronic active hepatitis	100%	13.3% at 1:160
	SS	80%	Drug induced lupus	100%	
	RA	60%	Myasthenia gravis	50%	
	PM	90%	Waldenström's macroglobulinemia	20%	FDR's of SLE patients 20–30%
	PAN	18%	Diabetes	25%	

Scl, scleroderma; SS, Sjögren's syndrome; RA, rheumatoid arthritis; PM, polymyositis; PAN, polyarteritis nodosa; FDR, first-degree relative; ARD, autoimmune rheumatic disease.
Modified from *Oxford Textbook of Rheumatology,* 2nd ed.

Thus, homogeneous staining and the presence of antihistone antibodies alone cannot distinguish between idiopathic and DIL when a patient has appropriate symptoms, having been exposed to a potential lupus-inducing drug. If other autoantibodies are present and the symptoms do not abate within a few months of stopping the drug, accompanied by a decline in the ANA, then DIL is unlikely.

MORE SPECIFIC DIAGNOSTIC TESTS

Once the presence of autoimmunity is suspected clinically and then reinforced with a positive ANA, more specific tests of antibody detection are required. Antibodies to the target antigen of interest are labeled with markers such as enzymes, fluorochromes, or radioisotopes in the tests commonly used, notably radioimmunoassay (RIA), ELISA, and Western blotting, which are more sensitive than immunodiffusion techniques.

RIA is similar to IFM in that a labeled antibody, conjugated with a radioisotope in this case, is used to detect a specific antigen. The technique is very sensitive, detecting antigen in the picogram range. An inherent drawback of RIA is the use of radioisotopes, which require careful handling and expensive equipment to monitor radioactive emissions. Hence, the ELISA was devised whereby antibodies against the antigen of interest are attached to an enzyme such as horseradish peroxidase or alkaline phosphatase instead of a radioisotope. Detection of the antibody (and thus antigen) is facilitated by the addition of a substrate and developer that will generate a color reaction if the enzyme-labeled antibody is present. The end-point color can be read in a spectrophotometer or ELISA reader to give a quantitative estimation of the bound antibody and hence antigen. Advantages over RIA include the lack of radioisotopes and speed, as a 96-well plate can be read in less than 1 minute.

Western (immuno)blotting takes proteins from an extract of cultured cells and separates them by polyacrylamide gel electrophoresis according to their charge. The separated proteins are then transferred electrophoretically to a nitrocellulose (NC) sheet that is a replica of the original gel and a solid support for antigen. The NC sheet can then be probed with either enzyme or radiolabeled antibody (73).

IDENTIFICATION OF LUPUS-RELATED ANTIBODIES

Of the disease-specific antibodies in SLE, it is those targeting dsDNA that carry the most diagnostic power and clinical application. Between 60% and 83% of lupus patients are found to have anti-dsDNA antibodies when tested by one of the currently available assays, and in some patients the titer of these antibodies is an excellent measure of disease activity. Among the currently available methods of detecting antibodies to dsDNA, the Farr (RIA) may be the most specific test for SLE and is the assay most likely to predict occurrence of disease flare, especially glomerulonephritis. The *Crithidia* assay detects anti-dsDNA antibodies by their ability to bind to the kinetoplast of *Crithidia luciliae*, a protozoan organism with a circular dsDNA structure at one pole, and subsequent immunofluorescence. This assay is technically demanding, requiring careful training of technicians to correctly identify the kinetoplast rather than the nucleus or polar body upon IFM, as shown in Fig. 20.4. A major advantage is that it detects antibodies to dsDNA almost exclusively as opposed to the Farr and ELISA, which may give positive results with single-stranded DNA (ssDNA). However, the ELISA is widely available and relatively easy to perform detecting both high- and low-affinity immunoglobulin G (IgG) antibodies to dsDNA (74).

Among the different ELISA kits available there are marked differences in sensitivity, specificity, and predictive values in diagnosing SLE and determining disease activity (75). Hence, laboratories may offer more than one test for detection of anti-dsDNA antibodies in certain instances;

A

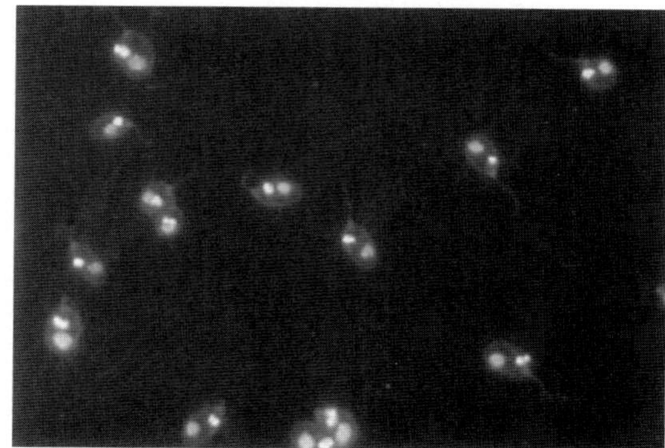

B

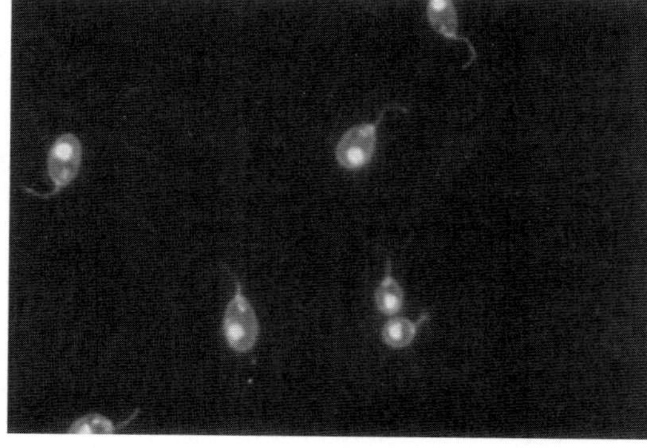

FIGURE 20.4. A: The *Crithidia luciliae* assay for antibodies to dsDNA is positive with immunofluorescence of the kinetoplast only. **B:** Fluorescence of the nuclei, in this example, or any structure other than the kinetoplast, is not indicative of the presence of anti-dsDNA antibodies.

ANA Negative

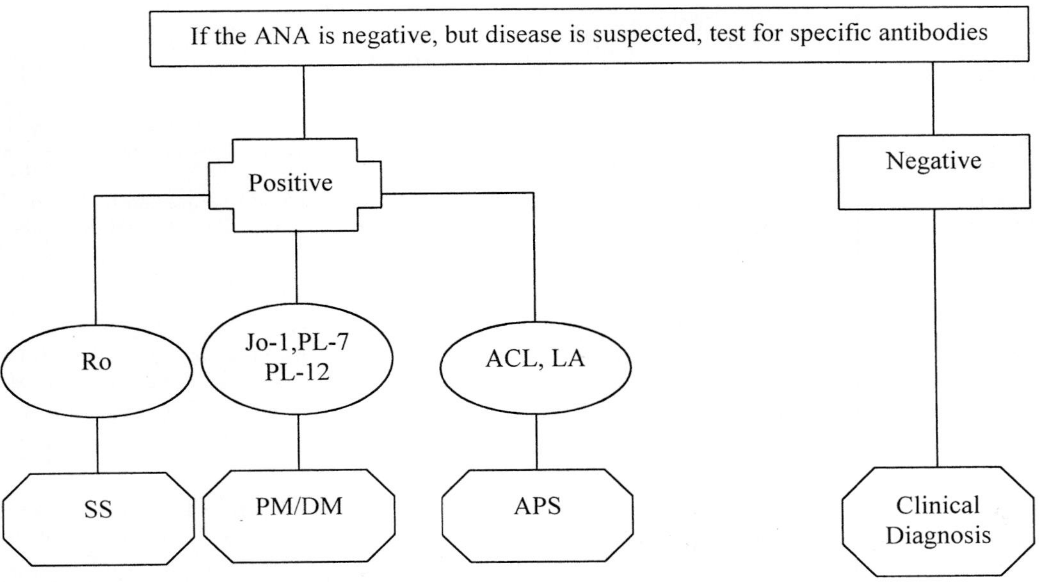

ANA Positive

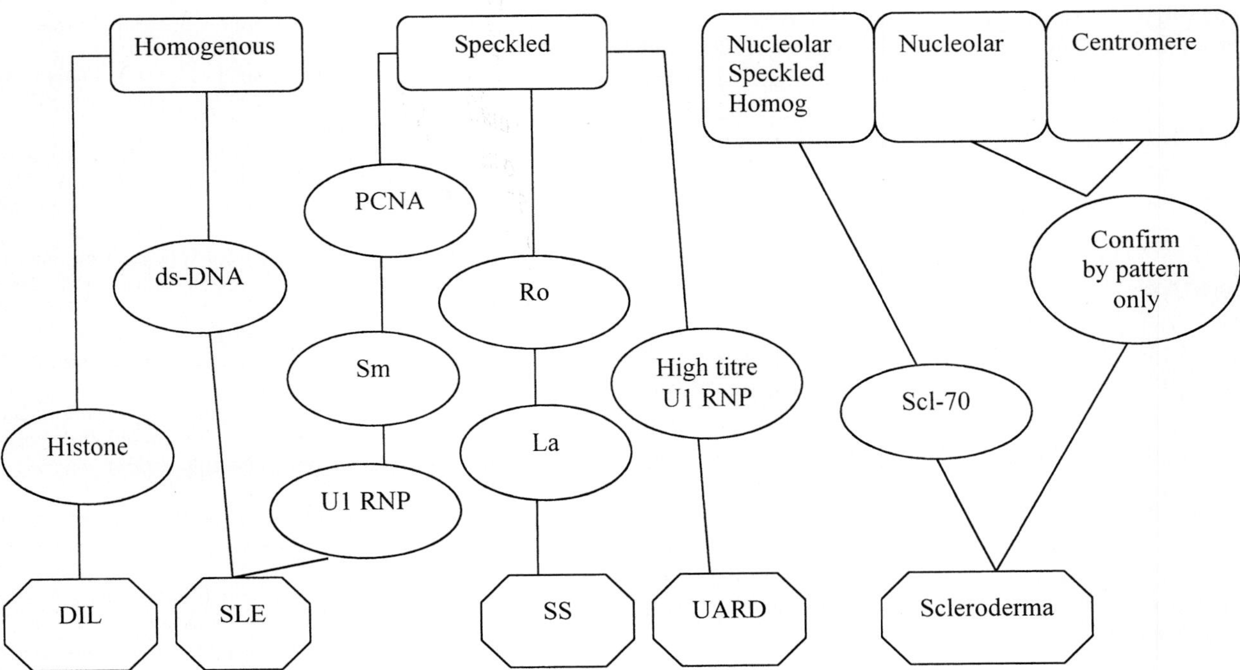

FIGURE 20.5. A practical guide to interpretation of the ANA test. (Modified from Morrow J, Nelson JL, Watts R, et al. *Autoimmune rheumatic disease*, 2nd ed. Oxford, England: Oxford University Press, 1999.)

for example, the *Crithidia* assay may be reserved for diagnosis, and the ELISA used to monitor antibody titers and thus reflect disease activity.

ANA-NEGATIVE LUPUS

True negative ANA tests in patients with lupus are now very rare, perhaps 2% of sera at most (76), with the advent of human tissue culture cells as the substrate. Previously, more patients were falsely labeled as being ANA negative, up to 5%, using rodent (mainly mouse and rat liver) tissue substrate. Autoantibodies, however, are detectable by ELISA against Ro and La antigens, originally found in 90% of ANA negative patients sera (77), and now, by using a more sensitive ELISA, they are found in virtually 100% of the same sera (78). The reason for this apparent dichotomy is the variable distribution of Ro and La antigens in cells of different species, with significant quantities of the antigen detected by IFM in cells of humans, monkeys, and guinea pigs, but low amounts, or none, found in cells of rat, mouse, and chicken (79).

A previously positive ANA test in patients with lupus may become negative with disease remission that occurs either spontaneously or following immunosuppressive treatment. Such ANA negativity can occur in 10% to 20% of cases, especially those lupus patients who experience renal failure.

The disappearance of previously positive ANA does not remove the usual need for careful vigilance of clinical and laboratory markers of disease, as the future course of the disease cannot be assumed to have burned out. Apart from anti-dsDNA antibodies and antiribosomal P antibodies (80), the titer of other autoantibodies and ANA is not a guide to disease activity.

SUMMARY

Identification of the presence and pattern of staining of ANA on IFM of HEp2 cells is an essential first step in the immunologic diagnosis of lupus. The subsequent detection of specific autoantibodies and their profile helps to cement the clinical diagnosis of SLE, in the case of anti-dsDNA and/or anti-Sm antibodies, or to suggest another ARD such as Scl if ACA or Scl-70 is found. A practical guide to interpretation of the ANA test is given in Fig. 20.5, to highlight the diagnostic decision pathway that must be taken each time an ANA test is ordered.

ACKNOWLEDGMENTS

We are very grateful to Professor Allan Wiik, Department of Autoimmunity, Statens Serum Institut, Copenhagen, Denmark, for providing us with the pictures of IFM upon HEp-2 cells.

REFERENCES

1. von Muhlen CA, Tan EM. Autoantibodies in the diagnosis of systemic rheumatic diseases. *Semin Arthritis Rheum* 1995;24:323–358.
2. Hargreaves MM, Richmond H, Morton R. Presentation of two bone marrow elements: the "Tart" cell and the "L. E. " cell. *Proc Mayo Clin* 1948;23:25–28.
3. Friou GJ, Finch SC, Detre KD. Interaction of nuclei and globulin from lupus erythematosus serum demonstrated with fluorescent antibody. *J Immunol* 1958;80:324–329.
4. Holborow J, Weir DM, Johnson GD. A serum factor in lupus erythematosus with affinity for tissue nuclei. *Br Med J* 1957;2:732–734.
5. Holman HR, Kunkel HG. Affinity between the lupus erythematosus serum factor and cell nuclei and nucleoprotein. *Science* 1957;126:162–163.
6. Tan EM, Cohen AS, Fries JF, et al. The 1982 revised criteria for the classification of systemic lupus erythematosus. *Arthritis Rheum* 1982;25:1271–1277.
7. Haserick JR, Lewis LL, Bortz DW. Blood Factor in acute disseminated lupus erythematosus 1. Determination of gamma globulin as specific plasma fraction. *Am J Med Sci* 1950;219:660–663.
8. Miescher P, Fauconnet M. L`absorption du facteur "L. E." par des noyaux cellulaires isolés. *Experientia* 1954;10:252–254.
9. Schett G, Steiner G, Smolen JS. Nuclear antigen histone H1 is primarily involved in lupus erythematosus cell formation. *Arthritis Rheum* 1998;41:1446–1455.
10. Friou GJ. The significance of the lupus globulin-nucleoprotein reaction. *Ann Intern Med* 1958;49:866–874.
11. Cohen AS, Reynolds WE, Franklin EC, et al. Preliminary criteria for the classification of systemic lupus erythematosus. *Bull Rheum Dis* 1971;21:643–648.
12. Toolan HW. Transplantable human neoplasms maintained in cortisone-treated laboratory animals: H. S. #1; H. Ep. #1; H. Ep. #2; H. Ep. #3; and H. Emb. Rh. #1*. *Cancer Res* 1954;14:660–666.
13. Moore AE, Sabachewsky L, Toolan HW. Culture characteristics of four permanent lines of human cancer cells. *Cancer Res* 1955;15:598–602.
14. Tan EM, Feltkamp TE, Smolen JS, et al. Range of antinuclear antibodies in "healthy" individuals [see comments]. *Arthritis Rheum* 1997;40:1601–1611.
15. Emlen W, O'Neill L. Clinical significance of antinuclear antibodies: comparison of detection with immunofluorescence and enzyme-linked immunosorbent assays. *Arthritis Rheum* 1997;40:1612–1618.
16. Tan EM. Antinuclear antibodies: diagnostic markers for autoimmune diseases and probes for cell biology. *Adv Immunol* 1989;44:93–151.
17. Fritzler MJ, Tan EM. Antibodies to histones in drug-induced and idiopathic lupus erythematosus. *J Clin Invest* 1978;62:560–567.
18. Rubin RL, Joslin FG, Tan EM. Specificity of anti-histone antibodies in systemic lupus erythematosus. *Arthritis Rheum* 1982;25:779–782.
19. Reeves WH, Chaudhary N, Salerno A, et al. Lamin B autoantibodies in sera of certain patients with systemic lupus erythematosus. *J Exp Med* 1987;165:750–762.
20. Dagenais A, Bibor-Hardy V, Senecal JL. A novel autoantibody causing a peripheral fluorescent antinuclear antibody pattern is

specific for nuclear pore complexes. *Arthritis Rheum* 1988;31: 1322–1327.

21. Courvalin JC, Lassoued K, Bartnik E, et al. The 210-kD nuclear envelope polypeptide recognized by human autoantibodies in primary biliary cirrhosis is the major glycoprotein of the nuclear pore. *J Clin Invest* 1990;86:279–285.
22. Nickowitz RE, Worman HJ. Autoantibodies from patients with primary biliary cirrhosis recognize a restricted region within the cytoplasmic tail of nuclear pore membrane glycoprotein Gp210. *J Exp Med* 1993;178:2237–2242.
23. Lassoued K, Guilly MN, Danon F, et al. Antinuclear autoantibodies specific for lamins. Characterization and clinical significance. *Ann Intern Med* 1988;108:829–833.
24. Friou GJ. Antinuclear antibodies: Diagnostic significance and methods. *Arthritis Rheum* 1967;10:151–159.
25. Tan EM, Kunkel HG. Characteristics of a soluble nuclear antigen precipitating with sera of patients with systemic lupus erythematosus. *J Immunol* 1966;96:464–471.
26. Williamson GG, Pennebaker J, Boyle JA. Clinical characteristics of patients with rheumatic disorders who possess antibodies against ribonucleoprotein particles. *Arthritis Rheum* 1983;26: 509–515.
27. Maddison PJ, Isenberg DA, Goulding NJ, et al. Anti La(SSB) identifies a distinctive subgroup of systemic lupus erythematosus. *Br J Rheumatol* 1988;27:27–31.
28. Tsokos GC, Pillemer SR, Klippel JH. Rheumatic disease syndromes associated with antibodies to the Ro (SS-A) ribonuclear protein. *Semin Arthritis Rheum* 1987;16:237–244.
29. Senecal JL, Oliver JM, Rothfield N. Anticytoskeletal autoantibodies in the connective tissue diseases. *Arthritis Rheum* 1985;28:889–898.
30. Senecal JL, Rauch J. Hybridoma lupus autoantibodies can bind major cytoskeletal filaments in the absence of DNA-binding activity. *Arthritis Rheum* 1988;31:864–875.
31. Francoeur AM, Peebles CL, Heckman KJ, et al. Identification of ribosomal protein autoantigens. *J Immunol* 1985;135: 2378–2384.
32. Elkon KB, Parnassa AP, Foster CL. Lupus autoantibodies target ribosomal P proteins. *J Exp Med* 1985;162:459–471.
33. Bonfa E, Golombek SJ, Kaufman LD, et al. Association between lupus psychosis and anti-ribosomal P protein antibodies. *N Engl J Med* 1987;317:265–271.
34. Schneebaum AB, Singleton JD, West SG, et al. Association of psychiatric manifestations with antibodies to ribosomal P proteins in systemic lupus erythematosus. *Am J Med* 1991;90:54–62.
35. Teh LS, Isenberg DA. Antiribosomal P protein antibodies in systemic lupus erythematosus. A reappraisal. *Arthritis Rheum* 1994; 37:307–315.
36. Yoshida S, Akizuki M, Mimori T, et al. The precipitating antibody to an acidic nuclear protein antigen, the Jo- 1, in connective tissue diseases. A marker for a subset of polymyositis with interstitial pulmonary fibrosis. *Arthritis Rheum* 1983;26 604–611.
37. Mathews MB, Reichlin M, Hughes GR, et al. Anti-threonyl-tRNA synthetase, a second myositis-related autoantibody. *J Exp Med* 1984;160:420–434.
38. Bunn CC, Bernstein RM, Mathews MB. Autoantibodies against alanyl-tRNA synthetase and tRNAAla coexist and are associated with myositis. *J Exp Med* 1986;163:1281–1291.
39. Targoff IN, Johnson AE, Miller FW. Antibody to signal recognition particle in polymyositis. *Arthritis Rheum* 1990;33: 1361–1370.
40. Targoff IN, Arnett FC, Berman L, et al. Anti-KJ: a new antibody associated with the syndrome of polymyositis and interstitial lung disease. *J Clin Invest* 1989;84:162–172.
41. Hirakata M, Mimori T, Akizuki M, et al. Autoantibodies to small nuclear and cytoplasmic ribonucleoproteins in Japanese patients with inflammatory muscle disease. *Arthritis Rheum* 1992;35: 449–456.
42. Douvas AS, Achten M, Tan EM. Identification of a nuclear protein (Scl-70) as a unique target of human antinuclear antibodies in scleroderma. *J Biol Chem* 1979;254:10514–10522.
43. Aeschlimann A, Meyer O, Bourgeois P, et al. Anti-Scl-70 antibodies detected by immunoblotting in progressive systemic sclerosis: specificity and clinical correlations. *Ann Rheum Dis* 1989; 48:992–997.
44. Weiner ES, Earnshaw WC, Senecal JL, et al. Clinical associations of anticentromere antibodies and antibodies to topoisomerase I. A study of 355 patients [see comments]. *Arthritis Rheum* 1988; 31:378–385.
45. Mimori T, Akizuki M, Yamagata H, et al. Characterization of a high molecular weight acidic nuclear protein recognized by autoantibodies in sera from patients with polymyositis- scleroderma overlap. *J Clin Invest* 1981;68:611–620.
46. Francoeur AM, Peebles CL, Gompper PT, et al. Identification of Ki (Ku, p70/p80) autoantigens and analysis of anti-Ki autoantibody reactivity. *J Immunol* 1986;136:1648–1653.
47. Reeves WH. Use of monoclonal antibodies for the characterization of novel DNA-binding proteins recognized by human autoimmune sera. *J Exp Med* 1985;161:18–39.
48. Mimori T, Hardin JA, Steitz JA. Characterization of the DNA-binding protein antigen Ku recognized by autoantibodies from patients with rheumatic disorders. *J Biol Chem* 1986;261: 2274–2278.
49. Yaneva M, Arnett FC. Antibodies against Ku protein in sera from patients with autoimmune diseases. *Clin Exp Immunol* 1989;76: 366–372.
50. Tojo T, Kaburaki J, Hayakawa M, et al. Precipitating antibody to a soluble nuclear antigen "Ki" with specificity for systemic lupus erythematosus. *Ryumachi* 1981;21:129–140.
51. Harmon CP, Peebles C, Tan EM. SL—a new precipitating system. *Arthritis Rheum* 1981;24:S122.
52. Bernstein RM, Hobbs RN, Lea DJ, et al. Patterns of antihistone antibody specificity in systemic rheumatic disease. I Systemic lupus erythematosus, mixed connective tissue disease, primary sicca syndrome, and rheumatoid arthritis with vasculitis. *Arthritis Rheum* 1985;28:285–293.
53. Yamanaka K, Takasaki Y, Nishida Y, et al. Detection and quantification of anti-Ki antibodies by enzyme-linked immunosorbent assay using recombinant Ki antigen. *Arthritis Rheum* 1992; 35:667–671.
54. Sakamoto M, Takasaki Y, Yamanaka K, et al. Purification and characterization of Ki antigen and detection of anti- Ki antibody by enzyme-linked immunosorbent assay in patients with systemic lupus erythematosus. *Arthritis Rheum* 1989;32: 1554–1562.
55. Miyachi K, Fritzler MJ, Tan EM. Autoantibody to a nuclear antigen in proliferating cells. *J Immunol* 1978;121:2228–2234.
56. Takasaki Y, Deng JS, Tan EM. A nuclear antigen associated with cell proliferation and blast transformation. *J Exp Med* 1981; 154:1899–1909.
57. Hassfeld W, Steiner G, Hartmuth K, et al. Demonstration of a new antinuclear antibody (anti-RA33) that is highly specific for rheumatoid arthritis. *Arthritis Rheum* 1989;32:1515–1520.
58. Steiner G, Hartmuth K, Skriner K, et al. Purification and partial sequencing of the nuclear autoantigen RA33 shows that it is indistinguishable from the A2 protein of the heterogeneous nuclear ribonucleoprotein complex. *J Clin Invest* 1992;90: 1061–1066.
59. Isenberg DA, Steiner G, Smolen JS. Clinical utility and serological connections of anti-RA33 antibodies in systemic lupus erythematosus [see comments]. *J Rheumatol* 1994;21:1260–1263.

60. Pollak VE. Antinuclear antibodies in families of patients with systemic lupus erythematosus. *N Engl J Med* 1964;271:165–171.
61. Miles S, Isenberg D. A review of serological abnormalities in relatives of SLE patients. *Lupus* 1993;2:145–150.
62. Hooper B, Whittingham S, Mathews JD, et al. Autoimmunity in a rural community. *Clin Exp Immunol* 1972;12:79–87.
63. Shoenfeld Y, Isenberg D. *The mosaic of autoimmunity (the factors associated with autoimmune disease)*. Amsterdam: Elsevier, 1989.
64. Smeenk R, Westgeest T, Swaak T. Antinuclear antibody determination: the present state of diagnostic and clinical relevance. *Scand J Rheumatol Suppl* 1985;56:78–92.
65. Juby A, Johnston C, Davis P. Specificity, sensitivity and diagnostic predictive value of selected laboratory generated autoantibody profiles in patients with connective tissue diseases. *J Rheumatol* 1991;18:354–358.
66. Thompson D, Juby A, Davis P. The clinical significance of autoantibody profiles in patients with systemic lupus erythematosus. *Lupus* 1993;2:15–19.
67. Burlingame RW, Rubin RL. Drug-induced anti-histone autoantibodies display two patterns of reactivity with substructures of chromatin. *J Clin Invest* 1991;88:680–690.
68. Rubin RL, Bell SA, Burlingame RW. Autoantibodies associated with lupus induced by diverse drugs target a similar epitope in the (H2A-H2B)-DNA complex. *J Clin Invest* 1992;90:165–173.
69. Bray VJ, West SG, Schultz KT, et al. Antihistone antibody profile in sulfasalazine induced lupus. *J Rheumatol* 1994;21:2157–2158.
70. Totoritis MC, Tan EM, McNally EM, et al. Association of antibody to histone complex H2A-H2B with symptomatic procainamide-induced lupus. *N Engl J Med* 1988;318:1431–1436.
71. Hardin JA, Thomas JO. Antibodies to histones in systemic lupus erythematosus: localization of prominent autoantigens on histones H1 and H2B. *Proc Natl Acad Sci USA* 1983;80:7410–7414.
72. Gioud M, Kaci MA, Monier JC. Histone antibodies in systemic lupus erythematosus. A possible diagnostic tool. *Arthritis Rheum* 1982;25:407–413.
73. Morrow J, Nelson JL, Watts R, et al. *Autoimmune rheumatic disease*, 2nd ed. Oxford, England: Oxford University Press, 1999.
74. Hahn BH. Antibodies to DNA. *N Engl J Med* 1998;338: 1359–1368.
75. Avina-Zubieta JA, Galindo-Rodriguez G, Kwan-Yeung L, et al. Clinical evaluation of various selected ELISA kits for the detection of anti-DNA antibodies. *Lupus* 1995;4:370–374.
76. Worrall JG, Snaith ML, Batchelor JR, et al. SLE: a rheumatological view. Analysis of the clinical features, serology and immunogenetics of 100 SLE patients during long-term follow-up. *Q J Med* 1990;74:319–330.
77. Maddison PJ, Provost TT, Reichlin M. Serological findings in patients with "ANA-negative" systemic lupus erythematosus. *Medicine (Baltimore)* 1981;60:87–94.
78. Reichlin M. ANA negative systemic lupus erythematosus sera revisited serologically. *Lupus* 2000;9:116–119.
79. Harmon CE, Deng JS, Peebles CL, et al. The importance of tissue substrate in the SS-A/Ro antigen-antibody system. *Arthritis Rheum* 1984;27:166–173.
80. Martin AL, Reichlin M. Fluctuations of antibody to ribosomal P proteins correlate with appearance and remission of nephritis in SLE. *Lupus* 1996;5:22–29.

21

ANTIBODIES TO DNA

BEVRA HANNAHS HAHN
BETTY P. TSAO

Antibodies to DNA (anti-DNA) are the classic autoantibodies that characterize systemic lupus erythematosus (SLE). High-avidity immunoglobulin G (IgG) antibodies to double-stranded DNA (dsDNA) play a major role in inducing some of the disease manifestations of SLE (especially nephritis), are relatively specific for the disease, and are good markers of disease activity.

THE HISTORY OF ANTIBODIES TO DNA

The lupus erythematosus (LE) cell phenomenon identified the first autoantibody recognized in patients with SLE (1). LE cells result from the action on nuclei of antibodies to DNA protein complexes; the major antigen recognized is a histone DNA complex (2). The altered nuclei are then ingested by phagocytic cells. LE cells can be formed by phagocytosis of apoptotic bodies induced by antinuclear antibodies (ANAs) (3).

The first reports of anti-DNA in the sera of patients with lupus appeared in 1957, discovered in several different laboratories almost simultaneously (2). The clinical importance of circulating anti-DNA was soon recognized. Certain subsets were found to be specific for SLE and correlated with disease activity and nephritis (4,5), and evidence mounted that anti-DNA causes some of the tissue lesions that are characteristic of SLE, especially lupus nephritis. Anti-DNA was eluted from tissue lesions (glomeruli, skin, choroid plexus) of patients and mice with SLE (6–9). In murine models of SLE, disease was accelerated by increasing anti-DNA responses and prevented by blocking them (6,10–14).

The development of monoclonal antibody (mAb) technology permitted expanded studies of DNA antibodies (15), which have provided new information regarding the characteristics of different antibody subsets, the presence of anti-DNA in unstimulated immune repertoires of healthy individuals, and the features of individual antibodies that contribute to their pathogenicity. The central role of these antibodies in the disease process in some patients seems clear.

ANTIBODIES TO DNA AS PART OF THE NORMAL IMMUNE REPERTOIRE: NATURAL AUTOANTIBODIES

There are many different individual antibodies to DNA. They differ in isotype, complement-fixing capabilities, avidity for DNA, antigenic specificities, charge, idiotypes (Ids), and V region sequences (reviewed in refs. 16–20) (Table 21.1). Healthy humans and mice make antibodies to DNA as part of their normal resting or natural immune repertoires (10,21–29). These natural autoantibodies are largely IgM class and react primarily with single-stranded DNA (ssDNA). They have low avidity for DNA and are weakly polyreactive. Analysis of the structure of natural anti-DNA shows that most are IgM encoded by germline DNA, with few or no somatic mutations. However, activation of the resting B-cell repertoire in mice and in humans yields not only IgM low-avidity anti-ssDNA but also some IgM and IgG subsets that bind dsDNA (10,22,23,25–29). Therefore, the ability of human and murine B cells to make antibodies to ssDNA and dsDNA is not forbidden but rather is normal. In fact, IgM and IgG antibodies to ssDNA can be found in many healthy individuals and in many disease states other than SLE that are associated with B-cell activation, such as infections, chronic inflammatory states, and aging. In contrast, IgG antibodies to dsDNA are more abundant in the repertoire of individuals with SLE than in healthy persons, and their presence in serum at high titers is indicative of SLE.

Polyreactivity is characteristic of natural autoantibodies. However, both IgM and IgG mAbs directed against ssDNA, dsDNA, or both can be quite specific for these antigens (30) or have multiple reactivities, including cross-reactivity with polynucleotides, Sm, La, the A and D polypeptides of ribonucleoprotein (snRNP), cytoskeletal proteins, histones, nucleosomes, laminin, phospholipids, the Fc of IgG, cell surface structures (on platelets, lymphocytes, and Raji cells), proteoglycans such as heparan sulfate, myelin, gangliosides, and bacterial polysaccharides and proteins (21,28,30–46). Some of these cross-reactivities probably contribute to the

TABLE 21.1. DIFFERENT SUBSETS OF ANTI-DNA

Probable nonpathogens (the normal repertoire)
IgM
IgG noncomplement fixing
Low avidity for ssDNA
Wide cross-reactivity (low avidity) to
Polynucleotides
Sm/RNP
Cytoskeleton
Histones
Fc of IgG
Laminin
Proteoglycans
Phospholipids
Cell surfaces
Myelin
Gangliosides
Bacteria
Polysaccharides
Phospholipids
Proteins
Probable pathogens (the SLE repertoire)
Complement-fixing Ig isotype (IgG1 and IgG3 in humans, IgG2a and IgG2b in mice, some IgM)
High avidity for dsDNA and ssDNA
Ability to bind directly to glomeruli
Cationic charge
High-avidity binding to
DNA
DNA/histone
Nucleosomes
Laminin
Heparan sulfate
Phospholipids
DNA receptors
C1q
Ability to form immune complexes of correct size and charge to avoid clearance and fix to GBM
Enrichment in certain idiotypes
IdGN2
16/6
32/15
31
O-81
Ability to penetrate cells and fix to cytoplasmic structures or to nucleus

dsDNA, double-stranded DNA; ssDNA, single-stranded DNA; GBM, glomerular basement membrane; Ig, immunoglobulin; RNP, ribonucleoprotein.

pathogenicity of individual antibodies, while others permit anti-DNA to bind undesirable foreign antigens.

Natural autoantibodies to DNA likely serve as a repertoire that, when a foreign antigen arrives, requires minimal somatic mutation to generate high-avidity antibodies against the bacterial or viral invader. Some IgG anti-DNA with pathogenic potential probably derives from a small number of somatic mutations in natural autoantibodies (47–50). Conversely, antibodies to bacteria can be precursors of antibodies to DNA, and these two types of antibody can share similar sequences. A single-point mutation changes the ability of an antibody to bind either pneumococcal phosphocholine or DNA (48), and some anti-DNA can bind bacteria directly, possibly via phospholipids (28, 29,44). Immunization of a lupus patient with pneumococcal vaccine produced antibodies with the capacity to bind different antigens; some were specific for the bacterial phosphocholine, some for DNA, and some bound both antigens (51). Similarly, immunization of mice with bacteria, bacterial DNA, or lipopolysaccharide can induce antibodies to DNA (10,33,34,52,53). Thus, the resting natural autoantibody repertoire serves as a sentinel that is designed to provide quick antibody protection against undesirable invaders of the host. Unfortunately, the natural repertoire also has the capacity to generate pathogenic autoantibodies; the difference between recognizing danger and recognizing self can be a matter of a single amino acid change.

EVIDENCE THAT SOME SUBSETS OF ANTIBODIES TO DNA ARE PATHOGENIC

The preceding discussion reviewed the early evidence that anti-DNA play a role in the pathogenesis of SLE. That evidence includes the following: (a) anti-DNA is located in sites of tissue damage in mice and patients with SLE; (b) large quantities of high-avidity IgG antibodies to dsDNA in the serum are strongly associated with active lupus nephritis and active clinical disease in humans and mice; (c) DNA administered as immunogen accelerates murine lupus nephritis; and (d) DNA administered as tolerogen delays the appearance of anti-DNA and nephritis in mice with lupus.

More direct evidence has come from experiments in which anti-DNA are administered to normal mice and cause renal dysfunction or frank clinical nephritis. For example, Dang and Harbeck (54) injected polyclonal antibodies from the serum of nephritic New Zealand black/white (NZB/NZW) F1 mice into young mice of the same strain, and they showed that cationic populations of serum anti-DNA lodged in glomeruli and induced nephritis earlier than in controls. Raz et al. (55) perfused rat kidneys with various mAb anti-DNA and showed that some bound directly to glomeruli and caused proteinuria. Tsao et al. (56) implanted B-cell hybridomas secreting mAb IgG anti-DNA into pristane-primed peritoneal cavities of healthy, young BALB/c mice; several mAbs deposited in glomeruli and induced proteinuria and azotemia. Madaio et al. (57) have identified mAb murine anti-DNA that, when transferred to healthy mice, binds to capillary loops of glomeruli and cause proteinuria. Ehrenstein et al. (58) inoculated severe combined immunodeficiency disease (SCID) mice with human mAb anti-DNA from patients with lupus; one mAb bound to glomeruli and induced proteinuria even though histologic damage was not evident. Later, Ravirajan and colleagues (59) showed that one human IgG anti-dsDNA mAb grown as a hybridoma in SCID mice caused proteinuria and granular Ig deposition in renal glomerular capillaries. Finally, Tsao et al. (60) made normal mice transgenic for genes encoding both heavy and light chains of a murine IgG anti-dsDNA mAb. B cells in transgenic mice secreted the mAb, IgG anti-dsDNA appeared in the serum, IgG was deposited in glomeruli, and proteinuria appeared. None of these events occurred in non-transgenic littermates. Other laboratories have made mice transgenic for genes encoding heavy or light chains which, when paired with multiple different endogenous light chains, bind DNA; those mice develop glomerular Ig deposits and proteinuria (61).

Several groups have shown that some mAb anti-DNA bind directly to glomeruli, and they have defined some of the components of glomerular basement membrane with which those mAbs cross-react. Although other antibodies can play a role in inducing the nephritis of SLE, certain subsets of anti-DNA clearly induce nephritis and can be classified as pathogens.

PATHOGENIC ANTI-DNA

It is generally accepted that antibodies to DNA that can fix to tissue (glomeruli, skin, blood vessels, erythrocyte membranes, platelet membranes, endothelial cells, etc.) are likely to cause damage. There are many mechanisms by which this tissue fixation occurs. If antibody-antigen interactions occur in the tissue and complement is activated, tissue damage results. Mechanisms for the tissue injury are as follows: (a) Antigens and antibodies can form circulating immune complexes of the correct size and charge to be trapped in basement membranes of glomeruli, skin, and blood vessels where they activate complement; (b) Antibodies to DNA can bind directly to DNA or DNA/histone/nucleosome complexes planted in target tissues, following which complement is activated; (c) Cationic subsets of anti-dsDNA can bind to polyanions in the proteoglycans of basement membranes on the basis of charge, again creating immune complexes *in situ*; (d) Antibodies to DNA, or antibodies complexed to DNA/histone, can bind to non-DNA antigens that are present in basement membranes; (e) Some anti-DNA binds to living cells, mediates antibody-dependent cell-mediated toxicity (ADCC), or enters cells and binds to cytoplasm or nuclei, altering cell functions; (f) Some antibodies to DNA have enzyme activities; (g) Some anti-DNA may induce apoptosis of target tissue with creation of apoptotic bodies containing nucleosomal and snRNP antigens, further driving autoantibody production and immune complex formation; and (h) DNA-reactive T and B lymphocytes participate directly in tissue damage.

These various abilities are related to the structure of each mAb, and the ability to bind DNA may be only a marker for other reactivities that account for the physiologic effects of a given mAb. More than one or the mechanisms listed in the preceding paragraph probably participate in inducing disease.

IMPORTANCE OF ISOTYPE, COMPLEMENT-FIXING ABILITY, AVIDITY FOR DNA, AND ABILITY TO FORM IMMUNE COMPLEXES

Several investigators have shown that subsets of anti-DNA that are associated with active disease and with nephritis (in both humans and mice) are predominantly of the IgG isotypes, which fix complement well (21,54). These are IgG2a and IgG2b in mice, and IgG1 and IgG3 in humans. Such antibodies usually bind both dsDNA and ssDNA; only a small proportion binds dsDNA alone.

Studies of polyclonal anti-DNA eluted from glomeruli of humans or mice with nephritis showed that glomerular populations of Ig are enriched in Ig with high avidity for DNA compared to anti-DNA in sera and urine (8,9,62). However, studies of mAb anti-DNA have shown less relationship between avidity for DNA and the ability of a transferred mAb to cause glomerulonephritis in normal mice (63,64). In fact, mutations introduced in VH regions of mAb that changed avidity for DNA did not correlate with changes in pathogenicity or ability to bind glomeruli *in vitro*. It is possible that avidity for cross-reacting antigens is more important than avidity for DNA in determining pathogenicity or that high avidity offers a mAb some pathogenic advantage, but this property alone may not be sufficient to induce disease.

The ability of anti-DNA to form immune complexes of the correct intermediate size favors the ability of that antibody to be pathogenic. Large antigen/antibody complexes are engulfed by the phagocytic system and removed; small complexes are excreted in the urine, so they do not cause disease. In addition to size, conformation of the complex, overall charge and charge of individual components of the complex, and ability to activate complement after being trapped in tissues are all important in pathogenicity. These properties are discussed in detail in Chapter 12.

THE IMPORTANCE OF CHARGE

Many regions of the glomerular basement membrane are polyanionic. Therefore, antigens, antibodies, or immune complexes with cationic charges can bind to glomerular basement membrane via charge (21,65–68). If a cationic anti-DNA is trapped by this mechanism and DNA is available, then an immune complex forms in the glomerular basement membrane, complement is activated, and damage occurs. One group has reported that one antibody with a cationic charge in an immune complex is sufficient to permit trapping in the glomerular basement membrane (68). Several investigators have reported enrichment of cationic anti-DNA populations in IgG of glomerular eluates from mice with lupus nephritis (21,54,65,66), although one group disagrees (69). A study of Japanese patients with lupus nephritis showed that cationic clonotypes of anti-DNA (pI 7.0 to 8.5) were found in glomeruli but not in circulating immune complexes (70). Studies of the ability of mAb anti-DNA to induce nephritis in mice have shown that some mAb with neutral pI (7.0 to 7.5) as well as mAb with cationic pI (7.5 to 8.5) can induce nephritis in normal mice (38,56). As with high avidity, the presence of cationic charge on a particular anti-DNA probably confers a pathogenic advantage, but some antibodies without cationic charge are perfectly capable of causing disease. Thus, predicting whether a particular mAb anti-DNA is a pathogen or not is difficult and depends on multiple features of that antibody.

THE IMPORTANCE OF IDIOTYPES

The idiotypic characteristics of anti-DNA also may contribute to pathogenicity (21,66,70–76). Idiotypes are antigenic sequences in the V regions of antibodies; they induce B- and T-cell antiidiotypic responses that are important in regulating antibody production.

Idiotypes and idiotypic networks are reviewed elsewhere in this volume. Public idiotypes that characterize many antibodies to DNA have been identified in both murine and human lupus. Certain idiotypes have been found in tissue lesions (IdGN2, 16/6, 32/15, 3I, 0-81) of patients with lupus (21,66,70–76). One human public idiotype or antiidiotype (the 16/6 system), when injected into certain strains of normal mice, can activate an idiotype-antiidiotype network. This results in production of multiple idiotype-positive autoantibodies (including anti-DNA), and the mice develop nephritis (77,78). In addition, experiments in murine models of SLE have shown that anti-DNA and nephritis can be suppressed by administration of antiidiotypes (79,80). Therefore, pathogenic anti-DNA subsets are enriched in certain idiotypic markers, and those idiotypes can be targets of regulation that permit the abnormal upregulation of pathogenic subsets of anti-DNA. One study showed that in patients with lupus nephritis, anti-DNA and antiidiotypes leak into the urine (62). The highest avidity anti-DNA and anti-Id were found in glomerular eluates, moderate avidity anti-DNA and anti-Id in serum, and low-avidity anti-DNA and anti-Id in urine. Thus, anti-DNA and anti-Ids directed against it displayed similar avidities and locations.

THE IMPORTANCE OF CROSS-REACTIVITY

The ability of anti-DNA to cause disease may result from cross-reactivity with structural components of glomeruli or other target tissue rather than (or in addition to) the binding of DNA planted in tissue or passive entrapment of DNA–anti-DNA complexes. For example, several investigators have shown that various mAb anti-DNAs that persist in glomeruli after transfer and cause renal dysfunction can bind laminin and proteoglycans such as heparan sulfate (either alone or complexed with antigen) (36,37,42,43,81,82).

Subsets of anti-DNA that bind DNA/histone complexes [including nucleosomes (NUCs)] may be particularly enriched in pathogens (38,43,46,82–85). Histones or NUCs are trapped in glomerular basement membrane, and anti-DNA can fix to those structures via planted histones. Some mAb anti-DNAs can bind to heparan sulfate in glomerular basement membrane only after they bind histone; thus, a complex of anti-DNA/DNA histone is required for pathogenesis (38). A recent study shows that approximately 70% of patients with SLE have antibodies to nucleosomes, and that IgG3 subclass of those antibodies correlates with disease activity and nephritis (86). In contrast, levels of nucleosomes are elevated in sera of patients with SLE but do not correlate with disease activity (87–89).

The source of DNA/histone that is planted in glomeruli might be NUC released by apoptotic cells during active SLE. NUC-size DNA is found in the circulation of such patients (86–89). Several investigators have shown that antibodies to NUC appear early in murine lupus; they suggest that NUCs are the antigens that induce antibodies that later mature/mutate to anti-dsDNA (83,84).

To study this further, an *in vitro* method was developed to estimate the pathogenicity of antibodies by incubating polyclonal or mAb Ig with permeabilized rat glomeruli isolated on filters, or with an extract of those glomerular basement membranes in an enzyme-linked immunosorbent assay (ELISA) (85,90–92). This work suggests that some anti-DNAs bind to glomeruli via DNA and/or DNA/histone or NUC combinations fixed to collagen type IV in glomerular basement membrane. In addition, several non–DNA-binding antibody populations can play a major role in the nephritis of SLE. In this regard, many investigators have reported that antibodies to the following antigens can be associated with nephritis in human and murine lupus: ssDNA, laminin, heparan sulfate, Ro (SSA), Sm/RNP, RNA, RNA polymerase I, gp70 (mice only), C1q, and ribosomes (36,81,92–98).

One laboratory has described a new type of antibody to DNA that binds DNA lining the cell membrane of cultured B lymphocytes: that DNA is different from nuclear DNA substrates used to detect and describe anti-dsDNA and anti-ssDNA (99). Its importance in biology remains to be seen.

THE POTENTIAL IMPORTANCE OF ANTIBODIES PENETRATING INTO LIVING CELLS

Several investigators have reported that some anti-DNA (including polyclonal populations isolated from the serum of patients or mAb from mice with SLE) can bind to the surface of living cells, enter those cells, and bind nuclear or cytoplasmic structures (104–111). There are probably at least three types of such anti-DNA subsets (109). One binds to cell surfaces and can mediate complement-induced cytotoxicity; the second penetrates cells and binds to cytoplasmic antigens; the third penetrates cells and binds to nuclei. In our library of murine mAb IgG anti-DNA, some pathogenic mAb (defined as causing nephritis in normal mice on transfer) have these properties, and others do not. F(ab)2 fragments of these anti-DNA also bind and enter cells, so they are not entering via Fc receptors. DNase treatment of cells and antibodies does not impair their ability to access the interior of cells, so DNA as a receptor is not a likely entry point. In fact, there are probably multiple receptors by which anti-dsDNA enters cells, one of which is brush-border myosin I (110). Anti-DNA entering via myosin receptors enters the cytoplasm, interacts with DNase-1, and inhibits endonuclease activity, before moving to the nucleus and attenuating apoptosis. The antibodies can then recycle back to the cell surface. After cell entry, several other abnormalities can occur, including cell activation in an abnormal pattern (111), and decrease of protein synthesis (109).

POTENTIAL ENZYME ACTIVITIES OF ANTI-DNA

Once anti-DNA enters living cells and interacts with intracellular substrates, it is also possible that some subsets act as catalysts for enzymes that degrade DNA via hydroxyl radicals (112,113).

All of these interactions between antibodies to dsDNA and living cells are likely to profoundly alter cell functions and to present altered antigens from damaged cells to the immune system to promote autoantibody expansion and T- and B-cell determinant spreading so that additional autoantigens are recognized.

POTENTIAL ROLE OF ANTIBODIES TO DNA PRODUCED BY RESPONSES TO APOPTOTIC CELLS

Increases in numbers of apoptotic cells can induce ANA, anticardiolipin, and anti-ssDNA in normal mice, with development of glomerular Ig deposits (114,115). Antibodies to DNA and to nucleosomes bind NUC released from hybridoma cells undergoing apoptosis. Since the generation of apoptotic cells in both lymphocytes and neutrophils is increased in patients with SLE, more antibodies to DNA and nucleosomes are induced (116,117). In addition, clearance of apoptotic cells is abnormally slow in patients with SLE, permitting persistence of these surface autoantigens (118). Therefore, we have the scenario in which damage to cells caused by lupus autoantibodies drives those cells into apoptosis, and the apoptotic state itself promotes production of more harmful antibodies to DNA, to cardiolipin and to snRNP, thus creating a vicious circle. Furthermore, the combination of nucleosome and IgG antinucleosome acts on normal peripheral blood mononuclear cells (PBMCs) *in vitro* to induce the release of interferon-α (IFN-α) (119). (This activity was associated more closely with anti-RNP than with anti-DNA.) Since IFN-α is immunostimulatory, it may play an additional role in keeping disease activated. Normal human PBMCs cultured with polyclonal or monoclonal antibodies to DNA from patients with active SLE showed diminished proliferation and enhanced secretion of interleukin-1β (IL-1β), IL-8, TNF-α, and IL-10 (120). Polyclonal IgG anti-DNA from SLE patients incubated *in vitro* with human umbilical vein endothelial cells caused increased expression of intercellular adhesion molecule-1 (ICAM-1) and vascular cell adhesion molecule-1 (VCAM-1) on those cells (121), which could be a mechanism for vascular damage. This is more evidence that additional activities of anti-DNA include influencing tissue damage by altering the release of proinflammatory cytokines or of molecules that mediate adhesion of potentially harmful phagocytic cells.

DIRECT ROLES OF T AND B LYMPHOCYTES IN CELL DAMAGE

Although we traditionally think of the role of B cells in lupus as a source of pathogenic autoantibodies, and those antibodies as being necessary for disease, B cells play an additional role. In recent experiments, Medical Research Laboratory (MRL)/Fas lymphoproliferative (*lpr*) mice expressing a mutant surface Ig but unable to secrete Ig still developed nephritis. The disease was characterized by cellular infiltration within the kidney, indicating that functional B cells produce adverse local effects, either by contributing directly to damage or by presenting peptide antigens that activate cytotoxic T cells (122).

T lymphocytes in the setting of lupus lesions also play a role beyond providing help for local autoantibody production. Multiple T cells and macrophages infiltrate the kidneys of patients and mice with lupus nephritis (123). Chemotactic factors (MCP-1) and adhesion molecules (ICAM-1) facilitate recruitment of these cells into areas of inflammation. Once there, the cells induce increased expression of major histocompatibility complex (MCH) class II and CD40L on renal tubular epithelial cells, coupled with upregulation of CD40L and IL-2R on infiltrating T cells. Doubtless these properties of infiltrating T cells contribute to the renal damage of SLE.

THE STRUCTURE OF ANTI-DNA

The structures of many human and murine mAbs to DNA have been determined (38,47–50,56,63,64,124–149) and

TABLE 21.2. STRUCTURE OF ANTI-DNA

Genes encoding immunoglobulin
- Germline DNA—no unique information
- Rearrangement of germline
  - No unique rearrangements
  - Many different VH, D, JH, VL, and JL can be used
  - Enriched in VH J558 in mice, VH3 in humans
- Somatic mutations—can be none, a few, or many

Amino acid sequences in heavy and light chains
- CDR of heavy and light chains are enriched in Arg, Asp, and Tyr
- Ser-Tyr found frequently in CDR1 of VH
- Tyr-Tyr-Gly-Gly-Ser-Tyr found frequently in CDR3 of VH

Region gene segments: VH, variable heavy; D, diversity; JH, joining heavy; VL, variable light; JL, joining light.

reviewed (16,17,19,20,59,149) (Table 21.2). As reviewed elsewhere in this volume, the heavy chains of Igs are encoded by rearrangements of variable (VH) region gene segments with diversity (D) and joining (JH) segments that combine with constant (CH) regions for the Ig isotype. Light chains are formed by rearrangements of VL and JL with C-κ or C-λ. Joining of the heavy and light chains forms an intact Ig molecule. Diversity in antibody binding is generated by (a) variations of the information contained in germline DNA within different individuals; (b) different rearrangements of V, D, and J segments for heavy chains, and of V and J segments for light chains; (c) addition of nucleic acids by terminal deoxyribonucleotidyl transferase (TdT) at the junctions between variable and constant regions in heavy or light chains; (d) junctional insertion of inverted mono- or dinucleotides that are independent of TdT, and (e) somatic mutations of single nucleic acids in rearranged heavy and light chains. In general, antigen-driven antibody responses undergo increasing numbers of somatic mutations with each cell division, and such mutations increase the affinity of the antibody for the stimulating antigen.

In the mAb anti-DNA studied to date, no unique germline DNA encoding Ig is used to make anti-DNA. Most DNA-binding mAbs use rearrangements of germline DNA that are similar to those used in antibodies to foreign antigens, especially bacteria (16,17,48,59,124,125,127–129, 141,145). Some mAb anti-DNAs are constructed from germline rearrangements with no or few mutations (138, 142), but most IgG anti-dsDNA contain somatic mutations (47,48,56,81,124,126–136,146,147,150–153). There is one example of a murine MAb directed against phosphocholine (i.e., a dominant response in BALB/c mice to immunization with pneumococcal polysaccharide) that underwent a productive single-point mutation that eradicated the ability to bind phosphocholine but introduced the ability to bind DNA (124,129). It seems likely that the resting IgM anti-DNA repertoire can be used to introduce somatic mutations that drive the immune response toward high-avidity IgG antibacterial or anti-DNA antibodies, and that high-avidity anti-DNA can arise from the mutation of antibacterial antibodies. These observations suggest that pathogenic IgG high-avidity anti-dsDNA can arise from stimulation with foreign antigens, such as bacteria, rather than from antigenic stimulation by mammalian self-DNA. This possibility is supported by the observation that immunization with phosphocholine coupled to protein carrier elicited anti-dsDNA antibodies in a normal mouse (145). Humans without SLE were immunized with pneumococcal vaccine (Pneumovax) and developed an antipneumococcal response that was characterized by a public idiotype found in patients with SLE; however, those idiotype-positive antibodies did not bind DNA. In contrast, a lupus patient immunized with pneumococcal vaccine developed B cells that secreted antibodies specific for phosphocholine, for DNA, or cross-reactive with both (51).

Certain structural characteristics are common to many mAb anti-DNAs. Although many different V, D, J heavy-chain regions and many different light chains can be used to construct anti-DNA, there is repeated use of certain VH and CDR3 regions (e.g., VH J558 in NZB/NZW and MRL/*lpr* mice, VH3 in human MAb anti-DNA) (130,131, 144,146,147,151,154). In fact, studies in MRL/*lpr* and NZB/NZW F1 lupus-prone mice suggest that each mouse makes autoantibodies from a small number of clonal B cells, which are then expanded and mutated to form anti-DNA (16,130,131,155).

To summarize, there is limited clonality of anti-DNA, but it is not stringent. Fifteen to 20 heavy-chain regions encode most anti-DNA. The CDR regions of heavy and light chains in anti-DNA often are enriched in arginine, asparagine, and tyrosine (130,131,137,139,155). These amino acids can form hydrogen bonds with the phosphate backbone of DNA. Studies of computer models and crystals of DNA/anti-DNA complexes have suggested that Arg, Asp, or Tyr project from CDR regions of the Ig molecule into the antigen-binding groove, where they can contribute to high-avidity binding of DNA (59,156).

Although not an absolute requirement, several laboratories have noted that the D regions of anti-DNA antibodies are read in an unusual frame. Certain amino acid motifs occur commonly in mAb anti-DNAs, such as Ser-Tyr in CDR1 of VH and other sequences in the D region of the heavy chain. Our observation (38) that the CDR regions of VH in pathogenic anti-DNA compared with nonpathogens is enriched in arginine, lysine, aspartate, and glutamate residues (i.e., positively and negatively charged amino acids) suggests that charge interactions play a role in pathogenicity, possibly by determining tissue structures with which the mAb can cross-react. Arginine residues in CDR and some framework regions of heavy and light chain are important to DNA binding in some anti-DNA, as shown by analysis of mutants in which R residues have been substituted, resulting in loss of binding or changed avidity for DNA (63,64,157). On the other hand, there are some mAb anti-DNAs that do not have R residues in the positions thought to influence DNA binding. For many mAb anti-DNAs, the heavy chain determines the ability to bind DNA, although only certain light chains in combination with that heavy chain permit the binding to occur (157,158). Most murine and human IgG high-avidity anti-dsDNAs have undergone numerous somatic mutations, suggesting that specific antigens are driving B-cell maturation and secretion (16,17,19,20,51,59,149,159).

In summary, there are no unique germline DNA sequences, heavy- or light-chain rearrangements, or amino acid motifs that are specific for anti-DNA. Many different heavy- and light-chain rearrangements can encode such antibodies. However, certain V region genes are used more frequently than would be expected, and certain amino acids or motifs are commonly found. The structural differences between pathogens and nonpathogens are not yet understood. Anti-DNA can arise spontaneously from germline DNA without antigenic stimulation; most IgG anti-dsDNAs are mutated and probably arise in response to many different antigenic stimuli, both self and foreign.

THE ORIGINS OF ANTI-DNA: GENETIC PREDISPOSITION, ANTIGENIC AND ENVIRONMENTAL TRIGGERS

The ability of an animal or person to make pathogenic, high-titer IgG antibodies to DNA (or DNA/histone) is influenced by genes. Other chapters in this volume detail the genetic predispositions to SLE in humans and in mice; only the summaries will be given here, as they pertain to anti-DNA. In general, the large genome studies of human SLE have not identified regions of genomic DNA that increase risk for anti-DNA. An exception to this is the work of Tsao and colleagues (160), which showed positive correlation between IgG antibodies to nucleosomes and the 1q41 region on human chromosome 1, a region that also contains a gene or genes that predispose to SLE. Several investigators have shown associations between human leukocyte antigen (HLA) molecules and anti-DNA in patients with SLE, specifically with HLA-DR3 (161), DR2 (162,163), and DR7 (164). Their respective linked HLA-DQ alleles may also responsible for the observed associations.

Studies in murine lupus have identified several candidate genes or loci associated with anti-DNA or antichromatin that occur on several different genes (100,165–171).

In mice with a New Zealand background, some of the ability to make anti-DNA depends on genes in the MHC class II region, with combinations such as H-2d/z being particularly susceptible. On chromosome 1, a gene region designated Sle1 contains a gene or genes that allow a mouse to break tolerance to nucleosome (100,168). That seems to be a critical gene; alone it cannot result in clinical immune nephritis, but when combined in a normal mouse with another predisposing gene, such as a gene related to T-cell hyperactivity (*Sle3*) or an autoimmunity accelerating gene on the Y chromosome of another lupus mouse model (BXSB), *Yaa*, clinical nephritis occurs in the majority of mice (170,171). In contrast, *Sle3* plus *Yaa* do not produce clinical nephritis. In several combinations, *Sle1* has been essential although not sufficient to induce clinical disease. As expected, the lupus-enhancing capacity of *Sle1* is opposed by a gene region from an unaffected mouse (NZW), designated *Slels*, located in or near the MHC region (171). The lesson from all of this exciting work is that antibodies to nucleosome and DNA probably require more than one gene for full expression that results in full-blown expression of the clinical disease.

POTENTIAL ENVIRONMENTAL CAUSES OF ABILITY TO MAKE ANTIBODIES TO DNA

In addition, to the genetic component, it is likely that certain environmental stimuli permit full expression of the gene, probably by initiating an immune reaction that then leads to formation of highly mutated and potentially pathogenic anti-nucleosome or anti-DNA. The possible antigens that might elicit IgG anti-dsDNA pathogenic antibodies are listed in Table 21.3. Possibilities include the following: (a) anti-DNA is induced by DNA of bacteria or viruses and cross-reacts with self-DNA; (b) self-DNA becomes altered (e.g., by viral infection) and therefore becomes immunogenic; (c) an antigen containing DNA plus protein is the initial immunogen, and some of the resultant reactivity happens to be directed toward naked DNA; (d) the initial immunogen is a peptide

TABLE 21.3. POSSIBLE ANTIGENS INDUCING ANTI-DNA

- Nucleosomes
  - May be made available in surface blebs of lymphocytes, neutrophils, or glomerular cells undergoing apoptosis; also released from apoptotic, but not necrotic, cells; there is some evidence that nucleosomal DNA is the initial DNA-containing antigen recognized by the immune system
- DNA/histone complexes, or DNA complexed with other proteins
- Altered self-DNA (e.g., enriched in CpG motifs)
- Bacterial DNA
- Viral DNA
- Bacterial polysaccharides
- Phospholipids
  - May be made available on surfaces of cells undergoing apoptosis, or in bacteria
- Other autoantigens (e.g., Sm, La)
  - B- and T-lymphocyte responses initially specific for immunodominant proteins in these Ags undergo degeneration and spreading so that the cell receptors recognize additional self-antigens, such as DNA
- Protective immune responses to external antigens (e.g., antibodies to phosphocholine of pneumococcus also bind DNA)
- Antibodies to external antigens with anti-Ids that bind DNA
  - Antibody to virus or bacteria may raise an antiidiotypic antibody that recognizes DNA; thus, protective response to an external antigen also generates autoreactive cells

from another self-antigen, and the immune response spreads to produce multiple autoantibodies, including anti-DNA; and (e) the initial immunogen is not self but has a conformation similar to that found in DNA, and the resultant anti-DNA recognizes a similar conformation.

One thinks first of infectious agents, given the examples of single mutations in anti-DNA or in antiphosphochloline antibodies resulting in an antibody of the opposite specificity. It is likely that several bacteria can participate. Although initial anti-DNA after bacterial immunization is anti-ssDNA, only a few mutations, or recombinations between H and L chains, are required to develop anti-dsDNA (53). Some anti-DNA cross-react with *Klebsiella* polysaccharides (28), with *Escherichia coli* galactosidase (41), and with phospholipids of streptococci and staphylococci (40). Further, the structure of many mAb anti-DNA molecules is similar to that of antibacterial antibodies (124,129,140,141,145). Therefore, it is possible that ordinary bacteria are the antigens that induce anti-DNA responses in humans. In contrast, MRL/*lpr* mice raised in a germ-free environment were not protected from disease, although if they were fed an ultrafiltered antigen-free diet their disease was less (172). It is probably useful to think of certain bacteria as capable of flaring if not inducing SLE, and as one of several environmental factors that can have that effect.

There has been recent renewed interest in viruses as etiologic agents of SLE and/or its autoantibodies, including anti-DNA. An interesting observation in children with SLE showed that the chance of the patients being infected with Epstein-Barr virus (EBV) is about 50-fold higher than the chance in matched controls of children without lupus attending the same clinics (173). Since this virus is so ubiquitous among adults, and no vaccines are currently available, it would be particularly prudent to pursue these initial data. Another virus that might be involved is polyomavirus, which has been carefully studied in SLE by one group (174–176). Polyoma virus has a transcription factor T antigen that as immunogen in mice induced antibodies to DNA [and to T antigen, TATA-binding protein, and the 3′,5′-cyclic adenosine monophosphate (cAMP) response element binding protein (CREB)]. The same investigators demonstrated frequent activation of polyoma virus in patients with SLE, as well as the same panel of autoantibodies. Among sera positive for anti-dsDNA, 60% were positive for T antigen. $CD4^+$ T cells from normal and SLE patients proliferate to T antigen and to T antigen complexed with nucleosomes. These $CD4^+$ T cells could help syngeneic B cells produce anti-DNA and anti–T antigen. The idea is that the polyoma virus reactivates, then presents T antigen to helper T cells, which activate B cells that respond to nucleosome–T antigen complexes, and then make anti-DNA and anti–T antigen. This interesting work awaits confirmation from other laboratories. In another example (148) BK virus administered to rabbits induced antibodies against self eukaryotic DNA if the infection became productive but not if it was contained.

Pristane is another external substance that can induce lupus when injected into genetically susceptible strains (177). BALB/c mice so treated develop IgG anti-DNA and anti-chromatin, as well as IgG anti-nRNP/Sm and -Su antibodies. Immune complex disease develops in glomeruli. Human exposure to pristane is exclusively by the oral route, whereas disease is induced in mice by intraperitoneal injections.

ANTIGENS FROM SELF MOLECULES THAT MAY INDUCE OR SUSTAIN ANTIBODIES TO DNA

As discussed above, there is currently great interest in the probability that many of the autoantigens that induce lupus autoantibodies, including pathogenic subsets, arise from apoptosis of autologous cells, particularly T and B lymphocytes. The surfaces of such cells contain blebs within which lie nucleosomal DNA/histone complexes of the size found in sera of patients with SLE (but not controls). Nucleosomal DNA is widely thought to be the initiating Ag that leads ultimately, as the B cell response matures and mutates, to IgG anti-dsDNA pathogenic antibodies. Apoptotic blebs also contain the snRNP and Ro antigens that stimulate autoantibodies in some patients. In addition, the cell membranes of cells undergoing apoptosis change conformation in a way that permits the antigenic "heads" of phospholipid molecules to flip toward the outside of the membrane, where they can be seen by the immune system. Apoptotic cells administered as immunogens to mice have induced antibodies to DNA, anti-RNP, anti-Ro, and anticardiolipin (114,115). Furthermore, patients with SLE have larger numbers of lymphocytes and neutrophils undergoing apoptosis than do matched healthy or diseased controls, and they have significantly less ability to phagocytose apoptotic bodies (116–118). Genetically engineered normal mice with genes encoding C1q or serum amyloid protein "knocked out" develop SLE-like disease with increased numbers of apoptotic bodies in tissues (101,178,179). Both C1q and SAP are required for normal removal of apoptotic bodies. It is reasonable to conclude that any condition that permits increases in apoptotic cells or allows them to persist longer than normal predisposes to SLE and to the production of antibodies to DNA and to nucleosomes. Peptides from nucleosome-related histones have been defined that activate T-cell help for antinucleosome and anti-DNA production (180).

Another autologous source of antigens that promote development of anti-DNA in individuals predisposed to SLE is the autoantibodies themselves. Several groups (181–187) have shown that certain peptides derived from autoantibodies, presented in MHC class II molecules by B cells or other antigen-presenting cells (APCs), are recognized by helper T cells. Those T cells are activated by the peptides, and in turn activate B cells making Ig containing the peptides. Thus, an antibody to dsDNA provides its own peptides that activate T-cell help for that B cell, resulting in sustained, rather than regulated production of a pathogenic autoantibody. T-cell stimulatory peptides have been demonstrated from the VH and VL areas of antibodies to DNA, from the Sm B/B′ peptides, and from the Ro antigen. The Sm B/B′ contains a highly stimulatory, proline-rich sequence that when used as an immunogen in mice, rabbits, or nonhuman primates can induce T cells, then B-cell responses to that peptide, then to related peptides, then to unrelated peptides on the same molecule, then to unrelated peptides on different molecules, culminating in IgG anti-dsDNA and proteinuria in some animals (188).

IMMUNOREGULATORY ABNORMALITIES THAT PERMIT SUSTAINED PRODUCTION OF PATHOGENIC ANTI-DNA IN SLE

Helper T cells are critical to SLE. They drive the IgM to IgG switch that enhances pathogenesis of autoantibodies, and they sustain autoantibody production and disease. Individuals with SLE have the ability to make pathogenic subsets of anti-DNA and either the ability to continually upregulate antibody production, the inability to downregulate it, or both. These mechanisms are reviewed in detail in Chapter 9. In the NZB × NZW mouse model of SLE, nephritis does not develop until young mice switch their IgM anti-DNA production to IgG anti-DNA (189). A major role of helper T cells in stimulating the Ig class switch has been shown (190), and, in fact, elimination of helper T cells virtually prevents disease in both the NZB × NZW and BXSB models of lupus (191–193). $CD4^+$ and $CD4^-CD8^-$ T cells have been cloned from NZB × SWR F1 mice that can make B cells from that animal secrete cationic (probably pathogenic) IgG anti-dsDNA (194). The T-cell receptors of those clones are enriched in positively and negatively charged amino acids in both T-cell receptor (TCR)-α and TCR-β chains (195,196), and some of the T cells are activated by nucleosomes (197). Pathogenic anti-DNAs react with DNA/histone and are enriched in charged amino acids in regions that contact antigen; many antigens with which they react are highly charged. Thus, charged amino acids in peptides from anti-DNA molecules are likely to be presented to TCRs containing oppositely charged amino acids. In that way, T-cell help is activated for antibodies to DNA. T-cell help is provided by many different types of cells in murine and human SLE. Helper T-cell phenotypes may be $CD4^+CD8^-$, $CD4–CD8^+$, or $CD4^-CD8^-$, and TCR may be α/β or γ/δ. If we understood why these cells are all skewed toward help, without normal regulation, we would be closer to understanding this disease. It is clear that a T cell or B cell initially specific for a single self antigen soon stimulates other T and B cells that greatly broaden the repertoire of reactivity toward self. This happens by two mechanisms: T- and B-cell degeneracy, in which the receptor on one cell can bind many antigens of different sequences; and T- and B-cell spreading, in which increasing numbers of cells with different but related specificities are recruited into an active state. As a result, the autoimmune repertoire can become quite diverse and a given patient can have autoantibodies to many apparently unrelated antigens (198–200).

Immune tolerance is a mechanism that controls autoreactivity in normal individuals. Normally, the ability to make IgG high-affinity anti-dsDNA is tightly downregulated. This results in part from multiple tolerance mechanisms in B- and T-cell compartments (207). Using normal mice that are transgenic for various mAb anti-DNAs, several investigators have shown that B cells expressing these antibodies are subject to all known tolerance mechanisms (201). In other words, B-cell deletion, anergy, and receptor editing are all used to eliminate B cells reacting with self-DNA. In normal mice transgenic for B cells secreting anti-DNA, some B cells are deleted in the bone marrow, those that reach the periphery undergo receptor editing (i.e., transgenic H chain is combined with endogenous L chains) until the B-cell receptor no longer binds self, and that B cell never enters the follicular regions of peripheral lymphoid tissue where it could encounter T-cell help and develop into an IgG anti-DNA–secreting cell. Therefore, it undergoes anergy and eventually dies (202,203). In contrast, if the transgene is introduced into MRL/Fas-*lpr* lupus-prone mice, self-reactive B cells reach the follicular zones of the spleen, T cells enter, and IgG anti-dsDNA is made. Those antibodies may contain H and L chain combinations that bind DNA with high aviditiy, and/or somatic mutations that also increase binding to self (204–206). This is a setting for disease.

Tolerance in T cells may be normal in lupus-prone mice. Deletion, anergy, and cytokine deviation occur in T cells of (NZB × NZW)F1 females (183,208). There is disagreement regarding abnormalities of tolerance in lupus T cells. Data are reviewed in Chapter 9.

Regulatory cells that suppress T-cell/B-cell interactions resulting in antiself antibodies also have been demonstrated in normal mice. In fact, they serve to prevent the appearance of diabetes in the nonobese diabetic (NOD) mouse, and it is only when the regulatory T cells disappear that disease emerges (reviewed in ref. 209). Suppressor cells exist in $CD4^+$ and $CD8^+$ compartments; some express CD25 surface markers and some are memory cells. Experiments have suggested that all mice are predisposed to autoimmunity, which is only held in check by natural, thymic-educated regulatory T cells. For example, when suppressor cells were blocked in BALB/c mice by injection of anti-I-Jd, the animals produced high-affinity anti-dsDNA encoded by germline genes (143). Where are these regulatory T cells in patients with SLE? The authors of Chapters 9 and 10 review their data suggesting that the evolution of regulatory T-cell precursors to effectors requires IL-2, TNF-α, and transforming growth factor-β (TGF-β), the first and last of which are often deficient in SLE patients. Solving the puzzle of the absence of regulatory T cells is an important challenge to lupus investigators.

In summary, B cells are hyperactive in humans and mice with SLE, and they make pathogenic subsets of anti-dsDNA that are infrequent in normal repertoires. T-cell help plays a major role in the upregulation of these undesirable antibody subsets and is stimulated by many autoantigens, including the antibodies themselves. In addition, abnormalities of downregulation are present, including inadequate clearance of immune complexes, defective suppression by regulatory T cells, and ineffective idiotype/antiidiotype networks (210). Each of these abnormalities is discussed in detail in other chapters.

THE ROLE AND NATURE OF DNA AND NUCLEOSOMAL ANTIGENS: STRUCTURE OF DNA

DNA occurs primarily as a B helix in solutions with physiologic tonicity and pH. The structure is shown in Fig. 21.1. Two polydeoxyribose-phosphate backbones spiral around central base pairs of purines and pyrimidines. The backbone is readily available to react with antibodies; the bases are contained in major and minor grooves. The binding sites of an anti-dsDNA can straddle the backbone and interact with bases in those grooves.

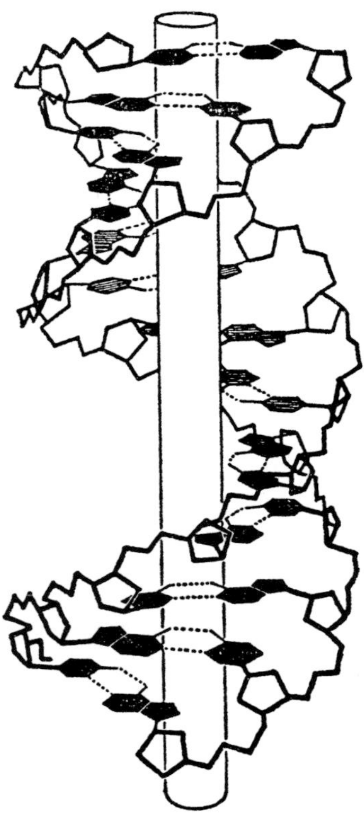

FIGURE 21.1. The DNA molecule in B helix conformation. Purine and pyrimidine bases in the center of the helix are *solid black*. Pentose sugars in backbone are open pentagons. Phosphate groups are along the *heavy black lines* on the outside of the helix. In SLE, anti-DNA may react with nucleosides, oligonucleotides, nucleotide sequences, or the sugar-phosphate backbone. (From Adams ROP, ed. *Davidson's the biochemistry of the nucleic acids*. New York: Academic Press, 1976, with permission.)

The structure of nucleosomes is shown in Chapter 22.

SPECIFICITIES OF ANTI-DNA

Anti-dsDNA can react with base pairs, including dG-dC and dA-dT. Anti-dsDNA can recognize the ribosephosphate backbone alone or particular conformations in dsDNA (28, 158,211–213). Multiple different conformations occur: dsDNA may form twisted, supercoiled, closed circular molecules; relaxed circular forms; left-handed Z-DNA segments; and cruciform structures. These polymorphisms are associated with different base-pair sequences and with the physicochemical characteristics of the environment. It is not known which of these reactivities is associated with the most pathogenic antibodies. However, variation in methylation of DNA, particularly with increased numbers of deoxymethylcytosines, increases the immunogenicity of DNA. GC-rich regions can be nuclease resistant, and these combinations increased immunogenicity. Such a combination is found nucleosomal DNA in apoptotic cells (214). The structure of the CDR3 sites of both heavy and light chains are critical for the binding of an antibody to Z-DNA (158).

When dsDNA is denatured, compact single chains are formed, which can present bases, nucleotide sequences, backbone, short regions of base-paired secondary structures, and short helices. Anti-ssDNA therefore can react with bases, nucleosides, nucleotides, oligonucleotides, and ribosephosphate backbone. Anti-ssDNA react predominantly with individual bases and even better with polynucleotides containing multiples of that base. The largest proportions of anti-ssDNA in sera react with guanosine and thymidine, but others recognize polyA, polyC, polyI, Z-DNA, ssRNA, RNA-DNA hybrids, and poly [adenosine diphosphate (ADP) ribose] (211,212).

Anti-DNA induced by immunization with bases, nucleosides, or oligonucleotides usually is highly specific for the immunogen. In contrast, spontaneous anti-DNAs that arise in individuals with SLE usually are polyspecific and react with multiple oligonucleotides and several forms of DNA. This wide reactivity could result from similar epitopes shared by multiple different molecules (probably conformational) or a single antibody-combining site having multiple contact regions for unrelated epitopes. An example of shared epitopes would be the cross-reactivity of many mAbs for DNA and cardiolipin (44,215). There are shared phosphodiester groups in the ribosephosphate backbone of DNA and in phospholipids.

Bacteria can supply DNA or lipopolysaccharides that induce anti-DNA (33,53,216). Pyun et al. (33) have shown that immunization of normal mice with *E. coli* DNA induces IgM and IgG anti-DNA. Also, mAb anti-DNAs from those mice have structural characteristics similar to those of spontaneous anti-DNA mAb, and some mAbs are capable of binding permealized rat glomeruli and of inducing nephritis in normal mice.

Krieg et al. (217) showed that unmethylated Cytosine phosphyrol Guanine (CpG) motifs in bacterial DNA can directly trigger B cells to proliferate and secrete antibodies. Because these motifs are more abundant in bacterial or viral genomes than in mammalian genomes, this property may confer on vertebrates an advantage to fight off microbial infection. These findings also suggest that the increased levels of hypomethylated CpG in DNA of patients with SLE may play a pathogenic role in inducing a polyclonal B-cell activation. In addition, hypomethylated CpG motifs in T cells promote their activation (218).

Desai et al. (219) showed that mammalian DNA (usually a weak immunogen) becomes strongly antigenic when combined with a highly charged fusion protein. In some studies, antibodies to nucleosomes or chromatin appear first in the anti-DNA repertoire of lupus mice; later antibodies to ssDNA and dsDNA appear (32,83–85). It has been suggested that the initiating antigens for most lupus autoantibodies are DNA and RNA combined with proteins. Nucleosomes, partly denatured DNA/histone complexes, and snRNP particles would be the likely candidates (32,83–85, 89,220). As antibodies mature and mutate, some become specific for various DNA/histone combinations and some for DNA alone. Many experts feel that antibodies to nucleosomes or chromatin core particles are important pathogens and, perhaps, the true anti-DNA response. DNA found in the circulation of patients with SLE is small in size [100 to 150 base pair (bp)], and units of 200 bp and their multiples (87,89,221). DNA of these sizes is usually found in nucleosomes. Cell apoptosis releases DNA of this size; cell necrosis does not. Therefore, in SLE, cell apoptosis may be induced by immunologic abnormalities, and the nucleosomes released from those cells provide the antigenic stimulus that results in somatically mutated, high-affinity IgG anti-DNA antibodies.

With regard to the initiating antigen being a peptide from a non–DNA-containing self antigen, Dang et al. (222) induced autoantibodies by immunizing normal animals with peptides from Ig molecules, and James et al. (223) injected rabbits with B/B′ peptides from the Sm antigen. Although the antibody responses were initially directed against immunodominant B/B′ peptides, the response spread to include other peptides as the rabbits aged and eventually expanded to include antinuclear and anti-DNA antibodies. Thus, peptides from non–DNA-containing self molecules can activate B and T cells into a degenerative phase when their antigen receptors recognize seemingly unrelated antigens. In fact, some MRL/Fas-*lpr* antibodies to Sm and to La also bind DNA (31).

The last hypothesis—that anti-DNA recognizes a conformation shared with the original, unknown immunogen—has been used to explain the ability of an anti-DNA to recognize molecules with no known structural similarity to DNA (224). This hypothesis will require progress in studies of three-dimensional conformations for verification. To date, one anti-ssDNA has been crystallized (156), but there are no reports of crystals containing anti-dsDNA with antigen.

DNA may be different in individuals with SLE from that in normal individuals. The quantities of DNA released by cultured lymphocytes from humans and mice with SLE are significantly greater than the quantities released by normal cells (225–227). The circulating DNA in patients with SLE also is richer in guanosine and cytosine than DNA from healthy controls (221), and such a change could increase the immunogenicity and ability to form Z-DNA.

DEGRADATION OF DNA

The degradation of DNA may be slower than normal in individuals with lupus, because their nucleases may be impaired. Based on studies in normal mice (227), DNA probably is cleared in two phases. First, large pieces of DNA (more than 15 bp) rapidly bind to various organs (primarily the liver for ssDNA and other soft tissues for dsDNA). Second, DNA is degraded in the circulation and in tissue by nucleases. ssDNA is cleared more rapidly than dsDNA (20 minutes vs. 40 minutes, respectively); the second, digestion phase of clearance is similar for both.

Several conditions may prolong the half-life of DNA. Hepatic uptake of DNA is saturable with excess DNA or excess immune complexes, which results in a prolonged half-life. If DNA is present in small size, organ binding is impaired. In patients with active disease, excess quantities of circulating DNA and of small immune complexes have been detected; therefore, clearance of antigenic DNA is probably impaired (227).

Another factor that allows DNA to persist in patients with SLE is its existence as protected fragments (228). Small DNA fragments (30 to 40 bp), are bound by the two arms of IgG anti-DNA and thus protected from both organ binding and the action of nucleases.

DNA may serve as a target antigen beyond its participation in immune complexes. There is a DNA receptor on a number of cells, including glomeruli (229,230), and DNA bound into that receptor might well be a target of pathogenic anti-DNA. In addition, the ability of DNA or DNA/histone to be implanted in tissues, particularly collagen, laminin, and heparan sulfate in basement membranes, may target antibodies to organs that are damaged in patients with SLE (35–38, 42–46,81,82,85,90–92,230,231).

In summary, DNA, DNA/histone complex, or small immune complexes containing protected fragments of DNA may persist for abnormally long periods in individuals with SLE for a variety of reasons. Such a situation could result in prolonged antigenic stimulation and in the availability of DNA to bind to target tissues or to circulating anti-DNA, thus perpetuating the disease process.

DNAse-1 is the major nuclease present in serum, urine, and secretions that degrades DNA, particularly at sites of high cell turnover. DNAse-1–deficient mice were generated. They developed ANA and Ig deposition in glomeruli, with clinical glomerulonephritis (232). These observations, coupled with the information that levels of DNAse-1 in plasma of patients with SLE is usually low, led to clinical studies in which recombinant human DNAse-1 was administered to patients with SLE. The trial contained 17 individuals who received a single IV dose of 25 to 125 μg of rhDNAse followed by ten subcutaneous doses or placebo. Only the intravenous dose achieved serum hydrolytic activity of DNA. Serum antibodies to DNA were unchanged, as were cytokine levels of soluble interleukin-2R (sIL-2R), IL-6, IL-10, and TNF-α (233).

THE CHARACTERISTICS OF IMMUNE COMPLEXES CONTAINING DNA AND ANTI-DNA

Immune complexes containing DNA have been found in the circulation of as many as 50% of patients with active SLE, depending on the sensitivity of the method (88,234,235). The DNA in these immune complexes probably consists primarily of nucleosomes (87,89,234,235). For other immune complexes, small soluble complexes in slight antigen excess that can fix complement are the most pathogenic. For DNA, complexes in slight antibody excess may be the most stable and therefore most pathogenic (235–237). The complexes should be bound by Fc and CR1 receptors and cleared by the mononuclear phagocyte system. However, during periods of active SLE, clearance of immune complexes is defective. The abnormalities are complex, as discussed in Chapter 12. Abnormalities include a combination of high quantities of complexes, decreased numbers of receptors, saturation of available receptors, and defective phagocytosis of the complexes fixed to receptors (238). Genetic abnormalities in quantities of CR1 receptors have been reported (239), but the low numbers on cells of patients with SLE probably reflect stripping of occupied receptors. No mutations in CR1 or in Fc receptors have yet been found in patients with SLE. However, recent studies shows that some patients, particularly African Americans with lupus nephritis, compared to healthy control individuals, are more likely to inherit an allele of the Fcγ2 receptor that is a less efficient binder/processor of immune complexes than the alternative allele (102,241). This receptor is particularly important for removing immune complexes containing IgG2, such as the dominant population of anti-C1q that is associated with nephritis (242). Alleles of FcγI-IIA that are inefficient binders of IgG1 and IgG3 are also more common in individuals with lupus nephritis (243). Therefore, inheritance of inefficient-binding-phagocytosing alleles of these Fcγ receptors could impair the clearance of most immune complexes that cause disease in SLE. IgG1 is usually the most abundant isotype in glomerular Ig deposits. As discussed above, immune complexes containing cationic antigen or antibody, or protected DNA fragments that cannot be bound by cells that clear DNA, are probably important pathogens. These features stabilize the complex and permit its persistence.

METHODS OF MEASURING ANTIBODIES TO DNA

Several techniques are available to measure anti-DNA in serum or plasma (240,244–246) (Table 21.4). The ones that are chosen by service or research laboratories are critical. Some detect primarily high-avidity subsets of anti-DNA that are enriched in pathogens; these tests have low sensitivity but strong association with nephritis and clinical disease activity. Others detect both low- and high-avidity anti-DNA; these are more sensitive but less likely to be associated with clinical correlations unless only high titers are considered to be meaningful. The following tests measure primarily high-avidity antibodies: precipitation, complement fixation, and the Farr assay. A second group of tests detects both high- and low-avidity antibodies: ELISA, *Crithidia luciliae*, hemagglutination, and radioimmunoassays with precipitation of DNA-containing immune complexes by polyethylene glycol (PEG) assay. In general, the first group is less sensitive than the second, being positive in only 50% to 60% of patients with SLE, but correlates bet-

TABLE 21.4. METHODS OF MEASURING ANTI-DNA

Test	Sensitive	Specific	Correlates with Disease Activity and Nephritis	Availability
Precipitation	+	+++	+++	Highly limited
Hemagglutination	++	+	+	Highly limited
Complement fixation	++	+++	+++	Limited
Farr assay	++	+++	+++	Limited
PEG assay	++	++	+	Limited
Crithidia luciliae immunofluorescence	++	+++	+	Good
ELISA	+++	++	+	Good

ELISA, enzyme-linked immunosorbent assay; PEG, polyethylene glycol.

ter with disease flares and high risk for glomerulonephritis. The second group is more sensitive, being positive in 70% to 85% of patients with SLE; however, they correlate less well with disease activity and manifestations. These differences account for some of the discrepancy in the literature regarding the clinical utility of anti-DNA testing.

The tests most commonly used in service laboratories are Farr, ELISA, and *C. luciliae*. In the Farr assay, radiolabeled DNA is added to diluted serum or plasma, and Ig is precipitated by ammonium sulfate. Radioactivity in the precipitate indicates binding of DNA by anti-DNA; unbound DNA is not precipitated by the ammonium sulfate. DNA can be purified to contain primarily dsDNA, although a few single-strand nicks develop during the assay. Both IgG and IgM high-avidity precipitating antibodies are captured in this assay, which probably is the best of the available tests to detect primarily high-avidity antibodies to DNA.

In the ELISA assay, DNA is bound to wells in plastic microtiter plates. In general, ssDNA sticks directly to the wells. The adherence of dsDNA is variable, and some laboratories coat the wells with negatively charged molecules such as protamine sulfate, poly-l-lysine, or methylated bovine serum albumin before dsDNA is added to ensure uniform entrapment of the antigen. However, there are commercial microtiter plates available to which dsDNA adheres well, without requirement for addition of charged lining molecules. Diluted patient plasma or sera are incubated with DNA in the wells. After several hours, the wells are washed and the bound Ig incubated with enzyme-labeled antihuman Ig, IgG, or IgM. The binding of the second antibody is detected by a color change following addition of a substrate on which the enzyme acts, the color being read in a spectrophotometer. This assay allows measurement of both low- and high-avidity antibodies and the detection of total IgG, IgG isotypes, IgM, and total populations of anti-DNA. The substrate fixed to the wells can be highly purified dsDNA (which can be from mammalian or bacterial sources); a few single-strand nicks develop during the incubations. Commercial substrates often contain significant quantities of ssDNA as well as dsDNA; therefore, low quantities of anti-DNA detected in this assay may be primarily directed against ssDNA. Clinical correlations are best if they are confined to the interpretation of high titers of anti-DNA detected in this manner. There is considerable variability in the sensitivity and specificity of various manufacturers' ELISA kits for the measurement of anti-DNA and other autoantibodies (246). It is therefore most useful to both clinicians and researchers if assays are done repeatedly in the same laboratory using the same procedure or kits from the same sources.

In Europe, one group has been analyzing the association between antibodies to nucleosomes (measured in ELISA) and clinical correlations. They have noted strong association between IgG3 anti-DNA, disease activity, and nephritis in their lupus patients (86). Another group is using recombinant human dsDNA as the antigen on ELISA plates (247). The strongest association with lupus disease activity was with IgA anti-dsDNA rather than other isotypes, and the IgA subset also was associated with vasculitis. These examples illustrate the importance of every detail of ELISA assays, beginning with the antigen used, in interpreting results. International standardization of these assays would be welcome.

The *C. luciliae* test takes advantage of the presence of a kinetoplast containing circular dsDNA in this flagellate. Test sera or plasma are incubated with the organisms on a glass slide. After washing, fluoresceinated antihuman Ig, IgG, or IgM are added. After appropriate incubation, Ig bound to the DNA structure is detected by examining the glass slide for fluorescence using an ultraviolet microscope. Although even this circular DNA structure can contain one or two single-strand nicks, this assay is the most specific for anti-dsDNA. Therefore, positive tests are highly specific for SLE. However, in our laboratories, the sensitivity is not as good as the ELISA assay. The *Crithidia* assay can be modified to detect complement-fixing antibody subsets, but both low- and high-avidity anti-dsDNA are measured. Titers of anti-DNA measured by this method have little correlation with clinical disease activity in our laboratories, but in other hands they are as good as clinical correlations with ELISA assays (248).

Recently, rapid-flow immunoassays, in which anti-dsDNAs are bound to alkaline-phosphatase–labeled DNA in a resin column and then identified by isoelectric points, are being developed (249,250). Whether they will be affordable and available in service laboratories, and whether measurements will have more clinical utility, remains to be studied.

In summary, several different assays for anti-dsDNA are available commercially; each has advantages and disadvantages. No standardized test is used uniformly in all service laboratories. The ideal anti-DNA assay would detect all IgG high-avidity, complement-fixing anti-dsDNA; however, none of the assays available in most service laboratories does so. Therefore, the physician should determine which assay is used in the laboratory to which the specimens are sent and understand the specificity, sensitivity, and clinical correlations of that method. With methods that detect most populations of anti-dsDNA (and some anti-ssDNA), weakly positive tests can be obtained in patients with chronic liver disease, rheumatoid arthritis, nonlupus connective tissue diseases, drug-induced lupus, infections, and aging.

MEASUREMENTS OF ANTIBODIES TO DSDNA: UTILITY FOR THE CLINICIAN

Detection of anti-dsDNA often is useful in the diagnosis and management of patients with SLE (Table 21.5). Their interpretation is limited by lack of a standardized assay to measure them, inability to equate results of assays with the

TABLE 21.5. CLINICAL UTILITY OF MEASURING ANTI-DNA

High titers of anti-dsDNA
- Have approximately 90% specificity for SLE
- Often indicate clinically active disease and increased risk for nephritis

Low titers of anti-dsDNA
- Can be detecting anti-ssDNA
- Can be found in
  - Drug-induced lupus
  - Rheumatoid arthritis
  - Sjögren's syndrome
  - Other CTD
  - Chronic infections
  - Chronic liver disease
  - Aging

CTD, connective tissue disease.

most pathogenic subsets of anti-DNA, and the fact that antibodies other than anti-DNA participate in the tissue lesions of SLE. Antibodies to ssDNA should not be measured, because they have no specificity for the disease.

Tests for antibodies to dsDNA are useful in establishing the diagnosis of SLE; 60% to 83% of patients with SLE have positive tests for these antibodies by the Farr, *Crithidia*, or ELISA assays at some time during their illness (245,248,251). The presence of anti-dsDNA fulfills a criterion for the classification of SLE diagnosis, as suggested by the American College of Rheumatology (252,253).

The ability of tests for anti-dsDNA to predict exacerbations of clinical disease, or various organ involvements, is controversial. Some studies suggest strong correlations between increasing levels of these antibodies and subsequence disease activation (245,248,254). Other studies suggest that such correlations are weak (255,256). A minority of patients have high titers of IgG anti-dsDNA for prolonged periods of time without developing exacerbations of disease or glomerulonephritis (257). In general, when tests for anti-dsDNA are performed at regular intervals using the same methods and materials, rising titers suggest that the risk of disease exacerbation, particularly of nephritis and/or vasculitis, is increased (248,255,256). Sometimes renal flares are preceded by drops in anti-DNA, probably because the antibodies are leaking into the urine. It comes as no surprise that the clinician must combine results of careful laboratory testing with symptoms and signs to make correct therapeutic decisions.

In summary, measurement of anti-dsDNA in sera has two useful clinical applications (Table 21.5). First, high titers of these antibodies have a specificity of more than 90% for SLE; therefore, they are useful in making the diagnosis. Second, rising levels should alert the clinician to the possibility of an imminent disease flare, and high levels (especially associated with low levels of serum complement) suggest increased risk for lupus nephritis. We recommend that in each patient with SLE, the physician establish whether the pattern of serum anti-DNA titers correlates with clinical manifestations and disease activity. If such correlations are present, serial measurements of anti-DNA are useful.

FUTURE DIRECTIONS: TARGETING ANTIBODIES TO DNA IN THERAPY OF SLE

Many effective, widely immunosuppressive therapies for SLE such as glucocorticoids and cytotoxic drugs are associated with falls in titers of anti-dsDNA that precede or accompany clinical improvement. There has been considerable interest in developing therapies that specifically target pathogenic autoantibodies and leave the normal immune repertoire intact.

There has been some success in experimental studies with LJP394, which is a DNA toleragen (258–261). LJP394 is a molecule in which four oligonucleotides are held on a tetrameric scaffold. The idea is to cross-link two Ig anti-DNA receptors on B cells; this gives a weak first signal without a second signal, so that the B cells are anergized (not activated) and stop producing anti-dsDNA. Administration as a toleragen was effective in BXSB lupus-prone mice. Recently, in a clinical trial in patients, the number of flares of nephritis was significantly reduced in the patients tolerized with LJP394 compared to those who received placebo—in the subset of patients with anti-dsDNA that bound the toleragen with high avidity (261). The toleragen was given once a week intravenously. It is likely that follow-up larger studies will take place soon, so that the utility of this treatment can be confirmed.

Other attempts to reduce anti-DNA antibody as disease treatment have included immunoadsorption of anti-DNA using columns designed to specifically trap anti-DNA and immune complexes (262–264). Passing SLE serum over phenylalanine or human anti-DNA (262,263), or dextran sulfate columns (264), reduced anti-DNA titers and was associated with clinical improvement in at least half of patients. Administration of DNAse-1 was not effective in initial studies. The future of therapies that target certain autoantibodies is exciting, since many of the autoantibodies of SLE are interconnected, and suppressing one might have beneficial effects on quantities of the others.

REFERENCES

1. Hargraves M, Richmond H, Morton R. Presentation of 2 bone marrow elements: "tart" cell and "L.E." cell. *Proc Staff Meet Mayo Clin* 1948;23:25–28.
2. Holborow J, Weir DM, Johnson GD. A serum factor in lupus erythematosus with affinity for tissue nuclei. *Br Med J* 1957;2: 732–734.
3. Schmidt-Acevedo S, Perez-Romano B, Ruiz-Arguelles A. "LE

cells" result from phagocytosis of apoptotic bodies induced by antinuclear antibodies. *J Autoimmun* 2000;15(1):15–20.
4. Rothfield NF, Stollar BD. The relation of immunoglobulin class, pattern of anti-nuclear antibody, and complement-fixing antibodies to DNA in sera from patients with systemic lupus erythematosus. *J Clin Invest* 1967;46(11):1785–1794.
5. Schur PH, Sandson J. Immunologic factors and clinical activity in systemic lupus erythematosus. *N Engl J Med* 1968;278(10): 533–538.
6. Lambert PH, Dixon FJ. Pathogenesis of the glomerulonephritis of NZB/W mice. *J Exp Med* 1968;127(3):507–522.
7. Tan E. Immunopathology and pathogenesis of cutaneous involvement in systemic lupus erythematosus. *J Invest Dermatol* 1976;67:360–365.
8. Winfield JB, Faiferman I, Koffler D. Avidity of anti-DNA antibodies in serum and IgG glomerular eluates from patients with systemic lupus erythematosus. Association of high avidity antinative DNA antibody with glomerulonephritis. *J Clin Invest* 1977;59(1):90–96.
9. Andrews BS, Eisenberg RA, Theofilopoulos AN, et al. Spontaneous murine lupus-like syndromes. Clinical and immunopathological manifestations in several strains. *J Exp Med* 1978; 148(5):1198–1215.
10. Smith HR, Green DR, Raveche ES, et al. Studies of the induction of anti-DNA in normal mice. *J Immunol* 1974;113(1): 292–297.
11. Borel Y, Lewis RM, Stollar BD. Prevention of murine lupus nephritis by carrier-dependent induction of immunologic tolerance to denatured DNA. *Science* 1973;182(107):76–78.
12. Parker LP, Hahn BH, Osterland CK. Modification of NZB-NZW F1 autoimmune disease by development of tolerance to DNA. *J Immunol* 1974;113(1):292–297.
13. Eshhar Z, Benacerraf B, Katz DH. Induction of tolerance to nucleic acid determinants by administration of a complex of nucleoside D-glutamic acid and D-lysine (D-GL). *J Immunol* 1975;114(2 pt 2):872–876.
14. Borel Y, Lewis RM, Andre-Schwartz J, et al. Treatment of lupus nephritis in adult (NZB + NZW)F1 mice by cortisone- facilitated tolerance to nucleic acid antigens. *J Clin Invest* 1978;61 (2):276–286.
15. Hahn BH, Ebling F, Freeman S, et al. Production of monoclonal murine antibodies to DNA by somatic cell hybrids. *Arthritis Rheum* 1980;23(8):942–945.
16. Marion TN, Krishnan MR, Desai DD, et al. Monoclonal anti-DNA antibodies: structure, specificity, and biology. *Methods* 1997;11(1):3–11.
17. Zouali M. The structure of human lupus anti-DNA antibodies. *Methods* 1997;11(1):27–35.
18. Hahn BH. Antibodies to DNA. *N Engl J Med* 1998;338(19): 1359–1368.
19. Rahman A, Latchman DS, Isenberg DA. Immunoglobulin variable region sequences of human monoclonal anti-DNA antibodies. *Semin Arthritis Rheum* 1998;28(3):141–154.
20. Radic MZ, Cocca BA, Seal SN. Initiation of systemic autoimmunity and sequence specific anti-DNA autoantibodies. *Crit Rev Immunol* 1999;19(2):117–126.
21. Ebling FM, Hahn BH. Pathogenic subsets of antibodies to DNA. *Int Rev Immunol* 1989;5(1):79–95.
22. Cairns E, St.Germain J, Bell DA. The in vitro production of anti-DNA antibody by cultured peripheral blood or tonsillar lymphoid cells from normal donors and SLE patients. *J Immunol* 1985;135(6):3839–3844.
23. Fish F, Ziff M. The in vitro and in vivo induction of anti-double-stranded DNA antibodies in normal and autoimmune mice. *J Immunol* 1982;128:409–414.
24. Hasselbacher P, LeRoy EC. Serum DNA binding activity in healthy subjects and in rheumatic disease. *Arthritis Rheum* 1974;17(1):63–71.
25. Hoch S, Schur PH, Schwaber J. Frequency of anti-DNA antibody producing cells from normals and patients with systemic lupus erythematosus. *Clin Immunol Immunopathol* 1983;27(1): 28–37.
26. Pisetsky DS, Jelinek DF, McAnally LM, et al. In vitro autoantibody production by normal adult and cord blood B cells. *J Clin Invest* 1990;85(3):899–903.
27. Rubin RL, Carr RI. Anti-DNA activity of IgG F(ab')2 from normal human serum. *J Immunol* 1979;122(4):1604–1607.
28. Schwartz RS, Stollar BD. Origins of anti-DNA autoantibodies. *J Clin Invest* 1985;75(2):321–327.
29. Steele EJ, Cunningham AJ. High proportion of Ig-producing cells making autoantibody in normal mice. *Nature* 1978;274 (5670):483–484.
30. Suenaga R, Mitamura K, Abdou NI. V gene sequences of lupus-derived human IgM anti-ssDNA antibody: implication for the importance of the location of DNA-binding amino acids [see comments]. *Clin Immunol Immunopathol* 1998;86(1):72–80.
31. Bloom DD, St. Clair EW, Pisetsky DS, et al. The anti-La response of a single MRL/Mp-lpr/lpr mouse: specificity for DNA and VH gene usage. *Eur J Immunol* 1994;24(6): 1332–1338.
32. Reeves WH, Satoh M, Wang J, et al. Systemic lupus erythematosus. Antibodies to DNA, DNA-binding proteins, and histones. *Rheum Dis Clin North Am* 1994;20(1):1–28.
33. Pyun EH, Pisetsky DS, Gilkeson GS. The fine specificity of monoclonal anti-DNA antibodies induced in normal mice by immunization with bacterial DNA. *J Autoimmun* 1993;6(1): 11–26.
34. Limpanasithikul W, Rya S, Diamond B. Cross-reactive antibodies have both protective and pathogenic potential. *J Immunol* 1995;155:967–973.
35. Jacob L, Lety MA, Louvard D, et al. Binding of a monoclonal anti-DNA autoantibody to identical proteins present at the surface of several human cell types involved in lupus pathogenesis. *J Clin Invest* 1985;75(1):315–317.
36. Sabbaga J, Line SR, Potocnjak P, et al. A murine nephritogenic monoclonal anti-DNA autoantibody binds directly to mouse laminin, the major non-collagenous protein component of the glomerular basement membrane. *Eur J Immunol* 1989;19(1): 137–143.
37. Faaber P, Rijke TP, van de Putte LB, et al. Cross-reactivity of human and murine anti-DNA antibodies with heparan sulfate. The major glycosaminoglycan in glomerular basement membranes. *J Clin Invest* 1986;77(6):1824–1830.
38. Ohnishi K, Ebling FM, Mitchell B, et al. Comparison of pathogenic and non-pathogenic murine antibodies to DNA: antigen binding and structural characteristics. *Int Immunol* 1994;6(6): 817–830.
39. Reichlin M, Martin A, Taylor-Albert E, et al. Lupus autoantibodies to native DNA cross-react with the A and D SnRNP polypeptides. *J Clin Invest* 1994;93(1):443–449.
40. Carroll P, Stafford D, Schwartz RS, et al. Murine monoclonal anti-DNA autoantibodies bind to endogenous bacteria. *J Immunol* 1985;135(2):1086–1090.
41. Pisetsky DS, Grudier JP. Polyspecific binding of Escherichia coli beta-galactosidase by murine antibodies to DNA. *J Immunol* 1989;143(11):3609–3613.
42. Faaber P, Capel PJ, Rijke GP, et al. Cross-reactivity of anti-DNA antibodies with proteoglycans. *Clin Exp Immunol* 1984;55(3): 502–508.
43. Brinkman K, Termaat R, Berden JH, et al. Anti-DNA antibodies and lupus nephritis: the complexity of crossreactivity [see comments]. *Immunol Today* 1990;11(7):232–234.

44. Lafer EM, Rauch J, Andrzejewski C Jr, et al. Polyspecific monoclonal lupus autoantibodies reactive with both polynucleotides and phospholipids. *J Exp Med* 1981;153(4):897–909.
45. Andre-Schwartz J, Datta SK, Shoenfeld Y, et al. Binding of cytoskeletal proteins by monoclonal anti-DNA lupus autoantibodies. *Clin Immunol Immunopathol* 1984;31(2):261–271.
46. Jacob L, Viard JP, Allenet B, et al. A monoclonal anti-double-stranded DNA autoantibody binds to a 94-kDa cell-surface protein on various cell types via nucleosomes or a DNA- histone complex. *Proc Natl Acad Sci USA* 1989;86(12): 4669–4673.
47. Shlomchik MJ, Marshak-Rothstein A, Wolfowicz CB, et al. The role of clonal selection and somatic mutation in autoimmunity. *Nature* 1987;328(6133):805–811.
48. Diamond B, Katz J, Paul E, et al. The role of somatic mutation in the pathogenic anti-DNA response. *Annu Rev Immunol* 1992;10:731–757.
49. Dersimonian H, Schwartz RS, Barrett KJ, et al. Relationship of human variable region heavy chain germ-line genes to genes encoding anti-DNA autoantibodies. *J Immunol* 1987;139(7): 2496–2501.
50. Naparstek Y, Andre-Schwartz J, Manser T, et al. A single germline VH gene segment of normal A/J mice encodes autoantibodies characteristic of systemic lupus erythematosus. *J Exp Med* 1986;164(2):614–626.
51. Kowal C, Weinstein A, Diamond B. Molecular mimicry between bacterial and self antigen in a patient with systemic lupus erythematosus. *Eur J Immunol* 1999;29(6):1901–1911.
52. Cavallo T, Granholm N. Bacterial lipopolysaccharide transforms mesangial into proliferative lupus nephritis without interfering with processing of pathogenic immune complexes in NZB/W mice. *Am J Pathol* 1991;137:971–978.
53. Pisetsky DS. The role of bacterial DNA in autoantibody induction. *Curr Top Microbiol Immunol* 2000;247:143–155.
54. Dang H, Harbeck RJ. The in vivo and in vitro glomerular deposition of isolated anti-double-stranded-DNA antibodies in NZB/W mice. *Clin Immunol Immunopathol* 1984;30(2): 265–278.
55. Raz E, Brezis M, Rosenmann E, et al. Anti-DNA antibodies bind directly to renal antigens and induce kidney dysfunction in the isolated perfused rat kidney. *J Immunol* 1989;142(9):3076–3082.
56. Tsao BP, Ebling FM, Roman C, et al. Structural characteristics of the variable regions of immunoglobulin genes encoding a pathogenic autoantibody in murine lupus. *J Clin Invest* 1990; 85(2):530–540.
57. Madaio MP, Carlson J, Cataldo J, et al. Murine monoclonal anti-DNA antibodies bind directly to glomerular antigens and form immune deposits. *J Immunol* 1987;138(9):2883–2889.
58. Ehrenstein MR, Katz DR, Griffiths MH, et al. Human IgG anti-DNA antibodies deposit in kidneys and induce proteinuria in SCID mice. *Kidney Int* 1995;48(3):705–711.
59. Ravirajan CT, Rahman MA, Papadaki L, et al. Genetic, structural and functional properties of an IgG DNA-binding monoclonal antibody from a lupus patient with nephritis [published erratum appears in *Eur J Immunol* 1999;29(9):3052]. *Eur J Immunol* 1998;28(1):339–350.
60. Tsao BP, Ohnishi K, Cheroutre H, et al. Failed self-tolerance and autoimmunity in IgG anti-DNA transgenic mice. *J Immunol* 1992;149(1):350–358.
61. Bynoe MS, Spatz L, Diamond B. Characterization of anti-DNA B cells that escape negative selection. *Eur J Immunol* 1999;29 (4):1304–1313.
62. Williams RC Jr, Malone CC, Miller RT, et al. Urinary loss of immunoglobulin G anti-F(ab)2 and anti-DNA antibody in systemic lupus erythematosus nephritis. *J Lab Clin Med* 1998;132 (3):210–222.
63. Katz J, Limpanasithikul W, Diamond B. Mutational analysis of an autoantibody: differential binding and pathogenicity. *J Exp Med* 1994;180:925–932.
64. Gilkeson GS, Bernstein K, Pippen AM, et al. The influence of variable-region somatic mutations on the specificity and pathogenicity of murine monoclonal anti-DNA antibodies. *Clin Immunol Immunopathol* 1995;76(1 pt 1):59–67.
65. Ebling F, Hahn BH. Restricted subpopulations of DNA antibodies in kidneys of mice with systemic lupus. Comparison of antibodies in serum and renal eluates. *Arthritis Rheum* 1980; 23(4):392–403.
66. Gavalchin J, Seder RA, Datta SK. The NZB × SWR model of lupus nephritis. I. Cross-reactive idiotypes of monoclonal anti-DNA antibodies in relation to antigenic specificity, charge, and allotype. Identification of interconnected idiotype families inherited from the normal SWR and the autoimmune NZB parents. *J Immunol* 1987;138(1):128–137.
67. Mannik M. Mechanisms of tissue deposition of immune complexes. *J Rheumatol* 1987;14(suppl 13):35–42.
68. Gauthier V, Mannik M. A small proportion of cationic antibodies in immune complexes is sufficient to mediate their deposition in glomeruli. *J Immunol* 1990;145:3348–3352.
69. Yoshida H, Yoshida M, Izui S, et al. Distinct clonotypes of anti-DNA antibodies in mice with lupus nephritis. *J Clin Invest* 1985;76(2):685–694.
70. Muryoi T, Sasaki T, Hatakeyama A, et al. Clonotypes of anti-DNA antibodies expressing specific idiotypes in immune complexes of patients with active lupus nephritis. *J Immunol* 1990; 144(10):3856–3861.
71. Kalunian KC, Panosian-Sahakian N, Ebling FM, et al. Idiotypic characteristics of immunoglobulins associated with systemic lupus erythematosus. Studies of antibodies deposited in glomeruli of humans. *Arthritis Rheum* 1989;32(5):513–522.
72. Hahn BH, Ebling FM. Idiotype restriction in murine lupus; high frequency of three public idiotypes on serum IgG in nephritic NZB/NZW F1 mice. *J Immunol* 1987;138(7): 2110–2118.
73. Isenberg DA, Shoenfeld Y, Madaio MP, et al. Anti-DNA antibody idiotypes in systemic lupus erythematosus. *Lancet* 1984;2(8400):417–422.
74. Isenberg D, Williams W, Axford J, et al. Comparison of 17 DNA antibody idiotypes in patients with autoimmune diseases, healthy relatives and spouses and normal controls—results of an international study from 10 laboratories. *J Autoimmun* 1990;3:393–414.
75. Solomon G, Schiffenbauer J, Keiser HD, et al. Use of monoclonal antibodies to identify shared idiotypes on human antibodies to native DNA from patients with systemic lupus erythematosus. *Proc Natl Acad Sci USA* 1983;80(3):850–854.
76. Weisbart RH, Noritake DT, Wong AL, et al. A conserved anti-DNA antibody idiotype associated with nephritis in murine and human systemic lupus erythematosus. *J Immunol* 1990;144 (7):2653–2658.
77. Mendlovic S, Brocke S, Shoenfeld Y, et al. Induction of a systemic lupus erythematosus-like disease in mice by a common human anti-DNA idiotype. *Proc Natl Acad Sci USA* 1988;85 (7):2260–2264.
78. Mendlovic S, Fricke H, Shoenfeld Y, et al. The role of anti-idiotypic antibodies in the induction of experimental systemic lupus erythematosus in mice. *Eur J Immunol* 1989;19(4):729–734.
79. Hahn B, Ebling F. Suppression of murine lupus nephritis by administration of an anti-idiotypic antibody to anti-DNA. *J Immunol* 1984;132:187–190.
80. Harata N, Sasaki T, Osaki H, et al. Therapeutic treatment of New Zealand mouse disease by a limited number of anti-idiotypic antibodies conjugated with neocarzinostatin. *J Clin Invest* 1990;86(3):769–776.

81. Foster MH, Sabbaga J, Line SR, et al. Molecular analysis of spontaneous nephrotropic anti-laminin antibodies in an autoimmune MRL-lpr/lpr mouse. *J Immunol* 1993;151(2): 814–824.
82. Schmiedeke TM, Stockl FW, Weber R, et al. Histones have high affinity for the glomerular basement membrane. Relevance for immune complex formation in lupus nephritis. *J Exp Med* 1989;169(6):1879–1894.
83. Burlingame RW, Boey ML, Starkebaum G, et al. The central role of chromatin in autoimmune responses to histones and DNA in systemic lupus erythematosus. *J Clin Invest* 1994;94 (1):184–192.
84. Amoura Z, Chabre H, Koutouzov S, et al. Nucleosome-restricted antibodies are detected before anti-dsDNA and/or antihistone antibodies in serum of MRL-Mp lpr/lpr and +/+ mice, and are present in kidney eluates of lupus mice with proteinuria. *Arthritis Rheum* 1994;37(11):1684–1688.
85. Bernstein KA, Valerio RD, Lefkowith JB. Glomerular binding activity in MRL lpr serum consists of antibodies that bind to a DNA/histone/type IV collagen complex. *J Immunol* 1995;154 (5):2424–2433.
86. Amoura Z, Koutouzov S, Chabre H, et al. Presence of antinucleosome autoantibodies in a restricted set of connective tissue diseases: antinucleosome antibodies of the IgG3 subclass are markers of renal pathogenicity in systemic lupus erythematosus. *Arthritis Rheum* 2000;43(1):76–84.
87. Amoura Z, Piette JC, Chabre H, et al. Circulating plasma levels of nucleosomes in patients with systemic lupus erythematosus: correlation with serum antinucleosome antibody titers and absence of clear association with disease activity. *Arthritis Rheum* 1997;40(12):2217–2225.
88. Nezlin R, Alarcon-Segovia D, Shoenfeld Y. Immunochemical determination of DNA in immune complexes present in the circulation of patients with systemic lupus erythematosus. *J Autoimmun* 1998;11(5):489–493.
89. Rumore PM, Steinman CR. Endogenous circulating DNA in systemic lupus erythematosus. Occurrence as multimeric complexes bound to histone. *J Clin Invest* 1990;86(1):69–74.
90. Bernstein K, Bolshoun D, Gilkeson G, et al. Detection of glomerular-binding immune elements in murine lupus using a tissue-based ELISA. *Clin Exp Immunol* 1993;91(3):449–455.
91. Bernstein KA, Bolshoun D, Lefkowith JB. Serum glomerular binding activity is highly correlated with renal disease in MRL/lpr mice. *Clin Exp Immunol* 1993;93(3):418–423.
92. Di Valerio R, Bernstein KA, Varghese E, et al. Murine lupus glomerulotropic monoclonal antibodies exhibit differing specificities but bind via a common mechanism. *J Immunol* 1995; 155(4):2258–2268.
93. Stetler DA, Cavallo T. Anti-RNA polymerase I antibodies: potential role in the induction and progression of murine lupus nephritis. *J Immunol* 1987;138(7):2119–2123.
94. Wasicek CA, Reichlin M. Clinical and serological differences between systemic lupus erythematosus patients with antibodies to Ro versus patients with antibodies to Ro and La. *J Clin Invest* 1982;69(4):835–843.
95. Schur P, Moroz L, Kunkel HG. Precipitating antibodies to ribosomes in the serum of patients with systemic lupus erythematosus. *Immunochemistry* 1967;4:447–452.
96. Maddison PJ, Reichlin M. Deposition of antibodies to a soluble cytoplasmic antigen in the kidneys of patients with systemic lupus erythematosus. *Arthritis Rheum* 1979;22(8):858–863.
97. Gallo R, Graves T, Granholm M, et al. Association of glycoprotein gp70 with progression or attenuation of murine lupus nephritis. *J Clin Lab Immunol* 1985;18:63–70.
98. Uwatoko S, Mannik M. Low-molecular weight C1q-binding immunoglobulin G in patients with systemic lupus erythematosus consists of autoantibodies to the collagen- like region of C1q. *J Clin Invest* 1988;82(3):816–824.
99. Servais G, Guillaume MP, Dumarey N, et al. Evidence of autoantibodies to cell membrane associated DNA (cultured lymphocytes): a new specific marker for rapid identification of systemic lupus erythematosus. *Ann Rheum Dis* 1998;57(10): 606–613.
100. Vyse TJ, Drake CG, Rozzo SJ, et al. Genetic linkage of IgG autoantibody production in relation to lupus nephritis in New Zealand hybrid mice. *J Clin Invest* 1996;98(8):1762–1772.
101. Walport MJ, Davies KA, Botto M. C1q and systemic lupus erythematosus. *Immunobiology* 1998;199(2):265–285.
102. Norsworthy P, Theodoridis E, Botto M, et al. Overrepresentation of the Fcgamma receptor type IIA R131/R131 genotype in caucasoid systemic lupus erythematosus patients with autoantibodies to C1q and glomerulonephritis. *Arthritis Rheum* 1999; 42(9):1828–1832.
103. Yamamoto AM, Amoura Z, Johannet C, et al. Quantitative radioligand assays using de novo-synthesized recombinant autoantigens in connective tissue diseases: new tools to approach the pathogenic significance of anti-RNP antibodies in rheumatic diseases. *Arthritis Rheum* 2000;43(3):689–698.
104. Alarcon-Segovia D, Lorente L. Antibody penetration into living cells. IV. Different effects of anti-native DNA and anti-ribonucleoprotein IgG on the cell cycle of activated T cells. *Clin Exp Immunol* 1983;52:365–369.
105. Okudaira K, Yoshizawa H, Williams RC Jr. Monoclonal murine anti-DNA antibody interacts with living mononuclear cells. *Arthritis Rheum* 1987;30(6):669–678.
106. Vlahakos D, Foster MH, Ucci AA, et al. Murine monoclonal anti-DNA antibodies penetrate cells, bind to nuclei, and induce glomerular proliferation and proteinuria in vivo. J *Am Soc Nephrol* 1992;2(8):1345–1354.
107. Koren E, Koscec M, Wolfson-Reichlin M, et al. Murine and human antibodies to native DNA that cross-react with the A and D SnRNP polypeptides cause direct injury of cultured kidney cells. *J Immunol* 1995;154(9):4857–4864.
108. Yanase K, Smith RM, Cizman B, et al. A subgroup of murine monoclonal anti-deoxyribonucleic acid antibodies traverse the cytoplasm and enter the nucleus in a time- and temperature-dependent manner. *Lab Invest* 1994;71(1):52–60.
109. Reichlin M. Cellular dysfunction induced by penetration of autoantibodies into living cells: cellular damage and dysfunction mediated by antibodies to dsDNA and ribosomal P proteins. *J Autoimmun* 1998;11(5):557–561.
110. Yanase K, Smith RM, Puccetti A, et al. Receptor-mediated cellular entry of nuclear localizing anti-DNA antibodies via myosin 1. *J Clin Invest* 1997;100(1):25–31.
111. Portales-Perez D, Alarcon-Segovia D, Llorente L, et al. Penetrating anti-DNA monoclonal antibodies induce activation of human peripheral blood mononuclear cells. *J Autoimmun* 1998; 11(5):563–571.
112. Watanabe N, Kubota T, Miyasaka N, et al. Enhancement of hydroxyl radical DNA cleavage by serum anti-dsDNA antibodies in SLE. *Lupus* 1998;7(2):108–112.
113. Kozyr AV, Kolesnikov AV, Aleksandrova ES, et al. Novel functional activities of anti-DNA autoantibodies from sera of patients with lymphoproliferative and autoimmune diseases. *Appl Biochem Biotechnol* 1998;75(1):45–61.
114. Mevorach D. The immune response to apoptotic cells. *Ann NY Acad Sci* 1999;87:191–198.
115. Mevorach D, Zhou JL, Song X, et al. Systemic exposure to irradiated apoptotic cells induces autoantibody production. *J Exp Med* 1998;188(2):387–392.
116. Courtney PA, Crockard AD, Williamson K, et al. Lymphocyte apoptosis in systemic lupus erythematosus: relationships with

Fas expression, serum soluble Fas and disease activity. *Lupus* 1999;8(7):508–513.
117. Courtney PA, Crockard AD, Williamson K, et al. Increased apoptotic peripheral blood neutrophils in systemic lupus erythematosus: relations with disease activity, antibodies to double stranded DNA, and neutropenia. *Ann Rheum Dis* 1999;58(5): 309–314.
118. Herrmann M, Voll RE, Zoller OM, et al. Impaired phagocytosis of apoptotic cell material by monocyte-derived macrophages from patients with systemic lupus erythematosus. *Arthritis Rheum* 1998;41(7):1241–1250.
119. Bave U, Alm GV, Ronnblom L. The combination of apoptotic U937 cells and lupus IgG is a potent IFN-alpha inducer. *J Immunol* 2000;165(6):3519–3526.
120. Sun KH, Yu CL, Tang SJ, et al. Monoclonal anti-double-stranded DNA autoantibody stimulates the expression and release of IL-1beta, IL-6, IL-8, IL-10 and TNF-alpha from normal human mononuclear cells involving in the lupus pathogenesis. *Immunology* 2000;99(3):352–360.
121. Lai KN, Leung JC, Lai KB, et al. Upregulation of adhesion molecule expression on endothelial cells by anti-DNA autoantibodies in systemic lupus erythematosus. *Clin Immunol Immunopathol* 1996;81(3):229–238.
122. Chan O, Hannum L, Haberman A, et al. A novel mouse with B cells but lacking serum antibody reveals an antibody-independent role for B cells in murine lupus. *J Exp Med* 1999; 189:1639–1648.
123. Kuroiwa T, Lee E. Cellular interactions in the pathogenesis of lupus nephritis: the role of T cells and macrophages in the amplification of the inflammatory process in the kidney. *Lupus* 1998;7:597–603.
124. Diamond B, Scharff M. Somatic mutation of T15 heavy chain gives rise to an antibody with autoantibody specificity. *Proc Natl Acad Sci USA* 1984;81:5841–5844.
125. O'Keefe TL, Bandyopadhyay S, Datta SK, et al. V region sequences of an idiotypically connected family of pathogenic anti-DNA autoantibodies. *J Immunol* 1990;144(11): 4275–4283.
126. van Es JH, Gmelig Meyling FH, van de Akker WR, et al. Somatic mutations in the variable regions of a human IgG anti-double-stranded DNA autoantibody suggest a role for antigen in the induction of systemic lupus erythematosus. *J Exp Med* 1991;173(2):461–470.
127. Behar SM, Scharff MD. Somatic diversification of the S107 (T15. VH11 germ-line gene that encodes the heavy-chain variable region of antibodies to double-stranded DNA in (NZB x NZW)F1 mice. *Proc Natl Acad Sci USA* 1988;85(11):3970–3974.
128. Davidson A, Manheimer-Lory A, Aranow C, et al. Molecular characterization of a somatically mutated anti-DNA antibody bearing two systemic lupus erythematosus-related idiotypes. *J Clin Invest* 1990;85(5):1401–1409.
129. Guisti A, Chien N, Zack D, et al. Somatic diversification of S107 from an anti-phosphocholine to an anti-DNA autoantibody is due to a single base change in its heavy chain variable region. *Proc Natl Acad Sci USA* 1987;84:2926–2930.
130. Shlomchik M, Mascelli M, Shan H, et al. Anti-DNA antibodies from autoimmune mice arise by clonal expansion and somatic mutation. *J Exp Med* 1990;171(1):265–292.
131. Shlomchik MJ, Aucoin AH, Pisetsky DS, et al. Structure and function of anti-DNA autoantibodies derived from a single autoimmune mouse. *Proc Natl Acad Sci USA* 1987;84(24): 9150–9154.
132. Behar S, Lustgarte K, Corbe S, et al. Characterization of somatically mutated S107 Vh11-encoded anti-DNA autoantibodies derived from autoimmune (NZB×NZW)F1 mice. *J Exp Med* 1991;173:731–736.
133. Behar SM, Corbet S, Diamond B, et al. The molecular origin of anti-DNA antibodies. *Int Rev Immunol* 1989;5(1):23–42.
134. Taki S, Hirose S, Kinoshita K, et al. Somatically mutated IgG anti-DNA antibody clonally related to germ-line encoded IgM anti-DNA antibody. *Eur J Immunol* 1992;22(4):987–992.
135. Eilat D. The role of germline gene expression and somatic mutation in the generation of autoantibodies to DNA. *Mol Immunol* 1990;27(3):203–210.
136. Bona CA. V genes encoding autoantibodies: molecular and phenotypic characteristics. *Annu Rev Immunol* 1988;6: 327–358.
137. Cairns E, Kwong PC, Misener V, et al. Analysis of variable region genes encoding a human anti-DNA antibody of normal origin. Implications for the molecular basis of human autoimmune responses. *J Immunol* 1989;143(2):685–691.
138. Chen PP, Liu MF, Sinha S, et al. A 16/6 idiotype-positive anti-DNA antibody is encoded by a conserved VH gene with no somatic mutation. *Arthritis Rheum* 1988;31(11):1429–1431.
139. Eilat D, Webster DM, Rees AR. V region sequences of anti-DNA and anti-RNA autoantibodies from NZB/NZW F1 mice. *J Immunol* 1988;141(5):1745–1753.
140. Kofler R, Dixon F, Theofilopoulos A. The genetic origin of autoantibodies (review). *Immunol Today* 1987;80:375–380.
141. Kofler R, Noonan DJ, Levy DE, et al. Genetic elements used for a murine lupus anti-DNA autoantibody are closely related to those for antibodies to exogenous antigens. *J Exp Med* 1985; 161(4):805–815.
142. Trepicchio W Jr, Maruya A, Barrett KJ. The heavy chain genes of a lupus anti-DNA autoantibody are encoded in the germ line of a nonautoimmune strain of mouse and conserved in strains of mice polymorphic for this gene locus. *J Immunol* 1987;139 (9):3139–3145.
143. Shefner R, Kleiner G, Turken A, et al. A novel class of anti-DNA antibodies identified in BALB/c mice. *J Exp Med* 1991; 173(2):287–296.
144. Panosian-Sahakian N, Klotz JL, Ebling F, et al. Diversity of Ig V gene segments found in anti-DNA autoantibodies from a single (NZB × NZW)F1 mouse. *J Immunol* 1989;142(12): 4500–4506.
145. Grayzel A, Solomon A, Aranow C, et al. Antibodies elicited by pneumococcal antigens bear an anti-DNA-associated idiotype. *J Clin Invest* 1991;87(3):842–846.
146. Marion TN, Bothwell AL, Briles DE, et al. IgG anti-DNA autoantibodies within an individual autoimmune mouse are the products of clonal selection. *J Immunol* 1989;142(12): 4269–4274.
147. Marion TN, Tillman DM, Jou NT. Interclonal and intraclonal diversity among anti-DNA antibodies from an (NZB × NZW)F1 mouse. *J Immunol* 1990;145(7):2322–2332.
148. Rekvig OP, Fredriksen K, Brannsether B, et al. Antibodies to eukaryotic, including autologous, native DNA are produced during BK virus infection, but not after immunization with non-infectious BK DNA. *Scand J Immunol* 1992;36(3): 487–495.
149. Vargas M, Gustilo K, D'Andrea D, et al. Structural features of nephritogenic lupus autoantibodies. *Methods* 1997;11:62–69.
150. Shibata S, Sasaki T, Hatakeyama A, et al. Clonal frequency analysis of B cells producing pathogenic anti-DNA antibody-associated idiotypes in systemic lupus erythematosus. *Clin Immunol Immunopathol* 1992;63(3):252–258.
151. Chastagner P, Demaison C, Theze J, et al. Clonotypic dominance and variable gene elements of pathogenic anti-DNA autoantibodies from a single patient with lupus. *Scand J Immunol* 1994;39(2):165–178.
152. Tillman DM, Jou NT, Hill RJ, et al. Both IgM and IgG anti-DNA antibodies are the products of clonally selective B cell

stimulation in (NZB × NZW)F1 mice. *J Exp Med* 1992;176(3): 761–779.

153. Winkler TH, Fehr H, Kalden JR. Analysis of immunoglobulin variable region genes from human IgG anti-DNA hybridomas. *Eur J Immunol* 1992;22(7):1719–1728.
154. Yaoita Y, Takahashi M, Azuma C, et al. Biased expression of variable region gene families of the immunoglobulin heavy chain in autoimmune-prone mice. *J Biochem (Tokyo)* 1988;104 (3):337–343.
155. Trepicchio W Jr, Barrett KJ. Eleven MRL-lpr/lpr anti-DNA autoantibodies are encoded by genes from four VH gene families: a potentially biased usage of VH genes. *J Immunol* 1987; 138(7):2323–2331.
156. Gibson AL, Herron JN, Ballard DW, et al. Crystallographic characterization of the Fab fragment of a monoclonal anti-ss-DNA antibody. *Mol Immunol* 1985;22(4):499–502.
157. Radic MZ, Mackle J, Erikson J, et al. Residues that mediate DNA binding of autoimmune antibodies. *J Immunol* 1993;150 (11):4966–4977.
158. Stollar BD. Molecular analysis of anti-DNA antibodies. *FASEB J* 1994;8(3):337–342.
159. Radic MZ, Weigert M. Genetic and structural evidence for antigen selection of anti-DNA antibodies. *Annu Rev Immunol* 1994;12:487–520.
160. Tsao BP, Cantor RM, Kalunian KC, et al. Evidence for linkage of a candidate chromosome 1 region to human systemic lupus erythematosus. *J Clin Invest* 1997;99(4):725–731.
161. Griffing WL, Moore SB, Luthra HS, et al. Associations of antibodies to native DNA with HLA-DRw3. A possible major histocompatibility complex-linked human immune response gene. *J Exp Med* 1980;152(2 pt 2):319s-325s.
162. Ahearn JM, Provost TT, Dorsch CA, et al. Interrelationships of HLA-DR, MB, and MT phenotypes, autoantibody expression, and clinical features in systemic lupus erythematosus. *Arthritis Rheum* 1982;25(9):1031–1040.
163. Alvarellos A, Ahearn JM, Provost TT, et al. Relationships of HLA-DR and MT antigens to autoantibody expression in systemic lupus erythematosus [letter]. *Arthritis Rheum* 1983;26 (12):1533–1535.
164. Schur PH, Meyer I, Garovoy M, et al. Associations between systemic lupus erythematosus and the major histocompatibility complex: clinical and immunological considerations. *Clin Immunol Immunopathol* 1982;24(2):263–275.
165. Gu L, Weinreb A, Wang XP, et al. Genetic determinants of autoimmune disease and coronary vasculitis in the MRL-lpr/lpr mouse model of systemic lupus erythematosus. *J Immunol* 1998;161(12):6999–7006.
166. Theofilopoulos AN, Kono DH. The genes of systemic autoimmunity. *Proc Assoc Am Physicians* 1999;111(3):228–240.
167. Vyse TJ, Halterman RK, Rozzo SJ, et al. Control of separate pathogenic autoantibody responses marks MHC gene contributions to murine lupus. *Proc Natl Acad Sci USA* 1999;96(14):8098–8103.
168. Mohan C, Alas E, Morel L, et al. Genetic dissection of SLE pathogenesis. Sle1 on murine chromosome 1 leads to a selective loss of tolerance to H2A/H2B/DNA subnucleosomes. *J Clin Invest* 1998;101(6):1362–1372.
169. Mohan C, Morel L, Yang P, et al. Genetic dissection of lupus pathogenesis: a recipe for nephrophilic autoantibodies. *J Clin Invest* 1999;103(12):1685–1695.
170. Morel L, Mohan C, Yu Y, et al. Multiplex inheritance of component phenotypes in a murine model of lupus. *Mamm Genome* 1999;10(2):176–181.
171. Morel L, Croker BP, Blenman KR, et al. Genetic reconstitution of systemic lupus erythematosus immunopathology with polycongenic murine strains. *Proc Natl Acad Sci USA* 2000;97(12): 6670–6675.
172. Maldonado MA, Kakkanaiah V, MacDonald GC, et al. The role of environmental antigens in the spontaneous development of autoimmunity in MRL-lpr mice. *J Immunol* 1999;162(11): 6322–6330.
173. James JA, Kaufman KM, Farris AD, et al. An increased prevalence of Epstein-Barr virus infection in young patients suggests a possible etiology for systemic lupus erythematosus. *J Clin Invest* 1997;100(12):3019–3026.
174. Rekvig OP, Moens U, Sundsfjord A, et al. Experimental expression in mice and spontaneous expression in human SLE of polyomavirus T-antigen. A molecular basis for induction of antibodies to DNA and eukaryotic transcription factors. *J Clin Invest* 1997;99(8):2045–2054.
175. Bredholt G, Olaussen E, Moens U, et al. Linked production of antibodies to mammalian DNA and to human polyomavirus large T antigen: footprints of a common molecular and cellular process? [published erratum appears in *Arthritis Rheum* 2000;43(4):929]. *Arthritis Rheum* 1999;42(12):2583–2592.
176. Andreassen K, Bredholt G, Moens U, et al. T cell lines specific for polyomavirus T-antigen recognize T-antigen complexed with nucleosomes: a molecular basis for anti-DNA antibody production. *Eur J Immunol* 1999;29(9):2715–2728.
177. Richards HB, Satoh M, Jennette JC, et al. Disparate T cell requirements of two subsets of lupus-specific autoantibodies in pristane-treated mice. *Clin Exp Immunol* 1999;115(3): 547–553.
178. Taylor PR, Carugati A, Fadok VA, et al. A hierarchical role for classical pathway complement proteins in the clearance of apoptotic cells in vivo. *J Exp Med* 2000;192(3):359–366.
179. Bickerstaff MC, Botto M, Hutchinson WL, et al. Serum amyloid P component controls chromatin degradation and prevents antinuclear autoimmunity [see comments]. *Nat Med* 1999;5(6): 694–697.
180. Lu L, Kaliyaperumal A, Boumpas DT, et al. Major peptide autoepitopes for nucleosome-specific T cells of human lupus. *J Clin Invest* 1999;104(3):345–355.
181. Ebling FM, Tsao BP, Singh RR, et al. A peptide derived from an autoantibody can stimulate T cells in the (NZB x NZW)F1 mouse model of systemic lupus erythematosus. *Arthritis Rheum* 1993;36(3):355–364.
182. Singh RR, Kumar V, Ebling FM, et al. T cell determinants from autoantibodies to DNA can upregulate autoimmunity in murine systemic lupus erythematosus. *J Exp Med* 1995;181(6): 2017–2027.
183. Singh RR, Ebling FM, Sercarz EE, et al. Immune tolerance to autoantibody-derived peptides delays development of autoimmunity in murine lupus. *J Clin Invest* 1995;96(6):2990–2996.
184. Gaynor B, Putterman C, Valadon P, et al. Peptide inhibition of glomerular deposition of an anti-DNA antibody. *Proc Natl Acad Sci USA* 1997;94(5):1955–1960.
185. Putterman C, Deocharan B, Diamond B. Molecular analysis of the autoantibody response in peptide-induced autoimmunity. *J Immunol* 2000;164(5):2542–2549.
186. Brosh N, Dayan M, Fridkin M, et al. A peptide based on the CDR3 of an anti-DNA antibody of experimental SLE origin is also a dominant T-cell epitope in (NZB×NZW)F1 lupus-prone mice. *Immunol Lett* 2000;72(1):61–68.
187. Hahn B, Singh R, Wong W, et al. Treatment with a consensus peptide based on amino acid sequences in autoantibodies prevents T cell activation by autoantigens and delays disease onset in murine lupus. *Arthritis Rheum* 2001;44(2):432–441
188. Arbuckle MR, Gross T, Scofield RH, et al. Lupus humoral autoimmunity induced in a primate model by short peptide immunization. *J Invest Med* 1998;46(2):58–65.
189. Talal N. Disordered immunologic regulation and autoimmunity. *Transplant Rev* 1976;31:240–263.

190. Ando DG, Sercarz EE, Hahn BH. Mechanisms of T and B cell collaboration in the in vitro production of anti-DNA antibodies in the NZB/NZW F1 murine SLE model. *J Immunol* 1987; 138(10):3185–3190.
191. Wofsy D, Seaman WE. Successful treatment of autoimmunity in NZB/NZW F1 mice with monoclonal antibody to L3T4. *J Exp Med* 1985;161(2):378–391.
192. Wofsy D, Seaman WE. Reversal of advanced murine lupus in NZB/NZW F1 mice by treatment with monoclonal antibody to L3T4. *J Immunol* 1987;138(10):3247–3253.
193. Wofsy D. Administration of monoclonal anti-T cell antibodies retards murine lupus in BXSB mice. *J Immunol* 1986;136(12): 4554–4560.
194. Datta S, Patel H, Berry D. Induction of cationic shift in IgG anti-DNA autoantibodies. Role of T helper cells with classical and novel phenotype in three models of lupus nephritis. *J Exp Med* 1987;165:1252–1268.
195. Rajagopalan S, Mao C, Datta SK. Pathogenic autoantibody-inducing gamma/delta T helper cells from patients with lupus nephritis express unusual T cell receptors. *Clin Immunol Immunopathol* 1992;62(3):344–350.
196. Mao C, Osman GE, Adams S, et al. T cell receptor alpha-chain repertoire of pathogenic autoantibody-inducing T cells in lupus mice. *J Immunol* 1994;152(3):1462–1470.
197. Mohan C, Adams S, Stanik V, et al. Nucleosome: a major immunogen for pathogenic autoantibody-inducing T cells of lupus. *J Exp Med* 1993;177(5):1367–1381.
198. Singh RR, Hahn BH, Tsao BP, et al. Evidence for multiple mechanisms of polyclonal T cell activation in murine lupus. *J Clin Invest* 1998;102(10):1841–1849.
199. Fatenejad S, Mamula MJ, Craft J. Role of intermolecular/intrastructural B- and T-cell determinants in the diversification of autoantibodies to ribonucleoprotein particles. *Proc Natl Acad Sci USA* 1993;90(24):12010–12014.
200. Topfer F, Gordon T, McCluskey J. Intra- and intermolecular spreading of autoimmunity involving the nuclear self-antigens La (SS-B. and Ro (SS-A). *Proc Natl Acad Sci USA* 1995;92(3): 875–879.
201. Tsao B, Hahn B. Ig-transgenic mice as models for studying the regulation and role of anti-DNA antibodies in murine lupus. *Immunomethods* 1992;1:185–190.
202. Chen C, Prak EL, Weigert M. Editing disease-associated autoantibodies. *Immunity* 1997;6(1):97–105.
203. Mandik-Nayak L, Nayak S, Sokol C, et al. The origin of anti-nuclear antibodies in bcl-2 transgenic mice. *Int Immunol* 2000; 12(3):353–364.
204. Rathmell JC, Goodnow CC. Effects of the lpr mutation on elimination and inactivation of self- reactive B cells. *J Immunol* 1994;153(6):2831–2842.
205. Roark JH, Kuntz CL, Nguyen KA, et al. B cell selection and allelic exclusion of an anti-DNA Ig transgene in MRL-lpr/lpr mice. *J Immunol* 1995;154(9):4444–4455.
206. Brard F, Shannon M, Prak EL, et al. Somatic mutation and light chain rearrangement generate autoimmunity in anti-single-stranded DNA transgenic MRL/lpr mice. *J Exp Med* 1999;190 (5):691–704.
207. Hartley SB, Crosbie J, Brink R, et al. Elimination from peripheral lymphoid tissues of self-reactive B lymphocytes recognizing membrane-bound antigens. *Nature* 1991;353(6346):765–769.
208. Singh RR, Hahn BH, Sercarz EE. Neonatal peptide exposure can prime T cells and, upon subsequent immunization, induce their immune deviation: implications for antibody vs. T cell-mediated autoimmunity [see comments]. *J Exp Med* 1996;183 (4):1613–1621.
209. Shevach EM. Regulatory T cells in autoimmunity. *Annu Rev Immunol* 2000;18:423–449.
210. Williams WM, Isenberg DA. Naturally occurring anti-idiotypic antibodies reactive with anti-DNA antibodies in systemic lupus erythematosus. *Lupus* 1998;7(3):164–175.
211. Munns TW, Liszewski MK, Hahn BH. Antibody-nucleic acid complexes. Conformational and base specificities associated with spontaneously occurring poly- and monoclonal anti-DNA antibodies from autoimmune mice. *Biochemistry* 1984;23(13): 2964–2970.
212. Stollar BD, Zon G, Pastor RW. A recognition site on synthetic helical oligonucleotides for monoclonal anti-native DNA autoantibody. *Proc Natl Acad Sci USA* 1986;83(12): 4469–4473.
213. Pisetsky DS, Reich CF III. The binding of anti-DNA antibodies to phosphorothioate oligonucleotides in a solid phase immunoassay. *Mol Immunol* 1998;35(18):1161–1170.
214. Huck S, Deveaud E, Namane A, et al. Abnormal DNA methylation and deoxycytosine-deoxyguanine content in nucleosomes from lymphocytes undergoing apoptosis. *FASEB J* 1999;13 (11):1415–1422.
215. Koike T, Tomioka H, Kumagai A. Antibodies cross-reactive with DNA and cardiolipin in patients with systemic lupus erythematosus. *Clin Exp Immunol* 1982;50(2):298–302.
216. Izui S, Lambert PH, Fournie GJ, et al. Features of systemic lupus erythematosus in mice injected with bacterial lipopolysaccharides: identification of circulating DNA and renal localization of DNA-anti-DNA complexes. *J Exp Med* 1977;145(5): 1115–1130.
217. Krieg AM, Yi AK, Matson S, et al. CpG motifs in bacterial DNA trigger direct B-cell activation. Nature 1995;374(6522): 546–549.
218. Yung RL, Richardson BC. Role of T cell DNA methylation in lupus syndromes. *Lupus* 1994;3(6):487–491.
219. Desai DD, Krishnan MR, Swindle JT, et al. Antigen-specific induction of antibodies against native mammalian DNA in nonautoimmune mice. *J Immunol* 1993;151(3):1614–1626.
220. Hardin JA. The lupus autoantigens and the pathogenesis of systemic lupus erythematosus. *Arthritis Rheum* 1986;29(4): 457–460.
221. Sano H, Imokawa M, Steinberg AD, et al. Accumulation of guanine-cytosine-enriched low M.W. DNA fragments in lymphocytes of patients with systemic lupus erythematosus. *J Immunol* 1983;130(1):187–190.
222. Dang H, Ogawa N, Takei M, et al. Induction of lupus-associated autoantibodies by immunization with native and recombinant Ig polypeptides expressing a cross-reactive idiotype 4B4. *J Immunol* 1993;151(12):7260–7267.
223. James JA, Gross T, Scofield RH, et al. Immunoglobulin epitope spreading and autoimmune disease after peptide immunization: Sm B/B′-derived PPPGMRPP and PPPGIRGP induce spliceosome autoimmunity. *J Exp Med* 1995;181(2):453–461.
224. Zack DJ, Yamamoto K, Wong AL, et al. DNA mimics a self-protein that may be a target for some anti-DNA antibodies in systemic lupus erythematosus. *J Immunol* 1995;154(4):1987–1994.
225. Golan DT, Borel Y. Spontaneous increase of DNA turnover in murine systemic lupus erythematosus. *Eur J Immunol* 1983;13 (5):430–433.
226. Pancer LB, Milazzo MF, Morris VL, et al. Immunogenicity and characterization of supernatant DNA released by murine spleen cells. *J Immunol* 1981;127(1):98–104.
227. Emlen W, Mannik M. Effect of DNA size and strandedness on the in vivo clearance and organ localization of DNA. *Clin Exp Immunol* 1984;56(1):185–192.
228. Emlen W, Ansari R, Burdick G. DNA-anti-DNA immune complexes. Antibody protection of a discrete DNA fragment from DNase digestion in vitro. *J Clin Invest* 1984;74(1): 185–190.

229. Bennett RM, Kotzin BL, Merritt MJ. DNA receptor dysfunction in systemic lupus erythematosus and kindred disorders. Induction by anti-DNA antibodies, antihistone antibodies, and antireceptor antibodies. *J Exp Med* 1987;166(4):850–863.
230. Horgan C, Johnson RJ, Gauthier J, et al. Binding of double-stranded DNA to glomeruli of rats in vivo. *Arthritis Rheum* 1989;32(3):298–305.
231. Izui S, Lambert PH, Miescher PA. In vitro demonstration of a particular affinity of glomerular basement membrane and collagen for DNA. A possible basis for a local formation of DNA-anti-DNA complexes in systemic lupus erythematosus. *J Exp Med* 1976;144(2):428–443.
232. Napirei M, Karsunky H, Zevnik B, et al. Features of systemic lupus erythematosus in Dnase1-deficient mice. *Nat Genet* 2000;25(2):177–181.
233. Davis JC Jr, Manzi S, Yarboro C, et al. Recombinant human Dnase I (rhDNase) in patients with lupus nephritis. *Lupus* 1999;8(1):68–76.
234. Bruneau C, Benveniste J. Circulating DNA: anti-DNA complexes in systemic lupus erythematosus. Detection and characterization by ultracentrifugation. *J Clin Invest* 1979;64(1):191–198.
235. Fournie G. Circulating DNA and lupus nephritis (editorial review). *Kidney Int* 1988;33:487–497.
236. Taylor RP, Weber D, Broccoli AV, et al. Stability of DNA/anti-DNA complexes. *J Immunol* 1979;122(1):115–120.
237. Lennek R, Baldwin AS Jr, Waller SJ, et al. Studies of the physical biochemistry and complement-fixing properties of DNA/anti-DNA immune complexes. *J Immunol* 1981;127(2):602–608.
238. Frank MM, Hamburger MI, Lawley TJ, et al. Defective reticuloendothelial system Fc-receptor function in systemic lupus erythematosus. *N Engl J Med* 1979;300(10):518–523.
239. Wilson JG, Wong WW, Schur PH, et al. Mode of inheritance of decreased C3b receptors on erythrocytes of patients with systemic lupus erythematosus. *N Engl J Med* 1982;307(16):981–986.
240. Reichlin M. ANAs and antibodies to DNA: their use in clinical diagnosis. *Bull Rheum Dis* 1993;42(7):3–5.
241. Salmon JE, Millard S, Schachter LA, et al. Fc gamma RIIA alleles are heritable risk factors for lupus nephritis in African Americans. *J Clin Invest* 1996;97(5):1348–1354.
242. Haseley LA, Wisnieski JJ, Denburg MR, et al. Antibodies to C1q in systemic lupus erythematosus: characteristics and relation to Fc gamma RIIA alleles. *Kidney Int* 1997;52(5):1375–1380.
243. Wu J, Edberg JC, Redecha PB, et al. A novel polymorphism of FcgammaRIIIa (CD16. alters receptor function and predisposes to autoimmune disease. *J Clin Invest* 1997;100(5):1059–1070.
244. Smeenk R, Hylkema M. Detection of antibodies to DNA: a technical assessment. *Mol Biol Rep* 1992;17(1):71–79.
245. Smeenk RJ, van den Brink HG, Brinkman K, et al. Anti-dsDNA: choice of assay in relation to clinical value. *Rheumatol Int* 1991;11(3):101–107.
246. Tan EM, Smolen JS, McDougal JS, et al. A critical evaluation of enzyme immunoassays for detection of antinuclear autoantibodies of defined specificities. I. Precision, sensitivity, and specificity. *Arthritis Rheum* 1999;42(3):455–464.
247. Witte T, Hartung K, Matthias T, et al. Association of IgA anti-dsDNA antibodies with vasculitis and disease activity in systemic lupus erythematosus. SLE Study Group. *Rheumatol Int* 1998;18(2):63–69.
248. ter Borg EJ, Horst G, Hummel EJ, et al. Measurement of increases in anti-double-stranded DNA antibody levels as a predictor of disease exacerbation in systemic lupus erythematosus. A long-term, prospective study. *Arthritis Rheum* 1990;33(5):634–643.
249. Lim T, Nakamura N, Matsunaga T. Use of anion exchange resin-packed capillary column for rapid detection of anti-double-stranded DNA antibody in systemic lupus erythematosus serum. *Biotechnol Bioeng* 2000;68(5):571–575.
250. Lim T, Komoda Y, Nakamura N, et al. Automated detection of anti-double-stranded DNA antibody in systemic lupus erythematosus serum by flow immunoassay. *Anal Chem* 1999;71(7):1298–1302.
251. Weinstein A, Bordwell B, Stone B, et al. Antibodies to native DNA and serum complement (C3) levels. Application to diagnosis and classification of systemic lupus erythematosus. *Am J Med* 1983;74(2):206–216.
252. Tan EM, Cohen AS, Fries JF, et al. The 1982 revised criteria for the classification of systemic lupus erythematosus. *Arthritis Rheum* 1982;25(11):1271–1277.
253. Hochberg MC. Updating the American College of Rheumatology revised criteria for the classification of systemic lupus erythematosus [letter]. *Arthritis Rheum* 1997;40(9):1725.
254. Bootsma H, Spronk P, Derksen R, et al. Prevention of relapses in systemic lupus erythematosus. *Lancet* 1995;345(8965):1595–1599.
255. Esdaile JM, Abrahamowicz M, Joseph L, et al. Laboratory tests as predictors of disease exacerbations in systemic lupus erythematosus. Why some tests fail [see comments]. *Arthritis Rheum* 1996;39(3):370–378.
256. Petri M, Genovese M, Engle E, et al. Definition, incidence, and clinical description of flare in systemic lupus erythematosus. A prospective cohort study. *Arthritis Rheum* 1991;34(8):937–944.
257. Gladman DD, Urowitz MB, Keystone EC. Serologically active clinically quiescent systemic lupus erythematosus: a discordance between clinical and serologic features. *Am J Med* 1979;66(2):210–215.
258. Coutts SM, Plunkett ML, Iverson GM, et al. Pharmacological intervention in antibody mediated disease. *Lupus* 1996;5(2):158–159.
259. Jones DS, Barstad PA, Feild MJ, et al. Immunospecific reduction of antioligonucleotide antibody-forming cells with a tetrakis-oligonucleotide conjugate (LJP 394), a therapeutic candidate for the treatment of lupus nephritis. *J Med Chem* 1995;38(12):2138–2144.
260. Weisman MH, Bluestein HG, Berner CM, et al. Reduction in circulating dsDNA antibody titer after administration of LJP 394. *J Rheumatol* 1997;24(2):314–318.
261. Alarcon-Segovia D, Tumlin J, Furie R, et al. SLE trial shows fewer renal flares in LJP 394-treated patients with high-affinity antibodies to LJP 394: 90-05 trial results. *Arthritis Rheum* 2000;43:S272.
262. Gaubitz M, Seidel M, Kummer S, et al. Prospective randomized trial of two different immunoadsorbers in severe systemic lupus erythematosus. *J Autoimmun* 1998;11(5):495–501.
263. Koll RA. Ig-Therasorb immunoadsorption for selective removal of human immunoglobulins in diseases associated with pathogenic antibodies of all classes and IgG subclasses, immune complexes, and fragments of immunoglobulins. *Ther Apheresis* 1998;2(2):147–52.
264. Matsuki Y, Suzuki K, Kawakami M, et al. High-avidity anti-DNA antibody removal from the serum of systemic lupus erythematosus patients by adsorption using dextran sulfate cellulose columns. *J Clin Apheresis* 1996 11(1):30–5.

22

ANTIBODIES TO HISTONE AND THE ROLE OF THE NUCLEOSOME

MARVIN J. FRITZLER

HISTONES AND NUCLEOSOMES

In 1884, Albrecht Kossel isolated a basic, proteinaceous material from a water and ether lysate of goose erythrocyte nuclei (1). This material was called histone. Ten years later, Leon Lilienfeld described the extraction of calf thymocyte histones and suggested that histone was a highly basic protein, as evidenced by its solubility in acidic water. In 1908, the International Nomenclature Body listed histones as a class of proteins along with albumins and other proteins. In the following half-century, histones received little interest until 1950, when Stedman (2) compared the histone from a wide variety of species and suggested that it was not a homogeneous protein. The following year, paper chromatography was used to distinguish two classes of histones: the arginine-rich main histones, and the lysine-rich subsidiary histones (3). These findings sparked an increase in histone research, eventually leading to publication of the first primary structure of calf thymus histone 4 (H4) in 1968 (4) and pea embryo H4 in 1969 (5).

The renewed interest in the biochemistry and cell biology of histones in the 1950s and 1960s coincided with the description and popularization of the lupus erythematosus (LE) cell phenomenon and the LE cell test in systemic lupus erythematosus (SLE). Eventually, it became apparent that the LE cell formed *in vivo* (6), and the LE cell phenomenon, demonstrated *in vitro* (7,8), was dependent on the histone H1 and mediated by histone antibodies (9,10). In the next three decades, these observations were followed by a proliferation of observations that histones are targets of the immune response in SLE, drug-induced lupus (DIL), and other diseases (11–13) (Table 22.1).

The histones are the best understood of the structural proteins in the eukaryotic nucleus (14–17). Nonhistone chromosomal proteins (NHCPs), such as high mobility group proteins, low mobility group proteins, chromosome scaffold proteins, centromere proteins, and ubiquitin, are present in quantities of approximately 100 to 1,000 molecules per nucleus (14,18). In dramatic contrast, the mass of each histone is 60 million molecules per cell and is approximately equal to the cellular DNA content (14). However, attention to histones as autoantigens postdated extensive studies of DNA and other nonhistone autoantigens such as Sm and other proteins associated with small nuclear ribonucleoprotein (snRNP).

In 1974, the nomenclature of histones was agreed upon and is the one that is accepted today: histones H1, H2A, H2B, H3, and H4 (19). Based on their primary structure, the five types of histones can be divided into three main groups. Two of the three groups, referred to as the core or nucleosomal histones, are the slightly lysine-rich histones H2A and H2B and the arginine-rich histones H3 and H4 (Fig. 22.1). The third and least conserved group is the lysine-rich histones H1 and H1 variants. The amino acid sequences of all histone classes from a variety of plant and animal tissues have been determined. The high proportion of positively charged amino acids of these relatively small proteins helps them bind tightly to DNA. Because histones are tightly bound to DNA, they are believed to participate in the control of gene expression, cell division, and packaging of eukaryotic DNA. DNA in other cellular organelles (mitochondria, chloroplasts, kinetoplasts) is not complexed with histones.

The Nucleosome

If the DNA in a single nucleus were stretched out, it would span the nucleus thousands of times. Histones play a key role in packaging this DNA into a single nucleus in an orderly way (14,15). The packaging of DNA is complex because not all DNA is folded in the same way. The manner in which portions of DNA are uniquely folded in specific cells appears to influence gene activation.

The basic repeating structural subunit of eukaryotic chromatin is known as the nucleosome. Having the appearance of beads on a string in the electron microscope, the nucleosome consists of approximately 200 base pair (bp) of DNA helix wound around an octameric complex of two

TABLE 22.1. HUMAN DISEASES AND ANIMAL MODELS ASSOCIATED WITH HISTONE AUTOANTIBODIES

Disease	Frequency (%)	References
Rheumatic diseases		
SLE	24–95	12,13,109,111,134,135,137,138,152,154,156–162,210–212,236–239
DIL-procainamide	67–100	12,13,111,126,160,163,167,208,240,241
DIL-hydralazine	50–100	48,112,136,137
DIA	22–81	138,160,164,167,242–244
RA	0–80	68,152,178,184,186,208,218,220,245
Vasculitis	75	124,152,192
Felty's syndrome	79	187,218
JCA	42–75	47,175–183
MCTD/UCTD	90	125,152
Sjögren's syndrome	67	152
Scleroderma spectrum	20–67	170,171,198–205
Immune and infectious diseases		
Monoclonal gammopathy	14	190
Neoplasmic disease	79	208
HIV	N/A	97
Gastrointestinal diseases		
PBC	50–60	206,207
Hepatic cirrhosis	0–50	206,207
Ulcerative colitis	N/A	197
Animal models		
Murine lupus	25–80	103,114,173,246–249
Canine lupus	62–74	250,251
Murine graft-vs.-host	80	252,253
Avian scleroderma	12–20	254

DIA, drug-induced autoimmunity; DIL, drug-induced lupus; JCA, juvenile chronic arthritis; MCTD, mixed connective tissue disease; N/A, not available; PBC, primary biliary cirrhosis; RA, rheumatoid arthritis; UCTD, undifferentiated connective tissue disease.

molecules each of histones H2A, H2B, H3, and H4 (14,17,20,21) (Fig. 22.1). A tetrameric complex of two molecules each of H3 and H4 comprises the interior of the nucleosomal core particle (Fig. 22.1), and a dimer of H2A-H2B sits on each face of the nucleosome. The path that DNA takes around the nucleosome core reduces its length by 40-fold (14,17). Histone H1 is thought to occupy a position on the top of the nucleosome and may serve to bind the incoming and outgoing strands of DNA (Fig. 22.2). The amino terminal portions of the histones have high concentrations of positively charged amino acids and are particularly accessible to proteases such as trypsin and antibodies (17,22).

The Core Particles And Octameric Complex

Brief digestion of chromatin with micrococcal nuclease cleaves the linker DNA between nucleosomes and produces a characteristic "adder," when the material is fractionated by gel electrophoresis (14,23,24) (Fig. 22.1). This ladder is generated by chromatin fragments composed of discrete increments of nucleosomes (14). Thus, a monomeric fragment contains DNA of a single unit length (~200 bp); a dimeric fragment contains DNA twice the unit length (~400 bp), and so on. In addition to the DNA, each monomeric fragment consists of a molecule of H1 and two molecules of each core histone (14,23–25). Additional digestion of the nucleosome releases more DNA and H1, resulting in a structure referred to as the core particle. The core particle is made up of approximately 146 bp of DNA and an octamer containing two molecules of H2A, H2B, H3, and H4 (14,17).

When nucleosome core particles are suspended in 2 mol/L NaCl at neutral pH, the DNA is dissociated, leaving an octameric complex that contains two molecules of the core histones H2A, H2B, H3, and H4 (Fig. 22.1). In solutions of low ionic strength or nonneutral pH, the octamer dissociates further to form a tetramer of H3-H4 and two dimers of H2A-H2B, although some evidence indicates that this dissociation may not be straightforward (26).

Nonhistone Chromosomal Proteins

The mechanisms that are responsible for the dynamic process of chromatin condensation and decondensation are not entirely understood. While the interactions between DNA and histone result in a 40-fold shortening of the DNA, there is a further 250-fold shortening that must be accounted for as well. This additional compaction is

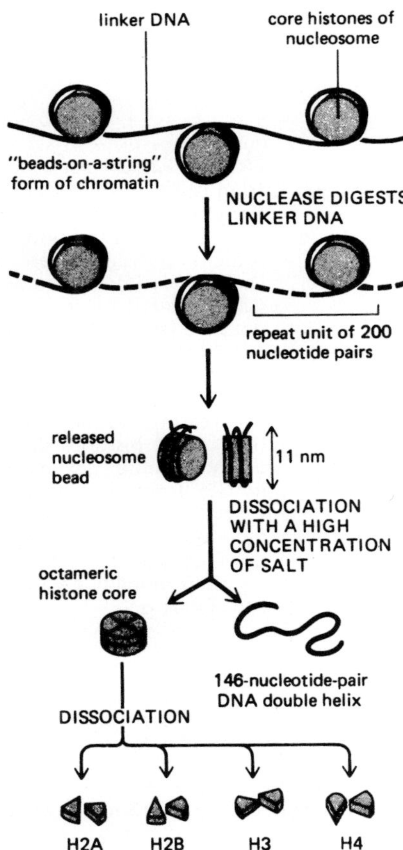

FIGURE 22.1. The structure of the nucleosome. The nucleosome consists of two full turns of DNA wound around a core of histones, plus adjacent linker DNA. The nucleosome bead can be released from chromatin by digestion of the linker DNA with micrococcal nuclease. In each nucleosome bead, approximately 146 nucleotide pairs of DNA remain wound around an octameric histone core. The histone core is composed of two each of histones H2A, H2B, H3, and H4. (From Chambon P, Elgin S, Felsenfeld G, et al. The cell nucleus. In: Alberts B, Bray D, Lewis J, et al., eds. *Molecular biology of the cell,* 2nd ed. New York: Garland, 1989:459–481, with permission.)

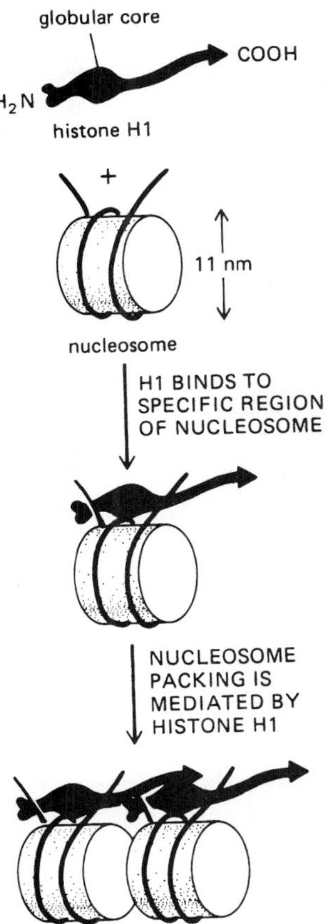

FIGURE 22.2. The structure and function of H1. H1 helps pack adjacent nucleosomes together. The globular core of H1 binds to each nucleosome near the site where the DNA helix enters and leaves the octameric complex. When H1 is removed, an extra 20 DNA nucleotide pairs are exposed and can be removed by micrococcal nuclease digestion. (From Chambon P, Elgin S, Felsenfeld G, et al. The cell nucleus. In: Alberts B, Bray D, Lewis J, et al., eds. *Molecular biology of the cell,* 2nd ed. New York: Garland, 1989:459–481, with permission.)

thought to be caused in large part by NHCPs that bind to chromatin at every 60 to 100 kilobase (kb) and anchor the loops of chromatin to their periphery (27). Some of these proteins have been identified as scaffold 1 (170 kd) and centromere proteins (CENPs) (27–31). Although many proteins play a role in chromatin condensation, the exact mechanisms leading to the initiation and termination of this dynamic process have yet to be determined. Even less information is available on the mechanisms leading to chromosome decondensation. One protein involved in this process is nucleolin (32,33); this protein, which has a highly acidic domain, displaces H1 from chromatin presumably by competing for H1 binding to DNA. Of interest, autoantibodies directed against nucleolin have been described in SLE and other rheumatic disease sera (34,35).

Histone H1 And Variants

Histone H1, which is the most variable of the histones, has an approximate molecular weight of 21.5 kd (Fig. 22.3) and has been found in all cells with the exception of yeast. H1 is a family of outer or linker histones (Fig. 22.2) that consists of H1, $H1^0$, H5, and other variants (14,36). The number of H1 variants can vary from tissue to tissue and from species to species (36,37). However, three major domains can be distinguished within the primary structure of all H1 variants: an amino terminal region that is highly basic, variable, and rich in alanine and proline; a central globular domain that is hydrophobic and nonvariable; and a carboxy terminal region that is highly basic and variable.

H1 is believed to stabilize the two complete turns of DNA in the nucleosome by binding at a point where the nucleic acid enters and leaves (14). This binding is essential

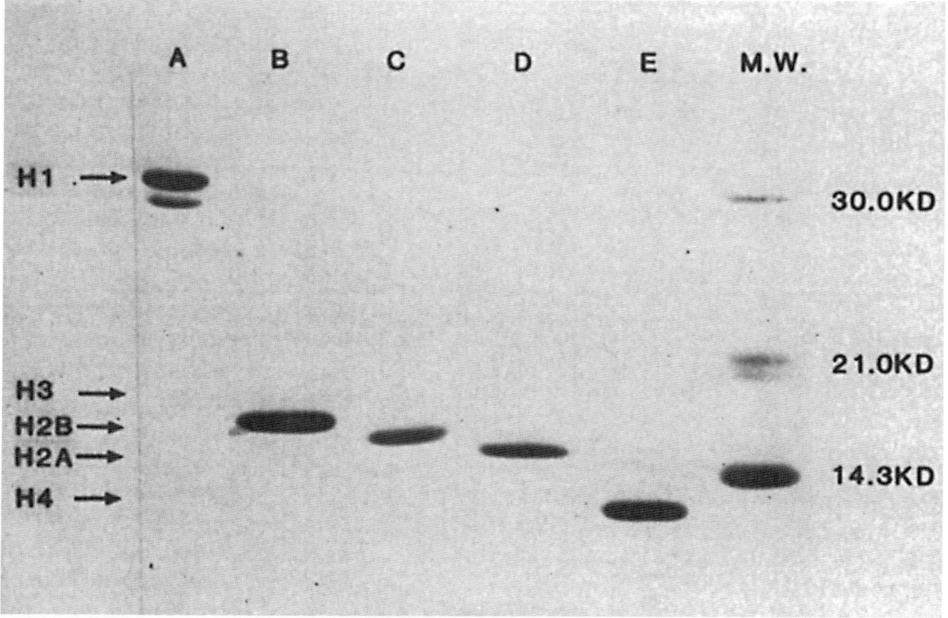

FIGURE 22.3. Histones extracted from calf thymus nuclei can be fractionated into the five main groups, as illustrated in this photograph of a sodium dodecyl sulfate (SDS) gel. Lane A: H1 [molecular weight ratio (M_r) = 33 kd] often represented as doublet; lane B: H3 (M_r = 18 kd); lane C: H2B (M_r = 17 kd); lane D: H2A (M_r = 15.5 kd); lane E: H4 (M_r = 13 kd); M.W., molecular weight markers. One reason why the relative mobility (M_r) of the histones differs in SDS–polyacrylamide gel electrophoresis (PAGE) from the actual molecular weights is that the basic amino acids, especially in H1, bind to SDS used in the electrophoresis, thereby retarding their mobility through the polyacrylamide gel.

for the formation of higher-order structures (15,17,38–41) (Fig. 22.2). Peptides from the globular and carboxy terminal domains of H1 have been shown to be just as effective as the intact protein in inducing higher-order structures (40). Because the globular domain of H1 alone cannot induce chromatin folding, the carboxy terminal domain of the molecule is believed to play a primary role in DNA packaging. Evidence suggests that the globular domain serves to locate H1 in the nucleosome at the point where the DNA strands leave the chromatosome, and that the carboxy terminal domain is necessary for stabilization of the fold (17).

Vertebrate species have from four to six different H1 subtypes that are derived from a set of primary amino acid sequence variants (36). The functional significance of having multiple subtypes is not fully understood, although it is speculated that they are responsible for the different transcriptional potentials of eukaryotic cells (17). The function of H1 can be better understood when examined in the context of its variants, $H1^0$ and H5. $H1^0$ is a mammalian protein that is present mainly in quiescent, nonreplicating cells, and there appears to be a direct correlation between the presence of $H1^0$ and the termination of cell division.

H5 is a variant of H1 and is present only in transcriptionally inactive cells of some species (42). At one time, H5 was thought to be present in mammals but it is most commonly associated with the nucleated erythrocytes of birds, reptiles, amphibians, and fish. H5 confers high stability and transcriptional inactivity to chromatin. Immunocytochemical studies have been used to identify interactions of H5 with structural and functional components of chromatin (43). H5 demonstrates limited sequence homology with an H1 subfraction from bovine thymus but extensive homology with the globular domain and terminal portion of the carboxy terminus of $H1^0$ (42,44). Therefore, observations of polyclonal and monoclonal antibodies directed against H5 (44–46) could be explained based on their cross-reactivity with $H1^0$.

Although H5 and $H1^0$ share sequence identity, it appears that not all reactivity with H5 can be accounted for by cross-reactivity with $H1^0$. In studies of SLE, DIL, and juvenile rheumatoid arthritis (JRA) sera where H5 reactivity was demonstrated, no reactivity with $H1^0$ was observed (Table 22.2) (47). Subsequent studies have suggested that SLE and DIL sera react with conformational epitopes on H5 domains on H5 (48). Therefore, in diseases like SLE, where conformational epitopes are the target of the autoantibody

TABLE 22.2. REACTIVITY OF HISTONE CLASSES WITH AUTOANTIBODIES FROM PATIENTS WITH SYSTEMIC RHEUMATIC DISEASES[a]

Disease	H2A-H2B/DNA	H1	H2B	H2A	H3	H4
SLE	5	5	4	2	1	1
PIL	10	5	4	2	1	1
HIL	4	1	3	2	5	5
JCA	1	5	2	1	1	1
RA	2	3	1	1	1	1
SSc	3	1	2	1	2	0

[a]Unit of reactivity are based on the least reaction assigned an arbitrary unit of 1 and the highest reactivity an arbitrary unit of 10. Data compiled and extracted from references in Table 22.1.
JCA, juvenile chronic arthritis; HIL, hydralazine-induced lupus; PIL, procainamide-induced lupus; RA, rheumatoid arthritis; SSc, systemic sclerosis.

response, comparison of sequences from closely related or widely divergent proteins may provide little meaningful information to explain cross-reactive antibodies.

Core Histones: H2A, H2B, H3, And H4

The slightly lysine-rich histones H2A and H2B have two domains that include an amino terminus made up of predominantly basic residues and a carboxy terminus that is rich in hydrophobic residues (49). Histones H2A and H2B have molecular weights of approximately 14 kd (Fig. 22.3) and are considered to be the most variable of the core histones (14,17). The arginine-rich histones H3 and H4 are the most highly conserved histones, and like H2A and H2B, they contain two domains: a basic amino terminal region, and a hydrophobic carboxy terminal region. Histones H3 and H4 have molecular weights of approximately 15 and 11 kd, respectively (Fig. 22.3), and they interact with each other to form an H3-H4 tetramer (Fig. 22.1) (14,17,49).

Like all eukaryotic gene messages, histone messenger RNAs are translated in the cytoplasm. After transport of newly synthesized histones across the nuclear membrane, they are combined with older histones into an octameric nucleosome (14,17). For example, newly synthesized histones H3 and H4 deposit as a tetramer and will associate only with old histones H2A and H2B. Similarly, newly synthesized histones H2A and H2B will deposit only as a dimer associated with old histones H2A, H2B, H3, and H4. During formation of the octamer, the core histones are deposited onto the DNA.

The role of core histones in stabilization of the nucleosome and the folding of chromatin is not clearly understood (14,17). One method that has been employed to analyze this role uses selective trypsinization and radiolabeling (50), and these studies have shown that after removal of the histone tails (generally the amino terminal regions of the core histones), stability of the nucleosome core particle was not affected (50). However, studies of the thermal stability of nucleosomes indicate that the amino terminal tails of H2B and H3 play a significant structural role (17,26).

POSTSYNTHETIC MODIFICATION OF HISTONES

Postsynthetic modifications of histones are important because they may be crucial in our understanding of the autoimmune responses that are directed against these proteins. For example, it is possible that drugs or other environmental agents that have been implicated in the pathogenesis of SLE trigger the induction of postsynthetic modifications of histones. As described earlier, all four core histones have randomly coiled, unstructured amino terminal tails and globular-structured carboxy terminal domains. The tails of the histones are of particular interest, because they include the dominant sites that undergo posttranslational modifications, which include ubiquitination, methylation, acetylation, phosphorylation, and adenosine diphosphate (ADP) ribosylation (17,49,51–54).

Acetylation

Acetylation occurs at specific lysine residues located in the amino terminal half of the core histones (53), and effectively neutralizes the positive charge of histones. This suggests that acetylation modulates the interaction of histone amino termini with the negatively charged DNA backbone, although acetylation alone does not change the structure or stability of nucleosomes (24). Increased acetylation of histones is correlated with transcriptional activity. Antibodies specific for acetylated histones also have been used to study acetylation in transcriptionally active chromatin.

Methylation

Methylation is a relatively stable modification and has been reported in all histones (49). Methylation occurs after DNA synthesis in the late S or G2 phase and after chromatin assembly, suggesting that this modification is not essential for the assembly of chromatin. On the other hand, methylation has been suggested to be important in chromatin condensation, other mitotic events, and gene transcription.

Phosphorylation

Unlike most other modifications, phosphorylation of histidine, lysine, serine, and threonine residues occurs in all of the histones (49). Phosphorylation, which reduces the net positive charge of the N-terminal region of the core histones and the N- and C-termini of H1, is thought to alter histone-DNA interaction (55). It is still not known whether the loosening of DNA-histone interaction after histone phosphorylation is sufficient to account for the enhanced template activity in DNA (55). The distribution and function of phosphorylated histone has been studied with antibodies that are highly specific for phosphorylated H1 (56).

Poly(ADP)Ribosylation

Poly(ADP)ribosylation is another important posttranslational modification of histones (57,58). The covalent addition of an ADP-ribose moiety of nicotinamide adenine dinucleotide (NAD) to proteins is catalyzed by poly(ADP)ribose polymerase (PADPRP) (54,59). The major acceptor proteins for poly(ADP)ribose are H1 and H2B, although ribosylation of H2A and H3 also have been reported. Modification by poly(ADP)ribosylation has been postulated to play a role in DNA replication, DNA repair, DNA amplification, cell differentiation, and apoptosis. Correlation of the rate and extent of poly(ADP)ribosylation with DNA repair activity and relaxation of chromatin structure has been experimentally confirmed (58,60). An increase in the activity of poly(ADP)ribose synthetase has also been correlated with the appearance of DNA strand breaks produced by nucleases and other agents (59). This is interesting in light of observations that metabolites of drugs that are associated with DIL induce extensive DNA strand breakage (61) and increase PADPRP activity in certain cells (62). In addition, ADP ribosylation, which essentially adds a ribose-phosphate moiety to acceptor proteins, may increase the immunogenicity of histones. Evidence supporting this is based on the observation that free histones are weakly immunogenic, but when coupled to ribose nucleic acids [i.e., transfer RNA (tRNA)] they are are highly immunogenic (63–65).

Ubiquitination

Ubiquitin, which is a protein of 76 amino acids found in all cells, has been shown to be bound to lysine 119 of H2A and lysine 120 of H2B (51). The major arrangement of ubiquitin in the polyubiquitinated histone H2A appears to be a chain of at least four ubiquitin molecules bound to the amino group of lysine 119 (66). Because ubiquitination in the cytoplasm is involved in controlled proteolysis, it is thought that ubiquitinated histones are involved in the same process (67). Ubiquitinated histones also may play a role in maintaining the structure of transcriptionally active chromatin. The observation that antibodies to ubiquitin and ubiquitinated histone are found in some SLE sera (51,68,69) provides supporting evidence for the concept that the nucleosome is an important immunogen in SLE.

Summary

The histones are small proteins with a large content of positively charged amino acids lysine and arginine. The histones may be divided into three groups based on their amino acid content. H1 is lysine rich and has the most interspecies amino acid sequence variability. H2A and H2B are slightly lysine rich and moderately conserved throughout evolution. H3 and H4 are arginine rich and are the most highly conserved of the histones. The fundamental subunit of chromatin is the nucleosome, which is composed of a core particle in which 146 bp of helical DNA are wrapped around an octamer of two H2A-H2B dimers that surround an H3-H4 tetramer. This complex of histones is surrounded by a third subunit composed of approximately two turns of double-stranded DNA (dsDNA). The structure of the nucleosome is sealed by a molecule of H1 that is able to associate with other H1 molecules on adjacent nucleosomes, forming a compact chromatin mass. The variable length of DNA between adjacent nucleosomes is referred to as linker DNA, and further compaction of the polynucleosome and compaction of the chromatin results in the familiar, higher-ordered structures known as chromosomes.

INDUCTION OF HISTONE AUTOANTIBODIES

The mechanisms that underlie the induction of histone antibodies are not clearly understood. Even when an inciting agent such as procainamide or hydralazine is identified, the events that lead to induction of histone antibodies are not clear. The immunogenicity of histones is remarkable considering that they are highly conserved among species.

A number of theories have been proposed to account for the origin of histone antibodies. It should be appreciated that none of these theories is independent, and features of each may result in the production of histone antibodies. The first theory is that environmental agents, drugs, or chemicals bind to endogenous macromolecules and alter their physical properties, causing them to become antigenic; in this model, the inciting agent may act as a hapten or a carrier. The second theory is that autoantibody production results from a process referred to as molecular mimicry. The third is that the autoantibody response to histone is generated and driven by endogenous nucleosomes. The fourth is that autoantibody production is primarily the outcome of an aberration in control of the immune network and cellular dysregulation.

Altered Antigen

The altered antigen hypothesis suggests that drugs or other environmental agents bind to nucleoprotein and then cause some portion of the macromolecule to become immunogenic or form an antibody recognition site (70). Details of this theory are discussed in Chapter 42.

Molecular Mimicry

Molecular mimicry can be defined as the products from dissimilar genes that share structural similarity or immune identity (71). For example, linear or conformational epitopes on macromolecules from different organisms (i.e., human and viral proteins or interspecies molecular mimicry) or from different cellular compartments (i.e., nucleus, cytoplasm, and cell surface or intraspecies molecular mimicry) that bear striking similarity can be said to demonstrate molecular mimicry. The macromolecules might be nucleic acids, proteins, glycoproteins, lipoproteins, or phospholipids. Similarities between proteins have been described based on immunologic reactions at the humoral or cellular level or by identifying similar amino acid sequences of antigens.

Molecular mimicry as a mechanism of inducing autoimmunity has been proposed by a number of authors (72–78). In the past, viruses and other microorganisms have been the favorite topic of research aimed at identifying the cause of autoimmune disease through the mechanism of interspecies molecular mimicry (72,75,78,79). Indeed, histones and histone-like proteins are found in yeast (80,81), bacteria (82–85), and viruses (86).

The conventional view of histones is that they are restricted to the nucleus, but as discussed earlier, histones are synthesized in the cytoplasm and transported to the nucleus, where they are assembled into nucleosomes. The stores of cytoplasmic histones are not large, and histone antibodies are not commonly associated with cytoplasmic staining by immunofluorescence (Fig. 22.4). There is evidence that certain nuclear and cytoplasmic structures share sequence similarity and antigenic reactivity with histones. For example, the centromeric protein CENP-A, which reacts with scleroderma sera (11,87), has been shown to share significant sequence and structural identity with H3 and macro-H2A (29,31,88). An H1-like molecule has been identified in the nuclear membrane (89), and human monoclonal histone antibodies, which react with cytoplasmic microfilaments (90) and antibodies to myeloperoxidase, which is a highly basic cytoplasmic protein, are seen with high frequency in the sera of hydralazine-induced lupus (91). Further, there is evidence that the cell surface of lymphocytes and other cells bear DNA and histones (92–96).

Although the prevailing concept is that molecular mimicry operates at the level of antigens in divergent species, it is equally possible that molecular mimicry may be related to similar proteins within a species (e.g., intraspecies molecular mimicry) (71). The features of histone and nucleosomal antigens described earlier support the concept of intracellular molecular mimicry, and these characteristics are illustrated by a number of other autoantigens, including DNA, Ro/SSA, To/Th, and others (71).

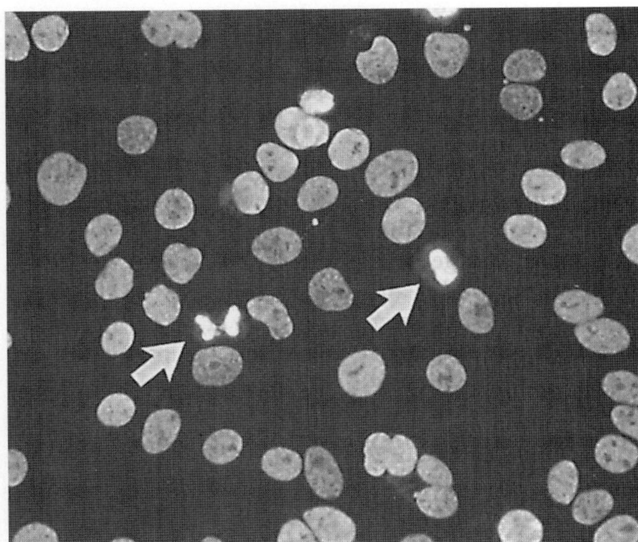

FIGURE 22.4. Indirect immunofluorescence (IIF) of autoantibodies from a patient with SLE produces a homogeneous pattern of nuclear staining on human epithelial (HEp-2) cells. Note that staining is particularly intense over chromosomes of dividing cells (*arrows*) and that the cytoplasm displays no detectable staining.

Knowledge about the role of viruses or other infectious agents in the induction of histone antibodies has not advanced rapidly. A few observations, however, are noteworthy. Histone antibodies have been described in patients with human immunodeficiency virus (HIV) (97) or mycobacterial (68) infections. A human polyomavirus containing dsDNA and host-cell histones, has been shown to terminate tolerance to dsDNA and histone antigens (98, 99). The reactivity of antibodies in this animal model was primarily directed toward virus structural proteins, dsDNA and single-stranded DNA (ssDNA), and H1 and H3. Although the autoantibody response was transient, it reappeared after a subsequent exposure to virus in one of the rabbits. These studies suggest that the anti-DNA and antihistone antibodies that are induced in this model are not a result of nonspecific polyclonal B-cell activation. Further, this model provides a convenient merging of the molecular mimicry and immune dysregulation theories.

In another animal model of viral-related histone antibody induction, rabbits infected with the rinderpest virus also developed anti-DNA and histone antibodies (100). The histone responses were directed predominantly toward H2A-H2B/DNA or H2B/DNA complexes in some rabbits. Because histone-reactive antibodies appeared in only some rabbits, these investigators suggested that the genetic background was a factor in the induction of the autoantibody response. More recently, it was demonstrated that termination of T-cell tolerance to histones could be achieved when histones were presented with polyoma T antigen complexed to nucleosomes (101).

Nucleosome-Driven Responses

There is compelling evidence that the genesis of the autoantibody response to histones and other nuclear antigens is initiated and driven by endogenous autoantigens (12,102). A study of the appearance of antichromatin antibodies in murine lupus suggested a T-cell–dependent immunization with chromatin (103), and nucleosomes were a major immunogen for pathogenic autoantibody-inducing T cells in lupus-prone mice (104). Other studies indicate that nucleosome-specific antibodies appeared earlier in murine models of SLE than antibodies to histones or DNA alone (105). Studies of the DNA circulating in SLE have concluded that it was of host origin, and its sensitivity to DNAse I but resistance to S1 nuclease suggested that it was dsDNA (106). Further, circulating DNA in the serum of patients with SLE was complexed to histones (107), and antihistone antibodies precipitated circulating DNA (106). The size of the DNA was approximately 120 to 200 bp, or roughly the size of DNA bound to core particles (24). The identification of autoantibodies that react with determinants present only on native DNA-histone complexes strongly supports the view that endogenous antigens (e.g., nucleosomes) play a role in the emergence of autoreactive antibodies (108), and this has led to the conclusion that the nucleosome has a central role in the genesis of histone autoantibodies (109).

The strong reactivity of DIL and SLE sera with the H2A-H2B/DNA complex, H1, and H2B compared with other histones is supporting evidence that nucleosomes, rather than free histones, act as immunogens in SLE or DIL (Table 22.2). In the intact nucleosome, H1, H2A, and H2B occupy particularly exposed external positions (14,17). In studies where the exposure of histones in native chromatin was measured by the adsorption of antibodies specific for individual histone by chromatin, it was shown that H1 and H2B were more available than H3 or H4 to interact with homologous antibody. Typically, free histones are weakly immunogenic, but when coupled to a nucleic acid, they are highly immunogenic (63,65,110). Immunization of rabbits with avian erythrocyte nucleosomes resulted in the production of antihistone antibodies, represented by the strongest response to H5 and followed in intensity by H2B, H2A, H3, and H4 (65). These observations are similar to the hierarchical binding activity of SLE, JRA, and DIL antibodies (Table 22.2) (47,111). However, whether the nucleosome itself or its digestion products were responsible for the antihistone antibodies is unclear.

The suggestion that the nucleosome is the immunogen in SLE and DIL is also supported by maps of the histones antigenic domains (discussed below). The domains have been localized to the extreme amino terminal segments of H2B and H4 and the amino and/or carboxy terminal ends of histone H3 and H2A (111,112). These domains are exposed on the nucleosomal structure, which would provide an appropriately exposed epitope to the immune system.

In addition to the evidence supporting the endogenous autoantigen-driven hypothesis, it is important to point out some difficulties with the nucleosome-driven concept and some possible resolutions. Earlier reference was made to observations that histone or histone-like proteins are located in multiple cellular compartments, including the cell surface of certain cells. Histone or histone-like proteins almost certainly are bound to DNA in these sites (113), and these observations suggest other pathways that might lead to a nucleosome-driven autoantibody response and provide some cause for reappraisal of the role of molecular mimicry. For one thing, these observations provide an alternative to the concept that the autoantigen is nuclear in origin, although there is ample means through the mechanism of apoptosis by which intracellular antigens are exposed to the immune system (see Chapter 8). The observation that some, and perhaps all, nuclear antigens are represented widely throughout intercellular and intracellular compartments gives support to the concept that molecular mimicry may operate at an intracellular rather than an interspecies level (71). An attractive part of this concept is that it may give more insight into the pathogenic role of autoantibodies, especially if nuclear proteins are represented or mimicked as cell surface or cytoplasmic structures with similar physiologic and functional properties. This raises the possibility that the pathophysiology of SLE includes the recognition of cell surface proteins by antinucleosomal antibodies, which can lead to an inflammatory response. The key questions that remains are: What triggers the response? And what breaks tolerance to nucleosomes?

Summary

There is compelling evidence to support the hypothesis that antihistone antibodies are driven by endogenous nucleosomes. It is not clear if components of the nucleosome, under the influence of drugs, toxic agents that are drug metabolites, environmental agents, or other factors, are able to break tolerance to this macromolecular complex. Less compelling evidence suggests that viruses or other infectious agents may initiate the loss of tolerance to the nucleosome, and through unknown mechanisms eventually lead to a prolonged autoantibody response to histones and other components of chromatin. The role of genetic factors and immune dysregulation is not discussed at length here, but the reader is referred to Chapters 5 to 18.

HISTONE ANTIBODY GENES

Antihistone antibodies can be found in all major immunoglobulin classes, but there is little agreement as to the predominant isotype. A clearer understanding of the origin and induction of histone autoantibodies may come from studies that identify the sequences of their variable (V) region genes. Earlier studies have indicated that some DNA antibodies, a common serologic feature of SLE, arise from unmutated germline genes, whereas others contain multiple somatic mutations (see Chapters 19 and 21). In a study of murine lupus it was shown that a specific locus on chromosome 1 (Sle1) leads to a selective loss of tolerance to H2A/H2B/DNA nucleosomes (114).

Reports of the nucleotide sequences of murine antihistone monoclonal antibodies demonstrated that these antibodies were not clonally related and that diverse V, D, and J genes were represented (115). Of interest, seven of the eight antibodies had VH segments encoded by genes from the J558 family. This is a remarkable finding, because J558 represents approximately 50 of the VH gene repertoire and is commonly used among autoantibodies of various specificities (116). The isoelectric points (pI) of two IgG histone antibodies ranged from 6.0 to 7.0. The second complementarity-determining region (CDR) of the VH gene of MRA12 (the most acidic and the strongest histone-reactive antibody) included only two positively charged, but five negatively charged, amino acid residues. This feature is unusual, because the CDR of most VH J558 genes is not composed predominantly of acidic residues. In a study of human monoclonal antihistone antibodies, similar physicochemical features were noted (117). A simplistic view of the role of these negatively charged residues is that they are responsible for binding to the basic region of histones. However, because the monoclonal MRA12 bound specifically to H1 and not other histones, factors other than charge-charge interactions likely are important for antibody specificity and binding.

The information that arises from the early studies of the V genes of histone antibodies bears remarkable resemblance to the studies of anti-DNA antibodies. For example, the anionic isoelectric points of the histone antibodies that react with H1 parallels observations that anionic antigens such as DNA elicit cationic anti-DNA antibodies (118–120). Also, the CDR sequence of the heavy chain of the histone monoclonal antibody MRA12 differed from an IgG1 antinitrophenyl antibody by only six amino acid residues (115); this observation is reminiscent of the report of a base substitution in the CDR of the antiphosphorylcholine antibody that resulted in DNA antibody-binding activity (121,122).

LABORATORY DETECTION OF HISTONE AUTOANTIBODIES

To appreciate data on the clinical and pathologic significance of histone autoantibodies, an understanding of the techniques and methods that are used to demonstrate them is important. In most clinical laboratories, an indirect immunofluorescence (IIF) assay is used as a screening test to identify antinuclear antibodies (ANAs) (123). In SLE most histone autoantibodies are detected by this screening test and are commonly correlated with a homogeneous or diffuse staining pattern (Fig. 22.4). However, the clinician should appreciate two exceptions to this generalization. First, the homogeneous or diffuse pattern also is seen with other autoantibodies, notably those directed against dsDNA (87). Second, sera that have antibodies to certain histone classes (e.g., H1, H3, H4) or hidden determinants (cryptotopes) on native or fixed histones may show only weak or negative ANAs (47,124–126). Therefore, the identification of histone antibodies must rely on more specific assays.

The seminal studies of Kunkel et al. (127) used a complement depletion assay to identify free histones as autoantigens. Many of the studies that followed continued to rely on unfractionated histones. A double immunodiffusion technique (128) and a complement fixation assay (129) demonstrated reactivity of SLE antibodies with unfractionated deoxyribonucleoprotein. These early investigations suggested that histone antibody titers in SLE fluctuated in concert with disease activity, were predominantly reactive with H1, but occurred infrequently and were of low titer (127,130,131). One explanation for these conclusions was that histones themselves demonstrated procomplementary activity (132).

The lack of sensitivity of the complement fixation assays used in the early studies of histone autoantibodies led to a general lack of interest in histone antibodies until Tan et al. (133) modified an IIF assay to demonstrate them. This assay, which used cryopreserved sections of rodent kidney as substrate, employed dilute acid to extract histones and other proteins from the nuclei. Purified histones then could be reconstituted onto the retained nuclear DNA by incubating the acid-extracted substrate in solubilized histones. Conventional IIF was then used to demonstrate histone reactivity. For example, sera containing antihistone antibodies demonstrated positive staining on untreated and reconstituted sections but not on acid-extracted sections. By comparison, sera that contained antibodies to dsDNA were positive on the untreated, the acid-extracted, and the reconstituted sections. This assay was used to demonstrate that high titers of histone antibodies are found in patients with SLE (134,135) and procainamide-induced lupus (135). It later became clear that this assay had limitations, because it detected primarily antibodies to H2A, H2B, and H2A-H2B complexes. Sera containing antibodies to H1, H3, or H4 are relatively nonreactive with reconstituted histone substrates, because these proteins are not adequately reconstituted under the experimental conditions of this assay (112,126,136,137).

In the years following introduction of the extraction-reconstitution assay, solid-phase assays became the predominant method for demonstrating histone antibodies. The most popular techniques have remained enzyme-linked immunosorbent assays (ELISAs) (12,103,109). These assays are relatively easy to establish because purified histone, histone complexes, and chromatin components are easily adsorbed to the polystyrene. Enzyme-conjugated, class-specific antibodies are then used to provide a quantitative and qualitative analysis of antihistone reactivity. Western blotting (i.e., immunoblotting) assays followed the ELISA techniques (111,138) (Fig. 22.3). These techniques have required substantial refinement because of the highly cationic nature of histones and their propensity to bind a variety of proteins, most notably C-reactive protein and α_2-macroglobulin (63,139–144). In addition, it is not clear if all epitopes are available for binding after the proteins are blotted, because higher-order structures may be altered after the denaturing treatment used to prepare proteins for electrophoresis (145–147). However, some evidence has suggested that secondary structures may be restored when histones and other proteins are transferred to the nitrocellulose paper used in the immunoblotting experiments (148–150).

Despite these advances in histone antibody assays, certain technical problems remain. Discrepancies reported in the frequency and titers of histone antibodies within disease groups likely are related to a number of factors, including the selection of sera, diagnostic criteria, ethnic or regional variation, purity of antigen preparations, and prescribed therapeutic agents, all providing an important source for intraobserver variation. As described earlier, the protocols that are employed to detect histone antibodies are primary among these factors.

Another significant variable is the use of different secondary antibodies as detecting reagents. Some studies have used polyvalent antisera, others immunoglobulin class-specific reagents, and still others protein A. The potential discordant results with protein A are important, because it does not bind to all immunoglobulin molecules with equal avidity.

Other technical concerns include the effect of histone denaturation on antigenicity, the solubility of histones and nucleohistones in biologic fluids, and the susceptibility of purified histones to degradation by serum proteases during the performance of assays (142). Differences in procedures to determine the cutoff between normal and pathologic sera likely are another variable that accounts for intralaboratory variation. Most studies also have used histones prepared from calf thymus, chicken erythrocytes, and other animal sources; ideally, human histones should be used for studies of true histone autoantibodies.

Despite these concerns and variables, there is remarkably good agreement on the frequency of histone antibodies in systemic rheumatic diseases. As with many other areas in clinical medicine, attempts to standardize these variables through interinstitutional collaboration are a mandate of the ANA Subcommittee of the International Union of Immunological Societies. For a thorough discussion of histone antibodies, refer to reviews published elsewhere on the subject (12,13,151).

DISEASES AND ANIMAL MODELS ASSOCIATED WITH HISTONE AUTOANTIBODIES

SLE

Histone antibodies have been found in 24% to 95% of patients with SLE (Table 22.1), and these antibodies are directed against all classes of histones, particularly H1 and H2B (12,111,136,151,152). In some studies, H1 (136,153) or H2B (68) did not show predominant reactivity, whereas H3 did (152–154). As discussed earlier, there are a number of reasons for these interobserver differences.

The correlation of clinical features and disease activity with histone antibody titers or classes is not clearly established. When sera from SLE patients with monospecific histone antibodies (i.e., absence of dsDNA and other nuclear antibodies) were compared to those having other ANAs, it was found that the former have a higher frequency of joint disease and a lower incidence of renal disease, central nervous system disease, alopecia, anemia, and hypocomplemententemia (134). Some reports have suggested a correlation of histone antibodies with SLE activity (68,129,155,156), skin and/or joint involvement (155, 157), renal disease (158), and neuropsychiatric manifestations of SLE (159). Other studies attempting to correlate histone antibodies with specific clinical symptoms or disease activity have not shown any clear-cut associations (68,134,152,160–162). Muller et al. (68) observed a correlation of disease activity with antibodies to the core histones but not with H1; also of interest, an inverse correlation of disease activity and antiubiquitin antibodies was observed in the same study.

Drug-Induced Lupus And Drug-Induced Autoimmunity

Histone antibodies have been reported in 67% to 100% of patients with DIL (12) (Table 22.1). The drugs most commonly implicated in DIL include procainamide, hydralazine, quinidine, and isoniazid, although a variety of other drugs have been implicated as well (see Chapter 42). DIL is characterized by the presence of IgG antibodies to H2AH2B/DNA complexes (163,164). This profile is distinguished from that observed in SLE, because antibodies to dsDNA, Sm, U1-RNP, Ro/SSA, La/SSB antigens, and others that are characteristic of the autoimmune state typically are absent in DIL (87).

Patients who are treated with procainamide eventually develop antihistone antibodies, but symptomatic disease occurs in only 10% to 20% (165). Thus, most antihistone antibodies are apparently benign, and examination of their class and fine specificity has revealed that antihistone antibodies in asymptomatic patients are predominantly immunoglobulin M (IgM) and display broad reactivity with all the individual histones (136,166,167). In contrast, patients with symptomatic procainamide-induced lupus develop predominantly IgG antihistone antibodies that, rather than reacting predominantly with individual histones, displays pronounced reactivity with a H2A-H2B complex (126,163,164,166,168,169). Antibodies to this complex have a high (>90%) sensitivity and specificity for symptomatic procainamide-induced lupus compared to asymptomatic patients, and an even higher specificity when an H2A-H2B/DNA complex is used as the antigen (163,164,169). Antibodies to the H2A-H2B complexes are remarkable, because they appear to be a feature of the immune response in SLE (170), other DIL syndromes (169), the scleroderma spectrum of diseases (170,171), and murine (172,173) as well as canine (174) models of SLE. Chapter 42 provides a comprehensive review of the reactivity of histone antibodies in DIL.

Juvenile Chronic Arthritis

The presence of antihistone antibodies has been thoroughly studied in juvenile chronic arthritis (JCA) (47,175–182). Most studies agree that histone antibodies are found in more than 40% of JCA sera, are predominantly IgM, and are most commonly directed against H1 and H3 (Table 22.1). In early studies, when the acid extraction-reconstitution technique was used, JCA sera were found to bind histones infrequently (183). Other studies using immunoblot techniques demonstrated that the predominant reactivity of JCA sera was with a 33-kd doublet thought to be H1 (175). Weaker reactivity to lower molecular weight bands was attributed to antibodies binding the core histones. A study using ELISA for the detection of antibodies to only the core histones reported that the overall frequency of antibodies to histones in JRA was 44%, and that 62% of the sera bound to the amino terminus of H3. An interesting observation in this study was that not all sera that bound the 1 to 21 residues of H3 demonstrated reactivity to the intact histones.

The studies of histone antibodies in JCA were of interest because of their potential to aid in the subclassification of this disease. Histone antibodies have been reported in 67% to 93% of patients with JCA and uveitis (47,175,176), compared to 33% of patients without uveitis (177). However, either a weak or no association with uveitis was observed in other studies (175,178,182). When other clinical subsets were compared, histone antibodies tended to be more common in the pauci- or polyarticular subset than in the systemic onset (i.e., Still's disease) subset (47,175). Although the association of antihistone antibodies with HLA-A2 created optimism that histone antibodies might identify a subset of patients with JCA, the evidence of earlier studies as well as a thorough subsequent study (182) do not favor an association of histone antibodies, of any specificity, with patterns of disease onset or the course of disease.

Rheumatoid Arthritis

The frequency of histone antibodies in rheumatoid arthritis (RA) has been reported to be as high as 80%. One of the first studies, by Aitcheson et al. (184), found that 14% of unselected patients with RA and 24% of patients with RA and a positive ANA had histone antibodies as demonstrated by the extraction-reconstitution assay. Other studies have reported similar frequencies in unselected patients with RA (Table 22.1) but higher frequencies in patients with RA and a positive ANA (185,186). Unlike patients with SLE and DIL, the titer of histone antibodies tends to be low.

Felty's Syndrome

Campion et al. (187) reported histone antibodies in the sera of 20 of 32 patients (63%) with Felty's syndrome. The frequency of antihistone antibodies in this study was compared to 12% frequency in RA and the 54% frequency in SLE. The antibodies in this syndrome appear to be directed against conformational histone determinants, because reactivity was lost when the histones were denatured in detergent. The high frequency of histone antibodies in Felty's syndrome is of interest because they commonly have high levels of rheumatoid factor, an autoantibody believed to cross-react with histones (184,188), especially H3 (185).

Glomerulonephritis

Goshen et al. (189) reported histone antibodies in 17% of patients with IgA nephropathy, 11% with mesangiocapillary glomerulonephritis, and 20% with membranoproliferative glomerulonephritis. Because the study populations were small, the incidence of histone antibodies in these diseases did not reach statistical significance even though the normal control population had no histone antibodies at all.

Monoclonal Gammopathies

In a study of 249 patients with monoclonal gammopathies, Shoenfeld et al. (190) found that 34 (13.7%) were positive for histone antibodies. When monoclonal antibodies were purified from 12 sera, all but one demonstrated antihistone activity. The observation that most of these antibodies also demonstrated anti-DNA activity, as measured by the *Crithidia luciliae* assay, raises the interesting possibility that these antibodies may have similar reactivity as monoclonal antibodies isolated from murine lupus (173).

Vasculitides

Antibodies to histones have been reported in 75% of patients with RA and vasculitis (152), and antibodies to H2B have been reported in a man with vasculitis (124). These reports are of interest because both vasculitis (191,192) and SLE (193–196) have been associated with the presence of myeloperoxidase antibodies and, like histones, myeloperoxidase is a highly basic (pI >11) protein. This raises the possibility that myeloperoxidase antibodies cross-react with histone, and vice versa. Evidence supporting this notion is based on observations that antibodies to neutrophil myeloperoxidase, which is one of the antigens in the neutrophil cytoplasm recognized by antineutrophil antibodies, are found in patients on hydralazine (91,194), a syndrome (i.e., hydralazine-induced lupus syndrome) that is characterized by histone antibodies. More recently, it was reported that anti-H1 antibodies that react with a PKKAK motif predominate in peripheral antineutophil cytoplasmic antibody (pANCA)-positive ulcerative colitis patients (197).

Scleroderma Spectrum Of Diseases

Antibodies to histones are found in 20% to 67% of sera from the scleroderma spectrum of diseases (170,171,

198–205). In one study, the reactivity of the scleroderma spectrum of diseases was relatively restricted to H2A-H2B/DNA (170,205) in 62% of patients. Of particular interest, patients with localized scleroderma appear to have a particularly high frequency of antihistone reactivity (170,203,204), and other reports have demonstrated that sera from patients with localized scleroderma had antibodies directed against H1 and H3 (171,200). Reports suggesting that patients with scleroderma who have concomitant histone antibodies have a higher frequency of pulmonary fibrosis (202), a more severe form of the disease, and a poor clinical outcome (201) have not been substantiated in another study (203). As in studies of SLE and JCA, reasons for these differences likely are related to patient selection and technical aspects of the antihistone assays.

Other Diseases

Histone antibodies have been reported in other diseases, including primary biliary cirrhosis and other chronic liver disease (206,207), Sjögren's syndrome (152), and patients with neoplastic disease selected based on the basis of a positive ANA (208). In a recent study of 46 polymyositis/dermatomyositis patients, 17% were found to have antihistone antibodies (209). In this study the predominant reactivity was with H1.

Summary

Numerous studies have conclusively shown that antibodies to all classes of mammalian histones, H1, H2A, H2B, H3, and H4, are predominantly, but not exclusively, present in SLE and DIL (Table 22.1). Studies of the clinical correlates of histone antibodies suggest several conclusions. First, antihistone antibodies are not a specific marker for a single disease. However, the determination of histone reactivity, especially IgG antibodies to H2A-H2B/DNA complexes, can be used as a distinguishing feature of DIL. Second, the presence of histone antibodies likely is not correlated with disease activity.

HISTONE DETERMINANTS AND EPITOPES

Investigation of the histone epitopes that are reactive with SLE and DIL autoantibodies has been undertaken by a number of investigators, and there is general agreement that SLE and DIL antibodies bind to all classes of intact histone, with H1 being the most reactive and H4 the least (111,210). The epitope mapping studies have used peptides derived from the enzymatic and chemical cleavage of core histones. By using this approach, it can be concluded that most DIL and SLE sera bind to determinants in the amino and carboxyl termini but not to those in the central hydrophobic domain (111,137,147,211) (Fig. 22.5). For example, the reactive epitope of H2B lies within peptides 1 to 20 (137,210). Although similar analyses have provided a less clear picture of H2A, the evidence suggests that the epitopes are present in peptides 1 to 11 and 119 to 129. When viewed in the context of intact chromatin, the epitopes on H2A and H2B are in relatively exposed areas of the nucleosome (14,22). Epitopes on H3 were mapped

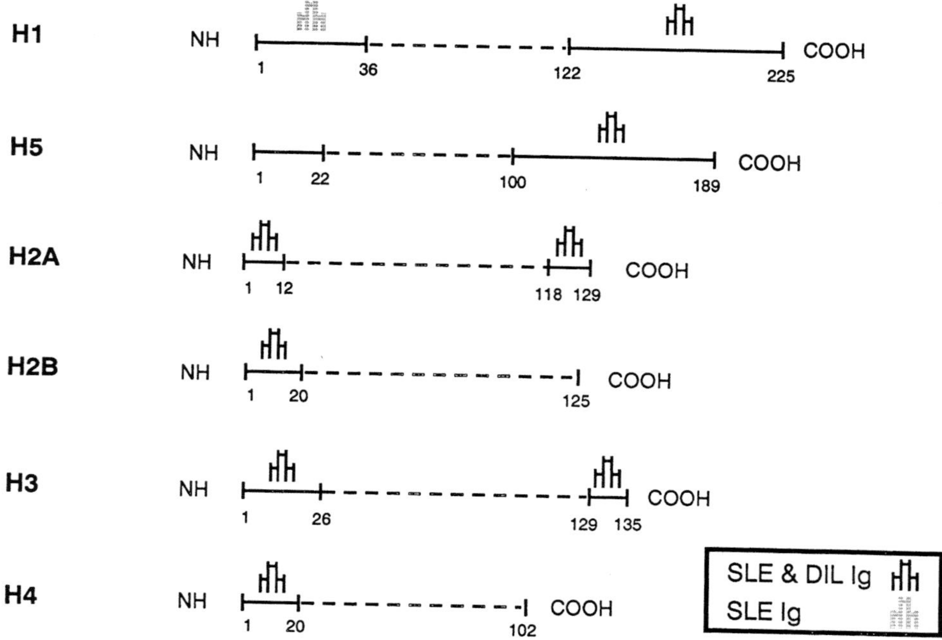

FIGURE 22.5. Histone domains bound by SLE and drug-induced lupus (DIL) antibodies.

to amino terminal residues 1 to 26 and the carboxy terminal 6 amino acids, whereas residues 1 to 29 of H4 were the most reactive (111,112,137,178,210). Last, the epitopes on H1 and H5 are localized in last 15 to 80 carboxy terminal residues (48,147,210,211,212), and some studies have demonstrated significant reactivity with H1 and H5 amino terminal peptides (48,147,155). A conclusion from many of these studies is that the histone epitopes reacting with DIL sera are no less restricted than those reacting with SLE sera.

More recently the histone epitopes reacting with murine and human T cells have been characterized (213,214). In the murine Medical Research Laboratory lymphoproliferative (MRL/*lpr*) model, analysis of peptides bound to I-A^k and I-E^k showed that a peptide homologous to a portion of H2A representing amino acids 84 to 104, (HLQLAIRDEELNKLLGKVT), bore an appropriate motif necessary for I-E^k binding (213). Another conclusion of this study is that H2A may serve as a donor of peptides that represent potential epitopes for autoreactive T cells. H2A, a component of the nucleosomes, can provide epitopes that serve as cognate T-cell determinants for autoantibodies to other histones and even to DNA.

In the study of human T cell epitopes, peptides 10 to 33 of H2B, 16 to 39, 49 to 63, and 71 to 94 of H4, 91 to 105 of H3, and 49 to 63 of H2A are among the immunodominant epitopes (214). All these autoepitopes had multiple human leukocyte antigen (HLA)-DR binding motifs, and the epitopes were generally located in histone regions recognized by autoantibodies, suggesting their immunodominance. In addition, native nucleosomes and peptides 16 to 39 and 71 to 94 of H4 and 91 to 105 of H3 demonstrated an enhanced interferon-γ response, whereas peptides 34 to 48 of H2A favored an interleukin-10 (IL-10) and/or IL-4 response.

The results summarized here are a simplification of a large body of data in which discrepancies do exist. As with the assays for histone antibodies themselves, the reactivity with histone epitopes is fraught with similar limitations and interobserver variability. The significance and limitations of epitope mapping studies in relation to the etiology and pathogenesis of SLE is discussed below. However, a model of histone autoantibody production that emerges from these and related studies is that nucleosomes are taken into B cells by virtue of reactivity of the DNA-specific Ig receptor of the autoreactive B cell. The nucleosomes are then processed and peptides derived from histones are bound and presented by major histocompatibility complex (MHC) class II molecules of the B cell (104). The autoreactive $CD4^+$ T cell then interacts with the peptide–class II complex and delivers the helper signals that stimulate B cells to proliferate and differentiate into different populations of plasma cells that secrete autoantibodies to various components of the nucleosomes, including dsDNA (213).

HISTONES AND THE LE CELL

The relationship between antibodies to histones and SLE is of interest, because most evidence suggests that the binding of histone autoantibodies to histones is responsible for the LE cell phenomenon (8,10,11,215). A central role for histones was suggested when Holman and Kunkel (216), and then Holborow and Weir (217), demonstrated abrogation of the LE cell phenomenon after histones were replaced by protamine. In addition, the LE cell factor and certain ANAs were absorbed by DNAse-digested deoxyribonucleoprotein (DNP) (8). These early studies implied that DNP antibodies were directed against DNA-histone complexes and that this reactivity was responsible for the LE cell phenomenon. Additional evidence for the accuracy of these observations was provided by Hannestad et al. (215), who demonstrated that histones were responsible for the LE cell phenomenon. More recently, it has been conclusively shown that H1 is the primary histone involved in this phenomenon (10,11). These observations have been substantiated by clinical observations, because LE cells and histone antibodies have been associated with other diseases such as DIL (see Chapter 42) and rheumatoid arthritis (184,186,218).

ARE HISTONE AND NUCLEOSOME AUTOANTIBODIES PATHOGENIC?

The deposition of immune complexes and activation of a wide range of mediators, including complement, in target organs has been implicated as one of the primary mechanisms of tissue inflammation and injury in SLE (see Chapters 12 through 14). A key historical concept in the development of lupus nephritis has centered on a pathogenic role for anti-dsDNA and anti-dsDNA–DNA complexes (219). More recent evidence has suggested a key role for histones, nucleosomes, and their cognate autoantibodies. This attention was inevitable because of the following observations.

Nucleosomes are an immunogen for T cells (104) and stimulate a proliferative response in B cells (113), thus resulting in the formation of pathogenic antibodies (104). Histones most likely are bound to circulating DNA and are present in circulating anti-DNA–DNA complexes (107). Histone antibodies commonly coexist with antibodies to dsDNA (158,161,220), and specific epitopes are found on histone-DNA complexes (105,108,173). In autoimmune MRL and New Zealand black (NZB) mice, the autoantibody response is first directed against histones, whereas later in the disease anti-DNA antibodies appear (103,221). Experimental models suggested that DNA is rapidly cleared and broken down in the circulation, making it unlikely that intact DNA can persist long enough to bind antibody (106,222–224). Although DNA antibodies can bind to glomerular antigens (225), histones appear to be an important component in the binding of DNA antibodies (225), and anti-DNA–nucleosome complexes to certain cells (92,93) and to the glomerular basement membrane (140,226–230).

These observations have led to the postulate that histone-DNA–anti-DNA complexes bind to histones that are preferentially bound in the glomerulus. This is supported by studies showing that the binding of anti-DNA antibodies to glomerular basement membranes is enhanced by the sequential perfusion of purified histones and then DNA (225). By comparison, anti-DNA antibodies perfused in the absence of histone tend to localize in the mesangium. It has been suggested that DNA antibodies bind to two different glomerular structures, the glomerular capillary wall and the mesangium, both areas in which immune deposits are found in SLE (225). Based on some studies, glomerular heparan sulfate is a candidate ligand for histones (140,227,231,232), and the origin of nucleosomes, DNA, and histone DNA that participate in these pathogenic processes could be nuclear material released during apoptosis (113,233–235). For a review of the role of apoptosis in the pathophysiology of SLE, see to Chapter 8.

REFERENCES

1. Doenecke D, Karlson P. Albrecht Kossel and the discovery of histones. *Trends Biochem Sci* 1984;9:404–405.
2. Stedman E. Cell specificity of histones. *Nature* 1950;166: 780–781.
3. Stedman E. The basic proteins of cell nuclei. *Philos Trans R Soc Lond [Biol]* 1951;235:565–566.
4. DeLange RJ, Smith EL, Fambrough DM, et al. Amino acid sequence of histone IV: presence of epsilon-N-acetyllysine. *Proc Natl Acad Sci USA* 1968;61:1145–1146.
5. DeLange RJ, Fambrough DM, Smith EL, et al. Calf and pea histone IV. III. Complete amino acid sequence of pea seedling histone IV: comparison with homologous calf thymus histone. *J Biol Chem* 1969;244:5669–5697.
6. Hargraves MM, Richmond H, Morton R. Presentation of two bone marrow elements: the tart cells and the L.E. cell. *Mayo Clin Proc* 1948;27:25–28.
7. Hamburger RN. Induction of the lupus erythematosus (L.E.) cell in vitro in peripheral blood. *Yale J Biol Med* 1950;407–410.
8. Holman R, Deicher HR. The reaction of the lupus erythematosus (L.E.) cell factor with deoxyribonucleoprotein of the cell nucleus. *J Clin Invest* 1959;38:2059–2072.
9. Friou GJ. Identification of the nuclear component of the interaction of lupus erythematosus globulin and nuclei. *J Immunol* 1958;80:476–481.
10. Schett G, Steiner G, Smolen JS. Nuclear antigen histone H1 is primarily involved in lupus erythematosus cell formation. *Arthritis Rheum* 1998;41:1446–1455.
11. Schett G, Rubin RL, Steiner G, et al. The lupus erythematosus cell phenomenon: comparative analysis of anti-chromatin antibody specificity in lupus erythematosus cell-positive and -negative sera. *Arthritis Rheum* 2000;43:420–428.
12. Burlingame RW. The clinical utility of antihistone antibodies. Autoantibodies reactive with chromatin in systemic lupus erythematosus and drug-induced lupus. *Clin Lab Med* 1997;17: 367–378.
13. Shen GQ, Shoenfeld Y, Peter JB. Anti-DNA, anti-histone and antinucleosome antibodies in systemic lupus erythematosus and drug-induced lupus. *Clin Rev Allergy Immunol* 1998;16: 321–334.
14. Lewin B. Nucleosomes. In: Lewin B, ed. *Genes*, 7th ed. New York: Oxford University Press, 2000:567–615.
15. Bray B, Lewis J, Raff M, et al., eds. *Molecular biology of the cell*, 3rd ed. New York: Garland, 1994:342–354.
16. Workman JL, Buchman AR. Multiple functions of nucleosomes and regulatory factors in transcription. *Trends Biochem Sci* 1993;18:90–95.
17. Zlatanova J. Histone H1 and the regulation of transcription of eukaryotic genes. *Trends Biochem Sci* 1995;15:273–276.
18. Wiland E, Siemieniako B, Trzeciak WH. Binding of low mobility group protein from rat liver chromatin with histones studied by chemical cross-linking. *Biochem Biophys Res Commun* 1990; 166:11–21.
19. Bradbury EM. *The structure and function of chromatin*. Amsterdam: Associated Scientific, 1975:14.
20. Felsenfeld G, McGhee JD. Structure of the 30 nm chromatin fiber. *Cell* 1986;44:375–377.
21. Luger K, Mader AW, Richmond RK, et al. Crystal structure of the nucleosomes are particle at 2.8 resolution. *Nature* 1997; 389:251–260.
22. Stollar BD. The antigenic potential and specificity of nucleic acids, nucleoproteins, and their modified derivatives. *Arthritis Rheum* 1981;24:1010–1017.
23. McGhee JD. The structure of interphase chromatin. In: Risley MS, ed. *Chromosome structure and function*. New York: Van Nostrand Reinhold, 1986:138.
24. Zlatnova J, Leuba SH, van Holde K. Chromatin structure revisited. *Crit Rev Eukaryot Gene Expr* 1999;9:245–255.
25. Simpson RT. Nucleosome positioning in vivo and in vitro. *Bioessays* 1986;4:172–176.
26. Wang BC, Rose J, Arents G, et al. The octameric histone core of the nucleosome. Structural issues resolved. *J Mol Biol* 1994; 236:179–188.
27. Earnshaw WC. Mitotic chromosome structure. *Bioessays* 1988; 9:147–150.
28. Maney T, Ginkel LM, Hunter AW, et al. The kinetochore of higher eukaryotes: a molecular view. *Int Rev Cytol* 2000;194: 67–131.
29. Van Hooser AA, Mancini MA, Allis CD, et al. The mammalian centromere: structural domains and attenuation of chromatin modeling. *FASEB J* 1999;13(suppl 12):S216–S220.
30. Rattner JB. The structure of the mammalian centromere. *Bioessays* 1991;13:51–56.
31. Wolffe AP. Centromeric chromatin: histone deviants. *Curr Biol* 1995;5:452–454.
32. Luji SCS, Zumei N, Shi Z, et al. Involvement of a nucleolar component, perichromonucleolin, in the condensation and decondensation of chromosomes. *Proc Natl Acad Sci USA* 1987; 84:7953–7956.
33. Kharrat A, Derancourt J, Doree M, et al. Synergistic effect of histone H1 and nucleolin on chromatin condensation in mitosis: role of phosphorylated heteromer. *Biochemistry* 1991;30: 10329–10336.
34. Minota S, Jarjour WN, Suzuki N, et al. Autoantibodies to nucleolin in systemic lupus erythematosus and other diseases. *J Immunol* 1991;146:2249–2252.
35. Jarjour WN, Minota S, Roubey RAS, et al. Autoantibodies to nucleolin cross-react with histone H1 in systemic lupus erythematosus. *Mol Biol Rep* 1992;16:263–266.
36. Parseghian MH, Henschen AH, Krieglstein KG, et al. A proposal for a coherent mammalian histone H1 nomenclature correlated with amino acid sequences. *Protein Sci* 1994;3:575–587.
37. Parseghian MH, Harris DA, Rishwain DR, et al. Characteriza-

tion of a set of antibodies specific for three histone H1 subtypes. *Chromosoma* 1994;103:198–208.
38. Buttinelli M, Panetta G, Rhodes D, et al. The role of histone H1 in chromatin condensation and transcriptional repression. *Genetica* 1999;106:117–124.
39. Kohlstaedt LA, Cole RD. Specific interaction between H1 histone and high mobility protein HMG1. *Biochemistry* 1994; 33:570–575.
40. Crane-Robinson C. How do linker histones mediate differential gene expression? *Bioessays* 1999;21:367–371.
41. Kornberg RD, Lorch Y. Chromatic structure and transcription. *Annu Rev Cell Biol* 1992;8:563–587.
42. Cole RD. Microheterogeneity in H1 and its consequences. *Int J Pept Protein Res* 1987;30:433–449.
43. Thomas JO. Histone H1: location and role. *Curr Opin Cell Biol* 1999;11:312–317.
44. Mendelson E, Smith BJ, Bustin M. Mapping the binding of monoclonal antibodies to H5. *Biochemistry* 1984;23: 3466–3471.
45. Monestier M, Fasy TM, Debbas ME, et al. Specificities of IgM and IgG anti-histone H1 autoantibodies in autoimmune mice. *Clin Exp Immunol*1990;81:39–44.
46. Yasuda H, Logan KA, Bradbury EM. Antibody against globular domain of H1 histone. *FEBS Lett* 1984;166:263–266.
47. Pauls JD, Silverman E, Laxer RM, et al. Antibodies to histones H1 and H5 in sera of patients with juvenile rheumatoid arthritis. *Arthritis Rheum* 1989;32:877–883.
48. Pauls JD, Edworthy SM, Fritzler MJ. Epitope mapping of histone 5 (H5) with systemic lupus erythematosus, procainamide-induced lupus and hydralazine-induced lupus sera. *Mol Immunol* 1993;30:709–719.
49. Spencer VA, Davie JR. Role of covalent modifications of histones in regulating gene expression. *Gene* 1999;240:1–12.
50. Ausio J, Dong F, van Holde KE. Use of selectively trypsinized nucleosome core particles to analyze the role of the histone tails in the stabilization of the nucleosome. *J Mol Biol* 1989; 206:451–463.
51. Muller S. Ubiquitin. In: van Venrooij WJ, Maini RN, eds. *Manual of biological markers of disease*. Boston: Kluwer Academic, 1994:111.
52. Dixon GH, Candido EPM, Honda BM, et al. The biological roles of post-synthetic modifications of basic nuclear proteins. *Ciba Symp Struct Funct Chromatin* 1975;28:229–258.
53. Kouzarides T. Acetylation: a regulatory modification to rival phosphorylation? *EMBO J* 2000;19:1176–1179.
54. Althaus FR, Hfferer L, Kleczkowska HE, et al. Histone shuttling by poly ADP-ribosylation. *Mol Cell Biochem* 1994;138: 53–59.
55. Fasy TM, Inoue A, Johnson EM, et al. Phosphorylation of H1 and H5 histones by cyclic AMP-dependent protein kinase reduces DNA binding. *Biochim Biophys Acta* 1979;564: 322–334.
56. Lu JM, Dadd CA, Mizzen CA, et al. Generation and characterization of novel antibodies highly selective for phosphorylated linker histone H1 in tetrahymena and HeLa cells. *Chromasoma* 1994;103:111–121.
57. Ueda K, Hayaishi O. ADP-ribosylation. *Annu Rev Biochem* 1985;54:73–100.
58. Gaal JC, Pearson CK. Eukaryotic nuclear ADP-ribosylation reactions. *Biochem J* 1985;230:1–18.
59. Boulikas T, Bastin B, Boulikas P, et al. Increase in histone poly(ADP-ribosylation) in mitogen-activated lymphoid cells. *Exp Cell Res* 1990;187:77–84.
60. Huletsky A, de Murcia G, Muller S, et al. The effect of poly(ADP-ribosyl)ation on native and H1-depleted chromatin. *J Biol Chem* 1989;264:8878–8886.
61. Rubin RL, Uetrect JP, Jones JE. Cytotoxicity of oxidative metabolites of procainamide. *J Pharmacol Exp Ther* 1987;242: 833–841.
62. Ayer LM, Edworthy SM, Fritzler MJ. Effect of procainamide and hydralazine on poly(ADP-ribosylation) in cell lines. *Lupus* 1993;2:167–172.
63. Mendelson E, Bustin M. Monoclonal antibodies against distinct determinants of histone H5 bind to chromatin. *Biochemistry* 1984;23:3459–3466.
64. Atanassov C, Briand JP, Bonnier D, et al. New Zealand white rabbits immunized with RNA-complexed total histones develop an autoimmune-like response. *Clin Exp Immunol* 1991;86: 124–133.
65. Einck L, Dibble R, Frado LLY, et al. Nucleosomes as antigens: characterization of determinants and cross-reactivity. *Exp Cell Res* 1982;54:320–332.
66. Nickel BE, Davie JR. Structure of polyubiquitinated histone H2A. *Biochemistry* 1989;28:964–968.
67. Hershko A. Ubiquitin-mediated protein degradation. *J Biol Chem* 1988;263:15237–15240.
68. Muller S, Barakat S, Watts R, et al. Longitudinal analysis of antibodies to histones, Sm-D peptides and ubiquitin in the serum of patients with systemic lupus erythematosus, rheumatoid arthritis and tuberculosis. *Clin Exp Rheumatol* 1990;8: 445–453.
69. Muller S, Briand JP, Van Regenmortel MHV. Presence of antibodies to ubiquitin during the autoimmune response associated with systemic lupus erythematosus. *Proc Natl Acad Sci USA* 1988;85:8176–8180.
70. Rubin RL, Burlingame RW. Biochemical mechanisms in autoimmunity. *Biochem Soc Trans* 1991;19:153–159.
71. Fritzler MJ, Salazar M. The diversity and origin of rheumatologic autoantibodies. *Clin Microbiol Rev* 1991;4:256–269.
72. Oldstone MBA. Virus-induced autoimmunity: molecular mimicry as a route to autoimmune disease. *J Autoimmun* 1989;2: 187–194.
73. Kalden JR, Gay S. Retroviruses and autoimmune rheumatic diseases. *Clin Exp Immunol*1994;98:1–5.
74. Behar SM, Porcelli SA. Mechanisms of autoimmune disease induction; the role of the immune response to microbial pathogens. *Arthritis Rheum* 1995;38:458–476.
75. Perl A. Mechanisms of viral pathogenesis in rheumatic diseases. *Ann Rheum Dis* 1999;58:454–461.
76. Nissen P, Kjeldgaard M, Nyborg J. Macromolecular mimicry. *EMBO J* 2000;19:489–495.
77. Baum H, Butler P, Davies H, et al. Autoimmune disease and molecular mimicry: an hypothesis. *Trends Biol Sci* 1993;18: 140–144.
78. Horwitz MS, Sarvetnick N. Viruses, host responses and autoimmunity. *Immunol Rev* 1999;169:241–253.
79. Watts RA, Isenberg DA. Autoantibodies and antibacterial antibodies: from both sides now. *Ann Rheum Dis* 1990;49:961–965.
80. Singh VK, Yamaki K, Donoso LA, et al. Molecular mimicry: yeast histone H3-induced experimental autoimmune uveitis. *J Immunol* 1989;142:1512–1517.
81. Singh VK, Yamaki K, Donoso L, et al. Sequence homology between yeast histone H3 and uveitopathogenic site of S-antigen: lymphocyte cross-reaction and adoptive transfer of the disease. *Cell Immunol* 1989;119:211–221.
82. Pettijohn DE. Histone-like proteins and bacterial chromosomes structure. *J Virol Chem* 1988;263:12793–12796.
83. Hirvas L, Coleman J, Koski P, et al. Bacterial "histone-like protein I" (HLP-I) is an outer membrane constituent? *FEBS Lett* 1990;262:123–126.
84. Drlica K, Rouviere-Yaniv J. Histone like proteins of bacteria. *Microbiol Rev* 1987;51:301–319.

85. Eriksen N, Kumar SB, Fukuchi K, et al. Molecular mimicry: histone H3 and mycobacterial protein epitopes. *Proc Natl Acad Sci USA* 1995;92:2150–2153.
86. Serrano M, Gutirrez C, Freire R, et al. Phage x29 protein p6: a viral histone-like protein. *Biochimie* 1994;76:981–991.
87. von Muhlen CA, Tan EM. Autoantibodies in the diagnosis of systemic rheumatic disease. *Semin Arthritis Rheum* 1995;24: 323–258.
88. Palmer DK, O'Day K, Trong HL, et al. Purification of the centromere-specific protein CENP-A and demonstration that it is a distinctive histone. *Proc Natl Acad Sci USA* 1991;88: 3734–3738.
89. VenKatraman JT, Gohill J, Fritzler MJ, et al. A histone 1–like antigen is a component of the nuclear envelope. *Biochem Biophys Res Commun* 1988;156:675–680.
90. Miller BJ, Pauls JD, Fritzler MJ. Human monoclonal antibodies demonstrate polyspecificity for histones and the cytoskeleton. *J Autoimmun* 1991;4:665–679.
91. Nassberger L, Johansson AC, Bjorck S, et al. Antibodies to neutrophil granulocyte myeloperoxidase and elastase: autoimmune responses in glomerulonephritis due to hydralazine treatment. *J Intern Med* 1991;229:261–265.
92. Jacob L, Viard J, Allenet B, et al. A monoclonal anti-double-stranded DNA autoantibody binds to a 94-kDa cell surface protein on various cell types via nucleosomes or a DNA-histone complex. *Proc Natl Acad Sci USA* 1989;86:4669–4673.
93. Rekvig OP. Intrinsic cell membrane antigens recognized by antichromatin autoantibodies. *Scand J Immunol* 1989;29:7–13.
94. Bennett RM, Davis J, Campbell S, et al. Lactoferrin binds to cell membrane DNA (association of surface DNA with an enriched population of B cells and monocytes). *J Clin Invest* 1983;71:611–618.
95. Bennett RM, Davis J, Merritt M. Anti-DNA antibodies react with DNA expressed on the surface of monocytes and the cell surface. *J Rheumatol* 1986;13:679–685.
96. Rekvig OP, Muller S, Briand JP, et al. Human antinuclear autoantibodies crossreacting with the plasma membrane and the N-terminal region of histone H2B. *Immunol Invest* 1987; 16:535–547.
97. Viard J-P, Chabre H, Bach J-F. Autoantibodies to nucleosomes in HIV-1–infected patients. *J AIDS* 1994;7:1286–1287.
98. Rekvig OP, Moens U, Fredriksen K, et al. Human polyoma virus BK and immunogenicity of mammalian DNA: a conceptual framework. *Methods* 1997;11:44–54.
99. Fredriksen K, Traavik T, Flaegstad T, et al. BK virus terminates tolerance to dsDNA and histone antigens in vivo. *Immunol Invest* 1990;19:133–151.
100. Imaoka K, Kanai Y, Yoshikawa Y, et al. Temporary breakdown of immunological tolerance to dsDNA and nucleohistone antigens in rabbits infected with rinderpest virus. *Clin Exp Immunol* 1990;82:522–526.
101. Andreassen K, Moens U, Nossent A, et al. Termination of human T cell tolerance to histones by presentation of histones and polomavirus T antigen provided that T antigen is complexed with nucleosomes. *Arthritis Rheum* 1999;42:2449–2460.
102. Hardin JA. The lupus autoantigens and the pathogenesis of systemic lupus erythematosus. *Arthritis Rheum* 1986;29:457–460.
103. Burlingame RW, Rubin RL, Balderas RS, et al. Genesis and evolution of antichromatin autoantibodies in murine lupus implicates T-dependent immunization with self antigen. *J Clin Invest* 1993;91:1687–1696.
104. Mohan C, Adams S, Stanik V, et al. Nucleosome: a major immunogen for pathogenic autoantibody-inducing T cells of lupus. *J Exp Med* 1993;177:1367–1381.
105. Amoura Z, Chabre H, Koutouzov S, et al. Nucleosome-restricted antibodies are detected before anti-dsDNA and/or antihistone antibodies in serum of MRL-Mp lpr/lpr and +/+ mice, and are present in kidney eluates of lupus mice with proteinuria. *Arthritis Rheum* 1994;37:1684–1688.
106. Fourni GJ. Circulating DNA and lupus nephritis. *Kidney Int* 1988;33:487–497.
107. Rumore PM, Steinman CR. Endogenous circulating DNA in systemic lupus erythematosus. Occurrence as multimeric complexes bound to histone. *J Clin Invest* 1990;86:69–74.
108. Losman JA, Fasy TM, Novick KE, et al. Nucleosome-specific antibody from an autoimmune MRL/Mp-lpr/lpr mouse. *Arthritis Rheum* 1993;36:552–560.
109. Burlingame RW, Boey ML, Starkebaum G, et al. The central role of chromatin in autoimmune responses to histones and DNA in systemic lupus erythematosus. *J Clin Invest* 1994; 94:184–192.
110. Hengartner C, Lagueux J, Poirier GG. Analysis of the activation of poly (ADP-ribose) polymerase by various types of DNA. *Biochem Cell Biol* 1991;69:577–580.
111. Gohill J, Cary PD, Couppez M, et al. Antibodies from patients with drug-induced and idiopathic lupus erythematosus react with epitopes restricted to the amino and carboxyl termini of histone. *J Immunol* 1985;135:3116–3121.
112. Craft JE, Radding JA, Harding MW, et al. Autoantigenic histone epitopes: a comparison between procainamide- and hydralazine-induced lupus. *Arthritis Rheum* 1987;30:689–694.
113. Bell DA, Morrison B, VandenBygaart P. Immunogenic DNA-related factors. Nucleosomes spontaneously released from normal murine lymphoid cells stimulate proliferation and immunoglobulin synthesis of normal mouse and human B lymphocytes. *J Clin Invest* 1990;85:1487–1496.
114. Mohan C, Alas E, Morel L, et al. Genetic dissection of SLE pathogenesis. Sle1 on murine chromosome 1 leads to a selective loss of tolerance to H2A/H2B/DNA subnucleosomes. *J Clin Invest* 1998;101:1362–1372.
115. Monestier M. Variable region genes of anti-histone autoantibodies from a MRL/Mp-lpr/lpr mouse. *Eur J Immunol* 1991; 21:1725–1731.
116. Theofilopoulos AN. The basis of autoimmunity: part II. Genetic predisposition. *Immunol Today* 1995;16:150–159.
117. Tuaillon N, Watts RA, Isenberg DA, et al. Sequence analysis and fine specificity of two human monoclonal antibodies to histone H1. *Mol Immunol* 1994;31:269–277.
118. Davidson A, Smith A, Katz J, et al. A cross-reactive idiotype on anti-DNA antibodies defines a H chain determinant present almost exclusively on IgG antibodies. *J Immunol* 1989;143: 174–180.
119. Hahn BH, Ebling FM. A public idiotypic determinant is present on spontaneous cationic IgG antibodies to DNA from mice of unrelated lupus-prone strains. *J Immunol* 1984;133: 3015–3021.
120. Bell DA, Hahn B, Harkiss G. Idiotypes, antibodies and immunopathology. *Lupus* 1992;1:335–337.
121. Davidson A, Shefner R, Livneh A, et al. The role of somatic mutation of immunoglobulin genes in autoimmunity. *Annu Rev Immunol* 1987;5:85–108.
122. Diamond B, Scharff MD. Somatic mutation of the T15 heavy chain gives rise to an antibody with autoantibody specificity. *Proc Natl Acad Sci USA* 1984;81:5841–5844.
123. Fritzler MJ. Immunofluorescent antinuclear antibody test. In: Rose NR, de Macario EC, Folds JD, et al., eds. *Manual of clinical laboratory immunology*, 5th ed. Washington, DC: American Society for Microbiology, 1997:920–927.
124. Caturla A, Colome JA, Bustos A, et al. Occurrence of antibodies to protease-treated histones in a patient with vasculitis. *Clin Immunol Immunopathol* 1991;60:65–71.
125. Molden DP, Klipple GL, Peebles CL, et al. IgM anti-histone H3

antibodies associated with undifferentiated rheumatic disease syndromes. *Arthritis Rheum* 1986;29:39–46.
126. Portanova JP, Rubin RL, Joslin FG, et al. Reactivity of anti-histone antibodies induced by procainamide and hydralazine. *Clin Immunol Immunopathol* 1982;25:67–79.
127. Kunkel HG, Holman HR, Deicher HRG. Multiple autoantibodies to cell constituents in systemic lupus erythematosus. *Ciba Found Symp* 1960;1:429–437.
128. Tan EM. An immunologic precipitin system between soluble nucleoprotein and serum antibody in systemic lupus erythematosus. *J Clin Invest* 1967;46:735–745.
129. Rothfield NF, Stollar BD. The relation of immunoglobulin class, pattern of anti-nuclear antibody, and complement-fixing antibodies to DNA in sera from patients with systemic lupus erythematosus. *J Clin Invest* 1967;46:1785–1794.
130. Stollar BD. Varying specificity of systemic lupus erythematosus sera for histone fractions and a periodate-sensitive antigen associated with histone. *J Immunol* 1969;103:804–808.
131. Stollar BD. Reactions of systemic lupus erythematosus sera with histone fractions and histone-DNA complexes. *Arthritis Rheum* 1971;14:485–491.
132. Hekman A, Sluyser M. Antigenic determinants on lysine-rich histone fractions. *Biochim Biophys Acta* 1973;295:613–620.
133. Tan EM, Robinson J, Robitaille P. Studies on antibodies to histones by immunofluorescence. *Scand J Immunol* 1976;5:811–818.
134. Fritzler MJ, Ryan JP, Kinsella TD. Clinical features of SLE patients with antihistone antibodies. *J Rheumatol* 1982;9:46–51.
135. Fritzler MJ, Tan EM. Antibodies to histones in drug-induced and idiopathic lupus erythematosus. *J Clin Invest* 1978;62:560–567.
136. Hobbs RN, Clayton A-L, Bernstein RM. Antibodies to the five histones and poly(adenosine diphosphate-ribose) in drug induced lupus: implications for pathogenesis. *Ann Rheum Dis* 1987;46:408–416.
137. Portanova JP, Arndt RE, Tan EM, et al. Anti-histone antibodies in idiopathic and drug-induced lupus recognize distinct intrahistone regions. *J Immunol* 1987;138:446–451.
138. Rubin RL, Waga S. Anti-histone antibodies in systemic lupus erythematosus. *J Rheumatol* 1987;14:118–126.
139. DuClos TW, Marnell L, Zlock LR, et al. Analysis of the binding of C-reactive protein to chromatin subunits. *J Immunol* 1991;146:1220–1225.
140. Schmiedeke TMJ, Stockl FW, Weber R, et al. Histones have high affinity for the glomerular basement membrane. *J Exp Med* 1989;169:1879–1894.
141. Subiza JL, Caturla A, Pascual-Salcedo D, et al. DNA-anti-DNA complexes account for part of the antihistone activity found in patients with systemic lupus erythematosus. *Arthritis Rheum* 1989;32:406–412.
142. Waga S, Tan EM, Rubin RL. Identification and isolation of soluble histones from bovine milk and serum. *Biochem J* 1987;244:675–682.
143. Bustos A, Boimorto R, Subiza JL, et al. Inhibition of histone/anti-histone reactivity by histone-binding serum components; differential effect on anti-H1 versus anti-H2B antibodies. *Clin Exp Immunol* 1994;95:408–414.
144. DuClos TW, Zlock LT, Marnell L. Definition of a C-reactive protein binding determinant on histones. *J Biol Chem* 1991;266:2167–2171.
145. Bestagno M, Cerino A, Riva S, et al. Improvements of Western blotting to detect monoclonal antibodies. *Biochem Biophys Res Commun* 1987;146:1509–1514.
146. Stott DI. Immunoblotting and dot blotting. *J Immunol Methods* 1989;119:153–187.
147. Stemmer C, Briand J-P, Muller S. Mapping of linear epitopes of human histone H1 recognized by rabbit anti-H1/H5 antisera and antibodies from autoimmune patients. *Mol Immunol* 1994;31:1037–1046.
148. Gershoni JM, Palade GE. Protein blotting: principles and applications. *Anal Biochem* 1983;131:1–15.
149. Towbin H, Gordon J. Immunoblotting and dot immunobinding current status and outlook. *J Immunol Methods* 1984;72:313–340.
150. Towbin H, Staehelin T, Gordon J. Immunoblotting in the clinical laboratory. *J Clin Chem Clin Biochem* 1989;27:495–501.
151. Monestier M. Autoantibodies to nucleosomes and histone-DNA complexes. *Methods* 1997;11:36–43.
152. Bernstein RM, Hobbs RN, Lea DJ, et al. Patterns of antihistone antibody specificity in systemic rheumatic disease. *Arthritis Rheum* 1985;28:2–85.
153. Shoenfeld Y, Segol G, Segol O, et al. Detection of antibodies to total histones and their subfractions in systemic lupus erythematosus patients and their asymptomatic relatives. *Arthritis Rheum* 1987;30:169–175.
154. Shoenfeld Y, Segol O. Anti-histone antibodies in SLE and other autoimmune diseases. *Clin Exp Immunol* 1989;7:265–271.
155. Konstantinov K, Russanova V, Russeva V. Antibodies to histones and disease activity in systemic lupus erythematosus: a comparative study with an enzyme-linked immunosorbent assay and immunoblotting. *Arch Dermatol Res* 1986;278:410–415.
156. Gioud M, Kaci MA, Monier JC. Histone antibodies in systemic lupus erythematosus. A possible diagnostic tool. *Arthritis Rheum* 1982;25:407–413.
157. Ait-kaci A, Monier J, Mamelle N. Enzyme-linked immunosorbent assay for anti-histone antibodies and their presence in systemic lupus erythematosus. *J Immunol Methods* 1981;44:311–322.
158. Kohda S, Kanayama Y, Okamura M, et al. Clinical significance of antibodies to histones in systemic lupus erythematosus. *J Rheumatol* 1989;16:24–28.
159. Fishbein E, Alarcon-Segovia D, Vega JM. Antibodies to histones in systemic lupus erythematosus. *Clin Exp Immunol* 1979;36:145–150.
160. Epstein A, Greenberg M, Halbert S, et al. The clinical application of an ELISA technique for the detection of histone antibodies. *J Rheumatol* 1986;13:304–307.
161. Krippner H, Springer B, Merle S, et al. Antibodies to histones of the IgG and IgM class in systemic lupus erythematosus. *Clin Exp Immunol* 1984;58:49–56.
162. Gompertz NR, Isenberg DA, Turner BM. Correlation between clinical features of systemic lupus erythematosus and levels of antihistone antibodies of the IgG, IgA, and IgM isotypes. *Ann Rheum Dis* 1990;49:524–527.
163. Rubin RL, Burlingame RW, Arnott JE, et al. IgG but not other classes of anti-(H2A-H2B)-DNA is an early sign of procainamide-induced lupus. *J Immunol* 1995;154:2483–2493.
164. Rubin RL, Bell SA, Burlingame RW. Autoantibodies associated with lupus induced by diverse drugs target a similar epitope in the (H2A-H2B)-DNA complex. *J Clin Invest* 1992;90:165–173.
165. Totoritis MC, Tan EM, McNally EM, et al. Association of antibody to histone complex H2A-H2B with symptomatic procainamide-induced lupus. *N Engl J Med* 1988;318:1431–1462.
166. Rubin RL, Joslin FG, Tan EM. A solid-phase radioimmunoassay for anti-histone antibodies in human sera: comparison with an immunofluorescence assay. *Scand J Immunol* 1982;15:63–70.
167. Rubin RL, McNally EM, Nusinow SR, et al. IgG antibodies to the histone complex H2A-H2B characterize procainamide-induced lupus. *Clin Immunol Immunopathol* 1985;36:49–59.

168. Rubin RL, Burlingame RW, Bell SA. Specific anti-histone antibody common to lupus induced by diverse drugs. *Arthritis Rheum* 1991;34:S104(abst).
169. Burlingame RW, Rubin RL. Drug-induced anti-histone autoantibodies display two patterns of reactivity with substructures of chromatin. *J Clin Invest* 1991;88:680–690.
170. Wallace DJ, Lin H, Shen GQ, et al. Antibodies to histone (H2A-H2B)-DNA complexes in the absence of antibodies to double-stranded DNA or to (H2A-H2B) complexes are more sensitive and specific for scleroderma-related disorders than for lupus. *Arthritis Rheum* 1994;37:1795–1797.
171. Ihn H, Soma Y, Igarashi A, et al. Anti-histone antibodies in patients with localized scleroderma. *Arthritis Rheum* 1993;36:1137–1141.
172. Burlingame RW, Rubin RL, Balderas RS, Theofilopoulos AN. Genesis and evolution of antichromatin antibodies in murine lupus implicates T-dependent immunization with self antigen. *J Clin Invest* 1993;91:1687–1696.
173. Losman MJ, Fasy TM, Novick KE, et al. Monoclonal autoantibodies to subnucleosomes from a MRL/Mp mouse. Oligoclonality of the antibody response and recognition of a determinant composed of histones H2A, H2B, and DNA. *J Immunol* 1992;148:1561–1569.
174. Monestier M, Novick KE, Karam ET, et al. Autoantibodies to histone, DNA and nucleosome antigens in canine systemic lupus erythematosus. *Clin Exp Immunol*1995;99:37–41.
175. Malleson P, Petty RE, Fung M, et al. Reactivity of antinuclear antibodies with histones and other antigens in juvenile rheumatoid arthritis. *Arthritis Rheum* 1989;32:9–19.
176. Monestier M, Losman JA, Fasy TM, et al. Antihistone antibodies in antinuclear antibody-positive juvenile arthritis. *Arthritis Rheum* 1990;33:1836–1841.
177. Stensen M, Fredriksen K, Kass E, et al. Identification of antihistone antibodies in subsets of juvenile chronic arthritis. *Ann Rheum Dis* 1989;48:114–117.
178. Tuaillon N, Muller S, Pasquali JL, et al. Antibodies from patients with rheumatoid arthritis and juvenile chronic arthritis analyzed with core histone synthetic peptides. *Int Arch Allergy Appl Immunol* 1990;91:297–305.
179. Burlingame RW, Rubin RL, Rosenberg AM. Autoantibodies to chromatin components in juvenile rheumatoid arthritis. *Arthritis Rheum* 1993;36:836–841.
180. Leak AM, Woo P. Juvenile chronic arthritis, chronic iridocyclitis, and reactivity to histones. *Ann Rheum Dis* 1991;50:653–657.
181. Malleson PN, Fung MY, Petty RE, et al. Autoantibodies in chronic arthritis of childhood: relations with each other and with histocompatibility antigens. *Ann Rheum Dis* 1992;51:1301–1306.
182. Stemmer C, Tuaillon N, Prieur A-M, et al. Mapping of B-cell epitopes recognized by antibodies to histones in subsets of juvenile chronic arthritis. *Clin Immunol Immunopathol* 1995;76:82–89.
183. Haynes DC, Gershwin ME, Robbins DL, et al. Autoantibody profiles in juvenile arthritis. *J Rheumatol* 1986;13:358–363.
184. Aitcheson CT, Peebles C, Joslin F, et al. Characteristics of antinuclear antibodies in rheumatoid arthritis. *Arthritis Rheum* 1980;1980:528–538.
185. Martin T, Knapp AM, Muller S, et al. Polyclonal human rheumatoid factors cross-reacting with histone H3: characterization of an idiotope on the H3 binding site. *J Clin Immunol* 1990;10:211–219.
186. Muzellec Y, Le Goff P, Jouquan J, et al. Antibodies to histones in rheumatoid arthritis. *Diagn Clin Immunol* 1988;5:326–331.
187. Campion G, Maddison PJ, Goulding N, et al. The Felty syndrome: a case-matched study of clinical manifestations and outcome, serologic features, and immunogenetic associations. *Medicine (Baltimore)* 1990;69:69–80.
188. Pasquali JL, Azerad G, Martin T, et al. The double reactivity of a human monoclonal rheumatoid factor to IgG and histones is related to distinct binding sites. *Eur J Immunol* 1988;18:1127–1130.
189. Goshen E, Livne A, Nagy J, et al. Antinuclear autoantibodies in sera of patients with IgA nephropathy. *Nephron* 1990;55:33–36.
190. Shoenfeld Y, Pick AL, Danzinger Y, et al. Immunoglobulin changes in systemic lupus erythematosus. *Ann Allergy* 1977;39:99–111.
191. Baslund B, Wiik A. Anti-neutrophil cytoplasmic autoantibodies (ANCA) and vasculitis. *Clin Rev Allergy* 1994;12:297–304.
192. Esnault LM, Short AK, Audrain MAP, et al. Autoantibodies to lactoferrin and histone in systemic vasculitis identified by anti-myelo-peroxidase solid phase assays. *Kidney Int* 1994;46:153–160.
193. Pauzner R, Urowitz M, Gladman D, et al. Antineutrophil cytoplasmic antibodies in systemic lupus erythematosus. *J Rheumatol* 1994;21:1670–1673.
194. Nassberger L, Sjoholm AG, Jonsson H, et al. Autoantibodies against neutrophil cytoplasm components in systemic lupus erythematosus and in hydralazine-induced lupus. *Clin Exp Immunol*1990;81:380–383.
195. Schnabel A, Csernok E, Isenberg DA, et al. Antineutrophil cytoplasmic antibodies in systemic lupus erythematosus: prevalence, specificities, and clinical significance. *Arthritis Rheum* 1995;38:633–637.
196. Lee SS, Lawton JMW. Antimyeloperoxidase antibody in systemic lupus erythematosus. *J Intern Med* 1992;232:283–286.
197. Eggena M, Cohavy O, Parseghian MH, et al. Identification of histone H1 as a cognate antigen of the ulcerative colitis-associated marker antibody pANCA. *J Autoimmun* 2000;14:83–97.
198. Sato S, Fujimoto M, Ihn H, et al. Clinical characteristics associated with antihistone antibodies in patients with localized scleroderma. *J Am Acad Dermatol* 1994;31:567–571.
199. Ayer LM, Senecal J, Martin L, et al. Antibodies to high mobility group (HMG) proteins in systemic sclerosis. *J Rheumatol* 1994;21:2071–2075.
200. Garcia-de la Torre I, Castello-Sendra J, et al. Autoantibodies in Parry-Romberg syndrome: a serologic study of 14 patients. *J Rheumatol* 1995;22:73–77.
201. Martin L, Pauls JD, Ryan JP, et al. Identification of a subset of patients with scleroderma with severe pulmonary and vascular disease by the presence of autoantibodies to centromere and histone. *Ann Rheum Dis* 1993;52:780–784.
202. Sato S, Ihn H, Kikuchi K, et al. Antihistone antibodies in systemic sclerosis. *Arthritis Rheum* 1994;37:391–394.
203. Ihn H, Soma Y, Igarashi A, et al. Antihistone antibodies in patients with localized scleroderma. *Arthritis Rheum* 1993;1137–1141.
204. Sato S, Fujimoto M, Ihn H, et al. Antigen specificity of antihistone antibodies in localized scleroderma. *Arch Dermatol* 1994;130:1273–1277.
205. Hasegawa M, Sato S, Kikuchi K, et al. Antigen specificity of antihistone antibodies in systemic sclerosis. *Ann Rheum Dis* 1998;57:470–475.
206. Konikoff F, Swissa M, Shoenfeld Y. Autoantibodies to histones and their subfractions in chronic liver diseases. *Clin Immunol Immunopathol* 1989;51:77–82.
207. Penner E, Muller S, Zimmermann D, et al. High prevalence of antibodies to histones among patients with primary biliary cirrhosis. *Clin Exp Immunol*1987;70:47–52.
208. Klajman A, Kafri B, Shohat T, et al. The prevalence of antibodies to histones induced by procainamide in old people, in can-

cer patients, and in rheumatoid-like disease. *Clin Immunol Immunopathol* 1983;27:1–8.
209. Kubo M, Ihn H, Yazawa N, et al. Prevalence and antigen specificity of anti-histone antibodies in patients with polymyositis/dermatomyositis. *J Invest Dermatol* 1999;112:711–715.
210. Thomas JO, Wilson CM, Hardin JA. The major core histone antigenic determinants in systemic lupus erythematosus are in the trypsin-sensitive regions. *FEBS Lett* 1984;169:90–96.
211. Gohill J, Fritzler MJ. Antibodies in procainamide-induced and systemic lupus erythematosus bind the C-terminus of histone 1 (H1). *Mol Immunol* 1987;24:275–285.
212. Costa O, Tchouatcha-Tchouassom JC, Roux B, et al. Anti-H1 histone antibodies in systemic lupus erythematosus: epitope localization after immunoblotting of chymotrypsin-digested H1. *Clin Exp Immunol* 1986;63:608–613.
213. Freed JH, Marrs A, VanderWall J, et al. MHC Class II-bound self peptides from autoimmune MRL/lpr mice reveal potential T cell epitopes for autoantibody production in murine systemic lupus erythematosus. *J Immunol* 2000;164:4697–4705.
214. Lu L, Kaliyaperumal, Boumpas DT, et al. Major peptide autoepitopes for nucleosome-specific T cells of human lupus. *J Clin Invest* 1999;104:345–355.
215. Hannestad K, Rekvig OP, Husebekk A. Cross-reacting rheumatoid factors and lupus erythematosus (LE) factors. *Springer Semin Immunopathol* 1981;4:133–160.
216. Holman HR, Kunkel HG. Affinity between the lupus erythematosus serum factor and cell nuclei and nucleoprotein. *Science* 1957;126:162–163.
217. Holborow EJ, Weir DM. Histone: an essential component for the lupus erythematosus antinuclear reaction. *Lancet* 1959;1:809–810.
218. Cohen MG, Webb J. Antihistone antibodies in rheumatoid arthritis and Felty's syndrome. *Arthritis Rheum* 1989;32:1319–1324.
219. Theofilopoulos AN, Dixon FJ. Murine models of systemic lupus erythematosus. *Adv Immunol* 1985;37:358–369.
220. Costa O, Monier JC. Antihistone antibodies detected by ELISA and immunoblotting in systemic lupus erythematosus and rheumatoid arthritis. *J Rheumatol* 1986;13:722–755.
221. Brick JE, Ong S-H, Bathon JM, et al. Anti-histone antibodies in the serum of autoimmune MRL and NZB/NZW F1 mice. *Clin Immunol Immunopathol* 1990;54:372–381.
222. Emlen W, Burdick G. Clearance and organ localization of small DNA anti-DNA immune complexes in mice. *J Immunol* 1988;140:1816–1822.
223. Emlen W, Mannik M. Effect of DNA size and strandedness on the in vivo clearance and organ localization of DNA. *Clin Exp Immunol* 1984;56:185–192.
224. Ben-Chetrit E, Dunsky EH, Wollner S, et al. In vivo clearance and tissue uptake of an anti-DNA monoclonal antibody and its complexes with DNA. *Clin Exp Immunol* 1985;60:1–59.
225. Termaat R-M, Assmann KJM, Dijkman HBPM, et al. Anti-DNA antibodies can bind to the glomerulus via two distinct mechanisms. *Kidney Int* 1992;42:1363–1371.
226. Termaat R, Brinkman K, Nossent JC, et al. Anti-heparan sulphate reactivity in sera from patients with systemic lupus erythematosus with renal or non-renal manifestations. *Clin Exp Immunol* 1990;82:268–274.
227. Schmiedeke T, Stoeckl F, Muller S, et al. Glomerular immune deposits in murine lupus models may contain histones. *Clin Exp Immunol* 1992;90:453–458.
228. Kramers K, Hylkema M, Termaat R, et al. Histones in lupus nephritis. *Exp Nephrol* 1993;1:224–228.
229. Brinkman K, Termaat R, Berden JMH, et al. Anti-DNA antibodies and lupus nephritis: the complexity of crossreactivity. *Immunol Today* 1990;11:232–234.
230. van Bruggen MC, Kramers C, Hylkema MN, et al. Pathophysiology of lupus nephritis: the role of nucleosomes. *Neth J Med* 1994;45:273–279.
231. Stockl F, Muller S, Batsford S, et al. A role for histones and ubiquitin in lupus nephritis? *Clin Nephrol* 1994;41:10–17.
232. Hylkema MN, Zwet IVD, Kramers C, et al. No evidence for an independent role of anti-heparan sulphate reactivity apart from anti-DNA in lupus nephritis. *Clin Exp Immunol* 1995;101:55–59.
233. Tax WJM, Kramers C, van Bruggen MCJ, et al. Apoptosis, nucleosomes, and nephritis in systemic lupus erythematosus. *Kidney Int* 1995;48:666–673.
234. Franek F, Dolnikova J. Nucleosomes occurring in protein-free hybridoma cell culture. Evidence for programmed cell death. *FEBS Lett* 1991;284:285–287.
235. Tan EM. Autoimmunity and apoptosis. *J Exp Med* 1994;179:1083–1086.
236. Rubin RL, Joslin FG, Tan EM. Specificity of anti-histone antibodies in systemic lupus erythematosus. *Arthritis Rheum* 1982;25:779–782.
237. Cohen MG, Pollard KM, Webb J. Antibodies to histones in systemic lupus erythematosus: prevalence, specificity, and relationship to clinical and laboratory features. *Ann Rheum Dis* 1992;51:61–66.
238. Muller S, Bonnier D, Thiry M, et al. Reactivity of autoantibodies in systemic lupus erythematosus with synthetic core histone peptides. *Int Arch Allergy Appl Immunol* 1989;89:288–296.
239. Fritzler MJ, Gohill J, Ayer LM. Antibodies from patients with certain systemic rheumatic diseases react with histone epitopes. *Protides Biol Fluids* 1985;33:191–194.
240. Grossman L, Barland P. Histone reactivity of drug-induced antinuclear antibodies. A comparison of symptomatic and asymptomatic patients. *Arthritis Rheum* 1981;24:9–27.
241. Mongey AB, Donovan-Brand R, Thomas TJ, et al. Serologic evaluation of patients receiving procainamide. *Arthritis Rheum* 1992;35:219–223.
242. Monestier M, Novick KE, Losman MJ. D-penicillamine- and quinidine-induced antinuclear antibodies in A.SW (H-2s) mice: similarities with autoantibodies in spontaneous and heavy metal-induced autoimmunity. *Eur J Immunol* 1994;24:723–730.
243. Rubin RL. Autoantibody specificity in drug-induced lupus and neutrophil-mediated metabolism of lupus-inducing drugs. *Curr Biol* 1992;25:223–234.
244. Vazquez-del Mercado M, Casiano CA, Rubin RL. IgA antihistone antibodies in isoniazid-treated tuberculosis patients. *Autoimmunity* 1995;20:105–111.
245. Bustin M, Einck L, Reisch J. Autoantibodies to nucleosomal proteins: antibodies to HMG-17 in autoimmune diseases. *Science* 1982;215:1245–1247.
246. Pollard KM, Chan EKL, Rubin RL, et al. Monoclonal autoantibodies to nuclear antigens from murine graft-versus-host disease. *Clin Immunol Immunopathol* 1987;44:31–40.
247. Gioud M, Kotzin BL, Rubin RL, et al. In vivo and in vitro production of anti-histone antibodies in NZB/NZW mice. *J Immunol* 1983;131:2–69.
248. Kotzin BL, Lafferty JA, Portanova JP, et al. Monoclonal anti-histone autoantibodies derived from murine models of lupus. *J Immunol* 1984;133:2554–2559.
249. Monestier M, Fasy TM, Losman MJ, et al. Structure and binding properties of monoclonal antibodies to core histones from autoimmune mice. *Mol Immunol* 1993;30:1069–1075.
250. Brinet A, Fournel C, Faure JR, et al. Anti-histone antibodies (ELISA and immunoblot) in canine lupus erythematosus. *Clin Exp Immunol* 1988;74:105–109.

251. Monier JC, Ritter J, Caux C, et al. Canine systemic lupus erythematosus. II: antinuclear antibodies. *Lupus* 1992;1:287–293.
252. Portanova JP, Claman HN, Kotzin BL. Autoimmunization in murine graft-vs-host disease. I. Selective production of antibodies to histones and DNA. *J Immunol* 1985;135:3850–3856.
253. Rubin RL, Tang F-L, Tsay G, et al. Pseudoautoimmunity in normal mice: anti-histone antibodies elicited by immunization versus induction during graft-versus-host reaction. *Clin Immunol Immunopathol* 1990;54:320–332.
254. Gruschwitz MS, Shoenfeld Y, Krupp M, et al. Antinuclear antibody profile in UCD line 200 chickens: a model for progressive systemic sclerosis. *Int Arch Allergy Immunol* 1993;100:307–313.

23

ANTIBODIES TO RO/SSA AND LA/SSB

MORRIS REICHLIN
JOHN B. HARLEY

Anti-Ro and anti-La are important autoantibodies in systemic lupus erythematosus (SLE). Respectively, they are found in just less than one half and nearly one fifth of these patients in concentrations sufficient for precipitin formation. These autoantibodies also are closely allied with particular clinical findings. They are such an intrinsic component of disease expression that one is led to the conclusion that an understanding of the immune response to these (or to any one of the other major autoantigens) would reveal the mechanism of the autoimmune dysregulation of lupus, if not the etiology of the disease as well.

HISTORY AND DEVELOPMENT

A precipitin, likely to have been anti-Ro or anti-La, was first described over 40 years ago in a patient with Sjögren's syndrome (1). This observation was expanded on by Anderson et al. (2), who defined both antigens, which they called *SjT* and *SjD*. In addition, they observed a "lupus" precipitin that in retrospect is likely to have been an anti–nuclear ribonucleoprotein (nRNP) or anti-Sm specificity. Unfortunately, these observations lay fallow until the anti-Ro and anti-La specificities were independently described by Reichlin and colleagues (3,4). Anti-Ro and anti-La autoantibodies, as well as the autoantigens they bind, have been under continuous investigation since then. They also have been described as Sjögren's syndrome A (SS-A) and Sjögren's syndrome B (SS-B) antigens (5,6). An Ouchterlony immunodiffusion showing an example of the anti-Ro and anti-La responses is presented in Fig. 23.1. Beyond this discovery, the most fundamental contribution has been the marriage of autoimmune serology with molecular biologic approaches for the analysis of these antigens (7).

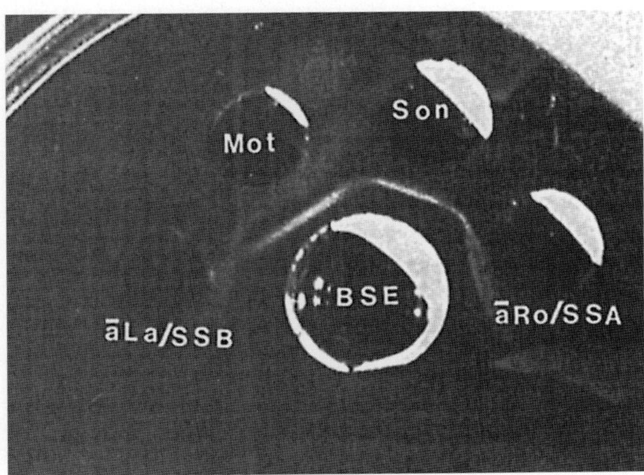

FIGURE 23.1. Anti-Ro and anti-La precipitins. The mother (Mot) has both anti-Ro and anti-La autoantibodies, while the affected son (Son) has only a faint anti-Ro precipitin. Precipitins from reference anti-La (aLa/SSB) and anti-Ro (aRo/SSA) sera also are presented against a bovine spleen extract (BSE). The anti-La precipitin is light and diffused in this example. This pedigree is described in Reichlin et al. (44).

CLINICAL RELATIONSHIPS

The clinical relevance of anti-Ro has been particularly well established. The data are less compelling for anti-La, although clearly this autoantibody also is important. The associations of clinical findings with anti-Ro and anti-La, as presented in Table 23.1, do not in themselves constitute direct evidence of an immunopathogenic role of the autoantibody in any aspect of the disease. Nevertheless, and at the very least, these associations are important as aids in diagnosis and prognosis.

Photosensitive skin rash in lupus as an association with anti-Ro was first appreciated by Maddison et al. (8) and has been confirmed by Mond et al. (9). Lee and David (10) as well as Lee and Weston (11) also have established that anti-Ro is specifically deposited in human skin, and therefore is likely to be directly involved in injury to the skin.

Chest radiographs showing the changes of interstitial pneumonitis have been found to be associated with anti-Ro (12). There is no evidence directly implicating anti-Ro in the pulmonary disease of lupus, however, but the association of anti-Ro with pulmonary disease has been previously appreciated (13).

TABLE 23.1. ASSOCIATIONS WITH ANTI-RO AND ANTI-LA AUTOANTIBODIES IN SYSTEMIC LUPUS ERYTHEMATOSUS AND RELATED DISORDERS[a]

Specificity	Clinical or Genetic Association
Anti-Ro	Photosensitive skin rash (lupus)
	Interstitial pneumonitis (lupus)
	Thrombocytopenia (lupus, Sjögren's syndrome)
	Lymphopenia (lupus, Sjögren's syndrome)
	Nephritis (lupus)
	C2 complement deficiency (lupus)
	HLA-DQ1/2
	T-cell receptor β gene (lupus)
	Vasculitis (Sjögren's syndrome)
	Thrombocytopenic purpura (Sjögren's syndrome, subacute cutaneous lupus)
	Primary biliary cirrhosis
Anti-Ro and anti-La	Absence of nephritis (lupus)
	HLA-B8, DR3 (lupus)
	HLA-DQ1/2 (Sjögren's syndrome)
	Rheumatoid factor (lupus, Sjögren's syndrome)
	Sjögren's syndrome
	Subacute cutaneous lupus erythematosus
	Neonatal lupus dermatitis
	Complete congenital heart block

[a]Associations are presented for systemic lupus erythematosus (lupus) unless the data are derived from patients with another diagnosis, such as Sjögren's syndrome. While rheumatoid factor, Sjögren's syndrome, subacute cutaneous lupus erythematosus, neonatal lupus dermatitis, and complete congenital heart block are frequently associated with both anti-Ro and anti-La precipitins, they also all occur in association with anti-Ro without anti-La.
HLA, human leukocyte antigen.

Idiopathic thrombocytopenic purpura is well known to present before lupus can be diagnosed in some patients. These patients tend to have anti-Ro precipitins (14–16). Both anti-Ro and a positive antinuclear antibody test may be found at presentation with immune thrombocytopenia and precede fulfilling the classification criteria for lupus by as much as 14 years (14). How long before presentation with immune thrombocytopenic purpura these patients develop anti-Ro is not known.

Indeed, the temporal relationship of the appearance of anti-Ro or anti-La to the clinical presentation with lupus or Sjögren's syndrome is not known. Anti-Ro or anti-La appears after diagnosis only in the rare patient. In addition, most mothers with anti-Ro and anti-La who have infants with congenital heart block or neonatal lupus dermatitis have never had clinical manifestations of any of the disorders associated with these autoantibodies (17,18). Many mothers, however, develop Sjögren's or lupus in the years following birth of the affected infant (19,20). This leads one to suspect that anti-Ro and anti-La autoantibodies may arise before the clinical illness appears. Perhaps in many cases these autoantibodies are present for years before the patient becomes ill.

In addition to thrombocytopenia, other hematologic cytopenias have been associated with anti-Ro. Patients with lupus who in any way satisfy the hematologic criterion for classification of SLE (21), but particularly those with lymphopenia, tend to have anti-Ro (22). In Sjögren's syndrome, thrombocytopenia, anemia, and lymphopenia are associated with anti-Ro (23). In rheumatoid arthritis, although anti-Ro is uncommon [i.e., approximately 5% of patients (24)], this autoantibody is associated with leukopenia when it is present (25). One study showed that anti-Ro binds directly to the granulocyte surface and is closely associated with granulocytopenia (26).

There are data supporting a role for anti-Ro in nephritis as well. In a series of patients with anti-Ro precipitin, only those who had anti-Ro without an anti-La precipitin developed renal disease (27). Subsequent work has confirmed that patients with anti-La tend to be spared renal disease (22). Acid-eluted immunoglobulin from the renal tissue of two patients with anti-Ro precipitin contained anti-Ro that had been concentrated in the antibody deposited in the kidney (28). More recent data have shown that anti-Ro, anti-La, and anti-DNA all are concentrated in renal tissue (29). This is prima facie evidence to support a direct role for anti-Ro and other autoantibodies in the nephritis of some patients. Anti-Ro deposited in the tissue either as an immune complex or by virtue of binding to a specific antigen has the potential to be phlogistic and to mediate the inflammatory response that follows antibody binding.

COMPLETE CONGENITAL HEART BLOCK

Over the past two decades, a compelling association has been demonstrated between complete congenital heart block and both anti-Ro and anti-La precipitating autoantibodies (17,30,31). The anti-Ro immunoglobulin G (IgG) clearly originates with the mother, who may be asymptomatic for an autoimmune rheumatic disorder. In a few cases, normal fetal cardiac conduction has been demonstrated before the third trimester (32,33). Heart block often appears late in the second trimester or early in the third trimester, coincident with the active transport of maternal IgG across the placenta.

Complete congenital heart block is found in approximately one of every 20,000 births (34). In the largest series of congenital heart block cases, anti-Ro and/or anti-La was found in 83% (17). Survey studies estimate that an anti-Ro precipitin may be present in as many as 1% of pregnant women (35,36). An expectant mother with an anti-Ro precipitin has an increased risk of bearing a child with complete congenital heart block, but even so, this risk remains small.

The mechanism of heart block is unclear. Cardiac conduction tissue is bound by anti-Ro more avidly than other cardiac cell types (37). Data from a set of fraternal twins who were discordant for heart block have shown depletion of anti-Ro in the serum of the affected twin, which is consistent with the possibility that anti-Ro is being specifically deposited in cardiac tissue (38). This observation strongly suggests that critical contributions are made toward the generation of heart block by the fetus in a way that varies among potentially affected pregnancies. Specific concentration of anti-Ro (both anti–60-kd Ro and anti–52-kd Ro) in cardiac tissue, but not in other tissues, has been demonstrated (39).

One theory of pathogenesis holds that the basic process is a nonspecific endomyocarditis that involves the atrioventricular node by extension at a time when the node is anatomically vulnerable (38). If true, then many fetuses of mothers with anti-Ro autoantibodies may have the endomyocarditis, while only a fraction of these involve the atrioventricular node and develop heart block.

Much progress has been made in understanding the pathogenesis of complete heart block related to anti-Ro/SSA antibodies. Boutjdir and colleagues (40) showed that anti–52-kd Ro/SSA antibodies induce complete atrioventricular (AV) block in the human fetal heart perfused by the Langendorff technique and inhibit L-type Ca^{2+} currents at the whole-cell and single-channel level. In addition, these workers immunized female BALB/c mice with recombinant 52-kd Ro/SSA protein and these antibodies crossed the placenta during pregnancy and were associated with varying degrees of AV conduction abnormalities, including complete AV block, in the pups (40). Similar results were reported by Viana et al. (41), in which affinity purified anti–52-kd Ro/SSA antibodies could induce complete AV block in isolated whole rabbit hearts. Finally, Miranda-Carus et al. (42) showed in mice that complete AV block was only seen in offspring from mothers immunized with 52-kd Ro/SSA, but not La/SSB or 60-kd Ro/SSA, although lesser AV conduction abnormalities were noted with the latter two antigens.

There are at least three ways that complete congenital heart block is relevant to lupus. First, pregnant female patients with lupus and anti-Ro, by virtue of having this autoantibody, have a one in 20 risk of having a child with complete congenital heart block (43). Second, the mothers of children with heart block are at an increased risk of developing a systemic autoimmune rheumatic disorder, even if the mother is asymptomatic when the child is born (19). Indeed, we have seen a patient whose lupus developed 26 years after the delivery of an infant with congenital heart block and that coincided with her retiring from Ohio to bask in the sunshine of Florida (44). Third, a study of adult patients with lupus has revealed an increased prevalence of conduction abnormalities among patients with anti-Ro precipitins (45).

NEONATAL LUPUS DERMATITIS

Infants of mothers with anti-Ro also may develop neonatal dermatitis. This rash most often appears after birth. Areas that are exposed to sunlight predominate but are not exclusively involved. Skin lesions often are similar to those found in subacute cutaneous lupus with arcuate erythematous macules or papulosquamous lesions. Occasionally, they may leave hypopigmented skin, but the lesions generally resolve without sequelae. In infants, all lesions that appear usually develop and resolve together. As the maternal IgG is cleared from the infant's circulation, the rash also resolves. In addition, in those infants who are not affected at or very soon after birth, the likelihood of developing the rash diminishes as maternal IgG is metabolized. Maternal IgG is almost undetectable in the infant by 6 months of age, and the onset of neonatal lupus dermatitis is unheard of at this stage. A few cases of neonatal dermatitis have been reportedly associated with an anti-nRNP precipitin in the absence of an anti-Ro precipitin (46).

SUBACUTE CUTANEOUS LUPUS ERYTHEMATOSUS

The diagnosis of subacute cutaneous lupus erythematosus is established by the presence of one of the two typical and usually photosensitive rashes, annular or papulosquamous (Fig. 23.2), along with consistent histology. Approximately

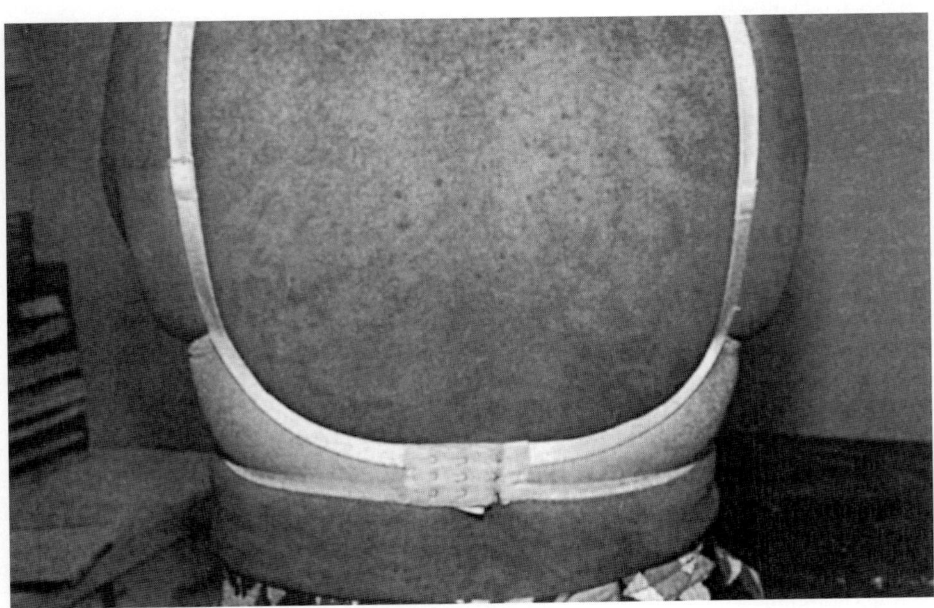

FIGURE 23.2. The rash of subacute cutaneous lupus erythematosus, showing erythematous macules and papulosquamous lesions. The typical arcuate lesions can be appreciated on the back of this middle-aged woman at presentation.

75% of patients with subacute cutaneous lupus have anti-Ro precipitins (47). These patients may or may not satisfy the classification criteria for systemic lupus (21). The lesions are erythematous and may or may not be raised. In some patients, the lesions have central clearing. Lesions at all the different stages of maturity may be present simultaneously. Some of these patients develop petechiae or purpura, particularly of the lower extremities, biopsy specimens of which often reveal small vessel vasculitis. Those with vasculitis seem to be a subgroup with greater hypergammaglobulinemia who are more likely than the remaining patients to have Sjögren's syndrome.

SJÖGREN'S SYNDROME

Of the disorders that are associated with anti-Ro and anti-La, perhaps none is more intriguing than Sjögren's syndrome. Depending on the assay performed and the population selected, from 40% to over 95% of these patients have anti-Ro, and from 15% to over 85% have anti-La (48). Dry eyes and dry mouth associated with a lymphocytic infiltrate of the salivary or lacrimal glands are not uncommon in a number of autoimmune rheumatic disorders, including SLE, rheumatoid arthritis, progressive systemic sclerosis, primary biliary cirrhosis, and autoimmune myositis. Hence, Sjögren's syndrome is a feature shared by a minor proportion of the patients with each of these disorders, which suggests that these diseases also must have fundamental aspects in common.

Primary Sjögren's syndrome is considered to be present when the diagnostic criteria for Sjögren's syndrome are satisfied (49) in the absence of another rheumatic disease with autoimmune features. Because the etiology and pathogenesis of all these diseases are unknown, and because there is great latitude in applying the diagnostic standards, the relative composition of patient groups is likely to vary greatly between investigators. This situation does not seem to have been helped by the current criteria for classification of rheumatoid arthritis (50), which are more broadly inclusive than the previous criteria (51).

There are a number of patients whose predominant disease process over time is Sjögren's syndrome but who then develop features that are consistent with SLE (52–54). As a group, they are highly enriched for human leukocyte antigen (HLA)-DR3 and commonly have both anti-Ro and anti-La. The usefulness of the distinction between primary and secondary Sjögren's syndrome is lost in this situation. Indeed, these patients are commonly referred to as having lupus-Sjögren's overlap disease. The important point is that these and other patients with lupus or Sjögren's syndrome form a continuous spectrum of disease expression, from classic primary Sjögren's syndrome through the overlap with shared features to a more typical lupus process. The failure of existing nosology to distinctly separate patients demonstrates the inadequacy of present diagnostic practices, and it provides some of the impetus to understand etiology and pathogenesis.

COMPLEMENT DEFICIENCY STATUS

SLE also is associated with hereditary deficiencies of the early components of the classic complement cascade (55,56). Patients with complement component C2 deficiency tend to have an anti-Ro precipitin but not an anti-La precipitin. Anti-Ro may be more common in homozygous patients with C2 deficiency than in the remainder of patients with lupus (57). Patients with lupus and C2 complement component deficiency also tend to have a mild form of lupus with cutaneous manifestations, but with neither anti–double-stranded DNA (anti-dsDNA) autoantibody nor nephritis. Patients with lupus and the other early complement component deficiencies also have anti-Ro without an anti-La precipitin, but this has not been evaluated in a large enough sample to be conclusive (56).

TISSUE CONCENTRATION OF ANTI-RO AND ANTI-LA

Anti-Ro and anti-La clearly are related to autoimmune rheumatic disease expression. In only a few situations has strong evidence been obtained for their phlogistic potential. In individual tissues, anti-Ro has been shown to be concentrated in the kidney, heart, and parotid gland (28,29,39,58). Affinity-enriched anti-Ro has been shown to deposit specifically in human skin transplanted onto nude and severe combined immunodeficiency disease (SCID) mice (10,11).

IMMUNOGENETICS OF ANTI-RO AND ANTI-LA

Immunogenetic associations with individual autoantibodies have led to model building in an effort to understand the possible molecular events in the context of what has been learned about the immune response. The first relationship to be appreciated has been the association of anti-Ro with HLA-DR3 (59,60). Subsequently, it has been appreciated that anti-Ro also is related to HLA-DR2 in both lupus and Sjögren's syndrome (61,62).

These multiple associations have been reconciled in two ways. First, a gene interaction effect has been defined between HLA-DQw1 and HLA-DQw2 such that patients with lupus or Sjögren's syndrome who have both of these alleles tend to have anti-Ro. This has been extended in lupus to show that particular subsets of the DQA1 and DQB2 genes mediate this effect, which therefore is consistent with a gene complementation mechanism (63). One of the attractive possibilities that could explain these results is a DQ molecule composed of the predicted DQA1 and DQB2 genes and encoded by different chromosomes. There is not direct evidence for or against such a molecule in lupus or Sjögren's patients. Others have performed experiments in cell lines and have obtained data suggesting that the predicted molecule is not favored (64).

Reveille et al. (65) have taken a more inclusive approach by attempting to define the primary sequence of HLA-DQ that is common to all patients with anti-Ro relative to that of a control population. They also have mapped the most powerful associations to the DQ locus. Nearly all patients with an anti-Ro response had a glutamine at amino acid position 34 of at least one of their DQ α-chains and a leucine at amino acid position 26 of at least one of their DQ β-chains.

The HLA associations with the anti-La response are a little different. In primary Sjögren's syndrome, anti-La is related to HLA-B8, DR3, and DR2 (48,66,67), much as for anti-Ro. Indeed, the association of anti-La with the HLA-DQ1/w2 heterozygous state was as powerful as it was for anti-Ro (68). In lupus, however, the strongest association is with the B8, DR3 haplotype (22). The basis for this discrepancy is not known.

MODELS OF PATHOGENESIS

Humoral autoimmunity is revealed by the presence of autoantibodies. It is much more difficult to be confident that human diseases with lymphocytic infiltrates but without autoantibodies also are autoimmune, but work in animal models has provided convincing and overwhelming evidence that this mechanism of disease pathogenesis is a practical possibility. Here, the prevailing suspicion is that T lymphocytes are mediating autoimmunity without stimulating B lymphocytes to differentiate and produce autoantibodies. T lymphocytes appear to determine not only whether a cellular, as opposed to an antibody, response results from immunogen exposure, but also in many circumstances whether tolerance is maintained or broken. For these and other reasons, most investigators suspect that T lymphocytes have an obligate role in the immunoregulatory decision to synthesize autoantibody against protein autoantigens. Defining this role in human lupus has been difficult, as it has been in other inflammatory, and possibly autoimmune, disorders of unknown etiology. For example, in lupus, there is no evidence to suspect the linkage of lupus with α, β, or γ T-lymphocyte receptor genes in multiplex families (69).

On the other hand, just as the histocompatibility associations are different for risk of disease than they are for production of individual autoantibodies, there may be analogous differences at the level of the T-cell receptor. Recent work has shown that alleles of the T-cell receptor β-chain gene are related to the presence of anti-Ro in lupus (70). Interestingly, the association is most significant for those patients who have an anti-Ro precipitin without an anti-La precipitin, and it does not exist for those who have both anti-Ro and anti-La precipitins. Preliminary analysis is consistent with synergy between the T-cell receptor association and the HLA-DQ alleles that are associated with anti-Ro (71). Other work with the 70-kd U1 ribonucleoprotein has shown that lymphocytes proliferate after exposure to this peptide when it is presented as a fusion protein, and that a region from the carboxyl terminus is more stimulatory than other regions of the molecule (72).

These data are consistent with a model of the generation of lupus autoantibodies in general, and of anti-Ro in particular, that requires the participation of HLA-DQ and T-cell receptor alleles along with the autoantigen to form a trimolecular complex (Fig. 23.3). Human Ro is suspected to be directly involved, because Ro from other species is less antigenic with human autoantibodies (73). From these data the conclusion that the anti-Ro autoimmune response is Ro autoantigen-driven in lupus is compelling. Similar conclusions have been reached using other experimental strategies for the anti-Sm and anti-DNA responses in lupus (74,75). Accordingly, autoantigen-driven autoimmune responses appear to be the general rule in lupus.

Some of the genetic risk factors for the generation of individual autoantibodies have been defined. Associations with clinical manifestations also are known. The question

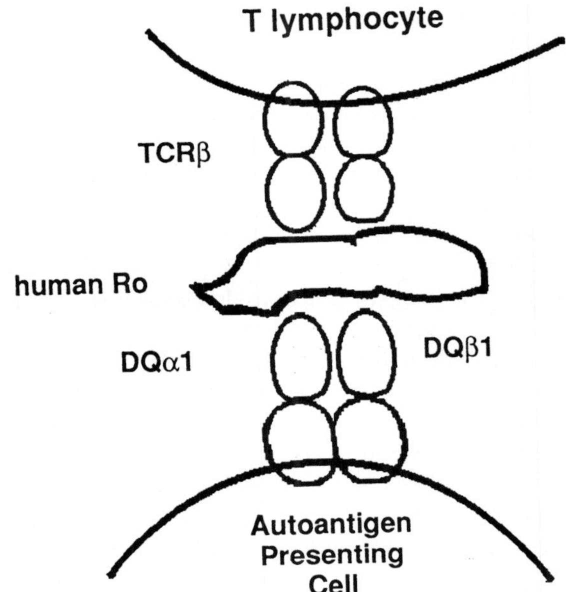

FIGURE 23.3. The trimolecular complex model for autoantigen presentation of the human Ro autoantigen based on associations of anti-Ro with alleles at human leukocyte antigen (HLA)-DQ and the β peptide of the T-lymphocyte receptor.

TABLE 23.2. LOGISTIC REGRESSION MODEL OF RENAL DISEASE IN 40 PATIENTS WITH LUPUSA

		Improvement		Goodness of Fit			
Step	Term	ξ^2	*p*	ξ^2	*p*	Coefficient	Standard Error
1	Anti-La	8.7	.003	33	.50	−1.22	0.52
2	Anti-dsDNA	6.9	.008	26	.79	2.75	1.19

[a]Anti-La is presented as the $\log_{10}$ of the ELISA units of the La solid-phase binding activity (range, 2.00–7.03). Anti-dsDNA is a dichotomous variable (1, present; 0, never detected). The standard error of the mean of the coefficient is given.
dsDNA, double-stranded DNA; ELISA, enzyme-linked immunosorbent assay.
From Harley JB, Sestak AL, Willis LG, et al. A model for disease heterogeneity in systemic lupus erythematosus. Relationships between histocompatibility antigens, autoantibodies, and lymphopenia or renal disease. *Arthritis Rheum* 1989;32:826–836, with permission.

that remains to be determined, however, is how the clinical features, immunogenetics, and autoantibodies are interrelated in lupus, although one would suspect that relationships should flow from the genetic features to the autoantibodies and from autoantibodies to the disease manifestations. This concept of the disease predicts, for example, that HLA alleles generally are related to clinical manifestations through the autoantibodies, and that the relationships of autoantibodies with HLA alleles and of autoantibodies with clinical manifestations will be stronger than those of HLA alleles with clinical manifestations.

This hypothesis was confirmed in a group of 40 patients with lupus in whom the anti-La, anti-Ro, anti-Sm, anti-nRNP, anti–single-stranded DNA (anti-ssDNA), and anti-dsDNA were measured (22). The first four specificities were detected by gel diffusion. Antibodies to ssDNA were detected by radioimmunoassay and anti-dsDNA antibodies were detected by the *Crithidia* assay. Primary relationships were found between HLA-DQw1/w2 and anti-Ro, and between HLA-B8, DR3, and anti-La. Primary associations were found between anti-Ro and lymphopenia, and between anti-La and the absence of nephritis. Nephritis was present if either proteinuria exceeded 0.5 g per 24 hours or cellular casts were present in the urine. No statistically relevant relationships were present between any of the HLA antigens that were determined and any criterion for the classification of lupus (21). Logistic regression analysis established that the presence of lymphopenia was best explained by considering the combined contributions of anti-Ro and anti-ssDNA (22).

The relationship of anti-La with the absence of nephritis was analyzed by an analogous approach (22). The literature inconsistently shows an association of anti-dsDNA with nephritis, although there is convincing evidence that some anti-dsDNA antibodies are deposited in the kidney (76–80). On the other hand, both anti-La and anti-nRNP have been associated with a decreased incidence of nephritis in lupus (27,81,82). In this group of 40 patients with lupus, there was no simple association between anti-dsDNA and nephritis (22). Logistic regression analysis, however, produces an interesting result (Table 23.2). The association of anti-La with the absence of nephritis is powerful; however, once this effect is incorporated into the logistic model, then anti-dsDNA makes an important contribution. Here, anti-La and anti-dsDNA have opposing effects, which is demonstrated in the resulting logistic equation presented in Fig. 23.4. These data support a mechanism of disease expression in which the clinical manifesta-

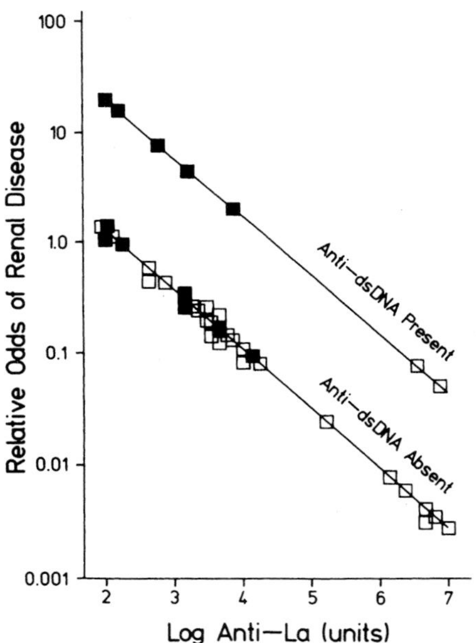

FIGURE 23.4. Relative odds of lupus nephritis in 40 patients with lupus as modeled from the anti-La and anti–double-stranded DNA (anti-dsDNA) antibody levels. Anti-La titer is expressed as the $\log_{10}$ of the relative binding in a solid-phase assay using purified bovine La. The presence or absence of anti-dsDNA is indicated. The presence (*closed squares*) or absence (*open squares*) of renal disease is indicated as well. The relative odds of renal disease are calculated from the logistic regression model presented in Table 23.2 (n = 40): ln (relative odds of renal disease) = −1.22 (anti-La) + 2.75 (anti-dsDNA) + 2.67. (From Harley JB, Sestak AL, Willis LG, et al. A model for disease heterogeneity in systemic lupus erythematosus. Relationships between histocompatibility antigens, autoantibodies, and lymphopenia or renal disease. *Arthritis Rheum* 1989;32:826–836, with permission.)

tions result from complicated interactions of various kinds of autoantibodies. The autoantibodies in turn are strongly influenced by the particular HLA and T-cell receptor alleles that are present. One mechanism to explain these relationships is the recent demonstration that subsets of anti-La antibodies are in fact antiidiotypes to anti-dsDNA (83).

ASSAYS FOR DETECTING ANTI-RO AND ANTI-LA

In clinical practice, Ouchterlony double immunodiffusion is the traditional method of determining whether anti-Ro or anti-La is present (Fig. 23.1). Most data relating these serologies to clinical manifestations have been developed using either this technique or the closely related procedure of counterimmunoelectrophoresis. Double immunodiffusion is specific and sufficiently sensitive for nearly all clinical applications. Unfortunately, the procedure usually requires 2 days to complete, and its performance requires specialized training. Not infrequently, an anti-Ro precipitin is missed, either because poor-quality reagents have been used or because an inexperienced person is performing the test.

These difficulties and inefficiencies have provided an incentive for the development and marketing of alternative methodologies. Immunoprecipitation, immunoblotting, and solid-phase enzyme-linked immunosorbent assays (ELISAs) are available in research laboratories. Anti-Ro and anti-La ELISAs have been marketed to clinicians and clinical laboratories and these assays have largely supplanted the more traditional methodologies for clinical assessment. These assays appear to provide as much as a 10- to 100-fold increase in sensitivity over double immunodiffusion. There is greater potential for interfering and artifactual binding in ELISA, and consequently the specificity of these assays is reduced relative to double immunodiffusion. The increased sensitivity means that half or more of patients with lupus, and perhaps over three quarters of patients with Sjögren's syndrome, are positive for anti-Ro in these assays. The proportion of patients who are positive for anti-La often is doubled, from 10% to 20% in lupus and from 15% to 40% in Sjögren's syndrome, by the application of the routinely available assays.

The antigenicity of the Ro antigen is adversely affected by denaturation and often is not detected whether the antigen is fixed *in situ* (e.g., in a cell line for the antinuclear antibody test) or by another method (e.g., by boiling in sodium dodecyl sulfate for the Western blot test). Indeed, the Ro antigen as expressed by bacterial systems produces an antigen that has a similar profound reduction in antigenicity as seen in the denatured material. Thus, Western blotting or reliance on Ro antigen in Western blots or on expression in a bacterial system from a recombinant complementary DNA (cDNA) will provide misleading results unless special precautions or adjustments are made.

Another ingenious assay is available for the detection of anti-Ro. Three groups have transfected cell lines with the coding sequence of the 60-kd Ro protein behind a promoter that increases the production of Ro protein in the cell (84–86). With the increased Ro antigen available, the problems that are associated with fixation may be overcome (84). Indeed, HEp-2 slides with overexpressed Ro are now commercially available (HEp-2 2000).

The importance of identifying patients who have anti-Ro or anti-La by an ELISA is problematic for those who do not form precipitins. A significant proportion of normal individuals may fall into this category. At present, this level of anti-Ro does not assist in formulating diagnosis or prognosis. The ready availability and relative ease of performing these solid-phase assays dictates their increasing use. Nevertheless, whatever assay the clinician chooses, he or she should fully understand the meaning of the results and the limitations on their interpretation.

The levels of anti-Ro and anti-La vary over time by as much as 10- to 20-fold during the course of the disease, but the relevance of this to disease expression is not known. Mildly affected patients have been known, or inferred, to have had anti-Ro or anti-La precipitins for decades. It is rare to observe the disappearance of an anti-Ro or anti-La precipitin after disease onset unless the patient has had aggressive cytotoxic therapy, corticosteroids at high doses for an extended period, heavy proteinuria, or renal failure.

MOLECULAR CONSIDERATIONS

Important progress also has been made in defining the molecular properties of the Ro and La antigens. All four human Ro-associated RNAs, known as hY RNAs, have been sequenced (Fig. 23.5). Each is a product of RNA polymerase III and is from 84 to 112 bases in length. The hY RNAs have a triphosphate 5′ terminus and a polyuridine 3′ terminus (87,88). Two highly conserved regions of 24 bases, one half from the 3′ end and one half from the 5′ end, are found in each hY RNA sequence (89). Part of this conserved region is thought to bind to the Ro protein by virtue of its being protected from RNAse digestion of the intact ribonuclear particle (88). From two to four Y RNAs have been isolated from every other vertebrate species evaluated (90), leading to the impression of substantial heterogeneity in Y RNAs between species. The Y3 RNA appears to be the most conserved among vertebrate species (91).

The peptide with a molecular weight of approximately 60 kd is the major antigenic peptide in the Ro RNA protein particle (92). Two sequences of this peptide have been obtained, which are essentially identical except for a small region of sequence divergence at the amino terminus (93,94). The 60-kd Ro peptide has a putative ribonucleoprotein binding domain and a zinc finger. Itoh et al. (95)

```
hY1 GGCUGGUCCGAAGGUAGUGAGUUAUCUCAAUUGAUUGUUCACAGUCAGUUACAGAUCGAA
hY3 GGCUGGUCCGAGUGCAGUGGUGUUUA.CAACUAAUUGAUCACAACCAGUUACAGAUUU..
hY4 GGCUGGUCCGAUGGUAGUGGGUUAUC...AGAACUUAUUAACAUU.AGUGUCA...CUAA
hY5 AGUUGGUCCGAGUGUUGUGGGUUAU..........UGUUA......AGUU...GAUUUAA

                                                   112
hY1 CUCCUUGUUCUACUCUUUCCCCCUUCUCACUACUGCACUUGACUAGUCUUU
hY3 CU..UUGUUC....CUU.CUCCACU.CCCACUGCUUCACUUGACUAGCCUUU
hY4 AG..UUGGUAUACAA...CCCCCC.....ACUGCUAAAUUUGACU.GGCUU
hY5 CA..UUG......UC..UCCCCCC.....ACAACCGCGCUUGACUA.GCUUGCUGUUUU
```

A

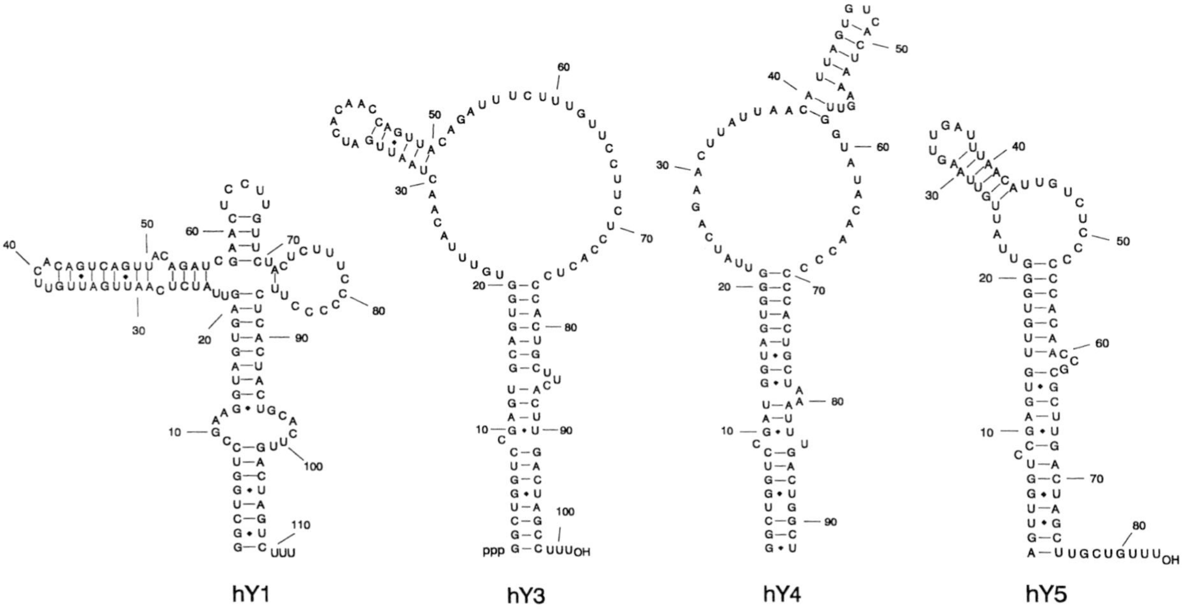

B

FIGURE 23.5. hY RNAs. **A:** Sequence comparison of the four Y RNAs. Periods indicate gaps in the sequence arranged to maximize sequence alignment. **B:** Proposed secondary structures of the hY RNAs. (Adapted from Farris AD. *Phylogenetic analysis of Ro ribonucleoprotein associated small RNAs* [dissertation]. Oklahoma City, OK: University of Oklahoma Health Sciences Center, 1995:119, for hY1; Farris AD, O'Brien CA, Harley JB. Y3 is the most conserved small RNA component of Ro ribonucleoprotein complexes in vertebrate species. *Gene* 1995;154:193–198, for hY3 and hY4; and O'Brien CA, Margelot K, Wolin SL. Xenopus Ro ribonucleoproteins: members of an evolutionarily conserved class of cytoplasmic ribonucleoproteins. *Proc Natl Acad Sci USA* 1993;90:7250–7254, for hY5.)

have presented evidence for two antigenically related forms of 60-kd Ro. Of the Y RNAs, only hY5 is antigenic (96).

A number of other polypeptides have been related to anti-Ro autoantibodies, including 54-kd Ro and 60-kd Ro, which are both found in red cells; 52-kd Ro, a 57-kd polypeptide; and calreticulin. With La, these constitute a family of autoantigens. Except for calreticulin (97–99), antibodies that bind these autoantigens are found virtually only in sera that contain precipitating levels of anti-Ro autoantibodies.

A 52-kd peptide has been identified from lymphocytes by immunoblot (100), and its cDNA has been cloned and sequenced (101,102). Although one study detected a molecular association of the 52-kd Ro with the 60-kd Ro protein (103), this has not been confirmed, and most existing data support there being no stable molecular association between 52-kd Ro and the 60-kd Ro (104–107). The Ro hY RNAs are immunoprecipitated in association with 60-kd Ro (107,108). While some anti-Ro and anti-La sera immunoprecipitate the 52-kd protein, most appear to contain antibodies against the denatured form of 52-kd Ro found in Western blot (107,108). The 52-kd Ro gene may be important beyond its being a target of autoimmunity, because an allele of the 52-kd Ro gene is associated with lupus in blacks (109,110).

In erythrocytes, 60-kd and 54-kd peptides are variably identified in immunoblot by different sera containing anti-

Ro (111). The 54-kd erythrocyte Ro peptide appears to be antigenically related to the 52-kd lymphocyte Ro (101). Interestingly, only hY1 and hY4 RNAs are immunoprecipitated from human erythrocytes, where they are slightly smaller than in other human cell types (89). This difference probably results from the shorter polyuridine 3′ end on the Y RNAs found in erythrocytes. The Y RNAs in human platelets are demonstrated to be restricted to hY3 and hY4 (112).

A 46-kd protein has been identified and sequenced using patient sera that contain anti-Ro activity. This sequence appears to be the human form of calreticulin, which is a calcium-binding protein (113). No clinical associations with this autoantibody have been established.

Maddison et al. (114) defined another specificity found in sera with anti-Ro autoantibodies: anti-p57. These antibodies are found in approximately 10% of patients with lupus and in nearly 40% of mothers of infants with complete congenital heart block or neonatal lupus dermatitis.

Ro particles also have been studied without exposure to denaturing conditions to allow an evaluation of *in vivo* Ro particle composition. In gel filtration, these particles range from 230 to 350 kd, thus supporting the position that there may be more than one peptide in a Ro particle (115). One of these particles appears to contain the hY5 RNA and not the other hY RNAs (96,115).

At least one of these isolated Ro particles also contains the La peptide, thereby providing a structural basis for the association of anti-Ro and anti-La autoantibodies in patient serum. The La peptide contains 408 amino acids and has a predicted molecular weight of 46.7 kd (116–118). La also has an 80 amino acid conserved element referred to as the *RNA recognition motif* (119). The carboxyl end of the protein is methionine free and phosphorylated, while the amino end is methionine rich (120). The La peptide appears to bind any RNA with a polyuridine 3′ end (121,122). In addition to the Y RNAs, these include the precursors of 7S, 5S, U6, and precursors of transfer RNAs. The bound RNAs generally are the immature transcription products of RNA polymerase III, except for U1-RNA, which is an RNA polymerase II product that binds La (123).

Some virus-encoded RNAs also bind La from adenovirus, Epstein-Barr virus, and vesicular stomatitis virus (124–126). In addition, La appears to play important roles in the expression of genes from poliovirus and human immunodeficiency virus (127,128).

There is evidence for La playing multiple roles in the molecular economy of the cell, while Ro has been implicated in only the discard pathway for 5S RNA (129). La may function as a shuttle protein to carry RNA transcripts from the nucleus to the cytoplasm (130,131), and other investigators have obtained evidence that La is a termination factor for RNA polymerase III (132,133). La has been shown to melt an RNA-DNA hybrid in a reaction that requires adenosine triphosphate (ATP) hydrolysis (134) and to bind double-stranded RNA, thereby influencing interferon-inducible protein kinase (135). Perhaps the most intriguing data show that La increases the efficiency and fidelity of internal translation (128,136,137).

La proteins are found in widely divergent species, from humans to yeast. In both, the La protein binds polyuridine termini of RNA (138). Despite all the activities found for La and the evolutionary implications of its presence throughout eukaryotic life, yeast are viable despite the destruction of the La protein gene (138,139).

FINE SPECIFICITY OF ANTI-RO AND ANTI-LA

With more detailed structural information now available, attention has turned to the fine specificity of anti-Ro and anti-La autoantibodies. By expressing fragments of the recombinant La cDNA clone, a number of groups have shown multiple epitopes on the La peptide that are distributed throughout the primary structure (116,140–145).

The 60-kd Ro peptide also appears to have multiple linear epitopes (146,147). In addition, there is evidence of multiple epitopes throughout the 52-kd Ro molecule (145,148), suggesting this is a general finding in lupus autoimmunity.

In both anti-Ro and anti-La autoantibodies, IgG1 predominates, with the other subclasses of IgG being variably represented (149–151). Anti-La is composed predominantly of IgG1k antibodies, while anti-Sm is not subclass restricted (149).

Unexpectedly, the antigenic peptides of 60-kd Ro tend to share short sequence homology with the nucleocapsid protein of vesicular stomatitis virus (146,147). Humans infected with vesicular stomatitis virus tend to have low levels of anti-Ro (152), and animals immunized with the cross-reactive nucleocapsid from vesicular stomatitis produce antibodies that bind 60-kd Ro (153).

There are many other hints about the origin of anti-Ro and anti-La autoantibodies. Sera with these antibodies and anti-dsDNA cross-react with the denatured Sm D and nRNP A polypeptides (154,155), thereby providing some unity for lupus autoimmunity across the major known protein autoantigen specificities. Antibodies that bind to hY5 RNA, but not the other hY RNAs, have been detected (96). Because Ro ribonuclear particles containing hY5 RNA can be isolated as distinct particles, some suspect that this may be the original autoantigen (96).

Mechanisms explaining maturation of the autoimmune response are under intensive inquiry. Epitope spreading has been shown for anti-La antibodies (156,157) and for the Sm B/B′, where this maturation can be induced by immunization with a single peptide. Such a situation is also found in the restricted autoimmune response of the few patients with sera available from early in the disease process (158). Perhaps, defining the initial autoimmune response will provide important clues to etiology and pathogenesis.

ACKNOWLEDGMENTS

We gratefully thank our many colleagues who have contributed to the work discussed herein. Our efforts are supported by National Institutes of Health grants AI14717, AI31584, AR42460, AR42474, AR31133, and AR43975, and by the U.S. Department of Veterans Affairs.

REFERENCES

1. Jones BR. Lacrimal and salivary precipitating antibodies in Sjögren's syndrome. *Lancet* 1958;2:773–776.
2. Anderson JR, Gray KG, Beck JS, et al. Precipitating autoantibodies in the connective tissue diseases. *Ann Rheum Dis* 1962; 21:360–369.
3. Clark G, Reichlin M, Tomasi TB. Characterization of a soluble cytoplasmic antigen reactive with sera from patients with systemic lupus erythematosus. *J Immunol* 1969;102:117–120.
4. Mattioli M, Reichlin M. Heterogeneity of RNA protein antigens reactive with sera of patients with systemic lupus erythematosus. Description of a cytoplasmic nonribosomal antigen. *Arthritis Rheum* 1974;17:421–429.
5. Alspaugh M, Maddison PJ. Resolution of the identity of certain antigen-antibody systems in systemic lupus erythematosus and Sjögren's syndrome. *Arthritis Rheum* 1979;22:796–798.
6. Alspaugh MA, Tan EM. Antibodies to cellular antigens in Sjögren's syndrome. *J Clin Invest* 1975;55:1067–1073.
7. Lerner MR, Boyle JA, Mount SN, et al. Are snRNPs involved in splicing? *Nature* 1980;283:220–224.
8. Maddison PJ, Mogavero H, Reichlin M. Antibodies to nuclear ribonucleoprotein. *J Rheumatol* 1978;5:407–411.
9. Mond CB, Peterson MG, Rothfield NF. Correlation of anti-Ro antibody with photosensitivity rash in systemic lupus erythematosus patients. *Arthritis Rheum* 1989;32:202–204.
10. Lee LA, David KM. Cutaneous lupus erythematosus. *Curr Probl Dermatol* 1989;1:161–200.
11. Lee LA, Weston WL. New findings in neonatal lupus syndrome. *Am J Dis Child* 1984;138:233–236.
12. Hedgpeth MT, Boulware DW. Interstitial pneumonitis in antinuclear antibody-negative systemic lupus erythematosus: a new clinical manifestation and possible association with anti-Ro (SS-A) antibodies. *Arthritis Rheum* 1988;31:545–548.
13. Smolen JS, Morimoto C, Steinberg AD, et al. Systemic lupus erythematosus: delineation of subpopulations by clinical serologic and T cell subset analysis. *Am J Med* 1985;289:139–148.
14. Adachi M, Mita S, Obana M, et al. Thrombocytopenia subsequently develops systemic lupus erythematosus. Can anti-SSA antibody predict the next event? *Jpn J Med* 1990;29:481–486.
15. Anderson MJ, Peebles CL, McMillar R, et al. Fluorescent antinuclear antibodies and anti-SSA/Ro in patients with immune thrombocytopenia developing systemic lupus erythematosus. *Ann Intern Med* 1985;103:548–551.
16. Morley KD, Bernstein RM, Bunn CC, et al. Thrombocytopenia and anti-Ro. *Lancet* 1981;2:940.
17. Scott JS, Maddison PJ, Taylor PJ, et al. Connective-tissue disease, antibodies to ribonucleoprotein, and congenital heart block. *N Engl J Med* 1983;39:209–212.
18. Watson RM, Lane AT, Barnett NK, et al. Neonatal lupus erythematosus: a clinical, serological and immunogenetic study with review of the literature. *Medicine* 1984;63:362–378.
19. McCune AB, Weston WL, Lee LA. Maternal and fetal outcome in neonatal lupus erythematosus. *Ann Intern Med* 1987;106: 518–523.
20. Julkun H, Kurki P, Kaaja R, et al. Isolated congenital heart block. Long-term outcome of mothers and characterization of the immune response to SS-A/Ro and to SS-B/La. *Arthritis Rheum* 1993;36:1588–1598.
21. Tan EM, Cohen AS, Fries JF, et al. Special article: the 1982 revised criteria for the classification of systemic lupus erythematosus. *Arthritis Rheum* 1982;25:1271–1277.
22. Harley JB, Sestak AL, Willis LG, et al. A model for disease heterogeneity in systemic lupus erythematosus. Relationships between histocompatibility antigens, autoantibodies, and lymphopenia or renal disease. *Arthritis Rheum* 1989;32:826–836.
23. Alexander EL, Arnett FC, Provost TT, et al. Sjögren's syndrome association of anti-Ro (SSA) antibodies with vasculitis, hematologic abnormalities, and serologic hyperreactivity. *Ann Intern Med* 1983;98:155–159.
24. Bernstein RM, Bunn CC, Hughes GRV, et al. Cellular protein and RNA antigens in autoimmune disease. *Mol Biol Med* 1984; 2:105–120.
25. Boire G, Menard HA. Clinical significance of anti-Ro (SSA) antibody in rheumatoid arthritis. *J Rheumatol* 1988;15: 391–394.
26. Kurien BT, Moore KL, Scofield RH. Neutrophils and anti-Ro/SSA. *Ann NY Acad Sci* 1997;815:481–484.
27. Wasicek CA, Reichlin M. Clinical and serological differences between systemic lupus erythematosus patients with antibodies in Ro versus patients without antibodies to Ro and La. *J Clin Invest* 1982;69:835–843.
28. Maddison PJ, Reichlin M. Deposition of antibodies to a soluble cytoplasmic antigen in the kidneys of patients with systemic lupus erythematosus. *Arthritis Rheum* 1979;22:858–863.
29. Skinner RP, Maddison PJ. Analysis of polyethylene glycol precipitates from SLE sera: antibody enrichment in association with disease activity. *Clin Exp Rheum* 1990;8:553–560.
30. Franco HL, Weston WL, Peebles C, et al. Autoantibodies directed against sicca syndromes antigens in neonatal lupus syndrome. *J Am Acad Dermatol* 1981;4:67–72.
31. Kephart DC, Hood AF, Provost TT. Neonatal lupus erythematosus: new serological findings. *J Invest Dermatol* 1981;77: 331–333.
32. Buyon J, Roubey R, Swersky S, et al. Complete congenial heart block: risk of occurrence and therapeutic approach to prevention. *J Rheumatol* 1988;15:1104–1108.
33. Truccone NJ, Mariona FG. Prenatal diagnosis and outcome of congenial complete heart block: the role of fetal echocardiography. *Fetal Ther* 1986;1:210–216.
34. Michaelson M, Engle MA. Congenital complete heart block: an international study of the natural history. *Cardiovasc Clin North Am* 1972;4(3):85–101.
35. Calmes BA, Bartholomew BA. SSA-A(Ro) antibody in random mother-infant pairs. *J Clin Pathol* 1985;38:73–75.
36. Taylor PV, Taylor KF, Norman A, et al. Prevalence of maternal Ro(SS-A) and La(SS-B) autoantibodies in relation to congenital heart block. *Br J Rheumatol* 1988;27:128–132.
37. Deng JS, Bair LW, Shen-Schwarz S, et al. Localization of Ro(SS-A) antigen in the cardiac conduction system. *Arthritis Rheum* 1987;301:1232–1238.
38. Harley JB, Kaine JL, Fox OF, et al. Ro (SS-A) antibody and antigen in a patient with congenital complete heart block. *Arthritis Rheum* 1985;28:1321–1325.
39. Reichlin M, Brucato A, Frank MB, et al. Concentration of

autoantibodies to native 60-kD Ro/SS-A and denatured 52-kD Ro/SS-A in eluates from the heart of a child who died with congenital complete heart block. *Arthritis Rheum* 1994;37: 1698–1703.
40. Boutjdir M, Chen L, Zhang ZH, et al. Arrhythmogenicity of IgG and anti52-kd SSA/Ro affinity purified antibodies from mothers of children with congenital heart block. *Circ Res* 1997; 80:354–362.
41. Viana VS, Garcia S, Nascimento JH, et al. Induction of in vitro heart block is not restricted to affinity purified anti-52 Kda Ro/SSA antibodies from mother of a child with neonatal lupus. *Lupus* 1998;7:141–147.
42. Miranda-Carus ME, Boutjdir M, Tseng CE, et al. Induction of antibodies reactive with SSA/Ro-SSB/La and development of congenital heart block in a murine model. *J Immunol* 1998; 161:5886–5892.
43. Ramsey-Goldman R, Hom D, Deng J-S, et al. Anti-SS-A antibodies and fetal outcome in maternal systemic lupus erythematosus. *Arthritis Rheum* 1986;29:1269–1273.
44. Reichlin M, Friday K, Harley JB. Complete congenital heart block followed by the development of antibodies to Ro/SSA in adult life: serological clinical and HLA studies in an informative family. *Am J Med* 1988;84:339–344.
45. Logar D, Kveder T, Rozman B, et al. Possible association between anti-Ro antibodies and myocarditis or cardiac conduction defects in adults with systemic lupus erythematosus. *Ann Rheum Dis* 1990;49:627–629.
46. Provost TT, Watson R, Gammon WR, et al. The neonatal lupus syndrome associated with U1RNP (nRNP) antibodies. *N Engl J Med* 1987;315:1135–1139.
47. Sontheimer RD, Maddison PJ, Reichlin M, et al. Serologic and HLA associations in subacute cutaneous lupus erythematosus: a clinical subset of lupus erythematosus. *Ann Intern Med* 1982; 97:664–671.
48. Harley JB, Alexander EL, Arnett FC, et al. Anti-Ro/SSA and anti-La/SSB in patients with Sjögren's syndrome. *Arthritis Rheum* 1986;29:196–206.
49. Manthorpe R, Andersen V, Jensen OA, et al. Editorial comments to the four sets of criteria for Sjögren's syndrome. *Scand J Rheumatol* 1986;61(suppl):31–35.
50. Arnett FC, Edworthy SM, Bloch DA, et al. The American Rheumatism Association 1987 revised criteria for the classification of rheumatoid arthritis. *Arthritis Rheum* 1988;31:315–324.
51. Ropes MW, Bennett GA, Cobb S, et al. 1958 revision of diagnostic criteria for rheumatoid arthritis. *Bull Rheum Dis* 1958; 9:175–176.
52. Alexander EL, McNicholl J, Watson RM, et al. The immunogenetic relationship between anti-Ro(SS-A)/La(SS-B) antibody positive Sjögren's/lupus erythematosus overlap syndrome and the neonatal lupus syndrome. *J Invest Dermatol* 1989;93: 751–756.
53. Provost TT, Talal N, Bias W, et al. Ro (SS-A) positive Sjögren's/lupus erythematosus (SC/LE) overlap patients are associated with the HLA-DR3 and/or DRw6 phenotypes. *J Invest Dermatol* 1988;91:369–371.
54. Provost TT, Talal N, Harley JB, et al. The relationship between anti-Ro (SS-A) antibody-positive Sjögren's syndrome and anti-Ro (SS-A) antibody-positive lupus erythematosus. *Arch Dermatol* 1988;124:63–71.
55. Agnello V. Complement deficiency and systemic lupus erythematosus. In: Lahita RG, ed. *Systemic lupus erythematosus*. New York: Wiley, 1987:565–592.
56. Meyer O, Hauptmann G, Tappeiner G, et al. Genetic deficiency of C4, C2 or C1q and lupus syndromes: association with anti-Ro (SSA) antibodies. *Clin Exp Immunol* 1985;62:678–684.
57. Provost TT, Arnett FC, Reichlin M. Homozygous C2 deficiency, lupus erythematosus and anti-Ro(SS-A) antibodies. *Arthritis Rheum* 1983;26:1279–1282.
58. Penner E, Reichlin M. Primary biliary cirrhosis associated with Sjögren's syndrome: evidence for circulating and tissue-deposited Ro/anti-Ro immune complexes. *Arthritis Rheum* 1982;25:1250–1253.
59. Bell DA, Maddison PJ. Serologic subsets in systemic lupus erythematosus: an examination of autoantibodies in relationship to clinical features of disease and HLA antigens. *Arthritis Rheum* 1980;23:1268–1273.
60. Maddison PJ, Bell DA. HLA antigens in relationship to serologic subsets of systemic lupus erythematosus. *Arthritis Rheum* 1980;23:714–715.
61. Ahearn JM, Provost TT, Dorsch CA, et al. Interrelationships of HLA-DR, MB and MT phenotypes, autoantibody expression, and clinical features in systemic lupus erythematosus. *Arthritis Rheum* 1982;25:1031–1040.
62. Alvarellos A, Ahearn JM, Provost TT, et al. Relationships of HLA-DR and MT antigens to autoantibody expression in SLE. *Arthritis Rheum* 1983;26:1533–1535.
63. Fujisaku A, Frank MB, Neas B, et al. HLA-DQ gene complementation and other histocompatibility relationships in man with the anti-Ro/SSA autoantibody response in systemic lupus erythematosus. *J Clin Invest* 1990;86:606–611.
64. Kwok WW, Thurtle P, Nepom GT. A genetically controlled pairing anomaly between HLA-DQ alpha and HLA-DQ beta chains. *J Immunol* 1989;143:3598–3601.
65. Reveille JD, MacLeod MJ, Whittington K, et al. Specific amino acid residues in the second hypervariable region of HLA-DQA1 and DQB1 chain genes promote the Ro (SS-A)/La (SS-B) autoantibody responses. *J Immunol* 1991;146:3871–3876.
66. Whittingham S, Mackay IR, Tait BD. Autoantibodies to small nuclear ribonucleoproteins. A strong association between anti-SS-B(La), HLA-B8 and Sjögren's syndrome. *Aust NZ J Med* 1983;23:565–570.
67. Wilson RW, Provost TT, Bias WB, et al. Sjögren's syndrome. Influence of multiple HLA-D region alloantigens on clinical and serologic expression. *Arthritis Rheum* 1984;27:1245–1253.
68. Harley JB, Reichlin M, Arnett FC, et al. Gene interaction at the HLA-DQ locus enhances autoantibody production in primary Sjögren's syndrome. *Science* 1986;232:1145–1147.
69. Wong DW, Bentwich Z, Martinez-Tarquino C, et al. Nonlinkage of the T cell receptor α, β, and γ; genes to systemic lupus erythematosus in multiplex families. *Arthritis Rheum* 1988;31: 1371–1376.
70. Frank MB, McArthur R, Harley JB, et al. Anti-Ro (SSA) autoantibodies are associated with T cell receptor β genes in systemic lupus erythematosus patients. *J Clin Invest* 1990;85: 33–39.
71. Scofield RH, Frank MB, McArthur R, et al. Cooperative association of T cell β receptor and HLA-DQ alleles in the production of anti-Ro in systemic lupus erythematosus. *Clin Immunol Immunopathol* 1994;72:335–341.
72. O'Brien RM, Cram DS, Coppel RL, et al. T-cell epitopes on the 70-kDa protein of the (U1) RNP complex in autoimmune disorders. *J Autoimmun* 1990;3:747–757.
73. Reichlin M, Rader M, Harley JB. Autoimmune responses to Ro/SSA is directed to the human antigen. *Clin Exp Immunol* 1989;76:373–377.
74. Eisenberg RA, Dyer K, Craven SY, et al. Subclass restriction and polyclonality of the systemic erythematosus marker antibody anti-Sm. *J Clin Invest* 1985;75:1270–1277.
75. Pisetsky DS, Grudier JP, Gilkeson GS. A role for immunogenic DNA in the pathogenesis of systemic lupus erythematosus. *Arthritis Rheum* 1990;33:153–159.
76. Ebling FM, Ando DG, Panosian-Sahakian N, et al. Idiotypic

spreading promotes the production of pathogenic autoantibodies. *J Autoimmun* 1988;1:47–61.
77. Hahn BH, Kalunian KC, Fronek Z, et al. Idiotypic characteristics of immunoglobulins associated with human systemic lupus erythematosus. *Arthritis Rheum* 1990;33:978–984.
78. Koffler D, Kunkel HG. Mechanisms of renal injury in systemic lupus erythematosus. *Am J Med* 1968;45:165–169.
79. Koffler D, Schur PH, Kunkel HG. Immunological studies concerning the nephritis of systemic lupus erythematosus. *J Exp Med* 1967;126:607–623.
80. Winfield JB, Faiferman I, Koffler D. Avidity of anti-DNA antibodies in serum and IgG glomerular eluates from patients with systemic lupus erythematosus. Association of high avidity antinative DNA antibody with glomerulonephritis. *J Clin Invest* 1977;59:90–96.
81. Reichlin M, Mattioli M. Correlation of a precipitating reaction to an RNA protein antigen and a low prevalence of nephritis in patients with systemic lupus erythematosus. *N Engl J Med* 1972;286:908–911.
82. Reichlin M, van Venrooij WJ. Autoantibodies to the URNP particles: relationship to clinical diagnosis and nephritis. *Clin Exp Immunol* 1991;83:286–290.
83. Zhang W, Reichlin M. Some autoantibodies to Ro/SS-A and La/SS-B are anti-idiotypes to anti-double stranded DNA. *Arthritis Rheum* 1996;39:522–531.
84. Keech CL, McCluskey J, Gordon TP. Transfection and overexpression of the human 60-kDa Ro/SS-A autoantigen in HEp-2 cells. *Clin Immunol Immunopathol* 1994;73:146–151.
85. Fritzler MJ, Miller BJ. Detection of autoantibodies to SS-A/Ro by indirect immunofluorescence using a transfected and overexpressed human 60 kD Ro autoantigen in HEp-2 cells. *J Clin Lab Anal* 1995;9:218–224.
86. Chan EKL, Hamel JC, Tan EM, et al. Functional interaction of 52-kD and 60-kD SS-A/Ro autoantigens in transfection analysis. *Arthritis Rheum* 1995;38:S277(abst).
87. Kato N, Hiro OH, Fumio H. Nucleotide sequence of 45S RNA (C8 or hY5) from HeLa cells. *Biochem Biophys Res Commun* 1982;108:363–370.
88. Wolin SL, Steitz JA. The Ro small cytoplasmic ribonucleoproteins: identification of the antigenic protein and its binding site on the Ro RNAs. *Proc Natl Acad Sci USA* 1984;81:1996–2000.
89. O'Brien CA, Harley JB. A subset of Y RNAs are associated with erythrocyte Ro ribonucleoproteins. *EMBO J* 1990;9: 3683–3689.
90. Mamula MJ, O'Brien CA, Harley JB, et al. The Ro ribonucleoprotein particle: induction of autoantibodies and the detection of Ro RNAs among species. *Clin Immunol Immunopathol* 1989; 52:435–446.
91. Farris AD, O'Brien CA, Harley JB. Y3 is the most conserved small RNA component of Ro ribonucleoprotein complexes in vertebrate species. *Gene* 1995;154:193–198.
92. Yamagata H, Harley JB, Reichlin M. Molecular properties of the Ro/SS-A antigen and enzyme-linked immunosorbent assay for quantitation of antibody. *J Clin Invest* 1984;74:625–633.
93. Ben-Chetrit E, Gandy BJ, Tan EM, et al. Isolation and characterization of a cDNA clone encoding the 60-kD component of the human SS-A/Ro ribonucleoprotein autoantigen. *J Clin Invest* 1989;83:1284–1292.
94. Deutscher SL, Harley JB, Keene JD. Molecular analysis of the 60 kd human Ro ribonucleoprotein. *Proc Natl Acad Sci USA* 1988;85:9479–9483.
95. Itoh Y, Rader MD, Reichlin M. Heterogeneity of the Ro/SSA antigen and autoanti-Ro/SSA response: evidence of the four antigenically distinct forms. *Clin Exp Immunol* 1990;81:45–51.
96. Boulanger C, Chabot B, Menard HA, et al. Autoantibodies in human anti-Ro sera specifically recognize deproteinized hY5 Ro RNA. *Clin Exp Immunol* 1995;99:29–36.
97. Lieu T-S, Zappi EG, McCauliffe DP, et al. Frequency of antibodies to human calreticulin(CR) in precipitating Ro/SS-A autoantibody (SSA-Ro)-positive sera. *Arthritis Rheum* 1991; 34: S102(abst).
98. Rokeach LA, Haselby JA, Meilof JF, et al. Characterization of the autoantigen calreticulin. *J Immunol* 1991;147:3031–3039.
99. Fritzler MJ, Miller BJ, Chan EKL. Studies of SS-A/Ro autoantibody reactivity with calreticulin. *Arthritis Rheum* 1992;35: S171(abst).
100. Ben-Chetrit E, Chan EKL, Sullivan KF, et al. A 52-kD protein is a novel component of the SS-A/Ro antigenic particle. *J Exp Med* 1988;167:1560–1571.
101. Itoh K, Itoh Y, Frank MB. Protein heterogeneity of the human ribonucleoprotein: the 52 and 60 kD Ro/SSA autoantigens are encoded by separate genes. *J Clin Invest* 1991;87:177–186.
102. Chan EKL, Hamel JC, Buyon JP, et al. Molecular definition and sequence motifs of the 52-kD component of human SS-A/Ro autoantigen. *J Clin Invest* 1991;87:68–76.
103. Slobbe RL, Pluk W, van Venrooij WJ, et al. Ro ribonucleoprotein assembly in vitro. Identification of RNA-protein and protein-protein interactions. *J Mol Biol* 1992;227:361–366.
104. Kelekar A, Saitta MR, Keene JD. Molecular composition of Ro small ribonucleoprotein complexes in human cells. Intracellular localization of the 60- and 52-kD proteins. *J Clin Invest* 1994; 93:1637–1644.
105. Boire G, Gendron M, Monast N, et al. Purification of antigenically intact Ro ribonucleoproteins: biochemical and immunological evidence that the 52-kD protein is not a Ro protein. *Clin Exp Immunol* 1995;100:489–498.
106. Peek R, Pruijn GJ, van Venrooij WJ. Epitope specificity determines the ability of anti-Ro52 autoantibodies to precipitate Ro ribonucleoprotein particles. *J Immunol* 1994;153:4321–4329.
107. Itoh Y, Reichlin M. Autoantibodies to the Ro/SSA antigen are conformation dependent. I: Anti-60 kD antibodies are mainly directed to the native protein; anti-52 kD antibodies are mainly directed to the denatured protein. *Autoimmunity* 1992;14: 57–65.
108. Itoh Y, Itoh K, Frank MB, et al. Autoantibodies to the Ro/SSA autoantigen are conformation dependent. II: Antibodies to the denatured form of 52 kD Ro/SSA are a cross reacting subset of antibodies to the native 60 kD Ro/SSA molecule. *Autoimmunity* 1992;14:89–95.
109. Tsugu H, Horowitz R, Gibson N, et al. The location of a disease-associated polymorphism and genomic structure of the human 52-kDa Ro/SSA locus (SSA1). *Genomics* 1994;24: 541–548.
110. Frank MB, Itoh K, Fujisaku A, et al. The mapping of the human 52-kD Ro/SSA autoantigen gene to human chromosome 11, and its polymorphisms. *Am J Hum Genet* 1993;52: 183–191.
111. Rader MD, O'Brien CO, Liu Y, et al. The heterogeneity of the Ro/SSA antigen: different molecular forms in lymphocytes and red blood cells. *J Clin Invest* 1989;83:1556–1562.
112. Itoh Y, Reichlin M. Ro/SS-A antigen in human platelets: different distributions of the isoforms of Ro/SS-A protein and the Ro/SS-A binding RNA. *Arthritis Rheum* 1991;34:888–893.
113. McCauliffe DP, Zappi E, Lieu TS, et al. A human Ro/SS-A autoantigen is the homologue of calreticulin and is highly homologous with onchocercal RAL-1 antigen and an aplasia memory molecule. *J Clin Invest* 1990;86:332–335.
114. Maddison PJ, Lee L, Reichlin M, et al. Anti-p57: a novel association with neonatal lupus. *Clin Exp Immunol* 1995;99:42–48.
115. Boire G, Craft J. Human Ro ribonucleoprotein particles: char-

acterization of native structure and stable association with the La polypeptide. *J Clin Invest* 1990;85:1182–1190.
116. Chambers JC, Denan D, Martin BJ, et al. Genomic structure and amino acid sequence domains of the human La autoantigen. *J Biol Chem* 1988;263(34):18043–18051.
117. Chambers JC, Keene JD. Isolation and analysis of cDNA clones expressing human lupus antigen. *Proc Natl Acad Sci USA* 1985; 82:2115–2119.
118. Chan EKL, Sullivan KF, Tan EM. Ribonucleoprotein SS-B/La belongs to a protein family with consensus sequences for RNA-binding. *Nucleic Acids Res* 1989;17:2233–2244.
119. Query CC, Bently RC, Keene JD. A common RNA recognition motif identified within a defined U1 RNA binding domain of the 70K U1 snRNP protein. *Cell* 1989;57:89–101.
120. Chan EKL, Francoeur AM, Tan EM. Epitopes, structural domains, and asymmetry of amino acid residues in SS-B/La nuclear protein. *J Immunol* 1986;136:3744–3749.
121. Mathews MB, Francoeur AM. La antigen recognizes and binds to the 3′ oligouridylate tail of a small RNA. *Mol Cell Biol* 1984; 4:1134–1140.
122. Stephano JE. Purified lupus antigen La recognizes an oligouridylate stretch common to the 3′ termini of RNA polymerase III transcripts. *Cell* 1984;36:145–154.
123. Modore SJ, Wieben ED, Pederson T. Eukaryotic small ribonucleoproteins: anti-La human autoantibodies react with U1 RNA-protein complexes. *J Biol Chem* 1984;259:1929–1933.
124. Kurilla MG, Keene JD. The leader RNA of vesicular stomatitis virus is bound by a cellular protein reactive with anti-La lupus antibodies. *Cell* 1983;34:837–845.
125. Lerner MR, Andrews NC, Miller G, et al. Two small RNAs encoded by Epstein-Barr virus and complexed with protein are precipitated by antibodies from patients with systemic lupus erythematosus. *Proc Natl Acad Sci USA* 1981;78:805–809.
126. Rosa MA, Gottlieb E, Lerner MR, et al. Striking similarities are exhibited by two small Epstein-Barr virus-encoded ribonucleic acids and the adenovirus-associated ribonucleic acids VAI and VAII. *Mol Cell Biol* 1981;1: 785–796.
127. Svitkin YV, Pause A, Sonenberg N. La autoantigen alleviates translational repression by the 5 leader sequence of the human immunodeficiency virus type 1 mRNA. *J Virol* 1994;68: 7001–7007.
128. Meerovitch K, Svitkin YV, Lee HS, et al. La autoantigen enhances and corrects aberrant translation of poliovirus RNA in reticulocyte lysate. *J Virol* 1993;67:3798–3807.
129. O'Brien CA, Wolin SL. A possible role for the 60-kD Ro autoantigen in a discard pathway for defective 5S rRNA precursors. *Genes Dev* 1994;8:2891–2903.
130. Bachmann M, Falke D, Schroder HC, et al. Intracellular distribution of the La antigen in CV-1 cells after herpes simplex virus type 1 infection compared with the localization of U small nuclear ribonucleoprotein particles. *J Gen Virol* 1989;70: 881–891.
131. Bachmann M, Pfiefer K, Schroder HC, et al. The La antigen shuttles between the nucleus and cytoplasm in CV-1 cells. *Mol Cell Biochem* 1989;85:103–114.
132. Gottlieb E, Steitz JA. The RNA binding protein La influences both the accuracy and the efficiency of RNA polymerase III transcription in vitro. *EMBO J* 1989;8:841–850.
133. Gottlieb E, Steitz JA. Function of the mammalian La protein: evidence for this action in transcription termination by RNA polymerase III. *EMBO J* 1989;8:851–861.
134. Bachmann M, Pfiefer K, Schroder HC, et al. Characterization of the autoantigen La as a nucleic acid-dependent ATPase/dATPase with melting properties. *Cell* 1990;60:85–93.
135. Xiao Q, Sharp TV, Jeffrey IW, et al. The La antigen inhibits the activation of the interferon-inducible protein kinase PKR by sequestering and unwinding double-stranded RNA. *Nucleic Acids Res* 1994;22:2512–2518.
136. Chang YN, Kenan DJ, Keene JD, et al. Direct interactions between autoantigen La and human immunodeficiency virus leader RNA. *J Virol* 1994;68:7008–7020. [Published erratum appears in *J Virol* 1995;69:618.]
137. Svitkin YV, Meerovitch K, Lee HS, et al. Internal translation initiation on poliovirus RNA: further characterization of La function in poliovirus translation in vitro. *J Virol* 1994;68: 1544–1550.
138. Lin-Marq N, Clarkson SG. A yeast RNA binding protein that resembles the human autoantigen La. *J Mol Biol* 1995;245: 81–85.
139. Yoo CJ, Wolin SL. La proteins from Drosophila melanogaster and Saccharomyces cerevisiae: a yeast homolog of the La autoantigen is dispensable for growth. *Mol Cell Biol* 1994;14: 5412–5424.
140. Kohsaka H, Yamamoto K, Fujii H, et al. Fine epitope mapping of the human SS-B/La protein. Identification of a distinct autoepitope homologous to a viral gag polyprotein. *J Clin Invest* 1990;85:1566–1574.
141. Rauh AJ, Hornig H, Luhrmann R. At least three distinct B cell epitopes reside in the C-terminal half of La protein, as determined by a recombinant DNA approach. *Eur J Immunol* 1988; 18:2049–2057.
142. St. Clair EW, Pisetsky DS, Reich CG, et al. Analysis if the autoantibody binding to different regions of the human La antigen expressed in recombinant proteins. *J Immunol* 1988;141: 4173–4180.
143. Sturgess AD, Peterson MG, McNeilage LJ, et al. Characteristics and epitope mapping of a cloned human autoantigen La. *J Immunol* 1988;140:3212–3218.
144. Rischmueller M, McNeilage LJ, McCluskey J, et al. Human autoantibodies directed against the RNA recognition motif of La (SS-B) bind to a conformational epitope present on the intact La (SS-B)/Ro (SS-A) ribonucleoprotein particle. *Clin Exp Immunol* 1995;101:39–44.
145. McCauliffe DP, Yin H, Wang LX, et al. Autoimmune sera react with multiple epitopes on recombinant 52 and 60 kDa Ro(SSA) proteins. *J Rheumatol* 1994;21:1073–1080.
146. Scofield RH, Dickey WD, Jackson KW, et al. A common autoepitope near the carboxyl terminus of the 60 kD Ro ribonucleoprotein: sequence similarity with a viral protein. *J Clin Immunol* 1991;11:378–388.
147. Scofield RH, Harley JB. Autoantigenicity of Ro/SSA antigen is related to a nucleocapsid protein of vesicular stomatitis virus. *Proc Natl Acad Sci USA* 1991;88:3343–3347.
148. Kato T, Sasakawa H, Suzuki S, et al. Autoepitopes of the 52-kD SS-A/Ro molecule. *Arthritis Rheum* 1995;38:990–998.
149. Meilof JF, Hebeda KM, de Jong J, et al. Analysis of heavy and light chain use of lupus-associated anti-La/SS-B and anti-Sm autoantibodies reveals two distinct underlying immunoregulatory mechanisms. *Res Immunol* 1992;143:711–720.
150. Wahren M, Ringertz NR, Pettersson I. IgM and IgG subclass distribution of human anti-Ro/SSA 60 kDa autoantibodies. *Scand J Immunol* 1994;39:179–183.
151. Lindstrom FD, Eriksson P, Tejle K, et al. IgG subclasses of anti-SS-A/Ro in patients with primary Sjögren's syndrome. *Clin Immunol Immunopathol* 1994;73:358–361.
152. Hardgrave KL, Neas B, Scofield RH, et al. Antibodies to vesicular stomatitis virus proteins in patients with systemic lupus erythematosus and normals. *Arthritis Rheum* 1993;36:962–970.
153. Huang SC, Pan Z, Kurien BT, et al. Immunization with vesicular stomatitis virus nucleocapsid protein induces autoantibod-

ies to the 60 kD Ro ribonucleoprotein particle. *J Invest Med* 1995;43:151–158.

154. Zhang W, Reichlin M. IgM anti-A and D SnRNP proteins and IgM anti-dsDNA are closely associated in SLE sera. *Clin Immunol Immunopathol* 1995;74:70–76.
155. Reichlin M, Martin A, Taylor-Albert E, et al. Lupus autoantibodies to native DNA cross react with the A and D SnRNP polypeptides. *J Clin Invest* 1994;93:443–449.
156. Topfer F, Gordon T, McCluskey J. Intra- and intermolecular spreading of autoimmunity involving the nuclear self-antigens La (SS-B) and Ro (SS-A). *Proc Natl Acad Sci USA* 1995;92:875–879.
157. Tseng CE, Chan EK, Miranda E, et al. The 52 kd protein as a target of intermolecular spreading of the immune response to components of the SS-A/Ro-SS-B/La complex. *Arthritis Rheum* 1997;40:936–944.
158. James JA, Gross T, Scofield RH, et al. Immunoglobulin epitope spreading and autoimmune disease after peptide immunization. *J Exp Med* 1995;181:453–461.

24

ANTI-snRNP ANTIBODIES

JOSEPH E. CRAFT

Autoantibodies to the U series of small nuclear ribonucleoproteins (U snRNPs) are prominent features of the humoral immune response in patients with systemic lupus erythematosus (SLE). These autoantibodies, which include the anti-RNP and anti-Sm specificities, are quite useful as diagnostic markers in SLE and related connective tissue diseases. Moreover, sera that bind the U snRNPs have proved to be invaluable as probes of gene expression and nuclear structure. These antibodies also have attracted considerable attention because of the possibility that they hold clues to the basic etiologic mechanisms for connective tissue diseases; however, this hope has not yet been realized.

This chapter briefly reviews the history of discovery of these specificities, summarizes present knowledge of their structure and function, and describes clinical uses of anti-U1 RNP and anti-Sm antibodies. In addition, current ideas regarding the genesis of these autoantibodies are addressed.

DISCOVERY OF AUTOANTIBODIES TO snRNPs

Antibodies to the Sm antigen, named after a prototype serum, were first identified by Tan and Kunkel (1) in 1966 using immunodiffusion. The specificity known as nRNP (nuclear RNP; originally called anti-Mo after the prototype serum) was identified in the sera of patients with SLE by Mattioli and Reichlin (2) in 1971. The term *RNP* stems from the early observation that its antigenic activity could be destroyed by treatment with ribonuclease and trypsin (2). Thus, it was a ribonucleoprotein or RNA protein antigen (3), whereas the Sm antigen was resistant to such treatment (1). Also in 1971, Sharp et al. (4) described a group of patients with a syndrome that was characterized by features of SLE, inflammatory muscle disease, scleroderma, and the absence of renal disease, which they called mixed connective tissue disease (MCTD). The sera of these patients contained high titers of antibodies to extractable nuclear antigens (ENAs) as measured by passive hemagglutination. Subsequent studies showed that ENA contained both the Sm and the nRNP antigens (3,5–7), and that the patients described by Sharp et al. (6) were reacting with the latter component.

It is important to note that the original discovery of these specificities was based on application of the techniques of hemagglutination and immunodiffusion, and that the present clinical associations are based largely on studies that were conducted with these methodologies. Interestingly, the careful, early studies of Mattioli and Reichlin (8), while based on the relatively insensitive technique of immunodiffusion, revealed that the nRNP and Sm antigens were physically associated. The molecular nature of these antigens became clear in 1979, when Lerner and Steitz (9) demonstrated that both the Sm and nRNP antigens were located on the U1 snRNP (thus the often-used modifications of the term *anti-nRNP* to *anti-U1 RNP*, or *anti-U1 snRNP antibodies*), a complex of a small nuclear RNA, the U1 RNA, and associated polypeptides. While the U1 RNA itself may be targeted by autoantibodies, the polypeptide components of the U1 snRNP bear the nRNP and Sm antigenic determinants. In addition to being a principal target of the autoimmune response in SLE, this particle, and a series of closely related U snRNP particles, plays a key role in the splicing of premessenger RNA, as described later (10–12).

STRUCTURE AND PROTEIN COMPONENTS OF THE Sm snRNPs

The U snRNPs all are intranuclear and composed of a small RNA [small nuclear RNA (snRNA)] and at least several polypeptides (13) (Table 24.1). The RNA components were initially called U snRNAs, because the most abundant of them had a high uridine content. These RNAs are still grouped together, because with the exception of the U6 snRNA, they have a unique, 5-terminal trimethylguanosine cap (14); in other words, the 5 G residue of the U RNAs has an unusual modification with three methyl groups in comparison to messenger RNAs (mRNAs), which have monomethyl caps. At least 13 U snRNAs (i.e., U1 to U13) have been found in mammalian cells, and several others

TABLE 24.1. POLYPEPTIDE COMPONENTS OF THE ABUNDANT Sm snRNPs IN HUMAN CELLS[a]

Particle	Protein Components	Antibody Reactivity
U1 snRNP	*70K, A, C*[b], B′/B, D1–D3, E–G[a]	Anti-Sm, anti-U1 snRNP
U2 snRNP	*A′, B″*[c], B′/B, D1–D3, E–G[a]	Anti-Sm, anti-U2 snRNP
U5 snRNP	*8 proteins*[d], B′/B, D1–D3, E–G[a]	Anti-Sm, anti-U5 snRNP
U4/U6 snRNPs	*150 kd*[d], B′/B, D1–D3, E–G[a]	Anti-Sm, anti-U4/U6 snRNP
U7 snRNP	*18 kd*[d], B′/B, D1–D3, E–G[a]	Anti-Sm, anti-U7 snRNP
U11/U12 snRNPs	*62, 65, 140 kd*[d], B′/B, D1–D3, E–G[a]	Anti-Sm, anti-U11 snRNP

[a]The B′/B and D–G proteins are common to all Sm snRNPs, including U1, U2, U5, U4/U6, U7, and U11/U12 (9,13,19). Each of the abundant snRNPs listed here also contains unique proteins (*in italics*). Anti-Sm antibodies principally bind the B′/B and D1–D3 (20,21) proteins that are common to all Sm snRNPs, although they sometimes bind E (87). Occasional sera also bind F and G (143). The B′ protein is a tissue-specific variant of B and is not found in nonhuman species; for example, the proteins that are common to Sm snRNPs in mouse cells are B, D1–D3, and E–G. The N polypeptide is found on Sm snRNPs in neural tissues in at least humans and rodents (24,27–29).
[b]Anti-U1 snRNP antibodies bind the 70K, A, and/or C proteins of the U1 snRNP (87).
[c]Anti-U2 snRNP antibodies bind the A′ and B" proteins of the U2 snRNP (49,88,89).
[d]The U5 snRNP contains eight unique proteins (52), including polypeptides of 100, 102, and a doublet of 200 kd; antigenic epitopes on U5 snRNPs are as yet undefined. The exact frequency of anti-U5 snRNP antibodies also is unknown at present, but these antibodies likely are quite unusual (90). The U4/U6 snRNP apparently contains one unique antigenic protein that is bound by anti-U4/U6 autoantibodies, with the molecular weight of this polypeptide reported as either 120 or 150 kd (50,51). The U7 snRNP contains one unique 18-kd protein (53), and the U11 snRNP contains unique proteins of 62, 65, and 140 kd (54). Like anti-U5 snRNPs, antibodies to the U4/U6, U7, and U11/U12 snRNPs are rare.
snRNP, small nuclear ribonucleoprotein.

have been tentatively identified (15). Most of these snRNAs have been shown to exist within snRNP particles (i.e., complexes of RNA and proteins). Three of these snRNAs, U4, U5, and U6, are part of the same tri-snRNP particle but, when biochemically purified, exist as the U5 monoparticle and the U4/U6 duplex particle and are so referred to in the literature. Most U11 and U12 snRNPs also appear to exist as a di-snRNP particle. Three of the U snRNPs, the abundant U3 snRNP and the less abundant U8 and U13 snRNPs, are found in the nucleolus (16,17), as are multiple other, lower-abundance U RNAs that are encoded within introns of mRNA coding genes (18). Those snRNPs found in the nucleolus now more typically are referred to as snoRNPs (small nucleolar RNPs).

The most abundant U snRNPs, the U1, U2, U4/U6, and U5 particles, share a number of polypeptides that associate into a common structure and are referred to as the Sm core proteins (9,13,19) (Table 24.1). This name reflects their recognition by anti-Sm antibodies. The intranucleolar U3, U8, and U13 snRNPs do not contain these core proteins; instead, they contain a common protein fibrillarin, which is a target of autoantibodies in scleroderma (16,17). In human cells, the Sm core group consists of polypeptides B/B (29 and 28 kd), D1 (typically referred to D), D2, D3 (approximately 16 to 18 kd), E (12 kd), F (11 kd), and G (9 kd; perhaps consisting of two proteins) (9,13,19–21), and a newly described protein of 69 kd (22). Thus, by polyacrylamide gel electrophoresis, the B protein is the largest of the Sm group, and G is the smallest. Of note, the B polypeptide is not found in nonhuman species (9,19,23–26), and its expression is tissue specific in human cells, where it is absent in brain (24,27). In the latter tissue, the Sm snRNPs contain a polypeptide referred to as N (27–29), which has close homology with B and B but is encoded by a separate gene (24). The tissue-specific variations of these common Sm proteins may reflect the differential splicing needs of cells.

The common polypeptides of Sm snRNPs are highly conserved evolutionarily, as would be expected considering the crucial role of these particles in splicing premessenger RNA. For example, the B and D polypeptides are found in a variety of eukaryotic species, including humans (19,30), rodents (9,19), *Xenopus* (23), and *Drosophila* (26). When sought, these proteins also are found in all tissues and cell lines from these species (9,19,23–28). Proteins of similar size to the B and D polypeptides and immunologically reactive with anti-Sm antibodies also are found in plants (31). In addition, human anti-Sm antibodies immunoprecipitate U snRNAs from the cells of species as diverse as humans to *Drosophila* to yeasts (32,33), indicating that the epitopes bound by these antibodies, which are constituted by proteins bound to the RNAs, are conserved in all eukaryotes. Recent evidence indicates that all Sm proteins share a structural motif that is composed of a conserved fold and secondary structure, a commonality that likely accounts for the ability of human anti-Sm antibodies to bind these polypeptides from such widely divergent species (34).

The Sm core of polypeptides binds to their U RNAs at a conserved, single-stranded nucleotide stretch consisting of purineA(U)nGpurine, a sequence that is referred to as the Sm binding site (35) (Fig. 24.1). It is uncertain whether the Sm core proteins bind this nucleotide motif directly,

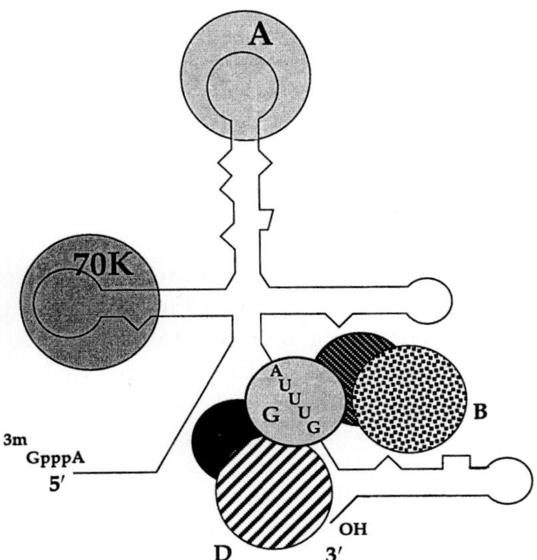

FIGURE 24.1. Schematic of the abundant U1 snRNP, as originally proposed by Lutz-Freyermuth and Keene (144) as well as Query et al. (145). This snRNP, like all U snRNPs involved in splicing premessenger RNA, contains a common Sm core group of proteins (in human cells, B, B, D1D3, and EG). These core proteins bind to a conserved, single-strand RNA region purineA(U)nGpurine via the G protein (44). Additionally, each snRNP has unique proteins. For the U1 snRNP, these include the 70K and A proteins that bind to the first- and second-stem loops of the U1 RNA, respectively (58,59). Along with the C polypeptide, these proteins are the targets of anti-U1 snRNP (anti-nRNP or anti-RNP) antibodies. The binding site of the U1 snRNP protein C is not precisely known and thus is not shown. (Adapted from Craft J. Antibodies to snRNPs in SLE. *Rheum Dis Clin* 1992;18:311–336, with permission.)

because the B, N, D, and E proteins lack an amino acid sequence (27,36–40) called an RNA recognition motif (41) [or RNP consensus sequence (42)] that is found in certain proteins that bind RNA directly (43). The core protein G may play a role in direct RNA binding via direct binding to the Sm binding site (44). Like the proteins that bind it, the Sm binding site is highly conserved evolutionarily; for example, this RNA sequence is found in organisms as diverse as humans and yeast (*Sacchromyces cerevisiae*) (45) as well as in certain viral RNAs (46).

In addition to the common core proteins, individual Sm snRNPs also contain unique polypeptides (13) (Table 24.1). For example, the U1 snRNP contains polypeptides known as 70K, A, and C (19,47,48). The U2 snRNP contains polypeptides A and B, so named because they were identified after the A and B/B proteins and they closely migrate to these polypeptides on polyacrylamide gels (47–49). The U4/U6 snRNPs contain at least one unique protein, which is reported to be of either 150 or 120 kd (50,51). The U5 snRNPs, when found in large 20S particles, also contain eight unique proteins (52), U7 contains an 18-kd protein (53), and U11 has specific proteins of 62-, 65-, and 140-kd (54). In addition, in snRNP complexes that are prepared as part of active splicing extracts (discussed below), other specific proteins associated with U2 (55) and the U4/U6.U5 tri-snRNPs (56) can be identified. Like the Sm core polypeptides, the snRNP-specific proteins also appear to be highly conserved. For example, an A-protein homologue is found in plants (31), and a protein that corresponds to the 70K protein is found in yeast (*S. cerevisiae*) (57).

The 70K and A proteins of the U1 snRNP bind directly to the first- and second-stem loops of the U1 RNA, respectively (41,58–62) (Fig. 24.1). Both of these polypeptides contain the RNA-recognition motif mentioned earlier. This motif also is found in the B protein, which binds directly to the U2 RNA. This interaction is enhanced by binding of B by the A protein, likely via a repetitive leucine motif found in A (63–66). The binding of the C protein to the U1 RNA appears to require other snRNP proteins for association with the U1 particle (67). The primary structure of most proteins of the U1 snRNP, including the 70K (68–70), A (71), and C (72,73) proteins, and the B/B (38–40), N (27–29), D (36), and E (37) polypeptides that are common to all Sm snRNPs, has now been determined; the unique proteins of the U2 snRNP, A (74), and B (75) also have been cloned. For further reviews, see Lhrmann et al. (76) as well as van Venrooij and Sillekens (77).

FUNCTION OF THE U snRNPs

The U1, U2, U5, and U4/U6 snRNPs are the most abundant [amounts range from 2×10^5 copies per mammalian cell for U5 and U4/U6 to 1×10^6 copies per mammalian cell for the U1 snRNP (14)] and play a central role in the splicing of premessenger RNA (11,12,78). Genes of higher organisms contain regions, called introns, that are noncoding and that separate the coding regions, called exons. Although the noncoding regions are transcribed wholesale along with the coding regions into premessenger RNA, the introns must be removed for effective translation of the mRNA into protein. The process of intron removal is called splicing, and it is mediated in the nucleus by the abundant Sm snRNPs via recognition of conserved (i.e., canonical) nucleotide sequences in the premessenger RNA before export of the mature mRNA to the cytoplasm for translation into proteins on ribosomes (11,12,78).

The less abundant U7 snRNP (2.5×10^4 copies per mammalian cell) participates in the processing of 3′ ends of histone mRNAs (79). The less abundant U11 and U12 snRNPs (10^3–10^4 copies per mammalian cell) function in concert with the U5 snRNP to splice a minor class of introns in premessenger RNA that contain noncanonical splice-site sequences (80). The nucleolar U3 snRNP is involved in ribosomal RNA processing (81), as are the closely related U8 and U13 particles. The U9 and U10 RNAs are likely components of Sm snRNPs, but they have not been further characterized (14).

INTRACELLULAR ASSEMBLY OF Sm snRNP PARTICLES

Sm snRNP assembly, with the exception of the U6 particle, begins in the cytoplasm (82–84). Formation of these particles begins with transcription of the appropriate U small RNAs in the nucleus, a step that is mediated via RNA polymerase II, with the exception that the U6 RNA is synthesized by RNA polymerase III. RNA polymerase II is the enzyme complex that also transcribes mRNA, while RNA polymerase III transcribes transfer RNAs (tRNAs), 5S ribosomal RNAs, and other small RNAs, including the Ro RNAs. The U RNAs are transported to the cytoplasm, where they interact with snRNP polypeptides in an ordered assembly process. The Sm core proteins (DG, along with B and B) first associate as a group in cytoplasmic pools. Binding of the resulting complex to the U snRNAs via the Sm binding site (Fig. 24.1) is associated with conversion of the 5-guanosine residue of the latter molecules from a monomethyl to a trimethyl form (referred to as a trimethyl guanosine cap). Both of these steps are required for entry of the assembled snRNPs into the nucleus. Additional individual proteins such as 70K, A, and/or C of the U1 particle either enter the nucleus independently before binding their respective snRNAs or are incorporated into the snRNP while the new complex remains in the cytoplasm. Presumably, this highly programmed assembly pathway ensures that partially assembled snRNP complexes will not interact with premessenger RNA. An exception to cytoplasmic assembly pathway of the abundant snRNPs is the U6 particle, whose RNA as an RNA polymerase III transcript (discussed above) never leaves the nucleus; hence, this snRNP and the U4/U6 di-snRNP assemble in the nucleus (85,86).

ANTIGENIC POLYPEPTIDES OF THE U snRNPs

Dominant autoimmune reactions in patients with SLE often are directed against the abundant snRNPs. The anti-Sm response involves production of antibodies that immunoprecipitate the U1, U2, U4/U6, and U5 snRNPs through interactions with some combination of the B, B, N, D1D3, and E polypeptides that are shared among these particles (9,28,87). In contrast, anti-U1 snRNP antibodies bind the 70K, A, and/or C proteins of the U1 snRNP (87), while anti-U2 RNP antibodies recognize the A and B polypeptides of the U2 particle (49,88,89) (Table 24.1). Similarly, autoantibodies bind the proteins that are specific to the U4/U6 (50,51), U5 (90), U7 (53), and U11 snRNPs (54), although these specificities appear to be quite rare. Thus, as discussed later, these latter antibodies immunoprecipitate individual snRNPs because they recognize unique proteins of each respective snRNP. In contrast, the nucleolar U3, U8, and U13 snRNPs lack the common Sm proteins, but they share the polypeptide fibrillarin and are immunoprecipitable with antibodies that bind this polypeptide (17).

DETECTION OF ANTI-Sm AND ANTI-U1 RNP ANTIBODIES

Anti-Sm and anti-U1 RNP antibodies stain the nucleus of cells in a fine, speckled pattern, with sparing of nucleoli, when examined in indirect immunofluorescence (Fig. 24.2). This staining pattern reflects the uniform location of the U1 snRNPs in the nucleoplasm. Certain anti-U1 snRNP and anti-Sm sera also appear to stain the nucleus with brighter intensity in more discrete, larger speckles on the background of diffuse speckling (J. Craft, unpublished observation), possibly reflecting that the major components of the splicing machinery exist in discrete speckles of interchromatin granules within the nucleus and coiled bodies (91–94). Similarly, sera specific for the U2, U5, and U4/U6 snRNPs also produce an identical speckled staining pattern (50,51,90), which is consistent with the role that these particles play in premessenger RNA splicing.

In the past, and to a certain extent today, laboratories have relied on immunodiffusion for the routine detection of anti-Sm and anti-U1 RNP antibodies. The sensitivity of immunodiffusion can be enhanced with use of counterimmunoelectrophoresis (95). This method is of particular use in the detection of anti-Sm and anti-U1 RNP antibodies. It is important to recall that the currently accepted clinical associations of these antibodies with various diseases largely are based on data developed with immunodiffusion (95). In immunodiffusion, a prototype anti-Sm or anti-U1 RNP serum is placed into a well that is cut into agarose. The soluble fraction of a tissue extract (e.g., rabbit or calf thymus or spleen) prepared by sonication in a saline buffer is placed

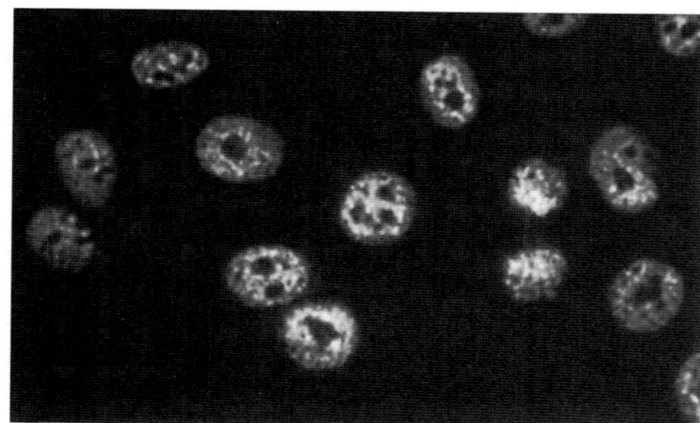

FIGURE 24.2. Indirect immunofluorescence of a human anti-Sm serum diluted 1:40; note the fine, speckled staining. Anti-U1 snRNP and U2 snRNP sera would produce an identical pattern of immunofluorescence. (From Craft J. Antibodies to snRNPs in SLE. *Rheum Dis Clin* 1992;18:311–336, with permission.)

in an adjacent well. During a 24- to 48-hour incubation period, diffusion brings the antibodies together with their respective antigens (i.e., ENAs), and as they bind, a lattice structure develops that appears as a visible, precipitin band. Antibodies in a particular serum can be identified through comparison with a serum of known specificity. In other words, if the two sera are binding the same antigen, the precipitin lines will fuse to form a line of identity; otherwise, they will spur across one another. When anti-U1 RNP antibodies are compared with anti-Sm antibodies, a line of partial identity often is observed (i.e., the Sm line spurs over the U1 RNP line, but the latter fuses with the Sm line). This pattern occurs when some soluble particles contain both antigens (bound by anti-Sm and anti-U1 RNP sera) and others contain Sm determinants alone (bound by anti-Sm sera).

More recently, enzyme-linked immunosorbent assays (ELISAs) for the detection of anti-Sm and anti-U1 RNP antibodies have been developed and have come into commercial use. In these assays, a highly pure antigen is allowed to adhere to the surface of wells in a plastic tray. Dilute patient serum is then added, and antibodies that bind the antigen on the plastic surface can be detected by the use of a second, antihuman antibody that is tagged with an enzyme that catalyzes a color change in an indicator substrate. Originally, these assays depended on biochemically or affinity-purified antigens; however, recombinant forms of the snRNP polypeptides that now are available have been substituted into some commercial preparations.

ELISA methods have the advantages of speed (results are available within hours rather than the 1 to 2 days required for immunodiffusion) and sensitivity (approximating that of radioimmunoassays). They also are easier and safer to perform than most radioimmunoassays. Their major limitations are the requirement for a pure antigen to serve as substrate and a somewhat higher rate of false-positive results compared with immunodiffusion.

IMMUNOPRECIPITATION AND IMMUNOBLOT ASSAYS FOR THE DETECTION OF ANTIBODIES TO THE Sm snRNPs

Antibodies that bind polypeptides present on an individual snRNP can be used to specifically remove, or immunoprecipitate, that particle from solution and thus ascertain its function. A practical application of such an experiment was the use of sera from patients with lupus to inhibit premessenger RNA splicing by the selective removal of individual snRNPs from splicing extracts. Such experiments helped to determine the role of the individual snRNPs in the splicing pathway.

The protein components of the Sm snRNPs also were initially demonstrated using immunoprecipitation assays (9,19,87). Immunodiffusion data previously had shown that the Sm and RNP determinants were physically associated, but that they were different antigens (2,8). These observations were explained by the finding from immunoprecipitation experiments that both of these determinants were located on the U1 snRNP. In these experiments, both anti-Sm and anti-U1 RNP antibodies were used to immunoprecipitate radiolabeled snRNPs. In such experiments, which are commonly used in research laboratories, cells are labeled *in vivo* with 35S-methionine, which places a radioactive tag in all cellular proteins. The radiolabeled cell extracts then are mixed with human sera containing anti-Sm or anti-U1 RNP antibodies (or sera of other specificities) bound to a particulate carrier, such as protein A-sepharose (96). After binding of the antibody to its antigenic target, the antibody–antigen complex can be immunoprecipitated via the particulate carrier. Then, immunoprecipitated antigens bearing the 35S-methionine tag can be detected by polyacrylamide gel electrophoresis and autoradiography.

An example of such an experiment is shown in Fig. 24.3. Immunoprecipitates formed with an anti-U1 RNP serum and with anti-Sm serum are shown in lanes 2 and 3, respectively. Both immunoprecipitate from solution all the components of the U1 snRNP, because their antigenic targets (B, B, D, and E for anti-Sm antibodies, and the 70K, A, and C proteins for anti-U1 RNP antibodies) (Table 24.1) are associated via their common RNA backbone (Fig. 24.1). The 70K protein and the D2 and D3 proteins are not visualized under the conditions of this experiment. The N protein also is absent in these nonneural cells.

Cells also can be labeled *in vivo* with 32P to tag RNAs with radioactivity (96). In a fashion similar to that described for immunoprecipitation of 35S-methionine-labeled proteins, autoantibodies then can be used to immunoprecipitate selective RNAs via their associated antigenic proteins. Recall that autoantibodies usually are directed toward the protein components of the snRNP complex rather than at the RNA itself, although the latter does occur (97). After immunoprecipitation, bound RNA(s) can be visualized by gel fractionation followed by exposure of the gel to radiographic film. Because anti-U1 RNP antibodies only bind the 70K, A, and C proteins, which are unique to the U1 snRNP (Fig. 24.1 and Table 24.1), the U1 RNA component is visualized on the gel when these antibodies are used to form immunoprecipitates (Fig. 24.4). Note that this serum also immunoprecipitates the U2 RNA via low titers of antibodies directed toward the antigenic A and B proteins of the U2 snRNP (Table 24.1). An immunoprecipitate formed with a serum containing high titers of anti-U2 snRNP antibodies also is shown in Fig. 24.4 (lane 5). This anti-U2 snRNP serum also contains anti-U1 RNP antibodies in low titer, so the U1 RNA also is seen in immunoprecipitates that are formed with this serum. In contrast, anti-Sm antibodies immunoprecipitate

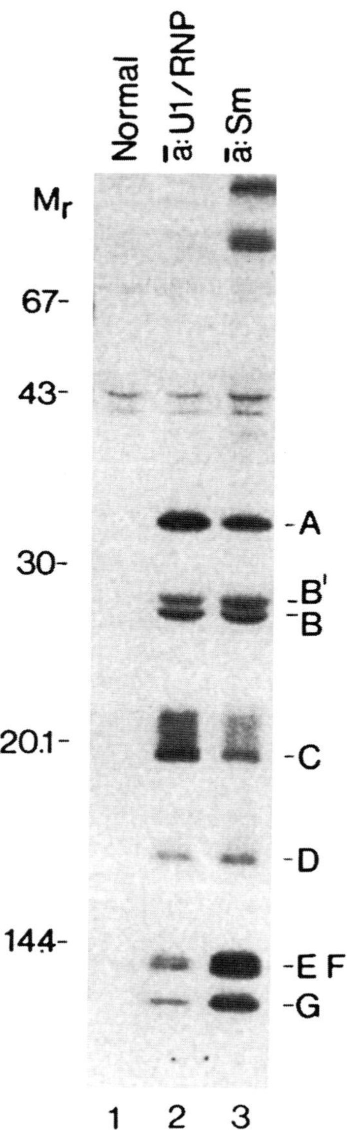

FIGURE 24.3. Immunoprecipitation of 35S-methionine-labeled HeLa cell extracts with human antisera. Cells were labeled *in vivo* with 35S-methionine, followed by sonication and centrifugation to remove particulate debris. Sera from patients with SLE were mixed with protein A sepharose beads, allowing the immunoglobulin G (IgG) fraction of sera to bind specifically to the beads. IgG-coated sepharose beads then were incubated with radiolabeled cell extracts. Bound proteins were then fractionated by gel fractionation and detected by autoradiography. Lane 1 shows an immunoprecipitate formed with a normal control serum, whereas lanes 2 and 3 show immunoprecipitates formed with anti-U1 RNP and anti-Sm sera, respectively. Although these sera bind different polypeptide components of the U1 snRNP, they both immunoprecipitate all the proteins of this particle via their link on the U1 RNA backbone. The 70K protein is not labeled under the conditions used here and therefore is not seen in the immunoprecipitates. Similarly, the D2 and D3 proteins are not visualized under the gel conditions used. (From Craft J. Antibodies to snRNPs in SLE. *Rheum Dis Clin* 1992;18:311–336, with permission.)

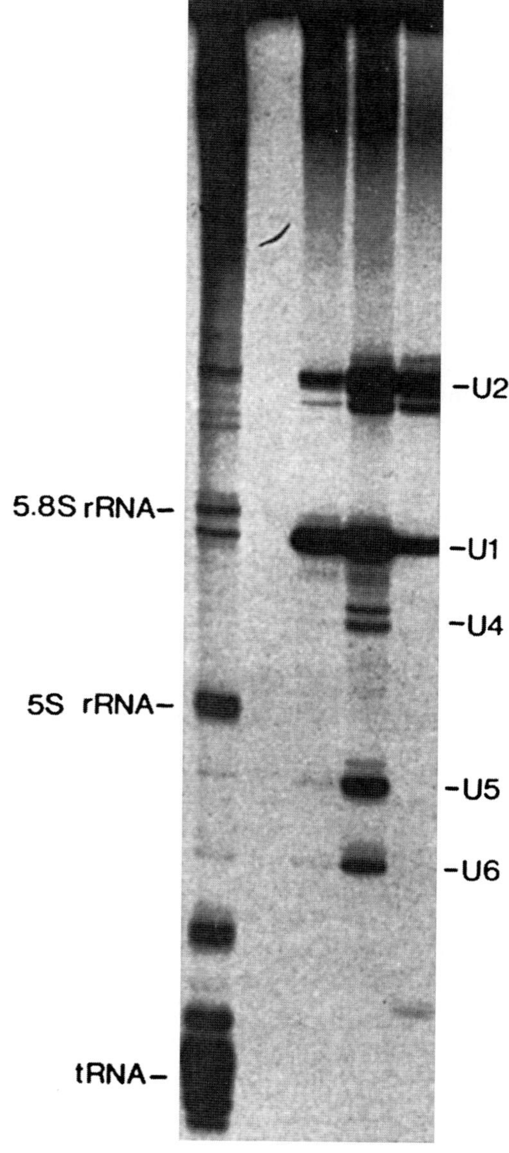

FIGURE 24.4. Immunoprecipitation of 32P-labeled HeLa cell extracts with human antisera. Cells were labeled *in vivo* with 32P, followed by sonication and centrifugation to remove particulate debris. Sera from patients with SLE were mixed with protein A sepharose beads, allowing the IgG fraction of sera to bind specifically to the beads. IgG-coated sepharose beads then were incubated with radiolabeled cell extracts. snRNP particles bound by the IgG via antigenic polypeptides were then extracted to remove protein and the radiolabeled RNAs recovered, followed by gel fractionation and autoradiography. Shown in lane 1 are total radiolabeled RNAs present in the soluble cell extract, including the abundant Sm snRNAs. Lane 2 shows the immunoprecipitate formed with a normal control serum. Lanes 3 through 5 show immunoprecipitates formed with an anti-U1 RNP serum, an anti-Sm serum, and an anti-U2 snRNP serum, respectively. Note that the anti-U1 serum primarily immunoprecipitates the U1 RNA, because this specificity binds the 70K, A, and/or C polypeptides that are unique to the U1 snRNP. In contrast, the anti-U2 snRNP serum, via antibodies that target the A and B proteins, only immunoprecipitates the U2 snRNA; this serum also contains a low titer of anti-U1 RNP antibodies. Finally, the anti-Sm serum immunoprecipitates all the abundant Sm snRNPs via the Sm core proteins that are common to all the Sm snRNAs. (From Craft J. Antibodies to snRNPs in SLE. *Rheum Dis Clin* 1992;18:311–336, with permission.)

all the Sm snRNAs via epitopes that are found on the common B/B, D (D1D3), and E proteins (Fig. 24.4). The amount of each of the Sm snRNAs (i.e., U1, U2, U4, U5, and U6) in the immunoprecipitate at least partly reflects their relative abundance within the nucleus, as discussed above.

Radioimmunoprecipitation assays can be used as a very sensitive means to screen sera for the presence of anti-Sm and anti-U1 RNP antibodies, as well as for other antibodies directed against ribonucleoproteins, such as anti-Ro, anti-La, anti-Jo-1, and anti-U3. Immunoprecipitation assays are extremely sensitive and specific, because the radiolabeled antigen can be detected in minute quantity and visualized directly. A major disadvantage of immunoprecipitation assays is that they typically require use of radioactivity. Although this latter problem now can be circumvented through use of very sensitive staining procedures to identify immunoprecipitates in gels (96), these assays are somewhat laborious compared with ELISA or immunodiffusion; thus, they are usually limited to use by research laboratories.

Immunoblots also can be used for the detection of anti-Sm and anti-U1 RNP antibodies (87). Cell nuclei, a source of snRNPs or purified snRNPs, can be fractionated on polyacrylamide gels, followed by transfer to nitrocellulose and probing with diluted patient sera. Bound antibodies can be detected with a second antibody that is coupled to an enzyme that produces a color when its substrate is added, or via a second antibody that can be detected with a ^{125}I tag. A major advantage of immunoblots is their specificity, because the antigenic protein targets of these antibodies can be visualized directly. Additionally, in comparison to immunoprecipitation assays, immunoblots can provide information about which polypeptide carries the specific epitope that is being recognized (because the antigens are probed with antisera after electrophoretic separation), whereas immunoprecipitation reveals only the total protein or RNA composition of the bound antigen (87). For example, antibodies that are specific for the B or D proteins on the U1 snRNP will immunoprecipitate all the polypeptide components of this particle via their association on an U1 snRNA backbone (Figs. 24.1 and 24.3). In general, however, immunoblots are not any more sensitive than ELISAs, and their performance is more laborious. Like immunoprecipitation assays, immunoblots for the detection of anti-Sm and anti-U1 RNP antibodies typically are limited to research laboratories.

CLINICAL ASSOCIATION OF ANTI-Sm ANTIBODIES

Anti-Sm antibodies are an important diagnostic marker for SLE (98) (Table 24.2). When sera are examined in immunodiffusion, these antibodies are found in approximately 25% of all patients with lupus, and their presence has been included as part of the revised American College of Rheumatology criteria for diagnosis of this disorder (99). In comparison to immunodiffusion, ELISAs increase detection of these antibodies (100–103) by approximately 10% (101,103) to twofold (100), without sacrificing their specificity as a disease marker for SLE (101,103). Anti-Sm antibodies are more common in blacks and Asians compared with those of European descent (102,103), and in the United States SLE population, they occur about twice as often in the former as in the latter group (102). Overall, the incidence of these antibodies ranges from approximately 10% to 20% in white patients with SLE, compared with 30% to 40%, or more, of Asian and black patients, respectively (101,104). Although anti-Sm antibody titers may fluctuate over time (105–107), it is unusual for them to disappear completely when measured by sensitive immunoprecipitation assays (106); however, they may become undetectable by standard immunodiffusion tests (105).

TABLE 24.2. ASSOCIATION OF DISEASES AND ANTIBODIES TO THE Sm snRNPs

Antibody	Disease or Clinical Syndrome
Anti-Sm	SLE[a]
Anti-U1 snRNP	SLE[a] MCTD[b]
Anti-70K[c]	MCTD, SLE (paucity of nephritis)
Anti-A[c]	SLE
Anti-C[c]	Unclear
Anti-U2 snRNP	MCTD, SLE, or scleroderma with myositis
Anti-U4/U6 snRNP	Unknown (rare specificity)
Anti-U5 snRNP	Unknown (rare specificity)

[a]In SLE, anti-Sm antibodies frequently occur with anti-U1 snRNP; the latter antibodies may occur alone.
[b]In MCTD, anti-U1 snRNP antibodies are found alone and typically in high titer.
[c]The anti-U1 snRNP response is comprised of three separate antibody populations: anti-70K, anti-A, and anti-C.
Adapted from Craft J. Antibodies to snRNPs in SLE. *Rheum Dis Clin* 1992;18:311–336, with permission.

Several clinical studies have sought to correlate anti-Sm antibodies with disease activity and individual disease parameters. Early studies using immunodiffusion assays suggested that patients with these antibodies may have milder renal disease and less central nervous system involvement than patients with anti-DNA antibodies (108). Other studies have found that rising anti-Sm titers are predictive of disease flares (105) or more active disease (109). In a subsequent study based on ELISA, however, these antibodies did not correlate with particular disease manifestations (103). A large study involving over 100 Japanese patients found that anti-Sm antibodies, when detected by ELISA, correlated with a low frequency of progression to end-stage renal disease (and thus with milder renal disease), despite a high prevalence of late-onset proteinuria and a poorer prognosis overall than patients without anti-Sm (101). This finding was supported by an evaluation of group of U.S. patients that suggested these antibodies, when detected by ELISA, were associated with renal disease, the progression of which was not defined (107).

The sum total of current evidence indicates that the presence of anti-Sm antibodies is a very helpful adjunct in diagnosing SLE. On balance, however, their role in predicting or following the course of illness is much less clearly defined (110). Even so, in certain populations these antibodies could possibly identify a group of patients with a propensity to develop certain disease manifestations.

CLINICAL ASSOCIATION OF ANTI-U1 RNP ANTIBODIES

Anti-U1 RNP antibodies are found in approximately 30% to 40% of patients with SLE whose sera are tested in immunodiffusion (98,102,109,111) (Table 24.2). These antibodies may occur alone but often are present in conjunction with other specificities. They almost always are demonstrable in patients who have anti-Sm antibodies; conversely, the latter specificity rarely occurs without anti-U1 RNP antibodies (8,87,100). This pattern suggests that when the U1 snRNP particle acts as an autoimmunogen, initial responses are induced against U1 RNP determinants and are propagated, particularly in patients with SLE, to include Sm determinants, which is a notion that finds support in experimental data (112,113). Thus, an ability to expand autoimmune responses to a wide array of epitopes on the U1 snRNP appears to characterize SLE.

The major clinical association of anti-U1 RNP antibodies is with MCTD, where they typically occur in high titers and are not associated with other specificities (6,100,114) (Table 24.2). Indeed, this illness is defined by the presence of these antibodies. Anti-U1 RNP antibodies also may occur in a small fraction of patients with Sjögren's syndrome, rheumatoid arthritis, scleroderma, and polymyositis (98,100,114). Like anti-Sm, anti-U1 RNP antibodies are more common in black patients with SLE than in those of European background (102).

The three unique proteins of the U1 snRNP (i.e., 70K, A, and C) do not share known cross-reactive epitopes (88) and are recognized by at least three separate antibody populations (referred to as anti-70K, anti-A, and anti-C), which may occur either together or singly in a given patient (87). In other words, all three antibodies contribute to the anti-U1 RNP response. ELISAs that detect antibodies to individual 70K, A, and C proteins have now been established, and they demonstrate these antibodies in a small percentage of patients whose sera are negative on immunodiffusion (111).

Antibodies to the 70K protein, which are detectable in immunoblots, occur in 75% to 95% of patients with MCTD who are preselected because they have the anti-U1 RNP specificity as determined by immunodiffusion or by counterimmunoelectrophoresis (115–117) (Table 24.2). These antibodies may be less frequent in comparable groups of patients with SLE, in which anti-70K antibodies detectable by immunoblot appear to occur in as few as one fifth to as many as one half of individuals (115–117). However, ELISAs, based on either gel-purified 70K polypeptides or recombinant 70K fusion proteins expressed in *Escherichia coli*, reveal that up to 85% of patients with SLE, with anti-U1 RNP antibodies detectable by immunodiffusion, will have anti-70K antibodies (107,111). Among patients who are not preselected for the anti-U1 RNP specificity, anti-70K antibodies are found in approximately 12% of patients with SLE (118) and in occasional patients with rheumatoid arthritis, polymyositis, and scleroderma (111). When patients with MCTD and SLE are grouped together, anti-70K antibodies appear to correlate with myositis, esophageal hypomotility, Raynaud's phenomenon, lack of nephritis, and the human leukocyte antigen (HLA)-DR4 phenotype (107,117,119). Longitudinal studies have indicated that anti-70K antibody titers vary over time, but it is uncertain whether these levels reflect underlying disease activity (107,111,116,120,121). There is no experimental evidence that the antibodies themselves are involved in tissue injury. Thus, anti-70K antibodies, and anti-U1 snRNP antibodies in general, occur in both MCTD and SLE, may be markers for the former diagnosis when present in high titer, and may correlate with overlap features in patients who are otherwise thought to have SLE (122).

Antibodies to the A polypeptide also are quite common in patients who have anti-U1 RNP antibodies. Among patient populations selected for the presence of anti-U1 RNP, anti-A and anti-70K antibodies occur with approximately the same overall frequency when measured by immunoblots (87). However, among patients selected because they have SLE, anti-A antibodies appear to be twice as common as anti-70K antibodies (116,118), appearing in approximately 23% of such patients overall (118) or in approximately 75% of patients with lupus who have anti-U1 RNP antibodies by immunodiffusion (107). Presently, it is unclear whether anti-A antibodies are associated with specific disease manifestations (107). Like antibodies to the 70K polypeptide, those against A also vary over time, and these changes in titer do not necessarily reflect disease activity (107,121).

Antibodies to the C polypeptide occur with almost the same frequency as anti-70K and anti-A antibodies in patients with either MCTD or SLE who are preselected for the anti-U1 RNP specificity (87,116,123–125). Clinical associations of these antibodies beyond those for the anti-U1 snRNP response, however, have not been recognized as yet.

In summary, it appears that antibodies to all three unique proteins of the U1 snRNP contribute to the anti-U1 RNP response, as measured by immunodiffusion or other assays that do not detect antibodies to the specific proteins. The contributions of the anti-70K and anti-A response to the overall anti-U1 RNP response may vary depending on disease (i.e., MCTD vs. SLE) as well as, perhaps, on the manifestations of SLE.

CLINICAL ASSOCIATION OF ANTI-U2 RNP ANTIBODIES

Anti-U2 RNP antibodies were first described by Mimori et al. (49) in a patient with scleroderma-polymyositis overlap syndrome. Habets et al. (88) subsequently identified four patients whose sera contained these antibodies, although they did not find a specific disease association. However, later studies did find that these antibodies were associated with overlap syndromes (89,116), occurring in approximately 15% of patients with MCTD (89,116) and approximately the same frequency in patients with SLE or scleroderma plus myositis (89) (Table 24.2). Like anti-U1 RNP or anti-Sm, these antibodies produce a speckled immunofluorescence pattern (49,88,89); however, they can be distinguished by immunodiffusion, where they give partial identity with control anti-Sm sera (49). In the latter assay, they have lines of nonidentity with control anti-U1 RNP sera unless they contain these latter antibodies in addition to anti-U2 RNP. The best available methods to confirm the presence of anti-U2 RNP antibodies are immunoprecipitation or immunoblotting.

OTHER ANTI-snRNP ANTIBODIES

Antibodies against the U4/U6, U5, U7, and U11 snRNP have been described, as have antibodies to the trimethylguanosine cap structure of the U RNAs per se. While all these specificities are apparently quite rare, they maybe found in individuals with overlap syndromes or with features of systemic sclerosis, reminiscent of the clinical associations of the more common anti-U1 and anti-U2 snRNP specificities described earlier. For example, anti-U4/U6 snRNP-specific antibodies have been uniquely described in one patient with scleroderma and in another with Sjögren's syndrome (50,51). Similarly, one patient with an overlap syndrome has been described with anti-U5 snRNP antibodies (90). Anti-U7 snRNP antibodies have been found in a small series of patients with SLE (53), and anti-U11 snRNP antibodies have been found in one scleroderma serum in association with antitrimethylguanosine cap activity (54). The latter antibodies also have been found in a few patients with systemic sclerosis (126).

GENESIS OF THE ANTI-U1 RNP AND ANTI-SM RESPONSES

Accumulating information about the spectrum of antibodies to the Sm snRNPs and their relationship to the architecture of these particles make it possible to speculate about the underlying mechanisms accounting for production of these autoimmune responses. Several lines of evidence support the idea that anti-Sm and anti-U1 RNP responses arise as a result of antigen drive by the U1 snRNP (127). In other words, it seems likely that these responses are engendered by T-cell–dependent B-cell activation, a process that is initiated by presentation of these antigens as peptides by major histocompatibility complex (MHC) class II molecules.

The support for this scenario includes the following data and rationale: anti-Sm and anti-U1 RNP antibodies often occur in very high titer, may represent the majority of detectable autoantibodies that are present in a patient, and are responsible for a significant proportion of the total serum immunoglobulin (128). All of these features are similar to immune responses that are seen after the immunization of animals with exogenous antigens. Although SLE is characterized by B-cell hyperactivity with polyclonal immunoglobulin (Ig) synthesis, events that appear to precede specific autoantibody production (129), genetic analysis of anti-snRNP antibodies suggests they are selected by self-snRNP antigens (130). This latter conclusion is supported by the more extensive analysis of anti-DNA antibodies that also indicates they likely are selected by DNA (131), analogous to the selection of antibodies after conventional immune responses to a foreign antigen. While the physical nature of self antigens in lupus are unknown, analysis of autoantibody patterns that arise in both human and murine lupus suggest that intact particles, such as native self snRNPs or chromatin (DNA and associated proteins, including histones), serve as antigens for selection of B-cell clones for activation and autoantibody synthesis. For example, in SLE and lupus in Medical Research Laboratory (MRL) mice, nearly all mice with anti-Sm have anti-U1 snRNP antibodies, and individual antibodies to the U1 snRNP proteins 70K and A typically occur together in a given patient (132). While these data do not preclude the notion that disrupted snRNPs may be autoantigens, the findings that anti-snRNP antibodies occur in grouped arrays in both humans and mice (133) is consistent with the hypothesis that as particles, snRNPs serve as autoantigens for B cells. This hypothesis is supported by work showing that intact snRNPs are required for tandem generation of anti-snRNP autoantibodies in normal mice after abrogation of T-cell tolerance to one snRNP protein; disrupted snRNP particles did not support antibody expansion into grouped arrays (112). Such intact particles presumably are available to the immune system as part of apoptotic bodies (134), which after uptake by B cells or other antigen-presenting cells can potentially serve to activate grouped sets of T cells. The latter in turn then can provide help to multiple sets of B cells that after maturation make antibodies that target the individual components of the snRNP, or chromatin, particle (113).

The T-cell dependence of the anti-U1 RNP and anti-Sm response also is supported by several observations. Anti-snRNP-specific T cells have been isolated from normal individuals and from patients with SLE (135–137). Anti-snRNP antibodies also are restricted to T-dependent isotypes (138); however, it is not known if such T cells can provide cognate help. Likewise, ribosomal peptide specific CD4+ T cells have been isolated from patients with SLE and antiribosomal antibodies, although direct evidence for specific help has not been demonstrated (139). In comparison, however, CD4+ T-cell lines derived from patients with lupus and nephritis have been shown to help pathogenic anti-DNA production in *vitro* and to proliferate when mixed with self–B cells in an MHC class II–restricted fashion, suggesting the possibility that anti-DNA help was cognate (140,141). Moreover, in preliminary studies, these T cells appear to respond to peptides of chromatin proteins (142), fitting with the notion that they help anti-DNA B cells.

Although all these lines of evidence suggest that the anti-Sm and anti-U1 RNP responses are secondary to response to self-U1 snRNP particles, it should be emphasized that direct evidence for this scenario is not currently available. To support this view, evidence that shows processing by antigen-presenting cells and presentation of peptides derived from self-U1 snRNP proteins, with subsequent activation of autoreactive T cells with autoreactive B-cell help, is necessary.

ACKNOWLEDGMENTS

This work is supported in part by grants from the National Institutes of Health (AR40072 and AR42475), the Arthritis Foundation and its Connecticut chapter, the Connecticut chapter of the Lupus Foundation, and donations to Yale Rheumatology in the memories of Irene Feltman, Albert L. Harlow, and Chantal Marquis.

REFERENCES

1. Tan EM, Kunkel HG. Characteristics of a soluble nuclear antigen precipitating with sera of patients with systemic lupus erythematosus. *J Immunol* 1966;96:464–471.
2. Mattioli M, Reichlin M. Characterization of a soluble nuclear ribonucleoprotein antigen reactive with SLE sera. *J Immunol* 1971;107:1281–1290.
3. Reichlin M, Mattioli M. Correlation of a precipitating reaction to an RNA protein antigen and a low prevalence of nephritis in patients with systemic lupus. *N Engl J Med* 1972;286:908–911.
4. Sharp GC, Irvin WS, Laroque RL, et al. Association of autoantibodies to different nuclear antigens with clinical patterns of rheumatic disease and responsiveness to therapy. *J Clin Invest* 1971;50:350–359.
5. Northway JD, Tan EM. Differentiation of antinuclear antibodies giving speckled staining patterns in immunofluorescence. *Clin Immunol Immunopathol* 1972;1:140–154.
6. Sharp GC, Irvin WS, Tan EM, et al. Mixed connective tissue disease: an apparently distinct rheumatic disease syndrome associated with a specific antibody to an extractable nuclear antigen (ENA). *Am J Med* 1972;52:148–159.
7. Sharp GC, Irvin WS, Northway JD. Specificity of antibodies to extractable nuclear antigens (ENA) in mixed connective tissue disease (MCTD) and systemic lupus erythematosus (SLE). *Arthritis Rheum* 1972;15:125.
8. Mattioli M, Reichlin M. Physical association of two nuclear antigens and mutual occurrence of their antibodies: the relationship of the Sm and RNAprotein (Mo) systems in SLE sera. *J Immunol* 1973;110:1318–1324.
9. Lerner MR, Steitz A. Antibodies to small nuclear RNAs complexed with proteins are produced by patients with systemic lupus erythematosus. *Proc Natl Acad Sci USA* 1979;76: 5495–5499.
10. Lerner MR, Boyle JA, Mount SM, et al. Are snRNPs involved in splicing? *Nature* 1980;283:220–224.
11. Steitz JA. Snurps. *Sci Am* 1988;June:56–63.
12. Steitz JA, Black DL, Gerke V, et al. Functions of the abundant U-snRNPs. In: Birnstiel ML, ed. *Structure and function of major and minor small nuclear ribonuclear ribonucleoprotein particles.* Heidelberg: Springer-Verlag, 1988:115–154.
13. Lhrmann R. snRNP Proteins. In: Birnstiel ML, ed. *Structure and function of major and minor small nuclear ribonuclear ribonucleoprotein particles.* Heidelberg: Springer-Verlag, 1988: 71–99.
14. Reddy R, Busch H. Small nuclear RNAs: RNA sequences, structure, and modifications. In: Birnstiel ML, ed. *Structure and function of major and minor small nuclear ribonuclear ribonucleoprotein particles.* Heidelberg: Springer-Verlag, 1988:137.
15. Montzka K, Steitz JA. Additional low-abundance human small nuclear ribonucleoproteins: U11, U12, etc. *Proc Natl Acad Sci USA* 1988;85:8885–8889.
16. Lischwe MA, Ochs RL, Reddy R, et al. Purification and partial characterization of a nucleolar scleroderma antigen (Mr = 34,000; +8.5) rich in NG NG dimethylarginine. *J Biol Chem* 1985;260:14304–14310.
17. Tyc K, Steitz JA. U3, U8, and U13 comprise a new class of mammalian snRNPs localized in the cell nucleolus. *EMBO J* 1989;8:3113–3119.
18. Filipowicz W, Kiss T. Structure and function of nucleolar snRNPs. *Mol Biol Rep* 1993;18:149–156.
19. Hinterberger M, Pettersson I, Steitz JA. Isolation of small nuclear ribonucleoproteins containing U1, U2, U4, U5, and U6 RNAs. *J Biol Chem* 1983;258:2604–2613.
20. Andersen J, Feeney RJ, Zieve GW. Identification and characterization of the small nuclear ribonucleoprotein particle D' core protein. *Mol Cell Biol* 1990;10:4480–4485.
21. Lehmeier T, Foulaki K, Lhrmann R. Evidence for three distinct D proteins, which react differentially with anti-Sm autoantibodies, in the cores of the major snRNPs U1, U2, U4/U6 and U5. *Nucleic Acids Res* 1990;18:6475–6484.
22. Hackl W, Fischer U, Lhrmann R. A 69-kD protein that associates reversibly with the Sm core domain of several spliceosomal snRNP species. *J Cell Biol* 1994;124:261–272.
23. Zeller R, Nyffenegger T, De Robertis EM. Nucleocytoplasmic distribution of snRNPs and stockpiled snRNA-binding proteins during oogenesis and early development in Xenopus laevis. *Cell* 1983;32:425–434.
24. Schmauss C, Lerner MR. The closely related small nuclear ribonucleoprotein polypeptides N and B/B are distinguishable by antibodies as well as by differences in their mRNAs and gene structures. *J Biol Chem* 1990;265:10733–10739.
25. Griffith AJ, Schmauss C, Craft J. Murine gene encoding the highly conserved Sm B protein contains a nonfunctional alternative 3 splice site. *Gene* 1992;114:195–201.
26. Brunet C, Quan T, Craft J. Comparison of the Drosophila

melanogaster, human and murine Sm B cDNAs: evolutionary conservation. *Gene* 1993;124:269–273.
27. McAllister G, Roby-Shemkovitz A, Amara SG, et al. cDNA sequence of the rat U snRNP-associated protein N: description of a potential Sm epitope. *EMBO J* 1989;8:1177–1181.
28. McAllister G, Amara SG, Lerner MR. Tissue-specific expression and cDNA cloning of N: a novel snRNP-associated polypeptide. *Proc Natl Acad Sci USA* 1988;85:5296–5300.
29. Schmauss C, McAllister G, Ohosone Y, et al. A comparison of snRNP-associated autoantigens: human N, rat N, and human B/B. *Nucleic Acids Res* 1989;17:1733–1743.
30. Matter L, Wilhelm JA, Nyffenegger T, et al. Molecular characterisation of ribonucleoprotein antigens bound by antinuclear antibodies: a diagnostic evaluation. *Arthritis Rheum* 1982;25: 1278–1283.
31. Plfi Z, Bach M, Solymosy F, et al. Purification of the major UsnRNPs from broad bean nuclear extracts and characterization of their protein constituents. *Nucleic Acids Res* 1989;17: 1445–1458.
32. Tollervey D, Mattaj IW. Fungal small nuclear ribonucleoproteins share properties with plant and vertebrate U-snRNPs. *EMBO J* 1990;6:469–476.
33. Wright-Sandor L, Reichlin M, Tobin SL. Alteration by heat shock and immunological characterization of Drosophila small nuclear ribonucleoproteins. *J Cell Biol* 1990;108:2007–2016.
34. Sraphin B. Sm and Sm-like proteins belong to a large family: identification of proteins of the U6 as well as the U1, U2, U4, and U5 snRNPs. *EMBO J* 1995;14:2089–2098.
35. Branlant C, Krol A, Ebel JP, et al. U2 RNA shares a structural domain with U1, U4, and U5 RNAs. *EMBO J* 1982;1: 1259–1265.
36. Rokeach LA, Haselby JA, Hoch SA. Molecular cloning of a cDNA encoding the human Sm-D autoantigen. *Proc Natl Acad Sci USA* 1988;85:4832–4836.
37. Stanford DR, Kehl M, Perry CA, et al. The complete primary structure of the human snRNP E protein. *Nucleic Acids Res* 1988;16:10593–10605.
38. van Dam A, Winkel I, Zijlstra-Baalbergen J, et al. Cloned human snRNP proteins B and B′ differ only in their carboxy-terminal part. *EMBO J* 1989;8:3853–3860.
39. Ohosone Y, Mimori T, Griffith A, et al. Molecular cloning of cDNA encoding Sm autoantigen: derivation of a cDNA for a B polypeptide of the U series of small nuclear ribonucleoprotein particles. *Proc Natl Acad Sci USA* 1989;86:4249–4253.
40. OhosoneY, MimoriT, Griffith A, et al. Molecular cloning of cDNA encoding Sm autoantigen: derivation of a cDNA for a B polypeptide of the U series of small nuclear ribonucleoprotein particles (correction). *Proc Natl Acad Sci USA* 1989;86: 4249–4253.
41. Query CC, Bentley RC, Keene JD. A common RNA recognition motif identified within a defined U1 RNA binding domain of the 70K U1 snRNP protein. *Cell* 1989;57:89–101.
42. Bandziulis RJ, Swanson MS, Dreyfuss G. RNA binding proteins as developmental regulators. *Genes Dev* 1989;3:431–437.
43. Keene JD, Query CC. Nuclear RNA binding proteins. In: Moldave K, Cohn W, eds. *Progress in nucleic acid research and molecular biology.*Orlando: Academic, 1991:179–202.
44. Heinrichs V, Hackl W, Lhrmann R. Direct binding of small ribonucleoprotein G to the Sm site of small nuclear RNA. Ultraviolet light cross-linking of protein G to the AAU stretch within the Sm site (AAUUUGUGG) of U1 small nuclear ribonucleoprotein reconstituted in vitro. *J Mol Biol* 1992;227: 15–28.
45. Riedel N, Wolin S, Guthrie C. A subset of yeast snRNA's contains functional binding sites for the highly conserved Sm antigen. *Science* 1987;235:328–331.
46. Lee SI, Murthy SCS, Trimble JJ, et al. Four novel U RNAs are encoded by a herpesvirus. *Cell* 1988;54:599–607.
47. Kinlaw CS, Dusing-Swartz SK, Berget SM. Human U1 and U2 small nuclear ribonucleoproteins contain common and unique polypeptides. *Mol Cell Biol* 1982;2:1159–1166.
48. Kinlaw CS, Robberson BL, Berget SM. Fractionation and characterization of human small nuclear ribonucleoproteins containing U1 and U2 RNAs. *J Biol Chem* 1983;258:7181–7189.
49. Mimori T, Hinterberger M, Pettersson I, et al. Autoantibodies to the U2 small nuclear ribonucleoprotein in a patient with scleroderma-polymyositis overlap syndrome. *J Biol Chem* 1984; 259:560–565.
50. Mimori T, Fujii T, Hama N, et al. Newly identified autoantibodies to U4/U6 small nuclear ribonucleoprotein particle in a patient with primary Sjögren's syndrome. *Arthritis Rheum* 1991; 34:S46.
51. Okano Y, Medsger T. Newly identified U4/U6 snRNP-binding proteins by serum autoantibodies from a patient with systemic sclerosis. *J Immunol* 1991;146:535–542.
52. Bach M, Winkelmann G, Lhrmann R. 20S small nuclear ribonucleoprotein U5 shows a surprisingly complex protein composition. *Proc Natl Acad Sci USA* 1989;86:6038–6042.
53. Pironcheva G, Russev G. Characterization of the protein moiety of U7 small nuclear RNP particles. *Microbios* 1994;77: 41–46.
54. Gilliam A, Steitz J. Rare scleroderma autoantibodies to the U11 small nuclear ribonucleoprotein and to the trimethylguanosine cap of U small nuclear RNAs. *Proc Natl Acad Sci USA* 1993;90: 6781–6785.
55. Behrens SE, Tyc K, Kastner B, et al. Small nuclear ribonucleoprotein (RNP) U2 contains numerous additional proteins and has a bipartite RNP structure under splicing conditions. *Mol Cell Biol* 1993;13:307–319.
56. Behrens SE, Lhrmann R. Immunoaffinity purification of a [U4/U6.U5]tri-snRNP from human cells. *Genes Dev* 1991;5:1439–1452.
57. Smith V, Barrell BG. Cloning of a yeast U1 snRNP 70K protein homologue: functional conservation of an RNA-binding domain between humans and yeast. *EMBO J* 1991;10: 2627–2634.
58. Lutz-Freyermuth C, Keene JD. The U1 RNA-binding site of the U1 small nuclear ribonucleoprotein (snRNP)-associated A protein suggests a similarity with U2 snRNPs. *Mol Cell Biol* 1989;9:2975–2982.
59. Query CC, Bentley RC, Keene JD. A specific 31-nucleotide domain of U1 RNA directly interacts with the 70K small nuclear ribonucleoprotein component. *Mol Cell Biol* 1989;9: 4872–4881.
60. Scherly D, Boelens W, van Venrooij WJ, et al. Identification of the RNA binding segment of human U1 A protein and definition of its binding site on U1 snRNA. *EMBO J* 1989;8: 4163–4170.
61. Surowy CS, van Santen VL, Scheib-Wixted SM, et al. Direct, sequence-specific binding of the human U1-70K ribonucleoprotein antigen protein to loop I of U1 small nuclear RNA. *Mol Cell Biol* 1989;9:4179–4186.
62. Lutz-Freyermuth C, Query CC, Keene JD. Quantitative determination that one of two potential RNA-binding domains of the A protein component of the U1 small nuclear ribonucleoprotein complex binds with high affinity to stem-loop II of U1 RNA. *Proc Natl Acad Sci USA* 1990:87:6393–6397.
63. Scherly D, Boelens W, Dathan NA, et al. Major determinants of the specificity of interaction between small nuclear ribonucleoproteins U1A and U2Band their cognate RNAs. *Nature* 1990;345:502–506.
64. Scherly D, Dathan NA, Boelens W, et al. The U2B RNP motif

as a site of protein-protein interaction. *EMBO J* 1990;9: 3675–3681.
65. Bentley R, Keene J. Recognition of U1 and U2 small nuclear RNAs can be altered by a 5-amino acid segment in the U2 small nuclear ribonucleoprotein particle (snRNP) B protein and through interactions with U2 snRNP-A protein. *Mol Cell Biol* 1991;11:1829–1839.
66. Fresco LD, Harper DS, Keene JD. Leucine periodicity of U2 small nuclear ribonucleoprotein particle (snRNP) A protein is implicated in snRNP assembly via protein-protein interactions. *Mol Cell Biol* 1991;11:1578–1589.
67. Nelissen RLH, Heinrichs V, Habets WJ, et al. Zinc-finger like structure in U1-specific protein C is essential for specific binding to U1 snRNP. *Nucleic Acids Res* 1991;19:449–454.
68. Theissen H, Etzerodt M, Reuter R, et al. Cloning of the human cDNA for the U1 RNA-associated 70K protein. *EMBO J* 1986;5:3209–3217.
69. Query CC, Keene JD. A human autoimmune protein associated with U1 RNA contains a region of homology that is cross-reactive with retroviral p30gag antigen. *Cell* 1987;51:211–220.
70. Spritz RA, Strunk K, Surowy CS, et al. The human U1-70K protein: cDNA cloning, chromosomal localization, expression, alternative splicing and RNA-binding. *Nucleic Acids Res* 1987; 15:10373–10391.
71. Sillekens PTG, Habets WJ, Beijer RP, et al. cDNA cloning of the human U1 snRNP associated A protein: extensive homology between U1 and U2 snRNP-specific proteins. *EMBO J* 1987;6:3841–3848.
72. Sillekens PTG, Beijer RP, Habets WJ, et al. Human U1 snRNP-specific C protein: complete cDNA and protein sequence and identification of a multigene family in mammals. *Nucleic Acids Res* 1988;16:8307–8321.
73. Yamamoto K, Miura H, Moroi Y, et al. Isolation and characterization of a complementary DNA expressing human U1 small nuclear ribonucleoprotein C polypeptide. *J Immunol* 1988;140: 311–317.
74. Sillekens PTG, Beijer RP, Habets WJ, et al. Molecular cloing of the cDNA for the human U2 snRNP-specific A protein. *Nucleic Acids Res* 1989;17:1893–1906.
75. Habets WJ, Sillekens PTG, Hoet MH, et al. Analysis of a cDNA clone expressing a human autoimmune antigen: full-length sequence of the U2 small nuclear RNA-associated B antigen. *Proc Natl Acad Sci USA* 1987;84:2421–2425.
76. Lhrmann R, Kastner B, Bach M. Structure of spliceosomal snRNPs and their role in pre-mRNA splicing. *Biochim Biophy Acta* 1990;1087:265–292.
77. van Venrooij WJ, Sillekens PTG. Small nuclear RNA associated proteins: autoantigens in connective tissue diseases. *Clin Exp Rheum* 1989;7:635–645.
78. Sharp PA. Split genes and RNA splicing. *Cell* 1994;77: 805–815.
79. Mowry KL, Steitz JA. Identification of the human U7 snRNP as one of the several factors involved in the 3′ end maturation of histone premessenger RNAs. *Science* 1987;238:1682–1687.
80. Tarn W-Y, Steitz J. A novel spliceosome containing U11, U12, and U5 snRNPs excises a minor class (AT-AC) intro in vitro. *Cell* 1996;84:801–811.
81. Kass S, Tyc K, Steitz JA, et al. The U3 small nucleolar ribonucleoprotein functions in the first step of preribosomal RNA processing. *Cell* 1990;60:897–908.
82. Mattaj IW. Functions of the abundant U-snRNPs. In: Birnstiel ML, ed. *Structure and function of major and minor small nuclear ribonuclear ribonucleoprotein particles.* Heidelberg: Springer-Verlag, 1988:100–114.
83. Zieve GW, Sauterer RW. Cell biology of the snRNP particles. *CRC Crit Rev Biochem Mol Biol* 1990;25:146.
84. Nigg EA, Baeuerle PA, Lhrmann R. Nuclear import-export: in search of signals and mechanisms. *Cell* 1991;66:15–22.
85. Vankan P, McGuigan C, Mattaj I. Domains of U4 and U6 snRNAs required for snRNP assembly and splicing complementation in Xenopus oocytes. *EMBO J* 1990;9:3397–3404.
86. Wersig C, Guddat U. Pieler T, et al. Assembly and nuclear transport of the U4 and U4/U6 snRNPs. *Exp Cell Res* 1992; 199:373–377.
87. Pettersson I, Hinterberger M, Mimori T, et al. The structure of mammalian small nuclear ribonucleoproteins. *J Biol Chem* 1984;259:5907–5914.
88. Habets WJ, Hoet M, Bringmann P, et al. Autoantibodies to ribonucleoprotein particles containing U2 small nuclear RNA. *EMBO J* 1985;4:1545–1550.
89. Craft J, Mimori T, Olsen TL, et al. The U2 small nuclear ribonucleoprotein particle as an autoantigen: analysis with sera from patients with overlap syndrome. *J Clin Invest* 1988;8:1716–1724.
90. Okano Y, Targoff IN, Oddis CV, et al. Anti-U5 snRNP antibodies: a rare anti-U snRNP specificity. *Clin Immunol Immunopathol* 1996;81(1):41–47.
91. Fu XD, Maniatis T. Factor required for mammalian spliceosome assembly is localized to discrete regions in the nucleus. *Nature* 1990;343:437–441.
92. Carmo-Fonseca M, Tollervey D, Pepperkok R, et al. Mammalian nuclei contain foci which are highly enriched in components of the pre-mRNA splicing machinery. *EMBO J* 1991;10:195–206.
93. Gall JG. Spliceosomes and snurposomes. *Science* 1991;252: 1499–1500.
94. Spector DL. Macromolecular domains within the cell nucleus. *Annu Rev Cell Biol* 1993;9:265–315.
95. Reichlin M. Antinuclear antibodies. In: Kelley W, Harris E, Ruddy S, et al., eds. *Textbook of rheumatology*, 3rd ed. Philadelphia: WB Saunders, 1989:208–225.
96. Craft J, Hardin JA. Immunoprecipitation assays for the detection of soluble nuclear and cytoplasmic nucleoproteins. In: Rose N, Friedman H, Fahey J, eds. *Manual of clinical laboratory immunology*, 4th ed. Washington, DC: American Society of Microbiology, 1992:747–754.
97. van Venrooij W, Hoet R, Castrop J, et al. Anti-(U1) small nuclear RNA antibodies in anti-small nuclear ribonucleoprotein sera from patients with connective tissue diseases. *J Clin Invest* 1990;86:2154–2160.
98. Notman DD, Kurata N, Tan EM. Profiles of antinuclear antibodies in systemic rheumatic diseases. *Ann Intern Med* 1975;83: 464–469.
99. Tan EM, Cohen AS, Fries JF, et al. The 1982 revised criteria for the classification of systemic lupus erythematosus. *Arthritis Rheum* 1982;25:1271–1277.
100. Reeves WH, Fisher DE, Lahita RG, et al. Autoimmune sera reactive with Sm antigen contain high levels of RNP-like antibodies. *J Clin Invest* 1985;75:580–587.
101. Homma M, Mimori T, Takeda Y, et al. Autoantibodies to the Sm antigen: immunological approach to clinical aspects of systemic lupus erythematosus. *J Rheumatol* 1987;14(suppl 13): 188–193.
102. Arnett FC, Hamilton RG, Roebber MG, et al. Increased frequencies of Sm and nRNP autoantibodies in American blacks compared to whites with systemic lupus erythematosus. *J Rheumatol* 1988;15:1773–1776.
103. Field M, Williams DG, Charles P, et al. Specificity of anti-Sm antibodies by ELISA for systemic lupus erythematosus: increased sensitivity of detection using purified peptide antigens. *Ann Rheum Dis* 1988;47:820–825.
104. Abuaf N, Johanet C, Chretien P, et al. Detection of autoanti-

bodies to Sm antigen in systemic lupus erythematosus by immunodiffusion, ELISA and immunoblotting: variability of incidence related to assays and ethnic origin of patients. *Eur J Clin Invest* 1990;20:354–359.
105. Barada FA Jr, Andrews BS, Davis JS IV, et al. Antibodies to Sm in patients with systemic lupus erythematosus. *Arthritis Rheum* 1981;24:1236–1244.
106. Fisher DE, Reeves WH, Wisniewolski R, et al. Temporal shifts from Sm to ribonucleoprotein reactivity in systemic lupus erythematosus. *Arthritis Rheum* 1985;28:1348–1355.
107. Takeda Y, Wang GS, Wang RJ, et al. Enzyme-linked immunosorbent assay using isolated (U) small nuclear ribonucleoprotein polypeptides as antigens to investigate the clinical significance of autoantibodies to these polypeptides. *Clin Immunol Immunopathol* 1989;50:213–230.
108. Winn DM, Wolfe JF, Lindberg DA, et al. Identification of a clinical subset of systemic lupus erythematosus by antibodies to the Sm antigen. *Arthritis Rheum* 1979;22:1334–1337.
109. Boey ML, Peebles CL, Tsay G, et al. Clinical and autoantibody correlations in Orientals with systemic lupus erythematosus. *Ann Rheum Dis* 1988;47:918–923.
110. Gulko PS, Reveille JD, Koopman WJ, et al. Survival impact of autoantibodies in systemic lupus erythematosus. *J Rheumatol* 1994;21:224–228.
111. St. Clair EW, Query CC, Bentley R, et al. Expression of autoantibodies to recombinant (U1) RNP-associated 70K antigen in systemic lupus erythematosus. *Clin Immunol Immunopathol* 1990;54:266–280.
112. Fatenejad S, Mamula MJ, Craft J. Role of intermolecular/intrastructural B and T cell determinants in the diversification of autoantibodies to ribonucleoprotein particles. *Proc Natl Acad Sci USA* 1993;90:12010–12014.
113. James JA, Gross T, Scofield RH, et al. Immunoglobulin epitope spreading and autoimmune disease after peptide immunization. *J Exp Med* 1995;185:453–459.
114. Sharp GC, Irvin WS, May CM, et al. Association of antibodies to ribonucleoprotein and Sm antigens with mixed connective-tissue disease, systemic lupus erythematosus and other rheumatic diseases. *N Engl J Med* 1976;295:1149–1154.
115. Habets WJ, de Rooij DJ, Salden MH, et al. Antibodies against distinct nuclear matrix proteins are characteristic for mixed connective tissue disease. *Clin Exp Immunol* 1983;54:265–276.
116. Pettersson I, Wang G, Smith EI, et al. The use of immunoblotting and immunoprecipitation of (U) small nuclear ribonucleoproteins in the analysis of sera of patients with mixed connective tissue disease and systemic lupus erythematosus. *Arthritis Rheum* 1986;29:986–996.
117. Reichlin M, van Venrooij WJ. Autoantibodies to the URNP particles: relationship to clinical diagnosis and nephritis. *Clin Exp Immunol* 1991;83:286–290.
118. Ehrfeld H, Renz M, Seelig HP, et al. Antibodies to recombinant U1-70K and U1–a protein in systemic lupus erythematosus (SLE). *Mol Biol Rep* 1991;15:190.
119. Hoffman RW, Rettenmaier LJ, Takeda Y, et al. Human autoantibodies against the 70-kd polypeptide of U1 small nuclear RNP are associated with HLA-DR4 among connective tissue disease patients. *Arthritis Rheum* 1990;33:666–673.
120. Houtman PM, Kallenberg CGM, Limburg PC, et al. Fluctuations in anti-nRNP levels in patients with mixed connective disease are related to disease activity as part of a polyclonal B cell response. *Ann Rheum Dis* 1986;45:800–808.
121. de Rooij DJ, Habets WJ, van de Putte LB, et al. Use of recombinant RNP peptides 70K and A in an ELISA for measurement of antibodies in mixed connective tissue disease: a longitudinal follow up of 18 patients. *Ann Rheum Dis* 1990;49:391–395.
122. Snowden N, Hay E, Holt PJL, et al. Clinical course of patients with anti-RNP antibodies. *J Rheumatol* 1993;20:1256–1258.
123. Combe B, Rucheton M, Graafland H, et al. Clinical significance of anti-RNP and anti-Sm autoantibodies as determined by immunoblotting and immunoprecipitation in sera from patients with connective tissue diseases. *Clin Exp Immunol* 1989;75:18–24.
124. Habets WJ, Hoet MH, van Venrooij W. Epitope patterns of anti-RNP antibodies in rheumatic diseases. Evidence for an antigen-driven autoimmune response. *Arthritis Rheum* 1990;33:834–841.
125. Lundberg I, Nyman U, Hedfors E. Clinical manifestations and anti-(U1)snRNP antibodies: a prospective study of 29 anti-RNP antibody positive patients. *Br J Rheumatol* 1992;31:811–817.
126. Okano Y, Medsger TA. Novel human autoantibodies reactive with 5-terminal trimethylguanosine cap structures of U small nuclear RNA. *J Immunol* 1992;149:1093–1098.
127. Hardin JA. The lupus autoantigens and the pathogenesis of systemic lupus erythematosus. *Arthritis Rheum* 1986;29:457–460.
128. Maddison PJ, Reichlin M. Quantitation of precipitating antibodies to certain soluble nuclear antigens in SLE. *Arthritis Rheum* 1977;20:819–824.
129. Klinman DM, Eisenberg R, Steinberg AD. Development of the autoimmune B cell repertoire in MRL-lpr/lpr mice. *J Immunol* 1990;144:506–511.
130. Bloom DD, Davignon J, Retter MW, et al. V region gene analysis of anti-Sm hybridomas from MRL/Mp-lpr/lpr mice. *J Immunol* 1993;150:1591–1610.
131. Diamond B, Katz JB, Paul E, et al. The role of somatic mutation in the pathogenic anti-DNA response. *Annu Rev Immunol* 1992;10:731–757.
132. Craft J. Antibodies to snRNPs in SLE. *Rheum Dis Clin* 1992;18:311–336.
133. Fatenejad S, Brooks W, Schwartz A, et al. The pattern of anti-snRNP antibodies in MRL-lpr mice suggests that the intact U1 snRNP is their autoimmunogenic target. *J Immunol* 1994;152:5523–5531.
134. Casciola-Rosen LA, Anhalt G, Rosen A. Autoantigens targeted in systemic lupus erythematosus are clustered in two populations of surface structures on apoptotic keratinocytes. *J Exp Med* 1994;179:1317–1330.
135. O'Brien RM, Cram DS, Coppel RS, et al. T cell epitopes on the 70kDa protein of the U1 (RNP) complex in autoimmune rheumatologic disorders. *J Autoimmun* 1990;3:747–753.
136. Hoffman RW, Takeda Y, Sharp GC, et al. Human T cell clones reactive against U-small nuclear ribonucleoprotein autoantigens from connective tissue disease patients and healthy individuals. *J Immunol* 1993;151:6460–6469.
137. Okubo M, Yamamoto K, Kato T, et al. Detection and epitope analysis of autoantigen-reactive T cells to U1-small nuclear ribonucleoprotein A protein in autoimmune disease patients. *J Immunol* 1993;151:1108–1115.
138. Eisenberg R, Dyer K, Craven SY, et al. Subclass restriction and polyclonality of the systemic lupus erythematosus marker antibody anti-Sm. *J Clin Invest* 1985;75:1270–1277.
139. Crow MK, DelGiudice-Asch G, Zehetbauer JB, et al. Autoantigen-specific T cell proliferation induced by the ribosomal P2 protein in patients with systemic lupus erythematosus. *J Clin Invest* 1994;94:345–352.
140. Rajagopalan S, Zordan T, Tsokos GC, et al. Pathogenic anti-DNA autoantibody-inducing T helper cell lines from patients with active lupus nephritis: Isolation of CD4-8-T helper cell lines that express the gd T-cell antigen receptor. *Proc Natl Acad Sci USA* 1990;87:7020–7024.
141. Shivakumar S, Tsokos GC, Datta SK. T cell receptor a/b

expressing double-negative (CD4–/CD8–) and CD4;pl T helper cells in humans augment the production of pathogenic anti-DNA autoantibodies associated with lupus nephritis. *J Immunol* 1989;143:103–112.

142. Desai-Mehta A, Mao C, Rajogopalan S, et al. Structure and specificity of receptors expressed by pathogenic anti-DNA autoantibody-inducing T cells in human lupus. *Arthritis Rheum* 1994;37:S282.

143. Reuter R, Rothe S, Habets W, et al. Autoantibody production against the U small nuclear ribonucleoprotein particle proteins E, F, and G in patients with connective tissue diseases. *Eur J Immunol* 1990;20:437–440.

144. Lutz-Freyermuth C, Keene JD. The U1 RNA binding site of the U1 small nuclear ribonucleoprotein (snRNP)-associated A protein suggests a similarity with U2 snRNPs. *Mol Cell Biol* 1989;9:2975–2982.

145. Query CC, Bentley R, Keene JD. A specific 31-nucleotide domain of U1 RNA directly interacts with the 70K small nuclear ribonucleoprotein component. *Mol Cell Biol* 1989;9:4872–4881.

25

THE LUPUS ANTICOAGULANT AND ANTIPHOSPHOLIPID ANTIBODIES

GALE A. MCCARTY

The antiphospholipid antibody syndrome (APS) is characterized by an ever-widening spectrum of clinical correlates, screening and confirmatory tests detecting diverse antigenic specificities, well-established and evolving models of *in vivo* pathogenesis, and various treatments (1–3). Clinical features of antiphospholipid antibodies (aPLs), specificities detected by enzyme immunoassays (EIAs), and management are considered in Chapter 52, but are discussed in detail here for that set of aPLs that are classically, but ironically, called lupus anticoagulants (LACs), and defined by coagulation-based tests.

HISTORICAL PERSPECTIVES

Circulating anticoagulants (CACs) are ubiquitous inhibitors of coagulation that are detected by abrogation of *in vitro* coagulation tests and *in vivo* coagulation. Specific CACs are most often but not always naturally occurring or acquired immunoglobulins (Igs) that either recognize epitopes on various coagulation factors at active sites and thus inhibit functional activity (e.g., an antibody to factor VIII), or do not recognize epitopes associated with the active site and are not always associated with pathology, e.g., the subset of LAC patients who have antibodies to prothrombin (aPT), which can be clinically silent, associated with bleeding, or rarely thrombosis. Nonspecific CACs include various LACs, paraproteins, or fibrin split products. LAC is defined here as a mixture of immunoglobulins (most commonly IgG/M/A) that interfere with one or more phospholipid-dependent coagulation tests, originally identified in patients with systemic lupus erythematosus (SLE). The multidisciplinary work on LACs that burgeoned from 1948 to 1983 (Table 25.1) served to explain and interrelate three prior discoveries: (a) reaginic antibodies reactive to ethanol tissue extracts in syphilitic sera in 1906 (i.e., the first aPL recognizing the mixture of the neutral phospholipid choline, cholesterol, and cardiolipin); (b) biologic false-positive serologic tests for syphilis (BFP-STS) in 1938; and (c) cardiolipin (i.e., a negatively charged phospholipid [PL] as its major antigenic component in 1941 (4–20).

From the initial description by Conley et al. (7) in 1948, the chronology of LAC reflects confusion due to limitations of available technology, as well as a lack of recognition of the complex symptomatology that eventually came to be associated with APS. Clinical associations such as bleeding (7), thrombosis (12,18,20), the BFP-STS (8), and fetal loss (9,20) were recognized but incompletely interrelated, even before Laurell and Nilsson (10) demonstrated that the factor responsible for LAC activity was an immunoglobulin, an observation extended to both IgG and IgM isotypes by Yin and Gaston (13). That these clinical features and laboratory components (Table 25.1) occurred in patients with SLE and with non-SLE diseases was shown by Bowie et al. (12) and Schleider et al. (16), and they encompass most major elements of what now is considered to be the spectrum of the primary and secondary APS (12,16,20). Even before the naming of this CAC as "LAC" by Feinstein and Rapaport (14), several major areas reflecting pathophysiology and test variability were known; these include prothrombin-like cofactor activity (11), phospholipid dependence (7,11,15,17–19), and the common occurrence of paradoxic findings in LAC tests (17). The Scientific and Standardization Committees on Thrombosis and Hemostasis spearheaded by hematologists and laboratory investigators worldwide since the 1980s has facilitated some consensus recommendations in nomenclature and technology; analogously, the heterogeneity of aPLs in general as detected by EIAs has been addressed by the aPL standardization committees and workshops organized by E. Nigel Harris, M.D., since 1988. This chronology ironically foreshadows the continuing controversies about the interrelationships of LAC and aPL (8,10,13,14), the necessary and sufficient cofactors (11), and phospholipid-protein antigenic targets (8,15,19).

TABLE 25.1. CIRCULATING ANTICOAGULANT AND LUPUS ANTICOAGULANT CHRONOLOGY

1948	Conley et al. (7)	CAC and bleeding
1952	Conley and Hartmann (8)	CAC and BFP-STS
1954	Beaumont (9)	CAC and fetal loss
1957	Laurell and Nilsson (10)	CAC = immunoglobulin absorbed by cardiolipin
1959	Loeliger (11)	CAC cofactor-prothrombin
1963	Bowie et al. (12)	CAC and thrombosis in SLE
1965	Yin and Gaston (13)	CAC = IgG or IgM
1972	Feinstein and Rapaport (14)	CAC is a LAC
1974	Feltkamp et al. (15)	LAC is phospholipid-dependent
1976	Schleider et al. (16)	LAC and non-SLE diseases
1978	Exner et al. (17)	LAC and paradoxic reactions
1980	Soulier and Boffa (18)	LAC and thrombosis
1983	Triplett et al. (19)	LAC and PNP
1983	Boey et al. (20)	LAC and SLE and thrombosis

BFP-STS, biologic false-positive serologic tests for syphilis; CAC, circulating anticoagulant; Ig, immunoglobulin; LAC, lupus anticoagulant; PNP, platelet neutralization procedure.

CONDITIONS ASSOCIATED WITH LAC POSITIVITY

That LAC is a misnomer and attempts should be made to simply rename the entity as "a positive coagulation based test" is supported by several tenets: (a) the majority of "LAC"-associated conditions are not associated with lupus, and represent the primary syndrome, "lupus like disease" in patients who do not meet criteria for the diagnosis of SLE, but may be evolving primary APS patients who will develop thromboses, as did several of the patients with positive aPL/LACs recently published by Lockshin et al. (21) in their validation study of the Sapporo criteria; (b) thrombosis is more common than bleeding, and the number of patients who are being identified as having aPL by LAC or other aPL tests may alert the clinician to consider special circumstances such as combined clinical conditions (46).

CLINICAL SITUATIONS FOR TESTING

Clinical presentations prompting coagulation testing primarily involve patients with unexplained bleeding or thrombosis, asymptomatic or symptomatic prolonged screening tests, or acquired coagulation abnormalities [dysproteinemias, lymphomas, other neoplasia, infections (chronic bacterial, HIV, parvovirus), or drugs]. The goal of testing is to differentiate the presence of a true phospholipid-dependent LAC from that of primary coagulation factor deficiencies [most commonly, factors VIII, IX, or XI, acquired immunoglobulin inhibitor(s) of these factors, or apparent coagulopathies due to binding of "LAC" to various plasma proteins that bind to phospholipid surfaces]. The important differential here is the risk of thrombosis in the LAC group versus that of bleeding, which more commonly is seen with the factor-deficient patients (4–6). The astute clinician will already have ruled out historical or age-related factors suggesting causes of venous thrombosis that may exist independently of LAC or aPL positivity (e.g., protein S/C/antithrombin III deficiencies, activated protein C resistance because of the factor V Leiden mutation and activated protein C resistance, paroxysmal nocturnal hemoglobinuria, oral contraceptive use, nephrotic syndrome) or vaso-occlusive disease states where vascular damage exteriorizes altered self components that might function as an "antigen driven state" (e.g., hypertension, diabetes, smoking, intracardiac thrombi, Buerger's disease, hyperhomocysteinemia).

A recent review of the epidemiology of LAC positivity by Petri (44) shows that (a) in normals where LAC and one aPL test was performed simultaneously, approximately 6% were positive for aPL vs. 4% for LAC; (b) in three studies of pregnant women, the LAC was slightly more frequently positive 1.2% to 3.8% vs. 1.0% to 2.2% for aPL; and (c) in 1,000 patients from the Eurolupus Study, 15% of patients were LAC positive and simultaneously 24% were anticardiolipin (aCL) positive. A consensus of other studies systematically evaluating conditions associated with LAC positivity shows that approximately 45% occur in established or evolving SLE (21–23), 15% in the peripartum state (24), and 12% in drug exposures, primarily procainamide (25,26), phenothiazines (27,28), chlorpromazine (29), and, rarely, procainamide and hydralazine (30,31). The remainder occurs in adults and children with viral infections (often transient), human immunodeficiency virus (HIV) disease (either sustained or intermittent), and in hematogenous or solid malignancies (32,33), or they are discovered in normal individuals undergoing preoperative assessment.

Clinical Cautions

An important clinical subset are patients with hemophilia who acquired HIV via blood products and develop aPL or LAC that is uncommonly associated with thrombosis but risk bleeding caused by specific factor deficiencies (34). Rarely, immunoglobulins directed at von Willebrand factor (35), factor VIII (36), factor IX (37), factor XI (38), and fibrin polymerization (39) occur in SLE. Increasing reports of LAC and/or aPL positivity with concurrent antibodies to specific coagulation factors should alert rheumatologists, hematologists, and both hospital and reference laboratory directors to the importance of consultative comanagement in these patients (40–42,46).

Prevalence Of LAC

The prevalence of LAC activity in normal individuals as well as in patient populations varies widely because of several factors: (a) the vagaries of methodology and lack of adherence to standardization for performance of the most commonly used

TABLE 25.2. COMPARATIVE ASPECTS OF MAJOR LAC TESTS

	aPTT	KCT	dRVVT	TTI (dPT)	Textarin time
Test choice	1st	2nd	2nd	2nd	2nd
Sensitivity for LAC	Very	Intermediate	Very	Intermediate	Very
Screen and confirm LAC	Y/N	Y/N	Y/Y	Y	Y/Y
Phospholipid source	Cephalin	None	Thrombofax	TF/thromoplastin	None/platelets
Initiator	Silica/kaolin	Kaolin	Russell's viper venom	(See text)	*Pseudonaja textilis* and *Ecaris* venoms
Normal (secs)	25–35	60–100	25–30	Ratio, <1.3	20–40
Use in Pregnancy	N	Y	Y	Y	Y
Resistance to factor deficiency/inhibition	Variable	Variable	Most resistant (except low X, V)	(See text)	Except V
Sensitivity to heparin	Y	Y	N	N	(See text)
Mechanized test	Y	Y	Y	Potential	Potential
Specificity	Low	High	High	High	(See text)

aPTT, activated partial thromboplastin time; KCT, kaolin clot time; dRVVT, dilate Russell's viper venom test; TTI (dPT), tissue thromboplastin inhibition test (dilute prothrombin time).

test worldwide, the activated partial thromboplastin time (aPTT), and other screening and confirmatory CAC tests (43,44); and (b) the sparseness of studies in which both normal and patient plasma and sera were co-investigated for LAC and aPL, respectively, with sensitive and specific screening as well as confirmatory tests that demonstrated PL-dependency or where a platelet neutralization procedure (PNP) was performed (45,46) (Table 25.2). In SLE, the prevalence of LAC varies from less than 10% to approximately 40% relative to the sensitivity and specificity of the individual screening and/or confirmatory test procedures used (46) (Table 25.2). Other studies cumulatively show higher percentages for aCL (69%) versus LAC (48%) positivity in SLE sera analyzed concurrently by multiple methods; when populations are examined based on investigation at the time of a thrombotic event, the percentages are proportionally higher in some studies and in others they are lower, due to aPLs being involved in tissue deposition and/or immune complexes (47,48). Of note is that when patients are retested within 2 months of an index event, there is a demonstrable, incremental benefit in diagnosis, especially for LAC testing; performance of a repeat test and a second, different test increases the chance of demonstrating an aPL or a LAC (49). That LAC and aPL are likely subsets of antibodies recognizing related but different antigenic determinants is indisputable, and there is a wide range of concordance (0% to 60%) between the functional (e.g., LAC) and the immunologically (e.g., BFP-STS, aPL) derived test procedures. These figures are general guidelines in that during testing, many factors such as the nature of the patient population and test-related variables should be considered on an individual basis.

LABORATORY DIAGNOSIS OF LAC

The classic coagulation scheme is shown in Fig. 25.1 and involves dynamic interactions among cellular, protein, phospholipid, and calcium ions that are localized and controlled in space and time. That procoagulant reactions occur faster than fibrinolytic reactions is an important concept to recall as the molecular basis for thrombosis evolves.

Since 1964, coagulation has been thought to be initiated by the intrinsic pathway (i.e., contact factor components) or the extrinsic pathway [i.e., cell membrane proteins and tissue factor (TF)], with either pathway resulting in factor Xa generation and eventual thrombin formation

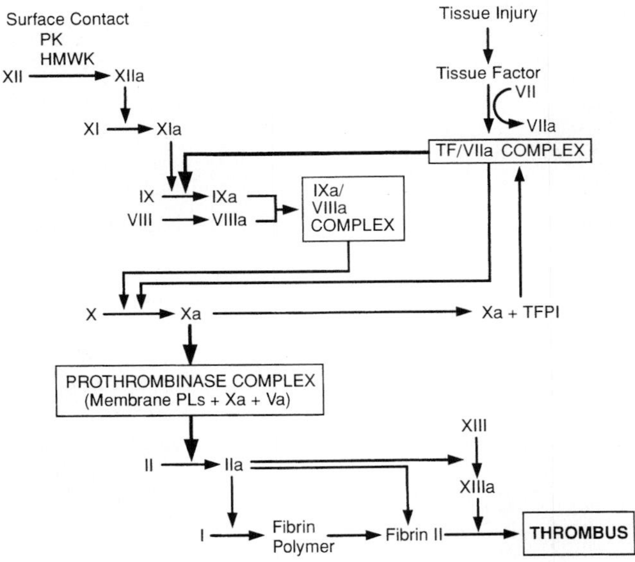

FIGURE 25.1. The coagulation scheme updated from 1964 to the present, with the three main phospholipid-dependent complexes highlighted in *closed boxes* (the two classic tenase complexes, tissue factor/factor VIIa and factor IXa/factor VIIIa, and the prothrombinase complex; membrane phospholipids, factor Xa, and factor Va). For simplicity, calcium and magnesium ions are not shown, but they are integral parts of many coagulation reactions. The end of the cascade results in thrombosis.

(50,51). Testing for the intrinsic pathway involved the aPTT, and for the extrinsic pathway the prothrombin time (PT). In 1996, the accepted scheme involved TF VIIa complexes initiating coagulation via factor X, sustaining the process via factor IXa activation of factor VII, and completing the process by activation of factor XI. The two classic tenase complexes and the prothrombinase complex are depicted in boxes in Fig. 25.2 for emphasis; these represent three of the four major phospholipid-dependent coagulation processes.

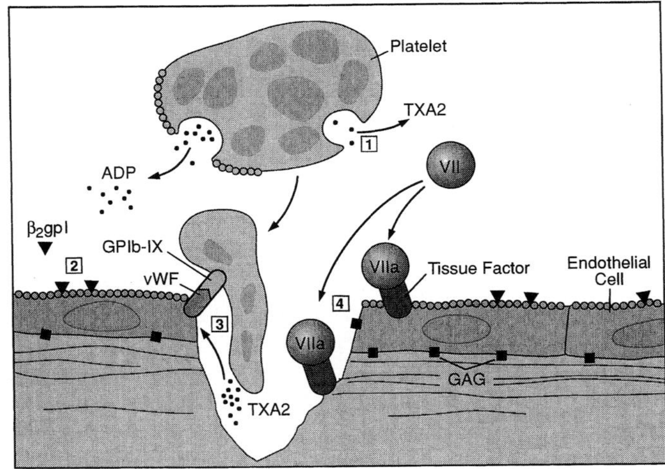

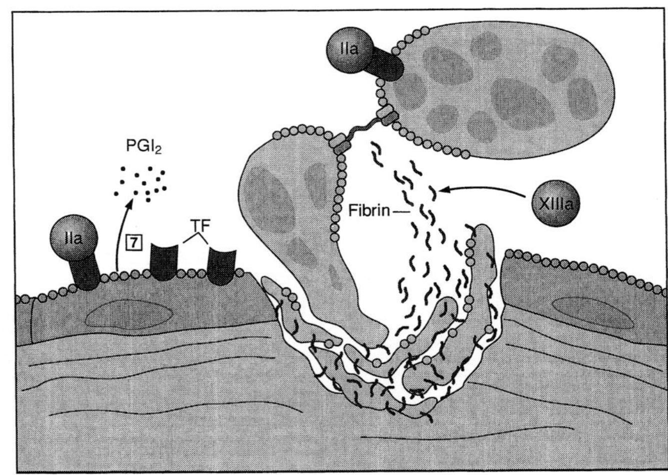

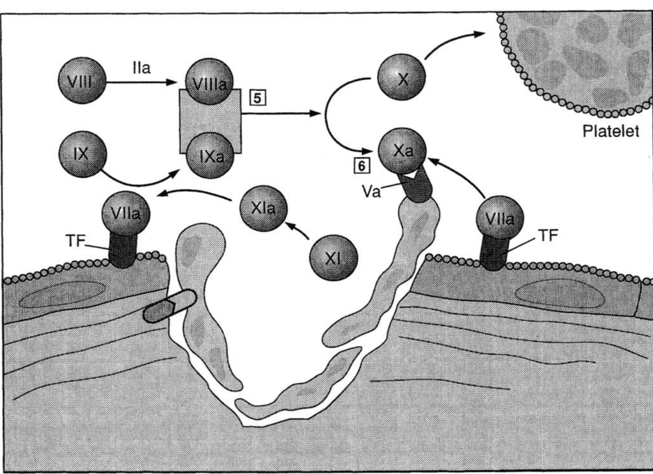

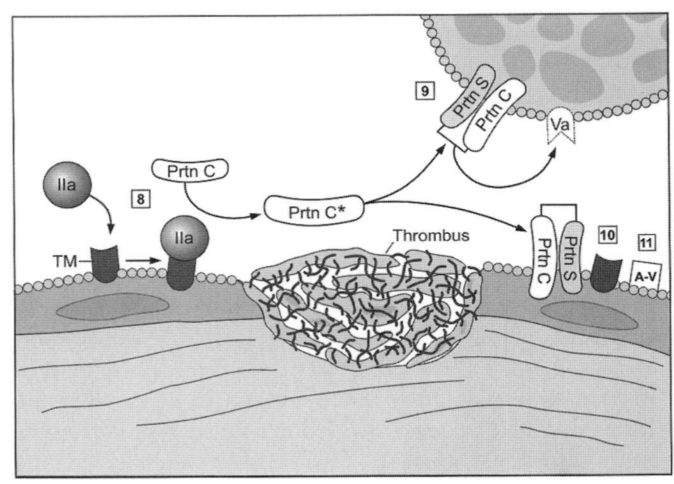

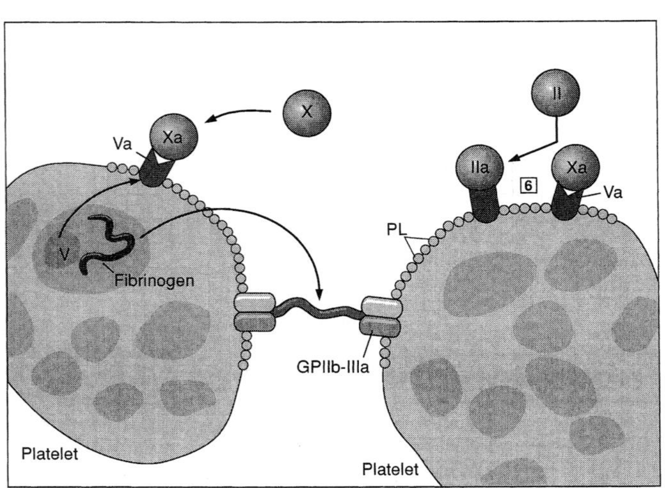

FIGURE 25.2. The coagulation scheme occurring at a localized site of vascular injury or altered self. The luminal side is up; the basement membrane side is down. For this series, phospholipids (PLs) on cell membranes are designated by *open circles* on the luminal side; β_2-glycoprotein I (2gpI) by a *black triangle*; glycosaminoglycans (GAGs) in subendothelial areas by a *black square*; coagulation factors by *shaded and numbered circles*, often bound to tissue factor (TF), with activated coagulation factor fragments as specified and shown by stippled receptors. The *small-boxed* numbers 1 to 11 refer to areas where lupus anticoagulants (LACs) and antiphospholipid antibodies (aPLs) have either been proven to interact with components of the coagulation scheme or where they are suspected to exert their influence on PL-dependent binding reactions. **A–D**: The steps in Fig. 25.1 culminate in the formation of a thrombus at the site of a vessel injury or altered self. **E:** The fourth main PL-dependent complex is added, that of protein S/C and thrombomodulin (TM; depicted with a previously used stippled receptor symbol, but here specified as being thrombomodulin). The annexin V shield has been added (A-V). Thus, LACs and aPLs also may work in effecting the return to an anticoagulant surface after procoagulant effector molecules have resulted in thrombosis. TF, tissue factor; TXA_2, thromboxane A_2; vWF, von Willebrand factor.

Endothelial cell or platelet damage or activation exposes negatively charged inner membrane leaflets or reorganizes phospholipid arrays. The vitamin K–dependent clotting factors bind to these charged phospholipid surfaces, and platelet receptors allow adherence to subendothelial connective tissue and other sites (Fig. 25.2A–D). The endothelial cell surface itself modulates its procoagulant versus anticoagulant properties via thrombomodulin and the activated protein C/protein S complex [i.e., the fourth phospholipid-dependent complex (Fig. 25.2E)]. Coagulation therefore is localized to sites of vessel injury and restricted there by binding to negatively charged phospholipid/membrane components that are not normally accessible. Recently, the elucidation of the thrombomodulatory role of annexin V as a regulatory "shield" that clusters on exposed PL-rich surfaces and abrogates the binding of aPL or LAC to PLs in the maternal-fetal unit will likely be shown to be operative at other endothelial cell sites (51a).

Thus, several phospholipid-dependent complexes have the capacity to be influenced by LACs or different aPLs. Additionally, the natural anticoagulant β_2-glycoprotein I ($\beta_2$gpI, or apolipoprotein H) has affinity for anionic phospholipid as well as other coagulation components; phospholipid flip-flop or loss of membrane asymmetry that exteriorizes or exposes phosphatidylserine (PS), or other phospholipids, via the translocase reaction after membrane perturbation or injury might contribute to immunogenicity by revelation and/or creation of neoepitopes, perhaps related to $\beta_2$gpI binding to cardiolipin (CL), which might drive LAC/aPL production (52). Thus, there are multifactorial ways in which these antibodies might interact *in vivo* to generate a procoagulant surface, which might then continue to drive phospholipid-dependent coagulation reactions. Recent vascular injury models in the presence of aPLs or LACs have shown augmentation of cell functions and thrombosis size or frequency (see Chapter 52).

RATIONALE FOR SCREENING TESTS

The minimal laboratory assessment for all coagulation abnormalities includes an aPTT, a PT, and a platelet count as a first step (53). The second step is the determination of LAC by demonstrating that the prolongation of the screening test results from an antibody and not a quantitative or qualitative coagulation factor deficit or inhibition. Mixing normal plasma with patient plasma does not correct the aPTT prolongation to normal with most LACs, whereas mixing with normal plasma usually does partially or completely correct aPTT prolongation by the provision of normal clotting factors. This is not infallible, as some aPLs act at multiple levels or on multiple factors in the coagulation scheme.

The definition of a screening test is an assay that is based on a single concentration of phospholipid (54). The major tests compared are the aPTT, the kaolin clot time (KCT), the dilute Russell's viper venom test (dRVVT), the tissue thromboplastin inhibition test [TTI; otherwise known as the dilute prothrombin time (PT)], and the Textarin time test (Table 25.3). Other tests include the plasma clot time (PCT), and new integrated systems where multiple reagents are incorporated in reaction mixtures (46,54).

A source of confusion for nonhematologists interpreting the literature is use of the descriptive phrase that a test component is "sensitive to the presence of the LAC"; often, this is misinterpreted as the test has high sensitivity. When referring to aPTT reagents, reagent sensitivity means that the abnormal aPTT results from the presence of a LAC, while reagent responsiveness means the degree of test prolongation (46,53). Thus, reagents often are classified in terms of paired sensitivity/responsiveness, and as laboratories strive to improve tests in different size study populations, inconsistencies in comparative results occur. This is the basis for both past (46) as well as current (55–57) recommendations that even if the screening aPTT is normal, an additional screening test is recommended.

Because LACs are heterogeneous, no single test detects all LAC, and no one test approximates 100% sensitivity or

TABLE 25.3. PROFILING OF LAC/aPL

Antibody	Characteristics and Function
LAC	Inhibit phospholipid-dependent coagulation Reactions Recognize phospholipid-bound PT
aCL	Type A Inhibit phospholipid-dependent reaction by increasing β2gp1-phospholipid binding Recognize β2gp1-phospholipid complex Type B LAC
Anti-free β2gp1	Inhibit phospholipid-dependent reaction in β2gp1-dependent manner
Antiprotein S & activated protein C	Inhibit anticoagulant function of both Recognize proteins S and C after phospholipid binding
aPL (? True)	Inhibit phospholipid-dependent reaction without cofactors ? True
Other "aPL"	?
?Apoptosis	May require prothrombin, other factors
Antiprotein S & activated protein C	Inhibit anticoagulant function of both Recognize protein S & C after phospholipid binding
aPE (Zwitterionic-Positive + Negative Charge)	Inhibit phospholipid-dependent reaction without cofactors High and low molecular weight kininogens?
Other "aPL" (Negative Charge, Neutral Charge)	aPS, aPC

aCL, anticardiolipin; aPL, antiphospholipid; PT, prothrombin time.

100% specificity. Caveats and special circumstances are clarified in this text to reflect these methodologic considerations as an evolving area; while a majority of experts now agree that two tests need to be performed (one screening test and a confirmatory test), there are some who espouse that perhaps a third test be added, but they remain in the minority at this time. An overview of some comparative aspects of LAC screening and confirmatory testing is provided by Fig. 25.3 and represents a consensus from clinical experience and the current literature (46,54–58).

The laboratory criteria for LAC testing, as established by the Scientific and Standardization Committee Subcommittee for the Standardization of Lupus Anticoagulants in 1991 (57), have been simplified by Exner et al. (57) to represent the minimally acceptable criteria to define LAC: (a) an *in vitro*, phospholipid-dependent coagulation test must be prolonged; (b) an inhibitor (or LAC) must be demonstrable as the cause by mixing studies using appropriate ratios of patient-to-normal plasma; and (c) the inhibitor (or LAC) must be differentiated as being directed at a phospholipid, preferably a hexagonal phase II PL, not at a specific coagulation factor (46,54—56,58a). However, recent data reviewed by Exner (5) show that correction of test abnormality by PL is more specific for LACs than the platelet neutralization procedure that has been "recommended" since 1984. The most recent recommendations from the subcommittee, summarized by Brandt et al. (58) in late 1995, are similar and state appropriately that despite excellent and careful research, both the ordering physician and the patient must be aware that aPLs are very heterogeneous, and that even well-standardized LAC assays may have a range of sensitivity for the detection of certain subgroups of LACs.

In addition, the subcommittee recommends the following: (a) two or more different screening tests should be performed for LAC, one of which should be a low phospholipid concentration test (KCT, dRVVT, dilute aPTT, daPPT, dPT); (b) the presence of inhibitor activity should be determined by incorporation of a mixing step (i.e., patient plasma's effect on pooled normal plasma) in the initial screening test, using a well-characterized, pooled normal plasma that has ratios; (c) documentation of multiple abnormal screening tests is not presumptive evidence of a LAC until phospholipid dependence is established; (d) confirmatory tests should be based on methodology similar to screening tests (Fig. 25.3); (e) a PT and an aPTT should be performed before screening LAC tests to

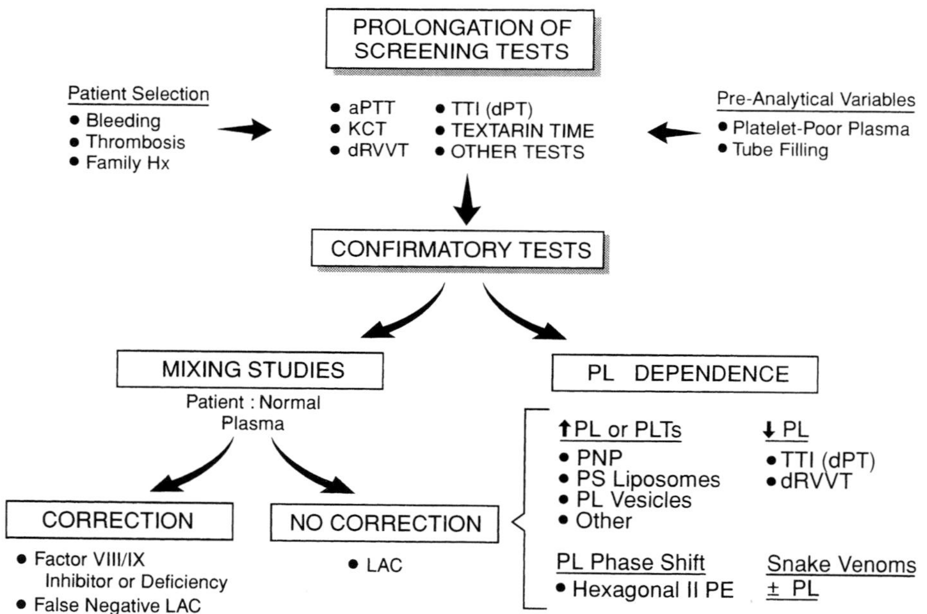

FIGURE 25.3. The laboratory evaluation of circulating anticoagulants, with the main procedures highlighted in *closed boxes* (demonstration of a prolonged screening test, performance of a confirmatory test, usually not the same test as the screen, with mixing studies of patient and normal plasma, and demonstration of phospholipid dependence by one of a variety of means). The presence of a LAC often is determined when the mixing study does not correct to normal, thus separating LAC from coagulation factor inhibitors or deficiencies. Phospholipid dependence is now favored over platelet neutralization procedures.

rule out other coagulation factor disorders that might affect LAC determination, and they should be based on clinical history; (f) heparin presence should be determined by a thrombin time before screening or confirmatory LAC tests if the tests used are sensitive to heparin; (g) concurrent positivity of patient sera for aPL enzyme-linked immunosorbent assay (ELISA) is not considered to be a confirmatory test for the presence of LAC by one method; and (h) the current LAC nomenclature should be retained until a more definitive understanding is available regarding its pathophysiology, although there is universal awareness of the need to consider shedding the "LAC" designation (58). Lastly, the committee has not readdressed the need to consider that some LAC are time dependent, such as factor VIII inhibitors because of the time it takes for factor VIII antigen to dissociate from von Willebrand factor.

Thus, there are many bases from both past (46) and current (57,58) recommendations supporting the premise that even if the screening aPTT is normal, an additional screening test is recommended. Both aPL and aPTT tests appear to be warranted.

Preanalytic Variables

Preparation and handling of patient and normal plasma used for both screening and confirmatory studies (e.g., mixing studies or phospholipid dependence) may be affected by the following: (a) less than 50% filling of the anticoagulated tube with patient blood does not afford the proper dilutionary effect; (b) the type of anticoagulant that is used in the tube may be a source of variation; (c) temperature during processing and handling, as membrane microvesicles might be created during a freeze-thaw cycle, gives an *in situ* PNP and thus a false-negative test result; (d) the pH of the mixture as it changes over incubation time may range from physiologic to 8.2, at which level factor V is likely to be selectively destroyed; (e) the presence of platelets or platelet fragments (which provide a source of factor V, other procoagulants, and platelet factor 4) that decrease the sensitivity of tests using low phospholipid concentrations because they bind aPLs–gentle centrifugation (10 minutes, 5,000 to 10,000*g*) and/or filtration (pore size 0.22 μm) is recommended to avoid platelet fragmentation and release of platelet factors via activation that can augment coagulation or affect von Willebrand factor assays (5,58).

A recent study comparing commercial reagents for the detection of LA using a photo-optical array versus a mechanical coagulometer showed that considerable variation in sensitivity and specificity was noted for the same reagent used on the different analyzers, as well as between reagents. Thus, there remains a need to address optimization of reagents for specific analyzer types.

aPTT Test

The sensitivity of the aPTT varies proportionally with the nature of the commercial reagents, including the activator, and the source, amount, composition, and physical state of the phospholipid. That excess phospholipid shortens the prolonged aPTT because of LAC is the basis for the development of tests on this model, and the aPTT is more sensitive than the PT to the presence of LAC. Phosphatidylserine (PS) concentration and lipid phase (either bilayer or hexagonal phase II conformation) (59), either in the phospholipid in aPTT reagents or the phospholipid in tissue factor reagents, may be operative here. Modifications to increase sensitivity have included using a dilute phospholipid or increasing the dilution of the aPTT reagents (daPTT) (5), but studies have shown that increasing the incubation time rather than the phospholipid concentration may be more important (i.e., dual-incubation aPTT) (58).

That LAC may show time dependency, a feature that previously was relegated to factor deficiency or inhibitor states, has been recently recognized, and extended to include effects related to the pH of the mixture, which varies with time. Addition of 0.05 M HEPES buffer in one study looking at the aPTT over time showed that a stable pH using Platelin as the reagent was achieved (57). Comparative assessments have shown that several reagents (i.e., actin FSL, automated aPTT, and Thrombosil) are sensitive to LAC (60–62). Recent advances such as the Staclot-LA reagent have incorporated a heparin blocker and hexagonal phase II lipids in the incubation mixture for increased specificity, but mechanically this test is more difficult. Some IgM LAC may be missed with this test as well. While rising factor VIII levels have often limited the usefulness of aPTT during pregnancy in prior studies (46,53), Blanco et al. (60) showed that the standard aPTT was more useful during pregnancy than the daPTT. False-positive aPTTs occur with contact factor deficiencies, heparin, factor VII inhibitors, and factor IIX/VIII deficiencies (4).

KCT Test

The KCT test is an aPTT without a platelet lipid source, and the activator is provided by kaolin (clay). Current recommendations state that a 2% suspension in water is a more sensitive text mixture, as sodium chloride hastens the precipitation of kaolin out of suspension. Preparation of PPP is most critical for the KCT (46,53,58). Its sensitivity is intermediate between that of a sensitive aPTT and the dRVVT, and it is considered to be a test with high specificity. The modified KCT is considered to be useful in the detection of low-titer LACs. Like the aPTT, KCT can have false-positive results under the same conditions as noted earlier. Exner (5) has improved its performance with 4:1 dilutions of plasma, and the test now has been automated because of the ability to decrease the kaolin concentration from 12 to less than 1, thus permitting photoelectric quantification. Additionally, in paired samples with KCT and DRVVT (LA Screen, Gradipore, Sydney, Australia), a platelet count of 1×10^9/L will obviate a positive KCT but will not affect the dRVVT results.

dRVVT Test

Developed by Thiagarajan and colleagues, this test is increasingly used worldwide both investigationally and in clinical usage, and it is unique in being a screening as well as a confirmatory test (46,53,58). Sources of both phospholipid and venom may affect the test, and it now can be performed in a single vial. It requires low phospholipid concentrations. The venom activates factor X, bypasses factors VIII, IX, and contact factors, and eliminates some of the poorly understood effects in LAC testing that can either lengthen or shorten the tests. Polybrene or other heparin inhibitors may be added, which will not give false-positive results, but without these additives the dRVVT may yield false positives with patients who have been on heparin. Sensitive reagents include the LA-Confirm and the DRVV-Confirm.

Like the previous two tests, the dRVVT is sensitive to factor VII inhibitors or factor IX/VII deficiencies, but it is prolonged only in very high-titer factor VIII inhibitors. Therefore, in reality, it is the most resistant (6). The dRVVT is useful during pregnancy as it is independent of the naturally occurring increase in some clotting factors, and does not give false-positive results with contact deficiencies. In the most recent recommendations, it is considered to be the next test after an aPTT (58). In our experience with 392 patients followed between 2 and 4 months longitudinally from 1996 to mid-2000, two caveats have emerged: (a) 20% of all patients will only be positive by an LAC test; (b) in paired simultaneously drawn sera/plasma samples, the DRVVT was five times more likely to identify an aPL than the standardized aPTT (McCarty, Indiana APS Database Project, 1996–2000).

TTI (dPT) Test

This test is a dilute PT performed with varying dilutions of tissue factor (TF) or thromboplastin and expressed as a ratio of patient-to-normal PT. A major source of variation is the lack of a standardized normal plasma, which is a common complaint with many of these tests. Because the TTI assesses all three critical phospholipid-dependent coagulation reactions, it seems ideal for a LAC screening test. Like some aPTT variations, however, IgM LAC may be missed. Like the dRVVT, it does not give false-positive results with contact deficiencies, and heparin inhibitors have been added to the reagents to increase the utility of this test. Direct data on use in pregnancy have not been reported, but the test is likely to be useful in pregnancy. Recombinant human TF modifications by Zanon et al. (63) and Arnout et al. (64) are attempts to provide a uniform reagent for the TTI. The TTI due to its use of TF as a reagent may be optimized to more selectively identify anti–β_2-glycoprotein I antibodies, as recent studies have shown that this specific aPL may enhance tissue factor activity on monocytes.

Textarin Time Tests

Venom from *Pseudonaja textilis* and *Echis carinatus* snakes is used in these tests, popularized by Triplett et al. (65), which were developed as a confirmatory test but actually violate the definition of a confirmatory test in that phospholipid is not augmented to demonstrate correction (58). The basis for this test is the difference in the phospholipid requirements of the two venoms. Currently, it is considered to be the most specific test available for LAC, and interest in its development is based on a high specificity for phospholipid effects on the prothrombinase complex. The Textarin time is compared with the Ecarin time here. These tests are resistant to factor inhibitors or deficiencies, except for factor V.

Other LAC Tests

In contrast to the above functional tests, an ELISA using partial thromboplastin derived from human brain as the antigen was developed for detection of LACs (64). This assay circumvents some of the disadvantages of coagulation assays and is highly sensitive and specific. A synthetic reagent called Synthesil in preliminary tests compared well to rabbit thromboplastin. In addition, Schjetlein and Wisloff (66) have developed an integrated test system, adapted for computer analysis, that uses aPTT and dRVVT comparison between normal plasma and a mixing test with high PL. Finally, the plasma clot time (PCT) requires fresh plasma and is unaffected by the presence of platelet membrane fragments in reagent preparations, but is not generally performed (5,6).

Rationale For Confirmatory Tests

The observation that excess phospholipid substantially shortens the prolonged aPTT because of LAC has been exploited to distinguish LAC from other CACs. As shown in Fig. 25.3, the platelet neutralization procedure (PNP) (46,53,58), PS liposomes, and rabbit brain phospholipid are common ways to demonstrate phospholipid dependence. The PNP has been particularly recommended since its inception in the early 1980s as a confirmatory test for aPTT-based tests and the dRVVT. Platelet vesicles are particularly suited for the dRVVT and KCT. Phospholipid dilutions are best matched with the TTI (dPT) and the dRVVT. Hexagonal phase II phospholipid also is used to confirm aPTT results.

Special Cases

Despite appropriate precautions, discrepancies often occur with these tests, and paradoxic results are sometimes the legacy of LAC testing. Several clinical situations may arise to challenge the clinician and the consulting hematologist or laboratory director.

Specific factor inhibitors may cause false-positive results with confirmatory LAC tests. The performance of factor assays using two or more dilutions of patient plasma may be helpful if the clinical history and screening aPTT and PT results are not. LACs often have a dilutional effect on several specific factor activities, whereas specific factor inhibitors are associated with a low level of one factor that does not change with dilution. The LAC can artifactually decrease the values by impairing the reactivity of the PL reagents. One approach is to perform several of the specific, one-stage clotting factor assays based on the aPTT technique (e.g., factors VIII, IX, and XI) (46,57,58).

Strong factor inhibitors may cause dilutional effects on levels of other factors to which they are not directed specifically. Thus, the absence of a dilutional effect is not presumptive evidence that LAC is not present.

High-titer LACs may artifactually appear as a factor deficiency when a sensitive aPTT is used, without the dilutional effect mentioned earlier. In this setting, specific factor antigenic assays should be performed.

The hypoprothrombinemia-LAC syndrome is an important clinical entity because the prothrombin deficiency resulting from this LAC-like antibody that binds to prothrombin *in vivo* may result in significant bleeding. Hypoprothrombinemia might also result from direct-acting anti-PT antibodies. Additionally, binding in immune complexes if active aPL antibodies are proximal is possible. This is the modern correlate of the classic LAC misnomer, although its existence was reported in 1959 by Loeliger (11).Prothrombin-LAC immune complexes cause an artifactual hypoprothrombinemia by their normal removal from the circulation, but prothrombin function in the *in vitro* assays is normal (67). The clinical clue here is the finding of a substantially prolonged PT, beyond the range that is noted for LAC (e.g., 18–20 seconds). Prothrombin antigenic activity is present but the level is decreased and abnormal mobility may be electrophoretically present (68). SLE, viral infections, drugs, and idiopathic etiologies have been associated with the production of this syndrome (69). Prothrombin antibodies have all reacted with epitopes on the carboxy terminal segment of the prothrombin molecule (67). Whether these are distinctive antiprothrombin antibodies or represent part of the antigenic target spectrum of LAC/aPL reactivity with epitopes on prothrombin and anionic phospholipids, however, remains unclear (70).

Summary

The innate heterogeneity of aPLs and the features of APS are mirrored by the necessity to perform several levels of screening and confirmatory testing, and the vagaries of LAC screening and confirmatory tests remain protean despite significant new knowledge regarding multifactorial mechanisms by which aPLs interfere with coagulation. Large meta-analyses are difficult because of the rare performance of simultaneous or longitudinal standardized studies, so summary statements regarding overall sensitivity and specificity remain incorrect and misleading if taken out of the context of the individual test. As has been noted for the EIA-based aPL tests since the publication of the Sapporo criteria, the trend is toward the performance of two tests for LAC (aPTT and DRVVT), coupled with the caveats for addressing preanalytical variables such as sample obtainment and reagent matching for type of analyzer. Appropriate studies regarding the positive predictive values of individual as well as panels of tests are needed. General guidelines have been used to generate Fig. 25.3, and specific caveats regarding individual tests are addressed in Table 25.2.

The update from the Scientific and Standardization Subcommittee (58) supports performing two screening tests (i.e., an aPTT plus another test, such as dRVVT) and further evaluating those tests results either sequentially or concurrently. If both an aPTT and dRVVT are abnormal, a mixing study of patient and normal plasma is done. If the mixing study is abnormal, then progression to demonstration of phospholipid dependence is performed, and if positive, LAC is confirmed. If the initial mixing study corrects to normal, then an incubated mixing study is performed. If the incubated mixing study fails to correct to normal, then the demonstration of phospholipid dependence is next. If it corrects to normal, then specific factor assays are done. Although no specific protocols are as yet agreed on for mixing studies, these tests are relatively easy to perform in most laboratories and may be helpful cost-savers if standards and units for LAC indices or calibrations evolve.

MECHANISMS OF LAC ACTION

A consideration of proven and putative mechanisms of action for LAC supports the contention that they are separable activities from other aPLs in some ways (13) (see Chapter 52). The reader is referred to Fig. 25.3, in which both proven and putative mechanisms of action that are relevant to coagulation components and vascular injury models are indicated by numbered squares. Although there exist murine induction and vascular injury models that produce with some fidelity the major features of APS and a fulfillment (to some extent) of Koch's postulates for their contributions to pathogenicity (see Chapters 27 and 57), the full *in vivo* correlates of these likely mechanisms are still not fully understood. Two reviews (71,72) examined the hypotheses that concepts regarding the relevant antigens should be extended beyond phospholipids only (i.e., the antiphospholipid antibody protein syndromes), and Harris et al. (73) and Koike et al. (74) have parried and rechallenged this topic in interesting exchanges.

PHOSPHOLIPID BINDING

Anionic phospholipid binding initially was demonstrated for an IgM monoclonal LAC (75) and, since then, for sera and plasma samples using affinity purification (76–79). Studies using affinity-purified patient IgGs and improvements in column chromatography of LAC plasma have fostered the reexamination of anionic phospholipid binding. The discovery of 2gpI (discussed below) has prompted this reevaluation, and some data are still under discussion. The presumed form of the phospholipid was a lamellar array but subsequently was shown to be a different phase form changed by calcium and PS. When critically examined, the data for direct cardiolipin binding in the absence of 2gpI or other lipid-protein interactions have been based primarily on the initial IgM monoclonal LAC (75,78,79). Perhaps other anionic phospholipids such as PS will prove to be more important or that the true epitopes represent phospholipid–protein-lipid combinations that are recognized differentially by LAC and aPLs (Fig. 25.2A).

COFACTORS FOR LAC: 2GPI AND PROTHROMBIN

LACs were shown to be chromatographically separable into two different populations using phospholipid liposome preparations (79–83). The identification of 2gpI, a natural anticoagulant (see Chapter 27), as the cofactor responsible for a prolonged PTT or KCT of patient plasma lengthening further with the addition of normal plasma (i.e., the source of $\beta_2$gpI) has allowed the profiling of aPLs into different sets (Table 25.2; Fig. 25.2A). Many aPLs and some LACs also have been shown to require $\beta_2$gpI for binding (82,83). These type A antibodies (Table 25.3) enhance the inhibition of prothrombin conversion by $\beta_2$gpI; thus, the LAC effect in plasma results from enhancement of $\beta_2$gpI binding (80–83). Although this research has opened several new areas of mechanistic consideration, there are still some areas of controversy (71–74,80,84). However, the irony that is intrinsically associated with LACs continues in that although $\beta_2$gpI is a natural anticoagulant, patients who are genetically deficient in $\beta_2$gpI paradoxically do not appear to be at risk for thrombosis (71,72,84).

PROTHROMBINASE COMPLEX AND OTHER PHOSPHOLIPID-DEPENDENT COAGULATION REACTIONS

LACs have been shown to interfere with phospholipid-dependent coagulation reactions in the presence of human plasma (79—83). Three potential sites exist where LAC might bind and shift the balance between an anticoagulant and a procoagulant surface on endothelial cells or platelets (Fig. 25.2B). Because LAC affects all phospholipid-dependent reactions, its site of action is at least at the level of the prothrombinase complex. The inhibition is specific for human, but not for bovine, prothrombin and required phospholipid vesicles (83). Thus, this population of LAC is different from the antiprothrombin LAC described later. The anticoagulant effect of LAC likely results from binding to the phospholipid-bound human prothrombin complex once calcium has also bound. That this reaction could occur on platelet surfaces was shown by the substitution of activated platelets or platelet-derived vesicles as phospholipid sources (79,84,85). An IgM monoclonal LAC was shown to inhibit factor X activation by the intrinsic tenase complex, thus confirming previous direct LAC binding to anionic phospholipids.

Prothrombin binding of LAC and the hypoprothrombinemia-LAC syndrome have been discussed previously.

ENDOTHELIAL CELL/PLATELET-PROTEIN S/PROTEIN C AND THROMBOMODULIN INTERACTIONS

Prostaglandins are major products of endothelial cells and platelets, and their production is important in maintaining the neutrality of a coagulant surface. LACs (and aPLs) have been shown to stimulate prostacyclin release from endothelial cells in both patients with and without thrombosis (71,72,79). Thromboxane A_2 has been shown to inhibit endothelial cell production of procoagulant molecules and thus plays a role via its balance with prostacyclin (PGI_2) (Fig. 25.2A). Once tissue injury occurs, TF on the cell surface, and glycosaminoglycans (GAGs) from the subendothelium may become exposed, and GAGs are important in determining the anticoagulant properties of the endothelial cell surface (Fig. 25.2A,D). Platelets are thought to bind LAC (as well as aPL), but most LACs may require only platelet activation to bind, independently of 2gpI, although some LAC may require the cofactor, as does aPL (84,85). It currently is unclear whether this binding generates procoagulant effects. When thrombin binds to thrombomodulin on the surface of endothelial cells, an anticoagulant milieu is generated, protein C is activated, and, once complexed with protein S, is capable of inhibiting factors Va and VIIIa. Currently, LACs are thought by some investigators to inhibit thrombomodulin-mediated activation of protein C, although this has been questioned (71,72,79,84,86,87) (Fig. 25.2E).

OTHER ANTIPHOSPHOLIPID ANTIBODY ELISA TESTS AND THEIR PHOSPHOLIPID TARGETS

A concensus statement on the preliminary classification criteria for definite antiphospholipid antibody syndrome in 1999 now referred to as the Sapporo Criteria represented the extensive work of an international panel of physician-investigators and laboratory researchers to put forth general guidelines based on the most widely used tests (the IgG/M aCL enzymeimmunoassay (ELISAs) as described in Chapter 55, and one or more LAC tests as detailed in this chapter and meeting specifications in references 55–58) (88). There are some caveats: a) as with most clinical guidelines, the criteria may not be applicable in an individual patient, who may not make these particular antibodies or have only these manifestations of APS; b) that proven thrombotic events were required to be temporally relevant to positive tests, and c) strict exclusions were refined for the diagnosis of APS-related fetal loss (88). Despite the widely known studies since 1990 showing that β2gpI binding to CL forming a neoepitope is the most likely antigenic target of aPLs, β2gp1 positivity is not yet a criterion, as this test is not standardized to the same extent that IgG/M aCL has been and in most reports very low percentages of APS patients exhibit soley this antibody. Despite use of the Harris standards for IgG/M ELISAs in second- and third-generation kits, various commercial and hospital labs use different criteria for the definition of aPL positivity. Some of the variability in aPL assays has been shown to be related to the provision of adequate B2gpI in the diluents in the ELISA tests, which initially used fetal or newborn bovine serum as blocking agents or patient sera diluents (88–91). Most of the negatively charged PLs (CL and PS) require β2gpI as a cofactor. Buffers containing only β2gpI do not detect aPL that are dependent on other PL-binding proteins such as prothrombin or protein C, or those such as aPE that require the low or high molecular weight kininogens (LMWK-HMWK), and are clinically relevant to patients, being associated with the same APS clinical criteria as cited above (91). The incremental value of adding IgA aPS and IgA aPE testing to IgG and IgM aCL ELISA testing in 5632 patients with APS-associated events has been well demonstrated to additionally identify patients who would otherwise be considered "seronegative" and therefore not be identified for treatment by McIntyre et al. (92). IgA isotype testing and β2gp1 testing has been suggested by Harris as the next steps to consider in IgG/M aCL/LAC negative patients with APS symptoms in a recent review; the prevalence of IgA aCL responses may also be related to ethnicity rather than methodology (90). Testing for various aPLs is evolving rapidly, as is the clinical spectrum of APS-related features not yet validated as clinical criteria by Sapporo Criteria, but are being considered for future inclusion by this Committee.

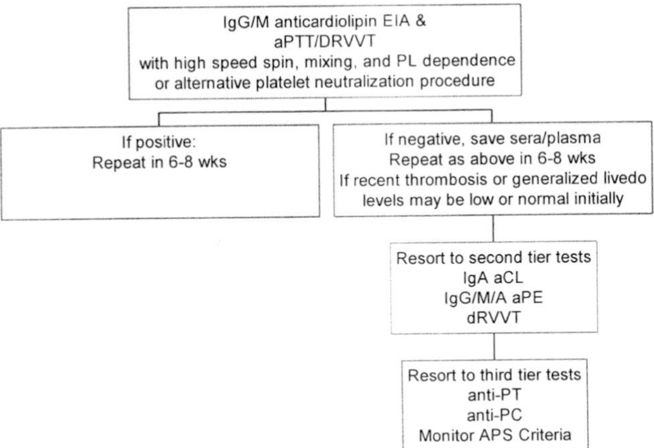

FIGURE 25.4. A proposal for the sequential evaluation of LAC/aPL is presented.

ANIMAL MODELS

Most work on APS has involved the passive or active immunization of purified human IgG aCL or purified PL antigens into non-autoimmune prone or naive mice. aPLs are not exclusively produced by autoimmune mice such as the MRL/lpr and the (NZW x BXSB)F1 strains, but develop in the non-obese diabetic (NOD) mice; several recent reviews address this subject in detail (93,94). Demonstration of thrombocytopenia, autoimmune hemolytic anemia, decreased fertility due to involution of murine pregnancies, and placental thrombotic microangiopathy have been found for CL and PS antibodies by active induction (reviewed in refs. 93 and 94). Active induction studies with β2gpI show decreased fecundity, elevated APTTs, and hemolytic anemia, but no clinical thromboses: some mouse models develop aCL, aPS, aPI (phosphatidylinositol) in response. In most experiments, CL alone is not immunogenic by itself in most of the early studies but the response is enhanced by its cofactor. The spontaneously-developing aPL mice produce functional antibodies but may not faithfully reproduce human pathology-only male (W/B) F1 mice develop arterial thrombosis, and aCL have been detected in mouse strains without clinical APS features. Another approach has been to induce an endothelial cell pinch injury by clamping femoral or cremasteric veins, infuse aCL or other aPLs, and evaluate the kinetics of thrombus formation, size, and platelet content, showing aPLs do induce thrombosis at sites of vascular injury (95).

When immunized with β2gpI, mice made antibodies to this antigen and to aCL; when immunized with human

IgG, murine aCL and anti-human IgG were produced, and mean thrombus area was significantly greater in these groups than controls immunized with human serum albumin. These murine aCLs were thrombogenic analogously to the passively immunized mice in other models, showing thrombogenicity is related to aCL specificity rather than to the source of the aCL. Recently, this group has shown that some human IgG monoclonal aCL and aPS antibodies, and the 15 amino acid sequence GDKV binding site epitope of β2gpI in the pinch model activates endothelium as measured by the upregulation of vascular endothelial cell adhesion molecule 1 (VCAM-1) on cultured endothelia (96). A recent analysis of hybridomas from a (NZW x BXSB) F1 male showed binding to 3 supramolecular complexes of anionic PLs and protein: CL-β2gpI, PS-annexin V, and nucleosomes, and H and L chain analyses showed recurrent H and/or L chain rearrangements (97). That aCL monoclonal antibodies cross react with nucleosomes may explain the frequent coincidence of APS and SLE (secondary APS) and primary APS patients with antinuclear antibodies. These models are important in both pathogenesis and evaluation of treatment modalities for APS.

SUMMARY

Lupus anticoagulants are a heterogeneous set of aPLs with the potential to reflect *in vitro* actions with *in vivo* consequences. Endothelial cell or platelet membrane injury or activation could result in an enhanced procoagulant surface that is permissive for the binding of prothrombin, 2gpI, or protein S and activated protein C to exposed anionic phospholipids. In a manner analogous to the creation of a neoepitope or altered reactivity of other domains of 2gpI, these components then might be recognized as immunogenic and continue to drive the production of LACs/aPLs, which likely are part of the natural repertoire already. This scenario would explain the protean nature of LAC effects, in that the shift to the procoagulant state would then drive phospholipid-dependent coagulation reactions and cause thrombosis. That qualitative and quantitative differences in regional vascular beds exist might be evoked to explain why thrombosis (while sometimes mimetic in site) can range in scope from trivial and localized to catastrophic and generalized. A proposed sequential evaluation flow diagram for LAC/aPL that represents my opinion but not a formal recommendation from any governing body is represented in Fig. 25.4. Although cost containment is important, consideration of the cost of morbidity, and possibly mortality, is balanced only by that which might be prevented by appropriate therapy, also a controversial area (see Chapter 27). Progress in the methodology of LAC testing, with judicious adoption of mixing study protocols as inherent parts of screening tests rather than their current relegation to confirmatory testing, and perhaps continued profiling of LAC/aPL for phospholipid and 2gpI specificities, should contribute to improving studies enough to better address positive predictive values that will help to identify at-risk patients for expectant treatment.

ACKNOWLEDGMENTS

I gratefully acknowledge many colleagues in antiphospholipid antibody research worldwide who again provided critical but thoughtful discussion. The devotion of Drs. Bevra H. Hahn and Daniel J. Wallace to the success of this book is gratefully appreciated. Dana Clerkin, Dahlgren Memorial Library, Georgetown University, and Rose H. Davis, Division of Rheumatology and Immunology, University of Virginia, assisted in online searches. David Klemm, Georgetown University Educational Media, is again thanked for graphic artistry.

REFERENCES

1. Amigo MC, Khamashta MA. Antiphospholipid antibody syndrome in systemic lupus erythematosus. *Rheum Dis Clin North Am* 2000;26:331–348.
2. Harris EN. The antiphospholipid antibody syndrome: diagnosis, management, and pathogenesis. *Clin Rev Allergy Immunol* 1995; 13:39–48.
3. Triplett DA. Use of the dilute Russell Viper Venom time: Its importance and pitfalls. *J Autoimmun* 2000;15:173–178.
4. Triplett DA. The many faces of lupus anticoagulants. *Lupus* 1998;7;S1822.
5. Exner T. Conceptions and misconceptions in testing for lupus anticoagulants. *J Autoimmun* 2000;16:179–184.
6. Horrelou MH, Samama MM. Detection of lupus anticoagulants. *Clin Rev Allergy Immunol* 1995;13:1924.
7. Conley CL, Rathbun HK, Morse, WI, et al. Circulating anticoagulant as a cause of hemorrhagic diathesis in man. *Bull Johns Hopkins Hosp* 1948;83:288–296.
8. Conley CL, Hartmann RC. A haemorrhagic disorder caused by circulating anticoagulant in patients with disseminated lupus erythematosus. *J Clin Invest* 1952;31:621–622.
9. Beaumont JL. Syndrome hemorrhagique acquis du a un anticoagulant circulant. *Sangre* 1954;25:115.
10. Laurell AB, Nilsson IM. Hypergammaglobulinaemia, circulating anticoagulant and biologic false positive Wasserman reaction: a study of two cases. *J Lab Clin Med* 1957;49:694–707.
11. Loeliger EA. Prothrombin as cofactor of the circulating anticoagulant in systemic lupus erythematosus. *Thromb Diath Haemorrh* 1959;3:237–256.
12. Bowie EJW, Thompson JH, Pascuzzi CA, et al. Thrombosis in systemic lupus erythematosus despite circulating anticoagulants. *J Clin Invest* 1963;62:416–430.
13. Yin ET, Gaston LW. Purification and kinetic studies on a circulating anticoagulant in a suspected case of systemic lupus erythematosus. *Thromb Diath Haemorrh* 1965;14:88–114.
14. Feinstein DE, Rapaport SI. Acquired inhibitors of blood coagulation. *Prog Hemost Thromb* 1972;1:75–95.
15. Feltkamp JJ, Kerkhoven P, Loeliger EA. Circulating anticoagulant in systemic lupus erythematosus. *Thromb Haemost* 1974;2: 253–259.

16. Schleider MA, Nachman RL, Jaffe EA, et al. A clinical study of the lupus anticoagulant. *Blood* 1976;48:499–509.
17. Exner T, Richard KA, Kronenberg H. A sensitive test demonstrating lupus anticoagulant and its behavioural patterns. *Br J Haematol* 1978;40:143–151.
18. Soulier JP, Boffa MC. Avortements à repetition, thromboses, et anticoagulant circulant anti-thromboplastin. *Nouv Presse Med* 1980;9:859–864.
19. Triplett DA, Brandt JT, Kaczor D, et al. Laboratory diagnosis of lupus inhibition: a comparison of the tissue thromboplastin inhibition procedure with a new platelet neutralization procedure. *Am J Clin Pathol* 1983;79:678–682.
20. Boey ML, Colaco CB, Gharavi AE, et al. Thrombosis in systemic lupus erythematosus: striking association with the presence of circulating lupus anticoagulant. *Br Med J* 1983;287:1021–1023.
21. Lockshin MD, Sammaritano LR, Schwartzman S. Validation of the Sapporo Criteria for antiphospholipid antibody syndrome. *Arthritis Rheum* 2000;43:430–43.
22. Calaco CB, Elkon KB. The lupus anticoagulant. *Arthritis Rheum* 1985;28:67–74.
23. Shapiro SS, Thiagarajan P. Lupus anticoagulants. *Prog Hemostat Thromb* 1982;6:263–285.
24. Derue G, Englert H, Harris EN, et al. Fetal loss in systemic lupus: association with anticardiolipin antibodies. *J Obstet Gynaecol Neonatal Nurs* 1985;2:207–209.
25. Davis S, Furie BC, Griffin JH, et al. Circulating inhibitors of blood coagulation associated with procainamide-induced lupus erythematosus. *Am J Hematol* 1978;4:401–407.
26. Baer AN, Woosley RL, Pincus T. Further evidence for the lack of association between acetylator phenotype and systemic lupus erythematosus. *Arthritis Rheum* 1986;29:843–850.
27. Zarrabi MH, Zucker S, Miller F, et al. Immunologic and coagulation disorders in chlorpromazine-treated patients. *Ann Intern Med* 1979;91:194–199.
28. Green D, Lechner K. A survey on 215 non-haemophilic patients with inhibitors to factor VIII. *Thromb Haemost* 1981;45: 200–203.
29. Triplett DA, Brandt JA, Maas RL. The laboratory heterogeneity of lupus anticoagulants. *Arch Pathol Lab Med* 1985;109:946–951.
30. Kunkel LA. Acquired circulating anticoagulants. *Hematol Oncol Clin North Am* 1992;8:1341–1357.
31. Echaniz-Laguna A, Thiriaux A, Ruolt-Olivesi I, et al. Lupus anticoagulant induced by the combination of valproate and lamotrigine. *Epilepsia* 1999;40:161–163.
32. Brodeur GM, O'Neill PJ, Williams JA. Acquired inhibitors of coagulation in nonhemophiliac children. *J Pediatr* 1980;96: 439–443.
33. Canoso RT, Zon LT, Groopman JE. Anticardiolipin antibodies associated with HTLV-III infection. *Br J Haematol* 1987;65: 495–497.
34. Cohen AJ, Philips TM, Kessler CM. Circulating coagulation inhibitors in the acquired immunodeficiency syndrome. *Ann Intern Med* 1986;104:175–180.
35. Simone JV, Cornet JA, Abildagaard CF. Acquired von Willebrand's syndrome in systemic lupus erythematosus. *Blood* 1968; 31:803–812.
36. Robbey SJ, Lewis EJ, Schur PJ, et al. Circulating anticoagulants to factor VIII. *Am J Med* 1957;49:575–579.
37. Feinstein DI, Francis RB. The lupus anticoagulant and anticardiolipin antibodies. In: Hahn BH, Wallace DJ, eds. *Dubois' lupus erythematosus*, 4th ed. Philadelphia: Lea & Febiger, 1993:246–268.
38. Thompson AR. Structure, function, and molecular defects of factor IX. *Blood* 1986;67:655–709.
39. Feinstein DI, Rapaport SI. Lupus anticoagulant and other hemostatic problems. In: Wallace DJ, Dubois EL, eds. *Lupus erythematosus*. Philadelphia: Lea & Febiger, 1987:271.
40. McNeil HP, Chesterman CN, Krilis SA. Immunology and clinical importance of antiphospholipid antibodies. *Adv Immunol* 1994;49:193–280.
41. Reyes, H, Dearing L, Bick RL, et al. Laboratory diagnosis of antiphospholipid antibodies. *Clin Lab Med* 1995;15:63–84.
42. Triplett DA. Antiphospholipid antibodies: laboratory detection and clinical relevance. *Thromb Res* 1995;78:131.
43. Lupus Anticoagulant Working Party. Guidelines on testing for the lupus anticoagulant. *J Clin Pathol* 1991;44:885–889.
44. Petri M. Diagnosis of antiphospholipid antibodies. *Rheum Clin North Am* 1994;20:443–469.
45. Haemostasis Committee of the Societe Francaise de Biologie Clinique. Laboratory heterogeneity of the lupus anticoagulant, a multicentre study using different clotting assays on a panel of 78 samples. *Thromb Res* 1992;66:349–364.
46. Forastiero RR, Cerrato GS, Carreras LO. Evaluation of recently described tests for detection of lupus anticoagulants. *Thromb Haemost* 1994;72:728–733.
47. Fligelstone II, Cachia PG, Ralis H, et al. Lupus anticoagulant in patients with peripheral vascular disease: a prospective study. *Eur J Vasc Endovasc Surg* 1995;9:277–283.
48. Zanon E, Saracino MA, Simioni P, et al. Prevalence of antiphospholipid antibodies and lupus anticoagulant in juvenile patients with objectively documented deep vein thrombosis. *Clin Appl Thromb Hemost* 1996;2:69–73.
49. Rai RS, Regan L, Clifford K, et al. Antiphospholipid antibodies and beta2-glycoprotein I in 500 women with recurrent miscarriage-results of a comprehensive screening approach. *Hum Reprod* 1995;10:200–212.
50. Davie EW, Ratnoff OD. Waterfall sequence for intrinsic blood clotting. *Science* 1964;145:1310–1312.
51. Luchtman-Jones L, Broze GJ. The current status of coagulation. *Ann Med* 1995;27:45–52.

51a. Rand JH. Antiphospholipid antibody-mediated disruption of the anrexin-V antithrombotic shield: a thrombogenic mechanism for the antiphospholipid syndrome. *J Autoimmun* 2000;15: 107–111.

52. Comfurious P, Seden JMG, Tilly RHJ, et al. Loss of membrane phospholipid asymmetry in platelets and red cells may be associated with calcium-induced shedding of plasma membrane and inhibition of aminophospholipid translocase. *Biochim Biophys Acta* 1990;1026:153–160.
53. Hemker HC, Hamulyak K, Kessels H. Hemostasis and thrombosis. In: Noe DA, Rock RC, eds. *Laboratory medicine: the selection and interpretation of laboratory studies*. Philadelphia: Williams & Wilkins, 1993:236–253.
54. Mannucci PM, Canciani MT, Mari D, et al. The variable sensitivity of partial thromboplastin and prothrombin time reagents in the demonstration of lupus-like anticoagulants. *Scand J Haematol* 1979;22:423–432.
55. Exner T. Conceptions and misconceptions in testing for lupus anticoagulants. *J Autoimmun* 2000;15:179–183.
56. Kaczor DA, Bickford NM, Triplett DA. Evaluation of different mixing study reagents and dilution effect in lupus anticoagulant testing. *Am J Clin Pathol* 1991;95:408–411.
57. Exner T, Triplett DA, Taberner D, et al. Guidelines for testing and revised criteria for lupus anticoagulants. *Thromb Haemost* 1991;65:320–325.
58. Brandt JT, Triplett DA, Alving B, et al. Scientific and Standardization Committee Communications: criteria for the diagnosis of lupus anticoagulants-an update. *Thromb Haemost* 1995;74: 1185–1190.

58a. Rauch J, Subang R, D'Agrillo P, et al. Apoptosis and the antiphospholipid syndrome. *J Autoimmun* 200-;15:231–235.

59. Narayanan S. Preanalytical aspects of coagulation testing. *Haematologica* 1995;80(suppl to no. 2):16.

60. Blanco AN, Grand BE, Pieroni G, et al. Behavior of diluted activated partial thromboplastin time in pregnant women with a lupus anticoagulant. *Am J Clin Pathol* 1993;100:99–102.
61. Stevenson KJ, Easton AC, Curry A, et al. The reliability of activated partial thromboplastin time methods and the relationship to lipid composition and ultrastructure. *Thromb Haemost* 1986; 55:250–258.
62. Kelsey PR, Stevenson KJ, Poller L. The diagnosis of lupus anticoagulants by the activated partial thromboplastin time-the central role of phosphatidyl serine. *Thromb Haemost* 1984;52172–175.
63. Zanon E, Simion P, Saracina MA, et al. Recombinant thromboplastin (Innovin) inhibition assay for detection of lupus anticoagulants. *Thromb Haemost* 1993;69:12–20(abst).
64. Arnout J, Vanrusselt M, Huybrachts E, et al. Optimization of the dilute prothrombin time for the detection of the lupus anticoagulant by use of a recombinant human tissue thromboplastin. *Thromb Haemost* 1993;69:12–22(abst).
65. Triplett DA, Stocker KF, Unger GA, et al. The Textarin/Ecarin ratio: a confirmatory test for lupus anticoagulants. *Thromb Haemost* 1993;70:925–931.
66. Schjetlein R, Wisloff F. An evaluation of two commercial test procedures for the detection of lupus anticoagulants. *Am J Clin Pathol* 1993;103:108–111.
67. Rapaport SI, Ames SB, Duvall BJ. A plasma coagulation defect in systemic lupus erythematosus arising from hypoprothrombinemia combined with antiprothrombinase activity. *Blood* 1960;15:212–227.
68. Fleck RA, Rapaport SI, Rao VM. Antiprothrombin antibodies and the lupus anticoagulant. *Blood* 1988;72:512–519.
69. Erkan D, Bateman H, Lockshin MD. Lupus anticoagulant-hypoprothrombinemia syndrome associated with systemic lupus erythematosus: report of 2 cases and review of the literature. *Lupus* 1999;8:5604.
70. Bajaj SP, Rapaport SI, Fierer DS, et al. A mechanism for the hypoprothrombinemia-lupus anticoagulant syndrome. *Blood* 1983;61:684–692.
71. Roubey RAS. Autoantibodies to phospholipid-binding plasma proteins: a new view of lupus anticoagulants and other antiphospholipid antibodies. *Blood* 1994;84:2854–2867.
72. Cines DB, McCrae KR. The antiphospholipid-protein syndrome. *J Clin Immunol* 1995:15(suppl 1):86S–100S.
73. Harris EN, Pierangeli S, Gharavi A, et al. Phospholipid binding antibodies warrant continued investigation. *Blood* 1995;85: 2276–2277.
74. Koike T, Tsusumi A, Ichikawa K, et al. Antigenic specificity of the anticardiolipin antibodies. *Blood* 1995;85:2277–2278.
75. Thiagarajan P, Shapiro SS, De Marco L. Monoclonal immunoglobulin M inhibitor with phospholipid specificity: mechanism of a lupus anticoagulant. *J Clin Invest* 1980;66:397–405.
76. Pierangeli S, Harris EN, Gharavi AE, et al. Are immunoglobulins with lupus anticoagulant activity specific for phospholipids? *Br J Haematol* 1993;85:124–132.
77. Pengo V, Biasolo A. Purification of anticardiolipin and lupus anticoagulant activities by using cardiolipin immobilized on agarose beads. *Thromb Res* 1993;72:423–430.
78. Goldsmith GH, Pierangeli SS, Branch DW, et al. Inhibition of prothrombin activation by antiphospholipid antibodies and 2gpI. *Br J Haematol* 1996;92:435–441.
79. Harris EN. Anticardiolipin antibodies: specificity and function. *Lupus* 1994;3:217–222.
80. Matsuura E, Igarashi Y, Fujimoto M. Anticardiolipin cofactor(s) and differential diagnosis of autoimmune disease. *Lancet* 1990; 336:177–178.
81. McNeil HP, Simpson RJ, Chesterman CN, et al. Anti-phospholipid antibodies are directed against a complex antigen that includes a lipid-binding inhibitor of coagulation: 2-glycoprotein I (apolipoprotein H). *Proc Natl Acad Sci USA* 1990;87:4120–4124.
82. Bevers EM, Galli M, Barbui, et al. Lupus anticoagulant immunoglobulins are not directed to phospholipids only but to a complex of lipid-bound human prothrombin. *Thromb Haemost* 1991;66: 629–632.
83. Galli M, Bevers EM. Inhibition of phospholipid-dependent coagulation reactions by antiphospholipid antibodies-possible mechanisms of action. *Lupus* 1994;3:223–228.
84. Hunt JE, Adelstein S, Krilis SA. New basic aspects of the antiphospholipid antibody syndrome. *Clin Exp Rheumatol* 1994;12: 661–668.
85. Shi W, Chong BH, Hogg PJ, et al. Anticardiolipin antibodies block the inhibition by 2gpI of the factor Xa generating activity. *Thromb Haemost* 1993;48:499–509.
86. Oosting JD, Deerksen RHWM, Bobbink IWG, et al. Antiphospholipid antibodies directed against a combination of phospholipids with prothrombin, protein C or protein S: an explanation for their pathogenetic mechanisms. *Blood* 1993;81:2618–2625.
87. de Groot PG, Derksen RHWM. Protein C pathway, antiphospholipid antibodies, and thrombosis. *Lupus* 1994;3:229–233.
88. Wilson WA, et al. International concensus statement on preliminary classification criteria for definite antiphospholipid antibody syndrome. *Arthritis Rheum* 1999;42:1309–1311.
89. Pierangeli SS, Harris EN. Advances in antiphospholipid antibody testing. *Clinical and Applied Immunology Reviews* 2000;1:59–72.
90. Harris EN, Pierangeli SS. 'Equivocal' antiphospholipid antibody syndrome. *J Autoimmunity* 2000;15:81–85.
91. McIntyre JA, Wagenknecht DR. Antiphosphatidylethanolamine antibodies. *J Autoimmunity* 2000;15:185–193.
92. McIntyre JA, Wagenknecht DR. Antiphospholipid antibodies-risk assessments for solid organ, bone marrow, and tissue transplantation. *Rheum Clin N Am* 2001:3:900–921.
93. Radway-Bright EL, Isenberg DA. Animal models of the antiphospholipid antibody syndrome. *Rheumatology (Oxford)* 1999; 38:591–601.
94. Sherer Y, Shoenfeld Y. Antiphospholipid antibody syndrome: insights from animal models. *Current Opinion Hematol* 2000; 7:321–214.
95. Piergangeli SS, Harris EN. Functional analyses of patient-derived IgG monoclonal anticardiolipin antibodies using in vivo thrombosis and in vivo microcirculation models. *Thromb Haemost* 2000;84:388–395.
96. Gharavi AE, Pierangeli SS, Colden-Stanfield M, et al. GDKV-induced antiphospholipid antibodies enhance thrombosis and activate endothelial cells in vivo and in vitro. *J Immunol* 1999;163:2922–2927.
97. Gilbert D, Lopez B, Parain J, et al: Overlap of the anticardiolipin and antinucleosome responses of the (NZWxBXSB)F1 mouse strain: a new pattern of cross-reactivity for lupus-related autoantibodies. *Eur J Immuno*l 2000:30:3271–3280.

26

AUTOANTIBODIES, AUTOANTIGENS, AND NERVOUS SYSTEM

PATRICIA M. MOORE

Autoantibody formation is a *sine qua non* in systemic lupus erythematosus (SLE). Specific autoantibodies may be pathogenic, markers of disease, or neither. Some antibodies have a "housekeeping function" and likely participate in feedback immunoregulation. Recently, there are suggestions that antibodies may participate in tissue repair. When antibodies are pathogenic, they may exert these effects in several ways. In the cutaneous and renal manifestations of SLE, most pathogenic autoantibodies exert their effects by immune-complex formation with subsequent recruitment of an inflammatory cascade. Direct effects of antibody binding to cognate antigen are well described in the hematologic abnormalities of SLE (1, 2).

In neurologic disorders, autoantibodies participate in disease processes at several levels of the neuraxis. The myoneural junction, peripheral nerves, autonomic nerves, nerve roots, spinal cord, brainstem, basal ganglia, cerebellum, limbic system, and cortex are all regions implicated in autoantibody-associated dysfunction. In some situations, the data do reveal a pathogenic role for antibodies and the mechanisms of the antibody-mediated damage is well explored. In other cases there is evidence for a specific, well-defined population of antibodies that are markers for disease although mechanisms for immunopathogenicity are not defined. More recently, we detect antibodies to products of cells within the nervous system, such as cytokines and growth factors; this opens new areas of experimental design in determining how to detect potential changes in function from these antibodies (3).

The neurologic consequences of antibodies in SLE have remained an intriguing but largely unsubstantiated topic (4). In other neurologic diseases, autoantibody-mediated neurologic dysfunction is well delineated, clearly associated with specific disorders, or of uncertain relevance. The clearest progress has been in those diseases that have fulfilled standard criteria as shown in Table 26.1.

Most clearly defined among the antibody-mediated neurologic disorders are those where the autoantibody binds to and alters the function of a specific ion channel or receptor (5). Other more indirect mechanisms of antibody-mediated neurologic disease occur but whether these changes also occur with spontaneously occurring autoantibodies in autoimmune disease is not clear.

To begin the review and analysis of the autoantibodies in neuropsychiatric-SLE (NP-SLE), we first will mention some of the unique aspects of the interactions between the nervous and immune systems; we then will examine how roles for antibodies have been established in other neurologic disorders.

The mechanisms of neurologic injury are complex because of (i) the enormous intricacies of the nervous system, which actively consists of many subsystems interacting on several different levels, (ii) the extensive array of molecules including neurotransmitters, hormones, and cytokines that affect targets within the nervous system distal from their stimulus, (iii) adaptive responses of the nervous system, and (iv) relatively few final common pathways that result in specific neuronal injury.

Some diverse manifestations of NP-SLE could share common mechanisms of injury. Excitatory amino-acid (EAA) toxicity is an example of this process, which is unique to the nervous system (6). Glutamate, the principal excitatory neurotransmitter in the brain, mediates many normal neurologic functions. However, overstimulation of the glutamate receptors initiates an excessive influx of calcium into neurons and mediates specific cell damage. Whether the cell recovers or dies depends on many processes including location of injury and other molecules present in the local *milieu.* Notably, glucocorticoids either endogenously increased through stress or pharmacologically administered, increase the damage in this process (7). There are many pathologic abnormalities including seizures, stroke, toxins, and degenerative processes that utilize EAA-mediated cell death. Proving that a specific event is responsible for a change in neurologic function is a daunting task.

Within the central nervous system (CNS) there are several ways that antibodies could affect neuronal function. Direct binding to a cognate antigen that controls an ion

TABLE 26.1. A CRITERIA FOR ESTABLISHED AUTOANTIBODIES THAT CAUSE CLINICAL DISEASE

1. Correlate autoantibodies with specific clinical abnormalities.
2. Determine that the antibodies are present in the target tissue, within the CNS.
3. Define the fine specificities of the autoantigen.
4. Determine an effect of the antibodies of the target tissue *in vitro* and *in vivo*.

CNS, central nervous system.

channel or receptor is certainly the simplest model to define a role for the antibody. However in the nervous system, antibodies may also mediate damage through immune-complex deposition with subsequent inflammation, and by effects on the vasculature or coagulation pathways, which subsequently cause tissue ischemia and loss of neurons. Further complicating the investigation of autoantibody-induced changes in CNS function is the presence of a least one indirect pathway affecting both neurologic function and immunoregulation; this is through modulation of the hypothalamic-pituitary-adrenal (HPA) axis and hypothalamic-sympathetic pathways. There is evidence that generalized, systemic-immune activation resulting from large autoantibody loads in SLE is a stressor and stimulates the HPA axis (8). Acutely, this is a normal mechanism to minimize the damaging effects of inflammation. However, chronic activation of the HPA axis has neurologic side effects that are evident in well-studied diseases including posttraumatic stress disorder. Because a critical component of the neurophysiology is the consequence of glucocorticoid binding to high- and low-affinity receptors in the brain, the short- and long-term consequences of receptor regulation is important for life-long disorders (9). Brain structures bearing the brunt of injury in chronic stress are the hippocampus and amygdala and their connections. Clinical features of chronic stress include abnormalities such as anxiety, memory loss, and behavior disturbances; their similarities with features of SLE are noteworthy.

A variety of mechanisms are proposed as potential causes of involvement of the nervous system in SLE. Certainly strokes, including both large-vessel and microvasculature diseases, occur but they do not explain the majority of abnormalities in the nervous system in patients with SLE (10). The paucity of cell loss and tissue destruction evident in the brains of patients with SLE diminishes the likelihood of a cytotoxic process. The prominence of cognitive, emotional, and behavioral abnormalities as well as the movement disorders and ataxias suggest that functional changes in regions or systems within the CNS happen. In other diseases, we have models of hormonal, cytokine, and antibody-mediated changes in function. Any of these can affect the frontal cortices, limbic system, and hypothalamus, as receptors for a variety of hormones and cytokines are present (11). However, the focus of this chapter is antibody-mediated changes in neurologic function. Prior to reviewing studies of antibodies reactive with brain tissue in SLE, it is useful to examine studies of other potentially antibody-neurologic disorders.

IMMUNE FEATURES OF THE CNS

Inflammation occurs far less frequently in the CNS than in many other tissues. This is attributed to a relative immune privilege of the CNS, which means that under normal circumstances the CNS parenchyma has limited exposure to immune-effector cells. This relative immune privilege of the CNS exists because of (i) the blood-brain and blood-cerebrospinal fluid (CSF) barriers, (ii) low levels of class I and II antigens expressed on neurons and glia, (iii) reduced lymphocyte trafficking within the CNS, and (iv) production of immunosuppressant cytokines (i.e., TGF-β) by glial cells. Consequences of this include the rarity of neutrophils within the CNS, a usual IgG partition between the serum and CSF at a ratio of about 1000:1 when the blood-brain barrier (BBB) is intact, and a decreased response to foreign tissue within the CNS.

However, the CNS and immune systems actually interact closely. Two aspects are worth mentioning. Lymphocytes and other immune cells do normally traffic into the CNS and the CNS has a huge modifying effect on the immune system largely through neuro-hormones. T lymphocytes, activated in the tissue of the immune system, routinely cross through the BBB into the parenchyma (12). There they either encounter an antigen or they depart. In their egress it is thought that they return to the circulation, although an apoptotic mechanism cannot be excluded yet. B lymphocytes also traffic into the CNS and if they encounter their antigen, they arrest their migration, expand, and mature into plasma cells secreting antibodies to their antigen. This is the mechanism for the CSF oligoclonal bands seen in numerous infectious and inflammatory diseases. It is not clear if T cells in the CNS are necessary for the final differentiation of B cells to occur.

In an animal model, the intrathecal antibody Ab response to antigen introduced into the normal brain develops beginning at day 14. If the animals are preimmunized systemically with the antigen prior to the intraparenchymal antigen dose, the intrathecal antibody response is even faster, by postimmunization day 5. Isoelectric focusing of CSF reveals banding patterns consistent with local Ab production. Immunohistochemic studies at the infusion site assessed Ag-specific B cells, T cells, plasma cells, and activated antigen-presenting cells (APCs) (13).

Critical features of the afferent side of brain-immune interaction appears in (i) cells in the periventricular structures and areas postrema that detect immune activation secretion of cytokines, (ii) vagal afferents from the abdomen to the brainstem, and (iii) glucocorticoid receptors (GR) and mineralocorticoid receptors (MR) in the hippocampus, cingulated, and other forebrain structures that respond to levels of circulating glucocorticoids. CNS modulation of the immune system occurs through the powerful effects of the HPA axis and the hypothalamic-sympathetic responses. Intermediaries in these effector pathways are cytokines particularly IL-1 and IL-6, prostaglandins, neurotransmitters including serotonin, and hormones including prolactin. Chronic activation of these pathways can lead to damage of regulatory cells (particularly in the hippocampus) that may affect normal neurologic function and as well immune regulation.

AUTOANTIBODIES AND THE MYONEURAL JUNCTION

Myasthenia Gravis

The best-studied example of an antibody-mediated neurologic disorder is that of myasthenia gravis, a disease characterized by particular patterns of muscular weakness and fatigability. Autoimmune myasthenia gravis (MG) is a B cell–mediated disease in which the target autoantigen is the acetylcholine receptor (AChR) at the neuromuscular junction (14). The AChR is an oligomeric membrane protein made up of homologous $\alpha_2\beta\gamma\delta$ chains arranged around a central ion pore. In normal muscle, the nerve action potential leads to release of acetylcholine (ACh) from the motor-nerve ending, and binding of ACh to the AChR on the postsynaptic membrane induces a depolarization, the end-plate potential (15).

Autoantibodies to several regions of the AChR appear with the majority being to native rather than denatured molecule. Most of the determinants are on the (α subunit, although individual MG patients have antibodies to varying immunodominant antigenic regions. Patients do respond to multiple determinants and epitope-spreading occurs (16).

The effects of the AChR-specific B cells, T cells, and systemically circulating antibody are delineated *in vivo* and *in vitro*. Further, the effects of antibodies *in vitro* are delineated. In MG and the animal model, experimental allergic encephalomyelitis (EAMG), investigators have identified three major effector mechanisms by which anti-AChR antibodies appear to induce altered neuromuscular transmission. The first mechanism involves anti-AChR antibodies binding to or near the pharmacologically active binding site and functioning as inhibitors (competitive or noncompetitive) of ACh binding, thereby blocking neuromuscular function. The second mechanism, referred to as AChR modulation, is a consequence of the bivalent nature of the F(ab′)2 portion of the antibody molecule. Antibody molecules, at conditions of antigen excess, are able to cross-link adjacent AChR molecules in the muscle end-plate membrane. The cross-linking has been demonstrated to increase the rate of AChR turnover in the membrane, resulting in a lowered steady-state concentration of AChR. The third mechanism involves antibody binding with subsequent complement fixation leading to end-plate membrane lysis (17). In chronic human MG, this last mechanism may play a predominant role. Antibody-mediated pathology at the postsynaptic muscle membrane leads to deficits in neuromuscular transmission and progressive weakness. The process can be reproduced in experimental animals by both immunization with the antigen and passive transfer of antibodies (18–20).

Treatment of the diseases centers on the autoimmune aspects with focus on removing an associated cause by thymectomy, plasmapheresis, corticosteroids, and intravenous immunoglobulin helpful in many of the patients.

The depth of understanding the immunopathogenic processes in myasthenia can be attributed to careful investigator observations, accessible neuroanatomic target that permitted study of physiologic changes in function *in vivo*, and the existence of naturally occurring ligands that bound to the target. In no other potential antibody-mediated neurologic disorder are so many of the steps detailing pathogenicity available.

Lambert-Eaton Myasthenic Syndrome

Lambert-Eaton myasthenic syndrome (LEMS) is an autoimmune disease of neuromuscular transmission in which antibodies directed against voltage-gated calcium channels (VGCCs) in the motor nerves play a central role in causing a deficient quantal release of acetylcholine (21). LEMS is clinically associated with fatigable muscle weakness, loss of tendon reflexes, and autonomic dysfunction. Electrophysiologic and biochemical studies indicate that the somatic symptoms are caused by a reduction in the evoked release of acetylcholine from motor nerve terminals (22). Multiple VGCC types have been generally classified as L, N, P/Q, R, and T according to their electrophysiologic and pharmacologic properties. A majority of LEMS patients carry the specific antibody against the P/Q-type VGCC receptor (23–25). Experimentally, these antibodies bind to and induce a down-regulation of VGCCs, resulting in a reduction in the nerve-evoked, Ca2+-dependent release of acetylcholine from motor nerve terminals *in vitro*. *In vivo* support for this comes from morphologic studies demonstrating a disorganization and decrease in number of nerve-terminal active zones (believed to be the VGCCs) at the skeletal neuromuscular junction in human tissue and in tissue from mice injected with LEMS IgG. It also is possible to transfer the electrophysiologic abnormalities to mice by injecting them with purified IgG from LEMS patients (26, 27).

Approximately 60% of patients have an associated small-cell lung carcinoma (SCLC), a tumor that is thought to be neuroendocrine in origin. This strong association with cancer makes LEMS a member of the group of paraneoplastic disorders. Calcium flux measured using Ca2+, and whole-cell calcium currents measured by patch clamping, are reduced in several cell types including SCLC tumor cells when exposed to LEMS IgG, and tumor VGCCs appear to provoke the antibody response in SCLC-associated LEMS (28).

The motor end plate is not the only target of these autoantibodies. LEMS patients have clinically prominent autonomic nervous system abnormalities, which also may be from the autoantibodies. IgG from LEMS patients inhibit one or more components of transmitter release from both parasympathetic and sympathetic neurons. Thus, it appears that antibodies to the P/Q-type VGCC also regulate the transmitter release from parasympathetic nerves. However, there also is evidence that the nature of the calcium channels down regulated by the LEMS IgG vary from patient to patient so there may be individual mechanisms for the weakness (5, 29).

Further evidence that LEMS is autoantibody-mediated includes the clinical response to plasma exchange and to immunosuppressive drug treatment although the underlying disease remains the determinant of recovery.

ANTIBODIES TO THE AUTONOMIC NERVOUS SYSTEM

Dysfunction of the nervous system is prominent in many neurologic disorders of both the central and peripheral nervous systems. Idiopathic autonomic neuropathy is a severe, subacute disorder with prominent symptoms of orthostatic hypotension, gastrointestinal dysmotility, and abnormal pupillary responses to light and accommodation. In both the postviral and paraneoplastic forms of this disorder, there is a presumed autoimmune basis (30–32). It is clinically indistinguishable from the subacute autonomic neuropathies that may accompany lung cancer or other tumors and certain degenerative diseases. Nonetheless, in some patients autoantibodies specific for nicotinic acetylcholine receptors in the autonomic ganglia occur as serologic markers of a form of autoimmune autonomic neuropathy and potentially are pathogenic.

Ganglionic receptor-binding antibodies were found in 19 of 46 patients with idiopathic or paraneoplastic autonomic neuropathy (41%), in 6 of 67 patients with postural tachycardia syndrome, idiopathic gastrointestinal dysmotility, or diabetic autonomic neuropathy (9%), and in none of 44 patients with other autonomic disorders. High levels of the binding antibodies correlated with more severe autonomic dysfunction (including the presence of tonic pupils). There is some evidence that these antibodies have specific binding or blocking actions at the ganglionic receptor although the specific mechanisms of these effects are not delineated (33).

There is a correlation of these antibodies with clinical effects. High levels of ganglionic receptor-binding antibody correlated significantly with the severity of autonomic dysfunction, and the level of such antibodies decreased or became undetectable with improvement of autonomic function. These findings suggest that the autoantibodies contribute to the pathogenesis of subacute autonomic failure.

There is yet no animal model of dysfunction associated with these antibodies.

ANTIBODIES TO CENTRAL NERVOUS SYSTEM ANTIGENS

A plethora of antibodies to CNS targets are described in a variety of disorders including Alzheimer's, Huntington's and Parkinson's diseases. In none of these diseases is a disease mechanism defined so it appears that the antibodies could be an epi-phenomenon or housekeeping antibodies (34–36). However, several disorders do indicate a strong link between autoantibody, antigen, and clinical disorder. An intriguing one is the disturbance of rapid eye movement (REM) sleep associated with antibodies to the locus ceruleus (37).

Paraneoplastic Syndromes

A strong association between antibodies and specific antigens occurs in the paraneoplastic syndromes. These syndromes have been defined both on the basis of the neurologic abnormalities and of their target antigens, which have been defined regionally within the CNS and in the tumor tissue (38–40). The more frequently encountered autoantigens are shown in Table 26.2. A large proportion of patients with paraneoplastic disorders can be grouped into an entity known as paraneoplastic encephalomyelitis (PEM). Nearly all patients display signs and symptoms of multifocal

TABLE 26.2. AUTOANTIBODIES AND THE PARANEOPLASTIC SYNDROMES

Antibody	Clinical Syndrome	Associated Tumor	Immunocytochemical Pattern
Anti-Hu (ANNA-1)	Encephalomyelitis, sensory neuronopathy	Small cell lung	Pan neuronal
Anti-Ri (ANNA-2)	Opsoclonus-myoclonus	Breast, ovarian	CNS neurons
APCA (Anti-Yo)	Cerebellar degeneration	Breast, ovarian	Purkinje cell cytoplasm
Anti-CAR	Retinal degeneration	Small cell lung	Photoreceptor cell nuclear layer
Anti-Ma1	Brainstem and cerebellar dysfunction		Nucleoli of neurons and testicular germ cells

involvement of the CNS and dorsal-root ganglia. The most common clinical manifestation of PEM is a disabling subacute sensory neuronopathy (SSN); other patients have predominant involvement of other parts of the CNS, leading to a clinical diagnosis of subacute cerebellar degeneration, limbic encephalitis, brainstem encephalitis, paraneoplastic motor neuron disease, or autonomic system failure (41, 42). The most common clinical course of PEM/SSN is for patients to deteriorate over a period of weeks to months and then to stabilize at a level of severe neurologic disability (39, 43).

The bulk of recent research on autoimmunity in neurologic paraneoplastic syndromes has focused on the specific presence of circulating antineuronal antibodies in some affected patients. There are good, but not perfect correlations among paraneoplastic syndromes, antineuronal antibody specificities, and the associated tumor types (Table 26.2). A number of protein autoantigens have been identified and cloned by using sera from these patients to screen human cDNA expression libraries.

A high percentage of patients with PEM/SSN have polyclonal IgG anti-Hu antibodies (also called type 1 antineuronal nuclear antibodies or ANNA-1). Anti-Hu antibodies produce diffuse staining of the nuclei and to a lesser degree the cytoplasm of all neurons in human brain, spinal cord, dorsal-root ganglia, and autonomic ganglia. In immunoblots of human neuronal extracts, anti-Hu antibodies react with a group of closely spaced proteins with apparent molecular weight of 35 to 40 kd. Intrathecal synthesis of anti-Hu antibodies out of proportion to the serum titer is common and probably is more prevalent among patients with clinically overt PEM plus SSN than among patients with relatively "pure" SSN. High-titer anti-Hu antibodies have been reported in a few patients with sensory neuronopathy and encephalomyelitis in whom no tumor was detected, even at autopsy. Depending on the methodology used, low serum titers of anti-Hu antibodies can be detected in 20% to 50% of patients with small-cell lung carcinoma, but without clinically overt PEM/SSN (44).

Anti-Hu antibodies react with a group of very closely related RNA-binding proteins that are believed to play an essential role in posttranscriptional processing of genes that participate in the development, maturation, and maintenance of neurons. The HuD and Hel-N 1 proteins can bind to the 3′-untranslated regulatory region of mRNA encoding several oncoproteins and cytokines, including c-fos and c-myc. Alternative splicing of mRNA transcripts produces multiple isoforms of the Hu autoantigen proteins, which probably differ in their neuronal distribution and antigenicity. It is not yet known whether some of the polyclonal anti-Hu antibody response is targeted specifically to one neuronal autoantigen or whether individual PEM/SSN patients' anti-Hu antibodies react preferentially with one Hu autoantigen over another. Differences in the fine specificity of the anti-Hu autoimmune response among different individuals may in part explain the clinical heterogeneity of patients with PEM/SSN (45).

To date, there is not a successful experimental model for PEM/SSN. Passive transfer of human anti-Hu antibodies into mice fails to produce any histopathologic changes in the cerebellum, spinal cord, or dorsal-root ganglia. Active immunization with the antigen does produce antibodies but does not cause disease (46). A monoclonal antibody against the HuD protein has been reported to cause apoptosis in human neuroblastoma cells. Conversely, in another study, patients' anti-Hu IgG was specifically taken up into the nucleus and cytoplasm of NCI-H69 human small-cell lung carcinoma cells, but did not inhibit cell proliferation nor cause complement-dependent lysis or antibody-dependent, cell-mediated cytotoxicity other than Ag (47).

Small-cell lung carcinoma is by far the tumor most commonly associated with PEM, with a scattering of patients with a variety of other neoplasms. Anti-neuronal antibodies are a useful clinical tool, both for diagnosing a patient's condition as paraneoplastic and for guiding a search for the underlying tumor. These antineuronal antibody assays do have important practical clinical limitations: (i) a small percentage of patients have high-titer, antineuronal autoantibodies and yet never develop a demonstrable tumor; (ii) several of the autoantibodies are present at low titers in tumor patients without any accompanying clinical manifestations; (iii) a considerable proportion of patients with the paraneoplastic syndromes described below either do not have demonstrable antineuronal antibodies or have atypical antibodies that may not be detected in commercially available assays (48, 49).

Patients with PEM/SSN and anti-Hu antibodies rarely improve with prednisone, intravenous immunoglobulin (IVIG), or cyclophosphamide therapy, despite reductions in serum autoantibody titers, probably fewer than 10% (50, 51). The disappointing response of most patients with PEM/SSN or paraneoplastic cerebellar degeneration (PCD) to immunosuppressive therapies is open to several possible interpretations and does not necessarily refute an autoimmune etiology. It is possible that plasmapheresis or systemic immunosuppressive drugs do not adequately treat an autoimmune response that started in the periphery, but then became established and "sequestered" within the CNS. This is supported by the finding that plasmapheresis in patients with PEM/SSN or PCD reduces serum anti-Hu or anti-Purkinje cell antibodies (APCA) titers, but often fails to affect the level of autoantibodies in the CSE. Unfortunately, an alternative explanation is that, at the time of diagnosis, many patients with PEM/SSN or PCD already have suffered irreversible neuronal damage or loss. This is supported by the typical monophasic clinical course in which patients deteriorate subacutely and then "level off" at a level of severe disability.

PCD is a subacute and progressive pancerebellar dysfunction that also may include symptoms or signs of a multifocal PEM, including lethargy, cognitive deterioration, bulbar palsy, and limb weakness. Ninety percent of PCD have small-cell lung carcinoma, Hodgkin's lymphoma, or carcinomas of the breast, ovary, or female genital tract. The most-prevalent autoantibodies in patients with PCD are high-titer, polyclonal IgG APCA, also called "anti-Yo" antibodies. In most patients, the APCA titers are disproportionately higher in the CSF than in serum, indicating intrathecal synthesis or selective concentration of the antibodies within the CNS (52). APCA characteristically stain the cytoplasm and proximal dendrites of Purkinje cells in a coarsely clumped pattern. Except for faint staining of neurons in the molecular and granular layers of the cerebellar cortex, these antibodies do not stain other neurons in the CNS or any extraneural tissues. In immunoblots of isolated human Purkinje cells, the APCA react specifically with a 58- to 62-kd protein.

The role of APCA remains unknown. To date, all attempts at reproducing PCD in an experimental model have been unsuccessful. APCA IgG injected into the lateral ventricles or peritoneal cavity of rats or guinea pigs is taken up into the cytoplasm of Purkinje cells and other cerebellar neurons, but the animals show no clinical effects or neuropathologic changes (53). The actual intracellular fate of immunoglobulin molecules taken up by Purkinje cells is unknown. Mice immunized with recombinant PCD-17 protein mount a good APCA response, but show no clinical or pathologic signs of disease, and have only minimal uptake of antibodies into Purkinje cells (52, 54).

Another autoimmune disorder, carcinoma-associated retinopathy, is characterized by bilateral dimming or blurring of vision often with impaired color vision. More than 90% of patients have a small lung cell carcinoma. The prominent autoantibody in this disorder is against recoverin, also called anti-CAR (cancer-associated retinopathy) autoantibodies. In contrast to the studies of PEM and PCD, there has been success in establishing an animal model for CAR (55). Rats immunized with a segment of recoverin develop antirecoverin antibodies, uveoretinitis with cellular infiltrates, and degeneration of photoreceptors. The same histopathologic changes can be reproduced by passive transfer of stimulated lymphocytes from rats immunized with recoverin into naive animals, indicating that a combination of antibody-mediated injury and cellular immune effector cells is at work.

Finally, a limbic and brainstem encephalitis occurs in patients with testicular cancer. In this disorder, 10 of 13 patients had autoantibodies to an antigen named Ma2. Ma2 is distributed in the brain, largely in the hippocampus, amygdala, diencephalic structures, and the dentate of the cerebellum (56). These antibodies also are reported in a patient with breast cancer (57). As in other paraneoplastic diseases, autoantibodies within the CNS were high. Although Ma2 is cloned, as yet there are no animal studies.

Stiff-Person Syndrome

An unusual disorder with an intriguing connection to a specific antigen is the stiff-person syndrome or stiff-man syndrome (SMS), a rare disorder of the CNS, which is characterized clinically by fluctuating and progressive muscle rigidity and spasms. The diagnosis relies also on the electrophysiologic evidence of the presence of continuous motor unit activity, without evidence of neuromyotonia, extrapyramidal or pyramidal dysfunction, or focal lesions of the spinal cord. Rigidity and spasms may dominate in the axial muscles, or in one or more distal limbs at clinical examination. Barker et al. distinguished between (i) stiff-person syndrome: rigidity and spasms of the lumbar paraspinal, abdominal, and occasionally proximal leg muscles, and (ii) stiff-limb syndrome on clinical and electrophysiologic grounds. The patients with stiff-person syndrome responded to γ-aminobutyric acid (GABA) -ergic drugs, remained ambulant, and almost all had unique autoantibodies. Although there was overlap, fewer patients with stiff-limb syndrome had autoantibodies (58).

Further understanding of the pathogenesis of SMS was gained with the description of polyclonal and oligoclonal patterns of IgG antibody elevations in the CSF of the majority of patients with SMS, suggesting local production within the BBB (59). Using immunocytochemic assays, these antibodies were identified as targeting the GABA-ergic neurons and their nerve terminals, as well as the beta cells of the pancreas. The dominant autoantigen recognized by these autoantibodies was the γ-aminobutyric acid (GABA)-synthesizing enzyme, glutamic acid decarboxylase (GAD). Fifty to 60% of these patients have autoantibodies in the serum and CSF directed against GAD. A high proportion of these patients have other autoimmune diseases including diabetes mellitus. Antibodies against the two isoforms of GAD, GAD-65 and GAD-67 predominate (60, 61).

Antibodies to GAD are frequent in patients with idiopathic diabetes mellitus (59). Nonetheless, despite the frequent occurrence of these anti-GAD antibodies, SMS is an extremely rare condition. This is explained on the basis of both the epitopes identified and the titers in the specific diseases. First, the titer of anti-GAD autoantibodies in IDDM and SMS differs by orders of magnitude as great as 100 to 500 fold. Second, sera from patients with IDDM recognize conformational epitopes of GAD, whereas SMS patient sera recognize a combination of linear and conformational epitopes. SMS sera uniformly recognize denatured GAD-65 on Western blots, yet such reactions are seen rarely with sera from patients with IDDM. Epitope specificity demonstrated in SMS sera may reflect epitope spreading that occurs in SMS patients but not IDDM patients (62, 63).

The relevance of GAD autoantibody production to SMS still is being elucidated, because 40% of SMS patients are GAD-antibody negative. It is proposed that the autoantibodies could inhibit GABA synthesis (64) or potentiate a functional impairment of GABA-ergic transmission by blocking membrane-associated GAD during the exocytosis of GABA. Also, a recent study shows impairment of cerebellar-inhibitory synapses (65). Interestingly, clinical support for a role of the autoantibodies in human disease pathogenesis comes from a clinical neuroradiographic test, magnetic resonance spectroscopy (MRS). Despite normal conventional magnetic resonance imaging (MRI), proton MRS has assessed regional levels of γ-aminobutyric acid in the brain of normal persons and those with stiff-person syndrome. Ratios of N-acetylaspartate, choline, and glutamate to creatine are regionally comparable in patients and controls. However, decreased GABA levels in the motor cortex and posterior occipital cortex were observed in patients with stiff-person syndrome. Ratios of GABA to creatine in the right and left sensorimotor cortices of patients were significantly lower than those in healthy participants corresponding to a 30% to 40% decrease; $p < .01$). A smaller decrease in ratios of GABA to creatine also was observed in the posterior occipital region corresponding to an 18% decrease; $p < .05$). The spectroscopic evidence of diminished GABA levels in patients supports the hypothesis that in the stiff-person syndrome, anti-GAD antibodies interfere with the regional synthesis of GABA and play a major role in the clinical motor symptoms (66).

A minority of patients (5% to 10%) affected by SMS and cancer (usually women with breast cancer) have autoantibodies directed against another autoantigen, the 128 kd autoantigen identified as amphiphysin I, a protein associated with synaptic vesicles. A considerable proportion of patients (around 40%) affected by this chronic disorder show no signs of autoimmunity and may thus represent a different subgroup of patients (67).

Patients with stiff-person syndrome often respond to GABA-ergic medications such as vigabatrin. The response to immunosuppressive therapy including plasmapheresis and immunosuppressive therapy is variable (68–70).

Multiple Sclerosis

Multiple sclerosis (MS) is an inflammatory and demyelinating disease of the CNS, characterized by infiltrating CD4+ T cells and large amounts of intrathecally synthesized oligoclonal immunoglobulins (Igs). The role of the oligoclonal bands (persistent Igs with a specificity varying among individuals) within the CSF remains enigmatic. Some recent work suggests that these antibodies could contribute to repair rather than tissue dysfunction.

In the experimental models of MS such as experimental allergic encephalomyelitis (EAE), as in the human disease, the predominant immunopathogenic mechanism is cell mediated largely through T lymphocytes and macrophages. However, in one primate model of MS, demyelination develops from antibodies to myelin oligodendrocyte glycoprotein (MOG) (71, 72). In the common marmoset *Callithrix jacchus*, demyelination can be induced by immunization with either whole myelin or the extracellular domain of a MOG but not by the quantitatively major myelin proteins, myelin-basic protein, or proteolipid protein. These latter proteins induce inflammation but little or no demyelination. In the presence of encephalitogenic (e.g., disease-inducing) T cells, the fully demyelinated lesion can be reconstructed by systemic administration of IgG purified from whole myelin-, or MOG-immunized animals, and equally by a monoclonal antibody against MOG, but not by control IgG (73, 74). Complement and macrophages do not need to be present at this stage for these effects to occur. Thus, in this disorder the pathology is dependent upon the presence of autoantibodies. The likely sequence of events is that small amounts of antibody directed against specific myelin epitopes may be sufficient to stimulate the initial myelinolysis possibly through neutral proteases, even in the absence of complement and macrophages. This then may leave the myelin sheath much more open to attack by other mechanisms. For instance, new antigenic epitopes may be exposed, such as myelin basic protein (MBP) and proteolipid protein (PLP), and recognized by encephalitogenic T cells. Specific T-cell responses then trigger an inflammatory cascade that opens the BBB to other circulating antibodies and serum complement.

The local production of complement-derived proinflammatory factors further amplifies the local inflammatory response. The histopathology of the lesions induced by this combination of immune effector mechanisms does resemble that seen in MS (75, 76).

There is *in vitro* support for the effect of antibodies. Anti-MOG mAb 8-18C5 antibodies produce demyelination in aggregating brain-cell cultures. In contrast, polyclonal antibodies raised against MBP, PLP, or myelin-associated glycoprotein (MAG) have no such demyelinating effects on cultured CNS (77).

Despite the animal model and evidence for anti-MOG antibodies in patients with MS, it is not clear if these antibodies are important in the onset of disease. By the time MS is recognized in patients, there is a complicated system of pro- and antiinflammatory mechanisms within the CNS.

ANTIBODIES IN SYSTEMIC AUTOIMMUNITY

Sjögren's Syndrome

Primary Sjögren's syndrome (SS) is a systemic autoimmune disease that is characterized by keratoconjunctivitis sicca and xerostomia resulting from lymphocytic infiltrates in the lacrimal and salivary glands. Extraglandular manifestations include a variety of organ systems. Neurologic abnormalities occur with varying frequency in different series (78–82). Cranial and peripheral neuropathies were an early and persistent observation in the study of Sjögren's syndrome. The mechanism is not clear but frequently involves some form of vascular inflammation. The autonomic nervous system is currently an important area for the study of autoimmune mechanisms. Abnormalities of parasympathetic neurotransmission may contribute to the glandular dysfunction in Sjögren's syndrome (83–87). There are two basic types of acetylcholine receptors: nicotinic and muscarinic. Nicotinic receptors are present in skeletal muscle. Muscarinic receptors are present in autonomic neurons and in neurons of the hippocampus and cerebral cortex. Autonomic nervous-system disturbances are recognized in patients with SS although the mechanisms are not clear. Because muscarinic receptors are important in salivary flow, investigators question whether an autoimmune mechanism directed at a muscarinic would contribute to sicca symptoms. It has been proposed that autoantibodies inhibit the action of parasympathetic neurotransmission at the muscarinic receptor postganglionic parasympathetic neurons innervating the lacrimal and salivary glands. Antibodies to muscarinic receptors (M3) are identified by radioligand-binding studies in some patients with primary SS. The functional effects of these antibodies are being studied (88). Serum and IgG from these patients were able to abolish bladder muscle contraction in response to nerve stimulation and to carbachol (89). Autoantibodies thus may act as antagonists at the M3-muscarinic receptor and interfere with parasympathetic neurotransmission to smooth muscle.

Perhaps the most prominent abnormality in SS is the dorsal-root ganglionitis (90). Although there is a similarity with the autoantibody-mediated ganglionitis in paraneoplastic disease, the role of autoantibodies in SS is not determined.

Although clinical abnormalities of the CNS are recognized in Sjögren's syndrome, the frequency and pathogeneses of these features are not yet defined.

AUTOANTIBODIES AND NEUROLOGIC DISEASE IN SLE

The neurologic abnormalities in SLE are broad and difficult to classify (91). Autoantibodies have long been suspected of playing a role in the pathogenesis of neurologic abnormalities in SLE but as yet none of the reported antibodies is established as pathogenic. It may be the enormous multilevel complexity of the nervous systems and the limited access of tissue that elude identification of autoantibody-mediated effects. However, compared with studies in other diseases, it seems clear that we are not choosing clinical subsets well enough. Combining all neurologic abnormalities in SLE together to look for a mechanism or even association of autoantibodies dilutes any data that might be present in a smaller better-chosen sample. Even within the "cognitive disorders" there are so many potential neuroanatomic localizations and systems, grouping dissimilar patients increases the difficulty in identifying specific causes. The key to establishing an immunopathogenic role for antibodies in NP-SLE will be to determine the effects of specific autoantibodies on brain function. Thus, future studies should be designed to examine autoantibody-mediated changes in physiologic pathways.

TABLE 26.3. ANTIBODIES ASSOCIATED WITH SYSTEMIC LUPUS ERYTHEMATOSUS

Lymphocyte
Neuroblastoma cell membranes
Brain plasma membranes
Antiphospholipid antibodies (APA)
Ribosomal P
Glycolipid
Lupus brain antigen 1 (Lba1)

There are several plausible mechanisms whereby antibodies could exert effects on brain function producing clinical abnormalities similar to those of NP-SLE. Given the preponderance of abnormalities in frontal lobe and limbic function, movement disorders, ataxias, and vascular disease, mechanisms worthy of study, would include the following.

In emotional/cognitive abnormalities, look for binding directly to ion channels or receptors on neurons (particularly cortical or hippocampal cells).

In chorea, studies of antibodies affecting release of dopamine

In ataxias, search for antibodies to structures found in the paraneoplastic syndromes.

In vascular disease and coagulation, *in vivo* use of APA to study effects on tissue perfusion by MRI.

Autoantibodies reported to be associated with NP-SLE are shown in Table 26.3.

ANTIBODIES AND ACCESS TO CENTRAL NERVOUS SYSTEM TISSUE

With the exception of antibodies thought to work directly on the luminal side of the vasculature and induce ischemia, antibodies directly causing neurologic abnormalities must be demonstrably present in the CNS. Thus, unless the clinical features are associated with a stroke, antibody binding to target tissue is required as with other tissues.

Serum autoantibodies do pass into the CNS in pathophysiologic situations when the BBB is disrupted. The antibodies present in the CSF at this time are likely transient. However, in normal circumstances, B cells traffic into the CNS and if they encounter an appropriate antigen can set up residence and differentiate. Thus, although the BBB and blood-CSF barriers are normally closed to large, nonspecific molecules in CNS diseases determined to be antibody mediated, the presence of specific CSF antibodies exceeds those in the serum. CSF studies in patients with SLE reveal increased intrathecal immunoglobulin synthesis and/or oligoclonal bands occurring in about half of the patients with encephalopathies, seizures, and psychiatric abnormalities however, the specificities of the antibodies and their duration are not well defined (92–95).

AUTOANTIBODIES ASSOCIATED WITH NEUROPSYCHIATRIC-SLE

Several different populations of biologically interesting circulating autoantibodies correlate with the presence of neuro-psychiatric abnormalities in patients with SLE. Early studies identified a lymphocytotoxic antibody cross-reactive with brain tissue in patients with active neurologic disease (96) including patients with cognitive impairment, although later studies failed to correlate a temporal profile of antibody with disease activity (97). Many studies identify serum autoantibodies reactive with brain or neuroblastoma tissue. The antibodies often are called antineuronal although the cell type and regional localization are not always defined. CNS cells other than neurons, such as glia, also are potential targets. The presence of serum antibodies binding to specific targets in sections of brain cortex, to brain-derived plasma membranes and cultured neuroblastoma cells (98, 99) also correlated with neurologic abnormalities particularly encephalopathies. Of note, neuroblastoma cells, which are derived from peripheral nervous system cells, are not a good choice of target when looking for CNS antigens. Further, a cytotoxicity assay is not a good choice in a disease model without CNS cytotoxicity. There are other targets investigated. Antibodies with binding activity to CNS targets are reported in both the CSF and brain eluates of patients with neuro-SLE.

More specific molecules targeted by antibodies include gangliosides, asialo GM1, and ribosomal P proteins, particularly 60S ribosomal subunit phosphoproteins PO, P1, and P2 (100–103) although these are not molecules specific to the CNS. Antibodies to ribosomal P have a well-defined target antigen that exists in three forms P0, P1, and P2. The frequency with which anti-P antibodies occur in SLE patients is low, ranging from 5% to 20% (104). The access of antibodies to the intracellular antigens ribosomal P would be considered a problem, but studies do show antibodies to ribosomal P protein (38 kd) also are immunoreactive with cell surfaces including those of neuroblastoma cells (105). A further difficulty is that the concentration of antiribosomal P antibodies is much lower in the CSF than in the serum unlike the situation with the paraneoplastic antibodies described above. More recently, anti-P antibodies have been associated with lupus, hepatitis, and nephritis.

Antiphospholipid antibodies (APL), detected by the presence of either an *in vitro* lupus anticoagulant or anticardiolipin antibody (aCL) binding, have been associated with cognitive dysfunction in some cross-sectional studies. However, because both APL levels and cognitive function in SLE patients are known to fluctuate over time, a longitudinal analysis is required in order to more accurately determine an etiologic association (106, 107).

An antibody that we have detected in the serum and CSF in murine SLE also is present in patients. This autoantigen Lba1 has been sequenced but the target protein is not yet delineated. The transcript for the protein is present only in the brain and within the brain in the limbic system predominantly in the cingulate, hippocampus, orbitofrontal regions, and hypothalamus. Further work needs to be done to determine if the antibodies induce changes in neuronal function (108).

Clinical Features Of NP-SLE Potentially Due Autoantibody Mediated Abnormalities

If we shift analyses from the specific autoantibodies to disease groups where there might be an effect of antibodies, there are several interesting studies. There are several studies that have either narrowed the focus of clinical feature or subdivided a larger series into smaller groups.

Movement disorders, particularly *chorea,* occur sufficiently often in SLE that the onset of chorea in a young woman often suggests the diagnosis. The clinical features of chorea, rapid, brief, involuntary, and irregular movements, may be generalized or limited to the extremities, trunk, or face. Slower, writhing movements superimposed upon the chorea are choreoathetosis. The anatomic substrate for chorea is subcortical, usually in the caudate, putamen, globus pallidus, or subthalamic nucleus. Neither the cause nor the mechanism of the intermittent chorea in SLE is known. Despite early reports that chorea was associated with an antibody to the caudate nucleus and recent reports of an association with antiphospholipid antibodies, the pathogenesis is uncertain (109, 110). One study investigating metabolic images in the striatum of four patients with SLE and chorea did not discern striatal hypometabolism as a correlate of chorea. The intermittent nature of the process, the absence of structural damage, and the rather prompt response to plasmapheresis are consistent with a direct autoantibody-mediated mechanism.

Seizures

Although there was an early report associating seizures with autoantibody activity, there is little recent data. However, in patients with intractable seizures, plasmapheresis has been effective suggesting that some patients may have an autoimmune component (111).

Psychoses are a broad classification of disorders that implicate a behavioral or thought process disorder that impairs the individual's ability to function. Acquired, transient psychoses are encountered in toxic, metabolic, and autoimmune disorders. In SLE, the association of psychosis and autoantibodies to the ribosomal P protein (anti-P) first was characterized in 1985. Clinically, the association between anti-ribosomal P and psychoses and depression has been both confirmed (112) and refuted (113). The CSF levels of antibody are lower than the serum in several series raising questions about access of autoantibody if, indeed, they are pathogenic (112). More recently, studies determining whether the type of antigen used in the assay could be related to the variable correlation of anti-P with psychosis have been examined. Using either recombinant fusion protein or synthetic peptide, there are still conflicting results about the association of anti-P with psychoses or other CNS events (113, 114).

Cognitive abnormalities are frequently described in patients with SLE but the term is broad and could encompass involvement of several different regions and systems.

Neuropsychologic assessment examines the performance of individuals on a range of tests that evaluate different areas of cognition, such as attention, memory, and language function (115–117). These tests have been found to be sensitive in detecting mild cerebral dysfunction and have been widely applied in SLE. The task of identifying nonfocal neurologic problems through neuropsychologic assessment also is heavily reliant on the choice of tests used in the assessment. However, full batteries that can appropriately localize disturbances takes 6 to 8 hours of testing. Shorter batteries can be used but only after they have been validated against longer batteries as specific and appropriate for the individual disease (118). Suggestions made by the Ad Hoc Committee bypassed a rigorous testing that would have been necessary to validate the results.

The association of cognitive impairment and anticardiolipin antibodies has been reexamined recently. Although ACL antibody titers are known to fluctuate during the course of the disease, a recent study does examine an association between persistently elevated levels of ACL and change in cognitive performance in 51 SLE patients. In this study, SLE patients with persistently elevated IgG ACL values over a 2- to 3-year period, as opposed to those with negative or inconsistently raised titers, were found to have significantly poorer performance on cognitive tasks. The mechanism is not examined but it is thought that persistently high titers of ACL are associated with a greater risk of thrombotic events and this could contribute to cognitive decline (107). CSF antibodies were not determined. Nor was there other evidence to suggest that multifocal ischemia occurred.

The disparity between these findings and those of other studies that failed to show any relationship between poor cognitive functioning and level of autoantibody also may be attributed to the way in which poor cognitive functioning was classified. Although the term "cognitive impairment" is widely used in much of the literature on SLE today, there is no consensus on how to define cognitive impairment. As stated above, the tasks are not validated for SLE, nor are methods for evaluating the effect of depression or poor motor performance included. Any number of methods can be used to define cognitive impairment, such as poor scores on one task or poor scores on two or more tasks, with variations in threshold for defining a poor score ranging from one to two standard deviations below an agreed-upon normative score for the task. This may account in part for the fact that the reported prevalence rates of cognitive impairment in SLE range from 15% to 66%. Emotional abnormalities are conspicuous in patients with chronic diseases but both anxiety and depression are prominent in SLE (119). A role of antibodies in these patients is not yet examined.

Inflammation And Autoantibodies As A Stressor

Consequences of persistent activation of the HPA axis are interesting. It is not yet clear whether the response of the HPA in SLE is appropriate for the disease stimulus or inappropriate and contributes to the perpetuation of disease (120, 121). There are several reasons to hypothesize that the HPA axis, and particularly a regulatory limb from the hippocampus is involved in the genesis of symptoms of NP-SLE: (i) cytokines IL-1 and IL-6, two known activators of the hypothalamus, are elevated in the CSF of patients with SLE (122); (ii) prolactin appears elevated and bromocriptine (although toxic) may influence disease activity (123–125); (iii) seizures are a frequent and often presenting feature of SLE, and imaging abnormalities in the temporal lobe are prominent; (iv) autoantibodies reactive with neuronal targets in general and hippocampal and hypothalamic neurons in particular occur in human and murine SLE (126); and (v) particular patterns of cognitive and behavioral changes in human disease implicate dysfunction in the hippocampus and prefrontal structures (127, 128).

If dysfunction of the HPA axis was associated with NP-SLE, potential mechanisms could include high levels of circulating antibodies producing a stress response, specific autoantibodies that might target specific regions within the CNS, or chronically elevated levels of cortisol. Further contributing to the dysregulation of the stress axis is the vulnerability of the hippocampus to seizures, hypoxic or ischemic injury, and damage caused by glucocorticoids. Among the important roles of these cells are their prominent regulatory influences on inflammation, as well as reproductive and autonomic nervous system function. Studies investigating the integrity of this region of the brain in patients with SLE are proceeding.

REFERENCES

1. Mimori T. Autoantibodies in connective tissue diseases: clinical significance and analysis of target autoantigens. *Internal Medicine* 1999;38:523–532.
2. Isenberg DA. Autoantibodies: markers of disease or pathogenic?

Annals of the New York Academy of Sciences 1997;823: 256–262.

3. Micera A, Properzi F, Triaca V, et al. Nerve growth factor antibody exacerbates neuropathological signs of experimental allergic encephalomyelitis in adult lewis rats. *J Neuroimmunol* 2000;104:116–123.
4. Moore PM, Lisak RP. Systemic lupus erythematosus: immunopathogenesis of neurologic dysfunction. Springer Semin Immunopathol 1995;17:43–60.
5. Vincent A, Mills K. Genetic and antibody-mediated channelopathies at the neuromuscular junction. *Electroencephalogr Clin Neurophysiol Suppl* 1999;50:250–258.
6. Choi DW. Excitotoxic cell death. *J Neurobiol* 1992;23: 1261–1276.
7. McEwen BS. Protective and damaging effects of stress mediators: central role of the brain. *Prog Brain Res* 2000;122:25–34.
8. Bennett R, Hughes GR, Bywaters EG, et al. Neuropsychiatric problems in systemic lupus erythematosus. *British Medical Journal* 1972;4:342–345.
9. Shanks N, Windle RJ, Perks PA, et al. Early-life exposure to endotoxin alters hypothalamic-pituitary-adrenal function and predisposition to inflammation. *Proc Natl Acad Sci USA* 2000; 97:5645–5650.
10. McLean BN. Neurological involvement in systemic lupus erythematosus. *Curr Opin Neurol* 1998;11:247–251.
11. McEwen BS, Alves SE. Estrogen actions in the central nervous system. *Endocr Rev* 1999;20:279–307.
12. Williams KC, Hickey WF. Traffic of hematogenous cells through the central nervous system. *Curr Top Microbiol Immunol* 1995;202:221–245.
13. Knopf PM, C.J., Cserr HF, et al. Antigen-dependent intrathecal antibody synthesis in the normal rat brain: tissue entry and local retention of antigen-specific B cells. *J Immunol* 1998; 161:692–701.
14. Drachman DB. Myasthenia gravis. *N Engl J Med* 1994;330: 1797–1810.
15. Lindstrom JM. Acetylcholine receptors and myasthenia. *Muscle Nerve* 2000;23:453–477.
16. Vincent A, Willcox N, Hill M, et al. Determinant spreading and immune responses to acetylcholine receptors in myasthenia gravis. *Immunol Rev* 1998;164:157–168.
17. Ruff RL, Lennon VA. End-plate voltage-gated sodium channels are lost in clinical and experimental myasthenia gravis. *Ann Neurol* 1998;43:370–379.
18. Infante AJ, Kraig E. Myasthenia gravis and its animal model: T cell receptor expression in an antibody mediated autoimmune disease. *Int Rev Immunol* 1999;18:83–109.
19. Yoshikawa H, Satoh K, Iwasa K, et al. In vitro production of antiacetylcholine receptor antibody and IgG by peripheral blood lymphocytes of patients with myasthenia gravis. *Ann NY Acad Sci* 1998;841:351–354.
20. Christadoss P, Kaul R, Shenoy M, et al. Establishment of a mouse model of myasthenia gravis which mimics human myasthenia gravis pathogenesis for immune intervention. *Adv Exp Med Biol* 1995;383:195–199.
21. Tim RW, Massey JM, Sanders DB. Lambert-Eaton myasthenic syndrome: electrodiagnostic findings and response to treatment. *Neurology* 2000;54:2176–2178.
22. Maddison P, Newsom-Davis J, Mills KR. Distribution of electrophysiological abnormality in Lambert-Eaton myasthenic syndrome. J Neurol Neurosurg Psychiatry 1998;65:213–217.
23. Motomura M, Lang B, Johnston I, et al. Incidence of serum anti-P/O-type and anti-N-type calcium channel autoantibodies in the Lambert-Eaton myasthenic syndrome. *J Neurol Sci* 1997; 147:35–42.
24. Takamori M, Iwasa K, Komai K. Antigenic sites of the voltage-gated calcium channel in Lambert-Eaton myasthenic syndrome. *Ann Ny Acad Sci* 1998;841:625–635.
25. Verschuuren JJ, Dalmau J, Tunkel R, et al. Antibodies against the calcium channel beta-subunit in Lambert-Eaton myasthenic syndrome. *Neurology* 1998;50:475–479.
26. Lambert EH, Lennon VA. Selected IgG rapidly induces Lambert-Eaton myasthenic syndrome in mice: complement independence and EMG abnormalities. *Muscle Nerve* 1988;11: 1133–1145.
27. Kim YI, Middlekauff EH, Viglione MP, et al. An autoimmune animal model of the Lambert-Eaton syndrome. *Ann Ny Acad Sci* 1998;841:670–676.
28. Engisch KL, Rich MM, Cook N, et al. Lambert-Eaton antibodies promote activity-dependent enhancement of exocytosis in bovine adrenal chromaffin cells. *Ann Ny Acad Sci* 1999; 868:213–216.
29. O'Suilleabhain P, Low PA, Lennon VA. Autonomic dysfunction in the Lambert-Eaton myasthenic syndrome: serologic and clinical correlates. *Neurology* 1998;50:88–93.
30. Low PA. Autonomic neuropathies. *Curr Opin Neurol* 1998;11: 531–537.
31. Dupond JL, Gil H, Bouhaddi M, et al. Acute dysautonomia secondary to autoimmune diseases: efficacy of intravenous immunoglobulin and correlation with a stimulation of plasma norepinephrine levels. *Clin Exper Rheumatol* 1999;17:733–736.
32. Vernino S, Adamski J, Kryzer TJ, et al. Neuronal nicotinic ACh receptor antibody in subacute autonomic neuropathy and cancer-related syndromes. *Neurology* 1998;50:1806–1813.
33. Vernino S, Low PA, Fealey RD, et al. Autoantibodies to ganglionic acetylcholine receptors in autoimmune autonomic neuropathies. *N Engl J Med* 2000;343:847–855.
34. Chapman J, Alroy G, Weiss Z, et al. Anti-neuronal antibodies similar to those found in Alzheimer's disease induce memory dysfunction in rats. *Neuroscience* 1991;40:297–305.
35. Watts H, Kennedy PG, Thomas M. The significance of anti-neuronal antibodies in Alzheimer's disease. *J Neuroimmunol* 1981;1:107–116.
36. Husby G, Wedege E, Williams RCJ. Characterization of brain proteins reacting in vitro with anti-neuronal antibodies in patients with Huntington's disease. *Clin Immunol Immunopathol* 1978;11:131–141.
37. Schenck CH, Ullevig CM, Mahowald MW, et al. A controlled study of serum anti-locus ceruleus antibodies in REM sleep behavior disorder. *Sleep* 1997;20:349–351.
38. Dropcho EJ. Principles of paraneoplastic syndromes. *Ann Ny Acad Sci* 1998;841:246–261.
39. Dalmau J, Gultekin HS, Posner JB. Paraneoplastic neurologic syndromes: pathogenesis and physiopathology. *Brain Pathol* 1999;9:275–284.
40. Scaravilli F, An SF, Groves M, et al. The neuropathology of paraneoplastic syndromes. *Brain Pathol* 1999;9:251–260.
41. Gultekin SH, Rosenfeld MR, Voltz R, et al. Paraneoplastic limbic encephalitis: neurological symptoms, immunological findings and tumour association in 50 patients. *Brain* 2000;123: 1481–1494.
42. Ichimura M, Yamamoto M, Kobayashi Y, et al. Tissue distribution of pathological lesions and Hu antigen expression in paraneoplastic sensory neuronopathy. *Acta Neuropathol (Berl)* 1998; 95:641–648.
43. Keime-Guibert F, Graus F, Broet P, et al. Clinical outcome of patients with anti-Hu-associated encephalomyelitis after treatment of the tumor. *Neurology* 1999;53:1719–1723.
44. Dalmau J, Graus F, Rosenblum MK, et al. Anti-Hu—associated paraneoplastic encephalomyelitis/sensory neuronopathy. A clinical study of 71 patients. *Medicine* 1992;71:59–72.
45. Sodeyama N, Ishida K, Jaeckle KA, et al. Pattern of epitopic

reactivity of the anti-Hu antibody on HuD with and without paraneoplastic syndrome. *J Neurol Neurosurg Psychiatry* 1999; 66:97–99.

46. P.A., Manley GT, Posner JB. Immunization with the paraneoplastic encephalomyelitis antigen HuD does not cause neurologic disease in mice. *Neurology* 1995;45:1873–1878.
47. Verschuuren JJ, Dalmau J, Hoard R, et al. Paraneoplastic anti-Hu serum: studies on human tumor cell lines. *J Neuroimmunol* 1997;79:202–210.
48. Voltz RD, Posner JB, Dalmau J, et al. Paraneoplastic encephalomyelitis: an update of the effects of the anti-Hu immune response on the nervous system and tumour. *J Neurol Neurosurg Psychiatry* 1997;63:133–136.
49. Sillevis SP, Kinoshita A, De Leeuw B, et al. Paraneoplastic cerebellar ataxia due to autoantibodies against a glutamate receptor. *N Engl J Med* 2000;342:21–27.
50. Oh SJ, Dropcho EJ, Claussen GC. Anti-Hu-associated paraneoplastic sensory neuropathy responding to early aggressive immunotherapy: report of two cases and review of literature. *Muscle Nerve* 1997;20:1576–1582.
51. Inuzuka T. Autoantibodies in paraneoplastic neurological syndrome. *Am J Med Sci* 2000;319:217–226.
52. Greenlee JE, Dalmau J, Lyons T, et al. Association of anti-Yo (type I) antibody with paraneoplastic cerebellar degeneration in the setting of transitional cell carcinoma of the bladder: detection of Yo antigen in tumor tissue and fall in antibody titers following tumor removal. *Ann Neurol* 1999;45:805–809.
53. Graus F, Illa I, Agusti M, et al. Effect of intraventricular injection of an anti-Purkinje cell antibody (anti-Yo) in a guinea pig model. *J Neurol Sci* 1991;106:82–87.
54. Tanaka K, Tanaka M, Igarashi S, et al. Trial to establish an animal model of paraneoplastic cerebellar degeneration with anti-Yo antibody. 2. Passive transfer of murine mononuclear cells activated with recombinant Yo protein to paraneoplastic cerebellar degeneration lymphocytes in severe combined immunodeficiency mice. *Clin Neurol Neurosurg* 1995;97:101–105.
55. Goldstein SM, Syed NA, Milam AH, et al. Cancer-associated retinopathy. *Arch Ophthalmol* 1999;117:1641–1645.
56. Dalmau J, Gultekin SH, Voltz R, et al. Ma1, a novel neuron- and testis-specific protein, is recognized by the serum of patients with paraneoplastic neurological disorders [see comments]. *Brain* 1999;122:27–39.
57. Sutton I, Winer J, Rowlands D, et al. Limbic encephalitis and antibodies to Ma2: a paraneoplastic presentation of breast cancer. *J Neurol Neurosurg Psychiatry* 2000;69:266–268.
58. Barker RA, Revesz T, Thom M, et al. Review of 23 patients affected by the stiff man syndrome: clinical subdivision into stiff trunk (man) syndrome, stiff limb syndrome, and progressive encephalomyelitis with rigidity. *J Neurol Neurosurg Psychiatry* 1998;65:633–640.
59. Solimena M, Folli F, Denis-Donini S, et al. Autoantibodies to glutamic acid decarboxylase in a patient with stiff-man syndrome, epilepsy, and type I diabetes mellitus. *N Engl J Med* 1988;318:1012–1020.
60. Vincent A, Grimaldi LM, Martino G, et al. Antibodies to 125I-glutamic acid decarboxylase in patients with stiff man syndrome. *J Neurol Neurosurg Psychiatry* 1997;62:395–397.
61. Butler MH, Solimena M, Dirkx RJ, et al. Identification of a dominant epitope of glutamic acid decarboxylase (GAD-65) recognized by autoantibodies in stiff-man syndrome. *J Exp Med* 1993;178:2097–2106.
62. Lohmann T, Hawa M, Leslie RD, et al. Immune reactivity to glutamic acid decarboxylase 65 in stiffman syndrome and type 1 diabetes mellitus. *Lancet* 2000;356:31–35.
63. Sohnlein P, Muller M, Syren K, et al. Epitope spreading and a varying but not disease-specific GAD65 antibody response in Type I diabetes. The Childhood Diabetes in Finland Study Group. *Diabetologia* 2000;43:210–217.
64. Dinkel K, Meinck HM, Jury KM, et al. Inhibition of gamma-aminobutyric acid synthesis by glutamic acid decarboxylase autoantibodies in stiff-man syndrome. *Ann Neurol* 1998;44: 194–201.
65. Mitoma H, Song SY, Ishida K, et al. Presynaptic impairment of cerebellar inhibitory synapses by an autoantibody to glutamate decarboxylase. *J Neurol Sci* 2000;175:40–44.
66. Levy LM, Dalakas MC, Floeter MK. The stiff-person syndrome: an autoimmune disorder affecting neurotransmission of gamma-aminobutyric acid. *Ann Intern Med* 1999;131: 522–530.
67. Rosin L, DeCamilli P, Butler M, et al. Stiff-man syndrome in a woman with breast cancer: an uncommon central nervous system paraneoplastic syndrome. *Neurology* 1998;50:94–98.
68. Prevett MC, Brown P, Duncan JS. Improvement of stiff-man syndrome with vigabatrin. *Neurology* 1997;48:1133–1134.
69. Khanlou H, Eiger G. Long-term remission of refractory stiff-man syndrome after treatment with intravenous immunoglobulin. *Mayo Clin Proc* 1999;74:1231–1232.
70. Hayashi A, Nakamagoe K, Ohkoshi N, et al. Double filtration plasma exchange and immunoadsorption therapy in a case of stiff-man syndrome with negative anti-GAD antibody. *J Med* 1999;30:321–327.
71. Massacesi L, Genain CP, Lee-Parritz D, et al. Active and passively induced experimental autoimmune encephalomyelitis in common marmosets: a new model for multiple sclerosis. *Ann Neurol* 1995;37:519–530.
72. Genain CP, Nguyen MH, Letvin NL, et al. Antibody facilitation of multiple sclerosis-like lesions in a nonhuman primate. *J Clin Invest* 1995;96:2966–2974.
73. Adelmann M, Wood J, Benzel I, et al. The N-terminal domain of the myelin oligodendrocyte glycoprotein (MOG) induces acute demyelinating experimental autoimmune encephalomyelitis in the Lewis rat. *J Neuroimmunol* 1995;63:17–27.
74. Stefferl A, Brehm U, Storch M, et al. Myelin oligodendrocyte glycoprotein induces experimental autoimmune encephalomyelitis in the "resistant" Brown Norway rat: disease susceptibility is determined by MHC and MHC-linked effects on the B cell response. *J Immunol* 1999;163:40–49.
75. Genain CP, Cannella B, Hauser SL, et al. Identification of autoantibodies associated with myelin damage in multiple sclerosis. *Nat Med* 1999;5:170–175.
76. Slavin A, Ewing C, Liu J, et al. Induction of a multiple sclerosis-like disease in mice with an immunodominant epitope of myelin oligodendrocyte glycoprotein. *Autoimmunity* 1998;28: 109–120.
77. Cai D, Shen Y, De Bellard M, et al. Prior exposure to neurotrophins blocks inhibition of axonal regeneration by MAG and myelin via a cAMP-dependent mechanism. *Neuron* 1999; 22:89–101.
78. Cox PD, Hales RE. CNS Sjogren's syndrome: an underrecognized and underappreciated neuropsychiatric disorder. *J Neuropsychiatry Clin Neurosci* 1999;11:241–247.
79. Belin C, Moroni C, Caillat-Vigneron N, et al. Central nervous system involvement in Sjogren's syndrome: evidence from neuropsychological testing and HMPAO-SPECT. *Ann Med Interne (Paris)* 1999;150:598–604.
80. Govoni M, Bajocchi G, Rizzo N, et al. Neurological involvement in primary Sjogren's syndrome: clinical and instrumental evaluation in a cohort of Italian patients. *Clin Rheumatol* 1999; 18:299–303.
81. Coates T, Slavotinek JP, Rischmueller M, et al. Cerebral white matter lesions in primary Sjogren's syndrome: a controlled study. *J Rheumatol* 1999;26:1301–1305.

82. Manabe Y, Sasaki C, Warita H, et al. Sjogren's syndrome with acute transverse myelopathy as the initial manifestation. *J Neurol Sci* 2000;176:158–161.
83. Hakala M, Niemela RK. Does autonomic nervous impairment have a role in pathophysiology of Sjogren's syndrome. *Lancet* 2000;355:1032–1033.
84. Kovacs L, Torok T, Bari F, et al. Impaired microvascular response to cholinergic stimuli in primary Sjogren's syndrome. *Ann Rheum Dis* 2000;59:48–53.
85. Bachmeyer C, Zuber M, Dupont S, et al. Adie syndrome as the initial sign of primary Sjogren syndrome. *Am J Ophthalmol* 1997;123:691–692.
86. Wright RA, Grant IA, Low PA. Autonomic neuropathy associated with sicca complex. *J Auton Nerv Syst* 1999;75:70–76.
87. Borda E, Leiros CP, Bacman S, et al. Sjogren autoantibodies modify neonatal cardiac function via M1 muscarinic acetylcholine receptor activation. *Int J Cardiol* 1999;70:23–32.
88. Bacman S, Perez LC, Sterin-Borda L, et al. Autoantibodies against lacrimal gland M3 muscarinic acetylcholine receptors in patients with primary Sjogren's syndrome. *Invest Ophthalmol Vis Sci* 1998;39:151–156.
89. Waterman SA, Gordon TP, Rischmueller M. Inhibitory effects of muscarinic receptor autoantibodies on parasympathetic neurotransmission in Sjogren's syndrome. *Arthritis Rheum* 2000;43: 1647–1654.
90. Malinow K, Yannakakis GD, Glusman SM, et al. Subacute sensory neuronopathy secondary to dorsal root ganglionitis in primary Sjogren's syndrome. *Ann Neurol* 1986;20:535—537.
91. West SG, Emlen W, Wener MH, et al. Neuropsychiatric lupus erythematosus: a 10-year prospective study on the value of diagnostic tests. *Am J Med* 1995;99:153–163.
92. Hirohata S, Miyamoto T. Increased intrathecal immunoglobulin synthesis of both kappa and lambda types in patients with systemic lupus erythematosus and central nervous system involvement. *J Rheumatol* 1986;13:715–721.
93. Golombek SJ, Graus F, Elkon KB. Autoantibodies in the cerebrospinal fluid of patients with systemic lupus erythematosus. *Arthritis Rheum* 1986;29:1090–1097.
94. Winfield JB, Shaw M, Silverman LM, et al. Intrathecal IgG synthesis and blood-brain barrier impairment in patients with systemic lupus erythematosus and central nervous system dysfunction. *Am J Med* 1983;74:837–844.
95. Mevorach D, Raz E, Steiner I. Evidence for intrathecal synthesis of autoantibodies in systemic lupus erythematosus with neurological involvement. *Lupus* 1994;3:117–121.
96. Denburg SD, Behmann SA, Carbotte RM, et al. Lymphocyte antigens in neuropsychiatric systemic lupus erythematosus. Relationship of lymphocyte antibody specificities to clinical disease. *Arthritis Rheum* 1994;37:369–375.
97. Hanly JG, Fisk JD, Eastwood B. Brain reactive autoantibodies and cognitive impairment in systemic lupus erythematosus. *Lupus* 1994;3:193–199.
98. Hanly JG, Hong C. Antibodies to brain integral membrane proteins in systemic lupus erythematosus. *J Immunol Meth* 1993;161:107–118.
99. Bluestein HG, Woods VLJ. Antineuronal antibodies in systemic lupus erythematosus. *Arthritis Rheum* 1982;25:773–778.
100. Weiner SM, Klein R, Berg PA. A longitudinal study of autoantibodies against central nervous system tissue and gangliosides in connective tissue diseases. *Rheumatol Int* 2000;19:83–88.
101. Galeazzi M, Annunziata P, Sebastiani GD, et al. Anti-ganglioside antibodies in a large cohort of European patients with systemic lupus erythematosus: clinical, serological, and HLA class II gene associations. European Concerted Action on the Immunogenetics of SLE. *J Rheumatol* 2000;27:135–141.
102. Chen Y, Wu F, Hou L, et al. Antiganglioside antibodies in cerebrospinal fluid of children with neuropsychiatric lupus erythematosus. *Chin Med J (Engl)* 1997;110:594–597.
103. Elkon KB, Bonfa E, Weissbach H, et al. Antiribosomal antibodies in SLE, infection, and following deliberate immunization. *Adv Exp Med Biol* 1994;347:81–92.
104. Arnett FC, Reveille JD, Moutsopoulos HM, et al. Ribosomal P autoantibodies in systemic lupus erythematosus. Frequencies in different ethnic groups and clinical and immunogenetic associations. *Arthritis Rheum* 1996;39:1833–1839.
105. Koren E, Reichlin MW, Koscec M, et al. Autoantibodies to the ribosomal P proteins react with a plasma membrane-related target on human cells. *J Clin Invest* 1992;89:1236–1241.
106. Hanly JG, Hong C, Smith S, et al. A prospective analysis of cognitive function and anticardiolipin antibodies in systemic lupus erythematosus. *Arthritis Rheum* 1999;42:728–734.
107. Hanly JG, Cassell K, Fisk JD. Cognitive function in systemic lupus erythematosus: results of a 5-year prospective study. *Arthritis Rheum* 1997;40:1542–1543.
108. King PH, Redden D, Palmgren JS, et al. Hu antigen specificities of ANNA-I autoantibodies in paraneoplastic neurological disease. *J Autoimmun* 1999;13:435–443.
109. Okun MS, Jummani RR, Carney PR. Antiphospholipid-associated recurrent chorea and ballism in a child with cerebral palsy. *Pediatric Neurol* 2000;23:62–63.
110. Masala C, Morino S, Zangari P, et al. Chorea in primary antiphospholipid syndrome. *Clin Neurol Neurosurg* 1996;98: 247–248.
111. Lousa M, Sanchez-Alonso S, Rodriguez-Diaz R, et al. Status epilepticus with neuron-reactive serum antibodies: response to plasma exchange. *Neurology* 2000;54:2163–2165.
112. Schneebaum AB, Singleton JD, West SG, et al. Association of psychiatric manifestations with antibodies to ribosomal P proteins in systemic lupus erythematosus. *Am J Med*1991; 90:54–62.
113. Hirohata S, Isshi K, Toyoshima S. Association between serum IgG antibodies to recombinant ribosomal P0 fusion protein and neuropsychiatric systemic lupus erythematosus. *Arthritis Rheum* 1998;41:745–747.
114. Yoshio T, Masuyama JI, Minota S, et al. Correlation of serum IgG antibodies to recombinant P0 fusion protein with IgG antibodies to carboxyl-terminal 22 synthetic peptides and carboxyl-terminal 22 amino acid-deleted recombinant P0 fusion protein in patients with systemic lupus erythematosus. *Arthritis Rheum* 1997;40:1364–1365.
115. Kozora E, Thompson LL, West SG, et al. Analysis of cognitive and psychological deficits in systemic lupus erythematosus patients without overt central nervous system disease. *Arthritis Rheum* 1996;39:2035–2045.
116. Carbotte RM, Denburg SD, Denburg JA. Cognitive dysfunction in systemic lupus erythematosus is independent of active disease. *J Rheumatol* 1995;22:863–867.
117. Carlomagno S, Migliaresi S, Ambrosone L, et al. Cognitive impairment in systemic lupus erythematosus: a follow-up study. *J Neurol* 2000;247:273–279.
118. Grant I, Heaton RK, Marcotte TD. Evaluating the neurocognitive complications of SLE. Lessons from HIV disease. *Ann Ny Acad Sci* 1997;823:18–43.
119. Miguel EC, Pereira RM, Pereira CA, et al. Psychiatric manifestations of systemic lupus erythematosus: clinical features, symptoms, and signs of central nervous system activity in 43 patients. *Medicine* 1994;73:224–232.
120. Zietz B, Reber T, Oertel M, et al. Altered function of the hypothalamic stress axes in patients with moderately active systemic lupus erythematosus. II. Dissociation between androstenedione, cortisol, or dehydroepiandrosterone and interleukin 6 or tumor necrosis factor. *J Rheumatol* 2000;27:911–918.

121. Shanks N, Moore PM, Perks P, et al. Alterations in hypothalamic-pituitary-adrenal function correlated with the onset of murine SLE in MRL +/+ and lpr/lpr mice. *Brain Behav Immun* 1999;13:348–360.
122. Hirohata S, Miyamoto T. Elevated levels of interleukin-6 in cerebrospinal fluid from patients with systemic lupus erythematosus and central nervous system involvement. *Arthritis Rheum* 1990;33:644–649.
123. Walker SE, Allen SH, Hoffman RW, et al. Prolactin: a stimulator of disease activity in systemic lupus erythematosus. *Lupus* 1995;4:3–9.
124. McMurray RW, Weidensaul D, Allen SH, et al. Efficacy of bromocriptine in an open label therapeutic trial for systemic lupus erythematosus. *J Rheumatol* 1995;22:2084–2091.
125. Fox RA, Moore PM, Isenberg DA. Neuroendocrine changes in systemic lupus erythematosus and Sjogren's syndrome. *Baillieres Clin Rheumatol* 1996;10:333–347.
126. Moore PM, Vo T, Carlock LR. Identification and cloning of a brain autoantigen in neuro-behavioral SLE. *J Neuroimmunol* 1998;82:116–125.
127. Moore PM. Neuropsychiatric systemic lupus erythematosus. Stress, stroke, and seizures. *Ann Ny Acad Sci* 1997;823:1–17.
128. Stubgen JP. Nervous system lupus mimics limbic encephalitis. *Lupus* 1998;7:557–560.

27

OTHER SEROLOGIC ABNORMALITIES IN SYSTEMIC LUPUS ERYTHEMATOSUS

FRANCISCO P. QUISMORIO, JR.

ANTIERYTHROCYTE ANTIBODIES

Antibodies to red blood cells (RBCs) are detected by the antiglobulin (i.e., Coombs') test, of which there are two variations. The direct Coombs' test measures the presence of antibodies that are bound to the surface of circulating RBCs. The antiglobulin reagent, usually rabbit or goat antibody to human gamma globulin, is added to a saline suspension of washed erythrocytes of the patient, and if the erythrocytes are coated with antibodies, cell agglutination ensues. The indirect Coombs' test measures for free anti-RBC antibody in the serum of the patient. Test serum is incubated with suspension of a mixture of washed normal group O red cells that express most of the known RBC antigens; thereafter, the cells are allowed to react with antihuman gamma globulin. Cell agglutination indicates the presence of free anti-RBC antibodies in the patient's serum.

Antiwhole human gamma globulin usually is employed as the antiglobulin reagent, but monospecific antisera to human IgG and other IgG classes, IgG subclasses, C3, and C4 also are being used. In certain situations, immune complexes that are unrelated to RBC antigens may bind to erythrocytes, giving rise to a positive direct Coombs' test.

Washed RBC from healthy nonanemic subjects has less than 14 fg IgG per 10,000 cells. Hypergammaglobulinemia of various etiology results in an increase in surface IgG, causing a positive direct Coombs' test but with no evidence of significant hemolysis. Immunoglobulin eluted from the RBCs of patients with hypergammaglobulinemia patients and the corresponding serum are negative for specific anti-RBC antibody activity (1). On the other hand, RBC eluates of patients with systemic lupus erythematosus (SLE) and polyclonal hypergammaglobulinemia as well as a positive direct Coombs' test contain anti-RBC autoantibodies. This has been interpreted to mean that the net effect of hypergammaglobulinemia on the Coombs' test is obscured by the bound anti-RBC antibodies (2).

The limited sensitivity of the antiglobulin test has led to the development of other methods with improved sensitivity, such as the enzyme-linked immunosorbent assay (ELISA) and radioassay (35); however, in most clinical laboratories, the Coombs' test remains the standard test for anti-RBC antibodies.

Characteristics Of Anti-Red Blood Cell Antibodies In Systemic Lupus Erythematosus

Autoantibodies to RBCs are classified into two major types (5) according to their thermal requirements: warm antibodies react optimally with surface membrane antigens at 37°C (6, 7), and cold-type autoantibodies react more avidly with RBC antigens at 0 to −5°C than at higher temperatures (8, 9).

Autoantibodies to RBC in SLE as well as in idiopathic autoimmune hemolytic anemia (AIHA) are predominantly warm antibodies. Warm antibodies most commonly belong to the IgG class (8). All four subclasses of IgG are represented, although IgG1 is the predominant IgG subclass while IgG2 and IgG3 are found less frequently. Warm anti-RBC antibodies belonging to IgG4 subclass are uncommon. Cold-reacting antibodies to RBCs are mostly IgM antibodies and rarely of the IgG class. A few cases of patients with SLE and hemolytic anemia associated with cold agglutinins have been reported (9, 10); the agglutinin titers in some of the patients are relatively low (10).

Warm antibodies that are bound to the surface of RBCs in vivo can be eluted and examined for biologic properties. in vitro, warm antibodies do not fix complement when allowed to react with normal allogeneic erythrocytes; however, these antibodies often are detected bound in vivo to autologous RBCs together with complement components (6, 11). in vitro, warm antibodies do not cause red-cell agglutination, cell lysis, or alteration of RBC membranes (6).

Specificity Of Anti-RBC Antibodies

In patients with idiopathic AIHA, the warm antibodies react with antigenic determinants of the Rh complex (12,

13). The specificity of warm antibodies in SLE is not completely known; however, it has been noted that warm antibodies eluted from erythrocytes containing both IgG and complement on their surface (including that from patients with idiopathic AIHA) react with Rh null cells (14, 16).

Recent investigations employing more sensitive immunochemical techniques have shown that warm antibodies (including those seen in SLE) are heterogeneous, reacting with a variety of antigens on the RBC membrane. Two minor RBC proteins that appear to be members of the Rh family as well as two major integral membrane glycoproteins (Band 3, an anion transporter and glycophorin A) have been identified as target antigens of warm anti-RBC antibodies (17, 18).

Several studies have demonstrated a significant association between anticardiolipin (aCL) antibodies and AIHA in SLE (19, 20). Sthoeger et al. (21) reported that immunoglobulin eluted from the RBCs of patients with lupus contained aCL antibody activity, suggesting that in some patients, aCL antibodies may act as anti-RBC autoantibodies, causing hemolysis. IgG aCL antibodies may bind to phospholipids of the Rh system or to the phosphatidylcholine moiety of RBC membranes.

Prevalence Of Anti-RBC Antibodies In SLE

Mongan et al. (22) examined the frequency of a positive direct Coombs' test in patients with various types of systemic rheumatic diseases. Five of 103 patients with rheumatoid arthritis (RA) and 15 (65) of 23 patients with SLE had a positive test. None of six patients with systemic sclerosis and two with polyarteritis nodosa were positive. In addition, two of three cases of thrombotic thrombocytopenic purpura and only one of 103 subjects with nonrheumatic conditions were positive. Worlledge (11) found positive antiglobulin tests in 16 (44) of 35 patients with SLE. Among normal blood donors, the frequency of a positive Coombs' test was estimated to be one in 14,000 (23).

Despite the high frequency of positive direct antiglobulin tests among patients with SLE and RA, Mongan et al. (22) found no clinical evidence of active hemolysis. This observation illustrates the frequent dissociation between abnormal serologic findings and the occurrence of tissue injury. A positive direct Coombs' test in the absence of hemolysis should be regarded as one of the multiple serologic abnormalities that frequently are seen in SLE.

Pattern Of Reaction With Antiglobulinserum

With the use of antisera of different specificities, three patterns of reactivity are commonly identified in the direct Coombs' test: (i) type I: IgG, IgM, IgA, either singly or in combination is present on the RBC surface; (ii) type II: both immunoglobulin and complement components are bound on the RBC surface; and (iii) type III: RBCs are coated with complement components (C3, C4) alone. Type I is the pattern most commonly found in patients with idiopathic AIHA, while types II and III are the patterns generally associated with SLE (11, 24, 25).

Of 180 patients with warm-type AIHA, Worlledge (26) found that 83 patients (46) had IgG coating alone on their RBCs, 64 (36) had both IgG and complement, and 33 (18) had complement coating alone. Of the 17 patients with SLE who were included in her series, none had bound IgG alone, 12 showed bound IgG and complement, and the remaining five had complement reactivity alone. Chaplin and Avioli (8) suggested that a diagnosis of SLE is unlikely in a patient with immune hemolytic anemia if complement components are not detectable on the RBC surface.

Among patients with SLE who have a positive direct Coombs' test but no evidence of overt hemolysis, 12 of 13 showed complement reactivity alone, three had both IgG and complement, and none showed IgG alone (26). Of 103 patients with RA tested, five had a positive direct Coombs' test, and all showed complement reactivity alone (22). The pattern of red-cell autosensitization in RA was confirmed by Gilliland and Turner (27), who found that 12 of 75 consecutive patients with RA who were tested reacted with anti-C antiserum exclusively. Two independent investigations established that RBCs coated with complement components alone, as determined by the standard direct Coombs' test, contain IgG antibody as well, suggesting that complement deposition is in fact antibody mediated (28, 29). Gilliland et al. (28) devised a sensitive, complement-fixing antibody consumption test, based on the principle of the antiglobulin test that detected as few as 20 IgG molecules on the red-cell surface. On the other hand, MacKenzie and Creevy (29) detected IgG antibody on the surface of complement-coated RBCs when the standard Coombs' test was performed at 4° but not at 37°C. The IgG antibody was not eluted from RBCs at 37°C; however, it apparently underwent a thermal-dependent conformational change so that agglutination with the Coombs' antiglobulin reagent did not occur. Patients with SLE and combined warm-reacting IgG and cold-reacting IgM anti-RBC antibodies have been reported (30, 31) (see Chapter 43, Infections in Systemic Lupus Erythematosus).

Pathophysiology Of Immune Hemolytic Anemia

The pathogenesis of RBC damage by anti-RBC autoantibodies has been extensively investigated (32,35). Erythrocytes that are sensitized with warm-reactive IgG antibodies are cleared from the circulation by macrophages in the splenic sinusoids. Macrophages express surface receptors for the Fc portion of the IgG molecule and C3b fragment of complement. The macrophage Fc receptors bind erythrocytes with bound IgG anti-RBC antibody, causing membrane damage, spherocytosis, and phagocytosis of some

RBCs. Microspherocytes have a shortened life span because of their increased rigidity and increased osmotic fragility. As the amount of surface-bound antibody increases, splenic trapping becomes more efficient, and red-cell survival shortens significantly. When the density of bound IgG antibody is substantial, complement activation occurs. RBCs coated with IgG and complement are cleared by two distinct macrophage receptors, the C3b and Fc receptors, causing an accelerated clearance of RBCs from the circulation that results in extravascular hemolysis. Sequestration of sensitized RBCs by hepatic macrophages with complement but no Fc receptors also may occur at this stage.

The IgG subclass of the anti-RBC antibody is an important determinant in RBC destruction, because splenic macrophages have IgG Fc receptors for IgG1 and IgG3 subclasses. The macrophage FcR avidity for IgG3 is greater than that for IgG2 antibodies. RBCs with critical quantities of IgG1 and/or IgG3 antibodies on their surface are destroyed. It has been calculated that RBCs coated with IgG1 antibody alone or with additional IgG2 and IgG4 antibodies require at least 2,000 molecules per each RBC to initiate phagocytosis or rosette formation with monocytes in vitro. In contrast, as few as 230 molecules of IgG3 anti-RBC antibodies per each RBC are required for binding to monocytes (36). Moreover, the clearance of RBCs that are sensitized with IgG antibody and complement is accelerated, and IgG1 and IgG3 antibodies fix complement efficiently while IgG2 antibodies are less efficient and IgG4 antibodies do not activate complement.

Erythrocytes coated with increased amounts of IgM and IgA in addition to warm IgG anti-RBC antibodies are more predisposed to hemolysis than are RBCs coated with IgG antibodies alone (37). Erythrocytes coated with IgM anti-RBC antibody, as in the case of cold hemagglutinin disease, are cleared by a mechanism that is dependent on complement activation. IgM-coated RBCs bind to C3b receptors of macrophages and are cleared rapidly in the liver (38, 39). When the amount of IgM antibody on the RBC surface is high, complement activation is rapid and extensive so that the terminal components of complement become activated, resulting in intravascular hemolysis (Table 27.1).

TABLE 27.1. ANTIERYTHROCYTE ANTIBODIES IN SYSTEMIC LUPUS ERYTHEMATOSUS (SLE)

1. A positive direct Coombs' test in the absence of active hemolysis is a frequent serologic finding.
2. The direct Coombs' test frequently shows reactivity with complement alone or with immunoglobulin plus complement.
3. Antierythrocyte antibodies in SLE are IgG antibodies, warm type, and react with a variety of antigens on the RBC surface.
4. These antibodies can be associated with significant hemolysis in some patients.

RBC, red blood cell.

PLATELET ANTIBODIES

A special relationship exists between SLE and chronic immune thrombocytopenic purpura (ITP), both of which primarily afflict young women. Some patients with thrombocytopenic purpura that is labeled as idiopathic at the onset later develop classic SLE (40, 41), suggesting that ITP may be an early manifestation of the disease. Further, a thrombocytopenic purpura that is indistinguishable from chronic ITP may develop during the course of SLE. Thrombocytopenia in SLE, as in chronic ITP, is caused by increased peripheral destruction of platelets brought about by autoimmune mechanisms. Platelet survival studies in SLE with 51Cr-labeled platelets have demonstrated shortened life span (42).

In 1953, Harrington et al. (43) transfused normal human volunteers with plasma from patients with chronic ITP and noted a significant and prompt drop in platelet counts. Autologous plasma from chronic ITP subjects, obtained during disease exacerbations and then stored, produced thrombocytopenia when reinfused into the same patients during periods of disease remission (44). The humoral antibody nature of the antiplatelet factor in this disorder has been established, and Shulman et al. (44) showed that the factor was a 7S gamma globulin, reactive to autologous as well as to allogeneic platelets, and produced in vivo effects both quantitatively and qualitatively similar to those exhibited by known antiplatelet antibodies. These findings indicate that the platelet-depressing factor in the plasma is an antiplatelet antibody.

Similar plasma transfusion experiments have not been performed in patients with SLE and thrombocytopenia. However, Nathan and Snapper (45) reported an analogous situation in a premature infant born of a mother with SLE who at the time of delivery had thrombocytopenia. At birth, the infant had low platelet counts, which persisted until 3 weeks of age. Both mother and infant had platelet agglutinins and positive lupus erythematosus (LE)-cell tests. It was suggested that transplacental transfer of both platelet antibody and antinuclear antibody (ANA) had occurred from the mother to the baby.

Tests For Antiplatelet Antibodies In Systemic Lupus Erythematosus

Although the transfusion experiments provided a strong argument for the autoimmune nature of chronic ITP, some investigators remain unconvinced, because reliable in vitro tests for the detection of antiplatelet antibodies are not available. Over the years, many in vitro tests have been introduced, indicating that a test of reasonable specificity, reproducibility, and sensitivity has yet to become widely accepted. Of the many in vitro tests for antiplatelet antibodies, few have been employed in SLE. Those that have include platelet agglutination (46, 47), direct antiglobulin consumption test

(48, 49), dextran agglutination test (50), platelet factor III method (51), the indirect immunofluorescence method (52-54), direct platelet immunofluorescence test, immunobead (55), and more recently the monoclonal antibody-specific immobilization of platelet antigens (MAIPA) (56, 57).

Karpatkin and Siskind (58) introduced the platelet factor III immunoinjury technique to detect antiplatelet antibodies in SLE and chronic ITP. The method is based on the property of antiplatelet antibodies to damage normal platelets, releasing factor III. In turn, this factor is made available to the coagulation cascade, and its effect is measured as a shortening of the clotting time. The gamma globulin fraction of serum isolated by ammonium sulfate precipitation rather than whole serum was tested for antiplatelet antibodies, and with this sensitive method, they found platelet antibodies in 65 of patients with chronic ITP (of whom 96 were thrombocytopenic at the time of testing). The antiplatelet antibody was removed with prior incubation of the serum using rabbit antihuman IgG or absorption with normal human platelets. Further, the antiplatelet activity can be eluted from normal platelets after prior incubation with positive, but not with negative, serum (51). Karpatkin and Lackner (59) suggested that patients with SLE who test positive for antiplatelet antibodies but have normal platelet counts represent a subset of patients with a compensated thrombocytolytic state, in which an increased turnover of platelets is compensated for by increased platelet production. On the other hand, Kutti and et al. (60) showed that the abnormal values of platelet factor III assay in nonthrombopenic patients with SLE correlated with the amount of circulating immune complexes, suggesting that the assay measured not only antiplatelet antibodies but also immune complexes that presumably bind to surface Fc receptors.

The direct antiglobulin consumption test detects the presence of gamma globulin that is fixed onto the surface of platelets. Used extensively by early workers, this test appears to be sensitive, but it is technically complex and may yield false-positive results (61). Van de Wiel et al. (49) found that 13 of 23 patients with chronic ITP and all of six patients with SLE and thrombocytopenia were positive by this test. Dausett et al. (48) reported that 46 of 93 patients with chronic ITP and 23 of 24 patients with SLE were positive.

Pujol et al. (54) found a high prevalence (62%) of antiplatelet antibodies in 90 consecutive patients with SLE, especially in those with active disease, using a platelet immunofluorescence method. The antibodies were predominantly IgG, although IgM and IgA isotypes also were detected in some patients. Except for thrombocytopenia, the presence of platelet antibodies was not associated with other disease manifestations.

Platelet-Bound Igg In SLE

In 1975, Dixon et al. (62) introduced a quantitative method of measuring the IgG bound on the surface of platelets that is based on the inhibition of complement lysis. All of 17 patients with chronic ITP showed an elevated level of platelet-associated IgG when compared with that of healthy controls. Moreover, an inverse relationship between platelet count and the concentration of platelet-associated IgG was observed both before and during drug therapy. These observations were soon confirmed by several investigators using other methods of measuring platelet-bound IgG (63, 64).

Platelet-associated IgG has been shown to be increased in practically all patients with SLE and thrombocytopenia (65–68). Kelton et al. (67) reported an inverse correlation between platelet count and platelet-associated IgG in 10 thrombocytopenic patients with SLE. Mulshine et al. (68) confirmed this inverse relationship and further observed that patients with SLE and normal platelet counts had platelet-associated IgG levels even lower than those seen in normal controls. Conversely, Bonacossa et al. (69) found an elevated level of platelet-bound IgG in patients with SLE and normal platelet counts. Subjects with high amounts of platelet-associated IgG had significantly more anti-DNA antibodies than those with normal or slightly elevated levels of platelet-bound IgG. However, they found no correlation between disease activity and platelet-bound IgG.

The IgG antiplatelet antibodies in the sera of patients with chronic ITP appear to be restricted to the IgG3 subclass (70), whereas in SLE sera, all four IgG subclasses are represented (71). Conversely, all four IgG subclasses are bound *in vivo* to platelets of patients with chronic ITP, suggesting that circulating antiplatelet IgG and platelet-associated IgG may represent different populations of platelet antibodies (72, 73). The nature of the platelet-associated IgG is not completely known. It may represent IgG antibody bound to platelet-specific surface antigens (i.e., autoantigens), IgG antibody bound to HLA or blood group antigens or to exogenous antigens absorbed on the surface of platelets, IgG nonspecifically fixed to damaged platelets, or circulating immune complexes attached to platelet surface Fc receptors (63, 74).

McMillan (75) showed that IgG platelet antibodies that are synthesized by splenic lymphocyte cultures of patients with chronic ITP bind to platelets through their Fab terminus, indicating a specific antibody reaction. Moreover, eluates from platelets of the same patients contain IgG that bind to normal allogeneic platelets. Kelton et al. (76) reported that the increased amounts of platelet-associated IgG in malaria were partly caused by the binding of IgG-specific antibody to malarial antigens absorbed on the surface of platelets. Thrombocytopenic purpura in patients infected with human immunodeficiency virus is associated with increased platelet-associated IgG. Walsh et al. (77) presented evidence to show that the platelet-associated IgG in these patients does not result from bound antiplatelet antibodies but rather from the deposition of complement and immune complexes onto the surface of platelets. Samuel et al. (78) reported higher amounts of platelet-associated IgG, C3 and C4 in thrombocytopenia-associated immune complex disease including SLE, human immunodeficiency virus (HIV) infection, and chronic liver disease than in classic ITP.

The nature of platelet-associated IgG in SLE has not been fully studied, but it may in part represent bound immune complexes (63). This is supported by the observation that the antiplatelet antibody found in SLE sera fixes complement, unlike that found in the sera of patients with chronic ITP, which is noncomplement fixing (71). Moreover, preformed complexes of DNAanti-DNA antibodies bind to the surface of platelets (79). Puram et al. (80) noted a positive relationship between platelet counts in SLE with immune complexlike material in serum, as measured by polyethylene glycol precipitation, but not with platelet-associated IgG. On the other hand, no correlation was evident between the level of circulating immune complexes as measured by C1q binding (69) or Raji-cell assay (59) and the amount of platelet-bound IgG in SLE, indicating that platelet-bound IgG is not entirely caused by antigenantibody complexes. Kurata et al. (81) reported an ether elution method of differentiating between platelet-specific antibodies and bound immune complexes, and they showed that eluates from platelets of patients with SLE contain specific antiplatelet antibodies.

Elevated levels of platelet-associated IgG are not necessarily diagnostic of chronic ITP or thrombocytopenia as a result of SLE. High levels can be seen in patients with thrombocytopenia that is considered to be nonimmune in origin (63) as well as in some patients with normal platelet counts (69). Conversely, a diagnosis of ITP is unlikely in a patient with thrombocytopenia if the platelet-associated IgG level is low or normal.

Specificity Of Antiplatelet Antibodies In SLE

To date, a limited number of studies have examined the antigenic specificity of autoantibodies to platelets in SLE (82–84). Multiple platelet antigens, including surface membrane and cytoplasmic proteins, have been identified, implying heterogeneity of these antibodies in SLE.

Howe and Lynch (83) examined the binding specificities of circulating antiplatelet antibodies in SLE by Western blotting. All patients with SLE who were thrombocytopenic and had increased amounts of platelet-bound IgG had serum antibodies that reacted with platelet protein fractions having molecular weights of 120 and 80 kd. Patients with SLE and normal platelet counts but with elevated platelet-associated IgG also were positive for serum antiplatelet antibodies. Absorption of sera with whole platelets or platelet lysates removed the antibody activity. The binding pattern was found to be relatively specific for SLE and was not seen in healthy controls. Sera from patients with chronic ITP reacted with multiple platelet fractions but with no consistent pattern, unlike that seen in SLE, suggesting that the specificities of platelet antibodies in the two conditions are different.

Using a similar methodology, Kaplan et al. (84) confirmed the presence of serum antibodies to platelets in three of ten thrombocytopenic patients with SLE. The antigens involved were cytoplasmic proteins from normal platelets with molecular weights of 108 and 66 kd, respectively. Tomiyama et al. (85) identified the 120 kd antigen to be vinculin, a cytoplasmic platelet protein. Antivinculin antibodies were found to be prevalent not only in patients with immune thrombocytopenia (70) but also in healthy subjects (40), suggesting that these are naturally occurring antibodies. The pathogenetic role of these antibodies remains to be determined.

In chronic ITP, target antigens of circulating antiplatelet antibodies as well as platelet-bound IgG have been identified by immunoblotting and by using monoclonal antibodies. Antigenic epitopes on the GPIIb-IIIa complex (CD41/CD61) have been the most frequently observed, while GP Ib/IX and GPIa/IIa antigens also have been reported (86, 87, 88). These glycoproteins belong to a complex of membrane proteins on the surface of platelets, termed integrins, that function as receptors for fibrinogen, fibronectin, collagen, and other extracellular matrix components that are important in hemostasis.

Berchtold et al. (82) examined the specificity of antiplatelet antibodies in patients with disease-related immune thrombocytopenia, including SLE, other connective tissue diseases, and lymphomas. Autoantibodies against platelet GPIIb-IIIa complex were found in patients with SLE and in mixed connective tissue disease and Sjogren's syndrome, showing that the specificity of the antiplatelet antibodies in some patients with systemic rheumatic diseases is similar to that seen in patients with chronic ITP (Table 27.2). The presence of specific antibodies against GP IIb-IIIa and to other platelet glycoproteins in SLE has been confirmed by other investigators (55, 56, 89). Serum antibodies to platelet membrane antigens (GP IIb-IIa, GP Ib-

TABLE 27.2. PLATELET ANTIBODIES IN SYSTEMIC LUPUS ERYTHEMATOSUS (SLE)

1. *In vitro* tests for platelet antibodies, such as immunofluorescence, direct antiglobulin consumption test, and monoclonal antibody-specific immobilizatoion of platelet antigens frequently are positive in SLE. These tests are of limited clinical application.
2. Tests that measure platelet-associated IgG are widely used and show elevated values in practically all patients with SLE and thrombocytopenia as well as in some patients with normal platelet count.
3. The nature of platelet-associated IgG is not completely known, but it probably represents specific antiplatelet antibodies and bound immune complexes.

ICX, GP Ia-IIa, and GP IV) were found to more prevalent in thrombocytopenic SLE patients than in those patients with normal platelet counts (89), however other investigators have failed to confirm this association (56). Prospective studies are needed to determine the clinical significance of these antibodies in SLE.

Antiphospholipid Antibodies And Antiplatelet Antibodies

The presence of antiphospholipid antibodies, including aCL, and lupus anticoagulant in SLE is strongly associated with thrombocytopenia (see Chapter 28, Pathomechanisms of Cutaneous Lupus Erythematosus). For this reason, it has been hypothesized that aCL may cross-react with platelet phospholipids, resulting in inactivation and/or subsequent sequestration in the reticuloendothelial system. Rupin et al. (89) examined the significance of specific platelet antibodies and aCL in patients with SLE and thrombocytopenia, and although one half of their patients with low platelet counts tested positive for aCL, the thrombocytopenia correlated better with the presence of serum IgG antibody to an 80-kd platelet antigen. Moreover, absorption of the serum with platelets removed the aCL activity in only one half of the sera with antiplatelet antibodies. Jouhikainen et al. (91) examined 71 consecutive patients with SLE for platelet antibodies by immunoblotting. The most common antibody found reacted with a 65-kd platelet antigen, and its presence was significantly associated with lupus anticoagulant, a history of thrombocytopenia, and thrombosis, especially arterial occlusions. Out et al. (92) observed that IgG eluted from the platelets of patients with SLE had antibody activity against negatively charged phospholipids. Nevertheless, there was no evidence of the *in vivo* activation of platelets, and platelet aggregation was not impaired. By adsorption experiments, Lipp et al. (55) have shown that antiphospholipid antibodies and antiglycoprotein antibodies (GPIIb-IIA and GPIb-IX) in chronic ITP and in SLE with thrombocytopenia have distinct specificities and do not cross-react.

These data indicate a heterogeneity of platelet antibodies in SLE, some of which cross-react with cardiolipin phospholipids and some with specific platelet glycoproteins, as well as other membrane and cytoplasmic antigens. Further studies to characterize the antigens and to clarify the relative importance of the different antibodies in the pathogenesis of the thrombocytopenia are needed.

ANTINEUTROPHIL ANTIBODIES

The frequent occurrence of leukopenia in SLE, possibly mediated by immunologic processes similar to those described in autoimmune hemolytic anemia or autoimmune thrombocytopenia, led to investigations on the presence of antileukocyte antibodies. Various conventional serologic methods, such as agglutination, complement fixation, antiglobulin consumption test, and cytotoxicity, have been used (93). Early studies employed whole leukocyte preparations rather than purified fractions (e.g., lymphocyte subsets) as substrate, and differences in their specificity and sensitivity make it difficult to compare results of the various tests. Further, the presence of isoantibodies against leukocytes, which may be a consequence of multiple pregnancies and/or blood transfusions, must be differentiated from genuine leukocyte antibodies when interpreting the results.

Technical improvements in the fractionation of peripheral blood leukocytes led to the development of new procedures to detect antibodies to lymphocytes. In 1970, Mittal et al. (94) employed the lymphocyte microcytotoxicity test, which was developed for histocompatibility testing, for the detection of cytotoxic antibodies to lymphocytes in SLE. They found a high prevalence of specific lymphocytotoxic antibodies in SLE, and this observation soon was confirmed independently by other workers (95–97) (see Chapter 26, Autoantibodies, Autoantigens, and Nervous System). In contrast, techniques to detect specific immune reactions to granulocytes have been more difficult to standardize (98).

Tests for antineutrophil antibodies fall into two major types: immunochemical and functional (98). The former detects immunoglobulins that are bound to the surface of the patient's neutrophils (i.e., direct test) or free antibodies in the serum (i.e., indirect test) using normal allogeneic neutrophils as substrate. When interpreting the results of these tests, immune complexes binding via Fc and complement receptors on leukocytes should be excluded from the binding of specific antineutrophil antibodies. The latter type measures *in vitro* sequelae of granulocyte antibodies such as lysis of sensitized cells, phagocytosis, and so on. Flourescence flow cytometry has been adapted for measuring IgG antineutrophil antibodies, and a study using this method found that sera from nonneutropenic patients with SLE as well as patients with other connective tissue diseases show significant binding (99).

Both IgM- and IgG-specific antineutrophil autoantibodies have been found in SLE. Drew and Terasaki (100) described cytotoxic granulocyte-specific antibodies in 53 of 57 patients with SLE using a panel of 70 granulocytes from random normal persons. The antibodies were of IgM class, complement fixing, exhibited optimum activity at 4°C, and were present in ten healthy, nonimmunized individuals. The clinical significance of these antibodies in SLE was not examined. Starkebaum et al. (101) studied the mechanism of neutropenia in a patient with SLE and found increased amounts of IgG bound on the surface of polymorphonuclear neutrophils (PMNs). The patient's serum caused opsonization of normal neutrophils for ingestion by other neutrophils. In addition, fractionation of the serum showed that both immune complexes and monomeric IgG antineutrophil bound to PMNs; however, only the latter caused opsonization of neutrophils.

The F(ab)2 fragment of the IgG reacted to the PMNs, confirming the true antibody activity (102). Although IgG neutrophil-binding activity of serum was found to be common in SLE, there was no association between the level and neutropenia (102). Two independent groups of investigators confirmed the absence of correlation between neutrophil count in SLE and the titer of PMN-binding IgG in the serum (103–104). In contrast, there is some correlation between antilymphocyte antibody titers and lymphopenia (see Chapter 29, Cutaneous Manifestations of Lupus Erythematosus). However, the ability of SLE sera to opsonize normal PMNs to be phagocytosed by monocytes (103), as well as the capacity of serum antineutrophil antibodies to fix C3 on allogeneic normal PMNs, were both found to be correlated inversely with neutrophil count in SLE.

Specificity Of Antineutrophil Antibodies

The specificity of antineutrophil antibodies in SLE was examined by Sipos et al. (105) using Western immunoblots. The antibodies reacted with two membrane antigens with molecular weights of 50 to 60 kd and of 30 kd, respectively. Moreover, the antineutrophil antibodies inhibited the binding of mouse monoclonal antibodies to CD15 (granulocyte antigen) and CD16 (FcR) to normal neutrophils. Whether the antigens seen in the immunoblots are identical to CD15 or CD16, however, remains to be clarified.

The lack of correlation between titer of antineutrophil antibodies and neutrophil count suggests that factors other than antineutrophil antibodies are important in the pathogenesis of neutropenia in SLE. Antibody-coated PMNs may remain in the circulation longer because of the defective reticuloendothelial function in SLE. The role of antibody avidity, specificity, and the density of membrane antigens may be important. A study of neutrophil kinetics is needed to determine whether peripheral destruction of neutrophils in SLE is compensated for by increased production, such that the net result is a normal peripheral neutrophil count (Table 27.3).

Kurien et al. (106) found a correlation between neutropenia and the presence of anti-Ro antibodies in SLE. Anti-Ro antibodies were shown to bind to neutrophils and thus, can potentially induce cell injury via complement activation. However, they found that the antigen bound on the surface of neutrophils was not the 60-kd Ro but instead a 64-kd membrane protein called "D1", an antigen associated with autoimmune thyroid disease. Inhibition studies showed serologic cross-reactivity between the two antigens, implying that anti-Ro antibodies may be important in the pathogenesis of granulocytopenia.

TABLE 27.3. ANTINEUTROPHIL ANTIBODIES IN SYSTEMIC LUPUS ERYTHEMATOSUS (SLE)

1. Circulating antineutrophil antibodies are prevalent in SLE; however, the antibody titer does not correlate with the neutrophil count.
2. Ability of SLE sera to opsonize as well as to fix C3 on normal allogeneic PMNs is inversely correlated with the neutrophil count.
3. Most antineutrophil antibodies are directed to surface antigens on polymorphonuclear cells; however, some react with cytoplasm of PMNs. P-ANCAs may be found, but not C-ANCAs.

ANCA, antigen(s) of human neutrophils and monocytes; PMN, polymorphonuclear neutrophils.

Antineutrophil Cytoplasmic Antibodies

Autoantibodies directed against cytoplasmic antigen(s) of human neutrophils and monocytes (ANCA) are associated with Wegener's granulomatosis, microscopic polyangiitis, and other primary systemic small-vessel vasculitides (107, 108). These antibodies are detected by the indirect immunofluorescent test using ethanol-fixed normal neutrophils as substrate. Four fluorescent patterns are seen: a classic cytoplasmic (C-ANCA), atypical C-ANCA, a perinuclear with or without nuclear extension (P-ANCA), and atypical ANCA. (109). C-ANCA are detected in most patients with Wegener's granulomatosis and react with proteinase 3, although other antigens also are involved. P-ANCAs are found in patients with idiopathic, necrotizing, crescentic glomerulonephritis and polyarteritis nodosa and react predominantly with myeloperoxidase, a lysosomal enzyme, although other antigens such as elastase, cathepsin G, lactoferrin, and azurocidin are involved as well (110, 108). ANA may interfere with interpretation of the immunofluorescent test for P-ANCA (111). All serum samples containing ANCA should be tested for specific antibodies to proteinase-3 and myeloperoxidase by ELISA.

None of 96 patients with SLE studied by Nassberger et al. (112) using the immunofluorescent test had C-ANCA, while 93 had ANA. Antimyeloperoxidase antibodies were found in 21 of the patients by a specific ELISA test. Serum titers generally were low, and presence of the antibody did not correlate with any particular disease feature. Other investigators have reported serum titer of antimyeloperoxidase antibodies in 9% of patients with lupus (113). Both antibodies to elastase and to myeloperoxidase were found to be prevalent in hydralazine-induced LE (112).

Lactoferrin is a single-chain glycoprotein that is present in many body secretions and derived primarily from neutrophils; it is located in the secondary granules of these cells. IgG antilactoferrin antibodies are reported in five to 39 of patients with SLE (114, 115), and IgM antilactoferrin antibodies are present in ten of these patients (115). IgG antilactoferrin antibodies are more prevalent in patients with active disease and appear to be associated with adenopathy and crescentic glomerulonephritis (114).

Schnabel et al. (116) found ANCA in 40 of 157 (25%) patients with SLE. Only P-ANCA was found. The specificities of the SLE antibodies were directed to lactoferrin, elastase, and lyzozyme. No reactivity to myeloperoxidase or to proteinase 3 was detected. More importantly, there was no correlation between P-ANCA with organ system involvement, including lupus vasculitis. Other investigators confirmed the lack of correlation between ANCA, disease activity, and clinical features of SLE (111, 117). In contrast, a study of a large cohort of European patients with SLE showed correlation of ANCA and antilactoferrin with certain clinical manifestations including serositis, livedo reticualris, thrombosis, and arthritis. However, anticardiolipin and anti-Ro antibodies were more closely correlated than ANCA with these features (118). Antibodies to lysozyme were found in one third of 44 patients with SLE in another study (119).

A 5-year prospective controlled study of ANCA in a large number of patients with various connective-tissue diseases including SLE and healthy controls showed a high prevalence of P-ANCA and atypical ANCA. P-ANCA was associated with the presence of antinuclear antibodies. None had C-ANCA and specific antibodies to proteinase-3 rarely were found (120).

Thus, the presence of C-ANCA and antibodies to proteinase-3 suggests a systemic vasculitic disease other than SLE. P-ANCA, however, can be found in patients with SLE as well as in patients with other conditions.

RHEUMATOID FACTORS

Rheumatoid factors (RFs) comprise a heterogenous group of antibodies that are reactive with antigenic determinants on the Fc portion of human or animal IgG. Although RFs belonging to the IgM class are the most commonly measured isotype by clinical tests, RFs belonging to the IgA, IgG, IgD, and IgE classes have been identified (121, 122). RFs can react with autologous and isologous as well as homologous IgG.

Serum RFs are measured by a variety of serologic methods, including agglutination, ELISA, radioimmunoassay, and nephelometry. Agglutination tests such as the latex fixation test preferentially measure IgM RFs that are reactive with human IgG. The sheep-cell agglutination test (SCAT) measures IgM RFs using rabbit IgG as an antigen. Clinical laboratories prefer nephelometry over the latex fixation test, because the former is automated and less labor intensive.

Prevalence Of RFS In SLE

The prevalence of RFs in large series of patients with SLE as measured by the latex fixation test varies from 20 to 60 (mean, 33). Singer (123) reviewed several earlier reports and found that 20.5 of tested patients with SLE were positive. Estes and Christian (124) found a positive latex fixation test in 21 of their 150 patients. The serum antibody titer was relatively low, and unlike RA, in which the titer persists, most of their patients did not have a sustained titer. Lee et al. (125) reported positive tests for RFs in 36.7 of 110 patients with SLE. In 31.2 of their patients, the titer was equal to or greater than 1:160, and in 28.8, the serum titer was greater than 1:320. On the other hand, Feinglass et al. (126) described a higher frequency of RFs among their patients with SLE; 61 of their 122 patients had a positive latex fixation test. In agreement with other studies, the RF titers were modest, with a titer of 1:80 seen in one half of the patients. Further, the serum titer fluctuated intermittently in patients in whom serial determinations were performed.

The SCAT for RFs is less sensitive than the latex fixation test, but a positive SCAT is considered to be more characteristic of RA (122). None of 25 patients with SLE studied by Cathcart et al. (127) had a positive SCAT, and only three patients had borderline titers of less than 1:32.

RFs belonging to isotypes other than IgM are not commonly seen in SLE. If present, they tend to have lower serum titers than those observed in patients with RA. IgG RFs, which are implicated in the pathogenesis of synovitis and extraarticular lesions of RA such as vasculitis, generally are absent in SLE (128, 129). IgE RFs that also are associated with the extraarticular manifestations of RA are not seen in SLE (130, 131). Dunne et al. (132) found elevated levels of IgA RFs in the sera of patients with RA, Sjgren's syndrome, and SLE. The serum level of IgA RFs in SLE was lower than that in RA.

The major RF cross-reactive idiotype (RF-CRI) is a public idiotype defined by human IgM RF paraproteins. RF-CRI is expressed in adult and juvenile RA. In SLE, Bonagura et al. (133) found RF-CRI to correlate with the presence of anti–double-stranded DNA (anti-dsDNA) antibodies and disease activity.

Potential Significance Of Rheumatoid Factors In Systemic Lupus Erythematosus

In vitro experiments as well as studies in experimental animal models point to a dual effect of RFs on immune-mediated tissue injury. On one hand, RFs have been shown to exert protective effects by competing with complement for binding to immune complexes (134, 135). RFs binding to antigenantibody complexes may result in more efficient removal from the circulation by the reticuloendothelial system (136, 137). Bolton et al. (138) showed that RFs blocked the attachment of C3 to aggregated IgG and the formation of C3b capable of reacting with the C3b receptors of glomeruli *in vitro*. This phenomenon potentially can shield the glomerulus from deposition of pathogenic immune complexes.

Conversely, others have found RFs to enhance immune-mediated tissue injury in different experimental animal models (139). Floyd and Tesar (139) showed that the administration of IgM RFs aggravated cutaneous Arthus reaction in animals. RFs and immune complexes injected into the mesenteric arteries of rats induced thrombosis and hemorrhage (140). Another series of experiments (141–143) showed that RFs bind *in situ* to immune complexes that are bound to renal glomeruli in experimental glomerulonephritis. These investigators postulated that bound RFs subsequently act as an immunosorbent, trapping circulating antigenantibody complexes that may be unrelated to the initial renal insult and, by fixing complement, contribute to the chronicity of the renal disease. Birchmore et al. (144) noted that RFs enhanced the binding of DNAanti-DNA immune complexes to C3b receptors on red blood cells *in vitro* by fixing complement by way of its own Fc region. Their finding suggests that RFs may potentiate renal injury in SLE.

Miyazaki et al. (145) found IgM, IgA, and IgG RFs in the serum of five patients with diffuse lupus nephritis, but not in two patients with membranous lupus nephritis. More importantly, they observed the binding of fluorescein-labeled normal human IgG and Fc fragment, but not F(ab)2 fragment, to the renal glomeruli in diffuse lupus glomerulonephritis. No binding was observed in membranous lupus nephritis or in IgA nephropathy. They interpreted this to mean RF activity was present in the glomerular deposits that bind the labeled IgG, suggesting that RFs may be important in the development of diffuse lupus nephritis. This study confirms earlier observations by Agnello et al. (146), who showed glomerular deposits of IgM RFs in lupus nephritis by reacting fluorescein-labeled aggregated human IgG and antiidiotypic antibody to RFs with renal biopsy specimens.

Clinical Correlates Of Rheumatoid Factors In Systemic Lupus Erythematosus

Which of the many and varied biologic effects of RFs *in vitro* or in experimental models are important in the pathogenesis of lesions in SLE remains to be seen. Nevertheless, several investigators have examined clinical correlates of RFs in SLE. In 1966, Davis and Bollet (147) noted that nephritis was less prevalent in a group of patients with SLE who were RF positive by the latex fixation test. They suggested that RFs exerted a protective role *in vivo* in SLE and other diseases of immune complex deposition. A retrospective analysis of their patients confirmed their initial observation, and in addition, they found that patients with SLE who are RF negative and cryoglobulin positive are likely to develop renal disease, whereas those who are RF positive and cryoglobulin negative are unlikely to do so (148). Hill et al. (149) found that patients with SLE and nephritis who were RF positive (by latex fixation test) had milder morphologic renal lesions compared with RF-negative patients with SLE and nephritis. This protective effect of RFs on lupus nephritis was likewise observed in a study using the SCAT for measuring RFs (150), and Corke (151) found that in patients with SLE, proteinuria was less frequent in RF-positive than in RF-negative patients. Mustakallio et al. (152) described a negative correlation between RFs and anemia, skin disease, and the LE-cell test. Moreover, the RF-positive patients with SLE tended to have a more benign and chronic clinical course. A multicenter European study of 1,000 patients with SLE found RF in 180 patients (18) and was associated with higher prevalence of discoid skin rash, sicca syndrome, and a lower prevalence of nephropathy (28 vs. 41) (153).

In the foregoing studies, the tests used for detecting RFs preferentially measured IgM RFs. Tarkowski and Westerberg (154) used an ELISA assay to measure the different isotypes of RFs in SLE and found that the presence and serum level of IgG RFs, IgA RFs, and IgM RFs correlated significantly with the absence of renal disease.

Witte et al. (155) confirmed this negative association and in addition found that the presence of IgA RF defined a clinical subset characterized by sicca syndrome, anti-Ro and anti-La antibodies and HLA DR3.

Other investigators, however, have failed to confirm a protective role of RFs in SLE nephritis or in other organ involvement (156) Kantor et al. (157) measured RFs in 51 consecutive patients with SLE and found that the frequency as well as the antibody titer of RFs in those with nephritis did not differ from those without clinical renal disease. Baldwin et al. (158) confirmed these observations and found that the presence of RFs was not associated with histologic type of nephritis. Estes and Christian (124) reported that the frequency of renal disease as well as the 5-year survival rate of RF-positive patients with SLE did not differ from those of the general SLE population. Two other studies using the SCAT for RFs (159) and radioimmunoassay for IgM, IgA, and IgG RF isotypes (160) failed to find a protective effect from RFs on the development of nephritis (see Chapter 50, Lupus Nephritis: Pathology, Pathogenesis, Clinical Correlations, and Prognosis).

Certain observations not only refute the protective role of RFs but in fact point to their participation in the pathogenesis of tissue lesions in SLE. Cryoglobulins, which represent a subset of circulating immune complexes in SLE, often contain RF activity. Agnello et al. (146) identified RFs in the glomerular immune deposits of patients with SLE and nephritis, hypocomplementemia, and cryoglobulinemia. Deposition of antiglobulins (including RFs) in the renal glomeruli was observed in lupus nephritis and in other types of glomerulonephritis, and their presence appeared to be associated with a relatively severe renal injury (161, 162). My own group has found that immune deposits in the walls of pulmonary arteries in patients with SLE and pulmonary hypertension were eluted when incubated with aggregated human IgG, suggesting the presence of RFs in the vascular immune deposits (163).

In addition to renal disease, a correlation between RFs and other clinical features of SLE has been examined.

Moutsopoulos et al. (164) described a high frequency of RFs in patients with SLE and histologic evidence of sicca syndrome on lip biopsy. The prevalence of RFs in 35 patients with SLE positive for anti-Ro/SSA antibody (66) was significantly higher than that in 77 such patients negative for anti-Ro/SSA antibody (7). Zizic et al. (165) reported a high frequency of RFs among patients with SLE presenting with acute abdomen secondary to vasculitis and/or serositis. My own group as well as other investigators have found a high prevalence of RFs in patients with SLE presenting with pulmonary hypertension (163, 166).

Conversely, Feinglass et al. (126) observed no correlation between RFs and neuropsychiatric involvement in SLE. Patients with SLE and a persistently positive latex fixation test for RFs tended to have less severe clinical manifestations of the disease, were less likely to have received high-dose steroids or cytotoxic drugs for treatment, and were less likely to have had an episode of herpes zoster than patients with SLE who had persistently negative or inconsistently positive tests for RFs (167).

The discrepancy in the results of various investigations on the relationship between RFs and lupus nephritis or SLE in general probably is caused by several factors such as differences in the methods used to measure RFs, selection of patients, ascertainment of activity of the renal disease, and the retrospective design of most of the studies. In addition, the titer of the RFs may fluctuate or even disappear along the course of the illness, thus the timing of the test will affect the result of the study. Moreover, it now is well recognized that RFs are heterogenous with respect to the immunoglobulin class, reactivity with IgG of different species, complement-fixing property, avidity, and other characteristics. Conceivably, varying types of RFs may differ in their effects on renal disease and other tissue lesions. My own group's observations, showing that IgM RFs specific for rabbit IgG correlate positively with arthritis and negatively with other clinical manifestations, suggest a dual effect of RF (168).

Rheumatoid Factors Cross-Reactive With Nuclear Antigens

In 1963, McCormick and Day (169) observed that exhaustive absorption of certain sera containing both RF and ANA activities with aggregated gamma globulin removed the RF activity and was accompanied by a substantial loss of ANA titer. They suspected that the phenomenon was caused by the presence of IgG ANAs associated with the IgM RFs as an immune complex. Subsequently, Hannestad (170) and Hannestad and Johannessen (171) established that this was not caused by complexed IgG ANAs, but rather by the dual reactivity of certain polyclonal IgM RFs with both IgG and nuclear antigens. Other investigators have confirmed these findings (172) and showed that isolated IgM RFs reacts with DNAhistone complex (173, 174), with histones (175), and/or with nonhistone nuclear polypeptides (176). Cross-reactive IgM RFs have been found most frequently in patients with RA and in some cases of overlap syndromes and mixed connective-tissue disease (173). Kinoshita et al. (177) found IgM RFs that are cross-reactive with single-stranded DNA to be prevalent in a variety of rheumatic diseases, including SLE; however, the serum titer was highest among patients with RA and extraarticular features. Johnson (172) suggested that the cross-reactive IgM RFs are of limited immunopathogenic significance, because such antibodies are noncomplement fixing, react optimally at pH 8 or 9, and fail to bind at pH 6.5. The explanation for the reactivity of human RF with histones is not entirely clear, but recent evidence suggests multifunctional combining regions on RF for human IgG and histones with distinct binding sites located in the variable regions (178) (Table 27.4).

TABLE 27.4. RHEUMATOID FACTORS (RFS) IN SYSTEMIC LUPUS ERYTHEMATOSUS (SLE)

1. The latex fixation test for IgM RFs is positive in 33% of patients with SLE. Serum titers generally are lower than those seen in patients with RA, tend to fluctuate, and may become negative.
2. RFs have been identified in serum cryoglobulins and glomerular deposits of some patients with SLE.
3. The hypothesis that renal disease tends to be less frequent and less severe in RF-positive than in RF-negative patients with SLE has not been confirmed consistently by other investigators and remains controversial.
4. IgM RFs that are cross-reactive with nuclear antigens, including ssDNA and histone, are found in SLE, RA, and other rheumatic conditions.

ssDNA, single-stranded DNA.

CRYOGLOBULINS IN SYSTEMIC LUPUS ERYTHEMATOSUS

It has long been recognized that serum specimens from certain groups of patients develop a precipitate spontaneously when they are allowed to incubate in a test tube at low temperatures. Lerner et al. (179) described this phenomenon in patients with leukemia, pneumonia, bacterial endocarditis, and other diagnoses. Having identified gamma globulin as the serum protein fraction that reversibly precipitates at 5°C, the term cryoglobulin was introduced to refer to the cold-insoluble precipitates.

Frequency Of Cryoglobulins In SLE

Barr et al. (180) examined sera from patients with various diagnoses as well as from normal subjects for cryoprecipitation. Sera from eight of 121 patients, but none from 57 healthy controls, had significant amounts of cryoglobulins. Three of the six patients with SLE in this early series had cryoglobulins. Christian et al. (181) reported the presence of cryoglobulins in 10 of 12 patients with SLE, with protein concentrations ranging from 7 to 38 mg/dL. In a larger series, Stastny and Ziff (182) studied 137 sera from 31 patients with SLE; 37 sera from 11 patients had cryoglobulins. Lee and Rivero (183) observed cryoglobulinemia in nine of 57 SLE sera, while Barnett et al. (184) found cryoglobulins in 16 of 18 unselected SLE sera.

Components Of Cryoglobulins

Immunochemical analysis of the cryoprecipitate (185) has revealed three major types of cryoglobulins. Type I cryoglobulins consist of a single monoclonal immunoglobulin: IgG, IgM, IgA, or Bence Jones protein. Type I cryoglobulins are associated with lymphoproliferative disorders. Type II cryoglobulins are mixed cryoglobulins with one of the components being a monoclonal immunoglobulin. Monoclonal IgM with polyclonal IgG is the most common combination, and frequently, the monoclonal component has antiimmunoglobulin (i.e., RF) activity. Type II cryoglobulins are found in patients with chronic hepatitis C infection, lymphoproliferative diseases, Sjogren' syndrome, and autoimmune disorders. Type III cryoglobulins are mixed cryoglobulins with polyclonal components. This type is the most common and is associated with infections and autoimmune disorders such as SLE, RA, and systemic sclerosis. Types II and III may contain RF, other autoantibodies, and complement components C1q, C3, and C4.

Hanauer and Christian (186) analyzed isolated serum cryoprecipitates from six subjects with SLE and observed that these consisted largely of IgG, IgM, and C1q. When the washed cryoglobulins were used as immunogens in rabbits, the resulting antiserum reacted with IgG, IgM, C1q, and 2-macroglobulin. Some of the antisera also reacted with C4, C3, and IgA.

Barnett et al. (187) found IgG and IgM in all 156 SLE cryoprecipitates they studied. Eleven contained IgA and C3. Stastny and Ziff (182) reported that IgM was not a prominent component in SLE cryoprecipitates and that the complex consisted mainly of IgG and C1q. Although IgG was the predominant immunoglobulin, relatively more IgM than IgG was concentrated when compared with the corresponding immunoglobulin levels (188).

The formation of cryoprecipitates in SLE sera requires the presence of C1q (181). Prior incubation of SLE serum at 56°C for 30 minutes to inactivate complement resulted in the loss of cryoprecipitability, which was restored when either fresh human serum or purified C1q was added to the test serum.

Fibronectin, which is a normal plasma protein and a major cell surface membrane protein of fibroblasts, is a component of cryoglobulins from patients with connective tissue diseases and other illnesses (189–191) Plasma fibronectin can bind to other molecules, such as collagen, fibrin, and heparin, and the binding may result in formation of a precipitate at low temperatures. Kono et al. (192) showed that fibronectin is capable of binding to C1q, including C1q that is fixed to immune complexes. Because fibronectin and C1q frequently coprecipitate in SLE cryoglobulins, this reaction and/or binding of fibronectin to other serum proteins may be important in the formation of cryoglobulins.

Clinical Correlates Of Cryoglobulinemia In SLE

Cryoglobulinemia is associated with clinical disease activity. Eight of 11 patients with cryoglobulins reported by Stastny and Ziff (182) had active nephritis, and the remaining three had evidence of extrarenal involvement. Nine of the 12 patients with cryoglobulins studied by Christian et al. (181) had active nephritis. Cryoglobulinemia in SLE also has been associated with reduced serum levels of C3 and C1q (193). Cryoglobulins and RF have independent and opposite association with lupus myelitis (148).

Cryoglobulins As Circulating Immune Complexes

The association between cryoglobulinemia, disease activity, and hypocomplementemia in SLE led to investigations on the potential pathogenicity of the cryoprecipitates. Mixed cryoglobulins are considered to represent circulating immune complexes for several reasons. In certain conditions, such as essential mixed cryoglobulinemia, the property of cryoprecipitability does not reside on either moiety of the cryoglobulin; it requires combination of the separated components (194). Complement components are required for cryoprecipitability, and further, isolated cryoglobulins have the property of activating the complement system (195, 196). Cryoglobulins isolated from the sera of patients with lupus nephritis activate the complement system *in vitro* either through the classic or alternative pathway (197).

Despite similarities in immunoglobulin content, SLE cryoglobulins differ from RA cryoglobulins in their complement-binding property. Whereas SLE cryoglobulins frequently bind C1q *in vitro*, isolated RA cryoglobulins do not (188). This difference may reflect varying properties of the antigenantibody systems that involved in cryoglobulin formation in the two conditions.

Antibody Activity Of SLE Cryoglobulins

The deposition of ANAs and their corresponding antigens in target organs has been implicated in the pathogenesis of organ injury in SLE. Cryoprecipitates in patients with SLE during periods of disease activity may represent circulating immune complexes of ANAs and nuclear antigens. Lee and

Rivero (183) found no ANA activity in the cryoprecipitates of nine SLE sera that contained high titers of ANAs. Stastny and Ziff (182) reported ANA IgG component in two out of three SLE cryoglobulins tested; however, they failed to find a preferential concentration of ANAs in the cryoglobulins. Conversely, Winfield et al. (195) found that SLE cryoglobulins were highly enriched with antibodies to single-stranded DNA (ssDNA) and double-stranded DNA (dsDNA) and, less frequently, with antiribonucleoprotein antibodies relative to the concentration of these autoantibodies in the corresponding sera. Erhart et al. (188) confirmed these findings and reported that 95 of isolated SLE cryoglobulins studied contained antibodies to dsDNA.

Hanauer and Christian (186) found anti-IgG antibody (i.e., RF) in SLE cryoglobulins, and this finding has been confirmed by several investigators (146, 199–201). In addition, RF activity was found to be preferentially enriched in the cryoprecipitates when compared with the antibody activity of the matching serum specimen (199, 200). Similarly, cold-reactive IgM antilymphocyte antibodies were found to be selectively concentrated in SLE cryoglobulins (199, 200). Lymphocytotoxic activity of SLE cryoglobulins did not correlate with clinical severity of the disease, serum complement level, or serum titer of anti-DNA antibody (201).

Specific Antigens In SLE Cryoglobulins

To identify specific antigens that may be complexed with corresponding antibody in the cryoprecipitate, experimental animals were immunized with cryoprecipitates isolated from patients with SLE (186). After absorption with pooled normal human serum, anti-SLE cryoglobulin antisera did not recognize any unique antigens, except for two antisera that contained antibody activity against intrinsic determinants in IgM molecules. Using a similar approach, Klippel et al. (202) detected reactivity of anti-SLE cryoglobulin antiserum against lymphocytes, suggesting that lymphocyte membrane antigens or antigens that cross-react with cell surface determinants were present in SLE cryoprecipitates. McPhaul and Montgomery (203) found that anti-SLE cryoglobulin antisera reacted not only against nuclear antigens but also with reticulin and idiotypic determinants of immunoglobulin deposits in the renal glomeruli. These observations indicate the multiplicity of antigenantibody systems that are involved in the formation of cryoglobulins in SLE.

Lee and Rivero (183) reported the presence of DNA in SLE cryoprecipitates in only one of nine specimens using ultraviolet light absorption, diphenylamine reaction, and immunoprecipitation. Employing specific antiserum to ssDNA, Barnett et al. (184) identified DNA in two of 16 SLE cryoprecipitates. The DNA was demonstrable only with prior heating of the specimen, presumably to denature the DNA. In contrast, Davis et al. (204) identified DNA in most SLE cryoglobulins they tested, but only after digestion of the precipitate with pronase, suggesting the DNA was bound to anti-DNA antibodies and thus was inaccessible to biochemical or immunologic detection. The major portion of the DNAanti-DNA antibody system in cryoglobulin from patients with lupus nephritis consists predominantly of low-molecular-weight complexes (205).

The presence of DNA in cryoprecipitates is not specific for SLE. DNA also has been identified in cryoglobulins isolated from patients with bacterial endocarditis, Sjgren's syndrome, and non-SLE glomerulonephritis (206, 207). Free DNA has been demonstrated in the sera of normal individuals (206), patients receiving high doses of corticosteroids for a variety of medical conditions, and patients undergoing cardiac surgery (208, 209). Not only was DNA found in non-SLE cryoglobulins, but Roberts and Lewis (210, 211) identified anti-DNA activity in cryoglobulins isolated from patients with nonlupus glomerulonephritis, bacterial infections, and essential cryoglobulinemia. IgG anti-DNA antibody was demonstrable in cryoglobulins after preincubation of the precipitate in acid buffer or after digestion with deoxyribonuclease, suggesting that anti-DNA antibody in the cryoglobulin was bound to antigen.

It now is recognized that the syndrome of mixed cryoglobulinemia is strongly associated with chronic hepatitis C infection (212, 213). Hepatitis C virus, polyclonal IgG, and monoclonal RF have been identified in isolated cryoprecipitates, and these represent pathogenic immune complexes that become deposited in the blood vessels of target organs. Studies have shown no association between hepatitis C infection and SLE, and hepatitis C infection is not the primary etiology of cryoglobulinemia in lupus patients (214).

Pathogenetic Significance Of Cryoglobulins

In addition to complement activation, mixed cryoglobulins possess other biologic properties that suggest a potential pathogenic role. Intradermal injection of redissolved cryoglobulins in unsensitized animals caused localized skin edema, erythema, and hemorrhage within 24 hours, and intravenous administration caused either anaphylaxis or a glomerulitis (215). Whitsed and Penny (216) described the development of a cutaneous vasculitis following intradermal injection of autologous cryoglobulin into the clinically normal skin of a patient with mixed cryoglobulinemia. Deposition of cryoglobulin in target organs *in vivo* is supported by the demonstration of a distinctive crystalline fibrillar structure in renal glomeruli that was identical to that found in the serum cryoglobulins of the same patient with essential mixed cryoglobulinemia. Using an antiidiotypic antibody, Agnello et al. (146) demonstrated the deposition of IgM RF moiety of cryoglobulin in the renal glomeruli of a patient with SLE nephritis.

Cryoglobulins may contribute to the susceptibility of patients with SLE to bacterial infections. Nivend et al.

TABLE 27.5. CRYOGLOBULINS IN SYSTEMIC LUPUS ERYTHEMATOSUS (SLE)

1. Serum cryoglobulins in SLE usually are type III (mixed polyclonal) consisting of immunoglobulins, complement components, and fibronectin.
2. Elevated levels of serum cryoglobulins are associated with hypocomplementemia and clinical disease activity, especially active nephritis.
3. Cryoglobulins represent cold-precipitable, circulating immune complexes. ANAs (including anti-DNA), antilymphocyte antibodies, RFs, as well as DNA and lymphocyte antigens have been identified in SLE cryoglobulins.

ANA, antinuclear antibody; RF, rheumatoid factor.

(217) found that the impairment of opsonization of *Staphylococcus aureus* by SLE serum was associated with cryoglobulinemia. When the cryoglobulin fraction of the immune complexes was removed from the SLE serum, normal opsonic capacity was observed. Moreover, reduction of opsonic property was transferred with SLE cryoglobulins to normal serum. The binding of cryoglobulins to protein A of *Staphylococcus* sp. probably blocked contact between surface receptors of phagocytic cells and opsonized organisms, resulting in defective phagocytosis and killing (Table 27.5).

THE LUPUS ERYTHEMATOSUS CELL

In February 1946, Dr. Malcolm M. Hargraves, a hematologist at the Mayo Clinic, examined bone marrow aspirate from a boy with an obscure medical problem. Part of his report (130) read:

"The outstanding thing in this bone marrow is the phagocytic reticuloendothelial cells which contain a blue-staining material which we have not previously observed. Some cells are markedly filled with this material gathered together in round vacuoles or droplets. An occasional cell has been ruptured, with the material in discrete globules scattered out among the other cells. This material stains from a light blue to a very dark, almost indigo blue. There is an occasional reticuloendothelial cell that has other phagocytized material as well as that noted above, but most of the reticuloendothelial cells involved seem to be specifically concerned with this material and do not show other phagocytic activities."

On learning that the patient probably had SLE, Dr. Hargraves went on to examine bone-marrow specimens in the next 4 days from two other patients with definite SLE. He observed that the striking feature is the marked phagocytic activity of neutrophils containing a muddy purple homogenous material. Some of the cells are so filled with the material that the nucleus is crowded to the periphery.

This is the initial description of the LE cell, and 2 years later, Hargraves et al. (218) reported their experience in 25 patients with SLE and noted the frequent appearance of the LE cell in acute cases. The inclusion body of the LE cells as well as the extracellular material stained with Feulgen stain showed that both contained DNA and were presumed to be nuclear in origin. Hargraves et al. postulated that phagocytosis of the material resulted in the formation of LE cells.

The LE-cell phenomenon occurs *in vitro* during the incubation of peripheral blood or bone marrow aspirate. It is completed in two distinct stages (Fig. 27.1), with the initial phase involving the immunologic reaction of the LE-cell factor that is present in the serum of patients with the nuclear material of damaged or traumatized leukocytes. Trauma allows the nuclear penetration of the LE-cell factor, and the reaction leads to nuclear swelling accompanied by the disintegration of the normal chromatin pattern and basophilia. The altered nucleus then detaches itself from the cytoplasm and appears as a free extracellular LE body. In the second stage, the LE body is engulfed by a neutrophil (or occasionally a monocyte) in the presence of complement. The cytoplasm remains outside and is not taken up by the phagocyte (219). When stained with Wright's stain, the globular inclusion body appears as a homogenous, pale blue to deep purplish material, pushing the nucleus of the phagocyte to one side of the cell (Fig. 27.2).

In 1951, Lee et al. (220) observed a striking morphologic resemblance of the LE-cell inclusion body to the hematoxylin bodies found in the tissues of patients with SLE at autopsy. The latter, described earlier by Klemperer et al. (221), consisted of altered nuclear material containing DNA in a depolymerized state. The LE-cell inclusion body and the tissue-bound hematoxylin body were found to have diminished affinity for methyl green, which is a dye that binds stoichiometrically with DNA. Studies by Godman

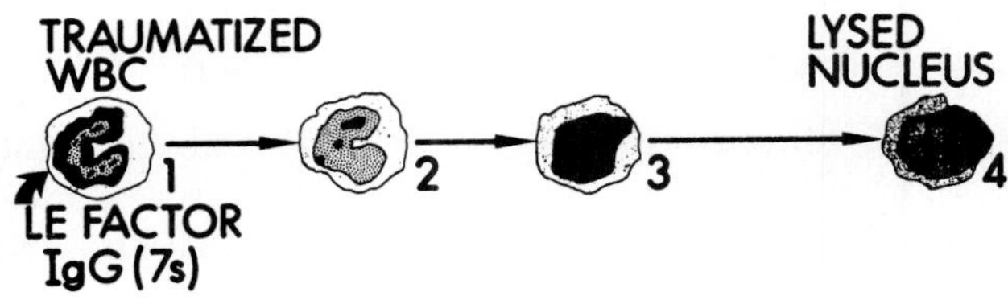

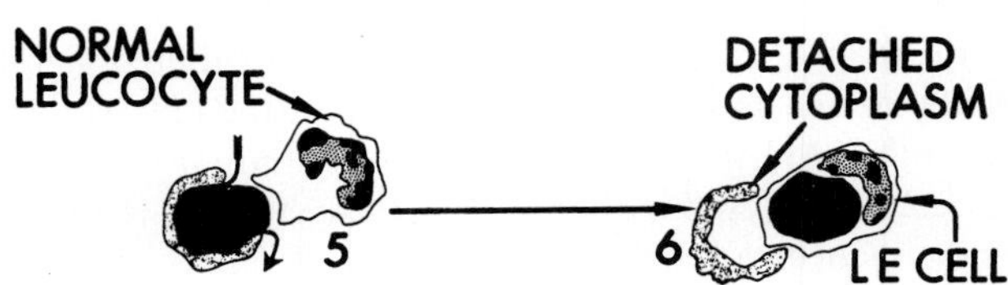

FIGURE 27.1. Scheme of the lupus erythematosus cell formation.

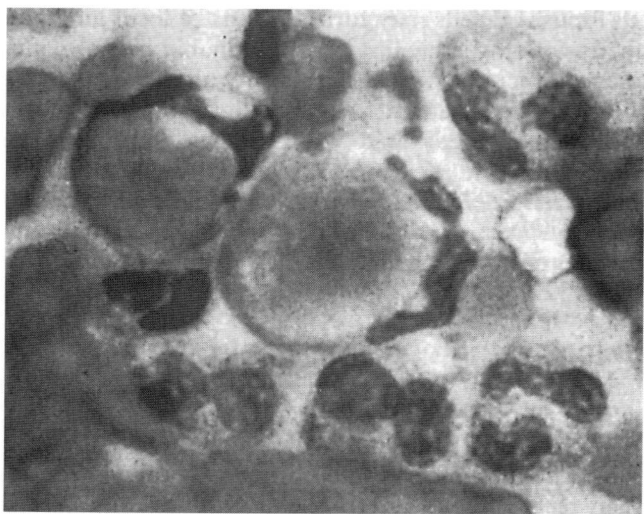

FIGURE 27.2. Two typical lupus erythematosus cells (1,700).

and Deitch (222) have established that the diminished affinity is not a result of DNA polymerization but rather of interference by proteins that are bound to the DNA moiety of the inclusion body.

Lupus Erythematosus-Cell Factor

Haserick et al. (223) fractionated SLE plasma by electrophoresis and identified the serum factor that participated in the LE-cell phenomenon as gamma globulin, implying that it is an antibody. Other investigators, using ultracentrifugation and chromatography separation methods, confirmed the LE factor to be a serum 7S gamma globulin (224, 225), while the 19S was inactive. Subsequent studies established that IgG but not IgM antibody to deoxyribonucleoprotein induces LE-cell formation *in vitro* (226).

Lupus Erythematosus-Cell Antigen

In 1960, Miescher and Fauconnet (227) noted that the capacity of SLE serum to induce LE cells *in vitro* diminished when the serum was preabsorbed with nuclei isolated from human leukocytes. This observation as well as the information that the LE-cell factor is a gamma globulin led to definitive investigations that established the ANA activity of the LE-cell factor. Application of the fluorescent antibody technique by Friou et al. (228) contributed significantly to our understanding the nature of the LE-cell factor and other ANAs. In a series of elegant studies, Holman et al. (229–231) established that the LE-cell factor is an antibody to deoxyribonucleoprotein of cell nuclei, requiring both DNA and histone for the reaction.

More than 50 years after its description, Schett et al. (232), using highly purified antigens and a series of immunoprecipitation and immunoblotting and blocking experiments, recently has identified histone H1 as the major antigen involved in the LE-cell phenomenon. In addition, they have shown that a positive LE-cell prep correlated not only with antihistone 1 antibody measured by ELISA test, but also with active disease with major organ involvement. (232, 233).

Role Of Complement In Lupus Erythematosus-Cell Formation

In 1959, Aisenberg (234) reported that the incubation of SLE serum at 56°C for 30 minutes diminished its capacity to induce LE-cell formation in an indirect LE-cell test. Instead of classical LE cells, the preparation instead showed homogenous, globular, purplish extracellular material. Addition of fresh human serum to isolated cell nuclei complexed with LE-cell factor caused formation of LE cells in the presence of viable phagocytes. This observation suggested that a heat-labile factor in normal serum is required for completion of the LE cell. It remained for Golden and McDuffie (226) and MacDuffie et al. (235) to establish the importance of complement in the LE-cell phenomenon. Frozen and thawed human leukocytes were incubated with gamma-globulin fraction of SLE serum containing anti-deoxyribonucleoprotein antibody. Viable leukocytes then were added to the system to complete the second, or phagocytic, stage of the LE-cell phenomenon. Typical LE cells formed even after thorough washing of the phagocytes and the leukocyte nuclei with saline. These investigators assumed that small amounts of complement remained adherent to the viable phagocytes. Nevertheless, when antiserum to human C3 was added to the system, there was inhibition of LE-cell formation; addition of excess fresh human serum abrogated the inhibitory effect of anti-C3 antiserum. Thus, complement clearly is required for the second stage of the LE-cell phenomenon, and the amount that is required probably is relatively small.

Extracellular Nuclear Material

Extracellular basophilic aggregates of amorphous or ovoid shape sometimes are seen in LE-cell preparations. This extracellular material (ECM), sometimes referred to as a hematoxylin body, may occur either alone or accompanied by typical LE cells. It has been assumed that ECMs represent products of the initial stage of the LE-cell phenomenon (i.e., complex of the LE-cell factor and nucleoprotein) left unphagocytosed. Arterberry et al. (236) found hematoxylin bodies without typical LE cells in 358 out of 3,000 patients with various diagnoses who underwent an LE-cell test. Three morphologic types were identified: (i) homogenous round hematoxylin body, (ii) a lacy type, and (iii) an amorphous variety. The homogenous round body was the most common, being found in 259 patients. Forty-five percent of patients in this group had definite SLE, and another 46% had RA or some disease variant.

By block titration of serum, Golden and McDuffie (226) have shown that the number of LE cells produced by lupus serum decreases as the number of ECMs increases while keeping the amount of complement and number of viable phagocytes constant in the indirect LE-cell test. IgG and IgM antideoxyribonucleoprotein antibodies were purified, and both antibody preparations produced ECMs. In contrast, only IgG antibody had the property to induce the classic LE cell. McDuffie et al. (235) suggest that the inability to induce typical LE cells may be related to the lack of complement-fixing property of IgM antideoxyribonucleoprotein antibody.

In Vivo Occurrence Of Lupus Erythematosus Cells

The LE-cell factor and most other ANAs are not capable of penetrating intact and viable cells to react with their corresponding antigens in the nuclei. Lachmann (219) observed no morphologic changes in actively dividing HeLa cells when grown in tissue culture medium containing lupus serum. Rapp (238) showed that ANAs reacted with the nuclei of air-dried, but not viable, HeLa cells. Direct smears of the peripheral blood of patients with SLE showed absence of *in vivo* binding of immunoglobulin with the nuclei of leukocytes (239). However, *in vivo* LE cells occasionally have been described in direct smears of pericardial fluid (240), pleural fluid (241), joint fluid (242), ascitic fluid (243), and cerebrospinal fluid (244) of patients with lupus. LE cells may form in areas of local inflammation, as within the pleural cavity, probably because of the presence of leukocytes that are subtly altered or damaged to allow nuclear penetration by the IgG antideoxyribonucleoprotein antibody to form LE bodies. These damaged leukocytes may appear to be active and viable by morphologic criteria (245). Phagocytosis of the LE bodies by polymorphonuclear leukocytes or by macrophages will complete the reaction to form classic, and sometimes atypical, LE cells (246).

Clinical Significance Of The Lupus Erythematosus Cell

The LE-cell test has largely been abandoned as a routine clinical test and supplanted by the fluorescent test for ANAs. The LE-cell test is labor intensive, and it requires a skilled technician to interpret the cytology. Atypical LE cells are seen not infrequently in clot preparations, and some observers may report this as a positive test while others will not unless classic LE cells also are present. Among the many modifications that were developed to increase the yield and/or to improve the cytology, the heparinized rotary glass bead method, the 2-hour clot test, and the combined rotated and washed clot technique were the major procedures used for several years. The American Society of Clinical Pathologists recently has endorsed that the LE-cell test (CPT No. 85544) be abandoned in favor of more definitive, quantitative immunologic tests for SLE (247).

The frequency of a positive LE-cell test in SLE varies with the method of testing used, the frequency of performing the test, and the duration of time that the patient is studied. At some point during the course of the illness, the rotary glass bead LE-cell test was positive in 75.7 of 520 patients with SLE who were studied by Dubois and Tuffanelli (248). With combined rotary glass-bead and washed-clot methods, LE cells were found in approximately 90 of the patients.

Despite the high frequency in SLE, it now is well recognized that a positive LE-cell test is not entirely specific for the disease. Positive LE-cell tests have been reported in five to ten of adult patients with RA and in a smaller percentage of patients with systemic sclerosis, polymyositis, polyarteritis nodosa, and mixed connective-tissue disease (93, 249–252). LE cells have been described in drug reactions secondary to penicillin (253–257), tetracycline (258), chlorpromazine (259), anticonvulsants (252), hydralazine (252), and procainamide (260) (see Chapter 47, The Mother in Systemic Lupus Erythematosus). LE cells have been found in a case of intermittent hydrarthrosis with positive ANAs (261), in lupoid hepatitis (262–264), in two cases of lymphoma with no autopsy evidence of SLE (265), and in DiGuglielmo's disease (acute erythroleukemia) (266).

Positive Lupus Erythematosus-Cell Test With Negative ANAS

There have been occasional reports of cases in which the LE-cell test is positive despite a negative fluorescent test for ANAs (266). Koller et al. (267) found 20 cases among a large group of patients tested for LE cells. Five met the criteria for SLE, seven had RA, and three had drug reactions. Wallace and Metzger (268) described two patients with biopsy-proven, cutaneous mild SLE with major organ involvement who had positive LE-cell and negative ANA tests using both rat liver and Hep-2 cells.

The explanation for this discrepancy in most of the cases that have been studied is not entirely clear (266). Nevertheless, when the clinical picture of a patient is compatible with or highly suspicious for SLE and the standard fluorescent test for ANA (FANA) is negative (after using multiple substrates), an LE-cell test should be ordered to corroborate the diagnosis (269). In addition, other tests that may be of value in this situation include the lupus band test on nonlesional skin and serologic tests for anti-Ro/SSA antibody and ELISA test for antihistone 1 antibody.

Table 27.6 summarizes information about the LE cells. Because positive LE cell tests are rare in patients without rheumatic disease, its presence in a patient with a low-titer, positive ANA may be confirmatory of lupus. (The reader is

TABLE 27.6. THE LUPUS ERYTHEMATOSUS (LE) CELL

1. The LE cell is induced *in vitro* by an IgG antibody to deoxyribonucleoprotein (LE-cell factor) and has specificity for histone H1
2. The LE-cell factor reacts with the nuclear material of traumatized white blood cells to form a hematoxylin body. Phagocytosis of the hematoxylin body by a viable phagocyte in the presence of complement leads to the formation of classic LE cells.
3. *In vivo* LE cells may be seen in pleural, pericardial, synovial, ascitic, blister fluid, and the cerebrospinal fluid of patients with systemic lupus erythematosus.
4. The LE-cell test is positive in 90% of all patients with SLE at some time during the disease course. A positive LE-cell test may be seen in other conditions, including rheumatoid arthritis, scleroderma, mixed connective tissue disease, lupoid hepatitis, and drug-induced LE

referred to pages 211 to 226 of the third edition of this textbook for a detailed description of LE-cell methodologies.)

ANTIENDOTHELIAL CELL ANTIBODIES

Antiendothelial cell antibodies (AECA) were first reported in 1971 by Linqvist and Osterland (270) using an indirect immunofluorescent test with mouse kidney sections as substrate. Since then, AECA have been reported in SLE, systemic vasculitis, other connective tissue diseases and inflammatory conditions (271). Several different techniques are used to measure AECA including cellular ELISA, cytofluorometry, microcytotoxicity, Western blot analysis using cell extracts, and immunoprecipitation of radiolabelled endothelial proteins. Human umbilical vein endothelial cells commonly are used as substrate.

AECA are a heterogenous group of antibodies that bind to a number of vascular endothelium cell antigens including surface-membrane proteins, nuclear and cytoplasmic antigens. However, nuclear and cytoplasmic components may represent contaminants released or exposed when endothelial cells are disrupted or fixed to prepare the antigen preparation in certain test systems for AECA. Westphal et al. (272) showed that an ELISA test using fixed cultured endothelial cells detected antibodies not only to cell surface antigens but to intracellular components including DNA, histones, and cytoskeletelal proteins. On the other hand, flow cytometry analysis using unfixed endothelial cells detected antibodies to endothelial cell surface antigens.

AECA bind to endothelial cells from arteries, veins, and human and murine endothelial cell lines, and cross-react with fibroblasts and peripheral blood mononuclear cells (273, 274). The specific target antigens in endothelial cells recognized by AECA are not known. Del Papa et al. (275) found AECA in SLE sera reacted with a heterogenous series of endothelial-cell surface antigens including four proteins with molecular weights of 200, 180, 155, and 25 kd. Further characterization of these antigens is needed to better understand the pathogenic significance of AECA in SLE.

Clinical Association Of AECA In Systemic Lupus Erythematosus

AECA are prevalent in SLE and have been reported by various investigators in 39% to 93% of patients (276). The wide range of prevalence rate is in part a result of the difference in the test method used and in the selection of patients. D'Cruz and associates (277) showed that AECA were associated with active lupus nephritis and the highest serum antibody titers were found in patients with both nephritis and vasculitis. There was no correlation between AECA levels and anti-dsDNA, antineutrophil cytoplasmic antibodies, and other antinuclear antibodies. The association of AECA and lupus nephritis has been confirmed by other investigators (274).

Arterial and venous thrombosis and anticardiolipin antibodies also have been reported to be associated with AECA in SLE (271), however other investigators have failed to observe correlation with anticardiolipin antibodies (277). Yoshio et al. (279) found elevated titers of AECA in SLE patients with pulmonary hypertension, Raynaud's phenomenon, and digital vasculitis.

A prospective study in a small group of SLE patients for 25 months showed that the serum level of AECA can serve as a marker of disease activity. In some patients, a rise in the serum titer of AECA was the only serologic marker of disease exacerbation when the serum C3 and anti-dsDNA levels remained unchanged (280).

Pathogenic Signficance Of AECA In SLE

The clinical association between AECA, active nephritis, and vasculitis led investigators to propose a role of AECA in the pathogenesis of vascular damage in SLE. Carvalho and coworkers (281) have shown that purified IgG isolated from SLE sera containing AECA up-regulated the expression of adhesion molecules and leukocyte adhesion to endothelial cells. AECA induced the release of interleukin-1 and another mediator that stimulates endothelial cells in an autocrine manner. AECA in patients with Wegener's granulomatosis also have been shown to exhibit similar *in vitro* activity and in addition induced the secretion of IL-1beta, IL-6, IL-8, and MCP-1 (282). Based on these observations, it is proposed that AECA induce vascular damage in SLE and other systemic vasculitides by activating endothelial cells and facilitating leukocyte recruitment and adhesion.

REFERENCES

1. Huh YO, Liu FJ, Rogge K, et al. Positive direct antiglobulin test and high serum immunoglobulin G values. *Am J Clin Pathol* 1988;89:197–200.
2. Heddle NM, Kelton JG, Turchyn KL, et al. Hypergammaglobulinemia can be associated with a positive direct antiglobulin test, a non-reactive eluate and no evidence of hemolysis. *Transfusion* 1988;28:29–33.
3. Hansen OP, Hansen TM, Jans H, et al. Red blood cell membrane-bound IgG: demonstration of antibodies in patients with autoimmune hemolytic anemia and immune complexes in patients with rheumatic diseases. *Clin Lab Haematol* 1984;6:341–349.
4. Leikola J, Perkins HA. Enzyme-linked antiglobulin test: an accurate and simple method to quantify red cell antibodies. *Transfusion* 1980;20:138–144.
5. Yam P, Petz LD, Spath P. Detection of IgG sensitization of red cells with I125 staphylococcal protein A. *Am J Hematol* 1982;12:337–346.
6. Axelson JA, LoBuglio AF. Immune hemolytic anemia. *Med Clin North Am* 1980;64:597–606.
7. Schreiber AD. Autoimmune hemolytic anemia. *Pediatr Clin North Am* 1980;27:253–267.
8. Chaplin H, Avioli LV. Autoimmune hemolytic anemia. *Arch Intern Med* 1977;137:346–352.
9. Dubois EL. Acquired hemolytic anemia as presenting syndrome of lupus erythematosus disseminatus. *Am J Med* 1952;22:197–204.
10. Videbaek A. Auto-immune haemolytic anaemia in systemic lupus erythematosus. *Acta Med Scand* 1962;171:187–194.
11. Worlledge SM. Annotation: the interpretation of a positive direct antiglobulin test. *Br J Haematol* 1978;39:157–168.
12. Dacie JV. Autoimmune hemolytic anemia. *Arch Intern Med* 1975;135:1293–1308.
13. Vos GH, Petz LD, Fudenberg HH. Specificity and immunoglobulin characteristics of autoantibodies in acquired hemolytic anemia. *J Immunol* 1971;106:1172–1176.
14. Leddy JP, Peterson P, Yeaw MA, et al. Patterns of serologic specificity of human gamma G erythrocyte autoantibodies: correlation of antibody specificity with complement-fixing behavior. *J Immunol* 1970;105:677–683.
15. Budman DR, Steinberg AD. Hematologic aspects of systemic lupus erythematosus. Current concepts. *Ann Intern Med* 1977;86:220–226.
16. Cines DB. Antibodies reactive with surface membranes of cellular elements in the blood. *Hum Pathol* 1983;14:429–441.
17. Barker RN, Casswell KM, Reid ME, et al. Identification of autoantigens in autoimmune hemolytic anaemia by a non-radioisotope immunoprecipitation method. *Br J Haematol* 1992;82:126–132.
18. Leddy JP, Falany JL, Kissel GE, et al. Erythrocyte membrane proteins reactive with human (warm reacting) anti-red cell autoantibodies. *J Clin Invest* 1993;91:1672–1680.
19. Fong KY, Loizou S, Boey ML, et al. Anticardiolipin antibodies, haemolytic anaemia and thrombocytopenia in systemic lupus erythematosus. *Br J Rheumatol* 1992;31:453–455.
20. Deleze M, Alarcon-Segovia D, Oria CV, et al. Hemocytopenia in systemic lupus erythematosus. Relationship to antiphospholipid antibodies. *J Rheumatol* 1989;16:926–930.
21. Sthoeger Z, Sthoeger D, Green L, et al. The role of anticardiolipin autoantibodies in the pathogeneis of autoimmune hemolytic anemia in systemic lupus erythematosus. *J Rheumatol* 1993;20:2058–2061.
22. Mongan ES, Leddy JP, Atwater EC, et al. Direct antiglobulin (Coombs) reactions in patients with connective tissue diseases. *Arthritis Rheum* 1967;10:502–508.
23. Gorst DW, Rawlinson VI, Merry RH, et al. Positive direct antiglobulin test in normal individuals. *Vox Sang* 1989;398:99–105.
24. Eyster ME, Jenkins DE Jr. Erythrocyte coating substances in patients with positive direct antiglobulin reactions. *Am J Med* 1969;46:360–371.
25. Rosse WF. The antiglobulin test in autoimmune hemolytic anemia. *Annu Rev Med* 1975;26:331–337.
26. Worlledge S. Auto-immunity and blood diseases. *Practitioner* 1967;199:171–179.
27. Gilliland BC, Turner E. Mechanism of complement binding by the red cell in rheumatoid arthritis. *Arthritis Rheum* 1969;12:498–503.
28. Gilliland BC, Leddy JP, Vaughan JH. The detection of cell-bound antibody on complement-coated human red cells. *J Clin Invest* 1970;49:898–906.
29. MacKenzie MR, Creevy CC. Hemolytic anemia with cold detectable IgG antibodies. *Blood* 1970;36:549–558.
30. Shulman IA, Branch DR, Nelson JM, et al. Autoimmune hemolytic anemia with both cold and warm autoantibodies. *JAMA* 1985;253;1746–1748.
31. Sokol RJ, Hewill S, Stamps BK. Autoimmune hemolysis: an 18 year study of 865 cases referred to a regional transfusion center. *Br J Med* 1981;282:2023–2027.
32. Frank MM, Schreiber AD, Atkinson JP, et al. Pathophysiology of immune hemolytic anemia. *Ann Intern Med* 1977;87:210–222.
33. Hillyer CD, Berkman EM, Schwartz RS. Autoimmune hemolytic anemia and cold agglutinin disease: autoantibodies, mechanisms and therapy. *Clin Aspects Autoimmun* 1990;5:22–32.
34. Rosse WF. The mechanisms of destruction of antibody-altered cells. *Clin Lab Med* 1982;2:211–219.
35. Sokol RJ, Booker DJ, Stamps R. The pathology of autoimmune haemolytic anaemia. *J Clin Pathol* 1992;42:1047–1052.
36. Zupanski B, Thompson EE, Merry AH. Fc receptors for IgG1 and IgG3 on human mononuclear cells — an evaluation with known levels of erythrocyte-count IgG. *Vox Sang* 1986;50:97–103.
37. Sokol RJ, Hewitt S, Booker DJ, et al. Red cell autoantibodies, multiple immunoglobuiln classes and autoimmune hemolysis. *Transfusion* 1990;30:714–717.
38. Schreiber AD, Frank MM. The role of antibody and complement in the immune clearance and destruction of erythrocytes. I. *In vivo* effects of IgG and IgM complement fixing sites. *J Clin Invest* 1972;51:575–582.
39. Schreiber AD, Frank MM. The roles of antibody and complement in the immune clearance and destruction of erythrocytes. II. Molecular nature of IgG and IgM complement fixing sites and effects of their interaction with serum. *J Clin Invest* 1972;51:583–589.
40. Baldini MG. Idiopathic thrombocytopenic purpura and the ITP syndrome. *Med Clin North Am* 1972;56:47–64.
41. Karpatkin S. Autoimmune thrombocytopenic purpura. *Blood* 1980;56:329–343.
42. Cohen P, Gardner FH, Barnett GO. Reclassification of the thrombocytopenias by the Cr51 labeling method for measuring platelet life span. *N Engl J Med* 1961;264:1294–1295.
43. Harrington WJ, Sprague CC, Minnich V, et al. Immunologic mechanisms in idiopathic and neonatal thrombocytopenic purpura. *Ann Intern Med* 1953;38:433–469.
44. Shulman NR, Marder VJ, Weinrach RS. Similarities between known antiplatelet antibodies and the factor responsible for thrombocytopenia in idiopathic purpura, physiologic, serologic and isotopic studies. *Ann N y Acad Sci* 1965;124:499–542.
45. Nathan DJ, Snapper I. Simultaneous placental transfer of fac-

tors responsible for L.E. cell formation and thrombocytopenia. *Am J Med* 1958;25:647–653.
46. Harrington WJ, Minnich V, Arimura C. The auto-immune thrombocytopenias. *Prog Hematol* 1956;1:166–192.
47. Weinreich J. Thrombocytopenias and platelet antibodies. *Vox Sang* 1957;2:294–300.
48. Dausset J, Colombani J, Colombani M. Study of leucopenias and thrombocytopenias by the direct antiglobulin consumption test on leucocytes and/or platelets. *Blood* 1961;18:672–690.
49. Van de Wiel TWM, Van de Wiel-Dorfmeyer H, Van Loghem JJ. Studies on platelet antibodies in man. *Vox Sang* 1961;6: 641–668.
50. Hanna N, Nelken D. A two-stage agglutination test for the detection of antithrombocyte antibodies. *Vox Sang* 1970;18: 342–348.
51. Karpatkin S, Strick N, Karpatkin M, et al. Cumulative experience in the detection of antiplatelet antibody in 234 patients with idiopathic thrombocytopenic purpura, systemic lupus erythematosus and other clinical disorders. *Am J Med* 1972; 52:776–785.
52. Pizzi F, Cararra PM, Aldeghi A, et al. Immunofluorescence of megakaryocytes in the thrombocytopenic purpuras. *Blood* 1966;27:521–526.
53. Von dem Brone AEG Jr, Helmerhorst FM, Van Leeuwen EF, et al. Autoimmune thrombocytopenia: detection of platelet autoantibodies with the suspension immunofluorescence test. *Br J Haematol* 1980;45:319–327.
54. Pujol M, Ribera A, Vilardell M, et al. High prevalence of platelet autoantibodies in patients with systemic lupus erythematosus. *Br J Haematol* 1995;89:137–141.
55. Lipp E, Von Felten A, Sax H, et al. Antibodies against platelet glycoproteins and antiphospholipid antibodies in autoimmune thrombocytopenia. *Eur J Haematol* 1998; 60:283–288.
56. Cordiano I, Salvan F, Randi ML, et al. Antiplatelet glycoprotein autoantibodies in patients with autoimmune diseases with and without thrombocytopenia. *J Clin Immunol* 1996;16:340–347.
57. Joutsi L, Kekomaki R. Comparison of the direct platelet immunofluorescence (direct PIFT) with a modified direct monoclonal antibody-specific immobilization of platelet antigens (direct MAIPA) in detection of platelet-associated IgG. *Br J Haematol* 1997;96:204–209.
58. Karpatkin S, Siskind GW. *In vitro* detection of platelet antibody in patients with idiopathic thrombocytopenic purpura and SLE. *Blood* 1969;33:795–812.
59. Karpatkin SI, Lackner HL. Association of antiplatelet antibody with functional platelet disorders, autoimmune thrombocytopenic purpura, systemic lupus erythematosus and thrombopathy. *Am J Med* 1975;59:599–604.
60. Kutti J, Safai-Kutti S, Good RA. The platelet factor 3 assay and circulating immune complexes as studied on non-thrombocytopenic patients with systemic lupus erythematosus. *Scand J Haematol* 1982;29:31–35.
61. Miescher PA. Autoantibodies against thrombocytes and leukocytes. In: Miescher PA, Muller-Eberhard HJ, eds. *Textbook of immunopathology, vol II*. New York: Grune & Stratton, 1969: 500–506.
62. Dixon R, Rosse W, Ebbert L. Quantitative determination of antibody in idiopathic thrombocytopenic purpura. Correlation of serum and platelet-bound antibody with clinical response. *N Engl J Med* 1975;292:230–236.
63. Kelton JG. The measurement of platelet-bound immunoglobulins: an overview of the methods and the biological relevance of platelet-associated IgG. *Prog Hematol* 1983;13:183–199.
64. Kelton JG, Gibbons S. Autoimmune platelet destruction. Idiopathic thrombocytopenic purpura. *Semin Thromb Hemost* 1982;8:83–104.
65. Faig D, Karpatkin S. Cumulative experience with a simplified solid-phase radioimmunoassay for the detection of bound antiplatelet IgG, serum auto-allo-, and drug-dependent antibodies. *Blood* 1982;60:807–813.
66. Hedge UM, Gordon-Smith EC, Worlledge S. Platelet antibodies in thrombocytopenic patients. *Br J Haematol* 1977;35: 113–182.
67. Kelton JG, Giles AR, Neame PB, et al. Comparison of two direct assays for platelet-associated IgG (PAIgG) in assessment of immune and nonimmune thrombocytopenia. *Blood* 1980; 55:424–429.
68. Mulshine J, Lucas FV, Clough JD. Platelet-bound IgG in systemic lupus erythematosus with and without thrombocytopenia. *J Immunol Methods* 1981;45:275–281.
69. Bonacossa IA, Chalmers IM, Rayner HL, et al. Platelet bound IgG levels in patients with systemic lupus erythematosus. *J Rheumatol* 1985;12:78–80.
70. Karpatkin S, Schur PH, Strick N, et al. Heavy chain subclass of human anti-platelet antibodies. *Clin Immunol Immunopath* 1973;2:18.
71. Dixon RH, Rosse WF. Platelet antibody in auto-immune thrombocytopenia. *Br J Haematol* 1975;31:129–134.
72. Hymes K, Schur PH, Karpatkin S. Heavy-chain subclass of bound antiplatelet IgG autoimmune hemolytic anemia. *Blood* 1980;56:84–87.
73. Rosse WF, Adams JP, Yount WJ. Subclasses of IgG antibodies in immune thrombocytopenic purpura (ITP). *Br J Haematol* 1980;46:109–114.
74. Karas SP, Rosse WF, Kurlander RJ. Characterization of IgG-FC receptor on human platelets. *Blood* 1982;60:1277–1282.
75. McMillan R. Chronic idiopathic thrombocytopenic purpura. *N Engl J Med* 1981;304:1135–1147.
76. Kelton JG, Keystone J, Moore J, et al. Immune mediated thrombocytopenia of malaria. *J Clin Invest* 1983;71:832–836.
77. Walsh CM, Nardi M, Karpatkin S. On the mechanism of thrombocytopenic purpura in sexually active homosexual men. *N Engl J Med* 1984;311:635–639.
78. Samuel H, Nardi M, Karpatkin M, et al. Differentiation of autoimmune thrombocytopenia from thrombocytopenia associated with immune complex disease: systemic lupus erythematosus, hepatitis-cirrhosis and HIV-1 infection by platelet and serum immunological measurements. *Br J Haematol* 1999;105: 1086–1091.
79. Clark WF, Tevaarwerk GJM, Reid BD. Human platelet-immune complex interaction in plasma. *J Lab Clin Med* 1982; 100:917–931.
80. Puram V, Giuliani D, Morse BS. Circulating immune complexes and platelet IgG in various diseases. *Clin Exp Immunol* 1984;58:672–676.
81. Kurata Y, Hayashi S, Kosugi S, et al. Elevated platelet-associated IgG in SLE patients due to anti-platelet autoantibody: differentiation between autoantibodies and immune complexes by ether elution. *Br J Haematol* 1993;85:723–728.
82. Berchtold P, Harris JP, Tani P, et al. Autoantibodies to platelet glycoproteins in patients with disease-related immune thrombocytopenia. *Br J Haematol* 1989;73:365–368.
83. Howe SE, Lynch DM. Platelet antibody binding in systemic lupus erythematosus. *J Rheumatol* 1987;14:482–486.
84. Kaplan C, Champeix P, Blanchar D, et al. Platelet antibodies in systemic lupus erythematosus. *Br J Haematol* 1990;67:89–93.
85. Tomiyama Y, Kekomaki R, McFarland J, et al. Antivinculin antibodies in sera of patients with immune thrombocytopenia and in sera of normal subjects. *Blood* 1992;79:161–168.
86. Woods VL, Oh EH, Mason D, et al. Autoantibodies against the platelet glycoprotein IIb/IIIa complex in patients with chronic ITP. *Blood* 1984;63:368–373.

87. Ikehara S, Mizutani H, Kurata Y. Autoimmune thrombocytoenic purpura. *Crit Rev Oncol Hematol* 1993;19:33–45.
88. Warner MN, Moore JC, Warkentin TE, et al. A prospective study of protein-specific assays used to investigate idiopathic thrombocytopenic purpura. *Br J Haematol* 1999;104:442–447.
89. Macchi L, Rispal P, Clofent-Sanchez G, et al. Anti-platelet antibodies in patients with systemic lupus erythematosus and the primary antiphospholipid antibody syndrome: their relationship with the observed thrombocytopenia. *Br J Haematol* 1997; 98:336–341.
90. Rupin A, Gruel Y, Poumier-Gashard P, et al. Thrombocytopenia in systemic lupus erythematosus: association with antiplatelet and anticardiolipin antibodies. *Clin Immunol Immunopathol* 1990;55:418–426.
91. Jouhikainen T, Keomaki R, Leirisalo-Repo M, et al. Platelet autoantibodies detected by immunoblotting in systemic lupus erythematous: association with the lupus anticoagulant, and with history of thrombosis and thrombocytopenia. *Eur J Haematol* 1990;44:234–239.
92. Out HJ, De Groot PG, Van Vliet M, et al. Antibodies to platelets in patients with antiphospholipid antibodies. *Blood* 1991;77:2655–2659.
93. Quismorio FP Jr, Friou GJ. Serological factors in systemic lupus erythematosus and their pathogenetic significance. *CRC Crit Rev Clin Lab Sci* 1979;1:639–684.
94. Mittal KK, Rossen RD, Sharp JT, et al. Lymphocyte cytotoxic antibodies in SLE. *Nature* 1970;225:1255–1256.
95. Nies KM, Brown JC, Dubois EL, et al. Histocompatibility (HLA) antigens and lymphocytotoxic antibodies in systemic lupus erythematosus (SLE). *Arthritis Rheum* 1974;17:397–402.
96. Stastny P, Ziff M. Antibodies against cell membrane constituents in systemic lupus erythematosus and related diseases. I. Cytotoxic effect of serum from patients with systemic lupus erythematosus for allogeneic and for autologous lymphocytes. *Clin Exp Immunol* 1971;8:543–550.
97. Terasaki PI, Mottironi VD, Barnett EV. Cytotoxins in disease. Autocytotoxins in lupus. *N Engl J Med* 1970;283:724–728.
98. Logue GL, Shimm DS. Autoimmune granulocytopenia. *Annu Rev Med* 1980;31:191–200.
99. Maher GM, Hartman KR. Detection of antineutrophil autoantibodies by flow cytometry: use of unfixed neutrophils as antigenic targets. *J Clin Lab Anal* 1993;7:334–340.
100. Drew SI, Terasaki PI. Autoimmune cytotoxic granulocyte antibodies in normal persons and various diseases. *Blood* 1978;52: 941–952.
101. Starkebaum G, Price TH, Lee MY, et al. Autoimmune neutropenia in systemic lupus erythematosus. *Arthritis Rheum* 1978;21:504–515.
102. Starkebaum G, Arend WP. Neutrophil-binding immunoglobulin G in systemic erythematosus. *J Clin Invest* 1979;64:902–912.
103. Hadley AG, Byron MA, Chapel HM, et al. Anti-granulocyte opsonic activity in sera from patients with systemic lupus erythematosus. *Br J Haematol* 1987;65:61–65.
104. Rustagi AK, Currie MS, Logue GL. Complement-activating antineutrophil antibody in systemic lupus erythematosus. *Am J Med* 1985;78:971–977.
105. Sipos A, Csortos C, Sipka S, et al. The antigen/receptor specificity of antigranulocyte antibodies in patient with SLE. *Immunol Lett* 1988;19:329–334.
106. Kurien BT, Newland J, Paczkowski C, et al. Association of neutropenia in systemic lupus erythematosus (SLE) with anti-Ro and binding of an immunologically cross-reactive neutrophil membrane antigen. *Clin Exp Immunol* 2000;120:209–217.
107. Nolle B, Specks U, Ludemann J, et al. Anticytoplasmic autoantibodies: their immunodiagnostic value in Wegener granulomatosis. *Ann Intern Med* 1989;111:28–40.
108. Hoffman GS, Specks U. Antineutrophil cytoplasmic antibodies. *Arthritis Rheum* 1998;41:1521–1537.
109. Savige J, Gillis D, Bensen E, et al. International Consensus statement on testing and reporting of antineutrophil cytoplasmic antibodies (ANCA). *Am J Pathol* 1999;111:507–513.
110. Jennett JC, Falk RJ. Antineurophil cytoplasmic autoantibodies and associated diseases. A review. *Am J Kidney Dis* 1990;15: 517–529.
111. Spronk PE, Bootsma H, Horst G, et al. Antineutrophil cytoplasmic antibodies in systemic lupus erythematosus. *Br J Rheumatol* 1996;35:625–631.
112. Nassberger L, Sjoholm AG, Johsson H, et al. Autoantibodies against neutrophil cytoplasm components in systemic lupus erythematosus and in hydralazine-induced lupus. *Clin Exp Immunol* 1990;81:380–383.
113. Lee SS, Lawton JMW. Antimyeloperoxidase antibody in systemic lupus erythematosus. *J Intern Med* 1992;232:283–286.
114. Lee SS, Lawton JMW, Chan CE, et al. Antilactoferrin antibody in systemic lupus erythematosus. *Br J Rheumatol* 1992;31: 669–673.
115. Nassberger L, Hultquist R, Sturfelt G. Occurrence of anti-lactoferrin antibodies in patients with systemic lupus erythematosus, hydralazine-induced lupus and rheumatoid arthritis. *Scand J Rheumatol* 1994;23:206–210.
116. Schnabel A, Csernok E, Isenberg DA, et al. Antineutrophil cytoplasmic antibodies in systemic lupus erythematosus: prevalence, specificities and clinical significance. *Arthritis Rheum* 1995;31:669–675.
117. Pauzner R, Urowitz M, Gladman D, et al. Antineutrophil cytoplasmic antibodies in systemic lupus erythematosus. *J Rheumatol* 1994;21:1670–1673.
118. Galeazzi M, Morozzi G, Sebastiani GD, et al. Anti-neutrophil cytoplasmic antibodies in 566 European patients with systemic lupus erythematosus: prevalence, clinical associations and correlation with other autoantibodies. *Clin Exp Rheumatol* 1998;16: 541–546.
119. Wiik A, Stummann L, Kjeldsen L, et al. The diversity of perinuclear antineutrophil cytoplasmic antibodies (pANCA) antigens. *Clin Exp Immunol* 1995;101(suppl 1):15–17.
120. Merkel PA, Polisson RP, Chang Y, et al. Prevalence of antineutrophil cytoplasmic antibodies in a large inception cohort of patients with connective tissue disease. *Ann Intern Med* 1997; 126:866–873.
121. Handley AJ. Thrombocytopenia and LE cells after oxyphenbutazone. *Lancet* 1971;i:245–246.
122. Williams RC. Rheumatoid factors. *Hum Pathol* 1983;14: 386–391.
123. Singer JM. The latex fixation test in rheumatic diseases. *Am J Med* 1961;31:766–779.
124. Estes D, Christian CL. The natural history of systemic lupus erythematosus by prospective analysis. *Medicine* 1971;50: 85–95.
125. Lee P, Urowitz MB, Bookman AA, et al. Systemic lupus erythematosus: a review of 110 cases with reference to nephritis, central nervous system, infections, aseptic necrosis and prognosis. *Q J Med* 1977;46:1–32.
126. Feinglass EJ, Arnett FC, Dorsch CA, et al. Neuropsychiatric manifestations of systemic lupus erythematosus: diagnosis, clinical spectrum, and relationship to other feature so the disease. Medicine 1976;55:323–339.
127. Cathcart ES, O'Sullivan JB, Lincoln G. Standardization of the sheep cell agglutination test. The use of pooled reference sera and hemagglutination trays. *Arthritis Rheum* 1965;8:530–537.
128. Pope RM, McDuffy SJ. IgG rheumatoid factor. *Arthritis Rheum* 1979;22:968–998.
129. Wernick R, Lospalluto JJ, Fink CW, et al. Serum IgG and IgM

rheumatoid factors by solid phase radioimmunoassay. *Arthritis Rheum* 1981;24:1501–1511.
130. Hargraves MM. Discovery of the LE cell and its morphology. *Mayo Clin Proc* 1969;44:579–599.
131. Zuraw BL, O'Hair CH, Vaughan JH, et al. Immunoglobulin E-rheumatoid factor in the serum of patients with rheumatoid arthritis, asthma, and other diseases. *J Clin Invest* 1981;68: 1610–1613.
132. Dunne JV, Carson DA, Spiegelberg HL, et al. IgA rheumatoid factor in the sera and saliva of patients with rheumatoid arthritis and Sjogren's syndrome. *Ann Rheum Dis* 1979;38:161–165.
133. Bonagura VR, Ilowite NT, Hatam L, et al. Expression of the major rheumatoid factor cross-reactive idiotype in pediatric patients with systemic lupus erythematosus. *Clin Immunol Immunopathol* 1991;60:232–243.
134. Davis JS, Bollet AJ. Protection of a complement-sensitive enzyme system by rheumatoid factor. *J Immunol* 1964;92: 139–144.
135. Zvaifler NJ, Block DJ. Rheumatoid factor an inhibitor of the complement fixation reaction (abstract). *Arthritis Rheum* 1962; 5:1–27.
136. Parker RL, Schmid FR. Phagocytosis of particular complexes of gamma globulin and rheumatoid factor. *J Immunol* 1962;88: 519–525.
137. Van Snick JL, Van Roost E, Markowetz R, et al. Enhancement by IgM rheumatoid factor of *in vitro* ingestion of macrophages and *in vivo* clearance of aggregated IgG or antigen antibody complexes. *Eur J Immunol* 1978;8:279–285.
138. Bolton WK, Schrock JH, Davis JS. Rheumatoid factor inhibition of *in vitro* binding of IgG complexes in the human glomerulus. *Arthritis Rheum* 1982;25:297–303.
139. Floyd M, Tesar JT. The role of IgM rheumatoid factor in experimental immune vasculitis. *Clin Exp Immunol* 1979;36: 165–174.
140. Baum J, Stastny P, Ziff M. Effect of rheumatoid factor and antigen-antibody complexes on the vessels of the rat mesentery. *J Immunol* 1964;93:985–995.
141. Ford PM. Interaction of rheumatoid factor with immune complexes in experimental glomerulonephritis—possible role of antiglobulins in chronicity. *J Rheumatol* 1983;10(suppl 11): 81–84.
142. Ford PM, Kosatka I. The effect of human IgM rheumatoid factor on renal glomerular immune complex deposition in passive serum sickness in the mouse. *Immunology* 1982;46:761–768.
143. Ford PM, Kosatka I. In situ immune complex formation in the mouse glomerulus: reactivity with human IgM rheumatoid factor and the effect on subsequent immune complex deposition. *Clin Exp Immunol* 1983;51:285–291.
144. Birchmore DA, Taylor RP, Waller SJ, et al. Interaction between rheumatoid factor and antibody/DNA complexes. *Arthritis Rheum* 1981;24:527–533.
145. Miyazaki M, Endoh M, Suga T, et al. Rheumatoid factors and glomerulonephritis. *Clin Exp Immunol* 1990;81:250–255.
146. Agnello V, Koffler D, Eisenberg JW, et al. Clq precipitins in the sera of patients with systemic lupus erythematosus and other hypocomplementemic states: characterization of high and low molecular weight types. *J Exp Med* 1971;134(suppl):228S–241S.
147. Davis JS, Bollet AJ. Complement levels, rheumatoid factor and renal disease in SLE (abstract). *Arthritis Rheum* 1966;9: 499–500.
148. Howard TW, Iannini MJ, Burge JJ, et al. Rheumatoid factor, cryoglobulinemia, anti-DNA, and renal disease in patients with systemic lupus erythematosus. *J Rheumatol* 1991;18:826–830.
149. Hill GS, Hinglais N, Tron F, et al. Systemic lupus erythematosus. Morphologic correlations with immunologic and clinical data at the time of biopsy. *Am J Med* 1978;64:61–79.
150. Helin H, Korpela M, Mustonen J, et al. Rheumatoid factor in rheumatoid arthritis associated renal disease in lupus nephritis. *Ann Rheum Dis* 1986;45:508–511.
151. Corke CE. Rheumatoid factor and renal disease in systemic lupus erythematosus. *Rheumatol Rehab* 1987;17:76–78.
152. Mustakallio KK, Lassus A, Putkonen T, et al. Cryoglobulins and rheumatoid factor in systemic lupus erythematosus. *Acta Derm Venereol (Stockh)* 1967;47:241–248.
153. Cervera R, Khamashta MA, Font J, et al. Systemic lupus erythematosus: clinical and immunologic patterns of disease expression in a cohort of 1000 patients. *Medicine* 1991;72: 113–124.
154. Tarkowski A, Westerberg G. Rheumatoid factor isotypes and renal disease in systemic lupus erythematosus. *Scand J Rheumatol* 1987;16:309–312.
155. Witte T, Hartung K, Sachse C, et al. Rheumatoid factors in systemic lupus erythematosus: association with clinical and laboratory parameters. *Rheumatol Int* 2000;19:107–111.
156. Zoli A, Altomonte L, Caricchio R, et al. Rheumatoid Factor in patients with systemic lupus erythematosus. *Clin Rheumatol* 1996;15:312–313.
157. Kantor GL, Bickel YB, Barnett EV. Coexistence of systemic lupus erythematosus and rheumatoid arthritis. Report of a case and review of the literature, and clinical, pathologic and serologic observations. *Am J Med* 1969;47:433–444.
158. Baldwin DS, Lowenstein J, Rothfield NF, et al. The clinical course of the proliferative and membranous forms of lupus nephritis. *Ann Intern Med* 1970;73:929–942.
159. Pinillos RM, Solle JMN, Roura XJ, et al. Rheumatoid factor in patients with systemic lupus erythematosus. *Ann Rheum Dis* 1987;46:877–878.
160. Stokes-Turner L, Mones M, Addison I, et al. Does rheumatoid factor protect lupus nephritis from the development of nephritis. *Ann Rheum Dis* 1989;48:14–16.
161. Rossen RD, Reisberg MA, Sharp JT, et al. Antiglobulins and glomerulonephritis. *J Clin Invest* 1975;56:427–437.
162. Rossen RD, Rickaway RH, Reisberg MA, et al. Renal localization of antiglobulins in glomerulonephritis and after renal transplantation. *Arthritis Rheum* 1977;20:947–961.
163. Quismorio FP Jr, Sharma O, Koss M, et al. Immunopathologic and clinical studies in pulmonary hypertension associated with systemic lupus erythematosus. *Semin Arthritis Rheum* 1984;13: 349–359.
164. Moutsopoulos HM, Klippel JH, Pavlidis N, et al. Corrective histologic and serologic findings of sicca syndrome in patients with systemic lupus erythematosus. *Arthritis Rheum* 1980;23: 36–40.
165. Zizic TM, Classen JN, Stevens MB. Acute abdominal complications of systemic lupus erythematosus and polyarteritis nodosa. *Am J Med* 1982;73:525–531.
166. Shen JY, Chen SL, Wu YX, et al. Pulmonary hypertension in systemic lupus erythematosus. *Rheumatol Int* 1999;18:147–151.
167. Feldman D, Feldman D, Ginzler E, et al. Rheumatoid factor in patients with systemic lupus erythematosus. *J Rheumatol* 1989;16:618–622.
168. Sankoorikal A, Stimmler M, Quismorio FP Jr. Contrasting effects of IgM rheumatoid factor on clinical manifestations of SLE (abstract). *Arthritis Rheum* 1990;34:S129.
169. McCormick JN, Day J. The association of rheumatoid factor with antinuclear factor activity. *Lancet* 1963;2:554–557.
170. Hannestad K. Certain rheumatoid factors react with both IgG and an antigen associated with cell nuclei. *Scand J Immunol* 1978;7:127–136.
171. Hannestad K, Johannessen A. Polyclonal human antibodies to IgG (rheumatoid factors) which cross-react with cell nuclei. *Scand J Immunol* 1976;5:541–547.

172. Johnson PM. IgM rheumatoid factors cross-reactive with IgG and a cell nuclear antigen: apparent masking in original serum. *Scand J Immunol* 1979;9:461–466.
173. Agnello V, Arbetter A, De Kasep GI, et al. Evidence for a subset of rheumatoid factors that cross-react with DNA-histone and have a distinct cross-idiotype. *J Exp Med* 1980;151:1514–1527.
174. Aitcheson CT, Peebles C, Joslin F, et al. Characteristics of antinuclear antibodies in rheumatoid arthritis. Reactivity of rheumatoid factor with a histone-dependent nuclear antigen. *Arthritis Rheum* 1980;23:528–538.
175. Hobbs RN, Lea DJ, Phua KK, et al. Binding of isolated rheumatoid factors to histone proteins and basic polycations. *Ann Rheum Dis* 1983;42:435–438.
176. Mason JC, Venables PJW, Smith PR, et al. Characterization of non-histone nuclear proteins cross reactive with purified rheumatoid factors. *Ann Rheum Dis* 1985;44:287–293.
177. Kinoshita M, Aotsuka S, Yokohari R. Cross-reactive rheumatoid factors in rheumatoid arthritis with extra-articular disease. *Clin Exp Immunol* 1990;79:72–77.
178. Martin T, Knapp AM, Muller S, et al. Polyclonal human rheumatoid factors cross-reacting with histone H3: characterization of an idiotype on the H3 binding site. *J Clin Immunol* 1990;10:211–219.
179. Lerner A, Barnum C, Watson J. Studies on cryoglobulins: II. The spontaneous precipitaton of protein from serum at 5C in various disease states. *Am J Med Sci* 1947;214:15–21.
180. Barr DP, Reader GG, Wheeler CH. Cryoglobulinemia: report of two cases with discussion of clinical manifestations, incidence and significance. *Ann Intern Med* 1950;32:6–29.
181. Christian CL, Hatfield WB, Chase PH. Systemic lupus erythematosus, cryoprecipitation of sera. *J Clin Invest* 1963;48:823–829.
182. Stastny P, Ziff M. Cold-insoluble complexes and complement levels in SLE. *N Engl J Med* 1969;280:1376–1381.
183. Lee SL, Rivero I. Cryoglobulins in SLE as circulating immune complexes (abstract). *Arthritis Rheum* 1964;7:3–21.
184. Barnett EV, Kantor G, Bickel YB, et al. Systemic lupus erythematosus. *CA Med* 1969;111:467–481.
185. Brouet JC, Clauvel JP, Danon F, et al. Biologic and clinical significance of cryoglobulins: a report of 86 cases. *Am J Med* 1976;57:7–75.
186. Hanauer LB, Christian CL. Studies of cryoproteins in SLE. *J Clin Invest* 1967:46:400–408.
187. Barnett EV, Bluestone R, Cracchiolo A III, et al. Cryoglobulinemia and disease. *Ann Intern Med* 1970;73:95–107.
188. Erhardt CC, Mumford P, Maini RN. Differences in immunochemical characteristics of cryoglobulins in rheumatoid arthritis and systemic lupus erythematosus and their complement-binding properties. *Ann Rheum Dis* 1984;43:451–455.
189. Anderson B, Rucker M, Entwisle R, et al. Plasma fibronectin is a component of cryoglobulins from patients with connective tissue and other diseases. *Ann Rheum Dis* 1981;40:50–54.
190. Beaulieu AD, Valet JP, Strevey J. The influence of fibronectin on cryoprecipitate formation in rheumatoid arthritis and systemic lupus erythematosus. *Arthritis Rheum* 1981;24:1383–1388.
191. Wood G, Rucker M, Davis JR, et al. Interaction of plasma fibronectin with selected cryoglobulins. *Clin Exp Immunol* 1980;40:358–364.
192. Kono I, Sakurai T, Kabashima T, et al. Fibronectin binds to Clq: possible mechanisms for their co-precipitation in cryoglobulins from patients with systemic lupus erythematosus. *Clin Exp Immunol* 1983;52:305–310.
193. Winfield JB. Cryoglobulinemia. *Hum Pathol* 1983;14:350–354.
194. Lospalluto J, Dorward B, Miller W Jr, et al. Cryoglobulinemia based on interaction between a gamma macroglobulin and 79 gamma globulin. *Am J Med* 1952;32:142–147.
195. Muller S, Rother U, Westerhausen M. Complement activation by cryoglobulin. *Clin Exp Immunol* 1976;23:233–241.
196. Rother U, Rother K, Flad HD, et al. Bithermic complement activation in cryoglobulinemic serum. *Eur J Clin Invest* 1972;2:59–65.
197. Adu D, Williams DG. Complement activating cryoglobulins in the nephritis of systemic lupus erythematosus. *Clin Exp Immunol* 1984;55:495–501.
198. Winfield JB, Koffler D, Kunkel HG. Specific concentration of polynucleotide immune complexes in cryoprecipitates of patients with systemic lupus erythematosus. *J Clin Invest* 1975;56:563–570.
199. McPhaul JJ Jr. Cryoimmunoglobulinemia in patients with primary renal disease and systemic lupus erythematous. I. IgG and DNA binding assessed by co-precipitation. *Clin Exp Immunol* 1978;31:131–140.
200. Winfield JB, Winchester RJ, Wernet P, et al. Specific concentrations of anti-lymphocyte antibodies in the serum cryoprecipitates of patients with systemic lupus erythematosus. *Clin Exp Immunol* 1975;19:399–406.
201. Zvaifler NJ, Bluestein HG. Lymphocytotoxic antibody activity in cryoprecipitates from serum of patients with SLE. *Arthritis Rheum* 1976;19:844–850.
202. Klippel JH, Bluestein HG, Zvaifler NJ. Lymphocyte reactivity of antisera to cryoproteins in systemic lupus erythematosus. *Clin Immunol Immunopathol* 1979;12:52–61.
203. McPhaul JJ Jr, Montgomery WR. Cryoimmunoglobulinemia in patients with renal disease. II. Attempts to demonstrate that cryoprecipitates contain autoantibodies and/or antigen. *Clin Exp Immunol* 1981;44:560–566.
204. Davis JS, Godfrey SM, Winfield JB. Direct evidence for circulating DNA/anti-DNA complexes in systemic lupus erythematosus. *Arthritis Rheum* 1978;21:17–22.
205. Roberts JL, Robinson MF, Lewis EJ. Low molecular weight plasma cryoprecipititable anti-native DNA: polynucleotide complexes in lupus glomerulonephritis. *Clin Immunol Immunopathol* 1981;19:75–90.
206. Barnett EV. Detection of nuclear antigens (DNA) in normal and pathologic fluids by quantitative complement fixation. *Arthritis Rheum* 1968;11:407–417.
207. Bluestone R, Goldberg LS, Cracchilo A, et al. Detection and characterization of DNA in mixed IgG-IgM cryoglobulins. *Int Arch Appl Allergy Immunol* 1970;39:16–26.
208. Davis GL, Davis JS. Detection of circulating DNA by counterimmunoelectrophoresis (CIE). *Arthritis Rheum* 1973;16:52–58.
209. Hughes GRV, Cohen SA, Lightfoot RW, et al. The release of DNA into serum and synovial fluid. *Arthritis Rheum* 1971;14:259–266.
210. Roberts JL, Lewis EJ. Identification of anti-native DNA antibodies to cryoglobulinemic states. *Am J Med* 1978;65:437–445.
211. Roberts JL, Lewis EJ. Immunochemical demonstration of cryoprecipitable anti-native DNA antibody and DNA in the serum of patients with glomerulonephritis. *J Immunol* 1980;124:127–133.
212. Pasero GP, Bombardieri S, Ferri C. From internal medicine to rheumatology and back: the example of mixed cyroglobulinemia. *Clin Exper Rheumatol* 1995;13:1–5.
213. Abel G, Zhang Q, Agnello V. Hepatitis C virus infection in type II mixed cryoglobulinemia. *Arthritis Rheum* 1993;36:1341–1349.
214. Marchesoni A, Podico M, Battafarano N, et al. Hepatitis C virus antibodies and systemic lupus erythematosus. *Clin Exp Rheuamtol* 1995;13:267–273.

215. McIntosh RM, Kulvinskas C, Kaufman DB. Cryoglobulins. II. The biological and chemical properties of cryoproteins in acute post streptococcal glomerulonephritis. *Int Arch Allergy Appl Immunol* 1971;41:700–715.
216. Whitsed HM, Penny R. IgA/IgG cryoglobulinemia with vasculitis. *Clin Exp Immunol* 1971;9:183–191.
217. Nived D, Linder C, Odeberg H, et al. Reduced opsonisation of protein A containing Staphylococcus aureus in sera with cryoglobulins from patients with active systemic lupus erythematosus. *Ann Rheum Dis* 1985;44:252–259.
218. Hargraves MM, Richmond H, Morton R. Presentation of 2 bone marrow elements: tart cell and L.E. cell. *Proc Staff Meet Mayo Clin* 1948;23:25–28.
219. Robineaux R, Pinet J. The Hargraves cell. Description, significance, and research techniques (in French). *Rev Prat* 1965;15: 2523–2530.
220. Lee SL, Michael SR, Vural IL. The L.E. (lupus erythematosus) cell: clinical and chemical studies. *Am J Med* 1951;10:446–452.
221. Klemperer P, Gueft B, Lee SL, et al. Cytochemical changes of acute lupus erythematosus. *Arch Pathol* 1950;49:503–516.
222. Godman GC, Deitch AD. A cytochemical study of the L.E. bodies of systemic lupus erythematosus. *J Exp Med* 1957;106: 575–616.
223. Haserick JR, Lewis LA, Bortz DW. Blood factor in acute disseminated lupus erythematosus: determination of gamma globulin as specific plasma fraction. *Am J Med Sci* 1950;219:660–663.
224. Fallett GH, Lospalluto J, Ziff M. Chromatographic and electrophoretic studies of the LE factor. *Arthritis Rheum* 1958;1: 419–425.
225. Goodman HC, Fahey JL, Malmgren RA. Serum factors in lupus erythematosus and other diseases reacting with cell nuclei and nucleoprotein extracts: electrophoretic, ultracentrifugal and chromatographic studies. *J Clin Invest* 1960;36:1595–1603.
226. Golden HE, McDuffie FC. Role of lupus erythematosus factor and accessory serum factors in production of extracellular nuclear material. *Ann Intern Med* 1967;67:780–790.
227. Miescher P, Fauconnet M. Absorption of the L.E. factor by isolated cell nuclei (in French). *Experientia* 1960;85:27–39.
228. Friou GJ, Finch SC, Detre KD. Interaction of nuclei and globulin from lupus erythematosus serum demonstrated with fluorescent antibody. *J Immunol* 1958;80:324–329.
229. Holman HR, Deicher HR. The reaction of the L.E. cell factor with deoxyribonucleoprotein of the cell nucleus. *J Clin Invest* 1959;38:2059–2072.
230. Holman HR, Deicher HR, Kunkel HG. The L.E. cell and the L.E. serum factors. *Bull N Y Acad Med* 1959;35:409–418.
231. Holman HR, Kunkel HG. Affinity between the lupus erythematosus serum factor and cell nuclei and nucleoprotein. *Science* 1957;126:162–163.
232. Schett G, Steiner G, Smolen JS. Nuclear antigen histone H1 is primarily involved in lupus erythematosus cell formation. *Arthritis Rheum* 1998;41:1446–1455.
233. Schett G, Rubin R, Steiner G, et al. The lupus erythematosus cell phenomenon: comparative analysis of antichromatic antibody specificity in lupus erythematosus cell-positive and –negative sera. *Arthritis Rheum* 2000;43:420–428.
234. Aisenberg AC. Studies on the mechanism of the lupus erythematosus (L.E.) phenomenon. *J Clin Invest* 1959;38:325–335.
235. McDuffie FC, Blondin C, Golden HE. Immunologic factors in lupus erythematosus cell formation. *May Clin Proc* 2969;44: 620–629.
236. Arterberry JD, Drexler E, Dubois EI. Significance of hematoxylin bodies in lupus erythematosus cell preparations. *JAMA* 1964;187:389–395.
237. Lachmann PJ. An attempt to characterize the lupus erythematosus cell antigen. *Immunology* 1961;4:153–163.
238. Rapp F. Localization of antinuclear factors from lupus erythematosus sera in tissue culture. *J Immunol* 1962;88:732–740.
239. Zweiman B, Hildreth K. *In vivo* and *in vitro* anti-nuclear reaction in lupus patients. *Arthritis Rheum* 1968;11:660–662.
240. Seaman AJ, Christerson JW. Demonstration of L.E. cells in pericardial fluid. Report of a case. *JAMA* 1952;149:145–147.
241. Pandya MR, Agus B, Grady RF. *In vivo* LE phenomenon in pleural fluid. *Arthritis Rheum* 1976;19:962–966.
242. Hunder GG, McDuffie FC. Hypocomplementemia in rheumatoid arthritis. *Am J Med* 1973;54:461–472.
243. Metzger AL, Coyne M, Lee S, et al. *In vivo* LE formation in peritonitis due to systemic lupus erythematosus. *J Rheumatol* 1974;1:130–133.
244. Nosanchuk JS, Kim CW. Lupus erythematosus cells in CSF. *JAMA* 1976;236:2883–2884.
245. Dyer HR, Zweiman B. *In vivo* LE cells. *Arthritis Rheum* 1969; 12:64.
246. Feng CS. Atypical lupus erythematosus cells in pleural fluid. *Pathology* 1989;19:317–319.
247. Conn RB. Practice parameterthe lupus erythematous cell test. An obsolete test now superseded by definitive immunologic tests. *Am J Clin Pathol* 1994;101:65–66.
248. Dubois EL, Tuffanelli DL. Clinical manifestations of systemic lupus erythematosus. Computer analysis of 520 cases. *JAMA* 1964;190:104–111.
249. Tuffanelli DL, Winkelmann RK. Systemic scleroderma. A clinical study of 727 cases. *Arch Dermatol* 1961;84:359–371.
250. Dubois EL, Chandor S, Friou GJ, et al. Progressive systemic sclerosis (PSS) and localized scleroderma (morphea) with positive LE cell test and unusual systemic manifestations compatible with systemic lupus erythematosus: presentation of 14 cases including one set of identical twins, one with scleroderma and the other with SLE. *Medicine* 1971;50:199–220.
251. Sharp GC, Irvin WS, May CM, et al. Association of antibodies to nucleoprotein and Sm antigens with mixed connective tissue disease, systemic lupus erythematosus, and other rheumatic diseaes. *N Engl J Med* 1976;295:1149–1154.
252. Dubois EL, ed. *Lupus erythematosus. A review of the current status of discoid and systemic lupus erythematosus and their variants, 2nd ed.* Rev. Los Angeles: USC Press, 1976.
253. Barbier F. The L.E. cell. Is it specific for systemic lupus erythematosus? (in French). *Acta Med Scand* 1953;147:325–330.
254. Berman L, Axelrod AR, Goodman HL, et al. So-called lupus erythematosus inclusion phenomenon of bone marrow and blood: morphologic and serologic studies. *Am J Clin Pathol* 1950;20:403–418.
255. Monto RW, Rizek RA, Rupe CE, et al. The L.E. cell. Significance and relation to collagen disease. In: Mills LC, Moyer JH, eds. *Inflammation and diseases of connective tissue. A Hahnemann symposium.* Philadelphia: WB Saunders, 1961:200–205.
256. Paull AM. Occurrence of the L.E. phenomenon in a patient with a severe penicillin reaction. *N Engl J Med* 1955;252: 128–129.
257. Walsh JR, Zimmerman HJ. Demonstration of the L.E. phenomenon in patients with penicillin hypersensitivity. *Blood* 1985;8:65–71.
258. Domz CA, McNamara DH, Holzapfel HF. Tetracycline provocation in lupus erythematosus. *Ann Intern Med* 1959;50: 1217–1226.
259. Quismorio FP Jr, Bjarnason DF, Dubois EL, et al. Chlorpromazine-induced antinuclear antibodies (abstract). *Arthritis Rheum* 1972;15:4–51.
260. Dubois EL. Procainamide induction of a systemic lupus erythematosus-like syndrome. Presentation of six cases, review of the literature, and analysis and follow-up of reported cases. *Medicine* 1969;48:217–228.

261. Seibold JR, Medsger TA Jr, Buckingham RB, et al. Central nervous system (CNS) involvement in systemic lupus erythematosus (SLE). Clinical features and response to therapy (abstract). *Arthritis Rheum* 1981;24(suppl 4):S70.
262. Mackay IR. Autoimmunity and the liver. *Clin Aspects Autoimmun* 1988;2:8–17.
263. Reynolds TB, Edmonson HA, Peters RL, et al. Lupoid hepatitis. *Ann Intern Med* 1964;61:650–666.
264. Soloway RD, Summerskill WHJ, Baggenstoss AH, et al. Lupoid hepatitis, a nonentity in the spectrum of chronic active liver disease. *Gastroenterology* 1972;63:458–465.
265. Howqua J, Mackay IR. L.E. cells in lymphoma. *Blood* 1963;22:191–198.
266. Finkel HE, Brauer MJ, Taub RN, et al. Immunologic aberrations in the Di Guglielmo syndrome. *Blood* 1966;28:634–369.
267. Koller SR, Johnson CL, Moncure CW, et al. Lupus erythematosus cell preparation-Antinuclear factor incongruity. A review of diagnostic tests for systemic lupus erythematosus. *Am J Clin Path* 1976;66:495–505.
268. Wallace DJ, Metzger AL. Positive LE preps and negative ANAs in brothers with systemic lupus erythematosus (SLE): is there still a role for the LE cell prep? A literature review. *J Rheumatol* 1992;19:497.
269. Wallace DJ. Lupus erythematosus cell test. *Am J Clin Pathol* 1995;104:110–111.
270. Linqvist KJ, Osterland CK. Human antibodies to vascular endothelium. *Clin Exp Immunol* 1971;9:753–759.
271. Navarro M, Cervera R, Font J, et al. Anti-endothelial cell antibodies in systemic autoimmune diseases: prevalence and clinical significance. *Lupus* 1997;6:521–526.
272. Westphal JR, Boerbooms AM TH, Schalkwijk CJM, et al. Antiendothelial cells antibodies in sera of patients with autoimmune diseases: comparison between ELISA and FACS analysis. *Clin Exp Immunol* 1994;96:444–449.
273. Meroni PL, D'Cruz D, Khamasta M, et al. Anti-endothelial cell antibodies: only for scientists or for clinicians too. *Clin Exp Immunol* 1996;104:199–202.
274. Van der Zee JM, Siegert CEH, De Vreede TA, et al. Characterization of anti-endothelial cell antibodies in systemic lupus erythematosus. *Clin Exp Immunol* 1991;84:238–244.
275. Del Papa N, Conforti G, Gambini D, et al. Characterization of endothelial surface proteins recognized by anti-endothelial antibodies in primary and secondary autoimmune vasculitis. *Clin Immunol Immunopathol* 1994;70:211–216.
276. Belizna C, Tervaert JWC. Specificity, pathogenicity and clinical value of antiendothelial cell antibodies. *Sem Arthritis Rheum* 1997;27:98–108.
277. D'Cruz DP, Houssiau FA, Ramirez G, et al. Antibodies to endothelial cells in systemic lupus erythematosus: a potential marker for nephritis and vasculitis. *Clin Exp Immunol* 1991;85:254–261.
278. Perry GJ, Elston T, Khouri Na, et al. Antiendothelial cell antibodies in lupus: correlations with renal injury and circulating markers of endothelial damage. *Q J Med* 1993;86:727–734.
279. Yoshio T, Masuyama J, Sumiya M, et al. Antiendothelial cell antibodies and their relation to pulmonary hypertension in systemic lupus erythematosus. *J Rheumatol* 1994;21:2058–2063.
280. Chan TM, Cheng IKP. A prospective study of anti-endothelial cell antibodies in patients with systemic lupus erythematosus. *Clin Immunol Immunopathol* 1996;78:41–46.
281. Carvalho D, Savage C, Isenberg D, et al. IgG anti-endothelial cell autoantibodies from patients with systemic lupus erythematosus or systemic vasculitis stimulate the release of two endothelial cell-derived mediators, which enhance adhesion molecule expression and leukocyte adhesion in an autocrine manner. *Arthritis Rheum* 1999;42:631–640.
282. Del Papa N, Guidali L, Sironi M, et al. Anti-endothelial cell IgG antibodies from patients with Wegener's granulomatosis bind to human endothelial cells *in vitro* and induce adhesion molecule expression and cytokine secretion. *Arthritis Rheum* 1996;39:758–766.

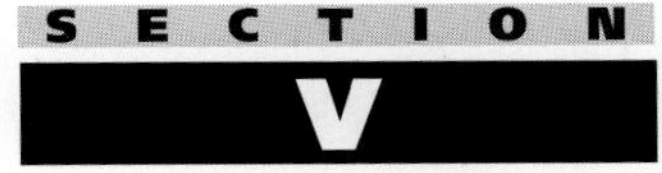

CUTANEOUS LUPUS

28

PATHOMECHANISMS OF CUTANEOUS LUPUS ERYTHEMATOSUS

JAN P. DUTZ
RICHARD D. SONTHEIMER

Abnormal cutaneous reactivity to sunlight is such a seminal clinical feature of lupus erythematosus (LE) that it is one of the 11 criteria proposed by the American Rheumatism Association in 1982 for a case definition of systemic lupus erythematosus (SLE) (1). Photosensitivity also is a cardinal feature of the cutaneous and neonatal forms of lupus erythematosus. This strong clinical association has led to the postulate that abnormal photoreactivity participates in the pathogenesis of cutaneous lesions in lupus erythematosus. In this review we will discuss the evidence for abnormal photoreactivity in lupus erythematosus and speculate on the cellular, molecular, and genetic factors that may underlie this abnormality. Most of our current understanding of cutaneous photoreactivity is derived from animal studies. As there is yet no convincing animal model of cutaneous lupus erythematosus, many studies remain descriptive in nature. To arrive at an understanding of the potential mechanisms underlying the development of cutaneous lupus, we will discuss the possible interrelated roles of ultraviolet light-mediated induction of apoptosis and inflammation as well as immunomodulation. We will in addition consider the role and importance of humoral and cellular factors and also discuss the roles of blood vessels as targets and participants in the disease process. Finally, we will comment on the participation of soluble cytokines and cofactors of inflammation in lesion induction. An incorporation of recent advances in the fields of photobiology, immunology, cell biology, and genetics then will allow the construction of a current model of the pathophysiology of cutaneous lupus.

CLINICAL PHOTOSENSITIVITY IN LUPUS

Skin lesions are common in SLE and are found in up to 90% of patients (2). Lupus-specific cutaneous findings such as malar rash [acute cutaneous lupus erythematosus (ACLE)] and discoid lupus [chronic cutaneous lupus erythematosus (CCLE)] were found in 64% and 31% of patients in a large cohort (2), respectively. Skin disease is the first symptom of disease in 23% to 28% of patients with SLE (3). There is a clear relationship between sunlight exposure and the manifestations of cutaneous LE and cutaneous lesions tend to occur in sun-exposed skin. Cazenave, in the original 1851 description of LE stated that outdoor workers were predisposed (4). Isolated case reports suggested that lesions could be induced by light (5). In 1965, Epstein used a repeated light exposure technique to demonstrate that ultraviolet (UV) radiation could induce skin lesions in patients with LE (6). This observation was confirmed quickly by two other groups (7, 8). In addition to lesion induction, which often was delayed by up to 2 weeks, a decreased threshold for the induction of erythema and prolonged erythema after UV irradiation were noted (9, 10). Thus, patients with either systemic lupus or cutaneous lupus were shown to develop prolonged skin redness at lower doses of UV light than normal controls.

ACTION SPECTRUM OF CUTANEOUS LUPUS ERYTHEMATOSUS

Ultraviolet light is commonly divided into germicidal UV light (UVC), midrange UV light or sunburn UV light (UVB) and long-wave UV light (UVA) also termed near UV or black light (Fig. 28.1). This separation is important as the differing wavelengths have varying biologic effects (vide infra). Although UVC has been used in many *in vitro* studies of the cellular response to UV irradiation, this spectrum of UV light is completely blocked by the earth's atmosphere and is of dubious pathophysiological relevance. Early investigators (6–8, 11, 12), defined an action spectrum in the UVB range (290 to 320 nm) for the cutaneous forms of LE. More recent studies have demonstrated that UVA (320 to 400 nm) also can contribute to the induction of skin lesions. Lehmann and colleagues performed extensive photoprovocation studies in 1990 (13). They were able

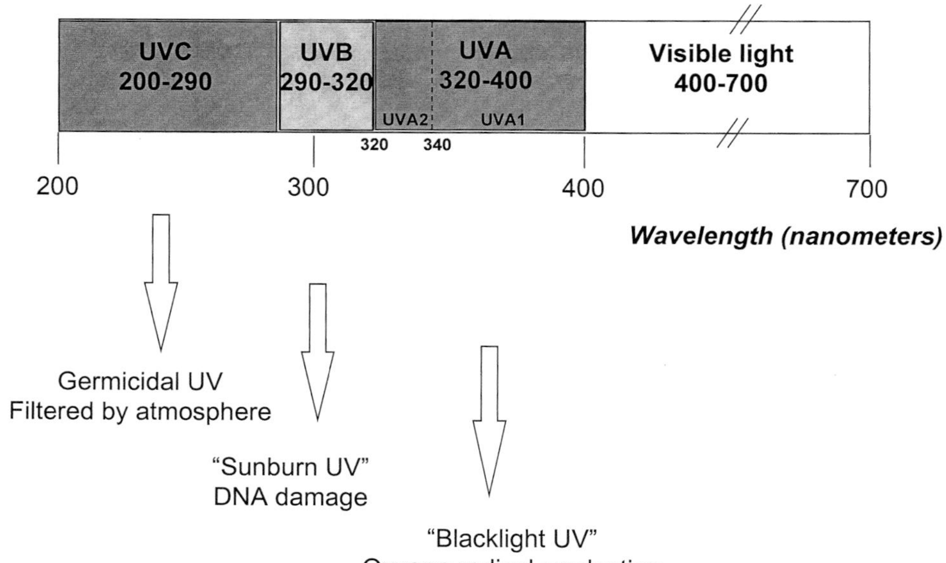

FIGURE 28.1. The spectrum of ultraviolet light irradiation by wavelength. Ultraviolet light is commonly divided into germicidal UV light (UVC), midrange UV light or sunburn light (UVB) and long-wave UV light (UVA) also termed near UV or black light. Both UVB and UVA can induce skin lesions in photosensitive lupus erythematosus. UVA-1 is light limited to the longer wavelength spectrum of UVA and has been used therapeutically in systemic lupus erythematosus.

to induce lesions in 64% of patients with subacute cutaneous lupus erythematosus (SCLE), the most photosensitive form of cutaneous lupus, and in 42% and 25% of patients with CCLE and SLE respectively. Of those with UV induced lesions, 53% were induced by a combination of UVB and UVA, 14% by UVA alone and 33% by UVB alone. Abnormally prolonged erythema was also noted in SLE patients after exposure to UVA (14). Although UVA-induced erythema in normal skin requires 1,000 times more energy than from UVB (12), daily exposure to UVA is much greater than UVB, and at the level of the dermal capillaries, the UVA effect, as a result of greater penetrance, is much stronger that UVB (Fig. 28.2). Thus UV light of varying wavelengths can induce abnormal skin responses in lupus patients and can induce cutaneous lesions.

Role Of Ultraviolet In Exacerbation Of SLE

It often is stated that sunlight cannot only aggravate cutaneous LE but can potentiate systemic features of disease. Up to 73% of patients with SLE report photosensitivity (15). However, phototesting with standardized protocols correlates poorly with patient-reported photosensitivity (16). This may be because of the delayed nature of the phenomena observed on phototesting. Although patients report that several disease symptoms (including weakness, fatigue, and joint pain) are increased by sun exposure (15),

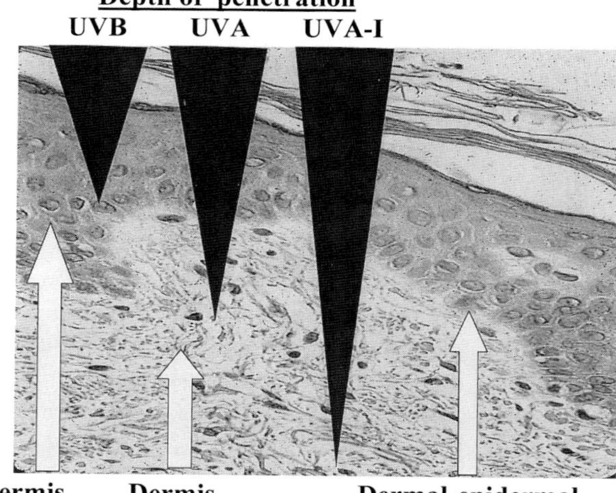

FIGURE 28.2. Photomicrograph of normal skin depicting the depth of penetration of the various forms of ultraviolet radiation (UVR). The skin is formed by an epidermal compartment that includes the stratum corneum (horny layer), the epidermis proper, and a basement membrane zone. Keratinocytes (skin cells), melanocytes (pigment cells), and Langerhans cells (dendritic cells) are found in this compartment. The dermal compartment includes the vasculature of the skin and connective tissue. Penetration of UVR is directly proportional to the wavelength of the radiation. UVB is absorbed primarily in the epidermis. UVA penetrates the dermis and can affect the skin vasculature. UVA1 has the potential to penetrate the skin more deeply that UVA of shorter wavelength.

variation in disease activity related to sun exposure using objective variables has not been shown in large cohort studies. The available evidence is largely anecdotal. Repeated single patient observations indicate that sunlight may precipitate disease *de novo* or aggravate existing disease. Phototherapy for presumed psoriasis has led to aggravation of the lupus lesions (17). Tanning-bed use also has been reported to exacerbate SLE (18). Two recent studies show that although cutaneous manifestations are more common in the summer months, systemic disease activity is increased in the 3 to 6 months following maximal potential sun exposure. This has led these authors to suggest that summer UV light exposure may lead to systemic flares several months later (19, 20).

Polymorphous Light Eruption As A Predisposing Feature Of LE Photosensitivity

Is there direct clinical evidence of a predisposing sensitivity to UV irradiation in patients with LE? Polymorphous light eruption (PLE) is a common photodermatosis affecting up to 10% of the population (21). There is a lag time of 2 hours to 5 days between sun exposure and the development of a pruritic, erythematous eruption on the skin. Selected patients with PLE have been noted to have severe photosensitivity as defined by the persistence of photo-induced lesions. These patients were noted to have positive antinuclear antibodies in significant titers and have been proposed to be a "forme fruste" of photosensitive LE (22). Nyberg recently assessed 337 consecutive lupus patients (with either cutaneous or systemic LE) recruited from dermatology departments in Finland and Sweden and found that almost 50% gave a history of photosensitivity consistent with PLE (23) and this predated the clinical onset of LE by many years. In a separate study, they went on to photoprovoke lesions in their photosensitive LE patients and produced lesions of clinical PLE with a histology consistent with PLE in about half of these patients (24). Immunohistochemical analysis shows upregulated intercellular adhesion molecule-1 (ICAM-1) staining on basilar keratinocytes in both PLE (25) and cutaneous LE (26). This molecule can enhance inflammatory cell infiltration. It is thus possible that there is a mechanistic link between abnormal photosensitivity (as manifest by a PLE-like eruption) and susceptibility to LE. As these studies were completed only on a mixed Finnish and Swedish population, applicability to other populations is still unknown. Furthermore, it should be pointed out that studies of long-term cohorts of patients with PLE have not documented an increased risk of LE in these populations (27, 28). Thus a less common disease (LE) may be preceded by an increased incidence of a more common photosensitive condition (PLE) but the presence of PLE-like photosensitivity alone does not predict lupus.

A SELECTIVE SENSITIVITY TO UV LIGHT IN LE?

Clinical observations suggestive of a role for UV light in the pathogenesis of systemic lupus erythematosus and lupus skin disease have been supported by mechanistic studies. Autoantibodies to DNA and DNA-associated proteins characterize systemic LE. In early studies, UV-irradiated DNA but not native DNA was shown to induce a humoral immune response in animals. Repeated injections of UV-irradiated DNA (UV-DNA) into rabbits resulted in renal disease characterized by proteinuria and renal immunoglobulin deposition (29). Similar results were obtained in mice and some of the immunopathological and histopathological changes associated with cutaneous LE were then reproduced by exposing the skin of UV-DNA immunized mice to UV radiation (30). One of the changes induced in DNA by UV is the formation of thymidine dimers. Thymidine dimers were found in the skin of UV-irradiated mice and UV-DNA antibodies reacted to these thymidine dimers (31, 32). Such immune responses to UV-altered DNA have also been found in LE patients (33). From this concept of an immune response to UV-DNA, evolved the idea that patients with LE may have an impaired ability to repair UV-damaged DNA with subsequent persistence of potentially immunogenic UV-damaged DNA. Studies using fibroblasts from patients with LE showed that these cells were more susceptible to the cytotoxic activity of UVB (34) as well as UVA (35) than fibroblasts from controls. This susceptibility was manifested as an increase in cellular lethality following UV exposure. This enhanced cellular toxicity to UV was not from defects in DNA repair and has not yet been adequately explained (36).

UV-altered DNA can induce lupuslike disease in animals and LE patients may exhibit increased levels of UV-altered DNA. Does UV light also accelerate disease in animal models? Repeated exposure to UV light can accelerate the spontaneous systemic lupus of certain murine strains. Exposure of BXSB autoimmune lupus mice to UVB has been shown to induce the release of autoantigens, to promote antibody production and to promote early death (37). This could not be reproduced in other lupus strains such as the NZB/NZW model (38) or the MRL/lpr mouse (37) suggesting that UV light may have a variable role in the genesis and acceleration of lupus depending on the genetic background. Nevertheless, these observations, both clinical and mechanistic, have been used to justify continued photoprotection for patients with systemic lupus (39, 40).

BIOLOGICAL RESPONSES TO ULTRAVIOLET LIGHT

Ultraviolet light has multiple effects on living tissue. Potential molecular targets of ultraviolet light include not only

TABLE 28.1. BIOLOGIC EFFECTS OF ULTRAVIOLET RADIATION

Characteristic	UVB	UVA
Absorption by molecules	DNA, amino acids, melanin, urocanoic acid	Melanin
Direct DNA damage	Increased	Minimal
Free-radical production	Minimal	Increased
Depth of penetration	Epidermal	Dermal
Epidermal effects	Stratum corneum thickening, intermediate and delayed apoptosis, keratinocyte cytokine transcription and release	Immediate apoptosis
Langerhans cell effects	Inactivation, emigration	Minimal
Endothelial effects	Papillary vessel damage	Dermal vessel damage and activation

UVA, ultraviolet A; UVB, ultraviolet B.

DNA, but RNA, proteins and lipids. The biologic effects of UV light on the skin are summarized in Table 28.1. In addition to alteration of DNA, cytoskeletal reorganization was noted in keratinocytes (skin cells) after UV irradiation (41). An early study by LeFeber revealed that UV light can induce the binding of antibodies to selected nuclear antigens on cultured human keratinocytes (42). The specificity of these antibodies was not defined but it is now known that they are commonly directed against Ro/SSA, La/SSB, ribonucleoprotein and Smith (Sm) antigens and are the antibodies associated with LE and photosensitivity. Norris later noted increased antibody binding to keratinocytes following *in vivo* UV irradiation of human skin (43). This was confirmed independently by Golan who observed binding of anti-Ro/SSA positive sera to cultured keratinocytes (44). These results could be explained by UV-induced translocation of antigens to the cell surface with or without the death of the cell, or by other alterations in the antigens allowing the binding of auto-antibodies taken up by the living cell (45). In 1994, Casciola-Rosen and colleagues demonstrated that when keratinocytes grown in cell culture are irradiated with UVB, they actively cleave their DNA and die by a process termed apoptosis (46). During this process, the antigens recognized by autoantibodies such as Ro/SSA, and calreticulin are concentrated in structures termed blebs or apoptotic bodies found at the cell surface. Larger blebs arise from the nucleus and harbor Ro/SSA, La/SSB, and other nuclear material. These investigators (47) and others (48) have proposed that these bleb-associated antigens may then be phagocytosed, packaged, and presented to lymphocytes, thereby stimulating autoimmune responses.

ULTRAVIOLET LIGHT, APOPTOSIS AND THE SKIN

Apoptosis and necrosis are the two major mechanisms of cell death. Apoptosis is an ordered means of noninflammatory cell removal in which a central biochemical program initiates the dismantling of cells by nuclear fragmentation, formation of an apoptotic envelope, and shrinking of the cell into fragments leading to phagocytosis by parenchymal cells as well as phagocytes (49–51). In necrosis, cells are passive targets of extensive membrane damage leading to cell lysis and release of contents. Apoptosis can be further categorized into "immediate" apoptosis or preprogrammed cell death, and "intermediate" and "delayed" apoptosis or programmed cell death [reviewed by (52)]. Immediate apoptosis is protein synthesis independent, occurs rapidly after triggering (53) and is the result of singlet-oxygen damage to mitochondrial membranes. Intermediate apoptosis is commonly the result of activation of a membrane receptor with a death domain such as Fas [reviewed in (54)]. Delayed apoptosis requires several hours for execution and is protein synthesis dependent. This can be the result of DNA damage (55) or from lack of essential survival signals (56).

Keratinocyte Apoptosis And Ultraviolet Light

Keratinocytes die by programmed cell death as part of their normal program of differentiation (57–59). This occurs normally in the granular cell layer of the epidermis, at the interface with the stratum corneum. The molecular machinery controlling this programmed cell death in keratinocytes is complex and still poorly understood (60). Basilar keratinocytes have been found to be relatively resistant to apoptosis induced by a variety of stimuli (61). This may be as a result of the expression of proteins that specifically inhibit apoptosis such as bcl-2, survivin (62), and other inhibitors of apoptosis (IAPs) [reviewed in (63)]. Ultraviolet light has long been known to induce apoptotic death in suprabasilar keratinocytes; such cells were called "sunburn cells" by morphologists (64). UV light now is known to induce apoptosis by multiple mechanisms. Long-wave ultraviolet light (UVA1; 380 to 400 nm) can induce "immediate" apoptotic death through singlet-oxygen damage to mitochondrial membranes (65). UVB can induce direct, ligand-independent activation of membrane death receptors such as Fas (66) as well as FasL (Fas ligand) upregulation and subsequent Fas-FasL binding (67). Tumor necrosis factor-α (TNF-α) release and consequent ligation of the TNF receptor p55 (TNFR1) also has been shown to be an important mediator of UVB-induced keratinocyte apoptosis (68, 69). Finally, UVB can induce keratinocyte apoptosis secondary to DNA damage (70). Once the signal for apoptosis is triggered, specific enzymes within the cell begin the dismantling process. These enzymes now are collectively called caspases, an anacronym for *c*ysteine *asp*arate protein*ases* (71). These enzymes are known to be important in UV-induced cell death because specific inhibitors of these enzymes prevent the UV-induced death of keratinocytes (72).

Apoptosis In Cutaneous Lupus Erythematosus

The potential importance of apoptosis in the pathogenesis of cutaneous lupus is underscored by a number of recent observations. Using terminal deoxynucleotidyl transferase-mediated UTP nick-end labeling (TUNEL) staining to detect nuclei with DNA damage, Norris demonstrated the presence of an increased number of apoptotic keratinocytes in the basal zone of CCLE lesions and in the suprabasal zone of SCLE lesions (61). An increase in the number of apoptotic cells in lesional skin from patients with cutaneous LE since has been confirmed and has been associated with increased p53 protein expression as determined by immunohistochemistry (73, 74). The nuclear phosphoprotein p53 is a tumor suppressor that is upregulated in response to UV-induced DNA damage (75) and in response to the cytokines TNF-α (68) and interferon-γ (IFN-γ) (76). Upregulation of p53 in suprabasilar keratinocytes can initiate cell death by apoptosis (77). The increased number of apoptotic cells therefore could be a result of an increased rate of apoptosis induction mediated directly by UV light or as a consequence of UV-induced cytokine release. Apoptosis also can be induced by cellular cytotoxic mechanisms. Cytotoxic T lymphocytes (CTL) and natural killer (NK) cells can induce apoptosis through multiple mechanisms [reviewed in (78)] including the release of perforin and granzymes (76); cytokine release [IFN-γ, tumor necrosis factor (TNF)-α, TNF-β, interleukin (IL)-1] (79); and triggering of Fas by FasL (80). The presence of leukocytes in proximity to the apoptotic cells (61) and the presence of FasL positive macrophages in proximity to apoptotic cells in lesional hair follicles (81) suggest a role for such cellular apoptotic mechanisms in established lesions.

An increased number of apoptotic cells are noted in lesional LE skin. Can this have systemic as well as local consequences? There is evidence that the biochemical processes of apoptosis generate novel antigens that are uniquely targeted by autoantibodies. Casciola-Rosen et al. have shown that the caspases activated during apoptosis cleave intracellular proteins into fragments that are bound by autoantibodies from some patients with LE (82). Further, proteins specifically phosphorylated by stress-induced apoptosis are targeted by antibodies from LE patient sera (83, 84). From these observations, it has been inferred that the process of apoptosis is important in the initiation of autoimmune responses. Recently, it has been shown that patients with LE skin disease have autoantibodies that preferentially recognize apoptotic-modified U1-70-kd RNP antigen when compared to patients without skin disease (85). This provides further *in vivo* evidence that immune recognition of modified forms of self antigen occurs in cutaneous LE and suggests that this immune recognition and the processing of apoptotic-derived antigens may participate in the pathogenesis of the disease.

Granzyme B, a serine protease found principally in the cytotoxic granules of CTL and NK cells, also can induce cell death by apoptosis in susceptible target cells. Granzyme B can cleave cellular proteins into unique fragments not detected in other forms of apoptosis. Such cleavage products, specific for cytotoxic-granule induced death, also are bound by antibodies present in LE sera (86). Interestingly, expression of granzyme B has been detected in keratinocytes, suggesting that these molecules may participate in cutaneous defense mechanisms (87) and perhaps in keratinocyte death. In this case, specific correlation of autoantibodies to granzyme B-generated epitopes with cutaneous LE has not yet been made. Novel autoantigens can be generated by apoptosis that is either stress-induced (UV light, viral infection, or other trigger) or secondary to cellular immune mechanisms. The generation and concentration of such neoantigens could pose a challenge to self-tolerance (88). Whether the increased keratinocyte apoptosis noted in cutaneous LE leads directly to the formation of autoantibodies specific to apoptosis-derived byproducts is still speculation.

Abnormalities Of Ultraviolet-Induced Keratinocyte Apoptosis As A Predisposing Factor In Cutaneous Lupus Erythematosus

Although detection of an increased number of apoptotic cells in LE epidermis may underlie an increase in apoptosis, either an increase in the rate of apoptotic death or a decrease in the rate of clearance of apoptotic debris could lead to the observed increase in apoptotic cell number. Phagocytosis by macrophages or parenchymal cells is the final event in the clearing of cells undergoing apoptosis (50, 51). A number of observations suggest that clearance of apoptotic debris may be impaired in LE. Interestingly, the surface blebs of apoptotic keratinocytes bind C1q, an early component of the complement cascade (89). The only C1q-binding protein that has been identified in apoptotic blebs to date is calreticulin (46), and autoantibodies to calreticulin can interfere with this binding (90). The binding of C1q to apoptotic cells has been postulated to facilitate the clearance of these cells by macrophages that express a C1q cell surface receptor (91). A potential role for C1q in the clearance of apoptotic debris and in the genesis of cutaneous LE is suggested by two observations. First, patients with C1q deficiency develop LE-like photosensitive eruptions (92). Second, mice with C1q deficiency develop an SLE-like disease associated with an accumulation of apoptotic cells in the kidney (93). Moreover, a recent study in humans has demonstrated that the clearance of apoptotic lymphocytes by macrophages is indeed impaired in some patients with SLE (94). What remains unclear is if this impaired clearance is secondary to a defect in the recognition and the binding of apoptotic particles or in macrophage phagocytosis. It is also unknown if this defect extends to the phagocytosis of other cell types such as keratinocytes. Sunburn cells normally are cleared rapidly and disappear within 24 to 48 hours in murine skin (95, 96). Whether this is the result of shedding or of phagocytosis by either neighboring keratinocytes or macrophages is unclear. Detailed studies of sunburn-cell clearance in humans have not yet been published but the mechanisms by which such apoptotic cells are recognized and cleared *in vivo* are an area of active investigation.

Macrophages are the organism's primary remover of cellular debris. Macrophages that have ingested apoptotic cells *in vitro* secrete factors such as transforming growth factor -β and prostaglandin E-2 (PGE-2). These factors can inhibit the release of proinflammatory cytokines such as TNF-α by neighboring cells. In addition to removal of cellular debris, macrophages may therefore actively promote tolerance and inhibit proinflammatory cytokine production (97). Dendritic cells (DC), in contrast, are professional antigen-presenting cells present in the skin that have been shown both to acquire antigen from apoptotic cells and then to prime naive T cells in an antigen-specific fashion (98). Thus, depending on the nature of the phagocytic cell with which the apoptotic cell interacts, autoimmunity or tolerance may ensue. High numbers of apoptotic cells have been shown to act as a trigger for local DC maturation and to promote antigen presentation to class I and class II MHC-restricted T cells in a murine system (99). An abundance of apoptotic cells, either from excessive amount of death induction by UV or other mechanisms or from a defect in clearance could permit tolerance to apoptotic antigens to be broken. The potential role of apoptotic mechanisms in the initiation and perpetuation of photosensitive LE is summarized in Figure 28.3.

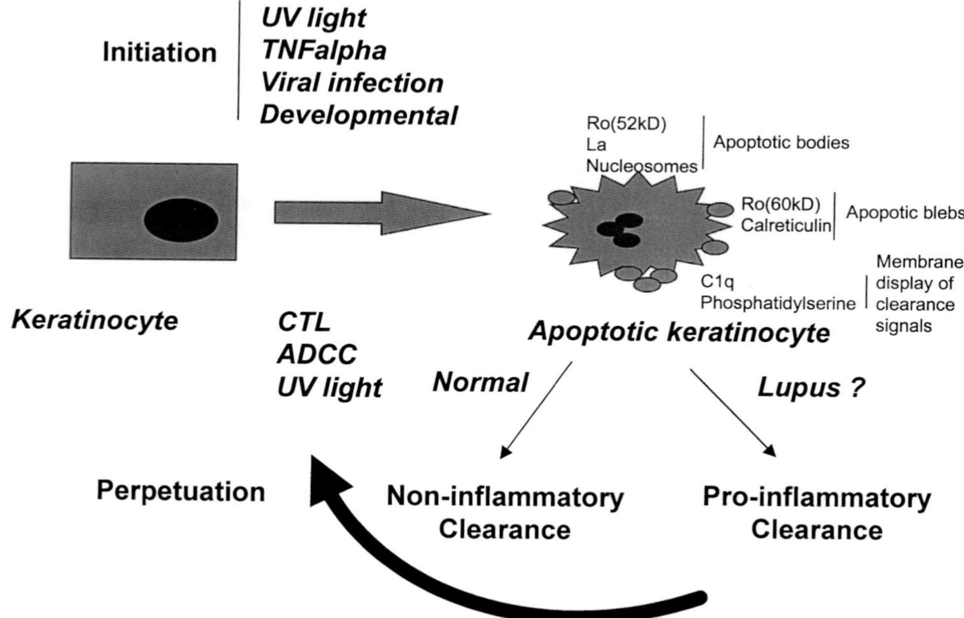

FIGURE 28.3. Potential role of keratinocyte apoptosis in the pathogenesis of photosensitive lupus erythematosus. Apoptosis is an ordered means of cell death. Apoptosis can be initiated in keratinocytes by ultraviolet (UV) radiation (UVB as well as UVA), by viruses, by cytokines (TNFα), by growth-factor withdrawal, by differentiation, and by cytotoxic cellular assault. Apoptosis leads to small bleb formation in which Ro antigen and calreticulin are concentrated. Larger apoptotic bodies contain other potential autoantigens including Ro antigen (60 kd), La, nucleosomes, and 70-kd RNP antigen. Apoptosis leads to the exposure of phosphtidylserine on the cell surface and to the binding of c1q. The presence of apoptotic cell in a proinflammatory environment may lead to uptake and processing by antigen-presenting cells leading the priming and boosting of T cells and B cells to self-antigen.

ULTRAVIOLET LIGHT AS INFLAMMATORY STIMULUS

Erythema (redness) is a normal response to UV light and is mediated by multiple eicosanoids, vasoactive mediators, neuropeptides, and cytokines released from keratinocytes, mast cells, endothelial cells, and fibroblasts (100, 101). (The wide range of mediators released by UV light in the skin is listed in Table 28.2). As discussed, UV light can induce prolonged erythema and cutaneous lesions in patients with LE. UV light is not only an executioner, killing keratinocytes by apoptosis, it also is a generator of neoantigens (such as UV-DNA).

Cytokine Release

UV light can induce cutaneous inflammation by promoting the release of inflammatory mediators and cytokines by inducing adhesion molecule display and by releasing chemokines to attract inflammatory cells into the skin [reviewed by Bennion and Norris (102)]. Both UVB and UVA can participate in lesion induction and act by differing mechanisms. UVB induces the release of the primary cytokines IL-1α and TNF-α from the epidermis, initiating a cascade of inflammatory events. UVB induces IL-1α gene transcription in keratinocytes (103) and elevates circulating levels of IL-1α bioactivity (104). Likewise, UVB induces the release of TNF-α from keratinocytes (105). This may be partly dependent on the photoisomerisation of *trans* to *cis* urocanoic acid in the differentiated epidermis (106). TNF-α release has been noted to be greatest in terminally differentiated keratinocytes in culture (107) and is thus proposed to be maximal in the superior layers of the epidermis. IL-1α and TNF-α are "primary cytokines" which induce the release of a number of other proinflammatory cytokines from the epidermis [reviewed in (108)]. For example, IL-1α and TNF-α induce the secondary release of IL-6, prostaglandin E-2, IL-8, and granulocyte-monocyte colony-stimulating factor (GM-CSF) by keratinocytes (109, 110). These molecules are costimulatory factors for lymphocyte activation by antigens or superantigens, stimulate Langerhans cell function (the Langerhans cell is the resident DC of the skin), stimulate collagenase production, and act as pyrogens and stimulators of acute-phase reactants. In addition, IL-8 and GM-CSF are chemotactic and induce inflammatory cell migration into the skin (111). Both IL-1α and TNF-α also induce adhesion molecule expression such as ICAM-1. Importantly, TNF-α can induce activation of Langerhans cells, the professional antigen presenting cells of the epidermis, via binding of the TNF p75 receptor (TNFR2) on these cells (112). This results in migration of these cells to the regional lymph nodes where they can participate in immune responses (113). In addition to IL-1α and TNF-α release, UVB can stimulate the release of IL-10 (114–117) and IL-6 directly (118). IL-10 has been shown to mediate local (119) as well as systemic UV-induced immunosuppression (120).

TABLE 28.2. MEDIATOR RELEASE BY ULTRAVIOLET RADIATION

Source of Mediator	UVB	UVA
Keratinocyte	IL-1α, TNF-α	
	GM-CSF, IL-6, IL-8	IL-8
	IL-10	IL-10, IL-12
	TGF-α	
	PGE_2, $PGF_{2\alpha}$	PGE_2, $PGF_{2\alpha}$
Mast cell	TNF-α	
	LTC4, LTD4, PGD	
	Histamine	
Endothelial cell	TNF-α, PCl_2	PCl_2
Langerhans cell		IL-12

Ultraviolet radiation results in the release of interleukins (IL), prostaglandins (PG), prostacyclin (PC), leukotrienes (LT), and other mediators.
UVA, ultraviolet A; UVB, ultraviolet B.

Transgenic overexpression of IL-6 in murine keratinocytes has been associated with an increase in the thickness of the stratum corneum but not with significant cutaneous inflammation when expressed alone (121). Both IL-10 and IL-6 have further been shown to induce local heat-shock protein synthesis (122, 123). UVB induced primary cytokine production and release is likely the result of UVB-induced DNA damage: UV-damaged DNA, specifically UV thymidine dimer formation, induces DNA repair enzymes that also regulate cytokine transcriptional activity (124).

In contrast to UVB, UVA upregulates ICAM-1 in keratinocytes directly by producing oxygen free radicals that affect gene transcription (125). UVA also upregulates IL-8 and IL-10 production in keratinocytes and FasL expression in dermal mononuclear cells (126, 127). The longer wavelength of UVA allows it to penetrate into the dermis and to upregulate vascular endothelial ICAM-1 and E selectin thereby increasing leukocyte-vascular adhesion (128). Acute low-dose UVA administration, but not UVB, also results in IL-12 production by keratinocytes (129, 130). UVA results in a rapid increase in interferon-γ (IFN-γ) levels in the skin, the source of which may be resident epidermal T cells (130). This IFN-γ has been postulated to potentiate IL-12 release (130). IL-12 is a potent immunostimulant that can abrogate tolerance induced by low-dose UVB (131).

Ultraviolet Light And Th-1/Th-2 Cytokine Balance

Overall, exposure to UVB radiation correlates with a predominance in cytokines that promote T helper 2 (Th2) immune responses at the expense of T helper 1 (Th1) immune responses and that may result in photoimmunosuppression (132). While potentially suppressing cellular immune responses, Th2 responses generally promote antibody production (133). Exposure to physiologic levels of

UVA radiation alone, or together with UVB (like natural sunlight), results in the local predominance cytokines that promote Th1 immune responses. These Th1 responses are "immunopotentiating" and result in strong cellular immune responses including $CD8^+$ cytotoxic T-cell responses (133). Whether patients with cutaneous LE have a unique primary or secondary sensitivity to UV light-induced cytokine changes is not yet clear. Significant interindividual variability in UV light-induced ICAM-1 expression and TNF-α release has been noted in keratinocyte cell lines (107) and this suggests that there may be genetic variability in the human skin response to UV.

Possible Benefit Of Ultraviolet In Lupus Erythematosus Patients

Although the above discussion has focused on the potential inflammatory effects of UV light, recent work has suggested that selective UV radiation may have salutatory effects in LE. UVA irradiation of NZB/NZW mice has resulted in increased survival and decreased levels of circulating anti-DNA antibodies (134). Subsequently, a randomized, double-blind cross-over study of UVA1 light (light limited to the longer wavelength spectrum of UVA, 340 to 400 nm) compared to visible light showed significant clinical and serologic improvements in SLE patients treated with UVA1 light (135). The investigators have proposed that the combination of "immediate apoptosis" induction (potentially preventing autoantigen translocation into blebs), the induction of the antiinflammatory cytokine IL-10 by UVA1, and a potential reduction of proinflammatory IL-12 may mediate these effects (136).

HUMORAL FACTORS IN CUTANEOUS LUPUS ERYTHEMATOSUS

Autoantibody production is a *sine-qua non* of SLE and the autoantibodies can be pathogenic. Extracutaneous lupuslike disease can be induced in animals by the introduction of anti-DNA antibodies either transgenically (137) or by intravenous injection (138). Autoantibodies can initiate cellular cytotoxicity and activate the complement cascade and also can promote the recognition of epitopes related to the original autoantigen through a process termed epitope spreading.

Immunopathology Of Cutaneous LE

Immunofluorescence studies of cutaneous LE lesions show lesional deposition of immunoglobulins (Fig. 28.4). In 80% to 90% of CCLE or ACLE, and in 50% to 60% of SCLE, a thick band of immunoglobulins and complement components is deposited along the dermo-epidermal junction (139). These complexes have been localized on the upper dermal collagen fibers and along the lamina densa of the epidermal basement membrane zone (140). As these deposits also are found in clinically normal skin of patients with SLE, their role in the local induction of cutaneous tissue injury is still unclear (141). Further, the specificities of these skin basement membrane-deposited antibodies has not been defined.

Ro/SS-A And La/SS-B Autoantibodies And LE Photosensitivity

Several specific autoantibodies have a special relationship to cutaneous LE. SCLE was recognized as a distinct and uniquely photosensitive subset of cutaneous LE by Sontheimer et al. (142). This form of cutaneous disease is strongly associated with a particular autoantibody specificity, anti-Ro/SSA (143); Ro/SSA antibodies have been observed in frequencies ranging from 40% to 100% of SCLE patients by immunodiffusion techniques (144). Neonatal LE also is strongly associated with an anti-Ro response (145). In this disorder, infants have maternally acquired IgG Ro/SSA antibodies and develop SCLE-like skin lesions. As the maternally derived Ro/SSA antibodies are cleared from the infant's circulation several months after

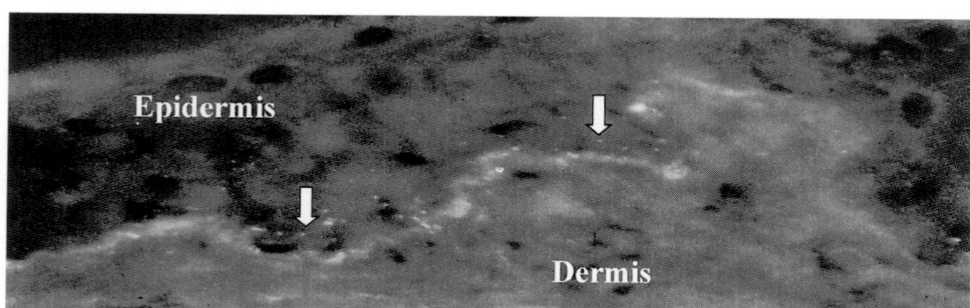

FIGURE 28.4. (See color plate.) Immunopathology of subacute cutaneous lupus. Direct immunofluorescence analysis for the presence of IgG reveals a "dustlike" distribution of IgG deposits in the suprabasilar keratinocytes (arrowheads mark specific IgG "dust" deposits). There is also IgG deposition in the basement membrane zone.

birth, the skin lesions resolve (146). The anti-Ro antibody specificity has been implicated in animals as a direct cause of heart block, another manifestation of neonatal LE (147–150). It has been proposed that Ro/SSA and La/SSB antibodies bind human cardiocytes only after appropriate developmental apoptosis and that *in vivo* opsonized apoptotic cardiocytes then promote an inflammatory response damaging surrounding tissue (151). Anti-Ro/SSA antibody infusion can lead to the deposition of anti-Ro/SSA antibodies onto human skin grafts in severe combined immundeficient (SCID) mice (152). The deposition pattern is identical to "dustlike particles" of immunoglobulin deposition over the cytoplasm and nuclei of cells in the lower epidermis and upper dermis seen in adults with SCLE and babies with NLE and first described by Nieboer (153) (see also Fig. 28.3). The cellular pathology of SCLE however, is not reproduced in the SCID mouse model arguing that autoantibodies may be participatory, but other factors must be present as well. In favor of this, no difference has been noted in the frequency of Ro/SSA autoantibodies among lupus patients with positive or negative phototest reactions (9, 14). In addition, titers of antibodies to Ro/SSA do not always correlate with skin activity (154). The presence of levels of Ro/SSA antibodies similar to SCLE in disorders such as Sjogren's syndrome (not typically associated with cutaneous lesions) also argues that factors other than the serologic presence and local Ro/SSA antibody deposition must participate in the genesis of LE skin disease.

The Ro/SS-A Autoantigen System

The originally described Ro antigen is a protein of 60 kd that may be bound *in vivo* to four small RNA molecules called "Y RNA" or "hY RNA" (155). Subsequent studies have indicated that the hY RNA molecules also can be targets of autoantibody production in SLE patients (156). The term "Ro" derives from the first two letters of the last name of the index patient from whom the antibody was characterized. It is identical to an antigen characterized from patients with Sjögren's syndrome and given the name "SSA" (157). It is now known that Ro/SSA autoantibodies can variably bind to at least four antigenically distinct polypeptide components of the Ro/SSA ribonucleoprotein (158) in addition to the hY RNA molecules themselves. The function of the 60-kd antigen still is unknown but it has been proposed that it may be involved in ribosome synthesis, assembly, or transport (159) or that it may be part of a salvage pathway for mutant rRNA precursors (160). A recent study has linked a bacterial homologue of Ro/SSA to a UV-resistant phenotype in bacteria (161). Based on these observations, Ro/SSA may bind to UV damaged RNA and protect the cell from UV damage.

Reactivity against a 52 kd polypeptide is another antibody specificity commonly found in anti-Ro/SSA positive sera (162). The function of the 52 kd Ro/SSA antigen is likewise still unknown but the protein recently has been shown to interact with the deubiquinating enzyme UNP, suggesting an involvement in the ubiquitin pathway (163). A physical association between the 52-kd and 60-kd proteins has been demonstrated by immunoprecipitation assays (164). A protein-protein interaction between these two polypeptides recently has been confirmed (165). Calreticulin, a 46-kd calcium-binding protein also has been reported to bind both hY RNA and 52-kd Ro (166) and may play a role in facilitating the binding of 60 kd Ro/SSA to hY RNA. Calreticulin binds calcium in the endoplasmic reticulum and has been found to have multiple functions including the inhibition of C1q-mediated immune functions (167, 168). Calreticulin also has been shown to have *in vivo* peptide-binding activity and to facilitate the priming of CTL against such bound peptides (169).

The La/SS-B Autoantigen System

The La/SSB antigen is a 48 kd protein that participates in the control of RNA polymerase III transcription termination (170). Recently, La/SSB has been shown to control the synthesis of the x-linked inhibitor of apoptosis protein (XIAP), a key inhibitor of apoptosis, that is upregulated in cells under physical stress (171). La/SSB also is associated with 60 kd Ro, likely through mutual binding to hY RNA (172). The functions and cellular redistribution of calreticulin (173), the 52-kd and 60-kd Ro/SSA polypeptides (174–176), and the La antigen (175) all have been associated with the heat-shock response. The heat-shock response is characterized by the production and activation of ubiquitous cellular proteins that detect and bind proteins damaged by heat or other physiologically stressful stimuli (177). The potential involvement of the variable cutaneous LE-associated autoantibody antigens with the heat-shock response may relate to the general importance of this response to cellular stresses or may be a function of a potentially unique relationship of this response to the abrogation of self-tolerance. Heat shock proteins (HSP), which are induced in heat-shock responses, have been shown to promote cellular immune responses by both chaperoning peptides into cellular antigen processing compartments and by directly activating antigen-presenting cells (178, 179). HSP induction by UV light has been correlated to the increased binding of Ro/SSA and La/SSB antibodies in keratinocytes *in vitro* (175). Finally, increased HSP70 expression is increased in both sun-exposed and sun-protected skin of SLE patients (180).

Epitope Spreading

Epitope spreading is the process by which specific immune responses that arise to particular determinants on a macromolecule diversify over time (181). B cells, by virtue of their immunoglobulin receptors, can process and concentrate antigen prior to T-cell presentation and are central to this process. This spread of immune responses can occur to epitopes within the primary macromolecule (*intra*molecular epitope spreading) or to physically associated molecules (*inter*molecular epitope spreading). Both inter- and *intra*molecular epitope spreading have been reported in cases of murine immunization with peptides of 60 kd Ro/SSA, 52 kd Ro/SSA, and La (182–184). This is consistent with a physical linking of these antigens (185). Spreading of the immune response for 52 kd Ro/SSA and 60 kd Ro/SSA (but not La/SSB) to calreticulin is consistent with the notion that calreticulin may associate with a subpopulation of Ro/SSA particles from which La/SSB already has dissociated (184). The observation that human anti-Ro/SSA immune responses segregate with either anticalreticulin responses or anti-La/SSB responses (186) also is consistent with a differential compartmentalization of Ro/SSA and La/SSB antigens at the time of initiation of the immune response. The secondary recruitment of antibodies to the inducible heat shock proteins Grp78 and HSP70, following immunization of mice with either 52-kd Ro/SSA, 60-kd Ro/SSA, but not La/SSB, suggests physical association and co-localization of these proteins with the Ro/SSA polypeptides under conditions such as apoptosis, that may promote autoimmunization (174). In addition to providing evidence for the physical association of autoantigens, the phenomenon of epitope spreading to specific antigens associated with cutaneous LE in these animal models suggests that such epitope spreading may occur in human disease. These autoantibodies thereby may enhance and perpetuate cell-mediated autoimmune inflammation.

Interaction Of Ro/SS-A And La/SS-B Autoantibodies And Human Skin

There is compelling evidence that antibodies to Ro/SSA and La /SSB bind to human epidermis *in vivo* (152). The binding of these antibodies to keratinocytes *in vitro* can be enhanced by UV radiation in the presence (46) or absence (187) of apoptosis. Estrogens (188), heat shock (175), and viral-induced apoptosis (189) also can enhance binding. What are the potential consequences of this binding? The predominant IgG subclass that is deposited in lesions is IgG_1, a form that is known to activate complement and initiate antibody-dependent cellular cytotoxicity (ADCC) (190). The presence of complement membrane attack complex at the dermal-epidermal junction (DEJ) of cutaneous LE lesions further suggests an antibody-mediated pathogenesis for the cell damage seen in cutaneous LE (191). The presence of the complement membrane attack complex (C5b-9) in only the lesional skin of patients with SLE, SCLE, or CCLE (192, 193) suggests that this complex may then play a role in the pathogenesis of the lesions. Furukawa et al. have shown that keratinocytes from patients with lupus are more susceptible to binding of anti-Ro/SSA antibodies following UV exposure than controls and that such cells can be lysed by ADCC when sera and peripheral blood leukocytes from patients are added to the keratinocytes (194, 195). This increased binding may be from an increased susceptibility to UV-induced apoptosis or from other causes of increased Ro/SSA antigen availability (44). Considerable interindividual variation in levels of keratinocyte Ro/SSA and La/SSB epitope expression has been noted (196) and expression is higher in lupus patients with documented photosensitivity (197). Despite this evidence, anti-Ro/SSA, La/SSB, and other autoantibodies may not have an initiating role in the clinical lesions of cutaneous lupus because the deposition of immunoglobulin and complement components as detected by fluorescence microscopy generally follows the appearance of perivascular inflammation in photoprovoked lesions (8, 13). Keratinocytes generally are susceptible to ADCC but are able to resist cytotoxic damage by the complement membrane attack complex (198). Although anti-Ro/SSA antibodies can potentiate ADCC *in vitro* (199), natural killer cells are the most common mediators of ADCC and these are seen rarely in cutaneous lupus infiltrates (200, 201). It remains possible that other cell types, including monocytes or lymphocytes, are participating in ADCC but this has not been confirmed *in vivo*.

While the anti Ro/SSA response is clearly associated with SCLE, another clinical type of cutaneous lupus, CCLE is not exquisitely photosensitive. The majority of CCLE patients do not have anti-Ro/SSA responses as detected by standard immunodiffusion techniques. In addition, epidermal IgG deposits are found rarely, and immunoglobulin deposition is limited to the DEJ (144). When sensitive ELISA techniques were used, 11 out of 15 CCLE patients were found to have low-level IgG anti-Ro/SSA antibodies. Other, as yet undefined antibody sensitivities or cell-mediated responses may be paramount in CCLE.

CELLULAR FACTORS

Immunogenetics

Anti-Ro/SSA antibody responses have been linked to susceptibility loci associated with Class II MHC alleles. There is a strong association between SCLE, anti-Ro/SSA antibodies, and the HLA-B8, DR-3, DRw52 phenotypes (202). Associations between Ro antibody responses and DQA1 alleles, DQ2 alleles, and HLA-DR3 in different populations suggest that specific MHC class II molecules participate in the anti-Ro response (203–205). Diversification of the Ro/SSA and LA/SSB antibody response also has been linked to specific HLA class II phenotypes (206). This would imply the participation of Ro/SSA antigen-specific T cells in the generation of the Ro/SSA antibody response. Although 52 kd Ro/SSA-specific T cells have been described in the salivary glands of Sjögren's patients (207), no antigen-specific T cells have been described in cutaneous

LE. Murine T-cell epitopes have been defined in a number of lupus autoantigen systems including the La/SSB autoantigen (208) and the Ro/SSA antigen (209). The specificity and role of similar autoantigen-specific T cells in humans is an obvious area of ongoing investigation.

T Cells And Murine Models Of Cutaneous LE

As in the examples above, there is growing evidence that the highly specific humoral immune response to autoantigens in SLE is T-cell dependent (210). Murine models of cutaneous LE include the spontaneously occurring and UV accelerated forms of disease in MRL/lpr mice, graft-versus-host disease, and NZB/NZW mice [reviewed in (211)]. None of these accurately recapitulate the cutaneous pathology seen in human disease. They nevertheless have been useful in a dissection of the potential cellular mechanisms of autoimmune inflammation.

The NZB/NZW mouse offers a model of immune globulin deposition at the DEJ, but these animals do not develop clinical cutaneous inflammation (212). The acute phase of graft-versus-host disease generated by minor histocompatibility disparity simulates the histopathology of cutaneous lupus (213) but immunoglobulin deposition at DEJ is uncommon.

MRL/lpr mice develop alopecia and scab formation associated with histopathological changes similar to cutaneous lupus including DEJ immunoglobulin deposition (214, 215). These lesions are characterized by a T-cell inflammatory infiltrate. The important accelerator role of the lpr mutation on the MRL background has been documented in backcross experiments. The lpr mutation results in deficient Fas expression and this interferes with the apoptotic death of potentially self-reactive B and T cells (216). Both conventional ($\alpha\beta$) and nonclassical ($\gamma\delta$) T cells have been shown to participate in the MRL/lpr disease phenotype including the skin disease (217, 218) and autoantigen-specific $\alpha\beta$ T cells are absolutely required for full penetrance of disease (219). The spontaneous activation of T cells in MRL/lpr mice is highly B-cell dependent (220) but is dissociated from antibody production (221) suggesting that antigen processing and presentation to T cells by B cells is important (222).

Recently, the critical role of the costimulatory molecules B7-1(CD80) and B7-2 (CD86) in this model has been shown. MRL/lpr mice deficient in both of these molecules have diminished skin lesions and do not develop renal pathology (223). These molecules provide essential signals for T-cell activation and immunoglobulin class switching, again establishing a crucial role for B and T cells in this disease.

Role Of Activated T Cells In Human Cutaneous Lupus Erythematosus

The pathology of cutaneous lupus is one of a lichenoid tissue reaction in which the basal keratinocytes are the primary focus of injury (224) (Fig. 28.5). This injury is associated with keratinocyte hyperproliferation, with normal early differentiation and premature terminal differentiation (225). The inflammatory-cell infiltrate is characterized by mononuclear cells at the DEJ as well as around blood vessels and dermal appendages. Inflammatory cells in the infiltrate of established cutaneous LE lesions are predominantly CD3 positive cells with CD4 positive cells present in higher numbers than CD8 cells [reviewed in (139)]. The study of photo-induced lesions has allowed an analysis of early histological changes and their evolution. In early lesions, this analysis has demonstrated $CD4^+$ T cells predominantly at the DEJ associated with rare HLA class II expression by keratinocytes. In spontaneous lesions and late photo-induced lesions, an increased number of $CD8^+$ T cells was observed,

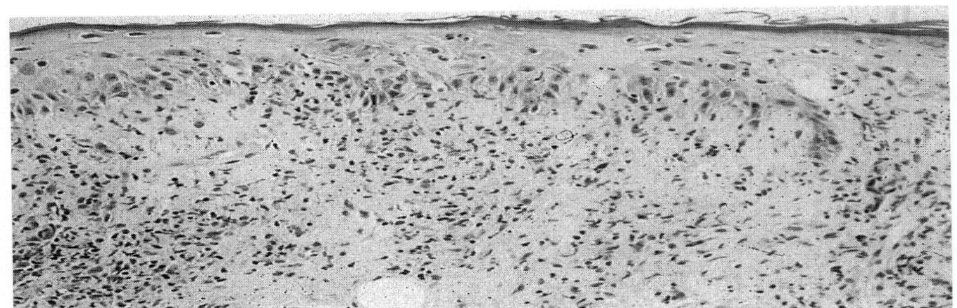

FIGURE 28.5. (See color plate.) Photomicrograph of a biopsy of subacute cutaneous lupus. There is disarray in the maturation pattern of the keratinocytes. There is evidence of hyperkeratosis (increase the thickness of the horny-cell layer). The basement membrane zone is disorganized with a mononuclear cell infiltrate and thickening of the basement membrane zone. There is a dermal mononuclear cell infiltrate that is predominantly perivascular. The mononuclear cells are predominantly CD4 T cells, many showing an activation phenotype, and macrophages.

epidermal class II MHC expression was increased and the number of Langerhans cells was reduced (226–229). The decrease in Langerhans cell number may reflect DC activation and migration into the regional lymph nodes. The predominant type of T cell in established inflammatory infiltrates remains controversial. Volc-Platzer et al. have suggested that T cells of a specific γδ T-cell receptor phenotype are preferentially expanded within the infiltrates (230). They proposed that these cells may recognize heat shock proteins induced or translocated in keratinocytes by UV or stress. Fivenson et al. however, reported that γδ T cells are virtually absent in the infiltrates (231). The Vβ usage of infiltrating T cells in lesions of cutaneous LE recently was compared to that in peripheral blood and in other inflammatory skin conditions (232). The percentage of Vβ8.1 $CD3^+$ cells was elevated in skin lesion from both CCLE and ACLE when compared to patients with other inflammatory skin disease. There was a significant skew to this Vβ type when compared to peripheral blood. This selective expansion is consistent with an antigen-driven response. Sequencing of TCR clonotypes derived from the inflammatory infiltrates further suggests antigen-induced clonal accumulation (233). The expression of class II MHC molecules and CD28 by infiltrating T cells and expression of B7-1(CD80) and B7-2(CD86) costimulatory molecules by antigen-presenting cells in the lesional but not nonlesional skin suggests ongoing active and productive antigen presentation to T cells in cutaneous LE (234).

COFACTORS IN CUTANEOUS LUPUS ERYTHEMATOSUS

Ultraviolet Effects On Cutaneous Vasculature

Observational studies in humans and animal models have furthered our understanding of the roles of autoantibodies and cellular mechanisms in cutaneous lupus. Dermal blood vessels are involved in all forms of cutaneous lupus as targets for the cytokines and other mediators released from keratinocytes. These vessels also are affected directly by UV light. The potential importance of UV light in contributing to dermal and perivascular inflammation is underscored by the exquisite photosensitivity of lupus tumidus, a dermal variant of cutaneous LE without epidermal or interface changes (226, 235). In a model of UV-induced erythema in the guinea pig, infusion of sera from patients with SCLE greatly enhanced UV-induced blood flow and this was greatest with sera containing high titers of anti-Ro/SSA (236). This observation highlights the potential interactions of the various soluble factors present in circulation of patients with cutaneous LE with the vasculature. Passive transfer of serum from patients with vesiculobullous LE into guinea pigs followed by UV irradiation also results in lesion induction (237) providing further evidence that circulating factors contribute to LE photosensitivity.

Vascular Activation

Enhanced expression of adhesion molecules on the surface of endothelial cells is an essential point of control for leukocyte attachment and migration through the endothelial barrier into cutaneous tissues [reviewed by (238, 239)]. A subpopulation of human memory T cells preferentially recirculates to the skin. These cells interact via cutaneous lymphocyte adhesion molecules (CLA) on their surface with E-selectin molecules on dermal microvascular endothelial cells. E-selectin can be upregulated by UVB (240) and its expression is increased in CCLE and SLE photoinduced lesions (241). Elevated levels of soluble E-selectin in LE patients with widespread and active cutaneous disease further suggests and important role for endothelial-cell activation in the pathogenesis of disease (242). Intracellular adhesion molecule 1 (ICAM-1) expression by endothelial cells is a crucial step in the initiation of endothelial T-cell binding, which occurs via LFA-1. ICAM-1 expression also facilitates T-cell adhesion to keratinocytes (243). Endothelial ICAM-1 also is upregulated following UV irradiation, and this is stimulated by TNF-α and IFN-γ (244). In the MRL/lpr mouse model of SLE, TNF-α and IL-1 sequentially induce endothelial ICAM-1 *in vivo* with disease evolution (245). Vascular cell adhesion molecule (VCAM)-1 is necessary for leukocyte emigration from the microvasculature and is the ligand for VLA-4 on leukocytes. Immunohistochemical studies have confirmed that the endothelium underlying cutaneous lupus lesions is activated: VCAM-1 is expressed both in lesional and nonlesional cutaneous endothelium in active systemic lupus (246) and levels of VCAM-1 are increased in lesional skin (241, 247). ICAM-1 is expressed by the endothelial cells in lesional skin of most patients with CCLE or SCLE (248). The role of these molecular interactions in facilitating leukocyte migration into the skin is summarized in Figure 28.6. Chemokines doubtless also have a key role in the recruitment of inflammatory cells to lesional skin but their specific expression and regulation in cutaneous LE has not yet been studied.

Nitric Oxide

The clinically normal appearing skin of patients with active SLE demonstrates elevated levels of inducible nitric oxide synthase (iNOS) in both the epidermis and adjacent vascular endothelium (249). Aberrant regulation of iNOS expression also has been noted in photoinduced lesion of cutaneous lupus (250). Healthy controls were shown to have short-term expression (Days 1 to 2) of iNOS after either UVA or UVB irradiation. Patients with cutaneous

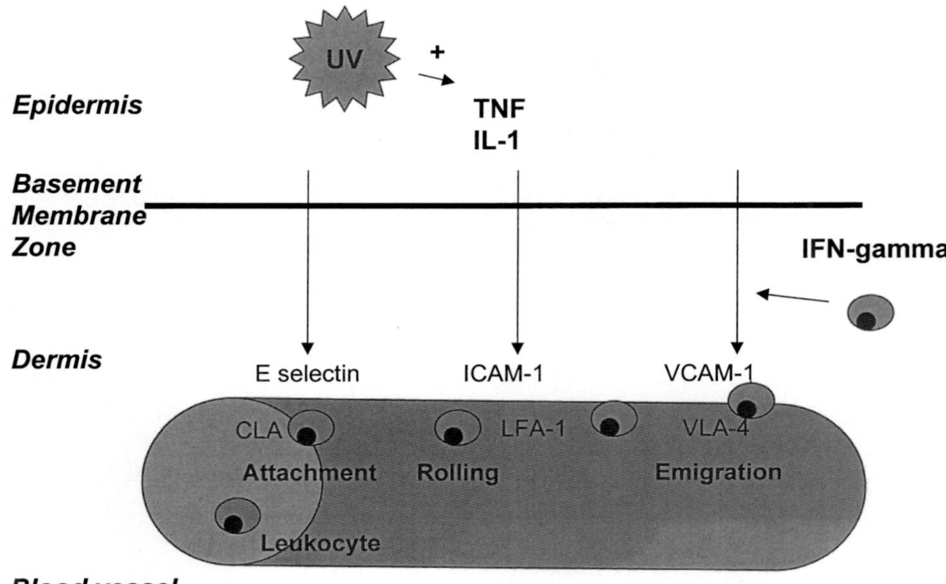

FIGURE 28.6. Ultraviolet (UV)-induced leukocyte migration into the skin. UV radiation induces cytokine release in cutaneous tissues. These cytokines then induce adhesion molecule expression on endothelial cells and leukocytes promoting inflammatory cell recruitment to the skin. Likewise, cytokines released by the inflammatory cells can enhance and perpetuate this recruitment. The selectins and adhesion molecules depicted all have been shown to be upregulated in cutaneous lupus erythematosus.

LE were noted to have significantly delayed but prolonged expression (days 3 to 24) of iNOS. Both IL-1 and TNF-α promote the expression of iNOS (251) and this abnormal expression in cutaneous LE may be secondary to a genetic dysregulation of these cytokines (see below). Synthesis of iNOS leads to nitric oxide (NO) production, which is known to promote apoptosis and have multiple proinflammatory effects. When applied to normal human skin, NO induced accumulation of $CD4^+$ and $CD8^+$ T cells, expression of ICAM-1 and VCAM-1, and accumulation of p53, followed by apoptosis (252). Altered expression of this molecule may link dysregulated apoptosis and inflammation.

Cytokines

An appropriate cytokine *milieu* can facilitate and modulate immune responses. Abnormalities in the production and function of cytokines could underlie the abnormal photoreactivity noted in cutaneous LE. Analysis of interleukin-2, -4, -5 and -10 and IFN-γ mRNA levels in lesions of cutaneous LE has revealed increased local levels of IL-5 and significant levels of IL-10 and IFN-γ (253). These results indicate a mixed cytokine pattern favoring cell adhesion and cellular inflammation via IFN-γ-induced ICAM-1 expression and a T-helper 2 response, favoring antibody production, with IL-5 and IL-10.

TNF-α

TNF-α is a primary cytokine that can be induced in keratinocytes (105) and in dermal fibroblasts by UVB and possibly UVA (254, 255). TNF-α has numerous effector functions and has been termed a master regulator of leukocyte movement (256). Abnormal TNF-α expression can promote autoimmunity. Prolonged overexpression of TNF-α in the pancreas of mice has been shown to initiate organ-specific autoimmune disease (257). In the skin, TNF-α can induce rapid Ro/SSA and La/SSB antigen translocation and surface expression in keratinocytes (258). In mice, transgenic overproduction of TNF-α by the epidermis, results in: (i) epidermal basal-cell degeneration; (ii) a pleomorphic dermal leukocyte infiltrate with macrophage engulfment of degenerating cells; (iii) hyperkeratosis, and (iv) ultimately, a graft-versus-hostlike histology (259). Some of these features are reminiscent of cutaneous lupus. Unfortunately, these mice also have high levels of TNF-α in the serum and soon die of cachexia, which has presumably prevented further analysis for features of autoimmunity. In the MRL/lpr mouse model of lupus, systemic TNF-α (and IL-1) levels are elevated and induce endothelial adhesion molecule expression (245). Raised circulating levels of TNF-α may correlate with disease activity in human systemic lupus (260). A polymorphic variant in the TNF-α promoter in humans (TNF-α 308A) is associated with increased production of TNF-α (261). The presence of this promoter is associated with an increased risk of SLE in African Americans (261). It is an independent susceptibility factor for systemic lupus in Dutch Caucasians (262). TNF-α production in keratinocytes shows interindividual variability and it has been proposed that this variability may underlie a predisposition to cutaneous lupus (26, 107). Recently, this concept has found support in that the TNF-α 308A promoter polymorphism associated with increased TNF-α production has been shown to be highly associated with photosensitive cutaneous LE in Caucasians (263). Direct involvement of TNF-α in the pathogenesis of cutaneous LE inflammation could explain the clinical benefit of thalidomide in this setting (264–266). Thalidomide is known to decrease TNF-α production, possibly via an increase in the rate of TNF-α mRNA degradation (267, 268).

IL-1

Another early response to UV light is the production of and release of IL-1 by keratinocytes. Like TNF-α, IL-1 has broad proinflammatory activities (269). IL-1α predominates in keratinocytes while IL-1β is the predominant form in monocytes, macrophages, and dendritic cells. Transgenic overexpression of IL-1α by basal keratinocytes in mice results in hair loss, scaling, and focal inflammatory lesions (270). Keratinocytes also contain an excess of IL-1 receptor antagonist, which binds to the IL-1 receptor and inhibits IL-1–induced activation (271). This molecule is particularly polymorphic and a significant increase of a null allele has been reported in SLE patients (272), especially those with photosensitivity (273). A correlation with CCLE also has been published in abstract form (274).

Interleukin-10.

IL-10 is a key mediator of UV induced immune suppression (120). IL-10 also can promote B-cell activation (275). Polymorphisms within the IL-10 gene promoter associated with high levels of expression of this cytokine have been associated with anti-Ro/SSA sero-positivity (276). Abnormalities in either constitutive or UV-induced cytokine expression or the genes governing these factors thus may be central to the cutaneous-lupus phenotype. The associations of gene polymorphisms with disease described so far remain preliminary in nature and will need to be confirmed in multiple populations.

Interferon γ

Interferon γ is detected in normal skin after low-dose UVA exposure (130) and elevated IFN-γ mRNA levels are noted in lesions of cutaneous LE (253). This cytokine recently has been shown to be pivotal in the induction of keratinocyte apoptosis in two skin inflammatory conditions: allergic contact dermatitis and atopic dermatitis (277). In these conditions, T-cell derived IFN-γ promotes keratinocyte apoptosis by enhancing the expression the Fas death-inducing molecule on the keratinocytes (277). Overexpression of IFN-γ alone in the suprabasal skin of transgenic mice by the use of the involucrin promoter (a protein restricted to suprabasal keratinizing epithelium) results in a model of systemic lupus with the production of antinuclear antibodies and immune-complex glomerulonephritis (278, 279). The mice also develop scaly skin, alopecia, and cutaneous inflammation — suggestive but not characteristic of cutaneous LE. This murine model demonstrates increased keratinocyte apoptosis and requires the presence of αβ T cells (280). This is currently the most provocative experimental evidence that the upregulation of cutaneous immune responses through cytokine overexpression can promote T-cell–mediated local and systemic lupuslike disease.

Complement

Homozygous deficiencies of the complement components C2, and C4 have been associated with both SCLE and systemic LE (281, 282), and most patients with homozygous C2 or C4 complement deficiency possess anti-Ro/SSA antibodies. Likewise, most individuals with a complete deficiency of C1q or C1r/C1s develop systemic LE [reviewed by (283)]. These patients also have prominent photosensitive cutaneous involvement. Such deficiencies may enhance the lupus phenotype by decreasing the clearance of apoptotic cells, thereby allowing immune-cell activation. Such abnormalities thus may both initiate and potentiate cutaneous lupus.

A MODEL OF PATHOGENESIS OF CUTANEOUS LUPUS ERYTHEMATOSUS

David Norris has proposed a four-step model for the pathogenesis of cutaneous lupus (43): (i) exposure to UV light induces the release of proinflammatory epidermal and dermal mediators such as IL-1 and TNF-α; (ii) these mediators induce changes in the dermal and epidermal cells including the induction of adhesion molecules and the promotion of translocation of normally intracellular autoantigens such as Ro/SSA to the surface of epidermal cells; (iii) autoantibodies then bind to the translocated autoantigens and (iv) keratinocyte cytotoxicity ensues as the result of lymphoid cells that are recruited from the circulation via an antibody-dependent cellular cytotoxicity mechanism. According to this model, several factors are required concurrently for the development of cutaneous LE: (i) Abnormal susceptibility to UV light, resulting in altered cytokine expression and possibly increased keratinocyte apoptosis induction; (ii) The presence of antibodies with appropriate specificities, targeting keratinocyte components upregulated by stress; (iii) The presence of activated lymphocytes, specific for autodeterminants.

Since this model was first proposed, a great deal of new data has accumulated [reviewed herein and in (284–286)]. Clinical and experimental data now suggest that apoptosis may be an important mechanism leading to autoantigen display in cutaneous LE and that UV light may be an important initiator of apoptosis. Abnormalities may exist in either apoptosis induction or in apoptotic cell clearance that result in an increased load of apoptotic cells. In addition to promoting cell death and neoantigen generation (such as UV-DNA), UV light induces and modulates inflammatory mediator release. Genetic abnormalities in TNF-α, IL1 receptor antagonist, and IL-10 have been linked tentatively to cutaneous lupus. The dysregulation of such cytokines may allow the upregulation of adhesion molecules, chemokines, and costimulatory molecules to allow self-antigen recognition and the initiation of an immune response in genetically predisposed individuals. The autoantibodies linked with cutaneous LE are directed at antigens involved in cellular-stress responses and in the heat-shock response. Autoantibody production and directed T-cell responses may perpetuate and amplify autoantigen recognition as well as keratinocyte toxicity leading to the clinical hallmarks of cutaneous LE disease. The salient points of this revised model are shown in Figure 28.7. Ongoing research will no doubt shed light on the *in vivo* role of cellular apoptosis in disease induction and perpetuation, the primary or secondary pathophysiologic role of specific autoantibodies, and the nature of the underlying genetic makeup that predisposes to disease.

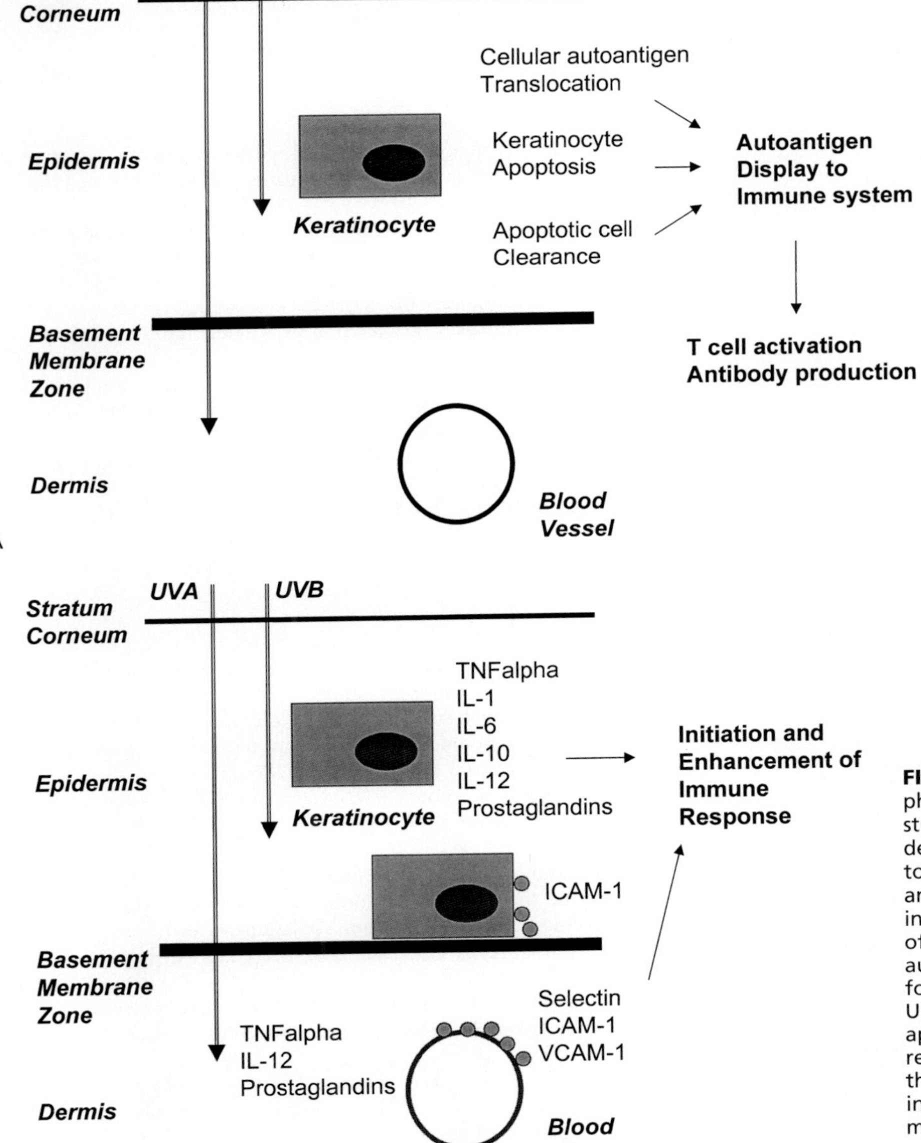

FIGURE 28.7. A model of the pathogenesis of photosensitive lupus erythematosus. Recent studies of photosensitive lupus patients have demonstrated an increased number of apoptotic keratinocytes in both established lesions and following photoprovocation. Either increased apoptosis or a delay in the clearance of apoptotic cells could result in an increase in autoantigen packaging and processing in a form accessible to the immune system **(A)**. Ultraviolet radiation can induce keratinocyte apoptosis and also can stimulate local cytokine release. This cytokine release then can lead to the observed increase in local mediators of inflammation including selectins, adhesion molecules, and prostanoids **(B)**. *(Continued on next page)*

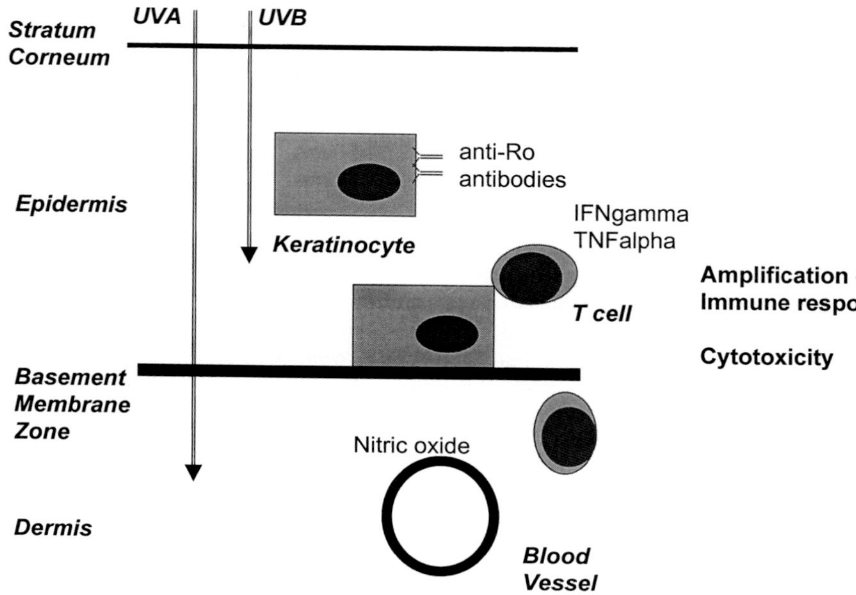

FIGURE 28.7. *(Continued).* The end result is a stimulation of the immune system to to produce antibodies and possibly prime T cells directed against stress-induced or stress-altered molecules (Ro antigen, La antigen, calreticulin). These agents of the immune system then act to promote further inflammation and tissue damage by processes such as epitope spreading mediated by antibodies and B cells, and cellular cytotoxic mechanisms mediated by T cells, natural-killer cells, and monocyte-macrophages **(C)**.

ACKNOWLEDGMENTS

This work was supported by NIH grant AR19101. Dr. Sontheimer holds the John S. Strauss Chair in Dermatology at the University of Iowa College of Medicine.

REFERENCES

1. Tan EM, Cohen AS, Fries JF, et al. The 1982 revised criteria for the classification of systemic lupus erythematosus. *Arthritis Rheum* 1982;25:1271–1277.
2. Petri M. Dermatologic lupus: Hopkins Lupus Cohort. *Semin Cutan Med Surg* 1998;17:219–227.
3. Pistiner M, Wallace DJ, Nessim S, et al. Lupus erythematosus in the 1980s: a survey of 570 patients. *Semin Arthritis Rheum* 1991;21:55–64.
4. Wallace DJ, Lyon I. Pierre Cazenave and the first detailed modern description of lupus erythematosus. *Semin Arthritis Rheum* 1999;28:305–333.
5. Kesten B, Slatkin M. Disease related to light sensitivity. *Arch Dermatol* 1953;67:284–301.
6. Epstein J, Tuffanelli D, Dubois E. Light sensitivity in lupus erythematosus. *Arch Dermatol* 1965;91:483–485.
7. Baer R, Harber L. Photobiology of lupus erythematosus. *Arch Dermatol* 1965;92:124–127.
8. Cripps D, Rankin J. Action spectra of lupus erythematosus and experimental immunofluorescence. *Arch Dermatol* 1973;107: 563–567.
9. Wolska H, Blaszczyk M, Jablonska S. Phototests in patients with various forms of lupus erythematosus. *Int J Dermatol* 1989;28:98–103.
10. Doria A, Biasinutto C, Ghirardello A, et al. Photosensitivity in systemic lupus erythematosus: laboratory testing of ARA/ACR definition. *Lupus* 1996;5:263–268.
11. Freeman R, Knox J. Cutaneous lesions of lupus erythaemosus induced by monochromatic light. *Arch Dermatol* 1973;100: 677–682.
12. Kochevar I. Action spectrum and mechanism of UV-radiation induced injury in lupus erythematosus. *J Invest Dermatol* 1985; 85:140S–143S.
13. Lehmann P, Holzle E, Kind P, et al. Experimental reproduction of skin lesions in lupus erythematosus by UVA and UVB radiation [see comments]. *J Am Acad Dermatol* 1990;22:181–187.
14. Nived O, Johansen PB, Sturfelt G. Standardized ultraviolet-A exposure provokes skin reaction in systemic lupus erythematosus. *Lupus* 1993;2:247–250.
15. Wysenbeek AJ, Block DA, Fries JF. Prevalence and expression of photosensitivity in systemic lupus erythematosus. *Ann Rheum Dis* 1989;48:461–463.
16. Walchner M, Messer G, Kind P. Phototesting and photoprotection in LE. *Lupus* 1997;6:167–174.
17. Dowdy MJ, Nigra TP, Barth WF. Subacute cutaneous lupus erythematosus during PUVA therapy for psoriasis: case report and review of the literature. *Arthritis Rheum* 1989;32:343–346.
18. Stern RS, Docken W. An exacerbation of SLE after visiting a tanning salon [letter]. *JAMA* 1986;255:3120.
19. Krause I, Shraga I, Molad Y, et al. Seasons of the Year and Activity of SLE and Behcets-Disease. *Scand J Rheumatol* 1997;26: 435–439.
20. Leone J, Pennaforte JL, Delhinger V, et al. Influence of seasons on risk of flare-up of systemic lupus: retrospective study of 66 patients. *Rev Med Interne* 1997;18:286–291.
21. Van Praag MC, Boom BW, Vermeer BJ. Diagnosis and treatment of polymorphous light eruption. *Int J Dermatol* 1994;33: 233–239.
22. Petzelbauer P, Binder M, Nikolakis P, et al. Severe sun sensitivity and the presence of antinuclear antibodies in patients with polymorphous light eruption-like lesions. A form fruste of photosensitive lupus erythematosus? [see comments]. *J Am Acad Dermatol* 1992;26:68–74.
23. Nyberg F, Hasan T, Puska P, et al. Occurrence of polymorphous light eruption in lupus erythematosus. *Br J Dermatol* 1997;136: 217–221.
24. Hasan T, Nyberg F, Stephansson E, et al. Photosensitivity in lupus erythematosus, UV photoprovocation results compared with history of photosensitivity and clinical findings. *Br J Dermatol* 1997;136:699–705.

25. Verheyen AM, Lambert JR, Van Marck EA, et al. Polymorphic light eruption—an immunopathological study of provoked lesions. *Clin Exp Dermatol* 1995;20:297–303.
26. Bennion SD, Middleton MH, David-Bajar KM, et al. In three types of interface dermatitis, different patterns of expression of intercellular adhesion molecule-1 (ICAM-1) indicate different triggers of disease. *J Invest Dermatol* 1995;105(suppl 1): 71S–79S.
27. Jansen CT, Karvonen J. Polymorphous light eruption. A seven-year follow-up evaluation of 114 patients. *Arch Dermatol* 1984; 120:862–865.
28. Hasan T, Ranki A, Jansen CT, et al. Disease associations in polymorphous light eruption. A long-term follow-up study of 94 patients. *Arch Dermatol* 1998;134:1081–1085.
29. Natali GP, Tan EM. Experimental renal disease induced by DNA-anti-DNA immune complexes. *J Clin Invest* 1972;51: 345–355.
30. Natali PG, Tan EM. Experimental skin lesions in mice resembling systemic lupus erythematosus. *Arthritis Rheum* 1973;16: 579–589.
31. Natali PG, Tan EM. Immunological detection of thymidine photoproduct formation in vivo. *Radiat Res* 1971;46:506–518.
32. Tan EM, Stoughton RB. Ultraviolet light alteration of cellular deoxyribonucleic acid in vivo. *Proc Natl Acad Sci U S A* 1969;62:708–714.
33. Davis P, Russell AS, Percy JS. Antibodies to UV light denatured DNA in systemic lupus erythematosus: detection by filter radioimmunoassay and clinical correlations. *J Rheumatol* 1976;3:375–379.
34. Golan TD, Foltyn V, Roueff A. Increased susceptibility to in vitro ultraviolet B radiation in fibroblasts and lymphocytes cultured from systemic lupus erythematosus patients. *Clin Immunol Immunopathol* 1991;58:289–304.
35. Zamansky GB, Minka DF, Deal CL, et al. The in vitro photosensitivity of systemic lupus erythematosus skin fibroblasts. *J Immunol* 1985;134:1571–1576.
36. Rosenstein BS, Rosenstein RB, Zamansky GB. Repair of DNA damage induced in systemic lupus erythematosus skin fibroblasts by simulated sunlight. *J Invest Dermatol* 1992;98:469–474.
37. Ansel JC, Mountz J, Steinberg AD, et al. Effects of UV radiation on autoimmune strains of mice: increased mortality and accelerated autoimmunity in BXSB male mice. *J Invest Dermatol* 1985;85:181–186.
38. Davis P, Percy JS. Effect of ultraviolet light on disease characteristics of NZB/W mice. *J Rheumatol* 1978;5:125–128.
39. Millard TP, Hawk JL, McGregor JM. Photosensitivity in lupus. *Lupus* 2000;9:3–10.
40. Yell J, Wojnarowska F. Diagnosis and management of systemic lupus erythematosus. Sun protection is vital [letter; comment]. *BMJ* 1993;307:939.
41. Zamansky GB, Chou IN. Disruption of keratin intermediate filaments by ultraviolet radiation in cultured human keratinocytes. *Photochem Photobiol* 1990;52:903–906.
42. LeFeber WP, Norris DA, Ryan SR, et al. Ultraviolet light induces binding of antibodies to selected nuclear antigens on cultured human keratinocytes. *J Clin Invest* 1984;74:1545-1551.
43. Norris DA. Pathomechanisms of photosensitive lupus erythematosus. *J Invest Dermatol* 1993;100:58S–68S.
44. Golan TD, Elkon KB, Gharavi AE, et al. Enhanced membrane binding of autoantibodies to cultured keratinocytes of systemic lupus erythematosus patients after ultraviolet B/ultraviolet A irradiation. *J Clin Invest* 1992;90:1067–1076.
45. Golan TD, Sigal D, Sabo E, et al. The penetrating potential of autoantibodies into live cells in vitro coincides with the in vivo staining of epidermal nuclei. *Lupus* 1997;6:18–26.
46. Casciola-Rosen LA, Anhalt G, Rosen A. Autoantigens targeted in systemic lupus erythematosus are clustered in two populations of surface structures on apoptotic keratinocytes [see comments]. *J Exp Med* 1994;179:1317–1330.
47. Casciola-Rosen L, Rosen A. Ultraviolet light-induced keratinocyte apoptosis: a potential mechanism for the induction of skin lesions and autoantibody production in LE. *Lupus* 1997;6: 175–180.
48. Tan EM. Autoimmunity and apoptosis [comment]. *J Exp Med* 1994;179:1083–1086.
49. Vaux DL. Toward an understanding of the molecular mechanisms of physiological cell death. *Proc Natl Acad Sci U S A/* 1993;90:786–789.
50. Savill J, Fadok V, Henson P, et al. Phagocyte recognition of cells undergoing apoptosis. *Immunol Today* 1993;14:131–136.
51. Savill J. Apoptosis. Phagocytic docking without shocking [news; comment]. *Nature* 1998;392:442–443.
52. Godar DE. Light and death: photons and apoptosis. *J Investig Dermatol Symp Proc* 1999;4:17–23.
53. Godar DE. Preprogrammed and programmed cell death mechanisms of apoptosis: UV-induced immediate and delayed apoptosis. *Photochem Photobiol* 1996;63:825–830.
54. Ashkenazi A, Dixit VM. Death receptors: signaling and modulation. *Science* 1998;281:1305–1308.
55. Kasibhatla S, Brunner T, Genestier L, et al. DNA damaging agents induce expression of Fas ligand and subsequent apoptosis in T lymphocytes via the activation of NF-kappa B and AP-1. *Mol Cell* 1998;1:543–51.
56. Akbar AN, Salmon M. Cellular environments and apoptosis: tissue microenvironments control activated T-cell death. *Immunol Today* 1997;18:72–76.
57. Weedon D, Strutton G. Apoptosis as the mechanism of the involution of hair follicles in catagen transformation. *Acta Derm Venereol* 1981;61:335–339.
58. Budtz PE, Spies I. Epidermal tissue homeostasis: apoptosis and cell emigration as mechanisms of controlled cell deletion in the epidermis of the toad, Bufo bufo. *Cell Tissue Res* 1989;256 475–486.
59. McCall CA, Cohen JJ. Programmed cell death in terminally differentiating keratinocytes: role of endogenous endonuclease [see comments]. *J Invest Dermatol* 1991;97:111–114.
60. Seitz CS, Freiberg RA, Hinata K, et al. NF-kappaB determines localization and features of cell death in epidermis. *J Clin Invest* 2000;105:253–260.
61. Norris DA, Whang K, David-Bajar K, et al. The influence of ultraviolet light on immunological cytotoxicity in the skin. *Photochem Photobiol* 1997;65:636–646.
62. Chiodino C, Cesinaro AM, Ottani D, et al. Communication: expression of the novel inhibitor of apoptosis survivin in normal and neoplastic skin. *J Invest Dermatol* 1999;113:415–418.
63. Deveraux QL, Reed JC. IAP family proteins—suppressors of apoptosis. *Genes Dev* 1999;13:239–252.
64. Daniels FJ. Histochemical responses of human skin following ultraviolet radiation. *J Invest Dermatol* 1961;37:351–356.
65. Godar DE. UVA1 radiation triggers two different final apoptotic pathways. *J Invest Dermatol* 1999;112:3–12.
66. Aragane Y, Kulms D, Metze D, et al. Ultraviolet light induces apoptosis via direct activation of CD95 (Fas/APO-1) independently of its ligand CD95L. *J Cell Biol* 1998;140:171–182.
67. Hill LL, Ouhtit A, Loughlin SM, et al. Fas ligand: a sensor for DNA damage critical in skin cancer etiology. *Science* 1999;285:898–900.
68. Schwarz A, Bhardwaj R, Aragane Y, et al. Ultraviolet-B-induced apoptosis of keratinocytes: evidence for partial involvement of tumor necrosis factor-alpha in the formation of sunburn cells. *J Invest Dermatol* 1995;104:922–927.

69. Zhuang L, Wang B, Shinder GA, et al. TNF receptor p55 plays a pivotal role in murine keratinocyte apoptosis induced by ultraviolet B irradiation. *J Immunol* 1999;162:1440–1447.
70. Kulms D, Poppelmann B, Yarosh D, et al. Nuclear and cell membrane effects contribute independently to the induction of apoptosis in human cells exposed to UVB radiation. *Proc Natl Acad Sci U S A* 1999;96:7974–7979.
71. Alnemri ES, Livingston DJ, Nicholson DW, et al. Human ICE/CED-3 protease nomenclature [letter]. *Cell* 1996;87:171.
72. Takahashi H, Kinouchi M, Iizuka H. Interleukin-1beta-converting enzyme and CPP32 are involved in ultraviolet B-induced apoptosis of SV40-transformed human keratinocytes. *Biochem Biophys Res Commun* 1997;236:194–198.
73. Chung JH, Kwon OS, Eun HC, et al. Apoptosis in the pathogenesis of cutaneous lupus erythematosus. *Am J Dermatopathol* 1998;20:233–241.
74. Pablos JL, Santiago B, Galindo M, et al. Keratinocyte apoptosis and p53 expression in cutaneous lupus and dermatomyositis. *J Pathol* 1999;188:63–68.
75. Smith ML, Fornace AJ, Jr. p53-mediated protective responses to Uv irradiation. *Proc Natl Acad Sci U S A* 1997;94: 12255–12257.
76. Brysk MM, Selvanayagam P, Arany I, et al. Induction of apoptotic nuclei by interferon-gamma and by predesquamin in cultured keratinocytes. *J Interferon Cytokine Res* 1995;15: 1029–1035.
77. Tron VA, Trotter MJ, Tang L, et al. p53-regulated apoptosis is differentiation dependent in ultraviolet B-irradiated mouse keratinocytes. *Am J Pathol* 1998;153:579–585.
78. Henkart PA. Lymphocyte-mediated cytotoxicity: two pathways and multiple effector molecules. *Immunity* 1994;1:343–346.
79. Wright SC, Kumar P, Tam AW, et al. Apoptosis and DNA fragmentation precede TNF-induced cytolysis in U937 cells. *J Cell Biochem* 1992;48:344–355.
80. Lowin B, Hahne M, Mattmann C, et al. Cytolytic T-cell cytotoxicity is mediated through perforin and Fas lytic pathways. *Nature* 1994;370:650–652.
81. Nakajima M, Nakajima A, Kayagaki N, et al. Expression of Fas ligand and its receptor in cutaneous lupus: implication in tissue injury. *Clin Immunol Immunopathol* 1997;83:223–229.
82. Casciola-Rosen LA, Anhalt GJ, Rosen A. DNA-dependent protein kinase is one of a subset of autoantigens specifically cleaved early during apoptosis. *J Exp Med* 1995;182:1625–1634.
83. Utz PJ, Hottelet M, Schur PH, et al. Proteins phosphorylated during stress-induced apoptosis are common targets for autoantibody production in patients with systemic lupus erythematosus. *J Exp Med* 1997;185:843–854.
84. Utz PJ, Anderson P. Posttranslational protein modifications, apoptosis, and the bypass of tolerance to autoantigens. *Arthritis Rheum* 1998;41:1152–1160.
85. Greidinger EL, Casciola-Rosen L, Morris SM, et al. Autoantibody recognition of distinctly modified forms of the U1-70-kd antigen is associated with different clinical disease manifestations. *Arthr Rheum* 2000;43:881–888.
86. Casciola-Rosen L, Andrade F, Ulanet D, Wong WB, Rosen A. Cleavage by granzyme B is strongly predictive of autoantigen status: implications for initiation of autoimmunity. *J Exp Med* 1999;190:815–826.
87. Berthou C, Michel L, Soulie A, et al. Acquisition of granzyme B and Fas ligand proteins by human keratinocytes contributes to epidermal cell defense. *J Immunol* 1997;159:5293–5300.
88. Rosen A, Casciola-Rosen L. Autoantigens as substrates for apoptotic proteases: implications for the pathogenesis of systemic autoimmune disease. *Cell Death Differ* 1999;6:6–12.
89. Korb LC, Ahearn JM. C1q binds directly and specifically to surface blebs of apoptotic human keratinocytes: complement deficiency and systemic lupus erythematosus revisited. *J Immunol* 1997;158:4525–4528.
90. Eggleton P, Ward FJ, Johnson S, et al. Fine specificity of autoantibodies to calreticulin: epitope mapping and characterization. *Clin Exp Immunol* 2000;120:384–391.
91. Nepomuceno RR, Henschen-Edman AH, Burgess WH, et al. cDna cloning and primary structure analysis of C1qR(P), the human C1q/Mbl/Spa receptor that mediates enhanced phagocytosis in vitro. *Immunity* 1997;6:119–129.
92. Bowness P, Davies KA, Norsworthy PJ, et al. Hereditary C1q deficiency and systemic lupus erythematosus. *Qjm* 1994;87: 455–464.
93. Botto M, Dell'Agnola C, Bygrave AE, et al. Homozygous C1q deficiency causes glomerulonephritis associated with multiple apoptotic bodies [see comments]. *Nat Genet* 1998;19:56–59.
94. Herrmann M, Voll RE, Zoller OM, et al. Impaired phagocytosis of apoptotic cell material by monocyte-derived macrophages from patients with systemic lupus erythematosus. *Arthritis Rheum* 1998;41:1241–1250.
95. Okamoto H, Mizuno K, Itoh T, et al. Evaluation of apoptotic cells induced by ultraviolet light B radiation in epidermal sheets stained by the TUNEL technique. *J Invest Dermatol* 1999;113: 802–807.
96. Woodcock A, Magnus IA. The sunburn cell in mouse skin: preliminary quantitative studies on its production. *Br J Dermatol* 1976;95:459–468.
97. Fadok VA, Bratton DL, Konowal A, et al. Macrophages that have ingested apoptotic cells in vitro inhibit proinflammatory cytokine production through autocrine/paracrine mechanisms involving TGF-beta, PGE2, and PAF. *J Clin Invest* 1998;101: 890–898.
98. Albert ML, Sauter B, Bhardwaj N. Dendritic cells acquire antigen from apoptotic cells and induce class I-restricted CTLs. *Nature* 1998;392:86–89.
99. Rovere P, Vallinoto C, Bondanza A, et al. Cutting Edge — Bystander Apoptosis Triggers Dendritic Cell Maturation and Antigen-Presenting Function. *J Immunol* 1998;161:4467–4471.
100. Gilchrest BA, Soter NA, Stoff JS, et al. The human sunburn reaction: histologic and biochemical studies. *J Am Acad Dermatol* 1981;5:411–422.
101. Hruza LL, Pentland AP. Mechanisms of UV-induced inflammation. *J Invest Dermatol* 1993;100:35S–41S.
102. Bennion SD, Norris DA. Ultraviolet light modulation of autoantigens, epidermal cytokines and adhesion molecules as contributing factors of the pathogenesis of cutaneous LE. *Lupus* 1997;6:181–192.
103. Kupper TS, Chua AO, Flood P, et al. Interleukin 1 gene expression in cultured human keratinocytes is augmented by ultraviolet irradiation. *J Clin Invest* 1987;80:430–436.
104. Granstein RD, Sauder DN. Whole-body exposure to ultraviolet radiation results in increased serum interleukin-1 activity in humans. *Lymphokine Res* 1987;6:187–193.
105. Kock A, Schwarz T, Kirnbauer R, et al. Human keratinocytes are a source for tumor necrosis factor alpha: evidence for synthesis and release upon stimulation with endotoxin or ultraviolet light. *J Exp Med* 1990;172:1609–1614.
106. Kurimoto I, Streilein JW. cis-urocanic acid suppression of contact hypersensitivity induction is mediated via tumor necrosis factor-alpha. *J Immunol* 1992;148:3072–3078.
107. Middleton MH, Norris DA. Cytokine-induced ICAM-1 expression in human keratinocytes is highly variable in keratinocyte strains from different donors. *J Invest Dermatol* 1995; 104:489–496.
108. Ansel J, Perry P, Brown J, et al. Cytokine modulation of keratinocyte cytokines. *J Invest Dermatol* 1990;94(suppl 6): 101S–107S.

109. Kupper TS. Mechanisms of cutaneous inflammation. Interactions between epidermal cytokines, adhesion molecules, and leukocytes [published erratum appears in Arch Dermatol 1989 Dec;125(12):1643]. *Arch Dermatol* 1989;125:1406–1412.
110. Luger TA, Schwarz T. Evidence for an epidermal cytokine network. *J Invest Dermatol* 1990;95(suppl 6):100S–104S.
111. Schroder JM. Cytokine networks in the skin. *J Invest Dermatol* 1995;105(suppl 1):20S–24S.
112. Wang B, Fujisawa H, Zhuang L, et al. Depressed Langerhans cell migration and reduced contact hypersensitivity response in mice lacking TNF receptor p75. *J Immunol* 1997;159: 6148–6155.
113. Banchereau J, Steinman RM. Dendritic cells and the control of immunity. *Nature* 1998;392:245–252.
114. Ullrich SE. Mechanism involved in the systemic suppression of antigen-presenting cell function by UV irradiation. Keratinocyte-derived IL-10 modulates antigen-presenting cell function of splenic adherent cells. *J Immunol* 1994;152:3410–3416.
115. Beissert S, Hosoi J, Kuhn R, et al. Impaired immunosuppressive response to ultraviolet radiation in interleukin-10-deficient mice. *J Invest Dermatol* 1996;107:553–557.
116. Beissert S, Ullrich SE, Hosoi J, et al. Supernatants from UVB radiation-exposed keratinocytes inhibit Langerhans cell presentation of tumor-associated antigens via IL-10 content. *J Leukoc Biol* 1995;58:234–240.
117. Beissert S, Hosoi J, Grabbe S, et al. IL-10 inhibits tumor antigen presentation by epidermal antigen-presenting cells. *J Immunol* 1995;154:1280–1286.
118. de Vos S, Brach M, Budnik A, et al. Post-transcriptional regulation of interleukin-6 gene expression in human keratinocytes by ultraviolet B radiation. *J Invest Dermatol* 1994;103:92–96.
119. Wang B, Zhuang L, Fujisawa H, et al. Enhanced epidermal Langerhans cell migration in IL-10 knockout mice. *J Immunol* 1999;162:277–283.
120. Rivas JM, Ullrich SE. Systemic suppression of delayed-type hypersensitivity by supernatants from UV-irradiated keratinocytes. An essential role for keratinocyte-derived IL-10. *J Immunol* 1992;149:3865–3871.
121. Turksen K, Kupper T, Degenstein L, et al. Interleukin 6: insights to its function in skin by overexpression in transgenic mice. *Proc Natl Acad Sci U S A* 1992;89:5068–5072.
122. Ripley BJ, Stephanou A, Isenberg DA, et al. Interleukin-10 activates heat-shock protein 90beta gene expression. *Immunology* 1999;97:226–231.
123. Stephanou A, Latchman DS. Transcriptional regulation of the heat shock protein genes by STAT family transcription factors. *Gene Expr* 1999;7:311–319.
124. Nishigori C, Yarosh DB, Ullrich SE, et al. Evidence that DNA damage triggers interleukin 10 cytokine production in UV-irradiated murine keratinocytes. *Proc Natl Acad Sci U S A* 1996; 93:10354–10359.
125. Grether-Beck S, Olaizola-Horn S, Schmitt H, et al. Activation of transcription factor AP-2 mediates UVA radiation- and singlet oxygen-induced expression of the human intercellular adhesion molecule 1 gene. *Proc Natl Acad Sci U S A* 1996;93: 14586–14591.
126. Morita A, Werfel T, Stege H, et al. Evidence that singlet oxygen-induced human T helper cell apoptosis is the basic mechanism of ultraviolet-A radiation phototherapy. *J Exp Med* 1997;186: 1763–1768.
127. Morita A, Grewe M, Grether-Beck S, et al. Induction of proinflammatory cytokines in human epidermoid carcinoma cells by in vitro ultraviolet A1 irradiation. *Photochem Photobiol* 1997; 65:630–635.
128. Heckmann M, Pirthauer M, Plewig G. Adhesion of leukocytes to dermal endothelial cells is induced after single-dose, but reduced after repeated doses of UVA. *J Invest Dermatol* 1997; 109:710–715.
129. Kondo S, Jimbow K. Dose-dependent induction of IL-12 but not IL-10 from human keratinocytes after exposure to ultraviolet light A. *J Cell Physiol* 1998;177:493–498.
130. Shen J, Bao S, Reeve VE. Modulation of IL-10, IL-12, and IFN-gamma in the epidermis of hairless mice by UVA (320-400 nm) and UVB (280-320 nm) radiation. *J Invest Dermatol* 1999;113:1059–1064.
131. Schwarz A, Grabbe S, Aragane Y, et al. Interleukin-12 prevents ultraviolet B-induced local immunosuppression and overcomes UVB-induced tolerance. *J Invest Dermatol* 1996;106: 1187–1191.
132. Ullrich SE. Does exposure to UV radiation induce a shift to a Th-2-like immune reaction? *Photochem Photobiol* 1996;64: 254–258.
133. Abbas AK, Murphy KM, Sher A. Functional diversity of helper T lymphocytes. *Nature* 1996;383:787–793.
134. McGrath H, Jr., Bak E, Michalski JP. Ultraviolet-A light prolongs survival and improves immune function in (New Zealand black x New Zealand white) F1 hybrid mice. *Arthritis Rheum* 1987;30:557–561.
135. McGrath H, Martinez-Osuna P, Lee FA. Ultraviolet-A1 (340-400 nm) irradiation therapy in systemic lupus erythematosus. *Lupus* 1996;5:269–274.
136. McGrath H, Jr. Ultraviolet A1 (340-400 nm) irradiation and systemic lupus erythematosus. *J Investig Dermatol Symp Proc* 1999;4:79–84.
137. Tsao BP, Ohnishi K, Cheroutre H, et al. Failed self-tolerance and autoimmunity in IgG anti-DNA transgenic mice. *J Immunol* 1992;149:350–358.
138. Mendlovic S, Brocke S, Shoenfeld Y, et al. Induction of a systemic lupus erythematosus-like disease in mice by a common human anti-DNA idiotype. *Proc Natl Acad Sci U S A* 1988;85: 2260–2264.
139. David-Bajar KM, Davis BM. Pathology, immunopathology, and immunohistochemistry in cutaneous lupus erythematosus. *Lupus* 1997;6:145–157.
140. Ueki H, Wolff HH, Braun-Falco O. Cutaneous localization of human gamma-globulins in lupus erythematosus. An electron-microscopical study using the peroxidase-labeled antibody technique. *Arch Dermatol Forsch* 1974;248:297–314.
141. Gilliam JN. The significance of cutaneous immunoglobulin deposits in lupus erythematosus and NZB/NZW F1 hybrid mice. *J Invest Dermatol* 1975;65:154–161.
142. Sontheimer RD, Thomas JR, Gilliam JN. Subacute cutaneous lupus erythematosus: a cutaneous marker for a distinct lupus erythematosus subset. *Arch Dermatol* 1979;115:1409–1415.
143. Sontheimer RD, Maddison PJ, Reichlin M, et al. Serologic and HLA associations in subacute cutaneous lupus erythematosus, a clinical subset of lupus erythematosus. *Ann Intern Med* 1982; 97:664–671.
144. Lee LA, Roberts CM, Frank MB, et al. The autoantibody response to Ro/SSA in cutaneous lupus erythematosus [see comments]. *Arch Dermatol* 1994;130:1262–1268.
145. Weston WL, Harmon C, Peebles C, et al. A serological marker for neonatal lupus erythematosus. *Br J Dermatol* 1982;107: 377–382.
146. Lee LA. Neonatal lupus erythematosus. *J Invest Dermatol* 1993;100:9S–13S.
147. Alexander E, Buyon JP, Provost TT, et al. Anti-Ro/SS-A antibodies in the pathophysiology of congenital heart block in neonatal lupus syndrome, an experimental model. In vitro electrophysiologic and immunocytochemical studies. *Arthritis Rheum* 1992;35:176–189.
148. Miranda-Carus ME, Boutjdir M, Tseng CE, et al. Induction of

antibodies reactive with SSA/Ro-SSB/La and development of congenital heart block in a murine model. *J Immunol* 1998;161: 5886–5892.
149. Boutjdir M, Chen L, Zhang ZH, et al. Serum and immunoglobulin G from the mother of a child with congenital heart block induce conduction abnormalities and inhibit L-type calcium channels in a rat heart model. *Pediatr Res* 1998;44: 11–19.
150. Garcia S, Nascimento JH, Bonfa E, et al. Cellular mechanism of the conduction abnormalities induced by serum from anti-Ro/SSA-positive patients in rabbit hearts. *J Clin Invest* 1994;93: 718–724.
151. Buyon J. Congenital heart block: Autoimmune associated or autoimmune mediated? *Immunologist* 1999;7:98–104.
152. Lee LA, Gaither KK, Coulter SN, et al. Pattern of cutaneous immunoglobulin G deposition in subacute cutaneous lupus erythematosus is reproduced by infusing purified anti-Ro (SSA) autoantibodies into human skin-grafted mice. *J Clin Invest* 1989;83:1556–1562.
153. Nieboer C, Tak-Diamand Z, Van Leeuwen-Wallau HE. Dust-like particles: a specific direct immunofluorescence pattern in sub-acute cutaneous lupus erythematosus [letter] [see comments]. *Br J Dermatol* 1988;118:725–729.
154. Purcell SM, Lieu TS, Davis BM, et al. Relationship between circulating anti-Ro/SS-A antibody levels and skin disease activity in subacute cutaneous lupus erythematosus. *Br J Dermatol* 1987;117:277–287.
155. Clark G, Reichlin M, Tomasi TB, Jr. Characterization of a soluble cytoplasmic antigen reactive with sera from patients with systemic lupus erythmatosus. *J Immunol* 1969;102:117–122.
156. Boulanger C, Chabot B, Menard HA, et al. Autoantibodies in human anti-Ro sera specifically recognize deproteinized hY5 Ro RNA [see comments]. *Clin Exp Immunol* 1995;99:29–36.
157. Alspaugh MA, Tan EM. Antibodies to cellular antigens in Sjogren's syndrome. *J Clin Invest* 1975;55:1067–1073.
158. McCauliffe DP, Sontheimer RD. Molecular characterization of the Ro/SS-A autoantigens. *J Invest Dermatol* 1993;100:73S–79S.
159. Farris AD, Puvion-Dutilleul F, Puvion E, et al. The ultrastructural localization of 60-kDa Ro protein and human cytoplasmic RNAs: association with novel electron-dense bodies. *Proc Natl Acad Sci U S A* 1997;94:3040–3045.
160. CA OB, Wolin SL. A possible role for the 60-kD Ro autoantigen in a discard pathway for defective 5S rRNA precursors. *Genes Dev* 1994;8:2891–2903.
161. Chen X, Quinn AM, Wolin SL. Ro ribonucleoproteins contribute to the resistance of Deinococcus radiodurans to ultraviolet irradiation. *Genes Dev* 2000;14:777–782.
162. Ben-Chetrit E, Chan EK, Sullivan KF, et al. A 52-kD protein is a novel component of the SS-A/Ro antigenic particle. *J Exp Med* 1988;167:1560–1571.
163. DiDonato F, Chan E, Askenase A, et al. Interaction between 52kDSSA/Ro and deubiquinating enzyme UNP; a clue to function [abstract]. *Arthritis Rheumat* 1999;42:S109.
164. Slobbe RL, Pluk W, van Venrooij WJ, et al. Ro ribonucleoprotein assembly in vitro. Identification of RNA-protein and protein-protein interactions. *J Mol Biol* 1992;227:361–366.
165. Scofield RH, Kurien BT, Zhang F, et al. Protein-protein interaction of the Ro-ribonucleoprotein particle using multiple antigenic peptides. *Mol Immunol* 1999;36:1093–1106.
166. Cheng ST, Nguyen TQ, Yang YS, et al. Calreticulin binds hYRNA and the 52-kDa polypeptide component of the Ro/SS-A ribonucleoprotein autoantigen. *J Immunol* 1996;156: 4484–4491.
167. Eggleton P, Reid KB, Kishore U, et al. Clinical relevance of calreticulin in systemic lupus erythematosus. *Lupus* 1997;6: 564–571.
168. Eggleton P, Llewellyn DH. Pathophysiological roles of calreticulin in autoimmune disease. *Scand J Immunol* 1999;49: 466–473.
169. Nair S, Wearsch PA, Mitchell DA, et al. Calreticulin displays in vivo peptide-binding activity and can elicit CTL responses against bound peptides. *J Immunol* 1999;162:6426–6432.
170. Gottlieb E, Steitz JA. Function of the mammalian La protein: evidence for its action in transcription termination by RNA polymerase III. *EMBO J* 1989;8:851–861.
171. Holcik M, Korneluk R. Functional characterization of the X-linked inhibitor of apoptosis (XIAP) IRES element: the role of La autoantigen in XIAP translation. *Mol Cell Biol* 2000; 20(13):4648-4657.
172. Hendrick JP, Wolin SL, Rinke J, et al. Ro small cytoplasmic ribonucleoproteins are a subclass of La ribonucleoproteins: further characterization of the Ro and La small ribonucleoproteins from uninfected mammalian cells. *Mol Cell Biol* 1981;1: 1138–1149.
173. Nguyen TO, Capra JD, Sontheimer RD. Calreticulin is transcriptionally upregulated by heat shock, calcium and heavy metals. *Mol Immunol* 1996;33:379–386.
174. Kinoshita G, Purcell AW, Keech CL, et al. Molecular chaperones are targets of autoimmunity in Ro(SS-A) immune mice. *Clin Exp Immunol* 1999;115:268–274.
175. Furukawa F, Ikai K, Matsuyoshi N, et al. Relationship between heat shock protein induction and the binding of antibodies to the extractable nuclear antigens on cultured human keratinocytes. *J Invest Dermatol* 1993;101:191–195.
176. Igarashi T, Itoh Y, Fukunaga Y, et al. Stress-induced cell surface expression and antigenic alteration of the Ro/SSA autoantigen. *Autoimmunity* 1995;22:33–42.
177. Ellis J. Stress proteins as molecular chaperones. In: van Eden W, Young D, eds. *Stress proteins in medicine*. New York: Marcel Dekker, 1996:126.
178. Srivastava PK, Menoret A, Basu S, et al. Heat shock proteins come of age: primitive functions acquire new roles in an adaptive world. *Immunity* 1998;8:657–665.
179. Birk OS, Gur SL, Elias D, et al. The 60-kDa heat shock protein modulates allograft rejection. *Proc Natl Acad Sci U S A* 1999; 96:5159–5163.
180. Ghoreishi M, Katayama I, Yokozeki H, et al. Analysis of 70 KD heat shock protein (HSP70) expression in the lesional skin of lupus erythematosus (LE) and LE related diseases. *J Dermatol* 1993;20:400–405.
181. Mamula MJ. Epitope spreading: the role of self peptides and autoantigen processing by B lymphocytes. *Immunol Rev* 1998;164:231–239.
182. Scofield RH, Henry WE, Kurien BT, et al. Immunization with short peptides from the sequence of the systemic lupus erythematosus-associated 60-kDa Ro autoantigen results in anti-Ro ribonucleoprotein autoimmunity. *J Immunol* 1996;156: 4059–4066.
183. Keech CL, Gordon TP, McCluskey J. The immune response to 52-kDa Ro and 60-kDa Ro is linked in experimental autoimmunity. *J Immunol* 1996;157:3694–3699.
184. Kinoshita G, Keech CL, Sontheimer RD, et al. Spreading of the immune response from 52 kDaRo and 60 kDaRo to calreticulin in experimental autoimmunity. *Lupus* 1998;7:7–11.
185. McCluskey J, Farris AD, Keech CL, et al. Determinant spreading: lessons from animal models and human disease. *Immunol Rev* 1998;164:209–229.
186. Scofield RH, Racila DM, Gordon TP, et al. Anti-calreticulin segregates anti-Ro sera in systemic lupus erythematosus: anti-calreticulin is present in sera with anti-Ro alone but not in anti-Ro sera with anti-La or anti-ribonucleoprotein. *J Rheumatol* 2000;27:128–134.

187. Furukawa F, Kashihara-Sawami M, Lyons MB, et al. Binding of antibodies to the extractable nuclear antigens SS-A/Ro and SS-B/La is induced on the surface of human keratinocytes by ultraviolet light (UVL): implications for the pathogenesis of photosensitive cutaneous lupus [see comments]. *J Invest Dermatol* 1990;94:77–85.
188. Furukawa F, Lyons MB, Lee LA, et al. Estradiol enhances binding to cultured human keratinocytes of antibodies specific for SS-A/Ro and SS-B/La. Another possible mechanism for estradiol influence of lupus erythematosus. *J Immunol* 1988;141:1480–1488.
189. Rosen A, Casciola-Rosen L, Ahearn J. Novel packages of viral and self-antigens are generated during apoptosis. *J Exp Med* 1995;181:1557–1561.
190. Bennion SD, Ferris C, Lieu TS, et al. IgG subclasses in the serum and skin in subacute cutaneous lupus erythematosus and neonatal lupus erythematosus. *J Invest Dermatol* 1990;95:643–646.
191. Biesecker G, Lavin L, Ziskind M, et al. Cutaneous localization of the membrane attack complex in discoid and systemic lupus erythematosus. *N Engl J Med* 1982;306:264–270.
192. Helm KF, Peters MS. Deposition of membrane attack complex in cutaneous lesions of lupus erythematosus [see comments]. *J Am Acad Dermatol* 1993;28:687–691.
193. Magro CM, Crowson AN, Harrist TJ. The use of antibody to C5b-9 in the subclassification of lupus erythematosus. *Br J Dermatol* 1996;134:855–862.
194. Furukawa F, Kanauchi H, Imamura S. Susceptibility to UVB light in cultured keratinocytes of cutaneous lupus erythematosus. *Dermatology* 1994;189(suppl 1):18–23.
195. Furukawa F, Itoh T, Wakita H, et al. Keratinocytes from patients with lupus erythematosus show enhanced cytotoxicity to ultraviolet radiation and to antibody-mediated cytotoxicity. *Clin Exp Immunol* 1999;118:164–170.
196. Niimi Y, Ioannides D, Buyon J, et al. Heterogeneity in the expression of Ro and La antigens in human skin. *Arthritis Rheum* 1995;38:1271–1276.
197. Ioannides D, Golden BD, Buyon JP, et al. Expression of SS-A/Ro and SS-B/La antigens in skin biopsy specimens of patients with photosensitive forms of lupus erythematosus [In Process Citation]. *Arch Dermatol* 2000;136:340–346.
198. Norris DA, Ryan SB, Kissinger RM, et al. Systematic comparison of antibody-mediated mechanisms of keratinocyte lysis in vitro. *J Immunol* 1985;135:1073–1079.
199. Norris DA, Ryan SR, Fritz KA, et al. The role of RNP, Sm, and SS-A/Ro-specific antisera from patients with lupus erythematosus in inducing antibody-dependent cellular cytotoxicity (ADCC) of targets coated with nonhistone nuclear antigens. *Clin Immunol Immunopathol* 1984;31:311–320.
200. Viljaranta S, Ranki A, Kariniemi AL, et al. Distribution of natural killer cells and lymphocyte subclasses in Jessner's lymphocytic infiltration of the skin and in cutaneous lesions of discoid and systemic lupus erythematosus. *Br J Dermatol* 1987;116:831–838.
201. Velthuis PJ, van Weelden H, van Wichen D, et al. Immunohistopathology of light-induced skin lesions in lupus erythematosus. *Acta Derm Venereol* 1990;70:93–98.
202. Bell DA, Maddison PJ. Serologic subsets in systemic lupus erythematosus: an examination of autoantibodies in relationship to clinical features of disease and HLA antigens. *Arthritis Rheum* 1980;23:1268–1273.
203. Scofield RH, Harley JB. Association of anti-Ro/SS-A autoantibodies with glutamine in position 34 of DQA1 and leucine in position 26 of DQB1. *Arthritis Rheum* 1994;37:961–962.
204. McCauliffe DP, Faircloth E, Wang L, et al. Similar Ro/SS-A autoantibody epitope and titer responses in annular erythema of Sjogren's syndrome and subacute cutaneous lupus erythematosus. *Arch Dermatol* 1996;132:528–531.
205. Miyagawa S, Shinohara K, Fujita T, et al. Neonatal lupus erythematosus: analysis of HLA class II alleles in mothers and siblings from seven Japanese families. *J Am Acad Dermatol* 1997;36:186–190.
206. Rischmueller M, Lester S, Chen Z, et al. HLA class II phenotype controls diversification of the autoantibody response in primary Sjögren's syndrome (pSS). *Clin Exp Immunol* 1998;111:365–371.
207. Namekawa T, Kuroda K, Kato T, et al. Identification of Ro(SSA) 52 kDa reactive T cells in labial salivary glands from patients with Sjögren's syndrome. *J Rheumatol* 1995;22:2092–2099.
208. Reynolds P, Gordon TP, Purcell AW, et al. Hierarchical self-tolerance to T cell determinants within the ubiquitous nuclear self-antigen La (SS-B) permits induction of systemic autoimmunity in normal mice. *J Exp Med* 1996;184:1857–1870.
209. Deshmukh US, Lewis JE, Gaskin F, et al. Immune responses to Ro60 and its peptides in mice. I. The nature of the immunogen and endogenous autoantigen determine the specificities of the induced autoantibodies. *J Exp Med* 1999;189:531–540.
210. Burlingame RW, Rubin RL, Balderas RS, et al. Genesis and evolution of antichromatin autoantibodies in murine lupus implicates T-dependent immunization with self antigen. *J Clin Invest* 1993;91:1687–1696.
211. Furukawa F. Animal models of cutaneous lupus erythematosus and lupus erythematosus photosensitivity. *Lupus* 1997;6:193–202.
212. Sontheimer RD, Gilliam JN. Regional variation in the deposition of subepidermal immunoglobulin in NZB/W F1 mice: association with epidermal DNA synthesis. *J Invest Dermatol* 1979;72:25–28.
213. Charley MR, Bangert JL, Hamilton BL, et al. Murine graft-versus-host skin disease: a chronologic and quantitative analysis of two histologic patterns. *J Invest Dermatol* 1983;81:412–417.
214. Furukawa F, Tanaka H, Sekita K, et al. Dermatopathological studies on skin lesions of MRL mice. *Arch Dermatol Res* 1984;276:186–194.
215. Kanauchi H, Furukawa F, Imamura S. Characterization of cutaneous infiltrates in MRL/lpr mice monitored from onset to the full development of lupus erythematosus-like skin lesions. *J Invest Dermatol* 1991;96:478–483.
216. Takahashi T, Tanaka M, Brannan CI, et al. Generalized lymphoproliferative disease in mice, caused by a point mutation in the Fas ligand. *Cell* 1994;76:969–976.
217. Peng SL, McNiff JM, Madaio MP, et al. Alpha beta T cell regulation and Cd40 ligand dependence in murine systemic autoimmunity. *J Immunol* 1997;158:2464–2470.
218. Peng SL, Madaio MP, Hayday AC, et al. Propagation and regulation of systemic autoimmunity by gammadelta T cells. *J Immunol* 1996;157:5689–5698.
219. Peng SL, Fatenejad S, Craft J. Induction of nonpathologic, humoral autoimmunity in lupus-prone mice by a class II-restricted, transgenic alpha beta T cell. Separation of autoantigen-specific and -nonspecific help. *J Immunol* 1996;157:5225–5230.
220. Chan O, Shlomchik MJ. New Role For B Cells in Systemic Autoimmunity—B Cells Promote Spontaneous T Cell Activation in Mrl-Ipr/Ipr Mice. *J Immunol* 1998;160:51–59.
221. Chan OT, Hannum LG, Haberman AM, et al. A novel mouse with B cells but lacking serum antibody reveals an antibody-independent role for B cells in murine lupus. *J Exp Med* 1999;189:1639–1648.
222. Lanzavecchia A. Antigen-specific interaction between T and B cells. *Nature* 1985;314:537–539.

223. Kinoshita K, Tesch G, Schwarting A, et al. Costimulation by B7-1 and B7-2 is required for autoimmune disease in MRL-Faslpr mice. *J Immunol* 2000;164:6046–6056.
224. Pinkus H. Lichenoid tissue reactions. A speculative review of the clinical spectrum of epidermal basal cell damage with special reference to erythema dyschromicum perstans. *Arch Dermatol* 1973;107:840–846.
225. de Jong EM, van Erp PE, Ruiter DJ, et al. Immunohistochemical detection of proliferation and differentiation in discoid lupus erythematosus. *J Am Acad Dermatol* 1991;25:1032–1038.
226. Kind P, Lehmann P, Plewig G. Phototesting in lupus erythematosus. *J Invest Dermatol* 1993;100:53S–57S.
227. Sontheimer RD, Bergstresser PR. Epidermal Langerhans cell involvement in cutaneous lupus erythematosus. *J Invest Dermatol* 1982;79:237–243.
228. Andrews BS, Schenk A, Barr R, et al. Immunopathology of cutaneous human lupus erythematosus defined by murine monoclonal antibodies. *J Am Acad Dermatol* 1986;15:474–481.
229. Shiohara T, Moriya N, Tanaka Y, et al. Immunopathologic study of lichenoid skin diseases: correlation between HLA-DR-positive keratinocytes or Langerhans cells and epidermotropic T cells [see comments]. *J Am Acad Dermatol* 1988;18:67–74.
230. Volc-Platzer B, Anegg B, Milota S, et al. Accumulation of gamma delta T cells in chronic cutaneous lupus erythematosus. *J Invest Dermatol* 1993;100:84S–91S.
231. Fivenson DP, Rheins LA, Nordlund JJ, et al. Thy-1 and T-cell receptor antigen expression in mycosis fungoides and benign inflammatory dermatoses. *J Natl Cancer Inst* 1991;83:1088–1092.
232. Furukawa F, Tokura Y, Matsushita K, et al. Selective expansions of T cells expressing V beta 8 and V beta 13 in skin lesions of patients with chronic cutaneous lupus erythematosus. *J Dermatol* 1996;23:670–676.
233. Kita Y, Kuroda K, Mimori T, et al. T cell receptor clonotypes in skin lesions from patients with systemic lupus erythematosus. *J Invest Dermatol* 1998;110:41–46.
234. Denfeld RW, Kind P, Sontheimer RD, et al. In situ expression of B7 and CD28 receptor families in skin lesions of patients with lupus erythematosus. *Arthritis Rheum* 1997;40:814–821.
235. Kind P, Lehmann P. [Photobiology of lupus erythematosus]. *Hautarzt* 1990;41:66–71.
236. Davis TL, Lyde CB, Davis BM, et al. Perturbation of experimental ultraviolet light-induced erythema by passive transfer of serum from subacute cutaneous lupus erythematosus patients. *J Invest Dermatol* 1989;92:573–577.
237. Iacobelli D, Bianchi L, Hashimoto K. Passive transfer of photosensitivity by intradermal injection of vesiculobullous lupus erythematosus serum and ultraviolet light irradiation in the guinea pig. *Photodermatol* 1987;4:288–295.
238. Springer TA. Traffic signals for lymphocyte recirculation and leukocyte emigration: the multistep paradigm. *Cell* 1994;76: 301–314.
239. Robert C, Kupper TS. Inflammatory skin diseases, T cells, and immune surveillance. *N Engl J Med* 1999;341:1817–1828.
240. Norris P, Poston RN, Thomas DS, et al. The expression of endothelial leukocyte adhesion molecule-1 (ELAM-1), intercellular adhesion molecule-1 (ICAM-1), and vascular cell adhesion molecule-1 (VCAM-1) in experimental cutaneous inflammation: a comparison of ultraviolet B erythema and delayed hypersensitivity. *J Invest Dermatol* 1991;96:763–770.
241. Nyberg F, Hasan T, Skoglund C, et al. Early events in ultraviolet light-induced skin lesions in lupus erythematosus: expression patterns of adhesion molecules ICAM-1, VCAM-1 and E-selectin. *Acta Derm Venereol* 1999;79:431–436.
242. Nyberg F, Acevedo F, Stephansson E. Different patterns of soluble adhesion molecules in systemic and cutaneous lupus erythematosus. *Exp Dermatol* 1997;6:230–235.
243. Dustin ML, Singer KH, Tuck DT, et al. Adhesion of T lymphoblasts to epidermal keratinocytes is regulated by interferon gamma and is mediated by intercellular adhesion molecule 1 (ICAM-1). *J Exp Med* 1988;167:1323–1340.
244. Barker JN, Sarma V, Mitra RS, et al. Marked synergism between tumor necrosis factor-alpha and interferon-gamma in regulation of keratinocyte-derived adhesion molecules and chemotactic factors. *J Clin Invest* 1990;85:605–608.
245. McHale JF, Harari OA, Marshall D, et al. TNF-alpha and IL-1 sequentially induce endothelial ICAM-1 and VCAM-1 expression in MRL/lpr lupus-prone mice. *J Immunol* 1999;163: 3993–4000.
246. Belmont HM, Buyon J, Giorno R, et al. Up-regulation of endothelial cell adhesion molecules characterizes disease activity in systemic lupus erythematosus. The Shwartzman phenomenon revisited. *Arthritis Rheum* 1994;37:376–383.
247. Jones SM, Mathew CM, Dixey J, et al. VCAM-1 expression on endothelium in lesions from cutaneous lupus erythematosus is increased compared with systemic and localized scleroderma. *Br J Dermatol* 1996;135:678–686.
248. Tebbe B, Mazur L, Stadler R, et al. Immunohistochemical analysis of chronic discoid and subacute cutaneous lupus erythematosus—relation to immunopathological mechanisms. *Br J Dermatol* 1995;132:25–31.
249. Belmont HM, Levartovsky D, Goel A, et al. Increased nitric oxide production accompanied by the up-regulation of inducible nitric oxide synthase in vascular endothelium from patients with systemic lupus erythematosus. *Arthritis Rheum* 1997;40:1810–1816.
250. Kuhn A, Fehsel K, Lehmann P, et al. Aberrant timing in epidermal expression of inducible nitric oxide synthase after UV irradiation in cutaneous lupus erythematosus. *J Invest Dermatol* 1998;111:149–153.
251. Farrell AJ, Blake DR. Nitric oxide. *Ann Rheum Dis* 1996;55: 7–20.
252. Ormerod AD, Copeland P, Hay I, et al. The inflammatory and cytotoxic effects of a nitric oxide releasing cream on normal skin. *J Invest Dermatol* 1999;113:392–397.
253. Stein LF, Saed GM, Fivenson DP. T-cell cytokine network in cutaneous lupus erythematosus. *J Am Acad Dermatol* 1997;36: 191–196.
254. de Kossodo S, Cruz PD, Jr., Dougherty I, et al. Expression of the tumor necrosis factor gene by dermal fibroblasts in response to ultraviolet irradiation or lipopolysaccharide. *J Invest Dermatol* 1995;104:318–322.
255. Avalos-Diaz E, Alvarado-Flores E, Herrera-Esparza R. UV-A irradiation induces transcription of IL-6 and TNF alpha genes in human keratinocytes and dermal fibroblasts. *Rev Rhum Engl Ed* 1999;66:13–19.
256. Sedgwick JD, Riminton DS, Cyster JG, Korner H. Tumor necrosis factor: a master-regulator of leukocyte movement. *Immunol Today* 2000;21:110–113.
257. Green EA, Flavell RA. The temporal importance of TNFalpha expression in the development of diabetes. *Immunity* 2000;12: 459–469.
258. Dorner T, Hucko M, Mayet WJ, et al. Enhanced membrane expression of the 52 kDa Ro(SS-A) and La(SS-B) antigens by human keratinocytes induced by TNF alpha. *Ann Rheum Dis* 1995;54:904–909.
259. Cheng J, Turksen K, Yu QC, et al. Cachexia and graft-vs.-host-disease-type skin changes in keratin promoter-driven TNF alpha transgenic mice. *Genes Dev* 1992;6:1444–1456.
260. Davas EM, Tsirogianni A, Kappou I, et al. Serum IL-6, TNFalpha, p55 srTNFalpha, p75srTNFalpha, srIL-2alpha levels and disease activity in systemic lupus erythematosus. *Clin Rheumatol* 1999;18:17–22.

261. Sullivan KE, Wooten C, Schmeckpeper BJ, et al. A promoter polymorphism of tumor necrosis factor alpha associated with systemic lupus erythematosus in African-Americans. *Arthritis Rheum* 1997;40:2207–2211.
262. Rood MJ, van Krugten MV, Zanelli E, et al. TNF-308A and HLA-DR3 alleles contribute independently to susceptibility to systemic lupus erythematosus. *Arthritis Rheum* 2000;43:129–134.
263. Werth V, Sullivan K. Strong association of a promoter polymorphism of tumor necrosis factor-alpha with a photosensitive form of cutaneous lupus erythematosus [Abstract]. *Arthritis Rheumat* 1999;42:S105.
264. Warren KJ, Nopper AJ, Crosby DL. Thalidomide for recalcitrant discoid lesions in a patient with systemic lupus erythematosus. *J Am Acad Dermatol* 1998;39:293–295.
265. Stevens RJ, Andujar C, Edwards CJ, et al. Thalidomide in the treatment of the cutaneous manifestations of lupus erythematosus: experience in sixteen consecutive patients. *Br J Rheumatol* 1997;36:353–359.
266. Duong DJ, Spigel GT, Moxley RT, 3rd, et al. American experience with low-dose thalidomide therapy for severe cutaneous lupus erythematosus. *Arch Dermatol* 1999;135:1079–1087.
267. Sampaio EP, Sarno EN, Galilly R, et al. Thalidomide selectively inhibits tumor necrosis factor alpha production by stimulated human monocytes. *J Exp Med* 1991;173:699–703.
268. McHugh SM, Rowland TL. Thalidomide and derivatives: immunological investigations of tumour necrosis factor-alpha (TNF-alpha) inhibition suggest drugs capable of selective gene regulation. *Clin Exp Immunol* 1997;110:151–154.
269. Murphy JE, Robert C, Kupper TS. Interleukin-1 and cutaneous inflammation: a crucial link between innate and acquired immunity. *J Invest Dermatol* 2000;114:602–608.
270. Groves RW, Mizutani H, Kieffer JD, et al. Inflammatory skin disease in transgenic mice that express high levels of interleukin 1 alpha in basal epidermis. *Proc Natl Acad Sci U S A* 1995;92:11874–11878.
271. Bigler CF, Norris DA, Weston WL, et al. Interleukin-1 receptor antagonist production by human keratinocytes. *J Invest Dermatol* 1992;98:38–44.
272. Suzuki H, Matsui Y, Kashiwagi H. Interleukin-1 receptor antagonist gene polymorphism in Japanese patients with systemic lupus erythematosus. *Arthritis Rheum* 1997;40:389–390.
273. Blakemore AI, Tarlow JK, Cork MJ, et al. Interleukin-1 receptor antagonist gene polymorphism as a disease severity factor in systemic lupus erythematosus. *Arthritis Rheum* 1994;37:1380–1385.
274. Cork M, Tarlow J, Blakemore A, et al. Genetics of interleukin one receptor antagonist in inflammatory skin diseases [Abstract 202]. *J Invest Dermatol* 1993;100:522.
275. al-Janadi M, al-Dalaan A, al-Balla S, et al. Interleukin-10 (IL-10) secretion in systemic lupus erythematosus and rheumatoid arthritis: IL-10-dependent CD4+CD45RO+ T cell-B cell antibody synthesis. *J Clin Immunol* 1996;16:198–207.
276. Lazarus M, Hajeer AH, Turner D, et al. Genetic variation in the interleukin 10 gene promoter and systemic lupus erythematosus [see comments]. *J Rheumatol* 1997;24:2314–2317.
277. Trautmann A, Akdis M, Kleemann D, et al. T cell-mediated Fas-induced keratinocyte apoptosis plays a key pathogenetic role in eczematous dermatitis. *J Clin Invest* 2000;106:25–35.
278. Carroll JM, Crompton T, Seery JP, et al. Transgenic mice expressing IFN-gamma in the epidermis have eczema, hair hypopigmentation, and hair loss. *J Invest Dermatol* 1997;108:412–422.
279. Seery JP, Carroll JM, Cattell V, et al. Antinuclear autoantibodies and lupus nephritis in transgenic mice expressing interferon gamma in the epidermis. *J Exp Med* 1997;186:1451–1459.
280. Seery JP, Wang EC, Cattell V, et al. A central role for alpha beta T cells in the pathogenesis of murine lupus. *J Immunol* 1999;162:7241–7248.
281. Provost TT, Arnett FC, Reichlin M. Homozygous C2 deficiency, lupus erythematosus, and anti-Ro (SSA) antibodies. *Arthritis Rheum* 1983;26:1279–1282.
282. Howard PF, Hochberg MC, Bias WB, et al. Relationship between C4 null genes, HLA-D region antigens, and genetic susceptibility to systemic lupus erythematosus in Caucasian and black Americans. *Am J Med* 1986;81:187–193.
283. Walport MJ, Davies KA, Morley BJ. Complement deficiency and autoimmunity. *Ann N Y Acad Sci* 1997;815:267–281.
284. Lee LA, Farris AD. Photosensitivity diseases: cutaneous lupus erythematosus. *J Investig Dermatol Symp Proc* 1999;4:73–78.
285. Werth VP, Dutz JP, Sontheimer RD. Pathogenetic mechanisms and treatment of cutaneous lupus erythematosus. *Curr Opin Rheumatol* 1997;9:400–409.
286. Sontheimer RD. Photoimmunology of lupus erythematosus and dermatomyositis: a speculative review. *Photochem Photobiol* 1996;63:583–594.

29

CUTANEOUS MANIFESTATIONS OF LUPUS ERYTHEMATOSUS

RICHARD D. SONTHEIMER
DANIEL P. MCCAULIFFE

Realizing that the classification of cutaneous lupus erythematosus (LE) remains somewhat controversial, the authors have chosen to use the Gilliam classification system for LE skin disease (1) to organize the material in this chapter (Table 29.1). Following the introductory discussions related to history and definition/classification, the remainder of the chapter will be divided into two sections—LE-Specific Skin Disease and LE-Nonspecific Skin Disease—according to the Gilliam classification scheme. See Table 29.2 for an overview of the organization of this chapter. Some of the LE-nonspecific diseases, including vasculitis, Raynaud's phenomena, erythromelalgia, and rheumatoid nodules will be covered in Chapter 30. The pathogenic mechanisms that may contribute to the development of cutaneous LE were covered in Chapter 28.

TABLE 29.1. THE GILLIAM CLASSIFICATION OF LUPUS ERYTHEMATOSUS (LE)-ASSOCIATED SKIN LESIONS

I. HISTOPATHOLOGICALLY SPECIFIC (LE-SPECIFIC)
- A. Acute cutaneous LE
  - 1) Localized
  - 2) Generalized
- B. Subacute cutaneous LE
  - 1) Annular
  - 2) Papulosquamous
- C. Chronic cutaneous LE
  - 1) "Classical" DLE
    - a) Localized
    - b) Generalized
  - 2) Hypertrophic (verrucous) DLE
  - 3) Lupus profundus (LE panniculitis)
  - 4) Mucosal LE
  - 5) LE tumidus
  - 6) Chilblains LE (perniotic LE)
  - 7) DLE-lichen planus overlap

II. HISTOPATHOLOGICALLY NONSPECIFIC (LE-NONSPECIFIC)
- A. Cutaneous vascular disease
  - 1) Vasculitis
    - a) Leukocytoclastic
      - (1) Palpable purpura
      - (2) Urticarial vasculitis
    - b) Periarteritis nodosa-like
  - 2) Vasculopathy
    - a) Dego's disease-like
    - b) Atrophy blanche-like
  - 3) Periungual telangiectasia
  - 4) Livedo reticularis
  - 5) Thrombophlebitis
  - 6) Raynaud's phenomenon
  - 7) Erythromelalgia
- B. Alopecia (nonscarring)
  - 1) "Lupus hair"
  - 2) Telogen effluvium
  - 3) Alopecia aerata
- C. Sclerodactyly
  - Sclerodermatous skin changes in LE patients is rather uncommon.
- D. Rheumatoid nodules
- E. Calcinosis cutis
- F. LE nonspecific bullous lesions
  - 1) Epidermolysis bullosa acquisita
  - 2) Dermatitis herpetiformis-like bullous LE
  - 3) Pemphigus erythematosus
  - 4) Bullous pemphigoid
  - 5) Porphyria cutanea tarda
- G. Urticaria
- H. Papulo-nodular mucinosis
- I. Cutis laxa/anetoderma
- J. Acanthosis nigricans (Type B insulin resistance)
- K. Erythema multiforme
- L. Leg ulcers
- M. Lichen planus

DLE, discoid lupus erythematosus; LE, lupus erythematosus.

TABLE 29.2. CHAPTER ORGANIZATION

I. Historical Perspective
II. Definition and Classification
III. LE-Specific Skin Disease
  A. Epidemiology
  B. Cutaneous manifestations
  C. Relationship with systemic disease features
    1. Risk of developing SLE
    2. Lupus band test
  D. Pathology and immunopathology
  E. Laboratory findings
  F. Differential diagnosis
  G. Management
  H. Prognosis
IV. LE-Nonspecific Skin Disease

LE, lupus erythematosus; SLE, systemic lupus erythematosus.

HISTORICAL PERSPECTIVE

In his more comprehensive review of the history of LE in *Dubois' Lupus Erythematosus, 5th edition*, Thomas Benedek points out that this disease initially was recognized by its visible cutaneous manifestations long before its systemic manifestations were known to exist (2) (see Chapter 1). In this section, we will attempt only to highlight the people and events that relate primarily to the evolution of thought concerning the cutaneous manifestations of this protean disease process [Those more interested in this area are referred to Dr. Benedek's excellent chapter on this subject (2) and to a previous overview of this area by one of the authors (RDS) derived in part from an abstraction of this work (3) and other authoritative treatments of this subject (4).].

1851. Cazenave first used the term "lupus érythèmateaux" in referring to Biett's earlier description of what appears to have been discoid LE (DLE) skin lesions (5). The term "lupus érythèmateaux" helped to further distinguish this entity as a cutaneous malady that was distinct from cutaneous tuberculosis (lupus vulgaris) with which it had been earlier confused. Cazenave stated that LE preferentially occurred in outdoor workers and that exacerbations were related to cold, heat, fire, and the action of air.

1875. Kaposi further expanded Hebra's earlier description of what is now recognized as the systemic manifestations of LE and employed the "butterfly" simile first used by Hebra to describe the facial skin lesions of LE (6). He also commented upon the relationship between DLE skin lesions and the systemic manifestations of this disease, noting that DLE can, on occasion, progress to SLE.

Hutchinson (7) and later Osler, at the turn of the century (8), emphasized the multisystem nature of LE and the patient-to-patient variation with which its cutaneous and systemic manifestations are expressed. Lehmann and Ruzicka (9) have pointed out the later went on to say that LE patients did not tolerate sun well (10).

Payne first treated DLE with the natural antimalarial, quinine (11).

1913. Lehmann and Ruzicka (9) also have noted that Pussey commented on the exacerbating effects of sunlight on cutaneous LE in a young woman (12).

Brocq's initial description of "symmetrical erythema centrifugum" (13), probably representing the earliest delineation of what Gilliam later referred to as "subacute cutaneous LE" (SCLE), the bridging form of LE-specific skin disease in his revised classification of cutaneous LE (14).

1929. Lehmann and Ruzicka have pointed out that Fuhs reported the exacerbating effect of an artificial light source on a patient with "lupus erythematosus subacutus," a term that appears to be referring to what we recognize today as SCLE (15).

1934. O'Leary's introduction of the term "disseminated DLE" as part of his new classification scheme that included both its cutaneous and systemic manifestations (16). The term "disseminated" in his classification scheme was used somewhat ambiguously in referring both to a widespread distribution of LE skin lesions and the transition from disease limited to skin to the systemic illness that we now recognize as SLE. Thus, several forms of widespread LE-specific skin disease (i.e., generalized DLE and SCLE) were thereafter often lumped together under the designation "disseminated DLE" or "subacute-disseminated LE," thereby obscuring the clinical and laboratory correlates of each of these clinically distinctive types of cutaneous LE. As a result, when the large LE population studies were later presented in which the clinical features of LE patients were correlated with the newly identified autoimmune serological manifestations of the disease, the distinction between patients having generalized DLE and SCLE often was blurred.

1936. Freidberg's presentation of the heretical idea that the systemic manifestations of LE could occur in the absence of any type of skin lesion (17).

1951. Introduction of the use of synthetic antimalarial, quinacrine (18) and corticosteroids (19) for the treatment of LE.

1948. Hargraves description of the LE-cell factor (20) and Friou's subsequent description of the antinuclear antibody assay in 1957 (21) ushered in the era of serological-clinical correlation in LE.

1963. Neville Rowell's description of EM-like lesions occurring in LE patients in the context of autoantibodies to the Sjögren's syndrome antigen Sj-T that is now thought to represent the La/SS-B specificity (22). Dr. Rowell's other work has contributed significantly to our current understanding of various aspects of cutaneous LE including chilblains lupus (perniotic LE) and classical DLE.

1963. Burnham and coworkers' identification of the "lupus band" (23).

1963. Edmund Dubois and Denny Tuffanelli present their landmark description of 520 consecutive SLE patients, 29% of whom had DLE skin lesions (24). Dubois was among the first to use the "spectrum" analogy for LE, emphasizing that this illness represented a disease continuum extending from localized DLE at the more benign pole to fully expressed SLE at the more severely affected pole. He also emphasized the fact that various transitional forms commonly occurred within this spectrum including the appearance of SLE in patients who had initially presented with DLE lesions alone as well as the development of DLE lesions in patients with preexisting SLE. These concepts were emphasized in the first edition of his classical book (25), which is currently in its fourth edition (26). Dubois' spectrum concept influenced Jim Gilliam's thinking concerning the classification of cutaneous LE.

1969. Morris Reichlin and coworkers' description of anti-Ro/SS-A antibodies (27), later to be identified as the serological marker for SCLE and neonatal LE.

1975. James N. Gilliam extended Edmund Dubois' spectrum analogy focusing especially upon the relationships that exist between the various cutaneous and systemic manifestations of LE (28). He also stressed the value of the various forms of cutaneous LE as markers for subsetting LE (the exercise of identifying more homogeneous subgroups of LE patients based upon the sharing of common clinical, pathological, and laboratory features) that had become popular by the 1970s (29).

1976. Publication of comprehensive monograph by Marian W. Ropes (30) detailing the experience gained from a large number of SLE patients followed over several decades in the inpatient and outpatient settings at Massachusetts General Hospital. Careful observations concerning the mucocutaneous manifestations of this disease were reported.

1977. Barba and Gonzalez presented one of the earliest reports on the beneficial effects of thalidomide on cutaneous LE (31). The tremendous impact of thalidomide on cutaneous LE inflammation subsequently was documented by a number of other workers [reviewed in (32)]. Thalidomide subsequently has been shown to inhibit TNF-α gene expression. These observations taken together with the modern work indicating abnormal TNF-α expression in photosensitive cutaneous LE such as SCLE could lead to new therapeutic approaches.

1979. Gilliam and coworkers' characterization of the immunogenetically homogeneous LE subset marked by the presence of SCLE skin lesions (33–35). These were virtually the same group of patients being described concurrently by Thomas Provost and his colleagues under the designation of "ANA-negative SLE" (36). The concept of SCLE originally was introduced by Gilliam as a component of a new classification of cutaneous LE that emphasized the clinical differences that exist between different types of histopathologically specific LE skin lesions (29). Gilliam's earlier work at Stanford with the dermatopathologist, Alvin Cox, and later at University of Texas Southwestern with Robert Freeman greatly influenced his thinking in this area.

Description of anti-Ro/SS-A autoantibody as the serological marker for neonatal LE by groups led by Bill Weston and Tom Provost (37).

1990. Lehmann, Kind, and coworkers redefine LE photosensitivity in modern photobiological terms documenting that SCLE is among the most photosensitive subsets of cutaneous LE and that ultraviolet A (UVA) plays a significant role in SCLE photosensitivity (38, 39).

1984. Norris and coworkers show that ultraviolet B (UVB) radiation modulates Ro/SS-A autoantigens to the surface of human epidermal keratinocytes and propose a model for the pathogenesis of Ro/SS-A autoantibody-associated photosensitive cutaneous LE involving antibody-dependent, cell-mediated cytotoxicity (40, 41).

1993. Attempt to systematically classify the clinical forms of cutaneous LE (42, 43).

1994. Casciola-Rosen et al. first demonstrated that autoantigens (Ro/SS-A, calreticulin) that are targeted in SLE are clustered in two populations of surface structures on UVB-induced apoptotic keratinocytes.

1995. Systematic characterization of cutaneous LE subsets in a relatively homogenous ethnic population (44, 45).

2000. Modern characterizations of the subsets of LE tumidus (46) and LE profundus/panniculitis (47).

Werth et al. initially reported a specific genetic marker for SCLE, the presence of the -308A TNF-α promoter polymorphism (48).

DEFINITION AND CLASSIFICATION

LE is a systemic autoimmune disorder associated with polyclonal B-cell activation that is thought to result from an interplay of genetic, environmental, and hormonal elements. It is convenient to consider the heterogenous clinical expression of this disorder as constituting a disease continuum or spectrum extending from a limited cutaneous disorder to a life-threatening systemic disease process.

The term "discoid LE" (DLE) often was used in the past to generically designate the subgroup of LE patients whose disease was expressed only in the skin (49). The use of the term "DLE" in this sense can create confusion because this same term also is commonly used to identify one of several clinically distinctive forms of LE-specific skin disease. In the following discussion, the term "DLE" will be used in the latter, more restricted sense to refer only to a certain clinical form of chronic cutaneous LE. The term "cutaneous LE" will be used in an umbrella fashion in this chapter to refer to all skin lesions that have some form of association with LE.

The term "SLE" has been used in the past synonymously with the term "LE" to generically designate all patients suffering from this autoimmune disease process (unfortunately, many in the present continue to use the term in this manner). However, in this sense, the term "SLE" unfairly stigmatizes those LE patients whose disease is expressed clinically only in their skin throughout their entire disease course. The term "SLE" will be used in this discussion to refer only to the systemic manifestations of the fundamental underlying disease process, LE. It must be remembered that the large majority of patients with SLE will express some form of cutaneous LE during the course of their disease.

The American College of Rheumatology has formulated a set of revised clinical and laboratory criteria for the classification of SLE primarily for the purpose of providing some degree of uniformity to the patient populations of clinical studies (50). This classification system is used commonly by clinicians to establish a diagnosis of SLE in a given patient. However, this system is not perfect. For example, based on the devised criteria, a patient can be classified as SLE based on skin findings only (i.e, the four criteria being photosensitivity, oral ulcers, discoid rash, and malar rash). It also is unfortunate that this classification did not include histopathologic evidence of cutaneous LE as a diagnostic criterion (e.g., evidence of vacuolar degeneration in the basal layer of the epidermis).

The LE disease spectrum can be subdivided in a number of ways—clinically, serologically, or pathologically. Using this approach, various patterns (or subsets) of illness can be identified, i.e., some patients will share common patterns of clinical, immunological, and pathological abnormalities. One example would be SCLE. Patients who present with SCLE skin lesions have a clinically and pathologically distinctive form of cutaneous LE, frequently produce anti-Ro/SS-A autoantibodies, and share a common HLA phenotype (HLA-B8, DR3, DRw52, DQ 1/2) (51).

The clinical expression of skin involvement in LE is very common and extremely heterogenous (Table 29.1). Because the type of skin involvement in LE can be reflective of the underlying pattern of SLE activity, it is important to have a common language when referring to LE skin lesions. Much attention has been paid to the issue of classifying LE from the dermatological perspective in the past and there continues to be considerable debate in this area (52). For the purpose of this discussion, we will use the classification system developed by Jim Gilliam, which divides the skin lesions that can be encountered in LE patients into those that are histologically specific for LE (i.e., LE-specific skin disease) and those that are not histologically specific for this disease (i.e., LE-nonspecific skin disease) (29). The histologically specific skin lesions share the following elements of a lichenoid tissue reaction (53): hyperkeratosis; epidermal atrophy; liquefactive (vacuolar, hydropic) degeneration of the epidermal basal-cell layer; a mononuclear cell infiltrate focused at the dermal-epidermal junction, perivascular areas, and perifollicular areas; thickening of the epidermal-basement membrane; and melanin-pigment incontinence. There are three broad categories of LE-specific skin disease: acute cutaneous LE (ACLE), subacute cutaneous LE (SCLE), and chronic cutaneous LE (CCLE). LE-nonspecific skin lesions such as cutaneous vasculitis have histopathologic changes that are seen in conditions other than LE and thus are not specific for this disorder.

It is important to note, however, that other cutaneous disorders can have LE-like histopathology. These disorders include dermatomyositis, graft-versus-host disease, erythema multiforme, drug eruptions, and polymorphous light eruption, which sometimes can clinically mimic the gross morphologic features of cutaneous LE. An experienced dermatologist usually can differentiate between these various disorders by analyzing additional information from the patient's history, physical examination, and laboratory evaluation.

With any arbitrary subdivision of a disease continuum such as LE, overlapping features can occur. For example, patients who have predominately SCLE lesions also can develop scarring DLE or ACLE lesions at some point in their course. However, in most patients, one form of LE-specific skin involvement will predominate.

An occasional patient will be encountered who has skin lesions that demonstrate LE-specific histopathology but whose cutaneous disease does not conform fully to one of the categories of LE-specific skin disease under the Gilliam classification scheme. The few such patients that have been encountered have been considered to have a clinically generic variety of LE-specific skin disease. It has been the impression of one of the authors (RDS) that this situation arises more commonly in African American patients.

It also should be remembered that LE patients not infrequently develop unrelated common dermatological disorders that are not the direct result of LE activity in the skin. Harm to patients can result when skin disorders are misdiagnosed as cutaneous LE causing patients to be subjected to unnecessary tests and/or potentially toxic therapies. In their study of 84 consecutive SLE patients, Weinstein et al. found that (42%) had dermatoses attributable to SLE while 58 (69%) had dermatoses that were not directly attributable to SLE (54). Some conditions can simulate the clinical appearance of different forms of cutaneous LE. One example would be acne rosacea simulating the clinical appearance of ACLE on the face (55). In addition, cutaneous complications of treatment of SLE such as corticosteroid-induced acne vulgaris might be attributed to the underlying systemic autoimmune process by observers less familiar with the cutaneous manifestations of this disorder.

LUPUS ERYTHEMATOSUS-SPECIFIC SKIN DISEASE

Epidemiology

There is very little population-based data concerning the epidemiology of LE—cutaneous or systemic. Most studies are reported by rheumatologists or dermatologists working separately, and as a result, selection bias often is present in the data that are commonly reported. In most large clinical studies of selected LE patients, the skin is second only to joints as the most frequently affected organ system, and skin disease is the second-most common way that LE initially presents clinically (56). This also was true for a population-based cohort of 80 patients (57). In some study populations, cutaneous disease has been the most common disease manifestation (58).

Together, all forms of cutaneous LE have a significant socioeconomic impact within the United States. It has been suggested that cutaneous LE is the third-most common cause of industrial disability from dermatological disease, with 45% of cutaneous LE patients experiencing some degree of vocational handicap (59). It is most informative to discuss the epidemiology of the three major types of LE-specific skin disease in more detail.

Acute Cutaneous Lupus Erythematosus

In most large clinical studies carried out by rheumatologists or internists, ACLE is reported under the designations "malar rash" or "butterfly rash" (i.e., presumably ACLE) and "rash," "maculopapular rash," or "photosensitive lupus dermatitis" (presumably generalized ACLE). In such studies, the skin lesions usually are not biopsied and thus it is difficult to know whether they in fact represent LE-specific skin disease. Because dermatologists usually do not primarily mange such patients because of the strong association between ACLE and systemic LE activity, little data concerning this form of LE-specific skin disease is available in the dermatological literature. Because of its strong association with SLE, the epidemiology of ACLE might be expected to closely parallel that of unselected SLE patients, which recently has been comprehensively reviewed (60).

Demographics

Malar rash or butterfly rash has been reported in 20%–60% of large LE patient cohorts (58). Limited data suggest that the "maculopapular rash" of SLE is present in about 35% of SLE patients (56). Malar rash is more common in women than men (56). Because photosensitivity is seen more frequently in Whites than African Americans (61), one might infer that the same could be true for ACLE. Malar rash has been suggested to be associated with a younger age of disease onset (56). A clinically nonspecific maculopapular rash resembling a drug eruption but felt to be related to SLE was present in 59% of the 81 patients studied by Wysenbeek et al. (62); however, because biopsy data were not presented, it cannot be certain whether this "rash" was related to generalized ACLE.

Genetic Associations

Curiously, little effort has been made to determine whether ACLE has any specific HLA associations. ACLE lesions usually occur in the context of SLE and SLE has been associated with HLA-DR2 and -DR3 (63). Familial associations and concordance in twins suggest that SLE has an important genetic component (63).

Environmental Factors

Exposure to natural or UV irradiation is a frequent precipitating factor for SLE patients (64), especially those who produce anti-Ro/SS-A autoantibody (65). Chemicals such as L-canavanine present in alfalfa sprouts can induce a SLE-like illness (60). Numerous drugs have been implicated in inducing various features of SLE (66), although the skin often is spared in classical drug-induced SLE. Infections, especially with subtle types of viruses, have long been suspected to be capable of precipitating and/or exacerbating SLE (67).

Subacute Cutaneous Lupus Erythematosus

Demographics

SCLE patients comprised 9% of the total LE patient population examined by Sontheimer et al. (33). Others have found SCLE lesions in 7% to 27% of their LE patient populations (68). SCLE is primarily a disease of white females of all ages. Seventy percent of the original cohort of SCLE patients were female and 85% were white (33). The mean age of this group of patients was 43.3 years with a range from 17 to 67 years. Others have reported similar racial and sexual demographic data (68).

Genetic Associations

The majority of studies have found that at least one half of their SCLE patients have the HLA-DR3 phenotype (69), although some groups have found a lower frequency of HLA-DR3 (70). HLA-DR3 normally is found in only 25% of the United States white population (71). One group has suggested that the HLA-DR3 phenotype is most strongly associated with the annular form of SCLE (72) and that annular SCLE lesions denote the most homogenenous subgroup of SCLE patients immunogenetically (72). HLA-DR2 also has been associated with SCLE (73). SCLE patients with overlapping features of SCLE and Sjögren's syndrome are more likely have the HLA-B8, DR3, DRW6, DQ2, and DRW52 extended haplotype (74). It has been suggested that the HLA-DR antigen associations of SCLE relate more to the anti-Ro/SS-A antibody response in these patients than to the SCLE skin lesions (73). Patients with the extended haplotype HLA-B8, DR3, DRW6, DQ2, and DRW52 produce very high levels of Ro/SS-A autoantibodies (75). High Ro/SS-A antibody titers also have been associated in individuals with HLA-DQw1/DQw2 (75). More recently, Werth et al. have reported a specific genetic marker for SCLE—the presence of the -308A TNF-α promoter polymorphism (76).

Genetically based deficiencies in various complement components including C2, C3, C4, and C5 have been associated with SCLE and/or DLE (77). In addition, genetic deficiency of C1q is a very strong risk factor for photosensitive SLE (78, 79).

Environmental Factors

Earlier studies [data reviewed in (80)] and the more recent data (81) have indicated that a large majority of SCLE patients are highly sensitive to ultraviolet irradiation. SCLE also has developed following radiation therapy (82) and UVA therapy in combination with oral psoralen (83). A number of drugs, many of which are photosensitizers, have been implicated in inducing SCLE. These drugs include aldactone (84), angiotensin-converting enzyme inhibitors (captopril, cilazapril) (85, 86), calcium-channel blockers (verapamil, diltiazem, nifedipine) (87), hydrochlorothiazide (88), interferon-α (89), procainamide (90), d-penicillamine (80), sulfonylureas (80), terbinafine (91), oxyprenolol (92), griseofulvin (93), piroxicam (94), naproxen (95), and PUVA (83). One patient developed annular SCLE after taking the combination of cinnarizine and thiethylperazine (96). The implication that the antihisamine cinnarizine might induce SCLE is of additional interest in light of the recent report of antihistamine-induced SCLE-like dermatitis (97). One of the authors (DPM) has witnessed a patient who developed SCLE shortly after starting the gastric acid/proton-pump inhibitor omeprazole that resolved after discontinuing this medicine. The patient noted a recurrence of her lesions 1 to 2 years later after starting the proton-pump inhibitor lansoprazole (unpubl. observation). The other author (RDS) is aware of a case of omperazole (Prilosec, Astra Merck) - induced annular SCLE in a male (personal communication, Dr. Mark DeMay, Sioux City, Iowa; April, 2000).

Chronic Cutaneous Lupus Erythematosus

No reliable population-based data exist pertaining to the true prevalence or incidence of classical DLE (the most common form of CCLE) presenting in the absence of systemic LE activity. Such patients tend to be underrepresented in studies reported by rheumatologists and internists and over represented by those reported by dermatologists. In addition, the epidemiological data that is available pertaining to DLE is hard to interpret. Studies prior to 1970 did not stratify patients according to the American Rheumatism Association's (American College of Rheumatology) classification criteria for SLE. Additionally, these workers did not have access to the various laboratory parameters that gauge the presence and degree of activity of systemic autoimmunity. Also, prior to 1979, investigators did not distinguish between DLE and SCLE, usually lumping these two varieties of cutaneous LE together under the generic designations of "DLE" or "disseminated DLE." Thus, it can be difficult to gain an accurate view of the prevalence of or incidence of DLE from the data presented in studies prior to that time.

Demographics

Based upon data from the available studies, the following points can be made concerning the epidemiology of DLE, as distinguished from SCLE. DLE skin lesions are present in 15% to 30% of variously selected study populations of SLE (58). Approximately 5% to 10% of SLE populations have DLE skin lesions as their presenting disease manifestation (24). For every patient affected primarily with DLE, seven will be affected primarily by SLE (98). The most common age of onset of DLE is between 20 and 40 years in both males and females (99). DLE lesions, however, can appear in infancy as well as the elderly. The female:male ratio for DLE has been reported to be between 3:2 to 3:1 (100, 101)which is much lower than that of SLE. Any race can be affected and most of the classical studies have found DLE to be more frequent in whites (102). Some earlier studies suggested that African Americans were relatively protected from DLE; however, Hochberg and coworkers have presented data that argue that DLE might actually be more prevalent in African Americans (61).

Genetic Associations

Knop et al. found significant increases of HLA-B7, B8, Cw7, DR2, DR3, DQW1, and a significant decrease in HLA-A2 in a large group of German DLE patients (103). The combinations of HLA-Cw7, DR3, DQW1, and HLA-B7, Cw7, DR3 conferred the maximum relative risk (7.4) for DLE. Partial C2 and C4 complement deficiencies have been reported in LE panniculitis (104–106).

Environmental Factors

Skin lesions are precipitated or aggravated by ultraviolet irradiation, especially UVB, in approximately half of patients with DLE. Several reports have suggested that smoking may predispose patients to develop DLE (107–109). We have observed several patients whose previously refractory DLE lesions improved spontaneously in a dramatic fashion following the cessation of cigarette smoking. Nonspecific injury to the skin can precipitate the development of DLE activity within the areas of trauma (i.e., the Köebner/isomorphic phenomenon) (110–112). In contrast to many drug-induced SCLE reports, there is a lack of drug-induced DLE reports in the literature.

Cutaneous Manifestations

Acute Cutaneous Lupus Erythematosus

ACLE can present in either a localized or generalized distribution. Localized ACLE (the classic "butterfly rash" or "malar rash" of SLE) is the most common pattern (Fig. 29.1). Localized ACLE typically is characterized by confluent, symmetrical erythema and edema centered over the malar eminences (unilateral involvement with ACLE has been described (30)). Inflammation extending over the bridge of the nose completes the body of the classic butterfly. However, the nasolabial folds typically are spared. The forehead and V area of the neck can be similarly involved. Facial swelling may be severe in some patients with ACLE (113). Occassionally, ACLE begins on the face as small, discrete macular and/or papular lesions that later become confluent and hyperkeratotic (114) (Fig. 29.2).

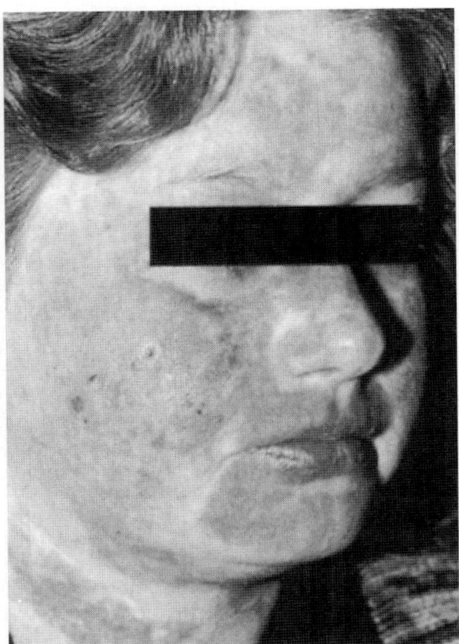

FIGURE 29.1. (See color plate.) Localized acute cutaneous lupus erythematosus (ACLE). ACLE confined to the face and neck is classified under the Gilliam scheme as localized ACLE. The most typical presentation, as seen in this case, is that of a confluent erythema that can be associated with some degree of induration because of edema formation. As the inflammation subsides, postinflammatory hyper- or hypopigmentation can remain; however, atrophic dermal scarring is not seen.

Generalized ACLE is less common than DLE. It presents as a more widespread morbilliform or exanthematous eruption (Fig. 29.3). This presentation has been referred to in the past as the "maculopapular rash" or "photosensitive lupus dermatitis."

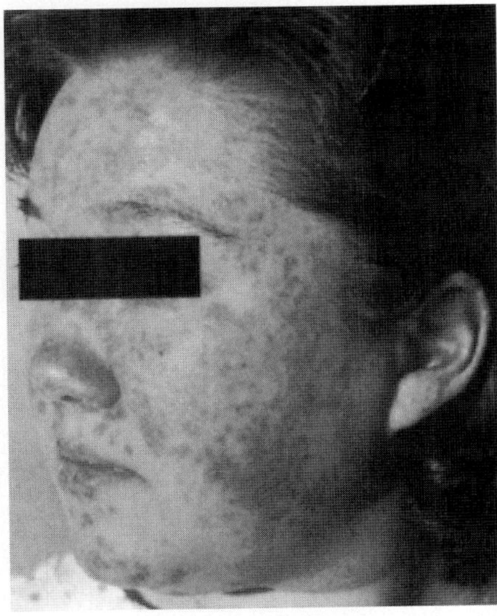

FIGURE 29.2. (See color plate.) Macular/papular acute cutaneous lupus erythematosus (ACLE). ACLE less commonly presents as a macular and/or papular erythema, as demonstrated in this young woman who ultimately died from systemic lupus erythematosus.

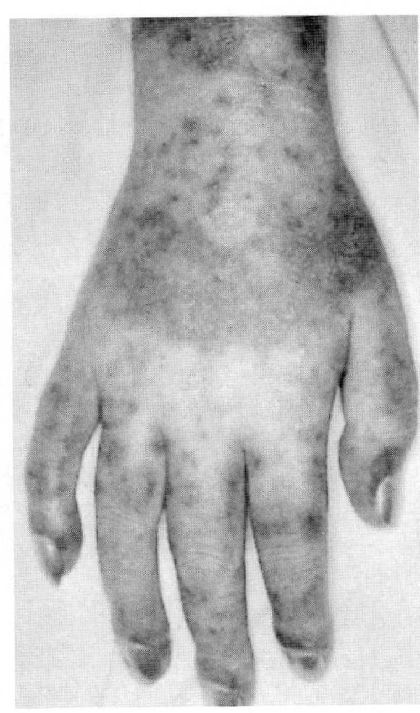

FIGURE 29.3. Generalized acute cutaneous lupus erythematosus (ACLE). ACLE that presents both above and below the neck is classified as generalized ACLE. Note the macular erythema over the extensor aspect of the wrists that becomes confluent over the dorsal aspect of the hand and interphalangeal areas.

Some patients experience an extremely acute form of ACLE that can simulate toxic epidermal necrolysis. This form of bullous LE results from dissolution of the epidermal basal-cell layer as a result of intense lichenoid inflammation (115) (Fig. 29.4) . Su presents a framework for considering how this form of bullous LE skin change relates to the other clinical patterns of bullous cutaneous injury that can be seen in LE patients (116). The other bullous skin lesions that occur in LE are discussed separately below and listed in Table 29.3.

ACLE is very photosensitive and can be quite transient, lasting only several days or weeks. Occasionally, lesions will wax and wane over a period of several hours and some patients will experience more prolonged disease activity. Postinflammatory pigmentary change is most prominent in LE patients with darkly pigmented skin (Fig. 29.5). ACLE lesions do not result in scarring. Patients with localized ACLE occasionally will have SCLE lesions elsewhere on their body, however, the simultaneous occurrence of ACLE and active DLE is very unusual.

Subacute Cutaneous Lupus Erythematosus

SCLE was first discussed as a distinct disease entity by Gilliam in 1977 (14) and expanded further in 1981 (29). SCLE skin lesions have been referred to in the past under a number of other designations including symmetric erythema centrifugum, disseminated DLE, autoimmune annular erythema, subacute-disseminated LE, superficial-disseminated LE, psoriasiform LE, pityriasiform LE, and

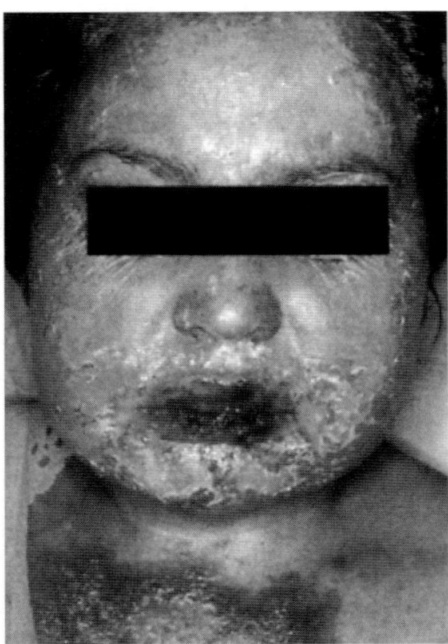

FIGURE 29.4. Acute cutaneous lupus erythematosus (ACLE) simulating the appearance of toxic epidermal necrolysis. Note the hemorrhagic crusting of the lips and the erosions over the V-area of the neck and upper chest. These skin changes developed during an acute flare of this patient's systemic lupus erythematosus that followed her decision to abruptly discontinue all medications. Therefore, there was no possibility that her toxic epidermal necrolysislike skin changes resulted from a drug hypersensitivity reaction.

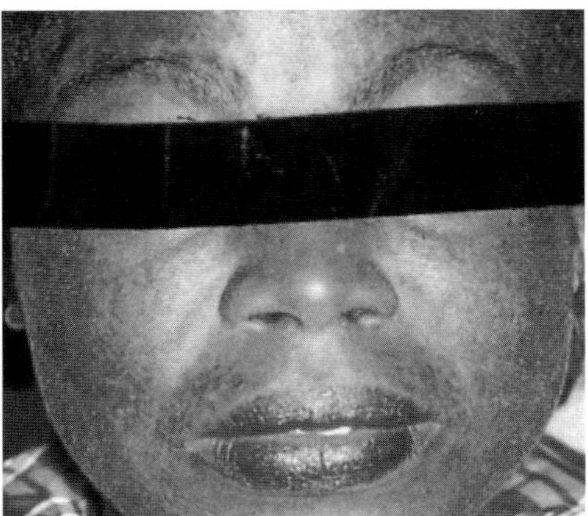

FIGURE 29.5. Hyperpigmented acute cutaneous lupus erythematosus (ACLE). Hyperpigmentation often can soon follow the onset of ACLE inflammation in darkly pigmented individuals. This rather stoic patient's only presenting complaint was darkening of the skin of her face. However, her evaluation revealed the presence of active systemic lupus erythematosus, including renal involvement. Soon after starting prednisone and hydroxychloroquine, she developed an acute abdominal crisis, resulting in an unrevealing exploratory laparotomy. The source of her abdominal pain subsequently was realized to have been antimalarial agentinduced hepatotoxicity in the setting of clinical silent porphyria cutanea tarda.

maculopapular-photosensitive LE [original data reviewed in (33)]. The entity "LE gyratum repens" now is also considered to be synonymous with annular SCLE (117). The original cohort of SCLE patients presented in 1979 (33) and the others that have followed indicate that SCLE is a distinct subset of cutaneous LE having characteristic clinical, serologic, and genetic features (69).

SCLE consists of nonscarring papulosquamous or annular skin lesions having an LE-specific histopathology (118) that occurs in a characteristic photodistribution (33). Approximately 85% of all SCLE patients report photosensitivity (119), although some ethnic groups report this less frequently. While circulating autoantibodies to the Ro/SS-A ribonucleoprotein particle supports this diagnosis (35), their presence is not required to make a diagnosis of SCLE according to its original definition (33).

TABLE 29.3. BULLOUS SKIN LESIONS THAT CAN BE SEEN IN LE PATIENTS

LE-Specific ("Classical" Bullous LE)
Toxic epidermal necrolysislike ACLE and SCLE
Vesiculobullous annular SCLE
Bullous DLE
LE-Nonspecific
"Bullous SLE"
Dermatitis herpetiformislike cutaneous LE
Epidermolysis bullosa acquisitalike cutaneous LE
Bullous disorders anecdotally reported to occur in LE patients
Bullous pemphigoid
Pemphigus erythematosus
Porphyria cutanea tarda

ACLE, acute cutaneous lupus erythematosus; DLE, discoid lupus erythematosus; LE, lupus erythematosus; SCLE, subacute cutaneous lupus erythematosus; SLE, systemic lupus erythematosus.

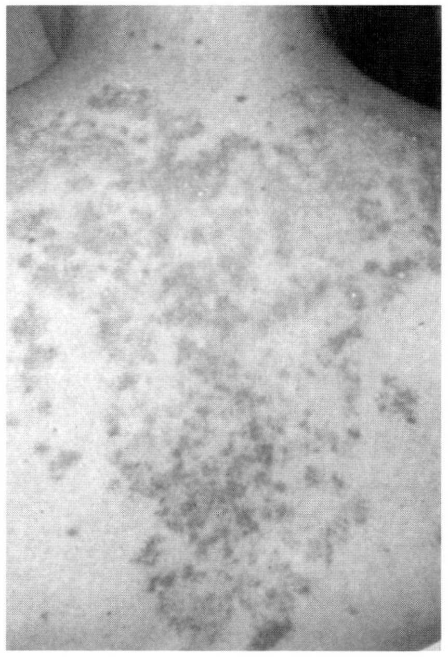

FIGURE 29.6. Papulosquamous subacute cutaneous lupus erythematosus on the mid- and upper back of a patient with no extracutaneous manifestations of systemic lupus erythematosus. Note the superficial scale and tendency for the individual lesions to merge into a retiform pattern.

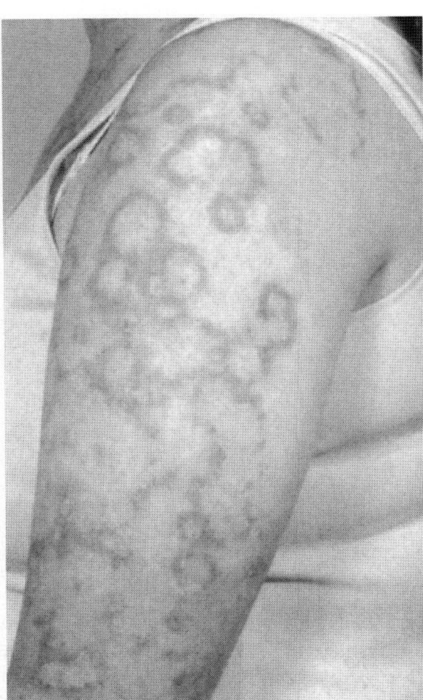

FIGURE 29.7. (See color plate.) Annular subacute cutaneous lupus erythematosus. Note the polycyclic array resulting from the confluence of the individual annular lesions. This young woman ultimately died from complications of chronic active lupus.

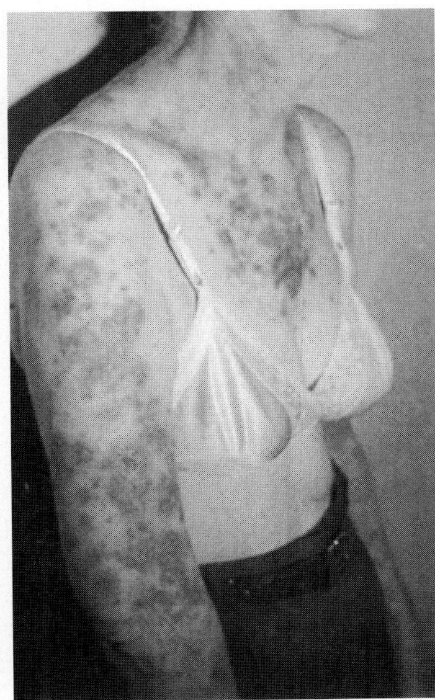

FIGURE 29.8. (See color plate.) Characteristic photodistribution of subacute cutaneous lupus erythematosus (SCLE). Curiously, the face of this patient with hydrochlorothiazide-induced SCLE was not affected. In the experience of one of the authors (RDS), sparing of the face in patients with SCLE has been the rule rather than the exception.

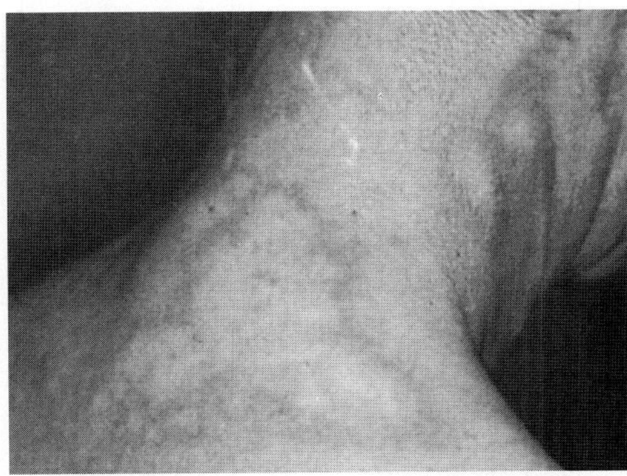

FIGURE 29.9. Annular subacute cutaneous lupus erythematosus (SCLE) with central hypopigmentation. As opposed to other types of annular skin lesions, the central portions of annular SCLE lesions characteristically display hypopigmentation in areas where the inflammation has subsided, reflecting the pigment-compartment injury pattern commonly seen on biopsy specimens. Although not visible in this photograph, telangiectasia also frequently can be observed in the inactive central areas of annular SCLE lesions.

SCLE lesions present initially as erythematous macules or papules that evolve into scaly, papulosquamous or annular/polycyclic plaques (Figs. 29.6, 29.7). Approximately 50% of patients have predominately papulosquamous- or psoriasis-form lesions, (Fig. 29.6), while the other half have the annular/polycyclic form (Fig. 29.7). A few patients may develop both types of lesions. Some workers have observed a predominance of papulosquamous lesions (70) while others have noted an abundance of the annular/polycyclic form (120). SCLE lesions characteristically occur in sun-exposed areas (i.e., upper back, shoulders, extensor aspects of the arms, V area of the neck, and less commonly, on the face) (Figs. 29.8, 29.9).

Infrequently, SCLE lesions present initially with an appearance of erythema multiforme (Fig. 29.10) (121). Occasionally, arcuate lesions are seen resembling erythema annulare centrifugum (Fig. 29.11). Such cases can simulate the appearance of Rowell's syndrome (erythema multi-

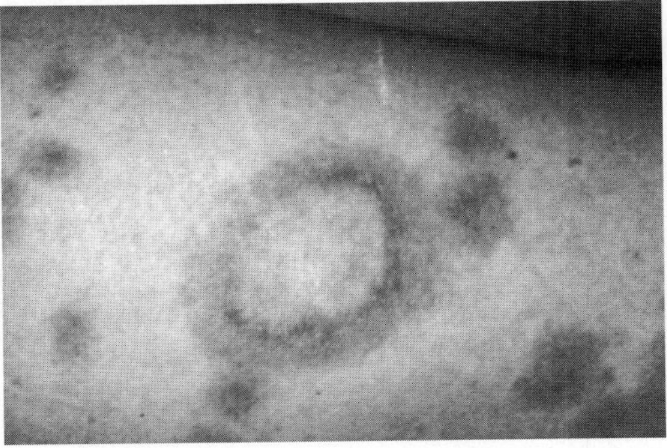

FIGURE 29.10. Annular subacute cutaneous lupus erythematosus (SCLE) presenting with an appearance highly similar to that of erythema multiforme. Note the targetoid appearance of the small primary lesions surrounding the more established annular SCLE lesion in the center.

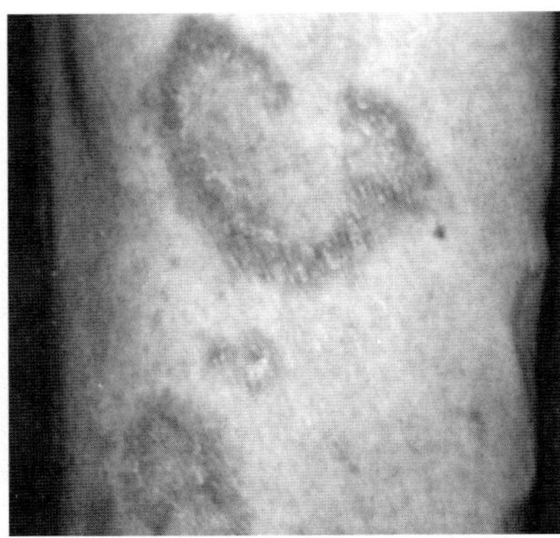

FIGURE 29.11. An arcuate lesion of biopsy-confirmed subacute cutaneous lupus erythematosus (SCLE) simulating the appearance of erythema annulare centrifugum. While the fine scale at the trailing edge of the actively inflamed border is characteristic of erythema annulare centrifugum, it also can be seen in arcuate and annular lesions of SCLE.

formelike lesions occurring in SLE patients in the presence of La/SS-B autoantibodies (22). As a result of hyperacute basal-cell-layer injury, the active edge of annular SCLE lesions on rare occasion undergoes a vesicular change that breaks down to produce a striking crusted appearance (Fig. 29.12) (122). On at least one occasion, such lesions have progressed to mimic toxic epidermal necrolysis (123). One SCLE patient was reported to initially present with exfoliative erythroderma (124) while another presented with a curious acral distribution of annular lesions (125). Pityriasiform (80) (Fig. 29.13), poikilodermatous (126), and exanthematous (121) variants of SCLE have been mentioned anecdotally on rare occasion.

Lesions typically heal without scarring but can sometimes leave long-lasting or permanent vitiligolike leukoderma and telangiectasias (Figs. 29.9, 29.14). In one case, annular SCLE lesions were observed over time to progress to plaques of morphea (127).

Patients with SCLE lesions also may develop ACLE (Fig. 29.15) or classical DLE (Fig. 29.16). Localized facial ACLE lesions have been seen in 20% of the SCLE patients examined by one of the authors (RDS). Others have reported ACLE lesions in 7% to 100% of SCLE patients (120). Figure 29.17 illustrates the patterns of overlap that can occur between the three forms of LE-specific skin disease. ACLE skin lesions tend to be more transient than SCLE and heal with less pigmentary change. They tend to be more edematous and less scaly than SCLE lesions. ACLE more commonly affects the malar areas of the face. The experience of one of the authors (RDS) and others (81) suggests that SCLE affects the face much less often.

Various reports have noted that 0 to 29% of SCLE patients manifest DLE lesions sometime during their clinical course (128). Nineteen percent of the original cohort of SCLE patients had classical DLE lesions (33). DLE lesions can predate the onset of SCLE lesions. DLE lesions in patients with SCLE usually are confined to the head and neck but may be more widely distributed (Fig. 29.16). DLE lesions in this setting generally are associated with a greater degree of hyper- and hypopigmentation, may display atrophic dermal scarring, are more characteristically associated with follicular plugging and adherent scale. DLE

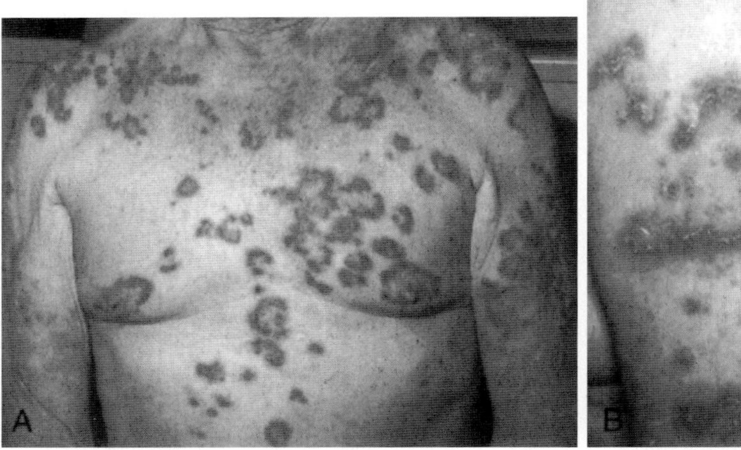

FIGURE 29.12. (See color plate.) Vesicobullous annular subacute cutaneous lupus erythematosus (SCLE). On rare occasions, the active advancing border of annular SCLE lesions undergoes a vesiculobullous change because of extensive liquefactive degeneration of the epidermal basal cell layer **(A)**. As these vesicular elements break down, crusts can form (more evident on the closer view shown in **B**). At times, such eroded areas can become secondarily infected with gram-positive bacteria. Intact pustules occasionally can be seen intermixed with vesicles at the border of annular SCLE lesions such as this.

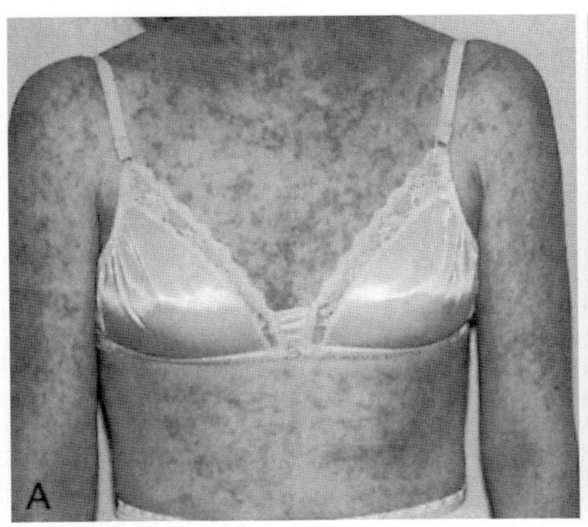

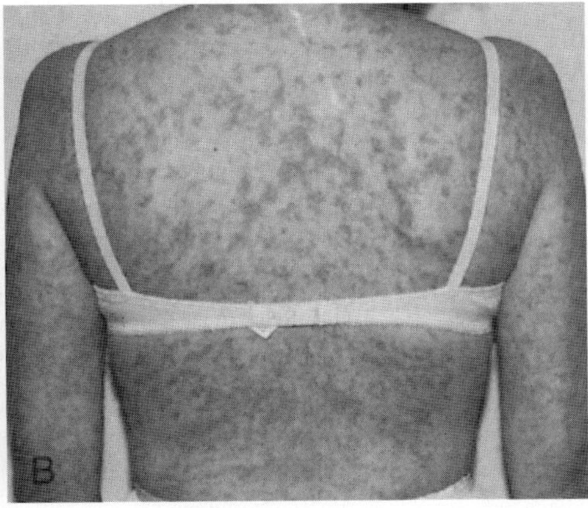

FIGURE 29.13. (See color plate.) Pityriasiform subacute lupus erythematosus. This anti-Ro(SS-A) antibody-positive patient had a generalized eruption of local, minimally scaling, nonscarring lesions demonstrating lupus erythematosus-specific skin disease on biopsy.

lesions are characteristically indurated whereas SCLE is not (81).

A number of other skin lesions that are not histopathologically specific for LE can be found in SCLE patients [data reviewed in (80)]. The most frequently encountered of these include alopecia, painless mucous-membrane lesions, livedo reticularis, periungual telangiectasias, vasculitis, and Raynaud's phenomenon (129). Cutaneous sclerosis (130) and calcinosis (131) may be seen rarely in SCLE patients. Multiple HPV-11-associated squamous-cell carcinomas of the skin were noted in one SCLE patient (132).

Chronic Cutaneous Lupus Erythematosus

Classical DLE

The most common form of chronic cutaneous LE is classical DLE (hereafter, the unqualified term "DLE" will be used to refer to this form of DLE lesion). DLE lesions of this type begin as flat or slightly elevated, well-demarcated, red-purple macules or papules with a scaly surface. Early DLE lesions most commonly evolve into larger, coin-shaped (i.e., "discoid") erythematous plaques covered by a

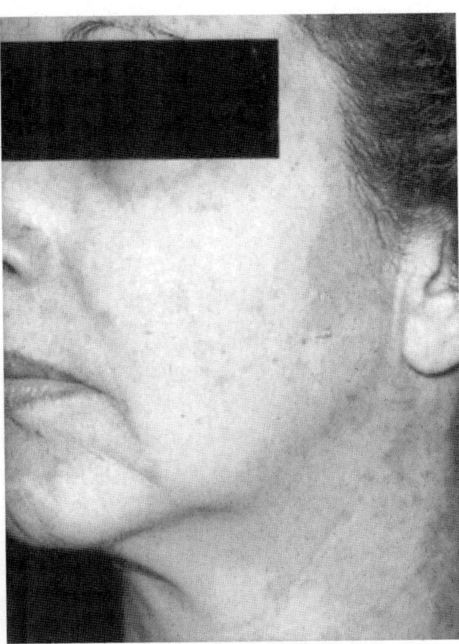

FIGURE 29.14. Subacute lupus erythematosus of the neck and face resolving with permanent vitiligolike depigmentation.

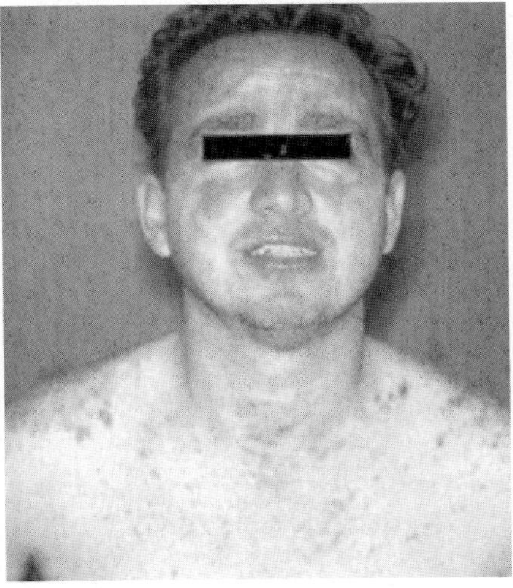

FIGURE 29.15. (See color plate.) Facial acute cutaneous lupus erythematosus (ACLE) occurring in a patient with subacute cutaneous lupus erythematosus (SCLE). This man had experienced uncomplicated papulosquamous SCLE for several years before developing confluent malar erythema at a point in his illness where he experienced clear evidence of extracutaneous SLE activity, including nephritis. It has been the experience of one of the authors (RDS) that the superimposition of ACLE on SCLE is a worrisome prognostic sign regarding the risk for developing extracutaneous manifestations of SLE.

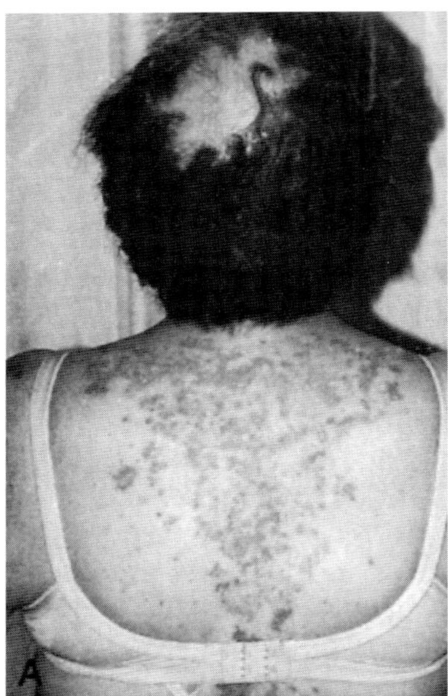

FIGURE 29.16. (See color plate.) Coexistence of subacute cutaneous lupus erythematosus (SCLE) and discoid lupus erythematosus (DLE). Approximately 20% of patients with SCLE will develop classical scarring DLE skin lesions at some point. This patient presented initially with DLE of her scalp and, several years later, developed typical nonscarring papulosquamous SCLE lesions on her back **(A)**. Her cutaneous disease was extremely resistant to therapy, and over the ensuing 5 years, she experienced progression of her DLE scalp involvement, resulting in extensive scarring alopecia **(B)**. The SLCE activity on her back smoldered throughout this period, resulting in the development of superficial atrophy **(C)**. This is one of two such cases observed by one of the authors (RDS) in which dermal atrophy developed within long-smoldering papulosquamous SCLE lesions. Such a progression has not been observed in annular SCLE lesions.

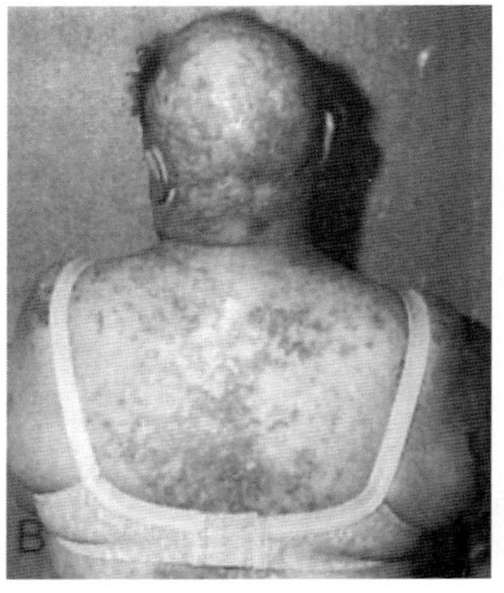

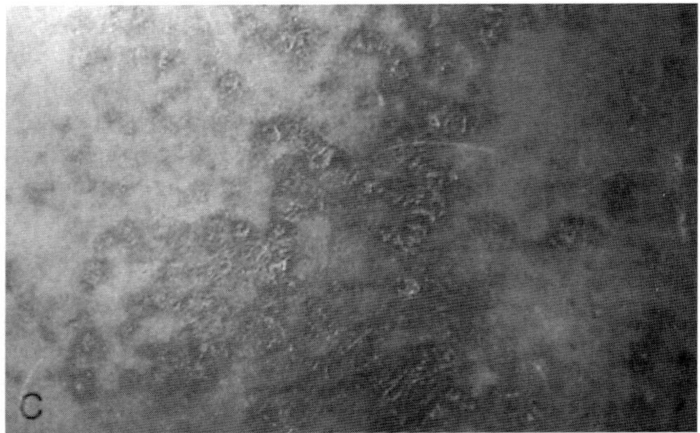

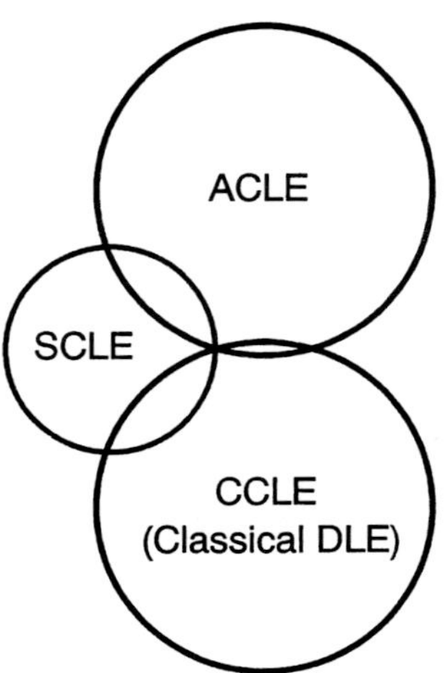

FIGURE 29.17. Potential for overlap between the three major forms of lupus erythematosus-specific skin disease.

prominent, adherent scale that extends into dilated hair follicles (Fig. 29.18). These discoid plaques can enlarge and merge to form even larger, confluent, disfiguring plaques (Figs. 29.19).

Involvement of hair follicles is a prominent clinical feature of DLE lesions. Scales accumulate in dilated follicular openings, which soon become devoid of hair (Fig. 29.20). When the adherent scale is peeled back from more advanced lesions, follicle-sized keratotic spikes similar in appearance to carpet tacks can be seen to project from the undersurface of the scale (i.e., the carpet-tack sign) (Fig. 29.20).

Erythema and hyperpigmentation are present during the initial phase of DLE lesions. The lesions slowly expand with active inflammation and hyperpigmentation at the periphery leaving depressed central scarring, telangiectasia, and depigmentation. The central atrophic scarring is highly characteristic (Fig. 29.18, 29.19). Pigment changes alone

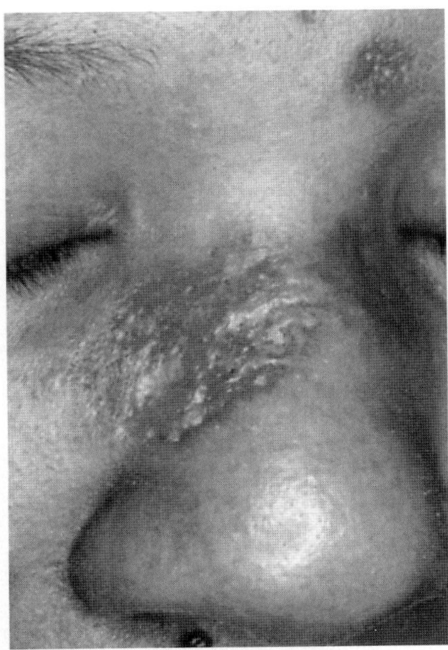

FIGURE 29.18. Classical discoid lupus erythematosus lesion. Note the erythema (indicating disease activity), keratin-plugged follicles, and dermal atrophy. This is a relatively early lesion that lacks the typical adherent scale usually accompanying more established lesions.

do not constitute scarring when referring to cutaneous LE lesions. In some ethnic backgrounds such as Asian Indians, the DLE histopathology can present clinically as isolated areas of macular hyperpigmentation (133).

Typical DLE lesions occur most often on the face, scalp, ears, V-area of the neck, and extensor aspects of the arms. Any area of the face can be affected, including the eyebrows (Fig. 29.19), eyelids (Fig. 29.21), nose (Fig. 29.18, 29.19), and lips (Fig. 29.19, 29.22). A symmetrical, butterfly-shaped DLE plaque occasionally will be found over the malar areas and bridge of the nose. Such DLE lesions are not to be confused with the more transient, edematous-erythema reactions that occur over the same distribution in ACLE lesions. As with ACLE, DLE usually spares the nasolabial folds. Perioral DLE lesions can occur and often resolve with a striking acneiform pattern of pitted scarring (Fig. 29.23). DLE often involves the external ear including the outer portion of the external auditory canal. The earliest lesions in this area present as dilated, hyperpigmented follicles (Fig. 29.24).

Scalp involvement occurs in 60% of DLE patients, and is the only area involved in approximately 10% (134) (Fig. 29.20). Irreversible scarring alopecia from permanent follicular destruction occurred in 34% of patients in one recent series (135). The *irreversible, scarring* alopecia that occurs as the result of persistent DLE activity in a localized area differs from the more widespread, *reversible, nonscarring* alopecia that SLE patients often develop during periods of disease activity.

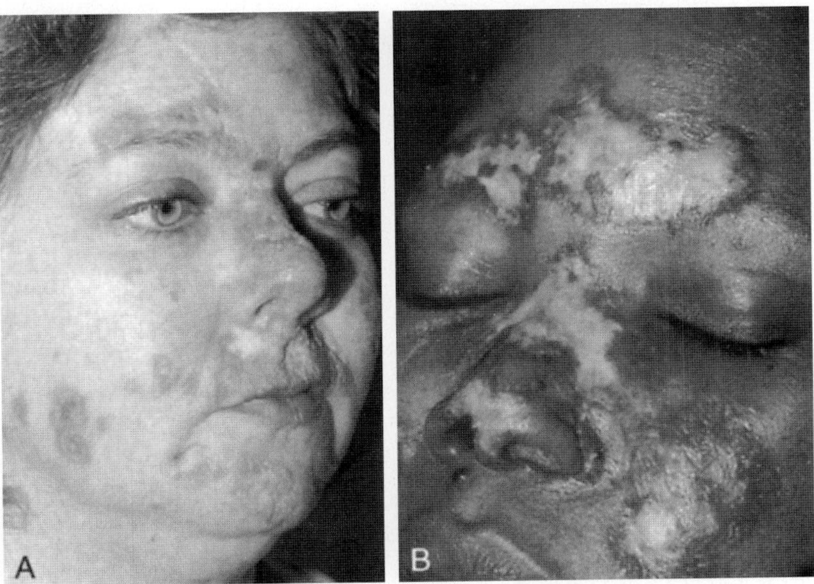

FIGURE 29.19. More extensive examples of therapeutically refractory facial discoid lupus erythematosus lesions that produce large areas of disfigurement on confluence. The characteristic pattern of hyperpigmentation at the active border and hypopigmentation at the inactive center is especially evident in African American patients **(B)**. Facial involvement of this sort can produce extreme psychosocial disability. The proper application of corrective camouflage cosmetics can be of great psychologic benefit to such patients.

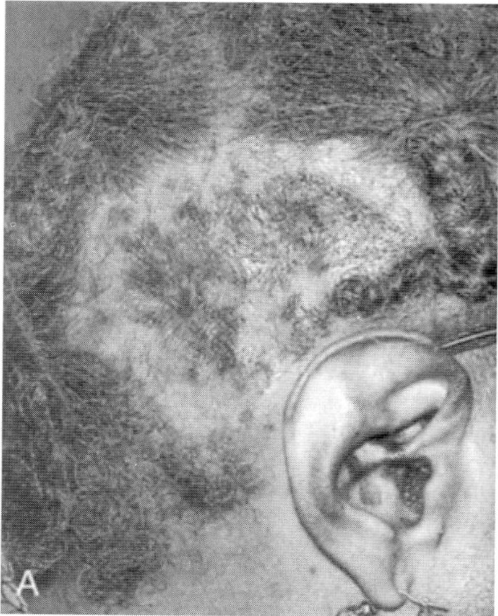

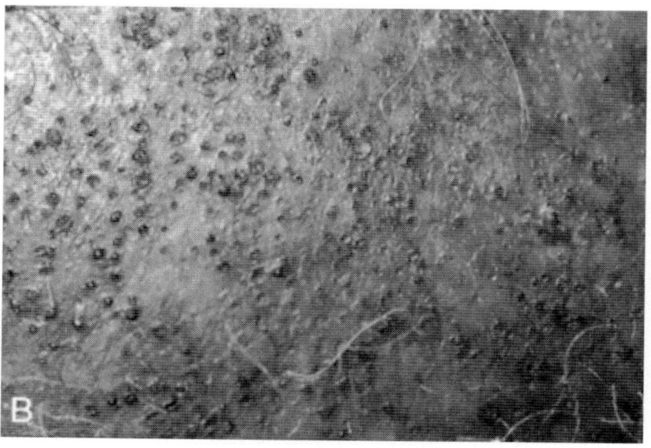

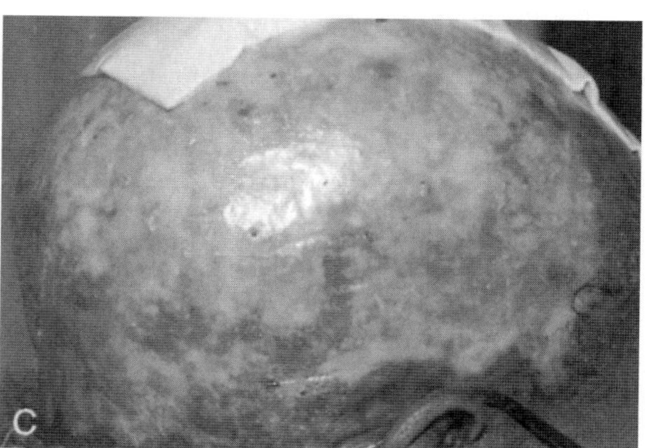

FIGURE 29.20. Discoid lupus erythematosus (DLE) of the scalp. **A,** A relatively early lesion. At this stage, the alopecia might be reversible to some degree with effective treatment. **B,** Close-up of the pattern of keratin-plugged follicles that can be observed in such lesions. **C,** A patient in whom the DLE disease process has progressed to the point of total, irreversible scarring alopecia. The areas of crusting represent a superimposed secondary bacterial infection.

DLE lesions that occur only on the head or neck are referred to as "localized DLE." DLE lesions occurring both above and below the neck are referred to as "generalized DLE." The presence of DLE lesions below the neck only is extremely uncommon. When DLE lesions occurring below the neck are most commonly found on the extensor aspects of the arms, forearms, and hands (Fig. 29.25), although DLE lesions can occur at virtually any site on the body, including completely sun-protected sites such as the perineal area (Fig. 29.26. Unusual locations can reflect the fact that DLE, as well as other forms of LE skin disease activity, can follow in the wake of any form of trauma to the skin (i.e., the Köebner or isomorphic response) (Fig. 29.27).

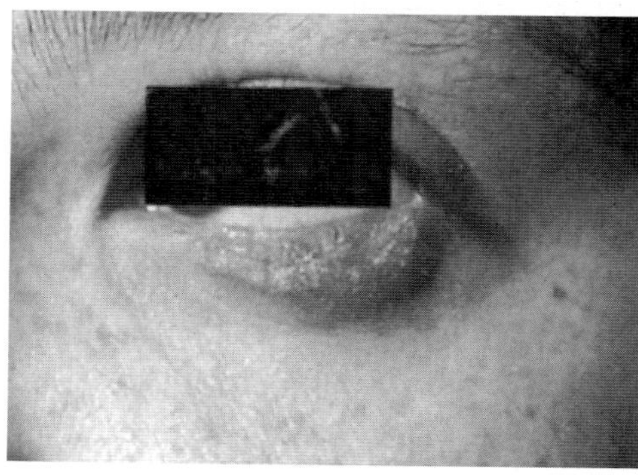

FIGURE 29.21. Discoid lupus erythematosus of the lower eyelid resulting in loss of the eyelashes.

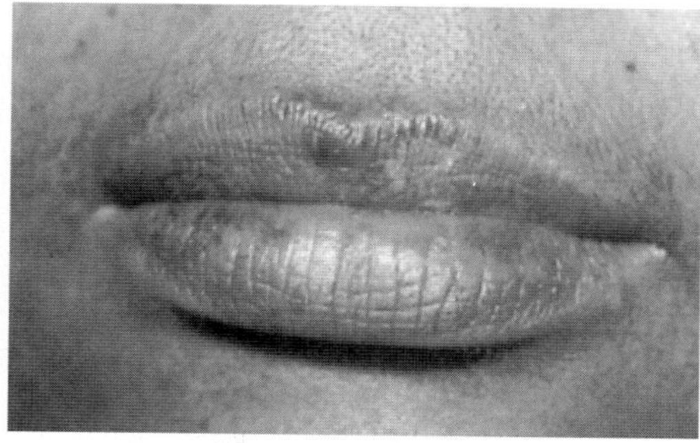

FIGURE 29.22. Discoid lupus erythematosus of the vermillion border of the upper lip. Although the lower lip is more exposed to sunlight, the upper lip for some reason more often is affected with lupus erythematosus-specific skin disease.

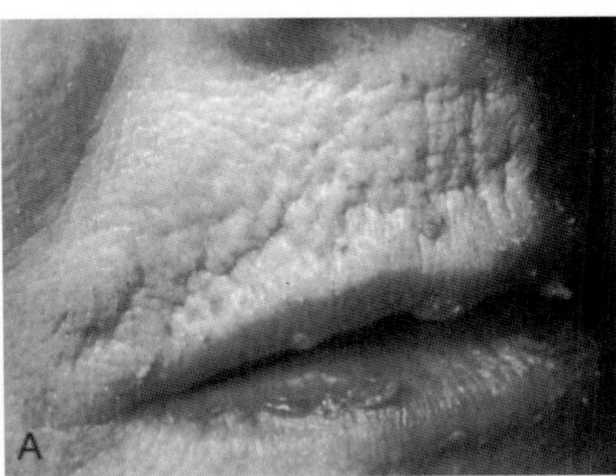

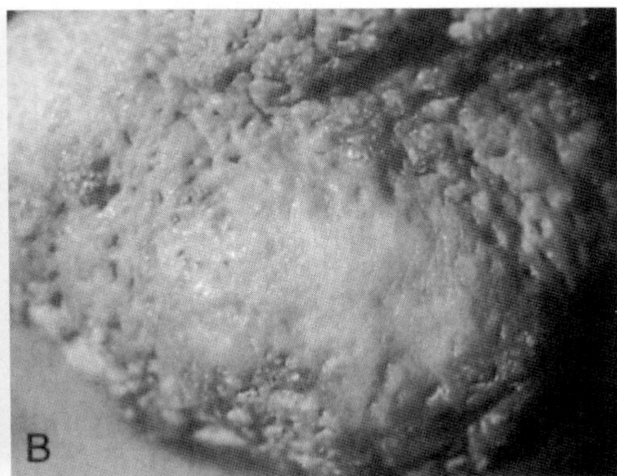

FIGURE 29.23. (See color plate.) **A,** Perioral pitted scarring resulting from prior discoid lupus erythematosus involvement. **B,** This pattern of scarring over the chin of a different patient was improved by dermabrasion. Note that smoother surface and appearance of the central part of the photograph that was treated as a test area. This patient was on antimalarial treatment at the time of the dermabrasion to minimize the chance for kebnerization.

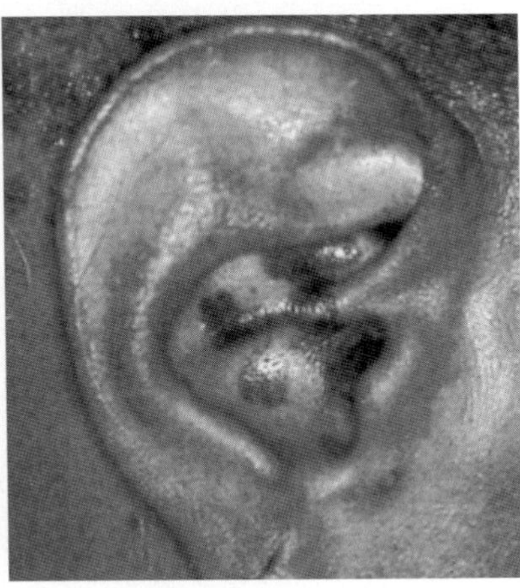

FIGURE 29.24. Discoid lupus erythematosus (DLE) involvement of the ear. Note the patulous, keratin-plugged follicles within areas of hyperpigmentation in the conchae. This pattern of clinical involvement is highly specific for DLE.

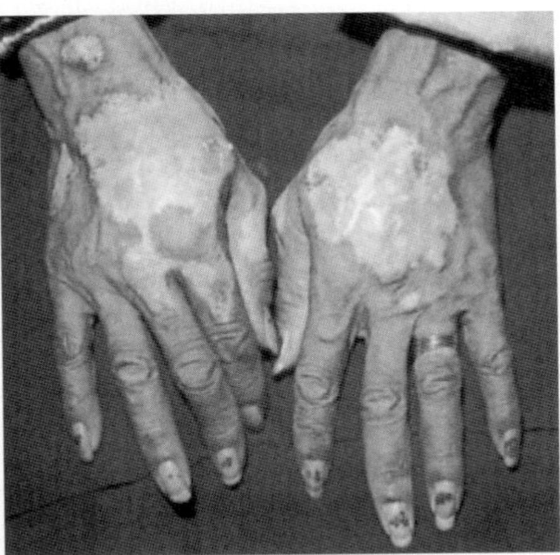

FIGURE 29.25. Discoid lupus erythematosus (DLE) lesions of the dorsal hands indicating generalized DLE. There is a somewhat higher risk of developing systemic lupus erythematosus in patients with generalized DLE compared to those patients with localized DLE (i.e., head and neck involvement only).

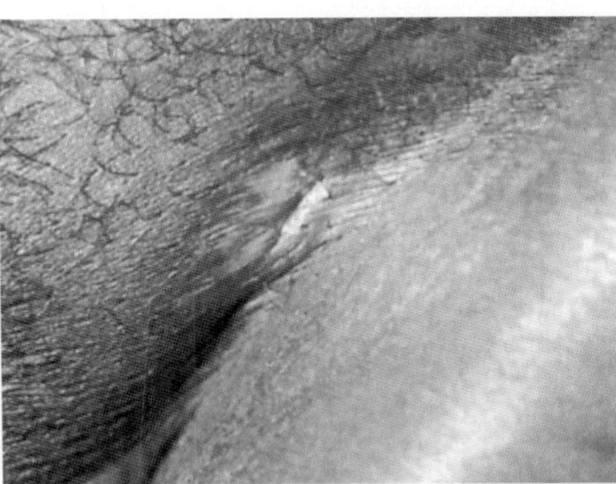

FIGURE 29.26. Biopsy-confirmed discoid lupus erythematosus lesion of the inguinal fold.

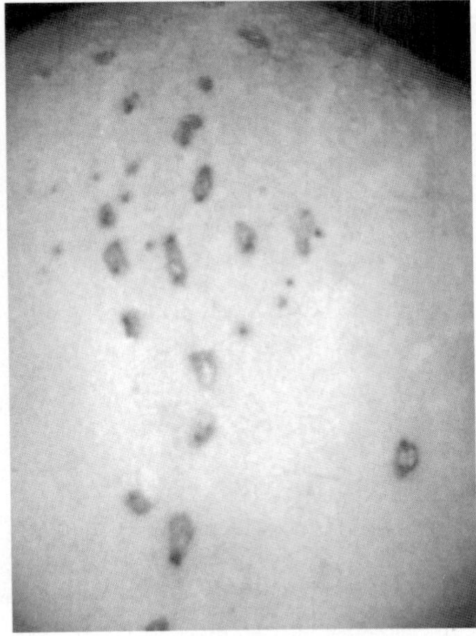

FIGURE 29.27. Köebnerized discoid lupus erythematosus (DLE). DLE lesions occurring in areas of neurotic excoriation. Note the linear shape of some of these lesions.

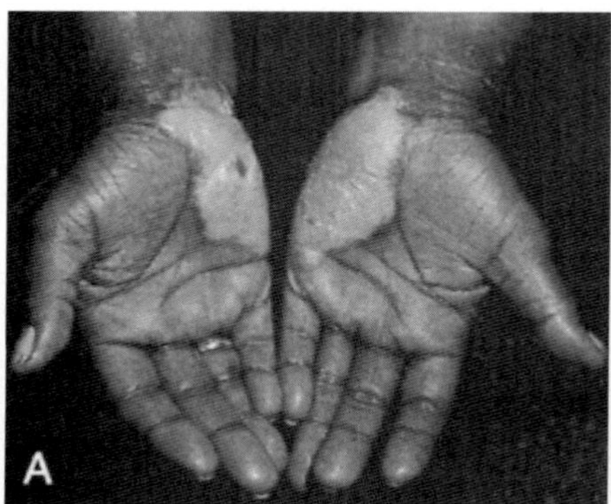

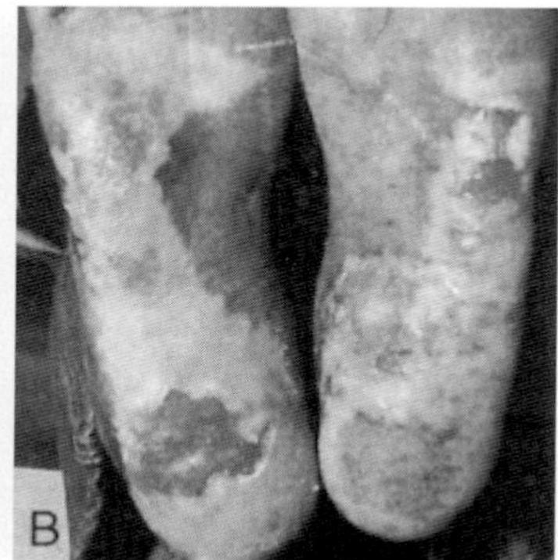

FIGURE 29.28. (See color plate.) Palmar-plantar discoid lupus erythematosus (DLE). DLE involvement of the palms of the hands **(A)** and soles of the feet **(B)** can present a very difficult management problem. Erosions that can develop in such areas can cause extreme pain and result in occupational disability **(B)**.

Painful, erosive palmar-plantar DLE involvement can predominate in some cases producing significant disability and presenting an especially difficult management problem (136) (Fig. 29.28). On occasion, DLE lesions can remain as small, discrete, follicule-based papules having a diameter of less than one centimeter or less. Such "follicular DLE" lesions often are seen around the elbow (Fig. 29.29), but can occur elsewhere as well.

Linear DLE lesions rarely have been reported and may be more common in children (137, 138), usually following Blaschko's lines (139).

DLE lesions can be potentiated by sunlight exposure however, this occurs less frequently than with ACLE and SCLE. Patients often are unaware that UV irradiation exacerbates or precipitates their skin disease, perhaps from the fact that there may be a 1- to 2-week lag time from the time of light exposure until the skin lesions develop (38). It is predominately UV-B that aggravates DLE lesions, although increasing evidence suggests that the longer UV-A wavelengths also can be deleterious in some LE patients (140). However, in as many as 50% of patients, sun exposure does not appear to be related to the cause of their DLE lesions. DLE lesions in the hair-bearing scalp, external auditory canal, or perineal areas are examples where this form of cutaneous LE is not related to light exposure.

DLE also can localize to the nail unit (141). Focal lesions of DLE occurring over the nail fold can produce nail-plate dystrophy (Fig. 29.30). The nail unit can be impacted by other forms of cutaneous LE as well as SLE-producing nailfold erythema and telangiectasia, red lunulae, clubbing, paronychia, pitting, leukonychia striata, and onycholysis [primary data reviewed in (3)].

Hypertrophic Discoid Lupus Erythematosus

Hypertrophic DLE (i.e., hyperkeratotic DLE, verrucous DLE) is a rare variant of chronic cutaneous LE in which the hyperkeratosis that normally is present in classical DLE lesions is greatly exaggerated (Fig. 29.31). These lesions can

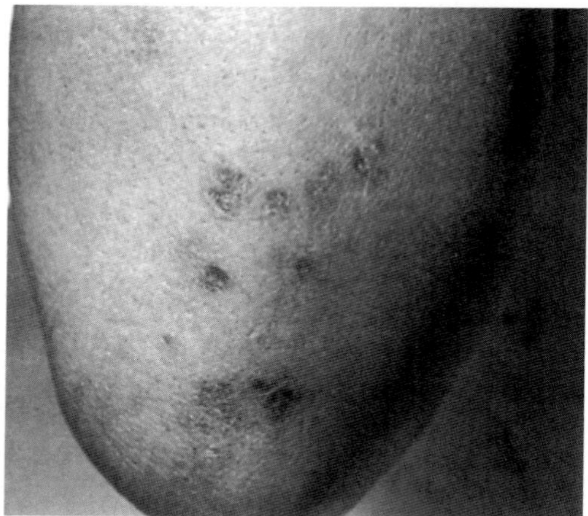

FIGURE 29.29. Discoid lupus erythematosus presenting as discrete follicular lesions around the elbow, the most common site for this pattern of involvement.

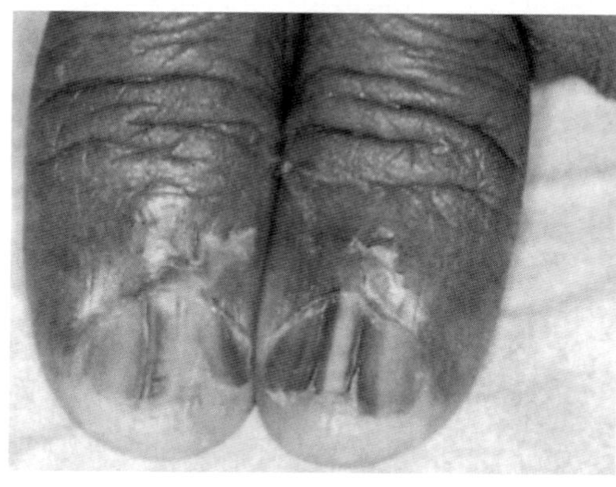

FIGURE 29.30. Symmetric discoid lupus erythematosus lesions of the nail fold producing medial nailplate dystrophy. None of the other fingernails were affected.

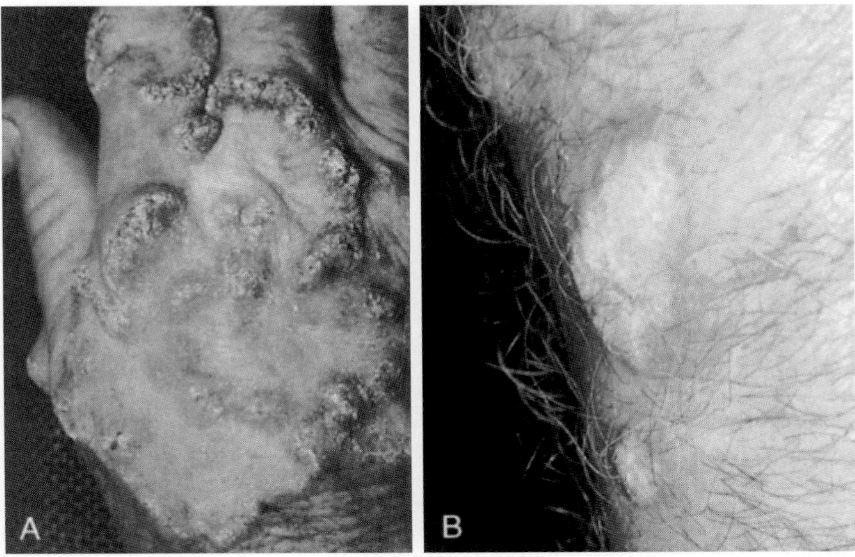

FIGURE 29.31. Two clinical patterns of hypertrophic (verrucous) discoid lupus erythematosus (DLE). **A,** A pattern where warty hyperkeratosis occurs at the active edge of an active DLE lesion. **B,** A DLE lesion that is entirely covered by a thickened shield of hyperkeratosis, presenting a clinical appearance that could be mistaken for other common dermatoses such as keratoacanthoma, squamous-cell carcinoma, or pruigo nodularis.

occur at any site that classical DLE lesions develop, although the extensor aspects of the extremities, the upper back and the face are the areas most frequently affected. The histopathology sometimes reveals features of squamous-cell carcinoma or keratoacanthoma, which can lead clinicians to make the wrong diagnosis (142, 143). However, it is important to realize that squamous-cell carcinoma sometimes can develop in DLE lesions and can metastasize (144, 145). When multiple widespread lesions with histopathologic features of squamous-cell carcinoma or keratoacanthoma are present, one should consider a diagnosis of hypertrophic LE. Overlapping features of hypertrophic LE and lichen planus also have been described (146). Fortunately, patients with hypertrophic DLE lesions often have classical DLE lesions elsewhere on their body that helps clinicians make the correct diagnosis.

The entity "LE hypertrophicus *et profundus*," that was described originally by Bechet in 1942 (147) appears to represent a very rare form of hypertrophic DLE affecting the face associated with the additional features of violaceous (or dull red), indurated, rolled borders, and striking central, crateriform atrophy. The name of this entity is somewhat ambiguous because its pathology does not include a significant degree of LE panniculitis.

LE Profundus/LE Panniculitis

Historically referred to as Kaposi-Irgang disease (148), this rare form of chronic cutaneous LE is characterized by inflammatory lesions in the lower dermis and subcutaneous tissue. Approximately 70% of the patients with this type of chronic cutaneous LE also have typical DLE lesions often overlying the panniculitis lesions (149). The term "LE profundus" has been used by some [including one of the authors (RDS)] to arbitrarily designate those patients who have both LE panniculitis and DLE lesions. However, traditionalists might considered this to be an artificial distinction.

The lesions present as deep, firm, 1- to 3-cm diameter nodules often with normal-appearing overlying skin (150). The skin ultimately becomes attached to the firm, subcutaneous nodular lesions and is drawn inward to produce deep, saucerized depressions as the lesions mature (Fig. 29.32). The head, proximal upper arms, chest, buttocks, and thighs are the sites of predominant involvement. Confluent involvement of the face can simulate the appearance of lipoatrophy (Fig. 29.33). LE profundus also can present as periorbital edema (151, 152).

Linear involvement of the extremities also has been observed (153). Dystrophic calcification within older lesions of LE profundus is common and at times can be a prominent clinical feature of the disease requiring surgical excision. In addition, LE panniculitis may produce breast nodules that can mimic carcinoma clinically and radiologically (154).

Mucosal DLE

It long has been recognized that mucosal-membrane involvement can occur in chronic cutaneous LE patients (155). Recent studies by Burge and coworkers have confirmed that the prevalence of mucous-membrane involve-

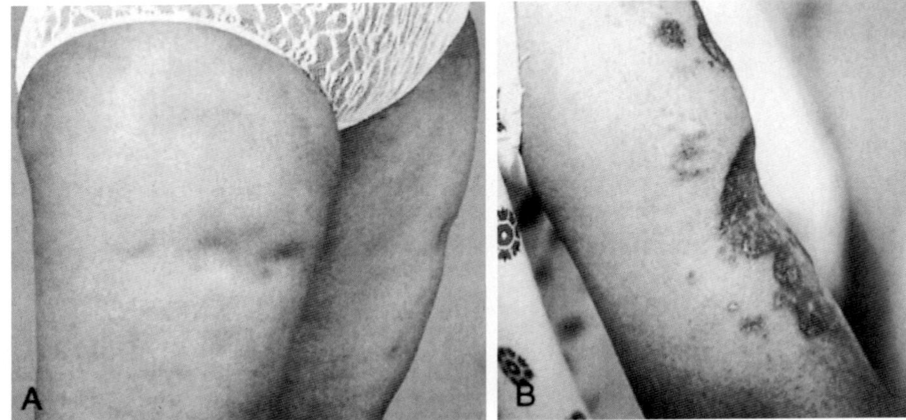

FIGURE 29.32. Lupus erythematosus (LE) panniculitis/profundus. **A,** An example of LE panniculitis without overlying discoid lupus erythematosus (DLE). The primary lesion is a firm subcutaneous nodule that is associated with saucerized areas of atrophy at the surface of the skin. **B,** The combination of LE panniculitis with overlying DLE involvement, referred to as LE profundus.

ment in chronic, cutaneous LE is about 25% (156). While the oral mucosa is most frequently involved, nasal, conjunctival, and genital mucosal surfaces also can be affected.

Within the mouth, the buccal mucosal surfaces are most commonly involved, with the palate, alveolar processes, and tongue being sites of less-frequent involvement. Individual lesions begin as painless, erythematous patches later maturing to a chronic plaque that can present an appearance quite similar to that of lichen planus (Fig. 29.34). The chronic buccal-mucosal plaques have a sharply marginated, irregularly scalloped white border with radiating white striae and telangiectasia (156). The surface of these plaques overlying the palatal mucosa often has a well-defined meshwork of raised hyperkeratotic white strands that encircle zones of punctate erythema, which gives a "honeycomb" appearance (156). The center of older lesions can become depressed and occasionally undergoes painful ulceration. Well-defined chronic DLE plaques also can appear on the vermillion border of the lips (Fig. 29.22). At times, DLE involvement of the lips can present as a diffuse cheilitis, especially on the more sun-exposed lower lip. Although lesions can appear on the tongue, this location is quite rare (156).

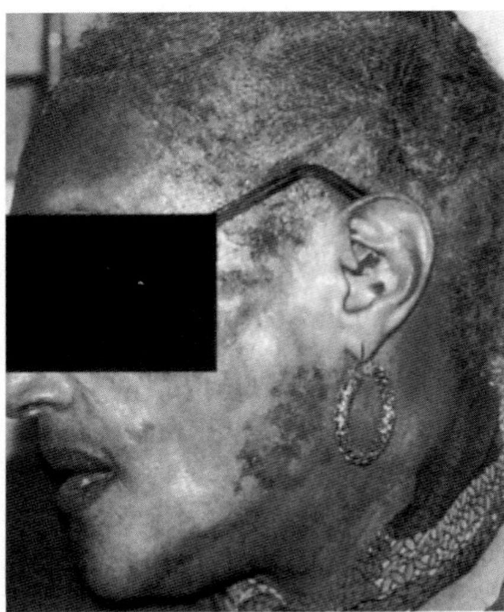

FIGURE 29.33. Lipoatrophy of the face resulting from lupus erythematosus profundus.

Chronic oral-mucosal DLE lesions occasionally can degenerate into squamous-cell carcinoma (157), similar to cutaneous DLE lesions. Any area of asymmetrical nodular induration within a mucosal DLE lesion should be carefully evaluated for the possibility of malignant degeneration.

Discrete DLE plaques also can develop on the nasal, conjunctival, and genital mucosa (156). Nasal septum perforation is relatively rare and is more often associated with SLE than DLE (158). However, nasal-mucosal involvement recently has been suggested to be relatively common in LE patients (159). Conjunctival DLE lesions begin as small areas of nondescript inflammation most commonly affecting the palpebral conjunctivae or the margin of the eyelid. The lower lid is affected more often than the upper lid. As the early lesions progress, scarring becomes more evident and can produce permanent loss of eyelashes and ectropion (Fig. 29.21). DLE involvement of the eyelid can produce considerable disability (160). It recently has been suggested that corneal, stromal keratitis also can occur as a result of DLE ocular involvement (161). Although quite rare, anogenital mucosal DLE lesions also have been observed (156).

Chilblains Lupus/Lupus Pernio

Some LE patients develop red-purple patches and plaques on their toes, fingers, and face that are precipitated by cold, damp climates. Such lesions are highly reminiscent of sim-

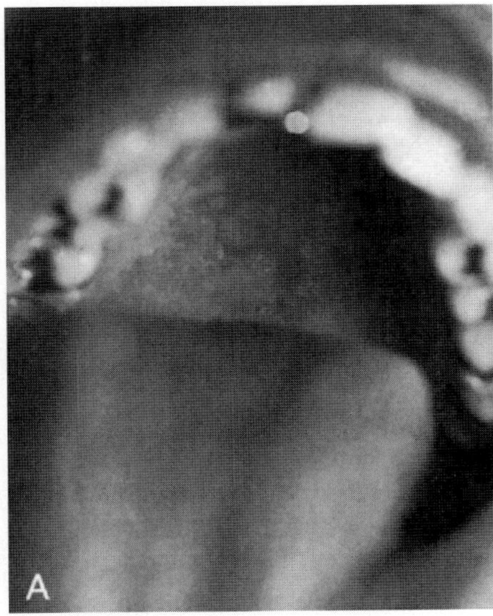

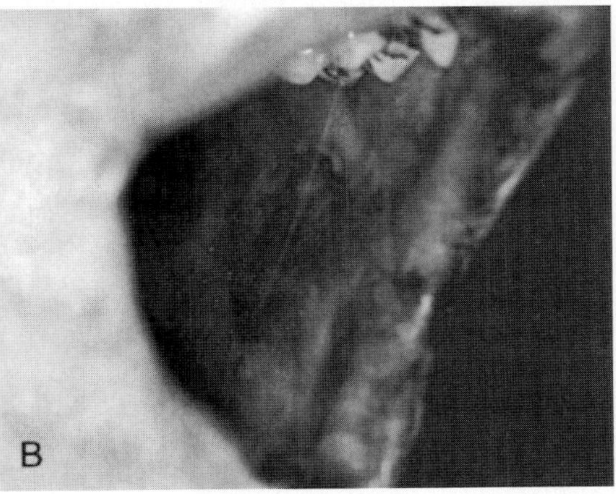

FIGURE 29.34. (See color plate.) Discoid lupus erythematosus (DLE) of the oral mucosa. **A,** Typical appearance of a lesion on the hard palate. Note the honeycomb appearance. These lesions show a typical lupus erythematosus-specific histopathology and usually are painless. **B,** Margins of a DLE lesion on the buccal mucosa of another patient are demarcated by staining with a toluidine blue mouthwash. This patient ultimately developed a squamous-cell carcinoma within a different area of chronic DLE involvement on his buccosal mucosa.

ple chilblains or pernio lesions (162). As these lesions evolve, however, they take on the typical appearance of DLE lesions clinically and histopathologically. The terms "chilblains lupus" and "perniotic LE" have been used to describe such lesions (Fig. 29.35). Unfortunately, the term "lupus pernio" also has been used for such lesions, however, this term is more properly used to designate a form of cutaneous sarcoidosis (163). Chilblains lupus patients often have typical DLE lesions on the face and head (162).

A recent study found Ro/SS-A antibodies in the sera of eight out of nine chilblain lupus patients, suggesting that these antibodies might be a useful clinical marker of this disorder (164). The majority of these patients also complained of photosensitivity and Raynaud's phenomenon.

Lupus Erythematosus Tumidus

The accumulation of excessive dermal mucin early in the course of a cutaneous LE lesion can result in the succulent, edematous, urticaria-appearing plaques of LE tumidus (Fig. 29.36). The characteristic epidermal histological changes of DLE often are not as prominent in lupus tumidus lesions. When this occurs, confusion often arises concerning the diagnosis. There has been one case report of possible hydrochlorothiazide-induced tumid LE (165).

Kuhn et al. recently have reported a series of 40 LE tumidus patients and have traced the line of thought relating to this clinical entity from its apparent original description by Gougerot and Bournier in France in 1930 (46) (166). Two other smaller patient cohorts of LE tumidus also have appeared recently (166, 167). It now is clear that terms

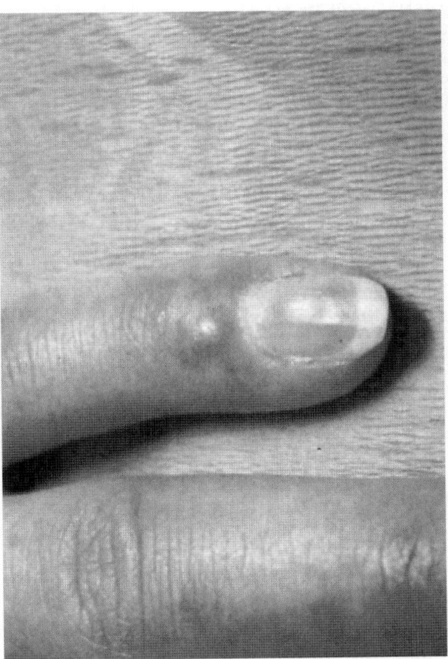

FIGURE 29.35. Chilblains lupus erythematosus (LE) (perniotic LE). Note the rather nondescript appearance of this early lesion. At this stage, the pathology might be nonspecific; however, with time, such lesions can present a typical discoid lupus erythematosus histopathology.

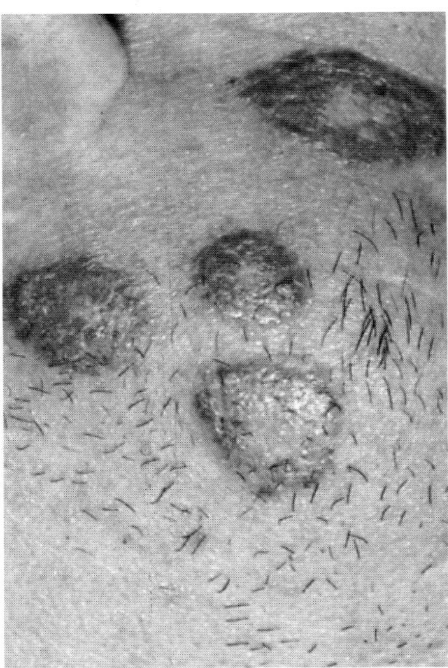

FIGURE 29.36. Lupus tumidus. This form of chronic cutaneous lupus erythematosus (CCLE), which is very rare in the authors' experience, presents succulent, elevated plaques occurring in a sun-exposed distribution. In this case, which is not typical of all cases of lupus tumidus, there was a pattern of surface-color change reminiscent of Wickham's striae. However, the biopsy specimen did not show changes of lichen planus, nor were LE-specific skin disease changes clearly present at the dermalepidermal junction. The predominant pathologic change was mononuclear cell infiltration around the superficial and deep dermal blood vessels. It is quite likely that lupus tumidus lesions and lesions described by other investigators under different designations such as urticarial plaque lupus erythematosus represent the same disease process (personal communication, Irwin M. Braverman, MD).

such as the "urticarial plaque" form of LE (168), "lupus tumidus" (167, 169), and "tumid LE" (166) in the modern English literature have been functionally equivalent to the classical term "LE tumidus" described by Gougerot and Bournier in 1930 and others since.

LE tumidus patients accounted for 16% of their total population of cutaneous LE patients examined by Kuhn et al. LE tumidus has accounted for a much lower percentage of the total number of cutaneous LE lesions seen by the workers outside Germany including the United States (150, 167, 170, 171). In addition, in epidemiologic studies of large series of SLE patients in which cutaneous lesions have been recorded, lesions consistent with LE tumidus are mentioned rarely (24, 44, 54, 172). This plus the dearth of specific published experience on LE tumidus from the United States suggests the possibility that the epidemiology of LE tumidus might differ somewhat between Western Europe and the United States. Alternatively, some of these latter workers might not have recognized LE tumidus as a distinct form of cutaneous LE or have included patients with LE tumidus under other designations such as "urticaria" in the context of SLE.

Other intriguing aspects of the large LE tumidus case series presented by Kuhn et al. include male predominance, negative lesional direct immunofluorescence, and virtual absence of associated SLE disease activity. However, the other two recently published cases series of LE tumidus, although much smaller in patient number, did not find a male predominance and some of their patients had LE tumidus occurring in the context of discoid LE and systemic LE (173, 173). Further study of the cutaneous LE subset is needed.

The systematic phototesting studies performed by Kuhn et al. revealed a rather strong presence of UVA in the action spectrum of LE tumidus. This is in agreement with earlier such work (174). The extreme photosensitivity noted in their patients occurred in the virtual absence of epidermal changes and Ro/SS-A antibody production. These findings suggest the possibility that there is a fundamentally different mechanism of photosensitivity in LE tumidus compared to SCLE. However, it is interesting to note that when Lehmann et al. (38) challenged the nonlesional skin of SCLE patients with UVA alone, only dermal changes of LE-specific skin disease were noted.

Table 29.4 presents a comparison of the selected clinical and laboratory features of patients presenting with ACLE, SCLE, and classical DLE skin lesions.

Relationship Between Cutaneous And Systemic Disease

Figure 29.37 illustrates the different relationships that exist between the three major forms of LE-specific skin disease and the systemic autoimmune manifestations of LE.

Acute Cutaneous Lupus Erythematosus

Because the "malar rash" or "butterfly rash" is so common in patients with SLE and because such lesions are considered to be a fundamental component of the clinical expression of SLE disease activity, few workers have directly examined the relationship that exists between ACLE and SLE disease activity.

Ropes noted that the "butterfly rash" of SLE often waxed and waned in parallel with underlying SLE disease activity (30). However, Dr. Ropes was unable to demonstrate a positive correlation between skin disease activity and evidence of LE nephritis. Curiously, a significant negative correlation was noted with psychosis and serum protein electrophoresis abnormalities (30). Vlachoyiannopoulos et al. found that flaring of the "rash" of SLE frequently accompanies flares of SLE activity (58). Wysenbeek et al. also have recently demonstrated that the generalized "nonspecific rash" of SLE (presumably generalized ACLE) correlated positively with lymphadenopathy, antinative DNA antibody, low-comple-

TABLE 29.4. COMPARISON OF FORMS OF LE-SPECIFIC SKIN DISEASE

Disease Features	ACLE	SCLE	Classical DLE
Clinical features of skin lesions:			
Induration	0	0	+++
Scarring	0	0	+++
Pigment changes	+	++	+++
Follicular plugging	0	0	+++
Hyperkeratosis	+	++	+++
Histopathology:			
Thickened basement	0	+	+++
Membrane:			
Lichenoid infiltrate	+	++	+++
Periappendaggeal inflammation	0	+	+++
Lupus band:			
Lesional	++	++	+++
Nonlesional	++	+	0
Antinuclear antibodies	+++	++	+
Ro/SS-A antibodies:			
By immunodiffusion	+	+++	0
By ELISA	++	+++	+
Antinative DNA antibodies	+++	+	0
Hypocomplementemia	+++	+	+
Risk for developing SLE	+++	++	+

+++ Strongly associated.
++ Moderately associated.
+ Weakly associated.
0 Negative, no association; ACLE, acute cutaneous lupus erythematosus; DLE, discoid lupus erythematosus; ELISA, enzyme-linked immunosorbent assay; SCLE, subacute cutaneous lupus erythematosus; SLE, systemic lupus erythematosus.

ment levels, and higher prednisone doses (62). However, these workers found no such correlation with renal disease, central nervous system disease, or SLE disease activity index.

It has always been our impression that either localized or generalized ACLE is associated with a high risk for aggressive SLE activity, including the risk of LE nephritis.

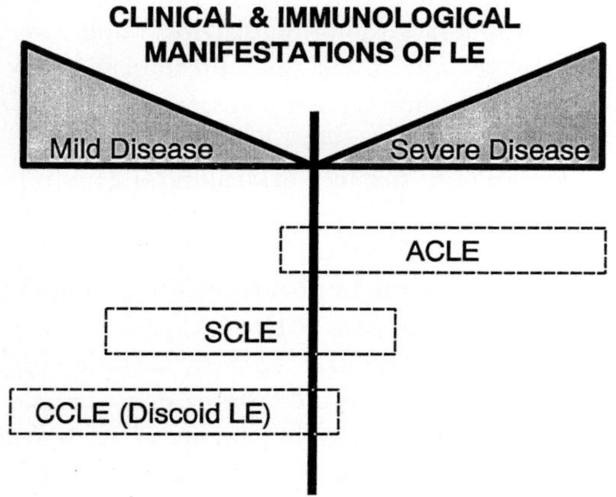

FIGURE 29.37. Relative risks for systemic lupus erythematosus disease activity that are associated with the three major forms of lupus erythematosus-specific skin disease.

Subacute Cutaneous Lupus Erythematosus

Approximately one half of SCLE patients meet the American College of Rheumatology's revised criteria for the classification of SLE (50) [data reviewed in (80)]. However, it has been the experience of most observers that severe SLE (i.e., LE nephritis, central nervous system disease) develops in only 10% of SCLE patients (data reviewed in (80). While most SCLE patients who develop four or more SLE classification criteria tend to have a relatively mild disease course overall, there are reports of such patients who have had severe and sometimes fatal outcomes, usually from renal and central nervous system involvement (175). There is some indication that patients with the papulosquamous variety of SCLE might be at more risk of developing renal involvement (68).

Sontheimer and coworkers identified five patients in a cohort of 47 individuals with SCLE that had evidence of lupus nephritis (176). All five of these patients had the papulosquamous type of SCLE, leukopenia, high-titer antinuclear antibody (ANA) (>1:640) and anti-double-stranded (ds) DNA antibodies. All five also developed ACLE lesions at some point during their disease course and all had been refractory to antimalarial treatment. Another report noted that SCLE patients with renal disease were more likely to have the papulosquamous type of lesions (177). Men with papulosquamous SCLE may have higher risk of severe SLE (68). SCLE can overlap with other autoimmune disorders. Some patients with SCLE will later manifest clear evidence of Sjögren's syndrome while some patients whose illness begins as Sjögren's syndrome who later develop SCLE lesions. Three to 12% of patients who present with SCLE skin lesions will later developed Sjögren's syndrome (34). It is interesting to note in this regard that both SCLE and Sjögren's syndrome have been associated with the same immunogenetic background-circulating Ro/SS-A and La/SS-B autoantibodies and the presence of the HLA-B8, DR3, DRW6, DQ2, and DRW52 extended haplotype.

A number of Japanese patients having Sjögren's syndrome and Ro/SS-A and La/SS-B autoantibodies have been reported to have an annular erythema reaction that appears somewhat similar clinically to annular SCLE although biopsies of the lesions have revealed histopathologic findings somewhat distinct from SCLE (178). While some consider this to be a distinct entity (i.e., annular erythema of Sjögren's syndrome), it is possible that genetic differences between Occidentals and Whites could account for this difference in disease expression. For example, the HLA-DR3 allele is distinctly unusual in the citizens of Japan.

Roughly one third of SCLE patients produce rheumatoid factor (80). It is therefore not surprising that SCLE patients have been noted to subsequently develop rheumatoid arthritis (RA) on occasion (179). In addition, patients presenting with RA can subsequently developed SCLE lesions. One group reported that of 12 RA patients who produced Ro/SS-A autoantibodies, two had SCLE skin lesions (180). An association between SCLE and antithyroid autoantibodies and Hashimoto's thyroiditis also has been reported (181).

More recent reports concerning the epidemiology of SCLE for the most part have confirmed the earlier work in this area.

There have been case reports suggesting an occasional association between SCLE and malignancy (breast, lung, gastric, uterus, and lymphoma) (182–184). In some of these reports, the SCLE lesions have been suggested to represent a paraneoplastic manifestation of the underlying malignancy. Other disorders that have been anecdotally related to SCLE have been Sweet's syndrome (185), porphyria cutanea tarda (186), gluten-sensitive enteropathy (187), and Crohn's disease (188). The infrequency of these associated conditions mitigates against anything more than a casual association. However, it should be kept in mind that the usual dose of aminoquinoline antimalarial agents used in the management of SCLE (or DLE) can cause significant hepatotoxicity in patients who might have underlying subclinical porphyria cutanea tarda.

Chronic Cutaneous Lupus Erythematosus

The relationship that exists between classical DLE and SLE has been the subject of debate throughout the 20th century. Daniel Wallace recently has presented a comprehensive overview of this subject, which systematically and thoughtfully addresses the following issues (102).

What Is The Risk For Patients Presenting With Classical DLE Subsequently Developing SLE?

Five percent to 10% of patients presenting with classical DLE lesions subsequently will develop unequivocal evidence of SLE (102). Considerable effort has been made to identify clinical or laboratory features that might correlate with such a pattern of disease progression. One clinical feature that can be useful in this regard is the extent and distribution of the DLE lesions. Generalized DLE patients (i.e., lesions both above and below the neck) have a higher rate of immunological abnormalities and risk for progressing to SLE compared to localized DLE patients (171). In addition, generalized DLE patients are at higher risk for developing the more severe manifestations of SLE (171). In some instances, SLE patients may develop DLE skin lesions late in the course of their disease when their SLE disease activity has fully remitted (189).

Other physical findings that should alert one to the possibility of underlying systemic disease are diffuse, nonscarring alopecia, generalized lymphadenopathy, periungual nailfold telangiectasia, Raynaud's phenomenon, SCLE, and LE-nonspecific skin lesions such as vasculitis (134).

The following laboratory findings have been reported to be risk factors for the development of SLE in DLE patients: unexplained anemia, marked leukopenia, false-positive tests for syphilis, persistently positive high-titer antinuclear antibody assay, anti-single-stranded DNA antibody, hypergammaglobulinemia, an elevated erythrocyte sedimentation rate (especially of greater than 50 mm/hour), and immune deposits at the dermal-epidermal junction of nonlesional skin (i.e., a positive lupus band test) (171).

A recent multivariate study of 51 SLE patients and 245 patients with SCLE and/or DLE revealed that those patients with evidence of nephropathy (e.g. proteinuria, hematuria), arthralgias, or an ANA titer 1:320 were at significantly greater risk of having systemic disease (190). This analysis found that the erythrocyte sedimentation rate, anti-dsDNA antibodies, photosensitivity, and recurrent headaches were not useful in distinguishing between patients with or without systemic disease. Recent work also has suggested that elevated soluble interleukin 2 (IL-2) receptor levels might also be a risk factor for SLE in patients with DLE (191).

What Are The Clinical Implications Of Classical DLE Lesions Occurring In SLE Patients?

Roughly one fourth of SLE patients will develop DLE lesions at some point in the course of their disease. Some work has suggested that such patients tend to have less severe forms of SLE with life-threatening complications such as diffuse proliferative glomerulonephritis are being uncommon in these patients and survival is increased when compared to SLE patients without DLE lesions (192).

What Are The Risks For Developing Systemic Disease Associated With Other Forms Of Chronic Cutaneous LE?

Hypertrophic DLE patients do not appear to have a greater risk for developing SLE than do patients with classical DLE lesions (193). Several reports have indicated that approximately 50% of the patients with LE profundus/panniculitis have a relatively mild form of SLE (147). In a recent retrospective review of 40 LE panniculitis patients, only 10% met the ACR criteria for SLE (194). In an earlier study only 25% of 16 LE panniculitis patients that were followed over a decade on average ever developed SLE (195). The systemic features of patients with LE panniculitis/profundus tend to be less severe, similar to those in SLE patients who have DLE skin lesions (147). Severe nephritis is an uncommon complication in SLE patients with LE panniculitis. In one study, 3 of 15 (20%) patients presenting with chilblain LE later developed SLE (162).

The risk for systemic disease activity in LE patients having mucosal involvement is a function of the type of mucosal lesion that is present. Superficial, transient oral or nasal mucosal ulcerations having a relatively nonspecific histopathology are commonly seen in patients with active SLE (Fig. 29.38) (such mucosal lesions represent one of the 11 American College of Rheumatology's revised classification criteria for SLE). Chronic mucosal LE plaques, however, are seen most commonly in LE patients who do not have life-threatening SLE. The more severe manifestations of SLE such as renal disease appear to be quite uncommon in SLE patients who develop chronic mucosal plaques (156).

Fig. 29.39 illustrates the relative risks for systemic disease activity that are associated with the various clinical varieties of chronic cutaneous LE.

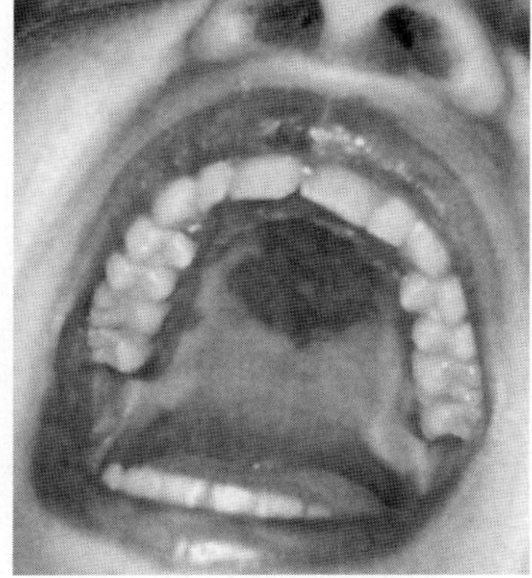

FIGURE 29.38. Oral mucosal ulceration in systemic lupus erythematosus (SLE). As seen in this case, superficial ulcers often occur in the junctional area of the hard and soft palates; however, ulceration of the gingival, buccal, and lingual mucosa also occur. In the early stages of such lesions, the histopathology often is nonspecific. While difficult to see in this photograph, this young woman with active SLE, including nephritis, also had ulceration of the nasal mucosa. Oral and nasal mucosal ulceration in this setting can be associated with severe pain, or it can be painless.

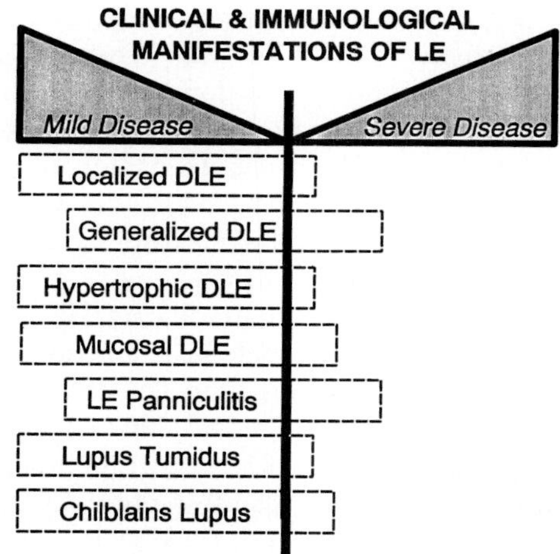

FIGURE 29.39. Relative risks for systemic lupus erythematosus disease activity that are associated with the various clinical varieties of chronic cutaneous lupus erythematosus (CCLE).

The Lupus Band Test

No discussion of the relationship between the cutaneous and systemic manifestations of LE would be complete without addressing the lupus band test.

Burnham and coworkers using direct immunofluorescence microscopy first identified by the presence of immunoglobulins and complement components in a continuous bandlike array at the dermal-epidermal junction of lesional skin biopsies from LE patients (23). This phenomenon, subsequently referred to as the "lupus band" (196), initially was felt to be quite specific for LE; however, subsequent work has documented that the lupus band can be found in a number of skin disorders other than those caused by LE (197).

Cormane (198) later described similar findings in biopsies from clinically normal skin of SLE patients in the complete absence of any signs of cutaneous inflammation. Because DLE patients lacked this finding in their nonlesional skin, it was suggested that such results might have diagnostic specificity for SLE. The search for immunoreactant deposition in nonlesional skin of LE patients subsequently has been referred to by many as the "lupus band test" (LBT).

Controversies concerning terminology have clouded this field from the beginning. While some workers use the term "LBT" to refer to LE lesional as well as nonlesional immunopathological findings (199), others reserve this designation for reference to the results of immunopathological examination of nonlesional skin (200). Less confusion might exist in this area if the terms "lesional LBT" and "nonlesional LBT" were uniformly adopted by those working in this area.

The immunopathological findings in nonlesional skin of LE patients must be distinguished from those present in LE lesional skin biopsies. Issues related to immunopathological findings in LE-specific skin lesions (i.e., the lesional LBT) will be discussed later in this chapter in the Pathology/Immunopathology section. The remainder of this discussion will be limited to the presence or absence of immunoreactants at the dermal-epidermal junction of *nonlesional* skin (i.e., the nonlesional LBT).

All three major immunoglobulin classes (IgG, IgM, and IgA) and a variety of complement components including constituents of the membrane attack complex have been identified in these dermal-epidermal junction deposits (197). Recent studies have suggested that the presence of membrane attack complex in lesional skin is relatively sensitive and specific for LE (201). The immunoglobulin-staining pattern of immunoreactants in nonlesional LE skin under low power generally is described as being granular. Upon high-power magnification, the pattern of fluorescence has been variously described as appearing homogeneous, stippled, fibrillar, shaggy, lumpy-bumpy, linear, or thready [details related to the appearance and significance of these various patterns recently have been reviewed (202)]. Ultrastructurally, these immunoreactants are seen to be deposited on and below the *lamina densa* of the dermal-epidermal junction (203). The intensity of the staining and the number of immunoreactants present in these deposits can vary considerably (199). Most authorities require a continuous pattern of immunoreactant deposition along the dermal-epidermal junction for a positive nonlesional LBT. Numerous studies have suggested that a discontinuous or interrupted nonlesional LBT can be seen in a number of other disorders and thus is much less specific for SLE (197). In addition, the presence of IgM alone appears to be very nonspecific (197).

The diagnostic and prognostic significance of the nonlesional LBT has been the subject of much controversy over the past two decades. In-depth analyses of these issues are available elsewhere (199). The following summary points can serve to acquaint the reader with the clinically relevant issues pertaining to the nonlesional LBT:

1. Standardization. It is quite curious that a test such as this that has been used clinically for well over two decades has been so poorly standardized. Only recently have large numbers of clinically normal individuals been studied to determine the incidence of a false-positive nonlesional LBT in both sun-exposed and nonexposed skin regions. Such studies have suggested that as many as 20% of healthy young adults have a positive LBT in sun-exposed nonlesional skin regions such as the lateral aspect of the neck whereas virtually none are positive in sun-protected nonlesional sites such as the buttocks (204). Thus, considerable caution must be taken when interpreting the results of immunopathological findings in both lesional and nonlesional biopsies taken from fully sun-exposed skin sites (e.g., face, neck, extensor aspect of forearm and hand) or partially sun-exposed skin sites (flexor aspect of the forearm, deltoid region) with respect to the diagnosis of cutaneous or systemic LE.

   Autofluorescence of dermal collagen and elastin fibers at low power can give the appearance of a positive nonlesional LBT [i.e., the "fibrillar pseudoband" (196)]. At higher power, the artifactual nature of this false-positive finding becomes apparent. A false-negative, nonlesional LBT can occur when high levels of extravascular dermal IgG is present. This finding, which correlates with hypergammaglobulinemia, can obscure the distinctness of the lupus band at the dermal-epidermal junction (205).

   It also is important to understand that considerable anatomical regional variation exists with respect to the nonlesional LBT. It has been suggested that there is a cephalo-caudal gradient in the frequency of a positive lesional LBT in DLE lesions, with lesions on the head more often being positive than those on the trunk (199). There are indications that a similar phenomenon might exist with the LBT in nonlesional skin of NZB/W mice, a murine model of SLE (33). Firm data addressing this issue in human LE patients have not yet been presented.
2. Diagnostic specificity. Because the strongest clinical association of the nonlesional LBT has been with SLE, it is not surprising that classical DLE patients without clinical or laboratory evidence of extracutaneous disease have been uniformly nonlesional LBT negative (134). Only about 25% of SLE patients who have DLE lesions have a positive, nonlesional LBT (134). Approximately 25% of SCLE patients (an LE subset that frequently has mild symptoms of SLE) are nonlesional LBT positive in relatively sun-protected flexor forearm skin (33). As noted earlier, the diagnostic specificity of the nonlesional LBT for SLE has become a point of controversy. Factoring in the profile of individual immunoreactants present in a positive nonlesional LBT has been suggested to be one approach to enhancing the specificity of this test. Several studies have suggested that when three or more immunoreactants are present in the nonlesional LBT, the diagnostic specificity for SLE is very high (206). These observations taken together with the fact that actinically damaged skin can yield false-positive results (204) would suggest that a positive nonlesional LBT (confirmed under high-power observation to exclude the artifacts such as the fibrillar pseudoband) in fully sun-protected skin from the buttock or inner aspect of the upper arm that consists of three or more immunoglobulin or complement components might have the greatest specificity for SLE. Under these conditions, a positive nonlesional LBT can serve as a very useful piece of additional diagnostic information in those difficult cases of SLE where the clinical and laboratory manifestations of this disorder are being expressed atypically.

3. Prognostic significance. While the nonlesional LBT was initially adopted because of its perceived diagnostic specificity for SLE, subsequent work suggested that it also correlated positively with a more aggressive course of systemic disease including the development of lupus nephritis (207). The presence of IgG in the nonlesional LBT was suggested to be more indicative of severe SLE than the presence of IgM alone (208). The idea that the nonlesional LBT had prognostic value also became a point of contention. However, a prospective follow-up study has confirmed the predictive value of a positive nonlesional LBT (209). Whether the nonlesional LBT provides incremental value over more generally available and less invasive tests such as circulating ds DNA antibody levels in prognosis assessment is not clear; however, there are those who continue to feel that this is the case (206). It is the authors' opinion that a properly interpreted nonlesional LBT has its greatest utility as an additional diagnostic maneuver in patients with atypical clinical and laboratory presentations of SLE.

Pathology And Immunopathology

Acute Cutaneous Lupus Erythematosus

Histopathology

The histologic picture in ACLE is generally less impressive than that seen in SCLE and DLE lesions. The dermal cellular infiltrate is often relatively sparse. The most prominent changes are edema of the upper dermis and focal liquefactive degeneration of the epidermal basal-cell layer. In the most severe forms of ACLE, epidermal necrosis may occur, producing a histopathologic pattern strongly resembling toxic-epidermal necrolysis.

Immunopathology

Curiously, there is very little published data concerning direct immunofluorescence findings in ACLE. In one study, 5 of 5 (100%) skin biopsies from ACLE (i.e., "diffuse erythema") lesions were reported to be lesional lupus band test (LBT) positive (210). More recent work has indicated that the lesional lupus band test is positive in 60% of patient having the "malar rash" of SLE (54).

Subacute Cutaneous Lupus Erythematosus

Histopathology

While the histopathology of SCLE is clearly that of LE-specific skin disease, it may be impossible to clearly differentiate SCLE from ACLE and DLE. Characteristically, ACLE, SCLE, and DLE have variable degrees of hyperkeratosis, basal-cell degeneration, dermal edema, and mononuclear cell infiltration around the dermal-epidermal junction extending into the dermis. In SCLE, there is focal basal-cell injury and disorientation with liquefaction degeneration, sparse upper-dermal mononuclear-cell infiltrate that may partially obscure the dermal-epidermal junction, dermal edema, and rarely epidermal necrosis (118). The mononuclear infiltrate usually is limited to perivascular and adnexal structures in the upper third of the dermis and the epidermis may be mildly atrophic. Vesicular changes can occur in SCLE lesions, particularly at the active border of annular SCLE lesions (211). It has been suggested that such patients are more likely be HLA-DR3 and have Ro/SS-A autoantibodies (211).

SCLE lesions generally have less hyperkeratosis, follicular plugging, mononuclear cell infiltration of adnexal structures, and dermal melanophages compared to DLE lesions. Qualitative differences in the histopathology of SCLE versus DLE have been noted (212); however, not all agree on this point (213). Bangert and coworkers were unable to differentiate papulosquamous from annular SCLE by blinded histopathological examination (118).

Immunopathology

As in other LE-specific lesions, immune deposits can be detected frequently by immunofluorescence staining in SCLE skin lesions. The initial studies indicated that these deposits consist of immunoglobulin (IgM, IgG, and/or IgA) and complement components arranged in a granular bandlike pattern along the dermal-epidermal junction (33). Approximately 60% of SCLE lesions from the original cohort of SCLE patients had such deposits, compared to somewhat higher percentages for ACLE and DLE lesions. Others have found similar results in SCLE skin lesions (211) while some workers have found even higher frequencies (133). Thus, the presence of immune deposits at the dermal-epidermal junction can help confirm a diagnosis of SCLE, but its absence does not necessarily rule it out. These immune deposits are not specific for LE as similar deposits can be found in normal or sun-damaged skin (204) and in other non-LE dermatologic conditions (197).

Nonlesional deltoid and flexor forearm skin biopsies from the original group of SCLE patients contained junctional immune deposits in 46% and 26%, respectively (33). The prognostic significance of such deposits has not yet been determined.

Nieboer et al. have reported finding a "dust-like particle" pattern of IgG deposition deposited in and around the epidermal basal keratinocytes and subepidermal regions in 30% of SCLE lesional skin biopsies (214). This group suggested that this pattern of immunoglobulin deposition is specific for SCLE although its presence did not correlate with the presence of circulating Ro/SS-A autoantibodies. Others have noted this same immunofluorescence pattern in SCLE patients (215). A recent review of 4,374 skin-biopsy specimens submitted for direct immunofluorescence exam revealed 66 samples from 60 patients with "dust-like particles." Fifty-three percent of these patients had SCLE, but only 36% of these 60 patients had Ro/SS-A autoantibodies (216).

It is curious, however, that one of the authors (RDS) as well as a number of other observers (206) have not been impressed by this pattern of immunofluorescence in SCLE lesional biopsies, suggesting that it might be somewhat technique dependent. This dustlike pattern of IgG is similar to that found in human skin explants grafted onto nude mice that resulted from intravenous infusion of human Ro/SS-A autoimmune sera (217). One of the authors (RDS) has noted a similar pattern of IgG and IgM deposition in guinea-pig skin following intradermal injections of human Ro/SS-A autoimmune sera (personal, unpubl. observation).

Chronic Cutaneous Lupus Erythematosus

Classical Discoid Lupus Erythematosus

The epidermal basal cell layer is the principal site of injury in all three forms of LE-specific skin disease (118). In classical DLE, there is also prominent hyperkeratosis and follicular plugging. The nucleated layer of the epidermis generally is not thickened and may be somewhat atrophic. Epidermal basal-layer changes include: loss of the normal organization and orientation of basal cells, edema with vacuole formation between and sometimes within basal cells (i.e., liquefaction or vacuolar degeneration), partial obliteration of the dermal-epidermal junction by a mononuclear-cell infiltrate, thickening of the epidermal-basement membrane, increased melanin-pigment formation, and interruption of pigment transfer between melanocytes and keratinocytes leading to the accumulation of melanin by phagocytosis in dermal macrophages.

The dermal histopathologic changes are less specific. A mononuclear-cell infiltrate composed predominantly of T lymphocytes and macrophages is present most predominately in the periappendageal and perivascular areas. Plasma cells occasionally are seen in the more chronic lesions and dermal mucin deposition can at times be quite prominent. The chronic scarring DLE lesions more often have a denser inflammatory cell infiltrate that extends well into the deeper reticular dermis and/or subcutis. In contrast, ACLE and SCLE lesions contain a less dense inflammatory infiltrate that is confined to the upper dermis but still shows the distinctive pattern of injury along the dermal-epidermal junction (118). The periappendageal inflammation that is characteristic of DLE is less prominent in SCLE and ACLE.

Direct immunofluorescence examination of biopsy specimens taken from DLE lesions often reveals a thick, continuous band of immunoreactants along the dermal-epidermal junction (199). This band also extends along the basement membrane of the hair follicle, a finding that is not often seen in those other disorders that have been reported to have similar dermal-epidermal junction immunoreactants deposited in a bandlike pattern. Multiple immunoglobulin classes (IgG, IgA, IgM) usually are present within this band and various complement components (C3, C4, Clq, properdin, factor B, and the membrane attack complex, $C_{5b\text{-}C9}$) also can present in many of these lesions (201).

Early reports suggested that over 90% of DLE lesions had lesional immunoreactants at the dermal-epidermal junction (210), however, subsequent studies have reported somewhat lower frequencies (199). The frequency with which immunoreactants are found in DLE lesions also appears to vary with the anatomic region from which the biopsy is taken. In one study, lesions on the head, neck, and arms were more often positive (80%) than those on the trunk (20%) (218). The frequency of bandlike immunoreactant deposition at the dermal-epidermal junction appears also to be a function of the age of the lesion being examined with older lesions (i.e., greater than 3 months) being more often positive than younger ones (i.e., less than 1 month) (219). Ultrastructural localization of immunoglobulin at the dermal-epidermal junction has confirmed that these proteins are deposited on the upper dermal collagen fibers and along the *lamina densa* of the epidermal basement membrane zone (203).

Hypertrophic Discoid Lupus Erythematosus

The histopathology and immunopathology is similar to that of classical DLE lesions except for a much greater degree of epidermal acanthosis and hyperkeratosis. The histopathology sometimes reveals features of squamous-cell carcinoma or keratoacanthoma, which can lead clinicians to make the wrong diagnosis (23, 24). Overlap between the histologic features of hypertrophic LE and lichen planus have been described (146).

Lupus Erythematosus Panniculitis/Profundus

LE panniculitis is the only LE-specific skin lesion that spares the epidermis; however, Dr. James Gilliam felt that the pathological changes within the subcutaneous tissue were characteristic enough to classify this entity as a form of LE-specific skin disease.

Absence of the characteristic epidermal and dermal changes of LE can make the histologic diagnosis difficult and controversy has existed in the past as to the specificity of the histopathological changes of LE panniculitis when overlying changes of DLE are not present at the dermal-epidermal junction. The histologic features are that of a lobular lymphocytic panniculitis: perivascular infiltration with lymphocytes, plasma cells, and histiocytes in the deep dermis and subcutaneous fat (including lymphoid nodule formation); vessel-wall thickening and invasion by mononuclear cells ("lymphocytic vasculitis"); absence of polymorphonuclear leukocytes; hyaline-fat necrosis, prominent fibrinoid degeneration of collagen; as well as mucinous degeneration and calcification in old, established lesions (220). Immunoglobulin and complement deposits usually are found in blood-vessel walls of the deep dermis and subcutis by direct immunofluorescence staining of biopsy specimens (149). Immunoglobulin deposits at the dermal-epidermal junction may or may not be present depending on the site biopsied, the presence or absence of accompanying SLE, and the presence or absence of overlying changes of DLE at the dermal-epidermal junction.

Mucosal Discoid Lupus Erythematosus

Except for the differences related to the absence of hair follicles and *stratum corneum* in mucous membranes, the microscopic changes are highly reminiscent of those seen in cutaneous DLE lesions (221).

Laboratory Findings

Acute Cutaneous Lupus Erythematosus

Little data are available concerning specific laboratory associations of ACLE. Wysenbeek et al. recently have reported that anti-dsDNA antibodies and low complement levels were more common in patients who had the nonspecific "rash" of SLE (presumably generalized ACLE) (62). An overview of the autoantibody that can be encountered in LE patients is presented in Table 29.5.

Subacute Cutaneous Lupus Erythematosus

Autoantibodies

ANAs have been detected in 60% to 81% of SCLE patients when human-tissue substrate was used (128), but only in 49% to 55% of patients when mouse or rat substrates were used (211). Ro/SS-A antibodies have been observed in frequencies ranging from 40% to 100% of patients by immunodiffusion techniques (222) [earlier data reviewed in (80)]. Very higher percentages of patients are anti-Ro/SS-A positive by the more sensitive enzyme-linked immunosorbent assay (ELISA) (222). Some have suggested recently that anti-Ro/SS-A precipitins more often are associated with annular SCLE patients (72) although this has not been the experience of the authors. Most SCLE patient series report finding La/SS-B antibodies by immunodiffusion in 12% to 42% of their SCLE patients (223), however, two series outside of the United States found that considerably higher percentages of their patients had these antibodies (120). A comparison of the frequency of lab abnormalities seen in SCLE to those seen in ACLE and DLE is presented in Table 29.4.

False-positive VDRL reactions, indicative of antiphospholipid antibodies, have been detected in anywhere from 7% to 33% of SCLE patients (80). Anticardiolipin antibodies have been detected by ELISA in approximately 10% to 16% of patients (224). Rheumatoid factor has been present in approximately one third of SCLE patients (80), however, relatively few SCLE patients have developed RA (179). Sm, dsDNA, and U_1RNP antibodies have been reported to occur in approximately 10% of SCLE patients [data reviewed in (80)]. One report has found anti-U_1RNP antibodies in eight of their 15 patients (53%) (225), though others have noted a much lower frequency (35). Antilymphocyte antibodies were found in 33% of patients in one study (35). Antithyroid antibodies have been reported in 18% (177) and 44% (226) of SCLE patients. A comparison of the frequency of autoantibodies in SCLE and classical DLE patients is presented in Table 29.4.

TABLE 29.5. AUTOANTIBODIES ENCOUNTERED IN SLE PATIENTS

Antigen	Autoantibody Frequency		Specificity	Clinical Association
	ID[1]	SPA/RIA/IIF[2]		
High disease specificity				
dsDNA		40–60%	Native DNA	LE nephritis
Sm	25%		Ribonucleoprotein	–
rRNP	10%		Ribosomal P protein	CNS LE
PCNA	3%		Cyclin	–
Low disease specificity				
ssDNA		60%–80%	Denatured DNA	Risk for SLE in DLE patients
Histones		50%–70%	Histones	Drug-induced SLE
Calreticulin		40%	Calreticulin	SLE
U1RNP	25%	30%–40%	Ribonucleoprotein	Overlap CTD[3] (MCTD)
Ro/SS-A	25%	50%	Ribonucleoprotein	SCLE, SSj[4], neonatal LE
La/SS-B	10%	30%	Ribonucleoprotein	SSj, SCLE
Ku	10%		Transcription factor	Overlap CTD

[1]immunodiffusion
[2]solid phase immunoassay (i.e., ELISA), radioimmunoassay, or indirect immunofluorescence assay
[3]connective tissue disease
[4]Sjögren's syndrome
CNS, central nervous system; DLE, discoid lupus erythematosus; SCLE, subacute cutaneous lupus erythematosus; SLE, systemic lupus erythematosus.

Other Laboratory Findings

Patients with SCLE, particularly those with systemic involvement, may have a number of laboratory abnormalities. Various studies have found the following: anemia, leukopenia, thrombocytopenia, an elevated erythrocyte sedimentation rate, hypergammaglobulinemia, proteinuria, hematuria, urine casts, elevated serum creatine and blood urea nitrogen, and depressed complement levels [data reviewed in (80)]. Levels of complement components such as C2 or C4 can be depressed as a result of genetic deficiency (227).

Chronic Cutaneous Lupus Erythematosus

Autoantibodies

Only a small percentage of patients with classical DLE who have no evidence of systemic disease by history or physical examination will have detectable immunologic abnormalities (134). Antinuclear antibodies may be detected in low titer in as many as 30% to 40% of DLE patients; however, less than 5% will have the higher levels that are characteristically seen in severe SLE. While antibodies to single-stranded DNA are not uncommon in DLE, antibodies to dsDNA are distinctly uncommon (228). Precipitating antibodies to U_1RNP sometimes are found in patients whose disease course is dominated by DLE lesions, however, such patients usually have evidence of mild SLE or overlapping connective-tissue disease (171). Ro/SS-A precipitins also can be seen occasionally in DLE patients (222). The presence of precipitating Sm and La/SS-B antibodies are, however, distinctly unusual in patients with isolated DLE lesions (229). Fewer than 10% of DLE patients have IgG anticardiolipin antibodies (230).

Antinuclear antibodies are present in 70% to 75% of patients with LE profundus/panniculitis, but anti-dsDNA antibodies are uncommon (147).

Other Laboratory Abnormalities

A small percentage of DLE patients will have a biologic false-positive serologic test for syphilis (VDRL), positive rheumatoid factor tests, slight depressions in serum-complement levels, modest elevations in gamma globulin, and modest leukopenia. The significance of such findings will be discussed below.

Differential Diagnosis

Acute Cutaneous Lupus Erythematosus

There are a number of dermatoses unrelated to LE that can produce a red face (55, 231, 232). Among those more commonly confused with ACLE are acne rosacea, dermatomyositis, and seborrheic dermatitis. Facial swelling may be severe in patients with ACLE and SLE, sometimes simulating the facial skin changes that are characteristic of dermatomyositis (113). Generalized ACLE can be confused with other causes of widespread exanthematosus reactions such as drug hypersensitivity reactions as well as erythema multiforme.

Subacute Cutaneous Lupus Erythematosus

The cutaneous lesions of papulosquamous SCLE can be most closely mimicked by psoriasis (particularly photosensitive psoriasis). Occasionally, they also can be confused with *pityriasis rubra pilaris* (233) and crusted scabies (234). Seborrheic dermatitis, polymorphous-light eruption, dermatophyte infections, nummular eczema, contact dermatitis, dermatomyositis, and cutaneous T-cell lymphoma/mycosis fungoides also can be confused with SCLE on occasion. Annular SCLE lesions are more apt to be misdiagnosed as granuloma annulare (235), erythema multiforme, or types of figurate erythemas such as erythema annulare centrifigum and erythema gyratum repens. The photodistribution of SCLE lesions and the LE-specific histopathology often are crucial in helping the clinician differentiate SCLE from these other skin diseases. The presence of circulating Ro/SS-A autoantibodies can serve to further support a diagnosis of SCLE.

Chronic Cutaneous Lupus Erythematosus

Classical Discoid Lupus Erythematosus

With respect to diagnosis, discoid-shaped skin lesions that have erythema and hyperpigmentation at their active borders and depigmentation, telangiectasia, and atrophy at the centers are very unlikely to result from dermatological disorders other than cutaneous LE. However, there are other dermatoses that can produce persistent red plaques on the face that at times can be confused with DLE.

Polymorphous light eruption (PMLE), as the name implies, is an exclusively photo-triggered dermatosis that can be expressed in several clinical forms, including succulent red plaques that occasionally can mimic the earlier phases of evolving DLE lesions. PMLE lesions, however, clinically lack the keratinaceous follicular plugging, telangiectasia, and atrophy that are characteristic of DLE lesions. Histopathologically, PMLE usually lacks the prominent liquefaction degeneration of the epidermal basal-cell layer and basement membrane thickening that is characteristic of DLE lesions. In the dermis, the lymphoid-cell infiltrate is predominately perivascular in PMLE and does not involve the cutaneous appendages as in DLE. Immunoglobulins and complement components are not deposited at the dermal-epidermal junction in PMLE as in DLE. Ro/SS-A autoantibodies have been detected in 3.5% to 14% of PMLE sera (236–238). ANA titers 1:80 were found in 14% (28 of 198) of PMLE patient sera (237), six of whom were Ro positive. Three of the 198 patients met the American College of Rheumatology criteria for SLE, one of whom was Ro positive. Some of these patients may have had cutaneous LE rather than PMLE, as histopathological exam of lesions from six of these patients revealed vacuolar changes of the basal keratinocytes. However, none of these patients developed typical SCLE lesions, and PMLE lesions can show LE-like histopathology (239, 240). At times, it can be difficult to differentiate cutaneous LE from PMLE. The history of a recurrent photodistributed eruption that begins in spring and improves or resolves during the summer months supports the diagnosis of PMLE over cutaneous LE.

Granuloma faciale also can present as indolent, red-brown, to purple facial plaques that can be very resistant to all forms of treatment. Hyperkeratosis, follicular plugging and atrophy are not seen in this disorder. The epidermis is spared by the histopathologic process seen in granuloma faciale and the pattern of dermal inflammation is quite distinct from that seen in DLE lesions.

Sarcoidosis, Jessner's benign-lymphocytic infiltration of the skin, pseudolymphoma of Spiegler-Fendt (syn., Spiegler-Fendt sarcoid), lymphocytoma cutis, angiolymphoid hyperplasia with eosinophilia, lymphoma cutis, lupus vulgaris (241), and tertiary syphilis (242) are other disorders that can clinically simulate some phases of DLE lesions and at times present diagnostic confusion. The histopathologies of these conditions are quite distinct from DLE and each is usually negative for immunoglobulin and complement components at the dermal-epidermal junction upon direct immunofluorescence examination.

Hypertrophic Discoid Lupus Erythematosus

Uitto and coworkers (142) have pointed out that the verrucous, hyperkeratotic character of these lesions could be mistaken for keratoacanthoma, squamous-cell carcinoma, prurigo nodularis, or hypertrophic lichen planus.

Lupus Erythematosus Profundus/Panniculitis

The differential diagnosis of patients with lupus panniculitis includes Weber-Christian panniculitis, factitial panniculitis, Talwin-induced panniculitis, pancreatic panniculitis, traumatic panniculitis, morphea profundus, eosinophilic fascitis, sarcoidosis, subcutaneous granuloma annulare, and rheumatoid nodules. Deep excisional biopsy often is required to distinguish LE panniculitis from these other disorders, particularly when classical DLE lesions are not present.

Mucosal Discoid Lupus Erythematosus

With respect to differential diagnosis, oral lichen planus presents the closest clinical appearance to that of oral mucosal DLE. A biopsy can be useful to differentiate between these two disorders, but often is not necessary.

Management

Acute Cutaneous Lupus Erythematosus

ACLE lesions respond to the more aggressive regimens of systemic corticosteroids and other immunosuppressive agents (e.g., azathioprine, cyclophosphamide) that often are required to manage the more severe systemic manifestations of LE that often accompany this form of LE-specific skin disease. Increasing evidence suggests that drugs such as hydroxychloroquine can have a steroid-sparing effect on SLE (243). This is likely to be true for ACLE as well.

Subacute Cutaneous Lupus Erythematosus

The management of patients with SCLE should include evaluation to rule out underlying systemic disease at the time of diagnosis, then again at 6- to 12-month intervals, unless the patient develops symptoms that dictate an earlier reassessment (244). The initial evaluation should include a history, review of systems, and physical exam to elicit symptoms and signs of underlying systemic disease (i.e., arthritis, serositis, central nervous system disease, renal disease). Initial laboratory evaluation should include, at minimum, a complete blood count, platelet count, erythrocyte sedimentation rate, urinalysis, and blood-chemistry profile. Additional determinations that can be of help include C3, C4, and CH50.

The initial management of all SCLE patients should include education regarding protection from sun and artificial sources of UV light, and the elimination of potentially provocative photosensitiving drugs such as hydrochlorothiazide, griesofulvin, and piroxicam if at all possible. With regards to specific medical therapy, local measures should be maximized first then systemic agents employed if significant disease activity continues.

Sun Protection

Patients should be advised to avoid direct sun exposure, particularly during the midday hours and during the summer months when the UV component of sunlight is least attenuated by the atmosphere. A useful rule of thumb is that if one's shadow is longer than one is tall, there is relatively less danger from UV radiation exposure. Tightly woven clothing with vented panels for comfort in hot environments and hats should be worn in conjunction with broad-spectrum sunscreens to achieve maximal shielding from sunlight. Several clothing lines offering maximized UV protection currently are being marketed and are easily accessed through the internet [e.g., Solumbra Ultra Sun Protective Clothing (sunprecautions.com); MasqueRays (sunproof.com); Sun Protective Clothing (sunprotective-clothing.com)]. Such specialty clothing also is marketed for fishermen and those going on safaris.

Patients should select broad-spectrum sunscreens that contain agents that block UVB with a sun protective factor (SPF) of 30 or greater. It has been found that much lower amounts of sunscreens actually are used in real-life situations compared to the amounts employed under lab conditions for determining the SPF rating of a specific sunscreen product. Therefore, when a photosensitive patient uses a

SPF 30 sunscreen in real life, they often get a real-life SPF of about 15, the minimum necessary for adequate protection for a LE patient. Sunscreen products containing Parsol 1789 (avobenzone), zinc oxide, or titanium dioxide provide the broadest degree of UVA protection (245) and such products may have added value in SCLE patients (246). Products also should be selected that are most resistant to being washed off by sweating or bathing. Sunscreens should be applied at least 30 minutes before sun exposure and reapplied after bathing or appreciable perspiration. Stick-type sunscreens that are formulated for use on the lips also can be applied around the eyes to avoid the eye irritation that often occurs when other products are applied to this area. Several reviews addressing comparative sunscreen efficacy have been published (245).

A number of companies offer UV light-blocking films can be applied to home and automobile windows. More information on these products can be obtained through the internet [e.g., Solis films from Southwall Technologies (southwall.com); North Solar Screen (northsolarscreen.com)]. Several of these companies offer films or plastic shields that can be placed over fluorescent light bulbs to block the small but finite amount of UV irradiation that can leak from such sources (247).

Corrective camouflage cosmetics such as Dermablend (Johnson Products) and Covermark (Covermark Cosmetics) offer the dual benefit of being highly effective physical sunscreens as well as aesthetically pleasing cosmetic masking agents for patients suffering psychologically from therapeutically-refractory, chronic, disfiguring skin disease as can result from cutaneous LE.

Local Corticosteroids

Initial treatment usually includes the use of a potent topical corticosteroid like clobetasol propionate 0.05% (Temovate, Glaxo Wellcome), betamethasone dipropionate 0.05% (Diprolene, Schering), halobetasol proprionate 0.05% (Ultravate, Westwood-Squibb) or diflorosone diacetate 0.05% (Psorcon, Dermik). Twice-daily application of these products to lesional skin for two weeks followed by a two-week rest period can minimize the risk of local complications such as steroid atrophy and telangiectasia. Cutaneous LE represents one of the very few clinical situations where such potent topical fluorinated corticosteroids can be recommended for use on atrophy-prone areas such as the face, because the alternatives are unchecked, disfiguring skin disease, or the potential side for effects from systemic therapy. Unfortunately, topical corticosteroids alone do not provide adequate improvement for the large majority of SCLE patients. Most SCLE patients' lesions are too numerous to be managed by intralesional corticosteroid injections and oral corticosteroids should be avoided as long as possible when treating this chronic cutaneous condition.

Antimalarials

While a number of systemic medications have been reported to be of benefit to SCLE patients, by far the most useful are the aminoquinoline antimalarial agents. The authors as well as others (248) have found that approximately 80% of SCLE patients will respond to single-agent or combined antimalarial therapy. The three agents most frequently prescribed for SCLE patients are hydroxychloroquine sulfate (Plaquenil-Sanofi Pharmaceuticals), chloroquine phosphate (Aralen-Sanofi Pharmaceuticals), and quinacrine hydrochloride (Compounding Labs of America) (quinacrine was previously available in the United States under the brand name, Atabrine (Winthrop Labs). In general, hydroxychloroquine is best tolerated with the least side effects. The generic form of quinacrine dihydrochloride that has been available from compounding pharmacies in the United States over the past decade appears to be functionally equivalent to Atabrine in the treatment of LE-specific skin disease (personal observation, RDS).

When using either hydroxychloroquine and chloroquine, ophthalmologic examination is required to minimize the risk of retinal toxicity (quinacrine has not been confirmed to be retinopathic). A baseline ophthalmologic evaluation should be obtained before starting antimalarial therapy to document any preexisting changes. This should be repeated in 6- to 12-month intervals while on therapy. This evaluation should, at minimum, include a fundoscopic exam, visual field testing (including central fields with a red object), and visual acuity testing. Use of the self-administered Amsler Grid at home to detect the earliest evidence of visual-field defects has become popular. Retinal changes can become irreversible if not detected early. It has been suggested that the risk of retinal toxicity is minimized when the total daily dose of hydroxychloroquine does not exceed 6 mg/kg/day (4 mg/kg/day for chloroquine) (249). There does not appear to be an upper limit on the "safe" total lifetime dose of these drugs if these daily maximum dosing recommendations are not exceeded.

Periodic assessments of hematological and hepatic function should be obtained during antimalarial therapy to identify the occasional patient who will suffer an idiosynchrytic reaction. Quinacrine hydrochloride is more likely to induce hemolysis in glucose-6-phosphate dehydrogenase-deficient patients than is hydroxychloroquine or chloroquine (250). Neurotoxicity and muscular toxicity can occur but was much more of a problem in the past when higher daily doses of these drugs were used.

Antimalarial agents can induce a number of dermatologic changes. All can cause a blue-black pigmentation of the skin (particularly in the sun-exposed areas), the palatal mucosa, and the nails. They also can rarely cause bleaching of lightly pigmented hair. Quinacrine frequently causes diffuse yellowing of the skin, sclera, and bodily secretions that are fully reversible on discontinuation of the drug. On occasion, quinacrine and other antimalarials can produce a lichenoid drug reaction that can be the harbinger of severe bone-marrow toxicity (251).

Therapy with hydroxychloroquine alone at 400 mg/day initially should be tried. If there is no significant improvement by 2 months, quinacrine, 100 mg/day, can be added to the hydroxychloroquine (252). If the response is inadequate after 4 to 6 weeks of hydroxychloroquine plus quinacrine, chloroquine 250 mg/day can be substituted for the hydroxychloroquine while continuing the quinacrine (an occasional cutaneous LE patient will respond better to chloroquine than hydroxychloroquine). Once disease activity is controlled, the hydroxychloroquine can be decreased to 200 mg/day for maintenance.

Two studies have confirmed earlier suspicions that smoking may interfere with the efficacy of antimalarials in treating DLE and SCLE (108, 109). Both authors have witnessed dramatic improvement in DLE skin lesions in antimalarial-resistant patients soon after they have quit smoking. Therefore, one has additional reasons to encourage cutaneous LE patients to quit this dangerous habit.

Dapsone

Dapsone (diaminodiphenylsulfone—Jacobus Pharmaceutical Co.) is best for treating the occasional patient having LE-nonspecific vesiculobullous skin lesions that can occur in SLE patients ("bullous SLE") (253). Within days, 100 mg/day of this drug can provide significant improvement. Hematologic, renal, and hepatic toxicity can occur with this drug and requires frequent monitoring. The authors have had relatively little positive experience in treating SCLE patients with this agent, although others have reported benefit in isolated cases within a few weeks after starting therapy (227).

Retinoids

The synthetic retinoids isotretinoin (Accutane, Roche Laboratories), etretinate (Tegison, Roche Laboratories), and acitretin (Soriatane, Roche Laboratories) at approximately one half to 1 mg/kg/day have been shown to significantly improve SCLE lesions (254). (Please note that etretinate is no longer available, and has been replaced by acitretin.) These agents also have been advocated for hypertrophic DLE (255). The great potential for teratogenic effects with the retinoids make it imperative that fertile females are using contraceptive techniques according to guidelines set forth specifically for patients on retinoids. A common dose-related side effect is mucocutaneous dryness. It is advisable to have patients use sunscreens judiciously while being treated with these agents to minimize their tendency to aggravate photosensitivity. Drug-induced hepatitis and hypertriglceridemia can occur with these agents and require periodic laboratory evaluation. On occasion, these drugs also can induce bony changes consistent with the diffuse idiopathic skeletal hyperostosis (DISH) syndrome.

Clofazimine

Crovoto reported the successful use of clofazamine (Lamprene, Geigy Pharmaceuticals) in a patient with annular SCLE in 1981 (256). He used a dose of 100 mg/day and noted clearing of the lesions within a few weeks. At this dosage, clofazimine generally is well tolerated, though gastrointestinal intolerance can be a problem. At higher doses, clofazamine rarely has been reported to precipitate in mesenteric arteries resulting in major abdominal catastrophes such as splenic infarction (257). A pink to brownish-black skin pigmentation develops in most patients on long-term clofazimine therapy. This pigmentation resolves over months to years after discontinuing the drug. Similar discoloration of bodily secretions also frequently occurs.

Thalidomide

Thalidomide, 50 to 200 mg/day, can be very effective in otherwise-refractory SCLE and DLE (32, 258–263). In general, about 75% of cutaneous LE patients will respond to antimalarial monotherapy or combination therapy. It now appears that thalidomide can produce good-to-excellent results in 75% of antimalarial-refractory cutaneous LE.

Because of its notorious teratogenicity (264), special precautions should be taken when prescribing thalidomide. It recently has become available in the United States under the brand name Thalomid (Celgene Corporation). Prescribing physicians and dispensing pharmacies first must register with Celgene Corporation. Once this has been accomplished, Celgene Corporation will send the physician specially developed materials [System for Thalidomide Education and Prescribing Safety (STEPS)] to educate patients to help them avoid birth defects.

Thalidomide can produce irreversible sensory neurotopathies in treated patients (265, 266). Baseline and periodic peripheral nerve conduction studies (i.e., measurements of sensory nerve-action potential amplitudes) have been recommended in hopes of detecting neuropathy early so that the thalidomide can be discontinued before more severe, irreversible neuropathy develops. The role of nerve conduction studies in monitoring thalidomide-treated patients still is not well defined.

Other occasional side effects include a transient myoclonic jerking reactions of the extremities, neutropenia, and secondary amenorrhea as a result of ovarian failure (267).

Gold

Oral gold [auranofin (Ridaura, Connetics Corporation)] or parenteral gold [aurothioglucose (Solganal, Schering)] therapy has been successfully used in those cutaneous LE patients whose disease is resistant to the less toxic forms of therapy (268). Gold frequently has mucocutaneous toxicity and less commonly has hematologic, renal, and pulmonary toxicity that may require its discontinuance.

Alpha Interferon

Earlier clinical observations had suggested that endogenously produced interferon might be of benefit in SCLE (269). Recombinant interferon alpha 2A (Roferon-A, Roche) has been used to treat four SCLE patients (270). The dosage ranged from 18 to 120 × 10^6 units injected weekly for 4 to 13 weeks. Two patients had a complete response, one had a partial response, and one patient had no response to treatment. All three patients that responded to treatment later relapsed 4 to 12 weeks after treatment was stopped. Others have noted similar effects (271). Intralesional interferon alpha has been reported to be of value in DLE (272). However, the risk of inducing or exacerbating systemic autoimmune reactions probably outweighs any benefits of alpha interferon in this setting.

Systemic Corticosteroids And Other Immunosuppressive Agents

Systemic corticosteroids and cytotoxic agents are reserved for patients with more severe disease who have failed the less toxic forms of therapy discussed above. A patient occasionally may be encountered whose disease is so severe that these more potent agents may be used earlier in the disease course, even before the patient is given a complete trial of the less toxic agents.

Methylprednisolone given in "pulse doses" (1 g intravenously for three consecutive days) has been reported to provide improvement in SCLE patients with systemic LE (273). Anecdotally, cyclophosphamide and methotrexate (248, 274) as well as azathioprine (275) have been suggested to be of benefit in refractory SCLE. Because of the potential for severe immunosuppression, risk of cancer induction, bone marrow, and mucous-membrane toxicity, these agents should be reserved for patients with severe disease and used only as a last resort in patients with severe cutaneous LE alone.

UVA-I Phototherapy

Preliminary animal work has suggested that UVA might dampen the autoimmune abnormalities in experimental SLE (276). In addition, work from two centers has suggested that SCLE patients might actually benefit from very low doses of whole-body UVA-I (340 to 400 nm) irradiation (277). However, the true value that this somewhat controversial form of treatment will ultimately play remains to be confirmed by controlled studies in larger groups of patients. Caution should be taken in interpreting these data in view of the increasing evidence that UVA (278), including long-wave UVA (140), can play an exacerbating role in the cutaneous manifestations of SLE. Recent experimental evidence in a murine model of SLE argues for further caution in this area (279).

A suggested algorithm for using the various systemic agents discussed above is presented in (Fig. 29.40). These recommendations are based upon the authors' personal experience pertaining to the relative efficacy and safety of this group of drugs.

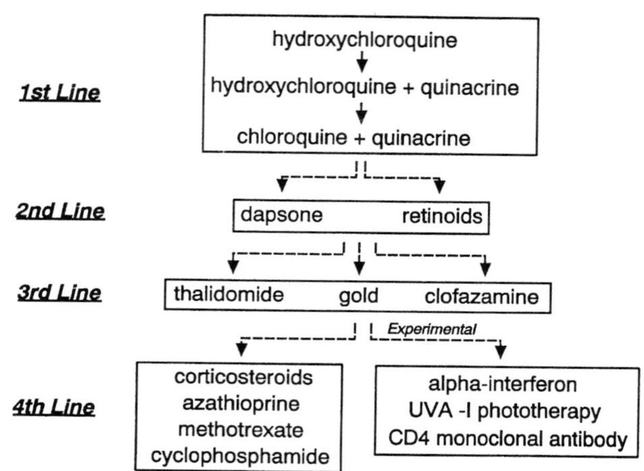

FIGURE 29.40. Suggested algorithm for use of systemic medical agents in the management of subacute cutaneous lupus erythematosus and chronic cutaneous lupus erythematosus.

Chronic Cutaneous LE

The initial approach to the medical management of DLE lesions is basically the same as that described above for SCLE lesions. For the most part, both forms of cutaneous LE respond similarly to medical therapy. Local therapy, especially intralesional corticosteroids (e.g., triamcinolone acetonide suspension, 3 to 5 mg/mL for the face with higher concentrations allowable elsewhere), often is more useful in the management of DLE compared to SCLE because one often is treating fewer individual lesions in a DLE patient compared to a SCLE patient. In addition, we, and others (252), have been particularly impressed that combination antimalarial treatment (hydroxychloroquine or chloroquine plus quinacrine) has been more effective in a number of our DLE patients who did not respond to hydroxychloroquine alone. As stated earlier, two studies have indicated that smoking may interfere with the efficacy of antimalarials in treating DLE and SCLE (108, 109). These findings, and the fact that both authors have witnessed dramatic improvement in DLE skin lesions in antimalarial-resistant patients soon after they have stopped smoking, make it advisable for all cutaneous LE smokers to quit smoking. It is possible that the dramatic effects that cigarette smoking can have on hepatic microsomal enzyme induction (280) could alter the metabolism of the aminoquinoline antimalarials so as to blunt their effect on cutaneous LE. Alternatively, compounds present in cigarette smoke might be capable of directly exacerbating LE-specific cutaneous inflammation.

As with SCLE, drugs such as dapsone (281), retinoids (281), clofazamine (282), thalidomide (263, 264), gold

(268), methotrexate (283, 284), and azathioprine (281), can be of value in DLE when antimalarials have failed.

That small number of hypertrophic DLE lesions that does not respond to single-agent or combined antimalarial therapy has been reported to respond to treatment with systemic retinoids such as isotretinoin (Accutane) (255). Untreated, LE panniculitis/profundus is indolently progressive with ulceration often eventually supervening. Intralesional corticosteroid therapy should be approached with great caution because even this minimal form of trauma can cause LE panniculitis lesions to break down and ulcerate. Even a carefully executed diagnostic skin biopsy can, at times, produce chronic ulceration in these lesions. Most cases of LE panniculitis/profundus can be managed successfully with single-agent or combined antimalarial therapy, however, some will require more aggressive treatment with systemic corticosteroids (147). Thalidomide (285) and gold (286) also have been used in refractory LE panniculitis/profundus patients in the past. Azathioptine has been advocated for those patients having antimalarial-resistant palmar/plantar DLE (275).

Once DLE lesions have progressed to the point of irreversible dystrophic scarring, the use of properly personalized and applied corrective camouflage cosmetics (e.g., Covermark, Dermablend) and properly fitted hair pieces can offer temporary refuge from the devastating emotional impact that this disfiguring disease process can produce.

Once scarring develops within a DLE lesion, little can be done to reverse this process. While disease activity is present, the trauma of plastic surgery procedures carry the risk of further exacerbating disease activity (i.e., the Köebner or isomorphic phenomenon). However, recent reports have suggested that procedures such as dermabrasion, hair transplantation, and autologous fat transplantation might occasionally be safely carried out in areas of scarring that are devoid of active inflammation (287). There is some evidence to suggest that the risk of disease reactivation is lessened if the patient is concurrently on medical therapy (e.g., antimalarials) to blunt the Köebner response. The best overall strategy for the management of DLE, however, is always one of *early*, aggressive, medical management to suppress the inflammatory disease process before scarring and alopecia has developed.

Prognosis

The risks of developing systemic manifestations of LE have already been discussed under the sections dealing with the relationship between the cutaneous and systemic manifestations of the various types of LE-specific skin disease. In this section, we will deal with the outcome of the skin lesions themselves as well as the available morbidity and mortality data concerning these forms of cutaneous LE.

Acute Cutaneous Lupus Erythematosus

Localized ACLE lesions can wax and wane in parallel with the underlying SLE activity (30), often leaving pigment changes in their wake but not producing atrophic dermal scarring.

The authors are unaware of mortality data associated specifically with ACLE. As previously discussed, ACLE often is considered to be an integral expression of underlying SLE and as such, little effort has been made to determine if such patients fare better or worse than those who do not develop ACLE.

Subacute Cutaneous Lupus Erythematosus

Having been recognized as a distinct disease entity for only 15 years, the long-term outcome associated with SCLE lesions has yet to be determined. In the authors' experience, most patients appear to have intermittent recurrences over long periods of time. Some have unremitting lesions that smolder in the same location for years. A superficial form of atrophy has been noted to develop in the lesions of several such patients (personal observation) (Fig. 29.16). Other patients appear to enjoy long-term, if not permanent, remissions of their skin disease.

In short-term follow-up studies, approximately 15% of the SCLE patients studied by one of the authors (RDS) developed ACLE lesions and evidence of active SLE including lupus nephritis (121). This subgroup of patients was marked by the presence of high-titer ANA, leukopenia, and/or anti-dsDNA (176). An interim report from a long-term follow up study involving the original cohort of SCLE patients at University of Texas, Southwestern Medical Center in Dallas, Texas, indicates that the relatively mild disease course that these patients enjoy over the short term appears to hold for longer periods of time (up to 20 years) (288). One of the authors (RDS) is aware of only one death directly attributable to SLE in over 130 SCLE patients that he has examined personally (personal unpubl. observation).

More recent reports of the epidemiology of additional SCLE cohorts from different parts of the world have supported the view that this is a subset of LE patients with relatively low risk of developing life-threatening forms of SLE (289, 290). Additional long-term follow up studies will be required to determine the true risk of severe systemic disease in patients presenting with SCLE skin lesions.

Chronic Cutaneous Lupus Erythematosus

Left untreated, the majority of patients with classical DLE lesions tend to suffer an indolently progressive disease that can spread to produce large areas of dystrophic cutaneous scarring and scarring alopecia that can be disabling emotionally if not physically. In one recent series of 86 chronic cutaneous LE patients having a mean disease duration of 15.1

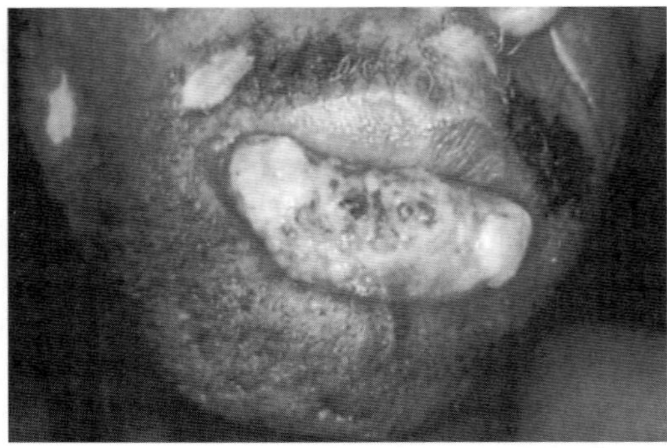

FIGURE 29.41. Squamous-cell carcinoma developing in the discoid lupus erythematosus lesions of the lower lip.

years, 57% had some form of destructive or deforming scarring while 35% had pigmentary disturbances (291). Spontaneous remission is observed occasionally (171) and the disease activity can recrudesce within the site of older inactive lesions. Squamous-cell carcinoma occasionally develops in chronic smoldering DLE lesions (Fig. 29.41) (292).

Death from SLE disease activity is distinctly uncommon in patients who present initially with localized DLE. As previously discussed, generalized DLE does carry a higher risk of associated SLE activity.

LUPUS ERYTHEMATOSUS-NONSPECIFIC SKIN DISEASE

A large number of cutaneous lesions that are found in LE patients are not specific for LE, that is, they also occur in patients that don't have or never develop LE (Table 29.1). Such skin lesions usually are found in the context of SLE or a significant risk thereof. Nonspecific skin findings in LE include vasculitis, photosensitivity reactions, alopecia, soft-tissue calcification, bullous lesions, urticaria, cutaneous mucinoses, skin necrosis, ulcerations, and nail changes. Some of the LE-nonspecific diseases, including vasculitis, Raynaud's phenomena, erythromelalgia, and rheumatoid nodules will be covered in Chapter 36.

Photosensitivity

Patients with LE, particularly ACLE and SCLE, are more likely to complain of photosensitivity reactions than are patients with other rheumatic disorders (a review of the pathogenetic basis of such photosensitivity has been presented in the previous chapter). These reactions include exaggerated sunburn reactions that do not necessarily show the characteristic LE-specific histopathology, although LE-specific skin lesions often can be induced after UVA and/or UVB light exposure (293, 294). Treatment of photosensitivity reactions includes the photoprotective measures reviewed earlier in this chapter.

Alopecia

One study found alopecia in 54% of 74 SLE patients (295). A study of 57 pediatric SLE patients found alopecia in 32% of the patients (296). As discussed earlier in this chapter, scarring alopecia frequently occurs in DLE lesions. Nonscarring alopecia, that is usually reversible, also occurs in LE patients. One study reported nonscarring alopecia in 40% of 73 SLE patients (297). Diffuse nonscarring alopecia may develop secondary to telogen effluvium that can result from steroid withdrawal or physical or mental stress. Some patients develop course, dry "lupus hair" that has increased fragility resulting in broken hairs that may be more prominent over the frontal hairline (Fig. 29.42). Dubois noted such "lupus hair" in 6% of 520 SLE patients (24). Alopecia areata has been reported in LE and in other autoimmune disorders. One study found alopecia areata in 10% of 39 LE patients (298). A number of systemic drugs including some of those employed in LE patients can induce diffuse hair loss. An example would be cyclophosphamide.

Calcinosis Cutis

Calcinosis cutis is much less common in LE than in juvenile dermatomyositis and systemic sclerosis (299). Calcinosis occurring in SLE has occurred often in the setting of normal calcium metabolism and renal function. Calcinosis cutis also has been reported in SCLE (131) and DLE (300, 301). The calcifications are commonly found on the extremities and often are asymptomatic. Sometimes the overlying skin can ulcerate and the calcified material can be extruded as a white toothpastelike or pebblelike material. Patients with superficial lesions should protect these areas from trauma with padded bandages. Some improvement of calcinosis cutis has been noted anecdotally in patients treated with aluminum hydroxide (302), calcium-channel blockers (303), colchicine (304), probenicid (305), and low-dose warfarin (306). Surgical treatment has been reported to provide additional benefit in some cases (302, 307).

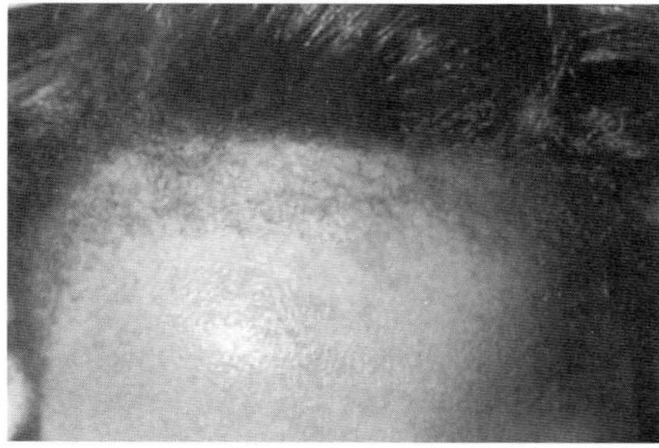

FIGURE 29.42. Lupus hair. Note the sparse, unruly hair at the anterior hair line. The abnormal appearance of the hair in this area is somewhat accentuated by the fact that this patient has a hair weave, giving an artificially healthy appearance to the remainder of her hair.

LE Nonspecific Bullous Lesions

Confusion persists concerning the nosology and classification of the bullous skin changes that can occur in LE (49). Like nonbullous LE skin disease, the variety of bullous skin lesions that occur in LE patients can be divided into those that do and those that do not have a LE-specific histopathology (Table 29.3). Bullae may develop in LE-specific skin lesions such as ACLE and SCLE as a direct extension of the vacuolar degeneration of the epidermal basal layer (116). Skin cleavage occurs as a result of dissolution of the basal-cell layer, resulting in a subepidermal cleavage plane. In both ACLE (115) (Fig. 29.4) and SCLE (123), large areas of sheetlike cleavage occasionally develop, resulting in the clinical appearance of toxic epidermal necrolysis. Documentation of LE as the causal factor in this type of bullous skin change can be difficult because such patients also are frequently on systemic medication and toxic epidermal necrolysis most commonly develops as a result of drug hypersensitivity reaction. In some SCLE patients, vesiculobullous changes develop at the active advancing edge of annular SCLE lesions (123) (Fig. 29.12). Subepidermal bullous changes also have been reported to rarely occur in DLE lesions (308).

The entity commonly described as "bullous SLE" represents an example of LE-nonspecific bullous skin disease. Active SLE patients occasionally will develop a severe, generalized vesiculo-bullous eruption that resembles dermatitis herpetiformis (DH) or epidermolysis bullosa acquisita (EBA) (309) (Fig. 29.43). The histology of these lesions shows marked neutrophilic infiltration with papillary microabscess formation similar to DH and the inflammatory variant of EBA. The direct immunofluorescence findings however, are more consistent with those seen in SLE. Autoantibodies against type VII collagen (the EBA antigen), a normal constituent of anchoring fibrils of the sublamina densa zone, are present in some such patients (310).

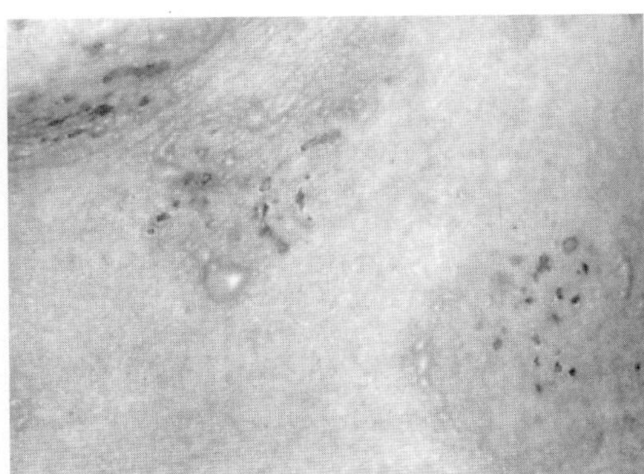

FIGURE 29.43. Epidermolysis bullosa acquisita lesions in a patient with systemic lupus erythematosus (SLE). The appearance of these lesions preceded by 2 years the development of this patient's SLE, which included membranoproliferative glomerulonephritis.

This type of lesion occasionally can represent the initial manifestation of SLE and often occurs in the context of very active SLE including lupus nephritis (311). The rather vague term "bullous SLE" often has been used to describe such lesions (310), however, we feel that the more descriptive terms "DH-like cutaneous LE" or "EBA-like cutaneous LE" are more appropriate because other forms of bullous skin lesions can occur in SLE patients.

Examples of bullous skin diseases that have been linked anecdotally to cutaneous LE and SLE include bullous pemphigoid (312), dermatitis herpetiformis (313), and porphyria cutanea tarda (314). In many of these reports, it is not clear whether the bullous skin changes are the result of the LE autoimmune process or develop as a mere chance occurrence in patients who also have LE and pemphigus erythematosus. Pemphigus erythematosus also has been linked to LE. Patients with pemphigus erythematosus often have immunological evidence of LE-like autoimmunity, circulating antinuclear antibodies and immunoglobulin/complement deposition at the dermal-epidermal junction (i.e., the Senear-Usher syndrome) (315). However, such patients rarely develop significant clinical manifestations of SLE.

Urticaria

Urticaria is sometimes associated with LE. One study found chronic urticaria in 44% of 73 SLE patients (172). This study also reported that some patients noted that their urticaria worsened on sun exposure. Urticaria typically presents with an acute onset of edematous erythematous papules and plaques that itch. It must be differentiated from urticarial vasculitis (see Chapter 36, Psychopathology in the Patient with Lupus). Urticarial vasculitic lesions are more apt to be painful, nonblanching (e.g., purpuric), and remain in the same location for at least several days, while urticarial lesions tend to be pruritic, blanching, and more evanescent. A skin biopsy can be helpful in differentiating between the two.

Treatment of urticaria includes discontinuing any suspected drugs or foods, in addition to the use of antihistamines and other antipruritics. If the urticaria persists beyond several weeks, it is prudent to perform a more extensive workup to rule out other underlying conditions that may be associated with chronic urticaria (i.e., occult infections and malignancies). Urticarial vasculitis can be difficult to treat. Numerous agents have been reported to be beneficial including antihistamines, nonsteroidal antiinflammatory agents, dapsone, antimalarials, systemic corticosteroids, and cytotoxic agents (see Chapter 36, Psychopathology in the Patient with Lupus).

Cutaneous Mucinoses

Small amounts of mucin deposition are sometimes found in LE-specific skin lesions, particularly in biopsies from

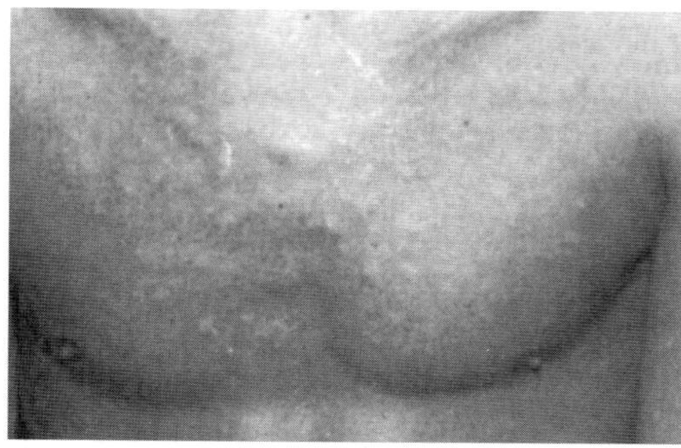

FIGURE 29.44. (See color plate.) Papular and nodular dermal mucinosis in a patient with systemic lupus erythematosus, including pleural effusions and glomerulonephritis.

chronic cutaneous LE lesions. However, some LE patients will manifest papulonodular cutaneous lesions with abundant amounts of mucin in the absence of the classic vacuolar changes in the basal layer of the epidermis (66, 67, 316, 317). These lesions can appear as indurated erythematous papules, nodules, or plaques, typically on the trunk and/or arms (Fig. 29.44). Histopathological exam of these lesions reveals diffuse dermal mucin deposits but lacks the classic vacuolar changes typically seen in LE-specific skin lesions. Some of these patients have LE-specific lesions elsewhere.

The pathogenesis of these lesions remains uncertain, although one report found that fibroblasts isolated from an LE patient with cutaneous mucinosis produced larger amounts of glycosaminoglycan than normal fibroblasts, and the production of this glycosaminoglcan was stimulated by the patient's serum (318). Similar lesions also have been reported in patients with dermatomyositis and scleroderma (319). There have been anecdotal reports of massive cutaneous (320) and periorbital (321) mucinosis in LE. One LE patient presented with nodular cutaneous mucinosis that 3 years later developed into atrophie blanchelike skin lesions (322), with evidence of an underlying vasculopathy, as has been found in other cases (323). Cutaneous mucinoses often are responsive to antimalarial or prednisone therapy.

Skin Necrosis/Ulceration And Antiphospholipid Antibody-Associated Skin Lesions

Cutaneous necrosis as well as leg and digital ulcers can result from vasculitis/vasculopathy and in some patients have been associated with circulating antiphospholipid antibodies (324) (Fig. 29.45). These antibodies also have been associated with other cutaneous lesions including LE-specific skin disease, livedo reticularis, livedo vasculitis (vasculopathy), necrotizing vasculitis, thrombophlebitis, erythematous macules, purpura, ecchymoses, painful skin nodules, subungual splinter hemorrhages, and anetoderma (Fig. 29.46) (325).

Skin necrosis also can result from calciphylaxis in SLE patients with renal failure. These lesions typically present with painful indurated areas of cutaneous hemorrhage that rapidly become necrotic and ulcerate. Radiographic or histopathologic evidence of cutaneous calcification can help diagnose this disorder. It is important to remember that cutaneous vasculitis, necrosis, and ulcerations also can be induced by certain medications (e.g., propylthiouracil, warfarin, hydroxyurea).

Oral Ulcers And Candidiasis

Oral ulcers are a commonly found in patients with LE. They are present in roughly 25% to 45% of SLE patients (326, 327) and roughly 25% of DLE patients (156). Although these lesions can show LE-specific histopathologic changes, particularly in DLE patients, they often are nonspecific. The location and asymptomatic nature of LE-related oral ulcers (Fig. 29.38) can help differentiate them

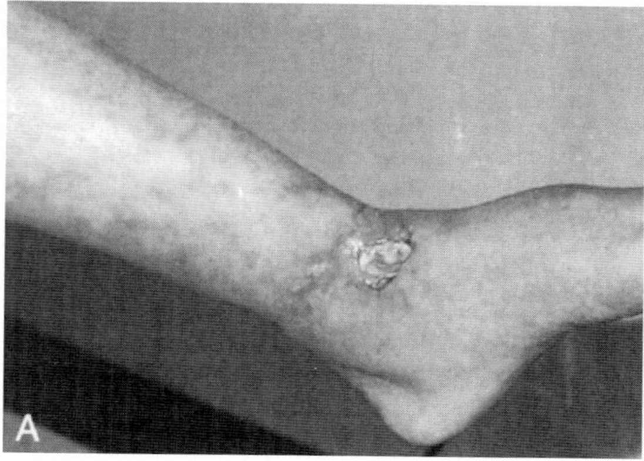

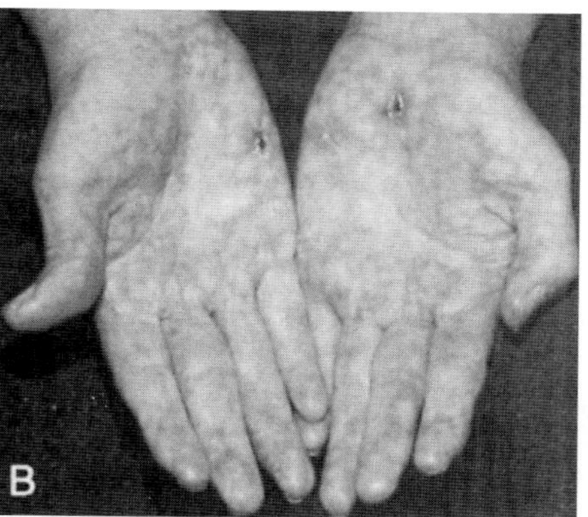

FIGURE 29.45. (See color plate.) **A,** Livedo reticularis and ulceration of the leg in a patient with systemic lupus erythematosus and high-titer IgG anticardiolipin antibodies. **B,** Similar changes on the hands of the same patient.

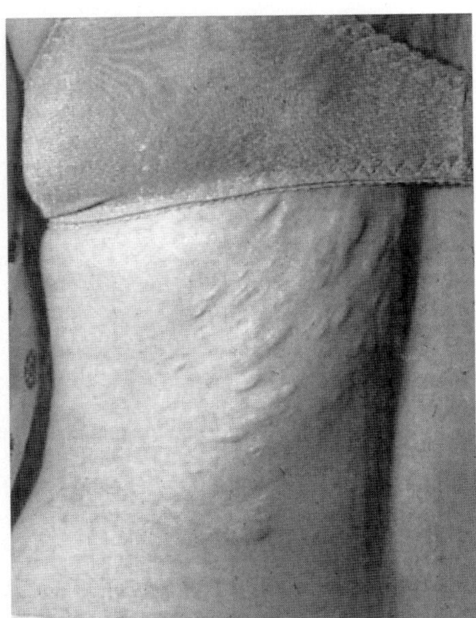

FIGURE 29.46. (See color plate.) Anetoderma in a patient who had typical discoid lupus erythematosus lesions on other parts of her body.

from other types of oral ulcers such as apthous stomatitis, lichen planus, herpes simplex, or drug-induced ulcers (e.g., methotrexate or gold). LE-related ulcerations are more apt to be on the hard palate. One study found them on the hard palate in 89% of 182 SLE patients (326). The non–LE-related oral ulcers usually are quite painful, whereas oftentimes LE-related ulcers are rather asymptomatic. One study found that oral ulcers were asymptomatic in 89% of 182 SLE patients (326). LE-related oral ulcers often improve with treatment of the other systemic or cutaneous manifestations of LE. Symptomatic lesions also can be treated topically with various agents alone or in combination, including corticosteroids, tetracycline, dipenhydramine, and viscous xylocaine.

LE patients on immunosuppressive drugs are more inclined to develop oral candidiasis that usually presents as white plaques on the buccal mucosa and tongue that can be scrapped off easily. The diagnosis can be confirmed by direct microscopic examination and culture. This condition can be treated with systemic azole therapy or with topical agents including nystatin oral suspension and clotrimazole troches.

Nail Changes

A number of nail changes have been noted in LE patients. One study reported nail changes in 31% of 165 SLE patients, the most common change being onycholysis (328). One study reported finding diffuse, dark blue-black nail dyschromia in 52% of 33 African American SLE patients, apparently from increased melanin deposition (329).

Red lunula have been reported in LE (330, 331). One study found red lunulae in 11 of 56 (20%) patients with SLE or cutaneous LE, usually in association with periungual erythema or chilblains (331). Dilated capillaries of the nailfolds have been found in LE patients but less frequently than in dermatomyositis (including clinically amyopathic dermatomyositis) or systemic sclerosis.

Cutaneous Manifestations Of Overlapping Autoimmune Disorders

LE patients often may present with clinical features that overlap with other autoimmune disorders such as Sjögren's syndrome and systemic sclerosis. It is therefore not surprising that LE patients sometimes can present with cutaneous manifestations of other autoimmune disorders, including sicca signs and scerodermatous skin changes, such as sclerodactyly. Anti-U1RNP antibodies have been found frequently in sera from patients with SLE-systemic sclerosis overlap syndrome (332).

Drug-Related Skin Disorders

A wide variety of skin lesions can be induced by medications, including SCLE as discussed above. Many nonspecific skin lesions that are associated with LE also can be caused by medications, including photosensitivity reactions, alopecia, vasculitis, urticaria, bullous skin lesions, and erythema multiforme. *The Drug Eruption Reference Manual,* which is updated annually by Jerome Z. Litt, is a useful resource that lists the cutaneous side effects of numerous medications that have been cited in the literature.

Drugs that are often administered to LE patients not infrequently induce skin lesions. Nonsteroidal antiinflammatory agents frequently are associated with pruritis, urticaria, and/or edema. Photosensitivity reactions, oral ulcerations, alopecia, purpura, erythema multiforme, toxic epidermal necrosis, vasculitis, exacerbation of psoriasis, and fixed drug eruptions also have been associated with the use of these agents.

Systemic corticosteroids are commonly associated with acneiform lesions, ecchymoses, and stria formation. Facial erythema, acanthosis nigricans, hypertrichosis, black hairy tongue, and steroid-withdrawal panniculitis are less frequently associated with the use of these agents. Depigmentation, atrophy, and skin necrosis have occurred at corticosteroid injection sites. The immunosuppressive effects of these medications can result in bacterial, viral, and fungal skin infections.

Antimalarials can cause ecchymotic blue-black pigmentary changes in the skin, particularly on photoexposed areas, oral mucosa, nails, and anterior shins. Bleaching of body hair also can be seen. Quinacrine can cause a yellow discoloration of the skin, sclera, and body secretions and might be misdiagnosed as jaundice. Quinacrine also can cause lichenoid reactions (thickening of the skin often with increased pigmentation and accentuated skin markings). The pigmentary changes usually will resolve within several months after stopping the antimalarial agent, however the pigmentation of the oral mucosa may be irreversible.

Both parenteral and oral-gold preparations can cause pruritus, stomatitis, exfoliative dermatitis, lichen planus-like, and pityriasis rosealike skin reactions. Chyrisiasis is the term that refers to the slate-gray pigmentary skin change that occurs in gold-treated patients. The dose-dependent color change is most marked in sun-exposed areas and may be permanent. Gold compounds also may cause drug-induced LE, alopecia, purpura, vasculitis, erythema nodosum, and brown-nail discoloration.

Physicians always should consider the possibility that a drug might be inducing cutaneous disease in patients that present with skin problems. A history that a drug was recently started within weeks before a skin change was noted might implicate an offending medication. However, it is important to realize that some drug-induced skin conditions do not become apparent until after months, and sometimes years, of treatment with a particular medication. Delayed cutaneous hypersensitivity reactions to Dilantin and a number of other drugs characteristically appear at 3 to 6 weeks following initiation of the drug [delayed drug-induced multiorgan hypersensitivity syndrome (DIDMOHS) (333); drug rash with eosinophilia and systemic symptoms (DRESS) (334)]. In addition, hydroxyurea-induced dermatomyositislike skin disease might become apparent only after the patient has been treated with hydroxyurea for several years (335, 336).

Miscellaneous

There is some controversy over whether lichen planus occurs simultaneously in some cutaneous LE patients or whether some cutaneous LE lesions are mimicking lichen planus (337). In one case, lesions of SCLE appeared to evolve into those of lichen planus (338). One study concluded that some LE patients do, in fact, have both skin disorders, based on clinical, histopathological, and immunopathological findings (339). The histopathology of lichen planus can sometimes mimic that of LE-specific skin lesions so that it may not always be so easy to differentiate between the two when the clinical appearance of the skin lesions is not classic for either.

Acanthosis nigricans has been reported in SLE in the absence of glucose intolerance (340), as well as in the presence of antiinsulin receptor antibodies (Type B insulin resistance). Acanthosis nigricans also has been associated with lupoid hepatitis (341).

LE patients may develop erythema multiforme from drugs or other causes. It is important to remember that sometimes SCLE can mimic erythema multiforme and one might wonder if the initial report of Rowell's syndrome (e.g., erythema multiforme along with chilblains and DLE) might not have been SCLE rather than erythema multiforme (22).

ACKNOWLEDGMENTS

This work was supported in part by NIH grant AR19101.

REFERENCES

1. Gilliam JN, Sontheimer RD. Skin manifestations of SLE. *Clinics in Rheumatic Diseases* 1982;8:207–218.
2. Benedek TG. Historical background of discoid and systemic lupus erythematosus. In: Wallace DJ, Hahn BH, eds. *Dubois' lupus erythematosus.* Baltimore: Williams & Wilkins, 1997: 3–16.
3. Sontheimer RD. Clinical manifestations of cutaneous lupus erythematosus. In: Wallace DJ, Hans BH, eds. *Dubois' lupus erythematosus.* Philadelphia and London: Lea & Febiger, 1993: 285–301.
4. Smith CD, Cyr M. The history of lupus erythematosus from Hipprocates to Osler. *Rheum Dis Clin N Am* 1988;14:1–14.
5. Cazenave PLA, Chausit M. Du lupus. *Ann Malad Peau Syph* 1852;4:113–117.
6. Hebra F, Kaposi M. *On diseases of the skin, including the exanathemata.* London: The New Sydenham Society, 1875.
7. Hutchinson J. *On lupus and its treatment. British Medical Journal,* 1880;1:650.
8. Osler W. On the visceral complications of erythema exudativum multiforme. *Am J Med Sci* 1895;100:629–646.
9. Lehmann P, Ruzicka T. Sunscreens and photoprotection and lupus erythematosus. *Dermatol Therapy.* In press.
10. Hutchinson J. Harveian lectures on lupus. *Br Med J* 1888; 1:113–118.
11. Payne JF. A postgraduate lecture on lupus erythematosus. *Clin J* 1894;4:223–229.
12. Pusey WA. Attacks of lupus erythematosus following exposure to sunlight or other weather factors. *Arch Dermatol Syphol* 1915; 34:388.
13. Kiel H. Conception of lupus erythematosus and its morphologic variants. With particular references to systemic lupus erythematosus. *Arch Dermatol* 1937;36:729–757.
14. Gilliam JN. The cutaneous signs of lupus erythematosus. *Continuing Education for the Family Physician* 1977;6:34–70.
15. Fuhs H. Lupus erythematosus subacutus mit ausgesprochener Überempfindlichkeit gegen Quarzlicht. *Zb Hautkr* 1929;30: 308–309.
16. O'Leary PA. Disseminated lupus erythematosus. *Minn Med* 1934;17:637–644.
17. Friedberg CK, Gross L, Wallach K. Nonbacterial thrombotic endocarditis associated with prolonged fever, arthritis, inflammation of serous membranes and wide-spread vascular lesions. *Arch Intern Med* 1936;56:662–672.
18. Page F. Treatment of lupus erythematosus with mepacrine. *Lancet* 1951;ii:755–758.
19. Hench PS. The reversibility of certain rheumatic and non-rheumatic conditions by the use of cortisone or of the pituitary adrenocorticotrophic hormone. *Ann Intern Med* 1952;36:1–38.
20. Hargraves M, Richmond H, Morton R. Presentation of two bone marrow elements: The "tart" cell and the "LE" cell. *Mayo Clin Proc* 1948;23:25–28.

21. Friou GJ. Clinical applicatio of lupus serum: nucleoprotein reaction using fluorescent antibody technique. *J Clin Invest* 1957;36:890. Abstract.
22. Rowell NR, Swanson-Beck J, Andrson JR. Lupus erythematosus and erythema multiforme-like lesions. *Arch Dermatol* 1963;88:176–180.
23. Burnham TK, Neblett TR, Fine G. The application of the fluorescent antibody technique to the investigation of lupus erythematosus and varioius dermatoses. *J Invest Dermatol* 1963;41: 451–456.
24. Dubois EL, Tuffanelli DL. Clinical manifestations of systemic lupus erythematosus. *JAMA* 1964;190:104–111.
25. Dubois E. The relationship between discoid and systemic lupus erythematosus. In: Dubois EL, editor. *Lupus erythematosus.* New York: McGraw Hill Book Co., 1966.
26. Wallace DJ, Hahn BH. *Dubois' lupus erythematosus. 4 ed.* Philadelphia, London: Lea & Febiger, 1993.
27. Clark G, Reichlin M, Tomasi TB. Characterization of a soluble cytoplasmic antigen reactive with sera from a patient with systemic lupus erythematosus. *J Immunol* 1969;102:117–122.
28. Prystowsky SD, Gilliam JN. Discoid lupus erythematosus as part of a larger disease spectrum: Correlation of clinical features with laboratory findings in lupus erythematosus. *Arch Dermatol* 1975;11:1448–1452.
29. Gilliam JN, Sontheimer RD. Distinctive cutaneous subsets in the spectrum of lupus erythematosus. *J Am Acad Dermatol* 1981;4:471–475.
30. Ropes MW. *Systemic Lupus Erythematosus.* Cambridge and London: Harvard University Press, 1976.
31. Barba RJ, Franco GF. [Fixed lupus erythematosus (its treatment with thalidomide)]. [Spanish]. *Medicina Cutanea Ibero–Latino-Americana* 1977;5:279–285.
32. Duong DJ, Spigel GT, Moxley RT, et al. American experience with low-dose thalidomide therapy for severe cutaneous lupus erythematosus. *Arch Dermatol* 1999;135:1079–1087.
33. Sontheimer RD, Thomas JR, Gilliam JN. Subacute cutaneous lupus erythematosus: a cutaneous marker for a distinct lupus erythematosus subset. *Arch Dermatol* 1979;115:1409–1415.
34. Sontheimer RD, Stastny P, Gilliam JN. Human histocompatibility antigen associations in subacute cutaneous lupus erythematosus. *J Clin Invest* 1981;67:312–316.
35. Sontheimer RD, Maddison PJ, Reichlin M, et al. Serologic and HLA associations in subacute cutaneous lupus erythematosus, a clinical subset of lupus erythematosus. *Ann Intern Med* 1982;97:644–671.
36. Maddison PJ, Provost TT, Reichlin M. Serological findings in patients with "ANA-negative" systemic lupus erythematosus. *Medicine* 1981;60:87–94.
37. Franco HL, Weston WL, Pebble C, et al. Autoantibodies directed against sicca syndrome antigens in the neonatal lupus syndrome. *J Am Acad Dermatol* 1981;4:67–72.
38. Lehmann P, Hölzle E, Kind P, et al. Experimental reproduction of skin lesions in lupus erythematosus by UVA and UVB radiation. *J Am Acad Dermatol* 1990;22:181–187.
39. Kind P, Lehmann P, Plewig G. Phototesting in lupus erythematosus. *J Invest Dermatol* 1993;100:53S–57S.
40. LeFeber WP, Norris DA, Ryan SR, et al. Ultraviolet light induces binding of antibodies to selected nuclear antigens on cultured human keratinocytes. *J Clin Invest* 1984;74: 1545–1551.
41. Norris DA. Pathomechanisms of photosensitive lupus erythematosus. *J Invest Dermatol* 1993;100:58S–68S.
42. Beutner EH, Blaszczyk M, Jablonska S, et al. Preliminary, dermatologic first step criteria for lupus erythematosus and second step criteria for systemic lupus erythematosus. *Int J Dermatol* 1993;32:645–651.
43. Beutner EH, Jablonska S, Whie DB, et al. Dermatologic criteria for classifying the major forms of cutaneous lupus erythematosus: methods for systematic discriminant analysis and questions on the interpretation of findings. *Clin Dermatol* 1992;10:443–456.
44. Watanabe T, Tsuchida T. Classification of lupus erythematosus based upon cutaneous manifestations. Dermatological, systemic and laboratory findings in 191 patients. *Dermatology* 1995; 190:277–283.
45. Watanabe T, Tsuchida T. Lupus erythematosus profundus: a cutaneous marker for a distinct clinical subset? *Brit J Dermatol* 1996;134:123–125.
46. Kuhn A, Richter-Hintz D, Osliso C, et al. Lupus erythematosus tumidus: A neglected subset of cutaneous lupus erythematosus. Report of 40 cases. *Arch Dermatol* 2000;136: 1033–1041.
47. Boehm I, Wenzel J, Uerlich M, et al. Lupus erythematosus profundus Kaposi-Irgang: Classification on the basis of a review of 180 cases. *J Am Acad Dermatol.* In press.
48. Werth VP, Zhang W, Dortzbach K, et al. Association of a promoter polymorphism of tumor necrosis factor-alpha with subacute cutaneous lupus erythematosus and distinct photoregulation of transcription. *J Invest Dermatol* 2000;115:726–730.
49. Sontheimer RD. The lexicon of cutaneous lupus erythematosus —a review and personal perspective on the nomenclature and classification of the cutaneous manifestations of lupus erythematosus. *Lupus* 1997;6:84–95.
50. Tan EM, Cohen AS, Fries JF, et al. The 1982 revised criteria for the classification of systemic lupus erythematosus. *Arthritis Rheum* 1982;25:1271–1277.
51. Sontheimer RD. Subacute cutaneous lupus erythematosus: a decade's perspective. *Med Clin North Am* 1989;73:1073.
52. Rothfield NF, Braverman IM, Moschella S, et al. Classification of Lupus Erythematosus. An Open Forum. *Fitzpatrick's J Clin Dermatol* 1994;1:9–12.
53. Pinkus MD. Lichenoid Tissue Reactions. A speculative review of the clinical spectrum of epidermal basal cell damage with special reference to erythema dyschromicum perstans. *Arch Dermatol* 1973;107:840–844.
54. Weinstein C, Miller MH, Axtens R, et al. Lupus and non-lupus cutaneous manifestations in systemic lupus erythematosus. *Aust NZ J Med* 1987;17:501–506.
55. Black AA, McCauliffe DP, Sontheimer RD. Prevalence of acne rosacea in a rheumatic skin disease subspecialty clinic. *Lupus* 1992;1:229–237.
56. Cervera R, Khamashta MA, Font J, et al. Systemic lupus erythematosus: Clinical and immunologic patterns of disease expresison in a cohort of 1,000 patients. *Medicine* 1993;72: 113–124.
57. Jonsson H, Nived O, Sturfelt G. The effect of age on clinical and serological manifestations in unselected patients with systemic lupus erythematosus. *J Rheumatol* 1988;15:505–509.
58. Vlachoyiannopoulos PG, Karassa FB, Karakostas KX, et al. Systemic lupus erythematosus in Greece. Clinical features, evolution and outcome: a descriptive analysis of 292 patients. *Lupus* 1993;2:303–312.
59. O'Quinn S, Cole J, Many H. Problems of disability in patients with chronic skin diseases. *Arch Dermatol* 1972;105:35–40.
60. Hochberg MC. The Epidemiology of Systemic Lupus Erythematosus. In: Wallace DJ, Hahn BH, eds. *Dubois' lupus erythematosus.* Philadelphia and London: Lea & Febiger, 1993:49–57.
61. Hochberg MC, Boyd RB, Ahearn JM, et al. Systemic lupus erythematosus: A review of clinicolaboratory features and immunogenetic markers in 150 patients with emphasis on demographic subsets. *Medicine* 1985;64:285.
62. Wysenbeek AJ, Guedj D, Amit M, et al. Rash in systemic lupus

erythematosus: prevalence and relation to cutaneous and non-cutaneous disease manifestations. *Ann Rheum Dis* 1992;51: 717–719.
63. Arnett FC, Jr. The Genetic Basis of Lupus Erythematosus. In: Wallace DJ, Hahn BH, eds. *Dubois' lupus erythematosus.* Philadelphia and London: Lea & Febiger, 1993:36.
64. Wysenbeek AJ, Block DA, Fries JF. Prevalence and expression of photosensitivity in systemic lupus erythematosus. *Ann Rheumat Dis* 1989;48:461–463.
65. Mond CB, Peterson MGE, Rothfield NF. Correlation of anti-Ro antibody with photosensiivity rash in systemic lupus erythematosus patients. *Arthritis Rheum* 1989;32:202–204.
66. Fritzler MJ, Rubin RL. Drug-Induced Lupus. In: Wallace DJ, Hahn BH, editors. *Dubois' lupus erythematosus.* Philadelphia and London: Lea & Febiger, 1993:442–453.
67. Wallace DJ. Infections in Systemic Lupus Erythematosus. In: Wallace DJ, Hahn BH, eds. *Dubois' lupus erythematosus.* Philadelphia and London: Lea & Febiger, 1993:454–456.
68. Cohen MR, Crosby D. Systemic disease in subacute cutaneous lupus erythematosus: a controlled comparison with systemic lupus erythematosus. *J Rheumatol* 1994;21:1665–1669.
69. Vazquez-Doval J, Ruiz de Erenchun F, Sanchez-Ibarrola A, et al. Subacute cutaneous lupus erythematosus—clinical, histopathological and immunophenotypical study of five cases. *J Invest Allerg* 1992;2:27–32.
70. Drosos AA, Dimou GS, Siamopoulou-Mavridou A, et al. Subacute cutaneous lupus erythematosus in Greece. A clinical, serological and genetic study. *Ann Med Interne Paris* 1990;141: 421–424.
71. Ahearn JM, Provost TT, Dorsch CA, et al. Interrelationships of HLA-DR, MB andMT phenotypes, autoantibody expression, and clinical features in systemic lupus erythematosus. *Arthritis Rheum* 1982;25:1031–1040.
72. Bielsa I, Herrero C, Ercilla G, et al. Immunogenetic findings in cutaneous lupus erythematosus. *J Am Acad Dermatol* 1991;25: 251–257.
73. Watson RM, Talwar P, Alexander E, et al. Subacute cutaneous lupus erythematosus-immunogenetic associations. *J Autoimmun* 1991;4:73–85.
74. Provost TT, Talal N, Bias W, et al. Ro/SS-A SS-A positive Sjögren's/lupus erythematosus overlap patients are associated with the HLA-DR3 and/or DRW6 phenotypes. *J Invest Dermatol* 1988;91:369–371.
75. Harley JP, Reichlin M, Arnett FC, et al. Gene interaction at the HLA-DQ locus enhances autoantibody production in primary Sjögren's syndrome. *Science* 1986;232:1145–1147.
76. Werth VP, Sullivan KE. Strong association of a promoter polymorphism of tumor necrosis factor-alpha (TNF-a) with a photosensitive form of cutaneous lupus erythematosus. *Arthritis Rheum* 1999;42(suppl 9):S105. Abstract.
77. Asghar SS, Venneker GT, Van Meegen M, et al. Hereditary deficiency of C5 in association with discoid lupus erythematosus. *J Am Acad Dermatol* 1991;24:376–378.
78. Walport MJ, Davies KA, Botto M. Clq and systemic lupus erythematosus. *Immunobiology* 1998;199:265–285.
79. Korb LC, Ahearn JM. C1q binds directly and specifically to surface blebs of apoptotic human keratinocytes—complement deficiency and systemic lupus erythematosus revisited. *J Immunol* 1997;158:4525–4528.
80. Sontheimer RD. Subacute cutaneous lupus erythematosus: a decade's perspective. *Med Clin North Am* 1989;73:1073–1090.
81. David-Bajar KM, Bennion SD, DeSpain JD, et al. Clinical, histologic, and immunofluorescent distinctions between subacute cutaneous lupus erythematosus and discoid lupus erythematosus. *J Invest Dermatol* 1992;99:251–257.
82. Balbanova MB, Botev IN, Michailova JI. Subacute cutaneous lupus erythematosus induced by radiation therapy. *Br J Dermatol* 1997;137:648–649.
83. McGrath H, Jr, Scopelitis E, Nesbitt LT, Jr. Subacute cutaneous lupus erythematosus during psoralen ultraviolet A therapy [letter]. *Arthritis Rheum* 1990;33:302–303.
84. Leroy DA, Dompmartin A, Le Jean SGJLMJC, et al. Toxidermie A L'aldactone a type d'erytheme annulaire centrifuge lupique. *Ann Dermatol Venereol* 1987;114:1237–1240.
85. Patri P, Nigro A, Rebora A. Lupus erythematosus-like eruption from captopril. *Acta Derm Venereol* 1985;65:447–448.
86. Fernandez-Diaz ML, Herranz P, Suarez-Marrero MC, et al. Subacute cutaneous lupus erythematosus associated with cilizapril. *Lancet* 1995;345:398.
87. Crowson AN, Magro CM. Subacute cutaneous lupus erythematosus arising in the setting of calcium channel blocker therapy. *Human Pathol* 1997;28:67–73.
88. Fine RM. Subacute cutaneous lupus erythematosus associated with hydrochlorothiazide therapy. *Int J Dermatol* 1989;28: 375–376.
89. Nousari HC, Kimyai-Asadi A, Tausk FA. Subacute cutaneous lupus erythematosus associated with interferon beta-1a. *Lancet* 1998;352:1825–1826.
90. Sheretz EF. Lichen planus following procainamide induced lupus erythematosus. *Cutis* 1988;42:51–53.
91. Brooke R, Coulson IH, al-Dawoud A. Terbinafine-induced subacute cutaneous lupus erythematosus. *Br J Dermatol* 1998; 139:1132–1133.
92. Gange KW, Levene GM. A distinctive eruption in patients receiving oxprenolol. *Clin Exper Dermatol* 1979;4:87–97.
93. Miyagawa S, Okuchi T, Shiomi Y, et al. Subacute cutaneous lupus erythematosus lesions precipitated by griseofulvin. *J Am Acad Dermatol* 1989;21:343–346.
94. Roura M, Lopez-Gil F, Umbert P. Systemic lupus erythematosus exacerbated by piroxicam. *Dermatologica* 1991;182: 56–58.
95. Wishart JM. Reticulosarcoma of the vulva complicating dermatomyositis treated by immunosuppression. *Proceedings of the Royal Socociety of Medicine* 1973;66:330.
96. Toll A, Campopisa P, Gonzalezcastro J, et al. Subacute cutaneous lupus erythematosus associated with cinnarizine and thiethylperazine therapy. *Lupus* 1998;7:364–366.
97. Crowson AN, Magro CM. Lichenoid and subacute cutaneous lupus erythematosus-like dermatitis associated with antihistamine therapy. *J Cutan Pathol* 1999;26:95–99.
98. Pistiner M, Wallace DJ, Nessim S, et al. Lupus erythematosus in the 1980s: A survey of 570 patients. *Sem Arth Rheum* 1991; 21:55–64.
99. Shrank AB, Doniach D. Discoid lupus erythematosus. Correlation of clinical features with serum auto-antibody pattern. *Arch Dermatol* 1963;87:677–685.
100. Marten RH, Blackburn EK. Lupus erythematosus: a five year followup of 77 cases. *Arch Dermatol* 1961;83:430–436.
101. O'Laughlin S, Schroeter AL, Jordon RE. A study of lupus erythematosus with particular reference to generalized discoid lupus. *Br J Dermatol* 1978;99:1–11.
102. Wallace DJ. The relationship between discoid and systmic lupus erythematosus. In: Wallace DJ, Hahn BH, Quismorio FPJrAE, et al., eds. *Dubois' lupus erythematosus.* Philadelphia and London: Lea & Febiger, 1993:310–312.
103. Knop J, Bonsmann G, Kind P, et al. Antigens of the major histocompatibility complex in patients with chronic discoid lupus erythematosus. *Br J Dermatol* 1990;122:723–728.
104. Taieb A, Hehunstre JP, Goetz J, et al. Lupus erythematosus panniculitits with partial deficiency of C2 and C4 in child. *Arch Derm* 1986;122:576–582.
105. Burrows NP, Walport MJ, Hammond AH, et al. Lupus erythe-

matosus profundus with partial C4 deficiency responding to thalidomide. *Br J Dermatol* 1991;125:62–67.
106. Nousari HC, Kimyai-Asadi A, Provost TT. Generalized lupus erythematosus profundus in a patient with genetic partial deficiency of C4. *J Am Acad Dermatol* 1999;41:362–364.
107. Gallego H, Crutchfield CE, Lewis EJ, et al. Report of an association between discoid lupus erythematosus and smoking. *Cutis* 1999;63:231–234.
108. Rahman P, Gladman DD, Urowitz MB. Smoking interferes with efficacy of antimalarial therapy in cutaneous lupus. *J Rheumatol* 1998;25:1716–1719.
109. Jewell M, McCauliffe DP. Cutaneous lupus erythematosus patients that smoke are less responsive to antimalarial treatment. *J Am Acad Dermatol* 2000;42:983–987.
110. Barnett JH. Discoid lupus erythematosus exacerbated by contact dermatitis. *Cutis* 1990;46:430–432.
111. Temesvari E, Horvath A, Kramer M, et al. Isomorphic skin reaction with DCNB in SLE and DLE. *Contact Dermatitis* 1979;5:85–89.
112. Abdel-Aal H, Abdel-Aal MA. Koebner phenomenon and unusual manifestation of discoid lupus erythematosus. *J Egypt Med Assoc* 1972;55:704–708.
113. Norden D, Weinberg J, Schumacher HR, et al. Bilateral periorbital edema in systemic lupus erythematosus. *J Rheumatol* 1993;20:2158–2160.
114. McHugh NJ, Maddison PJ, MacCleod TIF, et al. Papular lesions and cutaneous lupus erythematosus: a comparative clinical and histological study using monoclonal antibodies. *J Rheumatol* 1988;15:1097–1103.
115. Gilliam JN, Sontheimer RD. Subacute cutaneous lupus erythematosus. *Clin Rheumat Dis* 1982;8:343–352.
116. Su WP, Alegre VA. Bullous lesions in cutaneous lupus erythematosus. *Chang Keng I Hsueh* 1991;14:15–21.
117. Manganoni Am, Facchetti F, Pasolini G, et al. Guess What? Lupus erythematosus gyratum repens. *Eur J Dermatol* 1994;4:63–64.
118. Bangert JL, Freeman RG, Sontheimer RD, et al. Subacute cutaneous lupus erythematosus and discoid lupus erythematosus. Comparative histopathologic findings. *Arch Dermatol* 1984;120:332–337.
119. Hymes SR, Russell TJ, Jordon RE. The anti-Ro antibody system. *Int J Dermatol* 1986;25:1–7.
120. Shou-yi S, Shu-fang F, Kang-huang L, et al. Clinical study of 30 cases of subacute cutaneous lupus erythematosus. *Chin Med J* 1987;100:45–48.
121. Sontheimer RD. Subacute cutaneous lupus erythematosus. *Clin Dermatol* 1985;3:58–68.
122. Beilsa I, Herrero C, Font J, et al. Lupus erythematosus and toxic epidermal necrolysis. J Am Acad Dermatol 1987;16:1265–1267.
123. Bielsa I, Herrero C, Font J, et al. Lupus erythematosus and toxic epidermal necrolysis. *J Am Acad Dermatol* 1987;16:1265–1267.
124. DeSpain J, Clark DP. Subacute cutaneous lupus erythematosus presenting aserythroderma. *J Am Acad Dermatol* 1988;19:388–392.
125. Scheinman PL. Acral subacute cutaneous lupus erythematosus: an unusual variant. *J Am Acad Dermatol* 1994;30:800–801.
126. Pramatarov K, Vassileva S, Miteva L. Subacute cutaneous lupus erythematosus presenting with generalized poikiloderma. *J Am Acad Dermatol* 2000;42:286–288.
127. Rao BK, Coldiron B, Freeman RG, et al. Subacute cutaneous lupus erythematosus lesions progressing to morphea. *J Am Acad Dermatol* 1990;23:1019–1022.
128. Callen JP, Klein J. Subacute cutaneous lupus erythematosus. Clinical, serologic, immunogenetic, and therapeutic considerations in 72 patients. *Arthritis Rheum* 1988;31:1007–1013.
129. Sanchez-Perez J, Fernandez-Herrera J, Sols M, et al. Leucocytoclastic vasculitis in subacute cutaneous lupus erythematosus. *Br J Dermatol* 1993;128:469–470.
130. Rao BK, Coldiron BM, Freeman RF, et al. Subacute cutaneous lupus erythematosus lesions progressing to morphea. *J Am Acad Dermatol* 1990;23:1019–1022.
131. Marzano AV, Kolesnikova LV, Gasparini G, et al. Dystrophic calcinosis cutis in subacute cutaneous lupus. *Dermatology* 1999;198:90–92.
132. Cohen LM, Tyring SK, Rády P, et al. Human papillomavirus type II in multiple squamous cell carcinomas in a patient with subacute cutaneous lupus erythematosus. *J Am Acad Dermatol* 1992;26(suppl):840–845.
133. George R, Mathai R, Kurian S. Cutaneous lupus erythematosus in India: immunofluorescence profile. *Int J Dermatol* 1992;31:265–269.
134. Prystowsky SD, Herndon JH, Gilliam JN. Chronic cutaneous lupus erythematosus (DLE): a clinical and laboratory investigation of 80 patients. *Medicine* 1975;55:183–191.
135. Wilson CL, Burge SM, Dean D, et al. Scarring alopecia in discoid lupus erythematosus. *Br J Dermatol* 1992;126:307–314.
136. Parrish LC, Kennedy RJ, Hurley HJ. Palmar lesions in lupus erythematosus. *Arch Dermatol* 1967;96:273–276.
137. Green JJ, Baker DJ. Linear childhood discoid lupus erythematosus following the lines of Blaschko: a case report with review of linear manifestations of lupus erythematosus. *Pediatr Dermatol* 1999;16:128–133.
138. Abe M, Ishikawa O, Miyachi Y. Linear cutaneous lupus erythematosus following the lines of Blaschko. *Br J Dermatol* 1998;139:307–310.
139. Bolognia JL, Orlow SJGA. Lines of Blaschoko. *J Am Acad Dermatol* 1994;31:157–190.
140. Nived O, Johansen PB, Sturfelt G. Standardized ultraviolet-A exposure provokes skin reaction in systemic lupus erythematosus. *Lupus* 1993;2:247–250.
141. Kanwar J, Dhar S, Ghosh S. Involvement of nails in discoid lupus erythematosus. *J Assoc Physicians India* 1993;41:543.
142. Uitto J, Santa-Cruz DJ, Eisen AJ, et al. Verrucous lesions in patients with discoid lupus erythematosus: clinical, histopathological, and immunofluorescence studies. *Br J Dermatol* 1978;98:507–520.
143. Perniciaro C, Randle HW, Perry HO. Hypertrophic discoid lupus erythematosus resembling squamous cell carcinoma. *Dermatol Surg* 1995;21:255–257.
144. Caruso WR, Stewart ML, Nanda VK, et al. Squamous cell carcinoma of the skin in black patients with discoid lupus erythematosus. *J Rheumatol* 1987;14:156–159.
145. Sulisa VI, Kao GF. Squamous-cell carcinoma of the scalp arising in lesions of discoid lupus erythematosus. *Am J Dermatopath* 1988;10:137–141.
146. Camisa C. Lichen planus and related conditions. *Adv Dermatol* 1987;2:47–69.
147. Winkelmann RK, Peters MS. Lupus panniculitis. *Dermatol Update* 1982;135.
148. Irgang S. Lupus erythematosus profundus. Report of an example with clinical resemblance to Darier-Roussy sarcoid. *Arch Dermat & Syph* 1940;42:97–108.
149. Tuffanelli DL. Lupus erythematosus panniculitis (profundus). Clinical and immunological studies. *Arch Dermatol* 1971;103:231–242.
150. Tuffanelli DL. Lupus erythematosus. *Arch Dermatol* 1972;106:553–566.
151. Jordan DR, McDonald H, Olberg B, et al. Orbital panniculitis as the initial manifestation of systemic lupus erythematosus. *Opht Plast Reconst Surg* 1993;9:71–75.
152. Nowinski T, Bernardino V, Naidoff M, et al. Ocular involve-

ment in lupus erythematosus profundus (panniculitis). *Ophthalmology* 1982;1149–1154.
153. Tada J, Arata J, Katayama H. Linear lupus erythematosus profundus in a child. *J Am Acad Dermatol* 1991;24:871–874.
154. Harris RB, Winkelmann RK. Lupus mastitis. *Arch Dermatol* 1978;114:410–412.
155. Tuffanelli DL, Dubois EL. Cutaneous manifestations of systemic lupus erythematosus. *Arch Dermatol* 1964;90:377–386.
156. Burge SM, Frith PA, Juniper RP, et al. Mucosal involvement in systemic and chronic cutaneous lupus erythematosus. *Br J Dermatol* 1989;121:727–741.
157. Andreasen JO, Poulsen HE. Oral discoid and systemic lupus erythematosus. I. Clinical Investigation. *Acta Odont Scand* 1964;22:295–310.
158. Vachtenheim J, Grossman J. Perforation of the nasal septum in systemic lupus erythematosus. *Br Med J* 1969;2:98.
159. Robson AK, Burge SM, Millard PR. Nasal mucosal involvement in lupus erythematosus. *Clin Otolaryngol* 1992;17: 341–343.
160. Bettis VM, Vaughn RY, Guill MA. Erythematous plaques on the eyelids. Discoid lupus erythematosus (DLE). *Arch Dermatol* 1993;129:497–500.
161. Raizman NB, Baum J. Discoid lupus keratitis. *Arch Ophthalmol* 1989;107:545–547.
162. Doutre MS, Beylot C, Beylot J, et al. Chilblain lupus erythematosus: report of 15 cases [see comments]. *Dermatology* 1992; 184:26–28.
163. James DG. Sarcoidosis of the skin. In: Fitzpatrick TB, Eisen AZ, Wolff K, et al., eds. *Dermatology and general medicine.* New York: McGraw Hill Book Company, 1987.
164. Franceschini F, Calzavara-Pinton P, Quinzanini M, et al. Chilblain lupus erythematosus is associated with antibodies to SSA/Ro. *Lupus* 1998;8:215–219.
165. Brown CW, Deg JS. Thiazide diureteics induce cutaneous lupus-like adverse reaction. *J Toxicol Clin Toxicol* 1995;33: 729–733.
166. Ruiz H, Sanchez JL. Tumid lupus erythematosus. *Am J Dermatopathol* 1999;21:356–360.
167. Dekle CL, Mannes KD, Davis LS, et al. Lupus tumidus. *J Am Acad Dermatol* 1999;41:250–253.
168. Braverman IM. Cutaneous signs of systemic disease. *Medical Times* 1977;105:82–95.
169. Wan IC, Ki CC, Il SJ. Lupus tumidus involving facial skin, nasal cavity, throat and eye (with 1 color plate). *Dermatologica* 1983;166:38–39.
170. Lee LA, David KM. Cutaneous lupus erythematosus. *Curr Probl Dermatol* 1989;1:161–200.
171. Callen JP. Chronic cutaneous lupus erythematosus: clinical, laboratory, therapeutic, and prognostic examination of 62 patients. *Arch Dermatol* 1982;118:412–416.
172. Yell JA, Mbuagbaw J, Burge SM. Cutaneous manifestations of systemic lupus erythematosus. *Brit J Dermatol* 1996;135: 355–362.
173. Makhoul E, Abadjian G, Bendaly-Halaby E, et al. [Tuberculous lupus. Apropos of a case of tuberculous lupus tumidus]. *J Med Libanais—Lebanese Med J* 1997;45:43–45.
174. Kind P, Goetz G. Klinik und differential diagnose des cutanen lupus erythematodes. *Z Hautkr* 1987;62:1337–1347.
175. Gudmundsen K, Otridge B, Murphy GM. Fulminant fatal lupus erythematosus. *Br J Dermatol* 1992;126:303–304.
176. Sontheimer RD. Clinical significance of subacute cutaneous lupus erythematosus skin lesions. *J Dermatol* 1985;12:205–212.
177. Callen JP, Kulick KB, Stelzer G, et al. Subacute cutenaous lupus erythematosus. Clinical, serologic, and immunogenetic studies of 49 patients seen in a non-referral seting. *J Am Acad Dermatol* 1986;15:1227–1237. 178. Katayama I, Yamamoto T, Otoyama K, et al. Clinical and immunological analysis of annular erythema associated with Sjögren's syndrome. *Dermatology* 1994; 189(suppl 1):14–17.
179. Cohen S, Stastny P, Sontheimer RD. Concurrence of subacute cutaneous lupus erythematosus and rheumatoid arthritis. *Arthritis Rheum* 1986;29:421–425.
180. Boire G, Menard HA. Clinical significance of anti-Ro(SSA) antibody in rheumatoid arthritis. *J Rheumatol* 1988;15: 391–394.
181. Ilan Y, Ben Yehuda A. Subacute cutaneous lupus associated with Hashimoto's thyroiditis. *Neth J Med* 1991;39:105–107.
182. Brenner S, Golan H, Gat A, et al. Paraneoplastic subacute cutanelus lupus erythematosus—report of a case associated with cancer of the lung. *Dermatology* 1997;194:172–174.
183. Castanet J, Taillan B, Lacour JP, et al. Subacute cutaneous lupus erythematosus associated with Hodgkin's disease. *Clin Rheumatol* 1995;14:692–694.
184. McKenna KE, Hayes D, McMillan JC. Subacute cutaneous lupus erythematosus-like gyrate erythema and hypertrichosis lanuginosa acquisita associated with uterine adenocarcinoma. *Br J Dermatol* 1992;127:443–444.
185. Levenstein MM, Fisher BK, Fisher LL, et al. Simultaneous occurrence of subacute cutaneous lupus erythematosus and Sweet's syndrome. A marker of Sjogren's syndrome? *Int J Dermatol* 1991;30:640–643.
186. Callen JP, Ross L. Subacue cutaneous lupus erythematosus and porphyria cutanea tarda. Report of a case. *J Am Acad Dermatol* 1981;5:269–273.
187. Messenger AG, Church RE. Subacute cutaneous lupus erythematosus and malabsorption. *Br J Dermatol* 1986;115(suppl 30): 56–57.
188. Ashworth J. Subacute cutaneous lupus erythematosus in a patient with Crohn's disease. *Clin Exp Dermatol* 1992;17:135–136.
189. Ganor S, Sagagen F. Systemic lupus erythematosus changing to the chronic discoid type. *Dermatologica* 1962;125:81-92.
190. Tebbe B, Mansmann U, Wollina U, et al. Markers in cutaneous lupus erythematosus indicating systemic involvement—a multicenter study on 296 patients. *Acta Dermato-Venereologica* 1997;77:305–308.
191. Blum C, Zillikens D, Tony HP, et al. Soluble interleukin 2 receptor as activity parameter in serum of systemic and discoid lupus erythematosus. *Hautarzt* 1993;44:290–295.
192. Prystowsky SD, Gilliam JN. Discoid lupus erythematosus as part of a larger disease spectrum. Correlation of clinical features with laboratory findings in lupus erythematosus. *Arch Dermatol* 1975;111:1448–1452.
193. Spann CR, Callen JP, Klein JB, et al. Clinical, serological and immunogenetic studies in patients with chronic cutaneous (discoid) lupus erythematosus who have verucous and/or hypertrophic skin lesions. *J Rheumatol* 1988;15:256–261.
194. Martens PB, Moder KG, Ahmed I. Lupus panniculitis: clinical perspectives from a case series. *J Rheumatol* 1999;26:68–72.
195. Watanabe T, Tsuchida T. Lupus erythematosus profundus: a cutaneous marker for a distinct subset? *Br J Dermatol* 1996; 134:123–125.
196. Burnham TK, Fine G. The immunofluorescence "band" test for lupus erythematosus. I. Morphologic variations of localized immunoglobulins at the dermal-epidermal junction in lupus erythematosus. *Arch Dermatol* 1969;99:413–420.
197. Dahl MV, Gilliam JN. Direct immunofluorescence in lupus erythematosus. In: Beutner EH, Chorzelski TP, Kumar V, eds. *Immunopathology of the skin.* New York: John Wiley and Sons, 1987.
198. Cormane RH. Band globulin in the skin of patients withchronic discoid lupus erythematosus and systemic lupus erythematosus. *Lancet* 1964;1:534–535.

199. Weigand DA. Cutaneous immunofluorescence. *Med Clin North Am* 1989;73:1263–1274.
200. Dahl MV. Lupus erythematosus and systemic sclerosis. In: Dahl MV, ed. *Clinical immunodermatology*. Boca Raton, FL: Yearbook Medical Publishers, Inc., 1988.
201. Helm KF, Peters MS. Deposition of membrane attack complex in cutaneous lesions of lupus erythematosus. *J Am Acad Dermatol* 1993;28:687–691.
202. Burnham TK, Mohr RH. *Atlas of Diagnostic Immunofluorescence. Descriptive Morphology and Diagnostic Significance of Direct and Indirect Cutaneous Immunofluorescence of the Nuclear Immunofluorescent Patterns. 1st ed.* Evanston, IL: American Academy of Dermatology, 1991.
203. Ueki H, Wolf HH, Braun-Falco O. Cutaneous localization of human globulins in lupus erythematosus. Electron microscopy study using the peroxidase-labeled antibody technique. *Arch Dermatol Res* 1974;248:297–314.
204. Fabre VC, Lear S, Reichlin M, et al. Twenty percent of biopsy specimens from sun-exposed skin of normal young adults demonstrates positive immunofluorescence. *Arch Dermatol* 1991;127:1006–1111.
205. Brown C, Lieu T-S, Sontheimer RD. Correlation between dermal interstitial immunoglobulin G and hypergammaglobulinemia. *J Invest Dermatol* 1991;97:373–377.
206. Velthuis PJ, Kater L, Van der Tweel I, et al. Immunofluorescence microscopy of healthy skin from patients with systemic lupus erythematosus: more than just the lupus band. *Ann Rheum Dis* 1992;51:720–725.
207. Carvalho MF, Coelho RA. Lupus band test: diagnostic value in disseminated lupus erythematosus (Portuguese). *Acta Medica Portuguesa* 1991;4:242–248.
208. Pennebaker JB, Gilliam JN, Ziff M. Immunoglobulin classes of DNA binding activity in serum and skin in systemic lupus erythematosus. *J Clin Invest* 1977;60:1331–1338.
209. Davis BM, Gilliam JN. Prognostic significance of subepidermal immune deposits in uninvolved skin of patients with systemic lupus erythematosus: a 10-year longitudinal study. *J Invest Dermatol* 1984;83:242–247.
210. Pohle EL, Tuffanelli DL. Study of cutaneous lupus erythematosus by immunohistochemical methods. *Arch Dermatol* 1968;97:520–526.
211. Herrero C, Bielsa I, Font J, et al. Subacute cutaneous lupus erythematosus: clinical pathologic findings in 13 cases. *J Am Acad Dermatol* 1988;19:1057–1062.
212. Bielsa I, Herrero C, Collado A, et al. Histopathologic findings in cutaneous lupus erythematosus. *Arch Dermatol* 1994;130:54–58.
213. Hood AF, Jerden MS, Moore W, et al. Histopathologic comparison of the subsets of lupus erythematosus. *Arch Dermatol* 1990;126:52–55.
214. Nieboer C, Tak-Diamand Z, VanLeeuwen-Wallau AG. Dust-like particles: a specific direct immunofluorescence pattern in subacute cutaneous lupus erythematosus. *Br J Dermatol* 1988;118:725–734.
215. Valeski JE, Kumar V, Forman AB, et al. A characteristic cutaneous direct immunofluorescent pattern associated with Ro(SS-A) antibodies in subacute cutaneous lupus erythematosus. *J Am Acad Dermatol* 1992;27:194–198.
216. Lipsker D, Dicesare MP, Cribier D, et al. The significance of the 'dust-like particles' pattern of immunofluorescence. *Br J Dermatol* 1998;138:1039–1042.
217. Lee LA, Gaither Kg, Coulter SN, et al. The pattern of cutaneous immunoglobulin G deposition in subacute cutaneous lupus erythematosus is reproduced by infusing purified anti-Ro(SSA) antibodies into human skin grafted mice. *J Clin Invest* 1989;83:1556–1563.
218. Weigand DA. Lupus band test: anatomically regional variations in discoid lupus erythematosus. *J Am Acad Dermatol* 1986;14:426–428.
219. Dahl MV. Usefulness of direct immunofluorescence in patients with lupus erythematosus. *Arch Dermatol* 1983;119:1010–1017.
220. Sanchez NP, Peters MS, Winkelman RK. The histopathology of lupus erythematosus panniculitis. *J Am Acad Dermatol* 1981;5:673–680.
221. Schiodt M. Oral discoid lupus erythematosus. III. A histopathologic study of sixty-six patients. *Oral Surg* 1984;57:281–293.
222. Lee LA, Roberts CM, Frank MB, et al. The autoantibody response to Ro/SSA in cutaneous lupus erythematosus. *Arch Dermatol* 1994;130:1262–1268.
223. Johansson-Stephansson E, Koskimes S, Partanen J, et al. Subacute cutaneous lupus erythematosus: Genetic markers and clinical and immunological findings in patients. *Arch Dermatol* 1989;125:791–796.
224. Fonseca E, Alvarez R, Gonzalez MR, et al. Prevalence of anticardiolipin antibodies in subacute cutaneous lupus erythematosus. *Lupus* 1992;1:265–268.
225. Marschalko M, Dobozy E, Daroczy J, et al. Subacute cutaneous lupus erythematosus: a study of 15 cases. *Orvosi Hetilap* 1989;130:2623–2628.
226. Konstadoulakis MM, Kroubouzos G, Tosca A, et al. Thyroid autoantibodies in the subsets of lupus erythematosus: correlation with other autoantibodies and thyroid function. *Thyroidol Clin Exp* 1993;5:1–7.
227. Holtman JH, Neustadt DH, Klein J, et al. Dapsone is an effective therapy for the skin lesions of subacute cutaneous lupus erythematosus and urticarial vasculitis in a patient with C2 deficiency. *J Rheumatol* 1990;17:1222–1225.
228. Callen JP, Fowler JF, Kulick KB. Serologic and clinical features of patients with discoid lupus erythematosus: relationship of antibodies to single-stranded deoxyribonucleic acid and of other antinuclear antibody subsets to clinical manifestations. *J Am Acad Dermatol* 1985;13:748–755.
229. Provost TT, Ratrie H. Autoantibodies and autoantigens in lupus erythematosus and Sjögren's syndrome. *Curr Probl Dermatol* 1990;2:150–208.
230. Mayou SC, Wojnarowska F, Lovell CR, et al. Anticardiolipin and antinuclear antibodies in discoid lupus erythematosus—their clinical significance. *Clin Exp Dermatol* 1988;13:389–392.
231. Stonecipher MR, Callen JP, Jorizzo JL. The red face: dermatomyositis. *Clin Dermatol* 1993;11:261–273.
232. Jablonska S, Blaszczyk-Kostanecka M, Chorzelski T, et al. The red face: lupus erythematosus. *Clin Dermatol* 1993;11:253–260.
233. Boyd AS, Zemtsov A, Neldner KH. Pityriasis rubra pilaris presenting as subacute cutaneous lupus erythematosus. *Cutis* 1993;52:177–179.
234. Chen DY, Lan JL. Crusted scabies in systematic lupus erythematosus: a case report. *Chung Hua Min Kuo Wei Sheng Wu Chi Mien I Hsueh Tsa Chih [Chin J Microbiol Immunol Taipei]* 1993;26:44–50.
235. Tarlow JK, Clay FE, Cork MJ, et al. Severity of alopecia areata is associated with a polymorphism in the interleukin-1 receptor antagonist gene. *J Invest Dermatol* 1994;103:387–390.
236. Petzelbauer P, Binder M, Nikolakis P, et al. Severe sun sensitivity and the presence of antinuclear antibodies in patients with polymorphous light eruption-like lesions. A form fruste of photosensitive lupus erythematosus? *J Am Acad Dermatol* 1992;26:68–74.
237. Kiss M, Husz S, Dobozy A. The occurrence of antinuclear, anti-SSA/Ro and anti-SSB/La antibodies in patients with polymorphous light eruption. *Acta Derm Venereol* 1991;71:341–343.

238. Murphy GM, Hawk JLM. The prevalence of antinuclear antibodies in patients with apparent polymorphic light eruption. *Br J Dermatol* 1991;125:448–451.
239. Holzle E, Plewig G, von Kries R, et al. Polymorphous light eruption. *J Invest Dermatol* 1987;88:32S–38S.
240. Epstein JH. Polymorphous light eruption. *J Am Acad Dermatol* 1980;3:329–343.
241. Sehgal VN, Jain S, Jain VK. Lupus vulgaris simulating discoid lupus erythematosus. *Int J Dermatol* 1991;30:498–499.
242. Chung G, Kantor GR, Whipple S. Tertiary syphilis of the face. *J Am Acad Dermatol* 1991;24:832–835.
243. A randomized study of the effect of withdrawing hydroxychloroquine sulfate in systemic lupus erythematosus. Canadian Hydroxychloroquine Study Group. *N Engl J Med* 1991;324: 150–154.
244. Sontheimer RD. Lupus Erythematosus. In: Provost TT, Farmer ER, eds. *Current therapy in dermatology* Philadelphia: B.C. Decker, Inc., 1988:123–128.
245. Lowe NJ. Photoprotection. *Semin Dermatol* 1990;9:78–83.
246. Callen JP, Roth DE, McGrath C, et al. Safety and efficacy of a broad-spectrum sunscreen in patients with discoid or subacute cutaneous lupus erythematosus. *Cutis* 1991;47:130–132, 135–136.
247. Sontheimer RD. Fluorescent light photosensitivity in patients with systemic lupus erythematosus. *Arthritis Rheumat* 1993; 36:428–431.
248. Furner BB. Treatment of subacute cutaneous lupus erythematosus. *Int J Dermatol* 1990;29:542–547.
249. Lanham JG, Hughes GRV. Antimalarial therapy in SLE. *Clin Rheumat Disease* 1982;8:279–299.
250. Trenholme GM, Carson PE. Therapy and prophylaxis of malaria. *JAMA* 1978;240:2293–2295.
251. Wallace DJ. The use of quinacrine (Atabrine). In rheumatic diseases: a re-examination. *Sem Arth Rheum* 1989;18:282–297.
252. Feldmann R, Salomon D, Saurat J-H. The association of the two antimalarials chloroquine and quinacrine for treatment-resistant chronic and subacute cutaneous lupus erythematosus. *Dermatology* 1994;189:425–427.
253. Ruzicka T, Meurer M, Braun-Falco O. Treatment of cutaneous lupus erythematosus with etretinate. *Acta Derm Venereol (Stockh)* 1985;65:324–329.
254. Furner BB. Subacute cutaneous lupus erythematosus response to isotretinoin. *Int J Dermatol* 1990;29:587–590.
255. Green SG, Piette WW. Successful treatment of hypertrophic lupus erythematosus with isotretinoin. *J Am Acad Dermatol* 1987;17:364–368.
256. Crovato F. Clofazimine in the treatment of annular lupus erythematosus. *Arch Dermatol* 1981;117:249–250.
257. McDougall AC, Horsfall WR, Hede JE, et al. Splenic infarction and tissue accumulation of crystals associated with the use of clofazamine (Lamprene B663) in the treatment of pyoderma gangrenosus. *Br J Dermatol* 1980;102:227–230.
258. Stevens RJ, Andujar C, Edwards CJ, et al. Thalidomide in the teatment of cutaneous manifestations of lupus erythematosus —experience in sixteen consecutive patients. *Br J Rheumatol* 1997;36:353–359.
259. Georgala S, Katoulis AC, Hasapi V, et al. Thalidomide treatment for hypertrophic lupus erythematosus. *Clin Exp Dermatol* 1998;23:141.
260. Warren KJ, Nopper AJ, Crosby DL. Thalidomide for recalcitrant discoid lesions in a patient with systemic lupus erythematosus. *J Am Acad Dermatol* 1998;39:293–295.
261. Sato EI, Assis LS, Lourenzi VP, et al. Long-term thalidomide use in refractory cutaneous lesions of systemic lupus erythematosus. *Revista da Associacao Medica Brasileira* 1998;44: 289–293.
262. Ordi-Ros J, Cortes F, Cucurull E, et al. Thalidomide in the treatment of cutaneous lupus refractory to conventional therapy. *J Phycology* 2000;27:1429–1433.
263. Stevens RJ, Andujar C, Edwards CJ, et al. Thalidomide in the treatment of the cutaneous manifestations of lupus erythematosus: experience in sixteen consecutive patients. *Br J Rheumatol* 1997;36:353–359.
264. Holm AL, Bowers KE, McMeekin TO, et al. Chronic cutaneous lupus erythematosus treated with thalidomide. *Arch Dermatol* 1993;129:1548–1550.
265. Knopp J, Bonsmann G, Happle R, et al. Thalidomide in the treatment of sixty cases of chronic discoid lupus erythematosus. *Br J Dermatol* 1983;108:461–466.
266. Ochonisky S, Verroust J, Bastuji-Garin S, et al. Thalidomide neuropathy incidence and clinicoelectrophysiologic findings in 42 patients. *Arch Derm* 1994;130:66–69.
267. Ordi J, Cortes F, Martinez N, et al. Thalidomide induces amenorrhea in patients with lupus disease. *Arthritis Rheumat* 1998;41:2273–2275.
268. Dalziel K, Going G, Cartwright PH, et al. Treatment of chronic discoid lupus erythematosus with an oral gold compound (Auranofin). *Br J Dermatol* 1986;115:211–216.
269. Charley MR, Sontheimer RD. Clearing of subacute cutaneous lupus erythematosus around molluscum contagiosum lesions. *J Amer Acad Dermatol* 1982;6:529–533.
270. Nicolas J-F, Thivolet J, Kanitakis J, et al. Response of discoid and subacute cutaneous lupus erythematosus to recombinant interferon alpha 2a. *J Invest Dermatol* 1990;95:142S–145S.
271. Thivolet J, Nicolas JF, Kanitakis J, et al. Recombinant interferon 2a is effective in the treatment of discoid and subacute cutaneous lupus erythematosus. *Br J Dermatol* 1990;122: 405–409.
272. de Jong EM, van Erp PE, Ruiter DJ, et al. Immunohistochemical detection of proliferation and differentiation in discoid lupus erythematosus. *J Am Acad Dermatol* 1991;25:1032–1038.
273. Goldberg JW, Lidsky MD. Pulse methylprednisolone therapy for persistent subacute cutaneous lupus. *Arthritis Rheum* 1984;27:837–838.
274. Boehm IB, Boehm GA, Bauer R. Management of cutaneous lupus erythematosus with low-dose methotrexate: indication for modulation of inflammatory mechanisms. *Rheumatol Int* 1998;18:59–62.
275. Callen JP, Spencer LV, Bhatnagar Burruss J, et al. Azathioprine: an effective, corticosteroid-sparing therapy for patients with recalcitrant cutaneous lupus erythematosus or with recalcitrant cutaneous leukocytoclastic vasculitis. *Arch Dermatol* 1991;127: 515–522.
276. McGrath H, Jr., Bak E, Zimny ML, et al. Fluorescent light decreases autoimmunity and improves immunity in B/W mice. *J Clin Lab Immunol* 1990;32:113–116.
277. Sonnichsen N, Meffert H, Kunzelmann V, et al. UV-A-1 therapy of subacute cutaneous lupus erythematosus. *Hautarzt* 1993; 44:723–725.
278. Lehmann P, Holzle E, Kind P, et al. Experimental reproduction of skin lesions in lupus erythematosus by UVA and UVB radiation. *J Am Acad Dermatol* 1990;22:181–187.
279. Cai W, Werth VP. Differential effects of UVA1 and UVB on skin lesions at MRL/lpr lupus mice. *J Invest Dermatol* 2000; 114:884.
280. Miller LG. Cigarettes and drug therapy: pharmacokinetic and pharmacodynamic considerations. *Clin Pharm* 1990;9:125–135.
281. Callen JP. Treatment of cutaneous lesions in patients with lupus erythematosus. *Dermatol Clin* 1994;12:201–206.
282. Kossard S, Doherty E, McColl I, et al. Autofluorescence of clofazimine in discoid lupus erythematosus. *J Am Acad Dermatol* 1987;17:867–871.

283. Goldstein E, Carey W. Discoid lupus erythematosus: successful treatment with oral methotrexate. *Arch Dermatol* 1994;130: 938–939.
284. Boehm IB, Boehm GA, Bauer R. Management of cutaneous lupus erythematosus with low-dose methotrexate: indication for modulation of inflammatory mechanisms. *Rheumatol Int* 1998; 18:59–62.
285. Sorg C. Macrophages in acute and chronic inflammation. *Chest* 1991;100(suppl):173S–175S.
286. Irgang S. Lupus erythematosus profundus. Report of an example with clinical resemblance to Darier-Roussy sarcoid. *Arch Dermat Syph* 1940;42:98–108.
287. Pinski KS, Roenigk HH, Jr. Autologous fat transplantation. Long-term follow-up. *J Dermatol Surg Oncol* 1992;18:179–184.
288. Nguyen TQ, Black AA, Zappi E, et al. Subacute cutaneous lupus erythematosus: Interim analysis of a long term prospective follow-up study. *J Invest Dermatol* 1998;110:591. Abstract.
289. Chlebus E, Wolska H, Blaszczyk M, et al. Subacute cutaneous lupus erythematosus versus systemic lupus erythematosus—diagnostic criteria and therpeutic options. *J Am Acad Dermatol* 1998;38:405–412.
290. Parodi A, Caproni M, Cardinali C, et al. Clinical, histological and immunopathological features of 58 patients with subacute cutaneous lupus erythematosus—a review by the Italian Group of Immunodermatology leg ulcers in patients with myeloproliferative disorders: disease- or treatment-related? *Dermatology* 2000;200:6–10.
291. de Berker D, Dissaneyeka M, Burge S. The sequelae of chronic cutaneous lupus erythematosus. *Lupus* 1992;1:181–186.
292. Sherman RN, Lee CW, Flynn KJ. Cutaneous squamous cell carcinoma in black patients with chronic discoid lupus erythematosus. *Int J Dermatol* 1993;32:677–679.
293. Lehmann P, Holze E, Kind P, et al. Experimental reproductio of skin lesions in lupus erytehmatosus by UV-A and UV-B radiation. *J Am Acad Dermatol* 1990;22:181.
294. Wolska H, Blaszczyk M, Jablonska S. Phototests in patients with various forms of lupus erythematosus. *Int J Derm* 1989; 28:98–103.
295. Wysenbeek AJ, Leibovici L, Amit M, et al. Alopecia in systemic lupus erythematosus. Relation to disease manifestations. *J Rheumatol* 1991;18:1185–1186.
296. Wananukul S, Watana D, Pongprasit P. Cutaneous manifestations of childhood systemic lupus erythematosus. *Pediatr Dermatol* 1998;15:342–346.
297. Yell JA, Mbuagbaw J, Burge SM. Cutaneous manifestations of systemic lupus erythematosus. *Br J Dermatol* 1996;135: 355–362.
298. Werth VP, White WL, Sanchez MR, et al. Incidence of alopecia areata in lupus erythematosus. *Arch Dermatol* 1992;128:368–371.
299. Rothe M, Grant-Kels JM, Rothfield NF. Extensive calcinosis cutis with systemic lupus erythematosus. *Arch Dermatol* 1990; 126:1060.
300. Kabir JDI, Malkinson FD. Lupus erythematosus and calcinosis cutis. *Arch Dermatol* 1969;100:17–22.
301. Johansson E, Kanerva L, Niemi KM, et al. Diffuse soft tissue calcifications (calcinosis cutis) in a patient with discoid lupus erythematosus. *Clin Exp Dermatol* 1988;13:193–196.
302. Park YM, Lee SJ, Kang H, et al. Large subcutaneous calcification in systemic lupus erythematosus: treatment with oral aluminum hydroxide administration followed by surgical excision. *J Korean Med Sci* 1999;14:589–592.
303. Palmieri GM, Sebes JI, Aelion JA, et al. Treatment of calcinosis with diltiazem. *Arth Rheum* 1995;38:1646–1654.
304. Vereecken P, Stallenberg B, Tas S, et al. Ulcerated dystrophic calcinosis cutis secondary to localized linear scleroderma. *Int J Clin Pract* 1998;52:593–594.
305. Skuterud E, Sydnes OA, Haavik TK. Calcinosis in dermatomyositis treated with probenecid. *Scand J Rheumatol* 1981;10: 92–94.
306. Matsuoka Y, Miyajima S, Okada N. A case of calcinosis universalis successfully treated with low-dose warfarin. *J Dermatol* 1998;25:716–720.
307. Cousins MA, Jones DB, Whyte MP, et al. Surgical management of calcinosis cutis universalis in systemic lupus erythematosus. *Arthritis Rheum* 1997;40:570–572.
308. Nagy E, Balogh E. Bullous form of chronic discoid lupus erythematodes accompanied by LE cell symptoms. *Dermatologica* 1961;122:6–10.
309. Boh E, Roberts LJ, Lieu TS, et al. Epidermolysis bullosa acquisita preceding the development of systemic lupus erythematosus. *J Am Acad Dermatol* 1990;22:587–593.
310. Barton DD, Fine JD, Gammon WR, et al. Bullous systemic lupus erythematosus: an unusual clinical course and detectable circulating antibodies to the epidermolysis bullosa acquisita antigen. *J Am Acad Dermatol* 1986;16:369–373.
311. Boh E, Roberts LJ, Lieu T-S, et al. Epidermolysis bullosa acquisita preceding the development of systemic lupus erythematosus. *J Am Acad Dermatol* 1990;22:587–593.
312. Miller JF, Dawhan TF, Chapel TA. Co-existent bullous pemphigoid in systemic lupus erythematosus. *Cutis* 1985;21: 368–373.
313. Davies MG, Marks R, Waddington E. Simultaneous sysemic lupus erythematosus and dermatitis herpetiformis. *J Invest Dermatol* 1984;83:242–247.
314. Weatherhead L, Adam J. Discoid lupus erythematosus. Coexistence with porphyria cutanea tarda. *Int J Dermatol* 1985;24: 453–455.
315. Cruz PD, Jr., Coldiron BM, Sontheimer RD. Concurrent features of cutaneous lupus erythematosus and pemphigus erythematosus following myasthenia gravis and thymoma. *J Am Acad Dermatol* 1987;16:472–480.
316. Fowler JF, Callen JP. Cutaneous mucinosis associated with lupus erythematosus. *J Rheumatol* 1984;11:380–383.
317. Kano Y, Sagawa Y, Yagita A, et al. Nodular cutaneous lupus mucinosis: report of a case and review of previously reported cases. *Cutis* 1996;57:441–444.
318. Pandya AG, Sontheimer RD, Cockerell CJ, et al. Papulonodular mucinosis associated with systemic lupus erythematosus: possible mechanisms of increased glycosaminoglycan accumulation. *J Am Acad Dermatol* 1995;32:199–205.
319. Rongiolette F, Revora A. The new cutaneous mucinosis: a review with an up-to-date classification of cutaneous mucinosis. *J Am Acad Dermatol* 1991;24:265.
320. Maruyama M, Miyaychi S, Hashimoto K. Massive cutaneous mucinosis associated with systemic lupus erythematosus. *Br J Dermatol* 1997;137:450–453.
321. Williams WL, Ramos-Caro FA. Acute periorbital mucinosis in discoid lupus erythematosus. *J Am Acad Dermatol* 1999;41: 871–873.
322. Egawa H, Abe-Matsuura Y, Tada J, et al. Nodular cutaneous lupus mucinosis associated with atrophie blanchelike lesions in a patient with systemic lupus erythematosus. *J Dermatol* 1994; 21:674–679.
323. Kanda N, Tsuchida T, Watanabe T, et al. Cutaneous lupus mucinosis: a review of our cases and the possible pathogenesis. *J Cutan Pathol* 1997;24:553–558.
324. Jou IM, Liu MF, Chao SC. Widespread cutaneous necrosis associated with antiphospholipid syndrome. *Clin Rheumatol* 1996;15:394–398.
325. Gibson GE, Su WP, Pittelkow MR. Antiphospholipid syndrome and the skin. *J Am Acad Dermatol* 1997;36:970–982.
326. Urman JD, Lowenstein MB, Abeles M, et al. Oral mucosal

ulceration in systemic lupus erythematosus. *Arthritis Rheumat* 1978;21:58–62.
327. Jonsson R, Heyden G, Westberg NG. Oral mucosal lesions in systemic lupus erythematosus: a clinical, histopthological and immunopathological study. *J Rheumatol* 1984;11:38–42.
328. Urowitz MB, Gladman DD, Chalmers A, et al. Nail lesions in systemic lupus erythematosus. *J Rheumatol* 1978;5:551–557.
329. Vaughn RY, Bailey JP, Jr., Field RS, et al. Diffuse nail dyschromia in black patients with systemic lupus erythematosus. *J Rheumatol* 1990;17:640–643.
330. Garcia-Pathos V, Bartralot R, Ordi J, et al. Systemic lupus erythematosus presenting with red lunulae. *J Am Acad Dermatol* 1997;36:834–836.
331. Wollina U, Barta U, Uhlemann C, et al. Lupus erythematosus-associated red lunula. *J Am Acad Dermatol* 1999;419–421.
332. Kamitani T, Nguyen HP, Kito K, et al. Covalent modification of PML by the sentrin family of ubiquitin-like proteins. *J Biol Chem* 1998;273:117–120.
333. Sontheimer RD, Houpt KR. DIDMOHS—a proposed standardized nomenclature for the drug-induced delayed multiorgan hypersensitivity syndrome. *Arch Dermatol* 1998;134:874–875.
334. Bocquet H, Roujeau JC. Severe drug-induced skin reactions [French]. *Revue Francaise d Allergologie et d Immunologie Clinique* 1997;37:651–659.
335. Senet P, Aractingi S, Porneuf M, et al. Hydroxyurea-induced dermatomyositis-like eruption. *Br J Dermatol* 1995;133:455–459.
336. Dauod MS, Gibson LE, Pittelkow MR. Hydroxyurea dermopathy: a unique lichenoid eruption complication long-term therapy with hydroxyurea. *J Am Acad Dermatol* 1997;36:178–182.
337. Callen JP. Discoid lupus erythematosus—variants and clinical associations. *Lupus Erythematosus*. Philadelphia: J.P. Lippincott, 1985.
338. Grabbe S, Kolde G. Coexisting lichen planus and subacute cutaneous lupus erythematosus. *Clin Exp Dermatol* 1995;20:249–254.
339. VanDerHorst JC, Cirkel PKS, Niebore C. Mixed lichen planus —lupus erythematosus disease—a distinct entity? Clinical, histopathological, and immunopathological studies in 6 patients. *Clin Exp Dermatol* 1983;8:631–640.
340. Baird JS, Johnson JL, Elliot-Mills D, et al. Systemic lupus erythematosus with acanthosis nigricans, hyperpigmentation, and insulin receptor antibody. *Lupus* 1997;6:275–278.
341. Tuffanelli DL. Acanthosis nigricans with lupoid hepatitis. *JAMA* 1964;189:584–585.

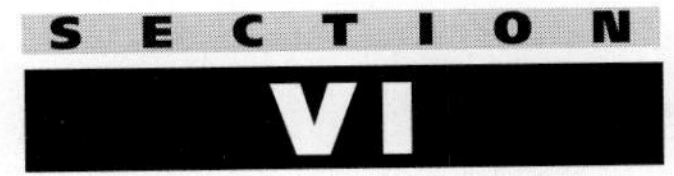

CLINICAL AND LABORATORY FEATURES

30

THE CLINICAL PRESENTATION OF SYSTEMIC LUPUS ERYTHEMATOSUS

DANIEL J. WALLACE

Before the description of the lupus erythematosus (LE) cell by Hargraves et al. (1) in 1948, systemic lupus erythematosus (SLE) was considered to be a rare, fulminant disease occurring in young women, with classic rash and a fatal termination in months. The illness now is conceptualized as a chronic disorder of a pleomorphic nature. No classic pattern exists, and the diagnosis must be based on an overall view of the clinical picture with the aid of serologic and laboratory studies and, if required, biopsies or other diagnostic procedures. The typical case, with the classic butterfly-area eruption, is seen only occasionally. This chapter presents an overview of the clinical presentation of SLE; the following chapters detail its involvement in various organ systems.

HISTORY

The most important part of the examination of a patient who is suspected of having this disorder is the history; it must be obtained in painstaking detail, along with a review of systems. Earlier, seemingly unimportant events often provide clues to the correct diagnosis. It is best to take a chronologic history of all possible pertinent events and to carry out a complete systems review. The family history also is important, because between 10% and 20% of patients have a relative, from first cousin to grandparent, with SLE (2, 3).

All of the items in Table 30.1 and Figure 30.1 should be covered. The physician should inquire specifically about the effects of sun exposure on the patient's skin and their general sense of well being. Other important questions concern hair loss, fracturing of frontal hair, positive serologic tests for syphilis, seizures, blood clots, miscarriage(s), adenopathy, dry eyes or mouth, anemia, leukopenia, thrombocytopenia, pleuritis, pleural effusion, pericarditis, myalgia and arthralgia with or without overt joint swelling, diffuse puffiness of the hands without localization to joints, Raynaud's phenomenon, and leg ulcers.

The transitory nature of the polyarthralgia and arthritis during the early phases of SLE should be emphasized. Patients frequently complain of morning stiffness, with diffuse puffiness of the fingers and dorsa of the hands. These conditions may subside 10 minutes to several hours after awakening. Fleeting pains may be present in both joints and muscles. At the time of physical examination, which usually is later in the day, no objective abnormalities are seen. Early in the course of the disease, antinuclear antibody (ANA) may be positive, although the sedimentation rate and other routine laboratory tests may be normal. Consequently, it is important that SLE be considered in equivocal cases, and that further studies be performed. (Caution must be exercised in interpreting previously positive ANA tests. The test is performed on various substrates and is positive in low titers for 2% to 5% of healthy persons, especially in older individuals.) Difficulties in early diagnosis were summarized in a review of 40 cases (4), in which patients presented problems in the diagnosis of migratory polyarthralgia, functional illness, or mild illness with nonspecific, systemic symptoms. (See Chapter 46, Differential Diagnosis and Disease Associations, for a detailed discussion of the differential diagnosis.)

It sometimes is useful to have patients fill out a detailed medical-history questionnaire during their first visit, which should take less than 30 minutes to complete. This allows detection of subtle pyschosocial or sensitive issues that otherwise would not be found. Having patients write down what bothers them, in their own words, can be revealing. Filling out a questionnaire also decreases the possibility that important information might be inadvertently omitted.

CHIEF COMPLAINT

Many variations are seen in the presenting complaint that brings a patient to the physician. Diagnosis is rendered difficult by the protean manifestations of the disease. The

TABLE 30.1. CUMULATIVE PERCENTAGE INCIDENCE OF SLE MANIFESTATIONS

Manifestations	Harvey et al. (49) 1954 (105 cases)	Dubois and Tuffanelli (50) 1964 (520 cases)	Estes and Christian (67) 1971 (140 cases)	Fries and Holman (39) 1977 (193 cases)	Hochberg et al. (14) 1985 (150 cases)	Pistiner et al. (3) 1991 (464 cases)	Eurolupus (62) 1992 (704 cases)	Jacobsen et al. (45) 1998 (513 cases)
I. Systemic Sx								
A. Fever	86	84	—	55	—	41	52	
B. Weight loss	71	51	—	31	—	—	—	
II. Musculoskeletal								
A. Arthritis and arthralgia	90	92	95	53	76	91	84	67
B. Subcutaneous nodules	10	5	11	—	12	—	—	
C. Myalgias	—	48	—	42	—	79	—	
D. Aseptic bone necrosis	—	5	—	—	24	5	—	
III. Cardiorespiratory								
A. Cardiomegaly	15	16	—	10	—	—	—	
B. Pericarditis	45	31	19	6	23	2	—	20
C. Myocarditis	40	8	8	—	—	12	—	3
D. Cardiac failure	8	5	11	—	—	3	—	
E. Systolic heart murmur	44	20	—	38	—	12	—	
F. Diastolic heart murmur	—	1	—	2	—	1	—	
G. Libman-Sacks valvulitis	32	—	—	—	—	1	—	3
H. Hypertension	14	25	46	—	—	25	—	23
I. Pleurisy	56	45	48	41	57	31	—	31
J. Plural effusion	16	30	40	16	—	12	—	
K. Lupus pneumonia	22	1	9	—	—	6	—	8
IV. Cutaneous-vascular								
A. Skin lesions, all types	85	72	81	67	—	55	—	
B. Butterfly area lesions	39	57	39	10	61	34	58	48
C. Alopecia	3	21	39	45	45	31	—	23
D. Oral/nasal ulcers	14	9	7	18	23	19	24	11
E. Photosensitivity	11	33	—	—	45	37	45	43
F. Urticaria	7	7	13	—	—	4	—	
G. Raynaud's	10	18	21	17	44	25	34	32
H. Discoid lesions	—	29	9	10	15	23	10	14
V. Nervous system								
A. CNS damage, all types	—	26	59	—	39	—	27	13
B. Peripheral neuritis	—	12	7	—	21	5	—	6
C. Psychosis	19	12	37	—	16	5	—	6
D. Seizures	17	14	26	8	13	6	—	9
VI. Ocular lesions								
A. Cytoid bodies	24	10	—	—	—	4	—	
B. Uveitis	—	1	—	2	—	1	—	
VII. Genitourinary								
A. Proteinuria/abnormal sediment	65	46	53	47	—	31	39	45
B. Nephrotic syndrome	—	23	26	—	13	14	—	
VIII. Gastrointestinal								
A. Dysphagia	6	2	—	—	—	8	—	
B. Severe nausea	14	53	—	36	—	7	—	
C. Diarrhea	8	6	—	25	—	8	—	
D. Ascites	—	11	9	—	—	—	—	
E. Abdominal pain	10	19	16	34	—	8	—	
F. Bowel hemorrhage	5	6	—	6	—	1	—	
IX. Hemic-lymphatic								
A. Adenopathy	34	59	36	23	—	10	12	
B. Anemia (<11 g)	78	57	73	38	57	30	—	
C. Hemolytic anemia	—	—	12	—	8	8	8	
D. Leukopenia (<4,500)	—	43	66	35	41	51	—	42
E. Thrombocytopenia (<100,000)	26	7	19	—	30	16	22	24
X. Serologic								
A. Hypoalbuminemia	58	32	77	—	30	—	—	
B. False + VDRL	15	11	29	—	26	—	—	10
C. ⊕ LE PREP	82	82	78	—	71	42	—	62
D. ⊕ ANA	—	—	87	95	—	96	96	98
E. Low C3	—	—	—	40	59	39	—	87
F. ⊕ Anti-DNA	—	—	—	39	28	40	78	7
G. ⊕ Anti-Sm	—	—	—	26	17	6	10	
H. ⊕ Anti-SSA (Ro)	—	—	—	—	32	19	25	
I. ⊕ Anti-RNP	—	—	—	—	34	14	13	
J. ⊕ Anticardiolipin	—	—	—	—	—	38	—	

CNS, Central nervous system; VDRL, Venereal disease research laboratory (a syphilis test).

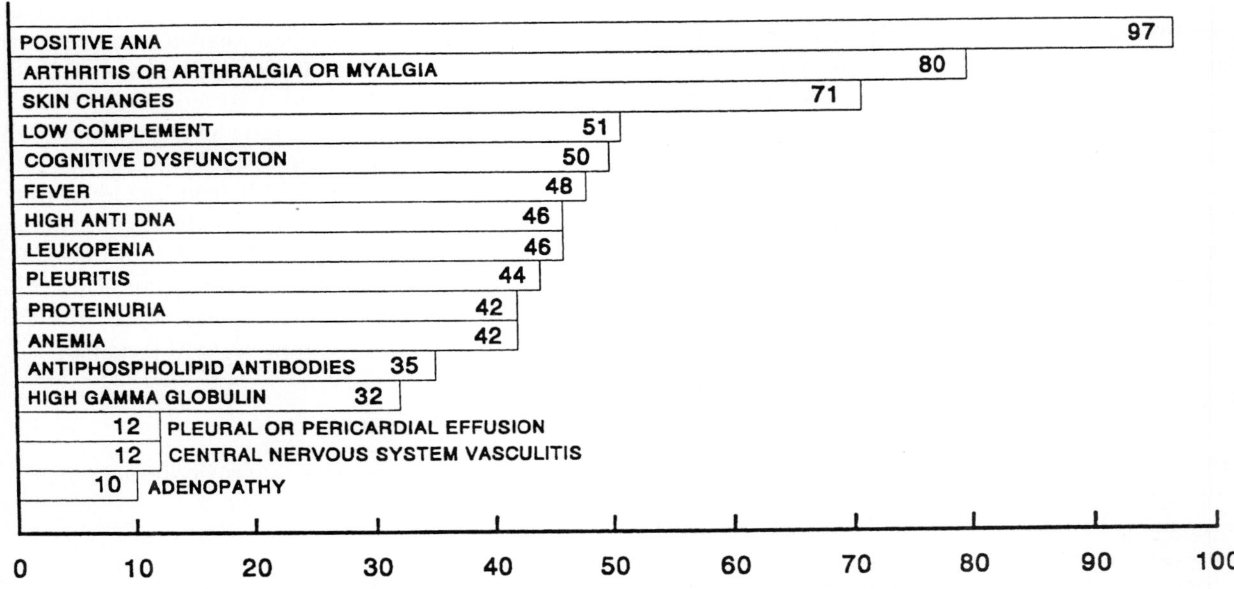

FIGURE 30.1. Cumulative percentage incidence of 16 clinical and laboratory manifestations of systemic lupus erythematosus, based on approximately 2,000 patients evaluated in seven studies since 1975.

classic presentation of butterfly rash and arthritis in a young woman occurs in a minority of patients. Initially, any system may be affected and heal; months or years later, the same or another system may become involved. Table 30.2 lists the chief complaints noted at the initial diagnosis of SLE in several large studies. The two major areas of involvement are joint and cutaneous systems, followed by the nonspecific complaints of fatigue, fever, and malaise. The presentation of 101 children who were followed at the Mayo Clinic was similar to that of adults (5). In addition, Ropes

TABLE 30.2. FIRST SYSTEM INVOLVED AS DETERMINED BY HISTORY (%)

Manifestation	Dubois and Tuffanelli (50) (520 cases)	Harvey et al. (49) (105 cases)	Haserick (69) (275 cases)	Larsen et al. (70) (200 cases)	Norris et al. (5) (101 cases)
Arthritis and arthralgia	46	47	55	59	48
Discoid lupus	11	0	4	0	13
Butterfly area eruptions and blush	6 }	20	17 }	14	—
Eruptions on other parts of body (nonspecific dermatitis)	2 }		0 }		
Fever	4	2	0	1 }	24
Fatigue, malaise, weakness	4	17	0	0 }	
Renal involvement	3	5	3	6	—
Pleurisy	3	5	2	2	—
Edema and anasarca	1	0	0	0	2
Positive STS	2	5	8	4	—
Cervical adenopathy	2	0	0	0	—
Anemia	2	4	0	0	—
Raynaud's phenomenon	2	3	5	1	—
Myalgia	2	0	0	0	—
Photosensitivity reaction	1	4	4	0	—
Pericarditis	1	1	0	2	—
Plural effusion	1	0	2	0	—
Epilepsy	1	0	3	0	—
Generalized adenopathy	1	2	0	1	—
Purpura	—	—	—	—	9
Mouth ulcers	—	—	—	—	3

STS, biologic false positive for syphilis.

(6) found that joints were the first system to be involved in 27% of 142 patients, followed by fever, weight loss, and malaise (25%), and then skin rash (20%). Grigor et al. (7) followed 50 patients with lupus; the initial manifestations were arthritis or arthralgia (62%), cutaneous (20%), fever and malaise, thrombocytopenia, hemolytic anemia, and neuropsychiatric symptoms (4% each), and recurrent thrombophlebitis (2%). If present, organ-system damage evolves early. Rivest et al. followed 200 lupus patients and showed evidence for organ-system damage a mean 3.8 years after disease onset (8).

VARIATIONS IN CLINICAL PRESENTATION

The presentation and clinical characteristics of SLE are presented in detail in the following chapters. Age and sex may cause variations in the appearance of the disease; these distinctions are summarized here. Features of incomplete lupus, other rheumatic diseases and undifferentiated connective-tissue disease are covered in Chapter 51, Clinical and Laboratory Features of Lupus Nephritis.

Proto Or Latent Lupus

When does lupus begin? Sixteen healthy Finnish women who stored sera in connection with a maternity welfare program developed SLE years later. Ten (62.5%) were ANA positive at the time of collection, compared with 6% of controls (9). 43 individuals diagnosed with SLE while serving in the United States military had previously donated blood to the Army/Navy Serum Repository. ANAs, as well as other autoantibodies, were positive an average of 3.2 years prior to diagnosis (10).

A 1981 survey of our 609 private patients who were diagnosed between 1950 and 1980 revealed a 4.1-year interval between the onset of symptoms and the diagnosis of SLE (11). Our survey of 464 patients with idiopathic SLE who were seen between 1980 and 1989 documented a 2.1-year interval (3). Is the disease changing, or have increased physician awareness and newer diagnostic and serologic testing made it possible to diagnose SLE earlier? In the 0- to 19-year age group, it took only a mean of 3 months to make the diagnosis; in patients over 60 years, the more subtle presentation of idiopathic SLE took 3.2 years to detect, on average. One third of 44 patients who were referred to our group with a positive ANA to rule out lupus but who did not fulfill American College of Rheumatology (ACR) criteria for the disease at the time of the visit had clear-cut SLE 6 months later (12). Urowitz's group identified 22 patients with a constellation of features that were suggestive of SLE but who did not fulfill ACR criteria (13). Over a 5-year observation period, seven patients (32%) evolved into SLE. Few had organ-threatening disease, and no predictive factors distinguished the seven who developed SLE from the 15 who did not. Hochberg's Johns Hopkins-based group reported a 1-year interval among 150 patients who were seen between 1980 and 1984 (14). The Eurolupus cohort of 1,000 patients reported a mean 2-year period between the onset of symptoms and diagnosis in 1993 (15). Improved diagnostic techniques have allowed for more rapid diagnosis. In Limerick, Ireland, the mean time from symptoms to diagnosis has decreased from 102.8 months to 11.5 months between the 1970s and 1990s (16). In summary, nonorgan-threatening lupus, especially in older patients, can be difficult to diagnose initially; in addition, it may be difficult to determine when SLE started.

Lupus In Children

See Chapter 41, Systemic Lupus Erythematosus in Childhood and Adolescence.

Late-Onset Lupus

Defined as disease with onset in patients over the age of 50 years, late-onset lupus often is insidious (17), with a polymyalgialike or rheumatoid arthritislike pattern (18), and it may be difficult to distinguish from autoimmune thyroiditis (5) or primary Sjögren's syndrome (19). It comprises 6% to 20% of all cases (20) and includes more men than any other group, except young children (Table 30.3). The clinical course generally is benign, and the disease is more easily controlled with medication. One of our patients had active disease at age 90 (21), and onset has been reported at age 92 (22). The relatively small number of patients with late-onset lupus in large, published series led Ward and Pollison (23) to perform a meta-analysis based on nine studies of its clinical and laboratory features. Their 1989 effort compared 170 late-onset patients with 1,612 younger-onset patients. They concluded that the older-onset subset had more serositis, interstitial lung disease, Sjögren's syndrome, and anti-La/SSB. A significantly lower incidence of alopecia, Raynaud's phenomenon, fever, lymphadenopathy, hypocomplementemia, and neuropsychiatric disease was present (24). Only one of the reviewed

TABLE 30.3. SEX RATIOS BY AGE AT AGE OF ONSET OR FIRST DIAGNOSIS OF SLE

Age at Onset or First Diagnosis (yr)	Female:Male Ratio
0–4	1.4:1
5–9	2.3:1
10–14	5.8:1
15–19	5.4:1
20–29	7.5:1
30–39	8.1:1
40–49	5.2:1
50–59	3.9:1
60 and above	2.2:1

studies was population based (25). These findings have been confirmed among European (15) and Asian populations (26–30). Additional reports have suggested that HLA-DR3 is more common in whites with late-onset lupus (14), autoantibodies other than ANA are much less common in late-onset patients (31, 32), serositis is the most frequent presenting feature (33, 34), late-onset lupus is more frequent in whites than African Americans (35), and African Americans with late-onset lupus have a worse prognosis than whites with late-onset disease (36). Braunstein et al. (37) evaluated the joint films of 24 patients with SLE onset over the age of 50 years. No differences were noted in the amount of osteoporosis, erosions, or soft-tissue calcification, but soft-tissue swelling was significantly increased in the older group. In summary, most studies have shown that patients with SLE onset after the age of 50 years have more serositis, pulmonary parenchymal disease, and Sjögren's syndrome, less central nervous system involvement and nephritis, and a better prognosis.

Male Lupus

Although males constitute only 4 to 18% of those with SLE, their clinical presentation is similar to that observed in women. Hochberg et al. (14) noted a mean age of onset in men of 40.4 years (vs. 31.8 in women) among a 150-patient cohort. Except for a statistically significant increase in peripheral neuropathy, no other clinical, laboratory, or HLA phenotypic differences, could be found.

If we restrict our review to studies including at least 30 males, Ward and Studenski (38) compared 62 men with 299 women who were followed at Duke University between 1969 and 1983; 23 clinical and laboratory variables were analyzed. The only significant differences were more seizures and renal disease in the men. Pistiner et al. (3) compared 125 clinical and laboratory parameters among 30 men and 434 women who were seen in our office between 1980 and 1989. Only four significant differences were observed ($p<.01$): men had less alopecia and fibromyalgia but more nephritis and hypocomplementemia. Fries and Holman (39) observed that men had more anti-DNA and skin disease; Urowitz's group (40) found that men had more pleuritis but less photosensitivity, alopecia, and thrombocytopenia. The 92 males in the Eurolupus cohort (15) had more arthritis and less serositis but no other differences. This includes 30 males who were studied in more detail by Font et al. (41) in Spain. Sixty-one Chinese male patients with lupus had less arthritis and leukopenia and anti-Ro(SSA) than matched females (42). Forty-one males followed by the Hopkins Lupus Cohort had more thrombotic episodes, lower complement, more hemolytic anemia and seizures (43). 72 males in Taiwan had more renal and skin diseases than females but less arthritis and adenopathy (44). Fifty-nine Danish males had more serositis, nephropathy and atherosclerotic complications than 454 females (45). Alarcon-Segovia's group in Mexico City compared 107 males with 1,209 females (46). They had a higher prevalence of anti-double standed (ds) DNA antibodies, renal disease, and vascular thromboses and took higher doses of corticosteroids. A study of 30 male Turks (compared with 100 females) with SLE also confirms this (47). The reader is referred to Isenberg's critical review of the so-far-difficult search for unifying features for male lupus (48).

CONSTITUTIONAL SYMPTOMS

The generalized symptoms of fever, weight loss, malaise, and fatigue do not fit into any organ-system classification; therefore, they are discussed here.

Fever

Fever secondary to active disease was recorded at some time in 86% of Harvey's patients who were seen in the early 1950s (49), in 84% of Dubois' 520 patients between 1950 and 1963 (50), in 55% of 193 patients at Stanford University in the 1960s and 1970s (39), 52% of the Eurolupus cohort (15), and in 41% of Wallace's 464 patients seen between 1980 and 1989 (3). This consistent, decreasing trend probably reflects better understanding of the disease-and the greater availability of nonsteroidal antiinflammatory drugs (NSAIDs). No fever curve or pattern is characteristic. SLE can present with fever as its sole manifestation (51). Active SLE can result in temperatures as high as 106°F (41°C). It can be difficult to distinguish the fever of SLE from that caused by complicating infections. A review of 617 patients with fever of unknown origin from five classic studies found SLE to be the cause in 0% to 5% of cases (52).

Fever in SLE results from endogenous pyrogens that are produced largely by polymorphonuclear leukocytes and monocyte/macrophages. These include tumor necrosis factor alpha; interleukin (IL) -1, -2, and -6; interferons, and arachidonic acid products. IL-1, in particular, promotes the release of arachidonic acid and, ultimately, prostaglandin E2 (PGE2). PGE2 is known to exert a direct pyrogenic effect on the hypothalamic thermoregulatory center (53, 54).

Stahl et al. (55) at the National Institutes of Health studied 106 hospitalized patients with SLE. In 63 patients (38%), 83 febrile episodes were recorded; 60% resulted from SLE activity, 23% from infection (bacteremia was present in one half of these and was fatal in one third), and 17% from other causes (primarily postoperative fevers and drug reactions). The single most useful feature identifying infection was the presence of shaking chills. Leukocytosis (especially in the absence of steroid therapy), neutrophilia, and normal anti-DNA levels also were helpful. The SLE components associated with fever were dermatitis, arthritis, and pleuropericarditis. Although often associated with SLE, a daily low-grade fever, up to 100°F (37.8°C), may be overlooked unless patients are specifically asked to check their temperatures daily. Inoue et al. (56) followed 49 patients with SLE through 74 febrile episodes and found that 25 episodes were secondary to infection. Discriminant analysis showed that 95% of 74 febrile episodes could be correctly classified as to the cause of fever when a combination of white blood cell count (low with SLE, normal to high with infection) and alpha-2-globulin levels (high with SLE, normal with infection) are used as variables. A close correlation between interferon-alpha (but not IL-1 or tumor necrosis factor) and degree of fever was observed in 25 untreated patients with SLE (57).

Temperature elevation in an illness that is characterized by a high incidence of this finding should not prevent the physician from carefully searching for other causes. The frequent occurrence of infection in patients with SLE often warrants blood cultures, urine cultures, and chest radiographs. Urinary tract infections are common in young women, who may be asymptomatic. Opportunistic infections and drug reactions should be considered. The cause of the temperature elevation should be investigated before suppressing this helpful clinical finding by administering or increasing the dose of salicylates, NSAIDs or corticosteroids.

Anorexia And Change In Weight

Anorexia and an insidious onset of weight loss over a period of months were noted in 51% of patients in the Dubois series (50), in 71% of patients in Harvey's group (49), in 31% of 193 patients followed by Fries and Holman (39), in 63% of Rothfield's 209 patients (58), and in 35% of children with SLE (59). It was a clinical finding in 9% of 704 European patients with SLE who were evaluated at a routine visit (60). The degree of weight loss almost always is less than 10% and most immediately precedes the diagnosis of SLE. Weight gain in SLE usually results from nephrotic syndrome, ascites, and tricyclic antidepressant or corticosteroid therapy.

Malaise And Fatigue

A sense of malaise and fatigue is common in patients with SLE, especially during periods of disease activity. They feel tired and achy but initially find difficulty in pinpointing the problem. Low-grade fevers, anemia, or any source of inflammation can result in fatigue, as can emotional stress, fibromyalgia, or depression. The administration of certain cytokines, such as IL-2 and interferon-alpha induce fatigue (61), and SLE is associated with cytokine dysregulation. Rothfield (58) noted moderate to severe fatigue in 81% of 209 patients, and Fries and Holman (39) noted fatigue in 82% of 193 patients. Fifty-nine patients who were followed at the National Institutes of Health filled out a fatigue questionnaire (62). Their mean fatigue severity (on a scale of 1 to 7) was 4.6. Of these, 53% reported fatigue to be their most disabling symptom, although it did not correlate with any laboratory measure. Three surveys published in the late 1990s suggested that fibromyalgia was the most important component of fatigue in lupus patients (63–65) Goldenberg's review of the literature suggests that the prevalence of fatigue in patients seen in primary-care settings ranges from 14 to 25% and costs $1 billion a year in diagnostic evaluations in the United States (66). (See Chapter 53, Principles of Therapy and Local Measures, for a discussion of the management of fatigue.)

REFERENCES

1. Hargraves MM, Richmond H, Morton R. Presentation of 2 bone marrow elements: tart cell and L.E. cell. *Proc Staff Meet Mayo Clin* 1948;23:25–28.
2. Buckman KJ, Moore SK, Ebbin AJ, et al. Familial systemic lupus erythematosus. *Arch Intern Med* 1978;138:1674–1676.
3. Pistiner M, Wallace DJ, Nessim S, et al. Lupus erythematosus in the 1980s: a survey of 570 patients. *Semin Arthritis Rheum* 1991; 21:55–64.
4. Carpenter RR, Sturgill BC. The course of systemic lupus erythematosus. *J Chronic Dis* 1966;19:117–131.
5. Norris DG, Colon AR, Stickler GB. Systemic lupus erythematosus in children: the complex problems of diagnosis and treatment encountered in 101 such patients at the Mayo Clinic. *Clin Pediatr* (Phila) 1977;16:744–778.
6. Ropes MW. *Systemic lupus erythematosus.* Cambridge, MA: Harvard University Press, 1976.
7. Grigor R, Edmonds J, Lewkonia R, et al. Systemic lupus erythematosus. A prospective analysis. *Ann Rheum Dis* 1978;37: 121–128.
8. Rivest C, Lew RA, Welsing MJ, et al. Association between clinical factors, socioeconomic status, and organ damage in recent onset systemic lupus erythematosus. *J Rheumatol* 2000;27: 680–684.
9. Aho K, Koskela P, Makitalo R, et al. Antinuclear antibodies heralding the onset of systemic lupus erythematosus. *J Rheumatol* 1992;19:1377–1379.
10. Arbuckle MR, Dennis GL, Neas BR, et al. Autoantibodies are commonly present years before the onset of clinical illness in lupus. *Arthritis Rheum* 1999;42: S383 (abstract).
11. Wallace DJ, Podell T, Weiner J, et al. Systemic lupus erythematosus—survival patterns. Experience with 609 patients. *JAMA* 1981;245:934–938.
12. Wallace DJ, Schwartz E, Chi-Lin H, et al. The rule out lupus rheumatology consultation: clinical outcomes and perspectives. *J Clin Rheumat* 1995;1:158–164.
13. Ganczarczyk L, Urowitz MB, Gladman DD, et al. *J Rheumatol* 1989;16:475–478.
14. Hochberg MC, Boyd RE, Ahearn JM, et al. Systemic lupus erythematosus: a review of clinico-laboratory features and immunogenetic markers in 150 patients with emphasis on demographic subsets. *Medicine* 1985;64:285–295.
15. Cervera R, Khamashta MA, Font J, et al. European Working Party on Systemic Lupus Erythematosus. Systemic lupus erythematosus: clinical and immunologic patterns of disease expression in a cohort of 1000 patients. *Medicine* 1993;72:113–124.

16. Cocoran D, O'Sullivan M, Wall JG. Clinical specturm and diagnosis of systemic lupus in the Republic of Ireland. *Medical Sci Res* 1999;27:769–771.
17. Font J, Pallares L, Cervera R, et al. Systemic lupus erythematosus in the elderly: clinical and immunological characteristics. *Ann Rheum Dis* 1991;56:702–705.
18. Maragou M, Siotsiou F, Sfondouris H, et al. Late-onset systemic lupus erythematosus presenting as polymyalgia rheumatica. *Clin Rheumatol* 1989;8:91–97.
19. Bell DA. SLE in the elderly—is it really SLE or systemic Sjögren's syndrome? *J Rheumatol* 1988;15:723–724.
20. Stevens MB. Systemic lupus erythematosus: clinical issues. *Springer Semin Immunopathol* 1986;9:251–270.
21. Wallace DJ. Active idiopathic systemic lupus erythematosus in a 90-year-old woman requiring corticosteroid therapy. *J Rheumatol* 1991;18:1611–1612.
22. Ikeda K, Ishibashi T, Noji H, et al. A 92-year old man with systemic lupus erythematosus who developed acute lupus pneumonitis. *J Rheumatol* 2000;27:234–237.
23. Ward MM, Polisson RP. A meta-analysis of the clinical manifestations of older-onset systemic lupus erythematosus. *Arthritis Rheum* 1989;32:1226–1232.
24. Ward MM, Studenski S. Age associated clinical manifestations of systemic lupus erythematosus: a multivariate regression analysis. *J Rheumatol* 1990;17:476–481.
25. Jonsson H, Nived O, Sturfelt G. The effect of age on clinical and serological manifestations in unselected patients with systemic lupus erythematosus. *J Rheumatol* 1988;15:505–509.
26. Koh ET, Boey ML. Late onset lupus: a clinical and immunological study in a predominantly Chinese population. *J Rheumatol* 1994;21:1463–1467.
27. Shaikh SH, Wang F. Late-onset systemic lupus erythematosus: clinical and immunological characteristics. *Med J Malaysia* 1995; 50:25–31.
28. Ho CTK, Mok CC, Lau CS, et al. Late onset systemic lupus erythematosus in southern Chinese. *Ann Rheum Dis* 1998;57: 437–440.
29. Mak SK, Lam EKM, Wong AKM. Clinical profile of patients with late-onset SLE: not a benign subgoup. *Lupus* 1998;7:23–28.
30. Pu SJ, Luo SF, Wu YJJ, et al. The clinical features and prognosis of lupus with disease onset at age 65 and older. *Lupus* 2000;9: 96–100.
31. Wysenbeek AJ, Mandel DR, Mayes MD, et al. Autoantibodies in systemic lupus erythematosus of late onset. *Cleve Clin Q* 1985; 52:119–122.
32. Domenech I, Aydintug O, Cervera R, et al. Systemic lupus in 50 year olds. *Postgrad Med J* 1992;68:440–444.
33. Baker SB, Rovira JR, Campion EW, et al. Late onset lupus erythematosus. *Am J Med* 1979;66:727–732.
34. Dimant J, Ginzler EM, Schlesigner M, et al. Systemic lupus erythematosus in the older age group: computer analysis. *J Am Geriatr Soc* 1979;27:58–61.
35. Ballou SP, Khan MA, Kushner I. Clinical features of systemic lupus erythematosus: differences related to race and age of onset. *Arthritis Rheum* 1982;25:55–60.
36. Studenski SA, Bembe ML, Caldwell DS, et al. Late onset systemic lupus erythematosus—race and sex factors (abstract). *Clin Res* 1984;32:469A.
37. Braunstein EM, Weisman BN, Sosman JJ, et al. Radiologic findings in late-onset systemic lupus erythematosus. *AJR Am J Roentgenol* 1983;140:587–589.
38. Ward MM, Studenski S. Systemic lupus erythematosus in men: a multivariate analysis of gender differences in clinical manifestations. *J Rheumatol* 1990;17:220–224.
39. Fries J, Holman H. *Systemic lupus erythematosus: a clinical analysis*. Philadelphia: WB Saunders, 1975.
40. Miller MH, Urowitz MB, Gladman DD, et al. Chronic adhesive lupus serositis as a complication of systemic lupus erythematosus. Refractory chest pain and small bowel obstruction. *Arch Intern Med* 1984;144:1863–1864.
41. Font J, Cervera R, Navarro M, et al. Systemic lupus erythematosus in men: clinical and immunological characteristics. *Ann Rheum Dis* 1992;51:1050–1052.
42. Koh WH, Fong KY, Boey ML, et al. Systemic lupus erythematosus in 61 Oriental males. A study of clinical and laboratory manifestations. *Br J Rheumatol* 1994;33:339–342.
43. Petri M. Male lupus differs from female lupus in presentation and outcome. *Arthritis Rheum* 1997;40:S162.
44. Chang D-M, Chang C-C, Kuo S-Y, et al. The clinical features and prognosis of male lupus in Taiwan. *Lupus* 1998;7:462–468.
45. Jacobsen S, Petersen J, Ullman S, et al. A multicentre study of 513 Danish patients with systemic lupus erythematosus: I. Disease manifestations and analyses of clinical subsets. *Clin Rheumatol* 1998;17:468–477.
46. Molina JF, Drenkard C, Molina J, et al. Systemic lupus erythematosus in males. A study of 107 Latin American males. *Medicine* 1996;75:124–130.
47. Keskin G, Tokgoz G, Duzgun N, et al. Systemic lupus erythematosus in Turkish men. *Clin Exper Rheumatol* 2000;18: 114–115.
48. Isenberg DA. Male lupus and the Loch Ness syndrome. *Br J Rheumatol* 1994;33:307–308.
49. McGehee HA, Shulman LE, Tumulty AP, et al. Systemic lupus erythematosus: review of the literature and clinical analysis of 138 cases. *Medicine* 1954;33:291–437.
50. Dubois EL, Tuffanelli DL. Clinical manifestations of systemic lupus erythematosus. Computer analysis of 520 cases. *JAMA* 1964;190:104–111.
51. Petersdorf RG, Beeson PB. Fever of unexplained origin: report on 100 cases. *Medicine* 1961;40:1–30.
52. Knockaert DC, Vanneste LJ, Vanneste SB, et al. Fever of unknown origin in the 1980s. An update of the diagnostic spectrum. *Arch Intern Med* 1992;152:51–55.
53. Mackowiak PA. Fever: modern insights into an ancient clinical sign. *Contemp Intern Med* 1992;April:17–28.
54. Sapar CB, Breda CD. The neurologic basis of fever. *N Engl J Med* 1994;330:1880–1886.
55. Stahl NI, Klippel JH, Decker JL. Fever in systemic lupus erythematosus. *Am J Med* 1979;67:935–940.
56. Inoue T, Takeda T, Koda S, et al. Differential diagnosis of fever in systemic lupus erythematosus using discriminant analysis. *Rheumatol Int* 1986;6:69–77.
57. Kanayama Y, Kim T, Inariba H, et al. Possible involvement of interferon alpha in the pathogenesis of fever in systemic lupus erythematosus. *Ann Rheum Dis* 1989;48:861–863.
58. Rothfield N. Clinical features of systemic lupus erythematosus. In: Kelly WN, Harris ED, Ruddy S, et al., eds. *Textbook of rheumatology*. Philadelphia: WB Saunders, 1981:1106–1132.
59. Szer IS, Jacobs JC. Systemic lupus erythematosus in childhood. In: Lahita R, ed. *Systemic lupus erythematosus*. New York: Wiley & Sons, 1987:383–413.
60. Vitali C, Bencivelli W, Isenberg DA, et al. European Concensus Study Group for Disease Activity in SLE. Disease activity in systemic lupus erythematosus: report of the Concensus Study Group of the European Workshop for Rheumatology Research. A descriptive analysis of 704 European lupus patients. *Clin Exp Rheumatol* 1992;10:527–539.
61. Wallace DJ. Fibromyalgia and interleukin-2 therapy for malignancy. *Ann Inter Med* 1988;109:909.
62. Krupp LB, LaRocca NG, Muir J, et al. A study of fatigue in systemic lupus erythematosus. *J Rheumatol* 1990;17:1450–1452.
63. Bruce IN, Mak VC, Hallett DC, et al. Factors associated with

fatigue in patients with systemic lupus erythematosus. *Ann Rheum Dis* 1999;58:379–381.
64. Tench CM, Mc Curdie I, White PD, et al. The prevalence and association of fatigue in outpatients with SLE. *Arthritis Rheum* 1998;41:S332.
65. Taylor J, Skan J, Erb N, et al. Lupus patients with fatigue: is there a link with the fibromyalgia syndrome? *Arthritis Rheum* 1998;41: S332.
66. Goldenberg DL. Fatigue in rheumatic disease. *Bull Rheum Dis* 1995;44:4–8.
67. Estes D, Christian CL. The natural history of systemic lupus erythematosus by prospective analysis. *Medicine* 1971;50:85–95.
68. Tan EM, Cohen AS, Fries JF, et al. Special article: the 1982 revised criteria for the classification of systemic lupus erythematosus. *Arthritis Rheum* 1982;25:1271–1277.
69. Haserick JR. Unpublished observations.
70. Larsen RA, Solheim BG. Family studies in systemic lupus erythematosus. V. Presence of antinuclear factors (ANTFs) in relatives and spouses of selected SLE probands. *Acta Med Scand* 1972;543(suppl):55–64.

31

THE MUSCULOSKELETAL SYSTEM

DANIEL J. WALLACE

Joints, muscles, and their supporting structures are the most commonly involved system in systemic lupus erythematosus (SLE), affecting 53% to 95% of patients (see Chapter 30, Table 30.1). Kaposi (1), in 1872, first described the joint manifestations. Most commonly, musculoskeletal symptoms are the chief complaint in lupus (see Chapter 30, Table 30.2), and articular pain is the initial symptom in 50% of patients (2). The biochemical mediators of joint inflammation in SLE and the pathophysiology of this arthritis have not been well studied.

JOINTS: SYMPTOMS, SIGNS, DEFORMITY, AND RADIOGRAPHIC FINDINGS

The chief joint manifestations are stiffness, pain, and inflammation. The pattern of arthritis is recurrent, often evanescent, and can be deforming. Morning stiffness occurs in 46% to 73% of patients (3–5). Fries and Holman (6) found arthritis in 53% of their 193 patients, nodules in 3%, wrist swelling in 31%, metacarpophalangeal (MCP) swelling in 31%, and proximal interphalangeal (PIP) swelling in 40% at any point. Grigor et al. (7) described nondeforming arthritis or arthralgia in 88% of their patients, deforming arthritis in 10%, erosions in 6%, avascular necrosis in 6%, myalgias or myositis in 32%, and tendon contractures in 12%. Petri (8) has associated musculoskeletal damage in SLE with blacks and those of lower socioeconomic status.

AREAS AFFECTED

All major and minor joints may be affected, including the wrists, knees, ankles, elbows, and shoulders, in that order of prevalence (5). Most patients with SLE eventually develop some PIP and MCP involvement, and complaints of joint pain without objective physical findings for long periods may be noted. Once symptoms of discomfort became objectively apparent, morning stiffness characteristic of typical rheumatoid arthritis usually is seen. Marked, diffuse puffiness of the hands also often occurs. Stress fractures caused by corticosteroid-induced osteoporosis can produce swelling and mimic synovitis (9).

Hand

Persistent, rheumatoid-like deformities may occur in the hand, as they did in 35% of Dubois and Tuffanelli's (3) 520 patients, with thickening of the PIP joints, ulnar deviation, and subluxation. Armas-Cruz et al. (10) found similar changes in 22% of 108 patients. Those changes often may appear insidiously over the course of many years while the patient is in an apparent clinical remission. The primary lesion appears to be inflammation involving synovial tissues, with minimal or belated destruction of cartilage and bone. Bywaters (11) stated that whenever a patient with rheumatoid-like arthritis remained free of erosions for 2 years or longer, the diagnosis of SLE is more likely, although this concept does not necessarily apply to children (12). He was the first to emphasize the similarity between the fibrosing synovitis of SLE and that reported by Jaccoud in recurrent rheumatic fever (13). Silver and Steinbrocker (14) noted that when synovial swelling persisted, a lessened tendency toward destruction of the cartilage occurred compared with that seen in rheumatoid arthritis (RA).

Hand deformities can include ulnar deviation and subluxation, swan-neck deformities (in 3% to 38%), and subluxation of the thumb interphalangeal joints (4,15–19). Erosions are rare (seen in approximately 4%). Some authors have noted positive correlations among deforming arthritis, Sjögren's syndrome, anti-SSA, C-reactive protein, and the presence of rheumatoid factor (15,18,20–27) and negative correlations with hypertension (28). Jaccoud's reversible, subluxing, nondeforming arthropathy is seen in 3% to 14% of patients with SLE (16,17,19). Table 31.1 summarizes the differential diagnosis between SLE and RA of the hand, and Fig. 31.1 demonstrate some of the abnormalities mentioned here. Jaccoud's arthropathy was found in 43% of 939 patients with SLE and is associated with a benign prognosis (29).

TABLE 31.1. COMPARISON OF HAND INVOLVEMENT IN SYSTEMIC LUPUS ERYTHEMATOSUS (SLE) AND RHEUMATOID ARTHRITIS (RA)

Parameter	SLE	RA
Raynaud's phenomenon	Approximately 30%	Rare
Joint pain	Mild	May be severe
Recurrent synovitis	In 10–30%	Common
Joint deformity	Caused by loss of soft-tissue support	Caused by loss of soft tissue support and articular surface destruction
Thumb IP joint hyperextension	Not associated with MP joint flexion contracture	Often associated with MP joint flexion contracture
Ulnar drift of fingers	Almost always reversible	Often irreversible, with subluxed MP joints
Wrist	May be lax; normal function	Often subluxed, with carpal bone destruction
Erosive changes	Rare	Common
Cause of deformity	Uncertain; occurs after supporting soft tissue structures are weakened	Synovitis, pannus formation; cartilage and bone destruction

IP, interphalangeal; MP, metacarpophalangeal.

Whether or not primary antiphospholipid syndrome without SLE is associated with an inflammatory arthritis is the subject of some debate (30). A Dutch group correlated Jaccoud's arthropathy with anticardiolipin antibodies, fetal loss, and thrombosis (31). It does not require surgical treatment, because grip strength is usually intact. In 1981, Dray et al. (32) treated ten patients with subluxation excision, MCP arthroplasties, and joint stabilization by ligamentous reconstruction; unfortunately, 70% of the tendon relocations failed to maintain correction. An excellent review of hand surgery consideration in SLE has been published (33).

Hand Imaging Studies

Several reports have examined the radiographic findings of the lupus hand in detail. Weissman et al. (34) evaluated 59 patients, and 34 demonstrated abnormalities. Of these, ten had acral sclerosis (these probably had mixed connective tissue disease), seven had alignment abnormalities, and one showed an erosion. Leskinen's group (35,36) reviewed joint radiographs of 124 patients with SLE, and cystic bone lesions were found in 51 (41%). Most were subchondral and located in the small joints of the hands and feet, and a vasculitic cause was proposed. In a multicentered European study, ten of 60 lupus patients with erosive disease (vs. 28% without) had anti-RA33 antibodies (p <.05) (37). About half with SLE demonstrate evidence for inflammatory arthritis of the hands as determined by uptake on a technetium NDP (TcMDP) bone scan (38).

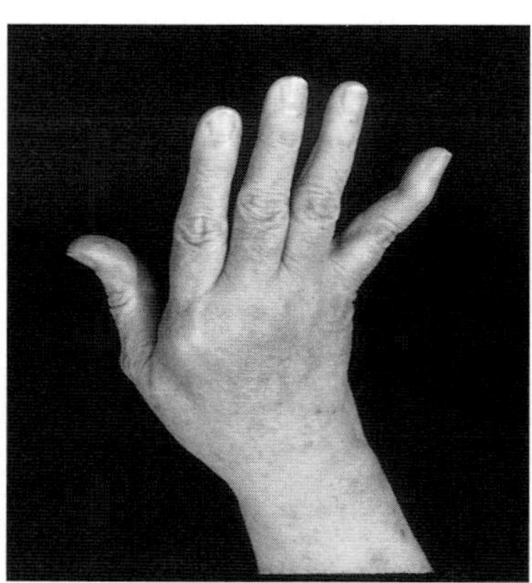

FIGURE 31.1. Jaccoud's arthropathy.

Rarely, a resorptive arthropathy resembling the opera-glass hand syndrome has been reported (39,40), as has periosteal elevation secondary to ischemic bone disease or, perhaps, vasculitis (41).

Knees

Jaccoud-like arthropathy (i.e., reversible subluxation) has been observed in the knees (42–44). Deep venous thrombosis in a patient with antiphospholipid antibodies may be difficult to differentiate from a Baker's cyst, both of which are observed in SLE (45). At least one case of chrondrocalcinosis involving the knee joint associated with SLE has been reported (46), and it certainly is more common.

Feet

Mizutani and Quismorio (47) noted hallux valgus, metatarsophalangeal subluxation, hammertoes, and forefoot widening without erosions or cystic changes in patients with SLE. This is similar to the Jaccoud type of arthropathy in the hands. Other studies have confirmed these findings (48). The deformities result in painful bunions and callosities, and several podiatry publications have reviewed the issues of proper foot care in those with SLE (49,50).

Neck

Several cases of atlantoaxial subluxation have been reported (51,52). One report postulated that patients who are treated with corticosteroids have increased ligamentous laxity, which promotes the rupture of ligamentous and capsular supporting structures (52), but it seems equally likely that laxity of ligaments in the neck have the same physiologic bond as laxity in any other joint. In another report, 5 of 59 patients with lupus had atlantoaxial subluxation. All were asymptomatic. Subluxation was associated with longer disease duration, Jaccoud's arthropathy, and chronic renal failure (51).

Sacroiliac Joint

Several studies of almost 100 patients suggested that over half of all patients with active SLE have radiographic sacroiliitis or increased uptake on joint scanning. I believe this figure is too high. Seronegative spondyloarthropathies were excluded, and most patients had no sacroiliac symptoms (53–58). A French survey of 41 SLE patients found radiographic unilateral sacroiliitis in six (15%). Only one individual was symptomatic (59).

Hips

Although hip synovitis is not uncommon, any complaints of isolated severe hip pain should lead one to suspect avascular necrosis (discussed below).

Shoulders

Jaccoud's arthropathy can be found in the shoulders (60).

Temporomandibular Joint

Jonsson et al. (61) evaluated temporomandibular joint (TMJ) involvement in 37 patients with SLE and compared them to a control group of 37 healthy age- and sex-matched individuals. Of those with SLE referred to an oral surgeon, 59% had severe past TMJ symptoms (vs. 14% of controls), and 14% had present severe symptoms (vs. 3% of controls). Clinical examination revealed TMJ signs, such as clicking, crepitation, jaw fatigue or stiffness, facial pain, tenderness to palpation, pain on movement of the mandible, locking, or dislocation, to be present in 41% (vs. none of the controls). In addition, of the patients with SLE, 30% had abnormal radiographs (vs. 9% of controls) that included condyle flattening and osteophytes; 11% had erosion, confirming other reports (62,63); and 72.5% had renal disease (vs. only 27.5% of the non–TMJ-involved patients with SLE). Although symptoms may be referred to this joint, limitation of the ability to open the jaw is rare unless coexistent scleroderma is present (64,65).

Synovial Histopathology

SLE is characterized by a mild to moderate inflammatory synovitis that is similar in character but less angry-appearing than that in RA (10,66). Bywaters (11,13) reported the presence of chronic synovitis with a fibrotic process in SLE in patients with Jaccoud-type deformities. Only three groups have examined the synovial histopathology of SLE in any detail.

Goldenberg and Cohen (67) studied 13 patients with lupus: 92% had synovial membrane hyperplasia, 100% had microvascular changes, 83% had surface fibrin deposits, and most had a perivascular infiltrate. Several of the biopsy specimens were indistinguishable from those of RA.

Labowitz and Schumacher (23) studied synovial biopsy specimens from seven patients; superficial fibrinlike material was seen in four, and focal or diffuse synovial lining proliferation in six. Five had a primary perivascular inflammatory reaction with predominantly mononuclear cells, and vasculitis was noted in only one patient. Synovial and vascular lesions were found in two patients, who had no objective signs of joint inflammation. On electron microscopy, fibrin was noted in three of four specimens. Type A (i.e., phagocytic), type B (i.e., synthetic), and intermediate cells were seen, but there was no clear predominance. Two patients had platelets and fibrinlike material obliterating small-vessel lumens. Vascular endothelial inclusions of a viruslike type were observed in two patients.

Natour et al. (68) reviewed 30 knee synovial biopsies. The most frequent findings were synoviocyte hyperplasia, minimal inflammation, edema, congestion, vascular proliferation, fibrinoid necrosis, intimal fibrous hyperplasia, and fibrin on the synovial surface.

In conclusion, the synovial histopathology of SLE does not appear to be specific, and it cannot clearly be differentiated from that of RA. Despite the extensive connective tissue change, little cartilage and bone destruction seems to occur. This gross finding tends to separate the deforming arthritis associated with SLE from that typically seen in RA.

Synovial Cysts

Large synovial cysts are uncommonly reported in patients with SLE (69–71). My group has observed soft synovial cysts several millimeters in diameter appearing in the dorsum of PIP joints in patients with SLE following years of localized inflammation. These should be differentiated from rheumatoid nodules.

Synovial Fluid

Ropes (72) found that the volume of accessible synovial joint fluid (Table 31.2) ranged from 5 to 1,500 mL in 133 patients. It was unusually clear, but occasionally hemorrhagic, and could be a transudate or an exudate. Pekin and Zvaifler (73) reported synovial fluid findings in 26 patients with SLE, and viscosity was uniformly good. The white count was less than 2,000/mL in 19 and exceeded 10,000/mL in only two patients. Granulocytes were always

TABLE 31.2. CHARACTERISTICS OF SYNOVIAL FLUID IN SLE

Clear, yellow, normal viscosity, good mucin clot
White blood cell count: 2,000 to 15,000/mL, with primarily lymphocytic predominance
Low-titer ANAs may be present; LE cells occasionally are seen
Glucose level normal
Protein levels normal or increased
Complement levels normal or decreased

ANAs, antinuclear antibodies; LE, lupus erythematosus.

less than 50%, and the synovial fluid complement level was normal in 11. Of the 26 patients, ten were classified as having noninflammatory transudates. Most had nephrotic syndrome. The exudates had a high protein content but variable complement levels. Serum to synovial fluid complement ratios generally were elevated in contrast to the total protein or immunoglobulin G (IgG) ratios, suggesting consumption of complement at the synovial level.

Schumacher (74) and Schumacher and Howe (75) examined synovial fluid from 17 patients with SLE. All had a white count lower than 40,000/mL. In comparing SLE with RA, Hollander et al. (76) reported a mean white count of 5,000/mL for SLE (vs. 15,000 for RA) with 10% neutrophils (vs. 50 for RA) and a good mucin clot and high viscosity (vs. a poor mucin clot and low viscosity for RA). Pascual (77) found that 14 patients with SLE had a synovial fluid counts ranging from 3,000 to 19,300/mL, and Hasselbacher (78) confirmed the increased viscosity in SLE synovial fluid and generally found low C3 complement levels. Cell counts in joint fluids must be interpreted cautiously, because analysis of the same fluid is subject to a great deal of variability among laboratories (79).

Secondary joint infection or avascular necrosis of bone may occur infrequently in SLE. It should be suspected when a localized effusion persists despite antiinflammatory therapy (80–83).

Lupus erythematosus (LE) cells can be found *in vivo* in synovial fluid (80). They were present in six of nine patients in one report (84), in 8 of 17 fluids examined by Schumacher (74) and by Schumacher and Howe (75) with electron microscopy, in 44% of 18 patients (85), in 2 of 14 patients examined by Pascual (77), and in two of three patients with drug-induced lupus (86). Rarely, RA cells (i.e., ragocytes) may be found in SLE synovial fluid (87,88).

Antinuclear antibodies (ANAs) are difficult to measure in synovial fluid, which must be treated with hyaluronadase before analysis. ANAs are present in approximately 20 of synovial fluid samples from patients with either RA or SLE (23,89–91), irrespective of serum levels. The synovial fluid of those with drug-induced lupus is similar to that reported for idiopathic SLE (86). Lipid synovial effusions rarely occur (92). These observations are summarized in Table 31.2.

On electron microscopy, Schumacher's group (75,93) found meshworks or tubuloreticular structures in monocytes in seven patients. LE cells contained distinct chromatin filaments.

Subcutaneous Nodules

Described by Hebra (94) and Kaposi (1) in 1872, subcutaneous nodules are present in 5% to 12% in the large series listed in Table 30.1 (Chapter 30) and in 2% to 10% in other series (95–97). Most occur in small joints of the hand, but nodules as large as 2 cm in diameter frequently occur on the extensor tendons of the hand and wrist. They may be exceedingly tender and often are transitory. Hoarseness secondary to rheumatoid-like vocal cord nodules has been described (98). These nodules are associated with patients who have SLE and rheumatoid-like arthritis and positive rheumatoid factor and rarely are seen without these features (99–101).

Histologically, subcutaneous nodules are granulomas and need to be differentiated from lupus panniculitis (profundus) (102), erythema nodosum, and a benign mesenchymoma. In children, it is important to distinguish them from granuloma annulare. Several reviews of the histology of the nodules in SLE have appeared (95,103,104). Vascular damage, with structural disarray in areas having collagen degeneration, is found, along with fibrinoid deposits and lymphocytic infiltrates in vessel walls. This microvasculopathy is similar to that observed in rheumatoid nodules.

Tendinitis, Tendon Rupture, And Carpal Tunnel Syndrome

Synovitis can induce a carpal tunnel syndrome, which may be the initial manifestation of idiopathic SLE or drug-induced lupus (105,106). Numerous reports and reviews have been published regarding tendon ruptures in SLE (107–111). The following conclusions can be derived: (a) almost all occur in weight-bearing areas, especially in tendons about the knee (65%; most are infrapatellar) and ankle (Achilles tendon; 27%); (b) an increased association with trauma, males, long-term oral steroid administration, intraarticular injections, Jaccoud's deformity, and/or long disease duration is noted; and (c) most patients are in clinical remission at the time of rupture.

A definitive diagnosis can be made with magnetic resonance imaging (MRI) (112,113). Tendon biopsy specimens reveal degeneration, mononuclear infiltration, neovascularization, and vacuolar myopathy (114). One group has correlated hyperparathyroidism (especially in patients with severe renal disease) and hydroxyapatite and urate crystal deposition in the knee tendons, with resulting ligamentous laxity (115,116). Pritchard and Berney (110) observed four cases of tendon rupture (all patellar) in 180 patients followed over a 10-year period. Carpal tunnel syndrome was found in 48 (11%) of 436 patients with SLE seen at the University of Pittsburgh between 1972 and 1990 (117).

Calcinosis And Soft Tissue Swelling

Commonly observed in scleroderma, dermatomyositis, and crossover syndromes, soft-tissue calcifications rarely are seen in SLE (118,119). They were observed radiographically in 9 of 130 patients in one study in which SLE was not adequately defined (120). Otherwise, approximately 30 case reports have appeared in the literature. Calcinosis universalis has been noted (121), and deposits of calcium phosphate in muscle, subcutaneous nodules, and periarthritis can occur in those with discoid or systemic lupus (122–124). Literature reviews are available (125,126). Periarticular radiographic calcification was present in 13.5% of 52 SLE patients, and was more common in patients taking diuretics (127). Diltiazem, which is a calcium channel blocker, is the probable treatment of choice (128,129). Aluminum hydroxide may be helpful (130), though surgical removal may be necessary (131,132). Soft tissue edema without calcinosis has been reported (133).

Chondritis

See Chapter 37.

Osteoporosis

See Chapter 60.

Costochondritis

Patients with SLE frequently complain of discomfort at the costochondral junctions. Esophageal spasm, angina pectoris, and pericarditis must be ruled out.

Myalgia, Myositis, And Myopathy

Generalized myalgia and muscle tenderness (Table 31.3), most marked in the deltoid areas and quadriceps (proximal muscles), are common during exacerbations of the disease and have been observed in 40% to 48% of patients (3,6,134). Inflammatory myositis involving the proximal musculature occurs in 5% to 11% of patients (134–137) and can be confirmed by muscle biopsy, electromyographic (EMG) studies, and elevation of the serum creatine phosphokinase (CPK) or aldolase levels. Myoglobin levels also may be increased (137). The myositis responds to steroid therapy.

The differential diagnosis of proximal muscle weakness is a common problem in the management of patients with SLE. An inflammatory myositis must be differentiated from a drug-induced myopathy (glucocorticoid or antimalarial).

TABLE 31.3. LUPUS MYOSITIS AND MYOPATHY IN SLE

Myalgias occur in 40% to 80% of patients with SLE and are most marked in proximal muscles; weakness is a common symptom
Inflammatory myositis (often with an increased CPK level) has a cumulative incidence of 5% to 11%
Steroid- and antimalarial-induced myopathies must be excluded
EMG and muscle biopsy findings range from the normal to the classic patterns seen in dermato/polymyositis
Myalgias without myositis may respond to salicylates, NSAIDs, antimalarials, or 20 mg/d of prednisone or less
If diagnostic criteria are met for both SLE and dermato/polymyositis, treatment with 1 mg/kg/d of prednisone should be initiated

CPK, creatine phosphokinase; EMG, electromyogram; NSAIDs, nonsteroidal antiinflammatory drugs.

Muscle enzyme levels are only elevated in the former group, but many untreated patients with SLE and myalgias have normal muscle enzyme levels. Frequently, generalized weakness is so prominent that some patients initially are diagnosed as having dermatomyositis (138). Inflammatory myositis can develop at any time during the course of the disease (139–146). Three large groups of dermatomyositis/polymyositis patients demonstrated a 7%, 4%, and 1% concurrence of SLE (147–149). The skin lesions of dermatomyositis/polymyositis also can appear in patients with SLE (142,143).

Tsokos et al. (150) evaluated 228 patients with SLE at the National Institutes of Health (NIH). Of these, 18 (8%) had prominent muscle disease. The CPK level was elevated in one patient, and the aldolase level was higher in 11. In 72%, myositis was concomitant with disease onset. No evidence of myocarditis was found, and all responded to 20 mg or less of prednisone daily.

Foote et al. (151) followed 276 patients with SLE at the Mayo Clinic, and 11 met the diagnostic criteria for dermatomyositis/polymyositis. All were female, with a mean age of 29 years. In contrast to the NIH findings, the onset of myositis in these patients occurred 13 years after the onset of SLE. Also, Raynaud's phenomenon was more prevalent in this group. The patients were treated with 30 to 60 mg of prednisone daily, and one was given azathioprine. After 4 years, two were dead and six asymptomatic. Isenberg's group (152) compared 11 patients with SLE and myositis with 19 who had polymyositis. Over a 7-year period, both groups had chronic, relapsing courses and no differences could be noted.

Rhabdomyolysis has never been reported in SLE (153).

Electromyography

The principal EMG findings in polymyositis and dermatomyositis are (a) spontaneous fibrillation; (b) positive or sawtooth potentials; (c) small-amplitude, complex, polyphasic, or short-duration potentials; and (d) salvos of repetitive, high-frequency potentials. In patients with SLE, the EMG findings range from normal to those of classic dermatomyositis/polymyositis. Only four studies, however, have examined EMG findings in patients with SLE.

O'Leary et al. (154) found nonspecific EMG abnormalities in two of nine patients with SLE but in all with dermatomyositis. Erbsloh and Baedeker (155) performed EMGs on 15 patients with muscle symptoms, and their main findings were a decrease in mean potential duration to only 54% of normal, an increase in the mean phase frequency, and a corresponding decrease in the phase quotient. In only one patient were the findings normal. Tsokos et al. (150) performed EMGs on eight of their 18 patients with SLE and myopathy. Of these, five had normal findings, neuropathy was demonstrated in one, and the classic polyphasic peaks seen in polymyositis were noted in two. In a study of 35 unselected patients with SLE, EMGs were suggestive of a myopathy in 23 (156). Also, 34 Norwegian patients with SLE underwent extensive neurophysiologic testing: 62% complained of muscle weakness, and 33% had any EMGs and 21% any nerve conduction abnormalities, neither of which correlated with symptoms (157).

Depending on various parameters, such as observer interpretation, whether an outpatient or inpatient population was used, and whether patients had muscle symptoms, between 22% and 90% of patients with SLE have abnormal EMGs (2,150,154–156).

Muscle Biopsies

Muscle biopsy findings (Fig. 31.2) range from normal to interstitial inflammation, fibrillar necrosis, degeneration, and vacuolization with fibrosis as a late occurrence seen with dermatomyositis/polymyositis. First used in the 1930s (154,158), muscle biopsies can be helpful in distinguishing inflammatory from drug-induced myopathies, as well as in determining reversibility based on the degree of fibrotic changes.

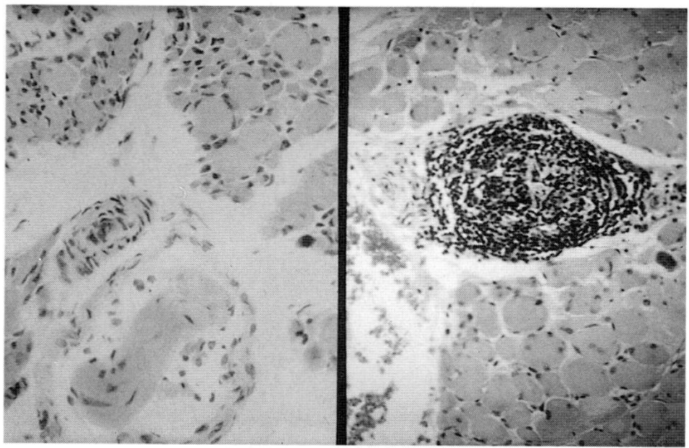

FIGURE 31.2. Lupus myositis.

Klemperer et al. (158) noted an inflammatory infiltrate in 5 of 30 cases of SLE, and Madden (159) noted the same in 6 of 21 biopsy specimens. The changes were nonspecific. Erbsloh and Baedeker (155) performed biopsies on 16 patients: two demonstrated impressive round cell infiltration, and 12 had parenchymal damage that occasionally included necrosis, along with a sparse interstitial infiltrate. Tsokos et al. (150) performed biopsies of 11 of 18 patients with SLE and myopathy: a mixed cellular, perivascular, and inflammatory reaction with interstitial inflammation without much muscle fiber degeneration was noted in six patients, and five had nonspecific changes or atrophy without inflammation.

Pearson (160) described muscle biopsies in 20 patients with various forms of SLE and noted rare, nonspecific fiber degeneration and interstitial myositis in ten patients, no change in three, and minor or insignificant muscle fiber vacuolization in seven (four taking steroids and two antimalarials). The vacuolar lesions were variable in extent and degree, sometimes being focal and scanty and on other occasions appearing widespread and extensive in individual fibers. These changes did not correlate with CPK levels, clinical measures of strength, or steroid administration. No vacuolar myopathy was noted among 16 biopsy specimens at the University of Toronto (161) and was seen in only one of 12 cases in another report (162). One case of inclusion body myositis has been observed in SLE (163). In the last few years, some centers have started performing less-invasive needle quadriceps biopsies. Lim et al. (164,165) also evaluated needle biopsy specimens from 55 patients with SLE. In these studies, lymphocytic vasculitis correlated with high sedimentation rates, inflammatory arthritis, and Sjögren's syndrome. Subclinical skeletal muscle lymphocytic vasculitis was present in 10 of 22 patients with active lupus and was not seen with inactive disease. Staining muscle tissue for immune fluorescence revealed evidence for deposits in 37% of 132 European patients (166).

Three studies have included ultrastructural examinations. Oxenhandler et al. (167) evaluated the immunopathologic characteristics of lupus myopathy in 19 patients. Type I fibers predominated in 44%, and type II fiber atrophy was seen in 33%. Eight patients had an inflammatory myositis. Immunoglobulin or complement staining was seen in 13 patients in sarcolemmal-basement membrane areas, five had myofibrillar IgG, five showed vascular immunoglobulin or complement deposits, and IgG-containing globules were seen in ten. The University of Toronto group (161) emphasized the universality of immunoglobulin deposition in 16 SLE muscle biopsies, despite the rarity of concurrent inflammation. Finol et al. (162) emphasized the presence of muscle atrophy, microtubular inclusions, and a bland mononuclear cell infiltrate in 12 biopsy specimens; necrotic changes were only present in one patient, who had an elevated CPK level. This group confirmed earlier suggestions by Norton et al. (168,169) that the microvascular circulation of skeletal muscle is decreased because of capillary basement membrane thickening. Pallis et al. (170) extended these findings and correlated thickening with impaired pulmonary gas exchange (as measured by diffusing capacity) and improvement with steroid therapy. Immunocytochemical studies have suggested increased levels of vascular cell adhesion molecule-1 (VCAM-1) in SLE muscle inflammatory infiltrates (171).

AVASCULAR NECROSIS OF BONE

First reported in SLE by Dubois and Cozen (172) in 1960, avascular necrosis (AVN), also known as aseptic necrosis or ischemic necrosis of bone, was observed in 26 (5) of Dubois' 520 patients (3), in twenty-five of Wallace's 464 patients (173), and in 24% to 30% of 150 and 103 patients at Johns Hopkins, which is an AVN referral center (174,175). Other studies have noted AVN in 4% to 9% of patients with SLE (176–186). AVN is a major source of morbidity and alteration in the quality of life in young women with lupus. This section reviews the pathophysiology, diagnostic testing, clinical presentation, and associations of AVN, as well as its treatment (Table 31.4).

Pathophysiology And Classification

The usual mechanism is death of subchondral bone, resulting in osseocartilaginous sequestration with adjacent secondary osteosclerosis. The term *osteochondritis dissecans* has been used to refer to small areas of this process, such as disease involving a segment of femoral head or condyle.

The initial pathologic lesion probably is obliteration of the blood supply of the epiphysis, followed by reactive hyperemia, which is seen on the radiograph as osteoporosis. At this stage, the necrotic bone is radiographically demarcated from viable bone, because the dead tissue does not take part in the decalcification. By contrast, the necrotic area appears increased in density compared with the osteoporotic bone around it. During the healing stage, as new blood vessels grow in and bone repair occurs, the newly formed bone is soft. With continued pressure on the surface, flattening may occur (e.g., on the medial and superior aspects of the femoral head). These irregularities in the contour of the articular surfaces cause definite and consistent adaptive changes that are manifested later as degenerative arthritis.

TABLE 31.4. AVASCULAR NECROSIS (AVN) OF BONE IN SLE

- AVN occurs in 5% to 10% of patients
- Most cases are associated with corticosteroid administration; the remainder probably are induced by Raynaud's phenomenon, a small-vessel vasculitis, fat emboli, or the antiphospholipid syndrome
- MRI is the diagnostic method of choice; CT and bone scans are less accurate and do not pick up preradiographic lesions as well; the radiographic appearance can be classified into four stages
- Multiple sites can be affected; the femoral head, tibial plateaus, and humeral head are the most common
- An association exists between AVN and Raynaud's phenomenon, increased steroid dosage, and duration of treatment
- Treatment includes limiting weight-bearing, administration of antiinflammatory analgesics, and core decompression for stage I and II lesions; reconstructive surgery usually is required for stage III and IV disease

AVN can have various types of causes (187,188): posttraumatic, nontraumatic, or idiopathic. Fractures, microfractures, or dislocations may cause AVN. Nontraumatic causes include embolic factors (e.g., as in sickle cell anemia, thalassemia, alcoholism, pancreatitis, and decompression states), small-vessel changes (e.g., as in SLE, polyarteritis, or Fabry's disease), and deposition ischemic necrosis (e.g., increased lipocytes caused by steroid therapy, Gaucher's disease, or Cushing's disease). Renal transplant patients who receive pulse steroids and high doses of steroids are especially susceptible. Conditions that are associated with idiopathic AVN include gout, pregnancy, prolonged immobilization, cytotoxic therapy, hyperparathyroidism, familial tendencies, lymphoma, metastatic carcinoma, and degenerative arthritis.

In SLE, Raynaud's phenomenon, vasculitis (189–191), fat emboli (192–194), corticosteroids, and defects in fibrinolysis (195) can induce ischemia that results in bony necrosis (196). That no cases of AVN were recorded before 1960 indicates the importance of the introduction of corticosteroids in the 1950s in regard to our perception of this entity.

Ficat and Arlet (197) have classified AVN using a radiographic scale. In stage 0, only hemodynamic changes have taken place. The patient is asymptomatic, and routine radiographs are normal. In stage I, minimal pain with mild restriction of motion may be present. Stage II is characterized by a dull, aching pain on weight-bearing, decreased range of motion, and a slight limp. Radiographs demonstrate diffuse osteoporosis, sclerosis, or cyst formation. By the time that stage III is reached, advanced radiographic changes are evident, and the patient has taken a quantum leap in restricted movement and pain. Subchondral bone collapse (the crescent sign) with normal joint space is present radiographically. Stage IV represents end-stage disease with osteoarthritis, as seen on the radiograph. Most patients are symptomatic and require surgery.

Diagnostic Techniques And Hemodynamic Studies

MRI can detect AVN months to years before it is evident on routine radiographs (Fig. 31.3). This has made earlier, noninvasive methods of detecting AVN obsolete. MRI

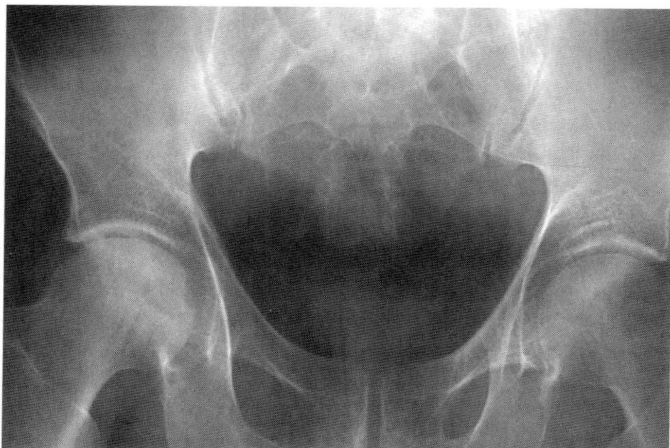

FIGURE 31.3. Avascular necrosis of the hip: plain film.

should be ordered for a patient with SLE who has hip pain and a normal radiograph if glucocorticoid therapy is being given. Plain x-rays are often unreadable and subject to marked observer variations (Fig 31.4) (198). Gallium scans (181) and technetium scans with pertechnetate or sulfur colloid (200–203) generally are accurate but can be subject to false-positive or false-negative interpretation. Scintigraphic images of radiographically negative osteonecrosis tend to contain a photopenic zone, whereas more advanced lesions have increased uptake (204). Several studies have compared bone scanning with MRI (205–210); the latter has better specificity and sensitivity, but both procedures can yield false-positive findings. Although computed tomography (CT) with multiplanar reformation (211) can be useful, MRI derives the same, or more, information with less effort and without exposing the patient to radiation.

On MRI, the reactive interface between live and dead bone at the periphery of AVN lesions has a characteristic double-line sign on T2-weighted images (212). A low-intensity band on T1-weighted images is an early, specific finding for AVN (213). Early changes at the femoral head can demonstrate bone marrow edema (214), and premature conversion to fatty marrow is evident in younger patients. In AVN, the femoral neck usually is surrounded by joint fluid. These findings have been confirmed in patients with SLE (205,208,215,216). Interestingly, the advent of MRI has allowed investigators to detect cases of incidental, asymptomatic, and nonprogressive AVN (243).

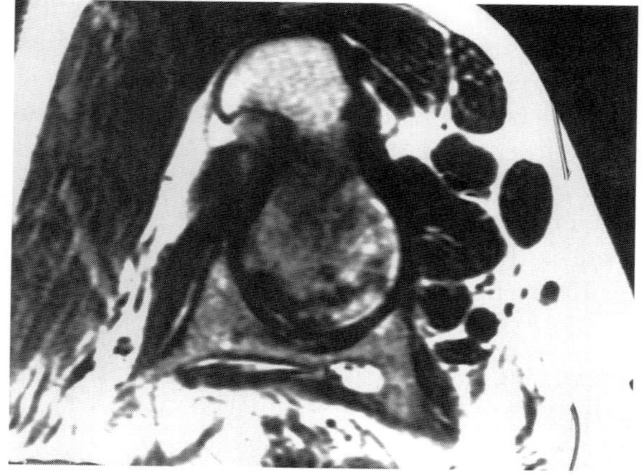

FIGURE 31.4. Avascular necrosis: T1-weighted magnetic resonance imaging.

Zizic et al. (217,218) at Johns Hopkins have used invasive techniques to obtain more information about the hemodynamics of AVN. They found increased baseline bone marrow pressure in most patients with SLE after carrying out a stress test (a greater than 10 mm Hg elevation after instillation of 5 mL of physiologic saline into the femoral head). Almost 90% of patients had abnormal intraosseous venography, as characterized by incomplete filling of the main extraosseous veins, diaphyseal reflux, and stasis of contrast material. Venography was abnormal in all stages of AVN, including preradiologic ones. In a follow-up study (219), bone marrow pressure, saline stress test, and/or ischemic intraosseous venography results were abnormal in 254 of 259 ischemic bones (98%) so evaluated, and AVN was detected in 93% of 55 radiologically normal bones. Using these parameters, 36 of 48 joints on the contralateral asymptomatic side had abnormalities, and 15 patients (42%) developed AVN over a 47-month follow-up period. Thus, hemodynamic measurements are of predictive value in identifying the at-risk joints (220), but this procedure is not widely available. Femoral head perfusion is decreased in lupus in general without AVN due to greater marrow fat content (221).

Clinical Associations In SLE

In SLE, AVN tends to occur at multiple sites. At the NIH, 90% of 31 cases were polyarticular, and 84% were symmetric (222). Of Dubois' 26 patients, 22 had bilateral femoral head involvement, one had unilateral involvement, and three had affected knees (223). Zizic's group (224–226) reported that 91 cases involved the femoral head and 83 occurred in multiple sites. Reports have appeared of 6, 8, 13, and even 28 different sites in a single patient (227–231). Although the hip is the most common site, AVN can involve other joints and often results in a delay in diagnosis. Three of 11 University of Connecticut patients studied by Urman's group (183) had AVN of the wrist. Most studies have recorded a mean onset of AVN in the fourth decade of life, with an average SLE disease duration of 4 to 7 years (103,232).

The diagnosis of AVN should be considered in any patient with SLE who has persistent pain in one or a few joints without evidence of disease activity in other systems, especially if glucocorticoids have been given. The association between vasculitis and AVN in the absence of steroid administration is well documented (189–191). Many studies have addressed the role of corticosteroids in inducing AVN in those with SLE, but early studies were hampered by control groups in which AVN was excluded based on normal radiographs (232,233). It has been suggested that increased doses of steroids (especially in the first year of treatment) and the duration of steroid therapy are correlated with a greater risk of AVN in SLE patients (224,225,234,235). Bolus steroids were not similarly associated (236,237). These dose-time relationships were confirmed in a meta-analysis of 22 papers (most patients without SLE) by Felson and Anderson (238), although this confirmation has been challenged (239). A widely cited, 1992 prospective study of AVN after high-dose steroid therapy is invalid, because the American College of Rheumatology (ACR) criteria were not used to define SLE and neither MRI nor CT scanning was employed (240). The clinical associations observed by our group are shown in Table 31.5

TABLE 31.5. COMPARISONS BETWEEN SYSTEMIC LUPUS ERYTHEMATOUS PATIENTS WITH AND WITHOUT AVASCULAR NECROSIS (AVN)

Characteristic	Percentage[a] of Patients With AVN (n = 26)	Percentage[a] of Patients Without AVN (n = 462)	p value[b]
Female	96.15	93.29	
Hispanic	7.69	7.61	
Black	19.23	10.85	
White	57.69	72.67	
On dialysis	11.54	5.15	
Living in 1991	95.15	95.02	
Mean age at diagnosis (years)	26.15	31.47	0.02
Mean follow-up (years)	9.28	5.94	
History of			
Fevers	53.85	41.34	
Arthritis	88.46	91.56	
Myalgias	76.92	79.44	
Pericarditis	23.08	11.90	
Hypertension	46.15	24.03	0.02
Pleural effusion	26.92	11.06	0.03
Pleuritic pain	34.62	30.30	
Skin rashes	73.08	52.60	
Raynaud's	26.92	26.42	
Headache	26.92	30.30	
Cerebritis	26.92	9.74	0.01
Nephritis	57.69	25.16	0.04
Thromboemboli	15.38	7.14	
Anemia	50.00	29.69	0.047
Hemolytic anemia	21.74	7.26	0.03
Leukopenia	50.00	50.55	
Thrombocytopenia	24.00	15.63	
Laboratory test results of			
Positive ANA	95.83	95.74	
Decreased C3	36.00	38.41	
Positive anti-DNA	40.00	40.05	
Positive anti-RNP	25.00	14.54	
Positive RA latex	23.52	22.62	
Positive anti-Ro (SSA)	19.05	17.76	
Anticardiolipin antibody	30.77	38.07	
Elevated sedimentation rate	65.22	54.38	
Treatment history of			
Trial of NSAIDs	88.46	70.77	
Rx hydroxychloroquine	44.00	61.76	
Use of systemic steroids	84.62	76.25	
High-dose oral steroids	50.00	35.75	
Pulse IV steroids	20.00	11.26	

[a]Percentage unless otherwise noted (ie, years).
[b]A p value of <.05 is considered to be statistically significant. Only significant p values are listed.
ANA, antinuclear antibody; C3, third component of complement; RN, ribonucleoprotein; RA, rheumatoid arthritis; Ro (SSA), Sjögren's syndrome A; NSAIDs, nonsteroidal antiinflammatory drugs; IV, intravenous.
From ref. 241.

(241). Mok et al (242) performed a similar survey and found many of the same associations.

SLE also has additional unique features that might predispose a patient to the development of AVN. Zizic (245) and Smith et al. (182) have both commented on the comparative rarity of AVN in steroid-dependent populations of patients with asthma, dermatologic disorders, and inflammatory bowel disease. AVN was found to be associated with Raynaud's phenomenon, central nervous system lupus, vasculitis, myositis, peripheral neuropathy, and elevated sedimentation rates (234,243,244). Others have only been able to suggest the association with Raynaud's phenomenon (179,182).

Does the presence of antiphospholipid antibodies predispose the patient to AVN? Since Asherson et al. (246) originally made the suggestion based on older and less accurate methods of detection, two studies have concurred with this finding (202,242) and five have not (186,221,241, 247,261). The Hopkins cohort has published studies with conflicting results (175,248). It is possible that antibodies to annexin-V may be important (249).

Treatment

Small areas of AVN can remain asymptomatic or heal spontaneously. Rare reports of spontaneous regression have appeared (250), but most patients with a clearly established diagnosis experience progressive disease if they are treated nonoperatively. Conservative management often is a holding action (especially in the hips) and consists of analgesics, nonsteroidal antiinflammatory drugs (NSAIDs), and limited or non–weight-bearing for several months (251). Alcohol use should be discouraged, and efforts to decrease steroid doses should be attempted.

A number of surgical techniques have been used successfully with AVN of the femoral head, including drilling or core decompression, free bone grafts (cortical or osteochondral allograft), vascularized bone grafts (muscle pedicle graft, free vascularized fibular graft, vascular anastomosis), osteotomy (varus or valgus angulation, rotation), and joint reconstruction (femoral head or total hip replacement) (251). Other joints are approached in a conceptually similar manner. The discussion here is limited to results that have been reported for SLE.

Early series documented excellent results with total hip replacement (252,253). Between 1971 and 1982, 39 of 43 prosthetic hip replacements performed at the Mayo Clinic on patients with SLE were for stage III or IV AVN (254). Of these, 29 patients had conventional hip replacements, and 14 had bipolar endoprosthetic replacements. Over a 66-month follow-up period, all were rated as having good or excellent results. Complications included delayed wound healing (15%) and superficial wound infection (10%). In our group, all seven patients who underwent total hip arthroplasties with at least a 10-year follow-up reported excellent results (241). Success rates are equal to patients with AVN and rheumatoid arthritis (257). Other groups also have reported greater than 90% long-term success rates (255–257). Joint arthroplasty in SLE has not been associated with increased rates of infection or lupus flare risks (258). Total knee arthroplasty for corticosteroid associated AVN yielded excellent results in only 11 of 25 patients treated at Johns Hopkins (175).

Whereas few disagree about the management of stage III and IV AVN, the indications for core decompression in earlier stages are controversial. First reported by Zizic et al. (217,260) as removal of an 11-mm diameter core of bone from the central axis of the femoral head, success was claimed in treating stages I, II, and III disease. Two studies of SLE failed to confirm these findings (164,197), however, and our results at UCLA Medical Center have been mixed. Zizic's (245) review of the literature (including other diseases) suggests a 77% success rate for preradiologic disease and a 52% success rate for stage II AVN. At Johns Hopkins, 68% of 31 patients undergoing core decompression for AVN required total hip replacements over a mean 12-year follow up period (259). The coring procedure probably is not indicated for patients with stage III or IV disease.

REFERENCES

1. Kaposi M. New reports on knowledge of lupus erythematosus (in German). *Arch Dermatol Syph* 1872;4:36–78.
2. Stevens MB. Musculoskeletal manifestations. In: Schur PH, ed. *The clinical management of systemic lupus erythematosus.* New York: Grune & Stratton, 1983:63–84.
3. Dubois EL, Tuffanelli DL. Clinical manifestations of systemic lupus erythematosus. Computer analysis of 520 cases. *JAMA* 1964;190:104–111.
4. Ropes MW. *Systemic lupus erythematosus.* Cambridge, MA: Harvard University Press, 1976.
5. Szczepanski L, Targonska B, Piotrowski M. Deforming arthropathy and Jaccoud's syndrome in patients with systemic lupus erythematosus. *Scand J Rheumatol* 1992;21:308–309.
6. Fries J, Holman H. *Systemic lupus erythematosus: a clinical analysis.* Philadelphia: WB Saunders, 1975.
7. Grigor R, Edmonds J, Lewkonia R, et al. Systemic lupus erythematosus. A prospective analysis. *Ann Rheum Dis* 1978;37: 121–128.
8. Petri M. Musculoskeletal complications of systemic lupus erythematosus in the Hopkins Lupus Cohort: an update. *Arthritis Care Res* 1995;8:137–145.
9. Buskila D, Gladman DD. Stress fractures of the legs and swelling of the ankles in a patient with lupus: a diagnostic dilemma. *Ann Rheum Dis* 1990;49:783–784.
10. Armas-Cruz R, Harnecker J, Ducach G, et al. Clinical diagnosis of systemic lupus erythematosus. *Am J Med* 1958;25: 409–419.
11. Bywaters EGL. Classification criteria for systemic lupus erythematosus, with particular reference in lupus-like syndromes. *Proc R Soc Med* 1967;60:463–464.
12. Martini A, Ravelli A, Viola S, et al. Systemic lupus erythematosus with Jaccoud's arthropathy mimicking juvenile rheumatoid arthritis. *Arthritis Rheum* 1987;30:1062–1064.

13. Bywaters EGL. Anatomic changes in Jaccoud's syndrome. *Arthritis Rheum* 1971;14:153(abst).
14. Silver M, Steinbrocker O. The musculoskeletal manifestations of systemic lupus erythematosus. *JAMA* 1961;176:100–111.
15. Alarcon-Segovia D, Abud-Mendoza C, Diaz-Jouanen E, et al. Deforming arthropathy of the hands in systemic lupus erythematosus. *J Rheumatol* 1988;15:65–69.
16. Bleifeld CJ, Inglis AE. The hand in systemic lupus erythematosus. *J Bone Joint Surg* 1974;56A:1207–1215.
17. Dreyfus JN, Schnitzer TJ. Pathogenesis and differential diagnosis of the swan-neck deformity. *Semin Arthritis Rheum* 1983;13: 200–211.
18. Esdaile JM, Danoff D, Rosenthall L, et al. Deforming arthritis in systemic lupus erythematosus. *Ann Rheum Dis* 1981;40:124–126.
19. Kahn MF. Jaccoud's syndrome in a rheumatology unit. *Clin Rheum Pract* 1986;Winter:153–155.
20. Girgis FL, Popple AW, Bruckner FE. Jaccoud's arthropathy. A case report and necropsy study. *Ann Rheum Dis* 1978;37: 561–565.
21. Klemp P, Majoos FL, Chalton D. Articular mobility in systemic lupus erythematosus (SLE). *Clin Rheumatol* 1987;6:202–207.
22. Kramer LS, Ruderman JE, Dubois EL, et al. Deforming, nonerosive arthritis of the hands in chronic systemic lupus erythematosus (SLE). *Arthritis Rheum* 1970;13:329–330(abst).
23. Labowitz R, Schumacher HR Jr. Articular manifestations of systemic lupus erythematosus. *Ann Intern Med* 1971;74:911–921.
24. Manthorpe R, Bendixen G, Schioler H, et al. Jaccoud's syndrome: a nosographic entity associated with systemic lupus erythematosus. *J Rheumatol* 1980;7:169–177.
25. Noonan CD, Odone DT, Englemann EP, et al. Roentgenographic manifestations of joint disease in systemic lupus erythematosus. *Radiology* 1963;80:837–843.
26. Spronk PE, ter Borg EJ, Kallenberg CGM. Patients with systemic lupus erythematosus and Jaccoud's arthropathy: a clinical subset with an increased C reactive protein response? *Ann Rheum Dis* 1991;51:358–361.
27. Francheschini F, Cretti L, Quinzanini M, et al. Deforming arthropathy of the hands in systemic lupus erythematosus is associated with antibodies to SSA/Ro and to SSB/La. *Lupus* 1993;3:419–422.
28. Kaplan D, Ginzler EM, Feldman J. Arthritis and hypertension in patients with systemic lupus erythematosus. *Arthritis Rheum* 1992;35:423–428.
29. Molina JF, Molina J, Gutierrez S, et al. Deforming arthropathy of the hands (Jaccoud's) in systemic lupus erythematosus (SLE): an independent subset of SLE? *Arthritis Rheum* 1995;38:S347(abst).
30. Queyrel V, Hachulla E, Cardon T. Arthritis in primary antiphospholipid syndrome? Piette JC, Asherson RA (reply) *J Rheumatol* 1996;23:1305–1306.
31. Van Vugt RM, Derksen RHWM, Kater L, et al. Deforming arthropathy or lupus and rhupus hands in systemic lupus erythematosus, *Ann Rheum Dis* 1998;57:540–544.
32. Dray GJ, Millender LM, Halebuff EA, et al. The surgical treatment of hand deformities in systemic lupus erythematosus. *J Hand Surg* 1981;6:339–342.
33. Nalebuff EA. Surgery of systemic lupus erythematosus arthritis of the hand. *Hand Clin* 1996;12:591–602.
34. Weissman BN, Rappoport AS, Sosman JL, et al. Radiographic findings in the hands of patients with systemic lupus erythematosus. *Radiology* 1978;126:313–317.
35. Laasonen L, Gripenberg M, Leskinen R, et al. A subset of systemic lupus erythematosus with progressive cystic bone lesions. *Ann Rheum Dis* 1990;49:118–120.
36. Leskinen RH, Skrifvars BV, Laasonen LS, et al. Bone lesions in systemic lupus erythematosus. *Radiology* 1984;153:349–352.
37. Richter Cohen M, Steiner G, Smolen JS, et al. Erosive arthritis in systemic lupus erythematosus: analysis of a distinct clinical and serological subset. *Br J Rheumatol* 1998;37:421–424.
38. Van de Wiele C, van den Bosch F, Mielants H, et al. Bone scintigraphy of the hands in early stage lupus erythematosus and rheumatoid arthritis, *J Rheumatol* 1997;24:1916–1921.
39. Muniain M, Spilberg I. Opera-glass deformity and tendon rupture in a patient with systemic lupus erythematosus. *Clin Rheumatol* 1985;4:335–339.
40. Swezey RL, Bjarnason DM, Alexander SJ, et al. Resorptive arthropathy and the opera-glass hand syndrome. *Semin Arthritis Rheum* 1972–1973;2:191–244.
41. Martinez-Cordero E, Lopez Zepeda J, Andrade-Ortega L, et al. Mutilans arthropathy in systemic lupus erythematosus. *Clin Exp Rheumatol* 1989;7:427–429.
42. de la Sota M, Maldonado-Cocco JA. Jaccoud's arthropathy in knees in systemic lupus erythematosus. *Clin Rheumatol* 1989; 8:416–417.
43. de la Sota M, Garcio-Morteo O, Maldonado-Cocco JA. Jaccoud's arthropathy of the knees in systemic lupus erythematosus. *Arthritis Rheum* 1985;28:825–827.
44. Glickstein M, Neustadter L, Dalinka M, et al. Periosteal reaction in systemic lupus erythematosus. *Skeletal Radiol* 1986;15: 610–612.
45. Reilly PA, Maddison PJ. Painful, swollen calf in a patient with SLE (letter). *Br J Rheumatol* 1987;26:319–320.
46. Moskowitz RW, Katz D. Chondrocalcinosis coincidental to other rheumatic disease. *Arch Intern Med* 1965;115:680–683.
47. Mizutani W, Quismorio FP. Lupus foot:deforming arthropathy of the feet in systemic lupus erythematosus. *J Rheumatol* 1984;11:80–82.
48. Morley KD, Leung A, Rynes RI. Lupus foot. *Br Med J (Clin Res)* 1982;284:557–558.
49. Beilstein DP, Hawkins ES. Pedal manifestations of systemic lupus erythematosus. *Clin Podiatr Med Surg* 1988;5:37–56.
50. Lagana FJ, McCarthy DJ. Podiatric implications of lupus erythematosus. *J Am Podiatr Med Assoc* 1988;78:577–583.
51. Babini SM, Cocco JA, Babini JC, et al. Atlantoaxial subluxation in systemic lupus erythematosus: further evidence of tendinous alterations. *J Rheumatol* 1990;17:173–177.
52. Klemp P, Meyers OL, Keyzer C. Atlanto-axial subluxation in systemic lupus erythematosus: a case report. *S Afr Med J* 1977; 52:531–532.
53. Kohli M, Bennett RM. Sacroiliitis in systemic lupus erythematosus. *J Rheumatol* 1994;21:170–171.
54. de Smet AA, Mahmood T, Robinson RG, et al. Elevated sacroiliac joint uptake ratios in systemic lupus erythematosus. *AJR* 1984;143:351–354.
55. Gosset D, Foucher C, Lecouffe P, et al. Asymptomatic sacroiliitis in systemic lupus erythematosus (letter). *J Rheumatol* 1988; 15:152–153.
56. Nassonova VA, Alekberova ZS, Folomeyev MY, et al. Sacroiliitis in male systemic lupus erythematosus. *Scand J Rheumatol* 1984;53(suppl):23–29.
57. Vivas J, Tiliakos NA. Sacroiliitis in male systemic lupus erythematosus. *Scand J Rheumatol* 1985;14:441.
58. Vivas J, Tiliakos NA. Sacroiliitis in male systemic lupus erythematosus. *Bol Assoc Med P R* 1985;77:271–272.
59. Leone J, Borela C, Cleenewerck N, et al. Prevalence of sacroiliac involvement in systemic lupus erythematosus. *Rev Rhum* 1997;64:517–522.
60. Siam ARM, Hammoudeh M. Jaccoud's arthropathy of the shoulders in systemic lupus erythematosus. *J Rheumatol* 1992; 19:980–981.
61. Jonsson R, Lindvall AM, Nyberg G. Temporomandibular joint involvement in systemic lupus erythematosus. *Arthritis Rheum* 1983;26:1506–1510.

62. Gelbracht D, Shapiro L. Temporomandibular joint erosions in patients with systemic lupus erythematosus (letter). *Arthritis Rheum* 1982;25:597.
63. Liebling MR, Gold RH. Erosions of the temporomandibular joint in systemic lupus erythematosus. *Arthritis Rheum* 1981; 29:948–950.
64. Dubois EL, Chandor S, Friou GJ, et al. Progressive systemic sclerosis (PSS) and localized scleroderma (morphea) with positive LE cell test and unusual systemic manifestations compatible with systemic lupus erythematosus (SLE): presentation of 14 cases including one set of identical twins, one with scleroderma and the other with SLE. Review of the literature. *Medicine* 1971;50:199–222.
65. Bade DM, Lovasko JH, Montana J, et al. Acute closed lock in a patient with lupus erythematosus: case review. *J Craniomandibular Disord* 1992;6:208–212.
66. Cruickshank B. Lesions of joints and tendon sheaths in systemic lupus erythematosus. *Ann Rheum Dis* 1959;18:111–119.
67. Goldenberg DL, Cohen AS. Synovial membrane histopathology in the differential diagnosis of rheumatoid arthritis, gout, pseudogout, systemic lupus erythematosus, infectious arthritis and degenerative joint disease. *Medicine* 1978;57:239–252.
68. Natour J, Montezzo LC, Moura LA, et al. A study of synovial membrane of patients with systemic lupus erythematosus (SLE). *Clin Exp Rheumatol* 1991;9:221–225.
69. Dubois EL, Friou GJ, Chandor S. Rheumatoid nodules and rheumatoid granuloma in systemic lupus erythematosus. *JAMA* 1972;220:515–518.
70. Harvey JP Jr, Corcos J. Large cysts in lower leg originating in the knee, occurring in patients with rheumatoid arthritis. *Arthritis Rheum* 1960;3:218–228.
71. Palmer DG. Synovial cysts in rheumatoid disease. *Ann Intern Med* 1969;70:61–68.
72. Ropes MW. *Systemic lupus erythematosus*. Cambridge, MA: Harvard University Press, 1976:19.
73. Pekin TJ Jr, Zvaifler NJ. Synovial fluid findings in systemic lupus erythematosus (SLE). *Arthritis Rheum* 1970;13:777–785.
74. Schumacher HJ. Electron microscopic study of synovial fluid cells in systemic lupus erythematosus. *Arthritis Rheum* 1978;21: 590(abst).
75. Schumacher HR Jr, Howe HS. Synovial fluid cells in systemic lupus erythematosus: light and electron microscopic studies. *Lupus* 1995;4:353–364.
76. Hollander JL, Jessar RA, McCarty DJ. Synovianalysis:an aid in arthritis diagnosis. *Bull Rheum Dis* 1961;12:263–264.
77. Pascual E. Analysis of synovial fluid from healthy knees. Comparison with fluid from asymptomatic knees in RA, SLE and gout. *Br J Rheumatol* 1992;31(suppl 2):219(abst).
78. Hasselbacher P. Immunoelectrophoretic assay for synovial fluid C3 with correction for synovial fluid globulin. *Arthritis Rheum* 1979;22:243–250.
79. Schumacher HR Jr, Sieck MS, Rothfuss S, et al. Reproducibility of synovial fluid analysis. A study among four laboratories. *Arthritis Rheum* 1986;29:770–774.
80. Barnes SS, Moffatt TW, Lane CW, et al. Studies on the L.E. phenomenon. *Arch Dermatol Syph* 1950;62:771–785.
81. Edelen JS, Lockshin MD, LeRoy EC. Gonococcal arthritis in two patients with active lupus erythematosus. A diagnostic problem. *Arthritis Rheum* 1971;14:557–559.
82. Morris JL, Zizic TM, Stevens MB. Proteus polyarthritis complicating systemic lupus erythematosus. *Johns Hopkins Med J* 1973;133:262–269.
83. Quismorio FP Jr, Dubois EL. Septic arthritis in systemic lupus erythematosus. *J Rheumatol* 1975;2:73–82.
84. Hunder GG, Pierre RV. In vivo LE cell formation in synovial fluid. *Arthritis Rheum* 1970;13:448–454.
85. Freemont AJ, Denton J, Chuck A, et al. Diagnostic value of synovial fluid microscopy: a reassessment and rationalization. *Ann Rheum Dis* 1991;50:101–107.
86. Vivino FB, Schumacher HR Jr. Synovial fluid characteristics and the lupus erythematosus cell phenomenon in drug-induced lupus. Findings in three patients and review of pertinent literature. *Arthritis Rheum* 1989;32:560–568.
87. Sones DA, McDuffie FC, Hunder GG. Clinical significance of the RA cell. *Arthritis Rheum* 1968;11:400–403.
88. Willkens RF, Healey LA Jr. The nonspecificity of synovial leukocyte inclusions. *J Lab Clin Med* 1966;68:628–635.
89. MacSween RNM, Dalakos TG, Jasani MK, et al. A clinicoimmunological study of serum and synovial fluid antinuclear factors in rheumatoid arthritis and other arthritides. *Clin Exp Immunol* 1968;3:17–24.
90. MacSween RNM, Dalakos TK, Jasani MK, et al. Antinuclear factors in synovial fluids. *Lancet* 1967;1:312–314.
91. Pollard KM, Furphy LJ, Webb J. Anti-Sm and anti-DNA antibodies in paired serum and synovial fluid samples from patients with SLE. *Rheumatol Int* 1988;8:197–204.
92. Ryan WE, Ellefson RD, Ward LE. Clinical conference: lipid synovial effusion. Unique occurrence in systemic lupus erythematosus. *Arthritis Rheum* 1973;16:759–764.
93. Howe HS, Schumacher HR. Light and electron microscopic (EM) studies on synovial fluid (SF) cells with systemic lupus erythematosus (SLE) (abstract). *Arthritis Rheum* 1993;36:S196.
94. Hebra F. *Hebra's Hautkrankheiten*. Vienna: Theill, 1845:B3.
95. Gonzalez T, Gantes M, Bustabad S, et al. Formation of rheumatoid nodules in systemic lupus erythematosus. *Med Clin (Barc)* 1985;85:711–714(English abst).
96. Moore CP, Willkens RF. The subcutaneous nodule: its significance in the diagnosis of rheumatic disease. *Semin Arthritis Rheum* 1977;7:63–79.
97. Ross SW, Wells BB. Systemic lupus erythematosus: review of the literature. *Am J Clin Pathol* 1953;23:139–160.
98. Schwartz IS, Grishman E. Rheumatoid nodules of the vocal cords as the initial manifestation of systemic lupus erythematosus. *JAMA* 1980;244:2751–2752.
99. Allison JH, Bettley FR. Rheumatoid arthritis with chronic leg ulceration. *Lancet* 1957;1:288–290.
100. Friedman IA, Sickley JF, Poske RM, et al. The L.E. phenomenon in rheumatoid arthritis. *Ann Intern Med* 1957;46: 1131–136.
101. Ziff M, Esserman P, McEwen C. Observations on the course and treatment of SLE. *Arthritis Rheum* 1956;7:332–350.
102. Tuffanelli DL. Lupus erythematosus panniculitis (profundus) clinical and immunologic studies. *Arch Dermatol* 1971;103: 231–242.
103. Dubois EL, ed. *Lupus erythematosus. A review of the current status of discoid and systemic lupus erythematosus and their variants*, 2nd ed. rev. Los Angeles: USC Press, 1976.
104. Larson DL. *Systemic lupus erythematosus*. Boston: Little, Brown, 1961.
105. Dubois EL. Procainamide induction of a systemic lupus erythematosus-like syndrome. Presentation of six cases, review of the literature, and analysis and follow-up of reported cases. *Medicine* 1969;48:217–228.
106. Sidiq M, Kirsner AB, Shoen RP. Carpal tunnel syndrome:first manifestation of systemic lupus erythematosus. *JAMA* 1972; 222:1416–1417.
107. Furie RA, Chartash EK. Tendon rupture in systemic lupus erythematosus. *Semin Arthritis Rheum* 1988;18:127–133.
108. Halpern AA, Horwitz BG, Nagel DA. Tendon ruptures associated with corticosteroid therapy. *West J Med* 1977;127:378–382.
109. Khan MA, Ballou SP. Tendon rupture in systemic lupus erythematosus. *J Rheumatol* 1981;8:308–310.

110. Pritchard CH, Berney S. Patellar tendon rupture in systemic lupus erythematosus. *J Rheumatol* 1989;16:786–788.
111. Potasman I, Bassan HM. Multiple tendon rupture in systemic lupus erythematosus: care report and review of the literature. *Ann Rheum Dis* 1984;43:347–348.
112. Gould ES, Taylor S, Naidich JB, et al. MR appearance of bilateral spontaneous patellar tendon rupture in systemic lupus erythematosus. *J Comput Assist Tomogr* 1987;11:1096–1097.
113. Formiga F, Moga I, Pac M, et al. Spontaneous tendinous breakage in systemic lupus erythematosus. Discussion of two cases. *Rev Clin Esp* 1993;192:175–177.
114. Potasman I, Bassan HM. Multiple tendon rupture in systemic lupus erythematosus: case report and review of the literature. *Ann Rheum Dis* 1984;43:348–347.
115. Babini SM, Arturi A, Marcos JC, et al. Laxity and rupture of the patellar tendon in systemic lupus erythematosus. Association with secondary hyperparathyroidism. *J Rheumatol* 1988;15: 1162–1165.
116. Babini SM, Cocco JA, de la Sota M, et al. Tendinous laxity and Jaccoud's syndrome in patients with systemic lupus erythematosus. Possible role of secondary hyperparathyroidism. *J Rheumatol* 1989;16:494–498.
117. Medsger TA Jr. Raynaud's, carpal tunnel associated but distinct (questions and answers). *J Musculoskeletal Med* 1991;8:15–16.
118. Carette S, Urowitz MB. Systemic lupus erythematosus and diffuse soft tissue calcifications. *Int J Dermatol* 1983;22:416–418.
119. Lawrence RC, Hochberg MC, Kelsey JL, et al. Estimates of prevalence of selected arthritis and musculoskeletal diseases in the United States. *J Rheumatol* 1989;16:427–441.
120. Budin JA, Feldman F. Soft tissue calcifications in systemic lupus erythematosus. *AJR* 1975;124:350–364.
121. Weiner AL. Disseminated lupus erythematosus treated by sulfanilamide:report of 4 cases. *Arch Dermatol Syph* 1940;441: 534–544.
122. Grinlinton FM, Vuletic JC, Gow PJ. Rapidly progressive calcific periarthritis occurring in a patient with lupus nephritis receiving chronic ambulatory peritoneal dialysis. *J Rheumatol* 1990;17:1100–1103.
123. Johansson E, Kanerva L, Niemi KM, et al. Diffuse soft tissue calcifications (calcinosis cutis) in a patient with discoid lupus erythematosus. *Clin Exp Dermatol* 1988;13:193–196.
124. Nomura M, Okada N, Okada M, et al. Large subcutaneous calcification in systemic lupus erythematosus. *Arch Dermatol* 1990;126:1057–1059.
125. Minami A, Suda K, Kaneda K, et al. Extensive subcutaneous calcification of the forearm in systemic lupus erythematosus. *J Hand Surg* 1994;19B:638–641.
126. Okada J, Nomura M, Shirataka M, Kondo H. Prevalence of soft tissue calcification in patients with SLE and effects of alfa CARCIDUL. *Lupus* 1999;8:456–461.
127. Sugimoto H, Hyodoh K, Kikuno M, et al. Periarticular calcification in systemic lupus erythematosus. *J Rheumatol* 1999;26: 574–579.
128. Palmieri GMA, Sebes JI, Aelion JA, et al. Treatment of calcinosis with diltiazem. *Arthritis Rheum* 1995;38:1646–1654.
129. Torralba TP, Li-Yu J, Navarra TGV. Successful use of diltiazem in calcinosis caused by connective tissue disease. *J Clin Rheumatol* 1999;54:74–78.
130. Park YM, Lee SJ, Kang H, et al. Subcutaneous calcification in systemic lupus erythematosus: treatment with oral aluminum hydroxide administration followed by surgical excision. *J Korean Med Sci* 1999;14:589–592.
131. Minami A, Suda K, Kaneda K, et al. Extensive calcinosis cutis with systemic lupus erythematosus. *J Hand Surg* 1994;19B: 638–641.
132. Cousins MAM, Jones DB, Whyte MP, et al. Surgical management of calcinosis cutis universalis in systemic lupus erythematosus, *Arthritis Rheum* 1997;40:570–572.
133. Mc Dermott EM, Powell RJ. Soft tissue involvement in systemic lupus erythematosus. *Br J Rheumatol* 1997;36:703–704
134. Isenberg DA, Snaith ML. Muscle disease in systemic lupus erythematosus: a study of its nature, frequency and cause. *J Rheumatol* 1981;8:917–924.
135. Estes D, Larson DL. Systemic lupus erythematosus and pregnancy. *Clin Obstet Gynecol* 1965;8:307–321.
136. Feinglass EJ, Arnett FC, Dorsch CA, et al. Neuropsychiatric manifestations of systemic lupus erythematosus: diagnosis, clinical spectrum, and relationship to other feature so the disease. *Medicine* 1976;55:323–339.
137. Kagen LJ. Myoglobinemia in inflammatory myopathies. *JAMA* 1977;237:2448–2452.
138. McCombe PA, McLeod JG, Pollad JD, et al. Peripheral sensorimotor and autonomic neuropathy associated with systemic lupus erythematosus. Clinical, pathological, and immunologic features. *Brain* 1987;110:533–549.
139. Degos R, Garnier G, Darnis F, et al. Subacute lupus erythematosus with signs of subacute dermatomyositis (electromyographic abnormalities) (in French). *Bull Soc Franc Dermatol Syph* 1949;56:114–116.
140. Graciansky P de. Two forms of dermatomyositis (in French). *Semin Hop Paris* 1949;25:1406–1413.
141. Graciansky P de. Remarks concerning six cases of dermatomyositis (in French). *Semin Hop Paris* 1953;29:1621–1633.
142. Keil H. Dermatomyositis and systemic lupus erythematosus:I. Clinical report of transitional cases, with consideration of lead as possible etiologic factor. *Arch Intern Med* 1940;66:109–139.
143. Keil H. Dermatomyositis and systemic lupus erythematosus: II. Comparative study of essential clinicopathologic features. *Arch Intern Med* 1940;66:339–383.
144. Pagel W, Treip CS. Viscero-cutaneous collagenosis:study of intermediate forms of dermatomyositis, scleroderma and disseminated lupus erythematosus. *J Clin Pathol* 1955;8:118.
145. Turner JC. Dermatomyositis. A study of 3 cases. *N Engl J Med* 1937;216:158–161.
146. White W. Lupus erythematosus. Polymyositis. *Proc R Soc Med* 1959;52:1035–1036.
147. DeVere R, Bradley WG. Polymyositis: its presentation, morbidity and mortality. *Brain* 1975;98:637–666.
148. Plotz PH, Dalakas M, Leff RL, et al. Current concepts in the idiopathic inflammatory myopathies: polymyositis, dermatomyositis, and related disorders. *Ann Intern Med* 1989;111:143–157.
149. Rowland LP, Clark C, Olarte M. Therapy for dermatomyositis and polymyositis. *Adv Neurol* 1977;17:63–97.
150. Tsokos GC, Moutsopoulos HM, Steinberg AD. Muscle involvement in systemic lupus erythematosus. *JAMA* 1981;246: 766–768.
151. Foote RA, Kimbrough SM, Stevens JC. Lupus myositis. *Muscle Nerve* 1982;5:65–68.
152. Garton MJ, Isenberg DA, Clinical features of lupus myositis versus idiopathic myositis: a review of 30 cases. *Br J Rheumatol* 1997;36:1067–1074.
153. Menon S, Round JM, Isenberg DA. Rhabdomyolysis in a patient with discoid lupus erythematosus. *J Rheumatol* 1994;21: 1967–1969.
154. O'Leary PA, Lambert EH, Sayre GP. Muscle studies in cutaneous disease. *J Invest Dermatol* 1955;24:301–310.
155. Erbsloh F, Baedeker WD. Lupus myopathy. A clinical, electromyographic and bioptic histological study (in German). *Dtsch Med Wochenschr* 1962;87:2464–2470.
156. Vilppula A. Muscular disorders in some collagen diseases. A clinical, electromyographic and biopsy study. *Acta Med Scand* 1972;540(suppl):147.

157. Omdal R, Mellgren SI, Henriksen OA, et al. Muscular weakness in systemic lupus erythematosus. *J Rheumatol* 1991;18:1364–1367.
158. Klemperer P, Pollack AD, Baehr G. Pathology of disseminated lupus erythematosus. *Arch Pathol* 1941;32:569–631.
159. Madden JF. Comparison of muscle biopsies and bone marrow examinations in dermatomyositis and lupus erythematosus. *Arch Dermatol Syph* 1950;62:192–205.
160. Pearson CM. Vacuolar myopathy in a patient with a positive LE cell preparation. Discussion. *Arthritis Rheum* 1967;10:147.
161. Russell ML, Hanna WM. Ultrastructural pathology of skeletal muscle in various rheumatic diseases. *J Rheumatol* 1988;15:445–453.
162. Finol HJ, Montagnani S, Marquez A, et al. Ultrastructural pathology of skeletal muscle in systemic lupus erythematosus. *J Rheumatol* 1990;17:210–219.
163. Yood RA, Smith TW. Inclusion body myositis and systemic lupus erythematosus. *J Rheumatol* 1985;12:568–570.
164. Lim KL, Abdul-Wahab R, Lowe J, et al. Muscle biopsy abnormalities in systemic lupus erythematosus: correlation with clinical and laboratory parameters. *Ann Rheum Dis* 1994;53:178–182.
165. Lim KL, Lowe J, Powell RJ. Skeletal muscle lymphocytic vasculitis in systemic lupus erythematosus: relation to disease activity. *Lupus* 1995;4:148–151.
166. Vizjak A, Perkovic T, Rozman B, et al. Skeletal muscle immune deposits in systemic lupus erythematosus. *Scand J Rheumatol* 1998;27:207–214.
167. Oxenhandler R, Hart MN, Bickel J, et al. Pathologic features of muscle in systemic lupus erythematosus: a biopsy series with comparative clinical and immunopathologic observations. *Hum Pathol* 1982;13:745–757.
168. Norton WL. Comparison of the microangiopathy of systemic lupus erythematosus, dermatomyositis, scleroderma, and diabetes mellitus. *Lab Invest* 1970;22:301–308.
169. Norton WL, Hurd ER, Lewis DC, et al. Evidence of microvascular injury in scleroderma and systemic lupus erythematosus: quantitative study of the microvascular bed. *J Lab Clin Med* 1968;71:919–933.
170. Pallis M, Hopkinson N, Lowe J, et al. An electron microscopic study of muscle capillary wall thickening in systemic lupus erythematosus. *Lupus* 1994;3:401–407.
171. Pallis M, Robson DK, Haskard DO, et al. Distribution of cell adhesion molecules in skeletal muscle from patients with SLE. *Ann Rheum Dis* 1993;52:667–671.
172. Dubois EL, Cozen L. Avascular (aseptic) bone necrosis associated with systemic lupus erythematosus. *JAMA* 1960;174:966–971.
173. Pistiner M, Wallace DJ, Nessim S, et al. Lupus erythematosus in the 1980s: a survey of 570 patients. *Semin Arthritis Rheum* 1991;21:55–61.
174. Hochberg MC, Boyd RE, Ahearn JM, et al. Systemic lupus erythematosus: a review of clinico-laboratory features and immunogenic markers in 150 patients with emphasis on demographic subsets. *Medicine* 1985;64:285–295.
175. Mont MA, Glueck CJ, Pacheco IH, et al. Risk factors for osteonecrosis in systemic lupus erythematosus. *J Rheumatol* 1997;24:654–662.
176. Abeles M, Urman JD, Weinstein A, et al. Systemic lupus erythematosus in the younger patient: survival studies. *J Rheumatol* 1980;7:515–522.
177. Diaz-Jouanen E, Abud-Mendoza C, Inglesias-Gamarra A, et al. Ischemic necrosis of bone in systemic lupus erythematosus. *Orthop Rev* 1985;14:303–309.
178. Dimant J, Ginzler EM, Diamond HS, et al. Computer analysis of factors influencing the appearance of aseptic necrosis in patients with SLE. *J Rheumatol* 1978;5:136–141.
179. Kalla AA, Learmonth ID, Klemp P. Early treatment of avascular necrosis in systemic lupus erythematosus. *Ann Rheum Dis* 1986;45:649–652.
180. Klippel JH, Gerberg LH, Pollak L, et al. Avascular necrosis in systemic lupus erythematosus: silent symmetric osteonecrosis. *Am J Med* 1979;67:83–87.
181. Lin RY, Landsman L, Krey PR, et al. Multiple dermatofibromas and systemic lupus erythematosus. *Cutis* 1986;37:45–49.
182. Smith FE, Sweet DE, Brunner CM, et al. Avascular necrosis in SLE. An apparent predilection for young patients. *Ann Rheum Dis* 1976;35:227–232.
183. Urman JD, Abeles M, Houghton AN, et al. Aseptic necrosis presenting as wrist pain in SLE. *Arthritis Rheum* 1977;20:825–828.
184. Vroninks P, Remans J, Kahn MF, et al. Aseptic bony necrosis in systemic lupus erythematosus. Report of 7 newcases (in French). *Semin Hop Paris* 1972;48:3001–3009.
185. Zizic TM. Systemic lupus erythematosus. X: corticosteroid therapy and its complications. *Md State Med J* 1984;33:370–381.
186. Rascu A, Manger K, Kraetsch HG, et al. Osteonecrosis in systemic lupus erythematosus, steroid-induced or a lupus-dependent manifestation? *Lupus* 1996;5:323–327.
187. Griffiths HJ. Etiology, pathogenesis and early diagnosis of ischemic necrosis of the hip. *JAMA* 1981;246:2615–2617.
188. Chang CC, Greenspan A, Gershwin ME. Osteonecrosis:current perspectives on pathogenesis and treatment. *Semin Arthritis Rheum* 1993;23:47–69.
189. Milch RA. Blood supply and the localization of tetracycline fluorescence in arthritic femoral heads. *Arthritis Rheum* 1963;6:377–380.
190. Siemsen JK, Brook J, Meister L. Lupus erythematosus and avascular bone necrosis: a clinical study of three cases and review of the literature. *Arthritis Rheum* 1962;5:492–501.
191. Velayos EE, Leidholt JD, Smyth CJ, et al. Arthropathy associated with steroid therapy. *Ann Intern Med* 1966;64:759–771.
192. Fisher DE, Bickel WH. Corticosteroid-induced avascular necrosis. A clinical study of 77 patients. *J Bone Joint Surg* 1971;53A:859–873.
193. Fisher DE, Bickel WH, Holley KE. Histologic demonstration of fat emboli in aseptic necrosis associated with hypercortisonism. *Mayo Clin Proc* 1969;44:252–259.
194. Jones JP, Engleman EP, Steinbach HL, et al. Fat embolization as a possible mechanism producing avascular necrosis. *Arthritis Rheum* 1965;8:448(abst).
195. Sheikh JS, Retzinger GS, Hess EV. Association of osteonecrosis in systemic lupus erythematosus with abnormalities in fibrinolysis. *Lupus* 1998;7:42–48.
196. Nagasawa K, Ishii Y, Mayumi T, et al. Avascular necrosis of bone in systemic lupus erythematosus: possible role of haemostatic abnormalities. *Ann Rheum Dis* 1989;48:672–676.
197. Ficat RP, Arlet J. Functional investigation of bone under normal conditions. In: Hungerford DS, ed. *Ischemia and necrosis of bone.* Baltimore: Williams & Wilkins, 1980:171–182.
198. Mahood J, Bogoch E, Gladman DD, et al. Osteonecrosis of the hip in SLE: observer and patient variation on six methods of assessing femoral head involvement. *J Orthop Rheumatol* 1995;8:37–42.
199. Mayer JW, Antoine JE, deHoratius RJ, et al. Aseptic necrosis in systemic lupus erythematosus: early detection by radionuclide scan. Report of case. *Rocky Mt Med J* 1977:74:324–326.
200. D'Ambrosio R, Riggins R, Stadalnick R, et al. 99m Tc Diphosphonate scintigraphy validated with tetracycline labelling. *Clin Orthop* 1976;121:143–145.
201. Lutzker LG, Alavi A. Bone and marrow imaging in sickle cell disease: diagnosis of infarction. *Semin Nucl Med* 1976;6:83–93.

202. Scoles PV, Yoon YS, Makley JT, et al. Nuclear magnetic resonance imaging in Legg-Calve-Perthes disease. *J Bone Joint Surg* 1984;66A:1357–1363.
203. Zizic TM, Conklin JJ, Hungerford DS, et al. Sensitivity of quantitative scintigraphy in the early detection of ischemic necrosis of bone. *Arthritis Rheum* 1981;24:S62(abst).
204. Maddison PJ, Provost TT, Reichlin M. Serological findings in patients with ANA-negative systemic lupus erythematosus. *Medicine* 1981;60:87–94.
205. Nagawsawa K, Tsukamoto H, Tada Y, et al. Imaging study on the mode of development and changes in avascular necrosis of the femoral head in systemic lupus erythematosus: long-term observations. *Br J Rheumatol* 1994;33:343–347.
206. Beltran J, Herman LJ, Burk JM, et al. Femoral head avascular necrosis MR imaging with clinical pathologic and radionuclide correlation. *Radiology* 1988;166:215–220.
207. Genez BM, Wilson MR, Houk RW, et al. Early osteonecrosis of the femoral head: detection in high-risk patients with MR imaging. *Radiology* 1988;168:521–524.
208. Kalunian KC, Hahn BH, Bassett L. Magnetic resonance imaging identifies early femoral head ischemic necrosis in patients receiving glucocorticoid therapy. *J Rheumatol* 1989;16: 959–963.
209. Robinson HJ Jr, Hartleben PD, Lund G, et al. Evaluation of magnetic resonance imaging in the diagnosis of osteonecrosis of the femoral head. Accuracy compared with radiographs, core biopsy, and intraosseous pressure measurements. *J Bone Joint Surg* 1989;71A:650–663.
210. Stulberg BN, Levine M, Bauer TW, et al. Multimodality approach to osteonecrosis of the femoral head. *Clin Orthop* 1989;240:181–193.
211. Sartoris DJ, Resnick D, Gershuni D, et al. Computed tomography with multiplanar reformation and 3-dimensional image analysis in the preoperative evaluation of ischemic necrosis of the femoral head. *J Rheumatol* 1986;13:153–163.
212. Mitchell DG, Steinberg MC, Dalinka MK, et al. Magnetic resonance imaging of the ischemic hip. Alterations within the osteonecrotic, viable and reactive zone. *Clin Orthop* 1989;244: 60–72.
213. Sugano N, Ohzono K, Masuhara K, et al. Prognostication of osteonecrosis of the femoral head in patients with systemic lupus erythematosus by magnetic resonance imaging. *Clin Orthop* 1994;35:190–199.
214. Turner DA, Templeton AC, Selzer PM, et al. Femoral capital osteonecrosis: MR finding of diffuse marrow abnormalities without focal lesions. *Radiology* 1989;171:135–140.
215. Ganczarczyk ML, Lee P, Fornasier VL. Early diagnosis of osteonecrosis in systemic lupus erythematosus with magnetic resonance imaging. Failure of core decompression. *J Rheumatol* 1986;13:814–817.
216. Zizic TM. Systemic lupus erythematosus. X. Corticosteroid therapy and its complications. *Md State Med J* 1984;33: 370–371.
217. Zizic TM, Hungerford DS, Stevens MB. Ischemic bone necrosis in systemic lupus erythematosus. II. The early diagnosis of ischemic necrosis of bone. *Medicine* 1980;59:134–142.
218. Zizic TM, Hungerford DS, Stevens MB. Ischemic bone necrosis in systemic lupus erythematosus. II. The treatment of ischemic necrosis of bone in systemic lupus erythematosus. *Medicine* 1980;59:143–148.
219. Zizic TM, Marcoux C, Hungerford DS, et al. The early diagnosis of ischemic necrosis of bone. *Arthritis Rheum* 1986;29: 1177–1186.
220. Zizic TM, Lewis CG, Marcoux C, et al. The predictive value of hemodynamic studies in preclinical ischemic necrosis of bone. *J Rheumatol* 1989;16:1559–1564.
221. Bluemke DA, Petri M, Zerhouni EA. Femoral head perfusion and composition: MR imaging and spectroscopic evaluation of patients with systemic lupus erythematosus and at risk for avascular necrosis. *Radiology* 1995;197:433–438
222. Klippel JH, Gerberg LH, Pollak L, et al. Avascular necrosis in systemic lupus erythematosus: silent symmetric osteonecrosis. *Am J Med* 1979;67:83–87.
223. Dubois EL, Tuffanelli DL. Clinical manifestations of systemic lupus erythematosus. Computer analysis of 520 cases. *JAMA* 1964;190:104–111.
224. Klipper AR, Stevens MB, Zizic TM, Hungerford DS. Ischemic recrosis of bone in systemic lupus erythematosus. *Medicine* 1976;251–257.
225. Zizic TM, Hungerford DS, Dansereau J-Y, et al. Corticosteroid associated ischemic necrosis of bone in SLE. *Arthritis Rheum* 1982;25(suppl):S82(abst).
226. Zizic TM, Marcoux C, Hungerford DS, et al. Corticosteroid therapy associated with ischemic necrosis of bone in systemic lupus erythematosus. *Am J Med* 1985;79:596–604.
227. Fishl B, Caspi D, Eventov I, et al. Multiple osteonecrotic lesions in systemic lupus erythematosus. *J Rheumatol* 1987;14: 601–604.
228. Lightfoot RW Jr, Hughes GRV. Significance of persisting serologic abnormalities in SLE. *Arthritis Rheum* 1976;19:837–843.
229. Nilsen KH. Systemic lupus erythematosus and avascular bone necrosis. *N Z Med J* 1977;85:472–475.
230. Ruderman M, McCarty DJ Jr. Arthritis rounds:(4). Aseptic necrosis in systemic lupus erythematosus. Report of a case involving six joints. *Arthritis Rheum* 1964;7:709–721.
231. Guillaume MP, Brandelet B, Peretz A. Unusual high frequency of multifocal lesions of osteonecrosis in a young patient with systemic lupus erythematosus. *Br J Rheumatol* 1998;37: 1248–1249.
232. Dimant J, Ginzler EM, Diamond HS, et al. Computer analysis of factors influencing the appearance of aseptic necrosis in patients with SLE. *J Rheumatol* 1978;5:136–141.
233. Klippel JH, Gerberg LH, Pollak L, et al. Avascular necrosis in systemic lupus erythematosus: silent symmetric osteonecrosis. *Am J Med* 1979;67:83–87.
234. Klipper AR, Stevens MB, Zizic TM, et al. Ischemic necrosis of bone in systemic lupus erythematosus. *Medicine* 1976;55: 251–157.
235. Weiner ES, Abeles M. Aseptic necrosis and glucocorticosteroids in systemic lupus erythematosus: a reevaluation. *J Rheumatol* 1989;16:604–608.
236. Milgliaresi S, Picillo U, Ambrosone L, et al. Avascular necrosis in patients with SLE: relation to corticosteroid therapy and anticardiolipin antibodies. *Lupus* 1994;3:37–41.
237. Williams IA, Mitchell AD, Rothman W, et al. Survey of the long-term incidence of osteonecrosis of the hip and adverse medical events in rheumatoid arthritis after high dose intravenous methylprednisolone. *Ann Rheum Dis* 1988;47:930–933.
238. Felson DT, Anderson JJ. Across-study evaluation of association between steroid dose and bolus steroids and avascular necrosis of bone. *Lancet* 1987;1:902–906.
239. Massardo L, Jacobelli S, Leissner M, et al. High-dose intravenous methylprednisolone therapy associated with osteonecrosis in patients with systemic lupus erythematosus. *Lupus* 1992; 1:401–405.
240. Ono K, Tohjuma T, Komazawa T. Risk factors of avascular necrosis of the femoral head in patients with systemic lupus erythematosus under high-dose corticosteroid therapy. *Clin Orthop* 1992;277:89–97.
241. Cozen L, Wallace DJ, Avascular necrosis in systemic lupus erythematosus: clinical associations and a 47-year perspective. *Am J Orthop* 1998;27:352–354.

242. Mok CC, Lau CS, Wong RWS. Risk factors for avascular bone necrosis in systemic lupus erythematosus. *Br J Rheumatol* 1998;37:895–900.
243. Aranow C, Zelicof S, Leslie D, et al. Clinically occult avascular necrosis of the hip in systemic lupus erythematosus. *J Rheumatol* 1997;24:2318–2322.
244. Freeman HJ, Kwan WCP. Non-corticosteroid associated osteonecrosis of the femoral heads in two patients with inflammatory bowel disease. *N Engl J Med* 1993;329:1314–1316.
245. Zizic TM. Avascular necrosis of bone. *Curr Opin Rheumatol* 1990;2:26–37.
246. Asherson RA, Liote F, Page B, et al. Avascular necrosis of bone and antiphospholipid antibodies in systemic lupus erythematosus. *J Rheumatol* 1993;20:284–288.
247. Dromer C, Marv V, Laroche M, et al. No link between avascular necrosis of the femoral head and antiphospholipid antibodies. *Rev Rhum* 1997;6:382–385.
248. Petri M, Baker J, Goldman D. Risk factors for avascular necrosis in SLE. *Arthritis Rheum* 1992;35:5110.
249. Sugiura K, Muro Y. Anti-annexin V antibodies and osteonecrosis in systemic lupus erythematosus. *J Rheumatol* 1998;25:2477.
250. Lee CK, Hansen HT, Weiss AB. The silent hip of idiopathic ischemic necrosis of the femoral head in adults. *J Bone Joint Surg* 1981;62A:795–780.
251. Lotke PA, Steinberg ME. Osteonecrosis of the hip and knee. *Bull Rheum Dis* 1985;35:18.
252. Baganz HM, Bailey WL. Systemic lupus erythematosus complicated by avascular necrosis of the hip. Medical and surgical management. *Del Med J* 1961;33:34–37.
253. Dubois E. Clinical picture of systemic lupus erythematosus. In: Dubois E, ed. *Lupus erythematosus.* Los Angeles: USC Press, 1974:232–379.
254. Hanssen AD, Cabanela ME, Michet CJ. Hip arthroplasty in patients with systemic lupus erythematosus. *J Bone Joint Surg* 1987;69A:807–814.
255. Huo MH, Salvati EA, Browne MG, et al. Primary total hip arthroplasty in systemic lupus erythematosus. *J Arthroplasty* 1992;7:51–56.
256. Low CK, Lai CH, Low YP. Results of total hip replacement in systemic lupus erythematosus. *Singapore Med J* 1991;32:391–392.
257. Zangger P, Gladman DD, Urowitz MB, et al. Outcome of total hip replacement for avascular necrosis in systemic lupus erythematosus. *J Rheumatol* 2000;27:919–923.
258. Maestrello S, Haiko G, Ahmed A, et al. Complications of total joint arthroscopy (TJA) in systemic lupus erythematosus (SLE). *Arthritis Rheum* 1994;37:R41(abst).
259. Mont MA, Myers TH, Krackow KA, et al. Core decompression for osteonecrosis of the femoral head in systemic lupus erythematosus. *Clin Orthop* 1997;(338):124–130.
260. Zizic TM, Thomas SC, Hungerford DS. Advanced ischemic necrosis of the hip treated by core decompression. *Arthritis Rheum* 1984:27(suppl):S31(abst).
261. Houssiau FA, N'Zeusseu Toukap A, Depresseux G, et al. Magnetic resonance imaging-directed osteonecrosis in systemic lupus erythematosus: lack of correlation with antiphospholipid antibodies. *Br J Rheumatol* 1998;37:448–453.

32

CARDIOVASCULAR MANIFESTATIONS OF SYSTEMIC LUPUS ERYTHEMATOSUS

DAVID D'CRUZ
MUNTHER KHAMASHTA
GRAHAM HUGHES

Cardiovascular manifestations in lupus patients range from mild symptoms of pericarditis to life-threatening complications such as angina, myocardial infarction, arrhythmias, valvular disease, embolic phenomena, cardiac failure, and sudden death. Furthermore, there is a growing appreciation that accelerated atheroma is a significant cause of morbidity and mortality. Patients are surviving for much longer than in the precorticosteroid era and the reasons for this increased risk of cardiovascular disease are being intensively studied.

Cardiac involvement in systemic lupus erythematosus (SLE) is common though it is not usually a presenting feature of the disease. This chapter presents a historical review, describes a clinical approach to the diagnosis of cardiovascular disease in SLE, and describes the main clinical manifestations of cardiovascular involvement.

HISTORICAL REVIEW

The most significant historical papers describing cardiac disease in lupus are those of Libman and Sacks (1) and Keefer and Felty (2) in 1924, Friedberg et al. (3) in 1936, Gross (4) in 1940, and Klemperer et al. (5) in 1941. In their landmark paper describing four necropsy studies, Libman and Sacks drew attention to the abnormal appearances on cardiac valves that they termed "atypical verrucous endocarditis." All four patients had pericardial friction rubs in life and three had precordial murmurs, though none had been diagnosed with SLE in life. Keefer and Felty described three further women with fatal lupus and cardiac involvement, one of whom may have had a superimposed infective endocarditis. Later, Friedberg et al. described sterile fibrin lesions on valves in four women with SLE but without the classic malar skin lesions, illustrating that cardiac disease may occur in the absence of the typical skin lesions of lupus. Gross (4) included in his paper patients previously reported by Libman and Sacks (1) and Baehr et al. (6), and described in detail 27 patients with lupus and their cardiac lesions. This was followed by 20 further necropsy studies in patients diagnosed with lupus in whom Klemperer et al. (5) described six with valvular verrucae consisting of sterile fibrin deposits, two others with valvular vegetations with microorganisms, and two with underlying rheumatic heart disease. Half their patients had necropsy evidence of pericardial disease. Indeed, these authors were the first to develop the term *connective tissue disease* to describe lupus and scleroderma (5,7).

Tumulty and Harvey (8) in 1949 described the clinical features of 32 patients with lupus, seven of whom had valvular verrucae (including one with superimposed bacterial endocarditis) and nine of whom had pericardial disease.

These historical papers are useful to compare with subsequent studies in which lupus patients were widely treated with corticosteroids. The most significant of these include the large study by Harvey et al. (9) of 138 patients including 52 who received corticosteroids, and the necropsy study of Bulkley and Roberts (10) in 1975. The frequency of valvular disease at necropsy has remained about 40% to 50% (7,10). However, whereas in the precorticosteroid era these lesions affected all valves, they are now predominantly left sided, mainly affecting the mitral valve. Furthermore, histologically the lesions have changed from being predominantly fibrin to mainly fibrous in nature (reviewed in ref. 11). In Bulkley and Roberts' necropsies, complete or partial healing was present in over half the patients. This suggests that corticosteroids may encourage healing of these lesions leading to fibrous thickening and occasional calcification of the affected valves that were not observed in the precorticosteroid era (10). The obvious downsides to corticosteroid therapy, however, are the increased risks of hypertension, diabetes, and dyslipidemia, resulting in accelerated atherosclerosis.

There have been several good reviews of the cardiac manifestations of SLE that thoroughly review these clinical problems since the advent of corticosteroid, immunosuppressive, and anticoagulant therapy in these patients (12–25).

THE CLINICAL ASSESSMENT OF CARDIOVASCULAR DISEASE IN LUPUS

The clinical assessment of cardiovascular disease in lupus patients is based on a careful history, thorough examination, and appropriate further investigations.

A useful screening question is, "Have you had any chest pains, heaviness, or breathlessness?" Positive answers to the question should be explored in detail. For example, pleuritic chest pains are a common symptom of lupus pleuritis. However, the pain of pericarditis may occasionally be differentiated from pleuritic pain by the fact that pericarditis is often less painful when the patient sits forward and is worse on lying flat or swallowing. A large pericardial effusion will result in dyspnea. It may be useful to estimate the severity of dyspnea in terms of exercise tolerance and activities of daily living. For example the patient may be housebound and unable to do simple tasks like washing and dressing, or may simply have mild limitations on walking because of breathlessness. Fevers, severe malaise, and sweats in such patients are an ominous symptom that should always be explored for the possibility of infection, especially bacterial endocarditis. Although tamponade is quite rare and cardiac failure a late manifestation, it is usually worth inquiring about symptoms of peripheral edema and orthopnea. The symptoms of ischemic heart disease are sufficiently characteristic to be diagnostic, though it is surprising how often symptoms of angina and myocardial infarction are ignored or missed in younger women and ethnic minorities (26). The symptoms of peripheral vascular disease such as claudication and peripheral ischemia may need to be specifically elicited especially in the older patient.

Clinical examination of these patients is often rewarding. There may be evidence of hyperlipidemia such as xanthelasma, especially in patients who have had nephrotic syndrome. Examination of the fingers may reveal the splinter hemorrhages of vasculitis, bacterial endocarditis, or antiphospholipid syndrome. Patients with tamponade have the characteristic features of generalized edema, small pulse volume with pulsus paradoxus, hypotension, and grossly elevated jugular venous pressure. Occasionally large pericardial effusions and tamponade may coexist with nephrotic syndrome. Patients with severe pulmonary hypertension or cardiac failure may be centrally and/or peripherally cyanosed. The precordium should be examined carefully for murmurs, friction rubs, and split or extra sounds using the classic clinical methods; it is often easy to miss these signs. The lungs should be examined for signs of cardiac failure or interstitial lung disease that may be associated with pulmonary hypertension. In this context it is worth examining the legs for previous evidence of deep venous thrombosis. The peripheral pulses should be carefully documented and where appropriate arterial bruits should be elicited and capillary return in the digits assessed, since these patients are at increased risk of peripheral vascular disease and occasionally aortic lesions. In hypertensive patients with antiphospholipid antibodies, there is an increased risk of renal artery stenosis, which may manifest with renal bruits.

INVESTIGATION OF CARDIOVASCULAR DISEASE IN SLE

Electrocardiography

The electrocardiogram is a simple bedside investigation that yields useful information on pericarditis, right or left ventricular hypertrophy, rhythm disturbances, myocarditis, and myocardial ischemia or infarction. However, none of these signs is specific for lupus, and many studies have reported a prevalence of abnormal electrocardiograms in lupus (10,13,16,24,27). Abnormal electrocardiograms may be seen in as many as 77% of patients (10,28) or as few as 17% (24) (Table 32.1). An interesting study showed a poor correlation between electrocardiographic and postmortem findings (15). In nine of the 30 SLE patients studied with normal electrocardiograms, four had postmortem lesions including pericarditis, myocarditis, and left ventricular hypertrophy (15). The prevalence of electrocardiogram abnormalities depends on when the recording is done and will naturally be higher in the presence of clinical evidence of cardiac disease and concomitant disease or therapy, which may be associated with electrolyte disturbances such as diuretic therapy.

Sinus tachycardia is the most frequent abnormal finding followed by nonspecific ST-T wave changes (10,16,27, 29,31). Conduction defects are uncommon, usually around 4% to 9% of series (16,27,29), but were seen in 7 of 35 patients in another series (10). Findings have included premature atrial contractions, atrioventricular block, bundle branch block, and complete heart block, and very rarely first-degree heart block (28). While congenital complete heart block is a classic feature of the neonatal lupus syndrome associated with Ro and La antibodies, there are occasional reports of heart block in adults, not all of whom were Ro positive (32–35). A study of 67 SLE patients, 36 of whom were Ro positive, concluded that myocarditis and conduction defects were reasonably common in adults with SLE and are associated with anti-Ro antibodies (36). However, the total num-

TABLE 32.1. PREVALENCE OF ABNORMAL ELECTROCARDIOGRAMS

Author	Number of Patients	Number (%) of Abnormal Electrocardiograms
Shearn (29)	73	45 (62)
Dubois and Tuffanelli (30)	520	34% of 291
Hejtmancik et al. (16)	137	71 (52)
Bulkley and Roberts (10)	35	27 (77)
Klinkhoff et al. (27)	47	15 (32)
Sturfelt et al. (24)	54	9 (17)

ber of myocarditis patients was only three, though the authors found no patients with complete atrioventricular block (36). A postmortem study of the conduction system described one of eight patients with sudden complete heart block and cardiac arrest. Histology showed focal degeneration and fibrosis of the sinus node caused by arteritis and occlusion of the central sinus node artery. Damage to the atrioventricular node was less extensive but showed focal degeneration secondary to small artery pathology (37). Furthermore, in a 12-year-old girl with complete heart block, lupus nephritis, and renal failure, the sinoatrial and atrioventricular nodes were completely replaced by fibroblastic and mononuclear cells with degenerative and necrotic changes in the small blood vessels and capillaries (38).

Echocardiography And Magnetic Resonance Imaging (MRI)

Two-dimensional, M-mode, and color flow Doppler echocardiography are excellent noninvasive tests for the diagnosis and monitoring of cardiac abnormalities in lupus patients. The techniques are especially useful for the detection of pericarditis and pericardial effusions, valvular lesions, ventricular dysfunction, hypokinetic areas, aortic lesions such as dissection or dilatation, and pulmonary hypertension. Serial studies are very helpful in assessing the progress of any lesions (46). Where transthoracic echocardiography is normal and a cardiac lesion is still suspected, transesophageal echocardiography may be more sensitive. This is especially true of valvular verrucae, which were found in 43% of 69 patients, compared to about 3% to 10% of patients when transthoracic techniques are used (Table 32.2) (24,27,28,39–48).

T1-weighted MRI has been used to detect myocardial abnormalities in SLE patients where other noninvasive cardiac investigations were negative, and it warrants further assessment (49).

INVESTIGATIONS FOR ISCHEMIC HEART DISEASE AND PERIPHERAL VASCULAR DISEASE

There is increasing evidence that premature atherosclerosis is a major complication of SLE, antiphospholipid antibodies, and therapy with corticosteroids. A number of fairly standard noninvasive techniques may be used to investigate ischemic cardiac syndromes including resting and exercise electrocardiography and technetium-99m sestamibi (Tc-99m MIBI) single photon emission computed tomography (SPECT) scans (50) prior to coronary angiography if indicated. Carotid color Doppler ultrasonography is a useful screening technique for early intima-medial thickening as a measure of the risk of atheroma (51), and ankle-brachial blood pressure indices may be used to assess lower limb peripheral vascular disease. Magnetic resonance imaging/angiography of the renal arteries may be used to detect early stenoses especially in patients with the antiphospholipid syndrome (52).

CARDIAC MANIFESTATIONS OF SLE

Pericarditis

Pericardial disease is the most common cardiac manifestation of SLE and was recognized by Keefer and Felty (2) in 1924. The prevalence of pericarditis ranges from 12% to 100% depending on how the studies are done and whether the patients were symptomatic. The highest prevalences are in autopsy and echocardiographic studies (53–62) (Table 32.3).

Acute pericarditis is rarely a presenting feature of lupus and commonly occurs as part of a generalized serositis (62) with pleurisy and pleural effusions. Clinically these patients present with substernal pleuritic-like pain that is worse on respiratory movements such as inspiration and coughing, and occasionally on swallowing. Pericarditic pain improves on bending forward and is worse on lying down. A pericardial friction rub may be heard but is uncommon. The pain may be mild to severe and signs include fever, tachycardia, and soft heart sounds, especially if there is a large effusion. If tamponade is present, there may be marked peripheral edema with grossly elevated jugular venous pressure. The jugular pulse is obvious and there is no y descent with a prominent x descent, and Kussmaul's sign and pulsus paradoxus may be elicited. Chest radiography often shows an enlarged cardiac silhouette, often with pleural effusion. An electrocardiogram may show the classic features of concave ST elevation or small complexes if the effusion is large (Fig. 32.1). Echocardiography is usually diagnostic and may guide pericardial aspiration.

Cardiac tamponade is relatively unusual given the high prevalence of pericardial disease in SLE. For example, only 2.5% of 395 patients in Kahl's (61) series had tamponade. It may occur at any stage in the disease course including at presentation (63–71). Tamponade is rarely fatal in SLE (61) and may complicate anticoagulation (71). On echocardiography, tamponade manifests as large pericardial effusions, reduced transverse dimensions and right ventricular diameter, early collapse of the right ventricular outflow tract, and indentation of the left atrial free wall (72). Cardiac tamponade is nearly always rapidly responsive to corticosteroid therapy and rarely needs surgical decompression.

Constrictive pericarditis is quite rare in SLE, and the literature is composed of case reports (16,73–78). Constrictive pericarditis may result from chronic fibrous thickening of the wall of the pericardial sac, causing impairment of normal diastolic filling of the heart. It may occur despite systemic corticosteroid therapy, the majority of patients are

TABLE 32.2. ECHOCARDIOGRAPHIC STUDIES IN SLE

First author	Klinkhoff	Badui	Galve	Crozier	Khamashta	Nihoyannopoulos	Leung
Year (reference)	1985 (27)	1985 (28)	1988 (39)	1990 (40)	1990 (41)	1990 (42)	1990 (43)
Type of study	Transthoracic	Transthoracic	Transthoracic	Transthoracic	Transthoracic	Transthoracic	Transthoracic
Number of patients	47	100	74	50	132	93	75
Abnormality[a]							
Pericardial effusion	9	39	—	54	—	20	28
Pericardial thickening	13	—	—	—	—	1	17
Valvular abnormality	21	9	24	—	23	28	—
Valvular verrucae	0		9	0	7	9	12
Valvular thickening	21		8	6	4	19	9
Left-sided regurgitation	0		3	50	30	—	25
Dilated ventricle	0		—	—	—	—	5
Depressed ventricular function	2	14	3	—	—	5	9
Thickened ventricular wall	—		—	—	—	—	12
Valve replacement	—		8	—	0.01	0	3
Normal heart	79	28	76	—	77	46	—
Antiphospholipid antibodies	n/a		n/a	n/a	38	54	31
Valve disease — associated with aPL		—	—	—	—	Yes	Yes
Control subjects?	Yes	No	Yes	Yes	Yes	Yes	Yes

First author	Cervera	Sturfelt	Ong	Roldan	Roldan	Giunta
Year (Ref)	1992 (44)	1992 (24)	1992 (45)	1992 (46)	1996 (47)	1993 (48)
Type of study	Transthoracic	Transthoracic	Transthoracic	Transesophageal	Transesophageal	Transthoracic
Number of patients	70	75	40 (inpatients)	64	69	75
Abnormality[a]						
Pericardial effusion	27	19	36		—	
Pericardial thickening	0	—	5		—	
Valvular abnormality	44	27	37		—	
Valvular verrucae	4	4	2.5		43	
Valvular thickening	17	23	38	50	51	12
Left-sided regurgitation	29	5	—	73	25	
Dilated ventricle	10	16	10		—	
Depressed ventricular function	1	7	10		—	31
Thickened ventricular wall	9	—	20		—	
Valve replacement	—	—	0		22	
Normal heart	43	—	27.5	—	39	
Antiphospholipid antibodies	33	32	26	32/64	—	50/75
Valve disease associated with aPL	Yes	Yes	No	No	—	Yes
Control subjects?	Yes	No	No	Yes	Yes	No

[a]Figures refer to percentages of study population with the abnormality.

TABLE 32.3. PREVALENCE OF PERICARDITIS

Authors	Reference	Year	Number of Patients	% with Pericarditis	Comment
Libman & Sacks	1	1924	4	100	
Gross	4	1940	23	61	Autopsy study
Humphreys	12	1948	21	43	Autopsy study
Griffith and Vural	53	1951	18	61	Autopsy study
Jessar et al.	54	1953	44	23	7/15 autopsies
Harvey et al.	9	1954	138	46	
Copeland et al.	55	1958	47	23	15/18 autopsies
Armas-Cruz et al.	56	1958	108	12	
Shearn	29	1959	83	31	7/16 autopsies
Brigden et al.	14	1960	27	74	Autopsy study
Kong et al.	15	1962	30	47	Autopsy study—4 tamponade
Dubois and Tuffanelli	30	1964	520	31	
Hejtmancik et al.	16	1964	142	17	11/16 autopsies—2 tamponade
James et al.	37	1965	8	100	Autopsy study
Estes and Christian	31	1971	150	19	2 tamponade
Bulkley and Roberts	10	1975	36	53	Autopsy study
Elkayam et al.	57	1977	32	6	Echo study
Collins et al.	58	1978	17	35	1/1 autopsy, echo study
Ito et al.	18	1979	48	46	Echo study
Chia et al.	19	1981	21	24	Echo study
Godeau et al.	59	1981	112	24	
Klinkhoff et al.	27	1985	47	21	Echo study
Badui et al.	28	1985	100	39	Echo study
Doherty et al.	60	1988	50	42	Echo study
Crozier et al.	40	1990	50	54	Echo study
Kahl et al.	61	1992	395	19	10 tamponade
Cervera et al.	62	1993	1,000	36	Serositis

A
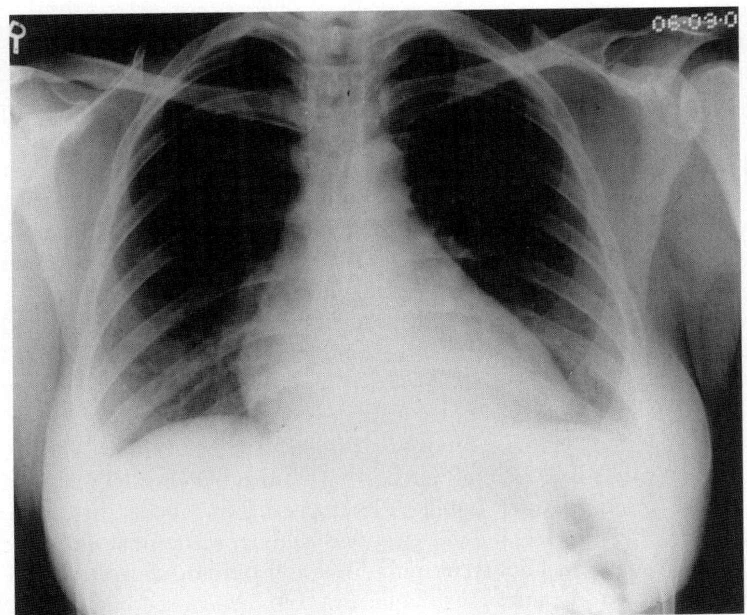

B
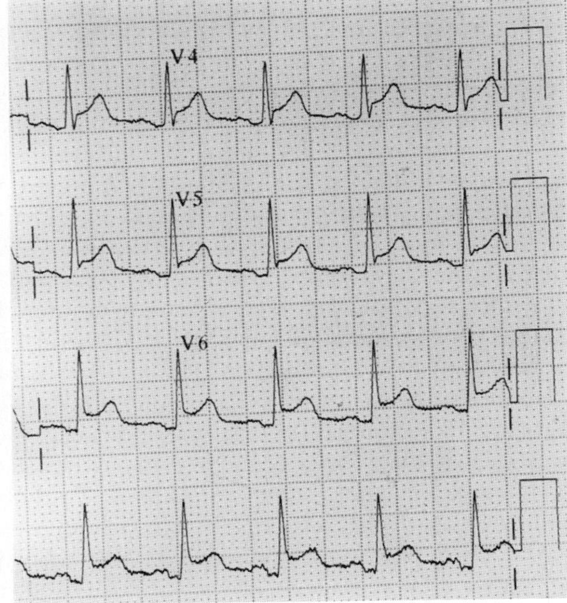

FIGURE 32.1. A: Chest radiograph showing cardiomegaly from a pericardial effusion resulting from pericarditis. **B:** Electrocardiogram from this patient showing the characteristic ST changes of pericarditis.

male, and pathologic findings include hyalinized fibrotic thickening of the pericardium and perivascular mononuclear infiltrates (73). Constrictive pericarditis also has been seen in patients with drug-induced lupus erythematosus (LE) resulting from procainamide and hydralazine (77,78).

Pathologic And Histologic Findings

The pathologic features of pericardial disease in SLE have been modified by corticosteroid therapy. Thus, prior to the advent of steroid therapy, autopsy studies showed focal or diffuse fibrinous pericarditis. Subsequently, a predominantly fibrous pericarditis has been observed more frequently (11).

Pericardial fluid in SLE is straw-colored and exudative with a high leukocyte cell count, with a predominance of polymorphonuclear cells. The mean white cell count in reported cases is 30,000 cells/mL, with a mean of 98% neutrophils (79). Rarely, the pericardial fluid is hemorrhagic (80). Typical LE cells can be identified in the centrifuged cell sediment, although this has now been superseded by the finding of antinuclear antibodies, anti-DNA antibodies, low complement levels, and immune complexes (80–85).

Treatment Of Pericardial Disease

The treatment of pericarditis in SLE depends on its severity. Minor pericardial effusions, for example, will not need specific therapy as they usually respond to general treatment for other aspects of the patients disease. Nonsteroidal anti-inflammatory drugs (NSAIDs) are the usual first-line therapy for pericarditis (86), though in our experience most patients require the addition of, or an increase in the dose of, corticosteroids to 20 to 30 mg daily. Antimalarials may be useful in the longer term. In critically ill patients, intravenous methylprednisolone is certainly helpful when a rapid effect is required, and intravenous immunoglobulins have also been used (87). A pericardial effusion developing in a patient with documented lupus does not need pericardiocentesis unless infection is suspected. In patients with chronic symptomatic constrictive pericarditis resistant to steroid therapy, pericardial resection may be helpful.

Septic pericarditis may occur in heavily immunosuppressed patients and is potentially fatal. The most common organism is *Staphylococcus aureus*, though *Salmonella* species, *Mycobacterium tuberculosis*, and *Candida albicans* have also been reported (88–91). These patients are usually extremely unwell with fevers and high white cell counts and erythrocyte sedimentation rate (ESR) levels. The C-reactive protein is usually grossly elevated in comparison to lupus patients with pure serositis, whose C-reactive protein levels are only mildly to modestly elevated. In this context, pericardiocentesis is certainly indicated but is associated with a high risk of complications. In a literature review, Berbir et al. (91) found that 5 of 24 procedures were complicated by death resulting from myocardial or coronary artery lacerations, so it is essential to have specialist cardiology supervision of these patients.

THE CONDUCTION SYSTEM AND SLE

The utility of the electrocardiogram in patients with SLE has been described above (Table 32.1). Most conduction abnormalities are not specific for lupus and may reflect coexisting coronary artery disease, idiopathic conduction system disease, or electrolyte imbalances.

Abnormalities of heart rate variability may be relatively common and are associated with autonomic dysfunction in SLE patients (92–95). For example, Lagana et al. (94) found abnormalities of the standard deviation of the RR intervals average in 78% of their 23 SLE patients, with significant differences in this and other variables compared to 14 healthy control volunteers (94).

MYOCARDITIS

Symptomatic myocarditis is relatively uncommon in SLE with a prevalence of around 10% to 14% (9,28,31). Subclinical involvement is almost certainly much more common, and autopsy studies, for example, suggest prevalences of between 40% and 50% (21). The precise prevalence in life however is difficult to ascertain. Sensitive techniques such as MRI and Ga-67 citrate scintigraphy may be useful but have not yet been studied in large numbers of SLE patients (49,96). Likewise, indium 111–antimyosin Fab imaging has been used to demonstrate myocardial involvement in two SLE patients but awaits larger studies (97).

The clinical presentation of lupus myocarditis resembles that of viral myocarditis. Symptoms include dyspnea, palpitations, and fevers, and patients may develop a tachycardia that is disproportional to the fever. The heart becomes diffusely enlarged, often with marked displacement of the apex beat. Other findings include murmurs, ventricular arrhythmias, gallop rhythm, and/or congestive heart failure. The diagnosis of lupus myocarditis needs to be differentiated from other causes of congestive heart failure such as coronary artery disease, anemia, hypertension, infection, valvular disease, and fluid and salt retention resulting from renal disease.

The pathogenesis of true lupus myocarditis is thought to be immune complex mediated with complement activation. Thus, granular deposits of complement and immunoglobulin have been demonstrated in myocardial blood vessel walls and within muscle bundles (98), especially in patients with active disease. Despite this extensive staining, myocardial histologic abnormalities were more focal and did not always correlate with the immunoglobulin and complement staining patterns (98). Others have found an association between myocarditis and skeletal myositis, especially in anti-ribonucleoprotein (anti-RNP)–positive patients, raising the possibility of a generalized disease process that affects striated muscle fibers (99,100). Claims have been made for an association between anti-Ro antibodies and myocarditis and conduction defects but have not been confirmed (101,102). Antimyocardial antibodies have been described in patients with SLE, though their significance is unclear (103).

Most of the information about the pathology of lupus myocarditis comes from autopsy studies and endomyocardial biopsies. Probably the largest autopsy report is that of Doherty and Siegel (21), who collated eight separate reports of 236 patients and found myocarditis in 100 (42%). The pathologic abnormalities consisted of small foci of interstitial plasma cell and lymphocyte infiltrates and, rarely, of a widespread, diffuse, interstitial inflammation. Fibrinoid change and hematoxylin bodies may occur (14), and small foci of patchy myocardial fibrosis are common in corticosteroid-treated patients (10).

Endomyocardial biopsies are certainly worth considering where the diagnosis of lupus myocarditis needs to be established (104,105). Biopsy may confirm the diagnosis and also give some indication of the extent of myocardial involvement (105,106). Rarely, antimalarials may cause cardiomyopathy, and endomyocardial biopsies may help to confirm this (107).

The treatment of lupus myocarditis is based on excluding other common causes such as viruses and drugs and then treating the underlying lupus disease activity. This is usually achieved with steroids and immunosuppressive agents, but plasmapheresis has previously been used (99,104,105).

CARDIAC FAILURE AND VENTRICULAR DYSFUNCTION

Over the last two decades, the widespread availability of echocardiography has demonstrated that abnormal ventricular function is a feature of SLE. Several studies have demonstrated depressed ventricular function in 2% to 10% of patients (24,27,39,42–45,108). For example, patients with stable lupus were found to have good preservation of systolic left ventricular function but impaired diastolic left ventricular function that worsened with age and likely represented lupus myocardial involvement (108). Similarly, Crozier et al. (40) showed that lupus patients had decreased left ventricular ejection fractions and diastolic compliance with increased left ventricular systolic dimensions compared to healthy controls.

A cardiac catheter study of five women with SLE who had no evidence of overt cardiac disease demonstrated impaired pump function, reduced contractility, increased myocardial wall stiffness, and decreased coronary artery reserve (109). A further study compared 25 SLE patients with 22 healthy controls and examined myocardial function noninvasively. The SLE patients had a shorter left ventricular ejection time, a longer pre-ejection period, and an increased ratio of pre-ejection period/left ventricular ejection time compared to controls, suggesting cardiac dysfunction (110). An important study by Winslow et al. (111) showed that over a 5-year period, increases in left ventricular mass index, mean wall thickness, and end-systolic volume, and decreases in ejection fraction were seen in 28 lupus patients compared with controls. These differences were related to the presence of hypertension and coronary artery disease. In some ways this study is reassuring in that although subclinical myocardial involvement appears to be common, it does not generally lead to overt clinical cardiac failure unless other factors, such as coronary artery disease or hypertension, are present. Furthermore, there is evidence that abnormal left ventricular systolic and diastolic dysfunction correlate with anti-DNA antibody titers and may improve with corticosteroid therapy, supporting the idea that active SLE patients have left ventricular dysfunction that may be caused by an immunopathologic mechanism (112).

CONGESTIVE HEART FAILURE

Severe biventricular cardiac failure directly resulting from lupus is relatively uncommon, and, when present, there are often other features such as hypertension or ischemic heart disease. Active lupus itself, especially in the context of glomerulonephritis and nephrotic syndrome, may make it difficult to establish an accurate diagnosis of cardiac failure since both nephrotic syndrome and cardiac failure may present with dyspnea, hypertension, generalized edema, pleural effusions, and ascites. Direct causes of cardiac failure resulting from lupus include valvular disease, pulmonary hypertension, myocarditis, pericarditis, coronary thrombosis, and severe anemia.

The prevalence of congestive cardiac failure in SLE is between 5% and 11% (14,16,28,30,31). The most common causes of cardiac failure in these studies included hypertension, myocarditis, and valvular heart disease, and in most patients a combination of these factors was present.

The treatment of these patients depends on controlling the causative factors such as hypertension and treating the underlying lupus disease activity. Where possible, angiotensin-converting enzyme inhibitors should be considered—they are among the most successful therapies for cardiovascular diseases. These agents not only are effective in treating hypertension and cardiac failure, but also have beneficial effects such antithrombotic and antiatherogenic properties; they also regulate smooth muscle proliferation and endothelial function, and reduce the rate of sudden death (113).

HYPERTENSION

Hypertension in lupus is most commonly seen with glomerulonephritis, the antiphospholipid syndrome, and corticosteroid use. The prevalence of hypertension, defined as readings of greater than 140/90 mm Hg, is around 25% in most studies (14,15,114) but may be as high as 45% (115).

In patients with lupus nephritis, there is a consensus that hypertension is a powerful independent predictor for deterioration in renal function, the development of end-stage renal failure, and death (114,116–118). Patients with the highest blood pressures had in one study 2.3 times the odds of renal deterioration at 12 months and 4.6 times the odds of end-stage renal failure compared to those with the lowest blood pressures (118). This remained so even after adjustment for age, sex, baseline serum creatinine, C3, erythrocyte sedimentation rate, hematocrit, anti-DNA antibodies, and proteinuria (118).

The treatment of hypertension should be intensive in patients with SLE, especially if they have glomerulonephritis. Malignant hypertension has been observed in lupus patients (16) and needs very careful but aggressive treatment. In the absence of renal artery stenosis, angiotensin-converting enzyme inhibitors should be considered wherever possible in view of their beneficial effects on blood pressure as well as in improving proteinuria, though potassium levels should be monitored. Since corticosteroids are so closely associated with hypertension, every effort should be made to reduce the dose of prednisone, if necessary by the addition of immunosuppressive agents. A variety of other agents may be used and, interestingly, although agents such as hydralazine, methyldopa, and some beta-blockers may cause drug induced lupus, they have successfully been used in SLE without exacerbating the disease (119). Methyldopa in particular has found application in the treatment of hypertension in lupus pregnancy (120).

LIBMAN-SACKS ENDOCARDITIS AND VALVULAR DISEASE

The most famous and characteristic lesion affecting cardiac valves in SLE is Libman-Sacks "atypical verrucous endocarditis" (1–4) (Fig. 32.2). The prevalence of these lesions in autopsy studies ranges from 13% to 74% (4,7,10,12, 15,16,30,121–123). The lesions consist of granular, pea-sized masses that may be found near the edge of the valve, on both surfaces of the valves, on the rings and commissures, and less frequently, on the chordae tendinae, papillary muscles, and atrial and ventricular mural endocardium (21). The vegetations can develop in any valve and often are multivalvular. Libman and Sacks (1) as well as Gross (4) found the verrucae most commonly in the tricuspid valve, but later studies found a higher frequency on the mitral valve (9,10), especially in the recess between the posterior valve leaflet and the ventricular wall (21).

Histologically, these vegetations are quite characteristic and differ from the lesions seen in rheumatic fever and bacterial endocarditis. Libman-Sacks vegetations consist of proliferating and degenerating cells, fibrin, fibrous tissues, and hematoxylin bodies. The involved leaflet contains granulation tissue, fibrin, and necrotic foci, and variable numbers of lymphocytes and plasma cells are seen. Shapiro et al. (121) described three zones in the verrucous lesions: (a) an outer exudative zone of fibrin, nuclear debris, and hematoxylin bodies; (b) a middle zone of proliferating capillaries and fibroblasts; and (c) an inner zone of neovascularization, with thin-walled junctional blood vessels. Vascular deposits of immunoglobulins and complement have been identified in the inner zone (121), and Bidani et al. (98) found gran-

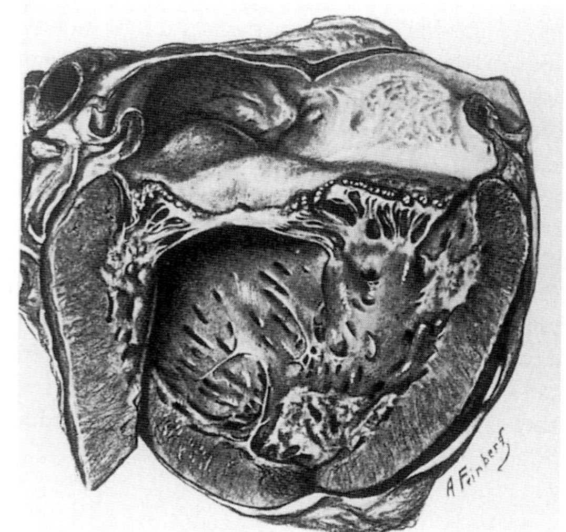

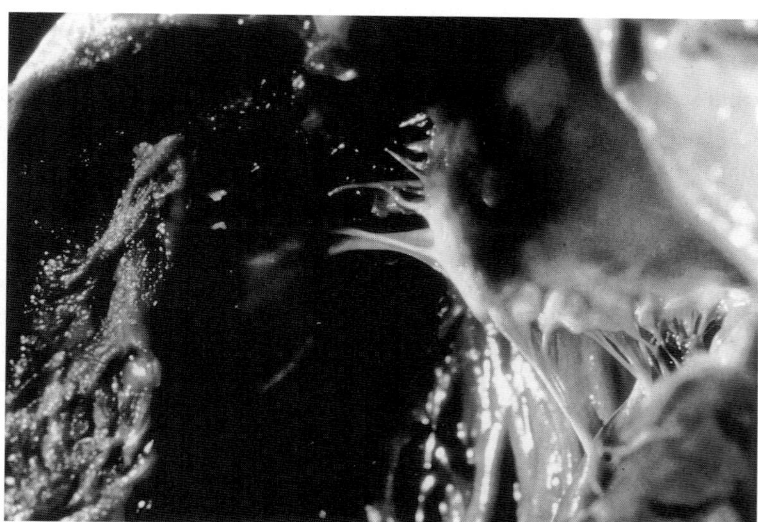

FIGURE 32.2. A: Drawing from Libman and Sacks' paper showing verrucous endocarditis. (From Libman E, Sacks B. A hitherto undescribed form of valvular and mural endocarditis. *Arch Intern Med* 1924;33:701–737, with permission). **B:** Postmortem specimen of verrucous endocarditis affecting the mitral valve leaflet.

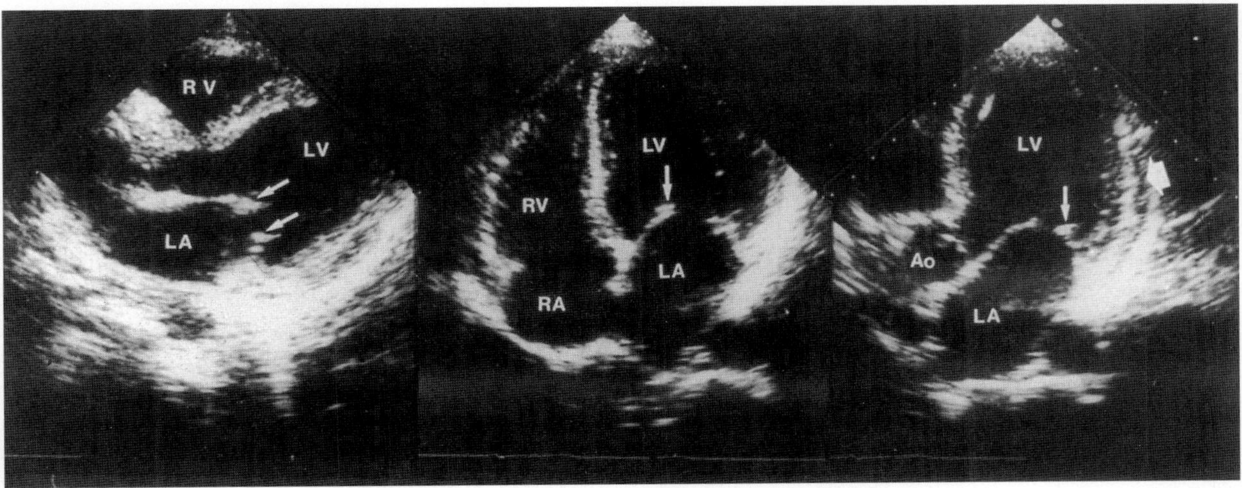

FIGURE 32.3. Echocardiography showing mitral valve vegetation.

ular immune deposits in the endocardial stroma at the base of the valve, along the valve leaflet, and in the vegetation. These deposits probably are immune complexes, which may be important in the pathogenesis of verrucous lesions (98,121).

Libman-Sacks endocarditis may be difficult to diagnose on clinical grounds. Clues to the diagnosis include splinter hemorrhages and cardiac murmurs, especially mitral regurgitation, in the context of active lupus with tachycardia, anemia, and fever. However, these are certainly not specific findings; in the paper by Griffith and Vural (122), for example, murmurs were heard in only two of six patients with Libman-Sacks endocarditis diagnosed at autopsy. Echocardiography should be considered whenever there is a suspicion of valvular disease, however subtle the clinical clues may be (Fig. 32.3). Libman-Sacks endocarditis rarely produces hemodynamic changes, but it has been associated with ruptured chordae tendinae (124), aortic stenosis resulting from massive thrombotic deposits on the valve (125), and cerebral emboli (126). Rarely, Libman-Sacks vegetation may mimic a large intracardiac tumor (127).

VALVULAR HEART DISEASE

The prevalence of valvular heart disease depends on the techniques used; transesophageal techniques are more sensitive than transthoracic methods, and clinical examination is the least sensitive. Table 32.2 shows that with transesophageal echocardiography, valvular verrucae are found in around 43% of patients compared to between 0 and 12% in studies using transthoracic methods.

There are several mechanisms by which valvular dysfunction may occur: (a) Healing with fibrosis of verrucae following steroid therapy results in regurgitation. Valvular stenosis may occasionally occur if the fibrosis results in severe leaflet thickening. (b) Large verrucous masses may result in valvular obstruction. (c) Infective endocarditis may complicate valvular damage, but this is relatively uncommon. (d) Ruptured chordae tendineae or papillary muscle dysfunction from previous myocardial infarction may result in mitral regurgitation. (e) Mitral valve prolapse is common in young women, the same population that is at risk for SLE.

In a small number of patients, valvular disease becomes clinically significant and results in hemodynamic problems requiring surgical intervention (Table 32.2). In most studies the commonest lesions requiring surgery are mitral (10,128–131) and aortic regurgitation (131–134). Less commonly, stenotic lesions of the mitral (129,130,135, 136), aortic (130,131,134,137–139), and tricuspid valves (140) may occur. In general, the prevalence of hemodynamically significant valve disease is around 3% to 4%, with 1% to 2% requiring valve surgery. However, one small prospective controlled study found that 18% of patients had clinically significant valve dysfunction, with 8% requiring surgery (39) (Table 32.2).

The first mitral valve replacement in a lupus patient appears to be that reported by Myerowitz et al. (141); the patient survived for 12 years. Surgical valve replacement in these patients is not without risk, however, and in one series of patients the mortality was 25% (129). Kalangos et al. (128) reviewed 14 patients reported in the literature in whom five of the excised valves contained verrucae, and 14 contained foci of fibrinoid necrosis and fibrous tissue in the valve leaflets and variable amounts of lymphocytic plasma cell infiltrates and calcific deposits. Three patients died in the early postoperative period and the authors suggest that mitral valve repair rather than replacement should be considered wherever possible. There remains some controversy over whether to use a mechanical valve or a bioprosthesis in these patients. In general, younger patients fare better with mechanical valves, and since these valves require anticoagulation, they would be of benefit in antiphospholipid-positive patients. Bioprostheses may become affected by valvulitis. Gordon et al. (142) described a man with lupus who underwent aortic valve replacement with a porcine bioprosthesis. This valve subsequently failed and at reoperation lupus valvulitis was noted on the porcine valve; the patient died following surgery.

Libman-Sacks endocarditis may be complicated by infective endocarditis. Doherty and Siegel's (21) review of the literature showed that 4.9% of autopsy-diagnosed Libman-Sacks endocarditis cases and 1.3% of clinically diagnosed cases were complicated by infective endocarditis. Endocarditis is a characteristic complication of dental procedures, and antibiotic prophylaxis is recommended before operative dental or other surgical procedures in all patients with SLE and clinical or echocardiographic evidence of valve disease. The need for prophylaxis is further supported by the disproportionately high frequency of mitral valve prolapse in SLE diagnosed by echocardiography (21,122). A number of patients have been described who have fevers, murmurs, splinter hemorrhages, and active lupus, but have negative blood cultures (143). In these patients, a high C-reactive protein is a good indicator of bacterial endocarditis.

Embolic phenomena are another obvious complication of valvular heart disease in lupus (143–145). For example, in the study by Khamashta et al. (41), nine patients with abnormal valves had cerebrovascular occlusions with strokes or transient ischemic attacks, and one stroke was fatal. There is certainly a compelling case for full anticoagulation with warfarin in any patient who has antiphospholipid antibodies and valvular disease on echocardiography and who has even the most transient of cerebrovascular events.

THE HEART AND ANTIPHOSPHOLIPID ANTIBODIES

Valvular lesions are the most common cardiac manifestations of patients with the antiphospholipid syndrome, now becoming known as Hughes syndrome (146). Two reports by Anderson et al. (147) and Ford et al. (148) of patients with the lupus anticoagulant and mitral valve disease were the first clues to the association between valvular disease and antiphospholipid antibodies. In Ford's paper, both patients underwent prosthetic valve replacement, and both had thrombus formation on the mitral valve. Chartash et al. (134) described 11 patients characterized by a tetrad of recurrent thrombotic disease, valvulitis, thrombocytopenia, and antiphospholipid (aPL) antibodies. Of these, eight patients had aortic insufficiency, three had isolated mitral regurgitation, and two had combined lesions. Furthermore, several studies have found a high prevalence of valvular heart disease in patients with the primary antiphospholipid antibody syndrome (39,149,150). None of the patients had features of SLE, but all had immunoglobulin G (IgG) anticardiolipin (aCL) antibodies (149,150).

A literature review of 13 studies by Nesher et al. (151) noted that valvular abnormalities are found in 36% of patients with the primary antiphospholipid syndrome, in 35% with SLE, and in 48% of patients with SLE and aPL. These abnormalities included leaflet thickening, vegetations, regurgitation, and stenoses. Significant morbidity from valvular dysfunction, mostly mitral regurgitation leading to congestive heart failure, occurs in 4% and 6% of SLE and primary antiphospholipid syndrome patients, respectively (151). A comparison of patients with the primary antiphospholipid syndrome and lupus patients with the antiphospholipid syndrome showed that endocardial valve disease was significantly more common in the lupus with antiphospholipid syndrome group (152). By comparison, a slightly different approach was taken by Gleason et al. (153), who compared ten primary antiphospholipid syndrome patients with 20 aPL-negative patients with SLE and 20 healthy controls. They still found a high prevalence of cardiac valvular lesions in 60% of the primary antiphospholipid syndrome and 40% of the SLE patients, though the numbers were small (153). A study by Espinola-Zavaleta et al. (154), using transesophageal echocardiography, found abnormal valves in 76% of 29 primary antiphospholipid syndrome patients. One year later, despite anticoagulation, the valvular lesions had either not regressed or worsened, with the appearance of new lesions in seven of the 13 who had repeat studies. A further study in primary antiphospholipid syndrome patients found cardiac disease in 83% of 40 patients, most commonly mitral valve thickening (155). This study suggested a correlation with the titer of anticardiolipin antibodies: 94% of patients with high titer aCL (>40 GPL) had mitral valve thickening, significantly higher than 42% of patients with low positive aCL (155).

Most studies, therefore, have shown a correlation between aPL and valvular lesions (Table 32.2). In addition, Leung et al. (43) found a positive correlation between aPL and valvular abnormalities and isolated left ventricular dysfunction. Giunta et al. (48) found major valvular involvement to be associated with longer disease duration and the presence of IgG aCL. Two other studies found correlations of IgG aCL with cardiac involvement in SLE (including pericardial, myocardial, and endomyocardial abnormalities) (42,156).

There are, however, some negative studies. Thus, other controlled studies have shown a high frequency of valvular disease, including the presence of vegetations, regardless of the presence or absence of aPL (45,46,126,157,158). Using transesophageal Doppler echocardiography, Roldan et al. (46) found no difference in the prevalence or severity of valvular lesions in patients with SLE and IgG aCL and in those who tested negative for these antibodies.

The precise role of aPL in the pathogenesis of valvular lesions in patients with SLE is unclear. The presence of vascular deposits of immunoglobulins including aPL and complement in the valvular lesions (96,119,159,160) suggest that antigen-antibody complexes may be important in the growth and proliferation of vegetations. Garcia-Torres et al. (161) suggested that interaction between circulating aPL and local factors on the cardiac valves may lead to endocardial damage, resulting in thrombosis, as well as subendocardial mononuclear cell infiltration resulting in fibrosis and calcification. An alternative explanation might be that capillary endothelium in the intravalvular vessels may be damaged by aPL, resulting in focal inflammation and thrombosis and later resulting in fibrosis and scarring (161).

The frequent occurrence of valvular diseases in patients with lupus but without aPL suggests that these antibodies may play a secondary role in lupus valvular diseases (153). However, Hojnik et al. (162) are persuasive in arguing that aPL has a significant pathogenetic role in the development of valve lesions and the associated thromboembolic complications, though why the endocardium appears to be selectively vulnerable to these antibodies remains unclear.

Other cardiovascular manifestations associated with aPL include myocardial infarction and intracardiac thrombus (163–165). For example, Asherson et al. (166) found a history of myocardial infarction in five of 70 patients (7%) in their study of primary antiphospholipid syndrome. In many of these reports, the left anterior descending artery was most frequently involved, usually without any evidence of atherosclerosis.

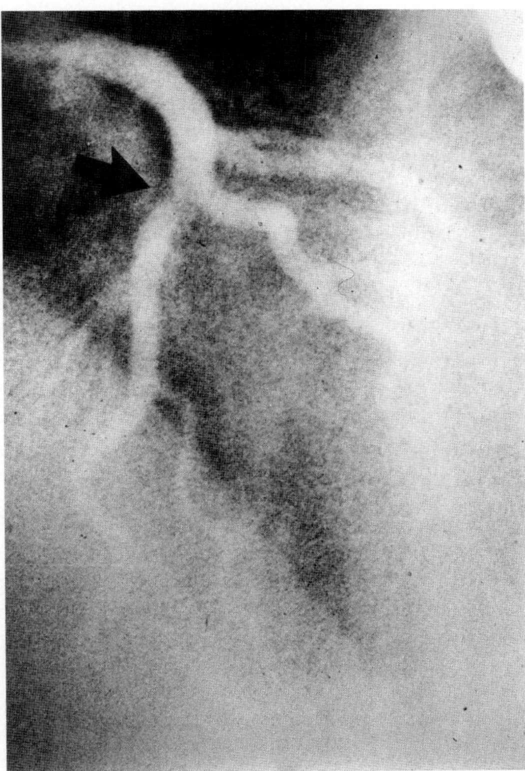

FIGURE 32.4. Atherosclerotic coronary artery disease in a patient with SLE.

ACCELERATED ATHEROMA

There is now convincing evidence that lupus patients are at risk of accelerated atheroma (Fig. 32.4). The reasons for this are almost certainly multifactorial and include long-term prednisolone and disease duration; patients with lupus are now living a great deal longer than they did in the precorticosteroid era. Furthermore, coronary atherosclerosis was virtually never reported prior to the advent of steroids (11). A postmortem study of 36 patients showed that 22% had at least one major coronary artery narrowing that was less than 50% of its cross-sectional area (10). All these patients were under 45 years of age and had received corticosteroids for more than 1 year. Even in the 17 patients who had received shorter courses of prednisolone, all had some degree of coronary arterial atherosclerotic plaques and cross-sectional area narrowing (10). Another postmortem study of corticosteroid treated patients also showed a high prevalence of coronary artery narrowings in 10 of 22 patients who had a mean age at death of 25 years (167). It is important to note that none of these patients had any evidence of coronary arteritis. These findings were confirmed by another autopsy study of 50 lupus patients matched with controls (168). Interestingly, in this study the mean intimal thickening ratio of the coronary arteries in the patients with SLE who did not receive corticosteroid therapy was larger than that of corticosteroid-treated patients. Thus, the authors suggested that inflammatory processes associated with SLE itself may promote coronary atherosclerosis (168). These studies are in marked contrast to those of Harvey et al. (9) and Copeland et al (55) from the 1950s in which apparently none of the patients had clinical evidence of myocardial ischemia and there were no deaths from myocardial infarction. Thus, while corticosteroids may well be causally related to atherosclerosis by increasing the risk of hyperlipidemia, hyperglycemia, hypertension, and obesity, they might also by a marker for more severe disease, especially if there is renal impairment.

Urowitz et al. (169) described a bimodal distribution of mortality in these patients: an early increase in death rates from infection and severe disease, and a later increase from accelerated atherosclerosis resulting in myocardial infarction. Much larger studies have come up with similar conclusions. For example, Wallace et al. (170) described 128 deaths in 609 patients followed for an average of 10 years. The most common causes of death were renal disease and sepsis, but 20% of the deaths were attributable to cardiovascular disease. Rosner et al. (171) reported deaths due to myocardial infarction in 3% of their 222 deaths of a total of 1,103 patients. Jonsson et al. (172) found that the incidence of coronary artery disease was nine times higher than expected for the Swedish control population, and again prolonged glucocorticoid treatment was related to cardiovascular mortality.

However, not all studies show this increase in cardiovascular death rates (158). More recently, Cervera et al. (173) reported a relatively low death rate of 45 deaths out of 1,000 patients (4.5%) followed for 5 years. There were only three coronary deaths (6.7% of all deaths), all of whom were antiphospholipid antibody positive. Indeed, antiphospholipid antibody–related thrombotic events accounted for 27% of all deaths.

Ward (174) assessed admission rates for cardiovascular morbidity and found that, compared with young women without SLE, young women with SLE were 2.3 times more likely to be hospitalized because of acute myocardial infarction, 3.8 times more likely to be hospitalized because of congestive heart failure, and 2.1 times more likely to be hospitalized because of cerebrovascular accidents. These differences lessened in older age groups. A further study by Manzi et al. found that women with lupus in the 35- to 44-year age group were over 50 times more likely to have a myocardial infarction compared to women of similar age in the Framingham Offspring Study (51). Furthermore, there is an increased prevalence of peripheral vascular disease in lupus patients (175).

Subclinical coronary artery disease may occur in up to 40% of lupus patients (176,177). Hosenpud et al. (176) found segmental perfusion abnormalities in 10 of 26 patients (38.5%) undergoing exercise thallium-201 cardiac scintigraphy. Five patients had reversible defects suggesting ischemia, four patients had persistent defects consistent with scar, and one patient had both reversible and persistent defects in two areas. In a larger study, Bruce et al. (189) found abnormal myocardial perfusion in 40% of 130 patients. A reversible defect was seen in 47 of the 52 (90%) abnormal studies, and abnormal perfusion studies were more common in patients with a clinical history of coronary artery disease, in patients with increasing age, and in postmenopausal women (177).

The possible risk factors for this accelerated atherosclerosis have been carefully studied (51,178). The classic risk factors for cardiovascular disease in the general population are also prevalent in lupus patients and include hyperlipidemia, diabetes mellitus, smoking, obesity, hypertension, and a sedentary lifestyle. Thus, in Manzi et al.'s (179) study of carotid plaque and intima-media wall thickness, variables significantly associated with focal plaque included age, duration of lupus, hypertension, body mass index, menopausal status, cholesterol levels, fibrinogen and C-reactive protein levels, SLE-related disease damage, and disease activity. Women with longer duration of prednisone use and a higher cumulative dose of prednisone as well as those with prior coronary events were more likely to have plaque (179). In Petri et al.'s (178) study, changes in prednisolone dose apparently led to changes in risk factors for coronary artery disease, even after adjustment for other variables known to affect these risk factors. However, hydroxychloroquine therapy was associated with lower serum cholesterol and so may ameliorate this effect to some extent.

A powerful risk factor for atherosclerosis in lupus may be renal disease, which may occur in up to 50% of patients. It is certainly well established that patients in end-stage renal disease from any cause, but especially diabetes mellitus, have markedly elevated risks of cardiovascular mortality; atherosclerotic vascular disease was present in 46% of dialysis patients in one such study (180).

Apart from these traditional risk factors, there is now increasing evidence that inflammation may have an important role in the generation of atherosclerotic plaque (181–183). In nonlupus population studies, it appears that high sensitivity C-reactive protein levels may be a good surrogate marker for low-grade inflammation that is a powerful predictor for atherosclerosis (182). It seems likely that inflammation involving the vascular endothelium may well have a role in the generation of atherosclerotic plaque in patients with lupus in addition to the traditional cardiovascular risk factors.

Another likely hypothesis involves aPL (184). The primary antiphospholipid syndrome is a relatively "clean" syndrome immunologically since these patients are not usually exposed to corticosteroids and do not develop glomerulonephritis, and there is much less evidence of an inflammatory immune response compared to that in lupus patients. There is some evidence that these patients may develop accelerated atheroma. For example, the renal artery stenoses seen in antiphospholipid syndrome patients may be a manifestation of atherosclerosis (52).

It is well established that low-density lipoproteins (LDL) and especially oxidized LDL has a central role in the pathogenesis of atherosclerosis. Since Vaarala and her colleagues (185) showed that some aPL could be absorbed by oxidized LDL, suggesting cross-reactivity (185), there has been tremendous interest, with several studies confirming and extending these observations (186,187). Certainly, oxidized LDL contains phospholipids and apolipoprotein B, which becomes antigenic after oxidative modification of LDL (188,189). Furthermore, β_2-glycoprotein-1, the aPL cofactor, is bound to oxidatively modified lipoproteins and may therefore be recognized by aPL (190), strengthening the link between aPL and oxidized LDL.

Whatever the precise pathogenesis of accelerated atheroma in lupus, it is clear that clinicians looking after these patients should pay close attention to reducing the known risk factors for atherosclerotic disease such as obesity, diabetes, smoking, hypertension, lipid levels, and previous coronary artery disease (191). The early use of steroid sparing agents such as antimalarials and immunosuppressive therapies will reduce the known effects of corticosteroids on lipid and glucose metabolism (192). Lipid lowering agents should also be considered, given the solid evidence of the ability of these agents to reduce myocardial infarction rates (193–195).

These agents may also have other beneficial effects on vascular endothelium that may be useful in lupus patients (196). In aPL-positive patients, there has been a trend for using low-dose aspirin to prevent thrombosis, although the evidence for this is poor. Nevertheless, if aPL is truly involved in the pathogenesis of accelerated atheroma, there is some sense in continuing this practice while further studies get under way. Homocysteine levels may also be relevant to the risk of stroke and arterial thrombosis in some patients with SLE, and folate supplementation may be useful (197,198). Regular exercise is undoubtedly beneficial in reducing cardiovascular risk, and it may also reduce the fatigue that is so common in SLE (199,200), and reduce the risk of osteoporosis associated with corticosteroids. Thus, lupus patients need to be proactively screened for atherosclerotic disease risk factors in order to reduce mortality from this increasingly important cause.

REFERENCES

1. Libman E, Sacks B. A hitherto undescribed form of valvular and mural endocarditis. *Arch Intern Med* 1924;33:701–737.
2. Keefer EB, Felty AR. Acute disseminated lupus erythematosus. *Bull Johns Hopkins Hosp* 1924;35:294–304.
3. Friedberg CK, Gross L, Wallach K. Nonbacterial thrombotic endocarditis associated with prolonged fever, arthritis, inflammation of serous membranes and widespread vascular lesions. *Arch Intern Med* 1936;58:641–661.
4. Gross L. Cardiac lesions in Libman-Sacks disease with consideration of its relationship to acute diffuse lupus erythematosus. *Am J Pathol* 1940;16:375–408.
5. Klemperer P, Pollack AD, Baehr G. Pathology of disseminated lupus erythematosus. *Arch Pathol* 1941;32:569–631.
6. Baehr G, Klemperer P, Schifrin A. A diffuse disease of the peripheral circulation (usually associated with lupus erythematosus and endocarditis). *Trans Assoc Am Physicians* 1935;50: 139–155.
7. Klemperer P, Pollack AD, Baehr G. Diffuse collagen disease: acute disseminated lupus erythematosus and diffuse scleroderma. *JAMA* 1942;119:331–331.
8. Tumulty PA, Harvey AM. The clinical course of disseminated lupus erythematosus: an evaluation of Osler's contribution. *Bull Johns Hopkins Hosp* 1949;85:47–73.
9. Harvey AM, Shulman LE, Tumulty PA, et al. Systemic lupus erythematosus: review of the literature and clinical analysis of 138 cases. *Medicine (Baltimore)* 1954;33:291–437.
10. Bulkley BH, Roberts WC. The heart in systemic lupus erythematosus and the changes induced in it by corticosteroid therapy. A study of 36 necropsy patients. *Am J Med* 1975;58:243–264.
11. Roberts WC, High ST. The heart in systemic lupus erythematosus. *Curr Probl Cardiol* 1999;24:4–56.
12. Humphreys EM. Cardiac lesions of acute disseminated lupus erythematosus. *Ann Intern Med* 1948;28:12–14.
13. Shearn MA. The heart in systemic lupus erythematosus. *Am Heart J* 1959;58:452–466.
14. Brigden W, Bywaters EG, Lessof MH, et al. The heart in systemic lupus erythematosus. *Br Heart J* 1960;22:1–16.
15. Kong TQ, Kellum RE, Haserick JR. Clinical diagnosis of cardiac involvement in systemic lupus erythematosus. A correlation of clinical and autopsy findings in thirty patients. *Circulation* 1962;26:7–11.
16. Hejtmancik MR, Wright JC, Quint R, et al. Cardiovascular manifestations of systemic lupus erythematosus. *Am Heart J* 1964;68:119–230.
17. Marks AD. The cardiovascular manifestations of systemic lupus erythematosus. *Am J Med Sci* 1972;264:254–265.
18. Ito M, Kagiyama Y, Moura I, et al. Cardiovascular manifestations of systemic lupus erythematosus. *Jpn Circ J* 1979;43: 985–994.
19. Chia BL, Mah EPK, Feng PH. Cardiovascular abnormalities in systemic lupus erythematosus. *J Clin Ultrasound* 1981;9: 237–243.
20. Ansari A, Larson PH, Bates HD. Cardiovascular manifestations of systemic lupus erythematosus: current perspective. *Prog Cardiovasc Dis* 1985;27:421–434.
21. Doherty NE, Siegel RJ. Cardiovascular manifestations of systemic lupus erythematosus. *Am Heart J* 1985;110:1257–1265.
22. Mandell BF. Cardiovascular involvement in systemic lupus erythematosus. *Semin Arthritis Rheum* 1987;17:126–141.
23. Cujec B, Sibley J, Haga M. Cardiac abnormalities in patients with systemic lupus erythematosus. *Can J Cardiol* 1991;7: 343–349.
24. Sturfelt G, Eskilsson J, Nived O, et al. Cardiovascular disease in systemic lupus erythematosus: a study of 75 patients from a defined population. *Medicine (Baltimore)* 1992;71:216–223.
25. De Inocencio J, Lovell DJ. Cardiac function in systemic lupus erythematosus. *J Rheumatol* 1994;21:2147–2156.
26. Pope JH, Aufderheide TP, Ruthazer R, et al. Missed diagnoses of acute cardiac ischemia in the emergency department. *N Engl J Med* 2000;342:1163–1170.
27. Klinkhoff AV, Thompson CR, Reid GD, et al. M-mode and two-dimensional echocardiographic abnormalities in systemic lupus erythematosus. *JAMA* 1985;253;3273–3277.
28. Badui E, Garcia-Rubi D, Robles E, et al. Cardiovascular manifestations in systemic lupus erythematosus. Prospective study of 100 patients. *Angiology* 1985;36:431–441.
29. Shearn MA. The heart in systemic lupus erythematosus. *Am Heart J* 1959;58:452–466.
30. Dubois EL, Tuffanelli DL. Clinical manifestations of systemic lupus erythematosus. Computer analysis of 520 cases. *JAMA* 1964;190:104–111.
31. Estes D, Christian CL. The natural history of systemic lupus erythematosus by prospective analysis. *Medicine (Baltimore)* 1971;50:85–95.
32. Fonseca E, Crespo M, Sobrino JA. Complete heart block in an adult with systemic lupus erythematosus. *Lupus* 1994;3: 129–131.
33. Martinez-Costa X, Ordi J, Barbera J, et al. High grade atrioventricular heart block in 2 adults with systemic lupus erythematosus. *J Rheumatol* 1991;18:1926–1928.
34. Bilazarian SD, Taylor AJ, Brezinski D, et al. High-grade atrioventricular heart block in an adult with systemic lupus erythematosus: the association of nuclear RNP (U1 RNP) antibodies, a case report, and review of the literature. *Arthritis Rheum* 1989; 32:1170–1174.
35. Mevorach D, Raz E, Shalev O, et al. Complete heart block and seizures in an adult with systemic lupus erythematosus. *Arthritis Rheum* 1993;36:259–262.
36. Logar D, Kveder T, Rozman B, et al. Possible association between anti-Ro antibodies and myocarditis or cardiac conduction defects in adults with systemic lupus erythematosus. *Ann Rheum Dis* 1990;49:627–629.
37. James TN, Rupe CE, Monto RW. Pathology of the cardiac conduction system in systemic lupus erythematosus. *Ann Intern Med* 1965;63:402–410.
38. Bharati S, de la Fuente DJ, Kallen RJ, et al. Conduction system in systemic lupus erythematosus with atrioventricular block. *Am J Cardiol* 1975;35:299–304.

39. Galve E, Candell-Riera J, Pigrau C, et al. Prevalence, morphologic types, and evolution of cardiac valvular disease in systemic lupus erythematosus. *N Engl J Med* 1988;319:817–823.
40. Crozier IG, Li E, Milne MJ, et al. Cardiac involvement in systemic lupus erythematosus detected by echocardiography. *Am J Cardiol* 1990;65:1145–1148.
41. Khamashta MA, Cervera R, Asherson RA, et al. Association of antibodies against phospholipids with heart valve disease in systemic lupus erythematosus. *Lancet* 1990;335:1541–1544.
42. Nihoyannopoulos P, Gomez PM, Joshi J, et al. Cardiac abnormalities in systemic lupus erythematosus. Association with raised anticardiolipin antibodies. *Circulation* 1990;82:369–375.
43. Leung WH, Wong KL, Lau CP, et al. Association between antiphospholipid antibodies and cardiac abnormalities in patients with systemic lupus erythematosus. *Am J Med* 1990;89:411–419.
44. Cervera R, Font J, Pare C, et al. Cardiac disease in systemic lupus erythematosus: prospective study of 70 patients. *Ann Rheum Dis* 1992;51:156–159.
45. Ong ML, Veerapen K, Chambers JB, et al. Cardiac abnormalities in systemic lupus erythematosus: prevalence and relationship to disease activity. *Int J Cardiol* 1992;34:69–74.
46. Roldan CA, Shively BK, Lau CC, et al. Systemic lupus erythematosus valve disease by transesophageal echocardiography and the role of antiphospholipid antibodies. *J Am Coll Cardiol* 1992;20:1127–1134.
47. Roldan CA, Shively BK, Crawford MH. An echocardiographic study of valvular heart disease associated with systemic lupus erythematosus. *N Engl J Med* 1996;335:1424–1430.
48. Giunta A, Picillo U, Maione S, et al. Spectrum of cardiac involvement in systemic lupus erythematosus: echocardiographic, echo-Doppler observations and immunological investigation. *Acta Cardiol* 1993;48:183–197.
49. Been M, Thomson BJ, Smith MA, et al. Myocardial involvement in systemic lupus erythematosus detected by magnetic resonance imaging. *Eur Heart J* 1988;9:1250–1256.
50. Lagana B, Schillaci O, Tubani L, et al. Lupus carditis: evaluation with technetium-99m MIBI myocardial SPECT and heart rate variability. *Angiology* 1999;50:143–148.
51. Manzi S, Meilahn EN, Rairie JE, et al. Age-specific incidence rates of myocardial infarction and angina in women with systemic lupus erythematosus: comparison with the Framingham Study. *Am J Epidemiol* 1997;145:408–415.
52. Godfrey T, Khamashta MA, Hughes GR. Antiphospholipid syndrome and renal artery stenosis. *Q J Med* 2000;93:127–129.
53. Griffith GC, Vural IL. Acute and subacute disseminated lupus erythematosus: correlation of clinical and postmortem findings in eighteen cases. *Circulation* 1951;3:492–500.
54. Jessar RA, Lamont-Havers RW, Ragan C. Natural history of lupus erythematosus disseminatus. *Ann Intern Med* 1953;38: 717–731.
55. Copeland GD, von Capellar D, Stern TN. Systemic lupus erythematosus: A clinical report of forty-seven cases with pathologic findings in eighteen. *Am J Med Sci* 1958;236:318–328.
56. Armas-Cruz R, Harnecker J, Ducach G, et al. Clinical diagnosis of systemic lupus erythematosus. *Am J Med* 1958;25: 409–419.
57. Elkayam U, Weiss S, Laniado S. Pericardial effusion and mitral valve involvement in systemic lupus erythematosus. Echocardiographic study. *Ann Rheum Dis* 1977;36:349–353.
58. Collins RL, Turner RA, Nomeir AM, et al. Cardiopulmonary manifestations of systemic lupus erythematosus. *J Rheumatol* 1978;5:299–306.
59. Godeau P, Guillevin L, Fechner J, et al. Manifestations cardiaques du lupus erythemateux aigu dissemine. 103 observations. *Nouv Presse Med* 1981;10:2175–2178.
60. Doherty NE 3d, Feldman G, Maurer G, et al. Echocardiographic findings in systemic lupus erythematosus. *Am J Cardiol* 1988;61:11–44.
61. Kahl LE. The spectrum of pericardial tamponade in systemic lupus erythematosus. Report of ten patients. *Arthritis Rheum* 1992;35:1343–1349.
62. Cervera R, Khamashta MA, Font J, et al. Systemic lupus erythematosus: clinical and immunologic patterns of disease expression in a cohort of 1,000 patients. The European Working Party on Systemic Lupus Erythematosus. *Medicine (Baltimore)* 1993;72:113–124.
63. Bergen SS. Pericardial effusion. A manifestation of systemic lupus erythematosus. *Circulating* 1960;22:144–150.
64. Carroll N, Barrett JA. Systemic lupus erythematosus presenting with cardiac tamponade. *Br Heart J* 1984;51:452–453.
65. Kelly TA. Cardiac tamponade in systemic lupus erythematosus. An unusual initial manifestation. *South Med J* 1987;80:514–515.
66. Lerer RJ. Cardiac tamponade as initial finding in systemic lupus erythematosus. *Am J Dis Child* 1972;124:436–437.
67. Omdal R, Dickstein K, Von Brandis C. Cardiac tamponade in systemic lupus erythematosus. *J Rheumatol* 1988;17:55–57.
68. Ehrenfeld M, Asman A, Spilberg O, et al. Cardiac tamponade as the presenting manifestation of systemic lupus erythematosus. *Am J Med* 1989;86:626–627.
69. Zashin SJ, Lipsky PE. Pericardial tamponade complicating systemic lupus erythematosus. *J Rheumatol* 1989;16:374–377.
70. Gulati S, Kumar L. Cardiac tamponade as an initial manifestation of systemic lupus erythematosus in early childhood. *Ann Rheum Dis* 1991;51:279–280.
71. Leung WH, Lau CP, Wong CK, et al. Fatal cardiac tamponade in systemic lupus erythematosus: a hazard of anticoagulation. *Am Heart J* 1990;119:422–434.
72. Moder KG, Miller TD, Tazelaar HD. Cardiac involvement in systemic lupus erythematosus. *Mayo Clin Proc* 1999;74: 275–284.
73. Jacobson EJ, Reza MJ. Constrictive pericarditis in systemic lupus erythematosus. *Arthritis Rheum* 1978;21:972–974.
74. Miller MH, Urowitz MB, Gladman DD, et al. Chronic adhesive lupus serositis as a complication of systemic lupus erythematosus. Refractory chest pain and small bowel obstruction. *Arch Intern Med* 1984;144:1863–1864.
75. Yurchak PM, Levine SA, Gorlin R. Constrictive pericarditis complicating disseminated lupus erythematosus. *Circulation* 1965;31:113–118.
76. Wolf RE, King JW, Brown TA. Antimyosin antibodies and constrictive pericarditis in lupus erythematosus. *J Rheumatol* 1988; 15:1284–1287.
77. Browning CA, Bishop RL, Heilpern RJ, et al. Accelerated constrictive pericarditis in procainamide-induced systemic lupus erythematosus. *Am J Cardiol* 1984;53:376–377.
78. Richards RM, Fulkerson WJ. Constrictive pericarditis due to hydralazine-induced lupus erythematosus. *Am J Med* 1990;88: 56N–59N.
79. Mandell BF. Pericardial effusion in patients with systemic lupus erythematosus. *Arthritis Rheum* 1993;36:1029–1030.
80. Askari AD. Pericardial tamponade with hemorrhagic fluid in systemic lupus erythematosus. *JAMA* 1978;33:111–116.
81. Seaman AJ, Christerson JW. Demonstration of L.E. cells in pericardial fluid. Report of a case. *JAMA* 1952;149:145–147.
82. Wolkove N, Frank H. Lupus pericarditis. *Can Med Assoc J* 1974;11:1331–1334.
83. Goldenberg DL, Leff G, Grayzel AI. Pericardial tamponade in systemic lupus erythematosus. *NY State Med J* 1975;75: 910–914.
84. Hunder GG, Mullen BJ, McDuffie FC. Complement in pericardial fluid lupus erythematosus. *Ann Intern Med* 1974;80: 453–458.

85. Quismorio FP Jr. Immune complexes in the pericardial fluid in systemic lupus erythematosus. *Arch Intern Med* 1980;140: 112–114.
86. Porcel JM, Selva A, Tornos MP, et al. Resolution of cardiac tamponade in systemic lupus erythematosus with indomethacin. *Chest* 1989;96:1193–1194.
87. Petersen HH, Nielsen H, Hansen M, et al. High dose immunoglobulin therapy in pericarditis caused by SLE. *Scand J Rheumatol* 1990;19:91–93.
88. Dorlon RE, Smith JM, Cook EH, et al. Staphylococcal pericardial effusion with tamponade in a patient with systemic lupus erythematosus. *J Rheumatol* 1982;9:813–814.
89. Knodell RG, Manders SJ. Staphylococcal pericarditis in a patient with systemic lupus erythematosus. *Chest* 1974;65: 103–105.
90. Sanchez-Guerrero J, Alarcon-Segovia D. Salmonella pericarditis with tamponade in systemic lupus erythematosus. *Br J Rheumatol* 1990;29:69–71.
91. Berbir N, Allen J, Dubois E. The risk of pericardiocentesis in SLE: case report and literature review (in French). *Rev Rhum* 1976;44:359–362.
92. Hosoya K, Takeda K, Masuda T, et al. Cross-bridge activation rate constant determined from systolic time intervals in patients with systemic lupus erythematosus. *J Cardiol* 1995;26:89–97.
93. Stein KS, McFarlane IC, Goldberg N, et al. Heart rate variability in patients with systemic lupus erythematosus. *Lupus* 1996; 5:44–48.
94. Lagana B, Tubani L, Maffeo N, et al. Heart rate variability and cardiac autonomic function in systemic lupus erythematosus. *Lupus* 1996;5:49–55.
95. Laversuch CJ, Seo H, Modarres H, et al. Reduction in heart rate variability in patients with systemic lupus erythematosus. *J Rheumatol* 1997;24:1540–1544.
96. Jolles PR, Tatum JL. SLE myocarditis. Detection by Ga-67 citrate scintigraphy. *Clin Nucl Med* 1996;21:284–286.
97. Morguet AJ, Sandrock D, Stille-Siegener M, et al. Indium 111-antimyosin Fab imaging to demonstrate myocardial involvement in systemic lupus erythematosus. *J Nucl Med* 1995;36: 1432–1435.
98. Bidani AK, Roberts JL, Schwartz MM, et al. Immunopathology of cardiac lesions in fatal systemic lupus erythematosus. *Am J Med* 1980;69:849–858.
99. Borenstein DG, Fye WB, Arnett FC, et al. The myocarditis of systemic lupus erythematosus. *Ann Intern Med* 1978;89: 619–624.
100. Lash AD, Wittman AL, Quismorio FP Jr. Myocarditis in mixed connective tissue disease: clinical and pathologic study of three cases and review of literature. *Semin Arthritis Rheum* 1986;15: 288–296.
101. Logar D, Kveder T, Rozman B, et al. Possible association between anti-Ro antibodies and myocarditis or cardiac conduction defects in adults with systemic lupus erythematosus. *Ann Rheum Dis* 1990;49:627–629.
102. O'Neill TW, Mahmoud A, Tooke A, et al. Is there a relationship between subclinical myocardial abnormalities, conduction defects and Ro/La antibodies in adults with systemic lupus erythematosus? *Clin Exp Rheumatol* 1993;11:409–412.
103. Das SK, Cassidy JT. Antiheart antibodies in patients with systemic lupus erythematosus. *Am J Med Sci* 1973;265:275–80.
104. Tamburino C, Fiore CE, Foti R, et al. Endomyocardial biopsy in diagnosis and management of cardiovascular manifestations of systemic lupus erythematosus. *Clin Rheumatol* 1989;8: 108–112.
105. Fairfax MJ, Osborn TG, Williams GA, et al. Endomyocardial biopsy in patients with systemic lupus erythematosus. *J Rheumatol* 1988;15:593–596.
106. Berg G, Bodet J, Webb K, et al. Systemic lupus erythematosus presenting as isolated congestive heart failure. *J Rheumatol* 1985;12:1182–1185.
107. Ratliff NB, Estes ML, Myles JL, et al. Diagnosis of chloroquine cardiomyopathy by endomyocardial biopsy. *N Engl J Med* 1987;316:191–193.
108. Enomoto K, Kaji Y, Mayumi T, et al. Left ventricular function in patients with stable systemic lupus erythematosus. *Jpn Heart J* 1991;32:445–453.
109. Strauer BE, Brune I, Schenk H, et al. Lupus cardiomyopathy: cardiac mechanics, hemodynamics and coronary blood flow in uncomplicated systemic lupus erythematosus. *Am Heart J* 1976; 92:715–722.
110. del Rio A, Vazquez JJ, Sobrino JA, et al. Myocardial involvement in systemic lupus erythematosus. A noninvasive study of left ventricular function. *Chest* 1978;74:414–417.
111. Winslow TM, Ossipov MA, Fazio GP, et al. The left ventricle in systemic lupus erythematosus: initial observations and a five-year follow-up in a university medical center population. *Am Heart J* 1993;125:1117–1122.
112. Murai K, Oku H, Takeuchi K, et al. Alterations in myocardial systolic and diastolic function in patients with active systemic lupus erythematosus. *Am Heart J* 1987;113:966–971.
113. Brown NJ, Vaughan DE. Angiotensin-converting enzyme inhibitors. *Circulation* 1998;97:1411–1420.
114. Schieppati A, Remuzzi G. Prevalence and significance of hypertension in systemic lupus erythematosus. *Am J Kidney Dis* 1993;21(suppl 2):58–60.
115. Budman DR, Steinberg AD. Hypertension and renal disease in systemic lupus erythematosus. *Ann Intern Med* 1976;136: 1003–1007.
116. Ginzler EM, Felson DT, Anthony JM, et al. Hypertension increases the risk of renal deterioration in systemic lupus erythematosus. *J Rheumatol* 1993;20:1694–1700.
117. D'Cruz D, Cuadrado MJ, Mujic F, et al. Immunosuppressive therapy in lupus nephritis. *Clin Exp Rheumatol* 1997;15: 275–282.
118. Ginzler EM, Felson DT, Anthony JM, et al. Hypertension increases the risk of renal deterioration in systemic lupus erythematosus. *J Rheumatol* 1993;20:1694–1700.
119. Reza MJ, Dornfeld L, Goldberg LS. Hydralazine therapy in hypertensive patients with idiopathic systemic lupus erythematosus. *Arthritis Rheum* 1975;18:335–338.
120. Buchanan NM, Khamashta MA, Morton KE, et al. A study of 100 high risk lupus pregnancies. *Am J Reprod Immunol* 1992; 28:192–194.
121. Shapiro RF, Gamble CN, Wiesner KB, et al. Immunopathogenesis of Libman Sachs endocarditis. Assessment by light and immunofluorescent microscopy in two cases. *Ann Rheum Dis* 1977;36:508–516.
122. Griffith GC, Vural IL. Acute and subacute disseminated lupus erythematosus: correlation of clinical and postmortem findings in eighteen cases. *Circulation* 1951;3:492–500.
123. Lehman TJA, McCurdy DK, Bernstein BH, et al. Systemic lupus erythematosus in the first decade of life. *Pediatrics* 1989; 83:235–239.
124. Kinney EJ, Wynn J, Ward S, et al. Ruptured chordae tendinea: its association with systemic lupus erythematosus. *Arch Pathol Lab Med* 1980;104:595–596.
125. Pritzker MR, Ernst JD, Caudill C, et al. Acquired aortic stenosis in systemic lupus erythematosus. *Ann Intern Med* 1980; 93:434–436.
126. Fox IS, Spence AM, Wheelis RF, et al. Cerebral embolism in Libman-Sacks endocarditis. *Neurology* 1980;30:487—491.
127. Applebe AF, Olson D, Mixon R, et al. Libman-sacks endocarditis mimicking intracardiac tumor. *Am J Cardiol* 1991;68:817–818.

128. Kalangos A, Panos A, Sezerman O. Mitral valve repair in lupus valvulitis—report of a case and review of the literature. *J Heart Valve Dis* 1995;4:202–207.
129. Dajee H, Hurley EJ, Szarnicki RJ. Cardiac valve replacement in systemic lupus erythematosus. A review. *J Thorac Cardiovasc Surg* 1983;85:718–726.
130. Straaton KV, Chatham WW, Reveille JD, et al. Clinically significant valvular heart disease in systemic lupus erythematosus. *Am J Med* 1988;85:645–650.
131. Alameddine AK, Schoen FJ, Yanagi H, et al. Aortic or mitral valve replacement in systemic lupus erythematosus. *Am J Cardiol* 1992;70:955–956.
132. Bernhard GC, Lange RL, Hensley GT. Aortic disease with valvular insufficiency as the principal manifestation of systemic lupus erythematosus. *Ann Intern Med* 1969;71:81–87.
133. Benotti JR, Sataline LR, Sloss LJ, et al. Aortic and mitral insufficiency complicating fulminant systemic lupus erythematosus. *Chest* 1984;86:140–143.
134. Chartash EK, Lans DM, Paget SA, et al. Aortic insufficiency and mitral regurgitation in patients with systemic lupus erythematosus and the antiphospholipid syndrome. *Am J Med* 1989; 86:407–412.
135. Paget SA, Bulkley BH, Grauer LE, et al. Mitral valve disease of systemic lupus erythematosus. A cause of severe congestive heart failure reversed by valve replacement. *Am J Med* 1975;59: 134–139.
136. Vaughton KC, Walker DR, Sturridge MF. Mitral valve replacement for mitral stenosis caused by Libman-Sacks endocarditis. *Br Heart J*1979;41:730–733.
137. Pritzker MR, Ernst JD, Caudill C, et al. Acquired aortic stenosis in systemic lupus erythematosus. *Ann Intern Med* 1980;93: 434–436.
138. Lerman BB, Thomas LC, Abrams GD, et al. Aortic stenosis associated with systemic lupus erythematosus. *Am J Med* 1982; 72:707–710.
139. Zimmermann B 3d, Lally EV, Sharma SC, et al. Severe aortic stenosis in systemic lupus erythematosus and mucopolysaccharidosis type II (Hunter's syndrome). *Clin Cardiol* 1988;11: 723–725.
140. Ames DE, Asherson RA, Coltart JD, et al. Systemic lupus erythematosus complicated by tricuspid stenosis and regurgitation: successful treatment by valve transplantation. *Ann Rheum Dis* 1992;51:120–122.
141. Myerowitz PD, Michaelis LL, McIntosh CL. Mitral valve replacement for mitral regurgitation due to Libman-Sacks endocarditis. Report of a case. *J Thorac Cardiovasc Surg* 1974; 67:869–874.
142. Gordon RJ, Weilbaecher D, Davy SM, et al. Valvulitis involving a bioprosthetic valve in a patient with systemic lupus erythematosus. *J Am Soc Echocardiogr* 1996;9:104–107.
143. Asherson RA, Gibson DG, Evans DW, et al. Diagnostic and therapeutic problems in two patients with antiphospholipid antibodies, heart valve lesions, and transient ischaemic attacks. *Ann Rheum Dis* 1988;47:947–953.
144. Fox IS, Spence AM, Wheelis RF, et al. Cerebral embolism in Libman-Sacks endocarditis. *Neurology* 1980;30:487–491.
145. Gorelick PB, Rusinowitz MS, Tiku M, et al. Embolic stroke complicating systemic lupus erythematosus. *Arch Neurol* 1985; 42:813–815.
146. Font J, Cervera R. Cardiac manifestations in the antiphospholipid syndrome. In: Khamashta MA, ed. *Hughes syndrome. Antiphospholipid syndrome.* New York: Springer 2000:32–42.
147. Anderson D, Bell D, Lodge R, et al. Recurrent cerebral ischemia and mitral valve vegetation in a patient with antiphospholipid antibodies. *J Rheumatol* 1987;14(4):839–841.
148. Ford PM, Ford SE, Lillicrap DP. Association of lupus anticoagulant with severe valvular heart disease in systemic lupus erythematosus. *J Rheumatol* 1988;15:597–600.
149. Cervera R, Khamashta MA, Font J, et al. High prevalence of significant heart valve lesions in patients with the "primary" antiphospholipid syndrome. *Lupus* 1991;1:43–47.
150. Brenner B, Blumenfeld Z, Markiewicz W, et al. Cardiac involvement in patients with primary antiphospholipid syndrome. *J Am Coll Cardiol* 1991;18:931–936.
151. Nesher G, Ilany J, Rosenmann D, et al. Valvular dysfunction in antiphospholipid syndrome: prevalence, clinical features, and treatment. *Semin Arthritis Rheum* 1997;27:27–35.
152. Vianna JL, Khamashta MA, Ordi-Ros J, et al. Comparison of the primary and secondary antiphospholipid syndrome: a European Multicenter Study of 114 patients. *Am J Med* 1994;96: 3–9.
153. Gleason CB, Stoddard MF, Wagner SG, et al. A comparison of cardiac valvular involvement in the primary antiphospholipid syndrome versus anticardiolipin-negative systemic lupus erythematosus. *Am Heart J* 1993;125:1123–1129.
154. Espinola-Zavaleta N, Vargas-Barron J, Colmenares-Galvis T, et al. Echocardiographic evaluation of patients with primary antiphospholipid syndrome. *Am Heart J* 1999;137:973–978.
155. Turiel M, Muzzupappa S, Gottardi B, et al. Evaluation of cardiac abnormalities and embolic sources in primary antiphospholipid syndrome by transesophageal echocardiography. *Lupus* 2000;9:406–412.
156. Cujec B, Sibley J, Haga M. Cardiac abnormalities in patients with systemic lupus erythematosus. *Can J Cardiol* 1991;7: 343–349.
157. Metz D, Jolly D, Graciet-Richard J, et al. Prevalence of valvular involvement in systemic lupus erythematosus and association with antiphospholipid syndrome: a matched echocardiographic study. *Cardiology* 1994;85:129–136.
158. Li EK, Crozier IG, Milne MJ, et al. Lack of association between anticardiolipin antibodies and heart valve disease in Chinese patients with systemic lupus erythematosus. *Lancet* 1990;336: 504–505.
159. Ziporen L, Goldberg I, Arad M, et al. Libman-Sacks endocarditis in the antiphospholipid syndrome: immunopathologic findings in deformed heart valves. *Lupus* 1996;5:196–205.
160. Amital H, Langevitz P, Levy Y, et al. Valvular deposition of antiphospholipid antibodies in the antiphospholipid syndrome: a clue to the origin of the disease. *Clin Exp Rheumatol* 1999;17: 99–102.
161. Garcia-Torres R, Amigo MC, de la Rosa A, et al. Valvular heart disease in primary antiphospholipid syndrome (PAPS): clinical and morphological findings. *Lupus* 1996;5:56–61.
162. Hojnik M, George J, Ziporen L, et al. Heart valve involvement (Libman-Sacks endocarditis) in the antiphospholipid syndrome. *Circulation* 1996;93:1579–1587.
163. Asherson RA, Khamashta MA, Baguley E, et al. Myocardial infarction and antiphospholipid antibodies in SLE and related disorders. *Q J Med* 1989;73:1103–1115.
164. Lubbe WF, Asherson RA. Intracardiac thrombus in systemic lupus erythematosus associated with lupus anticoagulant. *Arthritis Rheum* 1988;31:1453–1454.
165. Leventhal LJ, Borofsky MA, Bergey PD, et al. Antiphospholipid antibody syndrome with right atrial thrombosis mimicking an atrial myxoma. *Am J Med* 1989;87:111–113.
166. Asherson RA, Khamashta MA, Ordi-Ros J, et al. The "primary" antiphospholipid syndrome: major clinical and serological features. *Medicine (Baltimore)* 1989;68:366–374.
167. Haider YS, Roberts WC. Coronary arterial disease in systemic lupus erythematosus; quantification of degrees of narrowing in 22 necropsy patients (21 women) aged 16 to 37 years. *Am J Med* 1981;70:775–781.

168. Fukumoto S, Tsumagari T, Kinjo M, et al. Coronary atherosclerosis in patients with systemic lupus erythematosus at autopsy. *Acta Pathol Jpn* 1987;37:1–9.
169. Urowitz MB, Bookman AA, Koehler BE, et al. The bimodal mortality pattern of systemic lupus erythematosus. *Am J Med* 1976;60:221–225.
170. Wallace DJ, Podell T, Weiner J, et al. Systemic lupus erythematosus—survival patterns. Experience with 609 patients. *JAMA* 1981;245:934–938.
171. Rosner S, Ginzler EM, Diamond HS, et al. A multicenter study of outcome in systemic lupus erythematosus. II. Causes of death. *Arthritis Rheum* 1982;25:612–617.
172. Jonsson H, Nived O, Sturfelt G. Outcome in systemic lupus erythematosus: a prospective study of patients from a defined population. *Medicine (Baltimore)* 1989;68:141–150.
173. Cervera R, Khamashta MA, Font J, et al. Morbidity and mortality in systemic lupus erythematosus during a 5-year period. A multicenter prospective study of 1,000 patients. European Working Party on Systemic Lupus Erythematosus. *Medicine (Baltimore)* 1999;78:167–175.
174. Ward MM. Premature morbidity from cardiovascular and cerebrovascular diseases in women with systemic lupus erythematosus. *Arthritis Rheum* 1999;42:338–346.
175. McDonald J, Stewart J, Urowitz MB, et al. Peripheral vascular disease in patients with systemic lupus erythematosus. *Ann Rheum Dis* 1992;51:56–60.
176. Hosenpud JD, Montanaro A, Hart MV, et al. Myocardial perfusion abnormalities in asymptomatic patients with systemic lupus erythematosus. *Am J Med* 1984;77:286–292.
177. Bruce IN, Burns RJ, Gladman DD, et al. Single photon emission computed tomography dual isotope myocardial perfusion imaging in women with systemic lupus erythematosus. I. Prevalence and distribution of abnormalities. *J Rheumatol* 2000;27:2372–2377.
178. Petri M, Lakatta C, Magder L, et al. Effect of prednisone and hydroxychloroquine on coronary artery disease risk factors in systemic lupus erythematosus: a longitudinal data analysis. *Am J Med* 1994;96:254–259.
179. Manzi S, Selzer F, Sutton-Tyrrell K, et al. Prevalence and risk factors of carotid plaque in women with systemic lupus erythematosus. *Arthritis Rheum* 1999;42:51–60.
180. Manns BJ, Burgess ED, Hyndman ME, et al. Hyperhomocyst(e)inemia and the prevalence of atherosclerotic vascular disease in patients with end-stage renal disease. *Am J Kidney Dis* 1999;34:669–677.
181. Ross R. Atherosclerosis is an inflammatory disease. *Am Heart J* 1999;138(5 pt 2):S419–420.
182. Ridker PM, Cushman M, Stampfer MJ, et al. Inflammation, aspirin, and the risk of cardiovascular disease in apparently healthy men. *N Engl J Med* 1997;336:973–979.
183. Kuller LH, Tracy RP, Shaten J, et al. Relation of C-reactive protein and coronary heart disease in the MRFIT nested case-control study. Multiple Risk Factor Intervention Trial. *Am J Epidemiol* 1996;144:537–547.
184. George J, Shoenfeld Y. The anti-phospholipid (Hughes) syndrome: a crossroads of autoimmunity and atherosclerosis. *Lupus* 1997;6:559–560.
185. Vaarala O, Alfthan G, Jauhiainen M, et al. Crossreaction between antibodies to oxidised low-density lipoprotein and to cardiolipin in systemic lupus erythematosus. *Lancet* 1993;341(8850):923–925.
186. Amengual O, Atsumi T, Khamashta MA, et al. Autoantibodies against oxidized low-density lipoprotein in antiphospholipid syndrome. *Br J Rheumatol* 1997;36:964–968.
187. Romero FI, Amengual O, Atsumi T, et al. Arterial disease in lupus and secondary antiphospholipid syndrome: association with anti-beta2-glycoprotein I antibodies but not with antibodies against oxidized low-density lipoprotein. *Br J Rheumatol* 1998;37:883–888.
188. Witztum JL. The oxidation hypothesis of atherosclerosis. *Lancet* 1994;344(8925):793–795.
189. Palinski W, Yla-Herttuala S, Rosenfeld ME, et al. Antisera and monoclonal antibodies specific for epitopes generated during oxidative modification of low density lipoprotein. *Arteriosclerosis* 1990;10:325–335.
190. Matsuura E, Igarashi Y, Yasuda T, et al. Anticardiolipin antibodies recognize beta 2-glycoprotein I structure altered by interacting with an oxygen modified solid phase surface. *J Exp Med* 1994;179:457–462.
191. Bruce IN, Gladman DD, Urowitz MB. Detection and modification of risk factors for coronary artery disease in patients with systemic lupus erythematosus: a quality improvement study. *Clin Exp Rheumatol* 1998;16:435–440.
192. Hallegua DS, Wallace DJ. How accelerated atherosclerosis in SLE has changed our management of the disorder. *Lupus* 2000;9:228–231.
193. Scandinavian Simvastatin Survival Study Group. Randomised trial of cholesterol lowering in 4444 patients with coronary heart disease: the Scandinavian Simvastatin Survival Study (4S). *Lancet* 1994;344:1383–1389.
194. Manninen V, Elo MO, Frick MH, et al. Lipid alterations and decline in the incidence of coronary heart disease in the Helsinki Heart Study. *JAMA* 1988;260:641–651.
195. Tonkin AM, Colquhoun D, Emberson J, et al. Effects of pravastatin in 3260 patients with unstable angina: results from the LIPID study. *Lancet* 2000;356:1871–1875.
196. Sotiriou CG, Cheng JW. Beneficial effects of statins in coronary artery disease—beyond lowering cholesterol. *Ann Pharmacother* 2000;34:1432–1439.
197. Petri M, Roubenoff R, Dallal GE, et al. Plasma homocysteine as a risk factor for atherothrombotic events in systemic lupus erythematosus. *Lancet* 1996;348:1120–1124.
198. Fijnheer R, Roest M, Haas FJ, et al. Homocysteine, methylenetetrahydrofolate reductase polymorphism, antiphospholipid antibodies, and thromboembolic events in systemic lupus erythematosus: a retrospective cohort study. *J Rheumatol* 1998;25:1737–1742.
199. Daltroy LH, Robb-Nicholson C, Iversen MD, et al. Effectiveness of minimally supervised home aerobic training in patients with systemic rheumatic disease. *Br J Rheumatol* 1995;34:1064–1069.
200. Tench CM, McCurdie I, McCarthy J, et al. A randomised controlled trial of aerobic exercise on fatigue in systemic lupus erythematosus. *Rheumatology* 2000;40:79.

33

PULMONARY MANIFESTATIONS OF SYSTEMIC LUPUS ERYTHEMATOSUS

DAVID D'CRUZ
MUNTHER KHAMASHTA
GRAHAM HUGHES

The lungs may conveniently be considered in six main regions: the pleural space, the parenchyma, the pulmonary vasculature, the airways, the diaphragm, and the chest wall including the ribs and respiratory muscles. Systemic lupus erythematosus (SLE) and the adverse effects of various therapies may affect all these regions of the chest. Pulmonary involvement is common in SLE and will affect half of patients during the disease course and is part of the spectrum of presenting symptoms in 4% to 5% of patients (1). Furthermore, other complications of lupus such as cardiac failure or nephrotic syndrome may lead to lung involvement with the development of pleural effusions. Pulmonary involvement may increase the risk of mortality; in one study, lung involvement was one of several factors that was predictive for increased mortality (2).

The prevalence of pulmonary manifestations in SLE depends on the referral pattern to the unit where patients are studied, the population under scrutiny, and the methods used to detect pulmonary involvement. For example, the total cumulative prevalence of clinically apparent lung involvement was approximately 20%, with serositis seen in 45% of patients in a large cohort of patients (1). However, in a cross-sectional study of lung function, 90% of patients had subclinical abnormalities of pulmonary function tests (3).

This chapter describes the clinical features, investigation, pathologic features, and management of the various pulmonary manifestations of SLE.

HISTORICAL PERSPECTIVE

The contributions of Osler and Jadasson established that SLE was a distinct syndrome, and in 1904 Osler (4) described the occurrence of pneumonia in SLE. Further reports in the 1930s and 1940s described polyserositis, patchy lung consolidation, and other pulmonary changes including "atelectizing pneumonitis" in patients with SLE (5,6). Autopsy of these patients showed diffuse lung consolidation with hyaline alveolar thickening and marked obliterating cellular infiltration. Baggentoss extended these observations and observed a peculiar basophilic, mucinous edema of the alveolar walls and the peribronchial and perivascular tissues in association with interstitial pneumonitis and alveolar hemorrhage. These pathologic changes were distinct from the ordinary pyogenic and fibrinous bronchopneumonia that frequently complicates the terminal stages of SLE, but they were not pathognomonic of SLE (7). In atelectizing pneumonitis, the alveolar walls as well as the peribronchial and perivascular connective tissues appeared to be the primary sites of an inflammatory process that obliterated alveolar spaces.

In 1953 and 1954, two reports of radiographic studies in SLE emphasized the high frequency of pulmonary involvement. Israel (8) showed that nonspecific pneumonia occurred frequently, not only during the terminal stages of SLE but throughout the course of the disease. Garland and Sisson (9) reported lung parenchymal changes in one third of their patients and observed both pleural and cardiac abnormalities to be prevalent. Comprehensive reviews of the pulmonary manifestations of SLE in adults (10–12) and in children (13) have appeared.

PATHOLOGY

A wide variety of lesions have been described in the lungs, but none are specific for SLE. For example, an autopsy study of 54 patients showed the following pathologic abnormalities in more than 50% of cases: bronchopneumonia, hemorrhage, pleural effusion, edema, interstitial pneumonia, and congestion (7). Fibrinoid necrosis and hematoxylin bodies occasionally were seen (14), whereas bronchiolar dilatation and foci of panacinar emphysema often were found (15). Fayemi (16) noted a high frequency of occlusive vascular changes of varying severity in the lungs of 8 of 20 patients with SLE; these changes affected arterioles, arteries, and veins. The acute lesions consisted of fibrinoid necrosis and vasculitis, and the chronic lesions included intimal fibrosis, medial hypertrophy, alteration of the elastic laminae, and periadventitial fibrosis.

Haupt et al. (17) examined pathologic changes in the lungs of 120 patients seen at autopsy and correlated these with their clinical features. In contrast to the high frequency of lung involvement in a clinical series (10), they showed that many of the pathologic lesions were not caused by SLE itself but rather by secondary factors, such as congestive heart failure, infection, aspiration, and oxygen toxicity. Only 18% of the lung parenchymal lesions were found to be directly attributable to SLE.

Although informative, analyses of autopsy cases may not represent a cross section of the general population of lupus patients and probably underestimate the prevalence of lung involvement. Certainly in the clinical setting pulmonary abnormalities can change rapidly and subside either spontaneously or with drug therapy, so anatomic lesions may not be evident later at autopsy.

THE CLINICAL ASSESSMENT OF PULMONARY INVOLVEMENT

As with any other branch of medicine the clinical assessment of pulmonary disease in lupus patients is based on a careful history, thorough examination, and appropriate further investigations.

A useful screening question is, "Have you been short of breath or had chest pains?" The most common early symptom of serositis is pleuritic chest pains, which occur on both inspiration and expiration. There is nothing particular about the pain that differentiates lupus from other causes of pleurisy such as infection or pulmonary embolism. Resolution of pleuritic pain does not always imply improvement since the pain at a particular site of the chest may disappear if a significant pleural effusion develops. Dyspnea may be the presenting symptom of many of the other complications of lupus to affect the lung. A sudden onset is more likely to be due to pulmonary embolism, but the more usual presentation is an insidious onset of breathlessness. An estimate of the patient's walking distance is a useful guide to exercise tolerance and the extent of lung involvement. A careful history to exclude cardiac disease should be undertaken. Hemoptysis may be the presenting feature of infection, infarction, cardiac failure, or very rarely pulmonary hemorrhage.

The examination of the respiratory system should be part of a comprehensive clinical examination that includes blood pressure and urinalysis. For example, vasculitic lesions may indicate more widespread disease activity. Splinter hemorrhages raise the possibility of small vessel vasculitis or cardiac valvular disease in a breathless patient with SLE. Interestingly, although finger clubbing is common in patients with idiopathic fibrosing alveolitis, it is relatively unusual in patients with interstitial lung disease of lupus (12). The presence of central cyanosis should be noted and a careful search should be made for late inspiratory basal crepitations—a sensitive sign of interstitial lung disease that should prompt further investigation. Pleural rubs and effusions should be sought as indicated by a history of pleuritic pains, though other causes of pleural effusions should be considered such as infection, nephrotic syndrome, cardiac failure, and malignancy. A thorough cardiac assessment is essential, with particular attention to signs of cardiac valve disease, left or right ventricular failure, and pointers toward pulmonary hypertension.

INVESTIGATION OF PULMONARY INVOLVEMENT

Imaging

Chest Radiography In SLE

The chest radiograph is a simple and useful extension of the clinical examination of the patient with SLE. Previous films, when available, may give valuable information on disease progression or the appearance of new lesions.

Abnormalities on chest radiographs are reasonably common in patients with SLE. For example, in a prospective study of 50 unselected patients, abnormalities were found in 38% (18), and in a study of 43 patients who were examined specifically for pulmonary dysfunction, 23% had abnormal chest radiographs (19). In contrast, none of 70 nonsmoking patients with SLE who were free of respiratory complaints and enrolled in a study of pulmonary function had abnormal chest radiographs (20). Several factors may explain this difference in the prevalence of abnormalities, including patient selection, the many manifestations of the disease that may be transient, and the timing of the radiographic study.

Radiographic Findings

A wide variety of abnormalities may be seen in chest radiographs. Early studies documented radiographic changes in the pleura, lung parenchyma, and heart (21). However, none of these abnormalities are specific or diagnostic for SLE and may be seen in other conditions such as rheumatoid arthritis and systemic sclerosis.

Pleural changes as an isolated abnormality or in combination with cardiac or parenchymal lesions are the most common radiographic changes (21,22). The pleura may appear as a shaggy thickening of the pleural surface. Pleural effusions are usually small and, in 50% of patients, bilateral (12). With clearing of the effusion, residual pleural thickening may be seen. Parenchymal lesions are characterized by ill-defined focal patches, linear bands, infiltrates, and small nodules or plaques at the bases (22). Diffuse granular, reticular, or reticulonodular lesions throughout the lung fields, but especially at the bases, are found in a small number of patients with SLE and chronic interstitial fibrosis (10). Cardiomegaly, if present, is usually mild to moderate (21), and isolated cardiac enlargement is almost as frequent as isolated pleural disease. In patients with cardiomegaly, there are often other factors such as hypertension, pericarditis, valvular disease, myocardial involvement, and anemia to explain the cardiac enlargement (21). Elevated diaphragms are found in 5% to 18% of patients (18,19).

Early investigators often ascribed parenchymal changes in chest radiographs to primary lung involvement caused by SLE. The term *lupus pneumonitis* was used indiscriminately to encompass various types of pulmonary lesions and has been reported in 15% to 50% of patients (12,23). In 111 patients with SLE, Levin (23) found that radiographic parenchymal changes (infiltrates or small nodules) were mostly the result of secondary complications, such as infections, uremic pulmonary edema, and basilar atelectasis. Primary lupus pneumonitis was relatively rare, being found in only three (2.7%) patients, and the diagnosis therefore became one of exclusion.

High-Resolution Computed Tomography (CT) And Magnetic Resonance Imaging (MRI)

High-resolution CT (HRCT) is an essential tool in the evaluation of lung disease in SLE. Early inflammatory lesions may be visualized as alveolar or ground-glass shadowing, and later in the disease course fibrotic lesions may be visible as fixed reticular honeycombing. These appearances usually correlate with the clinical finding of late inspiratory crackles at the lung bases.

Two studies from the same group have demonstrated the usefulness of HRCT scans of the chest in determining the prevalence of pulmonary involvement (24,25). The most common CT findings were interstitial lung disease (ILD), bronchiectasis, mediastinal or axillary lymphadenopathy, and pleuropericardial abnormalities. No correlation was found between disease activity, duration of disease, chest symptoms, drug therapy, smoking history, and the presence of abnormal HRCT findings. Interestingly, no correlation was found between pulmonary function abnormalities and the presence or grade of interstitial lung disease or bronchiectasis as determined by HRCT, and the prevalence of pleuropulmonary disease was lower than in previous studies. Thus, HRCT evidence of airways disease and interstitial lung disease was frequently present despite an absence of symptoms, a normal chest radiograph, and normal pulmonary function testing. Furthermore, the study by Sant et al. (25) showed that 72% of HRCT scans were abnormal when only 34% of plain chest radiographs were abnormal.

When combined with contrast injections, CT pulmonary angiography is a highly accurate method of detecting pulmonary emboli where ventilation/perfusion (V/Q) scans give indeterminate results, especially if the clinical suspicion of pulmonary embolism is high. The use of D-dimer assays in this clinical situation may increase the predictive value of diagnosing pulmonary emboli considerably and is less invasive than the gold standard of pulmonary arterial angiography. However, if the V/Q scan is indeterminate, the CT angiogram is inconclusive, and the clinical suspicion of pulmonary embolism is high, then pulmonary arterial angiography should still be considered, especially if D-dimer assays are positive (26).

The role of MRI in the evaluation of pulmonary disease in lupus remains the subject of continuing studies. Case reports suggest that MRI may be useful in the evaluation of pulmonary artery thrombosis and pulmonary hemorrhage in SLE (27,28). In other fields MRI has been useful in assessing respiratory diaphragmatic and chest wall dynamics in pulmonary emphysema (29) and chronic infiltrative lung diseases (30). The major limitation of MRI of the lung parenchyma is image degradation due to breathing, though breath-hold techniques are now possible with faster acquisition times and gadolinium enhancement (30).

Pulmonary Function Tests

Simple spirometry gives useful information on the pattern of pulmonary involvement. The ratio of 1-second forced expiratory volume to forced vital capacity (FEV_1/FVC) distinguishes restrictive patterns, most often due to interstitial lung disease, from obstructive patterns due to lesions that may affect the larger airways as well as documenting lung volumes. The pulmonary transfer factor using a single breath carbon monoxide technique is particularly useful in the detection of early interstitial lung disease, documenting disease progression and monitoring responses to treatment.

Pulmonary Function Test Abnormalities

Pulmonary function test (PFT) abnormalities are exceedingly common in patients with SLE, even in those without respiratory complaints and with normal chest radiographic findings (18,19,31,32) (Table 33.1). In 1965, Huang et al. (32) studied 28 consecutive patients with SLE and found a high prevalence of physiologic abnormalities with a restrictive pattern. Reduction of the diffusing capacity was the most common finding with a mean value of 65% of the predicted value. Importantly, they observed a disparity between clinical and chest radiographic findings and PFT abnormalities.

In 1966, another study of PFTs in 20 patients with SLE and respiratory symptoms and described three major abnormalities: (a) restrictive disease, (b) airway obstruction, and (c) pulmonary vascular obstruction (33). Twelve of the

TABLE 33.1. RESPIRATORY FUNCTION STUDIES IN SYSTEMIC LUPUS ERYTHEMATOSUS (SLE)

Authors	Year	No. of Patients	Conclusions
Uncontrolled studies			
Huang and Lyons	1965	n = 20 with compared to n = 8 without lung disease	↓ DLCO in 57%, ↓ lung volumes; no correlations between PFT, CXR, or clinical findings
Gold and Jennings	1966	n = 20, 5 with lung	Restrictive pattern in 60%, obstructive symptoms in 10%. ↓ DLCO most common finding
Holgate et al.	1976	n = 30 SLE all with lung disease	All abnormal
Wohlgelernter et al.	1978	n = 10 (group 1) with and n = 14 (group 2) without lung symptoms or signs	↓ DLCO, arterial hypoxemia and/or restrictive pattern in 90% (group 1) and 71% (group 2); small airways disease in n = 10
Silberstein et al.	1980	n = 43	88% abnormal: ↓ DLCO (72%), ↓ lung volumes (44%), obstructive pattern (7%); no correlation between PFT and disease activity
Longitudinal studies			
Eichacker et al.	1988	n = 25 followed for 2–7 years	No changes in DLCO, forced vital capacity or lung volumes; reduction in small airway function unrelated to smoking
Cerveri et al.	1996	n = 15 children followed for 5 years	↓ TLCO 45% at baseline, 35% at follow-up; TLCO correlated with disease activity
Controlled studies			
Chick et al.	1976	n = 28 SLE and no lung symptoms, n = 28 controls	↓ DLCO, lung capacity and functional residual volume in SLE; smoking effects similar in both groups
Andonopoulos et al.	1988	n = 70 SLE nonsmokers, n = 70 control nonsmokers	Abnormal PFT in 63% SLE and 17% controls; isolated ↓ DLCO in 31% SLE and 0% in controls; small airways disease in 24% and 17%, respectively
Rolla et al.	1996	n = 24 SLE and n = 24 controls	↓ lung capacity, ↓ bronchial threshold to metacholine, increased AaO_2 gradient (n = 12); KCO correlated with disease activity

CXR, chest x-ray; DLCO, carbon monoxide diffusing capacity; KCO, pulmonary gas transfer; PFT, pulmonary function test; TCLO, total lung carbon monoxide diffusing capacity.

patients had evidence of restrictive disease, three had severe airway obstruction without pulmonary restriction, and five had pulmonary vascular obstruction. Three patients died, and the pathologic findings in the lungs correlated with the physiologic abnormalities observed during life.

Wohlgelernter et al. (3) found PFT abnormalities in 90% of their patients with SLE and a previous history of pleuritis and/or pneumonitis, and in 71% of their patients without pulmonary complaints. The most common abnormalities were a decreased carbon monoxide diffusing capacity of the lungs (DLCO), lack of response to breathing helium, restrictive ventilatory defect, and arterial hypoxemia. None of their patients with chronic discoid lupus erythematosus had an abnormal PFT, which is a finding consistent with the limited disease process in this condition. Rolla et al. (34) suggested a relationship between disease activity and KCO, indicating that systemic inflammation correlated with alveolar inflammation. Likewise, disease severity was related to airway patency and airway reactivity indices, suggesting cumulative damage to the airways in these patients (34). A similar study in children confirmed that transfer factor measurements were related to disease activity, and decreases in disease activity with treatment resulted in better pulmonary function (35). An interesting study described elevated nitric oxide (NO) levels in the exhaled air of lupus patients and correlation with disease activity in addition to pulmonary function testing (36). It was not clear, though, whether the NO arose from lung or systemic inflammation.

In a prospective study of 43 ambulatory, consecutive patients with SLE, Silberstein et al. (19) attempted to correlate PFT abnormalities with other measures of lupus activity. Pulmonary dysfunction was noted in 88% of patients. An impaired DLCO (72% of all patients), reduction in lung volume (49%), and hypoxia (44%) were the most common abnormalities that were found. No correlation was found between the type or severity of the abnormality and serum complement levels, anti-DNA antibody, lupus-band test, or nephritis. Patients with SLE and abnormal PFT results did not differ from those with normal PFT results in regard to their clinical or immunologic features. In contrast, Holgate et al. (37) reported that patients with SLE and prominent pleuropulmonary disease had a lower prevalence of lupus nephritis, suggesting that this is partly a result of the low frequency of anti-DNA antibodies in this group of patients. These two studies are not comparable, however, because the latter included only patients with SLE and pleuropulmonary disease.

Chick et al. (38) compared the PFT findings in 28 patients with SLE but without pulmonary involvement to those of healthy individuals matched for age, gender, and height. A restrictive pattern with reduced lung volume and vital capacity was seen in the SLE group. DLCO was reduced in patients with SLE in proportion to the reduction in lung volume, suggesting that this results from pleural thickening rather than from parenchymal disease. Cigarette smoking caused a reduction in flow at low lung volumes in both patients with SLE and normal controls.

Andonopoulos et al. (39) conducted the largest controlled study to date of PFTs in patients with SLE. They studied 70 lifelong nonsmoking SLE patients and an equal number of age- and sex-matched, nonsmoking healthy subjects. None of the patients had active pulmonary disease, and all had normal chest radiographs at the time of the study. An isolated reduction in the DLCO was the most prevalent abnormality found in the SLE patients. Isolated small airway disease, defined as less than 60% of the predicted value of the maximal flow at 25% of vital capacity, was common in both patients with SLE (24%) and controls (17%). Restrictive and obstructive patterns were uncommon in SLE, being seen in only 5.7% of patients. Overall, only 33% of the patients with SLE had normal PFT results, compared with 83% of the controls.

Eichacker et al. (40) evaluated the PFTs of 25 patients with SLE serially over a period of 2 to 7 years. Reductions in diffusing capacity, forced vital capacity, and total lung capacity did not change significantly with time. In contrast, small airway function decreased significantly with time and was unrelated to smoking history. The significance of this finding is not clear in view of Andonopoulos et al.'s (39) data that the prevalence of small airway disease in SLE patients is the same as that in healthy controls. Many of the studies of PFTs in patients with SLE that have been summarized here were uncontrolled, and did not consider the effects of cigarette smoking.

In the absence of respiratory symptoms, isolated abnormalities in PFT such as a reduced DLCO do not require treatment but should be monitored, and further investigation with HRCT chest scanning should be considered.

Nuclear Medicine Imaging

Ventilation/Perfusion (V/Q) Scans

In any patient with SLE presenting with breathlessness and pleuritic pains, the possibility of pulmonary embolism should be considered. V/Q scans offer a simple and reasonably reliable screening test for pulmonary embolism that can be used with CT pulmonary angiography where the results are indeterminate. V/Q scans may also be abnormal in the absence of pulmonary embolism, and severe pulmonary hypertension may produce an appearance of hypoperfusion in the peripheral areas of the lung. The combined use of D-dimer assays, V/Q scanning, and, where appropriate, CT pulmonary angiography may raise the accuracy in diagnosing pulmonary embolism (26) (Table 33.2).

Gallium-67 scans have been useful in the diagnosis and monitoring of patients with sarcoidosis, but there is little data on their use in the assessment of pulmonary disease in lupus. Witt et al. (41) studied lupus patients with interstitial lung disease and found an association between the presence of late inspiratory crackles clinically and increased uptake on gallium-67 scanning and abnormal bronchoalveolar lavage. However, abnormal gallium-67 scans were seen in only 37% of SLE patients compared to a prevalence of 74% with late inspiratory crackles and 95% of patients with abnormal CT chests, making the scans somewhat insensitive at picking up interstitial lung disease.

Arterial Blood Gases

Arterial blood gases give an accurate estimate of alveolar ventilation. It is essential in the assessment of pulmonary embolism, extensive pulmonary infiltration, severe pneumonia, pulmonary hemorrhage, and acute reversible hypoxemia where hypoxia (type I respiratory failure) may occur.

TABLE 33.2. COMPARISON OF TECHNIQUES IN THE DIAGNOSIS OF PULMONARY EMBOLISM

	Sensitivity	Specificity	Advantages	Disadvantages
D-dimer	85–100%	41%	High negative predictive value; cheap	Not compared to pulmonary angiography yet
Ventilation/perfusion				
High probability	41%	97%	Well validated, widely available	High proportion of nondiagnostic results
Highly/intermediate Probability	82%	52%		
Low probability	98%	10%		
Spiral CT	53–100%	81–97%	Well validated, widely available, detects other conditions	Cost, contrast load, subsegmental emboli may be missed
MR Angiography	50–100%	91–100%	Low contrast load, may be used to diagnose DVT	Cost, subsegmental emboli may be missed

CT, computed tomography; DVT, deep venous thrombosis; MR, magnetic resonance.

Bronchoscopy And Bronchoalveolar Lavage (BAL)

These techniques may be useful when evaluating the etiology of interstitial pulmonary shadowing in patients with lupus. BAL fluid may be examined to exclude opportunistic infections especially in immunosuppressed patients. In patients with suspected interstitial lung disease where CT chest images show ground-glass shadowing with a honeycomb appearance, elevated cell counts in BAL fluid may suggest alveolar inflammation and direct treatment with immunosuppressive agents once infection has been excluded.

The technique of BAL facilitates the analysis of cellular and soluble components from the epithelial surface of the lower respiratory tract. BAL has yielded valuable information about immune responses and the pathogenesis of lung injury in the connective tissue diseases, especially systemic sclerosis and rheumatoid arthritis (RA). BAL findings may be diagnostic in some diseases, such as infections; in others, however, findings are nonspecific but may contribute to the management of these diseases. For example, an increased number of BAL eosinophils were associated with progressive lung disease in idiopathic interstitial pulmonary fibrosis, RA, and scleroderma (42).

In a multicenter study designed to standardize the test procedure, BAL was performed in 24 patients with diffuse ILD secondary to rheumatic disorders, including SLE (43). The total number of cells in the BAL fluid was increased with the percentage increase in neutrophils and decrease in macrophages. Total protein, immunoglobulin M (IgM), IgG, and IgA, but not albumin, increased in concentration in the BAL fluid. Walaert et al. (44) studied BAL fluid in 61 patients with collagen vascular disease without respiratory symptoms, and included in their study were 11 patients with SLE, all of whom had normal PFT results. An abnormal differential count of BAL fluid leukocytes was found in 48 of patients, including three with SLE. In contrast to patients with RA and systemic sclerosis, who had a predominant polymorphonuclear alveolitis, patients with SLE showed a lymphocytic predominance. An increased percentage of BAL fluid eosinophils was also found in two patients with SLE and ILD (42). Similarly, Witt et al. (41) found elevated lymphocyte and neutrophil counts in the BAL fluid from 19 lupus patients.

Alveolar macrophages in BAL fluid from 17 patients with inactive SLE were found to be normal in number, viability, and respiratory burst activity, but had severely impaired antibacterial function (44). This dysfunction, which was observed in both steroid-treated and untreated patients, may contribute to the increased frequency of pulmonary infections in this disease.

Walaert et al. (45) introduced the concept of subclinical alveolitis in SLE and in other systemic rheumatic diseases, which is characterized by the accumulation of inflammatory and immune cells in the BAL fluid of patients without respiratory complaints, with a normal chest radiograph, and with or without significant PFT abnormalities. The clinical significance of subclinical alveolitis, however, is not clear since it is not known how many of these patients will develop overt interstitial lung disease.

Higher concentrations of soluble immune complexes have been observed in BAL fluid compared to the corresponding serum specimen from patients with ILD associated with rheumatic diseases, including SLE (46). Immune complexes were also seen within the cytoplasm of BAL neutrophils, indicating that locally formed immune complexes may induce an inflammatory response in the lungs of these patients.

Increased numbers of activated $CD8^+$. T lymphocytes and natural killer (NK) cells were found in the BAL fluid of lupus patients with abnormal pulmonary function tests and correlated with reduced carbon monoxide transfer factor and diffusing capacity values (47). In contrast, the number of $CD19^+$ B cells in the BAL fluid was lower than that seen in the fluid of healthy controls, despite the high percentage of these cells in SLE peripheral blood. These observations suggest a cell-mediated immune response in the lungs in SLE (47).

BAL, therefore, may be a potentially useful technique in the assessment and follow-up of patients with SLE and pulmonary involvement, especially in those with acute lupus pneumonitis and chronic diffuse ILD.

CLINICAL MANIFESTATIONS OF PULMONARY INVOLVEMENT IN LUPUS

Respiratory tract involvement occurs in about half of lupus patients over their disease course (12). The following sections describe the main features of lung disease in SLE.

Pleurisy

Prevalence

Pleurisy is the most common manifestation of pulmonary involvement in SLE, and the pleura is involved more commonly in lupus than in any other connective tissue disease. Several early studies documented the prevalence of pleural involvement. For example, in Dubois and Tuffanelli's (48) 520 patients, the cumulative incidence of recurrent pleuritic pain was 45% and that of pleural effusions was 30%. McGehee Harvey et al. (49) reported pleurisy in 56% of their patients with recurrent pleuritic episodes in 13%, while 16% had associated pleural effusions. Several other studies have documented high prevalences of pleuritis, ranging from 41% to 56% (18,50), being found more commonly in blacks than whites (51). Perhaps the largest study to date, that of 1,000 European lupus patients, found a prevalence at disease onset of serositis (including both pleural and pericardial inflammation) of 17% with a cumulative incidence of 36%, with pleuritis occurring more commonly in men than in women (52). Lung involvement defined as acute or chronic lupus pneumonitis was much less common, with a prevalence at disease onset of 3% and cumulative incidence of 7%—almost certainly an underestimate. The highest prevalence comes from a postmortem study: Ropes (53) described pleural changes in 93% of 58 patients with SLE at autopsy, with fluid in the pleural cavity in 33 cases.

Clinical Features

Pleurisy as the initial manifestation of SLE was noted by Dubois' (54) in 13 of 520 patients. Pleuritic symptoms may antedate other manifestations of lupus by months or even years, resulting in a delay in the diagnosis of SLE (55).

Pleuritic chest pain may be unilateral or bilateral, and is usually located at the costophrenic margins, either anteriorly or posteriorly. Attacks of pleuritic pain often last for several days, and, when associated with effusions, the pain may persist for weeks often accompanied by cough, dyspnea, or fever. The effusion generally occurs on the side of the chest pain (Fig. 33.1). Pleural effusions may also occur in patients with SLE and nephrotic syndrome; infections, such as tuberculosis; or cardiac failure (23). Massive bilateral pleural effusion is a rare presenting feature of the disease (56). It is important to remember that the differential diagnosis of pleuritic pain in a patient with lupus may include infection and pulmonary embolism, especially in the presence of antiphospholipid antibodies.

Pleural Fluid

The volume of pleural effusions usually is small to moderate (400 to 1,000 mL) and may be unilateral or bilateral.

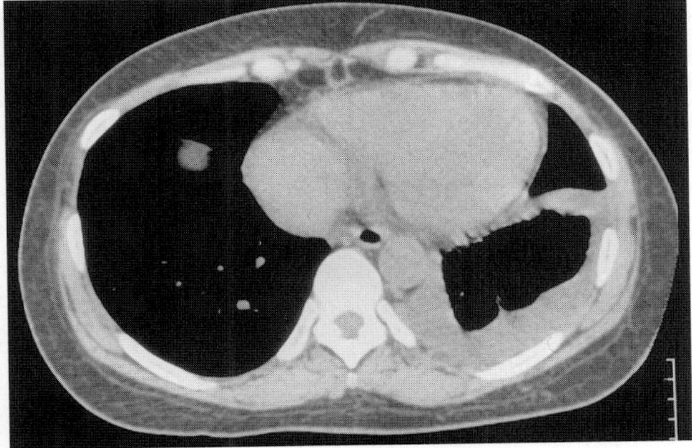

FIGURE 33.1. Computed tomography (CT) chest scan showing a large pleural effusion in a patient presenting with left-sided pleuritic chest pain and breathlessness.

Large pleural effusions are uncommon (10,57). Thoracocentesis is not always necessary in lupus patients unless the cause of the pleural effusion is uncertain and infection is suspected. The pleural fluid in SLE is usually exudative in character, although transudates have also been reported (10). The fluid can be yellow, amber, or slightly turbid in color. In a study of 14 patients with lupus pleuritis (57), the white cell count in the pleural fluids ranged from 325 to 14,950 cells/mL (mean, 4,895 cells/mL). Half the specimens showed a predominance of polymorphonuclear leukocytes, with cell counts ranging from 10% to 100% (mean, 57%). Kelley et al. (58) examined pleural effusions from ten patients with SLE and found atypical cells resembling plasma cells. The presence of these cells with other inflammatory cells, fibrinoid debris, erythrocytes, and few mesothelial cells and in the absence of pathogenic organisms or malignant cells constituted a pattern that was characteristic of SLE in eight of the ten patients studied.

In most patients with lupus pleuritis, the pleural fluid glucose concentration is greater than 60 mg/dL, with a pleural fluid/serum glucose ratio of greater than 0.5. Good et al. (57) found the mean pleural fluid/serum glucose ratio to be 0.3 or lower. This contrasts with the finding of low glucose levels in the pleural fluid of patients with RA and pleurisy, in whom the glucose concentration is less than 30 mg/dL in 75% of patients (59). Low glucose concentrations, or a low pleural fluid/serum glucose ratio, may also occur in those with malignant effusions, empyema, or tuberculosis (59). The pH of SLE pleural fluid usually is greater than 7.35. A few patients have a pH of less than 7.3, which is associated with a low pleural fluid glucose level (57,59).

Classic LE cells have been documented in smears of pleural fluids from patients with SLE (57,60,61). It has been suggested that the presence of *in vivo* LE cells in the pleural fluid is highly characteristic of SLE (62). However, the LE cell test is now largely obsolete and has been replaced by searching for antinuclear antibodies (ANAs) in pleural fluid (12).

The presence of ANAs in the pleural fluid may be a useful diagnostic test for patients with undiagnosed pleural effusions. For instance, Leechawengwong et al. (63) tested pleural fluid from 100 consecutive patients with pleural effusion and found positive ANA in all seven patients with SLE and in one patient with drug-induced LE, but not in patients with other diagnoses. Conversely, Small et al. (64) found that a positive ANA in the pleural fluid was not specific for SLE; it also was found in patients without SLE but with pleural effusions who tested positive for ANA in the blood. Khare et al. (65) found positive ANA in eight of 74 non-lupus pleural effusions (10.8%), including those associated with malignancy.

Good et al. (57) measured the ANA titer in paired samples of pleural fluid and serum of patients with SLE. In lupus pleuritis, the pleural fluid/serum ANA ratio was greater than 1. In contrast, the ratio was less than 1 in patients with SLE who had pleural effusions from other causes, such as congestive heart failure. Moreover, none of 67 patients with pleural effusions of different causes had a positive ANA.

Pathogenesis

The pathogenesis of pleural effusion in SLE differs from that of RA. For example, immune complexes in RA are thought to be produced locally in the pleura, whereas immune complexes are derived from the circulation in SLE. In addition, the concentration of soluble interleukin-2 (IL-2) receptor in the pleural fluid in RA is significantly higher than that in SLE. This suggests that a local T-cell–mediated immune reaction may be a more important mechanism in rheumatoid pleurisy than in lupus (66).

In an autopsy study, 54 of 58 patients (93%) in Ropes' series showed pleural involvement (53). Fluid was found in the pleural space in 33 patients, and adhesions were seen in 63%. Microscopic changes of varying degrees were observed in 24%; these consisted of accumulations of lymphocytes and macrophages, pleural thickening, perivascular fibrinoid necrosis with neutrophilic and mononuclear infiltrates, fibrinous exudate, and rare hematoxylin bodies. Pleural biopsy in one patient with SLE and bilateral effusions revealed noncaseating pleural granulomas (67).

Several early studies demonstrated reduced levels of hemolytic complement, C1q, C4, and C3 in pleural fluid from lupus patients when compared to pleural effusions from patients with cancer, heart failure, and other conditions (68–70). These complement levels remained low even after adjustment for the total protein content of the pleural fluid (69). However, low pleural fluid complement levels are not specific for SLE, and may occur in patients with RA or empyema (70,71).

There is some evidence that low pleural fluid complement levels in SLE results from activation of the complement cascade by immune complexes. Thus, conversion products that are generated by activation of the complement cascade are present in SLE pleural fluid (71,72), and immune complexes abound in SLE pleural fluid (71–73). Furthermore, perivascular deposits of immunoglobulins and complement components in the parietal pleura have been found in patients with lupus pleuritis (71). The nature of the immune complexes in SLE pleural fluid is not clear, though they may well be DNA–anti-DNA complexes (74).

None of the immunologic abnormalities that are described in pleural fluid is diagnostic of lupus pleuritis. Thus, the presence of immune complexes, complement activation products, and immune deposits in the parietal pleurae all have been reported in pleurisy associated with other rheumatic diseases, such as RA, as well as in non-rheumatic conditions, including cancer and empyema (64,71). This suggests that an immune-mediated mechanism(s) is a common pathway by which SLE and other diseases can cause pleurisy.

Treatment Of Lupus Pleurisy

Analgesics and nonsteroidal antiinflammatory drugs (NSAIDs) are useful treatments for mild lupus pleurisy. If the patient fails to improve or the symptoms are severe, systemic corticosteroids (10 to 20 mg of prednisone daily) are usually rapidly effective. Hydroxychloroquine may be added to provide longer-term benefit after tapering the prednisone dose. When present, the effusion begins to clear within days of beginning steroid therapy, though it may take several weeks for the radiographic changes to clear up completely. It is not necessary to consider chest tube drainage of these effusions. When clinical or radiographic changes are slow to improve, the addition of a steroid sparing agent such as azathioprine may be considered. In those very rare patients with chronic, unremitting lupus pleurisy that is refractory to medical therapy, pleurectomy (75), talc poudrage (76), and tetracycline pleurodesis (77,78) may be used. Intravenous immunoglobulin therapy was of limited value in a patient with lupus and refractory pleural effusion (79).

Acute Lupus Pneumonitis

Clinical Presentation

Acute lupus pneumonitis is an uncommon clinical manifestation of SLE. In Estes and Christian's (50) series of 150 patients, 48% had evidence of pulmonary involvement at some time during the course of their illness, but only 14 (9%) had acute lupus pneumonitis. Other studies found prevalences of between 1% and 7% in their series (18,21,23,52).

Patients with acute lupus pneumonitis usually present with fever, dyspnea, cough productive of scanty sputum, hemoptysis, tachypnea, and pleuritic chest pain (80). Physical findings commonly include basal crepitations, and, when severe, central cyanosis may be present. Chest radiographs demonstrate diffuse acinar infiltrates with a predilection for the bases in all patients and pleural effusion in 50% of patients (80) (Fig. 33.2). The vast majority of patients have some degree of arterial hypoxemia. The white cell count is usually normal, and anti-DNA antibodies are present in these patients with severe active lupus, often with other evidence of multisystem involvement. Multiple cultures and investigations for bacteria, fungi, and viruses are usually negative, and prompt diagnosis of lupus pneumonitis is essential, as the mortality rate may be as high as 50% (80).

Pathology

The histopathology of the lung in acute lupus pneumonitis has been examined in a few untreated patients; light micro-

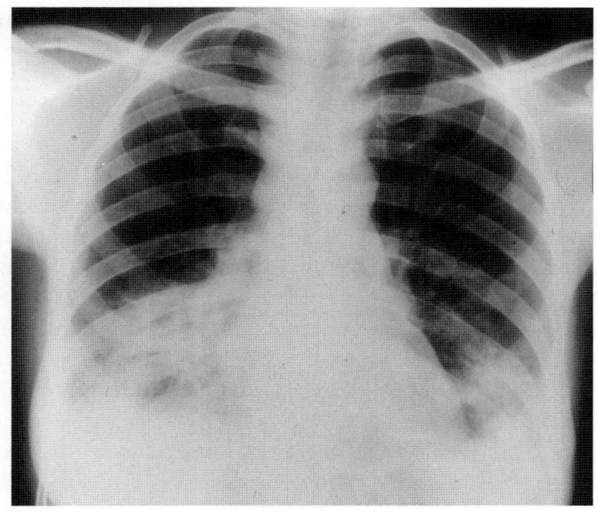

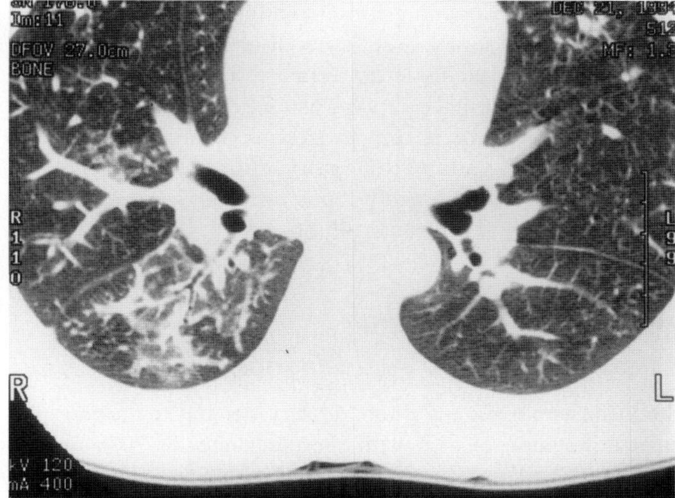

FIGURE 33.2. **A:** Chest radiograph in a patient with acute lupus pneumonitis. **B:** CT scan in this patient shows right-sided interstitial shadowing.

scopic changes are variable and nonspecific. An open-lung biopsy obtained before therapy in one of Matthay et al.'s (80) patients showed a diffuse interstitial lymphocytic infiltrate with prominent lymphoid nodules and bronchiolitis. Despite therapy, the patient died, and at autopsy alveolar hyaline membranes and persistent cell infiltrates were found. Other findings at the autopsy of four patients included acute alveolitis, interstitial edema, hyaline membranes, and arteriolar thrombosis. Pertschuk et al. (81) reported eight patients with SLE who presented with a clinical diagnosis of acute lupus pneumonitis and 50% had changes of interstitial pneumonia. The pathologic picture was considered to be nonspecific and similar to that seen in those patients with oxygen toxicity, viral pneumonia, or uremia. The other four patients showed other pathologic changes: bronchiolitis, pulmonary infarction, focal atelectasis, and cytomegalovirus pneumonia, respectively. Vasculitis was not observed in any patient in either study (80,81). Widespread thrombosis was found in the lungs and other organs at autopsy of a patient with acute lupus pneumonitis and disseminated intravascular coagulation (82).

The wide variety of histologic changes in the lungs suggests that acute lupus pneumonitis may result from different pathologic processes (10). Many of the patients studied had received prior treatment, however, including oxygen, high-dose steroids, or cytotoxic agents, which can affect lung pathology either directly or indirectly. Thus, some of the pathologic abnormalities in the lungs may be secondary changes rather than resulting directly from SLE.

Granular deposits of IgG, C3, and DNA have been found in the alveolar septa of two patients with acute lupus pneumonitis (83). Electron microscopy revealed electron-dense deposits in the septal interstitium and in the walls of alveolar capillaries. Immunoglobulin eluted from the lung tissue had ANA activity, including IgG anti-DNA antibody. Another study described deposits of immunoglobulin within the nuclei of alveolar lining cells and pleural mesothelial cells, rather than in the septal interstitium, in acute lupus pneumonitis (81). The concomitant presence of C3 within the nuclei suggested that this was an *in vivo* rather than an artifactual phenomenon. These immunopathologic observations are consistent with the deposition of antigen-antibody complexes and may be important in the pathogenesis of the lung injury.

Parenchymal pulmonary infiltrates that develop acutely in a patient with SLE should not be considered as acute lupus pneumonitis until infectious processes such as viral pneumonia, tuberculosis, and other bacterial pneumonias and fungal and *Pneumocystis carinii* infections have been completely excluded (10). An elevated C-reactive protein (CRP) in such patients should encourage a vigorous search for lung sepsis.

Treatment And Prognosis

High-dose corticosteroids including bolus intravenous methylprednisolone together with supportive measures such as oxygen and mechanical ventilation where necessary are still the mainstay of drug therapy for acute lupus pneumonitis, although no controlled trials have established their efficacy (10,83). Cytotoxic agents such as azathioprine are added to the regimen in patients who fail to respond to steroid therapy or who relapse on steroid dose tapering (80). Intravenous pulse cyclophosphamide combined with systemic corticosteroids has also been used successfully (84).

Acute lupus pneumonitis carries a poor prognosis. Of 12 patients reported by Matthay et al. (80), the mortality was 50% during the acute episode—from respiratory failure, opportunistic infection, and thromboembolism. All six surviving patients remained relatively well after more than a year of follow-up, but three developed residual interstitial infiltrates with abnormal pulmonary function tests, indicating that the acute process can progress to chronic interstitial lung disease. Adult respiratory distress syndrome (ARDS) may occur with acute lupus pneumonitis, greatly increasing the risk of mortality (85,86).

Pulmonary Hemorrhage

Clinical Presentation And Diagnosis

Pulmonary hemorrhage is a rare, devastating, and frequently fatal manifestation of SLE with mortality rates of 70% to 90% (87–93). For example, Abud-Mendoza et al. (88) described 12 patients with massive pulmonary hemorrhage among 750 patients with SLE (1.6%) of whom 11 died. A further study found 34 patients in a cohort of 630 patients, all of whom had severe respiratory failure (91). A higher prevalence of 3.7% of all inpatient admissions for SLE had pulmonary hemorrhage reported by Zamora et al (87). Autopsy studies found pulmonary hemorrhage to be the cause of death in 11% to 14% lupus fatalities (88,92). Several children with SLE and lung hemorrhage also have been reported (94–97). Single-case reports also describe pulmonary hemorrhage in pregnancy (98) and the antiphospholipid syndrome (99).

The clinical presentation is similar to that of acute lupus pneumonitis, with a sudden onset of fever, dyspnea, cough, blood-stained sputum, and occasionally frank hemoptysis. The clinical course is rapidly progressive over hours or days, with increasing tachypnea, arterial hypoxemia, tachycardia, acute respiratory distress, and frank hemoptysis. The hemoglobin and hematocrit drop suddenly, and chest radiographs show bilateral pulmonary infiltrates, with a predominantly alveolar pattern. The infiltrates are coarsely nodular, fluffy, or homogeneous in pattern, often extending to the bases but occasionally unilateral in distribution. Single breath diffusing capacity for carbon monoxide may well be raised due the presence of blood in the alveolar spaces, though patients are often too ill to undergo this investigation (100). Mechanical ventilation is frequently required for marked arterial hypoxia (87), and patients usually have clinical and laboratory evidence of multisystem involvement, including positive anti-DNA antibodies and hypocomplementemia. The mortality in these patients is 62%, rising to 78% to 100% if there is concomitant infection (87).

Frank hemoptysis does not always occur, even with massive intra-alveolar hemorrhage, so the clinical diagnosis is often delayed (88,92). For example, in a series of 140 patients with SLE, three developed pulmonary hemorrhage, and in two of these patients the diagnosis was made only at autopsy (93). In the absence of hemoptysis, a rapidly falling hematocrit and diffuse lung infiltrates in a patient with SLE should alert the clinician to the possibility of lung hemorrhage (88). Bronchoalveolar lavages are universally hemorrhagic, and transbronchial lung biopsies may be helpful (87). Although open lung biopsy is sometimes advocated, these patients are usually very unwell and are poor operative risks. MRI and CT have been reported to be helpful in the diagnosis of diffuse alveolar hemorrhage in SLE (101,102).

While pulmonary hemorrhage is very rarely the presenting feature of SLE, the majority of cases arise in patients with established lupus. The median disease duration of such patients ranges from 31 months to 3.2 years (87,92). Multisystem disease is often present in patients with pulmonary hemorrhage and renal disease is the most common occurrence. In one study, 94% of patients had both pulmonary hemorrhage and lupus nephritis (87), justifying the inclusion of SLE in the list of diseases associated with the pulmonary-renal vasculitic syndromes (103).

Pathology

The histopathology of the lung is that of diffuse, intra-alveolar hemorrhage with intact erythrocytes and hemosiderin-laden macrophages in the alveoli (87,92,104). Other microscopic findings include thickening of the alveolar septa, hyaline membrane formation, and fibrin deposits within the alveolar cavities. Evidence of vasculitis usually is not seen. A distinctive microangiitis that is characterized by acute inflammation and necrosis of alveolar capillaries, arterioles, and small muscular arteries also has been described in four patients (105), while in another study pulmonary capillaritis was seen in 80% of lung tissue specimens (87).

Electron microscopic studies in a small number of cases have shown type II alveolar-lining cell hyperplasia and electron-dense deposits in the alveolar septa within the basement membrane of alveolar capillaries and in the walls of small arteries (87,104,106–108). Direct immunofluorescence studies have demonstrated the presence of granular deposits of immunoglobulin, principally IgG, and complement components in the alveolar septa and in the walls of small blood vessels (104,106,107,109). Other investigators, however, have failed to find immune deposits in the alveolar septa in patients with SLE and pulmonary hemorrhage (104,110).

Pathogenesis

The pathogenesis of pulmonary hemorrhage in SLE is not known. Deposition of immune complexes in the alveolar septa and in blood vessels, with activation of the complement system, has been proposed as being the major mechanism, which is analogous to the lung changes that are seen in experimental models of chronic serum sickness. Brentjens et al. (111) described changes of interstitial pneumonitis with proliferation of septal cells, thickening of the alveolar septa, accumulation of leukocytes in capillaries, and alveolar hemorrhages in rabbits that were hyperimmunized with foreign serum protein. Conversely, Eagen et al. (104)

identified several factors that potentially contributed to the pathogenesis of lung hemorrhage in their patients with SLE, including bleeding diathesis, oxygen toxicity, infection, uremia, and shock lung. Desnoyers et al. (110) described a patient with SLE and cutaneous vasculitis, nephritis, and pulmonary hemorrhage but without the complicating factors described earlier that could cause nonspecific alveolar damage. No immune deposits were found in the alveolar septa, although they were present in the renal glomeruli. These authors suggested that pulmonary hemorrhage could occur in SLE by mechanism(s) other than immune complex deposition, such as vascular injury with disruption of the alveolar capillary membrane. Unlike Goodpasture's syndrome, in which pulmonary hemorrhage is characteristic, there is no association with smoking (87).

Treatment And Prognosis

The prognosis of massive pulmonary hemorrhage in patients with SLE is grave, despite treatment with high-dose systemic corticosteroids combined with a cytotoxic agent (10,80,88,104). Other investigators have reported a better prognosis, however. Six of eight patients (75%) with SLE and pulmonary alveolar hemorrhage who were reported by Schwab et al. (112) recovered. In another large study the overall survival rate was only 38% (91). The mortality rate of pediatric lupus cases with lung hemorrhage has been reported to be 50% (96).

The poor prognosis in these patients suggests that it may be advisable to employ a regimen of high-dose corticosteroids, cyclophosphamide, and perhaps plasmapheresis (113–115).

Erickson et al. (114) reported dramatic improvement in three patients who underwent intensive plasmapheresis combined with steroids and cyclophosphamide. A review of reported cases of pulmonary hemorrhage in SLE showed that the survival rate of those patients who received corticosteroids with or without cytotoxic agents was 43% (23 of 53 patients). In contrast, 7 of 11 patients (64%) who also underwent plasmapheresis survived (114). Complications (especially a high rate of serious infections) have been reported in patients receiving plasmapheresis combined with steroids and cyclophosphamide (116).

Carette et al. (117) reviewed more than 400 SLE patients who were followed over 10 years, of whom eight became acutely ill with diffuse lung infiltrates. Pulmonary hemorrhage was eventually diagnosed in six patients, of whom four had other complicating factors, including uremia, coagulopathy, and infection. Based on their experience, a practical management approach was suggested. Four major conditions should be considered in the differential diagnosis: (a) congestive heart failure, (b) noncardiogenic pulmonary edema, (c) infection, and (d) pulmonary hemorrhage. A careful clinical history should be taken, and a thorough physical examination performed. Evidence of lupus activity in other organ systems should be documented. If the diagnosis of congestive heart failure is unclear on clinical grounds, an echocardiogram or Swan-Ganz catheter should be considered. Infection and factors that are associated with noncardiogenic pulmonary edema, including uremia, pancreatitis, and side effects from drugs, should be excluded. If a definite diagnosis is not reached at this point, broad-spectrum antibiotics and high-dose corticosteroids should be considered while bronchoalveolar lavage, transbronchial lung biopsy, and brushings are obtained. If pathogenic organisms are not found after appropriate stains and cultures, antibiotics should be discontinued. Systemic corticosteroids should be continued until clinical improvement occurs, but if the patient fails to respond, an open-lung biopsy sample should be considered, bearing in mind the operative risks that this procedure entails.

Chronic Diffuse Interstitial Lung Disease

Clinical Presentation

Diffuse ILD is a well-recognized pulmonary manifestation of systemic rheumatic diseases, particularly systemic sclerosis, dermatomyositis, and RA. Somewhat surprisingly, it is much less common in SLE than in other connective tissue diseases. ILD in SLE was described in detail in 1973, by Eisenberg et al. (118). The prevalence of symptomatic ILD in SLE has been calculated to be approximately 3% (118,119). In an early prospective study of 150 patients, nine developed radiographic changes of pulmonary fibrosis, but it is unclear whether these patients were symptomatic or how severe the pulmonary functional abnormalities were (50). A retrospective study of 63 SLE patients noted 16 patients (25%) with ILD (120). The high prevalence was partly due to the inclusion of severely ill, hospitalized patients in their series.

The initial presentation of diffuse ILD in SLE can be one of two types. The more common is an insidious onset of a chronic nonproductive cough, dyspnea on exertion, and a history of recurrent pleuritic chest pain. Less commonly, ILD may develop in a patient following acute lupus pneumonitis: two studies suggest that between 43% and 50% of patients with acute lupus pneumonitis may go on to develop chronic diffuse ILD (80,120).

The presentation of ILD in SLE resembles that of lung disease in systemic sclerosis and RA. The most common clinical manifestations are persistent dyspnea on exertion, pleuritic chest pains, and nonproductive cough. ILD can occur at any time during the course of SLE, but in most patients it develops in those with long-standing disease. Multisystem involvement is relatively common, and patients usually test positive for both ANAs and anti-DNA antibodies.

In the study by Eisenberg et al. (118), the mean age of their 18 patients with SLE and ILD was 45.7 years, with a mean disease duration of 10.3 years. Pulmonary manifestations were present for a mean of 6 years. Initially, seven patients presented with pulmonary symptoms developing over weeks to months with dyspnea on exertion, and three with dyspnea at rest. Twelve complained of cough with scanty sputum, and a similar number had pleuritic chest pain. All patients had poor diaphragmatic movement, with diminished resonance to percussion over the lung bases. Cyanosis and clubbing were present in one patient, and 12 had basilar rales. All 18 had persistent, diffuse interstitial infiltrates on chest radiography that could not be attributed to other complication. Markedly elevated diaphragms were seen in eight patients, and diaphragmatic excursion was decreased in six as evaluated by chest radiography on deep inspiration and expiration. A pleural reaction was present in nine patients, and plate-like atelectasis in six, which was usually seen just above the diaphragm and persisted for several months to years. The diffusing capacity of the lung, as measured by the carbon monoxide method, was decreased below the predicted normal values in all but one patient.

Laboratory Evaluation

To investigate the possibility of pulmonary infarction, Eisenberg et al. (118), obtained ventilation-perfusion lung scans in 13 patients. Of these, eight had matched ventilation and perfusion defects occurring at the same site. In seven of 13 patients, ventilation-perfusion defects were noted in areas other than those occupied by long line shadows, effusions, or atelectasis.

Spirometry and lung-volume measurements were consistent with a restrictive defect or loss of lung volume without obstruction to air flow. Diffuse pulmonary interstitial infiltration typically results in this type of ventilatory defect. Infiltrated lung areas are less elastic and change their volume less with each breath. Underventilation results in under oxygenation of the blood perfusing these regions, and if this ventilation-perfusion mismatching is extensive, significant arterial hypoxemia may occur. Obstructive defects were not seen (118).

The arterial blood oxygen tension (PaO_2) was diminished in all patients, and the alveolar-arterial difference for oxygen ($PAO_2 - PaO_2$) increased significantly. The PaO_2 was lowest and the $PAO_2 - PaO_2$ difference greatest in patients with the most extensive pulmonary involvement, as noted in their radiographs. The oxyhemoglobin saturation, however, was above 94% in all but four patients, and ventilation-perfusion mismatching was responsible for these changes. Thickening and fibrosis of the interstitial wall and microinfarcts in the lung alter the elastic properties of the ventilatory lung units, leading to underventilation relative to perfusion. Lung biopsy in four patients showed nonspecific interstitial fibrosis, with chronic inflammation in two (118).

Boulware and Hedgpeth (120) found precipitating anti-Ro/SSA antibodies in 81% of patients with SLE and ILD compared to 38% in their general SLE population. In contrast, the frequency of other specific types of ANA, such as anti-U1 ribonucleoprotein (RNP), and anti-La/SSB, was not significantly increased. This possible association with anti-Ro/SSA has also been found by Mochizuki et al. (121) but not by Weinrib et al. (119), and the discrepancy may result from differences in patient selection.

There is evidence that chronic ILD occurs in a subset of lupus patients with features of scleroderma, including Raynaud's phenomenon, sclerodactyly, and nail-fold capillary abnormalities (122). In addition, there is an increased frequency of anti-U1 RNP and anti-U1 RNA antibodies in these patients. However, in this study, seven of the 19 patients with SLE and chronic ILD had concomitant connective tissue disease, including RA, scleroderma, and mixed connective tissue disease (MCTD) (122).

High-Resolution CT Scans

High-resolution CT (HRCT) scans of the lungs are essential in the diagnosis, assessment of disease activity in the lung parenchyma, and provision of prognostic information in patients suspected of having ILD associated with connective tissue diseases (123–126) (Fig. 33.3).

Johkoh et al. (127) compared HRCT lung scans and pulmonary function tests in idiopathic pulmonary fibrosis and ILD associated with connective tissue disease including SLE. The extent of morphologic changes correlated with the severity of impairment of the diffusing capacity (DLCO) in both patient groups. Steroid-responsive patients showed a ground-glass and alveolar consolidation and no honeycomb lesions on the HRCT scans. In contrast, patients who failed to respond to therapy had severe honeycomb lesions on the HRCT scans. A further study of 15 HRCT scans in ten lupus patients with respiratory symptoms found 14 of the 15 scans to be abnormal (128). The main finding was that of chronic lower zone interstitial lung disease with honeycombing, architectural distortion, paren-

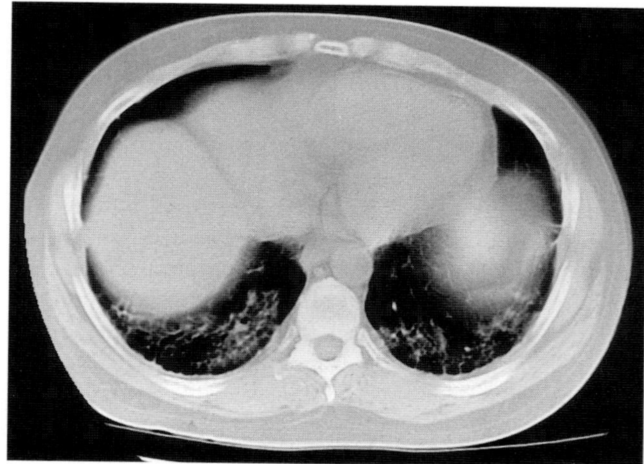

FIGURE 33.3. High-resolution CT chest scan showing bilateral basal interstitial fibrosis with honeycombing.

chymal bands, and pleural changes. Pleural thickening was seen in 87% of scans, and all patients had abnormal lung function tests, especially reduced carbon monoxide diffusion capacity.

Pathogenesis Of Chronic ILD

Studies in idiopathic pulmonary fibrosis and systemic sclerosis suggest a key role for cytokines and other mediators that are secreted by alveolar macrophages and inflammatory cells as well as resident structural cells of the lung. IL-1, tumor necrosis factor (TNF), endothelin, and especially growth and differentiating cytokines [transforming growth factor, platelet-derived growth factor (PDGF), and granulocyte-macrophage colony-stimulating factor (GM-CSF)] are believed to be important in the alteration of cell phenotypes in the lung, accumulation of inflammatory cells from the circulation, and increased collagen secretion by stimulated fibroblasts (129,130).

Chronic ILD is a predominantly T-lymphocyte–mediated immunologic reaction to some unknown antigen, in contrast to acute lupus pneumonitis, which primarily is an immune-complex–mediated condition (131). This study found increased numbers of activated $CD8^+$ T cells, $CD56^+/CD16^+/CD3^-$ NK cells, and other markers of T-cell activation in the BAL fluid of patients with SLE (131). These cellular abnormalities were associated with upregulated local production of oxygen radicals and with impaired pulmonary diffusing capacity. In addition, cells in the BAL fluid of patients with SLE and ILD spontaneously secrete increased amounts of PDGF and TNF, which can induce proliferation of fibroblasts (132).

Treatment And Prognosis

The clinical course of chronic ILD is variable in individual patients, but as a group, most patients follow a slow course, tending to improve or stabilize with time. In one study of 14 patients, all received high-dose prednisone (60 mg daily) for at least 4 weeks early in the course of the pulmonary disease (119). The diffusing capacity for carbon monoxide (DLCO) and inspiratory vital capacity (IVC) either improved or remained unchanged in most patients, and respiratory symptoms improved in all patients. Two died of progressive pulmonary fibrosis, however, and another succumbed to bacterial pneumonia (119). A study comparing patients with ILD associated with connective tissue diseases, including SLE, and those with idiopathic pulmonary fibrosis showed that lung function deteriorated significantly over 2 years in the idiopathic group, but remained essentially unchanged in the connective tissue diseases group (133).

Patients with SLE and symptomatic, chronic, progressive ILD should undergo assessment of the extent and activity of the lung disease with pulmonary function tests, gallium lung scan, BAL, and/or transbronchial biopsy. An open-lung biopsy is usually not indicated. HRCT scans of the lungs give useful information on the extent and activity of disease, and repeat HRCT may document changes, especially if the changes are predominantly of ground-glass alveolar shadowing. Serial pulmonary function tests are useful in monitoring the disease and the response to therapy (10).

In the presence of an active inflammatory process in the lung, and once infection has been excluded, high-dose prednisone (40 to 60 mg daily) for at least 6 to 8 weeks should be considered. The dose is tapered depending on the clinical and laboratory responses of the patient. Immunosuppressive agents such as azathioprine and intravenous cyclophosphamide may be needed in patients who fail to respond satisfactorily to steroids.

Corticosteroid therapy of ILD in lupus and other connective tissue diseases results in a decrease in total cell count, immune complexes, and immunoglobulin levels in BAL fluid (134). The efficacy of systemic corticosteroids and immunosuppressive agents in the treatment of ILD and SLE has not been validated by well-designed, controlled trials.

Pulmonary Embolism

Pleuritic chest pain and dyspnea are relatively common, and most patients with SLE presenting with these symptoms usually have pleurisy or pneumonitis. However, pulmonary embolism (PE) should always be considered especially if antiphospholipid antibodies are present or there is a previous history of PE. The predictive value of V/Q scans, D-dimer levels, and CT pulmonary angiography has been discussed above (Table 33.2), and it should be remembered that abnormal perfusion scans may occur in patients with active lung disease in the absence of PE. Nevertheless, if PE is suspected clinically in a patient with a low probability V/Q scan, angiography should be performed.

Peripheral deep venous thrombosis (DVT) is common in patients with SLE and predisposes to PE (13,48,50,135). Perhaps the most widely recognized risk factor for venous thromboembolism in SLE is the presence of circulating lupus anticoagulants and other antiphospholipid antibodies (136–138). In the European study of 1,000 patients, antiphospholipid antibodies including the lupus anticoagulant were significantly associated with thrombosis, fetal losses, thrombocytopenia, and livedo reticularis (52). Patients who develop DVT and/or PE in the context of antiphospholipid antibodies will usually require lifelong anticoagulation (139) (See Chapter 52 for a further discussion of thrombosis and antiphospholipid antibodies.)

Reversible Hypoxemia

A relatively rare syndrome of acute reversible hypoxemia in acutely ill patients with SLE but without evidence of parenchymal lung involvement may occur (140–142). The first description was by Abramson et al. (140); among 22 inpatients with acute disease exacerbation, six (27%) had this syndrome. Although some patients had mild pleuropulmonary symptoms, chest radiographs and lung scans were normal. The patients had hypoxemia and hypocapnia with a wide alveolar-arterial (A-a) gradient, which reversed with corticosteroid therapy. The pathogenesis of the syndrome is unclear, but a correlation between hypoxemia and the level of complement split products was noted, and others have suggested a relationship with disease activity (141). Complement activation may lead to diffuse pulmonary injury with the aggregation of neutrophils in the lungs similar to that seen in cardiopulmonary bypass, hemodialysis with cuprophane membranes, and ARDS.

Pulmonary Hypertension

Clinical Presentation

Severe, symptomatic pulmonary hypertension (PH) is a relatively rare manifestation of lung involvement in SLE, but mild subclinical cases are surprisingly common with prevalences of between 5% and 14% (reviewed in ref. 12).

Perez and Kramer (143) were the first to report four patients with severe PH in a group of 43 patients with SLE over a period of 2 years. Other studies, however, found rather lower prevalences (144). Of great interest is a 5-year follow-up study of a cohort of lupus patients that showed that the prevalence of PH rose from 14% to 43%, with the mean pulmonary artery pressures rising from 23.4 mm Hg to 27.5 mm Hg (145).

The clinical diagnosis of PH is difficult to make in early and mild cases, and only the severe cases, with right ventricular hypertrophy and/or congestive heart failure, have been reported in the literature. Pulmonary artery pressure at rest and during exercise is significantly higher in unselected patients with SLE as compared to normal subjects, probably secondary to increased pulmonary vascular resistance in lupus patients (146). A study of the prevalence and severity of PH in a group of 36 patients with SLE and healthy controls was undertaken by Simonson et al. (147) using two-dimensional and Doppler echocardiographic data to calculate pulmonary artery systolic pressure. Five patients (14%) and none of the controls had PH, as defined by a pulmonary artery pressure of greater than 30 mm Hg. This study suggests that PH is common in SLE, but usually mild in degree. Conceivably, mild cases of PH in SLE may improve with systemic corticosteroid and/or cytotoxic drug therapy given for other organ involvement, so that mild PH remains unrecognized.

The symptoms of PH in SLE are in general similar to those of patients with idiopathic or primary PH (144). In most of the reported cases, the symptoms of PH occurred within a few years of onset of the multisystem disease, with a mean duration of approximately 2.3 years (144). The most common complaints are dyspnea on exertion, chest pain, and chronic nonproductive cough. Chronic fatigue, weakness, palpitations, edema, and/or ascites may also occur. Symptoms usually develop insidiously and progress gradually. The physical findings may include a loud second pulmonary heart sound, systolic murmur, and right ventricular lift. Chest radiography findings include cardiomegaly with a prominent pulmonary artery and clear lung fields. Electrocardiography may show changes of right ventricular hypertrophy. Although PFTs may show restrictive abnormalities, these are mild in degree and disproportionate to the severity of the PH. Pulmonary angiograms in severe cases demonstrate symmetric dilatation of the central pulmonary artery trunk, with pruning of the peripheral blood vessels. Cardiac catheterization is the definitive investigation and demonstrates the characteristic elevation of the pulmonary artery pressure and normal wedge pressure without evidence of intracardiac or extracardiac shunting.

Pathology

The histopathology of the lung in patients with SLE and PH is that of plexiform lesions similar to those seen in primary PH (144). Medial hypertrophy and intimal fibrosis of the branches of the pulmonary artery may be seen. Thrombosis and vasculitis have also been reported in a few patients (144). Deposits of IgG, IgM, and C3 in the walls of the pulmonary blood vessels have been found (144). These immunoglobulin deposits, when eluted with acidic buffer, showed ANA activity, including anti-DNA antibody and rheumatoid factor activity (144). The putative antigen DNA also was found in the walls of blood vessels, indicating the deposition of immune complexes.

Pathogenesis

The pathogenesis of PH is not well understood, and it is likely that multiple etiologic factors are involved (148). For example, although immune deposits have been found in the large pulmonary vessels, it is not clear whether this is important in the pathogenesis or merely represents a secondary phenomenon. Vasculitis affecting the pulmonary artery is rarely seen and is unlikely to be a major cause of PH (149–151). Occasionally, PH can develop as a complication of diffuse pulmonary fibrosis.

Asherson et al. (152) reported a high frequency of anticardiolipin antibodies in patients with SLE and PH, indicating the possible causative role of recurrent thromboembolic phenomena, but others have not observed this association (149). In addition, other features of the antiphospholipid syndrome are uncommon in patients with SLE and PH (152), and thrombosis is not commonly seen in autopsied cases (144). Thrombosis of the pulmonary vessels has been confirmed in a small number of patients with antiphospholipid antibody syndrome with PH (153,154).

Miyata et al. (155) reported that patients with SLE or MCTD and anticardiolipin antibodies have higher mean pulmonary artery pressures than those without anticardiolipin antibodies. The high frequency of Raynaud's phenomenon in the PH group (up to 75%, compared to 25% to 40% of other lupus patients) suggests that PH may be a complication of pulmonary arterial vasospasm (147,152). Another intriguing study suggested a significant correlation between nail-fold capillary density and pulmonary gas transfer (KCO) in patients with SLE. It may be that in SLE, poor gas transfer may be dependent on alveolar capillary loss and that nail-fold capillary density may be a good indicator of alveolar capillary density (156). This group also assessed muscle biopsy specimens in relation to pulmonary involvement in lupus but found no strong correlation (157).

Recent investigations point to the possible role of endothelial dysfunction and abnormal vascular response in PH. One study showed an increase in the release of thromboxane A_2, a potent pulmonary vascular vasocontrictor and procoagulant, and a decrease in the release of prostacyclin in patients with both primary and secondary PH, including SLE (158). Antiendothelial cell antibodies, which are associated with lupus nephritis (159) have also been described in patients with SLE and PH (160).

Primary PH in children is associated with human leukocyte antigen (HLA)-DR3, DRw2, and DQw2, while PH in systemic sclerosis is associated with DRw52, suggesting a role for genetic factors (161,162). This is supported by a report of fatal PH in identical twins with lupus (163).

Prognosis And Treatment

The overall outcome of severe PH in SLE is poor. Of the patients reported in the literature, cardiac failure or sudden death presumably due to an arrhythmia were the most common modes of death. Although the presence of Raynaud's phenomenon is associated with a poorer outcome, the most accurate predictors are pulmonary artery pressure, right atrial pressure, and cardiac index (reviewed in ref. 12).

A trial of various vasodilator agents is certainly worth trying in these patients. For example, nifedipine was useful in patients with PH associated with MCTD and scleroderma (164). However, the effect on exercise tolerance and survival was not examined in this study. In primary PH, high doses of nifedipine and other calcium channel blockers have been shown to improve hemodynamic abnormalities and to prolong survival (165).

Other strategies include anticoagulants, systemic corticosteroids, or cytotoxic agents (reviewed in ref. 12). Some patients have experienced symptomatic improvement, although hemodynamic abnormalities remained unchanged with drug therapy (144,166,167). Improvements in cardiac hemodynamics have been reported in a few patients (168) and intermittent intravenous infusions of cyclophosphamide have resulted in partial improvement in hemodynamics in a patient with lupus and PH (169). Sequential administration of cyclophosphamide and cyclosporin A improved the hemodynamic and clinical course of a patient with MCTD and PH (170).

Short-term infusion of prostacyclin and prostaglandin E_1 has been tried successfully in the treatment of a patient with lupus and PH (171). Chronic prostaglandin infusion and other treatment modalities, including nitrous oxide, have been used in primary PH and may be applicable to SLE, but there is little evidence in support of these therapies in SLE at present.

Despite combinations of these drugs, most of the patients reported by Asherson et al. (152) died within 5 years after the diagnosis of PH. Two of their patients underwent heart-lung transplantation, with satisfactory results in one but poor results in the other because of chronic rejection (172).

Shrinking Lung Syndrome

In 1965, Hoffbrand and Beck (173) described a group of patients with SLE with breathlessness and reduced chest expansion, but no cyanosis, clubbing, or abnormal auscultatory findings. Many of the patients had a previous history of pleurisy. Chest radiography revealed clear lung fields but with an elevated diaphragm, which moved sluggishly and not paradoxically (Fig. 33.4). The vital capacity was extremely reduced. The authors coined the term *shrinking lung syndrome* and suggested that the main pathologic lesion is that of alveolar atelectasis secondary to deficiency of the surface tension reducing film that lines the normal alveoli. Gibson et al. (174) measured diaphragmatic function in these patients by determining the transdiaphragmatic pres-

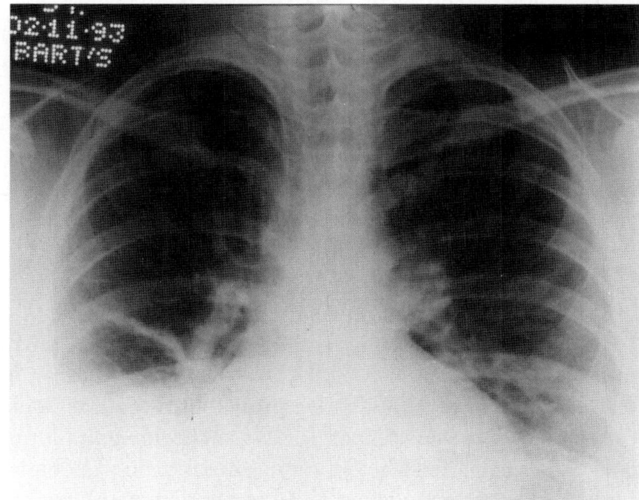

FIGURE 33.4. Chest radiograph showing raised right hemidiaphragm and a linear atelectasis in the right midzone.

sure using a double-balloon technique, and they found it to be grossly abnormal. This finding led them to suggest that diaphragmatic dysfunction, rather than parenchymal or pleural disease, accounts for the unexplained dyspnea in these patients. Martens et al. (175) concluded that the restrictive ventilatory defect in these patients results primarily from the weakness of expiratory and inspiratory muscles. Diaphragmatic dysfunction correlated with the degree of dyspnea but not with overall disease activity, proximal muscle weakness, or serologic markers. Contrary to these reports, however, Laroche et al. (176), using a wide range of tests for determining respiratory muscle strength, found no evidence of isolated weakness of the diaphragm in 12 patients with SLE and this syndrome. The discrepancy between their results and those of previous studies is not entirely clear, but it may result partly from patient selection and differences in the methods that were used to assess diaphragmatic function.

The pathogenesis of the diaphragmatic weakness in patients with SLE is not well understood. Wilcox et al. (177) found no evidence of phrenic nerve neuropathy as the cause of this weakness. Diffuse fibrosis of the diaphragm without evidence of acute inflammatory infiltrates was observed in one patient examined at autopsy (178), supporting an extrapulmonary, restrictive cause for this unusual syndrome. An electromyographic study of the diaphragm and external intercostal muscles demonstrated that fatigue of the respiratory muscles occurs at lower loads in patients with SLE as compared to those in healthy controls (179). Whether myopathy is an isolated process affecting primarily the diaphragm and other respiratory muscles or is part of a generalized muscle disease in SLE is not entirely clear. When the diagnosis of shrinking lung syndrome is suspected, measurements of transdiaphragmatic pressures and elastic recoil of the respiratory system should be considered.

The clinical course of the syndrome is a chronic, low-grade, restrictive defect. Follow-up of some patients over a period of several years has shown that the volume restriction is not progressive (174,175). In symptomatic patients, prednisone therapy (30 to 60 mg daily for several weeks) is clinically beneficial and tends to stabilize the PFT abnormalities (180–182). Agonist agents and theophylline may also be useful in the treatment of this syndrome (183,184).

Airway Obstruction

Severe airway obstruction has been reported in a small number of patients with SLE (185,186). Lung biopsy in one patient showed obliterative bronchiolitis and an acute inflammatory process that affected small bronchi and bronchioles, resulting in necrosis and eventual endobronchiolar proliferation of epithelial cells and peribronchial infiltration by lymphocytes. Dense plugs composed of alveolar debris and fibrin strands within the bronchioles caused partial or complete obstruction. Bronchiolitis obliterans with organizing pneumonia has been described in SLE (187).

Evidence of airway obstruction has been described in several controlled studies of PFT in patients with SLE (3,188–191). Some series did not take into consideration the effect of cigarette smoking, but in those that did it was evident that airway obstruction occurred even in nonsmoking patients with SLE. The frequency of airway obstruction is variable, primarily because of differences in the criteria that are used to define the abnormality and in the selection of patients. In the only controlled study of lifelong nonsmoking patients with SLE, Andonopoulos et al. (39) observed a high prevalence (24%) of isolated small airway disease in patients with SLE. The clinical significance of this observation remains unclear, however, because a similarly high frequency (17%) of small airway disease was found in their healthy, nonsmoking age- and sex-matched controls.

Very occasionally the upper airways have been affected in lupus. Case reports have described hypopharyngeal ulceration, laryngeal inflammation, vocal cord paralysis, epiglottitis, and subglottic stenosis (reviewed in ref. 12).

Infections And The Lung In SLE

Pulmonary infections are common in patients with lupus, especially in those taking corticosteroids and immunosuppressive therapies. Organisms include viruses, bacteria, mycobacteria, parasites, and opportunisitic fungal infections. For a more thorough review of infectious complications in SLE, see Chapter 43).

REFERENCES

1. Vitali C, Bencivelli W, Isenberg DA, et al., and the European Consensus Study Group for Disease Activity in SLE. Disease activity in systemic lupus erythematosus: report of the Consensus Study Group of the European Workshop for Rheumatology Research. I. A descriptive analysis of 704 European lupus patients. *Clin Exp Rheumatol* 1992;10:527–539.
2. Abu-Shakra M, Urowitz MB, Gladman DD, et al. Mortality studies in systemic lupus erythematosus. Results from a single center. I. Causes of death. *J Rheumatol* 1995;22:1259–1264.
3. Wohlgelernter D, Loke J, Matthay RA, et al. Systemic and discoid lupus erythematosus: analysis of pulmonary function. *Yale J Biol Med* 1978;51:157–164.
4. Osler W. On the visceral manifestations of the erythema group of skin diseases. *Am J Med Sci* 1904;127:123.
5. Rakov HL, Taylor JS. Acute disseminated lupus erythematosus without cutaneous manifestations and with heretofore undescribed pulmonary lesions. *Arch Intern Med* 1942;70:88–100.
6. Foldes J. Acute systemic lupus erythematosus. *Am J Clin Pathol* 1946;16:160–173.
7. Purnell DC, Baggentoss AH, Olsen AM. Pulmonary lesions in disseminated lupus erythematosus. *Ann Intern Med* 1955;42: 619–628.
8. Israel HL. Pulmonary manifestations of disseminated lupus erythematosus. *Am J Med Sci* 1953;226:387–392.

9. Garland LH, Sisson MA. Roentgen findings in collagen disease. *AJR* 1954;71:581–598.
10. Quismorio FP Jr. Clinical and pathologic features of lung involvement in systemic lupus erythematosus. *Semin Respir Dis* 1988;9:297–304.
11. Segal AM, Calabrese LH, Ahmad M, et al. The pulmonary manifestations of systemic lupus erythematosus. *Semin Arthritis Rheum* 1985;14:202–224.
12. Murin S, Wiedemann HP, Matthay RA. Pulmonary manifestations of systemic lupus erythematosus. *Clin Chest Med* 1998;19: 641–665.
13. Delgado EA, Malleson PN, Pirie GE, et al. Pulmonary manifestations of childhood onset systemic lupus erythematosus. *Semin Arthritis Rheum* 1990;29:285–293.
14. Olsen EGJ, Lever JV. Pulmonary changes in systemic lupus erythematosus. *Br J Dis Chest* 1972;66:71–77.
15. Gross M, Esterly JR, Earle RH. Pulmonary alterations in systemic lupus erythematosus. *Am Rev Respir Dis* 1972;105: 572–577.
16. Fayemi AO. The lung in systemic lupus erythematosus: a clinico-pathologic study of 20 cases. *Mt Sinai J Med* 1975;142: 110–118.
17. Haupt HM, Moore GW, Hutchins GM. The lung in systemic lupus erythematosus. Analysis of the pathologic changes in 120 patients. *Am J Med* 1981;71:791–798.
18. Grigor R, Edmonds J, Lewkonia R, et al. Systemic lupus erythematosus. A prospective analysis. *Ann Rheum Dis* 1978;37: 121–128.
19. Silberstein SL, Barland P, Grayzel AI, et al. Pulmonary dysfunction in systemic lupus erythematosus: prevalence, classification and correlation with other organ involvement. *J Rheumatol* 1980;7:187–195.
20. Andonopoulos AP, Constantopoulos SH, Galanopoulou V, et al. Pulmonary function of nonsmoking patients with systemic lupus erythematosus. *Chest* 1988;94:312–315.
21. Bulgrin JG, Dubois EL, Jacobson G. Chest roentgenographic changes in systemic lupus erythematosus. *Radiology* 1960;74: 42–49.
22. Gould DM, Daves ML. Roentgenologic findings in systemic lupus erythematosus. Analysis of 100 cases. *J Chronic Dis* 1955;2:136–145.
23. Levin DC. Proper interpretation of pulmonary roentgen changes in systemic lupus erythematosus. *AJR* 1971;11: 510–517.
24. Fenlon HM, Doran M, Sant SM, et al. High resolution CT chest in systemic lupus erythematosus. *AJR* 1996;166:301–307.
25. Sant SM, Doran M, Fenlon HM, et al. Pleuropulmonary abnormalities in patients with systemic lupus erythematosus: Assessment with high resolution computed tomography, chest radiography and pulmonary function tests. *Clin Exp Rheumatol* 1997;15:507–513.
26. Indik JH, Alpert JS. Detection of pulmonary embolism by D-dimer assay, spiral computed tomography and magnetic resonance imaging. *Prog Cardivasc Dis* 2000;42:261–272.
27. Hsu BY, Edwards DK 3rd, Trambert MA. Pulmonary hemorrhage complicating systemic lupus erythematosus: role of MR imaging in diagnosis. *AJR* 1992;158:519–520.
28. Roche-Bayard P, Rossi R, Mann JM, et al. Left pulmonary artery thrombosis in chlorpromazine-induced lupus. *Chest* 1990;98:1545.
29. Suga K, Tsukuda T, Awaya H, et al. Interactions of regional respiratory mechanics and pulmonary ventilatory impairment in pulmonary emphysema: assessment with dynamic MRI and xenon-133 single-photon emission CT. *Chest* 2000;117: 1646–1655.
30. Gaeta M, Blandino A, Scribano E, et al. Chronic infiltrative lung diseases: value of gadolinium-enhanced MRI in the evaluation of disease activity—early report. *Chest* 2000;117(4): 1173–1178.
31. Collins RL, Turner RA, Nomeir AM, et al. Cardiopulmonary manifestations of systemic lupus erythematosus. *J Rheumatol* 1978;5:299–305.
32. Huang CT, Henniger GR, Lyons HA. Pulmonary dysfunction in systemic lupus erythematosus. *N Engl J Med* 1965;272:288–293.
33. Gold WM, Jennings DB. Pulmonary function in patients with systemic lupus erythematosus. *Am Rev Respir Dis* 1966;93: 556–567.
34. Rolla G, Brussino L, Bertero MT, et al. Respiratory function in systemic lupus erythematosus: relation with activity and severity. *Lupus* 1996;5:38–43.
35. Cerveri I, Fanfulla F, Ravelli A, et al. Pulmonary function in children with systemic lupus erythematosus. *Thorax* 1996;510: 424–428.
36. Rolla G, Brussino L, Bertero MT, et al. Increased nitric oxide in exhaled air of patients with systemic lupus erythematosus. *J Rheumatol* 1997;24:1066–1071.
37. Holgate ST, Glass DN, Haslam P, et al. Respiratory involvement in systemic lupus erythematosus: a clinical and immunologic study. *Clin Exp Immunol* 1976;24:385–395.
38. Chick TW, de Horatius RJ, Skipper BE, et al. Pulmonary dysfunction in systemic lupus erythematosus without pulmonary symptoms. *J Rheumatol* 1976;3:262–268.
39. Andonopoulos AP, Constantopoulos SH, Galanopoulou V, et al. Pulmonary function of nonsmoking patients with systemic lupus erythematosus. *Chest* 1988;94:312–315.
40. Eichacker PQ, Pinsker K, Epstein A, et al. Serial pulmonary function testing in patients with systemic lupus erythematosus. *Chest* 1988;94:129–132.
41. Witt C, Dorner T, Hiepe F, et al. Diagnosis of alveolitis in interstitial lung manifestation in connective tissue diseases: importance of late inspiratory crackles, 67 gallium scan and bronchoalveolar lavage. *Lupus* 1996;5:606–612.
42. Peterson MW, Monick M, Hunninghake GW. Prognostic role of eosinophils in pulmonary fibrosis. *Chest* 1987;92:51–56.
43. BAL Cooperative Steering Committee. Bronchoalveolar lavage constituents in healthy individuals, idiopathic pulmonary fibrosis and selected comparison group. *Am Rev Respir Dis* 1990;141 (Suppl):S169–S202.
44. Walaert B, Aerts C, Bart F, et al. Alveolar macrophage dysfunction in systemic lupus erythematosus. *Am Rev Respir Dis* 1987; 136:293–297.
45. Walaert B, Dugas M, Dansin E, et al. Subclinical alveolitis in immunological systemic disorders: transition between health and disease? *Eur Respir J* 1990;3:1206–1216.
46. Jansen HM, Schutte AJH, Elema JD, et al. Local immune complexes and inflammatory response in patients with chronic interstitial pulmonary disorders associated with collagen vascular diseases. *Clin Exp Immunol* 1984;56:311–320.
47. Groen H, Aslander M, Bootsma H, et al. Bronchoalveolar lavage cell analysis and lung function impairment in patients with systemic lupus erythematosus. *Clin Exp Immunol* 1993; 94:127–133.
48. Dubois EL, Tuffanelli DL. Clinical manifestations of systemic lupus erythematosus. Computer analysis of 520 cases. *JAMA* 1964;190:104–111.
49. McGehee Harvey A, Shulman LE, Tumulty AP, et al. Systemic lupus erythematosus: review of the literature and clinical analysis of 138 cases. *Medicine* 1954;33:291–437.
50. Estes D, Christian CL. The natural history of systemic lupus erythematosus by prospective analysis. *Medicine* 1971;50: 85–95.

51. Ward MM, Studenski S. Clinical manifestations of systemic lupus erythematosus. Identification of racial and socioeconomic influences. *Arch Intern Med* 1990;150:849–853.
52. Cervera R, Khamashta MA, Font J, et al. Systemic lupus erythematosus: clinical and immunologic patterns of disease expression in a cohort of 1,000 patients. The European Working Party on Systemic Lupus Erythematosus. *Medicine (Baltimore)* 1993;72:113–124.
53. Ropes MW. *Systemic lupus erythematosus*. Cambridge, MA: Harvard University Press, 1976.
54. Dubois EL. Effect of LE cell test on clinical picture of systemic lupus erythematosus. *Ann Intern Med* 1953;38:1265–1294.
55. Winslow WA, Ploss LN, Loitman B. Pleuritis in systemic lupus erythematosus: its importance as an early manifestation in diagnosis. *Ann Intern Med* 1958;49:70–88.
56. Bouros D, Panagou P, Papandreou L, et al. Massive bilateral pleural effusion as the only first presentation of systemic lupus erythematosus. *Respiration* 1992;59:173–175.
57. Good JT, King TE, Antony VD, et al. Lupus pleuritis. Clinical features and pleural fluid characteristics with special reference to pleural fluid antinuclear antibodies. *Chest* 1983;84:714–718.
58. Kelley S, McGarry P, Hutson Y. A typical cells in pleural fluid characteristic of systemic lupus erythematosus. *Acta Cytol* 1971; 15:357–362.
59. Shan SA. The pleura. *Am Rev Respir Dis* 1988;138:184–234.
60. Pandya MR, Agus B, Grady RF. In vivo LE phenomenon in pleural fluid. *Arthritis Rheum* 1976;19:962–966.
61. Reda MG, Baigelman W. Pleural effusion in systemic lupus erythematosus. *Acta Cytol* 1980;24:553–557.
62. Carel RS, Shapiro MS, Shoham D, et al. Lupus erythematosus cells in pleural effusion: initial manifestation of procainamide induced lupus erythematosus. *Chest* 1977;72:670–672.
63. Leechawengwong M, Berger H, Sukumaran M. Diagnostic significance of antinuclear antibodies in pleural effusion. *Mt Sinai J Med* 1979;46:137–141.
64. Small P, Frank H, Kreisman H, et al. An immunological evaluation of pleural effusions in systemic lupus erythematosus. *Ann Allergy* 1982;49:101–103.
65. Khare V, Baethge B, Lang S, et al. Antinuclear antibodies in pleural fluid. *Chest* 1994;106:866–871.
66. Pettersson T, Soderbolom T, Nyberg P, et al. Pleural fluid soluble interleukin 2 receptor in rheumatoid arthritis and systemic lupus erythematosus. *J Rheumatol* 1994;21:1820–1824.
67. Datta SK, Gandhi VC, Lee HJ, et al. Granuloma in systemic lupus erythematosus. *S Afr Med J* 1972;46:1514–1516.
68. Hunder GG, McDuffie FC, Hepper NGG. Pleural fluid complement in systemic lupus erythematosus and rheumatoid arthritis. *Ann Intern Med* 1972;76:357–363.
69. Glovsky MM, Louie JS, Pitts WH Jr, et al. Reduction of pleural fluid complement activity in patients with systemic lupus erythematosus and rheumatoid arthritis. *Clin Immunol Immunopathol* 1976;6:31–41.
70. Peterson T, Klockars M, Hellstrom PE. Chemical and immunological features of pleural effusions: comparison between rheumatoid arthritis and other diseases. *Thorax* 1982;37:354–361.
71. Andrews BS, Arora NS, Shadforth MF, et al. The role of immune complexes in the pathogenesis of pleural effusions. *Am Rev Respir Dis* 1981;124:152–161.
72. Hunder GG, McDuffie FC, Huston KA, et al. Pleural fluid complement, complement conversion and immune complexes immunologic and nonimmunologic diseases. *J Lab Clin Med* 1977;90:971–980.
73. Halla JT, Schrohenloher RE, Volanakis JE. Immune complexes and other laboratory features of pleural effusions: a comparison of rheumatoid arthritis, systemic lupus erythematosus and other diseases. *Ann Intern Med* 1980;92:748–752.
74. Riska H, Fyhrquist F, Selander RK, et al. Systemic erythematosus and DNA antibodies in pleural effusions. *Scand J Rheumatol* 1978;7:159–160.
75. Bell R, Lawrence DS. Chronic pleurisy in systemic lupus erythematosus. *Br J Dis Chest* 1976;73:324–326.
76. Kaine JL. Refractory massive pleural effusion in systemic lupus erythematosus treated with talc poudrage. *Ann Rheum Dis* 1985;44:61–64.
77. Gilleece MH, Evans CC, Bucknall RC. Steroid resistant pleural effusion in the systemic lupus erythematosus treated with tetracycline pleurodesis. *Ann Rheum Dis* 1988;47:1031–1032.
78. McKnight KM, Adair NE, Agudelo CA. Successful use of tetracycline pleurodesis to treat massive pleural effusion secondary to systemic lupus erythematosus. *Arthritis Rheum* 1991;34: 1483–1484.
79. Ben-Cherit E, Putterman C, Naparstek Y. Lupus refractory pleural effusion: transient response to intravenous immunoglobulins. *J Rheumatol* 1991;18:1635–1637.
80. Matthay RA, Schwartz MI, Petty TL, et al. Pulmonary manifestations of systemic lupus erythematosus: review of twelve cases of acute lupus pneumonitis. *Medicine* 1975;54:397–409.
81. Pertschuk LP, Moccia LF, Rosen Y, et al. Acute pulmonary complications in systemic lupus erythematosus: immunofluorescence and light microscopic study. *Am J Clin Pathol* 1977;68: 553–557.
82. Chellingsworth M, Scott DG. Acute systemic lupus erythematosus with fatal pneumonitis and disseminated intravascular coagulation. *Ann Rheum Dis* 1985;44:67–69.
83. Inoue T, Kanayama Y, Ohe A, et al. Immunopathologic studies of pneumonitis in systemic lupus erythematosus. *Ann Intern Med* 1979;91:30–34.
84. Eiser AR, Shanies HM. Treatment of lupus interstitial lung disease with intravenous cyclophosphamide. *Arthritis Rheum* 1994; 37:428–431.
85. Domingo-Pedrol P, De la Serna A, Mancebo-Cortes J, et al. Adult respiratory distress syndrome caused by systemic lupus erythematosus. *Eur J Respir Dis* 1985;67:141–144.
86. Andonopoulos AP. Adult respiratory distress syndrome: an unrecognized premortem event in systemic lupus erythematosus. *Br J Rheumatol* 1991;30:346–348.
87. Zamora MR, Warner ML, Tuder R, et al. Diffuse alveolar hemorrhage and systemic lupus erythematosus. Clinical presentation, histology, survival, and outcome. *Medicine (Baltimore)* 1997;76:192–202.
88. Abud-Mendoza C, Diaz-Jouanen E, Alarcon-Segovia D. Fatal pulmonary hemorrhage in systemic lupus erythematosus. Occurrence without hemoptysis. *J Rheumatol* 1985;12: 558–561.
89. Kim WU, Min JK, Lee SH, et al. Causes of death in Korean patients with systemic lupus erythematosus: a single center retrospective study. *Clin Exp Rheumatol* 1999;17:539–545.
90. Liu MF, Lee JH, Weng TH, et al. Clinical experience of 13 cases with severe pulmonary hemorrhage in systemic lupus erythematosus with active nephritis. *Scand J Rheumatol* 1998;27:291–295.
91. Barile LA, Jara LJ, Medina-Rodriguez F, et al. Pulmonary hemorrhage in systemic lupus erythematosus. *Lupus* 1997;6: 445–448.
92. Mintz G, Galindo LF, Fernandez-Diez J, et al. Acute massive pulmonary hemorrhage in systemic lupus erythematosus. *J Rheumatol* 1978;5:39–50.
93. Marino CT, Pertschuk LP. Pulmonary hemorrhage in systemic lupus erythematosus. *Arch Intern Med* 1981;141:201–203.
94. Uziel Y, Laxer RM, Silverman ED. Persistent pulmonary hemorrhage as the sole initial clinical manifestation of pediatric systemic lupus erythematosus. *Clin Exp Rheumatol* 1997;15: 697–700.

95. Reznik VM, Griswold WR, Lemire JM, et al. Pulmonary hemorrhage in children with glomerulonephritis. *Pediatr Nephrol* 1995;9:83–86.
96. Miller RW, Salcedo JR, Fink RJ, et al. Pulmonary hemorrhage in pediatric patients with systemic lupus erythematosus. *J Pediatr* 1986;108:576–579.
97. Rajani KB, Ashbacher LV, Kinney TR. Pulmonary hemorrhage and systemic lupus erythematosus. *J Pediatr* 1978;93:810–812.
98. Keane MP, Van De Ven CJ, Lynch JP 3rd, et al. Systemic lupus during pregnancy with refractory alveolar haemorrhage: recovery following termination of pregnancy. *Lupus* 1997;6: 730–733.
99. Crausman RS, Achenbach GA, Pluss WT, et al. et al. Pulmonary capillaritis and alveolar hemorrhage associated with the antiphospholipid antibody syndrome. *J Rheumatol* 1995;22: 554–556.
100. Greening AP, Hughes JM. Serial estimations of carbon monoxide diffusing capacity in intrapulmonary haemorrhage. *Clin Sci (Colch)* 1981;60:507–512.
101. Hsu BY, Edwards DK III, Trambert MA. Pulmonary hemorrhage complicating systemic lupus erythematosus: role of MR imaging in diagnosis. *AJR* 1992;158:519–520.
102. Makino Y, Ogawa M, Ueda S, et al. CT appearance of diffuse alveolar hemorrhage in a patient with systemic lupus erythematosus. *Acta Radiol* 1993;34:634–635.
103. Bosch X, Font J. The pulmonary-renal syndrome: a poorly understood clinicopathologic condition. *Lupus* 1999;8: 258–262.
104. Eagen JW, Memoli VA, Roberts JL, et al. Pulmonary hemorrhage in systemic lupus erythematosus. *Medicine* 1978;57: 545–560.
105. Myers JL, Katzenstein AA. Microangiitis in lupus-induced pulmonary hemorrhage. *Am J Clin Pathol* 1986;85:552–556.
106. Castaneda S, Herrero-Beaumont G, Valenzuela A, et al. Massive pulmonary hemorrhage: fatal complication of systemic lupus erythematosus. *J Rheumatol* 1985;12:185–187.
107. Churg A, Franklin W, Chan KL, et al. Pulmonary hemorrhage and immune complex deposition in the lung: complications in a patient with systemic lupus erythematosus. *Arch Pathol Lab Med* 1980;104:388–391.
108. Gould DB, Soriano RZ. Acute alveolar hemorrhage in lupus erythematosus. *Ann Intern Med* 1975;83:836–837.
109. Rodriquez-Iturbe B, Garcia R, Rubio L, et al. Immunohistologic findings in systemic lupus erythematosus. *Arch Pathol Lab Med* 1977;101:342–344.
110. Desnoyers MR, Bernstein S, Cooper AG, et al. Pulmonary hemorrhage in lupus erythematosus without evidence of an immunologic cause. *Arch Intern Med* 1984;144:1398–1400.
111. Brentjens JR, O'Connell DW, Paulowski IB, et al. Experimental immune complex disease of the lung. *J Exp Med* 1974;140: 150–152.
112. Schwab EP, Schumacher HR, Breundlich B, et al. Pulmonary alveolar hemorrhage in systemic lupus erythematosus. *Semin Arthritis Rheum* 1993;23:8–15.
113. Millman RP, Cohen TB, Levinson AI, et al. Systemic lupus erythematosus complicated by acute pulmonary hemorrhage: recovery following plasmapheresis and cytotoxic therapy. *J Rheumatol* 1981;8:1021–1022.
114. Erickson RW, Franklin WA, Emlen W. Treatment of hemorrhagic lupus pneumonitis with plasmapheresis. *Semin Arthritis Rheum* 1994;24:114–123.
115. Huang DF, Tsai ST, Wang SR. Recovery of both acute massive pulmonary hemorrhage and acute renal failure in a systemic lupus erythematosus patient with lupus anticoagulant by the combined therapy of plasmapheresis plus cyclophosphamide. *Transfus Sci* 1994;15:283–288.
116. Euler HH, Schroeder JO, Harten P, et al. Treatment-free remission in severe systemic lupus erythematosus following synchronization of plasmapheresis with subsequent pulse cyclophosphamide. *Arthritis Rheum* 1994;37:1784–1794.
117. Carette S, Macher AM, Nussbaum A, et al. Severe, acute pulmonary disease in patients with systemic lupus erythematosus: ten years of experience of the National Institutes of Health. *Semin Arthritis Rheum* 1985;14:52–59.
118. Eisenberg H, Dubois EL, Sherwin RP, et al. Diffuse interstitial lung disease in systemic lupus erythematosus. *Ann Intern Med* 1973;79:37–45.
119. Weinrib L, Sharma OP, Quismorio FP Jr. A long term study of interstitial lung disease in systemic lupus erythematosus. *Semin Arthritis Rheum* 1990;16:479–481.
120. Boulware DW, Hedgpeth MT. Lupus pneumonitis and anti-SSA(Ro) antibodies. *J Rheumatol* 1989;16:479–481.
121. Mochizuki T, Aotsuka S, Satoh T. Clinical and laboratory features of lupus patients with complicating pulmonary disease. *Respir Med* 1999;93:95–101.
122. Groen H, TerBorg EJ, Postma DS, et al. Pulmonary function in systemic lupus erythematosus is related to distinct clinical, serologic and nailfold capillary patterns. *Am J Med* 1992;93: 619–627.
123. Du Bois RM. Diffuse lung disease: combined clinical and laboratory studies. *J R Coll Physicians Lond* 1994;28:338–346.
124. Wells AU, Hansell DM, Rubens MB, et al. The predictive value of appearances on thin-section computed tomography in fibrosing alveolitis. *Am Rev Respir Dis* 1993;148:1076–1082.
125. Wells AU, Hansell DM, Corrin B, et al. High resolution computed tomography as a predictor of lung histology in systemic sclerosis. *Thorax* 1992;47:738–742.
126. Nishimura K, Izumi T, Kitaichi M, et al. The diagnostic accuracy of high-resolution computed tomography in diffuse infiltrative lung diseases. *Chest* 1993;104:1149–1155.
127. Johkoh T, Ikezoe J, Kohno N, et al. High-resolution CT and pulmonary function tests in collagen vascular disease: comparison with idiopathic pulmonary fibrosis. *Eur J Radiol* 1994;18: 113–121.
128. Ooi GC, Ngan H, Peh WC, et al. Systemic lupus erythematosus patients with respiratory symptoms: the value of HRCT. *Clin Radiol* 1997;52:775–781.
129. Gauldie J, Jordana M, Cox G. Cytokines and pulmonary fibrosis. *Thorax* 1993;48:931–935.
130. Cambrey AD, Harrison NK, Dawes KE, et al. Increased levels of endothelin-1 in bronchoalveolar lavage fluid from patients with systemic sclerosis contribute to fibroblast mitogenic activity in vitro. *Am J Respir Cell Mol Biol* 1994;11:439–445.
131. Groen H, Aslander M, Bootsma H, et al. Bronchoalveolar lavage cell analysis and lung function impairment in patients with systemic lupus erythematosus. *Clin Exp Immunol* 1993;94: 127–133.
132. Thornton SC, Robbins JM, Penny R, et al. Fibroblast growth factors in connective tissue associated interstitial lung disease. *Clin Exp Immunol* 1992;90:447–452.
133. Agusti C, Xaubet A, Roca J, et al. Interstitial pulmonary fibrosis with and without associated collagen vascular disease: results of a two year follow up. *Thorax* 1992;47:1035–1040.
134. Jansen HM, Schutte AJH, Elema JD, et al. Local immune complexes and inflammatory response in patients with chronic interstitial pulmonary disorders associated with collagen vascular diseases. *Clin Exp Immunol* 1984;56:311–320.
135. Gladman DD, Urowitz MB. Venous syndromes and pulmonary embolism in systemic lupus erythematous. *Ann Rheum Dis* 1980;39:340–343.
136. Boey ML, Colaco CB, Gharavi AE, et al. Thrombosis in systemic lupus erythematosus: striking association with the pres-

ence of circulating lupus anticoagulant. *Br Med J (Clin Res)* 1983;287:1021–1023.

137. Harris EN, Gharavi AE, Boey ML, et al. Anticardiolipin antibodies: detection by radioimmunoassay and association with thrombosis in systemic lupus erythematosus. *Lancet* 1983;2: 1211–1214.
138. Hasselaar P, Derksen RHWM, Blokzijl L, et al. Risk factors of thrombosis in lupus patients. *Ann Rheum Dis* 1989;48: 933–940.
139. Khamashta MA, Cuadrado MJ, Mujic F, et al. The management of thrombosis in the antiphospholipid-antibody syndrome. *N Engl J Med* 1995;332:993–997.
140. Abramson SB, Dobro J, Eberle MA, et al. Acute reversible hypoxemia in systemic lupus erythematosus. *Ann Intern Med* 1991;114:941–947.
141. Martinez-Taboada VM, Blanco R, Armona J, et al. Acute reversible hypoxemia in systemic lupus erythematosus: a new syndrome or an index of disease activity? *Lupus* 1995;4: 259–262.
142. Susanto I, Peters JI. Acute lupus pneumonitis with normal chest radiograph. *Chest* 1997;111:1781–1783.
143. Perez HD, Kramer N. Pulmonary hypertension in systemic lupus erythematous: report of 4 cases and review of the literature. *Semin Arthritis Rheum* 1981;11:177–181.
144. Quismorio FP Jr, Sharma O, Koss M, et al. Immunopathologic and clinical studies in pulmonary hypertension associated with systemic lupus erythematosus. *Semin Arthritis Rheum* 1984; 13:349–359.
145. Winslow TM, Ossipov MA, Fazio GP, et al. Five-year follow-up study of the prevalence and progression of pulmonary hypertension in systemic lupus erythematosus. *Am Heart J* 1995; 129:510–515.
146. Winslow TM, Ossipow M, Redberg RF, et al. Exercise capacity and hemodynamics in systemic lupus erythematosus: a Doppler echocardiographic exercise study. *Am Heart J* 1993;126: 410–414.
147. Simonson JS, Schiller NB, Petri M, et al. Pulmonary hypertension in systemic lupus erythematosus. *J Rheumatol* 1989;16: 918–925.
148. Gomez-Reino JJ. Pulmonary hypertension in connective tissue disease. *Br J Rheumatol* 1993;33:796–798.
149. Badui E, Garcia-Rubi D, Robles E, et al. Cardiovascular manifestations in systemic erythematosus. Prospective study of 100 patients. *Angiology* 1985;36:431–440.
150. Rubin LA, Geran A, Rose TH, et al. A fatal pulmonary complication of lupus in pregnancy. *Arthritis Rheum* 1995;38: 710–714.
151. Roncoroni AJ, Alvarez C, Molinas F. Plexogenic arteriopathy associated with pulmonary vasculitis in systemic lupus erythematosus. *Respiration* 1991;59:52–56.
152. Asherson RA, Higenbottom TW, Dihn Xuan AT, et al. Pulmonary hypertension in a lupus clinic: experience with twenty-four patients. *J Rheumatol* 1990;17:1292–1298.
153. Brucato A, Baudo F, Barberis M, et al. Pulmonary hypertension secondary to thrombosis of the pulmonary vessels in a patient with antiphospholipid syndrome. *J Rheumatol* 1994;21: 942–944.
154. De Clerck LS, Michielsen PP, Ramael MR, et al. Portal and pulmonary vessel thrombosis associated with systemic lupus erythematosus and anticardiolipin antibodies. *J Rheumatol* 1991; 18:1919–1921.
155. Miyata M, Kida S, Kanno T, et al. Pulmonary hypertension in MCTD: report of two cases with anticardiolipin antibody. *Clin Rheumatol* 1992;11:195–201.
156. Pallis M, Hopkinson N, Powell R. Nailfold capillary density as a possible indicator of pulmonary capillary loss in systemic lupus erythematosus but not in mixed connective tissue disease. *J Rheumatol* 1991;18:1532–1536.
157. Evans SA, Hopkinson ND, Kinnear WJ, et al. Respiratory disease in systemic lupus erythematosus: correlation with results of laboratory tests and histological appearance of muscle biopsy specimens. *Thorax* 1992;47:957–960.
158. Christman BW, McPherson CD, Newman JH, et al. An imbalance between the excretion of thromboxane and prostacylin metabolites in pulmonary hypertension. *N Engl J Med* 1992; 327:70–75.
159. D'Cruz DP, Houssiau FA, Ramirez G, et al. Antiendothelial cell antibodies in systemic lupus erythematosus: A potential marker for nephritis and vasculitis. *Clin Exp Immunol* 1991;85:254–261.
160. Yoshio T, Masuyama J, Sumiya M, et al. Antiendothelial cell antibodies and their relation to pulmonary hypertension in systemic lupus erythematosus. *J Rheumatol* 1994;21:2058–63.
161. Barst RJ, Flaster ER, Menon A, et al. Evidence for the association of unexplained pulmonary hypertension in children with the major histocompatibility complex. *Circulation* 1992;85: 249–258.
162. Langevitz P, Buskila D, Gladman DD, et al. HLA alleles in systemic sclerosis: association with pulmonary hypertension and outcome. *Br J Rheumatol* 1992;31:609–613.
163. Wilson L, Tomita T, Braniecki M. Fatal pulmonary hypertension in identical twins with systemic lupus erythematosus. *Hum Pathol* 1991;22:295–297.
164. Alpert MA, Pressly TA, Mukerji V, et al. Acute and long-term effects of nifedipine on pulmonary and systemic hemodynamics in patients with pulmonary hypertension associated with diffuse systemic sclerosis, the CREST syndrome and mixed connective tissue disease. *Am J Cardiol* 1991;68:1687–1691.
165. Rich S, Kaufmann E, Levy PS. The effect of high doses of calcium channel blockers on survival in primary pulmonary hypertension. *N Engl J Med* 1992;327:76–81.
166. Gladman DD, Sternberg L. Pulmonary hypertension in systemic lupus erythematosus. *J Rheumatol* 1985;12:365–367.
167. Mahowald ML, Weir EK, Ridley DJ, et al. Pulmonary hypertension in systemic lupus erythematosus: effect of vasodilators on pulmonary hemodynamics. *J Rheumatol* 1985;12:773–777.
168. Machet L, Callens A, Machet MC, et al. Pulmonary hypertension in systemic lupus erythematosus: treatment with high dose nifedipine therapy. *Clin Exp Dermatol* 1993;18:486–487.
169. Groen H, Bootsma H, Postma DS, et al. Primary pulmonary hypertension in a patient with systemic lupus erythematosus: partial improvement with cyclophosphamide. *J Rheumatol* 1993;20:1055–1057.
170. Dahl M, Chalmers A, Wade J, et al. Ten year survival of a patient with advanced pulmonary hypertension and mixed connective tissue disease treated with immunosuppressive therapy. *J Rheumatol* 1992;19:1807–1809.
171. Ignaszewski AP, Percy JS, Humen DP. Successful treatment of pulmonary hypertension associated with SLE with prostaglandin I2 and prostaglandin E1. *J Rheumatol* 1993;20:595–596.
172. Levy RD, Guerraty AJ, Yacoub MH, et al. Prolonged survival after heart-lung transplantation in systemic lupus erythematosus. *Chest* 1993;104:1903–1905.
173. Hoffbrand BI, Beck ER. Unexplained dyspnoea and shrinking lungs in systemic lupus erythematosus. *Br Med J* 1965;1:1273–1277.
174. Gibson GJ, Edmonds JP, Hughes GRV. Diaphragm function and lung involvement in systemic lupus erythematosus. *Am J Med* 1977;63:926–932.
175. Martens J, Demedts M, Vanmeenen MT, et al. Respiratory muscle dysfunction in systemic lupus erythematous. *Chest* 1983;83:170–175.
176. Laroche CM, Mulvey DA, Hawkins PN, et al. Diaphragm

strength in the shrinking lung syndrome of systemic lupus erythematosus. *Q J Med* 1990;265:429–439.

177. Wilcox PG, Stein HB, Clarke SD, et al. Phrenic nerve function in patients with diaphragmatic weakness and systemic lupus erythematosus. *Chest* 1988;93:352–358.
178. Rubin LA, Urowitz MB. Shrinking lung syndrome in SLE: a clinical pathologic study. *J Rheumatol* 1983;10:973–976.
179. Worth H, Grahn S, Lakomek HJ, et al. Lung function disturbances versus respiratory muscle fatigue in patients with systemic lupus erythematosus. *Respiration* 1988;53:81–90.
180. Stevens WMR, Burdon JGW, Clemens LE, et al. The shrinking lung syndrome an infrequently recognized feature of systemic lupus erythematosus. *Aust NZ J Med* 1990;20:67–70.
181. Walz-Leblanc BA, Urowitz MB, Gladman DD, et al. The shrinking lungs syndrome in systemic lupus erythematosus improvement with corticosteroid therapy. *J Rheumatol* 1992;19:1970–1972.
182. Elkayam O, Segal R, Caspi D, et al. Restrictive lung disease due to diaphragmatic dysfunction in systemic lupus erythematosus, two case reports. *Clin Exp Rheumatol* 1992;10:267–269.
183. Thompson PJ, Dhillon DP, Ledingham J, et al. Shrinking lungs, diaphragmatic dysfunction and systemic lupus erythematosus. *Am Rev Respir Dis* 1985;132:926–928.
184. Van Veen S, Peeters AJ, Sterk PJ, et al. The shrinking lung syndrome in SLE, treatment with theophylline. *Clin Rheumatol* 1993;12:462–465.
185. Kallenback J, Zwi S, Goldman HI. Airway obstruction in a case of disseminated lupus erythematosus. *Thorax* 1978;33:814–815.
186. Kinney WW, Angelillo VA. Bronchiolitis in systemic lupus erythematosus. *Chest* 1982;82:646–648.
187. Gammon RB, Bridges TA, Al-Nezir H, et al. Bronchiolitis obliterans organizing pneumonia associated with systemic lupus erythematosus. *Chest* 1992;102:1171–1174.
188. Chick TW, de Horatius RJ, Skipper BE, et al. Pulmonary dysfunction in systemic lupus erythematosus without pulmonary symptoms. *J Rheumatol* 1976;3:262–268.
189. Collins RL, Turner RA, Nomeir AM, et al. Cardiopulmonary manifestations of systemic lupus erythematosus. *J Rheumatol* 1978;5:299–305.
190. Gold W, Jennings D. Pulmonary function in systemic lupus erythematosus. *Clin Res* 1964;12:291.
191. Huang CT, Lyons HA. Comparison of pulmonary function in patients with systemic lupus erythematosus, scleroderma and rheumatoid arthritis. *Am Rev Respir Dis* 1966;93:865–875.

34

SELECTED CUTANEOVASCULAR MANIFESTATIONS OF SYSTEMIC LUPUS ERYTHEMATOSUS

DANIEL J. WALLACE

Skin manifestations of lupus erythematosus (LE) are approached on several levels. The histopathologic classification includes acute cutaneous lupus (with active systemic disease), subacute cutaneous lupus, and chronic cutaneous LE [(which can be its own disorder or part of systemic lupus erythematosus (SLE)]. These are all lupus-specific lesions. Histopathologically, nonspecific lesions seen in lupus include cutaneovascular disease, alopecia, sclerodactyly, nodules, calcinosis, bullous lesions, urticaria, mucinosis, leg ulcers, and erythema multiforme. Most of these topics are covered in Section V, Cutaneous Lupus, which is written by our dermatology colleagues. From an editing standpoint, it was felt that the readers' appreciation of selected topics of cutaneous vascular disease could be enhanced by an internal medicine/rheumatologic approach in addition to the discussions in Chapters 28 and 29. Dr. Petri covers the cutaneous manifestations of antiphospholipid syndrome in Chapter 52, and a few other selected topics are reviewed here.

OVERVIEW

Skin manifestations represent some of the most common symptoms, signs, and pathologies that are noted in SLE. The lesions are pleomorphic and run the entire gamut of the dermatologic field, from erythema to bullae. Cutaneous involvement does not always occur in SLE, but it was present in 55% to 85% of patients in the large series detailed in Table 30.1. The skin presentation often can be subtle and can range from acute cutaneous lupus observed with multisystem, active disease to the classic, chronic cutaneous lesions in patients with SLE of varying activity. A typical history is a persistent or recurrent sunburn, butterfly area flush, or discoid lesions appearing years before any other manifestation of SLE. Harvey et al. (1) noted that 28% of patients in their series had cutaneous manifestations of SLE before systemic spread, with intervals as long as 14 years. Many patients first seek out a dermatologist, and if no systemic complaints are expressed, necessary laboratory evaluations often are delayed. Years later, when the disease disseminates and the patient seeks the aid of an internist, the skin lesions no longer may be present.

Table 34.1 lists the incidence of specific skin manifestations of SLE as observed in several large studies. Much of the variation resulted from patient selection. For example, Grigor et al. (2) evaluated a subgroup of patients with known SLE who had disease that was severe enough to warrant treatment at a tertiary referral center in Great Britain; as a result, the incidence of dermal vasculitis was 70%. All data on patients in these reports listed were derived by rheumatologists, not dermatologists. In the only study of its type, which was published in 1987, an Australian group had a dermatologist examine 84 consecutive patients attending a university SLE clinic (3). Cutaneous features attributable to SLE were mucous-membrane lesions (35%), malar erythema (22%), subacute cutaneous LE (22%), moderate or severe livedo reticularis (18%), vasculitis (palpable purpura or infarction, 18%), diffuse palmar erythema (17%), nail-fold erythema (16%), nail-fold telangiectasia (11%), discoid lesions (11%), lupus pernio (5%), and sclerodactyly (4%). These results differ considerably from those in Table 34.1, and they indicate the importance of accounting for the specific skills of different observers.

The incidence of dermal pathologies in SLE is not related to age. A review of the pediatric literature (4) and studies in elderly patients with SLE (5,6) described similar distributions to those in Table 34.1, although pure cutaneous lupus is rare in children (7).

The presence of a single cutaneous manifestation is statistically associated with other skin abnormalities, but not with disease-activity index, clinical parameters, or disease exacerbations (8). Brown et al. (9) have suggested that the close association between malar rash, discoid lupus, photosensitivity, and mouth sores calls into question their use as independent criteria for the classification of SLE.

TABLE 34.1. CUTANEOUS MANIFESTATIONS OF SLE

Parameter	Dubois and Tuffanelli (61)	Estes and Christian (64)	Lee et al. (99)	Grigor et al. (2)	Rothfield and Marino (98)	Pistiner et al. (100)
Cases (n)	520	150	110	50	375	464
Butterfly blush (%)	37	39	36	68	52	34
Photosensitivity (%)	33	—	50	28	71	37
Alopecia (%)	21	37	38	64	74	—
Raynaud's phenomenon (%)	18	21	46	32	20	24
Mouth ulcers (%)	9	7	—	34	40	19
Urticaria (%)	7	13	—	—	10	4
Dermal vasculitis (%)	—	21	—	70	20	—
Hyperpigmentation (%)	8	—	—	—	—	—
Leg ulcers (%)	6	—	—	—	—	—
Gangrene (%)	1	1	—	—	—	—
Bullae (%)	1	2	—	—	—	—
Panniculitis (%)	—	2	—	—	—	1

RAYNAUD'S PHENOMENON

Paroxysmal vasospasm of the fingers, or Raynaud's phenomenon, is a frequent abnormality in SLE. Raynaud's represents an abnormally regulated neuroendothelial control of vascular tone as a form of dysautonomia (10) (Fig. 34.1.) Here again, as with alopecia and fractured frontal hair, incidence varies with the observer's specific questioning of the patient. Raynaud's phenomenon was present at some time in 10% to 57% of the patients listed in Table 34.1. Because a history of Raynaud's phenomenon may be vague, nonspecific, and difficult to document, it was deleted from the 1982 revised American College of Rheumatology (ACR) criteria for SLE. Its prevalence takes the middle range between the 95% found in scleroderma (11) and the 3% seen with rheumatoid arthritis (12). Cholesterol emboli, cryoglobulinemia, digital infarcts from the lupus anticoagulant, and reflex sympathetic dystrophy can mimic Raynaud's phenomenon and must be excluded. The activity of Raynaud's usually is independent of SLE disease activity.

Raynaud's phenomenon is nonspecific and may be present years before the development of other changes caused by SLE, scleroderma, or dermatomyositis. De Takats and Fowler (13) reviewed 66 patients with Raynaud's phenomenon with follow-up for 1 to 25 years, and they observed that 32 subsequently developed scleroderma, two developed SLE, and one developed dermatomyositis. Three later reports repeated their survey and found that 0 of 96, 0 of 85, and 0 of 87 patients with Raynaud's phenomenon carried a diagnosis of SLE, with a mean 5-, 6-, and 9-years of follow-up, respectively (14–16). Studies of patients referred to rheumatologists because of Raynaud's phenomenon revealed that 5% to 9% had SLE (1, 17–19). Raynaud's phenomenon was the first manifestation of SLE in two of Dubois' patients (Table 30.2).

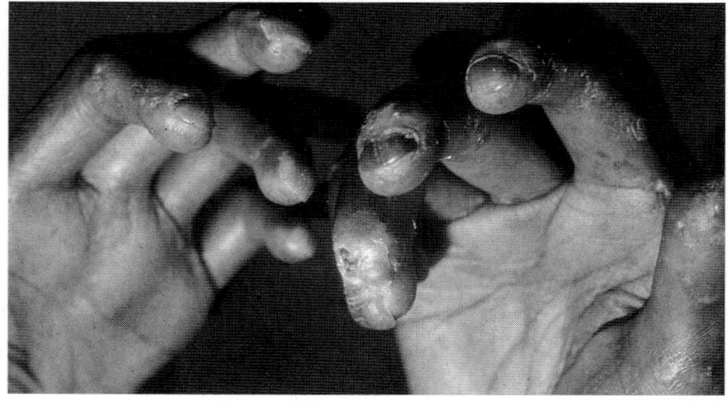

FIGURE 34.1. Severe Raynaud's phenomenon with digital gangrene.

Dimant et al. (20) compared 91 of their 276 patients with Raynaud's phenomenon to those without it. Those in the Raynaud's group had significantly more arthritis, malar rash, and photosensitivity and less renal disease, lower steroid requirements, and fewer deaths than those in the unaffected group. The Raynaud's phenomenon that is associated with SLE is similar to that seen in Raynaud's disease and is less severe than that in scleroderma (21). The vasospasm rarely leads to permanent damage; small ulcers on the fingers can occur following prolonged and frequent attacks. Raynaud's phenomenon usually operates independent of disease activity and is not steroid responsive. It may be associated with antibodies to hn-RNP protein A1 (22), migraine, and chest pain (23). Arteriograms of 10 patients with SLE and Raynaud's phenomenon showed severe vasospasm and severe digital artery involvement that did not correlate with disease activity (24). Evaluation of two studies (25, 26) leads to the conclusion that cold-pressor testing improved or did not change the diffusing capacities in patients with SLE and Raynaud's phenomenon and worsened it in those with primary Raynaud's phenomenon. One report was able to document a renal Raynaud's after cold exposure with 99m-technetium scanning (27). Another demonstrated Raynaud's phenomenon of the tongue (28), and a recent report suggests that Raynaud's in SLE is associated with pulmonary hypertensions (29). Single photon emission computed tomography (SPECT) brain-imaging correlates with hypoperfusion associated with Raynaud's in SLE (30).

The treatment of Raynaud's phenomenon is not different in those with concurrent SLE. Avoidance of cold or inciting drugs (e.g., beta-blockers, ergot alkaloids), along with wearing gloves, biofeedback (31), and use of vasodilators (e.g., nifedipine, nicardipine, nitroglycerin paste, nitroprusside) (32–34) may be advised. Steroids have no effect upon Raynaud's. Pentoxifylline (35) may be useful. Prostaglandin E1 infusions (36–38) improve digital ulcers and early gangrene in severe cases.

NAIL-FOLD MICROCAPILLAROSCOPY

In 1935, Baehr et al. (39) noted that the involved skin about the nail bed, when viewed under the capillary microscope, contained many more patent and dilated capillaries than normal. In 1968, Buchanan and Humpston (40) observed hemorrhage in 62% of 29 patients and abnormal capillary loops in 93%. These findings were confirmed by others (41–43).

Maricq and LeRoy (44) as well as Kenik et al. (45) have studied these phenomena extensively in connective tissue diseases. Capillary loops in SLE (independent of coexistent Raynaud's phenomenon) appear meandering and tortuous, with most having some disorganization and glomerulization (46, 47) (Fig. 34.2). They claimed that a trained, blinded observer could identify SLE 75% of the time. SLE patients have less frequent microvascular abnormalities (48). Three independent studies have given photomicrographs of patients with scleroderma, rheumatoid arthritis, SLE, and mixed connective tissue diseases to blinded observers. Lefford and Edwards (49) could not find any relation between capillary morphology and those clinical diagnoses. Granier et al. (50) noted that 64% of patients with mixed connective tissue disease had a scleroderma pattern and only 23% an SLE pattern, and McGill and Gow (51) found an 89% specificity and 80% sensitivity in selecting the correct diagnosis. Increased nail-fold capillary density may indicate pulmonary capillary loss in SLE (52) and correlate with anticardiolipin antibody along with the presence of microhemorrhages (53, 54). SLE patterns are similar to those seen in primary Sjögren's syndrome (55).

COMPLICATIONS OF CUTANEOUS VASCULITIS: ULCERATION AND GANGRENE

Cutaneous vasculitis is common in SLE and is reviewed in Chapter 29, Cutaneous Manifestations of Lupus Erythe-

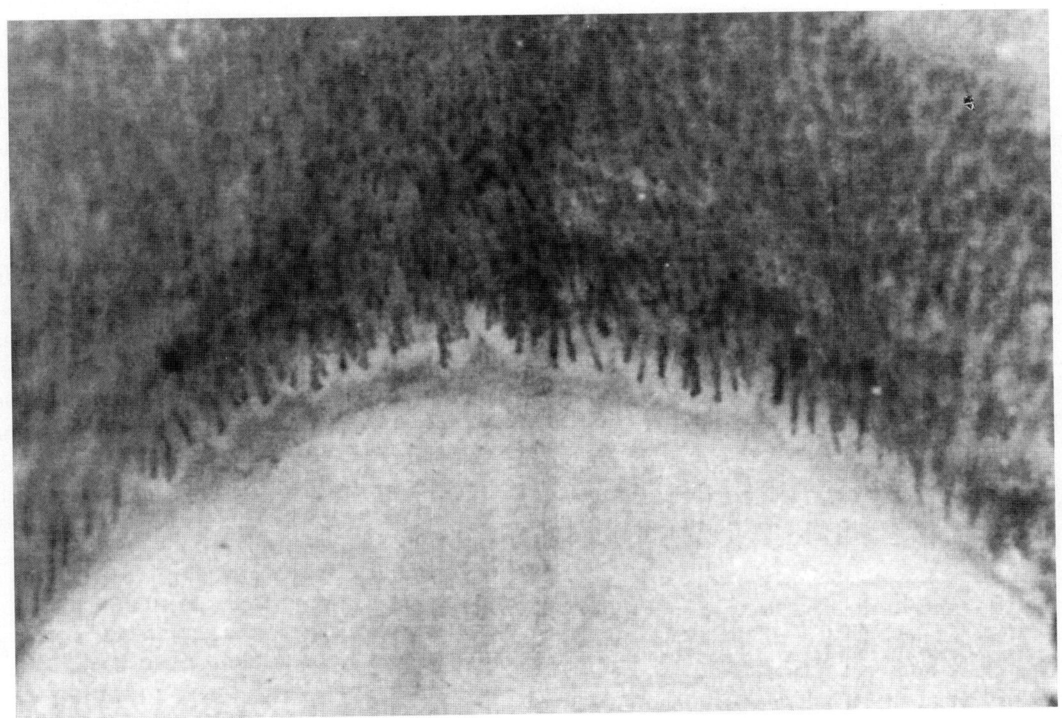

FIGURE 34.2. Nail-fold microcapillaroscopy in systemic lupus erythematosus. (Courtesy of Dr. J. Kenik.)

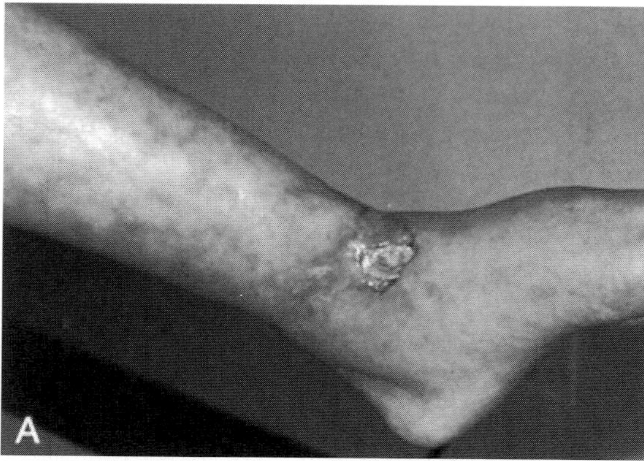

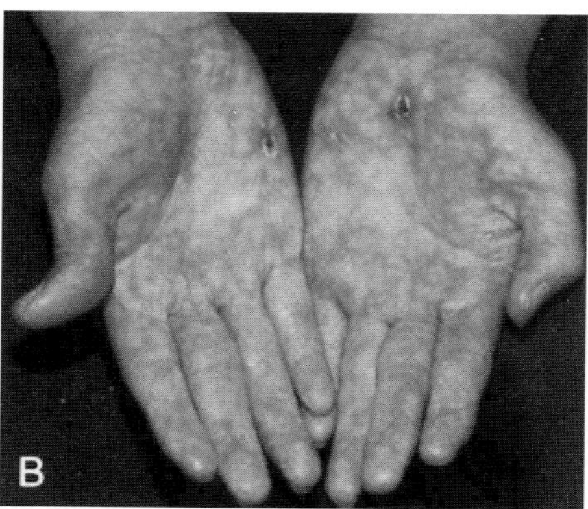

FIGURE 34.3. A, Livedo reticularis and ulceration of the leg of systemic lupus erythematosus patient with high-titer IgG anticardiolipin antibodies. **B**, Similar changes on the hands on this same patient.

matosus. A small percentage of these patients with active vasculitis may manifest necrotic ulcerations, digital and peripheral gangrene, and/or cutaneous infarctions. They frequently have a high-titer antinuclear antibody (ANA), elevated levels of serum anti-DNA and IgG, and reduced serum complement levels (56, 57). Direct immunofluorescence has demonstrated IgG, complement, and fibrinogen, with fibrin in the vessel walls surrounding the involved tissue (58–60).

Vasculitic leg ulcers were found in 29 of Dubois' 520 patients in 1963 (61) and in three of Brogadir and Mejers' patients (62), and 6.2% of Petri's Hopkins Cohort (63). Dermal vasculitis was present in 18 to 70 patients in the series listed in Table 34.1. Of Dubois' 520 patients, seven developed peripheral gangrene, as did three of Estes and Christian's 150 patients (64).

Ulcerations and gangrene can occur as a result of active vasculitis, the antiphospholipid syndrome, or both (65–69) (Fig. 34.3). Asherson et al. (66) followed six patients with gangrene of the extremities. Three had the antiphospholipid syndrome with no vasculitis, two had a classic immune-complex–mediated vasculitis without evidence of a lupus anticoagulant, and one had both. Similar findings were reported by Alarcon-Segovia et al. (65) and by Lockshin's group (70, 71). Additionally, the lupus anticoagulant rarely is associated with a syndrome of cutaneous necrosis, not unlike what has been reported in protein C deficiency states (72, 73). Cutaneous necrosis, antiphospholipid antibodies, livedo reticularis, and central nervous system findings have been termed *Sneddon's syndrome* (see Chapter 57, Immunosuppressive Drug Therapy). The differential diagnosis of cutaneous ulcerations requires ruling out ischemia from degenerative arterial disease, venous stasis, cryoglobulinemia, hyperviscosity syndrome, cholesterol emboli, and other hypercoagulable states. (Thrombosis is reviewed in Chapter 52, Clinical and Management Aspects of the Antiphospholipid Antibody Syndrome.)

The optimal treatment of peripheral vasculitis includes systemic corticosteroids, cyclophosphamide, and if necessary, plasmapheresis (70, 74, 75). If the antiphospholipid syndrome is present, anticoagulation is advised (70, 71). Short-term treatment with the prostaglandin E-derivative alprostadil-alpha-cyclodextrine is the most effective method of managing critical peripheral ischemia of the hands, feet, and legs (36–38, 76, see Chapter 59, Occasional, Innovative, and Experimental Therapies). Cutaneous vasculitis may respond to colchicine (see Chapter 59, Occasional, Innovative, and Experimental Therapies).

LIVEDO RETICULARIS

Livedo reticularis occurs because of disordered autonomically mediated blood flow through subpapillary and dermal blood vessels. It can be brought on by cold, connective-tissue diseases, fibromyalgia-cold agglutinins, and cryoglobulinemia. In SLE, it presents as a reticulated poikiloderma, most often on the arms and legs. Usually painless, livedo rarely can appear as a cutaneous vasculitis known as livedoid vasculitis. This reddish-purplish mottling on the skin blanches on pressure, is independent of temperature changes, and represents a vasospastic phenomenon of dermal-ascending arterioles (77–81). In the last decade, livedo reticularis has been shown in case-controlled studies to be unequivocally associated with cutaneous necrosis, central nervous disease, and the antiphospholipid syndrome (82–87). Livedo was observed in 11 of 66 patients with SLE in one report (88), and anticardiolipin antibodies were found in 81% of patients with SLE and livedo (see Chapter 29, Cutaneous Manifestations of Lupus Erythematosus). Unless livedoid vasculitis is present, no treatment is indicated.

ANTIPHOSPHOLIPID ANTIBODIES AND THE SKIN

See Chapter 52, Clinical and Management Aspects of the Antiphospholipid Antibody Syndrome.

PURPURA

Ecchymoses and petechiae may be noted depending on the platelet count and whether the patient has received steroid therapy. Cutaneous hemorrhages were seen in 9% to 21% of patients in various series (1, 9, 64). The most common cause of hemorrhagic lesions was steroid therapy, although salicylates and nonsteroidal antiinflammatory drugs (NSAIDs) also could induce them. NSAIDs can induce ecchymoses through their antiplatelet actions, and long-term steroid administration is associated with skin atrophy. Patients with untreated SLE occasionally report that they bruise easily, and many are thrombocytopenic. Occasionally, petechiae may occur because of active cutaneous vasculitis. Purpuric leg lesions should be differentiated from pigmentary changes resulting from long-term antimalarial therapy. Thrombotic thrombocytopenic purpura, idiopathic thrombocytopenic purpura, cryoglobulinemia, and other dysproteinemias may be seen in SLE and need to be ruled out.

ERYTHROMELALGIA

Erythromelalgia consists of burning distress of the extremities that is accompanied by increased redness and skin temperature, initiated by an increase in environmental skin temperature, and diminished by measures that cool the skin (89–91). Mostly seen in myelodysplastic disorders with thrombocytosis, erythromelalgia can occur in patients with SLE and normal platelet counts (77, 92–95). It usually is treated with antiplatelet agents (e.g., low-dose aspirin, dipyrimadole) or corticosteroids (96), but one report documented a dramatic response to clonazepam (94) and another suggested that propanolol with methysergide may be useful (97).

REFERENCES

1. McGehee Harvey A, Shulman LE, Tumulty AP, et al. Systemic lupus erythematosus: review of the literature and clinical analysis of 138 cases. *Medicine* 1954;33:291–437.
2. Grigor R, Edmonds J, Lewkonia R, et al. Systemic lupus erythematosus. A prospective analysis. *Ann Rheum Dis* 1978;37:121–128.
3. Weinstein C, Miller MH, Axtens R. Lupus and non-lupus cutaneous manifestations in systemic lupus erythematosus. *Aust N Z J Med* 1987;17:501–506.
4. Nepom BS, Schaller JG. Childhood systemic lupus erythematosus. *Prog Clin Rheumatol* 1984;1:33–69.
5. Baker SB, Rovira JR, Campion EW. Late onset lupus erythematosus. *Am J Med* 1979;66:727–732.
6. Dimant J, Ginzler EM, Schlesinger M, et al. Systemic lupus erythematosus in the older age group: computer analysis. *J Am Geriatr Soc* 1979;27:58–61.
7. George PM, Tunnessen WW, Jr. Childhood discoid lupus erythematosus. *Arch Dermatol* 1993;129:613–617.
8. Wysenbeek AJ, Guedj D, Amit M, et al. Rash in systemic lupus erythematosus: prevalence and relation to cutaneous and non-cutaneous disease manifestations. *Ann Rheum Dis* 1992;51:717–719.
9. Brown K, Petri M, Goldman D. Cutaneous manifestations of SLE: associations with other manifestations of SLE and with smoking (abstract). *Arthritis Rheum* 1995;38:R27.
10. Kahaleh B, Matucci-Cerinic MM. Raynaud's phenomenon and scleroderma. *Arthritis Rheum* 1995;38:14.
11. Rodnan GP. Scleroderma, calcinosis and eosinophilic fascitis. In: McCarty DJ, ed. *Arthritis and allied conditions* 9th ed. Philadelphia: Lea & Febiger, 1979:762–809.
12. Carroll GJ, Withers K, Bayliss CE. The prevalence of Raynaud's syndrome in rheumatoid arthritis. *Ann Rheum Dis* 1981;40:567–570.
13. De Takats G, Fowler EF. Raynaud's phenomenon. *JAMA* 179;1:1962–1968.
14. Gerbracht DD, Steen VD, Ziegler GL, et al. Evolution of primary Raynaud's phenomenon (Raynaud's disease) to connective-tissue disease. *Arthritis Rheum* 1985;28:87–92.
15. Kallenberg CG, Wouda AA, Hoet MH, et al. Development of connective tissue disease in patients with Raynaud's phenomenon: a six year follow up with emphasis on the predictive value of antinuclear antibodies as detected by immunoblotting. *Ann Rheum Dis* 1988;47:634–641.
16. Priollet P, Vayssairat M, Housset E. How to classify Raynaud's phenomenon. Long-term follow-up study of 73 cases. *Am J Med* 1987;83:494–498.
17. Blunt RJ, Porter JM. Raynaud syndrome. *Semin Arthritis Rheum* 1981;10:282–308.
18. Kallenberg CG, Wouda AA, The TH. Systemic involvement and immunologic findings in patients presenting with Raynaud's phenomenon. *Am J Med* 1980;69:675–680.
19. Velayos EE, Robinson H, Porciuncula FU, et al. Clinical correlation analysis of 137 patients with Raynaud's phenomenon. *Am J Med Sci* 1971;262:347–356.
20. Dimant J, Ginzler E, Schlesinger M, et al. The clinical significance of Raynaud's phenomenon in systemic lupus erythematosus. *Arthritis Rheum* 1979;22:815–819.
21. Rosal EJ, Maricq HR. Comparison of digital artery pressure responses to local cooling in Raynaud's phenomenon associated with systemic lupus erythematosus, systemic sclerosis and primary Raynaud's phenomenon (abstract). *Arthritis Rheum* 1989;32(suppl):R45.
22. Montecucco C, Caporali R, Cobianchi F, et al. Antibodies to hn-RNP protein A1 in systemic lupus erythematosus: clinical association with Raynaud's phenomenon and esophageal dysmotility. *Clin Exp Rheumatol* 1992;10:223–227.
23. O'Keefe ST, Tsapatsaris NP, Beetham WP, Jr. Increased prevalence of migraine and chest pain in patients with primary Raynaud disease. *Ann Intern Med* 1992;116:985–989.
24. Porter JM, Bardana EJ, Baur GM, et al. The clinical significance of Raynaud's syndrome. *Surgery* 1976;80:756–764.
25. Fahey PH, Utell MJ, Condemi JJ, et al. Raynaud's phenomenon of the lung. *Am J Med* 1984;76:263–269.
26. Wise RA, Wigley F, Newball HH, et al. The effect of cold exposure on diffusing capacity in patients with Raynaud's phenomenon. *Chest* 1982;81:695–698.
27. Yamauchi K, Suzuki Y, Arimori S. Renal Raynaud's phenomenon in systemic lupus erythematosus: measurement of the glomerular filtration rate with 99m-technetium-DTPA (letter). *Arthritis Rheum* 1989;32:1487–1488.
28. Bang FDC, Wantzin GL, Christensen JD. Raynaud's phenomenon with oral manifestations in systemic lupus erythematosus. *Dermatologica* 1985;170:263–264.
29. Lavras Costallat LT, Valente Coimbra AM. Raynaud's phenom-

enon in systemic lupus erythematosus. *Rev Rheum* (Eng Ed) 1995;62:349–353.
30. Ferraccioli G, di Pol E, di Gregorio F, et al. Changes in regional cerebral blood flow after a cold hand test in systemic lupus erythematosus patients with Raynaud's syndrome. *Lancet* 1999; 354:2135–2136.
31. Miller FW, Love LA. Prevention of predictable Raynaud's phenomenon by sublingual nifedipine (letter). *N Engl J Med* 1987; 317:1476.
32. Sappington JT, Fiorito EM. Thermal feedback in Raynaud's phenomenon secondary to systemic lupus erythematosus: long term remission of target symptoms. *Biofeedback Self Regul* 1985; 10:335–341.
33. Surwit RS, Gilgor RS, Allen LM, et al. A double-blind study of prazosin in the treatment of Raynaud's phenomenon in scleroderma. *Arch Dermatol* 1984;120:329–331.
34. Kaplan LI. Nitroprosside in systemic lupus erythematosus vasospasm. *Arthritis Rheum* 1992;35:1536–1537.
35. Goldberg J, Dlesk A. Successful treatment of Raynaud's phenomenon with pentoxifylline (letter). *Arthritis Rheum* 1986;29: 1055–1056.
36. The ICAI Study Group, Prostanoids for chronic critical leg ischemia. A randomized, controlled, open-label trial with prostaglandin E1. *Annals Intern Med* 1999;130:412–421.
37. Lange K, Ores R, Strauss W, et al. Steroid therapy of systemic lupus erythematosus based on immunologic considerations. *Arthritis Rheum* 1965;8:244–259.
38. Hauptman HW, Ruddy S, Roberts WN. Reveral of vasospastic component of lupus vasculopathy by infusion of prostaglandin E1. *J Rheumatol* 1991;18:1747–1752.
39. Baehr G, Klemperer P, Schifrin A. Diffuse disease of the peripheral circulation usually associated with lupus erythematosus and endocarditis. *Trans Assoc Am Physicians* 1935;50:139–155.
40. Buchanan IS, Humpston DJ. Nail-fold capillaries in connective-tissue disorders. *Lancet* 1968;i:845–847.
41. Minkin W, Rabhan NB. Office nailfold capillary microscopy using the ophthalmoscope. *J Am Acad Derm* 1982;7:190–193.
42. Redisch W, Messina GH, McEwen C. Capillaroscopic observations in rheumatic diseases. *Ann Rheum Dis* 1970;29:244–253.
43. Kabasakal Y, Elvins DM, Ring EFJ, et al. Quantitative nailfold capillaroscopy findings in a population with connective tissue disease and in normal healthy controls. *Annals Rheum Dis* 1996; 55:507–512.
44. Maricq HR, LeRoy EC. Patterns of finger capillary abnormalities in connective tissue disease by wide-field microscopy. *Arthritis Rheum* 1973;16:619–628.
45. Kenik JG, Maricq HR, Bole GG. Blind evaluation of the diagnostic specificity of nailfold capillary microscopy in the connective tissue diseases. *Arthritis Rheum* 1981;24:885–891.
46. Caspary L, Schmees C, Schoetensak I, et al. Alterations of the nailfold capillary morphology associated with Raynaud phenomenon in patients with systemic lupus erythematosus. *J Rheumatol* 1991;18:559–566.
47. Studer A, Hunziker T, Lutolf O, et al. Quantitative nailfold capillary microscopy in cutaneous and systemic lupus erythematosus and localized and systemic scleroderma. *J Am Acad Dermatol* 1991;24:941–945.
48. Von Bierbrauer A, Barth P, Willert J, et al. Electron microscopy and capillaroscopically guided nailfold biopsy in connective tissue diseases: detection of ultrastructural changes of the microcirculatory vessels. *Brit J Rheumatol* 1998;37:1272–1278.
49. Lefford F, Edwards JC. Nail fold capillary microscopy in connective tissue disease: a quantitative morphological analysis. *Ann Rheum Dis* 1986;45:741–749.
50. Granier F, Vayssairat M, Priollet P, et al. Nailfold capillary microscopy in mixed connective tissue diseases. Comparison with systemic sclerosis and systemic lupus erythematosus. *Arthritis Rheum* 1986;29:189–195.
51. McGill NW, Gow PJ. Nailfold capillaroscopy: a blinded study of its discriminatory value in scleroderma, systemic lupus erythematosus and rheumatoid arthritis. *Aust N Z J Med* 1986;16: 457–460.
52. Pallis M, Hopkinson N, Powell R. Nailfold capillary density as a possible indicator of pulmonary capillary loss in systemic lupus erythematosus but not in mixed connective tissue disease. *J Rheumatol* 1991;18:1532–1536.
53. Bongard O, Bounameaux H, Miescher P-A, et al. Association of anticardiolipin antibodies and abnormal nailfold capillaroscopy in patients with systemic lupus erythematosus. *Lupus* 1995;4: 142–144.
54. Candela M, Pansoni A, de Carolis ST, et al. Nailfold capillary microscopy in patients with antiphospholipid syndrome. *Recenti Prog Med* 1998;89:444–449.
55. Ohtsuka T. Nailfold capillary abnormalities in patient with Sjögren's syndrome and systemic lupus erythematosus. *Brit J Dermatol* 1997;136:94–96.
56. Kirsner AB, Diller JG, Sheon RP. Systemic lupus erythematosus with cutaneous ulceration. Correlation of immunologic factors with therapy and clinical activity. *JAMA* 1971;271:821–823.
57. Tufanelli DL, Kay DM. Morphological and immunological studies of necrotizing vasculitis in systemic lupus erythematosus (SLE) (abstract). *Clin Res* 1969;17:278.
58. Ansari A, Larson PH, Bates HD. Vascular manifestations of systemic lupus erythematosus. *Angiology* 1986;37:423–432.
59. Baart de La Faille-Kuype EH. *Lupus erythematosusan immunohistochemical and clinical study of 485 patients* [thesis]. Utrecht, Nev: Grafisch Bedriff Schotamus & Jens. Utrecht NV; 1969.
60. Hashimoto H, Tsuda H, Takasaki Y, et al. Digital ulcers/gangrene and immunoglobulin classes/complement fixation of anti-ds-DNA in systemic lupus erythematosus patients. *J Rheumatol* 1983;10:727–732.
61. Dubois EL, Tuffanelli DL. Clinical manifestations of systemic lupus erythematosus. Computer analysis of 520 cases. *JAMA* 1964;190:104–111
62. Brogadir SP, Mejers AR. Chronic leg ulceration in systemic lupus erythematosus. *J Rheumatol* 1979;6:204–209.
63. Petri M. Dermatologic lupus: Hopkins lupus cohort. *Seminars Cutaneous Med Surg* 1998;17:219–227.
64. Estes D, Christian CL. The natural history of systemic lupus erythematosus by prospective analysis. *Medicine* 1971;50: 85–95.
65. Alarcon-Segovia D, Cardiel MH, Reyes E. Antiphospholipid arterial vasculopathy. *J Rheumatol* 1989;16:762–767.
66. Asherson RA, Derksen RH, Harris EN, et al. Large vessel occlusion and gangrene in systemic lupus erythematosus and lupus-like disease. A report of six cases. *J Rheumatol* 1986;13:740–747.
67. Jindal BK, Martin MF, Gayner A. Gangrene developing after minor surgery in a patient with undiagnosed systemic lupus erythematosus and lupus anticoagulant. *Ann Rheum Dis* 1983; 42:347–349.
68. Johansson E, Niemi KM, Mustakallio KK. A peripheral vascular syndrome overlapping with systemic lupus erythematosus. *Dermatologica* 1977;15:257–267.
69. Sibley JT, Blocka KLN, Sheridan DP, et al. Familial systemic lupus erythematosus characterized by digital ischemia. *J Rheumatol* 1993;20:299–303.
70. Greisman SG, Thayaparan LS, Godwin TA, et al. Occlusive vasculopathy in systemic lupus erythematosus. Association with anticardiolipin antibody. *Arch Intern Med* 1991;151:389–392.
71. Harris EN, Bos K. An acute disseminated coagulopathy-vasculopathy associated with the antiphospholipid syndrome. *Arch Intern Med* 1991;15:231–233.

72. Alegre VA, Winklemann RK, Gastineau DA. Cutaneous thrombosis, cerebrovascular thrombosis and the lupus anticoagulant-the Sneddon syndrome. Report of 10 cases. *Int J Dermatol* 1990;29:45–49.
73. Frances C, Tribout B, Boisnic S, et al. Cutaneous necrosis associated with the lupus anticoagulant. *Dermatologica* 1989;178: 194–201.
74. Fruchter L, Gauthier B, Marino F. The use of plasmapheresis in a patient with systemic lupus erythematosus and necrotizing cutaneous ulcers (letter). *J Rheumatol* 1983;10:341–343.
75. Jinadal BK, Martin MF, Gayner G. Gangrene developing after minor surgery in a patient with undiagnosed systemic lupus erythematosus and the lupus anticoagulant. *Ann Rheum Dis* 1983;42:347–349.
76. Constans J, de Precigout V, Compe C, et al. Efficacy of prostacyclin perfusion for microangiopathy association with lupus. *La Presse Medicale* 1991;20.
77. Alarcon-Segovia D, Diaz-Jouanen E. Erythromalgia in systemic lupus erythematosus (case report). *Am J Med Sci* 1973;266: 149–151.
78. Alarcon-Segovia D, Osmundson PJ. Peripheral vascular syndromes associated with systemic lupus erythematosus. *Ann Intern Med* 1965;62:907–919.
79. Golden RL. Livedo reticularis in systemic lupus erythematosus. *Arch Dermatol* 1963;87:299–301.
80. Tuffanelli DL, Levan NE, Dubois EL. Unusual cutaneous disorders in familial lupus erythematosus. *Arch Dermatol* 1964;89: 324–327.
81. Winkelmann RK. Diagnosis and treatment of lupus erythematosus, dermatomyositis, and scleroderma, with emphasis on cutaneous findings. *J Chronic Dis* 1961;13:401–410.
82. Alegre VA, Gastineau DA, Winklemann RK. Skin lesions associated with circulating lupus anticoagulant. *Br J Dermatol* 1989; 120:419–429.
83. Englert HJ, Loizou S, Derue GG, et al. Clinical and immunologic features of livedo reticularis in lupus: a case-controlled study. *Am J Med* 1989;87:408–410.
84. Frances C, Boisnic S, Lefebvre C, et al. Rare cutaneous manifestations in the course of lupus: cutaneous skin necrosis. *Ann Dermatol Venereol* 1986;113:976–977.
85. McHugh NJ, Maymo J, Skinner RP, et al. Anticardiolipin antibodies, livedo reticularis, and major cerebrovascular and renal disease in systemic lupus erythematosus. *Ann Rheum Dis* 1988; 47:110–115.
86. Weinstein C, Miller MH, Axtens R, et al. Livedo reticularis associated with increased titers of anticardiolipin antibodies in systemic lupus erythematosus. *Arch Dermatol* 1987;123: 596–600.
87. Van Steenbergen W, Beyls J, Vermylen J, et al. Lupus anticoagulant and thrombosis of the hepatic veins (Budd-Chiari syndrome). Report of three patients and review of the literature. *J Hepatol* 1986;3:87–94.
88. Yasue T. Livedoid vasculitis and central nervous system involvement in systemic lupus erythematosus. *Arch Dermatol* 1986; 122:66–70.
89. Michiels JJ. Erythromelalgia in SLE (letter). *J Rheumatol* 1991; 18:481–482.
90. Kurzrock R, Cohen PR. Erythromelalgia: review of classical characteristics and pathophysiology. *Am J Med* 1991;91: 416–422.
91. Drenth JPH, Michiels JJ. Clinical characteristics and pathophysiology of erythromelalgia and erythermalgia. *Am J Med* 1992;93:111–112.
92. Alarcon-Segovia D, Babb RR, Fairbairn JF, 2nd. Systemic lupus erythematosus with erythromelalgia. *Arch Intern Med* 1963; 112:688–692.
93. Desser KB, Sartiano GP, Cooper JL. Lupus livedo and cutaneous infarction. *Angiology* 1969;20:261.
94. Kraus A. Erythromelalgia in a patient with systemic lupus erythematosus treated with clonazepam. *J Rheumatol* 1990;17:120.
95. Kraus A, Alarcon-Segovia D. Erythermalgia, erythromelalgia, or both? Conditions neglected by rheumatologists. *J Rheumatol* 1993;20:13.
96. Drenth JPH, Michiels JJ, van Joost T, et al. Secondary erythermalgia in systemic lupus erythematosus. *J Rheumatol* 1993;20: 144–146.
97. Abeles M. Erythromelalgia: successful treatment and ten year follow-up of five patients, *Arthritis Rheum* 1998;41:S233.
98. Rothfield N, Marino C. Studies of repeat skin biopsies of nonlesional skin in patients with systemic lupus erythematosus. *Arthritis Rheum* 1982;25:624–630.
99. Lee P, Urowitz MB, Bookman AA, et al. Systemic lupus erythematosus: a review of 110 cases with reference to nephritis, the nervous system, infections, aseptic necrosis and prognosis. *Q J Med* 1977;46:1–32.
100. Pistiner M, Wallace DJ, Nessim S, et al. Lupus erythematosus in the 1980s: a survey of 570 patients. *Semin Arthritis Rheum* 1991;21:55–64.

35

SYSTEMIC LUPUS ERYTHEMATOSUS AND THE NERVOUS SYSTEM

STERLING G. WEST

Neuropsychiatric manifestations of systemic lupus erythematosus (NP-SLE) are frequent, vary from mild to severe, and often are difficult to diagnose and distinguish from those of other diseases. Any location within the nervous system may be affected, with symptoms and signs ranging from mild cognitive dysfunction to seizures, strokes, and coma. At the initial development of neurologic manifestations, many patients have other medical conditions or are receiving medications, which can affect the central or peripheral nervous systems. The challenge to the clinician is to determine the exact cause of the nervous system dysfunction so that appropriate therapy can be instituted. This chapter describes the classification, etiopathogenesis, clinical signs and symptoms, laboratory and radiographic findings, differential diagnosis, and treatment of lupus involving the nervous system.

HISTORICAL CONSIDERATIONS

Neurologic involvement in SLE first was noted by Hebra and Kaposi (1) in 1875, who described stupor and coma as terminal manifestations of the disease. Osler (2–4), in several papers on the systemic effects of the erythema group of skin diseases, discussed associated cerebral changes and reported a patient who "imagines all sorts of things." In 1904, Baum (5) related active delirium, aphasia, and hemiparesis to probable disseminated lupus erythematosus (LE). During the next 40 years, the psychiatric and neurologic correlates of systemic lupus erythematosus (SLE) were recognized, but seldom discussed.

The first modern study of NP-SLE was conducted by Daly in 1945 (6). He correlated clinical symptoms with abnormal spinal fluid findings and with the pathologic finding of vasculitis. In 1948, Sedgwick and Von Hagen (7) discussed five cases in detail. In 1953, Dubois (8) described clinical neurologic subsets among 62 cases and, in 1954, Lewis et al. (9) were the first to focus on the importance of electroencephalographic findings and psychometric testing in patients with NP-SLE.

From the 1950s through the 1970s, hundreds of reports delineated the various manifestations of neurologic involvement in SLE. Over the last two decades, however, appreciation of the clinical significance of antineuronal, antiribosomal P, and antiphospholipid antibodies, as well as advances in brain imaging, have again altered our concept of NP-SLE.

CLASSIFICATION AND CLINICAL PRESENTATION

The incidence of neuropsychiatric manifestations in SLE ranges from 24% to 59% depending on the ascertainment methodology. It often is impossible to compare past studies of NP-SLE, because no standardized definition or classification system was used. Some reports included patients with minimal, nonspecific symptoms, while others restricted themselves to those with objective neurologic findings. Recently, an international, multidisciplinary committee developed case definitions, including diagnostic criteria and important exclusions, for 19 neuropsychiatric lupus syndromes (10) (Table 35.1). This nomenclature should help clinicians diagnose NP-SLE, as well as help investigators in future studies. The complete case definitions are available on the American College of Rheumatology worldwide web site at http://www.rheumatology.org/ar/ar.html.

SLE patients with NP-SLE can present with a myriad of diffuse and/or focal symptoms and signs involving the brain, spinal cord, or peripheral nervous system. The central nervous system (CNS) manifestations include headache, confusion, altered consciousness, seizures, focal or generalized neurologic deficits, ataxia, chorea and other movement disorders, papilledema, psychosis, and severe depression. Peripheral nervous system manifestations include cranial nerve dysfunction, acute weakness, paresthesias, and abnormalities of autonomic function. The pathologic abnormalities observed in the nervous system also are diverse (Table 35.2). Oftentimes, there is no clear-

TABLE 35.1. NEUROPSYCHIATRIC SYNDROMES OF SYSTEMIC LUPUS ERYTHEMATOSUS

Central nervous system
- Acute confusional state
- Cognitive dysfunction
- Psychosis
- Mood disorder
- Anxiety disorder
- Headache (including migraine and benign intracranial hypertension)
- Cerebrovascular disease
- Myelopathy
- Movement disorder
- Demyelinating syndrome
- Seizure disorders
- Aseptic meningitis

Peripheral nervous system
- Cranial neuropathy
- Polyneuropathy
- Plexopathy
- Mononeuropathy, single/multiplex
- Acute inflammatory demyelinating polyradiculo-neuropathy (Guillain-Barré syndrome)
- Autonomic disorder
- Myasthenia gravis

Adapted from ACR Ad Hoc Committee on Neuropsychiatric Lupus Nomenclature. The American College of Rheumatology Nomenclature and Case Definitions for Neuropsychiatric Lupus Syndromes. *Arthritis Rheum* 1999;42:599–608, with permission.

TABLE 35.2. PATHOLOGIC CLASSIFICATION OF CENTRAL NERVOUS SYSTEM CHANGES OBSERVED IN SYSTEMIC LUPUS ERYTHEMATOSUS

Vasculopathy
- Hyalinization
- Perivascular inflammation without infection
- Endothelial proliferation without infection
- Thrombosis
- Vasculitis

Infarction
- Microinfarcts
- Large infarcts

Hemorrhage
- Subarachnoid
- Microhemorrhages
- Subdural
- Intracerebral

Infection
- Meningitis
- Perivascular inflammation with infection
- Septic hemorrhages
- Focal cerebritis
- Vasculitis with infection

Adapted from Ellis SG, Verity MA. Central nervous system involvement in systemic lupus erythematosus: a review of neuropathologic findings in 57 cases, 1955–1977. *Semin Arthritis Rheum* 1979;8:212–221, with permission.

cut clinicopathologic relationship between CNS signs and localized CNS lesions. This section discusses the prevalence of NP-SLE as described in some of the principal surveys from the last 50 years (Table 35.3).

Important Surveys: 1950–1980

Of Dubois' 520 patients (11) who were followed between 1950 and 1963, 25% had some type of central or peripheral nervous system involvement. In a 1956 review of the cliniconeurologic changes that were observed in 24 of 100 patients with SLE followed at the Mayo Clinic, Clark and Bailey (12) reported changes that varied from convulsive seizures to monoplegia, and they revealed an entire gamut of neurologic findings. Signs and symptoms of neurologic disease alone were noted in 11 patients, and neurologic and psychiatric disease together were present in 13.

In 1966, O'Connor and Musher (13) reviewed 150 patients with SLE who were followed at Columbia Presbyterian Medical Center. Of these, four patients presented with NP-SLE. CNS disturbances were more frequent among patients who were followed through terminal illness. Sixty-seven percent of the 150 patients had psychiatric disorders, and 43% had neurologic disorders. Neurologic signs were seen at one time or another in 46 of the 150 patients.

In 1971, Estes and Christian (14) observed neuropsychiatric manifestations of SLE in 59% of 150 patients who were followed mostly in the 1960s. Disorders of mental function were found in 42% and grand-mal seizures in 26%. The neurologic manifestations were cranial nerve involvement (seven patients), oculomotor signs (six patients), and optic atrophy and blindness (three patients). Intention tremor was observed in eight patients and was associated with cogwheel rigidity in two patients. Hemiparesis occurred in eight patients, six of whom had chronic renal disease with hypertension and/or uremia. Peripheral neuropathy with predominantly sensory deficits developed in ten patients.

In 1975, Sergent et al. (15) reported on 52 episodes in 28 patients with SLE: ten had seizures, nine had encephalopathy, four had aseptic meningitis, seven had focal neurologic deficits, 15 had psychiatric abnormalities, and one had chorea. They found no evidence that large doses of steroids were helpful in treating these patients. Also in 1975, Klippel and Zvaifler (16) compiled a literature review of NP-SLE in 995 reported patients with SLE (one half of these were Dubois' 520 patients). Overall, neuropsychiatric abnormalities were found in 33%, seizures in 16%, neuropathy in 10%, psychopathology in 18%, and myelopathy and chorea in 4% each.

In 1976, a review of 140 patients with SLE at the Johns Hopkins Hospital revealed neuropsychiatric changes in 52% (17), and 63% of these had episodes in the first year of disease. Only two instances of documented steroid-induced psychosis occurred. Of these 140 patients, 84%

TABLE 35.3. NEUROLOGIC MANIFESTATIONS OF SYSTEMIC LUPUS ERYTHEMATOSUS IN SELECTED LARGE SERIES (%)

Parameter	Clark & Bailey 1956	Ester & Christian 1971	Ropes[a] 1976	Gibson & Myers 1976	Feinglass 1976	Lee 1977	Hochberg[b] 1985	Wallace 1990
No. of cases	100	150	150	81	140	110	150	464
CNS manifestations	24	59	–	51	52	40	55	50
Seizures	14	26	11	20	17	8	13	6
Cranial neuropathy	–	7	–	4	16	3	–	–
Vasculopathy	8	8	15	10	16	3	–	11
Peripheral neuropathy	3	7	5	2	15	8	21	5
Psychosis	17	16	28	27	14	16	16	5

[a]Ropes MW. *Systemic lupus erythematosus.* Cambridge, MA: Harvard University Press, 1976.
[b]Hochberg MC, Boyd RE, Ahearn JM, et al. Systemic lupus erythematosus: a review of clinico-laboratory features and immunogenetic in 150 patients with emphasis on demographic subsets. *Medicine* 1985:285–295.
CNS, Central nervous system

improved with treatment of SLE. A striking, positive correlation was noted among CNS involvement, vasculitis, and thrombocytopenia. Five- and 10-year survival rates for those in the CNS group were 94% and 82%, respectively.

Urowitz's group at the University of Toronto published two large SLE series (18, 19) that emphasized CNS findings; those with CNS disease had lower serum complement levels and more disease manifestations than those without CNS pathology. Grigor et al. (20) found neuropsychiatric symptoms in 50% of 50 patients. No correlations could be found with any other SLE manifestations, including vasculitis and thrombocytopenia.

Gibson and Myers (21) noted episodes of NP-SLE in 41 of 80 patients (51%) who were followed before 1976. More episodes were noted in African Americans, and an increased incidence of renal failure as well as a poorer survival were seen in this group as opposed to the non-CNS group. In contrast to most of the preceding reports, Seibold et al. (22) calculated that CNS involvement occurred at a mean of 4.3 years after the onset of disease in 26 patients.

Important Surveys: Since 1980

The 1980s saw a continuing decline in the reported frequency of classic NP-SLE. Pistiner et al. (23) observed 49 cases of cerebritis and, comparing patients who were evaluated from 1950 to 1963 with those between 1980 and 1989, this represented a decrease from 26% to 11%. Using the American College of Rheumatology definition for CNS-lupus as a criterion (i.e., seizures or psychosis), 30 patients (6%) had seizures and 24 (5%) psychotic episodes. The prevalence of significant CNS abnormalities was 27% in two European multicenter studies (24, 25) surveying 1,704 patients with lupus; 12% had these abnormalities at presentation. West et al. (26) noted CNS lupus in 50 of 184 patients (28%) in Colorado, and others (27–29) noted CNS disease in 48 of 266 patients (18%) in Saskatchewan, in 35 of 222 (16%) in Australia, in 22 of 53 (42%) in Italy, and in 171 of 1,203 (14%) in China (30).

The recognition of antineuronal, antiribosomal P, and antiphospholipid antibodies in the 1980s has affirmed the value of clinically classifying CNS episodes into "diffuse" and "focal" presentations. Several studies showed that serum and cerebrospinal fluid (CSF) antineuronal antibodies are found more commonly in patients with diffuse, global dysfunction such as acute confusion, altered level of consciousness, seizures, cognitive dysfunction, and psychiatric abnormalities (31–35). Bonfa and Elkon were first to associate antiribosomal P antibodies with psychosis and severe depression (36). Some investigators confirmed this association, while others did not (37). Antiphospholipid antibodies were associated with thromboembolic episodes leading to focal manifestations, including strokes, transverse myelitis, and chorea (38).

West et al. reported in a 10-year prospective study of 184 SLE patients that certain combinations of tests were most useful in establishing a diagnosis of severe NP-SLE, depending on whether the patient had a diffuse or focal presentation. Of these SLE patients, 52 developed NP-SLE and 14 had CNS dysfunction as a result of a nonlupus cause. Cases were divided into diffuse, focal, and complex (both diffuse and focal symptoms) presentations. SLE patients with diffuse presentations were more likely to have elevated CSF antineuronal antibodies, abnormal CSF IgG indices with oligoclonal bands, or serum antiribosomal P antibodies. Patients with focal symptoms had evidence of vasculitis or high-titer antiphospholipid antibodies with abnormal brain magnetic resonance imaging (MRI) showing multiple lesions (26). More recently, Isshi and Hirohata reported that serum antiribosomal P and CSF antineuronal antibodies were detected more frequently in lupus psychosis patients than in lupus patients with other symptoms of NP-SLE or lupus patients without NP-SLE (39).

Clinical surveys confirmed that NP-SLE can occur early in the course of SLE (40–41) and usually is associated with lupus that is clinically and serologically active (42). Two studies pointed out that secondary causes such as infection always need to be ruled out in SLE patients presenting with mental confusion or alterations in consciousness. Infections were found in 14 of 91 SLE patients with CNS dysfunction by Futrell et al. (43) and in 28% of 36 acute CNS presentations by Wong et al. (44).

Studies by the Denburgs and others (33–35) established that mild cognitive dysfunction is common in SLE patients and should be considered a subset of NP-SLE. Symptoms of cognitive dysfunction often were present in the absence of objective neurologic, clinical, laboratory, or neuroimaging abnormalities, but could be demonstrated on neuropsychologic testing. A significant percentage of these patients progressed to more severe neuropsychiatric disease.

Two Canadian studies that followed 900 patients with lupus for 15 to 20 years reported that most CNS events were self-limited, reversible, and not associated with a poor outcome (45, 46). However, patients with focal findings had a worse prognosis than patients with diffuse presentations (45).

CENTRAL NERVOUS SYSTEM DISEASE IN CHILDREN AND THE ELDERLY

Several groups have examined NP-SLE in children. Cassidy et al. (47) noted a 31% incidence in 58 children. Bahabri et al. (48) reported a 30% incidence in 60 Saudi children with SLE. Yancey et al. (49) found a 43% incidence in 37 children, and their literature review of 11 pediatric studies found a 33% incidence in 353 children (see Chapter 41).

CNS involvement in older age groups (i.e., >50 years) is reported to be milder and less frequent with an incidence between 6% and 19% (50–52). In one report, however, nine of ten patients who were diagnosed with SLE at an age of older than 50 years had neuropsychiatric manifestations. Of these, five had peripheral neuritis, three had cerebellar ataxia (53), and nearly all were steroid responsive. Two percent of 254 individuals, who were admitted to a psychogeriatric center in England over a 2-year period, turned out to have SLE (54).

Summary

SLE can involve the nervous system in many ways. Until recently, the presence of specific neuropathology causing seizures, stroke, and paresis was considered to constitute NP-SLE and was found in approximately 25% of patients. Over the last three decades, the incidence of these features has decreased as early intervention and the diagnosis and treatment of active SLE became more common. Over the last decade, however, the recognition of lupus headache and cognitive dysfunction as distinct syndromes, in the absence of specific neuropathology, has resulted in a net increase in the incidence of what many rheumatologists call "CNS lupus." NP-SLE now is regarded as being present in many patients with SLE at some point during the course of their disease. Specific neuropathology is seen in a minority and usually is short-term, but can lead to chronic neurologic deficits.

ETIOPATHOGENESIS

The Clinicopathologic Studies

Several autopsy series have reported detailed analyses of the neuropathology of patients with NP-SLE. Many of these studies are hampered by the inclusion of patients with secondary causes of CNS dysfunction, as well as patients with prolonged intervals between NP-SLE manifestations and death. Despite these limitations, these studies provide important insights into the pathogenesis of NP-SLE. Johnson and Richardson (55, 56) reviewed the brain sections of 24 patients observed at Massachusetts General Hospital in the 1960s. Neurologic and psychiatric manifestations were found in 18 patients (75%). In nine of these 18, neurologic involvement occurred during the last 6 weeks of life. Death was attributable to CNS disease in six patients (intracerebral hemorrhage in four, status epilepticus in two). Seizures were present in 54%, cranial nerve disorders in 42%, hemiparesis in 12%, paresis in 4%, peripheral neuropathy in 8%, and mental disorders in 33%. Significant gross brain abnormalities were found in ten of the 24 patients, including large intracerebral hemorrhages (three patients), multiple pontine hemorrhages (one patient), fresh hemorrhages (two patients), small areas of old infarction (four patients), and a small, subapical hemorrhage (one patient). Microscopic lesions were more common than macroscopic lesions; microinfarcts with increased pericapillary microglia were found in 20 of the 24 patients. Johnson and Richardson concluded that the nervous system involvement of SLE was caused primarily by vascular disease affecting small vessels and producing microinfarcts with hemorrhages. True vasculitis was rare; inflammatory cells within the vessel wall were found in only three of the 24 patients. In contrast, perivascular inflammation was more common. Destructive lesions in the wall of small vessels, which were described as fibrinoid degeneration, were found in five patients.

Funata (57) performed detailed neuropathologic evaluations on 26 patients with SLE. Twelve died as a result of uremia, and one half of these 12 had perivascular inflammation in the brain. Thrombi associated with endothelial swelling and proliferation and fibrinoid degeneration were noted in five patients.

Ellis and Verity (58) reviewed 57 autopsied SLE cases at UCLA Medical Center. Vasculopathy was observed in 65%, infarction in 44%, hemorrhage in 42%, and infection in 28%. In the vasculopathy group, hyalinization (54% of patients), perivascular inflammation (28%), endothelial proliferation (21%), thrombosis (7%), and vasculitis (8%) were found. The infarctions consisted mostly of microinfarcts. Hemorrhages included subarachnoid (30%), intracerebral (10%), and subdural (4%) hemorrhages, as well as microhemorrhages (19%). In those with infections, meningitis (18%), perivascular inflammation (14%), septic hemorrhages (5%), and focal cerebritis (3%) were seen. Many patients in this group had received combined corticosteroids and azathioprine therapy.

All of the studies discussed so far have antedated the availability of anticardiolipin antibody testing. They certainly may reflect the most severe end of the NP-SLE spectrum.

In 1988, Devinsky and coworkers reported autopsy results of 50 SLE patients (59). Neuropsychiatric manifestations had occurred in 74% of the patients. Half of the patients had microscopic lesions, with embolic brain infarcts (ten patients) and intracerebral infection (eight patients) being most common. A cardiac source was found in nine of the ten patients with embolic brain infarcts. A true vasculitis was not seen. Interestingly, 14 patients had clinical evidence of thrombotic thrombocytopenic purpura during the terminal phase of their illness. Unfortunately, the antiphospholipid antibody status of these patients was not reported, although Greisman et al. (60) have indicated in a subsequent report that many of them had antiphospholipid antibodies. Importantly, a correlation between the patients' neuropsychiatric manifestations and pathologic brain lesions could only be made in half of the patients. Recently, Hanly and coworkers associated brain microinfarcts with seizures in ten patients, but not with antiphospholipid, antiribosomal P, or antineuronal antibodies (61).

These autopsy series agree on several important points. First, there is no distinct typical or pathognomonic lesion that NP-SLE causes in the brain that is diagnostically specific, like the "wire loop" lesion of the kidney or the "onion-skin" lesion of the spleen. The degenerative and proliferative changes in the small cerebral vessels were not distinct from the vascular changes in hypertensive encephalopathy. The neuropathologic lesions of SLE, however, are characterized as more focal or more scattered and by the fact that they varied in age from region to region, rather than appearing to have occurred simultaneously. Finally, clinical manifestations may not be readily explained by pathologic findings. Some NP-SLE patients, particularly those with diffuse manifestations, may have normal or relatively unremarkable brain pathology.

Pathogenesis

The pathogenesis of NP-SLE is unknown. However, it is unlikely that a single pathogenetic mechanism is responsible for the myriad of neuropsychiatric manifestations seen in NP-SLE (Table 35.4). Diffuse cerebral manifestations

TABLE 35.4. PATHOGENETIC MECHANISMS CAUSING NEUROPSYCHIATRIC SYMPTOMS IN SYSTEMIC LUPUS ERYTHEMATOSUS

Primary	Secondary
Vascular occlusion/hemorrhage	Infection
Immune complex-mediated vasculitis	Medications
Immune complex-mediated anaphylatoxin release causing leukoagglutination	TTP
Antiphospholipid antibody-associated hypercoagulability/thrombosis	Hypertension
Emboli from cardiac source	Uremia
Cryoglobulinemia/hyperviscosity	Electrolyte imbalances
Autoantibody-mediated	Fever
Antineuronal antibodies	Thyroid disease
Choroid plexus dysfunction	Atherosclerotic strokes
Cytokine effects	Subdural hematoma
Other mechanisms	Berry aneurysm
Abnormal HPA axis response	Cerebral lymphoma
Abnormal noradrenergic response	Fibromyalgia
Nitric oxide/oxidative stress	Reactive depression
Excitatory amino-acid toxicity	Sleep apnea
	Other primary neurologic or psychiatric disease

HPA, hypothalamic-pituitary-adrenal; TTP, thrombotic thrombocytopenic purpura
Adapted from reference West SG. Neuropsychiatric lupus. *Rheum Dis Clin North Am* 1994;20:129–158, with permission.

that are often transient, reversible on therapy, and not consistently associated with abnormal brain pathology, most likely have a different pathogenesis from the focal symptoms, which are usually acute in onset, permanent even with therapy, and frequently associated with pathologic lesions at autopsy.

Vascular Occlusion

All clinicopathologic studies have reported that multiple vascular occlusions resulting in large and small infarcts and hemorrhages are commonly observed in the brains of patients with NP-SLE at autopsy (55–61). These studies report that less than 15% of these arterial occlusions can be attributed to immune-mediated vasculitis. This may be because the tight junctions between endothelial cells and the blood-brain barrier hinder deposition of immune complexes in the cerebral blood vessels. However, there have been several case reports of angiographically and/or histologically proven large and small vessel vasculitis occurring in SLE patients presenting with acute symptoms of NP-SLE (62–66). Rarely, an isolated phlebitis and venulitis can be observed. Cerebral vasculitis is a dramatic process that presents with fever, confusion, and headache, followed within hours to days by seizures, psychosis, and encephalomyelitis. If untreated, it can lead to coma and death. Cerebral changes usually are generalized. Laboratory investigation often reveals active, multisystem SLE with elevated serologies and decreased serum complement components. The CSF usually demonstrates pleocytosis, an elevated protein level, increased IgG, and an elevated Q-albumin, indicating disruption of the blood-brain barrier. MRI of the brain frequently reveals multiple ischemic gray- and white-matter lesions, and positron emission tomography (PET) scan reveals hypoperfusion (Fig. 35.1).

The most common lesion leading to vascular occlusion is a noninflammatory vasculopathy with marked endothelial proliferation, obliterative intimal fibrosis, thrombosis, and occasionally perivascular lymphocytes. The etiology of this bland vasculopathy is unclear. Some investigators have suggested these lesions are scarring from healed or treated vasculitis or represent a unique response of cerebral arterioles to immune reactants, which can occasionally be demonstrated in the blood vessel walls. Indeed, several animal models have shown that chronic, low levels of circulating immune complexes are associated with an endothelial and intimal-proliferative lesion and thrombosis in blood-vessel walls, rather than an inflammatory vasculopathy (67, 68). However, others have pointed out that this bland vasculopathy is similar to lesions observed in patients with antiphospholipid antibodies (60, 69) and in patients with thrombotic thrombocytopenic purpura (70). Antiphospholipid antibodies have been shown to activate endothelial cells, possibly leading to upregulation of adhesion molecules and release of coagulation proteins, which can contribute to the development of vasoocclusive thrombosis (71). Platelet deposition in this thrombus could result in release of platelet-derived growth factors, resulting in endothelial cell proliferation and intimal fibrosis, commonly observed in this bland vasculopathy. Immunohistochemical staining with monoclonal antibodies have demonstrated CD 31 (endothelial cells), factor VIII antigen, and CD 61 (platelet membrane glycoprotein IIIa) in these thickened vessels, indicating the local incorporation of them in the thrombus (72, 73). Finally, although uncommon, vasculitis has been reported to occur in patients with antiphospholipid antibodies (74). Perhaps antiphospholipid antibody activation of endothelial cells results in influx of leukocytes into the blood vessel walls via the upregulated adhesion molecules.

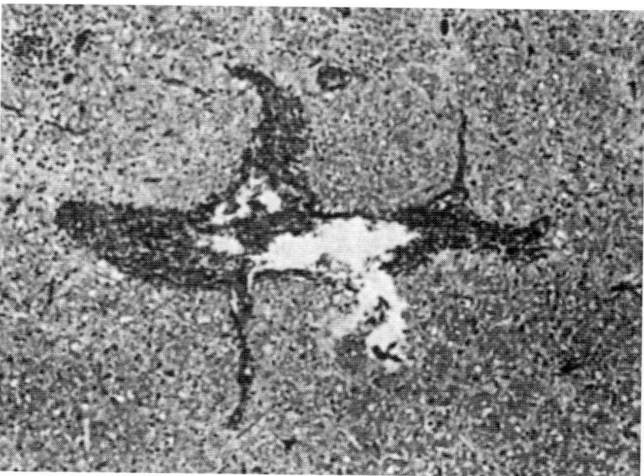

FIGURE 35.1. Periphlebitis in the floor of the third ventricle of the brain of a 13-year-old girl with convulsions caused by systemic lupus erythematosus (H&E; 85).

Clinically, Hughes and coworkers in the 1980s were first to correlate antiphospholipid antibodies with focal manifestations and seizures in NP-SLE patients (75, 76). Subsequently, Hughes' group observed neuropsychiatric manifestations in 96 of 340 SLE patients (28%) with 55% of patients with NP-SLE having antiphospholipid antibodies, compared to 20% of patients without NP-SLE (p <.001) (77). The most common clinical manifestations were transient ischemic attacks (TIAs) and strokes. Chorea, dementia, migraine headaches, transverse myelitis, seizures, cerebral-venous thrombosis (78), and anterior-spinal artery syndrome (79) also have been associated with antiphospholipid antibodies (80). Patients with antiphospholipid antibodies in NP-SLE frequently have livedo reticularis (81), although other clinical and laboratory manifestations of active lupus may or may not be present. The cerebrospinal fluid usually demonstrates elevated protein, but commonly a low white-blood-cell count. Antiphospholipid antibodies generally are not present in the cerebrospinal fluid (38). Brain MRI shows focal or generalized ischemic white-matter lesions (82, 83).

Other causes of vascular occlusion also have been described. Recently, activation of inflammatory cells by complement-mediated anaphylatoxins (C3a, C5a), resulting in leukothrombi-causing vessel occlusion, has been observed in the brains of some patients dying of acute cerebral lupus (84). These leukothrombi have been shown to cause infarction, in the absence of vasculitis, in the brain as well as other organs of SLE patients. Another cause of cerebrovascular occlusion is emboli, usually from a cardiac source. Emboli from Libman-Sacks vegetations can cause acute vascular occlusion resulting in strokes. A recent autopsy series has suggested that a cardiac source of emboli in NP-SLE patients may be more common than previously reported (59). Antiphospholipid antibodies have been associated with cerebral artery embolization with fragments from Libman-Sacks–like endocarditis and abnormal heart valves (85–88). Whether these antibodies can directly cause valvular damage, or only contribute to thrombus formation (which can subsequently embolize) on already damaged valves, is presently unclear. Finally, although not truly vascular occlusion, sludging as a result of cryoglobulinemia and hyperviscosity rarely has been reported in patients presenting with mental clouding, dizziness, and confusion (89–92).

Vascular Hemorrhage

Although microhemorrhages are common, larger subarachnoid, intracerebral, and subdural hemorrhages occur in 0.4% to 7.0% of NP-SLE patients. One survey of 500 patients with SLE revealed evidence for cerebrovascular disease in 15, being occlusive in 11 and hemorrhagic in four (93). Several cases of subarachnoid hemorrhage caused by a Berry aneurysm have been described in SLE. It is not known if these aneurysms are more common in SLE patients than in the general population (94–96). A small subset of SLE patients with antiphospholipid antibody have an increased bleeding tendency with neurologic consequences, but this group usually has an associated thrombocytopenia or hypoprothrombinemia. Other causes of cerebral hemorrhage, such as hypertension or thrombotic thrombocytopenic purpura, must be excluded.

Antineuronal Antibodies

Antineuronal antibodies injected into the ventricles of experimental animals cause a variety of neurologic symptoms, such as convulsions and impaired memory, suggesting that brain-reactive antibodies may cause certain NP-SLE manifestations (97–99). Several investigators have reported that up to 75% of SLE patients have elevated levels of serum antineuronal or antilymphocyte antibodies that cross-react with brain tissue (100–105). Some of these studies indicate that NP-SLE patients, particularly those with diffuse manifestations, have these antibodies more commonly than SLE patients without CNS dysfunction (102, 104, 105).

A variety of epitope specificities have been demonstrated as the targets for some of these antineuronal antibodies. Earlier studies showed some antibodies are directed against ganglioside GM_1 (106). More recent studies have demonstrated antineuronal antibodies directed against a 50-kd antigen in the plasma membrane of brain synaptic terminals (107), neurofilaments (108), and ribosomal P protein, which has homology with a 38-kd protein on the surface of human neuroblastoma cells (109). Interestingly, antineurofilament antibodies have been associated more closely with diffuse NP-SLE manifestations (108), whereas antiribosomal P antibodies have been demonstrated most often in NP-SLE patients with psychosis and depression (36). Recently, antiphospholipid antibodies have been shown to permeabilize and depolarize brain synaptoneurosomes (110). This suggests antiphospholipid antibodies have the ability to disrupt neuronal function by direct action on nerve terminals, possibly explaining the nonthrombotic CNS manifestations observed in some lupus patients with antiphospholipid antibodies. Furthermore, anti-β2 glycoprotein-1 antibodies have been reported to bind to astrocytes and neurons, both in culture and histologic sections, in 11 of 20 SLE patients with these antibodies (111).

Serum antineuronal antibodies may be useful markers for NP-SLE, but only can be considered pathogenic if they are demonstrated in the CSF and have the ability to bind directly to brain tissue. Investigators have found CSF IgG antineuronal antibodies in up to 90% of NP-SLE patients compared with less than 10% of SLE patients without CNS manifestations (26, 31, 32, 39, 113). Furthermore, the antineuronal-antibody activity was concentrated to a greater extent in the CSF of these patients relative to a paired serum sample. Similar to serum antineuronal antibodies, the presence and amount of these CSF antibodies correlated best with diffuse manifestations, such as acute confusion, psychosis, generalized seizures, and cognitive dysfunction (26, 31, 39, 112).

Several theories have been proposed to explain how these antineuronal antibodies are generated and get into the cerebrospinal fluid. As previously mentioned, some of the serum antilymphocyte antibodies are cross-reactive with brain tissue. Other serum antineuronal antibodies may have been generated by neuronal antigens released from the brain. Notably, as shown experimentally, the brain does have lymphatic drainage and antigens in the brain may cause a systemic immune response (114). Although normally the blood-brain barrier would prevent these antineuronal antibodies from coming into direct contact with cortical tissues, this barrier could be breached at sites of brain microinfarction caused by vascular occlusions, allowing influx of antineuronal antibodies from the serum. Additionally, ischemia without infarction and increased serotonin (from platelet thrombi) can facilitate immunoglobulin transport from the serum to cerebrospinal fluid (115). Finally, antineuronal antibodies may gain access to the CNS by passage through the choroid plexus.

An alternative explanation is that antineuronal antibodies do not come from the serum, but are derived from local production within the CNS. Recent studies have demonstrated that activated T cells, B cells, and monocytes/macrophages can get through the blood-brain barrier (116). Neuronal antigens, which are normally in an immunologically privileged site protected by the blood-brain barrier, may stimulate these immunocompetent cells within the CNS. Interleukin-6, which has been found to be elevated in the cerebrospinal fluid of patients with NP-SLE, may facilitate the differentiation of these cells into plasma cells capable of intrathecal synthesis of antineuronal antibodies. The demonstration of an elevated IgG index, oligoclonal bands, a normal Q-albumin ratio (suggesting an intact blood-brain barrier), and antineuronal antibodies in the cerebrospinal fluid in some NP-SLE patients, who lack serum antineuronal antibodies, supports this hypothesis (22, 26, 39, 117–122).

Antineuronal antibodies are hypothesized to be able to bind to neuronal membranes and interfere with cell function without causing nerve cell death or inflammation. Binding to neuronal ion channels could lead to recurrent depolarization, increasing susceptibility of the neuron to excitatory amino acid or oxidative, stress-mediated, nerve-cell injury. Alternatively, antineuronal antibodies could interfere with receptor ligand binding, resulting in neuronal dysfunction. Other immunopathogenic mechanisms also are possible. Each of these mechanisms would explain the reversibility of symptoms and the poor correlation of CNS pathologic changes with clinical manifestations seen in NP-SLE patients with antineuronal antibodies.

Choroid Plexus Dysfunction

The choroid plexus differs from the blood-brain barrier in that it has a fenestrated capillary bed and glial cells, which have receptors for immune complexes (123, 124). The choroid plexus is important in the production of CSF and provides a transport-mediated pathway for the influx of certain hormones, vitamins, and other molecules into the CSF. Postmortem examination has demonstrated IgG and complement deposits in the choroid plexus of some SLE patients (125, 126). This deposition could alter the secretory or transport properties of the choroid plexus or result in cytokine release into the CNS, resulting in neuronal dysfunction. However, the significance of choroidal immune reactant deposition remains unclear, because these deposits are seen in SLE patients with and without neurologic symptoms (126).

Cytokine Effects

Patients with active SLE can have elevated serum levels of interleukin-2, interleulin-10, and interferon gamma (see Chapter 10, Cytokine in the Pathogenesis of Systemic Lupus Erythematosus). Cytokines in the systemic circulation may affect the hypothalamus, which lacks the blood-brain barrier, and/or the cerebral microvasculature, resulting in upregulation of adhesion molecules (84). These effects, as well as others, can facilitate the recruitment of activated lymphocytes (T cells more than B cells), monocytes, and macrophages to pass through the blood-brain barrier into the CNS (116). Patients with active NP-SLE can have interleukin-1, interleukin-6, and interferon alpha elevated within their cerebrospinal fluid (127–131). These cytokines can be produced by several regions of the brain or by infiltrating immunocompetent cells from within the CNS (132). Interleukin-1 is important in neuronal injury and repair, causes release of neurotransmitters from brain structures, and through prostaglandin E causes corticotropin-releasing hormone (CRH) release from the hypothalamus (133). Interleukin-6 in the CNS can stimulate B cell differentiation into plasma cells with resultant intrathecal synthesis of immunoglobulin. Interleukin-6 also is important in neuronal differentiation, neuronal repair, and hypothalamic CRH release.

Systemic infusion of interleukin-2 and interferons for therapy of diseases, such as cancers and hepatitis, has resulted in several neurobehavioral side effects (134). Likewise, injection of interleukin-1 into the cerebrospinal fluid of experimental animals causes behavioral disturbances, anorexia, drowsiness, slow wave sleep, and coma with neuronal destruction (135). Thus, the contribution of these and other cytokine effects on the brain in NP-SLE needs to be considered and further investigated.

Neuroendocrine-Immune Systems

There is a complex intercommunication between the nervous, endocrine, and immune systems (136). Most important are the connections between the limbic system (hippocampus, amygdala) of the CNS with the hypothalamic-pituitary-adrenal (HPA) axis and the central noradrenergic and peripheral autonomic nervous systems. The function of these interconnected systems is to restore the body to basal state after being exposed to stress of physical, psychologic, or inflammatory stimuli (137). The degree an individual responds to stress depends on several physical, genetic, and environmental factors, such as age, gender, and reproductive status. Several investigators have postulated that an abnormal stress response partially explains the predilection for SLE to occur in young females in their reproductive years (see Chapter 17, Neuroendocrine Immune Interactions: Principles and Relevance to Systemic Lupus).

The systemic immune activation occurring in SLE could result in a chronic stress response, resulting in persistent activation of the HPA axis and noradrenergic systems. Chronically elevated glucocorticoid levels can result in hippocampal atrophy, resulting in abnormalities in spatial and declarative memory (138). Furthermore, excessive cortisol decreases the synaptic uptake of glutamate, resulting in increased glutamate levels, which could cause excitatory amino-acid–mediated neuronal injury (139). To what extent this plays a role in neuropsychiatric manifestations in SLE patients presently is unclear and is the subject of ongoing research (140).

Central Nervous System Tissue Injury

Oxidative stress and excitatory amino acid (EAA) toxicity are the two major mechanisms responsible for nerve-cell injury and death within the CNS. Oxidative stress causing nerve-cell injury and apoptosis involves the production of nitric oxide. Nitric oxide is produced by the interaction of the enzyme, nitric-oxide synthetase (NOS), and L-arginine (141). There are three major forms of NOS. Two of the isoforms are constitutively expressed (cNOS) (e.g., neuronal cNOS and endothelial cNOS). One of the isoforms is inducible (iNOS) and expressed by many cells, including those that can constitutively express cNOS. Constitutively expressed nitric-oxide synthetases produce small amounts of nitric oxide, which play a protective role in the nervous system and microvasculature. This protection is caused by the capacity of nitric oxide to inhibit platelet and neutrophil adhesion to endothelial cells, as well as to inhibit leukocyte superoxide anion production. In contrast to the cNOS isoforms, iNOS is expressed after exposure to various stimuli, including inflammatory cytokines such as interleukin-1. The inducible form of NOS binds to calmodulin and generates large and sustained amounts of nitric oxide. Nitric oxide is labile and, in the presence of oxygen, is metabolized rapidly to nitrate and nitrite. Nitric oxide also can react with superoxide anions, resulting in the production of the toxic hydroxyl radical, which leads to nerve-cell death. Nitric oxide also can promote oxidative injury via formation of peroxynitrous acid. Additionally, nitric oxide can directly nitrosylate the N-methyl-D-aspartate (NMDA) receptor, causing inactivation of membrane ion channels and nerve dysfunction (142). Recently, increased expression of iNOS by endothelial cells was found in patients with active SLE (143). This upregulation of vascular iNOS in SLE patients may be the result of immune complexes, complement components, cytokines, and/or antiphospholipid antibodies. This could result in excessive nitric-oxide production leading to nerve-cell injury as well as other toxicities.

EAA toxicity is the second mechanism for nerve-cell injury and death (144). Glutamate is the most important EAA neurotransmitter in the brain and is important in many normal neurologic functions. However, overproduction of glutamate, causing overstimulation of glutamate receptors, can result in excessive influx of positively charged ions and water, resulting in neuronal-cell swelling, injury, or death. Some neurons, such as those in the hippocampus, are more vulnerable to glutamate than other neurons. This most likely is because of variation in repertoire and density of glutamate receptors in different areas of the brain. Furthermore, stresses such as ischemia, recurrent depolarization (seizures), and cytokines within the CNS can make individual neurons more sensitive to EAA toxicity, even when exposed to only minor insults. The role EAA toxicity has in NP-SLE is unclear and an area of future research.

Summary

Although our understanding of the pathogenetic mechanisms involved in NP-SLE has advanced over the past two decades, it is still incomplete. Clearly, the cerebral vasculature plays an important role. If the vascular endothelium allows the deposition of immune complexes, then an inflammatory vasculitis can result. Alternatively, simultaneous activation of endothelial cells and neutrophil adhesion molecules by cytokines (interleukin-1) and biologically active complement split products (C5a desarg) can cause a local Shwartzman phenomenon, resulting in leukothrombosis and vasoocclusive plugs. Additionally, antiphospholipid antibodies are prothrombotic and may result in acute vasoocclusive thromboemboli or chronically cause endothelial-cell proliferation and intimal fibrosis, commonly observed in the bland vasculopathy seen in NP-SLE patients. Each of these mechanisms can lead to vascular occlusion (less commonly hemorrhage) leading to focal neurologic manifestations and seizures.

Antineuronal antibodies with specificity against lymphocytic, neuronal membrane, and neuronal intracellular antigens have been demonstrated to occur with increased frequency in the serum of NP-SLE patients. Some of these may breach the blood-brain barrier and gain entrance into the CSF. Alternatively, activated lymphocytes within the CNS may make antineuronal antibodies, which can bind to neuronal cells or receptors, resulting in neuronal dysfunction without nerve-cell death or inflammation. These antineuronal antibodies could lead to diffuse manifestations such as acute confusion, coma, and seizures.

Cytokine effects and abnormalities in the neuroendocrine-immune system undoubtedly play a role in some of the neuropsychiatric manifestations observed in NP-SLE patients. Cytokines such as interleukin-1 can upregulate endothelial adhesion molecules, contributing to the development of vasculitis or leukothrombi. Cytokines within the CSF have been shown to cause cognitive and behavioral disturbances commonly observed in SLE patients. Additionally, cytokines such as interleukin-1 can upregulate iNOS, resulting in excessive nitric-oxide production and nerve-cell injury. Furthermore, inflammatory cytokines within the CNS can sensitize neurons to be more prone to injury from EAA toxicity.

Finally, the chronic immune stimulation may stress normal homeostasis, resulting in abnormalities in the neuroendocrine-immune system. Persistent activation of the HPA axis may result in chronically elevated glucocorticoid levels, leading to hippocampal atrophy. Likewise, chronic activation of the sympathetic and autonomic nervous systems may cause vasoconstriction and alteration in cerebral blood flow. Both of these mechanisms could lead to the mild cognitive dysfunction, memory problems, and abnormalities in neuroimaging observed in many SLE patients.

CLINICAL MANIFESTATIONS

NP-SLE can involve the CNS, the peripheral/autonomic nervous system, and/or myoneural junction. An SLE patient can present with diffuse, focal, or a combination of symptoms (Table 35.1). The chief manifestations are symptoms of global dysfunction without any focal abnormalities, whereas focal symptoms are manifestations that can be attributed to a specific brain area. Clinical signs and symptoms can be mild and transient dysfunction to severe presentations, resulting in permanent neurologic sequelae and/or death. This diversity of manifestations and severity results from the several different immunopathogenic mechanisms that can affect various areas of an anatomically and physiologically complex nervous system. The clinician must always be aware that neurologic abnormalities in SLE patients may not be NP-SLE, but secondary to infection, electrolyte abnormalities, or numerous other causes (Table 35.4).

Many of the cognitive, level of consciousness, behavioral, and personality abnormalities observed in SLE patients are difficult to classify. In the past, these have been termed acute or chronic organic brain syndrome, which now has been abandoned. This has been replaced by the term "encephalopathy," which is diffuse-cerebral dysfunction associated with a disturbance in consciousness, cognition, mood, affect, and behavior. The ad-hoc American College of Rheumatology (ACR) committee on neuropsychiatric lupus nomenclature felt that encephalopathy was too generalized and decided to separate it into its more specific presentations (10). This committee's recommended classification has been used for the discussion of clinical manifestations.

Acute-Confusional State

Acute-confusional state is defined as disturbance of consciousness or level of arousal characterized by reduced ability to focus, maintain, or shift attention to external stimuli, and accompanied by disturbances of cognition, mood, affect, and/or behavior (10). This has been termed delirium in the DSM IV and ICD-9 diagnostic classifications. Disorganized thinking, loss of orientation, agitation, and delusions can be present. Symptoms may fluctuate or progress. An ominous sign is progression to a reduced level of consciousness, such as stupor or coma. Acute-confusional state is one of the most common presentations observed in up to 30% of NP-SLE patients (26). Vasculitis, leukothrombosis, and autoantibodies all have been described as causes of acute confusion. Notably, this also is a common presentation of SLE patients with neuropsychiatric disturbances caused by cerebral infections, medications, thrombotic thrombocytopenic purpura (TTP), and metabolic disturbances, which always must be excluded.

Cognitive Dysfunction

Cognitive dysfunction can range from mild cognitive impairment to dementia, where there are chronic abnormalities in multiple domains of attention, reasoning, memory, language, visual-spatial processing, psychomotor speed, and executive function (10). Mild-cognitive impairment first was noted in SLE patients without a history of NP-SLE by Goodwin and Goodwin (145). The Denburgs, as well as others, have extended this observation and report that up to 66% of adult SLE patients have mild cognitive impairment on comprehensive neuropsychological testing, compared to less than 20% of rheumatoid arthritis patients and normal controls (145–150). This dysfunction includes various deficits, as there is no specific SLE pattern of abnormalities (151). In the majority of patients, these abnormalities are subclinical and do not significantly impact their quality of life. In a five-year prospective study, Hanly et al. reported that only 20% of patients, who had mild cognitive impairment on neuropsychological tests, went on to develop clinically overt NP-SLE, while 19% resolved their cognitive dysfunction on follow-up testing without any therapy (152).

The pathogenesis of cognitive dysfunction in SLE is unclear. Most studies have demonstrated an association between cognitive impairment and active NP-SLE, but have not shown an association with active SLE, corticosteroid use, or psychological distress (147–158). However, Hay et al. reported that many SLE patients with mild cognitive abnormalities have psychiatric problems, which could cause the cognitive dysfunction (159, 160). An association has been reported by some investigators between cognitive abnormalities and elevated serum–anti-DNA antibodies, serum-antilymphocytotoxic/antineuronal antibodies, serum-antiphospholipid antibodies, and CSF IgG antineuronal antibodies, suggesting this dysfunction is a result of autoantibodies or cytokines (33–35, 161–164). However, antiribosomal P antibodies are not associated (150, 158), and some investigators have not confirmed the association between antilymphocytotoxic/antineuronal antibodies and mild cognitive impairment (158).

Many SLE patients (up to 88%) with a previous history of NP-SLE have significant cognitive dysfunction on neuropsychological testing (146). Some patients can progress to dementia with global cognitive dysfunction marked by impairment in short- and long-term memory and disturbances in judgment, abstract thinking, and other higher cortical functions. The degree of cognitive impairment may be severe, interfering with the patient's ability to live independently. Dementia can be a result of active NP-SLE, the result of scarring from previously active NP-SLE, or from multiple infarctions as a result of antiphospholipid antibodies (165, 166).

Most studies of cognitive impairment have used adult SLE patients as study subjects. However, Papero et al. (167) have reported cognitive impairment associated with antineuronal antibodies in children with SLE. Recently, a study of eight children with SLE demonstrated mean intellectual scores were in the low-to-average range and visual memory was depressed. Academic achievement was globally depressed and reading comprehension averaged 5 years below-grade placement (168).

Psychosis

Psychosis is defined as a severe disturbance in the perception of reality, characterized by delusions and/or hallucinations. Psychosis occurs in 5% to 30% of NP-SLE patients (Table 35.3). The sudden onset of psychosis in an SLE patient without a prior psychiatric history or precipitating cause usually is indicative of NP-SLE. Some investigators have reported an association between antiribosomal P antibodies and psychosis (169–173). Titers of these antibodies would rise with exacerbation of psychosis and decrease in response to corticosteroid therapy. Other studies have not found a correlation between these antibodies and psychosis (37, 174, 175) (see Chapter 36).

Mood And Anxiety Disorders

Severe affective disorders such as major depression and anxiety/panic disorders can be NP-SLE manifestations. Some previous studies have included these manifestations under the category of "lupus psychosis." Whether these psychiatric problems are a direct manifestation of NP-SLE, or a reaction to a chronic illness or other psychosocial factors, is unclear. However, antiribosomal P antibodies, cytokine effects, and alterations of the HPA and other neuroendocrine axes each have been associated with severe depression (137, 170), suggesting that mood disorders can be a manifestation of NP-SLE.

Previous studies have reported a high prevalence of nonpsychotic psychopathology in SLE patients (176). However, a recent review noted that previous studies were too methodologically limited to permit drawing confident conclusions about the prevalence and etiology of psychiatric abnormalities in SLE patients (177). An attempt was made to overcome some of these limitations in a population-based study reporting the prevalence of lifetime psychiatric disorders among all SLE patients in Iceland (178). Approximately 50% of SLE patients received one or more psychiatric diagnoses over the course of their disease. This was in agreement with a 46.5% prevalence of nonpsychotic, psychiatric disturbances in a cross-sectional study of 42 SLE patients, compared with 15.6% of healthy controls (179). Another study of 80 consecutively treated SLE patients found that psychiatric dysfunction was more closely associated with psychosocial factors than with measures of disease activity (180). These studies found depression, anxiety, phobias, and difficulty coping to be the most common psychiatric abnormalities. Determining if these abnormalities are from NP-SLE or emotional stress can be a challenge to the clinician. However, clearly, patients with good disease-coping strategies and better social support have significantly less depression and a better functional outcome, when followed over time (181) (see Chapter 36).

Headache

Headaches are common in SLE patients, occurring in up to 45% to 50% of patients (45, 182–185). Despite its frequency, the nature of headache in lupus was not addressed until 1975. At that time, Atkinson and Appenzeller described a headache syndrome that was distinct for SLE and independent of hypertension and other secondary causes of headache (186). Brandt and Lessel studied, in detail, 11 SLE patients that had "migrainous phenomenon." These patients' headaches were associated with disease activity, abnormal CSF findings, abnormal electroencephalograms (EEGs), and usually responded to corticosteroid treatment (187). Most investigators believe that headache, as a manifestation of NP-SLE, is characterized by an acute presentation during a lupus flare, frequent association with other neurologic complications and abnormal laboratory tests, and resolution during corticosteroid therapy, as the lupus disease activity improves.

Many SLE patients have headaches, which are not related to the disease activity or other manifestations of lupus. Several studies have shown these headaches to be either migrainous or tension-type headaches with approximately equal frequency (184, 188, 189). Earlier controlled and uncontrolled studies suggested that headache was increased in prevalence in SLE patients (188–190). However, selection criteria for patients and controls, methodology used to collect data, and lack of use of accepted criteria for definition of headache and its severity make the results of these studies difficult to interpret. Recently, Fernandez-Nebro et al. reported, in a well-controlled study, that the overall prevalence of headache, tension-type headache, and migraine was similar among SLE patients and healthy controls (184).

Migraine headaches occur in up to 20% to 25% of SLE patients, which is similar to a normal, healthy, young, female population. Recent studies suggest that migraine headache in the general population has a strong genetic component and is a result of an abnormality of the trigeminovascular system (191). Previous studies have suggested that migraine headache in SLE patients was associated with Raynaud's phenomenon, antiphospholipid antibodies, and/or thrombotic events (192–194). However, three controlled studies of over 275 patients have failed to confirm these observations (184, 195, 196).

Benign intracranial hypertension (pseudotumor cerebri) occasionally can occur in NP-SLE patients. Patients present with refractory headaches, papilledema, and no focal neurologic symptoms. Lumbar puncture reveals increased intracranial pressure (>200 mm H_2O), normal protein, and no white blood cells in the CSF. There have been less than 30 reported cases (197–200). Although it can occur in adults, most patients are adolescent females with severe SLE. Several patients had rapid corticosteroid withdrawal and one half had dural-venous sinus thrombosis as a potential cause of their pseudotumor cerebri. Up to 60% had clinical or laboratory evidence of hypercoagulability manifested by history of thromboembolic episodes, nephrotic syndrome, or elevated antiphospholipid antibodies (197). Therapy included multiple lumbar punctures and/or corticosteroids in all patients. Some patients also received acetazolamide, anticoagulants (two patients), or intravenous gammaglobulin (one patient).

Secondary causes must be ruled out in all patients before ascribing a severe headache to NP-SLE. The most common or important ones include: hypertension, infection, nonsteroidal antiinflammatory medications, antimalarial therapy, sleep apnea, subdural hematoma, and intracranial hemorrhage.

Cerebrovascular Disease

Cerebrovascular accidents occur in 5% to 15% of SLE patients (38, 40, 201, 202). Stroke syndromes secondary to NP-SLE can affect any area of the brain (203, 204). Patients can present acutely with TIAs, hemiplegia, aphasia, cortical blindness (205), or other deficits of cerebral function. Strokes usually occur within the first 5 years of the onset of SLE; and between 13% and 64% of patients, who have had a stroke, will have a recurrent stroke resulting in significant morbidity and a 28% to 40% mortality rate (40, 206).

The etiology of strokes in SLE can be from vasculitis, a noninflammatory vasculopathy, thrombosis associated with a coagulopathy, leukothrombosis, emboli from cardiac valvular lesions, and intraparenchymal or subarachnoid hemorrhage (see pathogenesis section). SLE patients with Sneddon's syndrome present with a combination of stroke and livedo reticularis. This syndrome has been associated with antiphospholipid antibodies (81). There also is evidence for accelerated atherosclerosis occurring in SLE patients, which can lead to early cerebrovascular disease (207).

Several investigators have identified risk factors for strokes in SLE patients. Futrell et al. reported that 94% of their 18 SLE patients with strokes had at least one of the following risk factors: age greater than 60, previous stroke or TIA, antiphospholipid antibodies, or cardiac valvular disease (40). The five SLE patients with both cardiac valvular disease and coagulopathy had a 100% risk of stroke, compared to the 77 SLE patients who did not have these risk factors and did not subsequently develop a stroke. Levine and Welch reported that over 50% of patients with antiphospholipid antibodies and strokes had hypertension, hyperlipidemia, diabetes mellitus, or smoked cigarettes, each of which can contribute to increased stroke risk (208). Early clinical experience suggests that the use of the specific cyclooxygenase-2 inhibitors in SLE patients with these risk factors may contribute to the risk of subsequent clotting. These studies point out that control of hypertension, elevated cholesterol, and blood-glucose levels, as well as smoking cessation, must be part of the treatment plan to prevent stroke or recurrence of stroke.

The diagnosis of cerebrovascular disease is made clinically and supported by neuroimaging studies. A computed tomography (CT) scan of the brain is capable of detecting cerebral hemorrhage and large infarcts, making it a useful study in screening SLE patients with acute neurologic deterioration. Cranial MRI with contrast is superior to CT scan in detecting smaller and frequently transient lesions. MRI typically shows hyperintense gray- and white-matter lesions on T2-weighted images, which account for the patient's clinical symptoms. Additional lesions in clinically silent areas also are frequently observed. Magnetic resonance angiography, carotid Doppler ultrasound, and echocardiogram are noninvasive procedures, which can be useful in detecting large-vessel vasculitis, thrombosis, or sources of emboli, leading to vascular occlusion and stroke. Angiograms are more likely to show abnormalities in patients with larger infarcts. CSF examination may show pleocytosis and high protein in patients with cerebral vasculitis or blood in patients with subarachnoid hemorrhage. Otherwise, the CSF examination usually is normal or demonstrates nonspecific abnormalities, such as a few cells and/or high protein.

Treatment of strokes in SLE patients is based on the suspected pathogenesis. Patients with suspected vasculitis are treated with corticosteroids and cytotoxic drugs, while those with a coagulopathy or cardiac emboli are treated with anticoagulation. Treatment of patients with strokes as a result of a noninflammatory vasculopathy is difficult because the pathogenesis of these vascular lesions is unclear. Although not proven to reduce stroke in SLE patients, most clinicians put these patients on aspirin or other platelet inhibitors and aggressively treat stroke risk factors. The value of corticosteroids in these patients is uncertain and potentially could contribute to stroke risk by increasing hypertension, cholesterol, and blood glucose. Patients, however, often are given corticosteroids to control other accompanying lupus manifestations.

Myelopathy

Spinal-cord myelopathy is an infrequent but devastating manifestation of NP-SLE. Patients present with progressive or sudden weakness or paralysis (paraplegia or quadriplegia), bilateral sensory deficits, and impaired sphincter control. It occurs in less than 1% of patients and can be the initial presentation of SLE (209, 210). Dubois (11) found lupus myelopathy in two of his 520 patients between 1950 and 1963, and Pistiner found myelopathy in two of his 464 SLE cohort followed between 1980 and 1989 (23). Alarcon-Segovia's group in Mexico reported four cases of myelopathy among 500 SLE patients (211). Spinal-cord myelopathy also can occur in pediatric and neonatal lupus (212, 213).

There have been several reviews of the reported cases of lupus myelopathy (210, 214–216). These reports agree that most patients (80%) are young females between ages 20 to 40 years old. Of the first 28 patients, myelopathy was the initial manifestation in three, and 11 had no prior diagnosis of SLE. Two were quadriplegic, seven paraparetic, and 19 paraplegic (214). Weakness, sensory loss, and impaired sphincter control were abnormal in all patients, while hyperreflexia was seen in less than 25% at initial presentation. These reviews report CSF abnormalities in the majority of patients, including elevated protein (>80%), pleocytosis (50% to 70%), and decreased glucose levels less than 30 mg% (50%). The CSF, however, can be normal and may contain elevated levels of myelin-basic protein (217). Of the nine patients who underwent myelograms, eight had normal studies. There have been several additional case reports and case series, which have reinforced these clinical findings.

The diagnosis of myelopathy is made clinically. MRI of the spinal cord can help confirm the diagnosis and exclude other causes of spinal cord compression, which may benefit from surgery. MRI in lupus myelopathy typically shows edema with abnormalities of T2-weighted images, which may be accompanied by spinal-cord enlargement in 75% of patients (218–220). Any level of the spinal cord can be involved (221). Notably, some patients may have a normal MRI, especially if the examination is delayed (>5 days) or the patient has received treatment (220). The differential diagnosis includes the following: compressive myelopathy [tumor, abscess, hematoma (222)], epidural lipomatosis (223), vertebral compression fracture (224), anterior spinal-artery syndrome (225), infection (herpes zoster, tuberculosis, polyoma JC virus) (226–228), and Guillain-Barré syndrome (229). The etiology of lupus myelopathy is multifactorial. Small series have reported neuropathologic changes to include arteritis (Fig. 35.2), perivascular-lymphocytic infiltrates and myelitis, thrombosis of small and big arteries and veins, ischemic necrosis of the cord, microhemorrhages, spinal-cord subdural hematomas, and myelomalacia of the cord (214, 230). Although vasculitis during an acute exacerbation of SLE has been reported, many patients do not have active SLE at the time of their presentation. Lavalle and others have reported that SLE patients with myelopathy frequently have antiphospholipid antibodies (76, 211, 231).

In their 1989 review, Propper and Bucknall emphasized the poor prognosis of the reported cases of lupus myelopathy (215). Of 26 patients, seven had a full recovery, nine a static

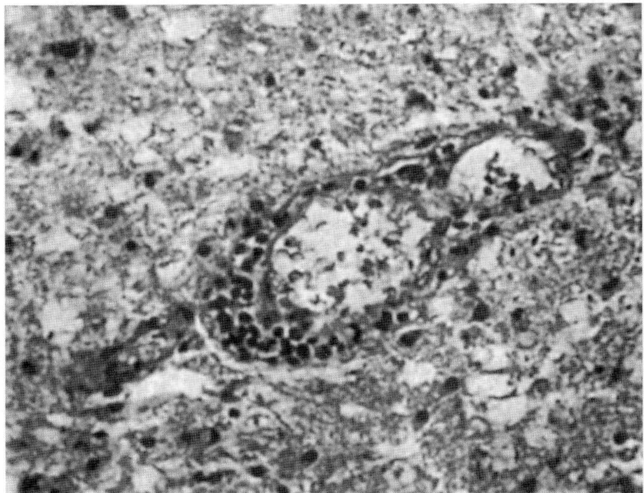

FIGURE 35.2. Acute arteritis and edema of surrounding tissue in the spinal cord of a 22-year-old patient with paraplegia caused by lupus vasculitis (H&E; 750).

or slowly deteriorating course, and ten died. Of eight patients who promptly received high-dose corticosteroids, five recovered, compared with only two of 18 who did not receive steroids. Conversely, Hachen and Chantraine (232) reviewed 28 cases and felt that steroids can worsen myelomalacia, which could lead to further motor and sensory losses.

More recent reports have emphasized that the use of pulsed methylprednisolone and cyclophosphamide may improve the prognosis of patients with lupus myelopathy (231, 233–235). This therapy must be used early, because 50% of patients will reach their peak severity of myelopathy symptoms within 3 to 5 days of onset. Early use of aggressive therapy has resulted in reversal of symptoms and stabilization in the majority of patients. In patients with significant titers of antiphospholipid antibodies, anticoagulation probably should be used, although studies are limited. Recurrences of myelopathy, particularly within the first year, are common. Rehabilitation measures to prevent pressure sores; preserve range of motion, strength, and mobility; and institute appropriate bladder management also should be initiated early.

Movement Disorders

Chorea, hemiballismus, cerebellar ataxia, and Parkinsonian-like rigidity/tremor are rare manifestations. Chorea is the most common, occurring in 1% to 4% of patients with SLE. Chorea is characterized by rapid, brief, involuntary, and irregular movements. It may be generalized or limited to the extremities, trunk, or face. Choreoathetosis is diagnosed when chorea is accompanied by slow, writhing movements of the affected extremity. Chorea occurs most commonly in young females, children, and during pregnancy (chorea gravidarum) or the postpartum period (236–240). It may be the initial presentation of SLE or precede other manifestations of SLE by as long as 7 years (236). Chorea usually occurs early in the course of SLE, tends to be bilateral, rarely is recurrent, and frequently is associated with other NP-SLE symptoms such as strokes. The CSF examination is frequently unremarkable (236). The symptoms of chorea usually last for several weeks, but rarely can last for up to 3 years (238).

Infarction of the subthalamic nucleus can result in hemiballismus (241). It rarely has been reported in SLE. Ballismus may be steroid responsive (242) or related to antiphospholipid antibodies (243). Cerebellar ataxia is reported in less than 1% of patients with SLE (244, 245). Patients have an inability to stop or end purposeful movements. The abnormalities may involve the trunk or extremities. The etiology is uncertain, but some cases may be from cerebellar/brainstem infarction (204, 246), antiphospholipid antibodies, or associated with Purkinje's cell antibodies (247). In patients with cerebellar atrophy associated with antibodies against Purkinje's cells, a paraneoplastic syndrome must be ruled out before attributing it to NP-SLE (248).

Tremor of all types has been reported in up to 5% of SLE patients during the course of their disease (249). However, Parkinsonianlike symptoms resulting from alterations of the substantia nigra are an extremely rare manifestation of NP-SLE. Miyoshi et al. (250) presented a case with a literature review of three previous reports. Recently, two adolescent females with severe, extrapyramidal Parkinsonism complicating SLE were reported (251). Patients presented with behavioral alterations (irritability or apathy), rigidity and progressive bradykinesia, and/or akinetic mutism. The EEG showed mild abnormalities, but single photon emission computed tomography (SPECT) cerebral scanning detected decreased regional cerebral blood flow at the basal ganglia. Treatment with dopamine-agonist drugs led to complete recovery within 3 months, along with normalization of the EEG and SPECT scans.

The etiology of chorea is unknown. Autopsy studies have not shown vasculitis (252). Multiple infarction of the basal ganglia (caudate, putamen, globus pallidus, or subthalamic nucleus) has been reported, which may lead to defective control of the thalamus, leading to abnormal movements. Recently, chorea has been associated with antiphospholipid antibodies, which can cause brain infarctions. In 1986, Hadron et al. reanalyzed the previously reported cases of chorea and determined that at least 20 of the patients had spontaneous abortions, false-positive serologic test results for syphilis, or evidence for the lupus anticoagulant (239). Asherson et al. observed chorea in 12 of 500 SLE patients (240). Of these 12 patients, nine had antiphospholipid antibodies and seven also had TIAs or cerebral infarcts. Others have confirmed this association (253, 254); and two case reports have claimed an association of chorea with antiphospholipid antibodies, SLE, and oral-contraceptive use (255, 256). Notably, however, Lafeuillade et al. (253) cautioned that not all patients with chorea have antiphospholipid antibodies or abnormal MRIs of the brain. A recent study of four patients with SLE and chorea failed to find basal ganglia hypometabolism, which should be found if the striatum had been infarcted (257). This suggests that, in some patients, other mechanisms such as antineuronal antibodies may be an alternative pathogenetic process.

There is a long differential diagnosis of illnesses rarely associated with chorea. Sydenham's chorea, secondary to rheumatic fever, is the most common and can be ruled out by obtaining antistreptococcal antibodies. However, the onset of chorea in a young woman with a positive antinuclear antibody (ANA) should suggest strongly SLE. The recommended treatment of chorea has been corticosteroids and neuroleptic drugs such as haloperidol. Some patients recover spontaneously, while others fail to respond to immunosuppressive therapy. Asherson et al. has recommended aspirin or anticoagulation in patients with chorea and antiphospholipid antibodies (240). More studies are needed, however.

Demyelinating Syndrome

A multiple sclerosis-like syndrome, sometimes called lupoid sclerosis, has been described in SLE patients (258–264). Interestingly, both multiple sclerosis and NP-SLE can share many features including clinical presentation, Lhermitte's sign (265), positive ANA, abnormal CSF with elevated IgG index and oligoclonal bands, and abnormal brain MRIs. Whether both diseases can coexist in one patient, or lupoid sclerosis is just an unusual presentation of NP-SLE, is unclear. Recently, antiphospholipid antibodies have been demonstrated in a number of patients with multiple sclerosis-like illnesses, suggesting these antibodies may be pathogenic in lupoid sclerosis (263–266).

Patients with definite multiple sclerosis have an acute, relapsing, demyelinating encephalomyelitis with discreet neurologic events distributed in place and time (267). Patients characteristically develop, at different time points, the following: limb weakness with sensory loss, transverse myelitis, optic neuritis, cranial nerve palsies often leading to diplopia, sphincter dysfunction, and/or brainstem or cerebellar abnormalities. Cognitive dysfunction and mood alterations also can be seen. CSF analysis shows elevated IgG index, multiple oligoclonal bands, and myelin basic protein (268). Brain MRI (269) shows discreet, low-density lesions often in the periventricular area as well as other areas of the white matter throughout the CNS. Lesions in the corpus callosum are particularly characteristic, because this is an area of relative avascularity, suggesting a demyelinating lesion instead of a vascular etiology. A previous retrospective study reported that 27% of 150 patients with multiple sclerosis had a positive ANA (270). However, a more recent, prospective study found that only one of 48 multiple sclerosis patients had a positive ANA (271). Multiple sclerosis patients with positive ANA should not have autoantibodies against specific antigens such as Sjögren's syndrome A (SS-A), Sjögren's syndrome B (SS-B), Smith, ribonuclear protein, or double-stranded DNA, nor should they have hypocomplementemia. Recently, two studies reported that multiple sclerosis patients occasionally have anticardiolipin antibodies (272, 273). Notably, these multiple sclerosis patients frequently had transverse myelitis, which is a known manifestation of antiphospholipid antibody syndrome. In summary, any multiple sclerosis patient with a positive ANA, hypocomplementemia, or antiphospholipid antibodies should be reevaluated for an alternative diagnosis such as primary antiphospholipid antibody syndrome, SLE, or Sjögren's syndrome.

Patients with antiphospholipid antibodies can have multiple sclerosis-like presentations (266, 274). They frequently have transverse myelitis with or without optic neuritis. They may have livedo reticularis of the skin. The MRI of these patients may be indistinguishable from multiple sclerosis (266, 275), however the pathophysiology is felt to be different. Patients with antiphospholipid antibodies develop their lesions as a result of vascular occlusion, while multiple sclerosis patients develop demyelinating plaques. Laboratory evaluation shows the patients have the lupus anticoagulant and/or anticardiolipin antibodies (IgG or IgM). When tested, they also have anti-β2 glycoprotein-1 antibodies, which are felt to be more specific for antiphospholipid antibody-mediated disease. CSF evaluation reveals the majority of these patients have normal IgG indexes, negative oligoclonal bands, and negative myelin basic protein antibodies (276, 279, 280). In SLE patients (irrespective of antiphospholipid antibody status) who have oligoclonal bands in their CSF, the average number of bands is less than the number seen in multiple sclerosis patients and may disappear with immunosuppressive therapy, which does not occur in multiple sclerosis (277–280).

The therapy of patients with lupoid sclerosis differs from multiple sclerosis therapy. Both patient populations may respond to immunosuppressive therapy. However, SLE patients with lupoid sclerosis resulting from vascular occlusion from antiphospholipid antibodies are best treated with anticoagulation. Therapies used for multiple sclerosis such as beta interferon or Copaxone (Teva Pharmaceutical Industries, Limited) have not been evaluated in lupoid sclerosis, but are unlikely to be effective.

Seizures

Seizures occur in 10% to 20% of patients with SLE (Table 35.3). They may occur prior to the development of other symptoms of SLE or at any time during its course (281–284). Generalized major-motor and partial-complex seizures are most common, although any kind of seizure can occur. Seizure episodes usually are self-limited, although status epilepticus can occur and frequently signals a preterminal event. Seizures may occur in isolation or accompany other neurologic symptoms.

The etiology of seizures in NP-SLE is multifactorial. Antineuronal antibodies, focal ischemia, and infarcts resulting from vascular occlusion from thrombosis and emboli, hemorrhage, and cytokine or neuroendocrine effects on the seizure threshold all have been implicated. Several studies have shown an association between antiphospholipid antibodies and seizures in SLE patients (285–287). There is increased risk of seizures with higher titers of antiphospholipid antibodies (287). Liou et al. have demonstrated that anticardiolipin antibodies from SLE patients with seizures can inhibit the γ-aminobutyric acid (GABA) receptor-ion channel complex system, and this may increase cellular excitability (288). Chapman et al. reported that antiphospholipid antibodies may bind, permeabilize, and depolarize brain synaptoneurosomes, possibly leading to neuronal dysfunction by a nonthrombotic mechanism (110). However, most seizures in patients with antiphospholipid antibodies probably are because of cerebral ischemia from cerebral microinfarctions. Secondary causes of seizures include: infections, medication effects, metabolic disturbances, hypoxemia, and hypertension, which must be ruled out in all SLE patients with seizures.

Most patients with seizures resulting from NP-SLE will respond to anticonvulsant medications. Although some anticonvulsants have been shown to cause a positive ANA and rarely clinical SLE, this is not a reason to withhold these medications when they are indicated for patients with established lupus. Seizure control is important because recurrent seizures increase the vulnerability of neurons to additional injury. Consequently, in patients with status epilepticus, recurrent seizures, or other neurologic manifestations, corticosteroids and other immunosuppressive medications may be used. SLE patients with high-titer antiphospholipid antibodies and seizures also should receive anticoagulation, especially if the brain MRI shows areas of microinfarction.

Aseptic Meningitis

SLE patients with aseptic meningitis present with fever, headache, meningeal signs, and CSF pleocytosis with normal CSF glucose (289–291). The pleocytosis is most commonly less than 200 to 300 cells/mm^3 and predominantly lymphocytes. Rarely, significantly higher cell counts with a neutrophil predominance can occur in severely ill patients. Infectious meningitis of any cause (292), subarachnoid hemorrhage, carcinomatous meningitis, sarcoidosis, and medication effects, such as from nonsteroidal antiinflammatory drugs (ibuprofen, tolmetin, indomethacin, and sulindac) as well as from intravenous gammaglobulin and azathioprine, must be excluded (293). The etiology of aseptic meningitis in NP-SLE is unclear, but patients usually respond to corticosteroid therapy.

Cranial Neuropathies

Cranial neuropathy occurs in 3% to 16% of SLE patients during the course of their disease. It usually occurs during active SLE, can be transient, and usually responds to corticosteroid therapy. Ptosis (294), third and sixth nerve palsies (295–297), internuclear ophthalmoplegia (298), trigeminal neuralgia (299, 300), and facial nerve palsies are the most common. Optic neuropathy causing blindness (301), tinnitus, vertigo, and sensorineural hearing loss are less common symptoms (302). The etiology of cranial neuropathies include vascular occlusion and focal meningitis. Autopsy studies have demonstrated lesions in the brainstem as well as the peripheral part of the cranial nerves (56). Some of these neuropathies have been associated with vasculitis and others with thrombosis associated with antiphospholipid antibodies (303). Keane reported a retrospective study describing eye movement abnormalities in 113 hospitalized SLE patients seen by a neuroophthalmology service over a 25-year period (304). Of 55 oculomotor abnormalities, 33 involved limitation of eye movements or abnormal eye position at rest. Many of the abnormalities were subtle or transient. Sixteen of these 33 patients had evidence of brainstem infarcts causing cranial-nerve dysfunction.

Other unusual presentations or causes of cranial nerve dysfunction in SLE have been reported. These include bilateral facial nerve palsy caused by angioedema (305), painful ophthalmoplegia (306), Brown's syndrome (307, 308), Miller-Fisher syndrome (309), cavernous sinus thrombosis (310), and visual disturbances resulting from lymphocytic hypophysitis (311).

PERIPHERAL POLYNEUROPATHIES

Peripheral nervous system involvement occurs in 2% to 21% of SLE patients (Table 35.3). Two recent cross-sectional studies of 30 and 31 patients, respectively, both found a 6.5% prevalence of peripheral sensorimotor neuropathy on extensive neuromuscular testing (312, 313). The most common presentation is a distal sensorimotor neuropathy (66% of patients) (312–317). Less commonly, patients can have mononeuritis multiplex (14, 318, 319), acute or chronic polyradiculopathy (320–322), and rarely, a plexopathy (323, 324). Peripheral nervous system involvement can be the initial presentation of SLE (314, 318). Symptoms can be severe or subtle and overlooked by the clinician.

Patients with distal, symmetric, peripheral polyneuropathy can present with a mild to severe sensory or sensorimotor fiber involvement. Patients mainly have small, nonmyelinated afferent fiber involvement and complain of numbness and dysesthesias. Neurologic testing shows cutaneous hypesthesia to pinprick, light touch, and temperature stimuli. Less commonly, there is large, myelinated afferent fiber involvement, which manifests as deficits of vibratory and proprioceptive sense, areflexia, and sensory ataxia (325) with variable motor dysfunction. When motor axons are affected, weakness and muscle atrophy are seen. Electrodiagnostic studies usually show features of a mixed axonal and demyelinating neuropathy. The pathogenesis of the peripheral neuropathy is unclear. Antineuronal antibodies and vasculitis (315–317) from deposition of immune complexes have both been implicated (326).

Mononeuritis multiplex presents as multifocal and random dysfunction of individual, noncontiguous nerve trunks. Patients frequently present with development of sensorimotor deficits in the upper or lower extremities (wrist or foot drop) with an asymmetric distribution (Fig. 35.3). Occasionally, it can be widespread and mimic a distal, symmetric polyneuropathy. It typically occurs in the setting of active SLE, often with other neurologic abnormalities (319). Neurodiagnostic studies usually show an axonal pattern with reduction in amplitude of evoked compound action potentials with relative preservation of nerve conduction velocities. The etiology is felt to be a vasculitis of the vasonervorum (326–328), although this can only be demonstrated on sural nerve biopsy in 50% of cases. Aggressive therapy with corticosteroids and intravenous pulse or daily oral cyclophosphamide with or without plasma exchange is recommended (318, 319, 328). Recovery of nerve function takes up to 1 year.

There have been few reported cases of SLE patients with an inflammatory polyradiculoneuropathy. There are two forms: the acute form resembles Guillain-Barré syndrome and the chronic form resembles chronic, inflammatory, demyelinating polyradiculoneuropathy (CIDP). Patients presenting acutely have an ascending, predominantly areflexic motor paralysis, which peaks in 10 to 14 days. There is little or no sensory loss, but there can be autonomic dysfunction. There is little loss of cutaneous sensation as small, nonmyelinated fibers are not involved. Involvement of large, myelinated, afferent fibers leads to loss of proprioception and vibratory sensation. There can be an associated autonomic dysfunction in some patients. There is no sphincter disturbance, which helps separate it from transverse myelitis. CSF examination reveals an elevated total protein with a white blood cell count less than 50. Electrodiagnostic studies reveal a demyelinating pattern with slowing of nerve conduction velocities, dispersion of evoked compound action potentials, conduction block, and marked prolongation of distal latencies. The pathogenesis is unknown. Unlike Guillain-Barré syndrome without SLE, patients have been treated successfully with corticosteroids. Recovery can occur within weeks if there has been no neuronal damage. There has been limited experience with the use of plasmapheresis (three cases) or intravenous gammaglobulin (no cases) in SLE patients with Guillain-Barré syndromelike symptoms (320). Rarely, a patient presenting with acute polyradiculopathy will have an axonal pattern on electrodiagnostic studies and evidence of vasculitis (329). These patients should be treated with corticosteroids and cyclophosphamide. Recovery will take many months, because there is axonal damage.

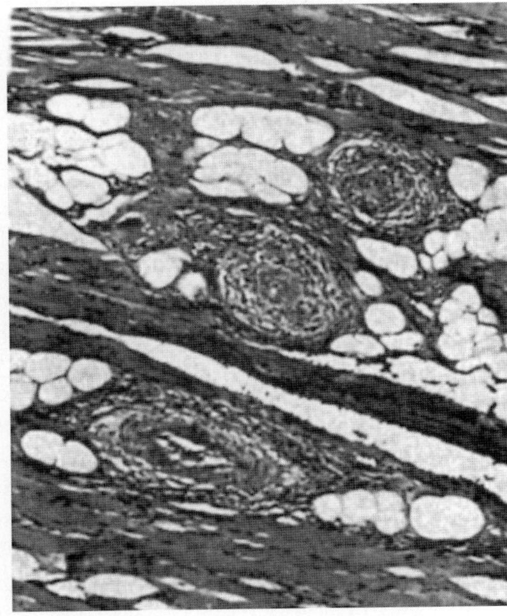

FIGURE 35.3. Vasculitis in gastrocnemius muscle biopsy of a patient with severe peripheral neuritis of legs and bilateral foot-drop (H&E; 150).

SLE patients with chronic, demyelinating polyradiculopathy resembling CIDP can present with recurrent episodes of acute, Guillain-Barré syndromelike symptoms, a mononeuritis multiplexlike pattern, or as a symmetric polyradiculopathy evolving over weeks to months. Electrodiagnostic studies frequently are confusing, showing a mixed axonal-demyelinating pattern. Nerve biopsy usually is not helpful, but may show inflammation. Therapy includes corticosteroids, plasmapheresis, cyclophosphamide, and intravenous gammaglobulin (321).

There are multiple secondary causes of peripheral nervous system involvement, which must be ruled out before attributing peripheral nerve dysfunction to NP-SLE. Uremia, diabetes mellitus, drug toxicities, vitamin deficiencies, heavy metal/solvent exposure, cancers and paraproteinemias, viral and other infections, sarcoidosis, alcohol and other toxins, hereditary neurologic diseases, and other causes must be considered and evaluated for in the SLE patient.

Autonomic Disorders

The autonomic nervous system probably is more commonly involved in SLE patients than previously reported. Acute autonomic neuropathy with profound dysfunction of the parasympathetic and/or sympathetic nervous system rarely has been reported in SLE (330, 331). Gastrointestinal (constipation), cardiovascular (orthostatic hypotension), genitourinary (sphincter/sphincteric, erectile/ejaculatory dysfunction), sweating (anhydrosis and heat intolerance), and pupillary abnormalities are evident and, when severe, respond to corticosteroids.

Sensitive tests of autonomic function show that mild dysfunction may be present, although clinically unappreciated. Recently, Straub and colleagues reported that 29% of 31 SLE patients had abnormal pupillometry, reflecting lesions of the pupillary parasympathetic nervous system (313). This may be from cytokine effects on the hypothalamic-autonomic nervous system (332). In addition, 9.7% of these 31 patients had abnormal cardiovascular autonomic nervous system findings using a standard battery of tests, age-matched norms, and modern definitions of autonomic dysfunction. This is in agreement with the 2% to 13% prevalence found in two controlled studies of 34 and 23 outpatient SLE patients, respectively (333, 334). Two older reports found a 20% to 40% prevalence of cardiovascular autonomic nervous system dysfunction. This is probably an overestimate, as these studies did not use age-matched norms or the new criteria for cardiovascular autonomic dysfunction (335, 336). Of note, corticosteroids can mask cardiovascular autonomic changes resulting from SLE (337).

Myasthenia Gravis And Related Disorders

Myasthenia gravis and SLE may coexist in the same patient (338). There have been over 50 reported cases. Myasthenia typically precedes the onset of SLE in the majority of these patients. In some cases, SLE develops shortly following thymectomy for the treatment of myasthenia gravis (339). Patients have typical manifestations of myasthenia with neuromuscular fatigue and weakness of bulbar or other voluntary muscles with repetitive muscular contractions. There is no impairment of sensation or loss of reflexes. Antibodies to the acetylcholine receptor can be demonstrated in 85% of myasthenia patients and are felt to cause neuromuscular symptoms by reducing the number of acetylcholine receptors at the neuromuscular junction. Diagnosis is made clinically and confirmed with electromyography and repetitive peripheral nerve stimulation at a rate of two per second showing a characteristic decremental response, which is reversed by the acetylcholinesterase drugs, edrophonium, or neostigmine (see Chapter 38).

There have been three SLE patients reported with Lambert-Eaton myasthenic syndrome (LEMS) (340). Patients present with weakness and hyporeflexia, which improves with exercise. Neurodiagnostic studies show a myopathic electromyogram (EMG) with low-amplitude compound muscle action potential, which increases in amplitude after exercise. High-frequency, repetitive stimulation demonstrates a 50% or more increment in the amplitude of the compound-motor action potential. There is no improvement of clinical or EMG findings with anticholinesterase drugs. The etiopathogenesis is suspected to be an IgG antibody against the voltage-gated calcium channels in the presynaptic neuromuscular junction. Plasmapheresis and immunosuppressive medications are effective therapy. There has been one case report recently of an SLE patient with neuromyotonia (341). This patient presented with persistent myokymia at rest, both clinically and on EMG. The suspected pathogenesis is an IgG antibody against the voltage-gated potassium channels in the presynaptic neuromuscular junction.

Other Neuropsychiatric Lupus Syndromes

There have been other NP-SLE syndromes reported. Schnider et al. reported a patient who developed the acute onset of severe amnesia. MRI of the brain showed isolated hippocampal damage (342). A case of limbic encephalopathy as a result of NP-SLE was reported in a young woman with SLE (343). The patient had fever, headache, encephalopathy, generalized seizures, and antiribosomal P antibodies in her cerebrospinal fluid. All tests for herpes simplex and paraneoplastic syndromes were negative. A case of the syndrome of inappropriate antidiuretic hormone (SIADH) was reported as the initial manifestation of SLE in an elderly woman with antiribosomal P antibodies (344). Other cases of NP-SLE with SIADH have been reported (345). Finally, there has been a recent case reported of reversible posterior leukoencephalopathy (346).

Differential Diagnosis Of Secondary Causes Of CNS Dysfunction In SLE Patients

Secondary causes of CNS dysfunction in SLE patients must always be ruled out before attributing symptoms to primary NP-SLE (Table 35.4) (42–44). The most common secondary causes include infections, medications, and metabolic disturbances. Equally important is the clinician must realize that the presence of an antinuclear antibody in a patient with neurologic symptoms does not imply that the patient has NP-SLE or, for that matter, SLE at all (347). Many other possibilities must be considered in the differential diagnosis.

Infections

SLE patients have an increased susceptibility to bacterial, viral, fungal, and parasitic infections from disease and medication effects on the immune system (292, 348). The neurologic manifestations of CNS infection can include confusion, lethargy, headache, neck pain, seizures, psychosis, and fever with or without focal or generalized sensory and motor deficits (42–44). Nearly every organism has been reported to infect patients with SLE (292). Tuberculosis, bacterial endocarditis (349), herpes simplex encephalitis, bacterial meningitis (Neisserial, Listeria, Nocardia, Salmonella, and syphilitic), and opportunistic CNS infections [Toxoplasma, Aspergillus, amoebic (350), and Cryptococcal] all have been reported as potentially mistaken for NP-SLE. Human polyoma virus JC has been demonstrated as the cause of progressive multifocal leukoencephalopathy in SLE patients (351, 352).

The most critical test to exclude CNS infection is a lumbar puncture with cerebrospinal fluid examination. Although CSF pleocytosis and elevated protein also can be seen in cerebral vasculitis, an associated low glucose, positive Gram stain and/or cultures, or polymerase chain reaction tests for viruses are diagnostic of CNS infections. CT scan with contrast or brain MRI may help to locate an abscess or focal area of involvement. Whenever infection is likely, broad-spectrum antibiotics that cross the blood-brain barrier should be initiated. After that, corticosteroid doses can be increased to treat possible NP-SLE while cultures are pending or to prevent Addisonian crisis during stress. Unfortunately, unsuspected CNS infections are all too commonly first diagnosed at time of postmortem examination.

Medications

Patients with lupus often take medications that are known to have CNS toxicity. Corticosteroids have been reported to cause psychosis, depression, mania, and delirium (353–355). Notably, mood alteration (depression/mania) is more common than psychosis. The majority of patients who develop psychiatric disturbances will do so within 2 weeks of starting or increasing the corticosteroid dose. Factors that have predicted psychiatric side effects from corticosteroids include high-dose intravenous methylprednisolone, doses of prednisone greater than 40 mg/day, and female gender. Age, previous psychiatric illness, and prior history of steroid psychosis were not predictive of corticosteroid-induced psychiatric side effects (354). Most patients improve within days to a few weeks by lowering and dividing the dose of corticosteroids. Antipsychotic medications (chlorpromazine, risperidone), lithium, and electroconvulsive therapy have been used successfully. Tricyclic antidepressants make symptoms worse and should be avoided (356). There is little experience with the use of selective serotonin reuptake inhibitors.

Antimalarial therapy has been associated with a variety of neurologic symptoms, including headaches, irritability, seizures, and neuromyopathy (see Chapter 55). Nonsteroidal antiinflammatory drugs (NSAIDs) can cause a variety of CNS side effects (357). Ibuprofen and rarely other NSAIDs have caused aseptic meningitis, particularly in SLE patients (293). Acute psychosis with disorientation, paranoia, or hallucinations can occur with indomethacin or sulindac. The indolacetic acid derivatives (indomethacin, tolmetin, and sulindac) also can induce headache. Cognitive dysfunction with memory impairment and depression can occur with indomethacin and less commonly with other NSAIDs, especially in elderly patients. Antihypertensive medications can cause fatigue and depression. Azathioprine can cause aseptic meningitis; intravenous gammaglobulin also has been reported to cause aseptic meningitis (293) and strokes (358). All treating physicians must obtain a careful drug history from their patients. Nearly all of these medications can be withheld for brief periods to determine causation.

Thrombotic Thrombocytopenic Purpura

Thrombotic thrombocytopenia purpura (TTP) is characterized by fever, thrombocytopenia, microangiopathic hemolytic anemia, neurologic symptoms, and renal involvement. The thrombocytopenia and hemolytic anemia are nonimmune mediated, which helps separate this from SLE. There have been approximately 30 cases of TTP and SLE occurring in the same individual (359). In the majority (62%) of cases, SLE preceded the development of TTP, while in 17% the two diseases developed simultaneously. Rarely, TTP preceded the onset of SLE. In 50% of cases, TTP complicated the course of active SLE, while in the remaining, it developed in SLE patients with inactive disease.

The etiology of TTP occurring in SLE may be similar to idiopathic TTP. Acute TTP recently has been found to be from IgG autoantibody against the metalloprotease responsible for cleavage of the monomeric subunits of von Willebrand factor (360). This allows for the accumulation of unusually large multimers of von Willebrand factors secreted by endothelial cells into the plasma. These multimers bind to platelet glycoprotein receptors, causing platelet adhesion and microthrombi. The treatment of acute TTP in SLE patients includes plasmapheresis to remove the autoantibody and large multimers of von Willebrand factor, followed by fresh frozen plasma to replace the metalloprotease. Antiplatelet agents, corticosteroids, and/or immunosuppressive drugs have been used, but are not as effective as plasmapheresis and plasma replacement. However, corticosteroids and immunosuppressives may be needed to prevent recurrence by suppressing autoantibody formation. Precipitating causes of idiopathic TTP include drugs such as ticlopidine and infection. These, however, rarely have been reported in patients with SLE complicated by TTP (359).

Other Causes Of CNS Dysfunction

Other secondary causes of CNS dysfunction that must be excluded include: hyponatremia, hypercalcemia, uremia, hypoxia, accelerated hypertension, fever, hypothyroidism, cerebral lymphoma (361), and subdural hematoma (362), as well as others. SLE patients have accelerated atherosclerosis, which can lead to stroke and hypertension, causing intracerebral hemorrhage. Berry aneurysms have been reported in SLE patients and can cause subarachnoid hemorrhage (94–96).

Fibromyalgia is observed commonly in SLE patients. Pistiner et al. reported that 20% of their SLE patients fulfilled established criteria for fibromyalgia (23). Middleton et al. confirmed these findings (363). Fatigue, myalgias, paresthesias, insomnia, and headaches are frequent in patients with fibromyalgia. Additionally, reactive depression with or without fibromyalgia also is commonly found in SLE patients. Living with SLE can involve lifestyle adjustments and create stress. This can lead to depression, anxiety, and functional symptoms such as sweating, palpitations, diarrhea, and hyperventilation, which are observed with increased frequency in patients with SLE (364). It is important to not confuse these symptoms with active NP-SLE.

Sleep apnea also can occur in SLE patients. Corticosteroid therapy leads to weight gain and weakness of respiratory muscles. This can lead to apnea/hypoventilation during sleep. Patients with sleep apnea complain of fatigue, headaches, and mental clouding, which can be misdiagnosed as NP-SLE. This is a common and under-diagnosed cause of mild CNS symptoms in SLE patients.

Positive ANA Without Lupus

There are patients with nonspecific complaints such as myalgias, arthralgias, fatigue, and headache, who are found by their primary care physician to have a low-titer ANA without other objective or laboratory findings of lupus. These patients may be sent for rheumatologic consultation to confirm a diagnosis of SLE or NP-SLE as a cause of their symptoms. Furthermore, there are patients with a drug-induced ANA from procainamide, phenothiazines, or other medications who may have or develop neuropsychiatric symptoms from causes other than SLE or drug-induced SLE (365, 366). Consequently, it is imperative to first confirm a diagnosis of SLE in any patient being sent for consultation to rule out NP-SLE.

CLINICAL AND LABORATORY EVALUATION

A methodological work-up is essential for the patient with SLE who presents with neuropsychiatric manifestations (26, 367, 368). A careful and thorough history and physical examination including a complete neurologic and mental status evaluation must be done on each patient. In addition, a variety of laboratory, CSF, neurodiagnostic studies, and when appropriate, cultures of bodily fluids are done to assess disease activity and to exclude other diseases that can cause neurologic symptoms. Earlier studies emphasized that certain clinical signs, such as retinal and dermal vasculitis or livedo reticularis, were more common in NP-SLE patients, particularly those with cerebrovascular disease (17). Furthermore, although NP-SLE can be the initial or sole active manifestation of SLE, many studies have reported that NP-SLE frequently occurs when SLE is clinically and serologically active (17–19, 21, 27). However, in all SLE patients with CNS dysfunction, additional tests will be necessary to confirm an NP-SLE diagnosis and exclude other causes (Tables 35.5–35.7) . Recently, an international, multidisciplinary committee made recommendations of the basic laboratory evaluation and diagnostic imaging, which should be obtained on all patients suspected of having NP-SLE (Table 35.5) (10). See Figure 35.4.

CLINICAL LABORATORY TESTS

Blood tests include a complete blood count, including platelet count and peripheral smear. The blood smear should be examined for schistocytes and thrombocytopenia to exclude TTP. Chemistries including electrolytes, creatinine, glucose, and liver-associated enzymes are obtained to exclude

TABLE 35.5. LABORATORY EVALUATION AND DIAGNOSTIC IMAGING OF SYSTEMIC LUPUS ERYTHEMATOSUS PATIENTS WITH NEUROPSYCHIATRIC MANIFESTATIONS

Complete blood count/peripheral blood smear
Chemistries: electrolytes, creatinine, glucose
Liver-associated enzymes
Urinalysis
C3/C4 and/or CH_{50}
Anti dsDNA antibodies
Antiphospholipid antibodies/anti β2 glycoprotein I
Cerebrospinal fluid: cell count, protein, glucose, IgG index, oligoclonal bands, VDRL, cultures
Brain magnetic resonance imaging with gadolinium
Electroencephalogram
Other tests when indicated
- Computerized tomography of brain
- Echocardiogram
- Magnetic resonance angiogram
- Angiogram
- Tests for hypercoagulability: protein C, protein S, SAT III, prothrombin mutation, factor V Leiden, homocysteine
- Antiribosomal P antibodies
- Cryoglobulins

Other tests—investigational
- Serum and CSF antineuronal antibodies
- Single-photon emission tomography
- Magnetic resonance spectroscopy
- Positron emission tomography

CSF, cerebrospinal fluid; dsDNA, double-stranded DNA; VDRL, Venereal Disease Research Laboratory
Adapted from ACR Ad Hoc Committee on Neuropsychiatric Lupus Nomenclature. The American College of Rheumatology Nomenclature and Case Definitions for Neuropsychiatric Lupus Syndromes. *Arthritis Rheum* 1999;42:599–608, with permission.

TABLE 35.6. FREQUENCY OF ABNORMAL LABORATORY TESTS COMMONLY USED IN THE EVALUATION OF NEUROPSYCHIATRIC LUPUS ERYTHEMATOSUS

Test	Frequency ofAbnormal Test Result Range (%)	Comment
Serologic		
Antineuronal antibodies	30–92	Diffuse manifestations
Antineurofilament antibodies	58	Diffuse manifestations
Antiribosomal-P antibodies	45–90	Psychosis/depression
Antiphospholipid antibodies	45–80	Focal manifestations, strokes
Cerebrospinal fluid		
Routine		
Pleocytosis	6–34	Rule out infection and NSAID meningitis
Increased protein	22–50	Nonspecific
Low glucose	3–8	Rule out infection, transverse myelitis
Special		
Antineuronal antibodies (IgG)	40–90	Diffuse manifestations, present in 40% with focal manifestations
Elevated Q albumin	8–33	Break in blood-brain barrier
Elevated IgG/IgM index	25–66	Diffuse manifestations
Oligoclonal band (≥2 bands)	20–82	Diffuse manifestations

NSAID, nonsteroidal antiinflammatory drug.
Adapted from West SG. Neuropsychiatric lupus. *Rheum Dis Clin North Am* 1994;20:129–158, with permission.

TABLE 35.7. FREQUENCY OF ABNORMAL DIAGNOSTIC TESTS COMMONLY USED IN THE EVALUATION OF NEUROPSYCHIATRIC LUPUS ERYTHEMATOSUS

Test	Frequency of Abnormal Test Results, Range (%)	Comment
Electroencephalogram	54–85	No specific abnormality. SLE pts without CNS Sxs can have abnormal EEG (48%).
Neuroimaging procedures		
Brain scan	8–19	Some studies report higher prevalence of abnormalities.
CT scan	27–71 (atrophy) 10–25 (infarct or hemorrhage)	Atrophy may be from corticosteroids. CT scan will miss 20% to 25% of definite clinical infarcts.
MRI scan		
All NPLE pts	77	No specific lesion, atrophy (28%–71%).
NPLE pts, diffuse Sxs only	<50	More likely abnormal if obtained within 48 hours of treatment
NPLE pts, focal Sxs	Up to 100	
SLE pts, CNS Sxs unrelated to NPLE	31	
SLE pts, (<age 45), no hx CNS Sxs	<5–10	
SPECT scan	44–88	Up to 67% of SLE pts with CNS events unrelated to NPLE have abnormal scans.
Angiography	10	More likely abnormal in embolic strokes.
Echocardiography	40	Definite valvular lesions more common in stroke pts. May have association with antiphospholipid antibodies.

CNS, central nervous system; Sxs, symptoms; pts, patients; EEG, electroencephalogram; CT, computed tomography; MRI, magnetic resonance imaging; NPLE, neuropsychiatric lupus erythematosus; SPECT, single-photo-emission computer tomography; hx, history.
Adapted from West SG. Neuropsychiatric lupus. *Rheum Dis Clin North Am* 1994;20:129–158, with permission.

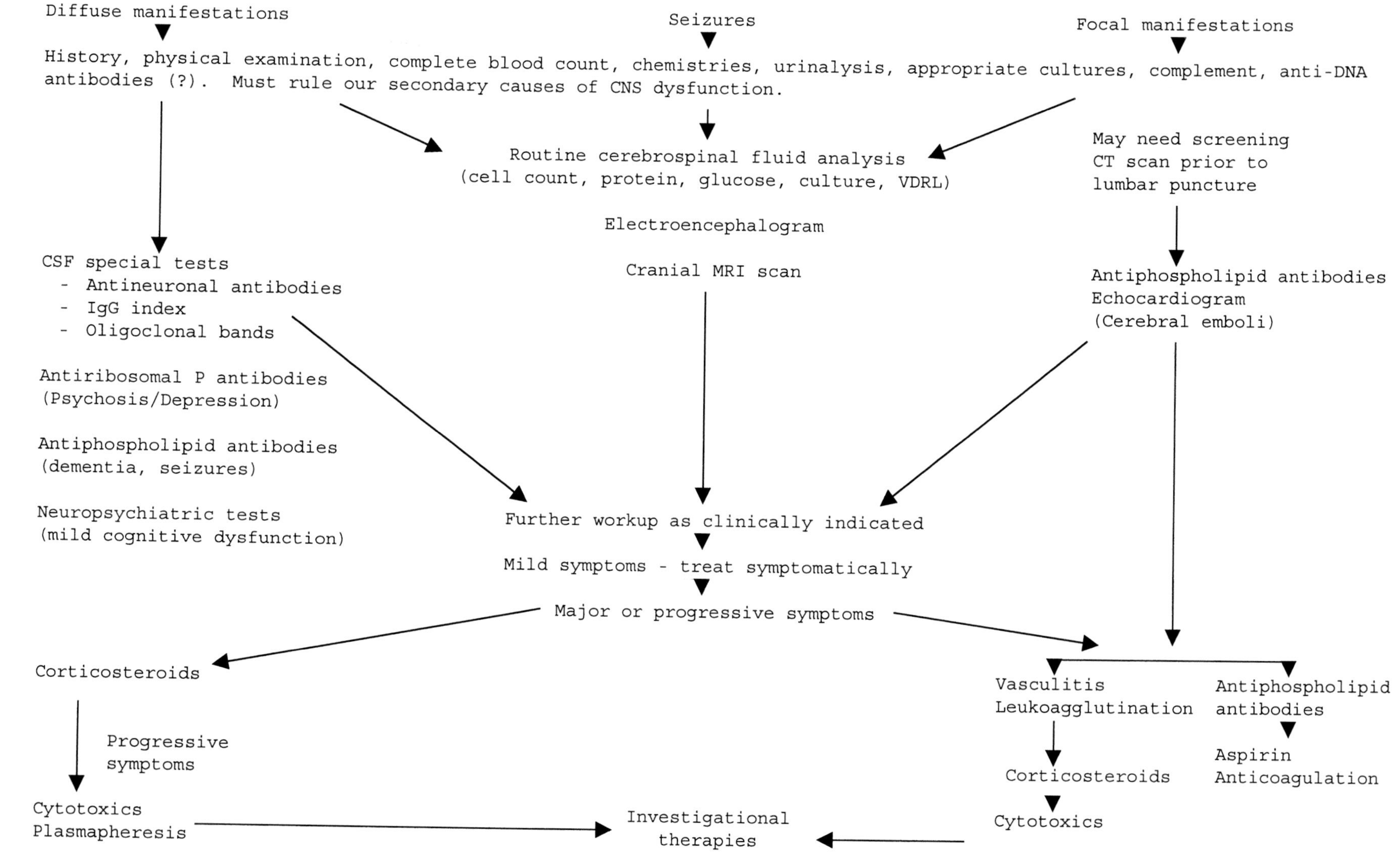

FIGURE 35.4. Algorithm for the evaluation and treatment of systemic lupus erythematosus patients with neuropsychiatric lupus erythematosus.

metabolic abnormalities, which can cause neurologic dysfunction. A urinalysis should be obtained for disease activity and to rule out infection. Complement (C3/C4 or CH50) determinations and antidouble-stranded DNA antibodies should be obtained to assess disease activity. Testing for antiphospholipid antibodies includes lupus anticoagulant, anticardiolipin antibodies, and anti-β2 glycoprotein-1 antibodies. Other tests for hypercoagulable states, including factor V Leiden, protein C and S levels, and serum antithrombin III levels, may be indicated in selected patients. Most patients with SLE will have an elevated erythrocyte sedimentation rate and a normal or mildly elevated C-reactive protein. A significantly elevated C-reactive protein usually indicates systemic vasculitis or infection. A fasting lipid profile and homocysteine levels are obtained to establish vascular risk factors. Serum antilymphocyte and antineuronal antibodies are considered investigational.

Antiribosomal P Antibodies

Antibodies to the C-terminal region of cytoplasmic ribosomal P protein are found in 12% to 16% of SLE patients and are among the most specific tests for SLE (169, 170, 174, 371). Bonfa et al. first observed these antibodies in 18 of 20 SLE patients with psychosis/major depression (169). Several other groups have related antiribosomal P antibodies to psychosis and severe depression (26, 39, 169–172, 370), but others have failed to confirm this association (37, 173, 174, 369, 372). Some investigators have found antiribosomal P associated with CNS disease in general, as opposed to psychosis in particular (175, 369). Serum levels of the antibody may correlate with the severity of the psychosis in selected patients (26, 39, 373), but also vary widely over time without any clinical associations. The antibody usually is not found in the CSF (26, 39), although it has been in some patients (374). SLE patients with mild depression and/or cognitive dysfunction do not have elevated ribosomal P levels (150, 158).

Iverson in a recent editorial summarized the available evidence concerning the value of testing for antiribosomal P antibodies (375). He noted that studies supported the specificity of antiribosomal P antibodies for SLE, and that these antibodies are not found in patients with neuropsychiatric conditions who do not have SLE. Additionally, several studies have shown that these antibodies are more prevalent in Oriental patients with SLE than Caucasians or African-Americans, regardless of whether these patients had neuropsychiatric manifestations. Combining the studies, Iverson estimated that the sensitivity of antiribosomal P antibodies to neuropsychiatric manifestations was 0.64 to 0.66, the positive predictive value was only 0.29, and the negative predictive value was 0.90. Therefore, he supported the opinion of Teh and Isenberg's review (37) that, "There is no value in measuring anti-P antibodies, either as a single determinate for identifying patients with lupus psychosis (or depression) or sequentially as a predictor of impending relapse of the lupus psychiatric disorder." This opinion, however, is not supported by all clinicians who care for patients with NP-SLE (26, 39). Some feel that the high specificity of this antibody for SLE makes it particularly useful as a diagnostic test in neuropsychiatric cases without a definite diagnosis of SLE (10). Furthermore, in an individual patient who does have NP-SLE and antiribosomal P antibodies, the titer of antibody may become undetectable with successful therapy (39, 170).

The mechanism of how an antibody against a cytoplasmic antigen can cause CNS dysfunction is unclear. However, recently ribosomal P antigens have been demonstrated on the surface of endothelial cells (376) and on the surface of human neuroblastoma cells (109). This suggests that these autoantibodies may bind to membrane surface antigens, instead of cytoplasmic ribosomal P proteins. Binding of antiribosomal P to neuronal cells might directly participate in neuronal dysfunction (110). The binding of antiribosomal P to these surface antigens might explain why antiribosomal P antibodies are not found free in the CSF of patients with NP-SLE, while antiribosomal P antibodies are found in their sera.

Antilymphocyte Antibodies

Antilymphocyte antibodies are not specific for SLE and can occur in other illnesses, including infections, malignancy, inflammatory bowel disease, and multiple sclerosis (377, 378). A subset of antilymphocyte antibodies, however, cross-reacts with neurons. Fever, neuropsychiatric symptoms, skin lesions, and hematologic abnormalities are the most common manifestations in patients with SLE and serum lymphocytotoxic antibodies (379, 380). Denburg's group has related cognitive dysfunction to the presence of serum IgM lymphocytotoxic antibodies in over 445 patients evaluated (164, 381–383). This may reflect the presence of the antineuronal subset; antilymphocyte antibodies cross-react with antineuronal antibodies. In a prospective study, Temesvari et al. (384) found a correlation between fluctuation in serum lymphocytotoxicity and relapses or remissions of neuropsychiatric involvement in individual patients with SLE (see Chapters 26 and 27).

Serum Antineuronal Antibodies

Serum antineuronal antibodies are more common in NP-SLE patients (30%–92%) than in SLE patients without CNS lupus (5%–20%)(31, 32, 100–105, 385). They are neither as sensitive nor as specific as CSF antineuronal antibody measurements. Nevertheless, neuroblastoma-binding serum autoantibodies are particularly frequent in NP-SLE patients with diffuse presentations, such as encephalopathy and cognitive dysfunction (32, 33, 385). A limited number of studies have investigated the fine specificity of some of these antibodies. Several membrane antigens have been identified as targets of these antineuronal antibodies. In neuroblastoma cells, a 97-kd membrane protein of unknown function is the target antigen for autoantibodies from a limited number of NP-SLE patients (386). An immunodominant, C-terminal epitope of ribosomal P antibody has been demonstrated on the surface of human neuroblastoma cells (109). Hanson et al. have found antibodies against a 50-kd antigen in the plasma membrane of brain synaptic terminals in 19 of 20 NP-SLE patients (107), while Denburg and Behmann documented the presence of antilymphocyte/antineuronal antibodies against a 52 kd antigen in patients with NP-SLE (387). Recently, Galeazzi et al. and others have found antiganglioside antibodies (GM_1) or antigalactocerebroside antibodies more commonly in SLE patients with NP-SLE (388–391). Several cytoplasmic antigens including ribosomal P, neurofilaments, and L-fimbrin have been reported as target antigens. Serum antineurofilament antibodies, which react against cytoskeletal neurofilament protein antigens, were found in 58% of patients with diffuse neuropsychiatric manifestations, compared to 20% with focal symptoms and 18% of controls (108). Antibodies to L-fimbrin expressed in cytoplasmic microfilaments of leukocytes also have been found increased in patients with NP-SLE (392). The significance of these targets, or how antibodies against them cause disease, is unclear. Each of these autoantibodies is more common in patients with diffuse, as opposed to focal, manifestations of NP-SLE.

Antiphospholipid Antibodies

Antiphospholipid antibodies are a heterogenous group of autoantibodies associated with thromboembolic events. The lupus anticoagulant and anticardiolipin antibodies are the ones best characterized. Lupus anticoagulant prolongs phospholipid-dependent coagulation assays, such as the activated partial thromboplastin time and the kaolin clotting time. Subsequently, more sensitive assays, particularly the dilute Russell viper venom time (dRVVT), have been used to detect and/or confirm the presence of a lupus anticoagulant, even in patients with normal activated PTT and clinical features of the antiphospholipid antibody syndrome. Anticardiolipin antibodies are detected by a standard enzyme-linked immunoabsorbent assay. In the meta-analysis by Love and Santora of 29 retrospective studies comprising greater than 1,000 patients with SLE, the average prevalence of lupus anticoagulants and anticardiolipin antibodies were 34% and 44%, respectively, with an overall incidence of thrombotic complications of 28% (393). Many studies combined primary antiphospholipid antibody syndrome patients with SLE patients with antiphospholipid antibodies, making interpretation of these studies difficult to apply to SLE patients only.

There have been several neurologic syndromes associated with antiphospholipid antibodies in patients with lupus (303). The most common are stroke, cerebral-venous sinus thrombosis (78), ocular ischemia, sensorineural hearing loss (302), dementia, seizures, chorea, and transverse myelopathy. Each one is felt to be a result of a thromboembolic event resulting in vascular occlusion. A major clinical question is why do some patients with antiphospholipid antibodies develop these neurologic syndromes, while others do not. SLE patients at greatest risk are those who have the lupus anticoagulant and/or high-titer IgG (and possibly IgM) anticardiolipin antibodies with β2 glycoprotein-1 specificity. Clinically, patients with antiphospholipid antibodies who have a history of a previous thromboembolic event, livedo reticularis, thrombocytopenia, or active lupus (vasculitis, hypocomplementemia, elevated antidouble-stranded DNA antibodies) are at increased risk for thrombosis (394–398). Furthermore, approximately one third of patients with antiphospholipid antibodies have abnormal echocardiograms, which demonstrate left-sided valvular lesions, which are a potential cardiac source for an embolic stroke (88, 399). SLE patients with antiphospholipid antibodies, who have cerebral microemboli detected by transcranial Doppler ultrasound, are more likely to develop cerebrovascular ischemic events (400). Up to 30% of SLE patients who develop a thromboembolic event are likely to develop a recurrent episode within 1 year of the initial event (401). The initial type of thromboembolic event (arterial versus venous) is the most likely type of event to recur in a given patient, although usually not in the same vascular territory (402).

The ability of antiphospholipid antibodies to cause thrombosis is likely enhanced by congenital abnormalities, including protein C and S deficiencies (particularly venous thrombosis), factor V Leiden mutation, prothrombin mutation, and SAT III deficiency. Furthermore, surgery and infection causing release of tissue factor may increase thrombotic risk. Finally, other cerebrovascular risk factors may be additive to the thrombotic risk conferred by antiphospholipid antibodies (403, 404). Cigarette smoking, hyperlipidemia, hypertension, diabetes mellitus, and hyperhomocystinemia are all correctable risk factors, which need to be identified and treated.

There are SLE patients with neurologic thromboembolic events who will lack antiphospholipid antibodies on testing during the acute event. This may be a false-negative result possibly from consumption of the antibody during the acute thrombotic episode. Consequently, these patients should be retested for these antibodies 6 to 8 weeks after the initial thrombotic event, because some patients will become positive for antiphospholipid antibodies at this time. However, approximately 10% of patients with an antiphospholipid antibodylike syndrome will remain negative for the lupus anticoagulant and anticardiolipin antibodies, even with repeated testing. Some of these patients may demonstrate antibodies against other negatively-charged noncardiolipin phospholipids, such as phosphatidylserine and phosphatidylinositol, or against specific phospholipid-binding proteins, including β2 glycoprotein-1, prothrombin, protein C, protein S, thrombomodulin, and kininogens (405). It is not clear how, or if, these autoantibodies put SLE patients at increased risk for thromboembolic events.

CEREBROSPINAL FLUID TESTS

CSF analysis is useful in all SLE patients with a change in neurologic status, particularly to exclude infection or other secondary causes of CNS dysfunction. In patients with NP-SLE, CSF results may be unremarkable. However, patients with NP-SLE may have abnormalities helpful in confirming the diagnosis and guiding management. The NP-SLE consensus panel recommended that routine CSF tests, IgG index, and oligoclonal bands be determined on all patients suspected of having NP-SLE (10).

Routine CSF Tests

Routine CSF tests include cell count with differential, protein, glucose, Gram stain, and other special stains, VDRL, and cultures. Pleocytosis and elevated protein are found in some patients with active NP-SLE. Protein abnormalities were found to be more common (range 22% to 50%) than pleocytosis (range 6% to 34%) in ten studies analyzing spinal fluid findings in 250 patients with NP-SLE (11, 17, 18, 21, 22, 49, 117, 406). Neutrophilic pleocytosis with elevated protein suggests cerebral vasculitis with ischemia, if infection is ruled out (407). Patients with antiphospholipid antibodies and neurologic thromboembolic events frequently have elevated protein with mild or no pleocytosis.

The CSF glucose level is rarely decreased in NP-SLE. It has been reported low in between 3% and 8% of patients (18, 21, 22). Patients with acute transverse myelopathy have been reported to have hypoglycorrhea more than patients with other manifestations of NP-SLE (214, 216), although they frequently have normal CSF glucose levels. CSF pleocytosis, elevated protein levels, and low glucose always should raise suspicion of an acute or chronic infection before attributing these abnormalities to NP-SLE.

Cerebrospinal Fluid Immunologic Tests

Several studies have noted that CSF IgG levels are elevated in 69% to 96% of NP-SLE patients (22, 32, 406). Bluestein and Zvaifler found that a CSF IgG level greater than 6 mg/dL almost always indicated NP-SLE, but was present in only 40% of their patients (32). An elevated CSF Q-albumin ratio, indicating a break in the blood-brain barrier, has been noted in up to one third of patients, especially those with progressive encephalopathy, transverse myelitis, and strokes (26, 117, 118). Several groups now have confirmed that an elevated IgG index and/or IgG oligoclonal bands are seen in up to 80% of patients, particularly those with diffuse manifestations, such as encephalopathy and psychosis (22, 26, 117–119, 122). Hirohata et al. also have found IgM and IgA indices elevated (119). Patients with focal manifestations, such as stroke as a result of antiphospholipid antibodies, typically do not have an elevated IgG index or oligoclonal bands, unless they also have a coexistent encephalopathy (complex presentation) (26). These abnormalities have been shown to normalize in some patients after successful therapy (26, 121).

Cerebrospinal Fluid Antineuronal Antibodies

Bluestein et al. (31, 32) found IgG antibodies to neurons in the CSF of 74% of 28 SLE patients with CNS involvement, as compared to only 11% of 18 SLE patients without CNS disease, using a radioimmunoassay with SK-N-SH neuroblastoma cells as the target. Furthermore, 90% of the patients with diffuse manifestations of psychosis, encephalopathy, or generalized seizures had elevated IgG antineuronal antibodies, compared to only 25% of patients with focal manifestations of hemiparesis or chorea. Notably, the antineuronal antibody was concentrated eightfold in the CSF, relative to its concentration in paired serum samples. In contrast, Kelly and Denburg, using a less sensitive hemadsorption assay, detected IgG antineuronal antibodies in only 17% of their patients with NP-SLE, using SK-N-ML neuroblastoma cells as a target (35). They correlated the presence of these antibodies with cognitive dysfunction; diffuse, nonfocal CNS manifestations; abnormal Q-albumin ratios; and active lupus with elevated antidouble-stranded DNA antibody levels (33–35).

More recently, West et al. and Isshi and Hirohata, using sensitive ELISA assays with neuroblastoma cells as the target antigen, found a high percentage of their patients with active NP-SLE had antineuronal antibodies in their CSF. West et al. (26) reported that 12 of 40 (30%) SLE patients with diffuse manifestations had antineuronal antibodies, while Isshi and Hirohata (39) found 39 of 41 (95%) NP-SLE patients had CSF IgG antineuronal antibodies. Moreover, Isshi found in the one patient they followed serially that the CSF antineuronal antibody activity markedly fell with successful therapy, but increased along with an elevation of CSF interleukin-6 during an exacerbation of NP-SLE (39).

Miscellaneous Determinations

Several other laboratory and immunologic tests have been reported to be helpful and/or abnormal in NP-SLE. Brook et al. found CSF lactic acid to be normal in those with NP-SLE, whereas it is increased in patients with bacterial meningitis (408). Occasionally, LE cells can be found in the CSF in patients with NP-SLE, but rarely are they looked for and documented (409). Myelin basic protein has been reported, particularly in myelopathy patients (217). Other CSF serologic tests reported to be elevated in NP-SLE include immune complexes (22), substance P (410), β2-microglobulin levels (411), cyclic GMP levels (412, 413), prostaglandin E2 (130), quinolinic acid (414), and CD4+ T cells (415). Most of these are single center reports or abstracts and generally not available to clinicians.

A past study reported that C4 levels in CSF decrease in those with acute NP-SLE (416). The C4 level turned out to be unstable in CSF, difficult to measure, and its value unconfirmed in other reports (406, 417–419). However, intrathecal C4 synthesis may be increased in NP-SLE patients with diffuse manifestations (420). Another group reported increased levels of SC5b in the CSF of patients with active NP-SLE, suggesting intrathecal complement activation (421). Autoantibodies rarely have been reported in the CSF, including antiribosomal P (374), antideoxyribonucleoprotein (422), antidouble-stranded DNA (406, 423), anticardiolipin antibodies (129), and anti-Ro/anti-La (423). Other groups have failed to detect some of these antibodies (26, 170).

Several cytokines have been reported to be elevated in the CSF of active NP-SLE patients. Four groups have found elevated interleukin-6 levels in patients with NP-SLE (127–130). This is of interest because interleukin-6 can contribute to B-cell differentiation into antibody-secreting plasma cells. Recently, Isshi and Hirohata reported a patient whose CSF interleukin-6 level and antineuronal antibodies increased during an exacerbation of NP-SLE, whereas the serum antineuronal antibody levels did not increase, suggesting intrathecal synthesis of antineuronal antibodies (39). Other cytokines reported to be elevated in the CSF of NP-SLE patients are interleukin-1 (127) and interferon alpha (424).

Summary

When a lumbar puncture is performed in SLE patients with CNS dysfunction, the CSF tests that should be ordered are cell count with differential, glucose and protein levels, VDRL, and Gram stain and cultures. In addition, CSF should be sent for antineuronal antibodies and a "multiple sclerosis panel," which includes a CSF IgG level, Q-albumin ratio, IgG index, oligoclonal bands, and a calculated IgG synthesis rate. Patients with diffuse manifestations frequently have elevated antineuronal antibodies and/or an elevated IgG index and oligoclonal bands, suggesting immunologic activity (26, 39). Patients with focal manifestations only usually do not have antineuronal antibodies, elevated IgG index, or oligoclonal bands, but may have an elevated Q-albumin ratio as a result of disruption of the blood-brain barrier. Patients with pleocytosis and elevated protein levels with negative cultures frequently have acute inflammation from vasculitis causing their focal symptoms. In contrast, patients with antiphospholipid antibodies causing thrombosis and focal symptoms usually have elevated protein levels, but mild or no pleocytosis in their CSF. Infection must be ruled in all patients with CNS dysfunction.

NEUROIMAGING STUDIES

There have been dramatic advancements in neuroradiographic procedures for a variety of neurologic diseases. Brain imaging is an important part of the evaluation of SLE patients with neurologic dysfunction. A recent, excellent review by leaders in the field summarized the scientific basis for the use of neuroimaging modalities in NP-SLE, points out their limitations, and makes recommendations for their use (425).

Computed Tomography

Earlier studies using CT scanning of the brain have noted abnormalities in 27% to 71% of NP-SLE patients (22, 426, 427). The predominant finding is cerebral atrophy, which is perisulcal in 50% (428–430). The etiology of this atrophy, which can occur within months (431), is unclear and does not correspond to any specific clinical sign/symptom. Some patients may have this atrophy because of alcoholism or corticosteroid therapy, and not NP-SLE (428, 432). CT scanning also can detect basal ganglia and periventricular calcifications (433–436) (Fig. 35.5).

In SLE patients with acute neurologic presentations, the CT scan is more likely to be abnormal in patients with focal symptoms. CT scanning can pick up large infarcts, intracerebral hemorrhage, or massive brain edema (437). It also is useful for excluding secondary causes of CNS dysfunction, such as brain abscess, mass lesion, subdural hematoma, and possibly meningitis or mycotic aneurysm. However, CT scanning is poor in its detection of small infarcts, focal cerebral edema, transverse myelitis, or other lesions, which can be seen on MRI of the brain and spinal cord. One study found that at least 20% of patients with clear-cut CNS episodes had normal CT scans (42).

CT scans are faster, but clearly inferior to MRI of the brain. They are most useful in SLE patients with acute neurologic deterioration to rapidly screen for large hemorrhages, infarcts, or mass lesions. CT scans also are useful in serially following an SLE patient with antiphospholipid

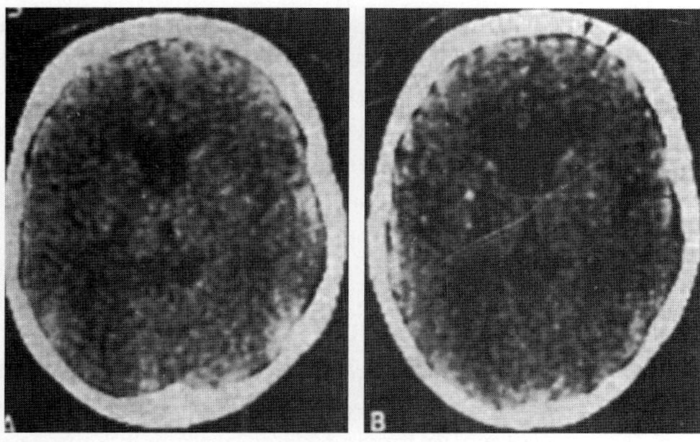

FIGURE 35.5. Perisulcal atrophy in a 27-year-old woman with psychosis. **A,** Computed tomography (CT) scan shows top normal lateral ventricles. **B,** After 1 year, CT scan shows enlargement of the ventricles, sulci (arrows), and fissures (open arrows) caused by atrophy. (Source: From Bilaniuk LT, Patel S, Zimmerman RA. Computed tomography of systemic lupus erythematosus. *Radiology* 1977;124:119, with permission.)

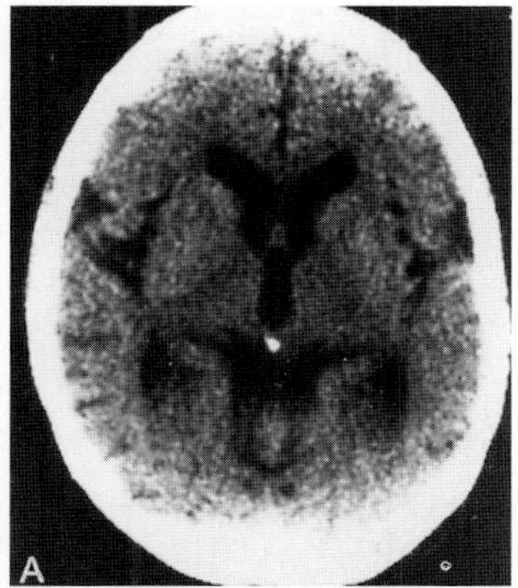

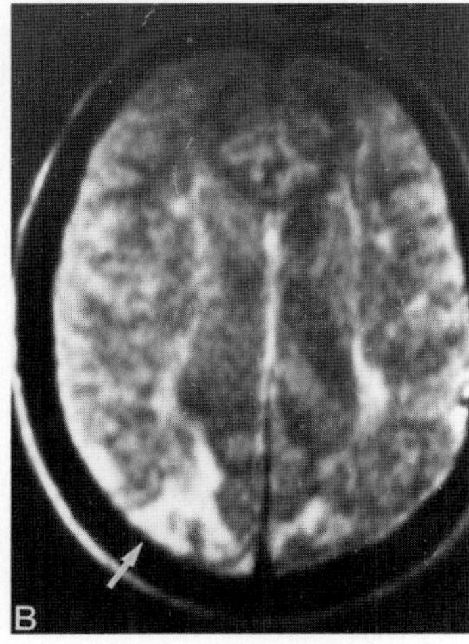

FIGURE 35.6. A, Computed tomography (CT) scan showing cerebral atrophy in a 42-year-old woman with systemic lupus erythematosus who presented with visual symptoms and organic brain syndrome. **B,** Magnetic resonance imaging (T2-weighted image: TR = 2,000, TE = 45) done at the same time showing occipital lobe (arrow) and other infarcts not observed on the CT scan (Diasonics MTS scanner was used.) From West SG. Neuropsychiatric lupus. *Rheum Dis Clin North Am* 1994;20:129–158, with permission.

antibodies and a large cerebral infarct, who is being anticoagulated, to make sure that the patient is not bleeding into the infarcted area. Finally, CT scan can be used if MRI is unavailable, not tolerated, or contraindicated (425).

Magnetic Resonance Imaging

MRI with gadolinium enhancement is the recommended imaging modality for evaluating patients with NP-SLE. It should be obtained, if possible, within 24 hours of the neurologic event and therapy, in order to pick up reversible, high-intensity lesions, which can resolve with corticosteroid therapy (438–440). Seven groups evaluated a total of 143 patients with SLE using concurrent CT and MRI (440–445). MRI was clearly superior for detecting edema, arterial and venous infarction, hemorrhage, and transverse myelitis, whereas CT scan was slightly better for detecting cerebral atrophy. Of great importance, between 25% and 80% of those with NP-SLE and a normal CT scan had an abnormal MRI (Fig. 35.6). However, there is no specific MRI-finding diagnostic of NP-SLE (441). In a prospective study, Stimmler et al. (441) found that SLE patients, who had CNS dysfunction that was produced by causes other than NP-SLE, exhibited similar MRI abnormalities to those with NP-SLE, thus limiting the diagnostic specificity of MRI.

Twenty-five to 50% of SLE patients without active NP-SLE can have MRI abnormalities (446–449). The most common abnormality is small (less than 1 cm), punctate, focal lesions in the white matter. The frequency and number of these lesions increases with patient age (greater than 50 years old), duration and severity of SLE, prior history of NP-SLE, migraine headaches, presence of antiphospholipid antibodies, and cardiovascular risk factors (hypertension, diabetes mellitus, smoking, hyperlipidemia, and prior history of myocardial infarction) (450, 451). These lesions are well demarcated, do not enhance with gadolinium, and do not disappear on serial MRIs, suggesting they are chronic lesions. These lesions are most likely small infarcts in white matter with secondary gliosis. Their relevance to neurologic function is unclear, although the more focal lesions present, the more neuronal loss is present (452). The clinician and radiologist must recognize that these lesions can occur and not misinterpret them as representing active NP-SLE.

MRI lesions are observed in 15% to 78% of patients with active NP-SLE (26, 425, 439–445). However, many of these lesions represent old injury rather than active disease. McCune et al. (438, 439) were first to describe three MRI patterns in patients with NP-SLE: areas of large infarction, small microinfarcts, and increased intensity in gray matter that could resolve in 2 to 3 weeks after the acute event. Patients with diffuse presentations, such as acute confusional state, psychosis, major depression, and headaches, frequently have a normal brain MRI, although unexpected abnormalities have been observed (26, 439, 441). NP-SLE patients with generalized seizures also may have a normal MRI. This may be because of timing of the MRI, as patients with seizures frequently have focal and punctate, high-intensity lesions on T2-weighted images in both white and gray matter, which can resolve rapidly on therapy (440, 453). In NP-SLE patients with focal manifestations, especially cerebrovascular accidents, brain MRI usually shows multiple large and small, high-intensity lesions on T2-weighted images, involving both the gray and white matter of the brain (26, 439, 441). These lesions occur in areas of the brain that correlate with the patients' symptoms as well as other areas that are clinically silent. The lesions particularly involving the white matter frequently are irreversible on repeat MRI, suggesting they are infarcts (438). The larger and more persistent MRI lesions can be observed on CT scans (437).

A major clinical conundrum is differentiating lesions that indicate active NP-SLE from chronic or nonspecific lesions (439, 446). Acute lesions indicating active NP-SLE typically lack discreet borders; are intermediate intensity on T2-weighted images; have a lacy, filamentous pattern; are located at the gray-white matter junction along the sulci and gyri assuming a semilunate shape; and/or are located in the white matter with overlying gray matter hyperintensity (425, 439). Furthermore, lesions that enhance with gadolinium (443), are new compared to old scans, correspond to new neurologic symptoms, and/or resolve on follow-up scans also indicate active NP-SLE lesions (439, 440). Many of these reversible lesions represent edema caused by a variety of possible pathogenetic mechanisms.

MRI abnormalities are present in up to 75% of SLE patients with the antiphospholipid antibody syndrome (454–457). The most common lesions are cerebral infarcts; small, focal lesions; and multiple sclerosislike lesions (266). SLE patients with antiphospholipid antibodies are more likely than other SLE patients to have a higher number and increased severity of these MRI abnormalities.

Some NP-SLE patients, particularly those with diffuse manifestations, may have a normal MRI of the brain. However, recent developments in MR technology have shown that these patients may have abnormalities on other MR techniques, which are not present on conventional MRI. MR relaxometry can provide quantitative data regarding the relaxation properties of water in different chemical environments induced by inflammatory diseases of the brain (453). The spin-spin relaxation time (T2) has been reported to be elevated in normal-appearing white matter in NP-SLE patients (453, 458). Sibbitt and coworkers recently showed that quantitative T2 measurements of frontal gray matter were abnormal in patients with diffuse, major neurologic manifestations, including seizures, psychosis, and coma, but not in patients with minor neurologic symptoms such as headaches, minor depression, and minor cognitive dysfunction (453). The prolongation of the T2 value suggesting acute cerebral edema was present even when the conventional MRI appeared normal. This MRI technique can be performed at any clinical MRI center that has the widely available T2 calculation software. Bigler et al. used specialized computer software analysis of conventional brain MRI of SLE patients to demonstrate subtle atrophy and white matter hyperintensities, which were not seen by experienced neuroradiologists on conventional MRI (459).

Three other modifications of conventional MRI techniques include diffusion MRI, perfusion MRI, and magnetization transfer imaging (MTI). Diffusion-weighted imaging on MRI is based on the slowdown in microscopic brain-water motion, which occurs within minutes of vessel occlusion. The slowdown in moving water protons is because of depolarization and edema resulting from the ischemia. Diffusion-weighted imaging shows abnormalities far sooner than changes appear on T2-weighted images (460). Perfusion imaging on MRI maps cerebral blood flow using rapid MRI scanning and an MR tracer bolus. Perfusion imaging detects changes in blood flow and volume in cortical and leptomeningeal vessels prior to any abnormalities appearing on T2-weighted images (461). MTI is an MRI technique that is more sensitive than MRI in quantifying structural brain damage (462, 463). Lower MTI values reflect abnormalities in brain parenchyma as well as atrophy. Bosma et al. recently reported that SLE patients with a history of NP-SLE had significantly lower MTI values, compared to SLE patients without a history of NP-SLE and healthy controls (463).

Magnetic Resonance Spectroscopy

Magnetic resonance spectroscopy (MRS) uses the same hardware and technology as MRI (464). MRI produces images based on water nuclei signals, while MRS provides information from hydrogen and phosphorus nuclei of other chemical compounds. Because water is more abundant than other chemical compounds, MRI provides better anatomic detail than MRS. However, MRS can demonstrate abnormalities in tissue metabolism before MRI shows the structural lesion. MRS abnormalities are displayed in spectra of peaks, reflecting the chemical structure and concentration of individual metabolites (Fig. 35.7) (425).

Proton MRS examines the spectrum of hydrogen (^{1}H) nuclei in brain tissue. Signals are obtained from N-acetylaspartic acid (NAA), creatinine, choline, lactate, inositol, glutamate and glutamine, and lipid/macromolecules. NAA is located exclusively in neurons. Choline is located in water-soluble choline compounds found in the cytoplasm of all cells and in membrane-bound phosphatidylcholine and sphingomyelin. Patients with NP-SLE have reduced NAA in gray and white matter, which appears normal on MRI. Decreased NAA also correlates with neurocognitive dysfunction, cerebral atrophy, antiphospholipid antibodies, and focal lesions, suggesting it is an accurate measure of brain injury in NP-SLE (465–470).

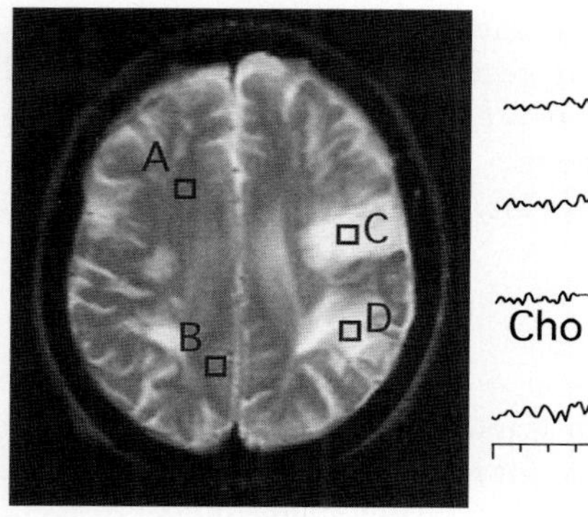

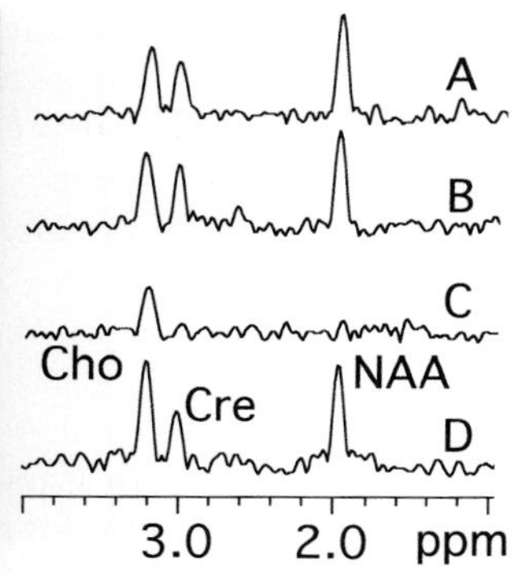

FIGURE 35.7. T2-weighted image of the brain of a neuropsychiatric systemic lupus erythematosus patient with multiple lesions, showing the locations of the spectroscopic voxels. Each voxel yields a separate magnetic resonance spectrum. The spectra reflect the neurochemistry in normal-appearing white matter **(A)**, normal-appearing gray matter **(B)**, and hyperintense lesions **(C** and **D)**. Spectra from voxels A, B, C, and D demonstrate decreased NAA and increased Cho. These abnormalities are accentuated in the lesions **(C** and **D)**, which demonstrate different spectroscopic patterns relative to NAA, Cre, and Cho, indicating considerable metabolic heterogeneity within the population of focal lesions. NAA, N-acetylaspartic acid; Cre, creatine; Cho, Choline. From Sibbitt WL, Sibbitt RR, Brooks WM. Neuroimaging in neuropsychiatric systemic lupus erythematosus. *Arthritis Rheum* 1999;42:2026–2038, with permission.

Patients with NP-SLE have increased choline in brain tissue, which appears normal on conventional MRI. Increased choline is also seen in NP-SLE patients with stroke, inflammation, and cognitive impairment. Notably, NP-SLE patients without an overt stroke have normal lactate spectra, suggesting that cerebral dysfunction can be by pathogenetic mechanisms other than vascular ischemia. The reversibility of these MRS abnormalities is unclear, with many NP-SLE patients continuing to have reduced NAA levels after the neurologic dysfunction has resolved on therapy (471).

Phosphorus MRS examines the phosphorus (^{31}P)-containing compounds of the brain. It displays ATP and phosphocreatine peaks, which are important in cellular energy metabolism. Patients with active NP-SLE demonstrate decreased ATP and phosphocreatine in deep white matter, which are reversible on corticosteroid therapy (472). This is consistent with neuronal injury from ischemia and other mechanisms.

Angiography

Cerebral angiography is frequently normal in NP-SLE patients, even in those with cerebral infarction on MRI (63–66, 473–476). This lack of sensitivity may be explained by the small size of vessels affected by lupus vasculopathy. Occasionally, vasculitis of larger-size arteries or cerebral emboli can be documented. However, angiograms are an invasive procedure with possible morbidity. A recent study reported angiograms in patients with suspected vasculitis were associated with transient neurologic deficits in 11.5%, which were persistent in 0.8% (477). MR angiography is a noninvasive alternative, which can demonstrate abnormalities in medium to large vessels. In patients with suspected emboli, carotid Doppler and echocardiogram (including transesophageal technique) should be done to rule out a source of emboli.

Radionuclide Brain Scans

Technetium brain scans are abnormal in less than 20% of patients with NP-SLE (17, 20–22), although two groups have found a higher sensitivity (478–480). Other neuroimaging techniques have largely replaced these scans in the evaluation of NP-SLE patients. However, other radionuclide tests, specifically PET and SPECT, may be helpful in the future.

Positron Emission Tomography

Positron emission tomography (PET) is a radionuclide technique using unstable isotopes of biologically important elements, which decay rapidly, releasing a positron burst. Glucose uptake and utilization is measured using 2-(^{18}F)-fluoro-2-deoxyglucose (^{18}FDG), while cerebral blood flow and oxygen consumption are measured using ^{15}O-labeled water and ^{15}O-labeled molecular oxygen, respectively (481–489). Two studies have demonstrated that 100% of patients with NP-SLE have multiple, focal areas of hyper or hypometabolism on ^{18}FDG-PET scans (481, 482). The hypometabolism abnormalities were located predominantly in the temporoparietooccipital region, which is located at the boundary of supply of all three major arteries to the brain and thought to be the most vulnerable zone of the cerebrum. Hypermetabolism was seen in the striatum. These abnormalities are seen in NP-SLE patients with normal CT and/or MRI scans (481–483, 486–488). Serial FDG-PET scans have demonstrated improvement in these areas of hypometabolism with treatment (490, 491). However, not all investigators have found abnormal glucose utilization on PET scans in SLE patients. Sailer et al. recently reported that glucose utilization was the same in SLE patients with or without NP-SLE and similar to age-matched, normal controls (492).

In 1978, Pinching et al. (493) demonstrated $^{15}O_2$-$C^{15}O_2$ perfusion deficits in patients with NP-SLE. Others also have found abnormalities in cerebral blood flow in focal areas throughout the cerebrum (425). Despite these findings, abnormalities of metabolism and perfusion found on PET scans in SLE patients should be interpreted with caution and in conjunction with MRI findings. There are multiple confounding variables, other than NP-SLE, which can lead to an abnormal PET scan in a patient with SLE (425).

Single-Photon Emission Computed Tomography

SPECT scans measure cerebral blood flow by using CT reconstruction to image single photons emitted by radiolabeled tracers, usually ^{99}mTc-HMPAO (489). Two patterns are typically observed. Patients with diffuse manifestations of NP-SLE show symmetric and widespread areas of decreased uptake at multiple sites, consistent with patchy hypoperfusion. NP-SLE patients with focal manifestations frequently have large, focal defects that are not as widespread (494–507). Perfusion abnormalities are most common in the parietal greater than frontal greater than temporal lobes greater than basal ganglia, which are supplied by the middle cerebral artery (495, 503). Although the majority of patients with NP-SLE (33% to 100%) will have an abnormal SPECT, up to 50% of SLE patients without clinically evident neurologic or psychiatric manifestations will also have abnormal SPECT scans (494–507). Furthermore, SPECT scans must be interpreted in conjunction with MRI findings, cannot separate new or reversible lesions from old or chronic ones, and do not separate active NP-SLE from secondary causes of neurologic dysfunction in SLE patients (425). Thus, using a single abnormal SPECT scan to diagnose active NP-SLE is not recommended, whereas a normal SPECT scan may indicate a lack of significant pathology. Unlike PET scanners, which require a cyclotron and thus are limited to a few university centers, SPECT scans are relatively inexpensive and available to the community physician. However, more research is necessary before this can be recommended as a diagnostic technique for NP-SLE.

Transcranial Doppler Ultrasound

Transcranial Doppler ultrasound (TCD) is a noninvasive measure of flow velocity for intracranial vessels (middle cerebral artery). It can be used for the detection of intracranial microemboli from carotid artery disease, artificial heart valves, and coagulopathies (508). Microembolic signal detection by TCD has correlated with prior brain infarcts and used to predict future cerebral ischemic events in patients with carotid stenosis (509). Specker et al. tested TCD in SLE patients with and without antiphospholipid antibodies. The positive predictive value of detectable microembolic signals for previous cerebral ischemic events was 0.93, whereas the negative predictive value was 0.94 (400). There was a significant correlation with high-titer IgG anticardiolipin antibodies. This study may add additional information to other clinical predictors for which SLE patients with antiphospholipid antibodies are at risk for recurrent cerebral ischemia and require anticoagulation. Furthermore, TCD results suggest that cerebral ischemia associated with antiphospholipid antibodies is more often due to microemboli than *in situ* vessel thrombosis.

Summary

Currently, MRI with gadolinium is the only imaging modality recommended for the evaluation of NP-SLE (10). CT scan is useful to rapidly rule out a large infarct or hemorrhage in an SLE patient with acute neurologic deterioration. MRI is superior to CT scan for detecting edema, infarcts, and hemorrhage. However, there is no MRI finding which is specific for NP-SLE. Furthermore, patients with NP-SLE, particularly those with diffuse manifestations, may have a normal conventional MRI. Conversely, SLE patients without NP-SLE may have abnormalities on MRI, which may be misinterpreted as NP-SLE. Thus, the results of MRI must be interpreted along with the clinical and other laboratory findings to establish a diagnosis of NP-SLE (26). Other MRI techniques, including MR relaxometry, MRS, diffusion MRI, perfusion MRI, and MTI are presently research tools. In the future, they may increase the sensitivity and specificity of conventional MRI and prove that all patients with NP-SLE will have demonstrable abnormalities. Although MRS cannot be used to specifically diagnose NP-SLE, it is very sensitive and specific for brain injury and may be very useful to confirm an organic basis for neurocognitive dysfunction in a patient suspected of having mild NP-SLE (425).

PET and SPECT scans are very sensitive but lack specificity, thus limiting their value in the diagnosis of NP-SLE. These modalities should be considered research neuroimaging procedures and not used in the clinical evaluation of patients with NP-SLE. However, a normal SPECT scan may rule against significant brain pathology in an SLE patient with nonspecific neuropsychiatric symptoms.

ELECTROENCEPHALOGRAPHY

Conventional EEG is abnormal in 60% to 91% of adult and pediatric patients with NP-SLE (17–22, 26, 49, 510, 511). The most common finding is diffuse slowing with increased beta and delta background activity. Focal abnormalities and seizure activity also can be seen. Unfortunately, the EEG findings are not specific for NP-SLE, and other disorders, including metabolic encephalopathies and drug effects, can give similar findings. Furthermore, up to 50% of SLE patients without active NP-SLE can have abnormal EEGs. Consequently, a single abnormal EEG has limited diagnostic value for NP-SLE. On occasion, however, an EEG may be very helpful, revealing unsuspected seizure activity, which was not apparent clinically. EEGs may be able to distinguish steroid-induced psychosis from NP-SLE (512).

Quantitative EEG (Q-EEG) has been found to be more sensitive and specific compared to conventional EEG (513, 514). Q-EEG is abnormal in 87% of patients with definite NP-SLE, 74% of patients with probable NP-SLE, and 28% of SLE patients without neuropsychiatric symptoms. Serial Q-EEG reportedly shows improvement with therapy.

Visual, brainstem, auditory, and somatosensory-evoked potentials have been reported to be useful in detecting subtle cortical dysfunction not detected with conventional EEG (515–518). Others have failed to demonstrate evoked potential to be of value (519). Further controlled studies on these modalities are needed to establish their usefulness in clinical practice.

TREATMENT

The therapy of NP-SLE differs depending upon the clinical presentation and suspected pathogenesis. A thorough clinical evaluation and appropriate diagnostic evaluation of any SLE patient with new neuropsychiatric symptoms is important to establish the extent of neurological impairment and brain injury, in order to assess future progression and response to therapy. Secondary causes of CNS dysfunction should be excluded quickly and all unnecessary medications should be stopped. Therapy should not be delayed pending test results. If it is unclear whether the CNS dysfunction is due to primary NP-SLE or a secondary cause, then the patient should be treated for both until diagnostic test results return (Fig. 35.4).

Central Nervous System Manifestations

The treatment of NP-SLE is empiric, as there have been no controlled clinical trials. The therapy should be tailored to the severity of the presentation and suspected etiology. Patients with mild, diffuse manifestations such as headaches, anxiety/dysphoria, paresthesias, or an isolated seizure may need only analgesics, psychotropic medications, and psychologic support, or antiseizure medications, respectively, and observed closely for any neurologic progression. A particularly difficult clinical situation is the SLE patient with a complaint of cognitive dysfunction but a clinically normal mental status examination. In these patients, serial psychometric testing may be helpful in establishing the presence, extent, and progression, if any, of impairment. Secondary causes, such as medications, thyroid disease, depression, and especially sleep apnea need to be excluded. Treatment should be supportive, including memory aids, unless progression can be documented. The use of immunosuppressive therapy in this clinical situation is limited (154).

NP-SLE patients with severe or progressive, diffuse presentations such as acute confusional state, psychosis, severe depression, and coma may benefit from immunosuppressive medications. Most clinicians recommend 1 mg/kg/day of prednisone in divided doses. For the most severe cases, pulse intravenous methylprednisolone (1 gm daily for 3 days) may be beneficial (520–522). Failure to respond within a few days may necessitate doubling of the prednisone dose. Another alternative is to switch from prednisone to dexamethasone (12 to 20 mg q.d.), which penetrates the blood-brain barrier better than other corticosteroid preparations. Continued failure to respond is an indication to add cytotoxic medications and/or a trial of plasmapheresis, particularly for comatose patients. Pulse intravenous cyclophosphamide (0.75 to 1.0 gm/m^2) given every 3 to 6 weeks has been reported to be beneficial in both adult and pediatric patients (523–526). Azathioprine also has been used, but with less impressive results. Patients with psychosis or depression should receive appropriate psychotropic medications to aid in the subsequent tapering of immunosuppressive medications.

NP-SLE patients presenting with focal manifestations demand an immediate and aggressive evaluation. If vasculitis is suspected, corticosteroids in high doses similar to patients with severe, diffuse manifestations are used. Cytotoxic medications should be used early in patients with vasculitis. Clinical experience suggests that cyclophosphamide is more effective than azathioprine, methotrexate, cyclosporine, or mycophenolate mofetil (CellCept, Hoffmann-La Roche Inc.) (527). Once the patient's NP-SLE is controlled on cyclophosphamide, another cytotoxic medication may be substituted to maintain remission. It is unknown if chronic antiplatelet therapy prevents thrombosis or atheroma formation in the damaged vessel, but it is often used.

Many patients with focal manifestations of NP-SLE have antiphospholipid antibodies. Because the suspected pathogenesis is thrombosis and not vasculitis, patients are treated with antiplatelet drugs, hydroxychloroquine for its mild anticoagulant effect, and/or anticoagulation. In patients with large or cardioembolic strokes, excessive heparinization is dangerous and may cause hemorrhage into the infarcted area. Consequently, particularly in patients with an elevated partial thromboplastin time as a result of the lupus anticoagulant, heparin levels should be followed as well as serial CT scans. Patients with significant thrombotic events should then receive warfarin to maintain an INR of 3.0 to 3.5 (528, 529). Patients with the lupus anticoagulant should also have periodic factor II and chromogenic factor X levels followed and maintained at 15% to 20% of normal to assure adequate anticoagulation (530). Some physicians also obtain a prothrombin fragment F1.2, which should be within the normal range if the patient is not clotting on anticoagulation therapy. Patients who continue to thrombose on anticoagulation may respond to intravenous gammaglobulin or plasmapheresis with immunosuppressive therapy (524).

NP-SLE patients with seizures should be treated with antiseizure medications. Patients presenting in status epilepticus or who have recurrent seizures should be treated with high-dose prednisone. Patients with seizures, cerebral infarcts, and antiphospholipid antibodies should be anticoagulated once seizures are controlled, although they are at increased risk for falls and cerebral trauma. Antiseizure medications may have side effects, which can mimic active lupus. Phenytoin can cause fever, adenopathy, and leukopenia. Ataxia and other neurologic symptoms can occur if the phenytoin level rises above therapeutic levels. Carbamazepine can cause severe leukopenia and must be monitored closely. SLE patients with seizures should remain on antiseizure medications for at least 1 year. If they have no recurrence of seizures, a normal MRI, and normal EEG, then antiseizure medications can be withdrawn, and the patient followed closely. Vehicle driving restrictions should be enforced.

Some patients with NP-SLE will not respond to, may not tolerate, or will have contraindications to aggressive therapy. In these patients, a variety of other therapies have been tried. One novel therapy is intrathecal methotrexate and dexamethasone (10 mg of each, weekly for 3 weeks). Two reports totaling 27 patients with diffuse manifestations of NP-SLE received this therapy with over 90% of patients responding (30, 531). Another therapy is intravenous immunoglobulin (IVIG). Six of seven patients with severe, acute NP-SLE responded to IVIG (532). IVIG should be given at a dose of 400 mg/kg/day for five consecutive days, instead of 1,000 mg/kg/day for two days, in order to lessen the chance of side effects such as thrombosis, fluid overload, renal function deterioration, and aseptic meningitis. A third therapy is plasmapheresis (533-537). For a critically ill patient, 40 to 60 mL of plasma/kg/day is removed for up to five consecutive days. For a more stable patient, 40 mL of plasma/kg/day three times a week for 3 weeks constitutes a therapeutic trial. Oftentimes, only 1 week of plasmapheresis is needed to stabilize the patient. Plasmapheresis is particularly useful for patients with cerebral vasculitis to allow time for the corticosteroids and cytotoxic medications to take effect. It is also used in patients with recurrent cerebral infarcts, associated with antiphospholipid antibodies, who fail anticoagulation. However, some investigators are using IVIG in this clinical situation to avoid the catheter-related thrombosis frequently seen in these patients (524, 538). Notably, immunosuppressive medications are continued during plasmapheresis to prevent rebound antibody production and/or disease flare. Frequent side effects of plasmapheresis are catheter-related problems and infection (539). Patients developing hypogammaglobulinemia should receive replacement immunoglobulin to help prevent infection. Another use for plasmapheresis is in SLE patients with hyperviscosity syndrome (viscosity >4) from circulating immune complexes, severe hypergammaglobulinemia, or cryoglobulinemia (cryocrits greater than 8%) who have symptoms of cerebral insufficiency. Finally, plasmapheresis with fresh frozen plasma replacement is the best therapy for SLE patients with TTP (540). Other therapies reported in isolated case reports to be successful in steroid-unresponsive NP-SLE are hyperbaric oxygen for cognitive impairment (541) and intrathecal CSF-pheresis (542). Hematopoietic stem cell transplantation (543) or high-dose cyclophosphamide therapy (544) may be considered for patients with severe and resistant NP-SLE.

Several difficult clinical situations warrant further comment. First is the SLE patient on corticosteroids who presents with neuropsychiatric symptoms that could be NP-SLE versus steroid psychosis. One approach is to double the dose of corticosteroids for three days while awaiting test results. If the psychotic episode is due to NP-SLE, it will respond to this therapy. Failure to improve lessens the likelihood of NP-SLE and the corticosteroids should be tapered to half of the original dose. If corticosteroids cannot be tapered, then antipsychotics such as haloperidol or lithium can be used (354, 545). Tricyclic antidepressants should be avoided (356). Another situation is the SLE patient with dementia from prior NP-SLE or from infarctions related to antiphospholipid antibodies. The dementia in these patients will not respond to corticosteroids and, in fact, may worsen. SLE patients with stable dementia should not be automatically assumed to have active NP-SLE and treated aggressively with immunosuppressive medications.

Two other difficult clinical situations are transverse myelitis and chorea. Transverse myelitis should be treated aggressively with corticosteroids and cyclophosphamide (231–235). Patients presenting acutely should receive intravenous pulse methylprednisolone followed by high-dose prednisone and intravenous monthly cyclophosphamide. Patients with chorea usually respond to corticosteroids and haloperidol. Those that do not respond may need cytotoxic medications and/or plasmapheresis.

Several neurologic syndromes, including stroke, transverse myelitis, chorea, seizures, and multiple sclerosislike syndromes, have been associated with antiphospholipid antibodies (303) as well as other pathogenetic mechanisms. When a patient presents with one of these manifestations, the antiphospholipid antibody results may take a few days to return. In the interim, we have treated these patients with corticosteroids and antiplatelet drugs until results of antiphospholipid antibodies return, particularly because vasculitis can coexist with antiphospholipid antibody-associated thrombosis (74). If the antiphospholipid antibodies are positive, the next decision is whether to continue with antiplatelet drugs or to anticoagulate. One approach has been to anticoagulate those patients with the lupus anticoagulant or high-titer (>40 to 50 GPL units) IgG anticardiolipin/anti-β2 glycoprotein-1 antibodies and/or other manifestations of the antiphospholipid antibody syndrome, including livedo reticularis, previous miscarriages, previous thrombotic episodes, and mild thrombocytopenia (529).

Peripheral Nervous System Manifestations

SLE patients with mild, nonprogressive paresthesias require only symptomatic therapy. Patients with cranial, peripheral, or autonomic neuropathy are treated with high-dose corticosteroids initially. Patients with Guillain-Barré or CIDP frequently have IVIG or plasmapheresis as additional therapy. Patients with mononeuritis multiplex resulting from vasculitis also should receive cytotoxic therapy such as cyclophosphamide. When using cyclophosphamide in patients with peripheral/autonomic nervous system involvement, it is important to determine if the patient has a neurogenic bladder, which may not eliminate the cyclophosphamide metabolites leading to hemorrhagic cystitis. SLE patients with myasthenia gravis are treated with medications, which increase the concentration of acetylcholine at the neuromuscular junction. Other therapy is similar to that given patients without SLE who have myasthenia. The role of thymectomy is controversial since SLE has been reported to flare after the thymus has been removed (339).

PROGNOSIS

The prognosis for NP-SLE patients remains guarded. Although many NP-SLE patients with diffuse symptoms appear to recover, recent studies using psychometric testing demonstrate that many patients are left with cognitive dysfunction suggesting residual CNS damage (146–148). Patients with focal manifestations may stabilize, but usually do not reverse their deficits during therapy. Recurrences of NP-SLE episodes occur in 30% to 40% of NP-SLE patients, leading to more residual dysfunction. Using the ACR-Systemic Lupus International Collaborating Clinics damage index, Petri has found neuropsychiatric damage steadily accrues and is the second-leading organ system that is damaged in the Hopkin's lupus cohort (546). With dialysis and transplantation enabling lupus patients with nephritis to survive longer, NP-SLE and its therapy may now be the leading cause of death with a 7% to 19% mortality rate (21, 30, 547, 548). Previous studies indicate that seizures, especially status epilepticus, stroke, and coma are particularly poor prognostic signs (14, 17, 547, 548), demanding aggressive evaluation and treatment to help prevent residual neurologic damage or death. Whether the therapy improves or contributes to long-term morbidity and mortality from conditions like atherosclerosis and cancer is unclear (549). Consequently, the clinician must make every effort to limit the toxicities of therapy by controlling hypertension, treating hyperlipidemia and hyperglycemia, utilizing osteoporosis prophylaxis, administering Pneumovax, advising against smoking, treating hyperhomocystinemia with appropriate vitamins, and using medications for Pneumocystis carinii prophylaxis.

REFERENCES

1. Hebra F, Kaposi M. *On diseases of the skin including the exanthemata.* Translated and edited by Tay W. London: The New Syndeham Society, 1875, v.4.
2. Osler W. On the visceral complications of erythema exudativum multiforme. *Am J Med Sci* 1895;110:629–646.
3. Osler W. The visceral lesions of the erythema group. *Br J Dermatol* 1900;12:227–245.
4. Osler W. On the visceral manifestations of the erythema group of skin diseases. *Am J Med Sci* 1904;127:123.
5. Baum WL. *The practical medicine year books.* Chicago: Year Book Publishers, 1904;10:89.
6. Daly D. Central nervous system in acute disseminated lupus erythematosus. *J Nerv Ment Dis* 1945;102:461–465.
7. Sedgwick RP, Von Hagen KO. Neurological manifestations of lupus erythematosus and periarteritis nodosa: report of 10 cases. *Bull Los Angeles Neurol Soc* 1948;13:129–142.
8. Dubois EL. Effect of LE cell test on clinical picture of systemic lupus erythematosus. *Ann Intern Med* 1953;38:1265–1294.
9. Lewis BI, Sinton BW, Knott JR. Central nervous system involvement in disorders of collagen. *Arch Intern Med* 1954;93: 315–327.
10. ACR Ad Hoc Committee on Neuropsychiatric Lupus Nomenclature. The American College of Rheumatology Nomenclature and Case Definitions for Neuropsychiatric Lupus Syndromes. *Arthritis Rheum* 1999;42:599–608.
11. Dubois EL, Tuffanelli DL. Clinical manifestations of systemic lupus erythematosus. Computer analysis of 520 cases. *JAMA* 1964;190:104–111.
12. Clark EC, Bailey AA. Neurological and psychiatric signs associated with systemic lupus erythematosus. *JAMA* 1956;160: 455–457.
13. O'Connor JF, Musher DM. Central nervous system involvement in systemic lupus erythematosus. A study of 150 cases. *Arch Neurol* 1966;14:157–164.
14. Estes D, Christian CL. The natural history of systemic lupus erythematosus by prospective analysis. *Medicine* 1971;50: 85–95.
15. Sergent JS, Lockshin MD, Klemperer MS, et al. Central nervous system disease in systemic lupus erythematosus therapy and prognosis. *Am J Med* 1975;58:644–654.
16. Klippel JH, Zvaifler NJ. Neuropsychiatric abnormalities in systemic lupus erythematosus. *Clin Rheum Dis* 1975;1:621–638.
17. Feinglass EJ, Arnett FC, Dorsch CA, et al. Neuropsychiatric manifestations of systemic lupus erythematosus: diagnosis, clinical spectrum, and relationship to other features of the disease. *Medicine* 1976;55:323–339.
18. Abel T, Gladman DD, Urowitz MB. Neuropsychiatric lupus. *J Rheumatol* 1980;7:325–332.
19. Lee P, Weston WL, Bookman AA, et al. Systemic lupus erythematosus: a review of 110 cases with reference to nephritis, the nervous system, infections, aseptic necrosis, and prognosis. *Q J Med* 1977;46:132.
20. Grigor R, Edmonds J, Lewkonia R, et al. Systemic lupus erythematosus. A prospective analysis. *Ann Rheum Dis* 1978;37: 121–128.
21. Gibson T, Myers AR. Nervous system involvement in systemic lupus erythematosus. *Ann Rheum Dis* 1975;35:398–406.
22. Seibold JR, Buckingham RB, Medsger TA Jr, et al. Cerebrospinal fluid immune complexes in systemic lupus involving the CNS. *Semin Arthritis Rheum* 1982;12:68–76.
23. Pistiner M, Wallace DJ, Nessim S, et al. Lupus erythematosus in the 1980s: a survey of 570 patients. *Semin Arthritis Rheum* 1991;21:55–64.

24. Vitali C, Bencivelli W, Isenberg DA, et al. Disease activity in systemic lupus erythematosus: report of the Consensus Study Group of the European Workshop for Rheumatology Research. I. A descriptive analysis of 704 European lupus patients. *Clin Exp Rheumatol* 1992;10:527–539.
25. Cervera R, Khamashta MA, Font J, et al. Systemic lupus erythematosus: clinical and immunologic patterns of disease expression in a cohort of 1000 patients. *Medicine* 1993;72: 113–124.
26. West SG, Emlen W, Wener MH, et al. Neuropsychiatric lupus erythematosus: a 10–year prospective study on the value of diagnostic tests. *Am J Med* 1995;99:153–163.
27. Buchbinder R, Hall S, Littlejohn GO, et al. Neuropsychiatric manifestations of systemic lupus erythematosus. *Aust N Z J Med* 1988;18:679–684.
28. Migliaresi S, Di Iorio G, Picillo U, et al. Neurological manifestations of systemic lupus erythematosus. Study of 53 cases. *Ann Ital Med Int* 1989;4:10–15.
29. Sibley JT, Olszynski WP, Decoteau WE, et al. The incidence and prognosis of central nervous system disease in systemic lupus erythematosus. *J Rheumatol* 1992;19:47–52.
30. Xuan Z, Yi D, Fu-Lin T, et al. Central nervous system involvement in systemic lupus erythematosus in a hospital-based study of 171 cases. *J Clin Rheumatol* 1999;5:314–319.
31. Bluestein HG, Williams GW, Steinberg AD. Cerebrospinal fluid antibodies to neuronal cells: association with neuropsychiatric manifestations of systemic lupus erythematosus. *Am J Med* 1981;70:240–246.
32. Bluestein HG, Zvaifler HG. Antibodies reactive with central nervous system antigens. *Hum Pathol* 1983;14:424–428.
33. Denburg JA, Carbotte RM, Denburg SD. Neuronal antibodies and cognitive function in systemic lupus erythematosus. *Neurology* 1987;37:464–467.
34. Hanly JG, Behmann S, Denburg SD, et al. The association between sequential changes in serum antineuronal antibodies and neuropsychiatric systemic lupus erythematosus. *Postgrad Med J* 1989;65:622–627.
35. Kelly MC, Denburg JA. Cerebrospinal fluid immunoglobulins and neuronal antibodies in neuropsychiatric systemic lupus erythematosus and related conditions. *J Rheumatol* 1987;14: 740–744.
36. Bonfa E, Elkon KB. Clinical and serologic associations of the anti-ribosomal P protein antibody. *Arthritis Rheum* 1986;29:981–985.
37. Teh LS, Isenberg DA. Anti-ribosomal P protein antibodies in systemic lupus erythematosus. A reappraisal. *Arthritis Rheum* 1994;37:307–315.
38. Fields RA, Sibbitt WL, Toubbeh H, et al. Neuropsychiatric lupus erythematosus, cerebral infarctions, and anticardiolipin antibodies. *Ann Rheum Dis* 1990;49:114–117.
39. Isshi K, Hirohata S. Differential roles of the anti-ribosomal P antibody and antineuronal antibody in the pathogenesis of central nervous system involvement in systemic lupus erythematosus. *Arthritis Rheum* 1998;41;1819–1827.
40. Futrell N, Millikan C. Frequency, etiology, and prevention of stroke in patients with systemic lupus erythematosus. *Stroke* 1989;20:583–591.
41. Gristanti MAA, Vergara EF, Cartier RL, et al. Central nervous system involvement in systemic lupus erythematosus. *Rev Med Chile* 1985;113:1194–1202.
42. Kaell AT, Shetty M, Lee BC, et al. The diversity of neurologic events in systemic lupus erythematosus. Prospective clinical and computed tomographic classification of 82 events in 71 patients. *Arch Neurol* 1986;43:273–276.
43. Futrell N, Schultz LR, Millikan C. Central nervous system disease in patients with systemic lupus erythematosus. *Neurology* 1992;42:1649–1657.
44. Wong KL, Woo EKS, Wong RWS. Neurologic manifestations of systemic lupus erythematosus: a prospective study. *Q J Med* 1991;294:857–870.
45. Kovacs JAJ, Urowitz MB, Gladman DD. Dilemmas in neuropsychiatric lupus. *Rheum Dis Clin North Am* 1993;19: 795–814.
46. Sibley JT, Olszynski WP, Decoteau WE, et al. The incidence and prognosis of central nervous system disease in systemic lupus erythematosus. *J Rheumatol* 1992;19:47–52.
47. Cassidy JT, Sullivan DB, Petty RE, et al. Lupus nephritis and encephalopathy. Proceedings of the Conference of Rheumatic Diseases in Childhood. *Arthritis Rheum* 1977;20(suppl 2): 315–322.
48. Bahabri S et al. Juvenile systemic lupus erythematosus in 60 Saudi children. *Ann Saudi Med* 1997;17:612–615.
49. Yancey CL, Doughty RA, Athreya BH. Central nervous system involvement in childhood systemic lupus erythematosus. *Arthritis Rheum* 1981;24:1389–1395.
50. Baker SB, Rovira JR, Campion EW, et al. Late onset lupus erythematosus. *Am J Med* 1979;66:727–732.
51. Dimant J, Ginzler EM, Schlesinger M, et al. Systemic lupus erythematosus in the older age group: computer analysis. *J Am Geriatr Soc* 1979;27:58–61.
52. McDonald K, Hutchinson M, Bresnihan B. The frequent occurrence of neurological disease in patients with late-onset systemic lupus erythematosus. *Br J Rheumatol* 1984;23: 186–189.
53. Eustace S, Hutchison M, Bresnihan B. Acute cerebrovascular episodes in systemic lupus erythematosus. *Q J Med* 1991;80: 739–750.
54. Dennis MS, Byrne EJ, Hopkinson N, et al. Neuropsychiatric systemic lupus erythematosus in elderly people: a case series. *J Neurol Neurosurg Psychiatry* 1992;55:1157–1161.
55. Johnson RT. Neurologic and neuropathologic observations in lupus erythematosus. *N Engl J Med* 1962;266:895.
56. Johnson RT, Richardson EP. The neurological manifestations of systemic lupus erythematosus. A clinical-pathological study of 24 cases and review of the literature. *Medicine* 1968;47:337–369.
57. Funata N. Cerebral vascular changes in systemic lupus erythematosus. *Bull Tokyo Med Dent Univ* 1979;26:91–112.
58. Ellis SG, Verity MA. Central nervous system involvement in systemic lupus erythematosus: a review of neuropathologic findings in 57 cases, 1955–1977. *Semin Arthritis Rheum* 1979; 8:212–221.
59. Devinsky O, Petito CK, Alonso DR. Clinical and neuropathological findings in systemic lupus erythematosus: the role of vasculitis, heart emboli, and thrombotic thrombocytopenic purpura. *Ann Neurol* 1988;23:380–384.
60. Greisman SG, Rose-Sunitha T, Godwin TA, et al. Occlusive vasculopathy in systemic lupus erythematosus. Association with anticardiolipin antibody. *Arch Intern Med* 1991;151:389–392.
61. Hanly JG, Walsh NMG, Sangalang V. Brain pathology in systemic lupus erythematosus. *J Rheumatol* 1992;19:732–741.
62. Smith RW, Ellison DW, Jenkins EA, et al. Cerebellum and brainstem vasculopathy in systemic lupus erythematosus: two clinico-pathologic cases. *Ann Rheum Dis* 1994;53:327–330.
63. Weiner DK, Allen NB. Large vessel vasculitis of the central nervous system in systemic lupus erythematosus: report and review of the literature. *J Rheumatol* 1991;18:748–751.
64. Kelley RE, Stokes N, Reyes P, et al. Cerebral transmural angiitis and ruptured aneurysm: a complication of systemic lupus erythematosus. *Arch Neurol* 1980;37:526–527.
65. Suzuki Y, Kitagawa Y, Matsuoka Y, et al. Severe cerebral and systemic necrotizing vasculitis developing during pregnancy in a case of systemic lupus erythematosus (case report). *J Rheumatol* 1990;17:1408–1411.

66. Bunning RD, Laureno R, Barth WF. Florid central nervous system vasculitis in a fatal case of systemic lupus erythematosus. *J Rheumatol* 1982;9:735–738.
67. Berden JHM, Hang L, McConahey PJ, et al. Analysis of vascular lesions in murine SLE. *J Immunol* 1983;130:1699.
68. Accinni L, Dixon FJ. Degenerative vascular disease and myocardial infarction in mice with lupus-like syndrome. *Am J Pathol* 1979;96:477.
69. Westerman EM, Miles JM, Backonja M, et al. Neuropathologic findings in multi–infarct dementia associated with anticardiolipin antibody. Evidence for endothelial injury as the primary event. *Arthritis Rheum* 1992;35:1038–1041.
70. Berkowitz LR, Dalldorf FG, Blatt PM. Thrombotic thrombocytopenic purpura. A pathology review. *JAMA* 1979;241: 1709–1710.
71. Pierangeli SS, Colden-Stanfield M, Liu X, et al. Antiphospholipid antibodies from antiphospholipid syndrome patients activate endothelial cells in vitro and in vivo. *Circulation* 1999; 99:1997–2002.
72. Ellison D, Gatter K, Heryet A, et al. Intramural platelet deposition in cerebral vasculopathy of systemic lupus erythematosus. *J Clin Pathol* 1993;46:37–40.
73. Borowska-Lehman J, Bakowska A, Michowska M, et al. Antiphospholipid syndrome in systemic lupus erythematosus—immunomorphological study of the central nervous system: case report. *Folia Neuropathologica* 1995;33:231–233.
74. Goldberger E, Elder RC, Schwartz RA, et al. Vasculitis in the antiphospholipid antibody syndrome. A cause of ischemia responding to corticosteroids. *Arthritis Rheum* 1992;35: 569–572.
75. Harris EN, Gharavi AE, Asherson RA, et al. Cerebral infarction in systemic lupus: association with anticardiolipin antibodies. *Clin Exp Rheumatol* 1984;2:47–51.
76. Harris EN, Gharavi AE, Mackworth-Young CG, et al. Lupoid sclerosis: a possible pathogenetic role for antiphospholipid antibodies. *Ann Rheum Dis* 1985;44:281–283.
77. Toubi E, Khamashta MA, Panarra A, et al. Association of antiphospholipid antibodies with central nervous system disease in systemic lupus erythematosus. *Am J Med* 1995;99:397–401.
78. Carhuapoma JR, Mitsias P, Levine SR. Cerebral venous thrombosis and anticardiolipin antibodies. *Stroke* 1997;28: 2363–2369.
79. Markusse HM, Haan J, Tan WD, et al. Anterior spinal artery syndrome in systemic lupus erythematosus. *Br J Rheumatol* 1989;28:344–346.
80. Brey RL, Gharavi AE, Lockshin MD. Neurologic complications of antiphospholipid antibodies. *Rheum Dis Clin North Am* 1993;19:833–850.
81. Levine SR, Langer SL, Albers JW, et al. Sneddon's syndrome: an antiphospholipid antibody syndrome? *Neurology* 1988;38: 798–800.
82. Molad Y, Sidi Y, Gornish M, et al. Lupus anticoagulant: correlation with magnetic resonance imaging of brain lesions. *J Rheumatol* 1992;19:556–561.
83. Weingarten K, Filippi C, Barbut D, et al. The neuroimaging features of the cardiolipin antibody syndrome. *Clinical Imaging* 1997;21:6–12.
84. Hopkins P, Belmont HM, Buyon J, et al. Increased levels of plasma anaphylatoxins in systemic lupus erythematosus predict flares of the disease and may elicit vascular injury in lupus cerebritis. *Arthritis Rheum* 1988;31:632–641.
85. Asherson RA, Gibson DG, Evans DW, et al. Diagnostic and therapeutic problems in two patients with antiphospholipid antibodies, heart valve lesions, and transient ischemic attacks. *Ann Rheum Dis* 1988;47:947–953.
86. Asherson RA, Lubbe WF. Cerebral and valve lesions in SLE: association with antiphospholipid antibodies. *J Rheumatol* 1988;15:539–543.
87. Young SM, Fisher M, Sigsbee A, et al. Cardiogenic brain embolism and lupus anticoagulant. *Ann Neurol* 1989;26: 390–392.
88. Moder KG, Miller TD, Tazelaar HD. Cardiac involvement in systemic lupus erythematosus. *Mayo Clin Proc* 1999;74: 275–284.
89. Adoue D, Arlet P, Duffaut M, et al. Major hyprotidemia (sic) with serum viscosity in systemic lupus erythematosus. *Sem Hop Paris* 1986;62:1261–1264.
90. Fukasawa T, Arai T, Naruse T, et al. Hyperviscosity syndrome in a patient with systemic lupus erythematosus. *Am J Med Sci* 1977;273:329–334.
91. Jara LJ, Capin NR, Lavalle C. Hyperviscosity syndrome as the initial manifestation of systemic lupus erythematosus. *J Rheumatol* 1989;16:225–230.
92. Shearn MA, Epstein WV, Engelman EP. Serum viscosity in rheumatic diseases and macroglobulinemia. *Arch Intern Med* 1963;112:684–687.
93. Tsokos GC, Tsokos M, le Riche NG, et al. A clinical and pathologic study of cerebrovascular disease in patients with systemic lupus erythematosus. *Semin Arthritis Rheum* 1986;16:70–78.
94. Hashimoto N, Handa H, Taki W. Ruptured cerebral aneurysms in patients with systemic lupus erythematosus. *Surg Neurol* 1986;26:512–516.
95. Nagayama Y, Kusudo K, Imura H. A case of central nervous system lupus associated with ruptured cerebral Berry aneurysm. *Jpn J Med* 1989;28:530–533.
96. Savitz MH, Katz SS, Lestch SD, et al. Mirror-image intracerebral hemorrhages in a patient with systemic lupus erythematosus. *Mt Sinai J Med* 1987;54:522–524.
97. Kobiler D, Fuch S, Samual D. The effects of antisynaptosomal plasma membrane antibodies on memory. *Brain Res* 1976;15: 129–137.
98. Rappaport MM, Karpiak SE, Mahadik SP. Biological activity of antibodies injected into the brain. *Fed Proc* 1978;38: 2391–2396.
99. Simon J, Simon O. Effect of passive transfer of anti-brain antibodies to a normal recipient. *Exp Neurol* 1975;47:523–534.
100. Bluestein HG, Zvaifler NJ. Brain-reactive lymphocytotoxic antibodies in the serum of patients with systemic lupus erythematosus. *J Clin Invest* 1976;57:509–516.
101. Bluestein HG. Neurocytotoxic antibodies in the serum of patients with systemic lupus erythematosus. *Proc Natl Acad Sci USA* 1978;75:3965–3970.
102. Bresnihan B, Oliver M, Williams B, et al. An antineuronal antibody cross-reacting with erythrocytes and lymphocytes in systemic lupus erythematosus. *Arthritis Rheum* 1979;22:313–320.
103. Quismorio FP, Friou GJ. Antibodies reactive with neurons in SLE patients with neuropsychiatric manifestations. *Int Arch Allergy* 1972;43:740.
104. Denburg JA, Carbotte RM, Denburg SD. Neuronal antibodies and cognitive function in systemic lupus erythematosus. *Neurology* 1987;37:464–467.
105. Wilson HA, Winfield JB, Lahita RG, et al. Association of IgG anti-brain antibodies with central nervous system dysfunction in systemic lupus erythematosus. *Arthritis Rheum* 1979;22: 458–462.
106. Hirano T, Hashimoto H, Shiokawa Y, et al. Anti-glycolipid autoantibody detected in the sera from systemic lupus erythematosus patients. *J Clin Invest* 1980;66:1437–1440.
107. Hanson VG, Horowitz M, Rosenbluth D, et al. Systemic lupus erythematosus patients with central nervous system involvement show autoantibodies to a 50-kd neuronal membrane protein. *J Exp Med* 1992;176:565–573.

108. Bell CL, Partington C, Robbins M, et al. Magnetic resonance imaging of central nervous system lesions in patients with lupus erythematosus: correlation with clinical remission and anti-neurofilament and anticardiolipin antibody titers. *Arthritis Rheum* 1991;34:432–441.
109. Koren E, Reichlin MW, Kosec M, et al. Autoantibodies to the ribosomal P proteins react with a plasma membrane-related target on human cells. *J Clin Invest* 1992;89:1236–1241.
110. Chapman J, Cohen-Armon M, Shoenfeld Y, et al. Antiphospholipid antibodies permeabilize and depolarize brain synaptoneurosomes. *Lupus* 1999;8:127–133.
111. Caronti B, Calderaro C, Alessandri C, et al. Serum anti-beta2-glycoprotein I antibodies from patients with antiphospholipid antibody syndrome bind central nervous system cells. *J Autoimmunity* 1998;11:425–429.
112. Kelly MC, Denburg JA. Cerebrospinal fluid immunoglobulins and neuronal antibodies in neuropsychiatric systemic lupus and related conditions. *J Rheumatol* 1987;14:740–744.
113. Inoue T, Okamura M, Amatsu K, et al. Antineuronal antibodies in brain tissue of patients with systemic lupus erythematosus. *Lancet* 1982;1:852.
114. Kida S, Weller RO, Zhang ET, et al. Anatomical pathways for lymphatic drainage of the brain and their pathological significance. *Neuropathol Appl Neurobiol* 1995;21:181.
115. Westergaard E. The blood-brain barrier to horseradish peroxidase under normal and experimental conditions. *Acta Neuropathol* 1977;39:181–187.
116. Hickey WF. Migration of hematogenous cells through the blood-brain barrier and the initiation of CNS inflammation. *Brain Pathol* 1991;1:97.
117. Winfield JB 3rd, Shaw M, Silverman LM, et al. Intrathecal IgG synthesis and blood–brain barrier impairment in patients with systemic lupus erythematosus and central nervous system dysfunction. *Am J Med* 1983;74:837–844.
118. McLean BN, Miller D, Thompson EJ. Oligoclonal banding of IgG in CSF, blood-brain barrier function, and MRI findings in patients with sarcoidosis, systemic lupus erythematosus, and Behçet's disease involving the central nervous system. *J Neurol Neurosurg Psychiatry* 1995;58:548–554.
119. Hirohata S, Hirose S, Miyamoto T. Cerebrospinal fluid IgM, IgA, and IgG indexes in systemic lupus erythematosus. Their use as estimates of central nervous system disease activity. *Arch Intern Med* 1985;145:1843–1846.
120. Hirohata S, Miyamoto T. Increased intrathecal immunoglobulin synthesis of both kappa and lambda types in patients with systemic lupus erythematosus and central nervous system involvement. *J Rheumatol* 1986;13:715–721.
121. Hirohata S, Taketani T. A serial study of changes in intrathecal immunoglobulin synthesis in a patient with central nervous system systemic lupus erythematosus. *J Rheumatol* 1987;14:1055–1057.
122. Ernerudh J, Olsson T, Lindstrom F, et al. Cerebrospinal fluid immunoglobulin abnormalities in systemic lupus erythematosus. *J Neurol Neurosury Psychiatry* 1985;48:807–813.
123. Nilsson C, Lindvall-Axelsson M, Owman C. Neuroendocrine regulatory mechanisms in the choroid plexus-cerebrospinal fluid system. *Brain Res Rev* 1992;17:109.
124. Peress NS, Roxburgh VA, Glenfand MC. Binding sites for immune components in the human choroid plexus. *Arthritis Rheum* 1981;24:520.
125. Atkins CS, Kondon J, Quismorio FP, et al. The choroid plexus in systemic lupus erythematosus. *Ann Int Med* 1972;76:65–72.
126. Boyer RS, Sun NCJ, Verity A, et al. Immunoperoxidase staining of the choroid plexus in systemic lupus erythematosus. *J Rheumatol* 1980;7:645–650.
127. Alcocer-Varela J, Aleman-Hoey D, Alarcon-Segovia D. Interleukin-1 and interleukin-6 activities are increased in the cerebrospinal fluid of patients with CNS lupus erythematosus and correlate with local late T-cell activation markers. *Lupus* 1992;1:111–117.
128. Hirohata S, Miyamoto T. Elevated levels of interleukin-6 in cerebrospinal fluid from patients with systemic lupus erythematosus and central nervous system involvement. *Arthritis Rheum* 1990;33:644–649.
129. Yeh TS, Wang CR, Jeng GW, et al. The study of anticardiolipin antibodies and interleukin-6 in cerebrospinal fluid and blood of Chinese patients with systemic lupus erythematosus and central nervous system involvement. *Autoimmunity* 1994;18:169–175.
130. Tsai CY, Wu TH, Tsai ST, et al. Cerebrospinal fluid interleukin-6, prostaglandin E2, and autoantibodies in patients with neuropsychiatric systemic lupus erythematosus and central nervous system infections. *Scand J Rheumatol* 1994;23:57–63.
131. Shiozawa S, Kuroki Y, Kim M, et al. Interferon-alpha in lupus psychosis. *Arthritis Rheum* 1992;35:417–422.
132. Benveniste EN. Inflammatory cytokines within the central nervous system: sources, function, and mechanism of action. *Am J Physiol* 1992;263:C1.
133. Besedovsky H, DelRey A, Sorkin E, et al. Immunoregulatory feedback between interleukin-1 and glucocorticoid hormones. *Science* 1986;233:652.
134. Denicoff KD, Rubinow DR, Papa MZ, et al. The neuropsychiatric effects of treatment with interleukin-2 and lymphokine-activated killer cells. *Ann Int Med* 1987;107:293.
135. Hellerstein MK, Meydani SN, Meydani M, et al. Interleuklin-1 induced anorexia in the rat. Influence of prostaglandins. *J Clin Invest* 1989;84:228.
136. Wilder RL. Neuroendocrine-immune system interactions and autoimmunity. *Annu Rev Immunol* 1995;13:307–338.
137. McEwen BS. Protective and damaging effects of stress mediators. *N Engl J Med* 1998;338:171–179.
138. Harbuz MS, Lightman SL. Stress and the hypothalamo-pituitary-adrenal axis: acute, chronic, and immunological activation. *Endocrinol* 1992;134:327.
139. Lowry MT, Gault L, Yamamoto BK. Adrenalectomy attenuates stress-induced elevations in extracellular glutamate concentrations in the hippocampus. *J Neurochem* 1993;61:195.
140. Shanks N, Moore PM, Perks P, et al. Alterations in hypothalamic-pituitary-adrenal function correlated with the onset of murine SLE in MRL+/+ and lpr/lpr mice. *Brain Behav Immun* 1999;13:348–360.
141. Clancy RM, Amin AR, Abramson SB. The role of nitric oxide in inflammation and immunity. *Arthritis Rheum* 1998;41:1141–1151.
142. Hausladen A, Privalle CT, Keng T, et al. Nitrosative stress: activation of the transcription factor Oxy R. *Cell* 1996;86:719–729.
143. Belmont HM, Levartovsky D, Goel A, et al. Increased nitric oxide production accompanied by the up-regulation of inducible nitric oxide synthase in vascular endothelium from patients with systemic lupus erythematosus. *Arthritis Rheum* 1997;40:1810–1816.
144. Lipton SA, Rosenberg PA. Excitatory amino acids as a final common pathway for neurological disorders. *N Engl J Med* 1994;330:613.
145. Goodwin JS, Goodwin JM. Cerebritis in lupus erythematosus. *Ann Intern Med* 1979;90:437–438.
146. Carbotte RM, Denburg SD, Denburg JA. Prevalence of cognitive impairment in systemic lupus erythematosus. *J Nerv Ment Dis* 1986;174:357–364.
147. Denburg SD, Carbotte RM, Denburg JA. Cognitive impairment in systemic lupus erythematosus: a neuropsychological study of individual and group deficits. *J Clin Exp Neuropsychol* 1987;9:323–339.

148. Hanly JG, Fisk JD, Sherwood G, et al. Cognitive impairment in patients with systemic lupus erythematosus. *J Rheumatol* 1992;19:562–567.
149. Ginsburg KS, Wright EA, Larson MG, et al. A controlled study of the prevalence of cognitive dysfunction in randomly selected patients with systemic lupus erythematosus. *Arthritis Rheum* 1992;35:776–782.
150. Kozora E, Thompson L, West S, et al. Analysis of cognitive and psychological deficits in systemic lupus erythematosus patients without overt central nervous system disease. *Arthritis Rheum* 1996;39:2035–2045.
151. Carbotte RM, Denburg SD, Denburg JA. Cognitive deficit associated with rheumatic diseases: neuropsychiatric perspectives. *Arthritis Rheum* 1995;38:1363–1374.
152. Hanly JG, Cassell K, Fisk JD. Cognitive function in systemic lupus erythematosus: results of a 5-year prospective study. *Arthritis Rheum* 1997;40:1542–1543.
153. Carbotte RM, Denburg SD, Denburg JA. Cognitive dysfunction in systemic lupus erythematosus is independent of active disease. *J Rheumatol* 1995;22:863–867.
154. Denburg SD, Carbotte RM, Denburg JA. Corticosteroids and neuropsychiatric functioning in patients with systemic lupus erythematosus. *Arthritis Rheum* 1994;37:1311–1320.
155. Fisk JD, Eastwood B, Sherwood G, et al. Patterns of cognitive impairment in patients with systemic lupus erythematosus. *Br J Rheumatol* 1993;32:458–462.
156. Hanly JG, Fisk JD, Sherwood G, et al. Clinical course of cognitive impairment in systemic lupus erythematosus. *J Rheumatol* 1994;21:1825–1831.
157. Hanly JG, Fisk JD, Eastwood B. Brain reactive autoantibodies and cognitive impairment in systemic lupus erythematosus. *Lupus* 1994;3:193–199.
158. Hanly JG, Walsh NM, Fisk JD, et al. Cognitive impairment and autoantibodies in systemic lupus erythematosus. *Br J Rheumatol* 1993;32:291–296.
159. Hay EM, Black D, Huddy A, et al. Psychiatric disorder and cognitive impairment in systemic lupus erythematosus. *Arthritis Rheum* 1992;35:411–416.
160. Hay EM, Huddy A, Black D, et al. A prospective study of psychiatric disorder and cognitive function in systemic lupus erythematosus. *Ann Rheum Dis* 1994;53:298--303.
161. Denburg SD, Carbotte RM, Ginsberg JS, et al. The relationship of antiphospholipid antibodies to cognitive function in patients with systemic lupus erythematosus. *JINS* 1997;3:377–386.
162. Hanly JG, Hong C, Smith S, et al. A prospective analysis of cognitive function and anticardiolipin antibodies in systemic lupus erythematosus. *Arthritis Rheum* 1999;42:728–734.
163. Menon S, Jameson-Shortall E, Newman SP, et al. A longitudinal study of anticardiolipin antibody levels and cognitive functioning in systemic lupus erythematosus. *Arthritis Rheum* 1999;42:735–741.
164. Long AA, Denburg SD, Carbotte RM, et al. Serum lymphocytotoxic antibodies and neurocognitive function in systemic lupus erythematosus. *Ann Rheum Dis* 1990;49:249–253.
165. Asherson RA, Mercey D, Phillips G, et al. Recurrent stroke and multi-infarct dementia in systemic lupus erythematosus: association with antiphospholipid antibodies. *Ann Rheum Dis* 1987;46:605–611.
166. Coull BM, Bourdette DN, Goodnight SH Jr, et al. Multiple cerebral infarctions and dementia associated with anticardiolipin antibodies. *Stroke* 1987;18:1107–1112.
167. Papero PH, Bluestein HG, White P, et al. Neuropsychologic deficits and antineuronal antibodies in pediatric systemic lupus erythematosus. *Clin Exp Rheumatol* 1990;8:417–424.
168. Wycokoff PM, Miller CC, Tucker LB, et al. Neuropsychological assessment of children and adolescents with SLE. *Lupus* 1995;4:217–220.
169. Bonfa E, Golombek SJ, Kaufman LD, et al. Association between lupus psychosis and anti-ribosomal P protein antibodies. *N Engl J Med* 1987;317:265–271.
170. Schneebaum AB, Singleton JD, West SG, et al. Association of psychiatric manifestations with antibodies to ribosomal P proteins in systemic lupus erythematosus. *Am J Med* 1991;90:54–62.
171. Nojima Y, Minota S, Yamada A, et al. Correlation of antibodies to ribosomal P protein with psychosis in patients with systemic lupus erythematosus. *Ann Rheum Dis* 1992;51:1053–1055.
172. Teh LS, Amos N, Black D, et al. Anti-P antibodies are associated with psychiatric and focal cerebral disorders in patients with systemic lupus erythematosus. *Br J Rheumatol* 1993;32:287–280.
173. Sato T, Uchiumi T, Ozawa T, et al. Antibodies against ribosomal proteins found with high frequency in patients with systemic lupus erythematosus with active disease. *J Rheumatol* 1991;18:1681–1684.
174. Teh LS, Bedwell AE, Isenberg DA, et al. Antibodies to protein P in systemic lupus erythematosus. *Ann Rheum Dis* 1992;51:489–494.
175. Takehara K, Nojima Y, Kikuchi K, et al. Systemic lupus erythematosus associated with anti-ribosomal P protein antibody. *Arch Dermatol* 1990;126:1184–1186.
176. Kremer JM, Rynes RI, Bartholomew LE, et al. Non-organic non-psychotic psychopathology (NONPP) in patients with systemic lupus erythematosus. *Semin Arthritis Rheum* 1981:11:182–189.
177. Iverson GL. Psychopathology associated with systemic lupus erythematosus: a methodological review. *Seminars Arthritis Rheum* 1993;22:242–251.
178. Lindal E, Thorlacius S, Steinsson K, et al. Psychiatric disorders among subjects with systemic lupus erythematosus in an unselected population. *Scan J Rheumatol* 1995;24:346–351.
179. Omdal R, Husby G, Mellgren SI. Mental health status in systemic lupus erythematosus. *Scan J Rheumatol* 1995;24:142–145.
180. Shortall E, Isenberg D, Newman SP. Factors associated with mood and mood disorders in SLE. *Lupus* 1995;4:272–279.
181. McCracken LM, Semenchuk EM, Goetsch VL. Cross-sectional and longitudinal analyses of coping responses and health status in persons with systemic lupus erythematosus. *Behav Med* 1995;20:179–187.
182. Omdal R, Mellgren SI, Husby G. Clinical neuropsychiatric and neuromuscular manifestations in systemic lupus erythematosus. *Scand J Rheumatol* 1988;17:113–117.
183. Hietaharju A, Jantti V, Korpela M, et al. Nervous system involvement in systemic lupus erythematosus, Sjögren's syndrome, and scleroderma. *Acta Neurol Scand* 1993;88:299–308.
184. Fernandez-Nebro A, Palacios-Munoz R, Gordillo J, et al. Chronic or recurrent headache in patients with systemic lupus erythematosus: a case control study. *Lupus* 1999;8:151–156.
185. King KK, Kornreich HK, Bernstein BH, et al. The clinical spectrum of systemic lupus erythematosus in childhood. Proceedings of the Conference on Rheumatic Diseases of Childhood. *Arthritis Rheum* 1977;20(suppl):287–294.
186. Atkinson RA, Appenzeller O. Headache in small vessel disease of the brain: a study of patients with systemic lupus erythematosus. *Headache* 1978;15:198–204.
187. Brandt KD, Lessel S. Migrainous phenomenon in systemic lupus erythematosus. *Arthritis Rheum* 1978;21:716.
188. Vazquez-Cruz J, Traboulssi H, Rodriguez-De la Serna A, et al. A prospective study of chronic or recurrent headache in systemic lupus erythematosus. *Headache* 1990;30:232–235.

189. Markus HS, Hopkinson N. Migraine and headache in systemic lupus erythematosus and their relationship with antibodies against phospholipids. *J Neurol* 1992;239:39–42.
190. Isenberg DA, Meyrick-Thomas D, Snaith ML, et al. A study of migraine in systemic lupus erythematosus. *Ann Rheum Dis* 1982;41:30–32.
191. Moskowitz MA, Macfarlane R. Neurovascular and molecular mechanisms in migraine headaches. *Cerebrovasc Brain Metab Rev* 1993;5:159.
192. Levine SR, Deegan MJ, Futrell N, et al. Cerebrovascular and neurologic disease associated with antiphospholipid antibodies: 48 cases. *Neurology* 1990;40:1181–1189.
193. Hogan MJ, Brunet DG, Ford PM, et al. Lupus anticoagulant, antiphospholipid antibodies, and migraine. *Can J Neurol Sci* 1988;15:420–425.
194. O'Keefe ST, Tsapatsaris NP, Beetham WP Jr. Increased prevalence of migraine and chest pain in patients with primary Raynaud's disease. *Ann Intern Med* 1992;116:985–989.
195. O'Keefe ST, Tsapatsaris NP, Beetham WP Jr. Association between Raynaud's phenomenon and migraine in a random population in hospital employees. *J Rheumatol* 1993;20: 1187–1188.
196. Montalban J, Cervera R, Font J, et al. Lack of association between anticardiolipin antibodies and migraine in systemic lupus erythematosus. *Neurology* 1992;42:681–682.
197. Green L, Vinker S, Amital H, et al. Pseudotumor cerebri in systemic lupus erythematosus. *Semin Arthritis Rheum* 1995;25: 103–108.
198. Weisberg LA, Chutorian AM. Pseudotumor cerebri of childhood. *Am J Dis Child* 1977;131:1243–1248.
199. Mortifee PRS, Bebb RA, Stein H. Communicating hydrocephalus in systemic lupus erythematosus with antiphospholipid antibody syndrome. *J Rheumatol* 1992;19:1299–1302.
200. Uhl MD, Werner BE, Romano TJ, et al. Normal pressure hydrocephalus in a patient with systemic lupus erythematosus (case report). *J Rheumatol* 1990;17:1689–1691.
201. Santos MJ, Reis P, da Silva JA, et al. Ischemic lesion of the CNS in patients with systemic lupus erythematosus. *Acta Med Port* 1994;7:201–206.
202. Kitagawa Y, Gotoh F, Koto A, et al. Stroke in systemic lupus erythematosus. *Stroke* 1990;21:1533–1539.
203. Ware AE, Mongey A-B. Lupus and cerebrovascular accidents. *Lupus* 1997;6:420–424.
204. Kwon SU, Koh JY, Kim JS. Vertebrobasilar artery territory infarction as an initial manifestation of systemic lupus erythematosus. *Clin Neurol Neurosurg* 1999;101:62–67.
205. Brandt K, Lessell S, Cohen AS. Cerebral disorders of vision in systemic lupus erythematosus. *Ann Int Med* 1975;83:163–169.
206. Mitsias P, Levine SR. Large cerebral vessel occlusive disease in systemic lupus erythematosus. *Neurology* 1994;44:385–393.
207. Bruce IN, Gladman DD, Urowitz MB. Premature atherosclerosis in systemic lupus erythematosus. *Rheum Dis Clin North Am* 2000;26:257–278.
208. Levine SR, Welch KM. The spectrum of neurologic disease associated with antiphospholipid antibodies: lupus anticoagulants and anticardiolipin antibodies. *Arch Neurol* 1987;44: 876–883.
209. Lopez Dupla M, Khamashta MA, Sanchez AD, et al. Transverse myelitis as a first manifestation of systemic lupus erythematosus: a case report. *Lupus* 1995;4:239–242.
210. Kovacs B, Lafferty TL, Brent LH, et al. Transverse myelopathy in systemic lupus erythematosus: an analysis of 14 cases and review of the literature. *Ann Rheum Dis* 2000;59:120–124.
211. Lavalle C, Pizarro S, Drenkard C, et al. Transverse myelitis: a manifestation of systemic lupus erythematosus strongly associated with antiphospholipid antibodies. *J Rheumatol* 1990;17: 34–37.
212. Kaye EM, Butler IJ. Myelopathy in neonatal and infantile lupus erythematosus. *Ann Neurol* 1985;18:392.
213. al-Mayouf SM, Bahabri S. Spinal cord involvement in pediatric systemic lupus erythematosus: case report and literature review. *Clin Exp Rheumatol* 1999;17:505–508.
214. Andrianakos AA, Duffy J, Suzuki M, et al. Transverse myelopathy in systemic lupus erythematosus. Report of three cases and review of the literature. *Ann Int Med* 1975;83:616–624.
215. Propper DJ, Bucknall RC. Acute transverse myelopathy complicating systemic lupus erythematosus. *Ann Rheum Dis* 1989; 48:512–515.
216. Warren RW, Kredich DW. Transverse myelitis and acute central nervous system manifestations of systemic lupus erythematosus. *Arthritis Rheum* 1984;27:1058–1060.
217. Daras M, Tuchman AJ, Chengoti MT. Myelin basic protein elevation in myelopathy due to systemic lupus erythematosus. *N Y State J Med* 1982;82:357–358.
218. Kenik JA, Krohn K, Kelly RB, et al. Transverse myelitis and optic neuritis in systemic lupus erythematosus: a case report with magnetic resonance imaging findings. *Arthritis Rheum* 1987;30:947–950.
219. Provenzale JM, Barboriak DP, Gaensler EHL, et al. Lupus-related myelitis: serial MR findings. *Am J Neuroradiol* 1994;15:1911–1917.
220. Boumpas DT, Patronas NJ, Dalaks MC, et al. Acute transverse myelitis in systemic lupus erythematosus: magnetic resonance imaging and review of the literature. *J Rheumatol* 1990;17: 89–92.
221. Mok CC, Lee KW, Wong RW, et al. Acute lupus myelitis affecting the conus medullaris. *Clin Exp Rheumatol* 1999;17: 123–124.
222. Goker B, Block JA. Spinal epidural hematoma complicating active systemic lupus erythematosus. *Arthritis Rheum* 1999;42: 577–578.
223. Crayton HE, Partington CR, Bell CL. Spinal cord compression by epidural lipomatosis in a patient with systemic lupus erythematosus. *Arthritis Rheum* 1991;34:482–484.
224. Henry AK, Brunner CM. Relapse of lupus transverse myelitis mimicked by vertebral fractures and spinal cord compression. *Arthritis Rheum* 1985;28:1307–1311.
225. Dell'Isola B, Vidailhet M, Gatfosse M, et al. Recovery of anterior spinal artery syndrome in a patient with systemic lupus erythematosus and antiphospholipid antibodies. *Br J Rheumatol* 1991;30:314–316.
226. Baethge BA, King JW, Husain F, et al. Herpes zoster myelitis occurring during treatment for systemic lupus erythematosus. *Am J Med Sci* 1989;298:264–266.
227. Drosos AA, Constantopoulos SH, Moutsopoulos HM. Tuberculosis spondylitis: a cause for paraplegia in lupus. *Rheumatol Int* 1985;5:185–186.
228. Stoner GL, Best PV, Mazio M, et al. Progressive multifocal leukoencephalopathy complicating systemic lupus erythematosus: distribution of JC virus in chronically demyelinated cerebellar lesions. *J Neuropathol Exp Neurol* 1988;47:307.
229. Robson MG, Walport MJ, Davies KA. Systemic lupus erythematosus and acute demyelinating polyneuropathy. *Br J Rheumatol* 1994;33:1074–1077.
230. Provenzale J, Bouldin TW. Lupus-related myelopathy: report of three cases and review of the literature. *J Neurol Neurosurg Psychiatry* 1992;55:830–835.
231. Chan K-F, Boey M-L. Transverse myelopathy in SLE: clinical features and functional outcomes. *Lupus* 1996;5:294–299.
232. Hachen HJ, Chantraine A. Spinal cord involvement in sys-

temic lupus erythematosus. *Paraplegia* 1979–1980;17: 337–346.
233. Harisdangkul V, Doorenbos D, Subramony SH. Lupus transverse myelopathy: better outcome with early recognition and aggressive high-dose intravenous corticosteroid pulse treatment. *J Neurol* 1995;24:326–329.
234. Berlanga B, Rubio FR, Moga I, et al. Response to intravenous cyclophosphamide treatment in lupus myelopathy. *J Rheumatol* 1992;19:829–830.
235. Barile L, Lavalle C. Transverse myelitis in systemic lupus erythematosus: the effect of IV pulse methylprednisolone and cyclophosphamide. *J Rheumatol* 1992;19:370–372.
236. Donaldson I, Mac G, Espiner EA. Disseminated lupus erythematosus presenting as chorea gravidarum. *Arch Neurol* 1971;24:240–244.
237. Groothuis JR, Groothuis DR, Mukhopadhyay D, et al. Lupus-associated chorea in childhood. *Am J Dis Child* 1977;131: 1131–1134.
238. Bruyn GW, Padberg G. Chorea and lupus erythematosus. A critical review. *Eur Neurol* 1984;23:435–448.
239. Hadron PY, Bouchez B, Wattel A, et al. Chorea, systemic lupus erythematosus, circulating anticoagulant. *J Rheumatol* 1986;13: 991–993.
240. Asherson RA, Derksen RH, Harris EN, et al. Chorea in systemic lupus erythematosus and lupus-like disease: association with antiphospholipid antibodies. *Semin Arthritis Rheum* 1987; 16:253–259.
241. Havsager AM, Carstensen NC. Ballism in systemic lupus erythematosus. *Ugesdrift for Lager* 1991;153:2301–2302.
242. Thompson SW. Ballistic movements of the arm in systemic lupus erythematosus. *Dis Nerv Syst* 1976;37:331–332.
243. Tam L-S, Cohen MG, Li EK. Hemiballismus in systemic lupus erythematosus: possible association with antiphospholipid antibodies. *Lupus* 1995;4:67–69.
244. Singh RR, Prasad K, Kumar A, et al. Cerebellar ataxia in systemic lupus erythematosus: three case reports. *Ann Rheum Dis* 1988;47:954–956.
245. Al-Arfaj HF, Naddaf HO. Cerebellar atrophy in systemic lupus erythematosus. *Lupus* 1995;4:412–414.
246. Smith RW, Ellison DW, Gallagher PJ, et al. Cerebellum and brainstem vasculopathy in systemic lupus erythematosus: two clinico-pathological cases. *Ann Rheum Dis* 1994;53:327.
247. Shimomura T, Kuno N, Takenaka T, et al. Purkinje cell antibody in lupus ataxia. *Lancet* 1993;342:375–376.
248. Dalmau J, Posner JB. Neurological paraneoplastic syndromes. *Springer Semin Immunopathol* 1996;18:85.
249. Venegoni E, Biasioli R, Lamperti E, et al. Tremor as an early manifestation of systemic lupus erythematosus. *Clin Exp Rheumatol* 1994;12:199–201.
250. Miyoshi Y, Atsumi T, Kitagawa H, et al. Parkinson-like symptoms as a manifestation of systemic lupus erythematosus. *Lupus* 1993;2:199–201.
251. Shahar E, Goshen E, Tauber Z, et al. Parkinsonian syndrome complicating systemic lupus erythematosus. *Pediatric Neurology* 1998;18:456–458.
252. Kuroe K, Kurahashi K, Nakano I, et al. A neuropathological study of a case of lupus erythematosus with chorea. *J Neurol Sci* 1994;123:59.
253. Lafeuillade A, Aubert L, Quilichini R. Systemic lupus and chorea. Two personal cases with a review of the literature. *Sem Hop Paris* 1988;64:3109–3116.
254. Khamashita MA, Gil A, Anciones B, et al. Chorea in systemic lupus erythematosus: association with antiphospholipid antibodies. *Ann Rheum Dis* 1988;47:681–683.
255. Iskander MK, Khan MA. Chorea as the initial presentation of oral contraceptive related systemic lupus erythematosus (letter). *J Rheumatol* 1989;16:850–851.
256. Mathur AK, Gatter RA. Chorea as the initial presentation of oral contraceptive induced systemic lupus erythematosus (letter). *J Rheumatol* 1988;15:1042–1043.
257. Guttman M, Lang AE, Garnett ES, et al. Regional cerebral glucose metabolism in SLE chorea: further evidence that striatal hypometabolism is not a correlate of chorea. *Mov Dis* 1987;2: 201.
258. Allen IV, Millar JHD, Kirk J, et al. Systemic lupus erythematosus clinically resembling multiple sclerosis and with unusual pathological and ultrastructural features. *J Neurol Neurosurg Psychiatry* 1979;42:392–401.
259. Fulford KWM, Catterall RD, Delhanty JJ, et al. A collagen disorder of the nervous system presenting as multiple sclerosis. *Brain* (part II) 1972;95:373–386.
260. Hutchinson M, Bresnihan B. Neurological lupus erythematosus with tonic seizures simulating multiple sclerosis (letter). *J Neurol Neurosurg Psychiatry* 1983;46:583–585.
261. Kaplan PE, Betts HB. Lupoid sclerosis: evaluation and treatment. *Arch Phys Med Rehab* 1977;58:24–28.
262. Moriwaka F, Tashiro K, Fukazawa T, et al. A case of systemic lupus erythematosus: its clinical and MRI resemblance to multiple sclerosis. *Jpn J Psychiatry Neurol* 1990;44:601–605.
263. Marullo S, Clauvel JP, Intrator L, et al. Lupoid sclerosis with antiphospholipid antibodies. *J Rheumatol* 1993;20:747–749.
264. Pender MP, Chalk JB. Connective tissue disease mimicking multiple sclerosis. *Aust N Z J Med* 1989;19:469–472.
265. Falga-Tirado C, Ordi-Ros J, Cucurull-Canosa E, et al. Lhermitte's sign in systemic lupus erythematosus. *Lupus* 1995;4:327–331.
266. Ijdo JW, Conti-Kelly AM, Greco P, et al. Antiphospholipid antibodies in patients with multiple sclerosis and MS-like disease illness: MS or APS? *Lupus* 1999;8:109–115.
267. Poser CM, Paty DW, Scheinberg L, et al. New diagnostic criteria for multiple sclerosis: guidelines for research protocols. *Ann Neurol* 1983;13:227–231.
268. Markowitz H, Kokmen E. Neurologic diseases and the cerebrospinal fluid immunoglobulin profile. *Mayo Clin Proc* 1983;58:273–274.
269. Gillman S. Imaging the brain. *N Engl J Med* 1998;338:8l2–820.
270. Barned S, Goodman AD, Mattson DH. Frequency of antinuclear antibodies in multiple sclerosis. *Neurology* 1995;45: 384–385.
271. Michielsens B, Walravens B, Vermylen J, et al. Diagnostic significance of antinuclear antibodies in neurological patients. *Acta Neurol Scand* 1991;84:102–106.
272. Rombos A, Evangelopoulou K, Leventakou A, et al. Serum IgG and IgM anticardiolipin antibodies in neurological diseases. *Acta Neurol Scand* 1990;81:234–245.
273. D'Olhaberriague L, Levine SR, Salowich-Palm L, et al. Specificity, isotype, and titer distribution of anticardiolipin antibodies in CNS diseases. *Neurology* 1998;51:1376–1380.
274. Cuadrado MJ, Khamashta MA, Ballesteros A, et al. Can neurologic manifestations of Hughes (antiphospholipid) syndrome be distinguished from multiple sclerosis? *Medicine* 2000;79:57–68.
275. Karussis D, Leker RR, Ashkenazi A, et al. A subgroup of multiple sclerosis patients with anticardiolipin antibodies and unusual clinical manifestations: do they represent a new nosological entity? *Ann Neurol* 1998;44:629–634.
276. Khalili A, Cooper RC. A study of immune responses to myelin and cardiolipin in patients with systemic lupus erythematosus. *Clin Exp Immunol* 1991;85:365–372.
277. Hirohata S, Taketani J. A serial study of changes in intrathecal immunoglobulin synthesis in a patient with central nervous system lupus erythematosus. *J Rheumatol* 1987;14:1055–1057.

278. Lopez-Dupla ML, Khamashta MA, Sanchez AD, et al. Transverse myelitis as a first presentation of systemic lupus erythematosus: a case report. *Lupus* 1995;4:239–242.
279. Bastianello S, Gasperini C, Ristori G, et al. Multiple sclerosis with negative cerebrospinal fluid. Magnetic resonance differential diagnosis. *Radiol Med* 1994;88:749–751.
280. Cole SR, Beck RW, Moke PS, et al. The predictive value of CSF oligoclonal banding for MS 5 years after optic neuritis. Optic Neuritis Study Group. *Neurology* 1998;51:885–887.
281. Russell PW, Haserick JR, Zuker EM. Epilepsy in systemic lupus erythematosus: effect of cortisone and ACTH. *Arch Intern Med* 1951;88:78–92.
282. Hagiwara M, Katayose K, Kan R, et al. The feature of epileptic seizures in systemic lupus erythematosus. *Jap J Psych Neurol* 1987;41:533–534.
283. Mackworth-Young CG, Hughes GRV. Epilepsy: an early symptom of systemic lupus erythematosus. *J Neurol Neurosurg Psychiatry* 1985;48:145.
284. Futrell N, Schultz LR, Millikan C. Central nervous system disease in patients with systemic lupus erythematosus. *Neurology* 1992;42:1649–1657.
285. Verrot D, San-Marco M, Dravet C, et al. Prevalence and significance of antinuclear and anticardiolipin antibodies in patients with epilepsy. *Am J Med* 1997;103:33–37.
286. Herranz MT, Rivier G, Khamashta MA, et al. Association between antiphospholipid antibodies and epilepsy in patients with systemic lupus erythematosus. *Arthritis Rheum* 1994;37:568–571.
287. Liou H-H, Wang C-R, Chen C-J, et al. Elevated levels of anticardiolipin antibodies and epilepsy in lupus patients. *Lupus* 1996;5:307–312.
288. Liou H-H et al. Anticardiolipin antisera from lupus patients with seizure reduce a GABA receptor-mediated chloride current in snail neurons. *Life Sci* 1994;54:1119–1125.
289. Canoso JJ, Cohen AS. Aseptic meningitis in systemic lupus erythematosus: report of three cases. *Arthritis Rheum* 1975;18: 369–374.
290. Welsby P, Smith C. Recurrent sterile meningitis as a manifestation of systemic lupus erythematosus. *Scand J Infect Dis* 1977;2: 149–150.
291. Lancman ME, Mesrupian H, Granillo RJ. Chronic aseptic meningitis in a patient with systemic lupus erythematosus. *Can J Neurol Sci* 1989;16:354–356.
292. Iliopoulos AG, Tsokos GC. Immunopathogenesis and spectrum of infections in systemic lupus erythematosus. *Seminars Arthritis Rheum* 1996;25:318–336.
293. Morris G, Garcia-Monco JC. The challenge of drug-induced aseptic meningitis. *Arch Intern Med* 1999;159:1185–1194.
294. Aragon Diez A, Garcia-Consuegra G, Sanchez-Camacho G, et al. Blepharoptosis and systemic lupus erythematosus. *Rev Clin Exp* 1987;181:173.
295. Ribaute E, Weill B, Ing H, et al. Oculomotor paralysis in disseminated lupus erythematosus (English abstract). *Ophthalmologie* 1989;3:125–128.
296. Rosenstein ED, Sobelman J, Kramer N. Isolated, pupil-sparing third nerve palsy as initial manifestation of systemic lupus erythematosus. *J Clin Neuro-opthalmol* 1989;9:285–288.
297. Yigit A, Bingol A, Mutluer N, et al. The one-and-a-half syndrome in systemic lupus erythematosus. *J Neuroophthalmol* 1996;16:274–276.
298. Cogen MS, Kline LB, Duvall ER. Bilateral internuclear ophthalmoplegia in systemic lupus erythematosus. *J Clin Neuro-ophthalmol* 1987;7:69–73.
299. Lundberg PO, Werner I. Trigeminal sensory neuropathy in systemic lupus erythematosus. *Acta Neurol Scand* 1972;48:330–340.
300. Garcia Ruiz PJ, Guerrero Sola A, Garcia Urra D. Sensory neuralgia of the trigeminal nerve and systemic lupus erythematosus. *Neurologia* 1988;3:248.
301. Jabs DA, Miller NR, Newman SA, et al. Optic neuropathy in systemic lupus erythematosus. *Arch Ophthalmol* 1986;104: 564–568.
302. Naarendorp M, Spiera H. Sudden sensorineural hearing loss in patients with systemic lupus erythematosus or lupus-like syndromes and antiphospholipid antibodies. *J Rheumatol* 1998;25: 589–592.
303. Levine SR, Brey RL. Neurological aspects of antiphospholipid antibody syndrome. *Lupus* 1996;5:347–353.
304. Keane JR. Eye movement abnormalities in systemic lupus erythematosus. *Arch Neurol* 1995;52:1145–1149.
305. Cuenca R, Simeon CP, Montablan J, et al. Facial nerve palsy due to angioedema in systemic lupus erythematosus. *Clin Exp Rheumatol* 1991;9:89–97.
306. McDonald E, Marino C, Cimponeriu D. Painful ophthalmoplegia in a patient with SLE. *Hosp Pract* 1992;27:41–44.
307. McGalliard J. Acquired Brown's syndrome in a patient with SLE. *Ann Rheum Dis* 1993;52:385–386.
308. Alonso-Valdivielso JL, Alvarez Lario B, Lopez J Alegre, et al. Acquired Brown's syndrome in a patient with systemic lupus erythematosus. *Ann Rheum Dis* 1993;52:63–64.
309. Bingisser R, Speich R, Fontana A, et al. Lupus erythematosus and the Miller-Fisher syndrome. *Arch Neurol* 1994;51: 828–830.
310. Melon O, Cohen BA, Sharma L. Cavernous sinus syndrome and systemic lupus erythematosus. *Neurology* 1992;42: 1842–1843.
311. Katano H, Umemura A, Kamiya K, et al. Visual disturbance by lymphocytic hypophysitis in a non-pregnant woman with systemic lupus erythematosus. *Lupus* 1998;7:554–556.
312. Omdal R, Mellgren SI, Husby G, et al. A controlled study of peripheral neuropathy in systemic lupus erythematosus. *Acta Neurol Scand* 1993;88: 41–46.
313. Straub RH, Zeuner M, Lock G, et al. Autonomic and sensorimotor neuropathy in patients with systemic lupus erythematosus and systemic sclerosis. *J Rheumatol* 1996;23:87–92.
314. Bergemer AM, Fouquet B, Goupille P, et al. Peripheral neuropathy as the initial manifestation of systemic lupus erythematosus. Report of a case. *Sem Hop Paris* 1987;63:1979–1982.
315. Bailey AA, Sayre GP, Clark EC. Neuritis associated with systemic lupus erythematosus: report of 5 cases with necropsy in 2. *Arch Neurol Psychiatry* 1956;75:251–259.
316. Scheinberg L. Polyneuritis in systemic lupus erythematosus: review of literature and report of case. *N Engl J Med* 1956;255: 416–421.
317. McCombe PA, McLeod JG, Pollard JD, et al. Peripheral sensorimotor and autonomic neuropathy associated with systemic lupus erythematosus. Clinical, pathological, and immunological features. *Brain* 1987;110:533–549.
318. Hughes RA, Cameron JS, Hall SM, et al. Multiple mononeuropathy as the initial presentation of systemic lupus erythematosus—nerve biopsy and response to plasma exchange. *J Neurol* 1982;228:239–247.
319. Martinez-Taboada VM, Blanco-Alonso R, Armona J, et al. Mononeuritis multiplex in systemic lupus erythematosus: response to pulse intravenous cyclophosphamide. *Lupus* 1996; 5:74–76.
320. Vaidya S, Jasin HE, Logan J. Systemic lupus erythematosus and Guillain–Barré syndrome. *J Clin Rheumatol* 1999;5:349–353.
321. Sigal LH. Chronic inflammatory polyneuropathy complicating SLE: successful treatment with monthly oral pulse cyclophosphamide. *J Rheumatol* 1989;16:1518–1519.
322. Millette TJ, Subramony SH, Wee AS, et al. Systemic lupus ery-

thematosus presenting with recurrent acute demyelinating polyneuropathy. *Eur Neurol* 1986;25:397–402.
323. Assal F, Blanche P, Lamy C, et al. Involvement of the brachial plexus in a patient with systemic lupus erythematosus. *La Press Medicale* 1993;22:598.
324. Block SL, Jarrett MP, Swerdlow M, et al. Brachial plexus neuropathy as the initial presentation of systemic lupus erythematosus. *Neurology* 1979;29:1633–1634.
325. Sadeh M, Sarova-Pinhas I, Ohry A. Sensory ataxia as an initial symptom of systemic lupus erythematosus (letter). *J Rheumatol* 1980;7:420–421.
326. Bodi L, Varadi P, Pokorny G, et al. Polyneuropathy with endoneurial immune complex deposition as the first manifestation of systemic lupus erythematosus. *Acta Neuropathol* 1998; 96:297–300.
327. Markusse HM, Vroom TM, Heurkens AH, et al. Polyneuropathy as the initial manifestation of necrotizing vasculitis and gangrene in systemic lupus erythematosus. *Neth J Med* 1991;38:204–208.
328. Enevoldson TP, Wiles CM. Severe vasculitic neuropathy in systemic lupus erythematosus and response to cyclophosphamide. *J Neurol Neurosurg Psychiatry* 1991;54:468–469.
329. Stefurak TL, Midroni G, Bilbao JM. Vasculitic polyradiculopathy in systemic lupus erythematosus. *J Neurol Neurosurg Psychiatry* 1999;66:658–661.
330. Hoyle C, Ewing DJ, Parker AC. Acute autonomic neuropathy in association with systemic upus erythematosus. *Ann Rheum Dis* 1985;44:420–424.
331. Jodo S, Sagawa A, Ogura N, et al. A case of systemic lupus erythematosus developing pan-dysautonomia. *Ryumachi* 1992;32: 58–65.
332. Straub RH, Gluck T, Zeuner M, et al. Association of pupillary parasympathetic hyperreflexia and systemic inflammation in patients with systemic lupus erythematosus. *Br J Rheumatol* 1998;37:665–670.
333. Tooke AF, Stuart RA, Maddison PJ. The prevalence of autonomic neuropathy in systemic lupus erythematosus (abstract). *Br J Rheumatol* 1990;30(suppl 1):22.
334. Omdal R, Jorde R, Mellgren SI, et al. Autonomic function in systemic lupus erythematosus. *Lupus* 1994;3:413–417.
335. Gledhill RF, Dessein PH. Autonomic neuropathy in systemic lupus erythematosus (letter). *J Neurol Neurosurg Psychiatry* 1988;51:1238–1240.
336. Magaro M, Mirone L, Altomonte L, et al. Lack of correlation between anticardiolipin antibodies and peripheral autonomic nerve involvement in systemic lupus erythematosus. *Clin Rheumatol* 1992;11:231–234.
337. Liote F, Osterland CK. Autonomic neuropathy in systemic lupus erythematosus: cardiovascular autonomic function assessment. *Ann Rheum Dis* 1994;53:671–674.
338. Vaiopoulos G, Sfikakis PP, Kapsimali V, et al. The association of systemic lupus erythematosus and myasthenia gravis. *Postgrad Med J* 1994;70:741–745.
339. Mevorach D, Perrot S, Buchanan E, et al. Appearance of systemic lupus erythematosus after thymectomy: four case reports and review of the literature. *Lupus* 1995;4:33–37.
340. Deodhar A, Norden J, So Y, et al. The association of systemic lupus erythematosus and Lambert-Eaton myasthenic syndrome. *J Rheumatol* 1996;23:1292–1294.
341. Magnani G, Nemni R, Leocani L, et al. Neuromyotonia, systemic lupus erythematosus, and acetylcholine-receptor antibodies. *J Neurology* 1998;245:182–185.
342. Schnider A, Bassetti C, Schnider A, et al. Very severe amnesia with acute onset after isolated hippocampal damage due to systemic lupus erythematosus. *J Neuro Neurosurg Psychiatry* 1995; 59:644–646.
343. Stubgen JP. Nervous system lupus mimics limbic encephalitis. *Lupus* 1998;7:557–560.
344. Mirsattari SM, Power C, Fine A, et al. Neuropsychiatric systemic lupus erythematosus and the syndrome of inappropriate secretion of antidiuretic hormone: a case report with very late onset systemic lupus erythematosus. *Br J Rheumatol* 1998; 37:1132–1134.
345. Martin Santos JM, Dib B, Terroba Larumbe MC, et al. Systemic lupus erythematosus and the syndrome of inappropriate secretion of antidiuretic hormone. *Clin Exp Rheumatol* 1996: 14:578–579.
346. Hinchey J, Chaves C, Appignani B, et al. A reversible posterior leukoencephalopathy syndrome. *N Engl J Med* 1996;334: 494–500.
347. Markusse HM, Vecht JC. Is neurologic disease with positive lupus serology sufficient for a diagnosis of systemic lupus erythematosus? *Br J Rheumatol* 1986;25:302–305.
348. Ginzler E, Diamond H, Kaplan D, et al. Computer analysis of factors influencing frequency of infection in systemic lupus erythematosus. *Arthritis Rheum* 1978;21:37–44.
349. Davis JA, Weisman MH, Dail DH. Vascular disease in infective endocarditis: report of immune-mediated events in skin and brain. *Arch Intern Med* 1978;138:480–483.
350. Koide J, Okusawa E, Ito T, et al. Granulomatous amoebic encephalitis caused by Acanthamoeba in a patient with systemic lupus erythematosus. *Clin Rheumatol* 1998;17:329–332.
351. Agostini HT, Ryschkewitch CF, Stoner GL. Complete genome of a JC virus genotype type 6 from the brain of an African American with progressive multifocal leukoencephalopathy. *J Human Virology* 1998;1:267–272.
352. Newton P, Aldridge RD, Lessels AM, et al. Progressive multifocal leukoencephalopathy complicating systemic lupus erythematosus. *Arthritis Rheum* 1986;29:337–343.
353. Ismail K, Wessely S. Psychiatric complications of corticosteroid therapy. *Br J Hosp Med* 1995;53:495–499.
354. Hall RCW, Popkin MK, Stickney SK, et al. Presentation of the steroid psychoses. *J Nerv Ment Dis* 1979;167:229–236.
355. Joffe RT, Denicoff KD, Rubinow DR, et al. Mood effects of alternate-day corticosteroid therapy in patients with systemic lupus erythematosus. *Gen Hosp Psychiatry* 1988;10:56–60.
356. Hall RCW, Popkin MK, Kirkpatrick B. Tricyclic exacerbation of steroid psychosis. *J Nerv Ment Dis* 1978;166:738–742.
357. Hoppmann RA, Peden JG, Ober SK. Central nervous system side effects of nonsteroidal anti-inflammatory drugs. *Arch Intern Med* 1991;151:1309–1313.
358. Go RS, Call TG. Deep venous thrombosis of the arm after intravenous immunoglobulin infusion: case report and literature review of intravenous immunoglobulin-related thrombotic complications. *Mayo Clin Proc* 2000;75:83–85.
359. Caramaschi P, Riccetti MM, Fratta Pasini A, et al. Systemic lupus erythematosus and thrombotic thrombocytopenic purpura. Report of three cases and review of the literature. *Lupus* 1998;7:37–41.
360. Tsai H-M, Lian EC-Y. Antibodies to von Willebrand factor-cleaving protease in acute thrombotic thrombocytopenic purpura. *N Engl J Med* 1998;339:1585–1594.
361. Tomabechi M, Daita G, Ohgami S, et al. A case of primary intracerebral malignant lymphoma in systemic lupus erythematosus. *No Shinke Geka* 1992;20:429–432.
362. Futran J, Shore A, Urowitz MB, et al. Subdural hematoma in systemic lupus erythematosus: report and review of the literature (case report). *J Rheumatol* 1987;14:378–381.
363. Middleton GD, McFarlin JE, Lipsky PE. The prevalence and clinical impact of fibromyalgia in systemic lupus erythematosus. *Arthritis Rheum* 1994;37:1181–1188.

364. Wallace DJ. The role of stress and trauma in rheumatoid arthritis and systemic lupus erythematosus. *Semin Arthritis Rheum* 1987;16:153–157.
365. von Brauchitsch H. Antinuclear factor in psychiatric disorders. *Am J Psychiatry* 1972;128:1552–1554.
366. Plantey F. Antinuclear factor in affective disorders. *Biol Psych* 1978;13:149–150.
367. McNicholl JM, Glynn D, Mongey A-B, et al. A prospective study of neurophysiologic, neurologic, and immunologic abnormalities in systemic lupus erythematosus. *J Rheumatol* 1994;21:1061–1066.
368. West SG. Neuropsychiatric lupus. *Rheum Dis Clin North Am* 1994;20:129–158.
369. Yoshio T, Masuyama J-I, Ikeda M, et al. Quantification of anti-ribosomal P0 protein antibodies by ELISA with recombinant P0 fusion protein and their association with central nervous system disease in systemic lupus erythematosus. *J Rheumatol* 1995;22:1681–1687.
370. Wantanabe T, Sato T, Uchiumi T, et al. Neuropsychiatric manifestations in patients with systemic lupus erythematosus: diagnostic and predictive value of longitudinal examination of anti-ribosomal P antibody. *Lupus* 1996;5:178–183.
371. Elkon KB, Parnassa AP, Foster CL. Lupus autoantibodies target ribosomal P proteins. *J Exp Med* 1985;162:459–471.
372. van Dam A, Nossent H, de Jong J, et al. Diagnostic value of antibodies against ribosomal phosphoproteins; a cross-sectional and longitudinal study. *J Rheumatol* 1991;18:1026–1034.
373. Derksen RH, van Dam AP, Gmelig Meyling FHJ, et al. A prospective study on anti–ribosomal P proteins in two cases of familial lupus and recurrent psychosis. *Ann Rheum Dis* 1990;49:779–782.
374. Golombek SJ, Graus F, Elkon KB. Autoantibodies in the cerebrospinal fluid of patients with systemic lupus erythematosus. *Arthritis Rheum* 1986;29:1090–1097.
375. Iverson GL. Are antibodies to ribosomal P proteins a clinically useful predictor of neuropsychiatric manifestations in patients with systemic lupus erythematosus? *Lupus* 1996;5:634–635.
376. Yoshio T, Masuyama J-I, Kano S. Anti-ribosomal P0 protein antibodies react with the surface of human umbilical vein endothelial cells. *J Rheumatol* 1996;23:1311–1312.
377. Dawkins RL, Witt C, Richmond J, et al. Lymphocytotoxic antibodies in disease. *Aust N Z J Med* 1978;8(suppl 1):81–86.
378. DeHoratius RJ. Lymphocytotoxic antibodies. *Prog Clin Immunol* 1980;4:151–174.
379. Butler WT, Sharp JT, Rossen RD, et al. Relationship of the clinical course of systemic lupus erythematosus to the presence of circulating lymphocytotoxic antibodies. *Arthritis Rheum* 1972; 15:231–238.
380. Nies KM, Brown JC, Dubois EL, et al. Histocompatibility (HLA) antigens and lymphocytotoxic antibodies in systemic lupus erythematosus (SLE). *Arthritis Rheum* 1974;17:397–402.
381. Denburg SD, Behmann SA, Carbotte RM, et al. Lymphocyte antigens in neuropsychiatric systemic lupus erythematosus. Relationship of lymphocyte antibody specificities to clinical disease. *Arthritis Rheum* 1994;37:369–375.
382. Denburg SD, Carbotte RM, Long AA, et al. Neuropsychological correlates of serum lymphocytotoxic antibodies in systemic lupus erythematosus. *Brain Behav Immun* 1988;2:222–234.
383. Long AA, Denburg DS, Carbotte RM, et al. Serum lymphocytotoxic antibodies and neurocognitive function in systemic lupus erythematosus. *Ann Rheum Dis* 1990;49:249–253.
384. Temesvari A, Denburg J, Denburg S, et al. Serum lymphocytotoxic antibodies in neuropsychiatric lupus: a serial study. *Clin Immunol Immunopathol* 1983;28:243–251.
385. How A, Dent PB, Liao S-K, et al. Antineuronal antibodies in neuropsychiatric systemic lupus erythematosus. *Arthritis Rheum* 1985;28:789–795.
386. Hanly JG, Rajaraman S, Behmann S, et al. A novel neuronal antigen identified by sera from patients with systemic lupus erythematosus. *Arthritis Rheum* 1988;31:1492.
387. Denburg JA, Behmann SA. Lymphocyte and neuronal antigens in neuropsychiatric lupus: presence of an elutable, immunoprecipitable lymphocyte/neuronal 52kd reactivity. *Ann Rheum Dis* 1994;53:304–308.
388. Costallat LTL, de Oliveira RM, Santiago MB, et al. Neuropsychiatric manifestations of systemic lupus erythematosus: the value of anticardiolipin, anti-ganglioside, and anti-galactocerebroside antibodies. *Clin Rheumatol* 1990;9:489–497.
389. Martinez X, Tintore M, Montalban J, et al. Antibodies against gangliosides in patients with SLE and neurological manifestations. *Lupus* 1992;1:299–302.
390. Sindern E, Stark E, Haas J, et al. Serum antibodies to GM1 and GM3-gangliosides in systemic lupus erythematosus with chronic inflammatory demyelinating polyradiculoneuropathy. *Acta Neurol Scand* 1991;83:399–402.
391. Galeazzi M, Annunziata P, Sebastiani GD, et al. Anti-ganglioside antibodies in a large cohort of European patients with systemic lupus erythematosus: clinical, serological, and HLA class II gene associations. *J Rheumatol* 2000;27:135–141.
392. De Mendonca Neto EC, Kumor A, Shadick N, et al. Antibodies to T- and L-isoforms of the cytoskeletal protein, fimbrin, in patients with systemic lupus erythematosus. *J Clin Invest* 1992; 90:1037–1042.
393. Love PE, Santora SA. Antiphospholipid antibodies: anticardiolipin and the lupus anticoagulant in systemic lupus erythematosus (SLE) and in non-SLE disorders. Prevalence and clinical significance. *Ann Int Med* 1990;112:682–698.
394. Finazzi G, Brancaccio V, Moia M, et al. Natural history and risk factors for thrombosis in 360 patients with antiphospholipid antibodies: a 4-year prospective study from the Italian registry. *Am J Med* 1996;100:530–536.
395. Levine SR, Brey RL, Sawaya KL, et al. Recurrent stroke and thrombo-occlusive events in the antiphospholipid syndrome. *Ann Neurol* 1995;38:119–124.
396. Levine SR, Salowich-Palm L, Sawaya KL, et al. IgG anticardiolipin antibody titer >40 GPL and the risk of subsequent thrombo-occlusive events and death: a prospective cohort study. *Stroke* 1997;28:1660–1665.
397. Roubey RAS, Maldonado MA, Byrd SN. Comparison of an enzyme-linked immunosorbent assay for antibodies to β_2-glycoprotein I and a conventional anticardiolipin immunoassay. *Arthritis Rheum* 1996;39:1606–1607.
398. Sanmarco M, Soler C, Christides C, et al. Prevalence and clinical significance of IgG isotype and anti-β_2 -glycoprotein I antibodies in antiphospholipid syndrome: a comparative study with anticardiolipin antibodies. *J Lab Clin Med* 1997;129:499–506.
399. Asherson RA, Hughes GR. The expanding spectrum of Libman Sacks endocarditis: the role of antiphospholipid antibodies. *Clin Exp Rheumatol* 1989;7:225–228.
400. Specker C, Rademacher J, Söhngen D, et al. Cerebral microemboli in patients with antiphospholipid syndrome. *Lupus* 1997; 6:638–644.
401. Levine SR, Brey RL, Joseph CLM, et al., for The Antiphospholipid Antibodies in Stroke Study Group. Risk of recurrent thromboembolic events in patients with focal cerebral ischemia and antiphospholipid antibodies. *Stroke* 1992:23(supp 1):1–29, 1–32.
402. Rosove MH, Brewer PMC. Antiphospholipid thrombosis: clinical course after the first thrombotic event in 70 patients. *Ann Int Med* 1992;117:303–308.
403. Verro P, Levine SR, Tietjen GE. Cerebrovascular ischemic events with high positive anticardiolipin antibodies. *Stroke* 1998;29:2245–2253.
404. Tanne D, D'Olhaberriague L, Schultz LR, et al. Anticardiolipin

antibodies and their associations with cerebrovascular risk factors. *Neurology* 1999;52:1368–1373.
405. Tanne D, Triplett DA, Levine SR. Antiphospholipid-protein antibodies and ischemic stroke. Not just cardiolipin any more. *Stroke* 1998;29:1755–1758.
406. Small P, Mass MF, Kohler PF, et al. Central nervous system involvement in SLE: diagnosis profile and clinical features. *Arthritis Rheum* 1977;20:869–878.
407. Abialmouona J, Shoemaker DW, Pullicino PM, et al. Marked cerebrospinal fluid pleocytosis in systemic lupus erythematosus related cerebral ischemia. *J Rheumatol* 1992;19:626–629.
408. Brook I, Controni G, Kassan SS, et al. Lactic acid levels in cerebrospinal fluid from patients with systemic lupus erythematosus. *J Rheumatol* 1979;6:691–693.
409. Nosanchuk JS, Kim CW. Lupus erythematosus cells in CSF. *JAMA* 1976;236:2883–2884.
410. Korn S, Barbieri EJ, DeHoratius RJ. Cerebrospinal fluid (CSF) substance P (SP) in neuropsychiatric systemic lupus erythematosus (NP–SLE). *Arthritis Rheum* 1989;32:R34.
411. Golombek SJ, Magid SK. Cerebrospinal fluid beta2-microglobulin in central nervous system lupus erythematosus (abstract). *Arthritis Rheum* 1985;28(suppl):S23.
412. Kassan SS, Kagen LJ. Elevated levels of cerebrospinal fluid guanosine 3,5-cyclic monophosphate (C-GMP) in systemic lupus erythematosus. *Am J Med* 1978;64:732–741.
413. Kassan SS, Kagen LJ. Central nervous system lupus erythematosus: measurement of cerebrospinal fluid cyclic GMP and other clinical markers of disease activity. *Arthritis Rheum* 1979;22:449–457.
414. Vogelgesang SA, Heyes MP, West SG, et al. Quinolinic acid in patients with systemic lupus erythematosus and neuropsychiatric manifestations. *J Rheumatol* 1996;23:850.
415. Cush JJ, Lightfoot E, Duby AD, et al. Cerebrospinal fluid (CSF) T cell clones from patients with active lupus cerebritis (abstract). *Arthritis Rheum* 1989;32(suppl 4):S120.
416. Petz LD, Sharp GC, Cooper NR, et al. Serum and cerebral spinal fluid complement and serum autoantibodies in systemic lupus erythematosus. *Medicine* 1971;50:259–275.
417. Baker M, Hadler NM, Whitaker JN, et al. Psychopathology in systemic lupus erythematosus. II. Relation to clinical observations, corticosteroid administration, and cerebrospinal fluid C4. *Semin Arthritis Rheum* 1973;2:111–126.
418. Hadler NM, Gerwin RD, Frank MM, et al. The fourth component of complement in the cerebrospinal fluid in SLE. *Arthritis Rheum* 1973;16:507–521.
419. Sergent JS, Lockshin MD, Klemperer MS, et al. Central nervous system disease in systemic lupus erythematosus. Therapy and prognosis. *Am J Med* 1975;58:644–654.
420. Jongen PJH, Boerbooms AM Th, Lamers KJB, et al. Diffuse CNS involvement in systemic lupus erythematosus: intrathecal synthesis of the 4th component of complement. *Neurology* 1990;40:1593–1596.
421. Sanders ME, Alexander EL, Koski CL, et al. Detection of activated terminal complement (C5b-9) in cerebrospinal fluid from patients with central nervous system involvement of primary Sjögren's syndrome or systemic lupus erythematosus. *J Immunol* 1987;138:2095–2099.
422. Stimmler MM, Quismorio FPQ Jr. Anti-deoxyribonucleoprotein antibodies in cerebrospinal fluid (CSF) in neuropsychiatric SLE (NP-SLE). *Arthritis Rheum* 1995;38:S301.
423. Mevorach D, Raz E, Steiner I. Evidence for intrathecal synthesis of autoantibodies in systemic lupus erythematosus with neurological involvement. *Lupus* 1994;3:117–121.
424. Shiozawa S, Kuroki Y, Kim Y, et al. Interferon-alpha in lupus psychosis. *Arthritis Rheum* 1992;35:417–422.
425. Sibbitt WL, Sibbitt RR, Brooks WM. Neuroimaging in neuropsychiatric systemic lupus erythematosus. *Arthritis Rheum* 1999;42:2026–2038.
426. Omdal R, Selseth B, Klow NE, et al. Clinical neurological, electrophysiological, and cerebral CT scan findings in systemic lupus erythematosus. *Scand J Rheumatol* 1989;18:283–289.
427. Yang WT, Daly BD, Hutchison R. Cranial computed tomography in the assessment of neurological complications in critically ill patients with systemic lupus erythematosus. *Anaesth Intensive Care* 1993;21:400–404.
428. Carette S, Urowitz MB, Grosman H, et al. Cranial computerized tomography in systemic lupus erythematosus. *J Rheumatol* 1982;9:855–859.
429. Gaylis NG, Altman RD, Ostrov S, et al. The selective value of computed tomography of the brain in cerebritis due to systemic lupus erythematosus. *J Rheumatol* 1982;9:850–854.
430. Reinitz E, Hubbard D, Zimmerman RD. Central nervous system disease in systemic lupus erythematosus: axial tomographic scan as an aid to differential diagnosis. *J Rheumatol* 1984;11:252–253.
431. Gordon T, Maddison PJ, Isenberg DA. Rapid development of cerebral atrophy in systemic lupus erythematosus. *Br J Rheum* 1986;25:296.
432. Bentson J, Rezon M, Winters J, et al. Steroids and apparent cerebral atrophy on computed tomography scans. *J Comput Assist Tomogr* 1978;2:16–23.
433. Daud AB, Nuruddin RN. Solitary paraventricular calcification in cerebral lupus erythematosus: a report of two cases. *Neuroradiology* 1988;30:84–85.
434. Nordstrom DM, West SG, Andersen PA. Basal ganglia calcifications in central nervous system lupus erythematosus. *Arthritis Rheum* 1985;28:1412–1416.
435. Yamamoto K, Nogaki H, Takase Y, et al. Systemic lupus erythematosus associated with marked intracranial calcification. *AJNR Am J Neuroradiol* 1992;13:1340–1342.
436. Raya PG, Aguado AG, Merlo MJS, et al. Massive cerebral calcification in systemic lupus erythematosus: report of an unusual case. *Lupus* 1994;3:133–135.
437. Weisberg LA. The cranial computed tomographic findings in patients with neurologic manifestations of systemic lupus erythematosus. *Comput Radiol* 1986;10:63–68.
438. Aisen AM, Gabrielsen TO, McCune WJ. MR imaging of systemic lupus erythematosus involving the brain. *AJR Am J Roentgenol* 1985;144:1027–1031.
439. McCune WJ, MacGuire A, Aisen A, et al. Identification of brain lesions in neuropsychiatric systemic lupus erythematosus by magnetic resonance scanning. *Arthritis Rheum* 1988;31:159–166.
440. Sibbitt WL Jr, Sibbitt RR, Griffey RH, et al. Magnetic resonance and computed tomographic imaging in the evaluation of acute neuropsychiatric disease in systemic lupus erythematosus. *Ann Rheum Dis* 1989;48:1014–1022.
441. Stimmler MM, Colletti PM, Quismorio FP Jr. Magnetic resonance imaging of the brain in neuropsychiatric systemic lupus erythematosus. *Semin Arthritis Rheum* 1993;22:345–349.
442. Jacobs L, Kinkel PR, Costello PB, et al. Central nervous system lupus erythematosus: the value of magnetic resonance imaging. *J Rheumatol* 1988;15:601–606.
443. Sessoms SL, Kovarsky J. Monthly intravenous cyclophosphamide in the treatment of severe systemic lupus erythematosus. *Clin Exp Rheumatol* 1984;2:247–251.
444. Suzuki K, Hara M, Nakajima S, et al. Analysis of systemic lupus erythematosus (SLE) involving the central nervous system by magnetic resonance imaging (MRI). *Ryumachi* 1989;29:88–96.
445. Vermess M, Bernstein RM, Bydder GM, et al. Nuclear magnetic resonance (NMR) imaging of the brain in systemic lupus erythematosus. *J Comput Assist Tomogr* 1983;7:461–467.

446. Jarek MJ, West SG, Baker MR, et al. Magnetic resonance imaging in systemic lupus erythematosus patients without a history of neuropsychiatric lupus erythematosus. *Arthritis Rheum* 1994; 37:1609–1613.
447. Nomura K, Yamano S, Ikeda Y, et al. Asymptomatic cerebrovascular lesions detected by magnetic resonance imaging in patients with systemic lupus erythematosus lacking a history of neuropsychiatric events. *Intern Med* 1999;38:789–795.
448. Gonzalez-Crespo MR, Blanco FJ, Ramos A, et al. Magnetic resonance imaging of the brain in systemic lupus erythematosus. *Br J Rheumatol* 1995;34:1055–1060.
449. Cauli A, Montaldo C, Peltz MT, et al. Abnormalities of magnetic resonance imaging of the central nervous system in patients with systemic lupus erythematosus correlate with disease severity. *Clin Rheumatol* 1994;13:615–618.
450. Awad IA, Spetzler RF, Hodak JA, et al. Incidental subcortical lesions identified on magnetic resonance imaging in the elderly. I. Correlation with age and cerebrovascular risk factors. *Stroke* 1986;17:1084–1089.
451. Katzman GL, Dagher AP, Patronas NJ. Incidental findings on brain magnetic resonance imaging from 1000 asymptomatic volunteers. *JAMA* 1999;282:36–39.
452. Friedman SD, Stidley CA, Brooks WM, et al. Brain injury and neurometabolic abnormalities in systemic lupus erythematosus. *Radiology* 1998;209:79–84.
453. Sibbitt WL, Brooks WM, Haseler LJ, et al. Spin-spin relaxation of brain tissues in systemic lupus erythematosus. *Arthritis Rheum* 1995;38:810–818.
454. Ishikawa O, Ohnishi K, Miyachi Y, et al. Cerebral lesions in systemic lupus erythematosus detected by magnetic resonance imaging. Relationship to anticardiolipin antibody. *J Rheumatol* 1994;21:87–90.
455. Weingarten K, Filippi C, Barbut D, et al. The neuroimaging features of cardiolipin antibody syndrome. *Clinical Imaging* 1997;21:6–12.
456. Hachulla E, Michon-Pasturel U, Leys D, et al. Cerebral magnetic resonance imaging in patients with or without antiphospholipid antibodies. *Lupus* 1998;7:124–131.
457. Provenzale JM, Barboriak DP, Allen NB, et al. Patients with antiphospholipid antibodies: CT and MR findings of the brain. *Am J Roentgenol* 1996;167:1573–1578.
458. Petropoulos H, Sibbitt WL Jr, Brooks WM. Automated T2 quantitation in neuropsychiatric lupus erythematosus: a marker of active disease. *J Magn Reson Imaging* 1999;9:39–43.
459. Kozora E, West SG, Kotzin BL, et al. Magnetic resonance imaging abnormalities and cognitive deficits in systemic lupus erythematosus without overt central nervous system disease. *Arthritis Rheum* 1998;41:41–47.
460. Welch KM, Nagesh V, Boska M, et al. Detection of cerebral ischemia in systemic lupus erythematosus by magnetic resonance techniques. *Ann NY Acad Sci* 1997;823:120.
461. Runge VM, Kirsch JE, Wells JW, et al. Repeat cerebral blood volume assessment with first-pass MR imaging. *J Magn Reson Imaging* 1994;4:457–461.
462. Rovaris M, Viti B, Ciboddo G, et al. Brain involvement in systemic immune-mediated diseases: magnetic resonance and magnetization transfer imaging study. *J Neurol Neurosurg Psychiatry* 2000;68:170–177.
463. Bosma GP, Rood MJ, Zwinderman AH, et al. Evidence of central nervous system damage in patients with neuropsychiatric systemic lupus erythematosus, demonstrated by magnetization transfer imaging. *Arthritis Rheum* 2000;43:48–54.
464. Matson GB, Weiner MW. Spectroscopy. In: Stark DD, Bradley WG Jr (editors). *Magnetic resonance imaging.* St. Louis: Mosby; 1999:181.
465. Sibbitt WL Jr, Sibbitt RR. Magnetic resonance spectroscopy and positron emission tomography scanning in neuropsychiatric systemic lupus erythematosus. *Rheum Dis Clin North Am* 1993;19:851–868.
466. Brooks WM, Sabet A, Sibbitt WL Jr, et al. Neurochemistry of brain lesions determined by spectroscopic imaging in systemic lupus erythematosus. *J Rheumatol* 1997;24:2323–2329.
467. Chinn RJS, Wilkinson ID, Hall-Craggs MA, et al. Magnetic resonance imaging of the brain and cerebral proton spectroscopy in patients with systemic lupus erythematosus. *Arthritis Rheum* 1997;40:36–46.
468. Davie CA, Feinstein A, Kartsounis LD, et al. Proton magnetic resonance spectroscopy of systemic lupus erythematosus involving the central nervous system. *J Neurol* 1995;242:522–528.
469. Sibbitt WL Jr, Haseler LJ, Griffey RH, et al. Analysis of cerebral structural changes in systemic lupus erythematosus by proton MR spectroscopy. *Am J Neuroradiol* 1994;15:923.
470. Brooks WM, Jung RE, Ford CC, et al. Relationship between neurometabolite derangement and neurocognitive dysfunction in systemic lupus erythematosus. *J Rheumatol* 1999;26:81–85.
471. Sibbitt WL Jr, Haseler LJ, Griffey RR, et al. Neurometabolism of active neuropsychiatric lupus determined with proton MR spectroscopy. *Am J Neuroradiol* 1997;18:1271–1277.
472. Griffey RH, Brown MS, Bankhurst AD, et al. Depletion of high-energy phosphates in the central nervous system of patients with systemic lupus erythematosus, as determined by phosphorus-31 nuclear magnetic resonance spectroscopy. *Arthritis Rheum* 1990;33:827–833.
473. Mitsias P, Levine SR. Large cerebral vessel occlusive disease in systemic lupus erythematosus. *Neurology* 1994;44:385–393.
474. Sakaki T, Morimoto T, Utsumi S. Cerebral transmural angiitis and ruptured cerebral aneurysms in patients with systemic lupus erythematosus. *Neurochirurgia* 1990;33:132–135.
475. Trevor RP, Sondhemier FK, Fessel WJ, et al. Angiographic demonstration of major cerebral vessel occlusion in systemic lupus erythematosus. *Neuroradiology* 1972;4:202–207.
476. Nagayama Y, Okamoto S, Konishi T, et al. Cerebral Berry aneurysms and systemic lupus erythematosus. *Neuroradiology* 1991;33:466.
477. Hellmann DB, Roubenoff R, Healy RA, et al. Central nervous system angiography: safety and predictors of a positive result in 125 consecutive patients evaluated for possible vasculitis. *J Rheumatol* 1992;19:568–572.
478. Bennahum DA, Messner RP, Shoop JD. Brain scan findings in central nervous system involvement by lupus erythematosus. *Ann Int Med* 1974;81:763–765.
479. Tan RF, Gladman DD, Urowitz MB, et al. Brain scan diagnosis of central nervous system involvement in systemic lupus erythematosus. *Ann Rheum Dis* 1978;37:357–362.
480. Kulesha D, Moldofsky H, Urowitz M, et al. Brain scan lateralization and psychiatric symptoms in systemic lupus erythematosus. *Biol Psychiatry* 1981;16:407–412.
481. Stoppe G, Wildhagen K, Seidel JW, et al. Positron emission tomography in neuropsychiatric lupus erythematosus. *Neurology* 1990;40:304–308.
482. Otte A, Weiner Sm, Peter HH, et al. Brain glucose utilization in systemic lupus erythematosus with neuropsychiatric symptoms: a controlled positron emission tomography study. *Eur J Nucl Med* 1997;24:787–791.
483. Meyer GJ, Schober O, Stoppe G, et al. Cerebral involvement in systemic lupus erythematosus (SLE): comparison of positron emission tomography (PET) with other imaging methods. *Psychiatry Res* 1989;29:367–368.
484. Guttman M, Lang AE, Garnett ES, et al. Regional cerebral glucose metabolism in SLE chorea: further evidence that striational

hypometabolism is not a correlate of chorea. *Mov Disord* 1987; 2:201–210.
485. Hirawa M, Nonaka C, Abe T, et al. Positron emission tomography in systemic lupus erythematosus: relation of cerebral vasculitis to PET findings. *Am J Nucl Med Radiol* 1983;4:541–543.
486. Komatsu N, Kodama K, Yamanouchi N, et al. Decreased regional cerebral metabolic rate for glucose in systemic lupus erythematosus patients with psychiatric symptoms. *Eur Neurol* 1999;42:41–48.
487. de Jong BM, Pruim J, Sinnige LG, et al. Regional specific changes of cerebral metabolism in systemic lupus erythematosus identified by positron emission tomography. *Eur Neurol* 1999; 41:187–193.
488. Kao CH, Ho YJ, Lan JL, et al. Discrepancy between regional cerebral blood flow and glucose metabolism of the brain in systemic lupus erythematosus patients with normal brain magnetic resonance imaging findings. *Arthritis Rheum* 1999;42:61–68.
489. Holman BL. Functional imaging in systemic lupus erythematosus: an accurate indicator of central nervous system involvement? *Arthritis Rheum* 1993;36:1193–1195.
490. Carbotte RM, Denburg SD, Denburg JA, et al. Fluctuating cognitive abnormalities and cerebral glucose metabolism in neuropsychiatric systemic lupus erythematosus. *J Neurol Neurosurg Psychiatry* 1992;55:1054–1059.
491. Otte A, Weiner SM, Hoergerle S, et al. Neuropsychiatric systemic lupus erythematosus before and after immunosuppressive treatment: a FDG PET study. *Lupus* 1998;7:57–59.
492. Sailer M, Burchert W, Ehrenheim C, et al. Positron emission tomography and magnetic resonance imaging for cerebral involvement in patients with systemic lupus erythematosus. *J Neurol* 1997;244:186–193.
493. Pinching AJ, Travers RL, Hughes GR, et al. Oxygen-15 brain scanning for detection of cerebral involvement in systemic lupus erythematosus. *Lancet* 1978;i:898–900.
494. Rogers MP, Waterhouse E, Nagel JS, et al. I–123 iofetamine SPECT scan in systemic lupus erythematosus with cognitive and other minor neuropsychiatric symptoms: a pilot study. *Lupus* 1992;1:215–219.
495. Colamussi P, Giganti M, Cittanti C, et al. Brain single-photon emission tomography with 99Tc-HMPAO in neuropsychiatric systemic lupus erythematosus: relations with EEG and MRI findings and clinical manifestations. *Eur J Nucl Med* 1995;22:17–24.
496. Kodama K, Okada S, Hino T, et al. Single photon emission computed tomography in systemic lupus erythematosus with psychiatric symptoms. *J Neurol Neurosurg Psychiatry* 1995;58: 307–311.
497. Rubbert A, Marienhagen J, Pirner K, et al. Single-photon-emission computed tomography analysis of cerebral blood flow in the evaluation of central nervous system involvement in patients with systemic lupus erythematosus. *Arthritis Rheum* 1993;36: 1253–1262.
498. Szer IS, Miller JH, Rawlings D, et al. Cerebral perfusion abnormalities in children with central nervous system manifestations of lupus detected by single photon emission computed tomography. *J Rheumatol* 1993;20:2143–2148.
499. Emmi L, Bramati M, de Cristofaro MTR, et al. MRI and SPECT investigations of the CNS in SLE patients. *Clin Exp Rheumatol* 1993;11:13–20.
500. Kovacs JAJ, Urowitz MB, Gladman DD, et al. The use of single photon emission computerized tomography in neuropsychiatric SLE: a pilot study. *J Rheumatol* 1995;22:1247–1253.
501. Russo R, Gilday D, Laxer RM, et al. Single photon emission computed tomography scanning in childhood systemic lupus erythematosus. *J Rheumatol* 1998;25:576–582.
502. Nossent JC, Hovestadt DH. Single-photon emission computed tomography of the brain in the evaluation of cerebral lupus. *Arthritis Rheum* 1991;34:1397.
503. Lin WY, Wang SJ, Yen TC, et al. Technetium-99m-HMPAO brain SPECT in systemic lupus erythematosus with CNS involvement. *J Nucl Med* 1997:38:1112–1115.
504. Reiff A, Miller J, Shaham B, et al. Childhood central nervous system lupus: longitudinal assessment using single photon emission computed tomography. *J Rheumatol* 1997;24:2461–2465.
505. Falcini F, De Cristofari MT, Ermini M, et al. Regional cerebral blood flow in juvenile systemic lupus erythematosus: a prospective SPECT study. *J Rheumatol* 1998; 25:583–588.
506. Shen YY, Kao CH, Ho YJ, et al. Regional cerebral blood flow in patients with systemic lupus erythematosus. *J Neuroimaging* 1999;9:160–164.
507. Kao CH, Lan JL, Changlai SP, et al. The role of FDG-PET, HMPAO-SPECT and MRI in the detection of brain involvement in patients with systemic lupus erythematosus. *Eur J Nucl Med* 1999;26:129–134.
508. Babikian V, Wechsler L. Recent developments in transcranial Doppler sonography. *J Neuroimaging* 1994;4:159–163.
509. Siebler M et al. Cerebral microembolism in symptomatic and asymptomatic high-grade internal carotid artery stenosis. *Neurology* 1994;44:615–618.
510. Matsukawa Y, Nishinarita S, Hayama T, et al. Clinical significance of electroencephalograph in patients with systemic lupus erythematosus. *Ryumachi* 1993;33:20–28.
511. Bourke BE, de M Rudolf N. The value of electroencephalogram in cerebral systemic lupus erythematosus (abstract). In: *XVI International Congress of Rheumatology*, May 1985, Sydney, Australia, F69.
512. Finn P, Rudolf N, Ade M. The electroencephalogram in systemic lupus erythematosus. *Lancet* 1978;i:1255.
513. Nobili F, Rodriguez G, Arrigo A, et al. Accuracy of 133-Xenon regional cerebral blood flow and quantitative electroencephalography in systemic lupus erythematosus. *Lupus* 1996;5: 93–102.
514. Ritchlin CT, Chabot RJ, Alper K, et al. Quantitative electroencephalography. A new approach to the diagnosis of cerebral dysfunction in systemic lupus erythematosus. *Arthritis Rheum* 1992;35:1330–1342.
515. Mongey AB, Glynn D, Hutchinson M, et al. Clinical neurophysiology in the assessment of neurological symptoms in systemic lupus erythematosus. *Rheumatol Int* 1987;7:49–52.
516. Borton TE, Eby TL, Bail EV, et al. Stimulus repetition rate effect on the auditory brainstem response in systemic lupus erythematosus. *Laryngoscope* 1992;102:335–339.
517. Ito J, Suwazono S, Kimura J, et al. Auditory event-related potentials in patients with systemic lupus erythematosus. *Eur Neurol* 1993;33:373–377.
518. Fradis M, Podoshin L, Ben-David J, et al. Brainstem auditory evoked potentials with increased stimulus rate in patients suffering from systemic lupus erythematosus. *Laryngoscope* 1989; 99:325–329.
519. Fierro B, Brighina F, Amico L, et al. Evoked potential study and radiological findings in patients with systemic lupus erythematosus. *Electromyogr Clin Neurophysiol* 1999;39:305–313.
520. Lishner M, Ravid M. Methyl-prednisolone pulse therapy of recurrent peritonitis and cerebritis in systemic lupus erythematosus. *Harefuah* 1986;111:425–426.
521. Price J, Klestov A, Beacham B, et al. A case of cerebral systemic lupus erythematosus treated with methylprednisolone pulse therapy. *Aust N Z J Psychiatry* 1985;19:184–188.
522. Fessel WJ. Megadose corticosteroid therapy in systemic lupus erythematosus. *J Rheumatol* 1980;7:486–500.
523. Boumpas DT, Yamada H, Patronas NJ, et al. Pulse cyclophos-

phamide in severe neuropsychiatric lupus. *Q J Med* 1991;296: 975–984.
524. Neuwelt CM, Lacks S, Kaye BR, et al. Role of intravenous cyclophosphamide in the treatment of severe neuropsychiatric systemic lupus erythematosus. *Am J Med* 1995;98:32–41.
525. Ramos PC, Mendez MJ, Ames PR, et al. Pulse cyclophosphamide in the treatment of neuropsychiatric systemic lupus erythematosus. *Clin Exp Rheumatol* 1996;14:295–299.
526. Baca V, Lavalle C, Garcia R, et al. Favorable response to intravenous methyl-prednisolone and cyclophosphamide in children with severe neuropsychiatric lupus. *J Rheumatol* 1999;26: 432–439.
527. Gaubitz M, Schorat A, Schotte H, et al. Mycophenolate mofetil for the treatment of systemic lupus erythematosus: an open pilot trial. *Lupus* 1999;8:731–736.
528. Khamashta MA, Cuadrado MJ, Mujic F, et al. The management of thrombosis in the antiphospholipid-antibody syndrome. *N Engl J Med* 1995;332:993–997.
529. Brey RL, Levine SR. Treatment of neurologic complications of antiphospholipid antibody syndrome. *Lupus* 1996;5:473–476.
530. Moll S, Ortel TL. Monitoring warfarin therapy in patients with lupus anticoagulants. *Ann Int Med* 1997;127:177–185.
531. Velsini G, Priori R, Francia A, et al. Central nervous system involvement in systemic lupus erythematosus: a new therapeutic approach with intrathecal dexamethasone and methotrexate. *Springer Semin Immunopathol* 1994;16:313–321.
532. Engel G, van Vollenhoven RF. Treatment of severe CNS lupus with intravenous immunoglobulin. *J Clin Rheumatol* 1999;5: 228–232.
533. Wallace DJ. Apheresis for lupus erythematosus. *Lupus* 1999;8: 174–180.
534. Bouvier M, Colson F, Tebib JG, et al. Clinical analysis of neuropsychiatric disorders in systemic lupus erythematosus. Report of fourteen personal cases. *Sem Hop Paris* 1990;66:711.
535. Smith GM, Leyland MJ. Plasma exchange for cerebral lupus erythematosus. *Lancet* 1987;i:103.
536. Unterweger B, Klein G, Fleishchhacker WW. Plasma exchange for cerebral lupus erythematosus (letter). *Biol Psychiatry* 1988;24:946–947.
537. Tanter Y, Rifle G, Chalopin JM, et al. Plasma exchange in central nervous system involvement of systemic lupus erythematosus. *Plasma Ther Transfus Technol* 1987;8:161–168.
538. Sturfelt G, Mousa F, Jonsson H, et al. Recurrent cerebral infarction and the antiphospholipid syndrome: effect of intravenous gammaglobulin in a patient with systemic lupus erythematosus. *Ann Rheum Dis* 1990;49:939–941.
539. Aringer M, Smolen JS, Graninger WB. Severe infections in plasmapheresis-treated systemic lupus erythematosus. *Arthritis Rheum* 1998;41:414–420.
540. Rock GA et al. Comparison of plasma exchange with plasma infusion in the treatment of thrombotic thrombocytopenic purpura. *N Engl J Med* 1991;325:393–397.
541. Wallace DJ, Silverman S, Goldstein J, et al. Use of hyperbaric oxygen in rheumatic diseases: case report and critical analysis. *Lupus* 1995;4:172–175.
542. Pfrausler B, Bosch S, Grubwieser G, et al. Multimodal therapy in life-threatening cerebral lupus erythematosus: the benefit of cerebrospinal fluid pheresis. *Int Arch Allergy Immunol* 1995; 107:592–594.
543. Marmont AM. Intense immunosuppression and stem cell transplantation or rescue for severe systemic lupus erythematosus. *Lupus* 1999;8:256–257.
544. Brodsky RA, Petri M, Douglas Smith B, et al. Immunoablative high-dose cyclophosphamide without stem-cell rescue for refractory, severe autoimmune disease. *Ann Intern Med* 1998; 12:1031–1035.
545. Terao T, Yoshimura R, Shiratuchi T, et al. Effects of lithium on steroid-induced depression. *Biol Psychiatry* 1997;41:1225–1226.
546. Petri M. Hopkins lupus cohort: 1999 update. *Rheum Dis Clin North Am* 2000;26:199–213.
547. Ginzler EM, Schorn K. Outcome and prognosis in systemic lupus erythematosus. *Rheum Dis Clin North Am* 1988;14:67–78.
548. Ward MM, Pyun E, Studenski S. Mortality risks associated with specific clinical manifestations of systemic lupus erythematosus. *Arch Int Med* 1996;156:1337–1344.
549. Rubin LA, Urowitz MB, Gladman DD. Mortality in systemic lupus erythematosus: the bimodal pattern revisited. *Q J Med* 1985;55:87–98.

36

PSYCHOPATHOLOGY IN THE PATIENT WITH LUPUS

HOWARD S. SHAPIRO

Abnormal behavior patterns were first described in patients with lupus by Hebra and Kaposi (1) in 1874 and by Osler (2) (i.e., stupor and recurrent coma) at the turn of the century. Daly (3) contributed the first detailed modern description of psychotic behavior in central nervous system (CNS) lupus in 1945. Within 5 years of that time, introduction of the lupus erythematosus (LE) cell test by Hargraves et al. (4) and the availability of corticosteroids considerably altered our understanding and approach to neuropsychiatric disorders in systemic lupus erythematosus (SLE). This chapter describes the highly variable psychopathologies (including the cognitive dysfunction and deficits) that are seen with SLE as well as their differential diagnosis, addresses the special concerns of lupus sufferers, and outlines a rational treatment program.

The psychological and neurobehavioral difficulties that are encountered in lupus can be classified as psychoses, mood disorders, specific organic brain syndromes, cognitive impairment, drug reactions (particularly to corticosteroids), functional disorders, disruptions in circadian biorhythms, and various disruptions of the autonomic nervous systems (5–18). Although certain descriptive overlapping occurs, the cause and pathogenesis of each of these entities generally are mutually exclusive and are discussed separately. These conditions must be distinguished, and recognized as being distinct, from the inevitable and ongoing unpleasant adjustment reactions that occur and recur during the life of the patient with lupus.

As of 1998, there is no universally accepted diagnostic criteria or classification of neuropsychiatric SLE (NPSLE). The revised American Rheumatology Association (ARA) criteria for NPSLE include only seizure psychosis (19), despite the widely diverse clinical manifestations and varying degree of severity (20,21).

Kassan and Lockshin (22) first proposed a classification system in 1979 and specified key dimensions such as chronology and isolated occurrence versus occurrence during systemic flare, etc., at a time when the use of magnetic resonance imaging (MRI) and other radioimaging techniques in SLE was limited. Eleven years later, Singer et al. (21) published a consensus list of "descriptors" or elements important to the diagnosis of NPSLE.

In 1999 the American College of Rheumatology (ACR) Ad Hoc Committee on Neuropsychiatric Lupus Nomenclature (24) reported the results of their "objective to develop a standardized nomenclature for the psychiatric syndromes of SLE (NPSLE)." An international, multidisciplinary committee representing rheumatology, neurology, psychiatry, neuropsychology, and hematology developed "case definitions," reporting standards and *diagnostic testing recommendations.*

Case definitions including diagnostic criteria, important exclusions, and methods of ascertainment were developed for 19 NPSLE syndromes. Recommendations for standard reporting requirements, minimum laboratory evaluation, and imaging techniques were formulated. A short neuropsychological test battery for the diagnosis of cognitive deficits was proposed. [The complete case definitions are available on the ACR World Wide Web site: http://www.rheumatology.org/ac/ar.html.]

The ACR Ad Hoc Committee on Neuropsychiatric Lupus Nomenclature developed reporting standards, recommendations for laboratory and imaging evaluation, and case definitions for 19 neuropsychiatric syndromes observed in SLE, and these have been approved by the board of directors of the ACR. The case definitions give a basic clinical description, along with a delineation on the rules and methods of ascertainment, exclusions, and associations. Structural definition of the brain [e.g., by computed tomography (CT), MRI, or other radioimaging techniques] and neurophysiologic studies [electroencephalogram (EEG), electromyography] serve as criteria for specific syndromes and are recommended in others to exclude conditions that can have the same clinical presentation in practice.

The new ACR nomenclature system is intended to expand the neuropsychiatric criteria of the ACR classification criteria for SLE and, with more study, could be done with confidence for some syndromes. Thus, subjects might be said to have a given neuropsychiatric lupus syndrome if they meet both the case definition for neuropsychiatric lupus and three or more of the ACR (non-NPSLE) criteria for SLE. Patients who meet the definition for a neuropsychiatric syndrome but not a sufficient number of ACR criteria for SLE are classified as having possible NPSLE. Like the ACR classification criteria for SLE, the classification criteria for NPSLE are intended for purposes of classification and reporting, and it should be emphasized that they are not meant to replace clinical judgment or to be used in making a clinical diagnosis in a given patient.

Laboratory and radiologic evaluation, including identification of antibodies to neuronal cell constituents, cytokines, and other immunochemical phenomena in neuropsychiatric lupus, has provided insights into potential mechanisms of disease. However, the data are not widely available, standardized, or strongly correlated with specific neuropsychiatric syndromes, the only exceptions being antiphospholipid antibodies and possibly antiribosomal P. Other than testing for antiphospholipid antibodies, the committee decided that these antibody tests should be viewed as investigational at this time.

The cerebrovascular diseases observed in SLE illustrate how neuropsychiatric syndromes might be rationally classified once pathogenic mechanisms are elucidated. The process marked by the presence of antiphospholipid antibodies suggests that not all SLE manifestations must be inflammatory and that such disparate syndromes as Sneddon's syndrome, transverse myelopathy, stroke, and chorea may have a common etiology. It is imperative to report antiphospholipid antibody status in every SLE patient.

The evolving technologies for imaging brain structure and function have the potential to rewrite the literature of neuropsychiatric lupus and may become gold standards for classification. Indeed, they have become the modern "tissue diagnosis." However, their increased sensitivity is also their weakness in that prognosis and clinical significance of subtle or unexpected findings such as unidentified bright objects and abnormalities on single photon emission computed tomography (SPECT) are unknown at this time. Current imaging technologies are continually improving, and the committee considered them to be an essential component of some case definitions (see Differential Diagnosis of Psychosis, below).

It is difficult to determine whether a lupus patient's depression, psychosis, cognitive impairment, or confused states are neuropsychiatric manifestation caused by SLE or psychological reactions to the stress of having a major, chronic, systemic illness. The syndromes should be defined to facilitate study of the question. The case definitions for anxiety, mood disorder, and psychosis require a clinical evaluation to exclude merely reactive psychological disturbances, and psychiatric consultation may be required. If the syndrome is judged to be a neuropsychiatric manifestation of SLE, the presence of marked psychosocial stress should be reported as an association. The committee adopted the terminology of the *Diagnostic and Statistical Manual of Mental Disorders*, 4th edition (DSM-IV) (25) wherever possible since use of the DSM has been widespread since 1952 and reflects an iterative process whose reliability has been studied extensively. Detailed, explicit criteria, methods of ascertainment, rationale, and a manual for its use are available. Its codes are consistent with the *International Classification of Diseases*, 9th revision, which provides additional advantages for research. The committee believed it would be inadvisable to develop new psychiatric nomenclature.

For all major psychiatric disorders, the DSM-IV distinguishes primary entities from secondary disease due to underlying medical conditions or substance abuse.

INCIDENCE

The incidence of psychiatric symptoms in several series of patients with lupus is shown in Table 36.1. The range in various reports is from 12% to 71%. This large variation results in part from who defined the psychopathology (e.g., psychiatrist, neurologist, internist), whether a hospitalized or an outpatient group was used, criteria for defining lupus, and the ethnic group, sex, age, and socioeconomic status of the study population. In 1975, Klippel and Zvaifler (26) reviewed the literature and, in a total of 995 patients with SLE, reported that 18 had disturbances in mental function. This is inclusive of Dubois' 520 patients, in whom a 12%

TABLE 36.1. INCIDENCE OF PSYCHIATRIC SYMPTOMS IN PATIENTS WITH LUPUS

Parameter	O'Connor (91)	Stern and Robbins (93)	Estes & Christian (9)	Guze (98)	Ganz et al. (333)	Baker (100)	Ropes (53)	Feinglass et al. (10)	Grigor et al. (11)	Hall et al. (102)
Patients in study (*n*)	40	53	150	101	68	17	142	150	50	50
Psychiatric symptoms (%)	65	64	42	12	71	41	28	16	40	44
Psychosis	55	52	16	5	15	15	8	14	0	25
Schizophrenia	17	12	10	5	7	9	8	6	0	2
Organic brain syndrome	28	30	21	9	22	15	3	14	18	10
Functional disorders	12	30	5	10	51	36	20	2	22	25

incidence of psychosis was reported (8) when, in fact, the incidence of minor disturbances in mental function was not reported and certainly was much higher.

Typically, neuropsychiatric lupus (NPL) in the literature is a heterogeneous alloy of neurologic and psychiatric symptoms, including seizures, vertigo, headaches, organic brain syndromes, neuropathies, psychosis, depression, and unusual adjustment reactions that cannot be attributed to any other cause (27–31). Failure to distinguish psychiatric from clearly organic brain syndromes contributes to this large variation (32). For example, in 1985, Nollet et al. (33) reported an overall incidence of psychiatric symptoms of 54% in a prospective study of 35 patients with SLE. Abel et al. (5) followed 66 SLE patients (prospectively) who had 77 episodes of NPL. In 1980, they reported that patients with NPL had more SLE manifestations than patients without NPL. [Serologic data and cerebrospinal fluid (CSF) analysis were not helpful in identifying an episode of NPL, whereas the EEG was abnormal in more than 50% and brain scans in more than 75% of patients.) In 74 episodes with a known outcome, 54 improved, 44 of which having been treated with increased doses of corticosteroids. Patients with NPL also had a higher incidence of deaths when compared to patients without NPL.

In 1988, Lim et al. (13) reported on the frequency and type of psychiatric disease in 40 patients suffering from SLE and 27 control subjects with rheumatoid arthritis (RA) or inflammatory bowel disease. The psychiatric morbidity at the time of interview was the same in both groups. The patients with SLE had experienced more episodes of psychiatric illness in the past, however, and psychotic symptoms occurred only in this group. One half of the patients with SLE had previous or current evidence of neurologic involvement. An association was found between neurologic disease and psychotic symptoms in patients with SLE, whereas anxiety and affective disturbances appeared to be closely related to environmental factors both in patients with SLE and in controls. No correlation was found between psychiatric and neurologic disease and clinical or laboratory indices of disease activity. In 1988, Darby and Schmidt (34) reported on 100 psychiatric consultations in a rheumatology unit. Of these, 80 consisted of patients with SLE (36), RA (29), and fibrositis (15). Most patients with SLE had organic brain syndromes that related to CNS involvement or corticosteroids, and most patients with RA had a depressive diagnosis. Patients with fibrositis showed no specific psychiatric diagnosis.

In 1988, Omdal et al. (35) reported an 83% incidence of NPL in 25 patients, but they subdivided psychiatric problems into 17 entities. It is believed that patients with SLE have more psychiatric symptoms than patients with most other medical illnesses, and that they often are as psychiatrically disturbed as psychiatric patient groups. In 1990, Mitchell and Thompson (36) reported that this belief did not prove to be true for outpatients with SLE. In their study, 22 outpatients with SLE, 81 general medical outpatients, and 40 psychiatric outpatients were screened with psychometric tests that were designed to access psychiatric symptoms and stress. The SLE outpatients' psychiatric symptoms and stresses were more similar to those reported by general medical outpatients rather than to those reported by psychiatric outpatients, except in a few areas, and patients with SLE were significantly less distressed than psychiatric patients in all areas except those relating directly to their SLE.

Psychiatric symptoms rarely are reported as an initial feature of SLE (37). Nevertheless, many patients have the feeling that psychiatric symptoms occurred before they were diagnosed as having SLE. This feeling was confirmed by an inquiry among members of the Dutch Lupus Patients Society: half of them had experienced psychiatric complaints before their SLE was diagnosed, and two thirds of these patients searched for professional help for these complaints. Sera from 2,121 patients who were admitted to a psychiatric hospital and from 500 controls matched for sex and age were tested for the presence of antinuclear antibodies (ANAs) and antibodies to DNA. ANAs were found in 3% of patients; they were also found in 3% of controls. Anti-DNA antibodies were found in 1% of both patients and controls. Two of 114 psychiatric patients with ANA and/or anti-DNA antibodies had SLE and/or Sjögren's syndrome. The authors concluded that SLE is not an important cause of admission to psychiatric hospitals. Thus, routine tests for the determination of ANAs and anti-DNA antibodies on admissions in these hospitals would not seem to be useful.

The exhaustive studies of Carbotte and the Denburgs (38) in the 1980s clearly and consistently showed, with great objectivity, the unexpectedly high incidence of cognitive impairment in patients with SLE and inactive or absent neuropsychiatric symptomatology. By administering a battery of neuropsychologic tests to 62 female patients with SLE (and to controls), an overall incidence of cognitive impairment of 66 was obtained in the SLE patient sample. Neither steroid medication nor psychologic distress could account for these findings.

Several reports in the literature (39,40) have emphasized that psychiatric and/or psychological distress (as contrasted with classic neurologic symptoms) may be the presenting symptoms of SLE (41). Consistently, studies from around the world report that depression is the most common psychiatric disorder [using the International Classification of Disorders-9 (ICD-9)] that is observed in patients with SLE (16,42–44).

Acute psychotic manifestations in SLE usually have been considered to occur early in the course of illness, although these findings primarily are based on studies with few patients and limited lengths of observation. Ward and Studenski (101) investigated the chronology of acute psychiatric disturbances in SLE. The time course of these episodes was examined in 36 patients over a median duration of observation of 72 months. Of 36 initial psychiatric episodes, 22 (61.1%) occurred within the first year of diagnosis of SLE, although several patients experienced the initial onset of psychiatric manifestations several years after the onset of SLE. Recurrent episodes occurred in 10 of 36 patients at a median of 8 months after the initial episode. Although tending to occur early in SLE, primary acute psychiatric events may first occur in patients with long durations of illness, and the time of onset of these episodes does not appear to be helpful in their differential diagnosis (39,40,45).

In 1993, Iverson (46) conducted an extensive methodologic review of the literature relating to the presence of psychiatric dysfunction in patients with lupus. He concluded there is no conclusive evidence that lupus causes nonpsychotic psychiatric dysfunction in their patients.

Clinicians and staff who work with mentally handicapped and communication-impaired patients should be especially sensitive to the possibility of cerebral involvement in patients with SLE. CNS complications in one mentally handicapped woman were not recognized early because of impaired communication (47). Although routine testing for SLE in psychiatric populations has consistently proved to be nonproductive (48), one must be alert to the possibility of SLE with the development of sudden, unexplained psychiatric symptoms wherever a large aggregate of younger women patients exists.

Hugo et al. (49) reported from Cape Town South Africa in 1996 that DSM-III criteria applied in the evaluation of 88 systemic lupus erythematosus patients revealed a point prevalence rate of 18.2% for psychiatric disorders, the most common diagnosis being adjustment disorder (11.4%). No patients had disorders compatible with a functional psychosis. Psychiatric morbidity was not associated with increased disease activity, corticosteroid use, brain MRI abnormalities, or EEG abnormalities. High scores on a life event scale were associated with psychiatric disorders, suggesting that psychological stress is etiologically important. Cognitive testing showed that poor performance on the Stroop Color-Word Inference Test was associated with psychiatric disorders.

In 1999, in a hospital-based study, Purandare et al. (49a) reported from India that they had investigated psychiatric morbidity in SLE patients. Thirty patients (23 consecutive outpatients and seven unselected inpatients) were prospectively assessed by a multidisciplinary team for the presence of psychiatric disorders and disease activity. Psychiatric assessment was done with structured interviews. Demographic information was recorded in a structured pro forma setting; all the patients completed the Presumptive Stressful Life Event Scale. A close relative was interviewed in every case. Patients who had psychiatric disorders were compared with the rest with respect to demographic variables, lupus disease activity, use of steroids, and stressful life events. The authors found a 50% prevalence of psychiatric disorders. The patients with psychiatric disorders were similar to those who had no psychopathology with respect to age, sex, duration of illness, lupus activity, and the use of steroids. However, they had experienced more stressful life events in the last year.

PREDISPOSING FACTORS AND THE ROLE OF STRESS

A combination of physical, environmental, biosocial, iatrogenic, and drug-related factors place patients with lupus at a greater risk for developing psychologic disorders. Hypertension and uremia were noted by Heine (50) to be implicated with more psychopathology. Various antihypertensive drugs, corticosteroids, digitalis, and antimalarial agents, among others, can alter mood and behavior patterns. The last two decades have witnessed an exponential rise in the use of various psychotropic agents (e.g., anxiolytics, benzodiazepines, tricyclic antidepressants, selective serotonin reuptake inhibitors, and monoamine oxidase inhibitors). These agents may impair cognition, alter impulse control, potentiate an unrecognized but preexisting deficit in cognition (51), amplify preexisting neurotic and personality problems, and reduce libido and sexual function.

McLary et al. (52) observed that in 13 of 14 patients studied, significant crises in interpersonal relationships preceded the onset of symptoms. Ropes (53) reported that disease flares in 41 of 45 patients were precipitated by psychogenic or environmental factors. Emotional disturbance, stress, and personality disorder also were investigated in the genesis of SLE in 20 women who were compared to matched controls who had suffered a severe accidental hemorrhage in late pregnancy (54). Emotional deprivation in childhood was reported more frequently by patients than by controls. Both mothers and fathers were perceived as being unsatisfactory by more patients than by controls. All patients (and 12 controls) reported that the onset of illness was preceded by stresses, particularly those relating to marriage and other interpersonal relationships. Pregnancy and childbirth, although not always perceived as stressful, were associated with exacerbations of SLE. Patients under 20 years of age reported a considerably lower incidence of emotional deprivation in childhood, and antecedent stress appeared to be less significant in these patients. It is evident that patients frequently try to attribute the onset of physical illness to some type of trauma (55). In 1994, Adams et al. (56) reported a study of 41 subjects from across the United States who were diagnosed with SLE. Regressions were conducted to evaluate the relation among stress, depression, anxiety, anger, and SLE symptom complaints. Negative weighting of major life events predicted symptom history. Significant hierarchical regressions using negative weighting of major life events, impact of daily stress, depressions, anxiety, and anger were found for severity of joint pain and abdominal distress. Subject analyses suggested that there was much individual variability in the strength of the stress illness relation. Thus, some individuals appeared to be stress responders, while others did not. Findings for the impact of minor life events and depression were consistent across the different levels of analyses. It was concluded that stress, depression, anxiety, and anger are associated with, and may exacerbate, self-reported symptomatology of patients with SLE.

Blumenfield (57) questioned 36 patients. Of these, 50% were certain that psychological factors triggered disease onset, and an additional 25% felt that it was possible. Once lupus is diagnosed, various factors increase the risk of neuropsychiatric impairment. In one study, only 3 of 140 patients had neuropsychiatric symptoms at diagnosis, but eventually, a 37% incidence was observed (10).

Ever since Solomon and Moos (58) first proposed in 1974 that mental stress flares autoimmune disease, a flurry of activity has indirectly confirmed much of their hypothesis, despite a few negative reports. Rogers et al. (59) summarized a series of studies suggesting that stress can exacerbate RA; decreased lymphocyte cytotoxicity, natural killer activity, and mitogenic responsiveness were seen in response to stress, along with diminished lymphocyte response to antigenic stimulation, skin homograft rejection, graft-versus-host response, and delayed hypersensitivity. It has been suggested that right cerebral laterality (i.e., left-handedness) is increased in patients with SLE (60,61), and Satz and Soper (62) analyzed the claims of an association among left-handedness, dyslexia, migraine, and autoimmune disease. They found that results and theories in various studies offered misleading implications about left-handedness and contained only minimal support for their conclusions. Geschwind's (63) pioneering studies, along with Schur's (64) findings, implicated cerebral lateralization, immune disease, hormonal influences (65), biologic mechanisms, and developmental learning disorders. Salcedo et al. (61) disputed any association of SLE with left-handedness (66–68).

Wallace (55), in his extensive review of the evidence of the role of stress and trauma in RA and SLE, concluded that stress can depress immune responsiveness, but that the pathologic mechanism(s) and consequences of this (e.g., increased susceptibility to infection, increased disease activity) are not clearly understood. It is uncertain how much or what type of stress is required to depress responsiveness, or even how different degrees of stress can be quantitated or reduced. Even though 8 million Americans have RA and SLE, we still have much to learn about the influences of stress and trauma on these disorders.

The weight of evidence from various studies strongly suggests a role for psychological stress in inducing, exacerbating, and affecting the ultimate outcome of SLE. Wallace (55) argued convincingly about the need for well-designed, controlled trials that are aimed specifically at deciding these issues. The role of physical trauma has never been investigated, and disease exacerbation that is induced by emotional stress has been strongly suggested but not yet verified in a scientifically acceptable fashion. The phrase *scientifically acceptable* means either definitive laboratory confirmation or studies meeting epidemiologic criteria. However, much, if not most, of medical science does not meet this standard. The large and consistent number of peer-reviewed articles showing an association between stress and exacerbations of SLE and other autoimmune diseases is more than sufficient for clinicians to rely on in their diagnosis and treatment. As an example, many years ago the relationship between cigarette smoking and lung cancer was recognized, notwithstanding that there were no clinical studies verifying by laboratory or epidemiologic means. Today, there is a great emphasis in all of medical education on the relationship and role that stress has on the course of medical conditions, especially autoimmune disorders.

The lack of laboratory or epidemiologic studies should *not* in any way negate or disprove what is in fact so commonly observed by clinicians, patients, and their families: the consistent finding of *unremitting* psychosocial stress as an exacerbating prelude to SLE "flares" in a significant number of cases.

Animal disease models are used to assess the immunotoxicologic potential of chemicals or drugs in autoimmune processes. They may provide good examples of the same immunologic processes that are involved in natural human autoimmune diseases such as lupus, diabetes, arthritis, thyroiditis, and encephalitis. Attempting to evaluate psychosocial stressors in animal models has no clear and definitive application to humans at this time. Farine (69) pointed out that, unfortunately, the diversity of their different possibilities of immunoregulation and outcome makes it very difficult to standardize a model for the purpose of the immunotoxicology study. Some drugs show controversial activities in different models. Indeed, in some models, the autoimmune disease occurs spontaneously; in others it has to be induced. The incidence and severity can change from one species to another and varies with sex and strain. Stress and infection can also exert a strong influence. As of now, it is impossible to suggest one ideal animal model to study autoimmune toxicity of chemicals or drugs.

Lupus experts such as Schur (70), Dubois, and Rothfield (71) have stated that emotional stress can aggravate disease activity, but only Ropes backed up this contention with any data by relating that 41 of 45 lupus flares observed in her 160 patient cohort were precipitated by emotional stress (53). Pamphlets distributed by the Arthritis Foundation, the American Lupus Society, and the Lupus Foundation of America reinforce this viewpoint with patients, who are cautioned to develop serious coping mechanisms and to take care of themselves so that their disease activity has less chance of flaring. Many patients who develop serious infections, experience major trauma, and have emotional crises do not experience a flare of the disease, however. Further, SLE may be exacerbated in the absence of provocative circumstances. While the exact frequency of disease aggravation following stressful incidents has not been established, there is a fairly common clinical impression among treating physicians, patients, and their families that unremitting psychosocial stress correlates significantly with the onset and exacerbation of symptoms and illness. It cannot be overemphasized that what constitutes a major psychological stressor for a given individual may not conform to the conventional and more dramatic notions of a stressor. The stressor must be understood as particularly noxious, threatening, and traumatic to that given individual, and often is only understood in context of that person's life experience and psychodynamics. Wallace and Metzger (72) examined the question "Can an earthquake cause flares of rheumatoid arthritis or lupus nephritis?" in a provocative and thoughtful article in 1994.

In 1966, Rogers and Fozdar (73), in noting the intricate and complex interactions between the immune system and psychological states, and the new discoveries and findings in psychoneuroimmunology, explore the effects of stress on the onset and course of autoimmune disorders. They elaborate on the autoimmune-mediated neuropsychiatric manifestations of SLE. They explore the role of various neurotransmitters and neuromodulators in the stress response.

A few important points regarding differential diagnosis are noteworthy. Many patients with SLE have a secondary fibromyalgia (61). Fibromyalgia can produce symptoms of joint pains and stiffness (74). Emotional stress (75,76) is a well-known provocateur of fibrositis symptoms (53,77). Similarly, reductions in corticosteroid dosages can cause withdrawal symptoms of joint pains, and they may produce a more labile emotional state. The clinician must be careful to distinguish SLE flares from active fibromyalgia or corticosteroid withdrawal. Much work has been done on the prevalence of fibromyalgia in systemic lupus patients (78–82).

The effects of psychosocial stress or physical trauma on the immune system have been the subject of extensive study (83–85). Correlations among laboratory data and physical and psychosocial aspects reveal enormous individual differences in patients with SLE, especially in the self-reported, subjective ratings of their physical symptoms and well-being (86). Except for the studies mentioned earlier, this has not been investigated in humans. Most patients with SLE have depressed immune responsiveness to begin with. That stress induces further depressed immune responsiveness in SLE, and that this results in more active disease remains a tenable but untested hypothesis.

Hinrichsen et al. (87) explored the influence of a 2-hour neuropsychological stress test on plasma catecholamines, cortisol, and the distribution of lymphocyte subpopulations in 14 patients with SLE, in 10 patients on prednisone treatment (without collagenosis), and in 14 sex- and age-matched healthy controls. Psychological stress induced comparably significant increases in plasma adrenaline and noradrenaline levels as compared with baseline values ($p < .05$) in all three groups, whereas plasma cortisol remained unchanged. The rise in plasma catecholamines was accompanied by a significant cell mobilization in healthy subjects and prednisone-treated patients, but not in patients with SLE. $CD19^+$ cells increased significantly in number from baseline in healthy subjects and prednisone-treated controls ($p < .05$), while remaining unchanged in patients with SLE. Patients with SLE showed reduced cell mobilization because of psychological stress, despite hormonal alterations paralleling those of healthy or prednisone-treated subjects without collagenosis.

In 1999 Pawlak et al. (88) demonstrated a distinct difference between the stress response of SLE patients and healthy controls. They analyzed heart rate, blood pressure, catecholamine concentration, lymphocyte subpopulations, natural killer (NK) cell activity, and expression of β_2-adrenoceptors on peripheral blood mononuclear cells (PBMCs) before, immediately after, and 1 hour after a public-speaking task in 15 SLE patients and 15 healthy subjects. Both groups demonstrated similar psychological, cardiovascular, and neuroendocrine responses to acute stress. However, NK ($CD16^+/CD56^+$) cell numbers transiently increased after stress exposure, with significantly less pronounced changes in SLE patients. In addition, NK activity increased in healthy controls ($n = 8$) but not in SLE patients ($n = 4$) after acute stress. Furthermore, the number of β_2-adrenoceptors on PBMCs significantly increased only in healthy subjects ($n = 8$) after stress but not in SLE patients ($n = 7$). These data indicate that SLE patients differ from healthy controls in stress-induced immune responses.

PSYCHOSIS

Psychosis is defined as a gross impairment in reality testing with disordered thinking and bizarre ideation, often including delusions and hallucinations, which usually results in an inability to carry out the ordinary demands of living. As noted in Table 36.1, the incidence of psychosis ranges from 0% to 55%. More common in hospitalized patients, its incidence probably has decreased over the last 30 years as more rapid diagnosis and effective treatment of SLE became possible. For example, in evolving the preliminary ARA criteria for SLE in 1971, 19 of 245 patients were psychotic, compared with only 13 of 176 patients who were used for the revised criteria in 1982 (19). Wallace noted psychosis in only 5 of 464 patients with SLE who were seen between 1980 and 1989 (172).

Literature Review

Comparisons of studies from different decades are clouded by changes in definitions and by criteria for the psychoses (i.e., thought and mood disorders), as reflected in the DSM-II, DSM-III, DSM-III-R, and DSM-IV of the American Psychiatric Association. Brody's (89) pioneer report included 42 patients, many of whom initially were seen in the last year of the presteroid era (1949) and were interviewed pretreatment. Of these, 52% were judged to be psychotic (most probably, these were organic psychoses). Clark and Bailey (90) reviewed the records of 100 patients with SLE at the Mayo Clinic from 1948 to 1955 and found severe psychiatric disturbances in 17.

O'Connor (91) studied 40 unselected patients with SLE who were admitted to Columbia Presbyterian Medical Center between 1950 and 1954. Of these, 21 patients had overt psychotic episodes during their hospitalizations; seven were schizophrenic in type. In general, these patients showed paranoid ideation, hallucinations, fear, mutism, and withdrawal from the environment. Also, three had psychotic depressions. The remaining 11 psychotic patients were given a diagnosis of acute brain syndrome. Five were intermittently comatose, usually in the terminal phase of the disease; the others showed the classic symptoms of an organic psychosis with disorientation, confabulation, and visual and auditory hallucinations. The length of the psychosis ranged from hours to 4 months. No correlation could be established between the individual psychiatric syndrome and the postmortem findings. Although 18 of the 21 psychotic patients were receiving cortisone at the time of development of this reaction, I believe that organic brain disease resulting from SLE and not steroids caused the psychosis in almost all of these patients.

Psychosis of all types occurred in 12 of 520 of Dubois and Tuffanelli's (8) patients from 1950 to 1963. Almost all resulted from cerebral vasculitis and responded to an initiation, or increase in the dose, of corticoids. A true steroid-induced psychosis was less frequent than the organic form. These hormones frequently produce euphoria or anxiety, insomnia, and restlessness, but rarely a true psychosis. Ropes (53) reported that only 11 of 40 patients with SLE who developed psychiatric problems were taking steroids at the time. The usual error made in therapy is to ascribe the psychosis or severe neurosis to medication and to withhold corticoid therapy. In McGehee Harvey et al.'s (92) 1954 study, 19 of all SLE patients with psychiatric problems were psychotic. Of these 19, only 13 were found to have SLE as the only demonstrable cause.

In 1960, Stern and Robbins (93) similarly reviewed 53 patients at Bellevue Hospital, who primarily were referred from the medical to the psychiatric service. Half of the patients were psychotic, 15 with manifestations of organic brain disease. Six had schizophrenia and unclassified psychosis, and two had psychotic depressions. In only three patients was it believed that steroids caused the psychosis. Mild to moderate depressions occurred in eight additional patients. Again, it was emphasized that the prime cause of the psychosis was organic brain disease, not steroid therapy.

Fessel and Solomon (94) reviewed the literature on the problem of psychoses and SLE. Of 227 patients, information was given about steroid therapy in 97, and in only 25 of these had there been coincident steroid treatment, again emphasizing the primary organic nature of the psychosis. Tumulty (95) and others (96,97) noted that CNS changes were seen frequently, even before the advent of steroids.

In the 1960s, Estes and Christian (9) observed organic mental symptoms in 21 of 150 patients, as evidenced by disorientation, hallucinations, or deterioration of mental function. Of these, 16 had functional psychoses, such as schizophrenia and affective reactions.

In 1967, Guze (98) reviewed the occurrence of psychiatric illness in 101 consecutive patients with SLE who were admitted to a university hospital and found 12 who had significant difficulties. The psychiatric diagnoses varied in different admissions of the same patients and were organic brain syndrome in nine, affective illnesses in ten, and schizophreniform disorders in five. In patients with the organic brain syndrome, marked fluctuations in both disorientation and degree of memory impairment were frequent. Guze suggested that mental disturbances were more common in black women (25% vs. 12% overall). I and others (99) have noted that organic psychiatric symptoms usually improve following steroid therapy.

Baker's (100) experience with 17 patients was similar to the findings just described. Heine (50) in Scandinavia noted a 24% incidence of psychoses, primarily on a toxic, organic basis. Those with hypertension and renal disease had a worse prognosis. In 1976, Feinglass et al. (10) observed psychosis to be an early feature of SLE, to be short-lived in duration, and to be associated with a good prognosis. Its principal manifestations were hallucinations, autism, and paranoia. Steroid psychosis rarely occurred (2 of 140 patients), and all other patients responded to increases in steroid doses.

Although acute psychiatric manifestations in SLE have been considered usually to occur early in the course of illness, Ward and Studenski (101) reported in 1991 on the time course of acute (i.e., psychotic) episodes. They reported first occurrence in patients with SLE and long duration of illness.

In 2000, Karassa et al. (101a) investigated risk factors for CNS involvement in SLE in 32 such patients individually matched 1:3 to 96 control SLE patients without CNS events. Univariate analysis showed that CNS involvement was significantly associated with the antiphospholipid syndrome (APS) as well as its features: arterial thrombosis, recurrent fetal loss, livedo reticularis, and immunoglobulin G (IgG) anticardiolipin (aCL) antibodies in high titers. Other potential associations included cutaneous vasculitic lesions, thrombocytopenia, positive ANA, anti-SSB/La, and low serum levels of C3 and C4 complement components, while articular manifestations and discoid rash were significantly less common in patients with neuropsychiatric (NP) disease. In multivariate modeling, CNS involvement was strongly associated with cutaneous vasculitic lesions [odds ratio (OR) 33, 95% confidence interval (CI) 1.5–720] and arterial thromboses (OR 13, 95% CI 0.82–220), and negatively related to the presence of articular manifestations (OR 0.015, 95% CI 0.00–0.17) and discoid rash (OR 0.004, 95% CI 0.00–0.35). Associations with APS-related arterial thromboses and vasculitis point to the importance and arterial vascular pathophysiology in the pathogenesis of NP disease in SLE. Patients with articular manifestations and discoid rash are at very low risk of NP events. Patients with an adverse SLE disease profile may require closer observation and may be the target group for studying preemptive interventions.

STEROIDS, MOOD, COGNITION, AND BEHAVIOR

Hall and Beresford (102) followed 56 patients with SLE, 44 of whom had psychiatric symptoms. Of these, 14 patients (25%) had a psychotic episode. Ten were associated with specific neurologic symptoms (including peripheral neuropathy in four and seizures in three), and three had a steroid psychosis. Of the 14 patients, ten improved with increases in their steroid doses, and by the time of publication, psychosis had resolved in all 14 patients. In his literature review, Rogers (103) estimated the incidence of steroid psychosis as 5% of all psychoses in SLE.

In 1990, Reckart and Eisendrath (104) reported on eight patients who had undergone more than 5 years of intermittent treatments with corticosteroids and then volunteered to be interviewed about their experiences. Seven patients stated that they were not warned by their physicians of the possible psychiatric side effects, and five patients did not inform their physicians when symptoms did occur. The patients complained of insomnia, depression, hypomania or euphoria, confusion, and memory problems. Based on these reports, the frequency of affective and cognitive side effects of exogenous corticosteroids may be much higher than has been previously reported.

Joffe et al. (105,106) assessed mood and cognition on consecutive days in 18 women with SLE who were on alternate-day corticosteroid therapy. No overall differences were observed between the on- and off-medication days, but ten patients showed marked worsening or improvement of either depression or anxiety on their off-medication day. After 2 weeks of prospective behavioral ratings, the observed mood changes in several women were confirmed.

Because several monoamines (especially dopamine) have been implicated in the regulation of mood, Joffe et al. also examined the relationship between alterations in mood and plasma homovanillic acid (HVA) levels in patients who were on alternate-day corticosteroid treatment. Although several patients had substantial alterations in mood, no significant differences in plasma HVA levels between the on- and off-medication days were found. Further, alterations in depression and anxiety levels were not related to plasma HVA levels.

In a 1979 study, Hall et al. (107) defined the symptoms of steroid psychosis in 14 patients who had no CNS lesions. This study suggested that patients receiving daily doses of greater than 40 mg of prednisone or its equivalent are at greater risk for developing a steroid psychosis. These reactions are twice as likely to occur during the first 5 days of treatment than subsequently. Premorbid personality, a history of a previous psychiatric disorder, or a history of a previous steroid psychosis does not clearly increase the patient's risk of developing a psychotic reaction during any given course of subsequent therapy.

The steroid psychosis that was observed by Hall et al. presented as a spectrum psychosis, with symptoms ranging from affective to schizophreniform to those of organic brain syndrome. No characteristic, stable presentation was observed in these 14 patients. The most prominent symptom constellation that was noted during the course of the illness consisted of emotional lability, anxiety, distractibility, pressured speech, sensory flooding insomnia, depression, perplexity, agitation, auditory and visual hallucinations, intermittent memory impairment, mutism, disturbances of body image, delusions, apathy, and hypomania. In 1984 Varney (108) documented reversible steroid dementia without steroid psychosis.

Several other critical literature reviews (109,110) as well as newer studies have provided longitudinal insights into the nature of steroid-induced mental changes. The incidence of steroid psychosis varies widely in the literature, ranging from 13% to 62%, with a weighted average of 27.6% for some steroid-induced mental changes, the vast majority of which are mild to moderate and do not herald the development of a full-blown psychosis or affective syndrome. The incidence of a severe psychiatric syndrome in the more than 2,500 patients reported in the literature so far has ranged from 1.6% to 50.0%, with a weighted average of 5.7%. The incidence of steroid psychoses in patients with lymphoma, multiple sclerosis, severe intractable asthma, ulcerative colitis, regional enteritis, idiopathic thrombocytopenic purpura, RA, and severe poison ivy or poison oak was estimated at between 3% and 6%. The patients who are most at risk for developing steroid psychosis are those with SLE (43) and pemphigus (21).

The type of psychiatric disturbance that is seen is difficult to classify because symptoms tend to change radically during the course of the illness. Overall, approximately 40% of patients present predominantly with a depressive disorder, 25% with mania, 5% with bipolar disorder (cyclical form), 15% with an agitated schizophreniform or paranoid psychosis, and 10% with an acute progressive delirium. Three fourths of all patients with steroid psychosis evidence affective symptoms at some time during the course of their illness. A frank psychotic state without mood disturbance occurs in 10% to 15% of patients, and some psychotic features (i.e., marked impairment of reality testing) that are associated with affective symptoms occur in 70% of patients.

The dose of steroid administered has a clear relationship to the likelihood of the patient developing a subsequent steroid psychosis. A statistically significant increase in the incidence of psychiatric disturbances with increasing daily doses of steroid has been found. Patients who were treated with a mean daily dose of prednisone below 40 mg/d in the Boston Collaborative Drug Surveillance Study (111) had an incidence of psychotic symptoms of 1.3%, whereas patients who were treated with doses between 41 and 80 mg/d had an incidence of 4.6%. Patients who received more than 80 mg/d of prednisone or its equivalent had an incidence of steroid psychosis of 18.4%. The average daily dose of steroids for patients who developed psychosis was 59.5 mg/d of prednisone or equivalent, compared with 31.1 mg/d for patients who did not develop adverse psychiatric effects.

Several studies have shown that no relationship exists between response to the first course of steroid treatment and response to a subsequent course. Litz (102) noted that even the most highly unstable patients do not experience any untoward emotional reaction after adrenocorticotropic hormone (ACTH) or cortisone therapy when compared with their more emotionally mature counterparts. Therefore, a patient's past psychiatric history is not a reliable predictor of developing a future steroid psychosis. The most frequent initial presentation of an impending steroid psychosis is a state of cerebral hyperexcitability, which is clearly perceived and reported by the patient (102). Patients characterize these states as being marked by increased irritability, lability of mood, profound dysphoria, hyperacusis, and pressured thought processes. These changes often precede other, more serious disturbances of cognition by 72 to 96 hours.

Once a steroid psychosis has been fully defined, it is likely to present as a spectrum psychosis, with the most prominent symptoms consisting of profound distractibility, pressured speech, anxiety, emotional lability, severe insomnia, sensory flooding, depression, perplexity, auditory and visual hallucinations, agitation, intermittent memory impairment, mutism, delusions, disturbances of body image, apathy, and hypomania. Before the advent of treatment with phenothiazines, it was noted that these conditions spontaneously remitted between 2 weeks and 7 months after the discontinuance of steroids, with 80% of cases reported in the literature having remitted untreated by the 6th week. Administration of phenothiazines dramatically reduces this period. The current duration of psychiatric symptoms in patients who develop a steroid psychosis and are treated with phenothiazines ranges in the literature from 1 to 150 days, with a mean duration until total recovery of 22 days.

According to Hall and Beresford (102), 92% of patients who have steroids tapered fully recover, and 84% of patients who are maintained on steroids but treated with antipsychotic medicines show full recovery from symptoms. In the 11 cases reported in the literature, electroconvulsive therapy has been universally effective in reversing the course of steroid psychosis.

Several studies also have shown that patients, even those with affective disorder produced by steroids, tend to do poorly when treated concurrently with tricyclic antidepressants and steroids. These patients may show an exacerbation of symptoms, even after the tapering of steroids, when tricyclics are used. Therefore, it is recommended that tricyclic and other antidepressant medications be withheld until after the patient's steroid psychosis has been appropriately treated with neuroleptics.

In that difficult clinical situation of the patient with SLE who is on corticosteroids and presents with neuropsychiatric symptom that could be caused by NPSLE versus steroid psychosis, West (112) suggests doubling the dose of corticosteroids for 3 days while awaiting test results (14). If the psychotic episode is caused by NPSLE, it usually will respond to this therapy. Failure to improve lessens the likelihood of lupus cerebritis, and the corticosteroids should be tapered to half of the original dose.

Various treatment approaches are available for steroid psychosis. The most widely used and effective strategy is to discontinue steroids, where possible, and to treat the patient with phenothiazines or other antipsychotic medications. Tricyclic antidepressants usually are avoided. The most frequently used drug regimens include thioridazine hydrochloride, 50 to 200 mg daily (113); oral chlorpromazine hydrochloride, 50 to 200 mg daily; oral haloperidol, 2 to 10 mg daily (103); or oranzapine, 10 to 20 mg daily × 10 to 14 days.

Falk et al. (102) have shown that prophylactic treatment with lithium carbonate may be useful to prevent the development of ACTH-induced psychosis. Excitement, hyperstimulation, and overstimulation should be kept to a minimum and anxiety reduced, if possible. If tolerated, anxiolytic agents may be helpful. Serum lithium levels may be elevated by concurrent use of cox-2 blocking agents.

If a steroid psychosis exists, Rogers (103) has advised judicious but rapid tapering of corticosteroids to adrenal replacement levels (i.e., 7.5 mg of prednisone equivalent daily). Unfortunately, some patients have multisystem disease that requires corticosteroids, and a compromise must be reached and alternative therapies considered. If it was difficult to determine whether the psychosis was steroid-induced, Dubois acutely stopped steroids in hospitalized patients; if the psychosis was steroid-induced, dramatic clearing usually occurred in 48 to 72 hours.

Reckart and Eisendrath (104) reported eight patients who had undergone greater than 5 years of intermittent treatments with corticosteroids and who volunteered to be interviewed about their experiences. Seven patients stated that their physicians did not warn them about or prepare them for the adverse reactions that occurred. The patients complained of insomnia, depression, hypomania or euphoria, confusion, and memory problems. Based on these reports, the frequency of affective and cognitive side effects of exogenous corticosteroids may be much higher than has been previously reported.

Manic-depressive psychosis is rare in patients with SLE but sometimes may be mimicked by corticosteroid administration. Catatonia also has been reported. Psychotic depression in SLE may be helped by shock therapy when all other modalities fail (39,53,114–116).

Wysenbeek et al. (117) described two patients with SLE who developed an acute psychosis and a cerebrovascular accident after pulse methylprednisolone therapy. A literature review revealed eight additional patients with SLE and acute CNS complications after pulse therapy.

Two reports from Japan are of special note. First, Matsukawa et al. (118), in a retrospective study of seven patients with SLE who attempted suicide, reported that five patients made their attempts during the tapering course of steroids. Five patients manifested psychosis, whereas two patients displayed no psychotic findings. Increasing the steroids improved their conditions. Further, signs of an imminent suicide attempt were missed in some cases. Second, Terao et al. (119) reported the effectiveness of lithium as an antidepressant in a patient with NPSLE who was receiving high-dose corticosteroids for cerebral infarction.

Kohen et al. (120) reported on the usefulness of serum and CSF determination of antibodies to P-ribosomal protein in distinguishing steroid-induced psychosis in SLE from lupus cerebritis. Worldwide investigations have reported on the significance of antibodies to ribosome P in the serum and CSF in NPSLE (27). In 1992, Shiozawa et al. (121) reported increased levels of interferon (IFN) in the CSF and sera of five of six patients with lupus psychosis, and in four of these five patients levels in the CSF were higher than those in the serum. IFN levels lowered when the manifestations of lupus psychosis subsided.

ORGANIC BRAIN SYNDROMES

Several nonpsychotic organic brain syndrome manifestations may occur in patients with SLE. Most obvious organic brain syndromes present as a toxic, psychotic type (as noted in the preceding section). In the absence of signs of organic brain impairment, psychosis is uncommon in patients with SLE.

Impairment In Cognition (Organic Amnestic Syndrome)

More common than previously recognized is organic mental syndrome, whose essential requirement is impairment of cognitive function. This can be expressed as defective short-term memory, diminished attention, and diminution or impairment of the following: concentration, capability for abstraction, problem solving, and visual-spatial functioning. Subtle changes in memory, concentration, and other cognitive functions often do not come to clinical attention unless formal mental status testing is done. Thus, it is difficult to estimate the incidence of nonpsychotic organic mental involvement.

The studies of Carbotte et al. (38) identified the unexpectedly high incidence of cognitive impairment in patients with SLE and either inactive or absent neuropsychiatric symptomatology. In their study, 86 women with SLE were grouped according to present or past history of neuropsychiatric symptomatology (i.e., active, inactive, or never). The performance of these three groups was compared to that of 35 normal women on an extensive battery of neuropsychological tests that sampled a wide range of cognitive functions. In addition to making group comparisons, the authors also devised a system for identifying individual impairment using decision rules for both quantitative and qualitative data. Results indicated that various cognitive deficits are present in patients with SLE when taken together as a group; that no significant association between cognitive impairment and emotional disturbance is present; that patients with resolved neuropsychiatric symptomatology are as impaired as patients with active neuropsychiatric symptoms, suggesting residual CNS involvement, despite no significant difference emerging on direct group comparisons; and that significantly more never-NPSLE patients are impaired than are controls on several summary scores, suggesting subclinical CNS involvement.

In 1990 Wolkowitz (122) elaborated the effects of corticosteroids on cognition, followed in 1994 by Newcome's (123) studies on glucocorticoid-induced impairment.

The major difficulty in determining the significance of antineuronal antibodies in NPSLE had been the lack of consistent clinical diagnostic approaches. In 1987, by using a new clinical classification of NPSLE, neuropsychologic assessments, and an assay for IgG antineuronal antibodies, the same authors (124) found a significant association between antibody positivity and cognitive impairment or nonfocal NPSLE. These observations indicate that antineuronal antibodies may play a role in NPSLE and emphasize the clinical importance of cognitive function in patients with SLE. There is no specific or characteristic cognitive deficit that is found in patients with SLE; rather, there is a wide spectrum, variety, and combinations of deficits. These deficits do not appear to be related to emotional stress or use of medications such as corticosteroids. Patients with

SLE and clinically acute CNS disease, serum anti-DNA and/or lymphocytes toxic antibodies, and CSF IgG antineuronal antibodies are more likely to have this impairment, suggesting that it is autoantibody mediated (124–126).

In 1990, the Denburg group (126) reevaluated the hypothesis that lymphocytotoxic antibodies are associated with neuropsychiatric involvement in SLE. In an unselected cohort of 98 women with SLE, a cross-sectional study was performed to analyze associations among standardized clinical, neurologic, and neuropsychological assessments and lymphocytotoxic antibodies as measured by microcytotoxic assay. Of these, 50 patients showed objective clinical evidence of continuing or past NPSLE, and 54 patients had cognitive impairment. In accordance with previous observations, 44% (24 of 54 patients) in the cognitively impaired group did not have clinically detectable evidence of NP-SLE. Although lymphocytotoxic antibodies were found to be only marginally more prevalent in those patients with a clinical diagnosis of NPSLE than in those without (32% vs. 23%, respectively), these antibodies were significantly associated with cognitive impairment ($X^2 = 5.42$; $p < .02$). No association was detected between lymphocytotoxic antibodies and overall systemic disease activity or other organ-system involvement, suggesting that the association between lymphocytotoxic antibodies and cognitive dysfunction in SLE is specific.

In another report by the same authors (127), 98 consecutive female patients with SLE underwent extensive standardized neuropsychological testing to evaluate CNS functioning in relation to serum lymphocyte antibodies, which are measured at the time of neuropsychological testing by a microcytotoxicity test. A significant association was observed between the presence of serum lymphocytotoxic antibodies (LCAs) and cognitive impairment in patients with SLE. The pattern of impairment that predominated in the LCA-positive patients involved deficits in anteriorly associated, primarily visual-spatial functions. These findings support the hypothesis of localization of a particular antigen-antibody interaction in the brain in SLE, thus suggesting the existence of immunologic control mechanisms for normal brain functioning.

Antineuronal antibodies have received worldwide attention, especially in regard to the pathogenesis of NPSLE (30% of reports regarding NPSLE in world medical literature over the last 6 years) (26,125,128–132). Serum antineuronal antibodies may be a useful marker for NPSLE, but they can only be considered pathogenic if they are demonstrated in the CSF and have the ability to bind directly to brain tissue. Investigators have found CSF IgG antineuronal antibodies in up to 90% of patients with NPSLE, compared with less than 10% of patients with SLE but without CNS manifestations. A variety of targets for these antineuronal antibodies have been reported (133–135). Recent studies have identified antineuronal antibodies against a 50-kd antigen in the plasma membrane of brain synaptic terminals (136), neurofilaments (137), and the ribosomal protein that has homology with a 38-kd protein on the surface of human neuroblastoma cells (138).

The antiphospholipid antibody has received much attention (130,139–148), as have the anticardiolipin antibodies (149–152). Russian workers (153) reported in 1992 the discovery of anticardiolipin antibody in 12 of 18 patients with SLE who were suffering from migraine-like headaches and in four of five patients with mental disorders. Eighty percent of the reactive antibodies were of the IgM isotype, whereas an IgG was only identified in 13 of the patients. Older reports focused on antiganglioside antibodies (136, 154–156), anti-SM (157) (with an interesting connection to schizophrenia), antimyosin antibodies (158), and antiribosomal-P antibody (159–162). Antiribosomal-P antibodies have been demonstrated most often in patients with NPSLE and psychosis and depression (162–164), whereas antineurofilament autoantibodies have been associated more closely with diffuse NPSLE clinical pictures (137). A still unanswered question is how do these antineuronal antibodies get past the blood–brain barrier and contact cortical tissue. Less frequently reported, but also of importance, are reports of NPSLE that is associated with the presence in CSF of interleukin-6 (IL-6) (165), prostaglandin E_2 (165,166), and studies correlating antineuronal antibodies in patients with NPSLE to EEG findings (167), to MRI findings (168), to serum levels with quantitative EEGs (167), and to evoked potentials (169,170).

One group of patients with lupus has organic brain syndrome because of scarring from previously active CNS disease or from multiple infarctions resulting from the lupus anticoagulant. Wallace (171) reported several situations in which these patients were treated with steroids for CNS lupus, when in fact no active disease was present that could be treated. Giving steroids often worsens the clinical picture, because it produces cortical atrophy (172).

The assessment of cognitive function in patients with SLE has been studied worldwide following the Denburgs' pioneering studies and reports (173,174). Fisk et al. (174) examined neuropsychological test performance in a representative sample of 70 female patients with SLE. The influence of current or past clinically overt CNS involvement, use of corticosteroid medications, and overall disease activity were evaluated. The results suggest two distinct patterns of cognitive dysfunction. Impaired or delayed recognition memory was associated with past or current nervous system involvement, suggesting the presence of a residual neurologic deficit. Increased disease activity was associated with impaired immediate memory and concentration, which may represent transient and diffuse CNS effects. Although corticosteroid use was associated with poor work-list recall, group differences were not statistically significant when disease activity was considered as a covariate in the analysis. Schur's group (175) compared cognitive dysfunction in randomly selected patients with SLE (n = 49) and with RA (n = 40). Extensive neuropsychological testing included associated learning, switching attention, continuous performance, associated recall, hand-eye coordination, pattern comparison, pattern memory, the Stroop Color-Word Inference Test, and the Symptom Checklist-90R. Patients with SLE had significantly poorer performance than patients with RA. Patients with SLE also reported more symptoms of cognitive difficulty, which appears to correlate with objective performance.

In 1996, Kozora and Thompson (176) reported on findings on cognitive and psychological functioning in relation to antiribosomal P protein autoantibodies in patients with SLE who had no previous history of CNS disease (non-CNS SLE). Comprehensive neuropsychological tests were administered to 51 non-CNS SLE patients; 31% of the RA patients and 11% of the control subjects were classified as cognitively impaired. Similar reductions in intelligence, attention, and fluency were detected in the non-CNS SLE and RA patients compared with controls. The non-CNS SLE patients showed a distinct deficit in learning compared with the RA and control groups. Forty-two percent of the non-CNS SLE patients demonstrated psychological distress, compared with 7% of the RA patients and 6% of the controls. In the patient groups, neither cognitive dysfunction nor psychological distress was associated with disease activity or prednisone dosage. Elevated serum levels of autoantibodies to ribosomal P protein were not associated with either psychological or cognitive abnormalities. These results suggest that certain cognitive deficits in non-CNS SLE patients may not be specific to the immunopathology of SLE. In contrast, it is possible that deficits in learning, as well as psychological distress without major psychiatric pathology, may be subtle manifestations of CNS lupus.

In October 2000, at the XIX Brazilian Congress in Neurology, Dr. Roger Walz said in an interview with Reuters Health that neuropsychiatric manifestations of SLE may be confirmed by elevated serum levels of S100B, a protein released in response to brain injury. At the Federal University of Rio Grande do Sul, S100B was measured in controls, patients with inactive lupus, patients with active lupus, and patients known to have neuropsychiatric manifestations of lupus.

The investigators found that the level of serum S100B in patients with neuropsychiatric manifestations was much higher than in controls and in patients with active or inactive lupus. Patients with active lupus and no neuropsychiatric manifestations had higher levels than controls; however, the difference was not as marked. One patient with lupus transverse myelitis had levels of serum S100B that were 40 times greater than the levels in controls.

"S100B is a protein that binds to calcium and is produced by astrocyte cells in the brain, where it is almost exclusively found. It is released in response to brain damage and it has already been used in detecting posttraumatic brain injury and neonatal defects such as intraventricular hemorrhage," Dr. Walz said in the interview. He added that S100B has potential use as a marker in spinal cord injuries as well.

"These results may lead to S100B being used as a sensitive marker of brain injury, and even spinal cord injury, in patients with lupus," Dr. Walz added.

Application Of Neuropsychological Testing

The aforementioned studies were done as a result of the application of special neuropsychological tests that use selected parameters to evaluate the behavioral expression of organic brain injury. Before the studies of the Denburgs and others, neuropsychological tests were not used widely or routinely with patients who had SLE.

Neuropsychological testing has the unique capability of assessing functional deficits irrespective of their origin, whether functional (i.e., no demonstrable lesion) or organic. According to Koffler (177), the major behavioral functions that are studied are cognitive and intellectual abilities, sensory and perceptual functions, motor and psychomotor abilities, language skills, spatial skills, and academic skills. Each sensory modality (i.e., auditory, tactile, visual) and each response mode (i.e., oral, written, motor) are tested, where applicable, in the examination of these functions.

The results of neuropsychological tests are used to assess the presence of neural injury and to determine the site, type, and duration of CNS dysfunction. They are derived from studying four major parameters: (a) the expected level of performance, (b) specific pathognomonic signs, (c) comparison of right and left brain function, and (d) pattern analysis. Psychological and emotional status was assessed in 36 SLE patients with the General Health Questionnaire-30 (GHQ-30) and the Minnesota Multiphasic Personality Inventory (MMPI) (178). The two tests were found to measure different aspects of psychological functioning. More than 50% of the patients could be classified as cases with mild psychiatric disturbances, according to the GHQ, and 28% had an abnormal score >70 on the MMPI depression subscale, indicating significant depression. Emotional disturbances such as problems with social functioning, personal discomfort in social situations, and depressive mood were frequent and associated with skin and joint abnormalities. This suggests additional etiologies for psychological dysfunction among SLE patients other than the direct CNS effect of SLE.

The two most widely used neuropsychological test batteries are the Halstead-Reitan and Luria-Nebraska (179, 180). Both are reported to detect the presence of organic brain damage with 80% to 90% accuracy (181). Their ability to assess CNS dysfunction in patients with ambiguous physical or psychological signs and to quantitate functional deficits has resulted in their increased use in clinical medicine.

Results of the Luria-Nebraska test have been closely correlated with those of the Halsted-Reitan test when used for the detection of brain injury (182). The Luria-Nebraska requires a relatively short period of testing time and only minor equipment, and it may be administered to both hospitalized patients and outpatients. The Boston Processing Approach, developed by Kaplan et al. (183), also may become an instrument of choice.

In 1990, Papero et al. (184) reported having studied 21 pediatric patients who met SLE criteria (12 moderate, nine mild disease activity) and who had no history of CNS damage unrelated to lupus. Comparison of these patients with SLE to a contrast group of 11 patients with juvenile RA (JRA) revealed decreased complex problem-solving ability for the SLE group. Individual, IQ-adjusted neuropsychological profile analysis yielded a significant difference in the number of specific neuropsychological deficits for the two groups, with impairment rates of 43% for patients with SLE and 18% for patients with JRA. A longer duration of lupus was associated with a lower cognitive status. Neuron-reactive antibody studies for IgG and IgM were negative. Results suggest that the incidence of higher cortical impairment may be as great for younger individuals with lupus as has been documented for older individuals (184).

Neuropsychological testing of patients with SLE has shown consistent abnormalities in the four clinical scales (i.e., visual, arithmetic, writing, intelligence). This pattern is different than that found in patients with diffuse cerebral dysfunction (e.g., Alzheimer's disease), which typically includes elevations on multiple scales, particularly those measuring memory and language. Diffuse disturbance secondary to metabolic disorders often is reflected in scales that are sensitive to attentional deficits, such as memory and acoustic discrimination. The pattern for patients with focal lesions varies depending on the site of the lesion. The functional deficits that are suggested by the pattern of elevated scales for patients with CNS lupus patients is analogous to the pattern of abnormal scales found in patients with lesions occurring in the parietal-occipital regions or their associated tracts.

Koffler (177) and Rogers (103) advocate the assessment of neuropsychological functioning in patients with SLE. Further impetus for the documentation of cognitive changes was provided by a single case study of serial neuropsychological testing with a patient who had SLE (185). This patient also was evaluated using regional cerebral blood flow (CBF) CT; each test demonstrated diffuse cortical dysfunction that was associated with the exacerbation of CNS symptoms.

Wekking et al. (186) argued that it has not been proven convincingly that the occurrence of cognitive impairment is uniquely related to patients with SLE as compared to patients with RA. In their opinion, the interpretation of cognitive disturbances in relation to the total clinical picture is not clear, especially in patients with SLE but without overt CNS disease. Moreover, Wekking et al. stated that the effects of cognitive dysfunction on treatment or prognosis in these patients have not been reported.

SLE effects three times as many nonwhite American women as American white women (186a). In addition to increased incidence and prevalence rates, nonwhite females with SLE experience excess mortality rates compared to other groups, reaching peak mortality at 45 to 54 years of age compared to 65 to 74 years of age in other groups.

In 1998 Breitbach et al. (186b) addressed the issue of race as a determinant in lower or reduced score on cognitive functioning tests. SLE patients may have a variety of neuropsychiatric syndromes. Assessment of cognitive functioning for these patients is complicated by increased prevalence and disease severity among groups obtaining lower scores on measures of cognitive functioning when the presence of SLE was added to the equation derived from demographic variables. No significant interaction was found between race and disease. These results suggest that increased frequency impairment in African Americans with SLE is due to the additive effects of psychosocial variables.

Poor performance on cognitive testing is common in SLE, but it is not progressive in most patients and may fluctuate or resolve without specific treatment (187). Cognitive impairment in patients without overt CNS SLE may result from generalized disease activity or psychiatric disorders that reduce speed, concentration, and motivation. This emphasizes once again the importance of recognizing and treating psychiatric disorder in these patients. Although mean cognitive scores are lower in patients with SLE and overt CNS involvement than in those without CNS involvement, an individual's cognitive score is a poor predictor for the presence of CNS involvement because of considerable overlap between groups. In 1994, Hay (187) suggested that the pattern of cognitive impairment, rather than simply its presence or absence, may be more helpful in identifying patients with CNS involvement. Cognitive impairment at one point in time is not predictive of future CNS events during 1 or 2 years of follow-up. Therefore, routine cognitive testing in SLE does not appear to be helpful either for identifying patients with current CNS involvement or for identifying those at future risk of this complication. In the absence of double-blind, randomized, controlled trials, treatment of neuropsychiatric SLE is based on clinical experience and anecdotal case reports. Aggressive immunosuppression with high-dose corticosteroids in conjunction with either azathioprine or cyclophosphamide may be indicated in patients with life-threatening CNS SLE, but based on current evidence it is not justified in those with subtle cognitive abnormalities.

In 1977, in another seminal article, Denburg et al. (187a) proposed a role for cognitive assessment in the identification of SLE-related depression. Psychological variables such as personality and coping have received only limited attention in SLE to date, in contrast to the large body of studies in RA. The studies examine issues related to cognitive function, including its assessment and prevalence, and confounding factors in interpreting cognitive problems as reflecting primary CNS involvement in SLE. Cognitive data in relation to other facets of the disease such as pain and fatigue, and subjective complaints are also discussed.

Organic affective syndromes and organic personality syndromes often are difficult to differentiate from functional disorders and could reflect low-grade CNS lupus activity, hypertension, uremia, or lower-dose corticosteroid effects. Their true incidence is difficult to estimate but probably is high. Treatment involves managing lupus activity and providing the support mechanisms discussed elsewhere in this chapter.

FUNCTIONAL DISORDERS

Ever since 1956, when Clark and Bailey (90) identified depression and anxiety as being the most common personality changes in patients with SLE, studies have been performed to characterize and classify these disorders in a way that could optimize management. The incidence of functional disorders in SLE is shown in Table 36.1. It ranges from 2% to 51% and probably is an underestimate. Only a few of the studies included detailed interviewing and diligent searches for subtle functional problems.

Depression is particularly common in patients with SLE (188). Most depression is reactive, although endogenous and psychotic depression also occur. Often, it is uncertain whether depression is to be expected because of the stresses, strains, continuous adjustments, and frequent sacrifices that are imposed by the illness. The person with lupus often is aware that states of depression may be induced by the lupus or various factors and forces in the patient's life that are unrelated to lupus.

Depression can be understood as a natural, although unpleasant, experience that can vary in intensity, duration, and the degree that it is tolerated by the individual, but, most important, also in the degree to which it interferes with the patient's ability to function and maintain a reasonable sense of well-being. Therapeutic assistance and intervention are indicated when the degree and duration of depression are disruptive to the individual's well-being and interfere with his or her overall functioning and adjustment (189).

The medical condition that we refer to as depression is not to be confused with the transitory, everyday, mild mood swing that everyone experiences during a difficult time. Although depressive illness is more common in people with chronic medical illness than in the general population, not everyone with a chronic medical illness (e.g., lupus) suffers from clinical depression (61). Clinical depression is characterized by physical and psychological symptoms: sadness and gloom, spells of crying (often without provocation), insomnia or restless sleep (or sleeping too much), loss of appetite (or eating too much), uneasiness or anxiety, irritability, feelings of guilt and remorse, lowered self-esteem, inability to concentrate, diminished memory and recall, indecisiveness, loss of interest in things that one formerly enjoyed, fatigue, and various physical symptoms, such as headache, palpitation, diminished sexual interest and/or performance, other body aches and pains, indigestion, and constipation or diarrhea.

Two of the most common psychological signs of clinical depression are hopelessness and helplessness. People who feel hopeless believe that their distressing symptoms may never get better, whereas people who feel helpless think they are beyond help, that no one cares enough to help them, or that no one could succeed in helping even if they tried.

Not all depressed people have all of these symptoms. Someone is considered to be clinically depressed, however, if he or she experiences a depressed mood, disturbance in sleep and appetite, and at least one or two related symptoms that persist for several weeks and are severe enough to disrupt normal daily life. Many people who come for treatment have been depressed for a good deal longer than this. Some people stay depressed for years, and life seems flat and meaningless to them. Thoughts of death and deformity often are present and, occasionally, turn into self-destructive urges.

Although many symptoms are associated with depression, seven indicate the depth and degree of depression: (a) a sense of failure, (b) loss of social interest, (c) a sense of punishment, (d) suicidal thoughts, (e) dissatisfaction, (f) indecision, and (g) crying.

Depressive illness in the medically ill often goes unrecognized, because it presents symptoms that are similar to those of the underlying medical condition. In lupus (SLE), depressive symptoms such as lethargy, loss of energy and interest, insomnia, pain intensification, and diminished libido can be attributed to the lupus condition. Unfortunately, many people with lupus refuse to acknowledge themselves to be in a depressed state. In fact, most depressive illness goes unrecognized and untreated until the later stages, when its severity becomes unbearable to the patient and/or until the family or physician can no longer ignore it. In fact, several studies have indicated that between 30% and 50% of major depressive illness goes undiagnosed in medical settings. Perhaps more disturbing is that many studies indicate that major depressive disorders in the medically ill are undertreated and/or inadequately treated even when recognized.

Physicians who are familiar with their patients' usual mood and personality, as well as with their lifestyle and situation, are more likely to recognize changes that are associated with depressive illness. Similarly, patients are more apt to open up about their feelings when they are encouraged to do so by a physician they are familiar with and trust. This is especially important for that group of depressed individuals without subjective complaints of unhappy mood, who often deny or resist the notion of emotional distress and who substitute various physical complaints. Physicians suspect masked depression in such patients, especially when they appear with a saddened facial expression, have lost interest in and are withdrawn from their usual activities, and are preoccupied with painful somatic complaints.

Failure to recognize and diagnose depression in the medically ill reinforces patients' beliefs that they have reason to feel depressed because they are sick and discourages their seeking appropriate help. This error ignores the fact that clinical depression in the physically ill generally responds well to standard psychiatric treatment, and that patients who are treated only for their physical illness suffer from the effects of depression needlessly. Depression should not be used as a symptom for sadness.

Effective treatment is available for depressive illness and usually consists of psychotropic medication or psychotherapy and most often a combination of both. Antidepressant medication is the major class of drugs used; the four categories are tricyclics, newer generation nontricyclic antidepressants [selective serotonin reuptake inhibitors (SSRIs)], monoamine oxidase inhibitors, and lithium. The effectiveness of these medications may be increased by using them in combination or by adding other medications. Not infrequently, depressed patients are undertreated and/or inadequately treated, reflecting therapeutic uncertainty and pessimism.

Adequate and aggressive treatment is vigilant and involves the cooperation of the patient. Such treatment may involve blood tests to determine the appropriate dosages of medication, open communication, trial and error, and a large ration of optimistic support in the form of encouragement, patience, availability, and perseverance. Any underlying organic factors that contribute to the depressive state must be identified and addressed. Antidepressant medications have various side effects and may intensify certain symptoms that are associated with lupus (e.g., increase in the drying of mucous membranes in Sjögren's syndrome) (190). When antidepressant medications are effective, a welcome improvement is noted in the patient's sense of well-being and in his or her overall attitude and adjustment.

Recovery from depression usually is a gradual process. Dramatic improvements cannot be expected in a few days; however, one begins to see some progress after a few weeks. Even when depression seems to clear quickly, relapse is not unusual when the medication is stopped. Therefore, medication should be continued for approximately 6 months or longer, and the dosage should be tapered slowly over a 3- to 4-week period when treatment is discontinued. Patients who are resistant to those treatments mentioned earlier have several other effective options.

Often, depressive illness involves a general slowing and clouding of mental functions (i.e., cognition), and many people with lupus worry about changes in their alertness, attention span, capability for concentration, orientation, memory and recall, reasoning abilities, use of language, and ability to do calculations. These troublesome and not infrequent disruptions in mental functioning tend to go underreported and rarely are confirmed as resulting from any specific structural change. Transient alterations in mental functioning improve as the depressive condition improves. In 1994, the Denburgs and Carbotte (191) reported improvement in cognition and mood following brief exposure to relatively low doses of corticosteroids in women with mild SLE; these improvements persist over repeated drug exposure.

Psychotherapy can be helpful in assisting depressed people to work through and understand their feelings, illness, and relationships, and to cope more effectively with stress and their life situation. The patient is best served when the primary-care physician maintains a close relationship with a psychiatrist or psychologist for consultation about and referral of depressed patients who present difficult diagnostic and treatment problems. Such a working relationship maximizes the quality of patient care and provides the most powerful approach to the management of depression.

In addition to the physical and organic aspects of the disease, this chronic illness so alters the life of these women that the incidence of divorce is well over 50%. Estes and Christian (9) found that eight patients had anxiety or depressive neurosis. These conditions were severe enough in two to require electroshock therapy. Psychiatric disturbances also were observed in the absence of other neurologic manifestations in 27 patients. Fries and Holman (67) noted depression in half of their 193 patients at any time in their disease course, but it was labeled as severe in only ten.

Hall (109) evaluated 56 patients. Of 25 with psychiatric symptoms, 19 had no set of single long-term symptoms, but 23 complained of insomnia, 21 of depressed mood, 18 of emotional lability, 18 of nervousness, 17 of confusion, and 16 of a decrease in concentration. Patients who were socially active and not isolated did better. Later in this chapter (see Special Concerns, Challenges, and Adjustments), it is noted that depression is treated with tricyclic or related antidepressants and that anxiety is treated with anxiolytics such as diazepam. Temesvari et al. (192) noted depression in 16 of 34 outpatients with SLE; three had made suicide attempts.

Liang et al. (193) administered the Minnesota Multiphasic Personality Inventory (MMPI) to 76 patients with SLE and to 23 patients and outpatients with RA. Despite these numbers, however, the study was admittedly biased: only 15% to 20% of those who were followed with these disorders were represented, and they consisted of volunteers who generally had multiple complaints. A statistically significant increase in hypochondriasis, hysteria, and depression scales was noted in those with SLE and RA. Those with SLE had a marked increase in fear of death compared with the RA group. A sense of fatigue and complaints of loss of independence were common. Nevertheless, 50% stated that at times they thought their disease had been a positive experience.

Kremer et al. (194) evaluated 37 patients and outpatients with SLE at the Albany Medical Center. Of these, 46% had current psychopathology; 41% were diagnosed as having nonorganic, nonpsychotic psychopathology; and only two patients were believed to be psychotic. Anxiety, tension, depression, and somatic concerns dominated. Abnormal MMPI test results were seen in 61%. Hysteria, depression, and hypochondriasis indices were abnormally high, but only to a small extent. No correlation was found among psychopathology, neurologic evaluations, and clinical activity.

According to Engle et al. (195), the Rheumatology Attitudes Index (RAI) is of proven reliability and usefulness in patients with SLE. In 1990, these authors reported that all three components of the learned-helplessness construct (i.e., motivational, cognitive, and emotional deficits) are likely to influence psychosocial adjustments in patients with SLE. This correlation was found across all domains except health care orientation and sexual adjustment. Thus, assessment of patients' efforts to engage in activities of daily living and to develop new coping behaviors is associated with, and may be predictive of, their overall psychosocial adjustment. Engle et al.'s data correlated perceived helplessness and longer duration of disease (196).

FACTITOUS ILLNESS AND POSITIVE ANA WITHOUT LUPUS

Levy et al. (197) presented two cases of young women with factitious illness who claimed to have SLE. Secondary gain and/or the search for an all-encompassing disease entity have led many patients with borderline-positive ANA and nonspecific complaints to seek rheumatologic consultation and to become disappointed when told that they do not have lupus. The overwhelming majority of these patients have fibromyalgia, a somatization disorder that is poorly understood—especially by nonrheumatologists. It represents 15% of lupus referrals. The picture is further complicated by the high incidence of secondary fibromyalgia in patients with established SLE who have difficulty coping with the stress of their disease.

Von Brauchitsch (198) observed that patients in psychiatric facilities have an increased incidence of positive ANA and proposed that SLE is more common in this group. Other studies noted the same finding; the issue was resolved when Dubois' group (199) found that this phenomenon is secondary to psychotropic therapy, especially with phenothiazine administration for abnormal behavior states. Conversely, the diagnosis of SLE may be missed, resulting in phenothiazine administration for abnormal behavior states. In addition to steroid withdrawal, narcotic withdrawal can produce arthralgias, fevers, and behavior disorders that sometimes may be mistaken for lupus in young women. This is seen primarily in large, urban, public hospital settings.

ORGANIC VERSUS FUNCTIONAL DISEASE

According to Bluestein (200), the medical (rather than psychiatric) orientation of investigators accounts for the limited analysis of functional psychiatric illness in SLE. Organic brain syndromes and functional disorders have a significant amount of overlap, and they often are difficult to differentiate. Patients who manifest seizures, fever, emotional lability, personality changes, impairment of judgment, and focal neurologic abnormalities tend to have more organicity.

Jacobs et al. (201) have devised a questionnaire and scale to differentiate between organic syndrome and functional disorders. Andre-Schwartz (202) noted in a literature review that patients with organic complaints have a much poorer prognosis than do those with only functional problems.

In 1981, Kremer et al. (194) reported a high incidence of patients with nonorganic, nonpsychotic psychopathology (NONPP). Diagnoses of depression, anxiety, mania, and conversion reactions have been made in up to 50% of patients. Adding standardized psychological tests, such as the MMPI and the Brief Psychiatric Rating Scale, to the psychiatric interview identifies an even higher incidence of NONPP in patients with lupus. In contrast to analyses of organic psychiatric illness, no significant correlation has been found between functional psychiatric disturbances affecting patients with SLE and their disease activity, either systemically or in the nervous system. Chronic illness often is accompanied by depression and other NONPP. Its frequency and perhaps its severity, however, may be markedly increased in SLE. Perhaps being told that you have lupus is more stressful than being labeled with some other chronic illness, or the disease process of SLE itself makes the patient more susceptible to the stresses of being chronically ill.

Certainly, the represented prognosis was thought to be much worse in the presteroid era, when study subjects often represented the sickest and most advanced cases of SLE, usually being hospitalized with years of multisystem illness. With the advent of corticosteroids, earlier diagnosis, and earlier therapeutic intervention, however, the prognosis has improved substantially. Even so, recognition of the relatively benign course of ANA-positive cases did not discourage a therapeutic pessimism in some health-care professionals, who probably reinforced (inadvertently) the worst fears of their newly diagnosed patients with lupus.

In 1960, Stern and Robbins (93) pointedly stated that one great problem in managing these patients is the evaluation of how much of an emotional response is reactive. In understanding the psychiatric responses to lupus, both the nature of the disease and the premorbid personality characteristics of the patients must be considered. SLE has devastating systemic effects. There is no definitive treatment, and the prognosis is poor. These features are anxiety provoking, and at least one third of the nonpsychotic patients have had a depressive reaction (203).

Not infrequently, patients report intense anxiety and despair after reading about the prognosis and outcome of SLE in an outdated medical text or after speaking with some well-meaning but uninformed expert. To avoid such reactions, as well as to establish a better rapport and cooperation with a naively diagnosed patient (often a new patient of the rheumatologist), it is essential during the initial medical counseling to educate the patient and, when appropriate, the family, with current and accurate information, to reassure them, and to allay their many unstated fears (204).

MEDICATION-INDUCED MENTAL CHANGES IN SLE

Behavioral and cognitive disturbances may be associated with the use of barbiturates, anticonvulsant agents, long- and short-acting benzodiazepines, and other psychotropic and psychoactive substances (205–208). Motor function also may be affected (209), and noncompliance, underreporting, self-medication and overmedication abuse, nonmedically supervised use, and medication withdrawal all have been reported to be associated with a myriad or psychiatric syndromes (210,211), have produced lingering or residual cognitive impairment recognition defects (212, 213), and have significantly influenced neuropsychological test performances (214–216).

Commonly reported adverse reactions (217) are hyperactivity, disturbed sleep, irritability, and emotional lability. Subtle behavioral disturbances, however, also may adversely affect performance and learning. Behavioral changes resulting from therapy with barbiturates and benzodiazepines tend to be idiosyncratic, as opposed to the dose-related effects that are seen with phenytoin and valproate therapy. Carbamazepine and valproate can affect mood and behavior negatively. Generally, however, this occurs less frequently than when other anticonvulsants are used; this is especially true in patients without CNS damage. The suspicion of a causal relationship between anticonvulsant therapy and impairment of cognitive skills in nontoxicated patients is gaining increasing support. Neuropsychological studies in acutely exposed normal volunteers, studies in epileptic patients receiving monotherapy, and crossover studies between drugs have incriminated barbiturates and hydantoin drugs. Although affected to a greater extent with higher drug dosages, memory and cognitive dysfunction have been reported with levels within the therapeutic range. Thus, serum drug levels cannot be considered as good predictors of which patients have subtle side effects. Carbamazepine and valproate seem to be relatively free of many adverse neuropsychological effects; anterograde amnesia (218), retrograde amnesia (219), and toxic ictal confusion (220–222) all have been reported following benzodiazepine use.

Schmidt et al. (223) presented the case of a 21-year-old woman who was suffering from bipolar affective disorder and who developed SLE with characteristic laboratory findings 18 months after starting carbamazepine maintenance treatment. SLE receded after the withdrawal of carbamazepine and treatment with antiinflammatory drugs. Although both the spontaneous occurrence of SLE and the psychosis as a sign of CNS involvement of SLE cannot be excluded, SLE could be considered as an adverse effect of carbamazepine in this case.

Studies of substance abuse have not been specific to SLE, but by extrapolation it is reasonable to assume that substance abuse occurs in patients with lupus. Experience with numerous patients has revealed the excessive use of alcohol and nicotine products, poor dietary practices, and various dependencies on analgesics (including opiates), prescribed and proprietary sleeping products and hypnotics, an assortment of so-called psychic energizers, and appetite suppressants such as Fen-Phen. A small percentage of patients with lupus subject themselves to unnecessary expense, and possible harm, by ingesting a vast array of health-food products and substances labeled as orthomolecular vitamins and homeopathic herbs. I have seen at least four patients on 10 g per day of vitamin C (224). These patients customarily do not report the ingestion of such products to their physician.

The many different medications used in SLE often produce side effects that alter the patient's thinking, mood, emotional control, and behavior. Any of these effects may be difficult to distinguish from a concurrent anxious or depressed condition or from lupus itself.

Because of the broad variation of organ system involvement from case to case in SLE, as well as variations in medication programs, underlying personalities, and psychosocial stresses associated with the chronic illness state, determining the cause of psychiatric side effects (PSEs) in SLE may be quite challenging. Complicating this is the fact that medications frequently interact with one another.

Liver or kidney involvement may have a profound effect on the psyche, since these organs are involved in the metabolism and filtering of medications from the blood.

Some drugs *decrease* other drugs' potency and effect, whereas others may *increase* other drugs' potency and effect. Of course, many medications do not interact with one another. Often, a medication that has some predictable side effect is used for a brief period of time, since its undesirable side effect is significantly outweighed by its desired benefit. Given this complicated picture, it helps to understand the various possible psychological effects of medications as well as potential drug interactions.

A detailed elaboration of various drugs, including special aspects, effects, and a discussion of the consequences of the uses of narcotics, analgesics, and the so called psychic energizers and CNS stimulants may be found in Chapter 32 of *The Challenges of Lupus* (225).

DIFFERENTIAL DIAGNOSIS OF PSYCHOSIS

Despite its infrequency, the sudden onset of psychosis in a patient with SLE without a prior psychiatric history or discernible precipitating cause usually is indicative of NPSLE. An association of lupus psychosis with antiribosomal-P antibodies (126,129,131,132,159,162,173,226) has been found by some investigators, suggesting that these symptoms may result from autoantibodies (162–164), including antigangliosides (136,151,154,155) and anti-SM antibodies (227).

Although the prime cause of psychotic episodes in SLE is organic brain disease, approximately 5% of cases may result from other factors, such as hypokalemia, water intoxication with hyponatremia, steroids themselves, and occasionally unusual reactions to antimalarial therapy. Due consideration must be given to each of these additional problems in the evaluation of every case. Complete blood chemistry profiles should be obtained in all patients.

Several patients have had water intoxication, with psychosis varying from hallucinations to catatonia, that was associated with advanced lupus nephropathy (228–230). Hyponatremia and water intoxication [inappropriate antidiuretic hormone (ADH) secretion] remain a relatively frequent cause of mental disturbance, especially in patients with lupus nephropathy. Central hyperventilation and inadequate ADH secretion (231) may develop.

Although they usually decrease emotional lability, improve depression, and increase energy levels, antimalarials may produce personality changes, convulsive seizures, nightmares, and psychoses. Usually, these have been associated with large doses, and other side effects often have been prominent before the mental ones (232).

Rudin (232a) hypothesized that the choroid plexus in SLE represents a combined transport dysfunction model for schizophrenia, as part of the blood–brain barrier guarding the periventricular primary personality brain or limbic system. This unlikely theory has not been subject to testing, however, and patients without SLE may have choroid plexus immune complex deposition.

From the preceding discussion, the diagnosis of NPL clearly is clinical and one of exclusion. Brain cross-reactive lymphocytotoxins and various neuronal antibodies may be measured; using a panel of substrates, one can identify a significant proportion of patients who are independently defined as having NPL and who demonstrate specific serum neuronal antibodies (233).

Use of newer imaging techniques, such as MRI, positron-emission tomography (PET), and brain electric activity monitoring (BEAM), for metabolic assessment of the CNS hold great promise. In 1990, Stoppe et al. (234) reported that they performed PET using 18F-labeled 2-F-2-desoxyglucose in 13 patients with SLE; ten of them had clinical signs of CNS involvement (i.e., NPL). All patients with neurologic symptoms showed pathologic changes on PET, always in accordance with their clinical state, and three patients without neuropsychiatric manifestations had normal PETs. CT of the brain and MRI proved to be less sensitive to both the presence and localization of CNS lesions. The authors concluded that the combination of PET and MRI constitutes the most useful diagnostic procedure for NPL. Reports from Sibbitt et al. (235) concluded that for the evaluation of acute NPL, MRI is useful and provides more information than cranial CT.

Cranial MRI (142,236–245) is superior to CT in detecting lesions caused by lupus cerebritis (235,242,246–251). Between 25% and 80% of patients with NPSLE and normal CT scans (245,252,253) have abnormal cranial MRIs. There is no specific MRI finding that is diagnostic of NPSLE, however, and MRI abnormalities differ depending on the neuropsychiatric manifestation (5,19). Stimmler et al. (242) reported in 1993 that as expected, MRI abnormalities were more common in patients with focal neurologic deficits (19 of 26) than in those patients without focal findings (15 of 38). Periventricular increased signal was a frequent MRI finding (10 of 64). Enlargement of the prepontine cistern was seen in 14 of 64, and it is an MRI finding not previously described in NPSLE. Patients with NPSLE and generalized seizures also may have a normal MRI, but they frequently have multiple, small, high-intensity lesions that may resolve on therapy (235,249). The reversibility of these lesions suggests they represent edema that probably is associated with small microinfarcts. Large lesions, especially cerebrovascular accidents (CVAs) (in both gray and white matter), which usually correlate with the patient's symptoms, frequently are irreversible on repeat MRIs (234,247,254–256).

According to Sibbitt et al. (257), neuroimaging has greatly advanced the understanding of NPSLE, which appears to be caused by acute and chronic brain injury induced by the complex pathologic processes of SLE with unique expression in the brain. Certain neuroimaging methods are clearly sensitive to NPSLE. However, the presence of both acute and chronic brain injury and the inability of contemporary neuroimaging methods to distinguish between these forms of injury is the major reason neuroimaging has severe limitations for diagnosing active NPSLE. Thus, only cautious recommendations for neuroimaging in NPSLE can be made on the basis of the literature, but each modality may have special uses in the proper clinical and research situation.

Angiography is to be discouraged, except in certain cases where medium-to-large vessel disease is suspected and other methods are not applicable. MR angiography should be used preferentially to radiocontrast angiography when possible because of greater safety and lesser expense. MRI is the anatomic imaging modality of choice for NPSLE, and when available should be used instead of CT. MR contrast studies, perfusion imaging, diffusion imaging, angiography, and relaxometry may improve the sensitivity of MRI for NPSLE, but have not been extensively studied. Although MRS cannot be used to specifically diagnose NPSLE, it is very sensitive and specific for brain injury in NPSLE, and may be useful to confirm an organic basis for neurocognitive decline, determine if a lesion on MRI represents serious or nonserious brain injury, determine the presence of anaerobic metabolism, and possibly confirm brain death. EEG and quantitative EEG (QEEG) should be used as problem-solving tools, most specifically when a seizure disorder is suspected among other applications. SPECT and PET may be sensitive for NPSLE, but have poor specificity for differentiating NPSLE versus non-NPSLE, reversible versus irreversible lesions, old versus new lesions, and NPSLE versus confounding disorders common to SLE. PET and SPECT also detect considerable background abnormalities of uncertain significance and must be combined with another imaging modality such as MRI or CT to be interpretable in the context of NPSLE. Thus, PET and SPECT cannot be recommended for the routine clinical evaluation of SLE patients with neurologic symptoms.

Currently only anatomic imaging, specifically MRI, can be recommended to evaluate NPSLE, but other techniques noted above may be useful in specific patients. It should be recommended that all neuroimaging studies in NPSLE not be overinterpreted by either the radiologist or the clinician, and that the limitations of each method be understood and accepted. Further controlled trials may help determine the best combination of methods to diagnose NPSLE, as advocated by West (see Chapter 35). In the interim, the above methods will have an increasing role in research and a real, but highly restricted, role in clinical diagnosis.

In 2000, Bosma et al. (258) noted that whether or not the clinical symptoms of NPSLE are usually reversible is still a matter of debate. Since magnetization transfer imaging (MTI) is more sensitive than conventional MRI in demonstrating brain damage, it has become a useful tool in the detection and quantification of diffuse brain orders such as multiple sclerosis. In this study, MTI was applied to investigate whether CNS damage is present in patients with a history of NPSLE.

Methods

Eleven female patients with a history of NPSLE and no previous or concurrent primary neurologic or psychiatric disease (ages 17 to 49 years), 11 female patients with SLE without a history of NPSLE (non-NPSLE; ages 15 to 51 years), and 10 healthy female controls (ages 17 to 47 years) underwent MTI. From these MTI scans, quantitative data on the uniformity of the brain parenchyma and atrophy were derived. One NPSLE and one non-NPSLE patient were excluded from this study due to infarctions detected with conventional MRI. MTI measures normalized for intracranial volume, reflecting abnormalities of the brain parenchyma as well as atrophy, were lower ($p < .005$) than the mean ratio of CSF to intracranial volume, indicative of atrophy, and were present in the NPSLE group compared with either the non-NPSLE patients or healthy controls. Still, the MTI measures solely reflecting uniformity of the brain parenchyma (normalized for brain volume) were also significantly ($p < .001$) lower in the NPSLE patients than in both control groups. This study demonstrates that using MTI, CNS damage can be demonstrated in patients with a history of NPSLE. MTI might, therefore, be an alternative and sensitive tool to detect brain injury in NPSLE, and might be useful in studying the natural history of the disease.

SPECT scan remains a sensitive tool during initial CNS events in children with CNS lupus documenting the presence of damage during short-term follow-up of 1 to 4 months. However, during long-term follow-up, abnormalities documented by SPECT no longer correlate with the patient's clinical course, limiting the usefulness of SPECT as a clinical tool in children who recover from CNS disease (259). Russo et al. (260) reported that although SPECT scanning was a highly sensitive method, it was *not* a specific method in correctly diagnosing diffuse CNS SLE in children. However, the presence of an abnormal SPECT scan in SLE patients with no history of overt CNS SLE may suggest that subclinical CNS disease may be more common in children than previously suggested (260). Worldwide MRI studies in SLE, and NPSLE tend to concur that MRI abnormalities are detected in neurologically asymptomatic SLE patients (261,262). However, one group (263) concluded that MRI analyses are not likely to provide additional clinical information on cognitively impaired SLE patients who have no other evidence of CNS involvement, although quantified MRI analysis did indicate "atypical" brain structure. In 1998, Swiss researchers (264) reported on a reversal of findings following prednisone treatment. They reported on a 53-year-old white man with decreased memory and visual disturbances who met four of the ARA criteria for the classification of SLE. He was investigated before and after 3 months of therapy using PET and F-18-fluoro-2-deoxy-D-glucose (FDG). Treatment consisted of prednisone (25 mg/day, tapered to 10 mg/day) and cyclophosphamide (daily 100 mg for 3 weeks followed by a drug-free interval of 1 week). For the control group, 15 clinically and neurologically healthy volunteers (five male, ten female, aged 48 ± 7 years) were investigated. All study participants additionally had a cranial MRI. In both controls and the SLE patient, cranial MRI was negative. However, the patient showed a significant hypometabolism in the parieto-occipital region on both sides and the parietal region on the right side before treatment. After treatment metabolism in these regions was within normal limits. Hence, FDG-PET could help to verify brain-onset of SLE earlier and may be a powerful tool for controlling SLE treatment.

A French (265) multispecialty group studied the prevalence of cerebral MRI changes in patients with primary antiphospholipid syndrome (PAPS), or with SLE, and the relationship of any MRI changes to the antiphospholipid antibodies. Twenty-nine consecutive SLE patients, 24 PAPS patients, and 31 controls were prospectively included in the study and underwent MRI scans over a 1-year period. MRI scans were analyzed separately by a neuroradiologist for white matter changes [periventricular hyperintensity (PVH) (0–6 scale), deep white matter hyperintensity (WMH) (0–24)], and one neurologist for cerebral atrophy (0–39 scale) and stroke subtypes. Statistical assessment consisted of a discriminant analysis performed with the SAS package with MRI data as the dependent variables and, as independent variables, age, sex, arterial hypertension, diabetes mellitus, cardiopathy, migraine, neurologic symptoms, antiphospholipid antibodies, SLE, steroid treatment.

Results

The prevalence of cerebral atrophy was increased in both SLE and PAPS groups relative to controls. PVH and WMH scores were significantly higher in SLE and PAPS than in controls. Focal infarct did not differ in the SLE group when compared with PAPS. PVH and WMH scores were significantly higher in patients with neurologic symptoms. Using a correlation test we found a weak significant correlation between cerebral atrophy and lupus anticoagulant. The multivariate analysis found only three independent variables related to PVH and WMH: age, the diagnosis of SLE, and cerebral atrophy. The authors concluded that age, presence of SLE, and presence of neurologic symptoms were independently related with WMH and PVH, but not antiphospholipid antibodies.

Sabet et al. (266), in an attempt to identify neurometabolite markers of cerebral injury in the antiphospholipid antibody syndrome of SLE, designed the following study. Forty-nine SLE patients [12 SLE patients with antiphospholipid antibody syndrome (aPLS)] and 23 control subjects were studied using MRI and spectroscopy. *N*-acetylaspartate/creatine (NAA/Cre) and choline/Cre (Cho/Cre) were measured in normal-appearing tissue. IgG and IgM antiphospholipid antibodies (aPLs) were measured by enzyme-linked immunsorbent assay. Higher levels of stroke, epilepsy, and IgG-aPL were more common in SLE-aPLS patients than in SLE patients ($p<.001$). NAA/Cre was lower ($p<.05$) and Cho/Cre higher ($p<.001$) in SLE-aPLS patients than in SLE patients without aPLS. Regression models showed NAA/Cre was most related to injury seen by imaging ($p<.01$), disease duration ($p<.05$), and prior neuropsychiatric SLE (NPSLE) ($p = .07$). Reduced NAA/Cre was most associated with the presence of aPLS ($p = .05$) The authors concluded that SLE and SLE-aPLS are actually a clinical continuum describing brain injury in SLE, with SLE-aPLS being characterized by increased aPL, NPSLE, stroke, epilepsy, and disturbed neurochemistry. An elevated IgG-aPL level is a potent risk factor for brain injury as measured by NAA/Cre in SLE that is independent of stroke and aPLS. However, thrombotic phenomena and the presence of aPL (aPLS) are most closely associated with increased Cho/Cre in SLE. These results suggest that aPLS exacerbates SLE, resulting in increased thrombotic and nonthrombotic brain injuries. Spectroscopy detects brain injury in SLE and may permit better understanding of the neurologic consequences of SLE and SLE-aPLS.

Over the last few years, more studies have focused on the regional cerebral blood flow, regional cerebral metabolic rate, and computed (automated image processing) evaluations in both active and nonactive neuropsychiatric lupus. A Japanese research team (267) using FDG-PET, MRI, and neuropsychological testing found that SLE psychiatric patients had significantly decreased regional cerebral metabolic rates for glucose in the prefrontal inferior parietal and anterior cingulate regions. This may be related to attentional deficits that are involved in various psychiatric symptoms in SLE. A Swiss and German group (268) suggested that the common finding of parieto-occipital hypometabolism in MRI-negative neuropsychiatric SLE is the consequence since this region is located at the boundary of blood supply of all three major arteries and could be the most vulnerable zone of the cerebrum and may be affected at an early stage of the cerebrovascular disease. A group from the Netherlands (269), using PET and FDG, performed statistical parametric mapping, showed a relative increase in metabolism in the striatum and regional decreases in the premotor cortex as common features in the patient group. Region of interest measurements of absolute FDG uptake confirmed these findings. The increased striatal activity may support the presence of a direct immune response against neuronal tissue in SLE, similar to the cross-reaction against inhibitory components in striatal tissue provoked by streptococcal antigens.

In 1999, a Chinese/Taiwanese research team (270) used technetium-99m (Tc-99m) hexamethylpropylenamine (HMPAO) brain images to detect basal ganglion and cerebral cortex regional blood flow (rCBF) in patients with SLE with brain involvement; 109 female patients with SLE were investigated using Tc-99m HMPAO brain images with fan-beam SPECT and surface three-dimensional (3D) display. These patients were separated into two subgroups: group 1, 74 cases with definite neuropsychiatric symptoms/signs;

and group 2, 35 cases without any neuropsychiatric symptoms/signs. Fan-beam SPECT demonstrated unilateral or bilateral hypoperfusion and basal ganglia or thalamus in 22% and 9% of patients in groups 1 and 2, respectively. Local hypoactivity anomalies were found in the brain cortex of 89% and 20% of patients in groups 1 and 2, respectively, using surface 3D display of the brain. In either group 1 or group 2 patients, the parietal and frontal areas are the most common areas and cerebellum and thalamus are the least common areas of brain involvement. This study suggests that in comparison with traditional brain imaging techniques, Tc-99 HMPAO brain imaging with fan-beam SPECT in combination with surface 3D display may provide objective information for detection of anomalies of rCBF in patients with SLE.

This same group (271) reported on using two updated brain-imaging modalities, HMPAO-SPECT and FDG-PET, *simultaneously* to detect rCBF and glucose metabolism of the brain in patients with SLE. Twenty-five female SLE patients, ages 25 to 40 years, were enrolled in this study and assigned to one of two groups. Group 1 consisted of 13 patients with neuropsychiatric manifestations (seven had major and six had minor manifestations). Group 2 consisted of 12 patients without neuropsychiatric manifestations. Serum levels of aCLs and antiribosomal P antibodies (anti-P) were measured. All patients had normal brain MRI findings. Ten healthy female volunteers also underwent brain MRI, HMPAO-SPECT, and FDG-PET for comparison. Results indicated that (Tc-99m)-HMPAO-SPECT revealed hypoperfusion lesions in 11 (44%) of 25 SLE patients, including nine (69%) of the 13 patients in group 1, all seven (100%) patients with major manifestations, two (33%) of the six patients with minor manifestations, and two (17%) of the 12 patients in group 2. Parietal lobes were the areas most commonly involved. FDG-PET revealed hypometabolism in seven (54%) of the group 1 patients, six (86%) of the seven patients with major manifestations, and one (17%) of the six patients with minor manifestations. Temporal lobes were the most commonly involved area. However, no significant hypometabolism brain lesions were found in group 2 patients. All four patients with headaches and dizziness or headaches alone had normal findings on HMPAO-SPECT and FDG-PET. Nine (36%) of the 25 patients were positive for aCL. However, the presence of aCL was not related to neuropsychiatric manifestations or to HMPAO-SPECT or FDG-PET findings. Five (20%) of the 25 patients had anti-P antibodies and psychosis/depression. The authors concluded that in patients with normal brain MRI findings, decreases in glucose metabolism coupled with decreases in rCBF are associated with serious NPSLE presentations, while normal glucose metabolism with decreases in rCBF may be found in SLE patients with or without NPSLE.

An automated image processing method (272) was developed to segment gray matter (gm), while minimizing the effects of confounding factors, specifically cerebral atrophy and volume averaging artifacts. The automated method effectively identifies gm, minimizes volume averaging artifacts, and produces results similar to the manual method. However, this method *markedly decreases analysis time* and will make quantitative relaxometry a valuable contribution to the clinical management of NPSLE. The brain edema characteristic of NPSLE as measured by manual quantitative MR relaxometry was compared to T2 calculated for gm by automated methods. Both methods demonstrated a marked increase in gm T2 in patients with major NPSLE.

SPECT is widely used in evaluations and research of NPSLE (239–241,244,254,273). Carbotte et al. (254) correlated neuropsychological changes and behavioral/cognitive deficits with alterations in regional brain glucose metabolism in three women with NPSLE over a substantial period of time. Changes in each patient's cognitive profile on reassessment paralleled changes on PET, which strongly argues that cognitive deficits in patients with SLE reflect primary CNS involvement. PET using phosphorus-31 has shown decreased adenosine triphosphate and phosphocreatine levels in patients with NPSLE that increase toward normal with therapy (274). PET scans commonly demonstrate areas of hypometabolism in the temporal and parietal lobes (234,254,275). Cerebral angiography usually is normal in NPSLE. Occasionally, vasculitis of large-sized arteries or cerebral emboli can be documented (276). In patients with cerebral emboli, M-mode, two-dimensional, Doppler, and transesophageal echocardiography should be done to rule out Libman-Sacks vegetation, mural thrombi, or another cardiac source of emboli.

Kushner et al. (277) studied the patterns of CBF over time in patients with SLE and varying neurologic manifestations, including headache, stroke, psychosis, and encephalopathy. CBF was least affected in patients with nonspecific symptoms such as headache or malaise, whereas patients with encephalopathy or psychosis exhibited the greatest reduction in CBF. Reports from Japan, Great Britain, and Scandinavia (278–280) have reflected intense interest in the application and correlation of neuropsychiatric disorders in SLE with developments in imaging systems, neuroimmunology, neuroendocrinology, neuropsychological function assessment, and PET scanning.

Several important reports of rather uncommon and atypical clinical pictures in NPL also have appeared. In 1987, Bambery et al. (281) described one case of a patient with SLE who developed the classic features of anorexia nervosa.

Bovin et al. (282) suggested that the reported low incidence of subdural symptoms in SLE may be more apparent than real. They cited the case history of a patient with SLE who presented with headaches, psychiatric disturbances, and increasing pain paraparesis. With surgical evacuation, the neuropsychiatric symptoms and headaches disappeared.

Gossat and Walls (283) reported on 14 patients in whom SLE was diagnosed for the first time after the age of 45 years. The onset was insidious and diagnosis delayed in most patients, with the mean duration of symptoms before diagnosis being 5 years. Clinical features in this group of patients differed from classic descriptions of SLE in regard to an unusually high incidence of neuropsychiatric disturbances and a low incidence of serositis. Diagnosis in this age group is difficult, and SLE probably goes unrecognized in a number of older patients with nonspecific complaints.

The diagnostician should not overlook other etiologies for neuropsychiatric changes in a patient with prior NPSLE, especially if they are on maintenance corticosteroids. The worldwide literature abounds with reports of CNS infections, such as cryptococcosis (284,285), toxoplasmosis, nocardiosis (286), listeria meningitis (287), aspergillosis (288), meningococcal meningitis (289), syphilitic meningitis (290), infection with the herpes virus (291), and various other esoteric infections.

CLINICAL AND LABORATORY EVALUATION

A well-designed mental status examination is imperative (292). It should include evaluation of orientation, recent and remote memory, level of consciousness, reality testing, and a neurologic examination (293). Psychological profiles such as the MMPI and the Wechsler Adult Intelligence Scale (WAIS) often are helpful, but the patient's performance can be affected by the concurrent administration of medication. Personality (traits) profiles on testing performance may be altered or masked by concurrent use of medications.

The neuropsychological testing described earlier can be a useful and highly sensitive instrument for identifying and monitoring cognitive function impairment and its progression or improvement for clinical, investigative, and legal purposes.

Neuroendocrine testing, such as the dexamethasone suppression test (DMST) and measurement of 24-catecholamine breakdown in homovanillic acid (HVA) studies, has led to an impressive body of research on biologic markers of depressive illness. Evidence suggests that abnormalities of the hypothalamic-pituitary-adrenal (HPA) axis in depression (resistance of dexamethasone suppression, spontaneous plasma cortisol secretion, abnormal metyrapone responses, β-endorphin and β-lipotropin secretion, and corticotropin-releasing factor challenge) tend to subside on clinical recovery (294). In particular, abnormal DMST results tend to normalize with antidepressant treatment; failure to do so often is associated with a poor prognosis, indicating that full recovery from depression should include normalization of the HPA axis (295–300). As a result, persistent nonsuppression despite antidepressant treatment or reversion to abnormal DMST results may be a prodromal sign of relapse in unipolar depression. Specific applications of these neuroendocrine tests to NPL have not been studied to any significant extent.

Thyroid testing, including thyroid-stimulating and thyroid-releasing hormone studies, may unmask a subclinical hypothyroidism. Typically, these patients are refractory to tricyclic antidepressants but respond favorably with the addition of thyroid products.

Lumbar puncture, neuroradiologic testing, EEG, and BEAM may be useful.

The EEG is of little value in assessing cerebral SLE, except for identifying epileptic activity and focal pathology. Waterloo et al. (301) evaluated 36 patients with SLE using cerebral CT, EEG, and a neuropsychological test battery. This Norwegian research team was investigating whether brain dysfunction as assessed by comprehensive neuropsychological investigation is associated with findings of routine investigation methods such as CT and EEG, which are available in most hospitals. Abnormal EEG was found in 19%, and CT revealed cerebral atrophy in 47% of SLE patients. Few neuropsychological functions were affected by the presence of abnormal EEG, cerebral atrophy, or infarcts. Significant associations were found only between cortical atrophy and impairment of tactile spatial problem solving and motor dexterity, and between cortical infarcts and motor dexterity in the dominant hand. Cerebral CT has little relevance in predicting brain dysfunction as established by neuropsychological assessment in SLE, except for detecting cortical atrophy and infarcts.

Glanz et al. (302) reviewed the records of 478 SLE patients. They noted that SLE is an immune-mediated multisystem disease that can affect the CNS. CNS manifestations occur in 25% to 75% of patients with SLE, and include seizures, stroke, headache, aseptic meningitis, transverse myelitis, psychosis, and cognitive dysfunction. CNS involvement in SLE is a major cause of patient morbidity, and a poor prognostic indicator.

Seizures have been reported in 15% to 20% of patients with SLE. Seizures may precede the onset of SLE, be the first manifestation of SLE, or develop during the course of the disease. Both generalized (i.e., tonic-clonic seizures and minor motor seizures) and focal seizures (i.e., simple partial seizures and complex partial seizures) have been reported. The precise prevalence of generalized versus focal seizures in patients with SLE is unknown. Generalized seizures tend to occur in patients with secondary involvement of the CNS due, for example, to renal disease or hypertension. Previous stroke syndromes have also been shown to predispose patients with SLE to the development of seizure disorders. The pathophysiology of primary seizures in patients with SLE is unclear. EEG abnormalities have been described in SLE patients with diverse CNS symptoms and in patients with no history of CNS disease. Both diffuse and focal EEG changes have been observed. The most commonly reported EEG abnormality is generalized slowing of the background.

Focal EEG abnormalities including focal slowing and epileptiform activity have also been described (303–308). These studies indicated that patients with SLE and seizure disorders demonstrated predominantly left temporolimbic EEG abnormalities. There is considerable evidence to suggest that immune-mediated mechanisms cause damage to specific neural structures in pseudo-SLE (PLE), herpes simplex virus encephalitis (HSVE), and Lyme encephalopathy. Similar immune-mediated damage may be occurring in patients with SLE. This damage appears to principally affect the left hemisphere. These findings are consistent with data from neuropsychological testing, and are currently being confirmed using a large-scale prospective study design and SLE patients with diverse neuropsychiatric symptoms such as seizures, psychosis, and cognitive dysfunction.

A fascinating application of transcranial Doppler use in SLE comes from Hungary, where Csepany et al. (309) report that the CNS is clinically affected in about half of their SLE patients. Mean blood flow velocities in the middle cerebral artery measured by transcranial Doppler ultrasound (TCD), before acetazolamide administration, were significantly higher in nine patients without neurologic symptoms and without MRI abnormalities (74.5 ± 3.1 cm/s; mean ± SEM) than in ten healthy controls (56 ± 2.8 cm/s) or in hemispheres of six SLE patients with neurologic symptoms (44.5 ± 2.6 cm/s). After acetazolamide, the response was significantly higher in symptom-free SLE patients (125 ± 4.6 cm/s) and lower in six patients with focal neurologic symptoms in the affected hemisphere (66.5 ± 3.1 cm/s) compared with healthy controls (87.3 ± 4.1 cm/s). These results suggest that the severity of impairment of the cerebral vessels is detectable by TCD in SLE patients. The acetazolamide test is suggested to be used in the follow-up of this disease.

SPECIAL CONCERNS, CHALLENGES, AND ADJUSTMENTS

From the onset of symptoms, the patient with lupus must adapt to a continuous series of unexpected physical, psychosocial, and emotional stresses and challenges. Usually, a person with SLE must adjust to a chronic illness with no cure, to an illness with a pattern of remissions and flares, often of brief duration, that generally occurs early in life and commonly after a prolonged period of elusive symptoms that have gone undiagnosed for some time. Before a specific diagnosis of lupus, the undiagnosed person and family and friends often even begin to wonder about the validity of the patient's actual complaints. A transient sense of elation and relief often is experienced when a specific diagnosis finally is established.

A common and problematic aspect of SLE is that the patient often does not look sick and often tries to conceal symptomatic complaints. This discourages support and empathy from those who are unfamiliar with the disease, although the patient is exhausted and feels terrible (310). Life's stresses often serve as explanations to the patient and family for all of the fatigue and emotional instability. Unexpressed, but commonly felt by the patient, is the fear of disfigurement, disability, and death; perhaps most often feared is being an invalid, unable to care for oneself and therefore dependent on others. These common feelings in the patient with lupus certainly are factors in the high incidence of depression, anxiety, and insomnia that are seen. Other factors also seem to be at work, however, because other types of chronic illness seem to be associated with depression and insomnia, although to a lesser degree.

The patient with lupus needs to cope with all aspects of modification in their goals and lifestyle that are dictated by their illness. The personality type seen so frequently in lupus—namely, a person who is outgoing, self-reliant, independent, and not given to complaint or passivity—can interfere with this coping. Unfortunately, such a person has a particularly difficult time in adjusting to the specific requirements of this illness—namely, frequent and careful medical monitoring, openness and honesty with the rheumatologist, and careful self-scrutiny and limit-setting on oneself. The struggle with self-esteem and depression can be, and often is, complicated by self-image and body-image problems (39). The stress of accepting this illness is followed by new challenges; the use of steroids often produces added physical changes and imposes limitations on an already fatigued patient. Fatigue, physical pain, and decreased muscle and joint mobility can lead to depression and withdrawal from normal activities, resulting in social isolation and personal disintegration, with loss of hope and suicidal despair.

During the prediagnosis phase of their illness, some younger patients try to cope with all of these stresses and tensions by doing what had worked so well for them before the onset of symptoms: actively pushing on even harder. This is common with the first abatement of symptoms, when patients push on until they burn out and drop. This can erode their self-confidence and self-image, intensify their anxiety and uncertainty, and often cloud their confidence in the physician's inability to make the diagnosis.

The return of symptoms begins to overcome any thoughts that patients might have about being just stressed out, or that their symptoms result from psychological forces. It ushers in the deep and growing conviction that despite what their physician cannot find, something is seriously and organically wrong. All of this commonly occurs in the prediagnosis phase. Most demoralizing after the uncertainty of the condition is the patient's loss of energy and fatigue, which leads to reduced and limited productivity.

Rogers (103) has noted that for many patients, the perceived injustice of an early recommendation for psychiatric treatment before the diagnosis of SLE may create wariness and resistance, suspicion, and even hostility about more appropriate and needed psychiatric intervention later (in the illness). As with any chronic illness, the relationship that is established with the primary physician is crucial in managing the patient's illness properly. The physician who is treating a patient with lupus can benefit by knowing about the patient's earlier treatment experience, including psychiatric experience. Patients often believe that their physician is not really listening in a nonjudgmental way. Often, patients report thinking that their physician ignores them as people. Because of the relative obscurity of SLE, family and friends generally are unfamiliar with it and are less able to relate to the patient. This leads to a sense of loss of independence and of control over their own lives and, when coupled with varying types and degrees of pain and marked fatigue, can lead to an increasing sense of emotional distance and isolation.

The stress early in the illness, especially that of accepting the illness, is followed by a series of new and unexpected challenges and impositions, such as the growing recognition that for the rest of their lives they will need to see doctors on a frequent and regular basis. This involves careful and frequent monitoring, incurs a substantial amount of medical expenses, and most likely requires steroids, with their associated physical and functional changes. More important, patients must modify many of their dreams and expectations and begin to accept increasing responsibility for a lifetime of limitations and financial burdens. The patient with lupus needs to cope, sooner or later, with all aspects of modifications in their lifestyle that are dictated by their particular illness, and this process takes time, work, and practice. As mentioned, this can be interfered with by the premorbid personality type that often is observed in lupus: a person who tends to be somewhat outgoing, self-controlled, achievement-oriented, self-reliant, independent, rather physical in their discharges of emotional tension, not given to complaint or passivity, and who, unfortunately, has a particularly difficult time in adjusting to an illness that reduces mobility, motor activity, attention span, and energy level while simultaneously contributing to a greater degree of dependency on others (311). This perceived dependency frequently induces guilt, anxiety, and depression, and it can lead to acting out, which translates into noncompliance and even treatment defiance. All this is occurring at a time in their lives when their healthy peers can anticipate such activities as exposure to the sun, uncomplicated pregnancies, substantially less need for rest, and relative freedom to explore their social and vocational interests and potentials; these peers tend to withdraw from the patient. Patients with lupus generally are ambivalent and hesitant to vocalize their fears, worries, and complaints to their physicians, families, and friends.

Adolescents in particular frequently are noncompliant. It often is difficult for them to fulfill these demands. Nashel and Ulmer (312) have noted that many do not take corticosteroids as advised because of their effects of weight gain, fluid retention, promotion of facial hair, acne, and easy bruisability. Fragile social relationships with friends can be altered by sun avoidance, hair loss, skin rash, and fatigability (313). They often have special concerns and questions when confronted with issues of dating, marriage, or childbearing. Compliance improves with a good physician–patient relationship and when the side effects of prescribed drugs (especially steroids) are discussed in detail before their use (314). Changing the lifestyle of the lupus patient is difficult. Often, physicians see their role as entirely treatment-oriented, and minimize the emotional component.

Because the time from onset of symptoms to diagnosis averages 3 years, many patients already are frustrated by the time they are told they have lupus. Their relationships with physicians already are strained. Initial feelings of relief, euphoria, and hopes for a quick cure occur after the diagnosis is made. A brief honeymoon with the diagnosing physician occurs and often is followed by a letdown as it becomes apparent that no quick fix is available. Some patients, particularly adolescents, try to deny that they have the disease, while others try to control their management by learning everything about it. They pressure the treating physician into therapeutic courses they might not otherwise undertake. Therefore, it is especially important that the lines of communication be kept open between patients and physicians to avoid irreparable damage. Appropriate relationships, according to Pincus et al. (315), can reverse the course of the illness and promote compliance and positive thinking as well as enhance the patient's satisfaction in activities of daily living [as assessed by the modified Stanford Health Assessment Questionnaire (HAQ)].

Crisis intervention becomes important when a sense of isolation, fear of death, and loss of independence occur. At this point, patients may feel that they are losing their minds and cannot control mood swings, and they may become unable to hold a job. Often, they are told they do not look sick when they feel exhausted and terrible. Those who retain their socialization skills, and especially those who attend group rap sessions sponsored by the various lupus societies (discussed later), tend to cope better. Such group discussions can dispel negative self-images and self-defeating attitudes and improve self-esteem. In addition, they facilitate the healthy release of feelings and emotions, encourage participants to confront and resolve their problems, and assist in consolidating and maintaining therapeutic gains. On the other hand, many patients who are leading a normal life find it depressing to hear of others' bad experiences with the illness. Unconscious guilt feelings that lupus is a punishment meted out by a supreme force must be abolished.

Despite these problems, most patients with lupus are outgoing, self-reliant, and independent. Most can handle their imposed handicaps well, maintain their jobs, and live fairly normal family lives. Some patients, however, box themselves into a corner with their defense mechanisms (316). Goodwin et al. (317) studied 25 patients with SLE who were treated by a group of four physicians and had those physicians rate those patients whom they liked the least. Of the 25 patients, ten were ranked by three physicians as the most disliked. They had more anxiety, hostility, and depression than the others, and generally were immature and uncooperative. An increased incidence of organic brain syndrome and suicidal ideation was noted in this group.

A chief compliant of patients with SLE is chronic fatigue (318). Periods of activity alternating with periods of rest often result in more being accomplished in a day than does working continuously (319). Self-employed individuals or those who can set their own pace (e.g., those who work out of their own home) often are the most productive. Demands for resolution of this problem results in patients being given thyroid preparations, iron, and sometimes amphetamines. Substance abuse may be a problem, but this is not as common as might be expected. Several pain-management centers surveyed in Los Angeles related that patients with SLE comprise a small percentage of their practice.

The patient with minimal organic brain disease represents a serious problem in management. Because of newly developing personality quirks, home life often becomes intolerable. Because the course of the illness is physically exhausting and produces personality changes, the incidence of divorce is exceedingly high. Judgment often is impaired. Patients may be in a state of limbo: not psychotic enough to be declared mentally incompetent, yet not really able to handle their own affairs effectively. Fruitlessly, many seek the help of psychoanalysts, especially before a definitive diagnosis. The physician managing the patient has a difficult time trying to decide how much of the patient's disordered thinking and behavior is due to brain dysfunction, and how much is due to nonorganic personality factors, and then what to tell the patient and the family. At times, the role of a functional overlay and organic process is so intertwined that it is impossible to distinguish these factors from each other (320). Many of these patients appear to be physically well while receiving steroid therapy, with relatively normal laboratory findings, but they complain of extreme lethargy and myalgia to the point of invalidism. Although extensive organic disease can be present with minimal findings, the evaluation and management of such problems can be trying for all concerned. Hochberg and Sutton (320) studied 106 ambulatory outpatients with SLE during 1985. The patients completed the Stanford HAQ and the Psychosocial Adjustment to Illness Scale (PAIS). Mean HAQ disability pain and global scores indicated a mild amount of impairment. Significant correlations were observed among increased disability, increased pain, worse global assessment, and poor psychosocial adjustment.

MARRIAGE, FAMILY, AND SEXUALITY

In dealing with a patient population consisting primarily of women of childbearing age, problems of marriage and pregnancy arise frequently for the physician who is called on for advice. In general, I have adopted a course of being frank with the patient in discussing the variability of the disease, with emphasis on the optimistic side.

Concerning marriage, it is advisable to review privately with the patient the limitations placed on her by the illness. These restrictions may vary from essentially none to tiring easily, which may interfere with a normal home life, and can progress to the point of long-term and expensive medication, repeated hospitalizations, and the need for continuous medical care. The chance of a spontaneous remission occurring at any time should be emphasized repeatedly, because these patients usually are depressed by the chronic nature of the disease and frightened by the little information that they have gathered from medical dictionaries and outdated medical texts (321). The risk of recurrences of a serious nature should be mentioned. If the patient is engaged to be married, then the fiancé can join the patient for a consultation with the physician, if the patient so desires. To avoid obvious problems, I never discuss prognosis with the fiancé alone or give him a worse outlook than I give to the patient, because if the engagement is broken off, as often happens, the patient may develop a mistrustful attitude toward the physician, which can interfere with future therapy.

Lupus is a family affair; it is important that the physician inquire about the patient's family life and background. Family members must learn to walk the fine line between not encouraging patients to become invalids and pushing them beyond their limitations. They must be informed about the nature of the disease, be able to anticipate physical and emotional changes, and respond in a supportive manner. Pfeiffer (322) has described clearly and concisely the various stages of disease development in women, along with the coping responses.

Sexual changes often occur during the lives of patients with SLE. The disease, side effects of medications, and/or depressions that many patients experience can contribute to a breakdown in sexual relationships. Patients often are reluctant to discuss these problems with their partner or physician, further contributing to the 50% divorce rate among patients with SLE. Antihypertensive medications can decrease libido; corticosteroids can alter appearance and may interfere with menstruation patterns and affect mood. Nonsteroidal drugs may cause edema. Tranquilizers and psychotropic drugs have more far-reaching effects.

The social functioning of 120 patients (114 women) with SLE was studied in British Columbia by Stein et al. (316). Of these, 61 women had 76 pregnancies after the onset of SLE; although fetal wastage was common, outcomes were otherwise satisfactory. Social difficulties worsened with disease exacerbations, drug reactions, and delay in diagnosis. After the onset of SLE, 33 completed their educations, and 63 with a work history were employed and 52 totally or partially self-supporting. Twenty patients experienced problems with self-image, four with sexual functioning, and 17 with lifestyle. SLE was not a barrier to marriage or a primary cause of divorce: 40 married after the onset of SLE, and 12.5% had a history of divorce. Stein et al. concluded that patients with SLE can function well socially, notwithstanding many varied limitations and readjustments, provided that these difficulties are recognized, accepted, and emotional support is provided. The authors emphasized the importance of psychological support and referral for counseling as factors in optimal psychosocial adjustment outcomes.

Curry et al. (323) investigated the impact of SLE and the mediating effects of psychosocial factors on women's sexual adjustments and concluded that sexual impairment is not inevitable among women with SLE. Their work underscores the positive role that medical providers play in helping to prevent sexual difficulties.

PATIENTS' RAP (SELF-HELP GROUPS)

Patients' self-help groups have become a national movement and now are common, with local and national SLE organizations (324). Patient rap groups are an adjunct to the total psychosocial and medical care of the person with lupus. Rap groups provide all sorts of intrinsic support, including emotional warmth, friendly commiseration, and a sense of closeness with other patients. These groups provide for the transmission of accurate and current medical information, an opportunity for venting one's feelings, and the inevitable selection of kindred spirits for friends, along with much more that contributes to the individual's welfare.

Group leaders actively guide the patients in an attempt to restore hope and to enhance their cooperation with physicians. Most important, perhaps, the group process seems to dispel and reverse negative self-images and self-defeating attitudes and behaviors. Regressive, noncompliant, and treatment-resisting behaviors often are modified or overcome.

Rap group participation seems to promote a greater sense of social involvement and self-control in the patient's mind. It contributes to greater hope, self-esteem, and intelligent and active redirection of energies into appropriate activities. The rap group promotes the acceptance of limitations without despair, and it fosters greater appreciation for and cooperation with the medical team.

In addition, the participants tend to develop more tolerance and acceptance of their friends, family, and themselves. They feel like they are more active participants in their own care and are contributing to the lupus cause by helping other members, usually the newer ones.

Recognizing common psychological fears and mechanisms so that they can be understood and shared, and their energies redirected into more realistic and appropriate attitudes and behavior, is essential to assisting the patient with lupus to cope and to contribute constructively. Patient rap groups have proven to be effective.

In 1993, Braden et al. (325) reported the beneficial effect and outcomes of patients with lupus who were involved in a given activity in the Systemic Lupus Erythematosus Self-Help (SLESH) course. Participants had significant increases in enabling skills and in the use of relaxation and exercise activities. Participants also had significantly less depression. Consistency between the amount of time spent in class and significant changes over time was demonstrated by analysis of treatment strength-response for perception of limitations, depression, enabling skill, and for use of rest, relaxation, heat, and exercise activities.

USE OF HYPNOSIS

Hypnosis (326) is a technique that health professionals have been using for at least 200 years. Esdaille used it in India in the late 19th century to control pain during surgery and reported incidentally that his infection rate was half of what was expected. Hypnosis has become more popular recently as physicians and researchers have come to understand the negative effects of stress on health and specifically on the immune system. Hypnosis has been approved by the American Medical Association and the American Psychological Association as an effective treatment technique to modulate stress and stress symptoms, to support and enhance deep relaxation in pain management and enhance the effects of certain medications.

THERAPEUTIC CONSIDERATIONS

Goals And Attitudes In Adjusting To SLE

The physician and family must recognize and understand that adjustment to a chronic illness is a gradual adaptation process, much like the emotional, psychosocial, and maturation aspects of the developmental process, with various phases, inevitable challenges, opportunities, and pitfalls. This adjustment is similar to the way in which good parents assist their child toward optimal growth. An open, relatively relaxed, and trusting relationship with the physician contributes directly toward a positive outcome. The adjustment capability and ego strength of the patient are enhanced by increased knowledge and education about their own condition. Toward this end, the physician's knowledge of the disease process and all aspects of the SLE illness experience, as well as an understanding of adjustment to chronic illness, are essential in assisting the patient (327). The physician should understand and transmit the following information to the patient and the important people in that patient's life:

1. Almost all patients with SLE experience intermittent periods of anxiety and depression, of varying intensity and duration, during the course of their illness.
2. If patients are to reach and maintain a comfortable emotional equilibrium with a satisfactory self-image and sense of hope, they must tolerate and understand these powerful emotions and develop a sense of control over their condition and their life.
3. Cure is not a goal worth pursuing; rather, the patient must learn to gain control of their condition and their life.
4. Self-monitoring of the condition is essential, and it represents an important step by patients toward contributing and participating in their own medical care. This is important, because they are in a cooperative relationship with their primary-care physician.
5. Illness is the best teacher, provided that it is listened to.
6. Pain is natural, inevitable, and tolerable, as long as it is controlled.
7. Families should be encouraged not to give advice, but rather to hear and understand the emotional concerns and feelings of the patient.
8. Patients must monitor their emotions as well as their body sensations.
9. Stress of all types exacerbates lupus. Stress is inevitable, so it cannot be avoided totally. However, the various stressors should be anticipated, identified, and controlled to whatever degree possible.
10. Hope, sublimations, and substitutions help to attenuate the continuous series of losses that occur with lupus.

Role Of Psychotherapy In SLE

In most cases of lupus, relapse is the rule, and that includes occasional psychological slips. Physicians, patients, and families must recognize that the value of psychotherapy in chronic illness is well established. The goals of psychotherapy remain the same whether or not the person has an illness. These goals are simply to encourage greater self-awareness, insight, and coping ability; to alleviate intrapsychic and interpersonal conflict; and to develop health-enhancing attitudes and behaviors.

Understanding The Chronically Ill

As a general rule, obvious neuropsychiatric manifestations in someone with chronic illness are treated in much the same way as in a person without a chronic illness with regard to the various chemical and physiologic limitations of the underlying physical condition and consideration for the use of concurrent medications. An organic basis for any neuropsychiatric manifestations must first be ruled out; this requires a careful medical and neurologic history and examination, with an emphasis on medication history, appropriate and thorough laboratory studies, and being prepared for the emergence of some new condition. One must be aware of drug dependency, masked depression, and masked suicide. Even when a definitive organic factor has been identified that contributes to the neuropsychiatric condition, psychological intervention usually is necessary and helpful, and a visit with the patient's family or even a visit to the home can prove illuminating. One must not be timid or conservative or use subclinical doses of psychopharmacologic agents if results are desired. Undertreatment can be more destructive than no treatment. Substance abuse, especially of alcohol, is more common than recognized. Liaison with the family is tricky but may prove helpful, especially if it can reinforce or establish support for the patient.

The powerful role of the doctor–patient relationship is explored in great depth in Aladjem's (328) *The Challenges of Lupus: Insights and Hope.* Balch (329) explores the specifics of the partnership between doctor and patient. Rogers (330) describes the doctor–patient relationship, while Schur (331) gives clear suggestions on optimizing the relationship. Shapiro (332) explores the relationship in light of the current changes in the medical delivery system and how to find and select a new physician. Shapiro describes specifically those traits and characteristics of a physician that are identifiable and important for the lupus patient.

The therapeutic goal for the SLE patient is to increase the sense of self-control and independence, and to promote participation with the health care team. I believe that the following factors contribute constructively and positively to therapeutic effectiveness with all patients:

1. Quality of life is a worthwhile goal, and the physician's therapeutic focus should be on that quality, both now and in the future.
2. Each inevitable loss or sense of loss by the patient should be neutralized in part by some replacement.
3. The process of medical treatment of the patient with lupus requires greater patience, tolerance, flexibility, and creativity from the physician than are needed in the treatment of other patients. It requires more common sense and acceptance of various, even strange, parameters than the more short-term conditions do.
4. The physician and the patient must develop a mutual honesty, respect, understanding of one another, and openness of communication to tolerate those aspects of the condition that are unclear, unpredictable, and often intolerable (but important).
5. Somatization and occasional opportunism with the use of illness is a human trait. It is inevitable, but by no means unforgivable or insurmountable.
6. Unpleasant emotional responses and mental distortions are an acceptable adaptation and will pass.

7. Despite incredible disruptions in one's lifestyle and existence, many patients recover their mental, emotional, spiritual, and, often, sexual sense of well-being. They then want to continue living, and to live well.
8. Realistic limit-setting is essential, both for the patient and psychotherapist.
9. Many chronically ill patients with severe neuropsychiatric pathology have been neglected, and essentially rejected, by a therapeutic pessimism that has led to undertreatment, therapeutic and familial abandonment, and deepening psychopathology and maladaptation.
10. Hopelessness is pathogenic.
11. Each medical condition has its own set of preconditions; these are as important to recognize as the ego strength, premorbid personality, and resources of the individual with a chronic illness.
12. Sexual libido and general aggressiveness are greatly reduced (i.e., tired).
13. A series of somatopsychic consequences of a specific condition is almost inevitable, and must be respected.
14. Terms and words mean different things to different patients.
15. Pain and immobility may be more stressful to the physician than to the patient, and patients tend to be highly sensitive to their physician's emotional responses.
16. Rarely should the physician attempt to deny or dispute the truth of a patient's accurate perception of their attitudes, feelings, or behavior.
17. The cornerstone of any good relationship is honest and open communication. Patients have the responsibility to tell the physician what really troubles them, and the physician has the responsibility to listen carefully. The physician must inquire not only about the physical condition but also, and perhaps more importantly, about the patient's inner feelings, relationships, and life situation. Communication is always a two-way street.
18. Physicians should not view psychotherapy as a substitute for vocational or social rehabilitation.

Dr. Shapiro's Recipe For Survival

The following recipe for survival for patients with lupus has been widely circulated and reprinted in the newsletters of the Lupus Foundation of America, the American Lupus Society, and other organizations that are devoted to issues concerning patients' coping with chronic illness. It concisely embodies my suggestions.

TO AVOID:

F STANDS FOR FATIGUE

L STANDS FOR LONESOMENESS and LONELINESS

A STANDS FOR ALCOHOL and DRUGS

R STANDS FOR RUMINATIONS (repetitive worrisome ideas)

E STANDS FOR EXHAUSTION

S STANDS FOR SELF-ABSORPTION and SELF-PITY

SEEK OUT:

R STANDS FOR REST, RELAX, RECREATE, and RAP REGULARLY

E STANDS FOR EXERCISE

L STANDS FOR LAUGHTER AS OFTEN AS POSSIBLE

A STANDS FOR AFFECTION, GIVEN and RECEIVED

X STANDS FOR EXCHANGES OF POSITIVE THOUGHTS FOR NEGATIVE THOUGHTS

E STANDS FOR EDUCATE YOURSELF ON YOUR CONDITION

S STANDS FOR SOCIALIZE WITH and OFFER SUPPORT TO OTHERS AS MUCH AS YOUR CONDITION ALLOWS and THEN A LITTLE MORE

R: Rest, relax, and recreate regularly. This does not mean just on weekends or holidays, but all the time, as a new life pattern. Now is the time to drop your workaholic tendencies. If you have neglected to incorporate "**R**" into your life so far, it is essential now that chronic illness has entered the picture.

E: Exercise! Not all of you can get out and jog or play tennis, but you should do what you can, at least several times a week, even if you are bound to a bed or a wheelchair. Ask your doctor to help you develop an exercise plan that is suited to your illness. Activity is important, even if it is just range-of-motion exercises.

L: Laughter can be crucial for your survival. You may be familiar with Norman Cousins, former editor of *Saturday Review*, who used laughter as a key part of his successful attempt to reach a remission of his illness. The same treatment can help us deal with our chronic illness. Laughter does not just make you feel good; it also causes you to take deep, relaxing breaths and, for a short time, clears your mind of other thoughts and emotions. And laughter begets laughter. What a wonderful habit to develop!

A: Affection, both given and received. SHARE YOURSELF. Pet a puppy, hug a child, love your spouse. Equally important, learn to ask for and receive affection in whatever way you feel comfortable. Don't be shy! Make it a constant in your life.

X: Exchange negative thoughts for positive thoughts, dwell on what you can change, not on what you can't. Think about how well you can be instead of how ill you might be.

E: Educate yourself about your chronic illness, and not only yourself. Take it upon yourself to gently and slowly educate those around you who care about your well-being.

S: Socialize with and offer support to others as much as your condition allows, plus a little more. If you keep yourself busy, you'll have less time to dwell on your pain and illness. It is hard to concentrate on two things at once. A particularly good way of keeping busy is to use your experiences to provide encouragement and support to others with a similar condition. By helping others, you help yourself even more.

REFERENCES

1. Hebra F, Kaposi M. *On diseases of the skin, including the exanthemata*, vol 4. Tay W, trans., Fagge CH, ed. London: New Sydenham Society 1866–1880, 1874.
2. Osler W. The visceral lesions of the erythema group. *Br J Dermatol* 1900;12:227–245.
3. Daly D. Central nervous system in acute disseminated lupus erythematosus. *J Nerv Ment Dis* 1945;102:461–465.
4. Hargraves MM, Richmond H, Morton R. Presentation of 2 bone marrow elements: tart cell and L.E. cell. *Proc Staff Meet Mayo Clin* 1948;23:25–28.
5. Abel T, Gladman DD, Urowitz MB. Neuropsychiatric lupus. *J Rheumatol* 1980;7:325–333.
6. Adelman DC, Saltiel E, Klinenberg JR. The neuropsychiatric manifestations of systemic lupus erythematosus: an overview. *Semin Arthritis Rheum* 1986;15:185–199.
7. Buchbinder R, Littlejohn GO, Hall S, et al. Neuropsychiatric manifestations of systemic lupus erythematosus. *Aust NZ J Med* 1988;18:679–684.
8. Dubois EL, Tuffanelli DL. Clinical manifestations of SLE: computer analysis of 520 cases. *JAMA* 1964;190:104–111.
9. Estes D, Christian CL. The natural history of systemic lupus erythematosus by prospective analysis. *Medicine* 1971;50: 85–95.
10. Feinglass EJ, Arnett FC, Dorsch CA, et al. Neuropsychiatric manifestations of systemic lupus erythematosus: diagnosis, clinical spectrum, and relationship to other features of the disease. *Medicine* 1976;55:323–339.
11. Grigor R, Edmonds J, Lewkonia R. Systemic lupus erythematosus. A prospective analysis. *Ann Rheum Dis* 1978;37: 121–128.
12. Lee P, Urowitz MB, Bookman AAM, et al. Systemic lupus erythematosus. A review of 110 cases with reference to nephritis, the nervous system, infections, aseptic necrosis and prognosis. *Q J Med* 1977;181–132.
13. Lim L, Ron MA, Ormerod IEC. Psychiatric and neurological manifestations in systemic lupus erythematosus. *Q J Med* 1988; 66:27–38.
14. McCune WJ, Golbus J. Neuropsychiatric lupus. *Rheum Dis Clin North Am* 1988;14:149–167.
15. Omdal R, Selseth B, Klow NE. Clinical neurological, electrophysiological, and cerebral CT scan findings in systemic lupus erythematosus. *Scand J Rheumatol* 1989;18:283–289.
16. Sibley JT, Olszynaski WP, Decoteau WE, et al. The incidence and prognosis of central nervous system disease in systemic lupus erythematosus. *J Rheumatol* 1992;19:47–52.
17. Wong KL, Woo EKW, Yu YL. Neurological manifestations of systemic lupus erythematosus: a prospective study. *Q J Med* 1991;81:857–870.
18. Llote F, Osterland CK. Autonomic neuropathy in SLE: cardiovascular autonomic function assessment. *Ann Rheum Dis* 1994; 53:671–674.
19. Tan EM, Cohen AS, Fries JF, et al. Special article: the 1982 revised criteria for the classification of systemic lupus erythematosus. *Arthritis Rheum* 1982;25:1271–1277.
20. Kassan SS, Kagen LJ. Central nervous system lupus erythematosus: measurement of cerebrospinal fluid cyclic GMP and other clinical markers of disease activity. *Arthritis Rheum* 1979; 22:449–457.
21. Singer J, Denburg JA, and the Ad Hoc Neuropsychiatric Lupus Workshop Group: diagnostic criteria for neuropsychiatric systemic lupus erythematosus: the results of a consensus meeting (workshop report). *J Rheumatol* 1990;17:1397–1402.
22. Kassan SS, Lockshin MD. Central nervous system lupus erythematosus: the need for classification. *Arthritis Rheum* 1979; 22:1382–1385.
23. Deleted in page proofs.
24. Ad Hoc Committee on Neuropsychiatric Lupus Nomenclature. The American College of Rheumatology nomenclature and case definitions for neuropsychiatric lupus syndromes. *Arthritis Rheum* 1999:42:599–608.
25. American Psychiatric Association. *Diagnostic and statistical manual of mental disorders*, 4th ed. (DSM-IV). Washington, DC: APA, 1994.
26. Klippel JH, Zvaifler NJ. Neuropsychiatric abnormalities in systemic lupus erythematosus. *Clin Rheum Dis* 1975;1:621–638.
27. Asherson RA, Denburg SD, Denburg JA, et al. Current concepts of neuropsychiatric systemic lupus erythematosus (NPSLE). *Postgrad Med J* 1993;69:602–608.
28. Barr WG, Merchut MP. Systemic lupus erythematosus with central nervous system involvement. *Psychiatr Clin North Am* 1992;15:439–454.
29. Putterman C, Naparstek Y. Neuropsychiatric involvement in systemic lupus erythematosus. *Isr J Med Sci* 1992;28:458–460.
30. Amital-Teplizki J, Bearman JE, Miele PW Jr, et al. A multidimensional autoantibody analysis specifying systemic lupus erythematosus patients with neuropsychiatric symptomatology. *Isr J Med Sci* 1992;28:422–427.
31. Mavrikakis ME, Antoniades LG, Germanides JB, et al. Organic brain syndrome with psychosis as an initial manifestation of systemic lupus erythematosus in an elderly woman. *Ann Rheum Dis* 1992;51:117–119.
32. Rimon R, Kronqvist K, Helve T. Overt psychopathology in systemic lupus erythematosus. *Scand J Rheumatol* 1988;27: 143–146.
33. Nollet D, Herreman G, Piette JC, et al. Psychic disorders in systemic lupus erythematosus. Prospective study of 35 cases. *Presse Med* 1985;14:401–404.
34. Darby PL, Schmidt PJ. Psychiatric consultations in rheumatology: a review of 100 cases. *Can J Psychiatry* 1988;33:290–293.
35. Omdal R, Mellgren SI, Husby G. Clinical neuropsychiatric and neuromuscular manifestations in systemic lupus erythematosus. *Scand J Rheumatol* 1988;17:113–117.
36. Mitchell WD, Thompson TL. Psychiatric distress in systemic lupus erythematosus outpatient. *Psychosomatics* 1990;31: 293–300.
37. van Dam AP, Wekking EM, Callewaert JA, et al. Psychiatric symptoms before systemic lupus erythematosus is diagnosed. *Rheumatol Int* 1994;14:57–62.
38. Carbotte RM, Denburg SD, Denburg JA. Prevalence of cognitive impairment in systemic lupus erythematosus. *J Nerv Ment Dis* 1986;174:357–364.
39. Langlo L. The efficiency of local application of chloroquine and mepacrine in preventing the effects of ultraviolet rays on human skin. *Acta Derm Venereol (Stockh)* 1975;37:85–87.
40. MacNeill A, Grennan DM, Ward D, et al. Psychiatric problems in SLE. *Br J Psychiatry* 1976;128:442–445.

41. van Dam A, Wekking EM, Ovmen HAPC. Psychiatric symptoms as features of systemic lupus erythematosus (reprint). *Psychother Psychosom* 1991;55:132–140.
42. Denburg SD, Denburg JA, Carbotte RM, et al. Cognitive deficits in systemic lupus erythematosus. *Rheum Dis Clin North Am* 1993;19:815–831.
43. Rubio Valladolid G, Olivares Zarco D, Orengo F, et al. Psychiatric manifestations in patients with erythematosus systemic lupus. *Actas Luso Esp Neurol Psiquiatr Cienc Afines* 1994;22:158–163.
44. Chin CN, Cheong I, Kong N. Psychiatric disorder in Malaysians with systemic lupus erythematosus. *Lupus* 1993;2:329–332.
45. Anonymous. Editorial. *J Rheumatol* 1988;15:959–964.
46. Iverson GL. Psychopathology associated with systemic lupus erythematosus: a methodological review. *Semin Arthritis Rheum* 1993;22:242–251.
47. Wilson DN. Systemic lupus erythematosus in a woman with mental handicap. *Br J Psychiatry* 1991;158:427–429.
48. Costa JP, Bajador IP, Alonso EP, et al. Prevalencia de lupus eritematoso generalizado en una poblacin psiquitrica. *Med Clin (Barc)* 1986;87:785–786.
49. Hugo FJ, Halland AM. DSM-III-R classification of psychiatric symptoms in systemic lupus erythematosus. *Psychosomatics* 1996;37(3):262–269.
49a. Purandare KN, Wagle AC, Parker SR. Psychiatric morbidity in patients with SLE. *QJM* 1999;92:283–286.
50. Heine BE. Psychiatric aspects of systemic lupus erythematosus. *Acta Psychiatry Scand* 1969;45:307.
51. Rummelt JD. Assessment of neuropsychological functioning in systemic lupus erythematosus. *Dissertation Abstracts International* 1990.
52. McClary AR, Meyer E, Weitzman EL. Observations on the role of depression in some patients with disseminated lupus erythematosus. *Psychosom Med* 1955;17:311–321.
53. Ropes MW. *Systemic lupus erythematosus.* Cambridge, MA: Harvard University Press, 1976:19.
54. Otto R, Mackay IR. Psycho-social and emotional disturbances to systemic lupus erythematosus. *Med J Aust* 1967;2:488–493.
55. Wallace DJ. The role of stress and trauma in rheumatoid arthritis and systemic lupus erythematosus. *Semin Arthritis Rheum* 1987;16:153–157.
56. Adams SG Jr, Dammers PM, Saia TL, et al. Stress, depression, and anxiety predict average symptom severity and daily symptom fluctuation in systemic lupus erythematosus. *J Behav Med* 1994;17:459–477.
57. Blumenfield M. Psychological aspects of systemic lupus erythematosus. *Prim Care* 1978;5:159–171.
58. Solomon GF, Moos RH. Emotions, immunity and disease. *Arch Gen Psychiatry* 1974;11:657.
59. Rogers MA, Dubey D, Reich P. The influence of the psyche and the brain on immunity and disease susceptibility: a critical review. *Psychosom Med* 1979;41:147.
60. Lahita RG, Chiorazzi N, Gibofsky A, et al. Familial systemic lupus erythematosus in males. *Arthritis Rheum* 1983;26:39–44.
61. Salcedo JR, Spiegler BJ, Gibson E, et al. The autoimmune disease systemic lupus erythematosus is not associated with left-handedness. *Cortex* 1985;21:645–647.
62. Satz P, Soper HV. Left-handedness, dyslexia, and autoimmune disorder: a critique. *J Clin Exp Neuropsychol* 1986;8:453–458.
63. Geschwind NBP. Left-handedness: association with immune disease, migraine, and developmental learning disorder. *Proc Natl Acad Sci USA* 1982;79:5097–5100.
64. Schur PH. Handedness in systemic lupus erythematosus. *Arthritis Rheum* 1986;29:419–420.
65. Verheul HAM, Stimson WH, den Hollander FL, et al. Effects of nandrolone, testosterone and their decanoate esters on murine lupus. *Clin Exp Immunol* 1981;44:11–17.
66. Hecaen H. *Les gaushers.* Paris: Presses Universitaires de France, 1984.
67. Fries JF, Holman H. *Systemic lupus erythematosus: a clinical analysis.* Philadelphia: WB Saunders, 1975.
68. Spiera H, Rothenberg RR. Myocardial infarction in four young patients with systemic lupus erythematosus. *J Rheumatol* 1983; 10:464.
69. Farine JC. Animal models in autoimmune disease in immunotoxicity assessment. *Toxicology* 1997;119(1):29–35.
70. Schur PH, ed. *The clinical management of systemic lupus erythematosus.* Orlando: Grune & Stratton, 1983.
71. Rothfield N. Clinical features of systemic lupus erythematosus. In: McCarty DJ, ed. *Arthritis and allied conditions,* 10th ed. Philadelphia: Lea & Febiger, 1985:1091.
72. Wallace DJ, Metzger AL. Can an earthquake cause flares of rheumatoid arthritis or lupus nephritis? *Arthritis Rheum* 1994; 37:1826–1828.
73. Rogers MP, Fozdar M. *Psychoneuroimmunology of autoimmune disorders.* Cambridge, MA: Department of Psychiatry, Harvard Medical School, 1966.
74. Dubois EL, ed. *Lupus erythematosus. A review of the current status of discoid and systemic lupus erythematosus and their variants,* 2nd ed rev. Los Angeles: USC Press, 1976.
75. Ahles TA, Yunus MB, Riley SD, et al. Psychological factors associated with primary fibromyalgia syndrome. *Arthritis Rheum* 1984;27:1101–1106.
76. Payne TC, Leavitt F, Garron DC, et al. Fibrositis and psychological disturbance. *Arthritis Rheum* 1982;25:213–217.
77. Smythe H. Fibrositis and other diffuse musculoskeletal syndromes. In: McCarty DJ, ed. *Arthritis and allied conditions.* Philadelphia: Lea & Febiger, 1985:481–489.
78. Wallace DJ. Prevalence of fibromyalgia in systemic lupus erythematosus patients: comment on the article by Middleton et al. *Arthritis Rheum* 1995;38:872.
79. Middleton GD, McFarlin JE, Lipsky PE. The prevalence and chemical impact of fibromyalgia in systemic lupus erythematosus. *Arthritis Rheum* 1994;37:1181–1188.
80. Romano TJ. Coexistence of fibromyalgia with systemic lupus erythematosus. *Am J Pain Management* 1992;2:211–214.
81. Wallace DJ, Shapiro S, Panush RS. Update of fibromyalgia syndrome. *Bull Rheum Dis* 1999;48(5).
82. Wallace DJ. What constitutes a fibromyalgia expert? *Arthritis Care Res* 1999;12:82–84.
83. Ader R, ed. *Psychoneuroimmunology.* New York: Academy, 1981.
84. Cooper EL. *Stress, immunity and aging.* New York: Dekker, 1984.
85. Solomon GF, Amkraut AA. Psychoneuroendocrinological effects of the immune response. *Annu Rev Microbiol* 1981;35: 155–184.
86. Wekking EM, Vingerhoets AJJM, van Dam JC, et al. Daily stressors and systemic lupus erythematosus: a longitudinal analysis. *Psychother Psychosom* 1991;55:108–113.
87. Hinrichsen H, Barth J, Ruckemann M, et al. Influence of prolonged neuropsychological testing on immunoregulatory cells and hormonal parameters in patients with systemic lupus erythematosus. *Rheumatol Int* 1992;12:47–51.
88. Pawlak CR, Jacobs R, Mikeska E, et al. Patients with systemic lupus erythematosus differ from healthy controls on their immunological response to acute psychological stress. *Brain Behav Immun* 1999;13(4):287–302.
89. Brody S. Psychological factors associated with disseminated lupus erythematosus and effects of cortisone and ACTH. *Psych Q* 1956;30:44.
90. Clark EC, Bailey AA. Neurological and psychiatric signs associated with systemic lupus erythematosus. *JAMA* 1956;160: 455–457.

91. O'Connor JF. Psychoses associated with systemic lupus erythematosus. *Ann Intern Med* 1959;51:5–26.
92. McGehee Harvey A, Shulman LE, Tumulty AP, et al. Systemic lupus erythematosus: review of the literature and clinical analysis of 138 cases. *Medicine* 1954;33:291–437.
93. Stern M, Robbins ES. Psychoses in systemic lupus erythematosus. *Arch Gen Psychiatry* 1960;3:205–212.
94. Fessel WJ, Solomon GF. Psychosis and systemic lupus erythematosus: review of the literature and case report. *CA Med* 1960; 92:266–270.
95. Tumulty PA. The clinical course of systemic lupus erythematosus. *JAMA* 1954;156:947–953.
96. Glazer GH. Lesions of the central nervous system in disseminated systemic lupus erythematosus. *Arch Neurol* 1952;67: 7–45.
97. Hanrahan GE. Three cases of disseminated lupus erythematosus with psychosis. *Can Med Assoc J* 1954;71:3–74.
98. Guze SB. The occurrence of psychiatric illness in systemic lupus erythematosus. *Am J Psychiatry* 1967;123:15–62.
99. Bach M, Winkelmann G, Lurhmann R. 20S small nuclear ribonucleoprotein U5 shows a surprisingly complex protein composition. *Proc Natl Acad Sci USA* 1989;86:6038–6042.
100. Baker M. Psychopathology in systemic lupus erythematosus. I. Psychiatric observations. *Semin Arthritis Rheum* 1973;3: 95–110.
101. Ward MM, Studenski S. The time course of acute psychiatric episodes in SLE. *J Rheumatol* 1991;18:535–539.
101a. Karassa FB, Ioanndis JP, Touloumi J, et al. Risk factors for central nervous system involvement in SLE. *QJM* 2000;93: 169–174.
102. Hall RCW, Beresford TP. Psychiatric manifestations of physical illness. In: Michels R, Cavenar JO, Brodie HKH, eds. *Psychiatry*, vol 2. Philadelphia: JB Lippincott, 1989:9.
103. Rogers M. Psychiatric aspects. In: Schur P, ed. *Clinical management of systemic lupus erythematosus*. New York: Grune & Stratton, 1983:189–210.
104. Reckart MD, Eisendrath SJ. Exogenous corticosteroid effects on mood and cognition: case presentations. *Int J Psychosom* 1990;37:58–61.
105. Joffe RT, Denicoff KD, Rubinow DR, et al. Mood effects of alternate-day corticosteroid therapy in patients with systemic lupus erythematosus. *Gen Hosp Psychiatry* 1988;10:56–60.
106. Joffe RT, Wolkowitz OM, Rubinow DR, et al. Alternate-day corticosteroid treatment, mood and plasma HVA in patients with systemic lupus erythematosus. *Neuropsychobiology* 1988; 19:17–19.
107. Hall RCW, Popkin MK, Stickney SK, et al. Presentation of the steroid psychoses. *J Nerv Ment Dis* 1979;167:229–236.
108. Varney NR. Reversible steroid dementias in patients without steroid psychosis. *Am J Psychiatry* 1984;141,(3):369–372.
109. Hall RCW. *Psychiatric presentations of medical illness: somatopsychic disorders*. New York: Septrum, 1980.
110. Lewis CD, Laemmli UK. Higher order metaphase chromosome structure: evidence for metalloprotein interactions. *Cell* 1982; 17:849–858.
111. Hall RCW. Psychiatric adverse drug reactions: steroid psychosis. *Clin Adv Psychiatr Disord* 1991;5:2.
112. West SG. Neuropsychiatric lupus. *Rheum Dis North Am* 1994; 20:129–158.
113. Hall RCW, Popkin MK, Kirkpatrick B. Tricyclic exacerbation of steroid psychosis. *J Nerv Ment Dis* 1978;166:738–742.
114. Cornwell CJ, Schmitt MH. Perceived health status, self-esteem and body image in women with rheumatoid arthritis or systemic lupus erythematosus. *Res Nurs Health* 1990;14:991–07.
115. Kronful Z, Schlesser M, Tsuang MT. Catatonia and systemic lupus erythematosus. *Dis Nerv Sys* 1977;38:7–29.
116. Kurokawa Y, Ueno T, Obara T, et al. Hyperkinetic mutism within the scope of consciousness disorder in a case of systemic lupus erythematosus. *Jpn J Psychiatry Neurol* 1989;43:1.
117. Wysenbeek AJ, Leibovici L, Zoldan J. Acute central nervous system complications after pulse steroid therapy in patients with systemic lupus erythematosus. *J Rheumatol* 1990;17:1695–1696.
118. Matsukawa Y, Sawada S, Hayama T, et al. Suicide in patients with SLE: a clinical analysis of seven suicidal patients. *Lupus* 1994;3:31–35.
119. Terao T, Mizuki T, Ohji T, et al. Antidepressant effect of lithium in patients with systemic lupus erythematosus and cerebral infarction treated with corticosteroid. *Br J Psychiatry* 1994;164: 109–111.
120. Kohen M, Asherson RA, Gharaui AE, et al. Lupus psychosis: differentiation from the steroid-induced state. *Clin Exp Rheumatol* 1993;11:323–326.
121. Shiozawa S, Kuroki Y, Kim M, et al. Interferon-alpha in lupus psychosis. *Arthritis Rheum* 1992;35:417–422.
122. Wolkowitz OW. Cognitive effects of corticosteroids. *Am J Psychiatry* 1990;147(10):1297–1303.
123. Newcome JW. Glucocorticoid-induced impairment. *J Neurosci* 1994;14(4):2047–2053.
124. Denburg SD, Carbotte RM, Denburg JA. Cognitive impairment is systemic lupus erythematosus: a neuropsychological study of individual and group deficits. *J Clin Exp Neuropsychol* 1987;9:323–339.
125. Hanly JG, Walsh NM, Fisk JD, et al. Cognitive impairment and autoantibodies in systemic lupus erythematosus. *Br J Rheumatol* 1993;32:291–296.
126. Long AA, Denburg DS, Carbotte RM, et al. Serum lymphocytotoxic antibodies and neurocognitive function in systemic lupus erythematosus. *Ann Rheum Dis* 1990;49:249–253.
127. Denburg SD, Carbotte RM, Long AA, et al. Neuropsychological correlates of serum lymphocytotoxic antibodies in systemic lupus erythematosus. *Brain Behav Immun* 1988;2:222–234.
128. Toussirot E, Figarella-Branger D, Disdier P, et al. Association of cerebral vasculitis with a lupus anticoagulant. A case with brain pathology. *Clin Rheumatol* 1994;13:624–627.
129. Denburg SD, Behmann SA, Carbotte RM, et al. Lymphocyte antigens in neuropsychiatric systemic lupus erythematosus. Relationship of lymphocyte antibody specificities to clinical disease. *Arthritis Rheum* 1994;37:369–375.
130. Teh LS, Hay EM, Amos N, et al. Anti-P antibodies are associated with psychiatric and focal cerebral disorders in patients with systemic lupus erythematosus. *Br J Rheumatol* 1993;32: 287–290.
131. Suenaga R, Abdou NI. Expression of inactive stage anti-dsDNA idiotypes on anti-ssDNA antibodies in lupus patient during active stage of lupus cerebritis. *J Autoimmun* 1992;5:379–392.
132. Hanly JG, Hong C, White TD. Brain synaptosomal antibodies in systemic lupus erythematosus. *Lupus* 1993;2:35–45.
133. Bluestein HG. Antibodies to neurons. In: Wallace DJ, Hahn BH, eds. *Dubois' lupus erythematosus*, 4th ed. Philadelphia: Lea & Febiger, 1993:260–263.
134. Bluestein HG, Williams GW, Steinberg AD. Cerebrospinal fluid antibodies to neuronal cells: association with neuropsychiatric manifestations of systemic lupus erythematosus. *Am J Med* 1981;70:240–246.
135. Kelly MC, Denburg JA. Cerebrospinal fluid immunoglobulins and neuronal antibodies in neuropsychiatric systemic lupus erythematosus and related conditions. *J Rheumatol* 1987;14: 740–744.
136. Hanson VG, Horowitz M, Rosenbluth D, et al. Systemic lupus erythematosus patients with central nervous system involvement show autoantibodies to a 50-KD neuronal membrane protein. *J Exp Med* 1992;176:565–573.

137. Robbins ML, Korngut SE, Bell CL. Antineurofilament antibody evaluation in neuropsychiatric systemic lupus erythematosus. Combination with anticardiolipin antibody assay and magnetic resonance imaging. *Arthritis Rheum* 1988;31:623–631.
138. Koren E, Reichlin MW, Kosec M. Autoantibodies to the ribosomal P proteins react with a plasma membrane-related target on human cells. *J Clin Invest* 1992;89:1236–1241.
139. Hachulla E, Leys D, Deleume JF, et al. Neurologic manifestations associated with antiphospholipid antibodies. Or what remains of neurolupus. *Rev Med Interne* 1995;16:121–130.
140. Jo ER, Shin HJ, Seo JH, et al. A case of cerebral infarction associated with positive antiphospholipid antibody in a systemic lupus patient. *Korean J Intern Med* 1994;9:43–46.
141. Fulham MJ, Gatenby P, Tuck RR. Focal cerebral ischemia and antiphospholipid antibodies: a case for cardiac embolism. *Acta Neurol Scand* 1994;90:417–423.
142. Cauli A, Montaldo C, Peltz MT, et al. Abnormalities of magnetic resonance imaging of the central nervous system in patients with systemic lupus erythematosus correlate with disease severity. *Clin Rheumatol* 1994;13:615–618.
143. Provenzale JM, Heinz ER, Ortel TL, et al. Antiphospholipid antibodies in patients without systemic lupus erythematosus: neuroradiologic findings. *Radiology* 1994;192:531–537.
144. Herranz MT, Rivier G, Khamashta MA, et al. Association between antiphospholipid antibodies and epilepsy in patients with systemic lupus erythematosus. *Arthritis Rheum* 1994;37: 568–571.
145. Sohngen D, Wehmeier A, Specker C, et al. Antiphospholipid antibodies in systemic lupus erythematosus and Sneddon's syndrome. *Semin Thromb Hemostasis* 1994;20:55–63.
146. Golstein M, Meyer O, Bourgeois P, et al. Neurological manifestations of systemic lupus erythematosus: role of antiphospholipid antibodies. *Clin Exp Rheumatol* 1993;11:373–379.
147. Watanabe T, Satoh M, Abe T, et al. Stroke and meningitis in a case of SLE with anti-phospholipid antibodies. *Acta Paediatr Jpn* 1993;35:423–425.
148. Marullo S, Clauvel JP, Intrator L, et al. Lupoid sclerosis with antiphospholipid and antimyelin antibodies. *J Rheumatol* 1993; 20:747–749.
149. Yeh TS, Wang CR, Jeng GW, et al. The study of anticardiolipin antibodies and interleukin-6 in cerebrospinal fluid and blood of Chinese patients with systemic lupus erythematosus and central nervous system involvement. *Autoimmunity* 1994;18:169–175.
150. Liou HH, Wang CR, Chou HC, et al. Anticardiolipin antisera from lupus patients with seizures reduce a GABA receptor-mediated chloride current in snail neurons. *Life Sci* 1994;54: 1119–1125.
151. Love PE, Santoro SA. Antiphospholipid antibodies: anticardiolipin and the lupus anticoagulant in systemic lupus erythematosus (SLE) and in non-SLE disorders. Prevalence and clinical significance. *Ann Intern Med* 1990;112:682–698.
152. Costallat LT, de Oliveira RM, Santiago MB, et al. Neuropsychiatric manifestations of systemic lupus erythematosus: the value of anticardiolipin, antigangliosides and antigalactocerebrosides antibodies. *Clin Rheumatol* 1990;9:489–497.
153. Travkina IV, Ivanova MM, Nasonov EL, et al. The clinico-immunological characteristics of central nervous system involvement in systemic lupus erythematosus: the relationship with antibodies to cardiolipin. *Terapevticheskii Arkhiv* 1992;64: 10–14.
154. Martinez X, Tintore M, Montalban J, et al. Antibodies against gangliosides in patients with SLE and neurological manifestations. *Lupus* 1992;1:299–302.
155. Pereira RM, Yoshinari NJ, De Oliveira RM, et al. Antiganglioside antibodies in patients with neuropsychiatric systemic lupus erythematosus. *Lupus* 1992;1:175–179.
156. Sindern E, Stark E, Haas J, et al. Serum antibodies to GM1 and GM3-gangliosides in systemic lupus erythematosus with chronic inflammatory demyelinating polyradiculoneuropathy. *Acta Neurol Scand* 1991;83(6):399–402.
157. Sirota P, Firer M, Schild K, et al. Increased anti-Sm antibodies in schizophrenic patients and their families. *Prog Neuropsychopharmacol Biol Psychiatry* 1993;17:793–800.
158. Matsunaga K, Kawai T, Kato K, et al. Antimyosin antibodies in CNS-lupus. *Tohoku J Exp Med* 1991;163:211–218.
159. Wichmann Schlipf I, Sanchez Roman J, Castillo Palma MJ, et al. Antiribosomal antibodies and the neurological manifestations in systemic lupus erythematosus. *Med Clin* 1993;100: 81–83.
160. Nojima Y, Minota S, Yamada A, et al. Correlation of antibodies to ribosomal P protein with psychosis in patients with systemic lupus erythematosus. *Ann Rheum Dis* 1992;51:1053–1055.
161. Teh LS. Antiribosomal P antibodies and lupus psychosis. *Ann Rheum Dis* 1992;51:1104.
162. Schneebaum AB, Singleton JD, West SG, et al. Association of psychiatric manifestations with antibodies to ribosomal P proteins in systemic lupus erythematosus. *Am J Med* 1991;90: 54–62.
163. Bonfa E, Elkon KB. Clinical and serologic associations of the antiribosomal P protein antibody. *Arthritis Rheum* 1986;29: 981–985.
164. Bonfa E, Golombek SJ, Kaufman LD. Association between lupus psychosis and anti-ribosomal P protein antibodies. *N Engl J Med* 1987;317:265–271.
165. Tsai CY, Wu TH, Tsai ST, et al. Cerebrospinal fluid interleukin-6, prostaglandin E2 and autoantibodies in patients with neuropsychiatric systemic lupus erythematosus and central nervous system infections. *Scand J Rheumatol* 1994:23:57–63.
166. Alcocer-Varela J, Aleman-Hoey D, Alarcon-Segovia D. Interleukin-1 and interleukin-6 activities are increased in the cerebrospinal fluid of patients with CNS lupus erythematosus and correlate with local late T-cell activation markers. *Lupus* 1992;1: 111–117.
167. Ritchlin CT, Chabot RJ, Alper K, et al. Quantitative electroencephalography. A new approach to the diagnosis of cerebral dysfunction in systemic lupus erythematosus. *Arthritis Rheum* 1992;35:1330–1342.
168. Molad Y, Sidi Y, Gornish M, et al. Lupus anticoagulant: correlation with magnetic resonance imaging of brain lesions. *J Rheumatol* 1992;19:556–561.
169. Fradis M, Podoshi L, Ben-David J. Brain stem auditory evoked potentials with increased stimulus rate in patients suffering from systemic lupus erythematosus. *Laryngoscope* 1989;99: 325–329.
170. Mongey AB, Glenn D, Hutchinson M. Clinical neurophysiology in the assessment of neurological symptoms in systemic lupus erythematosus. *Rheumatol Int* 1987;7:49–52.
171. Wallace D. Personal correspondence, September 1991.
172. Wallace D, Metzger A, Pistiner M, et al. Lupus erythematosus in the 1980: a survey of 570 patients. *Semin Arthritis Rheum* 1991;21:55–64.
173. Mulherin D, Doherty E, O'Connell A, et al. Assessment of cognitive function in patients with systemic lupus erythematosus. *Irish J Med Sci* 1993;162:9–12.
174. Fisk JD, Eastwood B, Sherwood G, et al. Patterns of cognitive impairment in patients with systemic lupus erythematosus. *Br J Rheumatol* 1993;32:458–462.
175. Ginsburg KS, Wright EA, Larson MG, et al. A controlled study of the prevalence of cognitive dysfunction in randomly selected patients with systemic lupus erythematosus. *Arthritis Rheum* 1992;35:776–782.
176. Kozora E, Thompson LL. Analysis of cognitive and psycholog-

ical deficits in systemic lupus erythematosus patients without overt central nervous disease. *Arthritis Rheum* 1996;39(12): 2035–2045.

177. Koffler S. The role of neuropsychological testing in systemic lupus erythematosus. In: Lahita RG, ed. *Systemic lupus erythematosus*. New York: Wiley, 1987:847–853.
178. Waterloo K, Omdal R. Emotional status in systemic lupus erythematosus. *Scand J Rheumatol* 1998;27(6):410–414.
179. Boll TJ. The Halstead-Reitan neuropsychology battery. In: Filskov SB, Boll TJ, eds. *Handbook of clinical neuropsychology*. New York: Wiley, 1981:5–77.
180. Reitan RM. *Manual for administration of neuropsychological test batteries for adults and children*. Indianapolis: privately printed, not dated.
181. Golden CJ, Moses JA, Fishburn FJ, et al. Cross-validation of the Luria-Nebraska neuropsychological battery for the presence, lateralization, and localization of brain damage. *J Consult Clin Psychol* 1981;49:491–507.
182. Vincente P, Kennelly MA, Golden CJ, et al. The relationship of the Halstead-Reitan neuropsychological battery and the Luria-Nebraska neuropsychological battery (preliminary report). *Clin Neuropsychol* 1980;2:140–141.
183. Kaplan E. A process approach to neuropsychology. In: Ball T, Briant K, eds. *Clinical neuropsychology and BF: research measurement and practice*. Washington, DC: American Psychological Association, 1988.
184. Papero PH, Bluestein HG, White P, et al. Neuropsychological deficits and antineuronal antibodies in pediatric systemic lupus erythematosus. *Clin Exp Rheumatol* 1990;8:417–424.
185. Sobota WL, Brickman CM, Doyle TH, et al. Serial neuropsychological examination during fluctuating systemic lupus erythematosus disease activity. In: Lahita R, ed. *Systemic lupus erythematosus*. New York: Wiley, 1987:847–853.
186. Wekking EM, Nossent JC, van Dam AP, et al. Cognitive and emotional disturbances in systemic lupus erythematosus. *Psychother Psychosom* 1991;55:126–131.
186a. Hochberg MC. The epidemiology of lupus. In: Wallace DJ, Hahn BH, eds. *Dubois' lupus erythematosus*, 4th ed. Philadelphia: Lea & Febiger, 1993:49–57.
186b. Breitbach SA, Alexander RW, Daltroy LH, et al. Determinants of cognitive performance in systemic lupus erythematosus. *J Clin Exp Neuropsychol* 1998;20(2):157–166.
187. Hay EM. Psychiatric disorder and cognitive impairment in SLE. *Lupus* 1994;3:145–148.
187a. Denburg SD, Carbotte RM, Denburg JA. Psychological aspects of systemic lupus erythematosus: cognitive fucntion, mood and self-report. *J Rheumatol* 1997;24:998–1003.
188. Shapiro HS. *Depression in lupus*. Official information pamphlet issued by the National Lupus Foundation of America Office. Washington, DC: no date.
189. Shapiro HS. Depression in lupus. *Lupus News* 1987;7:3.
190. Shapiro HS. Psychopharmacological effects and considerations of the various medications used in the treatment of SLE. In: *Proceedings of Lupus News*, vol 10. Washington, DC: Lupus Foundation of America, 1990:2.
191. Denburg SD, Carbotte RM, Denburg JA. Corticosteroids and neuropsychological functioning in patients with systemic lupus erythematosus. *Arthritis Rheum* 1994;37:1311–1320.
192. Temesvari A, Denburg J, Denburg S, et al. Serum lymphocytotoxic antibodies in neuropsychiatric lupus: a serial study. *Clin Immunol Immunopathol* 1983;28:243–251.
193. Liang M, Rogers M, Swafford J, Schur PH. The psychological impact of systemic lupus erythematosus and rheumatoid arthritis. *Arthritis Rheum* 1984;27:13–20.
194. Kremer JM, Rynes RI, Bartholomew LE, et al. Non-organic non-psychotic psychopathology (NONPP) in patients with systemic lupus erythematosus. *Semin Arthritis Rheum* 1981;11: 182–189.
195. Engle EW, Callahan CF, Pincus T, et al. Learn helplessness in systemic lupus erythematosus: analysis the rheumatology attitudes index. *Arthritis Rheum* 1990;33:281.
196. Lorig K, Lonkol L, Gonzalez V. Arthritis patient education: a review of the literature. *Patient Educ Counsel* 1987;10:207–252.
197. Levy M, Eldor A, Lotanc SZ, et al. Circulating anticoagulant and recurrent deep vein thrombosis in a 12-year-old girl. *Eur J Pediatr* 1983;140:343–345.
198. von Brauchitsch H. Antinuclear factor in psychiatric disorders. *Am J Psychiatry* 1972;128:1552–1554.
199. Quismorio FP Jr, Bjarnason DF, Kiely WF, et al. Antinuclear antibodies in chronic psychotic patients treated with chlorpromazine (brief communication). *Am J Psychiatry* 1975;132: 1204–1206.
200. Bluestein HG. Neuropsychiatric disease systemic lupus erythematosus. In: Lahita RG, ed. *Systemic lupus erythematosus*. New York: Wiley, 1987:593–614.
201. Jacobs J, Bernhard M, Delgado A, et al. Screening for organic mental syndromes in the mentally ill. *Ann Intern Med* 1977;86: 40.
202. Andre-Schwartz J, Datta SK, Shoenfeld Y, et al. Binding of cytoskeletal proteins by monoclonal anti-DNA lupus autoantibodies. *Clin Immunol Immunopathol* 1984;31:261–271.
203. Allen TW, Glicksman M. Psychological involvement in systemic lupus erythematosus: a psychometric approach. *Clin Rheumatol Pract* 1986;4:64–70.
204. Lewis HM, Frumess GM. Plaquenil in the treatment of discoid lupus erythematosus: preliminary report. *Arch Dermatol* 1956; 73:576–581.
205. Roehrs T, Zoric FJ, Sicklesteel JM, et al. Effects of hypnotics on memory. *J Clin Psychopharmacol* 1983;3:310–313.
206. Scharf M, Khosia N, Brocker N, et al. Differential amnestic properties of short and long-acting benzodiazepines. *J Clin Psychiatry* 1984;45:51–53.
207. Scharf MB, Khosia N, Lysaght R, et al. Anterograde amnesia with oral lorazepam. *J Clin Psychiatry* 1983;44:362–364.
208. Sha WC, Nelson CA, Newberry RD, et al. Selective expression of an antigen receptor on CD8-bearing T lymphocytes in transgenic mice. *Nature* 1988;335:271–274.
209. Hinrichs JV, Mewaldt SP, Ghoneim MM, et al. Diazepam and leading: assessment of acquisition deficits. *Pharmacol Biochem Behav* 1982;17:165–170.
210. Chandora DB. Delayed diazepam withdrawal syndrome: a case of auditory and visual hallucinations and seizures. *J Med Assoc GA* 1980;69:769–770.
211. Pishkin V, Lovallo WR, Fishkin SM, et al. Residual effects of temazepam and other hypnotic compounds on cognitive function. *J Clin Psychiatry* 1980;41:358–363.
212. Brown J, Lewis V, Brown M, et al. A comparison between transient amnesias induced by two drugs (diazepam or lorazepam) and amnesia of organic origin. *Neuropsychologia* 1982;20:55–70.
213. Levitt JI. Deterioration of renal function after discontinuation of long-term prednisone-azathioprine therapy in primary renal disease. *N Engl J Med* 1970;282:1125–1127.
214. Brooker AE, Wiens AN, Wiens DA. Impaired brain functions due to diazepam and meprobamate abuse in a 53-year-old-male. *J Nerv Ment Dis* 1984;172:498–501.
215. List AF, Doll DC. Thrombosis associated with procainamide-induced lupus anticoagulant. *Acta Hematol* 1989;82:50–52.
216. Roehrs T, McLenaghan A, Koshorek G, et al. Amnesic effects of lormetazepam. *Psychopharmacology* 1984;9(suppl 1):165–172.
217. Shapiro HS. Psychiatric side effects and problems associated with drugs used in the treatment of SLE. *Lupus* 1990;912.
218. Juhl RP, Daugherty VM, Kroboth PD. Incidence of next-day

anterograde amnesia caused by fluorazepam hydrochloride and triazolam. *Clin Pharm* 1984;3:622–625.
219. Liu S, Miller N, Waye JD. Retrograde amnesia effects of intravenous diazepam in endoscopy patients. *Gastrointest Endosc* 1984:30:340–342.
220. Van-Sweden B. Toxic ictal confusion in middle age: treatment with benzodiazepines. *J Neurol Neurosurg Psychiatry* 1985;48: 472–476.
221. Mac DS, Kumar R, Goodwin DW. Anterograde amnesia with oral lorazepam. *J Clin Psychiatry* 1985;46:137–138.
222. Sandyk R. Transient global amnesia induced by lorazepam. *Clin Neuropharmacol* 1985;8:297–298.
223. Schmidt S, Welcker M, Greil W, et al. Carbamazepine-induced systemic lupus erythematosus. *Br J Psychiatry* 1992;161: 560–561.
224. Shapiro H. Personal correspondence.
225. Shapiro H. *Psych side effects of medicines used in S.L.E. Challenges of lupus, insights and hope*. Boulder, CO: Avery Press, 1999: 163–169.
226. Denburg JA, Behmann SA. Lymphocyte and neuronal antigens in neuropsychiatric lupus: presence of an elutable, immunoprecipitable lymphocyte/neuronal 52kD reactivity. *Ann Rheumatic Dis* 1994;53:304–308.
227. Hirohata S, Kosaka M. Association of anti-Sm antibodies with organic brain syndrome secondary to systemic lupus erythematosus. *Lancet* 1994;343:796.
228. Bland JH. *Clinical recognition and management of disturbances of body fluids*, 2nd ed. Philadelphia: WB Saunders, 1956:101.
229. Decaux G, Unger J, Marneffe C. Psychosis, central hyperventilation and inappropriate secretion of antidiuretic hormone in systemic lupus erythematosus. *Postgrad Med J* 1981;57: 719–720.
230. Wynn V, Rob CG. Water intoxication: differential diagnosis of the hypotonic syndromes. *Lancet* 1954;1:587–594.
231. Kaplan AP, Curl FD, Decker JL. Central hyperventilation and inappropriate antidiuretic hormone secretion in systemic lupus erythematosus. *Am J Med* 1970;48:661–667.
232. Dubois EL. Systemic lupus erythematosus: recent advances in its diagnosis and treatment. *Ann Intern Med* 1951;45:163.
232a. Rudin DO. The choroid plexus and systemic disease in mental illness. I. Systemic lupus erythematosus: a combined transport dysfunction model for schizophrenia. *Biol Psych* 1981;16: 673–680.
233. How A, Den PD, Liao SK, et al. Antineuronal antibodies in neuropsychiatric systemic lupus erythematosus. *Arthritis Rheum* 1985;28:789–795.
234. Stoppe G, Wildhagen K, Seidel JW, et al. Positron emission tomography in neuropsychiatric lupus erythematosus. *Neurology* 1990;40:304–308.
235. Sibbitt WL Jr, Sibbitt RR, Griffey RH, et al. Magnetic resonance and computed tomographic imaging in the evaluation of acute neuropsychiatric disease in systemic lupus erythematosus. *Ann Rheum Dis* 1989;48:1014–1022.
236. Jarek MJ, West SG, Baker MR, et al. Magnetic resonance imaging in systemic lupus erythematosus patients without a history of neuropsychiatric lupus erythematosus. *Arthritis Rheum* 1994; 37:1609–1613.
237. Salmaggi A, Lamperti E, Eoli M, et al. Spinal cord involvement and systemic lupus erythematosus: clinical and magnetic resonance finding in 5 patients. *Clin Exp Rheumatol* 1994:12: 389–394.
238. Ishikawa O, Ohnishi K, Miyachi Y, et al. Cerebral lesions in systemic lupus erythematosus detected by magnetic resonance imaging. Relationship to anticardiolipin antibody. *J Rheumatol* 1994;21:87–90.
239. Rubbert A, Marienhagen J, Pirner K, et al. Single-photon-emission computed tomography analysis of cerebral blood flow in the evaluation of central nervous system involvement in patients with systemic lupus erythematosus. *Arthritis Rheum* 1993; 36(9):1253–1262.
240. Emmi L, Bramati M, De Cristofaro MT, et al. MRI and SPECT investigations of the CNS in SLE patients. *Clin Exp Rheumatol* 1993;11:13–20.
241. Sibbitt WK Jr, Sibbitt RR. Magnetic resonance spectroscopy and positron emission tomography scanning in neuropsychiatric systemic lupus erythematosus. *Rheum Dis Clin North Am* 1993;19:851–868.
242. Stimmler MM, Coletti PM, Quismorio FP Jr. Magnetic resonance imaging of the brain in neuropsychiatric systemic lupus erythematosus. *Semin Arthritis Rheum* 1993;22:335–349.
243. Lancman ME, Pomeraniec C, Norscini J. Magnetic resonance imaging findings in lupus ataxia. *Acta Neurol Scand* 1992;86: 425–426.
244. Rogers MP, Waterhouse E, Nagel JS, et al. I-123 iofetamine SPECT scan in systemic lupus erythematosus patients with cognitive and other minor neuropsychiatric symptoms: a pilot study. *Lupus* 1992;1:215–219.
245. Forrett-Kaminsky MC, Scherer C, Kaminsky P, et al. Magnetic resonance imaging in lupic chorea. *Rev Neurol* 1992;148: 383–384.
246. Aisen AM, Gabrielsen JO, McCune WJ. MR imaging of systemic lupus erythematosus involving the brain. *AJR* 1985;144: 1027–1031.
247. Bell CL, Partington C, Robbins M, et al. Magnetic resonance imaging of central nervous system lesions in patients with lupus erythematosus. Correlation with clinical remission and antineurofilament and anticardiolipin antibody titers. *Arthritis Rheum* 1991;34:432–441.
248. Jacobs L, Kinkel PR, Costello PB. Central nervous system lupus erythematosus: the value of magnetic resonance imaging. *J Rheumatol* 1988;15:601–606.
249. McCune WJ, MacGuire A, Aisen A. Identification of brain lesions in neuropsychiatric lupus erythematosus by magnetic resonance scanning. *Arthritis Rheum* 1988;31:159–166.
250. Sewell KL, Livneh A, Aranow CB. Magnetic resonance imaging versus computer tomographic scanning in neuropsychiatric systemic lupus erythematosus. *Am J Med* 1989;86:625–626.
251. Vermess M, Bernstein RM, Bydder GM. Nuclear magnetic resonance (NMR) imaging of the brain in systemic lupus erythematosus. *J Comput Assist Tomogr* 1983;7:461–467.
252. Caminero AB, Vivancos F, Diez Tejedor E, et al. Atypical neuroradiologic manifestation of systemic lupus erythematosus. *Arch Neurobiol* 1992;55:270–275.
253. Yang WT, Daly BD, Li EK, et al. Cranial computer tomography in the assessment of neurological complications in critically ill patients with systemic lupus erythematosus. *Anaesth Intensive Care* 1993;21:400–404.
254. Carbotte RM, Denburg SD, Denburg JA, et al. Fluctuating cognitive abnormalities and cerebral glucose metabolism in neuropsychiatric systemic lupus erythematosus. *J Neurol Neurosurg Psychiatry* 1992;55:1054–1059.
255. Ishikawa A, Okada J, Kondo H, et al. Abnormal findings of magnetic resonance imaging (MRI) in patients with systemic lupus erythematosus involving the brain. *Ryumachi* 1992;32: 191–199.
256. Miller DH, Buchanan N. Barker G, et al. Gadolinium-enhanced magnetic resonance imaging of the central nervous system in systemic lupus erythematosus. *J Neurol* 1992;239: 460–464.
257. Sibbitt JR, Sibbitt R, Brooks. Neuroimaging in neuropsychiatric systemic lupus erythematosus. *Arthritis Rheum* 1991; 42(10):2026–2038.

258. Bosma, Rood MJ, Zwinderman AH, et al. Evidence of central nervous system damage in patients with neuropsychiatric SLE, demonstrated by magnetization transfer imaging. *Arthritis Rheum* 2000;43(1):48–54.
259. Reiff A, Miller J, Shaham, et al. Childhood central nervous system lupus; longitudinal assessment using single photon emission computed tomography. *J Rheumatol* 1997;24:2461–2465.
260. Russo R, Gilday D, Laxer RM, et al. Single photon emission computed tomography scanning in childhood systemic lupus erythematosus. *J Rheumatol* 1998;25:576–582.
261. Gonzalez-Crespo MR, Blanco FJ, Ramos A, et al. Magnetic resonance imaging of the brain in SLE. *Br J Rheumatol* 1995;34: 1055–1060.
262. Chinn RJS, Wilkinson ID, Hall-Craggs MA, et al. Magnetic resonance imaging of the brain and cerebral proton spectroscopy in patients with SLE. *Arthritis Rheum* 1997;40(1):33–46.
263. Kozora E, West SG, Kotzin BL, et al. Magnetic resonance imaging abnormalities and cognitive deficits in SLE patients without overt central nervous system disease. *Arthritis Rheum* 1998l41(1):41–47.
264. Otte A, Weiner SM, Hoegerle S, et al. Neuropsychiatric systemic lupus erythematosus before and after immunosuppressive treatment: a FDG PET study. *Lupus* 1998;7:57–59.
265. Hachulla E, Michon-Pasturel U, Leys D, et al. Cerebral magnetic resonance imaging in patients with or without antiphospholipid antibodies. *Lupus* 1998;7:124–131.
266. Sabet A, Sibbitt WL, Stidley CA, et al. Neurometabolite markers of cerebral injury in the antiphospholipid antibody syndrome of SLE. *Stroke* 1998;29:2254–2260.
267. Komatsu N, Kodama K, Yamanouchi N, et al. Decreased regional cerebral metabolic rate for glucose in SLE patients with psychiatric symptoms. *Eur Neurol* 1999;42:41–48.
268. Otte A, Weiner SM, Peter HH, et al. Brain glucose utilization in SLE with neuropsychiatric symptoms: a controlled positron emission tomography study. *Eur J Nucl Med* 1997;24(7): 787–791.
269. de Jong BM, Pruim J, Sinnige LGF, et al. Regional specific changes of cerebral metabolism in SLE identified by positron emission tomography. *Eur Neurol* 1999;41:187–193.
270. Shen YY, Ho YJ, Kao CH, et al. Regional cerebral blood flow in patients with SLE. *J Neuroimag* 1999;9:160–164.
271. Kao CH, Ho YJ, Lan JL, et al. Discrepancy between regional cerebral blood flow and glucose metabolism of the brain in SLE patients with normal brain magnetic resonance imaging findings. *Arthritis Rheum* 1999;42(1):61–68.
272. Petropoulos H, Sibbitt WL, Brooks WM. Automated T(2) quantitation in neuropsychiatric lupus erythematosus: a marker of active disease. *J Magn Reson Imaging* 1999;9:39–43.
273. Szer IS, Miller JH, Rawlings D, et al. Cerebral perfusion abnormalities in children with central nervous system manifestations of lupus detected by single photon emission computer tomography. *J Rheumatol* 1993;20:2143–2148.
274. Griffey RH, Brown MS, Bankhurst AD. Depletion of high-energy phosphates in the central nervous system of patients with systemic lupus erythematosus, as determined by phosphorous-31 nuclear magnetic resonance spectroscopy. *Arthritis Rheum* 1990;33:827–833.
275. Hiraiwau M, Nonaka C, Abe T. Positron emission tomography in systemic lupus erythematosus: relation of cerebral vasculitis to PET finding. *AJNR* 1983;4:541–543.
276. Weiner DK, Allen NB. Large vessel vasculitis of the central nervous system in systemic lupus erythematosus: report and review of the literature. *J Rheumatol* 1991;18:748–751.
277. Kushner MJ, Tobin M, Fazekas F, et al. Cerebral blood flow variations in CNS lupus. *Neurology* 1990;40:99–102.
278. McCune WJ, MacGuire A, Aisen A, et al. Identification of brain lesions in neuropsychiatric systemic lupus erythematosus by magnetic resonance scanning. *Arthritis Rheum* 1988;31: 159–166.
279. Moriwaka F, Tashiro K, Fukazawa T, et al. A case of systemic lupus erythematosus: its clinical and MRI resemblance to multiple sclerosis. *Jpn J Psychiatry Neurol* 1990;44:601–605.
280. Sessoms SL, Kovarsky J. Monthly intravenous cyclophosphamide in the treatment of severe systemic lupus erythematosus. *Clin Exp Rheumatol* 1984;2:247–251.
281. Bambery P, Malhotra S, Kaun U, et al. Anorexia nervosa in a patient with systemic lupus erythematosus. *Rheumatol Int* 1987; 7:177–179.
282. Bovin G, Virstad S, Schrader H. Subdural hematoma presenting in systemic lupus erythematosus. *Cephalgia* 1990;10:25–29.
283. Gossat DM, Walls RS. Systemic lupus erythematosus in later life. *Med J Aust* 1982;1:297–299.
284. Zimmermann B 3rd, Speigel M, Lally EV. Cryptococcal meningitis in systemic lupus erythematosus. *Semin Arthritis Rheum* 1992;22:18–24.
285. Diaz Coto JF, Alpizar Campos R. Central nervous system cryptococcosis in 10 patients with systemic lupus erythematosus. *Rev Clin Esp* 1995;295:12–15.
286. Mok CC, Lau CS, Poon SP. Primary nocardial meningitis in systemic lupus erythematosus. *Br J Rheumatol* 1995;34: 178–181.
287. Soga T, Shirai A. Igarashi T, et al. A case of listeria meningitis associated with systemic lupus erythematosus. *Kansenshogaku Zasshi J Jpn Assoc Infect Dis* 1994;68:411–415.
288. Lammens M, Robberecht W, Waer M, et al. Purulent meningitis due to aspergillosis in a patient with systemic lupus erythematosus. *Clin Neurol Neurosurg* 1992;94:39–43.
289. Nilsson UR, Nilsson B, Storm KE, et al. Hereditary dysfunction of the third component of complement association with a systemic lupus erythematosus-like syndrome and meningococcal meningitis. *Arthritis Rheum* 1992;35:580–586.
290. Lewis S, Goldman R, Cronstein B. Acute syphilitic meningitis in a patient with systemic lupus erythematosus. *J Rheumatol* 1993;20:870–871.
291. Feinman MC, Friedberg MA, Schwartz JC, et al. Central nervous system herpes virus infection in systemic lupus erythematosus: diagnosis by endoretinal biopsy. *J Rheumatol* 1993;20: 1058–1061.
292. Nelson A, Fogel B. Faust D. Bedside cognitive screening instruments. *J Nerv Mental Dis* 1986;174:73–83.
293. Straub RL, Black FW. Mental status examination. In: *Organic brain syndrome.* 1990.
294. Fava GA, Sonino N. Hypothalamic-pituitary-adrenal axis disturbances in depression. *IRCS Med Sci* 1986;14:1058–1061.
295. Bowie PCW, Beaini AY. Normalization of dexamethasone suppression test: a correlate with clinical improvement in primary depressives. *Psychiatry* 1985;147:30–35.
296. Charles GA, Schittecatte M, Rush AJ, et al. Persistent cortisol non-suppression after clinical recovery predicts symptomatic relapse in unipolar depression. *J Affect Disord* 1989;17:271–278.
297. Holsboer F, Liebl R, Hofschuster E. Repeated dexamethasone suppression test during depressive illness. *J Affect Disord* 1982; 4:93–101.
298. Holsboer F, Steiger A, Maier W. Four cases of reversion to abnormal dexamethasone suppression test response as indicator of clinical relapse. *Biol Psychiatry* 1983;18:911–916.
299. Targum SD. Persistent neuroendocrine dysregulation in major depressive disorder: a marker for early relapse. *Biol Psychiatry* 1984;19:305–318.
300. Yerevanian BI, Olafsdottir H, Milanese E, et al. Normalization of the dexamethasone suppression test at discharge from hospital. *J Affect Disord* 1983;5:191–197.

301. Waterloo K, Omdal R, Jacobsen EA, et al. Cerebral computed tomography and electroencephalography compared with neuropsychological findings in systemic lupus erythematosus. *J Neurol* 1999;246:706–711.
302. Glanz BI, Schur PH, Koshbin. EEG abnormalities in systemic lupus erythematosus. *Clin Electroencephalogr* 1999;29(3):128–130.
303. Calabrese LV, Stern TA. Neuropsychiatric manifestations of SLE. *Psychosomatics* 1995;36:344–359.
304. Estes D, Christian CL. The natural history of systemic lupus erythematosus by prospective analysis. *Medicine* 1971;50:85–95.
305. Feinglass EJ, Amett FC, Dorsch CA, et al. Neuropsychiatric manifestations of SLE: diagnosis, clinical spectrum, and relationship to other features of the disease. *Medicine* 1976;55:323–339.
306. Kovacs J, Urowitz MB, Gladman DD. Dilemmas in neuropsychiatric lupus. *Rheum Dis Clin North Am* 1993;19:795–814.
307. Abel T, Gladman DD, Urowitz MB. Neuropsychiatric lupus. *J Rheumatol* 1980;7:325–333.
308. Johnson RT, Richardson EP. The neurological manifestations of SLE: a clinical-pathological study of 24 cases and review of the literature. *Medicine* 1968;47:337–369.
309. Csepany T, Valikovics A, Fulesdi B, et al. Transcranial Doppler may reveal asymptomatic cerebral vasculopathy in SLE. *Cerebrovasc Dis* 1995;5:178–181.
310. Shapiro HS. Personality traits that often interfere with the lupus patient's adjustment. Reprinted in *Lupus/Scleroderma Bulletin*, Australia (publication SAW 2654), April 1989.
311. Miller IW, Morman WH. Learned helplessness in humans: a review and attribution theory model. *Psychol Bull* 1979;86: 93–118.
312. Nashel D, Ulmer C. Systemic lupus erythematosus. Important considerations in the adolescent. *J Adolesc Health Care* 1982;2: 273.
313. Silber TJ, Chatoor I, White PH. Psychiatric manifestations of systemic lupus erythematosus in children and adolescents: a review. *Clin Pediatr* 1984;23:331–335.
314. Ascheim JH. The adolescent and systemic lupus erythematosus: a developmental and educational approach. *Issues Compr Pediatr Nurs* 1981;5:293–307.
315. Pincus T, Summey JA, Soraci SA, et al. Assessment of patient satisfaction in activities of daily living using a modified Stanford Health Assessment Questionnaire. *Arthritis Rheum* 1983;26: 1346–1353.
316. Stein H, Walters K, Dillon A, et al. Systemic lupus erythematosus: a medical and social profile. *J Rheumatol* 1986;13:570–576.
317. Goodwin J, Goodwin J, Kellner R. Psychiatric symptoms in disliked medical patients. *JAMA* 1979;241:11–17.
318. Krupp LB, LaRocca NG, Muir-Nash J, et al. The fatigue severity scale. Application to patients with multiple sclerosis and systemic lupus erythematosus. *Arch Neurol* 1989;46:1121–1123.
319. Joyce K, Berkebile C, Hastings C, et al. Heath status and disease activity in SLE. *Arthritis Care Res* 1989;2:65–69.
320. Hochberg MC, Sutton JD. Physical disability and psychosocial dysfunction in systemic lupus erythematosus. *J Rheumatol* 1988;15:959–964.
321. Esdaile JM, Sampalis JS, Lacaille D, et al. The relationship of socioeconomic status to subsequent health status in systemic lupus erythematosus. *Arthritis Rheum* 1988;31:423–427(abst).
322. Pfeiffer CA. The impact of gender-role socialization on women coping with a rheumatic disease. *Clin Rheumatol Pract* 1986; 1:75–80.
323. Curry SL, Levine SB, Corty E, et al. The impact of systemic lupus erythematosus on women's sexual functioning. *J Rheumatol* 1994;21:2254–2260.
324. Shapiro HS. Rap groups: aid to lupus management. *Newsletter of the British Columbia Association (Vancouver), The Lupus Lighthouse* 1986;7:4.
325. Braden CJ, McGlone K, Pennington F. Specific psychosocial and behavioral outcomes from the systemic lupus erythematosus self-help course. *Health Ed Q* 1993;20:29–41.
326. Shrier L. How and why hypnosis may help. *Lupus News* 1999; 19(3):1–11.
327. Shapiro HS. The physicians' ordeal on becoming a patient. Reprint *Minn News and Notes* (LFA), 1983:40, from an address before the National Lupus Foundation of America, Annual Meeting, July 1983.
328. Aladjem H. *The challenges of lupus: insights and hope.* New York: Avery Pub 1999;6:187–190.
329. Balch TS. *The challenges of lupus: insights, and hope.* New York: Avery Pub 1999;6:191–194.
330. Rogers MP. *The challenges of lupus: insights, and hope.* New York: Avery Pub 1999;6:195–197.
331. Schur PH. *The challenges of lupus: insights, and hope.* New York: Avery Pub 1999;6:205–211.
332. Shapiro HS. *The challenges of lupus: insights and hope.* New York: Avery Pub 1999;6:199–203.
333. Ganz VH, Gurland BJ, Beming WE, et al. The study of psychiatric symptoms of systemic lupus erythematosus. *Psychosom Med* 1972;34:207.

37

HEAD AND NECK FINDINGS IN SYSTEMIC LUPUS ERYTHEMATOSUS: SJÖGREN'S SYNDROME AND THE EYE, EAR, AND LARYNX

ROBERT FOX
PAUL MICHELSON
DANIEL J. WALLACE

HISTORY

The first descriptions of Sjögren's were reported by European clinicians between 1882 and 1925 (1). In 1892, Mikulicz observed a man with bilateral parotid and lachrymal gland enlargement that was associated with massive round-cell infiltration. In 1925, Gougerot described three patients with salivary and mucous-gland atrophy and insufficiency progressing to dryness. Two years later, Houwer emphasized the association of filamentary keratitis, which is the major ocular manifestation of the syndrome, with chronic arthritis. In 1933, Henrik Sjögren reported detailed clinical and histologic findings in 19 women with xerostomia and keratoconjunctivitis sicca, of whom 13 had chronic arthritis. In 1953, Morgan and Castleman (2) concluded that Sjögren's syndrome (SS) and Mikulicz's disease were the same entity. The distinction between primary and secondary SS was suggested by Bloch in 1960 (3).

The concurrence of SS and systemic lupus erythematosus (SLE) was described first by Morgan in 1954 (4), and numerous investigators in the 1950s and 1960s observed lupus erythematosus (LE) cells in patients with SS and lupuslike features. The incidence of SLE in patients with SS has been estimated to be about 20%.

SJÖGREN'S SYNDROME

SLE patients may exhibit a wide range of symptoms involving the head and neck. These include local manifestations of their systemic autoimmune disease, infectious processes related to immune suppression, and noninfectious complications from their medications. The differential diagnosis and treatment of these problems is often difficult.

This chapter will focus on SS, which is characterized by dry eyes (xerostomia) and dry mouth (xerostomia) resulting from lymphocytic infiltrates of the lacrimal and salivary glands (5). SS is divided into a primary form (1° SS) and secondary form (2° SS). In 2° SS, the sicca symptoms are associated with other well-defined autoimmune diseases such as rheumatoid arthritis (RA), SLE, progressive systemic sclerosis (PSS), polymyositis, or biliary cirrhosis. Dryness can result from many other causes including drugs with anticholinergic side effects (including certain herbal supplements) and is associated with infections such as hepatitis C or retroviruses, autonomic neuropathy, depression, and fibromyalgia.

In many instances, the patient may have low-titer, positive antinuclear antibodies (ANA) and have vague symptoms of dryness, fatigue, and myalgia. The differential diagnosis of these patients represents a challenge because these symptoms are so common in the population and "false positive" ANA titers frequently are found in the normal population (6). For example, low-titer antinuclear antibodies (1:40) are found in up to 23% of normals, and the misleading "cut off" values that come as an interpretation with these laboratory reports results in confusion of the patient and the referring physicians (6). Even at a higher titer ANA of 1:640, the actual risk for developing SLE (or SS) is less than 1 in 100 (7). Thus, it needs to be emphasized that an ANA may be used to confirm the clinical diagnosis of SLE or SS, but these tests lack the specificity to serve as a sole basis for diagnosis (7). Further, enzyme-linked assays (ELISAs) to detect antibodies to SS-A and SS-B antigens depend heavily on the quality of the antigen used in the assay and have great variability (discussed below) (8). There is a frequent misconception that commercial kits for detection of these autoantibodies utilized cloned gene products and thus are entirely reliable; in fact, difficulties with production of cloned antigens (particularly because of the importance of their structural folding and their glycosylation) has led to difficulty in their use in the clinical laboratory and most commercial assays continue to depend on antigens prepared by affinity chromatography (8). Thus, there is lack of reproducibility for the detection of antibody to SS-A and SS-B, resulting in further confusion in diagnosis when antibody titers are used as a primary tool for diagnosis. In summary, there are several "take home lessons" for rheumatologists: (i) all patients with complaints of dryness do not suffer from a systemic autoimmune disease but it is important that all patients with objective ocular and oral dryness deserve instruction in conservative treatment; and (ii) the most difficult diagnostic problem is the decision whether symptoms are from a systemic autoimmune process and thus require a more aggressive therapeutic intervention; and (iii) laboratory methods can be used to support a clinical diagnosis but should not be the sole basis for diagnosis.

Also, it is important to recognize that the clinical presentation and severity of SS appears to vary in different ethnic groups and in different parts of the world. For example, in ethnic groups such as Greek or Chinese SS patients there is a higher incidence of severe interstitial nephritis (patients often present with severe hypokalemia) (9) and the types of rashes (i.e., facial erythema annulare) is more common in Japanese SS patients (10) than seen in Caucasion SS patients. Different viruses [ranging from hepatitis C, HTLV-1, and human immunodeficiency virus (HIV)] that can mimic SS have very different incidence among these groups. As the world becomes increasingly filled with international travelers, a spectrum of patients and medications not used in the United States (particular herbal and "nutritional" medications) may increasingly lead to confusion in diagnosis.

TABLE 37.1. SAN DIEGO CRITERIA FOR DIAGNOSIS OF SJÖGREN'S SYNDROME*,**

I. Primary Sjögren's Syndrome (SS)
   A. Symptoms and objective signs of ocular dryness
      1. Schirmer's test <8 mm wetting per 5 minutes (without topical anesthetic) *and*
      2. Positive Rose Bengal or staining of cornea *or* conjunctiva to demonstrate keratoconjunctivitis sicca
   B. Symptoms and objective signs of dry mouth
      1. Decreased parotid flow rate using Lashley cups or other methods *and*
      2. Abnormal biopsy of minor salivary gland (focus score of ≥2 based on average of four evaluable lobules)
   C. Evidence of a systemic autoimmune disorder
      1. Elevated rheumatoid factor ≥1:320 *or*
      2. Elevated antinuclear antibody ≥1:320 *or*
      3. Presence of anti-SS-A (Ro) or anti-SS-B (La) antibodies
II. Secondary SS
   Characteristic signs and symptoms of SS (described above) plus clinical features sufficient to allow a diagnosis of RA, SLE, polymyositis, scleroderma, or biliary cirrhosis.
III. Exclusions
   Hepatitis C, HIV, HTLV-1, sarcoidosis, preexistent lymphoma, other known causes of keratitis sicca or salivary gland enlargement.

*Definite Sjögren's syndrome requires objective evidence of dryness of eyes/mouth and a systemic autoimmune process including a characteristic minor salivary gland biopsy.
**Probable Sjögren's syndrome does not require a minor salivary gland biopsy but can be diagnosed with demonstration of decreased salivary function (I-B-1)
HIV, human immunodeficiency virus; RA, rheumatoid arthritis; SLE, systemic lupus erythematosus
From Talal N. Sjögren's syndrome: historical overview and clinical spectrum of disease. *Rheum Dis Clin North Am* 1992;18:507–515, with permission.

The Controversy Regarding Diagnostic Criteria For Sjögren's Syndrome

Although the ophthalmic component [i.e., keratoconjunctivitis sicca (KCS)] is well defined, the criteria for classifying the oral component of SS remains controversial and thus no uniform classification system for SS exists (11). For example, two very different criteria for SS are listed in the most recent issue of the *Primer of Rheumatic Diseases* (one in the text and one in the appendix). On the one hand, the San Diego or San Francisco criteria (described below) for SS require objective evidence of KCS, xerostomia, the presence of autoantibodies, or histologic evidence such as minor salivary-gland biopsy (11). For diagnosis of "definite" SS, a characteristic minor salivary-gland biopsy is suggested for research protocols, but is not required for routine clinical diagnosis or management (Table 37.1). On the other hand, the original proposed SS criteria by the European Study Group (EEC criteria) (12) can be fulfilled in the absence of biopsy or autoantibodies (Table 37.2). A further difference between the San Diego and EEC criteria is the exclusion of patients with hepatitis C infection or retroviral infection in the San Diego criteria (but not in the EEC criteria). The incidence of SS in patients according to the San Diego criteria is about 0.5%, while the incidence using the EEC criteria is 3% to 5% of the adult population; thus there is almost a tenfold difference in patients fulfilling "criteria" (11). This lack of uniform classification criteria has led to confusion in clinical practice and in the research literature (13). For example, the incidence of a particular disease association (i.e., liver involvement, neurologic symptoms, or lymphoma) and the response to a particular therapy are directly affected by the inclusion and exclusion criteria for the study group.

A recent suggestion for modification of the EEC criteria (14) to require the presence of antibody against SS-A (Ro) antigen or a positive minor salivary-gland biopsy (focus score of 1 or greater) will lead to much closer agreement of criteria for diagnosis. However presently, rheumatologists must review published studies on treatment with careful attention to differences in inclusion and exclusion diagnostic criteria.

TABLE 37.2. PRELIMINARY CLASSIFICATION CRITERIA DEVELOPED BY THE EEC

I. Primary Sjögren's Syndrome (SS) (if at least 4 items present)
  A. Ocular symptoms (at least 1 present)
    1. Daily, persistent, troublesome dry eyes for more than 3 months
    2. Recurrent sensation of sand or gravel in the eyes
    3. Use of a tear substitute more than 3 times a day
  B. Oral symptoms (at least 1 present)
    1. Daily feeling of dry mouth for at least 3 months
    2. Recurrent feeling of swollen salivary glands as an adult
    3. Drink liquids to aid in washing down dry foods
  C. Objective evidence of dry eyes (at least 1 present)
    1. Schirmer I test
    2. Rose Bengal
    3. Lacrimal gland biopsy with focus score ≥1
  D. Objective evidence of salivary gland involvement (at least 1 present)
    1. Salivary gland scintography
    2. Parotid sialography
    3. Unstimulated whole sialometry (≤1.5 mL per 15 minutes)
  E. Laboratory Abnormality (at least 1 present)
    1. anti-SS-A or anti-SS-B antibody
    2. Antinuclear antibody (ANA)
    3. IgM rheumatoid factor (anti-IgG Fc)

From Vitali et al. (manuscript submitted).

Differential Diagnosis Of Primary Sjögren's Syndrome And Sjögren's Syndrome With Systemic Lupus Erythematosus

The rheumatologist often is faced with the diagnostic difficulty of distinguishing 1° SS from 2° SS associated with SLE. These patients frequently share similar symptoms (arthralgias, myalgias, fatigue, rashes, and visceral involvement from vasculitis) as well as laboratory tests including positive ANA and antibody to SS-A (Ro) (15). Indeed, it has been argued that SLE represents a spectrum of patients where subsets are "artificially" subdivided on the basis of their serology and the serology (i.e., antibody against SS-A, etc.) correlates better with their genotype than with their clinical features (16,17). If one accepts the premise that patients with SLE constitute a heterogeneous group of patients in terms of pattern of organ involvement and ANAs (17), then it reasonably can be argued that 1° SS patients represent a *forme fruste* of SLE where patients have only four of the necessary five criteria for diagnosis of SLE (5). The group of patients with 1° SS is genetically heterogeneous even among patients who have similar ethnic backgrounds. However, a significant proportion of Caucasion 1° SS patients have similar human leukocyte antigen (HLA) associations (HLA-DR3 and the linkage associated DQ alleles) that are found in a subset of SLE patients (18,19). Further, our experience with multiplex families (i.e., one member with 1° SS and another member with autoimmune disease such as RA, SLE, or scleroderma) in China (20) and in another study of a multiplex Caucasion family (21), family members (siblings, mothers, daughters) of 1° SS patients had an almost equal frequency of 1° SS or SLE. Similarly, in a large, multiplex family with multiple cases of SLE, family members with SS were noted (22). Thus, it might be postulated that certain genetic factors predispose to either 1° SS or a subset of SLE, while environmental (or gene recombination events) then propel the genetically susceptible patient down the clinical pathway of either 1° SS or SLE. In this regard, the close overlap of clinical symptoms of 1° SS and a subset of SLE would be expected. We would propose that SS develops in those patients with a more lymphocyte-aggressive disease, as manifested by the infiltration of lymphocytes (predominantly CD4+ T cells) into tissues normally lacking lymphoid infiltrates (i.e., lacrimal and salivary glands, as well as lung or renal parenchyma), as extension of this hypothesis is the increased frequency of lymphoma in SS patients (23). In comparison, many of the manifestations of SLE patients appear to result from pathogenetic antibodies that lead to immune-complex disease or specific antibodies against platelets or glomerular antigens. Although there is clearly a great deal of overlap in 1° SS and SLE in this regard, this is a relatively simple model for prognostically evaluating patients' symptoms (e.g., interstitial pneumonitis, interstitial nephritis, or increased lymphoma) with features of SS or SLE. Some differential points between primary SS and secondary SS with SLE are listed in Table 37.3.

TABLE 37.3. DIFFERENTIAL POINTS BETWEEN PRIMARY SJÖGREN'S AND SECONDARY SJÖGREN'S WITH SYSTEMIC LUPUS ERYTHEMATOSUS

1. Sjögren's syndrome (SS) is a systemic autoimmune disease characterized by objective signs of ocular and oral dryness.
2. It often is difficult to distinguish primary SS from patients with systemic lupus erythematosus (SLE) because a subset of SLE patients have secondary SS and have antibody to SS-A. Glomerulonephritis is more common in SLE and interstitial nephritis is more common in SS. Certain types of skin rashes are more common in SS patients (esp. hyperglobulemic purpura) than in SLE (malar rashes), while both may have vasculitis rashes.
3. It often is difficult to distinguish primary SS, secondary SS, and fibromyalgia, where sicca symptoms are common and low-titer antinuclear antibody (ANA) are relatively common (up to 20% of normal adults at titer 1:40 and 5% at titer 1:160); minor salivary gland biopsies and antibodies against SS-A help distinguish SS from fibromyalgia.
4. The lip biopsy must be read by individuals experienced in their evaluation, because only focal lymphocytic infiltrates should be quantitated and nonfocal infiltrates are nonspecific.
5. Hepatitis C patients often have sicca symptoms and a subset have a positive ANA.
6. Symptoms of ocular irritation may result from blepharitis in addition to acqueous tear deficiency and symptoms of oral discomfort may be from superimposed oral candida infections.

Presently, the label "Sjögren's syndrome" alerts the rheumatologist to the particular ocular and oral needs of the patient with sicca symptoms as well as to their particular problems of lymphoproliferative disorders. Thus, it is important for rheumatologists not to get bogged down in currently fashionable debates over classification criteria. The key point is that diseases are best classified by etiology and that the etiology of SLE and SS remains unknown; thus, we are left with classifying clusters of symptoms/signs and the key point is how to determine prognosis and treatment.

The pattern of rashes in 1° SS patients differs somewhat from those in most SLE patients. Malar rashes are more common in SLE, because of the presence of malar rash serving as criteria for SLE. However, the malar rash of SLE must be distinguished from rosacea, which can contribute to blepharitis and ocular symptoms mimicking 1° SS (24). Patients with 1° SS have a relatively higher incidence of hyperglobulinemic purpura based on retrospective studies (25); and the purpura may be associated with a type II mixed cryoglobulin (26) containing a monoclonal rheumatoid factor with a particular idiotype (27). In Japanese patients, particular types of rashes such as erythema annulare (particularly with location on the face) are more common in SS than SLE patients) (10,28). In the past, a psoriaform skin rash termed "subacute" lupus when associated with a negative ANA (done using mouse kidney substrate) and a positive anti-SS-A antibody (29). These patients had a high frequency of SS-like symptoms. In recent years, a different substrate for detection of ANAs (Hep 2 cells) has been used and patients with "subacute lupus" now are shown to have a positive ANA (30) and are frequently diagnosed as SS (31–33). A wide range of additional skin lesions is found in both SLE and SS, ranging from leukocytoclastic vasculitis to the purpura associated with low platelets (34).

Mouth (intraoral) lesions occur in both SS and SLE. However, the characteristic SLE lesion is an oral ulcer. The most common mouth lesion in SS patients is from oral candida (35). These lesions are recognized by the presence of angular cheilitis and erythematous patches (often resembling telangiectasias) on the hard palate (36). The use of corticosteroids and antibiotics predispose to oral candida in a patient with decreased salivary flow. Also, oral lesions in patients on methotrexate may not be a result of drug allergy but to oral candida.

Sjögren's Syndrome: Pathogenesis of Symptoms

It is important to recognize that SS patients complain about their dry, painful eyes and mouth, while rheumatologists talk about the patient's lacrimal and salivary glands, their autoantibodies and acute phase reactants. The patient is describing ocular symptoms because of increased friction as the eyelid (particularly the upper lid) passes over the orbital globe. When the tear film is inadequate and the "viscosity" of movement between the eyelid and globe is inadequate, the lid adheres to the surface layers of the globe and can actually pull epithelial cells away from the surface layer of the conjunctiva and cornea. It is these epithelial defects that are viewed clinically as "keratoconjunctivitis sicca" and corneal abrasions. As a result of the "insult" to the epithelial surface, an inflammatory response (release of cytokines and influx of inflammatory cells) occurs. As a result of the lack of adequate tear film, the "wounding" process continues and the normal healing process is impaired because an adequate tear film is required to provide "nutritive" and antiinflammatory substances. Thus in SS patients, exposure to certain environmental stresses can lead to KCS lesions, which are very slow to heal.

Similarly, the tongue and buccal mucosal surfaces require lubrication for the tongue to move around the mouth and for the actions of speaking and swallowing. However, there are important differences in the oral symptoms and the ocular symptoms. The eye is a "clean" environment (i.e., not colonized) while the mouth has high levels of resident aerobic and anaerobic organisms. A dry mouth is not necessarily a painful mouth. Common problems in the mouth involve changes in the microbial flora, especially with the emergence of chronic candidiasis (discussed below) or periodontal disease as a result of particular organisms. Further, there are important differences in the types of neural innervation, mucins, cytokines, and enzymes in the secretions of the mouth and the eye.

Normal lacrimal and salivary flow is regulated through feedback mechanisms shown schematically in Figure 37.1A. The mucosal surfaces of the eye and mouth are heavily innervated by unmyelinated fibers that carry afferent signals to the lacrimatory or salvatory nuclei located in the medulla. These medullary nuclei, which are part of the autonomic nervous system, are influenced by higher cortical inputs including taste, smell, anxiety, medications, and depression. The efferent neurons innervate both glandular cells and local blood vessels. The blood vessels provide not only water for tears and saliva, but also growth factors including hormones (e.g., insulin) and matrix proteins (e.g., fibronectin and vitronectin) of the lacrimal and salivary glands. In response to neural stimulation through muscarinic M3 receptors and vasoactive intestinal peptide (VIP) receptors, glandular acinar and ductal cells secrete water, proteins, and mucopolysacharides (mucins). This complex mixture forms a hydrated gel that lubricates the ocular surface (i.e., tears) and the oral mucosa (i.e., saliva). In the simplest model of SS (Fig. 37.1B), the lacrimal or salivary gland is incapable of adequate response to neural signals as a consequence of local immune infiltrates and their derived cytokines. The actual processes in SS or autonomic neuropathy are more complicated than indicated in these schematic diagrams, which are designed primarily to emphasize that salivation or lacrimation are part

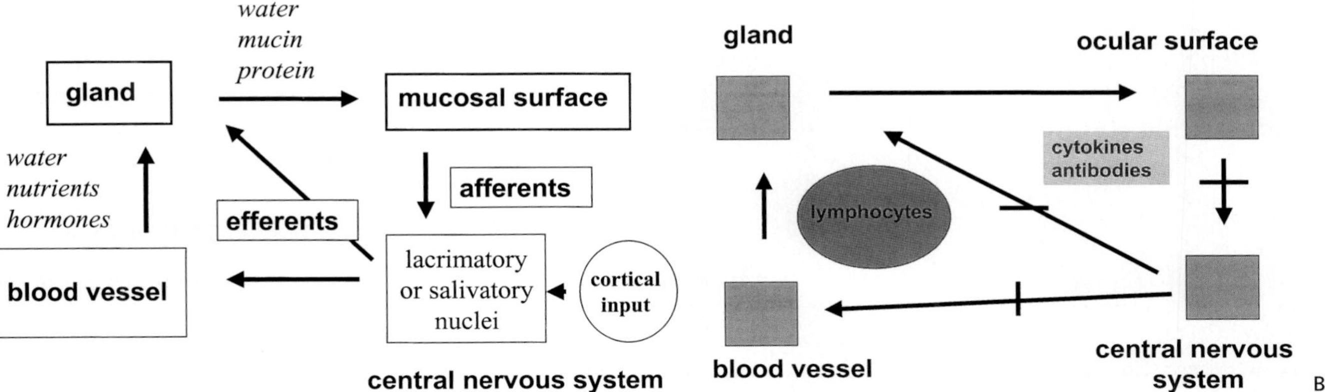

FIGURE 37.1. A, "circuit" that controls normal tear flow or salivation and interruption of the circuit in patients with Sjögren's syndrome. The stimulation of the ocular or oral mucosal surface leads to afferent nerve signals that reach the lacrimatory or salivatory nuclei in the medulla. Efferent neural signals stimulate both blood vessels and glandular epithelial cells. The medullary signal may be affected by cortical inputs that reflect stimuli such as taste, smell, anxiety, or depression. The efferent neural signal to the gland is mediated by acetylcholine. The gland contains recptors for acetylcholine of the muscarinic class, particularly M3 receptors (shown by arrow). **B,** In Sjögren's syndrome, lymphocytic infiltrates in the gland secrete cytokines that inhibit the release of neurotransmitter and the response of receptors that initiate glandular secretion.

of a regulatory circuit involving the central nervous system (37).

The stages in pathogenesis of SS include: (i) the change of small endothelial vessels to high endothelial venules that express adhesive molecules and release chemokines such as RANTES and lymphotactin; (ii) the migration of CD4+ T cells into the gland in the center of the lobule of the lacrimal or salivary gland where they form a cluster (or foci) of lymphocytes; (iii) release of cytokines including interferon gamma and tumor necrosis factor (TNF) -α by the T cells and interleukin 1 (IL-1) by the epithelial cells; (iv) upregulation of HLA-DR, DQ, and invariant chain (Ii) by the epithelial cells and perhaps costimulatory molecules such as B-7; (v) upregulation of perforin and granzyme that may lead to damage of ductal cells; (vi) increased expression of Fas on CD4+ T cells and Fas-ligand on the epithelial cells, that may lead to increased apoptotic death of epithelial cells; (vii) increased production of bcl-2 and bcl-x by the lymphocytes that helps prevent their own apoptosis; and (viii) clonal expansion of B-cell clones and increased risk of karyotypic translocation (t 14;18) associated with transformation to a non-Hodgkin's lymphoma (38). As a result of mutual stimulation of T cells, B cells, and epithelial cells, cytokines such as IL-1, IL-6, and TNF-α are released and lead to increases of acute phase reactants including ESR (fibrinogen) and c-reactive protein that are measured in clinical assays.

Several of the pathogenetic steps are summarized in Table 37.4.

The lymhocytic infiltrates in a minor salivary gland biopsy are shown in Figure 37.2A, in comparison to a normal gland (Fig. 2B). The infiltration of the lymphocytes (shown to be CD4+ T cells by immunohistology) under the basement membrane and in direct contact with the epithe-

TABLE 37.4. PATHOGENETIC FEATURES OF SJÖGREN'S SYNDROME

1. Sjögren's syndrome is a systemic autoimmune disease. The target organs (lacrimal or salivary glands) are accessible to biopsy, making this disease well suited for clinical-pathologic correlations.
2. Biopsies of lacrimal or salivary glands indicate that only about 50% of the acinar or ductal structures are destroyed. Thus, the severe dryness results from dysfunction of the residual glands. This may be the result of release of cytokines, metalloproteinases, or autoantibodies that interfere with glandular function or their response to neurotransmitters.
3. The predominant infiltrate in the glands is CD4+ T cells (memory phenotype) that release Th1-like cytokines. However, the lymphomas that develop with increased frequency are because of B-cell non-Hodgkin's lymphomas.
4. The epithelial cells are not merely innocent targets in the pathogenesis. In animal models, intrinsic defects in glandular development may play a role in generating tissue-specific autoantigens. Early in the disease, chemokines are secreted and later in the disease, the epithelial cells express class II histocompatibility antigens and secrete proinflammatory cytokines.

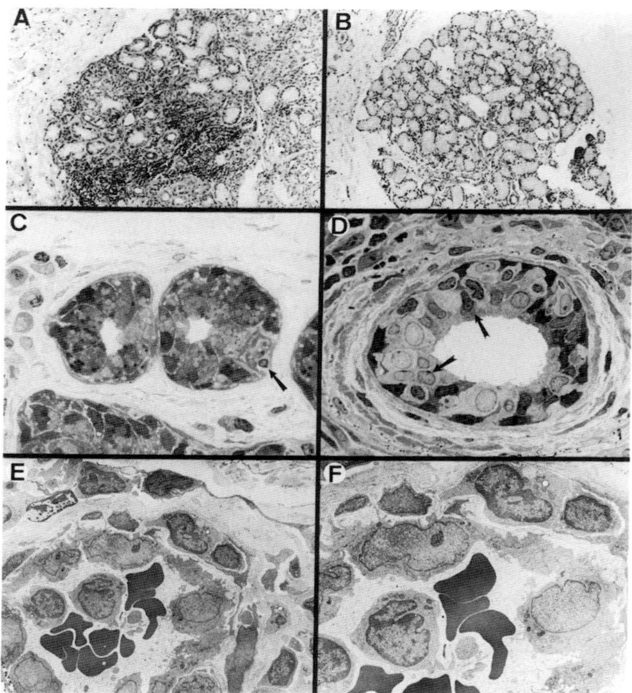

FIGURE 37.2. Minor salivary gland biopsy from patients with Sjögren's syndrome **(A)** and from a patient with fibromyalgia (a histologically normal biopsy) in **(B)**. Higher power views of the Sjögren's biopsy are shown in frames **(C)** and **(D)**, with low power electron microscopic views in frames **(E)** and **(F)**.

lial cells is shown in frames C and D. The changes in the high endothelial cells containing red blood cells (frames E and F) and adherent T-cells that are migrating through the vessel wall are seen under low power electron microscopy.

Evaluation of Symptoms in the Dry-Eye Patient

SS patients usually describe a burning or "foreign" body sensation in their eyes. The symptoms often are worse at the end of the day and are relieved by the use of over-the-counter artificial tears (which most patients have tried prior to seeing a rheumatologist). Symptoms of itching are poorly correlated with objective findings of keratoconjunctivitis (12). Patients may be relatively symptom free until their condition is precipitated by the use of medications with anticholinergic side effects (such as over-the-counter cold remedies or prescription medications) or environmental stress to the tear film (such as airline travel or exposure to dry winds). Often identification and alteration of the offending medication may be all that is required.

Contact lenses, especially the soft gas-permeable type, can contribute to corneal abrasions because adequate tear film may not be available to wash out foreign substances trapped under the lens. Thus, if contact lens are worn, they should be taken out at night and the patient needs to be cautioned about the risk of corneal abrasions. One study has suggested that SS patients should be offered photorefractive surgery (i.e., excimer laser keratectomy) if they do not tolerate contact lens (39); however, caution about the use of invasive procedures involving the cornea needs to be exercised until long-term follow-up of SS patients with refractive surgery (essentially a cosmetic procedure) is available.

Evaluation Of Symptoms Of Dry Eyes

When evaluating the patient with a complaint of dry eyes, it is important to determine if the objective signs of dry eyes are commensurate with the patient's symptoms. Methods to measure the integrity of the corneal surface and tear film include rose bengal, fluorescein staining, lissamine green staining, or the tear breakup time are described below. For example, the absence of a significantly abnormal exam using rose bengal (a test that is performed easily by the rheumatologist) should suggest a search for additional causes to explain the patient's ocular complaints. These may range from eye strain (poor refraction), blepharitis (irritation and low-grade infection of the Meibomian glands in the lids), blepharospasm (uncontrolled blinking from an increased local neural reflex circuit), or symptoms resulting from anxiety or depression (40).

Unstimulated tear flow is referred to as basal flow. This tear secretion derives from the minor tear glands located predominantly in the upper lid. They probably are stimulated by a local reflex arc involving neural receptors in the lid and probably do not involve neural loops that regulate the major salivary glands. This decrease in basal secretion correlates fairly well with symptoms of dryness but not closely with keratoconjunctivitis sicca. Decrease in basal tear flow is very common in the general population, especially the elderly, and does not signify an autoimmune condition. A decrease in basal tear flow also may be the initial symptom in SS patients. These symptoms of eye discomfort occur even though the patient can generate tears when they cry (i.e., supratentorial stimulation) or are exposed to certain stimuli such as onions (nasal lacrimal reflexes).

Tear volume usually is measured by the Schirmer's test; however, this test is performed routinely in several distinct ways and the results are often quite different. It is important for the rheumatologist to note the methods of quantitation of tear flow when evaluating patients clinically (or reports by their ophthalmologist) or reviewing the published literature. Many opthalmologists (and clinical studies) measure the Schirmer's I test with topical anesthetic (Ophthaine) and reflects the basal secretory rate of the minor lacrimal glands in the eyelids (i.e., not the major lacrimal glands). This test is sensitive but not specific and may be diminished for many reasons.

Most commonly, rheumatologists perform the Shirmer's I test in the absence of anesthetic. This value reflects both the minor glands and the stimulation of the major glands. However, the extent of stimulation of the major lacrimal glands is variable. This test is convenient, has less sensitivity, and has more specificity.

In addition to Schirmer's I test (either with or without anesthesia), the Schirmer's II test provides a rapid way to measure the maximal output of minor plus major lacrimal glands. The Schirmer's II test is performed by gently inserting the cotton end of a cotton swab into the nose, where it stimulates the nasolacrimal gland reflex (41). The volume of tearing is measured by Schirmer's paper strips without anesthesia. The stimulated tearing reflex involves a neural loop in which afferent fibers from the ocular surface travel to the midbrain (lacrimatory nucleus) where they stimulate efferent adrenergic and cholinergic nerves that travel back to the lacrimal gland (cholinergic) and its blood vessels (adrenergic) (42). A diminished Schirmer's II test has good specificity for SS, but lacks sensitivity to early stages of SS. The presence of an increased tearing on Schirmer's II test has been a good predictor of response to oral pilocarpine as a way to stimulate secretions, in the author's experience.

A wide range of tear volume flow (i.e., values on Schirmer's I test with anesthesia) occurs in SS patients as well as in normals, and is poorly correlated with signs and symptoms of KCS. Similarly, the volume of saliva produced as basal secretion or after stimulation correlates poorly with symptoms of dry mouth and objective signs of severe periodontal problems (43). This suggests that the qualitative content of tears and saliva (i.e., specific glycoproteins and mucins) plays an important role in the maintenance of ocular and oral mucosal integrity and that decreases in tear volume are not the sole cause of problems. An important implication of these findings is that the next generation of artificial tears, artificial salivas, and toothpastes may contain bioengineered products that provide these important functions lacking in the currently available products.

In addition to the volume of tears, the quality of the tear film is assessed by simple procedures such as rose bengal. This material is readily available from pharmacies that carry ocular supplies and a single drop is administered into the lower eyelid. After rinsing the rose bengal out with a preservative-free tear, the residual staining of the conjunctiva and cornea can be determined with an ophthalmoscope. Although this evaluation by the rheumatologist does not replace the more accurate evaluation of keratoconjunctivitis sicca by slit lamp performed by ophthalmologist, the test does provide a rapid method for assessing the significance of patient's complaints. The rose bengal should not be left in the patient's eye (before rinsing out with an artificial tear) for a prolonged period, as this may lead to local irritation. In comparison, lissamine green is reported to cause less irritation, but requires a slit lamp for adequate quantitation. The results obtained with both rose bengal and lissamine green methods are very dependent on the methods for performing the test and the "training" of the observer. In research studies (or in the evaluation of published studies by the rheumatologist), it is important to recognize limitations of the different methods and the variable between different observers.

Evaluation Of Symptoms Of Dry Mouth

The principal oral symptom of SS is mouth dryness with a broad range of severity. Not all patients complain of dryness specifically; many describe difficulty in swallowing food, problems in wearing dentures, changes in their sense of taste, increased incidence of dental caries, chronic burning symptoms, intolerance to acidic or spicy foods, and the inability to eat dry food or speak continuously for more than a few minutes. Nutrition may be compromised and patterns of sleep disturbed.

On examination of the mouth, the SS patient lacks the normal salivary pooling under the tongue and may have rapidly progressive caries. The mouth frequently exhibits petechial (i.e., small, red, nonpalpable) lesions on the hard palate and/or a lichen planuslike appearance (fine white, lacy strands) on the buccal mucosa. Also, these lesions only may be detected in the recesses of the buccal mucosa on careful examination. These petechial and lichen planuslike lesions result from chronic oral candidiasis infection in the SS patient; it is uncommon for an SS patient's mouth to exhibit the plaquelike appearance (thrush) found in severely immunocompromised patients. Another manifestation of oral candidiasis in the SS patient is angular cheilitis, a condition that must be treated at the same time as the buccal mucosal candidiasis.

Progressive periodontal disease should be suspected based on the increased need for dental restorations and the presence of cavities at the gum line. The loss of teeth and requirement for dentures at any age, but particularly in the younger patient, may have significant emotional and economic consequences. Patients with dentures may change their social patterns of interpersonal interactions. For example, their social life frequently involves eating meals with friends and the patient may feel uncomfortable about not being able to eat the same foods. Further, the patient's diet may be shifted over to preprocessed foods that often are higher in sugars and thus further accelerates the rate of their periodontal problems.

Systemic Manifestations Of Sjögren's Syndrome

Patent's with 1° SS as well as those with 2° SS associated with SLE may have a wide variety of systemic manifestations. As most of their manifestations are covered in other chapters, they simply are listed in Table 37.5. However, several of these manifestations (i.e., central nervous system, lymphoma) have been reported more commonly in 1° SS and will be discussed more fully below.

TABLE 37.5. EXTRAGLANDULAR MANIFESTATIONS IN PATIENTS WITH SJÖGREN'S SYNDROME

Respiratory	Chronic bronchitis secondary to dryness of upper and lower airway with mucus plugging
	Lymphocytic interstitial pneumonitis
	Pseudolymphoma with nodular infiltrates
	Lymphoma
	Pleural effusions
	Pulmonary hypertension
Gastrointestinal	Dysphagia associated with xerostomia
	Atrophic gastritis
	Liver disease including biliary cirrhosis and sclerosing cholangitis
Skin and mucous membranes	Candida—oral and vaginal
	Vaginal dryness
	Hyperglobulinemic purpura
	Raynaud's phenomenon
	Vasculitis
Endocrine, neurologic, and muscular	Thyroiditis
	Peripheral neuropathy involvement of hands and/or feet
	Mononeuritis multiplex
	Myositis
Hematologic	Neutropenia, anemia, thrombocytopenia
	Pseudolymphoma
	Lymphadenopathy
	Lymphoma and myeloma
Renal	Tubular-interstitial nephritis (TIN)
	Glomerulonephritis, in absence of antibodies to DNA
	Mixed cryoglobulinemia
	Amyloidosis
	Obstructive nephropathy as a result of enlarged periaortic lymph nodes
	Lymphoma
	Renal-artery vasculitis

Central Nervous System Symptoms of Sjögren's Syndrome

Similar to SLE (44), a wide variety of central nervous system manifestations has been reported in SS patients (45, 46). These range from vasculitic lesions of the central nervous system, thrombotic lesions associated with anticoagulants, affective disorders (47), autonomic neuropathy (48), myelopathy (49), cranial nerve neuropathy (50), dystonias (44), and autoimmune hearing loss (51,52). One of the main diagnostic problems for the clinician is that many patients with poorly defined neurologic diseases and a positive ANA (and perhaps a positive anti-SS-A antibody) are defined as having SS (or a *forme fruste* SS) even when they lack objective signs of keratoconjunctivitis sicca (53). It is again worth emphasizing that a relatively high normal proportion of the normal population have a false-positive ANA (6), the variation in results among assays for anti-SS-A antibody (8) and that positive ANA have been found in increased frequency in patients with other hematologic disorders that appear distinct from either SLE or SS.

Thus, rheumatologists often are faced with a patient with predominantly neurologic or affective disorder problems and a positive ANA for the question of whether immune suppressive therapy is indicated for SS. This problem is certainly most commonly encountered in the patient with symptoms of fibromyalgia where sicca symptoms are a prominent complaint. During litigation regarding the relationship of silicone breast implants and autoimmune disease (54), a slightly higher association (relative risk about 1.5) was found for SS than for SLE or scleroderma (relative risk about 1.0) (55). However, minor salivary-gland biopsies did not support the diagnosis of SS (56,57) in those patients studied and suggested that the cause of their dryness could be because of a mild autonomic neuropathy, perhaps associated with their fibromyalgia (58).

Several earlier studies suggested a relatively high frequency of demyelination in the central nervous system in primary SS patients (59,60). Although patients with sicca SS may develop symptoms and signs similar to multiple sclerosis patients, several issues remain unclear. First, the markedly increased frequency of demyelinating features was reported during a relatively short period at a single medical center. Longer-term follow-up studies in the same medical center did not confirm the earlier reports of a markedly increased frequency (61). The most likely explanation for the earlier reports derive from the later improved sensitivity of magnetic resonance imaging (MRI) brain scans where it was possible to better distinguish vascular lacunae from regions of demyelination and the improvement of assays for detection of antinuclear antibodies. Second, it was recognized that multiple sclerosis patients may develop dryness as a result of an associated autonomic neuropathy at the level of the central nervous system, rather than as a consequence of an autoimmune process involving the lacrimal or salivary glands (62).

Depression can present in many clinical forms including difficulty concentrating, poor appetite, or as a sleep disorder in both SLE and SS (63). The precise role of inflammation and hormone imbalances associated with SS as a contributing factor to depression remains unclear, but certainly depression is caused in part by chemical alterations in the brain (64,65). Stress, poor sleep, and chronic illness can all contribute to depression. When antidepressant medications are used to help regulate sleep patterns and treat fatigue, drugs with relatively less anticholinergic side effects [such as selective serotonin reuptake inhibitor (SSRI) agents that interfere with serotonin uptake] are preferred over tricyclic antidepressants (often given for fibromyalgia).

Systemic Medications And Sjögren's Patients

The overall approach to systemic therapy in the patient with SS is similar to that in the SLE patient. Disease manifestations are subdivided into nonvisceral (arthralgias, myalgias, skin, fatigue) and visceral (lung, heart, kidney, brain, peripheral nervous system). Nonvisceral manifestations generally are treated with salicylates, nonsteroidal agents, and often hydroxychloroquine. Particular attention to difficulty in swallowing pills in the SS patient is necessary because the decreased salivary content can lead to pills becoming stuck in the midesophagus with resultant erosions of the mucosa. Little improvement with salivary or lacrimal flow rates has been noted with NSAIDs, although some increase in tearing and salivation may occur after systemic corticosteroids. In terms of NSAIDs for the SS patients, indomethacin is the only agent readily available as a suppository for the patient with difficulty swallowing tablets. Flurbiprofen has been shown in a pilot study to decrease periodontal inflammation and resultant gum disease (66).

Among the slow-acting drugs, antimalarials (hydroxychloroquine) have proven useful in decreasing the arthralgias, myalgias, and lymphadenopathy in SS patients (67, 68), similar to its benefit in some SLE patients (69). We have used hydroxychloroquine (6 to 8 mg/kg/day) in SS patients where there is elevation of erythrocyte sedimentation rate (ESR) and polyclonal hyperglobulinemia, because these laboratory abnormalities suggest that symptoms of arthralgia and myalgia may have an inflammatory cause. In a European study (70), hydroxychloroquine improved ESR but did not increase tear-flow volumes. Comparison of drug benefit in SS patients in European and United States studies is strongly influenced by the very different inclusion criteria for diagnosis of SS (described above). When taken at the proper dose (6 to 8 mg/kg/day), hydroxychloroquine has a very good safety record, although there remains a remote possibility (probably less than 1/1,000) (71) of significant build-up in the eye. For this reason, periodic eye checks (generally every 6 to 12 months) are recommended so that the medicine can be discontinued if there is any significant build-up. In patients with cognitive features associated with SS, the use of atabrine has been advocated (69). However, the patients should be screened for G6PD deficiency prior to this drug and a "yellowing" of the skin is common. This skin changes can be partially ameliorated using oral vitamin A (solatene). These agents are not readily available from most pharmacies but can be obtained from compounding pharmacies.

For visceral involvement including vasculitic skin lesions, pneumonitis, neuropathy, and nephritis, corticosteroids are used in a manner similar to SLE patients. As in other autoimmune disorders, a key question is how to taper the corticosteroids because these agents have additional problems of accelerating their periodontal problems. Drugs such as hydroxychloroquine, azathioprine, and methotrexate are used to help taper the corticosteroids. In one study, methotrexate appeared most useful (72). It is likely that several of the newer agents approved for rheumatoid arthritis (leflunomide and TNF antagonist, etanercept) will prove useful in selected SS patients. In some SS patients, cyclosporin may be used (73), but the tendency towards interstitial nephritis in many Sjögren's patients limits the usefulness of the drug.

For life-threatening illness, cyclophosphamide occasionally is required. However, the increased frequency of lymphoma in SS patients (74) requires caution in the use of cyclophosphamide and has suggested its use as a pulse therapy rather than daily administration.

Topical Therapy for the Dry-Eye Patient

The mainstay of treatment for the dry-eye patient is the regular use of artificial tears (75). When evaluating a particular artificial-tear preparation (Table 37.6), the patient must carefully determine whether: (i) the tear gives benefit but does not last long enough, or (ii) the tear burns immediately upon installation. Artificial tears can be considered to have at least two distinct components: the moisturizing component and the preservative. If the tear is helpful but does not last long enough, then a more viscous tear (such as a higher concentration of hydroxymethylcellulose) or a different vehicle to concentrate the moisturizing element (such as a polymerlike dextran) is indicated.

If the tear burns soon after installation, then an irritant reaction to a preservative in the tear must be considered (76). These reactions were much more frequent in the past when benzalkonium chloride and thimerosal commonly were used in artificial tears. However, it should be remembered that these preservatives still are widely used in other ophthalmologic preparations (particularly topical antibiotics) and may contribute to ocular irritation. Irritation of the eyelids in some patients with blepharitis may be related

TABLE 37.6. THERAPEUTIC PRINCIPLES

1. Therapy includes topical replacement of lubrication (artificial tears and saliva), as well as preservation of tears by punctal occlusion.
2. Local inflammation of the ocular surface may be treated by use of antiinflammatory substances such as topical cyclosporin.
3. The normal tear film or saliva lubricants contain mucins as well as saliva. Although current therapies can replace aqueous secretions, they are still deficient in replacement of the mucin components.
4. New oral medications help stimulate muscarinic M3 secretions to lead to increased water content of secretions.
5. The overall treatment program for Sjögren's syndrome is similar to systemic lupus erythematosus with the use of corticosteroids (that can be used for short intervals), nonsteroidal agents, and slow-acting antirheumatic drugs (hydroxychloroquine, methotrexate, and perhaps newer agents such as leflunomide and tumor necrosis factor inhibitors) for chronic management of extraglandular manifestations, and the use of cytotoxic agents (i.e., cyclophosphamide) for life-threatening vasculitis.

to the preservatives present in some ocular lubricants (used at night), as well as the use of excessive amounts of lubricant at night that plug the Meibomian glands.

It is important for the patient to identify environmental factors and medications that contribute to dry-eye symptoms. For example, symptoms of dry eyes will be exacerbated by low-humidity environments such as airplanes, highly air-conditioned offices or department stores, and outdoor areas with strong dry winds. The increased use of tears *before* the onset of symptoms will be symptomatically helpful and prevent corneal abrasions. The use of cool-mist humidifiers at night (or even in the office) and wrap-around sunglasses when outdoors will help retard tear evaporation. Among patients who wear glasses, the optometrist can add moisture shields to the frames. In patients who like or need to be outdoors, ski goggles can provide a local "moisture chamber."

If the particular artificial tear seems helpful but benefit does not last long enough, punctal occlusion may be performed on a temporary or permanent basis (77). The puncta are the small openings at the medial aspects of the lids. Blockage of the puncta can be done with silicone plugs or by electrocautery (77). Previously, a trial of "temporary" punctal occlusion with collagen plugs (i.e., temporary occlusion that lasts several days) was advocated. However, clinical experience has indicated that adequate occlusion with collagen plugs only is achieved in a minority of patients and this procedure is no longer advocated as an adequate trial. In some patients, a prior punctal occlusion may reopen and this can be determined easily by instilling fluorescein in the patient's eye. If the puncta has reopened, the fluorescein will drain into the nasopharynx and the patient will experience the characteristic taste of fluorescein. This simple test will indicate the need (or absence) for repeat punctal occlusion.

Topical cyclosporin has been used to improve the keratoconjunctivitis in dogs with dry eyes. High levels of cyclosporin are achieved in the tear film but there is little absorption into the systemic circulation. The beneficial effects of cyclosporin are as a result of its ability to serve as an antiinflammatory agent. However, additional benefits may result from stimulation of prolactin receptors on the cell surface of corneal cell and lacrimal gland acinar cells (78). However, the diluents used to dissolve cyclosporin in the dog models was too irritating to use in SS patients in initial trials; more recently, Allergan has developed a new vehicle that has allowed cyclosporin to undergo phase III trials in KCS patients. These trials indicated that topical cyclosporin was significantly better than placebo or commercially available tears (M. Stern, pers. comm.) and that application to the Food and Drug Administration (FDA) currently is pending.

Adjuncts to therapy have included acetylcysteine 10% drops to break up mucuous strands, but these drops have the smell of rotten eggs and are thus objectionable to most patients (79). Vitamin A and related preparations have a theoretical role in the treatment of dry eye, because vitamin A-deficient patients have increased keratinization of the corneal surface (80); however, more recent studies have not supported the initial enthusiasm for this form of treatment (75).

Oral Therapy for the Dry-Eye Patient

Pilocarpine, an agonist for muscarinic M3 receptor, has been used as an oral preparation to stimulate the salivary and lacrimal-gland secretion. Initial studies in 1986 indicated the benefit of pilocarpine in SS patients (81). The effects on salivation were more marked than effects on lacrimal stimulation. Also of note, the relationship between subjective symptoms and objective measurements of saliva flow showed a weak correlation. These results were interpreted to indicate that pilocarpine stimulated "water" flow, while symptoms correlated with mucin secretion, which was not adequatedly quantitated in the studies. During recent years, a series of additional studies on oral pilocarpine have been presented (82,83,84) and led to approval to market for symptoms of dry mouth. The available dosage is 5 mg up to four times daily. The most common side effect is increased sweating or gastrointestinal intolerance, which generally is controlled by decreasing the dose.

A recent clinical study using a different oral-muscarinic agonist (cevimeline, SnowBrand SNI-2077) was presented in abstract form (85). In comparison to pilocarpine: (i) cevimeline has a longer half life (4 hours) than pilocarpine (1.5 hours); and (ii) cevimeline has a higher specificity for muscarinic M3 receptor (salivary and lacrimal gland) in comparison to muscarinic M2 (cardiac tissues) by about tenfold. This ratio of binding to M3 receptor (i.e., efficacy) and M2 receptor (i.e., toxicity) may prove important. In the clinical studies, an objective improvement in tear film as measured by exfoliative cytology was reported with cevimeline, which the same investigators had not seen in their prior studies with pilocarpine in the same population of study patients (85).

Systemic sialagogues have been used to increase salivation. Three agents have been studied in controlled trials. Bromhexine, a mucolytic agent, was not found to increase salivary flow rate but patients described subjective benefit (86). Anetholethrithione (Sialor) showed significant effects on saliva output in one study of SS patients with mild secretory hypofunction (87); however, a later study failed to find a significant response in patients with severe hypofunction (88). A series of controlled studies have indicated that pilocarpine exerts stimulatory properties in SS and postradiation therapy (81,89). The drug acts primarily as a muscarinic-cholinergic agonist with mild beta-adrenergic activity. In these studies, pilocarpine 5 mg three times a day increased salivary flow for several hours, in comparison with placebo (90). Side effects were common, including sweating, flushing, and increased urination (90). Further studies will be required to compare this treatment with other agents containing iodide (SSKI or organidin) that are occasionally helpful in some SS patients.

A dry mouth is not necessarily a painful mouth. It is common for a Sjögren's patient to develop a low-grade oral yeast infection (36). Predisposing factors include recent use of antibiotics and/or corticosteroids. Treatment of this problem is particularly difficult in the patient with dentures, because continued excoriation of the mucosal surface occurs. Many topical antifungal drugs (including Mycelex troches) are available, but these oral preparations suffer from a low content of antifungal agent and a high concentration of glucose (to improve the taste) and thus contribute to dental decay if used chronically (36). The reason for inclusion of dextrose (rather than aspartame as a "sweetener") was because of concern about long-term effects of aspartate by the FDA at the time when the drug was first introduced; attempts by the author to have Mycelex reformulated without dextrose by the manufacturer have not been successful. Nystatin and chlortrimazole (available as vaginal suppositories that can be sucked) are both helpful, but must be sucked for about 20 minutes twice daily for at least 6 weeks to prevent recurrence of oral candidiasis (91). Patients with very dry mouth will require periodic sips of water to help dissolve the troches. For angular cheilitis, topical antifungal creams are used two to three times per day for several weeks. This must be done concurrently with the treatment of intraoral candida treatment, because the angular cheilitis serves to reinfect the buccal mucosa (and vice versa).

To permit drug access to all intraoral mucosal sites, patients must remove their dentures while antifungtal tablets are dissolving. The dentures also must be treated to remove traces of candida, and the method of disinfectant must be discussed with the dentist. However, it usually is sufficient to soak the complete denture overnite in benzalkonium chloride (for example, a 1/700 dilution of the surgical-scrub solution, Zephrin). The dentures must be carefully cleaned with a toothbrush and nystatin powder must be applied to the fitting surfaces of the upper denture before reinserting the denture. In extreme cases, a short course of oral antifungal therapy (such as ketoconazole or fluconazole) may be required to control oral candidiasis.

The use of topical fluorides may help protect dental enamel. In some patients, a neutral fluoride drop may be applied by toothbrush or by their oral hygienist. In other patients, direct contact of the dental surfaces and the fluoride gel can be achieved by using "dental plates" at night to apply the fluoride. These "plates" are made specifically for each patient by their periodontist.

The use of correct technique of toothbrush to massage the gums and remove debris is important, because this normal function of saliva is diminished in SS patients. In some patients, a rotating toothbrush [such as Oratek (Oratek Products, Inc.)] is useful, together with regular oral hygiene from a technician experienced in dry-mouth care.

A variety of saliva substitutes are available. They differ in their flavoring agents and preservatives. MouthKote (Parnell Pharmaceuticals, Inc.) and Salivart (Xenex Laboratories, Inc.) sprays contain mucins, which are glycoproteins that help lubricate the mouth and thus provide relief for a longer time than simply rinsing with water (92). They can be obtained by calling 1-800-457-4276. After administration of these sprays, parotid flow rates are increased for 7 to 8 minutes in Sjögren's patients; however, the sense of "oral being" may last for several hours. Also, the use of oral balance gel at night may prove helpful and may be obtained by phone (1-800-922-5856). Electrical (vibrating) stimulation was used to stimulate saliva in some patients with mildly decreased flow rates (93), although the cost of the apparatus has precluded wide usage.

A single-blinded controlled trial was conducted to test the efficacy of low-dose oral human interferon-alpha (IFN-α) to improve salivary function in patients with SS (94). Fifty-six outpatients with primary and four patients with secondary SS were assigned randomly into treatment groups of either IFN-α or sucralfate (control). The IFN-α (150 IU) or sucralfate (250 mg) was given orally three times a day for 6 months. After 6 months of treatment, 15 of 30 (50%) IFN-α-treated patients had saliva production increases at least 100% above baseline, whereas only 1 of 30 (3.3%) sucralfate patients had a comparable increase (p = 0.001). Serial labial salivary-gland biopsies of nine IFN-α responder patients showed that lymphocytic infiltration was significantly decreased (p = 0.02) and the proportion of intact salivary-gland tissue was significantly increased (p = 0.004) after the IFN-α treatment. This agent is currently in double-blind trials.

Special Therapeutic Considerations in the Dry Eye Patient

Anesthesia and Surgery

SS patients have particular problems during the preoperative, perioperative, and postoperative periods. The normal preoperative instruction is no fluids by mouth after dinner or midnight on the day prior to surgery. In the absence of normal saliva flow, these patients have great discomfort that can be reduced by the use of artificial salivas. Because the main concern is aspiration of stomach contents during anesthesia, these patients can safely use oral mouth sprays such as MouthKote (described above) without increased risk. These also are useful in postoperative patients including those who are not able to take food by mouth.

Operating rooms and postoperative recovery areas are extremely low humidity, particularly as nonhumidified oxygen blows over a face mask. Therefore, SS patients have increased risk of developing corneal abrasions during surgery and in the postoperative setting. The decreased blink reflex of the patient during anesthesia also contributes to this problem. The administration of ocular lubricants prior to surgery and in the postoperative recovery suite will reduce the chance of this complication. The patient is advised to take their Refresh PM (Allergan) or Genteal (CIBA) ointment with them to the hospital. This will allow the ointment to be available for the anesthesiologist. It is increasingly common for hospitals to tell the patient to not bring their medications with them to the hospital (because all medications must be identified by the nurse for medical legal reasons) but specialty medications such as ocular or oral lubricants are not readily available in most hospitals. The patients should bring their medications in labeled containers to minimize the work in "logging in" their own medications. The patient may expect a certain resistance from the nurse when they present their own medications (more work for the nurse), but they should persist that their rheumatologist wanted them to have their ocular and oral lubricants available. (We have yet to see a first-morning case delayed while the anesthesiologist waited for the pharmacy to send them a tube of lubricant, so better for the patient to bring their own. Indeed, we often tape the chart shut with a tube of lubricant attached to make sure it is "seen" by the anesthesiologist).

Upper airway dryness of the SS patient may lead to mucus plug inspissation during the postoperative period, followed by obstructive pneumonias. The use of humidified oxygen and avoidance of medications that excessively dry the upper airways (i.e., used by anesthesia to control secretions) will help prevent this problem. Also, adequate hydration and respiratory therapy to keep airways clear is important. This problem has become more common because current practice is for one anesthesiologist to take the history and a different one to perform the procedure. Therefore, we advocate that the patient take the "special instructions at time of surgery" page in this chapter with them at the time of surgery.

An additional problem for the anesthesiologist is the poor state of teeth in the SS patient. Thus, a higher risk of damage to teeth during intubation must be considered. Not only can this lead to loss of the teeth and their subsequent aspiration, but these patients have great expense in preparing dentures to their remaining teeth that will be greatly affected by any further tooth loss.

Finally, assessment of the "fluid status" of the SS patient in the postoperative period may be relatively difficult. Normal clinical clues such as the moisture in the ocular and oral membranes may be quite misleading. Further, some SS patients have a tendency for interstitial nephritis, which prevents adequate urine concentration and fluid balance. This problem may be exacerbated by antibiotics such as aminoglycosides.

Ocular Lesions In SLE

Ocular manifestations of SLE are diverse and range from the relatively benign sicca syndrome to potentially destructive inflammatory conditions, including retinal vasculitis. Among 70 patients in a Singapore lupus clinic, only 7% had ophthalmic symptoms (97). However, 64% had an abnormal Shirmer's test, 20% had cataracts, and 3% had glaucoma. Active lupus, antiphospholipid antibody syndrome, and medications that are used to treat LE can cause ocular pathology. Immune-complex deposition has been found in the blood vessels of the conjunctiva, retina, choroid, sclera, ciliary body, in the basement membranes of the ciliary body and cornea, and in the peripheral nerves of the ciliary body and conjunctiva (96). This may manifest clinically as vasculitis. Retinal occlusive disease in association with the lupus anticoagulant is important to identify, because it is treated with antiplatelet therapy and anticoagulation as opposed to anti-inflammatory therapies. Medication may affect the eyes, and these changes must be differentiated from those that are induced by the disease process. Corticosteroids may induce blurred vision and cataracts. Further, they can raise intraocular pressure, which can cause glaucoma. Antimalarials such as hydroxychlorogen (at doses above 8 mg/kg/day) or chloroquine may cause retinotoxic changes (especially maculopathy) and occasionally deposit in the cornea. Antihypertensive agents also can alter ocular pressures.

Cutaneous Eye Lesions, Conjunctivitis, Corneal Lesions, And Orbital Myopathies

Although the literature emphasizes fundus or funduscopic lesions, changes may be seen from the periorbital tissues back to the retina. Lupus skin lesions have a propensity to appear about the eyelids. Several 1-mm diameter, slightly scaly, erythematous papules that are caused by SLE may resemble those of eczema, blepharitis, or infection about the lid. During acute phases of the disease, with extensive cutaneous involvement in the periorbital area, it is common to have periorbital edema. Recurrent conjunctivitis of viral, bacterial, or autoimmune origin is a frequent finding (10% of Dubois' 520 patients). In the Harvey et al. series (98), five patients out of 105 had conjunctivitis, with two of the follicular type; two also had episcleritis. Conjunctivitis was noted in 8% of 193 patients at Stanford University at any time during the disease course (99). A bulbar conjunctival biopsy with positive immunofluorescence (indicative of active SLE) may be useful (100). Biopsies from 11 patients with lupus conjunctival disease were compared to age-matched cataract patients at Harvard University (101). SLE was associated with inflammation (100%), immunoglobulin deposition (36%), increased CD4, natural killer-cell activity, and HLA-DR expression. Some cases of orbital inflammation associated with myositis and proptosis have been reported in SLE (102), and extraocular muscle swelling can be marked. Exophthalmos rarely has been observed.

Cranial neuropathies can present as ophthalmoplegias and be difficult to differentiate from multiple sclerosis (103, 104). Devic's neuromyelitis (transverse myelitis and optic neuritis) has been associated with SLE and antiphospholipid antibodies (105, 106). Adie's tonic pupil and blepharospasm have been noted during disease exacerbations (107–109). Keane evaluated 113 SLE patients at the University of Southern California for eye complaints (110). Thirty-three (29%) had limitation of eye movements, ptosis, or abnormal spontaneous eye movements. Most were transitory, and half were associated with brain-stem infarction. In a controlled study, lupus patients had significantly delayed eye movements (111).

The effects of SS on the eye were discussed earlier, but corneal infiltration and edema can occur in its absence (112,113). Spaeth (114) reviewed ocular findings in 24 patients with SLE. Corneal staining with fluorescein was present in 88% of the group, although the Schirmer's test was negative in all. Most characteristically, it was just inside the limbus, where the upper lid lay on the cornea. In most cases, staining was limited to three or four punctate spots in a line near the limbus; only 5 of 100 normal controls showed similar involvement. Gold et al. (115) observed similar findings in only 6.5% of 61 outpatients with SLE.

Uveitis And The Choroid

Many patients with uveitis have circulating autoantibodies and are referred to rheumatologists to rule out an underlying autoimmune disease. The prevalence of iritis in SLE ranges from 0.8% to 2.0% (116). The incidence of uveitis may be higher in childhood SLE, in which ocular findings of some type are found in 30% (117).

Jabs et al. (118) presented six cases of choroidal vascular disease and reviewed the literature. Involvement can lead to multifocal, serous elevations of retinal pigment epithelium and adjacent retinal sensory tissue, with resulting macular pathology and retinal detachment. Lupus arteritis of the eye is an immune-complex–mediated disorder, as documented by choroidal vasculitis, cellular infiltrates, and deposits of IgG prominence. Immune-complex deposition occurs primarily in the basement membrane and the pars plana of the choroid (119). Involved vessels correspond to sites of choroidal fluorescein leakage. This vasculitis is steroid responsive (120), but it can lead to rapid visual loss if untreated. Glaucoma is a known complication of steroid therapy and occasionally is observed in nonsteroid-treated LE (121,122).

Retinopathy And Optic Neuropathy

For over 50 years, ophthalmologists have recognized the white patches or cytoid bodies in patients with lupus (123, 124), which Roth first described in 1872 (125). Cytoid bodies, i.e., nerve-swollen B fiber 2° to microinfarcts in precapillary arterioles, are characterized histologically by hypertrophy or ganglioform degeneration of the nerve fibers. They occur in 5% to 15% of patients with SLE (126). Significant retinal vascular narrowing was recorded in 13% of Dubois' patients (126), both with and without hypertension. Ropes (127) described blurred vision in 26% of her 150 patients and cytoid bodies in 9% (which correlated with disease activity).

Urowitz's group (128) commented that 41 of 550 patients with SLE (7%) had retinopathy, of whom five had significant visual loss. This cohort was associated with active disease and a poor prognosis. Of these 41 patients, 34 had microangiopathy, three had papilledema, two had ischemic neuritis, two had occlusive disease, and one had retinal detachment. Kraus et al. (129) performed fluorescein angiography on 50 patients with SLE. Abnormalities were found in 13, with microaneurysms being the most frequent (observed in nine patients). Jabs' group (130) studied 11 patients with retinal occlusive disease in detail; 55% had some visual loss. In addition, most had a history of central nervous system lupus. Thirteen of 82 (15%) Spanish SLE patients had retinal vascular disease, 77% of whom had antiphospholipid antibodies (131). An excellent 1999 review is cited here (132). Retinal vasculitis is diagnosed with perivascular exudates and patches of fluorescein leakage along vessels (133). Retinal vasculitis may antedate the diagnosis of SLE, and visual loss may be the initial presentation of the disease. Vasculitis of the retinal capillaries, with local microinfarction of the superficial nerve fiber layers of the retina, usually is found (Fig. 37.3). Severe, occlusive, retinal-vascular disease is associated with extensive peripheral nonperfusion of the retina, secondary neovascularization, vitreous hemorrhage, and active central nervous system lupus (134,135).

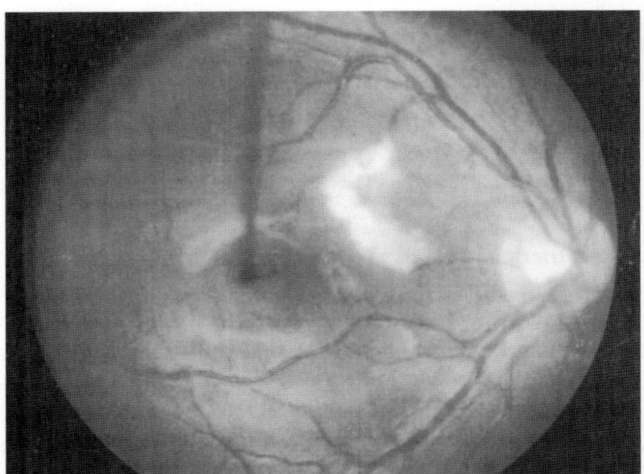

FIGURE 37.3. (See color plate.) Retinal vasculitis in an 18-year-old female. A large area of cotton-wool infarction is evident.

Optic neuritis can present as an ischemic neuropathy, retrobulbar neuritis, or both. Over 30 cases associated with SLE have been described in the literature (136), with a variable visual outcome. Transient monocular blindness was found in 6% of 175 SLE patients and reflected inflammation or migraine (137). Systemic corticosteroids traditionally have been used in the therapy of retinal vasculitis in patients with SLE. Nonetheless, corticosteroid-combination therapy, including azathioprine, methotrexate, or cyclophosphamide, has been used as corticosteroid-sparing strategy for retinal vasculitis with good results (138). Optic neuropathy also may be observed in patients with primary Sjögren's syndrome (139–141). A case of infectious retinitis in a compromised patient with lupus indicates the need for careful eye evaluations before pushing high-dose corticosteroids (142). Conversely, the case of a psychiatric patient with presumed hysteric blindness who had lupus retinitis emphasizes other important concerns (126). A pseudoretinitis pigmentosa also has been reported (143–145).

The eye toxicity of antimalarials and steroids is discussed in Chapters 55 and 56. Retinal vasculitis has been observed in both hydralazine- and procainamide-induced lupus (146,147).

In summary, patients with SLE who present with acute visual loss may have retinal or choroidal ischemia (from vasculitis or occlusion), serious retinal detachments, glaucoma, optic or retrobulbar neuritis, or even cortical infarcts of the brain (148,149). In some patients, the manifestations are associated with immune complex deposition in tissue. In others, they are associated with antiphospholipid antibodies; these have been reported in cases of retinal artery occlusion, diplopia, and ischemic neuropathy (150–153). Asherson et al. (150) observed seven cases of occlusive vascular disease affecting retinal and choroidal vessels among 84 patients with SLE and anticardiolipin antibody (9%). Because the therapies are different (i.e., immunosuppression vs. anticoagulation), it is useful to distinguish the two syndromes when possible (140,151–154).

The Ear: Hearing Deficits, Autoimmune Vestibulitis, And Chondritis

Involvement of the auditory organs in patients with SLE is uncommon, but it does occur. Autoimmune vestibulitis has been reported (155–161); Wallace (126) found it in 1 of 503 cases. Some have reported that vestibulitis responds to steroid therapy or plasmapheresis (156,158,159). Otitis or auditory nerve disease can be associated with severe hearing loss. Three studies performed audiometry in patients with SLE; in one, no abnormalities were found in 20 patients (160). Bowman et al. (161) prospectively studied 30 hospitalized patients with SLE by audiometry and found five with moderate to severe sensorineural hearing loss. In two patients, the hearing loss was caused by SLE; the remaining three had other causes. Forty females with SLE had decreased hearing acuity compared with a control group (162). There are ten case reports of antiphospholipid antibodies may induce hearing loss (163–165). Fries et al. (99) reported that 20% of patients with SLE had tinnitus. Although it usually is secondary to medication (e.g., salicylates, nonsteroidal antiinflammatory drugs, antimalarials), dizziness resulting from vestibulitis can be excluded by special testing (166). Eighty-four lupus patients followed in Brooklyn filled out a questionnaire. Thirty-one percent had aural symptoms, most of whom reported hearing loss with or without tinnitus (167). Fourteen temporal bones from seven lupus patients at the University of Minnesota were studied histologically and immunohistochemically. Eighty-six percent of the cochlea's showed blue staining of the striae vascularis, and most demonstrated loss of spiral ganglion cells with various degrees of hair-cell loss and atrophy of the stria vascularis (168).

Kitridou et al. (144) reported that 4 of 400 patients with SLE who were treated at LAC-USC Medical Center had relapsing auricular and nasal polychondritis that was steroid responsive. This supports occasional case reports of the concurrence of both diseases (145, 169). Harisdangkul and Johnson (170) reviewed 16 cases of coexisting relapsing polychondritis and SLE in the literature in 1994.

The Larynx

Laryngeal involvement caused by SLE is rare, and it can range from mild ulcerations, vocal cord paralysis, and edema to necrotizing vasculitis with airway obstruction. Teitel et al. (171) reported four cases and reviewed the literature; laryngeal edema was founded in 28% of cases and vocal cord paralysis in 11%. The clinical presentation of laryngeal involvement in patients with SLE follows a highly variable course, ranging from an asymptomatic state to severe, life-threatening upper-airway compromise. Teitel et al. divided these into nine overlapping categories: (1) mucosal inflammation, (2) infection, (3) vasculitis, (4) vocal cord paralysis, (5) cricoarytenoid arthritis, (6) subglottic stenosis, (7) inflammatory mass, (8) rheumatoid nodules, and (9) epiglottitis. In most of the cases, symptoms such as hoarseness, dyspnea, and vocal cord paralysis related to SLE resolved with corticosteroid treatment. Since this 1992 review, only scattered case presentations have appeared, which add little. Four of 158 patients with SLE followed in Calgary had life-threatening upper-airway complications (172).

REFERENCES

1. Talal N. Sjögren's syndrome: historical overview and clinical spectrum of disease. *Rheum Dis Clin North Am* 1992;18: 507–515.
2. Morgan WS, Castleman B. A clinicopathologic study of Mikulicz's disease. *Am J Pathol* 1953;29:471–503.
3. Bloch KJ, Wohl MJ, Ship II, et al. Sjögren's syndrome. I.

Serologic reactions in patients with Sjögren's syndrome with and without rheumatoid arthritis. *Arthritis Rheum* 1960;3: 287–297.

4. Morgan WS. Probable systemic nature of Mikulicz's disease and its relation to Sjögren's syndrome. *N Engl J Med* 1954;251: 5–10.
5. Fox R. Classification Criteria for Sjögren's syndrome. *Rheum Dis Clin North Am: Current Controversies in Rheumatology* 1994; 20:391–407.
6. Tan EM, TE Feltkamp, JS Smolen, et al. Range of antinuclear antibodies in "healthy" individuals. *Arthritis Rheum* 1997; 40: 1601-11.
7. Emlen W and O'Neill L. Clinical significance of antinuclear antibodies: comparison of detection with immunofluorescence and enzyme-linked immunosorbent assays. *Arthritis Rheum* 1997;40:1612–1618.
8. Tan EM, JS Smolen, JS McDougal, et al. A critical evaluation of enzyme immunoassays for detection of antinuclear autoantibodies of defined specificities. I. Precision, sensitivity, and specificity. *Arthritis Rheum* 1999;42:455–464.
9. Siamopoulos KC, Elisaf M, Moutsopoulos HM. Hypokalaemic paralysis as the presenting manifestation of primary Sjögren's syndrome. *Nephrol Dial Transplant* 1994;9:1176–1178.
10. Ruzicka T, J Faes, T Bergner, et al. Annular erythema associated with Sjögren's syndrome: a variant of systemic lupus erythematosus [see comments]. *J Am Acad Dermatol* 1991;25: 557–560.
11. Fox RI. Sjögren's syndrome. Controversies and progress. *Clin Lab Med* 1997;17:431–444.
12. Vitali C, Moutsopoulos HM, Bombardieri S. The European Community Study Group on diagnostic criteria for Sjögren's syndrome. Sensitivity and specificity of tests for ocular and oral involvement in Sjögren's syndrome. *Ann Rheum Dis* 1994;53: 637–647.
13. Fox R, Maruyami T, Tornwald J. Sjögren's syndrome: current issues in diagnosis and pathogenesis. *Curr Opin Rheumatol* 1999;10:446–456.
14. Vitali C, Bombardieri S. The Europian classification criteria for Sjögren's syndrome (SS): proposal for modification of the rules for classification suggested by the analysis of the receiver operating characteristic (ROCS) curve of the criteria performance. *J Rheum* 1997;24(suppl):S18.
15. Smolen JS, Butcher B, Fritzler MJ, et al. Reference sera for antinuclear antibodies. II. Further definition of antibody specificities in international antinuclear antibody reference sera by immunofluorescence and western blotting. *Arthritis Rheum* 1997;40:413–418.
16. Arnett F. Histocompatibility typing in the rheumatic diseases: diagnostic and prognostic implications. *Med Clin NA* 1994;20: 371–387.
17. Harley JB, Sestalk AL, Willia LG, et al. A model for disease heterogenecity in systemic lupus erythematosus. *Arthritis Rheum* 1989;32:826–36.
18. Guggenbuhl P, Jean S, Jego P, et al. Primary Sjögren's syndrome: role of the HLA-DRB1*0301-*1501 heterozygotes. *J Rheumatol* 1998;25:900–905.
19. Jean S, Quelvennec E, Alizadeh M, et al. DRB1*15 and DRB1*03 extended haplotype interaction in primary Sjögren's syndrome genetic susceptibility [In Process Citation]. *Clin Exp Rheumatol* 1998;16:725–728.
20. Kang HI, Fei H, Fox RI. Comparison of genetic factors in Chinese, Japanese and Caucasoid patients with Sjögren's syndrome. *Arthritis Rheum* 1991;34(suppl):S41.
21. Reveille J, Wilson R, Provost T, et al. Primary Sjögren's syndrome and other autoimmune diseases in families. *Ann Intern Med* 1984;101:748.
22. Sestak AL, Shaver TS, Moser KL, et al. Familial aggregation of lupus and autoimmunity in an unusual multiplex pedigree. *J Rheumatol* 1999;26:1495–1499.
23. Kassan SS, Thomas TL, Moutsopoulos HM, et al. Increased risk of lymphoma in sicca syndrome. *Ann Intern Med* 1978;89: 888–892.
24. Katayama I, Koyano T, Nishioka K. Prevalence of eyelid dermatitis in primary Sjögren's syndrome. *Int J Dermatol* 1994;33: 421–424.
25. Kyle R, Gleich G, Baynd E, et al. Benign hyperglobuliemic purpura of Waldenstrom. *Medicine* (Baltimore) 1971;50:113–123.
26. Ferri C, La Civita L, Longombardo G, et al. Mixed cryoglobulinaemia: a cross-road between autoimmune and lymphoproliferative disorders. *Lupus* 1998;7:275–279.
27. Fox RI, Chen PP, Carson DA, et al. Expression of a cross reactive idiotype on rheumatoid factor in patients with Sjögren's syndrome. *J Immunol* 1986;136:477–483.
28. Watanabe T, Tsuchida T, Ito Y, et al. Annular erythema associated with lupus erythematosus/Sjögren's syndrome. *J Am Acad Dermatol* 1997;36:214–218.
29. Bangert JL, Freeman RG, Sontheimer RD, et al. Subacute cutaneous lupus erythematosus and discoid lupus erythematosus. Comparative histopathologic findings. *Arch Dermatol* 1984; 120:332–337.
30. McCauliffe DP, Faircloth E, Wang L, et al. Similar Ro/SS-A autoantibody epitope and titer responses in annular erythema of Sjögren's syndrome and subacute cutaneous lupus erythematosus. *Arch Dermatol* 1996;132:528–531.
31. Bielsa I, Herrero C, Collado A, et al. Histopathologic findings in cutaneous lupus erythematosus. *Arch Dermatol* 1994;130:54–58.
32. Harper JI. Subacute cutaneous lupus erythematosus (SCLE): a distinct subset of LE. *Clin Exp Dermatol* 1982;7:209–212.
33. Provost TT, Watson R, Simmons OBE. Anti-Ro(SS-A) antibody positive Sjögren's/lupus erythematosus overlap syndrome. *Lupus* 1997;6:105–111.
34. Magro CM, Crowson AN. The cutaneous pathology associated with seropositivity for antibodies to SSA (Ro): a clinicopathologic study of 23 adult patients without subacute cutaneous lupus erythematosus. *Am J Dermatopathol* 1999;21: 129–137.
35. Daniels TE, Fox PC. Salivary and oral components of Sjögren's syndrome. *Rheum Dis Clinic North Am* 1992;18:571–589.
36. Daniels T. The association of patterns of lacrimal gland biopsy. *Arthritis Rheum* 1994;37:869–877.
37. Stern ME, Beuerman RW, Fox RI, et al. A unified theory of the role of the ocular surface in dry eye. *Adv Exp Med Biol* 1998; 438:643–651.
38. Fox R. Pathogenesis of Sjögren's syndrome. *Molecular Basis of Autoimmunity* 2001;(in press).
39. Toda I, Yagi Y, Hata S, et al. Eximer laser photorefractive keratectomy for patients with contact lens intoleranced caused by dry eye. *Br J Ophth* 1996;80:604–609.
40. Pflugfelder SC. Differential diagnosis of dry eye conditions. *Adv Dent Res* 1996;10:9–12.
41. Tsubota K. Tear dynamics and dry eye. *Prog Retin Eye Res* 1998; 17:565–596.
42. Stern ME, Beuerman RW, Fox RI, et al. The pathology of dry eye: the interaction between the ocular surface and lacrimal glands. *Cornea* 1998;17:584–589.
43. Atkinson JC, Travis WD, Pillemer S, et al. Major salivary gland function in primary Sjögren's syndrome and its relationship to clinical features. *J Rheumatol* 1990;17:318–322.
44. Olney RK. Neuropathies associated with connective tissue disease. *Semin Neurol* 1998;18:63–72.
45. De Backer H, Dehaene I. Central nervous system disease in primary Sjögren's syndrome. *Acta Neurol Belg* 1995;95:142–146.

46. Lafitte C. Neurological manifestations in Sjögren syndrome. *Arch Neurol* 2000;57:411–413.
47. Belin C, Moroni C, Caillat-Vigneron N, et al. Central nervous system involvement in Sjögren's syndrome: evidence from neuropsychological testing and HMPAO-SPECT. *Ann Med Interne* (Paris) 1999;150:598–604.
48. Mandl T, Jacobsson L, Lilja B, et al. Disturbances of autonomic nervous function in primary Sjögren's syndrome [corrected and republished article originally printed in *Scand J Rheumatol* 1997;26:253–258]. *Scand J Rheumatol* 1997;26:401–406.
49. Linardaki G, Skopouli FN, Koufos C, et al. Subclinical multisystemic autoimmunity presenting as a progressive myelopathy. *Lupus* 1997;6:675–677.
50. Gemignani F, Marbini A, Pavesi G, et al. Peripheral neuropathy associated with primary Sjögren's syndrome. *J Neurol Neurosurg Psychiatry* 1994;57:983–986.
51. Tumiati B, Casoli P, Parmeggiani A. Hearing loss in the Sjögren syndrome. *Ann Intern Med* 1997;126:450–453.
52. Stone JH, Francis HW. Immune-mediated inner ear disease. *Curr Opin Rheumatol* 2000;12:32–40.
53. Ioannidis JP, Moutsopoulos HM. Sjögren's syndrome: too many associations, too limited evidence. The enigmatic example of central nervous system involvement [comment]. *Semin Arthritis Rheum* 1999;29:1–3.
54. Solomon G. A clinical and laboratory profile of symptomatic women with silicone breast implants. *Semin Arthritis Rheum* 1994;24:29–37.
55. Janowsky EC, Kupper LL, Hulka BS. Meta-analyses of the relation between silicone breast implants and the risk of connective-tissue diseases. *N Engl J Med* 2000;342:781–790.
56. Freundlich B, Sandorfi N, Altman C, et al. Monocyte/macrophage infiltrates in the salivary glands of women with silicone breast implants. *Curr Top Microbiol Immunol* 1996;210: 323–326.
57. Freundlich B, Altman C, Snadorfi N, et al. A profile of symptomatic patients with silicone breast implants: a Sjögren's-like syndrome. *Semin Arthritis Rheum* 1994;24:44–53.
58. Martinez-Lavin M, Hermosillo AG. Autonomic nervous system dysfunction may explain the multisystem features of fibromyalgia [editorial] [In Process Citation]. *Semin Arthritis Rheum* 2000;29:197–199.
59. Alexander EL, Malinow K, Lejewski JE, et al. Primary Sjögren's syndrome with central nervous system disease mimicking multiple sclerosis. *Ann Intern Med* 1986;104:323–330.
60. Alexander EL, Lijewski JE, Jerdan MS, et al. Evidence of an immunopathogenic basis for central nervous system disease in primary Sjögren's syndrome. *Arthritis Rheum* 1986;29: 1223–1231.
61. Simmons-O'Brien E, Chen S, Watson A, et al. One hundred anti-Ro (SS-A) antibody positive patients: a 10-year follow-up. *Medicine* 1995;74:109–130.
62. Metz LM, Seland TP, Fritzler MJ. An analysis of the frequency of Sjögren's syndrome in a population of multiple sclerosis patients. *J Clin Lab Immunol* 1989;30:121–125.
63. Utset TO, Golden M, Siberry G, et al. Depressive symptoms in patients with systemic lupus erythematosus: association with central nervous system lupus and Sjögren's syndrome. *J Rheumatol* 1994;21:2039–2045.
64. Torpy DJ, Papanicolaou DA, Lotsikas AJ, et al. Responses of the sympathetic nervous system and the hypothalamic-pituitary-adrenal axis to interleukin-6: a pilot study in fibromyalgia. *Arthritis Rheum* 2000;43:872–880.
65. Pillemer SR, Bradley LA, Crofford LJ, et al. The neuroscience and endocrinology of fibromyalgia. *Arthritis Rheum* 1997;40: 1928–1939.
66. Curnock AP, Robson PA, Yea CM, et al. Potencies of leflunomide and HR325 as inhibitors of prostaglandin endoperoxide H synthase-1 and -2: comparison with nonsteroidal anti-inflammatory drugs. *J Pharmacol Exp Ther* 1997;282:339–347.
67. Fox RI, Chan E, Benton L, et al. Treatment of primary Sjögren's syndrome with hydroxychloroquine. *Amer J Med* 1988;85: 62–67.
68. Fox RI, Dixon R, Guarrasi V, et al. Treatment of primary Sjögren's syndrome with hydroxychloroquine: a retrospective, open-label study. *Lupus* 1996;5(suppl 1):S31–S36.
69. Wallace DJ. Antimalarial agents and lupus. *Rheum Dis Clin North Am 1994;20:243–263.*
70. Kruize A, Hene R, Kallenberg C, et al. Hydroxychloroquine treatment for primary Sjögren's syndrome: a two year double blind crossover trial. Ann Rheum Dis 1993;52:360–364.
71. Bernstein HN. Ocular safety of hydroxychloroquine. *Ann Ophthalmol* 1991;23:292–296.
72. Skopouli FN, Jagiello P, Tsifetaki N, et al. Methotrexate in primary Sjögren's syndrome. *Clin Exp Rheumatol* 1996;14: 555–558.
73. Dalavanga YA, Detrick B, Hooks JJ, et al. Effect of cyclosporin A (CyA) on the immunopathological lesion of the minor salivary glands from patients with Sjögren's syndrome. *Ann Rheum Dis* 1990;46:89–92.
74. Fox RI, Adamson TC III, Fong S, Robinson CA, et al. Lymphocyte phenotype and function of pseudolymphomas associated with Sjögren's syndrome. *J Clin Invest* 1983;72:52–62.
75. Friedlaender M. Ocular manifestations of Sjögren's syndrome. *Rheum Dis Clin North Am* 1992;18:591–609.
76. Wilson F. Adverse external ocular effects of topical ophthalmic medications. *Surv Ophthalmol* 1979;24:57–86.
77. Friedlaender MH, Fox RI. Punctal occlusion for the treatment of dry eye. *Adv Exp Med Biol* 1998;438:1017–1020.
78. Kaswan R. Characteristics of a canine model of KCS: effective treatment with topical cyclosporine. *Adv Exp Med Biol* 1994; 350:583–594.
79. Lemp M. General Measures in management of the dry eye. *Int Opththalmol Clin* 1988;27:36–46.
80. Tseng S. Topical tretinoin treatment for dry-eye disorders. *Int Ophthal Clin* 1987;27:47–57.
81. Fox PC, van der Ven PF, Baum BJ, et al. Pilocarpine for the treatment of xerostomia associated with salivary gland dysfunction. *Oral Surg Oral Med Oral Pathol* 1986;61:243–248.
82. Rhodus NL, Schuh MJ. Effects of pilocarpine on salivary flow in patients with Sjögren's syndrome [see comments]. *Oral Surg Oral Med Oral Pathol* 1991;72:545–549.
83. Rhodus NL. Oral pilocarpine HCl stimulates labial (minor) salivary gland flow in patients with Sjögren's syndrome. *Oral Dis* 1997;3:93–98.
84. Papas AS, Fernandez MM, Castano RA, et al. Oral pilocarpine for symptomatic relief of dry mouth and dry eyes in patients with Sjögrens syndrome. *Adv Exp Med Biol* 1998;438:973–978.
85. Fox R, Pentrone J, Condemi R, et al. Randomized, placebo controlled trial of SNI-2011, a novel M3 muscarinic receptor agonist, for the treatment of Sjögrenn's syndrome. *Arth Rheum* 1998;41(suppl):S288.
86. Fox P. Systemic therapy of salivary gland hypofunction. *J Am Dent Assoc* 1987;115:581–588.
87. Epstein J, Decoteau WE, Wilkinson A. Effect of Sialor in treatment of xerostomia in Sjögren's syndrome. *Oral Surg* 1983;56: 495–499.
88. Schiodt M, Oxholme P, Jacobsen A. Treatment of xerostomia in patients with primary Sjögren's syndrome with sulfarlem. *Scand J Rheum* 1986;61:250–253.
89. Fox P, Atkinson JC, Macynski AA. Pilocarpine treatment of sali-

vary gland hypofunction and dry mouth. *Arch Inter Med* 1991; 151:1149–1152.
90. Vivino FB, Al-Hashimi I, Khan Z, et al. Pilocarpine tablets for the treatment of dry mouth and dry eye symptoms in patients with Sjögren syndrome: a randomized, placebo-controlled, fixed-dose, multicenter trial. P92-01 Study Group [In Process Citation]. *Arch Intern Med* 1999;159:174–181.
91. Hernandez YL, Daniels TE. Oral candidiasis in Sjögren's syndrome: prevalence, clinical correlation and treatment. *Oral Surg Oral Med Oral Pathol* 1989;68:324–329.
92. Rhodus N, Schuh M. Effectiveness of three artifical salivas as assessed by mucoprotective relativity. *J Dental Res* 1991;70–82.
93. Steller M, Chou L, Daniels T. Electrical stimulation of salivary flow in patients with Sjögren's syndrome. *J Dental Res* 1988;67: 1334–1340.
94. Shiozawa S, Tanaka Y, Shiozawa K. Single-blinded controlled trial of low-dose oral IFN-alpha for the treatment of xerostomia in patients with Sjögren's syndrome. *J Interferon Cytokine Res* 1998;18:255–262.
95. Vitali C, Bombardieri S, Moutsopoulos HM, et al. Preliminary criteria for the classification of Sjögren's syndrome. *Arthritis Rheum* 1993;36:340–347.
96. Karpik AG, Schwartz MM, Dickey LE, et al. Ocular immune reactants in patients dying with systemic lupus erythematosus. *Clin Immunol Immunpathol* 1985;35:295–312.
97. Yap EY, Au Eong KG, Fong KY, et al. Ophthalmic manifestations in Asian patients with systemic lupus erythematosus. *Singapore Med J* 1998;39:557–559.
98. McGehee Harvey A, Shulman LE, Tumulty AP, et al. Systemic lupus erythematosus: review of the literature and clinical analysis of 138 cases. *Medicine* 1954;33:291–437.
99. Fries JF, Holman H. *Systemic lupus erythematosus: a clinical analysis.* Philadelphia, Pa: WB Saunders, 1975.
100. Frith P, Burge SM, Millard PR, et al. External ocular findings in lupus erythematosus: a clinical and immunopathological study. *Br J Ophthalmol* 1990;74:163–167.
101. Heilgenhaus A, Dutt JE, Foster CS. Histology and immunopathology of systemic lupus erythematosus affecting the conjunctiva. *Eye* 1996;10:425–432.
102. Norden D, Weinberg J, Schumacher HR, et al. Bilateral periorbital edema in systemic lupus erythematosus. *J Rheumatol* 1993; 20:2158–2160.
103. Evans OB, Lexow SS. Painful ophthalmoplegia in systemic lupus erythematosus. *Ann Neurol* 1978;4:584–585.
104. Jackson G, Miller M, Littlejohn G, et al. Bilateral internuclear ophthalmoplegia in systemic lupus erythematosus. *J Rheumatol* 1986;13:1161–1162.
105. Margaux J, Hayem G, Meyer O, et al. Systemic lupus erythematosus with optical neuromyelitis (Devic's syndrome). *Rev Rhum* (Eng Ed) 1999;66:102–105.
106. Bonnet F, Mercie P, Morfat P, et al. Devic's neuromyelitis optica during pregnancy in a patient with systemic lupus erythematosus. *Lupus* 1999;8:244–247.
107. Herson D, Krivitzky A, Douche C, et al. Familial lupus and Adie's tonic pupil. *Ann Med Interne* (Paris) 1989;140:56–57.
108. Jankovic J, Patten BM. Blepharospasm and autoimmune diseases. *Move Disord* 1987;2:159–163.
109. Rajagopalan N, Humphrey PR, Bucknall RC. Torticollis and blepharospasm in systemic lupus erythematosus. *Move Disord* 1989;4:345–348.
110. Keane JR. Eye movement abnormalities in systemic lupus erythematosus. *Arch Neurol* 1995;52:1145–1149.
111. Giacomini PG, Zoli A, Bruno E, et al. Voluntary occulomotoricity in systemic lupus erythematosus. *Clin Exp Rheumatol* 1997;15:579–585.
112. Raizman MB, Baum J. Discoid lupus keratitis. *Arch Ophthalmol* 1989;107:545–547.
113. Williams B, Hull DS. Lupus erythematosus keratoconjunctivitis. *South Med J* 1986;79:631–632.
114. Spaeth GL. Corneal staining in systemic lupus erythematosus. *N Engl J Med* 1967;276:1168–1171.
115. Gold DH, Morris DA, Henkind P. Ocular findings in systemic lupus erythematosus. *Br J Ophthalmol* 1972;56:800–804.
116. Drosos AA, Petris CA, Petroutsos GM, et al. Unusual eye manifestations in systemic lupus erythematosus patients. *Clin Rheumatol* 1989;8:49–53.
117. Schaller J. Lupus in childhood. *Clin Rheum Dis* 1982;8: 219–228.
118. Jabs DA, Henneken AM, Schachat AP, et al. Choroidopathy in systemic lupus erythematosus. *Arch Ophthalmol* 1988;106: 230–234.
119. Aronson AJ, Ordonez NG, Diddie KR, et al. Immune complex deposition in the eye in systemic lupus erythematosus. *Arch Intern Med* 1979;139:1312–1313.
120. Diddie KR, Aronson AJ, Ernest JT. Chorioretinopathy in a case of systemic lupus erythematosus. *Trans Am Ophthalmol Soc* 1977;75:122–131.
121. Wagemans MA, Bos PJ. Angle-closure glaucoma in a patient with systemic lupus erythematosus. *Doc Ophthalmol* 1989;72: 201–207.
122. Wisotsky BJ, Magat-Gordon CB, Puklin JE. Angle-closure glaucoma as an intitial presentation of systemic lupus erythematosus. *Ophthalmology* 1998;105:1170–1172.
123. Clifton F, Greer CH. Ocular changes in acute systemic lupus erythematosus. *Br J Ophthalmol* 1955;39:1–10.
124. Hollenhorst RW, Henderson JW. Ocular manifestations of diffuse collagen diseases. *Am J Med Sci* 1951;221:211–222.
125. Roth M. Contribution to knowledge of varicose hypertrophy of nerve fibers (in German). *Virchow Arch Path Anat* 1872;55: 197–217.
126. Wallace DJ. Head and neck findings in SLE: Sjögren's and the eye, ear and larynx. In: Wallace DJ, Hahn BH, eds. *Dubois' lupus erythematosus, 4th ed.* Philadelphia: Lea Febiger, 1993; 403–406.
127. Ropes MW. Systemic lupus erythematosus. Cambridge, Mass: Harvard University Press, 1976.
128. Stafford-Brady FJ, Urowitz MB, Gladman DD, et al. Lupus retinopathy. Patterns, associations and prognosis. *Arthritis Rheum* 1988;31:1105–1110.
129. Kraus A, Cervantes G, Barojas E, et al. Retinal vasculitis in mixed connective tissue disease. A fluoroangiographic study. *J Rheumatol* 1985;12:1122–1124.
130. Jabs DA, Fine SL, Hochberg MC, et al. Severe retinal vaso-occlusive disease in systemic lupus erythematosus. *Arch Ophthalmol* 1986;104:558–563.
131. Montehermoso A, Cervera R, Font J, et al. Association of antiphospholipid antibodies with retinal vascular disease in systemic lupus erythematosus. *Semin Arthritis Rheum* 1999;28: 326–332.
132. Giorgi D, Pace F, Giorgi A, et al. Retinopathy and systemic lupus erythematosus: Pathogenesis and approach to therapy. *Human Immunology* 1999;60:688–696.
133. Charles H. Retinal vasculitis. In: Tasman W, Jaeger EA, eds. *Duane's clinical ophthalmology*. Vol. 4. Philadelphia: JB Lippincott, 1991:1–17.
134. Hall S, Buettner H, Luthra HS. Occlusive retinal vascular disease in systemic lupus erythematosus. *J Rheumatol* 1984;11:846–850.
135. Jabs DA. The rheumatic diseases. In: Ryan SJ, Schachat AP, Murphy RB, et al., eds. *Retina*. St. Louis, Mo: Mosby, 1989: 457–480.

136. Jabs DA, Miller NR, Newman SA, et al. Optic neuropathy in systemic lupus erythematosus. *Arch Ophthalmol* 1986;104: 564–568.
137. Donders RC, Kappelle LJ, Derksen RH, et al. Transient monocular blindness and antiphospholipid antibodies in systemic lupus erythematosus. *Neurology* 1998;51:535–540.
138. Neumann R, Foster CS. Corticosteroid-sparing strategies in the treatment of retinal vasculitis in systemic lupus erythematosus. *Retina* 1995;15:206–212.
139. Rosler DH, Conway MD, Anaya JM, et al. Ischemic optic neuropathy and high-level anticardiolipin antibodies in primary Sjögren's syndrome. *Lupus* 1995;4:155–157.
140. Anaya JM. Optic nerve involvement in primary Sjögren's syndrome (in Spanish). *Rev Col Reumatol* 1995;2:38–41.
141. Cotter PB, Weiter JT. Retinopathy in a patient with systemic lupus erythematosus. *Ann Ophth* 1978;14:470–473.
142. Kitridou RC, Wittmann AL, Quismorio FP Jr. Chondritis in systemic lupus erythematosus: clinical and immunopathologic studies. *Clin Exp Rheumatol* 1987;5:349–353.
143. Small P, Frenkiel S. Relapsing polychondritis. A feature of systemic lupus erythematosus. *Arthritis Rheum* 1980;23:361–363.
144. Desatnik H, Ashkenazi I, Regenbogen L. Retinitis pigmentosa and discoid lupus erythematosus. *Metab Pediatr Syst Ophthalmol* 1992;15:9–11.
145. Sekimoto M, Hayasaka S, Noda S, et al. Pseudoretinitis pigmentosa in patients with systemic lupus erythematosus. *Ann Ophthalmol* 1993;25:264–266.
146. Doherty M, Maddison PJ, Grey RH. Hydralazine induced lupus syndrome with eye disease (abstract). *Br Med J (Clin Res)* 1985;290:675.
147. Nichols CJ, Mieler WF. Severe retinal vaso-occlusive disease secondary to procainamide-induced lupus. *Ophthalmology* 1989; 96:1535–1540.
148. Rubin BR, DeHoratius RJ. Acute visual loss in lupus erythematosus. *J Am Osteopath Assoc* 1989;89:73–77.
149. Van Coppenolle F, Vallat M, Smolick J, et al. Bilateral blindness caused by disseminated arterial lupus erythematosus (in French). *Bull Soc Ophthalmol Fr* 1989;89:207–209.
150. Asherson RA, Merry P, Acheson JF, et al. Antiphospholipid antibodies: a risk factor occlusive ocular vascular disease in systemic lupus erythematosus and the primary antiphospholipid syndrome. *Ann Rheum Dis* 1989;48:358–361.
151. Dessein PH, Gledhill RF, Asherson RA. Anticardiolipin antibody negative occlusive vascular retinopathy in systemic lupus erythematosus (letter). *Ann Rheum Dis* 1990;49:133–134.
152. Fitzpatrick EP, Chesen N, Rahn EK. The lupus anticoagulant and retinal vaso-occlusive disease. *Ann Ophthalmol* 1990;22: 148–152.
153. Kleiner RC, Najarian LV, Schatten S, et al. Vaso-occlusive retinopathy associated with antiphospholipid antibodies (lupus anticoagulant retinopathy). *Ophthalmology* 1989;96:896–904.
154. Snyers B, Lambert M, Hardy JP. Retinal and choroidal vaso-occlusive disease in systemic lupus erythematosus associated with antiphospholipid antibodies. *Retina* 1990;10:255–260.
155. Caldarelli DD, Rejowski JE, Corey JP. Sensorineural hearing loss in lupus erythematosus. *Am J Otol* 1986;7:210–213.
156. Hamblin TJ, Mufti GJ, Bracewell A. Severe deafness in systemic lupus erythematosus: its immediate relief by plasma exchange. *Br Med J (Clin Res)* 1982;284:1374.
157. Kovarsky J. Otorhinolaryngologic complications of rheumatic disease. *Semin Arthritis Rheum* 1984;14:141–150.
158. Luetje CM. Theoretical and practical implications for plasmapheresis in autoimmune inner ear disease. *Laryngoscope* 1989; 99:1137–1146.
159. Kobayashi S, Fujishiro N, Sugiyama K. Systemic lupus erythematosus with sensorineural hearing loss and improvement after plasmapheresis using the double filtration method. *Intern Med* 1992;31:778–781.
160. Narula AA, Powell RJ, Davis A. Frequency solving ability in systemic lupus erythematosus. *Br J Audiol* 1989;23:69–72.
161. Bowman CA, Linthicum FH Jr, Nelson RA, et al. Sensorineural hearing loss associated with systemic lupus erythematosus. *Otolaryngol Head Neck Surg* 1986;94:197–204.
162. Andonopoulos AP, Naxakis S, Goumas P, et al. Sensorineural hearing disorders in systemic lupus erythematosus. A controlled study. *Clin Exp Rheumatol* 1995;13:137–141.
163. Hisahi K, Komune S, Taira T, et al. Anticardiolipin antibody-induced sudden profound sensorineural hearing loss. *Am J Otolaryngol* 1993;14:275–277.
164. Naarendorp M, Speira H. Sudden sensorineural hearing loss in patients with systemic lupus erythematosus or lupus-like syndrome and antiphospholipid antibodies. *J Rheumatol* 1998;25: 589–592.
165. Toubi E, Ben-David J, Kessel A, et al. Autoimmune aberration in sudden sensorineural hearing loss: association with anti-cardiolipin antibodies. *Lupus* 1997;6:540–542.
166. Minnigerode B, Leitner C. Transient, directional changing spontaneous and provoked nystagmus in the course of lupus erythematodes visceralis (in German). *Klin Wochenschr* 1985; 63:230–232.
167. Sperling NM, Tehrani K, Liebling A, et al. Aural symptoms and hearing loss in patients with lupus. *Otolaryngol Head Neck Surg* 1998;118:762–765.
168. Sone M, Paparella MM, Schachiern PA, et al. Study of systemic lupus erythematosus in temporal bones. *Annals Oto Rhin Laryn* 1999;108:338–344.
169. Job-Deslandre C, Delrieu F, Delbarre F, et al. Relapsing polychondritis and systemic lupus erythematosus (letter). *J Rheumatol* 1983;10:666–668.
170. Harisdangkul V, Johnson WW. Association between relapsing polychondritis and systemic lupus erythematosus. *South Med J* 1994;87:753–757.
171. Teitel AD, Mackenzie R, Stern R, et al. Laryngeal involvement in systemic lupus erythematosus. *Semin Arthritis Rheum* 1992; 22:203–214.
172. Martin L, Edworthy SM, Ryan JP, et al. Upper airway disease in systemic lupus erythematosus: a report of 4 cases and a review of the literature. *J Rheumatol* 1992;19:1186–1190.

38

HEMATOLOGIC AND LYMPHOID ABNORMALITIES IN SYSTEMIC LUPUS ERYTHEMATOSUS

FRANCISCO P. QUISMORIO, JR.

LYMPHADENOPATHY

Lymphadenopathy, a common clinical manifestation of systemic lupus erythematosus (SLE), can be generalized or regional in distribution, especially in the cervical and axillary regions. Hilar adenopathy rarely is seen in SLE (1). In their series of 520 patients, Dubois and Tuffanelli (2) observed adenopathy in 59%, with axillary adenopathy in 42% and cervical adenopathy in 24%. Cervical adenopathy was an initial manifestation in 2% and generalized adenopathy in 1% of patients. The nodes usually were nontender and discrete, and they varied in size from shotty to 3 to 4 cm in diameter. The glandular enlargement was so pronounced in some patients that malignant lymphoma was suspected.

Lymphadenopathy was more common in children than in adults and most marked among black patients. Meislin and Rothfield (3) reported similar findings, with lymphadenopathy or hepatosplenomegaly in 69% of children as compared to 35% in adults with SLE. Among 698 adult patients with SLE collected from six large series in the literature, the frequency of regional and generalized lymphadenopathy ranged from 30% to 78%, with a mean prevalence of 50% (4–9).

Shapira et al. (10) observed SLE patients with lymphadenopathy to have more constitutional symptoms, lupus skin rash, hepatomegaly, splenomegaly, higher anti–double-stranded DNA (dsDNA) antibodies, and hypocomplementemia than those without lymphadenopathy.

HISTOPATHOLOGY OF THE LYMPH NODE

The characteristic finding in the lymph nodes of patients with SLE is a diffuse, reactive hyperplasia (11–13). Varying degrees of coagulative necrosis and lymphoid follicular hyperplasia are seen. Hyperplastic germinal centers with plasmacytosis and varying number of immunoblasts in the interfollicular areas are found. In the necrotic areas and within the sinuses are occasional extracellular amorphous bodies, 5 to 12 μm in diameter, that stain intensely with hematoxylin. These hematoxylin bodies contain aggregates of DNA, immunoglobulins, and polysaccharides (11), and when present, they are considered to be characteristic of lupus lymphadenitis (14). Cells resembling Reed-Sternberg cells also have been described in patients with SLE (15).

Medeiros et al. (16) examined the immunohistologic features of the lymph node in SLE and found both follicular and paracortical hyperplasia, with paracortical foci of necrosis. Two predominant cell populations within and surrounding the necrotic areas were identified: $CD11b^+CD15^+$ histiocytes, and $CD8^+CD3^+$ lymphocytes. The interfollicular regions in the nonnecrotic areas were populated by T cells, and the lymphoid follicles were composed of polytypic B cells. $CD4^+/CD3^+$ T lymphocytes outnumbered $CD8^+/CD3^+$ T-cells by a 3:1 ratio. The immunohistologic characteristics bear similarities to those of the necrotizing lymphadenitis of Kikuchi and Fujimoto.

Three histologic patterns of reactive follicular hyperplasia have been described by Kojima et al. (17) in SLE. These are histologic findings of multicentric Castleman's disease, T-zone dysplasia with hyperplastic follicles, and nonspecific follicular hyperplasia. This study emphasizes the variety of pathologic findings in lupus adenopathy.

Deftos and associates (18) reported an SLE patient with lymphadenopathy and hypercalcemia. There was no malignant transformation; however, there was an abundant expression of parathyroid hormone–related protein in the lymph nodes. This finding suggests that the hypercalcemia was due to increased production of the hormone.

KIKUCHI'S DISEASE AND SLE

Kikuchi's disease or histiocytic necrotizing lymphadenitis is a self-limited lupus-like illness of unknown cause in young women that is characterized by cervical adenopathy, fever, weight loss, and a prodrome of upper respiratory tract infection. Other than a mild leukopenia in 50% of patients, laboratory investigations generally are unremarkable. The disease may be confused clinically with SLE and histologically with malignant lymphoma (19). Diagnosis is based on the characteristic histologic changes in the lymph nodes with paracortical necrosis, mononuclear infiltrate, and absence of neutrophils and plasma cells (20). These morphologic changes may be indistinguishable from lupus lymphadenitis (21) and especially when the histology is atypical. The presence of hematoxylin bodies, prominent plasma cells, and deposition of DNA in the blood vessel wall in lupus lymphadenitis help differentiate it from Kikuchi's disease (20,22). Before a diagnosis of nodal Kikuchi's disease is made, serologic tests are necessary to exclude SLE.

Fatal cases of Kikuchi's disease are uncommon (23). Extranodal involvement is rare and has been documented in the skin, bone marrow, and myocardium. The skin rash in Kikuchi's disease is noncharacteristic and appears as single or multiple erythematous papules or plaques on the face, extremities, and trunk lasting for weeks to months and can mimic SLE. Spies et al. (24) described a constellation of histopathologic features in the cutaneous lesions of Kikuchi's disease including the presence of cells that stain with the CD68 marker for histiocytes.

Coexistent Kikuchi's disease and SLE have been reported in a few patients (25,26). The disease can occur along the course of SLE, simultaneously with the onset of SLE, or can precede the development of full-blown SLE (25,27,28). Two of 108 patients with Kikuchi's disease who were examined retrospectively developed SLE (20). The concurrent onset of mixed connective tissue disease and Kikuchi's disease also has been reported (29).

CASTLEMAN'S DISEASE AND SLE

Castleman's disease or angiofollicular lymph node hyperplasia is a rare lymphoproliferative disorder of unknown etiology characterized by lymphadenopathy with or without constitutional symptoms and clinically resembles malignant lymphoma. There are three histologic variants (hyaline vascular, plasma-cell, and mixed) and two clinical types (localized and multicentric) (30). The multicentric type can present with clinical features that may mimic systemic connective tissue disease including SLE (31–33). Castleman's disease should be considered in a patient with lupus-like presentation and with persistent lymphadenopathy despite corticosteroid therapy.

Kojima et al. (34) found histopathologic features of Castleman's disease in the lymph nodes of 5 of 19 (26%) of SLE patients presenting with peripheral lymphoadenopathy. The significance of these findings at this time is not clear.

LYMPHOGRAPHY IN SLE

Lymphography of the lower extremities was performed in SLE patients (35). Enlarged paraortic lymph nodes were seen in all patients, with a fine or coarse, evenly distributed, granulated appearance resembling that observed in the early stage of malignant lymphoma. Following prednisone therapy and clinical improvement, the lymphographic changes decreased. Similar lymphographic findings have been described in rheumatoid arthritis (RA), ankylosing spondylitis, and sarcoidosis, although the granulation in these disorders tends to be coarser and more heterogeneous.

THE SPLEEN IN SLE

Splenomegaly is not an uncommon finding in patients with SLE. In large series, the frequency of splenic enlargement ranges from 9% to as high as 46% (2,5,8,36–39). Dubois and Tuffanelli (2) found splenic enlargement in 9 of their 520 patients. When present, splenomegaly often is associated with hepatomegaly. In some patients, the spleen is so large that it can extend to the iliac crest (40).

The characteristic histopathologic picture of the spleen in SLE is periarterial fibrosis or onionskin lesion. First described in 1924 by Libman and Sacks (41), this lesion is defined as the presence of at least three to as many as 20 separated layers of the normally densely packed periarterial collagen of the penicillary or follicular arteries, producing the appearance of concentric rings. Larson (38) found the lesion in 40 of 51 SLE spleens (42) that were examined at autopsy. Calcified fibrous nodules that are continuous to the onionskin lesions have been described (43).

Although considered to be highly characteristic of SLE, periarterial fibrosis may be seen in a few other diseases. Kaiser (44) examined the specificity of the splenic lesion in 18 patients with SLE and 1,679 control cases at autopsy. Of these, 15 patients with SLE (45) and 53 of the control subjects (44) with various diagnoses were positive. In addition to SLE, the only group of patients in whom the lesion was found to be significantly more prevalent than in the rest of the controls was composed of those with essential thrombocytopenic purpura, with a frequency of 4 in 13 (43).

Isolated infarction of the spleen that is associated with circulating lupus anticoagulant and thrombosis may occur (46). Spontaneous rupture of the splenic artery in the absence of vasculitis also has been reported (47).

FUNCTIONAL ASPLENIA

Functional asplenia is a condition that is characterized by failure of the splenic uptake of radiolabeled sulfur colloid and the presence of Howell-Jolly bodies, Pappenheimer bodies, spherocytes, and poikilocytes in the peripheral blood smear. Functional asplenia is associated with a number of diseases, including sickle cell anemia, and it predisposes to infections, especially by pneumococci or other encapsulated organisms. In 1980, Dillon et al. (48) described its occurrence in a patient with lupus, and since then, several other cases have been reported (49,50). Most patients with SLE and functional asplenia who develop pneumococcal or salmonella bacterial sepsis die (49).

The condition is relatively uncommon in SLE. Of 70 patients who were screened by peripheral blood smear, five showed changes that were suggestive of functional hyposplenia; however, only three patients had no splenic uptake of the radiolabeled sulfur colloid, yielding a frequency of 4.3% (48). In another study, functional asplenia was found in two of 44 patients with SLE (4,6) who were studied by determining the presence of vacuolated red blood cells using phase-contrast microscopy, a method that is more reliable than examination of the peripheral blood smear for assessing splenic function (51).

The mechanism of functional hyposplenia in SLE is unclear. In those patients who died, the spleen showed atrophy without evidence of vasculitis (49). Functional hyposplenia also can be transient and reversible (49,52). It does not seem to be related to disease activity in SLE, and it may manifest clinically as an overwhelming infection in a patient who is in disease remission. Other mechanisms that have been proposed include thromboses of the splenic vessels, circulating serum factors, and reticuloendothelial blockade (50). The rare occurrence of congenital asplenism and SLE has been reported as well (53).

Because of the apparent high risk for pneumococcal infection, the peripheral blood smear of patients with SLE should be screened routinely for Howell-Jolly bodies. Polyvalent pneumococcal vaccine should be considered in patients with functional asplenia, because despite the splenic dysfunction, they can still mount an antibody response (49,54). In general, the antipneumococcal antibody titer is lower in patients with SLE than in vaccinated healthy subjects (55), and only half of the SLE patients develop a fourfold antibody response (56). Nevertheless, Uthman et al. (57) showed that the 23-valent pneumococcal vaccine is protective in SLE with autosplenectomy.

THE THYMUS GLAND IN SLE

Structure Of The Thymus

A central lymphoid organ, the thymus gland is critical in the development and differentiation of T cells and the induction of autoimmunity. Lymphocytes originate in the bone marrow and must migrate to the thymus to acquire immunocompetence. Microscopically, the thymus gland is composed of several lobules; each lobule consists of a lighter-staining medulla, which is populated predominantly by epithelial cells, and a darker-staining cortex, which is populated by lymphocytes. Hassall's corpuscles in the thymic medulla are mature epithelial cells that form concentric layers and become keratinized. Myoid cells with cross-striations are located adjacent to Hassall's corpuscles.

At puberty, when the thymus has reached its maximum size, the organ begins to undergo gradual physiologic involution, which is characterized by the loss of cortical thymocytes, spindling of epithelial cells, and an increase in adipose tissues. During periods of acute stress, cortical lymphocytes are rapidly depleted (i.e., stress involution) (58).

The size of the thymus in SLE, as assessed by pneumomediastinography, was found to be small, even in patients who had not received corticosteroids (59). Serial measurements in patients receiving prednisone showed a significant reduction in thymic size following steroid therapy. Most information on the histology of the thymus in SLE comes from early studies in 13 patients with SLE, which were conducted before thymic functions were fully understood (58,60). Changes that were associated with stress involution included a pronounced depletion of lymphocytes, resulting in cortical atrophy and disorganization of the medulla. Aggregates of epithelial cells and cystic Hassall's corpuscles were seen in the medulla. These abnormalities were not specific for SLE and also were seen in patients with long-standing terminal illness. An increased number of plasma cells, Russell bodies, and germinal centers in the thymus, similar to those found in patients with myasthenia gravis, was present, suggesting an immunologic reaction within the thymus (61).

The activity of thymic hormone decreases in patients with SLE, especially in those with clinically active disease (62,63). This decreased activity is a result of its low serum concentration rather than the presence of a circulating inhibitor.

Thymectomy has been performed in a small number of patients with SLE. No significant clinical improvement was noted, however, and the titer of the antinuclear antibodies (ANAs) remained unchanged (58,64).

MYASTHENIA GRAVIS AND SLE

Myasthenia gravis (MG) is a neuromuscular disorder that is characterized by a fluctuating weakness of the skeletal, bulbar, and respiratory muscles. Like SLE, MG has a predilection for young adults, with a female predominance. In MG, however, neuromuscular fatigue and an inability to sustain repeated muscular contractions are present. The basic defect is the reduction of available acetylcholine receptors (AChRs) at the neuromuscular junction because of an autoimmune process. Immunoglobulin G (IgG) antibodies to AChRs are present in 85% of patients.

The association between MG and SLE has fascinated investigators for some time. In 1963, Alarcon-Segovia et al. (65) reported the appearance of SLE in two patients several years after thymectomy for the treatment of MG, and they collected nine other patients from the literature. Since then, several reports of coexistent SLE and MG have appeared, although it is questionable whether some of these reported cases had definite SLE (66). Of 20 cases reviewed by Killian and Hoffman in 1980 (67), only 10 fulfilled the 1973 American Rheumatism Association (ARA) criteria for the classification of SLE. Ciaccio et al. (68) reported two patients with coexistent SLE and MG and found an additional 42 in the literature. Most of the 24 patients who were reported before 1972 failed to meet at least four of the 1982 ARA criteria, whereas 12 of the 20 patients reported after 1972 fulfilled these criteria.

Of the 44 reported patients with coexistent MG and SLE, MG preceded SLE in 32 (69), and in the remaining 12, MG followed SLE. In 13 patients, SLE developed following thymectomy for the treatment of MG (68). Polyarthritis and serositis were the most common presenting features of SLE. Malar skin rash was present in 20, discoid lupus erythematosus (LE) lesions in 11, and photosensitivity in seven. The disease that develops later tends to dominate the clinical picture and prognosis.

A study of the immunologic effects of thymectomy in MG showed that long-term thymectomized MG patients had mild T-cell lymphopenia, expansion of some Vβ T cells, polyclonal increase in serum immunoglobulins, and high levels of autoantibodies including anti-dsDNA and anticardiolipin antibodies. In contrast, these immunologic abnormalities were not seen in nonthymectomized and recently thymectomized MG patients. Two long-term thymectomized patients developed SLE and undifferentiated connective tissue diseases (70). Thus, thymectomy is effective in the treatment of MG, but the clinical data suggest that it may lead to the development of systemic autoimmunity in genetically predisposed subjects.

A patient with widespread cutaneous and mucosal eruption following MG and a thymoma with features of cutaneous LE and pemphigus erythematosus has been described (71). A pair of monozygotic twins who were concordant for MG underwent thymectomy, and one twin developed frank, severe SLE 18 years later. The other twin remained relatively well after thymectomy except for mild symptoms, leukopenia, and positive ANA (72). Primary antiphospholipid syndrome developed 2 years after thymectomy in a patients with MG (73).

Both SLE and MG are characterized by the presence of autoantibodies. ANAs are found in 30% of patients with MG, and IgG anticardiolipin antibodies are seen in 25%, especially those with thymic abnormalities (74). In addition, antibodies to organ-specific antigens, such as skeletal muscle, thyroid, and thymic cells, are abundant (75). The most characteristic serologic abnormality in MG is the presence of IgG antibodies to AChRs. No cross-reactivity between anti-DNA and AChRs antibody has been noted (76). SLE and MG differ in regard to certain cell-mediated immune functions. Whereas patients with SLE have decreased cellular immunity, as measured by skin testing, migratory inhibition factor production by mononuclear cells, and peripheral blood lymphocyte response to mitogens, patients with MG have a normal lymphocyte response to mitogens (77). Enumeration of lymphocyte subsets have yielded normal to abnormal numbers (75). Diaz-Jouanen (77) suggested that SLE and MG represent opposite extremes in the spectrum of abnormalities and modulations of the immune response by the thymus that may lead to autoimmunity.

The coexistence of autoimmune disorders in 721 patients with MG has been examined (78). Sixty-six other autoimmune diseases were found in 60 subjects (45), including three patients with SLE and five patients with RA. Oosterhuis and de Hass (79) found a 1% prevalence of SLE in a large series of patients with MG. Of their 142 patients with MG, two had SLE and seven RA, suggesting that RA and not SLE was more frequently associated with MG. Killian and Hoffman (67) found five cases of SLE among 1,604 cases of MG that were collated from five large series. Taking the prevalence rate of SLE as between 1/2,000 and 1/25,000 and that of MG as 1/20,000, they concluded that the five patients with SLE in the population of 1,604 patients with MG occurred other than by chance. These numbers would be even more significant if the patients with SLE who did not fulfill the ARA criteria were included in the computation. A population-based study of MG in Norway showed a prevalence rate of 9.6 per 100,000 inhabitants; SLE was found in 8.3 of the patients with MG, which was 200 times higher than the prevalence of SLE (0.039) in the general Scandinavian population (80).

Transient neonatal MG is a syndrome in infants that is mediated by the transplacental transfer of maternal IgG antibodies to AChRs, causing a weak suck, hypotonia, and difficulty in swallowing and respiration. A case of coexistent neonatal LE and transient MG in an infant who was born of a lupus mother with acetylcholine antibodies but without myasthenic symptoms has been reported (81).

Thymomas are uncommon neoplasms arising from thymic epithelial cells with variable morphology. They predominantly occur in adults, with no gender predilection (82). Of patients with thymoma, 40% have parathymic syndromes (83), the most common being MG, pure red cell aplasia, and adult-onset acquired hypogammaglobulinemia. Thymomas are found in 15% of patients with MG and also have been described in those with connective tissue diseases, including SLE. Of 598 patients with thymomas who were collected from the literature, eight had SLE (84). In some cases, thymoma and SLE have been associated with another disorder, such as progressive multifocal leukoencephalopathy (85), vacuolar myopathy (86), or red cell aplasia (87). The effect of removal of the thymoma on the clinical course of SLE is variable (88,89). Larsson (90) described a 62-year-

TABLE 38.1. LYMPHOID AND THYMIC ABNORMALITIES IN SYSTEMIC LUPUS ERYTHEMATOSUS (SLE)

Lymphadenopathy is seen in 30% to 78% of patients with SLE; the nodes are discrete and nontender; prominent enlargement of lymph nodes may develop particularly in children and blacks
The spleen is palpable in 9% to 46% of patients; an enlarged spleen is present in 67% of autopsy cases; the onionskin lesion in the splenic arterioles is a characteristic finding; hyposplenism is noted in <5%
Germinal centers consisting of focal collections of lymphocytes are noted in the thymic medulla of patients with SLE; myasthenia gravis and SLE occasionally coexist

old woman with SLE and coexistent thymoma; the tumor enlarged while the SLE improved. In contrast, a thymectomy in another patient temporarily reduced the clinical and laboratory manifestations of SLE (69).

In summary, SLE and MG occasionally may coexist, with the MG preceding SLE in 75% of patients. Thymectomy for MG appears to be a precipitating factor for development of SLE in some patients. Table 38.1 summarizes the lymphoid and thymic abnormalities that are seen in patients with SLE.

HEMATOLOGIC CHANGES

Hematologic abnormalities are exceedingly common in SLE and often are presenting manifestations of the disease. Sometimes, their features may mimic those of primary blood dyscrasias, and the nature of the underlying disorder can be completely overlooked unless SLE is considered in the differential diagnosis and specific diagnostic studies performed.

ANEMIA

Prevalence

Most patients with SLE develop anemia at some time during the course of their disease. Michael et al. (91) reported that 87 of 111 patients with SLE (78%) had a hemoglobin level of lower than 12 g/dL at diagnosis. Subsequently, 15 of 24 patients who had a normal hemoglobin level on presentation developed anemia. In general, anemia was moderate, but it was severe in some patients. The anemia usually was normochromic and normocytic, and it appeared to depend partly on the severity and duration of the illness. Three of their patients had autoimmune hemolytic anemia. The experience of other investigators has been similar to that of Michael et al. Hemoglobin of below 11 g/dL was present in 51% of Dubois and Tuffanelli's (2) 520 patients, in 73% of the 150 patients of Estes and Christian (5), and in 98% of the 275 patients of Haserick (36).

Classification

Anemia in SLE can be classified into two broad categories according to putative mechanisms: nonimmune and immune. The nonimmune-mediated group includes anemia of chronic disease, iron deficiency anemia, sideroblastic anemia, anemia of renal disease, drug-induced anemia, and anemia secondary to another disorder (e.g., sickle cell anemia). Immune-mediated anemias in SLE include autoimmune hemolytic anemia, drug-induced hemolytic anemia, aplastic anemia, pure red cell aplasia, and pernicious anemia.

A prospective study of 132 SLE patients with anemia (defined as hemoglobin of 12 g/dl or less in women and 13.5 g/dl or less in men) found the most common causes to be anemia of chronic disease (37%), iron deficiency anemia (36%) and autoimmune hemolytic anemia (14%). Other causes (13%) included pernicious anemia, chronic renal failure, cyclophosphamide-induced myelotoxicity, and miscellaneous conditions (92). It is not uncommon to see combination of two or more factors in the etiology of anemia in individual patients.

Tzioufas et al. (93) found serum antibodies to erythropoietin in 15% of SLE patients, and the presence of these antibodies was associated with severe anemia and active disease. Whether these antibodies can directly inhibit erythropoiesis in SLE or not remains to be investigated.

Anemia Of Chronic Disease

The most common type of anemia in SLE is anemia of chronic disease. The red cells on the peripheral blood smear are normochromic and normocytic. The serum iron concentration is reduced, and the total iron-binding capacity is unchanged or slightly low. A decrease in the iron saturation of transferrin is present. The bone marrow examination usually is normal, with adequate iron stores (91). The anemia develops slowly unless it becomes complicated by other factors, such as blood loss. The reticulocyte count is low for the degree of anemia (94).

Iron Metabolism

Iron metabolism was investigated by Burger et al. (95) in 11 patients with SLE using ^{59}Fe. Iron use was decreased in seven of these patients. Radioactivity over various organs differed from normal, with increased levels of radioactivity over the spleen and liver. The increased amount of absorbed iron did not appear to serve the purpose of hemoglobin synthesis but was stored instead. Plasma iron turnover, on the other hand, was elevated in most patients. The life span of erythrocytes was reduced in the absence of hemolysis. It was concluded that the anemia of chronic disease in patients with SLE may be attributed to insufficient bone marrow activity, shortened red-cell life span, and, possibly, poor uptake of iron.

Whittingham et al. (96) found low mean serum iron levels in SLE. Following the administration of prednisolone, a two- to fourfold rise in the serum iron level occurred. This increase in the serum iron concentration was not sustained. The mechanism of anemia of chronic disease is not well understood. Results of investigations on its pathogenesis in RA (97,98) indicate that multiple factors are involved, including impairment of iron release by the mononuclear phagocytic system, iron trapping by binding proteins, decreased erythropoietin responsiveness, and suppressive effects of cytokines on erythropoiesis.

The treatment of anemia of chronic disease in SLE is directed at the disease process. It does not warrant iron therapy or any specific intervention.

Iron Deficiency Anemia

Iron deficiency anemia is most commonly due to menorrhagia and to GI blood loss secondary to the chronic use of nonsteroidal antiinflammatory drugs (NSAIDs) and corticosteroids.

Differentiating between anemia due to iron deficiency and anemia of chronic disease may be difficult in some patients. In general, a low serum ferritin level is associated with depletion of body iron stores. However, in inflammatory conditions such as RA, ferritin is an acute-phase reactant and the serum level may become elevated. Thus, serum ferritin may be normal or elevated in an iron-deficient anemic RA patient. In SLE, the serum ferritin level is positively correlated with disease activity and high anti-dsDNA titer (99). Measurement of soluble transferrin receptor in the serum has recently been shown to be useful in differentiating the two causes of anemia (100).

Sickle Cell Anemia

Sickle cell anemia and SLE share common clinical manifestations, including arthralgias, chest pain, pleural effusion, cardiomegaly, nephropathy, strokes, and seizures. In addition, my group has found that patients with sickle cell hemoglinopathies have an increased prevalence of autoantibodies, including ANAs (42). The coexistence of SLE and sickle cell anemia has been reported (42,45,101–108), and in some of these patients, the recognition of SLE was delayed because of similarities in the clinical features of these conditions (106). Wilson et al. (107) postulated that abnormalities in the alternative pathway of complement in sickle cell hemoglobinopathy may predispose patients to immune complex disorders, including SLE, but no evidence has been found to show that SLE is more prevalent in those with sickle cell hemoglobinopathies. The risk for infectious complications is increased in both conditions. Hydroxyurea has been reported to reduce the severity and frequency of vaso-occlusive crises in a patient with sickle cell anemia and SLE (108).

Sideroblastic Anemia

A few cases of sideroblastic refractory anemia in SLE have been reported, including one terminating in erythroleukemia (109,110). Another patient who had refractory anemia with excess of blasts, which is a myelodysplastic syndrome, developed SLE (111). These cases probably are incidental and do not represent a true association with SLE.

Immune-Mediated Anemias

The inhibition of erythropoiesis by cellular and serum factors may be important in the pathogenesis of chronic anemia in patients with SLE. The number of erythroid colony-forming units (CFU-E), which are the late erythropoietic precursors, has been found to be significantly reduced in the bone marrow of anemic patients with SLE (112). Moreover, the formation of CFU-E was inhibited *in vitro* by autologous and allogeneic T lymphocytes from untreated subjects, but not by those from steroid-treated patients with SLE (112). The activity of monocytes to stimulate bone marrow fibroblasts to produce a hemopoietic growth factor was found to be diminished in SLE (113). Bone marrow stromal cells play an important role in hemopoiesis, and the diminished production of growth factor may be another cause of hemocytopenia in SLE.

Circulating inhibitors of erythropoiesis also have been described (114–119). Sera from patients with SLE and anemia of chronic disease suppressed CFU-E formation (117). Dainiak et al. (115) characterized the serum inhibitor as having the physical properties of an immunoglobulin, and its presence was associated with disease activity. The inhibitor was removed by plasma exchange and by steroid therapy.

Pure Red Cell Aplasia

Pure red cell aplasia (PRCA) is an autoimmune condition that is characterized by severe normochromic normocytic anemia, reticulocytopenia, and absence of red cell precursors in the bone marrow. Different pathogenetic mechanisms have been proposed for PRCA, including suppression of erythropoiesis by serum antibodies to erythroblasts, to CFU-Es, or to erythropoietin, and T-cell suppression of erythropoiesis.

Elevated serum titer of antibodies to erythropoietin has been reported in PRCA and SLE, and the antibody titer decreased with response to therapy (120). PRCA is associated with a number of autoimmune conditions, and a few cases of coexistent PRCA and SLE (and procainamide-induced LE) have been reported (121–124). Serum IgG from a patient with SLE and PRCA inhibited the growth of red cell precursors (114). Anticardiolipin antibodies also have been described in patients with SLE and PRCA (121).

Several therapeutic modalities have been used in the treatment of PRCA including corticosteroids, immunosuppressive agents, plasmapheresis, and lymphapheresis. SLE patient with PRCA has been treated successfully with recombinant erythropoietin (125) and high-dose intravenous (IV) gamma globulin (120).

Aplastic Anemia

Aplastic anemia rarely occurs in SLE secondary to the use of nitrogen mustard derivatives, azathioprine, antimalarials, or other agents, such as chloramphenicol (126) and dapsone (127). In a few published cases, the aplastic anemia was considered to be caused primarily by the underlying disease; however, the role of drugs cannot be completely excluded (116,128). Rarely, pancytopenia and aplastic anemia can be the initial manifestation of SLE antedating the other clinical features of the disease (129). Aplastic anemia has been reported in an infant with neonatal lupus erythematosus (130).

The presence of circulating antibodies to precursor bone marrow cells suggests that some cases of aplastic anemia may be the result of an autoimmune process. Brooks et al. (131) identified a complement-dependent IgG antibody that suppressed the growth of allogeneic granulocyte-macrophage progenitor cells *in vitro*. Bailey et al. (132) found a noncomplement IgG antibody that inhibited *in vitro* granulocyte-macrophage progenitor cells and erythroblast-forming units in a patient with SLE and aplastic anemia. The IgG antibody disappeared on recovery of the patient. Other investigators have suggested T-cell–mediated suppression of hematopoiesis in aplastic anemia.

Aplastic anemia has been reported in an infant with neonatal lupus erythematosus (131). Erythroid progenitor burst-forming units colonies were cultured from the patient's bone marrow. Removal of $CD8^+$ lymphocytes led to a marked increase in immature erythroid progenitors, suggesting that suppressor lymphocytes inhibited the development of immature erythroid progenitors.

Various regimens have been used successfully for the treatment of aplastic anemia that is associated with SLE. These include androgens, cyclophosphamide, antithymocyte globulin, and plasmapheresis in conjunction with systemic corticosteroids (132–135).

Bone Marrow Findings

Michael et al. (91) examined the bone marrow aspirates of 32 patients with SLE and found them to be normal in most. Plasma cells were increased (>2) in 13 patients. One patient had a hypoplastic marrow, and two patients with autoimmune hemolytic anemia had a hypercellular marrow. Similar findings have been reported by others (136).

Careful studies by Burkhardt (137) of bone marrow biopsy specimens in 21 patients with SLE have shown significant alterations in the blood vessels, cellular elements, and intercellular substance. Compared with those of control subjects, an increased frequency of the following changes in SLE was found:

1. Subintimal swelling of the arteries and arterioles, with evidence of the deposition of proteins in the vessel wall, was seen.
2. Endothelial swelling and dissociation were found in the sinusoids.
3. The ground substance was edematous, with fibrinoid and sclerosing changes.
4. A proliferation of histiocytes bearing cytoplasmic inclusions of iron-positive protein material was noted.
5. Diffuse plasma cell proliferation occurred, with the formation of Russell bodies.
6. There was a reduction of granulopoiesis with predominantly immature forms, and necrobioses with opal nuclei were observed.

Feng et al. (138) examined the bone marrow of 23 patients with lupus pancytopenia. The most common abnormalities, which were seen in nine patients (39%), were hypoplasia and dyserythropoiesis. The latter refers to nuclear budding and immaturity in the presence of full cytoplasmic hemoglobin. Lymphocytosis was found in five patients (22%). Other abnormal findings included gelatinous transformation, plasmacytosis, and marrow hyperplasia. Pereira et al. (139) found global hypocellularity (48%), increased reticulin proliferation (76%), and necrosis (19%) to be the most common abnormalities in the bone marrow in 21 SLE patients with peripheral cytopenias. An interesting finding is the presence of storage and hemophagocytic histiocytes in the bone marrow of SLE patients during episodes of hemocytopenia (140).

It should be noted that many of these morphologic changes are not specific for SLE; they also may be seen in those patients with RA and other diseases (137). Nevertheless, these findings, as well as the presence of autoantibodies and cellular factors that inhibit the growth of bone marrow precursor cells, suggest that the bone marrow is a major target organ in SLE.

Myelofibrosis

Myelofibrosis is a myeloproliferative disorder that is characterized by bone marrow fibrosis, splenomegaly, peripheral leukoerythroblastosis, and red cell poikilocytes. It frequently is associated with various benign and malignant disorders, and in some patients it appears to be a primary condition without an underlying disorder. Myelofibrosis occurring in the setting of SLE has been described in a few cases (114,141–146). Conversely, SLE is a rare etiology of myelofibrosis.

Paquette et al. (147) described eight patients with myelofibrosis and SLE. Myelofibrosis developed either before or concurrent with the diagnosis of lupus in five patients, while in the remaining three, myelofibrosis developed after the onset of SLE. Five patients fulfilled four or more American College of Rheumatology (ACR) criteria for SLE, and three patients met three criteria. All had positive ANAs, anti-DNA antibodies, and/or positive LE cell test. The patients presented with pancytopenia, and bone marrow biopsy showed fibrosis with increased amounts of fibrillar reticulin, collagen, and fibroblasts. Half of the patients had splenomegaly.

Steroid therapy improved the peripheral blood cytopenias in half of the patients with SLE and even reversed the myelofibrosis in a few (148–150). Compared to patients with idiopathic myelofibrosis and myeloid metaplasia, patients with SLE and this condition tended to be younger, had a lower frequency of splenomegaly, and were responsive to steroid and immunosuppressive therapy. High-dose gamma globulin has also been used successfully in the treatment of myelofibrosis in SLE (151).

Gelatinous Transformation Of The Bone Marrow

Gelatinous transformation of the bone marrow, which is a rare condition associated with cachexia caused by cancer, anorexia nervosa, tuberculosis, and other chronic illnesses, has been reported in 3 of 30 patients with SLE who had pancytopenia (152). Also, two patients with SLE were cachectic. Hyaluronic acid, which is a mucopolysaccharide, was present in the ground substance of the marrow associated with fat atrophy and cellular hypoplasia.

Acute Hemophagocytic Syndrome

SLE has been added to the list of diseases that are associated with acute hemophagocytic syndrome. Wong et al. (153) described six patients with SLE who presented with fever and severe pancytopenia related to reactive hemophagocytosis. This is a rare condition that is associated with various infections and neoplasms, especially lymphomas. It is characterized by pancytopenia and a bone marrow picture showing mature-looking histiocytes, many of which have phagocytosed erythrocytes, platelets, granulocytes, and erythroblasts. A study of 40 consecutive cases of reactive hemophagocytic syndrome in Hong Kong identified two patients with SLE (154).

Various modalities have been used for the treatment of hemophagocytic syndrome in SLE including corticosteroids, high-dose gamma globulin and plasmapheresis (154–156).

Pernicious Anemia And SLE

Pernicious anemia often is associated with other autoimmune disorders, such as Sjögren's syndrome and Hashimoto's thyroiditis, yet only a few cases of coexistent SLE and pernicious anemia have been reported (111, 157–160). The treatment of pernicious anemia when accompanied by SLE requires the administration of both vitamin B_{12} and systemic corticosteroids. Replacement therapy with vitamin B_{12} usually is not sufficient to reverse the hematologic abnormalities in patients with lupus and pernicious anemia (161).

Molad et al. (162) found that 18.6% of 43 female patients with SLE had abnormally low serum cobalamin levels, but none had pernicious anemia. As a group, SLE patients had lower mean levels of cobalamin than control subjects did. Low serum levels of transcobalamin II and unsaturated vitamin B_{12} capacity correlated with lupus disease activity (163).

Autoimmune Hemolytic Anemia

Autoimmune hemolytic anemia (AIHA) is not an uncommon cause of anemia in patients with SLE. Approximately 7% to 15% of those in large series developed AIHA (39,164,165). Among a group of 186 patients with SLE who were studied by Alger et al. (164), 17 (9%) had Coombs'-positive hemolytic anemia. Of these 17 patients, six had Evans' syndrome (i.e., the concurrence of AIHA and immune thrombocytopenic purpura). In a prospective study of 126 SLE patients, 16 (12.7%) developed AIHA, and three had Evans' syndrome (166).

AIHA may be the initial manifestation of SLE, occurring in 2% to 6% of patients (26,167). In five of ten patients who were studied by Videbaek (168), AIHA was the initial and dominant clinical feature of the disease for several months, and even years, before other manifestations of SLE appeared. AIHA developed during the course of SLE in the other patients.

Classification

AIHA can be classified into two major types with respect to the antierythrocyte antibody and the optimal temperature of antibody reactivity with antigens on the red cell surface. The warm type of AIHA is mediated by IgG antibodies that are capable of reacting with antigens optimally at 37°C. Cold agglutinin AIHA is mediated by IgM complement-fixing antibody, which binds optimally to red cell antigens at 4°C. (Chapter 27 discusses the immunology of antierythrocyte antibodies in SLE.)

Warm AIHA

Warm AIHA is the predominant type in patients with SLE. Red blood cells that are coated by the warm IgG antibodies are removed from the circulation, primarily by sequestration in the spleen. The antibody-coated red blood cells undergo membrane alteration *in vivo*, resulting in the formation of spherocytes. Matsumoto et al. (169) examined the fine structure of the spleen in AIHA during SLE and found that erythrocytes coated with IgG and complement were phagocytosed completely by splenic macrophages and, to a lesser extent, by sinus endothelial cells. In contrast, in the liver, only evidence of occasional phagocytosis of sensitized erythrocytes by the Kupffer cells was found, confirming that the spleen is the major site of red blood cell destruction.

The symptoms and clinical findings in AIHA are variable. Symptoms that are referable to the anemic state, such as weakness, dizziness, and fever, are common. Evidence of hemolysis, including jaundice and dark urine, may be found. AIHA in the setting of SLE develops gradually in most patients, but occasionally it may present as a rapidly progressive hemolytic crisis (167,168).

With a significant degree of hemolysis, anisocytosis and macrocytosis often are noted in the peripheral blood smear. Nucleated red blood cells are seen in patients with marked hemolysis. Occasionally, polychromatophilic red cells, stippled cells, and Howell-Jolly bodies are found. The bone marrow is hyperplastic, frequently with a shift to the left in the myeloid series (167). Reticulocyte counts are elevated in association with a significant degree of hemolysis after hemorrhage and during systemic corticosteroid therapy.

The serum haptoglobin level usually is reduced during active phases of hemolysis (170–172). In the presence of infection, cancer, or steroid treatment, the serum haptoglobin level rises; consequently, if hemolysis coexists with these factors, the serum level may be normal (170,172). This also is observed when bone marrow function is impaired.

AIHA With Positive ANA

Tan and Chaplin (173) found low-titer ANA in patients with idiopathic AIHA who did not have an underlying systemic connective tissue disease or lymphoproliferative disorder. No correlation was found among ANA and various clinical or serologic parameters. Favre et al. (174) described three patients with AIHA and one with immune thrombocytopenic purpura with positive ANA and anti-dsDNA antibodies who did not develop the full clinical picture of SLE after long-term follow-up. None had evidence of clinical renal disease, but on kidney biopsy all had mild mesangial proliferation of focal glomerulonephritis. Miescher et al. (175) enlarged their series to ten patients. All had AIHA and/or autoimmune thrombocytopenia with positive ANA and low-titer or negative anti-dsDNA antibodies. Two of their patients had mild arthralgias; however, none developed clinical features of SLE. The authors suggested that these patients represent a transitional form between SLE and AIHA and autoimmune thrombocytopenia.

SLE Subset With Hematocytopenia

Alger et al. (164) compared the features of 31 patients with SLE who presented with AIHA and/or immune thrombocytopenia to a group of 62 patients with SLE but without hematologic manifestations. The former group, which was younger and included a greater percentage of females, had a lower prevalence of fever, polyarthritis, serositis, cutaneous vasculitis, nephropathy, and central nervous system disease, and had fewer complement abnormalities. It was suggested that patients with SLE who develop AIHA and/or immune thrombocytopenia constitute two related subsets of lupus patients with a relatively better prognosis. The high frequency of antiphospholipid antibodies in SLE patients with hemocytopenia further supports this concept (176,177). In contrast, Nossent and Swaak (126) reported that hemolytic anemia, neutropenia, or lymphopenia did not influence the survival rate of patients with lupus. Moreover, late-onset thrombocytopenia was associated with a decreased probability of survival.

Kokori et al. (178) reported that the recurrence rate of hemolytic anemia in a group of SLE patients with AIHA was low among treated patients (4 per 100 persons-years). They also found an association between AIHA and IgG anticardiolipin antibodies and thrombosis.

Combined Warm And Cold AIHA

Sokol et al. (179) found that 7% of 865 patients with AIHA who were referred to a blood transfusion center had warm IgG and cold IgM anti–red cell antibodies, and that both antibodies contributed to the hemolysis. Of the patients in this group, 20% had SLE. The high frequency of SLE was confirmed by Shulman et al. (180), who found that 5 of 12 patients (42%) with combined warm and cold AIHA had SLE.

IgG and C3d usually are present on the patient's red blood cells. In the serum, both IgG warm antibodies and high-thermal-amplitude cold IgM autoagglutinins are detectable. The IgM antibodies are reactive over a broad temperature range, from 0° to 30°C or higher (180). Patients with this type of AIHA have severe hemolysis but generally are responsive to corticosteroid therapy (180).

Treatment

Medical Therapy

Systemic corticosteroids, 1 to 1.5 mg/kg of prednisone daily or its equivalent, are efficacious, and remain the mainstay of the treatment for AIHA in patients with SLE. It is preferable to administer steroids parenterally to the symptomatic and acutely ill patient and later switch to an oral preparation when the patient has stabilized and improved. The dose is maintained for at least 4 to 6 weeks and gradually tapered, provided that a continued and/or sustained response occurs. No controlled trials have been reported on the use of corticosteroids in the treatment of AIHA in SLE, but our clinical experience (and that of others) indicates that approximately 75% of patients respond satisfactorily to steroid therapy (181). The response rate is similar to the 76% reported in patients with idiopathic warm AIHA (181). All 16 patients with SLE and AIHA who were followed prospectively responded to steroid therapy (106).

In steroid-responsive patients who were studied by Priofsky (181), the clinical response was evident within a week. Stabilization of the hematocrit occurred within 30 to 90 days after the initiation of therapy.

In patients with severe and rapidly progressive hemolytic anemia, pulse methylprednisolone should be tried, 1 g intravenous for 3 consecutive days, followed by the conventional steroid dose (182). The reticulocyte count can be used to monitor the response to treatment and to detect any relapse as the steroid dose is tapered. A drop in the reticulocyte count is associated with a relapse in the hemolytic process.

Various treatment measures have been tried in patients who fail to respond to systemic corticosteroids or in those who continue to require a moderate to high dose of prednisone to control hemolysis. Most of the experiences have come from uncontrolled clinical studies. Priofsky (181) used azathioprine, 2 to 2.5 mg/kg, in conjunction with prednisone, 10 to 20 mg/d, in patients with AIHA who failed to respond to full therapeutic doses of prednisone. Danazol in conjunction with high-dose corticosteroids has been reported to be useful in the treatment of warm AIHA, including that associated with SLE (183). A combination of prednisone and danazol has been reported to be effective as a first line as well as for refractory AIHA including SLE (184). Plasmapheresis (185), high-dose IV gamma globulin (186), and vinca-laden platelets (187) have been used with some success in a small number of patients with idiopathic AIHA refractory to conventional therapy. Intravenous IgG has been shown to be effective in 40 of 73 patients with warm AIHA; thus, it is not recommended as a standard therapy but may be useful as an adjunctive therapy for selected patients, such as those with toxicity to other treatments (188).

Splenectomy

Splenectomy is used to treat patients with idiopathic warm AIHA who require a high maintenance dose of prednisone (20 mg/day or more), patients who have frequent relapses, or those with serious side effects to steroid therapy. In general, splenectomy as a treatment is less effective for warm AIHA than for immune thrombocytopenia. The response rate to splenectomy in those with idiopathic warm AIHA is 50% to 60% (189), with reduction in the steroid maintenance dose or amelioration of the hemolysis.

It was suggested by early workers that splenectomy for idiopathic immune thrombocytopenia or idiopathic AIHA somehow unmasks occult or latent lupus, thus causing a dissemination of the disease. Best and Darling (190) reviewed the pertinent evidence both for and against this controversial issue, and they concluded that splenectomy does not lead to the dissemination of SLE but, on the contrary, has a beneficial effect for many patients.

Early studies on a small number of cases suggested that splenectomy is not efficacious in the treatment of warm AIHA associated with SLE (2,168). More recent studies have shown that splenectomy is of some value in the treatment of selected cases, but that this benefit may not be long-lasting. Of seven patients with SLE and warm AIHA (five had concomitant immune thrombopenia) who underwent splenectomy, six showed a sustained increase in hematocrit of greater than 20% (191). Rivero et al. (192) compared the clinical course of 15 patients with SLE and AIHA and/or immune thrombocytopenia who underwent splenectomy and 15 SLE patients who were treated medically for the hemocytopenia. Splenectomy produced short-term benefit, but at follow-up, no clear-cut difference in the clinical course of the two groups was seen. The splenectomy group had a significantly higher frequency of cutaneous vasculitis and serious infections after surgery. More of the splenectomized patients eventually required immunosuppressive therapy than did those in the medically treated group at follow-up.

Patients with SLE and AIHA who fail to respond to systemic corticosteroids should be given immunosuppressive agents next. The role of other measures in these patients, including IV gamma globulin, plasmapheresis, or cyclosporine, remains to be defined. Splenectomy probably should be reserved for the patient with acute fulminant AIHA who fails to respond to aggressive medical treatment (192). Polyvalent pneumococcal vaccine should be given to splenectomized patients, such as those with functional asplenia.

Blood Groups And Transfusions In SLE

The distribution of ABO and Rh blood types of 138 patients with SLE who were studied by Dubois and Tuffanelli (2) was normal; 86 of the patients were Rh positive. Similar results were obtained by Leonhardt (193), who found no differences in the major blood groups of 54 patients with SLE, 221 of their relatives, and 5,668 healthy blood donors.

The prevalence of adverse reactions to blood transfusion has been low. In 82 patients 16% (2) studied by Dubois who received one or more blood transfusions, only three developed reactions, one developed urticaria, and two developed fever. Of McGehee Harvey et al.'s (8) patients, 39 (48%) received one or more blood transfusions. Over 200 blood transfusions were administered, and the frequency of untoward reactions was low. Occasionally, a brief febrile response or urticaria occurred, but these patients subsequently were transfused without recurrence of the reaction. In contrast, Michael et al. (91) commented that in their experience, transfusion reactions appeared to be more common in patients with SLE than in the general hospital population, but no statistical data were presented.

Blood transfusions should be avoided whenever possible, not only because of the risk of hepatitis and other infectious diseases but also because of the observation that patients with SLE develop isoantibodies against red cell antigens. Callender et al. (194,195) reported a patient with SLE who, in response to multiple blood transfusions, developed isoagglutinins to five different red cell antigens that usually are ignored by most individuals. Multiple types of isoagglutinins were found in the serum of another transfused patient with probable SLE (196). Another patient with SLE developed hemolytic anemia following multiple blood transfusions, with the appearance of three atypical hemagglutinins (197). A hemoglobinuric transfusion reaction resulting from Rh isosensitization has been described as well (198).

The antibody response of patients with SLE to blood group antigens has been examined following experimental immunization. The intravenous injection of 1 mL of incompatible whole blood led to the appearance of an unusually high isoagglutinin titer in a patient with SLE (199). Zingale et al. (200) immunized 15 SLE patients and matched controls with incompatible blood group substances. Patients with SLE developed higher titers of isohemagglutinin antibodies than the controls, as well as the transient appearance of a false-positive test for syphilis, circulating anticoagulants, antithyroglobulin, and antikidney antibodies. In contrast, the antibody production to various exogenous antigens following immunization in SLE has been either normal or depressed (201,202).

The few indications for blood transfusions in patients with SLE include those with acute massive bleeding, symptomatic patients with severe anemia, and a hemoglobin level falling to less than 6 g/dL, or those with concomitant severe heart disease or cerebrovascular ischemia. The response of patients with SLE and autoimmune hemolytic anemia to systemic corticosteroids generally is prompt and favorable, so that blood transfusion may not be necessary. Circulating antierythrocyte antibodies make blood cross-matching difficult (203).

Recombinant Erythropoietin Therapy

The anemia that is associated with chronic renal failure can be treated effectively with recombinant human erythropoietin, provided that sufficient iron stores are available (204). Used mainly for patients with end-stage kidney disease who are on maintenance hemodialysis, it is well tolerated except for the development or aggravation of hypertension in 25% and seizures in 2% of patients (205). The mechanisms underlying these adverse reactions are not clear. Whether patients with SLE who are on hemodialysis with anemia respond differently to erythropoietin therapy than patients without SLE has not been specifically investigated. My group has treated SLE patients on chronic hemodialysis before renal transplantation, and with good results.

Lim et al. (206) have shown that erythropoietin also is effective in ameliorating the anemia in a group of predialysis patients with chronic renal failure due to SLE and other conditions. Patients with SLE and end-stage renal disease who are on hemodialysis may become resistant to erythropoietin therapy if the underlying disease becomes active (207). Erythropoietin also has been found to be useful in a pregnant SLE patient with nephritis (208) as well as in patients with RA and anemia of chronic disease (209).

In vitro studies have shown that recombinant erythropoietin can increase the production of immunoglobulins by B cells, cause proliferation of bone marrow progenitor cells, and increase the expression of erythrocyte complement receptor type 1 (210). Theoretically, recombinant erythropoietin can be beneficial to patients with lupus by increasing clearance of immune complexes or be harmful by stimulating autoimmune responses. A longitudinal study of five patients with SLE but without renal failure who self-administered recombinant erythropoietin, however, showed no significant changes in anti-dsDNA, antiphospholipid antibody titers, C3, and renal function. One patient with anticardiolipin antibodies who was on estrogen replacement therapy developed thrombophlebitis that related temporally to erythropoietin therapy (211). Further studies are necessary to examine the possible relationship between erythropoietin therapy and thrombotic episodes in SLE.

THROMBOCYTOPENIA AND PLATELET DISORDERS

Frequency And Significance

Thrombocytopenia, which is defined as a platelet count of less than 150,000 cells/mL, is not an uncommon finding in SLE. The prevalence among seven large series in the literature has ranged from 7% to 52%, with a mean cumulative percentage of 14.5% (2,5,8,9,38,91,212) (see Chapter 30, Table 30.1).

The degree of thrombocytopenia is variable, but profound thrombocytopenia is uncommon. Mild thrombocytopenia often appears during an exacerbation of SLE without causing bleeding tendency. Platelet counts were available for 86 patients in McGehee Harvey et al.'s (8) series, and in 23 they were definitely depressed. Of the 12 who had platelet counts of less than 50,000/mL, patients were included in whom thrombocytopenia purpura was a predominant feature of their disease. Also, seven had counts of between 50,000 and

100,000/mL, and four had counts of between 100,000 and 150,000/mL. None of these patients had abnormal bleeding. In Larson's (38) series of 196 patients, 15 (8%) had platelet counts of below 100,000/mL on at least two occasions. Nine patients had purpuric lesions at the time that platelet counts were depressed, but six patients did not. An additional group of nine patients had purpuric skin rash as a prominent feature of their illness, but the platelet count in these patients was never found to be below 100,000/mL. In 112 patients with SLE who were studied for hemostatic functions, Gladman et al. (212) found 18 patients with a platelet count of less than 150,000/mL. In this group, ten patients had counts of below 100,000/mL, yet only one patient developed petechiae.

In association with thrombocytopenia, the usual coexistent laboratory abnormalities, such as a prolonged bleeding time and diminished clot retraction when the platelet count is below 50,000/mL, are noted. A positive tourniquet test may be present without any platelet deficit, however, and simply may reflect vascular fragility resulting from SLE or prolonged steroid therapy (213). Coexistent hemostatic defects often are observed in patients with SLE and low platelet counts (212). A correlation between the presence of anticardiolipin and other antiphospholipid antibodies and thrombocytopenia in SLE, as well as in chronic immune thrombocytopenic purpura, has been recognized (see Chapters 25 and 52).

The clinical significance of thrombocytopenia in SLE has been examined. A prospective study of 19 patients with platelet counts of less than 100,000/mL revealed two distinct clinical groups: patients who were thrombocytopenic only during severe multisystem disease flares, and patients with a chronic low platelet count and intermittent mild flares in other systems. None of the patients in either group developed severe bleeding; and whether acute or chronic, thrombocytopenia itself did not determine the subsequent course and prognosis of the patient (214). In two large studies on survivorship, the presence of thrombocytopenia appeared to be a significant risk factor for a worse prognosis in SLE (215,216). When the significance of thrombocytopenia was examined in a highly selective subset of patients with SLE and biopsy-proven nephritis, Clark et al. (217) found that thrombocytopenia was a useful index of disease activity.

Immune Thrombocytopenic Purpura

A special relationship exists between SLE and autoimmune thrombocytopenic purpura (also referred to as idiopathic or immune thrombocytopenic purpura; ITP), both of which primarily afflict young females. Some patients with ITP who initially are considered to be idiopathic later may develop a classic clinical picture of SLE. Further, a thrombocytopenic purpura, clinically indistinguishable from ITP, may occur along the course of SLE.

From 3% to 15% of patients with ITP go on to develop SLE (218). In a group of 62 adults with chronic ITP who were studied by Difino et al. (219), three patients (4.8%) developed SLE. Perez et al. (220) found that 6 of 18 patients with ITP (33%) tested positive for ANA at presentation, and that four of them developed classic SLE, within a mean duration of 2.3 years. A retrospective study of 117 patients with ITP showed a positive ANA in 24 patients, and four of them developed SLE (221). Patients with high-titer ANA tested positive for anti-Ro/SSA and anti-La/SSA antibody. Thus, patients with ITP and high-titer ANA and precipitating antibodies to Ro/SSA may develop later SLE (222). It is noteworthy that anti-Ro/SSA antibody is associated with thrombocytopenia in SLE (223). Firkin et al. (224) coined the term *lupoid thrombocytopenia* to refer to a group of patients with chronic ITP who were ANA positive but did not have other clinical or laboratory findings of SLE. None had anti-DNA, anti-Sm, or anti-Ro/SSA. The value of using this label is questionable, however, because the ANA-positive patients were similar in every other respect to those in the ANA-negative group.

In 1956, Dameshek and Reeves (221) emphasized the high frequency of SLE that occurs following splenectomy for apparent ITP. In a series of 51 consecutive patients, eight subsequently developed definite SLE, with two others being probable and six possible. Thus, at least 31 of the patients in this group eventually developed clinical manifestations of SLE, and 15 had definite SLE (225). A study of 115 ITP patients who underwent splenectomy revealed that 14 (12%) patients subsequently developed SLE. The high percentage may in part be due to a referral bias in a tertiary care center (226).

Other investigators have since disputed this claim and found that splenectomy in ITP does not lead to the development of SLE (190,227–229). In 1960, Doan et al. (228) reviewed their experience with 381 cases of thrombocytopenic purpura over a 28-year period and found that SLE caused the syndrome in 2% of patients. After splenectomy, the prevalence of new SLE cases was 1.2%. Splenectomy did not precipitate or disseminate the symptoms or signs of SLE in any patient, and the investigators believe that the hazards to life during acute hypersplenic thrombocytopenic crises outweigh the danger of developing subsequent SLE. Best and Darling (190) undertook a critical analysis of the existing data on this issue, and they concluded that splenectomy does not lead to the dissemination of latent SLE but actually is beneficial to some patients with drug-resistant cytopenias.

Clinical Presentation

The clinical manifestations of thrombocytopenia in SLE generally are similar to those seen in patients with ITP or other causes of thrombocytopenia, and they depend on the platelet count. When the platelet count is below

50,000/mL, spontaneous bleeding or purpura may occur. In addition to the platelet count, however, other factors, including qualitative platelet defects and platelet age, are important in the development of spontaneous bleeding (230). Bleeding usually presents as petechiae and/or ecchymoses, especially in the lower limbs, which experience increased capillary pressure. Nasal and buccal mucosal hemorrhage, heavy menstrual blood flow, epistaxis, and gum bleeding also may be present. Spontaneous bleeding into the brain is the most feared complication and can be fatal.

The immunologic properties of antiplatelet antibodies in ITP and SLE are discussed in Chapter 27.

Treatment

The mainstay of drug therapy is systemic corticosteroids, 1.0 to 1.5 mg/kg/d of prednisone equivalent. Corticosteroid therapy is considered to be the equivalent of medical splenectomy, because it prevents the sequestration of antibody-coated platelets in the spleen (230). In most patients, a clinical response is seen within 1 to 8 weeks. High-dose intravenous pulse methylprednisolone also has been used for profound thrombocytopenia in SLE, but its superiority over conventional steroid therapy has not been established (231). Moreover, repeated courses may result in a diminished platelet response (232).

In idiopathic ITP, splenectomy generally is recommended for patients who fail to respond to systemic corticosteroids or for those who require moderate doses of steroids to maintain the platelet count (230). Splenectomy removes the major site of destruction of damaged platelets and the source of antiplatelet antibodies. In SLE patients, however, it is preferable to try other agents before recommending splenectomy for steroid-resistant thrombocytopenia, because of the increased risk of severe infections following splenectomy and the apparent efficacy of other agents (192). Danazol, which is an androgenic steroid with few virilizing effects, has been shown to be effective in some patients with SLE and thrombocytopenia refractory to steroids, cytotoxic drugs, and/or splenectomy, and it is given at an average dose of 200 mg, three or four times a day. Often, however, danazol cannot be discontinued without recurrence of the thrombocytopenia (233,234). Danazol has been used in the therapy of thrombocytopenia associated with antiphospholipid antibody syndrome (235).

Intermittent intravenous cyclophosphamide was shown to be effective in the treatment of thrombocytopenia in seven patients with SLE refractory to splenectomy or steroids or requiring excessive doses of steroids (236,237). Other agents that have been reported to be useful in the treatment of thrombocytopenia, although in a limited number of patients with SLE, include azathioprine (238), cyclosporine (239), dapsone (240), and vincristine (241). In chronic ITP not associated with SLE, azathioprine has been found to be effective in 64 of patients who are refractory to steroids and/or splenectomy. Clinical response was delayed in many patients, requiring a course of at least 4 months on the drug (242). Combination chemotherapy using protocols in lymphoproliferative disorders has been found to be beneficial in some patients with refractory chronic ITP (243).

Extracorporeal immunoadsorption of plasma to remove IgG and circulating immune complexes using staphylococcal-A-silica columns has been reported to be effective in refractory ITP (244). The mechanism is unclear but the procedure may decrease platelet activation (245).

Intravenous gamma globulin also is effective, but its effect may not be long-lasting (246). As in idiopathic ITP, gamma globulin is most useful in the treatment of life-threatening bleeding or in preparing the patient for urgent surgery or elective cesarean section (247–249). A prospective, randomized, clinical trial showed that intravenous IgG offers no advantages over systemic corticosteroids as the primary form of therapy in untreated patients with ITP, including patients with SLE (250). My group also has used gamma globulin successfully as an adjunctive measure patients with SLE and thrombocytopenia who failed to respond optimally to corticosteroids and had a concomitant serious bacterial infection.

Maier et al. (251) studied the mechanism of action for intravenous IgG in SLE-associated thrombocytopenia. Five of seven patients with lupus who received IV IgG showed a greater than 50% increase in platelet count. The beneficial response was not dependent on the reduction of circulating platelet-binding IgG or circulating immune complexes, suggesting that blockade of the Fc receptor may be the major mechanism of action.

Anti-D immunoglobulin IV has been reported to be an effective treatment of nonsplenectomized children and adults with chronic or acute ITP in 70% of patients (252). The mechanism of action is not clear but in part it works via blockade of the reticuloendothelial system with autologous red blood cell antibody complexes. Treatment with anti-D immunoglobulin may be a means of preventing splenectomy and for long-term maintenance for ITP. Although its use in lupus thrombocytopenia has been described (253), there are no controlled drug trials in SLE.

The effectiveness of splenectomy in the treatment of steroid-resistant thrombocytopenia in SLE is controversial. Holman and Dineen (254) followed ten patients who underwent splenectomy for thrombocytopenia. Two died postoperatively, and eight had excellent results, with up to a 30-year follow-up. Breckenridge et al. (255) reported that 9 of 16 patients with SLE had normal platelet counts without medications a year after splenectomy. A similar experience was reported by others (226,256). Splenectomy in refractory thrombocytopenia associated with primary and SLE-related antiphospholipid syndrome showed a high rate of good and long-term response (257,258). In contrast, Hall et al. (259) found that only two of 14 splenectomized thrombocytopenic patients with SLE refractory to drug therapy went into remission at a mean follow-up of 6 years. Rivero et al. (192) found that splenectomy does not prevent recurrent episodes of thrombocytopenia in SLE.

When feasible, laparoscopic is preferred over open splenectomy because of fewer complications and shorter postoperative stay (260). Splenic irradiation has been reported to be effective in the treatment of older patients with steroid-resistant ITP, including SLE (261). This modality may be useful in selected older patients because of the high morbidity that is associated with splenectomy in this age group.

In summary, profound and persistent immune thrombocytopenia (less than 50,000/mL) in patients with SLE should be treated with systemic corticosteroids. Patients who become refractory to steroids or who experience undesirable side effects should be given a trial of azathioprine or danazol. Monthly intravenous cyclophosphamide therapy probably is preferable for patients with multisystem involvement, especially nephritis. Splenectomy may be necessary in some patients, although its long-term sequelae are not completely understood.

Amegakaryocytic Thrombocytopenia

Acquired thrombocytopenia that is associated with decreased numbers of megakaryocytes in the bone marrow, amegakaryocytic thrombocytopenia (AMT) is a rare disorder with different causes and pathogenetic mechanisms. A few cases of AMT associated with SLE have been reported (262,263). In a well-studied patient with SLE, peripheral T lymphocytes, but not serum, inhibited autologous colony-forming megakaryocytes *in vitro*, suggesting an underlying cell-medicated pathogenetic mechanism (264).

Acquired Abnormalities Of Platelet Function

Acquired abnormalities of platelet function include disorders of platelet adhesiveness to the vessel wall and subendothelial matrix, platelet aggregation, and platelet secretion. Platelet function, as measured by *in vitro* qualitative tests and by bleeding time, is affected by several factors, including aspirin and NSAIDs, common foods, spices, the presence of systemic conditions (including SLE and chronic renal failure, lymphoproliferative diseases, and other hematologic disorders), and circulating antiplatelet antibodies (265). These factors should be considered when interpreting the results of qualitative tests of platelet function in an individual patient.

Activation of normal platelets can be induced by adhesion to collagen and by soluble agonists such as epinephrine and adenosine diphosphate (ADP). The activation process involves a complex system of metabolic reactions acting in concert to stimulate platelet aggregation and granule secretion. Regan et al. (266) found that platelets from 12 of 21 patients with SLE failed to aggregate in response to collagen and showed impaired aggregation with ADP and epinephrine. These abnormalities are similar to those induced by aspirin, but none of their patients was on aspirin or any drug that is known to affect platelet function. Others have confirmed these abnormalities in SLE (267,268).

In 1980, Parbtani et al. (269) found that the concentration of serotonin and adenine nucleotides, as stored in the dense granules of platelets, was reduced in patients with acquired platelet function defects, including SLE. Weiss et al. (270) extended this observation and reported that levels of substances stored in platelet-dense granules, including thromboglobulin, were decreased in SLE. Because these findings were similar to those observed in patients with congenital storage pool deficiency, it has been suggested that the platelet defect in SLE represents an acquired storage pool disease. The reduction of the intraplatelet concentration of serotonin in SLE has been confirmed by other investigators (267–269,271–273). Although the concentration of plasma serotonin is normal in patients with SLE, the urinary excretion of serotonin is increased (268).

The low concentration of intraplatelet serotonin has been shown to correlate with disease activity and been taken to indicate *in vivo* platelet activation in SLE (268,273). This is supported further by the findings of elevated levels of plasma β-thromboglobulin and decreased amounts of platelet factors III and IV (212,274,275). β-Thromboglobulin, which is a specific constituent of granules, is released on stimulation of platelets.

The mechanism of *in vivo* platelet activation in SLE is not known. Parbtani et al. (269) suggested that the functional platelet defects result from the circulation of exhausted platelets following their *in vivo* exposure to factors that induce a release reaction, such as damaged endothelium, thrombin, and immune complexes. The globulin fraction of SLE sera has been shown to contain factors that cause the release of serotonin from normal platelets (271). These plasma factors probably include circulating immune complexes and specific antiplatelet antibodies. In addition, the level of platelet-activating factor (PAF), which is a mediator of inflammation with a wide range of biologic activities (including platelet activation), is increased in the plasma of patients with SLE and active disease (276). PAF, which is synthesized by a number of cell types after immunologic stimulation, including monocytes, macrophages, granulocytes, platelets, and endothelial cells, may be involved in SLE (277).

Studies in experimental models of immune complex glomerulonephritis have established that platelets participate in the pathogenesis of renal injury. Platelets can facilitate the deposition of immune complexes and augment the subsequent inflammatory response. The involvement of platelets in SLE nephritis also has been examined. By infusing radiolabeled autologous platelets to patients with diffuse lupus nephritis, Clark et al. (278) found the sequestration of platelets not only in the spleen and liver but also in the kidneys, suggesting intrarenal platelet consumption. Complexes of DNA and specific anti-DNA that are important in lupus glomerulonephritis have been identified on the surface of platelets of patients with SLE (279). Moreover, Duffus et al. (280) have localized platelet surface antigens and platelet factor IV at sites of glomerular injury in SLE.

Thrombotic Thrombocytopenic Purpura

Thrombotic thrombocytopenic purpura (TTP) is a diffuse disorder of the microcirculation of unknown cause that is characterized by a pentad of fever, thrombocytopenic purpura, microangiopathic hemolytic anemia (MAHA), fluctuating neurologic findings, and renal dysfunction. It is a rare disorder, usually seen in females 10 to 40 years of age, and may follow a prodrome of upper respiratory tract symptoms or arthralgias and myalgias (281). Patients present with nonspecific constitutional symptoms, including malaise, fatigue, weakness, and fever. Therefore, the other manifestations appear in rapid sequence, often baffling the clinician by the subtle appearance and diversity of features. Delays in establishing a correct diagnosis are not uncommon. Half of patients experience neurologic symptoms at presentation, most commonly headaches, confusion, and paresis. MAHA is diagnosed by the presence of fragmented red blood cells (i.e., schizocytes), nucleated red blood cells, an elevated lactate dehydrogenase (LDH) level, reticulocytosis, negative Coombs' test, indirect hyperbilirubinemia, and hemoglobulinuria. Severe thrombocytopenia is a characteristic finding. Coagulation parameters generally are normal or show only mild abnormalities, such as elevation of fibrin split products. Pathologically, intravascular microthrombi consisting of fibrin and platelet aggregates in capillaries and precapillary arterioles in several organs are found. No histologic evidence of vasculitis is seen. Systemic corticosteroids, antiplatelet agents, splenectomy, plasma infusions, and plasmapheresis are among the therapies that are used (282). Before 1965, cumulative experience showed that over 90% of patients succumbed to the disease (281). In the last 20 years, the introduction of effective therapy has led to a dramatic improvement in the survival rate to between 70% and 80% (281).

The association between TTP and SLE has been debated for years (283). In 1964, Levine and Shearn (284) reviewed the English-language literature, emphasizing the possible relationship to SLE. They presented two cases of their own showing overlapping features and analyzed 147 cases that were reported with adequate autopsy protocols. In 34 cases (23%), evidence of concomitant SLE was found. Libman-Sacks endocarditis was noted in 25 patients, onion-ring changes in the spleen in eight, wire-loop glomeruli in seven, and a positive LE-cell test in five. Patients with features of both SLE and TTP appeared to constitute a clinical variant and had a higher female predominance, a higher frequency of biologic false-positive tests for syphilis, elevated serum globulin levels, splenomegaly, arthritis and arthralgia, and pleuritis. Amorosi and Ultmann (285) found 13 cases of SLE among 271 cases of TTP reviewed. In contrast, other investigators concluded that the combination of SLE and TTP is rare (286).

There has been an increase in the number of published reports of the association (287–290). When prior reports were reviewed using the 1982 ACR criteria for SLE, Musio et al. (291) identified 41 reported patients with SLE associated TTP. The patients were divided into three groups: 30 (73%) patients who developed TTP after the diagnosis of SLE; six (15%) patients had TTP preceding SLE, and five (12%) patients presented simultaneously with TTP and SLE. TTP developed from 3 months to 25 years after the diagnosis of SLE in the first group. SLE antedated TTP for several years in three patients with hemolytic uremic syndrome variant (292,293). In half of the patients, TTP occurred in the setting of active SLE, while in the other half it occurred during an inactive phase (287). TTP can antedate the onset of SLE and also can occur as a terminal event in SLE (283,294–299). Dixit et al. (300) reported a patient with probable SLE, C2 deficiency, and chronic relapsing TTP.

The treatment of TTP associated with SLE is similar to that for idiopathic TTP. Systemic corticosteroids (301) and plasma infusion (302), with or without plasmapheresis, have been used successfully in a few cases. A Canadian study of 102 patients has shown that plasma exchange alone with fresh-frozen plasma is more effective than infusion in the treatment of TTP (303). Fourteen of 41 (34%) SLE patients with TTP died, and the mortality rates were significant in all forms of therapy: plasma exchange (32%), plasma infusion (20%), steroids alone (20%) (291).

The cause of TTP is not known. Several mechanisms have been proposed to explain the microvascular thrombosis, including the presence of serum platelet-aggregating factor, circulating immune complexes, endothelial injury, defects in the fibrinoloytic system, and prostacyclin abnormalities (304). Autoantibodies to microvascular endothelial cells (305) and to CD36, a single chain membrane polypeptide (also known as GPIV) that is expressed in platelets and endothelial cells, have been reported in TTP (306). In SLE, Itoh et al. (301) suggested the role of antiplatelet antibodies in the development of TTP in some patients. Tsai and Lian (307) found IgG antibodies that inhibited plasma protease that cleaves Van Willebrand factor in acute TTP. The defect in the proteolysis of multimers of Van Willebrand factor can lead to platelet thrombosis.

WHITE BLOOD CELL DISORDERS

White Cell Count And Leukopenia

The characteristic change in the leukocyte count in SLE, which first was observed in 1923 by Goeckerman (308), is a depression of the white blood cells to between 2,000 and 4,500/mL. In large series of SLE patients reported in the literature, leukopenia has been observed in over 50% (2,5,6,8,38).

Leukopenia, which is defined as a white blood cell count of below 4,500/mL, was noted in 43% of Dubois and Tuffanelli's (2) 520 patients and in 66% of Estes and Christian's (5) 150 patients. Severe leukopenia, with counts of below 2,000/mL, was uncommon. Of 122 patients with SLE who were studied serially by McGehee Harvey et al. (8), 75 patients had counts of below 5,000/mL. Larson (38) found that 18 of 200 patients had leukocyte counts of below 4,500/mL on two or more occasions, and that the usual range of leukopenia was between 2,500 and 3,500/mL. Among 111 hospitalized patients with SLE, Michael et al. (91) found a white blood cell count of below 500/mL in 66 (60%) patients at some time. In Ropes' (9) series of 142 patients, a white cell count of less than 4,000/mL was found in 67%, but in 12% the white cell count was always normal.

Leukopenia in SLE has been shown to be significantly associated with a high frequency of skin rash, lymphopenia, and elevated anti-DNA titer. Anemia, fatigue, arthritis, anemia, and elevated sedimentation rate also were more common in patients with leukopenia (309). A leukocyte count of 4,000/mL, and occasionally as low as 2,500 mL, may occur in patients with active and untreated discoid LE. This may arise after treatment of the skin lesions with antimalarials. Leukopenia and fever can be a rare manifestation of allergic reaction to prednisolone (310).

Differential White Cell Count

An increase of nonsegmented neutrophils in patients with SLE was first reported by Rose and Pillsbury (311). This increase was observed in patients with normal as well as elevated total white cell counts (91). Estes and Christian (5) noted a normal differential count in 50% of their patients with leukopenia. These data are similar to the findings of other investigators.

Of 111 patients who were studied by Michael et al. (91), 64% had an increase in nonsegmented neutrophils together with an increase in mature granulocytes. Also, 14 patients had one to seven myelocytes when first seen, and a few others showed a similar increase in later counts. This occurred more frequently in those with normal or low white cell counts than in those with elevated total leukocyte counts. Before the institution of therapy, 24 of 105 patients studied by McGehee Harvey et al. (8) had neutrophilic granulocyte counts of 80% to 89%, and 5% of patients had counts of over 90%.

Eosinophilia

In my experience, eosinophilia is uncommon in patients with SLE without concomitant parasite infection, allergic reaction, or some other known cause. Eosinophilia is not mentioned in several series of patients in the literature (5,7,309). In contrast, earlier workers observed that eosinophilia is not rare in SLE. In Larson's (38) series of 200 patients), ten had counts of 3% or more, and five patients had persistent eosinophilia in excess of 10%. McGehee Harvey et al. (8) found eosinophilia of 3% or more in 15 of 46 patients who were studied before therapy. Of these, two patients had counts of 17% and 24%, respectively, associated with extensive skin lesions and not attributable to causes other than SLE. Direct eosinophil counts were performed in 60 patients. Counts of less than 50/mL were found in 31 patients, of between 50 and 100/mL in 11, of between 100 and 200/mL in 10, of between 200 and 400/mL in six, and of more than 400/mL in only two. Ropes (9) observed a high prevalence of eosinophilia; an eosinophil count of more than 5% was seen in 21 of 142 patients at some time along the course of the illness. Michael et al. (91) noted an eosinophil count of over 3% in six of 111 untreated patients (15).

Two rare causes of eosinophilia, hypereosinophilic syndrome with diarrhea, and Loffler's endocarditis have been reported in SLE (312,313).

Basophils

Hunsiker and Brun (314) enumerated basophils in patients with various skin disorders and found a moderate reduction of basophils in those with discoid LE and a marked diminution in patients with SLE. Egido et al. (315) found the absolute basophil counts in SLE to be inversely related to anti-DNA antibodies and the level of circulating immune complexes and to be directly related to serum complement level. Basophils and tissue mast cells possess Fc receptors that are specific to IgE antibodies. If such antibodies are cross-linked by binding to antigen, basophils and mast cells degranulate, releasing granules that contain vasoactive substances and producing a hypersensitivity allergic reaction. High levels of IgE have been found on the surface of basophils in SLE patients. More important, SLE basophils underwent degranulation when incubated with soluble DNA antigen, suggesting the presence of cell-bound, specific IgE anti-DNA antibodies. Although glomerular deposits of IgE have been reported in SLE, the pathogenic role of these antibodies remains to be established.

Granulocytopenia

Granulocytopenia occurs infrequently in patients with SLE and can have a number of causes, including drug reaction, severe infection, decreased bone marrow production, and destruction mediated by antigranulocyte antibodies. At times, the total white blood cell count may decrease to levels as low as 1,000/mL without any apparent cause other than SLE. Nevertheless, in this situation, the physician should always be aware of the possibility that the granulocytopenia may be the result of medications used in SLE, such as antimalarials (8,316). A prospective study, however, showed a high prevalence (62%) of neutropenia at some time during the course of lupus, although it was severe [<1,000 polymorphonuclear neutrophils (PMNs) per mL] in only six of 126 patients (5%) who were studied (106).

My group has observed agranulocytosis in SLE caused by atabrine, levamisole, and triethylenemelamine (317). Agranulocytosis in SLE has occurred because of reaction to sulfadiazine (318). McDuffie (319) reported three patients with SLE who developed agranulocytosis secondary to medications that are not commonly associated with blood dyscrasias: hydroxychloroquine, dextropropoxyphene, and nitrofurantoin. Bone marrow examination showed the absence of myeloid precursors in two patients and aplastic changes in the third.

Both humoral and cell-mediated immune mechanisms are important in the pathogenesis of neutropenia in SLE. Starkebaum et al. (320) examined the *in vivo* neutrophil kinetics of a patient with lupus and severe neutropenia, and they found changes that were indicative of increased peripheral destruction of granulocytes combined with ineffective granulocytopoiesis by the bone marrow. Elevated levels of surface-bound IgG were detected on the patient's neutrophils. Monomeric IgG antibodies, but not immune complexes, isolated from the serum of the patient opsonized normal neutrophils for *in vitro* ingestion by other phagocytic cells. These observations provide a basis for the role of humoral factors in some cases of neutropenia. In addition, Hadley et al. (321) found an inverse correlation between the neutrophil count and the ability of SLE sera to opsonize granulocytes for recognition and clearance by human monocytes. Impairment of reticuloendothelial system function in SLE (322) may allow antibody-sensitized granulocytes to remain in the circulation.

Neutropenia in SLE has been reported to be associated with anti-Ro/SSA antibodies. Moreover, these antibodies bind to a 64-kd membrane protein that cross-react with the 60-kd Ro antigen, implying that anti-Ro/SSA antibodies may mediate neutropenia in SLE (323).

The number of progenitor cells of granulocyte and monocytes in the bone marrow [colony-forming unit culture (CFU-C)] has been found to be reduced in patients with SLE, and this correlated with the peripheral granulocyte and monocyte counts (112,324). Moreover, T lymphocytes suppressed the generation of autologous bone marrow CFU-C *in vitro*, suggesting a role of cell-mediated mechanisms in the impairment of granulopoiesis in SLE.

Courtney et al. (325) found an increased number of apoptotic neutrophils in SLE patients, especially those with anti-dsDNA and active disease as well as those with neutropenia. Whether increased neutrophil apoptosis contributes to neutropenia in SLE or not remains to be investigated.

Severe neutropenia in SLE is responsive to systemic corticosteroid therapy (326). Recombinant human granulocyte colony-stimulating factor (rhG-CSF) has been used successfully in combination with pulse methylprednisolone or with low-dose prednisone in the treatment of lupus neutropenia (326,327).

In the presence of infection in the patient who is not receiving systemic corticosteroids, leukocyte counts often may rise to between 15,000 and 20,000/mL. Unfortunately, other patients with SLE may have intercurrent infections without a demonstrable rise in the white cell count, so this valuable guide cannot be depended on in these cases. Marked leukocytosis with counts higher than 30,000/mL has been observed by my group and others in the presence of concomitant infections. During treatment with corticosteroids, the usual range of leukocytosis is 15,000 to 25,000/mL regardless of the initial white blood cell count.

Bone Marrow Granulocyte Reserve

The leukocytosis that occurs following the administration of endotoxin, etiocholanolone, or glucocorticoids primarily is caused by the release of PMNs from bone marrow reserves (328). The amount of PMN reserve is considered to be important in the host defense against infections, and it also serves as a guide in predicting the ability of the patient to tolerate a myelotoxic drug. Paulus et al. (329) found that the granulocyte reserve, as measured by etiocholanolone injection, in patients with SLE and nephritis was higher in those who were on azathioprine than in those on no medications or in patients on combined prednisone and azathioprine therapy. Kimball et al. (330) found that 62% of 59 patients with SLE had an abnormally low granulocyte reserve when challenged with etiocholanolone. No correlation among deficient granulocyte reserve and other clinical or laboratory parameters was found. Most of their patients were on corticosteroids, however, which now are known to challenge the bone marrow reserves (331), so that possibly the administration of etiocholanolone did not augment the maximally stimulated bone marrow, resulting in a subnormal response (338). This subnormal response to etiocholanolone of untreated patients with SLE suggests that the disease itself can suppress bone marrow reserves. Evidence suggesting the role of one or more circulating humoral factors for this abnormality has been described (330).

The number of bisegmented neutrophils (i.e., Pelger's anomaly) was significantly higher and the lymphocyte count lower in patients with leukopenia associated with SLE and other autoimmune disorders (332).

Lymphocyte Counts

Lymphopenia is one of the most common hematologic findings in SLE (6,333). Early investigators noted lymphopenia but failed to emphasize it, probably because relative percentages rather than absolute numbers of lymphocytes in the peripheral blood were used (8,91). The mechanism of lymphopenia in SLE is not clear. Delbarre et al. (334) followed lymphocyte counts in 19 patients with SLE, and they noted that lymphopenia developed in 84% during the acute stage and was associated with an increased sedimentation rate. At remission, the lymphocyte count increased and the sedimentation rate fell. Grigor et al. (6) found absolute lymphopenia to be more common than leukopenia.

Rivero et al. (333) examined the occurrence and significance of lymphopenia in 158 patients with SLE. At diagnosis, 75% of these patients had a significantly reduced absolute lymphocyte count, but on follow-up, additional patients became lymphopenic. Therefore, the total cumulative frequency of absolute lymphopenia was 93%. Lymphopenia was found to be independent of, although contributory to, leukopenia, so these two findings were not primarily interrelated. Absolute lymphopenia was correlated with disease activity, and patients with an absolute lymphocyte count of less than 1,500/mL at diagnosis had a higher frequency of fever, polyarthritis, and central nervous system involvement but a lower prevalence of thrombocytopenia and/or hemolytic anemia. Life-table analysis, however, showed no adverse influence of lymphopenia on survival of patients with lupus (106).

Table 38.2 summarizes the changes in red cells, platelets, and white cells in patients with SLE.

TABLE 38.2. RED CELLS, WHITE BLOOD CELLS AND PLATELETS IN SLE

Anemia occurs in over 50% of patients at some time during the course of the disease; anemia can result from one or a combination of factors including chronic disease, autoimmune hemolysis, iron deficiency, and chronic renal failure

Autoimmune hemolytic anemia characterized by the presence of warm-reacting immunoglobulin G (IgG) antibodies to erythrocytes develops in up to 16% of patients and may be the presenting manifestation of the disease; a combined warm- and cold-antibody type of autoimmune hemolytic anemia occurs occasionally

Leukopenia is common and may result from active disease or a drug reaction; Lymphopenia is a characteristic finding in untreated, active SLE; *in vitro* studies of granulocyte function generally are abnormal in SLE

Leukocytosis in SLE is associated with a concurrent infection or corticosteroid therapy

A platelet count of lower than 150,000 cells/mL is seen in 7% to 52% of patients (mean, 14%); *in vitro* platelet functions including aggregation in response to collagen are frequently abnormal in SLE

Autoimmune thrombocytopenic purpura is not uncommon in SLE; 3% to 15% of patients diagnosed as having idopathic autoimmune thrombocytopenic purpura go on to develop classic SLE

Thrombotic thrombocytopenic purpura is a rare, life-threatening complication of SLE

Granulocyte Function In SLE

To understand the importance of granulocyte function as a factor in the susceptibility of patients with SLE to infections, studies have been undertaken to examine the phagocytic, opsonizing, chemotactic, and oxidative functions of neutrophils and monocytes. Most of these studies have concluded that in general, granulocyte function in SLE is abnormal, but the specific qualitative and quantitative abnormalities reported in them were either inconsistent or contradictory.

Phagocytosis And Opsonization

Brandt and Hedberg (335) reported that the ability of neutrophils of SLE patients to ingest yeast particles is significantly lower than those of RA patients and of healthy subjects. Phagocytic activity was not reduced when normal granulocytes were suspended in normal plasma, and the lowest phagocytic activity tended to be associated with neutropenia. Orozco et al. (336) confirmed this observation and found that the phagocytosis of *Escherichia coli* by SLE leukocytes decreased by 62% in those with active disease. In contrast to Brandt et al. (335), they also observed that the phagocytic activity normalized if the SLE granulocytes were incubated with fresh normal serum rather than with SLE serum. The presence of a serum factor that inhibits phagocytosis in SLE also has been reported by others (337,338), although the nature of this factor is not known. Sera from SLE patients with active disease failed to support normal granulocytes in phagocytosis, indicating a defect in opsonic capability. The low serum complement level, rather than a deficiency in natural antibodies, was the limiting factor in the deficient serum opsonic activity of SLE sera (336). The initial rate of phagocytosis of lipopolysaccharide-coated paraffin droplets by neutrophils from untreated patients with active SLE was significantly lower than that in normal subjects (339). In contrast to these results, Al-Hadithy et al. (340) found the phagocytosis of *Candida* sp. by neutrophils of SLE patients to be normal when the patients were considered as a group, but 20 of their patients had impaired phagocytic values. In addition, Hallgren et al. (337) described an increased ability of SLE granulocytes to phagocytose IgG-coated latex particles in a serum-free system, to exclude the effects of circulating inhibitors.

Chemotaxis And Migration

The *in vitro* chemotactic response of the neutrophils in SLE, when compared as a group to that of healthy subjects, has been observed to be normal (341,342). Clark et al. (342) noted that the generation of chemotactic factors in SLE serum clearly was depressed, and that the defect correlated with an elevated titer of anti-DNA antibodies, low serum immunoglobulin level, and high frequency of infections. Alvarez et al. (341) showed that the generation of serum chemotactic activity by the classic pathway of complement, but not by the alternative pathway, was impaired in patients with SLE. Serum inhibitors of chemotaxis, including a specific inhibitor of C5-derived chemotactic activity, also have been found in SLE patients (340).

Oxidative Functions

Wenger and Bole (343) investigated the reduction of nitroblue tetrazolium (NBT) dye by peripheral blood leukocytes of patients with SLE, and they found the activity to be low in resting leukocytes. When the leukocytes were stimulated by allowing them to phagocytose latex particles, an incremental increase in NBT dye reduction, comparable to that seen in healthy individuals, was noted. On the other hand, neutrophils from patients with SLE who were infected failed to demonstrate the anticipated increase in NBT dye reduction. Others have confirmed the abnormal NBT dye reduction test results in patients with SLE (339,344). This test is considered to be a measure of the oxidative events associated with phagocytosis and intracellular killings, so it further supports the role of abnormal granulocyte function in the increased incidence of infection found in those with SLE.

The apparent inconsistencies in the studies of *in vitro* SLE granulocyte function by various investigators probably reflect differences in methodology and in the selection of patients. This also emphasizes the importance of other factors that affect these tests, such as the use of steroids and other drugs, activity of SLE, and the presence of inhibitory factors in the serum. The clinical significance of *in vitro* functional abnormalities is not entirely clear, but *in vivo* studies in SLE using the Rebuck skin window technique have shown abnormalities in granulocyte functions (345). Whether the observed abnormalities in granulocyte function are primary cellular defects or secondary to the disease process is not completely clear. Hurd et al. (346) have postulated that the ingestion of immune complexes by SLE neutrophils can alter their functions. *In vitro* exposure of normal granulocytes to SLE sera, especially those from patients with active disease, resulted in increased adhesiveness, aggregation, and oxygenation activity (347–349).

Neutrophils from patients with lupus, and especially those with active disease, express increased amounts of adhesive molecule β-integrin CD11b/CD18 but not L-selectin (350). Exposure in the circulation to complement products may lead to the intravascular activation of neutrophils (351). Activated neutrophils then can contribute to the development of vasculitis, transient pulmonary dysfunction, central nervous system involvement, and leukopenia, as well as to an increased susceptibility to infections.

REFERENCES

1. Tarzy BJ, Garcia C-R, Wallach EE, et al. Rheumatic disease, abnormal serology, and oral contraceptives. *Lancet* 1972;2:501–503.
2. Dubois EL, Tuffanelli DL. Clinical manifestations of systemic lupus erythematosus. Computer analysis of 520 cases. *JAMA* 1964;190:104–111.
3. Meislin AG, Rothfield N. Systemic lupus erythematosus in childhood. Analysis of 42 cases, with comparative data on 200 adult cases followed concurrently. *Pediatrics* 1968;42:37–49.
4. Arman-Cruz R, Harnecker J, Ducach G, et al. Clinical diagnosis of systemic lupus erythematosus. *Am J Med* 1958;25:409–419.
5. Estes D, Christian CL. The natural history of systemic lupus erythematosus by prospective analysis. *Medicine* 1971;50:85–95.
6. Grigor REJ, Lewkonia R, Bresnihan B, et al. Systemic lupus erythematosus: a prospective analysis. *Ann Rheum Dis* 1978;37:121–128.
7. Lee P, Urowitz MB, Bookman AA, et al. Systemic lupus erythematosus: a review of 110 cases with reference to nephritis, nervous system, infections, aseptic necrosis and prognosis. *Q J Med* 1977;46:132.
8. McGehee Harvey A, Shulman LE, Tumulty AP, et al. Systemic lupus erythematosus: review of the literature and clinical analysis of 138 cases. *Medicine* 1954;33:291–437.
9. Ropes MW. *Systemic lupus erythematosus*. Cambridge, MA: Harvard University Press, 1976.
10. Shapira Y, Weinberger A, Wysenbeek AJ. Lymphadenopathy in systemic lupus erythematosus. Prevalence and relation to disease manifestations. *Clin Rheumatol* 1996;15:335–338.
11. Case records of the Massachusetts General Hospital. Weekly clinicopathological exercises. Case 42-1979. *N Engl J Med* 1979;301:881–887.
12. Fox RA, Rosahn PD. Lymph nodes in disseminated lupus erythematosus. *Am J Pathol* 1943;19:73–99.
13. Klemperer P. Concept of collagen diseases. *Am J Pathol* 1950;26:505–519.
14. Schnitzer B. Reactive lymphoid hyperplasia in surgical pathology of the lymph nodes and related organs. In: Jaffe ES, ed. *Major problems in pathology series*. Philadelphia: WB Saunders, 1985;16:46.
15. Emberger J-M, Navarro M, Oules C, et al. Presence of Sternberg type cells in a case of lupus adenopathy (in French). *Nouv Presse Med* 1976;5:1994.
16. Medeiros LJ, Kaynor B, Harris NL. Lupus lymphadenitis: report of a case with immunohistologic studies on frozen section. *Hum Pathol* 1989;20:295–299.
17. Kojima M, Nakamura S, Morishita Y, et al. Reactive follicular hyperplasia in the lymph node lesions from systemic lupus erythematosus patients: a clinicopathologic and immunohistological study of 21 cases. *Pathol Int* 2000;50:304–312.
18. Deftos LJ, Burtown DW, Baird SM, et al. Hypercalcemia and systemic lupus erythematosus. *Arthritis Rheum* 1996; 39:2066–2069.
19. Dorfman DF. Histiocytic necrotizing lymphadenitis of Kikuchi and Fujimoto. *Arch Pathol Lab Med* 1987;111:1026–1029.
20. Dorfman RF, Berry GJ. Kikuchi's histiocytic necrotizing lymphadenitis: an analysis of 108 cases with emphasis on differential diagnosis. *Semin Diagn Pathol* 1988;5:329–345.
21. Eisner MD, Amory J, Mullaney B, et al. Necrotizing lymphadenitis associated with systemic lupus erythematosus. *Semin Arthritis Rheum* 1996;21:1–6.
22. Miliauskas JR. Systemic lupus erythematosus lymphadenitis. *Pathology* 1993;25:134–137.

23. Lin SH, Ko WS, Lee HS, et al. Kikuchi's disease associated with lupus-like syndrome: a fatal case. *J Rheumatol* 1992;19: 1995–1996.
24. Spies H, Foucar K, Thompson C, et al. The histopathology of cutaneous lesions of Kikuchi's disease (necrotizing lymphadenitis): a report of five cases. *Am J Surg Pathol* 1999;23:1040–1054.
25. Tumiati B, Bellelli A, Portioli I, et al. Kikuchi's disease in systemic lupus erythematosus: an independent or dependent event. *Clin Rheumatol* 1991;10:90–93.
26. Martinez-Vasquez C, Hughes G, Bordon J, et al. Histiocytic necrotizing lymphadenitis, Kikuchi-Fujimoto's disease, associated with systemic lupus erythematosus. *Q J Med* 1997; 90: 531–533.
27. Litwin MD, Kirkham B, Henderson DRF, et al. Histiocytic necrotizing lymphadenitis in systemic lupus erythematosus. *Ann Rheum Dis* 1992;51:805–807.
28. El-Ramahi KM, Karrar A, Ali MA. Kikuchi disease and its association with systemic lupus erythematosus. *Lupus* 1994;3: 409–411.
29. Gourley I, Bell AL, Biggart D. Kikuchi's disease as presenting feature of mixed connective tissue disease. *Clin Rheumatol* 1995;14:104–107.
30. Herrada J, Cabanilla F, Rice L, et al. The clinical behavior of localized and multicentric Castleman disease. *Ann Intern Med* 1998; 128:657–662.
31. Suwannaroj S, Elkins SL, McMurray RW. Systemic lupus erythematosus and Castleman's disease. *J Rheumatol* 1999;26: 1400–1403.
32. Simko R, Nagy K, Lombay B, et al. Multicentric Castleman disease and systemic lupus erythematosus phenotype in a boy with Klinefelter syndrome: long term disease stabilization with interferon therapy. *J Pediatr Hematol Oncol* 2000;22:180–183.
33. Gohlke F, Marker-Hermann E, Kanzler S, et al. Autoimmune findings resembling connective tissue disease in a patient with Castleman's disease. *Clin Rheumatol* 1997;16:87–92.
34. Kojima M, Nakamura S, Itoh H, et al. Systemic lupus erythematosus lymphadenopathy with histopathologic features of Castleman's disease. *Pathol Res Pract* 1997;193:565–571.
35. Wiljasalo M, Ikkala E. Lymphography in systemic lupus erythematosus. *Ann Clin Res* 1971;3:231–235.
36. Haserick JR. Modern concepts of systemic lupus erythematosus. A review of 126 cases. *J Chronic Dis* 1955;1:317–334.
37. Jessar RA, Lamont-Havers RW, Ragan C. Natural history of lupus erythematosus disseminatus. *Ann Intern Med* 1953;38: 717–731.
38. Larson DL. *Systemic lupus erythematosus*. Boston: Little, Brown, 1961.
39. Rothfield NF. Current approaches to SLE and its subsets. *DM* 1982;29:162.
40. Alarcon-Segovia D. Gross splenomegaly in SLE. *Arthritis Rheum* 1978;21:866.
41. Libman E, Sacks B. A hitherto undescribed form of valvular and mural endocarditis. *Arch Intern Med* 1924;33:701–737.
42. Quismorio FP Jr, Johnson C. Serum autoantibodies in patients with sickle cell anemia. *Am J Med Sci* 1984;287:13–15.
43. Kitamura H, Kitamura H, Ito T, et al. Systemic lupus erythematosus with multiple calcified fibrous nodules of the spleen. *Acta Pathol Jpn* 1985;35:213–226.
44. Kaiser IH. Specificity of periarterial fibrosis of the spleen in disseminated lupus erythematosus. *Bull Johns Hopkins Hosp* 1942; 71:31–42.
45. Wilson WA, Nicholson GR, Hughes GRV, et al. Systemic lupus erythematosus and sickle cell anemia. *Br Med J* 1976;1: 813–816.
46. Obraski TP, Stoller JK, Weinstein C, et al. Splenic infarction. *Cleve Clin J Med* 1989;56:174–176.
47. Rossner S, Ginzler E, Dimond H. Spontaneous rupture of the splenic artery and cerebrovascular accident with systemic lupus erythematosus. *NY State J Med* 1981;81:940–942.
48. Dillon AM, Stein HB, Kassen BO, et al. Hyposplenia in a patient with systemic lupus erythematosus. *J Rheumatol* 1980; 7:196–198.
49. Piliero P, Furie R. Functional asplenia in systemic lupus erythematosus. *Semin Arthritis Rheum* 1990;20:185–189.
50. Scerpella EG. Functional asplenia and pneumococcal sepsis in patients with systemic lupus erythematosus. *Clin Infect Dis* 1995;20:194–195.
51. Neilan BA, Barney SN. Hyposplenism in systemic lupus erythematosus. *J Rheumatol* 1983;10:332–334.
52. Malleson P, Petty RE, Nadel H, et al. Functional asplenia in childhood onset systemic lupus erythematosus. *J Rheumatol* 1988;15:1648–1652.
53. Liote F, Angle J, Gilmore N, et al. Asplenism and systemic lupus erythematosus. *Clin Rheumatol* 1995;14:220–223.
54. Poldre PA. Splenic hypofunction in systemic lupus erythematosus response to pneumococcal vaccine. *J Rheumatol* 1989;16: 1130–1131.
55. Jarrett MP, Schiffman G, Barland P, et al. Impaired response to pneumococcal vaccine in systemic lupus erythematosus. *Arthritis Rheum* 1980;23:1287–1293.
56. Battafarano D, Battafarano NJ, Larsen L, et al. Antigen-specific antibody responses in lupus patients following immunization. *Arthritis Rheum* 1998;41:1828–1834.
57. Uthman I, Soucy JP, Nicolet V, et al. Autosplenectomy in systemic lupus erythematosus. *J Rheumatol* 1996;23:1806–1810.
58. Mackay IR, Smalley M. Results of the thymectomy in SLE: observations on clinical course and serological reactions. *Clin Exp Immunol* 1966;1:129–138.
59. Suster S, Rosai J. Histology of the normal thymus. *Am J Surg Pathol* 1990;14:284–303.
60. Hutchins GM, Harvey AM. The thymus in systemic lupus erythematosus. *Bull Johns Hopkins Hosp* 1964;115:355–378.
61. Goldstein G, MacKay I. The thymus in SLE: a quantitative, histopathological analysis and comparison with stress involution. *Br Med J* 1967;2:475–478.
62. Hill GS, Hinglais N, Tron F, et al. Systemic lupus erythematosus. Morphologic correlations with immunologic and clinical data at the time of biopsy. *Am J Med* 1978;64:61–79.
63. Lewis VM, Twoney JJ, Steinberg AD, et al. Serum thymic hormone activity in systemic lupus erythematosus. *Clin Immunol Immunopathol* 1981;18:61–69.
64. Milne JA, Anderson JR, McSween RN, et al. Thymectomy in acute SLE and rheumatoid arthritis. *Br Med J* 1967;1:461–464.
65. Alarcon-Segovia D, Galbraith RF, Maldonado JE, et al. Systemic lupus erythematosus following thymectomy for myasthenia gravis. Report of two cases. *Lancet* 1963;2:662–665.
66. Vaiopoulos G, Sfikakis PP, Kapsimali V, et al. The association of systemic lupus erythematosus and myasthenia gravis. *Postgrad Med J* 1994;70:741–745.
67. Killian PJ, Hoffman GS. Coexistence of systemic lupus erythematosus and myasthenia gravis. *South Med J* 1980;73:244–246.
68. Ciaccio M, Parodi A, Regora A. Myasthenia gravis and lupus erythematosus. *Int J Dermatol* 1989;28:317–321.
69. Simeone JF, McCloud T, Putman CE, et al. Thymoma and systemic lupus erythematosus. *Thorax* 1975;30:670–679.
70. Gerli R, Paganelli R, Cossarizza A, et al. Long-term immunologic effects of thymectomy in patients with myasthenia gravis. *J Allergy Clin Immunol* 1999;103:865–872.
71. Cruz PD, Coldiron BM, Sontheimer RD. Concurrent features of cutaneous lupus erythematosus and pemphigus erythematosus following myasthenia gravis and thymoma. *J Am Acad Dermatol* 1987;16:472–476.

72. Grinlinton FA, Lynch NM, Hart HH. A pair of monozygotic twins who are concordant for myasthenia gravis but became discordant for systemic lupus erythematosus post-thymectomy. *Arthritis Rheum* 1991;34:916–919.
73. Shoenfeld Y, Lorber M, Yucel T, et al. Primary antiphospholipid syndrome emerging following thymectomy for myasthenia gravis: additional evidence for the kaleidoscope of autoimmunity. *Lupus* 1997;6:474–476.
74. Sanmarco M, Bernard D. Studies of IgG-class anticardiolipin antibodies in myasthenia gravis. *Autoimmunity* 1994;18:57–63.
75. Levinson AI, Zweiman B, Lisak RP. Immunopathogenesis and treatment of myasthenia gravis. *J Clin Immunol* 1987;7: 187–197.
76. Ben-Chetrit E, Pollack A, Flussaer D, et al. Coexistence of systemic lupus erythematosus and myasthenia gravis: two distinct populations of anti-DAN and anti-acetylcholine receptor antibodies. *Clin Exp Rheumatol* 1990;8:71–74.
77. Diaz-Jouanen E, de la Fuente JR, Llorente L, et al. Does the thymus play opposite roles in SLE and myasthenia gravis? *Arthritis Rheum* 1978;21:492–493.
78. Palmisani MR, Evoli A, Batocchi AP, et al. Myasthenia gravis and associated autoimmune diseases. *Muscle Nerve* 1994;20: 1234–1235.
79. Oosterhuis HJGH, de Haas WHD. Rheumatic diseases in patients with myasthenia gravis. *Acta Neurol Scand* 1968;44: 219–227.
80. Thoriacius S, Aarli JA, Riise T, et al. Associated disorders in myasthenia gravis: autoimmune diseases and their relation to thymectomy. *Acta Neurol Scand* 1989;80:290–295.
81. Rider LG, Sherry DD, Glass ST. Neonatal lupus erythematosus simulating transient myasthenia gravis at presentation. *J Pediatr* 1991;118:417–419.
82. Morgenthaler TI, Brown LR, Colby TV, et al. Thymoma. *Mayo Clin Proc* 1993;68:1110–1123.
83. Rosenow EC 3rd, Hurley BT. Disorders of the thymus. *Arch Intern Med* 1984;144:763–770.
84. Souadjian JV, Enriquez P, Silverstein MN, et al. The spectrum of diseases associated with thymoma. *Arch Intern Med* 1974; 134:374–379.
85. Malas D, Weiss S. Progressive multifocal leukoencephalopathy and cryptococcal meningitis with systemic lupus erythematosus and thymoma. *Ann Neurol* 1977;1:188–191.
86. Mastaglia FL, Papadimitrion JM, Dawkins RL, et al. Vacuolar myopathy associated with chloroquine, lupus erythematosus and thymoma. *J Neurol Sci* 1977;34:315–328.
87. Case records of the Massachusetts General Hospital. Weekly clinicopathological exercises. Case 46-1973. *N Engl J Med* 1973;288:729–733.
88. Zandman-Goddard G, Lorber M, Shoenfeld Y. Systemic lupus erythematosus and thymoma: a double-edged sword. *Int Arch Allergy Immunol* 1995;108:99–102.
89. Bozzolo E, Bellone M, Quaroni N, et al. Thymoma associated with systemic lupus erythematosus and immunologic abnormalities. *Lupus* 2000;9:151–154.
90. Larsson O. Thymoma and systemic lupus erythematosus in the same patient. *Lancet* 1963;2:665–666.
91. Michael SR, Vural IL, Bassen FA, et al. The hematologic aspects of disseminated (systemic) lupus erythematosus. *Blood* 1951;6: 1059–1072.
92. Voularelis M, Kokori S, Ioannidis JPA, et al. Anaemia in systemic lupus erythematosus: aetiological profile and role of erythropoietin. *Ann Rheum Dis* 2000;59:217–222.
93. Tzioufas AG, Kokori SI, Petrovas CI, et al. Autoantibodies to human recombinant erythropoietin in patients with systemic lupus erythematosus. Correlation with anemia. *Arthritis Rheum* 1997;40:2212–2216.
94. Richert-Boe KE. Hematologic complications of rheumatic disease. *Hematol Oncol Clin North Am* 1987;1:301–319.
95. Burger T, Brascgh G, Keszthelyl B. Iron metabolism and anemia in systemic lupus erythematosus and rheumatoid arthritis. *Acta Med Acad Sci Hung* 1967;23:95–104.
96. Whittingham S, Balazs NDH, Mackay IR. The effect of corticosteroid drugs on serum iron levels in systemic lupus erythematosus and rheumatoid arthritis. *Med J Aust* 1967;2:639–641.
97. Vreugdenhil G, Swaak AJG. Anaemia in rheumatoid arthritis: pathogenesis, diagnosis and treatment. *Rheumatol Int* 1990;9: 243–257.
98. Voulgari PV, Polios G, Papadopoulos GK, et al. Role of cytokines in the pathogenesis of anemia of chronic disease in rheumatoid arthritis. *Clin Immunol* 1999;92:153–160.
99. Nishiya K, Hashimoto K. Elevation of serum ferritin levels as a marker for active systemic lupus erythematosus. *Clin Exp Rheumatol* 1997;15:39–44.
100. Cook J. The measurement of serum transferrin receptor. *Am J Med Sci* 1999;318:269–279.
101. Gilliland BC, Leddy JP, Vaughan JH. The detection of cell-bound antibody on complement-coated human red cells. *J Clin Invest* 1970;49:898–906.
102. Karthikeyan G, Wallace SL, Blum L. Systemic lupus erythematosus and sickle cell disease. *Arthritis Rheum* 1978;21: 862–863.
103. Luban NLC, Boeck RL, Barr O. Sickle cell anemia and systemic lupus erythematosus. *J Pediatr* 1980;96:11–20.
104. Warrier RP, Sahney S, Walker H. Hemoglobin sickle cell disease and systemic lupus erythematosus. *J Natl Med Assoc* 1984;76: 1030–1031.
105. Weinblatt ME, Coblyn JS, Fox DA, et al. Efficacy of low-dose methotrexate in rheumatoid arthritis. *N Engl J Med* 1985;312: 818–822.
106. Katsanis E, Hsu E, Luke KH, et al. Systemic lupus erythematosus and sickle hemoglobinopathies: a report of two cases and review of the literature. *Am J Hematol* 1987;25:211–214.
107. Wilson WA, Hughes GRV, Lachman PJ. Deficiency of factor B of the complement system in sickle cell anemia. *Br Med J* 1976; 1:367–369.
108. Shetty A, Kumar S, Rajeev S, et al. Sickle cell anemia with systemic lupus erythematosus: response to hydroxyurea therapy. *J Pediatr Hematol Oncol* 1998;20:335–337.
109. Ballas SK. Sideroblastic refractory anemia in a patient with systemic lupus erythematosus (case report). *Am J Med Sci* 1973; 265;225–231.
110. Ng HS, Ng HW, Sinniah R, et al. A case of systemic lupus erythematosus with sideroblastic anemia terminating in erythroleukemia. *Ann Rheum Dis* 1981;40:422–426.
111. Levene NA, Buskila D, Dvilansky A, et al. Pernicious anemia in a patient with systemic lupus erythematosus. *Isr J Med Sci* 1987; 23:846–847.
112. Yamasaki K, Niho Y, Yanase T. Erythroid colony forming cells in systemic lupus erythematosus. *J Rheumatol* 1984;11: 167–171.
113. Otsuka T, Nagasawa K, Harada M, et al. Bone marrow microenvironment of patients with systemic lupus erythematosus. *J Rheumatol* 1993;20:967–971.
114. Cavalcant J, Shadduck RK, Winkelstein A, et al. Red cell hypoplasia and increased bone marrow reticulin in systemic lupus erythematosus: reversal with corticosteroid therapy. *Am J Haematol* 1978;5:253–263.
115. Dainiak N, Hardin J, Floyd V, et al. Humoral suppression of erythropoiesis in systemic lupus erythematosus (SLE) and rheumatoid arthritis. *Am J Med* 1980;69:537–544.
116. Fitchen JJ, Cline MJ, Saxon A, et al. Serum inhibitors of hematopoiesis in a patient with aplastic anemia and systemic

lupus erythematosus: recovery after plasmapheresis. *Am J Med* 1979;66:537–542.

117. Kallen PS, Nies KM, Louie JS, et al. Serum inhibition of erythropoiesis in systemic lupus erythematosus (abstract). *Arthritis Rheum* 1981;24(Suppl):S108.
118. Meyer RJ, Hoffman R, Zanjani ED. Autoimmune hemolytic anemia and periodic pure red cell aplasia in systemic lupus erythematosus: recovery after plasmapheresis. *Am J Med* 1978;65: 342–345.
119. Liu H, Ozaki K, Matsuzaki Y, et al. Suppression of haematopoiesis by IgG autoantibodies from patients with systemic lupus erythematosus. *Clin Exp Immunol* 1995;100: 480–485.
120. Linardaki GD, Boki KA, Fertakis A, et al. Pure red cell aplasia as presentation of systemic lupus erythematosus. *Scand J Rheumatol* 1999;28:189.
121. Agudelo CA, Wise CM, Lyles MF. Pure red cell aplasia in procainamide induced systemic lupus erythematosus: report and review of the literature. *J Rheumatol* 1988;15:1431–1432.
122. Francis DA. Pure red-cell aplasia: association with systemic lupus erythematosus with primary autoimmune hypothyroidism. *Br Med J (Clin Res)* 1982;284:85.
123. Franzen P, Friman C, Pettersson T, et al. Combined pure red cell aplasia and primary autoimmune hypothyroidism in systemic lupus erythematosus. *Arthritis Rheum* 1987;30:837–840.
124. Krantz SB, Moore WH, Zaentz SD. Studies of red cell aplasia. *J Clin Invest* 1973;52:324–336.
125. Orbach H, Ben-Yehuda D, Manor D, et al. Successful treatment of pure red cell aplasia in systemic lupus erythematosus with erythropoietin. *J Rheumatol* 1995;22:2166–2169.
126. Nossent JC, Swaak AJ. Pancytopenia in systemic lupus erythematosus related to azathioprine. *J Intern Med* 1990;227:69–72.
127. Meyerson MA, Cohen PR. Dapsone-induced aplastic anemia in a woman with bullous systemic lupus erythematosus. *Mayo Clin Proc* 1994;69:1159–1162.
128. Abdou NI, Verdirame JD, Amare M, et al. Heterogeneity of pathogenetic mechanisms in aplastic anemia. Efficacy based on in vitro results. *Ann Intern Med* 1981;95:43–50.
129. Chute JP, Hoffmeister K, Gotelingam J, et al. Aplastic anemia as the sole presentation of systemic lupus erythematosus. *Am J Hematol* 1996;51:237–239.
130. Wolach B, Choc L, Pomeranz A, et al. Aplastic anemia in neonatal lupus erythematosus. *Am J Dis Child* 1993;147: 941–944.
131. Brooks BJ Jr, Borxmeyer HE, Bryan CF, et al. Serum inhibitor in systemic lupus erythematosus associated with aplastic anemia. *Arch Intern Med* 1984;144:1474–1477.
132. Bailey FA, Lilly M, Bertoli LF, et al. An antibody that inhibits in vitro bone marrow proliferation in a patient systemic lupus erythematosus and aplastic anemia. *Arthritis Rheum* 1989;32: 901–906.
133. Stricker RB, Shuman MA. Aplastic anemia complicating systemic lupus erythematosus: response to androgens in two patients. *Am J Hematol* 1984;17:193–201.
134. Walport MJ, Hubbard WN, Hughes GR. Reversal of aplastic anaemia secondary to systemic lupus erythematosus by high-dose intravenous cyclophosphamide. *Br Med J (Clin Res)* 1982; 285:769–770.
135. Roffe C, Cahill MR, Samanta A, et al. Aplastic anemia in systemic lupus erythematosus: a cellular immune mechanism? Br *J Rheumatol* 1991;30:301–304.
136. Flood FT, Limarzi LR. Bone marrow studies in lupus erythematosus before and after ACTH and cortisone therapy. *J Lab Clin Med* 1950;36:823–833.
137. Burkhardt R. The bone marrow in systemic lupus erythematosus. *Semin Hematol* 1965;2:29–46.
138. Feng CS, Ng MH, Szeto RSC, et al. Bone marrow findings in lupus patients with pancytopenia. *Pathology* 1991;23:57.
139. Pereira RM, Velloso ER, Menezes Y, et al. Bone marrow findings in systemic lupus erythematosus patients with peripheral cytopenias. *Clin Rheumatol* 1998;17:219–222.
140. Morales-Polanco M, Jimenez-Balderas FJ, Yanez P. Storage histiocytes and hemophagocytosis; a common finding in the bone marrow of patients with active systemic lupus erythematosus. *Arch Med Res* 1996;27:57–62.
141. El Mouzan MI, Ahmad MAM, Saleh ALF, et al. Myelofibrosis and pancytopenia in systemic lupus erythematosus. *Acta Haematol* 1988;80:219–222.
142. Kaelin WG Jr, Spivak JL. Systemic lupus erythematosus and myelofibrosis. *Am J Med* 1986;81:935–940.
143. Laszlo MH, Alvarez A, Feldman F. Association of thrombotic thrombocytopenic purpura and disseminated lupus erythematosus (case report). *Ann Intern Med* 1955;42:1308–1320.
144. Matsuoka C, Liouris J, Andrianakos A, et al. Systemic lupus erythematosus and myelofibrosis. *Clin Rheumatol* 1989;8: 402–407.
145. Rosen PJ, Cramer AD, Dubois EL, et al. Systemic lupus erythematosus and myelofibrosis. A possible pathogenetic relationship. *Clin Res* 1973;21:565(abst).
146. Borba EF, Pereira RMR, Velloso EDRP, et al. Neutropenia associated with myelofibrosis in systemic lupus erythematosus. *Acta Haematol* 1993;89:82–85.
147. Paquette RL, Meshkinpour A, Rosen PJ. Autoimmune myelofibrosis: a steroid-responsive cause of bone marrow fibrosis associated with systemic lupus erythematosus. *Medicine* 1994;73: 145–152.
148. Inoue Y, Matsubara A, Okuya S, et al. Myelofibrosis and systemic lupus erythematosus: reversal of fibrosis with high dose corticosteroid therapy. *Acta Haematol* 1992;88:32–36.
149. Foley-Nolan D, Martin MFR, Rowbotham D, et al. Systemic lupus erythematosus presenting with myelofibrosis. *J Rheumatol* 1992;19:1303–1304.
150. Hirose W, Fukuya H, Anzai T, et al. Myelofibrosis and systemic lupus erythematosus. *J Rheumatol* 1993;20:2164–2165.
151. Abaron A, Levy Y, Bar-Dayan Y, et al. Successful treatment of early secondary myelofibrosis in SLE with IVIG. *Lupus* 1997;6: 408–411.
152. Ng MHL, Li EK, Feng CS. Gelatinous transformation of the bone marrow in systemic lupus erythematosus. *J Rheumatol* 1989;16:989–992.
153. Wong K, Hei P, Chan JC, et al. The acute lupus hematophagocytic syndrome. *Ann Intern Med* 1991;114:387–390.
154. Wong KF, Chan JKC. Reactive hemophagocytic syndrome: a clinicopathologic study of 40 patients in an oriental population. *Am J Med* 1992;93:177–180.
155. Matsumoto Y, Naniwa D, Banno S, et al. The efficacy of therapeutic plasmapheresis for the treatment of fatal hemophagocytic syndrome: two case reports. *Ther Apheresis* 1998;2: 300–304.
156. Gill SD, Spenser A, Cobcroft RG. High dose gamma globulin therapy in the reactive haemophagocytic syndrome. *Br J Haematol* 1994;88:204–208.
157. Costello C, Abdelaal M, Coomes EN. Pernicious anemia and systemic lupus erythematosus in a young woman. *J Rheumatol* 1985;12:798–799.
158. Feld S, Landau Z, Gefel D, et al. Pernicious anemia, Hashimoto's thyroiditis and Sjögren's in a woman with SLE and autoimmune hemolytic anemia (letter). *J Rheumatol* 1989;16: 258–259.
159. Korbet SM, Corwin HL. Pernicious anemia associated with systemic lupus erythematosus. *J Rheumatol* 1986;13:193–194.
160. Junca J, Cuxart A, Tural C, et al. Systemic lupus erythematosus

and pernicious anemia in an 82-year-old woman. *J Rheumatol* 1991;18:1924–1925.
161. Sukenik S, Buskila D. Treatment of pernicious anemia associated with systemic lupus erythematosus. *J Rheumatol* 1993;20: 592–293.
162. Molad Y, Rachmilewitz B, Sidi Y, et al. Serum cobalamin and transcobalamin levels in systemic lupus erythematosus. *Am J Med* 1990;88:141–144.
163. Laser U, Kierat L, Grob PJ, et al. Transcobalamin II, a serum protein reflecting autoimmune disease activity, the plasma dynamics, and the relationship to established parameters in systemic lupus erythematosus. *Clin Immunol Immunopathol* 1985; 36:345–357.
164. Alger M, Alarcon-Segovia D, Rivero SJ. Hemolytic anemia and thrombocytopenic purpura: two related subsets of systemic lupus erythematosus. *J Rheumatol* 1977;4:351–357.
165. Cohen AS, Reynolds WE, Franklin EC, et al. Preliminary criteria for the classification of systemic lupus erythematosus. *Bull Rheum Dis* 1971;21:643–648.
166. Nossent JC, Swaak AJG. Prevalence and significance of haematological abnormalities in patients with systemic lupus erythematosus. *Q J Med* 1991;291:605–612.
167. Dubois EL. Acquired hemolytic anemia as presenting syndrome of lupus erythematosus disseminatus. *Am J Med* 1952;22: 197–204.
168. Videbaek A. Auto-immune haemolytic anaemia in systemic lupus erythematosus. *Acta Med Scand* 1962;171:187–194.
169. Matsumoto N, Ishihara T, Fujii H, et al. Fine structure of the spleen in autoimmune hemolytic anemia associated with systemic lupus erythematosus. *Tohoku J Exp Med* 1978;124: 223–232.
170. Brus I, Lewis SM. The haptoglobin content of serum in haemolytic anaemia. *Br J Haematol* 1959;5:348–355.
171. Louderback AL, Shanbrom E. Hepatoglobulin electrophoresis. *JAMA* 1968;206:362–363.
172. Owen JA, De Gruchy GC, Smith H. Serum haptoglobins in haemolytic states. *J Clin Pathol* 1960;13:478–482.
173. Tan EM, Chaplin H Jr. Antinuclear antibodies in Coombs-positive acquired hemolytic anemia. *Vox Sang* 1968;15:161–170.
174. Favre H, Chatelanat F, Miescher PA. Autoimmune hematologic diseases associated with infraclinical systemic lupus erythematosus in four patients: a human equivalent of the NZB mice. *Am J Med* 1979;66:91–95.
175. Miescher PA, Tucci A, Beris P, et al. Autoimmune hemolytic anemia and/or thrombocytopenia associated with lupus parameters. *Semin Hematol* 1992;29:13–17.
176. Deleze M, Alarcon-Segovia D, Oria CV, et al. Hemocytopenia in systemic lupus erythematosus. Relationship to antiphospholipid antibodies. *J Rheumatol* 1989;16:926–930.
177. Fong KY, Loizou S, Boey ML, et al. Anticardiolipin antibodies, haemolytic anemia and thrombocytopenia in systemic lupus erythematosus. *Br J Rheumatol* 1992;31:453–455.
178. Kokori SIG, Ioannidis JPA, Voulgarelis M, et al. Autoimmune hemolytic anemia in patients with systemic lupus erythematosus. *Am J Med* 2000;108:198–204.
179. Sokol RJ, Hewill S, Stamps BK. Autoimmune hemolysis: an 18 year study of 865 cases referred to a regional transfusion center. *Br J Med* 1981;282:2023–2027.
180. Shulman IA, Branch DR, Nelson JM, et al. Autoimmune hemolytic anemia with both cold and warm autoantibodies. *JAMA* 1985:253;1746–1748.
181. Priofsky B. Immune haemolytic disease: the autoimmune haemolytic anemias. *Clin Haematol* 1975;4:167–180.
182. Jacob HS. Pulse steroids in hematologic disease. *Hosp Pract* 1985;5:87–94.
183. Ahn YS, Harrington WJ, Mylvaganam RM, et al. Danazol therapy for autoimmune hemolytic anemia. *Ann Intern Med* 1985; 102:298–301.
184. Pignon JM, Poirson E, Rochant H. Danazol in autoimmune hemolytic anemia. *Br J Haematol* 1993;83:343–345.
185. Von Keyserlingk H, Meyer-Sabellek W, Arnzt R, et al. Plasma exchanged treatment in autoimmune hemolytic anemia of the warm antibody type with renal failure. *Vox Sang* 1987;52: 598–600.
186. Majer RV, Hyde RD. High dose intravenous immunoglobulin in the treatment of autoimmune hemolytic anemia. *Clin Lab Haematol* 1988;10:391–395.
187. Ahn YS, Harrington WJ, Mylvaganam R, et al. Treatment of autoimmune hemolytic anemia with vinca loaded platelets. *JAMA* 1983;249:2189–2194.
188. Flores G, Cunningham-Rundles C, Newland AC, et al. Efficacy of intravenous immunoglobulin in the treatment of autoimmune hemolytic anemia: results in 73 patients. *Am J Hematol* 1993;44:237–242.
189. Murphy S, LoBuglio AF. Drug therapy of autoimmune hemolytic anemia. *Semin Haematol* 1976;13:323–337.
190. Best WR, Darling DR. A critical look at the splenectomy-SLE controversy. *Med Clin North Am* 1962;46:19–47.
191. Coon WW. Splenectomy for cytopenias associated with systemic lupus erythematosus. *Am J Surg* 1988;155:301–394.
192. Rivero SJ, Alger M, Alarcon-Segovia D. Splenectomy for hemocytopenia in systemic lupus erythematosus: a controlled reappraisal. *Arch Intern Med* 1979;139:773–776.
193. Leonhardt T. Family studies in systemic lupus erythematosus. *Acta Med Scand* 1964;176(suppl 416):1–156.
194. Callender S, Race RR, Paykoc ZV. Hypersensitivity to transfused blood. *Br Med J* 1945;2:83–84.
195. Callender ST, Race RR. Serological and genetical study of multiple antibodies formed in response to blood transfusion by a patient with lupus erythematosus diffusus. *Ann Eugenics* 1946; 13:102–117.
196. Waller RK, Race RR. Six blood-group antibodies in the serum of transfused patient. *Br Med J* 1951;1:225–226.
197. Kuhns WJ, Bauerlein TC. Exchange transfusion in hemolytic anemia complicating disseminated lupus erythematosus: report of case of acquired hemolytic disease associated with rare blood group antibodies following whole blood transfusions. *Arch Intern Med* 1953;92:284–292.
198. Baldwin GB. Acute disseminated lupus erythematosus with report of a fatal case. *Med J Aust* 1945;2:11–15.
199. Greger WP, Choy SH, Rantz LA. Experimental determination of the hypersensitive diathesis in man. *J Immunol* 1985;66: 445–450.
200. Zingale SB, Sanchez Avalos JC, Andrada JA, et al. Appearance of anticoagulant factors and certain autoimmune antibodies following antigenic stimulation and blood group substances in patients with systemic lupus erythematosus. *Arthritis Rheum* 1963;6:581–598.
201. Lee SL, Meiselas LE, Zingale SB, et al. Antibody production in systemic lupus erythematosus (SLE) and rheumatoid arthritis (RA). *J Clin Invest* 1960;39:1(abst).
202. Muschel LH. Systemic lupus erythematosus and normal antibodies. *Proc Soc Exp Biol Med* 1961;106;622–625.
203. Petz LD. Autoimmune hemolytic anemia. *Hum Pathol* 1983; 14:251–255.
204. Adamson JW, Eschbach JW. Treatment of the anemia of chronic renal failure with recombinant human erythropoietin. *Annu Rev Med* 1990;41:349–360.
205. Wong KC, Li PKT, Nicholls MG, et al. The adverse effects of recombinant human erythropoietin therapy. *Adverse Drug React Acute Poisoning Rev* 1990;9:183–206.
206. Lim VS, DeGowin RL, Zavala D, et al. Recombinant human

erythropoietin treatment in pre-dialysis patients. *Ann Intern Med* 1989;110:108–114.
207. Romero R, Novoa D, Perez-Freiria A, et al. Resistance to recombinant human erythropoietin in a hemodialysis patient with lupus reactivation. *Nephron* 1995;69:343–344.
208. Kontessis PS, Paraskevopoulos A, Papageorgiou I, et al. Successful use of recombinant human erythropoietin in a pregnant woman with lupus nephritis. *Am J Kidney Dis* 1995;26: 781–784.
209. Pincus T, Olsen NJ, Russel J, et al. Multicenter study of recombinant human erythropoietin in correction of anemia in rheumatoid arthritis. *Am J Med* 1990;89:161–166.
210. Hebert LA, Birmingham DJ, Dillon JJ, et al. Erythropoietin therapy in humans increases erythrocyte expression of complement receptor type 1 (CD35). *J Am Soc Nephrol* 1994;4: 1786–1791.
211. Hebert LA, Birmingham DJ, Shen XP, et al. Effect of recombinant erythropoietin therapy on autoimmunity in systemic lupus erythematosus. *Am J Kidney Dis* 1994;24:25–32.
212. Gladman D, Urowitz M, Tozman E, et al. Hemostatic abnormalities in systemic lupus erythematosus. *Q J Med* 1983;52: 424–433.
213. Dubois EL, Commons RR, Starr P, et al. Corticotropin and cortisone treatment for systemic lupus erythematosus. *JAMA* 1952; 149:9951.
214. Miller MH, Urowitz MB, Gladman DD. Significance of thrombocytopenia in systemic lupus erythematosus. *Arthritis Rheum* 1983;26;1181–1186.
215. Pistiner M, Wallace DJ, Nessim S, et al. Lupus erythematosus in the 1980s: a survey of 570 patients. *Semin Arthritis Rheum* 1991;21:55–64.
216. Reveille JD, Bartolucci A, Alarcon GS. Prognosis in systemic lupus erythematosus. Negative impact of increasing age at onset, black race, and thrombocytopenia, as well as causes of death. *Arthritis Rheum* 1990;33:37–48.
217. Clark WF, Linton AL, Cordy PE, et al. Immunologic findings, thrombocytopenia and disease activity in lupus nephritis. *Can Med J* 1978;118:1191–1195.
218. Karpatkin S. Autoimmune thrombocytopenic purpura. *Blood* 1980;56:329–343.
219. Difino SM, Lachant NA, Krishner JJH, et al. Adult idiopathic thrombocytopenic purpura. *Am J Med* 1980;69:430–442.
220. Perez HD, Katler E, Embury S. Idiopathic thrombocytopenic purpura with high titer speckled pattern antinuclear antibodies: possible marker for systemic lupus erythematosus. *Arthritis Rheum* 1985;28:596–597.
221. Dameshek W, Reeves WH. Exacerbation of lupus erythematosus following splenectomy in idiopathic thrombocytopenic purpura and autoimmune hemolytic anemia. *Am J Med* 1956;21: 560–566.
222. Anderson MJ, Peebles CL, McMillar R, et al. Fluorescent antinuclear antibodies and anti-SSA/Ro in patients with immune thrombocytopenia developing systemic lupus erythematosus. *Ann Intern Med* 1985;103:548–551.
223. Morley KD, Bernstein RM, Bunn CC, et al. Thrombocytopenia and anti-Ro. *Lancet* 1981;2:940.
224. Firkin BG, Buchanan RRC, Pfueller S, et al. Lupoid thrombocytopenia. *Aust NZ J Med* 1987;17:295–300.
225. Rabinowitz Y, Dameshek W. Systemic lupus erythematosus after idiopathic thrombocytopenic purpura: a review. A study of systemic lupus erythematosus occurring after 78 splenectomies for idiopathic thrombocytopenic purpura. *Ann Intern Med* 1960;52:1–28.
226. Mestanza-Peralta M, Ariza-Ariza R, Cardiel MH, et al. Thrombocytopenic purpura as initial manifestation of systemic lupus erythematosus. *J Rheumatol* 1997; 24:867–870.
227. Bunting WL, Kiely JM, Campbell DC. Idiopathic thrombocytopenic purpura. Treatment in adults. *Arch Intern Med* 1961; 108:733–738.
228. Doan CA, Bouroncle BA, Wiseman BK. Idiopathic and secondary thrombocytopenic purpura: clinical study and evaluation of 381 cases over a period of 28 years. *Ann Intern Med* 1960;53:861–876.
229. Meyers MC. Results of treatment in 71 patients with idiopathic thrombocytopenic purpura. *Am J Med Sci* 1961;242:295–302.
230. Karpatkin S. Autoimmune thrombocytopenic purpura. *Semin Hematol* 1985;22:260–288.
231. Eyanson S, Passo MH, Aldo-Benson MA, et al. Methylprednisolone pulse therapy for non-renal lupus erythematosus. *Ann Rheum Dis* 1980;39:377–380.
232. Mackworth-Young CG, Walport MJ, Hughes GRV. Thrombocytopenia in a case of systemic lupus erythematosus: repeated administration of pulse methylprednisolone. *Br J Rheumatol* 1984;23:298–300.
233. Marion C, Cook P. Danazol for lupus thrombocytopenia. *Arch Intern Med* 1988;108:703–706.
234. West SG, Johnson SC. Danazol for the treatment of refractory autoimmune thrombocytopenia in systemic lupus erythematosus. *Ann Intern Med* 1988;108:703–706.
235. Kavanaugh A. Danazol therapy in thrombocytopenia associated with the antiphospholipid antibody syndrome. *Ann Intern Med* 1994;121:767–768.
236. Boumpas DT, Barez S, Klippel JH, et al. Intermittent cyclophosphamide for the treatment of autoimmune thrombocytopenia in systemic lupus erythematosus. *Ann Intern Med* 1990;112:674–677.
237. Roach BA, Hutchinson GJ. Treatment of refractory, systemic lupus erythematosus-associated thrombocytopenia with lowdose intravenous cyclophosphamide. *Arthritis Rheum* 1993;36: 682–684.
238. Goegel KM, Gassel WD, Goebel FD. Evaluation of azathioprine in autoimmune thrombocytopenia and lupus erythematosus. *Scand J Haematol* 1973;10:28–34.
239. Matsumura O, Kawashima Y, Kato S, et al. Therapeutic effect of cyclosporin in thrombocytopenia associated with autoimmune disease. *Transplant Proc* 1988;20(suppl 4):317–322.
240. Moss C, Hamilton PJ. Thrombocytopenia in systemic lupus erythematosus responsive to dapsone. *Br Med J (Clin Res)* 1988; 297:266.
241. Ahn YS, Harrington WJ, Seelman RC, et al. Vincristine therapy of idiopathic and secondary thrombocytopenias. *N Engl J Med* 1974;291:376–380.
242. Quiquandon I, Fenaux P, Caulier MR, et al. Re-evaluation of azathioprine in the treatment of adult chronic idiopathic thrombocytopenic purpura: a report on 53 cases. *Br J Haematol* 1990;74:223–228.
243. Figueroa M, Gehlsen J, Hammound D, et al. Combination chemotherapy in refractory immune thrombocytopenic purpura. *N Engl J Med* 1993;328:1226–1229.
244. Snyder HW Jr, Cochran SK, Balint JP Jr, et al. Experience with protein A-immunoadsorption in treatment-resistant adult immunothrombocytopenia purpura. *Blood* 1992;79:2237–2245.
245. Cahill MR, Macey MG, Cavenagh JD, et al. Protein A immunoadsorption in chronic refractory ITP reverses increased platelet activation but fails to achieve sustained clinical benefit. *Br J Haematol* 1998;100:358–364.
246. Ter Borg EJ, Kallenberg CGM. Treatment of severe thrombocytopenia in systemic lupus erythematosus with intravenous gammaglobulin. *Ann Rheum Dis* 1992;51:1149–1151.
247. Newland AC. Annotation: the use and mechanism of action of intravenous immunoglobulin, an update. *Br J Haematol* 1989; 72:301–305.

248. Li E, Li C, Cohen MG. SLE-associated thrombocytopenia in pregnancy: successful outcome with combined IgG Infusion and platelet transfusion. *Br J Clin Pract* 1993;47:338–339.
249. Ruiz-Valverde MP, Segarra A, Tovar JL, et al. Treatment of systemic lupus erythematosus-associated thrombocytopenia with intravenous gamma globulin. *Nephron* 1994;67:500–501.
250. Jacobs P, Wood L, Novitzky N. Intravenous gamma globulin has no advantages over oral corticosteroids as primary therapy for adults with immune thrombocytopenia: a prospective randomized clinical trail. *Am J Med* 1994;97:55–59.
251. Maier WP, Gordon DS, Howard RF, et al. Intravenous immunoglobulin therapy in systemic lupus erythematosus-associated thrombocytopenia. *Arthritis Rheum* 1990;33:1233–1239.
252. Scaradavou A. Splenectomy-sparing, long-term maintenance with anti-D for chronic immune (idiopathic) thrombocytopenic purpura: the New York Hospital experience. *Semin Hematol* 2000;37(suppl 1):42–44.
253. Waintraub SE, Brody JI. Use of anti-D in immune thrombocytopenic purpura as a means to prevent splenectomy: case reports from two university hospital medical centers. *Semin Hematol* 2000;37(suppl 1):45–49.
254. Holman WR, Dineen P. The role of splenectomy in the treatment of thrombocytopenic purpura due to systemic lupus erythematosus. *Ann Surg* 1978;187:52–56.
255. Breckenridge RT, Moore RD, Ratnoff OD. A study of thrombocytopenia. New histologic criteria for the differentiation of idiopathic thrombocytopenia and thrombocytopenia associated with disseminated lupus erythematosus. *Blood* 1967;30:39–53.
256. Jacobs P, Wood L, Dent DM. Splenectomy and the thrombocytopenia of systemic lupus erythematosus. *Ann Intern Med* 1986;105:971–972.
257. Galindo M, Khamasta MA, Hughes GR. Splenectomy for refractory thrombocytopenia in antiphospholipid syndrome. *Rheumatology* 1999;38:848–853.
258. Hakim AJ, Machin SJ, Isenberg DA. Autoimmune thrombocytopenia in primary antiphospholipid syndrome and systemic lupus erythematosus: the response to splenectomy. *Semin Arthritis Rheum* 1998;28:20–25.
259. Hall S, McCormick JL, Griep PR, et al. Splenectomy does not cure the thrombocytopenia of systemic lupus erythematosus. *Ann Intern Med* 1985;102:325–330.
260. Park A, Marcaccio M, Sternbach M, et al. Laparoscopic versus open splenectomy. *Arch Surg* 1999;134:1263–1269.
261. Calverly DC, Jones GW, Kelton JG. Splenic irradiation for corticosteroid-resistant immune thrombocytopenia. *Ann Intern Med* 1992;116:977–981.
262. Griner PF, Hoyer LW. Megakaryocytic thrombocytopenia in systemic lupus erythematosus. *Arch Intern Med* 1970;125:328–332.
263. Manoharan A, Williams NT, Sparrow R. Acquired megakaryocytic thrombocytopenia: report of a case and review of literature. *Q J Med* 1989;70:234–252.
264. Nagasawa T, Sakurai T, Kashiwagi H, et al. Cell mediated megakaryocytic thrombocytopenia associated with systemic lupus erythematosus. *Blood* 1986;67:479–483.
265. George JN, Snaith SJ. Clinical importance of acquired abnormalities of platelet function. *N Engl J Med* 1991;324:2739.
266. Regan M, Lackner H, Karpatkin S. Platelet function and coagulation profile in lupus erythematosus: studies in 50 patients. *Ann Intern Med* 1974;81:462–468.
267. Dorsch CA, Meyerhoff J. Mechanisms of abnormal platelet aggregation in systemic lupus erythematosus. *Arthritis Rheum* 1982;25:966–973.
268. Kanai H, Tshuchida A, Yano S, et al. Intraplatelet and urinary serotonin concentrations in systemic lupus erythematosus with reference to its clinical manifestations. *J Med* 1989;20:371–377.
269. Parbtani A, Frampton G, Yewdall V, et al. Platelet and plasma serotonin in glomerulonephritis III. The nephritis of systemic lupus erythematosus. *Clin Nephrol* 1980;14:164–172.
270. Weiss HG, Rosove MH, Lages BA, et al. Acquired storage pool deficiency with increased platelet-associated IgG. *Am J Med* 1980;69:711–717.
271. Ginsberg HM, O'Malley M. Serum factors releasing serotonin from normal platelets: relation to the manifestation of systemic lupus erythematosus. *Ann Intern Med* 1977;87:564–569.
272. Meyerhoff J, Dorsch CA. Decreased platelet serotonin levels in systemic lupus erythematosus. *Arthritis Rheum* 1981;24:1495–1500.
273. Zeller J, Weissbarth E, Baruth B, et al. Serotonin content of platelets in inflammatory rheumatic disease. *Arthritis Rheum* 1983;26:532–540.
274. Dorsch C, Meyerhoff J. Elevated plasma beta-thromboglobulin levels in systemic lupus erythematosus. *Thromb Res* 1980;20:617–622.
275. Woo KT, Junor BJR, Salem H, et al. Beta thromboglobulin and platelet aggregation in glomerulonephritis. *Clin Nephrol* 1980;14:92–95.
276. Tetta C, Bussolino F, Modena V, et al. Release of platelet-activity factor in systemic lupus erythematosus. *Int Arch Allergy Immunol* 1990;91:244–256.
277. Camussi G, Tetta C, Coda R, et al. Release of platelet-activating factor in human pathology: evidence of the occurrence of basophil degranulation and release of platelet activating factor in systemic lupus erythematosus. *Lab Invest* 1981;44:241–251.
278. Clark WF, Lewis ML, Cameron JS, et al. Intrarenal platelet consumption in the diffuse proliferative nephritis of systemic lupus erythematosus. *Clin Sci Mol Med* 1975;49:247–252.
279. Frampton G, Perl S, Bennett A, et al. Platelet associated DNA and anti-DNA antibody in systemic lupus erythematosus. *Clin Exp Immunol* 1986;63:621–628.
280. Duffus P, Parbtani A, Frampton G, et al. Intraglomerular localization of platelet related antigens, platelet factor 4 and beta thromboglobulin in glomerulonephritis. *Clin Nephrol* 1981;17:288–297.
281. Ridolfi RL, Bell WR. Thrombotic thrombocytopenic purpura. *Medicine* 1981;60:413–428.
282. Rose M, Rowe JM, Eldor A. The changing course or thrombotic thrombocytopenic purpura and modern therapy. *Blood Rev* 1993;7:94–103.
283. Gatenby PA, Smith H, Krwan P, et al. Systemic lupus erythematosus and thrombotic thrombocytopenic purpura. A case report and review of the relationship. *J Rheumatol* 1981;8:504–508.
284. Levine S, Shearn MA. Thrombotic thrombocytopenic purpura and systemic lupus erythematosus. *Arch Intern Med* 1964;113:826–836.
285. Amorosi E, Ultmann J. Thrombotic thrombocytopenic purpura: report of 16 cases and review of the literature. *Medicine* 1966;45:139–159.
286. Fox DA, Faix JD, Coblyn J, et al. Thrombotic thrombocytopenic purpura and systemic lupus erythematosus. *Ann Rheum Dis* 1986;45:319–322.
287. Stricker RB, Davis JA, Gershow J, et al. Thrombotic thrombocytopenic purpura complicating systemic lupus erythematosus. Case report and literature review from the plasmapheresis era. *J Rheumatol* 1992;19:1469–1473.
288. Nesher G, Hanna VE, Moore TL, et al. Thrombotic microangiopathic hemolytic anemia in systemic lupus erythematosus. Semin *Arthritis Rheum* 1994;24:165–172.
289. Jain R, Chartash E, Susin M, et al. Systemic lupus erythemato-

sus complicated by thrombotic microangiopathy. *Semin Arthritis Rheum* 1994;24:173–182.

290. Hess DC, Sethi K, Awad E. Thrombotic thrombocytopenic purpura in systemic lupus erythematosus and antiphospholipid antibodies: effective treatment with plasma exchange and immunosuppression. *J Rheumatol* 1992;19:1474–1478.
291. Musio F, Bohen EM, Yuan CM, et al. Review of Thrombotic thrombocytopenic purpura in the setting of systemic lupus erythematosus. *Semin Arthritis Rheum* 1998;28:1–19.
292. Broun J, Sieper J, Schwarz A. Widespread vasculopathy with hemolytic uremic syndrome, perimyocarditis and cystic pancreatitis in a young woman with mixed connective tissue disease. *Rheumatol Int* 1993;13:31–36.
293. Miller JM, Pastorek JG. Thrombotic thrombocytopenic purpura and hemolytic uremic syndrome in pregnancy. *Clin Obstet Gynecol* 1991;34:64–71.
294. Alpert LI. Thrombotic thrombocytopenic purpura and systemic lupus erythematosus. Report of a case with immunofluorescence investigation of vascular lesions. *J Mt Sinai Hosp NY* 1968;35:165–173.
295. Cecere FA, Yoshinoya S, Pope RM. Fatal thrombotic thrombocytopenic purpura with systemic lupus erythematosus: circulating commune complexes. *Arthritis Rheum* 1981;24:550–553.
296. Dekker A, O'Brien ME, Cammarata RJ. The association of thrombotic thrombocytopenic purpura with systemic lupus erythematosus: a report of two cases with successful treatment of one. *Am J Med Sci* 1974;267:243–249.
297. Oen K, Petty RE, Schroeder ML, et al. Thrombotic thrombocytopenic purpura in a girl with systemic lupus erythematosus. *J Rheumatol* 1980;7:727–729.
298. Ramkissoon RA. Thrombotic thrombocytopenic purpura and systemic lupus erythematosus. *CA Med* 1966;104:212–214.
299. Reinter M, Cox J, Bernheim C, et al. Two cases of disseminated lupus erythematosus with terminal Moschowitz syndrome. *Schweiz Med Wochenschr* 1968;98:1691–1692.
300. Dixit R, Krieg AM, Atkinson JP. Thrombotic thrombocytopenic purpura developing during pregnancy in a C2-deficient patient with a history of systemic lupus erythematosus. *Arthritis Rheum* 1985;28:341–344.
301. Itoh Y, Sekine H, Hosono O, et al. Thrombotic thrombocytopenic purpura in two patients with systemic lupus erythematosus: clinical significance of antiplatelet antibodies. *Clin Immunol Immunopathol* 1990;57:125–136.
302. Gelfand J, Truong L, Stern L, et al. Thrombotic thrombocytopenic purpura in systemic lupus erythematosus. Treatment with plasma infusion. *Am J Kidney Dis* 1985;6:154–160.
303. Rock GA, Shumak KH, Buskard NA, et al., Canadian Apheresis Study Group. Comparison of plasma exchange with plasma infusion in the treatment of thrombotic thrombocytopenic purpura. *N Engl J Med* 1991;325:393–397.
304. Siddiqui FA, Lina EC-Y. Novel platelet-agglutinating protein from a thrombotic thrombocytopenic purpura plasma. *J Clin Invest* 1985;76:1330–1340.
305. Wright JF, Wang H, Hornstein A, et al. Characterization of platelet glycoproteins and platelet/endothelial cell antibodies in patients with thrombotic thrombocytopenic purpura. *Br J Haematol* 1999;107:546–555.
306. Schultz DR, Arnold PI, Jy W, et al. Anti-CD36 autoantibodies in thrombotic thrombocytopenic purpura and other thrombotic disorders: identification of an 85 kD form of CD 36 as target antigen. *Br J Haematol* 1998;103:849–857.
307. Tsai HM, Lian ECY. Antibodies to von Willebrand factor-cleaving protease in acute thrombotic thrombocytopenic purpura. *N Engl J Med* 1998; 339:1585–1594.
308. Goeckerman WH. Lupus erythematosus as a systemic disease. *JAMA* 1923;80:542–547.
309. Fries JF, Holman H. *Systemic lupus erythematosus: a clinical analysis*. Philadelphia: WB Saunders, 1975.
310. Maeshima E, Yamada Y, Yukawa S. Fever and leucopenia with steroids. *Lancet* 2000;355:198.
311. Rose E, Pillsbury DM. Lupus erythematosus (erythematoides) and ovarian function: observations on possible relationship with report of 6 cases. *Ann Intern Med* 1944;21:1022–1034.
312. Markusse HM, Schravenhoff R, Beerman H. Hypereosinophilic syndrome presenting with diarrhoea and anaemia in a patient with systemic lupus erythematosus. *Neth J Med* 1998; 52:79–81.
313. Thomeer M, Moerman P, Westhovens R, et al. Systemic lupus erythematosus, eosinophilia and Loffler's endocarditis. An unusual association. *Eur Resp J* 1999;13:930–933.
314. Hunsiker N, Brun R. Basophil counts in lupus erythematosus and in some other dermatoses. *Dermatologica* 1972;145: 291–298.
315. Egido J, Crespo MS, Lahoz C, et al. Evidence of an immediate hypersensitivity mechanism in systemic lupus erythematosus. *Ann Rheum Dis* 1980;39:321–327.
316. Dubois EL. Systemic lupus erythematosus: recent advances in its diagnosis and treatment. *Ann Intern Med* 1956;45:163–184.
317. Dubois EL. Nitrogen mustard in treatment of systemic lupus erythematosus. *Arch Intern Med* 1954;93:667–672.
318. Aegerter E, Long JH. The collagen diseases. *Am J Med Sci* 1949; 218:324–337.
319. McDuffie FC. Bone marrow depression after drug therapy in patients with systemic lupus erythematosus. *Ann Rheum Dis* 1965;24:289–292.
320. Starkebaum G, Price TH, Lee MY, et al. Autoimmune neutropenia in systemic lupus erythematosus. *Arthritis Rheum* 1978;21:504–512.
321. Hadley AG, Byron MA, Chapel HM, et al. Anti-granulocyte opsonic activity in sera from patients with systemic lupus erythematosus. *Br J Haematol* 1987;65:61–65.
322. Frank MM, Hamburger MI, Lawley TJ, et al. Defective reticuloendothelial system Fc-receptor function in systemic lupus erythematosus. *N Engl J Med* 1979;300:518–523.
323. Kurien BT, Newland J, Paczkowski C, et al. Association of neutropenia in systemic lupus erythematosus (SLE) with anti-Ro and binding of an immunologically cross-reactive neutrophil membrane antigen. *Clin Exp Immunol* 2000;120:209–217.
324. Arenas M, Abad A, Valverde V, et al. Selective inhibition of granulopoiesis with severe neutropenia in systemic lupus erythematosus. *Arthritis Rheum* 1992;35:979–980.
325. Courtney PA, Crockard AD, Williamson K, et al. Increased apoptotic peripheral blood neutrophils in systemic lupus erythematosus: relations with disease activity, antibodies to double stranded DNA, and neutropenia. *Ann Rheum Dis* 1999;58(5): 309–314.
326. Kondo H, Date Y, Sakai Y, et al. Effective simultaneous rhG-CSF and methylprednisolone pulse therapy in agranulocytosis associated with systemic lupus erythematosus. *Am J Hematol* 1994;46:157–158.
327. Euler HH, Harten P, Zeuner RA, et al. Recombinant human granulocyte colony stimulating factor in patients with systemic lupus erythematosus associated neutropenia and refractory infections. *J Rheumatol* 1997;24:215–237.
328. Dale DC, Fauci AS, Guerry D IV, et al. Comparison of agents producing a neutrophilic leukocytosis in man: hydrocortisone, prednisone, endotoxin and etiocholanolone. *J Clin Invest* 1975; 56:808–813.
329. Paulus HE, Okun R, Calabro JJ. Depression of bone marrow granulocyte reserves in systemic lupus erythematosus (SLE). *Arthritis Rheum* 1970;13:344(abst).
330. Kimball HR, Wolff SM, Talal N, et al. Marrow granulocyte

reserves in the rheumatic diseases. *Arthritis Rheum* 1973;16: 345–352.
331. Budman D, Steinberg AD. Bone marrow in lupus erythematosus. *Ann Intern Med* 1977;86:831–832.
332. Rivero I, Morales J. Bisegmental neutrophils and lymphocytes in diagnosis of leukopenia associated with systemic lupus erythematosus (SLE) (in Spanish). *Rev Med Chile* 1972;100: 526–528.
333. Rivero SJ, Diaz-Jouanen E, Alarcon-Segovia D. Lymphopenia in systemic lupus erythematosus. *Arthritis Rheum* 1978;21: 295–305.
334. Delbarre F, Pompidou A, Hahan A, et al. Study of lymphocytes during systemic lupus erythematosus. *Pathol Biol* 1971;19: 379–385.
335. Brandt L, Hedberg H. Impaired phagocytosis by peripheral blood granulocytes in systemic lupus erythematosus. *Scand J Haematol* 1969;6:348–353.
336. Orozco JH, Jasin HE, Ziff M. Defective phagocytosis in patients with systemic lupus erythematosus (SLE). *Arthritis Rheum* 1970;13:342(abst).
337. Hallgren R, Hakansson L, Venge P. Kinetic studies of phagocytosis. I. The serum independent particle uptake by PMN from patients with rheumatoid arthritis and systemic lupus erythematosus. *Arthritis Rheum* 1978;21:107–113.
338. Zurier RB. Reduction of phagocytosis and lysosomal enzyme release from human leukocytes by serum from patients with systemic lupus erythematosus. *Arthritis Rheum* 1976;19:73–78.
339. Landry M. Phagocytic function and cell mediated immunity in systemic lupus erythematosus. *Arch Dermatol* 1977;113: 147–154.
340. Al-Hadithy H, Isenberg DA, Addison IE, et al. Neurophil function in systemic lupus erythematosus and other collagen diseases. *Ann Rheumatol* 1982;41:33–38.
341. Alvarez I, Vazquez JJ, Fontan G, et al. Neutrophil chemotaxis and serum chemotactic in systemic lupus erythematosus. *Scand J Rheumatol* 1978;7:69–74.
342. Clark RA, Kimball HR, Decker JL. Neutrophil chemotaxis in systemic lupus erythematosus. *Ann Rheum Dis* 1974;33: 167–172.
343. Wenger ME, Bole GG. Nitrobule tetrazolium (NBT) dye reduction by peripheral leukocytes from patients with rheumatoid arthritis (RA) and systemic lupus erythematosus (SLE). *J Lab Clin Med* 1973;82:513–521.
344. Besana C, Lassarin A, Capsoni F, et al. Phagocyte function in systemic lupus erythematosus. *Lancet* 1975;2:918.
345. Gewurz H, Page AR, Pickering RJ, et al. Complement activity and inflammatory neutrophil exudation in man. *Int Arch Allergy* 1967;32:64–90.
346. Hurd ER, Jasin JE, Gilliam JN. Correlation of disease activity and C1-binding immune complexes with the neutrophil inclusions which form in the presence of SLE sera. *Clin Exp Immunol* 1980;40:283–291.
347. Abrahamson SB, Given WP, Edelson HS, et al. Neurophil aggregation induced by sera from patients with active systemic lupus erythematosus. *Arthritis Rheum* 1983;26:630–636.
348. Hashimoto Y, Ziff M, Hurd ER. Increased endothelial cell adherence aggregation and superoxide generation by neutrophils incubated in systemic lupus erythematosus and Felty's syndrome sera. *Arthritis Rheum* 1982;25:1409–1418.
349. Via CS, Allen RC, Blelton RC. Direct stimulation of neutrophil oxygen activity by serum from patients with systemic lupus erythematosus: a relationship to disease activity. *J Rheumatol* 1984; 11:745–753.
350. Molad Y, Buyon J, Anderson DC, et al. Intravascular neutrophil activation in systemic lupus erythematosus: dissociation between increased expression of CD11b/CD18 and diminished expression of L-selectin on neutrophils from patients with active SLE. *Clin Immunol Immunopathol* 1994;71:281–286.
351. Buyon JP, Shadick N, Berkman R, et al. Surface expression of GP165/95, the complement receptor CR3, as a marker of disease activity in systemic lupus erythematosus. *Clin Immunol Immunopathol* 1988;46:141–149.

39

THE USE OF EXOGENOUS ESTROGENS, ENDOCRINE SYSTEM, AND UROGENITAL TRACT

JILL P. BUYON
DANIEL J. WALLACE

The overwhelming preponderance of systemic lupus erythematosus (SLE) in women of child-bearing years has prompted numerous investigations into the disorder's hormonal effects and interactions. Complex interactions occur among neurotransmitters, sex hormones, and immune functions. The potential role of estrogenic hormones in permitting SLE to occur, as well as the role of androgenic hormones in protecting against it, are discussed both in this chapter and in Chapters 16 and 18. Issues that are related to the use of exogenous hormones, including oral contraceptives, ovulation induction, and hormonal replacement, are addressed in detail here.

THE USE OF EXOGENOUS ESTROGENS IN SYSTEMIC LUPUS ERYTHEMATOSUS

Four years since the writing of this chapter, it still remains true that oral contraceptives (OCs) containing synthetic estrogens and hormone replacement therapy (HRT) with conjugated estrogen alone or in combination with progesterone generally are not prescribed for women with SLE, because of the widely held view that these medications can activate disease. The situation is analogous to the way clinicians thought about pregnancy in SLE several decades ago: the biases high and the data slim. However, as in the case of pregnancy, trends are changing as new data from larger and better-designed studies become available. Historically (at least at the time of writing the previous chapter), the concern regarding exogenous estrogens has been based on the greater incidence of SLE in women than in men, biologic abnormalities of estrogen metabolism, murine models of lupus, several anecdotes of patients having disease flares while receiving exogenous hormones, and a single retrospective study in patients with preexisting renal disease. Despite these reservations, health issues specific to women, now more than ever, warrant attention and need to be confronted in patients with SLE. For both healthy women and those with SLE, there are clinical settings in which exogenous estrogens provide benefit. For the premenopausal woman, these include the provision of safe and effective birth control, the use of adjunctive hormonal manipulation to stimulate ovulation in patients with diminished fertility, and the consideration of OCs to preserve fertility in patients taking cyclophosphamide. It has even been suggested that OCs may be useful in controlling cyclical disease activity in certain SLE patients (1). Importantly, the high induced-abortion rate for "social and economic" reasons, approaching 23% of pregnancies in several reports of SLE, reflects a lack of an adequate birth-control program as an integral part of these patients' management, or the failure of the currently used methods (2–4). For the postmenopausal woman, the salutary effects of hormone replacement include treatment of hot flushes and vaginal dryness, prevention of osteoporosis and, albeit controversial, primary prevention of coronary artery disease (CAD).

The incidence of SLE is far greater in women than in men. During the reproductive years, the female-to-male ratio is at least 9:1, but this ratio diminishes during childhood and menopause (5). The inference is that female hormones are associated with SLE. Further indirect evidence is provided by the association with Klinefelter's syndrome (6,7) and by the finding that males with SLE have altered gonadotrophin and sex-steroid levels (8). In females and males with SLE, estrone metabolism appears to be skewed toward more feminizing 16-hydroxylated metabolites (9, 10). Additionally, females with SLE can oxidize testosterone to androstenedione at a greater rate than males, implying that the high levels of estrogens go unopposed by androgens (11,12). Finally, a pair of monozygotic twins discordant for SLE has been studied in which the unaffected twin under-

TABLE 39.1. COMPARATIVE PLASMA LEVELS OF 17β-ESTRADIOL (PG/ML)

Menstrual cycle[1]	
Peak (day 12–14, late follicular)	200–500
Nadir (day 1, early follicular)	40–100
Pregnancy[2,3]	
Peak (38–40 wk)	16,000–30,000
Ovulation induction[4]	1,000
Menopause[5]	5–20
Estrogen replacement[6]	
Premarin 0.625 mg	40–100
Transdermal (after 6 months of use)	40–100

[1]Vande Wiele, Dyrenfurth. *Pharmacological reviews,* Vol. 1. Baltimore: Williams & Wilkens, 1949.
[2]Levitz M, Young BK. Estrogens in pregnancy. *Vitamin Hormone* 1977;35:109.
[3]Buster JE. Estrogen metabolism. In: Sperott C, Simpson JL, eds. *Reproductive endocrinology, infertility and genetics.* Hagerstown, MD: Harper & Row, 1980:1.
[4]Quigley M. Pharmacologically enhanced follicular recruitment for in vitro fertilization. In: Collins R, ed. *Ovulation induction.* Berlin: Springer-Verlag, 1991:153–163.
[5]Good WR, Power MS, Campbell P, et al. A new transdermal delivery system for estradiol. *J Controlled Release* 1985;2:89–97.
[6]Castelo-Branco C, Martinez de Osaba MJ, Fortuny A, et al. Circulating hormone levels in menopausal women receiving different hormone replacement therapy regimens: a comparison. *J Reproductive Med* 1995;40:556–560.

went castration at age 21 for ovarian cancer, survived, and did not receive ovarian replacement for the following 23 years (13).

This chapter will focus on three broad categories: birth control, assisted reproduction, and hormone replacement. For reference, comparable biologic potencies of circulating 17β-estradiol during different physiologic and pharmacologic states are provided in Table 39.1.

Oral Contraceptives

General Considerations

Advice on the benefits and risks of exogenous estrogens is an important and difficult aspect of the care of women with SLE. Estrogens used in therapy are, for the most part, well absorbed through the skin, mucous membranes, and gastrointestinal (GI) tract. Although the absorption of most natural estrogens and their derivatives from the GI tract is efficient, oral effectiveness of natural estrogens is limited by hepatic metabolism (14). Estrogen metabolism involves interconversion to estrone sulfate, estrone, and estradiol within various intra- and extracellular compartments. Estradiol and estrone are largely converted to estrone sulfate, which constitutes the largest reservoir of estrogen in the body. Ninety percent of estrone sulfate circulates bound to albumin and is inactive (15). Estrone is cleared by conversion in the liver to estriol, epiestriol, and estrogen conjugates, which then are excreted by the kidney. The synthetic estrogen, ethinyl estradiol, is active orally because its inactivation in the liver and other tissues is very slow. It is the form of estrogen currently used in most OCs.

OCs, when taken properly, are the most effective nonsurgical method of birth control. The failure rate of the pill in compliant patients is the lowest of any available temporary contraceptive method (16). In 1988, approximately 10.7 million women in the United States were taking the pill, an increase from 8.4 million in 1982. For women choosing nonsurgical birth control, the pill is the method used by the majority of Caucasian and African-American women aged 15 to 44 years (17). It is important to give any woman who desires contraception the option of OCs. It has been clearly established that OCs are safe. While they had previously been reported to lead to diseases of the cardiovascular system, it has since been established that such occurrences are associated with advanced user age (over 35 years), smoking, and higher doses of estrogen previously used in many preparations. Additionally, OCs significantly protect the user from cancer of the ovary and endometrium (18).

Combination OCs induce a pharmacologic state, not a physiologic one. They contain both synthetic estrogen and progesterone components, which prevent conception through a number of mechanisms. Primarily, OCs prevent ovulation by inhibiting gonadotropin secretion via an effect on both pituitary and hypothalamic centers. The progesterone component suppresses luteinizing-hormone secretion; the estrogen component suppresses follicle-stimulating hormone secretion. Each hormone also exerts important effects peripherally. Estrogen provides stability to the endometrium to prevent breakthrough bleeding. Progesterone increases cervical mucus viscosity, decreases tubal peristalsis, and diminishes the ability of the endometrium to support the growth of an embryo. Each of these progestational effects is augmented by the estrogenic component of the pill (18).

Progestins have been suggested as an alternative to combination OCs in patients with SLE, and two studies found no increase in the rate of flares (19,20). The rationale for the use of an OC that contains only progestins is two-fold. In the NZB/NZW murine model of lupus, progesterone prolonged survival in castrated males, was less deleterious in castrated females than estrogen, but was associated with high levels of autoantibodies in both sexes (21). Additionally, progesterone has been demonstrated to have less adverse effects on clotting factors than estrogen (22), a concern particularly applicable to patients with antiphospholipid antibodies (aPL). Although OCs are available that contain only progestins, there are several disadvantages to their use. First, they are less effective in preventing pregnancy than the combination pill (17). Second, progestin-only pills are associated with a higher risk of ectopic pregnancies compared with the combination pill. Third, progestins may attenuate the beneficial effect of estrogen on lipoproteins (23,24). A further practical consideration is that pills containing only progestins can lead to menstruation at unpredictable intervals, resulting in a high rate of patient discontent as previously reported in lupus patients (20,25,26).

Levonorgestrel implants (Norplant System, Wyeth-Ayerst) are a long-term, highly effective form of birth control containing only progesterone. The progesterone (levonorgestrel) is placed into six thin sylastic capsules, which are surgically implanted into the subcutaneous tissue of the arm. Adequate levels of hormone then are released over 5 years, after which time the implants can be replaced. This system is appropriate for women who desire contraception but may have difficulty in complying with other birth-control methods. It is therefore useful in patients who are at high risk for unintended pregnancy, but also is associated with irregular menstrual bleeding during the first year of use.

Oral Contraceptives and Systemic Lupus Erythematosus

Given the experimental data linking female hormones and autoimmunity, it is not surprising that estrogen-containing OCs have been reported to induce, unmask, and exacerbate SLE in several case reports and a single retrospective investigation focusing on patients with renal disease (19,27–34) (Table 39.2). With regard to the first consideration, Sanchez-Guerrero and colleagues have examined the relationship between past use of OCs and the development of SLE in 121,645 women followed every 2 years as part of the Nurses' Health Study (35). Compared with never users of OCs, past users had a small but absolute risk (1.4) for the development of SLE. No relationship was observed between

TABLE 39.2. PUBLISHED LITERATURE ON EXOGENOUS ESTROGENS AND SYSTEMIC LUPUS ERYTHEMATOSUS

Author, Year	[Ref.]	Patients [N]	Type of Study	OCs or HRT	Flare Rate: Description
Mok, 1998	[134]	SLE [11]	Prospective, 23 controls	HRT	no difference in flare rate
Kreldstein, 1997	[133]	SLE [16]	Retrospective, 32 controls	HRT	no different in flare rate
Buyon, 1995	[36]	SLE [404]	Retrospective	OCs and/or HRT	7/55 who used OCs after dx SLE, 4/48 who used HRT after dx SLE
Arden, 1994	[130]	SLE [30]	Retrospective, 30 controls	HRT	no difference in flare rate
Julkunen, 1991	[25]	SLE [31]	Retrospective, Interview, 31 controls	30–50 μg ethinyl estradiol	4/31 [13%], same as controls
Furukawa, 1991	[33]	24 year old, healthy [1]	Case report 100 μg mestranol	500 μg etynodil	+ANA, rash, proteinuria, in 4 wks
Miller, 1987	[34]	16 year old, SLE [1]	Case report	30 μg ethinyl estradiol	pulmonary hypertension in 7 months
Barrett, 1986	[135]	64 year old, SLE [1]	Case report 500 μg norgestrel	625 μg estrogen	raised ANA, rash, arthritis, increased creatine
Lockshin, 1985	[136]	SLE ["several"]	Anecdotal reports	not provided	well tolerated
Todd, 1985	[27]	22 year old, hx arthritis [1]	Case report	30 μg ethinyl estradiol	pulmonary hypertension, dx SLE in 9 months
Mintz, 1984	[20]	SLE [10]	Prospective, 18 controls	norethisterone 200 mg IM/3 months	4 flares/48 pt months, same as control
		SLE [15]	Prospective, 18 controls	30 μg/day levonorgestrel	6 flares/122 pt months, same as control
Jungers, 1982	[19]	SLE renal [20]	Retrospective, Chart review, 31 controls	30–50 μg ethinyl estradiol	43% flare, 19% renal
		SLE renal [11]	Prospective	lynestrenol *OR* chlormadinone acetate	none
Garovich, 1980	[28]	18 yo, false + VDRL [1]	Case report	50 μg ethinyl estradiol	onset SLE in 4 wk
Travers, 1978	[29]	23 yo, false + VDRL [1]	Case report	50 μg ethinyl estradiol	malaise, arthralgia, fever, rash, dx SLE in 3 wk
Chapel, 1971	[30]	21 yo, SLE [1]	Case report	100 μg mestranol	arthritis in 10 days
		24 yo, SLE [1]	Case report	80 μg mostranol	cutaneous flare in 3 months
Hadida, 1968	[31]	discoid LE [1]	Case report	5 mg norethindrone	subacute LE in 15 days
Pimstone, 1966	[32]	23 yo, SLE [1]	Case report	50 μg ethinyl estradiol	arthritis, fever, cutaneous flare in 1 week

duration of OC use or time since first use and the risk of developing SLE. In three of the case reports cited in Table 39.2, the use of OCs was considered to have "unmasked" SLE in two women with false-positive tests for syphilis (28, 29) and in one woman with a history of an isolated episode of arthritis (27). In general, these reports cite a temporal association between the use of OCs and lupus flares with time to flare 1 week to 6 months after initiating drug. By contrast, in a more recent retrospective investigation, patients taking OCs experienced a low incidence of flare, which did not differ from a control group (25). In two other studies in women with SLE that included the use of OCs containing only progestins, there was no increase in the number of disease flares in the study group compared to patients who did not take these hormones (19,20). However, as might be predicted, the use of progesterone was limited by poor gynecologic tolerance. Two of the studies outlined in Table 39.2 merit closer attention.

In the retrospective study by Jungers (19), 20 lupus patients received 21 courses of OCs (50 μg ethinyl estradiol daily in 14 treatments and 30 μg in seven treatments). These patients all had renal involvement and were followed in the department of nephrology. During the first 3 months after starting OCs, exacerbations of lupus activity were observed in nine (43%). Five patients had only "minor" flares, and in four, a "major" flare was observed. The one patient who is highlighted in this study as demonstrating a "severe renal flare-up," had a kidney biopsy diagnosed as diffuse proliferative glomerulonephritis (DPGN), and was treated with high-dose corticosteroids 1 year prior to initiating OCs. Two months after the start of these medications, the patient had an increase in the titer of anti-DNA antibodies with a concomitant fall in serum complement levels. Repeat renal biopsy revealed DPGN with a high activity index. The flare reverted after discontinuing the OCs, but the patient also was treated with increased steroids. The patient controls for this study were 30 women previously treated with high-dose steroids, and 12-month periods were randomly chosen at similar intervals from the initial corticosteroid therapy. Recurrence of lupus activity was observed in only six controls. However, the authors correctly point out that "true statistical comparison was difficult."

A deleterious effect of OCs on disease activity was not corroborated in a retrospective study by Julkunen (25). Of 85 female lupus patients aged 18 to 44, 37 (44%) used or had used estrogen-containing OCs for a total of 41 hormonal courses. The spectrum of SLE ranged from almost asymptomatic to active renal disease. Proteinuria >500 mg/day was present in 14 (38%) of the 37 patients at some time during the course of their disease. The only estrogen used was ethinyl estradiol with a daily dose of 30 μg in 13 treatments, 50 μg in six treatments, 37.5 μg in two treatments, and 30 to 50 μg in 20 treatments. Thirty-two patients (38%) used or had used progestin-only contraceptives (continuous low-dose preparations containing lynestrenol, levonorgestrenol, or norethisterone) for a total of 33 hormonal courses. Disease activity was evaluated on a clinical basis and the medical records examined where possible. A flare-up was considered to be present "when a patient had clinical signs consistent with the worsening of SLE, and/or when medical treatment was introduced or increased." The rate of lupus exacerbations during the 12-month period after the start of OCs was compared with the corresponding rate during a 12-month period in 31 patients who had never used these medications. There were three flares of SLE during the first 12 months of therapy (flare-rate = 3/144 patient months) compared to five flares in patients not taking OCs (flare rate = 5/372 patient-months, p = NS). Details of the types of flares were not given. However, the authors point out that some of the side effects of the OCs could be interpreted as an exacerbation of SLE. Specifically, they did not consider elevation of liver enzymes, minor arthralgia, simple headache, or migraine as an exacerbation of SLE if these were the only signs or symptoms present.

The need for resolution of the issue of OCs in patients with SLE is further illustrated in a second publication by Julkunen et al. in March 1993 (26) who reported on current contraceptive practices in a group of 85 Finnish female SLE patients of reproductive age. Sexually active SLE patients used barrier and natural methods more often and OCs less often than healthy women. The authors offered the conclusion that this may "reflect the views of many gynecologists, general practitioners, and rheumatologists as regards OCs in SLE: they should be used with caution because of an increased risk of adverse effects." The risk of having a deep venous thrombosis (DVT) was higher in patients using than not using OCs (RR2.3, 95% C.5–10.3). One patient developed malignant hypertension 5 months after starting OCs. One patient with aPL had a DVT while taking pills containing only progesterone, an unexpected outcome because progesterone does not seem to significantly affect hemostatic parameters (22). No other major cardiovascular complications occurred. Exacerbation of lupus activity was not mentioned. As previously shown by Mintz et al. (20), the majority of patients who used progestin-only containing agents discontinued them because of poor gynecological tolerance.

In a retrospective multicenter survey on the past and present usage of OCs in women with SLE, 404 patients were surveyed from five medical centers (36). Two hundred twenty-four (55%) had used OCs at some time; however, only 51 (13%) were taking OCs at the time SLE was diagnosed. Fifty-five (14%) used OCs after their disease was diagnosed. Intriguingly, only seven (13%) of the 55 reported an exacerbation of disease activity, most confined to the musculoskeletal system. In a substudy at the Hospital for Joint Diseases, there were no significant differences observed between women with or without SLE with regard to the frequency of ever-use of OCs. In contrast, when women aged 35 years or younger were evaluated, significantly fewer women with established SLE were taking OCs at the time of interview compared to healthy women, p <.02. In agreement with the results of Julkunen (26), our observations, albeit based on patient recall, suggest that OCs generally are well tolerated in women with SLE but infrequently prescribed. Perhaps the lower rates of flare reflect differences in the dosage of estrogen; a decade ago, many women were taking 50 μg ethinyl estradiol while current preparations contain 30 to 35 μg. Interestingly, we see a complete swing of the pendulum in a brief report by Pando et al., in which three lupus patients with menstrual-related skin rashes experienced significant improvement in their skin disease after taking OCs (37).

Finally, it is noteworthy that reports of OC-related serological and clinical changes represent patients who presented with symptoms and therefore may be a selected population. Three separate studies, that together included over 250 apparently healthy women attending birth-control clinics, did not demonstrate a significant association between the use of OCs and the presence of antinuclear antibodies (ANA) (38–40). In a fourth study of healthy women reporting to birth-control clinics, the prevalence of a positive ANA was greater in a group of 210 women who were using OCs (13.4%) than in 174 women who had never used OCs (8.5%). However, no women developed symptoms of a rheumatic disease while taking OCs (41).

Thrombosis And Exogenous Estrogens

Estrogen has been associated with increased blood coagulability. In contrast, there is no epidemiologic evidence of an increased risk of thrombotic complications in users of progestin-only contraceptives (22). Retrospective and prospective studies on a large number of patients have shown that women who take combined OCs have an increased risk of venous thrombosis, but associations with various types of stroke and myocardial infarction are less consistent (42). This is an important consideration in SLE where substantial literature supports a measurable risk of thrombosis in patients with aPL. The additive risk of OCs and aPL is supported by the work of Asherson et al., describing 10 patients with aPL, all of whom developed vascular complications while taking OCs (43).

Several biologic properties of estrogens and aPL may contribute to thrombogenesis. It generally is accepted that arterial forms of thrombosis are mediated by platelets. Disturbances of the clotting cascade are more likely to result in venous thrombosis formation. Patients taking estrogens or combined OCs may have increased platelet aggregation (44), but these effects are apparently related to concomitant cigarette smoking (45). Estrogens can increase the concentration of coagulation factors VII, IX, X, XII and prothrombin (reviewed in 15), and decrease fibrinolysis (46). Most patients taking combined OCs have decreased partial thromboplastin times and prothrombin times, primarily as a result of increased levels of fibrinogen (22). Both estrogens and aPL can inhibit prostacyclin production by endothelial cells (47,48). However, although alterations occur in several factors that promote coagulation, they also occur in some anticoagulant and fibrinolytic factors (22). Synthetic estrogens are more "procoagulant" than natural preparations, and oral estrogen formulations influence coagulation to a greater degree than transdermal preparations, because the latter avoid the first-passage effect of oral estrogens (15). Importantly, the impact of estrogen on various clotting factors is dose dependent, with little if any effect at doses less than 50 μg of ethinyl estradiol (49). The U.S. Food and Drug Administration issued a bulletin stating that the rate of DVT in women taking low-dose OCs containing 20 to 40 μg ethinyl estradiol was four per 10,000, which approximates that of women not taking OCs, three per 10,000 (50).

Experimental data suggest that "antiphospholipid" antibodies are not directed against anionic phospholipids, as initially hypothesized, but are part of a larger group of autoantibodies that recognize phospholipid-binding proteins. At present, the best-characterized antigenic target is β2-glycoprotein I (β2GPI) (51–53). β2GPI, also designated apolipoprotein H, is associated with different lipoprotein fractions in normal human plasma such as chylomicrons and very-low-density and high-density lipoproteins (54). β2GPI inhibits contact activation of the intrinsic coagulation pathway (55), platelet prothrombinase activity (56), and ADP-induced platelet aggregation (57). Because β2GPI has been shown to possess multiple inhibitory functions in coagulation pathways, its interaction with aPL may eventually lead to an explanation for the thrombotic diathesis observed in patients with these antibodies. Preliminary data support a decrease in the circulating levels of β2GPI levels in the second trimester of pregnancy (58) but the effect of exogenous hormones on these levels is unknown. Despite favorable data on low dose estrogen OCs, it probably is advisable to avoid estrogen-containing OCs in patients with aPL until more definitive data are available on this subpopulation. General guidelines for the use of OCs in women with SLE are provided in Table 39.3.

TABLE 39.3. GUIDELINES FOR USE OF ORAL CONTRACEPTIVES IN WOMEN WITH SYSTEMIC LUPUS ERYTHEMATOSUS

1. Inactive or stable/moderate disease
2. No history of venous or arterial thrombosis
3. IgGaPL <40, IgMaPL <40, IgAaPL <50, no circulating lupus anticoagulant (unknown if presence of low-to-moderate titer of aPL in the absence of a previous thrombosis is contraindication)
4. Nonsmoker
5. Normotensive
6. For combined pill, use lowest dose of ethinyl estradiol (30–35 μg)
7. Consideration of pill containing progestin only

Oral Contraceptives and Antiestrogen Antibodies

Bucala et al. have investigated the induction of antiestrogen antibodies (59). These antibodies were found in 13 of 52 otherwise normal women who had ever taken OCs. The biochemical explanation for this is based on the fact that OCs contain an ethinyl-substituted estrogen to preserve the oral potency of the estrogen. These derivatives are metabolized by cytochrome P450 enzymes to reactive metabolites, which can readily add to proteins. The formation of estrogen-protein adducts can induce antibodies against either the A or the D ring of the steroid. Conjugates that are linked in the estrogen D ring are antigenically similar to 16αOHE-lysine adducts and therefore potentially cross-react with antibodies that recognize the estrogen A and B rings. Perhaps once antiestrogen antibodies are induced in susceptible individuals by 17α-ethinyl estradiol, their levels are perpetuated by the continuous presence of small amounts of endogenous, antigenically cross-reactive 16αOHE-protein adducts. This is intriguing, as increased levels of 16αOHE-modified proteins have been noted in patients with SLE (10,11). If these hypotheses are correct, it is not surprising that 26% of male and female SLE patients were found to possess circulating antiestrogen antibodies. While the formation of these antibodies might lead to immune complexes, their pathological role has not been elucidated. Bucala et al. have proposed that in sensitive SLE patients, OCs might contribute to antigen-antibody deposition by further stimulating the production of antiestrogen antibodies. Although there has been little subsequent investigation of this phenomenon, this possibility could theoretically be approached by measuring complement activation products in women taking OCs.

Assisted Reproduction Therapy And SLE

In addressing the consequences of exogenous estrogens in women with SLE, another clinical situation to consider is ovulation induction, in which ovarian stimulation is achieved by administration of clomiphine citrate (which acts on the hypothalamus as an antiestrogen to block negative feedback, resulting in a surge of follicle stimulating hormone and luteinizing hormone), gonadotropins, or gonadotropin-releasing hormones. The levels of circulating 17β-estradiol after such treatments may exceed peak menstrual levels by about two-fold and nadir levels by ten-fold (Table 39.1).

Again, the question arises as to whether the increased estrogen load might induce, unmask, or exacerbate preexisting SLE. Ben-Chetrit described three isolated cases in which SLE developed in two previously healthy women and one with Raynaud's phenomenon (60). It is curious that one of these women had a successful pregnancy antedating ovulation induction during which time she had no clinical signs of SLE. These anecdotal cases await larger epidemiologic studies.

Several recent publications address ovulation induction in women with established lupus. This is a relevant concern for patients in their later childbearing years who delay pregnancy until after attaining extended disease remission. In one study, a patient is described who developed transverse myelopathy and fatal pulmonary embolism (61). Huong and colleagues report that three of four lupus patients in remission developed a moderate flare of lupus within a few weeks after the onset of ovulation induction (62). All patients had aPL but no prior history of thrombotic events. One patient developed inferior vena cava and unilateral left renal-vein thrombosis. In a slightly larger retrospective study of seven women with SLE who underwent 16 cycles of OI/IVF, three experienced a mild increase in disease activity (63). Specifically the flares consisted of arthritis in one, discoid rash in another, and in a third patient a mild rash occurred following one ovulation induction and myositis, rash, vasculitis, and alopecia occurred after a second induction. The course of two additional patients was complicated by the ovarian-hyperstimulation syndrome [ovarian edema, electrolyte imbalance, diffuse capillary leak with resulting pleural effusions, ascites, occasionally accompanied by hypotension, hypercoaguability, thrombophlebitis, and hydrothorax (64,65)]. In this report, thromboses were not observed; however, none of these patients had aPL. Of note, this same study did include ten additional SLE patients with primary antiphospholipid syndrome (PAPS), none of whom had a thrombotic complication following ovulation induction. The authors attributed this safety profile to the fact that most of the patients received some form of prophylactic therapy. Although prospective studies on larger numbers of patients are clearly needed, data from Guballa and her colleagues (63) are reassuring that assisted reproductive therapy does not cause significant worsening of either SLE or PAPS.

Hormonal Therapy (ERT) In Postmenopausal Women

General Considerations

HRT (continuous conjugated estrogens alone or combined with continuous or cyclic progesterone) may be considered in all women who are hypoestrogenic. Symptoms appear when plasma estradiol concentrations decrease to less than 35 pg/mL. Specific indications for replacement include control of vasomotor hot flushes, atrophic vaginitis and urethritis, and prevention or retardation of postmenopausal and steroid-induced osteoporosis. In addition, there is ongoing debate whether postmenopausal estrogens can reduce the incidence of CAD, including myocardial infarction.

Atrophic vaginitis results from progressive thinning of the vaginal epithelium such that intercourse or douching may result in bleeding. Local bacterial invasion often causes vaginal pruritus and discharge. Tissue retraction occurs, which causes the vagina to become shortened and fused. Hot flushes, which may recur for a period of up to 5 years, can become very disturbing to hypoestrogenic patients, resulting in frustration and sleeplessness.

Osteoporosis is of considerable public-health importance, as it affects a large and expanding portion of an aging population worldwide (66). Postmenopausal osteoporosis is primarily a result of the accelerated bone loss that occurs in the years following the decline in estrogen (67). Estrogen deficiency is associated with increased osteoclastic bone resorption (68). While the precise pathogenetic mechanism for the effects of estrogen are undefined, it has been suggested that the effects of estrogens are both direct (69) and indirect. The latter may be from the suppression of bone-resorbing cytokines such as interleukin-1 and interleukin-6 (70,71). Estrogens also exert positive changes in calcium homeostasis by restoration of a defective synthesis of 1,25 (OH)2D and augmentation of intestinal calcium absorption (72). Estrogens not only prevent bone loss but also increase bone mass significantly at the lumbar spine, radius, and hips (73–77). Most of the increase in bone mass occurs during the first 12 months of therapy (76,77) and is consistent with an estrogen-mediated abrupt inhibition of bone resorption, during which time bone formation continues until a new steady state is achieved and bone density restabilizes (78).

Many additional risk factors are associated with the development of osteoporosis, including race, caffeine and alcohol intake, smoking history, body stature, exercise/inactivity, renal and thyroid diseases, and treatment with glucocorticoids (66). The latter variable assumes increased significance for women with SLE. Ramsey-Goldman et al. ascertained the frequency of fractures and associated risk factors by self-report in a retrospective cohort of 702 women with lupus followed up for 5,951 person-years (79). Fractures occurred in 12.3% of the patients, a nearly fivefold increase compared with women from the US population. Older age at diagnosis and longer duration of steroid use were important concomitant variables.

Limited trials of HRT use in glucocorticoid-treated postmenopausal patients have been conducted. One study of 15 asthmatic women treated with corticosteroids demonstrated that the combination of estrogen and progesterone therapy was associated with increased lumbar spine BMD after 1 year of treatment (80). Similar results were reported in women with rheumatoid arthritis who were taking prednisone and were randomized to receive HRT or placebo. Patients who received HRT had a significant increase in the lumbar spine BMD, but not in the femoral neck, compared with controls (81). The American College of Rheumatology task force on osteoporosis recommends that "postmenopausal women taking glucocorticoids should receive HRT if there are no contraindications" (82). Although studies have not been performed on glucocorticoid-treated premenopausal women, observational epidemiologic studies suggest that among women taking glucocorticoids, those taking OCs had higher adjusted BMD than those who did not (83).

In addition to abrogating increased bone breakdown, HRT may provide significant cardioprotective effects. In younger age groups, the incidence of atherosclerotic disease is much lower for women than for men. In western society, the death rate from CAD is five to eight times greater in men than in women 25 to 55 years of age (84). Following the menopause and its associated decrease in estrogen production, the rate of cardiovascular disease accelerates such that by age 65 the risk in women is equal to that of men. Earlier observational studies have demonstrated a survival advantage in postmenopausal women who are treated with HRT (85–91). Hong et al. found that HRT use was associated with an 87% reduction in the angiographic prevalence of CAD. Women receiving estrogen had a significantly lower mean total/high density lipoprotein (HDL) cholesterol ratio than did women not taking estrogen (90). Other studies have come to similar conclusions: healthy women who use estrogen have a 50% reduction in the risk of CAD compared with nonusers (91), with higher mean levels of HDL-cholesterol and lower mean levels of low-density lipoprotein (LDL) cholesterol (88). Transdermal estrogens do not appear to be as potent in affecting lipid parameters as orally active estrogens. However, when delivering high estrogen concentrations with transdermal formulations over time, an effect on serum lipids may be seen (92).

Whether the cardioprotective effects of estrogen are solely from improvement in lipid profile is currently unknown. Recent studies have linked plasma levels of plasminogen-activator inhibitor type 1 (PAI-1), an essential inhibitor of fibrinolysis in humans, to risk of cardiovascular disease. PAI-1 is an antagonist of fibrinolysis in humans, which rapidly and specifically inhibits both tissue plasminogen activator and urokinase plasminogen activator (93). PAI-1 has been demonstrated in endothelial and smooth-muscle cells of histologically normal arteries, and is present in increased quantities in all cellular components of atheromatous arteries (94). A greater risk of atherosclerosis is associated with increased plasma levels of PAI-1 (95–97). Higher levels of PAI-1 were noted in postmenopausal women compared to premenopausal women in the Framingham Offspring Study (98), which may be a factor contributing to the greater risk of atherosclerosis and its clinical consequences after menopause. Evidence that HRT reduces PAI-1 levels in postmenopausal women has been reported by several investigators (99–102). In a US-based study, Koh et al. demonstrated that conjugated estrogen, alone or combined with progestins, reduced PAI-1 levels by approximately 50% in postmenopausal women and was associated with enhanced systemic fibrinolysis (102). The greatest reduction in PAI-1 levels occurred in women with the highest baseline values. In a pilot study of 78 postmenopausal women with SLE, 21 (27%) had PAI-1 values above the upper limit of normal (43 ng/mL), although 14 of these 21 samples were drawn after 11:00 a.m. [generally, PAI-1 levels peak in the early morning and fall in late afternoon (103)] Both midday and afternoon mean values in these lupus patients were twice that reported for otherwise normal menopausal women (104). These data suggest that elevated PAI-1 levels may identify menopausal lupus patients at greater risk for cardiovascular disease (see below), even in those whose lupus is relatively inactive. The finding of an elevated morning level of PAI-1 may guide clinical decision-making, e.g., risk of CAD might outweigh risk of disease flare for a given patient.

Although many observational studies have found lower rates of CAD in women who take HRT than in those who do not, the results of a recent prospective randomized trial has raised considerable concerns (105). The Heart and Estrogen/progestin Replacement Study (HERS) included 2,763 postmenopausal women with established CAD. Overall, there were no significant differences between the placebo and HRT-groups in the occurrence of nonfatal myocardial infarction, coronary death, or secondary cardiovascular outcomes despite clear beneficial changes in lipid profiles. However, within the overall null effect, there was a statistically significant time trend, with more coronary events in the HRT group than placebo in year 1 and fewer in years 4 and 5. One explanation for these results is that the early increase in risk is attributable to an immediate prothrombotic effect of estrogens that is gradually outweighed by a favorable effect on the underlying progression of atherosclerosis such as the changes in lipoproteins. Because HERS focused on secondary prevention and did not evaluate the effects of HRT in women without CAD, this study is not generalizable to all women. Furthermore, a very recent update on a substudy from HERS revealed that levels of lipoprotein(a) [Lp(a)], an independent risk factor for CAD, were significantly decreased after treatment with estrogen and progestin compared to placebo (106). In a randomized subgroup comparison, women with low baseline Lp(a) levels had less benefit from HRT than women with high levels. In June 2000 another observational trial conducted in the United Kingdom, a population-based, case-control study nested in a cohort of women without CAD (age 50 to 74 years), demonstrated a beneficial effect of HRT after 1 year of use (107). It is clear that the relationship between HRT and cardiovascular protection remains a work in progress and we eagerly await the results of the National Institutes of Health (NIH) -sponsored long-term prospective Women's Health Initiative.

The results of HERS notwithstanding, the potential cardioprotective effects of postmenopausal estrogens are particularly applicable in SLE. Urowitz et al. have demonstrated a bimodal distribution of mortality in SLE with late deaths associated with atherosclerotic disorders (108). It has been established that the proportionate mortality from myocardial infarction is approximately 10 times greater in patients with SLE than in the general age- and sex-matched population (109,110), and the prevalence of nonfatal CAD in patients with SLE approaches 5% to 8% (109,111). Autopsy studies support the clinical data, as severe CAD is present in up to 40% of patients with SLE, compared with 2% of control subjects, matched for age at the time of death (112). Since the original writing of this chapter, published literature and presentations at scientific meetings of the American College of Rheumatology continue to strongly support accelerated atherosclerosis as an important cause of morbidity and mortality in SLE. Studies have identified hypercholesterolemia, hypertension, and lupus itself as risk factors in these patients. It also has become evident that glucocorticoid therapy contributes to the elevation of plasma lipids while antimalarials may result in a reduction of plasma cholesterol, LDL and VLDL, especially in steroid-induced hyperlipidemia. Studies of clinical outcomes for atherosclerotic disease, including angina and myocardial infarction, have shown a prevalence of 6% to 12% in a number of SLE cohorts (113,114). More sensitive investigations including carotid plaque and intima-media wall thickness (IMT) measured by B-mode ultrasound revealed that 40% of 175 women with SLE had focal plaque (115).

In contrast to the thrombogenic effects of estrogens noted with OCs, several earlier studies in which HRT was given to otherwise healthy women did not support this complication. Specifically, in women with surgical menopause who received estrogens for 3 months, there was no difference in platelet counts, fibrinogen levels, or fibrin degradation products (116). In the PEPI trial, all regimens lowered fibrinogen levels in comparison to placebo (117). In another study of women with natural menopause, HRT enhanced plasminogen activity without depressing the levels of antithrombin III (118). Biologic fibrinolysis was stimulated with estrogen treatment. However, five more recent observational studies reported a two- to four-fold increase in risk for idiopathic venous thromboembolism in postmenopausal women taking oral estrogen or estrogen plus progestin compared with nonusers (119–123). The overall risk of venous thromboembolism for women currently using HRT obtained from these studies was 2.6. This risk appears to be more prominent during the first year of HRT use, and in two studies the risk disappeared after the first year of therapy. In sum, evidence from these recent studies indicates that, among healthy postmenopausal women, between 1 and 2 additional cases of venous thromboembolism per 10,000 women can be annually attributed to current use of HRT (reviewed in 124). A further note of caution: investigators of HERS, cited above, reported that after 4.1 years of follow-up, 34 of 1,380 postmenopausal with previous CAD compared to 13 of 1,383 women in the placebo group experienced venous thromboembolic events (125). Not unexpectedly, the risk was increased among women with lower-extremity fracture, cancer, and prolonged hospitalizations. Risk was decreased with aspirin or statins.

HRT And SLE

The general rationale for considering HRT in women with SLE is outlined in Table 39.4. Although the levels of circulating 17β-estradiol reached while taking HRT are about a fifth of the peak menstrual cycle levels (Table 39.1), and HRT is roughly one fourth to one fifth the estrogenic potency of current "low-dose" OCs, the added "estrogen load" over barely detectable postmenopausal levels (Table 39.1) might induce, unmask, or exacerbate SLE.

In support of the first prediction, Sanchez-Guerrero and his colleagues have reported an increased relative risk for the development of SLE in a "naïve" cohort of nurses exposed to HRT (126). In this study, 69,435 menopausal women aged 30 to 55 years who did not have SLE or any connective-tissue disease were followed every 2 years from 1976 to 1990. Women currently using HRT accounted for 21.7% of the follow-up time; past hormone users accounted for 26.1%, and never users 52.2%. During 631,551 person-years of follow-up, 45 cases of SLE were confirmed, 15 cases in women who had never used HRT, and 30 cases in women who had ever used HRT. Compared with never users, ever users had an age-adjusted relative risk of 2.1 (95% CI, 1.1 to 4.0). A proportional increase in the risk for SLE was observed that was related to the duration of HRT. Based on the sex hormone hypothesis of SLE, the results of this study are intuitive. However, because this was an omnibus prospective observational study, not a randomized trial designed to test the association of postmenopausal estrogens and risk of SLE, confounders and biases are possible (127,128). Perhaps SLE was over-ascertained in women taking estrogens not only because they had more than the "at least one per year" physician visit, which characterized the unexposed cohort, but also because when seeking medical attention, symptomatology may have led to a blood test (ANA), given their estrogen use. Alternatively, those who developed unexplained mood swings, energy loss, low-grade fevers, facial flushing, and musculoskeletal complaints may have been diagnosed "postmenopausal syndrome" and given estrogen rather than diagnosed with late-onset SLE. It is curious that SLE did not become manifest during pregnancy (presuming all were not nulliparous) when estrogen levels exceed by 100-fold those achieved with HRT (Table 39.1). Perhaps the explanation lies in the

TABLE 39.4. RATIONALE FOR CONSIDERING HORMONE REPLACEMENT THERAPY IN WOMEN WITH SYSTEMIC LUPUS ERYTHEMATOSUS

Potential health benefits:

1. Reduction of menopausal symptoms (e.g., vasomotor flushing, genital dryness, emotional lability)
2. Prevention of postmenopausal (natural or cyclophosphamide-induced) and steroid-induced osteoporosis.
   Particular relevance in SLE:
   a. Corticosteroid correlates with increased diaphyseal:metaphyseal mass ratios, osteoporosis, increased fractures [**104a**].[1]
   b. Improved longevity of lupus patients.
3. HRT is associated with increased levels of HDL-cholesterol and decreased risk of CAD [albeit HERS Trial raises concern (**105, 106**)].[2]
   Particular relevance in SLE:
   a. Late deaths in SLE associated with atherosclerotic heart disease [**108**].[3]
   b. Mortality from MI is ten times greater in SLE than general age and sex-matched population [**109**].[4]
   c. Autopsies reveal CAD in up to 40% SLE versus 2% control [**112**].[5]
   d. Carotid plaque and IMT measured by B-mode ultrasound abnormal in 40% SLE [**115**].[6]

CAD, coronary artery disease; HDL, high-density lipoprotein; HERS, Heart and Estrogen/progestin Replacement Study; HRT, hormone replacement therapy; IMT, intima-media wall thickness; MI, myocardial infarction; SLE, systemic lupus erythematosus.

[1]Dykman TR, Gluck OS, Murphy WA, et al. Evaluation of factors associated with glucocorticoid-induced osteopenia in patients with rheumatic diseases. *Arthritis Rheum* 1985;28:361–368.

[2]Hulley S, Grady D, Bush T, et al. Randomized trial of estrogen plus progestin for secondary prevention of coronary heart disease in postmenopausal women. *JAMA* 1998;280:605–613, and Shlipak MG, Simon JA, Vittinghoff E, et al. Estrogen and progestin, lipoprotein (a), and the risk of recurrent coronary heart disease events after menopause. *JAMA* 2000;283:1845–1852.

[3]Urowitz MB, Bookman AA, Koehler BE, et al. The bimodal mortality pattern of systemic lupus erythematosus. *Am J Med* 1976;60:221–225.

[4]Rosner S, Ginzler EM, Diamond HS, et al. A multicenter study of outcome in systemic lupus erythematosus. II. Causes of death. *Arth Rheum* 1982;25:612–617.

[5]Haider YS, Roberts WC. Coronary arterial disease in systemic lupus erythematosus: quantification of degree of narrowing in 22 necropsy patients (21 women) aged 16 to 37 years. *Am J Med* 1981;70: 775–781.

[6]Manzi S, Selzer F, Sutton-Tyrrell K, et al. Prevalence and risk factors of carotid plaque in women with systemic lupus erythematosus. *Arthritis Rheum* 1999;42:51–60.

TABLE 39.5. RETROSPECTIVE STUDY ON SAFETY OF HORMONE REPLACEMENT THERAPY IN SYSTEMIC LUPUS ERYTHEMATOSUS: CLINICAL ASSESSMENT/DISEASE ACTIVITY*

Clinical Assessment/Disease Activity (12 months)			
	Users (n = 30)	Never Users (n = 30)	Significance
Nine meds	30%	13%	NS
Eight meds	11%	17%	NS
New meds	0%	3%	NS
Hospitalizations	7%	17%	NS
Disease flares	(2)	(6)	NS

Note: HRT users reported significant improvement in Depression ($p < .005$) Well Being ($p < .005$) Libido ($p < .01$)
*Adapted from Arden NK, Lloyd M, Spector TD, et al. Safety of hormone replacement therapy (HRT) in systemic lupus erythematosus (SLE). *Lupus* 1994;3:11–13.

fact that cortisol levels also rise during pregnancy and positively balance a potential immune-enhancing effect of the higher estrogen burden. Most important, this study did not evaluate patients with established SLE, and concerns that HRT will increase the flare rate in women with preexisting SLE may not be warranted.

In agreement with the results of Sanchez-Guerrero, Meier et al., using the United Kingdom-based General Practice Research Database (41 cases with SLE, 34 cases with discoid lupus, and 295 age-, sex- and practice-matched controls), reported that the risk of developing SLE or discoid lupus was significantly increased among current users exposed for two or more years (OR = 2.8) (129). The authors further suggest that progestogens may reduce the effect of estrogens on the risk of developing SLE or discoid lupus. However, the small sample size precludes any firm conclusions. An additional limitation of the data is the underrepresentation of minorities.

Arden and colleagues have reported on the use of HRT in postmenopausal women with established SLE (130). While the study was retrospective and included only 60 patients (age 34 to 60), the results are encouraging (Table 39.5). There was no increase in the rate of flares in 30 patients taking HRT compared to 30 age-matched patients who never used HRT. Moreover, the HRT group was significantly improved with regard to depression, migraines, well-being, and libido. Reassuringly, there was only one thromboembolic event in the user group, which occurred 5 weeks after discontinuation of HRT, despite seven patients having documented aPL (Table 39.6). This important observation is consistent with reports in the early 1990s that HRT (unlike OCs) does not appear to confer an increased risk of thrombosis in otherwise healthy women (131,132).

In two additional retrospective studies, the results are concordant with those reported by Arden et al. (130). In our multicenter retrospective patient survey described above (36), information on past and present usage of HRT was obtained in women followed at two of the sites. Fifty-five (59%) of the 94 postmenopausal patients at these centers had ever taken HRT, 23 (24%) at the time of diagnosis. Forty-eight women (51%) began or remained on HRT after the diagnosis of SLE, only four of whom reported exacerbations of disease activity. A significantly higher percentage of Caucasian women had taken or were taking HRT compared to other ethnic groups. Kreidstein and colleagues compared rates of flare in 16 postmenopausal patients with SLE who had been taking HRT and 32 controls matched for age at start of HRT and calendar year of follow-up (133). There was no statistically significant difference in flare as defined by any increase in the Systemic Lupus Erythematosus Disease Activity Index (SLEDAI) over 12 months.

In a limited prospective study (11 patients received HRT and 23 did not) reported by Mok et al., there was no significant increase in the rate of flares/patient-year between the

TABLE 39.6. RETROSPECTIVE STUDY ON SAFETY OF HRT IN SLE: THROMBOEMBOLIC EVENTS*

Thromboembolic Events (12 months)			
Users		Nonusers	
7 +thrombophilia screen	23 −thrombophilia screen	13 +thrombophilia screen	17 −thrombophilia screen
(7) No events	(1) TIA; (22) No events	(1) CVA; (12) No events	(1) (CVA); (1) TIA; (15) No events

*Adapted from Arden NK, Lloyd M, Spector TD, et al. Safety of hormone replacement therapy (HRT) in systemic lupus erythematosus (SLE). *Lupus* 1994;3:11–13.

groups (134). None of the 11 patients who received HRT developed thromboembolism during the observation period.

The Safety Of Estrogens In Lupus Erythematosus National Assessment (SELENA) Trial

Informed decisions concerning the use of HRT and OCs in women with SLE require prospective studies on large numbers of patients. The Safety of Estrogens in Lupus Erythematosus, National Assessment (SELENA) Trial comprises two separate, randomized, placebo-controlled studies being conducted at seventeen medical centers across the United States. In the HRT trial, postmenopausal (either natural or cyclophosphamide-induced) patients receive 0.625 mg conjugated estrogens daily for 12 months and 5 mg medroxyprogesterone acetate for 12 days of each month, or placebo. In the OC study, premenopausal women under the age of 40 receive triphasic ethinylestradiol/norethindrone (7 days of 35 μg ethinylestradiol and 0.5 mg norethindrone, 7 days of 35 μg ethinylestradiol and 0.75 μg norethindrone, 7 days of 35 μg ethinylestradiol and 1 mg norethindrone) for 12 cycles, or placebo. For both trials, patients are excluded if they have had any evidence of thrombosis or current documentation of a circulating anticoagulant or IgG aPL greater than 40. Patients with premenopausal myocardial infarction also are excluded. Each study requires 350 patients for completion. To date, 153 patients have been enrolled in the OC trial with 98 completed and 300 in the HRT trial with 210 completed. There have been nine severe flares and 127 mild/moderate flares per 97.8 patient years of study in the OC trial. In the HRT trial there have been 16 severe flares and 228 mild/moderate flares in 231 patient years of study. These overall flare rates do not exceed expected rates. In the OC trial one patient has had an ocular thrombosis, and one patient has had a DVT. In the HRT trial one patient had a stroke, and 2 patients have had DVTs. For both studies, treatment assignments have remained blinded. Results from this major effort should provide critical guidelines for future recommendations to postmenopausal lupus patients regarding the use of HRT.

Conclusions

Given the female preponderance of SLE in humans, adverse effects of female gender and sex hormones in murine lupus, and numerous reports (retrospective, often anecdotal and uncontrolled) describing a temporal association between estrogen exposure and development or exacerbation of SLE, it is tempting to accept that estrogens and SLE simply do not mix. While there are valid concerns regarding the use of exogenous estrogens in women with SLE, there are also potential health benefits to be considered. Several salutary effects of postmenopausal estrogens assume particular importance in SLE where the risks of osteoporosis, exaggerated by menopause (natural or cyclophosphamide-induced) and glucocorticoids, are substantial. Moreover, HRT is associated with a 40% reduction in the risk of CAD, higher levels of HDL-cholesterol and decreased LDL-cholesterol, benefits relevant in SLE. More recent studies, albeit retrospective and limited by less formal analyses of disease activity, suggest that OCs and HRT may be well tolerated. In counseling patients regarding lupus and pregnancy, there are now clinical predictors of pregnancy outcome, and patients in remission tend to have a good outcome. The same principles may be true regarding advice on the use of OCs and HRT: patients with inactive or stable/moderate disease and at low risk for thrombosis may benefit without a change in lupus activity. Large prospective, double-blind, placebo-controlled studies inclusive of all ethnic groups should provide the basis for more definitive recommendations.

MENSTRUAL IRREGULARITIES, GYNECOLOGIC ISSUES AND THE BREAST

Menstrual irregularities are common and range from menorrhagia to amenorrhea. Menorrhagia was found in 16 of Harvey's 106 patients (137), and was the initial manifestation of SLE in three. Dubois (138) observed menorrhagia in 12% of his 520 cases and associated it with thrombocytopenia or presence of the circulating lupus anticoagulant. Salicylate and nonsteroidal antiinflammatory drugs also can increase menstrual flow.

Amenorrhea is associated with SLE disease activity and immunosuppressive therapy (both glucocorticoid and cytotoxic) (139). Schaller (140) reported that 24% of females with childhood lupus had amenorrhea, and was noted in 27 of 160 with SLE who were studied by Fries et al. (141). Steroid administration can induce secondary amenorrhea or menorrhagia, the former of which is seen in the majority of patients with spontaneous Cushing's syndrome (142).

Steinberg and Steinberg (143) following 28 menstruating females with SLE through 991 cycles. Increased signs or symptoms of disease activity were observed in 172 (18%); in 140 (81%), these occurred in the 2 weeks before menstruation. Lahita et al. (144) observed that premenstrual flares of lupus were noted in 60% of patients, with resolution when menses began. The Johns Hopkins Lupus Cohort noted this in 45% (145). McDonagh et al. (146) hypothesized that shedding secretory endometrium (i.e., lymphoid tissue that is rich in CD8 cells and macrophages) can induce a "menstrual arthritis."

Isolated reports have correlated SLE with endometriosis (147), breast gigantism (148), cervical dysplasia (without immunosuppressive therapy) (149–151), cystic ovaries (152,153), uterine vasculitis (154), cervical cancer (155), and human pappilomavirus infection (156–158). The breast is a common site of lupus profundus, and mastitis can complicate it (159,160).

THE ENDOCRINE SYSTEM

Thyroid Disease

In 1956, Roitt et al. (161) first demonstrated that antibody to thyroglobulin is present in the serum of patients with Hashimoto's disease. Of their 27 patients, three had rheumatoid arthritis, and considerable interest was generated concerning the association of thyroiditis and other autoimmune disorders. Both White et al. (162) and Hijmans et al. (163) presented the first cases of concomitant thyroiditis and SLE in 1961. The presentation of additional case reports prompted two large-scale, controlled studies at Johns Hopkins in the 1960s, which demonstrated two and four cases of SLE out of 100 and 170 patients, respectively, with Hashimoto's disease (164,165). Subsequently, 74 autopsy-proven cases of Hashimoto's disease were matched with a control group: two patients with thyroiditis, but none of the controls, were found to have SLE. This slightly increased incidence of concurrence is of greater statistical significance if all autoimmune disorders are considered (166).

Detailed evaluations of thyroid function in patients with SLE have been the focus of six major studies and are summarized in Table 39.7 (167–172). Salient observations from these reports also suggest the following:

1. Hyperthyroidism usually antedates lupus, and the subsequent development of SLE occasionally may be induced by antithyroid medication (167,173–175).
2. The incidence of hypothyroidism is greater than that shown in Table 39.7, because patients with SLE have a greater incidence of elevated thyroid-stimulating hormone (TSH) levels but until recently were rarely tested for it (173–175).
3. The incidence of all thyroid disorders probably is greater in patients with SLE than in the general population when compared with the British National Health Service's estimate of the incidence of hyperthyroidism as 1.9 and of hypothyroidism as 1.0% (177).
4. Symptoms of thyroid disease can be confused with those of lupus.

These findings also apply to children with SLE (176, 177).

Kausman and Isenberg (178) measured thyroid function tests in 46 newly diagnosed patients with SLE a mean 6.2 years later. Thyroid serologies followed a fluctuating course; only 9% evolved new thyroid antibodies. Petri et al. (179) reported that 46% of patients with autoimmune thyroid disease have a positive ANA, but Gaches noted other autoimmune disease in 13.7% of 218 patients with autoimmune thyroid disease (180). Lupus and Sjögren's were the most common associations.

The only consistent additional clinical association in those with SLE and thyroid disease is Sjögren's syndrome. After several case reports noted concurrent SLE, Sjögren's syndrome, and Hashimoto's thyroiditis (181,182), a Scandinavian group evaluated 77 patients of lupus. Of these, eight of ten who had thyroid disease also had Sjögren's syndrome, compared with 6 of 67 without thyroid disorders ($p<.01$) (183). A antimicrosomal antigenantibody system, known as anti-Mic-1, has been described in patients with SLE and hyperthyroidism. Anti-Mic-1 was not present in patients with Hashimoto's disease or rheumatoid arthritis, but its clinical appearance still is controversial (184,185). Tsai et al. (186) suggested that thyroid peroxidase autoantibodies in SLE are distinct from those found in Hashimoto's thyroiditis. In addition, three of the nine published reports of patients with SLE and red cell aplasia also noted an association with hypothyroidism (187,188). Patients with SLE and anti-TSH antibodies have been reported as well (189, 190).

It is likely that the thyroid (and the lacrimal and salivary glands) can be a target of the same autoimmune abnormalities that result in SLE.

Diabetes

Type 1 diabetes mellitus is an autoimmune disorder that is caused largely by cytotoxic T cells that destroy pancreatic islet cells. Genetic predisposition has been defined, and antiislet antibodies occur. One survey found that 92 of 222 type 1 diabetics (41%) have a positive ANA (191). An atypical, mild, nonorgan-threatening SLE has been reported in up to 30% of patients with type 1 diabetes and insulin-receptor antibodies (192–196). Occasionally, patients with insulin-receptor antibodies may present with severe hypo-

TABLE 39.7. THYROID FUNCTION AND ANTIBODY STUDIES IN SYSTEMIC LUPUS ERYTHEMATOSUS

Parameter	Gordon and Isenberg (169)	Byron and Mowat (167)	Goh and Wang (168)	Miller et al. (171)	Ropes (170)	Boey et al. (172)
Cases (n)	41	64	319	332	142	129
Hypothyroid (%)	9.8	4.7	0.9	6.6	0.7	5.0
Hyperthyroid (%)	2.4	10.9	2.8	5.0	—	8.9
Hashimoto's disease (%)	—	—	0.6	—	2.1	3.9
Thyroid antibodies (%)	—	—	—	20	—	32.2

glycemia and require steroid therapy (197,198). Of our patients with SLE, 357 were treated with corticosteroids for more than 1 month, and steroid-induced diabetes developed in ten (199). Some of these patients might be more prone to developing antiinsulin antibodies (200).

The Johns Hopkins Lupus Cohort reported that 7% of patients with SLE were diabetics (201). Insulin resistance was common, and hydroxychloroquine use was associated with lower fasting insulin levels.

Adrenal Insufficiency And Cushing's Disease

The most common cause of adrenal insufficiency in patients with SLE is abrupt cessation of steroid therapy, but adrenal insufficiency secondary to cortical infarction in patients with the lupus anticoagulant can occur (202–207) (see Chapter 56). Rarely, adrenal failure also has been associated with amyloid and adrenal hemorrhage in patients with lupus (192,208–211). Cortisol levels are not elevated in nonsteroid-treated SLE, but the corticosterone level is increased (212,213). Cortisol is rapidly metabolized in patients with active disease (214). One patient with androgenital syndrome secondary to adrenal hyperplasia who developed SLE has been reported (215); no cases of autoimmune adrenalitis and SLE have appeared.

SLE activity has been reported to improve with the onset of Cushing's disease (216) and flare after a pituitary adenomectomy in a Cushing's disease patient (217).

Parathyroid Gland

Patients on renal dialysis develop secondary hyperparathyroidism, and this has been associated with an increased incidence of Jaccoud's arthropathy in those with SLE (218). Three reports of concurrent lupus and hypoparathyroidism have appeared (219–223). One case of active SLE associated with lymphadenopathy and parathyroid hormone-related protein (PTHrP) has been reported (224).

Hyperprolactinemia

Approximately 20% of patients with SLE have prolactinemia (225–227). On the whole, prolactin levels do not correlate with sex, age, disease activity, or serologic findings (228–233). When the subset of patients with elevated prolactins are examined, reports have suggested that those individuals have higher prolactin/cortisol ratios, take more corticosteroids, have antiprolactin autoantibodies, and more generalized or central nervous system activity. Some are responsive to bromocriptine therapy (see Chapters 39 and 59).

Fluid And Electrolyte Abnormalities

Antidiuretic Hormone

Scattered reports describing patients with the syndrome of inappropriate antidiuretic hormone (ADH) and SLE (220, 241–247) prompted Ginzler's group to perform an in-depth study of 36 stable patients with SLE and stable disease (248). The mean ADH level was elevated at 11.4 + 1.0 m/mL (normal, 0.4–1.4 m/mL). High levels were associated with a disease duration of more than 2 years, but not with clinical or serologic disease activity. A paradoxic increase in plasma ADH levels was noted in 50 of those who underwent a standard water-load challenge. It was concluded that SLE is associated with a state of primary neurohypophyseal hypersecretion of ADH. On the other hand, two reports of three cases of SLE and nephrogenic diabetes insipidus (249,250).

Renal Tubular Acidosis

Tu and Shearn (251) observed latent renal tubular acidosis (RTA) in 12 patients with SLE, but without clinical renal tubular dysfunction, as well as in patients with Sjögren's syndrome. RTA also has been reported in other autoimmune disorders (252–255). In RTA, impairment of renal acid secretion occurs out of proportion to reduction in the glomerular filtration rate. Clinically, it is manifested by hyperchloremic acidosis and an inability to excrete highly acid urine, and it often is associated with impaired renal concentrating ability. Potassium wasting may be seen (256). Subclinical cases are detected by an acid-loading test that is designed to detect acid excretion inappropriate to the induced metabolic acidosis. It has been hypothesized that autoantibodies to the intercalated cells, but not units of the H+-ATPase may play a pathogenic role in distal renal tubular acidosis (257). Ropes (170) found RTA in two of her 150 patients with SLE.

Hyporeninemic Hypoaldosteronism

Relatively few of our patients with lupus nephritis who are on diuretics require potassium replacement. De Fronzo (258) first noted this and determined that a primary defect in renal tubular potassium secretion, secondary to an immune complex mediated interstitial nephritis, might be responsible. Four case reports have confirmed the existence of a relative hyporeninemic hypoaldosteronism state in patients with SLE (259–262). These observations led Quismorio's group to study 142 patients with SLE; almost ten had unexplained hyperkalemia (213). Most of the hyperkalemic group had impaired renin and aldosterone responses to stimulation.

THE UROGENITAL TRACT

Lupus Cystitis

Interstitial cystitis is an uncommon but important manifestation of SLE. First described in patients with SLE in 1965 (263), it probably is an immune complex-mediated disorder that is associated with bladder vasculitis, a secretory diarrhea with malabsorption, and high titers of ANA (264–271). A literature review has appeared (272) stating that patients with idiopathic interstitial cystitis have an increased incidence of ANA (273). Isenberg's group performed serologic profiles on 34 patients with idiopathic interstitial cystitis (274). Antinuclear antibodies were positive in 25 (56.8%), and seven had SLE.

Significant bladder complaints were found in ten patients among 413 Koreans with SLE in a retrospective chart review (275). Lupus cystitis was noted in five, neurogenic bladder secondary to transverse myelitis in three, and cyclosphosphamide and tuberculous cystitis in one each. Weisman et al. (276) located immune deposits in the vessel walls of both the small intestine and the urinary bladder. His group later examined six patients in detail. Decreased bladder capacities, with thickened and irregular walls, were found, and five of the six had abdominal symptoms. In all patients, symptoms improved with high-dose steroid treatment. Others have reported neurogenic bladders associated with interstitial cystitis in patients with SLE (277,278).

Alarcon-Segovia et al. (279) found bladder abnormalities in 16 of 35 SLE necropsies; interstitial cystitis was found in 11, hemorrhage in nine, congestion in seven, vasculitis in five, and perivascular infiltrate in four. Interestingly, seven patients had pulmonary hemorrhages. Other causes of bladder pathology in SLE patients include myelopathy, cyclophosphamide administration, and inflammatory polyneuropathies. Intravesical instillation of dimethylsulfoxide (DMSO), elmiron, formalin, or high-dose steroid therapy are the probable treatments of choice for isolated lupus cystitis (280–283).

Jokinen et al. (284) performed immunofluorescence tests for tissue-bound immunoglobulin on urinary bladder biopsy specimens from 11 patients with discoid LE and from 14 patients with interstitial cystitis. Of the 11 with discoid LE, nine had immune deposits at the bladder basement membrane; none of the patients with interstitial cystitis had similar changes. Rarely, vasculitis can induce ureteral obstruction (285,286).

Antisperm Antibodies And Male Sexual Dysfunction

Antisperm antibodies represent a heterogeneous grouping that, when present in women, inhibits conception to varying degrees. In men, these antibodies are present in high levels after a vasectomy (287). Marcus and Hess (288) reported that 14 of 15 serum samples from female patients with SLE contained antisperm antibodies with a titer of greater than 1:8. Reichlin and Haas (289) found these antibodies in ten of 24 patients with SLE. The incidence of antisperm antibodies in males and females was the same. The presence of the antibody correlated with anti-DNA and increased disease activity.

Sexual dysfunction (i.e., decreased libido, erectile incompetence, failure to ejaculate) has been reported in 19% to 35% of a total of 64 males with SLE in two uncontrolled preliminary studies (290–292). Two case reports of testicular or penile vasculitis in SLE also have appeared (293,294).

HYPOTHERMIA

Four cases of severe hypothermia (temperature, <95°F or 35°C) have been described in patients with SLE (295–298). All occurred within 48 hours after the institution of corticosteroid therapy.

SUMMARY

1. Estrogen replacement therapy is not contraindicated in postmenopausal women with lupus who could benefit from it. The use of OCs is controversial but probably acceptable under certain circumstances. We do not recommend its use in patients with high titers of IgG antiphospholipid antibodies, migraine headaches, or moderate to severe hypertension.
2. Menstrual irregularity is common in women with SLE; amenorrhea is associated with disease activity, steroid administration, and chemotherapy.
3. The incidence of all major thyroid disorders (hyperthyroidism, hypothyroidism, autoimmune thyroiditis) is increased in SLE.
4. Patients taking steroids have an increased risk of developing diabetes. Type 1 autoimmune diabetes has an increased association with antinuclear antibody, and may display some lupuslike features.
5. Adrenal insufficiency in SLE is usually secondary to abrupt cessation of steroid therapy or infarction in patients with the antiphospholipid syndrome.
6. A small but significant number of lupus patients have renal tubular acidosis, hyporeninemic hypoaldosteronism with resulting hyperkalemia, or clinically relevant complications of antidiuretic hormone hypersecretion.
7. Lupus cystitis is noted infrequently; it is a classic immune complex-mediated vasculitis, and is associated with diarrhea.

REFERENCES

1. Petri M, Robinson C. Oral contraceptives and systemic lupus erythematosus. *Arthritis Rheum* 1997;40:797–803.

2. Lieb SM. The effect of systemic lupus erythematosus on fetal survival. pp 672-674. In: Fine LG, moderator. *Systemic lupus erythematosus in pregnancy.* Ann Intern Med 1981;94:667–677.
3. Tozman ECS, Urowitz MB, Gladman DD. Systemic lupus erythematosus and pregnancy. *J Rheum* 1980;7:624–632.
4. Zulman JI, Talal N, Hoffman GS, et al. Problems associated with the management of pregnancies in patients with SLE. *J Rheum* 1980;7:37–49.
5. Masi AT, Kaslow RA. Sex effects in systemic lupus erythematosus: a clue to pathogenesis. *Arth Rheum* 1978;21:480–484.
6. Lahita RG, Bradlow HL. Hormone metabolism in patients with Klinefelter's disease and SLE. *J Rheum* 1987;14:154–157.
7. Stern R, Fishman J, Brusman H, et al. Systemic lupus erythematosus associated with Klinefelter's syndrome. *Arth Rheum* 1977;20:18–22.
8. Inman RD. Immunologic sex differences and the female preponderance in systemic lupus erythematosus. *Arth Rheum* 1978; 21:849–852.
9. Lahita RG, Bradlow HL, Kunkel HG, etal. Alterations of estrogen metabolism in SLE. *Arth Rheum* 1979;22:1195–1198.
10. Lahita RG, Bradlow HL, Fishman J, et al. Estrogen metabolism in systemic lupus erythematosus: patients and family members. *Arth Rheum* 1982;25:843–846.
11. Lahita RG, Bradlow HL, Kunkel HG, et al. Increased oxidation of testosterone in systemic lupus erythematosus. *Arth Rheum* 1983;26:1517–1521.
12. Lahita RG, Bradlow HL, Ginzler E, et al. Low plasma androgens in women with systemic lupus erythematosus. *Arth Rheum* 1987;30:241–248.
13. Yocum MW, Grossman J, Waterhouse C, et al. Monozygotic twins discordant for systemic lupus erythematosus; comparison of immune response, autoantibodies, viral antibody titers, gamma globulin, and light chain metabolism. *Arth Rheum* 1975;18:193–l99.
14. Murad F, Kuret J. Estrogens and progestins. In: Gilman AG, Rall TW, Nies AS, et al., eds. *Goodman and Gilman's the pharmacological basis of therapeutics, 8th ed.* New York: McGraw-Hill, 1993:1384–1412.
15. Schwartz J, Freeman R, Frishman W. Clinical pharmacology of estrogens: cardiovascular actions and cardioprotective benefits of replacement therapy in postmenopausal women. *J Clin Pharmacol* 1995;35:314–329.
16. NCHS Advance Data, March 1990.
17. Trussell J, Kost K. Contraceptive failure in the United States: a critical review of the literature. *Studies in Family Planning* 1987; 18:237–283.
18. Speroff L, Glass R, Kase N. Clinical gynecologic endocrinology and infertility. Baltimore: Williams and Wilkins, 1989.
19. Jungers P, Dougados M, Pelissier C, et al. Influence of oral contraceptive therapy on activity of systemic lupus erythematosus. *Arth Rheum* 1982;25:618–623.
20. Mintz G, Gutierrez G, Deleze M, et al. Contraception with progestagens in systemic lupus erythematosus. *Contraception* 1984;30:29–38.
21. Roubinian J, Talal N, Siiteri PK, et al. Sex hormone modulation of autoimmunity in NZB/NZW mice. *Arth Rheum* 1979;11: 1162–1169.
22. Samsioe G. Coagulation and anticoagulation effects of contraceptive steroids. *Am J Obstet Gynecol* 1994;170:1523–1527.
23. Burkman RT, Robinson JC, Kruszon-Moran D, et al. Lipid and lipoprotein changes associated with oral contraceptive use. A randomized clinical trial. *Obstet Gynecol* 1988;71:33–38.
24. Bradley DD, Wingerd J, Petitti DB, et al. Serum high-density-lipoprotein cholesterol in women using oral contraceptives, estrogens and progestins. *New Engl J Med* 1978;299:17–20.
25. Julkunen HA. Oral contraceptives in systemic lupus erythematosus: side-effects and influence on the activity of SLE. *Scand J Rheum* 1991;20:427–433.
26. Julkunen HA, Kaaja R, Friman C. Contraceptive practice in women with systemic lupus erythematosus. *Br J Rheum* 1993; 32:227–230.
27. Todd GR, McAteer EJ, Jack CM, et al. Pulmonary hypertension, systemic lupus erythematosus, and the contraceptive pill. *Ann Rheum Dis* 1985;44:266–267.
28. Garovich M, Aguldo C, Pisko E. Oral contraceptives and systemic lupus erythematosus. *Arthritis Rheum* 1980;23: 1396–1398.
29. Travers RL, Hughes GRV. Oral contraceptive therapy and systemic lupus erythematosus. *J Rheum* 1978;5:448–451.
30. Chapel TA, Burns RE. Oral contraceptives and exacerbations of lupus erythematosus. *Am J Obstet Gynecol* 1971;110:366–369.
31. Hadida M, Sayag J. Lupus erythemateux subaigu apparu apres une cure de Norlutin chez une malade atteinte de lupus erythematreux chronique. *Soc Franc Derm Syph Bull* 1968;74: 616–621.
32. Pimstone BL. Systemic lupus erythematosus exacerbated by oral contraceptives. *S Afr J Obstet Gynaec* 1966;4:62–63.
33. Furukawa F, Tachibana T, Imamura S, et al. Oral contraceptive-induced lupus erythematosus in a Japanese woman. *J Derm* 1991;18:56–58.
34. Miller MH. Pulmonary hypertension, systemic lupus erythematosus, and the contraceptive pill: another report. *Ann Rheum Dis* 1987;46:159–161.
35. Sanchez-Guerrero J, Karlson EW, Liang MH, et al. Past use of oral contraceptives and the risk of developing systemic lupus erythematosus. *Arthritis Rheum* 1997;40:804–808.
36. Buyon JP, Kalunian KC, Skovron ML, et al. Can women with systemic lupus erythematosus safely use exogenous estrogens? *J Clin Rheum* 1995;1:205–212.
37. Pando JA, Gourley MF, Wilder RL, et al. Hormonal supplementation as treatment for cyclical rashes in patients with systemic lupus erythematosus. *J Rheumatol* 1995;22:2159–2162.
38. Tarzy BJ, Garcia CR, Wallach EE, et al. Rheumatic disease, abnormal serology and oral contraceptives. *Lancet* 1972;2: 501–503.
39. Dubois EL, Strain L, Ehn M, et al. LE cells after oral contraceptives. *Lancet* 1968;2:679.
40. McKenna CH, Wieman KC, Shulman LE. Oral contraceptives, rheumatic disease and autoantibodies. *Arth Rheum* 1969; 12: 313.
41. Kay DR, Bole GG, Ledger WJ. Antinuclear antibodies, rheumatoid factor and C-reactive protein in serum of normal women using oral contraceptives. *Arth Rheum* 1971;14: 239–248.
42. Realini JP, Goldzieher JW. Oral contraceptives and cardiovascular disease: a critique of the epidemiological studies. *Obstet Gynecol* 1985;152:729–798.
43. Asherson RA, Harris EN, Hughes GRV. Complications of oral contraceptives and antiphospholipid antibodies (letter). *Arthritis Rheum* 1988;31:575–576.
44. Bonnar J. Coagulation effects of oral contraception. *Am J Obstet Gynecol* 1987;157:1042–1048.
45. Strolin-Benedetti M, Gutty D, Strolin P. A comparative study of the effect of oral contraceptives and cigarette smoking on platelet adhesiveness. *Haemostasis* 1976;5:14–20.
46. Pizzo SV, Lewis JG, Campbell EE, et al. Fibrinolytic response and oral contraceptive associated thromboembolism. *Contraception* 1981;23:181–186.
47. Carreras LO, Vermylen JG. "Lupus" anticoagulant and thrombosis, possible role of inhibition of prostacyclin formation. *Thromb Haemost* 1982;48:28–40.
48. Ylikorkala O, Puolakka J, Viinikka L. Oestrogen-containing

oral contraceptives decrease prostacyclin production (letter). *Lancet* 1981;1:42.
49. Beller FK, Ebert C. Effects of oral contraceptives on blood coagulation, a review. *Obstet Gynecol Survey* 1985;40:425–436.
50. Anonymous. Improved safety with low-estrogen oral contraceptives. FDA Medical Bulletin, May 1994.
51. McNeil HP, Simpson RJ, Chesterman CN, et al. Antiphospholipid antibodies are directed against a complex antigen that includes a lipid-binding inhibitor of coagulation: beta2-glycoprotein I (apolipoprotein H). *Proc Natl Acad Sci USA* 1990;87: 4120–4124.
52. Galli M, Comfurius P, Maassen C, et al. Anticardiolipin antibodies (ACA) are directed not to cardiolipin but to a plasma protein cofactor. *Lancet* 1990;335:1544–1547.
53. Roubey RAS, Pratt C, Buyon JP, et al. Lupus anticoagulant activity of autoimmune antiphospholipid antibodies is dependent upon β2-glycoprotein I. *J Clin Invest* 1992;90:1100–1104.
54. Lee NS, Brewer HB, Osborne JCJ. Beta2-glycoprotein I. Molecular properties of an unusual apolipoprotein, apolipoprotein H. *J Biol Chem* 1983;258:4765–4770.
55. Schousboe I. Beta2-glycoprotein I: a plasma inhibitor of the contact activation of the intrinsic blood coagulation pathway. *Blood* 1985;66:1086–1091.
56. Nimpf J, Bevers EM, Bomans PH, et al. Prothrombinase activity of human platelet is inhibited by beta 2 glycoprotein I. *Biochem Biophys Acta* 1986;884:142–149.
57. Nimpf J, Wurm H, Kostner GM. Beta 2-glycoprotein I (apo-H) inhibits the release reaction of human platelet during ADP-induced aggregation. *Atherosclerosis* 1987;63:109–114.
58. Merrill JT, Buyon JP, Seligman S, et al. Pregnancy confers a natural protein S deficiency state and decreased β2glycoprotein I: clinical and pathologic evidence for a model of the antiphospholipid syndrome. *Arth Rheum* 1995;38:S211 (abstract).
59. Bucala R, Lahita RG, Fishman J, et al. Antioestrogen antibodies in users of oral contraceptives and in patients with systemic lupus erythematosus. *Clin Exp Med Immunol* 1987;67: 167–175.
60. Ben-Chetrit A, Ben-Chetrit E. Systemic lupus erythematosus induced by ovulation induction treatment. *Arth Rheum* 1994; 37:1614–1617.
61. Casoli P, Tumiati B, La Sala G. Fatal exacerbation of systemic lupus erythematosus after induction of ovulation. *J Rheumatol* 1997;24:1639–1640.
62. Huong DL, Wechsler B, Piette JC, et al. Risks of ovulation-induction therapy in systemic lupus erythematosus. *Br J Rheumatol* 1996;35:1184–1186.
63. Guballa N, Sammaritano L, Schwartzman S, et al. Ovulation induction and in vitro fertilization in systemic lupus erythematosus and antiphospholipid syndrome. *Arthritis Rheum* 2000;43:550–556.
64. Beerendonk CC, van Dop PA, Braat DD, et al. Ovarian hyperstimulation syndrome: facts and fallacies. *Obstet Gynecol Surv* 1998;43:439–449.
65. Isacs JD. Gonadotropin-releasing hormone analogs. In: Cowan BD, Seifer DB, eds. *Clinical reproductive medicine*. New York: Lippincott-Raven, 1997:225–229.
66. Consensus Development Conference. Diagnosis, prophylaxis, and treatment of osteoporosis. *Am J Med.* 1993; 94:646–650.
67. Dempster DW, Lindsay R. Pathogenesis of osteoporosis. *Lancet.* 1992;341:801–805.
68. Lindsay R, Hart DM, Forrest C, et al. Prevention of spinal osteoporosis in oophorectomised women. *Lancet.* 1980;2: 1151–1153.
69. Oursler MJ, Osdoby P, Pyfferoen J, et al. Avian osteoclasts as estrogen target cells. *Proc Natl Acad Sci USA* 1991;88: 6613–6617.
70. Pacifici R, Rifas L McCracken R, et al. Ovarian steroid treatment blocks a postmenopausal increase in blood monocyte interleukin-1 release. *Proc Natl Acad Sci USA* 1989;86: 2398–2402.
71. Jilka RL, Hangoc G, Girasole F, et al. Increased osteoclast development after estrogen loss-mediation by interleukin-6. *Science* 1992;257:88–91.
72. Gallagher JC, Riggs BL, Deluca HF. Effect of estrogen on calcium absorption and serum vitamin D metabolites in postmenopausal osteoporosis. *J Clin Endocrin Metab* 1980;51: 1359–1364.
73. Kiel DP, Felson DT, Anderson JJ, et al. Hip fracture and the use of estrogens in postmenopausal women. The Framingham study. *N Engl J Med* 1987;317:1169–1174.
74. Paganini-Hill A, Ross RK, Gerkins VR, et al. Menopausal estrogen therapy and hip fractures. *Ann Intern Med* 1981;95:28–31.
75. Ettinger B, Genant HK, Conn CE. Long-term estrogen replacement therapy prevents bone loss and fractures. *Ann Intern Med* 1985;102;319–24.
76. The Writing Group for the PEPI Trial. Effects of hormone therapy on bone mineral density: Results from the postmenopausal estrogen/progestin interventions (PEPI) trial. *J Am Med Assoc* 1996;276;1389–1396.
77. Lufkin EG, Riggs BL. Three-year follow-up on effects of transdermal estrogen (letter). *Ann Intern Med* 1996;125:77.
78. Insogna K, Concato J, Henrich J. Boning up on estrogen: new options, new concerns. *J Am Med Assoc* 1996;276;1430–1432.
79. Ramsey-Goldman R, Dunn JE, Huang CF, et al. Frequency of fractures in women with systemic lupus erythematosus: comparison with United States population data. *Arthritis Rheum* 1999;42:882–890.
80. Lukert BP, Johnson BE, Robinson RG. Estrogen and progesterone replacement therapy reduces glucocorticoid-induced bone loss. *J Bone Miner Res* 1992;7:1063–1069.
81. Hall GM, Daniels M, Doyle DV, et al. Effect of hormone replacement therapy on bone mass in rheumatoid arthritis patients treated with and without steroids. *Arthritis Rheum* 1994;37:1499–1505.
82. American College of Rheumatology Task Force on Osteoporosis Guidelines. Recommendations for the prevention and treatment of glucocorticoid-induced osteoporosis. *Arthritis Rheum* 1996;39:1791–1801.
83. Sowers MFR, Galuska DA. Epidemiology of bone mass in premenopausal women. *Epidemiol Rev* 1993;15:374–398.
84. Ryan KI. Estrogens and atherosclerosis. *Clin Obstet Gynecol* 1976;19:805–815.
85. Mason JE, Tosteson H, Ridker PM, et al. Review article: the primary prevention of myocardial infarction. *New Engl J Med* 1992;1325:1406–1416.
86. Wolf PH, Madans JH, Finucane FF, et al. Reduction of cardiovascular disease-related mortality among postmenopausal women who use hormones: evidence from a national cohort. *Am J Obstet Gynecol* 1991;164:489–494.
87. Barrett-Conner E, Wingard DL, Criqui MH. Postmenopausal estrogen use and heart disease risk factors in the 1980's. Rancho Bernardo, Calif., revisited. *J Am Med Assoc* 1989;261: 2095–2100.
88. Nabulsi AA, Folsom AR, White A, et al. Association of hormone-replacement therapy with various cardiovascular risk factors in postmenopausal women. *New Engl J Med* 1993;328: 1069–1075.
89. Grady D, Rubin S, Petitti DB, et al. Hormonal therapy to prevent disease and prolong life in postmenopausal women. *Ann Intern Med* 1992;117:1016–1037.
90. Hong MK, Romm PA, Reagan K, et al. Effects of estrogen replacement therapy on serum lipid values and angiographically

defined coronary artery disease in postmenopausal women. *Am J Cardiol* 1992;69:176–178.

91. Henderson BE, Paganini-Hill A, Ross RK. Decreased mortality in users of estrogen replacement therapy. *Arch Intern Med* 1991; 151:75–78.
92. Walsh BW, Schiff I, Rosner B, et al. Effects of postmenopausal estrogen replacement on the concentrations and metabolism of plasma lipoproteins. *New Engl J Med* 1991;325:1196–1204.
93. Sprengers ED, Kluft C. Plasminogen activator inhibitors. *Blood* 1987;69:381–387.
94. Lupu F, Bergonzelli GF, Heim DA. Localization and production of plasminogen activator inhibitor-1 in human healthy and atherosclerotic arteries. *Arterioscler Thromb* 1993;13:1090–1100.
95. Meade TW, Ruddock V, Stirling Y, et al. Fibrinolytic activity, clotting factors, and long-term incidence of ischemic heart disease in the Northwick Park Heart Study. *Lancet* 1993;342: 1076–1079.
96. Salomaa V, Stinson V, Kark JD, et al. Association of fibrinolytic parameters with early atherosclerosis: the ARIC Study. *Circulation* 1995;91:284–290.
97. Juhan-Vague E, Pyke SDM, Alessi MC, et al. Fibrinolytic factors and the risk of myocardial infarction or sudden death in patients with antina pectoris. *Circulation* 1996;94: 2057–2063.
98. Gebara OCE, Mittleman MA, Sutherland P, et al. Association between increased estrogen status and increased fibrinolytic potential in the Framingham offspring Study. *Circulation* 1995; 91:1952–1958.
99. Sporrong T, Mattson LA, Samsioe G, et al. Haemostatic changes during continuous oestradiol-progestogen treatment of postmenopausal women. *Br J Obstet Gynaecol* 1990;97: 939–944.
100. van Wersch JWJ, Ubachs JMH, van den Ende A, et al. The effect of two regimens of hormone replacement therapy on the haemostatic profile in postmenopausal women. *Eur J Clin Chem Clin Biochem* 1994;32;449–453.
101. Kroon UB, Silfverstolpe G, Tengborn L. The effects of transdermal estradiol and oral conjugated estrogens on haemostasis variables. *Thromb Haemost*1994;71:420–423.
102. Koh KK, Mincemoyer R, Bui MN, et al. Effects of hormone-replacement therapy on fibrinolysis in postmenopausal women. *N Engl J Med* 1997;336:683–690.
103. Sanchez-Guerrero J, Liang MH, Colditz GA. In response. Postmenopausal hormone therapy and systemic lupus erythematosus. *Ann Int Med* 1995;123:962 (letter).
104. Tseng C, Pertri M, Merrill J, et al. Plasma levels of plasminogen-activator inhibitor type 1 LPAI-1 in postmenopausal lupus patients [abstract]. *Arthritis Rheum* 1997;40(suppl):S302.
104a. Dykman TR, Gluck OS, Murphy WA, et al. Evaluation of factors associated with glucocorticoid-induced osteopenia in patients with rheumatic diseases. *Arthritis Rheum* 1985;28: 361–368.
105. Hulley S, Grady D, Bush T, et al. Randomized trial of estrogen plus progestin for secondary prevention of coronary heart disease in postmenopausal women. *JAMA* 1998;280:605–613.
106. Shlipak MG, Simon JA, Vittinghoff E, et al. Estrogen and progestin, lipoprotein(a), and the risk of recurrent coronary heart disease events after menopause. *JAMA* 2000;283:1845–1852.
107. Varas-Lorenzo C, Garcia-Rodriguea LA, Perez-Gutthahn S, et al. Hormone replacement therapy and incidence of acute myocardial infarction. A population-based nested case-control study. *Circulation* 2000;101:2572–2578.
108. Urowitz MB, Bookman AA, Koehler BE, et al. The bimodal mortality pattern of systemic lupus erythematosus. *Am J Med* 1976;60:221–225.
109. Rosner S, Ginzler EM, Diamond HS, et al. A multicenter study of outcome in systemic lupus erythematosus. II. Causes of death. *Arthritis Rheum* 1982;25:612–617.
110. Hejtmancik MR, Wright JC, Quint R. The cardiovascular manifestations of systemic lupus erythematosus. *Am Heart J* 1964; 68:119–130.
111. Petri M, Perez-Gutthann S, Spence D, et al. Risk factors for csoronary artery disease in patients with systemic lupus erythematosus. *Am J Med* 1992;93:513–519.
112. Haider YS, Roberts WC. Coronary arterial disease in systemic lupus erythematosus: quantification of degree of narrowing in 22 necropsy patients (21 women) aged 16 to 37 years. *Am J Med* 1981;70:775–781.
113. Urowitz MB, Gladman DD. Accelerated atheroma in lupus C background. *Lupus* 2000;9:161–165.
114. Petri M. Detection of coronary artery disease and the role of traditional risk factors in the Hopkins Lupus Cohort. *Lupus* 2000; 9:170–175.
115. Manzi S, Selzer F, Sutton-Tyrrell K, et al. Prevalence and risk factors of carotid plaque in women with systemic lupus erythematosus. *Arthritis Rheum* 1999;42:51–60.
116. Notelovitz M, Kitchens CS, Ware MD. Coagulation and fibrinolysis in estrogen-treated surgically menopausal women. *Obstet Gynecol* 1984;63:621–624.
117. The Writing Group for the PEPI Trial. Effects of estrogen or estrogen/progestin regimens on heart disease risk factors in postmenopausal women [the Postmenopausal Estrogen Progestin Intervention (PEPI) Trial]. *J Am Med Assoc* 1995;273: 199–208.
118. Notelovitz M, Kitchens C, Ware M, et al. Combination estrogen and progestogen replacement therapy does not adversely affect coagulation. *Obstet Gynecol* 1983;62:596–600.
119. Daly E, Vessey MP, Hawkins MM, et al. Risk of venous thromboembolism in users of hormone replacement therapy. *Lancet* 1996;348:977–980.
120. Jick H, Derby LE, Myers MW, et al. Risk of hospital admission for idiopathic venous thromboembolism among users of postmenopausal oestrogens. *Lancet* 1996;348:981–983.
121. Grodstein F, Stampfer MJ, Goldhaber SZ, et al. Prospective study of exogenous hormones and risk of pulmonary embolism in women. *Lancet* 1996:348:983–987.
122. Perez Gutthann S, Garcia Rodriguez LA, Castellsague J, et al. Hormone replacement therapy and risk of venous thromboembolism: population based case-control study. *Brit Med J* 1997; 314:796–800.
123. Varas-Lorenzo C, Garcia-Rodriguez L, Cattaruzzi C, et al. Hormone replacement therapy and the risk of hospitalization for venous thromboembolism: a population-based study in southern Europe. *Am J Epidemiol* 1998;147:387–390.
124. Castellsague J, Perez Gutthann S, Garcia Rodriguez LA. Recent epidemiological studies of the association between hormone replacement therapy and venous thromboembolism. A review. *Drug Saf* 1998;18:117–123.
125. Grady D, Wenger NK, Herrington D, et al. Postmenopausal hormone therapy increases risk for venous thromboembolic disease. The Heart and Estrogen/progestin Replacement Study. *Ann Intern Med* 2000 132:689–696.
126. Sanchez-Guerrero J, Liang MH, Karlson EW, et al. Postmenopausal estrogen therapy and the risk for developing systemic lupus erythematosus (SLE). *Annals Internal Med* 1995; 122:430–433.
127. Buyon JP, Kalunian KC, Belmont HM. Postmenopausal hormone therapy and systemic lupus erythematosus. *Annal Int Med* 1995;123:961 (letter).
128. Sanchez-Guerrero J, Liang MH, Colditz GA. In response. Postmenopausal hormone therapy and systemic lupus erythematosus. *Annal Int Med* 1995;123:962 (letter).

129. Meier CR, Sturkenboom MC, Cohen AS, et al. Postmenopausal estrogen replacement therapy and the risk of developing systemic lupus erythematosus or discoid lupus. *J Rheumatol* 1998;25:1515–1519.
130. Arden NK, Lloyd M, Spector TD, et al. Safety of hormone replacement therapy (HRT) in systemic lupus erythematosus (SLE). *Lupus* 1994;3:11–13.
131. Lobo RA. Editorial: Estrogen and the risk of coagulopathy. *Am J Med* 1992;92:275–282.
132. Devor M, Barrett-Connor E, Renvall M, et al. Estrogen replacement therapy and the risk of venous thrombosis. *Am J Med* 1992;92:275–282.
133. Kreidstein S, Urowitz MB, Gladman DD, et al. Hormone replacement therapy in systemic lupus erythematosus. *J Rheum* 1997;24:2149–2152.
134. Mok CC, Lau CS, Ho CT, et al. Safety of hormonal replacement therapy in postmenopausal patients with systemic lupus erythematosus. *Scand J Rheumatol* 1998;27:342–346.
135. Barrett C, Neylon N, Snaith ML. Case report: Oestrogen-induced systemic lupus erythematosus. *Br J Rheum* 1986;25: 300–301.
136. Lockshin MD. Lupus and pregnancy. *Clin Rheum Dis* 1985;11: 611–632.
137. McGehee Harvey A, Shulman LE, Tumulty AP, et al. Systemic lupus erythematosus: Review of the literature and clinical analysis of 138 cases. *Medicine* 1954 Dec;33:291– 437.
138. Wallace DJ, Dubois EL, editors. Dubois' Lupus Erythematosus. 3d ed. Philadelphia: Lea & Febiger, 1987.
139. Rothfield N. Systemic lupus erythematosus. Clinical and laboratory aspects. In: McCarty D, ed. *Arthritis and Allied Conditions, 9th ed.* Philadelphia: Lea & Febiger, 1979:691–715.
140. Fries JF, Sharp GC, McDevitt HO, et al. Cyclophosphamide therapy in systemic lupus erythematosus and polymyositis. *Arthritis Rheum* 1973;16:154–162.
141. Schaller J. Lupus in childhood. *Clin Rheum Dis* 1982;8: 219–228.
142. Plotz CM, Knowlton AI, Ragan C. Natural history of Cushing's syndrome. *Am J Med* 1952;13:597–614.
143. Steinberg AD, Steinberg BJ. Lupus disease activity associated with menstrual cycle (letter). *J Rheumatol* 1985;12:816–817.
144. Lahita RG, Bradlow HL, Kunkel HG, et al. Increased 16 alpha-hydroxylation of estradiol in systemic lupus erythematosus. *J Clin Endocrinol Metab* 1981;53:174–178.
145. Lim GS, Petri M, Goldman D. Menstruation and systemic lupus erythematosus (SLE). *Arthritis Rheum* 1993;36:R23.
146. Mc Donagh JE, Singh MM, Griffiths ID. Menstrual arthritis. *Annals Rheum Dis* 1993;52:65–66.
147. Smith S, Howell R, Scott L. Is endometriosis associated with systemic lupus erythematosus? *Int J Fertil* 1993;38:343–346.
148. Duffy DA, Denners ML, Molin MR. Systemic lupus erythematosus and breast gigantism. *J Rheumatol* 1995;22: 1214–1215.
149. Blumenfeld Z, Lorber M, Yoffe N, et al. Systemic lupus erythematosus: predisposition for uterine cervical dysplasia. *Lupus* 1994;3:59–61.
150. Eustace DLS. Systemic lupus erythmematosus and uterine cervical dysplasia (Editorial). *Lupus* 1994;3:3–4.
151. Aguirre MA, Jimena P, de Andres M, et al. Gynaecological abnormalities in women with systemic lupus erythematosus: a prospective controlled study. *Brit J Rheumatol* 1997;36:4.
152. Lahita RL, Merrill JT. Cystic ovaries and Stein-Leventhal syndrome in patients with systemic lupus erythematosus. *Arthritis Rheum* 1995;38:S392.
153. Praprotnik S, Orezekj J. Ovaries in systemic lupus erythematosus. *Lupus* 1995;4:41.
154. Fariozzi S, Muda AO, Amini M, et al. Systemic lupus erythematosus with membranous glomerulonephritis and uterine vasculitis. *Am J Kidney Dis* 1997;29:277–279.
155. Lima FR, Guerra D, Sella EMC, et al. Systemic lupus erythematosus (SLE) and cervical intraepithelial neoplasia. *Arthritis Rheum* 1998;41:S66.
156. Morris VH, Hakim A, Isenberg DA. Review of gynaecological abnormalities in patients with systemic lupus erythematosus. *Arthritis Rheum* 1997;40:S106.
157. Berthier S, Mougin C, Vercherin P, et al. Human papillomavirus infection and cervical cancer risk in women with lupus erythematosus. *Rev Med Interne* 1999;20:128–132.
158. Sanchez-Guererro J, Paredes-Paredes M, Avila-Casado MC, et al. Infection of the cervix due to papillomavirus (HPV) in SLE patients. *Arthritis Rheum* 1999;42:S304.
159. de Bandt M, Ribard P, Mayer O, et al. Lupus mastitis disclosing systemic lupus with antiphospholipid syndrome. *Ann Med Interne* 1993;144:147–150.
160. Cernea SS, Kihara SM, Sotto MN, et al. Lupus mastitis. *J Am Acad Dermatol* 1993;29:343–346.
161. Roitt IM, Doniach D, Campbell PN, et al. Auto-antibodies in Hashimoto's disease (lymphadenoid goiter): preliminary communications. *Lancet* 1956;ii:820–821.
162. White RG, Bass BH, Williams E. Lymphadenoid goiter and the syndrome of systemic lupus erythematosus. *Lancet* 1961;i: 368–373.
163. Hijmans W, Doniach D, Roitt IM, et al. Serological overlap between lupus erythematosus, rheumatoid arthritis, and thyroid auto-immune disease. *Br Med J* 1961;5257:909–914.
164. Masi AT, Hartmann WH, Hahn BH, et al. Hashimoto's disease. A clinicopathological study with matched controls. Lack of significant associations with other autoimmune disorders. *Lancet* 1965;i:123–126.
165. Mulhern LM, Masi AT, Shulman LE. Hashimoto's disease. A search for associated disorders in 170 clinically detected cases. *Lancet* 1966;ii:508–512.
166. Furszyfer J, Kurland LT, Woolner LB, et al. Hashimoto's thyroiditis in Olmsted County, Minnesota, 1935 through 1967. *Mayo Clin Proc* 1970;45:586–596.
167. Byron MA, Mowat AG. Thyroid disorders in systemic lupus erythematosus (letter). *Ann Rheum Dis* 1987;46:174–175.
168. Goh KL, Wang F. Thyroid disorders in systemic lupus erythematosus. *Ann Rheum Dis* 1986;45:579–583.
169. Gordon T, Isenberg D. The endocrinologic associations of the autoimmune rheumatic diseases. *Semin Arthritis Rheum* 1987; 17:58–70.
170. Ropes MW. Systemic lupus erythematosus. Cambridge, MA: Harvard University Press, 1976.
171. Miller FW, Moore GF, Weintraub BD, et al. Prevalence of thyroid disease and abnormal thyroid function test results in patients with systemic lupus erythematosus. *Arthritis Rheum* 1987;30:1124–1131.
172. Boey ML, Fong PH, Lee JSC, et al. Autoimmune thyroid disorders in SLE in Singapore. *Lupus* 1993;2:51–54.
173. Horton RC, Sheppard MC, Emery P. Propylthiouracil–induced systemic lupus erythematosus (letter). *Lancet* 1989;ii:568.
174. Sakata S, Nakamura S, Nagai K, et al. Two cases of systemic lupus erythematosus associated with hypothyroidism. *Jpn J Med* 1987;26:373–376.
175. Takuwa N, Kojima I, Ogata E. Lupus-like syndromea rare complication of thionamide treatment for Graves' disease. *Endocrinol Jpn* 1981;28:663–667.
176. Eberhard BA, Silverman ED, Eddy A, et al. Occurrence of thyroid abnormalities in childhood systemic lupus erythematosus (abstract). *Arthritis Rheum* 1990;33:S144.
177. Bajaj S, Bell MJ, Shumak S, et al. Antithyroid arthritis syndrome. *J Rheumatol* 1998;25:1235–1239.

178. Kausman D, Isenberg DA. Thyroid autoimmunity in systemic lupus erythematosus: the clinical significance of a fluctuating course. *Br J Rheumatol* 1995;34:361–364.
179. Petri M, Karlson EW, Cooper DS, et al. Autoantibody tests in autoimmune thyroid disease. *J Rheumatol* 1991;18:1529–1531.
180. Gaches F, Delaire L, Nadalon S, et al. Frequency of autoimmune diseases in 228 patients with autoimmune thyroid pathologies. *Rev Med Interne* 1998;19:173–179.
181. Feld S, Landau Z, Gefel D, et al. Pernicious anemia. Hashimoto's thyroiditis and Sjögren's in a woman with SLE and autoimmune hemolytic anemia (letter). *J Rheumatol* 1989;16: 258–259.
182. Galofre J, Bielsa I, Casademont J, et al. Papulonodular mucinosis and late-onset SLE associated with Hashimoto's thyroiditis and Sjögren's syndrome (letter). *Rev Clin Esp* 1989;184: 446–447.
183. Jonsson H, Nived O, Sturfelt G. Thyroid disorders are related to secondary Sjögren's syndrome in unselected systemic lupus erythematosus patients. *Arthritis Rheum* 1988;31:1079–1080.
184. Kohno Y, Naito N, Saito K, et al. Anti-thyroid peroxidase antibody activity in sera of patients with systemic lupus erythematosus. *Clin Exp Immunol* 1989;75:217–221.
185. Salazar-Paramo M, Garcia de la Torre I, Hernandez-Vazquez L, et al. Evidence of a new antigen-antibody system (anti-Mic-l) in patients with systemic lupus erythematosus and hyperthyroidism. *J Rheumatol* 1989;16:175–180.
186. Tsai RT, Chang TC, Wang CR, et al. Thyroid peroxidase autoantibodies and their effects on enzyme activity in patients with systemic lupus erythematosus. *Lupus* 1995;4:280–285.
187. Francis DA. Pure red-cell aplasia: association with systemic lupus erythematosus with primary autoimmune hypothyroidism (abstract). *Br Med J* (Clin Res) 1982;284:85.
188. Franzen P, Friman C, Pettersson T, et al. Combined pure red cell aplasia and primary autoimmune hypothyroidism in systemic lupus erythematosus. *Arthritis Rheum* 1987;30:837–840.
189. Sakata S, Yamamoto M, Takuno H, et al. A case of systemic lupus erythematosus (SLE) associated with anti-thyrotropin (TSH) autoantibodies. *Nippon Naika Gakkai Zasshi* 1989;78: 571–572.
190. Baker JR Jr, Miller FW, Steinberg AD, et al. Thyroid stimulating and thyrotrophin binding-inhibitory immunoglobulin activity in patients with systemic lupus erythematosus having thyroid function abnormalities. *Thyroid* 1991;1:229–234.
191. Helmke K, Otten A, Maser E, et al. Islet cell antibodies, circulating immune complexes and antinuclear antibodies in diabetes mellitus. *Horm Metab Res* 1987;19:312–315.
192. Da Costa GM, Forga Llenas L, Martinez Bruna MS, et al. Adrenal hemorrhage linked to systemic lupus erythematosus associated with the antiphospholipid syndrome. *Rev Clin Esp* 1992;191:54–55.
193. Di Paolo S, Lattanzi V, Guastamacchia E, et al. Extreme insulin resistance due to anti-insulin receptor antibodies: a direct demonstration of autoantibody secretion by peripheral lymphocytes. *Diabetes Res Clin Pract* 1990;9:65–73.
194. Howard RL, Beck LK, Schneebaum A. Systemic lupus erythematosus presenting as hypoglycemia with insulin receptor antibodies. *West J Med* 1989;151:324–325.
195. Kellett HA, Collier A, Taylor R, et al. Hyperandrogenism, insulin resistance, acanthosis nigricans and systemic lupus erythematosus associated with insulin receptor antibodies. *Metabolism* 1988;37:656–659.
196. Tsokos GC, Gorden P, Antonovych T, et al. Lupus nephritis and other autoimmune features in patients with diabetes mellitus due to autoantibody in insulin receptors. *Ann Intern Med* 1985; 102:176–181.
197. Moller DE, Ratner RE, Borenstein DG. Antibodies to the insulin receptor as a cause of autoimmune hypoglycemia in systemic lupus erythematosus. *Am J Med* 1988;84:334–338.
198. Varga J, Lopatin M, Boden G. Hypoglycemia due to antiinsulin receptor antibodies in systemic lupus erythematosus (case report). *J Rheumatol* 1990;17:1226–1229.
199. Pistiner M, Wallace DJ, Nessim S, et al. Lupus erythematosus in the 1980s: a survey of 570 patients. *Semin Arthritis Rheum* 1991;21:5564.
200. Thomas JW, Vertkin A, Nell LJ. Antiinsulin antibodies and clinical characteristics of patients with systemic lupus erythematosus and other connective tissue diseases with steroid induced diabetes. *J Rheumatol* 1987;14:732–735.
201. Petri M, Yoo SS. Predictors of glucose intolerance in systemic lupus erythematosus (abstract). *Arthritis Rheum* 1994;37:S323.
202. Alperin N, Babu S, Weinstein A. Acute adrenal insufficiency and the antiphospholipid syndrome (letter). *Ann Intern Med* 1989;111:950.
203. Carette S, Jobin F. Acute adrenal insufficiency as a manifestation of the cardiolipin syndrome? *Ann Rheum Dis* 1989;48: 430–431.
204. Carlisle EJ, Leslie W. Primary hypoadrenalism in a patient with the lupus anticoagulant. *J Rheumatol* 1990;17:1405–1407.
205. Grottolo A, Ferrari V, Mariano M, et al. Primary adrenal insufficiency, circulating lupus anticoagulant and anticardiolipin antibodies in a patient with multiple abortions and recurrent thrombotic episodes. *Haematologica* (Pavia) 1988;73:517–519.
206. Walz B, Ho Ping Kong H, Silver R. Adrenal failure and the primary antiphospholipid syndrome (case report). *J Rheumatol* 1990;17:836–837.
207. Koren S, Hanly JG. Adrenal failure in systemic lupus erythematosus. *J Rheumatol* 1997;24:1410–1412.
208. Eichner HL, Schambelan M, Biglieri EG. Systemic lupus erythematosus with adrenal insufficiency. *Am J Med* 1973;55: 700–705.
209. Levy EN, Ramsey-Goldman R, Kahl LE. Adrenal insufficiency in two women with anticardiolipin antibody. Cause and effect? *Arthritis Rheum* 1990;33:1842–1846.
210. Rigalleau V, Pommereau A, Martin L, et al. Unilateral adrenal hemorrhage in antiphospholipid syndrome associated with a lupus patient. *Presse Med* 1994;23:1092.
211. Thiagarajan D, Wongsurawat N. Systemic lupus erythematosus associated with adrenal insufficiency. *J Kans Med Soc* 1978;79: 565–566.
212. Hughes ER, Ely RS, Kelley VC. Plasma adrenocortical hormones in connective tissue diseases. *Am J Dis Child* 1962;104: 610–613.
213. Lee FO, Quismorio FP Jr, Troum OM, et al. Mechanisms of hyperkalemia in systemic lupus erythematosus. *Arch Intern Med* 1988;148:397–401.
214. Klein AM, Buskila D, Gladman D, et al. Cortisol catabolism by lymphocytes of patients with systemic lupus erythematosus and rheumatoid arthritis. *J Rheumatol* 1990;17:30–33.
215. Mohacsi G, Julesz J, Berger Z, et al. Bilateral renal malacoplakia in systemic lupus erythematosus and andrenogenital syndrome. *Int Urol Nephrol* 1989;21:31–38.
216. Arima K, Higuchi M, Yoshizawa S, et al. Improvement of systemic lupus erythematosus activity by the association of delayed onset Cushing's syndrome. *J Rheumatol* 1998;25:2456–2458.
217. Noguchi Y, Tamai H, Fujisawa K, et al. Systemic lupus erythematosus after pituitary adenomectomy in a patient with Cushing's disease. *Clin Endocrinol* 1998;48:670–672.
218. Babini SM, Cocco JA, de la Sota M, et al. Tendinous laxity and Jaccoud's syndrome in patients with systemic lupus erythematosus. Possible role of secondary hyperparathyroidism. *J Rheumatol* 1989;16:494–498.
219. Decaux G, Unger J, Marneffe C. Psychosis, central hyperventi-

lation and inappropriate secretion of antidiuretic hormone in systemic lupus erythematosus. *Postgrad Med J* 1981;57: 719–720.

220. Hajiroussou VJ. Hypoparathyroidism associated with systemic lupus erythematosus. *Postgrad Med J* 1981;57:597–598.
221. Hara K, Suzuki T, Tanaka M, et al. A case of pseudohypoparathyroidism type I with systemic lupus erythematosus. *Ryumachi* 1989;29:200–206.
222. Gazarian M, Laxer RM, Kooh S-W, et al. Hypoparathyroidism associated with systemic lupus erythematosus. *J Rheumatol* 1995;22:2156–2158.
223. Jara LJ, Gomez-Sanchez C, Silveira L, et al. Hyperprolactinemia in systemic lupus erythematosus (abstract). *Arthritis Rheum* 1991;34:R24.
224. Deftos LJ, Burton DW, Baird SM, et al. Hypercalcemia and systemic lupus erythematosus. *Arthritis Rheum* 1996;39: 2066–2069.
225. Pauzner R, Urowitz MB, Gladman DD, et al. Prolactin in systemic lupus erythematosus. *J Rheumatol* 1994;21:2064–2067.
226. Allen SH, Sharp GC, Wang G, et al. Prolactin levels and antinuclear antibody profiles in women tested for connective tissue disease. *Lupus* 1956;5:30–37.
227. Jara LJ, Gomez-Sanchez C, Silveira LH, et al. Hyperprolactinemia in systemic lupus erythematosus: association with disease activity. *Am J Med Sci* 1992;303:222–226.
228. Walker SE, Mc Murray RW, Houri JM, et al. Effects of prolactin in stimulating disease activity in systemic lupus erythematosus. *Annals of the New York Acad Sciences* 1998;840: 762–772.
229. Ostendorf B, Fischer R, Santen R, et al. Hyperprolactinemia in systemic lupus erythematosus? *Scand J Rheumatol* 1996;25: 97–102.
230. Buskila D, Lorber M, Neumann L, et al. No correlation between prolactin levels and clinical activity in patients with systemic lupus erythematosus. *J Rheumatol* 1996;23:629–632.
231. Mok CC, Lau CS. Lack of association between prolactin levels and clinical activity in patients with systemic lupus erythematosus. *J Rheumatol* 1996;23:2185–2186.
232. Mok CC, Lau CS, Wing Lee KA, et al. Hyperprolactinemia in males with systemic lupus erythematosus. *J Rheumatol* 1998;25: 2357–2363.
233. El-Garf A, Salah S, Shaarawy M, et al. Prolactin hormone in juvenile systemic lupus erythematosus: a possible relationship to disease activity and CNS manifestations. *J Rheumatol* 1996;23: 374–377.
234. Leanos-Miranda A, Pascoe-Lira D, Blanco-Favela F. Prolactin and systemic lupus erythematosus. *Brit J Rheumatol* 1998;37: 1029–1035.
235. Funauchi M, Ikoma S, Enomoto H, et al. Prolactin modulates the disease activity of systemic lupus erythematosus accompanied by prolactinoma. *Clin Exp Rheumatol* 1998;16: 479–482.
236. Rovensky J, Jurankova E, Rauova LU, et al. Relationship between endocrine, immune and clinical variables in patients with systemic lupus erythematosus. *J Rheumatol* 1997;24: 2330–2334.
237. Neidhart M. Elevated serum prolactin or elevated prolactin/cortisol ratio are associated with autoimmune processes in systemic lupus erythematosus and other connective tissue diseases. *J Rheumatol* 1996;23:476–481.
238. Alvarez-Nemegyei J, Cobarrubias-Cobos A, Escalante-Triay F, et al. Bromocriptine in systemic lupus erythematosus: a double-blind, randomized, placebo-controlled study. *Lupus* 1998;7: 414–419.
239. McMurray RW, Allen SH, Braum AL, et al. Longstanding hyperprolactinemia associated with systemic lupus erythematosus: possible hormonal stimulation of autoimmune disease. *J Rheumatol* 1994;21:843–850.
240. Walker SE, Reddy GH, Miller D, et al. Treatment of active systemic lupus erythematosus (SLE) with the prolactin (PRL) lowering drug bromocriptine (BC): comarison with hydroxychloroquine (HC) in a randomized, blinded one-year study. *Arthritis Rheum* 1999;42:S282 (abstract).
241. Elisaf MS, Milionis HJ, Drosos AA. Hyponatremia due to inappropriate secretion of antidiuretic hormone in a patient with systemic lupus erythematous. *Clin Exp Rheumatol* 1999;17: 223–226.
242. Mirsattari SM, Power C, Fine A, et al. Neuropsychiatric systemic lupus erythematosus and the syndrome of inappropriate secretion of antidiuretic hormone: a case report with very late onset systemic lupus erythematosus. *Brit J Rheumatol* 1998;37: 1132–1134.
243. Martin Santos JM, Dib B, Terroba Larumbe MC, et al. Systemic lupus erythematosus and the syndrome of inappropriate secretion of antidiuretic hormone. *Clin Exp Rheumatol* 1996; 14:578–579.
244. Agus B, Nayar S, Patel DJ, et al. Inappropriate secretion of ADH in a patient with systemic lupus erythematosus (letter). *Arthritis Rheum* 1983;26:237–238.
245. Kaplan AP, Curl FD, Decker JL. Central hyperventilation and inappropriate antidiuretic hormone secretion in systemic lupus erythematosus. *Am J Med* 1970;48:661–667.
246. Lowenthal LJ, Kobrin S, Callegari PC. Systemic lupus erythematosus and the sydrome of inappropriate secretion of ADH. *J Rheumatol* 1991;18:613–616.
247. Ben Hamid M, Bunker D, Baumelou A, et al. Inappropriate secretion of antidiuretic hormone (SIADH) in a patient with systemic lupus erythematosus (SLE): a case report. *Clin Nephrol* 1992;37:3435.
248. Trachtman H, Ginzler E, Tejani A, et al. Abnormal antidiuretic hormone secretion in patients with systemic lupus erythematosus. *Nephron* 1987;46:67–72.
249. Sanchez-Roman J, Castillo-Palma MJ, Ocana-Medina C, et al. Neurogenic diabetes insipidus in patients with systemic lupus erythematosus. *Annals Rheum Dis* 1998;57;261–262.
250. Tekin N, Kural N, Kocak AK, et al. Diabetes insipidus in a pediatric patient with systemic lupus erythematosus. *Turkish J Pediatr* 1997;39:281–284.
251. Tu WH, Shearn MA. Systemic lupus erythematosus and latent renal tubular dysfunction. *Ann Intern Med* 1967;67:100–109.
252. Carter NG, Whitworth JA, Mackay IR. Impaired urinary acidification—its incidence in diseases with autoimmune features. *Aust N Z J Med* 1971;1:39–43.
253. Caruana RJ, Barish CF, Buckalew VM Jr. Complete distal renal tubular acidosis in systemic lupus: clinical and laboratory findings. *Am J Kidney Dis* 1985;6:59–63.
254. Morris RC Jr. Renal tubular acidosis. Mechanisms, classification and implications. *N Engl J Med* 1969;281:1405–1413.
255. Bagga A, Jain Y, Srivastava RN, et al. Renal tubular acidosis preceding systemic lupus erythematosus. *Pediatr Nephrol* 1993;7: 735–736.
256. Nakhoul F, Plavnic Y, Lichtig H, et al. Hypokalemic flaccid paralysis as the presenting symptom of autoimmune interstitial nephropathy. *Isr J Med Sci* 1993;29:300–303.
257. Bastani B, Underhill D, Chu N, et al. Preservation of intercalated cell H+-ATPase in two patients with lupus nephritis and hyperkalemic distal renal tubular acidosis. *J Am Soc Nephrol* 1997;8:1109–1117.
258. De Fronzo RA, Cooke CR, Goldberg M, et al. Impaired renal tubular potassium secretion in systemic lupus erythematosus. *Ann Intern Med* 1977;86:268–271.
259. Aguirre C, Vallo A, Gonzalez de Zarate P, et al. Changes in

renin-aldosterone axis in systemic lupus erythematosus. *Med Clin* (Barcelona) 1988;91:206–210.
260. Graham S, Wilner H, Goodman D, et al. Hyperkalemia in lupus nephritis associated with hyporeninemic hypoaldosteronism (abstract). *Clin Res* 1980;28:62A.
261. Kozeny GA, Hurley RM, Fresco R, et al. Systemic lupus erythematosus presenting with hyporeninemic hypoaldosteronism in a 10 year old girl. *Am J Nephrol* 1986;6:321–324.
262. Lim L, Ron MA, Ormerod ID, et al. Psychiatric and neurological manifestations in systemic lupus erythematosus. *Q J Med* 1988;66:27–38.
263. Shipton EA. Hunner's ulcer (chronic interstitial cystitis). A manifestation of collagen disease. *Br J Urol* 1965;37:443–449.
264. Boye E, Morse M, Huttner I, et al. Immune complex-mediated interstitial cystitis as a major manifestation of systemic lupus erythematosus. *Clin Immunol Immunopathol* 1979;13:67–76.
265. de la Serna AR, Alarcon-Segovia D. Chronic interstitial cystitis as an initial major manifestation of systemic lupus erythematosus. *J Rheumatol* 1981;8:808–810.
266. Eberhard A, Shore A, Silverman E, et al. Bowel perforation and interstitial cystitis in childhood systemic lupus erythematosus. *J Rheumatol* 1991;18:746.
267. Kunimi K, Nagano K, Misaki T, et al. A case of lupus cystitis. *Hinyokika Kiyo* 1989;35:685–688.
268. Moriuchi J, Ichikawa Y, Takaya M, et al. Lupus cystitis and perforation of the small bowel in a patient with systemic lupus erythematosus and overlapping syndrome. *Clin Exp Rheumatol* 1989;7:533–536.
269. Vicencio GP, Chung-Park M, Ricanati E, et al. SLE with interstitial cystitis, reversible hydronephrosis and intestinal manifestations. *J Rheumatol* 1989;16:250–251.
270. De Arriba G, Velo M, Barrio V, et al. Association of interstitial lupus cystitis with systemic lupus erythematosus. *Clin Nephrol* 1993;39:287–288.
271. Nakauchi Y, Suehiro T, Tahara K, et al. Systemic lupus erythematosus relapse with lupus cystitis. *Clin Exp Rheumatol* 1995; 13:645–648.
272. Meulders Q, Michel C, Marteau P, et al. Association of chronic interstitial cystitis, protein-losing enteropathy and paralytic ileus with seronegative systemic lupus erythematosus: case report andreview of the literature. *Clin Nephrol* 1992;27: 239–244.
273. Jokinen EJ, Alfthan OS, Oravisto KJ. Antitissue antibodies in interstitial cystitis. *Clin Exp Immunol* 1972;11:333–339.
274. Christmas TJ, Le Page S, Maddison PJ, et al. Antinuclear antibodies in interstitial cystitis (IC) (abstract). *Br J Rheumatol* 1989;28(suppl 2):37.
275. Min JK, Byun JY, Lee SH, et al. Urinary bladder involvement in patients with systemic lupus erythematosus with review of the literature. *Korean J Internal Med* 2000;15:42–50.
276. Weisman MH, McDanald EC, Wilson CB. Studies of the pathogenesis of interstitial cystitis, obstructive uropathy and intestinal malabsorption in a patient with systemic lupus erythematosus. *Am J Med* 1981;70:875–881.
277. Amarenco P, Amarenco G, Malbec D, et al. Vesical neuropathy in acute disseminated lupus erythematosus, 2 cases. *Presse Med* 1988;17:1367.
278. Sugiyama T, Kiwamoto H, Esa A, et al. Neurogenic bladder in patients with SLE (English abstract). *Nippon Hinyokika Gakkai Zasshi* 1987;78:1613–1617.
279. Alarcon-Segovia D, Abud-Mendoza C, Reyes-Gutierrez E, et al. Involvement of the urinary bladder in systemic lupus erythematosus. A pathologic study. *J Rheumatol* 1984;11:208–210.
280. Sotolongo JR Jr, Swerdlow F, Schiff HI, et al. Successful treatment of lupus erythematosus cystitis with DMSO. *Urology* 1984;23:125–127.
281. Segawa C, Wada T, Yokoyama H. Efficacy of steroid pulse therapy in lupus cystitis. *J Rheumatol* 1995;22:2373–2374.
282. Goupille P, Jeannou J, Valat J-P. Lupus cystitis improved with oral prednisone therapy. *J Rheumatol* 1996; 23:1667.
283. Fu LW, Chen WP, Wang HH, et al. Formalin treatment of refractory hemorrhagic cystitis in systemic lupus erythematosus. *Pediatr Nephrol* 1998;12:788–789.
284. Jokinen EJ, Lassus A, Salo OP, et al. Discoid lupus erythematosus and interstitial cystitis. The presence of bound immunoglobulins in the bladder mucosa. *Ann Clin Res* 1972;4: 23–25.
285. Kim HJ, Park MH. Obstructive uropathy due to interstitital cystitis in a patient with systemic lupus erythematosus. *Clin Nephrol* 1996;45:205–208.
286. Baskin L, Mee S, Matthay M, et al. Ureteral obstruction caused by vasculitis. *J Urol* 1989;141:933–935.
287. Tung K. Immunopathology and male infertility. *Hosp Pract* (Off) 1988;23:191–206.
288. Marcus ZH, Hess EV. Antisperm antibodies in patients with systemic lupus erythematosus (letter). *Arthritis Rheum* 1980;24: 569–570.
289. Reichlin M, Haas GG Jr. Association of antisperm antibodies with lupus erythematosus (abstract). *Arthritis Rheum* 1985; 28(suppl):S67.
290. Folomeev M, Alekberova Z. Impotence in systemic lupus erythematosus. *J Rheumatol* 1990;17:117–118.
291. Inman RD, Jovanovic L, Markenson JA, et al. Systemic lupus erythematosus in men. Genetic and endocrine features. *Arch Intern Med* 1982;142:1813–1815.
292. Miller MH. Impotence in systemic lupus erythematosus. *J Rheumatol* 1990;17:118.
293. Kattwinkel N, Cook L, Agnello V. Overwhelming fatal infection in a young woman after intravenous cyclophosphamide therapy for lupus nephritis. *J Rheumatol* 1991;18:79–81.
294. Tripp BM, Chu F, Halwani F, et al. Necrotizing vasculitis of the penis in systemic lupus erythematosus. *J Urol* 1995;154:528–529.
295. Csuka ME, McCarty DJ. Transient hypothermia after corticosteroid treatment of subcutaneous lupus erythematosus (letter). *J Rheumatol* 1984;11:112–113.
296. Johnson RT, Richardson EP. The neurological manifestations of systemic lupus erythematosus. A clinical-pathological study of 24 cases and review of the literature. *Medicine* 1968;47: 337–369.
297. Kass GH. Hypothermia following cortisone administration. *Am J Med* 1955;18:146–149.
298. Kugler SL, Costakos DT, Aron AA, et al. Hypothermia and systemic lupus erythematosus (case report). *J Rheumatol* 1990;17: 680–681.

40

GASTROINTESTINAL AND HEPATIC MANIFESTATIONS

DAVID S. HALLEGUA
DANIEL J. WALLACE

GASTROINTESTINAL INVOLVEMENT

Although gastrointestinal (GI) manifestations are common in patients with systemic lupus erythematosus (SLE) (Table 40.1), their incidence varies with the interest and methods of the observer who is studying the illness. For example, two major studies failed to mention GI complications (1,2), and another made only brief reference to it (3). Abdominal symptoms and signs may be the result of SLE, medications that are used to treat SLE, or intercurrent processes.

HISTORICAL NOTES

Osler (4) was impressed with the frequency of GI manifestations or, as he called them, GI crises. He believed that they might mimic any type of abdominal condition. In 1939, Reifenstein et al. (5) found evidence of peritonitis in 13 to 18% autopsied SLE cases, with perihepatitis and enlargement of the liver in one third. The most feared GI complication of SLE is lupus enteritis, caused by vascular involvement of the bowel wall, with infarction or hemorrhage. The first modern description of this was by Klemperer (6) in 1941.

PREVALENCE

GI complaints were the initial presentation in 10% of Dubois' patients (7); 25% to 40% had protracted symptoms. Haserick's group (8) divided the GI symptoms of SLE among 87 patients into three groupings: none (63%), minor (29%), and major (8%). We have found this breakdown to be clinically useful. Subclinical involvement of the GI tract also is common. For example, Landing's group at Children's Hospital of Los Angeles found chronic mucosal infiltration in 96% of 26 autopsied children with SLE (9). Younger patients with lupus are more susceptible. Among 272 patients with SLE, the prevalence of GI manifestations ranged from 10% in children to none over the age of 50 (10). Sultan et al. published a recent review on GI manifestations in SLE and found anorexia to be the most common reported manifestation with a prevalence of 36% to 71% in published studies (11).

PHARYNGITIS, DYSPHAGIA, AND ESOPHAGITIS

Persistent sore throat is not an infrequent finding, especially in children (12). (Mucous membrane lesions and other features of oral pathology are discussed in Chapter 29.) Dysphagia occurs in 1% to 6% (7,13–18) and heartburn in 11% to 50% of patients (13,19). In a literature review, Zizic (17) related that although only 5% of patients with SLE complained of dysphagia, 25% had impaired esophageal peristalsis, compared with 67% of patients with scleroderma. Several studies using esophageal manometry noted aperistalsis or hypoperistalsis of the esophagus in approximately 10% of patients with SLE (18–23). Aperistalsis sometimes correlated with the presence of Raynaud's phenomenon. Gutierrez et al. (24) compared esophageal motility in 14 patients with SLE and 17 with mixed connective tissue disease (MCTD). A definite correlation was found between Raynaud's phenomenon and hypoperistalsis, with the latter being more common in MCTD. The SLE group had only a slightly decreased lower esophageal sphincter pressure. Esophageal motor dysfunction in SLE also can produce diffuse spasm and result in symptoms of chest pain (25). The aperistaltic group can show atony and dilatation of the esophagus on upper GI radiography (26).

Ramirez-Mata et al. (27) performed esophageal manometric studies in a group of unselected patients with SLE

TABLE 40.1. SYSTEMIC LUPUS ERYTHEMATOSUS AND THE GASTROINTESTINAL TRACT

1. Gastrointestinal (GI) symptoms are common in systemic lupus erythematosus (SLE). Secondary causes such as concurrent disease, stress, and medication must be ruled out.
2. Sore throat and oral ulcers are common.
3. Dysphagia is present in 2% to 6% of patients, especially in association with Raynaud's phenomenon.
4. Anorexia, nausea, vomiting, or diarrhea may be prominent in one third of patients when the disease is active. Chronic intestinal pseudoobstruction (CIPO) causes the above symptoms and is a disturbance of the enteric nervous system. Inflammatory bowel disease, infection, and concomitant drug administration must be ruled out as other causes.
5. The incidence of peptic ulcer disease was 6% in patients presenting with acute abdominal pain; it usually is caused by antiinflammatory medication.
6. Ascites is found in 8% to 11% of patients. If a result of nephrosis, cirrhosis, or congestive heart failure, it is a painless transudate. Exudative causes might be painful and include serosal inflammation. Patients with lupus peritonitis often are steroid-responsive.
7. Pancreatitis is a serious complication of SLE. It is associated with pancreatic vasculitis, activity of SLE in other systems, and rarely, with subcutaneous fat necrosis. Mild elevation of pancreatic enzyme levels may occur in SLE without pancreatitis; high levels suggest pancreatitis. Steroids are the treatment of choice, but they (along with thiazide diuretics and azathioprine) can induce pancreatitis.
8. Abdominal pain, distension, and tenderness warrant a search for ischemia or bowel ulceration especially in patients with a SLEDAI of 4 or more. In the outpatient setting, these signs may suggest the presence of small-bowel bacterial overgrowth (SIBO).
9. Malabsorption syndromes are rare but do occur.
10. Mesenteric or intestinal vasculitis is a life-threatening complication of SLE, usually associated with multisystem activity. High doses of steroids are required, and surgical intervention is indicated if extensive bowel infarction (with hemorrhage) and/or large intestinal perforations occur. Patients succumb from complications of obstruction, perforation, or infarction.

and noted abnormalities in 16. Absent or abnormally low contractions were found at the upper one third in seven patients, at the lower two thirds in three, in the entire esophagus in two, at the lower esophageal sphincter in two, and at the lower two thirds plus the lower sphincter in the remaining two. They found no relationship among the presence of esophageal dysfunction and activity, duration, or therapy of SLE. Interestingly, five of the 34 patients who had normal studies complained of dysphagia and heartburn. Upper esophageal skeletal muscle fiber atrophy also was found in two of 26 autopsies on children with SLE (9). One report confirmed these findings and suggested that hypoperistalsis or aperistalsis may be caused by an inflammatory reaction in the esophageal muscles or by ischemic or vasculitic damage to Auerbach's plexus (19). Esophageal imaging with gastrograffin, computed tomography (CT) scanning or endoscopy is required to make the diagnosis of esophageal ulceration or perforation from systemic vasculitis (18).

The treatment of esophageal symptoms is the same as that of Raynaud's esophagus. Small and frequent meals, avoidance of postprandial recumbency, and the administration of antacids, proton pump inhibitors, H2 antagonists, or parasympathomimetic agents play a therapeutic role.

ANOREXIA, NAUSEA, VOMITING, AND DIARRHEA

The most common cause of anorexia, nausea, vomiting, and diarrhea in SLE is related to the use of salicylates, nonsteroidal antiinflammatory drugs (NSAIDs), antimalarial drugs, corticosteroids, and cytotoxic agents. These symptoms even can occur for weeks after therapy is stopped. When caused by the disease, manifestations are persistent and are not explained by other factors.

Anorexia occurs in 49% to 82% of patients (7,13,28), especially if untreated. Nausea has been reported in 11% to 38% (7,13,15,28–30). When medications are excluded as a cause, however, the incidence is approximately 8% (16). Vomiting can be prominent (7,8,13,14,28–30); my own group has observed it as a symptom in 7% of patients (16). Diarrhea occurs in 4% to 21% of patients (7,13,14,28–30), and children have an increased incidence of all these symptoms (31).

MOTILITY DISORDERS

Recently, motility problems have been associated with SLE. Hirschsprung's disease has been reported in two patients with neonatal lupus (32). Chronic intestinal pseudo-obstruction (CIPO) reflects a dysfunction of the visceral smooth muscle or the enteric nervous system (31–34). Symptoms and signs of this complication in SLE include a subacute onset of abdominal pain and distension associated with vomiting and constipation and a distended tender abdomen with hypoactive or absent bowel sounds and lack of bowel sounds. Radiologic examination reveals dilated, fluid-filled bowel loops and occasionally bilateral ureteral dilatation with a reduced bladder capacity. Antroduodenal manometry demonstrates intestinal and esophageal hypomotility. Nojima et al. described two patients with CIPO who had antibodies to proliferating cell nuclear antigen (PCNA) but no other specific antibodies or clinical manifestations of SLE (37). Treatment of CIPO usually involves high doses of steroids, broad-spectrum antibiotics, and promotility drugs. Perlemuter et al. reported the use of octreotide in a dose of 50 μg twice a day subcutaneously in CIPO in SLE and scleroderma (38). The symptoms of CIPO resolved in the three patients receiving treatment within 48 hours. Recurrence of symptoms responded to increasing the dose of octreotide.

ABDOMINAL PAIN AND ACUTE ABDOMENS

Abdominal pain is found in 8% to 37% of patients with SLE (7,12–14,16,28), with the lowest incidence being reported in series that exclude medication-related symptoms. In 412 consecutive admissions to Cleveland hospitals for collagen vascular diseases (29), 63 patients had abdominal complaints; of these, 48 had SLE. Pain was present in 85%, and fever was noted on examination in 76% of patients and peritoneal signs in 10%. Corticosteroids were being given to 64%. An acute cause was determined in 33 patients, including duodenal or gastric ulcer, gastritis, and pancreatitis. Mesenteric vasculitis was present in three patients; in 16, the pain was of undetermined cause. Surgery was performed on 21 patients; in 11, it was exploratory. Al-Hakeem et al. identified 13 patients with a principal diagnosis of abdominal pain out of 88 patients with SLE who were admitted to the hospital during a 15-year period (39). Diagnoses accounting for abdominal pain included adhesions (three), diverticulitis (three), cholecystitis (two), perforated ulcer and colon, gastroenteritis, duodenitis, and inflammatory bowel disease (one each). Nine of the 13 patients required surgery. In another survey of 63 procedures, 16% morbidity and 6% surgical mortality rates were recorded (40). Min et al. studied the etiology of acute abdominal pain in patients visiting an emergency room (41). Twenty-six patients with SLE and abdominal pain made 44 visits to the emergency room. Twenty-seven (59.1%) of these visits were for ischemic bowel disease. Other diagnoses included pancreatitis, serositis, splenic infarction, angioedema, renal vein thrombosis, pelvic inflammatory disease, upper GI bleeding, and ectopic pregnancy. CT scanning and ultrasound help establish the diagnosis of ischemic bowel disease.

In the outpatient setting, abdominal pain in SLE may be from serositis, small-bowel bacterial overgrowth, or non-SLE causes. Serositis can present as an acute surgical abdomen as reported by Wakiyama et al. (42). Low et al. reported the characteristics of lupus serositis on barium x-ray and CT imaging (43). The small-bowel barium series showed segments of spiculation with tethering, angulation, and obstruction. CT scanning demonstrated ascites and asymmetric thickening of the small-bowel wall. Albano et al. investigated the prevalence of small intestinal bacterial overgrowth in 14 SLE patients using a lactulose hydrogen-breath test (44). Symptoms of small-bowel bacterial overgrowth such as bloating (50%), diarrhea (64%), constipation (42%), and abdominal pain (42%) were present in these SLE patients without any clear identifiable cause on history and physical examination. Breath hydrogen above 20 million parts per million with two distinct peaks of hydrogen production was diagnostic for small intestinal bacterial overgrowth (SIBO). Twelve patients (86%) were found to have SIBO by predefined criteria.

Abdominal pain and tenderness in patients with SLE can be the first manifestations of an intraabdominal disaster. Patients presenting with abdominal pain, even without tenderness, need an aggressive and comprehensive evaluation, including a complete blood count, amylase-level determination, blood-chemistry profiles, and abdominal radiography. If free air, moderate amount of free fluid, acidosis, or hyperamylasemia without pancreatitis is present, diagnostic laparoscopy should be performed. If pseudo-obstruction and/or thumbprinting of the bowel are seen without free peritoneal fluid, appropriate work-up and treatment should be instituted. Specialized tests, such as an upper GI, barium enema, CT, magnetic resonance imaging, gallium and indium white-cell scanning, and visceral angiography, may be helpful in specific cases.

Patients suspected of having an intraabdominal crisis should be placed on nothing by mouth and supported with intravenous fluids while undergoing these initial diagnostic evaluations. If peritonitis is suspected, broad-spectrum antibiotics should be administered. Symptoms of hypotension or third spacing warrant monitoring the urine output with a urinary catheter and inserting a central venous catheter or pulmonary artery catheter if required. Aggressive fluid replacement, antibiotics, and steroid stress dose coverage precedes laparoscopic or open surgical exploration. Steroid therapy can mask bowel ischemia and perforation. The best application of diagnostic laparoscopy is in the evaluation of a patient with equivocal findings. It can avoid an unnecessary laparotomy and offer an aggressive diagnostic approach.

PEPTIC ULCER DISEASE

The incidence of peptic ulcers in SLE has been reported as being from 4% to 21% (9,15,45,46), but these studies antedated the present era of endoscopy and gastroprotective therapy. Perforated ulcers have been reported (8,9,45,46) and were found in three (5.8%) out of 55 SLE patients presenting with an acute abdomen in a more recent report (47). Therapy with acetylated salicylates and NSAIDs probably is a more frequent cause of peptic ulcer disease than is active SLE. Siurala et al. (48) performed gastric biopsies on 17 patients with SLE; four had superficial gastritis and eight had atrophic gastritis in this 1965 report. Thirty years and ten gastroprotective agents later, this area is overdue for reexamination. Junca et al. investigated the prevalence of intrinsic factor and pernicious anemia in 30 patients with SLE and 45 control patients (49). Pernicious anemia characterized by the presence of low-serum cobalamin concentration, macrocytic anemia, and the presence of intrinsic factor antibody was found in only one patient (3.3%) though 23% had low cobalamin levels and 10% had intrinsic factor antibody out of the 30 patients with SLE. Archimandritis et al. reported a patient with SLE and vitiligo who presented with severe iron deficiency anemia as a result of a "watermelon stomach" (50). This condition is a result of gastric antral vascular ectasia and is associated with autoimmune disorders in up to 62% of patients with this disorder. The condition responds fairly well to moderate doses of prednisone for a few months but occasionally needs transendoscopic treatment or antrectomy. One case of Zollinger-Ellison syndrome with SLE has been recorded (51).

INFLAMMATORY BOWEL DISEASE

Ulcerative Colitis

Persistent diarrhea may result from ulcerative colitis that is rarely associated with SLE. Dubois noted concurrent disease in two of his 520 patients (7), and my own group has noted concurrent disease in two of our 464 patients with idiopathic SLE (16). Kurlander and Kirsner (52) elegantly documented the clinicopathologic correlations and remarked that lupus colitis and ulcerative colitis can be indistinguishable. Lupus colitis can be focalized to a single, small area (53). In 1965, Alarcon-Segovia et al. (54) reviewed the literature extensively and collected 19 cases of concomitant SLE and ulcerative colitis. They also presented eight additional patients in detail from their Mayo Clinic experience, which accounted for four of their SLE cases. In addition, 100 patients with ulcerative colitis were evaluated for SLE, which was found in three patients. In most, colitis preceded the onset of lupus. In this and other reports, symptoms and signs of lupus frequently began after the administration of sulfasalazine for treatment of inflammatory bowel disease (55,56). Folwaczny et al. found an increased prevalence of positive antinuclear antibody (ANA) in patients with Crohn's disease and ulcerative colitis compared to first-degree relatives and normal controls (57). Eighteen percent of Crohn's and 43% of ulcerative colitis patients had a positive ANA test whereas 13% of relatives of Crohn's patients and 24% of relatives of ulcerative colitis patients had a positive test. Two percent of healthy controls had a positive test.

Regional Ileitis

Concurrence of SLE and regional ileitis (i.e., Crohn's disease) is surprisingly rare and has been reported in only nine patients (58–65) (Fig. 40.1). Evidence that inflammatory-bowel disease may respond to methotrexate, azathioprine, anti-TNF therapy, and antimalarial drugs is intriguing, and this emphasizes the importance of initiating studies to delineate the relationship between inflammatory-bowel disease and SLE.

Collagenous Colitis

Collagenous colitis is a distinct disorder that is characterized by colonic lymphocytic infiltration of the surface epithelium. Patients have watery diarrhea but a normal endoscopic appearance and radiographic findings (66). This recently described condition responds to sulfasalazine and corticosteroids. Several reports have associated this condition with lupus (67–70).

One case of Canada-Cronkhite syndrome associated with SLE has appeared (71).

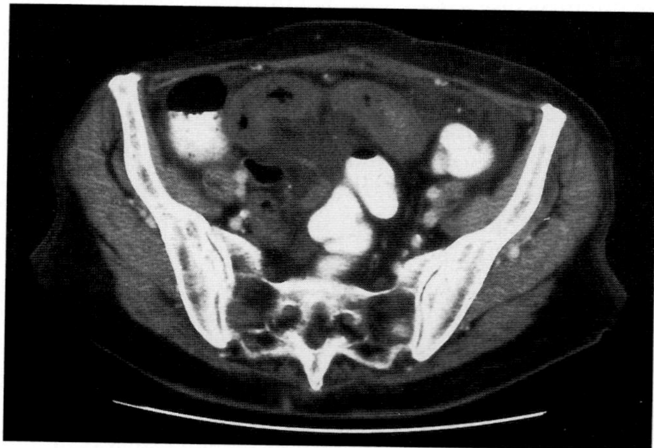

FIGURE 40.1. Lupus vasculitis involving mesenteric arteries causing bowel edema and necrosis of the small and large intestine. Histological examination showed vasculitis with small-vessel thrombosis. (Printed with permission from Cedars-Sinai Medical Center, Los Angeles.)

PROTEIN-LOSING ENTEROPATHY AND MALABSORPTION

The presence of severe diarrhea and marked hypoalbuminemia (reported to be as low as 0.8 g/dL) without proteinuria should raise the suspicion of a protein-losing enteropathy. Approximately 20 reports of clinically evident protein-losing enteropathy have been published, along with several literature reviews (47,55,72–77). Siurala et al. (47) studied the small intestine in patients with SLE and diarrhea. Among small intestinal biopsies in 19 cases, 12 were normal, and villous atrophy was noted in two. Radiographic signs as well as signs of intestinal malabsorption were found in seven patients. Subclinical cases can occur. Hizawa et al. described the radiologic findings in six SLE patients with PLE (78). He reported that there were two types of PLE, four patients presenting with acute onset of enteritis with abdominal pain, nausea, vomiting, and watery diarrhea, and the remaining two patients having mild diarrhea and developed progressive hypoalbuminemia. The first clinical presentation was associated with irregular spiculation and thickening, and thumb printing suggestive of ischemia, while the latter had thickened folds with nodules in them, which at biopsy were shown to be lymphangiectasia. Both groups responded well to steroids. The villi can be lustrous and swollen and may be of various sizes (81). Increased fecal excretion of intravenous radiolabeled albumin is the best quantitative study for following disease activity, although one report (82) has suggested that alpha1-antitrypsin clearance also can monitor response to therapy.

The cause of protein-losing enteropathy is unknown, but several theories have cited vascular damage, bacterial overgrowth, fat malabsorption, abnormalities in bile salt metabolism, thrombosis, and mesenteric venulitis as possibilities (79–81). Intestinal permeability may be altered in most patients with SLE as measured by Cr-51-labeled ethylenediaminetetraacetic acid (EDTA) resorption tests (83). Most patients have abdominal pain, and this can be the initial manifestation of their SLE (79). Cases have been reported of protein-losing enteropathy in association with Sjögren's (84) syndrome, interstitial cystitis (85), celiac disease (86), red blood cell aplasia (87), and as the initial manifestation of the disease (88). It may occur more often in children than in adults (89,90). Laboratory investigation may reveal normal lymphocyte counts, elevated serum cholesterol levels, low serum complement levels, antiribonucleoprotein (anti-RNP) antibody (91), and sterile paracentesis fluid with low white-cell counts (92). Lymphangiectasia is uncommon.

Response to corticosteroids is nearly universal, but some patients also may require a gluten-free diet (73,77,86,93, 94).

Mader et al. investigated a cohort of 21 SLE patients for malabsorption with a screening D-xylose absorption test, examination of the stool for fat droplets and with histological examination of a specimen of the duodenum obtained during endoscopy (95). Two patients (9.5%) had evidence of malabsorption manifested by an abnormal D-xylose absorption and excessive fecal fat excretion. Two other patients showed excessive fecal fat excretion. One of the patients with malabsorption had abnormal small bowel histology with flattened villi and an inflammatory infiltrate. There was no excessive deposition of immunoglobulins in the mucosa on immunoperoxidase staining. The etiology of the malabsorption was uncertain.

ASCITES AND PERITONITIS

Ascites can be the initial presentation of SLE. It occurs in 8% to 11% of patients, often as a manifestation of the nephrotic syndrome (15,30,96–98). Sterile peritonitis was observed in three of 704 European patients with lupus (99). In an excellent review of ascites in SLE, Schousboe et al. (100) classified ascites as either acute or chronic. Acute causes include lupus peritonitis, infarction, perforated viscus, pancreatitis, mesenteric vasculitis (101), and hemorrhagic and bacterial peritonitis (102). Chronic causes of ascites include lupus peritonitis, congestive heart failure, pericarditis, nephrotic syndrome, Budd-Chiari syndrome, protein-losing enteropathy, underlying malignancy (103), cirrhosis, and tuberculosis. Ascitic fluid can be inflammatory or noninflammatory. Noninflammatory lesions are always painless and associated with transudative fluid; most patients have nephrotic syndrome. Peritonitis usually is inflammatory and exudative. It generally is painful, but not always (98,104,105). Peritoneal tissue can contain immune complex deposits and inflammatory infiltrates (106,107). ANA, anti-DNA, and low complement levels can be present in peritoneal fluid (106,108,109). Reports also have appeared of concurrent familial Mediterranean fever (110,111) and of oligoclonal protein bands (112, 113) inducing ascites in patients with SLE. Fetal ascites in babies with Ro/SSA-positive mothers may result from congestive heart failure or from various immune mechanisms (114). Low et al. reported the characteristics of lupus serositis on barium x-ray and CT imaging (115). The small-bowel barium series showed segments of spiculation with tethering, angulation, and obstruction. CT scanning demonstrated ascites and asymmetric thickening of the small bowel wall.

Ascites caused by lupus peritonitis usually is steroid-responsive. Other causes may require additional interventions (100), including azathioprine (116) and cyclophosphamide (117). Gentle diuresis is an important adjunctive measure that often provides symptomatic relief, provided that renal function is not impaired by this approach.

PANCREATITIS

Pancreatitis can be the initial manifestation of SLE (118). First reported by Dubois in 1953 (28), it presents with severe epigastric pain radiating to the back, nausea, vomiting, an elevated serum amylase level, and dehydration. Seven of 704 European patients with SLE had a history of pancreatitis (99). Neither Fries and Holman (13) nor Ropes (14) noted pancreatitis in any of their combined experience with 350 patients. Ropes attributed this to the sparing use of steroids. Rothfield (119), however, observed pancreatitis in eight of 365 patients. Of 168 consecutive SLE admissions to the University of Alabama Medical Center, seven (4%) had pancreatitis; five of these seven succumbed (120).

Corticosteroids have been felt to play a role in causing pancreatitis in SLE patients. Hernandez-Cruz et al. reviewed their database of SLE patients and found 18 patients with 26 episodes of pancreatitis with an average SLEDAI score of 6.5 at the time of the acute pancreatitis episode (121). Eleven out of the 26 episodes were severe episodes and four patients died—three of pulmonary hemorrhage and one from septicemia. The most common cause was felt to be medication use (eight episodes) and hypertriglyceridemia, alcohol, and cholelithiasis were thought to be the etiology in four, two, and two patients, respectively. However, there were several case reports published about the occurrence of pancreatitis in patients with SLE with no other apparent cause (122,123,124). Saab et al. presented their data on eight patients with SLE and pancreatitis (125). The evidence showed that there could not be a role for steroid in the pathogenesis of pancreatitis in SLE. Steroid therapy often led to improvement of clinical findings and laboratory values in these individuals. Xochitl et al. compared the clinical and laboratory course of five consecutive SLE patients with no other obvious cause with five patients with biliary or alcoholic pancreatitis (126). Clinical resolution of pancreatitis in SLE patients took 6.8 days (range 3 to 15) whereas the illness lasted for only 4.2 days (range 1 to 7) in the control patients. Amylase and lipase enzyme elevation persisted in SLE patients for weeks after clinical resolution contrasting with earlier decreases to normal with other causes for pancreatitis.

Pancreatitis can be the initial presentation of SLE and may appear in childhood (127–129). Several cases of panniculitis and subcutaneous fat necrosis have been reported as being associated with SLE and pancreatitis (130–132), as has type I hyperlipidemia (133) with increased levels of chylomicrons and thrombi in pancreatic arteries because of antiphospholipid antibodies (134–137).

Corticosteroids, azathioprine, and thiazide diuretics are used in the treatment of SLE and may induce attacks of pancreatitis that are independent of the disease (138–140). Cases of pancreatic vasculitis were documented in the presteroid era (5). In 25 lupus necropsies, eight cases of pancreatitis were found (141–143). Four of these had pancreatitic vasculitis, and four were thought to have steroid-induced disease. Pancreatitis also can be caused by hypovolemia, ischemia, cholecystitis, alcoholism, carcinoma, and viral infections, all of which can occur in SLE.

Mild elevations of serum amylase levels may be noted in patients with SLE in the absence of pancreatitis. Hasselbacher et al. (144) studied 25 patients with SLE but without pancreatitis and 15 non-SLE controls. Amylase levels were elevated in five patients, and six had macroamylasemia, compared with none of the controls. The mean amylase level in the SLE group was 161.7 mg/dL, compared with 116.4 mg/dL in the control group; this difference was statistically significant. Macroamylasemia results from decreased renal clearance of an immunoglobulinamylase complex. The presence of a pathogenic autoantibody to amylase was proposed. Tsianos et al. (145) found elevated pancreatic and salivary amylase components in 11 of 36 unselected patients with SLE. Thirty-five percent of 20 children with SLE, most of whom were asymptomatic, had elevated serum cationic trypsinogen levels; this is indicative of subclinical pancreatic dysfunction (146). These reports have associated active SLE with elevated amylase levels without abdominal pain.

In their definitive study on lupus pancreatitis, Reynolds et al. (147) combined a literature survey with a review of 20 patients (75% were female). The mean age of their group was 34 years, and the mean disease duration was 3.75 years. The mean prednisone dose was 11 mg, and five patients also were taking azathioprine. Of the 20 patients, eight had recurrent attacks of pancreatitis, and amylase levels did not correlate with renal function or steroid doses. The mean duration of each episode was 15.5 days. The chief clue to the cause (i.e., lupus vs. drug induced) was that most of the patients with SLE-induced pancreatitis had multisystem SLE involvement (an average of 6.2 organ systems were involved) and responded well to increased steroid administration. Two literature reviews subsequently appeared (148, 149). One reported on 66 patients, 26 of whom were not taking steroids (146). Nearly 75% of the 66 patients had a fatal outcome.

Treatment includes immediate discontinuation of nonessential drugs that can induce pancreatitis (e.g., azathioprine, diuretics), intravenous hydration, nothing by mouth, antibiotics if needed, and sparing use of analgesics. The decision on whether to use corticosteroids is difficult if the patient has evidence of active SLE and is on high-dose glucocorticoid therapy. Careful observation is essential. Pancreatitis may induce diabetes (see Chapter 39).

MESENTERIC AND INTESTINAL VASCULITIS, MELENA, AND BOWEL HEMORRHAGE

Prevalence And Presentation

Mesenteric vasculitis, with or without infarction, is one of the most serious complications of SLE. Although Ropes

(15) found peritoneal involvement (from serositis) at autopsy in 63% of patients, with adhesion being common, only a small percentage had mesenteric vasculitis or acute abdomen. Vitali et al. (99) found that 1.1% of 704 European patients with lupus had intestinal vasculitis. Conversely, Landing's group noted ischemic bowel in 60% of 26 necropsies on children (9). Melena has been observed in from 1% to 6% of patients with SLE (7,13,14). Most mesenteric vasculitis presents with cramping or with constant abdominal pain, vomiting, and fever. Diffuse direct and rebound tenderness usually are present.

Four detailed and authoritative studies of lupus enteritis and other abdominal complications have been published (17,150–152). Zizic et al. (151) detailed five patients with large bowel perforation. All had active SLE and mesenteric or intestinal vasculitis. The presentation was insidious, with lower abdominal pain. Abdominal rigidity was present in only one patient. Most had nausea, vomiting, diarrhea, and bloody stools. All had tenderness, and most had rebound tenderness and distention. Bowel sounds were diminished or absent. Prior or concurrent administration of steroids masked symptoms in some, and it may have promoted the bowel wall thinning that led to perforation.

Chase et al. (150) recounted 15 cases of acute surgical abdomen in 140 patients with SLE. An increased incidence of peripheral vasculitis, central nervous system disease activity, ischemic necrosis of bone, thrombocytopenia, and rheumatoid factor was present. Of the 15 patients, 11 underwent exploratory laparatomies, nine were found to have vasculitis, and two were found to have polyserositis. Eight patients died, primarily from complications of infarction or perforation.

Shapeero et al. (153) reviewed the hospital records of 141 patients with SLE who were admitted to the Hospital of the University of Pennsylvania over a 20-year period. Of these, 68 had abdominal symptoms, and 20 were thought to have ischemic abdominal disease. In nine patients, this was confirmed radiographically by pseudo-obstruction of the gastric outlet, duodenal stasis, effacement of mucosal folds, spasticity, and thumb printing. Of these 20 patients, most had anorexia, nausea, vomiting, postprandial fullness, and abdominal pain. Only ten had melena, 35 had fevers, and 50 had guarding. In addition, 20 had leukocytosis, and 65 were anemic. All responded to steroid therapy.

Lupus enteritis can produce gastritis, mucosal ulceration, bowel edema with ileus, hemorrhagic ileitis, intussusception, perforation, and/or infarction (8,14,154–158). Spontaneous hemoperitoneum can be secondary to thrombocytopenia (159) or to ruptured aneurysms (160,161). Colonic diverticula (159) and mesenteric vasculitis (162, 163) may induce perforation. Antiphospholipid antibodies may play a prominent role in inducing intestinal infarction (163–167). Medina et al. studied the relationship between SLEDAI scores and the sources of an acute abdomen in 51 SLE patients (168). Patients with intraabdominal vasculitis (19 patients) or thrombosis (three patients) had higher SLEDAI scores than 14 active SLE patients with non-SLE related acute abdomens [mean 17.5 (range 13 to 24) versus 8.2 (range 5 to 11)]. Fifteen patients with inactive SLE (SLEDAI 1.7, range 0 to 4) had intraabdominal pathology that was diverse and not related to lupus. The authors emphasize early laporotomy in active SLE with high SLEDAI scores and an acute abdomen because the mortality in this subgroup was very high.

Laboratory, Pathogenetic, And Radiographic Findings

Laboratory evaluations are not particularly helpful. Acute-phase reactants and general indicators of active SLE usually are present. Paracentesis may be useful in ruling out pancreatitis or infection.

Apperloo-Renkema et al. (169,170) documented that patients with SLE have lower colonization resistance to indigenous bacteria of the intestinal tract. IgG-class antibacterial antibodies to fecal microflora are decreased in active SLE, which suggests sequestration in immune complexes that could play a role in mesenteric vasculitis. Small-intestinal bacterial overgrowth (SIBO) in SLE may be a result of decreased neutralizing antibodies to intestinal flora (44).

Radiographic changes include pseudo-obstruction of the gastric outlet, duodenal stasis, effacement of the mucosal folds, and thumbprinting. Thumbprinting represents bowel submucosal edema or hemorrhage on a barium or Gastrografin enema; this finding is relatively specific for ischemic bowel disease. Similar findings can be found using CT with contrast. CT of the abdomen has identified intraabdominal abscesses, lymphadenopathy, serositis, bowel-wall thickening, edematous and distended loops of bowel, pancreatic pseudocysts, and enlarged liver and spleens in patients with SLE (171–173). Ko et al. published their findings on radiological assessment of lupus mesenteric vasculitis (174). Of the 15 patients with mesenteric vasculitis, CT scans done within 3 to 4 days of the onset of abdominal pain revealed the characteristic palisade and comblike pattern of mesenteric blood vessels with vasculitis in 11 out of 15 patients. Peritoneal enhancement of ascitic fluid (11 patients), small-bowel wall thickening (ten patients) and a double halo or target sign (eight patients) were other common signs of mesenteric vasculitis (Fig. 40.1). Abdominal ultrasounds can show bowel-wall thickening (175). Gallium scans and indium-111 white-cell scans can light up areas of inflammation and sepsis (176).

The histologic characteristics and distribution of mesenteric vasculitis are similar to those that are seen in polyarteritis nodosa (151,177). The colon and small bowel often are involved with vasculitis in the submucosa. This results in ulcerated mucosa, submucosal edema, necrosis, and infarction (178). Two cases of appendiceal arteriolitis

(179) have been documented. Pneumatosis cystoides intestinalis may coexist with necrotizing vasculitis (180–185), and although usually benign, it occasionally can cause perforation.

Treatment And Outcome

The treatment of choice for lupus enteritis is 1 to 2 mg/kg/day of parenteral methylprednisolone (8,157, 186–190), or its equivalent, in addition to complete bowel rest. If a rapid response is not noted, surgical intervention may become necessary in cases of perforation or large areas of ischemia (153,157,187). Mesenteric vasculitis has a high mortality rate. One survey of patients with SLE undergoing surgery documented the widely held belief that in and of itself, steroid therapy increases the risk of postoperative complications (190). Grimbacher et al. reported successful treatment of relapsing intestinal vasculitis with intravenous pulse cyclophosphamide therapy (191). A summary of SLE and the GI tract is presented in Table 40.1.

LIVER ABNORMALITIES

Hepatomegaly

Enlargement of the liver was present in 10% to 32% of patients in the series listed in Table 40.1, with the frequency decreasing over the last three decades. An enlarged liver was present in 28 of 108 children with SLE who were studied by King et al. (12), and Ropes reported a palpable liver in one half of her patients (15). The liver usually extends 2 to 3 cm below the costal margin, but it occasionally can reach the iliac crest. Tenderness is uncommon unless viral hepatitis or peritonitis is present. Hepatomegaly and tenderness may be present with normal liver function tests. An enlarged liver can be histologically normal (192,193).

Jaundice

Jaundice was present in 1% to 4% of the patients listed in Table 40.1 and in nine (3%) of Rothfield's 375 patients (119). The most common causes of jaundice in SLE are hemolytic anemia and viral hepatitis; cirrhosis and obstructive jaundice from a biliary or pancreatic mass are responsible for the remainder.

Vascular Lesions: Hepatic Vasculitis, Portal Hypertension, The Budd-Chiari Syndrome, And Antiphospholipid Antibodies

Dubois described the first case of hepatic arteritis in 1953 (28). It was found in one of 58 necropsies reported by Ropes (15) and in 11 of 52 necropsies in Japan where it was specifically looked for (194) (Fig. 40.2). This rare complication of SLE (195) can be associated with ruptured hepatic aneurysms (196,197).

Five specific complications are attributable to antiphospholipid antibodies: (i) Budd-Chiari syndrome, (ii) hepatic veno-occlusive disease, (iii) nodular regenerative hyperplasia, (iv) liver infarction, and (v) transient elevation of hepatic enzymes resulting from multiple fibrin thrombi (198).

The Budd-Chiari syndrome is occlusion of the hepatic veins with secondary cirrhosis and ascites. It almost always is caused by thromboses in patients with antiphospholipid antibodies (199–207). This usually leads to portal hypertension, which rarely is seen by itself (208,209). In one

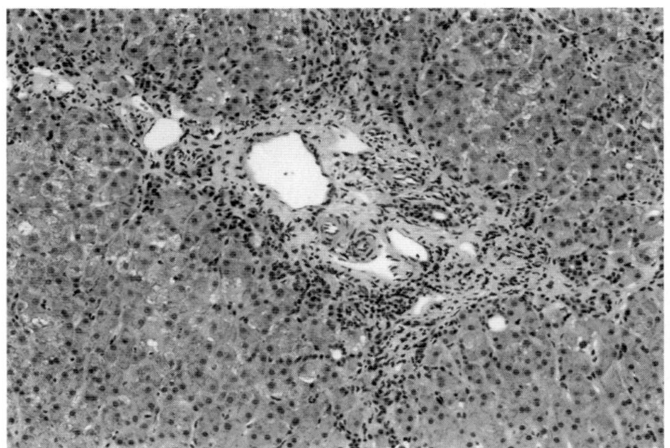

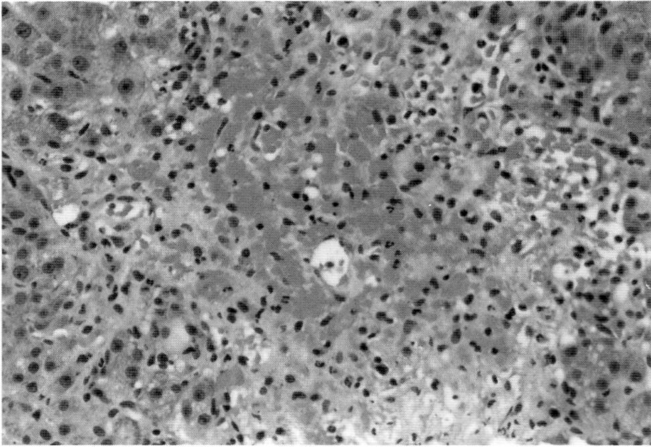

FIGURE 40.2. Biopsy of the liver in a 14-year-old Asian girl with classic systemic lupus erythematosus. Patient had a subacute onset of severe hepatitis (transaminases >tenfold) with negative hepatitis virus serologies and other hepatic autoantibodies and strongly positive antiribosomal P antibody. Patient had a complete recovery with high-dose steroids and azathioprine (H&E; 1:200). (Printed with permission from Cedars-Sinai Medical Center, Los Angeles.)

study, the disease was associated with antibody to proliferating-cell nuclear antigen (180). Hepatic infarction may be associated with pregnancy (210,211).

Neonatal Lupus Liver Disease

Lee et al. (212) found liver disease in four of 35 cases of neonatal lupus. Transient, although often severe, cholestasis was the principal finding, and no liver-specific antibodies were found. In a series of four cases (213), hepatic fibrosis was found along with giant-cell transformation, ductal obstruction, extramedullary hematopoiesis, and cholestasis.

Liver Function Test Abnormalities: Clinicopathologic Correlates

Liver function tests usually are obtained incidentally as part of blood chemistry panel. In SLE, nonspecific liver enzyme elevations are seen in a minority of patients and usually are of little significance. In our own experience, most liver function test abnormalities in SLE result from the administration of NSAIDs or methotrexate, or they are elevated because of increased muscle enzyme levels. Pathologic changes also are nonspecific and mild.

Rothfield (119) found elevated liver enzyme levels at diagnosis in 30% of patients with SLE, and Gibson and Myers (214) reviewed liver disease in 81 patients with SLE. Of these, 45 (55%) had abnormal liver function tests at some point, and 27% had enlarged livers. These abnormalities were accounted for by nonhepatic sources in nine patients, were drug-induced in 14, and from congestive heart failure in three. Of 19 biopsies that were reviewed, seven were normal, five had portal-inflammatory infiltrates, one had a fatty liver, and one had chronic active hepatitis. Only three of the 81 patients ever had transaminase levels exceeding 100 mg/dL. In another survey (215), elevations in liver function tests were associated with disease activity and liver membrane autoantibodies.

Altomonte et al. (216) compared 18 females with SLE but without known liver disease to 20 healthy controls. Significant differences included the following: delayed Bromsulphalein excretion (27%), elevated fasting serum bile acid levels (50%), and increased gamma-glutamyl transpeptidase levels (38%). Miller et al. (217) followed 260 patients with SLE and 100 controls for 12 months. Of the 60 patients with SLE and abnormal liver function testing, 41 could be traced to an identifiable cause (aspirin in 27, alcohol in six, and others in seven). In 12 of 15 patients with elevated transaminase levels, subclinical liver disease was a probable cause.

Runyon et al. (218) noted that 124 of 206 patients with SLE who they tested had abnormal liver-enzyme values; liver disease was identified in 43 patients. Biopsies were performed on 33 patients; 3 of the 206 patients died in hepatic failure. The ultimate diagnosis was steatosis in 12 patients, cirrhosis in four, chronic active hepatitis in three, chronic granulomatous hepatitis in three, centrilobular necrosis in three, chronic persistent hepatitis in two, and microabscess in two. None were positive for hepatitis B antigen. The pathology was thought to be drug-induced in 21% of patients. Corticosteroids were beneficial in eight of the 12 patients who received them. One third of 216 patients with SLE at Johns Hopkins had abnormal liver function tests over 1,717 visits, and elevations of their liver enzymes correlated with disease activity (219). On the other hand, severe liver disease can be present in patients with SLE and only minimal laboratory abnormalities (220).

Ropes (15) reported on 58 necropsies in SLE. Of these, 50% had an enlarged liver, moderate to marked fatty infiltration was observed in 44%, and portal congestion was noted in 47%. Hematoxylin bodies were seen in three, arteritis in one, and hemosiderosis in one. Fatty livers usually are associated with corticosteroid therapy, and several reports have commented on the presence of nodular regeneration and hyperplasia in SLE (201,221). The patients in these reports had normal liver function test results; this underdiagnosed finding could be secondary to steroid or danazol administration. Concentric membranous bodies in hepatocytes are found in hepatomas but occasionally are seen in lupus, and they reflect increased protein synthesis during regeneration (222).

Van Hoek reviewed the causes of elevated liver enzymes in SLE and found that medications such as nonsteroidal antiinflammatory medication, aspirin, or azathioprine was the most common etiology (223). Liver-function test abnormalities may result from non-liver–related causes such as unconjugated hyperbilirubinemia, hemolysis or hepatitis resulting from immunologic, infectious, or drug-related causes. Hepatitis resulting from SLE was most likely to be lobular and associated with autoantibodies such as anti-double–stranded DNA and antiribosomal P antibodies. In contrast, autoimmune hepatitis was more likely to be periportal (chronic active hepatitis) with rosetting of liver cells and dense lymphoid infiltrates and often has specific autoantibodies to anti-liver–specific protein or have anti-liver–kidney–microsomal antibody. Both conditions are associated with features of autoimmunity such as polyarthralgia, hypergammaglobulinemia, and a positive ANA.

In summary, most patients with SLE and elevated liver function tests have liver biopsy specimens that reveal nodules, mild fatty changes, or mild fibrosis. Rarely, features of chronic active hepatitis are found.

LUPUS HEPATITIS

Definition And Clinical Features

Lupus hepatitis may be defined as an insidious, rarely acute onset of transaminitis in patients who fulfill American College of Rheumatology (ACR) criteria for SLE, frequently have a positive test for ribosomal P antibody, and biopsy findings of lymphocytic infiltration of periportal areas with isolated areas of necrosis (223) (Fig. 40.2).

Our group found evidence for autoimmune hepatitis among 22 of 464 patients with SLE (4.7%) who fulfilled ACR criteria for SLE (16). Hepatitis was present in 2.4% of 704 European patients with lupus (99), and SLE was present in six (4.2%) of a group of Japanese patients with chronic active hepatitis (224). Chronic active hepatitis was found in 2.4 of 1,468 autopsied Japanese patients with lupus (194).

Patients usually present with nonspecific symptoms of fatigue, malaise, and anorexia. Jaundice is present in fulminant hepatitis. Mild liver enlargement, jaundice, or ascites in severe cases and other joint- and organ-threatening manifestations of SLE are found on physical exam.

Laboratory And Serologic Abnormalities

Elevations in serum glutamic-oxalocetic transminase (SGOT) and serum glutamate pyruvate transaminase (SGPT) usually are less than two- to threefold but in severe cases, marked elevation in transaminases (more than tenfold) with mild increase in bilirubin and alkaline phosphatase may be seen. Antibodies such as a positive ANA, doublestranded DNA, Smith, and hypergammaglobulinemia are seen. Antibody to Ribosomal P protein is a strong marker for lupus hepatitis (225,226). Patients with autoimmune hepatitis and primary biliary cirrhosis characterized by antibody to smooth muscle, liver-kidney microsomal and mitochondria rarely fulfill criteria for SLE. Of 89 patients with lupoid hepatitis who were followed at the Mayo Clinic, 43 had arthritis, ten had thrombocyotopenia, nine had pleurisy, and eight had leukopenia. Malar rash, pericarditis, neuritis, hemolytic anemia, and proteinuria were observed in two patients or less. Only nine fulfilled the ACR criteria for SLE (227,228). The overwhelming majority of patients are women, and an increased association with HLA haplotypes B8 and DR3 has been noted (229). In a comparison to 50 patients with SLE and 50 with chronic active hepatitis, 95% of the SLE group and 20% of the chronic active hepatitis group fulfilled ACR criteria for SLE (230).

TYPE I AUTOIMMUNE (LUPOID) HEPATITIS

In 1955, Joske and King (231) first called attention to the coexistence of LE cells in patients who had apparent viral hepatitis. Mackay et al. (232) continued their studies and, in 1956, coined the term lupoid hepatitis, believing it to be a manifestation of SLE. Despite steroid treatment, however, these patients all succumbed to liver failure an average of 3 years after presentation (233,234). Many early studies were conducted before the availability of ANA, smooth muscle antibody, antimitochondrial antibody, or hepatitis virus serologic tests. These reports are of historic interest and were reviewed on pages 91 to 93 of the second revised edition of this text (235). Mackay's 1990 review also is useful (236).

Definition And Clinical Features

Type I autoimmune (lupoid) hepatitis is defined serologically and histologically, and it is a subset of chronic active hepatitis (237). Histologic hepatic changes include periportal piecemeal necrosis, dense lymphoid infiltrates, and prominence of plasma cells. Serologically, patients have a positive ANA and high levels of gamma globulins, and antibodies to smooth muscle may be found. Chronic active hepatitis is associated with HLA-B8, DR3, and DR4, and it has many causes, including viral hepatitis A, B, or C; drug-induced hepatitis; Wilson's disease; alcoholism; primary biliary cirrhosis; and alpha1-antitrypsin deficiency, all of which must be ruled out (228,238).

Autoimmune hepatitis has an insidious onset. Generally found in a young or middle-aged female who complains of fatigue, malaise, anorexia, and low-grade fevers, there are usually no physical findings at first. Hepatosplenomegaly, jaundice, and signs of cirrhosis or liver failure occur late.

Sherlock (239) observed that 42% of patients with chronic active hepatitis have keratoconjunctivitis sicca and xerostomia. She thought that the incidence of ulcerative colitis, which is reported to be 10%, could be as high as 30%; it was found in five of Mackay's first 40 patients with lupoid hepatitis (233,234,240).

Laboratory And Serologic Abnormalities

Liver enzyme, gamma globulin, alkaline phosphatase, and bilirubin levels are elevated, the albumin level is decreased, and the prothrombin time may be prolonged (229,241, 242). LE preparations usually are positive, but they may become negative with claimed improvement (243). The ANA of autoimmune hepatitis has specificities for histones and granulocytes (229). ANAs are positive in approximately 10% of patients with nonautoimmune, chronic active hepatitis (243). Anti–single-stranded DNA (anti-ssDNA) is found in approximately 0% to 16% of patients with chronic active hepatitis (223,243–246). Up to 20% of those in both groups have anti-ssDNA. Other autoantibodies, such as anti-Sm, anti-RNP, anti-Ro/SSA, anti-La/SSB, and anticardiolipin antibody, are found in 0% to 5% of patients (244,246).

Smooth-muscle antibodies and antimitochondrial antibodies were present in 81 (30%) of Mackay's series (247) and in 64 (16%) of those reported by Leggett et al. (248). Antimitochondrial antibodies to M5 may cross-react with antibodies to phospholipids and yield false-positive readings in SLE (249). Smooth-muscle antibodies have specificity for actin (236). Antibodies to bile canaliculi have been claimed but not confirmed (247,250).

Other autoantibody systems that are found in autoimmune hepatitis include antibodies to liver-kidney-microsomal autoantigen, soluble cytoplasmic autoantigen, and M2 mitochondrial autoantigen. Five percent of patients with autoimmune hepatitis have false-positive antibodies for hepatitis C (239).

Association With Nephritis

Several studies have noted nephritis in patients with autoimmune hepatitis (251–253). Hepatitis B surface antigenemia is associated independently with glomerulonephritis (254). In one report (255), five patients with SLE who were hepatitis-B surface antigen positive underwent renal biopsy; lupus nephritis was present in two and antigen-associated nephritis in three. Renal tubular acidosis has been found in chronic active hepatitis (240,256, 257).

Treatment And Prognosis

Steroids remain the mainstay of treatment, prolonging life and making the patient more comfortable (229,240,258, 259). In a controlled study comparing prednisolone alone (40 mg daily at initiation of treatment and 15 mg daily maintenance), azathioprine alone (150–200 mg daily), and prednisolone azathioprine combined (10 mg and 100 mg daily, respectively), Mackay (260) reported that the relapse rate was lowest and overall survival longest in the combined-treatment group. All three regimens suppressed the disease, and indices of liver function showed improvement. Between-group comparisons for certain indices showed prednisolone alone to be superior to azathioprine alone. It was concluded that prolonged suppressive treatment has ameliorative effects while treatment is maintained, but that a long-term cure is infrequent.

Mistilis and Blackburn (261) recommended a daily dose of 60 mg of prednisone for the first 2 or 3 weeks, with gradual reduction over several months to a maintenance level of 5 to 20 mg daily. Steroids alone did not improve survival but did reduce early mortality. This group recommended a daily dose of 1.5 mg/kg of azathioprine to control disease activity, but other controlled studies have questioned the efficacy and safety of azathioprine (256).

Newer treatments for chronic, active hepatitis include interferon-, colchicine, and liver transplantation. Our group has shown that patients with SLE can safely undergo liver transplantation (262).

The prognosis of autoimmune hepatitis has improved. In 1968, the 5-year survival rate was reported by Mackay as being 65% (247). In 1988, he noted 80% 5-year and 70% 10-year survival rates with prednisolone and azathioprine therapy, respectively (239). Patients with autoimmune hepatitis have a slight, but definitely increased, risk of developing hepatocellular cancer, with approximately ten cases now documented in the literature (263,264).

OTHER CAUSES OF HEPATITIS IN SYSTEMIC LUPUS ERYTHEMATOSUS

SLE cohorts have the same incidence as control groups of hepatitis virus A or B antigens and antibodies (255,265). Autoimmune hepatitis rarely is observed in patients who are hepatitis B surface-antigen positive (242,265–267). Seventy-six patients with SLE in Singapore were tested for hepatitis B virus (HBV) infection; 15 (19.7%) had one or more of the three serologic markers for infection (267). This was comparable to the 19% positivity in 100 sex- and age-matched, healthy individuals. Lu et al. investigated the prevalence of hepatitis B in patients with SLE in Taiwan, which is a hyperendemic area for hepatitis B infection (269). The study also examined the level of interferons (IFNs) in both these disorders, which has been found to be low in both. The prevalence of HBV infection was lower than in the general population (3.5% versus 14.7%). The six patients out of the 173 SLE patients who had coexisting HBV infection and SLE had less active SLE with lesser degree of proteinuria and lower autoantibody levels than patients with SLE but no evidence of HBV infection. These patients and patients with HBV infection had near normal levels of IFN-gamma levels when compared to SLE patients. However, their levels of IFN-alpha were lower than in normal controls as well as patients with SLE. This suggests that subjects with low IFN-alpha levels are at increased risk for HBV infection and that IFN-gamma, which is probably induced by the HBV infection, ameliorates the activity of SLE patients who have coexistent HBV infection. Abu-Shakra and colleagues found no evidence of HBV infection in 96 SLE patients in Israel where the prevalence of HBV infection in the general population is 2% (268).

Some autoimmune hepatitis may be associated with the hepatitis C virus (HCV) (270). Antibodies to hepatitis C were found in four of 71 patients with SLE in an Italian clinic (271). Bronson et al. published a case report of a 35-year-old woman who developed an acute onset of SLE with manifestations of arthralgia, malar rash, low-titer double-stranded DNA antibody, negative tests for cryoglobulin and diffuse proliferative glomerulonephritis coincident with a HCV infection (272). McMurray et al. reviewed the serological and clinical manifestations associated with HCV infection (273). Autoantibodies that are specific for autoimmune hepatitis such as anti–smooth-muscle antibody are seen in up to 66% of patients with HCV infection (274). Nonspecific antibodies such as low-titer ANA (30%), anticardiolipin antibody (22%), and rheumatoid factor (76%) also are found in chronic HCV infection prompting the investigation of the prevalence of HCV infection in patients with SLE. Kowdley et al., Karakoc et al., and Abu-Shakra et al. investigated the prevalence of HCV infection in patients with SLE (268, 274,275). A total of 173 patients fulfilling ACR criteria for SLE had their assayed using enzyme immunoassay (EIA) and immunoblot assay. In one study, positive tests with either assay were confirmed by testing with a polymerase chain reaction (PCR) for HCV. Seven patients (4%) were positive for HCV by either assay but of the five patients with positive tests, only two patients had evidence of HCV in the serum by PCR testing. Thus, the true prevalence of HCV is probably close to that in the general population (0.5% to 1%). False-positive EIA and immunoblot assay can occur in SLE and PCR for HCV should be performed to confirm the presence of HCV infection.

Drug-induced autoimmune hepatitis has been reported after ingestion of the laxative oxyphenisatin (276) or after chlorpromazine (277). The picture can be confusing (without liver biopsy), especially because patients with lupus can develop viral hepatitis (as can any otherwise healthy person). Aspirin and NSAIDs are used to treat SLE but are hepatotoxic, and their effects can mimic those of chronic active hepatitis (278,279). Perihepatitis has been reported as well (280,281). Minocycline use has been reported to be associated with drug-induced lupus and autoimmune hepatitis in about 12 cases. An additional case of minocycline-induced SLE was described in Angulo et al. after taking the drug for 1 year for acne. A 22-year previously healthy woman developed arthritis, elevated liver function tests, and a positive ANA, anti–smooth-muscle antibody, and an antihistamine antibody (282). The hepatitis resolved after stopping the minocycline. The arthritis resolved after taking tapering doses of prednisone over 18 months.

Table 40.2 presents a summary of SLE and the liver.

BILIARY ABNORMALITIES: CHOLECYSTITIS, CHOLANGITIS, AND BILIARY CIRRHOSIS

Gallbladder disease is no more common in patients with SLE than it is in the general population. Cholecystitis and serositis can be difficult to tell apart (283). Cystic duct artery vasculitis commonly is seen in polyarteritis, but only a few reports have noted this in SLE (284–286). Kamimura et al. reported a case of acalculous cholecystitis in a SLE patient with abdominal pain and fever (287). Examination revealed positive Murphy's sign and pericholecystic edema with no gallstones on imaging. Treatment with corticosteroids resulted in rapid improvement of her symptoms and resolution of the pericholecystic edema in 5 days. The authors report that there were six previous cases of acalculous cholecystitis reported in SLE patients. The authors recommend surgical treatment if there is gall bladder distension on radiographs.

Three cases of sclerosing cholangitis and SLE have appeared (288,289).

Primary biliary cirrhosis (PBC) is associated with females who have features that are consistent with the CREST syndrome and antimitochondrial antibodies. Only ten patients with PBC who developed SLE later have been reported in the past (290–297). In one of the patients recently reported, the diagnosis of SLE antedated the diagnosis of PBC, which has not occurred in the previous cases.

TABLE 40.2. SYSTEMIC LUPUS ERYTHEMATOSUS AND THE LIVER

1. Hepatomegaly occurs in 10% to 31% of patients with systemic lupus erythematosus (SLE) and is seen in 50% at necropsy.
2. Jaundice is present in 1% to 4% of patients and is secondary to hemolysis, hepatitis, or pancreatitis.
3. Hepatic vasculitis is uncommon.
4. Budd-Chiari syndrome is associated with the presence of antiphospholipid antibodies.
5. Elevated liver enzyme levels are found in 30% to 60% of patients with SLE at some time. Most are caused by infections, salicylates, or NSAIDs. Enzyme levels greater than three times normal are rare.
6. Lupus hepatitis usually is insiduous in onset, varying in severity and frequently associated with ribosomal P antibody. These patients usually fulfill criteria for SLE and have biopsy findings of periportal infiltration of lymphocytes and isolated degeneration of hepatocytes.
7. Autoimmune hepatitis (lupoid hepatitis) is a form of chronic active hepatitis with malaise, arthralgia, fever, anorexia, jaundice, and negative hepatitis viral studies. Antimitochondrial and antismooth muscle antibodies often are present. Abnormalities associated with SLE, such as lupus erythematosus cells and antinuclear antibody are found. Most of these patients should be classified as being in a subset of chronic active hepatitis. Only 10% fulfill ACR criteria for SLE. Biopsy findings include piecemeal necrosis and are identical to chronic active viral hepatitis B and C.
8. The prevalence of Hepatitis B and C infection in SLE patients is not different to the prevalence in the general population.

REFERENCES

1. Grigor R, Edmonds J, Lewkonia R, et al. Systemic lupus erythematosus. A prospective analysis. *Ann Rheum Dis* 1978;37: 121–128.
2. Lee P, Urowitz MB, Bookman AA, et al. Systemic lupus erythematosus: a review of 110 cases with reference to nephritis, the nervous system, infections, aseptic necrosis and prognosis. *Q J Med* 1977;46:132.
3. Estes D, Christian CL. The natural history of systemic lupus erythematosus by prospective analysis. *Medicine* 171;50:85–95.
4. Osler W. On the visceral complications of erythema exudativum multiforme. *Am J Med Sci* 1895;110:629–646.
5. Reifenstein EC, Reifenstein EC Jr, Reifenstein GH. Variable symptom complex of undetermined etiology with fatal termination, including conditions described as visceral erythema group (Osler), disseminated lupus erythematosus atypical verrucous endocarditis (Libman-Sacks), fever of unknown origin (Christian) and diffuse peripheral vascular disease (Baehr and others). *Arch Intern Med* 1939;63:553–574.
6. Klemperer P, Pollack AD, Baehr G. Pathology of disseminated lupus erythematosus. *Arch Pathol* 1941;32:569–631.
7. Dubois EL, Tuffanelli DL. Clinical manifestations of systemic lupus erythematosus. Computer analysis of 520 cases. *JAMA* 1964;190:104–111.
8. Brown CH, Shirey EK, Haserick JR. Gastrointestinal manifestations of systemic lupus erythematosus. *Gastroenterology* 1956; 31:649–666.
9. Nadorra RL, Nakazato Y, Landing BH. Pathologic features of gastrointestinal tract lesions in childhood-onset systemic lupus erythematosus: study of 26 patients, with review of the literature. *Pediatr Pathol* 1987;7:245–259.
10. Costallat LTL, Coimbra AMV. Systemic lupus erythematosus: clinical and laboratory aspects related to age at disease onset. *Clin Exp Rheumatol* 1994;12:603–607.
11. Sultan SM, Ionnou Y, Isenberg DA. A review of gastrointestinal manifestations of systemic lupus erythematosus. *Rheumatol* 1999;38:917–932.
12. King KK, Kornreich HK, Bernstein BH, et al. The clinical spectrum of systemic lupus erythematosus in childhood. Proceedings of the Conference on Rheumatic Diseases of Childhood. *Arthritis Rheum* 1977;20(suppl):287–294.
13. Fries J, Holman H. *Systemic lupus erythematosus: a clinical analysis.* Philadelphia: WB Saunders, 1975.
14. McGehee Harvey A, Shulman LE, Tumulty AP, et al. Systemic lupus erythematosus: review of the literature and clinical analysis of 138 cases. *Medicine* 1954;33:291–437.
15. Ropes MW. *Systemic lupus erythematosus.* Cambridge, MA: Harvard University Press, 1976.
16. Pistiner M, Wallace DJ, Nessim S, et al. Lupus erythematosus in the 1980s: a survey of 570 patients. *Semin Arthritis Rheum* 1991;21:55–64.
17. Zizic TM. Gastrointestinal manifestations. In: P Schur, ed. *The clinical management of systemic lupus erythematosus.* New York: Grune & Stratton, 1983:153–166.
18. Fitzgerald RC, Triadafiliopoulos G. Esophageal manifestations of rheumatic disorders. *Semin Arthritis Rheum,* 1997;26: 641–666.
19. Castrucci G, Alimandi L, Fichera A, et al. Changes in esophageal motility in patients with systemic lupus erythematosus: an esophago-manometric study (English abstract). *Minerva Dietol Gastroenterol* 1990;36:37.
20. Clark M, Fountain RB. Oesophageal motility in connective tissue disease. *Br J Dermatol* 1967;79:449–452.
21. Stevens MB, Hookman P, Siegel CI, et al. The sclerodermatosus esophagus and Raynaud's phenomenon (abstract). *Arthritis Rheum* 1963;6:301–302.
22. Tatelman M, Keech MK. Esophageal motility in systemic lupus erythematosus, rheumatoid arthritis, and scleroderma. *Radiology* 1966;86:1041–1046.
23. Turner R, Lipshutz W, Miller W, et al. Esophageal dysfunction in collagen disease. *Am J Med Sci* 1973;265:191–199.
24. Gutierrez F, Valenzuela JE, Ehresmann GR, et al. Esophageal dysfunction in patients with mixed connective tissue diseases and systemic lupus erythematosus. *Dig Dis Sci* 1982;27: 592–597.
25. Peppercorn MA, Docken WP, Rosenberg S. Esophageal motor dysfunction in systemic lupus erythematosus. Two cases with unusual features. *JAMA* 1979;242:1895–1896.
26. Keats TE. The collagen diseases: a demonstration of the nonspecificity of their extrapulmonary manifestations. *AJR Am J Roentgenol* 1961;86:938–943.
27. Ramirez-Mata M, Reyes PA, Alarcon-Segovia D, et al. Esophageal motility in systemic lupus erythematosus. *Am J Dig Dis* 1974;19:132–136.
28. Dubois EL. Effect of LE cell test on clinical picture of systemic lupus erythematosus. *Ann Intern Med* 1953;38:1265–1294.
29. Flanigan RC, McDougal WS, Griffen WO. Abdominal complications of collagen vascular disease. *Am Surg* 1983;49:241–244.
30. Haserick JR. Unpublished data.
31. Glidden RS, Mantzouranis EC, Borel Y. Systemic lupus erythematosus in childhood: clinical manifestations and improved survival in fifty-five patients. *Clin Immunol Immunopathol* 1983;29:196–210.
32. Levartovsky D, Belmont HM, Buyon J, et al. Hirschprung's disease (HD): a novel form of neonatal lupus erythematosus? *Lupus* 1995;4(suppl 2):28.
33. Cacoub P, Benhamou Y, Barbet P, et al. Systemic lupus erythematosus and chronic intestinal pseudoobstruction. *J Rheumatol* 1993;20:377–381.
34. Perlemuter G, Chaussade S, Wechsler B, et al. Chronic intestinal pseudo-obstruction in systemic lupus erythematosus. *Gut* 1998;43:117–122.
35. Munyard P, Jaswon M. Systemic lupus erythematosus presenting as intestinal pseudo-obstruction. *J R Soc Med* 997;90: 48–49.
36. Mok Y, Lau CS, Wong RWS. Pseudointestinal obstruction in systemic lupus erythematosus. *Arth Rheum* 1997;40(suppl): S107.
37. Nojima Y, Mimura T, Hamasaki K, et al. Chronic intestinal pseudoobstruction associated with autoantibodies against profilerating cell nuclear antigen. *Arth Rheum* 1996;39:877–879.
38. Perlemuter G, Cacoub P, Chaussade S, et al. Octreotide treatment of chronic intestinal pseudoobstruction secondary to connective tissue diseases. *Arth Rheum* 1999;42:1545–1549.
39 Al-Hakeem MS, McMillen MA. Evaluation of abdominal pain in systemic lupus erythematosus. *Amer J Surg* 1998;176: 291–294.
40. Takahashi T, De la Garza L, Ponce de Leon S, et al. Risk factors for operative morbidity in patients with systemic lupus erythematosus: an analysis of 63 surgical procedures. *Am Surg* 1995;3: 260–264.
41. Min J, Park J, Kim S, et al. Acute abdominal pain in patients with systemic lupus erythematous entered in emergency room. *Arth Rheum* (abstract) 1997;40:S106.
42. Wakiyama S, Yoshimura K, Shimada M, et al. Lupus peritonitis mimicking acute surgical abdomen in a patient with systemic lupus erythematosus: report of a case. *Surg Today* 1996;26: 715–718.
43. Low VH, Robins PD, Sweeney DJ. Systemic lupus erythematosus serositis. *Australas Radiol* 1995;39:300–302.

44. Albano S, Hallegua DS, Wallace DJ, et al. Small intestinal bacterial overgrowth in systemic lupus erythematosus. *Arthritis Rheum* 1999;42(supplement):S305.
45. Dubois EL, Bulgrin JG, Jacobson G. The corticosteroid-induced peptic ulcer: a serial roentgenological survey of patients receiving high dosages. *Am J Gastroenterol* 1960;33: 435–453.
46. Dubois EL, Bulgrin JG, Jacobson G. The corticosteroid-induced peptic ulcer: a serial roentgenological survey of patients receiving high dosages. In: Mills LC, Moyer JH, eds. *Inflammation and diseases of connective tissue. A Hahnemann Symposium.* Philadelphia: WB Saunders, 1961:648–660.
47. Medina F, Ayala A, Jara LJ, et al. Acute abdomen in systemic lupus erythematosus: the importance of early laporotomy. *Amer J Med* 1987;103:100–105.
48. Siurala M, Julkunen H, Tolvonen S, et al. Digestive tract in collagen disease. *Acta Med Scand* 1965;178:13–25.
49. Junca J, Cuxart A, Olive A, et al. Anti-intrinsic Factor antibodies in lupus erythematosus. *Lupus* 1993;2:111–114.
50. Archimandritis A, Tsirantonaki M, Tzivras M, et al. Watermelon stomach in a patient with vitiligo and systemic lupus erythematosus. *Clin Exp Rheum* 1996;14:227–228.
51. Cadranel JF, Ruszniewski P, Lebiez E, et al. Neuro-lupus associated with Zollinger-Ellison syndrome with hepatic metastases: an incidental association? *Gastroenterol Clin Biol* 1991;15: 977–978.
52. Kurlander DJ, Kirsner JB. The association of chronic nonspecific inflammatory bowel disease with lupus erythematosus. *Ann Intern Med* 1964;60:799–813.
53. Palvio DH, Christensen KS. Systemic lupus erythematosus with rectal stenosis simulating tumor or diverticulosis (case report). *Acta Chir Scand* 1987;153:63–65.
54. Alarcon-Segovia D, Herskovic T, Dearing WH, et al. Lupus erythematosus cell phenomenon in patients with chronic ulcerative colitis. *Gut* 1965;6:39–47.
55. Alarcon-Segovia D, Cardiel MH. Connective tissue disorders and the bowel. *Baillieres Clin Rheumatol* 1989;3:371–392.
56. Font J, Bosch X, Ferrer J, et al. Systemic lupus erythematosus and ulcerative colitis (letter). *Lancet* 1988;i:770.
57. Folwaczny C, Noehl N, Endres SP, et al. Antinuclear antibodies in patients with inflammatory bowel disease. High prevalence in first-degree relatives. *Digestive Diseases and Sciences* 1997;42: 1593–1597.
58. Dubnow MH, McPherson JR, Bowie EJ. Lupus erythematosus presenting as an acute abdomen. *Minn Med* 1966;49:577–579.
59. Goldman DD, Ross T, Richardson B, et al. Bowel involvement in systemic lupus erythematosus: Crohn's disease or lupus vasculitis. *Arthritis Rheum* 1985;28:466–470.
60. Johnson DA, Diehl AM, Finkleman FD, et al. Crohn's disease and systemic lupus erythematosus. *Am J Gastroenterol* 1985;80: 869–870.
61. Knecht A, Rosenthal T, Many A, et al. Terminal ileitis in a patient with systemic lupus erythematosus. *Isr J Med Sci* 1985; 21:67–68.
62. Nagata M, Ogawa Y, Hisana S, et al. Crohn disease in systemic lupus erythematosus: a case report. *Eur J Pediatr* 1989;148: 525–526.
63. Shafer RB, Gregory DH. Systemic lupus erythematosus presenting as regional ileitis. *Minn Med* 1970;53:789–792.
64. Sugimoto M, Sato Y, Kumagai Y, et al. A case of systemic lupus erythematosus with lupus nephritis occurring in Crohn's disease. *Nippon Naika Gakkai Zasshi* 1989;78:583–584.
65. Constans J, Bernard PH, Bakhach S, et al. Crohn disease and systemic lupus erythematosus. *Presse Med* 1993;22:1193.
66. Bayless TM, Giardiello FM, Lazenby A, et al. Collagenous colitis. *Mayo Clin Proc* 1987;62:740–741.
67. Desmoulins F, Levy P, Boccaccio F, et al. Collagenous colitis associated with systemic lupus erythematosus: first case. *Gastroenterol Clin Biol* 1991;15:368.
68. Castanet J, Lacour J-P, Ortonne J-P. Arthritis, collagenous colitis and discoid lupus. *Ann Intern Med* 1994;120:89–90.
69. Boussen K, Mabrouk J, Ben Mami N, et al. Collagenous colitis with antinuclear antibody and chronic neutropenia. *Presse Med* 1992;21:1039.
70. Heckerling P, Urtubey A, Te J. Collagenous colitis and systemic lupus erythematosus. *Ann Intern Med* 1995;122:71–72.
71. Kubo T, Hirose S, Aoki S, et al. Canada-Cronkhite syndrome associated with systemic lupus erythematosus. *Arch Intern Med* 1986;146:995–996.
72. Azais-Noblinski B, Liscia G, Tubiana JM, et al. Acute systemic lupus erythematosus associated with protein-losing enteropathy (English abstract). *Ann Radiol* (Paris) 1988;31:183–187.
73. Braester A, Varkel Y, Horn Y. Malabsorption and systemic lupus erythematosus (letter). *Arch Intern Med* 1989;149:1901.
74. Perednia DA, Curosh NA. Lupus-associated protein-losing enteropathy. *Arch Intern Med* 1990;150:1806–1810.
75. Chung U, Oka M, Nakagawa Y, et al. A patients with protein-losing enteropathy associated with systemic lupus erythematosus. *Intern Med* 1992;31:521–524.
76. Sunheimer RL, Finck C, Mortazavi S, et al. Primary lupus-associated protein-losing enteropathy. *Ann Clin Lab Sci* 1994;24: 239–242.
77. Pelletier S, Ekert P, Landi B, et al. Exudative enteropathy in systemic lupus erythematosus. *Ann Gastroenterol Hepatol* 1992;28: 259–262.
78. Hizawa K, Iida M, Aoyagi K, et al. Double-contrast radiographic assessment of lupus-associated enteropathy. *Clin Radiol* 1998;53:925–929.
79. Bazinet P, Marin GA. Malabsorption in systemic lupus erythematosus. *Am J Dig Dis* 1971;16:460–466.
80. Casteneda S, Maldenhauen F, Herrero-Beaumont G, et al. Protein losing enteropathy as the initial manifestation of systemic lupus erythematosus (letter). *J Rheumatol* 1985;12:1210–1212.
81. Kobayashi K, Asakura H, Shinozawa T, et al. Protein-losing enteropathy in systemic lupus erythematosus. Observations by magnifying endoscopy. *Dig Dis Sci* 1989;34:1924–1928.
82. Benner KG, Montanaro A. Protein-losing enteropathy in systemic lupus erythematosus. Diagnosis and monitoring immunosuppressive therapy by alpha-1-antitrypsin clearance in stool. *Dig Dis Sci* 1989;34:132–135.
83. Wang SJ, Kao CH, Chen DU, et al. Intestinal permeability test in systemic lupus erythematosus. *Chinese Med J* 1992;49:2933.
84. Pena AS. Systemic lupus erythematosus, Sjögren's syndrome, and purpura in a patient with coeliac disease. *Neth J Med* 1987; 31:305–307.
85. Meulders Q, Michel C, Marteau P, et al. Association of chronic interstitial cystitis, protein-losing enteropathy and paralytic ileus with seronegative systemic lupus erythematosus: case report andreview of the literature. *Clin Nephrol* 1992;37:239–244.
86. Mukamel M, Rosenbach Y, Zahavi I, et al. Celiac disease associated with systemic lupus erythematosus. *Isr J Med Sci* 1994; 30:656–658.
87. Heck LW, Alarcon GS, Ball GV, et al. Pure red cell aplasia and protein-losing enteropathy in a patient with systemic lupus erythematosus. *Arthritis Rheum* 1985;28:1059–1061.
88. Lacasa JTM, Palacin AV, Minguez CC, et al. Intestinal malabsorption caused by bacterial overgrowth as the initial manifestation of systemic lupus erythematosus. *J Rheumatol* 1993;20: 919–920.
89. Hermann G. Intussusception secondary to mesenteric arteritis. Complication of systemic lupus erythematosus in a 5-year-old child. *JAMA* 1967;200:180–181.

90. Schaller J. Lupus in childhood. *Clin Rheum Dis* 1982;8: 219–228.
91. Edmunds SE, Ganju V, Beveridge BR, et al. Protein-losing enteropathy in systemic lupus erythematosus. *Aust N Z J Med* 1988;18:868–871.
92. Musher DR. Systemic lupus erythematosus. A cause of medical peritonitis. *Am J Surg* 1972;124:368–372.
93. Rustagi AK, Peppercorn MA. Gluten-sensitive enteropathy and systemic lupus erythematosus. *Arch Intern Med* 1988;148: 1583–1584.
94. Komatireddy GR, Marshall JB, Aqel R, et al. Association of systemic lupus erythematosus and gluten enteropathy. *South Med J* 1995;88:673–676.
95. Mader R, Adawi M, Schonfeld S. Malabsorption in systemic lupus erythematous. *Clin Exp Rheumatol* 1997:15:659–661.
96. Andreani T, Poupon R, Darnis F. Ascites disclosing systemic lupus erythematosus (abstract). *Gastroenterol Clin Biol* 1986;10: 845–847.
97. Averbuch M, Levo Y. Longstanding intractable ascites as the initial and predominant manifestation of systemic lupus erythematosus. *J Rheumatol* 1986;13:442–443.
98. Estes D, Christian CL. The natural history of systemic lupus erythematosus by prospective analysis. *Medicine* 1971;50:85–95.
99. Vitali C, Bencivelli W, Isenberg DA, et al. Disease activity in systemic lupus erythematosus: report of the Concensus Study Group of the European Workshop for Rheumatology Research. I. A descriptive analysis of 704 European lupus patients. *Clin Exp Rheumatol* 1992;10:527–539.
100. Schousboe JT, Koch AE, Chang RW. Chronic lupus peritonitis with ascites: review of the literature with a case report. *Semin Arthritis Rheum* 1988;18:121–126.
101. Jalil NS, Lee J, Hoffman B, et al. Lupus masquerading as CAPD peritonitis. *Adv Perit Dial* 1993;9:152–155.
102. Otano JB, Dominques LL, Goicoechea Fuentes AJL, et al. Spontaneous bacterial peritonitis in systemic lupus erythematosus. *Revista Clin Esp* 1993;192:147–148.
103. Aoshima M, Tanaka H, Takahashi M, et al. Meigs' syndrome due to Brenner tumor mimicking lupus peritonitis in a patient with systemic lupus erythematosus. *Am J Gastroenterol* 1995;90: 657–658.
104. Mier A, Weir W. Ascites in systemic lupus erythematosus. *Ann Rheum Dis* 1985;44:778–779.
105. Wilkens KW, Hoffman GS. Massive ascites in systemic lupus erythematosus. *J Rheumatol* 1985;12:571–574.
106. Bitran J, McShane D, Ellman MH. Arthritis rounds: ascites as the major manifestation of systemic lupus erythematosus. *Arthritis Rheum* 1976;19:782–785.
107. Ishiguro N, Tomino Y, Fujito K, et al. A case of massive ascites due to lupus peritonitis with a dramatic response to steroid pulse therapy. *Jpn J Med* 1989;28:608–611.
108. Jones PE, Rawchiffe P, White N, et al. Painless ascites in systemic lupus erythematosus. *Br Med J* 1977;1:1513.
109. Schocket AL, Lain D, Kohler PF, et al. Immune complex vasculitis as a cause of ascites and pleural effusions in systemic lupus erythematosus. *J Rheumatol* 1978;5:33–38.
110. Bakir F, Saaed B. Systemic lupus erythematosus and periodic peritonitis (FMF). *Br J Rheumatol* 1989;28:81–82.
111. Langevitz P, Livneh A, Zemer D, et al. SLE in patients with familial mediterranean fever (abstract). *Lupus* 1995;4(suppl 2): 11.
112. Miller FW, Santoro TJ, Papadopoulos NM. Idiopathic anasarca associated with oligoclonal gammopathy in systemic lupus erythematosus. *J Rheumatol* 1987;14:842–843.
113. Corbella X, Mitjavila F, Campoy E, et al. Chronic ascites in late onset systemic lupus erythematosus with antiphospholipid antibodies. *J Rheumatol* 1994;21:1141–1143.
114. Richards DS, Wagman AJ, Cabaniss ML. Ascites not due to congestive heart failure in a fetus with lupus-induced heart block. *Obstet Gynecol* 1990;76:957–959.
115. Low VH, Robins PD, Sweeney DJ. Systemic lupus erythematosus serositis. *Australas Radiol* 1995;39:300–302.
116. Kaklaminis P, Vayopoulos G, Stamatelos G, et al. Chronic lupus peritonitis with ascites. *Ann Rheum Dis* 1991;50:176–177.
117. Provenzano G, Rinaldi F, Le Moli S, et al. Chronic lupus peritonitis responsive to treatment with cyclophosphamide. *Br J Rheumatol* 1993;32:11–16.
118. Takasaki M, Yorimitsu Y, Takahashi I, et al. Systemic lupus erythematosus presenting with drug-unrelated acute pancreatitis as an initial manifestation. *Am J Gastroenterol* 1995;90: 1172–1173.
119. Rothfield N. Systemic lupus erythematosus. Clinical and laboratory aspects. In: McCarty D, ed. *Arthritis and allied conditions. 9th ed.* Philadelphia: Lea & Febiger, 1979:691–715.
120. DiVittorio G, Wees S, Coopman WJ, et al. Pancreatitis in systemic lupus erythematosus (abstract). *Arthritis Rheum* 1982; 25(suppl):S6.
121. Hernandez-Cruz B, Pascual V, Villa AR, et al. Twenty six episodes of acute pancreatitis in 18 patients with systemic lupus erythematosus. *Arth Rheum* 1998;4:S329.
122. Leong KP, Boey ML. Systemic lupus erythematosus (SLE) presenting as acute pancreatitis — a case report. *Singapore Med J* 1996;37:322–324.
123. Tahara K, Nishiya K, Nishioka T, et al. A case of systemic lupus erythematosus associated with severe acute pancreatitis. *Ryumachi* 1999;39:598–603.
124. Marum S, Veiga MZ, Silva F, et al. Lupus pancreatitis. *Acta Med Port* 1998;(8–9):779–782.
125. Saab S, Coor MP, Weisman MH. Corticosteroids and systemic lupus erythematosus pancreatitis. *J Rheumatol* 1998;25: 801–806.
126. Xochitl M, Carmen G, Medina F, et al. Enzymatic pattern in acute pancreatitis in systemic lupus erythematosus. *Arth Rheum* 1998;4:S330.
127. Giordano M, Gallo M, Chianese U, et al. Acute pancreatitis as the initial manifestation of systemic lupus erythematosus. *Z Rheumatol* 1986;45:60–63.
128. Mekori VA, Schneider M, Yaretzkty A, et al. Pancreatitis in systemic lupus erythematosusa case report and review of the literature. *Postgrad Med J* 1980;56:145–147.
129. Rupprecht T, Wenzel D, Michalk D. Pancreatitis as the first symptom of lupus erythematodes in childhood (English abstract). *Monatsschr Kinderheilkd* 1988;136:143–145.
130. Simons-Ling N, Schachner L, Pennys N, et al. Childhood systemic lupus erythematosus: association with pancreatitis, subcutaneous fat necrosis and calcinosis cutis. *Arch Dermatol* 1983; 119:491–494.
131. Saag KG, Niemann TH, Warner CA, et al. Subacute pancreatic fat necrosis associated with acute arthritis. *J Rheumatol* 1992;19: 630–632.
132. Feuer J, Speira H, Phelps RG, et al. Panniculitis of pancreatic disease masquerading as systemic lupus erythematosus panniculitis. *J Rheumatol* 1995;22:2170–2172.
133. Glueck CJ, Levy RI, Glueck HI, et al. Acquired type 1 hyperlipoproteinemia with systemic lupus erythematosus, dysglobulinemia and heparin resistance. *Am J Med* 1969;47:318–324.
134. Yeh T-S, Wang C-R, Lee Y-T, et al. Acute pancreatitis related to anticardiolipin antibodies in lupus patients visiting an emergency department. *Am J Emerg Med* 1993;11:230–232.
135. Hebbar M, Gosset D, Hatron PY, et al. Acute pancreatitis, systemic lupus and antiphospholipid syndrome. Two cases. *Rev Med Interne* 1995;15:146–147.
136. Wang C-R, Hsiet H-C, Lee G-L, et al. Pancreatitis related to

antiphospholipid antibody syndrome in a patient with systemic lupus erythematosus. *J Rheumatol* 1992;19:1123–1125.

137. Huong LT, Papo T, Laraki R, et al. Pancreatitis in systemic lupus erythematosus. 5 cases and a review of the literature. *Rev Med Interne* 1994;15:89–94.
138. Hamed I, Lindeman RD, Czerwinski AW. Acute pancreatitis following corticosteroid and azathioprine therapy (case report). *Am J Med Sci* 1978;276:211–219.
139. Oppenheimer EH, Boitnott JK. Pancreatitis in children following adrenal corticosteroid therapy. *Bull Johns Hopkins Hosp* 1960;107:297–306.
140. Paloyan D, Levin B, Simonowitz D. Azathioprine-associated acute pancreatitis. *Am J Dig Dis* 1977;22:839–840.
141. Paulino-Netto A, Dreiling DA. Pancreatitis in disseminated lupus erythematosus. *J Mt Sinai Hosp N Y* 1960;27:291–295.
142. Petri M. Pancreatitis in systemic lupus erythematosus: Still in search of a mechanism. *J Rheumatol* 1992;19:1014–1015.
143. Baron M, Brisson ML. Pancreatitis in systemic lupus erythematosus. *Arthritis Rheum* 1982;25:1006–1009.
144. Hasselbacher P, Myers AR, Passero FC. Serum amylase and macroamylase in patients with systemic lupus erythematosus. *Br J Rheumatol* 1988;27:198–201.
145. Tsianos EB, Tzioufas AG, Kita MD, et al. Serum isoamylases in patients with autoimmune rheumatoid diseases. *Clin Exp Rheumatol* 1984;2:235–238.
146. Eberhard A, Couper R, Durie P, et al. Exocrine pancreatic function in children with systemic lupus erythematosus. *J Rhematol* 1992;19:964–967.
147. Reynolds TB, Edmonson HA, Peters RL, et al. Lupoid hepatitis. *Ann Intern Med* 1964;61:650–666.
148. Eaker EY, Toskes PP. Case report: systemic lupus erythematosus presenting initially with acute pancreatitis and a review of the literature. *Am J Med Sci* 1989;297:38–41.
149. Watts RA, Isenberg DA. Pancreatic disease in the autoimmune rheumatic disorders. *Semin Arthritis Rheum* 1989;19:158–165.
150. Chase GJ, O'Shea PA, Collins E, et al. Protein-losing enteropathy in systemic lupus erythematosus. *Hum Pathol* 1981;3: 1053–1055.
151. Zizic TM, Classen JN, Stevens MB. Acute abdominal complications of systemic lupus erythematosus and polyarteritis nodosa. *Am J Med* 1982;73:525–531.
152. Zizic TM, Hungerford DS, Dansereau J-Y, et al. Corticosteroid associated ischemic necrosis of bone in SLE (abstract). *Arthritis Rheum* 1982;25(suppl):S82.
153. Shapeero LG, Myers A, Oberkircher PE, et al. Acute reversible lupus vasculitis of the gastrointestinal tract. *Radiology* 1974; 112:569–574.
154. Brown CH, Scanlon PJ, Haserick JR. Mesenteric arteritis with perforation of the jejunum in a patient with systemic lupus erythematosus. *Cleve Clin Q* 1964;31:169–178.
155. Bruce J, Sircus W. Disseminated lupus erythematosus of the alimentary tract. *Lancet* 1959;i:795–798.
156. Finkbiner RB, Decker JP. Ulceration and perforation of the intestine due to necrotizing arteriolitis. *N Engl J Med* 1963;268: 1418.
157. Hoffman BI, Katz WA. The gastrointestinal manifestations of systemic lupus erythematosus: a review of the literature. *Semin Arthritis Rheum* 1980;9:237–247.
158. Sonpal GM, Abramovici B. Acute abdomen in systemic lupus erythematosus with spontaneous hemoperitoneum. *J Rheumatol* 1987;14:636–637.
159. Korbet SM, Corwin HL, Patel SK, et al. Intraperitoneal hemorrhage associated with systemic lupus erythematosus. *J Rheumatol* 1987;14:398–400.
160. Yamaguchi M, Kumada K, Sugiyama H, et al. Hemoperitoneum due to a ruptured gastroepiploic artery aneurysm in systemic lupus erythematosus. A case report and literature review. *J Clin Gastroenterol* 1990;12:344–346.
161. Ho MS, Teh LB, Goh HS. Ischaemic colitis in systemic lupus erythematosusreport of case and review of the literature. *Ann Acad Med Singapore* 1987;16:501–503.
162. Molina Boix M, Ortega Gonzalez G, Perez Garcia B, et al. Perforation of the colon in systemic lupus erythematosus. *Rev Esp Enferm Dig* 1988;74:187–188.
163. Asherson RA, Morgan SH, Harris EN, et al. Arterial occlusion causing large bowel infarctiona reflection of clotting diathesis in SLE. *Clin Rheumatol* 1986;5:102–106.
164. Sasamura H, Nakamoto H, Ryuzaki M, et al. Repeated intestinal ulcerations in a patient with systemic lupus erythematosus and high serum antiphospholipid antibody levels. *South Med J* 1991;84:515–517.
165. Hamilton ME. Superior mesenteric artery thrombosis associated with antiphospholipid syndrome. *West J Med* 1991;155: 174–176.
166. Tincani A, Bozzetti F, Tardanico R, et al. Antiphospholipid antibodies and intestinal pathology. *J Rheumatol* 1993;20:2170.
167. Sanchez-Guererro J, Reyes E, Alarcon-Segovia D. Primary antiphospholipid syndrome as a cause of intestinal infarction. *J Rheumatol* 1992;19:623–625.
168. Medina F, Ayala A, Jara LJ, et al. Acute abdomen in systemic lupus erythematosus: The importance of early laporotomy. *Amer J Med* 1987;103:100–105.
169. Apperloo-Renkema HZ, Bootsma H, Mulder BI, et al. Host-microflora interaction in systemic lupus erythematotus (SLE): colonization resistance of the indigenous bacteria of the intestinal tract. *Epidemiol Infect* 1994;112:367–373.
170. Apperloo-Renkema HZ, Bootsma H, Mulder BI, et al. Host-microflora interaction in systemic lupus erythematosus (SLE): circulating antibodies to the indigenous bacteria of the intestinal tract. *Epidemiol Infect* 1994;133–141.
171. Boulter M, Brink A, Mathias C, et al. Unusual cranial and abdominal computed tomographic (CT) scan appearances in a case of systemic lupus erythematosus (SLE). *Ann Rheum Dis* 1987;46:162–165.
172. Heiberg E, Wolverson MK, Sundaram M, et al. Body computed tomography findings in systemic lupus erythematosus. *J Comput Tomogr* 1988;12:68–74.
173. Kirshy DM, Gordon DH, Atweh NA. Abdominal computed tomography in lupus mesenteric arteritis. *Comput Med Imaging Graphics* 1991;15:369–372.
174. Ko SF, Lee TY, Cheng TT, et al. CT findings at lupus mesenteric vasculitis. *Acta Radiologica* 1997;38:115–120.
175. Shiohira Y, Uehara H, Miyazato F, et al. Vasculitis-related acute abdomen in systemic lupus erythematosus ultrasound appearances in lupus patients with intra-abdominal vasculitis. *Ryumachi* 1993;33:235–241.
176. Spencer RP, Sziklas JJ, Rosenberg RJ. Waxing and waning of abdominal organ 67Ga uptake in a male with lupus: a potential for organ-specific therapy (letter). *Int J Rad Appl Instrum* 1987; 14:161–162.
177. Scully RE, Galdabini JJ, McNeely BU. Case records of the Massachusetts General Hospital. Weekly clinicopathological exercises. Case 171978. *N Engl J Med* 1978;198:1463–1470.
178. Helliwell TR, Flook D, Whitworth J, et al. Arteritis and venulitis in systemic lupus erythematosus resulting in massive lower intestinal haemorrhage. *Histopathology* 1985;9:1103–1113.
179. Derksen OS. Pneumatosis intestinalis in a female patient with systemic lupus erythematosus. *Radiol Clin* (Basel) 1978;47: 334–339.
180. Decrop E, Ponette E, Baert AL, et al. Pre-operative radiological diagnosis of acute necrotizing enteritis in systemic lupus erythematodes. *J Belge Radkiol* 1990;73:31–35.

181. Goldberg IM, McCord R, Schwartz AA. Right lower quadrant pain and systemic lupus erythematosus. *Am Surg* 1979;45: 52–53.
182. Kleinman P, Meyers MA, Abbott G, et al. Necrotizing enterocolitis with pneumatosis intestinalis in systemic lupus erythematosus and polyarteritis. *Radiology* 1976;121:595–598.
183. Lai KN, Lai FM, Lo S, et al. Is there a pathogenetic role of hepatitis B virus in lupus nephritis? *Arch Pathol Lab Med* 1987; 111:1851–1888.
184. Pruitt RE, Tumminello VV, Reveille JD. Pneumatosis cystoides intestinalis and benign peritoneum in a patient with antinuclear antibody negative systemic lupus erythematosus. *J Rheumatol* 1988;15:1575–1577.
185. Cabrera GE, Scopelitis E, Cuellar ML, et al. Pneumatosis cystoides intestinalis in systemic lupus erythematosus with intestinal vasculitis: treatment with high dose prednisone. *Clin Rheumatol* 1994;13:312–316.
186. Einhorn S, Horowitz Y, Einhorn M. Ischemic colitis in systemic lupus erythematosus. Treatment with corticosteroids. *Rev Rheum Mal Osteoartic* 1986;53:669.
187. Kistin MG, Kaplan MM, Harrington JT. Diffuse ischemic colitis associated with systemic lupus erythematosusresponse to subtotal colectomy. *Gastroenterology* 1978;75:1147–1151.
188. Morton RE, Miller AI, Kaplan R. Systemic lupus erythematosus: unusual presentation with gastric polyps and vasculitis. *South Med J* 1976;69:507–509.
189. Train J, Hertz I, Cohen BA, et al. Lupus vasculitis: reversal of radiographic findings after steroid therapy. *Am J Gastroenterol* 1981;76:460–463.
190. Papa MZ, Shiloni E, Vetto JT, et al. Surgical morbidity in patients with systemic lupus erythematosus. *Am J Surg* 1989; 157:295–298.
191. Grimbacher B, Huber M, von Kempis J, et al. Successful treatment of gastrointestinal vasculitis due to systemic erythematosus with intravenous cyclophosphamide: a clinical case report and review of the literature. *Br J Rheumatol* 1998;37:1023–8.
192. Klemperer P, Pollack AD, Baehr G. Diffuse collagen disease: acute disseminated lupus erythematosus and diffuse scleroderma. *JAMA* 1942;119:331–332.
193. Larson DL. *Systemic lupus erythematosus.* New York: Little and Brown, 1961.
194. Matsumoto T, Yoshimine T, Shimouchi K, et al. The liver in systemic lupus erythematosus: pathologic analysis of 52 cases and review of Japanese Autopsy Registry Data. *Hum Pathol* 1992;23:1151–1158.
195. Huang D-F, Yang A-H, Lin B-C, et al. Clinical manifestations of hepatic arteritis in systemic lupus erythematosus. *Lupus* 1995;4:152–154.
196. McCollum CN, Sloan ME, Davidson AM, et al. Ruptured hepatic aneurysm in systemic lupus erythematosus. *Ann Rheum Dis* 1979;38:396–398.
197. Trambert J, Reinitz E, Buchbinder S. Ruptured hepatic artery aneurysms in a patient with systemic lupus erythematosus (case report). *Cardiovasc Intervent Radiol* 1989;12:32–34.
198. Asherson RA, Khamashta MA, Hughes GRV. The hepatic complications of the antiphospholipid antibodies. *Clin Exp Rheumatol* 1991;9:341–344.
199. Disney TF, Sullivan SN, Haddad RC, et al. Budd-Chiari syndrome with inferior vena cava obstruction associated with systemic lupus erythematosus. *J Clin Gastroenterol* 1984;6: 253–256.
200. Hughes GR, Mackworth-Young C, Harris EN, et al. Veno-occulsive disease in systemic lupus erythematosus: possible association with anti-cardiolipin antibodies? (letter). *Arthritis Rheum* 1984;27:1071.
201. Klemp P, Timme AH, Sayers GM. Systemic lupus erythematosus and nodular regenerative hyperplasia of the liver. *Ann Rheum Dis* 1986;45:167–170.
202. Nakamura H, Uehara H, Okada T, et al. Occlusion of small hepatic veins associated with systemic lupus erythematosus with the lupus anticoagulant and anti-cardiolipin antibody. *Hepatogastroenterology* 1989;36:393–397.
203. Ordi J, Vargas V, Vilardell M, et al. Lupus anticoagulant and portal hypertension (letter). *Am J Med* 1988;84:566–568.
204. Pomeroy C, Knodell RG, Swaim WR, et al. Budd-Chiari syndrome in a patient with the lupus anticoagulant. *Gastroenterology* 1984;86:158–161.
205. Roudot-Thoraval F, Gouault-Heilmann M, Zafrani ES, et al. Budd-Chiari syndrome and the lupus anticoagulant. *Gastroenterology* 1985;87:605.
206. Van Steenbergen W, Beyls J, Vermylen J, et al. Lupus anticoagulant and thrombosis of the hepatic veins (Budd–Chiari syndrome). Report of three patients and review of the literature. *J Hepatol* 1986;3:87–94.
207. Takahashi C, Kumagai S, Tsubata R, et al. Portal hypertension associated with anticardiolipin antibodies in a case of systemic lupus erythematosus. *Lupus* 1995;4:232–235.
208. Drouhin F, Fischer D, Vadrot J, et al. Idiopathic portal hypertension associated with connective tissue disease similar to systemic lupus erythematosus (English abstract). *Gastroenterol Clin Biol* 1989;13:829–833.
209. Kato M, Noma K, Takeuchi Y, et al. A case of idiopathic portal hypertension supervening on SLE (systemic lupus erythematosus) a study of the possible role of SLE in the pathogenesis of IPH. *Nippon Naika Gakkai Zasshi* 1986;75:1836–1840.
210. Young N, Wong KP. Antibody to cardiolipin causing hepatic infarction in a post partum patient with systemic lupus erythematosus. *Australas Radiol* 1991;35:83–85.
211. Khoury G, Tobi M, Oren M, et al. Massive hepatic infarction in systemic lupus erythematosus. *Dig Dis Sci* 1990;35: 1557–1560.
212. Lee LA, Reichlin M, Ruyle SZ, et al. Neonatal lupus liver disease. *Lupus* 1993;2:333–338.
213. Laxer RM, Roberts EA, Gross KR. Liver disease and neonatal lupus erythematosus. *J Pediatr* 1990;116:238–242.
214. Gibson T, Myers AR. Subclinical liver disease in systemic lupus erythematosus. *J Rheumatol* 1981;8:752–759.
215. Kushimoto K, Nagasawa K, Ueda A, et al. Liver abnormalities and liver membrane autoantibodies in systemic lupus erythematosus. *Ann Rheum Dis* 1989;48:946–952.
216. Altomonte LA, Zoli A, Sommella L, et al. Concentration of serum bile acids as an index of hepatic damage in systemic lupus erythematosus. *Clin Rheumatol* 1984;3:209–212.
217. Miller MH, Urowitz MB, Gladman DD, et al. The liver in systemic lupus erythematosus. *Q J Med* 1984;53:401–409.
218. Runyon BA, LaBrecque DR, Anuras S. The spectrum of liver disease in systemic lupus erythematosus: report of 33 histologically-proved cases and review of the literature. *Am J Med* 1980; 69:187–194.
219. Petri M, Baker C, Goldman D. Liver function test (LFT) abnormalities in systemic lupus erythematosus (SLE) (abstract). *Arthritis Rheum* 1992;35(suppl):S329.
220. Atsumi T, Sagawa A, Amasaki Y, et al. Severe hepatic involvement without inflammatory changes in systemic lupus erythematosus: report of two cases and review of the literature. *Lupus* 1995;4:225–228.
221. Hubscher O, Elsner B. Nodular transformation of the liver in a patient with systemic lupus erythematosus (letter). *J Rheumatol* 1989;16:410–412.
222. Shapiro SH, Wessely Z, Lipper S. Concentric membranous bodies in hepatocytes from a patient with systemic lupus erythematosus. *Ultrastruct Pathol* 1985;8:241–247.

223. B. van Hoek. The spectrum of liver disease in systemic lupus erythematosus. *Netherlands Journal of Medicine* 1996;48: 244–253.
224. Horie Y, Kawasaki H, Hirayama C, et al. Chronic active lupoid hepatitis and HLA system: report of 6 cases. *Jpn J Med* 1991; 30:299–304.
225. Arnett FC, Reichlin M. Lupus hepatitis: an under-recognized disease feature associated with autoantibodies to ribosomal P. *Am J Med* 1995;99:465–472.
226. Koren E, Schnitz W, Reichlin M. Concommitant development of chronic active hepatitis and antibodies to ribosomal P proteins in a patient with systemic lupus erythematosus. *Arthritis Rheum* 1993;36:1325–1328.
227. Hall S, Czaja AJ, Ginsburg WW. How lupoid is lupoid hepatitis? (abstract). *Arthritis Rheum* 1984;27(suppl):S62.
228. Hall S, Czaja AJ, Kaufman DK, et al. How lupoid is lupoid hepatitis? *J Rheumatol* 1986;13:95–98.
229. Mackay IR. Autoimmunity and the liver. *Clin Aspects Autoimmun* 1988;2:817.
230. Chwalinska-Sadowski H, Milewski B, Maldyk H. Diagnostic troubles connected with differentiation of systemic lupus erythematosus against chronic hepatitis. *Mater Med Pol* 1977;9: 60–64.
231. Joske RA, King WE. LE-cell phenomenon in active chronic viral hepatitis. *Lancet* 1955;ii:477–480.
232. Mackay IR, Taft LI, Cowling DC. Lupoid hepatitis. *Lancet* 1956;ii:1323.
233. Mackay IR, Taft LI, Cowling DC. Lupoid hepatitis and the hepatic lesions of systemic lupus erythematosus. *Lancet* 1959;i: 6569.
234. Mackay IR, Wood IJ. Lupoid hepatitis: comparison of 22 cases with other types of chronic liver disease. *Q J Med* 1962;31: 485–507.
235. Dubois EL, ed. *Lupus erythematosus. A review of the current status of discoid and systemic lupus erythematosus and their variants, 2nd ed.* Rev. Los Angeles: USC Press, 1976.
236. Mackay IR. Auto-immune (lupoid) hepatitis: an entity in the spectrum of chronic active liver disease. *J Gastroenterol Hepatol* 1990;5:352–359.
237. Czaja AJ. Chronic active hepatitis: the challenge for new nomenclature. *Ann Intern Med* 1993;119:510–517.
238. Meyer zum Buschenfeldr K-H, Lohse AW. Autoimmune hepatitis. *N Engl J Med* 1995;333:110–116.
239. Sherlock S. Chronic active hepatitis. Definition, diagnosis and management. *Postgrad Med* 1971;50:206–211.
240. Taft LI, Mackay IR, Cowling DC. Autoclasia: a perpetuating mechanism in hepatitis. *Gastroenterology* 1960;38:563–566.
241. Mistilis SP. Active chronic hepatitis. In: Schiff L, ed. *Diseases of the liver, 3rd ed.* Philadelphia: JB Lippincott, 1969:645–671.
242. Soloway RD, Summerskill WHJ, Baggenstoss AH, et al. Lupoid hepatitis, a nonentity in the spectrum of chronic active liver disease. *Gastroenterology* 1972;63:458–465.
243. Gurian LE, Rogoff TM, Ware AJ, et al. The immunologic diagnosis of chronic active autoimmune hepatitis: distinction from systemic lupus erythematosus. *Hepatology* 1985;5:397–402.
244. Anderson PA, Harmon CE, Sjogren R. Anti-nuclear antibodies in chronic active hepatitis (abstract). *Arthritis Rheum* 1982; 25(suppl):S109.
245. Pollard KM, Steele R, Hogg S, et al. Measurement of serum DNA binding in chronic active hepatitis and systemic lupus erythematosus using the Farr assay. *Rheumatol Int* 1986;6:139–144.
246. Konikoff F, Isenberg DA, Barrison I, et al. Antinuclear autoantibodies in chronic liver diseases. *Hepatogastroenterology* 1989; 36:341–345.
247. Mackay IR. Lupoid hepatitis and primary biliary cirrhosis. Autoimmune diseases of the liver? *Bull Rheum Dis* 1968;18: 487–494.
248. Leggett B, Collins R, Prentice R, et al. CAH or SLE? *Hepatology* 1986;6:341–342.
249. Trujillo MA, Yebra M, Mulero J, et al. Antimitochondrial antibodies and the antiphospholipid syndrome (letter). *J Rheumatol* 1990;17:718–719.
250. Johnson GD, Holborow EJ, Glynn LE. Antibody to liver in lupoid hepatitis. *Lancet* 1966;ii:416–418.
251. Benner EJ, Gourley RT, Cooper RA, et al. Chronic active hepatitis with lupus nephritis. *Ann Intern Med* 1968;68: 405–413.
252. Silva H, Hall EW, Hill KR, et al. Renal involvement in active juvenile cirrhosis. *J Clin Pathol* 1965;18:157–163.
253. Taft LI, Mackay IR, Larkin L. Hepatitis complicated by manifestations of lupus erythematosus. *J Path Bac* (Lond) 1958;75: 399–404.
254. Golding PL, Smith M, Williams R. Multisystem involvement in chronic liver disease. Studies on the incidence and pathogenesis. *Am J Med* 1973;55:772–782.
255. Lai FM, Lai KN, Lee JC, et al. Hepatitis B virus-related glomerulopathy in patients with systemic lupus erythematosus. *Am J Clin Pathol* 1987;88:412–420.
256. Sherlock S. The immunology of liver disease. *Am J Med* 1970; 49:693–706.
257. Chng HH, Fock KM, Chew CN, et al. Hepatitis B virus infection in patients with systemic lupus erythematosus. *Singapore Med J* 1993:34:325–326.
258. Cook GC, Mulligan R, Sherlock S. Controlled prospective trial of corticosteroid therapy in active chronic hepatitis. *QJ Med* 1971;40:159–185.
259. Soloway RD, Baggenstoss AH, Elveback LR, et al. The treatment of chronic active liver disease (CALD) (abstract). *Gastroenterology* 1971;60:167.
260. Mackay IR. The effects in active chronic (lupoid) hepatitis of three long-term suppressive treatment regimes. *Gastroenterology* 1971;60:693.
261. Mistilis SP, Blackburn CRB. The treatment of active chronic hepatitis with 6-mercaptopurine and azathioprine. *Aust Ann Med* 1967;16:305–311.
262. Barthel HR, Wallace DJ, Klinenberg JR. Liver transplantation in patients with systemic lupus erythematosus. *Lupus* 1995;4: 15–17.
263. Lien CT, Kanel GC. Lupoid hepatitis and hepatocellular carcinoma (HCC) (abstract). *Hepatology* 1985;5:1051.
264. Satake Y, Takada K, Ikeda K, et al. A case of primary liver cell cancer complicating lupoid hepatitis. *Jpn J Med* 1988;27: 83–86.
265. Bonafede RP, van Staden M, Klemp P. Hepatitis B virus infection and liver function in patients with systemic lupus erythematosus. *J Rheumatol* 1986;13:1050–1052.
266. Bresnihan B, Jenkins W, Chadwick YS, et al. Chronic active hepatitis in a patient presenting with clinical and serological evidence of SLE. *J Rheumatol* 1979;6:38–42.
267. Lai FMN, Lai K-N, Lee JCK, et al. Hepatitis B virus-related glomerulopathology in patients with systemic lupus erythematosus. *Am J Clin Pathol* 1987;88:412–420.
268. Abu-Shakra M, El-Sana S, Margalith M, et al. Hepatitis B and C viruses serology in patients with SLE. *Lupus* 1997;6: 543–544.
269. Lu CL, Tsai S, Chan C, et al. Hepatitis B infection and changes in interferon-α and -χ production in patients with systemic lupus erythematosus in Taiwan. *J Gasteroenterology Hepatology.* 1997;12:272–276.
270. Nishiguchi S, Kuroki T, Ueda T, et al. Detection of hepatitis C

virus antibody in the absence of viral RNA in patients with autoimmune hepatitis. *Ann Intern Med* 1992;116:21–25.

271. Marchesoni A, Battafaranco N, Podico M, et al. Hepatitis C virus antibodies and systemic lupus erythematosus. *Clin Exp Rheumatol* 1995;13:267–273.
272. Bronson W, McMurray R. Hepatitis C Virus and Systemic Lupus Erythematosus. *J Clinical Rheumatology*. 1997;3: 153–156.
273. McMurray RW, Elbourne K. Hepatitis C virus infection and autoimmunity. *Seminars in Arthritis and Rheumatism* 1997;26: 689–701.
274. Kowdley KV, Subler DE, Scheffel J, et al. Hepatitis C virus antibodies in systemic lupus erythematosus. *J Clin Gastroenterol* 1997;25:437–439.
275. Karakoc Y, Dilek K, Akalyn H, et al. Prevalence of hepatitis C virus antibody in patients with systemic lupus erythematosus. Letters, Matters arising.
276. Reynolds TB, Peters RL, Yamada S. Chronic active and lupoid hepatitis caused by a laxative, oxyphenisatin. *N Engl J Med* 1971;285:813–820.
277. Russell RI, Allan JG, Patrick R. Active chronic hepatitis after chlorpromazine ingestion. *Br Med J* 1973;1:655–656.
278. Seaman WE, Ishak KG, Plotz PH. Aspirin-induced hepatotoxicity in patients with systemic lupus erythematosus. *Ann Intern Med* 1974;80:18.
279. Seaman WE, Plotz PH. Effect of aspirin on liver tests in patients with RA or SLE and in normal volunteers. *Arthritis Rheum* 1976;19:155–160.
280. Bonnin A, Besancenot JF, Caillot D, et al. Perihepatitis and lupus erythematosus. *Rev Med Interne* 1985;6:301–302.
281. Emilie D, Wechsler B, Belmatoug N, et al. Perihepatitis and lupus. *Rev Med Interne* 1985;6:462–463.
282. Angulo JM, Sigal LH, Espinoza LR. Minocycline induced Lupus and Autoimmune Hepatitis. *J Rheumatol* 1999;26:1420–1421.
283. Martinez D, Lowe R. Case report: systemic lupus erythematosus (SLE) serositis mimicking acute cholecystitis. *Clin Radiol* 1991;44:434–435.
284. Newbold KM, Allum WH, Downing R, et al. Vasculitis of the gall bladder in rheumatoid arthritis and systemic lupus erythematosus. *Clin Rheumatol* 1987;6:287–289.
285. Raijman I, Schrager M. Hemorrhagic acalculous cholecystitis in systemic lupus erythematosus (letter). *Am J Gastroenterol* 1989; 84:445–447.
286. Swanepoel CR, Floyd A, Allison H, et al. Acute acalculous cholecystitis complicating systemic lupus erythematosus: case report and review. *Br Med J (Clin Res)* 1983;286:251–252.
287. Kamimura T, Mimori A, Takeda A, et al. Acute acalculous cholecystitis in systemic lupus erythematosus: a case report and review of the literature. *Lupus* 1998;7:361–363.
288. Lamy P, Valla D, Bourgeois P, et al. Primary sclerosing cholangitis and systemic lupus erythematosus. *Gastroenterol Clin Biol* 1988;12:962–964.
289. Audan A, Bruley des Varannes S, Georgelin T, et al. Primary sclerosing cholangitis and systemic lupus erythematosus. *Gastroenterol Clin Biol* 1995;19:123–126.
290. Clark M, Sack K. Deforming arthropathy complicating primary biliary cirrhosis. *J Rheumatol* 1991;18:619–621.
291. Iliffe GD, Naidoo S, Hunter T. Primary biliary cirrhosis associated with systemic lupus erythematosus. *Dig Dis Sci* 1982;27: 274–278.
292. Krulik M, Aylberait D, Vittexoq D, et al. Primary biliary cirrhosis associated with systemic lupus erythematosus: case report. *La Nouvelle Presse Medicale* 1980;8:31–34.
293. Saki S, Tanaka K, Fujisawa M, et al. A patient with asymptomatic primary biliary cirrhosis in association with Sjögren syndrome developing features of systemic lupus erythematosus. *Nippon Shokakibyo Gakkai Zasshi* 1986;83:2445–2449.
294. Nachbar F, Korting HC, Hoffmann RM, et al. Unusual coexistence of systemic lupus erythematosus and primary biliary cirrhosis. *Dermatology* 1994;188:313–317.
295. Islam S, Riordan JW, McDonald JA. A rare association of primary biliary cirrhosis and systemic lupus erythematosus and review of the literature. *J Gastroenterol and Hepatology* 1999:14: 431–435.
296. Shifter T, Lewinski UH. Primary biliary cirrhosis and systemic lupus erythematosus. A rare association. *Clinical and Experimental Rheumatology* 1997;15:313–314.
297. Michel F, Toussirot E, Wendling D. Primary biliary cirrhosis and systemic lupus erythematosus. A new case report. *Rev. Rheum (Engl. Ed.)* 1998;65:504–507.

41

SYSTEMIC LUPUS ERYTHEMATOSUS IN CHILDHOOD AND ADOLESCENCE

THOMAS J.A. LEHMAN

Children and adolescents with systemic lupus erythematosus (SLE) represent both a special challenge and a special opportunity. Early onset allows us to observe the natural history of SLE and investigate potential etiologies, free from the confounding factors that frequently are present in older patients (1). The impact of SLE on children and adolescents, however, often is profound. Recognition of the special considerations that relate to ongoing physical and emotional growth directly influences the choice of medications and the likelihood of success. Satisfactory outcome for a child or adolescent with SLE is not 5- or 10-year survival, into the earliest years of adulthood, but 50- or 60-year survival, which more closely approximates the normal human lifespan.

Awareness of the complex interaction between the child's illness and the needs of his or her family is critical to successful care. Children and adolescents are emotionally immature individuals just beginning to formulate their concept of self. They are extremely vulnerable to the psychologic impact of both chronic illness and medications that dramatically alter their appearance (Fig. 41.1). Family and peer-group pressures, which are difficult even for normal children, may be overwhelming for the child or adolescent with SLE. The interaction of these special needs with the complexities of SLE makes caring for children and adolescents with SLE a unique process. Optimal results require excellent medical care coupled with multidisciplinary patient and family education and support.

Childhood-onset SLE often is described as more severe than adult-onset disease (2), and early age of onset has been correlated with a worse prognosis (3). Other studies, however, have suggested an improved prognosis for children and adolescents with SLE (4,5). In published series, a large proportion of both children and adolescents with SLE have significant renal or central nervous system (CNS) involvement (6–14), but many cases of mild SLE in children and adolescents probably go unreported, either because they are not recognized or they never warrant referral to specialized centers. Delayed diagnosis because physicians failed to consider SLE in the differential diagnosis of a young or male child is one of the greatest risks to children and adolescents with SLE. Severe damage to the evolving self-image and sense of worth is another complication of SLE that is unique to children and adolescents. Both of these problems may profoundly affect the prognosis.

English-language reports of children with SLE appeared as early as 1892 (15). Sequeira and Balean (16), writing from the London Hospital in 1902, noted that the disease commences early in life in a much larger proportion of cases than is commonly believed. Eight children with SLE were among 71 cases they reported. Further reports of SLE in childhood continued to appear throughout the 1920s, 1930s, and 1940s (17–22).

The modern era began in the 1950s and 1960s, when series of children with SLE began to be published. Zetterstrom and Berglund (23) described ten patients in 1956, and Gribetz and Henley (24) described an additional 15 in 1959. Between 1960 and 1968, more than 150 additional children with SLE were described (2,8,12,25). The total number of children with SLE in published series now exceeds 500 (5–7,9,11,13,14,26–28).

In the presteroid era, childhood-onset SLE was a rapidly evolving, and usually fatal, multisystem disease. Since the 1960s, however, corticosteroids and improved pediatric care have resulted in greatly enhanced survival (4,29). SLE now is a common diagnosis in every large pediatric rheumatology program. Systematic management and vigorous treatment protocols are rapidly improving the outlook for children with even the most severe disease (30,31). With proper care, most children and adolescents with SLE now have an excellent prognosis.

EPIDEMIOLOGY

Despite the many published cases of childhood SLE, its true incidence and prevalence are unknown (32). Fessel's 1973 survey of 126,000 members of the Kaiser Permanente

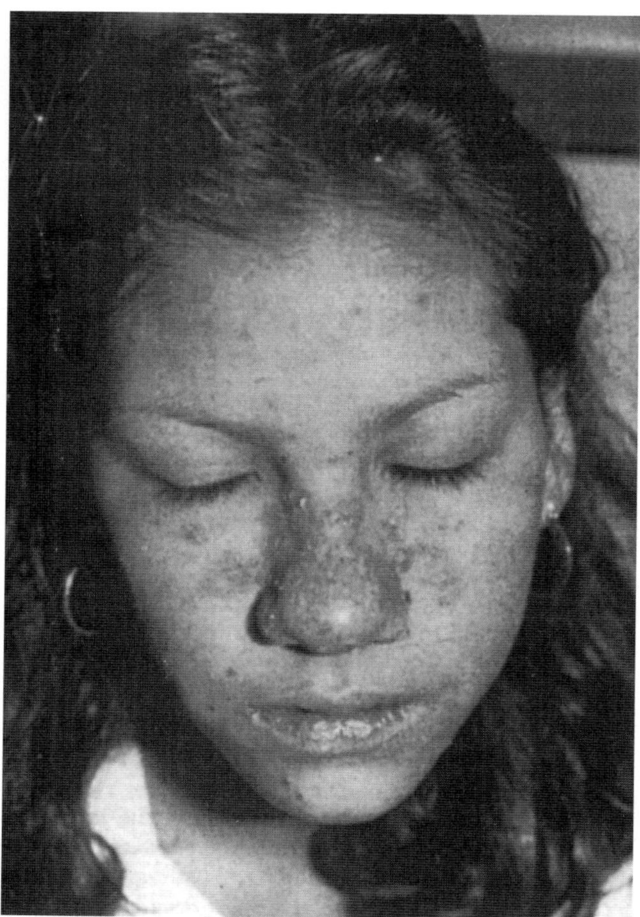

FIGURE 41.1. Markedly altered facial appearance resulting from skin manifestations in a teenage female with systemic lupus erythematosus.

plan did not report any patients with onset of SLE before 15 years of age (33). Siegel and Lee (34) estimated the annual incidence of SLE in childhood to be 0.6 per 100,000. Hochberg (35) found a similar incidence in Baltimore. Studies coordinating multiple regional pediatric rheumatology centers in New England and in Canada found a similar annual incidence of approximately 0.4 per 100,000 (35,37). The Canadian study (37) was complicated by wide differences in the incidence of SLE in the data from various reporting institutions. Every effort to provide an accurate determination of the incidence of SLE has been complicated by the recognized variations in racial incidence and geographic referral patterns. Although better numbers have been provided by countries where every child with a specific diagnosis is reported to a central registry, these countries have lacked the ethnic diversity that is found in larger countries, making their data inapplicable. Efforts to develop a central registry for children with SLE to provide demographically more diverse information are underway.

Because of the difficulties in assessing the true incidence of SLE, the prevalence of childhood SLE can only be estimated. Figures from the regional referral center in Los Angeles suggest there are between 5,000 and 10,000 children with SLE in the United States (5). A similar estimate arises from the assumption that children with SLE are 0.10 as common as children with juvenile rheumatoid arthritis (JRA) (32). [The corresponding prevalence of SLE is five to ten per 100,000 children (38–41), again suggesting 5000 to 10,000 children with SLE in the United States.] Unfortunately, these figures represent only a first approximation of the true prevalence of SLE in children and adolescents.

The influences of sex and racial origin on the occurrence and manifestations of SLE are widely recognized (5,34,42, 43). In childhood, the influence of race is striking. The age- and sex-adjusted prevalence of SLE in black, Asian, and Hispanic children were more than threefold that of white children at one large center (5). Female sex, age, and race were even more striking influences when the incidence of SLE among pre- and postpubertal children was considered. For all male children, the frequency of SLE rose from 1 per 100,000 male children aged 1 through 9 years to 1.61 per 100,000 male children aged 10 through 19 years (i.e., a 60% increase with puberty). For white females, the increase with puberty was from 1.27 to 4.40 per 100,000 (246%); for black females, 3.72 to 19.86 per 100,000 (434%); and for Asian females, 6.16 to 31.14 per 100,000 (406%). In contrast, the increase for Hispanic females was only 4.62 to 13.00 per 100,000 (181%) (5). Although based on a limited sample, these data suggest a marked variation in the influence of sex hormones on the predisposition to SLE among different races.

CAUSATIVE FACTORS

The cause of SLE remains unknown. The availability of parents and siblings who live in the same household as children with SLE, however, provides a unique opportunity to evaluate environmental and genetic hypotheses. Many studies have demonstrated an increased frequency of immunologic abnormalities in first-degree relatives of both adults and children with SLE (44–56). These studies have been interpreted as evidence both of an infectious cause and of a genetic predisposition. Current evidence suggests that both environmental and genetic factors are important with preliminary data suggesting that Epstein Barr virus infection may have a pivotal role in the susceptible host (1). (These theories are discussed in detail in other chapters.)

Much of the evidence for a genetic predisposition to SLE has come from studies of twin and sibling pairs. Many twin pairs have onset of SLE in childhood or adolescence. Identical twins with the onset of SLE as early as 3 years of age have been reported (57). The percentage of identical twins who are concordant for lupus may be as high as 70 (58), but this figure has been challenged. When both twins develop SLE, they typically have the onset of disease at a similar and earlier age when compared to non-identical in siblings who develop SLE (16.5 + 7.9 vs. 26.2 + 20.5 years) (59).

Additional evidence for a genetic component of SLE has come from the study of immunologic abnormalities in family members of children with SLE. Expression of this genetic component appears to be promoted by female sex hormones. In a study of 34 families having children with SLE, Ro/SSA antibody-positive mothers were more likely than Ro/SSA negative mothers to have Ro/SSA antibody-positive daughters (7/11 vs. 4/18, $P < .05$ probands excluded). There was no association between Ro/SSA antibody-positive fathers and sons: however, Ro/SSA antibody-positive fathers had fewer male children than expected (5 sons/12 daughters for Ro/SSA antibody-positive fathers vs. 19 sons/19 daughters for Ro/SSA antibody-negative fathers, $P < .05$) (60). The explanation for the decreased number of male offspring remains under investigation.

The frequent occurrence of serologic abnormalities in the families of children with SLE strongly supports the "supergene" hypothesis. Formulated in response to the occurrence of multiple autoimmune diseases within some families (61,62), the "supergene" hypothesis proposes the existence of a single gene that predisposes to autoimmune disease. The subsequent occurrence of autoimmune disease in carriers of this gene is determined both by its interaction with the remainder of the genome and by environmental events. Efforts to evaluate this hypothesis have been hampered by the absence of a means for identifying carriers of the supergene. The increased frequency and amount of antibodies to Ro/SSA in mothers of children with SLE may be evidence of this supergene expression in otherwise well individuals (50). Ro/SSA antibody expression is linked to histocompatibility antigens in patients with SLE and Sjögren's syndrome (63). Efforts to link Ro/SSA expression to a specific haplotype in children with SLE and their families continue.

Antiphospholipid antibodies are an additional immunologic abnormality, which occurs with increased frequency in children with SLE and in their family members (64,65). Because the antiphospholipid syndrome often appears to be independent of SLE, the explanation for this association is unclear. The report of Mujic et al. (66) describing an adolescent with evidence of antiphospholipid antibodies at age 16 but who did not manifest SLE until 17 years later is a reminder that SLE may evolve over an extended period of time.

An increased frequency of SLE in childhood occurs in children with defects of the immune system. This is especially true of genetic defects in the complement system (most often C2 or C4 deficiency) (59,74). Such an association may occur because the genes controlling C4 synthesis are closely linked to the HLA histocompatibility complex, or because the complement defect directly increases the likelihood of autoimmune disease (69–75). HLA linkages in this region have been demonstrated for adults with SLE, but they have not been independently evaluated in children (76,77). A Turkish family has been reported in which homozygous C1q deficiency was associated with the development of SLE in one sibling and IgA nephropathy in another (78). Interestingly a common pattern of hypergammaglobulinemia, cytopenias, and rash which may be associated with other findings suggestive of SLE has been described in a group of individuals with CD95 (Fas/APO-1) mutations (79).

IgA deficiency is another defect of immune function that occurs more frequently than expected among children with SLE (6,80,81). In one study (80), IgA deficiency was found in only 0.03 of the normal population but in 4.6 of children with SLE. The association of SLE in childhood with defects in the immune system strongly suggests that defective antigen processing predisposes to the development of SLE. The development of discoid lupus (and in one case, SLE in children with chronic granulomatous disease and their mothers) is another observation suggesting an association between defective antigen processing and the development of SLE (73,82,83).

Despite the associations between defective immunoglobulin and complement function and SLE, treatment with intravenous immunoglobulin therapy has not been of benefit. Most patients with SLE are hypergammaglobulinemic, even if IgA-deficient. Further, because IgA is a secretory immunoglobulin, intravenous immunoglobulin therapy does not restore effective mucosal immunity, and administering intravenous immunoglobulin to IgA-deficient individuals may be associated with dangerous allergic reactions.

Children and adolescents with SLE are a valuable resource for large-scale efforts to understand the genetics and molecular biology of this disease. The opportunity to study SLE in populations such as young white males (who lack the known predisposing factors) may facilitate the identification of new risk factors. Each risk factor is a piece in the puzzle that ultimately will lead to understanding the pathogenesis of SLE (50).

CLINICAL MANIFESTATIONS

Unexplained fever, malaise, and weight loss are the most common manifestations of SLE in children and adolescents. However, because these symptoms may be associated with many chronic illnesses, the physician should actively seek evidence of arthritis or a photosensitive rash, hematuria or proteinuria, hypergammaglobulinemia, and hypocomplementemia. Any of these findings should prompt consideration of SLE, but one cannot rely on their presence. On initial evaluation, the patient and family often do not describe findings such as arthritis of the small joints of the hands, alopecia, or photosensitivity. Unless they are specifically questioned, they do not relate these to the primary complaint. The reported frequency of many complaints varies widely among series of children with SLE, and this variation reflects not only selection and referral criteria but also the care with which the complaint was sought and validated by the investigators (Table 41.1) (84).

Most children with SLE present with chronic illness, but some children and adolescents with SLE are acutely ill at presentation. These children may present with seizures, psychosis, uremia, profound anemia, pulmonary hemorrhage, or sepsis as the initial manifestation (85). Often, the diagnosis of SLE is not considered until the clinicians note that the child is not recovering as expected despite adequate therapy for the presenting event.

Confirming the diagnosis of SLE in children and adolescents is based on criteria developed by the American Rheumatism Association (ARA) for use in adults (80). Classification as definite SLE is based on the fulfillment of four criteria, but the diagnosis should not be discarded automatically in children who meet only three. While the ARA criteria are useful guidelines, fulfillment of four criteria does not exclude other diagnoses; likewise, failure to fulfill four does not exclude SLE. Antinuclear antibody (ANA) testing is useful, but a positive test is not sufficient for the diagnosis of SLE in childhood. ANA-positive children who fulfill at least one other criterion should be periodically reevaluated. Definite SLE may manifest decades after the initial presentation (87).

TABLE 41.1. CLINICAL MANIFESTATIONS OF SYSTEMIC LUPUS ERYTHEMATOSUS IN CHILDREN AND ADULTS[a]

	Cases (n)		
Parameter	Cassidy et al. (6)	King et al. (12)	Pistiner[b] et al.
Renal involvement	86	61	28
Hypertension	28	—	25
Musculoskeletal findings	76	79	91
Cutaneous	76	70	55
Photosensitivity	16	—	37
Hair loss	20	—	31
Oral, nasal ulceration	16	—	19
Cardiac involvement	47	17	12
Pulmonary involvement	36	19	12
CNS involvement	31	13	11
Anemia	47	—	30
Leukopenia	71	—	51
Thrombocytopenia	24	—	16

[a]The findings from Cassidy et al. and King et al. represent two large pediatric series; those from Pistiner et al. represent a large adult series.
[b]From Pistiner M, Wallace DJ, Nessim S, Metzger AL, Klinenberg JR. Lupus erythematosus in the 1980s: a survey of 570 patients. *Semin Arthritis Rheum* 1991;21:55–64.

RENAL DISEASE

Renal disease is evident in approximately two thirds of children and adolescents with SLE (2,6–14,88). Renal manifestations range from mild glomerulitis with a normal urine sediment to sudden renal failure (85,89). The most common signs of renal involvement are hematuria, proteinuria, and hypertension. Although children and their families may complain of malaise, headache, swollen feet, and/or swollen eyelids (if nephrotic syndrome is present), the signs of renal involvement commonly are silent in childhood.

Renal biopsy of children and adolescents with SLE without regard to clinical manifestations demonstrates varying degrees of renal involvement in nearly every case (89,91). Although most children with a normal urine sediment have only mild glomerulitis, diffuse proliferative glomerulonephritis (DPGN) may be present. The significance of silent DPGN is uncertain. Series reporting follow-up of silent nephritis in SLE have described a benign prognosis (89–91), and this makes proper interpretation of such biopsies and the importance of detecting silent DPGN uncertain. Most investigators agree that renal biopsy may be deferred if the creatinine clearance and urinalysis are normal. However, renal biopsy should be performed whenever necessary to confirm the diagnosis, to investigate unexplained changes in renal function, and when considering or monitoring the effects of aggressive therapy (31,92).

Renal involvement in childhood SLE is categorized according to the World Health Organization (WHO) criteria (93). Mild glomerulitis is the most benign form, followed by focal segmental glomerulonephritis and membranous glomerulonephritis (94). DPGN carries the greatest risk of chronic renal failure. DPGN was the most frequent abnormality in children who underwent biopsy because of abnormal urine sediment (57), but in a series in which all children with SLE underwent biopsy, only 20% of children had DPGN (4,7,11,13,29,95). Combining the data from several large series, 42% of children (108 of 256) had DPGN at the time of initial biopsy, 26% had either mild glomerulitis or no abnormality, 25% had focal glomerulitis, and 6% had membranous glomerulonephritis.

Focal glomerulonephritis and membranous glomerulonephritis generally are benign, but either may progress to DPGN, with ultimate renal failure (4,10,13,29,93,96–98). Repeat renal biopsy should be performed in these patients if renal function continues to deteriorate or they manifest persistent hypocomplementemia. Long-term studies indicate that renal scarring (i.e., chronicity index) is a better predictor of ultimate outcome than the WHO classification (93,98,99). In the absence of scarring, active disease (including glomerular crescents) is not automatically associated with a poor prognosis (97,98); however, good outcome for these children is contingent on aggressive management of their renal disease to prevent the development of scarring (discussed later). Most children with SLE do not develop renal disease after the first 2 years following diagnosis (2,7), but one third of those who ultimately do develop significant renal disease lack evidence of renal involvement at presentation.

The sudden onset of renal failure in a child with SLE may result from active nephritis (85), but alternative explanations must be appropriately excluded. Renal vein thrombosis and renal artery thrombosis are other causes of sudden renal deterioration in children with SLE, and both are more frequent in association with anticardiolipin antibodies (100,101). Drugs and self- or family-administered health-food supplements that interfere with glomerular filtration or are directly nephrotoxic also must be considered when seeking the cause of sudden onset renal failure. A mild rise in the blood urea nitrogen level (BUN) usually follows the initiation of acetylsalicylic acid or other nonsteroidal anti-inflammatory drugs (NSAIDs) in patients with renal involvement, but some children with SLE are unusually sensitive to their effects. An unexpectedly sharp rise in the BUN following initiation of NSAIDs should prompt further investigation for previously unsuspected renal involvement.

Mild clinical manifestations of renal involvement usually are well controlled with corticosteroids and diuretics. Persistent renal disease may require immunosuppressive therapy (102). Chronic glomerular scarring is prevented by cyclophosphamide over the intermediate term (31,103). The major concern of the physician caring for a child with lupus nephritis is preserving sufficient renal function to support normal growth and development. For adolescent females, this includes the preservation of adequate renal function to support pregnancy. These concerns dictate intervention before significant renal compromise has occurred.

Current treatment regimens for children and adolescents with SLE have led to a steady improvement in 5- and 10-year renal function survival (30). It is not yet clear, however, whether these improvements result in significantly enhanced survival 20 and 30 years following diagnosis. Maintaining adequate renal function is important for children and adolescents with SLE. In contrast to adults, they do poorly on long-term dialysis (93). Children with SLE coming to dialysis often die of sepsis or other complications within the first year.

Children whose proteinuria and hematuria improve with corticosteroid therapy but whose creatinine clearance slowly deteriorates are of particular concern. Often, these children do well over a 5-year period but progress to renal failure between 5 and 10 years following diagnosis. Routine monitoring of creatinine clearance and, if deterioration is evident, early intervention, are important. In the event of chronic deterioration, the clinician should intervene aggressively while adequate function can still be preserved. Adult series suggest that maintaining a creatinine clearance of 70 mL/min per 1.75 m2 is adequate (103,104), but intervention at this point may not preserve sufficient renal function for the satisfactory growth and development of children and adolescents.

Optimal therapy for children and adolescents with lupus nephritis remains uncertain. In large part, this results from the failure of many investigators to properly stratify the patients in their studies (94). The systematic use of intermittent intravenous cyclophosphamide has been successful in children with DPGN and useful for children with membranous glomerulonephritis (31,102). Others have reported excellent results with the combined use of large doses of prednisone and, when necessary, azathioprine (9,29,105). When 10-year renal survival is considered, the systematic use of intravenous cyclophosphamide appears to offer the best outcome. Individual physicians who proclaim excellent results in their institution with other regimens rarely have prospective data to support their claims. This situation is made even more difficult by the consistent failure of reporting centers to stratify patients according to age, race, sex, and severity of disease despite the fact that these factors are all recognized to impact survival.

At present, a large-scale study of staging criteria for children with SLE is underway (94). Use of these criteria should improve our ability to assess the various therapeutic regimens that have been advocated for children with lupus nephritis. Routine use of intravenous cyclophosphamide has many advantages, including accurate assessment of patient compliance and clinical status at each dosage interval. Poor compliance is a major determinant of poor outcome (106). In addition, periodic inpatient cyclophosphamide therapy allows the physician to monitor renal function status and clinical status before each immunosuppressive drug dosage, thus minimizing complications.

All of the recommended regimens for treatment of lupus nephritis fail in some patients. Continued efforts to improve care are necessary for these children and adolescents, who may relentlessly progress to renal failure and, often, death. Systematic therapy modeled on the experience of pediatric oncologists may hold the key to enhanced survival for children and adolescents with severe lupus nephritis (107,108). Evolution of current therapeutic regimens to include multiple agents that are given at fixed intervals to induce a remission of disease, followed by prolonged maintenance therapy, is under investigation.

Low-dose oral methotrexate has been an effective adjunctive therapy in a few children (109), but it has not proven to be successful when used in isolation. Low-dose oral methotrexate may be a beneficial addition to immunosuppressive regimens to provide improved maintenance after the induction phase (e.g., children who have reached 3-month dosage intervals on cyclophosphamide). Higher dosages of intravenous methotrexate have been used in protocols for the treatment of children who have failed conventional immunosuppressive therapy. Presently, four children at the Hospital for Special Surgery who failed therapy with intravenous cyclophosphamide alone have received intensive chemotherapy combining monthly boluses of 1 g/M2 of cyclophosphamide with 300 mg/M2 of methotrexate given intravenously on the same day. All of these patients have responded to therapy and their disease remains well controlled. However, the long-term safety and utility of this regimen remain uncertain. In selected patients with continuing disease activity, it also may be useful to incorporate concurrent intravenous methylprednisolone (30 mg/kg/dose, up to a maximum of 1 g/dose).

Autologous stem-cell transplantation has been proposed and utilized for a variety of autoimmune diseases including some children with SLE (110–112a). This technique may hold great promise, but this technique is associated with a significant mortality and the majority of the reported responses have not persisted over time. Whether the beneficial effect results from the stem-cell transplantation or is from the immunosuppressive chemotherapy given at the time of stem-cell transplant is under active investigation.

CENTRAL NERVOUS SYSTEM MANIFESTATIONS

Psychosis, sudden personality change, seizures, chorea, transverse myelitis, peripheral neuropathy, and pseudotumor cerebri all may be presenting manifestations of SLE in childhood (113–124). Most series have reported CNS involvement in 20 to 30 of children (2,6,11,13,29). If carefully sought, mild evidence of CNS involvement is present in up to 45 of children and adolescents (23,124). In every instance appropriate investigation should be undertaken to exclude stroke as the etiology of sudden CNS changes, even in the patient who is not known to be anticardiolipin antibody-positive.

Subtle CNS changes, including impaired judgment and poor short-term memory, are the most common CNS manifestations of SLE (115,120,125,126). These alterations often are ascribed to steroid therapy or situational stress, but they occur with greater frequency in SLE than in other chronic childhood rheumatic diseases that require similar corticosteroid therapy. Adolescents with SLE often have difficulty complying with their medications or appointments, and they often alienate friends and family in ways that are inconsistent with their prior behavior. Physicians must be acutely aware of these changes, because they may have disastrous consequences. A trial of increased corticosteroids may be beneficial in children with SLE whose behavior has become erratic or uncharacteristic, even in the absence of objective findings. Others have argued for reducing the corticosteroids in such circumstances, but this rarely is effective.

Delirium, hallucinations, seizures, and coma are the most common objective neurologic signs in childhood. Psychosis that is unrelated to corticosteroids typically occurs in 4 to 10 of children (2,7,13,28,29,124). Caeiro et al. (6) reported significant neuropsychiatric findings in 30 of children in an English series. The reported frequency of neuropsychiatric manifestations in children and adolescents with SLE is lower than that in adults (127). This may be a true finding, but it more likely represents a decreased appreciation of neuropsychiatric involvement in childhood.

Chorea is more frequent in children than in adults with SLE (127). Although it is infrequent, it has been documented as being the initial manifestation of childhood SLE in multiple reports (118,123,128–130), perhaps because it is such a striking finding. Of children with SLE, 4% to 10% are affected by chorea at some point (2,7,23,28,29,124). This increased incidence may reflect an increased sensitivity of the basal ganglia to damage by autoreactive antibodies or vascular events accompanying SLE in childhood (131).

Most often, acute CNS involvement occurs early in the natural history of childhood SLE (132). Frequently, it first becomes evident during, or worsens immediately after, initiation of corticosteroid therapy. The explanation for this is uncertain, but these symptoms frequently resolve with pulse methylprednisolone therapy. Late-onset CNS involvement more often results from stroke, uremia, or an infectious process (133).

Both sudden onset of optic neuritis and acute sensorineural hearing loss may occur in children with SLE (134,135). However, the most striking CNS damage in children and adolescents with SLE typically results from seizures or strokes, including cerebral vein thrombosis. These complications may occur in the presence or absence of anticardiolipin antibodies (136–138).

Cognitive defects and aberrant behavior present a more difficult management problem. Aberrant behavior may have dramatic effects on social acceptance, grades, and compliance, thereby directly affecting both self-image and long-term prognosis. Efforts to ascribe behavioral change to a single cause rarely are successful (115,120,125).

Nonspecific problems in children with diffuse CNS involvement most likely represent the combined effects of SLE, situational factors, and corticosteroid therapy. When such symptoms are present, increasing the corticosteroid dosage more often is successful than a dramatic reduction.

No single objective test for the presence of CNS-SLE is accurate in childhood. Computed tomography (CT) of children and adolescents with SLE who have received long-term corticosteroids commonly demonstrates diffuse cortical atrophy (139–141). Alterations in cerebrospinal fluid protein or sugar levels or cell count cannot be relied on (115,124,132), but these studies often are necessary to exclude infection and other explanations for altered CNS function (133). Single-photon emission CT may be a more sensitive test for cerebral perfusion abnormalities in these children (142), but other studies suggest that magnetic resonance imaging (MRI) is more sensitive (143). Antibodies to ribosomal P have been found to correlate with CNS manifestations of SLE in adults, but their presence correlates less reliably with CNS disease in children and adolescents (144,145).

Treatment of CNS manifestations in children and adolescents with SLE is a challenge. Because the manifestations may result from corticosteroid therapy, physicians frequently hesitate to increase the dosage; nonetheless, this often is the most effective therapy. For severe CNS manifestations, pulse methylprednisolone therapy often is effective. When other measures fail, intravenous cyclophosphamide frequently is beneficial. Children with short-term psychosis or coma often respond to therapy, but when significant impairment has been present for long periods, the prognosis is guarded. It is important to respond aggressively when faced with continuing evidence of CNS deterioration. Chronic "mild" problems for which intervention is not felt to be warranted often progress to dementia over time.

PSYCHOSOCIAL CONCERNS

Psychologic reactions that relate to the many issues affecting children and adolescents with SLE often are confusing. Adolescents who are afflicted with chronic disease are caught between their need to establish an independent personality and the dependency of the sick role. Just as they are struggling to assert their independence, they must be taken for doctor's visits, forced to undergo examinations and blood tests, and required to take unpleasant medications. This situation is intensified by the almost universal need for dosages of corticosteroids that increase acne and produce obvious cushingoid facies. It is the unusual adolescent who does not rebel under these circumstances. This rebellion may take the form of noncompliance with scheduled physician visits, overt or covert medication noncompliance, or familial disruption. The physician who expects the adolescent with SLE to act like an adult should expect an unsatisfactory patient-physician relationship.

Anger frequently is the adolescent's predominant response to his or her situation. It is important to remember that there is no well-defined target for this anger. The adolescent obviously is angry about having SLE, but the disease has no direct embodiment. The physician, the medications, and the required examinations, however, all are direct manifestations of the disease and thus easy targets for the adolescent's rage. This may be expressed overtly by refusing to cooperate, but it is more difficult to deal with when covert and unrecognized.

There is no single, successful method for dealing with adolescent rebellion in the setting of chronic illness. Because adolescents frequently believe that important information is being kept from them, it is important to emphasize honesty, trust, and integrity. The physician cannot demand these from the adolescent patient without promising to provide them in return. Often, the situation is handled best by excusing the family from the room, because there may be many issues that the adolescent is afraid to voice in front of parents or siblings. It often is useful to ask the patient directly what the physician or family has done to provoke the behavior. Frequently, it takes only a few minutes of conversation to elicit a recognition that the anger is primarily over being ill. Dealing with this honestly and directly is a key step in developing a healthy patient-physician-family relationship.

For some children, no amount of discussion and reassurance is sufficient. Often, this is in response to unspoken fears or needs in the family of which the physician may not be aware. In these circumstances, it is best to recommend family counseling. Individual counseling of the adolescent furthers their feeling of having been singled out and often is counterproductive (unless it develops out of initial family-centered care). Situations in which both honest discussion and family counseling fail are unusual. When they do occur, it is important to determine whether the adolescent behavior may be a manifestation of unrecognized cerebritis, for which increased medication may be required. If a satisfactory patient-family-physician relationship cannot be established despite every possible effort, then referral to another physician or center may be indicated. Because this forces the adolescent and family to reevaluate their conduct and initiate new relationships, it may be beneficial even when no additional steps are taken.

PULMONARY MANIFESTATIONS

Pleurisy and pleural effusions are the most common pulmonary manifestations (146,147). Severe manifestations, including pneumothorax, pneumonia, chronic restrictive lung disease, pulmonary hypertension, and acute pulmonary hemorrhage, may occur (146–153). Pleuritic chest pain, pleural effusions, and chronic interstitial infiltrates affect from 10% to 30% of children with SLE (2,6,11,13, 14,28,29). When a series of Canadian children with SLE was reviewed for manifestations of respiratory involvement, 17 of 24 patients (77%) had evidence of pulmonary involvement (146).

Chronic pulmonary involvement may result in slowly progressive diaphragmatic dysfunction and restrictive lung disease. These changes appear as malaise and dyspnea on exertion (146,148,152,154). Diaphragmatic dysfunction may contribute to frequent infection (146,148). Diaphragmatic involvement also may be more common than previously recognized. Changes ranging from wide variation in fiber size to calcinosis were common in autopsy specimens of children dying from SLE (149). It is useful to note both pulse rate and respirations as part of the routine examination. Gradual increases in either or both parameters recorded over time may be the earliest clue to developing cardiac or pulmonary dysfunction, which are not clinically evident to either the patient or physician.

Significant restrictive lung disease may be present in children with normal chest radiographs. A study of 15 children with SLE by Trapani et al. found pulmonary involvement in six who were without pulmonary symptoms (155). Children with dyspnea or tachypnea at rest should be monitored with periodic pulmonary function testing. As the ability to ameliorate renal and CNS manifestations of SLE in children and adolescents improves, chronic pulmonary involvement is becoming an increasing concern.

The most common fatal complication of pulmonary involvement in children and adolescents with SLE is pneumonia (150). Pneumonia was the primary cause of death for nine of 26 children with SLE coming to autopsy in one reported series; pulmonary hemorrhage contributed to the death of five others. In contrast, renal failure and CNS involvement were the primary causes of death in only four and three children, respectively.

Pulmonary hypertension, denoted by accentuation of the second heart sound, is an ominous finding in children and adolescents with SLE. Once established, it progresses steadily to right-sided heart failure and death (148). Pulmonary hemorrhage may occur in the setting of preexisting pulmonary hypertension or in isolation (148,151,152, 154). Sudden, unexplained pallor and tachypnea often indicate the onset of pulmonary hemorrhage (144), which if left untreated is rapidly fatal.

Minor manifestations of pulmonary involvement normally respond to corticosteroids (146,147,156). Deaths from pneumonia, in which *Escherichia coli*, *Klebsiella* sp., or *Staphylococcus aureus* were the predominant organisms, illustrate the need for broad-spectrum antibiotic coverage (150). Pneumocystis carinii and other nonbacterial organisms may be present (157). When pneumonia is superimposed on active pulmonary SLE, the contributions of infection and active SLE cannot be differentiated with certainty. Both antibiotics and increased doses of corticosteroids may be appropriate.

Children with pulmonary hypertension may benefit symptomatically from the addition of calcium channel blocking agents to reduce pulmonary vascular resistance. No therapy is known to reverse the course of this complication. Cytotoxic drugs have been ineffective, except in rare anecdotal reports. Pneumonia is a frequent complication in children with established pulmonary hypertension and may progress rapidly to sepsis. Massive pulmonary hemorrhage may respond to large doses of corticosteroids with ventilator support and, perhaps, plasmapheresis or extracorporeal membrane oxygenation (151,157).

MUSCULOSKELETAL MANIFESTATIONS

The arthritis of SLE generally is nondeforming and responds well to antiinflammatory medications. Significant arthritis at presentation is found in 40% to 60% of children and adolescents with SLE, and it occurs in over 80% of children with SLE at some point (2,6,7,11,13,14,29,40). Usually, the arthritis affects the small joints of the hands and feet, with swelling and pain on motion. Asymptomatic knee effusions frequently are present in children with active disease who may not have arthritis elsewhere.

Rarely, children with well-documented JRA and erosive changes develop definite SLE (158). These children appear to have two independent diseases. The frequency of this occurrence suggests that SLE and JRA share a common genetic predisposition.

Avascular necrosis is the most significant musculoskeletal complication of SLE in children and adolescents, and it may result from SLE alone, corticosteroid therapy, or their interaction. A cross-sectional radiographic study of 35 children with SLE found evidence of avascular necrosis in 40% (159). However, these children were drawn from a program that routinely uses high-dose corticosteroids (i.e., 2 mg/kg/day). The frequency of avascular necrosis in a general population of children and adolescents with SLE is unknown.

Avascular necrosis usually affects the hips and knees of children with SLE. Children report gradual onset of progressive discomfort in the affected joints, and the initial evaluation may prove negative. MRI and, later, routine radiography ultimately reveal evidence of osteonecrosis. Although no clear association of avascular necrosis with the total dosage of corticosteroids or their mode of administration has been found, the incidence of avascular necrosis is far higher in children who have received corticosteroids (159,160).

Meaningful muscle involvement is rare in children with SLE. Diffuse weakness may be the result of steroid myopathy (161). Mild elevations of serum creatinine phosphokinase levels often are seen but rarely are associated with clinical weakness. Antibodies to the acetylcholinesterase receptor may produce a myasthenia gravislike picture, and transplacental passage of antibodies to this receptor is reported to have caused weakness in the child of a mother with SLE (162). Dermatomyositis, which may be associated with a positive ANA, arthritis, a heliotropic rash, and significant proximal muscle weakness, must be excluded if significant weakness is present. The presence of antibodies to double stranded DNA does not automatically exclude the diagnosis of dermatomyositis, but hypocomplementemia is not expected in children with this condition.

DERMATOLOGIC MANIFESTATIONS

Rashes occur frequently in children with SLE (2,6,7,11,13, 14,28,29), but only 30% to 50% ever manifest the typical butterfly rash (11,28) (Fig. 41.2). Vasculitic involvement of the hard palate frequently accompanies the facial rash of SLE, and these lesions are a useful confirmatory sign if the

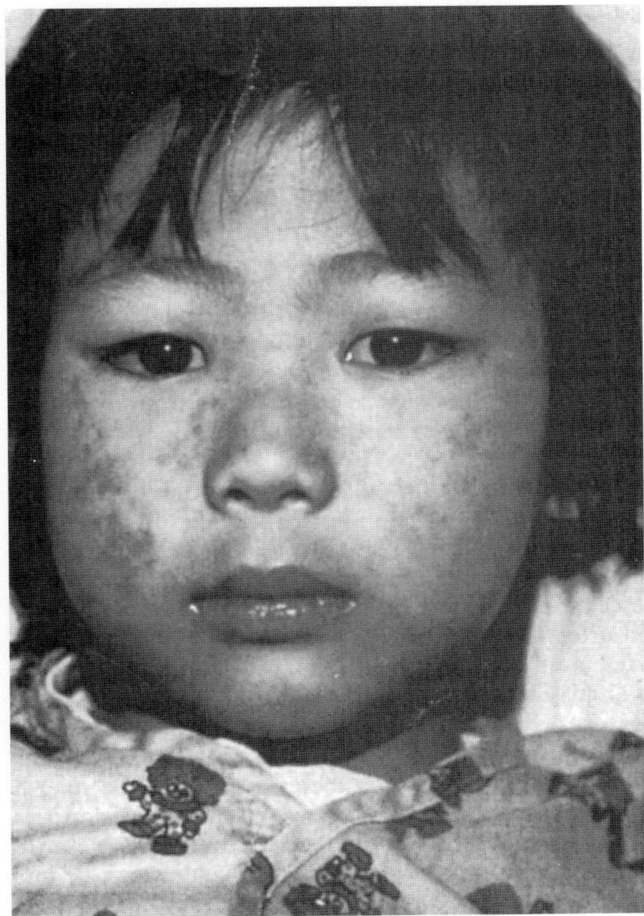

FIGURE 41.2. Typical bilateral malar rash in a young Asian female with systemic lupus erythematosus.

cause of the facial rash is in question. Cutaneous lesions may take the form of recurrent urticaria, bullae, vasculitic nodules, or chronic ulceration. Vasculitic lesions frequently are a manifestation of active disease. Other dermatologic manifestations may wax and wane without exacerbation of systemic disease.

Bullous lesions resembling bullous pemphigoid are the predominant manifestations of SLE in some children (163). Boys with this manifestation predominate. Often, they have mild systemic disease, and renal involvement is rare. Little information is available about these children in the literature. Dapsone often is helpful but has not been uniformly useful (164).

Dermatologic manifestations usually are not of long-term significance. Most respond to treatment without significant scarring. All the dermatologic lesions of SLE may be aggravated by sun exposure, and children with SLE should be counseled to use sun-blocking agents and to avoid unnecessary sun exposure, which may provoke increased systemic disease activity. Definite photosensitivity occurs in 16% of children (7).

It is important to discuss photosensitivity and its attendant precautions with great sensitivity. Adolescents often resent being told they cannot go to the beach or other all day outdoor activities (e.g., theme parks) with their friends. One must make every effort to accentuate the positive. For example we encourage our patients to participate in these activities in the evening when the risk of significant ultraviolet exposure is less. However, we recommend long sleeves, hats, and sun block at all times. One also must be sure to emphasize the exact nature of the risk. A recent patient suffered severe skin irritation after going to a tanning salon. They professed not to understand that this too was ultraviolet exposure and included in the photosensitivity precautions explained to them.

Discoid lupus erythematosus (DLE) is unusual in childhood. Most children referred for DLE have systemic manifestations when questioned and examined carefully. Some children with DLE progress to SLE, but this is rare (151). Isolated DLE is of concern because of associated disfigurement and psychologic effects.

CARDIAC MANIFESTATIONS

Cardiac manifestations rarely are prominent in children and adolescents with SLE, but occasionally, they are catastrophic (166). Pericarditis, myocarditis, and mild valvular involvement are common (6,7,13,14,167–169). Clinically evident pericarditis or myocarditis occurs in 10% of children (11,13,14,28), but occasional series report a higher frequency (2,7,150). Children with SLE may develop cardiac tamponade, but this complication is uncommon (170).

Many children with SLE are anemic and develop flow murmurs. Libman-Sacks endocarditis may occur in childhood, however, and this predisposes to bacterial endocarditis. In large series of patients with SLE, bacterial endocarditis occurs with a greater-than-expected frequency (150, 156,171). All children with significant valvular lesions must receive antibiotic coverage for dentistry and other invasive procedures; some recommend routine bacterial endocarditis prophylaxis for all patients with SLE.

Premature myocardial infarctions occur in adolescents and young adults with SLE in the settings of coronary arteritis, septic thrombosis, and prolonged corticosteroid therapy (97,156,172–176). The association of prolonged corticosteroid therapy with premature myocardial infarction raises significant questions about the long-term safety of high-dose corticosteroid regimens.

GASTROINTESTINAL MANIFESTATIONS

Mild gastrointestinal involvement is common in children and adolescents with SLE; 30% to 40% manifest hepatomegaly or splenomegaly at diagnosis (7,13,14). Chronic abdominal pain, anorexia, weight loss, and malaise also are frequent presenting complaints (2,7,11,13,14,29) that often resolve with corticosteroid therapy. Abdominal pain that is unresponsive to corticosteroids may result from small-vessel vasculitis that may not be detected by routine testing (177). These children may respond to a further increase in their corticosteroid dosage (14). Retroperitoneal fibrosis is a rare cause of abdominal pain in children with SLE (178). More often, abdominal pain is the result of pancreatitis that is induced either by SLE, corticosteroids, or both (2,13,179,183). Fulminant pancreatitis resulting in death has occurred.

Pneumatosis cystoides intestinalis may be discovered radiographically in patients who have complained of abdominal pain without evident explanation for weeks or months (13,182–184). This may be the result of chronic ischemia. Frank bowel ischemia often is found at autopsy (182). Although severe ischemia probably is a terminal event, its frequency suggests that the bowel frequently is compromised by lesser degrees of vascular insufficiency during life. This may be the explanation for some children with unexplained chronic abdominal pain.

Less frequent gastrointestinal manifestations of SLE include hepatitis and ileitis (2,182). Protein-losing enteropathy and marked hyperlipoproteinemia (185,186) also have been reported. The relationship of these manifestations to SLE is uncertain. Gastrointestinal irritation secondary to drugs used in treating SLE is frequent, and aspirin-induced hepatotoxicity is particularly common. Severe gastritis and ulcers may occur as well.

Although infarction of the spleen may produce acute abdominal pain, splenic involvement in SLE usually is asymptomatic. Functional asplenia is a very worrisome complication, because it is associated with increased susceptibility to infection (187). The presence of Howell-Jolly bodies on the peripheral smear should alert clinicians to the possibility of functional asplenia and prompt hospitalization if the child is febrile without adequate explanation.

INFECTION

Infection is a major cause of both morbidity and mortality for children and adolescents with SLE (2,6,11,13,29). Platt et al. (29) documented 55 separate infections occurring in 70 patients over a mean follow-up of 9 years. Sepsis was a contributing cause of death in 25% to 85% of deaths in various series (2,6,11,13,29), and it was a cited factor in 35 of 83 deaths (42%) occurring in 374 children collected from six large studies (2,6,11,13,29).

The increased frequency of sepsis most likely results from the combined effects of SLE and the drugs that are used to mediate it (188,189). The frequency of infection increases with increasing steroid dosage (188). Not only do bacterial infections increase, but opportunistic infections and infections caused by viruses, fungi, and related organisms are more common in children with SLE (29,150). The indiscriminate use of immunosuppressive drugs also may contribute to the increased incidence of infection; however, careful use of periodic intravenous cyclophosphamide accompanied by a reduced dosage of corticosteroids often leads to a reduced frequency of infections. In contrast to children taking a prescribed daily dosage of azathioprine or other immunosuppressive agents, children receiving periodic intravenous cyclophosphamide therapy can be intensively screened prior to receiving each dosage of the immunosuppressive agent. For all children with SLE potentially fatal infections, including both bacterial endocarditis and meningitis, occur with a greater-than-expected frequency (133,171). Functional asplenia, decreased phagocytosis, poor complement metabolism, and corticosteroid effects all may contribute to this problem.

HEMATOLOGIC MANIFESTATIONS

The most common hematologic manifestation of SLE in children and adolescents is anemia. Usually, this is not a Coombs'-positive hemolytic anemia with a reticulocytosis; rather, it is a microcytic anemia of chronic disease. Leukopenia and thrombocytopenia are common but not invariably present. Sickle cell anemia is not directly associated with SLE, but it is common in African Americans, who have an increased incidence of SLE. When SLE and sickle cell disease occur together, the similarity of symptoms between the two illnesses may produce confusion. If the physician cannot distinguish the etiology of problems with certainty, he or she may have to treat as appropriate to both conditions.

Children often are seen who have ANAs and thrombocytopenia, which has been labeled idiopathic thrombocytopenic purpura (ITP). A false-positive biologic test result for syphilis or prolonged partial thromboplastin time (PTT) in this setting may suggest SLE. Children with ITP may have antibodies to Sm, Ro, La, or RNP. All children with serologic markers such as these should be carefully followed and periodically reevaluated for evidence of systemic disease including periodic testing for hypocomplementemia, renal impairment, and proteinuria or hematuria. Some of these children ultimately develop SLE (190) (Table 41.2). In the absence of other manifestations of SLE, therapy for these children is similar to that for ITP alone.

Menorrhagia may be the presenting feature of SLE in teenage females. Prolonged bleeding or a prolonged PTT resulting from the lupus anticoagulant may be the initial manifestation of SLE in a patient who is being screened for other reasons. However, these findings alone do not establish the diagnosis of SLE. Management of these complications is the same for children and adolescents as for adults.

TABLE 41.2. INCIDENCE OF SEROLOGIC ANTIBODIES IN 92 CHILDREN WITH SYSTEMIC LUPUS ERYTHEMATOSUS[a]

	Incidence (%)	
Antibody	**Onchterlony**	**ELISA**
Ro/SSA	16	46
La/SSB	11	17
Sm (RNP)	27	58

[a]The presence of these antibodies did not correlate with disease activity, except that Ro/SSA antibodies by Ouchterlony were significantly more common in children younger than 10 years of age (11 of 28 vs. 4 of 64, $P < .001$). Children younger than 10 years of age also had a significantly higher mean ELISA titer of Ro/SSA antibodies.
Abbreviation: ELISA—Enzyme-linked immunosorbent assay.

Anticardiolipin antibodies (aCL) occur in children with SLE with a similar frequency to that of adults (64,65,191). They are associated with an increased risk of thrombosis and CNS disease (192,193). Children with high titer aCL, lupus anticoagulant, and thrombocytopenia may be the group at highest risk of thrombosis (194). Others have suggested that SLE patients with the SA1 anti-DNA idiotype may be at increased risk of vascular complications in the setting of aCL (195). The risk for children with low titer aCL in the absence of lupus anticoagulant appears to be low (196). Low-dose aspirin therapy may be beneficial in reducing the risk. Children have been reported who presented with acute thrombosis and were found to be anticardiolipin antibody-positive but who did not have additional findings to support the diagnosis of SLE (197). Proper categorization of such children is uncertain, because over time, some have gone on to develop SLE (66).

LABORATORY EVALUATION

No laboratory feature of SLE in children and adolescents is unique to this age group. For clinicians, the diagnosis of SLE is strongly suggested by the constellation of hypergammaglobulinemia, leukopenia, anemia, and thrombocytopenia. A positive ANA is confirmatory, but none of these findings is essential.

ANAs are present in over 90% of children and adolescents with SLE (6,11,14,169,198). Antibodies to various other nuclear and cytoplasmic antigens also are found (49, 199–206). One study that compared the incidence of antibodies to DNA, Sm, and RNP found a lower frequency in children with SLE than in a simultaneously studied population of adult patients with SLE (49). Antibodies to Ro/SSA and La/SSB were found in similar numbers of adult- and childhood-onset patients. These antibodies also are found with increased frequency in the relatives of children with SLE (49). Their presence in asymptomatic relatives has been variously interpreted as being evidence of environmental exposure or genetic predisposition. Recent findings suggest that one may be genetically predisposed to manifest anti-Ro antibodies in response to viral infections such as Epstein-Barr virus suggesting that both environmental exposure and genetic predisposition play an important role in the development of SLE.

Antibodies against double-stranded DNA (dsDNA) are both sensitive and specific for active SLE in childhood (199,201) but may occur in other conditions (199). Decreased serum levels of the third component of complement (207) correlate well with active SLE in childhood, but neither decreased C3 levels nor antibodies to dsDNA can be relied on as a specific indicator of active renal disease (199,208).

Decreased C4 levels often are correlated with decreases in C3, but they may occur in isolation. Decreased C4 levels also frequently are found in the relatives of children with SLE. This may be evidence of the C4 null allele, a manifestation of subclinical disease, or both (30,69,209,210).

Hypergammaglobulinemia frequently is present in children with SLE but also may be found in various chronic inflammatory states (2,6,11). IgA deficiency occasionally is seen, as is panhypogammaglobulinemia (6,80,81). Panhypogammaglobulinemia is a common complication of cyclophosphamide therapy, but it also occurs in patients with SLE who have not received immunosuppressive agents (81).

False-positive test results for syphilis formerly were found in many children with SLE (2,14), but more recent studies report fewer false-positive results (6,11). In the United States, it is important to warn the family that positive results may be reported to the public health department. Unwarranted investigation can be halted if questions are referred to the physician. The diagnosis of SLE, however, does not exclude the possibility of treponemal disease. False-positive fluorescent treponemal antibody (FTA) test results may occur because of nonspecific agglutination resulting from hypergammaglobulinemia (211), but FTA-positive individuals in whom the possibility of treponemal disease cannot be reliably excluded should receive appropriate therapy.

THERAPY

NSAIDs provide useful control of the arthritis and musculoskeletal manifestations of SLE in children and adolescents (Table 41.3). Renal function and blood pressure must be monitored because of their known effects on glomerular filtration, but significant undesired effects are infrequent. Acetylsalicylic acid (i.e., aspirin) often is used in low dosage (5 mg/kg/day) in children with anticardiolipin antibodies. Antiinflammatory doses of aspirin (80 mg/kg/day) have been advocated, but children with SLE are very susceptible to salicylate-induced hepatotoxicity. Alternate NSAIDs are preferable.

TABLE 41.3. IMMUNOSUPPRESSIVE TREATMENT OF CHILDHOOD SLE

Drug(s)[a]	Suggested Dosage	Useful For	Remarks
NSAIDs, hydroxychloroquine	—	Mild disease	Monitor for idiosyncratic effects of NSAIDs on renal and central nervous system (CNS) function
Prednisone	1–2 mg/kg/d	More severe or unresponsive disease	Rarely exceed 80 mg/day; may be divided up to q.i.d., if necessary
Methylprednisolone	30 mg/kg/d, IV	Acute manifestations of CNS or renal disease	Maximum: 1,000 mg for 3 days
Cyclophosphamide	500–1000 mg/m²/mo for 7 months, then every 3 months for 30 additional months	DPGN	May be helpful for some children with severe nephrotic syndrome or CNS disease

[a]Other agents have been used, with differing reports of their efficacy. DPGN—diffuse proliferative glomerulonephritis.

Plaquenil (Sanofi) (hydroxychloroquine) and chloroquine routinely are used in children and adolescents with SLE (2,7,8,11,12,14). They are believed to have a useful steroid-sparing effect at a dose of 7 mg/kg/day. Although rare ocular toxicity is a concern, it was not reported in children or adolescents in any of these series (Table 41.4).

Intravenous pulse methylprednisolone (30 mg/kg daily, up to 1 g) given as an intravenous infusion has been used to control flares of nephritis (212) or CNS disease. Therapy was associated with dramatic short-term improvement in renal disease, but was not superior over the longer-term, to daily prednisone (212). Long-term benefit from pulse methylprednisolone is more likely in children with acute CNS involvement and other manifestations of SLE that appear to result from an acute event. Although rare, side effects may occur with pulse methylprednisolone, including significant hypotension, hypertension, and pancreatitis. Deaths have rarely occurred.

TABLE 41.4. DOSAGES OF MEDICATIONS COMMONLY USED FOR CHILDREN WITH SLEA

NSAIDs
- Naproxen 10–15 mg/kg divided b.i.d. (Usual maximum, 500 mg b.i.d.)
- Tolmetin 20–40 mg/kg divided b.i.d. (Usual maximum, 600 mg b.i.d.)
- Diclofenac 1–3 mg/kg divided b.i.d. (Usual maximum, 75 mg b.i.d.)
- Ibuprofen 20–40 mg/kg divided t.i.d. or q.i.d. (Usual maximum, 800 mg t.i.d.) may be associated with idiosyncratic reactions in SLE.

Other Drugs
- Hydroxychloroquine 7 mg/kg up to 200 mg/d (Some centers use 400 mg/d maximum dose)
- Dapsone 1 mg/kg up to 100 mg/d

Immunosuppressives
- Azathioprine 1–3 mg/kg/d (Usual maximum 100 mg/d)
- Cyclophosphamide (See text for intravenous administration. Not recommended p.o. because of hemorrhagic cystitis risk)
- Methotrexate 10 mg/m²/wk (Safety and efficacy in SLE not yet established)

[a]These typically are used dosages only. Full prescribing information provided by the manufacturer should be consulted for possible side effects, interactions, and other consequences of the use of these medications.

In the 1970s, most children were treated with high-dose corticosteroids (2 mg/kg/day) followed by a gradual tapering once their disease came under control (2,72,11,14,28). Children with continuing active disease and evidence of renal involvement received immunosuppressive agents (7,9, 13,29). Cushingoid facies, cataracts, avascular necrosis, and other complications were common (9, 11, 28).

In the late 1980s, systematic use of intravenous cyclophosphamide became common. It has been argued that corticosteroids are preferable to cytotoxic agents, because corticosteroids do not have life-threatening side effects. However, overt suicide resulting from the psychosocial stresses of Cushingoid facies and chronic disease has occurred, and covert suicide in the form of noncompliance (e.g., stopped corticosteroids against medical advice) is not uncommon (29).

Although the therapeutic role of cytotoxic drugs remains controversial, data supporting their safety and efficacy have become increasingly convincing (31,213–215). Concerns regarding sterility, risk of infections, and risk of neoplasia have limited their use to children with significant disease activity that is unresponsive to acceptable doses of corticosteroids (6,7,9,10,13,14,29,102,216). Immunosuppressives have been used in those with CNS disease, with varying results (6). Although a few centers report good results using high-dose prednisone and azathioprine over both 5- and 10-year periods (9,29), others have had less success with this regimen. Controlled trials in adult patients with SLE have found cyclophosphamide to be as effective as, and less toxic than, the combination of cyclophosphamide and azathioprine (102,103). Proper stratification of patients at study entry may be the key to resolving these issues (Table 41.5). We have

TABLE 41.5. STAGING CRITERIA FOR SLE

Stage 0	Patients with serologic evidence of SLE without clinical manifestations
0	Positive ANA without other manifestations
0a	Positive ANA plus false positive VDRL; or anticardiolipin antibodies; or antibodies to Ro, La, or RNP
0b	Positive ANA plus antibodies to Sm or anti-DNA antibodies.
Stage 1	
1	Serologic evidence of SLE plus at least one nonserologic criterion from the ACR criteria for the diagnosis of SLE, but without sufficient findings to fulfill criteria for a definite diagnosis of SLE or constitutional symptoms. (Note that any patient who fulfills the ACR criteria, or has >25 RBC/HPF or 1+ or greater protein by dipstick on urinalysis automatically is classified stage 3 or higher.)
1a	Criteria for stage 1 plus an elevated total protein (>8 g, or Hb <11.0 g/dL (without hemolytic anemia).
1b	The above plus an ESR >25 mm/H Westergren
Stage 2	
2	Serologic evidence of SLE plus at least one nonserologic criteria for the diagnosis of SLE with recurrent fever, weight loss, or other significant constitutional symptoms.
2a	The above plus hypocomplementemia (C3 <80% of lowest normal value)
2b	The above criteria plus an elevated total protein (>8 g, or Hb <11.0 g/dL (without hemolytic anemia)
Stage 3	
3	Any patient who fulfills the ACR criteria for the diagnosis of definite SLE, or patients with renal involvement who do not fulfill the ACR criteria for a definite diagnosis of SLE
3a	The criteria for stage 3 plus hypocomplementemia (C3 <80% of lowest normal value)
3b	The criteria for stage 3 plus an elevated total protein level (>8 g, or Hb <11.0 g/dL (without hemolytic anemia)
Stage 4	
4	Definite SLE with renal involvement characterized by consistent finding of >5 RBC/HPF or >500 mg total protein in a 24-h urine specimen (normal serum creatinine and creatinine clearance). These patients would be expected to have either minimal glomerulitis or focal segmental nephritis on biopsy
4a	These criteria plus hypocomplementemia (C3 <80% of lowest normal value)
4b	These criteria plus an elevated total protein (>8 g, or Hb <11.0 g/dL (without hemolytic anemia)
Stage 5	
5	Definite SLE with membranous glomerulonephritis on biopsy and >2.0 g total protein in a 24-h urine specimen
5a	These criteria with clinical evidence of nephrotic syndrome including serum albumin <3.0 g/dL or cholesterol >300. (Note presence of persistent hypertension with diastolic blood pressure >90 mm Hg without treatment automatically indicates stage 7.)
5b	These criteria with pitting edema
Stage 6	
6	Definite SLE with renal biopsy demonstrated diffuse proliferative glomerulonephritis; or seizure, or other neurologic manifestations (e.g., cerebritis) sufficient to warrant hospitalization
6a	These criteria plus hypocomplementemia (C3 <80% of lowest normal value)
6b	These criteria plus an elevated total protein (>8 g, or Hb <11.0 g/dL (without hemolytic anemia)
Stage 7	
7	Definite SLE with CrCl <100 mL/min/1.75 m^2 or serum Cr >1.5
7a	The above plus hypocomplementemia (C3 <80% of lowest normal value) or diastolic blood pressure consistently over 90 mm Hg before therapy
7b	These criteria plus an elevated total protein (>8 g, or Hb <11.0 g/dL (without hemolytic anemia)
Stage 8	
8	Definite SLE with CrCl <50 mL/min/1.75 m^2 or serum Cr >2.0
8a	plus hypocomplementemia (C3 <80% of lowest normal value) or diastolic blood pressure consistently over 90 mm Hg before therapy
8b	These criteria plus an elevated total protein (>8 g, or Hb <11.0 g/dL (without hemolytic anemia)
Stage 9	
9	Definite SLE with CrCl <30 mls/min/1.75 m^2 or serum Cr >3.0
9a	These criteria plus hypocomplementemia (C3 less than 80% of lowest normal value) or diastolic blood pressure consistently over 90 mm Hg prior to therapy
9b	These criteria plus an elevated total protein (>8 g, or Hb less than 11.0 g/dL (without hemolytic anemia)
Stage 10	Definite SLE with end stage renal failure requiring dialysis; or chronic psychotic or neurologic state unresponsive to corticosteroid or immunosuppressive drug therapy

Abbreviation: HPF—High-powered field.
Source: Adapted from Lehman and Mouradian (86); with permission.

found the systematic use of cyclophosphamide to be associated with a far greater and faster improvement in clinical parameters, and sense of well being, while allowing a more rapid reduction in corticosteroid dosage. A large number of children initially treated with systematic intravenous cyclophosphamide for a period of three years, are now off all immunosuppressive agents and disease free.

For children and adolescents with SLE, the desire to avoid iatrogenic injury must be balanced against the goal of sustained survival. Cyclophosphamide administered with vigorous intravenous hydration and careful inpatient monitoring has proven to be both safe and effective (31,102). Although sterility and late-onset neoplasia are theoretic risks, neither has been documented in children receiving cyclophosphamide with rigorous intravenous hydration. In contrast, avascular necrosis, cataracts, and Cushingoid facies commonly are experienced by children receiving high doses of corticosteroids over a prolonged period.

At the Hospital for Special Surgery in New York City, children who fail to respond adequately to corticosteroid therapy receive intravenous cyclophosphamide according to a well-defined protocol. Children initially receive 500 mg/m^2 of cyclophosphamide, followed by monthly increases to 750 mg/m^2, and then 1,000 mg/m^2 if the white blood cell count does not fall below 2000/mL at its nadir. (It should be noted that 875 mg/m^2 often is the maximum dose that does not produce too great a fall in white count for children smaller than 1 m^2. In addition, the dosage should not exceed 40 mg/kg, because larger doses have been associated with cardiac toxicity in oncologic studies.) The induction phase of cyclophosphamide therapy continues with monthly cyclophosphamide infusions for a total of seven doses. Many children do not show evidence of major improvement until after the third monthly dose. If a child has deteriorated despite 6 months of therapy with cyclophosphamide, however, further therapy may not be warranted.

Children who respond well to monthly cyclophosphamide continue on therapy at 3-month intervals at the same dosage for an additional 10 maintenance doses. After 36 months of therapy, a repeat renal biopsy is performed and the cyclophosphamide discontinued if no evidence of active disease is found. Some children demonstrate renewed disease activity (e.g., decreasing hemoglobin, decreasing complement levels, falling creatinine clearance, increasing hematuria or proteinuria) following the transition from monthly therapy to therapy every 3 months. These children are treated with three additional monthly doses of cyclophosphamide, following which therapy every 3 months is resumed. Acute flares are managed with intravenous bolus doses of methylprednisolone for 3 days (30 mg/kg/day, up to a maximum of 1,000 mg) as necessary.

Most children who complete 36 months of therapy are withdrawn from cyclophosphamide and do well on low-dose corticosteroids. Some of these initial children are now alive, more than 15 years later, off all medications despite having biopsy-proven DPGN when therapy was initiated. Children who respond to monthly cyclophosphamide but who deteriorate whenever the frequency of therapy is decreased to every 3 months or flare after the initial course of cyclophosphamide has been completed, represent a different situation. Children with persistent disease activity without established chronic renal damage currently are treated with an aggressive program of combination therapy, using both intravenous cyclophosphamide and intravenous methotrexate. For those with only moderate disease activity but persistent hypocomplementemia, therapy with mycophenolate mofetil (up to 1 gram bid) may be beneficial. For those children with severe disease recurrence, we have combined a 9-month course of intravenous cyclophosphamide with high-dose intravenous methotrexate (300 mg/m2). This regimen has allowed us to bring four previously resistant patients under good disease control. In these children, methotrexate should be initiated carefully at 50 mg/m^2 or less and gradually increased if significant renal compromise is present. They should receive daily folic acid, and may require folinic acid "rescue" if there is significant renal compromise. Creatinine clearance of less than 60 mL/minute may be associated with increased risk of methotrexate toxicity.

The major risks associated with the aggressive use of cytotoxic agents are bone-marrow suppression (often complicated by infection), hemorrhagic cystitis, infertility, and the induction of neoplastic disease (early or late). Infectious complications can be minimized by careful evaluation before the administration of each dose of cyclophosphamide and a high index of suspicion for infection if the patient experiences difficulty during the period of maximal marrow suppression following each dose. Cystitis, infertility, and the induction of neoplastic disease are the remaining concerns. In my experience, none of these has occurred among children receiving intravenous cyclophosphamide with in-hospital hydration, during a 3-year course of therapy. One child with severe recalcitrant disease who received 62 grams of cyclophosphamide over an 8-year period developed a renal papillary-cell carcinoma, which was removed *in situ*. Presently, any similar patient would be treated with the combination of intravenous cyclophosphamide and intravenous methotrexate to limit the total dose of cyclophosphamide received. Children failing such regimens may be candidates for autologous stem cell transplantation (see below).

Studies of older patients with SLE indicate that the risk of sterility following cytotoxic drug therapy increases with increasing age. Premenarchal children may have some protection. In children with amenorrhea that is secondary to active SLE, menses often return during cyclophosphamide therapy. Several successful pregnancies have been reported following cyclophosphamide therapy in adolescents, and one pregnancy that originated during cyclophosphamide therapy (despite counseling) was successfully carried to term without difficulty. (No further cytotoxics were given after the pregnancy was discovered.) No definitive data about the risks of infertility or neoplasia are available, however, for children with SLE. Both have occurred in children who received cyclophosphamide as part of multidrug regimens for neoplastic disease. Families should be warned about these concerns before therapy is begun, and patients should be selected accordingly.

The ratio of risk to benefit for cytotoxic drugs in children and adolescents with SLE is minimized by appropriate patient selection. Progressively deteriorating creatinine clearance, prolonged hypertension (> 6 months), and significant nonhemolytic anemia identify children who are at high risk of ultimate renal failure (93). These findings may occur without significant evidence of extra-renal disease activity, and such children should be aggressively treated. With corticosteroid therapy alone, many children progress inexorably to renal failure. Controlled studies at the Hospital for Special Surgery and at the National Institutes of Health have indicated that routine use of intravenous cyclophosphamide prevents or retards this deterioration (31,103,104,213,217).

Methotrexate, cyclosporine, and intravenous gamma globulin all have been used in small numbers of children with SLE (109,218,219). Sufficient data have not been obtained to judge their efficacy. Recently, autologous stem-cell transplantation has received extensive attention for the treatment of rheumatic diseases including SLE and some teenagers are included in the reported series (111,112,220, 221). There are some who question whether to good responses reported are due to the stem-cell transplantation or the preparative immunosuppressive regimen alone (222).

Most investigators who have taken care of children with SLE over an extended period are aware of children who were inadvertently profoundly immunosuppressed as a result of unexpected sensitivity to a drug or drug interactions. Many of them went into remission of their disease, but few remained in remission for longer than 24 months. Whether the benefits of autologous stem-cell transplantation will endure is unclear. The early European BMT consortium results already describe patients with SLE who have relapsed following autologous stem-cell transplantation. It increasingly is recognized that SLE is a chronic, recurrent disease that may require prolonged therapy, even in the absence of active disease. However, for the patient with continued active disease in the face of intensive chemotherapy these regimens may be warranted. Significant improvements in the therapy of children with SLE will require careful collaborative studies.

PROGNOSIS

The prognosis for children and adolescents with SLE has improved dramatically over the past 20 years (108). With improved antiinflammatory therapy as well as improved pediatric care, 10-year survival rates now are approaching 90% (11,29). Nonetheless, significant numbers of children continue to progress to chronic renal failure and/or death (93) (Tables 41.6 and 41.7) .

TABLE 41.6. INCIDENCE OF ADVERSE OUTCOMES IN 72 CHILDREN WITH SYSTEMIC LUPUS ERYTHEMATOSUS

Outcome	Incidence (%)
Renal failure	15
Severe central nervous system disease	11
Stroke	1
Chronic thrombocytopenia	7
Chronic active disease	56
Death	18

Often, children and adolescents with SLE do poorly because of the child's, and the family's, inability to cope with the chronic, relapsing nature of the disease. Success requires a sustained relationship among the child, family, and the treating facility. Institutions serving stable populations with good socioeconomic status and easy access to care consistently report superior survival to those serving disadvantaged populations (11,29,93,106,223). Poor understanding of the importance of medications for silent manifestations of SLE, such as hypertension, remains a familiar cause of morbidity. These preventable deaths have become increasingly frustrating, as our ability to control the manifestations of SLE has improved.

The quality of survival must be addressed in efforts to improve the outcome for children and adolescents with SLE. Long-term survival of a Cushingoid adolescent with aseptic necrosis who requires dialysis may not be satisfactory to the patient. Platt et al. (29) described three young adults who died more than 10 years following diagnosis; two of the three died after they had discontinued their medications against medical advice.

Although end-stage renal failure and dialysis have been associated with decreased SLE activity in some reports (224, 225), both children and adolescents requiring chronic dialysis often fare poorly. In one series, nine of 16 children with SLE succumbed within 5 years of beginning dialysis (93).

TABLE 41.7. PREDICTORS OF POOR PROGNOSIS IN CHILDHOOD SYSTEMIC LUPUS ERYTHEMATOSUS

1. Persistent anemia: Hb <10 g for >6 mo
2. Persistent hypertension: diastolic BP >90 mm Hg for >6 mo
3. Persistent hematuria: >20 RBC/HPF for >6 mo
4. Pulmonary hypertension
5. Recurrent emergency admissions

Abbreviation: HPF—High-powered field.

For children and adolescents with SLE, a satisfactory outcome is measured in decades. Our goal should be to report 90% 50-year survival. Children without renal disease who have survived 5 years are at low risk. Children with renal disease of any type, however, remain at risk. Gradual progression to renal failure over 5 to 10 years or more, despite clinically inactive disease, has been reported in both children and adults with SLE (28,96,196). Healthcare professionals dealing with children and adolescents who have SLE must strive to aid patients and their families through a normally difficult period under even more difficult circumstances. Every effort must be made to guarantee the availability of appropriate services. Not only must medical therapy be aggressive, so should patient and family education to ensure their compliance. With the increasing presence of specialized pediatric centers for children with rheumatic diseases and growing numbers of collaborative studies to determine optimal therapy, survival measured in decades now should become the norm.

SUMMARY

The information in this chapter can be summarized as follows:

1. Children and adolescents represent both a special challenge and opportunity. Success in caring for this group requires awareness of the complex interactions among the child's illness, the needs of their family, and their own needs as developing individuals.
2. Childhood-onset SLE has been recognized since the early 1900s. Although it frequently is described as a more severe disease than adult SLE, this may result from failure to properly diagnose many mild cases.
3. No thorough studies of the epidemiology of SLE in childhood have been completed. It is estimated that the annual incidence is approximately 0.6 per 100,000, and that between 5,000 and 10,000 US children have SLE today. The incidence of SLE is much higher in females than in males and in nonwhites than in whites.
4. The cause of SLE remains unknown, but the high frequency of immunologic abnormalities among family members of children with SLE suggests that a combination of genetic and environmental factors plays an important role. The presence of Ro/SSA in a large proportion of the mothers of young children with SLE may indicate predisposing genetic factors in the family. SLE also is more frequent in children who have defects of the immune system, suggesting that defective antigen processing may predispose to the development of SLE.
5. The most common clinical manifestations of SLE are fever, malaise, and weight loss, but these are nonspecific manifestations of many chronic ailments. The typical butterfly rash is present only in about one third of children with SLE. Diagnosis is based on fulfillment of the ARA criteria, just as in adults.
6. Renal disease occurs in two thirds of children with SLE in most reported series. Although the renal disease may be mild, severe DPGN remains a leading cause of morbidity in childhood SLE. Mild renal disease often can be controlled with corticosteroids, but active renal disease that does not respond fully to corticosteroids and DPGN with a falling creatinine clearance requires therapy with cytotoxic agents. Children with active SLE do poorly on dialysis.
7. All of the CNS manifestations that are described in adults with SLE also occur in children. Behavioral disturbances, which may be ascribed to acting out by an adolescent with SLE, often represent CNS disease that may respond to increased therapy. Chorea also is seen more commonly among children with SLE.
8. Pulmonary involvement in childhood SLE takes many forms, including pleurisy, pleural effusions, pulmonary fibrosis, and pulmonary hemorrhage. Diaphragmatic dysfunction is common and may be the underlying factor predisposing to recurrent episodes of pneumonia. Pulmonary hypertension often is a life-threatening complication. Abnormal pulmonary function may be present despite a normal chest radiograph.
9. Musculoskeletal manifestations of SLE include arthritis and mild inflammatory myopathy, and they often are predominant at presentation. Both are responsive to corticosteroid therapy, however, and rarely contribute to long-term morbidity. The exception is avascular necrosis, which may occur as a complication of SLE with or without corticosteroid therapy and ultimately requires ultimate joint replacement.
10. Dermatologic involvement is common in childhood SLE but rarely is a significant problem except when the face is prominently disfigured, causing psychologic problems (Fig. 41.1). DLE is unusual in childhood.
11. Cardiac manifestations of SLE include pericarditis and myocarditis, sometimes with recurrent effusions. These usually can be controlled with NSAIDs or low-dose corticosteroids. Valvular involvement is common and may predispose to bacterial endocarditis. Careful consideration should be given to antibiotic prophylaxis whenever bacteremia is expected. Premature myocardial infarctions have occurred in young adults, with significant atherosclerosis following prolonged corticosteroid therapy.
12. Gastrointestinal manifestations of childhood SLE are varied. Nonspecific findings such as chronic abdominal pain and anorexia are frequent, and significant bowel infarction may occur. Pneumatosis intestinalis may result from recurrent microvascular insults.
13. Infection is a major cause of morbidity and mortality in children and adolescents with SLE. Active SLE pre-

disposes to infection. Often, it is unclear whether a child's rapid deterioration is the result of infection or of active SLE. In this setting, increased doses of both corticosteroids and antibiotics may be necessary. Reticuloendothelial system overload and functional asplenia may predispose to rapid progression of sepsis in children with active SLE.

14. Hematologic manifestations are common in children and adolescents with SLE. Most are nonspecific. Thrombocytopenia is a frequent presenting complaint, particularly in young males, and menorrhagia also may be a significant problem in adolescent females. As in adults, the presence of anticardiolipin antibodies predisposes to clotting dysfunction and stroke in children.
15. Laboratory manifestations of childhood SLE are identical to those of adults. One unique concern is awareness that a positive serologic result for syphilis in a child or adolescent is reported to the school district and warrants prompt investigation by public welfare authorities. Families should be warned about this possibility, and inquiries should be promptly diverted to the physician.
16. Therapy for childhood-onset SLE is similar to that for adults. Because of the increased burdens of growth and development on renal function, however, it may be important to institute aggressive intervention earlier in children with DPGN. The goal must be to develop therapies that provide acceptable 50-year survival, not 5- or 10-year survival, for children and adolescents with SLE. The systematic administration of cytotoxic drugs may provide superior quality of life and long-term survival.

REFERENCES

1. James JA, Kaufman KM, Farris AD, et al. An increased prevalence of Epstein–Barr virus infection in young patients suggests a possible etiology for systemic lupus erythematosus. *Journal of Clinical Investigation* 1997;100:3019–3026.
2. Meislin AG, Rothfield N. Systemic lupus erythematosus in childhood. Analysis of 42 cases, with comparative data on 200 adult cases followed concurrently. *Pediatrics* 1968;42:37–49.
3. Ginzler EM, Diamond HS, Weiner M, et al. A multicenter study of outcomes of systemic lupus erythematosus. I. Entry variables as predictors of progress. *Arthritis Rheum* 1982;25: 601–611.
4. Abeles M, Urman JD, Weinstein A, et al. Systemic lupus erythematosus in the younger patient: survival studies. *J Rheumatol* 1980;7:515–522.
5. Lehman TJA, McCurdy D, Spencer C, et al. Prognostic value of antibodies to Ro/SSA, SSB/La, and RNP in children with systemic lupus erythematosus (abstract). *Arthritis Rheum* 1990; 33(suppl):S154.
6. Caeiro F, Michielson FMC, Bernstein R, et al. Systemic lupus erythematosus in childhood. *Ann Rheum Dis* 1981;40: 325–331.
7. Cassidy JT, Sullivan DB, Petty RE, et al. Lupus nephritis and encephalopathy. Proceedings of the conference of rheumatic diseases in childhood. *Arthritis Rheum* 1977;20(suppl 2): 315–322.
8. Cook CD, Wedgwood RJP, Craig JM, et al. Systemic lupus erythematosus. Description of 37 cases in children and a discussion of endocrine therapy in 32 of the cases. *Pediatrics* 1960;26: 570–585.
9. Fish AJ, Blau EB, Westberg NG, et al. Systemic lupus erythematosus within the first two decades of life. *Am J Med* 1977;62: 99–117.
10. Garin EH, Donnelly WH, Fenell RS, et al. Nephritis in systemic lupus erythematosus in children. *J Pediatr* 1976;89: 366–371.
11. Glidden RS, Mantzouranis EC, Borel Y. Systemic lupus erythematosus in childhood: clinical manifestations and improved survival in fifty-five patients. *Clin Immunol Immunopathol* 1983;29:196–210.
12. Jacobs JC. Systemic lupus erythematosus in childhood. Report of 35 cases with discussion of seven apparently induced by anticonvulsant medication, and of prognosis and treatment. *Pediatrics* 1963;32:257–264.
13. King KK, Kornreich HK, Bernstein BH, et al. The clinical spectrum of systemic lupus erythematosus in childhood. Proceedings of the conference on rheumatic diseases of childhood. *Arthritis Rheum* 1977;20 (suppl):287294.
14. Walravens P, Chase HP. The prognosis of childhood systemic lupus erythematosus. *Am J Dis Child* 1976;130:929–933.
15. Stowers JH. Lupus erythematosus in a child. *Br J Dermatol* 1892;20:236. (Cited in Stewart CC, Goeckerman WH. Lupus erythematosus disseminatus acutus in a juvenile. *Am J Dis Child* 1931;42:864–869.)
16. Sequeira JH, Balean H. Lupus erythematosus: a clinical study of seventy-one cases. *Br J Dermatol* 1902;14:367–379.
17. Denzer BS, Blumenthal S. Acute lupus erythematosus disseminatus. *Am J Dis Child* 1937;53:525–540.
18. Downing JG, Messina SJ. Acute disseminated lupus erythematosus associated with finger lesions resembling lupus pernio. *N Engl J Med* 1942;227:408–409.
19. Jacobs HJ. Acute disseminated lupus erythematosus with hemolytic anemia in a 10-year-old child. *J Pediatr* 1953;42: 728–730.
20. Lyon JM. Acute lupus erythematosus. *Am J Dis Child* 1993;45: 572–583.
21. Pehrson M. Lupus erythematosus disseminatus treated with ACTH. *Acta Paediatr* 1952;41:478–483.
22. Stewart CC, Goeckerman WH. Lupus erythematosus disseminatus acutus in a juvenile. *Am J Dis Child* 1931;42:864–869.
23. Zetterstrom R, Berglund G. Systemic lupus erythematosus in childhood: a clinical study. *Acta Paediatr* 1956;45:189–203.
24. Gribetz D, Henley WL. Systemic lupus erythematosus in childhood. *J Mt Sinai Hosp* 1959;26:289–296.
25. Peterson RDA, Vernier RL, Good RA. Lupus erythematosus. *Pediatr Clin North Am* 1963;10:941–975.
26. Coleman WP 3rd, Coleman WP, Derbes VI, et al. Collagen disease in children. A review of 71 cases. *JAMA* 1977;237: 1095–1100.
27. Gold AP, Yahr MD. Childhood lupus erythematosus. *Trans Am Neurol Assoc* 1960;85:96–102.
28. Norris DG, Colon AR, Stickler GB. Systemic lupus erythematosus in children: the complex problems of diagnosis and treatment encountered in 101 such patients at the Mayo Clinic. *Clin Pediatr* (Phila) 1977;16:774–778.
29. Platt JL, Burke BA, Fish AJ, et al. Systemic lupus erythematosus in the first two decades of life. *Am J Kidney Dis* 1982; 2(suppl 1):212–222.
30. Lehman TJA. Long-term outcome of systemic lupus erythe-

matosus in childhood: what is the prognosis? *Rheum Dis Clin North Am* 1991;17:921–930.
31. Lehman TJA, Onel KB. Intermittent intravenous cyclophosphamide arrests progression of the renal chronicity index in childhood systemic lupus erythematosus. *J Pediatrics* 2000;136: 243–247
32. Singsen BH. Epidemiology of rheumatic diseases: rheumatic diseases of childhood. *Rheum Dis Clin North Am* 1990;16: 581–599.
33. Fessel WJ. Systemic lupus erythematosus in the community. Incidence, prevalence, outcome, and first symptoms; the high prevalence in black women. *Arch Intern Med* 1974;134: 1027–1035.
34. Siegel M, Lee SL. The epidemiology of systemic lupus erythematosus. *Semin Arthritis Rheum* 1973;3:154.
35. Hochberg MC. The incidence of systemic lupus erythematosus in Baltimore, Maryland, 1970–1977. *Arthritis Rheum* 1985;28: 80–86.
36. Denardo BA, Tucker LB, Miller LC, et al. Demography of a regional pediatric rheumatology patient population. *J Rheumatol* 1994;21:1553–1561.
37. Malleson PN. The incidence of childhood rheumatic diseases in Canada (abstract). *Clin Exp Rheumatol* 1995;13:538.
38. Baum J. Epidemiology of juvenile rheumatoid arthritis. *Arthritis Rheum* 1977;20:158–160.
39. Gare A, Fasth A, Anderson J, et al. Incidence and prevalence of juvenile chronic arthritis. *Ann Rheum Dis* 1987;46:277–281.
40. Gewanter HL, Baum J. The frequency of juvenile arthritis. *J Rheumatol* 1989;16:556–557.
41. Towner SR, Michet CJ, O'Fallon WM, et al. The epidemiology of juvenile arthritis in Rochester, Minnesota, 19601970. *Arthritis Rheum* 1983;26:1208–1213.
42. Sequeira W, Polisky RB, Alrenga DP. Neutrophilic dermatosis (Sweet's syndrome). Association with a hydralazine-induced lupus syndrome. *Am J Med* 1986;81:558–560.
43. Gedalia A, Molina JF, Molina J, et al. Childhood-onset systemic lupus erythematosus: a comparative study of African Americans and Latin Americans. *Journal of the National Medical Association* 1999;91:497–501.
44. Cleland LG, Bell DA, Williams M, et al. Familial lupus. Family studies of HLA and serologic findings. *Arthritis Rheum* 1978; 21:183–191.
45. LaRochelle G, Lacks S, Borenstein D. IV cyclophosphamide therapy of steroid resistant neuropsychiatric SLE (NPSLE) (abstract). *Arthritis Rheum* 1990;33(suppl 5):R21.
46. Larsen RA. Family studies in systemic lupus erythematosus. I. A proband material from central eastern Norway. *Acta Med Scand Suppl* 1972;543:11–19.
47. Larsen RA. Family studies in systemic lupus erythematosus. III. Presence of LE factor in relatives and spouses. *Acta Med Scand Suppl* 1972;543:31–41.
48. Larsen RA, Godal T. Family studies in systemic lupus erythematosus (SLE). IX. Thyroid diseases and antibodies. *J Chronic Dis* 1972;25:225–233.
49. Lehman TJA, Hanson V, Singsen BH, et al. The role of antibodies directed against double-stranded DNA in the manifestations of sytemic lupus erythematosus in childhood. *J Pediatr* 1980;96:657–661.
50. Lehman TJA, Reichlin M, Harley JB. Familial concordance for antibodies to Ro/SSA among female relatives of children with systemic lupus erythematosus. Evidence for the "supergene" hypothesis? (abstract). *Arthritis Rheum* 1990;33 (suppl):S125.
51. Leohirun L, Thuvasethakul P, Sumethkul V, et al. Urinary neopterin in patients with systemic lupus erythematosus. *Clin Chem* 1991;37:47–50.
52. Lowenstein MB, Rothfield NF. Family study of systemic lupus erythematosus: analysis of the clinical history, skin immunofluorescence, and serologic parameters. *Arthritis Rheum* 1977;20: 1293–1303.
53. Masi AT. Family, twin, and genetic studies: a general review illustrated by systemic lupus erythematosus. Population studies of the rheumatic diseases. In: Bennet PH, Wood PHN, eds. *Proceedings of the Third International Symposium, New York*. International Congress Series No. 148. Amsterdam: Excerpta Medica, 1968:267–286.
54. Morteo OG, Franklin EC, McEwen C, et al. Clinical and laboratory studies of relatives with systemic lupus erythematosus. *Arthritis Rheum* 1961;4;356–361.
55. Pollak VE. Antinuclear antibodies in families of patients with systemic lupus erythematosus. *N Engl J Med* 1964;271: 165–171.
56. Solheim BG, Larsen RA. Family studies in systemic lupus erythematosus. IV. Presence of antinuclear factors (ANFs) in the total populations of relatives and spouses, and the correlation to rheumatic disease. *Acta Med Scand Suppl* 1972;543:43–53.
57. Lie TH, Rothfield NF. An evaluation of the preliminary criteria for the diagnosis of systemic lupus erythematosus. *Arthritis Rheum* 1972;15:532–534.
58. Block SR, Winfield JB, Lockshin MD, et al. Studies of twins with systemic lupus erythematosus. A review of the literature and presentation of 12 additional sets. *Am J Med* 1975;59: 533–552.
59. Kaplan D. The onset of disease in twins and siblings with systemic lupus erythematosus. *J Rheumatol* 1984;11:648–652.
60. Lehman TJA, Palmeri ST, Hastings C, et al. Bacterial endocarditis complicating systemic lupus erythematosus. *J Rheumatol* 1983;10:655–658.
61. Hochberg MC. The applicat'on of genetic epidemiology to systemic lupus erythematosus. *J Rheumatol* 1987;14:867–869.
62. Sestak AL, Shaver TS, Moser KL, et al. Familial aggregation of lupus and autoimmunity in an unusual multiples pedigree. *J Rheumatol* 1999;26:1495–1499.
63. Harley JB, Reichlin M, Arnett FC, et al. Gene interaction at the HLA-DQ locus enhances autoantibody production in primary Sjögren's syndrome. *Science* 1986;232:1145–1147.
64. Molta C, Meyer O, Dosquet C, et al. Childhood onset systemic lupus erythematosus: antiphospholipid antibodies in 37 patients and their first-degree relatives. *Pediatrics* 1993;92: 849–853.
65. Ravello A, Coporali R, Fuccia GD, et al. Anticardiolipin antibodies in pediatric systemic lupus erythematosus. *Arch Pediatr Adolesc Med* 1994;148:398–402.
66. Mujic F, Cuadrado MJ, Lloyd M, et al. Primary antiphospholipid syndrome evolving into systemic lupus erythematosus. *J Rheumatol* 1995;22:1589–1592.
67. Agnello V, DeBracco MME, Kunkel HG. Hereditary C2 deficiency with some manifestations of systemic lupus erythematosus. *J Immunol* 1972;108:837–840.
68. Douglass M, Lamberg SI, Lorincz AL, et al. Lupus erythematosus-like syndrome with a familial deficiency of C2. *Arch Dermatol* 1976;112:671–674.
69. Fiedler AHL, Walport MJ, Batchelor JR, et al. Family study of the major histocompatibility complex in patients with systemic lupus erythematosus: importance of null alleles of C4A and C4B in determining disease susceptibility. *Br Med J (Clin Res)* 1983;286:425–428.
70. Gewurz A, Lint TF, Robert JL, et al. Homozygous C2 deficiency with fulminant lupus erythematosus. *Arthritis Rheum* 1978;21:28–36.
71. Glass D, Raum D, Gibson D, et al. Inherited deficiency of the second component of complement. Rheumatic disease associations. *J Clin Invest* 1976;58:853–861.

72. Ochs HD, Rosenfeld SI, Thomas ED, et al. Linkage between the gene (or genes) controlling synthesis of the fourth component of complement and the major histocompatibility complex. *N Engl J Med* 1977;296:470–475.
73. Schaller J. Illness resembling lupus erythematosus in mothers of boys with chronic granulomatous disease. *Ann Intern Med* 1972;76:747–750.
74. Stern R, Fu SM, Fotino M, et al. Hereditary C2-deficiency. *Arthritis Rheum* 1976;19:517–522.
75. Schaller JG, Gilliland BG, Ochs HD, et al. Severe systemic lupus erythematosus with nephritis in a boy with deficiency of the fourth component of complement. *Arthritis Rheum* 1977; 20:1519–1525.
76. Nies KM, Brown JC, Dubois EL, et al. Histocompatibility (HLA) antigens and lymphocytotoxic antibodies in systemic lupus erythematosus (SLE). *Arthritis Rheum* 1974;17:397–402.
77. Welch TR, Beischel LS, Balakrishnan K, et al. Major histocompatibility complex extended haplotypes in systemic lupus erythematosus. *Dis Markers* 1988;6:247–255.
78. Topaloglu R, Bakkaloglu A, Slingsby JH, et al. Molecular basis of hereditary C1q deficiency associated with SLE and IgA nephropathy in a Turkish family. *Kidney International* 1996;50: 635–642.
79. Vaishnaw AK, Toubi E, Ohsako S, et al. The spectrum of apoptotic defects and clinical manifestations, including systemic lupus erythematosus, in humans with CD95 (Fas/APO–1) mutations. *Arthritis Rheum* 1999;42:1833–1842.
80. Cassidy JT, Burt A, Petty R, et al. Selective IgA deficiency in connective tissue diseases. *N Engl J Med* 1969;280:275.
81. Cronin ME, Balow JE, Tsokos GC. Immunoglobulin deficiency in patients with systemic lupus erythematosus. *Clin Exp Rheumatol* 1989;7:359–364.
82. Barton LL, Johnson CR. Discoid lupus erythematosus and X-linked chronic granulomatous disease. *Pediatr Dermatol* 1986;3: 376–379.
83. Manzi S, Urbach AH, McCune AB, et al. Systemic lupus erythematosus in a boy with chronic granulomatous disease: case report and review of the literature (brief report). *Arthritis Rheum* 1991;34:101–105.
84. Iqbal S, Sher MR, Good RA, et al. Diversity in presenting manifestations of systemic lupus erythematosus in children. *J Pediatr* 1999;135:500–505.
85. Phadke K, Trachtman H, Nicastri A, et al. Acute renal failure as the initial manifestation of systemic lupus erythematosus in children. *J Pediatr* 1984;105:38–41.
86. Tan EM, Cohen AS, Fries JF, et al. Special article: the 1982 revised criteria for the classification of systemic lupus erythematosus. *Arthritis Rheum* 1982;25:1271–1277.
87. Gianviti A, Barsotti P, Barbera V, et al. Delayed onset of systemic lupus erythematosus in patients with "full-house" nephropathy. *Pediatric Nephrology* 1999;13:683–687.
88. Morris MC, Cameron JS, Chantler C, et al. Systemic lupus erythematosus with nephritis. *Arch Dis Child* 1981;56:779–783.
89. Font J, Torras A, Cevera R, et al. Silent renal disease in systemic lupus erythematosus. *Clin Nephrol* 1987;27:283–288.
90. O'Dell JR, Hays RC, Guggenheim SJ, et al. Systemic lupus erythematosus without clinical renal abnormalities: renal biopsy findings and clinical course. *Ann Rheum Dis* 1985;44:415–419.
91. Stamenkovic I, Favre H, Donath A, et al. Renal biopsy in SLE irrespective of clinical findings: long-term follow-up. *Clin Nephrol* 1986;26:109–115.
92. Malleson PN. The role of renal biopsy in childhood onset systemic lupus erythematosus: a viewpoint. *Clin Exp Rheumatol* 1989;7:563–566.
93. McCurdy DK, Lehman TJA, Bernstein B, et al. Lupus nephritis: prognostic factors in children. *Pediatrics* 1992;89:240–246.
94. Lehman TJA, Mouradian JA. Systemic lupus erythematosus. In: Holliday MA, Barrat TM, Avner ED, eds. *Pediatric nephrology, 3rd ed.* Baltimore: Williams & Wilkins, 1994:849–870.
95. Leechawengwong M, Berger H, Sukumaran M. Diagnostic significance of antinuclear antibodies in pleural effusion. *Mt Sinai J Med* 1979;46:137–139.
96. Dumas R. Lupus nephritis. *Arch Dis Child* 1985;60:126–128.
97. Miller MN, Baumal R, Poucell S, et al. Incidence and prognostic importance of glomerular crescents in renal diseases of childhood. *Am J Nephrol* 1984;4:244–247.
98. Rush PJ, Baumal R, Shore A, et al. Correlation of renal histology with outcome in children with lupus nephritis. *Kidney Int* 1986;29:1066–1071.
99. Austin HA 3rd, Muenz LR, Joyce KM, et al. Prognostic factors in lupus nephritis: contribution of renal histologic data. *Am J Med* 1983;75:382–391.
100. Asherson RA, Lanham JG, Hull RG, et al. Renal vein thrombosis in systemic lupus erythematosus: association with the "lupus anticoagulant". *Clin Exp Rheumatol* 1989;2:75–79.
101. Ostuni PA, Lazzarin P, Pengo V, et al. Renal artery thrombosis and hypertension in a 13 year old girl with antiphospholipid syndrome. *Ann Rheum Dis* 1990;49:184–187.
102. Lehman TJA, Reichlin M, Santner TJ, et al. Maternal antibodies to Ro (SS;n-A) are associated with both early onset of disease and male sex among children with systemic lupus erythematosus. *Arthritis Rheum* 1989;32:1414–1420.
103. Balow JE, Austin HA 3rd, Muenz LR, et al. Effect of treatment on the evolution of renal abnormalities in lupus nephritis. *N Engl J Med* 1984;311:491–495.
104. Austin HA 3rd, Klippel JH, Balow JE, et al. Therapy of lupus nephritis. Controlled trial of prednisone and cytotoxic drugs. *N Engl J Med* 1986;314:614–619.
105. Urizar RE, Tinglof B, McIntosh R, et al. Immunosuppressive therapy of proliferative glomerulonephritis in children. *Am J Dis Child* 1969;118:411–425.
106. Levy M, Montes de Oca M, Claude-Babron M. Unfavorable outcomes (end-stage renal failure/death) in childhood onset systemic lupus erythematosus. *Clin Exp Rheumatol* 1994;12(suppl 10):S63–S68.
107. Lehman TJ, Sherry DD, Wagner-Weiner L, et al. Intermittent intravenous cyclophosphamide therapy for lupus nephritis. *J Pediatr* 1989;114:1055–1060.
108. Lehman TJA. Current concepts in immunosupressive drug therapy of systemic lupus erythematosus. *J Rheumatol* 1992;33:20–22.
109. Abud-Mendoza C, Sturbaum AK, Vazquea-Compean R, et al. Methotrexate therapy in childhood systemic lupus erythematosus. *J Rheumatol* 1993:20:731–733.
110. Burt RK. BMT for severe autoimmune diseases: an idea whose time has come. *Oncology* 2000;11:1001–1014.
111. Musso M, Porretto F, Crescimanno A, et al. Autologous peripheral blood stem cell and progenitor (CD34++) cell transplantation for systemic lupus erythematosus complicated by Evans syndrome. *Lupus* 1998;7:492–494.
112. Schachna L, Ryan PF, Schwarer AP. Malignancy associated remission of systemic lupus erythematosus maintained by autologous peripheral blood stem cell transplantation. *Arthritis Rheum* 1998;41:2271–2272.
112a. Wulffroat NM, Sanders EAM, Kamphuis SSM, et al. Prolonged remission without treatment after autologous stem cell transplanation for refractory childhood systemic lupus erythematosus. *Arthritis Rheum* 2001;44:728–731.
113. Cruickshank B. Lesions of joints and tendon sheaths in systemic lupus erythematosus. *Ann Rheum Dis* 1959;18:111–119.
114. Del Guidice GC, Scher CA, Athreya BH, et al. Pseudotumor cerebri and childhood systemic lupus erythematosus. *J Rheumatol* 1986;13:748–752.

115. Dietze HJ, Voegele GE. Neuropsychiatric manifestations associated with systemic lupus erythematosus in children. *Psychiatr Q* 1966;40:59–70.
116. Feinglass EJ, Arnett FC, Dorsch CA, et al. Neuropsychiatric manifestations of systemic lupus erythematosus; diagnosis, clinical spectrum, and relationship to other features of the disease. *Medicine* 1976;55:323–339.
117. Gibson T, Myers AR. Nervous system involvement in systemic lupus erythematosus. *Ann Rheum Dis* 1975;35:398–406.
118. Herd JK, Medhi M, Uzendoski DM, et al. Chorea associated with systemic lupus erythematosus. *Pediatrics* 1978;61:308–315.
119. Linn JE, Hardin JG, Halla JT. A controlled study of ANA; plRF- arthritis. *Arthritis Rheum* 1978;21:645–651.
120. Long AA, Denburg DS, Carbotte RM, et al. Serum lymphocytotoxic antibodies and neurocognitive function in systemic lupus erythematosus. *Ann Rheum Dis* 1990;49:249–253.
121. Papero PH, Bluestein HG, White P, et al. Neuropsychologic deficits and antineuronal antibodies in pediatric systemic lupus erythematosus. *Clin Exp Rheumatol* 1990;8:417–424.
122. Warren RW, Kredich DW. Transverse myelitis and acute central nervous system manifestations of systemic lupus erythematosus. *Arthritis Rheum* 1984;27:1058–1060.
123. Weintraub MI. Chorea in childhood systemic lupus erythematosus (letter). *JAMA* 1977;283:855.
124. Yancey CL, Doughty RA, Athreya BH. Central nervous system involvement in childhood systemic lupus erythematosus. *Arthritis Rheum* 1981;24:1389–1395.
125. Carbotte RM, Denburg SD, Denburg JA. Prevalence of cognitive impairment in systemic lupus erythematosus. *J Nerv Ment Dis* 1986;174:357–364.
126. Wyckoff PM, Miller LC, Tucker LB, et al. Neuropsychological assessment of children and adolescents with systemic lupus erythematosus. *Lupus* 1994;4:217–220.
127. Swaak AJG. Central nervous system involvement in systemic lupus erythematosus. *Neth J Med* 1986;29:221–228.
128. Arisaka O, Obinata K, Sasaki H, et al. Chorea as an initial manifestation of systemic lupus erythematosus. *Clin Pediatr* 1984;23:298–300.
129. Bruyn GW, Padberg G. Chorea and lupus erythematosus. A critical review. *Eur Neurol* 1984;23:435–448.
130. Groothuis JR, Groothuis DR, Mukhopadhyay D, et al. Lupus-associated chorea in childhood. *Am J Dis Child* 1977;131:1131–1134.
131. Asherson RA, Derksen RH, Harris EN, et al. Chorea in systemic lupus erythematosus and lupus-like disease: association with antiphospholipid antibodies. *Semin Arthritis Rheum* 1987;16:253–259.
132. Buchbinder R, Hall S, Littlejohn GO, et al. Neuropsychiatric manifestations of systemic lupus erythematosus. *Aust N Z J Med* 1988;18:679–684.
133. Lehman P, Holzle E, Kind P, et al. Experimental reproduction of skin lesions in lupus erythematosus by UVA and UVB radiation. *J Am Acad Dermatol* 1990;22:181–187.
134. Ahmadieh H, Roodpeyma S, Azarmina M, et al. Bilateral simultaneous optic neuritis in childhood systemic lupus erythematosus. *J Neuro-ophthalmol* 1994;14:84–86.
135. Hisashi K, Komune S, Taira T, et al. Anticardioplipin antibody-induced sudden profound sensorineural hearing loss. *Am J Otolaryngol* 1993;14:275–277.
136. Cunningham S, Conway E. Systemic lupus erythematosus presenting as an intracranial bleed. *Ann Emerg Med* 1991;20:810–812.
137. Dungan DD, Jay MS. Stroke in an early adolescent with systemic lupus erythematosus and coexistent antiphospholipid antibodies. *Pediatrics* 1992;1:96–99.
138. Uziel Y, Laxer RM, Blaser S, et al. Cerebral vein thrombosis in childhood systemic lupus erythematosus. *J Pediatr* 1995;126:722–727.
139. Bentson J, Reza M, Winter J, et al. Steroids and apparent cerebral atrophy on computed tomography scans. *J Comput Assist Tomogr* 1978;2:16–23.
140. Carette S, Urowitz MB, Grosman H, et al. Cranial computerized tomography in systemic lupus erythematosus. *J Rheumatol* 1982;9:855–859.
141. Gonzalez-Scarano F, Lisak RP, Bilaniuk LT, et al. Cranial computed tomography in the diagnosis of systemic lupus erythematosus. *Ann Neurol* 1979;5:158–165.
142. Szer I, Miller JH, Rawlings D, et al. Cerebral perfusion abnormalities in children with central nervous system manifestations of lupus detected by single photon emission computed tomography. *J Rheumatol* 1993;20:2143–2148.
143. Nomura K, Yamano S, Ikeda Y, et al. Asymptomatic cerebrovascular lesions detected by magnetic resonance imaging in patients with systemic lupus erythematosus lacking a history of neuropsychiatric events. *Internal Medicine* 1999;38:785–795.
144. Bonfa E, Golombek SJ, Kaufman LD, et al. Association between lupus psychosis and anti-ribosomal P protein antibodies. *N Engl J Med* 1987;317:265–271.
145. Reichlin M, Broyles TF, Hubscher O, et al. Prevalence of Autoantibodies to Ribosomal P Proteins in Juvenile-Onset Systemic Lupus Erythemtosus compared with the adult disease. *Arthritis Rheum* 1999;42:69–75.
146. Delgado EA, Malleson PN, Pirie GE, et al. Pulmonary manifestations of childhood onset systemic lupus erythematosus. *Semin Arthritis Rheum* 1990;29:285–293.
147. Pohlgeers AP, Eid MS, Schikler KN, et al. Systemic lupus erythematosus: pulmonary presentation in childhood. *South Med J* 1990;83:712–714.
148. DeJongste JC, Neijens HJ, Duiverman EJ, et al. Respiratory tract disease in systemic lupus erythematosus. *Arch Dis Child* 1986;61:478–483.
149. Matthay RA, Schwartz MI, Petty TL, et al. Pulmonary manifestations of systemic lupus erythematosus: review of twelve cases of acute lupus pneumonitis. *Medicine* 1975;54:397–409.
150. Nadorra RL, Landing BH. Pulmonary lesions in childhood onset systemic lupus erythematosus. *Pediatr Pathol* 1987;7:118.
151. Rajani KB, Ashbacher LV, Kinney TR. Pulmonary hemorrhage and systemic lupus erythematosus. *J Pediatr* 1978;93:810–812.
152. Ramirez RE, Glasier C, Kirks D, et al. Pulmonary hemorrhage associated with systemic lupus erythematosus in children. *Radiology* 1984;152:409–412.
153. Singsen BH, Platzker CG. Pulmonary involvement in the rheumatic disorders of childhood. In: Kendig EL, Chernick V, eds. *Disorders of the respiratory tract in children, 4th ed.* Philadelphia: WB Saunders, 1983:846–872.
154. Miller RW, Salcedo JR, Fink RJ, et al. Pulmonary hemorrhage in pediatric patients with systemic lupus erythematosus. *J Pediatr* 1986;108:576–579.
155. Trapani S, Camiciottoli G, Ermini M, et al. Pulmonary involvement in juvenile systemic lupus erythematosus: a study on long function in patients asymptomatic for respiratory disease. *Lupus* 1998;7:545–550.
156. Speira H, Rothenberg RR. Myocardial infarction in four young patients with systemic lupus erythematosus. *J Rheumatol* 1983;10:464–466.
157. Garty BZ, Stark H, Yaniv I, et al. Pulmonary nocardiosis in a child with systemic lupus erythematosus. *Pediatr Infect Dis* 1985;4:66–68.
158. Ragsdale CG, Petty RE, Cassidy JT, et al. The clinical progression of apparent juvenile rheumatoid arthritis to systemic lupus erythematosus. *J Rheumatol* 1980;7:50–55.

159. Bergstein J, Wiens C, Fish AJ, et al. Avascular necrosis of bone in systemic lupus erythematosus. *J Pediatr* 1974;85:31–35.
160. Dimant J, Ginzler EM, Diamond HS, et al. Computer analysis of factors influencing the appearance of aseptic necrosis in patients with SLE. *J Rheumatol* 1978;5:136–141.
161. Isenberg DA, Snaith ML. Muscle disease in systemic lupus erythematosus: a study of its nature, frequency and cause. *J Rheumatol* 1981;8:917–924.
162. Rider LG, Sherry DD, Glass ST. Neonatal lupus erythematosus simulating transient myasthenia gravis at presentation. *J Pediatr* 1991;118:417–419.
163. Lamy P, Valla D, Bourgeois P, et al. Primary sclerosing cholangitis and systemic lupus erythematosus. *Gastroenterol Clin Biol* 1988;12:962–964.
164. Alarcon GS, Sams WM Jr, Barton DD, et al. Bullous lupus erythematosus rash worsened by Dapsone. *Arthritis Rheum* 1984; 27:1072–1072.
165. Cassidy JT, Petty RE. *Textbook of pediatric rheumatology, 2nd ed.* New York: Churchill Livingstone, 1990.
166. Aiuto LT, Stambouly JJ, Boxer RA. Cardiac tamponade in an adolescent female. *Clin Pediatr* 1993;32:566–567.
167. De Inoncencio J, Lovell DJ. Cardiac function in systemic lupus erythematosus. *J Rheumatol* 1994;21:2147–2156.
168. Weinberg A, Kaplan JG, Myers AR. Extensive soft tissue calcification (calcinosis universalis) in systemic lupus erythematosus. *Ann Rheum Dis* 1979;38:384–386.
169. Wood G, Rucker M, Davis JR, et al. Interaction of plasma fibronectin with selected cryoglobulins. *Clin Exp Immunol* 1980;40:358–364.
170. Le Page SH, Williams W, Parkhouse D, et al. Relation between lymphocytotoxic antibodies, anti-DNA antibodies and a common anti-DNA antibody idiotype PR4 in patients with systemic lupus erythematosus, their relatives and spouses. *Clin Exp Immunol* 1989;77:314–318.
171. Lehman TJA, McCurdy DK, Bernstein BH, et al. Systemic lupus erythematosus in the first decade of life. *Pediatrics* 1989; 83:235–239.
172. Bor I. Myocardial infarction and ischemic heart disease in infants and children. *Arch Dis Child* 1969;44:268–281.
173. Englund JA, Lucas RV. Cardiac complications in children with systemic lupus erythematosus. *Pediatrics* 1983;72:724–730.
174. Friedman DM, Lazarus HM, Fierman AH. Acute myocardial infarction in pediatric systemic lupus erythematosus. *J Pediatr* 1990;117:263–266.
175. Homcy CJ, Liberthson RR, Fallon JT, et al. Ischemic heart disease in systemic lupus erythematosus in the young patient: report of 6 cases. *Am J Cardiol* 1982;49:478–484.
176. Ishikawa S, Segar WE, Gilbert EF, et al. Myocardial infarction in a child with systemic lupus erythematosus. *Am J Dis Child* 1978;132:696–699.
177. Eberhard A, Shore A, Silverman E, et al. Bowel perforation and interstitial cystitis in childhood systemic lupus erythematosus. *J Rheumatol* 1991;18:746–747.
178. Bashour B. Systemic lupus erythematosus with retroperitoneal fibrosis and thrombosis of the inferior vena cava. *South Med J* 1993;86:1309–1310.
179. Eberhard A, Couper R, Durie P, et al. Exocrine pancreatic function in children with systemic lupus erythematosus. *J Rheumatol* 1992;19:964–967.
180. Buntain WL, Wood JB, Woolley MM. Pancreatitis in childhood. *J Pediatr Surg* 1978;12:143–149.
181. Fonkalsrud EW, Henney P, Riemenschneider TA, et al. Management of pancreatitis in infants and children. *Am J Surg* 1968; 116:198–203.
182. Nadorra RL, Nakazato Y, Landing BH. Pathologic features of gastrointestinal tract lesions in childhood-onset systemic lupus erythematosus: study of 26 patients, with review of the literature. *Pediatr Pathol* 1987;7:245–259.
183. Simons-Ling N, Schachner L, Pennys N, et al. Childhood systemic lupus erythematosus: association with pancreatitis, subcutaneous fat necrosis and calcinosis cutis. *Arch Dermatol* 1983; 119:491–494.
184. Binstadt DH, L'Heureux PR. Pneumatosis cystoides intestinalis in childhood systemic lupus erythematosus. *Minn Med* 1977; 60:408–409.
185. Alverson DC, Chase HP. Systemic lupus erythematosus in childhood presenting as hyperlipoproteinemia. *J Pediatr* 1977; 91:72–75.
186. Tsukahara M, Matsuo K, Kojima H. Protein-losing enteropathy in a boy with systemic lupus erythematosus. *J Pediatr* 1990;97: 778–780.
187. Malleson P, Petty RE, Nadel H, et al. Functional asplenia in childhood onset systemic lupus erythematosus. *J Rheumatol* 1988;15:1648–1652.
188. Ginzler E, Diamond H, Kaplan D, et al. Computer analysis of factors influencing frequency of infection in systemic lupus erythematosus. *Arthritis Rheum* 1978;21:37–44.
189. Staples PJ, Gerdin DN, Decker JL, et al. Incidence of infection in systemic lupus erythematosus. *Arthritis Rheum* 1974;17:110.
190. Miyagawa S, Inagaki Y, Okada N, et al. A novel anti-ENA antibody in sera of patients with choldhood idiopathic thrombocytompenic pupura. *J Dermtaol* 1991;18:69–73.
191. Gedalia A, Molina JF, Garcia CO, et al. Anticardiolipin antibodies in childhood rheumatic disorders. *Lupus* 1998;7: 551–553.
192. Fields RA, Sibbitt WL, Toubbeh H, et al. Neuropsychiatric lupus erythematosus, cerebral infarctions, and anticardiolipin antibodies. *Ann Rheum Dis* 1990;49:114–117.
193. Shergy WJ, Kredich DW, Pisetsky DS. The relationship of anticardiolipin antibodies to disease manifestations in pediatric systemic lupus erythematosus. *J Rheumatol* 1988;15:1389–1394.
194. Nojima J, Suehisa E, Kuratsune H, et al. High prevalence of thrombocytopenia in SLE patients with a high level of anticardiolipin antibodies combined with lupus anticoagulant. *Am J Hematol* 1998;58:55–60.
195. Galeazzi M, Bellisai F, Sebastiani GD, et al. Association of 16/6 and SA1 anti-DNA idiotypes with anticardiolipin antibodies and clinical manifestations in a large cohort of SLE patients. *Clin Experimental Rheum* 1998;16:717–720.
196. Berube C, Mitchell L, Silverman E, et al. The relationship of antiphospholipid antibodies to thrombotic events in pediatric patients with systemic lupus erythematosus; a cross-sectional study. *Pediatric Research* 1998;44:351–356.
197. Ravelli A, Caporali C, Bianchi E, et al. Anticardiolipin syndrome in childhood: a report of two cases. *Clin Exp Rheumatol* 1990;8:95–98.
198. Gillespie JP, Lindsley CB, Linshaw MA, et al. Childhood systemic lupus erythematosus with negative antinuclear antibody test. *J Pediatr* 1981;98:578–581.
199. Lehman TJA, Curd JG, Zvaifer NJ, et al. The association of antinuclear antibodies, antilymphocyte antibodies, and C4 activation among the relatives of children with systemic lupus erythematosus: preferential activation of complement in sisters. *Arthritis Rheum* 1982;25:556–561.
200. Lehman TJA, Hanson V, Zvaifler N, et al. Antibodies to nonhistone nuclear antigens and antilymphocyte antibodies among children and adults with systemic lupus erythematosus and their relatives. *J Rheumatol* 984;11:644–647.
201. Pincus T, Hughes GRV, Pincus D, et al. Antibodies to DNA in childhood systemic lupus erythematosus. *J Pediatr* 1971;78: 981–984.
202. Barron KS, Silverman ED, Gonzales J, et al. Clinical, serologic,

and immunogenetic studies in childhood-onset systemic lupus erythematosus. *Arthritis Rheum* 1993;36:348–354.
203. Wong SN, Shah R, Dillon MJ. Antineutrophil cytoplasmic antibodies in childhood systemic lupus erythematosus. *Eur J Pediatr* 1995;154:43–45.
204. Bakkaloglu A, Topaloglu R, Saatci U, et al. Antineutrophil cytoplasmic antibodies in childhood systemic lupus erythematosus. *Clin Rheumatol* 1998;17:265–267.
205. Faure-Fontenia MA, Rodriguez-Suarez RS, Arias-Velasquez R, et al. Antineutrophil cytoplasmic antibodies in systemic lupus erythematosus in childhood. *J Rheumatol* 1999;26:2480–2481.
206. Conroy SE, Tucker L, Latchman DS, et al. Incidence of anti Hsp 90 and 70 antibodies in children with SLE, juvenile dermatomyositis, and juvenile chronic arthritis. *Clin Experimental Rheumatol* 1996;14:99–104.
207. Caggiano V, Fernando LP, Schneider JM, et al. Thrombotic thrombocytopenic purpura. Report of fourteen cases-occurrence during pregnancy and response to plasma exchange. *J Clin Apheresis* 1983;1:71–85.
208. Singsen BH, Bernstein BH, King KK, et al. Systemic lupus erythematosus in childhood: correlations between changes in disease activity and serum complement levels. *J Pediatr* 1976;89: 358–365.
209. Howard PF, Hochberg MC, Bias WB, et al. Relationship between C4 null genes, HLA–D region antigens and genetic susceptibility to systemic lupus erythematosus in Caucasians and black Americans. *Am J Med* 1986;81:187–193.
210. Kemp ME, Atkinson JP, Skanes VM, et al. Deletion of C4A genes in patients with systemic lupus erythematosus. *Arthritis Rheum* 1987;30:1015–1022.
211. McKenna CH, Schroeter AL, Kierland RR, et al. The fluorescent treponemal antibody absorbed (FTA-ABS) test beading phenomenon in connective tissue diseases. *Mayo Clin Proc* 1973;48:545–548.
212. Barron KS, Person DA, Brewer EJ, et al. Pulse methylprednisolone therapy in diffuse proliferative lupus nephritis. *J Pediatr* 1982;101:137–141.
213. Balow JE. Therapeutic trials in lupus nephritis. *Nephron* 1981; 27:171–176.
214. Hughes GRV. The treatment of SLE. *Clin Rheum Dis* 1982;8: 299–313.
215. Lehman TJA. A practical guide to systemic lupus erythematosus in childhood. *Pediatr Clin North Am* 1995;42:1223–1228.
216. Wallace DJ, Goldfinger D, Bluestone R, et al. Plasmapheresis in lupus nephritis with nephrotic syndrome. A long-term follow-up. *J Clin Apheresis* 1982;1:42–45.
217. Carette S, Klippel JH, Decker JL, et al. Controlled studies of oral immunosuppressive drugs in lupus nephritis. A long term follow-up. *Ann Intern Med* 1983;99:18.
218. Akashi K, Nagasawa K, Mayumi T, et al. Successful treatment of refractory systemic lupus erythematosus with intravenous immunoglobulins. *J Rheumatol* 1990;17:375–379.
219. Rothenberg RJ, Graziano FM, Grandone JT, et al. The use of methotrexate in steroid-resistant systemic lupus erythematosus. *Arthritis Rheum* 1988;31:612–615.
220. Marmont AM, van Lint MT, Gualandi F, et al. Autologous marrow stem cell transplantation for severe systemic lupus erythematosus of long duration. *Lupus* 1997;6:545–548.
221. Traynor A, Burt RK. Hematopoetic stem cell transplantation for active systemic lupus erythematosus. *Rheumatology* 1999;38: 767–772.
222. Brodsky RA, Petri M, Smith BD, et al. Immunoablative high-dose cyclophosphamide without stem cell rescue for refractory, severe autoimmune disease. *Ann Intern Med* 12998;129: 1031–1035.
223. Petri M, Perez-Guttham S, Longenecker C, et al. The association of black race with morbidity in patients with systemic lupus erythematosus is explained by socioeconomic status and compliance (abstract). *Arthritis Rheum* 1990;33(suppl):S83.
224. Coplon NS, Diskin CJ, Peterson J, et al. The long-term clinical course of systemic lupus erythematosus in end-stage renal disease. *N Engl J Med* 1983;308:186–190.
225. Kimberly RP, Lockshin MD, Sherman RL, et al. End-stage lupus nephritis. *Medicine* 1981;60:277–287.

42

DRUG-INDUCED LUPUS

ROBERT L. RUBIN

HISTORICAL PERSPECTIVE

Within 1 year after the introduction of hydralazine to control malignant hypertension in 1952, the first report appeared of a late onset "collagen disease" resembling systemic lupus erythematosus (SLE) in 17 out of 211 hydralazine-treated patients (1). However, because the treatment regimen of these patients was combined with hexamethonium chloride, the first definitive association between hydralazine and lupus-like disease should be attributed to Dustan and her colleagues (2) at the Cleveland Clinic, in which 13 out of 139 patients became ill after receiving hydralazine 400 to 800 mg per day for an average of 12 months. In their follow-up paper in 1954, Perry and Schroeder (3) demonstrated that hexamethonium ion was not implicated in the lupus-like reaction of the 17 patients described by Morrow et al. (1) because patients fully recovered after discontinuation of only hydralazine. Although procainamide was introduced for the treatment of cardiac arrhythmia at about the same time, it was not until 1962 that Ladd (4) reported a patient who developed lupus-like features after 6 months of procainamide therapy. During the next 3 years another 11 cases of procainamide-induced lupus were reported (5). By 1966 a scattering of cases of lupus-like disease as a side effect of therapy with isoniazid, diphenylhydantoin, sulfamethoxypyradazine, primidone, and tetracycline appeared. It is now clear that patients on a diverse array of drugs can develop autoantibodies and clinical features similar to those seen in patients with idiopathic SLE. Since this subject was reviewed 5 years ago, at least three additional drugs have been reported to induce lupus-like abnormalities, suggesting that the spectrum of drugs with the capacity to induce lupus will continue to increase.

It is important to distinguish drug-induced lupus-like disease from the more common condition of drug-induced autoimmunity. When patients receiving drug therapy develop autoantibodies or other laboratory features of autoimmunity such as elevated immunoglobulin levels but are clinically asymptomatic, the term "drug-induced autoimmunity" (DIA) should be used. In contrast a minority of drug-treated patients develop *de novo* clinical signs and symptoms similar to the spectrum of features associated with idiopathic SLE. This syndrome is referred to as drug-related lupus or drug-induced lupus (DIL). While DIA may be a more homeostatically regulated form of DIL as suggested by the quantitative differences in their overt autoimmune abnormalities as discussed below, most asymptomatic drug-treated patients with persistently high levels of autoantibodies do not progress into developing lupus-like symptoms (6).

DRUGS IMPLICATED IN DRUG-INDUCED LUPUS

Table 42.1 lists currently used drugs reported to be associated with a lupus-like syndrome. In all cases drugs that induce lupus also induce autoantibodies in a much higher frequency. Excluded from this list are drugs implicated only in the exacerbation of SLE or with the onset of chronic SLE prior to diagnosis, as discussed below. Also excluded are drugs that induce non-multisystem cell, tissue, or organ abnormalities such as cytopenias or cutaneous manifestations, although these may have an autoimmune etiology similar to DIL, as discussed below. Also not shown are drugs that were initially reported to be associated with a lupus-like syndrome, but no confirmation has appeared despite many decades of prescriptions with countless patients. However, several infrequently used drugs are included in which only a single case report and/or only an autoantibody association has been reported, to heighten vigilance for these possible lupus-inducing drugs. Eight drugs listed in the previous edition have been removed from this table because they are no longer in use. Finally, not included are macromolecular immunotherapeutics that have potential for induction of autoimmunity such as interferon-α, interleukin-2, interferon-γ, and anti–tumor necrosis factor-α (reviewed in ref. 7) because the mechanism underlying this phenomenon is probably different from classical DIL.

Thus, 41 drugs currently in use have a propensity for inducing autoantibodies and occasionally a lupus-like syn-

TABLE 42.1. DRUGS REPORTED TO INDUCE LUPUS-LIKE DISEASE AND ASSOCIATED AUTOANTIBODIES

Agent[a]	Risk[b]	Reference
Antiarrhythmics		
Procainamide (Pronestyl)	High	4,8–34
Quinidine (Quinaglute)	Moderate	33,35–47
Disopyramide (Norpace)	Very low	48
Propafenone (Rythmol)	Very low	49
Antihypertensives		50–52
Hydralazine (Apresoline)	High	2,3,33,53–99
Methyldopa (Aldomet)	Low	52,100–109
Captopril (Capoten)	Low	110–115
Acebutolol (Sectral)	Low	108,116–120
Enalapril (Vasotec)	Very low	121,122
Clonidine (Catapres)	Very low	122
Atenolol (Tenormin)	Very low	123
Labetalol (Normodyne, Trandate)	Very low	124,125
Pindolol (Visken)	Very low	126
Minoxidil (Loniten)	Very low	127
Prazosin (Minipress)	Very low	128–130
Antipsychotics		131,132
Chlorpromazine (Thorazine)	Low	33,131,133–150
Perphenazine (Trilafon)	Very low	151
Phenelzine (Nardil)	Very low	152
Chlorprothixene (Taractan)	Very low	153
Lithium carbonate (Eskalith)	Very low	154–157
Anticonvulsants		158–162
Carbamazepine (Tegretol)	Low	163–170
Phenytoin (Dilantin)	Very low	171–173
Trimethadione (Tridone)	Very low	162
Primidone (Mysoline)	Very low	174–176
Ethosuximide (Zarontin)	Very low	177–180
Antibiotics		
Isoniazid/INH	Low	108,181–198
Minocycline (Minocin)	Low	199–206
Nitrofurantoin (Macrodantin)	Very low	207
Anti-Inflammatories and Antirheumatics		
D-Penicillamine (Cuprimine)	Low	108,208–227
Sulfasalazine (Azulfidine)	Low	228–240
Phenylbutazone (Butazolidin)	Very low	241–242
Zafirlukast (Accolate)	Very low	243
Mesalamine/5-aminosalicylate	Very low	244
Diuretics		
Chlorthalidone (Hygroton)	Very low	109
Hydrochlorothiazide (Diuchlor H)	Very low	245,246
Antihyperlipidemics		
Lovastatin (Mevacor)	Very low	247
Simvastatin (Zocor)	Very low	248
Miscellaneous		
Propylthiouracil (Propyl-thyracil)	Low	249–252
Levodopa (Dopar)	Very low	100,253
Aminoglutethimide (Cytadren)	Very low	254
Timolol eye drops (Timoptic)	Very low	255

[a]Commonly used brand names are enclosed in parentheses.
[b]Risk refers to likelihood for lupus-like disease, not autoantibody induction, which is usually much more common.

drome. Table 42.1 divides these drugs into therapeutic classes and indicates their approximate risk levels based on the number of reports. By far the highest risk drugs are procainamide and hydralazine, with approximately 20% incidence for procainamide and 5% to 8% for hydralazine during 1 year of therapy at currently used doses. The risk for developing lupus-like disease for the remainder of the drugs is much lower, considerably less than 1% of treated patients. Quinidine can be considered moderate risk while sulfasalazine, chlorpromazine, penicillamine, methyldopa, carbamazepine, acebutalol, isoniazid, captopril, propylthiouracil, and minocycline are relatively low risk. The remaining 28 drugs should be considered very low risk based on the paucity of case reports in the literature. Obviously, the perception of risk is not rigorous since it depends on dose and frequency of prescriptions as well as occasion to publish case reports, and should not be equated with a fundamental, lupus-inducing propensity. Some drugs of very low risk may be falsely implicated or are currently of negligible risk because customary treatment doses have been decreased, but most reports on drug-induced lupus are convincing because cessation of therapy usually results in prompt resolution of symptoms and eventually autoantibodies. It should be appreciated that criteria for reaching a diagnosis of drug-induced lupus-like disease are not as rigorous as those for diagnosis of SLE (see Diagnostic Criteria for Drug-Induced Lupus, below).

As early as 1957, it was suggested that anticonvulsants can induce lupus-like features (256). However, manifestations of convulsive disorders may precede typical SLE by many years, and some anticonvulsants are associated with only renal or cutaneous disease (258). It is also difficult to identify the drug that may be responsible for DIL or DIA reactions because many of these patients are using more than one drug including an additional anticonvulsant medication. Wallace and Dubois (258) have doubted many of the reports suggesting a causative relationship between anticonvulsants and DIL, and some of the anticonvulsants in Table 42.1 may be unfairly implicated. However, DIL associated with the use of phenytoin (diphenylhydantoin) and carbamazepine is well documented.

As with anticonvulsant therapy, patients who develop DIL or DIA associated with antituberculous drugs are on more than one medication. Triple therapy with isoniazid (INH), *para*-aminosalicylic (PAS) acid, and streptomycin was once standard practice. The best evidence, however, points to isoniazid as the drug most likely to cause DIA or DIL (195). The major manifestation of autoimmunity in patients on isoniazid appears to be the development of low-titer antinuclear antibodies (ANAs), and clinically diagnosed DIL is rare (258). Interestingly, antihistone antibodies in these patients are predominantly immunoglobulin A (IgA), suggestive of the involvement of the mucosal immune system in isoniazid-induced autoimmunity (198).

A broad variety of therapeutic purposes are encompassed by lupus-inducing drugs including control of convulsion disorders, psychoses, hyperthyroidism, hypertension, fungal and bacterial infections, heart arrhythmias, edema, and even antiinflammatory agents. Consequently, the structures of these drugs show wide disparity and this is reflected in their diverse biochemical action as summarized in Table 42.2. Although some of these drugs are aromatic amines (procainamide, practolol, and sulfpyridine, a metabolite of sulfasalazine) or aromatic hydrazines (hydralazine, isoniazid), there is no common denominator of a pharmacologic, therapeutic, or chemical nature that links the drugs with capacity to induce lupus-like disease. Nevertheless, the remarkable similarity in clinical features and laboratory findings in lupus induced by this collection of drugs strongly suggests that the same mechanism underlies the process regardless of the inciting agent. How this process may be related to drug chemistry is discussed later (see Oxidative Drug Metabolism).

TABLE 42.2. PHARMACOLOGIC ACTIONS OF LUPUS-INDUCING DRUGS

Mechanism of Action	Drug
Monamine oxidase inhibitor	Phenelzine
α- and β-Adrenergic antagonists and agonists	Atenolol, timolol, labetol, clonidine, pindolol, practolol, chloroprothixene, methyldopa
Myocardial anticholinergic agents	Procainamide, quinidine
Cyclooxygenase inhibitor	Phenylbutazone, mesalamine
Bacterial flavoprotein substrate	Nitrofurantoin
Bacterial cell wall synthesis inhibitor	Isoniazid
Myocardial depressive agents	Procainamide, propafenone, disopyramide
Sodium reabsorption inhibitors	Hydrochlorothiazide, chlorthalidone
HMG-CoA reductase inhibitor	Lovastatin, simvastatin
Arteriole vasodilators	Minoxidil, hydralazine
Neuron function modifiers/effectors	Mephenytoin, diphenylhydantoin, ethosuximide, carbamazepine
Postsynaptic dopaminergic receptor agonists	Chloropromazine, perphenazine, chlorprothixine
Thyroid peroxidase competitive inhibitor	Propylthiouracil
Angiotensin-converting enzyme inhibitors	Captopril, enalapril

HMG-CoA, high-mobility group–coenzyme A.

TABLE 42.3. PROSPECTIVE STUDIES OF DRUG-INDUCED LUPUS

Drug	Approx Dose (gram/day)	Average Duration (yrs)	ANA Incidence	Drug-Induced Lupus Incidence	Reference
Procainamide	2–4	1	75%	15–20%	11,15,25,26,28,32
Hydralazine	0.1–0.3	3	15–45%	5–10%	9,53,56,66,86,259
Isoniazid	0.35	0.6	22%	<1/102[a]	195
Methyldopa	1–2	2	19%	<1/53[a]	106
Levodopa	1.5–8.0	1	11%	<1/80[a]	253
Estrogen/progesterone	0.05/1[b]	1.3	<1/80[a]	<1/80[a]	260

[a]No patients developed symptoms; the denominator is the number of patients in the prospective study.
[b]mg/day.

Prospective Studies

Relatively few prospective studies have been undertaken to establish the true incidences of induction of lupus and ANA by drugs (Table 42.3). Because clinicians' choice of drugs and their doses depend in part on the country in which they practice, there is considerable geographic variability on the incidence of DIL. Even within the United Kingdom the incidence of hydralazine-induced lupus was reported to be 6.7% after 3 years of treatment (86) and 4.3% after 13 years (76). Women treated with a daily dose of 200 mg hydralazine showed a 3-year incidence of DIL of 19.4% (86). Most patients develop symptoms between 6 months and 2 years of treatment, but it is not uncommon for a patient to require more than 3 years of treatment with a total intake of more than 1 kg hydralazine before symptoms become manifest (56). With procainamide the typical patient [i.e., the arithmetic median (261)] develops symptoms after 10 months of treatment. However, variations in therapeutic response to control ventricular arrhythmias as well as differences in drug clearance and metabolism (see Acetylator Phenotype, below) result in dose requirements that vary from 0.25 to 6 g procainamide/day. As a result, approximately 25% of patients do not develop symptoms until more than 2 years, and some as long as 6 years, of continuous treatment with procainamide (15,21,28,262). Discrepancies in the literature on the incidence of procainamide-induced lupus (25,26,28) and especially hydralazine-induced lupus (56,76,86) appear to be related to the use of lower doses of these drugs in recent years just to minimize the chances of lupus-like disease. Prospective studies of isoniazid, α-methyldopa, L-dopa, and oral contraceptives failed to reveal a single case of lupus-like illness during the observation period. Thus, the incidence of lupus induced by these latter drugs must be less than 1% but is probably considerably lower.

Autoantibody induction is relatively common with approximately one fifth of patients treated with isoniazid and methyldopa and one tenth of patients treated with L-dopa developing ANAs during one half to 2 years of treatment. Studies of patients receiving procainamide therapy have shown that 75% of patients develop ANA within 1 year of treatment (11,25) and almost 100% develop ANA after 2 years (26,263). Most of these patients remain asymptomatic. The incidence of ANA positivity in patients who remain asymptomatic during approximately 3 years of treatment with hydralazine has been reported as low as 15% (66) to as high as 44% (259). Although formal prospective studies have not been performed, several other medications shown in Table 42.1 also have a high propensity for inducing ANA, anti–denatured DNA, and/or anticardiolipin antibodies, especially chlorpromazine, in which prevalences of 15% to 40% have been reported (136–138), and acebutalol, with reported ANA prevalences from 15% to 89% (50,51,119,120,128,264). It should be appreciated that the fine specificity and predominant isotype of the ANA in asymptomatic patients is generally not the same as in patients with symptomatic DIL (see Anti-[(H2A-H2B)-DNA] Antibodies), and there is no evidence that patients who convert to ANA positivity are more likely to develop symptomatic disease.

Rechallenge Studies

Between 1954 and 1973, reports appeared on the rapid reoccurrence of symptoms of DIL upon the reintroduction of hydralazine (3,9,56,267,268), procainamide (265,266), isoniazid (269), penicillamine (227), and chlorpromazine (141). These studies contributed to the notion that DIL behaves like a hypersensitivity reaction or that DIL occurs in patients predisposed to this side effect. However, examination of these reports reveals that in most cases, reintroduction of the implicated drug occurred just a few weeks after therapy was discontinued because of DIL (Table 42.4). Typically, these patients displayed symptom recurrence within 1 to 2 days after resuming therapy. It is now clear that although subjective symptoms of DIL may resolve in a few weeks, serologic abnormalities, especially antihistone antibodies, persist for much longer. Thus, immune abnormalities in most of these patients probably had not normalized when rechallenged with the drug, suggesting that a combination of autoantibody and another, unknown factor dependent on the presence of the drug is required for the pathology of DIL. In perhaps the most thorough study of this phenomenon in 11 patients with hydralazine-induced lupus after a "long" (though unstated) washout period, Perry (56) reported that three patients had symptom recurrence within

TABLE 42.4. REAPPEARANCE OF LUPUS-LIKE SYMPTOMS AFTER RECHALLENGE WITH THE LUPUS-INDUCING DRUG

	First Drug-Induced Lupus Episode			Second Drug-Induced Lupus Episode		
Drug	Dose/Day	Time for Symptoms Manifestation	Washout Period	Dose/Day	Time for Symptoms Manifestation	Reference
Procainamide	4–5 g	20 months	8 days	2 g	36 hours	265
Procainamide	1 g	25 months	3 months	1 g	"Promptly"	266
Hydralazine	0.25 g	12 months	Few days	Not stated	"Immediately"	3
Hydralazine	0.5 g	10 months	6 weeks	0.15 g	1–2 days	267
Hydralazine	0.4 g	14 months	2–3 weeks	0.6 g	12 days	268
Isoniazid	0.3 g	14 months	2 weeks	0.3 g	1 day	269
Penicillamine	2 g	27 months	18 months	0.5 g	None during 12 months	227
Chlorpromazine	0.4 g	13 months	6 weeks	0.2 g	1–2 days	141
Quinidine	0.5 g	3 weeks	1 week	0.5 g	4 days	37

1 day, two within 14 days, two within 2 months, and one after 7 months, and three never developed symptom recurrence during the second treatment period of 1 to 5 years. It remains debatable whether variability in symptom recurrence reflects differences in putative predisposing factors for development of DIL or differences in time for the hyperimmune state to return to normal. Clearly, however, this process does not reflect a drug hypersensitivity reaction that is characteristically drug dose independent and recurs immediately after rechallenge with the inciting agent (270).

OTHER LATE-ONSET TOXIC DRUG REACTIONS

Drugs That May Exacerbate SLE

The report of Hoffman (271) in 1945 describing a 19-year-old army recruit who developed cutaneous, hematologic, and renal disease with features of SLE after treatment with topical and oral sulfadiazine is often cited as the first description of DIL. In actuality this patient had a hypersensitivity-like reaction to sulfadiazine associated with exacerbation of preclinical SLE or with the onset SLE. This and subsequent similar reports [although only one involving an oral sulfa drug (272)] helped to entrench the view that many cases of idiopathic SLE are "unmasked" during drug therapy in patients with a lupus diathesis (158). This idea is difficult to discount or prove. Various drugs have been noted to have a temporal relationship with the exacerbation of SLE or with the onset of chronic SLE prior to diagnosis (258). In the latter cases SLE remains after withdrawal of the implicated agent. In the most recent case-controlled study of this phenomenon, 12% of SLE patients with drug allergies were considered to display disease exacerbation, predominately lupus rash (273,274). Since SLE patients are significantly more prone to develop drug allergies especially to antibiotics such as sulfonamides, penicillin/cephalosporin, and erythromycin (273), these agents should be avoided in patients with SLE (275). Two SLE patients who developed lupus flares after ciprofloxacin treatment required hospitalization (276), and severe clinical relapses temporally associated with therapy with sulfonamides have been reported in the older literature (277).

Drugs that appear to exacerbate SLE can be classified as antibiotics, anticonvulsants, hormones, nonsteroidal anti-inflammatory drugs (NSAIDs), and dermatologic agents. Sulfonamides (278), tetracyclines (279), griseofulvin, (280–282), piroxicam (283), and benoxaprofen (284) are reported to be photosensitizers of varying frequency. Rash or dermatitis related to drugs typically has a history of rapid onset and behaves as a drug hypersensitivity-type reaction that may be triggered by exposure to ultraviolet light (285). The majority of adverse drug reactions in previously diagnosed SLE patients are of this category (273,274). Another possibly related category of patients are those with acute or subacute cutaneous lupus erythematosus related to photoactive medications; these patients may have systemic disease and can fulfill criteria for a diagnosis of SLE (286). Some of these drugs are also associated with typical DIL and are included in Table 42.1. Drug-induced aseptic meningitis in SLE patients due to therapy with ibuprofen (287) and other NSAIDs [e.g., sulindac (288), tolmetin (289), diclofenac (290)] is an important consideration for the physician involved in the care of SLE patients who present with signs of meningeal irritation. Hypersensitivity reactions that have been interpreted as initiating or aggravating factors in SLE are associated with hydralazine (58), sulfonamides (271,272,278,291,292), penicillin (273,278), PAS acid (293), hydrochlorothiazide (246), cimetidine (294), phenylbutazone, (241,295), mesantoin (256), and various NSAIDs (258,296). Unknown or suspected environmental chemicals are also occasionally implicated as causal agents in SLE and related diseases (see Chapter 3).

Whether or not an environmental or pharmaceutical agent might aggravate or unmask incipient SLE should be considered a clinical problem distinct from DIL because, by definition, symptoms of DIL resolve after discontinuation of therapy, although in severe cases full recovery may require up to 1 year. [Although this view is not in accord with the influential study of Alarcon-Segovia et al. (58), in which 60% of patients with hydralazine-induced lupus had persistence of several symptoms 0.5 to 9 years after withdrawal of hydralazine, three fourths of these patients were reported to have preexisting rhematologic problems.] If drugs or environmental agents are truly causative in initiating or aggravating SLE, the mechanistic basis is probably different from that of DIL because the steady-state blood levels of bona fide lupus-inducing drugs must generally be sustained for many months to years (i.e., medications two to six times daily) for development of DIL. In contrast, for most cases believed to be aggravated or unmasked, exposure is of very low level or infrequent when the suspected agent is environmental or of relatively short duration when a drug is implicated. The association between drugs and the exacerbation or onset of SLE resembles the lupus flares following exposure to sunlight, exercise, or pregnancy.

Some reports have suggested that the incidence of SLE is increased after taking oral contraceptives, and that remissions follow cessation of their use (297,298). These findings could not be substantiated (258,260,299). Gold therapeutics such as disodium aurothiomalate frequently appear on lists of drugs associated with SLE induction or exacerbation. However, although late-onset toxic reactions to gold requiring discontinuation of therapy occur in up to one third of treated patients, the vast majority of episodes occur during the first few months of therapy and are limited to skin reactions or buccal irritation; rash occurs in about half the toxic gold reactions, and it is of a generalized or upper body distribution (300). Approximately 1% of treated patients develop leukopenia, thrombocytopenia, or proteinuria (300). These abnormalities are generally considered immune-mediated (301), but they fall outside the usual presenting symptoms and clinical progression of SLE (302) or DIL, and no report of gold-induced lupus has appeared despite over six decades of treatment experience. Gold toxicity does not appear to behave as a classic delayed-type hypersensitivity reaction in that only one of 30 patients with gold reactions had rapid recurrence of skin symptoms upon rechallenge with gold therapy (300).

Drug-Induced Immune Hemolytic Anemia

Long-term therapy with some drugs is associated with development of hemolytic anemia due to antibodies bound to red blood cells (RBCs) *in vivo* (direct Coombs' test positivity). In the penicillin-type, antibody to the drug binds to RBCs as a result of adsorption of the drug or its metabolite to the RBC membrane. In the methyldopa type, the drug is not required for (and does not affect) antibody binding, and anti-RBC antibodies typically have specificity for the rhesus locus or other intrinsic RBC antigens. These antibodies rarely produce frank hemolytic anemia possibly because their isotype or low avidity does not support complement fixation. Hemolytic anemia is commonly associated with the stibophen-type of drug-induced antibodies (as is quinidine and quinine) in which immune complexes consisting of the drug or drug metabolite bind to RBC presumably via Fc or complement receptors.

The mechanism underlying the penicillin-type of anti-RBC response is frequently used as the basis for models for autoantibody elicitation in DIL (see Mechanisms, below). Interestingly, the autoantibodies associated with DIL behave more like the methyldopa-type of immune response in that the likelihood for autoantibody appearance is dose dependent, but the drug is not required for antibody binding to its target antigen. In fact, many of the drugs associated with Coombs' test positivity of this drug-independent type [methyldopa, L-dopa, mefanamic acid (Ponstel), procainamide, chlorpromazine, and streptomycin (303)] are also known to cause DIA or DIL (Table 42.1), although there is generally no correlation between positive Coombs' test and ANA or DIL. However, patients with methyldopa-induced hemolytic anemia have been reported to have positive lupus erythematosus (LE) cells and ANAs (51,102,104, 105,107,304). As with the autoantibodies associated with DIL, Coombs' positivity gradually disappears after cessation of therapy, and individuals with a history of methyldopa-induced anti-RBC do not display significantly increased propensity for induction of anti-RBC upon reinstitution of therapy with the same drug (100). The mechanism for induction of this type of anti-RBC is unknown. However, despite the drug-independence of anti-RBC binding, a drug-altered RBC model is commonly invoked (303), and this model is commonly incorrectly applied to the origin of autoantibodies associated with DIA and DIL.

EPIDEMIOLOGY

The incidence of DIL has been estimated as 15,000 to 20,000 new cases annually in the United States (305). However, most of these cases were due to procainamide, a drug that has now largely been replaced by other antiarrhythmics. Therefore, the incidence of DIL is now probably considerably lower but is unknown. The incidence of DIL in other countries is unknown but has been estimated to be 10% that of idiopathic SLE (258). Lee et al. (306) reviewed the medical histories of 285 consecutive SLE case records and found that drugs were a possible causative factor in 12.4%. Fries and Holman (307) identified 12 DIL cases in a population of 198 lupus patients. In a recent retrospective study of 30 patients with elevated antimyeloperoxidase antibodies and vasculitis usually involving the kidney, lungs, and/or skin, 60% were exposed to a lupus-inducing drug for 1 to 10 years, usually hydralazine or propylthiouracil, suggesting that the majority of patients with high-titer antimyeloperoxidase antibodies may be drug induced (308). The frequency of DIL may be underestimated because most cases are mild, and only a small proportion are correctly diagnosed or seen by a rheumatologist. Because drugs such as isoniazid are more frequently administered in certain countries, studies in such countries are important to provide a more thorough epidemiologic picture of DIL.

The age of patients developing DIL reflects the age of the population undergoing treatment with the implicated drug. Because procainamide and hydralazine, the most common lupus-inducing drugs, tend to be administered to the older population displaying cardiac arrhythmias and hypertension, respectively, DIL usually occurs in people of age 50 or older.

Two epidemiologic features distinguish DIL from SLE. First, the high female-to-male predominance seen in SLE (9:1 to 7:1) is not seen in DIL largely because the majority of patients treated with the major lupus-inducing drugs are men. Nevertheless, procainamide- (25,30) and hydralazine-induced lupus (68,76,86,99) appear to be disproportionately more common in females. In the study of Totoritis et al. (30) the female to male ratio of procainamide-treated patients who developed lupus-like symptoms was 0.52 compared to a ratio of 0.19 for those who remained asymptomatic. A similar twofold to fourfold predominance of women over men for development of hydralazine-induced lupus has been reported (68,76,86). In the study of Cameron and Ramsay (86), the overall incidence of hydralazine-induced lupus during a 4-year observation period was 11.6% in women and 2.8% in men. In this same study, women treated with a daily dose of 200 mg hydralazine had a 19.4% incidence of hydralazine-induced lupus over a 3-year period. This is in contrast to the development of ANA in patients treated with hydralazine over a 3-year period, during which no gender differences were noted (99). Second, unlike SLE, the frequency of hydralazine-induced lupus in blacks was reported to be four- (9) to sixfold (56) lower than in whites. African Americans seem to be protected from lupus induced by procainamide as well (6).

CLINICAL AND LABORATORY FEATURES

The clinical and laboratory features of procainamide- and hydralazine-induced lupus are shown in Table 42.5 and compared with SLE. Musculoskeletal complaints are com-

TABLE 42.5. PREVALENCE OF CLINICAL AND LABORATORY ABNORMALITIES IN DRUG-INDUCED LUPUS AND SLE

Feature	Hydralazine-Induced Lupus[a]	Procainamide-Induced Lupus[b]	Systemic Lupus Erythematosus[c]
Symptoms			
Arthralgia	80%	85% }	
Arthritis	50–100%	20% }	80%
Pleuritis, pleural effusion	<5%	50%	44%
Fever, weight loss	40–50%	45%	48%
Myalgia	<5%	35%	60%
Hepatosplenomegaly	15%	25%	5–10%
Pericarditis	<5%	15%	20%
Rash	25%	<5%	71%
Glomerulonephritis	5–10%	<5%	42%
CNS disease	>5%	>5%	32%
Signs			
ANA	>95%	>95%	97%
LE cell	>50%	80%	71%
Antihistone[d]	>95%	>95%	54%
Anti-[(H2A-H2B)-DNA][d]	43%	96%	70%
Antidenatured DNA[d]	50–90%	50%	82%
Antinative DNA	<5%	<5%	28–67%
Anticardiolipin	5–15%	5–20%	35%
Rheumatoid factor	20%	30%	25–30%
Anemia	35%	20%	42%
Elevated ESR	60%	60–80%	>50%
Leukopenia	5–25%	15%	46%
+Coombs' test	<5%	25%	25%
Elevated gammaglobulins	10–50%	25%	32%
Hypocomplementemia	<5%	<5%	51%

[a]Data compiled from Alarcón-Segovia et al. (59), Hahn et al. (57), Cameron and Ramsay (86), and Russell et al. (76).
[b]Data compiled from Weinstein (309), Harmon and Portanova (310), Russell (311), and Hess and Mongey (312).
[c]Derived in part from Wallace (302).
[d]From refs. 33, 313, 314.
Each prevalence represents a consensus value ±5 percentage points. Abnormalities occurring in fewer than 5% of patients are not listed.
ESR, erythrocyte sedimentation rate.

monly observed, with arthralgia heading the list for both drugs. Arthritis is a less common feature with lupus induced by procainamide (20%) than by hydralazine (50% to 100%), whereas serositis (pleuritis and/or pericarditis) and/or myalgia are more common presenting features of procainamide-induced lupus. By contrast, hydralazine-induced lupus is associated with a higher frequency of skin rashes. However, in any one patient, lupus induced by procainamide, hydralazine, or other drugs cannot be distinguished by clinical features. The onset of symptoms can be slow or acute, although an interval of 1 to 2 months typically passes before the diagnosis is made (9,11,25,26,28,30,99).

Because arthralgia is such a common feature of patients in the age group at risk, the presence of other features, such as pleuritis, pleural effusion, fever, splenomegaly, skin rash, pericarditis, and certain autoantibodies should alert the clinician to consider the diagnosis of DIL. Approximately 50% of patients have constitutional symptoms of fever, weight loss, and fatigue. The symptoms of DIL usually resolve within days to weeks after discontinuing the offending drug, and therefore this maneuver provides a key (although retrospective) diagnostic tool.

In addition to classic DIL with associated antihistone antibodies and polyarthritis (33,41,44), Cohen et al. (37) reported that quinidine was associated with a mild drug reaction characterized only by polyarthralgias within 7 days to 3 months after initiation of therapy. These patients were ANA and antihistone antibody negative, and showed prompt recurrence of symptoms upon rechallenge with quinidine.

Lupus-like disease associated with minocycline is also atypical. Patients frequently present with symmetrical polyarthritis and may have evidence of hepatitis (elevated liver transaminases) and pneumonitis (due to pulmonary lymphocytic infiltrates) (200,201,205). These patients may not have ANA but appear to frequently have perinuclear antineutrophil cytoplasmic antibodies (pANCAs) due to antimyeloperoxidase (206). Nevertheless, as with classic DIL, symptoms and signs resolve after discontinuation of minocycline.

The frequency of serologic abnormalities in lupus induced by procainamide and hydralazine are essentially identical (Table 42.5). The immune response in this setting is characteristic and restricted. The most commonly observed abnormality is a positive ANA, which is largely due to histone-reactive antibodies (315,316). These antibodies are presumably responsible for the positive LE cells reported in the synovial fluid of two patients with procainamide-induced lupus (317), although recent studies could not produce LE cells in the indirect LE cell test using sera from patients with procainamide-induced lupus but only with DIL and SLE sera containing anti-H1 antibodies (318). Although generally of low titer, antibodies to denatured (but not native) DNA are also common in DIL. Less common laboratory features include rheumatoid factor (procainamide) (319), circulating immune complexes (320–322), and antineutrophil cytoplasmic antibodies [hydralazine (70,71), propylthiouracil (308, 323) and minocycline (206)], positive Coombs' test [methyldopa (106), chlorpromazine (144), and procainamide (319)], complement activation [procainamide (261,324,325)], hypocomplementemia (quinidine) (37), and a positive lupus band test (217). Phospholipid and cardiolipin antibodies, circulating anticoagulant activity, and biologic false-positive serologic test for syphilis (STS) results are discussed below. It should be appreciated that many of these laboratory abnormalities are not linked to symptomatic DIL. Thus, appearance of antibodies to RBC, denatured DNA, and total histones (but not a histone-DNA complex described below) is independent of lupus-like symptoms. Nevertheless, like the clinical features, these autoantibodies are truly drug-induced, and they gradually subside after drug therapy is discontinued.

Other laboratory features noted in a minority of patients include a mild anemia, leukopenia, and thrombocytopenia (13,19,261,305,319,326), a hypergammaglobulinemia that is not as frequent as in SLE (13,17,19,20,24,261,326,327), and an elevated erythrocyte sedimentation rate (ESR) (34, 41,320), which commonly reverts toward normal as symptoms resolve (37,41,326). Pancytopenia has been reported in association with procainamide therapy (328,329), but it is unlikely that these patients had DIL. Agranulocytosis or severe neutropenia develops in about 0.6% of procainamide-treated patients (330), but this condition is serologically and clinically distinct from DIL (331). Hydralazine-induced lupus has been reported to be associated with acute neutrophilic dermatosis (Sweet's syndrome) (81,332).

Although the spectrum of clinical abnormalities in DIL is indistinguishable from that observed in SLE, the severity of disease is usually milder in DIL. The number of symptoms and their intensities tend to increase with the duration of therapy, but patients who have inadvertently remained on procainamide for up to 2 years after onset of polyarthralgias did not progress to fulminant status (5). Interestingly, patients with more severe clinical problems and higher autoantibody levels tended to be treated with procainamide for shorter duration than those with milder DIL (32), suggesting the existence of clinical subsets differing in susceptibility to DIL. Patients with established SLE have been treated with procainamide for long durations without exacerbation of symptoms (307). These observations are contrary to the expectations of the hypothesis that drugs unmask a predisposition to SLE (158), and help to establish the view that DIL is a fundamentally different disease from SLE.

HISTONE AUTOANTIBODIES

Histone-reactive antibodies were discovered to be commonly present in patients with procainamide-induced lupus based on binding in a histone reconstituted ANA assay (315). Although patients with hydralazine-induced lupus (63) and asymptomatic drug treated patients (180,333) also have ANA, they tend to be negative for antihistone antibodies by the histone reconstituted ANA assay. However, with the advent of solid-phase immunoassays using pure histones, it was found that most patients with DIL and asymptomatic patients with ANA (i.e., DIA patients) induced by a variety of drugs including procainamide, hydralazine, chlorpromazine, acebutalol, and isoniazid also have antihistone antibodies (33,63,119,198, 334). Formal demonstration that histone-reactive antibodies constituted the bulk of the ANA was provided by chromatin-absorption studies (316).

Histones consist of five dissimilar proteins, and the fine specificity of antihistone antibodies in SLE, DIL, and DIA has been examined in detail. Considerable disagreements on the characteristic antihistone antibody profile in DIL accumulated (detailed in refs. 335, pp. 254–259, and 336, pp. 877–878). However, these reports generally indicated that antihistone antibodies react with only limited regions of the protein, especially their N- and/or C-terminal tails, possibly reflecting the solvent accessibility of these regions within the nucleosome. The diagnostic value of antihistone antibodies is limited. A positive test for antihistone antibodies may help to confirm a suspicion of DIL, but the conventional assay for antihistone antibodies cannot distinguish patients with DIL from patients who develop ANA yet remain asymptomatic (i.e., DIA). In fact, recent studies suggest that Ig binding to solid-phase histone may occur by non-cognate binding of the Fc Ig region rather than through specific antibody (337).

Anti-[(H2A-H2B)-DNA] Antibodies

Histones exist in the cell not as individual proteins but as a huge macromolecular complex termed chromatin, which is formed by highly organized histone-histone and histone-DNA interactions. The repeating unit of chromatin structure is the core particle of the nucleosome, which consists of a (H3-H4-H2A-H2B)$_2$ histone octamer wrapped with approximately two turns of DNA (Fig. 42.1).

The pronounced antigenicity of the H2A-H2B complex, a subunit of the nucleosome, was first detected in SLE patients (340) and subsequently found to dominate the serology of patients with procainamide-induced lupus (6, 29,30,341,342). These antibodies also react with the components H2A and H2B (30,31), but the magnitude of antibody binding to the H2A-H2B complex is often fivefold greater than to the individual histones. A systematic study of the antigenicity of nucleosome subunits revealed that the (H2A-H2B)-DNA complex contained the complete epitope for these antibodies and could largely account for the capacity of procainamide-induced lupus sera to bind to nucleosomes, chromatin, and nuclei (33).

IgG anti-[(H2A-H2B)-DNA] antibodies occur in over 90% of patients who develop procainamide-induced lupus (33,108) and have been detected in individual patients with

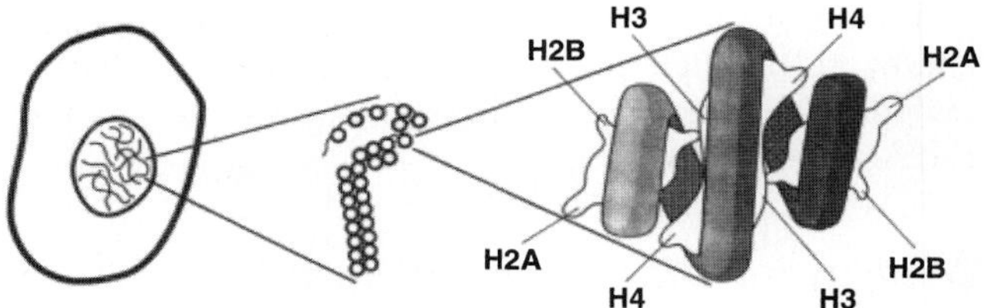

FIGURE 42.1. Organization of histones in chromatin. The core particle of the nucleosome (*right*) consists of eight histone molecules arranged in a tripartite structure [two H2A-H2B dimers and one (H3–H4)$_2$ tetramer] around which is wrapped 146 base pairs of DNA. For clarity, the core particle is depicted in an artificially loosened form; the actual structure is compact, and the DNA largely covers everything but the H2A-H2B side faces (338,339). A continuous strand of DNA connects each core particle to its adjacent core particles, forming the "beads-on-a-string" polynucleosomes fiber (*center*). After higher ordered supercoiling mediated in part by histone H1, the chromatin fiber becomes visible in the light microscope as a mitotic chromosome (*left*).

lupus induced by penicillamine (108,214), isoniazid (108, 196), acebutalol (108), methlydopa (105), sulfasalazine (230), and ophthalmic timolol (230). However, only approximately 50% of patients with quinidine- and 35% with hydralazine-induced lupus have detectable anti-[(H2A-H2B)-DNA] (Table 42.6). IgG anti-[(H2A-H2B)-DNA] has a sensitivity for procainamide-induced lupus of 84% at the time of diagnosis and a prognostic value of 70% one year before recognition of symptoms (32).

The use of an IgG-specific detecting reagent in testing for anti-[(H2A-H2B)-DNA] is important because procainamide-treated patients who remain asymptomatic commonly produce IgM and/or IgA antibodies of this specificity (31,32). There is no evidence that patients with these classes of drug-induced antibodies (and who are ANA positive) have an increased risk for converting to IgG anti-[(H2A-H2B)-DNA] and symptomatic drug-induced lupus. In addition, asymptomatic, procainamide-treated patients who develop DIA commonly have low levels of IgG antibodies to the DNA-free H2A-H2B complex (30,31,342,

TABLE 42.6. PREVALENCE OF IgG ANTI-[(H2A-H2B)-DNA] IN LUPUS INDUCED BY VARIOUS DRUGS

Lupus-Inducing Drug	Patients with Elevated Anti-[(H2A-H2B)-DNA] (%)	Reference
Procainamide	23/24 (96%)	33,108
Quinidine	9/17 (53%)	33,108
Hydralazine	6/14 (43%)	33
Penicillamine	1/1 (100%)	108,214
Isoniazid	1/1 (100%)	108,196
Acebutalol	1/1 (100%)	108
Methyldopa	2/2 (100%)	105,108
Timolol	1/1 (100%)	255
Sulfasalazine	2/2 (100%)	230

343), due to antibodies to the individual histones H2A and/or H2B. Therefore, a sensitive test for DIL that will exclude DIA patients requires employing the complete (H2A-H2B)-DNA complex.

Denatured DNA Autoantibodies

Denatured (single-stranded) DNA (dDNA) autoantibodies are found in up to 50% of DIL sera (19,24,29,31,57,59, 66,108,344,345). These autoantibodies probably have multiple reactivities, which have also been identified as binding to the nucleoside guanosine (30,346), polyriboadenylic acid (31,66), the phospholipid cardiolipin (347), and unusual conformations of DNA such as Z-DNA (31,348). Even antibodies directed to lymphocytes described in hydralazine- (62) and procainamide-induced lupus (349,350) may be related to the dDNA (or possibly chromatin) reactivity, because lymphocyte membranes can bind DNA (351). Anti-dDNA antibodies bearing the 16/6 and 32/15 idiotypes have been reported in one third of procainamide-induced lupus patients (352), idiotypes that are also commonly expressed in idiopathic SLE. However, the clinical significance of anti-dDNA is doubtful, because these antibodies are commonly seen in asymptomatic patients and in those with a wide variety of rheumatic and inflammatory conditions (353).

Antibodies To Drugs

Antibodies to the offending drugs have been reported in lupus induced by procainamide (354) and hydralazine (57). Other studies have been unable to detect drug-specific antibodies in patients treated with various lupus-inducing drugs (17,316,344,355). In a prospective study of patients treated with hydralazine, only 1 of 27 sera bound to the drug (66). The significance of antibodies to drugs is unclear because they have been reported in varying amounts in asymptomatic and symptomatic patients. In addition, it is unlikely that drug-binding antibodies represent cross-reactions with anti-dDNA or antichromatin autoantibodies (69,355,356).

Phospholipid Antibodies

The observation that DIA patients can have antiphospholipid (cardiolipin) antibodies, circulating anticoagulants, or biologic false-positive STS activity is noteworthy because much attention has focused on the clinical and pathogenic significance of these autoantibodies. The presence of the lupus anticoagulant (LAC) or of cardiolipin antibodies has been described in patients on hydralazine (357,358), procainamide, (359–363), chlorpromazine (137,140,143–145, 364–366), quinidine, and quinine (366). In one study, up to 75% of patients treated with chlorpromazine for up to 2.5 years developed a lupus anticoagulant (144). Canoso and deOliveira (137) reported that 54 of 93 chlorpromazine-treated psychiatric patients had IgM LAC activity. Of the 54 LAC-positive patients, 31 also had IgM cardiolipin antibodies, four also had IgG cardiolipin antibodies, and five had cardiolipin antibodies alone. During a mean follow-up period of 5 years, thrombotic events occurred in three patients (one with LAC, two with IgM cardiolipin antibodies). In a Canadian study, Lillicrap et al. (147) evaluated 97 psychotic patients treated with chlorpromazine, fluphenazine, or promazine. Of these, 25% developed a positive ANA, 4% had elevated titers of antibodies to cardiolipin and phosphatidylserine, and 5% had elevated titers of antibodies to phosphatidylinositol. None of the patients developed features of SLE or evidence of thrombotic events. Drug-induced LAC in a group of 13 patients had a narrower range of specificities than LAC in SLE or in primary antiphospholipid syndrome, rarely reacting with phosphatidylserine or phosphatidylcholine (366). None of these patients had thrombosis, indicating that there is no increased risk of thrombotic events associated with chlorpromazine- or quinidine-induced LAC. The antibody isotype in drug-induced LAC is usually IgM (137,140,144) as was the associated ANAs (138). It is likely that these observations also apply to procainamide and hydralazine, because thrombosis appears to be a rare clinical event in lupus induced by these drugs as well (367). The clinician should be cautious, however, because recurrent thrombotic events have been reported in phenothiazine- (149) and occasional procainamide-induced (359,363) lupus patients. It has not been determined whether the antiphospholipid antibodies associated with DIL interact with β_2-glycoprotein I, a correlative feature of SLE patients with a history of thromboembolisms (368).

The origin of lupus anticoagulants and cardiolipin antibodies in patients on various drugs, especially those in the phenothiazine group, is unknown. The pharmacologic action of drugs such as procainamide and chlorpromazine (Table 42.2) depends in part on their membranotropic nature, intercalation into plasma membranes, and interaction with phospholipids or lipoproteins (365,369,370). Based on these features, it has been postulated that the binding of the drug lipid moieties exposes cryptic epitopes or creates neoantigens that then serve as the stimulus for the production of antiphospholipid antibodies (365). However, since antiphospholipid antibodies are common in SLE patients (see Chapter 25), induction of lupus anticoagulants in DIL probably does not involve a drug-altered antigen mechanism.

Other Autoantibodies

Rheumatoid factor (RF) has been reported in procainamide-induced lupus patients (19). Prospective studies suggest that RF is not drug induced, and might merely reflect the increased prevalence of this autoantibody in the population treated with the drug (55,322). One study has reported antibodies in DIL sera directed against poly(adenosine diphosphate [ADP]-ribose) (371). Nässberger et al. (70,71,372) first demonstrated neutrophil myeloperoxidase (MPO) and elastase antibodies in hydralazine-induced lupus patients, and this has been confirmed (373); these specificities as well as antiproteinase-3 antibodies were also reported in patients treated with propylthiouracil (308,323), and anti-MPO antibodies were observed in patients with lupus induced by sulfasalazine (237) and minocycline (206). These observations are of considerable interest because these antibodies contribute to the pANCA and cytoplasmic ANCA (cANCA) neutrophil staining patterns that is associated with vasculitis of the capillaries and Wegener's granulomatosis, respectively (374). The occurrence of glomerulonephritis in some patients with hydralazine-induced lupus (Table 42.5) may be related to anti-MPO antibodies (308,372,373). Although anti-MPO antibodies occur in >50% of patients with hydralazine-induced lupus they are not found in lupus induced by procainamide (unpublished observations), consistent with the absence of kidney disease in procainamide-induced lupus. Antinuclear ribonucleoprotein (RNP) antibodies were reported after short-term (prophylactic) procainamide treatment (262). This observation has not been confirmed, and anti-RNP antibodies have not been observed in DIL (17,315,316,344). Cold-reactive lymphocytotoxic antibodies (LCTAs) have been reported in procainamide-induced lupus (349,350), but these reactivities were also detected in procainamide-treated patients at initiation of therapy and in asymptomatic procainamide-treated patients (66,316,322), so they are unrelated to DIL. LCTAs were also reported in four of seven patients with hydralazine-induced lupus, but also in 13 of 40 asymptomatic hydralazine-treated patients (62,259). Antibodies to high-mobility group (HMG) proteins, especially HMG-14 and -17, were detected in approximately half the patients treated with procainamide, hydralazine, and quinidine whether or not they expressed symptomatic DIL (375). This finding is of interest because the HMG proteins bind to the core particle of the nucleosome especially on transcriptionally active chromatin, consistent with the central role of chromatin in the autoantibody response in drug-treated patients.

NATURE OF THE IMMUNE RESPONSE IN DRUG-INDUCED LUPUS

Humoral Response

Numerous features of DIL point to the activation of the humoral immune system as its principal overt abnormality. As discussed above, the autoimmune response in DIL is largely restricted to antibodies reactive with (H2A-H2B)-DNA in native chromatin and to denatured histone and DNA components of nonnative chromatin. IgM, IgA, and IgG anti-[(H2A-H2B)-DNA] antibodies often appear to arise simultaneously during procainamide treatment, although patients who remain asymptomatic fail to develop IgG of these specificities (32). In a normal humoral immune response, recognition of a foreign antigen results in rapid clonal expansion of B cells, isotype switching to IgG, and somatic mutation to higher affinity antibodies. With drug-induced autoantibodies there appears to be a slow development of autoantibodies of the IgG, IgA, and IgM isotypes or the perpetuation of IgM autoantibodies for many years in asymptomatic, procainamide-treated patients (6,32), suggesting a weak adaptive immune response and/or evidence of homeostatic downregulation of autoimmunity. Nevertheless, the restriction in the immune response to chromatin-derived antigens suggests that B cells develop with immunoglobulin receptors for certain parts of chromatin, possibly the highly solvent exposed (H2A-H2B)-DNA region. In mouse models of SLE autoantibody secretion has been shown to require T-cell help (see Chapters 9 and 18), and drug-induced autoantibodies are likely to have a similar requirement. In fact initiation of autoimmunity by drugs may be at the T-cell level (see Mechanisms, below) with activation of autoreactive B cells merely a manifestation of this process. This view is supported by the observation that serum autoantibodies have an apparent half-life of 2.5 to 5.0 months after withdrawal of procainamide (32), approximately five times longer than the stability of immunoglobulin in the circulation, suggesting persistent, autoreactive T-cell help independent of the drug. Also, increased numbers of $CD4^+$ T cells of the $CD29^+$, activated phenotype along with soluble interleukin-2 receptor were detected in the pleural effusion of a patient with procainamide-induced lupus (20), consistent with the involvement of T-cell help in DIL.

Cellular Immune Response

Studies of *in vivo* cellular immune abnormalities in procainamide- and hydralazine-treated patients have been minimal and conflicting. Forrester et al. (376) observed increased spontaneous IgM and especially IgG secretion by circulating B cells from procainamide-induced lupus patients compared to B cells from patients with DIA or from normals, but whether polyclonal B-cell activation was being measured in patients with DIL or these were plasma cells secreting specific autoantibody was not distinguished. This result is consistent with older studies that failed to detect antibody-secreting cells in the circulation of procainamide-treated, asymptomatic patients (377,378). Although some or most of these patients would be expected to have serum ANAs (i.e., display DIA), whether these B-cell assays are too insensitive or antibody-secreting cells are primarily noncirculating and reside in lymphoid organs is unclear. One study reported that B cells from procainamide-treated patients were hyperresponsive to pokeweed mitogen (378) while just the opposite effect (377) or no difference (379) was seen by others. Reports of B-cell responses from procainamide-treated patients to procainamide *in vitro* have also been discrepant, with some detecting an increase (349,380) and others no effect (381,382). Only marginal or no capacity of hydralazine to activate peripheral blood lymphocytes from patients with hydralazine-induced lupus was observed (57), although another study reported that lymphocytes from 50% of asymptomatic hydralazine-treated patients showed a three- to fourfold stimulation index in the presence of hydralazine-albumin conjugates (66). Taken together, these older observations argue against the development of drug-specific T or B cells that would have been expected in a drug hypersensitivity response, consistent with other features of DIL such as its slow kinetics (delay of months to years from the onset of drug therapy to the development of autoantibodies and clinical symptoms), correlation with drug dose, and the inconsistent recurrence of symptoms upon drug rechallenge.

DIAGNOSTIC CRITERIA FOR DRUG-INDUCED LUPUS

Specific criteria for the diagnosis of DIL have not been formally established. Although some of the criteria for the classification of SLE are applicable to DIL, the requirement for four manifestations as established by the American College of Rheumatology (383) is overly rigid for DIL and is obviously not useful for distinguishing between drug-induced and idiopathic SLE. Patients with DIL often do not fulfill criteria for SLE, and a diagnosis of DIL can readily be missed if SLE diagnostic criteria are strictly applied. In particular symptoms common to SLE such as malar or discoid rash, photosensitivity, oral ulcers, alopecia, and renal or neurologic disorders are very unusual in DIL. Patients frequently present with mild or few lupus-like symptoms that typically worsen the longer the patient is maintained on the implicated drug, so that patients could readily be underdiagnosed if SLE criteria are strictly applied.

Guidelines for a diagnosis of DLE are shown in Table 42.7.

Elaboration Of Diagnostic Guidelines

Treatment Duration

Drug-induced lupus usually occurs after several months or years of continuous therapy and should not be confused with the short-term toxic side effects that are often suffered by patients treated with pharmaceuticals. Time for manifestation of lupus-like symptoms varies greatly among drug-treated patients; for procainamide, a median of 10 months was calculated, although one fourth of the 50 patients did not develop symptoms until 2 years or more of therapy (261); for hydralazine, the majority of patients require 6 months' to 2 years' exposure (56), but it is not uncommon for a patient to be treated for longer than 3 years before symptoms become manifested. This variation may be largely due to differences in the steady-state drug concentrations employed to maintain therapeutic control, but genetic factors may also be involved as discussed below.

Symptoms

In some patients, symptoms gradually appear and worsen over the course of many months of treatment with the implicated drug, whereas in others symptom onset is rapid. In one study of 21 patients, diagnosis of procainamide-induced lupus was based on one symptom in 20% of patients, two symptoms in 25%, and three or more symptoms in 55% of patients (30). Some suggestion of a drug-specific symptomatology in addition to the usual musculoskeletal and constitutional symptoms is suggested by the literature, with pleuritis and pericarditis common to procainamide-induced lupus, polyarthritis common to quinidine- and minocycline-induced lupus, glomerulonephritis and rash reported in hydralazine-induced lupus and autoimmune hepatitis in lupus related to minocycline (200,201). Lung involvement in procainamide-induced lupus occurs in approximately 50% of patients and consists of pleuritis, pleural effusions, and/or pulmonary infiltrates; pericardial effusions are also common. In most patients symptoms are mild although indistinguishable from SLE and consist of fever, malaise, weight loss, polyarticular arthralgias, and symmetric myalgias.

Probable Exclusionary Or Unrelated Symptoms

Central nervous system (CNS) disease is distinctly uncommon in drug-induced lupus, but because of possible inde-

TABLE 42.7. GUIDELINES FOR IDENTIFYING DRUG-INDUCED LUPUS

1. Continuous treatment with a known lupus-inducing drug for at least 1 month and usually much longer.
2. Presenting symptoms:
   Common: arthralgias, myalgias, malaise, fever, serositis (pleuropericarditis, especially with procainamide), polyarthritis (especially with quinidine and minicycline).
   Rare: rash or other dermatologic problems, glomerulonephritis (primarily with hydralazine).
3. Unrelated symptoms suggestive of SLE: multisystem involvement especially neurologic, renal, and skin symptoms.
4. Laboratory profile:
   Common: ANA that is due to antihistone antibodies especially IgG anti-[(H2A-H2B)-DNA], leukopenia, thrombocytopenia, and mild anemia, increased ESR.
   Absent or rare: antibodies to native DNA, Sm, RNP, SSA/Ro, SSB/La, hypocomplementemia.
5. Improvement and permanent resolution of symptoms generally within days or weeks after discontinuation of therapy. Serologic findings, especially autoantibody levels, often require months to resolve.

pendent neurotoxic effects of drugs or the occurrence of stroke, convulsions, or dementia syndromes in the elderly that are commonly treated with these drugs, CNS disease should not be an exclusion criterion. Similarly, although serious kidney disease is hardly ever reported for most lupus-inducing drugs, glomerulonephritis has been associated with hydralazine-induced lupus (83,88,89,95,372) so it should also not be a formal exclusion criterion. In the latter cases, it is difficult to distinguish hydralazine-induced glomerulonephritis from that related to the underlying hypertension for which hydralazine was administered. Mucocutaneous manifestations are also rare in DIL. Although a history of rheumatologic disease independent of the suspected drug tends to negate a diagnosis of DIL, a patient can have two diseases. This situation is characteristic of patients with various forms of arthritis who also develop DIL from penicillamine, sulfasalazine, or minocycline therapy. In these difficult cases serologic findings are especially informative.

Laboratory Abnormalities

Most patients with DIL have ANAs that are largely restricted to histone-containing antigens (315). IgG antibody to the (H2A-H2B)-DNA complex is an especially sensitive marker for lupus induced by a large variety of drugs except hydralazine. This test is particularly useful for distinguishing asymptomatic drug-treated patients who develop benign ANA (i.e., DIA) from patients with symptomatic DIL because only the latter have IgG anti-[(H2A-H2B)-DNA] antibodies (32). Some patients with DIL also have mild leukopenia, thrombocytopenia, and/or anemia and elevated sedimentation rate but rarely hypocomplementemia. Approximately 1% of procainamide-treated patients will present with neutropenia, but these patients do not have classic DIL (330,331). Although antihistone and anti-[(H2A-H2B)-DNA] antibodies are also common in SLE (313), these patients are rarely monospecific for this activity. Therefore, when a diagnosis of SLE or DIL cannot be clearly distinguished on clinical grounds, the presence of antibodies to native DNA, Sm, RNP, SSA/Ro, SSB/La, or other nuclear antigens should be considered as evidence against a diagnosis of DIL.

Symptom Resolution

Resolution of symptoms and laboratory abnormalities by withdrawing the offending drug is a defining feature of DIL. This simple manipulation and follow-up is a retrospective diagnosis but can be very reassuring. Although there is a strong temptation to treat patients suspected of DIL with antiinflammatory agents (see Treatment, below), this maneuver may confound the diagnosis and should not be required for recovery from DIL. Although autoantibody activity also resolves after discontinuation of therapy, these abnormalities often take much longer than symptom resolution and can still be present 1 to 2 years after withdrawal of therapy. However, quantitative measurements of autoantibodies should show a systematic decline in activity once the causative agent is withdrawn.

Differential Diagnosis

One concern of clinicians is how to differentiate DIL from SLE, and from other systemic rheumatic diseases. The reasons for this concern are threefold. First, the elderly SLE patient often does not present with the classic features of SLE (e.g., butterfly rash, glomerulonephritis) (384,385). Indeed, the clinical features of SLE in the elderly and DIL have significant overlap. Second, the treatment of DIL is generally straightforward, requiring only withdrawal of the drug and short-term antiinflammatory therapy, whereas the treatment of SLE can involve the prolonged use of corticosteroids or other immune modulators. Third, the outcome of DIL is better than SLE because these patients rarely, if ever, develop renal or neurologic disease. As discussed above, SLE is usually characterized by a much broader array of autoantibodies than is DIL, so the serologic profile can be very helpful in these difficult cases.

Because the clinical features of DIL are protean, a differential diagnosis should be considered (326). Viral syndromes and infectious diseases may present with arthralgia, fever, and pleuropericarditis. Dressler's syndrome should be considered in a patient with a previous myocardial infarction. An additional ischemic myocardial event may present with fever and pericarditis. The postpericardiotomy syndrome, which may present after cardiac surgery and is similar to Dressler's syndrome, can be confused with DIL because these patients are often treated with antiarrhythmics such as procainamide. Other diagnoses to be considered in the appropriate setting are rheumatoid arthritis, polymyalgia rheumatica, underlying malignancy, adverse or hypersensitive drug reactions, and graft-versus-host disease.

TREATMENT

Once the diagnosis of DIL has been established, the first step is discontinuation of the offending drug. Treatment with antiinflammatory agents, including corticosteroids, may be indicated for those with severe manifestations of the disease such as pericarditis with tamponade, inflammatory pleural effusions, or debilitating polyarthritis. The judicious use of NSAIDs and corticosteroids in the elderly is important because of potential side effects. The prolonged use of high doses of corticosteroids, or the use of chloroquine, hydroxychloroquine, or immunosuppressive agents is not indicated in the treatment of DIL. If DIL is associated with the rare feature of glomerulonephritis, as reported with hydralazine-induced lupus (83,88,89,95,372), corticosteroids can be used. Although some DIL patients have been restarted on procainamide or hydralazine without incident, this is not advisable if insufficient time (which may be as long as 1 year) has elapsed since the first episode of DIL (see Rechallenge Studies, above).

Clinicians are often consulted to consider the safety of drugs associated with DIL in the treatment of patients with idiopathic SLE. The use of hydralazine to treat hypertension in SLE patients has not been associated with exacerbations of the disease (258). Prockop (265) described an SLE patient treated for myotonia with 4 g procainamide per day for 15 months with no exacerbation of SLE despite the occurrence of lupus flares before and after the period of drug administration. The use of anticonvulsants to treat seizure disorders in SLE patients has not been associated with flares or acceleration of disease activity. Isoniazid has been given to SLE patients on corticosteroids without aggravating lupus (326). Despite the apparent safety of these drugs in the setting of SLE, the clinician should use the drugs judiciously, and carefully document the clinical and serologic status of the patient being considered for treatment.

GENETIC FACTORS

HLA Phenotype

The immunogenetic factors that underlie DIL are of interest because only a small proportion of drug-treated patients develop symptomatic disease, and the immune response is restricted to a relatively narrow range of autoantigens. These observations implicate a role for major histocompatibility complex (MHC) encoded class II human leukocyte antigens (HLAs), which are required for T-cell–dependent antibody responses. In a recent study of 13 patients with minocycline-induced lupus, all the patients had either HLA-DR4 or HLA-DR2 of subtypes that share a structural similarity (p <.01 vs. normals) (206). A study of 25 hydralazine-induced lupus patients by Batchelor et al. (68,386) showed a 73% frequency of HLA-DR4 versus a frequency of 25% in asymptomatic patients, representing a relative risk of 8.1. Another study using some of these same patients found a 70% frequency of HLA-DR4 in hydralazine-induced lupus patients (76). HLA-DR4 has been reported in individual patients with penicillamine-induced lupus (211,212) and hydralazine-induced Sweet's syndrome (332). However, hydralazine-induced lupus patients from Australia (85) and a limited study of American procainamide-induced lupus patients (30) failed to find a significantly increased incidence of any HLA markers. Reexamination of the hydralazine-induced lupus patients in the English study for complement protein phenotypes demonstrated that 76% of these patients had one or more C4 null alleles compared to 43% of normal controls (p <.01) (74). The genes encoding the C4 complement proteins are situated between the HLA-B and HLA-DR loci, and the C4 null/DR4 haplotype displays linkage disequilibrium in Caucasians. Therefore, the reported association of hydralazine-induced lupus with HLA-DR4 is probably a result of the C4 null trait (387), and linkage disequilibrium between HLA-DR4 and C4 may not occur in the Australian study group.

In chlorpromazine-treated patients HLA-B44 was a significant risk factor in the induction of ANA (relative risk = 3.6) (139) and LAC (relative risk = 2.1) (388), and HLA-DR7 was also weakly associated with chlorpromazine-induced LAC (388). Among procainamide-treated patients there was a significant association between HLA-DQw7 and IgG antibodies to histones and H2A-H2B (343). These results may suggest that these MHC class II antigens have a propensity to present histone peptides to T cells. However, since most patients treated with hydralazine or procainamide develop ANA, it is unlikely that only one or a few HLA allotypes are necessary for autoantibody induction by these drugs. More controlled studies using DNA typing for MHC class II alleles rather than the less accurate serologic typing are required to determine whether MHC genes are important in the development of DIL.

Complement

The complement genes are part of the MHC class III region, and C4A and C4B are encoded by separate loci. Individuals with genetic deficiencies in one, and especially both, C4 genes have greatly increased susceptibility to SLE (389) (see Chapter 13), presumably due to insufficient classical pathway activation, resulting in poor immune complex clearance. As mentioned above, 76% of hydralazine-induced lupus patients had one or more C4 null alleles compared to 43% of normal subjects (74), suggesting that a congenital defect in immune complex clearance may also predispose to DIL. It has not been determined, however, whether patients treated with hydralazine who remain asymptomatic have a low frequency of C4 null alleles. Similarly, it is not clear whether the occasional hypocomplementemia associated with procainamide-induced lupus (390) may be related to C4 deficiency. In most patients with DIL, serum complement levels are within the normal range (321). Interestingly, the null alleles of either C4A or C4B were also significantly more frequent in patients with procainamide-induced lupus than in normals at $p = .05$ (343).

A small but significant reduction (p <.01) in the mean number of type 1 complement receptors for C3b on erythrocytes (CR1) was observed in patients with a prior history of hydralazine-induced lupus, and these individuals tended to have elevated circulating immune complexes (321). However, based on restriction fragment polymorphism analysis, there was no difference between symptomatic and asymptomatic hydralazine-treated patients in the frequency of the allele encoding the low expression CR1 phenotype (391), indicating that hydralazine-induced lupus patients may have acquired a deficiency (perhaps due to persisting immune complexes) in CR1 expression. However, measurements of Fc-receptor–mediated immune clearance in patients treated with chlorpromazine, procainamide, penicillamine, or hydralazine with or without associated symptomatic disease demonstrated no differences and normal clearance function (320). These data suggest that, unlike in SLE, handling of circulating immune complexes by the reticuloendothelial system in DIL is not overloaded, possibly explaining the lack of kidney and CNS disease in DIL.

Acetylator Phenotype

The acetylator phenotype is the best described genetically determined predisposing factor in DIL, but its significance is often misunderstood. The studies of Perry and colleagues (53) demonstrated that the level of hepatic acetyltransferase activity was inversely associated with the likelihood for development of DIL. The acetyl group of acetyl–coenzyme A (CoA) can be transferred to the amino group of many small molecules by the action of acetyltransferases. North American white and black populations can be almost evenly divided into slow or fast acetylators based on their acetyltransferase activity. The acetylator phenotype can be determined by administering a tablet of dapsone, isoniazid, or caffeine to a patient and analyzing the serum or urine for acetylated and unacetylated drug. A preferable method is to determine acetylator genotype by amplifying lymphocyte genomic DNA by polymerase chain reaction followed by restriction nuclease digestion. Slow acetylators are homozygous for a recessive gene that controls hepatic acetyltransferase activity and have an approximately twofold higher serum level of unacetylated drugs at equivalent therapeutic doses.

Compared to rapid acetylators, autoantibodies and clinical symptoms develop more quickly and in higher frequency during the treatment of slow acetylators with hydralazine (53,68) and procainamide (26), although in a recent study seven out of nine patients (78%) with procainamide-induced lupus were rapid acetylators (6). Development of clinical symptoms can occur in up to 20% of rapid acetylators (76), but both the dose and duration of drug administration are generally higher in these patients (26). These studies generally support the hypothesis that the steady-state concentration of unacetylated procainamide and hydralazine and the duration of exposure are important elements in the development of DIL. Such observations have led to the use of *N*-acetylprocainamide (NAPA) in the successful control of cardiac arrhythmias while bringing about the remission of procainamide-induced lupus (392). NAPA did not induce lupus, ANA, or anti-dDNA (27,393). Furthermore, if the procainamide dose was adjusted so that all patients have the same steady-state plasma concentration by increasing the dose for rapid acetylators, no difference was observed between slow and rapid acetylators in the time for development of ANA or DIL (28). However, a recent study did not observe a tendency for the use of higher procainamide dose in rapid acetylators (6).

The importance of the free amino/hydrazino group in these drugs in the development of autoantibodies and lupus has been interpreted in two ways. A commonly held view is that these chemical moieties play a direct role in the induction of autoimmunity, and acetylation prevents this action. Alternatively, *in vivo* metabolism (other than acetylation) of the drug at this moiety generates the active, autoimmunity-inducing compound, and that *N*-acetylation blocks drug metabolism. With this view the putative reactive metabolites, rather than the parent molecule, would interact with a key immune target, leading to induction of autoimmunity (see Oxidative Drug Metabolism, below). The association of the slow acetylator phenotype with symptomatic DIL can then be explained by a higher steady-state concentration of the metabolizable form of the drug. Although isoniazid, like hydralazine, is a substrate for hepatic acetyltransferase, there is no difference in the development of ANA in fast and slow acetylators on INH therapy (187). The lack of an association between acetylator phenotype and induction of ANA by isoniazid (187) or by captopril (112), as well as idiopathic SLE (394), indicates that the slow acetylator phenotype is not a general predisposing factor for the autoimmune state, nor is it genetically linked to a putative autoimmunity-inducing or autoimmunity-accelerating gene.

Gender And Race

The preferential induction of lupus in Caucasian females by procainamide and hydralazine is discussed under Epidemiology.

OXIDATIVE DRUG METABOLISM

The following features of drug-induced autoimmunity are difficult to explain by a direct action of the ingested, parent compound on some component of the immune system:

1. Lupus-inducing drugs are highly diverse in chemical structure (Fig. 42.2) and pharmacologic action (Table 42.2), yet the laboratory and clinical features of lupus induced by all the drugs are essentially the same.
2. Except for their pharmacologic action, lupus-inducing drugs are largely inert at normal doses; nonspecific or generalized toxicity would preclude their use as therapeutic agents. DIL is an idiosyncratic drug reaction not predicted by any known property of the implicated drugs.
3. Drugs reach a steady-state concentration within a few hours, but drug-induced autoimmunity and lupus require many months for manifestation.

The requirement for metabolic transformation of the ingested drug to a reactive compound would account for many of the features of DIL. *In vivo* metabolism of dissimilar drugs to a product with a common, reactive property

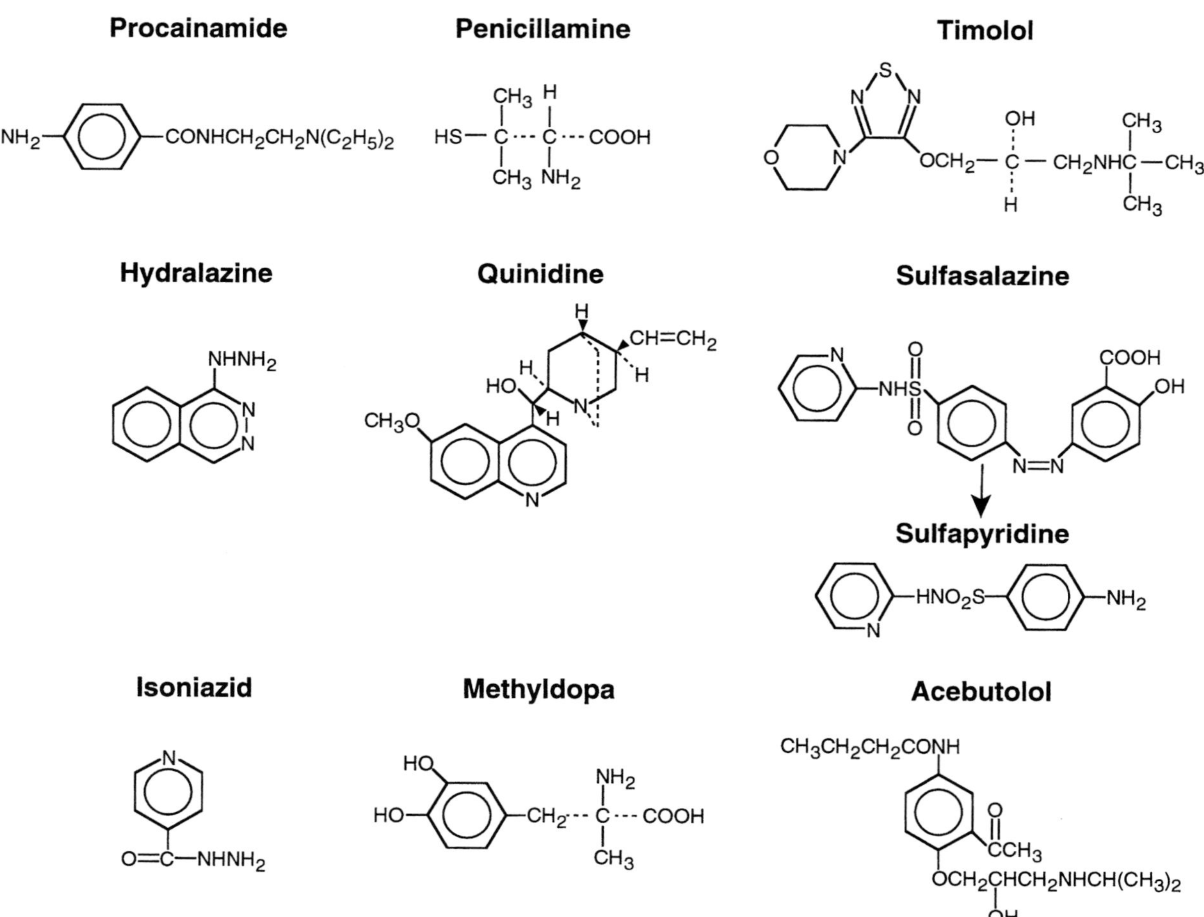

FIGURE 42.2. Structures of drugs reported to induce lupus and anti-[(H2A-H2B)-DNA] antibodies. Sulfasalazine undergoes hydrolysis in the intestine to 5-aminosalicylic acid and sulfapyridine, which is absorbed and the candidate agent for inducing lupus. Although four drugs are aromatic amines (procainamide and sulfapyridine) or hydrazines (hydralazine and isoniazid), the chemical structures of drugs with capacity to induce lupus are highly diverse.

could explain how compounds with widely different pharmacologic and chemical characteristics could produce the same adverse reaction. The low probability for a productive metabolic event could explain the long lag time for autoimmunity to unfold.

Incubation of procainamide with human or rat liver microsomes that contain the "mixed function oxidases" results in the formation of an unstable product, procainamide-hydroxylamine (PAHA) (395,396), and PAHA can be detected after the perfusion of rat liver with procainamide in a blood-free environment (397). Hydralazine and isoniazid are also susceptible to hepatic oxidative metabolism (398,399). PAHA enters RBCs, and oxyhemoglobin enhances its biologic activity (381,397), presumably by converting PAHA to nitroso-procainamide (400,401). Hepatic metabolism of drugs to reactive products demonstrates that the chemistry exists for generation of potentially toxic compounds, but these products typically bind to microsomes or macromolecules near their site of formation and fail to exit the liver in reactive forms. Although rats treated with procainamide showed increased liver lipid peroxide levels and antioxidant activity (402), hepatotoxicity is not associated with drug-induced autoimmunity or lupus, making it unlikely that sufficient amounts of reactive metabolites of lupus-inducing drugs are generated in the liver to interact with resident lymphocytes or inflammatory cells. Although drug metabolites might bind to self antigen in the liver, there is not enough structural information in such small molecules to specifically interact with the chromatin-derived targets that characterize the autoimmune response in DIL.

Phagocytic leukocytes including neutrophils, monocytes, macrophages, and skin Langerhans cells have drug metabolizing capacity due to the presence within these cells of various enzymes with promiscuous substrate properties such as myeloperoxidase, prostaglandin H synthase or, less commonly, the cytochrome P-450s. Rubin et al. (403) showed that activated peripheral blood neutrophils have capacity to metabolize procainamide to PAHA in the extra-

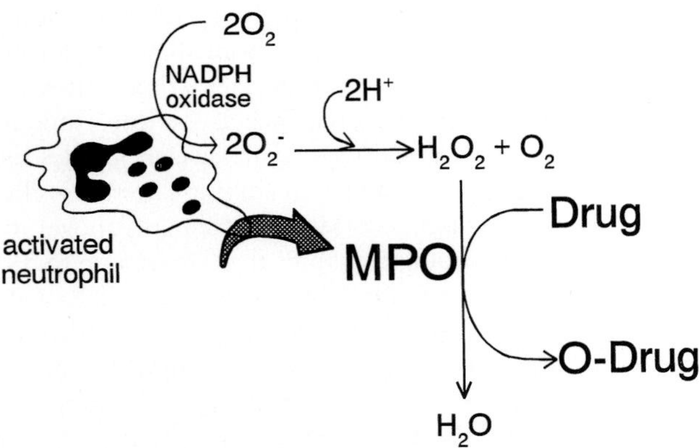

FIGURE 42.3. Mechanism for transformation of drugs by activated neutrophils (see text).

cellular milieu; the role of the respiratory burst and degranulation events associated with neutrophil and macrophage activation was confirmed (404) and analyzed in detail (405). Neutrophils are clearly the greatest drug-metabolizing engine outside the liver because of their preponderance in the circulation, apparently unlimited hematopoietic regenerative capacity, ability to freely circulate and populate essentially any organ or tissue including lymphoid tissue where autoimmunity presumably develops, and capacity to generate in response to stimulants a robust extracellular oxidizing machinery. It is this latter feature that is particularly important because generation of reactive drug metabolites outside a cell sets up a condition for delivering these agents some distance from their immediate site of formation.

Essentially all pharmacologic classes of lupus-inducing drugs (Table 42.1) but not their non–lupus-inducing analogues have been demonstrated to undergo oxidative metabolism by activated neutrophils including procainamide, hydralazine, phenytoin, quinidine, dapsone, propylthiouracil, penicillamine, chlorpromazine, isoniazid, and carbamazepine (404–417). The general mechanism responsible for drug transformation is shown in Fig. 42.3. Activation of neutrophils by opsonized particles or certain soluble factors triggers the ectoenzyme reduced nicotinamide adenine dinucleotide phosphate (NADPH) oxidase to produce superoxide anion (O_2^-) in the extracellular environment. O_2^- spontaneously dismutates to hydrogen peroxide (H_2O_2). Degranulation often follows, releasing myeloperoxidase (MPO). If a drug with an appropriate functional group is present, it will participate in electron transfer with the H_2O_2-MPO intermediate. Consequently, the functional group accepts an oxygen atom from H_2O_2, resulting in a new compound. Neutrophil-mediated drug metabolism by this mechanism requires the enzymatic action of MPO, as evidenced by the competitive inhibition of MPO activity by all lupus-inducing drugs tested and the correlation of this property with neutrophil-dependent drug cytotoxicity (Table 42.8) (416). The instability of these drug metabolites precludes their detection *in vivo*, but *in vitro* generated reactive oxidative intermediates of procainamide (400,401,418), hydralazine (413), chlorpromazine (414), and isoniazid (399) have been identified. Reactive intermediates of lupus-inducing drugs are strong candidates for triggering autoimmunity.

Although it is difficult to prove that neutrophil-mediated bioactivation of drugs occurs *in vivo*, the frequent finding of anti-MPO antibodies in patients with lupus induced by

TABLE 42.8. CORRELATION BETWEEN LUPUS-INDUCING PROPENSITY AND NEUTROPHIL-DEPENDENT DRUG METABOLISM MEDIATED BY MYELOPEROXIDASE (MPO) (DERIVED FROM REF. 416)

Drug	Lupus-Inducing Incidence (%)	Neutrophil-Mediated Cytotoxicity (%)[a]	Inhibition of MPO Activity (%)[a]
Procainamide	15–20	76 ± 11	17 ± 5
N-Acetylprocainamide	0	–3 ± 3	3 ± 2
Hydralazine	5–10	37 ± 4	95 ± 5
Phthalazine	N.T.	–3 ± 1	2 ± 1
Quinidine	<1	26 ± 4	21 ± 7
Quinilone	N.T.	1 ± 1	0 ± 3
Chlorpromazine	<1	30 ± 7	29 ± 8
Promazine	N.T.	–5 ± 1	3 ± 5
Isoniazid	<1	24 ± 3	40 ± 5
Isonicotinamide	N.T.	1 ± 1	1 ± 3
Propylthiouracil	<1	63 ± 11	87 ± 1
Propyluracil	N.T.	–4 ± 2	0 ± 2

[a]Neutrophil-dependent drug cytotoxicity measures the capacity of the indicated drug in the presence of activated neutrophils to affect the viability of a target cell line and is expressed as the percent of cells killed by the drug metabolite. Inhibition of MPO activity measures the capacity of the drug to act as a competitive inhibitor of the enzymatic activity of MPO. Both *in vitro* assays were measured at a drug concentration of 10 μM.
N.T., not tested.

hydralazine (308,372,373), propylthiouracil (308,323), and minocycline (206) is consistent with an autoimmune reaction initiated by drug bioactivation mediated by neutrophil-derived MPO. Indirect evidence that neutrophil-mediated drug metabolism is required for induction of autoimmunity is suggested by the strong correlation between MPO-mediated oxidative drug transformation and propensity of the drug to induce lupus (Table 42.8). Nitro-procainamide, a further oxidation product of PAHA (400,401), has been detected in the urine of procainamide-treated patients (343,419). Urinary metabolites of hydralazine have also been described (55,420). Murine T-cells sensitized to oxidative metabolites of procainamide (421), propylthiouracil or gold thiomalate (422, 423) displayed specific responses to lysates of phagocytic cells derived from mice subjected to long-term treatment with the respective parent compound, but did not respond to the parent compound itself. These data suggest that lupus-inducing drugs undergo oxidative metabolism *in vivo*, implicating these products in the induction of autoimmunity. *N*-acetylation of hydralazine and procainamide competes with *N*-oxidation of these drugs, accounting for the lower probability for development of autoimmunity in people with the rapid acetylation phenotype.

PATHOGENESIS

Since symptoms and serologic features of DIL overlap with those of idiopathic SLE, it is presumed that similar pathogenic factors underlie both syndromes. However, immune complex formation and deposition in vital organs, one of the mechanisms believed to operate in SLE, have not been well documented in DIL. Immune complexes have been reported in DIL (320–322), but their composition, correlation with disease activity, and pathogenic potential have not been evaluated. Evidence supporting the involvement of immune complexes in disease pathogenesis includes the observations that complement breakdown products (e.g., C3d and C4d) were detected in DIL (261,325). C4d/C4 ratios were significantly elevated in five of six procainamide-induced lupus patients (261), and, in a prospective study, C4d gradually increased during the development of DIL and returned to normal 2.5 months after discontinuation of procainamide treatment (324). Immune complexes involving IgG anti-[(H2A-H2B)-DNA] and a chromatin-derived antigen would be a candidate mediator of complement activation and subsequent inflammatory reactions. This possibility is consistent with the finding that anti-[(H2A-H2B)-DNA] activity is predominantly IgG1 and IgG3 (424), immunoglobulin subclasses that are potent activators of the classical complement pathway when engaged by antigen. Detection of LE cells in procainamide-induced lupus (317) also suggests the presence of complement-fixing autoantibodies. Although early studies of antihistone antibodies using indirect immunofluorescence failed to detect complement binding (425,426), a subsequent study demonstrated deposition of C3, C4, and properdin mediated by antihistone antibodies (427). However, the lack of renal disease in DIL suggests that other factor(s) such as the form, amount, or location of the target antigen, other autoantibodies such as anti-DNA, or abnormalities in immune complex clearance as previously discussed (see Complement, above) may account for the pathologic features that are unique to SLE.

Hydralazine and isoniazid inhibit C4, especially C4A, binding activity *in vitro*, and it has been suggested, therefore, that these drugs may interfere with immune complex clearance by inhibiting classical pathway activation (428, 429). Although these effects were only observed at drug concentrations that were 10- to 100-fold higher than therapeutic plasma levels in humans, penicillamine inhibition of C4A binding may fall within therapeutically relevant concentrations (429). Of particular interest was the finding by Sim et al. (430) that PAHA inhibits C3 or C4 activity at concentrations tenfold lower than that of procainamide. However, this effect still required concentrations of PAHA not pharmacologically obtainable, making it unlikely that an acquired C3 or C4 deficiency contributes to DIL

ANIMAL MODELS

Compared to human standards, all strains of mice are slow acetylators (431) and therefore should be susceptible to autoantibody elicitation upon exposure to lupus-inducing drugs. On the other hand, drug clearance rates in mice are at least ten times faster than in humans (432), so at equivalent weight-adjusted oral doses mice will have much lower steady-state blood levels of delivered drug. The measured elimination half-life for procainamide in 20 strains of mice varied from 23.5 to 54.7 minutes (433), compared to 180 to 300 minutes in humans (434). Use of excess drug concentrations in the drinking water is limited by the natural aversion of mice to higher oral doses.

Continuous oral administration of isoniazid or hydralazine for 6 to 8 months in C57BL/6 mice was reported by Cannat and Seligmann (188,435) to result in ANA induction in 34% to 46% of mice. Ten Veen and Feltkamp (436,437) reported similar findings and extended positive results to procainamide and to two other mouse strains. Tannen and Weber (438,439) also were able to elicit ANA by procainamide in A/J mice, but, contrary to the earlier reports, observed suppression of spontaneous ANA appearance during 9 months' exposure of C57BL/6 mice to procainamide. Injection of procainamide three times per week for 30 weeks failed to elicit ANA in mice, rats, rabbits, or guinea pigs (440). Although provocative, the murine models in which a lupus-inducing drug is administered in the drinking water are impractical because of the long duration required to develop even a partial response, the common spontaneous seroconversion of aging mice to ANA positivity and the inability to develop steady-state blood levels of the drug that are comparable to therapeutic doses in humans. Monoclonal antichromatin antibodies derived from mice receiving quinidine or penicillamine in their drinking water for 5 to 8 months were reported (441), but it is not certain that these autoantibodies were truly drug induced. Uniform mean plasma levels of 2.1 ± 0.7 μg/mL (7.4 μM) procainamide, which is at the lower end of the human therapeutic level, were obtained by delivering the drug via implanted osmotic pumps, but the mice failed to develop autoantibodies during the 7 weeks of exposure that this protocol could be sustained (433,442).

Oral administration of propylthiouracil into mongrel cats for 2 months resulted in ANA, direct anti-RBC antibodies, and lupus-like symptoms in approximately half the animals (443). Discontinuation of propylthiouracil or replacement with propyluracil caused resolution of symptoms and signs within 1 to 4 weeks (443), indicating that this was a bona fide drug-induced lupus-like syndrome. Induction of autoimmunity was drug dose dependent, and, as in human DIL (see Rechallenge Studies, above), cats that had previously developed propylthiouracil-induced lupus followed by a 3-month washout period were not hyperresponsive to challenge with propylthiouracil (i.e., they failed to redevelop disease at lower challenge doses) (444). Interestingly, the ANA was predominantly due to antinative DNA antibodies; antihistone antibodies were not detected (444). Therefore, this syndrome has features of both drug-induced and idiopathic lupus and may be a unique feline animal model.

A lupus-like pathology including autoantibodies and glomerulonephritis has been produced in mice by injection of splenocytes treated with procainamide *in vitro* (445). For this effect to be manifested, splenocytes were allogeneically activated and treated *in vitro* with procainamide prior to their adoptive transfer monthly for 6 months into syngeneic mice. A conalbumin-specific T-cell clone treated with procainamide or hydralazine but not their structural analogues produced a similar *in vivo* pathology (446–448), suggesting that autoimmunity in this animal model was a consequence of non–antigen-specific T-cell activation as discussed below.

A number of lupus-inducing drugs (hydralazine, chlorpromazine, carbamazepine, phenylbutazone, and nitrofurantoin) will cause significant enlargement of the draining popliteal lymph node when injected subcutaneously into the hind foot pad of mice (421–423,449). In this popliteal lymph node assay (PLNA) T cells apparently respond to drug-altered self proteins. Interestingly, procainamide, isoniazid, and propylthiouracil were negative in this assay (421,449,450), unless oxidatively metabolized by rat liver microsomes (450) or peritoneal macrophage (421) or if the metabolite itself such as PAHA or propyluracil 2-sulfonate was injected (421). The requirement for a drug metabolite is in good agreement with the *in vitro* studies demonstrating neutrophil- or macrophage-mediated metabolism of the same drugs (see Oxidative Drug Metabolism, above). The possible significance of this animal model in the context of DIL is discussed below.

Injection of PAHA into the thymus of normal adult mice resulted in the delayed appearance and long-lasting production of IgG anti-[(H2A-H2B)-DNA] antibodies, similar to those found in patients with drug-induced lupus (451). Transfer into naive mice of autoreactive peripheral T cells derived from PAHA-injected animals elicited a similar autoantibody profile, indicating that autoreactive T cells that emigrated from the thymus to the periphery accounted for autoantibody production in this system (452). The cellular basis for autoantibody production in this mouse model is discussed below.

MECHANISMS

Most of the older experimental studies on DIL explored the significance of the presumed capacity of lupus-inducing drugs to form stable complexes with self-macromolecules or to directly stimulate lymphocytes. The premise underlying much of this work was apparently based on previously described immune reactions to xenobiotics such as the penicillin-type of drug hypersensitivity (allergic) reaction mediated by antibodies or the delayed-type hypersensitivity reaction associated with allergic contact dermatitis mediated by T cells. Autoantibodies might develop if an immune response to the drug in the form of a hapten or to a self antigen altered by the drug induces antibodies that cross-react with or cause spreading of the immune response to native self-macromolecules. For the most part these experiments have not been illuminating because nonpharmacologic concentrations of drugs or artificial drug-macromolecular complexes together with immunologic adjuvants were employed (reviewed in ref. 336). A more recent examination of the specificities of antibodies elicited in rabbits by immunization with drug-albumin complexes revealed no cross-reaction between denatured DNA or histones and antibodies to procainamide or its oxidative metabolites (355). However, several groups are pursuing variants of this hypothesis at the T-cell level as discussed below.

Studies over the past 5 to 10 years attempting to determine which component(s) of the immune system are important in the initiation of drug-induced lupus and exactly how autoimmunity is triggered by drugs or drug metabolites are organized into the following four general mechanistic hypotheses:

Drug Metabolites Act As Haptens For Drug-Specific T Cells

Immune responses require presentation of the xenobiotic on either class I or class II molecules of the MHC on antigen-presenting cells, and most drugs are ignored by the immune system in part because their molecular mass is too small to enter this machinery. However, if a drug or its metabolite can form a stable bond to self molecules, it (as a hapten) or a combined epitope generated by the drug-self molecule complex may be recognized by antigen receptors on B and/or T cells. Such a phenomenon appears to be the basis of the immunoreactivity of many drugs in the PLNA reported by Gleichmann and others (421–423,449,450, 453) (see Animal Models, above). Since monocytes, macrophages, and Langerhans cells can present antigens to T cells, they have received special attention as a potential source of both drug biotransformation producing drug conjugates as well as immune presentation of the conjugate to initiate an immune response (292). These professional antigen-presenting cells could also take up drug conjugates produced in their immediate microenvironment by other cells such as neutrophils. Oxidative metabolites of carbamazepine, chlorpromazine, hydralazine, phenytoin, procainamide, and propylthiouracil have been demonstrated to form covalent bonds with cellular proteins. Alternatively, B cells within the microenvironment of a drug-specific T-cell response might become activated by cytokine-mediated bystander mechanisms.

Unfortunately for this hypothesis, mice that developed enlarged lymph nodes in response to lupus-inducing drugs or their oxidative metabolites failed to develop autoreactive T cells or autoantibodies, indicating that drug-specific T cells do not typically lead to autoimmunity. In addition the autoantibodies that arise in people with DIL or drug-induced cytopenias are limited in specificity, a feature not consistent with a bystander activation scenario. However, if an incipient autoimmune response were independently under way, and if the drug as a hapten becomes expressed on the MHC of autoreactive B cells, it is possible that drug-specific T cells could accelerate development of autoimmunity. Presentation of a drug on the MHC could occur after the endocytosis and intracellular processing of the drug bound to the cognate self antigen recognized by an autoreactive B cell or by binding directly to the MHC through a noncovalent association (454).

Drug Metabolites Cause Cell Death

Cytopenias associated with certain drugs (see Clinical And Laboratory Features, above) may be related to the capacity (based on *in vitro* studies) of various reactive drug metabolites to directly cause cell death. This would be a non–immune-mediated process. Demonstration that PAHA under certain *in vitro* conditions can directly kill a wide variety of cells at pharmacologically relevant concentrations (381,401,416,418) or enhance reactive oxygen species generation by murine macrophage (455) and human neutrophils (381) is consistent with this view. Recent reports implicate apoptosis rather than necrotic cell death in cytotoxicity mediated by sulfamethoxazole hydroxylamine (456) or by the nitrenium ion of clozapine (457). Cell death may be initiated by damage to the plasma or mitochondrial membrane or by covalent binding to critical intracellular molecules or may be due to redox cycling with NADH/NADPH, depleting the cell of its energy stores as suggested by the correlation between cell reducing potential and sensitivity to PAHA cytotoxicity (401). Cytotoxic drug metabolites generated by neutrophils *in vitro* have been demonstrated for amodiaquine, carbamazepine, chlorpromazine, clozapine, hydralazine, isoniazid, procainamide, propylthiouracil, quinidine, and sulfonamides at therapeutically feasible concentrations. Cytopenia could occur if reactive drug metabolites were produced via extracellular myeloperoxidase (Fig. 42.3) by mature neutrophils that recirculated into the bone marrow or by immature promyelocytes undergoing granulopoiesis, and these metabolites were cytotoxic to stem cells that were precursors of the formed elements of the blood. In addition, certain hematopoietic cell lineages sensitized by an immune-mediated mechanism because of drug binding to the cell surface could be destroyed by an otherwise subtoxic concentration of a reactive drug metabolite. Lymphocytes from patients with a history of agranulocytosis secondary to clozapine therapy were somewhat more sensitive to the cytotoxic effects of oxidative metabolites of clozapine than normals or patients who did not develop agranulocytosis (458,459), possibly related to differences in drug bioinactivation by intracellular glutathione or cysteine (460).

Although it is possible that this type of direct cytotoxicity of drug metabolites could be an independent pathogenic mechanism especially in certain susceptible populations, such a process cannot explain the bulk of the immune abnormalities in DIL.

It is also formally possible that drug toxicity alters degradation, clearance, or processing of self materials by antigen-presenting cells, producing abnormal macromolecular forms or unusual peptides. These "cryptic" T-cell autoepitopes may induce classical adaptive immune responses because immune tolerance to such unusual forms of self materials was never established. Autoreactive B cells preexisting in the immune repertoire could present such cryptic epitopes to T cells, resulting in B-cell activation and autoantibody secretion. Alternatively, repetitive macromolecular structures released from dying cells could theoretically elicit T-independent autoimmune responses. This type of scenario has been proposed to account for autoantibodies associated with diverse medications, environmental agents, and viruses, but there remains little in the way of experimental support.

Drugs Nonspecifically Activate Lymphocytes

A study of Adams et al. (381) suggested that PAHA at 2 μM had the capacity to enhance pokeweed mitogen–mediated lymphocyte proliferation and increase the number of

Ig plaque-forming cells, but these observations have not been verified. A later study reported an approximately twofold increase in poly(ADP-ribosylation) level in the lymphocyte Wil-2 cell line exposed to micromolar levels of procainamide or hydralazine (461). Mouse splenocytes exposed to procainamide or hydralazine while activated *in vitro* displayed an increased proliferative response to autologous antigen-presenting cells without the need for cognate antigen, killed autologous macrophage, and promoted B-cell differentiation into antibody-secreting cells (462–465). Autoantibodies and glomerulonephritis were produced after adoptive transfer of such drug-treated cells into mice (445,446). The autoreactive nature of drug-treated cells was shown by Richardson and colleagues (446,464–466) to be due to the inhibition by procainamide or hydralazine of DNA methyltransferase in $CD4^+$ T cells. As a result, with each round of cell division undermethylation of deoxycytosine residues in CpG pairs occurs in the genomic DNA. Hypomethylation of promoter sequences is associated with enhanced gene transcription, and drug-treated T cells showed increased expression of lymphocyte function antigen-1 (LFA-1), an important adhesion molecule that helps stabilize the interaction between T cells and antigen-presenting cells. Perhaps longer contact between the T-cell receptor on T cells and the MHC on antigen-presenting cells promotes T-cell activation upon contact with low-affinity self antigens.

One concern about these studies is that the immunopathologic features of this mouse model do not resemble DIL but are similar to the global autoimmune characteristics of a graft-versus-host reaction when adoptively transferred semi-allogeneic T cells recognize histoincompatible MHC molecules in the host (467). This syndrome is more like SLE, while DIL displays much more limited autoimmune features (Table 42.5). In addition, multiple exposures to large numbers of lymphocytes overexpressing LFA-1 due to drug presence during cell division were required to produce these phenomena. Normal immune responses to infectious agents (that might occur coincident with medication with a lupus-inducing drug) would be expected to be associated with a much more limited, oligoclonal T-cell activation. However, it is possible that in DIL autoreactive T cells developing through an independent mechanism become more aggressive due to such a drug-induced LFA-1 overexpression process, thereby aggravating disease in DIL.

Drug Metabolites Disrupt Immune Tolerance Machinery

Rather than stimulating mature T cells, drug metabolites when present during T-cell development in the thymus may prevent the *de novo* acquisition of self tolerance. T cells originate in the thymus where they are selected to ensure that only cells that are nonresponsive to self are released into the periphery. The possibility that lupus-inducing drugs interfere in this process had been generally ignored because it was widely assumed that there is no thymic function in the adult. However, recent studies demonstrated that T cells are generated in the thymus throughout life (468). Kretz-Rommel and Rubin (451,452) showed that injection of PAHA into the thymus but not into any part of the peripheral immune system of normal adult mice resulted in the delayed appearance and long-lasting production of anti-[(H2A-H2B)-DNA] autoantibodies, similar to the autoantibodies that characterize patients with DIL. Observations in this animal model and in an *in vitro* model of T-cell tolerance (469) indicated that PAHA did not reverse self tolerance of the mature thymocyte and did not prevent deletion of high-affinity autoreactive T cells in the thymus. Instead, PAHA apparently interfered with the establishment of tolerance to endogenous self antigens that are normally presented by the MHC on thymic epithelial cells during the positive selection of thymocytes (470). As a result mature T cells are produced that are capable of undergoing spontaneous activation when they encounter similar self antigens in the periphery. These studies suggest that the restricted autoantibody production associated with DIL reflects the specificity of T cells undergoing development and attempting to establish tolerance to self antigens in the presence of reactive drug metabolites in the thymus.

There are several major issues remaining about this system. Currently there is no evidence that reactive metabolites of procainamide can be produced in the thymus by circulating or resident phagocytic cells and that metabolites of other lupus-inducing drugs can also initiate autoimmunity by this mechanism. It would also be helpful to know that DIL patients, who are commonly in their sixth or seventh decade of life, have evidence of thymic function. Ultimately, identification of the molecular targets in developing thymocytes that are compromised by reactive drug metabolites will be needed to make this a convincing story.

ACKNOWLEDGMENTS

This work was supported in part by National Institutes of Health grants ES06334 and AI45978.

REFERENCES

1. Morrow JD, Schroeder HA, Perry HM Jr. Studies on the control of hypertension by hyphex. II. Toxic reactions and side effects. *Circulation* 1953;8:829–839.
2. Dustan HP, Taylor RD, Corcoran AC, et al. Rheumatic and febrile syndrome during prolonged hydralazine treatment. *JAMA* 1954;154:23–29.
3. Perry HM, Schroeder HA. Syndrome simulating collagen disease caused by hydralazine (Apresoline). *JAMA* 1954;154:670–673.
4. Ladd AT. Procainamide-induced lupus erythematosus. *N Engl J Med* 1962;267:1357–1358.

5. Sanford HS, Michaelson AK, Halpern MM. Procainamide induced lupus erythematosus syndrome. *Dis Chest* 1967;51: 172–176.
6. Mongey AB, Sim E, Risch A, et al. Acetylation status is associated with serological changes but not clinically significant disease in patients receiving procainamide. *J Rheumatol* 1999;26: 1721–1726.
7. Ioannou Y, Isenberg DA. Current evidence for the induction of autoimmune rheumatic manifestations by cytokine therapy. *Arthritis Rheum* 2000;43:1431–1442.
8. Fakhro AM, Ritchie RF, Lown B. Lupus-like syndrome induced by procainamide. *Am J Cardiol* 1967;20:367–373.
9. Condemi JJ, Moore-Jones D, Vaughan JH, et al. Antinuclear antibodies following hydralazine toxicity. *N Engl J Med* 1967; 276:486–490.
10. Rutherford BD. Procainamide induced systemic lupus erythematosus. *NZ Med J* 1968;68:235–240.
11. Blomgren SE, Condemi JJ, Bignall MC, et al. Antinuclear antibody induced by procainamide: a prospective study. *N Engl J Med* 1969;281:64–66.
12. Byrd RB, Schanzer B. Pulmonary sequelae in procainamide induced lupus-like syndrome. *Dis Chest* 1969;55:170–172.
13. Dubois EL. Procainamide induction of a systemic lupus erythematosus-like syndrome. Presentation of six cases, review of the literature, and analysis and follow-up of reported cases. *Medicine* 1969;48:217–228.
14. Gunther R, Asamer H, Dittrich P. The reversible procainamide-induced lupus erythematosus syndrome. *Dtsch Med Wochenschr* 1969;94:2338–2342.
15. Molina J, Dubois EL, Bilitch M, et al. Procainamide-induced serologic changes in asymptomatic patients. *Arthritis Rheum* 1969;12:608–614.
16. Condemi JJ, Blomgren SE, Vaughan JH. The procainamide-induced lupus syndrome. *Bull Rheum Dis* 1970;20:604.
17. Klajman A, Camin-Belsky N, Kimchi A, et al. Occurrence, immunoglobulin pattern and specificity of antinuclear antibodies in sera of procainamide treated patients. *Clin Exp Immunol* 1970;7:641–649.
18. Sheldon PJ, Williams WR. Procainamide-induced systemic lupus erythematosus. *Ann Rheum Dis* 1970;29:236–243.
19. Blomgren SE, Condemi JJ, Vaughan JH. Procainamide-induced lupus erythematosus. *Am J Med* 1972;52:338–348.
20. Klimas NG, Patarca R, Perez G, et al. Case report: distinctive immune abnormalities in a patient with procainamide-induced lupus and serositis. *Am J Med* 1992;303:99–104.
21. Hope RR, Bates LA. The frequency of procainamide-induced systemic lupus erythematosus. *Med J Aust* 1972;2:298–303.
22. Klajman A, Farkas R, Ben-Efraim S. Reactions of procainamide-induced antinuclear antibodies with fractions derived from calf thymus nuclei. *Int Arch Allergy* 1972;43: 630–638.
23. Swarbrick ET, Gray IR. Systemic lupus erythematosus during treatment with procainamide. *Br Heart J* 1972;34:284–288.
24. Winfield JB, Davis JS. Anti-DNA antibody in procainamide-induced lupus erythematosus. *Arthritis Rheum* 1974;17: 97–110.
25. Henningsen NC, Cederberg A, Hanson A, et al. Effects of long-term treatment with procainamide. *Acta Med Scand* 1975;198: 475–482.
26. Woosley RL, Drayer DE, Reidenberg MM, et al. Effect of acetylator phenotype on the rate at which procainamide induces antinuclear antibodies and the lupus syndrome. *N Engl J Med* 1978;298:1157–1159.
27. Lahita R, Kluger J, Drayer DE, et al. Antibodies to nuclear antigens in patients treated with procainamide or acetylprocainamide. *N Engl J Med* 1979;301:1382–1385.
28. Sonnhag C, Karlsson E, Hed J. Procainamide-induced lupus erythematosus-like syndrome in relation to acetylator phenotype and plasma levels of procainamide. *Acta Med Scand* 1979; 206:245–251.
29. Rubin RL, McNally EM, Nusinow SR, et al. IgG antibodies to the histone complex H2A-H2B characterize procainamide-induced lupus. *Clin Immunol Immunopathol* 1985;36:49–59.
30. Totoritis MC, Tan EM, McNally EM, et al. Association of antibody to histone complex H2A-H2B with symptomatic procainamide-induced lupus. *N Engl J Med* 1988;318:1431–1436.
31. Mongey A-B, Donovan-Brand R, Thomas TJ, et al. Serologic evaluation of patients receiving procainamide. *Arthritis Rheum* 1992;35:219–223.
32. Rubin RL, Burlingame RW, Arnott JE, et al. IgG but not other classes of anti-[(H2A-H2B)-DNA] is an early sign of procainamide-induced lupus. *J Immunol* 1995;154:2483–2493.
33. Burlingame RW, Rubin RL. Drug-induced anti-histone autoantibodies display two patterns of reactivity with substructures of chromatin. *J Clin Invest* 1991;88:680–690.
34. Gorsulowsky DC, Bank PW, Golberg AD, et al. Antinuclear antibodies as indicators for the procainamide-induced systemic lupus erythematosus-like syndrome and its clinical presentation. *J Am Acad Dermatol* 1985;12:245–253.
35. Amadio P Jr, Cummings DM, Dashow L. Procainamide, quinidine, and lupus erythematosus. *Ann Intern Med* 1985;102:419.
36. Anderson FP, Wanerka GR. Drug-induced systemic lupus erythematosus due to quinidine. *Conn Med* 1972;36:84–85.
37. Cohen MG, Kevat S, Prowse MV, et al. Two distinct quinidine induced rheumatic syndromes. *Ann Intern Med* 1988;108: 369–371.
38. Donoho CR, Pascual E, Abruzzo JL, et al. Quinidine-induced lupus erythematosus. *Arthritis Rheum* 1974;17:322.
39. Kim SY, Benowitz NL. Poisoning due to class IA antiarrhythmic drugs, quinidine, procainamide and disopyramide. *Drug Safety* 1990;5:393–420.
40. Krainin MJ, Clark JI. Quinidine-induced lupus erythematosus (letter). *Arch Intern Med* 1985;145:1740–1741.
41. Lavie CH, Biundo J, Quinet BJ, et al. Systemic lupus erythematosus (SLE) induced by quinidine. *Arch Intern Med* 1985;145:700–702.
42. McCormack GD, Barth WF. Quinidine induced lupus syndrome. *Semin Arthritis Rheum* 1985;15:73–79.
43. Tweed JM. Quinidine and SLE-like illness. *NZ Med J* 1977;86: 40.
44. West SG, McMahon M, Portanova JP. Quinidine-induced lupus erythematosus. *Ann Intern Med* 1984;100:840–842.
45. Yudis M, Meehan JJ. Quinidine-induced lupus nephritis. *JAMA* 1976;235:2000.
46. Barrier J, Grolleau JY, Choimet P. Lupus induced by quinidine, detected by thrombopenic purpura (letter). *Nouv Presse Med* 1981;10:2991–2992.
47. Bar El Y, Shimoni Z, Flatau E. Qunidine-induced lupus erythematosus. *Am Heart J* 1986;111:1209–1210.
48. Wanner WR, Irvin WS. Disopyramide and antinuclear antibodies (letter). *Am Heart J* 1981;101:687–689.
49. Guindo J, Rodriquez de la Serna A, Borja J, et al. Propafenone and a syndrome of the lupus erythematosus type. *Ann Intern Med* 1986;140:589.
50. Wilson JD. Antinuclear antibodies and cardiovascular drugs. *Drugs* 1980;19:292–305.
51. Booth RJ, Wilson J, Bullock J. Beta-adrenergic-receptor blockers and antinuclear antibodies in hypertension. *Clin Pharmacol Ther* 1982;31:555–558.
52. Wilson JD, Bullock JY, Sutherland DC, et al. Antinuclear antibodies in patients receiving non-practolol beta blockers. *Br Med J* 1978;1:14–16.

53. Perry HMJ, Tan EM, Carmody S, et al. Relationship of acetyl transferase activity to antinuclear antibodies and toxic symptoms in hypertensive patients treated with hydralazine. *J Lab Clin Med* 1970;76:114–125.
54. Carey RM, Coleman M, Feder A. Pericardial tamponade: a major presenting manifestation of hydralazine-induced lupus syndrome. *Am J Med* 1973;54:84–87.
55. Litwin A, Adams LE, Hess EV, et al. Hydralazine urinary metabolites in systemic lupus erythematosus. *Arthritis Rheum* 1973;16:217–220.
56. Perry HM Jr. Late toxicity of hydralazine resembling systemic lupus erythematosus or rheumatoid arthritis. *Am J Med* 1973; 54:58–72.
57. Hahn BH, Sharp GC, Irvin WS, et al. Immune response to hydralazine and nuclear antigens in hydralazine-induced lupus erythematosus. *Ann Intern Med* 1972;76:365–374.
58. Alarcon-Segovia D, Worthington JW, Ward LE, et al. Lupus diathesis and the hydralazine syndrome. *N Engl J Med* 1965; 272:462–466.
59. Alarcón-Segovia D, Wakim KG, Worthington JW, et al. Clinical and experimental studies on the hydralazine syndrome and its relationship to systemic lupus erythematosus. *Medicine* 1967;46:1–33.
60. Ohe A, Koda S, Negoro N. A case of hydralazine-induced lupus erythematosus with circulating antibodies to native DNA. *Osaka City Med J* 1982;28:149–151.
61. Weinstein J. Hypocomplementemia in hydralazine-associated systemic lupus erythematosus. *Am J Med* 1978;65:553.
62. Ryan PFJ, Hughes GRV, Bernstein R, et al. Lymphocytotoxic antibodies in hydralazine-induced lupus erythematosus. *Lancet* 1979;2:1248–1249.
63. Portanova JP, Rubin RL, Joslin FG, et al. Reactivity of anti-histone antibodies induced by procainamide and hydralazine. *Clin Immunol Immunopathol* 1982;25:67–79.
64. Ramsay LE, Silas J, Freestone S. Hydralazine antinuclear antibodies and the lupus syndrome (letter). *Br Med J* 1982;284: 1711.
65. Litwin A, Adams LE, Zimmer H, et al. Immunologic effects of hydralazine in hypertensive patients. *Arthritis Rheum* 1981;24: 1074–1077.
66. Litwin A, Adams LE, Zimmer H, et al. Prospective study of immunologic effects of hydralazine in hypertensive patients. *Clin Pharmacol Ther* 1981;29:447–456.
67. Neville E, Graham PY, Brewis RA. Orogenital ulcers, SLE and hydralazine. *Postgrad Med J* 1981;57:378–379.
68. Batchelor JR, Welsh KL, Tinoco RM, et al. Hydralazine-induced systemic lupus erythematosus: influence of HLA-DR and sex on susceptibility. *Lancet* 1980;1:1107–1109.
69. Carpenter JR, McDuffie FC, Sheps SG, et al. Prospective study of immune response to hydralazine and development of anti-deoxyribonucleoprotein in patients receiving hydralazine. *Am J Med* 1980;69:395–400.
70. Nässberger L, Johansson AC, Björck S, et al. Antibodies to neutrophil granulocyte myeloperoxidase and elastase: autoimmune responses in glomerulonephritis and due to hydralazine treatment. *J Intern Med* 1991;229:261–265.
71. Nässberger L, Sjöholm AG, Jonsson H, et al. Autoantibodies against neutrophil cytoplasm components in systemic lupus erythematosus and in hydralazine-induced lupus. *Clin Exp Immunol* 1990;81:380–383.
72. Mitchell JA, Sim RB, Sim E. CR1 polymorphism in hydralazine-induced systemic lupus erythematosus. *Clin Exp Immunol* 1989;78:354–358.
73. Palsson L, Weiner L, Englund G, et al. Cadralazine challenge in patients with previous hydralazine-induced lupus. *Clin Pharmacol Ther* 1989;46:177–181.
74. Speirs C, Chapel H, Fielder AHL, et al. Complement system protein C4 and susceptibility to hydralazine-induced systemic lupus erythematosus. *Lancet* 1989;1:922–924.
75. Craft JE, Radding JA, Harding MW, et al. Autoantigenic histone epitopes: a comparison between procainamide- and hydralazine-induced lupus. *Arthritis Rheum* 1987;30:689–694.
76. Russell GI, Bing RF, Jones JAG, et al. Hydralazine sensitivity: clinical features, autoantibody changes and HLA-DR phenotype. *Q J Med* 1987;65:845–852.
77. Servitje O, Ribera M, Juanola X, et al. Acute neutrophilic dermatosis associated with hydralazine-induced lupus. *Arch Dermatol* 1987;123:1435–1436.
78. Anandadas JA, Simpson P. Cardiac tamponade, associated with hydralazine therapy, in a patient with rapid acetylator status. *Br J Clin Pract* 1986;40:305–306.
79. Asherson RA, Benbow AG, Speirs CJ, et al. Pulmonary hypertension in hydralazine induced systemic lupus erythematosus: association with C4 null allele. *Ann Rheum Dis* 1986;45: 771–773.
80. Innes A, Rennie JA, Cato GR. Drug-induced lupus caused by very-low-dose hydralazine (letter). *Br J Rheumatol* 1986;25:225.
81. Sequeira W, Polisky RB, Alrenga DP. Neutrophilic dermatosis (Sweet's syndrome). Association with a hydralazine-induced lupus syndrome. *Am J Med* 1986;81:558–560.
82. Widgren BR, Andersson OK, Berglund GL. Adverse effects of prolonged treatment with hydralazine—a retrospective study. *Lakartidningen* 1986;83:2825–2828.
83. Bjorck S, Svalander C, Westberg G. Hydralazine-associated glomerulonephritis. *Acta Med Scand* 1985;218:261–269.
84. Doherty M, Maddison PJ, Grey RH. Hydralazine induced lupus syndrome with eye disease. *Br Med J Clin Res Ed* 1985; 290:675.
85. Brand C, Davidson A, Littlejohn G, et al. Hydralazine-induced lupus: no association with HLA-DR4. *Lancet* 1984;1:462.
86. Cameron HA, Ramsay LE. The lupus syndrome induced by hydralazine: a common complication with low dose treatment. *Br Med J* 1984;289:410–412.
87. French WJ. Hydralazine-induced lupus syndrome. *Alabama J Med Sci* 1984;21:427–430.
88. Ihle BU, Whitworth JA, Dowling JP, Kincaid-Smith P. Hydralazine and lupus nephritis. *Clin Nephrol* 1984;22: 230–238.
89. Naparstek Y, Kopolovic J, Tur-Kaspa R, et al. Focal glomerulonephritis in the course of hydralazine-induced lupus syndrome. *Arthritis Rheum* 1984;27:822–825.
90. Peterson LL. Hydralazine-induced systemic lupus erythematosus presenting as pyoderma gangrenosum-like ulcers. *J Am Acad Dermatol* 1984;10:379–384.
91. Ramsay LE, Cameron HA. The lupus syndrome induced by hydralazine (letter). *Br Med J* 1984;289:1310–1311.
92. Weiser GA, Farouhar FA, White WB. Hydralazine hoarseness: a new appearance of drug-induced systemic lupus erythematosus. *Arch Intern Med* 1984;144:2271–2272.
93. Kincaid-Smith P, Whitworth JA. Hydralazine-associated glomerulonephritis (letter). *Lancet* 1983;2:348.
94. Macleod WN. Anaemia in the hydralazine-induced lupus syndrome. *Scott Med J* 1983;28:181–182.
95. Shapiro KS, Pinn VW, Harrington JT, et al. Immune complex glomerulonephritis in hydralazine-induced SLE. *Am J Kidney Dis* 1984;3:270–274.
96. Shoenfeld Y, Isenberg D. Transient monoclonal gammopathy in hydralazine induced lupus erythematosus (letter). *Br Med J* 1983;286:224–224.
97. Aylward PE, Tonkin AM, Bune A. Cardiac tamponade in hydralazine-induced systemic lupus erythematosus. *Aust NZ J Med* 1982;12:546–547.

98. Freestone S, Ramsay LE. Transient monoclonal gammopathy in hydralazine-induced lupus erythematosus. *Br Med J* 1982;285: 1536–1537.
99. Mansilla-Tinoco R, Harland SJ, Ryan PJ, et al. Hydralazine, antinuclear antibodies, and the lupus syndrome. *Br Med J* 1982; 284:936–939.
100. Breckenridge A, Dollery CT, Worlledge SM, et al. Positive direct Coombs tests and antinuclear factor in patients treated with methyldopa. *Lancet* 1967;2:1265–1267.
101. Dupont A, Six R. Lupus-like syndrome induced by methyldopa. *Br Med J* 1982;285:693–694.
102. Harth M. LE cells and positive direct Coombs' test induced by methyldopa. *Can Med Assoc J* 1968;99:277–280.
103. Homberg JC, Abuaf N, Plouin PF. Antinuclear antibodies and lupus induced during treatment of arterial hypertension. Role of beta blockers and alpha-methyldopa. *J Pharmacol* 1983;14: 61–66.
104. Mackay IR, Cowling DC, Hurley TH. Drug induced autoimmune disease: hemolytic anemia and lupus cells after treatment with methyldopa. *Med J Aust* 1968;2:1047–1050.
105. Nordstrom DM, West SG, Rubin RL. Methyldopa-induced systemic lupus erythematosus. *Arthritis Rheum* 1989;32: 205–208.
106. Perry HM Jr, Chaplin H Jr, Carmody S, et al. Immunologic findings in patients receiving methyldopa: a prospective study. *J Lab Clin Med* 1971;78:905–917.
107. Sherman JD, Love DE, Harrington JF. Anemia, positive lupus and rheumatoid factors with methyldopa. Report of 3 cases. *Arch Intern Med* 1967;120:321–326.
108. Rubin RL, Bell SA, Burlingame RW. Autoantibodies associated with lupus induced by diverse drugs target a similar epitope in the (H2A-H2B)-DNA complex. *J Clin Invest* 1992;90: 165–173.
109. Feltkamp TEW, Mees EJD, Nieuwenhuis MG. Autoantibodies related to treatment with chlorthalidone and a-methyldopa. *Acta Med Scand* 1970;187:219–223.
110. Case DB, Atlas SA, Laragh J, et al. Clinical experience with blockade of the renin-angiotensin-aldosterone system by an oral converting-enzyme inhibitor (SQ14,225,captopril) in hypertensive patients. *Prog Cardiovasc Dis* 1978;21:195–206.
111. Patri P, Nigro A, Rebora A. Lupus erythematosus-like eruption from captopril. *Acta Derm Venereol* 1985;65:447–448.
112. Reidenberg MM, Chase DB, Drayer DE, et al. Development of antinuclear antibody in patients treated with high doses of captopril. *Arthritis Rheum* 1984;27:579–581.
113. Kallenberg CG. Antibodies during captopril treatment. *Arthritis Rheum* 1985;28:597–598.
114. Sieber C, Grimm E, Follath F. Captopril and systemic lupus erythematosus syndrome. *Br Med J* 1990;301:669.
115. Samanta A, Burden AC. Fever, myalgia, and arthralgia in a patient on captopril and allopurinol. *Lancet* 1984;1:679.
116. Bigot MC, Trenque T, Moulin M. Acebutolol and a lupus syndrome. Apropos of a case. *Therapie* 1984;39:571–575.
117. Hourdebaigt-Larrusse P, Ziza JM, Grivaux M. A new case of lupus induced by acebutolol. *Ann Cardiol Angeiol* 1985;34: 421–423.
118. Record NB Jr. Acebutolol-induced pleuropulmonary lupus syndrome. *Ann Intern Med* 1981;95:326–327.
119. Querin S, Feuillet-Fieux M-N, Jacob L, et al. Specificity of acebutolol-induced antinuclear antibodies. *J Immunopharmacol* 1986;8:633–649.
120. Bloomqist JN, Laddu A, Engler R. Adverse effects of acebutolol in chronic stable angina: drug-induced positive antinuclear antibody. *J Cardiovasc Pharmacol* 1984;6:735–738.
121. Schwartz D, Pines A, Averbuch M, et al. Enalapril-induced antinuclear antibodies. *Lancet* 1990;336:187.
122. Witman G, Davis R. A lupus erythematosus syndrome induced by clonidine hydrochloride. *R I Med J* 1981;64:147–150.
123. Gouet D, Marchaud R, Aucouturier P. Atenolol induced systemic lupus erythematosus syndrome. *J Rheumatol* 1986;13:11–32.
124. Brown RC, Cooke J, Losowsky MS. SLE syndrome, probably induced by labetalol. *Postgrad Med J* 1981;57:189–190.
125. Griffiths ID, Richardson J. Lupus-type illness associated with labetalol. *Br Med J* 1979;2:496–497.
126. Bensaid J, Aldigier JC, Gualde N. Systemic lupus erythematosus syndrome induced by pindolol. *Br Med J* 1979;1: 1603–1604.
127. Tunkel AR, Shuman M, Popkin M, et al. Minoxidil-induced systemic lupus erythematosus. *Arch Intern Med* 1987; 147:599–600.
128. Wilson JD, Booth RJ, Bullock JY. Antinuclear factor in patients on prazosin (letter). *Br Med J* 1979;1:553–554.
129. Marshall AJ, McGraw ME, Barritt DW. Positive antinuclear factor tests with prazocin. *Br Med J* 1979;1:165–166.
130. Melkild A, Gaarder PI. Does prazocin induce formation of antinuclear factor? (letter). *Br Med J* 1979;1:620–621.
131. Fabius AJ, Gaulhofer WK. Systemic lupus erythematosus induced by psychotropic drugs. *Acta Rheumatol Scand* 1971;17: 137–147.
132. Grupper C, Marcel GA. Lupus erythematosus and psychotropic drugs. *Bull Soc Fr Dermatol Syphilgr* 1965;72:714–721.
133. Alberti-Flor JJ. Chlorpromazine-induced lupus-like illness. *Am Fam Physician* 1983;27:151–152.
134. Ananth JV, Minn K. Chlorpromazine-induced systemic lupus erythematosus. *Can Med Assoc J* 1973;108:680.
135. Alarcon-Segovia D, Fishbein E, Cetina JA, et al. Antigen specificity of chlorpromazine-induced antinuclear antibodies. *Clin Exp Immunol* 1973;15:543–548.
136. Berglund S, Gottfries C-G, Gottfries I, et al. Chlorpromazine-induced antinuclear factors. *Acta Med Scand* 1970;187:67–74.
137. Canoso RT, deOliveira RM. Chlorpromazine-induced anti-cardiolipin antibodies and lupus anticoagulant: absence of thrombosis. *Am J Hematol* 1988;27:272–275.
138. Canoso RT, de Oliveira RM. Characterization and antigenic specificity of chlorpromazine-induced antinuclear antibodies. *J Lab Clin Med* 1986;108:213–216.
139. Canoso RT, Lewis ME, Yunis EJ. Association of HLA-Bw44 with chlorpromazine-induced autoantibodies. *Clin Immunol Immunopathol* 1982;25:278–282.
140. Canoso RT, Sise HS. Chlorpromazine-induced lupus anticoagulant and associated immunologic abnormalities. *Am J Hematol* 1982;13:121–129.
141. Dubois EL, Tallman E, Wonka RA. Chlorpromazine induced systemic lupus erythematosus (SLE). Case report and review of the literature. *JAMA* 1972;221:595–596.
142. Quismorio FPJ, Bjarnson DF, Kiely WF, et al. Antinuclear antibodies in chronic psychotic patients treated with chlorpromazine. *Am J Psychiatry* 1975;132:1204–1206.
143. Tollefson G, Rodysill K, Cusulos M. A circulating lupus-like coagulation inhibitor induced by chlorpromazine. *J Clin Psych Pharmacol* 1984;4:49–51.
144. Zarrabi MH, Zucker S, Miller F, et al. Immunologic and coagulation disorders in chlorpromazine-treated patients. *Ann Intern Med* 1979;91:194–199.
145. Zucker S, Zarrabi MH, Romano GS, et al. IgM inhibitors of the contact phase of coagulation in chlorpromazine treated patients. *Br J Hematol* 1978;40:447–457.
146. Zarrabi MH, Kaufman L, Gruber B, et al. Further characterization of the serologic immune response to chlorpromazine. *Blood* 1988;72:1007(abst).
147. Lillicrap DP, Pinto M, Benford K, et al. Heterogeneity of laboratory test results for antiphospholipid antibodies in patients

treated with chlorpromazine and other phenothiazines. *Am J Clin Pharm* 1990;6:771–775.

148. Gallien M, Schnetzler J-P, Morin J. Antinuclear antibodies and lupus induced by phenothiazines in 600 hospitalized patients. *Ann Med Psychol* 1975;1:237–248.
149. Steen VD, Ramsey-Goldman R. Phenothiazine-induced systemic lupus erythematosus with superior vena cava syndrome: case report and review of the literature. *Arthritis Rheum* 1988; 31:923–926.
150. Pavlidakey GP, Hashimoto K, Heller GL, et al. Chlorpromazine-induced lupuslike disease. *J Am Acad Dermatol* 1985; 13:109–115.
151. Gold MS, Sweeney DR. Perphenazine-induced systemic lupus erythematosus-like syndrome. *J Nerv Ment Dis* 1978;166: 442–445.
152. Swartz C. Lupus-like reaction to phenelzine. *JAMA* 1978;239: 2693.
153. McNevin S, MacKay M. Clorprothixene-induced systemic lupus erythematosus. *J Clin Psychopharmacol* 1982;2:411–412.
154. Ghose K, Coppen A, Hurdle AD, et al. Antinuclear antibodies, affective disorders and lithium therapy. *Pharmakopsychiatry Neuropsychopharmakol* 1977;10:243–245.
155. Presley AP, Kahn A, Williamson N. Antinuclear antibodies in patients on lithium carbonate. *Br Med J* 1976;2:280–281.
156. Shukla VR, Borison RL. Lithium and lupus-like syndrome (letter). *JAMA* 1982;248:921–922.
157. Whalley LJ, Roberts DF, Wentzel J, et al. Antinuclear antibodies and histocompatibility antigens in patients on long-term lithium therapy. *J Affect Disord* 1981;3:123–130.
158. Alarcon-Segovia D. Drug-induced lupus syndrome. *Mayo Clin Proc* 1967;44:664–681.
159. Alarcon-Segovia D, Fishbein E, Reyes PA, et al. Antinuclear antibodies in patients on anticonvulsant therapy. *Clin Exp Immunol* 1972;12:39–47.
160. Andersen P, Mosekilder L. Immunoglobulin levels and autoantibodies in epileptics in long-term anticonvulsant therapy. *Acta Med Scand* 1977;201:69–74.
161. Dorfmann H, Kahn M-F, deSeze S. Iatrogenic lupus erythematosus induced by anticonvulsants. *Semin Hop Paris* 1972; 48:2991–3000.
162. Jacobs JC. Systemic lupus erythematosus in childhood. Report of 35 cases with discussion of seven apparently induced by anticonvulsant medication, and of prognosis and treatment. *Pediatrics* 1963;32:257–264.
163. AlBalla S, Fritzler MJ, Davis P. A case of drug-induced lupus due to carbamazepine. *J Rheumatol* 1987;14:599–600.
164. Bateman DE. Carbamazepine induced systemic lupus erythematosus: case report. *Br Med J (Clin Res)* 1985;291:632–633.
165. DeGiorgio CM, Rabinowics AL, Olivas RD. Carbamazepine-induced antinuclear antibodies and systemic lupus erythematosus-like syndrome. *Epilepsia* 1991;32:128–129.
166. Jenryczko A, Drozdz M, Magner K. Carbamazepine induced systemic lupus erythematosus (letter). *Br Med J* 1985;291: 1198–1200.
167. Kolstee HJ. A patient with disseminated lupus erythematosus caused by the use of carbamazepine (Tegretol). *Ned Tijdsch Geneeskd* 1983;127:1588–1590.
168. Pacifici R, Paris L, DiCarlo S, et al. Immunologic aspects of carbamazepine treatment in epileptic patients. *Epilepsia* 1991;32: 122–127.
169. Beurey J, Weber M, Delrous JL, et al. Acute lupus erythematosus perhaps induced by tegretol (carbamazepine). *Bull Soc Fr Dermatol Syphilgr* 1972;79:186.
170. Paladini G, Tonazzi C, Maring L. Pulmonary eosinophilia and lupus-like syndrome secondary to carbamazepine. *J Clin Pharm Res* 1982;2(suppl):43.
171. Alarcon-Segovia D, Palacios R. Differences in immunoregulatory T cell circuits between diphenylhydantoin-related and spontaneously occurring systemic lupus erythematosus. *Arthritis Rheum* 1981;24:1086–1092.
172. Amadori G, Fiore D. Diagnostic problems in hydantoin immunopathy. Review of literature and description of 3 cases. *Minerva Med* 1984;75:2503–2509.
173. Rallison ML, Carlisle JW, Lee REJ, et al. Lupus erythematosus and Steven's Johnson syndrome. Occurrence as reactions to anticonvulsant therapy. *Am J Dis Child* 1961;101:725–738.
174. Ahuja GK, Schumacher GA. Drug-induced systemic lupus erythematosus, primidone as a possible cause. *JAMA* 1966;198: 669–671.
175. Cochran M, Nordin BE. Panhypopituitarism, testicular atrophy, alactasia, corticosteroid-induced osteoporosis and systemic lupus erythematosus induced by methoin. *Proc R Soc Med* 1968; 61:656.
176. Damm J, Sonnichsen N. Clinical examinations of chronic lupus erythematosus. *Dermatol Wschr* 1964;150:268.
177. Alter BP. Systemic lupus erythematosus and ethosuccimide. *J Pediatr* 1970;77:1093–1095.
178. Dabbous IA, Idriss HM. Occurrence of systemic lupus erythematosus in association with ethosuccimide therapy. Case report. *J Pediatr* 1970;76:617–620.
179. Livingston S, Rodriguez H, Greene CA, et al. Systemic lupus erythematosus. Occurrence in association with ethosuximide therapy. *JAMA* 1968;203:731–732.
180. Grossman L, Barland P. Histone reactivity of drug-induced anti-nuclear antibodies. *Arthritis Rheum* 1981;24:927–930.
181. Debeyre N, Kahn MF, deSeze S. Lupoid syndrome after absorption of isoniazid. Study of 6 cases. *Semin Hop Paris* 1967;43: 3063–3071.
182. Dutt AK, Shaw T. Isonicotinic acid hydrazine (INH) induced syndrome of lupus erythematosus. *Indian J Chest Dis Allied Sci* 1976;18:146–151.
183. Esocollar-Castellon F, Moya-Mir MS, Martin-Martin F. Disseminated lupus erythematosus induced by isoniazid manifesting as prolonged fever. Presentation of a case. *Rev Clin Esp* 1983;169:209–210.
184. Evans DAP, Bullen MF, Houston J, et al. Antinuclear factor in rapid and slow acetylator patients with isoniazid. *J Med Genet* 1972;9:53–56.
185. Godeau P, Aukert M, Imbert JD, et al. SLE and active isoniazid levels in 47 cases. *Ann Med Intern* 1973;124:181–186.
186. Granja CDB, Santiago MB, Viana VST, et al. Caracterizaçao clínico-laboratorial de auto-anticorpos induzidos por isoniazida. *Rev Paul Med* 1990;108:57–60.
187. Alarcón-Segovia D, Fishbein E, Alcala H. Isoniazid acetylation rate and development of antinuclear antibodies upon isoniazid treatment. *Arthritis Rheum* 1971;14:748–752.
188. Cannat A, Seligmann M. Possible induction of antinuclear antibodies by isoniazid. *Lancet* 1966;1:185–187.
189. Bickers JN, Buechner HA, Hood BJ, et al. Hypersensitivity reaction to antituberculosis drugs with hepatitis, lupus phenomenon, and myocardial infarction. *N Engl J Med* 1961;265: 131–132.
190. Dhand R, Gilhotra R, Sehgal S, et al. Incidence of isoniazid-induced antinuclear antibodies in patients of tuberculosis. *Indian J Med Res* 1987;85:503–507.
191. Hubscher O, Garcia-Morteo O, Arana RM. Isoniazid and antinuclear antibodies (letter). *Ann Intern Med* 1978;89:1011.
192. Lindqvist KJ, Coleman RE, Osterland CK. Autoantibodies in chronic pulmonary tuberculosis. *J Chron Dis* 1970;22: 717–725.
193. Muller S, Barakat S, Watts R, et al. Longitudinal analysis of antibodies to histones, Sm-D peptides and ubiquitin in the

serum of patients with systemic lupus erythematosus, rheumatoid arthritis and tuberculosis. *Clin Exp Rheumatol* 1990;8: 445–453.
194. Price-Evans DA, Bullen MF, Houston J, et al. Antinuclear factors in rapid and slow acetylator patients treated with isoniazid. *J Med Genet* 1972;9:53–56.
195. Rothfield NF, Bierer WF, Garfield JW. Isoniazid induction of antinuclear antibodies. A prospective study. *Ann Intern Med* 1978;88:650–652.
196. Salazar-Paramo M, Rubin RL, Garcia-de la Torre I. Isoniazid-induced systemic lupus erythematosus. *Ann Rheum Dis* 1992; 51:1085–1087.
197. Sela O, El-Roeiy A, Isenberg DA, et al. A common anti-DNA idiotype in sera of patients with active pulmonary tuberculosis. *Arthritis Rheum* 1987;30:50–56.
198. Vázquez-Del Mercado M, Casiano CA, Rubin RL. IgA antihistone antibodies in isoniazid-treated tuberculosis patients. *Autoimmunity* 1995;20:105–111.
199. Matsuura T, Shimizu Y, Fujimoto H, et al. Minocycline-related lupus. *Lancet* 1992;340:1553.
200. Knights SE, Leandro MJ, Khamashta MA, et al. Minocycline-induced arthritis. *Clin Exp Rheumatol* 1998;16:587–590.
201. Gough A, Chapman S, Wagstaff K, et al. Minocycline induced autoimmune hepatitis and systemic lupus erythematosus-like syndrome. *Br Med J* 1996;312:169–173.
202. Bulgen DY. Minocycline-related lupus. *Br J Rheumatol* 1995; 34:398.
203. Quilty B, McHugh N. Lupus-like syndrome associated with the use of minocycline. *Br J Rheumatol* 1994;33:1197–1198.
204. Byrne PAC, Williams BD, Pritchard MH. Minocycline-related lupus. *Br J Rheumatol* 1994;33:674–676.
205. Christodoulou CS, Emmanuel P, Ray RA, et al. Respiratory distress due to minocycline-induced pulmonary lupus. *Chest* 1999; 115:1471–1473.
206. Dunphy J, Oliver M, Rands AL, et al. Antineutrophil cytoplasmic antibodies and HLA class II alleles in minocycline-induced lupus-like syndrome. *Br J Dermatol* 2000;142:461–467.
207. Holmberg L, Boman G, Bottiger LE, et al. Adverse reactions to nitrofurantoin. Analysis of 921 reports. *Am J Med* 1980;69: 733–738.
208. Burns DA, Sarkany I. Penicillamine-induced discoid lupus erythematosus. *Clin Exp Dermatol* 1979;4:389–392.
209. Caille B, Harpey P-J, Lejeune C, et al. Lupoid syndrome due to D-penicillamine associated with Wilson's disease. Clinical study of a case. *Ann Med Interne (Paris)* 1971;122:255–260.
210. Camus JP, Homberg JC, Crouzet J, et al. Autoantibody formation in D-penicillamine-treated rheumatoid arthritis. *J Rheumatol* 1981;7:80–83.
211. Chalmers A, Thompson D, Stein HE. Systemic lupus erythematosus during penicillamine therapy for rheumatoid arthritis. *Ann Intern Med* 1982;97:659–663.
212. Chin GL, Kong NCT, Lee BC, et al. Penicillamine induced lupus-like syndrome in a patient with classical rheumatoid arthritis. *J Rheumatol* 1991;947–948.
213. Crawhall JC. Proteinuria in D-penicillamine treated RA. *J Rheumatol* 1981;7(suppl):161–163.
214. Enzenauer RJ, West SG, Rubin RL. D-penicillamine-induced systemic lupus erythematosus. *Arthritis Rheum* 1990;33: 1582–1585.
215. Harkcom TM, Conn DI, Holley KE. D-penicillamine and lupus erythematosus-like syndrome (letter). *Ann Intern Med* 1978; 89:1012.
216. Kalina P, Prochazkova L, Hauftova D. A syndrome similar to systemic lupus erythematosus caused by penicillamine in patients with Wilson's disease. *Bratisl Lek Listy* 1985;84:336–340.
217. Kirby JD, Dieppe PA, Huskisson EC, et al. D-penicillamine and immune complex deposition. *Ann Rheum Dis* 1979;38: 344–346.
218. LeBihan G, Birembaut JC, Bourreille J. Primary biliary cirrhosis and lupus: role of D-penicillamine? (letter). *Gastroenterol Clin Biol* 1982;6:405–406.
219. Oliver I, Liberman UA, DeVries A. Lupus-like syndrome induced by penicillamine in cystinuria. *JAMA* 1972;220: 588–588.
220. Tsankov NK, Lazarova AZ, Vasileva SG, et al. Lupus erythematosus-like eruption due to D-penicillamine in progressive systemic sclerosis. *Int J Dermatol* 1990;29:571–574.
221. Walshe JM. Penicillamine-induced SLE (letter). *Lancet* 1981;2: 1416–1416.
222. Pinals RS. Diffuse fasciculations induced by D-penicillamine. *J Rheumatol* 1983;10:809–810.
223. Webb J, Pollard KM. Induction of DNA-antibodies by d-penicillamine. *Clin Exp Rheumatol* 1985;3:213–219.
224. Morel E, Feuillet-Fieux MN, Garabedian BV-D, et al. Autoantibodies in D-penicillamine-induced myasthenia gravis: a comparison with idiopathic myasthenia and rheumatoid arthritis. *Clin Immunol Immunopathol* 1991;58:318–330.
225. Weinstein A. D-penicillamine-induced lupus erythematosus. *Arthritis Rheum* 1991;34:1343–1344.
226. Christie DJ, Mullen PC, Aster RH. Fab-mediated binding of drug-dependent antibodies to platelets in quinidine- and quinine-induced thrombocytopenia. *J Clin Invest* 1985;75: 310–314.
227. Elsas LJ, Hayslett JP, Spargo BH, et al. Wilson's disease with reversible renal tubular dysfunction. Correlation with proximal tubular ultrastructure. *Ann Intern Med* 1971;75:427–433.
228. Griffiths I, Kane S. Sulfasalazine-induced lupus syndrome in ulcerative colitis. *Br Med J* 1977;2:1188–1189.
229. Carr-Locke DL. Sulfasalazine-induced lupus syndrome in a patient with Crohn's disease. *Am J Gastroenterol* 1982;77: 614–616.
230. Bray VJ, West SG, Schultz KT, et al. Antihistone antibody profile in sulfasalazine induced lupus. *J Rheumatol* 1994;21: 2157–2158.
231. Olenginski TP, Harrington TM, Carlson JP. Transverse myelitis secondary to sulfasalazine (letter). *J Rheumatol* 1991;18:304.
232. Rafferty P, Young AC, Haeney MR. Sulphasalazine-induced cerebral lupus erythematosus. *Postgrad Med J* 1982;58:98–99.
233. Vanheule BA, Carswell F. Sulphasalazine-induced systemic lupus erythematosus in a child. *Eur J Pediatr* 1983;140:66–68.
234. Laversuch CJ, Collins DA, Charles PJ, et al. Sulphasalazine-induced autoimmune abnormalities in patients with rheumatic disease. *Br J Rheumatol* 1995;34:435–439.
235. Veale DJ, Ho M, Morley KD. Sulphasalazine-induced lupus in psoriatic arthritis. *Br J Rheumatol* 1995;34:383–384.
236. De Keyser F, Mielants H, Praet J, et al. Changes in antinuclear serology in patients with spondylarthropathy under sulphasalazine treatment. *Br J Rheumatol* 1993;32:521–526.
237. Caulier M, Dromer C, Andrieu V, et al. Sulphasalazine-induced lupus in rheumatoid arthritis. *J Rheumatol* 1994;21:750–751.
238. Wildhagen K, Hartung K, Hammer M. Drug-related lupus in a patient with rheumatoid arthritis under sulfasalazine treatment. *Clin Rheumatol* 1993;12:265–267.
239. Walker DM, Carty JE. Sulphasalazine-induced systemic lupus erythematosus in a patient with erosive arthritis. *Br J Rheumatol* 1994;33:175–176.
240. Siam AR, Hammoudeh M. Sulfasalazine-induced systemic lupus erythematosus in a patient with rheumatoid arthritis (letter). *J Rheumatol* 1993;20:207.
241. Handley AJ. Thrombocytopenia and L.E. cells after oxyphenbutazone. *Lancet* 1971;1:245–246.
242. Gráyson MF, Martin VM, Markham RL. Antinative DNA anti-

bodies as a reaction to pyrazole drugs. *Ann Rheum Dis* 1975; 34:373–375.

243. Finkel TH, Hunter DJ, Paisley JE, et al. Drug-induced lupus in a child after treatment with zafirlukast (Accolate). *J Allergy Clin Immunol* 1999;103:533–534.
244. Kirkpatrick AW, Bookman AA, Habal F. Lupus-like syndrome caused by 5-aminosalicylic acid in patients with inflammatory bowel disease. *Can J Gastroenterol* 1999;13:159–162.
245. Goodrich AL, Kohn SR. Hydrochlorothiazide-induced lupus erythematosus: a new variant? *J Am Acad Dermatol* 1993;28: 1001–1002.
246. Reed BR, Huff JC, Jones SK, et al. Subacute cutaneous lupus erythematosus associated with hydrochlorothiazide therapy. *Ann Intern Med* 1985;103:49–51.
247. Ahmad S. Lovastatin-induced lupus erythematosus. *Arch Intern Med* 1991;151:1667–1668.
248. Ahmad A, Fletcher MT, Roy TM. Simvastatin-induced lupus-like syndrome. *Tenn Med* 2000;93:21–22.
249. Amrhein JA, Kenny FM, Ross D. Granulocytopenia,lupus-like syndrome and other complications of propylthiouracil therapy. *J Pediatr* 1970;76:54–63.
250. Berkman EM, Orlin J, Wolfsdorf J. An antineutrophil antibody associated with propylthiouracil (PTU) induced lupus-like syndrome. *Transfusion* 1983;23:135–138.
251. Best MM, Duncan CH. A lupus-like syndrome following propylthiouracil administration. *J Ky Med Assoc* 1964;62:47.
252. Miyakawa M, Sato K, Sato Y. Presentation of a case of Graves' disease with neutropenia and splenomegaly: propylthiouracil-induced autoimmune neutropenia and review of the literature on the drug-induced lupus-like syndrome. *Nippon Naika Gakkai Zasshi* 1984;73:538–545.
253. Henry RE, Goldberg LS, Sturgeon P, et al. Serological abnormalities associated with L-dopa therapy. *Vox Sang* 1971;20: 306–316.
254. McCraken M, Benson EA, Hickling P. Systemic lupus erythematosus induced by aminoglutethimide. *Br Med J* 1980;281: 1254.
255. Zamber R, Martens H, Rubin RL, et al. Drug-induced lupus due to ophthalmic timolol. *J Rheumatol* 1992;19:977–979.
256. Lindqvist T. Lupus erythematosus disseminatus after administration of mesantoin. Report of two cases. *Acta Med Scand* 1957;158:131–138.
257. Tan EM, Kunkel HG. Characteristics of a soluble nuclear antigen precipitating with sera of patients with systemic lupus erythematosus. *J Immunol* 1966;96:464–471.
258. Wallace DJ, Dubois EL. Drugs that exacerbate and induce systemic lupus erythematosus. In: Wallace DJ, Dubois EL, eds. *Dubois' lupus erythematosus*, 3rd ed. Philadelphia: Lea & Febiger, 1987:450–469.
259. Hughes GRV, Rynes RI, Gharavi A, et al. The heterogeneity of serologic findings and predisposing host factors in drug-induced lupus erythematosus. *Arthritis Rheum* 1981;24:1070–1073.
260. Tarzy BJ, Wallach EE, Garcia C-R, et al. Rheumatic disease, abnormal serology, and oral contraceptives. *Lancet* 1972;2: 501–503.
261. Rubin RL. Autoimmune reactions induced by procainamide and hydralazine. In: Kammuller M, Bloksma M, Seimen W, eds. *Autoimmunity and toxicology: immune disregulation induced by drugs and chemicals*. Amsterdam: Elsevier, 1989:119–150.
262. Winfield JB, Koffler D, Kunkel HG. Development of antibodies to ribonucleoprotein following short-term therapy with procainamide. *Arthritis Rheum* 1975;18:531–534.
263. Kosowsky BD, Taylor J, Lown B, et al. Long-term use of procainamide following acute myocardial infarction. *Circulation* 1973;47:1204–1210.
264. Cody RJ, Calabrese LH, Clough JD, et al. Development of antinuclear antibodies during acebutolol therapy. *Clin Pharmacol Ther* 1979;25:800–805.
265. Prockop LD. Myotonia, procaine amide, and lupus-like syndrome. *Arch Neurol* 1966;14:326–330.
266. Mehta BR. Lupus-like syndrome after procainamide. *Hawaii Med J* 1968;28:120–121.
267. Slonim NB. Arthralgia, headache, prostration, and fever during hydralazine therapy. *JAMA* 1954;154:1419.
268. Reinhardt DJ, Waldron JM. Lupus erythematosus-like syndrome complicating hydralazine (apresoline) therapy. *JAMA* 1954;155:1491–1492.
269. Masel MA. A lupus-like reaction to antituberculosis drugs. *Med J Aust* 1967;2:738–740.
270. Pohl LR, Satoh H, Christ DD, et al. The immunologic and metabolic basis of drug hypersensitivities. *Annu Rev Pharmacol* 1988;28:367–387.
271. Hoffman BJ. Sensitivity to sulfadiazine resembling acute disseminated lupus erythematosus. *Arch Dermatol Syph* 1945;51: 190–192.
272. Honey M. Systemic lupus erythematosus presenting with sulphonamide hypersensitivity reaction. *Br Med J* 1956;1: 1272–1275.
273. Petri M, Allbritton J. Antibiotic allergy in systemic lupus erythematosus. *J Rheumatol* 1992;19:265–269.
274. Wang C-R, Chuang C-Y, Chen C-Y. Drug allergy in Chinese patients with systemic lupus erythematosus. *J Rheumatol* 1993; 20:399–400.
275. Wallace DJ, Hahn BH. Adjunctive measures and issues: allergies, antibiotics, vaccines, hormones and osteoporosis. In: Wallace DJ, Hahn BH, eds. *Dubois' lupus erythematosus*, 5th ed. Baltimore: Williams & Wilkins, 1997:1203–1212.
276. Mysler E, Paget SA, Kimberly R. Ciprofloxacin reactions mimicking lupus flares. *Arthritis Rheum* 1994;37:1112–1113.
277. Cohen P, Gardner BH. Sulfonamide reactions in systemic lupus erythematosus. *JAMA* 1966;197:163–165.
278. Gold S. Role of sulphonamides and penicillin in the pathogenesis of systemic lupus erythematosus. *Lancet* 1951;1(260):268–272.
279. Domz CA, McNamara DH, Holzapfel HF. Tetracycline provocation in lupus erythematosus. *Ann Intern Med* 1959;50: 1217–1226.
280. Alexander S. Lupus erythematosus in two patients after griseofulvin treatment of *Trichophyton rubrum* infection. *Br J Dermatol* 1962;74:72–74.
281. Anderson WA, Torre D. Griseofulvin and lupus erythematosus. *J Med Soc NJ* 1982;63:161–162.
282. Watsky MS, Lynfield YL. Lupus erythematosus exacerbated by griseofulvin. *Cutis* 1976;17:361–363.
283. Bigby M, Stern R. Cutaneous reactions to nonsteroidal anti-inflammatory drugs. A review. *J Am Acad Dermatol* 1985;5: 866–876.
284. Smythe HAe. Prostaglandins and benoxaprofen (editorial). Proceedings of the International Symposium on Benoxaprofen. *J Rheumatol* 1980;6(suppl 1):1–3.
285. Toll A, Campo-Pisa P, Gonzalez-Castro J, et al. Subacute cutaneous lupus erythematosus associated with cinnarizine and thiethylperazine therapy. *Lupus* 1998;7:364–366.
286. Sontheimer RD, Provost TT. Cutaneous manifestations of lupus erythematosus. In: Wallace DJ, Hahn BH eds. *Dubois' lupus erythematosus*, 5th ed. Baltimore: Williams & Wilkins, 1997:569–623.
287. Widener HL, Littman BH. Ibuprofen induced meningitis in systemic lupus erythematosus. *JAMA* 1978;239:1062–1064.
288. Ballas ZK, Donta ST. Sulindac-induced aseptic meningitis. *Arch Intern Med* 1982;142:165–166.
289. Ruppert GB, Barth WF. Tolmetin-induced aseptic meningitis. *JAMA* 1981;245:67–68.

290. Codding C, Targoff IN, McCarty GA. Aseptic meningitis in association with diclofenac treatment in a patient with systemic lupus erythematosus. *Arthritis Rheum* 1991;34:1340–1341.
291. Rallison ML, O'Brien J, Good RA. Severe reactions to long-acting sulfonamides. Erythema multiforme exudativum and lupus erythematosus following administration of sulfamethoxypyridazine and sulfadimethoxine. *Pediatrics* 1961;28:908–917.
292. Griem P, Wulferink M, Sachs B, et al. Allergic and autoimmune reactions to xenobiotics: how do they arise? *Immunol Today* 1998;19:133–141.
293. Simpson DG, Walker JH. Hypersensitivity to para-aminosalicylic acid. *Am J Med* 1960;29:297–306.
294. Davidson BL, Gilliam JN, Lipsky PE. Cimetidine-associated exacerbation of cutaneous lupus erythematosus. *Arch Intern Med* 1982;142:166–167.
295. Farid N, Anderson J. S.L.E.-like reaction after phenylbutazone (letter). *Lancet* 1971;1:1022–1023.
296. Sonnenblick M, Abraham AS. Ibuprofen hypersensitivity in systemic lupus erythematosus. *Br Med J* 1978;1:619–620.
297. Kay DR, Bole GG Jr, Ledger WJ. Antinuclear antibodies, rheumatoid factor and C-reactive protein in serum of normal women using oral contraceptives. *Arthritis Rheum* 1971;14: 239–248.
298. Bole GG Jr, Friedlaender MH, Smith CK. Rheumatic symptoms and serological abnormalities induced by oral contraceptives. *Lancet* 1969;1:323–326.
299. Travers RL, Hughes GR. Oral contraceptive therapy and systemic lupus erythematosus. *J Rheumatol* 1978;5:448–451.
300. Lockie LM, Smith DM. Forty-seven years experience with gold therapy in 1,019 rheumatoid arthritis patients. *Semin Arthritis Rheum* 1985;14:238–246.
301. Romagnoli P, Spinas GA, Sinigaglia F. Gold-specific T cells in rheumatoid arthritis patients treated with gold. *J Clin Invest* 1992;89:254–258.
302. Wallace DJ. The clinical presentation of systemic lupus erythematosus. In: Wallace DJ, Hahn BH eds. *Dubois' lupus erythematosus*, 4th ed. Philadelphia: Lea & Febiger, 1993:317–321.
303. Petz LD. Autoimmune and drug-induced immune hemolytic anemia. In: Rose NR, de Macario EC, Fahey JL, et al., eds. *Manual of clinical laboratory immunology*, 4th ed. Washington, DC: American Society for Microbiology, 1992:325–343.
304. Hodge JV, Casey TP. Methyldopa and the direct antiglobulin (Coombs') test. *N Z Med J* 1968;68:240–246.
305. Hess EV, Mongey A-B. Drug-related lupus: the same as or different from idiopathic disease? In: Lahita RG, ed. *Systemic lupus erythematosus*, 2nd ed. New York: Churchill Livingstone, 1993:893–904.
306. Lee SL, Rivero I, Siegel M. Activation of systemic lupus erythematosus by drugs. *Arch Intern Med* 1966;117:620–626.
307. Fries JF, Holman HR. *Systemic lupus erythematosus: a clinical analysis. Major problems in internal medicine*, 6th ed. Philadelphia: WB Saunders, 1975.
308. Choi HK, Merkel PA, Walker AM, et al. Drug-associated antineutrophil cytoplasmic antibody-positive vasculitis: prevalence among patients with high titers of antimyeloperoxidase antibodies. *Arthritis Rheum* 2000;43:405–413.
309. Weinstein A. Drug-induced lupus erythematosus. *Prog Clin Immunol* 1980;4:1–21.
310. Harmon CE, Portanova JP. Drug-induced lupus: clinical and serological studies. *Clin Rheum Dis* 1982;8:121–135.
311. Russell AS. Drug-induced autoimmune disease. *Clin Immunol Allergy* 1981;1:57–76.
312. Hess EV, Mongey A-B. Drug-related lupus. *Bull Rheum Dis* 1991;40:1–8.
313. Burlingame RW, Boey ML, Starkebaum G, et al. The central role of chromatin in autoimmune responses to histones and DNA in systemic lupus erythematosus. *J Clin Invest* 1994;94: 184–192.
314. Suzuki T, Burlingame RW, Casiano CA, et al. Antihistone antibodies in systemic lupus erythematosus: assay dependency and effects of ubiquitination and serum DNA. *J Rheumatol* 1994; 21:1081–1091.
315. Fritzler MJ, Tan EM. Antibodies to histones in drug-induced and idiopathic lupus erythematosus. *J Clin Invest* 1978;62: 560–567.
316. Rubin RL, Reimer G, McNally EM, et al. Procainamide elicits a selective autoantibody immune response. *Clin Exp Immunol* 1986;63:58–67.
317. Vivino FB, Schumacher HRJ. Synovial fluid characteristics and the lupus erythematosus cell phenomenon in drug-induced lupus. *Arthritis Rheum* 1989;32:560–568.
318. Schett G, Rubin RL, Steiner G, et al. The lupus erythematosus cell phenomenon: comparative analysis of antichromatin antibody specificity in lupus erythematosus cell-positive and -negative sera. *Arthritis Rheum* 2000;43:420–428.
319. Kleinman S, Nelson R, Smith L, et al. Positive direct antiglobulin tests and immune hemolytic anemia in patients receiving procainamide. *N Engl J Med* 1984;311:809–812.
320. Fields TR, Zarrabi MH, Gerardi EN, et al. Reticuloendothelial system Fc receptor function in the drug induced lupus erythematosus syndrome. *J Rheumatol* 1986;13:726–731.
321. Mitchell JA, Batchelor JR, Chapel H, et al. Erythrocyte complement receptor type 1 (CR1) expression and circulating immune complex (CIC) levels in hydralazine-induced SLE. *Clin Exp Immunol* 1987;68:446–456.
322. Becker M, Klajman A, Moalem T, et al. Circulating immune complexes in sera from patients receiving procainamide. *Clin Immunol Immunopathol* 1979;12:220–227.
323. Dolman KM, Gans RO, Vervaat TJ, et al. Vasculitis and antineutrophil cytoplasmic autoantibodies associated with propylthiouracil therapy. *Lancet* 1993;342:651–652.
324. Rubin RL, Nusinow SR, Johnson AD, et al. Serological changes during induction of lupus-like disease by procainamide. *Am J Med* 1986;80:999–1002.
325. Brandslund I, Ibsen HHW, Klitgaard NA, et al. Plasma concentrations of complement split product C3d and immune complexes after procainamide induced production of antinuclear antibodies. *Acta Med Scand* 1986;220:431–435.
326. Solinger AM. Drug-related lupus. Clinical and etiological considerations. *Rheum Dis Clin North Am* 1988;14:187–202.
327. Davies P, Bailey PJ, Goldenberg MM. The role of arachidonic acid oxygenation products in pain and inflammation. *Annu Rev Immunol* 1984;2:335–357.
328. Gill KS, Hayne OA, Zayed E. Another case of procainamide-induced pancytopenia (letter). *Am J Hematol* 1989;31:298–298.
329. Shields AF, Berenson JA. Procainamide-associated pancytopenia. *Am J Hematol* 1988;27:299–301.
330. Meyers DG, Gonzalez ER, Peters LL, et al. Severe neutropenia associated with procainamide: comparison of sustained release and conventional preparations. *Am Heart J* 1985;109: 1393–1395.
331. Starkebaum G, Kenyon CM, Simrell CG, et al. Procainamide-induced agranulocytosis differs serologically and clinically from procainamide-induced lupus. *Clin Immunol Immunopathol* 1996;78:112–119.
332. Ramsey-Goldman R, Franz T, Solano FX, et al. Hyralazine induced lupus and Sweet's syndrome. Report and review of the literature. *J Rheumatol* 1990;17:682–684.
333. Epstein A, Barland P. The diagnostic value of antihistone antibodies in drug-induced lupus erythematosus. *Arthritis Rheum* 1985;28:158–162.
334. Rubin RL, Joslin FJ, Tan EM. A solid-phase radioimmunoassay

for antihistone antibodies in human sera: comparison with an immunofluorescence assay. *Scand J Immunol* 1982;15:63–70.
335. Rubin RL. Antihistone antibodies. In: Lahita RG, ed. *Systemic lupus erythematosus*, 2nd ed. New York: Churchill Livingstone, 1992:247–271.
336. Rubin RL. Drug-induced lupus. In: Wallace DJ, Hahn BH, eds. *Dubois' lupus erythematosus*, 5th ed. Baltimore: Williams & Wilkins, 1997:871–901.
337. Gussin HA, Tselentis HN, Teodorescu M. Non-cognate binding to histones of IgG from patients with idiopathic systemic lupus erythematosus. *Clin Immunol* 2000;96:150–161.
338. Arents G, Moudrianakis EN. Topography of the histone octamer surface: repeating structural motifs utilized in the docking of nucleosomal DNA. *Proc Natl Acad Sci USA* 1993; 90:10489–10493.
339. Luger K, Mader AW, Richmond RK, et al. Crystal structure of the nucleosome core particle at 2.8 A resolution. *Nature* 1997; 389:251–260.
340. Rubin RL, Joslin FG, Tan EM. Specificity of antihistone antibodies in systemic lupus erythematosus. *Arthritis Rheum* 1982; 25:779–782.
341. Portanova JP, Arndt RE, Tan EM, et al. Antihistone antibodies in idiopathic and drug-induced lupus recognize distinct intrahistone regions. *J Immunol* 1987;138:446–451.
342. Lau CC, Du Clos TW. Anti-[(H2A/2B)-DNA] IgG supports the diagnosis of procainamide-induced arthritis or pleuritis. *Arthritis Rheum* 1999;42:1300–1301.
343. Adams LE, Balakrishnan K, Roberts SM, et al. Genetic, immunologic and biotransformation studies of patients on procainamide. *Lupus* 1993;2:89–98.
344. Klajman A, Farkas R, Gold E, et al. Procainamide-induced antibodies to nucleoprotein, denatured and native DNA in human subjects. *Clin Immunol Immunopathol* 1975;3:525–530.
345. Koffler D, Carr RI, Agnello V, et al. Antibodies to polynucleotides in human sera: antigenic specificity and relation to disease. *J Exp Med* 1971;134:294–312.
346. Weisbart RH, Yee WS, Colburn KK, et al. Antiguanosine antibodies: a new marker for procainamide-induced systemic lupus erythematosus. *Ann Intern Med* 1986;104:310–313.
347. Lafer EM, Rauch J, Andrzejewski C Jr, et al. Polyspecific monoclonal lupus autoantibodies reactive with both polynucleotides and phospholipids. *J Exp Med* 1981;153:897–909.
348. Thomas TJ, Seibold JR, Adams LE, et al. Hydralazine induces Z-DNA conformation in a polynucleotide and elicits anti(Z-DNA) antibodies in treated patients. *Biochem J* 1993;294:419–425.
349. Bluestein HG, Zvaifler NJ, Weisman MH, et al. Lymphocyte alteration by procainamide: relation to drug-induced lupus erythematosus syndrome. *Lancet* 1979;2:816–819.
350. Bluestein HG, Redelman D, Zvaifler NJ. Procainamide lymphocyte reactions: a possible explanation for drug-induced autoimmunity. *Arthritis Rheum* 1981;24:1019–1023.
351. Bennett RM, Davis J, Campbell S, et al. Lactoferrin binds to cell membrane DNA. *J Clin Invest* 1983;71:611–618.
352. Shoenfeld Y, Vilner Y, Reshef T, et al. Increased presence of common systemic lupus erythematosus (SLE) anti-DNA idiotypes (16/6 Id, 32/15 Id) is induced by procainamide. *J Clin Immunol* 1987;7:410–419.
353. Tan EM. Antinuclear antibodies: diagnostic markers for autoimmune diseases and probes for cell biology. *Adv Immunol* 1989;44:93–151.
354. Russell AS, Ziff M. Natural antibodies to procainamide. *Clin Exp Immunol* 1968;3:901–909.
355. Adams LE, Roberts SM, Donovan-Brand R, et al. Study of procainamide hapten-specific antibodies in rabbits and humans. Int *J Immunopharmacol* 1993;15:887–897.
356. McDuffie FC. Relationship between immune response to hydralazine and to deoxyribonucleoprotein in patients receiving hydralazine. *Arthritis Rheum* 1981;24:1079–1081.
357. Mongey AB, Hess EV. Drug-related lupus. *Curr Opin Rheumatol* 1989;1:353–359.
358. Anderson B, Stillman MT. False-positive FTA-ABS in hydralazine induced lupus. *JAMA* 1978;239:1392–1393.
359. Asherson RA, Zulman J, Hughes GRV. Pulmonary thromboembolism associated with procainamide-induced lupus syndrome and anticardiolipin antibodies. *Ann Rheum Dis* 1989;48: 232–235.
360. Chokron R, Robert A, Rozensztajn L. Procainamide-induced lupus with circulating anticoagulant (letter). *Nouv Presse Med* 1982;11:2568–2568.
361. Davis S, Furie BC, Griffin JH, et al. Circulating inhibitors of blood coagulation associated with procainamide-induced lupus erythematosus. *Am J Hematol* 1978;4:401–407.
362. Edwards RL, Rick ME, Wakem CJ. Studies on a circulating anticoagulant in procainamide-induced lupus erythematosus. *Arch Intern Med* 1981;141:1688–1690.
363. Triplett DA, Brandt JT, Musgrave KA, et al. The relationship between lupus anticoagulants and antibodies to phospholipid. *JAMA* 1988;259:550–554.
364. Derksen RHMW, Kater L. Lupus anticoagulant: revival of an old phenomenon. *Clin Exp Rheumatol* 1991;3:349–357.
365. McNeil HP, Chesterman CN, Krilis SA. Immunology and clinical importance of antiphospholipid antibodies. *Adv Immunol* 1991;49:193–280.
366. Drouvalakis KA, Buchanan RR. Phospholipid specificity of autoimmune and drug induced lupus anticoagulants; association of phosphatidylethanolamine reactivity with thrombosis in autoimmune disease. *J Rheumatol* 1998;25:290–295.
367. Gastineau DA, Holcomb GR. Lupus anticoagulant in drug-induced systemic lupus erythematosus (SLE). *Arch Intern Med* 1985;145:1926–1927.
368. Kaburaki J, Kuwana M, Yamamoto M, et al. Disease distribution of beta-2 glycoprotein I-dependent anticardiolipin antibodies in rheumatic diseases. *Lupus* 1995;4(suppl 1):S27–S31.
369. Butikofer P, Lin ZW, Kuypers FA, et al. Chlorpromazine inhibits vesiculation, alters phosphoinositide turnover and changes deformability of ATP-depleted RBC's. *Blood* 1989;73: 1699–1704.
370. Mori T, Takai Y, Minakuchi R, et al. Inhibitory action of chlorpromazine, dibucaine and other phospholipid-interacting drugs on calcium-activated phospholipid dependent protein kinase. *J Biol Chem* 1980;255:8378–8380.
371. Hobbs RN, Clayton A-L, Bernstein RM. Antibodies to the five histones and poly(adenosine diphosphate-ribose) in drug induced lupus: implications for pathogenesis. *Ann Rheum Dis* 1987;46:408–416.
372. Torffvit O, Thysell H, Nassberger L. Occurrence of autoantibodies directed against myeloperoxidase and elastase in patients treated with hydralazine and presenting with glomerulonephritis. *Hum Exp Toxicol* 1994;13:563–567.
373. Cambridge G, Wallace H, Bernstein RM, et al. Autoantibodies to myeloperoxidase in idiopathic and drug-induced systemic lupus erythematosus and vasculitis. *Br J Rheumatol* 1994;33: 109–114.
374. Jennette JC, Wilkman AS, Falk RJ. Anti-neutrophil cytoplasmic autoantibody-associated glomerulonephritis and vasculitis. *Am J Pathol* 1989;135:921–930.
375. Ayer LM, Rubin RL, Dixon GH, et al. Antibodies from patients with drug-induced autoimmunity react with high mobility group (HMG) proteins. *Arthritis Rheum* 1994;37:98–103.
376. Forrester J, Golbus J, Brede D, et al. B cell activation in patients with active procainamide induced lupus. *J Rheumatol* 1988;15: 1384–1388.

377. Yu CL, Ziff M. Effects of long-term procainamide therapy on immunoglobulin synthesis. *Arthritis Rheum* 1985;28:276–284.
378. Miller KB, Salem D. Immune regulatory abnormalities produced by procainamide. *Am J Med* 1982;73:487–492.
379. Green BJ, Wyse DG, Duff HJ, et al. Procainamide in vivo modulates suppressor T cell activity. *Clin Invest Med* 1988;11: 425–429.
380. Ochi T, Goldings EA, Lipsky PE, et al. Immunomodulatory effect of procainamide in man. *J Clin Invest* 1983;71:36–45.
381. Adams LE, Sanders CE Jr, Budinsky RA, et al. Immunomodulatory effects of procainamide metabolites: their implications in drug-related lupus. *J Lab Clin Med* 1989;113:482–492.
382. Tannen RH, Cunningham-Rundles S. Inhibition of Con A mitogenesis by serum from procainamide-treated patients and patients with systemic lupus erythematosus. *Immunol Commun* 1982;11:33–45.
383. Tan EM, Cohen AS, Fries JF, et al. The 1982 revised criteria for the classification of systemic lupus erythematosus. *Arthritis Rheum* 1982;25(11):1271–1277.
384. Cattogio LJ, Skinner RP, Smith G, et al. Systemic lupus erythematosus in the elderly: clinical and serological characteristics. *J Rheumatol* 1984;11:175–181.
385. Ward MM, Polisson RP. A meta-analysis of the clinical manifestations of older-onset systemic lupus erythematosus. *Arthritis Rheum* 1989;32:1226–1232.
386. Spears CJ, Batchelor JR. Drug-induced autoimmune disease. *Adv Nephrol* 1987;16:219–230.
387. Batchelor JR. Autoantibodies and HLA-DR phenotype in hydralazine induced lupus. *Anonymous Proceedings of the Second International Conference on Systemic Lupus Erythematosus*, 26th-30th November, Singapore, Professional Postgraduate Services, International, 1989:166–168.
388. Vargas-Alarcon G, Yamamoto-Furusho JK, Zuniga J, et al. HLA-DR7 in association with chlorpromazine-induced lupus anticoagulant (LA). *J Autoimmun* 1997;10:579–583.
389. Howard PF, Hochberg MC, Bias WB, et al. Relationship between C4 null genes, HLA-D region antigens, and genetic susceptibility in systemic lupus erythematosus in Caucasian and black Americans. *Am J Med* 1986;81:187–193.
390. Utsinger PD, Zvaifler NJ, Bluestein HG. Hypocomplementemia in procainamide-associated systemic lupus erythematosus. *Ann Intern Med* 1976;84:293.
391. Mitchell JA, Sim RB, Sim E. CR1 polymorphism in hydralazine-induced systemic lupus erythematosus: DNA restriction fragment length polymorphism. *Clin Exp Immunol* 1989;78:354–358.
392. Stec GP, Lertora JJL, Atkinson AJ Jr, et al. Remission of procainamide-induced lupus erythematosus with N-acetylprocainamide therapy. *Ann Intern Med* 1979;90:799–801.
393. Roden DM, Reele SB, Higgins SB, et al. Antiarrhythmic efficacy, pharmacokinetics and safety of N-acetylprocainamide in human subjects: comparison with procainamide. *Am J Cardiol* 1980;46:463–468.
394. Baer AN, Woosley RL, Pincus T. Further evidence for the lack of association between acetylator phenotype and systemic lupus erythematosus. *Arthritis Rheum* 1986;29:508–514.
395. Uetrecht JP, Sweetman BJ, Woosley RL, et al. Metabolism of procainamide to a hydroxylamine by rat and human hepatic microsomes. *Drug Metab Dispos* 1984;12:77–81.
396. Budinsky RA, Roberts SM, Coates EA, et al. The formation of hydroxylamine by rat and human liver microsomes. *Drug Metab Dispos* 1987;15:37–43.
397. Roberts SM, Adams LE, Donovan-Brand R, et al. Procainamide hydroxylamine lymphocyte toxicity—1. Evidence for participation by hemoglobin. *Int J Immunopharmacol* 1989;11:419–427.
398. Streeter AJ, Timbrell JA. Enzyme-mediated covalent binding of hydralazine to rat liver microsomes. *Drug Metab Dispos* 1983; 11:179–183.
399. Hein DW, Weber WW. Metabolism of procainamide, hydralazine, and isoniazid in relation to autoimmune(-like) reactions. In: Kammueller ME, Bloksma N, Seinen W, eds. *Autoimmunity and toxicology: immune disregulation induced by drugs and chemicals*. Amsterdam: Elsevier Science, 1989: 239–265.
400. Uetrecht JP. Reactivity and possible significance of hydroxylamine and nitroso metabolites of procainamide. *J Pharmacol Exp Ther* 1985;232:420–425.
401. Rubin RL, Uetrecht JP, Jones JE. Cytotoxicity of oxidative metabolites of procainamide. *J Pharmacol Exp Ther* 1987;242: 833–841.
402. Magner-Wröbel K, Toborek M, Drözdz M, et al. Increase in antioxidant activity in procainamide-treated rats. *Pharmacol Toxicol* 1993;72:94–97.
403. Rubin RL, Uetrecht JP, Jones JE. Metabolism of procainamide to the reactive hydroxylamine by leukocytes. *Fed Proc* 1987;46: 1380(abst).
404. Uetrecht JP, Zahid N, Rubin RL. Metabolism of procainamide to a hydroxylamine by human neutrophils and mononuclear leukocytes. *Chem Res Toxicol* 1988;1:74–78.
405. Rubin RL, Curnutte JT. Metabolism of procainamide to the cytotoxic hydroxylamine by neutrophils activated in vitro. *J Clin Invest* 1989;83:1336–1343.
406. Uetrecht J, Zahid N. N-chlorination of phenytoin by myeloperoxidase to a reactive metabolite. *Chem Res Toxicol* 1988;1: 148–151.
407. Uetrecht J, Zahid N, Shear NH, et al. Metabolism of dapsone to a hydroxylamine by human neutrophils and mononuclear cells. *J Pharmacol Exp Ther* 1988;245:274–279.
408. Van Zyl JM, Basson K, Uebel RA, et al. Isoniazid-mediated irreversible inhibition of the myeloperoxidase antimicrobial system of the human neutrophil and the effect of thyronines. *Biochem Pharmacol* 1989;38:2363–2373.
409. Mahlis E, Christophidis N. Modulation of the iodination reaction in normal human neutrophils and in whole blood by penicillamine, congeners and intracellular enzyme catalase and superoxide dismutase. *Clin Exp Rheumatol* 1989;7:365–371.
410. Van Zyl JM, Basson K, Kriegler A, et al. Activation of chlorpromazine by the myeloperoxidase system of the human neutrophil. *Biochem Pharmacol* 1990;40:947–954.
411. Lee E, Miki Y, Katsura H, et al. Mechanism of inactivation of myeloperoxidase by propylthiouracil. *Biochem Pharmacol* 1990; 39:1467–1471.
412. Waldhauser L, Uetrecht J. Oxidation of propylthiouracil to reactive metabolites by activated neutrophils. Implications for agranulocytosis. *Drug Metab Dispos* 1991;19:354–359.
413. Hofstra AH, Matassa LC, Uetrecht JP. Metabolism of hydralazine by activated leukocytes: implications for hydralazine induced lupus. *J Rheumatol* 1991;18:1673–1680.
414. Kelder PP, De Moal NJ, 't Hart BA, et al. Metabolic activation of chlorpromazine by stimulated human polymorphonuclear leukocytes. Induction of covalent binding of chlorpromazine to nucleic acids and proteins. *Chem Biol Interact* 1991;79:15–30.
415. Hofstra AH, Li-Muller SMA, Uetrecht JP. Metabolism of isoniazid by activated leukocytes. Possible role in drug-induced lupus. *Drug Metab Dispos* 1992;20:205–210.
416. Jiang X, Khursigara G, Rubin RL. Transformation of lupus-inducing drugs to cytotoxic products by activated neutrophils. *Science* 1994;266:810–813.
417. Furst SM, Sukhai P, McClelland RA, et al. Covalent binding of carbamazepine oxidative metabolites to neutrophils. *Drug Metab Dispos* 1995;23:590–594.
418. Wheeler JF, Lunte CE, Heineman WR, et al. Rapid communi-

cations: electrochemical determination of N-oxidized procainamide metabolites and functional assessment of effects on murine cells in vitro. *Proc Soc Exp Biol Med* 1988;188:381–386.
419. Wheeler JF, Adams LE, Mongey A-B, et al. Determination of metabolically derived nitroprocainamide in the urine of procainamide-dosed humans and rats by liquid chromatography with electrochemical detection. *Drug Metab Dispos* 1991;19: 691–695.
420. Timbrell JA, Facchini V, Harland SJ, et al. Hydralazine-induced lupus: is there a toxic metabolic pathway? *Eur J Clin Pharmacol* 1984;27:555–559.
421. Kubicka-Muranyi M, Goebels R, Goebel C, et al. T lymphocytes ignore procainamide, but respond to its reactive metabolites in peritoneal cells: demonstration by the adoptive transfer popliteal lymph node assay. *Toxicol Appl Pharmacol* 1993;122 (1):88–94.
422. Schuhmann D, Kubicka-Muranyi M, Mirtschewa J, et al. Adverse immune reactions to gold. I. Chronic treatment with an Au(I) drug sensitizes mouse spleen cells not to Au(I), but to Au(III) and induces autoantibody formation. *J Immunol* 1990; 145:2132–2139.
423. Goebel C, Kubicka-Muranyi M, Tonn T, et al. Phagocytes render chemicals immunogenic: oxidation of gold(I) to the T cell-sensitizing gold(III) metabolite generated by mononuclear phagocytes. *Arch Toxicol* 1995;69:450–459.
424. Rubin RL, Tang F-L, Chan EKL, et al. IgG subclasses of autoantibodies in systemic lupus erythematosus, Sjogren's syndrome, and drug-induced autoimmunity. *J Immunol* 1986;137: 2528–2534.
425. Fritzler M, Ryan P, Kinsella TD. Clinical features of systemic lupus erythematosus patients with antihistone antibodies. *J Rheumatol* 1982;9(1):46–51.
426. Klajman A, Farkas R, Ben-Efraim S. Complement-fixing activity of antinuclear antibodies induced by procainamide treatment. *Isr J Med Sci* 1973;9:627–630.
427. Kanayama Y, Peebles C, Tan EM, et al. Complement activating abilities of defined antinuclear antibodies. *Arthritis Rheum* 1986;29:748–754.
428. Sim E, Law S-K. Hydralazine binds covalently to complement component C4. Different reactivity of C4A and C4B gene products. *FEBS Lett* 1985;184:323–327.
429. Sim E. Drug-induced immune complex disease. *Biochem Soc Trans* 1991;19:164–170.
430. Sim E, Stanley L, Gill EW, et al. Metabolites of procainamide and practolol inhibit complement components C3 and C4. *Biochem J* 1988;251:323–326.
431. Roberts SM, Budinsky RA, Adams LE, et al. Procainamide acetylation in strains of rat and mouse. *Drug Metab Dispos* 1985;13:517–519.
432. Freireich EJ, Gehan EA, Rall DP, et al. Quantitative comparison of toxicity of anticancer agents in mouse, rat, hamster, dog, monkey and man. *Cancer Chemother Rep* 1966;50:219–244.
433. Rubin RL, Aucoin DP. Murine model for procainamide-induced autoimmunity. *Arthritis Rheum* 1988;31:S39(abst).
434. Mark LC, Kayden HJ, Steele JM, et al. The physiological disposition and cardiac effects of procainamide. *J Pharmacol Exp Ther* 1951;102:5–15.
435. Cannat A, Seligmann M. Induction by isoniazid and hydralazine of antinuclear factors in mice. *Clin Exp Immunol* 1968;3:99–105.
436. Ten Veen JH, Feltkamp TEW. Studies on drug induced lupus erythematosus in mice. I. Drug induced antinuclear antibodies (ANA). *Clin Exp Immunol* 1972;11:265–276.
437. Ten Veen JH. Studies on drug-induced lupus erythematosus in mice. II. Drug-induced smooth muscle and skeletal muscle antibodies. *Clin Exp Immunol* 1973;15:375–384.
438. Weber WW, Tannen RH. Pharmacogenetic studies on the drug-related lupus syndrome. Differences in antinuclear antibody development and drug-induced DNA damage in rapid and slow acetylator animal models. *Arthritis Rheum* 1981;24:979–986.
439. Tannen RH, Weber WW. Antinuclear antibodies related to acetylator phenotype in mice. *J Pharmacol Exp Ther* 1980;213: 485–490.
440. Whittingham S, Mackay IR, Whitworth JA, et al. Antinuclear antibody response to procainamide in man and laboratory animals. *Am Heart J* 1972;84:228–234.
441. Monestier M, Novick KE, Losman MJ. D-penicillamine- and quinidine-induced antinuclear antibodies in A.SW (H-2S) mice: similarities with autoantibodies in spontaneous and heavy metal-induced autoimmunity. *Eur J Immunol* 1994;24:723–730.
442. Bell SA, Hobbs MV, Rubin RL. Isotype-restricted hyperimmunity in a murine model of the toxic oil syndrome. *J Immunol* 1992;148(11):3369–3376.
443. Aucoin DP, Peterson ME, Hurvitz AI, et al. Propylthiouracil-induced immune-mediated disease in the cat. *J Pharmacol Exp Ther* 1985;234:13–18.
444. Aucoin DP, Rubin RL, Peterson ME, et al. Dose dependent induction of anti-native DNA antibodies by propylthiouracil in cats. *Arthritis Rheum* 1988;31:688–692.
445. Quddus J, Johnson KJ, Gavalchin J, et al. Treating activated CD4+ T cells with either of two distinct DNA methyltransferase inhibitors, 5-azacytidine or procainamide, is sufficient to induce a lupus-like disease in syngeneic mice. *J Clin Invest* 1993;92:38–52.
446. Yung RL, Quddus J, Chrisp CE, et al. Mechanisms of drug-induced lupus. I. Cloned Th2 cells modified with DNA methylation inhibitors in vitro cause autoimmunity in vivo. *J Immunol* 1995;154:3025–3035.
447. Yung R, Chang S, Hemati N, et al. Mechanisms of drug-induced lupus. IV. Comparison of procainamide and hydralazine with analogs in vitro and in vivo. *Arthritis Rheum* 1997;40:1436–1443.
448. Yung R, Powers D, Johnson K, et al. Mechanisms of drug-induced lupus. II. T cells overexpressing lymphocyte function-associated antigen 1 become autoreactive and cause a lupuslike disease in syngeneic mice. *J Clin Invest* 1996;97:2866–2871.
449. Kammüller ME, Thomas C, De Bakker JM, et al. The popliteal lymph node assay in mice to screen for the immune disregulation potential of chemicals—a preliminary study. *Int J Immunopharmacol* 1989;11:293–300.
450. Katsutani N, Shionoya H. Popliteal lymph node enlargement induced by procainamide. *Int J Immunopharmacol* 1992;14: 681–686.
451. Kretz-Rommel A, Duncan SR, Rubin RL. Autoimmunity caused by disruption of central T cell tolerance: a murine model of drug-induced lupus. *J Clin Invest* 1997;99:1888–1896.
452. Kretz-Rommel A, Rubin RL. Persistence of autoreactive T cell drive in required to elicit anti-chromatin antibodies in a murine model of drug-induced lupus. *J Immunol* 1999;162:813–820.
453. Goebel C, Vogel C, Wulferink M, et al. Procainamide, a drug causing lupus, induces prostaglandin H synthase-2 and formation of T cell-sensitizing drug metabolites in mouse macrophages. *Chem Res Toxicol* 1999;12:488–500.
454. von Greyerz S, Burkhart C, Pichler WJ. Molecular basis of drug recognition by specific T-cell receptors. *Intern Arch Allergy Immunol* 2000;119:173–180.
455. Adams LE, Roberts SM, Carter JM, et al. Effects of procainamide hydroxylamine on generation of reactive oxygen species by macrophages and production of cytokines. *Int J Immunopharmacol* 1990;12:809–819.
456. Hess DA, Sisson ME, Suria H, et al. Cytotoxicity of sulfonamide reactive metabolites: apoptosis and selective toxicity of

CD8(+) cells by the hydroxylamine of sulfamethoxazole. *FASEB J* 1999;13:1688–1698.

457. Williams DP, Pirmohamed M, Naisbitt DJ, et al. Induction of metabolism-dependent and -independent neutrophil apoptosis by clozapine. *Mol Pharmacol* 2000;58:207–216.
458. Tschen AC, Rieder MJ, Oyewumi LK, et al. The cytotoxicity of clozapine metabolites: implications for predicting clozapine-induced agranulocytosis. *Clin Pharmacol Ther* 1999;65:526–532.
459. Gardner I, Leeder JS, Chin T, et al. A comparison of the covalent binding of clozapine and olanzapine to human neutrophils in vitro and in vivo. *Mol Pharmacol* 1998;53:999–1008.
460. Williams DP, Pirmohamed M, Naisbitt DJ, et al. Neutrophil cytotoxicity of the chemically reactive metabolite(s) of clozapine: possible role in agranulocytosis. *J Pharmacol Exp Ther* 1997;283:1375–1382.
461. Ayer LM, Edworthy SM, Fritzler MJ. Effect of procainamide and hydralazine on poly (ADP-ribosylation) in cell lines. *Lupus* 1993;2:167–172.
462. Richardson BC, Liebling MR, Hudson JL. CD4+ cells treated with DNA methylation inhibitors induce autologous B cell differentiation. *Clin Immunol Immunopathol* 1990;55:368–381.
463. Richardson B, Powers D, Hooper F, et al. Lymphocyte function-associated antigen 1 overexpression and T cell autoreactivity. *Arthritis Rheum* 1994;9:1363–1372.
464. Cornacchia E, Golbus J, Maybaum J, et al. Hydralazine and procainamide inhibit T cell DNA methylation and induce autoreactivity. *J Immunol* 1988;140:2197–2200.
465. Richardson B, Cornacchia E, Golbus J, et al. N-acetylprocainamide is a less potent inducer of T cell autoreactivity than procainamide. *Arthritis Rheum* 1988;31:995–999.
466. Scheinbart LS, Johnson MA, Gross LA, et al. Procainamide inhibits DNA methyltransferase in a human T cell line. *J Rheumatol* 1991;18:530–534.
467. Gleichmann E, Pals ST, Rolink AG, et al. Graft-versus-host reactions: cues to the etiopathology of a spectrum of immunological diseases. *Immunol Today* 1984;5:324–332.
468. Douek DC, McFarland RD, Keiser PH, et al. Changes in thymic function with age and during the treatment of HIV infection. *Nature* 1998;396:690–695.
469. Kretz-Rommel A, Rubin RL. A metabolite of the lupus-inducing drug procainamide prevents anergy induction in T cell clones. *J Immunol* 1997;158:4465–4470.
470. Kretz-Rommel A, Rubin RL. Disruption of positive selection of thymocytes causes autoimmunity. *Nat Med* 2000;6:298–305.

43

INFECTIONS IN SYSTEMIC LUPUS ERYTHEMATOSUS

ELLEN M. GINZLER

Infection is a major source of morbidity and mortality in patients with systemic lupus erythematosus (SLE). The literature includes anecdotal reports of sepsis from common and unusual organisms as well as compilations of infections in both small and large series. Although the most frequent infections continue to be attributed to pyogenic organisms such as *Staphylococcus* sp. and *Escherichia coli*, opportunistic pathogens such as uncommon bacteria, deep-seated fungal organisms, viruses, and protozoans have been well described, including infection at multiple sites and multiple organisms at a single site. Features of SLE itself, including many forms of immunologic dysfunction, appear to play a role in an increased susceptibility to infection, which may be further affected by treatment modalities such as corticosteroids and other immunosuppressive agents. At times, the actions of microbial agents on the host are difficult to differentiate from those of a lupus flare and, by themselves, may aggravate the disease. This chapter reviews infections in SLE, discusses differential diagnosis, and describes the infectious agents that most frequently are found in these patients.

SLE MORTALITY FROM INFECTION

In 1987, Hellmann et al. (1) reviewed mortality studies from a 40-year period. Among the 3,175 patients included in their report, there were 641 deaths, 170 (27%) of which resulted from infection. A fairly constant death rate caused by infection has persisted since the preantibiotic era of the 1930s to 1940s, when Klemperer et al. (2) attributed 40% of the deaths in their patients with SLE to infection, generally with pyogenic organisms. Even with advances in treatment of the underlying disease, a large U.S. multicenter study of 1,103 patients with SLE found that 33% of the 222 deaths were directly caused by infection, and infection was a contributing cause in an additional 10% (3). When clinical and demographic features such as age, socioeconomic status, and race were considered, the leading cause of death in all groups in Reveille et al.'s (4) series of 389 patients followed from 1975 to 1985 in Birmingham, Alabama, was infection; 35 of 89 deaths (39%) were from this cause. In developing countries such as Jamaica, infection has been the major cause of death among patients with SLE, being directly responsible for the fatal course in 20 of 55 patients (36%) at the University Hospital of the West Indies from 1972 to 1985 (5). Nossent (6) observed that 50% of the 22 fatalities in his series of 68 Caribbean patients with SLE who were treated between 1980 and 1990 also resulted from sepsis; 25% of those with fatal infections had only mildly active SLE at the time of death. Similarly, a 1993 report from Thailand documented infection as the cause of death in 23 of 77 patients with SLE from a cohort of 537, with opportunistic organisms and other common bacterial pathogens being implicated equally (7). In European and Asian series reported in the late 1990s, despite wide ranges in overall case fatality rates of 4.5% to 24%, the proportion of deaths attributed to infection was similar, ranging from 20.5% to 32.5% (8–11).

RATES OF INFECTION IN SLE

The incidence of infection in SLE is a reflection of overall morbidity, and it has considerable prognostic significance. In a series of 223 patients followed at Downstate Medical Center in New York from 1966 to 1976, 150 patients had 384 infections diagnosed over 655 patient-years, for an overall infection rate of 59 per 100 patient-years (12). The bacterial infection rate was 25 per 100 patient-years. The rate of nonspecific viral infections was 28 per 100 patient-years. Twenty-eight opportunistic infections were identified in 23 patients. Twelve had oral candidiasis, and three other patients with oral thrush also had evidence of systemic infection. Two of 11 patients with deep-seated fungal infections had multiple organisms at a single site, two had coincident bacterial infection at the same site, and one had a single fungal organism at two sites. In a Swedish epidemiologic study reported in 1985, Nived et al. (13) found an overall infection rate of 142 per 100 patient-years of SLE. More than half of these infections were of suspected viral origin, and approximately 40% were bacterial. A high incidence of mucocutaneous infections was noted, often caused by *Staphylococcus aureus*.

The 1974 report of hospitalized SLE patients by Staples et al. (14) identified an overall culture-verified infection rate of 1.22 per 100 hospital days. The most common infection site was the urinary tract. Nearly half of the patients who developed infections had multiple episodes, with recurrent sites frequently involving the opportunistic organism *Candida albicans*. A 1991 review of infections in hospitalized patients at the University of Toronto found an infection rate of 1.94 per 100 hospital days (15). Nearly half of these infections were deemed to be major, requiring intravenous antibiotics; sites included pneumonia, septic arthritis, bacteremia, pyelonephritis, abdominal abscesses, endometritis, and esophageal candidiasis. In the United States multicenter lupus study, infections were responsible for 29% of all but obstetric hospitalizations (3), whereas 14% of the 1989 and 1990 hospitalizations in the Hopkins Lupus Cohort resulted from infection (16).

FACTORS INFLUENCING SUSCEPTIBILITY OF PATIENTS TO INFECTION

Many investigators have examined the risk factors that predispose to infection in SLE patients. Most agree that treatment with corticosteroids as well as some manifestations of active SLE itself play an important role. Staples et al. (14) found that the infection rate in hospitalized patients increased from 0.43 to 1.63 per 100 hospital days with an increase in steroid dose from zero to more than 50 mg/d. In the Downstate study, a fivefold increase in the frequency of all infections was found, ranging from 35 to 179 per 100 patient-years as average prednisone dose increased from zero to greater than 40 mg/d (12). The same trend was observed with bacterial infections (10/100 patient-years, increasing to 87/100 patient-years) and opportunistic infections (range, 142/100 patient-years).

The physiologic and pharmacologic actions of corticosteroids predispose to infection by affecting host responses to microorganisms. These include a decreased inflammatory response, decreased effector cell response in cell-mediated immunity, lysis of lymphoid follicles, and decreased immunoglobulin synthesis (17). Frenkel (18) reviewed the role of corticosteroids as predisposing factors in fungal diseases and concluded that inhibition of cellular host responses, particularly impaired proliferation of epithelioid and giant cells, and decreased digestive capability of these cells and macrophages were responsible. The role of steroids in the development of opportunistic infections was examined in a case-control study of 797 SLE patients hospitalized at Bellevue/New York University Medical Center; 26 patients with a total of 32 opportunistic infections were compared to 26 patients without opportunistic infections (19). Prednisone was a major risk factor for the development of opportunistic infection, with the most common organisms including *Salmonella, Candida, Strongyloides*, and *Aspergillus* sp. The mortality rate was highest among patients who had both opportunistic infection and active disease. The need to aggressively investigate the possibility of occult opportunistic infection was underscored by Hellmann et al. (1), who reviewed 44 lupus-related deaths at Moffitt Hospital in San Francisco between 1969 and 1986, where opportunistic infections occurred in 15 patients (34%) and caused death in 10. Antemortem diagnosis was made in only three of these 15 patients; *Candida* and *Pneumocystis* sp. were the most common organisms.

Prolonged corticosteroid administration further increases the risk of infection by causing chronic changes in tissues, such as skin atrophy, which in turn allow increased access of microorganisms into the circulation. A regimen of alternate-day steroid administration is believed to decrease the pharmacologic risk of infection; this was confirmed in a 1993 Spanish study that showed a significant decrease in infection rate ($p < .001$) among patients receiving an alternate-day dose compared with those on daily steroids (20).

Other immunosuppressive agents, especially azathioprine and cyclophosphamide, also have been implicated as risk factors for infection in patients with SLE, frequently in anecdotal reports and in the setting of aggressive treatment for disease exacerbations (7,21–26). When corrected for steroid dose, however, azathioprine use in the Downstate population was not associated with an increased risk of bacterial, opportunistic, or nonspecific viral infections (12). A French study of cytolytic therapy in rheumatic disease failed to find an increased risk of infection, with the exception of herpes virus, which was associated with a 10% to 20% incidence of infection compared with 2% in patients not treated with immunosuppressive agents (27). Similarly, a prospective study of infections in hospitalized patients with SLE in Singapore did not show an association of cytotoxic therapy and infection (28). On the other hand, Aringer et al. (29) observed that seven of nine patients treated with plasmapheresis in addition to intravenous cyclophosphamide had serious bacterial or viral infections, compared to only two of 12 patients with serious infections in the cyclophosphamide alone group.

CLINICAL FEATURES AND IMMUNOLOGIC DYSFUNCTION IN SLE AS RISKS FOR INFECTION

Even in the absence of corticosteroid treatment, infections are common in patients with SLE. Ropes (30) used steroids sparingly, and rarely if ever gave immunosuppressive agents, yet 108 of 137 patients (79%) had serious infections during their disease course. These infections usually were associated with disease exacerbations. In the Downstate study, new exacerbations of disease were associated with increased infection rates, but the correction for steroid dose eliminated this effect (12). This study also found that specific renal measures, most notably active urinary sediment, were a significant predictor of infection, whereas presence of the nephrotic syndrome and uremia were associated with an increased, but not statistically significant, incidence of bacterial and opportunistic infections. Among renal parameters, including blood urea nitrogen (BUN), creatinine clearance, urine sediment, and 24-hour protein excretion, Staples et al. (14) found BUN to have the strongest association with infection, suggesting that poor renal function is more important than active renal inflammation. Studies of hospitalized patients have shown that overall disease activity, measured by either the SLE Disease Activity Index (SLEDAI) or the Lupus Activity Index (LAI), correlates well with the incidence of infection (15,16).

Even among patients with SLE in clinical remission, an increased tendency to develop bacterial and opportunistic infections has been documented. Staples et al. (14) compared infection rates in SLE to those in patients with rheumatoid arthritis and idiopathic nephrotic syndrome, controlling for steroid dose. Infections were ten times more frequent among patients with SLE than in the other two groups. In Nived et al.'s (13) population-based study, which included many mild cases, a significant increase in bacterial infections was observed among patients with SLE as compared to an age- and gender-matched cohort of patients with rheumatoid arthritis and to a similarly matched cohort of normal controls. The incidence of fungal and viral infections was similar in patients with SLE and controls.

Among patients with end-stage renal failure receiving chronic maintenance hemodialysis, the incidence and severity of infections continue to be influenced by underlying SLE. Jarrett et al. (31) found that 4 of 14 patients with SLE undergoing long-term dialysis at Northwestern University died of infection, compared with only one infectious death in 62 non-SLE patients on hemodialysis.

Many abnormalities, including immunoglobulin deficiency, acquired and inherited complement deficiencies, defects in chemotaxis, phagocytic activity, and delayed hypersensitivity, may account for this susceptibility to infection. As the prototype immune complex disease, activation and consumption of complement have been well characterized in SLE, and the role of specific complement components has been defined (32). For example, fixation of C3 to bacterial cell walls is essential for phagocytosis and subsequent digestion of microorganisms. C3b, which is an activation product of C3, is critical to the opsonization of bacteria before phagocytosis. C3-deficient individuals therefore are at risk for recurrent and/or disseminated bacterial infections (33,34). Hereditary deficiencies in the production of various complement components also have been described in patients with SLE or lupus-like syndromes. Autosomal-recessive defects in C1q, C1r, and C2 production and homozygous deficiencies of C2 have been associated with repeated skin and upper airway infections, recurrent *Haemophilus influenzae* septicemia, and bacterial meningitis (35–37). Recurrent pulmonary infections in a family with lupus-like disease has been linked to an autosomal recessive, human leukocyte antigen (HLA)-associated total deficiency of C4 (38). Granulocyte phagocytic function was found to be normal in these family members; however, a serum defect, which was corrected by the addition of purified C4, appears to have been responsible for the abnormal phagocytosis and intracellular killing. Deficiency of complement components C5–9 (i.e., the membrane attack complex) makes individuals especially prone to infections with encapsulated organisms such as *Neisseria* sp., for which phagocytosis tends to be normal but bacterial lysis is impaired (39,40). Recently, homozygosity for variant alleles in the coding portion of the mannose-binding lectin (MBL) gene in patients with SLE has been shown to be associated with increased susceptibility to infections (odds ratio 8.6) (41). MBL is a serum protein structurally similar to C1q, which binds to antibodies and protein structures on bacteria and viruses. Homozygosity for MBL variant alleles was observed in 7.7% of SLE patients compared to 2.8% of controls by Garred et al. (41). Among homozygotes with SLE, the time interval from SLE diagnosis to the first infection was shorter, and the annual number of infections was four times higher than in patients homozygous or heterozygous for the normal allele (41).

Acquired functional defects in complement components that are associated with disease activity also have been described. Perez et al. (42) observed an increased incidence of infections in patients with SLE in whom they identified a serum inhibitor of C5-derived chemotactic activity. When levels of this inhibitor decreased as disease activity lessened, the incidence of infection also fell. A National Institutes of Health report also correlated a decrease in serum generation of chemotactic factors with infection in 23 patients with SLE (43).

Other studies have found impaired *in vitro* antibacterial activity from alveolar macrophages obtained at bronchioalveolar lavage (44), decreased *S. aureus* intracellular destruction capability (45), impaired opsonic capability (46,47), and defective degradation of bacterial DNA by phagocytes in patients with both discoid and systemic lupus (48), independent of steroid therapy.

Handling of microorganisms also may be influenced by abnormalities of reticuloendothelial function. Saturation of Fc receptors on liver and spleen cells by circulating immune complexes may prevent the clearance of opsonized bacteria (49). Fries et al. (50) demonstrated, however, that Fc receptors on the cell surface of monocytes from patients with SLE actually are increased in number, suggesting that a primary defect in Fc receptor function exists. Such a mechanism might explain the observations of overwhelming pneumococcal bacteremia (51,52) and the chronic *Salmonella* carrier state in some patients with SLE, leading to *Salmonella* arthritis and osteomyelitis (53,54). Functional asplenia (i.e., the complete absence of uptake of intravenously administered, radiolabeled sulfur colloid unrelated to splenic size) has been identified in seven to ten of the screened series of patients with SLE, and it has been implicated in the development of pneumococcal and salmonella septicemia (55).

Abnormalities of cellular immunity in patients with SLE appear to contribute to the risk of opportunistic infections. The incidence of herpes zoster is increased in patients with SLE compared to normal individuals; the rate among Japanese patients with SLE is especially high. Nagasawa et al. (56) found a 43% overall incidence of herpes zoster in their patients, with an annual incidence of 9%. Despite significantly higher antibody titers against herpes zoster than those seen in non-SLE subjects, only 30% of the patients with SLE showed positive delayed hypersensitivity skin reactions to varicella-zoster antigen. In contrast, 100% of normal individuals had a positive skin reaction.

SPECIFIC TYPES OF INFECTION

Bacterial Infections

The most frequent sites for bacterial infections in patients with SLE are similar to those in individuals without lupus, including the urinary and respiratory tracts and the skin (12–14,57). The organisms most often cultured include *S. aureus, E. coli, Klebsiella* sp., and *Pseudomonas* sp. (13,28). In general, gram-positive cocci and gram-negative bacilli are most often implicated as an infectious cause of death (5, 58). Bacteremia is common, especially in hospitalized patients with SLE (7,23); other sites of infection also have been well described and may account for some of the difficulty in distinguishing sepsis from exacerbations of SLE. For example, anecdotal cases of septic bacterial arthritis continue to be reported (50,53,58–68). Bacterial seeding resulting in septic discitis may put a patient at risk for serious neurologic deficit (69). Bursal abscesses also may mimic musculoskeletal problems such as sciatica (70,71).

Commonly diagnosed bacterial organisms, even among otherwise healthy individuals, appear to occur more frequently in unusual locations in patients with SLE. Purulent pericarditis is a rare phenomenon, yet it has been described in at least 14 patients with SLE, most often resulting from *Staphylococcus* sp. (72–74), and in one case which resulted in tamponade being caused by *Neisseria gonorrhoeae* (58). Bacterial epiglottitis, facial cellulitis, and multiple soft tissue abscesses have been described as well (75–77).

Opportunistic bacterial infections also occur with increased frequency in patients with SLE. Among the most common are *Salmonella* sp., especially *S. typimurium* and *S. enteritidis* (53,54,78–92). Occasionally *Salmonella* infection can coincide with the initial presentation of the disease, and aspects of the infection can mimic features of SLE (76,79). Hospitalized lupus vs. nonlupus patients have an increased risk for *Salmonella* infections (80), which can manifest not only as diarrheal illnesses but also as gas-producing leg abscesses (81), septic arthritis (53,54,82) especially at sites of former avascular necrosis (92), osteomyelitis (82,83), and spondylodiscitis (84). Patients with glomerulonephritis may have an increased susceptibility to becoming *Salmonella* carriers (53).

Infection with *Listeria monocytogenes* is uncommon in healthy adults, occurring predominantly in young children, the aged, and immunocompromised individuals. In two series of seven and eight patients with SLE, listerial infection usually presented as meningitis or bacteremia without a known focus, and it most often was associated with active disease, high-dose prednisone with or without other immunosuppressive drugs, or renal failure (24,93). Despite aggressive antibiotic therapy, a fatal course is not uncommon (25).

Active tuberculosis can mimic the manifestations of SLE, thus delaying diagnosis and appropriate treatment. Feng and Tan (94) found tuberculosis in 16 of 311 patients with SLE (5%) who were followed in Singapore between 1963 and 1979. Presentation with miliary (95) and far-advanced pulmonary disease was common. Seven of the Singapore cases were fatal, five of which were attributed directly to mycobacterial infection. Atypical mycobacterial infections have been reported rarely in patients with SLE and tend to be limited to the skin (96–98). The presentation may mimic lupus profundus, delaying appropriate diagnosis and treatment.

Other unusual bacterial infections reported in patients with SLE include five cases of Legionnaires's disease (99–102), *Campylobacter* endocarditis (103), toxic shock syndrome (104), *Pseudomonas pseudomallei* meningitis (105), and a documented tick bite with high antibody levels against *Borrelia burgdorferi* that coincided with the initial presentation of lupus (106). A 1992 report suggested that genitourinary colonization with mycoplasma organisms is common in women with SLE, documenting 22 of 49 urine specimens (45%) to be culture positive for *Ureaplasma urealyticum* or *Mycoplasma hominis* (107). It also should be remembered that while false-positive serologic tests for syphilis are an expected feature of SLE, concomitant infection with *Treponema pallidum* may occur (108), sometimes with signs and symptoms that may mimic those of active SLE (109). Distinguishing false-positive from true-positive serologic tests for syphilis in SLE patients has been problematic in part because of interference with the presence of antiphospholipid antibodies; the fluorescent treponemal antibody absorption (FTA-Abs) test is not considered to be an accurate confirmatory test for syphilis in such patients. Murphy et al. (110) have proposed the treponemal Western blot test as the gold standard, based on its combination of sensitivity and specificity.

Viral Infections

Herpes zoster is the most common specific viral infection that is diagnosed in patients with SLE. In Western countries, its reported incidence ranges from 3% to 21% (12, 111–114), which is somewhat increased over that observed in the general population (21) but considerably less than the 43% incidence diagnosed among Japanese patients with SLE (56). Treatment with corticosteroids and cytotoxic agents significantly increases the risk of herpes zoster; however, 65% of zoster episodes in Kahl's 1994 series occurred during mild or inactive SLE (113). In each of two series, dissemination occurred in 11% (112,113). Two reports of central nervous system herpes zoster mimicking active lupus have appeared (114,115); in one, visual loss and an unusual pattern of retinitis developed. Endoretinal biopsy established the diagnosis of herpesvirus infection, and the patient was successfully treated with acyclovir (115). Herpes simplex also is common in SLE and is particularly associated with esophageal and perianal lesions (116,117). If untreated, disseminated infection may progress to hepatic necrosis, coma, and death (118). Even in the absence of clinical manifestations of infection, antibody titers indicative of herpesvirus-6 infection were found in 55% of 56 patients with SLE in a 1991 study (119).

Cytomegalovirus (CMV) is uncommon. The usual presentation is pulmonary infection, which may be fatal (120–122). CMV has been identified in active SLE in the absence of immunosuppressive therapy (123), and unusual presentations including cutaneous vasculitis have been reported (124).

The role of human papilloma virus (HPV), which has been implicated in causing clinical disease ranging from warts to malignancy, has been examined in SLE. HPV titers were elevated in 45% of patients with SLE (compared to 12% of controls), in a 1977 study (125). Although a high prevalence of cutaneous warts did not correlate with immunosuppressive treatment in a 1993 series (126), an increased risk of uterine cervical atypia in women with SLE receiving cytotoxic agents was observed (127), and this in turn has been linked to a predisposition to infection with HPV, which may induce oncogenic mutations (128).

The association of parvovirus B19 (HPV-B19) with SLE is controversial. Especially in the pediatric population, presentation of the two diseases may be strikingly similar. Moore et al. (129) described six of seven children with HPV-B19 infection who had malar rash (the classic "slapped cheek" erythema) and positive antinuclear antibodies in titers of 1:40 or greater; all had prolonged arthralgias and fatigue. Although the overall course was generally self-limited, some patients had symptoms for up to 120 weeks. Although it has been suggested that HPV-B19 infection may actually trigger SLE (130), Bengtsson et al. (131) found no evidence that HPV-B19 infection was more prevalent among 99 SLE patients (88% of all new cases seen from 1981 to 1995 in a specific health care district in Sweden) compared to age- and sex-matched healthy controls.

(See the differential diagnosis section in Chapter 46 for a discussion of infection with human immunodeficiency virus and SLE).

Fungal Infections

Candida infection is a common complication in patients with SLE, most often presenting with oral thrush (12). Extension to the esophagus with mucosal invasion occurs in association with steroid and cytotoxic therapy. Peripheral blood lymphocytes from patients who are receiving high doses of prednisone have been shown to have markedly depressed *in vitro* lymphocyte transformation to antigenic stimulation by *Candida* sp. (132). Half of the patients with esophageal moniliasis do not have oral lesions (133,134). Esophageal candidiasis may coexist with herpes simplex (116).

The development of deep fungal infections in SLE patients is generally associated with corticosteroid and immunosuppressive therapy, and is most often due to *Candida* sp. or cryptococcus (135), frequently with a fatal outcome. Reports of visceral candidiasis include pericarditis with tamponade (136) and hepatic involvement (137). Cryptococcal infection is not uncommon and usually produces a terminal meningitis, with or without pulmonary changes (138–142). An insidious onset of persistent headache often is the earliest manifestation. It may also present with hepatic (143) or cutaneous (144) involvement. Zygomycosis (formerly known as "mucormycosis") is a severe infection that has been associated with central nervous system complications, thrombotic thrombocytopenic purpura, and a high mortality rate (145–147). Infection with *Aspergillus* sp. most often involves the lungs (137,148,149), presenting with fever and cough in an immunosuppressed patient. The finding of hyphae in the sputum should be confirmed with a tissue diagnosis demonstrating budding hyphae; long-term therapy with amphotericin B and/or fluorocytosine or itraconozole may improve survival. Fatal aspergillus meningitis (150) and septicemia (21,151) also have been documented in patients with SLE. Coccidiodomycosis has been reported in four patients as a complication of steroid-treated lupus (152–155). Other documented fungal infections in SLE include *Nocardia* of subcutaneous tissues, pneumonitis, laryngitis, encephalitis, and meningitis (156–163), disseminated histoplasmosis (164), and maduromycosis (165).

Parasitic Infections

Hyperinfection with *Strongyloides stercoralis* may occur in immunosuppressed patients. The syndrome is characterized by profound malabsorption, diarrhea, electrolyte disturbance, gram-negative or opportunistic fungal sepsis, coma, and death. It can mimic an SLE flare, and eosinophilia may be absent as a result of steroid treatment (166,167). Visceral leishmaniasis has been reported in one SLE patient (168), as has paragonimiasis (169).

Protozoan Infections

Pneumocystis carinii pneumonia (PCP) has been reported in patients with SLE since the 1960s, almost exclusively in the setting of aggressive treatment of active disease with high-dose corticosteroids and cytotoxic drugs (1,12,14,26,120, 170–176). Porges et al. (26) found that an additional important risk factor for PCP was severe lymphopenia; four of six patients in their series had lymphocyte counts of less than 350/mL. This is consistent with a single reported case of PCP in an untreated patient with SLE and severe lymphopenia (177).

Toxoplasmosis has been found in neonates with SLE (178) and in both lymphopenic (179) and immunosuppressed (180) patients. It may be difficult to identify, because the symptoms of central nervous system infection mimic lupus cerebritis (181), whereas false-positive antibody titers can be seen in patients with SLE (182). Further, toxoplasma infection may enhance the production of autoantibodies, which may interfere with the standard dye test that is used for diagnosis (183).

IMMUNIZATION AND ANTIBIOTICS

See Chapter 60.

A PRACTICAL APPROACH TO INFECTION IN SLE

Despite case series and anecdotal reports of unusual infections, each patient with SLE must be considered individually when infection is suspected. There is no "cookbook" approach to diagnosis and treatment; however, a number of important principles can provide guidance in determining a plan of action:

- Patients with SLE develop community-acquired infections just like individuals in the general population. Especially with classic or usual presentations, common bacterial and viral infections should be high on the list of differential diagnoses. Appropriate treatment of these common infections should help to avoid the risk of toxicity (often potentiated by renal or hematologic abnormalities resulting from active lupus) from unnecessary antimicrobial agents.
- Because the symptoms of SLE and of infection often are similar, a high index of suspicion is important; therefore, culture early and often. Advise the laboratory to hold specimens for fungal cultures, and freeze acute serum to match with convalescent serum in the event that antibody titers may be useful.
- While corticosteroids and cytotoxic agents increase the risk of infection, it is equally true that sick patients with active lupus are far less likely to recover from serious infections. Once a patient has been placed on an appropriate regimen for the suspected or documented infection, treatment of the underlying SLE activity should proceed with vigor.
- In difficult or recalcitrant cases, especially with persistent fever or increasing organ dysfunction (e.g., hepatic abnormalities, pulmonary infiltrates), a tissue diagnosis may be essential. Percutaneous or endoscopic biopsy procedures may be sufficient, but open surgical procedures may be necessary. These may be guided by radiographic procedures (e.g., computed tomography, magnetic resonance imaging) or by nuclear imaging (e.g., bone scans for suspected osteomyelitis).

SUMMARY

To summarize the major points of this chapter:

1. Infections are a major source of morbidity and mortality in patients with SLE.
2. Patients with SLE are susceptible to infection; treatment with corticosteroids increases this susceptibility in a dose-dependent fashion.
3. The respiratory and urinary tracts are the most common sites of infection in outpatients.
4. Patients on steroids are at a particularly increased risk for opportunistic infections. The most common organisms include herpes, *Candida* sp., *Salmonella* sp., *Cryptococcus* sp., and *Toxoplasma* sp.
5. Presentations of SLE often are difficult to differentiate from those of infection. The most helpful clues to infection are the presence of shaking chills, leukocytosis (unless steroids are being given), and the absence of active SLE in multiple systems.

REFERENCES

1. Hellmann DB, Petri M, Whiting-O'Keefe Q. Fatal infections in systemic lupus erythematosus: the role of opportunistic organisms. *Medicine* 1987;66:341–348.
2. Klemperer P. Pollack AD, Baehr G. Pathology of disseminated lupus erythematosus. *Arch Pathol* 1941;32:569–631.
3. Rosner S, Ginzler EM, Diamond HS, et al. A multicenter study of outcome in systemic lupus erythematosus. II. Causes of death. *Arthritis Rheum* 1982;25:612–617.
4. Reveille JD, Bartolucci A, Alarcon GS. Prognosis in systemic lupus erythematosus. Negative impact of increasing age at onset, black race, and thrombocytopenia, as well as causes of death. *Arthritis Rheum* 1990;33:3748.
5. Harris EN, Williams E, Shah DJ, et al. Mortality of Jamaican patients with systemic lupus erythematosus. *Br J Rheumatol* 1989;28:113–117.

6. Nossent JC. Course and prognostic value of Systemic Lupus Erythematosus Disease Activity Index in black Caribbean patients. *Semin Arthritis Rheum* 1993;23:16–21.
7. Janwityanuchit S, Totemchokchyakarn K, Krachangwongchai K, et al. Infection in systemic lupus erythematosus. *J Med Assoc Thai* 1993;76:542–548.
8. Jacobsen S, Petersen J, Ullman S, et al. Mortality and death of 513 Danish patients with lupus erythematosus. *Scand J Rheumatol* 1999;28:75–80.
9. Blanco FJ, Gomez-Reino JJ, de la Mata J, et al. Survival analysis of 306 European Spanish patients with systemic lupus erythematosus. *Lupus* 1998;7:159–163.
10. Cervera R, Khamashta MA, Font J, et al. Morbidity and mortality in systemic lupus erythematosus during a 5-year period. A multicenter prospective study of 1,000 patients. European Working Party on Systemic Lupus Erythematosus. *Medicine (Baltimore)* 1999;78:167–175.
11. Kim WU, Min JK, Lee SH, et al. Causes of death in Korean patients with systemic lupus erythematosus: a single center retrospective study. *Clin Exp Rheumatol* 1999;17:539–545.
12. Ginzler E, Diamond H, Kaplan D, et al. Computer analysis of factors influencing frequency of infection in systemic lupus erythematosus. *Arthritis Rheum* 1978;21:37–44.
13. Nived O, Sturfelt G, Wolhein F. Systemic lupus erythematosus and infection: a controlled and prospective study including an epidemiologic group. *Q J Med* 1985;218:271–287.
14. Staples PJ, Gerding DN, Decker JL, et al. Incidence of infection in systemic lupus erythematosus. *Arthritis Rheum* 1974;17:110.
15. Watanabe Duffy KN, Duffy CM, Gladman DD. Infection and disease activity in SLE: a review of hospitalized patients. *J Rheumatol* 1991;18:1180–1184.
16. Petri M, Genovese M. Incidence of and risk factors for hospitalizations in systemic lupus erythematosus: a prospective study of the Hopkins Lupus Cohort. *J Rheumatol* 1992;19:1559–1565.
17. Boumpas DT, Paliogianni F, Anastassiou ED, et al. Gluococorticosteroid action on the immune system: molecular and cellular aspects. *Clin Exp Rheumatol* 1991;9:413–423.
18. Frenkel JK. Role of corticosteroids as predisposing factors in fungal diseases. *Lab Invest* 1962;11:1192–1208.
19. Ritchlin C, Dobro J, Senie R, et al. Opportunistic infections in patients with systemic lupus erythematosus. *Arthritis Rheum* 1989;32(suppl):S115(abst).
20. Formiga Perez F, Moga Sampere I, Canet Gonzalez R, et al. Infection and systemic lupus erythematosus: analysis of a series of 145 patients. *Rev Clin Esp* 1993;193:105–109.
21. Dolin R, Reichman RC, Mazur MH, et al. Herpes zoster-varicella infections in immunosuppressed patients. *Ann Intern Med* 1978;89:375–388.
22. Kattwinkel N, Cook L, Agnello. Overwhelming fatal infection in a young woman after intravenous cyclophosphamide therapy for lupus nephritis. *J Rheumatol* 1991;18:7981.
23. Lee P, Urowitz MB, Bookman AAM, et al. Systemic lupus erythematosus. A review of 110 cases with reference to nephritis, the nervous system, infections, aseptic necrosis and prognosis. *Q J Med* 1977;66:132.
24. Kraus A, Cabral AR, Sifuentes-Osnorio J, et al. Listeriosis in patients with connective tissue disease. *J Rheumatol* 1994;21:635–638.
25. Giunta G, Piazza I. Fatal septicemia due to *Listeria monocytogenes* in a patient with systemic lupus erythematosus receiving cyclosporin and high prednisone doses. *Neth J Med* 1992;40:197–199.
26. Porges AJ, Beattie SL, Ritchlin C, et al. Patients with systemic lupus erythematosus at risk for *Pneumocystis carinii* pneumonia. *J Rheumatol* 1992;19:1191–1194.
27. Kahn MF, Vitale C, Grimaldi A. Infections and immunosuppressive agents in rheumatology. *Sem Hop Paris* 1976;52:1374–1376.
28. Oh HM, Chng HH, Boey ML, et al. Infections in systemic lupus erythematosus. *Singapore Med J* 1993;34:406–408.
29. Aringer M, Smolen JS, Graninger WB. Severe infections in plasmapheresis-treated systemic lupus erythematosus. *Arthritis Rheum* 1998;41:414–420.
30. Ropes MW. *Systemic lupus erythematosus*. Cambridge, MA: Harvard University Press, 1976.
31. Jarrett MP, Santhanam S, Del Greco F. The clinical course of end-stage renal disease in systemic lupus erythematosus. *Arch Intern Med* 1983;143:1353–1356.
32. Bartholomew WR, Shanahan TC. Complement components and receptors: deficiencies and disease associations. *Immunol Series* 1990;52:33–51.
33. Garty BZ, Nitzan M, Danon YL. Systemic meningococcal infections in patients with acquired complement deficiency. *Pediatr Allergy Immunol* 1993;4:69.
34. Feliciano R, Swedler W, Varga J. Infection with uncommon subgroup Y *Neisseria meningitides* in patients with systemic lupus erythematosus. *Clin Exp Rheumatol* 1999;17:737–740.
35. Lee SL, Wallace SL, Barone R, et al. Familial deficiency of two subunits of the first component of complement. C1r and C1s associated with a lupus erythematosus-like disease. *Arthritis Rheum* 1978;21:958–967.
36. Hyatt AC, Altenburger KN, Johnston RB, et al. Increased susceptibility to severe pyogenic infections in patients with an inherited deficiency of the second component of complement. *J Pediatr* 1981;98:417–419.
37. Thong YH, Simpson DA, Muller-Eberhard HJ. Homozygous deficiency of the second component of complement presenting with bacterial meningitis. *Arch Dis Child* 1989;55:471–473.
38. Mascart-Lemone F, Hauptmann G, Goetz J, et al. Genetic deficiency of C4 presenting with recurrent infections and a SLE-like disease. *Am J Med* 1983;75:295–304.
39. Nusinow SR, Zurow BL, Curd JG. The hereditary and acquired deficiencies of complement. *Med Clin North Am* 1985;69:487–504.
40. Takeda I, Igarashi S, Nishimaki T, et al. A case of systemic lupus erythematosus in late component (c9) complement deficiency. *Ryumachi* 1994;34:628–632.
41. Garred P, Madsen HO, Halberg P, et al. Mannose-binding lectin polymorphisms and susceptibility to infection in systemic lupus erythematosus. *Arthritis Rheum* 1999;42:2145–2152.
42. Perez HD, Andron RI, Goldstein IM. Infection in patients with systemic lupus erythematosus. Association with a serum inhibitor of complement-derived chemotactic activity. *Arthritis Rheum* 1979;22:1326–1333.
43. Clark RA, Kimball HR, Decker JL. Neutrophil chemotaxis in systemic lupus erythematosus. *Ann Rheum Dis* 1974;33:167–172.
44. Wallaert B, Aerts C, Bart F, et al. Impaired in vitro bacterial activity from alveolar macrophages in systemic lupus erythematosus. *Annu Rev Respir Dis* 1986;133:A138(abst).
45. Martinez-Cairo Cueto S, Ramirez-Lacayo ML, Veladiz-Saint-Martin P, et al. Deterioration of intracellular destruction capacity of *S. aureus* in children with systemic lupus erythematosus. *Arch Invest Med (Mex)* 1986;17:25–36.
46. Jasin HE, Orozco JH, Ziff M. Serum heat labile opsonins in systemic lupus erythematosus. *J Clin Invest* 1974;53:343–353.
47. Nived O, Linder C, Odeberg H, et al. Reduced opsonisation of protein A containing *Staphylococcus aureus* in sera with cryoglobulins from patients with active systemic lupus erythematosus. *Ann Rheum Dis* 1985;44:252–259.
48. Roberts PJ, Isenberg DA, Segal AW. Defective degradation of bacterial DNA by phagocytes from patients with systemic and discoid lupus erythematosus. *Clin Exp Immunol* 1987;69:68–78.

49. Frank MM, Hamburger MI, Lawley TJ, et al. Defective reticuloendothelial system Fc-receptor function in systemic lupus erythematosus. *N Engl J Med* 1979;300:518–523.
50. Fries LF, Mullins WM, Cho KR, et al. Monocyte receptors for the Fc portion of IgG are increased in systemic lupus erythematosus. *J Immunol* 1984;132:695–700.
51. Petros D, West S. Overwhelming pneumococcal bacteraemia in systemic lupus erythematosus. *Ann Rheum Dis* 1989;48:333–335.
52. van der Straeton C, Wei N, Rothschild J, et al. Rapidly fatal pneumococcal septicemia in systemic lupus erythematosus. *J Rheumatol* 1987;14:1177–1180.
53. Medina F, Fraga A, Lavalle C. Salmonella septic arthritis in systemic lupus erythematosus. The importance of chronic carrier state. *J Rheumatol* 1989;16:203–208.
54. van de Laar MAFJ, Meenhorst PL, van Soesbergen RM, et al. Polyarticular *Salmonella* bacterial arthritis in a patient with systemic lupus erythematosus. *J Rheumatol* 1989;16:231–234.
55. Piliero P, Furie R. Functional asplenia in systemic lupus erythematosus. *Semin Arthritis Rheum* 1990;20:185–189.
56. Nagasawa K, Yamauchi Y, Tada Y, et al. High incidence of herpes zoster in patients with systemic lupus erythematosus: an immunological analysis. *Ann Rheum Dis* 1990;49:630–633.
57. del Castillo M, Toblli JE, Rueda HJ, et al. Infection and systemic lupus erythematosus. *Presna Med Argentina* 1988;75: 49–60.
58. Harisdangkul V, Nilganuwonge S, Rockhold L. Cause of death in systemic lupus erythematosus: a pattern based on age at onset. *South Med J* 1987;80:1249–1253.
59. Coe MD, Hamer DH, Levy CS, et al. Gonococcal pericarditis with tamponade in a patient with systemic lupus erythematosus. *Arthritis Rheum* 1990;33:1438–1441.
60. Edelen JS, Lockshin MD, Leroy EC. Gonococcal arthritis patients with active systemic lupus erythematosus. A diagnostic problem. *Arthritis Rheum* 1971;14:557–559.
61. Mitchell SR, Nguyen PQ, Katz P. Increased risk of neisserial infections in systemic lupus erythematosus. *Semin Arthritis Rheum* 1990;20:174–184.
62. Schenfeld L, Gray RG, Poppo MJ, et al. Bacterial monarthritis due to *Neisseria meningitidis* in systemic lupus erythematosus. *J Rheumatol* 1981;8:145–148.
63. Carratala J, Moreno R, Cabellos C, et al. *Neisseria* meningitis monarthritis revealing systemic lupus erythematosus (letter). *J Rheumatol* 1988;15:532–533.
64. Morris JL, Zizic TM, Stevens MB. Proteus polyarthritis complicating systemic lupus erythematosus. *Johns Hopkins Med J* 1973;133:262–269.
65. Webster J, Williams BD, Smith AP, et al. Systemic lupus erythematosus presenting as pneumococcal septicemia and septic arthritis. *Ann Rheum Dis* 1990;49:181–183.
66. San Miguel VV, Lavery JP, York JC, et al. Achromobacter zylosoxidans septic arthritis in a patient with systemic lupus erythematosus (letter). *Arthritis Rheum* 1991;34:1484–1485.
67. Clough W, Cassell GH, Duffy LB, et al. Septic arthritis and bacteremia due to *Mycoplasma* resistant to antimicrobial therapy in a patient with systemic lupus erythematosus. *Clin Infect Dis* 1992;15:402–407.
68. Quismorio FP, Dubois EL. Septic arthritis in systemic lupus erythematosus. *J Rheumatol* 1975;2:73–82.
69. Hunter T, Plummer FA. Infectious arthritis complicating systemic lupus erythematosus. *Can Med Assoc J* 1980;122:791–793.
70. Mader R, Tanzman M, Schonfeld S. *Pseudomonas aeruginosa* arthritis and discitis in systemic lupus erythematosus. *Harefuah* 1990;118:149–150.
71. Shames JL, Fast A. Gluteal abscess causing sciatica in a patient with systemic lupus erythematosus. *Arch Phys Med Rehabil* 1989;70:410–411.
72. Lambie P, Kaufman R, Beardmore T. Septic ischial bursitis in systemic lupus erythematosus presenting as a perirectal mass. *J Rheumatol* 1989;16:1497–1499.
73. Knodell RG, Manders SJ. Staphylococcal pericarditis in a patients with systemic lupus erythematosus. *Chest* 1974;65:103–105.
74. Dorlon RE, Smith JM, Cook EH, et al. Staphylococcal pericardial effusion with tamponade in a patient with systemic lupus erythematosus (letter). *J Rheumatol* 1982;9:813–814.
75. Sanchez-Guerrero J, Alarcon-Segovia D. Salmonella pericarditis with tamponade in systemic lupus erythematosus. *Br J Rheumatol* 1990;29:69–71.
76. Derkson RHWM, Overbeek BP, Poeschmann PH. Serious bacterial cellulitis of the periorbital area in 2 patients with systemic lupus erythematosus. *J Rheumatol* 1988;15:840–844.
77. Shalit M, Gross DJ, Levo Y. Pneumococcal epiglottitis in systemic lupus erythematosus on high dose corticosteroids. *Ann Rheum Dis* 1982;41:615–616.
78. DiNubile MJ, Albornoz, MA, Shumacher RJ, et al. Pneumococcal soft-tissue infections: possible association with connective tissue diseases. *J Infect Dis* 1991;163:897–900.
79. Martinez Lacasa JTM, Palacin AV, Ferranz VP, et al. Systemic lupus erythematosus presenting as *Salmonella enteritidis* bacteremia (letter). *J Rheumatol* 1991;18:785.
80. Li EK, Cohen MG, Ho AK, et al. *Salmonella* bacteraemia occurring concurrently with the first presentation of systemic lupus erythematosus. *Br J Rheumatol* 1993;32:66–67.
81. Abramson S, Kramer SB, Radin A, et al. *Salmonella* bacteremia in systemic lupus erythematosus. Eight-year experience at a municipal hospital. *Arthritis Rheum* 1985;28:75–79.
82. Shamiss A, Thaler M, Nussinovitch N, et al. Multiple *Salmonella enteritidis* leg abscesses in a patient with systemic lupus erythematosus. *Postgrad Med J* 1990;66:486–488.
83. Hamza M, Elleuch M, Meddeb S, et al. Arthritis and osteomyelitis caused by *Salmonella typhimurium.* In a case of disseminated lupus erythematosus. *Rev Rheum Mal Osteoartic* 1990;57:670.
84. Satter MA, Molly J. Salmonella osteomyelitis in a patient with SLE. *J Infect* 1984;9:93–96.
85. Choukroun G, Quint L, Amoura Z, et al. *Salmonella typhimurium* spondylodiscitis in systemic lupus erythematosus. *Ann Med Interne (Paris)* 1988;139:446–447.
86. Guthaner DF, Stathers GM. *Salmonella typhimurium* and septicaemia complicating disseminated lupus erythematosus. *Med J Aust* 1969;2:11–56.
87. Lovy MR, Ryan PF, Hughes GR. Concurrent systemic lupus erythematosus and salmonellosis. *J Rheumatol* 1981;8:605–612.
88. Frayha RA, Jizi I, Saadeh G. *Salmonella typhimurium* bacteriuria. An increased infection rate in systemic lupus erythematosus. *Arch Intern Med* 1985;145:645–647.
89. Simeon-Aznar CP, Cuenca-Luque R, Solans-Laque R, et al. Fulminant soft tissue infection by *Salmonella enteritidis* in SLE (letter). *J Rheumatol* 1990;17:1570–1571.
90. Shahram F, Akbarian M, Davatchi F. *Salmonella* infection in systemic lupus erythematosus. *Lupus* 1993;2:55–59.
91. Pablos JL, Aragon A, Gomez-Reino JJ. Salmonellosis and systemic lupus erythematosus. Report of ten cases. *Br J Rheumatol* 1994;33:129–132.
92. Chen JY, Luo SF, Wu YJ, et al. *Salmonella* septic arthritis in systemic lupus erythematosus and other systemic diseases. *Clin Rheumatol* 1998;17:282–287.
93. Harisdangkul V, Songcharoen S, Lin AC. Listerial infections in patients with systemic lupus erythematosus. *South Med J* 1992; 85:957–960.
94. Feng PH, Tan TH. Tuberculosis in patients with systemic lupus erythematosus. *Ann Rheum Dis* 1982;41:11–14.
95. Raj SM, Hunt J. Systemic lupus erythematosus and miliary

tuberculosis in a prepubertal girl: a case report. *Med J Malayasia* 1990;45:347–348.

96. Enzenauer RJ, McKoy J, Vincent D, et al. Disseminated cutaneous and synovial *Mycobacterium marinum* infection in a patient with systemic lupus erythematosus. *South Med J* 1990; 83:471–474.
97. Kakinuma H, Suzuki H. *Mycobacterium avium* complex infection limited to the skin in a patient with systemic lupus erythematosus. *Br J Dermatol* 1994;130:785–790.
98. Czelusta A, Moore AY. Cutaneous *Mycobacterium kansasii* infection in a patient with systemic lupus erythematosus: case report and review. *J Am Acad Dermatol* 1999;40:359–363.
99. Edelstein PH. Legionnaires' disease (letter). *Arthritis Rheum* 1978;22:806.
100. Jacox RF, Stuard ID. Legionnaires' disease in a patient with systemic lupus erythematosus. *Arthritis Rheum* 1978;21:975–977.
101. Senear FE, Usher B. An unusual type of pemphigus combining features of lupus erythematosus. *Arch Dermatol Syph* 1926;13: 761–781.
102. Wendling D, Saint-Hillier Y, Hory B, et al. Legionnaire's disease in a patient with lupus (letter). *Rev Rheum Mal Osteoartic* 1986; 53:137.
103. Dzau VJ, Schur PH, Weinstein L. *Vibrio* fetus endocarditis in a patient with systemic lupus erythematosus. *Am J Med Sci* 1976; 272:331–334.
104. Findlay RF, Odom RB. Toxic shock syndrome in a patient with systemic lupus erythematosus. *Int J Dermatol* 1982;21: 140–141.
105. Christenson-Bravo B, Rodriguez JE, Vazquez G, et al. *Pseudomonas pseudomallei* (meloidosis): acute septicemia and meningitis in patients with systemic lupus erythematosus. *Bol Assoc Med P R* 1986;78:347–349.
106. Federlin K, Becker H. *Borrelia* infection and systemic lupus erythematosus (English abstract). *Immun Infekt* 1989;17:195–198.
107. Ginsburg KS, Kundsin RB, Walter CW, et al. *Ureaplasma urealyticum* and *Mycoplasma hominis* in women with systemic lupus erythematosus. *Arthritis Rheum* 1992;35:429–433.
108. Dhillon VB, Keeling DM, Ridgway GL, et al. Treponemal infection coexisting with systemic lupus erythematosus. *Br J Rheumatol* 1992;31:345–348.
109. Lewis S, Goldman R, Cronstein B. Acute syphilitic meningitis in a patients with systemic lupus erythematosus. *J Rheumatol* 1993;20:870–871.
110. Murphy FT, George R, Kubota K, et al. The use of Western blotting as the confirmatory test for syphilis in patients with rheumatic disease. *J Rheumatol* 1999;26:2448–2453.
111. Dubois EL, Wierzchowiecki M, Cox MB, et al. Duration and death in systemic lupus erythematosus. An analysis of 249 cases. *JAMA* 1974;227:1399–1402.
112. Moutsopoulos HM, Gallagher JD, Decker JL, et al. Herpes zoster in patients with systemic lupus erythematosus. *Arthritis Rheum* 1978;21:798–802.
113. Kahl LE. Herpes zoster infections in systemic lupus erythematosus: risk factors and outcome. *J Rheumatol* 1994;21: 84–86.
114. Baethge BA, King JW, Husain F, et al. Herpes zoster myelitis occurring during treatment for systemic lupus erythematosus. *Am J Med Sci* 1989;298:264–266.
115. Feinman MC, Friedberg MA, Schwartz JC, et al. Central nervous system herpesvirus infection in systemic lupus erythematosus: diagnosis by endoretinal biopsy. *J Rheumatol* 1993;20: 1058–1061.
116. Beecham JE, Abd-Elrazak M. Concomitant herpes-monilial esophagitis in a patient with systemic lupus erythematosus: successful systemic antiviral treatment. *Saudi Med J* 1987;8: 419–422.
117. Kalb RE, Grossman ME. Chronic perianal herpes simplex in immunocompromised hosts. *Am J Med* 1986;80:486–490.
118. Luchi ME, Feldman M, Williams WV. Fatal disseminated herpes simplex. II. Infection in a patient with systemic lupus erythematosus. *J Rheumatol* 1995;22:799–800.
119. Krueger GR, Sander C, Hoffmann A, et al. Isolation of human herpesvirus-6 (HHV-6) from patients with collagen vascular diseases. *In Vivo* 1991;5:217–225.
120. Leong KH, Boey ML, Feng PH. Coexisting *Pneumocystis carinii* pneumonia, cytomegalovirus pneumonitis and salmonellosis in systemic lupus erythematosus. *Ann Rheum Dis* 1991;50:811–812.
121. Sanchez-Roman J, Varela-Aguilar JM, Fraile I, et al. Cytomegalic inclusion disease in a patient with systemic lupus. *Rev Clin Esp* 1991;188:34–36.
122. Kwong YL, Wong KL, Kung IT, et al. Concomitant alveolar haemorrhage and cytomegalovirus infection in a patient with systemic lupus erythematosus. *Postgrad Med J* 1988;64:56–59.
123. Ku SC, Yu CJ, Chang YL, et al. Disseminated cytomegalovirus disease in a patient with systemic lupus erythematosus not undergoing immunosuppressive therapy. *J Formos Med Assoc* 1999;98:855–858.
124. Bulpitt KJ, Brahn E. Systemic lupus erythematosus and concurrent cytomegalic vasculitis: diagnosis by antemortem skin biopsy. *J Rheumatol* 1989;16:677–680.
125. Johansson E, Pyrhonen S, Rostila T. Wart and wart virus antibodies in patients with systemic lupus erythematosus. *Br Med J* 1977;1:74–75(abst).
126. Yell JA, Burge SM. Warts and lupus erythematosus. *Lupus* 1993;2:21–23.
127. Blumenfeld Z, Lorber M, Yoffe N, et al. Systemic lupus erythematosus: predisposition for uterine cervical dysplasia. *Lupus* 1994;3:59–61.
128. Eustace DLS. Systemic lupus erythematosus and uterine cervical neoplasia (editorial). *Lupus* 1994;3:34.
129. Moore TL, Bandlamudi R, Alam SM, et al. Parvovirus infection mimicking systemic lupus erythematosus in a pediatric population. *Semin Arthritis Rheum* 1999;28:314–318.
130. Trapani S, Ermini M, Falcini F. Human parvovirus B19 infection: its relationship with systemic lupus erythematosus. *Semin Arthritis Rheum* 1999;28:319–325.
131. Bengtsson A, Widell A, Elmstahl S, et al. No serological indications that systemic lupus erythematosus is linked to exposure to human parovirus B19. *Ann Rheum Dis* 2000;59:64–66.
132. Folb PI, Trounce JR. Immunological aspects of candida infection complicating steroid and immunosuppressive drug therapy. *Lancet* 1970;2:1112–1114.
133. Goldberg HI, Dodds WJ. Cobblestone esophagus due to monilial infection. *AJR* 1968;104:608–612.
134. Sheft DJ, Shrago G. Esophageal moniliasis. The spectrum of the disease. *JAMA* 1970;213:1859–1862.
135. Sieving RR, Kauffman CA, Watanakunakorn C. Deep fungal infection in systemic lupus erythematosus: three cases reported, literature reviewed. *J Rheumatol* 1975;2:61–72.
136. Kaufman LD, Seifert FC, Eilbott DJ, et al. *Candida* pericarditis and tamponade in a patient with systemic lupus erythematosus. *Arch Intern Med* 1988;148:715–726.
137. Kimura M, Udgawa S, Shoji A, et al. Pulmonary aspergillosis due to *Aspergillus terreus* combined with staphylococcal pneumonia and hepatic candidiasis. *Mycopathologia* 1990;111:47–53.
138. Al-Rasheed SA, Al-Fawaz IM. Cryptococcal meningitis in a child with systemic lupus erythematosus. *Ann Trop Paediatr* 1990;10:323–326.
139. Collins DN, Oppenheim IA, Edwards MR. Cryptococcoses associated with systemic lupus erythematosus. Light and electron microscopic observations on a morphologic variant. *Arch Pathol* 1971;91:78–88.

140. Mok CC, Lau CS, Yuen KY. Cryptococcol meningitis presenting concurrently with systemic lupus erythematosus. *Clin Esp Rheumatol* 1998;16:169–171.
141. Kimura K, Hatakeyama M, Miyagi J, et al. A case of systemic lupus erythematosus with cryptococcal meningitis successfully treated with amphotericin B and 5-FC. *Nippon Naika Gakkai Zasshi* 1986;75:406–413.
142. Zimmerman B III, Spiegel M, Lally EV. Cryptococcal meningitis in systemic lupus erythematosus. *Semin Arthritis Rheum* 1992;22:18–24.
143. Fong KY, Poh WT, Ng HS. Cryptococcoses of the liver in a systemic lupus erythematosus patient. *Singapore Med J* 1988;29:309–310.
144. Kruyswijk MR, Keuning JJ. Cutaneous cryptococcoses in a patient receiving immunosuppressive drugs for systemic lupus erythematosus. *Dermatologica* 1980;161:280–284.
145. Bloxham CA, Carr S, Ryan DW, et al. Disseminated zygomycosis and systemic lupus erythematosus (clinical conference). *Intensive Care Med* 1990;16:201–207.
146. Fingerote RJ, Seigel S, Atkinson MH, et al. Disseminated zygomycosis associated with systemic lupus erythematosus (case report). *J Rheumatol* 1990;17:1692–1694.
147. Wong KL, Tai YT, Loke SL, et al. Disseminated zygomycosis masquerading as cerebral lupus erythematosus. *Am J Clin Pathol* 1986;86:546–549.
148. Collazos J, Martinez E, Flores M, et al. Aspergillus pneumonia successfully treated with itraconazole in a patient with systemic lupus erythematosus. *Clin Invest* 1994;72:920–921.
149. Gonzalez-Crespo MR, Gomez-Reino JJ. Invasive aspergillosis in systemic lupus erythematosus. *Semin Arthritis Rheum* 1995;24:304–314.
150. Lammens M, Robberecht W, Waer M, et al. Purulent meningitis due to aspergillosis in a patient with systemic lupus erythematosus. *Clin Neurol Neurosurg* 1992;94:39–43.
151. Qi-Ling W, Jia-ning Y, Zhong-rong H. A case of fulminant systemic lupus erythematosus complicated by severe aspergillar septicemia confirmed by pathologic findings. *Chinese Med J* 1986;99:493–497.
152. Andersen FG, Guckian JC. Systemic lupus erythematosus associated with fatal pulmonary coccidioidomycosis. *Tex Rep Biol Med* 1968;16:93–99.
153. Berry CZ, Goldberg IC, Shepard WL. Systemic lupus erythematosus complicated by coccidioidomycosis. *JAMA* 1968;206:1083–1085.
154. Conger J, Farrell T, Douglas S. Lupus nephritis complicated by fatal disseminated coccidioidomycosis. *Calif Med* 1973;118:60–65.
155. Jones FJ Jr, Spivey CG Jr. Spread of pulmonary coccidioidomycosis associated with steroid therapy: report of a case with a lupus-like reaction to anti-tuberculosis chemotherapy. *J Lancet* 1966;86:226–230.
156. Santen RJ, Wright IS. Systemic lupus erythematosus associated with pulmonary nocardiosis. *Arch Intern Med* 1967;119:202–205.
157. Gorevic PD, Katler EI, Agus B. Pulmonary nocardiosis. Occurrence in men with systemic lupus erythematosus. *Arch Intern Med* 1980;140:361–363.
158. Grossman CB, Bragg DG, Armstrong D. Roentgen manifestations of pulmonary nocardiosis. *Radiology* 1970;96:325–330.
159. Petri M, Katzenstein P, Hellmann D. Laryngeal infection in lupus: report of nocardiosis and review of laryngeal involvement in lupus. *J Rheumatol* 1985;15:1014–1015.
160. Ishibashi Y, Watanabe R, Hommura S, et al. Endogenous *Nocardia asteroides* endophthalmitis in a patient with systemic lupus erythematosus. *Br J Ophthalmol* 1990;74:433–436.
161. Ludmerer KM, Kissane JM. Headache, mental status changes, and death in a 36–year-old woman with lupus. *Am J Med* 1989;86:94–102.
162. Mok CC, Lau CS, Poon SP. Primary nocardial meningitis in systemic lupus erythematosus. *Br J Rheumatol* 1995;34:178–181.
163. Balbir-Gurman A, Schapira D, Nahir AM. Primary subcutaneous nocardial infection in an SLE patient. *Lupus* 1999;8:164–167.
164. Hansen KE, St Clair EW. Disseminated histoplasmosis in systemic lupus erythematosus: case report and review of the literature. *Semin Arthritis Rheum* 1998;28:193–199.
165. Lippman SM, Arnett FC, Conley CL, et al. Genetic factors predisposing to autoimmune diseases. Autoimmune hemolytic anemia, chronic thrombocytopenic purpura, and systemic lupus erythematosus. *Am J Med* 1982;73:827–840.
166. Livneh A, Coman EA, Cho S, et al. *Strongyloides stercoralis* hyperinfection mimicking systemic lupus erythematosus flare (letter). *Arthritis Rheum* 1988;31:930–931.
167. Rivera E, Maldonado N, Velez-Garcia E, et al. Hyperinfection syndrome with *Strongyloides stercoralis*. *Ann Intern Med* 1970;72:199–204.
168. Wallis PJ, Clark CJ. Visceral leishmaniasis complicating systemic lupus erythematosus. *Ann Rheum Dis* 1983;42:201–202.
169. Kraus A, Guerra-Bautista G, Chavarria P. Paragonimiasis: an infrequent but treatable cause of hemoptysis in systemic lupus erythematosus (case report). *J Rheumatol* 1990;17:244–246.
170. Ruskin J, Remington JS. The compromised host and infection. I. *Pneumocystis carinii* pneumonia. *JAMA* 1967;202:1070–1074.
171. Ruskin J, Remington JS. *Pneumocystis carinii* pneumonia. *JAMA* 1968;203:162–163.
172. Fortenberry JD, Shew ML. Fatal *Pneumocystis carinii* in an adolescent with systemic lupus erythematosus. *J Adolesc Health Care* 1989;10:570–572.
173. Decker JL, Klippel JH, Plotz PH, et al. Cyclophosphamide or azathioprine in lupus glomerulonephritis. *Ann Intern Med* 1975;83:606–615.
174. Pohl MA, Lan SP, Berl T, and the Lupus Nephritis Collaborative Study Group. Plasmapheresis does not increase the risk for infection in immunosuppressed patients with severe lupus nephritis. *Ann Intern Med* 1991;114:924–929.
175. Liam CK, Wang F. *Pneumocystis carinii* pneumonia in patients with systemic lupus erythematosus. *Lupus* 1992;1:379–385.
176. Chayakul P, Thammakumpee G, Mitarnun W. Lung cavities from *Pneumocystis carinii* in a patient with systemic lupus erythematosus. *J Med Assoc Thai* 1991;74:310–312.
177. Nguyen TB, Galezowski N, Taksin AL, et al. *Pneumocystis carinii* infection disclosing untreated systemic lupus erythematosus. *Rev Med Interne* 1995;16:146–149.
178. Wechsler B, Le Thi Huong Du, Vignes B, et al. Toxoplasmosis and disseminated lupus erythematosus: four case reports and a review of the literature (English abstract). *Ann Med Interne (Paris)* 1986;137:324–330.
179. Klein B, Kalden JR. Toxoplasmic encephalitis with fatal outcome as an opportunistic infection in systemic lupus erythematosus. *Akt Rheumatol* 1989;14:62–66.
180. Dubin HV, Courter MH, Harrell ER. Toxoplasmosis. A complication of corticosteroid and cyclophosphamide-treated lupus erythematosus. *Arch Dermatol* 1971;104:547–550.
181. Zamir D, Amar M, Groisman G, et al. Toxoplasma infection in systemic lupus erythematosus mimicking lupus cerebritis. *Mayo Clin Proc* 1999;74:575–578.
182. Wilcox MH, Powell RJ, Pugh SF, et al. Toxoplasmosis and systemic lupus erythematosus. *Ann Rheum Dis* 1990;49:254–257.
183. Noel I, Balfour AH, Wilcox MH. Toxoplasma infection and systemic lupus erythematosus: analysis of the serological response by immunoblotting. *J Clin Pathol* 1993;46:628–632.

44

SERUM AND PLASMA PROTEIN ABNORMALITIES AND OTHER CLINICAL LABORATORY DETERMINATIONS IN SYSTEMIC LUPUS ERYTHEMATOSUS

DANIEL J. WALLACE

Abnormalities in plasma proteins are observed in most patients with systemic lupus erythematosus (SLE). Certain clinical manifestations of the disease, such as edema secondary to hypoalbuminemia, can be attributed directly to these aberrations. This chapter reviews nonserologic laboratory abnormalities and discusses their clinical relationships and importance.

HYPOALBUMINEMIA

In 1943, Coburn and Moore (1) first reported on the determination of proteins in SLE and found a low albumin and high globulin fraction in 17 patients. Scores of other reports have confirmed these findings. Albumin levels lower than 3.5 g/dL were found in 50% of Dubois and Tuffanelli's (2) 398 patients, in 50% of McGehee Harvey et al.'s (3) 105 patients, in 47% of Ogryzlo et al.'s (4) 36 patients, and in 34% of Ropes' (5) 106 patients. In 29 of Dubois and Tuffanelli's (2) patients, the albumin level was less than 2 g/dL; all were nephrotic. Pollak et al. (6) were able to correlate albumin levels with disease activity. Fries and Holman (7) found a mean serum albumin level of 3.4 g/dL in 193 patients. Low serum albumin levels are observed in those with SLE complicated by nephrotic syndrome, protein-losing enteropathies, malnutrition, and chronic disease. The absolute catabolic rate of albumin is increased in active SLE (8).

SERUM GLOBULINS

SLE is characterized by a polyclonal gammopathy representing a nonspecific, immunologic, antibody response. Hyperglobulinemia was found in 32% of Dubois and Tuffanelli's (2) 398 patients, in 58% of McGehee Harvey et al.'s (3) 105 patients, in 76% of Ropes' (5) 106 patients, and in 30% of Hochberg et al.'s (9) 150 patients. Certain globulin fractions that exhibit specific abnormalities are described later. Elevated serum globulin levels may be present with (as in lupus nephritis) or without (as in Sjögren's syndrome) low serum albumin levels.

α-Globulins: α_1-Acid Glycoproteins, Fetoprotein, α_1-Antitrypsin, And α_1-Antichymotrypsin

Pollak et al. (6) noted the mean level of α_1-globulin to be in the upper limits of the normal range. Patients with the highest levels had proteinuria, regardless of their disease activity. α_1-Globulin levels were elevated in 19 (17%) of Dubois' 110 patients (10) and in 8% of Ropes' (5) 106 patients. α_1-Globulins often are acute-phase reactants, which are glycoproteins made in the liver that defend against cellular injury. Others function as carriers and are decreased with cellular injury. Petri et al. (11) found that most pregnant women with SLE have elevated α-fetoprotein levels, but this was not associated with neural tube defects (11).

Denko and Gabriel (12) found α_1-glycoprotein (orosomucoid) levels to be increased by 69% to 90% in 48 patients, and other groups have confirmed this (13–16). They also observed a 25% mean increase in α_1-antitrypsin levels in their patients. Gladman et al. (17) noted elevated levels in 5% and decreased amounts in 11% of 112 patients. A Chinese and a Swedish group were unable to find any significant differences (18,19).

α_1-Antitrypsin is the dominant protease inhibitor in plasma. SLE is not associated with any specific α_1-antitrypsin phenotype (20,21). α_1-Antitrypsin deficiency has been hypothesized to be a promoting factor of autoimmunization (22). One study evaluated 33 patients with SLE and found that α_1-chymotrypsin and α_1-antitrypsin levels are higher in those with inactive disease (14), but another study found no abnormalities (18). Lacki et al. (23) correlated increased immunoglobulin A (IgA)–α_1-antitrypsin complex with SLE and central nervous system disease.

Plasma neutrophil elastase and lactoferrin levels also may be slightly elevated in patients with SLE (24).

α_2-Globulins: Ceruloplasmin, Haptoglobin, α_2-Macroglobulin-Ha-Glycoprotein

Elevations in the α_2-globulin fractions were noted in 19 of Dubois' (10) 110 patients, in 19 of Ropes' (5) 73 patients, and in 33% of Ogryzlo et al.'s (4) patients. Pollak et al. (6) found the highest levels in patients with active disease and considerable proteinuria. In contrast, the mean level was not elevated in patients with inactive disease and no proteinuria. This may represent selective retention by a damaged kidney of the high molecular weight α_2-globulin. Ogryzlo et al. (4) group confirmed this, but their findings have been challenged (25). Serum α_2-HA-glycoprotein is a negative acute-phase reactant that is active in bone mineralization and resorption; its levels probably are decreased in active SLE (26).

Ceruloplasmin, which is both an acute-phase reactant and carrier protein, is increased by 20% to 40% in patients with SLE (12). α_2-Macroglobulin is a protease inhibitor and is elevated in SLE (20,27,28). In one study, patients with SLE had a significant increase in haptoglobin type 2-2 (18). (See Chapter 25 for a discussion of antithrombin III.)

β-Globulins

β-Globulin levels were elevated in 18 of Dubois' (10) 110 patients. Pollak et al. (6) found that mean levels were not different than those of controls, but those with active disease had significantly decreased values (25). Transferrin, a β-globulin carrier molecule, was decreased in 20% of patients in one report (12) and normal in another (18). A β_2-macroglycoprotein (i.e., the Hakata antigen) has been associated with SLE (29). (See Chapters 13, 25, and 52 for a discussion of complement components, prothrombin, fibrinogen, plasminogen, and other clotting factors in the β-globulin region.)

Serum Lipids In SLE And Homocysteine

Hyperlipidemia is a significant problem in SLE and one of the leading causes of morbidity and mortality in the disease. An increasing number of patients are surviving the initial episodes of serious lupus, only to succumb 15 to 20 years later to the artherosclerotic and atheroembolic complications of corticosteroid use, antiphospholipid antibodies, and chronically high homocysteine levels. For example, the latter induces vascular-endothelial cell activation, vascular smooth muscle proliferation, and decreased endothelial cell growth (30). Folic acid therapy may prevent these complications.

β-Lipoproteins comprise a sizable component of the β-globulin mortality in the disease. β-Lipoproteins also comprise a sizable component of the β-globulin fraction. Our group (31) found significant hypercholesterolemia (>240 mg/dL) in 88 of 434 (20%) patients with idiopathic SLE, and hypertriglyceridemia (>200 mg/dL) in 17.6%. Seventy-three of 100 patients with SLE in Singapore had abnormal lipid profiles, usually because of renal disease or corticosteroid use (32). Within 3 years of diagnosis, 75% of 134 lupus patients followed in Toronto had hypercholesterolemia (33). Untreated SLE is associated with an endogenous dyslipidemia, increased very low density lipoprotein (VLDL), triglycerides, low high-density lipoprotein (HDL) levels, and altered chlylomicron metabolism (34,35).

The hyperlipidemic effect of corticosteroids has long been recognized and documented in patients with rheumatic disease. Ettinger et al. (36,37) reported that female patients with SLE who were not taking steroids have lipid levels similar to those of a control group; however, the administration of steroids leads to significant increases in triglyceride, cholesterol, apolipoprotein B, and low-density lipoprotein (LDL) cholesterol levels. Others have confirmed this (38,39). Apolipoprotein H levels are decreased in SLE (40). Because most patients with organ-threatening lupus are taking corticosteroids and most without organ-threatening disease are on antimalarials, these agents often interfere with baseline lipid determinations. Reports of types I, III, and V hyperlipidemia in patients with lupus have appeared (41–43), and nephrotic syndrome is associated with extremely high levels of cholesterol (especially high LDL cholesterol), low high-density lipoprotein-2, lipoprotein A, and triglycerides (44,45). Leptin is a protein made by fat cells that helps decrease appetite. A preliminary report suggests that its levels are increased in lupus (46).

Ilowite et al. (47) evaluated ten children with SLE and identified two distinct patterns of dyslipoproteinemia. Active disease was associated with a depressed HDL cholesterol level, and apoprotein A-I was associated with elevated VLDL cholesterol and triglyceride levels. After corticosteroid therapy, total cholesterol, VLDL cholesterol, and triglyceride levels were increased. Corticosteroid therapy of SLE is associated with accelerated atherosclerosis, with resulting increased mortality (48).

Recently, interest has focused on the interactions of phospholipid antibodies and serum lipids. Three groups have shown that although lipoprotein A levels are increased in SLE, they do not correlate with disease activity, thrombosis, anticardiolipin antibody, or steroid therapy (49–51), although two studies have disputed this (52,53). Apolipoprotein A-1 may correlate with anticardiolipin antibody (54), as might vascular disease associated with hypertriglyceridemia

(55). Cross-reactivity between antiphospholipid antibodies and antibodies to oxidized LDL has been reported (56–58), which may be clinically important in 10% to 20% of patients. Apolipoprotein antibodies may play a role in the decreased HDL levels that are seen in some patients with lupus and antiphospholipid syndrome (59–61).

Lupus sera itself has been postulated to be atherogenic, because SLE-derived immune complexes stimulate the accumulation of cholesterol in cultured smooth muscle cells (62). Active lupus may decrease HDL levels by suppressing lipoprotein lipase (39). Alternatively, the interactions of steroid use, anticardiolipin antibody, and lipids may explain the accelerated atherosclerosis found in SLE (63). Wallace et al. (64) reported that hydroxychloroquine can decrease LDL cholesterol, cholesterol, and triglyceride levels in patients with SLE by 15% to 20%. Hodis et al. (65) and Petri et al. (66) have confirmed this but also suggest a beneficial HDL effect. Petri et al. also studied this issue prospectively. (See Chapter 61 for more details.) Lipid-lowering agents such as gemfibrozil and lovastatin are effective in managing the hyperlipidemias of SLE (67,68), and additional consideration should be given to adding an antimalarial agent in steroid-dependent patients. Dietary treatment of hyperlipidemia alone in SLE has been disappointing (69).

Gamma Globulins

A broad polyclonal elevation of the gamma globulin fraction was observed in 61% of Dubois' (10) 110 patients, in 77% of Estes and Christian's (70) 150 patients, but in only 29% of Ropes' (5) 73 patients and 8% of Rothfield's 365 patients (71). Although associated with active disease and proteinuria, gamma globulin levels can be normal, even with significant disease activity (4,6,25,72,73).

Marked acquired hypogammaglobulinemia in SLE has been noted in 15 case reports, usually following high-dose corticosteroid and immunosuppressive therapy (74–82). This group of patients is especially susceptible to recurrent infections.

SERUM IMMUNOGLOBULINS

Immunoglobulin G And Its Subclasses

Mean serum levels of IgG are increased in patients with SLE compared to those in healthy controls (83). Evidence that this increase is polyclonal stems from the observation that isolated IgG elevation occurs in only 9% of patients with SLE (84). The IgG level tends to be elevated at diagnosis but normalizes with therapy. At any time, IgG was increased in 23% of 39 patients followed serially (85).

Levy (86) studied the mean survival half-life for IgG in patients with SLE. It averaged 8.2 days, compared with an average of 28 days in normal controls. An average of 10.1% of total-body IgG was catabolized daily, compared with a mean of 3.9% in normals. Despite normal serum IgG concentrations in patients with SLE, their synthetic rates were as much as four to five times normal, revealing far greater IgG antibody production in SLE than suggested merely by serum concentration. In a long-term serial study at the National Institutes of Health, 18 patients developed low IgG levels during the course of their disease, but it was transient in 110. Also, four developed recurrent infections. Excessive T-cell suppressor and decreased B-cell activity characterized this subset (87). Ward et al. (88) were unable to correlate IgG levels with age, sex, race, or duration of disease.

Several centers have evaluated patients with SLE for IgG subclasses. Among 20 children, significantly increased IgG1 and IgG3 subclasses were present, along with decreased IgG4; 48 adults with SLE had decreased IgG2 and IgG4 levels (89). Low IgG3 and IgG4 levels correlated with an increased rate of infection (90). Decreased IgG2 levels were found among 15 patients with SLE in Isenberg's group (91), compared with 20 controls. In another report, an increased IgG1 level was associated with a subgroup of patients having high-titer rheumatoid factor, antinuclear antibody, and low levels of anti–double-stranded DNA (92).

Immunoglobulin M

Elevated mean IgM levels were found by Alarcon-Segovia and Fishbein (83) in 481 serum samples from 106 patients compared with those from 106 controls. Schoenfeld et al. (85) noted that the IgM level often was decreased at diagnosis but normalized later. In 39 patients followed serially, the IgM level was elevated at any time in 18%. Three other large-scale studies found that very low IgM levels [>2 standard deviations (SD) below the mean] could be found in 20% of over 200 patients with SLE (93–95). Low IgM levels tended to correlate with disease duration but not with activity (88). Survival studies of IgM in SLE show a normal half-life (86).

A 7S β-M-globulin occurs in SLE, rheumatoid arthritis, and in the cord blood of apparently normal infants, but it is absent in normal human adult sera (96). This fraction was found by Rothfield (97) in 8 of 53 patients with SLE, four of whom were males, and in 32% of 31 men with SLE by Kaufman et al. (98). Low molecular weight IgM as a monomeric subunit probably comprises approximately 15% of the total IgM seen in patients with SLE (99).

In the hyper-IgM syndrome, patients have low IgG, IgA, and IgE with recurrent infections. The x-linked form is caused by mutations in the gene for CD40 ligand, and this has been reported in SLE patients (100).

Immunoglobulin A

IgA deficiency is found in from 1 in 400 to 1 in 3,800 adults. It has been observed in 3 of 72, 3 of 96, 0 of 181, 5 of 96, and 7 of 102 patients with SLE in five reports

(101–105), which suggests an increased incidence of this uncommon finding. Men and those with antibodies to Sm and La may have an increased incidence of IgA deficiency in SLE (98), as may Afro-Caribbeans (104,105). Although the serum IgA level usually is normal or slightly elevated in SLE (83,84,94), elevations of IgA were found in 30% of patients during the course of disease in one study (85). Saliva gamma A or secretory IgA levels may be reduced in patients with SLE and frequent attacks of respiratory disease (105). Blacks with SLE may have a higher IgA2 level than whites (106).

Immunoglobulin E

Increases in IgE levels may correlate roughly with disease activity in lupus erythematosus (107–110). Four cases of hyper-IgE syndrome, one following carbamazepine administration, have been reported in patients with SLE (111–114). A hyperimmunization phenomenon might by contributory to high IgE levels. (Chapter 60 reviews the relationship between IgE, lupus, and allergies.)

Paraproteinemia And Paraproteinuria

Of 415 patients with SLE followed in Toronto, nine (2.2%) had evidence of paraproteinemia (115). The monoclonal proteins were IgG (in six patients), IgA (in two), and IgM (in one). None had myeloma, and no consistent patterns could be discerned. Porcel et al. (116) noted a monoclonal gammopathy in four of 120 patients with SLE (3.3%). Approximately 30 cases have appeared in the literature (117). Characterized as transient, stable, or increasing, they are almost always benign. The large number of patients in this group treated with corticosteroids has led to the hypothesis that these agents might enhance production of immunoglobulin. Kappa/lambda ratios for serum IgG, IgA, and IgM in 40 patients with SLE were not different from those in healthy controls (118).

Unbound free urinary light chains are increased in lupus nephritis and represent quantitative markers of concurrent *in vivo* immunoglobulin synthesis and secretion (119,120). Tsai et al. (121) observed free kappa chains in 36% and free lambda chains in 43% of 23 patients with active lupus nephritis but in none of the patients with inactive lupus nephritis.

SEDIMENTATION RATE

Elevation of the sedimentation rate occurred in 84% of 463 of Dubois' (10) patients between 1950 and 1963 and in 94% of Arman-Cruz et al.'s (122) 108 patients, and Wallace's group (31) observed Westergren sedimentation rates to be greater than 30 mm/h in 236 of 434 patients (54%) tested. The mean Wintrobe sedimentation rate of Fries and Holman's (7) 193 patients was 39 mm/h; it was significantly associated with fevers, fatigue, alopecia, myalgias, and greater disease activity when elevated. Among 163 Italian SLE patients, the mean Westergren sedimentation rate was 37.26 ± 14.21 (1 SD) (123). Sedimentation rates can be high, with no obvious clinical activity, and normal with active disease. They usually are helpful in following the subset of patients for whom its rise and fall reflect other clinical and laboratory parameters. Occasionally, very high sedimentation rates in the absence of other findings lead to the performance of tests that ultimately result in the diagnosis of SLE (124).

The rapid sedimentation rate is partially attributable to the tendency of red cells to clump and form rouleaux, often because of the associated abnormal antibodies in SLE. When the Wintrobe method is used, rapid falling occasionally occurred, and the final value often was limited by the hematocrit. The Westergren method is more precise. [An excellent review of the subject can be found in Bedell and Bush (125).]

C-REACTIVE PROTEIN

C-reactive protein (CRP) is a serum component that binds to pneumococcal C-polysaccharide. It activates complement inhibits cytokine production and generates T-suppressor cells. It is composed of five identical nonglycosylated polypeptide units of 187 amino acid residues each that are noncovalently associated in a disk-like configuration. CRP is synthesized by hepatic parenchymal cells, weighs 120,000 daltons, and circulates in the gamma globulin fraction. It can act as an opsonin or agglutinin, and it mediates phagocytic activities while inhibiting immune responses. A putative evolutionary homology with immunoglobulin, complement, and human leukocyte antigen (HLA) has been suggested (126).

First described as being elevated in patients with SLE and infection by Hill (127) in 1951, other reports suggested that it was an accurate test for active SLE (128–131). Enthusiasm peaked in 1980 when an editorial in the journal *Arthritis and Rheumatism* suggested that it might be a good American Rheumatism Association classification criterion for SLE (132). Other studies, however, found the CRP level to be useful for neither SLE nor infection (133, 134). It soon became apparent that older methods for determining the CRP level were not accurate when rheumatoid factor also was present. Using the more reliable radioimmunodiffusion assay, Rothschild et al. (134) noted it to be elevated in 56% of 52 patients with SLE, with or without infection. It vaguely correlated with clinical activity but not with any organ system involvement, except for leukopenia. Bertouch et al. (135) observed elevated CRP levels in 55 of 70 patients with SLE; it was very high in 13, none of whom had infection. Morrow et al. (136) noted that CRP was present in 59% of 27 patients with SLE, especially in those with active disease. Zein et al. (137) found it in some patients without obvious explanation and observed numerous disease exacerbations in patients without any CRP changes. In another survey, only 9% of 34 patients with SLE had an elevated CRP level (138).

Pepys et al. (139) reviewed the subject at length. One of the strong advocates of its use, this group followed sedimentation rates and CRP binding in 429 measurements involving 124 patients with inactive, mildly active, and active SLE, and in SLE with infection. If one evaluates their data (as opposed to their conclusions), it is clear that the mean CRP level is not elevated, or is only slightly elevated, in the first three categories, but it is high with infection. Mean CRP levels were significantly greater than sedimentation rates with infection but significantly less with active disease. The CRP levels in individual patients with active disease or infection, however, ranged from absent to high. In other words, CRP was not useful in individual cases, although the mean values in patient groups were significantly elevated. The only positive conclusion that can be reached is that if the CRP level is very high (>60 mg/L), the chances of infection are greater (140,141), although Middleton et al. (142) have disputed this. Formiga et al. (143) compared CRPs in 14 infectious episodes vs. 77 lupus disease flares among 50 Spanish patients. Infections were associated with a higher CRP but the differences were not statistically significant. CRP values are high in those with rheumatoid arthritis and the seronegative spondyloarthropathies, but they are only modestly elevated in those with systemic vasculitis.

In conclusion, CRP is a misunderstood test of disease activity that is neither sensitive nor specific in SLE. It may be of some value, however, for ruling in infection and may be of some hitherto undescribed value in following patients with SLE.

β_2-MICROGLOBULIN

β_2-Microglobulin is a single-chain polypeptide (molecular weight, 11,800 daltons) that is found on the surface of most nucleated cells, especially T and B lymphocytes. A normal constituent of serum that is catabolized by the kidney, it is associated with the light chains of class I HLA antigens. Its serum values increase slightly with age and are elevated with decreased glomerular filtration rates and various rheumatic diseases. In SLE sera, anti–β_2-microglobulin antibodies inhibit *in vitro* mitogenic stimulation and lymphocyte proliferation (144). Eight well-designed studies have evaluated its clinical importance in SLE (145–152), and all came to similar conclusions. Overall, it has a 64% sensitivity and 87% specificity for assessing disease activity when compared to healthy controls. β_2-Microglobulin levels are increased with active disease, nephropathy, low C3 complement levels, elevated sedimentation rates, and anti-DNA. Its highest levels are seen in lupus nephritis, although azotemia with inactive disease also can result in larger values.

VISCOSITY AND FIBRINOGEN

Viscosity is an important determinant of blood flow. Plasma viscosity can be increased by elevations of high molecular weight globulins, such as fibrinogen and immunoglobulin. Four studies have shown that patients with SLE have slightly increased levels when compared to control groups (138,152–156). Fibrinogen is also an acute-phase reactant. Its levels also increase with SLE duration and may reflect the prematurity of vascular disease seen in the disorder. Rarely, complexes of IgG, and especially IgM rheumatoid factor, produce high levels of plasma viscosity and a clinical syndrome resembling that found in Waldenström's macroglobulinemia. This so-called hyperviscosity syndrome has been observed infrequently in SLE, and it is an indication for emergency plasmapheresis and steroid therapy (157–159).

MISCELLANEOUS LABORATORY ABNORMALITIES, CONNECTIVE TISSUE COMPONENTS, AND TRACE METALS

SLE is characterized by striking changes in the amorphous ground substance of tissues. Consisting largely of hyaluronic acid and chondroitin sulfuric acid, hexosamine constitutes approximately 40% of each of these mucopolysaccharides, and human serum contains definite amounts of bound hexosamine as glucose and galactosamine. Serum levels of hexosamine were increased in active disease in one report that followed 19 patients serially (160). Free and bound glycosaminoglycans, which consist mostly of slow sulfated chondroitin 4-sulfate, also are elevated with active disease (161). In addition, serum immunoreactive prolyl hydroxylase is an acute-phase reactant in SLE, and its increased levels may reflect greater connective tissue disease metabolism (162). On the other hand, serum sulfhydryl and serum histidine levels decrease in active disease (138,163). Urinary sialyated saccharides, serum sialic acid, and serum amyloid A protein may act as acute-phase reactants in SLE as well (164,165). Serum laminin P1 is one of the glycoproteins of basement membranesis found in high amounts with active disease (166,167). Zinc and selenium levels are normal in SLE (168). Calprotectin (L1 disease (147,148), which is a granulocytic and monocyte cytosolic protein released during activation of these cells, is said to be elevated in SLE (169,170). A marker for adenocarcinoma, CA 19.9, also can be increased with inflammatory joint disease (171), as can the ovarian cancer marker CA 125 (172–174). Several studies have suggested that serum thrombomodulin, a marker for endothelial cell injury, correlates with vasculitis and SLE activity (175–180). Nerve growth factor may be elevated in SLE as well as in rheumatoid arthritis (181, 182). Serum levels of a cytoplasmic enzyme in the pyrimidine salvage pathway, cytodine deaminase, and the enzyme for purine nucleosides, adenosine deaminase, are increased with active lupus as well (183–185). Endothelin-1 is a vasoconstrictor peptide that is present in active SLE in the plasma in high concentrations and may correlate with vascular injury and/or pulmonary hypertension (186,187), as are serum levels of the lysosomal enzyme β-glucuronidase (188) and the serine exoproteinase dipeptidyl peptidase IV (189). Single reports have claimed that cathepsin D activity (190) and plasma neopterin (191), ferritin (192), soluble vascular cell adhesion molecule-1 (VCAM-1) (193), tyrosine kinase receptor (194), matrix metalloproteinase-3 (195), serum levels of HLA class I antigen (196), katacalcin (197), serum leucine aminopeptidase (198), serum 3-nitrotyrosine (199), and plasma thrombospondin levels (200) are increased in SLE.

SUMMARY

1. Hypoalbuminemia occurs in patients with SLE and active disease, particularly nephrosis. Following its level serially is of prognostic value.
2. α_1- and α_2-globulins include acute-phase reactants that are increased and carrier proteins that are decreased in active SLE. β-Lipoprotein levels are elevated with nephrosis and corticosteroid therapy and decreased by antimalarial agents.
3. The IgG level is elevated with disease activity in patients who are not on steroids or immunosuppressive drugs. Its turnover is greatly increased. No IgG subclass is characteristic, and the IgM level is consistently decreased in 20% of patients.
4. Sedimentation rates are elevated with active SLE; disease activity thus can be followed in a subset of patients. In some patients, the sedimentation rate does not correlate with disease activity. The CRP level usually is normal or slightly elevated in SLE; high levels should raise suspicions of infection.
5. β_2-Microglobulin levels generally are increased in active SLE, especially if renal disease is present.
6. Although plasma viscosity is slightly increased in SLE, hyperviscosity syndrome is an extreme rarity.

REFERENCES

1. Coburn AF, Moore DH. The plasma proteins in disseminated lupus erythematosus. *Bull Johns Hopkins Hosp* 1943;73:196–221.
2. Dubois EL, Tuffanelli DL. Clinical manifestations of systemic lupus erythematosus. Computer analysis of 520 cases. *JAMA* 1964;190:104–111.
3. McGehee Harvey A, Shulman LE, Tumulty AP, et al. Systemic lupus erythematosus: review of the literature and clinical analysis of 138 cases. *Medicine* 1954;33:291–437.
4. Ogryzlo MA, Maclachlan M, Dauphinee JA, et al. The serum proteins in health and disease, filter paper electrophoresis. *Am J Med* 1959;27:596–616; *Med Serv J Canada* 1960;16:208–238.
5. Ropes MW. *Systemic lupus erythematosus.* Cambridge, MA: Harvard University Press, 1976.
6. Pollak VE, Mandema E, Doig AB, et al. Observations on electrophoresis of serum proteins from healthy North American Caucasian and Negro subjects and from patients with systemic lupus erythematosus. *J Lab Clin Med* 1961;58:353–365.
7. Fries J, Holman H. *Systemic lupus erythematosus: a clinical analysis.* Philadelphia: WB Saunders, 1975.
8. Niwa Y, Iio A, Niwa G, et al. Serum albumin metabolism in rheumatic diseases: relationship to corticosteroids and peptic ulcer. *J Clin Lab Immunol* 1990;31:11–16.
9. Hochberg MC, Boyd RE, Ahearn JM, et al. Systemic lupus erythematosus: a review of clinico-laboratory features and immunogenetic markers in 150 patients with emphasis on demographic subsets. *Medicine* 1985;64:285–295.
10. Dubois EL, ed. *Lupus erythematosus. A review of the current status of discoid and systemic lupus erythematosus and their variants,* 2nd ed. rev. Los Angeles: USC Press, 1976.
11. Petri M, Ho AC, Patel J, et al. Elevation of maternal alpha-fetoprotein in systemic lupus erythematosus: a controlled study. *J Rheumatol* 1995;22:1365–1368.
12. Denko CW, Gabriel P. Serum proteins-transferrin, ceruloplasmin, albumin, α_1 glycoprotein, and α_1 antitrypsin in rheumatic diseases. *J Rheumatol* 1979;6:664–672.
13. Bereikene IP, Matulis AA, Shevchenko OP, et al. Levels of C4 component of the complement, lactoferrin and leukocytic thermostable alpha glycoprotein during the treatment of patients with systemic rheumatic diseases. *Revmatologiia (Moskva)* 1989; 2:41–45.
14. Sturfelt G, Sjoholm AG. Complement components, complement activation and acute phase response in systemic lupus erythematosus. *Int Arch All Appl Immunol* 1984;75:75–83.
15. Greenspan EM. Survey of clinical significance of serum mucoprotein level. *Arch Intern Med* 1954;93:863–874.
16. Panja RK, Sengupta KP, Aikat BK. Seromucoid in lupus erythematosus scleroderma. *J Clin Pathol* 1964;17:658–659.
17. Gladman D, Urowitz M, Tozman E, et al. Hemostatic abnormalities in systemic lupus erythematosus. *Q J Med* 1983;52: 424–433.
18. Dalqvist SR, Beckman G, Beckman L. Serum protein markers in systemic lupus erythematosus. *Hum Hered* 1988;38:44–47.
19. Zhang XH, Yan YH, Liang ZQ, et al. Changes in neutrophil elastase and alpha 1-antitrypsin in systemic lupus erythematosus. *Proc Chin Acad Med Sci Peking Union Med Coll* 1989;4: 26–29.
20. Breit S, Clark P, Penny R. α_1 Protease inhibitor (1-antitrypsin) phenotypes in rheumatic diseases. *Aust N Z J Med* 1980;10:272.
21. Karsh J, Vergalla J, Jones EA. α_1 antitrypsin phenotypes in rheumatoid arthritis and systemic lupus erythematosus. *Arthritis Rheum* 1979;22:111–113.
22. Eulry F, Demaziere A, Crozes P, et al. Systemic lupus erythematosus with unilateral sacroiliitis, Jaccoud's arthropathy and α_1 antitrypsin deficiency. *Rev Rhum* (English edition) 1994;61: 270–272.
23. Lacki JK, Schochat T, Leszczynski P, et al. IgA-α_1-antitrypsin complex in systemic lupus erythematosus: preliminary report. *Lupus* 1995;4:221–224.
24. Adeyemi EO, Campos LB, Loizou S, et al. Plasma lactoferrin and neutrophil elastase in rheumatoid arthritis and systemic lupus erythematosus. *Br J Rheumatol* 1990;29:15–20.

25. Rees EG, Wilkinson M. Serum proteins in systemic lupus erythematosus. *Br Med J* 1959;5155:795–798.
26. Kalabay L, Jakab L, Cseh K, et al. Correlations between serum alpha 2-HA-glycoprotein and conventional laboratory parameters in systemic lupus erythematosus. *Acta Med Hung* 1990;47: 53–64.
27. Mach PS, Auscher C, Le Go A, et al. Study of alpha 2 macroglobulin, alpha 1 antitrypsin and their antitryptic activity in the serum in rheumatic disease and collagen diseases (in French). *Eur Etud Clin Biol* 1972;17:462–470.
28. Panzironi C, Silvestrini B, Mo MY, et al. An increase in the carbohydrate moiety of α_2-macroglobulin is associated with systemic lupus erythematosus. *Biochem Mol Biol Int* 1997;43: 1305–1322.
29. Yae Y, Inaba S, Sato H, et al. Isolation and characterization of a thermolabile β_2 macroglycoprotein (thermolabile substance or Hakata antigen) detected by precipitating (auto) antibody in sera of patients with systemic lupus erythematosus. *Biochim Biophys Acta* 1991;1078:369–376.
30. Petri M, Roubenoff R, Dallal GE, et al. Plasma homocysteine as a risk factor for atheroembolic events in systemic lupus erythematosus. *Lancet* 1996;348:1120–1124.
31. Pistiner M, Wallace DJ, Nessim S, et al. Lupus erythematosus in the 1980s: a survey of 570 patients. Semin *Arthritis Rheum* 1991;21:55–64.
32. Leong KH, Koh ET, Feng PH, et al. Lipid profiles in patients with systemic lupus erythematosus. *J Rheumatol* 1994;21: 1264–1267.
33. Bruce IN, Urowitz MB, Gladman DD, et al. Natural history of hypercholesterolemia in systemic lupus erythematosus. *J Rheumatol* 1999;26:2137–2143.
34. Borba EF, Bonfa E. Dyslipoproteinemias in systemic lupus erythematosus: influence of disease, activity and anticardiolipin antibodies. *Lupus* 1997;6:533–539.
35. Borba EF, Bonfa E, Vingare CGC, et al. Chylomicron metabolism is markedly altered in systemic lupus erythematosus, *Arthritis Rheum* 2000;43:1033–1040.
36. Ettinger WH, Goldberg AP, Appelbaum-Bowden D, et al. Dyslipoproteinemia in systemic lupus erythematosus. Effects of corticosteroids. *Am J Med* 1987;83:503–508.
37. Ettinger WH, Hazzard WR. Elevated apolipoprotein-B levels in corticosteroid-treated patients with systemic lupus erythematosus. *J Clin Endocrinol Metab* 1988;67:425–428.
38. Aranow C, Enoch L, Barland P. Lipoprotein profiles and corticosteroid treatment in systemic lupus erythematosus. *Arthritis Rheum* 1990;33(suppl):S12(abst).
39. Leong KH, Stirling CA, Reid J, et al. Lipid profiles of 38 SLE patients and their age and gender matched controls. *Br J Rheumatol* 1992;31(suppl):87.
40. Ichikawa Y, Takamatsu K, Shimizu H, et al. Serum apolipoprotein H levels in systemic lupus erythematosus are not influenced by antiphospholipid antibodies. *Lupus* 1992;1:145–149.
41. Alaverson DC, Chase HP. Systemic lupus erythematosus in childhood presenting as hyperlipoproteinemia. *J Pediatr* 1977; 91:72–75.
42. Stern MP, Kilterman OG, McDevitt H, et al. Acquired type 3 hyperlipoproteinemias. *Arch Intern Med* 1972;130:817.
43. Pauciullo P, de Simone B, Rubba P, et al. A case of association between type I hyperlipoproteinemia and systemic lupus erythematosus (SLE). Effects of steroid treatment. *J Endocrinol Invest* 1986;9:517–520.
44. Keane WF, Kasiske BL. Hyperlipidemia in the nephrotic syndrome. *N Engl J Med* 1990;323:603–604.
45. Wanner C, Rader D, Bartens W, et al. Elevated plasma lipotrotein (a) in patients with the nephrotic syndrome. *Ann Intern Med* 1993;119:263–269.
46. Kawai S, Kato M, Asunuma Y, et al. Elevated serum leptin levels in patients with systemic lupus erythematosus. *Arthritis Rheum* 1998;41:S247.
47. Ilowite NT, Samuel P, Ginzler E, et al. Dyslipoproteinemia in pediatric systemic lupus erythematosus. *Arthritis Rheum* 1988; 31:859–863.
48. Urowitz MB, Bookman AAM, Koehler BE, et al. The bimodal mortality pattern of systemic lupus erythematosus. *Am J Med* 1976;60:221–225.
49. Matsuda J, Gotoh M, Gohchi K, et al. Serum lipoprotein (a) level is increased in patients with systemic lupus erythematosus irrespective of positivity of antiphospholipid antibodies. *Thromb Res* 1994;73:84–94.
50. Borba EF, Bonfa E, Vinagre CG, et al. Lipoprotein (a) levels in systemic lupus erythematosus. *J Rheumatol* 1994;21:220–223.
51. Poderbarac T, McPherson R, Goldstein R. Lipid profiles and lipoprotein (a) levels in systemic lupus erythematosus and primary antiphospholipid antibody. *Arthritis Rheum* 1995;38: S169(abst).
52. Kawai S, Mizushima Y, Kaburaki J. Increased serum lipoprotein (a) levels in systemic lupus erythematosus with myocardial and cerebral infarction. *J Rheumatol* 1995;22:1210–1211.
53. Petri M, Miller J, Ebert RF, et al. Lipoprotein A (Lp(a)) is predictive of myocardial infarction in SLE. *Arthritis Rheum* 1995; 38:S220(abst).
54. Lahita RG, Rivkin E, Cavanagh I, et al. Low levels of total cholesterol, high-density lipoprotein, and apolipoprotein A1 in association with anticardiolipin antibodies in patients with systemic lupus erythematosus. *Arthritis Rheum* 1993;36:1566–1574.
55. MacGregor AJ, Dhillon VB, Binder A, et al. Fasting lipids and anticardiolipin antibodies as risk factors for vascular disease in systemic lupus erythematosus. *Ann Rheum Dis* 1992;51:152–155.
56. Vaarala O, Alfthan G, Jauhianen M, et al. Crossreaction between antibodies to oxidised low-density lipoprotein and to cardiolipin in systemic lupus erythematosus. *Lancet* 1993; 341:923–925.
57. Hasunuma Y, Matsuura E, Makita Z, et al. Involvement of β_2-glycoprotein I and anticardiolipin antibodies in oxidatively modified low density protein uptake by macrophages, *Clin Exp Immunol* 1997;107:569–573.
58. Amengual O, Atsumi T, Khamashta MA, et al. Autoantibodies against oxidized low-density lipoprotein in antiphospholipid syndrome. *Br J Rheumatol* 1996;36:964–968.
59. Merrill JT, Rivkin E, Shen C, et al. Selection of a gene for apolipoprotein A1 using autoantibodies from a patient with systemic lupus erythematosus. *Arthritis Rheum* 1995;38: 1655–1659.
60. Dimu AR, Merrill JT, Shen C, et al. Frequency of antibodies to the cholesterol transport protein apolipoprotein A1 in patients with SLE. *Lupus* 1998;7:355–360.
61. Okawa-Takatsuji M, Aotsuka S, Sumiya M, et al. Clinical significance of the serum lipoprotein (a) level in patients with systemic lupus erythematosus: its elevation during disease flare. *Clin Exp Rheumatol* 1996;14:531–536.
62. Kabakov AE, Tertov VV, Saenko VA, et al. The atherogenic effect of lupus sera: systemic lupus erythematosus-derived immune complexes stimulate the accumulation of cholesterol in cultured smooth muscle cells from human aorta. *Clin Immunol Immunopathol* 1992;63:214–220.
63. MacGregor AJ, Dhillon VB, Binder A, et al. Fasting lipids and anticardiolipin antibodies as risk factors for vascular disease in systemic lupus erythematosus. *Ann Rheum Dis* 1992;51:152–155.
64. Wallace DJ, Metzger AL, Stecher VJ, et al. Cholesterol-lowering effect of hydroxychloroquine in patients with rheumatic disease: reversal of deleterious effects of steroids on lipids. *Am J Med* 1990;89:322–326.

65. Hodis HN, Quismorio FP Jr, Wickham E, et al. The lipid, lipoprotein and apolipoprotein effects of hydroxychloroquine in patients with systemic lupus erythematosus. *J Rheumatol* 1993; 20:661–665.
66. Petri M, Lakatta C, Magder L, et al. Effect of prednisone and hydroxychloroquine upon hydroxychloroquine on coronary artery disease risk factors in systemic lupus erythematosus:a longitudinal data analysis. *Am J Med* 1994;96:254–259.
67. Scott D, Crawford K, Pucino F, et al. Treatment of hypercholesterolemia in systemic lupus with lovastatin. *Arthritis Rheum* 1992;35:S329(abst).
68. Hearth-Holmes M, Broadwell L, Baethge BA, et al. Treatment of hyperlipidemia with gemfibrozil in patients with systemic lupus erythematosus. *Arthritis Rheum* 1992;35:S153(abst).
69. Hearth-Holmes M, Baethge BA, Broadwell L, et al. Dietary treatment of hyperlipidemia in patients with systemic lupus erythematosus. *J Rheumatol* 1995;22:450–454.
70. Estes D, Christian CL. The natural history of systemic lupus erythematosus by prospective analysis. *Medicine* 1971;50: 85–95.
71. Rothfield N. Systemic lupus erythematosus. Clinical and laboratory aspects. In: McCarty D, ed. *Arthritis and allied conditions*, 9th ed. Philadelphia: Lea & Febiger, 1979:691–715.
72. Feldaker M, Brunsting LA, McKenzie BF. Paper electrophoresis of serum proteins in selected dermatoses. *J Invest Dermatol* 1956;26:293–310.
73. Seligmann M. Demonstration in the blood of patients with disseminated lupus erythematosus a substance determining a precipitation reaction with desoxyribonucleic acid. *C Rend Acad Sci (Paris)* 1957;244:243–245.
74. Ashman RF, White RH, Wiesenhutter C, et al. Panhypogammaglobulinemia in systemic lupus erythematosus: in vitro demonstration of multiple cellular defects. *J Allergy Clin Immunol* 1982;70:465–473.
75. Baum CG, Chiorazzi N, Frankel S, et al. Conversion of systemic lupus erythematosus to common variable hypogammaglobulinemia. *Am J Med* 1989;87:449–456.
76. Epstein RJ, Ogler RF, Gatenby PA. Lupus erythematosus and panhypogammaglobulinemia. *Ann Intern Med* 1984;100: 162–163.
77. Goldstein R, Izaguirre C, Smith CD, et al. Systemic lupus erythematosus and common absence of circulating B cells. *Arthritis Rheum* 1985;28:100–103.
78. Haserick JR. Modern concepts of systemic lupus erythematosus: review of 126 cases. *J Chronic Dis* 1955;1:317–334.
79. Stein A, Winkelstein A, Agarwal A. Concurrent systemic lupus erythematous and common variable hypogammaglobulinemia. *Arthritis Rheum* 1985;28:462–465.
80. Sussman GL, Rivera VJ, Kohler PF. Transition form systemic lupus erythematosus to common variable hypogammaglobulinema. *Ann Intern Med* 1986;99:32–35.
81. Weinstock I, Lee SL. Hypogammaglobulinemia in systemic lupus erythematosus: report of a case in a nine-year-old child. *J Dis Child* 1960;99:242–247.
82. Peral V, Vidau P, Herrera J, et al. Development of panhypogammaglobulinemia in a patient with systemic lupus erythematosus. *Nephrol Dial Transplant* 1994;9:709–712.
83. Alarcon-Segovia D, Fishbein E. Serum immunoglobulins in systemic lupus erythematosus. *Clin Sci* 1972;43:121–131.
84. Cass RM, Mongan ES, Jacox RF, et al. Immunoglobulins G, A, and M in systemic lupus erythematosus. Relationship to serum complement titer, latex titer, antinuclear antibody, and manifestations of clinical disease. *Ann Intern Med* 1968;69:749–756.
85. Schoenfeld Y, Pick AL, Danziger Y, et al. Immunoglobulin changes in systemic lupus erythematosus. *Ann Allergy* 1977;39: 99–111.
86. Levy G. Clinical pharmacokinetics of aspirin. *Pediatrics* 1978; 62:867–872.
87. Cronin ME, Balow JE, Tsokos GC. Immunoglobulin deficiency in patients with systemic lupus erythematosus. *Clin Exp Rheumatol* 1989;7:359–364.
88. Ward MM, Dawson DV, Pisetsky DS. Serum immunoglobulin levels in systemic lupus erythematosus: the effects of age, sex, race and disease duration. *J Rheumatol* 1991;18:540–544.
89. Olson NY, Lindsley CB, Peter JB. Immunoglobulin G subclasses in childhood systemic lupus erythematosus and systemic onset juvenile rheumatoid arthritis. *Arthritis Rheum* 1988;31 (suppl):R28(abst).
90. Tokano Y, Yagita H, Iida N, et al. Relation between the level of IgG subclasses and infections in patients with systemic lupus erythematosus. *Int Arch Allergy Appl Immunol* 1988;87:55–58.
91. Blanco F, Kalsi J, Ravirajan CT, et al. IgG subclasses in systemic lupus erythematosus and other autoimmune diseases. *Lupus* 1992;1:391–399.
92. Kay RA, Wood KJ, Bernstein RM, et al. An IgG subclass imbalance in connective tissue disease. *Ann Rheum Dis* 1988;47: 536–541.
93. Saiki O, Saeki Y, Tanaka T, et al. Development of selective IgM deficiency in systemic lupus erythematosus patients with disease of long duration. *Arthritis Rheum* 1987;30:1289–1292.
94. Senaldi G, Ireland R, Bellingham AJ, et al. IgM reduction in systemic lupus erythematosus. *Arthritis Rheum* 1988;31:12–13.
95. Sivri A, Hascelik Z. IgM deficiency in systemic lupus erythematosus. *Arthritis Rheum* 1995;38:1713–1714.
96. Stage DE, Mannik M. 7S gamma M-globulin in rheumatoid arthritis. Evaluation of its clinical significance. *Arthritis Rheum* 1971;14:400–450.
97. Rothfield NF. Current approaches to SLE and its subsets. *DM* 1982;29:162.
98. Kaufman LD, Heinicke MH, Hamburger M, et al. Male lupus: prevalence of IgA deficiency, 7S IgM and abnormalities of Fc-receptor function. *Clin Exp Rheumatol* 1991;9:265–269.
99. Roberts-Thompson PJ, Shepherd K, Bradley J, et al. Frequency and role of low molecular weight IgM in systemic lupus erythematosus. Study of patients from different ethnic origins. *Rheumatol Int* 1990;10:95–98.
100. Arai J, Yasukawa M, Takada K, et al. Non-X-linked hyper-IgM syndrome with systemic lupus erythematosus. *Clin Exp Rheumatol* 1998;16:84–86.
101. Kustimur S, Gulmezoglu E. Selective IgA deficiency in patients with systemic lupus erythematosus and rheumatoid arthritis. *Mikrobiyol Bul* 1985;19:190–199.
102. Rifle G, Bielfeld P, Chalopin JM, et al. Selective IgA deficiency and systemic lupus erythematosus. *Ann Med Interne (Paris)* 1988;139:134–137.
103. Carpenter M, Singleton JD, West SG. Systemic lupus erythematosus is not associated with selective immunoglobulin A deficiency. *Arthritis Rheum* 1993:36(suppl):R7(abst).
104. Erkeller-Yuskel FM, Rankin L, Isenberg DA. IgA deficiency: a predisposing factor for SLE? *Br J Rheumatol* 1993;32(suppl): 5(abst).
105. Rankin ECC, Isenberg DA. IgA deficiency and SLE: prevalence in a clinical population and a review of the literature, *Lupus* 1997;6:390–394.
106. Tomasi TB. The gamma A globulins: first line of defense. *Hosp Pract* 1967;2:26–35.
107. Conley ME, Coopman WJ. Serum IgA1 and IgA2 in normal adults and patients with systemic lupus erythematosus and hepatic disease. *Arthritis Rheum* 1983;26:390–397.
108. Goldman JA, Klimek GA, Ali R. Allergy in systemic lupus erythematosus, IgE levels and reaginic phenomenon. *Arthritis Rheum* 1976;19:669–676.

109. Rubin L, Urowitz MB, Pruzanski W. Systemic lupus erythematosus with paraproteinemia. *Arthritis Rheum* 1984;27:638–644.
110. Elkayam O, Tamir R, Pick AI, et al. Serum IgE concentrations, disease activity and atopic disorders in systemic lupus erythematosus. *Allergy* 1995;50:94–96.
111. Leyh F, Wendt V, Schever R. Systemic lupus erythematosus and hyperimmunoglobulinemia E syndrome in a 13 year old girl. *Zitautkr* 1985;61:611–614.
112. Schofer K, Feldges A, Baelocher K, et al. Systemic lupus erythematosus in *Staphylococcus aureus* hyperimmunoglobulinemia E syndrome. *Br Med J* 1983;287:524–526.
113. North J, Kotecha S, Houtman P, et al. Systemic lupus erythematosus complicating hyper IgE syndrome. *Br J Rheumatol* 1997;36:298–299.
114. Brugnoni D, Francheshini F, Airo P, et al. Discordance for systemic lupus erythematosus an hyper IgE syndrome in a pair of monozygotic twins. *Br J Rheumatol* 1998;37:807–808.
115. Rebhun J, Quismorio FP Jr, Dubois EL, et al. Systemic lupus erythematosus activity and IgE. *Ann Allergy* 1983;50:34–36.
116. Porcel JM, Ordl J, Tolosa C, et al. Monoclonal gammopathy in systemic lupus erythematosus. *Lupus* 1992;1:263–264.
117. Font J, Cervera R, Pallares L, et al. Systemic lupus erythematosus and monoclonal gammopathy. *Br J Rheumatol* 1988;27: 412–413.
118. Lam CW, Chul SH, Leung NW, et al. Light chain ratios of serum immunoglobulins in disease. *Clin Biochem* 1991;24: 283–287.
119. Epstein WV, Tan M. Increased of L-chain proteins in the sera of patients with systemic lupus erythematosus and the synovial fluids of patients with peripheral rheumatoid arthritis. *Arthritis Rheum* 1966;9:713–719.
120. Hooper JE, Sequeira W, Martellotto JN, et al. Clinical relapse in systemic lupus erythematosus: correlation with antecedent elevation of urinary free light chain immunoglobulin. *J Clin Immunol* 1989;9:338–350.
121. Tsai C-Y, Wu T-H, Sun K-H, et al. Increased excretion of soluble interleukin 2 receptors and free light chain immunoglobulins in the urine of patients with active lupus nephritis. *Ann Rheum Dis* 1992;51:168–172.
122. Arman-Cruz R, Harnecker J, Ducach G, et al. Clinical diagnosis of systemic lupus erythematosus. *Am J Med* 1958;25: 409–419.
123. Giacomello A, Quarantino CP, Zoppini A. Erythrocyte sedimentation rate within rheumatic disease clinics. *J Rheumatol* 1997;24:2263–2265.
124. Roche NF, Cohen MD, Persillin ST, et al. Elevated sedimentation rate (ESR) of 100/mm hr or more in a tertiary outpatient setting. *Arthritis Rheum* 1993;36(suppl):S116(abst).
125. Bedell SE, Bush BT. Erythrocyte sedimentation rate: from folklore to facts. *Am J Med* 1985;78:1001–1009.
126. Kinsella TD, Fritzler MJ. CRP: an immunoregulatory protein. *J Rheumatol* 1980;7:272–274.
127. Hill AGS. C-reactive protein in the chronic rheumatic diseases. *Lancet* 1951;261:807–811.
128. Becker GJ, Waldburger M, Hughes GR, et al. Value of serum C-reactive protein measurement in the investigation of fever in systemic lupus erythematosus. *Ann Rheum Dis* 1980;39:50–52.
129. Bravo MG, Alarcon-Segovia D. C reactive protein in the differential diagnosis between infection and disease reactivation in SLE. *J Rheumatol* 1981;8:291–294.
130. Honig S, Gorevic P, Weissmann G. C-reactive protein in systemic lupus erythematosus. *Arthritis Rheum* 1977;20:1065–1070.
131. Shetlar MR, Payne RW, Padron J, et al. Objective evaluation of patients with rheumatic diseases. I. Comparison of serum glycoprotein, cold hemagglutination, C-reactive protein and other tests with clinical evaluation. *J Lab Clin Med* 1956;48:94–200.
132. de Silva JA, Elkon KB, Hughes GR, et al. C-reactive protein levels in systemic lupus erythematosus: a classification criterion. *Arthritis Rheum* 1980;23:770–771.
133. Lauter SA, Espinoza LR, Osterland CK. The relationship between C-reactive protein and systemic lupus erythematosus. *Arthritis Rheum* 1979;22:1421–1424.
134. Rothschild BM, James KK, Jones JV, et al. Significance of elevated C-reactive protein in patients with SLE. *Arthritis Rheum* 1982;25(suppl):S82.
135. Bertouch JV, Roberts-Thompson PJ, Feng PH, et al. C-reactive protein and serologic indices of disease activity in systemic lupus erythematosus. *Ann Rheum Dis* 1983;42:655–658.
136. Morrow WJW, Isenberg DA, Parry HF, et al. C-reactive protein in sera from patients with systemic lupus erythematosus. *J Rheumatol* 1981;8:599–604.
137. Zein N, Ganuza C, Kushner I. Significance of C-reactive protein elevation in patients with systemic lupus erythematosus. *Arthritis Rheum* 1979;22:7–12.
138. Sitton NG, Dixon JS, Bird HA, et al. Serum biochemistry in rheumatoid arthritis, seronegative arthropathies, osteoarthritis, SLE and normal subjects. *Br J Rheumatol* 1987;26:131–135.
139. Pepys MB, Lanham JG, deBeer FC. C-reactive protein in SLE. *Clin Rheum Dis* 1982;8:91–103.
140. Hind CRK, Ng SC, Feng PH, et al. Serum C-reactive protein measurement in the detection of intercurrent infection in Oriental patients with systemic lupus erythematosus. *Ann Rheum Dis* 1985;44:260–261.
141. ter Borg EJ, Horst G, Limburg PC, et al. C-reactive protein levels during disease exacerbations and infections in systemic lupus erythematosus: a prospective longitudinal study. *J Rheumatol* 1990;17:1642–1648.
142. Middleton GD, McFarlin JE, Sipe JD, et al. C-reactive protein and systemic lupus erythematosus: elevation does not predict infection. *Arthritis Rheum* 1994;37(suppl):S321(abst).
143. Formiga F, Moga I, Pac M, et al. Is C-reactive protein useful in differentiating infection from disease exacerbation in systemic lupus erythematosus patients? *J Clin Rheumatol* 1998;4:177–180.
144. Meryhew NL, Zoschke DC, Messner RP. Anti β_2 microglobulin antibodies in systemic lupus erythematosus and ankylosing spondylitis: effects on in vitro lymphocyte function. *J Rheumatol* 1986;13:83–89.
145. Ervin PE, Strom T. β_2 Microglobulin and its binding activity in serum from patients with SLE. *Ann Rheum Dis* 1984;43: 267–274.
146. Falus A, Merety G, Glickman G, et al. β_2 Microglobulin containing IgG complexes in sera and synovial fluids of rheumatoid arthritis and systemic lupus erythematosus. *Scand J Immunol* 1980;13:25–34.
147. Font J, Coca A, Molina R, et al. Serum β_2 microglobulin as a marker of activity in systemic lupus erythematosus. *Scand J Rheumatol* 1986;15:201–205.
148. Konenkov VI, Prokofiev VF, Yu I, et al. Changes in the level of soluble HLA antigens and their light chains (β_2 microglobulin) in rheumatoid arthritis and systemic lupus erythematosus. *Ter Arkh*1986;7:57–59.
149. Valencia ME, Molano J, Vazquez JJ, et al. Determining β_2 macroglobulin levels in patients with systemic lupus erythematosus. A clinical and biochemical correlation. *Rev Clin Esp* 1987;181:310–313.
150. Weissel M, Scherak O, Fritzsche H, et al. Serum β_2 microglobulin and SLE. *Arthritis Rheum* 1976;19:968–972.
151. Yeung CK, Wong KL, Wong WS, et al. β_2 Microglobulin and systemic lupus erythematosus. *J Rheumatol* 1986;13:1053–1058.
152. Kochen J de A, Nobre MR, de Oliviera RM, et al. Anti β_2-microglobin antibodies in systemic lupus erythematosus. *Rev Hosp Clin Fac Sao Paolo* 1997;52:63–71.

153. Hazelton RA, Lowe GD, Forbes CD, et al. Increased blood and plasma viscosity in systemic lupus erythematosus. *J Rheumatol* 1985;12:616–617.
154. Ernst E, Hein A, Meuer M, et al. Blood rheology in lupus erythematosus. *Ann Rheum Dis* 1991;50:710–712
155. Reid HL, de Ceulaer K. Abnormal plasma and serum viscosity in systemic lupus erythematosus(SLE): a Jamaican study, *Clin Hemorheology Microcirc* 1999;20:175–180.
156. Ames PRJ, Alves J, Pap AF, et al. Fibrinogen in systemic lupus erythematosus: more than an acute phase reactant. *J Rheumatol* 2000;27:1190–1195.
157. Adoue D, Arlet P, Duffaut M, et al. Major hyprotidemia (sic) with serum viscosity in systemic lupus erythematosus. *Sem Hop Paris* 1986;62:1261–1264.
158. Fukasawa T, Arai T, Naruse T, et al. Hyperviscosity syndrome in a patient with systemic lupus erythematosus. *Am J Med Sci* 1977;273:329–334.
159. Jara LJ, Capin NR, Lavalle C. Hyperviscosity syndrome as the initial manifestation of systemic lupus erythematosus. *J Rheumatol* 1989;16:225–230.
160. Boas NF, Soffer LJ. Hexosamine level in lupus erythematosus. *Nutr Rev* 1951;9:219.
161. Friman C, Nordstrom D, Eronen I. Plasma glycosaminoglycans in systemic lupus erythematosus. *J Rheumatol* 1987;14: 1132–1134.
162. Kutti-Sarolainen ER, Kivirikko KI, Laitinen O. Serum immunoreactive propyl hydroxylase in inflammatory rheumatic diseases. *Ann Rheum Dis* 1980;39:217–221.
163. Lorber A, Bovy RA, Chang CC. Sulfhydryl deficiency in connective tissue disorders: correlation with disease activity and protein alterations. *Metabolism* 1971;20:446–455.
164. Maury CP, Teppo AM, Wegelius O. Relationship between urinary sialylated saccharides, serum amyloid A protein and C-reactive protein in rheumatoid arthritis and systemic lupus erythematosus. *Ann Rheum Dis* 1982;41:268–271.
165. Ota T, Uemura A, Eto S, et al. Clinical significance of serum sialic acid in rheumatoid arthritis and systemic lupus erythematosus. *Sangyo Ika Daigaku Zasshi* 1985;7:401–407.
166. Schneider M, Hengst K, Waldendorf M, et al. The value of serum laminin Pl in monitoring disease activity in patients with systemic lupus erythematosus. *Scand J Rheumatol* 1988;17: 417–422.
167. D'Cruz D, Schneider M, Khamashta MA, et al. Lamin P1 levels in lupus nephritis. *Arthritis Rheum* 1992;35(suppl):S109 (abst).
168. Almroth G, Westberg NG, Sandstrom BM. Normal zinc and selenium levels in patients with systemic lupus erythematosus. *J Rheumatol* 1985;12:633–634.
169. Haga H-J, Brun JG, Berntzen HB, et al. Calprotectin in patients with systemic lupus erythematosus: relation to clinical and laboratory parameters of disease activity. *Lupus* 1993;2: 47–50.
170. Routsias JG, Tzioufas AG, Sakarellos-Daitsiotis M, et al. Calreticulin synthetic peptide analogues: anti-peptide antibodies in autoimmune rheumatic diseases. *Clin Exp Immunol* 1993;91: 437–441.
171. Cantagrel A, Moulinier L, Belho K, et al. Elevated 19.9 levels in inflammatory joint disease with immune dysfunction (a report of 6 cases). *Rev Rhum* (English edition) 1994;61:530–536.
172. Moncayo R, Moncayo H. Serum levels of CA 125 are elevated in patients with active systemic lupus erythematosus. *Obstet Gynecol* 1991;77:932–934.
173. Miret C, Font J, Molina R, et al. Lack of correlation between tumor markers (CA 125 and SCC) and systemic lupus activity. *Anticancer Res* 1998;18:1341–1344.
174. Yucel AE, Calguneri M, Ruacan S. False positive pleural biopsy and CA 125 levels in serum and pleural effusion in systemic lupus erythematosus. *Clin Rheumatol* 1996;15:295–297.
175. Boehme MWJ, Nawroth PP, Kling E, et al. Serum thrombomodulin. A novel marker of disease activity in systemic lupus erythematosus. *Arthritis Rheum* 1994;37:572–577.
176. Ohdama S, Yoshizawa Y, Kubota T, et al. Plasma thrombomodulin as an indicator of thromboembolic disease in systemic lupus erythematosus. *Int J Cardiol* 1994;47(suppl):S1S6.
177. Hsu C-D, Chan DW, Iriye B, et al. Plasma thrombomodulin levels in women with systemic lupus erythematosus. *Am J Perinatol* 1995;12:27–29.
178. Mercie P, Seigneur M, Conri C, et al. Circulating thrombomodulin, a marker of acute systemic lupus erythematosus. *Presse Med* 1994;23:1450.
179. Cucurull E, Gharavi AE. Thrombomodulin: a new frontier for lupus research? *Clin Exp Rheumatol* 1997;15:1–4.
180. Kotajima L, Aotsuka S, Sato T. Clinical significance of serum thrombomodulin levels in patients with systemic rheumatic diseases. *Clin Exp Rheumatol* 1997;15:59–65.
181. Bracci-Lauiero L, Aloe L, Levi-Montalcini R, et al. Increased levels of NGF in sera of systemic lupus erythematosus patients. *Neuroreport* 1993;4:563–565.
182. Dicou E, Masson C, Jabbour W, et al. Increased frequency of NGF in sera of rheumatoid arthritis and systemic lupus erythematosus patients. *Neuroreport* 1993;5:321–324.
183. Skeith KJ, Wefuan J, Oswald R, et al. Serum cytidine deaminase as a measure of disease activity in rheumatoid arthritis and systemic lupus erythematosus. *J Rheumatol* 1993;20:1309–1315.
184. Nalini G, Hariprasad C, Chandrasekaran AN, et al. A comparative study of serum deaminases in systemic lupus erythematosus. *Br J Rheumatol* 1993;32:1118–1119.
185. Stancikova M, Lukac J, Istok R, et al. Serum adenosine deaminase activity and its isoenzyme pattern in patients with systemic lupus erythematosus. *Clin Exp Rheumatol* 1998;16:583–586.
186. Julkunen H, Saijonmaa O, Gronhagen-Riska C, et al. Raised plasma concentrations of endothelin-1 in systemic lupus erythematosus. *Ann Rheum Dis* 1991;50:526–527.
187. Yoshio T, Masuyama J, Mimori A, et al. Endothelin-1 release from cultured endothelial cells induced by sera from patients with systemic lupus erythematosus. *Ann Rheum Dis* 1995;54: 361–365.
188. Falkenback A, Unkelbach U, Gottschalk R, et al. Serum levels of beta-glucuronidase as potential indicator of disease activity in rheumatoid arthritis and systemic lupus erythematodes. *Med Klin* 1991;86:465–468.
189. Stancikova M, Lojda Z, Lukac J, et al. Dipeptidyl peptidase IV in patients with systemic lupus erythematosus. *Clin Exp Rheumatol* 1992;10:381–385.
190. Phi NC, Chien DK, Binh VV, et al. Cathepsin D-like activity in serum of patients with systemic lupus erythematosus. *J Lab Clin Immunol* 1990;29:185–188.
191. Hagihara M, Nagatsu T, Ohashi M, et al. Concentrations of neopterin and biopterin in serum from patients with rheumatoid arthritis or systemic lupus erythematosus and in synovial fluids from patients with rheumatoid or osteoarthritis. *Clin Chem* 1990;36:705.
192. Nishiya K, Hashimoto K. Elevation of serum ferritin levels as a marker for active systemic lupus erythematosus. *Clin Exp Rheumatol* 1997;15:39–44.
193. Ikeda Y, Fujimoto T, Ameno M, et al. Relationship between lupus nephritis activity and the serum level of soluble VCAM-1. *Lupus* 1997;7:347–354.
194. Kitoh T, Ishikawa H, Sawada S, et al. Significance of stem cell factor and soluble KIT in patients with systemic lupus erythematosus. *Clin Rheumatol* 1998;17:293–300.
195. Kotajima L, Aotsuka S, Fujimani M, et al. Increased levels of

matrix metalloproteinase-3 in sera from patients with active lupus nephritis. *Clin Exp Rheumatol* 1998;16:409–415.

196. Tsuchiya N, Shiota M, Yamaguchi A, et al. Elevated serum level of soluble HLA Class I antigens in patients with systemic lupus erythematosus. *Arthritis Rheum* 1996;39:792–796.
197. Navarro MA, Formiga F, Blanco A, et al. PDN-21 in premenopausal women with systemic lupus erythematosus treated with glucocorticoids. *J Rheumatol* 1995;22:2238–2230.
198. Inokuma S, Setoguchi K, Ohta T, et al. Serum leucine aminopeptidase as an activity indicator in systemic lupus erythematosus: a study of 46 consecutive cases. *Rheumatology* 1999;38:705–708.
199. Oates JC, Christensen EF, Reilly CM, et al. Prospective measure of serum 3-nitrotyrosine levels in systemic lupus erythematosus: correlation with disease activity. *Proc Assoc Am Phys* 1999;111: 611–621.
200. Huang S-W, Kao K-J. Plasma thrombospondin measurement in clinical practice. *Intern Med* 1990;11:52–70.

45

CLINICAL APPLICATION OF SEROLOGIC ABNORMALITIES IN SYSTEMIC LUPUS ERYTHEMATOSUS

FRANCISCO P. QUISMORIO, JR.

One hallmark of systemic lupus erythematosus (SLE) is the wide array of serologic abnormalities, including a polyclonal increase in serum gamma globulins, the presence of antinuclear antibodies (ANAs) and various serum organ-specific and nonorgan-specific autoantibodies, circulating immune complexes, and serum complement changes. The presence of some of these abnormalities is important in corroborating the clinical diagnosis of SLE, whereas others are useful in monitoring disease activity. Each abnormality is discussed in a separate chapter. This chapter focuses on the clinical application of selected serologic abnormalities in establishing the diagnosis, in assessing disease activity, and in predicting specific organ-system involvement and overall prognosis of the patient. Only serologic tests that generally are available in most clinical laboratories are included.

SEROLOGIC TESTS

Diagnosis Of Systemic Lupus Erythematosus

When the diagnosis of SLE is suspected or made on clinical grounds, the following serologic tests are considered to be helpful in corroborating the diagnosis (Table 45.1): fluorescent ANA test, ANA panel, serum-complement level, and Venereal Disease Research Laboratories (VDRL) or other comparable serologic test for syphilis. In certain situations, other serologic tests also are applicable, such as the Coombs' test in a patient presenting with hemolytic anemia, lupus anticoagulant test, and anticardiolipin antibody test in a patient with a history of thrombosis or multiple fetal loss.

Virtually all patients with active and untreated SLE test positive for ANA. Nevertheless, ANA is prevalent in other rheumatic and nonrheumatic disorders as well, including some conditions that may mimic the clinical picture of SLE. ANA also is found in healthy children and adults (1). Thus, by itself, a positive ANA has a low diagnostic specificity for the disease, but its value increases when the patient meets the clinical criteria for SLE. The indirect immunofluorescent test is the most commonly used method for detecting ANA, and the choice of substrate in this test is important. Sections of rodent liver or kidney and tissue culture cell lines (Hep-2 or KB cells) are used in most clinical laboratories. Certain types of ANA, such as anti-Ro/SSa and anticentromere antibodies, can be detected with these cell lines but not with rodent tissues (2). A positive serum should be titered to give a semiquantitative value to the antibody level. The fluorescent staining pattern also should be included, but in the presence of multiple types of ANA, the staining pattern may change as the serum is titered.

Test for ANA is a useful screening test when there is a high index of suspicion of SLE or other systemic rheumatic conditions. However, it should be noted that ANA can be seen in a number of nonrheumatic conditions as well as in some healthy individuals (3–5). A study of the clinical utility of ANA testing in a large teaching hospital revealed a high sensitivity of a positive ANA for SLE; however, the predictive value was low for SLE and for other systemic rheumatic diseases (6). Malleson et al. (7) concluded in a study of a pediatric population that a positive ANA test is a poor predictor of SLE or mixed connective tissue disease (MCTD). Many children with a positive ANA in their study did not have a rheumatic disease. The clinician should rec-

TABLE 45.1. SEROLOGIC TESTS USEFUL IN THE DIAGNOSIS OF SYSTEMIC LUPUS ERYTHEMATOSUS

1. Fluorescent antinuclear antibody (ANA)
2. ANA panel: anti-ds DNA, anti-Sm, anti-U1RNP, anti-Ro/SSA, anti-La/SSB
3. Serum complement level
4. VDRL
5. Anticardiolipin antibodies
6. Lupus anticoagulant
7. Coombs' test

ds DNA, double-stranded DNA; VDRL, Venereal Disease Research Laboratories.

ognize the significant limitations of a positive ANA when the patient in question does not have clinical features suggestive of SLE or other connective-tissue disease.

The ANA panel that is available in clinical laboratories includes ANA of defined specificity: anti–double-stranded DNA (anti-dsDNA), anti-Sm, anti-U1 RNP, anti-Ro/SSA, and anti-La/SSB. Some laboratories include antinucleoprotein, anticentromere, antihistone, and/or anti–single-stranded DNA (anti-ssDNA) in their panel. When the fluorescent ANA is positive in a patient who is suspected of having SLE, an ANA panel should be obtained. Anti-dsDNA and anti-Sm antibodies are considered to be highly diagnostic, and their presence almost confirms the clinical diagnosis. The other types of ANA in the panel have lesser value as diagnostic markers for SLE, except in special situations such as the presence of anti-Ro/SSa antibody in a patient with subacute cutaneous LE (SCLE) (individual ANA types are discussed later) or ANA-negative lupus.

The serum complement level generally is measured as concentration of C3 or C4, or as CH′50 or CH′100 hemolytic units. Although more commonly used in assessing disease activity, the presence of both hypocomplementemia and high titers of anti-dsDNA in a patient who is suspected of having SLE almost confirms diagnosis of the disease (8). In addition, a genetic deficiency of C1q, C2, or C4 may present clinically with an LE-like syndrome, and the combination of a low or absent CH50 and normal C3 level should raise the possibility of this diagnosis (9).

A biologic false-positive test for syphilis is one of the four immunologic abnormalities that are included in the American College of Rheumatology (ACR) criteria for the classification of SLE. Other antiphospholipid antibodies including the lupus anticoagulant and anticardiolipin antibodies are helpful in delineating a subset of patients who are prone to develop recurrent arterial or venous thrombosis and/or fetal loss (antiphospholipid syndrome).

Monitoring Disease Activity In Systemic Lupus Erythematosus

Serologic tests are widely used for assessing disease activity and predicting exacerbations (Table 45.2). Determinations of the serum titer of anti-dsDNA and of the complement level are the most common and, probably, the most useful serologic tests that are readily available to the clinician. Although applicable to most patients, both tests have important limitations. Anti-dsDNA antibodies and hypocomplementemia do not occur in all patients, and their correlation with disease activity is not absolute. A few patients can have persistently elevated anti-dsDNA antibody titers without developing evidence of clinical disease, even when followed for several months (10, 11). Serial measurement of the serum titer of anti-Sm and anti-Ro/SSA antibodies can be useful, particularly in those who test negative for anti-dsDNA antibodies.

TABLE 45.2. SEROLOGIC TESTS FOR ASSESSING DISEASE ACTIVITY IN SLE

1. Anti-double-stranded DNA antibodies
2. Serum complement level: C3, C4, C;prH50
3. Anti-Sm and other specific types of antinuclear antibody
4. Split products of complement
5. Circulating immune complexes
6. Serum cryoglobulins
7. Serum level of sIL-2R, adhesion molecules, cytokines

In analyzing reports about the predictive value of various serologic tests in SLE, several points should be stressed. The selection of patients varies widely, and the clinical criteria that are used to define active SLE are not uniform. The effect of previous or current drug therapy frequently is not addressed. Most studies are cross-sectional, comparing groups of patients, and only a few are well-designed, long-term, prospective studies. Conclusions often are derived from a single serum determination rather than from multiple specimens over a period of time. Different test systems are used by various investigators to measure a given serologic parameter. Thus, comparison of the results of various studies is not always feasible or appropriate. The use of uniform activity indices (e.g., SLAM and SLEDAI indices) in future prospective studies will help to correct these deficiencies.

Serologic abnormalities do not always occur before or during disease exacerbations, especially in clinically mild flare-ups. In a well-designed prospective cohort study of 185 patients with SLE, Petri et al. (12) demonstrated that lupus flare is quantifiable and that the incidence of a disease flare was approximately 0.65 per patient-year of follow-up. Most of the flares were minor, manifesting as fatigue, other constitutional symptoms, mucocutaneous lesions, and musculoskeletal complaints. Only ten of the flares were associated with the new appearance of anti-dsDNA antibodies, and only 17 with an increase in antibody titer. Depression of C3 and C4 were observed in 44 and 41 of the disease flares, respectively.

We, and others, have found the concentration of serum cryoglobulins to be a useful parameter that correlates with disease activity, especially in those with nephritis (13–16). Although technically simple, it is labor-intensive. Measurement of cryoglobulins requires careful handling of the specimen for proper interpretation of the results. Venous blood is allowed to clot at 37°C immediately after venipuncture. Following incubation at 4°C for 48 hours, the specimen is centrifuged in the cold and the precipitate saved. The precipitate is washed carefully with a low-ionic phosphate buffer, and the protein concentration is measured by standard methods.

The role of circulating immune complexes in monitoring disease activity in SLE remains controversial and unproven (17). The lack of a widely accepted standardized test system, the heterogeneity of immune complexes in SLE sera (18, 19), and the imprecise and inconsistent correlation with disease activity limit the application of circulating immune complexes in following the clinical course of the disease in individual patients. Of the numerous serologic tests for circulating immune complexes, the C1q solid-phase binding assay appears to be the most frequently used method in patients with SLE (20–24).

Two serologic tests with promising value are the measurements of products of complement activation and of soluble IL-2 receptors (25,26).

CLINICAL SIGNIFICANCE OF THE ANTI-DNA ANTIBODY

Diagnostic Value

Antibodies to DNA are classified according to their reactivity to native or double-stranded anti-dsDNA or to denatured or anti-ssDNA. The presence of anti-dsDNA is highly characteristic of idiopathic SLE and rarely is seen in other rheumatic conditions, including drug-induced LE (27,28). One of the four immunologic criteria for the classification of SLE by the ACR is the presence of anti-dsDNA. In contrast, anti-ssDNA antibodies, although prevalent in SLE, are found in many other disorders, including rheumatic and nonrheumatic conditions (29). Thus, in the clinical laboratory, anti-dsDNA, but not anti-ssDNA antibodies, is tested for routinely in the ANA panel.

In a large cohort prospective study, Weinstein et al. (8) found that high titers of anti-dsDNA and a low-serum C3 level are sensitive, and that each test had a high predictive value (115) for the diagnosis of SLE when applied to a patient population in which the diagnosis was clinically suspected. Moreover, the predictive value was even higher when both serologic abnormalities were present in an individual patient.

Clinical Tests For Anti-DsDNA

The four most commonly available tests for anti-dsDNA antibodies in the clinical laboratory are radioimmunoassay using either the Farr or the millipore-filter binding technique, enzyme-linked immunosorbent assay (ELISA), and the Crithidia luciliae immunofluorescence test. The radioimmunoassay is a sensitive technique, and approximately 60 to 70 of patients with SLE test positive for anti-dsDNA by use of this method (27,28). False-positive results occasionally are seen with this test because of the contamination of the DNA substrate with single-stranded forms. False-positive results have been reported with commercial kits (29). The ELISA test for anti-dsDNA is technically easy to perform, and is the least labor intensive. The serum titer can be readily measured and, more important, both high- and low-avidity anti-dsDNA antibodies can be detected. False-positive ELISA results can be seen when impure DNA is used as a substrate (30). The immunofluorescence test uses fixed smears of Crithidia luciliae, which is a nonpathogenic hemoflagellate containing a circular cytoplasmic organelle (called a kinetoplast) that consists of dsDNA. Serum anti-dsDNA, but not anti-ssDNA antibodies, bind to the kinetoplast. My own group has used this method to measure not only the titer of the antibody but also the immunoglobulin class and complement-fixing property of anti-dsDNA (31).

Qualitative properties of anti-dsDNA antibodies, including avidity, immunoglobulin class, and complement-fixing property, may affect the pathogenicity of the antibodies.

Because the three available tests for anti-dsDNA preferentially measure antibodies of different properties, some controversy has arisen as to which test yields the most useful information in assessing disease activity.

Ward et al. (32) compared the ELISA, Crithidia luciliae immunofluorescence test, and filter-binding radioimmunoassay in patients with SLE who were followed over a period of time. They found that in most patients, the changes in anti-dsDNA antibody levels measured over time parallel each other, and that the anti-dsDNA titer as measured by each assay is inversely correlated to the serum C3 concentration. Data from this study indicate that the repertoire of anti-dsDNA antibodies detected in an individual patient remains relatively constant over time, confirming the observation that high- and low-avidity anti-DNA antibodies do not move independently in an individual patient but rise and fall in a parallel pattern (33).

Smeenk et al. (34) compared four methods for measuring anti-dsDNA antibodies in a defined population of patients with SLE. They found good correlation between the Farr assay, a commercial radioimmunoassay kit, polyethelene glycol test, and Crithidia lucilae immunofluorescent test. As a diagnostic test, however, they recommend the Farr assay and Crithidia luciliae as having the highest specificity for SLE. Werle et al. (35) suggest that ELISA is a sensitive test that is well suited to screening for anti-dsDNA. However, positive sera should be confirmed by either Crithidia lucilae immunofluorescent test or by Farr assay, because they found positive ELISA in some patients with chronic liver disease, infections, and connective-tissue diseases other than SLE. Bootsma et al. (36) found the Farr assay have the highest specificity and sensitivity for the diagnosis of SLE when compared to the ELISA and Crithidia luciliae test. Moreover, SLE sera with IgM-class anti-dsDNA as measured by the ELISA were positive when tested by the Farr assay. In contrast, patients with other medical conditions who have IgM-class anti-dsDNA by the ELISA test were negative when tested with the Farr assay.

IgA anti-dsDNA antibodies have been reported to be associated with disease activity and a clinical subset of SLE patients with cutaneous vasculitis, acral necrosis, and erythema (37). In contrast, the presence and the serum level of IgM anti-ds DNA were not associated with disease activity or to particular clinical features of SLE (36). In a prospective study of 72 patients over a period of 19.6 months, Bootsma and coworkers (38) found that rises in the serum titer of the IgM anti-dsDNA, in contrast to rises of IgG anti-dsDNA, were not useful in predicting clinical relapses of SLE.

Telomeres are repetitive sequences of DNA at the end of eukaryotic chromosomes.

Wallace et al. (39) evaluated an ELISA test for antitelomere antibodies as a diagnostic test for SLE. Antitelomere antibodies were found to be more sensitive than the Farr assay for anti-dsDNA (71% vs. 50%) in a cohort of SLE patients. Further studies are needed to confirm the high sensitivity and specificity as well as its application in assessing lupus disease activity.

In summary, the most commonly available tests for anti-dsDNA antibodies yield comparable results over time in individual patients; however, as a diagnostic test, the Farr assay and Crithidia luciliae are preferred. In clinical practice, any of these tests can be used to follow the antibody titer sequentially in most patients with SLE. If a patient with clinically active lupus has repeatedly low serum levels of anti-dsDNA antibodies with one test, use of a different test system should be considered.

Assessment Of Disease Activity

A number of studies most retrospective, but a few prospective have examined the value of anti-dsDNA antibodies in predicting disease exacerbations and response to drug therapy. Table 45.3 summarizes the results of selected studies (21,35,40–46).

Retrospective Studies

Davis et al. (41) described a fairly good correlation between disease activity and anti-dsDNA antibodies as measured by

TABLE 45.3. ASSOCIATION OF ANTI-DOUBLE-STRANDED DNA AND DISEASE ACTIVITY

Source	No. of Patients	Method Used	Results and Comments
Retrospective studies			
Davis, 1977 (41)	23	Radioassay	Good correlation between disease activity but positive tests were seen in several patients in remission.
Swaak, 1979 (44)	78	Farr assay	Sharp drop in antibody titer especially if combined with low C3 and C1q; predictive of nephritis or major organ flare. Persistently high titer was not predictive.
Isenberg, 1988 (42)	39	ELISA	Severe lupus nephritis but not extrarenal involvement correlated with anti-double-stranded (ds) DNA and especially with antipoly (dT).
Lloyd, 1981 (21)	27 with 47 flares	*C. luciliae*	Only fair association with disease activity. Rising titer of anti-ds DNA coincided with 75% of renal 60% of extrarenal, and 30% to 50% of combined renal and extrarenal.
Adler, 1975 (40)	21 diffuse lupus nephritis	Farr assay	Persistently high anti-dsDNA despite drug therapy correlated with poor renal outcome. An initial high titer had no prognostic value.
Esdaile, 1996 (48)	202 with 83 flares	Farr assay	Fluctuation in anti-ds DNA, C3, C4, and C1q binding were poor predictors of disease flares.
Prospective studies			
Swaak, 1986 (45)	143, with 33 flares	Farr assay	All 33 flares preceded by a progressive rise and shapr drop of anti-ds DNA titer; 20 to 25 weeks prior to onset of nephritis; serum C4 decreased followed by C1q and C3.
ter Borg, 1990 (46)	72, with 27 flares	Farr assay, ELISA, *C. luciliae*	24 flares (89%) preceded by rise in anti-ds DNA by 8 to 10 weeks; anti-ds DNA was more predicitve than C3 or C4. Farr assay was the most sensitive test.
Minter, 1979 (43)	40	Radioassay filter	Half of active episodes associated with low C'H50 and high anti-ds DNA; isolated high anti-ds DNA or low C'H50 seen in inactive disease; most central nervous system episodes occurred with normal C'H50 and anti-ds DNA. Low C'H50 correlated better than high anti-dsDNA.
Bootsma, 1995 (47)	156	Farr assay	A rise in anti-ds DNA titer was treated with an increase in prednisone dose. This reduced the risk of a clinical relapse.
Zonana-Nacach, 1995 (194)	53	Farr assay	Odds ratio of three for flare in asymptomatic patients with high anti-ds DNA and odds ratio of two for low C3.
Bootsma, 1997 (38)	34 with 18 flares	ELISA and Farr assay	Rise in IgG anti-ds DNA but not IgM anti-ds DNA was predictive of disease flare.

ELISA, enzyme-linked immunosorbent assay.

a millipore radioassay. Several patients in clinical remission, however, had a mild to moderate elevation of anti-dsDNA antibody levels. Swaak et al. (44) found a sharp drop in anti-dsDNA antibody titer, usually preceded by a rise that correlated with lupus nephritis and other major organ involvement. In contrast, a continuously high antibody titer was not predictive of disease flare. Isenberg et al. (42) reported that severe lupus nephritis, but not central nervous system (CNS) and other extra-renal involvement, correlated with anti-dsDNA antibodies, especially with antipoly (dT) antibodies. Measurement of antibodies to different synthetic polynucleotides did not significantly add to the routine determination of anti-dsDNA antibodies. Lloyd and Schur (21) observed that anti-dsDNA antibody as measured by the Crithidia luciliae test correlates only fairly with disease activity. A rising antibody titer correlated with 75 of renal, 60 of extra-renal, and 30 to 50 of combined renal and extrarenal flares. In a study of patients with lupus nephritis who were treated with azathioprine and steroids, Adler et al. (40), using the Farr assay, found a persistently elevated anti-dsDNA to be predictive of a poor renal outcome.

Prospective Studies

A few long-term prospective studies have evaluated the clinical significance of anti-dsDNA antibodies both alone and in combination with serum complement level and other serologic parameters. Minter et al. (43) studied 70 patients longitudinally over 3 years. Only slightly more than one-half of the active-disease episodes were associated with both a low C′H%) and a high anti-dsDNA level as measured by the Farr assay. Many patients with clinically inactive disease had isolated elevated anti-dsDNA iters or low C′H50 level. Active lupus nephritis was associated with complement-fixing anti-dsDNA or a low C′H50. In contrast, most episodes of CNS disease occurred without significant changes in C′H50 level and anti-dsDNA antibody titer. Overall, the C′H50 parameter correlated better than the anti-dsDNA antibodies with disease activity.

In a longitudinal study of 143 patients with SLE, Swaak et al. (45) found that a progressive rise followed by a sharp drop in anti-dsDNA titer as measured by the Farr assay preceded all 33 major disease flares. A drop in the serum C4 level followed by a decrease in the serum C1q and C3 levels occurred 20 to 25 weeks before the onset of lupus nephritis.

Ter Borg et al. (46) reported that 89% of all disease flares that occurred in 72 patients with SLE studied serially were preceded by a rise in anti-dsDNA titer by 8 to 10 weeks. The anti-dsDNA antibody titer was more sensitive than serum C3 or C4 levels in predicting exacerbations. The Farr assay was superior to the Crithidia luciliae or ELISA test for the determination of anti-dsDNA antibodies. Based on these observations, a randomized, controlled trial was undertaken to determine if increasing the daily dose of prednisone after a rise in anti-dsDNA is detected can prevent relapses in SLE (47). A 25% increase in serum anti-dsDNA titer by the Farr method was considered to be significant. The cumulative risk of a major or minor relapse was significantly reduced in patients who received an additional dose of prednisolone.

Other investigators have found that anti-dsDNA and other serologic tests are not very useful in predicting disease flares. Esdaile et al. (48) analyzed retrospectively clinical and laboratory data from 202 SLE patients who were followed prospectively for a median period of 86.5 months. Using a modified SLE disease activity index, they concluded that fluctuations in the laboratory test values including anti-dsDNA, C3, C4, and C1q binding assay for immune complexes are poor predictors of disease exacerbations in SLE. For the four serologic tests, the sensitivity approximated 50% and the sensitivity was less than 75% (49). In this study, anti-dsDNA and other laboratory data were obtained every 3 months. In contrast, in the prospective studies that found anti-dsDNA to be predictive of disease flares (46,47), laboratory values were obtained more frequently every 4 to 6 weeks.

Summary

The quantitative determination of anti-dsDNA antibodies does not adequately predict disease flares in every patient. This is not unexpected considering the heterogeneity of the clinical disease and the anti-dsDNA antibodies. Several investigators have proposed that the qualitative properties of the anti-dsDNA antibodies, such as the complement-fixing property, avidity, dissociation constant, and immunoglobulin class, are more important determinants than the total antibody content in regard to pathogenecity and correlation with disease activity (59–54). Data from these studies are not readily available to the practicing clinician. Meanwhile, the anti-dsDNA antibody titer continues to be used widely as a serologic parameter for assessing disease activity. Combined with serum complement values, it is valuable in patients with lupus nephritis. In my experience, it is especially useful if the patient in question had a high anti-dsDNA and low serum complement in past exacerbations of the disease. Data from the prospective studies suggest that anti-dsDNA should be measured at frequent intervals, every 4 to 6 weeks to be predictive of disease flares. Considering the cost of laboratory testing, additional longitudinal studies are needed to confirm this finding.

CLINICAL SIGNIFICANCE OF THE ANTI-SM ANTIBODY

Anti-Sm antibody is present in only 30% of patients with SLE, but it has considerable diagnostic value as it is rarely found in other rheumatic diseases, such as MCTD, systemic sclerosis, and rheumatoid arthritis (55,56). Anti-Sm is included in the ACR criteria for the classification of SLE, and as an immunologic parameter, it carries the same weight as anti-dsDNA, positive LE-cell test, and false-positive serologic test for syphilis.

The anti-Sm antibody usually is measured in the clinical laboratory, by immunodiffusion, counterimmunoelectrophoresis (CIE), ELISA, and hemagglutination methods. The ELISA test, using highly purified antigens, is the most sensitive but less specific than the immunodiffusion and CIE (55,57). The lower specificity of the former is partly a result of the difficulty in preparing highly purified Sm antigen (58). The ELISA test is superior to other methods, however, in measuring the serum titer of the antibody. The use of recombinant Sm antigen and Sm polypeptides in ELISA is promising, but additional studies are needed to evaluate their clinical application (59–61).

Prevalence

Studies have shown that the prevalence of anti-Sm antibody in SLE varies among the different ethnic groups. In the United States, Arnett et al. (57) found anti-Sm and anti-RNP antibodies to be more common in African Americans (25% and 40%, respectively) than in whites (10% and 24%, respectively). Antibodies to Ro/SSA and La/SSB, however, occurred with equal frequencies in the two racial groups. The higher prevalence of anti-Sm and anti-U1 RNP in African Americans has been confirmed by others (62,64). The frequency of anti-Sm antibody in SLE apppears to be lower in France than in the United States (65). Anti-Sm was present in 12% (by immunodiffusion) and in 17% (by immunoblotting) of French patients with SLE; in contrast, the prevalence among French West Indies patients was five times higher: 39% by immunodiffusion and 50% by immunoblotting. In a smaller study, Field et al. (58) found a higher frequency of the antibody among patients with SLE originally from West Africa, the Carribean Islands, and Asia than among local whites in England. The prevalence of anti-Sm antibodies in a large number of European patients with SLE (93% whites) was 10.3% (65). The prevalence of anti-Sm in Thailand was 44% (66); in Mexico, 39.2% (67); in India, 13.7% (68) and in Malaysia 15% (69).

The selection of SLE patients and of controls, the antigen that is used, and the laboratory procedure are variable, so prevalence of anti-Sm antibodies may not be comparable among the cited studies.

Association With Organ Involvement

Whether the presence of anti-Sm antibodies defines a clinical subset of patients with SLE or carries a prognostic value in SLE remains controversial. Winfield (70) found a higher frequency of anti-Sm antibodies among patients with SLE and CNS dysfunction. Winn et al. (14) reported anti-Sm antibodies to be associated with milder CNS and renal disease. Other investigators, however, could not confirm these associations (71,72). Gripenberg et al. (73) found Raynaud's phenomenon to be more prevalent in patients with high titers of IgG anti-Sm antibodies. Yasuma et al. (74) found a positive correlation among serositis, interstitial pulmonary fibrosis, and IgG anti-Sm antibodies in a large cohort of Japanese patients. Huynh and associates (75) reported an increased frequency of anti-Sm antibodies in SLE patients with peripheral neuropathy. The discrepancies in these results may result from the variation in prevalence among various ethnic groups and differences in the sensitivity of the test system. More important, conclusions were based on a single serum specimen rather than on a sequential determination of the anti-Sm antibody.

Antibody Titer And Disease Activity

Few longitudinal studies on the usefulness of anti-Sm antibody titers in monitoring disease activity in patients with SLE have been performed. A prospective study of 14 patients with SLE and anti-Sm antibodies, over a period of 7 to 30 months, showed fluctuations in serum titer. A fourfold rise in titer predicted disease flare in 50% of aptients (but in only 28% of episodes) and correlated with exacerbation of the disease in 60%. The rise in titer occurred within 2 to 12 weeks preceding a major diseae flare (nephritis and CNS disease), but not in milder flares (arthritis, rash, or serositis) (74). Another study of 17 patients with SLE who were followed for 6 to 120 months showed a correlation between anti-Sm antibody and disease activity (73),

Summary

The anti-Sm antibody is considered specific for SLE, so it is a valuable serologic marker for diagnosis. It should be tested for in all patients with positive ANA who are suspected on clinical grounds of having SLE. Further studies are needed, however, to evaluate the value of anti-Sm antibody titer in monitoring disease activity, to determine whether it adds to the measurement of anti-dsDNA antibodies and other serologic tests, and to ascertain whether it may be more useful in blacks and other ethnic groups in whom the antibody is more prevalent.

SIGNIFICANCE OF ANTI-U1 RNP ANTIBODY IN SYSTEMIC LUPUS ERYTHEMATOSUS

Prevalence And Diagnostic Significance

Arnett et al. (57) found that the prevalence of anti-U1 RNP antibodies measured by the immunodiffusion and CIE tests, is higher in black patients (40%) than in white patients with SLE (23%). Using immunoprecipitation and autoradiography, Williamson et al. (63) found a higher frequency of anti-Sm (34% vs. 15%) but not anti-U1RNP (36% vs. 27%) in black compared to white SLE patients. The ELISA test is a sensitive test for anti-U1RNP, showing a prevalence of the antibody as high as 55% in patients with SLE (55). Anti-U1RNP antibodies were found in 20.1% of a large number of European patients with SLE who were collected from 14 different countries (65). A high frequency of anti-U1 RNP antibodies in SLE has been reported in Japanese patients (24%) (76) and in Malaysian patients (36%) (69).

Unlike anti-Sm antibodies, anti-U1RNP antibodies are not considered specific for SLE. They can be seen in patients with other systemic rheumatic conditions such as MCTD, rheumatoid arthritis, Sjögren's syndrome, systemic sclerosis, and polymyositis.

Clinical Association Of Anti-U1RNP Antibodies

The presence of high titers of anti-U1RNP antibodies is associated with MCTD, a clinical entity that is characterized by overlapping features of SLE, scleroderma, and polymyositis (27,28). Some investigators have proposed that in MCTD, anti-U1RNP should occur in the absence of other autoantibodies such as anti-Sm and anti-dsDNA (77), and that the occurrence of multiple types of ANA in an individual is more indicative of SLE. The issue of whether MCTD is a distinct rheumatic disease or merely a syndrome that may occur during the course of SLE or systemic sclerosis remains controversial. Some patients with MCTD eventually evolve into a more distinct rheumatic disease, such as definite systemic sclerosis (78,79). A study of the isotype of anti-U1RNP antibodies in Greek patients revealed a predominance of IgM antibodies in SLE. In contrast, IgG anti-U1RNP without IgM antibodies were found in MCTD (80).

In 1972, Reichlin and Mattioli (81) found that anti-U1RNP antibody is prevalent in SLE and is associated with a more benign disease. A cross-sectional study of 49 patients with SLE revealed that those with anti-U1RNP and anti-Sm antibodies have a higher frequency of scleroderma-associated features, such as Raynaud's phenomenon, sclerodactyly, interstitial changes in the chest radiograph, and nail-fold capillary abnormalities (82,83). Vasculitis, deforming, nonerosive, Jaccoud-type arthropathy of the hands and Raynaud's phenomenon also have been reported to be associated with anti-U1RNP in SLE by other investigators. (67,69,84).

Serum Antibody Titer

A few reports of longitudinal measurements of the serum titer of anti-U1RNP among patients with SLE have appeared. Nishikai et al. (85) showed that in some, but not all, patients with SLE, the anti-U1RNP titer appeared to fluctuate with disease activity. A prospective study of 71 patients with SLE and 40 separate clinical exacerbations showed that the measurement of antibodies to 70 kd and A polypeptides of the U1RNP complex was not useful in monitoring disease activity or predicting disease exacerbations (86). The presence of anti-U1RNP and/or anti-Sm did not appear to affect survivorship in SLE (87).

A prospective study of patients with anti-U1RNP antibodies showed that most patients with a persistently high serum titer evolve into a clinical picture of MCTD (88). A 10-year follow-up of a group of patients with rheumatic disease and anti-U1RNP antibodies showed clinical features of MCTD and a high frequency of erosive and deforming arthritis (89). A large proportion of patients with "undifferentiated connective tissue disease" who tested positive for anti-U1RNP subsequently developed MCTD (90).

Summary

Anti-U1RNP and anti-Sm antibodies commonly are found together in the sera of patients with SLE. Anti-U1RNP antibodies are not considered to be diagnostic of SLE; when present alone in a patient with systemic rheumatic disease (especially in high titer); the possibility of MCTD should be considered. Although the serum titer of anti-U1RNP may fluctuate in some patients, the determination of anti-dsDNA and complement are more useful in monitoring disease activity in patients with SLE.

ANTI-RO/SSA AND ANTI-LA/SSB ANTIBODIES IN SYSTEMIC LUPUS ERYTHEMATOSUS

Diagnostic Specificity

Anti-Ro/SSA antibodies are most commonly found in the sera of patients with primary Sjögren's syndrome and SLE, although they also occur in some patients with other systemic rheumatic diseases, including systemic sclerosis, rheumatoid arthritis, and polymyositis (27). In the clinical laboratory, anti-Ro/Ssa antibodies are detected by immunodiffusion in agarose gels or by CIE. They are present in 30% to 40% of patients with SLE and in 40% to 70% of patients with primary Sjögren's syndrome (28).

Immunoblotting, RNA precipitation, and ELISA have been developed to measure anti-Ro/SSA and anti-La/SSB antibodies. A comparative study of these methods (91,92) has shown that although the RNA precipitation has the highest sensitivity and specificity, the most convenient and practical clinical test is CIE for anti-Ro/SSA and immunoblotting for anti-La/SSB. ELISA tests using affinity-purified antigens and recombinant protein have become available (93,94).

Like anti-Ro/SSA antibodies, anti-La/SSB antibodies are found in patients with primary Sjögren's syndrome and

SLE. Precipitating anti-La/SSB antibodies are found in 12% of unselected patients with SLE (95).

Using various test systems, anti-Ro/SSA antibodies have been reported to occur in low titers in 15% of healthy individuals, especially those who are HLA-DR3 positive, and anti-La/SSB have been detected in 7.5% of normal subjects (55,96–98).

Disease Associations

Although anti-Ro/SSA antibodies do not have a high diagnostic specificity for SLE, their presence is associated with a number of clinical conditions. These include SCLE, neonatal lupus syndrome, homozygous C2 and C4 deficiency with SLE-like disease, ANA-negative SLE, photosensitivity in SLE, and interstitial pneumonitis.

SCLE is a distinct clinical subset of SLE. It is characterized by recurrent, erythematous, photosensitive, nonscarring skin lesions in a characteristic distribution involving the face, trunk, and arms, and by mild systemic disease. Anti-Ro/SSA antibodies are found in 63 to 90 of patients with SCLE (99–101). The major anti-Ro/SSA response in SCLE is directed against the native 60-kD Ro protein (102).

Neonatal lupus syndrome is an uncommon condition in infants born of SLE mothers. It is characterized by photosensitive, annular, discoid, or erythematous skin lesions of the face and trunk, which appear at or before 2 months of age and disappear by 6 to 12 months of age. Congenital heart block with or without structural cardiac defects is seen in 50 of patients. Almost all afflicted infants and their mothers have anti-Ro/SSA and/or anti-La/SSB antibodies (103–105). Buyon et al. (106) found that women with both antibodies, especially if the anti-Ro/SSA antibodies identify the 52-kd component, have an increased risk of giving birth to an infant with neonatal lupus syndrome. Unfortunately, most of the commercially available tests for anti-Ro/SSA antibodies do not distinguish between antibodies to the 52-kd and the 60-kd components.

The frequency of anti-Ro/SSA antibodies is increased in mothers of male children with SLE and in mothers of children with SLE that develops before the age of 10 years (107).

Homozygous C2 deficiency is characterized by a lupus-like illness with photosensitive cutaneous lesions reminiscent of those of SCLE and arthralgia but rare CNS and renal involvement. Anti-Ro/SSA antibodies are present in 50 to 75 of these patients (100,108). A genetic deficiency of C4, which may manifest clinically as SLE or a lupuslike syndrome, also is associated with anti-Ro/SSA antibodies (108). In one study, one of four patients with a genetic deficiency of C1q had anti-Ro/SSA antibodies (108).

ANA-negative SLE, first described by Fessel (109) and by Gladman et al. (110), refers to patients with clinical features that are compatible with those of SLE, except that their sera test negative for ANA by immunofluorescence using sections of rodent liver or kidney. In a study of 66 patients, Madison et al. (111) had SCLE. Precipitating anti-Ro/SSA antibodies were found in 41 patients, and anti-ssDNA antibodies were present in 18. Moreover, 66 of patients actually had a positive fluorescent ANA when KB epithelial tissue culture cells rather than mouse kidney sections were used as substrate. The Ro/SSA antigen appears to have a variable species distribution with significant amounts in certain cells, including a concentration in mouse, rat, and rabbit tissues (1).

Blomberg et al. (112) found that 25% of a group of patients suspected of having systemic rheumatic disease with anti-Ro/SSA antibodies by an ELISA test but with a negative standard ANA test had SLE or cutaneous SLE. Further characterization of the antibody revealed specificity for the Ro 52-kd protein (113). Using a sensitive ELISA test, Reichlin (114) found anti-Ro/SSA in all 66 patients with ANA negative SLE. Anti-La/SSB was detected in 46% and anti-U1RNP was present in 35%.

The presence of anti-Ro/SSA antibodies has been reported to correlate positively with photosensitivity in white patients with SLE (115). In contrast, among African Americans, anti-Ro/SSA antibodies appear to be inversely associated with photosensitivity (116). A probable relationship between anti-Ro/SSA antibodies and interstitial pneumonitis in SLE has been described (117), and deforming arthropathy in SLE has been reported to be associated with anti-Ro/SSA (especially the 52-kd component) and with anti-La/SSB antibodies (118).

SLE patients with anti-La/SSB antibodies usually have anti-Ro/SSA antibodies concomitantly, and they tend to be older at diagnosis (95,119). While lupus nephritis is positively associated with anti-dsDNA, it is inversely related with anti-La/SSB antibodies (120).

Hamilton and associates (95,121,122) suggested two serologic genetic subsets of SLE in whites, but not in African Americans, with different ages of onset. White patients with SLE and anti-Ro/SSA antibodies alone differ from those with both anti-Ro/SSA and anti-La/SSB antibodies. Those in the former group have a lower titer of anti-Ro/SSA antibodies, a younger age of onset, a higher frequency of anti-dsDNA and significant renal disease, and they are strongly associated with DR2 and DQw1. In contrast, those in the latter group are associated with an older age of onset, sicca complex, less renal involvement, and HLA-B8, Dr3, Drw52, and DQW2.

Serial Measurement Of Antibody Titer

Scopelitis et al. (123) reported fluctuating titers of anti-Ro/SSA antibodies in patients with SLE that appeared to correlate with disease activity and anti-dsDNA antibody levels. Moreover, some episodes of acute exacerbation were characterized by a rising titer in anti-Ro/SSA antibody in the absence of detectable anti-dsDNA antibodies. A longitudinal study of anti-Ro/SSA and anti-La/SSB in a lupus mother who gave birth to an infant with congenital heart block revealed fluctuations of serum antibody titers that were unrelated to disease activity or to immunosuppressive therapy (124). In addition, frequent measurements of these autoantibodies during pregnancy did not predict occurrence of congenital heart block. A two-year prospective study anti-Ro/SSA antibody by CIE method in SLE showed fluctuation in the serum antibody titer however there was no correlation with lupus disease activity (125). On the other hand, Wahren et al. (126), using a sensitive ELISA test in a small number of SLE patients, found correlation between disease activity and serum titer of anti-Ro/SSA and anti-La/SSB antibodies.

Summary

Anti-Ro/SSA antibodies are strongly correlated with the clinical subsets of SCLE, ANA-negative SLE, and lupuslike syndrome associated with a genetic deficiency of complement. Infants of SLE mothers with anti-Ro/SSB and anti-La/SSB antibodies have an increased risk of neonatal lupus syndrome, so pregnant patients with SLE should be tested for these antibodies. A sensitive ELISA test for anti-Ro/SSA antibodies is useful in the diagnosis of ANA negative SLE. Prospective studies are needed to evaluate the value of anti-Ro/SSA and anti-La/SSB antibodies in monitoring disease activity.

ANTI-HISTONE ANTIBODIES IN SYSTEMIC LUPUS ERYTHEMATOSUS

Prevalence And Diagnostic Specificity

Antihistone antibodies comprise a heterogeneous group of antibodies that are reactive with various subfractions or complexes. Although found mainly in patients with SLE, drug-induced LE, or rheumatoid arthritis, these antibodies have been described in those with other rheumatic conditions, malignancy, and liver disease (see Chapter 22). In SLE, these antibodies are directed against H1, H2B, H3, and H2A-H2B complex (127), although other specificities can occur. All isotypes of antihistone antibodies are common in SLE (128,129).

Several methods have been devised to measure antihistone antibodies, including ELISA, immunoblotting, complement fixation, and immunofluorescence (130). Depending on the method, substrate, and patient selection, the prevalence of antihistone antibodies in SLE has been reported to be from 21 to 90 (130).

Antihistone antibodies have limited diagnostic specificity for idiopathic SLE. The presence of these antibodies does not appear to be any more significant that that of anti-dsDNA or anti-Sm antibodies in corroborating the clinical diagnosis of the disease. Wallace et al. (131) found that antibodies to histone (H2A-H2B) DNA complex in the absence of anti-dsDNA antibodies are found more commonly in MCTD and scleroderma-related conditions than in SLE. (The diagnostic value of antihistone antibodies for drug-induced LE is discussed in Chapters 22 and 42.

Clinical Association

Few published studies have examined the relationship between the presence of antihistone antibodies and the clinical features of SLE. In a small number of patients with lupus, Fishbein et al. (132) found a significantly lower prevalence of CNS involvement among those with antihistone antibodies. Fritzler et al. (133) confirmed the lower frequency of neuropsychiatric disease and the lower prevalence of nephritis, alopecia, anemia, and hypocomplementemia in patients with SLE and antihistone antibodies, suggesting a milder form of the disease. In contrast, other investigators have failed to find any positive or negative correlation with specific clinical manifestations of the disease (128,134,135).

Similarly, the available data on the association between antihistone antibodies and disease activity are few and inconclusive. Fishbein et al. (132) found a significant drop in the serum antibody titer within a month after the initiation of steroid therapy for active SLE. Gioud et al. (134) reported a higher frequency of antihistone antibodies in patients with active disease (105) than in those who were in remission (23). A serial study in a small number of patients showed a correlation with disease activity (136). In untreated patients with lupus nephritis, antibodies to H2B correlated with renal, histologic, and clinical activity of the disease (136). Other investigators, however, have found no correlation among antihistone antibodies, disease activity, or activity index in the renal biopsy (129,133,135,137,138).

The discrepancies in the results of various studies have several causes, mainly differences in patient selection, the test system used, histone preparation, and inadequate study design.

Association With Anti-DNA Antibodies

Antihistone antibodies have been shown to correlate with the presence of anti-DNA antibodies (134,135) and circulating immune complexes (136). Subiza et al. (139) have established that some of the antihistone activity that is measured in SLE sera results from complexes of dsDNA anti-dsDNA, which bind to the histone substrate used in the assay. Stockl et al. (140) found that glomerular deposits of histones may bind to fixed anionic sites in the glomerular capillary wall, acting as a planted antigen that can induce immune complex formation *in situ*.

Association With Lupus Erythematosus Cell Test

Schett and associates (141) have identified serum antibodies to H1 as the major group of antinuclear antibodies responsible for the LE cell phenomenon in SLE. They also found that

SLE patients who have antihistone 1 antibodies had marked immune response to other histones and other nuclear proteins. Morever, these patients tended to have more severe organ involvement with nephritis and CNS disease (142).

Summary

Antihistone antibodies are of limited value in corroborating the clinical diagnosis of SLE. Serial determinations of these antibodies do not add significantly to the measurement of anti-dsDNA and other serologic parameters for assessing disease activity in patients with SLE. Well-designed prospective studies are needed to understand fully the clinicopathogenetic significance of antihistone 1 antibodies including assessment of disease activity.

SEROLOGIC PARAMETERS AND RENAL BIOPSY FINDINGS IN LUPUS NEPHRITIS

A number of studies (Table 45.4) have examined the relationship between renal biopsy findings and the serologic data obtained at biopsy (138,143–150). Could the histologic type of lupus nephritis, histologic activity, and chronicity indices be predicted by anti-dsDNA, C3, and/or serologic parameters? The results of various studies are not necessarily comparable because of differences in morphologic classification, parameters measured, and patient selection, including consideration of the effects of previous or current drug therapy. All studies except two (147,150) were based on a single kidney biopsy that was performed within a few months after onset of the renal abnormality.

Hill et al. (148) found an excellent correlation between serum levels of anti-dsDNA and C3 with the overall amount and distribution of immune deposits in the renal biopsy as assessed by immunofluorescence. In contrast, a poor association between the degree of epithelial proliferation and the histologic type of lupus nephritis was noted using the Baldwin classification system (151).

Houssiau et al. (149) reported a good correlation among the anti-dsDNA titer and the serum C3 (but not C4) level with functional severity of the renal disease and the World Health Organization (WHO) histologic classification of lupus nephritis. Patients with nephrotic syndrome or renal failure had a higher anti-dsDNA titer and a lower C3 level than those presenting with proteinuria alone and a normal serum creatinine level. Patients with class IV nephritis had a higher anti-dsDNA level than those with class III or V nephritis. In contrast, the serum C3 level did not correlate with the histologic type. Considerable overlap in values among the various clinical or histologic groups was found, however, so these associations are not applicable to the individual patient.

TABLE 45.4. CORRELATION OF SEROLOGIC ABNORMALITIES AND RENAL HISTOLOGY

Source	No. of Patients	Results and Comments
Hill, 1978 (148)	59 with 77 biopsies	Excellent correlation between anti-double-stranded (ds) DNA and C3 with overall amount and distribution of immune deposits; rheumatoid factor found in those with milder lesions; cryoglobulins correlated with more severe changes.
Hossiau, 1990 (149)	50	High anti-ds DNA and low C3 correlated with nephrotic syndrome with or without renal failure; class IV nephritis patients had higher anti-ds DNA titer than those with class III or V nephritis.
Nossent, 1991 (138)	35	High histologic activity index correlated with IgM antinuclear antibody and IgM anti-ds DNA. No correlation between histologic type and serologic abnormalities.
Clough, 1980 (143)	11	IgM anti-ds DNA was higher than IgG anti-ds DNA in class IV nephritis. IgG anti-ds DNA was higher than IgM anti-ds DNA in class III nephritis.
Hashimoto, 1983 (146)	20	Histologically active lesions, especially class IV nephritis, correlated with high titer and complement fixing IgG anti-ds DNA. Glomerular C3 deposits correlated with complement fixing IgG anti-ds DNA.
Feldman, 1982 (145)	34	Renal activity index but not chronicity index correlated with anti-ds DNA (Farr assay) and IgG anti-ds DNA by ELISA.
Esdaile, 1989 (144)	87	Low C3 was predictive of renal insufficiency, renal death and total SLE death; high anti-ds DNA associated with renal death and inversely related with non-renal death.
Hecht, 1976 (147)	31 with repeat biopsy	Persistently normal C3 was associated with stability or improvement of renal lesion of repeat biopsy in some but not all patients. Anti-ds DNA showed better correlation with clinical histologic improvement.
Pillemer, 1988 (150)	55 with repeat biopsy	Normalization of C3 correlated better than decrease in anti-ds DNA titer with activity index during repeat biopsy.
Okamura, 1993 (152)	40	IgG but not IgM anti-ds DNA by ELISA correlated with renal histologic activity score and amount of electron dense glomerular deposits.

Nossent et al. (138) observed no correlation among the WHO histologic classification and various serologic parameters (anti-dsDNA, other types of ANA, C3, C4, C1q, immune complexes, and anticardiolipin antibodies) in 35 patients with lupus nephritis. Conversely, using the National Institutes of Health renal histology index, the activity index correlated with serum titers of IgM ANA and IgM anti-dsDNA. Glomerular proliferation showed the best overall correlation with serologic parameters. Clough and Valenzuela (143) described a similar correlation between IgM anti-dsDNA and diffuse lupus nephritis.

Hashimoto et al. (146) reported a good correlation between histologically active lesions, especially in diffuse lupus nephritis, and high titers of IgG complement-fixing anti-dsDNA. Feldman et al. (145) obtained similar results, and they noted a good correlation between anti-dsDNA using the Farr binding assay and IgG anti-dsDNA using ELISA and renal activity, but not with the chronicity index. IgG, but not IgM, anti-dsDNA antibodies as measured by ELISA were found to correlate with the histological activity score and the amount of electron-dense deposits in 40 patients with untreated SLE who underwent kidney biopsy (152). The serum titer of anti-dsDNA antibodies was significantly higher in patients with class IV nephritis as compared to those with class I, II, or III (152).

In contrast to these studies, Pillemer et al. (150) correlated serologic tests and histologic changes over time in 55 patients who had both initial and repeat renal biopsies. All patients received various immunosuppressive drugs for nephritis during the interval. At the time of the second biopsy, the serum C3 level had improved in 78 and the anti-dsDNA level decreased in 85 of patients. Patients with a normal C3 level at the time of the second biopsy had a significantly lower activity index than those with a low C3 level. The activity index was not significantly affected by a decrease in anti-dsDNA antibody titer. The duration of hypocomplementemia, however, was less consistent as a prognostic indicator. Esdaile et al. (144) also found a low serum C3 level to be a valuable predictor of renal insufficiency, renal death, and total SLE death in a study of the long-term outcome of 87 patients with lupus nephritis. In a similar study of 31 patients with SLE and serial kidney biopsies, Hech et al. (147) showed that normalization of the serum C3 level and a drop in the anti-dsDNA titer following drug therapy are associated with stabilization or improvement of the renal disease.

A prospective study of 17 patients concluded that serum C3 levels are more sensitive and specific than serum C4 values for monitoring disease activity in lupus nephritis (153).

Summary

Kidney biopsy is useful in the management of patients with lupus nephritis. The histologic type of lupus nephritis and severity of renal damage as assessed by the activity and chronicity of the lesions are predictive of the outcome of lupus nephritis in most patients. None of the serologic parameters at the time of biopsy, either singly or in combination, can adequately and satisfactorily predict the histologic type or severity of the renal lesion in an individual patient. During drug therapy of lupus nephritis, a persistently low serum C3 level appears to be a better measure of active glomerular disease than an elevated anti-dsDNA antibody titer. As a corollary to this, the normalization of a previously low serum complement level is frequently associated with improvement or stabilization of the renal disease.

ACTIVATION PRODUCTS OF COMPLEMENT IN SYSTEMIC LUPUS ERYTHEMATOSUS

The *in vivo* activation of the complement system by complexes of anti-DNA and DNA antigen and other autoantibodies is central to the pathogenesis of the glomerular injury and, possibly, to other tissue damage in patients with SLE. Acute exacerbations of the disease often are associated with hypocomplementemia. Serial measurements of total hemolytic activity (i.e., CH50) and the serum concentrations of C3, C4, and C1q are widely used to assess disease activity.

Investigators have postulated that small-vessel injury in SLE may occur without evidence of immune complex mediation by the release of split products of complement activation, such as anaphylatoxins. These activation products, such as C3a, C5a, SC5b-9 can activate and attract inflammatory cells. This can lead to cell aggregation and vascular adherence, resulting in an occlusive vasculopathy and ischemia (25).

Correlation With Disease Activity

A number of studies have shown that measurement of the plasma concentration of activation products of complement, including iC3b neoantigen, C3a, C4a, C3d, C4d, and the terminal complex, C5b-9, can be useful in assessing disease activity and predicting exacerbations (154–161) (Table 45.5). The consensus of these various studies is that measurement of the activation products is superior to the determination of serum C3 or C4 values. Many patients with clinically active disease and normal serum C3 or C4 levels have elevated activation products of complement. Nevertheless, except for a few (154,156,162), most of these studies emphasized differences between patient groups (e.g., active vs. inactive) rather than longitudinal determinations in individual patients.

Three prospective studies examined the value of complement activation products and conventional measurements of complement in monitoring disease activity. Buyon et al.

TABLE 45.5. ACTIVATION OF COMPLEMENT AS A MEASURE OF DISEASE ACTIVITY IN SLE

Source	Activation product	No. of Patients	Results and Comments
Negoro, 1989 (158)	iC3b neoantigen	40 untreated	Plasma levels elevated in 83% of patients; highly correlated with disease activity and renal activity index.
Hopkins, 1988 (154)	C3a and C5a	40	C3a level increased in all patients; occurred 1 to 2 months prior to flare; marked elevation in cerebritis; C5a levels less sensitive.
Wild, 1990 (160)	C4a and C3a	24	C4a levels higher in patients with severe disease than in those with mild disease; C4a correlated with anti-double-stranded (ds) DNA and C1q assay for immune complexes; C4a superior to C3a.
Senaldi, 1988 (159)	C4d and C3d	48	C4d correlated better than C3d with disease activity; C3 and C4 did not correlate with disease activity.
Horigome, 1987 (155)	Terminal C attack complex (TCC)	54	TCC correlated with circulating immune complexes, C'H50, C4, C3, C5, and alternate pathway activity.
Garwryl, 1988 (156)	Terminal C complex (C5b-9)	22	Elevated TCC correlated with 89% of all flares.
Kerr, 1989 (157)	Factor B activation (Ba)	51	51% of patients with high Ba had severe multisystem disease; associated with cutaneous vasculitis; Ba correlated better than C4a and C3d with disease severity.
Buyun, 1992 (137)	BaBb, C4d, SC5b-9	86	C4d most sensitive in 86% with major flares.
Porcel, 1995 (163)	C3, C4, C3a, C4a iC3b	39	SC5b-9 most useful with 77% sensitivity and 80% specificity.
Mollnes, 1999 (165)	C4bc, Bb, C3a, C3bc, C5a, SC5b-9	21	Only SC5b-9 correlated with disease activity scores.
Nagy, 2000 (164)	C1rs-C1inh, C3b(Bb)P SC5b-9	65	C3b(Bb)P was highly specific and sensitive indictor of disease activity.

(137) reported that an elevated serum level of C4d had the most sensitivity, being found in 86 of patients who subsequently developed a major exacerbation. The specificity was low, however, such that 69 of the patients who did not flare during the study period had abnormally elevated C4d. Porcel et al. (163) found the terminal complement complex to be the most useful in monitoring disease activity, with 77% sensitivity and 80% specificity. Nagy et al. (164) compared the serum levels of C'H50, C4.C3 to the plasma levels of C1rs-C1inh, C3b(Bb)P, and SC5b-9 in 65 SLE patients. In a smaller number of patients studied serially, C3b(Bb)P, a complex formed during the activation of the alternative pathway, showed the highest difference between active and inactive disease and the best correlation with SLEDAI. Long-term study of a larger group of patients are needed to confirm these findings.

In the SLE patients without evidence of nephritis, Mollnes et al. (165) found that the routine measurement of complement including activation products is of limited importance in predicting disease flares. They measured conventional complement tests and plasma level of C1rs-C1inh, C4bc, Bb, C3a, C3bc, C5a, and SC5b-9. There were 27 flares in 21 patients but none developed nephritis during the study period. Only the plasma level of SC5b-9 correlated with disease activity at the time of the flare.

Measurement of C3d in the urine has been shown to be a sensitive indicator of complement activation and has been reported to be helpful in assessing disease activity in lupus nephritis (166,167).

Conventional measurements of complement and split products may be useful in evaluating disease flares during pregnancy and in differentiating a lupus flare from preeclampsia. The serum levels of CH50, C3, and C4 rise during pregnancy. In patients without SLE but with preeclampsia, the plasma concentration of complement split products, including Ba (i.e., activation product of the alternative pathway), C3a, C4d, and SC5b-9, is increased; however, CH50 generally remains normal. In pregnant patients with SLE and disease exacerbation, there is a reciprocal rise in complement split products and a drop in serum C3, C4, and CH50. A high ratio of CH50 to Ba has been suggested to differentiate patients with preeclampsia from those with active SLE (169,170).

Summary

Additional prospective studies are needed to compare the relative value (including cost-effectiveness) of the various complement activation products in assessing disease activity, major organ involvement such as nephritis, and in determining the possible effects of comorbid conditions, especially infections. A minor drawback of these assays is the need for special handling of the plasma specimen to prevent spurious activation of complement *in vitro*. The measurement of activation products of complement may be particularly useful in patients with isolated CNS involvement, who frequently do not exhibit hypocomplementemia (154).

SOLUBLE IL-2 RECEPTORS IN SYSTEMIC LUPUS ERYTHEMATOSUS

Following activation, resting T lymphocytes express receptors for IL-2 (IL-2R) on the cell surface, and a high-affinity IL-2R enables T lymphocytes to proliferate in response to the cytokine. The receptor can be shed or released *in vitro*, or physiologically *in vivo*, and can be detected in supernatants of cell cultures, in blood, and in body fluids. Elevated serum concentrations of soluble IL-2R (sIL-2R) have been found in patients with conditions that are characterized by immune-system activation, including SLE, rheumatoid arthritis, chronic infections, and malignancies.

Association With Disease Activity

We have found a positive correlation between serum levels of sIL-2R and immunologic markers of disease activity in SLE, including reduced serum C3 and high cryoglobulin levels (26). Sequential studies in patients with active SLE have revealed a decrease in serum sIL-2R levels concomitant with a clinical response to steroid therapy. Our findings have been confirmed and extended by other investigators (171–176).

A prospective study of 71 unselected patients with SLE by ter Borg et al. (171) showed an elevation of sIL-2R in 18 of 21 patients who developed clinical exacerbations, which correlated with changes in anti-dsDNA antibodies and with C3 and C4 values. Of these exacerbations, 75 were preceded by a rise in sIL-2R levels, but changes in anti-dsDNA and C3 levels tended to precede the increase in sIL-2R. The serum concentrations of sIL-2R in patients with inactive SLE were higher than those of healthy individuals, suggesting that an ongoing T cell-activation process was occurring in SLE, even during periods of clinical quiescence. The sIL-2R level increased further before disease exacerbation.

In lupus nephritis, Laut et al. (176) reported a correlation between sIL-2R and histologic activity and chronicity indices, along with presence of IgG and C3 in the kidney biopsy specimen. The serum level did not correlate with serum creatinine, suggesting that the high sIL-2R was not the result of decreased renal clearance. Significant elevation of sIL-2R occurred during lupus nephritis flare and appeared to more sensitive than anti-dsDNA and CH50 as a serologic marker.

Elevation of sIL-2R can occur in infections and should be taken into consideration in patients with lupus. Wong and Wong (177) found markedly elevated sIL-2R in patients with lupus and either active or inactive SLE and concurrent infection. Chronic infections, especially tuberculosis and candida infection, were associated with higher levels of sIL-2R than with pyogenic and herpes zoster infections.

Gilad et al (178) reported elevated levels of sIL-2R in the cerebrospinal fluid of patients with stroke as the initial manifestation of SLE. The levels were significantly higher than those seen in the CSF of non-lupus patients with ischemic strokes.

Summary

The serial measurement of sIL-2R is a sensitive test for assessing disease activity and predicting exacerbations of SLE. It probably is at least as sensitive as determination of the serum C3 level and anti-dsDNA titer, and it may be particularly valuable in patients with SLE who test negative for anti-dsDNA antibodies. Additional prospective studies are needed to confirm these results, to determine whether the sIL-2R measurement has an additive value with other serologic parameters, and to examine the effects of infections and other comorbid conditions in patients with SLE.

CIRCULATING ADHESION MOLECULES AND OTHER SOLUBLE FACTORS

The serum level of soluble factors, including interleukin-10, interleukin-6, soluble tumor necrosis factor receptor (sTNFR), intercellular adhesion molecule1 (ICAM-1), soluble CD8/CD4, E-selectin, and vascular cell adhesion molecule (VCAM-1) as a serologic marker of disease activity in SLE has been investigated.

Results of the various studies, however, have been inconsistent. Further prospective studies are needed to determine whether measurement of selected molecules, especially sTNFR (179) is superior to sIL2R and other serologic tests (180–189).

Application Of Multiple Serologic Measurements In Systemic Lupus Erythematosus

It is clear that no single serologic test can adequately assess or predict the clinical course of SLE in individual patients. A few studies have examined application of a panel of serologic reactions to improve sensitivity and correlation with disease activity.

In an early study, Schur and Sandson (190) concluded that a combination of complement-fixing anti-dsDNA and CH50 correlated better with active disease, especially lupus nephritis, than either of the serologic tests alone. In a more recent study, Lloyd and Schur (21) found that serial measurement of a combination of CH50, C3, C4, and circulating immune complexes by C1q-binding assay appears to be the most useful. Anti-dsDNA antibodies did not significantly increase the usefulness of this panel (see Chapter 13, Complement and Systemic Lupus Erythematosus).

In a prospective study of 48 unselected patients with SLE, Abrass et al. (20) found that circulating immune complexes, as determined by a solid-phase C1q-binding assay, correlate with active disease manifestations, particularly nephritis or arthritis, but not with skin or other organ involvement. A change in disease activity, prompting the physician to make a change in management, was predicted by the results of solid C1q-binding test. Neither C3 nor anti-dsDNA correlated with disease activity, and neither gave additional information when combined with use of the solid-phase C1q-binding test.

Using a battery of laboratory tests, Morrow et al. (191) failed to identify a single test that reliably distinguished between severely active, moderately active, and inactive disease groups of patients with SLE. Determination of circulating immune complexes by polyethylene glycol precipitation, platelet count, and erythrocyte sedimentation rate distinguished the active from the inactive disease group. Patients with severely active disease and involvement of three or more systems were different from the less active group by solid-phase C1q-binding assay for immune complexes, anti-dsDNA, CH50, and lymphocyte count, but patients with neuropsychiatric involvement and those with thrombocytopenia were the most difficult to sort out. Only 44 of patients could be classified accordingly into clinical grades when combinations of four out of five laboratory tests were used. Isenberg et al. (192) were unable to find a correlation between clinical disease activity and multiple serologic reactions to dsDNA, ssDNA, RNA, synthetic polynucleotides, and cardiolipin. In a retrospective study of complement and circulating immune complexes (as tested by five different assays) in 33 patients, Valentijn et al. (22) concluded that although disease activity correlates with serum levels of CH50, C3, or C1q (by binding assay), the sensitivity and predictive value of the serologic parameters are low. In 20 of patients, one or more parameters constantly was abnormal regardless of disease activity. On the other hand, in a small subset of patients, a patient-specific activity parameter could be identified.

In a cross-sectional study of 100 patients, Clough et al. (193) found that a combination of sIL-2R, Westergren sedimentation rate, and anti-dsDNA antibody by ELISA correlated best with disease activity as measured by SLAM index. In contrast, the serum levels of C4, iC3b, and Bb correlated poorly with disease activity.

A 12-month longitudinal study of 53 patients with lupus showed an incidence of disease flare of 0.69 per patient-year of follow-up and a good correlation with serologic abnormalities. Active nephritis was associated with high anti-dsDNA antibodies as measured by Farr method, low C3, and low C4. High anti-dsDNA level also was associated with musculoskeletal and cardiopulmonary involvement. The odds ratio for lupus flares in asymptomatic patients with high anti-dsDNA was three; for those with low serum C3, it was two (194).

CONCLUSIONS AND RECOMMENDATIONS (TABLE 45.6)

Many reports evaluating the application of serologic tests in the assessment and prediction of disease activity have been rife with shortcomings. No uniform index of clinical disease activity has been used, and certain groups of patients (e.g., those with nephritis) were either over- or under-represented in the test populations. Conclusions often were based on a single test sample, and length of the follow-up period was not adequate. Serologic tests were not standardized, so comparison of the various studies is not feasible. Despite these obvious faults, it is clear that no single serologic test available today is ideal and applicable to all patients with lupus. Considering the heterogeneity of the clinical disease, it is unlikely that a single such test will be found. Serologic abnormalities in a patient with active lupus nephritis are

TABLE 45.6. SUMMARY OF SEROLOGIC ABNORMALITIES IN SYSTEMIC LUPUS ERYTHEMATOSUS (SLE)

1. Anti-double-stranded (ds) DNA and anti-Sm antibodies are serologic markers of idiopathic SLE. Their presence in patients suspected of the disease on clinical grounds confirms the diagnosis.
2. Mixed connective-tissue disease should be considered in a patient with overlapping features of SLE, polymyositis, and scleroderma in the presence of a high titer of anti-U1RNP and the absence of anti-dsDNA and other specific types of antinuclear antibody (ANA).
3. Pregnant SLE patients should be tested for anti-Ro/SSA antibodies because their presence indicates a risk for neonatal lupus syndrome.
4. Anti-Ro/SSA antibodies are associated with SCLE, photosensitivity, ANA-negative SLE, and genetic deficiency of complement with LE-like clinical features.
5. Antihistone antibodies have limited diagnostic value for idiopathic SLE but are considered characteristic of drug-induced LE.
6. No single serologic test is predictive of disease exacerbation in SLE. The most useful parameters for assessing disease activity are anti-dsDNA and serum complement levels.
7. Measurements of the activation products of complement and sIL-2R are promising serologic markers predictive of disease severity and exacerbation.

LE, lupus erythematosus; SCLE, subacute cutaneous lupus erythematosus.

not necessarily the same as those in another patient with skin rash, fever, hematologic changes, and/or serositis.

Newer serologic tests, such as determination of complement split products, sIL-2R and other soluble factors, are undergoing further evaluation, and a combination of anti-dsDNA and serum complement now is generally used in clinical practice. The Farr binding test for anti-dsDNA probably is the most widely available test. The clinician should become familiar with the advantages and limitations of the particular assay that is used in the laboratory to which specimens are sent. In patients who continually do not have anti-dsDNA antibodies (even after using different assay methods), measuring the serum titer of some other ANA, such as anti-Sm or anti-Ro/SSa, may be useful (74). The serum C3 concentration is measured more frequently than CH50, although the latter probably is more a more sensitive parameter (21,191). In my experience, serial measurement of serum cryoglobulins is a useful parameter, but others may use a specific test for circulating immune complexes, such as the C1q solid-phase binding assay (20,21).

It must be remembered that there are some patients in clinical remission who have persistently abnormal serologic findings (10,11). Careful monitoring of specific organ functions, such as renal function, remains an important aspect in the assessment of disease activity and response to therapy.

REFERENCES

1. Forslid J, Heigl Z, Jonsson J, et al. The prevalence of antinuclear antibodies in healthy young persons and adults, comparing rat liver tissue sections with HEp-2 cells as antigen substrate. *Clin Exp Rheumatol* 1994;12:137–141.
2. Harmon CE, Deng JS, Peebles CL, et al. The importance of tissue substrate in the SSA/Ro antigen-antibody system. *Arthritis Rheum* 1984;27:116–173.
3. Illei GG, Klippel JH. Why is the ANA result positive. *Bull Rheum Dis* 1999; 48:1–5.
4. Tan EM, Feltkamp TEW, Smolen JS, et al. Range of antinuclear antibodies in "healthy" individuals. *Arthritis Rheum* 1997;40: 1601–1611.
5. De Vlam K, De Keyser F, Verbruggen G, et al. Detection and identification of antinuclear autoantibodies in the serum of normal blood donors. *Clin Exp Rheumatol* 1993;11:393–397.
6. Slater CA, Davis RB, Shmerling RH. Antinuclear antibody testing. A study of clinical utility. *Arch Intern Med* 1996;156: 141–1425.
7. Malleson PN, Sailer M, Mackinnon MJ. Usefulness of antinuclear antibody testing to screen for rheumatic diseases. *Arch Dis Child* 1997;77:299–304.
8. Weinstein A, Bordwell B, Stone B, et al. Antibodies to native DNA and serum complement (C3) levels. Application to diagnosis and classification of systemic lupus erythematosus. *Am J Med* 1983;74:206–216.
9. Schur PH. Genetics of complement deficiencies associated with lupus-like syndromes. *Arthritis Rheum* 1978;21(suppl): S153–S160.
10. Gladman DD, Urowitz MB, Keystone CC. Serologically active, clinically quiescent systemic lupus erythematosus. *Am J Med* 1979;66:210–215.
11. Walz-LeBlanc BA, Gladman DD, Urowitz EM. Serologically active clinically quiescent systemic lupus erythematosus. Predictors of clinical flares. *J Rheumatol* 1994;21:2239–2241.
12. Petri M, Genovese M, Engle E, et al. Definition, incidence and clinical description of flare in systemic lupus erythematosus. *Arthritis Rheum* 1991;34:937–944.
13. Stastny P, Ziff M. Cold-insoluble complexes and complement levels in SLE. *N Engl J Med* 1969;280:1376–1381.
14. Winn DM, Wolfe JF, Lindberg DA, et al. Identification of a clinical subset of systemic lupus erythematosus by antibodies to the Sm antigen. *J Clin Invest* 1979;22:1334–1337.
15. Howard TW, Iannini MJ, Burge JJ, et al. Rheumatoid factor, cryoglobulinemia, anti-DNA, and renal disease in patients with systemic lupus erythematosus. *J Rheumatol* 1991;18:826–830.
16. Quismorio FP Jr, Kaufman RL, Hoefs JC. Immune complexes and cryoproteins in ascitic fluid of patient with alcoholic liver disease. *Int Arch Allergy Appl Immunol* 1981;64:190–194.
17. Endo L, Croman LC, Panush RS. Clinical utility of assays for circulating immune complexes. *Med Clin North Am* 1985;69: 623–636.
18. Kilpatrick DC, Weston WL. Immune complex assays and their limitations. *Med Lab Sci* 1985;42:178–185.
19. Valentijn RM, Daha MR, Van Es LA. Clinical significance of laboratory investigations for immune complexes. *Clin Immunol Allergy* 1985;5:649–660.
20. Abrass CK, Nies KM, Louie JS, et al. Correlation and predictive accuracy of circulating immune complexes with disease activity in systemic lupus erythematosus. *Arthritis Rheum* 1980; 23:273–282.
21. Lloyd W, Schur PH. Immune complexes, complement, and anti-DNA in exacerbations of systemic lupus erythematosus (SLE). *Medicine* 1981;60:208–217.
22. Valentijn RM, Overhagen HV, Hazevoet HM, et al. The value of complement and immune complex determinations in monitoring disease activity in patients with systemic lupus erythematosus. *Arthritis Rheum* 1985;28:904–913.
23. Wener WH, Mannik M, Schwartz MM, et al. Relationship between renal pathology and the size of circulating immune complexes in patients with systemic lupus erythematosus. *Medicine* 1987;66:85–97.
24. Bernstein KA, Kahl E, Balow JE, et al. Serologic markers of lupus nephritis in patients: use of a tissue-based ELISA and evidence of immunopathogenic heterogeneity. *Clin Exp Immunol* 1994;98:60–65.
25. Abramson SB, Weissman G. Complement split products and the pathogenesis of SLE. *Hosp Pract* 1988;23:45–56.
26. Campen DH, Horwitz DA, Quismorio FP Jr, et al. Serum levels of interleukin-2 receptor and activity of rheumatic disease characterized by immune system activation. *Arthritis Rheum* 1988;31:1358–1364.
27. Tan EM. Antinuclear antibodies: diagnostic markers for autoimmune diseases and probes for cell biology. *Adv Immunol* 1989;44:93–151.
28. Mongey A, Hess EV. Antinuclear antibodies and disease specificity. *Adv Intern Med* 1991;36:151–169.
29. Kadlubowski M, Jackson M, Yap PL, et al. Lack of specificity for antibodies to double stranded DNA found in commercial kits. *J Clin Pathol* 1991;44:246–250.
30. Koffler D, Carr R, Agnello V, et al. Antibodies to human polynucleotides in human sera: antigenic specificity and relation to disease. *J Exp Med* 1971;134:294–312.
31. Beaulieu A, Quismorio FP Jr, Friou GJ, et al. IgG antibodies to double-stranded DNA in systemic lupus erythematosus sera. *Arthritis Rheum* 1979;22:565–570.
32. Ward MM, Pisetsky DS, Christenson VD. Antidouble stranded DNA antibody assays in systemic lupus erythematosus: correla-

tions of longitudinal antibody measurements. *J Rheumatol* 1989;16:609–613.

33. McGrath H Jr, Biundo JJ Jr. A longitudinal study of high and los avidity antibodies to double stranded DNA in systemic lupus erythematosus. *Arthritis Rheum* 1985;28:425–430.
34. Smeenk RJT, Van den Brink HG, Brinkman K, et al. Anti-dsDNA: choice of assay in relation in clinical value. *Rheumatol Int* 1991;11:101–107.
35. Werle E, Blazek M, Fiehn W. The clinical significance of measuring different anti-dsDNA antibodies by Farr assay, an enzyme immunoassay and a Crithidia lucilie immunofluorescence test. *Lupus* 1992;1:369–377.
36. Bootsma H, Spronk PE, Hummel EJ, et al. Anti-double stranded DNA antibodies in systemic lupus erythematosus: detection and clinical relevance of IgM-class antibodies. *Scand J Rheumatol* 1996;25:352–359.
37. Witte T, Hartung K, Matthias T, et al. Association of IgA anti-ds DNA antibodies with vasculitis and disease activity in systemic lupus erythematosus. *Rheumatol Int* 1998;18:63–69.
38. Bootsma H, Spronk PE, Ter Brog EJ, et al. The predicitive value of fluctuations of igM and IgG class anti-ds DNA antibodies for relapses in systemic lupus erythematosus. A prospective long term observation. *Ann Rheum Dis* 1997;56:661–666.
39. Wallace DJ, Salonen EM, Avantis-Aghajani E, et al. Anti-telomere antibodies in systemic lupus erythematosus: a novel ELISA test for anti-DNA with potential pathogenetic implications. *Lupus* 2000;9:328–332.
40. Adler MK, Baumgarten A, Hecht B, et al. Prognostic significance of DNA-binding capacity patterns in patients with lupus nephritis. *Ann Rheum Dis* 1975;34:444–450.
41. Davis P, Cumming RH, Verrier-Jones J. Relationship between Anti-DNA antibodies, complement consumption and circulating immune complexes in systemic lupus erythematosus. *Clin Exp Immunol* 1977;28:226–232.
42. Isenberg DA, Dudeney C, Williams W, et al. Disease activity in systemic lupus erythematosus related to a range of antibodies binding DNA and synthetic polynucleotides. *Ann Rheum Dis* 1988;47:717–724.
43. Miniter MF, Stollar BD, Agnello V. Reassessment of the clinical significance of native DNA antibodies in systemic lupus erythematosus. *Arthritis Rheum* 1979:959–968.
44. Swaak AJG, Aarden LA, Statius van Eps LW, et al. Anti-dsDNA and complement profiles as prognostic guides in systemic lupus erythematosus. *Arthritis Rheum* 1979;22:226–235.
45. Swaak AJG, Gorenwold J, Bronsveld W. Predictive value of complement profiles and anti-dsDNA in systemic lupus erythematosus. *Ann Rheum Dis* 1986;45:359–366.
46. ter Borg EJ, Horst G, Hummee EJ, et al. Measurement of increases in anti-double stranded DNA antibody levels as a predictor of disease exacerbation in systemic lupus erythematosus. *Arthritis Rheum* 1990;33:634–643.
47. Bootsma H, Spronk P, Derksen R, et al. Prevention of relapses in systemic lupus erythematosus. *Lancet* 1995;345:1595–1599.
48. Esdaile JM, Abrahamowicz M, Joseph L, et al. Laboratory tests as predictors of disease exacerbations in systemic lupus erythematosus: why some tests fail. *Arthritis Rheum* 1996;3:370–378.
49. Esdaile JM, Joseph L, Abrahamowicz M, et al. Routine immunologic tests in systemic lupus erythematosus: is there a need for more studies. *J Rheumatol* 1996;23:1891–1896.
50. Beaulieu A, Quismorio FP Jr, Kitridou RC, et al. Complement fixing antibodies to ds-DNA in SLE: a study using the immunofluorescent crithidia luciliae method. *J Rheumatol* 1979;6:389–396.
51. Cronin ME, Leair DW, Jaronski S, et al. Simultaneous use of multiple serologic tests in assessing clinical activity in systemic lupus erythematosus. *Clin Immunol Immunopathol* 1989;51:99–109.
52. Mackworth-Young CG, Chan JKH, Bunn CC, et al. Complement fixation by anti-dsdna antibodies in SLE: measurement by radioimmunoassay and relationship with disease activity. *Ann Rheum Dis* 1986;45:314–318.
53. Pearson L, Lightfoot RW Jr. Correlation of DNA-anti-DNA association rates with clinical activity in systemic lupus erythematosus. *J Immunol* 1981;126:16–19.
54. Sontheimer RD, Gilliam JN. DNA antibody class, subclass, and complement fixation in systemic lupus erythematosus with and without nephritis. *Clin Immunol Immunopathol* 1978;10: 459–467.
55. Maddisson PJ, Skinner RP, Vlahoyeannopoulos P, et al. Antibodies to nRNP, Sm, Ro (SSA), and La (SSB) detected by ELISA: their specificity and interrelationship in connective tissue disease sera. *Clin Exp Immunol* 1985;62:337–345.
56. Munves EF, Schur PH. Antibodies to Sm and RNP. Prognosticators of disease involvement. *Arthritis Rheum* 1983;26: 848–853.
57. Arnett FC, Hamilton RG, Roebber MG, et al. Increased frequencies of Sm and nRNP autoantibodies in American blacks compared to whites with systemic lupus erythematosus. *J Rheumatol* 1988;15:1773–1776.
58. Field M, Williams DG, Charles P, et al. Specificity of anti-Sm antibodies by ELISA for systemic lupus erythematosus: increase sensitivity of detection using purified peptide antigens. *Ann Rheum Dis* 1988;47:820–825.
59. Delpech A, Gilbert D, Daliphard S, et al. Antibodies to Sm, RNP and SSB detected by solid phase ELISAs using recombinant antigens: a comparison study with counterimmunoelectrophoresis and immunblotting. *J Clin Lab Anal* 1993;7: 197–202.
60. Muller S, Barakat S, Watts R, et al. Longitudinal analysis of antibodies to histones, Sm-D peptides and ubiquitin in the serum of patients with systemic lupus erythematosus, rheumatoid arthritis and tuberculosis. *Clin Exp Rheumatol* 1990;8: 445–453.
61. Petrovas CJ, Vlachoyiannopoulos PG, Tzioufas AG, et al. A major Sm epitope anchored to sequential oligopeptide carriers is a suitable antigenic substrate to detect ant-Sm antibodies. *J Immunol Methods* 1998;220:59–68.
62. Reveille JD, Bartolucci A, Alarcon GS. Prognosis in systemic lupus erythematosus. Negative impact of increasing age at onset, black race, and thrombocytopenia, as well as causes of death. *Arthritis Rheum* 1990;33:37–48.
63. Williamson GG, Pennebaker J, Boyle JA. Clinical characteristics of patients with rheumatic disorders who possess antibodies against ribonucleoprotein particles. *Arthritis Rheum* 1985;26: 509–515.
64. Abuaf N, Johanet C, Chretien P, et al. Detection of autoantibodies to Sm antigen in systemic lupus erythematosus but immunodiffusion, ELISA and immunoblotting: variability of incidence related to assays and ethnic origin of patients. *Eur J Clin Invest* 1990;20:354–359.
65. Vitali C, Bencivelli W, Isenberg DA, et al. Disease activity in systemic lupus erythematosus: report of the consensus study group for the European workshop for rheumatology research. *Clin Exp Rheumatol* 1992;10:527–539.
66. Janwityanuchit S, Verasertniyom O, Vanichapuntu M, et al. Anti-Sm: its predictive value in systemic lupus erythematosus. *Clin Rheumatol* 1993;12:350–353.
67. Martinez-Cordero E, Martinez-Miranda E, Negrete-Garcia MC, et al. Anti-dsDNA and Sm autoantibodies in systemic lupus erythematosus. *Clin Rheumatol* 1992;11:341–345.
68. Singh RR, Malaviya AN, Kailash S, et al. Clinical significance of anti-Sm antibody in systemic lupus erythematosus. *Indian J Med Res* 1991;94:206–210.

69. Wang CL, Ooi L, Wang F. Prevalence and clinical significance of antibodies to ribonucleoproteins in systemic lupus erythematosus in Malaysia. *Br J Rheumatol* 1996;35:129–132.
70. Winfield JB. Cryoglobulinemia. *Hum Pathol* 1983;14:350.
71. Barada FA Jr, Andrews BS, Davis JS IV, et al. Antibodies to Sm in patients with systemic lupus erythematosus. *Arthritis Rheum* 1981;24:1236–1244.
72. Reinitz E, Grayzel A, Barland P. Specificity of Sm antibody (letter). *Arthritis Rheum* 1980;23:868.
73. Gripenberg M, Teppo AM, Friman C. Antibodies to Sm and SS-A demonstrated by enzyme immunoassay. *Rheumatol Int* 1991;11:209–213.
74. Yasuda M, Takasaki Y, Matsumoto K, et al. Clinical significance of IgG anti-IgG antibodies in patients with systemic lupus erythematosus. *J Rheumatol* 1990;17:469–475.
75. Huynh C, Ho SL, Ka-Yeung RTF, et al. Peripheral neuropathy in systemic lupus erythematosus. *J Clin Neurophysiol* 1999;16: 164–168.
76. Ihn G, Yamane K, Yazawa N, et al. Distribution and antigen specificity of anti-U1RNP antibodies in patients with systemic sclerosis. *Clin Exp Immunol* 1999;117:383–387.
77. Sharp GC, Irvin WS, Tan EM, et al. Mixed connective tissue diseasean apparently distinct rheumatic disease syndrome associated with a specific antibody to an extractable nuclear antigen (ENA). *Am J Med* 1972;52:148–159.
78. Grant KD, Adams LE, Hess EV. Mixed connective tissue disease subset with sequential clinical and laboratory features. *J Rheumatol* 1981;8:587–598.
79. Nimelstein SH, Brody S, McShane D, et al. Mixed connective tissue disease: subsequent evaluation of the 25 original patients. *Medicine* 1980;59:239–248.
80. Vlachoyiannopoulos PG, Guialis A, Tzioufas AG, et al. Predominance of igM anti-U1RNP antibodies in patients with systemic lupus erythematosus. *Br J Rheumatol* 1996;35:534–541.
81. Reichlin M, Mattioli M. Description of a serologic reaction characteristic of polymyositis. *Clin Immunol Immunopathol* 1976;5:12–20.
82. ter Borg EJ, Groen H, Horst G, et al. Clinical associations of antiribonucleo-protein antibodies in patients with systemic lupus erythematosus. *Semin Arthritis Rheum* 1990;20:164–173.
83. Groen H, Ter Borg E, Postma DS, et al. Pulmonary function in systemic lupus erythematosus is related to distinct clinical, serologic and nailfold capillary patterns. *Am J Med* 1992;93: 619–627.
84. Reilly PA, Evison G, McHugh NJ, et al. Arthropathy of hands and feet in systemic lupus erythematosus. *J Rheumatol* 1990; 17:777–784.
85. Nishikai M, Okano Y, Mukohda Y, et al. Serial estimation of anti-RNP antibody titers in systemic lupus erythematosus, mixed connective tissue disease and rheumatoid arthritis. *J Clin Lab Immunol* 1984;13:15–19.
86. ter Borg E, Horst G, Limburg P, et al. Changes in levels of antibodies against 70 kDa and a polypeptides of the U1RNP complex in relation to exacerbations of systemic lupus erythematosus. *J Rheumatol* 1991;18:363–367.
87. Hochberg MC, Dorsch CA, Feinglass EJ, et al. Survivorship in systemic lupus erythematosus: effect of antibody to extractable nuclear antigen. *Arthritis Rheum* 1981;24:54–59.
88. Lundberg I, Hedfors E. Clinical course of patients with anti-RNP antibodies. *J Rheumatol* 1991;18:1511–1519.
89. Piirainen HI. Patients with arthritis and anti-U1RNP antibodies: a 10-year follow-up. *Br J Rheumatol* 1990;29:345–348.
90. Frandsen PB, Kriegbaum NJ, Ullman S, et al. Follow-up of 115 patients with high-titer U1RNP antibodies. *Clin Rheumatol* 1996;15:254–260.
91. Meilof JF, Bantjes I, De Jong J, et al. The detection of anti-Ro/SSA and anti-La/SSB antibodies: a comparison of counter-immunoelectrophoresis with immunoblot, ELISA, and RNA precipitation assays. *J Immunol Methods* 1990;133:215–226.
92. Manoussakis MN, Kistis KG, Liu X, et al. Detection of anti-Ro(SSA) antibodies in autoimmune diseases: comparison of five methods. *Br J Rheumatol* 1993;32:449–455.
93. St. Clair EW, Pisetsky DS, Reich CG, et al. Quantitative immunoassay of anti-La antibodies using purified recombinant La antigen. *Arthritis Rheum* 1988;31:506–514.
94. Smeenk RJT. Ro/SSA and La/SSB: autoantigens in Sj;auogren's syndrome. *Clin Rheumatol* 1995;14(suppl 1):11–16.
95. Hochberg MC, Boyd RE, Ahearn JM, et al. Systemic lupus erythematosus: a review of clinico-laboratory features and immunogenetic markers in 150 patients with emphasis on demographic subsets. *Medicine* 1985;64:285–295.
96. Gaither KK, Bias WB, Harley JB. The frequency of SLE autoantibodies in normal sera and correlations with class II HLA antigens (abstract). *Arthritis Rheum* 1987;30(suppl 4): S22.
97. Gaither KK, Fox OF, Yamagata H, et al. Implications of anti-Ro/Sj;auogren's syndrome A antigen autoantibody in normal sera for autoimmunity. *J Clin Invest* 1987;79:841–846.
98. Harley JB, Yamagata H, Reichlin M. Anti-La/SSB antibody is present in some normal sera and is coincident with anti-Ro/SSA precipitins in systemic lupus erythematosus. *J Rheumatol* 1984;11:309–314.
99. Gilliam JN, Sontheimer RD. Distinctive cutaneous subsets in the spectrum of lupus erythematosus. *J Am Acad Dermatol* 1981;4:471–475.
100. Hymes SR, Russell TJ, Jordon RE. The anti-Ro antibody system. *Int J Dermatol* 1986;25:17.
101. Sontheimer RD, Maddison PJ, Reichlin M, et al. Serologic and HLA associations in subacute cutaneous lupus erythematosus: a clinical subset of lupus erythematosus. *Ann Intern Med* 1982; 97:664–671.
102. Lopez-Longo FJ, Monteagudo I, Gonzalez CM, et al. Systemic lupus erythematosus: clinical expression and anti-Ro/SSA, a reposne in patients with and without lesions of subacute cutaneous lupus. *Lupus* 1997;6:32–39.
103. Franco HL, Weston WL, Peebles C, et al. Autoantibodies directed against sicca syndromes antigens in neonatal lupus syndrome. *J Am Acad Dermatol* 1981;4:67–72.
104. Landry M. Phagocyte function and cell-mediated immunity in systemic lupus erythematosus. *Arch Dermatol* 1977;113: 147–154.
105. Watson RM, Lane AT, Barnett NK, et al. Neonatal lupus erythematosus: a clinical, serological and immunogenetic study with review of the literature. *Medicine* 1984;63:362–378.
106. Buyon JP, Winchester RJ, Slade SS, et al. Identification of mothers at risk for congenital heart block and other neonatal lupus syndromes in their children. *Arthritis Rheum* 1993;36: 1263–1273.
107. Lehman TJA, Reichlin M, Harley JB. Familial concordance for antibodies to Ro/SSA among female relatives of children with systemic lupus erythematosus. Evidence for the "supergene" hypothesis? (abstract). *Arthritis Rheum* 1990;33(suppl):S125.
108. Meyer O, Hauptmann G, Tappeiner G, et al. Genetic deficiency of C4, C2 or C1q and lupus syndromes. Association with anti-Ro (SSA) antibodies. *Clin Exp Immunol* 1985;62: 678–684.
109. Fessell WJ. ANA-negative systemic lupus erythematosus. *Am J Med* 1978;64:80–86.
110. Gladman DD, Chalmers A, Urowitz MB. Systemic lupus erythematosus with negative LE cells and antinuclear factor. *J Rheumatol* 1978;5:142–147.
111. Maddison PJ, Provost TT, Reichlin M. Serological findings in

patients with "ANA-Negative" systemic lupus erythematosus. *Medicine* 1981;60:87–94.
112. Blomberg S, Ronnblom L, Wallgren AC, et al. Anti-SSA/Ro antibody determination by enzyme-linked immunosorbent assay as a supplement to standard immunofluorescence in antinuclear antibody screening. *Scand J Immunol* 2000;51:612–617.
113. Pourmand N, Blomberg S, Ronnblom L, et al. R0 52 kD autoantibodies are detected in a subset of ANA-negative SLE. *Scand J Rheumatol* 2000;29:116–123.
114. Reichlin M. ANA negative systemic lupus erythematosus sera revisited serologically. *Lupus* 2000;9:116–119.
115. Mond CB, Peterson MG, Rothfield NF. Correlation of anti-Ro antibody with photosensitivity rash in systemic lupus erythematosus patients. *Arthritis Rheum* 1989;32:202–204.
116. Sutej PG, Gear AJ, Morrison RC, et al. Photosensitivity and anti-Ro (SSA) antibodies in black patients with systemic lupus erythematosus (SLE). *Br J Dermatol* 1989;28:321–324.
117. Hedgpeth MT, Boulware DW. Interstitial pneumonitis in antinuclear antibody-negative systemic lupus erythematosus: a new clinical manifestation and possible association with anti-Ro (SS-A) antibodies. *Arthritis Rheum* 1988;31:545–548.
118. Franceschini F, Cretti L, Quinzanini M, et al. Deforming arthropathy of the hands in systemic lupus erythematosus is associated with antibodies to SSA/Ro and to SSB/La. *Lupus* 1994;3:419–422.
119. Catoggio LJ, Skinner RP, Smith G, et al. Systemic lupus erythematosus in the elderly: clinical and serological characteristics. *J Rheumatol* 1984;11:175–181.
120. Harley JB, Sestak AL, Willis LG, et al. A model for disease heterogeneity in systemic lupus erythematosus. Relationships between histocompatibility antigens, autoantibodies, and lymphopenia or renal disease. *Arthritis Rheum* 1989;32:826–836.
121. Hamilton RG, Harley JB, Bias WB, et al. Two Ro (SS-A) autoantibody responses in systemic lupus erythematosus correlation of HLA-DR/DQ specificities with quantitative expression of Ro (SS-A) autoantibody. *Arthritis Rheum* 1988;31: 496–505.
122. Wasichek CA, Reichlin M. Clinical and serological differences between systemic lupus erythematosus patients with antibodies in Ro versus patients without antibodies to Ro and La. *J Clin Invest* 1982;69:835–843.
123. Scopelitis E, Biundo JJ, Alspaugh MA. Anti-SSA antibody and other antinuclear antibodies in systemic lupus erythematosus. *Arthritis Rheum* 1980;23:287–293.
124. Berksen RHWM, Meilof JF. Anti-Ro/SSA and anti-La/SSB autoantibody levels in relation to systemic lupus erythematosus disease activity and congenital heart block. *Arthritis Rheum* 1992;35:953–959.
125. Praprotnik S, Bozic B, Kveder T, et al. Fluctuation of anti-Ro/SSA antibody levels in patients with SLE and Sjogren's syndrome: a prospective study. *Clin Exp Rheumatol* 1999;17: 63–68.
126. Wahren M, Tengner P, Gunnarsson I, et al. Ro/SSA and La/SSB antibody level variation in patients with Sjögren's syndrome and systemic lupus erythematosus. *J Autoimmunity* 1998;11:29–38.
127. Rubin RL, Nusinow SR, McNally EM, et al. Specificity of antihistone antibodies and relation to clinical symptoms in drug-induced lupus (abstract). *Arthritis Rheum* 1984;27(suppl):S44.
128. Cohen MG, Pollard KM, Webb J. Antibodies to histones in systemic lupus erythematosus: prevalence, specificity, and relationship to clinical and laboratory features. *Ann Rheum Dis* 1992; 51:61–66.
129. Suzuki T, Burlingame RW, Casiano CA, et al. Antihistone antibodies in systemic lupus erythematosus: assay dependency and effects of ubiquination and serum DNA. *J Rheumatol* 1994;21: 1081–1091.
130. Costa O, Monier JC. Antihistone antibodies detected by ELISA and immunoblotting in systemic lupus erythematosus and rheumatoid arthritis. *J Rheumatol* 1986;13:722–725.
131. Wallace DJ, Lin HC, Shen GQ, et al. Antibodies to histone (H2A-H2B)-DNA complexes in the absence of antibodies to double stranded DNA or to (H2A-H2B) complexes are more sensitive and specific for scleroderma-related disorders than for lupus. *Arthritis Rheum* 1994;37:1795–1797.
132. Fishbein E, Alarcon-Segovia D, Vega JM. Antibodies to histones in systemic lupus erythematosus. *Clin Exp Immunol* 1979;36:145–150.
133. Fritzler MJ, Ryan JP, Kinsella TD. Clinical features of SLE patients with antihistone antibodies. *J Rheumatol* 1982;9: 46–51.
134. Gioud M, Ait Kaci M, Monier JC. Histone antibodies in systemic lupus erythematosus. *Arthritis Rheum* 1982;25:407–413.
135. Krippner H, Springer B, Merle B, et al. Antibodies to histones of the IgG and IgM class in systemic lupus erythematosus. *Clin Exp Immunol* 1984;58:49–56.
136. Kohda S, Kanayama Y, Okamura M, et al. Clinical significance of antibodies to histones in systemic lupus erythematosus. *J Rheumatol* 1989;16:24–28.
137. Gompertz NR, Isenberg DA, Turner BM. Correlation between clinical features of systemic lupus erythematosus and levels of antihistone antibodies of the IgG, IgA, and IgM isotypes. *Ann Rheum Dis* 1990;49:524–527.
138. Nossent JC, Henzen-Logmans SC, Vroom TM, et al. Relation between serological data at the time of biopsy and renal histology in lupus nephritis. *Rheumatol Int* 1991;11:77–82.
139. Subiza JL, Caturla A, Pascual-Salcedo D, et al. DNA-anti-DNA complexes account for part of the antihistone activity found in patients with systemic lupus erythematosus. *Arthritis Rheum* 1989;32:406–412.
140. Stockl F, Muller S, Batsford S, et al., eds. A role for histones and ubiquitin in lupus nephritis? *Clin Nephrol* 1994;41:10–17.
141. Schett G, Steiner G, Smolen JS. Nuclear antigen histone H1 is primarily involved in lupus erythematosus cell formation. *Arthritis Rheum* 1998;41:1446–1455.
142. Schett G, Rubin RL, Steiner G, et al. The Lupus Erythematosus cell phenomenon: comparative analysis if antichromatin antibody specificity in lupus erythematosus cell-positive and -negative sera. *Arthritis Rheum* 2000;43:420–428.
143. Clough JD, Valenzuela R. Relationship of renal histopathology in SLE nephritis to immunologic class of anti-DNA. *Am J Med* 1980;68:80.
144. Esdaile JM, Levinton C, Federgreen W, et al. The clinical and renal biopsy predictors of long-term outcome in lupus nephritis: a study of 87 patients and review of the literature. *Q J Med* 1989;72:779–833.
145. Feldman MD, Huston DP, Karsh J, et al. Correlation of serum IgG, IgM and anti-native DNA antibodies with renal and clinical indexes of activity in systemic lupus erythematosus. *J Rheumatol* 1982;9:52–58.
146. Hashimoto H, Utagawa Y, Yamagata J, et al. The relationship of renal histopathological lesions to immunoglobulin classes and complement fixation of anti-native DNA antibodies in systemic lupus erythematosus. *Scand J Rheumatol* 1983;12:209–214.
147. Hecht B, Siegel N, Adler M, et al. Prognostic indices in lupus nephritis. *Medicine* 1976;55:163–181.
148. Hill GS, Hinglais N, Tron F, et al. Systemic lupus erythematosus. Morphologic correlations with immunologic and clinical data at the time of biopsy. *Am J Med* 1978;64:61–79.
149. Houssiau FA, D'Cruz D, Vianna J, et al. Lupus nephritis: the significance of serological tests at the time of biopsy. *Clin Exp Rheumatol* 1991;9:345–349.
150. Pillemer SR, Austin HA, Tsokos GC, et al. Lupus nephritis:

association between serology and renal biopsy measurements. *J Rheumatol* 1988;15:284–288.

151. Baldwin DS, Lowenstein J, Rothfield NF, et al. The clinical course of the proliferative and membranous forms of lupus nephritis. *Ann Intern Med* 1970;73:929–942.
152. Okamura M, Kamayama Y, Amastu K, et al. Significance of enzyme linked immunosorbent assay (ELISA) for antibodies to double stranded and single stranded DNA in patients with lupus nephritis: correlation with severity of renal histology. *Ann Rheum Dis* 1993;52:14–20.
153. Ricker DM, Heber LA, Rohde R, et al. Serum C3 levels are diagnostically more sensitive and specific for systemic lupus erythematosus activity than are serum C4 levels. *Am J Kidney Dis* 1991;18:678–685.
154. Hopkins P, Belmont HM, Buyon J, et al. Increased levels of plasma anaphylatoxins in systemic lupus erythematosus predict flares of the disease and may elicit vascular injury in lupus cerebritis. *Arthritis Rheum* 1988;31:632–641.
155. Horigome I, Seino J, Sudo K, et al. Terminal complement complex in plasma from patients with systemic lupus erythematosus and other glomerular disease. *Clin Exp Immunol* 1987;70: 417–424.
156. Garwryl MA, Chudwin DS, Longlois PF, et al. The terminal complement complex, C5b-9, a marker of disease activity in patients with systemic lupus erythematosus. *Arthritis Rheum* 1988;31:188–195.
157. Kerr LD, Adelsberg BR, Schulman P, et al. Factor B activation products in patients with systemic lupus erythematosus. A marker of severe disease activity. *Arthritis Rheum* 1989;32: 1406–1413.
158. Negoro N, Okamura M, Takeda T, et al. The clinical significance of iC3b neoantigen expression in plasma from patients withsystemic lupus erythematosus. *Arthritis Rheum* 1989;32: 1233–1242.
159. Senaldi G, Ireland R, Bellingham AJ, et al. IgM reduction in systemic lupus erythematosus. *Arthritis Rheum* 1988;31:1213.
160. Wild G, Watkins J, Ward A, et al. C4a anaphylatoxin levels an indicator of disease activity in systemic lupus erythematosus. *Clin Exp Immunol* 1990;80:167–170.
161. Rother E, Lang B, Coldewey R, et al. Complement split product C3d as an indicator of disease activity in systemic lupus erythematosus. *Clin Rheumatol* 1993;12:31–35.
162. Buyon JP, Tamerius J, Belmon HM, et al. Assessment of disease activity and impending flare in patients with systemic lupus erythematosus. Comparison of the use of complement split products and conventional measurements of complement. *Arthritis Rheum* 1992;35:1028–1037.
163. Porcel JM, Ordi J, Castro-Solomo A, et al. The value of complement activation products in the assessment of systemic lupus erythematosus flares. *Clin Immunol Immunopathol* 1995;74: 283–288.
164. Nagy G, Brozik M, Varga L, et al. Usefulness of detection of complement activation products in evaluating SLE activity. *Lupus* 2000;9:19–25.
165. Mollnes TE, Haga HJ, Brun JG, et al. Complement activation in patients with systemic lupus erythematosus without nephritis. *Rheumatol* 1999;933–940.
166. Manzi S, Rairie JE, Carpender AB, et al. Sensitivity and specificity of plasma and urine complement split products as indicators of lupus disease activity. *Arthritis Rheum* 1996;39: 1178–1188.
167. Negi VS, Aggarwal A, Dayal R, et al. Complement degradation product C3d in urine: marker of lupus nephritis. *J Rheumatol* 2000;27:380–383.
168. Buyon JP, Tamerius J, Ordorica S, et al. Activation of the alternative complement pathway accompanies disease flares in systemic lupus erythematosus during pregnancy. *Arthritis Rheum* 1992;35:55–61.
169. Abramson SB, Buyon JP. Activation of the complement pathway: comparison of normal pregnancy, preeclampsia and systemic lupus erythematosus during pregnancy. *Am J Reprod Immunol* 1992;28:183–187.
170. Selvaraj P, Rosse WF, Silber R, et al. The major Fc receptor in blood has a phosphatidylinositol anchor and is deficient in paroxysmal nocturnal haemoglobinuria. *Nature* 1988;333:565–567.
171. ter Borg EJ, Horst G, Limburg PC, et al. Changes in plasma levels of interleukin 2 receptor in relation to disease exacerbations and levels of anti-dsDNA and complement in systemic lupus erythematosus. *Clin Exp Immunol* 1990;82:21–26.
172. Lim KL, Jones AC, Brown NS, et al. Urine neopterin as a parameter of disease activity in patients with systemic lupus erythematosus: comparisons with serum sIL-2R and antibodies to dsDNA, erythrocyte sedimentation rate, and plasma C3, C4 and C3 degradation products. *Ann Rheum Dis* 1993;52:429–435.
173. Ward MM, Dooley MA, Christenson VD, et al. The relationship between soluble interleukin 2 receptor levels and antidouble strandedAu: antidouble stranded as in original? DNA antibody levels in patients with systemic lupus erythematosus. *J Rheumatol* 1991;18:234–240.
174. Wolf RE, Brelsford WG. Soluble interleukin-2 receptors in systemic lupus erythematosus. *Arthritis Rheum* 1988;31:729–733.
175. Sawada S, Hashimoto H, Iijma S, et al. Increased soluble IL-2 receptor in serum of patients with systemic lupus erythematosus. *Clin Rheumatol* 1993;12:204–209.
176. Laut J, Senitzer D, Petrucci R, et al. Soluble interleukin-2 receptor levels in lupus nephritis. *Clin Nephrol* 1992;38: 179–184.
177. Wong KL, Wong RPO. Serum soluble interleukin 2 receptor in systemic lupus erythematosus: effects of disease activity and infection. *Ann Rheum Dis* 1991;50:706–710.
178. Gilad R, Lampl Y, Eshel Y, et al. Cerebrospinal fluid soluble interleukin-2 receptor in cerebral lupus. *Br J Rheumatol* 1997; 36:190–193.
179. Duffin M, Quismorio FP Jr, Stimmler MM. Soluble TNF receptor in serum and cerebrospinal fluid in neuropsychiatric SLE. *Arthritis Rheum* 1994;37:333S.
180. Heilig B, Fiehn C, Brockhaus M, et al. Evaluation of soluble tumor necrosis factor (TNF) receptros and TNF receptor antibodies in patients with systemic lupus erythematosus, progressive systemic sclerosis, and mixed connective tissue disease. *J Clin Immunol* 1993;13:321–328.
181. Spronk PE, Ter Borg EJ, Huitema MG, et al. Changes in levels of soluble T-cell activation markers, sIL-2R, SCD4, sCD8, in relation to disease exacerbations in patients with systemic lupus erythematosus: a prospective study. *Ann Rheum Dis* 1994;53: 235–239.
182. Machold KP, Kiener HP, Graninger W, et al. Soluble intercellular adhesion molecule-1 (sICAM-1) in patients with rheumatoid arthritis and systemic lupus erythematosus. *Clin Immunol Immunopathol* 1993;68:74–78.
183. Mrowska C, Sieberth HG. Circulating adhesion moleucles ICAM-1, VCAM-1 and E-selectin in sytemic vasculitis: marked differences between Wegener's granulomatosis and systemic lupus erythematosus. *Clin Invest* 1994;72:762–768.
184. Sawada S, Hashimoto H, Iijima S, et al. Immmunologic significance of increased soluble CD8/CD4 molecules in patients with active systemic lupus erythematosus. *J Clin Lab Analysis* 1993;7:141–146.
185. Jannssen BA, Luqmani RA, Godon C, et al. Correlation of blood levels of soluble vascular cell adhesion molecule-1 with disease activity in systemic lupus erythematosus and vasculitis. *Br J Rheumatol* 1994;33:1112–1116.

186. Mason JC, Kapahi P, Haskard DO. Detection of increased levels of circulating intercellular adhesion molecule 1 in some patients with rheumatoid arthritis but not in patients with systemic lupus erythematosus: lack of correlation with levels of circulating vascular cell adhesion molecule 1. *Arthritis Rheum* 1993;36:519–527.
187. Kling E, Bieg S, Boehme M, et al. Circulating intercellular adhesion molecule 1 as a new activity marker in patients with systemic lupus erythematosus. *Clin Invest* 1993;71:299–304.
188. Park YB, Lee SK, Kim DS, et al. Elevated interleukin-10 correlated with disease activity in systemic lupus erythematosus. *Clin Exp Rheumatol* 1998;16:283–288.
189. Davas EM, Tsirogianni A, Kappou I, et al. 9Serum IL-6, TNF alpha p55, srTNF alpha p75, srTNF alpha, srIL-2alpha levels and disease activity in systemic lupus erythematosus. *Clin Rheumatol* 1999;18:17–22.
190. Schur PH, Sandson J. Immunologic factors and clinical activity in systemic lupus erythematosus. *N Engl J Med* 1968;278: 533–538.
191. Morrow WJW, Isenberg DA, Todd-Pokropek A, et al. Useful laboratory measurements in the management of systemic lupus erythematosus. *Q J Med* 1982;51:125–138.
192. Isenberg DA, Shoenfeld Y, Schwartz RS. Multiple serologic reactions and their relationship to clinical activity in systemic lupus erythematosus. *Arthritis Rheum* 1984;27:132–138.
193. Clough JD, Barna BP, Danao-Camara TC, et al. Serological detection of disease activity in SLE. *Clin Biochem* 1992;25: 201–208.
194. Zonana-Nacach A, Salas M, De Lourdes Sanchez M, et al. Measurement of clinical activity of systemic lupus erythematosus and laboratory abnormalities: a 12-month prospective study. *J Rheumatol* 1995;22:45–49.

46

DIFFERENTIAL DIAGNOSIS AND DISEASE ASSOCIATIONS

DANIEL J. WALLACE

Systemic lupus erythematosus (SLE) has replaced syphilis as the great imitator. Osler's classic remarks concerning the disease (1) might now be paraphrased to include SLE: Know syphilis and all its manifestations and relations and all things clinical will be added unto you. . . .

Syphilis simulates every other disease. It is the only disease necessary to know. One then becomes an expert dermatologist, an expert laryngologist, an expert alienist, psychiatrist, an expert oculist, and expert diagnostician.

SLE's mimicry of other diseases was noted by Harvey (2), who listed 24 different diagnoses made on his patients during the early stages of their disease. Usually, the greatest difficulty is separation of SLE from closely related connective tissue disorders. To make these differences readily apparent, the clinical data are summarized in Table 46.1.

IS IT REALLY LUPUS?

In addition to obtaining a detailed history, attempting to correlate any past features that might have been manifestations of SLE with the current illness, the physician must perform a thorough physical examination (see Chapter 30) and make a careful laboratory survey. This should include determination of the presence of antinuclear antibody (ANA), rheumatoid factor (RF), creatine phosphokinase (CPK), C3 complement, Westergren sedimentation rate, and also a complete blood count (with differential and platelet counts), blood-chemistry profile, Venereal Disease Research Laboratories (VDRL) test, partial thromboplastin time, urinalysis, chest radiography, and electrocardiography. If these tests are not diagnostic and SLE is strongly suspected, assays for anticardiolipin antibody, anti-Ro/SSA, anti-La/SSB, anti-DNA, anti-Sm, and antiribonucleoprotein (anti-RNP) should be done, as well as a serum-protein electrophoresis. The Mayo Clinic has advocated a cascade algorithm for screening positive ANAs (3). A positive ANA had a 10% predictive value for SLE at a university medical center (4) and a 23% value in a large consultative rheumatology practice (5). Along with a thorough clinical evaluation, a diagnosis can be derived 90% of the time.

Many people who are told they have or might have SLE do not. Hochberg et al. noted that only one third of patients who were told they had lupus by a physician actually fulfilled the American College of Rheumatology (ACR) criteria for SLE (6). One hundred forty-nine patients were referred to the University of Alabama for management and/or consultation for suspected SLE, 37 (25%) probably had only fibromyalgia and 15% had an undifferentiated or incomplete autoimmune syndrome (7). Factitious disorders mimicking SLE also have to be considered (8).

Our group evaluated 44 patients with a positive ANA and no other abnormal commonly derived tests or autoantibodies (i.e., Sm, RNP, Ro, La, Scl-70, RF, C3, C4, CPK) who did not fulfill the ACR criteria for SLE and were referred for a rule-out-lupus consultation (9). At 6 months, 43% fulfilled criteria for SLE, 32% had fibromyalgia, and 9% had seronegative rheumatoid arthritis (RA). Obtaining a bone scan, lupus-band test, serum-protein electrophoresis, and specific tests such as antineuronal antibodies, antibodies to histone-DNA complexes, or antiribosomal-P antibodies helped to make final determinations.

The differential diagnosis of connective tissue disorders is complicated by the overlap of coexisting rheumatic syndromes. Two large clinics have reported that 25 and 33 of their patients, respectively, had features of two connective-tissue disorders (10,11). Coexisting SLE and scleroderma, as well as SLE and polymyositis, have been found in a number of patients. If a positive anti-RNP is present, the overlap syndrome may represent a distinct entity termed mixed connective tissue disease (MCTD).

Complicating these issues is the recognition that autoimmune hemolytic anemia, idiopathic thrombocytopenic purpura, Sjögren's syndrome, or Raynaud's phenomenon can be isolated processes for years before evolving into an established connective-tissue disease. 30% of Isenberg's 215 British lupus patients also had at least one other autoimmune disorder (12). As early as 1956, Talbott and Ferrandis (13) observed frequent transitional forms from one rheumatic disease to

TABLE 46.1. DIFFERENTIAL DIAGNOSIS OF CONNECTIVE TISSUE DISORDERS

Parameter	SLE	RA	PSS	MCTD
Sex incidence	90% female	75% female	66% female	80% female
Age of majority	10–50 y	20–40 y	20–50 y	All ages
Family history	+ for LE or RA in 12% or more	Often +	0	Rarely +
Disease duration	Mo-y	Mo-y	Mo-y	Variable
First changes	Arthritis, rash	Arthritis	Skin	Arthritis, Raynaud's phenomenon
Cardiac involvement (clinical)	33%	65% at autopsy; clinically rare	+; perfusion and conduction abnormalities seen	Myocarditis in children
Skin and mucous membranes	Alopecia, butterfly erythema, scaling erythematous papules, ulcers	Subcutaneous nodules	Tightness of skin of hands, face, neck; hyperpigmentation of involved skin	Rashes of SLE, PSS, and dermatomyostitis
Ocular	Iritis, retinal vasculitis or infarcts; Sjögren's syndrome	Scleritis, Sjögren's syndrome	Sjögren's syndrome	Rare; Sjögren's syndrome
Adenopathy	Moderate	Minimal	0	Minimal
Pleurisy or lung disease	Most cases	Rare	Interstitial fibrosis common	30%
Pericarditis	30%	Clinically rare	Rare	25%
Generalized abdominal pain and tenderness	Often	0	Dysphagia common; bowel motility decreased	Dysphagia common
Hepatomegaly	Occasional	0	0	0
Splenomegaly	10%	Rare	0	0
Joints involved	All joints, esp. minor	All joints	Minor	Erosive arthritis in 30%
Arthritic deformity	Frequent, nonerosive	Often erosive	Often	20%
Myalgia	48%	Frequent	+20%	50%
Raynaud's phenomenon	26%	Occasional	Common	80%
CNS involvement	Personality changes, convulsions and localized deficits, fatigue	Rare	Rare	10%
Laboratory				
Urine abnormalities	46% at some time	0	Creatinuria	Lupus nephritis in 10–40%
WBC and differential	Leukopenia in 43%	Leukocytosis, acute phase	Normal	Leukopenia in 35%
Anemia	10% hemolytic; 56% < 11.0 g Hb	Normocytic	0	41%
Uremia	5–10%	0	Occasional	0
Hyperglobulinemia	Common	Frequent	40%	80%
LE cells	+ in 75%	+9% only	+5%	14%
ANA	+95%	+25%	+50% speckled, CREST-centromere	+100% speckled
Muscle biopsy	Usually 0	Usually 0	Myositis uncommon	Often positive
Skin biopsy	Suggestive +	0	Diagnostic	+ lupus band test or PSS
Remarks	No classic course; pattern of symptoms and findings suggest diagnosis; anti-DNA and low complement levels indicate systemic disease	RF in 80%	Progressive over years; may spontaneously remit Anti-Scl-70 in 30%	Swollen hands; anti-RNP

(continued)

TABLE 46.1. (*continued*)

Dermatomyositis and Polymositis	Polyarteritis Nodosa	Rheumatic Fever	Serum Sickness	Behçet's Syndrome
66% female	40% female	Equal	Equal	Mostly female
10–50 y	All ages	2–19 y	All ages	10–50 y
0	0	0	0	0
Mo-y	Variable	Mo-y	Weeks	Mo-y
Myalgia, skin changes, or weakness	Asthma, polyneuritis, abdominal pain, or fever	Arthritis	Urticaria	Orogenital ulcers
Occasional	Occasional	Most in acute phase	0	0
Periorbital edema, dusky erythema, Gottron's nodes	Hives, necrotic ulcerations, cutaneous and subcutaneous nodules	Erythema marginata, subcutaneous nodule	Hives, angioneurotic edema	Recurrent aphthous stomatitis, cutaneous vasculitis
0	Rarely, retinal hemorrhages and exudates	0	0	Uveitis in 66%
Rare	Minimal	Minimal	Minimal	0
Rare	0	0	0	0
Rare	0	Often	0	0
0	Often	Occasionally	Occasionally	Inflammatory bowel disease, occasionally
0	20%	+ with failure	0	0
Occasional	0	Rare without subacute bacterial endocarditis	0	0
Rare	Major	Major	All	55%
0	0	0	0	Rare
Marked	Common	Frequent	Rare	0
Common	Rare	0	0	0
0	25%	Chorea	0	22%
Creatinuria	Hematuria and red cell casts	0	0	0
Normal; eosinophila occasionally	Leukocytosis, eosinophilia in 18%	Leukocytosis	Leukocytosis, eosinophilia	0
Uncommon	50%	Normocytic	?	0
0	Common	0	0	0
0	Occasionally	0	0	Occasional
0	0	0	0	0
+30%	+20%	0	0	0
Usually +	Suggestive if +	0	0	0
Suggestive	Suggestive	0	Suggestive	0
20% of dermatomyositis cases associated with malignancy; proximal muscles involved; EMG may be diagnostic, CPK level elevations common	Association of asthma, eosinophilia, hypertension and polyneuritis suggests diagnosis; Biopsy or *p*-ANCA + in only 50%	Preceding streptococcal infection Diastolic heart murmur almost pathognomonic; elevated antistreptolysin titer		HLA-B5 associations, antibody to human mucosal cells

CNS, Central nervous system; EMG, electromyelography; *p*-ANCA, antineutrophil cystoplasmic antibody; WBC, white blood cell.

another. Some patients, who appear to have fulfilled all or most of the clinical criteria for a diagnosis of active RA, lose the exclusive features of this malady at some future time and manifest unmistakable SLE, polyarteritis, polymyositis, or scleroderma. Currently, it is not possible to determine whether the disorder was present from the beginning of symptoms and subsequently changed into another disorder.

Why is it necessary to differentiate among these conditions? Arriving at a specific diagnosis is necessary to understand the course and prognosis of the illness and to treat it effectively. For example, if gold therapy had been instituted in a patient who was thought to have RA and urinary or hematologic abnormalities developed, it would be assumed that they were a reaction to the treatment. If ANA had been initially sought and found, however, gold therapy might not have been used, and the changes noted would have been recognized as being evidence for progression of the underlying disease.

ANTINUCLEAR ANTIBODY-NEGATIVE LUPUS

Positive ANA is only one of 11 criteria that are used to define SLE according to the 1982 American Rheumatism Association (ARA) classification. As noted in Chapter 2, 4 of the 11 criteria must be present to make a diagnosis, but the ANA is so central to current concepts of SLE that many rheumatologists find it inconceivable for SLE to be present without it.

Several reports have documented the delayed appearance of ANA in patients suspected of having SLE. In view of my own group's studies (14,15) documenting a mean of 3 to 4 years between onset of symptoms and time of diagnosis, this is not surprising. Cairns et al. (16) reported 11 patients with lupus nephritis in whom a negative ANA persisted for years before becoming positive. Bohan (17) and Enriquez et al. (18) presented several well-documented cases. Persillin and Takeuchi (19) found ANA in the urine and pleural fluid of a patient with diffuse proliferative nephritis and nephrotic syndrome for some time before serum ANA was present. Low antibody concentrations in the serum secondary to loss in body fluids can be present, as was noted by Ferreiro et al. (20).

Numerous reports in the 1960s and 1970s examined the ANA-negative lupus subgroup, but only animal substrates for ANA were considered to be reliable at the time (21–25). Many patients actually had discoid or SCLE and did not meet ARA criteria, but the remaining number of ANA-negative patients with lupus was larger than necessary. This became documented when human cell line ANA substrates were introduced. Pollak et al. (26) observed ANA-negative lupus in nine of 112 patients, as did Leonhardt (27) in three of 71 patients in 1964, Zweiman et al. (28) in two of 28 patients with nephritis in 1968, Estes and Christian (29) in 13% of their 150 patients in 1971, Bartholomew (30) in five of 121 patients in 1974, Fries and Holman (31) in 2% of 193 patients in 1975, and Lee et al. (32) in five of 110 patients in 1977.

Provost's group evaluated 28 patients with SLE who had titers of 1:20 or less with a mouse liver substrate (21). Using a rat liver substrate, three (11%) had a positive ANA. With human spleen imprints, 16 (57%) were positive, nine (32%) were positive on a KB cell-line substrate, and eight (28%) were positive with an Hep-2 cell line. These results emphasize how a negative ANA can become positive merely by using another substrate, thereby converting ANA-negative lupus to ANA-positive lupus. Reichlin (33) has stated that with a KB or Hep-2 substrate, 98% of all patients with SLE are ANA-positive, because non-DNA–containing antigens such as Ro/SSA are better represented when these cell lines are studied. Unfortunately, human cell lines are less specific, although they are more sensitive. Larger numbers of healthy people have positive ANAs when human cell lines are used. Only 17 of 447 patients (3.8%) with idiopathic SLE who were tested between 1980 and 1989 on Hep-2 substrate were ANA-negative (34). They were evenly divided into three groups: (i) antiphospholipid syndrome, (ii) renal biopsy documented lupus in patients who had received steroids and chemotherapy, and (iii) skin biopsy positive patients who also fulfilled ARA criteria. Several reports also have documented patients with high-titer cardiolipin antibody, recurrent thromboses, and negative ANAs who fulfilled the ARA criteria for SLE (35,36).

Rothschild et al. (37) compared ten seronegative patients with SLE who met the ARA criteria with 42 seropositive patients. The former group included more whites and men. They were more leukopenic and had higher complement levels and less anti-DNA than the ANA-positive group. Technical inaccuracy, prozone phenomenon, variations in microscope quality, ANA hidden within circulating immune complexes (CICs), *in vivo* binding of ANA by tissues, substrate specificity, low-cutoff dilutions, and use of monospecific antisera are other causes of negative ANAs in patients with SLE. Occasionally, patients with positive LE-cell preparations and negative ANAs have been observed (38–40). Wide variations in the reproducibility of ANA tests and difficulties in standardization also are problems that have not yet been overcome (41,42).

A positive ANA often is found in patients with other disorders, even in seemingly healthy patients. A suburban rheumatology group studied 276 patients who were referred for a positive ANA without a diagnosis (43). After a comprehensive evaluation, 52 (18.8%) were diagnosed with SLE, 44 (15.9%) had an organ-specific autoimmune disease, 8.3% had an infectious disease, and 2.9% had neoplasia. No diagnosis was made in 13.4%.

In summary, if a KB or Hep-2 cell-line substrate is used to detect ANA, 90% of the ANA-negative patients who meet ARA criteria can be shown to be ANA-positive. If these substrates are not available, specific tests for anti-

Ro/SSA may be useful (44). Other ANA-negative patients with lupus may fulfill discoid LE (DLE), subacute cutaneous LE (SCLE), or juvenile RA (JRA) definitions without fulfilling ARA criteria. ANA-negative patients with lupus usually fall into three categories: (i) antiphospholipid syndrome, (ii) early disease, and (iii) previously positive ANA made negative by steroids, cytotoxic drugs, or uremia (45). True ANA-negative lupus probably comprises less than two of all SLE cases. Many patients who claim to have ANA-negative lupus do not have SLE (46).

CROSSOVER SYNDROMES: AN OVERVIEW

It has long been recognized that patients with SLE, RA, scleroderma, and dermato/polymyositis have overlapping features, and that the disease occasionally may evolve from one entity into another. In clinical services that see large numbers of patients with various rheumatic disorders, it soon becomes evident that many patients do not fit into typical nosologic classifications. In 1969, Sabo (47) used the term lanthanic or undifferentiated collagen disease for this group. As a result, the categorization of MCTD as a distinct disorder based on a single serologic finding (i.e., anti-RNP or anti-U1 RNP) that also is present in other disorders has been controversial.

For example, Hess' group (48) followed 23 patients with MCTD. Of these, four initially had a negative ANA that later became positive, anti-Sm antibody was transiently present in three, and antiextractable nuclear antigen (anti-ENA) levels underwent as much as tenfold titer fluctuations in nine patients. In addition, nine evolved into a more or less pure SLE, polymyositis, RA, or scleroderma. Ginsberg et al. (49) compared 83 patients with SLE to 71 who had overlap disease. The overlap group had a higher frequency of arthritis and Raynaud's phenomenon but a lower incidence of renal disease compared with the SLE group. The association was evident regardless of antibody patterns. Anti-U1 RNP and anti-Sm were not predictive of the diagnosis or prognosis. Anti-RNP also is found in SLE, scleroderma, and RA (50).

LeRoy et al. (51) as well as Black and Isenberg (52) rejected the notion of MCTD and, in an excellent review and editorial, advocated the use of undifferentiated connective-tissue disease syndrome for cases that are difficult to define. Fessel (53) also observed that definitions of MCTD overlapped those of SLE, and that anti-U1 RNP was found in 25% of his patients with SLE. He was unable to distinguish clinically between the two groups with anti-U1 RNP antibodies. Maddison et al. (54) considered MCTD to be SLE modified by anti-RNP. Kahn (55) has advocated calling MCTD a U1RNP 68-kd associated connective-tissue syndrome as opposed to a disease. Other noted rheumatologists have put forth a strong case for the existence of MCTD as a distinct entity; these are discussed in the next section.

UNDIFFERENTIATED CONNECTIVE-TISSUE DISEASE

Between 1982 and 1987, ten rheumatic disease centers enrolled 410 patients for a landmark study. All had symptoms for less than 1 year. Fifty-seven had rheumatoid arthritis, 57 SLE, 37 poly/dermatomyositis, 46 scleroderma, and 213 early "connective tissue disease." The latter was defined as patients with isolated Raynaud's phenomenon, unexplained polyarthritis, or isolated keratoconjunctivitis sicca and at least three of the following: Raynaud's, polyarthritis, sicca symptoms, myalgias, rash, pleurisy, pericarditis, central nervous system symptoms, pulmonary symptoms, peripheral neuropathy, false-positive test for syphilis, and elevated sedimentation rate. These patients have been monitored for nearly 20 years and the following observations have been made (56–60):

1. 20% with unexplained polyarthritis developed RA, one of 67 developed SLE.
2. Among 31 with isolated Raynaud's, one developed SLE.
3. Among 115 with undifferentiated connective-tissue disease (UCTD), 33 were still UCTD, 12 developed SLE, four developed RA
4. UCTD had an 87% 10 year survival compared with 56% for scleroderma
5. 13% of the UCTD patients evolved SLE. They were more likely to be younger, African American, have rashes and autoantibodies.

In other words, at 10 years, approximately one third with UCTD had no disorder, one third remained UCTD, and one third evolved a defined rheumatic disorder. Smaller-scale related efforts came to similar conclusions (61–63) and one provides an excellent review of earlier studies (178). The presence of malar rash, oral ulcers, elevated anti-DNA, or low C4 complement made the evolution to lupus more likely (64).

MIXED CONNECTIVE TISSUE DISEASE

In 1971, Sharp et al. (65,66) described an antibody to extractable nuclear antigens (ENA) whose presence appeared to correlate with either a benign form of SLE nephritis or MCTD. ENA were prepared from calf thymus nuclei, and presence of the antibody was determined by hemagglutination (65,67). Because patients with SLE frequently had similar ENA titers, attempts were made to differentiate between the two groups by enzymatic treatment of the tanned red cells with ribonuclease (RNase). In those with MCTD, the titers were reduced or abolished by treatment of ENA with RNase, whereas in SLE, the antibody titer was unaffected. This antibody, called anti-RNP, was further defined by immunoblotting, enzyme-linked immunosorbent assay, and immunoprecipitation techniques in the 1980s (68). In 1986,

Sharp's group reported that antibodies reacting with a 68-kd (or 70-kd) protein were associated with the anti-RNP specificity in MCTD and rarely occurred in SLE sera (69). This pattern persisted for years and only disappeared with a prolonged remission. Their work has been independently confirmed (70) and challenged (71,72). For example, a literature review (73) found that the predictive value of antibodies reactive against the 68-kd U1 RNP to be 38 to 69 for MCTD and 88% for SLE. This review also provides an excellent discussion of the changes in MCTD definitions and perceptions over a 22-year period. In 1999, Sharp and Hoffman (74) redefined MCTD as patients with autoantibodies against the 70-kd peptide of the U1 snRNP complex or autoantibody against the U1 RNA, have a common gene sequence encoded for MCTD or select genotypes of HLA-DR4 or HLA-DR2 and have common features of Raynaud's phenomenon, swollen hands, sclerodactyly, esophageal hypomotility, polyarthritis, or myositis (75). Smolen's group has suggested that differential epitope recognition of anti-A2/RA33 autoantibodies may be specific for MCTD (76).

Clinical Features

Table 46.2 delineates the clinical and laboratory features that were described in six of the most detailed studies of MCTD (34,77–81). Because an in-depth analysis of these features is beyond our scope here, these papers (as well as several other reports;82–86) are recommended. Articles cited in the following sections also are useful studies for review. The wide divergences noted in Table 46.2 for certain MCTD features can be explained by the inclusion in some studies of almost all patients with anti-RNP as having MCTD and others that excluded patients with obvious SLE. Fig. 46.1 compares the incidence of some of the signs, symptoms, and laboratory findings of patients with scleroderma, lupus, and MCTD. In most categories, MCTD occupies a middle ground between progressive systemic sclerosis (PSS) and SLE, except for a 100% incidence of ANA by definition and a greater incidence of myositis and Raynaud's phenomenon.

Of those with MCTD, 80 are female; their mean age at onset is 37 years. Familial aggregations have been reported (87,88). An increased prevalence of HLA-DR4 specificity has been confirmed (89,90).

Children

Children with MCTD have more nephritis, deforming arthritis, restrictive lung disease, motility disorders, central nervous system involvement, and also a worse prognosis than their adult counterparts (91–94). A literature review of

TABLE 46.2. COMPARISON OF CLINICAL AND LABORATORY FEATURES OF PATIENTS WITH MIXED CONNECTIVE TISSUE DISEASE

Parameter	Sharp et al. (64)	Prystowsky and Tuffanelli (62)	Rosenthal (63)	Bennett and O'Connell (60)	Kitridou et al. (61)	Pistiner et al. (31)
Cases (n)	100	46	40	20	30	23
Arthralgia/arthritis (%)	95	91	95	100	97	96
Raynaud's phenomenon (%)	85	81	75	75	83	70
Swollen hands (%)	66	45	88	75	60	—
Myalgia (%)	70	57	48	35	53	90
Lymphadenopathy (%)	40	30	30	50	17	17
Cutaneous LE (%)	38	51	50	5	83	39
Alopecia (%)	—	42	8	50	67	30
Fever (%)	33	—	55	45	—	57
Serositis (%)	27	32	23	50	53	26
Sjögren's syndrome (%)	7	19	10	20	23	—
Vascular headaches (%)	—	30	—	10	—	17
Neurologic lesions (%)	10	6	13	55	20	22
Nephritis (%)	10	21	10	20	40	13
Positive antinuclear antibody (%)	100	98	100	100	—	96
Hyperglobulinemia (%)	80	72	95	75	—	—
Anemia (%)	41	20	85	75	53	39
Leukopenia (%)	35	18	68	75	30	41
LE cells (%)	14	46	3	—	—	44
Positive rheumatoid factor (%)	55	48	93	2	—	22
Esophageal dysfunction (%)	73	58	15	47	60	22
Anti-nDNA (%)	12	24	13	100	10	40
Low serum complement level (%)	4	39	3	30	23	25
Positive lupus-band test (%)	—	34	—	—	—	—

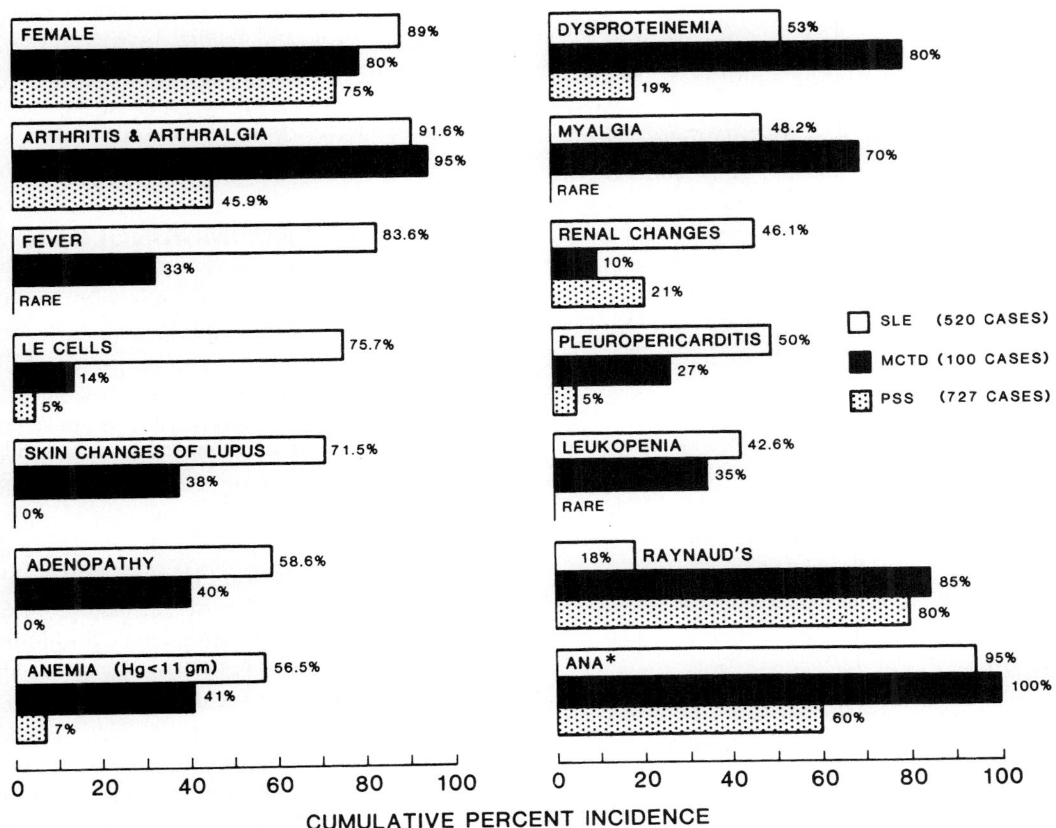

FIGURE 46.1. Cumulative incidence (%) of the most common clinical manifestations. (Source: data for systemic lupus erythematosus from Dubois EL, Tuffanelli DL. Clinical manifestations of systemic lupus erythematosus. *JAMA* 1964;190:104–111, with permission; for mixed connective tissue disease from Sharp GC, Irvin WS, Tan EM, et al. Mixed connective tissue disease—an apparently distinct rheumatic disease syndrome associated with a specific antibody to an extractable nuclear antigen (ENA). *Am J Med* 1972;52:148–159, with permission; and for progressive systemic sclerosis from Tuffanelli DL, Winklemann RK. Systemic scleroderma. A clinical study of 727 cases. *Arch Dermatol* 1961;84:359–371, and Tuffanelli DL, Winklemann RK. Scleroderma and its relationship to the collagenosis: dermatomyositis, lupus erythematosus, rheumatoid arthritis, and Sjögren's syndrome. *Am J Med Sci* 1962;242:133–146, with permission.)

274 patients with juvenile MCTD confirmed this (95). Seventeen (7.6%) died within 10 years.

Skin

Cutaneous lesions are found in most patients with MCTD. Sclerodermatous changes are seen in the hand, but they rarely extend beyond the wrist. Cutaneous LE changes are present in up to 50% of patients. Alopecia, pigment changes, telangiectasias, and cutaneous vasculitis may be present. Raynaud's phenomenon, which is noted in 85%, usually is one of the most prominent features of MCTD. Speckled (i.e., particulate) epidermal nuclear IgG deposition was seen in normal skin in 70% of 46 patients with MCTD and in 28% with SLE (79). Positive lupus-band test results may be found, and nail-fold capillaroscopy shows increased dilatation and dropout.

Joints And Muscles

Inflammatory arthritis almost always is seen; erosive arthritis is present radiographically in 25% to 60% of patients (96,97). Among the most common findings are swollen hands, which are seen in 45% to 88%. Diffuse soft-tissue finger swelling without sclerodactyly, especially in the morning, is common in SLE. Many patients initially present with a RA-like picture. Deforming arthritis is more common than in SLE (98). Over 50% of patients with

MCTD have elevated muscle enzyme levels at some point. Electromyographic and muscle biopsy findings range from SLE to polymyositis (99).

Cardiopulmonary System

Pericarditis has been described in one-third of patients but apparently is more common in children. Myocarditis is rare in adults (100). Pulmonary disease is evident in 80%, most of whom may be asymptomatic. Interstitial fibrosis, dyspnea, and decreased diffusing capability are common. In contrast to scleroderma, the lung involvement of MCTD usually is steroid responsive (101). Pulmonary hypertension is rare in adults but, unfortunately, is not uncommon in children (102–104).

Gastrointestinal System

Esophageal hypomotility is common, but dysphagia is not always evident (105,106). Changes that are similar to those of sclerodermal bowel have been reported, along with mesenteric vasculitis (107,108).

Nervous System

Neurologic lesions, which usually are minor, are seen in 10% to 15% of patients (109). The most common abnormality is trigeminal neuralgia. Changes that are identical to those seen in central nervous system SLE may occur (110). Vascular headaches may be pronounced (111).

Hematologic Disorders

Moderate anemia and leukopenia are common; thrombocytopenia is rare in adults but uncommon in children. Only two of our 23 patients had antiphospholipid antibodies. Hemolytic anemia is rare.

Renal Disease

Immune complex-mediated nephritis has been described in 10% to 40% of adults and 40% of children with MCTD. In most series, it usually is clinically inapparent in adults. Most lesions are mesangial or membranous (78,112,113), but these findings are not universal (114). Kitridou et al. (78) followed 11 patients with nephritis (out of 30 patients with MCTD) for a mean of 10 years. Of these, nine were nephrotic, and most were steroid responsive. Only three required dialysis.

Pregnancy

Normal fertility rates, decreased parity, increased fetal wastage, and a tendency toward postpartum disease exacerbation characterizes MCTD (115). These findings are similar to those observed in SLE.

Pathologic Lesions

Pathologic lesions are less inflammatory than in SLE. Intimal proliferation and medial hypertrophy of arteries and arterioles are evident. Skin biopsies suggest that the C5b-9 membrane attack complex may be the effector mechanism of endothelial and/or epithelial cell injury (116).

SEROLOGIC AND IMMUNOLOGIC STUDIES

By definition, almost all patients with MCTD are ANA-positive, usually with a speckled pattern, and have anti-RNP antibody. If anti-Sm also are present, SLE is the probable diagnosis. Rheumatoid factor is seen to 22% to 93%, anti-nDNA (native DNA) in 12% to 100%, and low serum complement in 3% to 39%. These widely divergent figures point out the different selection criteria that are used to define MCTD. Alarcon-Segovia and Cardiel (117) tested 593 patients with connective-tissue disease for three proposed criteria for MCTD (Table 46.3). Using their criteria, 80 patients with putative MCTD had a 99.6% specificity rate, but another comparative survey find Kahn's criteria for classification purposes (118).

Several studies have evaluated the importance of anti-RNP. One group correlated anti-RNP levels with disease activity and polyclonal B-cell responses (119). McCain et al. (120) screened 284 patients with rheumatic diseases. Two had anti-RNP, both with known MCTD, and no new cases were uncovered. Reichlin's group evaluated 43 patients with anti-RNP (23). Of these, 30 met the ARA criteria for SLE. Fifteen had both anti-RNP and anti-Sm, and only five had MCTD. Jonsson and Norberg (121) proposed that anti-RNP provides prophylaxis against serious vasculitis and nephropathy. Hamburger et al. (122) screened 378 sera and noted that 100% with MCTD, 15% with SLE, and 9% with PSS had anti-RNP. Two other reports have suggested that slightly under 50% of those with anti-RNP have MCTD (123,124).

Munves and Schur (125) evaluated 1,115 patients with positive ANA test results; 150 had anti-Sm and/or anti-RNP. None of the 42 with anti-Sm alone had MCTD, and 3% of the 76 patients with both antibodies had MCTD. Of the 150 patients, 66% were believed to have SLE. Similarly, only one of 25 patients followed by Clotet et al. (126) with anti-RNP alone failed to meet the ARA criteria for SLE.

Levels of CICs, as measured by the Raji cell assay, were elevated in 88% of 72 sera in 20 patients with MCTD, and these correlated with disease activity (127). A smaller-scale study reached similar conclusions (128). Reticuloendothelial system clearance of CICs probably is normal if anti-Sm is not present (129). Alarcon-Segovia's group (130) found free RNP in 10% of 299 MCTD sera at any time, but cumulatively present in 44% of 25 patients with MCTD, compared with 7% of 72 patients with SLE and 5% of 230

TABLE 46.3. DIAGNOSTIC CRITERIA FOR MIXED CONNECTIVE TISSUE DISEASE (MCTD)

Sharp et al. (52)	Kasukawa et al. (366)	Alarcón-Segovia and Villarreal (365)
A. Major criteria 1. Myositis, severe 2. Pulmonary involvement a. CO diffusing capacity <70% of normal values b. Pulmonary hypertension c. Proliferative vascular lesion or lung biopsy 3. Raynaud's phenomenon or esophageal hypomotility 4. Swollen hands observed, or sclerodactyly 5. Highest observed anti-ENA ≥1:10,000 and anti-U1 RNP + and anti-Sm— B. Minor criteria 1. Alopecia 2. Leukopenia 3. Anemia 4. Pleuritis 5. Pericarditis 6. Arthritis 7. Trigeminal neuropathy 8. Malar rash 9. Thrombocytopenia 10. Myositis, mild 11. Swollen hands	A. Common symptoms 1. Raynaud's phenomenon 2. Swollen fingers or hands B. Anti-nRNP antibody C. Mixed findings 1. SLE-like findings a. Polyarthritis b. Lymphadenopathy c. Facial erythema d. Pericarditis or pleuritis e. Leukopenia or thrombocytopenia 2. PSS-line findings a. Sclerodactyly b. Pulmonary fibrosis, restrictive change of lung, or reduced diffusion capacity c. Hypomotility or dilatation of esophagus 3. PM-like findings a. Muscle weakness b. Increased serum levels of myogenic enzymes (CPK) c. Myogenic pattern in EMG	A. Serologic: positive anti-RNP at a hemagglutination titer of 1:1,600 or higher B. Clinical Edema of the hands Synovitis Myositis Raynaud's phenomenon Acrosclerosis
	Requirements for Diagnosis of MCTD	
Four major criteria: anti-U1 RNP ≥1:4,000; exclusions; anti-Sm+ *or* Three major criteria; two major criteria from 1, 2, and 3 and two minor criteria with anti-U1 RNP ≥1:1,000 *or* Three major without anti-U1 RNP; two majors, one major, and three minors with anti-U1 RNP ≥100	A. Positive in either one of two common symptoms B. Positive anti-nRNP antibody C. Positive in one or more findings in two or three disease categories or 1, 2, and 3	A. Serologic B. At least three clinical findings C. Association of edema of the hands, Raynaud's phenomenon, and acrosclerosis requires at least one of the other two criteria

Source: Adopted from Alarcón-Segovia D and Cardiel MH: Comparison between 3 diagnostic criteria for mixed connective tissue disease. Study of 593 patients. *J Rheumatol* 1989;16:328–334, with permission.

patients with PSS. Free RNP was found, usually when anti-RNP titers fell or with steroid therapy.

COURSE AND PROGNOSIS

Most patients with MCTD are responsive to nonsteroidal antiinflammatory drugs, antimalarials, and salicylates, and those with systemic involvement usually are steroid responsive. Despite widespread acceptance of this statement, no controlled studies have been performed. MCTD is a dynamic, changing syndrome. Cases of discoid LE (131) or idiopathic Raynaud's phenomenon (132) evolving into MCTD are not uncommon. Alarcon-Segovia's group (112) commented that nine of their 40 patients with MCTD also met the criteria for four different connective-tissue diseases, and that 14 met the criteria for two connective-tissue diseases. Wolfe et al. (134) used the ACR database (ARAMIS) to compare 308 patients with MCTD to 262 patients with SLE. Significant differences (p<.01) that were demonstrated in patients with MCTD were a negative LE-cell test result, absent renal disease, and the presence of myositis and Raynaud's phenomenon.

Nimelstein et al. (135) reevaluated 22 of Sharp's original patients with MCTD 5 years later. Of these, eight had died—only two from disease-related problems—but this is still a much worse 5-year survival than in any SLE subset. Of the 14 patients who were alive, five had almost no symptoms, six had evolved into prominent PSS, and one had evolved into prominent RA. Fever, rashes, hepatosplenomegaly, adeonopathy, renal disease, and myositis were rare. Raynaud's phenomenon was universally present, but inflammatory arthritis was still seen in only three patients. Serum complement was normal in all patients, and anti-DNA was present in two. Anti-RNP titers varied greatly, with levels being independent of disease activity. Thus, those who survived generally improved, and their disease took on the appearance of a mild, chronic scleroderma.

The trend of MCTD to evolve into PSS has been observed by others (136). De Clerk et al. (137) followed 18 patients with MCTD for a mean of 4.6 years. Of these, six patients evolved into SLE, five evolved into scleroderma, and one evolved into RA. Of 44 patients who were followed by Lemmer et al. (138), seven died in a 5-year follow-up. Gendi et al. (89) followed 46 patients with MCTD for 10 years. Twelve (27%) evolved into SLE, 13 (29%) evolved into systemic sclerosis, and three (7%) evolved into RA. Eleven (24%) patients died. Nondifferentiation was associated with HLA-DR2 or DR4 (p = .007). Sharp (139) has cited a 7% mortality in 300 patients who were followed for a mean of 7 years. In 1999, his group reported a favorable outcome in 62% of 47 patients followed since 1969. This was associated with disappearance of anti-snRNP during prolonged remissions (140). These discrepancies in life-table findings emphasize the problems of following a disease that lacks a precise definition.

RHEUMATOID ARTHRITIS AND SYSTEMIC LUPUS ERYTHEMATOSUS

Differentiation

RA and SLE share many clinical and serologic features, an overlapping that was recognized in the 1950s and 1960s by the publication of hundreds of papers on RA with LE cells. (See pages 464 to 476 of the second edition of this book for an extensive review of these clinical and serologic features.) RA and SLE usually can be distinguished easily from each other, especially if the former is ANA-negative or erosive. When RA displays extraarticular involvement or is ANA-positive, however, it occasionally is difficult to differentiate from SLE. When a patient presents with a new inflammatory arthritis that has overlapping features of both diseases, it may take 6 to 12 months of clinical observation before a definitive diagnosis can be made.

Extraarticular RA may include serositis, Sjögren's syndrome, subcutaneous nodules, cutaneous vasculitis, anemia, and other features that are observed in SLE. Ropes (141) compared 142 patients with SLE to a cohort of patients with RA. The latter had a 6% incidence of LE cells, a one incidence of sun sensitivity (vs. 34% in SLE), and a four incidence of alopecia (vs. 46% in SLE). The incidence of thyroid antibodies is increased in both disorders (142). Four percent of 250 and of 365 patients with RA in each of two reports had reduced complement levels (143,144). Felty's syndrome consists of a positive ANA, splenomegaly, arthritis, leukopenia, and an increased incidence of cutaneous vasculitis. I have had a few patients with Felty's syndrome who were misdiagnosed as having lupus. Felty's syndrome is characterized by antigranulocyte (as opposed to antilymphocyte) antibodies and elevated complement levels (145). Close examination, however, reveals that the overwhelming majority of those with Felty's syndrome are middle-aged men, that anti-DNA is never present, and that most have circulating cryoglobulins (146–148). Central nervous system involvement and renal disease are absent. Another differentiating feature between RA and SLE is the lack of kidney involvement in those with RA. In what might be the definitive study, Davis et al. (149) reviewed the records of 5,232 patients with RA who were followed at UCLA between 1955 and 1977. Of these, 28 (0.5%) had renal disease of all types, only four of whom (0.1%) had glomerulonephritis. Also, three of the four met the ARA criteria for SLE, and one had MCTD. Davis et al.'s literature review of glomerulonephritis in RA (149) demonstrated that most of the cases could be accounted for by gold- or penicillamine-induced nephropathy, interstitial nephritis, amyloid, or diabetes. RF was present in 15% of 166 patients with SLE who were studied by Ginzler's group in detail (150), in 18% of Wolfe et al.'s 124 patients with lupus (129), and in 22.7% of 365 patients tested with idiopathic SLE who were followed by Wallace (unpubl. observations). Its presence is associated with milder disease.

Numerous investigators have looked for ANA in RA, and its incidence has ranged from 3% to 88%, with an average of 25% (152–154). A subset of RF-negative, ANA-positive RA has been described (155,156). Many of these patients have JRA; most have erosive disease and a good prognosis.

Coexistence Of Systemic Lupus Erythematosus And Rheumatoid Arthritis

Do SLE and RA coexist? It has long been known that patients may start with a diagnosis of RA or SLE that becomes SLE or RA over a period of years. Assuming that MCTD is not present, however, the true coexistence of these conditions is rare. Despite the frequent clinical overlap between RA and SLE features, the combination of advanced, deforming, erosive RA and a significant degree of biopsy-proven SLE is an extremely unusual finding.

Occasional case reports have appeared documenting a true coexistence (157–169). Of my own group's 464 patients with idiopathic SLE, one had classic seropositive, erosive, nodular RA with biopsy-documented proliferative SLE nephritis and nephrotic syndrome. The concurrence of SCLE in patients with RA who are Ro/SSA-positive is more common (170,171). Cohen and Webb (172) reported the development of SLE in 11 Australian patients with typical RA who were observed over a 17-year period, but the total number of patients with RA followed was not stated. Brand et al. (173) presented 11 coexisting cases; most had class II genetic determinations of both disorders. Panush et al. (174) have identified a true coexistence in six of 7,000 patients with RA who were evaluated over an 11-year period. It was concluded that rhupus did not occur more frequently (0.09%) than expected from the chance concurrence of SLE and RA (1.2%). Van Vollenhoven's group at Stanford found "rhupus" in 13 patients among 1,507 with RA and 893 with SLE (175). Seven appeared to have transformed from SLE to RA.

Juvenile Rheumatoid Arthritis And Systemic Lupus Erythematosus

JRA has been classified into systemic (i.e., Still's disease), oligoarticular, and polyarthritis subsets. Several large-scale studies have observed ANA in approximately 60% of patients with JRA, particularly oligoarticular disease in young girls with uveitis (176–177,179–180). One study has determined that ANA in this subset is directed against an RNP that requires both RNA and protein moieties for antigenic integrity (181). Despite the high frequency of ANA, other antibody systems, such as anti-RNP, anti-Sm, anti-Ro/SSA, anti-La/SSB, anti-nDNA, and anti-PM1, rarely are found.

Approximately 2.5% of patients with classic deforming polyarthritis originally diagnosed as JRA later develop multisystem lupus (182–184). In one study, two of 85 patients with JRA evolved into SLE both had anti-DNA while still carrying a JRA diagnosis (185). These distinctions often are clouded by the high incidence of ANA and the relatively low incidence of RF in JRA. ANA-negative childhood SLE also has been reported (186).

RELATIONSHIP OF SYSTEMIC LUPUS ERYTHEMATOSUS TO OTHER AUTOIMMUNE AND RHEUMATIC DISEASES

Scleroderma And Other Fibrosing Syndromes

Although ANA is present in most patients with scleroderma, other serologies associated with SLE are observed in a small minority with scleroderma. These include LE-cell preparations (187), antiphospholipid antibodies (188,189), and other nuclear antigens (190). Anticentromere antibodies usually are associated with the CREST (Calcinosis, Raynaud's, Esophagitis, Sclerodactyly, Telangiectasias) syndrome but can be found in up to 5% of patients with pure SLE (191). In contrast to SLE, familial occurrence of scleroderma is rare. Clinically, sclerodactyly, telangiectasias, calcinosis, and malignant hypertension with acute renal failure are almost unheard of in patients with SLE. It is important to differentiate among SLE, MCTD, and scleroderma, because the latter rarely is responsive to steroids or cytotoxic agents. Conversely, one would not attempt to treat SLE or MCTD with penicillamine.

Features that are relatively unique to both scleroderma and SLE are infrequently observed in patients who do not have MCTD. Dubois et al. (187) reviewed 14 cases of coexistent scleroderma and SLE in detail in 1971 and summarized the literature to date. Unfortunately, their work was hampered by the lack of accepted criteria for scleroderma, SLE, or MCTD. Since then, case reports have appeared of autoimmune hemolytic anemia (192,193), high levels of anti-nDNA (194), lupus nephritis (195,196), and discoid lupus (197–200) occurring in patients with scleroderma. Scleroderma may evolve into SLE and vice versa (201); morphea (202) and linear scleroderma can be seen with SLE (200,203,204). One case of neonatal LE with morphea (205) and four of *eosinophilic fasciitis* with SLE have been presented (206–209).

The extreme rarity of *retroperitoneal fibrosis* in SLE has been noted (206,210–212).

Polymyositis And Dermatomyositis

In contrast to SLE, patients with polydermatomyositis are less often women (83) and rarely have an autoimmune family history. Also, different skin lesions are present (i.e., Gottron's nodules and heliotrope rashes), a coexisting malignancy may occur, serositis is rare, and nephritis, liver inflammation, and hematologic abnormalities are absent. Lupus can present as a focal, acute myositis (213). Rarely, MCTD may evolve into a pure poly/dermatomyositis. A low-grade myositis with muscle enzyme levels two to three times normal may be seen in lupus that responds to low doses of corticosteroids. (See Chapter 31 for a detailed discussion of lupus myopathy and its comparison with other inflammatory myopathies.)

Systemic Vasculitis

Although *polyarteritis nodosa* is relatively rare, it can be mistaken for SLE. In contrast to patients with SLE, those with polyarteritis nodosa usually are men and include all age groups equally. Cutaneous vasculitis may be more prominent, as may eosinophilia, wheezing, and nerve and bowel symptoms. The ANA often is negative; two cases of coexistence of these entities has been reported (214,215). *Hypersensitivity angiitis* and *serum sickness* may mimic SLE at first but, ultimately, can be distinguished by a self-limited course, an absence of ANA, and rarity of severe visceral involvement. Ordering an antineutrophilic cytoplasmic antibody often can differentiate lupus from other forms of vasculitis (216).

Behcet's syndrome can mimic SLE with its uveitis, oral and genital ulcers, central nervous system involvement, and frank synovitis, but in Behcet's syndrome, the ANA is negative and certain ethnic predispositions (i.e., Japanese and

Turkish) as well as HLA predispositions (i.e., the B5 haplotypes) can be observed. I have little doubt that some ANA-negative patients with lupus actually have Behcet's syndrome. The lack of any diagnostic test for Behcet's syndrome further complicates the picture, and one case of coexistent disease has been reported (217).

One case of SLE in a child with *Kawasaki's disease* has been reported (218).

Large-Vessel Vasculitis

SLE is a disease of the small arteries and medium-sized arterioles, and it does not affect larger-caliber vessels. Large-vessel vasculitis is not associated with autoantibody formation. Elderly people more commonly develop *polymyalgia rheumatica* and *giant-cell arteritis*, however, and SLE occasionally is included in the differential diagnosis as musculoskeletal symptoms are present and an age-related positive ANA may be found (219,220). A true concurrence of giant-cell arteritis and SLE has been reported twice (221,222). *Takayasu's pulseless arteritis* is found in young women, who mostly are Japanese, but also in other Asian and Hispanic women. One Japanese literature review described ten cases of Takayasu's arteritis with coexistent SLE (223). Saxe and Altman (224) reviewed 18 cases in the literature and concluded that coexistence of these diseases was coincidental. The coexistence of large-vessel vasculitis with SLE is coincidental, possible, and rare (225,226).

Crystal-Induced Arthropathies

Although 29% of patients with SLE are hyperuricemic (usually secondary to nephritis, diuretics, or chemotherapy), clinical gout is rare (227). This could result from the predominance of menstruating females among those with active SLE. Fewer than 20 cases have been described in the literature (228–235); most were males taking diuretics. Wallace et al. (236) reviewed the negative association between gout and RA. Only three of their 464 patients with idiopathic SLE had clinical gout, including a 25-year-old woman with nephritis who had tophaceous deposits. One report reviewed three young women with SLE and tophaceous deposits; all were underexcretors of uric acid (237). It has been proposed that patients with SLE (who often have decreased synovial fluid complement levels) have a natural barrier to gout, because urate requires the presence of near-normal synovial fluid complement levels to induce inflammation (229).

The rarity of pseudogout in patients with SLE has been reviewed by Rodriquez et al. (238).

Fibromyalgia (Fibrositis) Syndrome

A secondary fibromyalgia fulfilling ACR criteria was first found in 22% of Wallace's 464 patients with idiopathic SLE (34,239), in 22% of 150 patients with SLE in Texas (240), and in 23.5% of 87 women with SLE in Australia (241), and in 8% to 25% among other groups (242–245). Brought on by inadequate coping mechanisms, emotional stress, physical trauma, and abrupt changes in steroid doses, the resulting fatigue, tender points, aching, and nonrestorative sleep can be difficult to differentiate from those of a lupus flare. Fibromyalgia symptoms are a major contributor to quality of life in lupus patients (246,247). In the absence of abnormal laboratory test results (e.g., Westergren sedimentation rate, C3 complement, and if necessary, bone scan to rule out inflammatory arthritis), physicians must reassure the patient, promote the use of physical measure (e.g., moist heat, gentle massage), and prescribe mild sedatives (particularly tricyclic antidepressants) to be taken at bedtime, but they should not increase the steroid doses (as they often are tempted to do).

Because the diagnosis of primary fibromyalgia frequently is missed or misunderstood by internists, patients with severe symptoms (e.g., fibromyalgia-related dysautomomia) sometimes believe that they have a serious, undiagnosed disorder (248). When confronted with normal laboratory results and an otherwise normal physical examination, a desperate physician might latch onto a low-titer, positive ANA (e.g., 1:10, 1:20) as evidence of early lupus (249). Their patients then might read SLE literature and become certain that they have SLE. Convincing this group that they do not have SLE is extremely difficult (250). Fourteen of 44 patients (32%) who were referred to our group with a positive ANA to rule out lupus and who underwent extensive autoantibody testing, bone scans, and/or lupus-band tests turned out to have fibromyalgia 6 months later (9).

Rheumatoid nodules occasionally can be mistaken for fibrositic nodules (251). Some groups have found discontinuous IgG deposits in the dermalepidermal junction of non-lesional skin (252,253) and suggested that fibrositis might be immune mediated. This can be differentiated from a positive lupus-band test in SLE, which generally shows continuous deposits of at least two proteins (e.g., IgG, IgM, IgA, C3, C4, C1q, fibrinogen) on immunofluorescence.

Dermatitis Herpetiformis

Thomas and Su (254) found nine patients with concomitant dermatitis herpetiformis and SLE who were followed at the Mayo Clinic from 1950 to 1981 and reviewed the literature. Five other reports have appeared, the most important of which are those of Aronson et al. (255) and Davies et al. (256).

The European Pseudolupus Epidemic

During the mid-1970s, a series of articles appeared reporting a bizarre, SLE-like syndrome among Western Europeans. Maas and Schubothe (257) described 21 patients who showed only antimitochondrial antibodies without evidence of liver disease, ANAs, or LE cells. The primary manifestation was chronic, recurrent attacks of pyrexia. In addition, varying combinations of polyarthritis, muscle aching, pericarditis and myocarditis, pleural effusions, and pulmonary infiltrates occurred. In this and other reports (258,259), the pseudolupus syndrome was found to occur in patients taking Venocuran, an extract of phenopyrazone, horse chestnut extract, and cardiac glycosides for venous disease. Maas et al. (260) analyzed the medication intake in 58 patients with this entity and found that 45 were taking Venocuran. None subsequently developed SLE.

Sarcoidosis

SLE and sarcoidosis share many immunologic features (261). Both manifest hyperglobulinemia, decreased skin test and lymphocyte responsiveness, lymphopenia, impaired antibody-dependent cellular cytotoxicity, and increased levels of CICs. Cryoglobulins and antilymphocyte antibodies may be present in both disorders, and up to 32 of patients with sarcoidosis may have a positive ANA. Differential diagnosis can be a problem (262,263), but despite these similarities, only six cases of coexistence have been reported in the English-language literature (261,262,264–267).

Amyloid

It would be expected that patients with SLE have an increased incidence of amyloid, as do those with RA or ankylosing spondylitis. Cathcart and Scheinberg (268) enumerated many reasons why SLE and amyloid should coexist. For example, both have a common pathogenetic pathway, and polyclonal B-cell proliferation is seen in both. Benson and Cohen (269) found serum levels of amyloid protein A to be elevated in 25 cases of active SLE (although these were one-half the levels seen in an RA group). This alpha-globulin is a precursor of the major protein constituent of secondary amyloid fibrils. Serum-amyloid P component also can be deposited in lupus tissues without evidence of clinical amyloid (270), and may be protective against lupus (271). Despite this, fewer than 20 cases of the coexistence of SLE and amyloidosis have been reported (272–290).

Seronegative Spondyloarthropathies

Nashel et al. (291) estimated that 500 concurrent cases of ankylosing spondylitis (AS) and SLE should be present in the United States, but this figure does not take into account the differences in catchment groups (AS–white males; SLE–females, especially nonwhites). They presented the first true case of coexistence and reviewed three cases reported earlier. None of these met both AS and SLE criteria, but one since has appeared (292). Kappes et al. (293) noted the difficulty in differential diagnosis, because patients with SLE may have sacroiliitis by bone scan and be HLA-B27 positive. Only one case of SLE and reactive arthritis and one case of discoid lupus in AS has been reported (294,295).

Several reviews have drawn attention to the coexistence of psoriasis and SLE (296–300). A 1980 report presented 23 cases of coexistence at the Mayo Clinic (ten met ARA criteria for SLE, and 13 had DLE) between 1950 and 1975 and reviewed 15 reports of 33 cases (11 of which antedated 1960) (298). Of these, 63% were female, SLE and psoriasis each appeared first one-half of the time, and 80% had discoid lesions that usually were distinct from psoriatic patches (appearing and disappearing independently), but seven of 27 biopsied lesions had pathologic features of both disorders. Discoid LE may flare with ultraviolet B or psoralen ultraviolet A (PUVA) therapy (296,297), and SCLE can be induced during PUVA treatments in patients who are Ro/SSA positive (299,300). Despite the not uncommon concurrence of LE and psoriasis, only one case of psoriatic arthritis and SLE has been reported, and no HLA studies were cited in any of these reports (301).

Association Of Systemic Lupus Erythematosus With Other Disorders

Several disorders have increased or decreased associations with SLE, and others can mimic its presentation and must be considered in the differential diagnosis. The relationship among Raynaud's phenomenon, HELLP syndrome, biliary cirrhosis multiple sclerosis, myasthenia gravis, thyroiditis, inflammatory-bowel disease, syphilis, Klinefelter's syndrome, sickle cell anemia, autoimmune hemolytic anemia, Sjögren's syndrome, thrombocytopenic purpura, pemphigus, chronic active hepatitis, and SLE are discussed in other chapters (see the index for specific listings). Additional associations and differential diagnostic considerations are reviewed here. The reader is referred to an excellent discussion by Lorberet al. (301) regarding the rationale for such associations.

Porphyria

Both porphyria and SLE are characterized by fever, rash, sun sensitivity, leukopenia, anemia, arthralgias, and central nervous system abnormalities. Although almost 50 concurrent cases have been reported, many of these patients have not fulfilled the established criteria for SLE, and almost all of their symptoms could be explained by porphyria alone (302–306). Two comprehensive evaluations of 55 and 158 patients with porphyria cutanea tarda patients (304,305) found that none met the ACR criteria for SLE, although 12 were ANA positive. One review of 38 patients with porphyria (267) found that eight of 15 with acute intermittent porphyria were ANA positive; one had SLE. Gibson and

McEvoy found that 15 of 676 patients with porphyria had concurrent SLE. Nine had discoid lupus, five had SLE and one had SCLE. Porphyria was precipitated by hydroxychloroquine therapy in two (307). Our group has had three concurrent cases among 2,000 lupus patients in 20 years. The ability of chloroquine to induce cutaneous porphyria further complicates the differential diagnosis.

Angioimmunoblastic Lymphadenopathy With Dysproteinemia

Angioimmunoblastic lymphadenopathy with dysproteinemia (AILD) is a hyperimmune state that presents with rash, polyclonal gammopathy, Coombs'-positive hemolytic anemia, hepatosplenomegaly, anergy, and decreased T-cell suppressor levels. It is fatal within months without treatment. AILD can resemble SLE (308–312) in that sicca syndrome, symmetric peripheral polyarthritis, and positive serologies can be observed (313,314). In their literature review, Rosenstein et al. (312) discussed several patients who followed the pattern of having an established autoimmune disease terminate with AILD, and they speculated that it represents a malignant transformation of immune-mediated disorders.

Carcinoma

The occurrence of malignancies in those with SLE is discussed in Chapter 61. The initial presentation of a patient with fevers, weight loss, adenopathy, and joint pains requires consideration of autoimmune and malignant disorders. Hypernephromas can present with necrotizing vasculitis, Raynaud's phenomenon, cryoglobulinemia, positive ANA, false-positive syphilis serologies, and elevated levels of CICs (315–317). Resection of the tumor usually reverses these findings. Mycosis fungoides can mimic chronic cutaneous lupus (318). A case of a woman with breast carcinoma and postradiation pneumonitis and serositis with a positive ANA and LE-cell preparation that disappeared after corticosteroid therapy also has been reported. Other malignancies are associated with ANAs (320). For example, 31% of 204 patients with hepatocellular carcinoma had a positive ANA (321). Patients with immunoblastic sarcoma (322), lymphoma (323–325), Burkitt's lymphoma (326), hairy-cell leukemia (327), ovarian carcinoma (328), adrenal adenoma (329), myelodysplastic syndromes (330,331), and Meigs' syndrome (332) were thought to have SLE on initial presentation. Tumor-associated antigen CA 19-9, which is a fairly specific marker for gastrointestinal adenocarcinomas, was positive in six of 19 patients with SLE in one report (333), and CA 125 in active SLE in another study (334).

Infectious Diseases

The propensity of patients with SLE to develop infections, and specific infectious associations with the disease, are discussed in Chapter 48, The Fetus in Systemic Lupus Erythematosus. Problems relating to differential diagnosis are presented here. Additionally, a variety of infections (e.g., toxoplasmosis, schistosomiasis, leishmaniasis) can present as SLE with autoantibodies (335–338).

Leprosy

Leprosy rarely occurs in association with SLE (339–341), but the presence of deforming arthritis, alopecia, rash, and neuropathy in both conditions can make the differential diagnosis confusing (342–346). A positive ANA or RF is found in three to 36% of leprosy cohorts, but other antibody systems are absent (342–346). Mackworth-Young et al. (347) have found a common idiotypic determinant that is shared by patients with SLE and lepromatous leprosy.

Tuberculosis

Tuberculosis and SLE have overlapping chest and central nervous system features, as well as symptoms of fever, malaise, and weight loss (348). Feng and Tan (349) found concurrent tuberculosis in 16 of 311 patients with SLE (5%) who were seen in Singapore between 1963 and 1979.

Viral Infections

Viral infections may display overlapping features with those of lupus on initial presentation, including intense fatigue. The chronicity of certain viral infections, such as the Epstein-Barr virus, cytomegalovirus, and viral hepatitis in young women, as well as the tendency of patients with SLE to develop infections, makes this a complex issue (350, 351). Infections with these viruses can induce a low-titer ANA, anticardiolipin antibody, rheumatoid factor, anti-DNA and cryoglobulin among others (352). Similarly, SLE may be associated with IgM antiviral antibodies (353,354, 448). A study of 44 patients with parvovirus B19 infection demonstrated an association with a transient, subclinical autoimmune state, complete with expression of anti-nDNA and antilymphocyte antibodies in most patients (355). This can be confused with SLE or may coexist or flare it (356–367). Increased antibody titers to Epstein-Barr viral capsid antigen, early antigen, and nuclear antigen and by PCR compared with those of controls have been noted in patients with SLE (368–371,450), and false-positive Monospot test results have been reported (372). Harley's group has suggested that Epstein-Barr virus can induce lupus (373) and that nearly all lupus patients have seroconverted. Winfield's group reported that the IgM in sera from children with acute infectious mononucleosis and hepatitis A is reactive with different antibody epitopes than from those with SLE (374). The measles virus genome along with elevated antibody titers has been found in lupus nephritis patients (375).

Human Immunodeficiency Virus And AIDS

The presentation of human immunodeficiency virus (HIV) infection can mimic that of autoimmune phenomena (376,377). Fevers, lymphadenopathy, rash, renal dysfunction, neurologic and hematologic disorders, sicca syndrome, and polyarthralgias can be observed. HIV positivity is associated with the presence of the lupus circulating anticoagulant (although thrombosis does not occur), hemolytic anemia, ANA, RF, CICs, immune thrombocytopenia, polyclonal hyperglobulinemia, and leukopenia. Anti-Ro/SSA and anti-La/SSB are not seen (378–382).

Barthels and Wallace discussed two cases, reviewed the literature, and presented an algorithm for following SLE patients with false-positive AIDS testing (383). Approximately 20 cases of concurrent AIDS and SLE have been presented (377,384–389). Interestingly, about half are males, have nephritis, are children (especially with congenital AIDS), and are African American. In a fascinating report, Fox and Isenberg followed a lupus patient who was infected with HIV while under their care (399). Stored sera showed the precise time of HIV seroconversion, which resulted in clinical improvement and the disappearance of autoantibodies. Kaye (400) hypothesized that SLE somehow may be protective of AIDS. Assuming that 500,000 Americans have SLE and that 150,000 have AIDS, at least 400 concurrent cases would be expected. This negative correlation becomes more impressive when one considers that if 10% of patients with SLE had autoimmune hemolytic anemia or other complications that required transfusions (e.g., uremia, surgery) between 1978 and 1983, when the US blood supply was unsafe, up to 50,000 should have been at risk of becoming infected with HIV (400), but not a single report has stated that any converted to HIV seropositivity (401).

Approximately 10% to 20% of patients with SLE will have intederminant reactivity patterns against various glycoproteins that are associated with HIV-1, human T-cell lymphotropic virus (HTLV)-1, and HTLV-2 (402–409). Occasional reports of concurrent disease have appeared (410–414); lupus activity may be suppressed (415).

Interestingly, many patients with HIV infections have antibodies to RNP. It has been suggested that immunization with anti-U1 snRNP potentially can block HIV infectivity (449,416). High IL-16 levels associated with SLE also might be protective (417).

Miscellaneous Disorders

Skin lesions of *chronic granulomatous disease* can mimic those of DLE (418–423) and coexist with SLE (424–425). *Thallium poisoning* can result in ANA formation and mimic SLE (426,427). *Down's syndrome* is associated with an inflammatory arthropathy that sometimes resembles SLE (428–430,440) and can coexist with it. Two cases of *lysinuric protein intolerance* (431,432) and prolidase (433) with SLE have been reported. One case each of *Hunter's syndrome* (434), *Osler-Weber-Rendu* (435), *amyotrophic lateral sclerosis* (436), *Fabry's disease* (437), *Moyamoya disease* (438), and *Werner's syndrome* (439) with SLE has appeared.

REFERENCES

1. Bean RB, Bean WB. *Sir William Osler: aphorisms from his bedside teachings and writings.* Collected by RB Bean and edited by WB Bean. New York: Henry Schuman, 1950.
2. McGehee Harvey A, Shulman LE, Tumulty AP, et al. Systemic lupus erythematosus: review of the literature and clinical analysis of 138 cases. *Medicine* 1954;33:291–437.
3. Homburger HA. Cascade testing for autoantibodies in connective tissue disease. *Mayo Clin Proc* 1995;70:183–184.
4. Slater CA, Shmerling RH. The predictive value of antinuclear antibody (ANA) testing (abstract). *Arthritis Rheum* 1994;37: S320.
5. Talbert MG, Moore SE. Clinical significance of a positive ANA: contrast with 2 year follow-up data (abstract). *Arthritis Rheum* 1994;37:S216.
6. Hochberg MC, Perlmutter DL, Medsger TA, et al. Prevalence of self-reported, physician-diagnosed systemic lupus erythematosus in the USA. *Lupus* 1995;4:454–456.
7. Calvo-Alen J, Bastian HM, Straaton KV, et al. Identification of patient subsets among those presumptively diagnosed with referred and/or followed up for systemic lupus erythematosus at a large tertiary care center. *Arthritis Rheum* 1995;38: 1475–1484.
8. Tlacuilo JA, Guevara-Gutierrez E, Garcia-de la Torre I. Factitious disorders mimicking systemic lupus erythematosus. *Clin Exp Rheumatol* 2000;18:89–93.
9. Wallace DJ, Schwartz E, Chi-Lin H, et al. The "rule out lupus" rheumatology consultation: clinical outcomes and perspectives. *J Clin Rheumatol* 1995;1:158–164.
10. Bencze G. Relationship of systemic lupus erythematosus (SLE) to rheumatoid arthritis (RA), discoid lupus erythematosus (DLE) and Sjögren's syndrome: a clinical study. *Acta Rheumatol Scand* 1970;16:191–196.
11. Wallace DJ, Dubois EL, eds. Differential diagnosis. In: *Dubois' lupus erythematosus, 3rd ed.* Philadelphia: Lea & Febiger, 1987: 470–487.
12. McDonagh JE, Isenberg DA. Development of additional autoimmune diseases in a population of patients with systemic lupus erythematosus. *Ann Rheum Dis* 2000;59:230–232.
13. Talbott JH, Ferrandis RM. Collagen diseases, including systemic lupus erythematosus, polyarteritis, dermatomyositis, systemic scleroderma, and thrombotic thrombocytopenic purpura. New York: Grune & Stratton, 1956.
14. Wallace DJ, Podell T, Weiner J, et al. Systemic lupus erythematosussurvival patterns. Experience with 609 patients. *JAMA* 1981;245:934–938.
15. Wallace DJ, Podell TE, Weiner JM, et al. Lupus nephritis. Experience with 230 patients in a private practice from 1950 to 1980. *Am J Med* 1982;72:209–220.
16. Cairns SA, Acheson EJ, Corbett CL, et al. The delayed appearance of an antinuclear factor and the diagnosis of systemic lupus erythematosus in glomerulonephritis. *Postgrad Med J* 1979;55: 723–727.
17. Bohan A. Seronegative systemic lupus erythematosus. *J Rheumatol* 1979;6:534–540.
18. Enriquez JL, Rajaraman S, Kalla A, et al. Isolated antinuclear antibody-negative lupus nephropathy in young children. *Child Nephrol Urol* 1988–1989;9:340–346.

19. Persellin RH, Takeuchi A. Antinuclear antibody-negative systemic lupus erythematosus: loss in body fluids. *J Rheumatol* 1980;7:547–550.
20. Ferreiro JE, Reiter WM, Saldana MJ. Systemic lupus erythematosus presenting as an chronic serositis with no demonstrable antinuclear antibodies. *Am J Med* 1984;76:1100–1105.
21. Dore N, Synkowski D, Provost TT. Antinuclear antibody determinations in Ro(SSA)-positive, antinuclear antibody-negative lupus and Sjögren's syndrome patients. *J Am Acad Dermatol* 1983;8:611–615.
22. Fessel WJ. ANA-negative systemic lupus erythematosus. *Am J Med* 1978;64:80–86.
23. Maddison PJ, Provost TT, Reichlin M. Serological findings in patients with 'ANA-negative' systemic lupus erythematosus. *Medicine* 1981;60:87–94.
24. Provost TT, Reichlin M. Antinuclear antibody-negative lupus erythematosus. *J Am Acad Dermatol* 1981;4:84–89.
25. Wasicek CA, Maddison PJ, Reichlin M. Occurrence of antibodies to single-stranded DNA in ANA negative patients. *Clin Exp Immunol* 1979;37:190–195.
26. Pollak VE, Pirani CL, Schwartz F. Natural history of the renal manifestations of systemic lupus erythematosus. *J Lab Clin Med* 1964;63:537–550.
27. Leonhardt T. Family studies in systemic lupus erythematosus. *Acta Med Scand Suppl* 1964;416.
28. Zweiman B, Kornblum J, Cornog J, et al. The prognosis of lupus nephritis. Role of clinical-pathological correlations. *Ann Intern Med* 1968;69:441–462.
29. Estes D, Christian CL. The natural history of systemic lupus erythematosus by prospective analysis. *Medicine* 1971;50: 85–95.
30. Bartholomew BA. Antinuclear antibody tests as a clinically selected screening procedure. *Am J Clin Pathol* 1974;61: 495–499.
31. Fries J, Holman H. *Systemic lupus erythematosus: a clinical analysis*. Philadelphia: WB Saunders, 1975.
32. Lee P, Urowitz MB, Bookman AA, et al. Systemic lupus erythematosus: a review of 110 cases with reference to nephritis, the nervous system, infections, aseptic necrosis and prognosis. *Q J Med* 1977;46:132.
33. Reichlin M. Diagnostic criteria and serology. In: Schur PH, ed. *The clinical management of systemic lupus erythematosus*. New York: Grune & Stratton, 1983.
34. Pistiner M, Wallace DJ, Nessim S, et al. Lupus erythematosus in the 1980s: a survey of 570 patients. *Semin Arthritis Rheum* 1991;21:55–64.
35. Case records of the Massachusetts General Hospital. Weekly clinicopathological exercises. Case 111990. *N Engl J Med* 1990; 322:754–769.
36. Meyer O, Piette JC, Bourgeois P, et al. Antiphospholipid antibodies: a disease marker in 25 patients with antinuclear antibody negative systemic lupus erythematosus (SLE): comparison with a group of 91 patients with antinuclear antibody positive SLE. *J Rheumatol* 1987;14:502–506.
37. Rothschild BM, Jones JV, Chesney C, et al. Relationship of clinical findings in systemic lupus erythematosus to seroreactivity. *Arthritis Rheum* 1983;26:45–51.
38. Koller SR, Johnson CL, Moncure CW, et al. Lupus erythematosus cell preparation-Antinuclear factor incongruity. A review of diagnostic tests for systemic lupus erythematosus. *Am J Clin Pathol* 1976;66:495–505.
39. Noz KC. ANA-negative systemic lupus erythematosus. *Br J Dermatol* 1993;129:345–346.
40. Nitsche A, Leiguarda RC, Maldonado Cocco JA, et al. Neurological features in overlap syndrome. *Clin Rheumatol* 1991;10: 5–9.
41. Beutner EH, Krasny S, Kumar V, et al. Prospects and problems in the definition and standardization of immunofluorescence. I. Present levels of reproducibility and disease specificity of antinuclear antibody tests. *Ann N Y Acad Sci* 1983;420:28–54.
42. Chaiamnuay P, Johnston C, Maier J, et al. Technique-related variation in results of FANA tests. *Ann Rheum Dis* 1984;43: 755–757.
43. Shiel WC Jr, Jason M. The diagnostic associations of patients with antinuclear antibodies referred to a community rheumatologist. *J Rheumatol* 1989;16:782–785.
44. Reichlin M. ANA negative systemic lupus erythematosus sera revisited serologically. *Lupus* 2000;9:116–119.
45. Moorhead SRJ, Lee AS. ANA negative systemic lupus erythematosus. *Br J Psychiat* 1994;164:682–683.
46. Fonseca E, Rubio G. Factitious lupus erythematosus. *Lupus* 1993;2:195–197.
47. Sabo I. The lanthanic or undifferentiated collagen disease. *Hiroshima J Med Sci* 1969;18:259–264.
48. Grant KD, Adams LE, Hess EV. Mixed connective tissue diseasea subset with sequential clinical and laboratory features. *J Rheumatol* 1981;8:587–598.
49. Ginsburg WW, Conn DL, Bunch TW, et al. Comparison of clinical and serologic markers in systemic lupus erythematosus and overlap syndrome: a review of 247 patients. *J Rheumatol* 1983;10:235–241.
50. Van den Hoogen FHJ, Boerbooms AMT, Spronk P, et al. Mixed connective tissue diseasea farewell? *Br J Rheumatol* 1993;32: 348–349.
51. LeRoy EC, Maricq HR, Kahaleh MB. Undifferentiated connective tissue syndromes. *Arthritis Rheum* 1980;23:341–343.
52. Black C, Isenberg DA. Mixed connective tissue disease: goodbye to all that. *Br J Rheumatol* 1992;31:695–700.
53. Fessel WJ. Mixed connective tissue diseases (letter). *N Engl J Med* 1977;296:450.
54. Maddison PJ, Mogavero H, Reichlin M. Antibodies to nuclear ribonucleoprotein. *J Rheumatol* 1978;5:407–411.
55. Kahn MF. UCTD or U1 RNP associated connective tissue syndrome. *Br J Rheumatol* 1993;32:348–349.
56. Alarcon GS, Williams GV, Singer JV, et al. Early undifferntiated connective tissue disease. 1. Early clinical manifestation in a large cohort of patients with undifferentiated connective tissue disease compared with cohorts of well established connective tissue disase. *J Rheumatol* 1991;18:1332–1339.
57. Alarcon GS, Wilkens RF, Ward JR, et al. Early undifferentiated connective tissue disease. IV. Musculoskeletal manifestations in a large cohort of patients with unidfferentiated connective tissue diseases compared with cohorts of patients with well established connective tissue diseases: Followup analyses in patients with unexplained polyarthritis and patients with rheumatoid arthritis at baseline. *Arthritis Rheum* 1996;39:403–414.
58. Williams HJ, Alarcon GS, Neuner R, et al. Early undifferentiated connective tissue disease. V. An inception cohort 5 years later: disease remissions and changes in diagnoses in well established and undifferentiated connective tissue diseases. *J Rheumatol* 1998;25:261–268.
59. Williams HJ, Alarcon GS, Joks R, et al. Early undifferentiated connective tissue disease (CTD): VI. An inception cohort after 10 years: disease remissions and changes in diagnoses in well established and unidfferentiated CTD. *J Rheumatol* 1999;26: 816–825.
60. Calvo-Alen J, Alarcon GS, Burgard SL, et al. Systemic lupus erythematosus: predictors of its occurrence among a cohort of patients with early undifferentiated connective tissue disease: multivariate analyses and identification of risk factors. *J Rheumatol* 1996;23:469–475.
61. Danieli MG, Fraticelli P, Franceschini F, et al. Five year follow-

up of 165 Italian patients with undifferentiated connective tissue diseases. *Clin Exper Rheumatol* 1999;17:585–591.
62. Mosca M, Tavoni A, Neri R, et al. Undifferentiated connective tissue diseases: the clinical and serological profiles of 91 patients followed for at least 1 year. *Lupus* 1998;7:95–100.
63. Vlachoyeannopoulos PG, Tzavara V, Dafni U, et al. Clinical features and evolution of antinuclear antibody positive individuals in a rheumatology outpatient clinic. *J Rheumatol* 1998;25: 886–891.
64. Vila LM, Mayor AM, Valentin AH, et al. Clinical outcome and predictors of disease evolution in patients with incomplete lupus erythematosus. *Lupus* 2000;9:110–115.
65. Sharp GC, Irvin WS, LaRoque RL, et al. Association of autoantibodies to different nuclear antigens with clinical patterns to rheumatic disease and responsiveness to therapy. *J Clin Invest* 1971;50:350–359.
66. Sharp GC, Irvin WS, Tan EM, et al. Mixed connective tissue disease-an apparently distinct rheumatic disease syndrome associated with a specific antibody to an extractable nuclear antigen (ENA). *Am J Med* 1972;52:148–159.
67. Holman HR. Partial purification and characterization of an extractable nuclear antigen which reacts with SLE sera. *Ann N Y Acad Sci* 1965;124:800–806.
68. Kallenberg CGM, ter Borg EJ, Jaarsma D, et al. Detection of autoantibodies to ribonucleoproteins by counter-immunoelectrophoresis, immunoblotting and RNA-immunoprecipitation: comparison of results. *Clin Exp Rheumatol* 1990;8:35–40.
69. Pettersson I, Wang G, Smith EI, et al. The use of immunoblotting and immunoprecipitation of (U) small nuclear ribonucleoproteins in the analysis of sera of patients with mixed connective tissue disease and systemic lupus erythematosus. A cross-sectional, longitudinal study. *Arthritis Rheum* 1986;29: 986–996.
70. Negoro N, Kanayama Y, Takeda T, et al. Clinical significance of U1-RNP immune complexes in mixed connective tissue disease and systemic lupus erythematosus. *Rheumatol Int* 1987;7:7–11.
71. McHugh N, James I, Maddison P. Clinical significance of antibodies to a 68kDa U1RNP polypeptide in connective tissue disease. *J Rheumatol* 1990;17:1320–1328.
72. Margaux J, Hayem G, Palazzo E, et al. Clinical usefulness of antibodies to U1snRNP proteins in mixed connective tissue disease and systemic lupus erythematosus. *Rev Rhum Engl Ed* 1998;65:378–386.
73. Citera G, Lazaro MA, Maldonado Cocco JA. Mixed connective tissue disease: fact or fiction? *Lupus* 1995;4:255–257.
74. Sharp GC, Hoffman RW. Clinical, immunologic and immunogenetic evidence that mixed connective tissue disease is a distinct entity: comment on the arttícle by Smolen and Steiner. *Arthritis Rheum* 1999;42:190–191.
75. Smolen JS, Steiner G. Mixed connective tissue disease. To be or not to be? *Arthritis Rheum* 1998;41:768–777.
76. Skriner K, Sommergruber WH, Tremmel V, et al. Anti-A2/RA33 autoantibodies are directed to the RNA binding region of the A2 protein of the heterogeneous nuclear ribonucleoprotein complex. Differential epitope recognition in rheumatoid arthritis, systemic lupus erythematosus, and mixed connective tissue disease. *J Clin Invest* 1997;100:127–135.
77. Bennett RM, O'Connell DJ. Mixed connective tissue disease: a clinicopathologic study of 20 cases. *Semin Arthritis Rheum* 1980;10:25–51.
78. Kitridou RC, Akmal M, Turkel SB, et al. Renal involvement in mixed connective tissue disease: a longitudinal clinicopathologic study. *Semin Arthritis Rheum* 1986;16:135–145.
79. Prystowsky SD, Tuffanelli DL. Speckled (particulate) epidermal nuclear IgG deposition in normal skin: correlation of clinical features and laboratory findings in 46 patients with a subset of connective tissue disease characterized by antibody to extractable nuclear antigen. *Arch Dermatol* 1978;114:705–710.
80. Rosenthal M. Sharp syndrome (mixed connective tissue disease): clinical and laboratory evaluation on 40 patients. *Eur J Rheumatol* 1979;2:237–242.
81. Sharp GC, Irvin WS, May CM, et al. Association of antibodies to ribonucleoprotein and Sm antigens with mixed connective-tissue disease, systemic lupus erythematosus and other rheumatic diseases. *N Engl J Med* 1976;295:1149–1154.
82. Kasukawa R, Sharp GC, eds. *Mixed connective tissue diseases and antinuclear antibodies.* Amsterdam: Elsevier, 1987.
83. Maddison PJ. Overlap syndromes, mixed connective tissue disease and eosinophilic fascitis. *Curr Opin Rheumatol* 1989;1: 523–528.
84. Prystowsky SD. Mixed connective tissue disease. *West J Med* 1980;132:288–293.
85. Sharp GC. Mixed connective tissue disease: current concepts. Proceedings of the conference commemorating the 25th anniversary, Research Fellowships Program, The Arthritis Foundation. *Arthritis Rheum* 1977;20(suppl 6):S181.
86. Sharp GC, Anderson PC. Current concepts in the classification of connective tissue diseases: overlap syndromes and mixed connective tissue disease (MCTD). *J Amer Acad Dermatol* 1980;2: 269–279.
87. Horn JR, Kapur JJ, Walter SE. Mixed connective tissue disease in siblings. *Arthritis Rheum* 1971;21:709–714.
88. Ramos-Niembro F, Alarcon-Segovia D. Familial aspects of mixed connective tissue disease (MCTD). I. Occurrence of systemic lupus erythematosus in another family member in two families and aggregation of MCTD in another family. *J Rheumatol* 1978;5:433–440.
89. Gendi NST, Welsh KI, van Vendroou JV, et al. HLA type as a predictor of mixed connective tissue disease differentiation. Ten year clinical and immunogenetic follow up of 46 patients. *Arthritis Rheum* 1995;38:259–266.
90. Hoffman RW, Shart GC. Is anti U1-RNP autoantibody positive connective tissue disease genetically distinct? *J Rheumatol* 1995; 22:586–588.
91. Singsen BH, Kornreich HK, Koster-King K, et al. Mixed connective tissue disease in children. Proceedings of the conference on rheumatic diseases in childhood. *Arthritis Rheum* 1976; 20(suppl):355–360.
92. Singsen BH, Swanson VL, Bernstein BH, et al. A histologic evaluation of mixed connective tissue disease of childhood. *Am J Med* 1980;68:710–717.
93. Stuckey M, Dawkins R, Zilko P, et al. MCTD in children: development of SLE with CNS involvement. *Aust N Z J Med* 1982;12:576.
94. Kotajima L, Aotsuka S, Sumiya M, et al. Clinical features of patients with juvenile onset mixed connective tissue disease: analysis of data collected in a nationwide collaborative study in Japan. *J Rheumatol* 1996;23:1088–1094.
95. Michaels H. Course of mixed connective tissue disease in children. *Ann Med* 1997;29:359–364.
96. Halla JT, Schrohenloher RE, Volanakis JE. Immune complexes and other laboratory features of pleural effusions: a comparison of rheumatoid arthritis, systemic lupus erythematosus and other diseases. *Ann Intern Med* 1980;92:748–752.
97. Ramos-Niembro F, Alarcon-Segovia D, Hernandez-Ortiz J. Articular manifestations of mixed connective tissue disease. *Arthritis Rheum* 1979;22:43–51.
98. Alarcon-Segovia D. Deforming arthropathy of the hands in SLE and the growing pains of MCTD. *J Rheumatol* 1991;18:632.
99. Oxenhandler R, Hart M, Corman L, et al. Pathology of skeletal muscle in mixed connective tissue disease. *Arthritis Rheum* 1977;20:985–988.

100. Alpert MA, Goldberg SH, Singsen BH, et al. Cardiovascular manifestations of mixed connective tissue disease in adults. *Circulation* 1983;68:1182–1193.
101. Lightfoot RW Jr, Lotke PA. Osteonecrosis of metacarpal heads in systemic lupus erythematosus. Value of radiostrontium scintimetry in differential diagnosis. *Arthritis Rheum* 1972;15: 486–492.
102. Jones MB, Osterholm RK, Wilson RB, et al. Fatal pulmonary hypertension and resolving immune-complex glomerulonephritis in mixed connective tissue disease. A case report and review of the literature. *Am J Med* 1978;65:855–863.
103. Rosenberg AM, Petty RE, Cumming GR, et al. Pulmonary hypertension in a child with mixed connective tissue disease. *J Rheumatol* 1979;6:700–704.
104. Wiener-Kronish JP, Solinger AM, Warnock ML, et al. Severe pulmonary involvement in mixed connective tissue disease. *Am Rev Respon Dis* 1981;124:499–503.
105. Doria A, Bonavina L, Anselmino M, et al. Esophageal involvement in mixed connective tissue disease. *J Rheumatol* 1991;18: 685–690.
106. Marshall JB, Kretschmar JM, Gerhardt DC, et al. Gastrointestinal manifestations of mixed connective tissue disease. *Gastroenterology* 1990;98:1232–1238.
107. Cooke CL, Lurie HI. Case report: fatal gastrointestinal hemorrhage in mixed connective tissue disease. *Arthritis Rheum* 1977; 20:1421–1427.
108. Norman DA, Fleischman RM. Gastrointestinal systemic sclerosis in serologic mixed connective tissue disease. *Arthritis Rheum* 1978;21:811–819.
109. Nitsche A, Leiguarda RC, Maldonado Cocco JA, et al. Neurological features of the overlap syndrome. *Clin Rheumatol* 1991; 10:5–9.
110. Bennett RM, Bong DM, Spargo BH. Neuropsychiatric problems in mixed connective tissue disease. *Am J Med* 1978;65: 955–962.
111. Bronshvag MM, Prystowsky SD, Traviesa DC. Vascular headaches in mixed connective tissue disease. *Headache* 1978; 18:154–160.
112. Bennett RM, Spargo BH. Immune complex nephropathy in mixed connective tissue disease. *Am J Med* 1977;63:534–541.
113. Glassock RJ, Goldstein DA. Recurrent acute renal failure in a patient with mixed connective tissue disease. *Am J Nephrol* 1982;2:282–290.
114. Kitridou RC, Akmal M, Ehresman GR, et al. Nephropathy in mixed connective tissue disease (abstract). *Arthritis Rheum* 1980; 23:704.
115. Kitridou RC. Pregnancy in mixed connective tissue disease, poly/dermatomyositis and scleroderma. *Clin Exper Rheumatol* 1988;6:173–178.
116. Magro CM, Crowson AN, Regauer S. Mixed connective tissue disease. A clinical, histological, and immunofluorescence study of eight cases. *Amer J Dermatopathol* 1997;19:206–213.
117. Alarcon-Segovia D, Cardiel MH. Comparison between 3 diagnostic criteria for mixed connective tissue disease. Study of 593 patients. *J Rheumatol* 1989;16:328–334.
118. Amigues JM, Cantagrel A, Abbal M, et al. Comparative study of 4 diagnostic criteria sets for mixed connective tissue disease in patients with anti-RNP antibodies. *J Rheumatol* 1996;23: 2055–2062.
119. Houtman PM, Kallenberg CG, Limburg PC, et al. The TH. Fluctuations in anti-NRNP levels in patients with mixed connective tissue disease are related to disease activity as part of a polyclonal B cell response. *Ann Rheum Dis* 1986;45:800–808.
120. McCain GA, Bell DA, Chodirker WB, et al. Antibody to extractable nuclear antigen in the rheumatic diseases. *J Rheumatol* 1978;5:399–406.
121. Jonsson J, Norberg R. Symptomatology and diagnosis in connective tissue disease. II. Evaluations and follow-up examinations in consequence of a speckled antinuclear immunofluorescence pattern. *Scand J Rheumatol* 1978;7:229–236.
122. Hamburger M, Hodes S, Barland P. The incidence and clinical significance of antibodies to extractable nuclear antigens. *Am J Med Sci* 1977;273:21–28.
123. Lazaro MA, Maldonado-Cocco JA, Catoggio LJ, et al. Clinical and serologic characteristics of patients with overlap syndrome: is mixed connective tissue disease a distinct clinical entity? *Medicine* 1989;68:58–65.
124. Rasmussen EK, Ullman S, Hoier-Madsen M, et al. Clinical implications of ribonucleoprotein antibody. *Arch Dermatol* 1987;123:601–605.
125. Munves EF, Schur PH. Antibodies to Sm and RNP. Prognosticators of disease involvement. *Arthritis Rheum* 1983;26:848–853.
126. Clotet B, Guardia J, Pigrau C, et al. Incidence and clinical significance of anti-ENA antibodies in systemic lupus erythematosus. Estimation by counter-immunoelectrophoresis. *Scand J Rheumatol* 1984;13:15–20.
127. Halla JT, Volanakis JE, Schrohenloher RE. Circulating immune complexes in mixed connective disease. *Arthritis Rheum* 1979; 22:484–489.
128. Cunningham PH, Andrews BS, Davis JS 4th. Immune complexes in progressive systemic sclerosis and mixed connective tissue disease. *J Rheumatol* 1980;7:301–308.
129. Hamburger MI, Moutsopoulus HM, Lawley TJ, et al. Reticuloendothelial system Fc receptor function in mixed connective tissue disease. *Arthritis Rheum* 1979;22:618–619.
130. Fishbein E, Ramon-Niembro F, Alacon-Segovia D. Free serum ribonucleoprotein in mixed connective tissue disease and other connective tissue diseases. *J Rheumatol* 1978;5:384–390.
131. Gilliam JN, Prystowsky SD. Conversion of discoid lupus erythematosus to mixed connective tissue disease. *J Rheumatol* 1977;4:165–169.
132. Ellman MH, Pachman L, Medof ME. Raynaud's phenomenon and initially seronegative mixed connective tissue disease. *J Rheumatol* 1981;8:632–634.
133. Alcocer-Varela J, Laffon A, Alarcon-Segovia D. Defective monocyte production of, and T lymphocyte response to, interleukin-1 in the peripheral blood of patients with systemic lupus erythematosus. *Clin Exp Immunol* 1983;55:125–132.
134. Wolfe JF, Takasugi S, Kingsland L, et al. Objective derivation of clinical discriminators for mixed connective tissue diseases. *Arthritis Rheum* 1979;22:675–676.
135. Nimelstein SH, Brody S, McShane D, et al. Mixed connective tissue disease: subsequent evaluation of the 25 original patients. *Medicine* 1980;59:239–248.
136. Manthorpe R, Teppo AM, Bendixen G, et al. Antibodies to SS-B in chronic inflammatory connective tissue diseases. Relationship with HLA-Dw2 and HLA-Dw3 antigens in primary Sjogren's syndrome. *Arthritis Rheum* 1982;25:662–667.
137. de Clerck LS, Meijers KA, Cats A. Is MCTD a distinct entity? Comparison of clinical and laboratory findings in MCTD, SLE, PSS and RA patients. *Clin Rheumatol* 1989;8:29–36.
138. Lemmer JP, Amy NH, Mallory JH, et al. Clinical characteristics and course in patients with high titer anti RNP antibodies. *J Rheumatol* 1982;9:536–542.
139. Sharp GC. Mixed connective tissue disease. In: McCarty D, ed. *Arthritis and allied conditions, 9th ed.* Philadelphia: Lea & Febiger, 1979:737–741.
140. Burdt MA, Hoffman RA, Deutscher SL, et al. Long-term outcome in mixed connective tissue disease. Longitudinal clinical and serological findings. *Arthritis Rheum* 1999;42:899–909.
141. Ropes MW. *Systemic lupus erythematosus*. Cambridge, MA: Harvard University Press, 1976.

142. Hijmans W, Doniach D, Roitt IM, et al. Serological overlap between lupus erythematosus, rheumatoid arthritis, and thyroid auto-immune disease. *Br Med J* 1961;4:909–914.
143. Franco AE, Schur PH. Hypocomplementemic rheumatoid arthritis (RA) (abstract). *Arthritis Rheum* 1971;14:162.
144. Hunder GG, McDuffie FC. Hypocomplementemia in rheumatoid arthritis. *Am J Med* 1973;54:461–472.
145. Denko CW, Zumpft CW. Chronic arthritis with splenomegaly and leukopenia. *Arthritis Rheum* 1962;5:478–491.
146. Goldberg J, Pinals RS. Felty syndrome. *Semin Arthritis Rheum* 1980;10:52–65.
147. Ruderman M, Miller LM, Pinals RS. Clinical and serologic observations on 27 patients with Felty's syndrome. *Arthritis Rheum* 1968;11:377–384.
148. Weisman M, Zvaifler NJ. Cryoimmunoglobulinemia in Felty's syndrome. *Arthritis Rheum* 1976;19:3110.
149. Davis JA, Cohen AH, Weisbart R, et al. Glomerulonephritis in rheumatoid arthritis. *Arthritis Rheum* 1979;22:1018–1023.
150. Feldman D, Feldman D, Ginzler E, et al. Rheumatoid factor in patients with systemic lupus erythematosus. *J Rheumatol* 1989;16:618–622.
151. Wolfe F, Cathey MA, Roberts FK. The latex test revisited. Rheumatoid factor testing 8,287 rheumatic disease patients. *Arthritis Rheum* 1991;34:951–958.
152. Barnett EV, Leddy JP, Condemi JJ, et al. Antinuclear factors in rheumatoid arthritis. *Ann N Y Acad Sci* 1965;124:896–903.
153. Elling P. On the incidence of antinuclear factors in rheumatoid arthritis. *Acta Rheumatol Scand* 1967;13:102–112.
154. Pollak VE. Antinuclear antibodies in families of patients with systemic lupus erythematosus. *N Engl J Med* 1964;271: 165–171.
155. Go T, Lockshin M. Latex-negative ANA-positive erosive arthritis. Prognosis more like SLE than RA (abstract). *Arthritis Rheum* 1975;18:401.
156. Linker-Israeli M, Quismorio FP Jr, Horwitz DA. CD8+ lymphocytes from patients with systemic lupus erythematosus sustain, rather than suppress, spontaneous polyclonal IgG production and synergies with CD4+ cells to support autoantibody synthesis. *Arthritis Rheum* 1990;33:1216–1225.
157. Barnett EV, Kantor G, Bickel YB, et al. Systemic lupus erythematosus. *CA Med* 1969;111:467–481.
158. Case records of the Massachusetts General Hospital. Weekly clinicopathological exercises. Case 291976. *N Engl J Med* 1976:295:156–163.
159. Dubois EL, ed. Lupus erythematosus. A review of the current status of discoid and systemic lupus erythematosus and their variants. 2nd ed. rev. Los Angeles: USC Press, 1976.
160. Fischman AS, Abeles M, Zanetti M, et al. The coexistence of rheumatoid arthritis and systemic lupus erythematosus: a case report and review of the literature. *J Rheumatol* 1981;8: 405–415.
161. Kantor GL, Bickel YB, Barnett EV. Coexistence of systemic lupus erythematosus and rheumatoid arthritis. Report of a case and review of the literature, and clinical, pathologic and serologic observations. *Am J Med* 1969;47:433–444.
162. Pons M, Nolla JM, Bover J, et al. Concurrence of rheumatoid arthritis and systemic lupus erythematosus. A case report with diffuse proliferative glomerulonephritis. *Nefrologia* 1991;9: 80–83.
163. Toone EC Jr, Irby R, Pierce EL. The L.E. cell in rheumatoid arthritis. *Am J Med Sci* 1960;240:599–608.
164. van den Brink H, Vroom TM, van de Laar MAF, et al. Superior vena cava syndrome caused by systemic lupus erythematosus in a patient with longstanding rheumatoid arthritis. *J Rheumatol* 1990;17:240–243.
165. Venegoni C, Chevallard M, Mele G, et al. The coexistence of rheumatoid arthritis and systemic lupus erythematosus. *Clin Rheumatol* 1987;6:439–445.
166. Satoh M, Yamagata H, Watanabe F, et al. A case of long-standing classical rheumatoid arthritis complicated by serological and clinical characteristics of SLE. *Scand J Rheumatol* 1993;22: 138–140.
167. Satoh M, Ajmani AK, Akizuki M. What is the definition for coexistent rheumatoid arthritis and systemic lupus erythematosus? *Lupus* 1994;3:137–138.
168. Jawad ASM, Habib S. The definition for coexistent rheumatoid arthritis and systemic lupus erythemtatosus. *Lupus* 1995;4: 166–167.
169. Bachmann S, Wunderlin B, Knusel O. Overlap syndrome of rheumatoid arthritis and systemic lupus erythematosusa case report and review of the literature. *Aktuelle Rheumatol* 1995;20: 149–154.
170. Cohen S, Stastny P, Sontheimer RD. Concurrence of subacute cutaneous lupus erythematosus and rheumatoid arthritis. *Arthritis Rheum* 1986;29:421–425.
171. Menard HA, Boire G, Lopez-Longo FJ, et al. Rhupus: an RA subset predicted and defined by the presence of anti-native Ro antibody (abstract). *Arthritis Rheum* 1989;32:S16.
172. Cohen MG, Webb J. Concurrence of rheumatoid arthritis and systemic lupus erythematosus: report of 11 cases. *Ann Rheum Dis* 1987;46:853–858.
173. Brand CA, Rowley MJ, Tait BD, et al. Coexistent rheumatoid arthritis and systemic lupus erythematosus: clinical, serological, and phenotypic features. *Ann Rheum Dis* 1992;51:173–176.
174. Panush RS, Edwards L, Longley S, et al. Rhupus syndrome. *Arch Intern Med* 1988;148:1633–1636.
175. Sundaramurthy SG, Karsevar MP, van Vollenhoven RF. Influence of hormonal events on disease expression in patients with the combination of systemic lupus erythematosus and rheumatoid arthritis. *J Clin Rheumatol* 1999;5:9–16.
176. Cassidy JT, Levinson JE, Bass JC, et al. A study of classification criteria for a diagnosis of juvenile rheumatoid arthritis. *Arthritis Rheum* 1986;29:274–281.
177. Chudwin DS, Ammann AJ, Cowan MJ, et al. Significance of a positive antinuclear antibody test in a pediatric population. *Am J Dis Child* 1983;137:1103–1106.
178. Mosca M, Neri R, Bombardieri S. Undifferentiated connective tissue disease (UCTD): A review of the literature and a proposal for preliminary classification criteria. *Clin Exper Rheumatol* 1999;17:615–620.
179. Moore TL, Osborn TG, Weiss TD, et al. Autoantibodies in juvenile arthritis. *Semin Arthritis Rheum* 1984;13:329–336.
180. Osborn TG, Patel NJ, Moore TI, et al. Use of the Hep-2 cell substrate in the detection of antinuclear antibodies in juvenile rheumatoid arthritis. *Arthritis Rheum* 1984;27:1286–1289.
181. Saulsbury FT. Antibody to ribonucleoprotein in pauciarticular juvenile rheumatoid arthritis. *J Rheumatol* 1988;15:295–297.
182. Nepom BS, Schaller JG. Childhood systemic lupus erythematosus. *Prog Clin Rheumatol* 1984;1:33–69.
183. Ragsdale CG, Petty RE, Cassidy JT, et al. The clinical progression of apparent juvenile rheumatoid arthritis to systemic lupus erythematosus. *J Rheumatol* 1980;7:50–55.
184. Saulsbury FT, Kesler RW, Kennaugh JM, et al. Overlap syndrome of juvenile rheumatoid arthritis and systemic lupus erythematosus. *J Rheumatol* 1982;9:610–612.
185. Rosenberg AM. The clinical associations of antinuclear antibodies in juvenile rheumatoid arthritis. *Clin Immunol Immunopathol* 1988;49:19–27.
186. Gillespie JP, Lindsley CB, Linshaw MA, et al. Childhood systemic lupus erythematosus with negative antinuclear antibody test. *J Pediatr* 1981;98:578–581.
187. Dubois EL, Chandor S, Friou GJ, et al. Progressive systemic

sclerosis (PSS) and localized scleroderma (morphea) with positive LE cell test and unusual systemic manifestations compatible with systemic lupus erythematosus (SLE): presentation of 14 cases including one set of identical twins, one with scleroderma and the other with SLE. Review of the literature. *Medicine* 1971;50:199–222.

188. Rowell NR, Tate GM. The lupus anticoagulant in systemic lupus erythematosus and systemic sclerosis. *Br J Dermatol* 1987; 117(suppl 32):13–14.
189. Seibold JR, Buckingham RB, Medsger TA Jr, et al. Cerebrospinal fluid immune complexes in systemic lupus involving the central nervous system. *Semin Arthritis Rheum* 1982;12:68–76.
190. Bennett RM. Scleroderma overlap syndromes. *Rheum Dis Clin North Am* 1990;16:185–198.
191. Wade P, Sack B, Schur PH. Anticentromere antibodies: clinical correlates. *J Rheumatol* 1988;15:1759–1763.
192. Ivey KJ, Hwang YF, Sheets RF. Scleroderma associated with thrombocytopenia and Coombs-positive hemolytic anemia. *Am J Med* 1971;51:815–817.
193. Rosenthal DS, Sack B. Autoimmune hemolytic anemia in scleroderma. *JAMA* 1971;216:2011–2012.
194. Hanson V, Drexler E, Kornreich H. DNA antibodies in childhood scleroderma. *Arthritis Rheum* 1970;17:798–801.
195. Kahn MF, Peltier AP, Degraeve B, et al. Successive connective tissue diseases: scleroderma, then lupus. Clinical and biological study of 4 cases (in French). *Ann Med Interne* 1977;128:1–8.
196. Mitchell AJ, Rusin LJ, Diaz LA. Circumscribed scleroderma with immunologic evidence of systemic lupus erythematosus. A report of a case and review of the literature. *Arch Dermatol* 1980;116:69–73.
197. Rowell NR. Discoid lupus erythematosus and systemic sclerosis. *Br J Dermatol* 1987;117(suppl 32):106–107.
198. Hayakawa K, Nagashima M. Systemic sclerosis associated with disseminated discoid lupus erythematosus. *Int J Dermatol* 1993; 32:440–441.
199. Sasaki T, Nakajima H. Systemic sclerosis (scleroderma) associated with discoid lupus erythematosus. *Dermatology* 1993;187: 178–181.
200. Umbert P, Winkelman RK. Concurrent localized scleroderma and discoid lupus erythematosus. Cutaneous "mixed" or "overlap" syndrome. *Arch Dermatol* 1978;114:1473–1478.
201. Roddi R, Riggio E, Gilbert PM, et al. Progressive hemifacial atrophy in a patient with lupus erythematosus. *Plastic Reconstr Surg* 1994;93:1067–1072.
202. Asherson RA, Angus H, Matthews J, et al. The progressive systemic sclerosis/systemic lupus overlap: an unusual clinical progression (case report). *Ann Rheum Dis* 1991;50:323–327.
203. Lee CW, Kwon CW, Yoo DH, et al. Linear scleroderma occurring in a patient with systemic lupus erythematosus. *J Korean Med Sci* 1994;9:197–199.
204. Goldenstein-Schainberg C, Rodrigues Pereira RM, Cossermelli W. Linear scleroderma and systemic lupus erythematosus (letter). *J Rheumatol* 1990;17:1427-1428.
205. Ohtaki N, Miyamoto C, Orita M, et al. Concurrent multiple morphea and neonatal lupus erythematosus in an infant boy born to a mother with SLE. *Br J Dermatol* 1986;115:85–90.
206. Garcia-Morteo O, Nitsche A, Maldonado-Cocco JA, et al. Eosinophilic fascitis and retroperitoneal fibrosis in a patient with systemic lupus erythematosus. *Arthritis Rheum* 1987;30: 1314–1315.
207. Sills EM. Systemic lupus erythematosus in a patient previously diagnosed as having Shulman disease (letter). *Arthritis Rheum* 1988;31:694–695.
208. Gallardo F, Vadillo M, Mitjavila F, et al. Systemic lupus erythematosus after eosinophilic fasciitis. A case report. *J Amer Acad Dermatol* 1998;38:283–285.
209. Baffoni L, Frisoni M, Maccaferri M, et al. Systemic lupus erythematosus and eosinophilic fasciitis. *Clin Rheumatol* 1995;14: 591–592.
210. Libman E, Sacks B. A hitherto undescribed form of valvular and mural endocarditis. *Arch Intern Med* 1924;33:701–737.
211. Uchino K, Hasegawa O, Matsumaru K, et al. A case of retroperitoneal fibrosis associ-ated with systemic lupus erythematosus. *Nippon Naika Gakkai Zasshi* 1986;75:666–669.
212. Bashour B. Systemic lupus erythematosus with retroperitoneal fibrosis and thrombosis of the inferior vena vaca. *South Med J* 1993;86:1309–1310.
213. Lawson TM, Borysiewicz LK, Camilleri JP, et al. Focal myositis mimicking acute psoas abscess. *Brit Med J* 1997;314:805–808.
214. Vivancos J, Solar-Carillo J, Rey JA, et al. Development of polyarteritis nodosa in the course of inactive systemic lupus erythematosus. *Lupus* 1995;4:494–495.
215. Gonzelez-Gay MA, Blanco R, Ferran C, et al. Successful treatment of polyarteritis nodosa related to systemic lupus erythematosus. *J Clin Rheumatol* 1996;2:366–368.
216. Ben-Chetrit E, Rahav G. Saved by a test result. *N Engl J Med* 1994;330:343–346.
217. Lee WS, Kim SJ, Ahn SK. Behcet's disease as a part of the symptom complex of SLE? *J Dermatol* 1996;23:196–199.
218. Lawson JP. The joint manifestations of the connective tissue diseases. *Semin Roentgenol* 1982;17:25–38.
219. Foley J. Systemic lupus erythematosus presenting as polymyalgia rheumatica. *Ann Rheum Dis* 1987;46:351.
220. Maragou M, Siotsiou F, Sfondouris H, et al. Late-onset systemic lupus erythematosus presenting as polymyalgia rheumatica. *Clin Rheumatol* 1989;8:91–97.
221. Bunker CB, Dowd PH. Giant cell arteritis and systemic lupus erythematosus. *Br J Dermatol* 1988;119:115–120.
222. Scharre D, Petri M, Engman E, et al. Large intracranial arteritis with giant cells in systemic lupus erythematosus. *Ann Intern Med* 1986;104:661–662.
223. Igarashi T, Nagaoka S, Matsunaga K, et al. Aortitis syndrome (Takayasu's arteritis) associated with systemic lupus erythematosus. *J Rheumatol* 1989;16:1579–1583.
224. Saxe PA, Altman RD. Takayasu's arteritis syndrome associated with systemic lupus erythematosus. *Semin Arthritis Rheum* 1992;21:295–305.
225. Saxe PA, Altman RD, Igarashi T, et al. Aortitis syndrome (Takayasu's arteritis) associated with SLE (letter). *J Rheumatol* 1990;17:1251–1252.
226. Harmon SM, Oltmanns KL, Min KW. Large vessel occlusion with vasculitis in systemic lupus erythematosus. *South Med J* 1991;84:1150–1154.
227. Frocht A, Leek JC, Robbins DL. Gout and hyperuricemia in systemic lupus erythematosus. *Br J Rheumatol* 1987;26: 303–306.
228. de Castro P, Jorizzo JL, Solomon AR, et al. Coexistent systemic lupus erythematosus and tophaceous gout. *J Am Acad Dermatol* 1985;13:650–654.
229. Greenfield DI, Fong JS, Barth WF. Systemic lupus erythematosus and gout. *Semin Arthritis Rheum* 1985;14:176–179.
230. Helliwell M, Crisp AJ, Grahame R. Co-existent tophaceous gout and systemic lupus erythematosus. *Rheumatol Rehab* 1982; 21:161–163.
231. Kurita Y, Tsuboi R, Numata K, et al. A case of multiple urate deposition, without gouty attacks, in a patient with systemic lupus erythematosus. *Cutis* 1989;43:273–275.
232. McDonald J, Fam A, Paton T, et al. Allopurinol hypersensitivity in a patient with coexistent systemic lupus erythematosus and tophaceous gout. *J Rheumatol* 1988;15:865–868.
233. Moidel RA, Good AE. Coexistent gout and systemic lupus erythematosus. *Arthritis Rheum* 1981;24:969–971.

234. Tsuboi R, Taneda A, Ogawa H. Coexistent systemic lupus erythematosus and urate deposition (letter). *J Am Acad Dermatol* 1986;15:1050–1051.
235. McMillen MA, Cunningham ME, Schoen R, et al. Gout in patients with systemic lupus erythematosus. *Br J Rheumatol* 1994;33:595–596.
236. Wallace DJ, Klinenberg JR, Morhaim D, et al. Coexistent gout and rheumatoid arthritis. Case report and literature review. *Arthritis Rheum* 1979;22:81–86.
237. Veerapen K, Schumacher HR, van Linthoudt D, et al. Tophaceous gout in young patients with systemic lupus erythematosus. *J Rheumatol* 1993;20:721–724.
238. Rodriquez MA, Paul H, Abadi I, et al. Multiple microcrystal deposition in a patient with systemic lupus erythematosus. *Ann Rheum Dis* 1984;43:498–502.
239. Wallace DJ. Prevalence of fibromyalgia in systemic lupus erythematosus patients: comment on the article by Middleton et al. *Arthritis Rheum* 1995;38:872.
240. Middleton GD, Mc Farlin JE, Lipsky PE. The prevalence and clinical impact of fibromyalgia in systemic lupus erythematosus. *Arthritis Rheum* 1994;37:1181–1188.
241. Morand EF, Miller MH, Whittingham S, et al. Fibromyalgia syndrome and disease activity in systemic lupus erythematosus. *Lupus* 1994;3:187–191.
242. Handa R, Aggarwal P, Wali JP, et al. Fibromyalgia in Indian patients with SLE. *Lupus* 1998;7:475–478.
243. Karaaslan Y, Ozturk M, Haznedaroglu S. Secondary fibromyalgia in Turkish patients with rheumatologic disorders. *Lupus* 1999;8:486–491.
244. Lopez-Osa A, Jimenez-Alonso J, Garcia-Sanchez A, et al. Fibromyalgia in Spanish patients with systemic lupus erythematosus. *Lupus* 1999;8:332–333.
245. Grafe A, Wollina U, Tebbe B, et al. Fibromyalgia in lupus erythematosus. *Acta Derm Venereol* 1999;79:62–64.
246. Gladman DD, Urowitz MB, Gough J, et al. Fibromyalgia is a major contributor to quality of life in lupus. *J Rheumatol* 1997; 24:2145–2148.
247. Akkasilpa S, Minor M, Goldman D, et al. Association of coping responses with fibromyalgia tender points in patients with systemic lupus erythematosus. *J Rheumatol* 2000;27:671–674.
248. Martinez-Lavin M, Leon A, Pindea C, et al. The dysautonomia of fibromyalgia may simulate lupus. *J Clin Rheumatol* 1999;5: 332–334.
249. Zonana-Nacach A, Alarcon GS, Reveille JD, et al. Clinical features of ANA positive and ANA negative patients with fibromyalgia. *J Clin Rheumatol* 1998;4:52–56.
250. Lluberas-Acosta G. Pseudolupus (letter). *South Med J* 1989;82: 1587.
251. Zuckner J, Baldassare H. The nonspecific rheumatoid subcutaneous nodule: its presence in fibrositis and scleroderma (case report). *Am J Med Sci* 1976;271:69–75.
252. Caro XJ. Immunofluorescent detection of IgG at the dermal-epidermal junction in patients with apparent fibrositis syndrome. *Arthritis Rheum* 1984;27:1174–1179.
253. Dinerman H, Goldenberg DL, Felson DT. A prospective evaluation of 118 patients with the fibromyalgia syndrome: prevalence of Raynaud's, phenomenon, sicca symptoms, ANA, low complement, and Ig deposition at the dermal-epidermal junction. *J Rheumatol* 1986;13:368–373.
254. Thomas JR 3rd, Su WP. Concurrence of lupus erythematosus and dermatitis herpetiformis. *Arch Dermatol* 1983;119: 740–745.
255. Aronson AJ, Soltani K, Aronson IK, et al. Systemic lupus erythematosus and dermatitis herpeteformis: concurrence with Marfan's syndrome. *Arch Dermatol* 1979;115:68–70.
256. Davies MG, Marks R, Waddington E. Simultaneous systemic lupus erythematosus and dermatitis herpeteformis. *Arch Dermatol* 1976;112:1292–1294.
257. Maas D, Schubothe H. Lupus erythematosus-like syndrome with antimitochondrial antibodies (in German). *Dtsch Med Wochenschr* 1973;98:131–139.
258. Grob PJ, Muller-Schoop JW, Hacki MA, et al. Drug-induced pseudolupus. *Lancet* 1975;2:144–148.
259. Guardia J, Richart C, Martinez-Vazquez JM, et al. Pseudolupus induced by a vasculotropic drug (English abstract). *Nouv Press Med* 1977;6:2873–2875.
260. Maas D, Schubothe H, Sennekamp J, et al. On the question of drug-induced pseudo-LE syndrome: preliminary results in 58 cases (in German). *Dtsch Med Wochenschr* 1975;100: 1551–1557.
261. Hunter T, Arnott JE, McCarthy DS. Feature of systemic lupus erythematosus and sarcoidosis occurring together. *Arthritis Rheum* 1980;23:364–366.
262. Soto-Aguilar MC, Boulware DW. Sarcoidosis presenting as antinuclear antibody positive glomerulonephritis. *Ann Rheum Dis* 1988;47:337–339.
263. Collins DA, Bourke BE. Systemic lupus erythematosus: an occasional misdiagnosis. *Annals Rheum Dis* 1996;55:421–422.
264. Harrison GN, Lipham M, Elguindi AS, et al. Acute sarcoidosis occurring in the course of systemic lupus erythematosus. *South Med J* 1979;72:1387–1388.
265. Needleman SW, Silber RA, Von Brecht JH, et al. Systemic lupus erythematosus complicated by disseminated sarcoidosis. Report of a case associated with circulating immune complexes. *Am J Clin Pathol* 1982;78:105–107.
266. Magasic MV, Venkatasehan VS, Vitting KE. Concurrent renal sarcoidosis and lupus nephritis. *Nephron* 1993;64:496–497.
267. Schnabel A, Barth J, Schubert F, et al. Pulmonary sarcoidosis coexisting with systemic lupus erythematosus. *Scand J Rheumatol* 1996;25:109–111.
268. Cathcart ES, Scheinberg MA. Systemic lupus erythematosus in a patient with amyloidosis. Discussion. *Arthritis Rheum* 1976; 19:254–255.
269. Benson MD, Cohen AS. Serum amyloid: a protein in amyloidosis, rheumatic and neoplastic diseases. *Arthritis Rheum* 1979; 22:36–42.
270. Breathnach SM, Kofler H, Sepp N, et al. Serum amyloid P component binds to cell nuclei in vitro and to in vivo deposits of extracellular chromatin in systemic lupus erythematosus. *J Exp Med* 1989;170:1433–1438.
271. Queffeulou G, Berentbaum F, Michel C, et al. AA amyoidosis in systemic lupus erythematosus: an unusual complication. *Nephrol Dial Transplant* 1998;13:1840–1848.
272. Alonso JF, Ramos M, Castilla J, et al. Renal amyloidosis and systemic lupus erythematosus without renal involvement. *Nefrologia* 1986;6:113–116.
273. Carstens PH, Ogden LL Jr, Peak WP. Renal amyloidosis associated with systemic lupus erythematosus. *Am J Clin Pathol* 1980; 74:835–838.
274. Chan CN, Li E, Lai FM, et al. An unusual case of systemic lupus erythematosus with isolated hypoglossal nerve palsy, fulminant acute pneumonitis and pulmonary amyloidosis. *Ann Rheum Dis* 1989;48:236–239.
275. Paul E, Carroll MC. SAP-less chromatin triggers systemic lupus erythematosus. *Nature Medicine* 1999;5:607–608.
276. King RW Jr, Falls WF Jr. Renal amyloidosis: development in a case of systemic lupus erythematosus (letter). *Clin Nephrol* 1976;6:497–499.
277. Nomura S, Kumagai N, Kanoh T, et al. Pulmonary amyloidosis associated with systemic lupus erythematosus (brief report). *Arthritis Rheum* 1986;29:680–682.
278. Pettersson T, Tornroth T, Totterman KJ, et al. AA amyloidosis

in systemic lupus erythematosus. *J Rheumatol* 1987;14: 835–838.

279. Schleissner LA, Sheehan WW, Orselli RC. Lupus erythematosus in a patient with amyloidosis, adrenal insufficiency, and subsequent immunoblastic sarcoma. Demonstration of the LE phenomenon in the lung. *Arthritis Rheum* 1976;19:249–255.
280. Sweet J, Bear RA, Lang AP. Amyloidosis and systemic lupus erythematosus. *Hum Pathol* 1981;12:853–856.
281. ter Borg EJ, Janssen S, van Rijswijk MH, et al. AA amyloidosis associated with systemic lupus erythematosus. *Rheumatol Int* 1988;8:141–143.
282. Webb S, Segura F, Cervantes F, et al. Systemic lupus erythematosus and amyloidosis. *Arthritis Rheum* 1979;22:554–556.
283. Wegelius O. Amyloidosis of the kidneys, adrenals and spleen as a complication of acute disseminated lupus erythematosus treated with ACTH and cortisone. *Acta Med Scand* 1956;156: 91–95.
284. Ellington KT, Troung L, Olivero JJ. Renal amyloidosis and systemic lupus erythematosus. *Am J Kidney Dis* 1993;21:676–678.
285. Betsuyaku T, Adachi T, Haneda H, et al. A secondary amyloidosis associated with systemic lupus erythematosus. *Intern Med* 1993;32:391–394.
286. Marenco JL, Sanchez-Burson J, Ruiz Campos J, et al. Pulmonary amyoidosis and unusual lung involvement in SLE. *Clin Rheumatol* 1994;13:525–527.
287. Demin AA, Semenova LA, Sentiakova TN, et al. Amyoidosis in systemic lupus erythematosus. *Klin Meditsina* 1992;70:61–66.
288. Garcia-Tobaruela A, Gil A, Lavilla P, et al. Hepatic amyoidosis associated with systemic lupus erythematosus. *Lupus* 1995;4: 75–77.
289. Orellana C, Collado A, Hernandez MV, et al. When does amyloidosis complicate systemic lupus erythematosus. *Lupus* 1995; 4:415–417.
290. Al-Hoqail I, Naddaf H, Al-Rikabi A, et al. Systemic lupus erythematosus and amyoidosis. *Clin Rheumatol* 1997;16:422–424.
291. Nashel DJ, Leonard A, Mann DL, et al. Ankylosing spondylitis and systemic lupus erythematosus. A rare HLA combination. *Arch Intern Med* 1982;142:1227–1228.
292. Olivieri I, Gemignani G, Balagi M, et al. Concomitant systemic lupus erythematosus and ankylosing spondylitis. *Ann Rheum Dis* 1990;49:323–324.
293. Kappes J, Schoepflin G, Bardana E, et al. Lupoid sacroarthropathy—a previously undescribed association. *Arthritis Rheum* 1980; 23:699–700.
294. Aisen PS, Cronstein BN, Kramer SB. Systemic lupus erythematosus in a patient with Reiter's syndrome. *Arthritis Rheum* 1983;26:1405–1408.
295. Moalla M, Elleuch M, Bergaoui N, et al. Association of ankylosing spondylitis, discoid lupus and a dermatofibrosarcoma. *Sem Hop Paris* 1987;63:1457–1461.
296. Eyanson S, Greist MC, Brandt KD, et al. Systemic lupus erythematosus: association with psoralen-ultraviolet-A treatment of psoriasis. *Arch Dermatol* 1979;115:54–56.
297. Kulick KB, Mogavero H Jr, Provost TT, et al. Serologic studies in patients with lupus erythematosus and psoriasis. *J Am Acad Dermatol* 1983;8:631–634.
298. Millus JL, Muller SA. The coexistence of psoriasis and lupus erythematosus: an analysis of 27 cases. *Arch Dermatol* 1980; 116:658–663.
299. Dowdy MJ, Nigra TP, Barth WF. Subacute cutaneous lupus erythematosus during PUVA therapy for psoriasis: case report and review of the literature. *Arthritis Rheum* 1989;32:343–346.
300. McGrath H Jr, Scopelitis E, Nesbitt LT Jr. Subacute cutaneous lupus erythematosus during psoralen ultraviolet A therapy (letter). *Arthritis Rheum* 1990;33:302–303.
301. Lorber M, Gershwin ME, Shoenfeld Y. The coexistence of systemic lupus erythematosus with other autoimmune diseases: the kaleidoscope of autoimmunity. *Semin Arthritis Rheum* 1994;24: 105–113.
302. Hetherington GW, Jetton RL, Knox JM. The association of lupus erythematosus and porphyria. *Br J Dermatol* 1970;82:118–124.
303. Rosemarin JI, Nigro EJ, Levere RD, et al. Systemic lupus erythematosus and acute intermittent porphyria: coincidence or association. *Arthritis Rheum* 1982;25:1134–1137.
304. Clemmensen O, Thomsen K. Porphyria cutanea tarda and systemic lupus erythematosus. *Arch Dermatol* 1982;118:160–162.
305. Griso D, Macri A, Biolcati G, et al. Does an association exist between PCT and SLE? Results of a study on autoantibodies in 158 patients affected with PCT. *Arch Dermatol Res* 1989;281: 291–292.
306. Allard SA, Charles PJ, Herrick AL, et al. Antinuclear antibodies and the diagnosis of systemic lupus erythematosus in patients with acute intermittent porphyria. *Ann Rheum Dis* 1990;49: 246–248.
307. Gibson GE, McEvoy MT. Coexistence of lupus erythematosus and porphyria cutanea tarda in 15 patients. *J Am Acad Dermatol* 1998;38:569–573.
308. Becker NJ, Borek D, Abdou NI. Angioimmunoblastic lymphadenopathy presenting as SLE with GI protein loss (letter). *J Rheumatol* 1988;15:1452–1454.
309. Gleichmann E, Van Elven F, Gleichman H. Immunoblastic, lymphadenopathy, systemic lupus erythematosus, and related disorders. Possible pathologenetic pathways. *Am J Clin Pathol* 1979;72(suppl 4):708–723.
310. Gusterson BA, Fitzharris BM. Angio-immunoblastic lymphadenopathy with lupus erythematosus cells. *Br J Haematol* 1979;43:149–150.
311. Pierce DA, Stern R, Jaffe R, et al. Immunoblastic sarcoma with features of Sjögren's syndrome and systemic lupus erythematosus in a patient with immunoblastic lymphadenopathy. *Arthritis Rheum* 1979;22:911–916.
312. Rosenstein ED, Wieczorek R, Raphael BG, et al. Systemic lupus erythematosus and angioimmunoblastic lymphadenopathy: case report and review of the literature. *Semin Arthritis Rheum* 1986;16:146–151.
313. Bignon YJ, Janin-Mercier A, Dubos Ult JJ, et al. Angioimmunoblastic lymphadenopathy with dysproteinemia (AILD) and sicca syndrome. *Ann Rheum Dis* 1986;45:519–522.
314. McHugh NJ, Campbell GJ, Landreth JJ, et al. Polyarthritis and angioimmunoblastic lymphadenopathy. *Ann Rheum Dis* 1987; 46:555–558.
315. Harisdangkul V, Benson CH, Myers A. Renal cell carcinoma presenting as necrotizing vasculitis with digital gangrene. *Intern Med* 1984;5:108–117.
316. Marcus RM, Grayzel AI. A lupus antibody syndrome associated with hypernephroma. *Arthritis Rheum* 1979;22:1396–1398.
317. Imai H, Nakano Y, Kiyosawa K, et al. Increasing titers and changing specificities of antinuclear antibodies in patients with chronic liver disease who develop hepatocellular carcinoma. *Cancer* 1993;71:26–35.
318. Friss AB, Cohen PR, Bruce S, et al. Chronic cutaneous lupus erythematosus mimicking mycosis fungoides. *J Am Acad Dermatol* 1995;33:891–895.
320. Stevanovic G, Cramer AD, Taylor CR, et al. Immunoblastic sarcoma in patients with systemic lupus erythematosus. *Arch Pathol Lab Med* 1983;107:589–592.
321. Covini G, von Muhlen CA, Pacchetti S, et al. Diversity of antinuclear antibody responses in hepatocellular carcinoma. *J Hepatology* 1997;26:1255–1265.
323. Asherson RA, Block S, Houssiau FA, et al. Systemic lupus erythematosus and lymphoma: association with an antiphospholipid syndrome. *J Rheumatol* 1991;18:277–279.

324. Legerton CW, Sergent JS. Intravascular malignant lymphoma mimicking central nervous system lupus. *Arthritis Rheum* 1993; 36:135–136.
325. Zuber M. Positive antinuclear antibodies in malignancies. *Annals Rheum Dis* 1992;51:573–574.
326. Posner MA, Gloster ES, Bonagura VR, et al. Burkitt's lymphoma in a patient with systemic lupus erythematosus. *J Rheumatol* 1990;17:380–382.
327. Strickland RW, Limmani A, Wall JG, et al. Hairy cell leukemia presenting as a lupus-like illness. *Arthritis Rheum* 1988;31: 566–568.
328. Freundlich B, Makover D, Maul GG. A novel antinuclear antibody associated with a lupus-like paraneoplastic syndrome. *Ann Intern Med* 1988;109:295–297.
329. Zuber M, Meisel R, Brandl B. A patient with a high titer of antinuclear antibody and a functioning adrenal tumor. *Clin Rheumatol* 1995;14:100–103.
330. Kuzmich PV, Ecker GA, Karsh J. Rheumatic manifestations in patients with myelodysplastic and myeloproliferative diseases. *J Rheumatol* 1994;21:1649–1654.
331. Kohli M, Bennett RM. An association of polymyalgia rheumatica and myelodysplastic syndromes. *J Rheumatol* 1994;21: 1357–1359.
332. Aoshima M, Tanaka H, Takahashi M, et al. Meigs syndrome due to Brenner tumor mimicking lupus peritonitis in a patient with systemic lupus erythematosus. *Am J Gastroenterol* 1995;90: 657–658.
333. Shimomura C, Eguchi K, Kawakami A, et al. Elevation of a tumor associated antigen CA 199 levels in patients with rheumatic diseases. *J Rheumatol* 1989;16:1410–1415.
334. Moncayo R, Moncayo H. Serum levels of CA 125 are elevated in patients with active systemic lupus erythematosus. *Obstet Gynecol* 1991;77:932–934.
335. Rahima D, Tarrab-Hazdai R, Blank M, et al. Anti-nuclear antibodies associated with schistosomiasis and anti-schistosomal antibodies associated with SLE. *Autoimmunity* 1994;17: 127–141.
336. Li EK, Cohen MG, Cheng AE. Salmonella bacteraemia occurring concurrently with the first presentation of systemic lupus erythematosus. *Br J Rheumatol* 1993;32:66–67.
337. Braun J, Sieper J, Schulte KL, et al. Visceral leishmaniasis mimicking a flare of systemic lupus erythematosus. *Clin Rheumatol* 1991;10:445–448.
338. Lyngberg KK, Vennervald BJ, Bygbjerg IC, et al. Toxaplasma pericarditis mimicking systemic lupus erythematosus. Diagnostic and treatment difficulties in one patient. *Ann Medicine* 1992;24:337–340.
339. Ohkawa S, Ozaki M, Izumi S. Lepromatous leprosy complicated with systemic lupus erythematosus. *Dermatologica* 1985; 170:80–83.
340. Posner DI, Guill MA 3rd. Coexistent leprosy and lupus erythematosus. *Cutis* 1987;39:136–138.
341. Zorbas P, Kontochristopoulos G, Detsi I, et al. Borderline tuberculoid leprosy coexisting with systemic lupus erythematosus. *J Eur Acad Dermatol Venereol* 1999;12:274–275.
342. Bonfa E, Llovet R, Scheinberg M, et al. Comparison between autoantibodies in malaria and leprosy with lupus. *Clin Exp Immunol* 1987;70:529–537.
343. Chavez-Legaspi M, Gomez-Vazquez A, Garcia-De La Torre I. Study of rheumatic manifestations and serologic abnormalities in patients with lepromatous leprosy. *J Rheumatol* 1985;12: 738–741.
344. Kitridou RC. Leprosy: the great imitator of rheumatic diseases (abstract). XVI International Congress of Rheumatology, Sydney, Australia, 1985:P247.
345. Lamarre D, Talbot B, De Murcia G, et al. Structural and functional analysis of poly(ADP ribose) polymerase: an immunological study. *Biochim Biophys Acta* 1988;950:147–160.
346. Miller RA, Wener MH, Harnisch JP, et al. The limited spectrum of antinuclear antibodies in leprosy. *J Rheumatol* 1987;14: 108–110.
347. Mackworth-Young CG, Sabbaga J, Schwartz RS. Idiotypic markers of polyclonal B cell activation: public idiotypes shared by monoclonal antibodies derived from patients with systemic lupus erythematosus and leprosy. *J Clin Invest* 1987;79:572–581.
348. Orth T, Filippi R, Schadmand-Fischer S, et al. Severe tuberculous meningoencephalitis in a 30 year old woman with active systemic lupus erythematosus. *J Clin Rheumatol* 1997;3: 230–233.
349. Feng PH, Tan TH. Tuberculosis in patients with systemic lupus erythematosus. *Ann Rheum Dis* 1982;41:11–14.
350. Bulpitt KJ, Brahn E. Systemic lupus erythematosus and concurrent cytomegalic vasculitis: diagnosis by antemortem skin biopsy. *J Rheumatol* 1989;16:677–680.
351. Jones JF, Ray CG, Minnich LL, et al. Evidence for active Epstein-Barr virus infection in patients with persistent, unexplained illnesses: elevated anti-early antigen antibodies. *Ann Intern Med* 1985;102:1–7.
352. Hansen KE, Bridges AJ. Autoantibodies and common viral illnesses. *Semin Arthritis Rheum* 1998;27:263–271.
353. Cannacan FPS, Constallat LTL, Bertolo MB, et al. False positive IgM antibody tests for human cytomegalovirus (HCMV) in patients with SLE. *Lupus* 1998;7:61–62.
354. Stratta P, Cavavese C, Ciccone G, et al. Correlation between cytomegalovirus infection and Raynaud's phenomenon in lupus nephritis. *Nephron* 1999;82:145–154.
355. Soloninka CA, Anderson MJ, Laskin CA. Anti-DNA and antilymphocyte antibodies during acute infection with human parvovirus B19. *J Rheumatol* 1989;16:777–781.
356. Chassagne P, Mejjad O, Gourmelen O, et al. Exacerbation of systemic lupus erythematosus during human parvovirus B19 infection. *Br J Rheumatol* 1993;32:158–159.
357. Kalish RA, Knopf AN, Gary GW, et al. Lupus-like presentation of human parvovirus B19 infection. *J Rheumatol* 1992;19: 169–171.
358. Nesher G, Osburn TG, Moore TL. Parvovirus mimicking systemic lupus erythematosus. *Semin Rheum Dis* 1995;24:297–303.
359. Moore TL, Bandlamudi R, Alam SM, et al. Parvovirus infection mimicking systemic lupus erythematosus in a pediatric population. *Semin Arthritis Rheum* 1999;28:314–318.
360. Loizou S, Cazabon JK, Walport MJ, et al. Similarities of specificity and cofactor dependence in serum antiphospholipid antibodies from patients with human parvovirus B19 infection and from those with systemic lupus erythematosus. *Arthritis Rheum* 1997;40:103–108.
361. Roblot P, Roblot F, Ramassamy A, et al. Lupus syndrome after parvovirus B19 infection. *Rev Rhum Engl Ed* 1997;64:849–851.
362. Nigro G, Piazze J, Taliani G, et al. Postpartum lupus erythematosus associated with parvovirus B19 infection. *J Rheumatol* 1997;24:968–970.
363. Estrup FF. Human parvovirus infection: rheumatic manifestations, angioedema, C1 esterase inhibitor deficiency, ANA positivity and possible onset of systemic lupus erythematosus. *J Rheumatol* 1996;23:1180–1185.
364. Glickstein SL. Lupus-like presentation of human parvovirus B19 infection. *J Rheumatol* 1993;20:1254.
365. Langgartner J, Andus T, Hemauer A, et al. Parvovirus B19 infection imitating an acute exacerbation of systemic lupus erythematosus. *Dtsch Med Wschr* 1999;124:859–862.
366. Hayashi T, Lee S, Ogasawara H, et al. Exacerbation of systemic lupus erythematosus related to cytomegalovirus infection. *Lupus* 1998;7:561–564.

367. Bengtsson A, Widell A, Elmstahl S, et al. No serological indications that systemic lupus erythematosus is linked with exposure to human parvovirus B 19. *Ann Rheum Dis* 2000;59:64–66.
368. Kitagawa H, Iho S, Yokochi T, et al. Detection of antibodies to the Epstein-Barr virus nuclear antigens in the sera from patients with systemic lupus erythematosus. *Immunol Lett* 1988;17:249–252.
369. Nagayama Y, Kazuyama Y. Serum anti-herpes virus antibody titre in patients with active systemic lupus erythematosus. *Int J Immunotherapy* 1987;3:59–64.
370. Sculley DG, Sculley TB, Pope JH. Reactions of sera from patients with rheumatoid arthritis, systemic lupus erythematosus and infectious mononucleosis to Epstein-Barr virus-induced polypeptides. *J Gen Virol* 1986;67:2253–2258.
371. Incaprera M, Rindi L, Bazzichi A, et al. Potential role of the Epstein-Barr virus in systemic lupus erythematosus autoimmunity. *Clin Exper Rheumatol* 1998;16:289–294.
372. Al-Jitawi SA, Hakooz BA, Kazimi SM. False positive Monospot test in systemic lupus erythematosus. *Br J Rheumatol* 1987;26:71.
373. James JA, Kaufman KM, Farris AD, et al. An increased prevalence of Epstein-Barr virus infection in young patients suggests a possible etiology for systemic lupus erythematosus. *J Clin Invest* 1997;100:3019–3026.
374. Cameron B, Minota S, Stein L, et al. Autoantibody interrelationships in acute viral disease and childhood systemic lupus erythematosus (abstract). *Arthritis Rheum* 1988;31(suppl):S20.
375. Filimonova RG, Bogomolova NN, Nevraeva EG, et al. Measles virus genome in patients with lupus nephritis and glomerulonephritis. *Nephron* 1994;67:488–489.
376. de Clerck LS, Couttenye MM, de Broe ME, et al. Acquired immunodeficiency mimicking Sjögren's syndrome and systemic lupus erythematosus. *Arthritis Rheum* 1988;31:272–275.
377. Kopelman RG, Zolla-Panzer S. Association of human immunodeficiency virus infection and autoimmune phenomena. *Am J Med* 1988;84:82–88.
378. Calabrese LH. The rheumatic manifestations of infection with the human immunodeficiency virus. *Semin Arthritis Rheum* 1989;18:225–239.
379. Cohen AJ, Philips TM, Kessler CM. Circulating coagulation inhibitors in the acquired immunodeficiency syndrome. *Ann Intern Med* 1986;104:175–180.
380. Stimmler MM, Quismorio FP Jr, McGehee WG, et al. Anticardiolipin antibodies in acquired immunodeficiency syndrome. *Arch Intern Med* 1989;149:1833–1835.
381. Montero A, Prato R, Jofren M. Systemic lupus erythematosus and AIDS, difficulties in the differential diagnosis. *Medicina* 1991;51:303–306.
382. Esteva MH, Blasini AM, Ogly D, et al. False positive results for antibody to HIV in two men with systemic lupus erythematosus. *Ann Rheum Dis* 1992;51:1071–1073.
383. Barthels HR, Wallace DJ. False-positive human immunodeficiency virus testing in patients with systemic lupus erythematosus. *Semin Arthritis Rheum* 1993;23:1–7.
384. D'Agati V, Seigle R. Coexistence of AIDS and lupus nephritis: a case report. *Am J Nephrol* 1990;10:243–247.
385. Furie R, Kaell A, Petrucci R, et al. Systemic lupus erythematosus complicated by infection with human immunodeficiency virus (HIV) (abstract). *Arthritis Rheum* 1988;31:S56.
386. Strauss J, Abitbol C, Zilleruelo G, et al. Renal disease in children with the acquired immunodeficiency syndrome. *N Engl J Med* 1989;321:625–630.
387. Lu I, Cohen PR, Grossman ME. Multiple dermatofibromas in a woman with HIV infection and systemic lupus erythematosus. *J Am Acad Derm* 1995;32:901–903.
388. Werninghaus K. Lupus-like eruption and human immunodeficiency virus infection. *Cutis* 1995;55:153–154.
389. Bambery P, Deodhar SD, Malhotra HS, et al. Blood transfusion related HBV and HIV infection in a patient with SLE. *Lupus* 1993;2:203–205.
390. Molina JF, Citera G, Rosler D, et al. Coexistence of human immunodeficiency virus infection and systemic lupus erythematosus. *J Rheumatol* 1995;23:347–350.
391. Itoh K, Nishioka Y, Hirohata S, et al. HIV induced systemic lupus erythematosus. *Lupus* 1994;3:205–206.
392. Maradona JA, Carton JA, Asensi V. Myasthenia gravis and systemic lupus erythematosus in association with human immunodeficiency virus infection. *Clin Infect Dis* 1995;20:1577–1578.
393. Fernandez-Miranda C, Rubio R, Pulido F. Development of acquired immune deficiency syndrome in a patient with systemic lupus erythematosus. *J Rheumatol* 1996;23:1308.
394. Contreras F, Green DF, Pardo V, et al. Systemic lupus erythemaotus in two adults with human immunodeficiency virus infection. *Amer J Kidney Dis* 1996;28:292–295.
395. Cimmino MA, de Maria A, Moggiana G, et al. HIV infection in a male patient with systemic lupus erythematosus. *Clin Exper Rheumatol* 1996;14:317–320.
396. Kudva YC, Peterson LS, Holley KE, et al. SLE nephropathy in a patient with HIV infection: Case report and review of the literature. *J Rheumatol* 1996;23:1811–1815.
397. D'Agati V, Seigle R. Coexistence of AIDS and lupus nephritis: a case report. *Am J Nephrol* 1990;10:243–247.
398. Chang BG, Markowitz GS, Seshan SV, et al. Renal manifestations of concurrent systemic lupus erythematosus and HIV infection. *Amer J Kid Dis* 1999;33:441–449.
399. Fox RA, Isenberg DA. Human immunodeficiency virus infection in systemic lupus erythematosus. *Arthritis Rheum* 1997;40: 1168–1172.
400. Kaye BR. Rheumatic manifestations of infection with human immunodeficiency virus (HIV). *Ann Intern Med* 1989;111: 158–167.
401. Wallace DJ. Lupus, acquired immunodeficiency syndrome, and antimalarial agents (letter). *Arthritis Rheum* 1991;34:372–373.
402. Soriano V, Ordi J, Grau J. Tests for HIV in lupus. *N Engl J Med* 1994;331:881.
403. Font J, Vidal J, Cervera R, et al. Lack of relationship between human immunodeficiency virus and systemic lupus erythematosus. *Lupus* 1995;4:47–49.
404. Higashi J, Kumagai S, Hatanaka M, et al. The presence of antibodies to p24gag protein of JRA-I in sera of patients with systemic lupus erythemtatosus. *Virus Genes* 1992;6:357–364.
405. Herrmann M, Baur A, Nebel-Schickel H, et al. Antibodies against p24 of HIV-1 in patients with systemic lupus erythematosus. *Viral Immunol* 1992;5:229–231.
406. Bermas BL, Petri M, Berzofsky JA, et al. Binding of glycoprotein 120 and peptides from the HIV-1 envelope by autoantibodies in mice with experimentally induced systemic lupus erythematosus and in patients with the disease. *AIDS Res Human Retrovirus* 1994;10:1071–1076.
407. Pinto LA, Dalgleish AG, Sumar N, et al. Panel anti-gp 120 monoclonal antibodies reacts with same nuclear proteins in uninfected cells as those recognized by autoantibodies from patients with systemic lupus erythematosus. *AIDS Res Hum Retrovirsus* 1994;10:823–838.
408. Scott TF, Goust JM, Strange CB, et al. SLE, thrombocytopenia, and JRA-1 (letter). *J Rheumatol* 1990;17:1565–1566.
409. Gui A, Inanc M, Yilmaz G, et al. Antibodies reactive with HIV-1 antigens in systemic lupus erythematosus. *Lupus* 1996;5:120–122.
410. Marlton P, Taylor K, Elliott S, et al. Monoclonal large granular lymphocyte proliferation in SLE with JRA-I seroreactivity. *Aust N Z J Med* 1992;22:54–55.
411. Montero A, Jofren M, Arpini R. HIV infection in a patient with chronic cutaneous lupus erythematosus. *Medicine* 1991;51: 545–547.

412. Kondo T, Matsui M. Migrating radiculopathyan unusual complication of systemic lupus erythematosus in an JRA-1 carrier. *Rinsho Shinkeigaku* 1994;34:466–469.
413. De Maria A, Cimmino MA. Diagnostic approach to possible HIV-1 infection in patients with systemic lupus erythematosus. *J Rheumatol* 1997;24:807–808.
414. Takayanagui OM, Moura LS, Petean FC, et al. Human T-lymphotropic virus type I-associated myelopathy/tropical spastsic paraparesis and systemic lupus erythematosus. *Neurology* 1997; 48:1469–1470.
415. Byrd VM, Sergent JS. Suppression of systemic lupus erythematosus by the human immunodeficiency virus. *J Rheumatol* 1996;23:1295–1296.
416. Gonzalez C, Lopez-Longo FJ, Samson J, et al. Antiribonucleoprotein antibodies in children with HIV infection: a comparative study with childhood-onset systemic lupus erythematosus. *AIDS Patient Care and STDs* 1998;12:21–28.
417. Sekigawa I, Lee S, Kaneko H, et al. The possible role of interleukin-16 in the low incidence of HIV infection in patients with systemic lupus erythematosus. *Lupus* 2000;9;155–157.
418. Brunsting R, Sillevis Smitt JH, van der Meer JW, et al. Discoid lupus erythematosus and other clinical manifestation in female carriers of chronic granulomatous disease. *Ned Tijdschr Geneeskd* 1988;132:18–21.
419. Strate M, Brandrup F, Wang P. Discoid lupus erythematosus-like skin lesions in a patient with autosomal recessive chronic granulomatous disease. *Clin Genet* 1986;30:184–190.
420. Hafner J, Enderlin A, Seger RA, et al. Discoid lupus erythematosus-like lesions in carriers of X-linked chronic granulomatosus disease. *Br J Dermatol* 1992;127:446–447.
421. Stalder JF, Dreno B, Bureau B, et al. Discoid lupus erythematosus-like lesions in an autosomal form of chronic granulomatous disease. *Br J Dermatol* 1986;114:251–254.
422. Sillevis Smitt JH, Weening RS, Krieg SR, et al. Discoid lupus erythematosus-like lesions in carriers of X-linked chronic granulomatous disease. *Br J Dermatol* 1990;122:643–650.
423. Lovas JGL, Issekutz A, Walsh N, et al. Lupus erythemtatosus-like oral mucosal and skin lesions in a carrier of chronic granulomatous disease. *Oral Surg Oral Med Oral Pathol Oral Radiol Endod* 1995;80:78–82.
424. Manzi S, Urbach AH, McCune AB, et al. Systemic lupus erythematosus in a boy with chronic granulomatous disease: case report and review of the literature (brief report). *Arthritis Rheum* 1991;34:101–105.
425. Cobeta-Garcia JC, Domingo-Morera JA, Montegudo-Saez I, et al. Autosomal chronic granulomatous disease and systemic lupus erythematosus and fatal outcome. *Brit J Rheumatol* 1998; 37:109–110.
426. Alarcon-Segovia D, Amigo MC, Reyes PA. Connective tissue disease features after thallium poisoning. *J Rheumatol* 1989;16: 171–174.
427. Montoya-Cabrera MA, Sauceda-Garcia JM, Escalante-Galindo P, et al. Thallium poisoning which stimulated systemic lupus erythematosus in a child. *Gaceta Medica de Mexico* 1991;127: 333–336.
428. Franklin CM, Torretti D. Systemic lupus erythematosus and Down's syndrome (letter). *Arthritis Rheum* 1985;28:598–599.
429. Yancey CL, Zmijewski C, Athreya BH, et al. Arthropathy of Down's syndrome. *Arthritis Rheum* 1984;27:929–934.
430. Bakkaloglu A, Ozen S, Besbas N, et al. Down syndrome associated with systemic lupus erythematosus: a mere coincidence or a significant association? *Clin Genet* 1994;46:322–323.
431. Parsons H, Snyder F, Bowen T, et al. Immune complex disease consistent with systemic lupus erythematosus in a patient with lysinuric protein intolerance. *J Inher Metab Dis* 1996;19: 627–634.
432. Kamoda T, Nagai Y, Shigeta M, et al. Lysinuric protein intolerance and systemic lupus erythematosus. *Eur J Pediatri* 1998; 157:130–131.
433. Shrinath M, Walter JH, Haeney M, et al. Prolidase deficiency and systemic lupus erythematosus. *Arch Dis Child* 1997;76: 441–444.
434. Zimmerman B, Lally EV, Sharma SC, et al. Severe aortic stenosis in systemic lupus erythematosus and mucopolysaccharidosis type II (Hunter's syndrome). *Clin Cardiol* 1988;11: 723–725.
435. Genereau T, Pasquier E, Cabane J, et al. Disseminated lupus erythematosus associated with Rendu-Osler disease. Antiphospholipid antibodies don't protect from hemorrhage. *Presse Med* 1992;21:129.
436. Forns X, Bosch X, Graus F, et al. Amyotrophic lateral sclerosis in a patient with systemic lupus erythematosus. *Lupus* 1993;2: 133–134.
437. Rahman P, Gladman DD, Wither J, et al. Coexistence of Fabry's disease and systemic lupus erythematosus. *Clin Exper Rheumatol* 1998;16:475–478.
438. Prelipcean V, Koch AE. Systemic lupus erythematosus associated with Moyamoya disease. Case report and review of the literature. *J Clin Rheumatol* 1998;4:328–332.
439. Kogure A, Ohshima Y, Watanabe N, et al. A case of Werner's syndrome associated with systemic lupus erythematosus. *Clin Rheumatol* 1995;14:199–203.
440. Dubois EL, Tuffanelli DL. Clinical manifestations of systemic lupus erythematosus. *JAMA* 1964;190:104–111.
441. Tuffanelli DL, Winklemann RK. Systemic scleroderma. A clinical study of 727 cases. *Arch Dermatol* 1961;84:359–371.
442. Tuffanelli DL, Winklemann RK. Scleroderma and its relationship to the collagenosis: dermatomyositis, lupus erythematosus, rheumatoid arthritis, and Sjögren's syndrome. *Am J Med Sci* 1962;242:133–146.
443. Sharp GC. Diagnostic criteria for classification of MCTD. In: Kasukawa R, Sharp GC, eds. *Mixed connective tissue diseases and antinuclear antibodies.* Amsterdam: Elsevier, 1987:23–32.
444. Kasukawa R, Tojo T, Miyawaki S. Preliminary diagnostic criteria for classification of mixed connective tissue disease. In: Kasukawa R, Sharp GC, eds. *Mixed connective tissue diseases and antinuclear antibodies.* Amsterdam: Elsevier, 1987:41–47.
445. Alarcon-Segovia D, Villarreal M. Classification and diagnostic criteria for mixed connective tissue diseases. In: Kasukawa R, Sharp GC, eds. *Mixed connective tissue diseases and antinuclear antibodies.* Amsterdam: Elsevier, 1987:33–40.
446. Feingold M, Schneller S. Down syndrome and systemic lupus erythematosus. *Clin Genet* 1995;48:277.
447. Kahn MF. Mixed connective tissue disease dispute. *Lupus* 1995; 4:258–259.
448. Benkiksen S, van Ghelue M, Rekvig OP, et al. A longitudinal study of human cytomegalovirus serology and viruria fails to detect active viral infection in 20 systemic lupus erythematosus patients. *Lupus* 2000;9:120–126.
449. Douvas A, Takehana Y, Ehresmann G, et al. Neutralization of HIV Type 1 infectivity by serum antibodies from a subset of autoimmune patients with mixed connective tissue disease. *AIDS Res Hum Retroviruses* 1996;12:1509–1517.
450. Dror Y, Blacher Y, Cohen P, et al. Systemic lupus erythematosus associated with acute Epstein-Barr virus infection. *Am J Kidney Dis* 1998;32:825–828.

47

THE MOTHER IN SYSTEMIC LUPUS ERYTHEMATOSUS

RODANTHI C. KITRIDOU

Systemic lupus erythematosus (SLE) primarily affects young women with normal fertility, who frequently get pregnant. The course of pregnancy in systemic lupus has changed materially in the last 50 years: In the 1950s, pregnancy in lupus was often fraught with serious disease flares, fetal death, and even maternal death. More recently, and especially over the last 20 years, pregnancy in lupus patients has become commonplace, and the outcome has improved remarkably. Before addressing lupus and pregnancy, we review briefly immunologic mechanisms in pregnancy, which seem intimately linked to the survival of the fetus, and sex hormone metabolism in SLE patients.

IMMUNOBIOLOGY OF NORMAL PREGNANCY

Maternal tolerance of the fetus and recurrent fetal loss have been the subjects of extensive research, which is in a state of flux. Pertinent protective events occur at the maternal-fetal interface and may or may not be reflected in peripheral blood. An excellent recent review of immune mechanisms in mammalian pregnancy examines the questions of fetal graft tolerance, fetal loss syndromes, preimplantation, implantation, and the inflammatory milieu in pregnancy (1). Prior to implantation, hormonal changes induced by ovulation are potent modulators of antigen-presenting cells and lymphocytes, and influence the maternal immune response. During insemination, transforming growth factor-β_1 (TGF-β_1), found in seminal fluid, stimulates production of granulocyte-macrophage colony-stimulating factor (GM-CSF) and recruitment of inflammatory cell infiltrates in the uterus (2).

During implantation of the fertilized ovum, the majority of lymphocytes infiltrating the decidua (70% to 80%) are distinctive uterine natural killer (NK) cells), which are $CD56^{++}CD16^{-}CD3^{-}$, and express various receptors (KIR2DL4 and CD94/NKG2) (3,4). The extravillous trophoblast (EVT), which is of fetal origin, invades the decidua, proceeds to the maternal spiral arteries, and destroys their muscular wall, in order to increase blood flow to the fetus. The EVT does not express classic human leukocyte antigens (HLAs), with the exception of HLA-C. Instead, EVT expresses nonclassic major histocompatibility complex (MHC) class I antigens HLA-G and HLA-E (5,6). HLA-G is unusual in that it has limited polymorphism and tissue-restricted expression on the trophoblast and certain solid tumors. Both HLA-G and HLA-E can bind to NK cells through their receptors (KIR2DL4 for HLA-G and CD94/NKG2 for HLA-E) and inhibit cell lysis (6,7). It is considered that through this recognition mechanism of HLA-G and HLA-E by NK cells, maternal NK cytotoxicity toward EVT is inhibited (5). Interleukin-10 (IL-10) enhances HLA-G gene transcription and expression in cultured trophoblast cells, and upregulates cell surface expression in blood monocytes, contrary to its usual downregulating effect on MHC I and MHC II expression (8). IL-10 secretion by the fetoplacental unit and its enhancement of HLA-G expression seems to protect the fetus from rejection.

Uterine decidua and the fetoplacental unit produce large numbers of cytokines, which contribute to a shift of the immune response from T helper-1 (Th1) to Th2: successful pregnancy has been considered akin to a Th2 type of response (9), where cytokines IL-10, IL-4, IL-5, IL-6, and IL-13 predominate. Recurrent spontaneous abortion of unknown cause ("pregnancy rejection") is mediated by a Th1 response (10), where interferon-γ (IFN-γ), tumor necrosis factor-α and -β (TNF-α, TNF-β), IL-2, and IL-12 predominate. The above have been substantiated by studies on endometrial tissue (11,12) and blood (13).

The role of progesterone, "the hormone of pregnancy," seems to be crucial in the maintenance of pregnancy; in studies of blood mononuclear cells of women with and without unexplained pregnancy loss, progesterone blocked Th1 immunity to trophoblast, and so did IL-10; progesterone upregulated TGF-β, but had no effect on Th2 cytokines (14).

In a series of elegant investigations, the function of progesterone-induced blocking factor (PIBF) has been elucidated. In the presence of progesterone, lymphocytes of pregnant women release PIBF, a 34-kd protein that controls cytokine production and CD56⁺ NK cell behavior: peripheral lymphocytes of healthy pregnant women had high PIBF and high IL-10; women at risk for pregnancy termination had increased IL-12 and low PIBF and IL-10 (15), increased serum TNF-α, and decreased PIBF on lymphocytes (16). Pregnant mice treated with anti-PIBF had decreased IL-10 production, increased IFN-γ production, and increased embryo loss (17). PIBF inhibits degranulation of NK cells (18) and modulates perforin expression in decidual lymphocytes, but not in peripheral lymphocytes (19), inhibiting NK cytotoxic activity. PIBF also inhibits arachidonic acid release from mononuclear cells, thus reducing IL-12 expression; inhibition of PIBF by specific antibody resulted in increase of IL-12 production from blood mononuclear cells, reversed by indomethacin treatment (20). All these functions of PIBF appear to favor maintenance of pregnancy.

Another mechanism of fetal protection is the expression of indoleamine 2,3-dioxygenase (IDO) on fetal-derived syncytiotrophoblasts at the maternal-fetal interface, an enzyme that catabolizes tryptophan (21). Inhibition of IDO in mice (inhibition of tryptophan catabolism) resulted in fetal rejection by maternal lymphocytes (22).

Two more immune mechanisms appear to confer immune privilege to the fetoplacental unit: The trophoblast expresses abundant Fas ligand, which puts any activated maternal lymphocyte expressing Fas, upon contact with the trophoblast, at risk to undergo apoptosis (programmed cell death) (23,24). In addition, complement regulatory proteins CD46 (formerly TLX), CD55, and CD59 are expressed on the syncytiotrophoblast epithelium, which is in direct contact with maternal blood (25). These substances are protective against cytolysis by the maternal complement system.

Estrogens, progestins, androgens, and corticosteroids are produced at a 4- to 100-fold greater-than-normal rate during pregnancy, and fall abruptly to normal within 2 days postpartum (Table 47.1) (26). Estrogens and progesterone are present at concentrations 50- to 100-fold in the third trimester. Work on the immunoregulatory properties of steroid sex hormones shows the following: 17β-estradiol (E2) significantly reduces neutrophil chemotaxis (to FMLP) through a receptor-dependent mechanism (27); in mice, estradiol reduces NK cell cytotoxicity in a dose-dependent manner, and augments polyclonal B-cell activation, probably through suppression of NK cells (28). *In vitro* experiments with adult male mononuclear cells under various stimuli (e.g., phytohemagglutinin (PHA), anti-CD3, IL-2) showed that estradiol and pituitary gonadotropins had a variety of effects on T-cell subsets, depending on the stimulus used (29): E2 significantly decreased CD4⁺ cells and increased CD8⁺ cells; prolactin had no subset-specific effects but enhanced proliferation of peripheral mononuclear blood cells (PMBCs), as did follicle-stimulating hormone (FSH) and luteinizing hormone (LH); FSH decreased CD4⁺ cells and enhanced CD8⁺ cells, especially CD8⁺CD28⁺; LH increased CD4⁺ cells. Human chorionic gonadotropin and somatotropin appear to suppress *in vitro* T-cell functions. Peripheral T-lymphocytes from pregnant women express human chorionic gonadotropin/LH receptor messenger RNA (mRNA) transcript and the receptor protein, suggesting that immunomodulatory effects are receptor-mediated (30). Some of the actions of progesterone were detailed earlier. Cortisol is present at a fourfold concentration in the third trimester, and the free cortisol index is elevated (26). This fact might have been responsible for some of the clinical amelioration seen in lupus pregnancy.

It would appear, then, that various immunomodulatory events occur during pregnancy, especially at the maternal-fetal interface, which regulate the maternal immune response and result in tolerance, survival, and growth of the embryo.

TABLE 47.1. PLASMA STEROID HORMONE LEVELS IN NONPREGNANT AND PREGNANT WOMEN (NG/ML)

Hormone	Nonpregnant	Trimester 1st	Trimester 2nd	Trimester 3rd	Postpartum 2nd Day
Estrone	0.1–0.3	1–2	3–8	5–20	0.5
Estradiol	0.2–0.5	2–4	5–10	10–30	0.5
Estriol	<0.1	0.2–1	2–4	5–15	<0.1
Progesterone	1–10	20–40	50–80	100–200	1
12α-OH progesterone	0.1–0.2	2–6	2	3–5	<0.5
Testosterone	0.4	1	1–2	3	1
Androstenedione	1–2	3	4	5–6	2
Cortisol	120	180	300	400–500	150

From Persellin RH. The effect of pregnancy on rheumatoid arthritis. *Bull Rheum Dis* 1977;27:922–927, with permission.

Summary

1. The fetoplacental unit is immunologically privileged by expressing (a) unique HLA antigens; (b) Fas Ligand, which protects it from Fas-expressing lymphocytes; and (c) complement regulatory proteins, which protect it from complement lysis action.
2. Successful pregnancy shows a shift to a Th2 response, with IL-10 playing a prominent role. Recurrent spontaneous abortion of unknown etiology is associated with a shift to Th1 response.
3. Progesterone at the maternal-fetal interface, through progesterone-induced blocking factor, inhibits the function of uterine NK cells, and may promote IL-10 secretion.
4. Expression of IDO on fetal-derived syncytiotrophoblasts at the maternal-fetal interface catabolizes tryptophan and inhibits fetal rejection by maternal lymphocytes.
5. Greatly increased levels of hormones such as progesterone, estrogen, cortisol, chorionic gonadotropin, and somatotropin may modulate cellular immunity at the maternal-fetal interface.

SEX HORMONE METABOLISM IN SYSTEMIC LUPUS ERYTHEMATOSUS

There is suggestive evidence that the immune-modulating effects of gonadal hormones occur through a thymus-hypothalamus-pituitary-gonadal axis (31). Thymic secretion of thymosin-β_4, and possibly other factors, affects the release of gonadotropin-releasing hormone (GnRH), which regulates the release of LH, resulting in ovarian development. Levels of thymosin-β_4 decrease in postmenopausal and ovariectomized women, suggesting possible modulation of thymic function by gonadal steroids. The hypothalamic-pituitary-ovarian axis in SLE is normal.

Abnormalities in the metabolism of sex hormones in SLE have been reported. To summarize, women and men with lupus, and their first-degree relatives, have a higher rate of C16[α] hydroxylation of estradiol to estrone and estriol, which retain estrogenic activity (32). In addition there is decreased C2 hydroxylation of estrogen, and increased C17 oxidation of testosterone, resulting in inactive metabolites (33). Women with lupus have decreased androgen levels, with the lowest levels found in women with active SLE (34). The net result is an overall increased estrogenic effect, which may give support to the use of dehydroepiandrosterone (DHEA), a weak androgen, in the treatment of mild SLE.

Prolactin (PRL) is considered necessary for immunocompetence. Prolactin levels are increased in a subset of lupus patients, and correlated with clinical and serologic disease activity (35). During lupus pregnancy, PRL was significantly higher than in control pregnant women, with highest levels late in pregnancy (36). Male SLE patients also had elevated serum PRL (37). A double-blind, placebo-controlled study of the prolactin antagonist bromocriptin in 66 SLE patients showed decreased PRL levels, Systemic Lupus Erythematosus Disease Activity Index (SLEDAI) score, and flare rates per patient/month (38). Of interest is that 33 women with increased PRL and no diagnosis of a rheumatic disease had increased prevalence of autoantibodies, including anti–double-stranded DNA (dsDNA), anti-Sm, and anti-Ro/SSA, compared to PRL-normal controls (39). Sex hormones in SLE are discussed in detail in Chapters 16 and 39.

DEFINITION OF TERMS

The following terms are used in this and Chapters 48 and 49 (40–43):

Fertility rate: Average number of pregnancies per pregnant woman.

Parity rate: Average number of viable infants per pregnant woman.

Adjusted fertility or **parity rate:** Corrected for years at risk for pregnancy (10-year intervals) (44).

Success rate or **success percentage:** The percentage of viable infants per group of patients (live births per total pregnancies × 100) (41).

Spontaneous abortion: Spontaneous termination of pregnancy prior to 20 weeks' gestation.

Elective or **induced ("therapeutic") abortion:** Voluntarily induced termination of pregnancy.

Stillbirth, or **intrauterine fetal death (IUFD):** Spontaneous termination of pregnancy after 20 weeks' gestation.

Fetal loss: Sum of spontaneous abortions and stillbirths; it has been also defined as the sum of spontaneous abortions, stillbirths, and perinatal deaths divided by the number of pregnancies minus elective abortions and expressed as a percentage (40).

Total fetal loss: Sum of abortions, stillbirths (IUFDs), and perinatal deaths.

Neonatal death: Death of a newborn within 30 days of birth.

Perinatal mortality: Sum of stillbirths and neonatal deaths.

Recurrent fetal loss or **recurrent spontaneous (habitual) abortion:** Three or more (45,46), or two or more (47), consecutive spontaneous abortions or intrauterine fetal deaths.

Recurrent spontaneous (habitual) aborter: A woman with recurrent fetal loss.

(Preterm) Premature rupture of membranes (PROM): Spontaneous rupture of membranes (amniorrhexis) before the onset of labor and before 37 weeks' gestation.

Intrauterine growth restriction (IUGR): Formerly intrauterine growth retardation; the newborn weight is below the 10th percentile for gestational age. Synonyms: small newborn for gestational age and intrauterine malnutrition.

Premature or preterm birth: Spontaneous termination of pregnancy with a live birth between 21 and 37 weeks of gestation.

Full-term or **term birth:** Spontaneous termination of pregnancy with a live birth between 38 and 40 weeks of gestation.

Pregnancy-induced hypertension (PIH): Presence of blood pressure ≥140/90 mm Hg on at least two occasions, 6 or more hours apart, during the second half of pregnancy in a previously normotensive woman (48).

Preeclampsia: PIH with proteinuria of >0.3 g/L in the absence of urinary tract infection (48), or abrupt onset of hypertension and proteinuria after 24 weeks of gestation (49,50).

Severe preeclampsia: Characterized by one or more of the following: blood pressure of at least 160 mm Hg systolic, or 110 mm Hg diastolic on two readings 6 hours apart; proteinuria ≥5 g/24 hours, oliguria (<400 mL/24 hours), cerebral or visual disturbances, pulmonary edema, or cyanosis (51).

Eclampsia: Severe preeclampsia with malignant hypertension, seizures, and renal failure.

PREGNANCY AND LUPUS INTERACTIONS—THE CONTROVERSY

The relationship of pregnancy and SLE activity has been controversial and contradictory since the earliest studies. The subject is fascinating, and there has been a virtual explosion in the number of studies addressing lupus pregnancy, both by rheumatologists and by obstetricians.

Reports from the 1950s recommended against pregnancy, and implied that it was not advisable and that termination should be offered (52,53). The numerous studies that followed, especially in the last 20 years, indicate that pregnancy in lupus patients can often have a successful outcome, if well timed and managed. Nevertheless, some controversy still exists, which arises from differences in study design, variability of SLE severity, the lack of uniformity in the definition of flares, and cultural and socioeconomic factors.

1. Study design: The majority of studies from the 1950s through the 1980s were uncontrolled and retrospective (41,52–80), with the exception of three studies that used controls (81–83). Since 1984, prospective and/or controlled studies have appeared, three in the 1980s (46,84,85), 11 (86,87,88–96) of the 19 published in the 1990s (86,87,88–98,100–104), and the two published in 2000 (105,106) (Table 47.2).
2. The great variability of SLE severity can skew study outcomes. For example, it has been well established that SLE nephritis is more severe and has a worse outcome in African-American and African-Caribbean patients (107, 108).
3. The variability in definition of flare ranges from the use of clinical indices of signs and symptoms and patient opinion, to complicated analysis of laboratory data, or the physician's decision to increase prednisone dosage. At this time the availability of lupus activity indices allows for a standardized approach (109,110). The frequency of flares within the "natural history" of SLE has been determined (81) and validated (46,86,87). In recognition of differential diagnostic dilemmas between SLE activity versus pre/eclamsia, which have certain symptoms and findings in common [headache, hypertension, proteinuria, seizures, red blood cells (RBCs) in urine], and versus pregnancy-associated problems (fatigue, edema, alopecia), certain modifications have been developed in the above activity measures for use in pregnancy (87a).
4. SLE patient populations vary greatly in terms of cultural diversity and educational-socioeconomic background, which influence their perception of disease severity, and determines their site of health care, ranging from private offices for patients of an affluent background to university, tertiary level hospitals for economically deprived patients (111).

On the other hand, greater diagnostic uniformity in patient selection has been achieved by the use of the SLE classification criteria, preliminary and revised, since 1971 and 1982, respectively (112,113). The availability of sophisticated and standardized laboratory tests [antinuclear antibody (ANA), complement C3 and C4, and antiphospholipid antibodies (APL)] has allowed the diagnosis and subsetting of patients, further contributing to the uniformity of patient selection and clinical follow-up. For these reasons, when analyzing the new data on lupus pregnancy, we should be mindful that patients diagnosed as SLE in studies reported since 1980 may be different from those diagnosed 30 to 50 years ago. In addition, nearly five decades of experience with the treatment of SLE patients in the poststeroid era have resulted in increased survival, a large patient population with controlled SLE, and, indeed, a modification of the natural history of the disease (114–116).

SLE ACTIVITY DURING PREGNANCY

It has been recognized for a quarter of a century that during menses a number of women with lupus have increased musculoskeletal symptoms and/or menstrual irregularities; amenorrhea with inability to conceive may be present during periods of severe disease activity or during high-dose

TABLE 47.2. COURSE OF SYSTEMIC LUPUS ERYTHEMATOSUS (SLE) IN PREGNANCY

Time Period	No. of Pregnancies	Flares All (%)	Flares Postpartum (%)	Remission (%)[a]	Maternal Death (%)	SLE Onset (%)
1950–1959	139	60	—	35	17.0	—
1960–1969	272	52	—	22	8.0	—
1970–1979	211	50	—	9	0.5	—
1980–1989	618	37	17	2	1.7	12.5
1990–1999	1,056 (2,275)*	43.6 (44.2)	11.8	0	0.26 (0.17)[b]	0.19
2000–	118	16.9 (48.2)	14.6	0	0.8	0
Studies in the 1980s						
Tozman et al. (66)	24	25	13	8	0	0
Houser et al. (67)	18	50	22	0	0	0
Zulman et al. (83)	24	54	22	0	8	8
Hayslett and Lynn (68)	65	39	13	5	4	—
Fine et al. (69)	52	23	20	0	2	<10
Varner et al. (71)	38	35	8	0	3	21
Gimovsky et al. (73)	77	23[d]	2[d]	0	0	20
Imbasciati et al. (74)	26	46	27	0	11	37
Lockshin et al. (84)[e,f]	33	27	—	0	0	—
Mintz et al. (46)[e,f]	92	60	20	0	0	—
Meehan et al. (78)	22	45	42	0	0	0
Bobrie et al. (77)	67	34	15	0	0	21
Lockshin et al. (85)[e]	80	21	0	0	0	8
Studies in the 1990s[c]						
Nossent and Swaak (97)	39	74	63	0	0	0
Wong et al. (86)[e,f]	29	58	0	0	0	0
Oviasu et al. (98)	53	2 (13)[g]	0	0	0	0
Petri et al. (87)[e,f]	74	36	—	0	0	0
Tincani et al. (88)[e]	25	44	0	0	0	0
Rubbert et al. (100)	21	95	—	0	0	0
Derksen et al. (89)[e]	35	17	0	0	0	0
Le-Thi-Huong et al. (90)[e]	103	45	9	0	2	0
Lima et al. (91)[e]	108	57	35	0	0	0
Ruiz-Irastorza et al. (92)[f]	78	65	—	0	0	0
Tomer et al. (93)[f]	54	14.5	Excluded	0	0	0
Le Huong et al. (94)[e,h]1	62	27	6	0	0	0
Johns et al. (101)	44	61	—	0	0	0
Rahman et al. (95)[a]	141	63	—	0	0	0
Carmona et al. (96)[e,h]2	60	28.3	9.4	0	0	3.3
Sittiwangkul et al. (102)[h]3	48	36	—	0	0	0
Kobayashi et al. (104)[h]4	82	20.7	4.9	0	0	0
Studies in 2000						
Georgiou et al. (105)[f]	59	13.5 (76)[g]	19[g]	0	2.1	0
De Bandt et al. (106)[e]	59	20.3	10.2	0	0	0

*2,275 pregnancies include studies without information on maternal flares (99,103,114,123,124), and pregnancies considered under nephritis (125–128).
[a]Spontaneous remission.
[b]Two deaths in 765 pregnant women with flare data (two deaths in over 1,200 reported pregnant women in the 1990s).
[c]Patients fulfilled American Rheumatism Association criteria for lupus before pregnancy.
[d]Exacerbations requiring hospitalization.
[e]Prospective studies.
[f]Controlled studies.
[g]See text.
[h]SLE inactive at conception: 1, in 100%; 2, in 90%; 3, in 94%; 4, in 95% of pregnancies.

steroid therapy (62,117). Antibody to corpus luteum has been recently described in 22% of 87 women with SLE and was associated with elevated levels of FSH, an early and specific sign of ovarian dysfunction (118). The investigators raised the possibility of autoimmune oophoritis in SLE. Pregnancy in SLE patients is a common event, since the prognosis has greatly improved with proper management, and patients function well within society and their families (76). Their fertility is normal, at 2 to 2.4 pregnancies per patient (41,55,73,82,97,119), not only in quiescent periods of the disease, but also during active episodes when approximately 10% of total reported pregnancies occur.

In the presteroid era exacerbations and remissions occurred almost equally during pregnancy, but severe postpartum flares were seen in virtually all patients (55). The course of pregnancy tended to be smoother in patients who conceived during a period of inactive lupus (60), and the value of steroid therapy in decreasing flares during pregnancy and postpartum was recognized in 1962: 16 of 33 patients on prednisone for part of the pregnancy had less flares during pregnancy (eight) and the 8 weeks postpartum (five), while 17 patients on no steroids had 15 and 11 flares, respectively (81). A sizable proportion of patients developed preeclampsia (1.8% to 20%) (56,57,62). It is still debated whether hypertension alone or with proteinuria during pregnancy represents pregnancy-induced hypertension, preeclampsia, or active lupus nephritis (83,84,119). The more acute the lupus, and the earlier the report, the worse was the outcome, with maternal death occurring in 10% to 25% of patients (52,57) (Table 47.2). In 1970, McGee and Makowski (61) advocated steroids for 6 weeks after delivery.

In the mid-1960s to mid-1970s, three major studies, from New York, Mexico City, and Los Angeles, respectively, were published: Estes and Larson (60) reported 79 pregnancies in 36 patients, Fraga et al. (82) reported 225 pregnancies in 53 patients, and Dubois (62) reported 217 pregnancies in 112 patients. The appropriate use of corticosteroids seemed to decrease pregnancy and postpartum flares to half of those in the 1950s (from 50–75% to 24–27%), and maternal mortality was very rare. The study by Fraga et al. from Mexico City was followed up by a prospective study by Mintz et al. (46).

Table 47.2 summarizes pregnancy data over the last 50 years categorized by decade, and in greater detail for the 1980s, 1990s, and the year 2000. The most striking change is a dramatic decrease in maternal mortality from 17% in the 1950s to 0.2% in the 1990s. Lupus flares during pregnancy range from 17% to 60%; however, in later reports the majority are mild and mostly musculocutaneous (46,89,97), with the exception of patients in whom disease began during pregnancy or postpartum. One third to one half of flares were in the postpartum period, and the rest were equally divided among trimesters. Patients whose SLE was inactive at conception had a lesser likelihood of disease flares, 9% to 35% (68,70). SLE onset during pregnancy is described only in one study (96) during the 1990s, because most studies are based on patients fulfilling the American College of Rheumatology (ACR) criteria (113).

Seven studies, spanning from 1962 to 1996, have examined the question of whether lupus flares are more frequent in pregnancy (46,81,83,84,86,92,120). Two studies used the patients as their own controls (81,83) and five used nonpregnant controls (46,84,86,92,120) (Table 47.3).

Garsenstein et al. (81) noted a clear-cut increase in flares during the first half of pregnancy (3.04/100 weeks at risk versus 0.91/100 weeks for the 32 weeks before pregnancy), a small increase during the second half of pregnancy (1.62/100 weeks), a sevenfold increase during the 2 months postpartum (6.31/100 weeks), and a return to baseline in the 9 to 40 weeks postpartum.

Zulman et al. (83) reported the percentage of flares per number of pregnancies during the 6 months preceding pregnancy (4%), each trimester (13%, 14%, and 55%, respectively), and during 6 months postpartum (23%). The flare rate during the third trimester and postpartum appears excessive.

Lockshin et al. (84) reported similar flares in 28 pregnant and 21 nonpregnant patients, with the exception of greater thrombocytopenia in the pregnant patients.

Mintz et al. (46) reported 55 flares in 909 months in their at-risk pregnant patients, not significantly different from the 19 flares in 468 months of their nonpregnant patients (p = NS). It is of note that all pregnant patients in this study, even without active lupus, were given 10 mg of prednisone daily.

Wong et al. (86), however, found the rate of flares in their pregnant patients to be twice that of their nonpregnant patients ($p < .02$).

In a prospective study of 40 pregnancies in 37 women, Petri et al. (120) defined flare as a change of over 1.0 in the physician's global assessment (scale of 0 to 3) since the preceding visit or during the previous 3 months. They noted 27 flares in 24 pregnancies, or 60%. The intrapregnancy flare rate of 1.6337 ± 0.30087 per person-year was significantly greater than the flare rate after delivery (0.6392, $p < .001$), and the rate in nonpregnant patients (0.6518, $p < .0001$). The majority of the flares were moderate (59%), or mild (30%), and only 11% were severe. In a prospective, controlled study from the University of Toronto of 79 lupus pregnancies, flares were twice as frequent in women with active SLE at conception (82%) than in women with inactive SLE at conception (41%), and inactive SLE at conception was deemed protective against flares (121).

A prospective, controlled study of 78 pregnancies in 68 SLE patients by Ruiz-Irastorza et al. (92) found that 65% of pregnant patients flared, versus 42% of the 50 nonpregnant SLE controls ($p = .015$). A flare was defined as an increase of ≥0.26 in the Lupus Activity Index (LAI). Flare rates per patient/month were 0.082 in the pregnant and 0.039 in the nonpregnant patients ($p = .0015$). A subset of

TABLE 47.3. FLARES (EXACERBATIONS) OF SLE IN PREGNANT AND NONPREGNANT PATIENTS

Study	Per 100 Weeks at Risk	Per Patient-Month	
Garsenstein et al. (81)			
32 weeks before pregnancy	0.91	0.04	
0–20 weeks of pregnancy	3.04	0.13	
21–40 weeks of pregnancy	1.62	0.07	
0–8 weeks postpartum	6.31	0.27	
9–40 weeks postpartum	0.84	0.04	
Study	**Flares/Pregnancies (%)**		
Zulman et al. (83)			
6 months before pregnancy	4		
1st trimester	13		
2nd trimester	14		
3rd trimester	55		
6 months postpartum	23		
Study		**Per Patient-Month**	
Wong et al. (86)			
Pregnant:	13 in 155 patient-months	0.08	*p* <.02
Nonpregnant:	218 in 5202 patient-months	0.04	
Petri et al. (120)			
Pregnant:	1.6337/patient-year	0.14	*p* <.0001
After delivery:	0.6392/patient-year	0.05	
Nonpregnant:	0.6518/patient-year	0.05	
Mintz et al. (46)			
Pregnant:	55 in 909 patient-months	0.06	*p* = NS
Nonpregnant:	19 in 468 patient-months	0.04	
Ruiz-Irastorza et al. (92)			
Pregnant:		0.08	*p* <.001
Nonpregnant:		0.04	
Pregnant vs. themselves after puerperium:		0.09	*p* = .0015
		0.05	
Lockshin et al. (84)			
Similar in 28 pregnant and 21 nonpregnant patients			
Greater thrombocytopenia in pregnant patients			

43 patients had higher flare rates during pregnancy versus after the puerperium, when SLE was controlled (0.093 vs. 0.049). Serious flares, affecting the kidneys and central nervous system, were equally distributed in the two groups.

Summary

1. There is lack of uniformity in the definition of flare.
2. Five studies have found increased flares during pregnancy and postpartum, and two studies found a similar risk of flare regardless of pregnancy status.
3. Flare rates are remarkably constant in the nonpregnant patients: when the data in the Garsenstein et al., Mintz et al., Petri et al., Wong et al., and Ruiz-Irastorza et al. studies are expressed as flares per patient-month, these rates are 0.04 to 0.05 (0.039565, 0.040598, 0.054316, 0.041907, and 0.039, respectively), about one flare for every 2 years (Table 47.3). This suggests that, over nearly four decades, the rate of flare in SLE has not changed.
4. All studies show that the severity of flares has lessened.
5. The differences in flares during pregnancy in these seven studies may be explained by differences in patient populations, definition of flare, and evolving therapeutic strategies over 38 years.

STUDIES IN THE 1980S (TABLE 47.2)

Studies with a minimum of ten lupus pregnancies are reviewed here, and fetal effects are reviewed in Chapter 48. Of 13 studies in the 1980s, ten are retrospective (66–69,71,73,74,77,78,83) and three are prospective with control groups (46,84,85). Maternal flares ranged from 21% to 60%, with a mean of 33%. The definition of flares was not uniform: Gimovsky et al. (73) defined an exacerbation as that which required hospitalization, whereas Mintz et al. (46), in their prospective study, accounted for even mild mucocutaneous and articular flares. Postpartum flares occurred in 2% to 42% of pregnancies, with a mean of 17%. Maternal deaths were few, primarily noted in a study of patients with SLE nephritis (74), and ranged from 0% to 11%, with a mean of 2%, well below that of the 1950s and 1960s. Spontaneous remissions were mentioned in only two reports (66,68). Onset of lupus during pregnancy or postpartum was noted in 0% to 37%, with a mean of 12%.

Prospective Studies

Three prospective studies on lupus pregnancy appeared in the 1980s (46,84,85). In 1984 Lockshin et al. (84) reported a multicenter study from New York City with 33 pregnancies compared to nonpregnant patients. A flare was defined as new signs from a previously inactive organ system, or an increase in corticosteroid dosage, or the treating physician's statement that a flare was present. In 21 pregnancies after elective and spontaneous abortions, five of eight instances of thrombocytopenia were attributed to SLE (24%), four patients developed new proteinuria that subsided after delivery (no renal biopsy), and corticosteroid dosage was increased in seven patients (33%). The authors found no significant differences between pregnant and nonpregnant groups in terms of flares, laboratory values [erythrocyte sedimentation rate (ESR), anti-DNA antibody, serum complement], and dosage of and number of patients treated with prednisone. These patients and controls seem to have mild SLE, as 40% did not require steroids during the observation period.

In a 9-year prospective study from Mexico City, Mintz et al. (46) reported 102 consecutive pregnancies in 75 patients in 1986. All patients were followed closely by a team of a rheumatologist, obstetrician, and neonatologist. No elective abortions were performed, and all patients received a minimum of 10 mg of prednisone daily from the time pregnancy was diagnosed to the end of postpartum. Of the 102 pregnancies, 10 started with active maternal disease, and in the remaining 92 a 60% flare rate was noted; 54% of flares occurred in the first trimester and 20% in the postpartum and postabortion periods. A matched group of women with SLE served as controls in this study and in a study of progestogens as contraceptives during the same 9 years (122). The pregnant patients had 55 flares in 909 patient-months and the controls had 19 in 468 patient-months, which is not statistically different (0.06 vs. 0.04 per patient/month). The authors concluded that the flare rate during pregnancy is not increased. The most frequent SLE flares were mucocutaneous and articular, while fever, serositis, and thrombophlebitis were mild; however, nine patients had episodes of nephritis activity and eight had central nervous system manifestations consisting of headache with electroencephalogram (EEG) changes in five, and grand mal seizures, chorea, and transient episodes of memory loss with dyslalia in one each of the remaining three patients. The disease activity was controlled by increasing prednisone to 15 to 45 mg daily, with the exception of seven patients: five patients with severe kidney disease were given 60 mg daily; one very ill patient with high fever, cutaneous vasculitis, and pericarditis required up to 300 mg daily; and one patient with thrombocytopenic purpura and hemolytic anemia was controlled with 200 mg of prednisone daily. No maternal deaths occurred in this study of seriously ill lupus patients.

In 1989, Lockshin (85) reported on 80 pregnancies, including 16 of the 33 in the 1984 study, without a control group. One third of the patients were on steroids at the time of pregnancy, which defines them as having mild disease, and, by global criteria, 26% had clinical evidence of active SLE during pregnancy.

LUPUS PREGNANCY STUDIES IN THE 1990S

The continued interest in SLE pregnancy produced 26 studies with 21 to 634 pregnancies each in the 1990s (86,87,88–104,114,123–128), for a total 2,275 pregnancies in more than 1,200 women: nine studies are prospective (86,87,88–91,94–96), four are controlled (86,87, 92,93), two are both prospective and controlled (86,87), and nine were retrospective (97–100,101–104,114) (Table 47.2). In four studies, the majority of pregnancies were conceived during inactive lupus at the prompting of the investigators: 100% (94), 90% (96), 94% (102), and 95% (104). Of the 20 studies, 17 report on maternal flares and are included in Table 47.2 (86,87,88–98,100–102,104). References 99, 103, 114, 123, and 124 have no information on maternal flares, and 125 to 128 are considered under nephritis. Flares were seen in 43.6% of pregnancies (44.2%, if 13% flares are calculated from ref. 98), with a range of 2% to 95% (13% to 95%). In the 2 months postpartum flares ranged from 0% to 63%, with four studies reporting no postpartum flares (86,88,89,98). All of these patients were well cared for, and the great majority were in remission at pregnancy onset. In the four studies with SLE inactivity at conception, flares were 27.3% on average (20.7% to 33%), and postpartum flares were 4.9% to 9.4% (94,96,102,104). In the remaining 13 studies, flares occurred in 49.4% on average. Two patients were reported with SLE onset in pregnancy, 3.3% of 60 pregnancies (96), or 0.19% of 1,056 pregnancies in the 1990s.

There were only two maternal deaths in these 17 series of 765 women, for the very low maternal death prevalence of 0.26%. However, if we account for all publications of lupus pregnancies reported in the 1990s, including those without information on maternal flares, the prevalence of maternal death is the lowest ever, 0.17%, or two deaths in over 1,200 women.

Prospective And Controlled Studies

Wong et al. (86) reported a prospective study from Hong Kong of 29 pregnancies in 22 patients. After 12 abortions, two spontaneous and ten elective, 15 patients had 17 successful pregnancies. Flares in 58% of patients included six episodes of renal disease, five of arthritis, and two of vasculitis. Steroid dose was maintained as needed until the 30th week of pregnancy, when it was increased to 10, 20, or 30 mg if the patients were taking less than 10, 10, or more than 10 mg daily, respectively. If disease activity required a higher dose, it was maintained until 4 weeks after delivery. No postpartum flares or maternal deaths occurred. The flare rate during pregnancy, 13 per 155 patient months, was significantly higher than that of the authors' nonpregnant patients (218 per 5,202 patient-months, $p < .02$).

Petri et al. (87), in their prospective study of 74 pregnancies, defined flare by the use of a visual analogue scale, graded from 0 to 3: of the 27 flares observed (36% flare rate), 11% were severe, necessitating a prednisone change of 43 ± 25 mg per day; 30% of flares were mild and 59% moderate.

Tincani et al. (88) assessed clinical activity by Systemic Lupus Activity Measure (SLAM) score (109) in their 25 pregnancies and found four renal flares out of 11, with skin, joint, thrombocytopenia, and neuropsychiatric flares accounting for the remainder. Most flares were treated with prednisone and azathioprine.

Derksen et al. (89) used the SLEDAI to assess lupus activity every month, from 6 months before pregnancy to 6 months postpartum. Flares occurred in six pregnancies, necessitating prednisone treatment in three patients with polymyositis, thrombocytopenia, and a combination of severe synovitis, vasculitis, and proteinuria. Increasing or new proteinuria without urine sediment abnormalities in an additional five patients was considered to be PIH and not treated.

In a multicenter study from France, Le-Thi-Huong et al. (90) observed flares in 34 of 75 patients with inactive lupus at conception (45%), with 9% of flares in postpartum and two deaths from opportunistic infection in mothers treated with steroids for nephrotic syndrome.

Lima et al. (91) reported 108 pregnancies in 90 SLE patients studied prospectively, with 74 flares in 62 pregnancies (57%). One third of flares (35%) occurred postpartum, with the second trimester having the majority, 38%. One in five flares (20%) was severe, 24% moderate, and 56% mild. Ten patients (9%) had active lupus at pregnancy onset and two had elective abortion. Active (n = 12) or prior nephritis (n = 2) was seen in 14 pregnancies and was present in five of six pre/eclampsia episodes. These patients were 79% white, and in 65% SLE manifestations were cutaneous and articular, with nephritis and hematologic and neuropsychiatric lupus in only 16%, 10%, and 9%, respectively. The patients were on prednisolone, azathioprine, and hydroxychloroquine, and dose modifications of these drugs were used to treat flares.

The controlled study by Ruiz-Irastorza was mentioned above (see SLE Activity During Pregnancy) and is from the same lupus research unit in London as the study by Lima et al. I am unaware of any patient duplication in these studies.

Tomer et al. (93) reported from Israel on 54 pregnancies of 46 SLE patients and 70 (non-SLE) pregnant controls, with only 14.5% flares during pregnancy, and the postpartum period was excluded from follow-up. The authors attributed the low flare rate to prophylactic prednisone that patients received; however, similar regimens did not prevent flares in the Mintz et al. (46) and Tincani et al. (88) studies.

Le Huong et al. (94), the same group as in ref. 90, reported 62 planned pregnancies in 38 women, who conceived after SLE inactivity for a year on ≤20 mg prednisone per day. Prednisone was maintained at ≥10 mg/day upon diagnosis of pregnancy and flares occurred in 27%, with 6% in postpartum. Flares were moderate, except for a patient with class IV nephritis. Preterm birth and cesarean section were common. Again, I do not know of any duplication of patients between refs. 90 and 94.

Rahman et al. (95) from the University of Toronto studied prospectively 141 pregnancies in 73 lupus patients and defined active lupus as SLEDAI ≥1. Flares were present in 63% of pregnancies, and renal flares were predictive of fetal loss. Patients were most commonly treated with steroids, antimalarials, and azathioprine.

Carmona et al. (96) from the University of Barcelona reported a prospective study of 60 pregnancies in 46 SLE patients, with inactive SLE at conception in 54 of 60 (90%). In 53 pregnancies, after three spontaneous abortions and four elective abortions, there were 28.3% flares (0.044/patient/month), 9.4% in postpartum, and most were moderate. Lupus nephritis in ten pregnancies was significantly associated with hypertension (50% vs. 11.6%) and smaller gestational age at delivery (35.9 vs. 37.3 weeks). Prednisone prophylaxis in the last month of pregnancy and first month of postpartum was used in 1985 to 1994 and abandoned in 1995. This is the only study in the 1990s that reports SLE diagnosed in pregnancy: two patients, 3.3%.

Retrospective Studies

Nossent and Swaak (97) from Holland reported 39 pregnancies in 19 patients, and found that 74% had mostly mild flares during pregnancy, and 63% during puerperium. Six patients had active SLE at conception and almost half (47%) with previously inactive disease had a flare. A few flares were severe: two patients developed new diffuse proliferative nephritis [class IV in the World Health Organization (WHO) classification], two serositis, and four thrombocytopenia. During the postpartum period, two patients developed serositis, one had convulsions with normal blood pressure, and four had thrombocytopenia without bleeding.

The largest retrospective series of lupus pregnancy was reported by Pistiner et al. (114) in a cohort of 570 private patients followed during the 1980s. Of 307 women with lupus, 227 (74%) had 634 pregnancies, (6 of which were twins, for a total of 640 embryos), with 439 live births (69%), 106 elective abortions (17%), and 95 spontaneous abortions (18% of 528 potentially viable pregnancies. There were 29 0f 227 women with recurrent abortion (13%), and most of those tested for anticardiolipin antibodies were positive. About half of the elective abortions were performed to protect the health of the mother. Pregnancy outcome in these patients was similar to those in 40 women with discoid lupus reported in the same article. These SLE patients had well-controlled lupus, with relatively less organ-threatening disease than most university clinic patients: 54% overall, with 28% nephritis and 11% neuropsychiatric disease. In the same metropolitan area, the indigent lupus population at the Los Angeles County–University of Southern California Medical Center had more than 50% prevalence of nephritis (111).

Rubbert et al. (100) from the University of Erlangen-Nurnberg, Germany, reported 21 pregnancies in 19 patients, who apparently had severe SLE, as 16 of 19 required immunosuppressive drugs before and during pregnancy. Mostly mild flares occurred in 95% of patients, severe flares were confined to patients with nephritis, and decreased C3 was the most sensitive marker of problems. Preterm delivery was common and preeclampsia complicated 3/19 pregnancies, with two neonatal deaths.

Johns et al. (101) from Australia reported 44 pregnancies in 28 patients with 61% flares in pregnancy. Again, overall pregnancy course and fetal outcome was worse in patients with renal flares.

Sittiwangkul et al. (102) from Chiang Mai University, Thailand, reported 48 pregnancies in 42 patients, with 94% of them inactive or quiescent at conception. Flares occurred in 36% of pregnancies and active nephritis had a poor fetal outcome.

Kobayashi et al. (104) from Hokkaido university, Japan, reported 82 pregnancies in 55 patients, 95% inactive at pregnancy onset. Flares were seen in 20.7%, with 4.9% in postpartum, and prednisone ≥15 mg/day was associated with premature delivery and preterm rupture of membranes.

STUDIES IN 2000

Two studies have appeared in 2000: Georgiou et al. (105), from the University of Ioannina, Greece, reported 59 pregnancies in 47 SLE patients, with 59 nonpregnant SLE controls and 59 healthy pregnant women (Table 47.2). Flares are described in eight of 59 pregnancies (13.6%), and six of eight had nephritis. The authors point out, however, that clinical features of SLE occurred during the first trimester in 57%, the second and third trimester in 13% each, and after delivery in 19%. The majority of patients were treated with ≤10 mg of prednisone/day, azathioprine, and hydroxychloroquine, and flares were treated with ≤60 mg of prednisone/day during pregnancy. There was one maternal death in a patient with severe nephritis.

De Bandt et al. (106) from Paris reported 59 pregnancies in 31 women, with 55 (93%) of pregnancies during "inactive" SLE (SLEDAI ≤4) and on ≤10 mg of prednisone/day. These patients would not be considered inactive by the Toronto group (95). There were 12 flares (20.3%), six severe ones during pregnancy (4/6 in active patients), and six mild ones postpartum.

Summary

The relationship of pregnancy and SLE activity can be summarized as follows:

1. Fertility in women with lupus is normal, except for amenorrhea and infertility during periods of severe disease activity.
2. Despite the variability of definition and assessment of disease activity and disease severity, flare assessment is increasingly done with standardized methods, the majority of patients have inactive or well-controlled disease at the onset of pregnancy, and therapy is prompt and decisive.
3. The average probability of flare during SLE pregnancy and postpartum is 40% to 50%, but, in contrast with studies of the 1950s, 1960s, and 1970s, most flares after 1980 are minor, with arthritis and cutaneous manifestations. Nevertheless, severe exacerbations occur in approximately 10% to 20% of pregnancies and, for this reason, this should be treated as a *high-risk pregnancy*.
3. Risk factors for flares include disease activity during the 3 to 6 months preceding conception and preexisting renal disease (see below). Conversely, conception during quiescence or remission is associated with a lesser risk for exacerbation (20% to 36%). Mild lupus rarely exacerbates during pregnancy.
4. Most studies avoid corticosteroid treatment for prevention of flares, and instead watch the patient very carefully and raise steroid dose at the slightest indication of flare.
5. There is a greater prevalence of preeclampsia or pregnancy-induced hypertension in lupus patients (see below).
6. Although recent reports concern mainly patients who fulfill American Rheumatology Association (ARA) criteria for SLE, onset of SLE during pregnancy or the postpartum period was seen in approximately 20% of patients (13% to 50%) in older reports, with a severe, catastrophic illness, and dire maternal and fetal outcome

(Table 47.2) (68,74,82,129). A high index of suspicion for SLE should prevail when a young woman, during pregnancy or the early postpartum period, has unexplained rashes, arthritis, alopecia, proteinuria with active urine sediment, psychosis, chorea, pleuropericarditis, or vasculitis, alone or in combination. Delay in diagnosis and management can be lethal.

COURSE OF LUPUS NEPHRITIS DURING PREGNANCY

Reports on lupus pregnancy from the 1950s and 1960s mention patients with nephritis, usually in the context of severe flare, increasing proteinuria, azotemia or acute anuric renal failure, hypertension, pre/eclampsia, onset of nephritis during pregnancy, and even maternal death (54,55,60,81). Active nephritis at conception, often not detected early nor treated aggressively, can put the mother and fetus at risk.

On the other hand, in the 1970s and 1980s, several papers reported an uneventful course of pregnancy, or a better prognosis, when renal function is normal, and lupus nephritis has been inactive for 3 to 6 months before conception (60,66,68–70,74,77). This trend has continued through the 1990s.

Table 47.4 summarizes available data from 19 series published from 1978 to 1999 that address lupus nephritis and pregnancy (46,63,65,67–70,73,74,77,83,86,88,96,98,99, 125–128). Although it is not a common practice, percutaneous needle biopsy can be performed during pregnancy under ultrasonic guidance (130).

In all, 605 pregnancies were reported in women with lupus nephritis. The prevalence of focal or diffuse proliferative nephritis was 40% to 100% (average, 64.6%), and nephrotic syndrome was present in 0% to 42% (average, 15.1%). The rate of flares in pregnancy was from 7.4% to 66% (average, 32%). Flare rates in 83 pregnancies with lupus nephritis activity at conception, were 48% to 66%

TABLE 47.4. COURSE OF LUPUS NEPHRITIS IN PREGNANCY

Study	Pregnancies (No.)	Proliferative Nephritis (%)	Nephrotic Syndrome (%)	Flare (%)	Preeclampsia (%)	Transient Renal Insufficiency (%) (Irreversible Renal Failure)
Thomas et al. (63)	13	64	31	55	—	23
Devoe and Taylor (65)	13	63	—	15	8	15
Houser et al. (67)	18	40	—	28	22	33
	10 inactive	—	—	20	20	20
	8 active	—	—	50	38	50
Hayslett and Lynn (68)	56	77	25	39	—	—
	31 inactive	43	10	32	6	10 (12)
	25 active	67	28	48	—	25 (11)
Zulman et al. (83)	19	58	11	63	32	13 (10)
Fine et al. (69)	37	—	—	23	—	32 (13.5)
Jungers et al. (70)	35	89	3	46	—	(4)
	11 inactive	100	9	9	—	(9)
	24 active	85	17	66	—	
Gimovsky et al. (73)	46	79	—	22	25	21 (16)
Imbasciati et al. (74)	26	58	42	46	—	37 (21)
Mintz et al. (46)	58 inactive	40	—	10	0	0
Bobrie et al. (77)	53	73	—	34	—	(11.4)
	27 inactive	—	—	7.4	—	5
	26 active	—	—	62	—	—
Wong et al. (86)	29	42	21	16	0	
Oviasu et al. (98)	47	66	—	13	0	11
Packham et al. (99)	64	—	17	48	5	19 (2)
Tincani et al. (88)	9	—	—	33	0	0
Julkunen et al. (125)	26 inactive	42	4	8	30	0
Font et al. (96,126)	10 nephritis	100	0	30	50 (HT)	0
	50 no nephritis	0	0	24	10 (HT)	0
Huong Du et al. (127)	25	76	12	32	16	8
Ramos et al. (128)	21	67	0	42.9	14.3	0

	No. Patients	Flares (%)	Preeclampsia (%)
Active nephritis at conception	83	56.5	38
Inactive nephritis at conception	163	14.4	14

HT, hypertension.
Data from refs. 46, 67, 68, 70, 77, and 125.

(average, 56.5%) (67,68,70,77); flares in 163 pregnancies with inactive lupus at conception from the above four series plus the Mintz and Julkunen reports were from 7.4% to 32% (average, 14.4%) (46,67,68,70,77,125).

Preeclampsia ranged from 0% to 38%, and hypertension was very common, up to 50%. Transient renal insufficiency occurred in 0% to 37% (up to 50% in active nephritis), and irreversible renal failure in 0% to 21% of patients (Table 47.4).

Some of the most notable studies with the most patients are reviewed here.

Devoe and Taylor (65) reported 13 pregnancies in eight women, five with biopsy-proven nephritis and two with severe flares with decreased renal function and preeclampsia. The authors credited serum complement C3 and C4 levels with prognostication of SLE flare. In a subsequent report of 18 pregnancies in 15 women with lupus and renal biopsies prior to conception, the authors found that decreased renal function, rather than severity of renal biopsy class, correlates with abnormal fetal outcome (131).

Lupus Nephritis And Pregnancy In The 1980s

In 1980, Houser et al. (67) reported 11 patients with lupus nephritis and 18 pregnancies; ten pregnancies in five patients with inactive SLE were uneventful, while eight pregnancies in six women with active disease included three with preeclampsia, severe in two, and disease exacerbation in a patient who developed class III lupus nephritis. All patients were receiving prednisone, and no maternal deaths occurred.

Hayslett and Lynn's (68) questionnaire study of 13 nephrology centers and individual nephrologists reported 47 patients with 65 pregnancies, with focal or diffuse proliferative nephritis on renal biopsy in 36 of 47. In nine instances (14%) SLE began during pregnancy and, in 56 pregnancies, manifestations of lupus nephritis preceded conception in 80%; worsening of nephritis was found in 39% of the mothers, 16 during pregnancy and six in the postpartum period. Of 25 pregnancies with active renal disease at conception, 12% improved, 48% worsened, and 40% remained unchanged. Pregnancy in patients with active SLE had a more hectic course, and successful outcome was reduced by 25%. Only nine of 16 patients with nephrotic syndrome had successful deliveries. When the serum creatinine level was lower than 1.5 mg/dL, nine of ten pregnancies resulted in live births, but in ten pregnancies with serum creatinine above 1.5 mg/dL, fetal loss was 50%. In four patients, however, with serum creatinine of 4 mg/dL or higher, pregnancies resulted in live births, indicating that a successful outcome is still possible despite severe renal failure.

Among the patients of Zulman et al. (83), 10 of 16 (62.5%) with prior nephritis had exacerbations during pregnancy. In 25% of patients, differentiation of acute presentation of lupus nephritis from toxemia was necessary. The authors suggested that the preeclamptic picture was a result of lupus nephritis.

Fine et al. (69) in 1981 observed that nearly one third of pregnancies (12 of 37) resulted in worse renal function, five of them irreversibly. No conception occurred in patients with even moderate renal insufficiency. The authors formulated a hemodialysis strategy for pregnant patients based on the physiology of pregnancy. Dialysis is indicated for a maternal blood urea nitrogen (BUN) of 50 mg/dL or greater and should maintain BUN under that level. Volume removal should be done through isolated ultrafiltration, blood pressure should be supported with albumin, the dialysate should contain glucose and bicarbonate, low-dose heparin should be used, and progesterone should be administered, because the endogenous progesterone is lost in the dialysate.

From Paris, Jungers et al. (70) reported a retrospective study of 36 patients with 104 pregnancies seen between 1962 and 1980. Of these, 26 occurred after SLE onset (14 women) and, in nine patients onset of lupus and nephritis occurred during pregnancy or postpartum (25% of patients). All patients had clinical renal disease, and biopsies showed five with mesangial or minimal disease, eight with focal proliferative, six with diffuse proliferative nephritis, and two with membranous nephropathy. Flares occurred in 12 of 26 pregnancies after SLE onset (46%), two of which (8%) progressed to irreversible renal failure. A full 66% of patients with active nephritis at the time of conception had a flare; in contrast, only 9% of patients with inactive disease during the 5 months before conception had a flare.

Gimovsky et al. (73) reviewed retrospectively 39 patients seen between 1973 and 1982 in the Department of Obstetrics and the Rheumatology Section at the University of Southern California; 46 pregnancies occurred in 19 SLE patients with nephritis, confirmed by renal biopsy in 15 (79%). Onset of lupus during pregnancy or postpartum occurred in 8 of 39 patients (21%). Hospitalization was required because of flare in 9%, 8%, 14%, and 4% of patients at risk during the three trimesters and postpartum, respectively. Of the ten cases of preeclampsia, six occurred in the patients with nephritis: 25% of 24 pregnancies, after six elective and 16 spontaneous abortions are subtracted from the 46 pregnancies. Of 19 patients, four (21%) developed a decrease in renal function within 2 years of delivery, and three required chronic hemodialysis (16%). Only 18 of 40 pregnancies (excluding induced abortions) were successful, with a total fetal loss of 55% in the renal group.

Imbasciati et al. (74) from the University of Milan, Italy, reported 19 SLE nephritis patients with 26 pregnancies and repeated kidney biopsies; 58% had diffuse proliferative glomerulonephritis, and 42% nephrotic syndrome. During 15 pregnancies in ten patients there were extrarenal or renal flares with no change in renal function; three patients had moderate deterioration of renal function, hypertension, and proteinuria during pregnancy, reversed in two by steroid therapy. The worst disease course was in seven patients with onset of SLE and nephritis during pregnancy: of these seven, four patients had mild nephritis but three, along with a fourth who had SLE for 1 year, developed anuric renal failure, with two maternal deaths. In all but two pregnancies, SLE was active and, by current standards, steroid dosage was low or of short duration, with inadequate control of maternal disease. Only in seven instances, mainly postpartum, did flaring patients receive high-dose steroid therapy (50 mg prednisone daily or more), which controlled SLE activity in most patients. This suggests that earlier therapeutic intervention was indicated. Multiple renal biopsies performed in seven patients showed that the majority (four patients) had progression of a minimal, focal proliferative, or membranous lesion to a diffuse proliferative nephritis. The converse occurred in two patients, in whom diffuse proliferative disease regressed to focal proliferative in one and to minimal lesion in the other patient. Fetal outcome was poor, with 61% live births (corrected for induced abortions).

In 1987, Bobrie et al. (77) again reviewed the patient population at the Hospital Necker in Paris and added 32 more pregnancies to their previous report (70). Of the 73 patients reviewed, eight first developed SLE manifestations during pregnancy, and six during the postpartum or postabortion periods, for a 19% prevalence of SLE onset in pregnancy; nephrotic syndrome with increased serum creatinine levels was seen in seven of these 14 patients. Subsequent kidney biopsies showed proliferative glomerulonephritis in all 14 patients (diffuse in 11); high-dose steroid therapy improved all but one patient, who progressed to renal failure in 2 years. In 35 women with 53 pregnancies after the onset of SLE, nephritis flare occurred in 18 (34%), either during pregnancy or postpartum (ten and eight cases, respectively). These exacerbations were more frequent in patients whose SLE was active at conception (16 of 26, 61.5%), than in patients with stable remissions (2 of 27, 7.4%). Corticosteroid therapy failed to reverse the course in four patients, who rapidly progressed to end-stage renal failure.

In the prospective study from Mexico City, 58 of 102 pregnancies occurred in patients with known, inactive SLE nephritis, and all but three had previous renal biopsies (43,46). Of 58 patients, 27 had mesangial lesions (47%), 13 had diffuse (22%), and nine had focal (16%) proliferative glomerulonephritis, five had membranous nephropathy (9%), one had membranoproliferative (1.7%), and three were undetermined (43). They were treated with 30 to 60 mg of prednisone daily, and were well 4 years later.

The rate at which patients with SLE without renal disease develop it is not known; in this study three cases occurred in 472 patient-months at risk during pregnancy and postpartum (0.006 new cases of nephritis/patient-month). The authors compared it with patients in the same study followed further for 1,537 patient/months, during which another five cases developed new nephritis (0.003/patient-month; p = NS). In these 58 pregnancies in patients with known SLE nephritis, six exacerbations occurred (10.3%), evenly distributed by trimester and postpartum period, and all responded to increases in prednisone dosage. These six patients had inactive renal disease for 2 to 5 years before pregnancy. On long-term follow-up of 75 total patients (40 to 65 months), renal function deterioration occurred in two of eight with diffuse proliferative and in one of seven patients with focal proliferative nephritis; five deaths occurred, only one from renal disease, 49 months after pregnancy. Of the remaining 44 pregnancies without previous kidney disease, renal involvement appeared for the first time in three patients (6.8%) during the second and third trimesters; subsequent biopsies showed two with mesangial and one with diffuse proliferative glomerulonephritis. All patients in this study had been previously diagnosed and were treated with at least 10 mg of prednisone daily during the entire pregnancy; also, all had mild, inactive kidney disease at the time of conception. Of these patients, six had experienced a bout of nephritis within 1 year of conception, but none exacerbated during pregnancy. The exacerbations were not related to the histologic biopsy class. The outcome of pregnancy in this study was not different for patients with or without kidney disease, and the authors related a better fetal outcome to inactive, well-controlled SLE, rather than to the absence of kidney disease.

Lupus Nephritis And Pregnancy In The 1990s

In the prospective study from Hong Kong (86), six nephritis relapses occurred in 13 patients, with increasing proteinuria in three and nephrotic syndrome in three. Two of the nephrotic patients remitted within 4 weeks after elective abortion and increased steroids, and the other four remitted with only increased doses of prednisone. Eight women with a history of preexisting diffuse proliferative renal disease had successful pregnancies, and it was suggested that this was possible because of proper prednisone therapy. The study noted a good maternal outcome in patients with severe disease, perhaps because of their treatment protocol with increasing doses of prednisone as pregnancy progressed.

In the 25 women with lupus nephritis reported by Oviasu et al. (98), a flare was seen in only one of 53 pregnancies, although six patients each had increased proteinuria and decreased creatinine clearance, and nine patients had more than trivial cutaneous lupus. Hypertension was present and controlled in 17 of 47 pregnancies (36%), excluding elective abortions, and absent in 30 of 47 (64%). No one developed renal failure, and cesarean section was necessary in 44% of the 39 completed pregnancies (11 of 17 as emergencies). Almost one third of the deliveries (28%) were preterm.

Among 64 pregnancies in 41 women with lupus nephritis reported by Packham et al. (99) from Australia, proteinuria was stable in ten pregnancies (16%), increased in 48% of pregnancies, with nephrotic syndrome in 17%, and was irreversible postpartum in 5% (three patients). Hypertension was present in 44%, was severe in 13%, and irreversible in nine patients (14%). Eclampsia occurred in three women (5%). Transient renal insufficiency was seen in 19% and renal failure in one patient (2%). Prematurity occurred in 19 of 43 live births (44%).

Of 25 pregnancies reported by Tincani et al. (88), nine occurred in seven women with nephritis. There were three nephritis flares in these patients and *de novo* nephritis in a fourth.

Julkunen et al. (125) presented 26 pregnancies in 16 patients with lupus nephritis: 42% of these patients had focal or diffuse proliferative nephritis, and were clinically inactive with normal renal function. Two patients flared (8%), one had nephrotic syndrome (4%), seven of the 23 completed pregnancies were complicated by preeclampsia (30%), and seven of 23 births (30%) were premature. There was no compromise of renal function in these patients.

Font et al. (96,126) from Barcelona reported ten pregnancies in nine patients with lupus nephritis and compared them to 50 pregnancies in 37 SLE patients without nephritis. Flares occurred in 30% of pregnancies, hypertension and preeclampsia were more prevalent in these patients than in patients without nephritis (50% vs. 11.6%), cesarean sections were more frequent (60% vs. 18%), and neonates were of lower gestational age and birth weight.

Huong Du et al. (127, same authors as ref. 90 and 94) from Paris reported 25 pregnancies in 16 women with biopsy-proven SLE nephritis, focal or diffuse proliferative in 76%. There was proteinuria in 32%, nephrotic syndrome in 12%, flares in 32%, preeclampsia in 16%, transient renal insufficiency in 8%, one maternal death (6.25%), and 15 premature births (60%). A second maternal death occurred 4 years after delivery. Treatment included prednisone, mean 22 mg/day, aspirin and heparin for antiphospholipid syndrome, azathioprine, and, after delivery, cyclophosphamide in two patients with renal flares.

Ramos et al. (128) from Mexico City reported 21 pregnant patients with lupus nephritis, proliferative (mostly class IV) in 67%, assessed by SLEDAI. Renal flare occurred in 42.9% (first and second trimester), preeclampsia in 14.3%, and fetal loss in 14.3%. No progression of renal disease was noted. Treatment included prednisone (mean 20 mg/day), aspirin, and heparin for antiphospholipid syndrome.

The outcome of SLE nephritis and pregnancy in the 1990s is far better than that of previous decades.

Preeclampsia In Lupus Pregnancy

Preeclampsia, defined as the abrupt onset of hypertension and proteinuria after 24 weeks of gestation, is found in 0.5% to 10% of all pregnancies, and is by far more common in the primigravida (49,50). Preeclampsia is caused by shallow placentation, insufficient development of the spiral arteries in the uteroplacental vasculature, which results in placental ischemia, oxidative stress, destruction of trophoblastic tissue, and infarction (132). It results in increased resistance of the uteroplacental circulation, atherosis of the placental vessels, systemic endothelial dysfunction, dyslipidemia, and ischemia with intrauterine growth restriction in the fetus and hypertension in the mother (133). In lupus pregnancy, up to 25% of patients develop significant proteinuria and hypertension in the second half of pregnancy. Opinions have varied widely as to whether this represents preeclampsia or active lupus nephritis (83,84,119). When this clinical picture is associated with low complement levels, and no hyperuricemia, it has often been interpreted as SLE nephritis flare (68,70,74,83). However, Lockshin et al. (84) noted no improvement with corticosteroids, and spontaneous improvement over several months postpartum, and regarded it as a "variant" of PIH. Although the issue of increased prevalence of preeclampsia versus nephritis flare in pregnant SLE patients has not been fully resolved (75,97), it is worthwhile to examine the frequency with which preeclampsia occurs in women with nephritis of other types.

In pregnancy with maternal renal disease other than lupus nephritis, hypertension develops in 41% of these women, with a higher risk for severe hypertension in women with diffuse proliferative nephritis or with nephrosclerosis (134). In these women, too, hypertension occurs most often during the third trimester (134,135). Women with prior chronic hypertension may develop preeclampsia in pregnancy, and then the term "superimposed preeclampsia" is used (133). In a renal biopsy study of 176 women with the clinical diagnosis of preeclampsia and without lupus, the typical histologic picture of glomerular endotheliosis was found in 96 of 176 patients (54.5%), 79 of whom (82%) were primigravidae, thus confirming that preeclampsia is uncommon in the multipara (136). Furthermore, the clinical diagnosis of preeclampsia was confirmed by the biopsy picture in 50% of primigravidae but only in 25% of multigravid women. Of the remaining patients, 10% had a mixed picture of glomerular endotheliosis plus nephrosclerosis, other renal disease, or both, 14% had nephrosclerosis with or without other renal disease, 17.6% had renal disease alone, and 4.5% had normal histology. Therefore, a clinical preeclamptic picture does not necessarily mean preeclampsia by histology.

A further cause for potential confusion of preeclampsia with lupus exacerbation is the HELLP syndrome (*h*emolysis, *e*levated *l*iver enzymes, *l*ow *p*latelets), which may complicate the course of severe preeclampsia in a minority of patients (51). Hemolysis and thrombocytopenia are due to disseminated intravascular coagulation with microangiopathic hemolytic anemia; 28 of 29 (97%) of Weinstein's patients with HELLP had characteristic blood smears with burr cells and schistocytes, and all had platelet counts under 100,000/mm^3. Elevated liver enzyme levels [serum glutamic–oxaloacetic transaminase (SGOT) and serum glutamic–pyruvic transaminase (SGPT)] were found in all 29 patients and an increased bilirubin level in 57%. The liver dysfunction is attributed to fibrin deposition with obstruction of the hepatic sinusoids, resulting in liver distention, subcapsular hematomas, infarction, and even rupture (137). Treatment of preeclampsia and prompt delivery by cesarean section is advocated because of grave danger to the mother and fetus (perinatal mortality, 9% to 60%).

Serum complement levels (C3) and anti-dsDNA can help differentiate between active lupus nephritis and preeclampsia. The C3 level is generally low in active nephritis, but normal in preeclampsia (138). Anti-dsDNA is strongly positive with complement-fixing activity in active proliferative lupus nephritis, and was negative in 40 patients with toxemia, even in six of 40 with a positive ANA (139). Renal biopsies before conception and postpartum in these patients may provide the definitive answer.

Another cause of proteinuria in lupus pregnancy is renal vein thrombosis. Proteinuria with severe flank pain and hematuria, especially in the presence of membranous nephropathy, a history of deep vein thrombosis, and positive antiphospholipid antibodies, should raise the possibility of renal vein thrombosis. Venography is contraindicated in a pregnant woman; a Doppler ultrasound examination of the renal veins can detect abnormal turbulence in the renal veins and other imaging techniques, if not contraindicated, could be applied, such as magnetic resonance imaging (MRI).

Preeclampsia: Risk Factors And Associated Disorders

In a study of 2,947 women with single pregnancies, risk factors for preeclampsia were, in order of importance, systolic hypertension, prepregnancy obesity, smoking history, and number of previous abortions or miscarriages (140). Additional factors include being primigravida, prior history of early onset preeclampsia, family history of preeclampsia, diabetes, and dyslipidemia. The association of antiphospholipid antibodies (APL) with preeclampsia has been pointed out in 1989 (141).

A study of 101 patients with severe early-onset preeclampsia (before 30 weeks), showed that associated disorders included chronic hypertension in 38.6%, APL in 29.4%, protein S deficiency in 24.7%, hyperhomocysteinemia in 17.7%, and activated protein C resistance in 16% (142). In 23 women with severe preeclampsia, anticardiolipin and lupus anticoagulant was significantly higher that in 43 controls (143).

The production of prostanoids in lupus, normal, and hypertensive pregnancies has been studied. In a controlled study of 14 pregnant lupus patients, Kaaja et al. (144) demonstrated that prostacyclin metabolite excretion was normal in early pregnancy, but reduced during late pregnancy in women without APL. In women with APL, prostacyclin metabolites were increased in early pregnancy, and more so (140% of normal) during the second half of pregnancy. Thromboxane production (as measured by thromboxane B_2 and 2,3-dinor-thromboxane B_2), was increased in lupus patients, especially when APL-positive and in the second half of the pregnancy. It seems that an increased ratio of thromboxane to prostacyclin is important in the genesis of hypertensive disorders of pregnancy. Therapy with aspirin, 50 mg per day, decreased thromboxane production, and did not affect prostacyclin production, resulting in an increased ratio of prostacyclin to thromboxane in the treated patients.

In a series of elegant studies, Peaceman and Rehnberg (145) showed that placental explants from normal pregnancies, incubated with immunoglobulin G (IgG) fractions of lupus anticoagulant-positive serum, showed similar to baseline prostacyclin production, while thromboxane production was significantly increased. A subsequent study by the same authors showed that, in the same *in vitro* system, addition of 10^{-4} aspirin did not affect prostacyclin production, while it decreased thromboxane production significantly (146). In contrast, addition of indomethacin at 10^{-7} caused significant decreases in the production of both prostacyclin and thromboxane, leaving their ratio unaffected.

Hawkins et al. (147) showed that stimulated thromboxane (TBX) production by monocytes of women with chronic hypertension was excessive, and basal secretion of TBX by platelets was high; women with PIH had high, but lesser, stimulated TBX production. Tsukimori et al. (148) reported the presence of a neutrophil activator in sera of preeclamptic women, which enhances superoxide production.

Abnormal uterine artery vascular resistance, as detected by Doppler flow velocity waveform at the 18th week of pregnancy, was associated with significant increase in preeclampsia, compared with normal resistance (11% versus 4%), and with adverse pregnancy outcome (45% versus 28%) (149). In this study there was no reduction of pregnancy complications by low-dose aspirin (100 mg/day).

The above studies on disturbed prostanoid metabolism in hypertensive women and lupus patients with APL would suggest that small doses of aspirin (ASA) in pregnancy can prevent preeclampsia. Numerous such studies suggest that low-dose aspirin is effective in a subset of patients with sensitivity to angiotensin-II, which can be identified with the rollover test, instead of the intravenous angiotensin infusion test (48,48a,150). ASA should be started between 10 and 14 weeks of gestation, because that is the time of onset of abnormal placentation that leads to preeclampsia (151). A trial of ketanserin (a selective serotonin-2 receptor antagonist) and aspirin versus placebo and aspirin (75 mg/day) showed promise, with significantly lower incidence of preeclampsia and severe hypertension (152).

Summary—Lupus Nephritis And Pregnancy

The interrelationship of pregnancy and lupus nephritis can be summarized as follows:

1. Patients with SLE nephritis have a 50% to 60% chance of nephritis flare during pregnancy or postpartum if they conceive during a period of active SLE. In contrast, patients with well-controlled SLE, who conceive after a 3- to 6-month period of remission, have only a 7% to 10% chance of nephritis exacerbation.
2. Nephritis flares during pregnancy and postpartum can be very severe, with anuric renal failure and even maternal death, or chronic renal failure. Vigilance for early detection and vigorous treatment of exacerbations is required.
3. No definitive relationship between the histologic class of lupus nephritis and the severity of flare during pregnancy has been established, but there seems to be a tendency for more severe exacerbations in patients with proliferative nephritis, WHO classes IV and III. Limited information on repeat kidney biopsies before and after SLE pregnancy has shown progression in four patients and regression in two.
4. Women with lupus nephritis are prone to "superimposed" preeclampsia, with the prevalence of a preeclamptic picture during SLE pregnancy greater than in normal pregnancy (up to 38% versus 0.5% to 10%). This clinical picture should be viewed as a possible nephritis exacerbation until proven otherwise, because of the possibility of acute anuric or chronic renal failure that may follow an exacerbation, and of the distinctly different therapeutic management indicated.
5. Preexisting hypertension and antiphospholipid antibodies are the two most common predisposing factors to preeclampsia.
6. In the setting of lupus nephritis and prior hypertension, with or without antiphospholipid antibodies, preventive treatment with low-dose aspirin should be initiated at the 10th to 14th week of pregnancy.
7. The onset of lupus with nephritis during pregnancy is often associated with a stormy course and acute anuric renal failure, and should be suspected in any young woman with a multisystem presentation that includes rashes, arthritis, and alopecia.
8. Renal vein thrombosis should be suspected, detected, and treated, especially in patients with antiphospholipid antibodies and/or membranous nephropathy.
9. Hemodialysis should be instituted during lupus pregnancy in patients with BUN levels of 50 mg/dL or greater.
10. In the presence of active lupus nephritis, especially diffuse proliferative, nephrotic syndrome, moderate to severe hypertension, and a serum creatinine level of 2 mg/dL or greater, pregnancy is contraindicated.

Bottom line: Pregnancy with lupus nephritis, even inactive, should be handled as a high-risk pregnancy.

LABORATORY FINDINGS, SEROLOGIC MARKERS, AND ANTIPHOSPHOLIPID ANTIBODIES

When used judiciously and in the context of the patient's clinical picture, certain laboratory tests in pregnant lupus patients are useful in predicting disease flare, or potential fetal problems. Monitoring of disease activity is achieved by the serial determination of complement levels, anti-dsDNA antibodies, circulating immune complexes, and urinalysis with microscopic exam. Fetal loss is high in patients with antiphospholipid antibodies, and neonatal lupus erythematosus is associated with anti-Ro/SSA, anti-La/SSB and, rarely, with anti-U1 ribonucleoprotein (RNP) antibodies.

Pregnancy Tests

Pregnancy test by radioimmunoassay may be false positive in SLE patients with nephrotic syndrome (153). False-positive urine pregnancy tests occurred in 14 of 140 (10%) nonpregnant lupus patients, including one male: 11 of the 14 had renal disease, eight with the nephrotic syndrome (154). The false-positive test presents as an atypical ring pattern and reflects a nonimmunologic interference with agglutination of human chorionic gonadotropin (HCG) by anti-HCG serum. Urine gamma globulins in concentrations of 1.7 to 16.6 mg/mL produced this phenomenon. Serum radioimmunoassay for β-HCG gives no false-positive results.

Pregnancy-Induced Laboratory Test Changes

The sedimentation rate increases in normal pregnancy and cannot be relied on for predicting disease activity (155). Average values by the Westergren method are 29 mm/h in the first, 42 mm/h in the second, and 36 mm/h in the third trimester. In 1956, Friedman and Rutherford (55) reported a high incidence of postpartum exacerbations in lupus patients with Westergren sedimentation rates in excess of 100 mm/h. In addition, creatinine clearance increases, immunoglobulin levels decrease but are still within normal limits (156), and the hemoglobin decreases; the latter two are attributed to hemodilution.

Complement

Several studies have shown that the C3 complement level rises in normal pregnancy but little, if at all, in SLE (155, 157). Failure of C3 to rise or declining levels have been associated with SLE exacerbation, with or without fetal morbidity. Zurier et al. (155) noted a 30% mean rise of C3 level in 20 normal pregnant women and concluded that a declining C3 during pregnancy was a valuable indicator of increased SLE activity. Zulman et al. (83) reached similar conclusions. The C3 level rose by 25% in a control group of normal pregnant women, while it only increased by 10% in a group of pregnant SLE patients (157). Ziegler and Medsger (158) confirmed the above findings at the same center, with a larger series; 87 of their patients who had a flat or declining C3 level had a significant increase in maternal problems, and in fetal morbidity and mortality. Devoe et al. (65,159) also noted that a falling C3 level was associated with increased SLE activity in the mother and with an increased risk of abortions.

The alternate complement pathway is also activated during lupus flares in pregnancy, and the level of Ba (activation product of the alternate pathway) is elevated, and is associated with low hemolytic complement (CH_{50}) values; the ratio of CH_{50} to Ba was significantly lower in lupus flares than in preeclampsia without SLE (160). In addition, despite high levels of C3, activation of the classic complement pathway in normal pregnancy has been shown (161). It has been suggested that hypocomplementemia in the pregnant lupus patient may be the result of a different mechanism than in the nonpregnant patient (162).

Lupus-Induced Laboratory Changes

Antinuclear Antibodies

Antinuclear antibody (ANA) tests have no specificity for disease activity in lupus. Studies of ANA in normal pregnant women have shown a similar prevalence as in the general population, between 1% and 5% (mean, 2.3%) (163–165). One report of 52% ANA positivity in normal pregnant patients (166) has been refuted by the above studies. A subsequent report compared 214 normal pregnant women with 50 age-matched controls and found 11% and 2% ANA positivity, respectively, which was significantly higher in pregnancy ($p < .05$) (167). Most positive ANAs were found in the third trimester. None of the ANA-positive subjects were symptomatic or took lupus-inducing drugs, and only two had anti-dsDNA. In an interesting study from Mexico, Garcia-de la Torre et al. (139) found a positive ANA in six of 20 habitual (recurrent) aborters (30%), in six of 40 toxemic patients (15%), and in two of 30 normal pregnant women (6.7%). Of the two ANA-positive habitual aborters with anti-dsDNA, one fulfilled four criteria for SLE; three more in this group had one to three criteria. Of the six preeclamptic patients with a positive ANA, three patients had one, and one patient had two criteria. The authors concluded that the high prevalence of ANA in women with recurrent abortion can help identify patients who will eventually develop lupus. We concur that ANA does not appear in pregnancy unless the patient is developing lupus.

Anti-dsDNA, especially the complement-fixing variety, has been recognized as a helpful marker for assessing the activity of lupus and lupus nephritis (168–170) and increasing anti-dsDNA levels or titers predict disease flare (171). IgG-class anti-dsDNA, when present in the mother's plasma, may cross the placenta: Grennan et al. (172) followed four systemic and one discoid lupus patients through pregnancy; they found anti-dsDNA in the four SLE patients and in the cord blood of the neonate whose mother had the highest DNA binding. In this baby, the DNA binding capacity fell from 96% in the cord blood to 52% at 2 weeks and to 9% (negative) at 8 weeks of age. Zulman et al. (83), however, did not detect anti-dsDNA in the cord blood of six neonates whose mothers had it. The appearance of complement-fixing anti-dsDNA, or an increase during pregnancy, should alert the physician to the possibility of new onset or flare of lupus nephritis.

The determination of anti-Ro/SSA and anti-La/SSB antibodies in the pregnant lupus patient is highly recommended because of their link to the neonatal lupus erythematosus syndrome (NLE) (173,174) (see Chapter 50). Anti-Ro/SSA is found in 25% to 40% of lupus patients and anti-La/SSB in 10% to 15%. The proportion of children with neonatal lupus in mothers positive for anti-Ro/SSA and/or anti-La/SSB is small, up to 8.8%, but it is worth looking for them, so as to counsel the patient appropriately.

Anti-U1RNP antibody is detected in 40% to 45% of lupus patients and is rarely associated with the neonatal lupus syndrome (175).

Cryoglobulins

It has been well established that cold-insoluble complexes (mixed cryoglobulins) are present in up to 30% of lupus patients' sera, and represent immune complexes. They are associated with decreased serum complement levels and with evidence of active lupus, especially nephritis (176). We have also found that increased levels of cryoglobulins correlate with disease activity.

Antiphospholipid Antibodies

One of the most important laboratory tests in lupus pregnancy is the determination of antiphospholipid antibodies (APL), the most common of which are anticardiolipin antibody (ACL), and lupus anticoagulant (LA or LAC) (47,177). Although separate and distinct, these antibodies and others (antibodies to β_2-glycoprotein I, to phosphatidylserine, phosphatidylinositol, etc.) to negatively charged membrane phospholipids frequently coexist.

Antiphospholipid antibodies have been linked to intravascular clotting, arterial or venous, recurrent fetal loss, livedo reticularis, immune thrombocytopenia, Coombs'-positive autoimmune hemolytic anemia, and false-positive tests for syphilis (167,178). In a review of 21 studies comprising over 1,000 lupus patients, circulating anticoagulant was found in 34% (7% to 73%), and anticardiolipin antibody in 44% (21% to 63%) (47). Patients with circulating anticoagulant have a prolonged activated partial thromboplastin time (APTT), which does not correct with a 1:1 dilution with normal serum. A quantitative determination is performed using the Exner test or the kaolin clotting time, or the Russel viper venom time (RVVT) (178–180). Anticardiolipin antibody can be detected by enzyme-linked immunosorbent assay (ELISA) or radioimmunoassay (177). (See also Chapter 25 and 48.)

There are numerous reports of the association of recurrent spontaneous abortion, fetal loss, and fetal distress with antiphospholipid antibodies in patients with and without lupus. In addition, intrauterine growth restriction (IUGR), prematurity, and preeclampsia have been associated with APL (142,143). Antibody to β_2-glycoprotein I is often found in association with anticardiolipin antibody and uncommonly alone. In a study of 424 women (152 healthy fertile controls, 141 with unexplained recurrent spontaneous abortions, 58 with unexplained fetal deaths, and 73 with antiphospholipid syndrome, testing for anti–β_2-glycoprotein I did not identify additional patients at risk for recurrent abortion or fetal loss (181). Thrombotic events have also been described with a functional or quantitative deficiency of protein C or protein S in association with antiphospholipid antibodies (182).

In 15 retrospective studies of 1,249 pregnancies in SLE and SLE-like illness, there were 479 pregnancies in APL-positive women and 770 pregnancies in APL-negative women (103,177,183–194). In the APL-positive pregnancies there was a mean fetal loss of 37% (range, 14% to 68%). In the APL-negative pregnancies, there was a mean fetal loss of 18% (range, 3% to 43%), not statistically significant.

In seven prospective studies of 892 lupus pregnancies, 301 occurred in APL-positive and 591 in APL-negative women. In the APL-positive pregnancies, mean fetal loss was 48% (range, 4% to 100%), and in the APL-negative, 9% (range, 0% to 20%) (195–201). Despite the large range, the significance of positive APL as a cause of fetal loss is irrefutable.

Similar facts emerge from studies of women with recurrent fetal loss but without lupus, women with normal pregnancies, and women with implantation failure from *in vitro* fertilization (see Chaps. 25 and 40).

A study from Japan is noteworthy in that Ishii et al. (191) described two subsets of lupus patients with IgG ACL antibodies. They found that 39 patients who were persistently positive for ACL, whether lupus was active or inactive, had the following significant differences from 29 patients who were positive only during active lupus: higher titers of ACL, more thromboses (33% vs. 3%), spontaneous abortions (41% vs. 7%), and lupus anticoagulant (45% vs. 8%), less nephritis (44% vs. 72%), and less anti-dsDNA positivity (72% vs. 97%). It may prove that fine differences within patients positive for ACL, as above, are important markers for ACL-associated morbidity.

IgG antiphospholipid antibody appears to be responsible for recurrent fetal loss (177), but no specific pathogenic subclass has been incriminated (202). The mechanism invoked for fetal loss is intravascular clotting, possibly through interference with endothelial prostacyclin production, which results in a small placenta with infarcts (197).

Thrombocytopenia during lupus pregnancy may be the result of association with antiphospholipid antibodies (162), and may signify lupus flare. Thrombocytopenia in the presence of preeclampsia, however, should prompt investigations for the HELLP syndrome (51), which needs to be differentiated from lupus flare.

Other Tests

It has been well established that cold-insoluble complexes (mixed cryoglobulins) are present in up to 30% of lupus patients' sera, and represent immune complexes. They are associated with decreased serum complement levels and with evidence of active lupus, especially nephritis (176). We have also found that increased levels of cryoglobulins correlate with disease activity.

Laboratory Monitoring In SLE Pregnancy

Recommendations for laboratory monitoring in SLE pregnancy can be summarized as follows:

1. Initial laboratory assessment of the pregnant lupus patient should include:

   Complete blood count (CBC) including platelets
   Urinalysis with microscopic examination
   Chemistry panel inclusive of BUN, creatinine, and blood glucose
   Coombs' test
   Venereal Disease Research Laboratory (VDRL) test, activated partial thromboplastin time (APTT), anticardiolipin
   Anti-dsDNA, anti-Ro/SSA, anti-La/SSB, anti-U1RNP
   Complement C3 and C4
   24-hour urine for protein and creatinine, in the event of nephritis

A positive screening APTT should be followed by appropriate investigations for the lupus anticoagulant. Highly positive levels of antiphospholipid antibodies should alert the rheumatologist and obstetrician to the possibility of spontaneous abortion or stillbirth, fetal distress, or preeclampsia.

Positive anti-Ro/SSA and/or anti-La/SSB and, to a lesser extent, a positive anti-U1RNP should alert these physicians to the possibility of neonatal lupus erythematosus. If the patient is nephrotic or on corticosteroids, serum lipid tests are also indicated. Patients with known nephritis should have frequent monitoring of blood pressure and an initial 24-hour urine collection for protein, creatinine, and creatinine clearance. At the University of Southern California we also obtain quantitative serum cryoglobulin levels as an indicator of circulatory immune complexes.

2. Monthly laboratory assessment during lupus pregnancy should include CBC, platelets, urinalysis, chemistry panel (as above), anti-dsDNA, C3, C4, and cryoglobulins or other measures of immune complexes. Patients with known lupus nephritis should also have 24-hour urine collections for protein, creatinine, and creatinine clearance.
3. In the event of a hematocrit decrease, the Coombs' test should be repeated and the peripheral smear reviewed. Increasing antibodies to dsDNA, especially if they are complement-fixing, decreasing complement C3 and C4, and increasing immune complexes, indicate active lupus or impending flare in over 80% of patients.

MANAGEMENT DURING PREGNANCY, DELIVERY, AND POSTPARTUM PERIOD

General Principles

Before pregnancy, the lupus patient should consider strongly planning her pregnancies after a remission of at least 6 months. Once pregnant, she requires special conjoint attention by the rheumatologist and obstetrician, who should have experience in systemic lupus and high-risk pregnancy management, respectively. At the onset of pregnancy, a thorough assessment of system involvement and disease severity and activity should be made. The pregnant woman, her husband or mate, and other family members should be counseled with regard to the pregnancy (see below). During the first half of pregnancy, the woman with SLE under control should be followed every month, with increased frequency of visits during the second half (every 2 to 3 weeks). Laboratory evaluation and monitoring should be performed as recommended above. Blood pressure should be monitored at every visit, and even more frequently, at home, in patients with known nephritis. Follow-up should be geared toward early detection and aggressive therapy of lupus flares during pregnancy and the postpartum period.

Follow-up of fetal development includes repeated ultrasound evaluation of growth of the fetal pole and fetal heart monitoring, and nonstress test (203,204) (see also Chaps. 48 and 49).

Women with nephritis, with or without a history of hypertension, should be considered for low-dose daily aspirin from the 10th or 14th week to week 36 of gestation, for prevention of preeclampsia.

Patients with high levels of antiphospholipid antibodies, and especially those with recurrent abortions, should be considered for treatment protocols that enhance the possibility of live births (see below). Cytotoxic drugs should be avoided during the first trimester and full doses of prostaglandin inhibitors should be used very sparingly. Steroid preparation for the stress of delivery is needed for patients on steroids for the 2 previous years. Cesarean section should be considered for certain maternal or fetal indications, such as maternal avascular necrosis (osteonecrosis) of the hips with inadequate hip abduction, fetal distress, abnormal nonstress test, and the usual obstetric indications (e.g., cephalopelvic disproportion, transverse presentation). A neonatologist should be available at delivery.

During the immediate postpartum period and for the next 2 months, the mother should be watched carefully for development of infection at the site of episiotomy or cesarean incision, endometritis, urinary tract infection, pneumonia, and disease exacerbation. Infection and exacerbation should be treated promptly and aggressively.

Use Of Medications During Pregnancy (Table 47.5)

The major drugs used to treat lupus are corticosteroids, nonsteroidal antiinflammatory drugs (NSAIDs, including salicylates), antimalarials, immunosuppressives/cytotoxics, and, in the case of associated antiphospholipid syndrome, anticoagulants. There is a justifiable tendency to use as few drugs as possible during gestation, but a smooth course for mother and fetus might dictate their use. The major concerns about medication use in pregnancy are the pharmacologic effects on the mother and fetus, effects on the length of gestation and labor, and developmental effects on the fetus (intrauterine growth, malformations, and survival). A valuable textbook on the use of drugs in pregnancy and lactation is available (205).

The Food and Drug Administration (FDA) has assigned categories of drugs in terms of fetal risk:

Category A: Controlled studies in women fail to show risk to the fetus in the first trimester or later. Possibility of fetal harm seems remote.

Category B: No controlled studies in pregnant women and no fetal risk in animal studies, or animal studies show adverse effect, not confirmed in controlled studies in women in first trimester and later.

Category C: Animal studies show teratogenic, embryocidal, or other fetal effects and there are no controlled studies in women, or there are no studies in women and animals. Category C drugs should be given only if benefit outweighs the potential fetal risk.

Category D: There is evidence of human fetal risk, but benefit from use in pregnant women may be acceptable in

TABLE 47.5. MEDICATION USE IN LUPUS PREGNANCY AND LACTATION

Medications Used in Lupus	FDA Category	Lactation Permitted, Maternal Dose
Corticosteroids	B	Yes, up to 20 mg/d
Azathioprine	D	No, no data
Cyclophosphamide	D	No, cytopenia in infant
Methotrexate	D	No
Cyclosporine	C	No
Mycofenolate mofetil	C	No data
Chlorambucil	D	No
Antimalarial ([hydroxy]chloroquine)	C	Yes per AAP
Low-dose aspirin	C	Probably yes
Heparin, enoxaparin	B	Yes
Warfarin	D, X_M	Yes
Intravenous immunoglobulin	C_M	Yes
NSAIDs	B, D[a]	Yes—short-acting NSAIDs
COX-2 inhibitors	C	No data
Misoprostol	X_M	No
Antihypertensive drugs allowed in pregnancy		
MethylDOPA	C	Yes
Labetalol	C_M	Yes
Nifedropine	C	Yes

AAP, American Academy of Pediatrics; FDA, Food and Drug Administration; NSAIDs, nonsteroidal antiinflammatory drugs.
[a]In third trimester.
$_M$, Category per manufacturer.

spite of risk (i.e., in life-threatening situations or serious disease).

Category X: Animal or human studies show fetal abnormalities, or there is evidence of fetal risk in humans, or both, AND the risk outweighs any possible benefit.

Subscript M: The manufacturer has assigned the fetal risk category.

A Web site is available, *www.motherisk.org*, of the Hospital for Sick Children in Toronto, Canada.

Corticosteroids Category B

In the early 1960s Garsenstein et al. (81) noted that steroid therapy decreased flares during pregnancy and the postpartum period, and this was confirmed in subsequent decades by McGee and Makowski (61) and by Fine et al. (69). More recent reports further assert that, active lupus or flares during pregnancy or postpartum should be controlled with aggressive steroid therapy (43,46,86,87). Dose selection depends on the extent and severity of system involvement. Nephritis of the more severe types (diffuse and focal proliferative), neuropsychiatric manifestations, autoimmune hemolytic anemia, thrombocytopenia, and extensive, severe vasculitis, cutaneous or visceral, require doses greater than or equal to 1 mg/kg/day of prednisone, or equivalent. Pleuropericarditis usually requires less, 0.5 to 0.8 mg/kg/day, while skin rashes and arthritis require 5 to 20 mg of prednisone daily, and/or antimalarials and NSAIDs. With life-threatening lupus manifestations, such as acute pneumonitis or pulmonary hemorrhage, intravenous pulse methylprednisolone at 500 to 1,000 mg per day for 3 to 5 days is justified.

Although Mintz et al. (46) and Wong et al. (86) put their pregnant patients on "prophylactic" steroids, and that may have prevented postpartum flares and maternal deaths, there is no hard evidence to prove that, and there is a tendency away from this practice (96).

Any woman treated with systemic steroids within 2 years of the anticipated delivery should be considered as potentially adrenal-insufficient, and should be given steroid stress coverage (steroid prep) during delivery. The most usual form consists of 100 mg hydrocortisone IV just prior to onset of delivery, and every 8 hours for the first day. During the next day the dose can be reduced to 50 mg every 8 hours and then adjusted to the patient's previous oral dose. If the patient is receiving more than 75 mg of prednisone daily, the appropriate hydrocortisone equivalent should be used in the first 2 days, and then the patient's steroid dose resumed.

Cortisol (206), prednisone (207), prednisolone (207), methylprednisolone (208), betamethasone (209), and dexamethasone (210,211) have all been shown to cross the placenta. With maternal administration of prednisone or prednisolone, fetal blood levels are approximately 10% of the mother's level; with methylprednisolone hemisuccinate, cord levels are 18% to 45% of the mother's, with a large standard deviation; with betamethasone, cord levels are approximately 33% and, with dexamethasone, are similar to the maternal level. Therefore, the use of prednisone or prednisolone to treat the mother is least likely to affect the fetus; conversely, if steroid therapy of the fetus is indicated, dexamethasone is the appropriate choice (212). There is evidence that placental oxidative enzymes (placental 11-hydroxygenase) inactivate *in vitro* cortisol and prednisolone, but not betamethasone or dexamethasone (206, 207,213,214).

Steroids are not teratogenic, despite reports of cleft palate in rabbits and mice (215,216). Such congenital abnormalities are extremely rare in humans. A review of 260 pregnancies with maternal steroid therapy showed spontaneous abortion, stillbirth, and prematurity comparable to the general, non–steroid-treated population (217). There were two infants with cleft palates (0.77%) and one with adrenocortical failure of 3 days' duration, who recovered. The prevalence of cleft lip with or without cleft palate in the United States varies, depending on race—1:300 in the Navajo, 1:400 to 600 in Asians, 1:750 to 800 in whites, and 1:1,500 to 2,000 in blacks (218). In the authors' large experience with lupus pregnancies under substantial steroid therapy, no clefts have been observed. A premature newborn to a mother receiving large doses of prednisone for sarcoidosis 24 days prior to delivery died of adrenal failure (219). The neonate had evidence of degeneration of the adrenal cortex with cystic changes, hemorrhage, and necrosis.

Intrauterine growth restriction (IUGR) and low birth weight have been reported with maternal steroid therapy (220). In the large prospective study by Mintz et al. (46), however, it seemed that IUGR was more a function of active maternal SLE than of steroid dose. Several studies have described prematurity in newborns of steroid-treated women. Hodgman et al. (221) reviewed the growth and development of 23 infants whose 19 mothers received 7.5 to 22.5 mg of prednisone daily during pregnancy because of lupus (n = 16) and rheumatoid arthritis (n = 3). Two of 20 children with first-trimester steroid exposure had major congenital defects without clefts. They were small for gestational age and prematurity was higher than in normal populations; the birth weight was below the 50th percentile in 14 of 19 infants (73.7%) and below the tenth percentile for five of them (26%). Follow-up at 6 months to 8 years showed normal height, weight, and developmental progress for 22 of 23, with the sole exception being one child with a major congenital defect, whose development was below the 3rd percentile.

A study of 55 steroid-treated asthma patients with 70 pregnancies on an average dose of 8.2 mg of prednisone/day found an increase in prematurity, which the authors did not attribute to steroids, but no increase in spontaneous abortion, congenital malformation, stillbirth, neonatal death, toxemia, or bleeding (222). It seems, however, that maternal steroid therapy may be linked to preterm rupture of membranes and preterm delivery (223). Prematurity appears to be multifactorial and related to maternal disease as well.

Induction or aggravation of diabetes mellitus and hypertension are known risks of steroid therapy. Overall, corticosteroid therapy seems innocuous in terms of fetal effects. It is the major factor in improved maternal survival between 1950 and 1980, with maternal mortality decreasing from 24% to 3% (40) and even lower (0.2%) in the 1990s.

Salicylates And Other NSAIDs Category C

COX-2 Inhibitors Category C

Salicylates and the newer NSAIDs have in common the capacity to interfere with prostaglandin formation through variable inhibition of cyclooxygenase. This inhibition includes prostaglandin action anywhere in the body, including uterine, platelet, and renal, and other prostaglandins. Thus, aspirin and NSAIDs inhibit uterine contractility and prolong labor and gestation (224). Aspirin irreversibly inhibits platelet aggregation, and the other NSAIDs have a reversible effect; both can cause bleeding during delivery (225). Given the immaturity of hepatic enzyme systems in the fetus and newborn, transplacentally delivered drugs may persist much longer. No human teratogenicity exists, at least with low-dose aspirin (205). Slone et al. (226) examined data on 50,282 mother-child pairs; 35,418 of the mothers had not taken aspirin during pregnancy. Of 14,864 who had taken aspirin, 9,736 had intermediate exposure and 5,128 were heavily exposed during the first 16 weeks of pregnancy. The observed and expected numbers of malformations were similar in the three groups.

Other NSAIDs have, to varying degrees, similar effects to those of aspirin in pregnancy. They readily cross the placenta, potentiate vasoconstriction under conditions of hypoxia, raise systemic vascular resistance, and have profound effects on fetal and neonatal circulation (227). Aspirin ingestion during pregnancy may cause *in utero* closure of the ductus arteriosus, with severe heart failure, tricuspid insufficiency, and acidosis, all of which disappeared the day after birth (228). Maternal indomethacin therapy was considered the cause of primary pulmonary hypertension in a newborn (229). Transient neonatal renal failure and oligohydramnios have also been described (230).

Other Indications For Salicylates And Other NSAIDs

The pharmacologic actions of prostaglandin inhibitors can be used to therapeutic advantage. For example, indomethacin has been successfully used to inhibit premature labor (231), and for the closure of patent ductus arteriosus (232).

Prevention Of Preeclampsia

The capacity of low aspirin doses (0.45 mg/kg/day) to inhibit thromboxane synthesis by platelets, while prostacyclin production by endothelium is unaffected (233), has promising applications in lupus pregnancy, preeclampsia and recurrent fetal loss. Preeclampsia seems to occur as a consequence of exaggerated placental production of thromboxane A_2, with normal or deficient prostacyclin production (144–147,234–236). In a double-blind, placebo-controlled study of 46 primigravidas at risk for development of preeclampsia, as determined by angiotensin-sensitivity at 28 weeks' gestation, 23 received 60 mg of aspirin daily, a dose that causes 90% inhibition of platelet thromboxane synthesis, and 23 received placebo (48). Only two of 21 patients (9.5%) in the aspirin group developed mild pregnancy-induced hypertension, while 12 of 23 women in the placebo group (52%) developed hypertension (PIH in four, preeclampsia in seven, and eclampsia in one). The necessity for cesarean sections was significantly greater in the placebo group. In a study of mostly multiparous women at high-risk for preeclampsia, 52 were treated with aspirin 150 mg/day and dipyridamole 300 mg/day, and 50 were untreated (237). Uncomplicated hypertension was similar in both groups (40% and 49%, respectively), but preeclampsia, fetal and neonatal loss, and severe IUGR occurred only in the untreated group (13%, 11%, and 9%, respectively).

The Australian Society for the study of hypertension in pregnancy has published a position paper recommending the use of low-dose aspirin in the following situations:

1. In women with prior fetal loss after the first trimester, with placental insufficiency;
2. In women with severe IUGR in a preceding pregnancy, either unexplained or due to preeclampsia;
3. In women with severe early-onset preeclampsia in a previous pregnancy necessitating delivery at or before 32 weeks' gestation (238).

Intrauterine Growth Restriction

There is further evidence supporting the use of low-dose aspirin for prevention of IUGR. A good review on the subject has been published (239). Wallenburg and Rotmans (240) treated 24 women with prior fetal growth restriction with low-dose aspirin and dipyridamole after 16 weeks' gestation, with reduction of fetal IUGR to 13% in treated versus 61% in untreated pregnancies. Two mothers had lupus anticoagulant.

Prevention Of Fetal Loss With Antiphospholipid Antibodies (Table 47.6)

Several reports and a review have addressed the prevention of recurrent fetal loss in patients with antiphospholipid antibodies (200,239–268). A variety of approaches have been used, including low-dose aspirin, 75, 81, or 150 mg/day, combinations of aspirin and 20 to 60 mg/day of prednisone (200,241–246,249,251,252,254–257,261,268), heparin alone (248), heparin and prednisone (247), heparin and aspirin (250,251,262–264), or aspirin, prednisone, and platelet antiaggregants (246,253). An interesting study from Italy used fish oil (eicosapentanoic acid and docosahexanoic acid, 5.1 g per day) in 22 pregnancies with success (258). Intravenous gamma globulin (IVIg) was used with low-dose aspirin, and with heparin (259,260,267). This treatment is discussed later.

These studies have reported an overall increase in live births (Table 47.6). Fetal loss in the over 1,100 untreated pregnancies was 76.2% to 100%, with only 7.9% mean live births (range, 0% to 23.8%). All treatments have resulted in increase of live births, to a mean of 72.3% (range, 28.6% to 100%).

Most of the studies with prednisone in doses of 40 to 60 mg per day were fraught with steroid complications, including cushingoid features, hypertension, and gestational diabetes.

The most effective treatment regimens have been those involving heparin, low-dose aspirin plus heparin, and low molecular weight heparin. The controlled study of aspirin 81 mg per day vs. aspirin plus heparin high dose (up to 30,000 IU per day) showed a definitive advantage of the combination (262,264). Comparison of aspirin plus heparin low dose (up to 12,000 IU/day) vs. aspirin plus heparin high dose (up to 30,000 IU per day) showed no advantage of the latter (76% vs. 80% live births) (263). Low molecular weight heparin is safe in pregnancy, can be given once a day, and showed a decided advantage over historic placebo controls (83.9 vs. 55.9 live births) (266). Several recent studies on APL-related fetal loss have excluded lupus patients. Such a pilot study compared aspirin plus heparin with IVIg vs. aspirin plus heparin plus albumin on 14 patients; there was no difference, with 100% live births with both regimens (267). A study on early fetal loss associated with APL compared aspirin 75 mg per day vs. placebo and found no difference, with 80% and 85% live birth rates, respectively. Heparin and low molecular weight heparin are category B drugs, do not cross the placenta, and are not harmful to the fetus. Both, however, can cause osteoporosis and thrombocytopenia. Concomitant calcium intake of 1.5 g/day and at least monthly CBC with platelet count is advised. Although warfarin has been used after organogenesis in mothers prone to recurrent fetal loss, it may be associated with malformations and fetal warfarin syndrome (205). Warfarin is FDA category D, X_M (Table 47.5).

Our high-risk obstetricians at Los Angeles County–University of Southern California Medical Center prefer the following regimen for anticoagulation during pregnancy:

For women with prior pregnancy complications, but no thrombosis, subcutaneous (SC) enoxaparin 0.5 mg/kg twice daily, calcium supplementation as above, and axial weight-bearing exercise, or unfractionated heparin, 10,000 IU SC twice daily, Ca^{2+}, and exercise.

For women who have clotted previously, enoxaparin SC 1 mg/kg twice daily, or adjusted dose of unfractionated heparin SC to prolong the partial thromboplastin time

TABLE 47.6. OUTCOME OF TREATMENT IN ANTIPHOSPHOLIPID-ASSOCIATED FETAL LOSS

		No. of Pregnancies		Live Births (%)	
First Author	**Therapy Used, mg/d U/d**	**Before Therapy**	**After Therapy**	**Before Therapy**	**After Therapy**
Lubbe (241,242)	Aspirin 75 + Prednisone 40–60	28	6	10.7	85.7
Branch (243)	Aspirin 81 + Prednisone 40–60	31	8	3.2	62.5
Gatenby (244)	Aspirin 75–150 + Prednisone 30–50 or 10–60	145	27	17.2	63
Ordi (245)	Aspirin 50 + Prednisone 20	18	9	0	78
Carp (246)	Aspirin 100–300 + Prednisone 10–40 ± Heparin 10,000 ± Dipyridamole 225	71	27	7	48
Semprini (247)	Heparin + Prednisone	27	14	3.7	64
Rosove (248)	Heparin 24,700	29	15	3.4	93.3
Silveira (249)	Aspirin 81 + Prednisone 40	32	12	15.6	100
Buchanan (250)	Aspirin 75, or ASA + heparin 10,000	101	87	18.7	63.2
Cowchock (251)	ASA 80 + Heparin 20,000	≥2/pt*	12	0	75
	ASA 80 + prednisone 40	≥2 pt*	8	0	75
Out (200)	Prednisone ≥40 ± ASA 40 ± heparin, or ASA or heparin	≥3/pt*	30	NS	73.3
Landy (252)	Prednisone 5–60 + ASA or + heparin, or single drug	126	33	23.8	90.9
Many (253)	ASA ± prednisone 30	102	52	6.8	51.9
	+ dipyridamole		23		43.5
	+ heparin		23		69.1
Stuart (254)	ASA + prednisone 10–30	24	7	4.2	28.6
Caruso (255)	ASA + prednisone 40	63	28	11.1	82.1
Al Momen (256)	ASA 100	33	9	9.1	55.6
	ASA + prednisone 40–60	80	13	13.8	53.8
	ASA + prednisone + IVIg	44	7	4.5	57.1
	(failed ASA + prednisone)	5	0		
Balasch (257)	ASA + prednisone 15–30	49	21	6.1	90.5
Rossi (258)	Fish oil (EPA + DHA 5.1 g)	≥3/pt*	22	NS	95.5
Kaaja (259)	IVIg 1 g/kg + ASA 75	14	4	7.1	100
Spinnato (260)	IVIg 0.4 g/kg ± ASA ± heparin	17	5	0	100
Harger (261)	ASA 81 + prednisone 10–60 Individualized, tapered	69	28	8.7	72.0
Kutteh (262)	ASA 81 vs.	≥3/pt*	25	NS	44.0
	ASA 81 + heparin 10,000–30,000	≥3/pt*	25	NS	80.0
Kutteh (263)	ASA 81 + heparin low dose (12,000)	≥3/pt*	25	NS	76.0
	ASA 81 + heparin high dose	≥3/pt*	25	NS	80.0
Rai (264)	ASA 75 vs.	≥3/pt*	45	NS	42.0
	ASA 75 + heparin 10,000	≥3/pt*	45	NS	71.0
Laskin (266)	Low molecular weight heparin vs historical	NS	46	NS	83.9
	placebo controls	NS	34	NS	55.9
Studies on patients with recurrent fetal loss, without lupus					
Laskin (265)	ASA 100 + prednisone 0.5–0.8/kg vs.	≥2/pt*	101	NS	65.0
(Pts w/autoabs)	Placebo	≥2/pt*	101	NS	56.0
Branch (267)	ASA 81 + heparin 15,000 + IVIg vs. }	31 for all pts	7	25.8	100.0
	ASA 81 + heparin 15,000 + albumin }		9		100.0
Pattison (268)	ASA 75 vs.	≥3/pt*	20	NS	80.0
(early fetal loss)	Placebo	*	20	NS	85.0

*Fetal losses/patient; NS, not specified.

(PTT) to 2, to 6 hours after the morning dose; all regimens are accompanied by daily low-dose aspirin.

It should be noted that not all pregnancies in mothers with antiphospholipid antibodies are doomed; four patients had uncomplicated pregnancies and delivered at term (269).

Summary: Salicylates

Large, antiinflammatory doses of aspirin and NSAIDs are not generally used in lupus patients and should be avoided during the last 2 to 4 weeks of pregnancy for fear of prolonging gestation and labor, increased maternal and fetal bleeding during delivery, and possible premature closure of ductus arteriosus. However, a great number of possibilities are open for low-dose aspirin therapy in susceptible patients, to assist in prevention of recurrent fetal loss, preeclampsia, and perhaps intrauterine growth retardation.

Summary: Prevention Of Fetal Loss Due To Antiphospholipid Antibodies

Women with prior IUFD related to antiphospholipid antibodies should be treated. Low-dose ASA should begin when the urine pregnancy test becomes positive, and heparin should be added when fetal heart beat is detectable, since most miscarriages occur before the 14th week of pregnancy, and should be continued until the 34th week of pregnancy (263,264). With prior late pregnancy complications, heparin could be continued until delivery. Unfractionated heparin, 5,000 to 6,000 IU, can be self-injected every 12 hours. I expect that low molecular weight heparin (enoxaparin, dalteparin) will eventually be used in preference to unfractionated heparin, although the cost of the former is a factor. Corticosteroids should only be given for lupus activity (251,265). Guidelines for the investigation and management of the antiphospholipid syndrome and excellent reviews have been published (270–272).

Antimalarial Drugs: FDA Category C

Antimalarial drugs have been used by pregnant women for years as prophylaxis in large-scale malaria eradication programs in Africa and Asia, mostly without problems (273). These reports have asserted that maternal malaria prophylaxis with chloroquine is safe in pregnancy and does not appear to induce premature labor or abortions. Even if the patient discontinues antimalarials early in the pregnancy, there are deposits in the liver and other organs from which the drug is slowly excreted (274).

One report of retinal degeneration in two infants as a consequence of malaria prophylaxis in the mother has appeared (275). No reports of fetal malformations associated with hydroxychloroquine (Plaquenil) per se have appeared.

Most of the admonitions against the use of antimalarials during pregnancy have cited a report of a woman with discoid lupus who intermittently took 500 mg of chloroquine daily (276). Of her seven pregnancies, three were conceived off the drug, and these children had no congenital defects; of four pregnancies conceived while on chloroquine, one child had hemihypertrophy of the body and a Wilms' tumor; one had neonatal seizures, deafness, ataxia, and vestibular paresis; one had mental retardation, deafness, ataxia, and vestibular paresis; and one pregnancy ended in spontaneous abortion at 3 months.

However, the recent literature points to the fact that several lupus pregnancies have been completed while the mother took antimalarials, without any fetal malformations.

In 36 pregnancies among 33 women with SLE who continued hydroxychloroquine during pregnancy, there were no teratogenic effects (277). Similarly, Levy et al. (278) reported their experience with 24 women who took chloroquine or hydroxychloroquine during the first trimester of 27 pregnancies, and reviewed the literature. Data were given for 18 women (11 women had SLE) who took antimalarials for a mean of 32 months before pregnancy (1 to 172 months), and for 21 pregnancies. No congenital malformations or developmental problems occurred in these children who were followed-up for a mean of 5.3 years (9 months to 19 years). In the authors' literature review, 215 pregnancies were reported under first-trimester antimalarial exposure, with only seven cases of congenital malformations (3.3%), which is no different from the general population.

Twenty pregnant lupus patients were randomized in a double- blind controlled study; ten were on hydroxychloroquine and ten on placebo. The mothers did not flare during pregnancy, and there were no congenital abnormalities in their children (279). Sixteen additional lupus patients received hydroxychloroquine throughout pregnancy without ocular or aural deficits in any of the children (280).

The patient should be informed about the few reports of congenital anomalies and about the antimalarial deposits in the liver, when deciding about the use of antimalarials during pregnancy. In our experience, most patients opt to discontinue medications during gestation.

Immunosuppressive-Cytotoxic Drugs

The most commonly used immunosuppressive drugs in SLE are azathioprine (FDA category D), cyclophosphamide (FDA category D), methotrexate (FDA category D), cyclosporine (FDA category C), and mycophenolate mofetil (FDA category C). Nitrogen mustard (FDA category D) and chlorambucil (FDA category D) are rarely, if ever, used. The first three are known to induce fetal malformations in animals. Cyclophosphamide, azathioprine, methotrexate, and chlorambucil have reportedly shown potential for human teratogenesis (205). Use of these drugs during fetal organogenesis (the first trimester) has the greatest potential for causing fetal demise or malformation. Two textbooks and an excellent review on the subject have been published (205,281,282).

Azathioprine crosses the placenta, but the fetus lacks the enzyme inosinate phosphorylase, which converts azathioprine to active metabolites (mercaptopurine); hence, only traces of mercaptopurine are found in cord blood (283). The drug causes decreases thymic shadow size, lymphocyte count, and IgG and IgM in the neonate (284), and can cause neonatal chromosomal abnormalities that may persist for up to a year. Cyclophosphamide is highly teratogenic in experimental animals, but its effects are species-specific. Methotrexate and nitrogen mustard induce skeletal, limb, palate, and central nervous system abnormalities in animals and occasionally in humans. The experience with cyclosporine in pregnancy is mostly in renal transplant recipients.

In humans the teratogenic effects of cytotoxic drugs do not appear to be as common. Stern and Johnson (281) have culled the experience of several authors with cytotoxic drugs given for neoplasias, transplants, or systemic lupus, alone or in combination. A total of 145 pregnancies occurred in women receiving single cytotoxic drugs, which included azathioprine, cyclophosphamide, 6-mercaptopurine, methotrexate, nitrogen mustard, and chlorambucil. Spontaneous abortions and fetal malformations were far more common when the drugs were taken in the first trimester (23% and 13%, respectively).

Among lupus, vasculitis, and rheumatoid arthritis patients on cytotoxic drugs, there is very little occurrence of fetal malformations. As a rule, patients are counseled to use effective contraception prior to starting immunosuppressive medication.

A review of three reports on the offspring of renal transplant recipients on azathioprine shows that the majority of the infants were normal, although fetal wastage was rather high. Of 36 pregnancies in mothers with renal transplants, 20 infants were normal, five were premature (four died of respiratory distress syndrome), and there were six spontaneous and five elective abortions. Of 57 pregnancies with fathers with renal transplants, 56 infants were normal, with three spontaneous abortions and one infant with a neural tube defect, perhaps attributable to paternal mutagenicity with thalidomide (285). Several additional reports of normal pregnancies and neonates in lupus and renal transplant patients who received azathioprine and prednisone have appeared. (68,69,78,286,287). Azathioprine interacts with warfarin. Either they should not be used concomitantly, or be used together with extreme caution (288).

Ramsey-Goldman et al. (286) reported on 23 lupus pregnancies with azathioprine, cyclophosphamide, or both, or methotrexate (two during and 21 before pregnancy). Ten of 23 had an adverse pregnancy outcome similar to outcomes before SLE diagnosis (286). Adverse outcomes included miscarriage (spontaneous abortion), stillbirth, prematurity, or neonatal complications, including congenital defects. No difference in neonatal complications was observed among 519 pregnancies before SLE, 117 pregnancies after SLE on no immunosuppressives, and 23 pregnancies on immunosuppressive therapy. Azathioprine dose should be reduced to half in the third trimester, otherwise the neonate develops hypogammaglobulinemia.

Daily oral cyclophosphamide causes amenorrhea within a year, usually with permanent ovarian failure (71%), and monthly intravenous "pulse" cyclophosphamide can also cause amenorrhea (45%), depending on the dose (289). The risk of amenorrhea depends on age and total dose: amenorrhea is greatest in women over 31 years of age, 62%, versus 12% when under 25 years of age, and 27% at 26 to 30 years of age (290). Patients receiving seven doses of IV cyclophosphamide had a 12% chance of amenorrhea, versus 39% in patients on long-term therapy (15 or more doses). It has been suggested that the administration of monthly IV cyclophosphamide be timed during menses, when the ovarian follicles are quiescent.

Maternal therapy with cyclophosphamide only in the first trimester was associated in three pregnancies with multiple abnormalities of the toes and extremities, palatine grooves, and hernias in one infant, a small hemangioma in another, and absent digits in one induced abortion. One pregnancy with cyclophosphamide late in the first trimester, and four pregnancies with chemotherapy including cyclophosphamide beyond the first trimester had a normal outcome (281). At the Los Angeles County–University of Southern California Medical Center, two of our lupus patients on monthly IV cyclophosphamide became pregnant; cyclophosphamide was immediately stopped on both. One woman proceeded with a normal pregnancy and had a normal infant at term. The other patient had a first-trimester spontaneous abortion but conceived two more times, after cessation of cyclophosphamide therapy, and, despite a mild exacerbation during both pregnancies, carried to term and had two healthy infants. At this time, 12 and 10 years later, the children have developed normally and are healthy. It is virtually impossible to foretell any risk of oncogenesis among such children. In the event of severe risk to the mother's life, such as in acute oliguric/anuric renal failure, I have used IV pulse cyclophosphamide on two occasions, with improvement in the mother and without ill effects to the fetus so far.

Nitrogen mustard has been used for the treatment of lupus nephritis in the past. In a report of 250 patients with nephritis, 18 of 44 women who had at least one course of nitrogen mustard had 11 successful pregnancies (111). Among the patients reviewed by Stern and Johnson (281), six pregnancies had exposure during the first trimester; there were two normal infants, three spontaneous abortions, and one elective abortion with a normal fetus, while four women treated after the first trimester had normal infants.

Two infants exposed to methotrexate in the first trimester had multiple cranial defects, malformed extremities, IUGR, and poor neonatal growth. Exposure after the first trimester in combination with other drugs resulted in eight normal infants. Methotrexate-induced malformations can reportedly be prevented by simultaneous treatment with citrovorum factor (folinic acid). Kozlowski et al. (291) reported eight women with rheumatoid arthritis who conceived during weekly methotrexate 7.5 mg. All except one stopped methotrexate within the first trimester. Of the ten pregnancies, five resulted in full-term normal infants, with three spontaneous and two elective abortions. Most of the patients received folate supplements.

Cyclosporine has been widely used to prevent rejection in organ transplantation; it can cross the placenta, and is excreted in milk. A total of 51 pregnancies in 48 women treated with cyclosporine during pregnancy have been reported, and 11 pregnancies have been conceived from men receiving the drug (292). Most of the women, 43 of 48, received cyclosporine after transplantation, especially of the kidney (39 of 43). Only one patient had systemic lupus. In these high-risk pregnancies, a number of antenatal maternal complications arose in 20 of 41 mothers (48.8%), including hypertension, pyelonephritis, uterine dystonia, diabetes mellitus, seizures, encephalopathy, and secondary hyperparathyroidism. Also, two spontaneous and six elective abortions occurred, one for fetal anencephaly. Of the 43 deliveries (95.6% live births), 15 were premature (34.9%), and 17 required forceps or cesarean section (39.5%). The mean birth weight for 29 of the babies was low (2,093 g). Of the 43 newborn, 34 were healthy (79%), two had birth defects, including absence of the corpus callosum, with seizures and death in one, and seven had various problems—neonatal jaundice, thrombocytopenia, leukopenia, or hypoglycemia with mild disseminated intravascular coagulation, asphyxia with intracerebral bleeding, oxygen dependence for 2 days, with subsequent cataracts, and mild hypoparathyroidism. On follow-up, one of 20 babies had slight growth retardation. Overall, 38 of the 43 liveborn who were exposed to cyclosporine throughout pregnancy did not have birth defects. Of the 11 pregnancies fathered by nine men on cyclosporine, two resulted in spontaneous abortions, and two pairs of twins were born. The 11 neonates were healthy. The fathers of the twins were being treated with cyclosporine for infertility resulting from an autoimmune disorder, and the remaining seven men were receiving it for renal transplantation. Three lupus patients treated during pregnancy have been reported, without any problems (293,294). In 197 pregnancies in 141 female kidney transplant recipients, there was preeclampsia in 29%, hypertension in 56%, preterm delivery in 54%, IUGR in 50%, and no fetal malformations were noted (295).

Mycophenolate mofetil (FDA category C) is an inosine monophosphate dehydrogenase inhibitor and is recently being used and studied for the treatment of lupus nephritis (296,297). No structural malformations were noted in the-offspring of 34 pregnancies (5 mothers, 29 fathers) (298). A child with first trimester exposure to mycophenolate, mofetil, tacrolimus, and prednisone, had hypoplastic nails and short fifth fingers (298a).

The decision to continue cytotoxic drugs during pregnancy depends on the need for disease control, and should be made jointly with the patient, while weighing the potential risks versus benefits. If continuation of pregnancy under cytotoxic therapy is desired, it is wise to have an amniocentesis done and the karyotype determined.

Miscellaneous Therapeutic Measures

Plasmapheresis

Plasmapheresis can be safely performed during pregnancy and has been used successfully in severe preeclampsia/eclampsia, and with refractory HELLP syndrome that does not improve after delivery in women who have APL syndrome and/or SLE (299–303). Lupus patients with severe disease have also been treated during pregnancy (304–306): in one, plasmapheresis improved vasculitis, and decreased steroid requirement; in a second, an extremely ill woman, striking improvement of myositis and overall disease occurred; in the third patient, plasmapheresis failed to reverse thrombocytopenia, with subsequent fetal demise. Two patients with recurrent fetal loss and anticardiolipin antibody were given plasmapheresis. In one, there was dramatic reduction of antiphospholipid antibody with successful pregnancy outcome (307). In the other, who had a multisystem disease with myositis, plasmapheresis was given because of fetal distress. The authors believed that they gained 2 more weeks of gestation, during which further fetal maturation occurred, which allowed fetal survival after cesarean section at 29 weeks (308). Immunoadsorbent plasmapheresis with dextran sulfate decreased lupus anticoagulant and anticardiolipin antibodies, with successful delivery in eight of nine lupus pregnancies (309,310). An excellent review on plasmapheresis in pregnancy has been published (311).

Intravenous Immunoglobulin (IVIg) Therapy

Ten papers have reported 34 women with four to nine fetal losses each, positive anticardiolipin antibodies, lupus anticoagulant, and preeclampsia in three (256,259,312–319). Treatment with IVIg, at times with the addition of low-dose aspirin, heparin, and steroids, resulted in live births. Immunoglobulin was given at 400 to 1,000 mg/kg/day for 2 to 5 days per month. In addition, a controlled study of IVIg vs. albumin in addition to heparin and aspirin was commented on previously (267). In the controlled study, all patients had 100% live births, which may be interpreted to mean that IVIg does not have much to add to heparin and aspirin therapy, or, that albumin is also effective in reducing repeated fetal loss due to APL antibodies. This expensive treatment seems worth considering in difficult clinical situations, such as prior fetal loss due to APL despite heparin therapy (up to ~30% of heparin treated patients do not respond), severe or early preeclampsia in prior pregnancy, or severe clinical lupus manifestations (severe thrombocytopenia, pulmonary alveolar hemorrhage, transverse myelitis, and perhaps anuric renal failure) (320). IVIg suppressed APL levels after each infusion (318). In an *in vitro* study, IVIg neutralized lupus anticoagulant activity in ten of 11 patient sera (321). The mechanism of IVIg action is probably due to antiidiotypic antibodies against antiphospholipid antibodies (322). A very good review recently was published (323).

Recommendations For Therapy In Lupus Pregnancy

1. The best assurance for a successful pregnancy is control of the mother's lupus. Maternal disease should be

assessed carefully for activity and severity months before, and at the onset of pregnancy, which should ideally be planned after several months of remission. The mother should be watched carefully for flares.

2. Maternal flares should be diagnosed early and treated aggressively with appropriate steroid dose. Unless there is a dire emergency, i.e., acute anuric renal failure, or pulmonary alveolar hemorrhage, cytotoxic drugs such as cyclophosphamide and methotrexate should be avoided during the first trimester. It appears that azathioprine in reduced doses, cyclosporine, can be use during pregnancy. More data are needed for mycophenolate mofetil in pregnancy. Mothers with nephritis at risk for hypertension and preeclampsia should be treated with low-dose aspirin (60 to 81 mg/day) until the 36th week of gestation.
3. The mother's status in terms of antiphospholipid antibody and anti-Ro/SSA, anti-La/SSB positivity should be known: the former, because of predisposition to fetal loss and IUGR, and the latter two because of the small risk for congenital heart block in the child (see also Chaps. 48 and 49).
4. Joint follow-up by the rheumatologist and high-risk obstetrician should be done every month for the first half of pregnancy, and more frequently thereafter (every 1 to 3 weeks), with blood pressure check, careful exam, repeat of CBC, urine, chemistry, quantitation of proteinuria in patients with nephritis, complement C3 and C4 levels, anti-dsDNA, and a measure of circulating immune complexes on a monthly basis. Patients with known prior problem pregnancies should be followed more often.
5. In the event of high-positive antiphospholipid antibody, especially of the IgG class, with a history of intravascular thrombosis or prior fetal loss, the patient should be enrolled in an effective antithrombotic protocol (heparin alone with or without low-dose aspirin, or low molecular weight heparin). Unless there is concomitant lupus activity, high-dose prednisone for APL alone should be avoided.

Breast-Feeding (Table 47.5)

All drugs are excreted in human milk, usually in trace but variable amounts (273,324–327). Factors influencing drug concentrations derived from milk in the infant have been delineated by Brooks and Needs (324). Maternal factors include fat and protein concentrations in milk, milk pH, mammary blood flow, and maternal drug metabolism (e.g., absorption, protein binding, and plasma clearance). Drug-related factors include molecular weight, lipid solubility, pK_a, elimination half-life, pharmacokinetics, dose amount, and interval. Infant factors include volume of milk consumed, feeding intervals relative to maternal drug intake, absorptive capability, and metabolic and deconjugating ability of the infant.

An index has been proposed to calculate infant exposure to drugs in breast milk, which takes into account milk to maternal plasma drug concentration and drug clearance in the infant (328).

After a single dose of 5 mg of prednisolone, 0.07% to 0.23% of the dose was found in maternal milk (325). Katz and Duncan (326) calculated that a child drinking 1 L of milk daily would receive 0.028 mg of prednisolone with a maternal dose of 7.5 mg (0.33%). Long-term treatment of the mother with 10 to 80 mg/day of prednisolone produces milk concentrations 5% to 25% of those in serum (327, 329). The milk/plasma ratio increases with increasing serum concentrations and it has been calculated that, at a maternal dose of 80 mg/day, the infant would be exposed to less than 0.1% of the maternal dose (327,330). The peak plasma level after oral intake is attained at 1.1 ± 0.7 hours; therefore, the exposure of the infant can be minimized by appropriate timing of nursing. No untoward effects in nursing infants have been reported (327,331), and maternal doses of up to 30 mg/day are probably safe.

Cyclophosphamide is found in substantial concentrations in human breast milk (332); thus, nursing is contraindicated in a mother who requires this drug. The milk level of methotrexate in a woman with choriocarcinoma of the uterus was 8% of the plasma level (333). With small weekly doses, such as those used in rheumatic diseases, there may be a greater measure of safety, but data are lacking. Only small amounts of azathioprine have been detected in breast milk (334). Overall, a great deal of good judgment and caution should be exercised. Until data such as those on cyclosporine are available, the need for maternal cytotoxic drug therapy would preclude breast-feeding.

Encouraging data are available for cyclosporine: in seven lactating transplanted mothers on cyclosporine, drug concentration in breast milk was similar to maternal trough level, but was below the detection limit in the infants, and their creatinine levels were normal (335).

Antimalarials are also found in small amounts in human milk (336,337). Nation et al. (337) have calculated that the infant would be exposed to about 2% of the maternal daily dose of hydroxychloroquine. Although there are very few problems with malaria prophylaxis in nursing mothers, doses used in lupus could expose the child to the risk of retinopathy.

In general, NSAIDs are weak acids and achieve low concentrations in the acidic pH of milk. After a single aspirin dose of 450 to 650 mg, 0.1% to 21% reaches the infant over a 24-hour period (338). Peak salicylate concentrations in milk occur about 2 hours after peak serum levels (339). However, if the mother takes antiinflammatory doses, in view of the immature neonatal metabolic processes, the infant may develop acidosis and bleeding diathesis. Furthermore, the infant can absorb free salicylic acid from the cleavage of salicylphenolic glucuronide in the milk (340). Trace amounts of naproxen, piroxicam, ibuprofen, and diclofenac have been reported in milk. Some of the NSAIDs have enterohepatic circulation (e.g., indomethacin, sulindac), and are not recommended during lactation. The position of the American Academy of Pediatrics on drugs in milk is stated in ref. 341.

Contraception

Uncontrolled and anecdotal reports have suggested that the older oral contraceptives containing larger doses of estrogens cause SLE flares (342,343). In a study by Jungers et al. (344) of 20 women with SLE nephritis, the use of preparations containing 30 to 50 μg of ethinyl estradiol was associated with exacerbation of disease in 43% within 3 months of beginning oral contraceptives. Nevertheless, many patients are reported to tolerate small-dose estrogen contraceptives ("mini-pills") without adverse effects (345). In retrospective studies by Julkunen et al. (346,347) and Buyon (348), substantial numbers of lupus patients are able to tolerate modern-day oral contraceptives without SLE flares or thromboembolism; flares were noted in 8% to 13% of patients receiving oral contraceptives or hormone replacement, respectively. Newer oral contraceptives contain <35 μg of ethinyl estradiol, and are preferable to 50 μg in the older preparations. Potential exceptions are women with antiphospholipid syndrome and history of thromboembolic episodes, or history of severe migraines, because thromboembolic phenomena have been associated with estrogen and anticardiolipin antibodies (349).

In contrast to estrogen-containing oral contraceptives, lupus flares did not occur in 11 patients receiving pure progestogens during a 30-month period. In a controlled study with progestogens (122) using either oral levonorgestrel 0.03 mg daily or norethisterone enanthate 200 mg IM every 3 months, the authors found no increase in flare rate when compared to a control group (6/122 patient/months and 4/48 patient/months respectively, same as the controls). Menstrual irregularity and spotting were common complaints among the patients. Commercially available progestational agents include oral norethindrone (norethisterone), norgestrel, levonorgestrel, ethynodiol diacetate, and lynestrenol (350). If long-term contraception (up to 5 years) is desired, a subdermal progestin implant (levonorgestrel) may be considered (351). In a lupus patient, the site of implantation should be carefully watched for any infection. Menstrual irregularity for 6 to 12 months from onset of use is common, and bleeding, amenorrhea, and, rarely, ectopic pregnancy may occur.

Mechanical barrier methods, such as the diaphragm or condom with spermicide cream or jelly, although considered cumbersome by some, are safe and effective. Intrauterine devices are associated with more frequent local infections (62), risk of endometritis, perforation, and menorrhagia, and are not recommended. At this time the results of a multicenter, double-blind, placebo-controlled study on the safety of oral contraceptives and of hormone replacement during menopause (SELENA study), are eagerly awaited. (See also Chapter 39.)

Lupus And Ovulation Induction

Ovulation induction (OI) is the first phase in assisted reproductive therapy (ART), followed by *in vitro* fertilization (IVF) and implantation of fertilized ova in the woman or a surrogate. Stimulation of ovulation is done with a variety of hormonal or nonhormonal manipulations and results in tremendously high plasma estradiol levels. Two types of problems related to OI have been described: development of flares in patients with known lupus, and *de novo* development of lupus. In addition, patients with APL syndrome have been reported to participate in OI. To further complicate matters, ovarian hyperstimulation syndrome (OHSS), which may occur in 0.2% to 23% of women undergoing ART, can mimic a lupus flare. OHSS appears to be mediated by a variety of cytokines and it consists of ovarian enlargement to 5 cm (grade 1); ovarian size of 5 to 12 cm, nausea, vomiting, diarrhea, and abdominal distention (grade 2); or massive ovarian size (>12 cm), ascites, pleural effusions, edema, hypotension, electrolyte imbalance, and hypercoagulability with phlebothrombosis (grade 3) (352). A total of four patients without prior SLE (one with Raynaud phenomenon) developed lupus, one with SLE and APL and other autoimmune syndromes, after OI (353,354). The development of SLE occurred after 6, 10, 8, and 27 cycles of OI. One of the patients developed rapidly progressive glomerulonephritis (353).

In eight of 12 patients, 11 with known SLE and one with discoid LE, flares developed, ranging from arthritis, malar rash, alopecia, and myalgia, to myositis, pericarditis, vasculitis, seizures, and transverse myelitis (355–357). The last patient died after a second attempt at conception with OI (357). One of the patients with SLE developed superior vena cava and left renal vein thrombosis (355). Of seven SLE patients reported from New York, three had flares and two OHSS (356). The same paper reported ten patients with APL syndrome and two with APL positivity undergoing OI while on antithrombotic therapy: one patient developed osteopenia secondary to heparin. Wechsler et al. (358) presented a review of the subject and proposed the following guidelines for SLE patients desirous of ART:

1. SLE remission without need for aggressive therapy for at least 12 months.
2. Absence of systemic hypertension, significant renal failure, pulmonary hypertension, frank heart valve disease, or major vascular past history.
3. Antiestrogens should be used (clomiphene and tamoxifen), followed by pulsatile GnRH, if the above fails. Gonadotropins have the greatest risk for OHSS.

Family Planning And Counseling

The patient with SLE and her partner must understand that she is just as fertile as any other woman in the general population, and that she is capable of having children; however, she has an increased likelihood of a high-risk pregnancy.

The woman with lupus should ideally plan her pregnancy during a sustained remission for several months. She, her partner, and the physician should assess her functional limitations and explore her emotional motivation prior to undertaking pregnancy and the responsibilities of raising a child. Her socioeconomic setting and spouse (mate) relationship are no less important. The rheumatologist and obstetrician should counsel the patient and family about chances of flare, fetal loss, prematurity, and intrauterine growth restriction (IUGR), and prepare her to cooperate with the rigorous follow-up necessary. Only in the event of severe renal, myocardial, or pulmonary compromise should elective abortion be considered. The patient and husband should be cautioned, however, about the possibility of exacerbation after elective abortion.

Couples should be made aware of the following points:

1. The normal fertility of women with lupus, and therefore the need for family planning, just as in individuals without lupus.
2. The best time to plan a pregnancy—during a 6 to 12 month inactive period of SLE, even though there is no guarantee that the disease will remain inactive. It should be emphasized that the chance of a flare with conception after remission is 10% or less.
3. The probability of a flare varies among series and depends on the severity of disease. The milder the disease, the lesser the chance of a flare.
4. The probability of hypertension or preeclampsia, especially in SLE nephritis patients, patients with antiphospholipid antibodies, and particularly in patients conceiving with active disease.
5. Increased abortion rates—double or triple that of the general population. In women with two or more fetal losses and the presence of antiphospholipid antibodies, the use of heparin and low-dose aspirin improves remarkably the possibilities of a successful pregnancy.
6. The risk of a stillbirth should be explained. The methods for monitoring fetal growth need to be clearly understood (see Chapters 48 and 49).
7. The potential necessity of and indications for cesarean section should be outlined (maternal aseptic necrosis of the hips with inadequate hip abduction, preeclampsia, fetal distress, abnormal nonstress test, and usual obstetric indications, including cephalopelvic disproportion, transverse presentation, and others).
8. The risk of prematurity may be as high as 60% in those with active disease, and the risk of intrauterine growth restriction may reach 30% of premature deliveries. The need for proper care of the newborn in adequate intensive care units should be stressed.
9. Women positive for anti-Ro/SSA and/or anti-La/SSB should be aware of the small risk of congenital heart block in the child. The general lupus population seems to have a 1% probability of congenital heart block in live births.
10. No risk of congenital malformations caused by prednisone has been noted, but cytotoxic drugs taken during the first trimester carry such a risk.
11. With close monitoring and aggressive treatment during pregnancy and the postpartum period, no long-term worsening of SLE should occur.

In the poststeroid era, the early diagnosis and appropriate therapy of lupus have led to tremendously increased survival rates of SLE patients—up to 97% for 5 years, 93% for 10 years, and 83% for 15 years (92). Similarly, with increased awareness of the potential problems for the mother and fetus, meticulous multidisciplinary follow-up, and effective disease control, most women with lupus can and do achieve motherhood.

ACKNOWLEDGMENTS

The author expresses gratitude to Dr. J. Lee Nelson for invaluable advice and to Lucy Stevenson, RN, for volunteering her help.

REFERENCES

1. Mellor AL, Munn DH. Immunology at the maternal-fetal interface: lessons for T cell tolerance and suppression. *Annu Rev Immunol* 2000;18:367–391.
2. Tremellen KP, Seamark RF, Robertson SA. Seminal transforming growth factor beta-1 stimulates granulocyte macrophage colony-stimulating factor production and inflammatory cell recruitment in the murine uterus. *Biol Reprod* 1998;58:1217–1225.
3. King A, Hiby SE, Gardner L, et al. Recognition of trophoblast HLA class I molecules by decidual NK cell receptors—a review. *Placenta* 2000;21(suppl A):S81–85.
4. Vince GS, Johnson PM. Leucocyte populations and cytokine regulation in human uteroplacental tissues. *Biochem Soc Trans* 2000;28:191–195.
5. Rouas-Freiss N, Paul P, Dausset J, et al. HLA-G promotes immune tolerance. *J Biol Regul Homeost Agents* 2000;14:93–98.
6. Rajagopalan S, Long EO. A human leukocyte antigen (HLA)-G-specific receptor expressed on all natural killer cells. *J Exp Med* 1999;189:1093–1100. Erratum in *J Exp Med* 2000;191: following 2027.
7. King A, Allan DS, Bowen M, et al. HLA-E is expressed in trophoblast and interacts with CD94/NKG2 receptors on decidual NK cells. *Eur J Immunol* 2000;30:1623–1631.
8. Moreau P, Adrian-Cabestre F, Menier C, et al. IL-10 selectively induces HLA-G expression in human trophoblasts and monocytes. *Int Immunol* 1999;11:803–811.
9. Wegmann TG, Lin H, Guilbert L, et al. Bidirectional cytokine interactions in the maternal-fetal relationship: is successful pregnancy a TH-2 phenomenon? *Immunol Today* 1993;14: 353–356.
10. Hill JA, Polgar K, Anderson DJ. T-helper 1 type immunity to troploblast in women with recurrent spontaneous abortion. *JAMA* 1995;273:1958–1959.

11. Lim KJH, Odukoya OA, Ajjan RA, et al. The role of T-helper cytokines in human reproduction. *Fertil Steril* 2000;73:136–142.
12. Bennett WA, Lagoo-Deenadayalan, Whitworth NS, et al. First trimester human chorionic villi express both immunoregulatory and inflammatory cytokines: a role for interleukin-10 in regulating the cytokine network of pregnancy. *Am J Reprod Immunol* 1999;41:70–78.
13. Marzi M, Vigano A, Trabattoni D, et al. Characterization of type 1 and type 2 cytokine production profile in physiologic and pathologic human pregnancy. *Clin Exp Immunol* 1996;106: 127–133.
14. Choi BC, Polgar K, Xiao L, et al. Progesterone inhibits in-vitro embryotoxic Th1 cytokine production to troploblast with recurrent pregnancy loss. *Hum Reprod* 2000;15:46–59.
15. Szereday L, Varga P, Szekeres-Bartho J. Cytokine production by lymphocytes in pregnancy. *Am J Reprod Immunol* 1997;38: 418–422.
16. Szekeres-Bartho J, Faust Z, Varga P, et al. The immunological pregnancy protective effect is manifested via controlling cytokine production. *Am J Reprod Immunol* 1996;35:348–351.
17. Szekeres-Bartho J, Par G, Szereday L, Smart CY, et al. Progesterone and non-specific immunologic mechanisms in pregnancy. *Am J Reprod Immunol* 1997;38:176–182.
18. Faust Z, Laskarin G, Rukavina D, et al. Progesterone-induced blocking factor inhibits degranulation of natural killer cells. *Am J Reprod Immunol*1999;42:71–75.
19. Laskarin G, Strbo N, Sotosek V, et al. Progesterone directly and indirectly affects perforin expression in cytolytic cells. *Am J Reprod Immunol* 1999;42:312–320.
20. Par G, Bartok B, Szekeres-Bartho J. Cyclooxygenase is involved in effects of progesterone-induced blocking factor on the production of interleukin 12. *Am J Obstet Gynecol* 2000;183: 126–130.
21. Kamimura, Eguchi K, Yonezawa M, et al. Localization and developmental change of indoleamine 2,3-dioxygenase activity in the human placenta. *Acta Med* 1991;45:135–139.
22. Munn DH, Zhou M, Attwood JT, et al. Prevention of allogeneic fetal rejection by tryptophan catabolism. *Science* 1998; 281:1191–1193.
23. Hammer A, Blaschitz A, Daxbock C, et al. Fas and Fas-ligand are expressed in the uteroplacental unit of first trimester pregnancy. *Am J Reprod Immunol* 1999;41:41–51.
24. Guller S, La Chapelle L. The role of placental Fas ligand in maintaining immune privilege at maternal-fetal interfaces. *Semin Reprod Endocrinol* 1999;17:39–44.
25. Holmes CH, Simpson KL, Okada H, et al. Complement regulatory proteins at the feto-maternal interface during human placental development: distribution of CD59 by comparison with membrane cofactor protein (CD46) and decay accelerating factor (CD55). *Eur J Immunol* 1992;22:1579–1585.
26. Persellin RH. The effect of pregnancy on rheumatoid arthritis. *Bull Rheum Dis* 1977;27:922–927.
27. Ito I, Hayashi T, Yamada K, et al. Physiological concentration of estradiol inhibits polymorphonuclear leukocyte chemotaxis via a receptor mediated system. *Life Sci* 1995;56:2247–2253.
28. Nilsson N. Carlsten H. Estrogen induces suppression of natural killer cell cytotoxicity and augmentation of polyclonal B cell activation. *Cell Immunol* 1994;158:131–139.
29. Athreya BH, Pletcher J, Zulian F, et al. Subset-specific effects of sex hormones and pituitary gonadotropins on human lymphocyte proliferation in vitro. *Clin Immunol Immunopathol* 1993; 66:201–211.(Erratum appears in *Clin Immunol Immunopathol* 1993;68:93.)
30. Lin J, Lojun S, Lei ZM, et al. Lymphocytes from pregnant women express human chorionic gonadotropin/luteinizing hormone receptor gene. *Mol Cell Endocrinol*1995;111:R13–17.
31. Goldsteyn EJ, Fritzler MJ. The role of the thymus-hypothalamus-pituitary-gonadal axis in normal immune processes and autoimmunity. *J Rheumatol* 1987;14:982–990.
32. Lahita RC, Bradlow HL, Fishman J, et al. Estrogen metabolism in systemic lupus erythematosus: patients and family members. *Arthritis Rheum* 1982;25:843–846.
33. Lahita RC, Bradlow HL, Fishman J, et al. Abnormal estrogen and androgen metabolism in the human with systemic lupus erythematosus. *Am J Kidney Dis* 1983;2(suppl 1):206–211.
34. Lahita RG, Bradlow L, Ginzler E, et al. Low androgen levels in females with active systemic lupus erythematosus. *Arthritis Rheum* 1984;30:241–248.
35. Jara LJ, Gomez-Sanchez C, Silveira LH, et al. Hyperprolactinemia in systemic lupus erythematosus (SLE). Association with immunological and clinical activity. *Am J Med Sci* 1992;303: 222–226.
36. Jara-Quesada L, Graef A, Lavalle C. Prolactin and gonadal hormones during pregnancy in systemic lupus erythematosus. *J Rheumatol* 1991;18:349–353.
37. Chang DM, Chang CC, Kuo SY, et al. Hormonal profiles and immunological studies of male lupus in Taiwan. *Clin Rheumatol* 1999;18:158–162.
38. Alvarez-Nemegyei J, Covarrubias-Cobos A, Escalante-Triay F, et al. Bromocriptine in systemic lupus erythematosus: a double-blind, randomized, placebo-controlled study. *Lupus* 1998;7:414–419.
39. Buskila D, Berezin M, Gur H, et al. Autoantibody profile in the sera of women with hyperprolactinemia. *J Autoimmun* 1995;8: 415–424.
40. Cecere FA, Persellin RH. The interaction of pregnancy and the rheumatic diseases. *Clin Rheum Dis* 1981;7:747–768.
41. Kaufman RL, Kitridou RC. Pregnancy in mixed connective tissue disease: comparison with systemic lupus erythematosus. *J Rheumatol* 1982;9:549–555.
42. Kitridou RC. Pregnancy in mixed connective tissue disease, poly/dermatomyositis and scleroderma. *Clin Exp Rheumatol* 1988;6:173–178.
43. Mintz G, Rodriquez-Alvarez E. Systemic lupus erythematosus. *Rheum Dis Clin North Am* 1989;15:255–278.
44. Bear R. Pregnancy and lupus nephropathy. *Obstet Gynecol* 1976; 47:715–718.
45. Creagh MD, Malia RG, Cooper SM, et al. Screening for lupus anticoagulant and anticardiolipin antibodies in women with fetal loss. *J Clin Pathol* 1991;44:45–47.
46. Mintz G, Niz J, Gutierrez G, et al. Prospective study of pregnancy in systemic lupus erythematosus. Results of a multidisciplinary approach. *J Rheumatol* 1986;13:732–739.
47. Love PE, Santoro SA. Antiphospholipid antibodies: anticardiolipin and the lupus anticoagulant in systemic lupus erythematosus (SLE) and in non-SLE disorders. Prevalence and clinical significance. *Ann Intern Med* 1990;112:682–698.
48. Wallenburg HCS, Makovitz JW, Dekker GA, et al. Low-dose aspirin prevents pregnancy-induced hypertension and preeclampsia in angiotensin-sensitive primigravidae. *Lancet* 1986;1:13.

48a. Schiff E, Peleg E, Goldenberg M, et al. The use of aspirin to prevent pregnancy-induced hypertension and lower the ratio of thromboxane A2 to prostacyclin in relatively high risk pregnancies. *N Engl J Med* 1989;321:351–356.

49. Brown MA, de Swiet M. Classification of hypertension in pregnancy. *Best Pract Res Clin Obstet Gynecol* 1999;13:27–39.
50. Broughton Pipkin F, Roberts JM. Hypertension in pregnancy. *J Hum Hypertens* 2000;14:705–724.
51. Weinstein L. Syndrome of hemolysis, elevated liver enzymes, and low platelet count: a severe consequence of hypertension in pregnancy. *Am J Obstet Gynecol* 1982;142:159–167.
52. Ellis FA, Bereston ES. Lupus erythematosus associated with pregnancy and menopause. *Arch Dermatol Syph* 1952;65:170–176.

53. Turner SJ, Levine L, Redman A. Lupus erythematosus and pregnancy. *Obstet Gynecol* 1956;8:601–609.
54. Murray FA. Lupus erythematosus in pregnancy. *J Obstet Gynecol Pr Emp* 1956;65:401–409.
55. Friedman EA, Rutherford JW. Pregnancy and lupus erythematosus. *Obstet Gynecol* 1956;8:601–610.
56. Madsen JR, Anderson BV. Lupus erythematosus and pregnancy. *Obstet Gynecol* 1961;8:492–494.
57. Donaldson LB, de Alvarez RR. Further observations on lupus erythematosus associated with pregnancy. *Am J Obstet Gynecol* 1962;83:1461–1473.
58. Dziubinski EH, Winkelmann RK, Wilson RB. Systemic lupus erythematosus and pregnancy. *Am J Obstet Gynecol* 1962;84: 1873–1877.
59. Mund A, Simson J, Rothfield NF. Effect of pregnancy on course of systemic lupus erythematosus. *JAMA* 1963;183:917–922.
60. Estes D, Larson DL. Systemic lupus erythematosus and pregnancy. *Clin Obstet Gynecol* 1965;8:307–321.
61. McGee CD, Makowski EL. Systemic lupus erythematosus in pregnancy. *Am J Obstet Gynecol* 1970;107:1008–1012.
62. Dubois EL, ed. *Lupus erythematosus. A review of the current status of discoid and systemic lupus erythematosus and their variants*, 2nd ed rev. Los Angeles: USC Press, 1976.
63. Thomas MM, Tischer CC, Robinson RR. Influence of pregnancy on lupus nephritis. *Kidney Int* 1978;14:665–669.
64. Zurier RB, Argyros TG, Urman JD, et al. Systemic lupus erythematosus. Management during pregnancy. *Obstet Gynecol* 1978;51:178–180.
65. Devoe LD, Taylor RL. Systemic lupus erythematosus in pregnancy. *Am J Obstet Gynecol* 1979;135:473–479.
66. Tozman ECS, Urowitz MB, Gladman DD. Systemic lupus erythematosus and pregnancy. *J Rheumatol* 1980;7:624–632.
67. Houser MT, Fish AJ, Tagatz GE, et al. Pregnancy and systemic lupus erythematosus. *Am J Obstet Gynecol* 1980;138:409–413.
68. Hayslett JP, Lynn RI. Effect of pregnancy in patients with lupus nephropathy. *Kidney Int* 1980;18:207–220.
69. Fine LG, Barnett EV, Danovitch GM, et al. Systemic lupus erythematosus in pregnancy. *Ann Intern Med* 1981;94:667–677.
70. Jungers P, Dougados M, Pelissier C, et al. Lupus nephropathy and pregnancy. *Arch Intern Med* 1982;142:771–776.
71. Varner MW, Meehan RT, Syrop CH, et al. Pregnancy in patients with systemic lupus erythematosus. *Am J Obstet Gynecol* 1983;145:1025–1040.
72. Hatakeyama M, Sumiya M, Gonda N, et al. Clinical study of systemic lupus erythematosus and pregnancy. *Ryumachi* 1983; 23:93–99.
73. Gimovsky ML, Montoro M, Paul RH. Pregnancy outcome in women with systemic lupus erythematosus. *Obstet Gynecol* 1984;63:686–692.
74. Imbasciati E, Surian M, Bottino S, et al. Lupus nephropathy and pregnancy. *Nephron* 1984;36:46–51.
75. Burkett G. Lupus nephropathy and pregnancy. *Clin Obstet Gynecol* 1985;28:310–323.
76. Stein H, Walters K, Dillon A, et al. Systemic lupus erythematosus: a medical and social profile. *J Rheumatol* 1986;13:570–576.
77. Bobrie G, Liote F, Houllier P, et al. Pregnancy in lupus nephritis and related disorders. *Am J Kidney Dis* 1987;9:339–343.
78. Meehan RT, Dorsey JK. Pregnancy among patients with systemic lupus erythematosus receiving immunosuppressive therapy. *J Rheumatol* 1987;14:252–258.
79. Gatenby PA. Systemic lupus erythematosus and pregnancy. *Aust NZ J Med* 1989;19:261–278.
80. Out HJ, Derksen RHWM, Christiaens GCML. Systemic lupus erythematosus and pregnancy. *Obstet Gynecol Surv* 1989;44: 585–591.
81. Garsenstein M, Pollack VE, Kark RM. Systemic lupus erythematosus and pregnancy. *N Engl J Med* 1962;267:165–169.
82. Fraga A, Mintz G, Orozco J, et al. Sterility and fertility rates, fetal wastage and maternal morbidity in systemic lupus erythematosus. *J Rheumatol* 1974;1:293–298.
83. Zulman JI, Talal N, Hoffman GS, et al. Problems associated with the management of pregnancies in patients with systemic lupus erythematosus. *J Rheumatol* 1980;7:37–49.
84. Lockshin MD, Reinitz E, Druzin ML, et al. Lupus pregnancy. Case-control prospective study demonstrating absence of lupus exacerbation during or after pregnancy. *Am J Med* 1984;77: 893–898.
85. Lockshin MD. Pregnancy does not cause systemic lupus erythematosus to worsen. *Arthritis Rheum* 1989;32:665–670.
86. Wong KL, Chan FY, Lee CHP. Outcome of pregnancy in patients with systemic lupus erythematosus. *Arch Intern Med* 1991;151:269–273.
87. Petri M, Howard D, Repke J, et al. The Hopkins Lupus Pregnancy Center: 1987–1991 update. *Am J Reprod Immunol* 1992; 28:188–191.
87a. Buyon JP, Kalunian KC, Ramsey-Goldman R, et al. Assessing disease activity in SLE patients during pregnancy. *Lupus* 1999; 8:677–684.
88. Tincani A, Faden D, Tarantini M, et al. Systemic lupus erythematosus and pregnancy: a prospective study. *Clin Exp Rheumatol* 1992;10:439–446.
89. Derksen RH, Bruinse HW, de Groot PG, et al. Pregnancy in systemic lupus erythematosus: a prospective study. *Lupus* 1994; 3:149–155.
90. Le-Thi-Huong D, Wechsler B, Piette JC, et al. Pregnancy and its outcome in systemic lupus erythematosus. *Q J Med* 1994; 87:721–729.
91. Lima F, Buchanan NMM, Khamashta MA, et al. Obstetric outcome in systemic lupus erythematosus. *Semin Arthritis Rheum* 1995;25:184–192.
92. Ruiz-Irastorza G, Lima F, Alves J, et al. Increased rate of lupus flare during pregnancy and the puerperium: a prospective study of 78 pregnancies. *Br J Rheumatol* 1996;35:133–138.
93. Tomer Y, Viegas OA, Swissa M, et al. Levels of lupus autoantibodies in pregnant SLE patients: correlations with disease activity and pregnancy outcome. *Clin Exp Rheumatol* 1996;14: 275–280.
94. Le Huong D, Wechsler B, Vauthier-Brouzes D, et al. Outcome of planned pregnancies in systemic lupus erythematosus: a prospective study on 62 pregnancies. *Br J Rheumatol* 1997;36: 772–777.
95. Rahman P, Gladman DD, Urowitz MB. Clinical predictors of fetal outcome in systemic lupus erythematosus. *J Rheumatol* 1998;25:1526–1530.
96. Carmona F, Font J, Cervera R, et al. Obstetrical outcome of pregnancy in patients with systemic lupus erythematosus. *Eur J Obstet Gynecol* 1999;83:137–142.
97. Nossent HC, Swaak TJG. Systemic lupus erythematosus. VI. Analysis of the interrelationship with pregnancy. *J Rheumatol* 1990;17:771–776.
98. Oviasu E, Hicks J, Cameron JS. The outcome of pregnancy in women with lupus nephritis. *Lupus* 1991;1:19–25.
99. Packham DK, Lam SS, Nicholls K, et al. Lupus nephritis and pregnancy. *Q J Med* 1992;83:315–324.
100. Rubbert A, Pirner K, Wildt L, et al. Pregnancy course and complications in patients with systemic lupus erythematosus. *Am J Reprod Immunol* 1992;28:205–207.
101. Johns KR, Morand EF, Littlejohn GO. Pregnancy outcome in systemic lupus erythematosus (SLE): a review of 54 cases. *Aust NZ J Med* 1998;28:18–22.
102. Sittiwangkul S, Louthrenoo W, Vithayassai P, et al. Pregnancy

outcome in Thai patients with systemic lupus erythematosus. *Asian Pac J Allergy Immunol* 1999;17:77–83.
103. Julkunen H, Jouhikainen T, Kaaja R, et al. Fetal outcome in lupus pregnancy: a retrospective case-control study of 242 pregnancies in 112 patients. *Lupus* 1993;2:125–131.
104. Kobayashi N, Yamada H, Kishida T, et al. Hypocomplementemia correlates with intrauterine growth retardation in systemic lupus erythematosus. *Am J Reprod Immunol* 1999;42: 153–159.
105. Georgiou PE, Politi EN, Katsimbri P, et al. Outcome of lupus pregnancy: a controlled study. *Rheumatology* 2000;39:1014–1019.
106. De Bandt M, Palazzo E, Belmatoug N, et al. Outcome of pregnancies in lupus: experience at one center. *Ann Med Interne* 2000;151:87–92.
107. Austin HA, Boumpas DT, Vaughan EM, et al. High-risk features of lupus nephritis: Importance of race and clinical and histologic factors in 166 patients. *Nephrol Dial Transplant* 1995; 10:16–20.
108. Dooley MA, Hogan S. Jennette C, et al. Cyclophosphamide therapy for lupus nephritis: Poor survival in black Americans. *Kidney Int* 1997;51:11–88.
109. Liang MH, Socher SA, Larson MG, et al. Reliability and validity of six systems for the clinical assessment of disease activity in systemic lupus erythematosus. *Arthritis Rheum* 1989;32: 1107–1118.
110. Petri M, Hellmann D, Hochberg M. Validity and reliability of lupus activity measures in the routine clinic setting. *J Rheumatol* 1992;19:53–59.
111. Wallace DJ, Podell T, Weiner J, et al. Systemic lupus erythematosus survival patterns. Experience with 609 patients. *JAMA* 1981;245:934–938.
112. Cohen AS, Reynolds WE, Franklin EC, et al. Preliminary criteria for the classification of systemic lupus erythematosus. *Bull Rheum Dis* 1971;21:643–648.
113. Tan EM, Cohen AS, Fries JF, et al. Special article: the 1982 revised criteria for the classification of systemic lupus erythematosus. *Arthritis Rheum* 1982;25:1271–1277.
114. Pistiner M, Wallace DJ, Nessim S, et al. Lupus erythematosus in the 1980s: a survey of 570 patients. *Semin Arthritis Rheum* 1991;21:55–64.
115. Reveille JD, Bartolucci A, Alarcon GS. Prognosis in systemic lupus erythematosus. Negative impact of increasing age at onset, black race, and thrombocytopenia, as well as causes of death. *Arthritis Rheum* 1990;33:37–48.
116. Studenski S, Allen NB, Caldwell DS, et al. Survival in systemic lupus erythematosus. A multivariate analysis of demographic factors. *Arthritis Rheum* 1987;30:1326–1332.
117. Rothfield N. Clinical features of systemic lupus erythematosus. In: Kelly WN, Harris ED, Ruddy S, et al., eds. *Textbook of rheumatology*. Philadelphia: WB Saunders, 1981:1106–1132.
118. Pasoto SG, Viana VS, Mendonca BB, et al. Anti-corpus luteum antibody: a novel serological marker for ovarian dysfunction in systemic lupus erythematosus? *J Rheumatol* 1999;26:1087–1093.
119. Grigor RR, Shervington PC, Hughes GRV, et al. Outcome of pregnancy in systemic lupus erythematosus. *Proc R Soc Med* 1977;70:99–100.
120. Petri M, Howard D, Repke J. Frequency of lupus flare in pregnancy. The Johns Hopkins Lupus Pregnancy Center experience. *Arthritis Rheum* 1991;34:1538–1545.
121. Urowitz MB, Gladman DD, Farewell VT, et al. Lupus and pregnancy studies. *Arthritis Rheum* 1993;36:1392–1397.
122. Mintz G, Gutierrez G, Deleze M, et al. Contraception with progestagens in systemic lupus erythematosus. *Contraception* 1984;30:29–38.
123. Petri M, Albritton J. Fetal outcome of lupus pregnancy: a retrospective case-control study of the Hopkins lupus cohort. *J Rheumatol* 1993;20:650–656.
124. Tamby Raja RL. Fetal salvage in maternal systemic lupus erythematosus. *Ann Acad Med Singapore* 1993;22:634–637.
125. Julkunen H, Kaaja R, Palosuo T, et al. Pregnancy in lupus nephropathy. *Acta Obstet Gynecol Scand* 1993;72:258–263.
126. Font J, Carmona F, Cervera R, et al. Influence of nephropathy in the outcome of lupus pregnancy: a comparative study. *Arthritis Rheum* 1998;41:S281.
127. Huong Du LT, Wechsler B, Vauthier-Brouzes D, et al. Pregnancy in women with past or current history of lupus nephritis. *Arthritis Rheum* 1998;41:S66.
128. Ramos A, Veloz G, Medina F, et al. The outcome of lupus nephritis and pregnancy. *Arthritis Rheum* 1999;42:S214.
129. Estes D, Christian CL. The natural history of systemic lupus erythematosus by prospective analysis. *Medicine* 1971;50: 85–95.
130. Krane NK, Thakur V, Wood H, et al. Evaluation of lupus nephritis during pregnancy by renal biopsy. *Am J Nephrol* 1995;15:186–191.
131. Devoe LD, Loy GL, Spargo BH. Renal histology and pregnancy performance in systemic lupus erythematosus. *Clin Exp Hypertens* 1983;B2:325–340.
132. Zhou Y, Damsky CH, Fisher SJ. Preeclampsia is associated with failure of human cytotrophoblast to mimic a vascular adhesion phenotype. *J Clin Invest* 1997;99:2152–2164.
133. Henriksen T. Complications of high risk pregnancies and their treatment. *Scand J Rheumatol* 1998;27(suppl 107):86–91.
134. Hou S. Pregnancy in women with chronic renal disease. *N Engl J Med* 1985;312:836–839.
135. Hou SH, Grossman SD, Madias NE. Pregnancy in women with renal disease and moderate renal insufficiency. *Am J Med* 1985; 78:185–194.
136. Fisher KA, Luger A, Spargo BH, et al. Hypertension in pregnancy: clinical-pathological correlations and remote prognosis. *Medicine* 1981;60:267–276.
137. Alsulyman OM, Castro MA, Zuckerman E, et al. Preeclampsia and liver infarction in early pregnancy associated with the antiphospholipid syndrome. *Obstet Gynecol* 1996;88:644–646.
138. Buyon JP, Cronstein BN, Morris M, et al. Serum complement values (C3 and C4) do differentiate between systemic lupus activity and preeclampsia. *Am J Med* 1986;81:194–200.
139. Garcia-de la Torre I, Hernandez-Vazquez L, Angulo-Vazquez J, et al. Prevalence of antinuclear antibodies in patients with habitual abortion and in normal and toxemic pregnancies. *Rheumatol Int* 1984;4:87–89.
140. Sibai BM, Gordon T, Thom E, et al. Risk factors for preeclampsia in healthy nulliparous women: a prospective multicenter study. The National Institute of Child Health and Human Development Network of Maternal-Fetal Medicine Units. *Am J Obstet Gynecol* 1995;172:642–648.
141. Branch DW, Andres R, Digre KB, et al. The association of antiphospholipid antibodies with severe preeclampsia. *Obstet Gynecol* 1989;73:541–545.
142. Dekker GA, de Vries JI, Doelitzsch PM, et al. Underlying disorders associated with severe early-onset preeclampsia. *Am J Obstet Gynecol* 1995;173:1042–1048.
143. Rafla N, Farquharson R. Lupus anticoagulant in preeclampsia and intra-uterine growth retardation. *Eur J Obstet Gynecol Reprod Biol* 1991;42:167–170.
144. Kaaja R, Julkunen H, Viinikka L, et al. Production of prostacyclin and thromboxane in lupus pregnancies: effect of small dose of aspirin. *Obstet Gynecol* 1993;81:327–331.
145. Peaceman AM, Rehnberg KA. The effect of immunoglobulin G fractions from patients with lupus anticoagulant on placental

prostacyclin and thromboxane production. *Am J Obstet Gynecol* 1993;169:1403–1406.
146. Peaceman AM, Rehnberg KA. The effect of aspirin and indomethacin on prostacyclin and thromboxane production by placental tissue incubated with immunoglobulin G fractions from patients with lupus anticoagulant. *Am J Obstet Gynecol* 1995;173:1391–1396.
147. Hawkins T, Jones MP, Gallery ED. Secretion of prostanoids by platelets and monocytes in normal and hypertensive pregnancies. *Am J Obstet Gynecol* 1993;168:661–667.
148. Tsukimori K, Maeda H, Ishida K, et al. The superoxide generation of neutrophils in normal and preeclamptic pregnancies. *Obstet Gynecol* 1993;81:536–540.
149. Morris JM, Fay RA, Ellwood DA, et al. A randomized controlled trial of aspirin in patients with abnormal uterine artery blood flow. *Obstet Gynecol* 1996;87:74–78.
150. Mills JL, DerSimonian R, Raymond E, et al. Prostacyclin and thromboxane changes predating clinical onset of preeclampsia. *JAMA* 1999;282:356.
151. Paller MS. Hypertension in pregnancy. *J Am Soc Nephrol* 1998; 9:314.
152. Steyn DW, Odendall HJ. Randomised controlled trial of ketanserin and aspirin in prevention of preeclampsia. *Lancet* 1997;30:12–67.
153. Regeste RT, Painter P. False-positive radioimmunoassay pregnancy test in nephrotic syndrome. *JAMA* 1981;246:1237–1238.
154. Wei N, Wu T, Klippel JH. False positive pregnancy tests in systemic lupus erythematosus. *J Rheumatol* 1982;9:303–304.
155. Zurier RB, Argyros TG, Urman JD, et al. Systemic lupus erythematosus. Management during pregnancy. *Obstet Gynecol* 1978;51:178–180.
156. Ailus KT. A follow-up study of immunoglobulin levels and autoantibodies in an unselected pregnant population. *Am J Reprod Immunol* 1994;31:189–196.
157. Chetlin SM, Medsger TA, Caritas SN, et al. Serum complement values during pregnancy in systemic lupus erythematosus. *Arthritis Rheum* 1977;20:111(abst).
158. Ziegler G, Medsger TA. Serial complement levels in SLE pregnancies. *Arthritis Rheum* 1984;27(suppl):S130(abst).
159. Devoe LD, Loy GL. Serum complement levels and perinatal outcome in pregnancies complicated by systemic lupus erythematosus. *Obstet Gynecol* 1984;63:796–800.
160. Buyon JP, Tamerius J, Ordorica S, et al. Activation of the alternative complement pathway accompanies disease flares in systemic lupus erythematosus during pregnancy. *Arthritis Rheum* 1992;35:55–61.
161. Hopkinson ND, Powell RJ. Classical complement activation induced by pregnancy: implications for management of connective tissue diseases. *J Clin Pathol* 1992;45:66–67.
162. Lockshin MD, Harpel PC, Druzin ML, et al. Lupus pregnancy. II. Unusual pattern of hypocomplementemia and thrombocytopenia in the pregnant patient. *Arthritis Rheum* 1985;28: 58–66.
163. Hess EV, Baum J. Antinuclear factor and LE cells in pregnant women. *Lancet* 1971;2:877–878.
164. Hinkle SC, Merkatz IR, Gyves MT, et al. Antinuclear factor and anti-DNA in sera of pregnant women. *Arthritis Rheum* 1979;22:201–202.
165. Reyes-Lopez PA, Santos G, Forsbach GB. Absence of ANA in pregnancy (letter). *Arthritis Rheum* 1980;23:378.
166. Polishuck WZ, Beyth Y, Izak G. Antinuclear factor and LE cells in pregnant women. *Lancet* 1971;2:270–271.
167. Farnam J, Lavastida MT, Grant JA, et al. Antinuclear antibodies in the serum of normal pregnant women: a prospective study. *J Allergy Clin Immunol* 1984;73:596–599.
168. Beaulieu A, Quismorio FP Jr, Kitridou RC, et al. Complement fixing antibodies to ds-DNA in SLE: a study using the immunofluorescent *Crithidia luciliae* method. *J Rheumatol* 1979;6:389–396.
169. Rothfield NF, Stollar BD. The relation of immunoglobulin class, pattern of anti-nuclear antibody, and complement-fixing antibodies to DNA in sera from patients with systemic lupus erythematosus. *J Clin Invest* 1967;46:1785–1794.
170. Tan EM, Schur PH, Carr RI, et al. Deoxyribonucleic acid (DNA) and antibodies to DNA in the serum of patients with systemic lupus erythematosus. *J Clin Invest* 1966;45:1732–1740.
171. ter Borg EJ, Horst G, Hummee EJ, et al. Measurement of increases in anti-double stranded DNA antibody levels as a predictor of disease exacerbation in systemic lupus erythematosus. *Arthritis Rheum* 1990;33:634–643.
172. Grennan DM, McCormick JN, Wojtacha D, et al. Immunological studies of the placenta in systemic lupus erythematosus. *Ann Rheum Dis* 1978;37:129–134.
173. Franco HL, Weston WL, Peebles C, et al. Autoantibodies directed against sicca syndromes antigens in neonatal lupus syndrome. *J Am Acad Dermatol* 1981;4:67–72.
174. Maddison PJ. Anti-Ro antibodies and neonatal lupus. *Clin Rheumatol* 1990;9:116–122.
175. Provost TT, Watson R, Gammon WR, et al. The neonatal lupus syndrome associated with U1RNP (nRNP) antibodies. *N Engl J Med* 1987;315:1135–1139.
176. Stastny P, Ziff M. Cold-insoluble complexes and complement levels in SLE. *N Engl J Med* 1969;280:1376–1381.
177. Harris EN, Chan JK, Asherson RA, et al. Thrombosis, recurrent fetal loss, and thrombocytopenia. Predictive value of the anticardiolipin antibody test. *Arch Intern Med* 1986;146:2153–2156.
178. Pierangeli SS, Gharavi AE, Harris EN. Testing for anti phospholipid antibodies: problems and solutions. *Clin Obstet Gynecol* 2001;44:48–57.
179. Exner T, Rickard KA, Kronenberg BH. A sensitive test demonstrating lupus anticoagulant and its behavioral patterns. *Br J Haematol* 1978;40:143–151.
180. Shapiro SS, Thiagarajan P. Lupus anticoagulants. *Prog Hemostat Thromb* 1982;6:263–269.
181. Lee RM, Emlen W, Scott JR, et al. Anti-beta (2)-glycoprotein I antibodies in women with recurrent spontaneous abortions, unexplained fetal death, and antiphospholipid syndrome. *Am J Obstet Gynecol* 1999;181:642–648.
182. Ruiz-Arguelles GJ, Ruiz-Arguelles A, Alarcon-Segovia D, et al. Natural anticoagulants in systemic lupus erythematosus. Deficiency of protein S bound to C4bp associates with recent history of venous thromboses, antiphospholipid antibodies, and the antiphospholipid syndrome. *J Rheumatol* 1991;18:552–558.
183. Boey ML, Colaco CB, Gharavi AE, et al. Thrombosis in systemic lupus erythematosus: striking association with the presence of circulating lupus anticoagulant. *Br Med J (Clin Res)* 1983;287:1021–1023.
184. Elias M, Eldor A. Thromboembolism in patients with the lupus-type circulating anticoagulant. *Arch Intern Med* 1984; 144:510–515.
185. Colaco CB, Elkon KB. The lupus anticoagulant. A disease marker in antinuclear antibody negative lupus that is cross-reactive with autoantibodies to double-stranded DNA. *Arthritis Rheum* 1985;28:67–74.
186. Petri M, Rheinschmidt M, Whiting-O'Keefe Q, et al. The frequency of lupus anticoagulant in systemic lupus erythematosus. A study of sixty consecutive patients by activated partial thromboplastin time, Russel viper venom time, and anticardiolipin antibody level. *Ann Intern Med* 1987;106:524–531.
187. Fort JG, Cowchock FS, Abruzzo JL, et al. Anticardiolipin anti-

bodies in patients with rheumatic diseases. *Arthritis Rheum* 1987;30:752–760.

188. Kalunian KC, Peter JB, Middlekauff HR, et al. Clinical significance of a simple test for anti-cardiolipin antibodies in patients with systemic lupus erythematosus. *Am J Med* 1988;85: 602–608.
189. Gharavi AE, Harris EN, Lockshin MD, et al. IgG subclass and light chain distribution of anticardiolipin and anti-DNA antibodies in systemic lupus erythematosus. *Ann Rheum Dis* 1988;47:286–290.
190. Deleze M, Alarcon-Segovia D, Valdes-Macho E, et al. Relationship between antiphospholipid antibodies and recurrent fetal loss in patients with systemic lupus erythematosus and apparently healthy women. *J Rheumatol* 1989;16:768–772.
191. Ishii Y, Nagasawa K, Mayumi T, et al. Clinical importance of persistence of anticardiolipin antibodies in systemic lupus erythematosus. *Ann Rheum Dis* 1990;49:387–390.
192. Vianna JL, Haga HJ, Pripathi P, et al. Reassessing the status of antiphospholipid syndrome in systemic lupus erythematosus. *Ann Rheum Dis* 1991;51:160–161.
193. Ramsey-Goldman R, Kutzer JE, Kuller LH, et al. Pregnancy outcome and anti-cardiolipin antibody in women with systemic lupus erythematosus. *Am J Epidemiol* 1993;138:1057–1066.
194. Kutteh WH, Lyda EC, Abraham SM, et al. Association of anticardiolipin antibodies and pregnancy loss in women with systemic lupus erythematosus. *Fertil Steril* 1993;60:449–455.
195. Lockshin MD, Druzin ML, Goei S, et al. Antibody to cardiolipin as a predictor of fetal distress or death in pregnant patients with systemic lupus erythematosus. *N Engl J Med* 1985;313:152–156.
196. Lockshin MD, Qamar T, Druzin ML, et al. Antibody to cardiolipin, lupus anticoagulant, and fetal death. *J Rheumatol* 1987; 14:259–262.
197. Hanly JG, Gladman DD, Rose TH, et al. Lupus pregnancy: a prospective study of placental changes. *Arthritis Rheum* 1988; 31:358–366.
198. Englert JH, Derue GM, Loizou S, et al. Pregnancy and lupus: prognostic indicators and response to treatment. *Q J Med* 1988; 66:125–136.
199. Koskela P, Vaarala O, Makitalo R, et al. Significance of false positive syphilis reactions and anticardiolipin antibodies in a nationwide series of pregnant women. *J Rheumatol* 1988;15: 70–73.
200. Out HJ, Bruinse HW, Christiaens Godelieve CML, et al. A prospective, controlled multicenter study on the obstetric risks of pregnant women with antiphospholipid antibodies. *Am J Obstet Gynecol* 1992;167:26–32.
201. Abu-Shakra M, Gladman DD, Urowitz MB, et al. Anticardiolipin antibodies in systemic lupus erythematosus: clinical and laboratory correlations. *Am J Med* 1995;99:624–628.
202. Qamar T, Levy RA, Sammaritano L, et al. Characteristics of high-titer IgG antiphospholipid antibody in systemic lupus erythematosus patients with and without fetal death. *Arthritis Rheum* 1990;33:501–504.
203. Druzin ML, Lockshin M, Edersheim TG, et al. Second trimester fetal monitoring and preterm delivery in pregnancies with systemic lupus erythematosus and/or circulating anticoagulant. *Am J Obstet Gynecol* 1987;157:1503–1510.
204. Evertson LR, Gauthier RJ, Shrifin BS. Antepartum fetal heart rate testing: I. Evolution of the non-stress test. *Am J Obstet Gynecol* 1979;133:29–33.
205. Briggs GG, Freeman RK, Yaffe SJ, eds. *Drugs in pregnancy and lactation: a reference guide to fetal and neonatal risk*, 5th ed. Baltimore: Williams & Wilkins, 1998.
206. Beitings IZ, Bayard F, Ances IG, et al. The metabolic clearance rate, blood production, interconversion and transplacental passage of cortisol and cortisone in pregnancy near term. *Pediatr Res* 1973;7:509–519.
207. Beitings IZ, Bayard F, Ances IG, et al. The transplacental passage of prednisone and prednisolone in pregnancy near term. *J Pediatr* 1972;81:936–945.
208. Anderson GG, Rotchell Y, Kaiser DG. Placental transfer of methylprednisolone following maternal intravenous administration. *Am J Obstet Gynecol* 1981;140:699–701.
209. Ballard PL, Grandberg P, Ballard RA. Glucocorticoid levels in maternal and cord serum after prenatal betamethasone therapy to prevent respiratory distress syndrome. *J Clin Invest* 1975;56: 1548–1554.
210. Funkhouser JD, Peevy KJ, Mockridge PB, et al. Distribution of dexamethasone between mother and fetus after maternal administration. *Pediatr Res* 1978;12:1053–1058.
211. Osathanondh A, Tulchinsky D, Kamali H, et al. Dexamethasone levels in treated pregnant women and newborn infants. *J Pediatr* 1977;90:617–620.
212. Buyon JP, Swersky SH, Fox HE, et al. Intrauterine therapy for presumptive fetal myocarditis with acquired heart block due to systemic lupus erythematosus. *Arthritis Rheum* 1987;30:44–49.
213. Bernal AL, Craft IL. Corticosteroid metabolism in vitro by human placenta, fetal membranes and decidua in early and late gestation. *Placenta* 1981;2:279–286.
214. Blanford AT, Murphy BEP. In vitro metabolism of prednisolone, dexamethasone, betamethasone and cortisol by the human placenta. *Am J Obstet Gynecol* 1977;127:264–267.
215. Fraser FC, Fainstat TD. Production of congenital defects in the offspring of pregnant mice treated with cortisone. *Pediatrics* 1951;8:527–530.
216. Kalter H, Warkany J. Experimental production of congenital abnormalities in mammals by metabolic procedure. *Physiol Rev* 1959;39:69–75.
217. Bongiovanni AM, McPadden AJ. Steroids during pregnancy and possible fetal consequences. *Fertil Steril*, 1960;11:181–186.
218. Chung CS, Marianthopoulos NC. Racial and prenatal factors in major congenital malformations. *Am J Hum Genet* 1968;20: 44–60.
219. Oppenheimer EH. Lesions of the adrenals of an infant following maternal corticosteroid therapy. *Bull Johns Hopkins Hosp* 1964;114:146–151.
220. Reinisch JM, Simon NG, Karow WG, et al. Prenatal exposure to prednisone in humans and animals retards intrauterine growth. *Science* 1978;202:436–438.
221. Hodgman JE, Elhassani S, Dubois EL. Growth and development of children born to steroid treated mothers. Presented to Western Society for Pediatric Research, Los Angeles, 1967.
222. Schatz M, Patterson R, Zeitz S, et al. Corticosteroid therapy for the pregnant asthmatic patient. *JAMA* 1975;223:804–807.
223. Johnson MJ, Petri M, Witter FR, et al. Evaluation of preterm delivery in a systemic lupus erythematosus pregnancy clinic. *Obstet Gynecol* 1995;86:396–399.
224. Lewis RB, Schulman JD. Influence of acetylsalicylic acid, an inhibitor of prostaglandin synthesis on the duration of human gestation and labor. *Lancet* 1973;2:1159–1161.
225. Stuart MJ, Gross SJ, Elrad H, et al. Effects of acetylsalicylic acid ingestion on maternal and neonatal hemostasis. *N Engl J Med* 1982;307:909–913.
226. Slone D, Heinonen OP, Kaufman D, et al. Aspirin and congenital malformations. *Lancet* 1976;1:1373–1375.
227. Levin DL, Fixler DE, Moriss FC, et al. Morphologic analysis of the pulmonary vascular bed in infants exposed in utero to prostaglandin synthetase inhibitors. *J Pediatr* 1978;92:478–484.
228. Areilla RA, Thilenius OG, Ranniger K. Congestive heart failure from suspected ductal closure in utero. *J Pediatr* 1969;75:74–78.
229. Manchester D, Margolis HS, Sheldon RE. Possible association

between maternal indomethacin therapy and primary pulmonary hypertension of the newborn. *Am J Obstet Gynecol* 1976;126:467–469.
230. Cantor B, Tyler T, Nelson RM. Oligohydramnios and transient neonatal anuria. A possible association with the maternal use of prostaglandin synthetase inhibitors. *J Reprod Med* 1980;24: 220–223.
231. Niebyl JR, Blake DA, White RD, et al. The inhibition of premature labor with indomethacin. *Am J Obstet Gynecol* 1980; 136:1014–1019.
232. Friedman WF, Hirschklau MJ, Printz MP, et al. Pharmacologic closure of the patent ductus arteriosus in the premature infant. *N Engl J Med* 1976;295:526–529.
233. Patrignani P, Filabozzi P, Patrono C. Selective cumulative inhibition of platelet thromboxane production by low-dose aspirin in healthy subjects. *J Clin Invest* 1982;69:1366–1372.
234. Hauth JC, Goldenberg RL, Parker CR Jr, et al. Maternal serum thromboxane B2 reduction versus pregnancy outcome in a low-dose aspirin trial. *Am J Obstet Gynecol* 1995;173:578–584.
235. Makila U-M, Viinikka L, Ylikorkala O. Increased thromboxane A2 production but normal prostacyclin by the placenta in hypertensive pregnancies. *Prostaglandins* 1984;27:87–95.
236. Walsh SW. Preeclampsia: an imbalance in placental prostacyclin and thromboxane production. *Am J Obstet Gynecol* 1985;152: 335–340.
237. Beaufils M, Donsimoni R, Uzan S, et al. Prevention of preeclampsia by early antiplatelet therapy. *Lancet* 1985;1:840–842.
238. Brennecke SP, Brown MA, Crowther CA, et al. Aspirin and prevention of preeclampsia. Position statement of the use of low-dose aspirin in pregnancy by the Australasian Society for the Study of hypertension in Pregnancy. *Aust NZ J Obstet Gynaecol* 1995;35:38–41.
239. Lubbe WF. Low-dose aspirin in prevention of toxemia of pregnancy. Does it have a place? *Drugs* 1987;34:515–518.
240. Wallenburg HCS, Rotmans P. Prevention of recurrent idiopathic fetal growth retardation by low-dose aspirin and dipyridamole. *Am J Obstet Gynecol* 1987;157:1230–1235.
241. Lubbe WF, Butler WS, Palmer SJ, et al. Fetal survival after prednisone suppression of maternal lupus anticoagulant. *Lancet* 1983;1:1361–1366.
242. Lubbe WF, Butler WS, Palmer SJ, et al. Lupus anticoagulant in pregnancy. *Br J Obstet Gynaecol* 1984;91:357–363.
243. Branch DW, Scott J, Kochenour N, et al. Obstetric complications associated with the lupus anticoagulant. *N Engl J Med* 1985;313:1322–1326.
244. Gatenby PA, Cameron K, Shearman RP. Pregnancy loss with antiphospholipid antibodies: improved outcome with aspirin containing treatment. *Aust NZ J Obstet Gynaecol* 1989;29: 294–298.
245. Ordi J, Barquinero J, Vilardell M, et al. Fetal loss treatment in patients with antiphospholipid antibodies. *Ann Rheum Dis* 1989; 48:798–802.
246. Carp HJ, Menashe Y, Frenkel Y, et al. Lupus anticoagulant. Significance in habitual first-trimester abortion. *J Reprod Med* 1993;38:549–552.
247. Semprini AE, Vucetich A, Garbo S, et al. Effect of prednisone and heparin treatment in 14 patients with poor reproductive efficiency related to lupus anticoagulant. *Fetal Ther* 1989;4: 73–76.
248. Rosove MH, Tabsh K, Wasserstrum N, et al. Heparin therapy and prevention of pregnancy loss in women with lupus anticoagulant or anticardiolipin antibodies. *Obstet Gynecol* 1990;75: 630–634.
249. Silveira LH, Hubble CL, Jara JL, et al. Prevention of anticardiolipin antibody-related pregnancy losses with prednisone and aspirin. *Am J Med* 1992;93:403–411.
250. Buchanan NMM, Khamashta MA, Morton KE, et al. A study of 100 high risk lupus pregnancies. *Am J Reprod Immunol* 1992;28:192–194.
251. Cowchock SF, Reece EA, Balaban D, et al. Repeated fetal losses associated with antiphospholipid antibodies: a collaborative randomized trial comparing prednisone with low dose heparin treatment. *Am J Obstet Gynecol* 1992;166:1318–1323.
252. Landy HJ, Kessler C, Kelly WK, et al. Obstetric performance in patients with the lupus anticoagulant and/or anticardiolipin antibodies. *Am J Perinatol* 1992;9:146–151.
253. Many A, Pauzner R, Carp H, et al. Treatment of patients with antiphospholipid antibodies during pregnancy. *Am J Reprod Immunol* 1992;28:216–218.
254. Stuart RA, Quinn MJ, McHugh NJ. Combined corticosteroid and aspirin treatment for the high risk lupus pregnancy. *Br J Obstet Gynaecol* 1993;100:601–602.
255. Caruso A, de Carolis S, Ferrazzani S, et al. Pregnancy outcome in relation to uterine artery flow velocity waveforms and clinical characteristics in women with antiphospholid syndrome. *Obstet Gynecol* 1993;82:970–977.
256. Al Momen AKM, Moghraby SA, El-Rab MOG, et al. Pregnancy outcome in women with antiphospholipid antibodies. *Clin Rheumatol* 1993;12:381–386.
257. Balasch J, Carmona F, Lopez-Soto A, et al. Low-dose aspirin for prevention of pregnancy losses in women with primary antiphospholipid syndrome. *Hum Reprod* 1993;8:2234–2239.
258. Rossi E, Costa M. Fish oil derivatives as a prophylaxis of recurrent miscarriage associated with antiphospholipid antibodies (APL): a pilot study. *Lupus* 1993;2:319–323.
259. Kaaja R, Julkunen H, Ammalea P, et al. Intravenous immunoglobulin treatment of pregnant patients with recurrent pregnancy losses associated with antiphospholipid antibodies. *Acta Obstet Gynecol Scand* 1993;72:63–66.
260. Spinnato JA, Clark AL, Pierangeli SS, et al. Intravenous immunoglobulin therapy for the antiphospholipid syndrome in pregnancy. *Am J Obstet Gynecol* 1995;172:690–694.
261. Harger JH, Laifer SA, Bontempo FA, et al. Low-Dose aspirin and prednisone treatment of pregnancy loss caused by lupus anticoagulants. *J Perinatol* 1995;15:463–469.
262. Kutteh WH. Antiphospholipid antibodies-associated recurrent pregnancy loss; treatment with heparin and low dose aspirin is superior to low-dose aspirin alone. *Am J Obstet Gynecol* 1996; 174:1584–1589.
263. Kutteh WH, Ermel LD. A clinical trial for the treatment of antiphospholipid antibody associated recurrent pregnancy loss with lower dose heparin and aspirin. *Am J Reprod Immunol* 1996;35:402–407.
264. Rai R, Cohen H, Dave M, et al. Randomized controlled trial of aspirin and aspirin plus heparin in pregnant women with recurrent miscarriage associated with phospholipid antibodies (or antiphospholipids). *BMJ* 1997;314:253–257.
265. Laskin, CA, Bombardier C, Hannah ME, et al. Prednisone and aspirin in women with autoantibodies and unexplained recurrent fetal loss. *N Engl J Med* 1997;337:148–153.
266. Laskin CA, Clark-Soloninka CA, Spitzer KA, et al. Pregnancy outcome following low molecular weight heparin therapy in women with the presence of prenatal lupus anticoagulant. *Arthritis Rheum* 1999;42:S368.
267. Branch DW, Peaceman AM, Druzin M, et al. A multicenter, placebo-controlled pilot study of intravenous immune globulin treatment of antiphospholipid syndrome during pregnancy. *Am J Obstet Gynecol* 2000;182:122–127.
268. Pattison NS, Chamley LW, Birdsall M, et al. Does aspirin have a role in improving pregnancy outcome for women with the antiphospholipid syndrome? A randomized controlled trial. *Am J Obstet Gynecol* 200;183:1008–1012.

269. Stafford-Brady FJ, Gladman DD, Urowitz MB. Successful pregnancy in systemic lupus erythematosus with an untreated lupus anticoagulant. *Arch Intern Med* 1988;148:1647–1648.
270. Greaves M, Cohen H, Machin SJ, et al. Guidelines on the investigation and management of the antiphospholipid syndrome. *Br J Haematol* 2000;109:704–715.
271. Kutteh WH. Antiphospholipid antibodies and reproduction. *J Reprod Immunol* 1997;35:151–171.
272. Welch S, Branch DW. Antiphospholipid syndrome in pregnancy. Obstetric concerns and treatment. *Rheum Dis Clin North Am* 1997;23:71–84.
273. Bruce-Chawat LJ. Malaria and pregnancy. *Br Med J* 1983;286: 1457–1458.
274. Mackenzie AH. Pharmacologic actions of 4-aminoquinoline compounds. *Am J Med* 1983;75(suppl 1A):510.
275. Panfique L, Magnard P. Degenerescence retinienne chez deux enfants consecutive a un traitement preventif antipalud; án chez la mère pendant la grossesse. *Bull Soc Ophthal Fr* 1969;69: 466–467.
276. Hart CW, Naunton RF. The ototoxicity of chloroquine phosphate. *Arch Otolaryngol* 1964;80:407–412.
277. Buchanan, NM, Toubi E, Khamashta MA, et al. Hydroxychloroquine and lupus pregnancy review of a series of 36 cases. *Ann Rheum Dis* 1996;55:486–488.
278. Levy M, Buskila D, Gladman DD, et al. Pregnancy outcome following first trimester exposure to chloroquine. *Am J Perinatol* 1991;8:174–178.
279. Levy RA, Jesus NR, Vilela V, et al. Hydroxychloroquine in lupus pregnancy double blind placebo controlled study. *Arthritis Rheum* 1998;41:S241.
280. Parke A. West B. Hydroxychloroquine in pregnant patients with systemic lupus erythematosus. *J Rheumatol* 1996;23:1715–1718.
281. Stern JL, Johnson TRB. Antineoplastic drugs and pregnancy. In: Niebyl JR, ed. *Drug use in pregnancy*. Philadelphia: Lea & Febiger, 1982:67–90.
282. Bermas BL, Hill JA. Effects of immunosuppressive drugs during pregnancy. *Arthritis Rheum* 1995;38:1722–1732.
283. Saarikoski S, Seppala M. Immunosuppression during pregnancy. Transmission of azathioprine and its metabolites from the mother to the fetus. *Am J Obstet Gynecol* 1973;115:1100–1106.
284. Cote CJ, Meuwissen HJ, Pickering RJ. Effects on the neonate of prednisone and azathioprine administered to the mother during pregnancy. *J Pediatr* 1974;85:324–328.
285. Davison JM, Lindheimer MD. Pregnancy in renal transplant recipients. *J Reprod Med* 1982;27:613–621.
286. Ramsey-Goldman R, Mientus JM, Kutzer JE, et al. Pregnancy outcome in women with systemic lupus erythematosus treated with immunosuppressive drugs. *J Rheumatol* 1993;20: 1152–1157.
287. Sharon E, Jones J, Diamond H, et al. Pregnancy and azathioprine in systemic lupus erythematosus. *Am J Obstet Gynecol* 1974;118:25–28.
288. Rivier G, Khamashta MA, Hughes GRV. Warfarin and azathioprine: a drug interaction does exist (letter). *Am J Med* 1993; 95:342.
289. Klippel JH. Morbidity and mortality, pp. 89–92, In: Balow JE, moderator, Austin HA 3rd, Tsokos GC, Antonovych TT, et al. Lupus nephritis. *Ann Intern Med* 1987;106:79–94.
290. Boumpas DT, Austin HA III, Vaughan E, et al. Risk for sustained amenorrhea in patients with systemic lupus erythematosus receiving intermittent pulse cyclophosphamide therapy. *Ann Intern Med* 1993;119:366–369.
291. Kozlowski RD, Steinbrunner JV, MacKenzie AH, et al. Outcome of first-trimester exposure to low-dose methotrexate in eight patients with rheumatic disease. *Am J Med* 1990;88: 589–592.
292. Grebenau MD. Personal communication.
293. Doria A, Di Lenardo L, Vario S, et al. Cyclosporin A in a pregnant patient affected with systemic lupus erythematosus. *Rheumatol Int* 1992;12:77–78.
294. Hussein MM, Mooij JM, Roujouleh H. Cyclosporine in the treatment of lupus nephritis including two patients treated during pregnancy. *Clin Nephrol* 1993;40(3):160–163.
295. Armenti VT, Ahlswede KM, Ahlswede DA, et al. Variables affecting birthweight and graft survival in 197 pregnancies in cyclosporine-treated female kidney transplant recipients. *Transplantation* 1995;59:476–479.
296. Dooley MA, Cosio FG, Nachman PH, et al. Mycophenolate mofetil therapy in lupus nephritis: Clinical observations. *J Am Soc Nephrol* 1999;10:833.
297. Chan TM, Li FK, Tang CS, et al. Efficacy of mycophenolate mofetil in patients with diffuse proliferative lupus nephritis. *N Engl J Med* 2000;343:1156.
298. Armenti VT, Wilson GA, Radomski JS, et al. Report from the National Transplantation Pregnancy Registry (NTPR): outcomes of pregnancy after transplanttaion. *Clinical Transplants* 1999:111–119.
298a. Pergola PE, Kancharla A, Riley DJ. Kidney transplantation during the first trimester pregnancy: immunosuppression with mycophenolate mofetil, tacrolimus, and prednisone. *Transplantation* 2001;71:994–997.
299. Apice AJ, Reti LL, Pepperell RJ, et al. Treatment of severe preeclampsia by plasma exchange. *Aust NZ J Obstet Gynecol* 1990;20:231–235.
300. Martin JN, Files JC, Blake PG, et al. Plasma exchange for preeclampsia. I. Postpartum use for severe preeclampsia-eclampsia with HELLP syndrome. *Am J Obstet Gynecol* 1990;162:126–137.
301. Kris M, White DA. Treatment of eclampsia by plasma exchange. *Plasma Ther* 1981;2:143–147.
302. Ornstein MH, Rand JH. An association between refractory HELLP syndrome and antiphospholipid antibodies during pregnancy; report of two cases. *J Rheumatol* 1994;21:1360–1364.
303. Saphier CJ, Repke JT. Hemolysis, elevated liver enzymes, and low platelets (HELLP) syndrome: a review of diagnosis and management. *Semin Perinatol* 1998;22:118–133.
304. Hubbard HC, Portnoy B. Systemic lupus erythematosus in pregnancy treated with plasmapheresis. *Br J Dermatol* 1979; 101:87–90.
305. Thompson BJ, Watson ML, Liston WA, et al. Plasmapheresis in a pregnancy complicated by acute systemic lupus erythematosus. Case report. *Br J Obstet Gynaecol* 1985;92:532–534.
306. Pritchard MH, Jessop JD, Trenchard P, et al. Systemic lupus erythematosus. Repeated abortions and thrombocytopenia. *Ann Rheum Dis* 1978;37:476–478.
307. Frampton G, Cameron JS, Thom M, et al. Successful removal of antiphospholipid antibody during pregnancy using plasma exchange and low-dose prednisone. *Lancet* 1987;2:1023–1024.
308. Fulcher D, Stewart G, Exner T, et al. Plasma exchange and the cardiolipin syndrome in pregnancy. *Lancet* 1989;2:171.
309. Kobayashi S, Tamura N, Tsuda H, et al. Immunoadsorbent plasmapheresis for a patient with antiphospholipid syndrome during pregnancy. *Ann Rheum Dis* 1992;51:399–401.
310. Nakamura Y, Yoshida K, Itoh S, et al. Immunoadsorption plasmapheresis as a treatment for pregnancy complicated by systemic lupus erythematosus with positive antiphospholipid antibodies. *Am J Reprod Immunol* 1999;41:307–311.
311. Wallace DJ. Apheresis for lupus erythematosus. *Lupus* 1999;8: 174–180.
312. Carreras LO, Perez G, Vega HR, et al. Lupus anticoagulant and recurrent fetal loss: successful treatment with gammaglobulin (letter). *Lancet* 1988;2:393–394.
313. Katz VL, Thorp JM Jr, Watson WJ, et al. Human immunoglobu-

lin therapy for preeclampsia associated with lupus anticoagulant and anticardiolipin antibody. *Obstet Gynecol* 1990;76:986–988.

314. Parke A, Maier D, Wilson D, et al. Intravenous gamma-globulin, antiphospholipid antibodies and pregnancy (letter). *Ann Intern Med* 1989;110:495–496.
315. Scott JR, Branch DW, Kochenour NK, et al. Intravenous immunoglobulin treatment of pregnant patients with recurrent pregnancy loss caused by antiphospholipid antibodies and Rh immunization. *Am J Obstet Gynecol* 1988;159:1055–1056.
316. Wapner RJ, Cowchock S, Shapiro SS. Successful treatment in two women with antiphospholipid antibodies and refractory pregnancy losses with intravenous immunoglobulin infusions. Am J *Obstet Gynecol* 1989;161:1271–1272.
317. Arnout J, Spitz B, Wittevrongel C, et al. High-dose intravenous immunoglobulin treatment of a pregnant patient with an antiphospholipid syndrome: immunological changes associated with a successful outcome. *Thromb Haemost* 1994;71: 741–747.
318. Kwak JY, Quilty EA, Gilman-Sachs A, et al. Intravenous immunoglobulin infusion therapy in women with recurrent spontaneous abortions of immune etiologies. *J Reprod Immunol* 1995;28:175–188.
319. Valensise H, Vaquero E, DeCarolis C, et al. Normal fetal growth in women with antiphospholipid syndrome treated with high-dose intravenous immunoglobulin. *Prenat Diagn* 1995;15: 509–517.
320. Cowchock S. Treatment of antiphospholipid syndrome in pregnancy. *Lupus* 1998;7 Suppl 2:S95–97.
321. Said PB, Martinuzzo ME, Carreras LO. Neutralization of lupus anticoagulant activity by human immunoglobulin in vitro. *Nouv Rev Fr Hematol* 1992;34:37–42.
322. Caccavo D, Vaccaro F, Ferri GM, et al. Anti-idiotypes against antiphospholipid antibodies are present in normal polyspecific immunoglobulins for therapeutic use. *J Autoimmun* 1994;7: 537–548.
323. Sherer Y, Levy Y, Shoenfeld Y. Intravenous immunoglobulin therapy of antiphospholipid syndrome. *Rheumatol (Oxf)* 2000; 39:421–426.
324. Brooks PM, Needs CJ. The use of antirheumatic medication during pregnancy and in the puerperium. *Rheum Dis Clin North Am* 1989;15:789–806.
325. McKenzie SA, Selley JA, Agnew JE. Secretion of prednisolone into breast milk. *Arch Dis Child* 1975;50:894–896.
326. Katz FH, Duncan DR. Entry of prednisolone into human milk. *N Engl J Med* 1975;293:1154–1160.
327. Ost L, Wettrel G, Bjorkhem I, et al. Prednisolone excretion in human milk. *J Pediatr* 1985;106:1008–1011.
328. Ito S, Koren G. A novel index for expressing exposure of the infant to drugs in breast milk. *Br J Clin Pharmacol* 1994;38:99–102.
329. Tauber U, Haack D, Nieuweboer B, et al. The pharmacokinetics of fluocortolone and prednisolone after intravenous and oral administration. *Int J Clin Pharmacol Ther Toxicol* 1984;22:48–55.
330. Sietsema WK. The absolute oral bioavailability of selected drugs. *Int J Clin Pharmacol Ther Toxicol* 1989;27:179–211.
331. Lawrence RA. *Breastfeeding: a guide for the medical profession*, 3rd ed. St. Louis: CV Mosby, 1989:256–284,571.
332. Wiernik PH, Duncan JH. Cyclophosphamide in human milk. *Lancet* 1971;1:912–914.
333. Johns DG, Rutherford LD, Leighton PG, et al. Secretion of methotrexate into human milk. *Am J Obstet Gynecol* 1972; 112:978–980.
334. Anderson PO. Drugs and breast feeding a review. *Drug Intell Clin Pharmacol* 1977;11:208–223.
335. Nyberg G, Haljamae U, Frisenette-Fich C, et al. Breast-feeding during treatment with cyclosporine. *Transplantation* 1998;65: 253–255.
336. Soares R, Paulini E, Pereira JP. Concentration and elimination of chloroquine by the placental circulation and milk in patients receiving chloroquine salt. *Bull Trop Dis* 1959;56:412–414.
337. Nation RL, Hacket LP, Dusci LJ, et al. Excretion of hydroxychloroquine in human milk. *Br J Clin Pharmacol* 1984;17: 368–369.
338. Berlin CM, Pascuzzi MJ, Yaffe SJ. Excretion of salicylate in human milk. *Clin Pharmacol Ther* 1980;27:245–248.
339. Findlay JW, DeAngelis RL, Kearney MF, et al. Analgesic drugs in breast milk and plasma. *Clin Pharmacol Ther* 1981;29: 625–633.
340. Levy G. Clinical pharmacokinetics of aspirin. *Pediatrics* 1978; 62:867.
341. American Academy of Pediatrics Committee on Drugs. The transfer of drugs and other chemicals into human miilk. *Pediatrics* 1994;93:137–150.
342. Chapel TA, Burns RE. Oral contraceptives and exacerbations of lupus erythematosus. *Am J Obstet Gynecol* 1971;110:366–369.
343. Garovich M, Agudelo C, Pisko E. Oral contraceptives and systemic lupus erythematosus. *Arthritis Rheum* 1980;23: 1396–1398.
344. Jungers P, Dougados M, Pelissier C, et al. Influence of oral contraceptive therapy on the activity of systemic lupus erythematosus. *Arthritis Rheum* 1982;25:618–623.
345. Wallace D. Personal communication.
346. Julkunen HA. Oral contraceptives in systemic lupus erythematosus: side-effects and influence on the activity of SLE. *Scand J Rheumatol* 1991;20:427–433.
347. Julkunen HA, Kaaja R, Friman C. Contraceptive practice in women with systemic lupus erythematosus. *Br J Rheumatol* 1993;32:227–230.
348. BuyonJP, Kalunian KC, Skovron ML, et al. Can women with systemic lupus safely use exogenous estrogens? *J Clin Rheumatol* 1995;1:205–212.
349. Asherson RA, Harris EN, Ghavari AE, et al. Systemic lupus erythematosus, antiphospholipid antibodies, chorea, and oral contraceptives (letter). *Arthritis Rheum* 1986;29:1535–1536.
350. Anonymous. Progestin-only pills. History, mechanism of action and effectiveness. *Contraceptive Technol* 1990–1992: 314–322.
351. Anonymous. A subdermal progestin implant for long-term contraception. *Med Letter* 1991;33:17–18.
352. Simon A, Revel A, Hurwitz A, et al. The pathogenesis of ovarian hyperstimulation syndrome: a continuing enigma. *J Assist Reprod Genet* 1998;15:202–209.
353. Ben-Chetrit A, Ben-Chetrit E. Systemic lupus erythematosus induced by ovulation induction treatment. *Arthritis Rheum* 1994;37:1614–1617.
354. Macut D, Micic D, Suvajdzic N, et al. Ovulation induction and early pregnancy loss in a woman susceptible to autoimmune diseases: a possible interrelationship. *Gynecol Endocrinol* 2000; 14:153–157.
355. Le Thi Huong D, Wechsler B, Piette JC, et al. Risk of ovulation-induction therapy in systemic lupus erythematosus. *Br J Rheumatol* 1996;35:1184–1186.
356. Guballa N, Sammaritano L, Schwartzman S, et al. Ovulation induction and in vitro fertilization in systemic lupus erythematosus and antiphospholipid syndrome. *Arthritis Rheum* 1999; 43:550–556.
357. Casoli P, Tumiati B, La Sala G. Fatal exacerbation of systemic lupus erythematosus after induction of ovulation. *J Rheumatol* 1997;24:1639–1640.
358. Wechsler B, Le Thi Huong D, Vauthier-Brouzes D, et al. Hormone stimulation and replacement therapy in women with rheumatic disease. *Scand J Rheumatol* 1998:27(suppl 107):53–59.

48

THE FETUS IN SYSTEMIC LUPUS ERYTHEMATOSUS

RODANTHI C. KITRIDOU
T. MURPHY GOODWIN

There are a variety of fetal and neonatal problems associated with lupus. This chapter will deal with fetal loss, its pathogenesis and treatment, prematurity, intrauterine growth restriction (IUGR), and management recommendations. For a definition of terms used, please see Chapter 47. Certain facts emerge through a plethora of studies over the last 50 years, although the populations studied may lack homogeneity, the study designs differ, and our practices have evolved toward earlier disease detection and more aggressive therapy. In the series antedating 1980, the outcome of pregnancy in patients with systemic lupus erythematosus (SLE) was very unsatisfactory: total fetal loss was triple the usual prevalence for normal populations, with increase in spontaneous abortions, stillbirths, and prematurity. As analyzed by Cecere and Persellin (1), there had been little change in the 30 years between 1950 and 1980 (Table 48.1). However, in the 1980s, 1990s, and 2000, there is better understanding of the causes of fetal loss and better fetal survival through improved pregnancy management (9–44).

FETAL OUTCOME IN SYSTEMIC LUPUS ERYTHEMATOSUS

A pregnancy may result in live birth, full-term or premature (preterm) delivery, or in fetal loss. A neonate may be of normal weight for age, or small for gestational age, the latter also known as IUGR. Fetal loss may be a result of spontaneous abortion (before the 20th week of pregnancy), or to intrauterine fetal death (stillbirth, after the 20th week of gestation).

Spontaneous Abortions

The prevalence of spontaneous abortions (SABs) in SLE pregnancy (Table 48.1) was 11.6% for the decade 1950 to 1959, 19.5% for the years 1960 to 1969, and 19.4% for the period 1970 to 1981. All these figures are derived from retrospective studies.

In most studies that compare pregnancy outcome before and after lupus onset, fetal loss was found to be increased even before disease onset (2–7). SABs ranged from 14% to 35%, with rates in normal general population reported at 7% to 12.5%. Full-term deliveries ranged from 64% to 86% (average 78%).

After onset of SLE, there was usually an increase in SABs, reported in 4% to 40%, or SLE onset during pregnancy. In the study by Fraga et al., 23.1% of 183 pregnancies before SLE onset ended in SABs, with 12.5% in 288 control pregnancies (3). After SLE onset, SABs rose to 40.5%. An exception is a study from Greece, where no increased fetal loss prior to disease onset was found (8).

Between 1980 and 1989, 16 reports on 689 lupus pregnancies appeared, three of them prospective (8–22). The mean prevalence of SABs was 15.6% (Table 48.1). The highest prevalence was 35% in a retrospective study (4), followed by 30% in a patient questionnaire study from Vancouver (17), while the lowest rates are 0% and 6% (8,9). In the prospective study by Mintz, the frequency of SABs was 16.6% (17 of 102 pregnancies) in Mexico City, significantly higher than the 6.7% of their controls (18).

Of 20 studies from the 1990s (23–42), ten are prospective (24,28–30,33–36,38,39), and two are prospective and controlled (24,28), with a total of 1,732 reported pregnancies. Spontaneous abortions range from a low of 5.4% (39) to a high of 30% (37), with a mean of 14.6% (Table 48.1). The reasons for the variations are not apparent, but may include socioeconomic, educational, and cultural diversity parameters.

The two studies from 2000, reporting 126 pregnancies (before elective abortions), differ in that spontaneous abortions, hence fetal loss, preterm births, and IUGR were much less in the study from Greece (43) than in the study from France (44). On the other hand, the former study had a large number of elective abortions, 17% (43).

Thus, with the exception of the latest sudy from France (44), the last 20 years show a stabilization of SABs around 15%, which is an improvement from the 19.5% rates of the

TABLE 48.1. FETAL OUTCOME OF SYSTEMIC LUPUS ERYTHEMATOSUS PREGNANCIES, EXCLUSIVE OF ELECTIVE ABORTIONS

Decade/ Time Period	Pregnancies Number	Spontaneous Abortions	Stillbirths (IUFD) (%)	Fetal Loss (%)	Prematurity (Preterm Birth)	IUGR
1950–1959	155	11.6	10.3	27.5	before 1980:	–
1960–1969	307	19.5	6.8	27.0	15.3	–
1970–1981	505	19.4	8.5	27.9	–	–
1980–1989	689	15.6	7.4	25.1	21.4	26.8
1990–1999	1732	14.6	4.6	19.2	33.3	17.2
2000–	101	20	2	22	26.9	16.2
Studies of the 1980s No. of Pregnancies						(percent)
Tozman[9]	18	6	6	11	11	–
Houser[10]	17	8	0	18	21	–
Zulman[11]	24	8	4	12	4	–
Hayslett[12]	55	15	9	25	5	–
Fine[13]	45	7	22	29	31	32
Varner[14]	34	9	6	15	10	35
Gimovsky[4]	65	35	11	46	22	34
Imbasciati[15]	24	25	8	33	42	10
Lockshin[16ab]	25	–	–	44	33	–
Stein[17]	54	30	7	37	–	–
Mintz[18ab]	102	17	5	23	63	23
Meehan[19]	18	17	0	17	17	–
Bobrie[20]	67	16	4	20	12	–
Siamopoulou-Mavridou[8]	14	0	14	14	7	–
McHugh[21]	47	–	–	34	–	–
Lockshin[22a]	80	–	–	24	–	–
Studies of the 1990s						
Nossent[23]	39	10	5	15	19	–
Wong[24a,b]	19	11	0	11	47	12
Pistiner[25]	528	18	–	18	–	–
Oviasu[26]	47	17	2	19	21	10
Packham[27]	57	9	12	21	33	–
Petri[28ab]	74	–	–	15	45	–
Tincani[29a]	25	16	0	16	20	27
TambyRaja[30a]	50	8	2	10	–	–
Julkunen[31]	105	19	2	21	–	–
Petri[32]	157	–	–	27	24	–
Derksen[33a]	35	23	3	26	–	–
LeThiHuong[34a]	94	16	3	19	51	–
Lima et al[35a]	106	6.6	9.4	16	42.7	31
Le Huong et al[36a]	60	16.7	3.3	20	60.4	–
Johns et al[37]	40	30	7.5	37.5	36	–
Rahman et al[38a]	121	28.1	2.5	30.6	24.4	7
Carmona et al[39a]	56	5.4	8.9	14.3	20.8	9.4
Sittiwangkul et al[40]	44	13.6	6.8	20.4	38.6	20
Kobayashi et al[41]	75	8	2.7	10.7	16.7	21.2
Huong Du et al[42]	24	8	8	16	64	NS
Studies of 2000						
Georgiou et al[43b]	49	15	2	17	5	4.1
De Bandt et al[44]	52	25	1.9	26.9	48.7	28.2

a, Prospective series; b, controlled series; NS, not specified.

1960s and 1970s, and much closer to normal population values.

The factors that appear responsible for SAB and overall fetal loss in lupus include antiphospholipid (APL) antibodies, disease activity, and lupus nephritis. These are discussed under the Fetal Loss section, below.

It is increasingly recognized that the death of a fetus of normal appearance on ultrasound after 10 weeks' gestation has a much stronger association with autoimmune mechanisms than does earlier loss. The very common early pregnancy loss is most often chromosomal or hormonal in nature. In practice, this means that we look for evidence of

APL antibodies, or subclinical SLE as a cause of pregnancy loss in the following settings:

1. Two or three losses less than 10 weeks' gestation
2. A single loss after 10 weeks' gestation of a normal-appearing fetus on prior ultrasound
3. Any loss with other events or findings suggestive of SLE or APL syndrome

The older data dividing spontaneous abortions and stillbirths by 20 weeks' gestation are still needed for comparison and trends, especially for regional and national statistical comparisons. In practice, however, these divisions are not meaningful.

Intrauterine Fetal Death (Stillbirth)

Intrauterine fetal death (IUFD) or stillbirth is the spontaneous termination of pregnancy after the 20th week of gestation. The frequency of stillbirths in the past (Table 48.1) was 10.3% from 1950 to 1959, 6.8% between 1960 and 1969, and 8.5% in the years 1970 to 1981 (1). In the 16 series reported from 1980 to 1989, there were 51 stillbirths among 689 pregnancies, or 7.4% (9–22). The prevalence in individual series varied from 0% (10,19) to 22% (13). Among 1,755 pregnancies reported in 20 studies from 1990 to 1999, excluding elective abortions, the prevalence of intrauterine fetal deaths was less than in previous time periods, 4.3%, ranging from 0% (24,28) to 12% in women with lupus nephritis and APL antibodies (27). The rate of stillbirths in SLE is higher than normal: for example, Nossent and Swaak found a prevalence of 5.1% (2 of 39 pregnancies), which is significantly higher than 0.6%, the rate for the Dutch population (23).

In the two series from 2,000, IUFD was seen in 2% of 101 pregnancies (43,44).

Neonatal Deaths

Neonatal deaths are excessive in SLE pregnancies, with the highest prevalence of 20% in the 1965 study by Estes and Larson (2), and of 25% in the 1978 study by Thomas et al. (45).

In 1950 to 1959 there were 5.8% neonatal deaths (nine of 155 uninterrupted pregnancies), in 1960 to 1969, 0.7% (two of 307), and in 1970 to 1981, zero of 505 pregnancies (1). Among the 16 series published between 1980 and 1989, there were 15 neonatal deaths in 689 pregnancies (2.2%) (4, 11,12,16,18). In the 20 reports from the 1990s, there were 18 neonatal deaths in 1,755 pregnancies (1.02%) (26,30,31, 33,39). Some of these were due to extreme prematurity, or to congenital heart block (39,44). This prevalence is over double the US neonatal death rate of 0.5%.

Fetal Loss (Table 48.1)

Fetal loss (or wastage) has been defined as the sum of spontaneous abortions and stillbirths. Cecere and Persellin also have defined it as the sum of spontaneous abortions, stillbirths, and perinatal deaths divided by the number of pregnancies minus elective abortions and expressed as a percentage (1). In Table 48.1, fetal loss includes neonatal deaths.

Excluding elective (induced, therapeutic) abortions, the prevalence of fetal loss in lupus patients remained stable in the three decades between 1950 and 1980, at 27% to 27.9%. From 1980–1989, fetal loss prevalence was 25.1%, and six series showed, for the first time, a decrease to under 20% (8,9–11,14,19). This trend continued into the 1990s, with the mean fetal loss at 18.7%, and 12 of 20 series showing fetal loss under 20% (23–26,28–30,34,35,39,41,42) (Table 48.1).

Etiology Of Fetal Loss

Activity of maternal lupus, nephritis, anti-Ro/SSA antibodies, and APL antibodies have been incriminated as etiologic factors of fetal loss in lupus.

Activity Of Lupus

In most reports, the spontaneous abortion rate seems independent of lupus activity or inactivity—for example, in the largest prospective study there is no statistical difference between spontaneous abortions or stillbirths in active SLE (13.7% and 6%) versus inactive lupus (19.6% and 3.9%) (18). Certain studies associate severe or nephritis flares with adverse pregnancy outcomes (see below). Lima et al., however, in their study of 108 pregnancies, concluded that flares during pregnancy did not increase the risk of fetal loss (35). In contrast, full-term delivery was seen in 12.5% of active lupus, and in 69% of inactive lupus pregnancies in the study by Georgiou (43). In most studies, disease activity was determined by experienced clinicians; more recently, it is assessed by validated lupus activity measurements [Systemic Lupus Erythematosus Disease Activity Index, (SLEDAI), Systemic Lupus Activity Measure (SLAM), and Lupus Activity Index (LAI)] (46,47). In recognition of differential diagnostic dilemmas between SLE activity versus preeclampsia, which have certain symptoms and findings in common (headache, hypertension, proteinuria, seizures, red blood cells (RBCs) in urine), versus pregnancy-associated problems (fatigue, edema, alopecia), certain modifications have been developed in the above activity measures for use in pregnancy (48).

Lupus Nephritis

Certain studies suggest that active lupus nephritis contributes to fetal loss. In the 1980s, Gimovsky et al. reported 40% spontaneous abortions and 12.5% IUFDs in women with lupus nephritis, with 28% and 2.5% respectively without (4). These patients were socioeconomically disadvantaged, with a great proportion (as much as 60% to 70%) of illegal aliens. Similar trends appeared in other studies (5,10,12,15).

In the last study, of 55 pregnancies with active lupus or nephritis at conception, live births were at 56% with nephrotic syndrome, 64% with active SLE, and 88% with quiescent SLE (12). Fetal loss was seen in one of 10 pregnancies with serum creatinine less than 1.5 mg/dL, and in 50% with creatinine more than 1.5 mg/dL. Hence, in the 1980s, severe lupus nephritis tended to be associated with greater fetal loss.

In the 1990s, several reports have addressed the role of active nephritis in the outcome of pregnancy: of 47 pregnancies in 25 women, most with stable lupus nephritis, there was fetal loss of 19% (eight spontaneous abortions, one IUFD) (26). All spontaneous abortions occurred in women with nephritis of class III–V. In hypertensive patients, fetal loss was double that of normotensive patients (29% vs.13%) (26). In the above studies, however, there were no determinations of APL antibodies. In the study of 57 pregnancies with lupus nephritis by Packham et al., fetal loss was slightly greater in women with diffuse and focal glomerulonephritis, than in women with membranous nephropathy. Nevertheless, the majority of fetal loss (three of five spontaneous abortions, all five stillbirths, and two of five neonatal deaths) occurred in mothers with the lupus anticoagulant (LAC) (27).

Five more studies from the 1990s merit attention: Rahman et al., in a study of 121 pregnancies, determined that active nephritis predicted fetal loss (13.4% live births with active nephritis, vs. 33% without active nephritis), and hypertension predicted prematurity and IUGR (23.8% preterm and IUGR babies with hypertensive mothers, vs. 6.6% without hypertensive mothers) (38). In this study, fetal loss with and without APL antibodies did not differ. In a study from Spain, hypertension occurred in one half of the ten pregnancies with, vs. 11.6% of 43 pregnancies without nephritis, and nephritis was significantly associated with lower gestational age at delivery, 35.9 vs. 37.3 weeks (39). Three additional studies related poor fetal outcome to nephritis flares (34,37,40), and one study linked small-for-date neonates to hypocomplementemia, even without flare (41).

Antiphospholipid Antibodies

Since Nilsson et al. (49) in 1975, Firkin et al. (50), and Soulier and Boffa (51) suggested a link between LAC and recurrent abortions, a tremendous collection of data has been amassed. Table 48.2 shows the fetal outcome in SLE and SLE-like illness in the presence or absence of antiphospholipid antibodies. In 15 retrospective studies of 1,249 pregnancies, there were 479 pregnancies in APL-positive women, and 770 pregnancies in APL-negative women (26,30,52–64). In the APL-positive pregnancies, there was a mean fetal loss of 37% (range, 14%–68%). In the APL-negative pregnancies, there was a mean loss of 18% (range, 3%–43%). Kutteh et al. have determined the prevalence of multiple abortions (two or more) in lupus, as 27% among anticardiolipin (ACL) -positive women and in only 3% of ACL-negative women (64). These authors showed that the percentage of fetal loss correlated with the level of ACL antibody: at ≤10 phospholipid units, fetal loss was 10%; at 10–20, 20%; at 21–80, 32%, and at 80 units, 60% (64).

In seven prospective studies of 892 lupus pregnancies, 301 occurred in APL-positive, and 591 in APL-negative women. In the APL-positive pregnancies, mean fetal loss was 48% (range, 4%–100%), and in the APL-negative, 9% (range, 0%–20%) (65–71). Despite the large range, the significance of positive APL as a cause of fetal loss seems irrefutable. APL positivity has been linked more so to midpregnancy and late fetal loss (27,56,72,73), but also is emerging as an important factor in early loss (see below, APL and Fetal Loss Without Lupus).

Risk factors for fetal loss include the LAC (27, 70), high-level IgG anticardiolipin, alone (55,60,64,65,68,72), or in combination with the LAC (74, 75), and a history of prior fetal loss (55,63,65). In lupus patients with both LAC and ACL (about 16% of 349 lupus patients), fetal loss was the highest, at 89% (75). It should be noted that APL levels may fluctuate, especially when low positive (61,76–78). Antibody to beta(2)-glycoprotein I often is found in association with ACL antibody and uncommonly alone. In a study of 424 women (152 healthy fertile controls, 141 with unexplained recurrent spontaneous abortions, 58 with unexplained fetal deaths, and 73 with APL syndrome), testing for anti-beta(2)-glycoprotein I did not identify additional patients at risk for recurrent abortion or fetal loss (79).

High APL positivity was predictive of fetal distress: nine lupus patients with midpregnancy fetal distress, manifested by abnormal fetal heart deceleration or fetal death, had over sevenfold anticardiolipin levels compared to 12 patients without fetal distress (65). Two studies provided further confirmation that high levels of IgG ACL, or lupus anticoagulant are associated with fetal death: the proportion of fetal deaths with IgG ACL of over 40 GPL international units was 46–65%, and with 0–39 GPL it was 17–19% (76); similarly, in women with high-positive APL (lupus anticoagulant, or more than 19 IgG binding units of ACL), fetal death was 27%, while with negative APL, IgM anticardiolipin only, or low-positive IgG ACL (>20 binding units), fetal death was 3–8% (76a).

Two studies have addressed the significance of elevated maternal alpha-fetoprotein (AFP) levels: in 13 of 60 pregnancies with APL antibodies, second trimester maternal AFP was elevated and was unexplained by fetal anomalies. Fetal death and perinatal loss were increased significantly over pregnancies with normal maternal AFP (62% vs. 6%, and 77% vs. 15%, respectively) (80). Petri et al. determined maternal AFP prospectively in 54 lupus, and 1,001 control pregnancies at the 16th–31st week of gestation (81): abnor-

TABLE 48.2. FETAL OUTCOME AND MATERNAL ANTIPHOSPHOLIPID ANTIBODIES IN SYSTEMIC LUPUS ERYTHEMATOSUS (SLE) AND SLE-LIKE ILLNESS

Author Retrospective Studies	No. APL Positive	% Fetal Loss	No. APL Negative	% Fetal Loss
Boey (52)	26	35	27	19
Elias (53)	16	25	–	–
Colaco (54)	17	18	32	3
Petri (56)	7	14	48	10
Fort (57)	9	22	13	31
Harris (55)	80	16	38	3
Kalunian (58)	19	68	24	42
Gharavi (59)	22	32	–	–
Deleze (60)	53	57	145	25
Ishii (61)	29	41	14	7
Vianna (62)	13	54	80	18
Ramsey-Goldman (63)	81	51	174	43
Kutteh (64)	31	39	94	11
Julkunen (31)	56	30	41	12
Mean		37%		18%
Prospective Studies				
Lockshin (65)	11	46	12	0
Lockshin (66)	13	77	37	5
Hanly (67)	4	100	7	0
Englert (68)	19	53	15	14
Koskela (69)	53	4	91	5
Out (70)	20	35	93	19
Abu-Shakra (71)	181	19	336	20
Mean		48%		9%

APL, antiphospholipid antibodies.

mal maternal AFP was significantly more frequent in lupus pregnancies (7.4% vs. 2.6%). The four patients with abnormal AFP had high ACL, preterm delivery, and were on more prednisone. Perhaps maternal AFP, in the absence of fetal anomalies, will be a valuable predictor of decreased fetal viability and preterm birth in APL-positive patients.

The pathogenesis of APL-related fetal loss is through placental vessel thrombosis with infarctions and fetal hypoxia. A potent natural anticoagulant system comprises protein C and protein S, which, in its free form, binds activated protein C to the surface of phospholipids, were factors Va and VIIIa undergo proteolytic inactivation. Deficiency of one of these proteins is associated with thrombotic events early in life. During pregnancy, functional and immunologic levels of protein S are decreased (82), and nephrotic syndrome is associated with decrease in free protein S (83). Three studies have addressed the status of protein S in women with APL: one found decreased functional protein S with normal free protein S in 6 of 16 nonpregnant women with LAC (84), another found decreased levels of free protein S in seven of 11 patients with fetal wastage and APL (85), and a third study found both free and total protein S decreased in 50 patients with LAC, as compared to controls (86). The same group has reported that ACL-positive patients probably have an acquired deficiency of protein S and C4b-binding protein (87). An inhibitor of the protein C pathway was found in a lupus patient with ACL, recurrent deep-vein thrombosis, fetal wastage, and seizures (88). Of a host of mutations of coagulation factors, factor V mutation (G1691), in association with APL, may confer even greater tendency to thrombosis. A great deal of further investigation is needed to clarify the potential role of proteins C and S, and factor mutations in fetal loss associated with lupus.

Antiphospholipid Antibodies And Fetal Loss Without Lupus

The significance of APL antibodies in fetal loss extends well beyond lupus and APL syndrome patients (see also Chapter 25, The Lupus Anticoagulant and Antiphospholipid Antibodies). The spectrum of obstretric problems associated with APL include (89) the following:

Recurrent pregnancy loss
Unexplained second or third trimester loss
Fetal death
Fetal growth restriction, especially severe, early onset
Oligohydramnios, otherwise unexplained
Placental abruption
Placental infarction
Unexplained high midpregnancy alpha-fetoprotein
Pregnancy-induced hypertension (PIH), especially severe and early onset
Pregnancy-related thrombosis, venous, or arterial.

Any of the above problems, especially if severe, of early onset, and otherwise unexplained, should prompt investigation for APL, even if the clinical picture does not point to lupus and the history does not include intravascular thrombosis.

There are now several studies in normal pregnancies, pregnancies with fetal loss, infertile women, and women with failure of *in vitro* fertilization, which incriminate APL. Table 48.3 summarizes findings up to 1996. As of 1997, APL was found in 5.3% of 7,278 normal obstetrical patients, 20% of 2,226 women with recurrent fetal loss, 24% of 3,343 women undergoing *in vitro* fertilization, and 37% of 1,579 women with SLE (89).

In part A of the table are shown five large studies of normal pregnancies, two of which are prospective (90–94). A total of 6,628 pregnant women, mostly consecutive patients in obstetric services, were tested for APL. Prevalence of positive APL varied from 1.25% (of >5 SD IgG ACL) (92) to 24.4% (94), for a mean of 8.2%. Fetal loss in these patients varied from zero (91) to 50% (92), with a mean of 25.8%. Four of the studies gave information on premature births and IUGR: APL-positive pregnancies had a 60% prevalence of preterm birth in Lockwood's study (90) and there was IUGR in 18% of neonates of women with prolonged APTT in Rix's study (93).

Part B of Table 48.3 examines the prevalence of positive APL in women with fetal losses. Eleven studies determined APL in 1,698 women with 1 to ≥3 fetal losses (56,70, 95–103). In women with ≥3 fetal losses, APL positivity ranged from 5.5% to 31% (56,70,95–100); with two or more fetal losses, it was 10.7% and 15% (97,101); with <2, 4.8% (95), and with one or no fetal loss, APL were present in 0%–11% (56,102,103). Eroglu and Scopelitis reported strictly on first trimester losses (99). Control subjects in references 96, 98, and 99 had 7%, 0% and 10% APL positivity and no fetal loss.

Part C of Table 48.3 shows that 17% of 41 infertile women had APL, in addition to other autoantibodies, versus 6% of

TABLE 48.3. FETAL OUTCOME AND MATERNAL ANTIPHOSPHOLIPID ANTIBODIES IN NON-LUPUS PREGNANCIES

A. Normal pregnancies

Author	No. Pregnancies	Percent (+) APL/Fetal Loss	Preterm/IUGR	(–) APL/Fetal Loss	Preterm/IUGR
Lockwood (90)	737	2.4/44	60	97.6/7	11/–
Harris (91)	1449	6.1/0	0/0	93.9/0.3	1.7/1.7
Perez (92)	1200	1.25/50 of >5 SD	–	98.8/–	–/–
Rix* (93)	2856	7 APPT/19	–/18	92.9/–	–/–
Lynch* (94)	389	24.4/15.8	5.3/0	75.6/6.5	7.8/0

B. Pregnancies with Fetal Loss

	No. of Women	No. of Losses	% APL (+)	Controls/APL
Petri (56)	44	≥3	9 LAC, 11 ACL	See below
Creagh (95)	35	≥3	31 (20 LAC, 17ACL)	See below
Parke (96)	81	≥3	16	88/7 no fetal loss
MacLean (97)	130	≥3	18.5	See below
Konidaris (98)	44	≥3	22.7	34 N/0
Out (70)	102	≥3	21 (5 LAC)	102 N/10 (0 LAC)
Eroglu (99)	72	≥3*	5.6 ACL	
Rai (100)	500	≥3	9.6 LAC, 5.5 ACL	
Balasch (101)	65	≥2	10.7 LAC	
MacLean (97)	113	2	15	
Creagh (95)	42	≤2	4.8	
Bocciolone (102)	99	1, late	4 LAC, 1 ACL	85 N pregnant/0
Petri (56)	40	≤1	0 LAC, 2.5 ACL	
Infante-Rivard (103)	331	1	5.1 LAC, 1.2 ACL	993 N preg./3.8 LAC, 1.5 ACL

C. APL in women with infertility or failure of in vitro fertilization (IVF)

Taylor (104)	41	Infertile	17 (10 ANA)	351 N pregnant/6 (3 ANA)
Birkenfeld (105)	56	IVF failure	30 (5.4 ANA)	
	14	IVF success	0	
	69	IVF candidates	10	
Geva (106)	21	IVF failure	14.2 (9.5 a-DNA)	
	21	IVF success	0	

*1st Trimester loss; ANA, antinuclear antibody; a-DNA, anti-double stranded DNA; ACL, anticardiolipin; APL, antiphospholipid antibodies; IUGR, intrauterine growth restriction; LAC, lupus anticoagulant; N, normal.

351 normal pregnant women (104). Two studies addressed APL in women with implantation failure in the process of *in vitro* fertilization (IVF): 17 of 56 such women (30%) were positive for APL, versus 0% of 14 IVF successes and 10% of 69 IVF candidates (105). The study by Geva et al. found 33.3% positive autoantibodies in 21 IVF failures, including 14.2% positive for ACL, vs. 0% positive in 21 IVF successes (106).

A controlled, nonrandomized study showed the prevalence of APL in 191 women undergoing IVF as 18.8%, 5.5% in 200 normal controls, 26% in 200 women with recurrent pregnancy loss, and 32% in 200 women with SLE (107). The investigators showed higher rates for implantation in the ASA and heparin-treated IVF group vs. the standard treatment for IVF group (25% vs. 19.4%), but no difference in terms of pregnancy and ongoing pregnancy rates.

In summary, APL antibodies appear to be the common factor in certain proportion of fetal loss in otherwise healthy women, in about 20% of recurrent aborters, and in 24% of implantation failures in IVF.

Treatment For Prevention Of Antiphospholipid-Related Fetal Loss (Table 48.4)

Since 1983, several publications have addressed the prevention of fetal loss associated with APL antibodies. In 29 studies reporting ten or more pregnancies, there has been improved fetal outcome (70,108–135). Fetal loss in the over 1,017 untreated pregnancies was 76.2%–100%, with only 7.9% mean live births (range, 0%–23.8%). All treatments have resulted in increase of live births, to a mean of 70.8% (range, 28.6%–100%) (Table 48.4). A total of at least 1,001 pregnancies were treated: the most common therapy, used in 401 pregnancies, was low-dose aspirin (75–100 mg/day) and corticosteroids (usually 40 mg of prednisone per day for 1 to 2 months with subsequent tapering), is no longer favored because of maternal side effects. The most effective treatment regimens have been those involving heparin, low-dose aspirin plus heparin, or low-molecular-weight heparin (115,117, 118,129–131,133,134). Comparison of aspirin plus low-dose heparin (up to 12,000 IU/day) vs. aspirin plus high-dose heparin (up to 30,000 IU per day) showed no advantage of the latter (76% vs. 80% live births) (130). Low-molecular-weight heparin is safe in pregnancy, can be given once a day, and showed a decided advantage over historical placebo controls [83.9 vs. 55.9 live births, (133)]. Heparin and low-molecular-weight heparin are category B drugs, do not cross the placenta, and are not harmful to the fetus, but heparin-induced osteoporosis and thrombocytopenia are the main concerns. Low-dose aspirin therapy alone resulted in 42–44% live births, versus 71–80% in combination with heparin (129, 131). Several recent studies on APL-related fetal loss have excluded lupus patients. Such a pilot study compared aspirin plus heparin and intravenous immunoglobulin (IVIg) to aspirin plus heparin and albumin on 14 patients: there was no difference, with 100% live births with both regimens (134). IVIg still can be effective and is reserved for use in failures of the ASA and heparin regimen. When women positive for APL underwent IVF while treated with ASA and heparin, there were 46% live births in treated IVF cycles, vs. 17% in untreated (135). Of 322 women with a single APL subtype treated with ASA and heparin, there were 17% live births with IVF in those with antiphosphatidylethanolamine (PE) or antiphosphatidylserine (PS), vs. 43% in women with other APL specificities. Of the women with PE and PS, 121 who did not achieve live births despite ASA and heparin, were given these plus IVIg: this treatment resulted in a 41% birth rate (135). This suggests that, in specific situations, addition of IVIg to ASA and heparin can provide further pregnancy success.

A study on early fetal loss associated with APL compared aspirin 75 mg per day vs. placebo and found no difference, with 80% and 85% live births, respectively (136).

TABLE 48.4. OUTCOME OF TREATMENT IN ANTIPHOSPHOLIPID-ASSOCIATED FETAL LOSS

	No. of Pregnancies		Live Births (%)	
Therapy used, mg/day	Before	After Therapy	Before	After Therapy
a. ASA 50–300 + prednisone 10–60	591	268	8.5 (0.7–17.2)	64.9 (28.6–100)
b. ASA + prednisone ± heparin ± dipyridamole	270	150	10.3 (3.7–23.8)	63.9 (48–90.9)
c. ASA 75–81 mg/d	>33	70	≥3/patient	44.3
d. ASA, or ASA + heparin	>134	149	9.9 (0–18.7)	71.6 (55.6–80)
e. Heparin	29	15	3.4	93.3
f. IVIg + ASA ± prednisone	75	16	3.9 (0–7.1)	85.7 (57.1–100)
g. Fish oil	≥3/pt	22	Not specified	95.5
h. Low–molecular-weight heparin	≥2/pt	46	Not specified	83.9

a. Data from references 108–112, 116, 118, 120–124, 128.
b. Data from references 70, 113, 114, 119, 120.
c. Data from references 129, 131.
d. Data from references 117, 118, 123, 129, 130, 131.
e. Data from reference 115.
f. Data from references 123, 126, 127.
g. Data from reference 125.
h. Data from reference 133.
ASA, aspirin (acetylsalicylic acid); IVIg, intravenous immunoglobulin.

For more details see Pregnancy Management for Optimal Fetal Survival, below, and Chapter 47.

Our preferred regimen for anticoagulation during pregnancy at the Los Angeles County and University of Southern California (LAC+USC) Medical Center is as follows:

As soon as pregnancy is confirmed, for women with prior pregnancy complications, but no thrombosis: subcutaneous enoxaparin (SC) 0.5mg/kg twice daily, calcium supplementation at 1.5 g daily, and axial weight-bearing exercise or, unfractionated heparin, 10,000 IU subcutaneously twice daily, calcium, and exercise.

For women who have clotted previously, SC enoxaparin 1 mg/kg twice daily, or adjusted dose of unfractionated heparin SC to prolong the partial thromboplastin time (PTT) to two, 6 hours after the morning dose; all regimens are accompanied by daily low-dose aspirin.

In summary, there is a substantial prevalence of spontaneous abortion, stillbirth, and overall fetal loss in lupus patients, which is linked mainly to maternal APL antibodies. There is a trend toward diminution of fetal loss during the 1990s, and live births have increased significantly in high-risk pregnancies treated with antiplatelet and anticoagulant agents.

Anti-Ro/SSA Antibodies

Hull et al. and Watson et al. have implied a possible role for anti-Ro/SSA antibodies in fetal loss in SLE (137,138). In a retrospective study of 50 anti-Ro/SSA-positive and 47 anti-U $_1$-RNP-positive women, 20 of the former and 33 of the latter fulfilled criteria for SLE (138). Of the anti-Ro/SSA-positive women, 34 had 84 pregnancies with 28% fetal wastage, which was similar to that of the anti-U $_1$-RNP group (19%). However, African American women with anti-Ro/SSA had a much higher fetal loss (71%). No information was given about the APL status of these patients. The subject was recently reassessed. Recurrent pregnancy loss was associated with antibody to Ro/SSA in women without SLE, who had Sjögren's syndrome or rheumatoid arthritis (23.7%) (139). The same investigators found that antibodies to Ro52, Ro60, p57, and thyroglobulin, were independent predictors of recurrent pregnancy loss in women with autoimmune diseases (140).

Other Observations

It is of interest that in the study by Nossent and Swaak the male:female sex ratio of offspring of lupus patients (male babies per 100 female babies) was 72.7 before, and 78.9 after onset of SLE: this is decreased compared to the normal of 105 for the Dutch population (23). This would imply greater fetal wastage of male offspring. In an attempt to explain the high female:male ratio in SLE, Oleinick examined the family histories of 198 lupus patients and their 581 siblings. He found that the ratio of male to total siblings born within 4 years of the birth of lupus patients was lower and suggested that excessive male fetal wastage may explain, in part, the female preponderance in SLE (141). In a further investigation, the author found that there was no excess mortality risk in early life for male siblings or offspring of lupus patients (142).

Other Treatment

Of special interest are two studies from the same center in Mexico City (3,18). In the retrospective study, fetal loss amounted to 40.5% (3). In the prospective study of 102 pregnancies, Mintz et al. used close maternal disease surveillance, with appropriate therapeutic intervention when needed, treatment of every pregnant woman with a minimum of 10 mg of prednisone per day, frequent obstetric follow-up of fetal development, early detection of fetal distress with immediate cesarean section, and utilization of newborn intensive care units: fetal wastage diminished to almost one half, 22.5% (18). In their prospective study, Wong et al. (24) used similar procedures as Mintz et al., but higher doses of prednisone: fetal wastage was only 10.5% (2 of 19). In recent studies, there is a trend away from such steroid "prophylaxis."

Elective (Induced, Therapeutic) Abortions

Elective (induced or therapeutic) abortions in lupus pregnancies are reported as high as 34% from Hong Kong (24), 25% from Toronto (9), 21% from Vancouver (17), and as low as 0% from Mexico City (18). In the US series, the prevalence ranges from 10% to 24% (14,16). These worldwide variations are probably a result of different local legislation regarding elective abortion, patient attitudes and socioeconomic setting, and physician attitudes, sophistication, and level of comfort with lupus pregnancy.

In certain early reports (13,143,144) therapeutic abortion was followed by severe flare of SLE, at times by death of the mother, or it failed to induce remission. More recently, the experience has been that patients tolerate the procedure, and that disease activity improves with corticosteroid or other treatment. Pistiner et al. reported 106 elective abortions in 634 pregnancies among 227 women with lupus, without ill effects (25). When appropriate, vigorous steroid treatment, rather than induced abortion, is medically indicated for suppression of disease activity during pregnancy. If an elective abortion is indicated for psychologic or social reasons, a careful evaluation of SLE activity should be undertaken, and steroid dosage adjusted accordingly before the procedure.

Prematurity (Preterm Birth) (Table 48.1)

Prematurity, or preterm birth generally is defined as birth before week 37 of gestation. Before 1980, the prematurity rate, defined as the percentage of premature infants among total neonates, was 15.3%, or 119 premature and 656 term births. The lowest rate was 6% (145), and the highest, 31% and 30% (13,146).

Thirteen of the 16 series in the 1980s contained adequate data on prematurity (4,8–16,18–20): of 508 pregnancies, 109 (21.4%) ended in preterm birth, which ranged from a low of 4% (11) to a high of 63% (18). In the 1990s, 16 of 20 series contained information on prematurity (23, 24,26–29,32,34–42): preterm birth ranged from a low of 16.7% (41) to 64% (42), with a mean of 33.3%. In the two series of 2,000, prematurity is quite disparate, 5% (43) and 48.7% (44).

In general, preterm birth trends have been increasing and are expected to increase further, as problems are identified on testing that lead to induction of preterm delivery. The authors believe that advances in maternal-fetal medicine are saving babies who would otherwise be lost as IUFDs or neonatal deaths.

Several authors have associated preterm births with active maternal lupus during pregnancy, including nephritis, active lupus during conception, APL antibodies, and maternal thromboxane B2, while others have not. Maternal preeclampsia, a known cause of prematurity, is discussed in Chapter 47. In addition, preterm, premature rupture of membranes (145) and steroid therapy (132) have been incriminated.

Maternal Lupus Activity, Nephritis, Hypertension, Corticosteroids

There are equal reports incriminating maternal SLE activity as a cause of prematurity (2,5,10,20,28,29,34), and as many consider prematurity unrelated to SLE flares (4,12,18,23, 24,31,42). For example, Petri et al. correlated preterm delivery with lupus activity (measured by physician's assessment, prednisone requirement, and low C3), and with hypertension (28). Of the ten preterm births in Oviasu's series, nine occurred in patients with the more severe forms of nephritis (26). In a prospective study from France, 48 of 94 pregnancies (51%) resulted in preterm births, which correlated with a history of fetal loss, active lupus at pregnancy onset, prednisone requirement of >20 mg/day, and hypertension (34). On the other hand, in the prospective study from Mexico City, there was no statistically significant difference between 68.1% premature births in active disease, and 48.7% in inactive SLE (18).

Rahman et al., in a study of 121 pregnancies, showed that hypertension predicted prematurity and IUGR (23.8% preterm and IUGR babies with, vs. 6.6% in nonhypertensive mothers), while active nephritis predicted fetal loss (13.4% live births with, vs. 33% without active nephritis) (38). In a study from Spain, hypertension occurred in half of the ten pregnancies with, vs. 11.6% of 43 pregnancies without nephritis, and nephritis was significantly associated with lower gestational age at delivery, 35.9 vs. 37.3 weeks (39).

In 66 lupus pregnancies reported by Johnson et al., premature rupture of membranes occurred in 39% of premature deliveries, and in 30.3% of term deliveries, and was the major cause of prematurity (147).

Very importantly, the role of steroid therapy in the cause of prematurity has been clarified by Laskin et al. (132): of 202 women with unexplained recurrent fetal loss, positive autoantibodies and no lupus, 101 were randomized to received ASA 100 mg/day and steroid, 0.5 to 0.8/mg/kg/day, and the remaining 101 patients, placebo. In the treatment group, preterm delivery occurred in 62% of patients, compared to 12% in the placebo group.

Therefore, premature birth is associated with maternal hypertension, premature rupture of membranes, and steroid therapy. SLE activity and nephritis appear to be important, but their role needs to be further clarified.

Antiphospholipid Antibodies And Preterm Birth

Several reports find increased preterm births in pregnancies of APL-positive women (90,116,122,148,166). In two studies, there was no correlation of preterm birth with maternal APL (27,31).

The role of maternal thromboxane (TBX2) production in preterm delivery has been investigated in 606 healthy women during their first pregnancy, who were assigned to take either aspirin, 60 mg/day, or placebo. A twofold or greater reduction in maternal serum TXB2 was associated with significantly less preterm delivery (5.7% vs. 10.7%) (149).

In summary, although there is no complete unanimity in the reported series, premature births are commonplace in lupus and tend to be associated with steroid therapy, and hypertension during pregnancy, preeclampsia, and premature rupture of membranes. The significance of APL antibodies, active maternal disease, and active nephritis as factors in preterm birth await further documentation.

Intrauterine Growth Restriction

Both birth and fetal weight are normally a function of the gestational age of the newborn or fetus, and growth curves have been developed to show this relationship (150). When weight is below the norm for gestational age, the condition has been alternatively called intrauterine growth restriction, small newborn for gestational age, or intrauterine malnutrition. By convention, IUGR means that weight is below the tenth percentile for gestational age. Very often, premature babies have low birth weight or IUGR.

Not all reports of SLE pregnancy have this information. From 1980 to 1989, five studies offered IUGR information (4,13–15,18): overall IUGR was present in 26.8% of pregnancies, with a range of 10% to 35%. In the 1990s, eight of 20 studies found overall 17.2% IUGR in 493 pregnancies (range, 7% to 31%) (24,26,29,35,38–41). In the two studies from 2000, IUGR was found in 4.1% and 28.2% (43,44).

IUGR often is associated with preterm birth: 66% of premature neonates had IUGR, compared to 28% of the term neonates (4); there was no apparent relationship to maternal disease activity. In the study by Mintz et al., 30% of the premature newborns had IUGR, compared to only 14% of the term neonates (18). This difference is statistically significant, and was associated with survival of the term neonates. In the study by Le-Thi-Huong, IUGR correlated with pregnancy of short duration, hypertension, low serum C3 or C4, and absence of anti-Ro/SSA antibodies (34).

Several publications point out the association of low birth weight and IUGR with maternal APL antibodies (93, 110,114–116,122,125). In fact, Caruso et al. found that birth weight was significantly lower when three tests were positive for APL [LAC, ACL, and Venereal Disease Research Laboratories (VDRL)] (122). In a study of 22 patients with IUGR and 43 healthy pregnant controls, ACL binding index was significantly higher in the former (151).

Out et al. found significantly lower birth weight in the APL-positive patients, but no difference in prevalence of IUGR between APL-positive and APL-negative women (24% vs. 21%) (70).

Treatment of APL-related recurrent pregnancy loss with antithrombotic therapy is associated with increased birth weight and reversal of IUGR: when Semprini et al. treated 14 recurrent aborters with heparin and prednisone, achieving a 64% rate of live births compared to 3.7% before treatment, the prevalence of low birth weight was reduced from 44% to 12% (114). Wallenburg and Rotmans treated 24 women with prior IUGR with low-dose aspirin and dipyridamole after 16 weeks' gestation, with reduction of fetal growth restriction to 13% in treated versus 61% in untreated pregnancies (152).

The role of maternal thromboxane B2 (TXB2) in IUGR was addressed by a study of 606 women in their first pregnancy, who were assigned to take either aspirin, 60 mg/day, or placebo. A twofold or greater reduction in TXB2 was associated with significantly less IUGR (2.9% vs. 7%) (149).

In summary, APL antibodies are emerging as an important factor in low fetal birth weight. There is also a clear trend toward greater IUGR in premature newborns, which, in some studies, tends to be associated with active maternal lupus.

Live Births

The overall proportion of live births in systemic lupus pregnancies (success rate) has varied from a low of 48% to a high of 89% (Table 48.1). In the 1950s mean live births were 72.5%, in the 1960s, 73%, in the 1970s, 72.1%, in the 1980s, 74.9%, and in the 1990s, 80.8%. The rate for cesarean sections in lupus births is as high as 44% to 89% (26,29,148,153). The major indication for cesarean section is fetal distress.

Pathogenesis Of Adverse Fetal Outcome

The nearly triple than normal prevalence of fetal loss and increased IUGR in systemic lupus has puzzled clinicians and investigators alike. Several findings from serologic and placental studies have been reported, and mechanisms have been proposed. All information available converges on APL antibodies being responsible for fetal loss. An interesting recent observation concerns the finding of increased antibodies against oxidized, low-density lipoprotein (ox-LDL) in lupus pregnancy and their predictive value for adverse fetal outcome (154). In 36 lupus pregnancies, increased anti-ox-LDL were found in the second and third trimester (29% and 19%, respectively): both were significantly associated with IUGR and preterm birth; in the second trimester, there was also association with preeclampsia, lupus flare, including nephritis and vasculitis, and hypertension. Elevation in the third trimester was associated with fetal distress. The authors suggest that elevated anti–ox-LDL may reflect increased lipid peroxidation, and be a marker for vascular damage, as in that which occurs in placental vessels.

Placental Studies

There are at least 20 reports concerning placentae of patients with lupus or APL syndrome (67,109,155–172). The largest studies were reported by Out et al. (161), Magid et al. (166), and Ogishima et al. (167), comprising 47, 40, and 47 placentae respectively.

Common findings in most studies include low placental weight, infarction [at times extensive (>20%)], thrombosis, ischemic-hypoxic change, decidual vasculopathy with fibrinoid change and atherosis, and chronic villitis. The majority of these studies had patients with SLE and APL, or just with APL syndrome (65,109,161–167,169–171). Magid et al. distinguished the following clinical risks and placental changes in SLE without APL: abortions, prematurity, and fetal growth restriction (IUGR), and corresponding placentae had decreased weight, ischemic-hypoxic change, decidual vasculopathy, decidual and fetal thrombi, and chronic villitis of implied unknown etiology; in SLE with APL there was fetal death in addition to abortions, prematurity, and IUGR, and placentae had extensive infarction, in addition to decreased weight, ischemic-hypoxic change, and decidual vasculopathy (166). Placental changes and adverse fetal events were not deemed to correlate with maternal SLE activity. Ogishima et al. noted the most severe placental infarctions, decidual vasculopathy, thrombosis, and fetal death to be associated with double APL positivity for ACL and LAC (167).

Interesting immunofluorescence and elution studies have been performed on lupus placentae with or without APL: granular IgG, C3, and fibrinogen deposits on placental vessels and stroma were found in five placentae (155), and linear and "tramline" deposits on trophoblast basement membranes, as described in normal placentae (173,174); in one patient with lupus nephritis and high DNA binding, granular deposits of IgG and C3 on the trophoblast membrane diminished appreciably after incubation with deoxyribonuclease (DNAse); another placental eluate had antinuclear antibody (ANA) activity. Large IgG, massive vascular IgM, and C3 deposits were found in decidual vasculopathy areas (156,157). Guzman et al. described ANA-like nuclear staining by IgG in five of five placentae, C3 in two, and IgG deposits along the amniotic membranes in a lupus band-like pattern (160). Hanly et al. found deposition of IgG and C3 in one SLE placenta and in a woman with positive ANA, anti-Ro/SSA, and anti-La/SSB, whose both pregnancies resulted in children with complete heart block (67). Erlendsson's two patients with SLE, LAC, ACL, and false-positive VDRL had very small, infarcted placentae with immunoglobulin deposition, necrotizing arteritis, severe IUGR, and fetal death; after treatment with low-dose ASA and 40 mg prednisone/day, they had successful pregnancies with minimal placental changes on biopsy (162). In La Rosa et al.'s study, beta-2 glycoprotein I, a natural anticoagulant and cofactor for APL antibodies, was found increased on the placental trophoblast surfaces of patients with persistently high APL titers, along with IgG deposition (163). IgG, IgM, IgA, C3, and fibrinogen deposits were found in the trophoblast membrane of nine placentae (168).

Two studies reported elution of APL from placentae of women with recurrent fetal loss (164,165). Chamley et al. eluted IgG ACL, ANA, and beta 2-glycoprotein I from placentae of four women with high serum ACL (164); beta-2 GP I was localized in syncytiotrophoblast.

Katano et al. eluted five types of APL from seven placentae of patients with IgG APL (three also had IgM APL) and a history of at least two fetal losses (165). One patient had SLE, and all were treated with prednisolone and aspirin. Only IgG APL were eluted from four of seven placentae, most commonly antiphosphatidyl inositol and antiphosphatidyl serine. Cord blood was negative for any APL. Fetal outcome was, one IUFD, four IUGR, and two neonates of normal weight. Infarcts and fibrinoid deposits were present in six of seven placentae, degeneration necrosis in four, and thrombosis in three. The number of pathological findings seemed to correlate inversely with placental and fetal birth weight (165).

A variety of cell-adhesion molecules was found in placentae from SLE and APL syndrome, not unlike the distribution in controls (170).

Striking decidual vasculopathy and extensive villous infarction occurred in the placenta of a first trimester miscarriage in a lupus patient with ACL (IgM and IgG) and lupus anticogulant (169).

The deposition of immunoglobulins, complement, anti-DNA, and ANA in the placenta, and in areas of vasculopathy/vasculitis, suggests that bland clotting is not the only mechanism of placental hypoperfusion and ischemia, and, hence, fetal ischemia, and that an immune-mediated mechanism may be at play as well.

Studies On Prostacyclin And Thromboxane

It is not entirely clear how antiphospholipid antibodies promote intravascular cloting. Proposed mechanisms include, inhibition of protein C, of antithrombin III, of beta2GPI, displacement of annexin V, and interference with the prostacyclin (PGI_2)/thromboxane (TXB2) balance. (175). Prostacyclin is a potent inhibitor of platelet aggregation, is produced by placental endothelium and human pregnant myometrium, is increased in human fetal vessels, and is considered an important regulator of fetal circulation. A balance in placental production of prostacyclin and thromboxane is considered essential for the changes in placental vessels necessary to allow trophoblast ingrowth. Indeed, preeclampsia seems to occur as a response to placental ischemia, with exaggerated placental production of thromboxane A2, and normal or deficient prostacyclin production (176,177).

Several studies point out that prostacyclin production is normal or increased, while thromboxane production is greatly exaggerated in patients with APL. In a controlled study of 14 pregnant lupus patients, Kaaja et al. demonstrated that prostacyclin metabolite excretion was normal in early pregnancy, but reduced during late pregnancy in women without APL (178). In women with APL, prostacyclin metabolites were increased in early pregnancy, and more so (approximately 140% of normal) during the second half of pregnancy. Thromboxane production (as measured by thromboxane B2 and 2,3-dinor-thromboxane B2), was increased in lupus patients, especially when APL positive and in the second half of the pregnancy. Therapy with aspirin, 50 mg per day, decreased thromboxane production, and did not affect prostacyclin production, resulting in an increased ratio of prostacyclin to thromboxane in the treated patients. Dudley et al. had found that baseline serum concentration of 6-keto-prostaglandin F1a, a metabolite of prostacyclin, was fourfold higher in APL-positive women, and that APL-positive serum did not impair production of prostacyclin by intact or damaged endothelium (179).

In a series of elegant studies, Peaceman and Rehnberg showed that placental explants from normal pregnancies, incubated with IgG fractions of LAC-positive serum, showed similar to baseline prostacyclin production, while thromboxane production was increased significantly (180). A subsequent study by the same authors showed that, in the same *in vitro* system, addition of 10^{-4} aspirin did not affect prostacyclin production, while it decreased thromboxane production significantly (181). In contrast, addition of indomethacin at 10^{-7} caused significant decreases in the production of both prostacyclin and thromboxane, leaving their ratio unaffected.

Other Antiphospholipid-Related Mechanisms

Giusti et al. have shown that the generation of procoagulant activity by monocytes was significantly increased in 18 women with LAC vs. 17 LAC-negative women, all of whom had recurrent abortions (182). The authors suggest that the beneficial effect of steroid therapy may occur through inhibition of monocyte procoagulant activity.

Another proposed mechanism of action is through cross-reactivity of 11% of ACL antibodies with heparin and heparan sulphate; these ACL may inhibit the heparin-dependent activation of antithrombin III up to 80% (183).

Other Autoantibodies

Other autoantibodies incriminated in fetal loss include lymphocytotoxic antibodies (137–140) and anti-Ro/SSA antibodies (see above).

Summary Of Pathogenesis Of Fetal Loss

Fetal loss in lupus patients is strongly related to maternal APL antibodies, with associated placental changes of small size with infarcts, hematomas, decidual vasculopathy or vasculitis with thrombosis, thickened trophoblast membrane, and immune deposits. The mechanisms seem to involve exaggerated thromboxane production and decrease of the ratio of prostacyclin to thromboxane, which may bring about platelet aggregation with intravascular thrombosis, resulting in conditions of relative ischemia for the fetus: this can at least in part explain the intrauterine growth restriction so common in this disease, and in APL patients without lupus. Interestingly, in three patients, cordocentesis showed predominantly metabolic acidosis than fetal hypoxia (155). Other autoantibodies as anti-DNA and anti-Ro/SSA may be contributing factors. Anti-DNA antibodies cross-reacting with laminin have been proposed as inhibitors of trophoblast attachment and migration, thus potentially implicated in early pregnancy loss (184).

PREGNANCY MANAGEMENT FOR OPTIMAL FETAL SURVIVAL

The value of multidisciplinary care, careful maternal and fetal monitoring, and judicious use of surgical delivery were amply demonstrated in the retrospective and prospective studies from Mexico City, where fetal wastage was reduced by almost half, from 40.5% to 22.5% (3,18). Modern obstetrics and neonatology offer tremendous advantages in fetal surveillance. Fetal ultrasound, Doppler studies of blood flow of the uterine and umbilical arteries (122,148, 153,185–188), the modified biophysical profile (189), fetal echocardiography (190,191), nonstress test (192,193) and contaction stress test (194) represent tremendous advances in obstetrical practice.

Early in the pregnancy, fetal ultrasound is used for accurate gestational dating, and for assessment of the growth of the fetus. Throughout pregnancy, ultrasound is used to assess fetal growth. In the third trimester, ultrasonic grading of placental maturity can predict fetal well being, with a grade 3 placenta foretelling low birth weight and even perinatal death (195). Evaluation and monitoring of the uterine and umbilical arterial blood flow by Doppler velocimetry or waveforms has an important place in the early (122, 141), and the third trimester evaluation of lupus pregnancies (153).

Kerslake et al. studied 56 pregnancies in 52 women with lupus and two with APL syndrome from the 14th week of gestation (148). Absence of umbilical-end, diastolic blood flow at 20 weeks' gestation with a surviving fetus, predicted early delivery with cesarean section; the presence of end diastolic blood flow and absence of ACL was consistent with a normotensive pregnancy, while the LAC predicted fetal death. In the study by Guzman et al., Doppler velocimetry was started at the first prenatal visit in 27 lupus pregnancies (185). Normal blood flow velocity in both arteries was associated with normal outcome in 18 pregnancies; reduced flow of the umbilical artery in five pregnancies predicted prematurity and low birth weight, and reduced flow velocity in both arteries had the worst outcome, with three of four perinatal losses and IUGR. Preeclampsia and active lupus nephritis was present in all nine women with abnormal velocimetry. Adams et al. initiated testing with all of the above parameters in 66 lupus pregnancies at the 20th to 26th week, and found that 21 complicated lupus pregnancies had lower birth weight and delivery without labor than 45 uncomplicated pregnancies (153). In 28 pregnancies with the lupus anticoagulant, IUGR was present in five of six fetuses with abnormal umbilical systolic/diastolic Doppler ratios, two of which also had abnormal uterine artery ratios; most of these also had nonreactive stress tests and abnormal biophysical profiles (186).

The biophysical profile consists of real-time ultrasonography, during which the fetal tone, movements, breathing movements, and amniotic fluid volume are scored; a nonstress test follows and a score of zero to ten is assigned, ten being optimal (189). At our institution, the modified biophysical profile is performed (196), which includes the nonstress test and amniotic fluid index, with the full biophysical profile as a back-up (194).

Fetal echocardiography is important for the detection of bradycardia, as in congenital heart block, fetal pericarditis, and myocarditis (191).

The mainstay of antepartum fetal heart testing is the nonstress test. During normal intrauterine fetal movement, the fetal heart accelerates. Failure to accelerate constitutes a nonreactive, or abnormal nonstress test. The earlier the gestational age, the greater the percentage of nonreactive nonstress tests: nonstress test is most meaningful after the 28th week of gestation (193). Fetal bradycardia during the nonstress test is associated with the risk of fetal distress during labor (190), and nonperiodic fetal heart decelerations at 20 to 28 weeks may detect the fetus at risk for intrauterine death (197).

The contraction stress test has been abandoned as cumbersome and difficult to perform.

Recommendations

The following are recommendations for management of lupus pregnancy to optimize fetal survival and diminish loss.

Mother

1. As recommended in Chapter 47, maternal disease should be assessed carefully for activity and severity at the outset of pregnancy, which ideally should be planned after 6 to 12 months of remission. The mother should be watched carefully for SLE flares.
2. Maternal flares should be diagnosed early and treated aggressively, depending upon severity, with appropriate steroid dose. Unless there is a dire emergency, i.e., acute anuric renal failure, cytotoxic drugs should be avoided during the first trimester. Mothers with nephritis at risk for hypertension and preeclampsia should be treated with low-dose aspirin (60 to 81 mg/day) until the 36th week of gestation, or until 1 week prior to delivery (to avoid excess bleeding).
3. The mother's status in terms of APL, and anti-Ro/SSA, anti-La/SSB positivity should be known; the former, because of predisposition to fetal loss and IUGR, and the latter two because of the small risk for congenital heart block in the child (see also Chapter 50, Lupus Nephritis: Pathology, Pathogenesis, Clinical Correlations, and Prognosis).
4. Joint follow-up by the rheumatologist and obstetrician should be done every month for the first half of pregnancy, and more frequently thereafter (every 1 to 3 weeks), with repeat of CBC, urine, chemistry, quantitation of proteinuria in patients with nephritis, complement C3 and C4 levels, anti-dsDNA, and a measure of circulating immune complexes on a monthly basis. The asymptomatic patient with normal initial tests may have lab testing every 3 months. Blood pressure should be monitored very carefully.
5. In the event of high-positive APL antibody, especially of the IgG class, or with a "double positive" for APL (both ACL and LAC positive), the patient should be enrolled in an effective antithrombotic protocol as soon as pregnancy is confirmed.

For women with prior pregnancy complications, but no thrombosis: subcutaneous enoxaparin (SC) 0.5mg/kg twice daily, calcium supplementation at 1.5 g daily and axial weight-bearing exercise or, unfractionated heparin, 10,000 IU subcutaneously twice daily, calcium, and exercise.

For women who have clotted previously, or prior fetal loss: SC enoxaparin 1 mg/kg twice daily, or adjusted dose of unfractionated heparin SC to prolong the PTT to two, 6 hours after the morning dose; all regimens are accompanied by daily low-dose aspirin.

6. Steroid stress doses should be given at the time of delivery, be it vaginal or by cesarean. Unless there is concomittant lupus activity, high-dose prednisone for APL alone should not be given, except as steroid prep.

Fetus

1. Accurate gestational dating is important because of the frequent IUGR and premature births in SLE. Menstrual dating should be confirmed by ultrasonography at the first prenatal visit.
2. Ultrasound evaluation of the growth of the fetus should be performed monthly. Delayed growth indicates an increased risk of fetal death in *utero* and should prompt a search for evidence of increased disease activity, or developing superimposed PIH. Doppler of the umbilical artery and middle cerebral artery is employed liberally at the time of the ultrasound for fetal growth.
3. In the event of positive anti-Ro/SSA and/or anti-La/SSB, fetal heart tones should be checked for 1 minute at every visit after the 16th week of gestation. Any abnormal heart rhythm should prompt a detailed fetal echocardiography to rule out developing heart block.
4. Antepartum testing for fetal well-being should be initiated between 24 and 34 weeks' gestation. In patients at highest risk, such as those with a history of fetal compromise, active SLE, or positive for both ACL and LAC, testing should be initiated near the cusp of viability, at 24 weeks. Those with quiescent who are APL and anti-Ro/SSA negative, may start testing at about 34 weeks with the modified biophysical profile (196). When testing is initiated before 32 weeks, the value of the nonstress test is to detect a change in serial testing, or to detect spontaneous deceleration. Umbilical artery doppler is used whenever low amniotic fluid volume, or fetal-growth restriction is suspected. Decreased amniotic fluid may presage IUGR or cord accidents leading to stillbirth.
5. An abnormal fetal heart tracing, or an amniotic-fluid index <5 cm is almost always an indication for prompt delivery, usually by cesarean section. When delivery is planned before 34 weeks gestation, it is our practice to administer precesarean and intraoperative, long-acting steroids (dexamethasone or betamethasone) to enhance fetal maturity (197).

Other drugs should be used with great care. Maternal thiazide diuretic therapy generally is safe in late pregnancy and rarely has been associated with severe neonatal thrombocytopenia (198). ACE inhibitors should not be used late in pregnancy because fetal and neonatal hypotension, anuria, and even renal failure may occur (198). For more information on antirheumatic drugs in pregnancy and lactation, see the section on use of medications in Chapter 47. As mentioned in that chapter, prednisone, prednisolone, and methylprednisolone are oxidized by placental enzymes, while dexamethasone and betamethasone are not and are utilized to treat fetus *in utero.*

Under dire circumstances, unusual and unconventional therapeutic interventions may be appropriate during pregnancy such as intravenous cyclophosphamide for maternal anuric renal failure, or intravenous gamma globulin for maternal SLE or fetal reasons.

It is reassuring to note that in over 2,800 lupus pregnancies reported in the last 45 years (Table 48.1), there were very few cases of congenital malformations, with the exception of congenital heart block (see Chapter 50, Lupus Nephritis: Pathology, Pathogenesis, Clinical Correlations, and Prognosis). These figures include infants whose mothers were on cytotoxic medications, mainly azathioprine and cyclophosphamide. Details are mentioned in Chapter 47.

REFERENCES

1. Cecere FA, Persellin RH. The interaction of pregnancy and the Rheumatic diseases. *Clin Rheum Dis* 1981;7:747–768.
2. Estes D, Larson DL. Systemic lupus erythematosus and pregnancy. *Clin Obstet Gynecol* 1965;8:307–321.
3. Fraga A, Mintz G, Orozco J, et al. Sterility and fertility rates, fetal wastage and maternal morbidity in systemic lupus erythematosus. *J Rheumatol* 1974;1:293–298.
4. Gimovsky ML, Montoro M, Paul RH. Pregnancy outcome in women with systemic lupus erythematosus. *Obstet Gynecol* 1984; 63:686–692.
5. Jungers P, Dougados M, Pelissier C, et al. Lupus nephropathy and pregnancy. *Arch Intern Med* 1982;142:771–776.
6. Kaufman RL, Kitridou RC. Pregnancy in mixed connective tissue disease: comparison with systemic lupus erythematosus. *J Rheumatol* 1982;9:549–555.
7. Mund A, Simson J, Rothfield NF. Effect of pregnancy on course of systemic lupus erythematosus. *JAMA* 1963;183:917–922.
8. Siamopoulou-Mavridou A, Manoussakis MN, Mavridis AK, et al. Outcome of pregnancy in patients with autoimmune rheumatic diseases before the disease onset. *Ann Rheum Dis* 1988;47:982–987.
9. Tozman ECS, Urowitz MB, Gladman DD. Systemic lupus erythematosus and pregnancy. *J Rheumatol* 1980;7:624–632.
10. Houser MT, Fish AJ, Tagatz GE, et al. Pregnancy and systemic lupus erythematosus. *Am J Obstet Gynecol* 1980;138:409–413.
11. Zulman JI, Talal N, Hoffman GS, et al. Problems associated with the management of pregnancies in patients with systemic lupus erythematosus. *J Rheumatol* 1980;7:37–49.
12. Hayslett JP, Lynn RI. Effect of pregnancy in patients with lupus nephropathy. *Kidney Int* 1980;18:207–220.
13. Fine LG, Barnett EV, Danovitch GM, et al. Systemic lupus erythematosus in pregnancy. *Ann Intern Med* 1981;94:667–677.
14. Varner MW, Meehan RT, Syrop CH, et al. Pregnancy in patients with systemic lupus erythematosus. *Am J Obstet Gynecol* 1982;145:1025–1040.
15. Imbasciati E, Surian M, Bottino S, et al. Lupus nephropathy and pregnancy. *Nephron* 1984;36:46–51.
16. Lockshin MD, Reinitz E, Druzin ML, et al. Lupus pregnancy. Case-control prospective study demonstrating absence of lupus exacerbation during or after pregnancy. *Am J Med* 1984;77: 893–898.
17. Stein H, Walters K, Dillon A, et al. Systemic lupus erythematosus: a medical and social profile. *J Rheumatol* 1986;13:570–576.
18. Mintz G, Niz J, Gutierrez G, et al. Prospective study of pregnancy in systemic lupus erythematosus. Results of a multidisciplinary approach. *J Rheumatol* 1986;13:732–739.
19. Meehan RT, Dorsey JK. Pregnancy among patients with systemic lupus erythematosus receiving immunosuppressive therapy. *J Rheumatol* 1987;14:252–258.
20. Bobrie G, Liote F, Houllier P, et al. Pregnancy in lupus nephritis and related disorders. *Am J Kidney Dis* 1987;9:339–343.
21. McHugh NJ, Reilly PA, McHugh LA. Pregnancy outcome and autoantibodies in connective tissue disease. *J Rheumatol* 1989; 16:42–46.
22. Lockshin MD. Pregnancy does not cause systemic lupus erythematosus to worsen. *Arthritis Rheum* 1989;32:665–670.
23. Nossent HC, Swaak TJG. Systemic lupus erythematosus. VI. Analysis of the interrelationship with pregnancy. *J Rheumatol* 1990;17:771–776.
24. Wong KL, Chan FY, Lee CHP. Outcome of pregnancy in patients with systemic lupus erythematosus. *Arch Intern Med* 1991;151:2690–2273.
25. Pistiner M, Wallace DJ, Nessim S, et al. Lupus erythematosus in the 1980s: a survey of 570 patients. *Semin Arthritis Rheum* 1991;21:55–64.
26. Oviasu E, Hicks J, Cameron JS. The outcome of pregnancy in women with lupus nephritis. *Lupus* 1991;1:19–25.
27. Packham DK, Lam SS, Nicholls K, et al. Lupus nephritis and pregnancy. *Q J Med* 1992;300:315–324.
28. Petri M, Howard D, Repke J, et al. The Hopkins Lupus Pregnancy Center: 1987–1991 update. *Am J Reprod Immunol* 1992;28:188–191.
29. Tincani A, Faden D, Tarantini M, et al. Systemic Lupus erythematosus and pregnancy: a prospective study. *Clin Exper Rheumatol* 1992;10:439–446.
30. TambyRaja RL. Fetal salvage in maternal systemic lupus erythematosus. *Ann Acad Med Singapore* 1993;22:634–637.
31. Julkunen H, Jouhikainen T, Kaaja R, et al. Fetal outcome in lupus pregnancy: a prospective case-control study of 242 pregnancies in 112 patients. *Lupus* 1993;2:125–131.
32. Petri M, Albritton J. Fetal outcome of lupus pregnancy: a retrospective case-control study of the Hopkins lupus cohort. *J Rheumatol* 1993;20:650–656.
33. Derksen RH, Bruinse HW, deGroot PG, et al. Pregnancy in systemic lupus erythematosus: a prospective study. *Lupus* 1994;3: 149–155.
34. Le-Thi-Huong D, Wechsler B, Piette JC, et al. *Q j Med* 1994; 87:721–729.
35. Lima F, Buchanan NM, Khamashta MA, et al. Obstetric Outcome in systemic lupus erythematosus. *Semin Arthritis Rheum* 1995;25:184–192.
36. Le Huong D, Wechsler B, Vauthier-Brouzes D, et al. Outcome of planned pregnancies in systemic lupus erythematosus: a prospective study of 62 pregnancies. *Br J Rheumatol* 1997;36: 772–777.
37. Johns KR, Morand EF, Littlejohn GO. Pregnancy outcome in systemic lupus erythematosus (SLE): a review of 54 cases. *Aust NZJ Med* 1998;28:18–22.
38. Rahman P, Gladman DD, Urowitz MB. Clinical predictors of fetal outcome in systemic lupus erythematosus. *J Rheumatol* 1998;25:1526–1530.

39. Carmona F, Font J, Cervera R, et al. Obstetrical outcome of pregnancy in patients with systemic lupus erythematosus. *Eur J Obstet Gynecol* 1999;83:137–142.
40. Sittiwangkul S, Louthrenoo W, Vithayasai P, et al. Pregnancy outcome in Thai patients with systemic lupus erythematosus. *Asian Pac J Aller Immun* 1999;17:77–83.
41. Kobayashi N, Yamada H, Kishida T, et al. Hypocomplementemia correlates with intraterine growth retardation in systemic lupus erythematosus. *Am J Reprod Immun* 1999;42:153–159.
42. Huong Du LT, Wechsler B, Vauthier-Brouzes D, et al. Pregnancy in women with past or current history of lupus nephritis. *Arthritis & Rheum* 1998;41:S66.
43. Georgiou PE, Politi EN, Katsimbri P, et al. Outcome of lupus pregnancy: a controlled study. *Rheumatology* 2000;39: 1014–1019.
44. De Bandt M, Palazzo E, Belmatoug N, et al. Outcome of pregnancies in lupus: experience at one center. *Annales de Med Interne* 2000;151:87–92.
45. Thomas MM, Tischer CC, Robinson RR. Influence of pregnancy on lupus nephritis. *Kidney Int* 1978;14:665.
46. Liang MH, Socher SA, Larson MG, et al. Reliability and validity of six systems for the clinical assessment of disease activity in systemic lupus erythematosus. *Arthritis Rheum* 1989;32: 1107–1118.
47. Petri M, Hellmann D, Hochberg M. Validity and reliability of lupus activity measures in the routine clinic setting. *J Rheumatol* 1992;19:53–59.
48. Buyon JP, Kalunian KC, Ramsey-Goldman R, et al. Assessing disease activity in SLE patients during pregnancy. *Lupus* 1999; 8:677–684.
49. Nilsson IM, Astedt B, Hedner U, et al. Intrauterine death and circulating anticoagulant ("antithromboplastin"). *Acta Med Scand* 1975;197:153–159.
50. Firkin BG, Howard MA, Radford N. Possible relationship between lupus inhibitor and recurrent abortion in young women [letter]. *Lancet* 1980;2:366.
51. Soulier JP, Boffa MC. Avortements a repetition, thrombose et anticoagulant circulant anti-thromboplastine. *Nouv Presse Med* 1980;9:859–864.
52. Boey ML, Colaco CB, Gharavi AE, et al. Thrombosis in systemic lupus erythematosus: striking association with the presence of circulating lupus anticoagulant. *Br Med J [Clin Res]* 1983;287:1021–1023.
53. Elias M, Eldor A. Thromboembolism in patients with the 'lupus'-type circulating anticoagulant. *Arch Intern Med* 1984; 144:510–515.
54. Colaco CB, Elkon KB. The lupus anticoagulant. A disease marker in antinuclear antibody negative lupus that is cross-reactive with autoantibodies to double-stranded DNA. *Arthritis Rheum* 1985;28:67–74.
55. Harris EN, Chan JK, Asherson RA, et al. Thrombosis, recurrent fetal loss, and thrombocytopenia. Predictive value of the anticardiolipin antibody test. *Arch Intern Med* 1986;146: 2153–2156.
56. Petri M, Rheinschmidt M, Whiting-O'Keefe Q, et al. The frequency of lupus anticoagulant in systemic lupus erythematosus. A study of sixty consecutive patients by activated partial thromboplastin time, Russel viper venom time, and anticardiolipin antibody level. *Ann Intern Med* 1987;106:524–531.
57. Fort JG, Cowchock FS, Abruzzo JL, et al. Anticardiolipin antibodies in patients with rheumatic diseases. *Arthritis Rheum* 1987;30:752–760.
58. Kalunian KC, Peter JB, Middlekauff HR, et al. Clinical significance of a simple test for anti-cardiolipin antibodies in patients with systemic lupus erythematosus. *Am J Med* 1988;85:602–608.
59. Gharavi AE, Harris EN, Lockshin MD, et al. IgG subclass and light chain distribution of anticardiolipin and anti-DNA antibodies in systemic lupus erythematosus. *Ann Rheum Dis* 1988; 47:286–290.
60. Deleze M, Alarcon-Segovia D, Valdes-Macho E, et al. Relationship between antiphospholipid antibodies and recurrent fetal loss in patients with systemic lupus erythematosus and apparently healthy women. *J Rheumatol* 1989;16:768–72.
61. Ishii Y, Nagasawa K, Mayumi T, et al. Clinical importance of persistence of anticardiolipin antibodies in sytemic lupus erythematosus. *Ann Rheum Dis* 1990;49:387–390.
62. Vianna JL, Haga HJ, Pripathi P, et al. Reassessing the status of antiphospholipid syndrome in systemic lupus erythematosus. *Ann Rheum Dis* 1991;51:160–161.
63. Ramsey-Goldman R, Kutzer JE, Kuller LH, et al. Pregnancy outcome and anti-cardiolipin antibody in women with systemic lupus erythematosus. *Am J Epidemiol* 1993;138:1057–1066.
64. Kutteh WH, Lyda EC, Abraham SM, et al. Association of anticardiolipin antibodies and pregnancy loss in women with systemic lupus erythematosus. *Fertil Steril* 1993;60:449–455.
65. Lockshin MD, Druzin ML, Goei S, et al. Antibody to cardiolipin as a predictor of fetal distress or death in pregnant patients with systemic lupus erythematosus. *N Engl J Med* 1985;313:152–156.
66. Lockshin MD, Qamar T, Druzin ML, et al. Antibody to cardiolipin, lupus anticoagulant, and fetal death. *J Rheumatol* 1987; 14:259–262.
67. Hanly JG, Gladman DD, Rose TH, et al. Lupus pregnancy: a prospective study of placental changes. *Arthritis Rheum* 1988; 31:358–66.
68. Englert HJ, Derue GM, Loizou S, et al. Pregnancy and lupus: prognostic indicators and response to treatment. *Q J Med* 1988; 66:125–136.
69. Koskela P, Vaarala O, Makitalo R, et al. Significance of false positive syphilis reactions and anticardiolipin antibodies in a nationwide series of pregnant women. *J Rheumatol* 1988;15:70–73.
70. Out HJ, Bruinse HW, Christiaens Godelieve CML, et al. A prospective, controlled multicenter study on the obstetric risks of pregnant women with antiphospholipid antibodies. *Am J Obstet Gynecol* 1992;167:26–32.
71. Abu-Shakra M, Gladman DD, Urowitz MB, et al. Anticardiolipin antibodies in systemic lupus erythematosus: clinical and laboratory correlations. *Am J Med* 1995;99:624–628.
72. Loizou S, Byron MA, Englert HJ, et al. Association of quantitative anticardiolipin antibody levels with fetal loss and time of loss in systemic lupus erythematosus. *Q J Med* 1988;68:525–531.
73. Cowchock S, Smith JB, Gocial B. Antibodies to phospholipids and nuclear antigens in patients with repeated abortions. *Am J Obstet Gynecol* 1986;155:1002–1010.
74. Ginsberg JS, Brill-Edwards P, Johnston M, et al. Relationship of antiphospholipid antibodies to pregnancy loss in patients with systemic lupus erythematosus: a cross-sectional study. *Blood* 1992;80:975–980.
75. Ninomiya C, Taniguchi O, Kato T, et al. Distribution and clinical significance of lupus anticoagulant and anticardiolipin antibody in 349 patients with systemic lupus erythematosus. *Intern Med* 1992;31:194–199.
76. Lockshin MD, Druzin ML, Qamar MA. Prednisone does not prevent recurrent fetal death in women with antiphospholipid antibody. *Am J Obstet Gynecol* 1989;169:439–443.

76a. Silver RM, Porter TF, van Leeuwen I, et al. Anticardiolipin antibodies: clinical consequences of low titers. *Obstet Gynecol* 1996;87:494–500.

77. Alarcon-Segovia D, Deleze M, Oria CV, et al. Antiphospholipid antibodies and the antiphospholipid syndrome in systemic lupus erythematosus. A prospective analysis of 500 consecutive patients. *Medicine* 1989;68:353–365.

78. Out HJ, de Groot PG, Hasselaar P. Fluctuations of anticardiolipin antibody levels in patients with systemic lupus erythematosus: a prospective study. *Ann Rheum Dis* 1989;48:1023–1028.
79. Lee RM, Emlen W, Scott JR, et al. Anti-beta (2)-glycoprotein I antibodies in women with recurrent spontaneous abortions, unexplained fetal death, and antiphospholipid syndrome. *Am J Obstet Gynecol* 1999;181:642–648.
80. Silver RM, Draper ML, Byrne JL, et al. Unexplained elevations of maternal serum alpha-fetoprotein in women with antiphospholipid antibodies: a harbinger of fetal death. *Obstet Gynecol* 1994;83:150–155.
81. Petri M, Ho AC, Patel J, et al. Elevation of maternal alpha-fetoprotein in systemic lupus erythematosus: a controlled study. *J Rheumatol* 1995;22:1365–1368.
82. Comp PC, Thurnau GR, Welsh J, et al. Functional and immunologic protein S levels are decreased during pregnancy. *Blood* 1986;68:881–885.
83. Vigano-D'Angelo S, D' Angelo A, Kaufman CL Jr, et al. Protein S deficiency occurs in the nephrotic syndrome. *Ann Intern Med* 1987;107:42–47.
84. Rossi E, Gatti L, Guarneri D, et al. Functional protein S in women with lupus anticoagulant inhibitor. *Thrombosis Res* 1992;65:253–262.
85. Parke AL, Weinstein RE, Bona RD, et al. The thrombotic diathesis associated with the presence of phospholipid antibodies may be due to low levels of free protein S. *Amer J Med* 1992; 93:49–56.
86. Korditch LC, Forastiero RR, Basilotta E, et al. Natural inhibitors of blood coagulation and fibrinolysis in patients with lupus anticogulants. *Blood Coagul Fibrinol* 1992;3:765–771.
87. Forastiero RR, Korditch LC, Basilotta E, et al. Differences in protein S and C4b-binding protein levels in different groups of patients with antiphospholipid antibodies. *Blood Coagul Fibrinol* 1994;5:609–616.
88. Amer L, Kisiel W, Searles RP, et al. Impairment of the protein C anticoagulant pathway in a patient with systemic lupus erythematosus, anticardiolipin antibodies and thrombosis. *Thrombosis Res* 1990;57:247–58.
89. Kutteh WH. Antiphospholipid antibodies and reproduction. *J Reprod Immunol* 1997;35:151–171.
90. Lockwood CJ, Romero R, Feinberg RF, et al. The prevalence and biologic significance of lupus anticoagulant and anticardiolipin antibodies in a general obstetric population. *Am J Obstet Gynecol* 1989;161:369–373.
91. Harris EN, Phil M, Spinnato JA. Should anticardiolipin tests be performed in otherwise healthy pregnant women? *Am J Obstet Gynecol* 1991;165:1272–1277.
92. Perez MC, Wilson WA, Brown HL, et al. Anticardiolipin antibodies in unselected pregnant women: relationship to fetal outcome. *J Perinatol* 1991;11:33–36.
93. Rix P, Stentoft J, Aunsholt NA, et al. Lupus anticoagulant and anticardiolipin antibodies in an obstetric population. *Acta Obstet et Gynecol Scand* 1992;71:605–609.
94. Lynch A, Marlar R, Murphy J, et al. Antiphospholipid antibodies in predicting adverse pregnancy outcome. *Ann Intern Med* 1994;120:470–475.
95. Creagh MD, Malia RG, Cooper SM, et al. Screening for lupus anticoagulant and anticardiolipin antibodies in women with fetal loss. *J Clin Pathol* 1991;44:45–47.
96. Parke AN, Wilson D, Maier D. The prevalence of antiphospholipid antibodies in women with recurrent spontaneous abortion, women with successful pregnancies, and women who have never been pregnant. *Arthritis Rheum* 1991;34:1231–1235.
97. MacLean MA, Cumming GP, McCall F, et al. The prevalence of lupus anticoagulant and anticardiolipin antibodies in women with a history of first trimester miscarriages. *Br J Obstet Gynaecol* 1994;101:103–106.
98. Konidaris S, Papadias K, Gregoriou O, et al. Immune dysfunction in patients with unexplained repeated abortions. *Intern J Gynaecol Obstet* 1994;45:221–226.
99. Eroglu GE, Scopelitis E. Antinuclear and antiphospholipid antibodies in healthy women with recurrent spontaneous abortion. *Am J Reprod Immun* 1994;31:1–6.
100. Rai RS, Regan L, Clifford K, et al. Antiphospholipid antibodies and beta-2 glycoprotein I in 500 women with recurrent miscarriage: results of a comprehensive screening approach. *Human Reprod* 1995;10:2001–2005.
101. Balasch J, Font J, Lopez-Soto A, et al. Antiphospholipid antibodies in unselected patients with repeated abortion. *Human Reprod* 1990;5:43–46.
102. Bocciolone L, Meroni P, Parazzini F, et al. Antiphospholipid antibodies and risk of intrauterine late fetal death. *Acta Obstet et Gynecol Scand* 1994;73:389–392.
103. Infante-Rivard C, David M, Gauthier R, et al. Lupus anticoagulants, anticardiolipin antibodies, and fetal loss. A case-control study. *N Engl J Med* 1991;325:1063–1066.
104. Taylor PV, Campbell JM, Scott JS. Presence of autoantibodies in women with unexplained infertility. *Am J Obstet Gynecol* 1989; 161:377–379.
105. Birkenfeld A, Mukaida T, Minichielo L, et al. Incidence of autoimmune antibodies in failed embryo transfer cycles. *AJRI* 1994;31:65–68.
106. Geva E, Yaron Y, Lessing JB, et al. Circulating autoimmune antibodies may be responsible for implantation failure in in vitro fertilization. *Fertil Steril* 1994;62:802–806.
107. Kutteh WH, Yetman DL, Chantilis SJ, et al. Effect of antiphospholipid antibodies in women undergoing in-vitro fertilization: role of heparin and aspirin. *Human Reproduction* 1997;12: 1171–1175.
108. Lubbe WF, Butler WS, Palmer SJ, et al. Fetal survival after prednisone suppression of maternal lupus anticoagulant. *Lancet* 1983;1:1361–1366.
109. Lubbe WF, Butler WS, Palmer SJ, et al. Lupus anticoagulant in pregnancy. *Br J Obstet Gynaecol* 1984;91:357–363.
110. Branch DW, Scott J, Kochenour N, et al. Obstetric complications associated with the lupus anticoagulant. *N Engl J Med* 1985;313:1322–1326.
111. Gatenby PA, Cameron K, Shearman RP. Pregnancy loss with antiphospholipid antibodies: improved outcome with aspirin containing treatment. *Aust N Z J Obstet Gynaecol* 1989;29: 294–298.
112. Ordi J, Barquinero J, Vilardell M, et al. Fetal loss treatment in patients with antiphospholipid antibodies. *Ann Rheum Dis* 1989;48:798–802.
113. Carp HJ, Menashe Y, Frenkel Y, et al. Lupus anticoagulant. Significance in habitual first-trimester abortion. *J Reprod Med* 1993;38:549–552.
114. Semprini AE, Vucetich A, Garbo S, et al. Effect of prednisone and heparin treatment in 14 patients with poor reproductive efficiency related to lupus anticoagulant. *Fetal Ther* 1989;4: 73–76.
115. Rosove MH, Tabsh K, Wasserstrum N, et al. Heparin therapy and prevention of pregnancy loss in women with lupus anticoagulant or anticardiolipin antibodies. *Obstet Gynecol* 1990;75: 630–634.
116. Silveira LH, Hubble CL, Jara JL, et al. Prevention of anticardiolipin antibody-related pregnancy losses with prednisone and aspirin. *Amer J Med* 1992;93:403–411.
117. Buchanan NMM, Khamashta MA, Morton KE, et al. A study of 100 high risk lupus pregnancies. *Amer J Reprod Immunol* 1992;28:192–194.

118. Cowchock SF, Reece EA, Balaban D, et al. Repeated fetal losses associated with antiphospholipid antibodies: a collaborative randomized trial comparing prednisone with low dose heparin treatment. *Am J Obstet Gynecol* 1992;166:1318–1323.
119. Landy HJ, Kessler C, Kelly WK, et al. Obstetric performance in patients with the lupus anticoagulant and/or anticardiolipin antibodies. *Am J Perinatol* 1992;9:146–151.
120. Many A, Pauzner R, Carp H, et al. Treatment of patients with antiphospholipid antibodies during pregnancy. *Am J Reprod Immunol* 1992;28:216–218.
121. Stuart RA, Quinn MJ, McHugh NJ. Combined corticosteroid and aspirin treatment for the high risk lupus pregnancy. *Br J Obstet Gynaecol* 1993;100:601–602.
122. Caruso A, de Carolis S, Ferrazzani S, et al. Pregnancy outcome in relation to uterine artery flow velocity waveforms and clinical characteristics in women with antiphospholid syndrome. *Obstet Gynecol* 1993;82:970–977.
123. Al Momen AKM, Moghraby SA, El-Rab MOG, et al. Pregnancy outocme in women with antiphospholipid antibodies. *Clin Rheumatol* 1993;12:381–386.
124. Balasch J, Carmona F, Lopez-Soto A, et al. Low-dose aspirin for prevention of pregnancy losses in women with primary antiphospholipid syndrome. *Human Reprod* 1993;8:2234–2239.
125. Rossi E, Costa M. Fish oil derivatives as a prophylaxis of recurrent miscarriage associated with antiphospholipid antibodies (APL): a pilot study. *Lupus* 1993;2:319–323.
126. Kaaja R, Julkunen H, Ammalea P, et al. Intravenous immunoglobulin treatment of pregnant patients with recurrent pregnancy losses associated with antiphospholipid antibodies. *Acta Obstet Gynecol Scand* 1993;72:63–66.
127. Spinnato JA, Clark AL, Pierangeli SS, et al. Intravenous immunoglobulin therapy for the antiphospholipid syndrome in pregnancy. *Am J Obstet Gynecol* 1995;172:690–694.
128. Harger JH, Laifer SA, Bontempo FA, et al. Low-Dose aspirin and prednisone treatment of pregnancy loss caused by lupus anticoagulants. *J Perinatol* 1995;15:463–469.
129. Kutteh WH. Antiphospholipid antibodies-associated recurrent pregnancy loss; treatment with heparin and low dose aspirin is superior to low-dose aspirin alone. *Am J Obstet Gynecol* 1996; 174:1584–1589.
130. Kutteh WH, Ermel LD. A clinical trial for the treatment of antiphospholipid antibody associated recurrent pregnancy loss with lower dose heparin and aspirin. *Am J Reprod Immunol* 1996;35:402–407.
131. Rai R, Cohen H, Dave M, et al. Randomized controlled trial of aspirin and aspirin plus heparin in pregnant women with recurrent miscarriage associated with phospholipd antibodies (or antiphospholipids). *BMJ* 1997;314:253–257.
132. Laskin CA, Bombardier C, Hannah ME, et al. Prednisone and aspirin in women with autoantibodies and unexplained recurrent fetal loss. *N Engl J Med* 1997;337:148–153.
133. Laskin CA, Clark-Soloninka CA, Spitzer KA, et al. Pregnancy outcome following low molecular weight heparin therapy in women with the presence of prenatal lupus anticoagulant. *Arthritis Rheum* 1999;42:S368.
134. Branch DW, Peaceman AM, Druzin M, et al. A multicenter, placebo-controlled pilot study of intravenous immune globulin treatment of antiphospholipid syndrome during pregnancy. *Am J Obstet Gynecol* 2000;182:122–127.
135. Sher G, Matzner W, Feinman M, et al. The selective use of heparin/aspirin therapy, alone or in combimation with intravenous immunoglobulin G, in the management of antiphospholid antibody positive women undergoing in vitro fertilization. *Amer J Reprod Immunol* 1998;40:74–82.
136. Pattison NS, Chamley LW, Birdsall M, et al. Does aspirin have a role in improving pregnancy outcome for women with the antiphospholipid syndrome? A randomized controlled trial. *Am J Obstet Gynecol* 2000;183:1008–1012.
137. Hull RG, Harris EN, Morgan SH, et al. Anti-Ro antibodies and abortions in women with SLE. *Lancet* 1983;2:1138.
138. Watson RM, Braunstein BL, Watson AJ, et al. Fetal wastage in women with anti-Ro(SSA) antibody. *J Rheumatol* 1986;13: 90–94.
139. Mavragani CP, Dafni UG, Tzioufas AG, et al. Pregnancy outcome and anti-Ro/SSA in autoimmune diseases: a retrospective cohort study. *Br J Rheumatol* 1998;37:740–745.
140. Mavragani CP, Ioannidis JP, Tzioufas AG, et al. Recurrent pregnancy loss and autoantibody profile in autoimmune diseases. *Rheumatol (Oxford)* 1999;38:1228–1233.
141. Oleinick A. Family studies in systemic lupus erythematosus. I. Prenatal factors. *Arthritis Rheum* 1969;12:10–16.
142. Oleinick A, Mantel N. Family studies in systemic lupus erythematosus. II. Mortality among siblings and offspring of index cases with a statistical appendix concerning life table analysis. *J Chron Dis* 1970;22:617.
143. Donaldson LB, de Alvarez RR. Further observations on lupus erythematosus associated with pregnancy. *Am J Obstet Gynecol* 1962;83:1461–1473.
144. Friedman EA, Rutherford JW. Pregnancy and lupus erythematosus. *Obstet Gynecol* 1956;8:601–610.
145. Dubois EL, ed. *Lupus Erythematosus. A Review of the Current Status of Discoid and Systemic Lupus Erythematosus and Their Variants, 2nd ed. revised.* Los Angeles: USC Press, 1976.
146. Grigor RR, Shervington PC, Hughes GRV, et al. Outcome of pregnancy in systemic lupus erythematosus. *Proc Roy Soc Med* 1977;70:99–100.
147. Johnson MJ, Petri M, Witter FR, et al. Evaluation of preterm delivery in a systemic lupus erythematosus pregnancy clinic. *Obstet Gynecol* 1995;86:396–399.
148. Kerslake S, Morton KE, Versi E, et al. Early Doppler studies in lupus pregnancy. *Amer J Reprod Immunol* 1992;28:172–175.
149. Hauth JC, Goldenberg RL, Parker CR Jr, et al. Maternal serum thromboxane B2 reduction versus pregnancy outcome in a low-dose aspirin trial. *Amer J Obstet Gynecol* 1995;173:578–584.
150. Dubowitz LMS, Dubowitz V, Goldberg C. Clinical assessment of gestational age in the newborn infants. *J Pediatr* 1970;77:1–4.
151. Rafla N, Farquarson R. Lupus anticoagulant in preeclampsia and intra-uterine growth retardation. *Europ J Obstet Gynecol Reprod Biol* 1991;42:167–170.
152. Wallenburg HCS, Rotmans P. Prevention of recurrent idiopathic fetal growth retardation by low-dose aspirin and dipyridamole. *Am J Obstet Gynecol* 1987;157:1230–1235.
153. Adams D, Druzin ML, Edersheim T, et al. Condition specific antepartum testing: Systemic lupus erythematosus and associated serologic abnormalities. *Amer J Reprod Immunol* 1992;28: 159–163.
154. Romero FI, Mendonca LLF, Tinahones FJ, et al. Autoantibodies against oxidized low-density lipoprotein in lupus pregnancy: a prospective study. *Arthritis Rheum* 1999;42:S147.
155. Grennan DM, McCormick JN, Wojtacha D, et al. Immunological studies of the placenta in systemic lupus erythematosus. *Ann Rheum Dis* 1978;37:129–134.
156. Abramowsky CR, Vegas ME, Swinehart G, et al. Decidual vasculopathy of the placenta in lupus erythematosus. *N Engl J Med* 1980;303:668–672.
157. Abramowsky CR. Lupus erythematosus, the placenta, and pregnancy: a natural experiment in immunologically mediated reproductive failure. *Prog Clin Biol Res* 1981;70:309–320.
158. De Wolf F, Carreras LO, Moerman P, et al. Decidual vasculopathy and extensive placental infarction in a patient with repeated thromboembolic accidents, recurrent fetal loss, and a lupus anticoagulant. *Am J Obstet Gynecol* 1982;142:829–834.

159. Labarrere CA, Catoggio LJ, Mullen EG, et al. Placental lesions in human autoimmune disease. *Am J Reprod Immunol Microbiol* 1986;12:78–86.
160. Guzman L, Avalos E, Ortiz R, et al. Placental abnormalities in systemic lupus erythematosus: in situ deposition of antinuclear antibodies. *J Rheumatol* 1987;14:924–929.
161. Out HJ, Kooijman CD, Bruinse HW, et al. Histopathologic findings in placentae from patients with intrauterine fetal death and antiphospholipid antibodies. *Europ J Obstet Gynecol Reprod Biol* 1991;41:179–186.
162. Erlendsson K, Steinsson K, Johannsson JH, et al. Relation of antiphospholipid antibody and placental bed inflammatory changes to the outcome of pregnancy in successive pregnancies of 2 women with systemic lupus erythematosus. *J Rheumatol* 1993;20:1779–1785.
163. La Rosa L, Meroni P, Tincani A, et al. beta-2 Glycoprotein and placental anticoagulant protein I in placentae from patients with antiphospholipid syndrome. *J Rheumatol* 1994;21: 1684–1693.
164. Chamley LW, Pattison NS, McKay EJ. Elution of anticardiolipin antibodies and their cofactor beta-2 glycoprotein I from the placentae of patients with poor obstetric history. *J Reprod Immunol* 1993;25:209–220.
165. Katano K, Aoki K, Ogasawara M, et al. Specific antiphospholipid antibodies (aPL) eluted from placentae of pregnant women with aPL-positive sera. *Lupus* 1995;4:304–308.
166. Magid MS, Kaplan C, Sammaritano LR, et al. Placental pathology in systemic lupus erythematosus: a prospective study. *Am J Obstet Gynecol* 1998;179:226–234.
167. Ogishima D, Matsumoto T, Nakamura Y, et al. Placental pathology in systemic lupus erythematosus with antiphospholipid antibodies. *Pathology International* 2000;50:224–229.
168. Ackerman J, Gonzalez EF, Gilbert-Barness E. Immunological studies of the placenta in maternal connective tissue disease. *Pediatr Dev Pathol* 1999;2:19–24.
169. Nayar R, Lage JM. Placental changes in a first trimester missed abortion in maternal systemic lupus erythematosus with antiphospholipid syndrome, a case report and review of the literature. *Hum Pathol* 1996;27:201–206.
170. Lakasing L, Campa JS, Parmar K, et al. Normal expression of cell adhesion molecules in placentae from women with systemic lupus erythematosus and the antiphospholipid syndrome. *Placenta* 2000;21:142–149.
171. Salafia CM, Parke AL. Placental pathology in systemic lupus erythematosus and the phospholipid antibody syndrome. *Rheum Dis Clin North Amer* 1997;23:85–97.
172. Levy RA, Avvad E, Oliveira J, et al. Placental pathology in antiphospholipid syndrome. *Lupus* 1998;7:S81–S85.
173. Faulk WP, Jeannet M, Creighton WD, et al. Immunological studies of the human placenta: characterization of immunoglobulins on trophoblastic basement membranes. *J Clin Invest* 1974;54:1011–1019.
174. McCormick JN, Faulk WP, Fox H, et al. Immunohistological and elution studies of the human placenta. *J Exp Med* 1971;133:1–18.
175. Carreras LO, Martinuzzo ME, Maclouf J. Antiphospholipid antibodies, eicosanoids and expression of endothelial cyclooxygenase-2. *Lupus* 1996;5:494–497.
176. Makila U-M, Viinikka L, Ylikorkala O. Increased thromboxane A2 production but normal prostacyclin by the placenta in hypertensive pregnancies. *Prostaglandins* 1984;27:87–95.
177. Walsh SW. Pre-eclampsia: an imbalance in placental prostacyclin and thromboxane production. *Am J Obstet Gynecol* 1985; 152:335–340.
178. Kaaja R, Julkunen H, Viinikka L, et al. Production of prostacyclin and thromboxane in lupus pregnancies: effect of small dose of aspirin. *Obstet Gynecol* 1993;81:327–331.
179. Dudley DJ, Mitchell DM, Branch DW. Pathophysiology of antiphospholipid antibodies: Absence of prostaglandin-mediated effects on cultured endothelium. *Am J Obstet Gynecol* 1990;162:953–959.
180. Peaceman AM, Rehnberg KA. The effect of immunoglobulin G fractions from patients with lupus anticoagulant on placental prostacyclin and thromboxane production. *Am J Obstet Gynecol* 1993;169:1403–1406.
181. Peaceman AM, Rehnberg KA. The effect of aspirin and indomethacin on prostacyclin and thromboxane production by placental tissue incubated with immunoglobulin G fractions from patients with lupus anticoagulant. *Am J Obstet Gynecol* 1995;173:1391–1396.
182. Giusti B, Gori AM, Attanasio M, et al. Lupus anticoagulant and monocyte procoagulant activity in polyabortive women. *Autoimmunity* 1993;15:299–304.
183. Chamley LW, McKay EJ, Pattison NS. Inhibition of heparin/antithrombin III cofactor activity by anticardiolipin antibodies: a mechanism for thrombosis. *Thrombosis Res* 1993; 71:103–111.
184. Qureshi F, Yang Y, Jaques SM, et al. Anti-DNA antibodies cross-reacting with laminin inhibit trophoblast attachment and migration: implications for recurrent pregnancy loss in SLE patients. *Am J Reprod Immunol* 2000;44:136–142.
185. Guzman E, Schulman H, Bracero L, et al. Uterine-umbilical artery Doppler velocimetry in pregnant women with systemic lupus erythematosus. *J Ultrasound Med* 1992;11:275–281.
186. Carroll BA. Obstetric duplex sonography in patients with lupus anticoagulant syndrome. *J Ultrasound Med* 1990;9:17–21.
187. Benifla JL, Tchobroutsky C, Uzan M, et al. Predictive value of uterine artery velocity waveforms in pregnancies complicated by systemic lupus erythematosus and the antiphospholipid syndrome. *Fetal Diagn Ther* 1992;7:195–202.
188. Weiner Z, Lorber M, Blumenfeld Z. Umbilical and uterine artery flow velocity waveforms in pregnant women with systemic lupus erythematosus treated with aspirin and glucocorticosteroids. *Amer J Reprod Immunol* 1992;28:168–171.
189. Manning FA, Platt LD, Sipos L. Antepartum fetal evaluation: Development of a fetal biophysical profile. *Am J Obstet Gynecol* 1980;136:787–795.
190. Druzin ML, Gratacos J, Keegan KA, et al. Antepartum fetal heart rate testing: the significance of fetal bradycardia. *Am J Obstet Gynecol* 1981;139:194–198.
191. Friedman DM. Fetal echocardiography in the assessment of lupus pregnancies. *Amer J Reprod Immunol* 1992;28:164–167.
192. Hage ML. Interpretation of nonstress tests. *Amer J Obstet Gynecol* 1985;153:490–495.
193. Druzin ML, Fox A, Kogut E, et al. The relationship of the nonstress test to gestational age. *Am J Obstet Gynecol* 1985;153: 386–389.
194. Nageotte MP, Towers CV, Asrat T, et al. The value of a negative antepartum test: contraction stress test and modified biophysical profile. *Obstet Gynecol* 1994;84:231–234.
195. Proud J, Grant AM. Third trimester placental grading by ultrasonography as a test of fetal wellbeing. *BMJ* 1987;294: 1641–1644.
196. Miller DA, Rabello YA, Paul RH. The modified biophysical profile: antepartum testing in the 1990s. *Am J Obstet Gynecol* 1996;174:812–817.
197. Druzin ML, Lockshin M, Edersheim TG, et al. Second trimester fetal monitoring and preterm delivery in pregnancies with systemic lupus erythematosus and/or circulating anticoagulant. *Am J Obstet Gynecol* 1987;157:1503–1510.
198. Briggs GG, Freeman RK, Yaffe SJ, eds. *Drugs in pregnancy and lactation: a reference guide to fetal and neonatal risk. 5th ed.* Baltimore: Williams & Wilkins, 1998.

49

THE NEONATAL LUPUS SYNDROME

RODANTHI C. KITRIDOU

Neonatal lupus erythematosus (NLE) is a syndrome of cutaneous lupus, congenital heart block (CHB), or both, and/or other systemic manifestations, which appears in children of women with systemic lupus, Sjögren's syndrome, other systemic rheumatic diseases, or asymptomatic mothers. The common finding in maternal sera is the presence of immunoglobulin G (IgG) class anti-Ro/SSA and/or anti-La/SSB. Maternal anti-U1 ribonucleoprotein (RNP) has rarely been associated with cutaneous NLE only. The first description of CHB or CCHB (complete congenital heart block) was in 1901 by Morquio (1), the association with systemic lupus erythematosus (SLE) was first recognized by Hogg (2), and the first description of cutaneous neonatal lupus and association with maternal SLE was made by McCuistion and Schoch (3). Among the earliest authors to describe congenital complete heart block were Aylward (4) in 1928, in two infants of a woman with Mikulicz's (Sjögren) syndrome, and Plant and Steven (5) in 1945, in an infant of a mother with SLE. Reports of CHB in the late 1970s rekindled interest in neonatal lupus (6–9), and during the last 23 years there have been tremendous advances in NLE pathogenesis, natural history, and maternal health. A voluminous literature has been amassed, including excellent reviews (10,11).

PREVALENCE

First Franco et al. (12), then Kephart et al. (13) and Miyagawa et al. (14) suggested in 1981 that maternal anti-Ro/SSA antibody, perhaps through transplacental passage, was responsible for the development of neonatal lupus. Evidence for the association of NLE with anti-Ro/SSA and anti-La/SSB has been well established during the last 20 years. In addition, there is evidence that selective antibody response to 52-kd Ro is responsible for cardiotoxic effects. For this reason, the prevalence of anti-Ro/SSA and anti-La/SSB in mothers with SLE and their offspring, and not only of the NLE syndrome, is reviewed here.

Prevalence Of Anti-Ro/SSA And Anti-La/SSB

In 12 studies of 11,895 normal individuals, including blood donors, pregnant women, and mother–infant pairs, a prevalence of 0% to 11% was found (15–26). The prevalence of anti-Ro/SSA by immunodiffusion or counterimmunoelectrophoresis varies from 0.1% to 2%, whereas by enzyme-linked immunosorbent assay (ELISA) it is found in 2.3% to 11% of normals individuals. Anti-La/SSB is less common, found in 0% to 1.8% of normals by immunodiffusion or counterimmunoelectrophoresis, and in 0% to 12.5% by ELISA (16,17,19,20,23,25). The prevalence of anti-Ro/SSA in normal pregnant women is 0.4% to 1% (15,21,25), and that of anti-La antibody, 0.7% of 445 normal pregnant women (24).

In 16 studies of 1,874 systemic lupus patients, anti-Ro/SSA was found by the two former methods in 14% to 52%, and by the more sensitive ELISA in 39% to 87%; an average, well-accepted prevalence is 40% (18,19,22,23, 26–37). Miyagawa et al. (38) determined the frequency of anti-Ro/SSA antibodies in 825 patients with systemic rheumatic diseases and found it to be significantly greater in women (74 of 670, 11%) than in men (5 of 155, 3.2%). The frequency of anti-La/SSB in SLE by immunodiffusion has been reported from 1.2% to 24%, and by ELISA from 21% to 38% (19,23,29,30,34–36). A generally accepted prevalence of anti-La/SSB in SLE is 15% to 20%. In patients with Sjögren's syndrome, anti-Ro/SSA prevalence is 40% to 45%, and anti-La/SSB, 15% to 20% (39).

It should be noted that anti-La/SSB is associated with anti-Ro/SSA in 99% or more of cases (34), whereas anti-Ro can be found alone. Rarely, cutaneous neonatal lupus has been associated with anti-U1RNP (40–43).

Prevalence Of Congenital Heart Block

The overall prevalence of CHB is estimated at 1 in 20,000 births, or 0.005% (44) (Table 49.1). The overall prevalence of neonatal lupus in live births of SLE mothers, derived

TABLE 49.1. NEONATAL LUPUS ERYTHEMATOSUS (NLE)

Prevalence of Congenital Heart Block: 1:20,000 Births		
	No.	Percent
NLE in unselected SLE births		
Mintz et al. (45)	1/86	1.2
Ramsey-Goldman et al. (33)	7/259	2.7
Overall	8/345	2.3
In SLE births without anti-Ro/SSA		
Ramsey-Goldman et al. (33)	1/180	0.6
In anti-Ro/SSA positive SLE		
Watson et al. (46)	1/67	1.5
McHugh et al. (47)	1/28	3.6
Maddison (48)	1/26	3.8
Ramsey-Goldman et al. (33)	6/79	7.6
Drosos et al. (51)	3/34	8.8
Lockshin et al. (49,50)	4/38	10.5
Nossent and Swaak. (52)	5/20	25.0
Overall	21/292	7.2

from the largest prospective study, is 1 in 86, or 1.2% (45). Ramsey-Goldman et al. (33) reported seven infants with NLE in 259 lupus pregnancies (2.7%): there was one NLE in 180 births without anti-Ro/SSA (0.6%) and 6 in 79 (7.6%) with anti-Ro, and the occurrence of heart block correlated with high titer of the antibody. These authors estimated the overall risk of a woman with lupus having a child with congenital heart block as 1:60, which increases to 1:20 in the presence of anti-Ro/SSA. In other series of lupus patients positive for anti-Ro/SSA, the prevalence of neonatal lupus has been reported as 1 in 67 births (1.5%) in the retrospective study by Watson et al. (46), 1 in 28 (3.6%) by McHugh et al. (47), 1 in 26 (3.8%) by Maddison (48), 4 in 38 (10.5%) by Lockshin et al. (49,50), 3 of 34 (8.8%) in mothers with lupus and Sjögren's syndrome, in a prospective study by Drosos et al. (51), and in 5 of 20 (25%) by Nossent and Swaak (52). In all, in the above reports there were 21 children with neonatal lupus in 292 live births in women with lupus or Sjögren's syndrome positive for anti-Ro/SSA, for an overall prevalence of 7.2%.

CLINICAL MANIFESTATIONS

By the year 2000, a total of 827 babies with neonatal lupus have been described, barring any duplication: 294 infants until 1991 (2–9,12–14,25,32,41,42,45,47–118), and 239 babies from 1992 to 2000 outside the registry (119–142,145, 147–149,153–155,165,167–170,172–180), for a subtotal of 533, and 294 from the registry (Table 49.2).

The Research Registry for Neonatal Lupus was established in September 1994 by the National Institute of

TABLE 49.2. MANIFESTATIONS OF NEONATAL LUPUS

	No.	Percent
Infants reported in 5th edition (228)[a]	294	
NLE reported outside registry 1992–2000[b]	239	
Subtotal	533	
Congenital heart block (CHB)	332	62.3
Cutaneous NLE (includes five with other)	165	31.0
CHB and cutaneous NLE	23	4.3
Other manifestations only	13	2.4
Manifestations in addition to CHB and cutaneous NLE[a]		
Hepatic/gastrointestinal	33	6.2
Hematologic	28	5.3
Neurologic	4	0.8
Pulmonary	4	0.8
Nephritis	2	0.4
Multiple thromboses w/ APL	2	0.4
Infants in NIAMS Registry as of September 2000 (143[c],144)	294	
Congenital heart block	184	62.6
Maternal antibodies positive	145	49.3
(maternal Abs negative/pending)	(22/17)	
Cutaneous NLE	72	24.5
Maternal antibodies positive	64	21.8
(maternal Abs negative/pending)	(1/7)	
CHB + cutaneous NLE	30	10.2
Hematologic/hepatic	6	2.0

[a]See text for references.
[b]References 119–142, 145, 147–149.
[c]Data presented by J. P. Buyon, MD, at the 2000 American College of Rheumatology meeting, reprinted with permission.
Abs, antibodies; APL, antiphospholipid antibody; NIAMS, National Institute of Arthritis, Musculoskeletal and Skin Diseases.

TABLE 49.3. SEX DISTRIBUTION IN NEONATAL LUPUS ERYTHEMATOSUS

	No. Females/Total	% Females
Congenital heart block		
Esscher and Scott (9)	42/67	62.7
McCue et al. (7)	12/22	54.5
McCune et al. (94)	9/14	64.3
Buyon et al. (144)	57/113	50.4
Eronen et al. (145)	60/91	65.9
Overall	180/307	58.6
Cutaneous NLE		
Neiman et al. (166)	37/57	64.9
Weston et al. (167)	14/18	77.8
Overall	51/75	68.0

Arthritis, Musculoskeletal and Skin Diseases (NIAMS) and is directed by Jill P. Buyon, M.D., at the Hospital for Joint Diseases in New York. Several data on NLE have been provided through publications from the registry. As of September 2000, 294 affected children and 251 mothers were enrolled (143)(Table 49.2).

Of the 533 infants, 332 (62.3%) had CHB, 165 had cutaneous NLE (31.0%), 23 had both heart block and cutaneous lesions (4.3%), and 13 (2.4%) had other manifestations of NLE, as seen below (Table 49.2).

Of the 294 infants of the research registry, 184 have CHB (62.6%), 72 have cutaneous NLE (24.5%), 30 have both CHB and cutaneous NLE (10.2%), and 6 (2%), have hematologic or hepatic manifestations (Table 49.2).

Congenital Heart Block

Congenital heart block is by far the most dangerous and life-threatening manifestation of neonatal lupus. The sex distribution in CHB is seen in Table 49.3. One half to nearly two thirds of CHB babies are female (7,9,94,144, 145). Hubscher et al. (123) distinguished two types of CHB according to age at detection: early detection, before 3 months of age (12 of 18 children), was associated with greater severity, requiring a pacemaker in 8 of 12, maternal connective tissue disease in 7 of 11 mothers, and positive anti-Ro and/or anti-La in 9/11; in six children with CHB diagnosed after 17 months of age, no mother had a rheumatic disease and only one had autoantibodies.

CHB is most commonly diagnosed *in utero* by routine ultrasonography and confirmed by echocardiogram. The time of diagnosis is the first occurrence of bradyarrhythmia (144,145), and that is rarely evident before 22 weeks of gestation (Table 49.4). Buyon et al. (144) and Waltuck and Buyon (146) detected CHB before 30 weeks in 82% and 85% of their patients, respectively, Eronen et al. (145) in 73% of their patients before 34 weeks of gestation, and Brucato et al. (147,148) in 69% *in utero* or at birth.

The CHB is complete by the time of birth in over 90% of reported cases. Other types of conduction defects described include first-degree atrioventricular (AV) block (144), second-degree block (12,71), 2:1 AV block (102), transient AV block (7,56), right bundle-branch block (13, 111,114), and sinus bradycardia (68). Several fascinating reports of postnatal intermittent arrhythmias and/or progressive heart block have appeared (7,40,72,73,144). McCue et al. (7) noted transient arrhythmias and varying block. Goldsmith (40) reported a male infant of an asymptomatic mother with arrhythmia and documented second-degree AV block at 10 weeks; at 7 months of age, an episode of tachycardia to 200 beats per minute with diaphoresis, unresponsiveness, and pulselessness was followed by development of CHB necessitating pacemaker implantation. Similar progression from second- to third-degree AV block was noted by Geggel et al. (72). In addition, development of sinus bradycardia, Mobitz type II, and intermittent complete heart block in a 9-year-old boy required pacemaker implantation (73). One of the children reported by Buyon et al. (144) had bradycardia *in utero*, borderline first-degree AV block at birth, then second-degree, and intermittent complete AV block at 18 months, requiring a pacemaker; another had second-degree block *in utero*, regressed to first-degree with therapy, and again reverted to second-degree AV block (144).

TABLE 49.4. DIAGNOSIS OF CONGENITAL HEART BLOCK (CHB) AND SHORT-TERM OUTCOME OF CHILDREN

			Death (%)			Pacemaker (%)			Dilated Cardiomyopathy (%)	
	No.	CHB Diagnosis (%) Before <34 Weeks	All	IUFD	0–1 Year	All	Neonatal	>30 Days	At 0–3 Months	3 Months–3 Years
Buyon et al. (144)	113	82	20	5	10	63	33	30	—	1
Eronen et al. (145)	91	73	16	1	11	93	53	40	10	11
Waltuck and Buyon (146)	55 (61)[a]	85	31	—	27	67	<3 months = 49			
Brucato et al. (147,148)	16	69[b]	19	6	6	50	—	—		

[a]61 includes six fetuses with *in utero* diagnosis of CHB.
[b]CHB diagnosed *in utero* or at birth.
IUFD, intrauterine fetal death.

In addition to intermittent, progressive arrhythmias with evolution to complete heart block, there is ample evidence of inflammatory processes in the heart of babies with CHB, including pericarditis with effusion (49,57,62,67,80,145), pericarditis with tamponade (99), myocarditis (49,55,57, 117,127), cardiomyopathy (6), endocarditis (126), and even pancarditis (126). A presumed viral myocarditis in a child with CHB might have actually been inflammatory (118). Recent studies support a very important role of neonatal carditis and late-onset dilated cardiomyopathy (DCM) in the morbidity and mortality of immune-mediated CHB (145,149,150). In the study by Eronen et al. (145), 21 of 90 children, or 23% (after exclusion of one death *in utero*) developed DCM, and 13 of the 21 died. In 16 of 21 patients, DCM was diagnosed before 1 year of age and was the major cause of death in this series (13 of 14 deaths), with 10 of the 14 deaths occurring before 12 months of age (one death by suicide is excluded) (145). Neonatal morbidity was noted in 58% of these infants, with the majority due to hydrops (severe swelling akin to anasarca due to heart failure) (27%), and heart failure without hydrops (21%). Eronen et al. also determined that poor prognosis, defined as clinically or pathologically evident congestive dilated cardiomyopathy, was associated with intrauterine hydrops, low fetal and neonatal heart rate (<55/minute), low birth weight, male sex, and neonatal problems attributable to prematurity or neonatal lupus (145). Buyon et al. (144) found that survival relates to gestational age at birth, with death in 52% of 27 babies born before 34 weeks of gestation, while only 9% of 86 children born at >34 weeks died. The authors suggest that "*in utero* injury can have continued sequelae despite clearance of [pathogenic] maternal antibodies from the neonatal circulation" (144). Because of intractable DCM, one of Buyon's patients and two of Eronen's underwent cardiac transplantation at 8 months and 3 years of age, respectively (144,145).

A variety of structural cardiac anomalies have been described in CHB, seen in 17% and 42% of the two largest series (144,145). These defects include, in order of approximate frequency, atrial septal defect (6,88,144,145), patent ductus arteriosus (6,9,81,94,111,144,145), ventricular septal defect (7,9,77,144, 145), corrected transposition (7,9, 55), patent foramen ovale (85), coarctation (7), possible tetralogy (64), hypoplastic right ventricle (7), dysplastic pulmonic valve (6,144), pulmonic stenosis (144), pulmonic regurgitation (86), anomalous pulmonary venous drainage (9), tricuspid insufficiency (7), mitral insufficiency (7,145), cardiomyopathy (150), and others.

Certain instances of CHB are unrelated to maternal rheumatic disease and autoantibodies (151,152). Gembruch et al. (151) diagnosed complete heart block prenatally in 21 fetuses, 18 (85.7%) of whom had associated cardiac defects, especially complete AV canal with atrial isomerism in five, and "corrected" great vessel transposition in four, with only one mother with SLE. In 11 fetuses, all of whom had cardiac defects, there was evidence of intrauterine congestive heart failure and nonimmune hydrops fetalis.

Both complete heart block and cutaneous NLE have been described in siblings and in successive pregnancies (7, 9,106,152–154), at a rate of 10% to 16% (144,145). Among 172 siblings in 65 families with two or more siblings reported in the above publications, 100 (58%) had NLE. A full 29 of the 65 families (44.6%) had two or more affected siblings, well above the prevalence in the general population. Of ten sets of twins, three were concordant (7, 145), and seven were discordant for congenital heart block (76,144,145), in spite of monozygosity in one set (144). Monozygous twins discordant for CHB had similar titers of anti-Ro/SSA and anti-La/SSB, and anti-52KD Ro specificity, suggesting that placental transfer of the antibody alone is not sufficient for CCHB (59). Buyon et al. (60) tested maternal and umbilical cord levels of anti-Ro/SSA and its subsets, and anti-La/SSB in 15 pregnancies with CCHB, and found similar titers in affected and unaffected pregnancies.

In the largest series, mortality in babies with CHB was from 15% to 31% (7,9,94,144–148), occurred mostly in the neonatal period, and was caused by congestive heart failure (144–147) or Adams-Stokes attack, in association with dilated cardiomyopathy (6,145,146), or myocarditis (117). Two publications from the same investigators show a much lower mortality, 8% and 11%, but about half of the children were diagnosed with CHB after 12 months of age (44), and the later study dealt with children who were >15 years old and contained no information of maternal autoimmune status (156).

Pacemakers are needed in 20% to 93% of the children (7,9,144,145,147), with more than half implanted in the neonatal period (144,145). In studies of the 1970s, pacemakers were implanted in 27% and 20.8% of CHB children (7,9), while in more recent reports the proportion with pacemakers has risen, suggesting, perhaps, a more proactive therapeutic approach: 67 of 107 (63%) of Buyon et al.'s (144) patients and 84 of 90 (93%) of Eronen et al.'s (145) patients received pacemakers. In the review by Reid et al. (155), only two patients reached age 50 without need of a pacemaker. A substantial proportion (20% to 30%) of CHB children undergo cardiac catheterization as a preamble to corrective cardiac surgery. Buyon et al. have reported no deaths due to CHB after age 3, with a survival of 79% at that age. Eronen et al. consider the prognosis good after age 4, with a cumulative probability of survival at 10 years old of 82%. Steroid therapy is discussed below (see Treatment of Neonatal Lupus).

In an elegant prospective electrocardiographic study of 28 infants born to mothers with systemic rheumatic diseases [SLE, Sjögren's syndrome, and undifferentiated connective tissue disease (UCTD)], 9 of 21 anti-Ro/SSA–positive infants (43%) had prolongation of the QTc interval without CHB (157); in contrast, the seven anti-Ro/SSA–negative infants did not show this abnormality. As prolongation of QTc is associated with increased risk for sudden death, the authors decided to treat the infants with beta-blockers to prevent potentially fatal arrhythmias. The same group of investigators has shown transient bradycardia in 3 of 21 (14.3%) anti-Ro–positive infants in the first 10 days of life (158), akin to experimentally induced bradycardia in mice pups (159). The subject is discussed further below (see Pathogenetic Mechanisms.)

A report by Yemini et al. (107) is suggestive of transplacental drug-induced lupus. A very low birth weight infant born to a woman with hydralazine-induced lupus died of pericardial effusion with tamponade, confirmed by autopsy. The mother had pregnancy-induced hypertension.

Autopsy studies of infants with CHB have almost uniformly shown dense connective tissue enveloping the conducting system (6,9,10,55,78,117,160–164), including the sinoatrial and atrioventricular nodes and bundle of His (7 of 7 hearts, 161), endo(myo)cardial fibroelastosis (5 of 7 hearts, 161), and in 7 of 9 hearts (9). At times there is a fibrous body around the AV bundle (6), epicarditis near the SA node (55), microcrystalline structures in the conducting system (160), and calcification of the heart, the conducting system, and valves (117). Inflammatory infiltrates of the conducting system were seen in 5 of 7 hearts (55,161, 162,164), and occasional myocarditis (6,55,117,161). In the 11 autopsies available from the Registry, aside from fibrotic changes, endocardial fibroelastosis and biventricular hypertrophy, there were tricuspid valve lesions suggestive of an inflammatory process, and inflammation of the SA and AV node in the least mature fetuses (25 and 29 weeks) (10). The relative scarcity of inflammatory change, therefore, may be a matter of timing.

Cutaneous Neonatal Lupus

As mentioned above, 25% to 31% of the reported neonatal lupus patients have cutaneous NLE, and the majority are females (65% to 76%) (63,114,124,165–169) (Table 49.3). There may be underreporting of cutaneous NLE as compared to CHB, because it is transient and a great proportion of mothers are asymptomatic. It is likely that annular erythema of newborns (14) and annular eruptions of infancy (84) represent cutaneous NLE. Cutaneous neonatal lupus was first described in 1954 by McCuistion and Schoch (3) in a 6-week-old daughter of a lupus patient, as possible discoid lupus erythematosus (DLE). A biopsy of the child's rash indeed showed findings similar to those seen in SLE and DLE (hyperkeratosis, follicular plugging, areas of acanthosis and atrophy, liquefactive degeneration of the basal layer, and perivascular lymphocytic infiltrate).

Since that report in 1954, over 230 cases of cutaneous neonatal lupus have been described. Skin biopsies in subsequent patients showed findings similar to subacute cutaneous lupus with mononuclear infiltrates in the upper dermis and basal layer change as above (63,103,110,114,168). Nitta and Ohashi (98) reported microtubular structures in the endothelial vessels of cutaneous NLE biopsy, and in the labial salivary gland biopsy of the infant's mother. An excellent review on cutaneous NLE has been published (170).

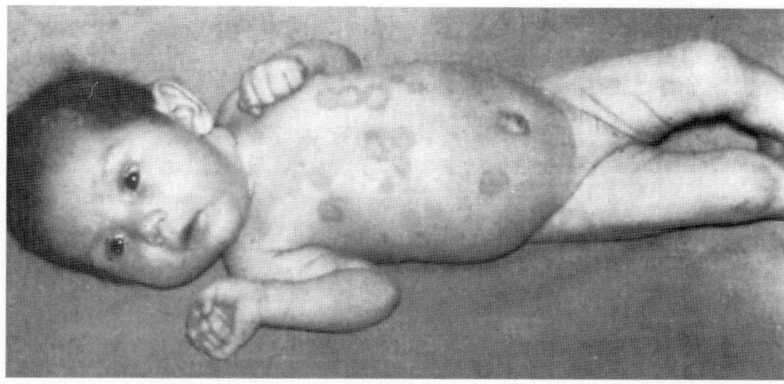

FIGURE 49.1. (See color plate.) Neonate with cutaneous neonatal lupus erythematosus (NLE).

The skin rash of cutaneous NLE consists of transient, annular, occasionally scaly, erythematous and telangiectatic lesions of the face, scalp, trunk, and extremities (Fig. 49.1). Vonderheid et al. (168) described a tendency of greater periorbital concentration of the lesions, which has been likened to an "eye-mask" or "owl-eye" (169). When the rash is annular, it resembles that of subacute cutaneous lupus erythematosus (171), and that of lupus with C2 complement component deficiency. Both of these variants of lupus have a high prevalence of anti-Ro/SSA. The rash usually appears shortly after birth, probably as a result of skin exposure to ultraviolet light. It was noted at birth in 23% of children (13 of 57) in the largest study of cutaneous NLE (166). It can be seen as late as 5 months of age (mean, 7 weeks). The rash is found on sun-exposed areas, and is highly photosensitive (53,89,91,114,170). In a report from Taiwan, an infant girl born to a mother with lupus developed cutaneous NLE after phototherapy for hyperbilirubinemia (91).

Cutaneous NLE typically lasts for 2 to 6 months and disappears without leaving a scar, or with minimal atrophy. In 25% of Neiman et al.'s (166) patients there was residual telangiectasia and dyspigmentation. The disappearance of the rash about the sixth month of age is consistent with the half-life of transplacentally acquired maternal IgG. For this reason, anti-Ro/SSA and anti-La/SSB positivity in the child depends on the age at which the testing is done and is not expected to persist for more than 5 to 6 months. NLE skin lesions, however, may persist for 10 months (122), and up to 28 months (172).

Data on the occurrence of cutaneous and cardiac neonatal lupus in siblings have been reviewed above (see Congenital Heart Block). Suffice it to say that 29 of 65 reported families (44.6%) had two or more siblings affected (7,9,94, 106,153,154). Of four sets of twins, two were concordant

(121,171), and two were discordant for cutaneous NLE (58,120). A set of triplets (two girls, one boy) with cutaneous NLE, thrombocytopenia, hepatic enzyme elevation, and anti-Ro antibodies was born to a mother with SLE (122). Thrombocytopenia was profound and persistent in one triplet, who also had positive anti–double-stranded (dsDNA), and necessitated intravenous steroid and gammaglobulin (IVIg) treatment.

The coexistence of CHB and cutaneous NLE is not common, found only in 23 of the 526 cases reported outside the registry (4.4%) (7,9,50,71,74,94,99,109,114), and in 30 of 294 cases from the registry (10.2%) (143).

Cutaneous NLE has been reported in three male infants, one female, and one of dizygotic twins in association with maternal anti-U1RNP antibodies, in the absence of anti-Ro/SSA and anti-La/SSB (40–43). To these we add a sixth (male) infant born to a systemic lupus patient at the Los Angeles County–University of Southern California Medical Center. The infant developed a few erythematous, macular, and annular lesions on the face and trunk shortly after birth, which disappeared over the ensuing month. Both mother and child had anti-U1RNP antibody and no anti-Ro/SSA or anti-La/SSB. It may be purely coincidental that four of the six infants were black males. In addition, four more infants with cutaneous NLE associated with maternal anti-U1RNP, for a total of ten (173,174).

Other Manifestations Of Neonatal Lupus

The first description of Coombs-positive hemolytic anemia, leukopenia, and thrombocytopenia in an infant born to a lupus patient with the same manifestations was reported by Seip (88) in 1960. Since then hepatic, hematologic, neurologic, pulmonary, renal, and thrombotic manifestations have been reported in neonates, usually in association with CHB, or cutaneous NLE, and maternal antibodies to Ro/SSA and/or to La/SSB (7–9,12,13,42,56,63,64,74,76,78,82,83, 87,94,96,97,102,104,114,134,135,138–143,175–177).

Hepatic and gastrointestinal involvement was seen in at least 33 of 529 infants (6.2%), hematologic involvement in 28 (5.3%), neurologic involvement in four (0.8%), pulmonary involvement in four (0.8%), nephritis in two (0.4%), and multiple thromboses (with seizures in one infant) in two due to maternal antiphospholipid antibody (APL) (0.4%). Anti-Ro/SSA, with or without anti-La/SSB, antibodies are found in the majority of these infants and almost all of their mothers. Of the 294 patients in the NLE registry, there were six (2%) with hematologic and hepatic manifestations (143).

Hepatic manifestations were seen in 4 of 35 of Lee et al.'s (176) patients, and in order of frequency include hepatomegaly, often accompanied by splenomegaly, transiently increased liver function tests, icterus, cholestasis, cirrhosis, and severe gastrointestinal hemorrhage. Liver biopsies and autopsies in some of the infants revealed noninfectious hepatitis, neonatal giant cell hepatitis, cholestasis, ductal and ductular hyperplasia, portal septal fibrosis, cirrhosis, excessive extramedullary hematopoiesis, and IgG deposits (175,176). Katayama et al. (82) reported an infant with cutaneous NLE, severe gastrointestinal hemorrhage, and a positive anticardiolipin antibody for more than 6 months. Her mother was asymptomatic, with anticardiolipin and anti-Ro/SSA antibodies.

Hematologic manifestations in NLE include thrombocytopenia, immune hemolytic anemia with Coombs' test positivity in mother and infant, leukopenia, and microangiopathic hemolytic anemia. One infant with cutaneous NLE had recurrent thrombocytopenia and microangiopathic anemia responsive to IVIg (138). Thrombocytopenia has been reviewed by Watson et al. (177) and is frequently accompanied by splenomegaly. Antiplatelet antibodies were negative in the mother–infant pair reported by Seip (88). At times, hemolytic anemia and thrombocytopenia were severe enough to require transfusions and steroid therapy of the infant (122).

Four infants had neurologic manifestations: one developed a myelopathy with residua at 16 months of age, in addition to cutaneous NLE and anti-Ro/SSA antibody (83); another had aseptic meningitis with CHB and anti-La/SSB (178); a third had seizures and hypocalcemia, in addition to rash, hemolytic anemia, and hepatosplenomegaly (96); a fourth infant, whose mother had lupus and acetylcholine receptor antibodies, had transient myasthenia gravis, confirmed by electromyography, cutaneous NLE, and the mother's acetylcholine receptor and anti-U1RNP antibodies, without anti-Ro or anti-La antibodies (42).

Pneumonitis was present in four infants, in addition to cutaneous NLE, thrombocytopenia, hemolytic anemia, and hepatic involvement (56,114,179,180). One of two infants with renal disease had membranous nephropathy, high-titer antinuclear antibodies (ANAs), and hypocomplementemia, along with congenital toxoplasmosis (139); the other infant had nephrotic syndrome (140). Of the two children with maternal APL, one had seizures with cerebral artery thrombosis due to maternal lupus anticoagulant, and the other, multiple arterial and aortic thrombi due to maternal anticardiolipin antibody (141,142).

PATHOGENETIC MECHANISMS

The transplacental passage of maternal IgG is well known: such passage of the lupus erythematosus (LE) cell factor [antideoxyribonucleoprotein (anti-DNP) antibody] was reported in 1957, producing positive LE cells in two healthy infants of lupus mothers, up to the seventh week of age (181). Seip (88) found an equivocal Coombs' test in a child with hemolytic anemia, whose mother also had it.

In 1981, Franco et al., then Kephart et al., and Miyagawa et al. (12–14) suggested that maternal anti-Ro/SSA antibody may be causally linked to NLE. Substantial accumulated evidence shows that transplacental passage of anti-Ro/SSA and/or anti-La/SSB, and, rarely, anti-U1RNP, possibly in concert with other factors, results in NLE (102, 182), truly a syndrome of passively acquired autoimmune injury (183).

As stated by Buyon and Brucato (10), for anti-Ro/SSA and anti-La/SSB to be causative for NLE, the following requirements must be satisfied: the candidate antigen must be present in the target fetal tissues, the maternal autoantibodies must be present in the fetal circulation, and the fetal antigens must be accessible to the maternal antibodies.

Ro/SSA And La/SSB Antigens In Fetal Tissues

The exact function of Ro/SSA and La/SSB is not known; Bachmann et al. (184) have found that Ro/SSA and La/SSB are associated with a fibrous network akin to cytokeratin, an intermediate filament system. La/SSB is probably a cofactor for RNA polymerase III (185) and binds adenoviral and Epstein-Barr viral (EBV) RNA (186).

Several lines of evidence show that Ro/SSA has been localized in fetal heart and neonatal skin, thus incriminating anti-Ro/SSA and anti-La/SSB in the genesis of CHB:

1. Harley et al. (75) described human leukocyte antigen (HLA)-identical twins discordant for congenital complete heart block, with anti-Ro/SSA titers in the affected twin 13-fold less than the normal twin, implying that it was bound to cardiac tissue. They also showed that Ro/SSA antigen is present in fetal heart aged 18 to 23 weeks and in adult heart.
2. Ro/SSA was identified by Deng et al. (187) in nuclei of conduction system cells and cardiac myofibers in hearts of 9 to 10 weeks' gestation, and by Lee et al. (154) in normal fetal myocardium, kidney, liver, and spleen, and in neonatal and adult, but not in fetal epidermis. Fraire-Velasquez et al. (187a) found Ro60 associated hyRNAs in nucleocytoplasmic areas of embryonic hearts at 8 to 12 weeks development, and in cytoplasmic areas of adult hearts.
3. Taylor et al. (163) demonstrated IgG antibodies against cardiac tissue in the sera of 51% of mothers of children with CHB, in three of eight CHB babies under 3 months old, and in none of normal controls; 81% of the mothers with anticardiac antibodies were positive for anti-Ro/SSA. The authors also found that anti-Ro/SSA titers in infants with NLE were lower than those in the mothers, whereas unaffected infants had titers similar to those in the mothers (25).
4. Litsey et al. (162), Taylor et al. (163), and Lee et al. (164) demonstrated immunoglobulin and complement component deposition in a total of four hearts from CHB. Litsey et al. showed diffuse staining for IgG in the epicardium, and for IgG and IgA in the endo- and myocardium of the right atrial appendage. Taylor et al. found diffuse cytoplasmic staining for IgG, IgM, IgA, and complement components in all cardiac tissue examined, including nodal tissue, bundle of His, Purkinje fibers, and myocardium at large. Lee et al. found particulate staining for IgG and C3 in all sections, but most intense and extensive in the atria.
5. Reichlin et al. (188) found the eluate from the heart of a child who died from CHB to be enriched for antibodies to 60-kd and 52-kd Ro/SSA, but not eluates from brain, kidney, and skin.
6. Buyon et al. (189) examined 22 fetal human hearts of 11 to 25 weeks gestation and three adult hearts for the Ro/SSA transcripts 52α and 52β and showed that 52β expression was maximal between 14 and 16 weeks of gestational age, when cardiac organogenesis occurs and maternal autoantibodies gain access to the fetal circulation; 52α dominated in fetal hearts aged 22 to 25 weeks and adult hearts (189).
7. In further work by Buyon and her group, cultures of fetal cardiac myocytes were established, with demonstration of intracellular Ro/SSA and La/SSB. Incubation with 17β-estradiol or progesterone did not increase the expression of Ro/SSA (190), contrary to cultured keratinocytes (191).

The following evidence shows that anti-Ro/SSA and anti-La/SSB interfere with cardiac function or cardiac myocyte function:

1. Alexander et al. (192) showed that anti-Ro/SSA– and anti-La/SSB–containing sera of mothers of CHB children preferentially inhibited *in vitro* the repolarization of neonatal, but not adult rabbit cardiac cells. They also showed immunocytochemical binding of sera and IgG-enriched fractions from anti-Ro/SSA–positive CHB mothers to neonatal rabbit cardiac tissue (193).
2. Boutjdir et al. (194) showed that IgG, and affinity-purified anti–52-kd Ro/SSA from mothers of children with CHB induce complete AV block in perfused human fetal heart, and inhibit L-type calcium currents in the whole myocardial cell. In addition, the authors developed an animal model of BALB/c mice immunized with recombinant anti-Ro/SSA, whose pups had AV conduction abnormalities, including complete AV block.
3. The same group perfused rat heart with purified IgG from a mother with anti-Ro/SSA and a child with CHB, causing bradycardia and AV block, AV block in AV node preparation, and inhibition of Ca^{2+} channels in cardiac myocytes (195).
4. Viana et al. (196) perfused isolated rabbit hearts with affinity purified anti–52-kd Ro/SSA from 20 SLE patients and one Sjögren patient who did not have children with CHB, and produced AV block with 6 of the 20 sera, demonstrating that prior CHB history was not necessary to produce experimental heart block.

5. Experimental lupus has been induced in BALB/c mice by immunization with human monoclonal anti-DNA antibody bearing the idiotype 16/6: among other antinuclear antibodies, the mice produce anti-La/SSB and anti-Ro/SSA, and some of their offspring have first-, second-, or third-degree heart block, or significant bradycardia and a wide QRS complex (197).

Evidence of accessibility of fetal cardiac antigens to maternal autoantibodies is provided by another elegant work from Dr. Buyon's group: Human fetal cardiac myocytes were cultured, then apoptosis was induced, and Ro/SSA and La/SSB were shown to translocate from the nucleus to the cell periphery, and to apoptotic blebs (10,198). Furthermore, apoptotic cardiocytes preincubated with antibodies to Ro/SSA and La/SSB, and cocultured with macrophages, induced secretion of tumor necrosis factor-α (TNF-α) from macrophages, thus promoting an inflammatory response, analogous, perhaps, to the conduction system and myocardial inflammation observed in some of the CHB hearts.

The following is a summary of evidence linking anti-Ro/SSA and anti-LA/SSB to cutaneous NLE:

1. Lee et al. (154) identified Ro/SSA in neonatal and adult, but not fetal epidermis, which may explain why cutaneous NLE occurs after birth and not *in utero*, and on the surface of serum-free cultured keratinocytes.
2. Lee et al. (199,200) and Lee and David (201) grafted nude athymic, and severe combined immunodeficiency disease (SCID) mice with normal human skin, injected anti-Ro/SSA in the peritoneal cavity, and showed particulate cytoplasmic deposition of IgG in the epidermis, and occasionally at the dermoepidermal junction, similar to that seen in patients with NLE or subcutaneous lupus erythematosus (SCLE). Absorption of the anti-Ro–containing serum with Ro/SSA antigen resulted in marked diminution of fluorescence (199–201). Anti-Ro/SSA from NLE mothers bound to skin grafts is predominantly of the IgG1 subclass (202).
3. By utilizing a panel of purified antibodies to 52- and 60-kd Ro/SSA, Yell et al. (203) demonstrated that the respective antigens have separate localization in the cytoplasm and nucleus of cultured human keratinocytes.
4. Low-dose ultraviolet B (UVB) irradiation induces binding by anti-Ro antibodies of Ro antigen expressed on the surface of cultured human keratinocytes (204–206). Enhanced membrane expression of the 52-kd Ro/SSA and La/SSB antigens by human keratinocytes is also induced by TNF-α (207). Furthermore, cultured keratinocytes of a patient with cutaneous NLE had greater surface expression of Ro/SSA and La/SSB molecules than normal skin, and UVB irradiation increased the expression by 2.5- to 3-fold (208); cytotoxicity of maternal and patient sera was complement-dependent and was enhanced by UVB irradiation for the NLE, but not for the normal keratinocytes. In guinea pigs, UV-induced microvascular flow rates of skin test sites were greatest with injections of anti-Ro/SSA–containing SCLE sera (209). In photosensitive SLE patients, the expression of 52-kd, 60-kd Ro/SSA and 48-kd La/SSB in skin biopsy specimens, was four- to tenfold higher than in nonphotosensitive patients, and correlated with the presence and titer of circulating antibodies to the above antigens (210). These data suggest a mechanism of induction of anti-Ro/SSA and anti-La/SSB autoantibodies and of photosensitivity in SLE and NLE.
5. Furukawa et al. (191) showed that 17β-estradiol enhances binding of anti-Ro and anti-La antibodies to cultured human keratinocytes, implying that estrogen may promote the expression of Ro and La antigens on keratinocytes. Wang and Chan (211) demonstrated that, at 17β-estradiol concentrations achieved in the third trimester of pregnancy, expression of 52- and 60-kd Ro/SSA increases fivefold in cultured keratinocytes. This may be a factor in the greater expression of cutaneous NLE in females.

In summary, the above section provides evidence for the presence of Ro/SSA and La/SSB antigens in fetal heart and neonatal skin, the tissues most often involved by NLE, and their accessibility to maternal autoantibodies.

Maternal Autoantibodies To Ro/SSA And La/SSB

In the previously mentioned reports and series, with an aggregate of over 827 NLE children reported (Table 49.2), anti-Ro/SSA was positive in approximately 85% to 100%, and anti-La/SSB in about 50% to 85%. Of 742 mothers reported (see Table 49.6), 90% to 100% were positive for anti-Ro/SSA, and up to 76% were positive for anti-La/SSB. Anti-Ro/SSA and anti-La/SSB are IgG antibodies; in all infants tested serially for anti-Ro and anti-La, the antibodies tended to disappear in 3 to 8 months, consistent with catabolism of transplacentally transmitted maternal IgG (25,182).

Several instances of NLE with anti-La/SSB alone have been reported, suggesting that this antibody alone can be responsible pathogenetically (25,57,70,89,115). Silverman et al. (109) consider the presence of both anti-Ro and anti-La important in the development of neonatal lupus: all 15 of their infants with CHB and six of eight infants with cutaneous NLE were positive for both antibodies, with only two cutaneous NLE infants positive for anti-Ro/SSA alone.

The fine specificities of the anti-Ro/SSA system have been explored by Buyon and others (10,183,189,212–214): the 52-kd component of the Ro/SSA particle and the 48-kd La/SSB elicit antibodies in 75% and 90%, respectively, of mothers of children with CHB. The authors suggested that the presence of both these antibodies confers an odds ratio of 35. In 57 mothers of CHB, 12 mothers of transient cutaneous or hepatic NLE, 152 SLE mothers of healthy infants, and 30 with autoimmune disease and fetal or neonatal loss, anti-Ro/SSA was present in 100% of CHB mothers, 91% of transient NLE mothers, and in 47% and 43%, respectively, in the other two groups (214). The prevalence of anti-La/SSB paralleled that of anti-Ro at 76%, 71%, 15%, and 7%, respectively. Among 31 mothers of children with CHB, Julkunen et al. (215) found 97% positivity for 52-kd anti-Ro/SSA, 77% for 60-kd, and 39% for La/SSB, and recommended that the best test for CHB risk is anti–52-kd Ro/SSA by immunoblot. The autoantibody profile of CHB mothers resembled more closely Sjögren's syndrome than SLE patients. In a study of 44 Finnish CHB mothers, the same investigators found that a positive 52-kd anti-Ro confers an odds ratio of 18.9, and was the only test to discern mothers at risk for a CHB child, from primary Sjögren's syndrome women (216). In studies over time, the anti-Ro and anti-La profile of NLE mothers remained stable (217).

The following observations are worth mentioning, although of not yet established significance: Anti-La antibodies cross-react with laminin, the major component of cardiac sarcolemmal membrane, and may have a new role in the development of CHB (218). Agalactosyl fractions of autoantibodies are the most pathogenic, and there is evidence that CHB infants have a higher percentage of agalactosyl anti-Ro (219). Wang et al. (220) described a 75-kd phosphoprotein associated with Ro/SSA, with high expression in human heart and specific antibodies in children with NLE. Maddison et al. (221) described IgG antibodies to a 57-kd protein in 10% of SLE sera, in association with anti-Ro/SSA, but in 38% of mothers of NLE children, cardiac or cutaneous. In the sera of CHB children and their mothers, Bacman et al. (222) described circulating antibodies against β-adrenergic and muscarinic cholinergic receptors, reactive with neonatal heart. Eftekhari et al. (223) found that anti-SSA/Ro52 antibodies block the cardiac 5-HT4 serotoninergic receptor due to molecular mimicry between the receptor and Ro-52. Obbiassi et al. (224) described antibodies to Purkinje fibers in CHB children, but also in patients with systemic rheumatic diseases. Orth et al. (225) described antibodies to calreticulin, a calcium-binding protein of the endoplasmic reticulum, in 9 of 18 children with CHB. Miyagawa et al. (226) reported antibodies to a cleavage product of α-fodrin in five cutaneous NLE, one CHB infant, and their mothers. Antibodies to endogenous retrovirus-3 (ERV-3), which encodes for an envelope protein expressed in placenta, were found in CHB mothers in higher levels than normal pregnancy, lupus, and Sjögren's syndrome; ERV-3 was found in fetal heart—the authors suggest a possible role in the pathogenesis of CHB (227).

In summary, it appears that maternal antibodies to Ro/SSA and La/SSB recognize their respective antigens in the immature cardiac conduction system and the fetal myocardium, gain access perhaps through apoptosis, cause *in utero* an inflammatory reaction of the conduction system and myo/pericardium, resulting in fibrosis of the conduction system with heart block and myocarditis. Similarly, the same maternal antibodies recognize antigens present in neonatal skin, which are expressed in greater density upon UV light exposure and high estradiol concentrations, and cause the dermal inflammation of cutaneous NLE.

HEALTH AND LONG-TERM OUTCOME OF MOTHERS

There is adequate information about maternal diagnosis on 748 mothers of the 827 children reported (Table 50–5). Of these, 281 mothers were summarized previously (228). From 1992 to 2000, 258 mothers were reported prior to the establishment of, and outside the Research Registry (123,124,132,145,147,229,230, and case reports), and 209 were reported through Registry publications (144,146,166).

Of 373 mothers of children with CHB, 203 (54%) had rheumatic diseases: 11% had SLE, 20% had Sjögren's syndrome or sicca symptoms, 20% had an undifferentiated autoimmune syndrome (or undifferentiated connective tissue disease, with arthralgia, photosensitivity, and Raynaud phenomenon), and 41% were asymptomatic, with anti-Ro/SSA and/or anti-La/SSB. In 236 of the 373 mothers there was follow-up information (132,145,146,225): an additional 49 mothers developed rheumatic diseases, which increased the total from 121 to 170 (72%) in the four studies above, with reduction of asymptomatic patients to 28% from 41%. Systemic lupus and UCTD patients increased to 20% and 26%, respectively (Table 49.5).

It is of note that in the Finnish (145,229) and the Italian studies (147) of CHB mothers, there are greater proportions of patients with Sjögren's syndrome (44%, 24% and 33%), while in the North American (U.S. and Canadian) studies of CHB and cutaneous NLE mothers, systemic lupus predominates (132,146,166,230). Whether this is a true regional difference or not remains to be established by longer-term studies.

A greater proportion of rheumatic disease vs. asymptomatic mothers is seen in cutaneous NLE: of 80 such mothers, 55 (69%) had a rheumatic disease at delivery of the child with NLE, with lupus in 39%, Sjögren's syndrome in 14%, UCTD/undifferentiated autoimmune syndrome (UAS) in 24%, and no symptoms in 31% (124,166,226). Follow-up (of at least 5 years in the registry) in 71 mothers showed that 11 more developed a rheumatic disease (83%), with lupus in 38%, Sjögren's in 18%, UCTD/UAS in 26%, and reduction of asymptomatic patients to 17% (166,230; Table 49.5). The greater proportion of rheumatic diseases in mothers of cutaneous NLE versus CHB infants was emphasized by two publications from the university of Toronto (132,230). A thoughtful editorial has addressed the issue of maternal health differences (231).

TABLE 49.5. INITIAL AND (FOLLOW-UP) MATERNAL DIAGNOSIS IN NEONATAL LUPUS

		All RD No. (%)		Percent (F/U %)			
	No.	Initial	F/U	SLE	Sjögren/Sicca	UCTD/UAS	Asymptomatic
Congenital heart block							
Buyon et al. (144)	105	63 (60)		NS	NS	NS	37 (24)
Eronen et al. (145)	82	55 (67)	72 (88)	11	44	12[a]	33 (12)
Press et al. (132)	64	22 (34)	28 (44)[b]	3 (9)	2 (5)	19 (16)	66 (56)
Waltuck and Buyon (146)	57	34 (60)	45 (79)	26 (33)	14 (16)	19 (30)	40 (21)
Brucato et al. (147)	15	12 (80)		7	33	40	20
Julkunen et al. (229)	33	10 (30)	25 (76)	6 (18)	6 (24)	19 (33)	52 (27)[c]
Hubscher et al. (123)	17	7 (41)					
Subtotal	373	203 (54)	170 (72) of 236	11 (20)	20 (16)	20 (26)	41 (28)
Cutaneous NLE							
Neiman et al. (166)	47	34 (72)	40 (85)	32 (48)	17 (19)	23 (19)	28 (13)
Lawrence et al. (230)	24	14 (58)	19 (79)	29 (29)	4 (17)	25 (33)	42 (21)
Ng et al. (124)	9	7 (78)		56	22	0	22
Subtotal	80	55 (69)	59 (83) of 71	39 (38)	14 (18)	24 (26)	31 (17)
Case reports[d]	14	7 (50)		29	0	21	50
Subtotal	467	265 (57)	229 (75) of 307	21 (27)	16 (17)	19 (26)	39 (25)
Data in 5th edition (228)[d]	281	174 (62)		39.5	13.2	9.3[e]	38
Total	743	439 (59)		30.3	14.6	14.2	38.5

F/U, at follow-up; UAS/UCTD, undifferentiated autoimmune syndrome/connective tissue disease; NS, not specified; RD, rheumatic disease.
[a]Includes 10% with rheumatoid arthritis.
[b]Includes 11% (14%) with miscellaneous rheumatic diseases.
[c]Includes 10% with autoimmune thyroid disease.
[d]Include CHB, cutaneous, and other NLE.
[e]Includes miscellaneous rheumatic diseases.

As seen above, with longer follow-up of NLE mothers, the proportion who develop rheumatic diseases increases, as noted in older studies; in the long-term study by McCune et al. (94), eight of the 11 asymptomatic mothers (73%) developed a systemic rheumatic disease in a span of 5 years. In Esscher and Scott's (9) series, which included NLE children as old as 30 years of age, 64% of mothers had a systemic rheumatic disease. The time interval to development of maternal disease was as long as 14 years in Kasinath and Katz's (81) report, and 26 years in Reichlin's (232) patients. In Waltuck and Buyon's (146) report, of 23 asymptomatic mothers followed for up to 20 years, almost half (11, 48%) developed a rheumatic disease, notably undifferentiated autoimmune syndrome, SLE, and Sjögren's syndrome. Other rheumatic diseases in these women include mixed connective tissue disease, hypocomplementemic vasculitis, and rheumatoid arthritis. In my opinion, it is a matter of timing of the study, with longer follow-up having the least proportion of asymptomatic mothers.

Genetics Of Mothers With NLE Children

Lee et al. (165) first studied the genetic makeup of mothers with NLE children, and found positive HLA-DR3 in five of six mothers tested (83%), with a relative risk of 32. All mothers were positive for HLA-B8, and MT2, and five of six for MB2 (the terminology has now changed). Watson et al. (114) found HLA-DR3 in five of ten mothers, with a relative risk of 8, and confirmed the other findings. Vazquez Rodriguez et al. (233) also found a 50% prevalence of DR3 in Madrid.

Alexander et al. (234) examined 21 mothers of NLE infants and compared them to 17 patients with Sjögren's syndrome–lupus overlap: 17 of 21 women (81%) had HLA-DR3, with a relative risk of 13.8; HLA-DQw2 was present in 95%, for the highest relative risk of 26.4; B8 was found in 81% with a relative risk of 12.2; and DRw52 was seen in 95%, with relative risk of 11.7. The extended haplotype HLA-B8, DR3, DQw2, DRw52 was present in 15 of 20 NLE mothers (75%) and conferred a relative risk of 11.3. Similar findings were noted in the Sjögren's syndrome–lupus overlap patients, and the authors concluded that these two groups were closely related immunogenetically.

It is well known that DR3 and DR2 are associated with the ability to produce antibody to Ro/SSA (19,235,236). Hamilton et al. (19) showed that patients with anti-Ro/SSA alone have a strong association with the linked HLA alleles DR2 and DQw1, and have lower levels of anti-Ro. Patients with both anti-Ro and anti/La are associated with the linked alleles B8, DR3, DRw52, and DQw2, and have higher levels of anti-Ro, more sicca complex, and less renal involvement.

In a study of 31 women (seven with CHB children and anti-Ro/SSA antibodies, 15 with anti-Ro but no CHB births, and nine without anti-Ro but with CHB births) Arnaiz-Villena et al. (237) confirmed the striking prevalence of DR3 in CHB mothers (100%), and suggested that class III antigens (complement genes), such as BfS and/or

C4AQ0B1, are increased in Ro-positive mothers of infants with heart block.

Julkunen et al. (215) reported that 31 CHB mothers had HLA-B8 and DR3 more often than 900 healthy controls (71% versus 10%, and 74% vs. 23%), for a relative risk (RR) of 9.8 each. Compared to SLE controls, CHB mothers had more often DR3 and DQ2 positivity (RR 4.1 and 3.1, respectively). Compared with Sjögren's syndrome patients, CHB mothers were less positive for HLA-B15 (RR 0.1).

In all, of 90 NLE mothers with HLA typing, 70 (77.8%) were positive for HLA-DR3 (114,165,215,233,234,237).

Miyagawa et al. (238) found differences in the genetic makeup of 26 Japanese NLE mothers, depending on the child's NLE lesion: maternal HLA-DR5 haplotype DRB1*1101-DQA1*0501-DQB1*0301 and individual class II alleles making up this haplotype were significantly associated with cutaneous NLE, while maternal HLA-DQB1*0602, carried on HLA-DR2 haplotypes, was associated with CHB; and HLA-DQA1 alleles with glutamine at position 34 of the first domain, which are associated with Ro/SSA response in other ethnic groups, was increased in cutaneous NLE mothers.

Watson et al. (239) studied C4 allotypes and genes in 18 NLE families: 15 mothers (83%) had C4 null phenotypes, versus 36% of controls. Eleven of 18 (61%) had C4A null allotypes; C4A gene duplication was seen in CHB mothers, while duplication of C4B was seen in cutaneous NLE mothers.

The prevalence of DR3 in children with NLE is approximately 43% and can be explained on the basis of the high prevalence in the mother.

TREATMENT OF NEONATAL LUPUS

Congenital Heart Block

Prenatal testing for anti-Ro/SSA and anti-La/SSB should probably be restricted to the population at risk, that is, women with SLE, or Sjögren's syndrome, other systemic rheumatic diseases, and women with UCTD or UAS, since they comprise 12% to 33% of NLE mothers (Table 49.5 and related references). In a mother positive for anti-Ro, especially 52-kd, and anti-La, there is a potential risk for neonatal lupus of 1.5% to 8%, as stated in greater detail under prevalence. A previous child with NLE, especially with heart block, puts future pregnancies at risk at 10% to 16%. Careful monitoring during gestation with fetal echocardiography should be instituted from the 16th week of pregnancy.

It would seem that the best treatment for congenital heart block is prevention, because attempts at treatment, once complete heart block is diagnosed, frequently are to no avail (57,117,153,230). However, there have been successes. Several attempts have been made to treat CHB *in utero* with fluorinated corticosteroids, such as dexamethasone or betamethasone, which do not get inactivated by placental hydroxylases (240).

Saleeb et al. (241) reported retrospectively the research registry therapeutic experience (241). In 50 pregnancies of 47 mothers positive for anti-Ro/SSA and/or anti-La/SSB, the diagnosis of CHB was made *in utero* with at least four echocardiograms. In 28 pregnancies, mothers were treated either with dexamethasone, 4 to 9 mg/day for 3 to 19 weeks, or with betamethasone, 12 to 24 mg/week for over 6 weeks, while in 22 pregnancies no fluorinated steroids were used. There was no reversal of third-degree block in 21 treated, and 18 untreated fetuses; alternating second- and third-degree block progressed to permanent third-degree block in three treated and two untreated fetuses; four treated fetuses with second-degree block reverted to first-degree by birth, two continued so at 4 years, one is in second-degree block, and the fourth alternates between first and second degree; two untreated fetuses with second degree progressed to third; 17 pericardial effusions *in utero* resolved and reappeared regardless of therapy, while two pleural effusions, six of eight ascites, and five of eight hydrops fetalis cleared with steroids. Pacemaker requirement and deaths were similar in treated and untreated fetuses (14 vs. 11 and 4 vs. 1). The authors concluded that fluorinated steroid treatment *in utero* should be considered for incomplete block or hydropic changes. It is unknown, however, whether third-degree CHB would reverse with immediate treatment upon diagnosis, as is suggested by two case reports (242,243).

Copel et al. (244) treated five mothers with dexamethasone after *in utero* diagnosis of CHB; in two cases (one complete CHB, one second degree), the degree of block lessened, and hydrops resolved in three fetuses. Buyon et al. (245) identified 19 pregnancies with fluorinated steroid treatment of the mother after *in utero* discovery of CHB. Pleuropericardial effusions resolved in eight fetuses, second-degree block reverted to sinus rhythm in one fetus, and two with third-degree block improved. Shinohara et al. (246) noted no CHB in 26 neonates whose mothers were treated with betamethasone before 16 weeks' gestation, while 15 of 61 neonates without, or with delayed (after 16 weeks of gestation) steroid therapy, had CHB. Vignati et al. (247) reported ten fetuses with CHB, five of whom developed heart failure. Maternal dexamethasone therapy in four stabilized the condition in three, and sympathomimetic drugs increased the heart rate in three, but with maternal discomfort in two.

Maternal sympathomimetic agents have been used to treat fetal bradycardia, and digoxin to treat fetal heart failure (145,248).

At least ten more CHB cases were treated *in utero* (57, 117,153,249–254). Four cases merit special mention as they included treatment with plasmapheresis to remove pathogenic anti-Ro/SSA and anti-La/SSB from the fetal circulation (57,117,249). In two, pericardial effusions and myocarditis subsided, but CHB persisted (57,117). The other two were treated prophylactically and aggressively because of prior fetal loss with CHB or bradycardia (57,249): Buyon et al. (57) treated a woman with Sjögren's syndrome, whose prior child with heart block had died, with plasmapheresis from week 19, prednisone at 23 weeks, changed to dexamethasone at 35 weeks; the woman had a live healthy baby through planned cesarean section, with anti-Ro and anti-La in the cord blood. The other mother, who had four unsuccessful pregnancies, including one with heart block and fetal bradycardia, was treated with 25 mg/day of prednisolone and plasmapheresis from the 12th week of gestation, with reduction in anti-Ro titers and a live infant with transient bradycardia, delivered at 31 weeks, with anti-Ro in the cord blood (249).

In utero pacing was possible, but not successful (253).

It is difficult to organize controlled studies because of the rarity of CHB; in addition, any withholding of therapeutic measures in such precarious pregnancies would be, in my opinion, inconsistent with the ethics of the profession. Under such circumstances, therapeutic heroism seems justified. It is self-evident that rigorous follow-up of such a pregnancy by a high-risk obstetrician, a perinatologist, and a rheumatologist, and the presence of a neonatologist at delivery, are essential. The need for pacemakers in the immediate neonatal period in over 50% of the infants, and in 67% to 93% overall, has been emphasized previously (144,145). A report of anesthetic problems with CHB has appeared (255).

A very well thought out decision tree for diagnosis and management of CHB has been proposed by Buyon and Brucato (10) and further refined by Buyon (143):

A. Laboratory evaluation
   1. Initial screening for anti-Ro and anti-La by ELISA. If both are negative, the pregnancy has no known risk for CHB. If positive,
   2. Test by immunoblot.
      A negative immunoblot defines a low-risk pregnancy (<2% probability of CHB).
      Positive 52-kd and 60-kd Ro and La antibodies define a moderate risk pregnancy (2% to 5%).
      Positive anti-Ro and anti-La as above plus previous NLE child with any manifestation constitutes a high-risk pregnancy (15% to 20%).
B. Monitoring
   1. For low-risk pregnancy: Fetal echocardiogram at week 24, continued auscultation.
   2. For moderate-risk pregnancy: Fetal echocardiogram every 2 weeks, from 16 to 30 weeks; most important to do echo at 16 and 24 weeks, and continued auscultation.
   3. For high-risk pregnancy: Fetal echocardiogram every week from 16 to 30 weeks; most important to do echo at 16 and 24 weeks, and continued auscultation.
      If echo shows prolonged mechanical PR interval or advanced degrees of block, then do
C. Therapeutic approach to CHB diagnosed *in utero* depends on the degree of block and associated fetal morbidity at presentation:
   1a. Third-degree, over 2 weeks from detection: evaluate by serial echocardiograms and obstetrical sonograms; no therapy is initiated.
   1b. Third-degree, less than 2 weeks from detection: start oral dexamethasone, 4 mg/day for 6 weeks. If no change, taper. If there is reversal to second-degree or better, continue until delivery, then taper.
   1c. Alternating second- and third-degree block: oral (PO) dexamethasone, 4 mg/day for 6 weeks. If it progresses to third-degree, taper. If it reverses to second-degree or better, continue until delivery, then taper.
   1d. Second-degree block, or,
   1e. Prolonged mechanical PR interval (first-degree block): oral dexamethasone, 4 mg/day until delivery, then taper, unless it progresses to third-degree for 6 weeks, then taper.
   2. Heart block associated with signs of myocarditis, congestive heart failure, and/or hydropic changes: PO dexamethasone 4 mg/day until improvement, then taper.
   3. Severely hydropic fetus: PO dexamethasone 4 mg/day, plus apheresis as a last resort to rapidly remove maternal antibodies, or deliver if lungs are mature.

Cutaneous NLE alone does not require much therapy beyond avoidance of sun exposure and use of sun block and hydrocortisone cream (170).

LONG-TERM PROGNOSIS OF THE CHILD WITH NLE

Early perinatal mortality in CHB was mentioned above. Late mortality may occur from arrhythmia (6,9), pacemaker failure (178), or congestive heart failure (93,103). A fascinating outcome is the occurrence of systemic rheumatic disease in children with neonatal lupus during adolescence or adulthood. Thirteen such children have been reported (see list below), seven with CHB and six with cutaneous NLE. Six of these children developed SLE, three juvenile rheumatoid arthritis, and one each Sjögren's syndrome, UCTD, Hashimoto thyroiditis, and Raynaud phenomenon (Table 49.6).

1. The original patient of McCuistion and Schoch (3), who had cutaneous NLE, presented at age 19 with hair loss, weight loss, malar rash, leukopenia, positive ANA, membranous nephropathy, and oral ulcers, fulfilling criteria for SLE (69). She did well on high doses of prednisone. Her mother had died of severe SLE.
2. A female infant with cutaneous NLE was born to a woman diagnosed with SLE at age 13 who died of SLE postpartum (79). At age 13 the child developed SLE

TABLE 49.6. RHEUMATIC AND OTHER IMMUNE-MEDIATED DISEASES IN NLE PATIENTS

Author	Sex	CHB	Cutaneous NLE	Age at Onset (Years)	Diagnosis	Mother's Diagnosis
Fox et al. (69)	F	–	+	19	SLE	SLE
Jackson and Gulliver (255)	F	–	+	13	SLE	SLE
Waterworth (256)	F	+	–	23	SLE	NS
Lanham et al. (86)	F	+	–	23	Sjögren	SLE
Lanham et al. (86)	F	+	–	19	SLE	SLE
Jordan et al. (80)	F	+	–	9 months	SLE	SLE
Esscher and Scott (9)	F	+	–	15	SLE	NS
McCue et al. (7)	M	+	–	4.5	JRA	NS
Hubscher et al. (257)	F	+	–	13	UCTD	SLE
Neiman et al. (166)	NS	–	+	2	JRA	NS
Neiman et al. (166)	NS	–	+	5	JRA	NS
Neiman et al. (166)	NS	–	+	7	Hashimoto	NS
Neiman et al. (166)	NS	–	+	NS	Raynaud	NS

Hashimoto, Hashimoto's autoimmune thyroiditis; JRA, juvenile rheumatoid arthritis; Raynaud, Raynaud's phenomenon; UCTD, unclassifiable connective tissue disease; NS, not specified.

with polyarthritis, a subcutaneous nodule, Coombs-positive hemolytic anemia, leukopenia, and nephritis, and required steroid therapy (255).

3. A 23-year-old woman with CHB developed Adams-Stokes attacks and was given a permanent pacemaker. During the operation, pericarditis with effusion was noted, and she further developed noninfectious pneumonitis, anemia, positive ANA, Raynaud's phenomenon, and polyarthritis. She was diagnosed with SLE and responded to prednisone and azathioprine (256).
4. A girl born to a mother with SLE had CHB, and at 23 years of age developed anemia, positive ANA, purpura, polyarthritis, dry eyes, and had a lip biopsy compatible with Sjögren's syndrome (86).
5. A girl with CHB and pulmonary regurgitation was born to a mother with SLE who died of a cerebrovascular accident at age 38 (86). At age 19 the patient developed arthritis and, after a spontaneous abortion, developed vasculitis, positive LE cells, ANA, and anti-DNA.
6. A girl with congenital complete heart block went on to develop severe systemic lupus with Libman-Sacks endocarditis, nephritis, and autoimmune thrombocytopenia at 9 months of age, and died at 12 months of age (80).
7. A girl with CHB, reported by Esscher and Scott (9), developed SLE at age 15.
8. A boy with CHB, reported by McCue et al. (7), developed juvenile rheumatoid arthritis at age 4½.
9. A girl born to a mother with SLE had CHB and at age 13 developed symptoms of UCTD with positive anti-Ro/SSA and anti-U1RNP (257).
10. A child with cutaneous NLE developed juvenile rheumatoid arthritis at age 2 (166).
11. A child with cutaneous NLE developed juvenile rheumatoid arthritis at age 5 (166).
12. A child with cutaneous NLE developed Hashimoto thyroiditis at age 7 (166).
13. A child with cutaneous NLE developed Raynaud phenomenon (166).

As a footnote we mention a report by Reichlin (232) of a fascinating family. An asymptomatic woman gave birth to a boy with complete heart block. Antibodies to Ro/SSA and La/SSB have developed in the son, age 33 at the time of the report, and his mother developed features of SLE and Sjögren's syndrome 26 years after the birth of her son. Neonatal lupus erythematosus is a capricious experiment of nature that is slowly being elucidated.

REFERENCES

1. Morquio L. Sur une maladie enfantile et familiale caracterisée par des modifications des pouls, des attaques syncopales et épileptiformes et la mort subite. *Arch Med Enfants* 1901;4:467.
2. Hogg GR. Congenital, acute lupus erythematosus associated with subendocardial fibroelastosis. Report of a case. *Am J Clin Pathol* 1954;28:648.
3. McCuistion CH, Schoch EP Jr. Possible discoid lupus erythematosus in newborn infant. Report of a case with subsequent development of acute systemic lupus erythematosus in mother. *Arch Dermatol* 1954;70:782–785.
4. Aylward RD. Congenital heart block. *Br Med J* 1928;1:943.
5. Plant RK, Steven RA. Complete A-V block in a fetus. Case report. *Am Heart J* 1945;30:615–618.
6. Chameides L, Truex RC, Vetter V, et al. Association of maternal systemic lupus erythematosus with congenital complete heart block. *N Engl J Med* 1977;297:1204–1207.
7. McCue CM, Mantakas ME, Tingelstad JB, et al. Congenital heart block in newborns of mothers with connective tissue disease. *Circulation* 1977;56:82–90.
8. Winkler RB, Nora AH, Nora JJ. Familial congenital complete heart block and maternal systemic lupus erythematosus. *Circulation* 1977;56:1103.
9. Esscher E, Scott JS. Congenital heart block and maternal systemic lupus erythematosus. *Br Med J* 1979;1:1235–1238.

10. Buyon JP, Brucato A. Neonatal lupus. *Semin Clin Immunol* 1998;(1):5–19.
11. Tseng CE, Buyon JP. Neonatal lupus syndromes. *Rheum Dis Clin North Am* 1997;23:31–54.
12. Franco HL, Weston WL, Peebles C, et al. Autoantibodies directed against sicca syndrome antigens in neonatal lupus syndrome. *J Am Acad Dermatol* 1981;4:67–72.
13. Kephart DC, Hood AF, Provost TT. Neonatal lupus erythematosus: new serological findings. *J Invest Dermatol* 1981;77: 331–333.
14. Miyagawa S, Kitamura W, Yoshioka J, et al. Placental transfer of anticytoplasmic antibodies in annular erythema of newborns. *Arch Dermatol* 1981;117:569–572.
15. Calmes BA, Bartholomew BA. SSA-A(Ro) antibody in random mother-infant pairs. *J Clin Pathol* 1985;38:73–75.
16. Fritzler MJ, Pauls JD, Kinsella TD, et al. Antinuclear, anticytoplasmic and anti-Sjögren's syndrome antigen A (SS-A/Ro) antibodies in female blood donors. *Clin Immunol Immunopathol* 1985;36:120–128.
17. Gaither KK, Fox OF, Yamagata H, et al. Implications of anti-Ro/Sjögren's syndrome A antigen autoantibody in normal sera for autoimmunity. *J Clin Invest* 1987;79:841–846.
18. Garcia-de la Torre I, Sanchez-Guerrero A, Salmon-de la Torre G, et al. Prevalence of anti-SSA(Ro) antibodies in a Mexican population of patients with various systemic rheumatic diseases. *J Rheumatol* 1987;14:479–481.
19. Hamilton RG, Harley JB, Bias WB, et al. Two Ro (SS-A) autoantibody responses in systemic lupus erythematosus correlation of HLA-DR/DQ specificities with quantitative expression of Ro (SS-A) autoantibody. *Arthritis Rheum* 1988;31: 496–505.
20. Harley JB, Yamagata H, Reichlin M. Anti-La/SSB antibody is present in some normal sera and is coincident with anti-Ro/SSA precipitins in systemic lupus erythematosus. *J Rheumatol* 1984; 11:309–314.
21. Harmon CE, Lee LA, Huff JC, et al. The frequency of antibodies to the SS-A/Ro antigen in pregnancy sera. *Arthritis Rheum* 1974;27(suppl 4):S20.
22. Maddison PJ, Mogavero H, Provost TT, et al. The clinical significance of autoantibodies to a soluble cytoplasmic antigen in systemic lupus erythematosus and other connective tissue diseases. *J Rheumatol* 1979;6:189–195.
23. Maddison PJ, Skinner RP, Vlahoyiannopoulos P, et al. Antibodies to nRNP, Sm, Ro (SSA), and La (SSB) detected by ELISA: their specificity and interrelationship in connective tissue disease sera. *Clin Exp Immunol* 1985;62:337–345.
24. Singsen BH, Nevon P, Wang G, et al. Anti-SSA and other antinuclear antibodies (ANA) in healthy pregnant women and in newborn cord bloods (abstract). *J Rheumatol* 1986;13:984.
25. Taylor PV, Taylor KF, Norman A, et al. Prevalence of maternal Ro(SS-A) and La(SS-B) autoantibodies in relation to congenital heart block. *Br J Rheumatol* 1988;27:128–132.
26. Bell DA, Komar R, Chordiker WB, et al. A comparison of serologic reactivity among SLE patients with or without anti-Ro(SSA) antibodies. *J Rheumatol* 1984;11:315–317.
27. Bell DA, Maddison PJ. Serologic subsets in systemic lupus erythematosus: an examination of autoantibodies in relationship to clinical features of disease and HLA antigens. *Arthritis Rheum* 1980;23:1268–1273.
28. Dennis GJ, West SG, Anderson PA. Identification of clinical subsets by serologic markers in systemic lupus erythematosus. *Arthritis Rheum* 1983;26(suppl):S13(abst).
29. Dillon CF, Jones JV, Reichlin M. Antibody to Ro in a population of patients with systemic lupus erythematosus: distribution, clinical and serological associations. *J Rheumatol* 1983;10:380.
30. Maddison PJ, Isenberg DA, Goulding NJ, et al. Anti-La(SSB) identifies a distinctive subgroup of systemic lupus erythematosus. *Br J Rheumatol* 1988;27:27–31.
31. Mond CB, Rothfield NF. Anti-Ro antibody correlates with photosensitive rash in SLE patients (abstract). *Arthritis Rheum* 1988;31(suppl):S55.
32. Parke AL, Rothfield NF. Congenital heart block, systemic lupus erythematosus, and anti-Ro antibodies. *Arthritis Rheum* 1985; 28:1077.
33. Ramsey-Goldman R, Hom D, Deng J-S, et al. Anti-SS-A antibodies and fetal outcome in maternal systemic lupus erythematosus. *Arthritis Rheum* 1986;29:1269–1273.
34. Reichlin M, Harley JB. Antibodies to Ro(SSA) and the heterogeneity of systemic lupus erythematosus. *J Rheumatol* 1987;14: 112.
35. Scopelitis E, Biundo JJ, Alspaugh MA. Anti-SSA antibody and other antinuclear antibodies in systemic lupus erythematosus. *Arthritis Rheum* 1980;23:287–293.
36. Synkowski DR, Reichlin M, Provost TT. Serum autoantibodies in systemic lupus erythematosus and correlation with cutaneous features. *J Rheumatol* 1982;9:380.
37. Wilson WA, Scopelitis E, Michalski JP. Association of HLA-DR with both antibody to SS-A (Ro) and disease susceptibility in blacks with systemic lupus erythematosus. *J Rheumatol* 1984; 11:653.
38. Miyagawa S, Dohi K, Yoshioka A, et al. Female predominance of immune response to SSA/Ro antigens and risk of neonatal lupus erythematosus. *Br J Dermatol* 1990;123:223–227.
39. Alexander EL, Hirsh TJ, Arnett FC, et al. Ro(SSA) and La(SSB) antibodies in the clinical spectrum of Sjögren's syndrome. *J Rheumatol* 1982;9:239–246.
40. Goldsmith DP. Neonatal rheumatic disorders. View of the pediatrician. *Rheum Dis Clin North Am* 1989;15:287–305.
41. Provost TT, Watson R, Gammon WR, et al. The neonatal lupus syndrome associated with U1 RNP (nRNP) antibodies. *N Engl J Med* 1987;315:1135–1139.
42. Rider LG, Sherry DD, Glass ST. Neonatal lupus erythematosus simulating transient myasthenia gravis at presentation. *J Pediatr* 1991;118:417–419.
43. Solomon BA, Laude TA, Shalita AR. Neonatal lupus erythematosus: discordant disease expression of U1 RNP-positive antibodies in fraternal twins—is this a subset of neonatal lupus erythematosus or a new distinct syndrome? *J Am Acad Dermatol* 1995;32:858–862.
44. Michaelsson M, Engle MA. Congenital complete heart block: an international study of the natural history. *Cardiovasc Clin North Am* 1972;4:85–101.
45. Mintz G, Niz J, Gutierrez G, et al. Prospective study of pregnancy in systemic lupus erythematosus. Results of a multidisciplinary approach. *J Rheumatol* 1986;13:732–739.
46. Watson RM, Braunstein BL, Watson AJ, et al. Fetal wastage in women with anti-Ro(SSA) antibody. *J Rheumatol* 1986;13: 90–94.
47. McHugh NJ, Reilly PA, McHugh LA. Pregnancy outcome and autoantibodies in connective tissue disease. *J Rheumatol* 1989; 16:42–46.
48. Maddison PJ. Anti-Ro antibodies and neonatal lupus. *Clin Rheumatol* 1990;9:116–122.
49. Lockshin MD, Bonfa E, Elkon K, et al. Neonatal lupus risk to newborns of mothers with systemic lupus erythematosus. *Arthritis Rheum* 1988;31:697–701.
50. Lockshin MD, Gibofsky A, Peebles CC, et al. Neonatal lupus erythematosus with heart block: family study of a patient with anti-SS-A and SS-B antibodies. *Arthritis Rheum* 1983;26: 210–213.
51. Drosos AA, Dimou GS, Siamopoulou-Mavridou A, et al. The neonatal lupus erythematosus syndrome in Greece and France,

a prospective study. In: *Hungarian Rheumatology Abstracts of the XIIth European Congress of Rheumatology*, 1991;32:50 (SW14–105).

52. Nossent HC, Swaak TJG. Systemic lupus erythematosus. VI. Analysis of the interrelationship with pregnancy. *J Rheumatol* 1990;17:771–776.
53. Barber KA, Jackson R. Neonatal lupus erythematosus: five new cases with HLA typing. *Can Med Assoc J* 1983;129:139.
54. Berube S, Lister G, Towes WH, et al. Congenital heart block and maternal systemic lupus erythematosus. *Am J Obstet Gynecol* 1978;130:595–596.
55. Bharati S, Swerdlow MA, Vitullo D, et al. Neonatal lupus with congenital atrioventricular block and myocarditis. *PACE Pacing Clin Electrophysiol* 1987;10:1058.
56. Bremers HH, Golitz LE, Weston WL, et al. Neonatal lupus erythematosus. *Cutis* 1979;24:287.
57. Buyon JP, Swersky SH, Fox HE, et al. Intrauterine therapy for presumptive fetal myocarditis with acquired heart block due to systemic lupus erythematosus. *Arthritis Rheum* 1987;30:44–49.
58. Callen JP, Fowler JF, Kulick KB, et al. Neonatal lupus erythematosus occurring in one fraternal twin. Serologic and immunogenetic studies. *Arthritis Rheum* 1985;28:271.
59. Watson RM, Scheel JN, Petri M, et al. Neonatal lupus erythematosus. Report of serological and immunogenetic studies in twins discordant for congenital heart block. *Br J Dermatol* 1994;130:342–348.
60. Buyon JP, Waltuck J, Caldwell K, et al. Relationship between maternal and neonatal levels of antibodies to 48-kda SSB(La), 52-kda SSA(Ro), and 60-kda SSA(Ro) in pregnancies complicated by congenital heart block. *J Rheumatol* 1994;21: 1943–1950.
61. Distelmeier MR, Hayne ST, Rada DC. Neonatal lupus: a case report. *Cutis* 1984;33:191.
62. Doshi N, Smith B, Klionsky B. Congenital pericarditis due to maternal lupus erythematosus. *J Pediatr* 1980;96:699–701.
63. Draznin TH, Esterly NB, Furey NL, et al. Neonatal lupus erythematosus. *J Am Acad Dermatol* 1979;1:437–442.
64. East WR, Lumpkin CR. Systemic lupus erythematosus in the newborn. *Minn Med* 1969;53:477.
65. Epstein HC, Litt JZ. Discoid lupus erythematosus in a newborn infant. *N Engl J Med* 1961;265:1106.
66. Fitzsimmons JS, Crawford MJ, Reeves WG. Congenital discoid lupus in the newborn. *J Med Genet* 1977;14:283–286.
67. Fox R, Hawkins DF. Fetal pericardial effusion in association with congenital heart block and maternal systemic lupus erythematosus. Case report. *Br J Obstet Gynecol* 1990;97:638–640.
68. Fox R, Lumb MR, Hawkins DF. Persistent fetal sinus bradycardia associated with maternal anti-Ro antibodies. Case report. *Br J Obstet Gynecol* 1990;7:1151–1153.
69. Fox RJ Jr, McCuistion CH, Schoch EP Jr. Systemic lupus erythematosus association with previous neonatal lupus erythematosus. *Arch Dermatol* 1979;115:340.
70. Franceschini F, Bertoli MT, Martinelli M, et al. The neonatal lupus erythematosus associated with isolated La(SSB) antibodies. *J Rheumatol* 1990;17:415–416.
71. Gawkrodger DJ, Beveridge GW. Neonatal lupus erythematosus in four successive siblings born to a mother with discoid lupus erythematosus. *Br J Dermatol* 1984;111:683.
72. Geggel RL, Tucker L, Szer I. Postnatal progression from second- to third-degree heart block in neonatal lupus syndrome. *J Pediatr* 1988;113:1049–1052.
73. McCarron DP, Hellmann DB, Traill TA, et al. Neonatal lupus erythematosus syndrome: late detection of isolated heart block. *J Rheumatol* 1993;20:1212–1214.
74. Hardy JD, Solomon S, Banwell GS, et al. Congenital complete heart block in the newborn associated with maternal systemic lupus erythematosus and other connective tissue disorders. *Arch Dis Child* 1979;54:713.
75. Harley JB, Kaine JL, Fox OF, et al. Ro (SS-A) antibody and antigen in a patient with congenital complete heart block. *Arthritis Rheum* 1985;28:1321–1325.
76. Hontani N, Horino K, Fukui J. Lupus erythematosus observed in a newborn infant. A case report and review of the literature. *Acta Pediatr Jpn* 1971;75:171.
77. Houssiau FA, Lebacq EG. Neonatal lupus erythematosus with congenital heart block associated with maternal systemic lupus erythematosus. *Clin Rheumatol* 1986;5:505.
78. Hull D, Binns BAO, Joyce D. Congenital heart block and widespread fibrosis due to maternal lupus erythematosus. *Arch Dis Child* 1966;41:688–690.
79. Jackson R. Discoid lupus in a newborn infant of a mother with lupus erythematosus. *Pediatrics* 1964;33:425–430.
80. Jordan JM, Valenstein P, Kredich DW. Systemic lupus erythematosus with Libman-Sacks endocarditis in a 9-month-old infant with neonatal lupus erythematosus and congenital heart block. *Pediatrics* 1989;84:574–577.
81. Kasinath BS, Katz AI. Delayed maternal lupus after delivery of offspring with congenital heart block. *Arch Intern Med* 1982; 142:2317.
82. Katayama I, Kondo S, Kawana S, et al. Neonatal lupus erythematosus with a high anticardiolipin antibody titer. *J Am Acad Dermatol* 1989;21:490–492.
83. Kaye EM, Butler IJ, Conley S. Myelopathy in neonatal and infantile lupus erythematosus. *J Neurol Neurosurg Psychiatry* 1987;50:923.
84. Kettler AH, Stone MS, Bruce S, et al. Annular eruptions of infancy and neonatal lupus erythematosus. *Arch Dermatol* 1987;123:298–199.
85. Kosmetatos N, Blackman MS, Elrad H, et al. Congenital complete heart block in the infant of a woman with collagen vascular disease. A case report. *J Reprod Med* 1979;22:213–216.
86. Lanham JG, Walport MJ, Hughes GRV. Congenital heart block and familial connective tissue disease. *J Rheumatol* 1983;10: 823–825.
87. Corona R, Angelo C, Cacciaguerra MG, et al. Neonatal lupus erythematosus. *Cutis* 2000;65:379–381.
88. Seip M. Systemic lupus erythematosus in pregnancy with haemolytic anaemia, leucopenia and thrombocytopenia in the mother and her newborn infant. *Arch Dis Child* 1960;35: 364–366.
89. Lee LA, Lillis PJ, Fritz KA, et al. Neonatal lupus in successive pregnancies. *J Am Acad Dermatol* 1983;9:401–406.
90. Lumpkin LR, Hall J, Hogan JD, et al. Neonatal lupus erythematosus. A report of three cases associated with anti-Ro/SSA antibodies. *Arch Dermatol* 1985;121:377–381.
91. Luo SF, Huang CC, Wang JW. Neonatal lupus erythematosus: report of a case. *J Formos Med Assoc* 1989;88:832–835.
92. Maddison JP, Sukhum P, Williamson DP, et al. Echocardiography and fetal heart sounds in the diagnosis of fetal heart block. *Am Heart J* 1979;98:505–509.
93. McCormack GD, Barth WF. Congenital complete heart block with maternal primary Sjögren's syndrome. *South Med J* 1985; 78:471.
94. McCune AB, Weston WL, Lee LA. Maternal and fetal outcome in neonatal lupus erythematosus. *Ann Intern Med* 1987;106: 518–523.
95. Moore PJ. Maternal systemic lupus erythematosus associated with fetal congenital heart block. A case report. *S Afr Med J* 1981;60:285–286.
96. Moudgil A, Kishore K, Srivastava RN. Neonatal lupus erythematosus, late onset hypocalcemia, and recurrent seizures. *Arch Dis Child* 1987;62:736.

97. Nice CM Jr. Congenital disseminated lupus erythematosus. *AJR* 1962;86:585–587.
98. Nitta Y, Ohashi M. Neonatal lupus syndrome and microtubular structures. *J Dermatol* 1989;16:54–58.
99. Nolan RJ, Shulman ST, Victorica BE. Congenital complete heart block associated with maternal mixed connective tissue disease. *J Pediatr* 1979;95:420–422.
100. Ohtaki N, Miyamoto C, Orita M, et al. Concurrent multiple morphea and neonatal lupus erythematosus in an infant boy born to a mother with SLE. *Br J Dermatol* 1986;115:85–90.
101. Paredes RA, Morgan H, Lachelin GC. Congenital heart block associated with maternal primary Sjögren's syndrome. Case report. *Br J Obstet Gynaecol* 1983;90:870.
102. Reed BR, Lee LA, Harmon C, et al. Autoantibodies to SS-A/Ro in infants with congenital heart block. *J Pediatr* 1983;103: 889–891.
103. Reed WB, May SB, Tuffanelli DL. Discoid lupus erythematosus in a newborn. *Arch Dermatol* 1967;96:64.
104. Rendall JR, Wilkinson JD. Neonatal lupus erythematosus. *Clin Exp Dermatol* 1978;3:69.
105. Romano C, Pongiglione R, Ruffa G, et al. Blocco atrioventricolare congenito di alto grado. *Minerva Pediatr* 1976;27: 1632–1649.
106. Scheib JS, Waxman J. Congenital heart block in successive pregnancies: a case report and evaluation of risk with therapeutic consideration. *Obstet Gynecol* 1989;73:481–484.
107. Yemini M, Shoham Z, Dgani R, et al. Lupus-like syndrome in a mother and newborn following administration of hydralazine: a case report. *Eur J Obstet Gynecol Reprod Biol* 1989;30: 193–197.
108. Shimizu T, Ino T, Nishimoto K, et al. Advanced atrioventricular block in a neonate with lupus erythematosus and anti-SSA antibodies. *Pediatr Cardiol* 1988;9:121–124.
109. Silverman E, Mamula M, Hardin JA, et al. Importance of the immune response to the Ro/La particle in the development of congenital heart block and neonatal lupus erythematosus. *J Rheumatol* 1991;18:120–124.
110. Soltani K, Pacernick LJ, Lorincz AL. Lupus erythematosus-like lesions in newborn infants. *Arch Dermatol* 1974;110:435.
111. Stephensen O, Cleland WP, Hallidie-Smith K. Congenital complete heart block and persistent ductus arteriosus associated with maternal systemic lupus erythematosus. *Br Heart J* 1981; 46:104–106.
112. Syed AA. Congenital heart block and hypothyroidism. *Arch Dis Child* 1978;53:256.
113. Veille JC, Sunderland C, Bennett RM. Complete heart block in a fetus associated with maternal Sjögren's syndrome. *Am J Obstet Gynecol* 1985;151:660.
114. Watson RM, Lane AT, Barnett NK, et al. Neonatal lupus erythematosus: a clinical, serological and immunogenetic study with review of the literature. *Medicine* 1984;63:362–378.
115. Weston WL, Harmon C, Peebles C, et al. A serological marker for neonatal lupus erythematosus. *Br J Dermatol* 1982;107:377–382.
116. Wright FS, Adams P Jr, Anderson RC. Congenital atrioventricular dissociation due to complete or advanced atrioventricular heart block. *Am J Dis Child* 1959;98:72.
117. Herreman G, Ferme I, Morel S, et al. Fetal death caused by myocarditis and isolated congenital complete heart block. *Presse Med* 1985;14:1547–1550.
118. Repke JT, Kuhajda F, Hochberg MC, et al. Fetal viral myocarditis and congenital complete heart block in a pregnancy complicated by systemic lupus erythematosus: a case report. *J Reprod Med* 1987;32:217–220.
119. Knolle P, Mayet W, Lohse AW, et al. et al. Complete congenital heart block in autoimmune hepatitis (SLA-positive). *J Hepatol* 1994;21:224–226.
120. Batard M, Sainte-Marie D, Clity E, et al. Cutaneous neonatal lupus erythematosus: discordant expression in identical twins. *Ann Dermatol Venereol* 2000;127(10):814–817.
121. Shimosegawa M, Akasaka T, Matsuta M. Neonatal lupus erythematosus occurring in identical twins. *J Dermatol* 1997;24: 578–582.
122. Yazici Y, Onel K, Sammaritano L. Neonatal lupus erythematosus in triplets. *J Rheumatol* 2000;27(3):807–809.
123. Hubscher O, Batista N, Rivero S, et al. Clinical and serological identification of two forms of complete heart block in children. *J Rheumatol* 1995;22:1352–1355.
124. Ng PP, Tay YK, Giam YC. Neonatal lupus erythematosus: our local experience. *Ann Acad Med Singapore* 2000;29(1):114–118.
125. Friedman DM, Zervoudakis I, Buyon JP. Perinatal monitoring of fetal well being in the presence of congenital heart block. *Am J Perinatol* 1998;15:669–673.
126. Ferrazzini G, Fasnacht M, Arbenz U, et al. Neonatal lupus erythematosus with congenital heart block and severe heart failure due to myocarditis and endocarditis of the mitral valve. *Intensive Care Med* 1996;22:464–466.
127. Falcini F, De Simone L, Donzelli G, et al. Congenital conduction defects in children born to asymptomatic mothers with anti-SSA/SSB antibodies. Report of two cases. *Ann Ital Med Int* 1998;13:169–172.
128. Gayad E, Haddad F, Tohme A, et al. Neonatal lupus erythematosus and atrial-ventricular block. A case report and review of the literature. *J Med Liban* 1998;46:36–39.
129. Louthrenoo W, Boonyaratavej S, Sittiwangkul R, et al. Anti-Ro/SSA positive undifferentiated connective tissue disease in a mother with a newborn with complete congenital heart block: a case report. *J Med Assoc Thai* 1998;81:633–636.
130. Fukazawa R, Seki T, Kamisago M, et al. A Ro/SSS-A auto-antibody positive mother's infant revealed congenital complete atrioventricular heart block, followed by insulin dependent diabetes mellitus and multiple organ failure. *Acta Pediatr Jpn* 1994; 36:427–430.
131. Gurakan B, Yalcin S, Tekinalp G, et al. Neonatal lupus syndrome: report of a case. *Turk J Pediatr* 1995;37:153–156.
132. Press J, Uziel Y, Laxer RM, et al. Long term outcome of mothers of children with complete congenital heart block. *Am J Med* 1996;100:328–332.
133. Hung CL, Lin CH, Mu SC, et al. Hydrops fetalis with complete heart block secondary to congenital lupus: report of one case. *Acta Paediatr Taiwan* 1999;40(4):265–267.
134. Selander B, Cedergren S, Domanski H. A case of severe neonatal lupus erythematosus without cardiac or cutaneous involvement. *Acta Pediatr* 1998:87:105–107.
135. Crowley E, Frieden IJ. Neonatal lupus erythematosus: an unusual congenital presentation with cutaneous atrophy, erosions, alopecia and pancytopenia. *Pediatr Dermatol* 1998;15:38–42.
136. Ruas E, Moreno A, Tellechea O, et al. Neonatal lupus erythematosus in an infant with Turner syndrome. *Pediatr Dermatol* 1996;13:298–302.
137. Freyschmidt-Paul P, Rieger CH, Happle R, et al. Neonatal lupus erythematosus and HELLP syndrome: is there a pathogenetic link? *Hautarzt* 1998;49:662–628.
138. Hariharan D, Manno CS, Seri I. Neonatal lupus erythematosus with microvascular hemolysis. *J Pediatr Hematol/Oncol* 2000;22 (4):351–354.
139. Lam C, Imundo L, Hirsch D, et al. Glomerulonephritis in a neonate with atypical congenital lupus and toxoplasmosis. *Pediatr Nephrol* 1999;13:850–853.
140. Westenend PJ. Congenital nephrotic syndrome in neonatal lupus syndrome. *J Pediatr* 1995;126:851.
141. de Klerk OL, de Vries TW, Sinnige LGF. An unusual cause of neonatal seizures in a newborn infant. *Pediatrics* 1997;100:E(8).

142. Tabbut S, Griswold WR, Ogino MT, et al. Multiple thromboses in a premature infant associated with maternal antiphospholipid syndrome. *J Perinatol* 1994;14:66–70.
143. Buyon JP. Neonatal lupus: bench to bedside and back. Presented at the 66th annual meeting of the American College of Rheumatology, October 2000.
144. Buyon J, Hiebert R, Copel J, et al. Autoimmune-associated congenital heart block: Demographics, mortality, morbidity and recurrence rates obtained from a national neonatal lupus registry. *J Am Coll Cardiol* 1998;31:1658–1666.
145. Eronen M, Siren MK, Ekblad H, et al. Short-and long-term outcome of children with congenital complete heart block diagnosed in utero or as a newborn. *Pediatrics* 2000;106:86–91.
146. Waltuck J, Buyon JP. Autoantibody-associated congenital heart block: outcome in mothers and children. *Ann Intern Med* 1994; 120:544–551.
147. Brucato A, Franceschini F, Gasparini M, et al. Isolated congenital complete heart block: long-term outcome of mothers, maternal antibody specificity and immunogenetic background. *J Rheumatol* 1995;22:533–540.
148. Brucato A, Gasparini M, Vignati G, et al. Isolated congenital complete heart block: long-term outcome of children and immunogenetic study. *J Rheumatol* 1995;22:541–543.
149. Agarwala B, Sheikh Z, Cibils LA. Congenital complete heart block. *J Natl Med Assoc* 1996;88:725–729.
150. Taylor-Albert E, Reichlin M, Toews W, et al. Delayed dilated cardiomyopathy as a manifestation of neonatal lupus: case reports, autoantibody analysis and management. *Pediatrics* 1997;99:733–735.
151. Gembruch U, Hansmann M, Redel DA, et al. Fetal complete heart block: antenatal diagnosis, significance and management. *Eur J Obstet Gynecol Reprod Biol* 1989;31:922.
152. Shenker L, Reed KL, Anderson CF, et al. Congenital heart block and cardiac anomalies in the absence of maternal connective tissue disease. *Am J Obstet Gynecol* 1987;157:248–253.
153. Petri M, Watson R, Hochberg MC. Anti-Ro antibodies and neonatal lupus. *Rheum Dis Clin North Am* 1989;15:335–360.
154. Lee LA, Harmon CE, Huff JC, et al. Demonstration of SSA/Ro antigen in human fetal tissues and in neonatal and adult skin. *J Invest Dermatol* 1985;85:143–146.
155. Reid JM, Coleman EN, Doig W. Complete congenital heart block. Report of 35 cases. *Br Heart J* 1982;48:236.
156. Michaelsson M, Jonzon A, Riesenfeld T. Isolated congenital complete atrio-ventricular block in adult life: a prospective study. *Circulation* 1995;92:442–449.
157. Cimaz R, Stramba-Badiale M, Brucato A, et al. QT interval prolongation in asymptomatic Anti-SSA/ro-positive infants without congenital heart block. *Arthritis Rheum* 2000;43: 1049–1053.
158. Brucato A, Cimaz R, Catelli L, et al. Anti-Ro-associated bradycardia in newborns. *Circulation* 2000;102:88.
159. Mazel JA, El-Sherif N, Buyon JP, et al. Electrocardiographic abnormalities in a murine model injected with IgG from mothers of children with congenital heart block. *Circulation* 1999; 99:1914–1918.
160. Carter JB, Blieden LC, Edwards JE. Congenital heart block: anatomic correlations and review of the literature. *Arch Pathol* 1974;97:51.
161. Meckler KA, Kapur RP. Congenital heart block and associated cardiac pathology in neonatal pulus syndrome. *Pediatr Dev Pathol* 1998;1:136–142.
162. Litsey SE, Noonan JA, O'Connor WN, et al. Maternal connective tissue disease and congenital heart block. Demonstration of immunoglobulin in cardiac tissue. *N Engl J Med* 1985;312: 98–100.
163. Taylor PV, Scott JS, Gerlis LM, et al. Maternal antibodies against fetal cardiac antigens in congenital complete heart block. *N Engl J Med* 1986;315:667–672.
164. Lee LA, Coulter S, Erner S, et al. Cardiac immunoglobulin deposition in congenital heart block associated with maternal anti-Ro autoantibodies. *Am J Med* 1987;83:793–796.
165. Lee LA, Bias WB, Arnett FC, et al. Immunogenetics of neonatal lupus syndrome. *Ann Intern Med* 1983;99:592–596.
166. Neiman AR, Lee LA, Weston WL, et al. Cutaneous manifestations of neonatal lupus without heart block: Characteristics of mothers and children enrolled in a national registry. *J Pediatr* 2000;137(5):674–680.
167. Weston WL, Morelli JG, Lee LA. The clinical spectrum of anti-Ro-positive cutaneous neonatal lupus erythematosus. *J Am Acad Dermatol* 1999;40(5 pt 1):675–681.
168. Vonderheid EC, Koblenzer PJ, Ming PML, et al. Neonatal lupus erythematosus. Report of four cases with review of the literature. *Arch Dermatol* 1976;112:698–705.
169. Thornton CM, Eichenfeld LF, Shinall EA, et al. Cutaneous telangiectases in neonatal lupus erythematosus. *J Am Acad Dermatol* 1995;33:19–25.
170. Lee LA, Weston WL. Cutaneous lupus erythematosus during the neonatal and childhood periods. *Lupus* 1997;6:132–138.
171. Sontheimer RD, Thomas JR, Gilliam JN. Subacute cutaneous lupus erythematosus: a cutaneous marker for a distinct lupus erythematosus subset. *Arch Dermatol* 1979;115:1409–1415.
172. Brustein D, Rodriguez JM, Minkin W, et al. Familial lupus erythematosus. *JAMA* 1977;238:2294–2296.
173. Dugan EM, Tunnessen WW, Honig PJ, et al. U1RNP antibody-positive neonatal lupus. A report of two cases with immunogenetic studies. *Arch Dermatol* 1992;128:1490–1494.
174. Sheth AP, Esterly NB, Ratoosh SL, et al. U1RNP positive neonatal lupus erythematosus: association with anti-La antibodies? *Br J Dermatol* 1995;132:520–526.
175. Laxer RM, Roberts EA, Gross KR, et al. Liver disease in neonatal lupus erythematosus. *J Pediatr* 1990;116:238–242.
176. Lee LA, Reichlin M, Ruyle SZ, et al. Neonatal lupus liver disease. *Lupus* 1993;2:333–338.
177. Watson RM, Kang JE, May M, et al. Thrombocytopenia in the neonatal lupus syndrome. *Arch Dermatol* 1988;124:560–563.
178. Buyon J, Roubey R, Swersky S, et al. Complete congenital heart block: risk of occurrence and therapeutic approach to prevention. *J Rheumatol* 1988;15:1104–1108.
179. Levy SB, Goldsmith LS, Morohashi M, et al. Tubuloreticular inclusions in neonatal lupus erythematosus. *JAMA* 1976;235: 2743–2744.
180. Fonseca E, Contreras F, Garcia-Frias E, et al. Neonatal lupus erythematosus with multisystem organ involvement preceding cutaneous lesions. *Lupus* 1991;1:49–50.
181. Berlyne GM, Short IA, Vickers CFH. Placental transmission of the LE factor. Report of two cases. *Lancet* 1957;273:1516.
182. Scott JS, Maddison PJ, Taylor PJ, et al. Connective-tissue disease, antibodies to ribonucleoprotein, and congenital heart block. *N Engl J Med* 1983;39:209–212.
183. Buyon JP, Winchester R. Congenital complete heart block: a human model of passively acquired autoimmune injury. *Arthritis Rheum* 1990;33:609–614.
184. Bachmann M, Mayet WJ, Schroder HC, et al. Association of La and Ro antigens with intracellular structures of HEp-2 carcinoma cells. *Proc Natl Acad Sci USA* 1986;83:7770.
185. Rinke J, Steitz JA. Precursor molecules of both human 5S ribosomal RNA and transfer RNAs are bound by a cellular protein reactive with anti-La lupus antibodies. *Cell* 1982;29:149.
186. McNeilage LJ, Whittingham S, Jaack I, et al. Molecular analysis of the RNA and protein components recognized by anti-La(SS-B) autoantibodies. *Clin Exp Immunol* 1985;62:685–695.

187. Deng JS, Bair LW, Schen-Schwartz S, et al. Localization of Ro (SSA) antigen in the cardiac conduction system. *Arthritis Rheum* 1987;30:1232–1238.

187a. Fraire-Velasquez A, Herrera-Esparza R, Villalobos-Hurtaclo R, Avalos-Piaz E. Ontogeny of Ro hyRNAs in human heart. *Scand J Rheumatol* 1999;28:100–105.

188. Reichlin M, Brucato A, Frank MB, et al. Concentration of autoantibodies to native 60-kD Ro/SSA and denatured 52-kD Ro/SSA in eluates from the heart of a child who died with congenital complete heart block. *Arthritis Rheum* 1994;37:1698–1703.

189. Buyon JP, Tseng CE, Di Donato F, et al. Cardiac expression of 52beta, an alternate transcript of the congenital heart block-associated 52kD SSA/Ro autoantigen, is maximal during fetal development. *Arthritis Rheum* 1997;40:655–660.

190. Tseng CE, Miranda E, Di Donato F, et al. MRNA and protein expression of SSA/Ro and SSB/La in human fetal cardiac myocytes cultured using a novel application of the Langendorff procedure. *Pediatr Res* 1999;45:260–269.

191. Furukawa F, Lyons MB, Lee L, et al. Estradiol enhances binding to cultured human keratinocytes of antibodies specific for SS-A/Ro and SS-B/La. Another possible mechanism for estradiol influence of lupus erythematosus. *J Immunol* 1988;141: 1480–1488.

192. Alexander EL, Buyon JP, Lane J, et al. et al. Anti-SSA/Ro SSB/La antibodies bind to neonatal rabbit cardiac cells and preferentially inhibit in vitro cardiac repolarization. *J Autoimmun* 1989;2:463–469.

193. Alexander E, Buyon JP, Provost TT, et al. Anti-Ro/SS-A antibodies in the pathophysiology of congenital heart block in neonatal lupus syndrome, an experimental model. In vitro electrophysiologic and immunocytochemical studies. *Arthritis Rheum* 1992;35:176–189.

194. Boutjdir M, Chen L, Zhang ZH, et al. Arrhythmogenicity of IgG and anti 52kD SSA/Ro affinity-purified antibodies from mothers of children with congenital heart block. *Circ Res* 1997; 80:354–362.

195. Boutjdir M, Chen L, Zhang ZH, et al. Serum and immunoglobulin G from the mother of a child with congenital heart block induce conduction abnormalities and inhibit L-type calcium channels in a rat heart model. *Pediatr Res* 1998;44: 11–19.

196. Viana VS, Garcia S, Nascimento JH, et al. Induction of in vitro heart block is not restricted to affinity purified anti 52kD Ro/SSA antibody from mothers of children with neonatal lupus. *Lupus* 1998;7:141–147.

197. Kalush F, Rimon E, Keller A, et al. Neonatal lupus erythematosus with cardiac involvement in the offspring of mothers with experimental systemic lupus erythematosus. *J Clin Immunol* 1994;14:314–322.

198. Miranda-Carus ME, Askanase AD, Clancey RM, et al. Anti-SSA/Ro and anti-SSB/La autoantibodies bind the surface of apoptotic fetal cardiocytes and promote secretion of TNF-alpha by macrophages. *J Immunol* 2000;165:5345–5351.

199. Lee LA, Weston WL, Krueger GG, et al. An animal model of antibody binding in cutaneous lupus. *Arthritis Rheum* 1986;29: 782–788.

200. Lee LA, Gaither KK, Coulter SN, et al. The pattern of cutaneous immunoglobulin G deposition in subacute cutaneous lupus erythematosus is reproduced by infusing purified anti-Ro (SSA) autoantibodies into human skin-grafted mice. *J Clin Invest* 1989;83:1556–1562.

201. Lee LA, David KM. Cutaneous lupus erythematosus. *Curr Probl Dermatol* 1989;1:161–200.

202. Bennion SD, Ferris C, Lieu TS, et al. IgG subclasses in the serum and skin in subacute cutaneous lupus erythematosus and neonatal lupus erythematosus. *J Invest Dermatol* 1990;95:643–646.

203. Yell JA, Wang L, Yin H, et al. Disparate locations of the 52- and 60-kD Ro/SSA antigens in cultured human keratinocytes. *J Invest Dermatol* 1996;107:622–626.

204. LeFeber WP, Norris DA, Ryan SB, et al. Ultraviolet light induces binding of antibodies to selected nuclear antigens on cultured human keratinocytes. *J Clin Invest* 1984;74:15–45.

205. Furukawa F, Kashihara-Sawami M, Lyons MB, et al. Binding of antibodies to the extractable nuclear antigens of SSA/Ro and SSB/La is induced on the surface of human keratinocytes by ultraviolet light (UVL): implications for the pathogenesis of photosensitive cutaneous lupus. *J Invest Dermatol* 1990;94:77.

206. Furukawa F. Antinuclear antibody-keratinocyte interactions in photosensitive cutaneous lupus erythematosus. *Histol Histopathol* 1999;14(2):627–633.

207. Dorner T, Hucko M, Mayet WJ, et al. Enhanced membrane expression of the 52kDRo (SSA) and La (SSB) antigens by human keratinocytes induced by TNF alpha. *Ann Rheum Dis* 1996;54:904.

208. Yu HS, Chiang CH, Kang JW, et al. The cytotoxic effect of neonatal lupus erythematosus and maternal sera on keratinocyte cultures is complement-dependent and can be augmented by ultraviolet irradiation. *Br J Dermatol* 1996;135: 297–301.

209. Davis TL, Lyde CB, Davis BM, et al. Perturbation of experimental ultraviolet light-induced erythema by passive transfer of serum from subacute cutaneous lupus erythematosus patients. *Soc Invest Dermatol* 1989;92:573–577.

210. Ioannides D, Golden BD, Buyon JP, et al. Expression of SSA/Ro and SSB/La antigens in skin biopsy specimens of patients with photosensitive forms of lupus erythematosus. *Arch Dermatol* 2000;136:340–346.

211. Wang D, Chan EK. 17beta-estradiol increases expression of 52kDa and 60kDa SSA/Ro autoantigens in human keratinocytes and breast cancer cell line MCF-7. *J Invest Dermatol* 1996;107:610–614.

212. Ben-Chetrit E, Chan EKL, Sullivan KF, et al. A 52-kD protein is a novel component of the SS-A/Ro antigenic particle. *J Exp Med* 1988;167:1560–1571.

213. Buyon JP, Ben-Chetrit E, Karp S, et al. Acquired congenital heart block. Pattern of maternal antibody response to biochemically defined antigens of the SSA/Ro-SSB/La system in neonatal lupus. *J Clin Invest* 1989;84:627–634.

214. Buyon JP, Winchester RJ, Slade SG, et al. Identification of mothers at risk for congenital heart block and other neonatal lupus syndromes in their children. Comparison of enzyme-linked immunosorbent assay and immunoblot for measurement of anti-SSA/Ro and anti-SSB/La antibodies. *Arthritis Rheum* 1993;36:1263–1273.

215. Julkunen H, Siren MK, Kaaja R, et al. Maternal HLA antigens and antibodies to SS-A/Ro and SS-B/La. Comparison with systemic lupus erythematosus and primary Sjögren's syndrome. *Br J Rheumatol* 1995;34:901–907.

216. Julkunen H, Kaaja R, Siren MK, et al. Immune-mediated congenital heart block (CHB): identifying and counseling patients at risk for having children with CHB. *Semin Arthritis Rheum* 1998;28:97–106.

217. Tseng CE, Di Donato F, Buyon JP. Stability of immunoblot profile of anti-SSA/Ro -SSB/La antibodies over time in mothers whose children have neonatal lupus. *Lupus* 1996;5:212–215.

218. Li JM, Horsfall AC, Maini RN. Anti-La(SSB)but not Ro52 (SSA) antibodies crossreact with laminin—a role in the pathogenesis of congenital heart block? *Clin Exp Immunol* 1995;99: 316–324.

219. Pilkington C, Taylor PV, Silverman E, et al. Agalactosyl IgG and maternofetal transmission of autoimmune neonatal lupus. *Rheumatol Int* 1996;16:89–94.

220. Wang D, Buyon JP, Zhu W, et al. Defining a novel 75kDa phosphoprotein associated with SSA/Ro and identification of distinct human autoantibodies. *J Clin Invest* 1999;104:1265–1275.
221. Maddison PJ, Lee L, Reichlin M, et al. Anti-p57: a novel association with neonatal lupus. *Clin Exp Immunol* 1995;99:42–48.
222. Bacman S, Sterin-Borda L, Camusso JJ, et al. Circulating antibodies against neurotransmitter receptor activities in children with congenital heart block and their mothers. *FASEB J* 1994; 8:1170–1176.
223. Eftekhari P, Salle L, Lezoualc'h F, et al. Anti-SSA/Ro52 autoantibodies blocking the cardiac 5-HT4 serotoninergic receptor could explain neonatal lupus congenital heart block. *Eur J Immunol* 2000;30:2782–2790.
224. Obbiassi M, Brucato A, Meroni PL, et al. Antibodies to cardiac Purkinje cells: further characterization in autoimmune diseases and atrioventricular heart block. *Clin Immunol Immunopathol* 1987;42:141–150.
225. Orth T, Dorner T, Meyer Zum Buschenfelde KH, et al. Complete congenital heart block is associated with increased autoantibody titers against calreticulin. *Eur J Clin Invest* 1996;26: 205–215.
226. Miyagawa S, Yanagi K, Yoshioka A, et al. Neonatal lupus erythematosus: maternal IgG antibodies bind to a recombinant NH2-terminal fusion protein encoded by human alpha-fodrin cDNA. *J Invest Dermatol* 1998;111:1189–1192.
227. Li JM, Fan WS, Horsfall AC, et al. The expression of human endogenous retrovirus-3 in fetal cardiac tissue and antibodies in congenital heart block. *Clin Exp Immunol* 1996;104:388–393.
228. Kitridou RC. The neonatal lupus syndrome. In: Wallace DJ, Hahn BH, eds. *Dubois' lupus erythematosus*, 5th ed. Baltimore: Williams & Wilkins, 1997:1023–1035.
229. Julkunen H, Kurki P, Kaaja R, et al. Isolated congenital heart block. Long term outcome of mothers and characterization of the immune response to SSA/Ro and to SSB/La. *Arthritis Rheum* 1993;36:1588–1598.
230. Lawrence S, Luy L, Laxer R, et al. The health of mothers of children with cutaneous neonatal lupus erythematosus differs from that of mothers of children with congenital heart block. *Am J Med* 2000;108(9):705–709.
231. Buyon JP. The heart and skin of neonatal lupus-does maternal health matter? *Am J Med* 2000;108:741–743.
232. Reichlin M. Antinuclear antibodies. In: Kelley W, Harris E, Ruddy S, et al., eds. *Textbook of rheumatology*, 3rd ed. Philadelphia: WB Saunders, 1989:208–225.
233. Vazquez Rodriguez JJ, Garcia Seoane J, Gial Aguado A, et al. Complete heart block and the HLA system. *Ann Intern Med* 1982;96:126.
234. Alexander EL, McNicholl J, Watson RM, et al. The immunogenetic relationship between anti-Ro(SS-A)/La(SS-B) antibody positive Sjögren's/lupus erythematosus overlap syndrome and the neonatal lupus syndrome. *J Invest Dermatol* 1989;93:751–756.
235. Ahearn JM, Provost TT, Dorsch CA, et al. Interrelationships of HLA-DR, MB and MT phenotypes, autoantibody expression, and clinical features in systemic lupus erythematosus. *Arthritis Rheum* 1982;25:1031–1040.
236. Alvarellos A, Ahearn JM, Provost TT, et al. Relationships of HLA-DR and MT antigens to autoantibody expression in SLE. *Arthritis Rheum* 1983;26:1533–1535.
237. Arnaiz-Villena A, Vasquez-Rodriguez JJ, Vicario JL, et al. Congenital heart block immunogenetics. Evidence for an additional role of HLA class II antigens and independence of Ro antibodies. *Arthritis Rheum* 1989;32:1421–1426.
238. Miyagawa S, Kidoguchi K, Kaneshige T, et al. Neonatal lupus erythematosus: analysis of HLA class I genes in Japanese child/mother pairs. *Lupus* 1999;8(9):751–754.
239. Watson RM, Scheel JN, Lee LA, et al. Neonatal lupus erythematosus syndrome: analysis of C4 allotypes and C4 genes in 18 families. *Medicine* 1992;71:84–95.
240. Blanford AT, Murphy BEP. In vitro metabolism of prednisolone, dexamethasone, betamethasone and cortisol by the human placenta. *Am J Obstet Gynecol* 1977;127:264–267.
241. Saleeb S, Copel J, Friedman D, et al. Comparison of treatment with fluorinated glucocorticoids to the natural history of autoantibody-associated congenital heart block: retrospective review of the research registry for neonatal lupus. *Arthritis Rheum* 1999;42(11):2335–2345.
242. Rosenthal D, Druzin M, Chin C, et al. A new therapeutic approach to the fetus with congenital complete heart block: preemptive, targeted therapy with dexamethasone. *Obstet Gynecol* 1998;92:689–691.
243. Ishimaru S, Izaki S, Kitamura K, et al. Neonatal lupus erythematosus: dissolution of atrioventricular block after administration of corticosteroid to the pregnant mother. *Dermatology* 1994;189(suppl 1):92–94.
244. Copel JA, Buyon JP, Kleinman CS. Successful in utero therapy of fetal heart block. *Am J Obstet Gynecol* 1995;173:1384–1390.
245. Buyon JP, Waltuck J, Kleinman C, et al. In utero identification and therapy of congenital heart block. *Lupus* 1995;4: 116–121.
246. Shinohara K, Miyagawa S, Fugita T, et al. Neonatal lupus erythematosus: results of maternal corticosteroid therapy. *Obstet Gynecol* 1999;93:952–957.
247. Vignati G, Brucato A, Pisoni MP, et al. Clinical course of preand port-natal isolated congenital atrioventricular block diagnosed in utero. *G Ital Cardiol* 1999;29:1478–1487.
248. Fukushige J, Takahashi N, Igarashi H, et al. Perinatal management of congenital complete atrioventricular block: report of nine cases. *Acta Pediatr Jpn* 1998;40:337–340.
249. Barclay CS, French MA, Ross LD, et al. Successful pregnancy following steroid therapy and plasma exchange in a woman with anti-Ro(SSA) antibodies. Case report. *Br J Obstet Gynaecol* 1987;94:369–371.
250. Chua S, Ostman-Smith I, Sellers S, et al. Congenital heart block with hydrops fetalis treated with high-dose dexamethasone: a case report. *Eur J Obstet Gynecol Reprod Biol* 1991;42: 155–158.
251. Rider LG, Buyon JP, Rutledge J, et al. Treatment of neonatal lupus: case report and review of the literature. *J Rheumatol* 1993;20:1208–1211.
252. Carreira PE, Gutierrez-Larraya F, Gomez-Reino JJ. Successful intrauterine therapy with dexamethasone for fetal myocarditis and heart block in a woman with systemic lupus erythematosus. *J Rheumatol* 1993;20:1204–1207.
253. Walkinshaw SA, Welch CR, McCormack J, et al. In utero pacing for fetal congenital heart block. *Fetal Diag Ther* 1994;9:183–185.
254. Pratilas V, Pratila M. Anesthesia in the presence of complete fetal atrioventricular heart block: an anesthetics dilemma. *Mt Sinai J Med* 1990;57:157–159.
255. Jackson R, Gulliver M. Neonatal lupus erythematosus progressing into systemic lupus erythematosus a 15 year follow-up. *Br J Dermatol* 1979;101:81–86.
256. Waterworth RF. Systemic lupus erythematosus occurring with congenital complete heart block. *NZ Med J* 1980;92:311–312.
257. Hubscher O, Carillo D, Reichlin M. Congenital heart block and subsequent connective tissue disorder in adolescence. *Lupus* 1997;6:283–284.

50

LUPUS NEPHRITIS: PATHOLOGY, PATHOGENESIS, CLINICAL CORRELATIONS, AND PROGNOSIS

MICHAEL KASHGARIAN

Both autopsy and biopsy studies of patients with the clinical diagnosis of systemic lupus erythematosus (SLE) have documented that renal involvement is a frequent and serious complication of the disease, making the renal biopsy an important part of the clinical management of these patients (1,2). Numerous reports have documented the unpredictable course of lupus nephritis and the role of the renal biopsy in the evaluation of individual patients with isolated and unusual clinical features (3–10). For example, some patients with other systemic manifestations but no clinical evidence of renal involvement have been found to have severe forms of lupus nephritis on renal biopsy (11–14). Other patients present initially with renal disease and exhibit systemic manifestations later in their course. Furthermore, the nature of the lesion on renal biopsy gives direct information relating to the severity of the autoimmune response within the kidney, thereby aiding in selecting the appropriate therapies and in predicting both the short-term and long-term outcome in individual patients. For these reasons, many clinicians advocate the renal biopsy as a routine part of the evaluation of all patients with SLE.

WORLD HEALTH ORGANIZATION CLASSIFICATION OF LUPUS NEPHRITIS

Over the last several decades, there have been major advances in our knowledge of the pathogenesis of immune-complex mediated glomerular injury, and this has been applied to the diagnostic interpretation of renal biopsies as well as to clinical pathologic correlations aimed at evaluating the natural history of disease and response to therapy. This approach has been particularly valuable in the case of lupus nephritis since its histology is varied and its pathogenesis is thought to be similar to that of various forms of experimental immune-complex glomerulonephritis. Thus, biopsy findings must be interpreted in the context of what we have learned from experimental models (15–19). The various patterns of lupus nephritis are best considered in the context of the potential pathogenic mechanisms that might be involved in their evolution. Analysis in this way not only gives a basis to correlate with clinical outcome but also offers a rationale for therapeutic manipulation. The classification scheme for lupus nephritis developed by the World Health Organization (WHO) provides a basis for this type of clinical application (Table 50.1) (20). It combines all the morphologic modalities of biopsy interpretation including light, immunofluorescence, and electron microscopic findings and thus represents a major improvement over previous classifications. The classification system along with a semiquantitative assessment of severity is now in general use and has been accepted by clinical nephrologists and renal pathologists alike. A more detailed subclassification has been suggested by the pathology advisory group of the International Study of Kidney Diseases in Children

TABLE 50.1. WHO CLASSIFICATION OF LUPUS NEPHRITIS

	Immunofluorescence		Electron Microscopy		
Patterns	Mesangial	Peripheral	Mesangial	Subendothelial	Subepithelial
I Normal	0	0	0	0	0
IIA Mesangial deposits	+	0	+	0	0
IIB Mesangial hypercellularity	+	0	+	0	0
III Focal-segmental GN (<50%)	++	+	++	+	+
IV Diffuse GN (>50%)	++	++	++	++	+
V Membranous GN	+	++	+	+	++

GN, glomerulonephritis.

TABLE 50.2. INTERNATIONAL STUDY OF KIDNEY DISEASE IN CHILDREN: CLASSIFICATION OF LUPUS NEPHRITIS

I. Normal
 A. Nil
 B. Normal by light microscopy but deposits present
II. Pure mesangiopathy
 A. Mild (+)
 B. Moderate (++)
III. Segmental and focal proliferative glomerulonephritis
 A. Active necrotizing
 B. Active and sclerosing
 C. Sclerosing
IV. Diffuse proliferative glomerulonephritis
 A. Without segmental necrotizing lesions
 B. With segmental necrotizing lesions
 C. With segmental active and sclerotic lesions
 D. Inactive, sclerotic
V. Diffuse membranous glomerulonephritis
 A. Pure membranous
 B. Associated with lesions in group IIA or IIB
 C. Associated with lesions in group IIIA, IIIB, or IIIC
 D. Associated with lesions in group IVA, IVB, IVC, or IVD
VI. Advanced sclerosing glomerulonephritis

(ISKDC) (21), but this seems to be of greater value for investigative purposes than for general clinical use (Table 50.2). It is best to use these classifications in the context of what we know about the potential pathogenic mechanisms that underlie the various lesions. These classifications do have the limitation of focusing on the glomerular lesions while attributing much less significance to tubular, interstitial, and vascular lesions. Nonetheless, they have been shown to be clinically useful and form a good structure for evaluation in individual patients.

HISTOPATHOLOGY AND PATHOGENESIS

Class I

In class I, the renal biopsy reveals essentially a normal kidney by light, electron, and immunofluorescence microscopy. Minor nonspecific changes such as irregular thickening of the basement membrane occasionally are observed on electron microscopy, but these changes usually are not associated with a functional abnormality. Since this class is defined in reality by the absence of morphologic evidence of glomerular damage, it denotes a lack of significant renal involvement in SLE. Although some reports suggest that all patients with SLE may have renal immune complex deposition even in the absence of clinical evidence, about 25% of affected patients exhibit no significant glomerular findings and thus could be categorized in this group.

Class II

Class II is composed of pure mesangial lesions (22,23). It has been subdivided into IIA and IIB. IIA contains lesions with minimal or no significant changes by light microscopy, although immunofluorescence may present evidence of immune deposits confined to the mesangium and the electron microscopy will reveal corresponding electron-dense deposits in this location. In IIB, light microscopy shows definite glomerular mesangial hypercellularity confined to the centrilobular areas away from the vascular pole (Fig. 50.1). There is no involvement of the peripheral glomerular capillary walls. Immunofluorescence reveals mesangial immunoglobulin deposition (Fig. 50.2), and electron microscopy discloses dense deposits confined to the mesangial regions (Fig. 50.3). In some cases deposits are occasionally seen in the paramesangial subendothelial areas. Tubular, interstitial, and vascular changes are usually insignificant. Patients with class II lesions generally have minimal clinical evidence of renal involvement with mild to moderate proteinuria and/or hematuria and little or no evidence of renal insufficiency (23). Rarely, full-blown nephrotic syndrome may be present, and this may predict a transformation to a more severe form of nephritis and the likelihood of progression to chronicity (24). It is likely that this lesion corresponds to the experimental lesion where the generation of relatively small numbers of stable immune complexes of intermediate size formed with antibodies having high affinity and high avidity accumulate in the mesangium as a result of the mesangial clearing system for removal of macromolecules (25). The relatively small number of complexes characteristic of this lesion prevents the mesangial system from becoming overloaded and allows the complexes to be sequestered in the mesangium, where they are subject to degradation and removal rather than remaining at sites where they could initiate an inflammatory response (26). This explanation of accumulation and restriction of immune complexes to the mesangium assigns

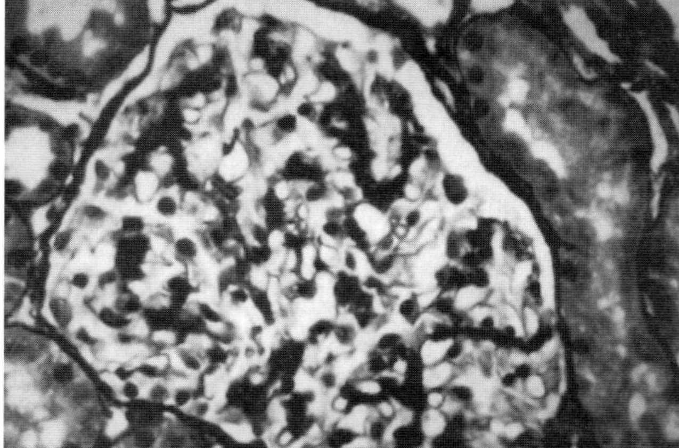

FIGURE 50.1. (See color plate.) Lupus glomerulonephritis, World Health Organization (WHO) class IIB. There is mild to moderate, but definite, mesangial hypercellularity confined to the centrilobular areas. The capillary loops are patent, and no evidence of inflammation is seen (H&E, ×300).

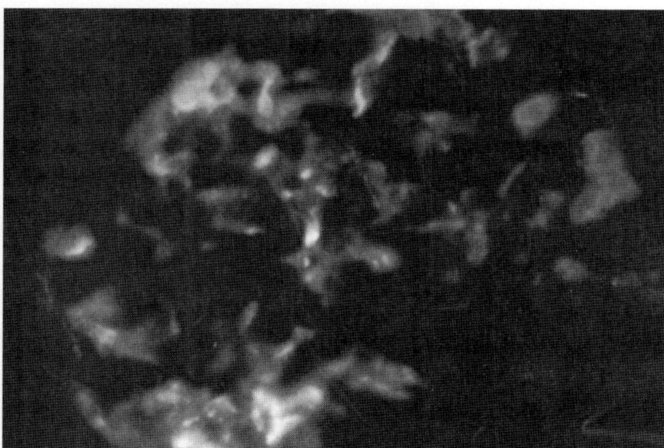

FIGURE 50.2. (See color plate.) Lupus nephritis, WHO class IIB. Immunofluorescence microscopy reveals mesangial immunoglobulin deposition. The peripheral capillary loops are free from immunoglobulins. Complement usually is present in a similar pattern.

no specific characteristics either to the nature of the antigen or to the nature of antibody (25–27). There is increasing evidence, however, that suggests that specific characteristics of both antigen and antibody are involved in localization of complexes to distinct glomerular sites. Fibronectin is an important component of the mesangial matrix, and given its capacity to interact with aggregates of immunoglobulins and immune complexes in the circulation, its presence in the mesangium may play a role in this type of localization (28). Regardless of the mechanisms involved in mesangial localization, the sequestration of such complexes to this site allows for their isolation from inflammatory mediators and results in a relatively benign noninflammatory lesion.

Class III

Class III is characterized by light microscopic findings of a focal and segmental glomerulonephritis (3,29). Less than 50% of the glomeruli that are involved show only focal damage occupying less than 50% of the glomerular surface. The segmental changes can be proliferative, necrotizing, sclerosing, or a combination of these alterations (Fig. 50.4). Segmental intracapillary and extracapillary cell proliferation with obliteration of the capillary lumina is sometimes found in addition to generalized mesangial widening. Segmental necrotic lesions may be associated with crescent formation that progress to segmental scars with focal capsular adhesions. These segmental lesions are usually superimposed on a minimal degree of mesangial hypercellularity (30,31).

Immunofluorescence and electron microscopic findings show major differences in comparison to class II. Immunofluorescence reveals peripheral granular as well as mesangial deposits of immunoglobulins (Fig. 50.5), and electron microscopy demonstrates subendothelial deposits in addition to the presence of mesangial deposits (Fig. 50.6). The similarity of the immunofluorescence and electron microscopic findings of class III to those of class IV suggests that these two classes actually may be variations of the same immunopathologic lesion and the focal nature of class III representing a quantitative rather than a qualitative difference. Class III has been broken down into three subclasses: active necrotizing lesions, necrotizing and sclerosing lesions, and purely sclerosing lesions. The clinical significance of this subclassification is not clear. The natural history of patients with class III lesions is similar to that of patients having class IV lesions, again suggesting that these two classes are a continuum of the same lesion (22,32).

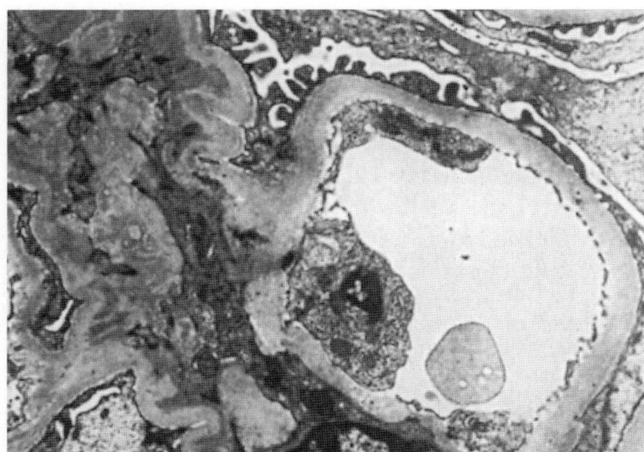

FIGURE 50.3. Lupus glomerulonephritis, WHO class IIB. Electron microscopy reveals abundant mesangial electron-dense deposits. The deposits are confined to the mesangial area, and the peripheral capillary loops show no evidence of immune complex deposition (×7,500).

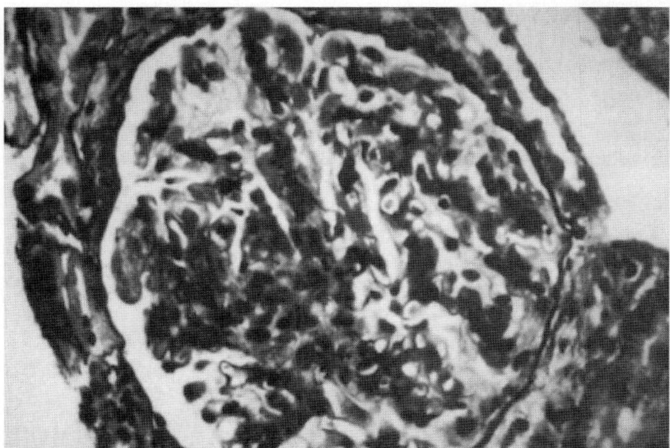

FIGURE 50.4. (See color plate.) Lupus glomerulonephritis, WHO class III. Light microscopy reveals a focal and segmental glomerulonephritis. There is a segment of focal necrosis associated with mesangial cell proliferation and infiltration with neutrophils. The remainder of the glomerulus shows only a moderate increase in mesangial cellularity (H&E, ×300).

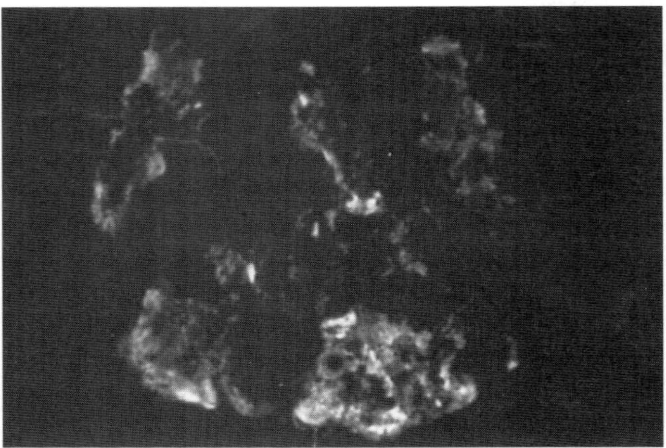

FIGURE 50.5. (See color plate.) Lupus glomerulonephritis, WHO class III. Immunofluorescence reveals peripheral granular as well as mesangial deposits of immunoglobulins. The immunoglobulin deposition is present diffusely throughout the glomerulus but is concentrated focally in the areas of segmental lesions.

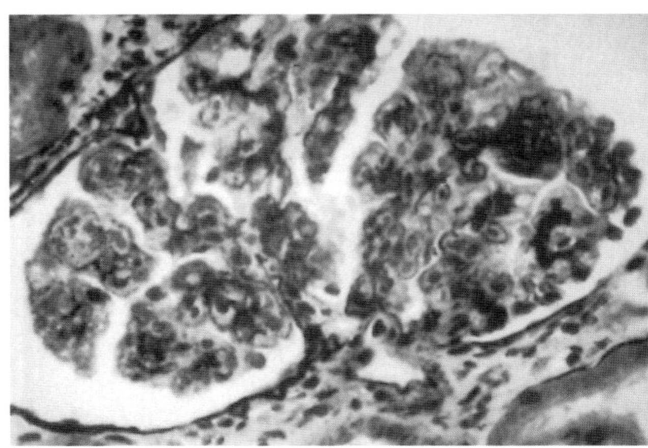

FIGURE 50.7. (See color plate.) Lupus glomerulonephritis, WHO class IV. There is diffuse hypercellularity throughout the glomerulus with lobular accentuation and mesangialization of the peripheral capillary loops. The peripheral walls are thickened and, in some areas, have a wire-loop appearance. Neutrophils also are seen in areas of proliferation (H&E, ×300).

Class IV

Histopathology

Class IV is the most common form of lupus nephritis and is characterized by a diffuse proliferative glomerulonephritis. The majority or all of the glomeruli are involved and each glomerulus shows diffuse hypercellularity (Fig. 50.7). As with class III, segmental areas of necrosis can occur, occasionally associated with focal areas of crescent formation. Nuclear debris represented by hemotoxyphil bodies can also be seen. Some segments of the peripheral capillary loop can be dramatically thickened by subendothelial deposition of immune complexes to form the so-called wire loop lesion. Some cases may demonstrate the presence of large intracapillary immune complex deposits forming so-called hyaline thrombi. Segmental areas of sclerosis are an indicator either of previous segmental necrosis or of chronicity. The variety of the lesions that can be encountered in this class range from diffuse mesangial hypercellularity without necrosis to a severe necrotizing and crescentic glomerulonephritis with focal and global areas of sclerosis. The four subclassifications of the ISKDC are useful in separating these different patterns into IVa, pure diffuse proliferative lesions; IVb, proliferative lesions with focal necrosis; IVc, proliferative lesions with necrosis and sclerosis; and IVd, proliferative lesions with sclerosis. About a quarter of cases exhibit lobular accentuation with mesangial extension around the peripheral loops, forming a pattern that is similar to other forms of mesangiocapillary glomerulonephritis.

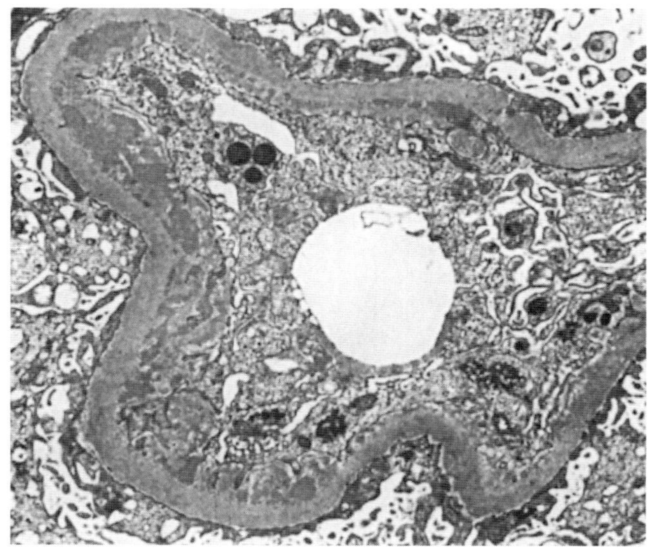

FIGURE 50.6. Lupus glomerulonephritis, WHO class III. Electron microscopy reveals abundant subendothelial deposits associated with endothelial cell swelling. Mesangial areas (not shown) also contain electron-dense deposits. Epimembranous deposits also may be seen in some capillary loops (×7,500).

Immunofluorescence microscopy reveals a coarsely granular pattern of immunoglobulin deposition both in the mesangium and in the peripheral capillary walls (Fig. 50.8). Multiple immunoglobulins are frequently encountered and are generally accompanied by evidence of activation of inflammatory mediators such as a deposition of complement components, fibrinogen, and properdin. This pattern has been called a "full house" pattern of immunoglobulin deposition.

Electron microscopic examination is similar to that seen with class III (Fig. 50.6). Large mesangial deposits accompany abundant subendothelial deposits. These deposits are generally larger and more abundant than in other classes of lupus nephritis. Epimembranous deposits are often present.

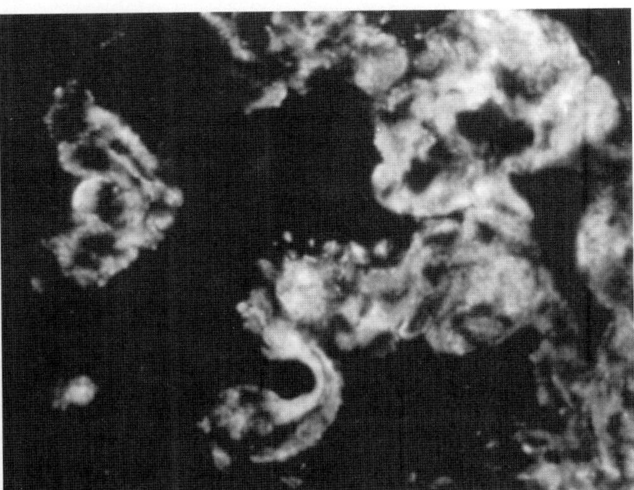

FIGURE 50.8. (See color plate.) Lupus glomerulonephritis, WHO class IV. Immunofluorescence microscopy reveals a coarsely granular pattern of immunoglobulin deposition both in the mesangium and in the peripheral capillary walls. The picture is similar to that seen in WHO class III. Multiple immunoglobulins frequently are seen and accompanied by complement components, fibrinogen, and properdin.

Mesangial hypercellularity with circumferential mesangial interposition is associated with the light microscopic pattern of a mesangiocapillary glomerulonephritis. Occasionally, the electron-dense deposits show an organized or crystalline pattern, which has been termed a fingerprint pattern. This organized appearance is most frequently seen in the presence of abundant endothelial deposits but can be present in all classes of lupus nephritis. The crystalline structure is thought by some to represent the presence of cryoglobulins because similar structures are seen in patients with idiopathic mixed cryoglobulinemia (33). They might also represent a pattern of crystalline DNA (34). Endothelial cell swelling and proliferation are prominent and occasional mitotic figures of glomerular cellular components suggest active proliferation and regeneration secondary to activation of inflammatory cytokines in growth factors. Intraendothelial tubular vesicular structures resembling myxoviruses have been identified in a majority of all patients with lupus nephropathy. The significance of these structures is unclear, but some evidence suggests that they are induced by the cytokine interferon-α (35,36).

Immunopathology

The localization of immune complexes to the subendothelial region where they have access to plasma inflammatory mediators is a critical step in initiating the severe glomerular nephritis seen in this form of lupus nephropathy. It is likely that large numbers of intermediate-sized or large complexes formed by high-affinity antibodies overcome the mesangial ability to clear these macromolecules (17,18,37). As a result, these complexes accumulate in a paramesangial subendothelial location and then ultimately in the peripheral capillary loops. Here they have access to circulating inflammatory mediators such as complement and platelets as well as cellular mediators of inflammation including monocyte macrophages and cytotoxic lymphocytes. The nature of the antigen and antibody may also contribute to the predominance of subendothelial localization in this class (25,27,38). Characteristics of certain antibodies such as cationic charge could permit binding of complexes that contain such antibodies to negative charges within the glomerular capillary wall, thus accounting for the nephrotropism. If the complexes are large and highly cationic, they will bind and fix to the closest anionic charges that are encountered at the subendothelial location. Following the initial binding of what might only be a small population of nephrotropic antibodies, activation of inflammatory cytokines can increase the permeability of the capillary wall, thus allowing other complexes to deposit. Some lupus antibodies have been identified to be cationic while others have been identified to cross-react with native glomerular components. Another significant factor is the activation of endothelial adhesion molecules including intercellular adhesion molecule (ICAM) and vascular cell adhesion molecule (VCAM) (39,40). Class III and class IV lesions represent the most severe form of glomerular involvement in patients with lupus because the deposited immune complexes have access to the humoral and cellular mediators of inflammation that are present in the circulation. Patients with class III or class IV pathologic lesions usually have evidence of significant clinical renal disease including proteinuria frequently in the nephrotic range, renal insufficiency, and an active urinary sediment. In some individual cases these lesions constitute the initial presentation of lupus erythematosus, and in rare instances these lesions are "silent." The nature of the immunopathogenesis underlying the renal lesion in patients with class III or class IV suggests an unfavorable prognosis, with a high percentage of such patients eventually progressing to renal failure despite aggressive treatment. A major consequence of severe glomerular inflammation with necrosis is the development of glomerular scarring and sclerosis, which results in decreasing glomerular filtration surface contributing to progressive renal scarring and loss of function.

Class V

The class V lesion describes a diffuse membranous glomerulonephropathy. Light microscopy reveals a generalized diffuse thickening of the peripheral capillary walls, which on silver methenamine-Masson stains exhibit a so-called spike and dome pattern (Fig. 50.9). The spikes are outward projections of membrane-like material between domes that correspond to the subepithelial and intramembranous deposits seen on immunofluorescence and electron microscopy. A variable

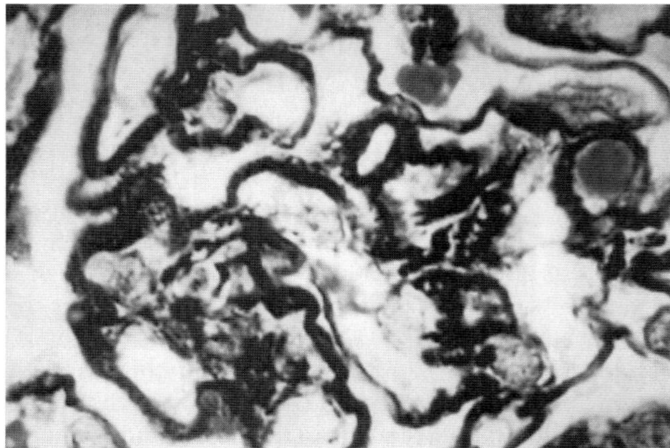

FIGURE 50.9. Lupus glomerulonephritis, WHO class V. Light microscopy reveals a diffuse membranous glomerulonephropathy. There is diffuse thickening of the peripheral capillary walls, which exhibit the so-called spike and dome pattern. The spikes are outward projections of silver-positive, basement membrane–like material between domes of red-staining material, which correspond to subepithelial and intramembranous deposits seen on electron microscopy (silver methenamine-Masson stain, ×1,000).

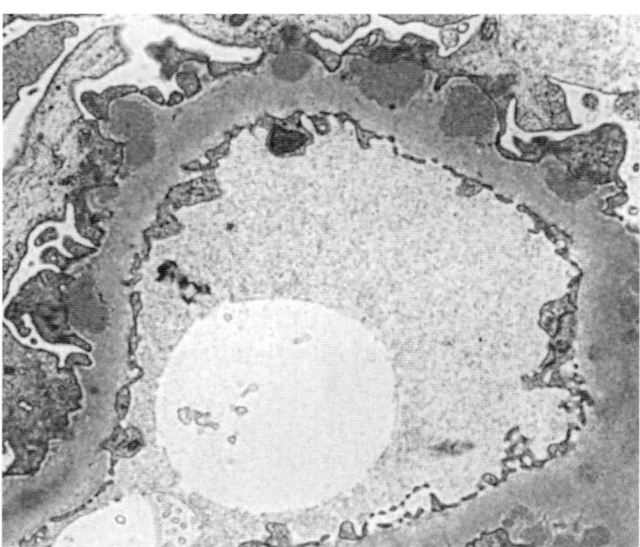

FIGURE 50.11. Lupus glomerulonephritis, WHO class V. Electron microscopy reveals abundant subepithelial deposits associated with basement membrane spikes. The deposits have varying electron density. Some intramembranous deposits also are present (×10,000).

degree of mesangial widening may be present involving an increase of both mesangial cells and mesangial matrix.

Immunofluorescence demonstrates a classic confluent peripheral granular deposition of immunoglobulins and occasionally by mesangial granular deposits (Fig. 50.10). Electron microscopy reveals a typical epimembranous nephropathy with subepithelial and intramembranous deposits of varying electron density (Fig. 50.11). The pattern is essentially identical to that seen in idiopathic membranous glomerulonephropathy except that mesangial deposits are occasionally present. The pathogenic mechanism leading to this pattern of injury is likely due to *in situ* formation of immune complexes (18). This suggests an immune response characterized by the presence of small unstable circulating immune complexes formed by low avidity and affinity antibodies in the presence of antigen excess. Under such conditions complexes may disassociate and the antigen or antibody log in the glomerular capillaries. Subsequently complexes are formed *in situ*, attaching to the target protein, which has been planted in the outer aspect of the glomerular basement membrane. The nature of the antigen becomes a major determinant in the pathogenesis of this lesion. The sera of all patients with lupus contain antibodies directed against the number of autoantigens including native and single-stranded DNA, histones, and small ribonuclear proteins of both nuclear and cytoplasmic origin. Of particular importance is that histones are highly cationic and potentially have a high affinity for the anionic sites of the glomerular basement membrane (38). Once bound to the glomerular basement membrane, they can act as a target antigen and a focus for *in situ* complex formation. Since such epimembranous deposits are also sequestered from access to circulating inflammatory mediators, the result is simply a change in glomerular permeability without evidence of an active inflammatory response. Such patients would be predicted to have heavy proteinuria as the most prominent clinical feature and an indolent course similar to that seen in patients with idiopathic membranous nephropathy (41).

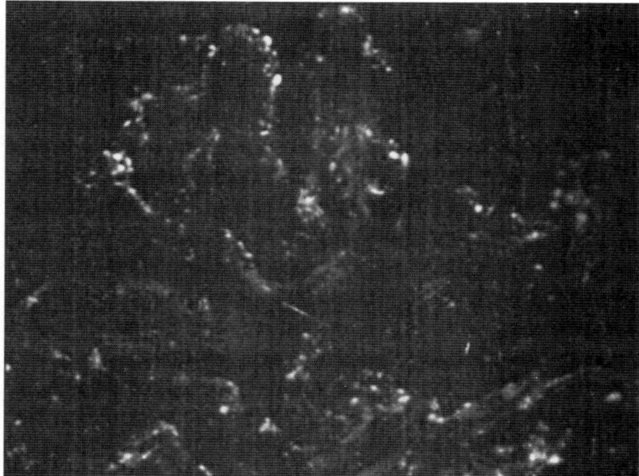

FIGURE 50.10. Lupus glomerulonephritis, WHO class V. Immunofluorescence demonstrates a classic, confluent, peripheral granular deposition of immunoglobulins, which can be associated with mesangial granular deposits. The immunoglobulins generally are confined to the peripheral capillary loops, and the immunoglobulin deposition generally is less extensive than that seen in class III or IV.

Some centers subclassify membranous lesions into pure membranous as class Va, with mesangial deposits as Vb, associated with lesions of class III as Vc, and associated with lesions of class IV as Vd. While this subclassification may more accurately describe the pathologic findings, it is not particularly useful from a clinical point of view since the presence of lesions of class III or IV with subendothelial deposits predicts a behavior like class III or IV and would dictate a more aggressive form of treatment than is generally used with a pure membranous lesion.

Class VI

This designation is given to those cases that have progressed to end-stage renal disease. Histologically, there is extensive glomerular sclerosis associated with interstitial fibrosis and tubular atrophy. Evidence of active immune complex deposition may be lacking with quite variable findings on immunofluorescence and electron microscopy. In some instances the degree of fibrosis and sclerosis is so marked that it is impossible to identify that active lupus nephritis preceded the end-stage findings. Patients in this category exhibit renal insufficiency often accompanied by hypertension.

MIXED PATTERNS AND TRANSFORMATION

Given the variability in the clinical and immunologic expression of disease that occurs in lupus erythematosus, it is likely that these classes and subclasses are not absolutely distinct clinical pathologic entities but rather represent different points in a continuum of disease. This is particularly evident in that the transformation of renal lesion from one class to another can occur both spontaneously and as a result of treatment. The exact incidence of spontaneous transformation is difficult to determine, as relatively few serial biopsy studies have been performed in untreated patients. A number of studies, however, suggest that transformation does occur commonly and is particularly noted after various treatment protocols (3,22,29,42). Transformation from class III to class IV disease has been reported so frequently that most nephropathologists consider them to be morphologic variants of a single class of lesion with common immunofluorescence and electron microscopic patterns. Transformation of diffuse proliferative glomerulonephritis to a predominately membranous glomerulonephropathy or to a mesangial pattern has been observed in patients undergoing remission during the course of treatment (29,43,44). The mechanism by which transformation occurs is not defined but may relate to the modification of the nature of the immune response or to the physical chemical characteristics of the immune complexes. Clinically, a spontaneous change in the morphologic pattern to the more severe forms of renal lesions such as class III or class IV may be heralded by a significant increase in proteinuria or a sudden deterioration in renal function. Conversely, transformation from class III to IV to mesangial lupus nephritis, class II to membranous lupus nephritis, or class V either spontaneously or after treatment is associated with improvement in both renal function and frequently the degree of proteinuria. Transformation from class II to the more serious class III or IV probably occurs in no more than 5% of patients with class II lesions on initial biopsy, confirming the impression that class II lesions are a more benign form of lupus nephritis and that patients with this lesion on initial biopsy will show little clinical evidence of progressive renal involvement. The transformation of the more severe and active forms of lupus nephritis (classes III and IV) induced by therapy relates primarily to modification of the immunologic basis of the renal lesion. Residual glomerular sclerotic lesions and interstitial fibrosis do not appear to be significantly altered by therapy and form a basis for progression by factors related not to active lupus nephritis but rather to hypertension and the functional overload on the residual nephrons.

IMMUNOFLUORESCENCE MICROSCOPIC FEATURES

One factor that has not been given enough consideration in the histopathologic evaluation of the glomerular lesion of patients with lupus nephritis is the role of the immunoglobulin isotope and subclass (45–47). Most studies of the immunofluorescence microscopic findings in lupus nephritis have emphasized the deposition rather than the classes of immunoglobulins found. A summary of the immunofluorescence microscopic findings from our own series of patients with lupus nephritis is presented in Table 50.3. Overall, immunoglobulin G (IgG) is present most frequently, followed by IgM and IgA. Less often, IgE is detected and is usually confined to the peripheral capillary wall. In WHO classes III and IV, peripheral granular and mesangial deposits appear concurrently. With equal frequency, IgM and IgG are detected in classes II and V disease. IgE is identified most frequently in class IV lupus nephritis and appears to be associated with necrosis in classes IVB and C. These findings are similar to those of other studies (3,21,22,29,42). IgG and IgM are the classes of immunoglobulin that are most commonly deposited,

TABLE 50.3. DISTRIBUTION OF IMMUNOGLOBINS IN LUPUS NEPHRITIS WHO CLASSES

	IgG	IgM	IgA	IgE
WHO Class II	33%	47%	14%	2%
WHO Classes III and IV	43%	27%	17%	10%
WHO Class V	41%	25%	22%	12%

and IgA, although found frequently, is not as common, nor is its distribution as extensive as that of the other two immunoglobulins. In one study, IgG2 was found more frequently than other subclasses (48). Because subclasses IgG2 and IgG4 do not readily activate complement, a mild lesion would be expected to occur with these subclasses rather than with IgG1 or IgG3. This analysis, however, showed a poor correlation between IgG subclass and the severity of the morphologic lesion. Deposition of IgE usually has not been identified specifically. In studies, however, it has been found infrequently and has been thought to reflect a part of the general autoimmune response associated with the clinical syndrome of SLE. Some reports have suggested that IgE deposits in lupus nephritis are associated with a poor prognosis (49–51). The so-called full-house pattern of multiple immunoglobulin deposition is characteristic of SLE and does not indicate any difference in severity of the lesion from a pattern of one immunoglobulin alone. Complement components including the membrane attack complex, fibrinogen, and properdin are usually associated with the presence of immunoglobulins, particularly in the more severe classes of disease. Less frequently, C4 is found in class II and class IV disease, and it correlates with a lower activity index. The pattern of deposition is usually coarsely granular and corresponds to the dense deposits seen by electron microscopy. Occasionally a pure linear pattern similar to that seen with antiglomerular basement membrane antibody is found, but no pathologic clinical implications for this type of depositions have been identified.

ADDITIONAL PATHOLOGIC FEATURES

Although the WHO classification is based primarily on the glomerular changes, it should be recognized that tubular interstitial and vascular lesions are an important part of the renal involvement and can contribute to the clinical picture. These additional pathologic features include vascular thrombosis, and proliferative and sclerotic vascular lesions including inflammatory vasculitis and tubular interstitial lesions. These complicating lesions occasionally are the predominant ones leading to clinical evidence of renal involvement. In addition, these lesions may become active or progress independently of the primary glomerular lesion and thus should be evaluated independently as additional comorbid factors that may relate to specific additional therapeutic maneuvers or have different prognostic significance.

VASCULAR LESIONS

Vascular lesions have not been taken into consideration in the establishment of the WHO classification or in the currently used activity and chronicity indices. Vascular lesions are common and may include intravascular thrombosis, arterial and arteriolosclerosis, and necrotizing vasculitis (52). Of particular importance is the occurrence of glomerular capillary thrombosis, signifying intravascular coagulation (53–58). A pattern similar to that seen in adult hemolytic uremic syndrome with multiple capillary and arteriolar thrombi containing fibrinogen has been associated with immune complex deposition and has been termed lupus vasculitis. In occasional instances, thrombotic micrangiopathy may occur in the absence of other manifestations of lupus nephritis (59). Plasminogen activators are depressed in some of these patients, whereas inhibitors of plasminogen activators are elevated (60). Studies have shown low levels of tissue type plasminogen activator and elevated levels of plasminogen inhibitor in patients with lupus nephropathy associated with glomerular capillary deposition of fibrin or thrombus formation. Since these alterations in plasma levels of tissue plasminogen activator and α_2-antiplasmin would be expected to retard fibrinolysis, they were corrected by administration of the fibrinolytic agent ancroid to patients with lupus glomerulonephritis (60). It is proposed that the disorder in fibrinolysis predisposes some patients with SLE to renal microvascular thrombi. Other authors have confirmed the association of glomerular thrombi with the presence of antiphospholipid antibodies (55,56). Patients with this lupus anticoagulant in their serum are subject to glomerular thrombosis and may mimic pauci-immune glomerulitis with necrosis and crescent formation (61), which might be independent of the presence of glomerular inflammation (54). In such patients, the glomerular thrombosis is sometimes the primary pathogenic event and likely causes the progression of renal disease without the participation of the accompanying immune responses.

Necrotizing vasculitis with vascular necrosis and leukocyte infiltration is a rare finding but appears to be a marker of poor prognosis in patients with lupus nephritis (62,63). The lesions can resemble the necrotizing arteriolitis seen with malignant hypertension and hemolytic uremic syndrome or a true vasculitis characterized by fibrinoid necrosis of small arteries and arterioles surrounded by an inflammatory infiltrate of the vessel wall. Electron microscopy sometimes reveals immune complex deposition in the vessel wall (64). These lesions reported in as many as 10% of patients with lupus nephritis generally are considered an additional morbid factor. Nephrosclerotic lesions with intimal fibroplasia and hyaline arteriolar sclerosis are encountered particularly in hypertensive patients. These lesions are also a major comorbid factor that not only contributes to the progression of renal failure but also may have an adverse effect on patient survival (65,66). A renal venous thrombosis is another vascular complication of lupus nephritis, but it is seen almost exclusively in patients with membranous lupus nephropathy complicated by the nephrotic syndrome (52,67,68).

TUBULOINTERSTITIAL DISEASE

Interstitial inflammation, fibrosis, and tubular epithelial changes are frequently encountered in all cases of lupus nephritis (69–71). Severe active tubulointerstitial nephritis is seen most commonly in patients with class III or class IV glomerular lesions. Although in most instances the interstitial inflammation is composed of lymphocytes and plasma cells, granulocytes and eosinophils are also frequently found and probably reflect the more active lesion. Tubulitis with infiltration of the tubules with lymphocytes similar to that seen in allograft rejection is often present. The infiltrating lymphocytes are predominantly T lymphocytes with a predominance of $CD8^+$ cells (72).

Immunofluorescence microscopy occasionally reveals granular peritubular deposits or rarely a linear deposition suggesting an antitubular basement membrane antibody (73,74). In most instances, the presence of interstitial disease without immune deposits suggests that several different mechanisms may be involved in the pathogenesis of this component of lupus nephritis. Of interest is the observation that tubular interstitial disease may progress independently of glomerular disease in some patients (75–77). It has been suggested that the infiltrate of T cells and monocytes may be an important determinant of the pathogenesis and progression of chronic injury in lupus nephritis by mediating interstitial injury (74).

ASSESSMENT OF SEVERITY AND CHRONICITY

Several studies have emphasized the important of using semiquantitative biopsy analyses to assess the activity and the severity of lupus nephritis (3,22,42,78,79). Disease activity has been related to the presence of necrosis, crescent formation, endocapillary and mesangial cellular proliferation, glomerular leukocytic infiltration, hyaline thrombi, and glomerular and interstitial inflammation (Table 50.4). Chronicity has been graded according to the degree of glomerulosclerosis and fibrosis as well as the amount of interstitial scarring and tubular atrophy. Although some authors have questioned the value of these indexes and their reproducibility (80–82), such an approach has been useful in studies of large groups of patients, and studies have suggested that quantification may be of value in assessing the prognosis in individual patients (12,22,45,62,65,83–89). Since the application of these indexes is observer and institution dependent, variations can occur between institutions. However, within an institution, where greater standardization of the application of criteria can be accomplished, these indices are of value in following patients, particularly those with serial or repeat biopsies.

TABLE 50.4. SEMIQUANTITATIVE ASSESSMENT OF ACTIVITY AND CHRONICITY[a]

Active indicators	Chronicity Indicators
Cellular proliferation	Glomerular sclerosis
Necrosis, karyorrhexis	Fibrous crescents
Cellular crescents	Interstitial fibrosis
Wire loops, hyaline thrombi	Tubular atrophy
Leukocytic infiltration	
Interstitial infiltration	

[a]Indicators are scored on a scale of 0 to 3, with necrosis, karyorrhexis, and cellular crescents weighted two times. The maximum for activity is 24, and the maximum for chronicity is 12.

SILENT LUPUS NEPHRITIS

Although clinical signs of renal involvement develop in 50% to 80% of patients, the disease is likely to involve the kidney in almost all patients from whom adequate data is available for analysis. Although the renal lesion is mild in most patients with clinically silent lupus nephritis, several reports have described severe proliferative glomerulonephritis with subendothelial deposits in the absence of proteinuria or abnormalities of the urinary sediment (11,13,14,29). Mahajan and co-workers (89a) performed renal biopsies in 27 patients with lupus erythematosus in whom careful evaluation of the urine specimens disclosed normal findings. The histopathologic changes in this series of patients included minimal glomerular damage in 11%, focal glomerular nephritis in 44%, and diffused glomerulonephritis in 44%. In the series of patients without clinical renal involvement, electron microscopy revealed electron-dense deposits in 16 of 19 patients examined, including three with diffuse proliferative glomerulonephritis. Although a consensus of opinion exists that more aggressive therapy is indicated in patients with diffuse proliferative and severe segmental lesions associated with overt signs of renal involvement, the clinical management of patients with similar pathologic changes in the absence of clinical evidence of renal involvement is less certain. Leehey and associates (90) studied 12 patients with clinically silent diffuse glomerulonephritis for intervals ranging from 5 to 11 years. They reported deteriorating renal function in three patients and an increase in urine protein excretion in four. One patient died of renal failure. The group with silent lupus nephritis had a seemingly good prognosis compared with a series of patients with overt renal disease in which eight of 37 patients progressed to end-stage renal disease. However, the authors noted that the number of patients analyzed was too small to say with certainty that the prognosis was improved in the group with silent renal involvement.

PATHOGENESIS

The pathogenesis of lupus nephritis is thought to be similar to that of experimental chronic immune complex associated glomerulonephritis. Several theories regarding the underlying immunologic mechanisms have been the subject of extensive reviews (15,91–93). The major immunologic mechanism appears to be a faulty regulation of the immune response system, resulting in an autoimmune disease with antibodies directed to nuclear proteins and cytoplasmic and plasma membrane constituents as well as specific plasma proteins. The defect in regulation has been attributed to an increase in helper T-cell function, lack of T-cell suppression, and/or polyclonal T-cell activation, any of which could lead to excess antibody production. In addition, although many of the antigens play specific roles in cell function, such as RNA slicing [small nuclear ribonucleoproteins (snRNPs)] DNA replication [proliferating cell nuclear antigen (PCNA)], and transcription (ssB/La) (93,94), it is unlikely that the autoantibodies inhibit their function but rather induce pathologic tissue reactions by acting as the autoantigen in the formation of immune complexes that initiate a subsequent inflammatory response (16,95). Another type of injury that has been implicated is intravascular thrombosis associated with the presence of antiphospholipid antibodies (54,55,57,58,96). In a report of 500 patients with SLE, antiphospholipid antibodies were found in 53%, with a significant correlation to thrombotic complications (56).

Initiation of the disease has been correlated with human leukocyte antigen (HLA)-dependent expression of HLAB7, HLAB8, and DRW2, and also is associated with increased susceptibility. HLA DRW2 and DQ1W are associated with younger onset and heightened response, whereas DQW2 is associated with older onset and Ro and La antibodies (41). Estrogen stimulation or possible induction with a latent viral infection has also been implicated (97). A number of animal models with some characteristics of human SLE have been studied, and information gained from these models has suggested that renal involvement is a prototype of experimental chronic immune complex–associated nephritis (15,16). The variety of lesions seen in lupus nephritis thus has been attributed to individual differences in the immune response in different patients or in an individual patient over the course of time. With differences in the logistics of the immune response, the different patterns of renal glomerular lesions can be seen, as was described previously. The nature of the antigen is also of importance since, for example, histones have been demonstrated to be highly cationic and thus have a high affinity for anionic sites of the glomerular basement membrane (38,95,98–100). Once bound to the glomerular basement membrane, they can act as a planted target antigen and a focus for *in situ* complex formation. The nature of the antibody can also be of importance depending on a variety of factors, which include the affinity and avidity of the antibodies; the class, subclass, and idiotype of the antibodies; the valence and phlogogenic activity of the complexes; as well as the overall charge. Binding of the anti-DNA antibody directly to glomerular structures has also been implicated in determining the severity of lesions (98,99,101). It has been suggested that DNA, particularly cationic histones, may accelerate or enhance immune complex deposition. A role for the interaction of the endothelium with lymphokines, monocyte macrophages, and cytotoxic lymphocytes has also been postulated (6,17,18,39,55,70,102,103).

CLINICAL PATHOLOGIC CORRELATIONS

Clinical studies of relatively large numbers of patients with lupus nephritis first appeared in the late 1950s [see Pollak and Pirani (6) for an early review]. Based on clinical signs of renal disease, the incidence of renal involvement in adult patients was found to be 50% to 80%. Clinical pathologic correlations demonstrated the significant relationship between the underlying histopathology and the patient's clinical course. In patients with what would now be classified as mesangial lupus glomerular nephritis (WHO class II) or membranous lupus nephritis (WHO class V), renal function was preserved for long periods, although the patients with the membranous lesion commonly exhibited persistent heavy proteinuria (6). In contrast, the clinical course of patients with focal segmental necrotizing glomerulonephritis (WHO class III) or diffuse proliferative glomerulonephritis (WHO class IV) usually had a rapidly progressive course, and the 2-year patient survival rate at that time was less than 30% despite the use of high-dose glucocorticoid therapy. In these reports, no significant tendency existed for transformation of one type of histologic lesion to another. Thus patients with mesangial proliferative WHO class II lesions did not appear to progress to class III or IV histology, the more severe forms of lupus renal involvement.

The correlation between renal histopathology and the clinical manifestations of renal disease was further explored by Baldwin and co-workers (3), and three types of renal injury were recognized by light microscopy, including focal proliferative glomerulonephritis, membranous glomerulonephropathy, and diffuse proliferative glomerulonephritis. The focal lesion was characterized by sharply delineated segmental proliferation of some tuffs involving 12% to 55% of glomeruli. In patients with this lesion, renal function tended to be preserved, although the nephrotic syndrome was present in two thirds of these patients, and all of them had proteinuria to some extent. The survival rate was 75% during the period of observation, and by life survival analysis the 5-year survival was estimated to be 70%. This group of patients under the current classification would be a mixture of WHO classes II and III. In those patients with membranous glomerulonephropathy, proteinuria was present in nearly all the patients and the nephrotic syndrome was evident in 70%. In agreement with previous reports, renal function was preserved in the majority, and the 5-year survival rate was 79%. Patients with diffuse proliferative glomerulonephritis were found to have a poor outlook in terms of morbidity and progression to renal failure. The nephrotic syndrome was present in more than 90% of these patients, and renal insufficiency was evident in 82%. Life table analysis indicated a 5-year survival rate of only 30%. Several subsequent reports have demonstrated similar findings (12,43,62,65,78,84,104–106, 118).

Other reports have emphasized the presence and location of electron-dense deposits in addition to the pattern of injury observed by light microscopy as important indices of the clinical course of lupus nephritis (5,42,65,107). In these analyses the presence of subendothelial electron-dense deposits (which in the current classification are characteristic of WHO classes III and IV) was correlated with an increased incidence of heavy proteinuria and renal insufficiency regardless of whether the pattern of hypercellularity was focal or diffuse. In contrast, localization of the deposits to the mesangial area (corresponding to WHO class II) or to the subepithelial location (corresponding to WHO class V) was associated with low rates of functional deterioration. Further evidence of the importance of the location of the deposits was provided by Hecht and his colleagues (29). In this series, 31 patients with proliferative glomerulonephritis and subendothelial deposits detected on the initial biopsy were treated with the same therapeutic regimen, which included low-dose prednisone and azathioprine. During follow-up, which averaged 40 months, a second renal biopsy demonstrated complete disappearance of subendothelial deposits in two thirds of these patients. At the end of the follow-up period, all of these patients had normal renal function and either no proteinuria or low levels of proteinuria. Of interest was the fact that on rebiopsy, the histopathologic lesion was transformed to either normal histology in 25% or to a membranous lesion in 75%. In patients with persistent subendothelial deposits, the disease course was characterized by renal deterioration as manifested by persistent proteinuria in excess of 3 g per day or an increase in serum creatinine of greater than 1.5 mg/dL or both.

More recently, several studies have emphasized the importance of using semiquantitative analysis of the biopsy to assess the severity of activity and chronicity (42,45,65,78, 85–88,96,108–118). Activity has been related to the presence of necrosis, cellular proliferation, leukocytic infiltration, and hyaline thrombi and glomeruli, as well as tubular damage and interstitial inflammation. Chronicity has been graded according to the degree of glomerulosclerosis and fibrosis as well as by the amount of interstitial and tubular atrophy. Both the activity and chronicity indices have been shown to have significant predictive value (43,78,110). Austin and co-workers (78) have reported that glomerulosclerosis and interstitial fibrosis are significant indicators of progression to renal failure (78). In their analysis of 102 adult patients who entered into treatment trials at the National Institutes of Health, disease chronicity at the time of entry into the study correlated with an increased incidence of renal insufficiency. As an extension of this study, Schwartz et al. (41) and Kant and associates (53) showed that thrombosis in the renal microvasculature of the kidney played an important role in the induction of chronic changes. The presence of glomerular thrombosis on the initial biopsy with predominant proliferative glomerulonephritis was found to correlate with glomerulosclerosis on subsequent biopsy. Banfi and co-workers (42) reported similar relationships between biopsy findings in clinical outcome. Alexopoulos et al. (72) have emphasized the importance of the interstitial cellular infiltrate in determining progression.

The widely variable outcome of patients with lupus nephritis has prompted clinicians to seek clinical and pathologic parameters by which to identify patients who are likely to have a poor outcome and thus warrant the most aggressive clinical approach. One study evaluated the prediction of experienced clinicians using clinical criteria they thought relevant, and compared these data with predictions based on a statistically derived computer-generated set of criteria (105). Predictions were made both with and without the inclusion of biopsy information. The criteria thought by clinicians to be most useful in predicting short-term outcome with serum creatinine at the time of biopsy, 24-hour urine protein, blood pressure, and serum complement. Those thought to be most useful for long-term prognosis were serum creatinine, 24-hour urine protein excretion, blood pressure, and hematuria. The computer-generated clinical model identified serum creatinine, age, and platelet count as the most important clinical predictors of short-term outcome and length of disease, and 24-hour urine protein excretion and serum complement as clinical indicators for long-term outcome. Although the predictions made by these clinicians were not improved on a statistical basis when biopsy data were added to the clinical information used, the predictions were more accurate and the level of confidence they expressed in their predictions was higher. The study concluded that experienced clinicians can indeed predict the response of patients with lupus nephritis using clinical and biopsy variables. The study also identified the important clinical and renal biopsy parameters that could have enhanced the clinicians' predictions but that were not utilized in the initial clinical evaluations. These included platelet count and the presence or absence of subendothelial deposits. It also identified criteria that were believed by the physicians to be important but contributed little to their prognostic accuracy.

Several recent studies have focused on the value of both histologic and clinical variables in determining prognosis (119–122). Austin et al. (120) found that black patients were significantly more likely to develop renal insufficiency than Caucasians with the same histology. Cellular crescents and interstitial fibrosis were the most important histologic features predictive of progression along with initial serum creatinine and hematocrit. Korbet et al. (119) identified similar criteria but also noted the importance of the presence of anti-Rho antibodies and failure to achieve remission after 4 weeks of therapy in predicting poor outcome. Moroni et al. (123) emphasized the potential role of repeat biopsies in evaluating the response to therapy, and noted that the presence of crescents and a chronicity index of greater than 5 are important predictors of progression.

Using elegant and sophisticated statistical analysis of the clinical and pathologic data from patients in our own series, Esdaile et al. (104) evaluated the value of a variety of prognostic indicators, and the short-term prognosis of lupus nephritis by assessing serum creatinine 12 months after renal biopsy. The significant clinical and laboratory predictors included the clinical signs of renal injury (serum, creatinine, and quantitative urine protein excretion), older age, and coexisting hypertension at the time of biopsy. Important biopsy criteria included the presence of a diffuse proliferative nephritis with a high activity score and subendothelial deposits. Indeed, the strongest predictor of short-term outcome was the finding of subendothelial deposits. These findings demonstrated definite incremental benefit of the renal biopsy in identifying patients in whom immunosuppressive agents might improve short-term outcome and confirm the incremental benefit of evaluating the presence of subendothelial biopsies. This was also noted by Whiting-O'Keefe and colleagues (124), and the importance of determining the activity index was emphasized by Magil and co-workers (83). Similarly, Austin and co-workers (78) found that the additional prognostic information offered by the renal biopsy to patients with severe active and chronic histologic changes was that they were at increased risk for developing renal insufficiency if not treated aggressively. In all of these studies these biopsy-related parameters contributed to decisions regarding the type and intensity of immunosuppressive therapy. Jacobsen et al. (121) found that the biopsy was of particular importance in patients with a normal serum creatinine.

The prognostic markers that Esdaile et al. (65,106) identified to predict a poor long-term outcome (renal insufficiency, dialysis dependency, or death due to lupus renal disease) included the duration of disease before biopsy, overall severity of disease, and the presence of vasculitis, hypertension, or a comorbid aliment. The best overall predictor appeared to be the extent of tubulointerstitial disease on biopsy. Cameron (69) came to similar conclusions for glomerular diseases in general. Similar findings were concluded from a study of the Italian Lupus Nephritis Study Group (62). Similar findings were found in a study of a series of children with lupus nephritis (118,125). Given the chronicity and fluctuating nature of the pathogenic processes in lupus, it is not surprising that prognostic factors can vary in their predictive power during the course of the disease. Using a technique called spline analysis, Esdaile et al. (111) showed that renal outcomes are predicted significantly by activity index, the tubulointerstitial index, and the amount of subendothelial deposits on renal biopsy throughout the course of disease, whereas laboratory findings that clinicians generally prefer as important predictors were useful prognostic indicators only in the early years postbiopsy. Measures of overall disease activity such as the Systemic Lupus Erythematosus Disease Activity Index (SLEDAI) and the LeRiche index proved useful only in later years. The response to therapy over 1 year was also found to be an important predictor of several long-term outcomes in lupus nephritis (115).

Taken together, all of these studies demonstrate that there is a distinct role for the renal biopsy in the management of patients with lupus nephritis. The benefit of early biopsy and the initiation of early treatment with immunosuppressive drugs were also confirmed in the analysis of our series of patients (112). We observed that patients with similar degrees of disease activity and biopsy findings who experienced a longer interval between disease onset and biopsy had a poorer long-term outcome. These findings forced the question as to whether delay of initiation of treatment with cytotoxic agents could adversely affected outcome. The rate of deterioration in serum creatinine and 24-hour urine protein over time from clinically evident disease onset to renal biopsy correlated with activity and chronicity indexes as well as with the abundance of subendothelial deposits, all of which are criteria for poor prognosis. This analysis suggests that early biopsy and initiation of treatment of patients with a class IV lesion and abundant subendothelial deposits is of benefit and the prompt use of immunosuppressive drugs is indicated. To the extent that the findings from renal biopsy provide a rationale for the use of potentially toxic drugs, the procedure appears worthwhile. Furthermore, an outcomes study by McInnes and colleagues (126) demonstrates that there is a significant positive economic impact with the early use of aggressive therapy in the modification of the clinical course of patients with lupus.

While the role of the renal biopsy in the initial evaluation of patients both in terms of choosing a therapeutic approach and in predicting short- and long-term outcome appears to be well established by these studies, the value of repeat biopsies to monitor response or progression is still controversial (123,127–129). In our series, nearly one half of the patients had a second biopsy at a median of 25 months after the first (110). A comparison of the two biopsies revealed that the prevalence of proliferative lupus glomerulonephritis of WHO classes III and IV decreased after treatment and that mesangial lupus nephritis of class II and membranous lupus nephritis of class IV increased. The activity index and subendothelial deposits declined, while in general the chronicity index and subepithelial deposits increased. While these changes reflect the response to therapy as well as an evolution of the disease process, we also observed that the relative change in the amount of mesangial or subendothelial deposits best identified the patients at risk for developing impairment and renal insufficiency and consequently dying. The results confirm the importance of immune complex deposition, as measured by electron microscopy, in the pathogenesis of lupus nephritis and in predicting the prognosis, and suggest that the control of this process by immunosuppressive therapy indeed alters the rate of renal functional deterioration.

SUMMARY

The clinical value of the renal biopsy in lupus nephritis appears to be well established, although some controversy still exists. Some authors continue to question its usefulness, whereas others recommend its use for every patient even in the absence of clinical and laboratory data involving renal involvement. In contrast, most investigators agree that it is impossible to predict the types of severity and activity of renal lesions from any combination of clinical and laboratory findings alone. Further advances are needed in the treatment of severe lupus erythematosus both to reduce the current mortality rate of 10% to 20% after 10 years and to decrease the development of renal insufficiency during dialysis, which occurs in nearly one fourth of patients. The close collaboration between the clinical nephrologist and the renal pathologist is most important in making appropriate therapeutic decisions in the application of new strategies. To the extent that the findings from renal biopsy provide a rationale for the use of potentially toxic drugs, the procedure appears more than worthwhile. This team approach will help to reduce the current mortality rate and to decrease the development of renal insufficiency requiring dialysis, which occurs in nearly one fourth of patients.

REFERENCES

1. Muehrcke RC, Kark RM, Pirani CL, et al. Lupus nephritis: a clinical and pathologic study based on renal biopsies. *Medicine* 1957;36:1–145.
2. Klemperer P, Pollack AD, Baehr G. Pathology of disseminated lupus erythematosus. *Arch Pathol* 1941;32:569–631.
3. Baldwin DS, Gluck MG, Lowenstein MJ, et al. Lupus nephritis: clinical causes as related to morphological forms and their transitions. *Am J Med* 1977;62:12–30.
4. Baldwin D, Lowenstein L, Rothfield N, et al. The clinical causes of the proliferative and membranous forms of lupus nephritis. *Ann Intern Med* 1970;73:929–942.
5. Comerford FR, Cohen AS. The nephropathy of systemic lupus erythematosus: an assessment of clinical, light and electron microscopic criteria. *Medicine* 1967;46:425–473.
6. Pollak V, Pirani C. Renal histologic findings in systemic lupus erythematosus. *Mayo Clin Proc* 1969;44:630–644.
7. Estes D, Christian CL. The natural history of systemic lupus erythematosus by prospective analysis. *Medicine* 1971;50:85–95.
8. Ginzler EM, Diamond HS, Weiner M, et al. A multicenter study of outcome of systemic lupus erythematosus. Entry variables as predictors of progress. *Arthritis Rheum* 1982;25:601–611.
9. Wallace DJ, Podell T, Weiner J, et al. Systemic lupus erythematosus—survival patterns. Experience with 609 patients. *JAMA* 1981;245(9):934–938.
10. Wallace DJ, Podell TE, Weiner JM, et al. Lupus nephritis. Experience with 230 patients in a private practice from 1950–1980. *Am J Med* 1982;72(2):209–220.
11. Woolf A, Croker B, Osafsky S, et al. Nephritis in children and young adults with systemic lupus erythematosus and normal urinary sediment. *Pediatrics* 1979;64:678–685.
12. Magil A, Puterman N, Ballon H, et al. Prognostic factors in diffuse lupus glomerulonephritis. *Kidney Int* 1988;34:511.
13. Eiser AR, Katz S, Swartz C. Clinically occult diffuse proliferative lupus nephritis: An age-related phenomena. *Arch Intern Med* 1979;139:1023–1025.
14. Bennett W, Bardana E, Houghton D, et al. Silent renal involvement in systemic lupus erythematosus. *Int Arch Appl Immunol* 1977;55:420–428.
15. Dixon F. The pathogenesis of murine systemic lupus erythematosus. *Am J Pathol* 1979;97:10–16.
16. Germuth F, Rodriguez E. *Immunopathology of the renal glomerulus*. Boston: Little, Brown, 1973:15–44.
17. Johnson R, Couser W, Chi E, et al. New mechanisms for glomerular injury. Myeloperoxidase-hydrogen peroxide-halide system. *J Clin Invest* 1987;79:1379–1387.
18. Johnson R, Alpers C, Pritzi P, et al. Platelet mediated neutrophil-dependent immune complex nephritis in the rat. *J Clin Invest* 1988;82:1225–1235.
19. McCulloch K, Powell J, Johnson K, et al. Enhancement by platelets of oxygen radical responses of human neutrophils. *Fed Proc* 1986;45:682–686.
20. McCluskey R. Lupus nephritis. In: Summers SC, ed. *Kidney pathology*. New York: Appleton-Century Crofts, 1975:456–459.
21. Churg J, Sobin JH. *Lupus nephritis: classification and atlas of glomerular diseases*. Tokyo: Igaku-Shoin, 1982:127–149.
22. Appel G, Silva F, Pirani C, et al. Renal involvement in systemic lupus erythematosus. *Medicine* 1978;57:371–410.
23. Domoto DT, Kashgarian M, Hayslett JP, et al. The significance of electron dense deposits in mild lupus nephritis. *Yale J Biol Med* 1980;53:314–324.
24. Stankeviciute N, Jao W, Bakir A, et al. Mesangial lupus nephritis with associated nephrotic syndrome. *J Am Soc Nephrol* 1997;8:1199–1204.
25. Vlahakos D, Foster M, Adams S, et al. Anti-DNA antibodies form immune deposits at distinct glomerular and vascular sites. *Kidney Int* 1992;41:1690–1700.
26. Kashgarian M, Sterzel R. The pathobiology of the mesangium. *Kidney Int* 1992;41:524–529.
27. Termaat R, Assmann K, Dijkman H, et al. Anti-DNA antibodies can bind to the glomerulus via two distinct mechanisms. *Kidney Int* 1992;42:1363–1371.
28. Rostagno A, Frangione B, Golo L. Biochemical studies of the interaction of fibronectin with Ig. *J Immunol* 1991;146:2687–2693.
29. Hecht B, Siegel N, Adler M, et al. Prognostic indices in lupus nephritis. *Medicine* 1976;55:163–181.
30. Monga G, Mazzucco G, di Belgiojoso B, et al. The presence and possible role of monocyte infiltration in human chronic proliferation glomerulonephritis. *Am J Pathol* 1979;94:271–284.
31. Schreiner GF, Cotran RS, Pardo V, et al. A mononuclear cell component in experimental immunological glomerulonephritis. *J Exp Med* 1978;147:369–384.
32. Hayslett J, Kashgarian M, Cook C, et al. The effect of azathioprine on lupus glomerulonephritis. *Medicine* 1972;49:393–412.
33. Grishman E, Porush J, Rosen S, et al. Lupus nephritis with organized deposits in the kidneys. *Lab Invest* 1967;16:393–412.
34. Kim Y, Choi Y, Reiner L. Ultrastructural fingerprint in cryo precipitate and glomerular deposits. A case report of systemic lupus erythematosus. *Hum Pathol* 1991;12:86–90.

35. Riche SA. Human lupus inclusions and interferon. *Science* 1981;213:772–774.
36. Schaff Z, Barry DW, Grimley PM. Cytochemistry of tubuloreticular structures in lymphocytes from patients with systemic lupus erythematosus and in cultures human lymphoid cells: comparison to a paramyxovirus. *Lab Invest* 1973;29:557–586.
37. Sakamoto H, Ooshima A. Activation of neutrophil phagocytosis of complement coated and IgG coated sheep erythrocytes by platelet release products. *Br J Haematol* 1985;60:173–181.
38. Schmiedeke T, Stockli F, Weber R, et al. Histones have high affinity for the glomerular basement membrane. *J Exp Med* 1989;169:1879–1894.
39. Bruijn J, Dinklo J. Distinct patterns of expression of ICAM-1, VCAM-1 and ELAM-1 in renal disease. *Lab Invest* 1993;69: 329–335.
40. Nishikawa K, Guo Y, Miyasaka M, et al. Antibodies to 1CAM-1/CFA-1 prevent crescent formations in rat autoimmune glomerulonephritis. *J Exp Med* 1993;177:667–677.
41. Schwartz MM, Kawala K, Roberts JL, et al. Clinical and pathological features of membranous glomerulonephritis of systemic lupus erythematosus. *Am J Nephrol* 1984;29:301–311.
42. Banfi G, Mazzucco G, Dibeldiojoso GB, et al. Morphological parameters in lupus nephritis: their relevance for classification and relationship with clinical and histological findings and outcome. *Q J Med* 1985;217:153–168.
43. Appel GB, Valeri A. The course and treatment of lupus nephritis. *Annu Rev Med* 1994;45:525–537.
44. Morel-Maroger L, Mery JP, Droz D, et al. The course of lupus nephritis: contribution of serial renal biopsies. *Adv Nephrol* 1976;6:79–118.
45. Donadio JV Jr, Hart GM, Bergstralh EJ, et al. Prognostic determinants in lupus nephritis: a long-term clinicopathologic study. *Lupus* 1995;4:109–115.
46. Haas M. IgG subclass deposits in glomeruli of lupus and nonlupus membranous nephropathies. *Am J Kidney Dis* 1994;23: 358–364.
47. Kashgarian M. New approaches to clinical pathological correlation in lupus nephritis. *Am J Kidney Dis* 1982;2:68–73.
48. Bannister KM, Horwarth GS, Clarkson AR, et al. Glomerular IgG subclass distribution in human glomerulonephritis. *Clin Nephrol* 1983;19:161–165.
49. Permin H, Wiik A. The prevalence of IgE antinuclear antibodies in rheumatoid arthritis and systemic lupus erythematosus. *Acta Pathol Microbiol Scand* 1978;86C:245–249.
50. Laurent J, Lagrue G, Sobel A. Increased serum IgE levels in patients with lupus nephritis [letter]. *Am J Nephrol* 1986;6: 413–414.
51. Tuma SN, Llach F, Sostrin S, et al. Glomerular IgE deposits in patients with lupus nephritis. *Am J Nephrol* 1981;1:31–36.
52. Appel GB, Pirani CL, D'Agati V. Renal vascular complications of systemic lupus erythematosus [editorial]. *J Am Soc Nephrol* 1994;4:1499–1515.
53. Kant K, Pollack V, Weiss M, et al. Glomerular thrombosis in systemic lupus erythematosus: prevalence and significance. *Medicine* 1981;60:71–86.
54. Farrugia E, Torres VE, Gastineau D, et al. Lupus anticoagulant in systemic lupus erythematosus: a clinical and renal pathological study. *Am J Kidney Dis* 1992;20:463–471.
55. Frampton G, Perry GJ, Chan TM, et al. Significance of anticardiolipin and antiendothelial cell antibodies in the nephritis of lupus. *Contrib Nephrol* 1992;99:7–16.
56. Frampton G, Hicks J, Cameron JS. Significance of anti-phospholipid antibodies in patients with lupus nephritis. *Kidney Int* 1991;39:1225–1231.
57. Hughson MD, Nadasdy T, McCarty GA, et al. Renal thrombotic microangiopathy in patients with systemic lupus erythematosus and the antiphospholipid syndrome. *Am J Kidney Dis* 1992;20:150–158.
58. Asherson R, MacKorth-Young C, Harris E, et al. Multiple venous and arterial thrombosis associated with the lupus anticoagulant and antibodies to cardiolipin in the absence of SLE. *Rheumatol Int* 1985;5:91.
59. Bridoux F, Vrtovsnik F, Noel C, et al. Renal thrombotic microangiopathy in systemic lupus erythematosus: clinical correlations and long-term renal survival [published erratum appears in *Nephrol Dial Transplant* 1998;13(5):1328]. *Nephrol Dial Transplant* 1998;13:298–304.
60. Glas-Greenwalt P, Kant KS, Dosekum A, et al. Ancrod: normalization of fibrinolytic enzyme abnormalities in patients with systemic lupus erythematosus and lupus nephritis. *J Lab Clin Med* 1985;105:99–107.
61. Charney DA, Nassar G, Truong L, et al. Pauci-immune proliferative and necrotizing glomerulonephritis with thrombotic microangiopathy in patients with systemic lupus erythematosus and lupus-like syndrome. *Am J Kidney Dis* 2000;35: 1193–1206.
62. Anonymous. Lupus nephritis: prognostic factors and probability of maintaining life-supporting renal function 10 years after the diagnosis. Gruppo Italiano per lo Studio della Nefrite Lupica (GISNEL). *Am J Kidney Dis* 1992;19:473–479.
63. Altieri P, Pani A, Bolasco P, et al. Is renal vasculitis in patients with systemic lupus erythematosus a bad prognostic factor? *Contrib Nephrol* 1992;99:72–78.
64. Meroni M, Torri Tarelli L, Tazzari S, et al. Renal ultrastructural findings in lupus vasculopathies. *Contrib Nephrol* 1992;99: 79–85.
65. Esdaile J, Levinton C, Federgreen W, et al. The clinical and renal biopsy predictors of long-term outcome in lupus nephritis: a study of 87 patients and review of the literature. *Q J Med* 1989;269:779–833.
66. Banfi G, Bertani T, Boevi V, et al. Renal vascular lesions as a marker of poor prognosis in patients with lupus nephritis. *Am J Kidney Dis* 1991;28:240–248.
67. Appel GB, Williams GX, Meltzer JI, et al. Renal vein thrombosis, nephrotic syndrome and systemic lupus erythematosus. *Ann Intern Med* 1976;85:310–317.
68. Bradley WG, Jacobs RP, Trew PA, et al. Renal vein thrombosis; occurrence in membranous glomerulonephropathy and lupus nephritis. *Radiology* 1981;139:571–576.
69. Cameron J. Interstitial changes in glomerulonephritis. In: Buccianti G, ed. *Prevention in nephrology*. Milan: Massion, 1987: 8–18.
70. Yamamoto T, Nagase M, Hishida A, et al. Interstitial inflammatory and chronic tubulointerstitial lesions in lupus nephritis: comparison with those in IgA nephropathy. *Lupus* 1993;2: 261–268.
71. Magil AB, Tyler M. Tubulo-interstitial disease in lupus nephritis: a morphometric study. *Histopathology* 1984;8:81–87.
72. Alexopoulos E, Seron D, Hartley RB, et al. Lupus nephritis: correlation of interstitial cells with glomerular function. *Kidney Int* 1990;37:100–109.
73. Schwartz MM, Fennel JS, Lewis EJ. Pathology of the renal tubule in systemic lupus erythematosus. *Hum Pathol* 1982;13: 534–547.
74. D'Agati VD, Appel GB, Estes D, et al. Monoclonal antibody identification of infiltrating leukocytes in lupus nephritis. *Kidney Int* 1986;30:573–581.
75. Gerl A, Samtleben W, Helmchen U, et al. [Interstitial lupus nephritis]. *Dtsch Med Wochenschr* 1992;117:782–786.
76. Cunningham E, Provost T, Brentjens J, et al. Acute renal failure

secondary to interstitial lupus nephritis. *Arch Intern Med* 1976; 138:1560–1562.

77. Tron F, Ganeval D, Droz D. Immunologically-mediated acute renal failure of non-glomerular origin in the course of systemic lupus erythematosus. *Am J Med* 1979;67:529–532.
78. Austin H, Muenz L, Joyce K, et al. Diffuse proliferative lupus nephritis: identification of specific pathologic features affecting renal outcome. *Kidney Int* 1984;25:689–695.
79. Coplon NS, Diskin CJ, Petersen J, et al. The long-term clinical course of systemic lupus erythematosus in end stage renal disease. *N Engl J Med* 1983;308:186–190.
80. Schwartz MM, Lan SP, Bernstein J, et al. Irreproducibility of the activity and chronicity indices limits their utility in the management of lupus nephritis. Lupus Nephritis Collaborative Study Group. *Am J Kidney Dis* 1993;21:374–377.
81. Schwartz MM, Lan SP, Bernstein J, et al. Role of pathology indices in the management of severe lupus glomerulonephritis. Lupus Nephritis Collaborative Study Group. *Kidney Int* 1992; 42:743–748.
82. Wernick RM, Smith DL, Houghton DC, et al. Reliability of histologic scoring for lupus nephritis: a community-based evaluation. *Ann Intern Med* 1993;119:805–811.
83. Magil A, Puterman M, Ballon H, et al. Prognostic factors in diffuse proliferative lupus glomerulonephritis. *Kidney Int* 1988; 34:511–517.
84. Nossent H, Henzer-Log S, Vroom T, et al. Contribution of renal biopsy data in predicting outcome in lupus nephritis. *Arthritis Rheum* 1990;33:970–977.
85. Cameron JS. Prediction of outcome in lupus nephritis [editorial]. *Lupus* 1992;1:197.
86. Bates WD, Halland AM, Tribe RD, et al. Lupus nephritis. Part I. Histopathological classification, activity and chronicity scores. *S Afr Med J* 1991;79:256–259.
87. Halland AM, Bates WD, Tribe RD, et al. Lupus nephritis. Part II. A clinicopathological correlation and study of outcome. *S Afr Med J* 1991;79:260–264.
88. McLaughlin J, Gladman DD, Urowitz MB, et al. Kidney biopsy in systemic lupus erythematosus. II. Survival analyses according to biopsy results. *Arthritis Rheum* 1991;34:1268–1273.
89. Gladman DD, Urowitz MB, Cole E, et al. Kidney biopsy in SLE: I. A clinical-morphologic evaluation. *Q J Med* 1989;73: 1125–1133.

89a. Mahajan SK, Ordonez NG, Feitelson PJ, et al. Lupus nephropathy without clinical renal involvement. *Medicine* 1977; 56:493–501

90. Leehey PJ, Katz AE, Azarum AH, et al. Silent diffuse lupus nephritis: long-term follow-up. *Am J Kidney Dis* 1982;2(suppl 1):188–196.
91. Koffler D, Shur P, Kunkel H. Immunological studies concerning the nephritis of systemic lupus erythematosus. *J Exp Med* 1967;126:607–623.
92. Kunkel H. The immunopathology of SLE. *Hosp Pract* 1980;15: 47–56.
93. Hardin J. The lupus autoantigen and the pathogenesis of systemic lupus erythematosus. *Arthritis Rheum* 1986;29: 457–463.
94. Tokano Y, Yasuma M, Harada S, et al. Clinical significance of anti-Sm and U1 RNP antibodies in patients with systemic lupus erythematosus and mixed connective tissue disease. *J Clin Immunol* 1991;11:317–325.
95. Fournier G. Circulation of DNA and lupus nephritis. *Kidney Int* 1988;33:487–497.
96. Esdaile JM, Joseph L, MacKenzie T, et al. The benefit of early treatment with immunosuppressive agents in lupus nephritis [see comments]. *J Rheumatol* 1994;21:2046–2051.
97. Leaker B, McGregor A, Griffiths M, et al. Insidious loss of renal function in patients with anticardiolipin antibodies and absence of overt nephritis. *Br J Rheumatol* 1991;30:422–425.
98. Batsford SR. Cationic antigens as mediators of inflammation. *APMIS* 1991;99:1–9.
99. Vlahakos DV, Foster MH, Adams S, et al. Anti-DNA antibodies form immune deposits at distinct glomerular and vascular sites. *Kidney Int* 1992;41:1690–1700.
100. Vogt A, Batsfdord S, Morioka T. Nephritogenic antibodies in lupus nephritis. *Tohoku J Exp Med* 1994;173:31–41.
101. van Bruggen MC, Kramers C, Hylkema MN, et al. Pathophysiology of lupus nephritis: the role of nucleosomes. *Neth J Med* 1994;45:273–279.
102. D'Cruz DP, Houssiau FA, Ramirez G, et al. Antibodies to endothelial cells in systemic lupus erythematosus: a potential marker for nephritis and vasculitis. *Clin Exp Immunol* 1991;85: 254–261.
103. Perry GJ, Elston T, Khouri NA, et al. Antiendothelial cell antibodies in lupus: correlations with renal injury and circulating markers of endothelial damage. *Q J Med* 1993;86: 727–734.
104. Esdaile J, Federgreen W, Quintal H, et al. Predictors of one year outcome in lupus nephritis: the importance of renal biopsy. *Q J Med* 1991;295:907–918.
105. Esdaile J, MacKensie T, Barre P, et al. Can experienced clinicians predict the outcome of lupus nephritis. *Lupus* 1992;1: 205–214.
106. Esdaile J, Joseph L, MacKenzie T, et al. The pathogenesis and prognosis of lupus nephritis: information from repeat renal biopsy. *Semin Arthritis Rheum* 1993;23:135–145.
107. Tateno S, Lobayashi Y, Shitematsu H, et al. Study of lupus nephritis: its classification and the significance of subendothelial deposits. *Q J Med* 1983;52:311–331.
108. Esdaile JM, Federgreen W, Quintal H, et al. Predictors of one year outcome in lupus nephritis: the importance of renal biopsy [see comments]. *Q J Med* 1991;81:907–918.
109. Esdaile JM, Mackenzie T, Barre P, et al. Can experienced clinicians predict the outcome of lupus nephritis? *Lupus* 1992;1: 205–214.
110. Esdaile JM, Joseph L, MacKenzie T, et al. The pathogenesis and prognosis of lupus nephritis: information from repeat renal biopsy. *Semin Arthritis Rheum* 1993;23:135–148.
111. Esdaile JM, Abrahamowicz M, MacKenzie T, et al. The time-dependence of long-term prediction in lupus nephritis. *Arthritis Rheum* 1994;37:3359–3368.
112. Esdaile JM, Joseph L, MacKenzie T, et al. The benefit of early treatment with immunosuppressive drugs in lupus nephritis [letter]. *J Rheumatol* 1995;22:1211.
113. Balow JE, Austin HAR, Boumpas DT. Treatment and prognosis of lupus nephritis [editorial; comment]. *J Rheumatol* 1994; 21:1985–1986.
114. Boumpas DT, Austin HA, Fessler BJ, et al. Systemic lupus erythematosus: emerging concepts. Part 1: renal, neuropsychiatric, cardiovascular, pulmonary, and hematologic disease. *Ann Intern Med* 1995;122:940–950.
115. Fraenkel L, MacKenzie T, Joseph L, et al. Response to treatment as a predictor of long-term outcome in patients with lupus nephritis. *J Rheumatol* 1994;21:2052–2057.
116. Krane NK, Thakur V, Wood H, et al. Evaluation of lupus nephritis during pregnancy by renal biopsy. *Am J Nephrol* 1995; 15:186–191.
117. Levey AS, Lan SP, Corwin HL, et al. Progression and remission of renal disease in the Lupus Nephritis Collaborative Study. Results of treatment with prednisone and short-term oral cyclophosphamide. *Ann Intern Med* 1992;116:114–123.

118. McCurdy DK, Lehman TJ, Bernstein B, et al. Lupus nephritis: prognostic factors in children [see comments]. *Pediatrics* 1992; 89:240–246.
119. Korbet SM, Lewis EJ, Schwartz MM, et al. Factors predictive of outcome in severe lupus nephritis. Lupus Nephritis Collaborative Study Group. *Am J Kidney Dis* 2000;35:904–914.
120. Austin HA 3rd, Boumpas DT, Vaughan EM, et al. High-risk features of lupus nephritis: importance of race and clinical and histological factors in 166 patients. *Nephrol Dial Transplant* 1995;10:1620–1628.
121. Jacobsen S, Starklint H, Petersen J, et al. Prognostic value of renal biopsy and clinical variables in patients with lupus nephritis and normal serum creatinine. *Scand J Rheumatol* 1999; 28: 288–299.
122. Balow JE, Austin HA 3rd. Progress in the treatment of proliferative lupus nephritis. *Curr Opin Nephrol Hypertens* 2000;9: 107–115.
123. Moroni G, Pasquali S, Quaglini S, et al. Clinical and prognostic value of serial renal biopsies in lupus nephritis. *Am J Kidney Dis* 1999;34:530–539.
124. Whiting-O'Keefe Q, Henke J, Shearn M, et al. The information content from renal biopsy in systemic lupus erythematosus. *Ann Intern Med* 1982;96:718–723.
125. Cameron JS. Lupus nephritis in childhood and adolescence. *Pediatr Nephrol* 1994;8:230–249.
126. McInnes PM, Schuttinga J, Sanslone WR, et al. The economic impact of treatment of severe lupus nephritis with prednisone and intravenous cyclophosphamide. *Arthritis Rheum* 1994;37: 1000–1006.
127. Esdaile JM. Current role of renal biopsy in patients with SLE. *Baillieres Clin Rheumatol* 1998;12:433–448.
128. Grande JP, Balow JE. Renal biopsy in lupus nephritis. *Lupus* 1998;7:611–617.
129. Ponticelli C, Moroni G. Renal biopsy in lupus nephritis—what for, when and how often? [editorial]. *Nephrol Dial Transplant* 1998;13:2452–2454.

51

CLINICAL AND LABORATORY FEATURES OF LUPUS NEPHRITIS

DANIEL J. WALLACE
BEVRA HANNAHS HAHN
JOHN H. KLIPPEL

Renal involvement in systemic lupus erythematosus (SLE) is one of the most serious complications of this disorder. Virtually all studies of prognosis have identified lupus nephritis as a predictor of poor outcome. Chronic glomerulonephritis was first described in four patients with SLE in 1922 (1). Baehr et al. (2) observed wire-loop lesions at autopsy in 13 of 23 patients with lupus in 1935 and associated it with the disease. In the late 1950s, pioneers in rheumatology, including Dixon, Holman, Mellors, Kunkel, Muller-Eberhard, and others (3–7), noted that positive LE-cell preps often were found in patients who had immune deposits in renal tissue. Introduction of the LE-cell prep in 1948 (8) allowed investigators to evaluate the prevalence of SLE in patients with idiopathic nephritis. Its bleak prognosis was improved by the availability of corticosteroids and nitrogen mustard in 1949 and by hemodialysis in 1960.

The immunopathogenesis, pathology, and clinicopathologic correlates of lupus nephritis are covered in Chapter 50, Clinical and Management Aspects of the Antiphospholipid Antibody Syndrome. Detailed discussions of specific treatment modalities for renal disease are covered separately. The reader is referred to Chapter 56, Systemic Corticosteroid Therapy in Systemic Lupus Erythematosus (corticosteroids and pulse steroids); Chapter 57, Immunosuppressive Drug Therapy (cyclophosphamide, nitrogen mustard, azathioprine, chlorambucil, mycophenolate mofetil, cyclosporin and methotrexate); Chapter 58, Nonpharmacologic Therapeutic Methods (apheresis, total lymphoid irradiation, hemodialysis, and transplantation); and Chapter 59, Occasional, Innovative, and Experimental Therapies (gamma globulin, 2-CDA). This chapter discusses the epidemiology, incidence, clinical features, and natural course, and it reviews the general management concepts of renal lupus.

DEFINITION, EPIDEMIOLOGY, AND PREVALENCE

In studies of patients who were diagnosed before the availability of the 1982 revised American College of Rheumatology (ACR) criteria for SLE, most patients with SLE were found to have histologic evidence of renal pathology on renal biopsy, although many patients had no clinical findings to suggest renal involvement. Although urine sediment and protein measurements, along with serum creatinine, C3 complement, and antidouble-stranded DNA (anti-dsDNA) determinations, are useful in analyzing the prognosis, course, and projected treatment, histologic nephritis can be present even if all these parameters are normal. Renal biopsies have shown early changes of SLE with normal urinalyses (9–18). This has been termed silent lupus nephropathy and usually is nonprogressive (11,17). Although these instances generally represent minimal disease histologically, diffuse, proliferative lesions occasionally have been found.

In a series of patients from the Wallace/Dubois practice studied from 1950 to 1991, the following criteria for lupus nephritis were found to have a greater than 95% sensitivity (19–21). One of the following must be present: (i) a renal biopsy showing class IIb mesangial, focal proliferative, diffuse proliferative, or membranous glomerulonephritis; (ii) a 30% decrease in creatinine clearance over a 1-year period in a patient with active lupus; and (iii) urine protein greater than 1 g in 24 hours. Alternatively, at least three of the following in a 12-month period allow us to make a diagnosis of nephritis in an SLE patient: (i) a serum albumin level greater than 3 g/dL; (ii) sustained 2 to 4+ proteinuria; (iii) oval fat bodies or granular, hyaline, or red cell casts in the urine; and (iv) persistent hematuria of greater than five red cell casts per high-power field in the urine. For each of these criteria, an alternative cause must be excluded. These criteria differ from the less extensive criteria of the ACR (Chapter 2, Definition, Classification, Activity, and Damage Indices). In the ACR criteria, renal disorders of SLE are defined as persistent proteinuria (>0.5 g/day or >-3+), or cellular casts of any kind.

With these or similar criteria, the prevalence of renal involvement varied from 29% to 65% among the eight series described in Table 51.1. Tertiary referral centers tended to have higher percentages of patients with renal disease, as did studies that were published before 1965 [when antinuclear antibodies (ANA) became widely available and identified more mild cases of SLE]. The true prevalence probably is approximately 40% (22). Nephritis is present in most children (see Chapter 41, Gastrointestinal and Hepatic Manifestations) and is rare in the elderly (23,24). Nephrotic syndrome (defined as a serum albumin <2.8 g/dL with >3.5 g of urine protein per 24 hours) was observed in 13% to 26% of all patients with SLE in the eight well-detailed series shown in Table 30.1; we have found (as have others) that about one half of our 128 patients with nephritis were nephrotic at some time during their disease course (20), African Americans are significantly more likely to develop renal insufficiency. They have more hypertension, interstitial fibrosis, hypocomplementemia, higher chronicity indices, and a poorer response to cyclophosphamide (25,26).

The mean age at disease onset in patients with nephritis in the Wallace series was 4 years younger than in those with SLE without nephritis (27 vs. 31 years of age and 230 vs. 379 patients, respectively) (21,27). Nossent et al. (28) also observed a similar difference in 110 Dutch patients. Most patients develop nephritis early in their disease (29); the oldest patient with SLE and new-onset nephritis was 80 (B Hahn, pers. comm.). Smaller-scale surveys have suggested that males have a relatively increased incidence or activity of renal disease (30–32). We have observed proportionately more men than women with renal disease among our 464 patients with SLE who were seen between 1980 and 1989, but this did not achieve statistical significance (19). Asians and blacks may have more nephritis than other racial groupings (19,33–35).

TABLE 51.1. FINDINGS IN PATIENTS WITH SYSTEMIC LUPUS ERYTHEMATOSUS AND NEPHRITIS (N = 128) COMPARED WITH THOSE WITHOUT NEPHRITIS (N = 336)[a]

More Frequent	Less Frequent
Family history of SLE	Other CNS sx
Anemia	Seizures
High sedimentation rate	Thrombocytopenia
High serum cholesterol	Fibromyalgia
High serum triglycerides	
Positive ANA	
High anti-dsDNA	
Low C3 complement	
Low C4 complement	

[a] $P < .01$.
ANA, antinuclear antibody; dsDNA, double-stranded DNA; SLE, systemic lupus erythematosus

Inheritance of the DR2 and B8 gene is associated with an increased risk of developing nephritis in some populations, and this risk is amplified if certain DQbeta genes also are present (see Chapter 6, The Genetics of Human Lupus). Inheritance of the DR4 gene reduces the risk for lupus nephritis (36) . Several studies have shown that allelic variants of the IgG Fcγ receptor RIIA and RIIIA, associated with poor binding and phagocytosis of IgG1 and IgG2 increase risk for lupus nephritis in several different ethnic populations (37). One could speculate that such individuals clear immune complexes less efficiently than persons who inherit other alleles for these receptors. However, the association has not been found in all populations (38), and it is likely that the predisposing allele must be inherited with other genes that increase risk in order to be associated with clinical nephritis.

CLINICAL AND LABORATORY PRESENTATION

In 3% to 6% of cases, renal disease manifestations constitute the initial presentation of SLE (39–42). This may occur before clinical symptoms of lupus are apparent. Cairns et al. (43) reported 11 ANA-negative patients whose onset of SLE began with clinical glomerulonephritis as the initial manifestation. All became ANA positive over a 6-year period. A similar group of 17 patients was described by Adu et al. (44), and three children by Gianuti et al. (45). ACR criteria may not be fulfilled at first even if the ANA is positive (46). Our group reviewed the literature and concluded that the overwhelming majority of clinically relevant nephritis is evident within 5 years of the diagnosis of SLE (47). Only five of our 230 patients with lupus nephritis who were seen between 1950 and 1980 had the onset of renal disease after 10 years. Others have confirmed this (28).

Klippel (48) has described five clinical types of lupus nephritis: (i) occult (or silent), (ii) chronic active nephritis, (iii) rapidly progressive (fulminant course) nephritis, (iv) nephrotic syndrome, and (v) progressive renal insufficiency in patients with repeatedly normal urinalyses. Glomerulosclerosis, hypertension, and occasionally, drugs (especially nonsteroidals) probably cause renal insufficiency in most of the latter group. Patients in this group, along with those with occult disease and chronic active nephritis, often are asymptomatic. Acute deterioration in renal function was observed in 36 (18.4%) of 196 SLE hospital admissions in the group followed by Yeung et al. (49). Infection and active central nervous system disease were frequent precipitating events, and recovery of renal function with aggressive management was reported in 76%. Others have confirmed these findings (50). Mildly nephrotic subjects may only have ankle edema on examination; frankly nephrotic states are associated with ascites, presacral edema, as well as pleural and pericardial effusions. Physical examinations often are deceptively normal except for blood pressure measurements in patients with isolated lupus nephritis. Patients with SLE have an increased incidence of renal tubular dysfunction, which is clinically characterized by a proximal or distal renal tubular acidosis (51). This is particularly evident in patients with Sjögren's syndrome. (See Chapters 39 and 50 for a discussion of renal physiology abnormalities in SLE.)

Numerous surveys have evaluated the prognostic importance of a variety of laboratory and serologic parameters (discussed later). Our group recorded 125 parameters and compared 128 patients with nephritis to 336 patients without renal disease who were seen between 1980 and 1989 (only parameters with p values <.01 shown) (27). Table 51.1 summarizes these findings. One hundred eighty of Piette's French group out of 436 with SLE reported in 1999 had nephritis. Renal patients had more malar rashes, psychosis, myocarditis, pericarditis, lymphadenopathy, hypertension, anti-DNA, and low C3 (22). Some investigators have proposed that rheumatoidlike arthritis is associated with a lower incidence of renal disease, especially if rheumatoid factor is present and the HLA-DR4 haplotype is present (55,56). However, we found no differences in the prevalence of rheumatoid factor among the nephritis versus the no-nephritis groups (21% vs. 23%, respectively). Walker et al. (32) noted that arthritis and arthralgia were the most common symptoms in a group of 45 patients with lupus nephritis who were followed in New Zealand. Usually, elevated Westergren sedimentation rates, low C3 complement, elevated anti-dsDNA levels, and low serum albumin levels are associated with more active nephritis.

Gallium scans demonstrate increased renal uptake with active disease (57) and roughly correlate with a biopsy activity index (52). Doppler ultrasounds are of little value, but elevated resistive indices correlate with a higher biopsy chronicity index (58,59).

MEASUREMENTS OF RENAL FUNCTION

The principal tests to evaluate renal function are blood urea nitrogen (BUN), serum creatinine, and creatinine clearance. The utility of the BUN is limited by its alteration with hydration status, bleeding, and hepatic and dietary conditions. In clinical practice, the most convenient serial measurement of renal function is the serum creatinine; in clinical research, a more reliable measure of glomerular filtration rate (GFR) is desirable in addition. Serum creatinine level can vary with body weight, muscle mass, and state of hydration, and it tends to overestimate renal function by as much as 20% as it does not account for proximal tubular creatinine secretion. Creatinine is hypersecreted by injured tubules in patients with glomerulopathy. Because creatinine is calculated on a logarithmic scale, a rise from 1 to 2 mg/dL represents a 50% change, while a rise from 6 to 7 mg/dL reflects a 3% change. Clinical investigators often must use the ratio 1/creatinine value for statistical analysis.

Because determining a true, reliable renal function is vital in SLE, GFR measurements have become the gold standard. Calculated by the standard formula $(U \times V)/P$, GFRs that are derived by inulin clearance, iothalamate clearance, and Tc99-DTPA clearance have proven to be reliable but expensive and inconvenient (60–62). Creatinine clearance, which is inexpensive and convenient to obtain, overestimates true GFR (60–62). One study suggests that giving cimetidine (400 mg) tablets four times a day for 2 days blocks tubular secretion of creatinine and provides a more reliable measure of GFR (62). Hughes' group recently suggested that chromium-51 labeled EDTA-GFR may be a better predictor of nephritis than GFR indices alone (63). Reductions of GFR out of proportion to renal plasma flow indicate a low filtration fraction and greater disease severity (64).

URINARY PROTEINS AND SEDIMENT

Ropes (65) was the first to attach importance to following urinary sediment and protein level. She noted that 15 of 68 patients (22%) who had proteinuria and were not given corticosteroids had spontaneous disappearance of the proteinuria up to 14 years later. Dubois' findings in 520 patients who were seen between 1950 and 1963 and who had multiple urine evaluations are summarized in Table 51.2 (66). Hematuria probably results from the escape of

TABLE 51.2. ABNORMAL URINARY FINDINGS IN 520 CASES OF SLE

	Cases (n)	%
Albuminuria	240	46.1
WBCs in urine (more than 6/HPF in clean specimen)	185	35.5
Hematuria	170	32.6
Granular casts	164	31.5
Hyaline casts	148	28.4
RBC casts	39	7.5
Fatty casts	32	6.1
Oval fat bodies	23	4.4
Double refractile bodies	10	1.9
Waxy casts	9	1.7
Mixed fatty casts	6	1.2

HPF, High-powered field; RBC, red blood cell; WBC, white blood cell.

red cells through a gap in the glomerular basement membrane (67). Other reports in patients with nephritis have found microscopic hematuria in 33% to 78% (19,68–72), fat bodies in 33% to 48% (20,71), cellular casts in 34% to 40% (70,73), and greater than 1 g of urinary protein per 24 hours in 26% to 87%. One report (74) has suggested that a random spot urine collection protein:creatinine ratio is just as reliable as a 24-hour urine collection.

Although the urinalysis may be normal despite abnormal findings on a renal biopsy, nearly all patients with clinically important renal disease have microscopic urine findings. The appearance of five leukocytes or red cells in a clean midstream urine specimen, especially with at least a trace of albumin, suggests active nephritis (75,76). As the process progresses, the amount of albumin gradually increases, as do the numbers of leukocytes and erythrocytes. At this point many patients often are considered to have urinary tract infections, and they frequently are given multiple courses of antibiotics (although the pyuria results from renal damage and not primary infection). Dubois observed bacterial cystitis or pyelonephritis in 22.5% of his 520 patients (66). Fries and Holman (71) reported dysuria in 14 of their 193 patients but stones or urethral discharge in only one. Ropes (77) reported urinary-tract infections in 47% of her 150 patients.

As lupus damage advances, hyaline and fine granular casts may appear. Later in the disease process, coarse granular casts, red-cell casts, and white-cell casts are found. If nephrotic syndrome is present, urinary protein may be as high as 30 g per 24 hours, with good renal function. The other classic findings of nephrosis, such as oval fat bodies in the urine, hypoalbuminemia, hyperlipidemia, and anasarca, also may be present.

With further progression of renal disease, the numbers of all types of casts increase, broad renal failure casts appear, and a telescoped sediment becomes evident. Herbert et al. (78) found that a relapse of lupus nephritis can be predicted best by cellular casts followed by hematuria and white cells in the urine; these are more reliable than a drop in C3 complement.

ANALYSIS OF URINE PROTEIN COMPONENTS

Albumin

Urine protein can be separated into albumin and gamma globulin fractions. Measurements of urinary albumin excretion by radioimmunoassay can pick up larger amounts than normally would be detected. They are not generally clinically helpful though diminution in albumin excretion correlates with clinical response to treatment (79–81). Microalbuminuria is associated with mesangial disease (81), does not predict the development of nephritis (82), while polymeric albumin is associated with more serious disease (83).

Gamma Globulins

Urinary protein electrophoresis demonstrates increased gamma-globulin levels during active disease; levels decrease with therapeutic response (84,85). No specific patterns are observed in SLE. Quantitative urine-protein analysis with can detect glomerular vs. nonglomerular proteinuria (86). Several groups have shown associations between levels of free immunoglobulin light chains and lupus nephritis activity (87–93).

Other Urinary Findings

Meryhew et al. (94) studied urinary ANAs. Positive tests were found in four of 25 patients with SLE (16%) as measured by incubating mouse kidney cells with concentrated urine. Thirty-two percent of patients were positive with Hep-2 cells. IgG ANA was most frequently seen; one half had more than one immunoglobulin class detected. Anti-Sm, antiribonucleoprotein (anti-RNP), anti-Ro/SSA, and anti-dsDNA also were detected. The presence of anti-dsDNA and ANA correlated with increased clinical severity. ANA might appear in the urine as a result of decreased tubular reabsorption, antigen deposition, or genitourinary tract inflammation, but it probably is representative of glomerular leakage.

Nephrotic syndrome is associated with false-positive urine pregnancy tests (95). Numerous reports have suggested that numerous urinary substances are increased with active lupus nephritis and are good markers of clinical activity. These include ferritin (96), anti-RNA polymerase I antibodies (97), neopterin (98–100), acid mucopolysaccharides (101), histuria (102), fibrin degradation products (103,104), several gastrointestinal enzymes (105), IL-6 (106,107), anti-DNA (108) soluble interleukin-2 receptors (92,109), urinary C4 (110), monocyte chemotactic and activating factor (111), retinal-binding protein (112), tumor necrosis factor-alpha and adhesion molecules (113) and low-molecular-weight C3 fragments (114,115).

Urinary prostaglandins, renal-tubular acidosis, aldosterone, the syndrome of inappropriate antidiuretic hormone, and renin activity measurements are discussed in Chapters 39, The Use of Exogenous Estrogens, Endocrine System, and Urogenital Tract, and 50, Lupus Nephritis: Pathology, Pathogenesis, Clinical Correlations, and Prognosis.

RENAL VEIN THROMBOSIS

Thrombosis of the renal veins complicating lupus nephritis was first reported in 1968 (116) and has been described in numerous cases since. It should be strongly considered in patients with nephrotic syndrome and/or the lupus anticoagulant whom present with flank pain and fever, thrombophlebitis, or pulmonary emboli (117–120). Bradley et al. (121) found renal-vein thrombosis in 11 of 280 patients with membranous glomerulonephritis or lupus glomerulonephritis. All 11 (three of whom had SLE) also had nephrotic syndrome, and ten had pulmonary emboli. Six of 625 Taiwanese SLE patients developed renal-vein thrombosis; all were nephrotic (122). Renal-vein thrombosis needs to be differentiated from renal arteriolar thrombi seen on biopsy that do not correlate with antiphospholipid antibodies (123,124).

Mintz et al. (123) performed inferior vena cava phlebography in 43 patients with SLE. Inferior vena cava or renal-vein thrombosis was found in 27% of 11 patients with nephrotic syndrome, 62% of 13 with a history of thrombophlebitis, and none of 20 controls with SLE. Mintz et al. concluded that a hypercoagulable state is a greater risk factor than the presence of nephrotic syndrome for renal vein thrombosis. Although the antiphospholipid antibodies predispose one to renal-vein thrombosis, their presence is not mandatory (125,126). Renal-vein thrombosis also has been reported in patients with SLE who have received renal allografts (127).

If reasonable clinical suspicions exist (e.g., flank pain, hematuria, oliguria, peripheral edema), a magnetic resonance angiogram or venogram should be performed. Renal-vein thrombosis must be treated promptly with anticoagulants. Renal failure and pulmonary emboli are its most serious complications. Purified Malayan pit-viper venom (ancrod) may be useful as a defibrinator (128), but it generally is not available. Thrombolytic therapies have been successfully used for renal vein thrombosis in patients without SLE (129–132).

ANTIPHOSPHOLIPID ANTIBODIES, RENAL THROMBOTIC MICROANGIOPATHY, AND LUPUS NEPHRITIS

See Chapter 50, Lupus Nephritis: Pathology, Pathogenesis, Clinical Correlations, and Prognosis, and Chapter 52, Clinical and Management Aspects of the Antiphospholipid Antibody Syndrome.

MANAGEMENT OF LUPUS NEPHRITIS

The management of lupus nephritis is controversial. The principal goals of therapy are, first, to improve or prevent the progressive loss of renal function. Second, because end-stage renal failure may be managed by dialysis or transplantation, treatment must do the patient as little harm as possible. Table 51.3 lists the toxicities of various therapies.

The general concepts and specific therapies outlined here have evolved over a 20- to 30-year period. We have been able to achieve a 10-year survival rate of over 80% with our approach. The guidelines are by no means absolute, however, and many highly qualified rheumatologists and nephrologists would treat lupus nephritis differently. The general concepts are:

TABLE 51.3. TOXICITIES OF AGGRESSIVE REGIMENS USED TO TREAT PROLIFERATIVE NEPHRITIS THAT MAY OCCUR >5% OF THE TIME

I. Prolonged high-dose oral prednisone therapy (1 mg/kg/day equivalent >6 weeks)
   - Accelerated development of cataracts, glaucoma, hypertension, osteoporosis
   - Diabetes mellitus
   - Avascular necrosis of bone
   - Diffuse ecchymoses
   - Weight gain and marked cushingoid appearance
   - Diplopia
   - Emotional lability, mood changes
   - Dyspepsia, ulcer risk
   - Increased infection risk
   - Menstrual irregularities

II. Cyclophosphamide (more common in oral doses)
   - Alopecia
   - Amenorrhea, infertility
   - Hemorrhagic cystitis
   - Risk of malignancy
   - Severe nausea and vomiting
   - Increased risk of infection
   - Teratogenicity
   - Anemia, leukopenia, thrombocytopenia

III. Azathioprine
   - Nausea and vomiting
   - Abnormal liver function tests
   - Increased risk of infection
   - Anemia, leukopenia, thrombocytopenia

1. All patients who present with lupus nephritis (as defined earlier in this chapter) should have a renal biopsy if there are no contraindications and a physician who is expert in biopsy is available. Because therapy often differs greatly for different biopsy patterns, tissue evaluation is desirable. If possible, activity and chronicity indices should be assessed from the histology. A renal biopsy may need to be repeated in patients with persistent nephritis in whom additional, more aggressive therapy is being considered.
2. Salt intake should be restricted if blood pressure is elevated. Fat intake should be restricted if hyperlipidemia is present or the patient is nephrotic. Protein intake should be restricted if renal function is impaired by over 40%. Calcium supplementation is given to minimize corticosteroid-induced osteoporosis (see Chapter 60, Adjunctive Measures and Issues: Allergies, Antibiotics, Vaccines, Osteoporosis, and Disability).
3. Loop diuretics are used to diminish edema when necessary, but if the creatinine level is greater than 3 mg/dL, they should be used with caution.
4. The authors place in order of importance the following parameters in evaluating renal activity: urine sediment appearance, serum creatinine, blood pressure, serum

albumin, 24-hour urine protein, C3 complement, anti-DNA, proteinuria estimated by urine dipstick, and creatinine clearance. These may be monitored as the clinical situation dictates. Daily measurement of serum creatinine may be useful in rapidly progressive disease; other parameters require 1 to 2 weeks to change.

5. The authors place in order of importance the following parameters in monitoring toxicity of corticosteroids, diuretics, and cytotoxic agents: blood pressure, complete blood count, platelet count, potassium, glucose, cholesterol, liver function tests, weight, muscle strength. These are closely monitored as the clinical situation requires.
6. Patients are instructed to avoid therapeutic doses of salicylates and nonsteroidal antiinflammatory agents, because they may impair renal function unless used for short periods at low doses with careful supervision.
7. Hypertension must be aggressively treated.
8. Pregnancy should be discouraged in patients with active nephritis, because it is associated with a greatly increased risk of renal failure.
9. Antimalarials may be given if there is active skin disease but will have no effect on nephritis.
10. Patients with antiphospholipid antibodies and nephritis have a poorer renal outcome, more histologic thrombotic microangiopathy, and increased complications with dialysis and transplantation. At a minimum, low-dose aspirin should be given; individuals with a history of a thrombotic event should be on lifelong warfarin or an equivalent thromboprophylactic regimen.

The following therapies are advised for specific biopsy patterns (Fig. 51.1):

1. Class I: No specific therapy is necessary.
2. Class II: Some mesangial lesions do not need therapy. In patients with class IIb patterns and over 1 g of proteinuria, high anti-dsDNA, and low C3 complement, we usually administer 20 mg of prednisone equivalent daily for 6 weeks to 3 months, followed by tapering and adjustment in accordance with the degree of clinical activity. Extrarenal lupus commonly is present and treated as is necessary.
3. Class III and IV: These are treated the same and have similar prognoses (Fig. 51.1). Because the risk of end-stage renal disease in 10 years may exceed 50%, aggressive management is advised. We recommend the following:
   A. Administration of 1 mg/kg/day of prednisone equivalent for at least 6 weeks, depending on clinical response. Cytotoxic drugs often take 3 to 4 months to become effective, and glucocorticoids stabilize the patient in the interim. Prednisone is tapered to alternate-day therapy as soon as feasible. When a level of 40 mg of prednisone daily equivalent dose is achieved, doses are then decreased by ten a week to a maintenance of 10 to 15 mg of prednisone equivalent daily or 20 to 30 mg every other day for at least 2 years.
   B. Prednisone treatment by itself can suppress proliferative disease, and cytotoxic drugs are not always needed, but this course of action is associated with more renal scarring and steroid related complications. Depending on the clinical situation, cytotoxic drugs should be added at the onset of therapy. Some published evidence suggests that the addition of cytotoxic drugs is associated with an increased probability of avoiding end-stage renal disease, as well as being steroid-sparing. Such benefit may require administration of cytotoxics for 2 years or longer in many patients. Intravenous cyclophosphamide administration of 750 mg/m^2 is given monthly for 6 months and tapered to every 2 to 3 months thereafter, depending on clinical response. We currently do not administer

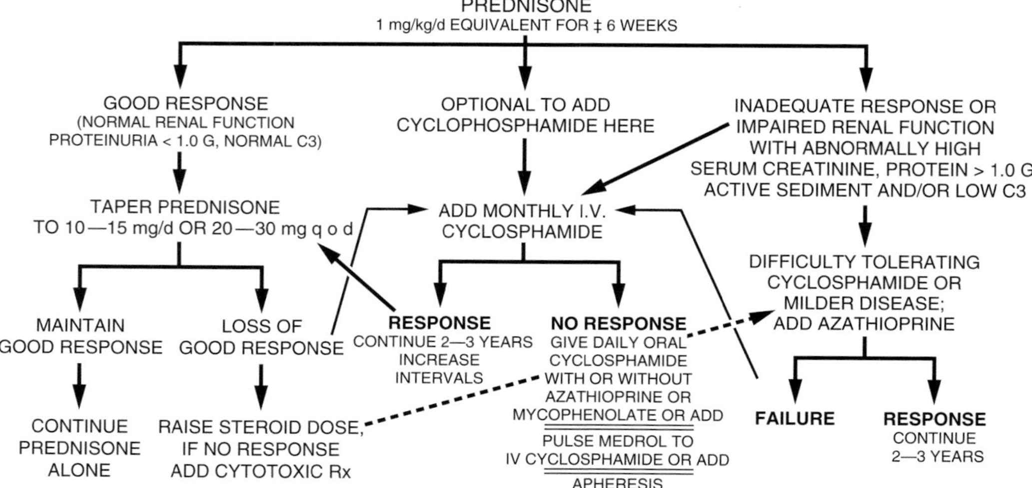

FIGURE 51.1. Algorithm for the treatment of proliferative (class III or IV) nephritis.

this therapy consecutively for more than 3 years. 2-Mercaptoethane sulfonate sodium (Mesna, Bristol-Myers Squibb Oncology/Immunology) can be given with each infusion to minimize bladder toxicity, and ondansetron (Zofran, Glaxo Wellcome Oncology/HIV) or gransitron (Kytril, SmithKline Beecham) can be given to minimize nausea.

C. Somewhere between 10% and 40% of patients, especially those who are nephrotic, will be refractory to prednisone plus intravenous cyclophosphamide (53). For issues in the treatment of lupus nephritis in children, see Chapter 41, Systemic Lupus Erythematosus in Childhood and Adolescence. Most of these patients will respond by 4 to 6 months but begin to worsen at 9 to 15 months. Among this subset, the following options are available:
   i. Repeating cycles of monthly intravenous cyclophosphamide for 6 months.
   ii. Monthly pulse doses of methylprednisolone may be added to the intravenous cyclophosphamide but should not be substituted for it (54).
   iii. Change to oral immunosuppressive with azathioprine, mycophenolate mofetil, cyclosporin, cyclophosphamide, or combinations of these drugs.
   iv. Adding apheresis, given 15 times over 6 weeks in volumes of 40 mg/kg/procedure with albumin replacement.
   v. Raising daily corticosteroid doses.

D. Acute flares with renal deterioration can be managed with pulse methylprednisolone or apheresis. The latter is especially useful if the patient has cryoglobulinemia, hyperviscosity, or thrombotic thrombocytopenic purpura.

E. Special circumstances may warrant adjustments or changes in the above regimen. These include:
   i. Corticosteroids: uncontrollable diabetes or hypertension, multiple sites of painful avascular necrosis, severe osteoporosis, steroid psychosis, life-threatening infection, severe myopathy.
   ii. Cyclophosphamide: refractory hemorrhagic cystitis despite Mesna therapy, severe nausea and/or vomiting, refusal to accept the possibility of infertility, prior radiation therapy, history of malignancy, cytopenia as a result of marrow suppression (cytopenias as a result of peripheral destruction are not contraindications).

F. Azathioprine or mycophenolate mofetil usually is the second-line agent of choice. Infrequently, chlorambucil, cyclosporin, 2-CDA or nitrogen mustard (133) may be advised.

G. Some experts use induction therapy with cyclophosphamide for at least 6 months and steroids followed by maintenance with azathioprine or myophenolate mofetil and steroids (134,135).

4. Class V: Patients are treated with 1 mg/kg/day of prednisone equivalent for 6 to 12 weeks, followed by its discontinuation if there is no response or tapering to a maintenance of 10 mg prednisone equivalent a day for 1 to 2 years if there is a response. Cytotoxic drugs generally are not used unless a proliferative component is present. Pure membranous lesions are uncommon, comprising less than 15 of all biopsies. Recently, evidence has been presented suggesting that cyclosporine is effective in managing membranous nephritis, though this is controversial (136,137).
5. Patients with a long-standing creatinine level over 3 mg/dL and/or a high chronicity index.
   A. Aggressive management usually is not advised unless a high activity index also is present or extrarenal disease warranting cytotoxic therapy is evident. It is better to plan for dialysis and/or transplantation.
   B. Patients usually are maintained on 5 to 10 mg of prednisone equivalent daily if needed to control extrarenal lupus.
   C. Salt and protein restrictions are enforced carefully. Blood pressure is closely monitored.
   D. Patients who should not be treated include those with significant renal scarring or other evidence of irreversible disease. There is little benefit in aggressively managing patients with a stable creatinine level above 5 mg/dL; it frequently produces more harm than good.

The reader is referred to Chapter 58, Nonpharmacologic Therapeutic Methods, for a discussion of the management of patients with lupus and end-stage renal disease (specifically, dialysis and transplantation).

WHEN SHOULD A RENAL BIOPSY BE PERFORMED?

Dubois felt there were only two undisputed reasons to obtain a renal biopsy: confirmation of diagnosis in equivocal cases and determination in advanced cases, when azotemia was present, as to whether further treatment was indicated. If diffuse scarring was present with little or no inflammation, conservative management would be the course of action. This view was upheld in 1978 by Fries et al. (138), who summarized the literature up to that date, examining 177 renal biopsies from several studies in detail. They concluded that biopsy information provided certain prognostic information but added little relevant clinical information. It was not cost-effective and had some inherent risks. Other reports appearing between 1978 and 1985 questioned the reliability of two observers coming to the same conclusion about a specific biopsy (139), failed to correlate a clinical nephritis index with histologic patterns (140), and showed that the World Health Organization (WHO) histologic classification was not a predictor of results of therapy at rebiopsy 12 months later (141). Smeeton et al. (142) concluded there was a small but definite risk of missing significant renal disease if a biopsy is not performed.

Several advances have resulted in our current enthusiasm for renal biopsy in most patients:

1. The development of Activity and Chronicity Indices by the National Institutes of Health (143–145). High chronicity scores clearly are associated with a poor outcome (146–148) and lack of response to immunosuppression. High activity indices, especially with more than 30% crescents, also are associated with poor outcomes but often are reversible (70,145,149) with aggressive treatment (Table 51.4). However, some have questioned their value (150) or reproducibility in a community setting (151).
2. Availability of an improved renal biopsy needle, which decreases the risk of significant bleeding.
3. Evidence that tubulointerstitial disease, which can be diagnosed only at biopsy, is of prognostic importance (152).
4. Documentation that clinically, mesangial disease can present identically to proliferative disease. Because the therapies are different and only biopsy can distinguish the two, biopsy is desirable. Mesangial disease does not require cytotoxic therapy (146,153).
5. Documentation that pure membranous disease has a different treatment and outcome than proliferative disease and can only be diagnosed by biopsy (146,154). Class Vc and Vd membranous nephritis may have a worse outcome than proliferative disease (155).
6. Three well-designed studies document that biopsy patterns have prognostic importance and help to predict outcomes (27,156,157).

We now recommend that all patients who fulfill the definition of lupus nephritis undergo an initial biopsy. Follow-up biopsies are indicated if therapy would be significantly altered as a result of the findings. Four separate editorials and/or commentaries by prominent investigators in the late 1990s support the above points in more detail (158–161). As reviewed in Chapter 50, up to 30% of patients undergoing second biopsies transform to different patterns; Chapter 50 reviews the various patterns and their clinicopathologic significance. The Mayo Clinic has recently published a concise summary of the mechanics of renal biopsy (162).

TABLE 51.4. RENAL PATHOLOGY SCORING SYSTEM[a]

Activity Index	Chronicity Index
Glomerular abnormalities	
1. Cellular proliferation	1. Glomerular sclerosis
2. Fibrinoid necrosis, karyorrhexis	2. Fibrous crescents
3. Cellular crescents	
4. Hyaline thrombi, wire loops	
5. Leukocyte infiltration	
Tubulointerstitial abnormalities	
1. Mononuclear cell infiltration	1. Interstitial fibrosis
	2. Tubular atrophy

[a]Fibrinoid necrosis and cellular crescents are weighted by a factor of 2. The maximum score of the activity index is 24; that of the chronicity index is 12. *Source:* From Austin et al. (69); with permission.

CLINICOPATHOLOGIC LABORATORY CORRELATES

The six major parameters that are used to follow lupus nephritis disease activity are: (i) serum creatinine, (ii) 24-hour urine for protein, (iii) creatinine clearance, (iv) C3 complement, (v) urine sediment, and (vi) anti-dsDNA. Each of these tests tells the clinician different things; therapeutic decisions are based on considering the results for all of these values. Clinical trials also use other outcome criteria that are less important in a community practice. These include rigorous definitions for remissions, flares, relapses, exacerbations and lupus activity scores (reviewed in reference (163).

Serum Creatinine, Or Creatinine Clearance

Serum creatinine or creatinine clearance reflects the level of renal function; it tells us little about disease activity. A persistent elevation in the serum creatinine to the abnormal range (1.4 mg/dL) implies that at least 40 of glomeruli are damaged. Normalization of the creatinine level is associated with a favorable prognosis (70,164). A creatinine clearance of less than 10 mL/hour, or a serum creatinine of over 7 mg/dL, usually is an indication for dialysis. As mentioned earlier, hydration status, severe infection, and certain medications (especially nonsteroidal antiinflammatory agents) can temporarily raise serum creatinine levels. Petri's group associated elevated serum creatinine with ages less than 20 or more than 40, disease duration and proteinuria but not socioeconomic status, race, autoantibodies or complement levels (165).

Twenty-Four-Hour Urine Proteins

Twenty-four-hour urine proteins are valuable to follow only if they are elevated (20,70,164). Levels below 200 mg per 24 hours are normal; values of up to 1,000 mg do not usually provide an indication for significant interventions and can be seen in healthy subjects after vigorous exercise. When more than 3,500 mg per 24 hours are recorded, the patient usually has nephrotic syndrome, and ankle edema is present. Anasarca can be observed in patients who have more than 7,000 mg per 24 hours. In general, 24-hour urine proteins do not correlate well with disease activity, although this is not always the case (70). We have had patients with membranous disease who have had nephrotic-range proteinuria continuously for more than 20 years and still have normal serum creatinines. Decreases in 24-hour urine protein values usually correlate with clinical improvement unless the serum creatinines are above 5 mg/dL; in this circumstance, dropping levels are a sign of renal failure.

Complement

Complement is a protein whose levels are reduced with inflammation. Various tests of complement are available in the clinical laboratory that are relevant to lupus nephritis: C3, C4, total hemolytic complement, antibodies to C1q and C3d:C4d ratios. (Chapters 13, Complement and Systemic Lupus Erythematosus, and 45, Clinical Application of Serologic Abnormalities in Systemic Lupus Erythematosus, review the biology and clinical importance of complement.) Low complement levels are associated with greater renal-disease activity (68,70,149,166–175). Falls in complement often predict disease exacerbation (70,149,171–173,175–178). The studies cited here suggest that the most specific test is C3, followed by total hemolytic complement and then C4. C3 correlates with activity indices on biopsy (179), and long-term normalization of complement is associated with a better prognosis (172).

Conversely, low complement levels also may denote congenital or acquired deficiencies of various components, and some patients have persistently low complement levels with no clinical evidence of disease activity. These patients are a minority, however. Gladman et al. (180) found 14 such patients in a group of 180 with SLE. Followed for a mean of 4.25 years, they had no symptoms and were on no medications, and none developed any evidence of lupus activity. Also, complement levels tend to normalize or be only slightly decreased in advanced renal failure.

Anti-dsDNA

Anti-dsDNA is elevated in most patients with active nephritis, although its precipitous decline can presage a flare (166–168,170,171,177,181–188). We prefer the enzyme immunoassays or the Farr assay to quantitate its presence. The Crithidia luciliae test also is available. Anti-DNA is found in 50% to 75% of patients with active nephritis; its levels often are normal in patients with pure membranous disease. Chapters 21, Antibodies to DNA, and 45, Clinical Application of Serologic Abnormalities in Systemic Lupus Erythematosus, review the biology and clinical importance of anti-DNA, which is not as reliable as C3 complement in assessing renal disease activity (149,189) and it may be elevated if extrarenal lupus activity is evident.

Other clinical correlates that might be useful in following renal disease activity have been sought. These include cryoglobulins (56,190), autoantibodies to poly(ADP)ribose (194), circulating immune complexes (167,192–194), IL-2-receptor levels (195), ANA patterns (196), antiendothelial-cell antibody levels (197), plasma thrombomodulin (198), antiheparan sulphate reactivity (199), decreased interleukin-1 receptor antagonist (200), antiribosomal P (201) and measurement of the activation and degradation components of complement (see Chapter 13, Complement and Systemic Lupus Erythematosus). These tests either are not universally available or are less reliable than those discussed earlier. No one test (except for a dramatic change in serum creatinine or C3 complement) usually allows the practitioner to take any particular course of action unless it is consistently abnormal or supported by other confirmatory laboratory tests and the clinical picture.

In summary, laboratory testing with serum creatinine, 24-hour urine protein and creatinine clearance, C3 complement levels, urine sediment abnormalities, and anti-dsDNA provide extremely useful information when used adjunctively with a careful patient history and physical examination, knowledge of the patient's disease, and clinical experience.

COURSE OF LUPUS NEPHRITIS

Over the last five decades, a tremendous change has evolved in the approach to lupus nephritis, and this has greatly altered its outcome (202).

Studies From 1950 To 1989

In the early 1950s, low-dose corticosteroids were used, with 5-year survival rates of close to zero (203). By the late 1950s and early 1960s, prolonged high-dose corticosteroids were employed (with a few centers using nitrogen mustard), and the overall 5-year survival rose to 25% (204). The mid to late 1960s were characterized by the availability of hemodialysis, moderate-dose steroid usage, and widespread use of high doses of azathioprine and oral cyclophosphamide. The overall 5-year survival then was 40% to 70%. By the early 1970s, physicians temporized their use of cytotoxic drugs and took advantage of newer antibiotics and antihypertensive agents, resulting in 60 to 80 5-year survivals. [In the Dubois/Wallace series (20), 10-year survivals for middle-class patients diagnosed in the decades beginning in 1950 were 65% and then 60% (1960), 76% (1970), and 92% (1980)]. The WHO classification system helped to stratify renal disease into pathologic subsets that helped tailor therapy. The 1980s saw the introduction of intermittent, parenteral cyclophosphamide combined with corticosteroids. Activity and chronicity indices were described, and interventions with pulse-dose corticosteroids and apheresis became more common (205,206). In 1989, Esdaile et al. (70) were able to document 85% and 73% 5- and 10-year survivals, respectively, among 87 patients followed for a mean of 8.4 years.

Recent And Cumulative Insights

Along the way, new insights were derived that allowed investigators to determine prognostic subsets and assess the impact of various therapies. Associated with a poorer outcome were nephrotic syndrome, WHO-defined class IV lesions, high chronicity indices, hypertension, interstitial disease, smoking, infections, thrombocytopenia, and childhood onset of nephritis (20,27,62,70,207–209). The National Institutes of Health group correlated corticosteroid therapy with progressive renal scarring and a worse prognosis than in those given corticosteroids plus cytotoxic treatments (205,206). Blacks, race, younger age at onset, low complements, anemia, and crescents on biopsy were similarly associated with a poor prognosis (210). Efforts also were made to correlate prognosis with biopsy pattern. McClusky (211) in 1975 and Pollak and Kant (212) in 1981 summarized several studies and found the 5-year survival rate of patients with minimal lesions to be 80% to 90%, with mesangial lesions to be 68%, mild proliferative lesions to be 40% to 80%, severe proliferative lesions to be 25% to 40%, and membranous lesions to be 60% to 80%. The worst prognostic subset of lupus nephritis is nephrotic syndrome, in which one half were dead within 10 years (20,213). The most common causes of death were and continue to be complications of renal disease and sepsis (22). Papers in the last few years for the first time have mentioned discontinuing therapy after successful treatment (214,215), and more emphasis is being placed on decreasing the risk of evolving end-stage renal disease. Despite all these advances, however, certain subsets of patients with focal or diffuse proliferative lesions and scarring glomerular and tubulointerstitial regions still have a 50% chance of evolving into end-stage renal disease within 5 years, and aggressive management appears to be warranted (27,216–219). Of 150 patients who were seen by one of us, 10%, 19%, and 30% developed end-stage disease at 5, 10, and 15 years, respectively (27). Piette's French group followed 180 lupus nephritis patients at a single center. In 1999, their 5-, 10-, and 15-year renal survivals were 95%, 89% and 76%, respectively (22). Mok et al. followed 183 nephritis patients in Hong Kong. In 1999, their 5, 10, and 15 year renal survivals were 94%, 92%, and 75% (220). Remissions after initial therapy for nephritis correlate with an improved renal and patient survival (221).

SUMMARY AND FUTURE DIRECTIONS

In summary, lupus nephritis has evolved from a frequently terminal process to one in which a fairly normal quality of life and good outcome are possible. First, the treating physician must accurately stage the disease with laboratory and tissue evaluations. Next, therapy is fashioned for the specific disease subsets that are involved. Third, both side effects and the complications of treatment must be managed, along with frequent assessments and modifications of therapy depending on the patient's response.

Since 1995, major advances in the management of lupus nephritis have been reported. These include: (i) the use of cyclosporin to treat membranous nephritis (137), and (ii) the use of mycophenolate mofetil (currently being evaluated in controlled trials) as an alternative to, or as an adjunct to cyclophosphamide treatment (222,223), and the introduction of biologic therapies into clinical trials. These include the polynucleotide toleragen LJP 394, anti-CD40 ligand antibody, anti-C5 monoclonal chimeric antibodies, anti-CD20 chimeric antibody, and CTLA4Ig and anti-DNAase (reviewed in references 224 and 225 and discussed in Chapter 62, Experimental Therapies in Systemic Lupus Erythematosus). It is our hope that the new millennium will see further advances in this difficult aspect of SLE, because substantial mortality and morbidity still occur.

REFERENCES

1. Keith NM, Rowntree LG. Study of renal complications of disseminated lupus erythematosus: report of four cases. *Trans Assoc Am Physicians* 1922;37:487–502.
2. Baehr G, Klemperer P, Schifrin A. Diffuse disease of the peripheral circulation usually associated with lupus erythematosus and endocarditis. *Trans Assoc Am Physicians* 1935;50:139–155.
3. Freedman P, Markowitz AS. Gamma globulin and complement in the diseased kidney. J *Clin Invest* 1962;41:328–334.
4. Friou GJ, Finch SC, Detre KD. Interaction of nuclei and globulin from lupus erythematosus serum demonstrated with fluorescent antibody. *J Immunol* 1958;80:324–329.
5. Lachmann PJ, Muller-Eberhard HJ, Kunkel HG, et al. The localization of in vivo bound complement in tissue sections. *J Exp Med* 1962;15:63–82.
6. Mellors RC, Ortega LC, Holman HR. Role of gamma globulins in pathogenesis of renal lesions in systemic lupus erythematosus and chronic membranous glomerulonephritis, with an observation on lupus erythematosus cell reaction. *J Exp Med* 1957;106: 191–202.
7. Vazquez JJ, Dixon FJ. Immunohistochemical analysis of lesions associated with fibrinoid change. *Arch Pathol* 1958;66:504–517.
8. Hargraves MM, Richmond H, Morton R. Presentation of 2 bone marrow elements: tart cell and L.E. cell. *Proc Staff Meet Mayo Clin* 1948;23:25–28.
9. Bennett WM, Bardana EJ, Houghton DC, et al. Silent renal involvement in systemic lupus erythematosus. *Int Arch Allergy Appl Immunol* 1977;55:420–428.
10. Eiser AR, Katz SM, Swartz C. Clinically occult diffuse proliferative lupus nephritis: an age related phenomenon. *Arch Intern Med* 1979;139:1022–1025.
11. Font J, Torras A, Cevera R, et al. Silent renal disease in systemic lupus erythematosus. *Clin Nephrol* 1987;27:283–288.
12. Hollcraft RM, Dubois EL, Lundberg GD, et al. Renal damage in systemic lupus erythematosus with normal renal function. *J Rheumatol* 1976;3:251–261.
13. Kark RM, Pollak VE, Soothill JF, et al. Simple test of renal function in health and disease. I. A reappraisal of their value in the light of serial renal biopsies. *Arch Intern Med* 1957;99:176–189.
14. Leehey DJ, Katz AI, Azaran AH, et al. Silent diffuse lupus nephritis: long term follow-up. *Am J Kidney Dis* 1982;2(suppl 1):188–196.
15. Mahajan SK, Ordonez NG, Feitelson PJ, et al. Lupus nephritis without clinical renal involvement. *Medicine* 1977;56:493–501.
16. Muehrcke RC, Kark RM, Pirani CL, et al. Lupus nephritis: a

clinical and pathologic study based on renal biopsies. *Medicine* 1957;36:11–45.

17. Rojas C, Jacobelli S, Massardo L, et al. Disseminated lupus erythematosus without abnormalities in urinary sediment. *Rev Med Chile* 1987;115:120–125.
18. Woolf A, Croker B, Osofski SG, et al. Nephritis in children and young adults with systemic lupus erythematosus and normal urinary sediment (abstract). *Kidney Int* 1978;14:667.
19. Pistiner M, Wallace DJ, Nessim S, et al. Lupus erythematosus in the 1980s: a survey of 570 patients. *Semin Arthritis Rheum* 1991;21:55–64.
20. Wallace DJ, Podell T, Weiner J, et al. Systemic lupus erythematosus survival patterns. Experience with 609 patients. *JAMA* 1981;245:934–938.
21. Wallace DJ, Podell TE, Weiner JM, et al. Lupus nephritis. Experience with 230 patients in a private practice from 1950 to 1980. *Am J Med* 1982;72:209–220.
22. Huong DLT, Papo T, Beaufils H, et al. Renal involvement in systemic lupus erythematosus. A study of 180 patients from a single center. *Medicine* 1999;78:148–166.
23. Baker SB, Rovira JR, Campion EW, et al. Late onset lupus erythematosus. *Am J Med* 1979;66:727–732.
24. Dimant J, Ginzler EM, Schlesinger M, et al. Systemic lupus erythematosus in the older age group: computer analysis. *J Am Geriatr Soc* 1979;27:58–61.
25. Dooley MA, Hogan S, Jennette C, et al. Cyclophosphamide therapy for lupus nephritis: poor renal survival in black Americans. *Kidney International* 1997;51:1188–1195.
26. Austin HA III, Boumpsas DT, Vaughan EM, et al. High-risk features of lupus nephritis: importance of race and clinical histological factors in 166 patients. *Nephrol Dial Transplant* 1995; 10:1620–1628.
27. Neumann K, Wallace DJ, Azen C, et al. Lupus in the 1980s: III. Influence of clinical variables, biopsy, and treatment on the outcome of 150 patients with lupus nephritis seen at a single center. *Semin Arthritis Rheum* 1995;25:47–55.
28. Nossent JC, Bronsveld W, Swaak AJ. Systemic lupus erythematosus. III. Observations on clinical renal involvement and follow up of renal function: Dutch experience with 110 patients studied prospectively. *Ann Rheum Dis* 1989;48:810–816.
29. Klippel JH. Predicting who will get lupus nephritis. *J Clin Rheumatol* 1995;1:257–259.
30. Blum A, Rubinow A, Galun E. Prominence of renal involvement in male patients with systemic lupus erythematosus (letter). *Clin Exp Rheumatol* 1991;9:206–207.
31. Tateno S, Hiki Y, Hamaguchi K, et al. Study of lupus nephritis in males. *Q J Med* 1991;81:1031–1039.
32. Walker RJ, Bailey RR, Swainson CP, et al. Lupus nephritis: a 13 year experience. *N Z Med J* 1986;99:894–896.
33. Lee HS, Spargo BH. A renal biopsy of lupus nephropathy in the United States and Korea. *Am J Kidney Dis* 1985;5:242–250.
34. McAlindon T, Giannotta L, Taub N, et al. Environmental factors predicting nephritis in systemic lupus erythematosus. *Ann Rheum Dis* 1993;52:720–724.
35. Hopkinson ND, Jenkinson C, Muir KR, et al. Racial group, socioeconomic status and the development of persistent proteinuria in systemic lupus erythematosus. *Ann Rheum Dis* 2000; 59:116–119.
36. Freedman BI, Spray BJ, Heise ER, et al. A race-controlled human leukocyte antigen frequency analysis in lupus nephritis. *Am J Kid Dis* 1993;21:378–382.
37. Salmon JE, Millard S, Schacter LA, et al. Fc-gammaRIIA alleles are heritable risk factors for lupus nephritis in African Americans. *J Clin Invest* 1996;97:1348–1354.
38. Akai Y, Sato H, Kurumatani N, et al. Association of an insertion polymorphism of angiotensin-converting enzyme gene with the activity of lupus nephritis. *Clin Nephrology* 1999;51: 141–146.
39. Estes D, Christian CL. The natural history of systemic lupus erythematosus by prospective analysis. *Medicine* 1971;50:85–95.
40. Haserick JR. Unpublished data.
41. Larsen RA, Solheim BG. Family studies in systemic lupus erythematosus. V. Presence of antinuclear factors (ANTFs) in relatives and spouses of selected SLE probands. *Acta Med Scand* 1972;543(suppl):55–64.
42. McGehee Harvey A, Shulman LE, Tumulty AP, et al. Systemic lupus erythematosus: review of the literature and clinical analysis of 138 cases. *Medicine* 1954;33:291–337.
43. Cairns SA, Acheson EJ, Corbett CL, et al. The delayed appearance of an antinuclear factor and the diagnosis of systemic lupus erythematosus in glomerulonephritis. *Postgrad Med J* 1979;55: 723–727.
44. Adu D, Williams DG. Complement activating cryoglobulins in the nephritis of systemic lupus erythematosus. *Clin Exp Immunol* 1984;55:495–501.
45. Gianviti A, Barsotti P, Barbera V, et al. Delayed onset of systemic lupus erythematosus in patients with "full house" nephropathy. *Pediatr Nephrol* 1999;13:683–687.
46. Fisher C, Gibb WRG, Cohen SL, et al. Lupus-like nephritis heralding the definitive manifestation of systemic lupus erythematosus. *Br J Rheumatol* 1984;24:256–262.
47. Adelman DC, Wallace DJ, Klinenberg JR. Thirty-four-year delayed-onset lupus nephritis: a case report. *Arthritis Rheum* 1987;30:479–480.
48. Klippel JH. How to alter the course of lupus nephritis. *J Musculoskeletal Dis* 1988;5:29–43.
49. Yeung CK, Ng WL, Wong WS, et al. Acute deterioration in renal function in systemic lupus erythematosus. *Q J Med* 1985; 56:393–402.
50. Henry R, Williams AV, McFadden NR, et al. Histopathologic evaluation of lupus patients with transient renal failure. *Am J Kidney Dis* 1986;8:417–421.
51. Kozeny GA, Barr W, Bansal VK, et al. Occurrence of renal tubular dysfunction in lupus nephritis. *Arch Intern Med* 1987; 147:891–895.
52. Lin WY, Lan JL, Wang SJ. Value of gallium-67 scintigraphy in monitoring the renal activity in lupus nephritis. *Scand J Rheumatol* 1998;27:42–45.
53. Belmont HM, Storch M, Buyon J, et al. New York University/ Hospital for Joint Diseases experience with intravenous cyclophosphamide treatment: efficacy in steroid unresponsive lupus nephritis. *Lupus* 1995;4:104–108.
54. Gourley MF, Austin HA III, Scott D, et al. Methylprednisolone and cyclophosphamide, alone or in combination, in patients with lupus nephritis. A randomized, controlled trial. *Annals Intern Med* 1996:125:549–557.
55. Helin H, Korpela M, Mustonen J, et al. Rheumatoid factor in rheumatoid arthritis associated renal disease in lupus nephritis. *Ann Rheum Dis* 1986;45:508–511.
56. Howard TW, Iannini MJ, Burge JJ. Rheumatoid factor, cryoglobulinemia, anti-DNA, and renal disease in patients with systemic lupus erythematosus. *J Rheumatol* 1991;18:826–830.
57. Bakir AA, Lopez-Majano V, Hyrhorczuk DO, et al. Appraisal of lupus nephritis by renal imaging with Gallium-67. *Am J Med* 1985;79:175–182.
58. Ozbek SS, Buyukberber S, Tolunay O, et al. Image-directed color Doppler ultrasonography of kidney in systemic lupus nephritis. *J Clin Ultrasound* 1995;23:17–20.
59. Platt JF, Rubin JM, Ellis JH. Lupus nephritis: predictive values of conventional and doppler US and comparison with serologic and biopsy parameters. *Radiology* 1997;203:82–86.
60. Petri M, Bockenstedt L, Colman J, et al. Serial assessment of

glomerular filtration rate in lupus nephropathy. *Kidney Int* 1988;34:832–839.

61. Ratain JS, Petri M, Hochberg MC, et al. Accuracy of creatinine clearance in measuring glomerular filtration rate in patients with systemic lupus erythematosus without clinical evidence of renal disease. *Arthritis Rheum* 1990;33:277–280.
62. Roubenoff R, Drew H, Moyer M, et al. Oral cimetidine improves the accuracy and precision of creatinine clearance in lupus nephritis. *Ann Intern Med* 1990;113:501–506.
63. Godfrey T, Cuadrado MJ, Fon C, et al. Chromium-51 ethyldiamine tetraacetic acid glomerular filtration rate (EDTA-GFR) a better predictor than biochemical calculated GFR for renal involvement in SLE patients with normal serum creatinine. *Arthritis Rheum* 1999;42:S213.
64. Nakano M, Ueno M, Hasegawa H, et al. Renal hemodynamic characteristics in patients with lupus nephritis. *Ann Rheum Dis* 1998;57:226–230.
65. Ropes MW. Observations on the natural course of disseminated lupus erythematosus. *Medicine* 1964;43:387–391.
66. Dubois EL, ed. Lupus erythematosus. A review of the current status of discoid and systemic lupus erythematosus and their variants. 2nd ed. rev. Los Angeles: USC Press, 1976.
67. Makino H, Kawasaki H, Murakami K, et al. Mechanism of haematuria in lupus nephritis. *Annals Rheum Dis* 1995;54: 934–935.
68. Appel GB, Silva FG, Pirani CL, et al. Renal involvement in systemic lupus erythematosus: a study of 56 patients emphasizing histologic classification. *Medicine* 1978;57:371–410.
69. Austin HA 3rd, Muenz LR, Joyce KM, et al. Prognostic factors in lupus nephritis: contribution of renal histologic data. *Am J Med* 1983;75:382–391.
70. Esdaile JM, Levinton C, Federgreen W, et al. The clinical and renal biopsy predictors of long-term outcome in lupus nephritis: a study of 87 patients and review of the literature. *Q J Med* 1989;72:779–833.
71. Fries J, Holman H. *Systemic lupus erythematosus: a clinical analysis*. Philadelphia: WB Saunders, 1975.
72. Wilson RM, Maher JF, Schreiner GE. Lupus nephritis: clinical and histologic survey. *Arch Intern Med* 1963;111:429–438.
73. Rothfield NF. Current approaches to SLE and its subsets. *DM* 1982;29:162.
74. Sessions S, Mehta K, Kovarsky J. Quantitation of proteinuria in systemic lupus erythematosus by random, spot urine collection. *Arthritis Rheum* 1983;26:918–920.
75. Rahman P, Gladman DD, Urowitz MB. Significance of isolated pyuria in SLE. *Arthritis Rheum* 1998:S282 (abstract).
76. Rahman P, Gladman DD, Urowitz MB. Significance of isolated hematuria in SLE. *Arthritis Rheum* 1998;S281 (abstract).
77. Ropes MW. *Systemic lupus erythematosus*. Cambridge, MA: Harvard University Press, 1976.
78. Herbert LA, Dillon JJ, Middendorf DF, et al. Relationship between appearance of urinary red blood cell/white blood cell casts and the onset of renal relapse in systemic lupus erythematosus. *Am J Kidney Dis* 1995;26:432–438.
79. Terai C, Nojima Y, Takano K. Determination of urinary albumin excretion by radioimmunoassay in patients with subclinical lupus nephritis. *Clin Nephrol* 1987;27:79–83.
80. Cottiero RA, Madalo MP, Levey AS. Glomerular filtration rate and urinary albumin excretion rate in systemic lupus erythematosus. *Nephron* 1995;69:140–146.
81. Valente de Almeida R, Rocha de Carvalho JG, de Azevedo VF, et al. Microalbuminuria and renal morphology in the evaluation of subclinical lupus nephritis. *Clin Nephrology* 1999;52:218–229.
82. Batlle-Gualda E, Martinez AC, Guerra RA, et al. Urinary albumin excretion in patients with systemic lupus erythematosus without renal disease. *Annals Rheum Dis* 1997;56:386–389.
83. Bazzi C, Petrini C, Sabadini E, et al. SDS-PAGE patterns and polymeric albumin in proteinuria of lupus glomerulonephritis. *Clin Nephrol* 1995;43:96–103.
84. Barcelo R, Pollak VE. A preliminary immunologic study of urinary proteins: the questionable value of protein clearances in kidney disease. *Can Med Assoc J* 1966;94:269–275.
85. Stevens MB, Knowles B. Significance of urinary gamma globulin in lupus nephritis. 1. Electrophoretic analysis. *N Engl J Med* 1962;267:1159–1166.
86. Boesken WH, Hsaio L, Stierle HE. Diagnostic relevance of quantitative and qualitative urine protein analyses in SLE. *Nieren und Hochdrukkrankheiten Jahrang* 1987;6:210–212.
87. Epstein WV. Immunologic events preceding clinical exacerbation of systemic lupus erythematosus. *Am J Med* 1973;54:631–636.
88. Epstein WV, Tan M. Effect of adrenocorticosteroid therapy on L-chain abnormalities of patients with systemic lupus erythematosus (abstract). *Arthritis Rheum* 1967;10:277.
89. Spriggs B, Epstein W. Clinical correlation of elevated urine L-chain concentrations in SLE (abstract). *Clin Res* 1973;21:213.
90. Cooper A, Bluestone R. Free immunoglobulin light chains in connective tissue diseases. *Ann Rheum Dis* 1968;27:537–543.
91. Hopper JE, Sequeira W, Martllotto J, et al. Clinical relapse in systemic lupus erythematosus: correlation with antecedent elevation of urinary free light-chain immunoglobulin. *J Clin Immunol* 1989;9:338–350.
92. Tsai C-Y, Wu T-H, Sun K-H, et al. Increased excretion of soluble interleukin 2 receptors and free light chain immunoglobulins in the urine of patients with active lupus nephritis. *Ann Rheum Dis* 1992;51:168–172.
93. Williams RC Jr, Malone CC, Miller RT, et al. Urinary loss of immunoglobulin G anti F (ab′)2 and anti-DNA antibody in systemic lupus erythematosus nephritis. *J Lab Clin Med* 1998;132:210–222.
94. Meryhew NL, Messner RD, Tan EM. Urinary excretion of antinuclear antibodies. *J Rheumatol* 1983;10:913–919.
95. Kountz DS, Kolander SA, Rozovsky A. False positive urinary pregnancy test in the nephrotic syndrome. *N Engl J Med* 1989; 321:1416.
96. Nishiya K, Kawabata F, Ota Z. Elevated urinary ferritin in lupus nephritis. *J Rheumatol* 1989;16:1513–1514.
97. Picking WL, Smith C, Petrucci R, et al. Anti-RNA polymerase I antibodies in the urine of patients with systemic lupus erythematosus. *J Rheumatol* 1990;1308–1313.
98. Lentz RD, Michael AF, Fried PS. Membranous transformation of lupus nephritis. *Clin Immunol Immunopathol* 1981;19:131–138.
99. Lim KL, Muir K, Powell RJ. Urine neopterin: a new parameter for serial monitoring of disease activity in patients with systemic lupus erythematosus. *Ann Rheum Dis* 1994;53: 743–748.
100. Lim KL, Jones AC, Brown NS, et al. Urine neopterin as a parameter of disease activity in patients with systemic lupus erythematosus: comparisons with serum sIL-2R and antibodies to dsDNA, erythrocyte sedimentation rate, and plasma C3, C4 and C3 degradation products. *Ann Rheum Dis* 1993;52:429–435.
101. Bitter T, Siegenthaler P, DePreux T, et al. Excretion in the urine of aminoacridine precipitable polyuronides (acid mucopolysaccharides) in patients with rheumatoid arthritis. *Ann Rheum Dis* 1970;29:427–433.
102. Antoine B, Ward PD. Histuria and fibrinuria in cases of systemic lupus erythematosus. *Clin Exp Immunol* 1970;6:153–159.
103. Kanyerezi BR, Lwanga SK, Bloch KJ. Fibrinogen degradation products in serum and urine of patients with systemic lupus erythematosus. Relation in renal disease and pathogenic mechanism. *Arthritis Rheuml* 1971;14:267–275.
104. Stevens MB, Zizic TM, Young N. Urinary fibrinogen fragments in lupus nephritis (abstract). *Arthritis Rheum* 1970;13:352.
105. Delektorskaya L, Janushkevich T, Okunev D. The significance of

the assays of urinary enzymes activity in patients with systemic lupus erythematosus. *Z Med Lab Diagn* 1990;31:375–379.
106. Iwano M, Dohi K, Hirata E, et al. Urinary levels of IL-6 in patients with active lupus nephritis. *Clin Nephrol* 1993;40:16–21.
107. Peterson E, Robertson AD, Emlen W. Serum and urinary interleukin-6 in systemic lupus erythematosus. *Lupus* 1996;5: 571–575.
108. Macanovic M, Hogarth MB, Lachmann PJ. Anti-DNA antibodies in the urine of lupus nephritis patients. *Nephrol Dial Transplant* 1999;14:1418–1424.
109. Roberti I, Dikman S, Speira H, et al. Comparative value of urinalysis, urine cytology and urine sIL2R in the assessment of renal disease in patients with systemic lupus erythematosus, *Clin Nephrol* 1996;46:176–182.
110. Ueda Y, Nagasawa K, Tsukamato H, et al. Urinary C4 excretion in systemic lupus erythematosus. *Clin Chim Acta* 1995;243: 11–23.
111. Wada T, Yokoyama H, Su SB, et al. Monitoring urinary levels of monocyte chemotactic and activating factor reflects disease activity of lupus nephritis. *Kidney International* 1996;49:761–767.
112. Guy JM, Brammah TB, Holt L. Urinary excretion of albumin and retinol binding protein in systemic lupus erythematosus. *Ann Clin Biochem* 1997;34:668–674.
113. Tesar V, Masek Z, Rychlilik I, et al. Cytokines and adhesion molecules in renal vasculitis and lupus nephritis. *Nephrol Dial Transplant* 1998;13:1662–1667.
114. Kelly RH, Carpenter AB, Sudol KS, et al. Complement C3 fragments in urine: detection in systemic lupus erythematosus patients by Western blotting. *Appl Theor Electrophoresis* 1993;3: 265–269.
115. Negi VS, Aggarwal A, Dayal R, et al. Complement degradation product C3d in Urine: Marker of Lupus Nephritis. *J Rheumatol* 2000;27:380–383.
116. Hamilton CR, Tumulty PA. Thrombosis of renal veins and inferior vena cava complicating lupus nephritis. *JAMA* 1968;206: 2315–2316.
117. Kant KS, Pollak VE, Weiss MA, et al. Glomerular thrombosis in systemic lupus erythematosus: prevalence and significance. *Medicine* 1981;60:71–86.
118. Llach F, Koffler A, Kinck E, et al. On the incidence of renal vein thrombosis in nephrotic syndrome. *Arch Intern Med* 1977;137: 333–336.
119. Millet VG, Usera G, de la Ossa JMA, et al. Renal vein thrombosis, nephrotic syndrome and focal lupus glomerulonephritis. *Br Med J* 1978;1:24–25.
120. Mintz G, Acevedo-Vazquez E, Gutierrez-Espinosa G, et al. Renal vein thrombosis and inferior vena cava thrombosis in systemic lupus erythematosus: frequency and risk factor. *Arthritis Rheum* 1984;27:539–544.
121. Bradley WG, Jacobs RP, Trew PA, et al. Renal vein thrombosis: occurrence in membranous glomerulonephropathy and lupus nephritis. *Radiology* 1981;139:571–576.
122. Lai NS, Lan JL. Renal vein thrombosis in Chinese patients with systemic lupus erythematosus. *Ann Rheum Dis* 1997;56:562–564.
123. Piette J-C, Cacoub P, Wechsler B. Renal manifestations of the antiphospholipid syndrome. *Semin Arthritis Rheum* 1994;23: 357–366.
124. Miranda JM, Garcia-Torres R, Jara LJ, et al. Renal biopsy of systemic lupus erythematosus: significance of glomerular thrombosis. Analysis of 108 cases. *Lupus* 1994;3:25–29.
125. Cagnoli L, Viglietta G, Madia G, et al. Acute bilateral renal vein thrombosis superimposed on calcified thrombus of the inferior vena cava in a patient with membranous lupus nephritis. *Nephrol Dial Transplant* 1990;(suppl 1):71–74.
126. Terabayashi H, Okuda K, Nomura F, et al. Transformation of inferior vena caval thrombosis to membranous obstruction in a patient with the lupus anticoagulant. *Gastroenterol* 1986;91: 219–224.
127. Liano F, Mampaso F, Garcia Martin F, et al. Allograft membranous glomerulonephritis and renal vein thrombosis in a patients with a lupus anticoagulant factor. *Nephrol Dial Transplant* 1988; 3:684–689.
128. Pollack VE, Glueck HI, Weiss MA, et al. Defibrination with ancrod in glomerulonephritis: effects on clinical and histologic findings and on blood coagulation. *Am J Nephrol* 1982;2: 195–207.
129. Lam KK, Lui CC. Successful treatment of acute inferior vena cava and unilateral renal vein thrombosis by local infusion of recombinant tissue plasminogen. *Amer J Kid Dis* 1998;32: 1075–1079.
130. Angle JF, Matsumoto AH, Al Shammari M, et al. Transcatheter regional urokinase therapy in the management of inferior vena cava thrombosis. *J Vasc Interventional Radiology* 1998;9:917–925.
131. Morrisey EC, Mc Donald BR, Rabetoy GM. Resolution of proteinuria secondary to bilateral renal vein thrombosis after treatment with systemic thrombolytic therapy. *Amer J Kid Dis* 1997;29:615–619.
132. Tamim W, Arous E. Thrombolytic therapy: the choice for iliac vein thrombosis in the presence of kidney transplant. *Annals Vascular Surgery* 1999;13:436–438.
133. Wallace DJ. Successful use of nitrogen mustard for cyclophosphamide resistant diffuse proliferative lupus glomerulonephritis. *J Rheumatol* 1995;22:801–802.
134. Chan TM, Li F-K, Wong RWS, et al. Sequential therapy for diffuse proliferative and membranous lupus nephritis: cyclophosphamide and prednisolone followed by azathioprine and prednisolone. *Nephron* 1995;71:321–327.
135. D'Cruz D, Cuadrado MJ, Mujic F, et al. Immunosuppressive therapy for lupus nephritis. *Clin Exper Rheumatol* 1997;15: 275–282.
136. Klein M, Radhakrishnan J, Appel G. Cyclosporine treatment of glomerular diseases. *Annual Rev Med* 1999;50:1–15.
137. Hallegua D, Wallace DJ, Metzger AL, et al. Cyclosporin for membranous lupus nephritis: experience with ten patients and review of the literature. *Lupus* 2000;9:241–251.
138. Fries JF, Porta J, Liang MH. Marginal benefit of renal biopsy in systemic lupus erythematosus. *Arch Intern Med* 1978;138: 1386–1389.
139. Whiting-O'Keefe Q, Riccardi PJ, Henke JE, et al. Recognition of information in renal biopsies of patients with lupus nephritis. *Ann Intern Med* 1982;96:723–727.
140. Sluiter HE, Kallenberg CGM, VanSon WJ, et al. When to perform a renal biopsy in systemic lupus erythematosus (SLE)? *Neth J Med* 1981;24:217–223.
141. Whiting-O'Keefe Q, Henke JE, Shearn MA, et al. The information content from renal biopsy in systemic lupus erythematosus: stepwise linear regression analysis. *Ann Intern Med* 1982;96:718–723.
142. Smeeton WMI, Doak PB, Simpson IJ, et al. Lupus nephritis: clinicopathological correlations. *N Z Med J* 1983;96:39–42.
143. Austin HA 3rd, Muenz LR, Joyce KM, et al. Diffuse proliferative lupus nephritis: identification of specific pathologic features affecting renal outcome. *Kidney Int* 1984;25:689–695.
144. Balow JE, Austin HA 3rd, Muenz LR, et al. Effect of treatment on the evolution of renal abnormalities in lupus nephritis. *N Engl J Med* 1984;311:491–495.
145. Moroni G, Pasquali S, Quaglini S, et al. Clinical and prognostic variables of serial renal biopsies in lupus nephritis. *Amer J Kid Dis* 1999;34:530–539.
146. McLaughlin J, Gladman DD, Urowitz MB, et al. Kidney biopsy in systemic lupus erythematosus: II. Survival analysis according to biopsy results. *Arthritis Rheum* 1991;34:1268–1273.

147. Nossent HC, Henzen-Logmans SC, Vroom TM, et al. Contribution of renal biopsy data in predicting outcome in lupus nephritis: analysis of 116 patients. *Arthritis Rheum* 1990;33:970–977.
148. McLaughlin JR, Bombardier C, Farewell VT. Kidney biopsy in systemic lupus erythematosus. III. Survival analysis controlling for clinical and laboratory variables. *Arthritis Rheum* 1995;37: 559–567.
149. Magil AB, Putterman ML, Ballon HS, et al. Prognostic factors in diffuse proliferative lupus glomerulonephritis. *Kidney Int* 1988;34:511–517.
150. Schwartz MM, Lan S-P, Bernstein J, et al. Role of pathology indices in the management of severe lupus glomerulonephritis. *Kidney Int* 1992;42:743–748.
151. Wernick RM, Smith DL, Houghton DC, et al. Reliability of histologic scoring for lupus nephritis: a community-based evaluation. *Ann Intern Med* 1993;119:805–811.
152. Park MH, D'Agati VD, Appel GB, et al. Tubulo-interstitial disease in lupus nephritis: relationship to immune deposits, interstitial inflammation, glomerular changes, renal function, and prognosis. *Nephron* 1986;44:309–319.
153. Gladman DD, Urowitz MB, Cole E, et al. Kidney biopsy in SLE. I. A clinical-morphologic evaluation. *Q J Med* 1989;73: 1125–1133.
154. Adler SG, Johnson K, Louie JS, et al. Lupus membranous glomerulonephritis: different prognostic subgroups obscured by imprecise histologic classification. *Modern Pathol* 1990;3: 186–191.
155. Sloan RP, Schwartz MM, Korbet SM, et al. Long-term outcome in systemic lupus erythematosus membranous glomerulonephritis. Lupus Nephritis Collaborative Study Group. *J Am Soc Nephrol* 1996;7:299–305.
156. McLaughlin J, Gladman DD, Urowitz MB, et al. Kidney biopsy in systemic lupus erythematosus. II. Survival analysis according to biopsy results. *Arthritis Rheum* 1991;34:1268–1273.
157. Esdaile JM, Joseph L, MacKenzie T, et al. The pathogenesis and prognosis of lupus nephritis: information from repeat biopsy. *Semin Arthritis Rheum* 1993;23:135–148.
158. Ponticelli C, Moroni G. Renal biopsy in lupus nephritis—what for, when and how often? *Nephrol Dial Transplant* 1998;13: 2452–2454.
159. Esdaile JM. Current role of renal biopsy in patients with SLE. *Balliere's Clinical Rheumatology* 1998;12:433–448.
160. Grande JP, Balow JE. Renal biopsy in lupus nephritis. *Lupus* 1998;7:611–617.
161. Kashgarian M. The role of the kidney biopsy in the treatment of lupus nephritis. *Renal Failure* 1996;18:763–773.
162. Radford MG, Donadio JV, Holley KE, et al. Renal biopsy in clinical practice. *May Clin Proc* 1994;69:983–984.
163. Boumpas DT, Balow JE. Outcome criteria for lupus nephritis trials: a critical review. *Lupus* 1998;7:622–629.
164. Edworthy SM, Bloch DA, McShane DJ, et al. A state model of renal function in systemic lupus erythematosus: its value in the prediction of outcome in 292 patients. *J Rheumatol* 1989;16: 29–35.
165. Rzany B, Coresh J, Whelton PK, et al. Risk factors for hypercreatinemia in patients with systemic lupus erythematosus. *Lupus* 1999;8:532–540.
166. Cameron JS, Turner DR, Ogg CS, et al. Systemic lupus with nephritis: a long-term study. *Q J Med* 1979;48:124.
167. Davis P, Cumming RH, Verrier-Jones J. Relationship between anti-DNA antibodies, complement consumption and circulating immune complexes in systemic lupus erythematosus. *Clin Exp Immunol* 1977;28:226–232.
168. Davis P, Percy JS, Russell AS. Correlation between levels of DNA antibodies and clinical disease activity in SLE. Retrospective evaluation. *Ann Rheum Dis* 1977;36:157–159.
169. Gotoff SP, Isaacs EW, Muehrcke RC, et al. Serum beta 1C globulin in glomerulonephritis and systemic lupus erythematosus. *Ann Intern Med* 1969;71:327–333.
170. Grennan DM, Moseley A, Sloane D, et al. The significance of serial measurement of serum antinative DNA antibodies and complement C3 and C4 components in the management of systemic lupus erythematosus. *Aust N Z J Med* 1977;7:625–629.
171. Houssiau FA, D'Cruz D, Vianna J, et al. Lupus nephritis: the significance of serologic tests at the time of biopsy. *Clin Exp Rheumatol* 1991;9:345–349.
172. Laitman RS, Glicklich D, Sablay LB, et al. Effect of long-term normalization of serum complement levels on the course of lupus nephritis. *Am J Med* 1989;87:132–138.
173. Lightfoot RW Jr, Hughes GRV. Significance of persisting serologic abnormalities in systemic lupus erythematosus. *Arthritis Rheum* 1976;19:837–843.
174. Schur PH, Sandson J. Immunologic factors and clinical activity in systemic lupus erythematosus. *N Engl J Med* 1968;278: 533–538.
175. Garin EH, Donnelly WH, Shulman ST, et al. The significance of serial measurements of serum complement C3 and C4 components and DNA binding capacity in patients with lupus nephritis. *Clin Nephrol* 1979;12:148–155.
176. Hill GS, Hinglais N, Tron F, et al. Systemic lupus erythematosus. Morphologic correlations with immunologic and clinical data at the time of biopsy. *Am J Med* 1978;64:61–79.
177. Lloyd W, Schur PH. Immune complexes, complement, and anti-DNA in exacerbations of systemic lupus erythematosus (SLE). *Medicine* 1981;60:208–217.
178. Swaak AJG, Groenwold J, Aarden LA, et al. Prognostic value of anti-ds DNA in SLE. *Ann Rheum Dis* 1982;41:388–395.
179. Pillemer SR, Austin HA, Tsokos GC, et al. Lupus nephritis: association between serology and renal biopsy measurements. *J Rheumatol* 1988;15:284–288.
180. Gladman DD, Urowitz MB, Keystone EC. Serologically active clinically quiescent systemic lupus erythematosus: a discordance between clinical and serological features. *Am J Med* 1979;66: 210–215.
181. Appel AE, Sablay LB, Golden RA, et al. The effect of normalization of serum complement and anti-DNA antibody on the course of lupus nephritis: a two-year prospective study. *Am J Med* 1978;64:274–283.
182. Ballou SP, Kushner I. Lupus patients who lack detectable anti-DNA. Clinical features and survival. *Arthritis Rheum* 1982;25: 1126–1129.
183. Hashimoto H, Utagawa Y, Yamagata J, et al. The relationship of renal histopathological lesions to immunoglobulin classes and complement fixation of anti-native DNA antibodies in systemic lupus erythematosus. *Scand J Rheumatol* 1983;12:209–214.
184. Lindstedt G, Lundberg PA, Westberg G, et al. SLE nephritis and positive tests for antibodies against native DNA but negative tests for antinuclear antibodies. *Lancet* 1977;ii:135.
185. Miniter MF, Stollar BD, Agnello V. Reassessment of the clinical significance of native DNA antibodies in systemic lupus erythematosus. *Arthritis Rheum* 1979;22:959–968.
186. Swaak AJG, Aarden LA, Statius van Eps LW, et al. Anti-dsDNA and complement profiles as prognostic guides in systemic lupus erythematosus. *Arthritis Rheum* 1979;22:226–235.
187. Swaak T, Smeenk R. Detection of anti-dsDNA as a diagnostic tool: a prospective study in 441 nonsystemic lupus erythematosus patients with anti-dsDNA antibody (anti-dsDNS). *Ann Rheum Dis* 1985;44:245–251.
188. Tron F, Bach J-F. Immunological tests in the diagnosis and prognosis of disseminated lupus erythematosus before treatment (in French). *Nouv Presse Med* 1977;6:2573–2578.
189. Clough JD, Couri J, Youssofian H, et al. Antibodies against

nuclear antigens: association with lupus nephritis. Cleve Clin Q 1986;53:259–265.

190. Roberts JL. Diagnosis of systemic lupus erythematosus and lupus nephritis. *Contrib Nephrol* 1983;35:150–169.
191. Morrow WJW, Isenberg DA, Parry HF, et al. Studies on autoantibodies to poly (adenosine diphosphate-ribose) in SLE and other autoimmune disease. *Ann Rheum Dis* 1982;41:396–402.
192. Levinsky RJ, Cameron JS, Soothill JF. Serum immune complexes and disease activity in lupus nephritis. *Lancet* 1977;i: 564–567.
193. Wener WH, Mannik M, Schwartz MM, et al. Relationship between renal pathology and the size of circulating immune complexes in patients with systemic lupus erythematosus. *Medicine* 1987;66:85–97.
194. Siegert CEH, Daha MR, Tseng CMES, et al. Predictive value of IgG autoantibodies against C1q for nephritis in systemic lupus erythematosus. *Ann Rheum Dis* 1993;52:851–856.
195. Laut J, Barland P, Glicklich D, et al. Soluble interleukin-2 receptor levels in lupus nephritis. *Clin Nephrol* 1992;38:179–184.
196. Akbar S, Tello AI, Luvira U, et al. Significance of antinuclear antibody (ANA) immunofluorescent patterns and titers in systemic lupus erythematosus nephritis. *Henry Ford Hosp Med J* 1988;36:121–129.
197. D'Cruz DD, Houssiau FA, Ramirez G, et al. Antibodies to endothelial cells in systemic lupus erythematosus: a potential marker for nephritis and vasculitis. *Clin Exp Immunol* 1991;85: 254–261.
198. Tomura S, Deguchi F, Ando R, et al. Plasma thrombomodulin in primary glomerular disease and lupus glomerulonephritis. *Nephron* 1994;67:185–189.
199. Kramers C, Termaat RM, ter Borg EJ, et al. Higher anti-heparan sulphate reactivity during systemic lupus erythematosus (SLE) disease exacerbations with renal manifestations: a long term prospective analysis. *Clin Exp Immunol* 1993;93:34–38.
200. Sturfelt G, Roux-Lumbard P, Wollheim FA, et al. Low levels of interleukin-1 receptor antagonist coincide with kidney involvement in systemic lupus erythematosus. *Brit J Rheumatol* 1997; 36:1283–1289.
201. Chindalore V, Neas B, Reichlin M. The association between anti-ribosomal P antibodies and active nephritis in systemic lupus erythematosus. *Clin Immunol Immunopathol* 1998;87: 292–296.
202. Coggins CH. Overview of treatment of lupus nephropathy. *Am J Kidney Dis* 1982;2(suppl 1):197–200.
203. Dubois EL, Commons RR, Starr P, et al. Corticotropin and cortisone treatment for systemic lupus erythematosus. *JAMA* 1952; 149:995–101.
204. Ben-Asher S. Recurrent acute lupus erythematosus disseminatus: report of case which has survived 23 years after onset of systemic manifestations. *Ann Intern Med* 1951;34:243–248.
205. Austin HA 3rd, Klippel JH, Balow JE, et al. Therapy of lupus nephritis. Controlled trial of prednisone and cytotoxic drugs. *N Engl J Med* 1986;314:614–619.
206. Steinberg AD, Steinberg SC. Long-term preservation of renal function in patients with lupus nephritis receiving treatment that includes cyclophosphamide versus those treated with prednisone only. *Arthritis Rheum* 1991;34:945–950.
207. Esdaile JM, Abramowicz M, MacKenzie T, et al. The time-dependence of long-term prediction in lupus nephritis. *Arthritis Rheum* 1994;37:359–368.
208. Ward MM, Studenski S. Clinical prognostic factors in lupus nephritis. The importance of hypertension and smoking. *Arch Intern Med* 1992;152:2082–2088.
209. Arce-Salinas CA, Villa AR, Martinez-Rueda JO, et al. Factors associated with chronic renal failure in 121 patients with diffuse proliferative nephritis: a case-control study. *Lupus* 1995;4:197–203.
210. Austin HA III, Boumpas DT, Vaughan EM, et al. Predicting renal outcomes in severe histologic nephritis: contributions of clinical and histologic data. *Kidney Int* 1994;45:544–550.
211. McCluskey RT. Lupus nephritis. In: Sommers SC, ed. *Kidney pathology decennial 1966–1975*. New York: Appleton-Century-Crofts, 1975:435–670.
212. Pollak VE, Kant KS. Nephritis in systemic lupus erythematosus. *Ricera Clinica Laboratorio* (Milano) 1981;11:1–10.
213. Appel GB, Cohen DJ, Pirani CL, et al. Long-term follow up of patients with lupus nephritis. A study based on the classification of the World Health Organization. *Am J Med* 1987;83:877–885.
214. Ponticelli C, Moroni G, Banfi G. Discontinuation of therapy in diffuse proliferative lupus nephritis. *Am J Med* 1988;85:275–276.
215. Schroeder JO, Euler HE, Loffler H. Synchronization of plasmapheresis and pulse cyclophosphamide in severe systemic lupus erythematosus. *Ann Intern Med* 1987;107:344–346.
216. Levey AS, Lin S-P, Corwin HL, et al. Progression and remission of renal disease in the Lupus Nephritis Collaborative Study. Results of treatment with prednisone and short-term oral cyclophosphamide. *Ann Intern Med* 1992;116:114–123.
217. Donadio JV Jr, Hart GM, Bergstralh DJ, et al. Prognostic determination in lupus nephritis: a long-term clinicopathologic study. *Lupus* 1995;4:109–115.
218. Matjavila F, Pac V, Moga I, et al. Clinicopathological correlations and prognostic factors in lupus nephritis. *Clin Exper Rheumatol* 1997;15:625–631.
219. Ionnidis JPA, Boka KA, Katsorida ME, et al. Remission, relapse and re-remission of proliferative nephritis treated with cyclophosphamide. *Kidney International* 2000;258–264.
220. Mok CC, Wong RW, Lau CS. Lupus nephritis in Southern Chinese patients: clinicopathologic findings and long-term outcome. *Amer J Kidney Dis* 1999;34:315–323.
221. Korbet SM, Lewis EJ, Schwartz MM, et al. Factors predictive of outcome in severe lupus nephritis. Lupus Nephritis Collaborative Study Group. *Amer J Kid Dis* 2000;35:905–914.
222. Pachinian N, Wallace DJ, Klinenberg JR. Mycophenolate mofetil for systemic lupus erythematosus. *J Clin Rheumatol* 199;4:374–376.
223. Dooley MA, Cosio FG, Nachman PH, et al. Mycophenolate mofetil in lupus nephritis. *J Am Soc Nephrol* 1999;10:833–839.
224. Tumlin JA, Lupus nephritis: novel immunosuppressive modalities and future directions. *Seminars Nephrol* 1999;19:67–76.
225. Illei GG, Klippel JH. Novel approaches in the treatment of lupus nephritis. *Lupus* 1998;7:644–648.

52

CLINICAL AND MANAGEMENT ASPECTS OF THE ANTIPHOSPHOLIPID ANTIBODY SYNDROME

MICHELLE PETRI

Antiphospholipid (APL) antibody syndrome now is recognized to be a misnomer. The field is more accurately described as antibody-mediated thrombosis, because multiple antibodies directed against plasma proteins, with or without attached phospholipid, can lead to hypercoagulability. These antibodies likely act by way of multiple mechanisms, which are addressed in Chapter 25. This chapter will review: (i) the APL and antiplasma-protein antibodies of clinical importance; (ii) laboratory assays that the clinician must interpret; (iii) epidemiology; (iv) clinical presentations; and (v) treatment.

CHARACTERISTICS OF ANTIPHOSPHOLIPID ANTIBODIES

The original triumvirate of APL antibodies included the false-positive test for syphilis, the lupus anticoagulant (LA), and anticardiolipin (aCL) antibody. The false-positive test for syphilis has not been associated with thrombosis in all studies, but will be described here, for completeness. The list of "new" APL and antiplasma-protein antibodies continues to lengthen. Several of these, including anti-β_2-glycoprotein I, and antiprothrombin, may have clinical utility, and will be discussed.

FALSE-POSITIVE TEST FOR SYPHILIS

The biologic false-positive test for syphilis was the first APL to be recognized (1). Patients with a false-positive test were found to be at risk (5% to 19%) for the development of lupus or another connective-tissue disease (1,2), but they did not seem to be at increased risk for thrombosis or pregnancy loss. The Venereal Disease Research Laboratory (VDRL) titer correlates with aCL levels only in sera from syphilis, not in sera from autoimmune patients (3). Mixing cardiolipin with phosphatidylcholine and cholesterol, as is done in the VDRL antigen, improves the binding of syphilitic APL antibodies, but it decreases the binding by autoimmune APL antibodies (3,4). It now is understood that aCL antibodies in patients with syphilis are not dependent on β_2-glycoprotein I (5). Patients may have the LA or aCL antibody and not have the false-positive test for syphilis, and vice versa. However, we have found a correlation of the false-positive test for syphilis with multiple other APL antibodies, including anti-β_2-glycoprotein I. In addition, in the Hopkins Lupus Cohort, a false-positive test for syphilis is predictive of later thrombosis.

LUPUS ANTICOAGULANT

A circulating anticoagulant in three patients (two of whom had probable autoimmune disease) was reported in 1948 by Conley et al. (6), who recognized that it blocked the conversion of prothrombin to thrombin. Although patients with LA who had a hemorrhagic diathesis tended to have a second coagulation defect (7), the term "lupus anticoagulant" became accepted. The second irony of this term is that as many as one half of patients with LA do not have lupus (8,9).

LAs, which are IgG or IgM immunoglobulins, potentially could inhibit any of four procoagulant-phospholipid complexes or two anticoagulant phospholipid-dependent reactions; however, the *in vitro* action appears to be inhibition of the prothrombinase reaction (10). LA assays do not actually measure a titer of antibody, but are functional tests. It has been recognized for some time that LAs were heterogeneous; no one assay is able to detect 100% of LAs. Two groups, one in which LA activity could be separated from aCL activity and one in which the LA and aCL activities were inseparable, have been found (11). In the first group, LA activity was dependent on human prothrombin (12). In the second group, LA was dependent on the plasma protein β_2-glycoprotein I (as is aCL antibody) (11).

The *in vitro* detection methods for LA may not be relevant to its *in vivo* action. LAs prolong clotting times *in vitro*, because they agglutinate phospholipids in the plasma, thereby preventing their participation as cofactors in coagulation steps. If a more physiologic surface, such as endothelial cells, is used for assembly of the prothrombinase complex, agglutination of phospholipids does not occur. For example, Oosting et al. (13) found that only four of 22 IgG fractions (18%) with LA activity were able to inhibit prothrombinase activity on endothelial cells.

In addition to the identification of coagulation proteins that combine with negatively charged phospholipids to form the epitopes that are targets for APL antibodies, the nature of the phospholipid that is involved in LA activity also has been studied. Both the physical nature and the phase behavior of the phospholipid are important. LA antibodies have a greater affinity for hexagonal phase than bilayer phospholipid (14,15).

If LAs can be subgrouped by the plasma-protein–phospholipid targets, it follows that thrombotic mechanisms in patients with different subgroups of LA might be different. Among the potential mechanisms that have been suggested are procoagulant activity of endothelial cells (mediated by thrombin generation, fibrinopeptide A generation, and/or platelet aggregation) (16,17), perturbation of the thromboxane-prostacyclin balance (18), and perturbation of the protein C, protein S, and thrombomodulin pathways (13,19). These are discussed in another chapter.

ANTICARDIOLIPIN ANTIBODY

Realizing that cardiolipin was the major antigenic component of the false-positive test for syphilis, Harris et al. (20), in the Graham Hughes laboratory, developed a radioimmunoassay for aCL antibody. Over time, an enzyme-linked immunosorbent assay (ELISA) replaced the radioimmunoassay and underwent several revisions to optimize diluents and buffers, create multiple standards for calibration curves, and shorten incubation times (4,21,22).

Cardiolipin, which is found in mitochondria, originally was thought unlikely to be the antigen against which the antibodies detected in solid-phase assays are directed *in vivo*. However, cardiolipin recently has been found to be a normal plasma component, with more than 94% found as part of VLDL, low-density lipoprotein (LDL), and high-density lipoprotein (HDL) fractions (23). Because APL antibodies cross-react with other negatively charged phospholipids (e.g., phosphatidylserine), cardiolipin can serve as a representative antigen in the solid-phase system (24,25). Phosphatidylserine also may serve as the antigen (26).

The rationale for the measurement of aCL isotypes (i.e., IgG, IgM, and IgA) was the finding in several studies that IgG aCL was the major predictor of thrombosis and pregnancy loss (27–29), although other groups have reported similar clinical associations with IgM aCL as well (30,31). However, polyclonal assays for aCL also have shown predictive value for thrombosis, both in cross-sectional studies (32) and in prospective ones (33). Recent work has demonstrated that IgM aCL is associated with not only hemolytic anemia (34–36), but also with thrombosis (31). Although the classification criteria for APS do not include IgA aCL, recent work suggests that some patients with APS manifestations may have IgA as their only isotype (37). In addition, in one series, IgA aCL was associated with vasculitis (38). The highest APL titers were of the IgA isotype in one study (39). Anti-β_2-glycoprotein I of IgA isotype has been associated with venous thrombosis, thrombocytopenia, valvular disease, livedo reticularis, and seizures (40). In contrast, one study found true IgA APL antibody in only two systemic lupus erythematosus (SLE) patients, both of whom also were positive for the IgG isotype (41). Some groups have reported the highest titer, regardless of isotype, as being the most predictive of APS complications (42,43).

Higher-titer IgG aCL antibody has shown a stronger association with thrombosis and pregnancy loss (27,28,44). Lower titers of aCL (often with concurrent LA, but not necessarily) also occur in patients with classic manifestations of APL antibody syndrome (32,43,45). Thus, although aCL antibody assays are able to quantify the antibody titer (as opposed to LA assays), it is not clear that the titer of aCL antibody is the only predictor of pathogenicity.

ANTI-β_2-GLYCOPROTEIN I

In 1990, three groups simultaneously reported that a plasma protein, β_2-glycoprotein I (also called apolipoprotein H), acted as a cofactor in the aCL antibody assays, improving the binding of aCL (45–47). This finding explained why investigators had previously noted that use of adult bovine serum (48) and fetal calf serum (49), both of which contain β_2-glycoprotein I, improved the performance of the assay. β_2-glycoprotein I has multiple roles *in vivo*, including the inhibition of ADP-induced platelet aggregation, activation of the intrinsic coagulation pathway, and activation of platelet prothrombinase activity (50–52). Although there was much initial discussion (53), it now is accepted that the true antigen against which most aCL antibodies are directed is a complex of negatively charged phospholipids with β_2-glycoprotein I (54). Recently, some (55) but not all (56,57) groups have identified antibodies that they believe are directed against β_2-glycoprotein I alone (58–60). An epitope in the fifth domain of β_2-glycoprotein I is exposed when assays use polystyrene plates that previously were oxygenated by gamma irradiation (61–63). Although levels of β_2-glycoprotein I are determined by genetic factors, race, sex, and age (64,65), levels do not seem to influence the antibody response or risk of thrombosis (66).

The binding of autoimmune aCL antibodies is enhanced by the presence of β_2-glycoprotein I, as opposed to aCL antibodies that are made in response to infections (47).

Thus, it now is possible to differentiate aCL caused by infections [with little association with thrombosis (67)] from those caused by autoimmunity, which are associated with the APL antibody syndrome (APS).

Even though β_2-glycoprotein I is the target of aCL antibodies, aCL and anti-β_2-glycoprotein I antibody results may be discrepant in individual patients. Patients can be positive for anti-β_2-glycoprotein I, but negative for aCL, if they have antibodies that recognize human epitopes, or β_2-glycoprotein I epitopes that are hidden when cardiolipin is bound. Conversely, patients can be positive for aCL, but negative for anti-β_2-glycoprotein I, if their antibodies recognize cardiolipin alone, epitopes in cardiolipin bound to β_2-glycoprotein I, or bovine epitopes (68). In one study, 11% of SLE patients made antibodies to β_2-glycoprotein I alone (69).

Multiple studies have suggested that anti-β_2-glycoprotein I may be a more specific marker than aCL for thrombotic events (55,58,70–74). Because it is unusual for a patient with APS to be negative for both aCL and LA, anti-β_2-glycoprotein I is not yet part of the routine work-up for patients with hypercoagulability.

It is not as clear if anti-β_2-glycoprotein I is a more specific marker than aCL for pregnancy morbidity. An association with pregnancy-induced hypertension, preeclampsia (75,76), and pregnancy loss (77) has been reported. However, several studies have found no association with pregnancy loss (78–81).

LUPUS ANTICOAGULANT AND ANTICARDIOLIPIN ANTIBODIES: SEPARATE BUT RELATED

With the development of assays for aCL antibodies, investigators initially wondered if these solid-phase immunoassays would detect the same antibodies as LA assays (82). Most studies found aCL antibody more frequently than LA in patients with lupus (32,83), even when sensitive assays for LA were used. The two antibodies are discordant in as many as 35% of patients (67,84). In our study, SLE patients followed prospectively over 5 years continue to show discordance for the two antibodies (Fig. 52.1). Proof that the two antibodies can be different ensued from separate isolation from patient plasmas using multiple techniques (12,85–87).

Studies of monoclonal antibodies suggested that LAs preferentially bound hexagonal-phase phospholipids (15). The chain length and degree of saturation of the fatty-acid chains also are critical determinants. Levy et al. (88) found that APL antibodies bound better to C18:1 phosphatidylglycerol than to C18:0 or C18:2, and that binding was greater to C18 than to C14:0 or C16:0 phosphatidylglycerol.

The demonstration that β_2-glycoprotein I (apolipoprotein H) is a requirement for autoimmune aCL antibody-binding in solid-phase assays (45, 46) was the next step in understanding the different specificities of aCL and LA antibodies.

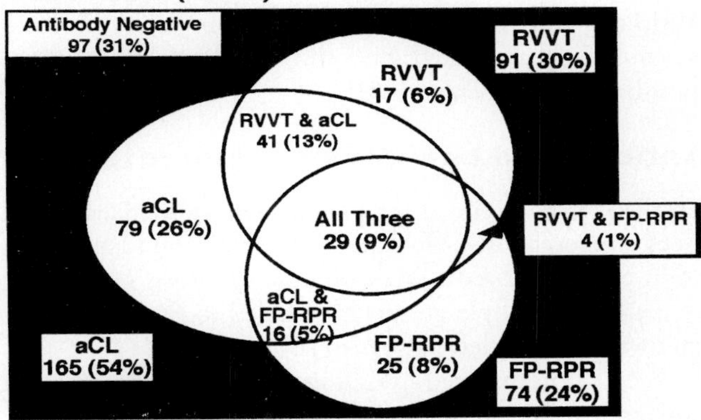

FIGURE 52.1. Venn diagram showing the percentage of patients in the Johns Hopkins Lupus Cohort who have had a positive acle antibody, LA (as determined by the modified RVVT assay, or a false-positive test for syphilis during proscpective followup. FP-RPR-false-positive rapid reagin test.

Although many LA antibodies also were dependent on β_2-glycoprotein I (17,89), some were directed against other plasma cofactors, including prothrombin (12).

Antiprothrombin

Antiprothrombin antibodies represent a subset of LAs. They have been found in 33% of SLE patients in one study (90). Several retrospective studies have shown an association with thrombosis (91–93). The prospective ATBC study of deep-venous thrombosis (94) and myocardial infarction (95) has shown an association, as well. However, multiple other studies, including our own, have failed to find an association with thrombotic events (96). Antiprothrombin antibodies most closely associate with the profile of LA detected by the kaolin clotting time (KCT), which is less associated with thrombosis than LA detected by the Russell viper venom time (RVVT) (97). In fact, antiprothrombin antibodies may cause hypoprothrominaemia and, therefore, bleeding (98).

Antiannexin

Annexin V is an anticoagulant in placental villi. Antiannexin V antibodies, by reducing annexin V at the maternal-fetal interface, may contribute to pregnancy losses in APS (99). Antiannexin V can have LA properties (100). The prevalence of antiannexin V in SLE patients ranges from 3.8% (101) to 19% (102). It has been found in association with both thrombosis and pregnancy loss (103).

Antiphosphatidyl Serine

Antiphosphatidyl serine has been found in 26% of SLE patients in one series (104).

Antithromboplastin

Antithromboplastin has been found in 35% of SLE patients. It is associated with thrombosis, pregnancy loss, and thrombocytopenia (105).

Antioxidized Low-density Lipoprotein

Oxidized LDL is one of the pivotal steps in the pathogenesis of atherosclerosis. Multiple studies have found an association of antioxidized LDL with atherosclerosis (106–113). In contrast, multiple groups have failed to find an association with atherosclerosis (114–116).

In SLE, antioxidized LDL is associated with arterial, but not venous thrombosis (117,118).

In prospective studies, antioxidized LDL has predicted myocardial infarction over 5 years in middle-aged men (108), myocardial infarction in men aged 50 years or older (119), and in middle-aged dyslipidemic men (106).

LABORATORY DETECTION OF LUPUS ANTICOAGULANT

Laboratory Definition

Laboratory criteria for LA almost certainly will continue to evolve as more knowledge about negatively charged phospholipid and plasma-protein neoantigens is obtained. The Scientific and Standardization Committee Subcommittee for the Standardization of LAs published criteria for the laboratory detection of LAs in 1995 (120). These criteria included the following:

1. Prolongation of phospholipid-dependent clotting tests [e.g., KCT, dilute RVVT, tissue-thromboplastin inhibition test, plasma-recalcification clotting time, or sensitive partial thromboplastin time (PTT)];
2. The clotting time of a mixture of test and normal plasma should be significantly longer than that of the normal mixed with various plasmas from patients without LA;
3. There should be a relative correction of the defect by the addition of lysed, washed platelets or, preferably, phospholipid liposomes containing phosphatidylserine or hexagonal-phase phospholipids; and
4. It should be nonspecific for any individual clotting factor, rapidly lose apparent activity on dilution of test plasmas with saline (i.e., nonparallel lines in factor assays), usually fast acting, associated with positive APL antibody ELISAs, and identified as an immunoglobulin whenever possible.

Some very practical summary recommendations also were made. The first was to use high-speed centrifugation (10 min at 5,000 g) and/or filtration to remove platelets. Platelet-poor plasma is essential to maximize the sensitivity of most assays, especially if frozen plasma is used (74). The second recommendation was to use a sensitive test to screen for LAs. The activated PTT (aPTT), for example, which is the most common screening test, often uses a thromboplastin reagent that is insensitive to LA. The third recommendation was to select an LA test that struck the right balance between sensitivity and specificity (121,122).

Triplett (123,124) has extracted what he considers to be minimal criteria for the laboratory diagnosis of LA: (i) an abnormality of an *in vitro* phospholipid-dependent coagulation test(s), (ii) demonstration of an inhibitor (i.e., anticoagulant) as the cause of the abnormal screening test (i.e., mixing step), and (iii) proof that the inhibitor is directed at phospholipid coagulation factors and not at specific coagulation factors. The use of two sensitive screening tests, such as a sensitive PTT and RVVT, may be preferable, because no one test is capable of detecting all LAs (125). The importance of using a battery of screening tests was demonstrated by McHugh et al. (126). Of 13 patients with LA, only four were abnormal on all three of the clotting assays that were employed (i.e., KCT, RVVT, and tissue-thromboplastin inhibition test). In addition, if a 1:1 patient to normal control plasma mixing study is not diagnostic, an additional mixing study with 4:1 patient to normal control plasma should be performed (124). Confirmatory tests that prove the inhibitor is directed at phospholipid include those that decrease the amount of phospholipid in the test system to accentuate the inhibitor effect (i.e., the RVVT), increase the amount of phospholipid to neutralize the LA [i.e., the platelet neutralization procedure (PNP)], or use specific hexagonal-phase phospholipids to neutralize LA (127).

INDIVIDUAL ASSAYS

aPTT

The sensitivity of detection of LA using the aPTT is highly dependent on the choice of reagents (122,128,129), activator, and phospholipid to be used as a platelet substitute (130). Both the phosphatidylserine concentration (131) and the physical state of the phospholipid (i.e., hexagonal or not) (127) can affect the sensitivity of the test. Most hospital laboratories have used aPTT reagents that were insensitive to LA, but sensitive aPTT reagents now are available commercially (132). Comparative studies have demonstrated that Actin FSL (American Dade), Automated APTT (Organon Teknika Corp.), and Thrombosil (Ortho Diagnostics) all are sensitive to LAs (125,130,133–135). A sensitive aPTT using a sensitive reagent is an excellent screening test (123). However, a sensitive aPTT may not be an appropriate screening test during pregnancy, because it is affected by rising factor VIII.

Modified (Dilute) Russell Viper Venom Time

The modified RVVT can be used as an initial, sensitive screening test for LA or as a confirmatory test (136). Its sensitivity has equaled or surpassed those of the KCT and tissue-thromboplastin inhibition tests in two studies (136,137), but it was not as sensitive as a sensitive aPTT in another (123).

In comparison to other tests for LA, the RVVT is relatively resistant to deficiencies of clotting factors and to clotting factor antibodies. It is unaffected by antibodies to factors VIII, IX, and XI, and it remains normal in plasma that is deficient in factors VII, IX, and XI. However, factor V or X levels below 0.4 U/mL do prolong the RVVT (136). The source of phospholipid can affect the RVVT (138), as can the source of venom. These factors can lead to variability in the method of performance and, therefore, the results of the RVVT (139). The RVVT method can be automated (140).

Kaolin Clotting Time

The KCT is an aPTT without added platelet substitute, with the kaolin acting as an activator and phospholipid surface (141). The KCT is affected by residual platelets and therefore requires a filtration step to remove platelets from the patient plasma (142). Originally, Exner et al. (143) performed multiple determinations of the KCT using different ratios of patient to normal plasma. A simplified KCT using just patient plasma has been developed, without important reduction in sensitivity or specificity (144). In some comparative studies, the KCT has not been as sensitive as a sensitive aPTT (123).

Platelet Neutralization Procedure

One approach to proving that an inhibitor is phospholipid dependent is to neutralize the inhibitor by increasing the amount of phospholipid in the assay [as in the platelet neutralization procedure (PNP)] or to accentuate the prolonged coagulation time by reducing the phospholipid (as in the tissue-thromboplastin inhibition time). The tissue-thromboplastin inhibition time is not widely used, however, because in most studies, it is both less sensitive and less specific than the PNP (129,133,137,145). The PNP can be combined with screening tests for LA by using freeze-thawed platelets with the sensitive aPTT or RVVT test to correct or shorten the abnormal clotting time (146).

THE ANTICOAGULATED PATIENT

No LA screening test is valid in the presence of heparin. In a patient who presents with a thrombotic event, plasma should be sent for LA testing before administration of heparin is begun. A more difficult problem is evaluation of the patient on warfarin. If the patient has moderate or high-titer aCL antibody, diagnosis of the APL antibody syndrome is secure, and the LA test is not necessary for diagnosis. In some patients, however, solid-phase assays for APL antibodies may be negative, and it may not be possible to stop anticoagulation to allow the LA testing to proceed. In this setting, mixing studies with normal plasma before LA testing (to correct deficiencies in vitamin K-dependent factors) or an LA test that already includes a mix with normal plasma (e.g., KCT or dilute aPTT) can be considered, although no consensus or criteria exist for the diagnosis of LA in this setting.

STANDARDIZATION OF LUPUS ANTICOAGULANT

Because of the heterogeneity of LA, it is unlikely that any one assay will be accepted as the preferred standard. Instead, a battery of the most sensitive tests (e.g., a sensitive aPTT and the RVVT) is the best approach to screening. The best assays will be those with predictive value (i.e., high relative risks) for future thrombosis or pregnancy loss. In the near future, assays for antibodies that are directed against individual complexes of negatively charged phospholipids and plasma proteins (e.g., β_2-glycoprotein I, prothrombin, and so on) may supercede other tests.

LABORATORY DETECTION OF ANTICARDIOLIPIN ANTIBODY

The aCL antibody assay, which is the most widely used solid-phase APL test, is a multistep procedure. In the first step, ELISA plates are coated with the negatively charged phospholipid, which usually is cardiolipin, although phosphatidylserine (26) and mixtures of phospholipid also are used (147). To prevent nonspecific antibody from binding to the plate, adult bovine serum, bovine serum albumin, or fetal calf serum are added and then washed from the plate. Diluted patient sera (the diluent should contain β_2-glycoprotein I, which is the cofactor for binding) then are incubated in the wells. After the incubation step, the wells are washed, and an enzyme-labeled antihuman antibody (e.g., anti-IgG, anti-IgM, anti-IgA, or polyclonal) is added. After washing, the enzyme substrate is added to develop the color reaction; the absorbance then is read.

The aCL antibody distribution is not Gaussian in most studies (32,148). Major differences have existed in the cutoff of negative from positive values in different laboratories. To facilitate calibration and comparative studies between laboratories, two international workshops have established and tested positive standards for the IgG and IgM isotypes, leading to the report of results in IgG isotype phospholipid (GPL) or IgM isotype phospholipid (MPL) units (21,22, 149). However, use of calibrated standards may not solve the problem of standardization, because the slopes of each standard change with the buffer that is used and are different for each standard (150).

EPIDEMIOLOGY OF ANTIPHOSPHOLIPID ANTIBODIES

Prevalence and Incidence of Antiphospholipid Antibodies in Normal Individuals

Published study designs primarily have been cross-sectional, with one ascertainment of aCL and/or LA status. Thus, the results represent the frequency or point prevalence of APL,

TABLE 52.1. FREQUENCY OF ANTIPHOSPHOLIPID ANTIBODIES IN NORMAL CONTROLS

Source of Control Population	LA (%)	Anticardiolipin (%)	Anti-β_2 GPI (%)	References
Blood donors	0.0–3.6	0.0–9.4		(151–155)
Pregnant women	0.0–13.7	0.0–9.9	1.0–3.0	(32, 35, 78, 148, 156–165)
Healthy women		7.5		(43)
Osteoarthritis		14.0		(166)
Neurologic disorders		1.2		(167)

not a true prevalence (i.e., prevalence equals the incidence multiplied by the duration) or incidence. Despite the methodologic issues discussed earlier, published studies are, in large part, quite consistent regarding the frequency of APL in normal individuals. Representative studies are shown in Table 52.1. The great majority of studies consisted of young women, whether pregnant or not. Most studies included aCL assays, but fewer included LA or anti-β_2-glycoprotein I.

Studies of prevalence (i.e., repeated measures of aCL or LA in normal individuals) are important. APL antibody titers fluctuate in patients with lupus over time because of disease activity and treatment, meaning that an assay performed at one point in time has less predictive value. If fluctuations occur within the normal population, this will influence the design of prospective studies on APL antibodies in normal individuals.

Frequency of Antiphospholipid Antibodies in the Elderly

Because both the frequency of antinuclear antibodies and antithyroid antibodies increases with age, it is not surprising that several studies have addressed the frequency of APL antibodies in the elderly. As these studies employed different definitions of a positive aCL [i.e., any positive versus highly positive (>5 SD from the mean)], they are not directly comparable. However, it does appear that a positive aCL is more common in the elderly (Table 52.2). A recent study found aCL in the elderly with chronic diseases but not in the healthy elderly (155).

Frequency of Antiphospholipid Antibodies in Systemic Lupus Erythematosus

The frequency of LA (Table 52.3), aCL antibody (Table 52.4), and anti-β_2-glycoprotein I (Table 52.5) in SLE has varied widely among studies. Some of this variation results from differing sensitivities of the assays, selection of patients, and bias introduced by retrospective study designs. Detection of APL antibodies in any cross-sectional study also may be influenced by transient production of the antibody. For example, Hedfors et al. (170) reported a woman who only made aCL antibodies transiently during early pregnancy. My own group (32) and others (171) have reported patients whose APL antibody titers or assays drop, or become negative, at the time of a thrombotic event.

In general, the LA assays appear to be more easily suppressed by treatment for active lupus (220), but treatment also may suppress aCL levels (42,205). Active lupus may increase the titer of either aCL antibody or LA (188,205, 215,221,222) Thus, it is not surprising that studies with multiple determinations of APL antibodies will find a higher prevalence of antibody positivity (42,216) or that many patients fluctuate from their entry category of negative, low positive, or high positive (222).

Occurrence of Antiphospholipid Antibodies in Diseases Other Than Systemic Lupus Erythematosus

APL antibodies commonly occur in infections, especially human immunodeficiency virus (HIV) and autoimmune deficiency syndrome (AIDS) (223–225), but in many other bacterial, protozoan, and viral illnesses as well. Most microbial APL antibodies are IgM isotype and nonpathogenic. Most of the infection-related APL antibodies are not dependent on β_2-glycoprotein I (226) or associated with APS. In one study, however, aCL was associated with cerebral perfusion defects in HIV-positive patients (224). One patient with AIDS and aCL developed a splenic infarction (227). Another patient with AIDS and a stroke had aCL (225). In

TABLE 52.2. ANTICARDIOLIPIN FREQUENCY IN THE ELDERLY

Study	Patient (n)	Mean Age (y)	aPL Positive (%)
Chakravarty et al., 1990 (168)	100	75.6	0 (aCL >5 SD)
Fields et al., 1989 (169)	300	70.0	12 (aCL IgG and IgM)
Manoussakis et al., 1987 (151)	64	80.0	50 (aCL)
Juby et al., 1998 (155)			
Healthy	63		0
Chronic disease	301		13.3

TABLE 52.3. FREQUENCY OF THE LUPUS ANTICOAGULANT IN PATIENTS WITH LUPUS

Series	Patients (n)	Assay Used	Frequency (%)
Clotting			
Lee & Sanders (172)	43	Whole blood or plasma clotting time	16
Meacham & Weisberger (173)	25	Clotting time	8
Zetterstrom & Berglund (174)	11	Clotting time	18
Margolius et al. (141)	23	Recalcified clotting time	13
Johansson & Lassus (175)	44	Racalcified and Quick times	31
Pauzner et al. (176)	66	Recalcified clotting time	49
Kaolin clotting time (KCT)			6
Exner et al. (143)	17	KCT, KPTT	65
Rosner et al. (177)	66	KCT	49
Padmakumar et al. (178)	55	KCT	13
Partial thromboplastin time (PTT)			59
Regan et al. (179)	50	PTT	6
Mintz et al. (180)	43	activated PTT (aPTT)	35
Averbuch et al. (181)	36	aPTT	19
Meyer et al. (182)	91	aPTT	49
Mayumi et al. (183)	106	aPTT	16
Kaolin partial thromboplastin time (KPTT)			
Boey et al. (184)	49	KPTT	51
Harris et al. (20)	59	KPTT	49
Bennett et al. (185)	67	KPTT	21
Colaco & Elkon (186)	52	KPTT	37
Russell viper venom time (RVVT)			26
Petri et al. (32)	60	RVVT	7
Multiple Assays			
Hasselaar et al. (16)	74	PTT phospholipid dilution test, KCT	49
Cervera et al. (153)	100	Prothrombin time, aPTT, KCT, RVVT, tissue thromboplastin inhibitor	30
McHugh et al. (126)	58	Kaolin-cephalin clotting time, RVVT, time thromboplastin inhibitor	22
Wong et al. (187)	91	aPTT, RVVT, platelet neutralization procedure, tissue thromboplastin inhibition	11
Cervera et al. (31)	1000	Multiple	9
Intragumtornchai et al. (188)	91	PTT, KCT, TTI, PNP	18
Sohngen et al. (189)	80	aPTT, KCT	19
Golstein et al. (190)	92	aPTT, dilute thromboplastin	22

a large study of 74 HIV-infected men, however, the presence of aCL (in 86%) or protein S deficiency (in 33%) was not associated with the development of thrombosis (223).

APL antibodies also occur in other autoimmune diseases, including connective-tissue diseases such as rheumatoid arthritis (228,229), Sjögren's syndrome (230), eosinophilic fasciitis (231), scleroderma (232–234), and related conditions such as hemolytic anemia (255) and idiopathic thrombocytopenic purpura (166,235–237). They also have been reported in small-vessel (238), medium-vessel [i.e., microscopic polyarteritis (239–241)], and large-vessel [i.e., giant-cell arteritis (242–244) and Takayasu's arteritis (245–247)] vasculitides. APL antibodies have been found in 38% of patients with sarcoidosis (248). Several reports of APL antibodies in Behcet's disease also exist (249–251), but there has been no consistent association with thrombotic disorders.

APL antibodies can occur with multiple malignant conditions (252,253). Whether they might be responsible for Trousseau's syndrome in these patients has not been adequately studied.

APL antibodies result from many of the drugs that are known to cause drug-induced lupus, including the major tranquilizers (254), procainamide, and thiazides (255). They have not been associated with thromboses in chlorpromazine-treated patients (256). However, aCL (both IgG and IgM) also can be found in drug-free, multiply affected families with schizophrenia (257).

APL antibodies have been found in 68% of a series of 25 patients with sickle cell anemia, suggesting that structural alterations in the red-cell membrane may be associated with autoantibody production (258).

Children who are on hemodialysis had a high frequency of aCL in one study. Those children with aCL had more fistula thromboses (259). In a study of 39 adult hemodialysis patients, however, the LA and aCL were β_2-glycoprotein I independent, suggesting that they would not be procoagulant (260). A large study of 84 patients with end-stage renal dis-

TABLE 52.4. FREQUENCY OF ANTICARDIOLIPIN ANTIBODY IN LUPUS PATIENTS[a]

Series	Patients (n)	Frequency (%)
Jones et al. (191)	200	17
Cervera et al. (31)	1000	20
Golstein et al. (190)	92	20
Hazeltine et al. (192)	65	22
Danao-Camara & Clough. (193)	47	23
McHugh et al. (194)	98	24
Axtens et al. (195)	127	24
Tubach et al. (196)	102	24
Petri et al. (32)	60	25
Kutteh et al. (197)	125	25
Wilson et al. (198)	44	27
McHugh et al. (126)	58	29
Buchanan et al. (199)	117	30
Guerin et al. (200)	20	30
Shimada et al. (201)	31	31
Cervera et al. (153)	100	36
Fanopoulos et al. (39)	48	37
Lopex-Soto et al. (202)	92	37
Toschi et al. (203)		37
Worrall et al. (204)	100	38
Alarcón-Segovia et al. (205)	500	39
Ishikawa et al. (206)	31	39
Meyer et al. (171)	108	40
Fort et al. (166)	30	40
Koike et al. (207)	24	42
Kalunian et al. (43)	85	42
Wilson et al. (208)	48	42
Kaburaki et al. (102)	140	44
Sebastiani et al. (209)	64	44
Wong et al. (210)	91	44
Savi et al. (211)	80	45
Faux et al. (212)	77	45
Knight & Peter et al. (213)	100	47
Hasselaar et al. (16)	74	47
Norberg et al. (214)	59	48
Tincani et al. (49)	51	49
Shergy et al. (215)	32	50
Sturfelt et al. (152)	59	54
Loizou et al. (28)	84	55
Harris et al. (20)	59	61
Picillo et al. (216)	102	86
Ravelli et al. (217)	30[b]	87

[a]Studies are ordered by frequency of anticardiolipin positivity.
[b]These patients were children.

TABLE 52.5. FREQUENCY OF ANTI-β_2 GLYCOPROTEIN I IN LUPUS PATIENTS

Series	Patients (n)	Frequency (%)
Viard, 1992 (55)	47	36
Kaburati, 1995 (218)	140	15
Romero, 1998 (219)	118	17
Fanopoulos, 1998 (39)	48	58
Tubach, 2000 (196)	102	19

ease found no association between thrombosis and aCL or LA (261). No thromboses occurred in the nine patients with IgG aCL or IgM aCL in a study of 42 patients who were dialyzed using cuprophane membranes (262).

Effects of Sex and Race

APS has been reported in several patients with Klinefelter's syndrome (263–266). The effect of race only has been adequately studied in African American and white populations; the frequency of LA and high-titer aCL is significantly less common in African Americans than in whites. Recent, unpublished studies will address the frequency of APL in Hispanic populations.

Genetic Factors

Familial

In descriptions of Sneddon syndrome, which is a syndrome that overlaps significantly with APS, studies have remarked on the frequent occurrence of more than one affected family member (267–269). Familial cases of LA and/or aCL antibody also have been reported (267,270–273). The increased frequency of lupus or other autoimmune disease (including idiopathic thrombocytopenic purpura and autoimmune thyroid disease) in the relatives of patients with SLE is well recognized. In one study of 37 pediatric patients with SLE and 107 first-degree relatives, the occurrence of APL in relatives was not always related to APL positivity in the probands, and none of the APL-positive relatives had thrombosis (274). Whether family members of patients with APS are more likely to have APS and/or autoimmune disease, and whether this results from an autosomal-dominant autoimmune gene that is incompletely penetrant, or a second APS gene, currently is under study in multiple centers. Murine models suggest that APL antibody syndrome is multigenic (275).

HLA

Multiple HLA-DR or DQ associations with APL antibodies have been described. In a study of 13 patients with the primary form of APS, HLA-DR4 ($p < .01$) and Drw53 ($p < .05$) were increased, but no correction was made for multiple comparisons (276). In a study of 20 patients with SLE and LA, an association with HLA-DQw7 (DQB1*0301), linked to HLA-DR5 and DR4 haplotypes, was found (and was increased versus that in normal controls; $p = .002$) (277). In previous studies of HLA and aCL, Savi et al. (211) found an increase of HLA-DR7 in Italian patients, and McHugh and Maddison (278) found an increase in HLA-DR4 in British patients with SLE (278). Our group's results failed to find any association of DQB1*0301 with either aCL or LA in SLE (279), and no HLA association with aCL positivity was found in a study of 139 patients with SLE (280). In a recent study, the association of aCL with DRB4 and DRB1 was investigated, with the conclusion that at the DRB1*04 locus, the *0402 allele is most common (281).

Complement Genes

One group has suggested that patients with either partial C4A or C4B null allotypes are more likely to have aCL antibody (198,282,283). In contrast, patients in the Hopkins Lupus Cohort study who were homozygous for C4A deficiency had a lower frequency of aCL and LA than patients with SLE who did not have this deficiency (284). In addition, the subgroup of patients with C4A deficiency who had a C4A deletion were less likely to have a positive polyclonal aCL antibody (p = .02) than those without the deletion.

Prospective Studies

Most studies of APL antibodies have been cross-sectional, with retrospective review of patients' case histories. One requirement to determine a pathogenic role for APL antibodies is to document their presence before the clinical event, whether it is fetal loss (285) or thrombosis (33). In the case of fetal loss, there is further documentation of pathogenic significance, in that multiple murine models of fetal loss associated with APL antibodies exist (286–289).

Multiple prospective studies in the general population have shown the predictive value of APL antibodies for a first episode of deep-venous thrombosis (290) or myocardial infarction (108, 119) as well as recurrent venous thrombosis (291) or stroke (292). Finazzi et al. found that 34 of 360 patients with APL had a thromboembolic event over 4 years (293).

Our prospective study, the Hopkins Lupus Cohort, has shown that both aCL and LA are predictive of later thrombosis (294). Most thrombotic events after cohort entry were arterial, with stroke leading the list. An occasional SLE patient makes APL antibodies for the first time after a thrombotic event. A second large study in SLE has shown that both LA and IgG aCL are associated with thrombosis (295).

PROGNOSIS AND NATURAL HISTORY

Several studies have suggested that recurrent thrombotic events will be in the same distribution as the initial event (296). In our experience, however, the distribution may cross over, from venous to arterial and arterial to venous. Many patients seem to peacefully coexist with their APL antibodies until a "second hit" occurs. However, several studies have failed to show that genetic hypercoagulability—specifically Factor V Leiden—is an additional risk factor in patients with APL who thrombosed (297,298).

Risk factors for thrombosis include the LA, high-titer aCL, and IgG isotype of aCL. A risk factor for recurrence includes persistence of APL antibodies for 6 months after the thrombotic event. However, there are no firm rules. IgM aCL, for example, also has been associated with venous thrombosis (299).

Seven recent studies, four of patients with APS and both arterial and venous events (300–303) and three of patients with APS and venous events (291,304,305), have addressed the natural history of recurrent thrombotic events in patients who already are diagnosed with APS. In the four studies that included patients with both arterial and venous thrombotic events, the risk of recurrence was high if the patient did not remain on adequate anticoagulation (300–303). There was a 50% risk of recurrent deep-venous thrombosis within 2 years in one study (304).

The natural history and prognosis of patients with APS who present with stroke have been studied extensively. In a retrospective review, Levine et al. (306–308) found a high frequency of recurrent events. In the Antiphospholipid Antibody and Stroke Study, the odds ratios for recurrent stroke or for all events (i.e., recurrent stroke, myocardial infarction, or death) were significantly higher in stroke patients with aCL than in those without aCL (292,309).

In a study of 139 patients with SLE, IgM aCL (present either in the past or as a persistent finding) was the only aCL isotype to be negatively associated with survival (280). A history of thromboembolic events had a strong negative association with survival, but thromboembolic events were not among the common causes of death. Further, the negative association of IgM aCL with survival was not related to the clinical criteria of APS. A second survival study of 667 patients with SLE found that APS led to decreased survival because of some (i.e., thrombocytopenia, arterial occlusions, and hemolytic anemias), but not all, APS manifestations (310). In a third study, LA was a predictor of mortality (because of vascular occlusions) in SLE (311). Further longitudinal cohort studies may clarify the predictive value of APL antibodies for morbidity and mortality in SLE.

CLASSIFICATION CRITERIA FOR ANTIPHOSPHOLIPID ANTIBODY SYNDROME

New classification criteria for APS were proposed at the International Conference in Sapporo, Japan (312) (Table 52.6). These classification criteria have superceded previously published criteria. The new criteria, in their simplest form, require either a thrombotic manifestation (venous, arterial, or vasculopathy) or pregnancy morbidity, in the setting of mild- to moderate-titer aCL or LA.

These new classification criteria differ from previous criteria in three major ways. First, vasculopathy now is included under thrombotic manifestation. This is an important clarification, because some patients with the cat-

TABLE 52.6. CRITERIA FOR CLASSIFICATION OF THE ANTIPHOSPHOLIPID ANTIBODY SYNDROME*

Clinical	Laboratory
Vascular thrombosis One or more clinical episodes of arterial, venous, or small- vessel thrombosis in any tissue or organ. Thrombosis must be confirmed by imaging, Doppler studies, or histopathology, with the exception of superficial-venous thrombosis. For histopathologic confirmation, thrombosis should be present without significant evidence of inflammation in the vessel wall.	Anticardiolipin antibody of IgG and/or IgM isotype in blood, present in medium or high titer, on two or more occasions, at least 6 weeks apart, measured by a standard enzyme-linked immunosorbent assay for β_2-glycoprotein I-dependent anticardiolipin antibodies.
Pregnancy morbidity a) One or more unexplained deaths of a morphologically normal fetus at or beyond the 10th week of gestation, with normal fetal morphology documented by ultrasound or by direct examination of the fetus, or b) One or more premature births of a morphologically normal neonate at or before the 34th week of gestation because of severe preeclampsia or eclampsia, or severe placental insufficiency or c) Three or more unexplained consecutive spontaneous abortions before the 10th week of gestation, with maternal anatomic, or hormonal abnormalities and paternal and maternal chromosomal causes excluded.	Lupus anticoagulant present in plasma on two or more occasions at least 6 weeks apart, detected according to the guidelines of the International Society on Thrombosis and Hemostasis.

*Patients with the syndrome should have at least one clinical plus one laboratory finding during their disease. The aPL test must be positive on at least two occasions more than 3 months apart.
Source: Wilson WA, Gharavi AE, Koike T, et al. International consensus statement on preliminary classification criteria for definite antiphospholipid syndrome: report of an international workshop. *Arthritis Rheum* 1999;42:1309–1311.

astrophic presentation of APS do not have a defined thrombosis in one named vessel, but present instead with vasculopathy, usually widespread. Second, the pregnancy criterion has been revised extensively. One late fetal loss, for example, now is sufficient for the diagnosis of APS. Much more controversial is the inclusion of severe preeclampsia or placental insufficiency as part of the pregnancy criteria, because not all studies have confirmed an association of APL antibodies with these outcomes. Third, thrombocytopenia is no longer a "stand alone" criterion for APS.

Even these new classification criteria fail to address some important clinical manifestations of APS. Currently, there is no way to classify nonthrombotic neurologic manifestations, such as chorea and transverse myelitis, or to classify cardiac valvular vegetations.

These new classification criteria have shown good sensitivity, specificity, and positive and negative predictive value in a validation study (313). However, only 61% of SLE patients with secondary APS were classified correctly.

Multiple issues remain unresolved in separating primary versus secondary APS. SLE is the disease overwhelmingly associated with secondary APS. Patients who have "lupus-like disease" may not fit primary or secondary classification well (314).

A further classification issue is the distinction of primary (i.e., without associated connective-tissue disease) (315–317) versus secondary (i.e., with associated connective-tissue disease, usually SLE) forms of APS. Some authors have argued, and quite convincingly, that no distinction need be made (53,318), because neither the clinical features nor the APL antibody specificities differ in the primary and the secondary forms. In one series representing three European referral centers, equal numbers of patients with primary and secondary APS were seen. The clinical features were similar, but heart-valvular disease, hemolytic anemia, hypocomplementemia, and neutropenia were more common in those with secondary APS (319).

Some overlap of primary and secondary APS is inevitable, and this may result from a shared genetic predisposition (320,321). A few patients with primary APS may evolve into secondary APS over time (322–324). Progression to secondary APS may be more frequent in young women (325).

DIFFERENTIAL DIAGNOSIS OF HYPERCOAGULABILITY

Major causes of genetic hypercoagulability include Factor V Leiden, the prothrombin mutation, protein C, protein S, and antithrombin III deficiency. Elevated levels of homocysteine can predispose to arterial thrombosis and to atherosclerosis.

Major acquired causes of hypercoagulability include pregnancy and postpartum, oral contraceptives and estrogen replacement therapy, nephrotic syndrome, diabetes mellitus, hyperlipidemia, obesity, postoperative state, vasculitis, and malignancy (326).

A different approach to hypercoagulability is to consider acute versus chronic presentations (APS can present in both ways) of thrombotic angiopathies (327). Acute presentations include hemolytic uremic syndrome/thrombotic thrombocytopenia purpura, allograft rejection, drugs (cyclosporin, FK506, and OKT3), chemotherapeutic agents (mitomycin, cis-platin, and bleomycin), HELLP syndrome (which can be associated with APS), malignant nephrosclerosis, systemic sclerosis, radiation nephritis, and HIV. Chronic presentations include healing hemolytic uremic syndrome, radiation nephropathy, transplantation nephropathy, dysfibrinogemias, and POEMS syndrome.

PREVALENCE OF ANTIPHOSPHOLIPID ANTIBODY SYNDROME

Retrospective or cross-sectional studies allow only an estimate of the prevalence of APS in patients who have APL antibodies. Patients with a clinical manifestation of APS but who are negative for APL at the time of the study may have had APL at the time of the event. In a recent editorial, Hughes (328) quoted an APS frequency of 35% in SLE. McNeil et al. (329) concluded that the frequency of thrombosis was 42% in APL-positive patients with SLE and 31% in all patients with APL. The review of Love and Santora listed 30% (330). These figures, however, may reflect selection bias, will be affected by length of follow-up, and are not adjusted for age, sex, or racial/ethnic background.

Frequency of Antiphospholipid Antibody Syndrome in Venous Thrombosis (Non-SLE)

In a study of 100 patients with verified venous thrombosis, 24 had aCL antibody, and four had LA (331). In a second study, 15% had APL antibodies (332). In a third study, 30% had APL (333). A lesser prevalence of 6% also has been reported (334). In the large Spanish multicenter study on thrombophilia (EMET) in 2,132 patients with venous thrombosis, only 4% had APL antibodies (335). Given new knowledge of the importance of factor V Leiden mutation as a cause of resistance to activated protein C, new and comprehensive studies of the frequency of various genetic or acquired predispositions to deep-venous thrombosis in the general population are needed. No association of APL antibodies has been found in upper extremity deep-venous thrombosis (336).

In patients with pulmonary emboli, 10% have had APL antibodies (337). APL antibodies are most frequently found in chronic thromboembolism (64%) (338).

Frequency of Antiphospholipid Antibody Syndrome in Arterial Thrombosis (Non-SLE)

Stroke

The most common arterial-thrombotic presentation of APS is stroke. The frequency of APL in unselected patients with thrombotic stroke has ranged from 5% to 29% (167,168, 339–344). Some studies (340,343), but not all (339,341), have found the frequency of APL in stroke patients to be significantly higher than that in controls.

The frequency of APL in younger stroke patients (<50 years of age) appears to be higher (345–351). In studies that included aCL antibody assays, the frequency of APL has ranged from 18% to 46%. Two studies, which used only LA assays (346,347), reported much lower frequencies, (2% to 4%). It is possible that aCL antibody is more prevalent than LA in stroke patients, but the use of insensitive LA assays also may explain the low reported frequencies.

Coronary Artery Disease

Myocardial infarction in APL antibody-positive patients without atherosclerosis supports a pathogenetic role for these antibodies (352–354). The role of APL antibodies in coronary-artery disease (or atherosclerotic disease in general), however, remains highly controversial. Certainly, there is a scientific basis for interest in this potential association (355,356). For example, the importance of oxidized LDL in the induction of atherosclerosis and cross-reaction between APL and oxidized LDL antibodies suggests a potential mechanism for the progression of atherosclerosis (357,358).

Several studies have found an association of aCL with myocardial infarction (359–361), either with graft occlusion (360,362) or in coronary-artery disease (363,364). In contrast, many large studies have failed to find either an association with coronary-atherosclerotic disease or with a higher rate of subsequent adverse events (365–371). In a nested, case-control study of middle-aged dyslipidemic men participating in the Helsinki Heart Study (108), however, aCL was significantly higher in those who had suffered a myocardial infarction or cardiac death. In the highest quartile of aCL, the relative risk for myocardial infarction was 2.0 (95% confidence interval, 1.1 to 3.5), independent of confounding factors. An association of aCL with antibodies to oxidized LDL also was found in this study.

ASSOCIATION OF LUPUS ANTICOAGULANT VERSUS ANTICARDIOLIPIN ANTIBODY WITH RISK OF ANTIPHOSPHOLIPID ANTIBODY SYNDROME

In eight studies that used different, but equally valid, LA assays, the LA test was a more specific associate of thrombosis in patients with lupus than was aCL (32,93,372–378). In patients with lupus and aCL, the simultaneous demonstration of LA also increases the specificity for APS manifestations (126). In a study that used the PTT (which my group has shown will fail to detect 50% of LAs), however, aCL was found to be a better predictor of fetal distress (285). Very few studies of fetal loss have taken into account that rising factor VIII levels during pregnancy will affect many of the commonly used assays for LA, including the aPTT. In this setting, the RVVT remains a valid assay (379).

A second, although related, question is if patients with both antibodies are at greater risk for APS. In two studies, patients with both antibodies had an increased risk of thrombosis over those with LA alone (374,380). Patients with both have been found to have more arterial thrombosis (381) and recurrent pregnancy losses (382). In contrast, Triplett et al. (67) did not find an increased risk of thrombosis with both autoantibodies.

In general, the greatest risk is associated with LA (versus aCL), higher titer aCL, IgG isotype of aCL, and persistence of either antibody for 6 months or longer (383,384).

MULTIFACTORIAL NATURE OF RISK FACTORS FOR THROMBOSIS IN SYSTEMIC LUPUS ERYTHEMATOSUS

The fluctuating titers of APL antibodies in patients with SLE, associated with disease activity or treatment, suggests that the thrombotic risk engendered by these antibodies might not be constant over time. In addition, it is important to recognize that patients with lupus can have multiple other risk factors for thrombosis. Hasselaar et al. (16) found reduced concentrations of antithrombin III, plasminogen, free protein S, and protein C in some patients. Mayumi et al. (183) found raised concentrations of fibrinopeptide 20A, and thromboxane B2 in some patients with lupus and LA.

In our group's prospective study of patients with lupus, we have emphasized the role of factors other than APL antibodies in predicting future thrombotic events. Serologic markers of disease activity (both a low serum C3 level and elevated antidouble-stranded DNA), hypertension, and hypercholesterolemia all are significantly associated with future thrombotic events (33,385).

CLINICAL PRESENTATION

Dermatologic Manifestations

The important role of the dermatologist in recognizing APS has been emphasized by Alegre et al. (386). In their series, 41% of patients had a skin lesion as the first sign of disease. Multisystem thrombotic events developed in 40% of their patients with cutaneous manifestations of APS.

Livedo reticularis is the hallmark dermatologic manifestation of APS (194,315,387–389). Its association with thrombosis was recognized before APS was described, first by Champion and Rook (390) in a patient with angina, claudication, and cerebral thrombosis, and then by Sneddon (391), who described six patients with livedo reticularis and cerebral ischemia. The name Sneddon syndrome continues to be used to describe the clinical syndrome of livedo reticularis and transient ischemic attacks, strokes, or other cerebral ischemia (392). Livedo reticularis also occurs in infectious illnesses, including syphilis and tuberculosis; other immunologic diseases, including polyarteritis nodosa and cryoglobulinemia; and in cholesterol crystal embolization (393). In a mild form, it is a normal variant in young women (394). Patients with lupus may have both cryoglobulins and APL antibodies, thus further confusing the differential diagnosis (395).

The pathology of the livedo reticularis in Sneddon syndrome is an endarteritis obliterans without vasculitis (390, 391,396). Some skin biopsy specimens have shown endothelial proliferation of deep dermal vessels, and some have been normal (397–399). Sneddon syndrome differs from APS in that the clinical presentation is one of livedo reticularis and predominantly cerebral-arterial thromboses rather than recurrent pregnancy loss, venous thrombosis, and thrombocytopenia. In fact, there are patients with Sneddon syndrome who do not have APL antibodies (393). However, many patients with Sneddon syndrome do have APL antibodies, such as one patient (400) who had central-retinal artery occlusion, cerebral ischemia, livedo reticularis, and aCL antibody.

The relationship between APL antibodies and vasculitis remains controversial. Most skin biopsies of livedo reticularis or other cutaneous manifestations of APS show bland, noninflammatory pathology, but reports of vasculitis exist (401). In some cases, this may reflect the coexistence of two different disease processes in a patient with lupus; in other cases, there appears to be a causal link. In the study by Weinstein et al. (388), patients with livedo reticularis had histologically proven vasculitis at sites that were unrelated to the livedo reticularis. Livedoid vasculitis has been associated with central nervous system involvement in lupus (402). When vasculitis occurs in livedo reticularis, it can be associated with ulceration (403,404).

A second, but less common, cutaneous manifestation of APS is leg ulceration, often resembling pyoderma gangrenosum (315,386,405–414). There appears to be a spectrum of pathology, with vascular thrombosis, capillary proliferation, endarteritis obliterans, and lymphocytic infiltration all playing a role (415).

Distal cutaneous ischemia, presenting as erythematous and purplish macules on fingers or toes, is another cutaneous manifestation of APS (412). Severe cutaneous necrosis also is reported (386,416–421). Cutaneous necrosis may be multifactorial, as in one patient with both protein S deficiency and APL antibodies (422). Cutaneous necrosis occurred in one patient treated with LMW heparin (423). Cutaneous necrosis can be the initial manifestation of APS (424).

Both superficial thrombophlebitis (386,389,425,426) and thrombosis of dermal vessels have been reported (386, 412). In the series of Alegre et al. (386), 34% of patients with LA had thrombophlebitis, and in this retrospective series, it was the most common cutaneous manifestation.

Davies and Triplett (427) have described a patient with LA and APL antibodies who developed the blue-toe syndrome when given corticosteroids for thrombocytopenia. Blue-toe syndrome is more classically associated with microembolism of fibrin-platelet debris or cholesterol crystals from proximal atherosclerotic lesions (428), or with warfarin, with destabilization of coagulation over ulcerated atherosclerotic plaques (428).

Subungual splinter hemorrhages also have been reported in patients with APL antibodies by several groups (429–432). Nail-fold capillary changes with hemorrhages and hemosiderin deposits can be seen (433).

Venous Thrombosis

Deep-venous thrombosis remains the most classic site of thrombosis in patients with LA. In the review by Lechner and Pabinger-Fasching (135), deep-venous thrombosis occurred in 64% of 25 patients with thrombosis and in 71.2% of 80 cases from the literature. This prevalence far exceeded that of arterial thrombosis: 25% of patients had cerebral thrombosis, and 16% had peripheral arterial thrombosis. Only four patients had both venous and arterial thrombosis. Venous thrombosis in other distributions certainly occurred, including the retinal and renal veins, but was less common. Superior mesenteric vein (434), renal vein (435), splenic vein (436), and hepatic venous thrombosis (437) also have been reported.

A special clinical concern in patients with APL antibodies and venous thrombosis is the pattern of recurrent thrombosis (438). In the series of six patients reported by Asherson et al. (438), five of the six second events were deep-venous thrombosis, but one was a myocardial infarction. All occurred 6 to 12 weeks after warfarin was stopped. Long delays between events are not unusual, however, such as the patient who started with a deep-venous thrombosis of the leg at age 24 only to develop Budd-Chiari syndrome 6 years later (439).

Neurologic Syndromes

After deep-venous thrombosis, cerebral events are the most commonly encountered thrombotic events in patients with APS. Levine and Welch (440) have reviewed the spectrum of neurologic disease in APS, which includes focal cerebral ischemia, ocular ischemia, transverse myelopathy, complicated migraines, chorea, seizures (usually secondary to cerebral ischemic events), apnea, multiinfarct dementia, ischemic encephalopathy, pseudotumor cerebri, and transient-global amnesia.

Neurologic disease in patients with APL antibodies who are selected from hospital clinics is not rare. Twenty-five of 80 patients with elevated aCL in one study had neurologic disease, with four patterns being found: (i) encephalopathy, (ii) multiple cerebral infarctions, (iii) migrainelike headaches, and (iv) visual abnormalities, including amaurosis fugax and ischemic-optic neuropathy (441). In a study of 48 patients with APL antibodies and both cerebral and visual problems, the most common presentations were transient cerebral ischemia (12 patients) or cerebral infarction (23 patients) (442). Severe vascular headache also was seen in 16 patients, as was visual disturbance (11 patients), seizures (five patients), vascular dementia (three patients), transient-global amnesia (three patients), and cerebral-venous thrombosis (two patients).

Methodologic issues abound in cross-sectional studies. One issue is persistence of APL antibodies. In a study of 120 patients with transient ischemic attack or stroke, 19 of 21 with aCL showed persistence, but only nine of 20 with a LA demonstrated by dilute prothrombin time (443).

Transient Ischemic Attacks

Landi et al. (444) reported two young women with LA and transient ischemic attacks who had normal cerebral arteriograms. Levine et al. (442) also found that patients with transient neurologic dysfunction tended to have normal cerebral angiograms; however, two of their patients with transient ischemic attacks or recurrent amaurosis fugax had ipsilateral carotid-artery stenosis of greater than 75%. Therefore, it is not clear from available reports whether cerebral angiograms should be done in all young patients with transient ischemic attacks and APL antibodies. Although the typical patient is younger than would be expected for the presentation of atherosclerotic neurologic disease, many patients have had other risk factors, including hypertension, diabetes, and smoking (444,445).

Cerebral Infarction

APS and Sneddon syndrome overlap in important ways. In one study, patients with Sneddon syndrome who did not have APL antibodies were more likely to have large livedo racemosa. Those with APL antibodies were more likely to have seizures, mitral regurgitation, and thrombocytopenia (446).

Cerebral infarcts in APS can occur in any territory and have been found in both the anterior and posterior circulation. They generally involve the superficial cerebrum, although deep infarcts also are seen (442). In a series of 15 patients, ten had anterior circulation infarcts, five had posterior circulation infarcts, and one had epilepsy (447). Magnetic resonance imaging (MRI) is consistently more sensitive than computed tomography in detecting infarcts in patients with APS (442). Some strokes in patients with APL antibodies are embolic, with mitral valve vegetations (i.e., Libman-Sacks endocarditis) and intracardiac clot being two possible sources (448).

Strokes in APS often are multiple, recurrent, and can lead to a multiinfarct dementia, as reported by Asherson et al. (449) in nine of their 35 patients with cerebrovascular disease (450–452). Encephalopathy also has been reported in patients with APS, and in some patients, it may occur before true infarction can be demonstrated on brain scan (453). Molad et al. (454) found that focal white-matter brain lesions on MRI were more common in patients with systemic lupus and the LA. Cerebral-venous thrombosis in two patients with LA also has been reported (455).

Cerebral atrophy has been noted in several studies and case reports of patients with APS. It is assumed that the mechanism is cerebral infarction (456,457). Cerebral hypoperfusion also has been reported in APS (458).

Multiple Sclerosis

The differentiation of neurologic APS from multiple sclerosis is not always possible. In one study, patients with multiple sclerosis had a higher severity score of white-matter lesions, whereas patients with APS had higher scores in the putamen (459).

Transverse Myelopathy

A small subset of patients with lupus has a syndrome, which sometimes is termed lupoid sclerosis, in which neurologic events such as optic neuritis and transverse myelitis occur, resembling multiple sclerosis (460). All four patients with transverse myelitis in the series of 500 patients with SLE reported by Lavalle et al. (461) had aCL antibody. Four other patients with lupus, transverse myelitis, and aCL antibody have been reported (462–465), as has anterior spinal-artery syndrome (466). Not all series have found an association with myelitis, including a recent study (467).

Ocular Symptoms

In addition to amaurosis fugax, multiple other ocular syndromes have been reported in patients with APL antibodies, including retinal artery occlusion (400), ischemic-optic neuropathy (468), occlusive-vascular retinopathy (469,470), and retinal-vein occlusion (471,472). A recent case-control study suggested an association with aCL, but not LA, for retinal vasculopathy (473).

Migraine

Severe, recurrent migraine episodes sometimes are reported in patients with APL antibodies who later go on to have a cerebral ischemic event (442,448). In one study, six of 16 patients with migrainous cerebral infarction had APL antibodies (474,475). However, other studies have failed to confirm any association of APL antibodies with migraine (476).

Apnea

One patient with lupus and two episodes of apnea as well as other evidence of brainstem dysfunction was found to have aCL antibody (477). She also had cerebrospinal fluid oligoclonal bands.

Chorea

Chorea, whether in patients with or without SLE, can be associated with APL antibodies (478–482). In a review of 12 patients with chorea, six had lupuslike disease and six had SLE (483). All of the patients in this series were women, but men and children also have been reported (484). In the Asherson et al. series (483), eight of the 12 patients with chorea had features of APS, including thrombocytopenia, recurrent pregnancy loss, and thrombosis, and most had APL antibodies. Four patients with APL antibodies developed cerebral infarcts, and three others had transient ischemic attacks. One patient developed dementia at the time that chorea appeared. Cardioembolic caudate infarction was the cause of chorea in one patient with LA (485).

In the largest case series of 50 patients with APS and chorea, other manifestations of APS were frequent, including 28% with stroke, 24% with venous thrombosis, 18% with pregnancy loss, 6% with peripheral arterial disease, 4% with myocardial infarction, and 44% with thrombocytopenia. Multiple treatment regimens were used, with the majority of patients responding to corticosteroids or haloperidol (486).

Cognitive Function

Experimental murine APS includes cognitive function abnormalities, such as hyperactivity, in its neurologic presentations (487).

Two major recent studies have suggested that persistence of APL antibodies is associated with cognitive dysfunction in humans. In one study, persistent IgG aCL was associated with problems in speed of attention and concentration (488). In the second study, both persistent IgG aCL and IgA aCL were associated with cognitive dysfunction, in the areas of psychomotor speed and conceptual reasoning/executive ability, respectively (489).

Cardiac Manifestations

Cardiac manifestations recently have been reviewed (490).

Angina and Myocardial Infarction

Both angina and myocardial infarction have been reported in association with APL antibodies, although these appear to be less frequent than neurologic-arterial events in APS (491). Coronary-artery disease secondary to premature atherosclerosis is a well-recognized complication of corticosteroid therapy in patients with lupus (492,493), but myocardial infarction without sufficient risk factors (494) and without atherosclerosis on coronary arteriography (491) is the usual presentation in young patients with APL antibodies. Often, thrombus is demonstrated as the cause of the ischemia (495,496).

Valvular Disease

Multiple groups have found an increased prevalence of valve vegetations and mitral regurgitation in patients with APL antibodies (352,497–503). In patients with cerebral events and APL antibodies, cardiac valvular vegetations are a potential source of emboli (448,497,504). APL antibodies were found in three of 15 patients with cyanotic congenital heart disease, and two of these three had thrombotic episodes and false-positive VDRL (505).

Intracardiac Thrombus

Intracardiac thrombus has been described in several patients with APL antibodies (506–510).

Coronary Vasculopathy

A patient has been reported with coronary-artery vasculopathy in the setting of APL antibodies (511). Vasculopathy secondary to APL antibodies is a well-recognized clinical presentation of APS (512–514).

Atherosclerosis

In a small series of patients, an association of atherosclerosis of the lower limbs with APL antibodies was reported (515). Three of these patients also had myocardial infarction. APL antibodies may have accelerated the development of atherosclerosis and subsequent cholesterol embolization in all of these patients.

Pregnancy Manifestations

Pregnancy Loss

In a review of 110 women with multiple obstetric complications, 5% had aCL (516).

The most specific association of APL antibodies is with late (midtrimester) pregnancy loss (517–520).

An association with early first-trimester losses has been much more difficult to confirm. In a recent case-control study of 93 women with first-trimester losses versus 190 controls, there was no association with APL antibodies (521). However, in a prospective study of 325 pregnancies, aCL and antiphosphatidylserine (but not anti-β_2-glycoprotein I) predicted pregnancy loss (80).

Pregnancy-Associated Thromboembolism

Both genetic causes of hypercoagulability and APL antibodies are associated with pregnancy thromboembolism (522,523).

Preeclampsia

Some studies have found an association of APL antibodies with severe preeclampsia (75,76,163,524–528) but others have failed to confirm this (529–531). HELLP syndrome has been reported in several case reports (532–534).

Intrauterine Growth Retardation

Most studies have not found an association of APL antibodies with intrauterine growth retardation (524,530,535–537).

Infertility

Several studies have suggested an increase in APL antibodies in infertility and *in vitro* fertilization (IVF) failures, but methodologic problems with study design hamper interpretation of these studies (538).

Pulmonary Manifestations

Pulmonary Emboli

Pulmonary emboli are a frequent complication of deep-venous thrombosis in patients with APS (135). When thoracic imaging was done in 88 patients with APS, 10% had pulmonary emboli (539).

Pulmonary Hypertension

Pulmonary hypertension has been reported in several patients with APL antibodies (540,541). In most, the mechanism has been pulmonary emboli (542,543), although *in situ* thrombosis remains a possibility (544,545).

Pulmonary Capillaritis With Hemorrhage

Pulmonary capillaritis is an unusual APS presentation usually manifested clinically by hemorrhage (546). Pulmonary hemorrhage is a recognized pulmonary manifestation of APS (547) and in one case was associated with microvascular pulmonary thrombosis, not capillaritis, which responded to methylprednisolone (548).

Pulmonary Alveolitis

There is one report of fibrosing alveolitis in an APS patient (549).

Pulmonary Vasculopathy

A noninflammatory vasculopathy can occur in the lungs with APS (550).

Pulmonary-Artery Thrombosis

Pulmonary-artery thrombosis has been reported (544), including a postpartum case (551).

Adult Respiratory-Distress Syndrome

Multiple cases of adult respiratory-distress syndrome in patients with APS have been reported (552,553).

Renal Manifestations

Glomerular Thrombi and Renal Insufficiency

Kant et al. (554) described two patients with lupus and LA who had thrombi in the glomerular capillaries and prominent vascular disease in the renal biopsy specimen. This work was extended in a second study of 23 biopsy specimens from 14 patients with LA (555). Thrombi were found in 14 of 18 specimens with LA, which was increased significantly over the rate in biopsy specimens without LA. In a series of 16 cases of primary APS, small-vessel occlusive lesions and focal cortical atrophy were found (556).

Renal biopsy findings in 12 women with LA, four of who had systemic lupus, showed a pattern of narrowing of the arteries because of recanalizing thrombi and cellular intimal proliferation (557). Renal function was impaired severely in four of these patients.

Hyalinosis of arterioles, fibrin thrombi of arterioles, and intimal proliferation in small- or medium-sized arteries was found on renal biopsy in four patients with APS (558). One patient with endothelial swelling of the glomerular capillary wall and intimal proliferation with focal luminal occlusion on renal biopsy had a deterioration in renal function when she was switched from coumarin to aspirin (559).

Accelerated Hypertension

Accelerated hypertension was reported in a 14-year-old girl with LA who had ischemic change on renal biopsy (560). Asherson (561) has emphasized the importance of hypertension as a feature of the catastrophic APL syndrome, which is a presentation of APS with multiorgan failure and prominent vasculopathy.

Renal-Artery Thrombosis

Renal-artery thrombosis leading to renovascular hypertension has been reported in a 13-year-old girl with APL antibodies (562).

Nephrotic Syndrome

Pérez-Vásquez et al. (563) have found a negative association between nephrotic syndrome and APS in patients with lupus. This may be partially explained by urinary loss of IgG (563). In dialysis patients, maintenance of graft access is more difficult.

Renal Transplant

APS may contribute to early graft loss (564) and other renal transplant morbidity (565) in SLE.

Endocrine Manifestations

Adrenal Failure

Adrenal failure now has been reported in multiple patients with APL antibodies (552,566,567). Multiple mechanisms may contribute, but hemorrhage or hemorrhagic infarction is the most common. Most of the adrenal hemorrhages reported so far have been spontaneous (484, 568–573), but some have been in the setting of anticoagulation (572,574–576). Another typical presentation appears to be postoperative or exertion-related hemorrhage (425,572,577–580). Adrenal infarction after cessation of warfarin therapy also has been reported as a cause of adrenal failure (574).

Gastrointestinal Manifestations

Portal- and Hepatic-Vein Thrombosis

APL antibodies are one of the major predisposing factors to both portal and hepatic vein thrombosis. In one study, 11% with portal-vein thrombosis and 19% with hepatic-vein thrombosis had an APL antibody (581). In a second study of 23 patients with portal-vein thrombosis, 17% had IgG aCL, 4% had IgM aCL, and one patient had a lupus anticoagulant (582). Hepatic-vessel thrombosis was reported in two patients with APS after liver transplant (583).

Other Arterial Manifestations

Arterial thrombi in virtually every known territory have been reported in patients with APL antibodies. Of particular note are aortic syndromes (584–586) and digital or extremity gangrene (587,588). Acute extremity arterial insufficiency has been reported secondary to emboli after pyelography (589).

Hematologic Manifestations

Thrombocytopenia

Thrombocytopenia is so well recognized as a manifestation of APS that it is was one of the former major criteria for the syndrome (27,590). Some LA antibodies bind and can induce a morphologic change in platelets (591,592). Similarly, aCL antibodies have been shown to bind to platelets (502). Thrombocytopenia in both patients with autoimmune disease (593) and patients with chronic-immune thrombocytopenia purpura (594) is associated with aCL antibody. Patients with SLE and with primary APL antibody syndrome make antibodies that react with a 50- to 70-kd internal platelet protein (595).

Some investigators (236), but not all (235), have found that the presence of APL antibodies in patients with thrombocytopenia is associated with fetal loss, thrombosis, and bleeding. Thrombocytopenia was more common in APS patients who had arterial thrombosis in one study (596). Although seven of 27 patients with immune thrombocytopenia purpura had APL antibodies, this did not separate this subgroup in clinically meaningful ways (597).

Hemolytic Anemia

Both aCL (especially IgM) and LA are associated with the positive Coombs' test and with hemolytic anemia (34–36, 192,598,599).

Bone-Marrow Necrosis

Rare cases of bone-marrow necrosis have been reported secondary to APS (600,601).

Hemorrhage

Patients with the lupus anticoagulant directed against prothrombin, on rare occasions, may develop clinically important hypoprothrombinemia leading to hemorrhage. This complication appears to occur more often in children (98,602).

Vascular Access

Multiple thromboses of vascular access have been reported in patients with APS. In one study, this was associated with antibodies to bovine thrombin (used by surgeons) (603).

Musculoskeletal

An association of APL antibodies with avascular necrosis of bone was not found in four large series of patients with SLE (205,604–606). In four other series, however, avascular necrosis was more frequent in patients with SLE and APL antibodies (607–610). In one case report, the catastrophic form of APS presented as multiple sites of avascular necrosis (611). Avascular necrosis also was found in a single vertebral body in an APS patient (612).

Neonatal Manifestations

Transplacental transfer of APL antibodies can lead to APS manifestations in neonates. There is one report of umbilical-cord thrombosis (613), several reports of stroke (614,615), seizures (616), multiple thromboses (617), and fatal aortic thrombosis (618).

Other consequences of placental insufficiency as a result of APS include growth restriction (517), although this has not been confirmed in all studies (618–620), and severe preeclampsia (525), also not confirmed in all studies (621).

Drug-Induced Lupus Anticoagulant

Several commonly used medications, including phenothiazines, procainamide, and hydralazine, can induce not just lupus but also drug-induced LAs. Many of these drug-induced LAs are IgM rather than IgG and, for some time, were regarded as benign. However, drug-induced LAs rarely may be associated with the thrombotic events that characterize APS (67,622).

TREATMENT

Newly Diagnosed, Asymptomatic Patients With APL Antibodies

Asymptomatic patients with APL antibodies either may remain untreated (623) or be treated with low-dose aspirin. There are no studies proving that low-dose aspirin will prevent future thrombosis, however. In fact, the Physician's Health Study did not find aspirin to be effective in preventing future deep-venous thrombosis or pulmonary emboli in male physicians (290). Reduction of other risk factors for thrombosis, including smoking cessation and avoidance of oral contraceptives, should be undertaken as well.

In patients with SLE and APL antibodies, our prospective cohort study has shown that the use of hydroxychloroquine reduces the odds ratio for future thrombosis (294,624). The mechanism is likely multifactorial, because hydroxychloroquine lowers titers of APL antibodies, controls disease activity (625), and may have a beneficial rheologic effect.

Management Of Acute Arterial Thrombosis

Treatment of an acute arterial event in a patient with APS must balance aggressive therapy to recanulate the vessel with the risk of hemorrhagic complications or of further thrombosis resulting from instrumentation of the vessel. Thrombolytics (626) and angioplasty (627,628) have been used successfully in individual cases. Heparin remains the usual therapy in most cases, however.

Management of Acute-/Chronic-Venous Thrombosis

Heparin or thrombolytics is the usual therapy for acute deep-venous thrombosis or pulmonary embolus. Thromboendarterectomy has been performed successfully in chronic pulmonary thromboembolism (629).

Long-Term Management After a Thrombotic Event

The high frequency of recurrent thrombotic events in APS has been demonstrated conclusively (300,308). Case reports or small series have suggested the utility of warfarin as a long-term treatment (322,444,448,449,630,631), and three large studies have addressed this issue in detail. Rosove and Brewer (300) reported that intensive warfarin with an international normalized ratio (INR) of three or greater was the most effective antithrombotic treatment. Khamashta et al. (301) reached a similar conclusion. Derksen et al. (304), in a study that was limited to venous thrombosis in APS, found the probability of no recurrence to be 100% with oral anticoagulation versus 22% with no treatment. The price to be paid for the intensive anticoagulation, however, is the increased risk of bleeding. If low-dose aspirin is added to the regimen, this will further increase the bleeding risk.

These case series did not address several important clinical issues. First, the need for high-intensity warfarin has not been demonstrated prospectively, or shown to be necessary for both arterial and venous thrombosis. Venous and arterial events were not separated in two of the case series (300,301). It often is assumed that recurrent thrombotic events occur in the same distribution, arterial or venous, and that APS can be divided into these two subgroups in terms of treatment. I have disagreed personally with this stance, because about 25% of our patients with recurrent thrombosis had initially venous thromboembolism and then "crossed over" with recurrent thrombosis on the arterial side of the circulation, or vice versa.

It is important to acknowledge, though, that there are studies suggesting low-intensity warfarin may be sufficient to prevent recurrent venous thromboembolism (632–634), but these studies did not specifically address APL antibody syndrome. Furthermore, there are studies (302,303,305) including a prospective one (291) showing that an INR below three, even below two, may be sufficient to prevent recurrent venous thromboembolism in APL antibody syndrome.

Second, patients whose thromboembolic event occurred with an identified precipitant, especially pregnancy or oral-contraceptive use, are not separately analyzed. If a known precipitant can be removed, does the patient still require long-term anticoagulation?

Third, the case series do not adequately address the addition of low-dose aspirin to warfarin. Is this helpful in those who present with arterial, rather than venous, thromboembolism?

Fourth, the potential beneficial role of hydroxychloroquine (which patients with secondary APS might be taking for SLE manifestations) on titers of APL antibodies (294) and thrombosis prophylaxis has not been a focus of the major case series.

Fifth, the special management concerns in the profoundly thrombocytopenic patient are not emphasized. I have advised that patients with a platelet count below 50,000 should not receive high-intensity warfarin. The platelet count should be raised above 50,000 (using intravenous immunoglobulin, prednisone, danocrine, etc.) and then routine (instead of high-intensity) warfarin can be begun.

Ultimately, case series cannot be the standard by which treatment is decided. Clinical trials comparing warfarin, low molecular weight heparin, aspirin, warfarin/aspirin, and aspirin/hydroxcychloroquine still are required.

There still is no consensus on the recommendation that patients with thrombosis caused by APS receive long-term anticoagulation with warfarin and achieve an INR of three to four (635). For example, in one study, 51% of patients with APS had no recurrence of thrombosis with no warfarin (636). One potential explanation for why patients with APS might need a higher-than-usual intensity of anticoagulation is if the INR underestimates the anticoagulant effect of warfarin when the patient has LA (637). Reduction of other factors that contribute to thrombotic risk should be a focus of treatment as well. The roles of low-dose corticosteroid therapy, immunosuppressive drugs, alkylating drugs, plasmapheresis, and intravenous immunoglobulin (638) in the treatment of APS are unknown.

PATIENTS WITH THROMBOCYTOPENIA AND ANTIPHOSPHOLIPID ANTIBODY SYNDROME

Thrombocytopenia does not protect patients with APS from either thrombosis or pregnancy loss. The patient with APS and both thrombosis and thrombocytopenia remains a special treatment challenge. In one report, heparin-induced thrombocytopenia developed in 56% of LA-positive patients who had pulmonary hypertension, further confusing the issue (337). Our group has recommended using prednisone, danocrine, intravenous immunoglobulin, or other therapies for thrombocytopenia to keep the platelet count above 50,000 cells/mL if therapy with heparin or warfarin is contemplated. There is a report of low-dose aspirin correcting thrombocytopenia, but this seems to be the exception (639). Careful introduction of warfarin (with less-intensive anticoagulation, such as an INR of 2 to 2.5) then can be considered. Splenectomy may be an option for patients with refractory life-threatening thrombocytopenia (640) but we have seen recurrences postsplenectomy.

TREATMENT OF CARDIAC VALVULAR DISEASE

Valvular vegetations occur most frequently on the mitral or aortic valve. They represent a major source of embolic transient ischemic attacks and strokes. Studies differ on the efficacy of treatment with anticoagulation alone. In a series of 13 patients, warfarin and antiplatelet therapy had no effect (641). Thus, corticosteroids may have a role in addition to anticoagulation (642).

TREATMENT FOR TRANSVERSE MYELITIS AND CHOREA

Transverse myelitis and chorea may represent largely nonthrombotic manifestations of APL antibodies. However, some patients have true cord or basal ganglia infarcts on MRI. Acute therapy usually is with intravenous methylprednisolone "pulse" therapy, 1,000 mg daily for 3 days, followed by high-dose corticosteroids with or without immunosuppressives (643). The addition of anticoagulation must be made on a case-by-case basis, taking into account the presence of any thrombosis on MRI or history of thrombosis elsewhere.

TREATMENT FOR CATASTROPHIC ANTIPHOSPHOLIPID ANTIBODY SYNDROME

Although rare, catastrophic APS has a high mortality (50%) in most series. Precipitating factors are found in 22%, including infections, drugs, surgery, and cessation of warfarin (317). We also have found oral contraceptives and pregnancy to be precipitants. Thrombocytopenia has been reported in 68% (317). Treatment includes heparin, to prevent additional thrombosis; corticosteroids with or without cyclophosphamide to prevent further production of APL antibodies; and plasmapheresis to remove circulating APL antibodies. Plasmapheresis appears to improve survival in case series (317), although it increases the risk of severe infections (644).

FUTURE AND EXPERIMENTAL THERAPIES

B-Cell Tolerance

The ideal prophylactic treatment would be to prevent production of APL antibodies, by the reintroduction of tolerance. The technology of B-cell tolerance has reached fruition in LJP394, a B-cell toleragen for anti-dsDNA. LJP394 has been shown to reduce anti-dsDNA in patients with SLE (645) and now is undergoing clinical trials to prevent lupus nephritis flares.

The great benefit of this approach is its ability to induce specific autoantibody tolerance, while sparing normal immune function. To induce tolerance, B cells are exposed to an antibody-binding epitope that leads to cross-linking of surface receptors. In the absence of T cell help, B cell anergy and apoptosis then occur.

Iverson and colleagues have identified a peptide epitope that binds anti-β_2 glycoprotein I–dependent aCL antibodies and covalently linked it to an organic platform. Multivalent presentation of this peptide epitope on the organic platform reduced antibody production in an immunized mouse model (646). To be effective clinically, cross-reaction of the B-cell epitope with the majority of anti-β_2 glycoprotein I antibodies in patients must occur.

Stem-Cell Transplantation

A more radical attempt to induce tolerance is stem-cell transplantation. Stem-cell transplantation has been introduced as a treatment for severe autoimmune disease, including SLE, in several centers worldwide. At the time this chapter was submitted, ten SLE patients had undergone stem-cell transplantation. Because of the short follow-up, no conclusions on its effectiveness can be drawn.

One 19-year-old woman with SLE and secondary APS later developed refractory Evans syndrome and underwent stem-cell transplantation. Her conditioning regimen consisted of cyclophosphamide, anti-T lymphocyte globulin, and prednisone, followed by transplantation with autologous CD34+ stem cells and progenitor cells. Eight months after stem-cell transplant, her APL antibody assays, both aCL and lupus anticoagulant, remained negative. This case report suggests a potential role for stem-cell transplantation for refractory APS (647).

Our group has raised concerns about the durability of the response to stem-cell transplantation: when long-term follow-up is available, relapses are common. We believe the explanation is the reintroduction of autoreactive lymphocytes as part of the stem-cell graft (648,649).

We have introduced high-dose immunoablative cyclophosphamide as a potential treatment for refractory SLE and/or APS. The conditioning regimen, high dose intravenous cyclophosphamide 50 mg/kg for 4 days, is similar to that used for stem-cell transplantation, but the patient's own stem cells (which are resistant to cyclophosphamide) are allowed to recover. This regimen avoids the possible reinfusion of autoreactive lymphocytes. Early results of the open-label series are encouraging (648), but long-term results in either SLE or APS are not yet available.

Intravenous Immunoglobulin

Commercial preparations of intravenous immunoglobulin (IVIG) have been found to contain both APL and anti-DNA autoantibodies in addition to their antiidiotypic antibodies, but the autoantibodies have not been found to be pathogenic (650). In fact, in murine models of APL antibody syndrome, IVIG has been beneficial (651). This beneficial effect of IVIG is likely mediated through multiple mechanisms, including antiidiotypes and IL-3 secretion (652).

IVIG remains of interest in APS for the following multiple reasons: it binds APL antibodies, down-regulates their production, and can raise the platelet count in thrombocytopenic patients. About 30% of women with APS and pregnancy loss fail treatment with heparin and aspirin, and require consideration of alternative treatments, such as IVIG.

However, the successful use of IVIG has been in case reports and small series, leading to the potential of publication bias. It often is combined with heparin, aspirin, and even prednisone, making it more difficult to assess the added benefit of IVIG. Multiple regimens have been used daily, although the two most common are 400 mg/kg for 5 days monthly or 1 g/kg/day for 2 days monthly (653). In a clinical trial, the addition of IVIG did not improve pregnancy outcome in APS (654). IVIG, because it is usually low risk, likely will continue to be used in the treatment of pregnant patients failing conventional therapy (655).

It is even more difficult to assess the role of IVIG in infertility. Multiple groups have shown an increase in APL antibodies in women with unexplained infertility and in women with recurrent IVF failures, but negative series also exist (656). In a large case-control study, heparin and aspirin improved IVF results. The addition of IVIG in women who had failed two consecutive IVF attempts with heparin and aspirin improved the birth rate to 41% from 17%, if antiphosphatidylserine or antiphosphatidylethanolamine were present (657). These results require confirmation from other groups, however, before IVIG can be recommended routinely to women with IVF failure and APL antibodies.

Other Experimental Therapies

In murine models of APS, several promising novel therapeutic approaches have been studied. Peptides that react specifically with anti-β_2-glycoprotein I monoclonal antibodies were identified and found to inhibit endothelial-cell activation and expression of adhesion molecules. These peptides prevented experimental APS in BALB/c mice (658).

A second novel approach in murine APS is to induce oral tolerance to low-dose β_2-glycoprotein I. If β_2-glycoprotein I was given orally before priming the BALB/c mice with β_2-glycoprotein I, it completely prevented experimental APS. However, it had less effect if given 70 days postimmunization. The induction of suppression was β_2-glycoprotein I specific, but also mediated by TGF-β (659).

REFERENCES

1. Moore JE, Mohr CF. Biologically false positive serologic tests for syphilis. *JAMA* 1952;150:467–473.
2. Moore JE, Lutz WB. The natural history of systemic lupus erythematosus: an approach to its study through chronic biologic false-positive reactors. *J Chronic Dis* 1955;1:297–316.
3. Loizou S, Mackworth-Young CG, Cofiner C, et al. Heterogeneity of binding reactivity to different phospholipids of antibodies from patients with systemic lupus erythematosus (SLE) and with syphilis. *Clin Exp Immunol* 1990;80:171–176.
4. Harris EN, Gharavi AE, Wasley GD, et al. Use of an enzyme-linked immunosorbent assay and of inhibition studies to distinguish between antibodies to cardiolipin from patients with syphilis or autoimmune disorders. *J Infect Dis* 1988;157:23–31.
5. Levy RA, Gharavi AE, Samaritano LR, et al. Characteristics of IgG APL antibodies in patients with systemic lupus erythematosus and syphilis. *J Rheumatol* 1992;17:1036–1040.
6. Conley CL, Rathbun HK, Morse II WI, et al. Circulating anticoagulant as a cause of hemorrhagic diathesis in man. *Bulletin Johns Hopkins Hosp* 1948;83:288–296.
7. Feinstein DI, Rapaport SI. Acquired inhibitors of blood coagulation. *Prog Hemostasis Thromb* 1972;1:75–95.
8. Schleider MA, Nachman RL, Jaffe EA, et al. A clinical study of the lupus anticoagulant. *Blood* 1976;48:499–509.
9. Boxer M, Ellman L, Carvalho A. The lupus anticoagulant. *Arthritis Rheum* 1976;19:1244–1248.
10. Triplett DA. Antiphospholipid antibodies: proposed mechanisms of action. *Am J Reprod Immunol* 1992;28:211–215.
11. Galli M, Barbui T, Comfurius P, et al. Anticoagulant activity of a distinct subtype of aCL antibodies is mediated by b2-glycoprotein I. Fifth International Symposium on Antiphospholipid Antibodies. San Antonio, Texas, 1992:S2.
12. Bevers EM, Galli M, Barbui T, et al. Lupus anticoagulant IgG's (LA) are not directed to phospholipids only, but to a complex of lipid-bound human prothrombin. *Thromb Haemostasis* 1991; 66:629–632.
13. Oosting JD, Derksen RHWM, Bobbink IWG, et al. Antiphospholipid antibodies directed against a combination of phospholipids with prothrombin, protein C or protein S—an explanation for their pathogenic mechanism? *Blood* 1993;81: 2618–2625.
14. Janoff AS, Rauch J. The structural specificity of anti-phospholipid antibodies in autoimmune disease. *Chem Phys Lipids* 1986; 40:315–332.
15. Rauch J, Tannenbaum M, Tannenbaum H, et al. Human hybridoma lupus anticoagulants distinguish between lamellar and hexagonal phase lipid systems. *J Biol Chem* 1986;261: 9672–9677.
16. Hasselaar P, Derksen RHWM, Blokzijl L, et al. Risk factors for thrombosis in lupus patients. *Ann Rheum Dis* 1989;48: 933–940.
17. Oosting JD, Derksen RHWM, Entjes TI, et al. Lupus anticoagulant activity is frequently dependent on the presence of b2-glycoprotein I. *Thromb Haemostasis* 1992;67:499–502.
18. Hasselaar P, Derksen RHWM, Blokzijl L, et al. Thrombosis associated with APL antibodies cannot be explained by effects on endothelial and platelet prostanoid synthesis. *Thromb Haemost* 1988;59:80–85.
19. Oosting JD, Derksen RHWM, Hackeng TM, et al. In vitro studies of APL antibodies and its cofactor, b2-glycoprotein I, show negligible effects on endothelial cell mediated protein C activation. *Thromb Haemost* 1991;66:666–671.
20. Harris EN, Gharavi AE, Boey ML, et al. Anticardiolipin antibodies: detection by radioimmunoassay and association with thrombosis in systemic lupus erythematosus. *Lancet* 1983;2: 1211–1214.
21. Harris EN, Gharavi AE, Patel SP, et al. Evaluation of the aCL antibody test: report of an international workshop held 4 April 1986. *Clin Exp Immunol* 1987;68:215–222.
22. Harris EN, Phil M. The second international aCL standardization workshop. The Kingston Antiphospholipid Antibody Study (KAPS) Group [Special Report]. *Am J Clin Pathol* 1990; 94:474–484.
23. Deguchi H, Fernandez JA, Hackeng TM, et al. Cardiolipin is a normal component of human plasma lipoproteins. *Proc Natl Acad Sci USA* 2000;97:1743–1748.
24. Inoue G, Nojima S. Immunochemical studies of phospholipids. IV. The reactivities of antisera against natural cardiolipin and synthetic cardiolipin analogues containing antigens. *Chem Phys Lipid* 1986;40:315–322.
25. Thiagarajan P, Shapiro SS, De Marco L. Monoclonal immunoglobulin Ml coagulation inhibitor with phospholipid specificity: mechanism of a lupus anticoagulant. *J Clin Invest* 1980;66:397–405.
26. Rote MS, Dostal-Johnson D, Branch WD. Antiphospholipid antibodies and recurrent pregnancy loss: correlation between

the activated partial thromboplastin time and antibodies against phosphatidylserine and cardiolipin. *Am J Obstet Gynecol* 1990; 163:575–584.

27. Harris EN, Chan JKH, Asherson RA, et al. Thrombosis, recurrent fetal loss, and thrombocytopenia: predictive value of the aCL antibody test. *Arch Intern Med* 1986;146:2153–2156.
28. Loizou S, Byron MA, Englert HJ, et al. Association of quantitative aCL antibody levels with fetal loss and time of loss in systemic lupus erythematosus. *Quart J Med* 1988;255:525–531.
29. Lockshin MD, Druzin ML, Qamar T. Prednisone does not prevent recurrent fetal death in women with APL antibody. *Amer J Obstet Gynecol* 1989;160:439–443.
30. Cronin ME, Biswas RM, Van der Straeton C, et al. IgG and IgM aCL antibodies in patients with lupus with aCL antibody associated clinical syndromes. *J Rheumatol* 1988;15:795–798.
31. Cervera R, Khamashta MA, Font J, et al. Systemic lupus erythematosus: clinical and immunologic patterns of disease expression in a cohort of 1,000 patients. *Medicine* 1993;72: 113–124.
32. Petri M, Rheinschmidt M, Whiting-O'Keefe Q, et al. The frequency of lupus anticoagulant in systemic lupus erythematosus: a study of 60 consecutive patients by activated partial thromboplastin time, Russell viper venom time, and aCL antibody. *Ann Int Med* 1987;106:524–531.
33. Petri M, Hochberg M, Hellmann D, et al. Incidence of and predictors of thrombotic events in SLE: protective role of hydroxychloroquine [abstract]. *Arthritis Rheum* 1992;35:S54.
34. Delezé M, Oria CV, Alarcón-Segovia D. Occurrence of both hemolytic anemia and thrombocytopenic purpura (Evan's syndrome) in systemic lupus erythematosus. Relationship to APL antibodies. *J Rheumatol* 1988;15:611–615.
35. Delezé M, Alarcón-Segovia D, Oria CV, et al. Hemocytopenia in systemic lupus erythematosus. Relationship to APL antibodies. *J Rheumatol* 1989;16:926–930.
36. Fong KY, Loizou S, Boey ML, et al. Anticardiolipin antibodies, haemolytic anaemia and thrombocytopenia in systemic lupus erythematosus. *Br J Rheumatol* 1992;31:453–455.
37. Greco TP, Amos MD, Conti-Kelly AM, et al. Testing for the APL syndrome: importance of IgA anti-b2-glycoprotein I. *Lupus* 2000;9:33–41.
38. Tajima C, Suzuki Y, Mizushima Y, et al. Clinical significance of immunoglobulin A APL antibodies: possible association with skin manifestations and small vessel vasculitis. *J Rheumatol* 1998; 25:1730–1736.
39. Fanopoulos D, Teodorescu MR, Varga J, et al. High frequency of abnormal levels of IgA anti-beta2-glycoprotein I antibodies in patients with systemic lupus erythematosus: relationship with APL syndrome. *J Rheumatol* 1998;25:675–680.
40. Lakos G, Kiss E, Regeczy N, et al. Isotype distribution and clinical relevance of anti-beta2-glycoprotein I (beta2-GPI) antibodies: importance of IgA isotype. *Clin Exp Immunol* 1999;117: 574–579.
41. Selva-O'Callaghan A, Ordi-Ros J, Monegal-Ferran F, et al. IgA aCL antibodies—relation with other APL antibodies and clinical significance. *Thromb Haemost* 1998;79:282–285.
42. Perez-Vasquez ME, Villa AR, Drenkard C, et al. Influence of disease duration, continued follow-up and further APL testing on the frequency and classification category of APL syndrome in a cohort of patients with systemic lupus erythematosus. *J Rheumatol* 1993;20:417–421.
43. Kalunian KC, Peter JB, Middlekauff HR, et al. Clinical significance of a single test for anti-cardiolipin antibodies in patients with systemic lupus erythematosus. *Am J Med* 1988;85:602–608.
44. Derue GJ, Englert HJ, Harris EN, et al. Fetal loss in systemic lupus erythematosus: association with aCL antibodies. *J Obstet Gynaecol* 1985;5:207–209.
45. McNeil HP, Simpson RJ, Chesterman CN, et al. Antiphospholipid antibodies are directed against a complex antigen that includes a lipid-binding inhibitor: b2-glycoprotein I (apolipoprotein H). *Proc Natl Acad Sci USA* 1990;87:4120–4124.
46. Galli M, Maassen C, Comfurius P, et al. Isolation and characterization of a plasmatic factor interacting with aCL antibodies. *Clin Exp Rheumatol* 1990;8:206.
47. Matsuura E, Igarashi Y, Fujimoto M, et al. Anticardiolipin cofactor(s) and differential diagnosis of autoimmune disease. *Lancet* 1990;1:177–178.
48. Gharavi AE, Harris EN, Asherson RA, et al. Anticardiolipin antibodies: isotype distribution and phospholipid specificity. *Ann Rheum Dis* 1987;46:1–6.
49. Tincani A, Meroni PL, Brucato A, et al. Anti-phospholipid and anti-mitochondrial type M5 antibodies in systemic lupus erythematosus. *Clin Exp Rheumatol* 1985;3:321–326.
50. Nimpf J, Bevers EM, Bomans PHH, et al. Prothrombinase activity of human platelets is inhibited by b2-glycoprotein-I. *Biochim Biophys Acta* 1986;884:142–149.
51. Schousboe I. b2-glycoprotein I: a plasma inhibitor of the contact activation of the intrinsic blood coagulation pathway. *Blood* 1985;66:1086–1091.
52. Nimpf J, Wurm H, Kostner GM. Interaction of b2-glycoprotein-I with human platelets: influence upon the ADP-induced aggregation. *Thromb Haemost* 1985;54:397–401.
53. Harris EN, Pierangeli S, Barquinero J, et al. Anticardiolipin antibodies and binding of anionic phospholipids and serum protein. *Lancet* 1990;336:505–506.
54. Shoenfeld Y, Meroni PL. The beta-2-glycoprotein I and APL antibodies. *Clin Exp Rheumatol* 1992;10:205–209.
55. Viard J-P, Amoura Z, Bach J-F. Association of anti-b2 glycoprotein I antibodies with lupus-type circulating anticoagulant and thrombosis in systemic lupus erythematosus. *Am J Med* 1992;93:181–186.
56. Jones JV. Antiphospholipid antibodies: new perspectives on antigenic specificity. *J Rheumatol* 1992;19:1774–1777.
57. Galli M, Comfurius P, Maassen C, et al. Anticardiolipin antibodies (ACA) directed not to cardiolipin but to a plasma protein cofactor. *Lancet* 1990;335:952–953.
58. Cabiedes J, Cabran AR, Alarcón-Segovia D. Clinical manifestations of the APL syndrome in patients with systemic lupus erythematosus associate more strongly with anti-b2-glycoprotein-I than with APL antibodies. *J Rheumatol* 1995;22:1899–1906.
59. Cabral AR, Cabiedes J, Alarcón-Segovia D. Antibodies to phospholipid-free b2-glycoprotein-I in patients with primary APL syndrome. *J Rheumatol* 1995;22:1894–1898.
60. Arvieux J, Roussel B, Ponard D, et al. IgG2 subclass restriction of anti-b2-glycoprotein I antibodies in autoimmune patients. *Clin Exp Immunol* 1994;95:310–315.
61. Matsuura E, Igarashi Y, Yasuda T, et al. Anticardiolipin antibodies recognize b2-glycoprotein I structure altered by interacting with an oxygen modified solid phase surface. *J Exp Med* 1994;179:457–462.
62. Roubey RAS, Eisenberg RA, Harper MF, et al. "Anticardiolipin" autoantibodies recognize b2-glycoprotein I in the absence of phospholipid. Importance of Ag density and bivalent binding. *J Immunol* 1995;154:954–960.
63. Ichikawa K, Khamashta MA, Koike T, et al. b2-glycoprotein I reactivity of monoclonal aCL antibodies from patients with the APL syndrome. *Arthritis Rheum* 1994;37:1453–1461.
64. Cleve H. Genetic studies on the deficiency of b2-glycoprotein I of human serum. *Humangenetik* 1968;5:294–304.
65. Cleve H, Rittner C. Further family studies on the genetic control of b2-glycoprotein I concentration in human serum. *Humangenetik* 1969;7:93–97.
66. De Benedetti E, Reber G, Miescher PA, et al. No increase in b2-

glycoprotein I levels in patients with APL antibodies [letter]. *Thromb Haemost* 1992;68:624.
67. Triplett DA, Brandt JT, Musgrave KA, et al. The relationship between lupus anticoagulants and antibodies to phospholipid. *JAMA* 1988;259:550–554.
68. Tincani A, Balestrieri G, Spatola L, et al. Anticardiolipin and anti-b2 glycoprotein I immunoassays in the diagnosis of APL syndrome. *Clin Exp Rheumatol* 1998;16:396–402.
69. Day HM, Thiagarajan P, Ahn C, et al. Autoantibodies to b2-glycoprotein I in systemic lupus erythematosus and primary APL antibody syndrome: clinical correlations in comparison with other APL antibody tests. *J Rheumatol* 1998;25:667–674.
70. Sanmarco M, Soler C, Christides C, et al. Prevalence and clinical significance of IgG isotype anti-b2-glycoprotein I antibodies in APL syndrome: a comparative study with aCL antibodies. *J Lab Clin Med* 1997;129:499–506.
71. Detkov, Gil-Aguado A, Lavilla P, et al. Do antibodies to b2-glycoprotein 1 contribute to the better characterization of the APL syndrome? *Lupus* 1999;8:430–438.
72. Tsutsumi A, Matsuura E, Ichikawa K, et al. Antibodies to b2-glycoprotein I and clinical manifestations in patients with systemic lupus erythematosus. *Arthritis Rheum* 1996;39:1466–1474.
73. Balestrieri G, Tincani A, Spatola L, et al. Anti-b2-glycoprotein I antibodies: a marker of APL syndrome? *Lupus* 1995;4:122–130.
74. Arvieux J, Roussel B, Colomb MG. [Antiphospholipid and anti beta 2-glycoprotein I antibodies]. *Ann Biol Clin* 1994;52: 381–385.
75. Katano K, Aoki A, Sasa H, et al. b2-Glycoprotein I-dependent aCL antibodies as a predictor of adverse pregnancy outcomes in healthy pregnant women. *Hum Reprod* 1996;11:509–512.
76. Faden D, Tincani A, Tanzi P, et al. Anti-b2 glycoprotein I antibodies in a general obstetric population: preliminary results on the prevalence and correlation with pregnancy outcome. Anti-b2 glycoprotein I antibodies are associated with some obstetrical complications, mainly preeclampsia-eclampsia. *Eur J Obstet Gynecol Reprod Biol* 1997;73:37–42.
77. Cuadrado MJ, Tinahones F, Camps MT, et al. Antiphospholipid, anti-b2-glycoprotein-I and anti-oxidized-low-density-lipoprotein antibodies in APL syndrome. *Q J Med* 1998;91: 619–626.
78. Lee RM, Emlen W, Scott JR, et al. Anti-b2-glycoprotein I antibodies in women with recurrent spontaneous abortion, unexplained fetal death, and APL syndrome. *Am J Obstet Gynecol* 1999;181:642–648.
79. Teixido M, Font J, Reverter JC, et al. Anti-b2-glycoprotein I antibodies: a useful marker for the APL syndrome. *Br J Rheumatol* 1997;36:113–116.
80. Lynch A, Byers T, Emlen W, et al. Association of antibodies to b2-glycoprotein 1 with pregnancy loss and pregnancy-induced hypertension: a prospective study in low-risk pregnancy. *Obstet Gynecol* 1999;93:193–198.
81. Balasch J, Reverter JC, Creus M, et al. Human reproductive failure is not a clinical feature associated with b2 glycoprotein-I antibodies in aCL and lupus anticoagulant seronegative patients (the APL/cofactor syndrome). *Hum Reprod* 1999;14: 1956–1959.
82. Harris EN, Gharavi AE, Hughes GRV. The anti-cardiolipin assay. In: Harris EN, Exner T, Hughes GRV, eds. *Phospholipid-Binding Antibodies* Boston: CRC Press, 1991:175–187.
83. Rosove MH, Brewer PMC, Runae A, et al. Simultaneous lupus anticoagulant and aCL assays and clinical detection of APLs. *Am J Hematol* 1989;32:148–149.
84. Lockshin MD. Anticardiolipin antibody (editorial). *Arthritis Rheum* 1987;30:471–472.
85. Exner T, Squahman N, Trudinger B. Separation of aCL antibodies from lupus anticoagulant on a phospholipid-coated polystyrene column. *Biochem Biophys Res Commun* 1988;2: 1001–1007.
86. McNeil HP, Chesterman CN, Krilis SA. Anticardiolipin antibodies and lupus anticoagulants comprise separate antibody subgroups with different phospholipid binding characteristics. *Br J Haematol* 1989;78:506–513.
87. Chamley LW, Pattison NS, McKay EJ. Separation of lupus anticoagulant from aCL antibodies by ion-exchange and gel filtration chromatography. *Haemostasis* 1991;21:25–29.
88. Levy RA, Gharavi AE, Sammaritano LR, et al. Fatty acid chain is a critical epitope for APL antibody. *J Clin Immunol* 1990;10: 141–145.
89. Roubey RAS, Pratt CW, Buyon JP, et al. Lupus anticoagulant activity of autoimmune APL antibodies is dependent upon beta2-glycoprotein-I. *J Clin Invest* 1992;90:1100–1104.
90. Guerin J, Smith O, White B, et al. Antibodies to prothrombin in APL syndrome and inflammatory disorders. *Br J Haematol* 1998;102:896–902.
91. Arvieux J, Darnige L, Caron C, et al. Development of an ELISA for autoantibodies to prothrombin showing their prevalence in patients with lupus anticoagulants. *Thromb Haemost* 1995;74: 1120–1125.
92. Puurunen M, Vaarala O, Julkunen H, et al. Antibodies to phospholipid-binding plasma proteins and occurrence of thrombosis in patients with systemic lupus erythematosus. *Clin Immunol Immunopathol* 1996;80:16–22.
93. Horbach DA, van Oort E, Donders RC, et al. Lupus anticoagulant is the strongest risk factor for both venous and arterial thrombosis in patients with systemic lupus erythematosus. Comparison between different assays for the detection of APL antibodies [see comments]. *Thromb Haemost* 1996;76:916–924.
94. Palosuo T, Virtamo J, Haukka J, et al. High antibody levels to prothrombin imply a risk of deep venous thrombosis and pulmonary embolism in middle-aged men—a nested case-control study. *Thromb Haemost* 1997;78:1178–1182.
95. Vaarala O, Puurunen M, Manttari M, et al. Antibodies to prothrombin imply a risk of myocardial infarction in middle-aged men. *Thromb Haemost* 1996;75:456–459.
96. Pengo V, Biasiolo A, Brocco T, et al. Autoantibodies to phospholipid-binding plasma proteins in patients with thrombosis and phospholipid-reactive antibodies. *Thromb Haemost* 1996; 75:721–724.
97. Galli M, Ruggeri L, Barbui T. Differential effects of anti-b2-glycoprotein I and antiprothrombin antibodies on the anticoagulant activity of activated protein C. *Blood* 1998;91:1999–2004.
98. Erkan D, Bateman H, Lockshin MD. Lupus anticoagulant-hypoprothrombinemia syndrome associated with systemic lupus erythematosus: report of 2 cases and review of literature. *Lupus* 1999;8:560–564.
99. Rand JH, Wu XX, Guller S, et al. Antiphospholipid immunoglobulin G antibodies reduce annexin-V levels on syncytiotrophoblast apical membranes and in culture media of placental villi. *Am J Obstet Gynecol* 1997;177:918–923.
100. Nakamura N, Kuragaki C, Shidara Y, et al. Antibody to annexin V has anti-phospholipid and lupus anticoagulant properties. *Am J Hematol* 1995;49:347–348.
101. Satoh A, Suzuki K, Takayama E, et al. Detection of anti-annexin IV and V antibodies in patients with APL syndrome and systemic lupus erythematosus. *J Rheumatol* 1999;26: 1715–1720.
102. Kaburaki J, Kuwana M, Yamamoto M, et al. Clinical significance of anti-annexin V antibodies in patients with systemic lupus erythematosus. *Am J Hematol* 1997;54:209–213.
103. Kaburaki J, Kuwana M, Ikeda Y. Anti-cardiolipin-b2-GPI complex antibodies in idiopathic thrombocytopenic purpura. *Intern Med* 1998;37:796.

104. Song KS, Park YS, Kim HK. Prevalence of anti-protein S antibodies in patients with systemic lupus erythematosus. *Arthritis Rheum* 2000;43:557–560.
105. Font J, Lopez-Soto A, Cervera R, et al. Antibodies to thromboplastin in systemic lupus erythematosus: isotype distribution and clinical significance in a series of 92 patients. *Thromb Res* 1997;86:37–48.
106. Puurunen M, Manttari M, Manninen V, et al. Antibody against oxidized low-density lipoprotein predicting myocardial infarction. *Arch Intern Med* 1994;154:2605–2609.
107. Erkkila AT, Narvanen O, Lehto S, et al. Autoantibodies against oxidized low-density lipoprotein and cardiolipin in patients with coronary heart disease. *Arterioscler Thromb Vasc Biol* 2000; 20:204–209.
108. Vaarala O, Manttari M, Manninen V, et al. Anti-cardiolipin antibodies and risk of myocardial infarction in a prospective cohort of middle-aged men. *Circulation* 1995;91:23–27.
109. Bellomo G, Maggi E, Poli M, et al. Autoantibodies against oxidatively modified low-density lipoproteins in NIDDM. *Diabetes* 1995;44:60–66.
110. Bergmark C, Wu R, de Faire U, et al. Patients with early-onset peripheral vascular disease have increased levels of autoantibodies against oxidized LDL. *Arterioscler Thromb Vasc Biol* 1995; 15:441–445.
111. Branch DW, Mitchell MD, Miller E, et al. Pre-eclampsia and serum antibodies to oxidised low-density lipoprotein. *Lancet* 1994;343:645–646.
112. Salonen JT, Yla-Herttuala S, Yamamoto R, et al. Autoantibody against oxidised LDL and progression of carotid atherosclerosis. *Lancet* 1992;339:883–887.
113. Maggi E, Chiesa R, Melissano G, et al. LDL oxidation in patients with severe carotid atherosclerosis. A study of in vitro and in vivo oxidation markers. *Arterioscler Thromb* 1994;14:1892–1899.
114. van de Vijver LP, Steyger R, van Poppel G, et al. Autoantibodies against MDA-LDL in subjects with severe and minor atherosclerosis and healthy population controls. *Atherosclerosis* 1996; 122:245–253.
115. Iribarren C, Folsom AR, Jacobs DR, Jr., et al. Association of serum vitamin levels, LDL susceptibility to oxidation, and autoantibodies against MDA-LDL with carotid atherosclerosis. A case-control study. The ARIC Study Investigators. Atherosclerosis Risk in Communities. *Arterioscler Thromb Vasc Biol* 1997;17:1171–1177.
116. Hulthe J, Wikstrand J, Lidell A, et al. Antibody titers against oxidized LDL are not elevated in patients with familial hypercholesterolemia. *Arterioscler Thromb Vasc Biol* 1998;18:1203–1211.
117. Amengual O, Atsumi T, Khamashta MA, et al. Autoantibodies against oxidized low-density lipoprotein in APL syndrome. *Br J Rheumatol* 1997;36:964–968.
118. Aho K, Vaarala O, Tenkanen L, et al. Antibodies binding to anionic phospholipids but not to oxidized low-density lipoprotein are associated with thrombosis in patients with systemic lupus erythematosus. *Clin Exp Rheumatol* 1996;14:499–506.
119. Wu R, Nityanand S, Berglund L, et al. Antibodies against cardiolipin and oxidatively modified LDL in 50-year-old men predict myocardial infarction. *Arterioscler Thromb Vasc Biol* 1997; 17:3159–3163.
120. Brandt JT, Triplett DA, Alving B, et al. Criteria for the diagnosis of lupus anticoagulants: an update. *Thromb Haemostasis* 1995;74:1185–1190.
121. McGlasson DL, Brey RL, Strickland MD, et al. Differences in kaolin clotting times and platelet counts resulting from variations in specimen processing. *Clin Lab Sci* 1989;2:109.
122. Green D, Hougie C, Kazmier FJ, et al. Report of the Working Party on acquired inhibitors of coagulation: studies on the "lupus" anticoagulant. *Thromb Haemost* 1983;49:144–146.
123. Triplett DA. Coagulation assays for the lupus anticoagulant: review and critique of current methodology. *Stroke* 1992;23: I11–I14.
124. Triplett DA, Brandt JT. Lupus anticoagulants: misnomer, paradox, riddle, epiphenomenon. *Haematologic Pathol* 1988;2: 121–143.
125. Triplett DA. Screening for the lupus anticoagulant. *Ric Clin Lab* 1989;19:379–389.
126. McHugh NJ, Moye DAH, James IE, et al. Lupus anticoagulant: clinical significance in aCL positive patients with systemic lupus erythematosus. *Ann Rheum Dis* 1991;50:548–552.
127. Rauch J, Tannenbaum M, Janoff AS. Distinguishing plasma lupus anticoagulants from anti-factor antibodies using hexagonal (II) phase phospholipids. *Thromb Haemostasis* 1989;62:892–896.
128. Mannucci PM, Canciani MT, Mari D, et al. The varied sensitivity of partial thromboplastin time reagents in the demonstration of the lupus-like anticoagulant. *Scand J Haematol* 1979; 22:423–432.
129. Brandt JT, Triplett DA, Musgrave K, et al. The sensitivity of different coagulation reagents to the presence of lupus anticoagulants. *Arch Pathol Lab Med* 1987;111:120–124.
130. Stevenson KJ, Easton AC, Curry A, et al. The reliability of activated partial thromboplastin time methods and the relationship to lipid composition and ultrastructure. *Thromb Haemost* 1986; 55:250–258.
131. Kelsey PR, Stevenson KJ, Poller L. The diagnosis of lupus anticoagulants by the activated partial thromboplastin time — the central role of phosphatidylserine. *Thromb Haemostasis* 1984; 52:172–175.
132. Adcock DM, Marlar RA. Activated partial thromboplastin time reagent sensitivity to the presence of the lupus anticoagulant. *Arch Pathol Lab Med* 1992;116:837–840.
133. Triplett DA, Brandt JT, Maas RL. The laboratory heterogeneity of lupus anticoagulants. *Arch Pathol Lab Med* 1985;109: 946–951.
134. Johns AS, Ockelford PA, Chamley L, et al. Comparison of tests for the lupus anticoagulant and phospholipid antibodies in systemic lupus erythematosus [abstract]. *Thromb Haemost* 1989; 62:380.
135. Lechner K, Pabinger-Fasching I. Lupus anticoagulants and thrombosis. A study of 25 cases and review of the literature. *Haemostasis* 1985;15:254–262.
136. Thiagarajan P, Pengo V, Shapiro SS. The use of the dilute Russell viper venom time for the diagnosis of lupus anticoagulants. *Blood* 1986;68:869–874.
137. Forastiero RR, Falcon CR, Carreras LO. Comparison of various screening and confirmatory tests for the detection of the lupus anticoagulant. *Haemostasis* 1990;20:208–214.
138. Brandt JT, Triplett DA. The effect of phospholipid on the detection of lupus anticoagulants by the dilute Russell viper venom time. *Arch Pathol Lab Med* 1989;113:1376–1378.
139. Exner T, Triplett DA, Taberner DA, et al. Comparison of test methods for the lupus anticoagulant: international survey on lupus anticoagulants-1 (ISLA-1). *Throm Haemostas* 1990;64: 478–484.
140. Petri M, Nelson L, Weimer F, et al. The automated modified Russell viper venom time test for the lupus anticoagulant. *J Rheumatol* 1991;18:1823–1825.
141. Margolis J. The kaolin clotting time: a rapid one stage method for diagnosis of coagulation defects. *J Clin Pathol* 1958;11: 406–409.
142. Exner T. Comparison of two simple tests for the lupus anticoagulant. *Am J Clin Pathol* 1985;83:215.
143. Exner T, Rickard KA, Kronenberg H. A sensitive test demonstrating lupus anticoagulant and its behavioural patterns. *Br J Haematol* 1978;40:143–151.

144. Gibson J, Starling E, Date C, et al. Simplified screening procedure for detecting lupus inhibitor. *J Clin Pathol* 1988;41: 226–228.
145. Lazarchick J, Kizer J. The laboratory diagnosis of lupus anticoagulants. *Arch Pathol Lab Med* 2989;113:177–180.
146. Kornberg A, Silber L, Yona R, et al. Clinical manifestations and laboratory findings in patients with lupus anticoagulants. *Eur J Haematol* 1989;42:90–95.
147. Harris EN, Pierangeli S, Simpson P. A more specific phospholipid antigen for the APL syndrome [abstract]. *Arthritis Rheum* 1990;33:S163.
148. Vaarala O, Palosuo T, Kleemola M, et al. Anticardiolipin response in acute infections. *Clin Immunol Immunopathol* 1986; 41:8–15.
149. Harris EN, Hughes GRV. Third international APL conference: barbecues, rum punches, and kaps. *Ann Rheum Dis* 1988;47: 612–614.
150. Reber G, Tremblet C, Bernard C, et al. Anticardiolipin antibodies and thrombosis: buffer's influence on the detection and quantitation of aCL antibody measured by ELISA. *Thromb Res* 1990;57:215–226.
151. Manoussakis MN, Tzioufas AG, Silis MP, et al. High prevalence of anti-cardiolipin and other autoantibodies in a healthy elderly population. *Clin Exp Immunol* 1987;69:557–565.
152. Sturfelt G, Nived O, Norberg R, et al. Anticardiolipin antibodies in patients with systemic lupus erythematosus. *Arthritis Rheum* 1987;30:383–388.
153. Cervera R, Font J, López-Soto A, et al. Isotype distribution of aCL antibodies in systemic lupus erythematosus: prospective analysis of a series of 100 patients. *Ann Rheum Dis* 1990;49: 109–113.
154. Shi W, Krilis SA, Chong BH, et al. Prevalence of lupus anticoagulant and aCL antibodies in a healthy population. *Aust N Z J Med*, 1990;20:231–236.
155. Juby AG, Davis P. Prevalence and disease associations of certain autoantibodies in elderly patients. *Clin Invest Med*, 1998;21: 4–11.
156. Lockwood CJ, Romero R, Feinberg RF, et al. The prevalence and biologic significance of lupus anticoagulant and aCL antibodies in a general obstetric population. *Am J Obstet Gynecol* 1989;161:369–373.
157. El-Roeiy A, Myers SA, Gleicher N. The prevalence of autoantibodies and lupus anticoagulant in healthy pregnant women. *Obstet Gynecol* 1990;75:390–396.
158. Harris EN, Spinnato JA. Should aCL tests be performed in otherwise healthy pregnant women? *Am J Obstet Gynecol* 1991; 165:1272–1277.
159. Infante-Rivard C, David M, Gauthier R, et al. Lupus anticoagulants, aCL antibodies, and fetal loss. A case-control study. *N Engl J Med* 1991;325:1063–1066.
160. Out HJ, Bruinse HW, Christiaens GC, et al. Prevalence of APL antibodies in patients with fetal loss. *Ann Rheum Dis* 1991;50: 553–557.
161. Perez MC, Wilson WA, Brown HL, et al. Anticardiolipin antibodies in unselected pregnant women in relationship to fetal outcome. *J Perinatol* 1991;11:33–36.
162. Soloninka CA, Laskin CA, Wither J, et al. Clinical utility and specificity of aCL antibodies. *J Rheumatol* 1991;18:1849–1855.
163. Pattison NS, Chamley LW, McKay EJ, et al. Antiphospholipid antibodies in pregnancy: prevalence and clinical associations. *Br J Obstet Gynaecol* 1993;100:909–913.
164. Stuart RA, Kornman LH, McHugh NJ. A prospective study of pregnancy outcome in women screened at a routine antenatal clinic for aCL antibodies. *Br J Obstet Gynaecol* 1993;100: 599–600.
165. Lynch A, Marlar R, Murphy J, et al. Antiphospholipid antibodies in predicting adverse pregnancy outcome; a prospective study. *Ann Intern Med* 1994;120:470–475.
166. Fort JG, Cowchock FS, Abruzzo JL, et al. Anticardiolipin antibodies in patients with rheumatic diseases. *Arthritis Rheum* 1987;30:752–760.
167. Kushner MJ. Prospective study of aCL antibodies in stroke. *Stroke* 1990;21:295–298.
168. Chakravarty KK, Al-Hillawi AH, Byron MA, et al. Anticardiolipin antibody associated ischaemic strokes in elderly patients without systemic lupus erythematosus. *Age Ageing* 1990;19: 114–118.
169. Fields RA, Toubbeh H, Searles RP, et al. The prevalence of aCL antibodies in a healthy elderly population and its association with antinuclear antibodies. *J Rheumatol* 1989;16:623–625.
170. Hedfors E, Lindahl G, Lindblad S. Anticardiolipin antibodies during pregnancy. *J Rheumatol* 1987;14:160–161.
171. Meyer O, Cyna L, Borda-Iriarte O, et al. Anticorps anti-phospholipides, thromboses et maladie lupique: interet du dosage des anticorps anti-cardiolipine par la methode ELISA. *Rev Rhum Mal Osteoartic* 1985;52:297–305.
172. Lee SL, Sanders M. A disorder of blood coagulation in systemic lupus erythematosus. *J Clin Invest* 1955;34:1814–1822.
173. Meacham GC, Weisberger AS. Unusual manifestations of disseminated lupus erythematosus. *Ann Intern Med* 1955;43: 143–152.
174. Zetterstrom R, Berglund G. Systemic lupus erythematosus in childhood: a clinical study. *Acta Paediatr* 1956;45:189–204.
175. Johansson EA, Lassus A. The occurrence of circulating anticoagulants in patients with syphilitic and biologically false positive antilipoidal antibodies. *Ann Clin Res* 1974;6:105–108.
176. Pauzner R, Rosner E, Many A. Circulating anticoagulant in systemic lupus erythematosus: clinical manifestations. *Acta Haemat* 1986;76:90–94.
177. Rosner E, Pauzner R, Lusky A, et al. Detection and quantitative evaluation of lupus circulating anticoagulant activity. *Thromb Haemost* 1987;57:144–147.
178. Padmakumar K, Singh RR, Rai R, et al. Lupus anticoagulants in systemic lupus erythematosus: prevalence and clinical associations. *Ann Rheum Dis* 1990;49:986–989.
179. Regan MG, Lackner H, Karpatkin S. Platelet function and coagulation profile in lupus erythematosus: studies in 50 patients. *Ann Intern Med* 1974;81:462–468.
180. Mintz G, Acevedo-Vazquez E, Gutierrez-Espinosa G, et al. Renal vein thrombosis and inferior vena cava thrombosis in systemic lupus erythematosus. *Arthritis Rheum* 1984;27:539–544.
181. Averbuch M, Koifman B, Levo Y. Lupus anticoagulant, thrombosis and thrombocytopenia in systemic lupus erythematosus. *Am J Med Sci* 1987;293:1–5.
182. Meyer O, Piette J-C, Bourgeois P, et al. Antiphospholipid antibodies: a disease marker in 25 patients with antinuclear antibody negative systemic lupus erythematosus (SLE). Comparison with a group of 91 patients with antinuclear antibody positive SLE. *J Rheumatol* 1987;14:502–506.
183. Mayumi T, Nagasawa K, Inoguchi T, et al. Haemostatic factors associated with vascular thrombosis in patients with systemic lupus erythematosus and the lupus anticoagulant. *Ann Rheum Dis* 1991;50:543–547.
184. Boey ML, Colaco CB, Gharavi AE, et al. Thrombosis in systemic lupus erythematosus: striking association with the presence of circulating lupus anticoagulant. *Br Med J (Clin Res Ed)* 1983;287:1021–1023.
185. Bennett RE, Calabrese LH, Lucas FV, et al. The association between anti-DNA antibodies and the lupus anticoagulant [abstract]. *Arthritis Rheum* 1984;27:S39.
186. Colaco CB, Elkon KB. The lupus anticoagulant: a disease marker in antinuclear antibody negative lupus that is cross-reac-

tive with autoantibodies to double-stranded DNA. *Arthritis Rheum* 1985;28:67–74.

187. Wong KL, Chan FY, Lee CP. Outcome of pregnancy in patients with systemic lupus erythematosus: a prospective study. *Arch Intern Med* 1991;151:269–273.
188. Intragumtornchai T, Akkawat B, Mahasandana S, et al. Lupus anticoagulant in Thai systemic lupus erythematosus patients. *Southeast Asian J Trop Med Public Health* 1993;24(suppl 1): 241–245.
189. Sohngen D, Specker C, Wehmeier A, et al. [Prevalence of lupus anticoagulant, autoimmune hemolysis, thrombocytopenia, and disorders of platelet function in unselected patients with SLE]. *Beitr Infusionther* 1992;30:469–473.
190. Golstein M, Meyer O, Bourgeois P, et al. Neurological manifestations of systemic lupus erythematosus: role of APL antibodies. *Clin Exper Rheumatol* 1993;11:373–379.
191. Jones HW, Ireland R, Senaldi G, et al. Anticardiolipin antibodies in patients from Malaysia with systemic lupus erythematosus. *Ann Rheum Dis* 1991;50:173–175.
192. Hazeltine M, Rauch J, Danoff D, et al. Antiphospholipid antibodies in systemic lupus erythematosus: evidence of an association with positive Coombs' and hypocomplementemia. *J Rheumatol* 1988;15:80–86.
193. Danao-Camara T, Clough JD. Anticardiolipin antibodies in systemic lupus erythematosus. *Cleve Clin J Med* 1989;56:525–528.
194. McHugh NJ, Maymo J, Skinner RP, et al. Anticardiolipin antibodies, livedo reticularis, and major cerebrovascular and renal disease in systemic lupus erythematosus. *Ann Rheum Dis* 1988; 47:110–115.
195. Axtens RS, Miller MH, Littlejohn GO, et al. Single aCL measurement in the routine management of patients with systemic lupus erythematosus. *J Rheumatol* 1994;21:91–93.
196. Tubach F, Hayem G, Marchand J-L, et al. IgG anti-b2-glycoprotein I antibodies in adult patients with systemic lupus erythematosus: prevalence and diagnostic value for the APL syndrome. *J Rheumatol* 2000;27:1437–1443.
197. Kutteh WH, Lyda EC, Abraham SM, et al. Association of aCL antibodies and pregnancy loss in women with systemic lupus erythematosus. *Fertil Steril* 1993;60:449–455.
198. Wilson WA, Perez MC, Michalski JP, et al. Cardiolipin antibodies and null alleles of C4 in black Americans with systemic lupus erythematosus. *J Rheumatol* 1988;15:1768–1772.
199. Buchanan RRC, Wardlaw JR, Riglar AG, et al. Antiphospholipid antibodies in the connective tissue diseases: their relation to the APL syndrome and forme fruste disease. *J Rheumatol* 1989;16:757–761.
200. Guerin J, Feighery C, Sim RB, et al. Antibodies to beta2-glycoprotein I — a specific marker for the APL syndrome. *Clin Exp Immunol* 1997;109:304–309.
201. Shimada K, Koike T, Ichikawa K, et al. IgG class anti-cardiolipin antibody as a possible marker for evaluating fetal risk in patients with systemic lupus erythematosus. *J Autoimmunity* 1989;2:843–849.
202. Lopez-Soto A, Cervera R, Font J, et al. Isotype distribution and clinical significance of antibodies to cardiolipin, phosphatidic acid, phosphatidylinositol and phosphatidylserine in systemic lupus erythematosus: prospective analysis of a series of 92 patients. *Clin Exp Rheumatol* 1997;15:143–149.
203. Toschi V, Motta A, Castelli C, et al. Prevalence and clinical significance of APL antibodies to noncardiolipin antigens in systemic lupus erythematosus. *Haemostasis* 1993;23:275–283.
204. Worrall JG, Snaith ML, Batchelor JR, et al. SLE: a rheumatological view. Analysis of the clinical features, serology and immunogenetics of 100 SLE patients during long-term follow-up. *Q J Med* 1990;74:319–330.
205. Alarcón-Segovia D, Delezé M, Oria CV, et al. Antiphospholipid antibodies and the APL syndrome in systemic lupus erythematosus: a prospective analysis of 500 consecutive patients. *Medicine* 1989;68:353–374.
206. Ishikawa O, Ohnishi K, Miyachi Y, et al. Cerebral lesions in systemic lupus erythematosus detected by magnetic resonance imaging. Relationship to aCL antibody. *J Rheumatol* 1994;21: 87–90.
207. Koike T, Sueishi M, Funaki H, et al. Anti-phospholipid antibodies and biological false positive serological test for syphilis in patients with systemic lupus erythematosus. *Clin Exp Immunol* 1984;56:193–199.
208. Wilson HA, Askari AD, Neiderhiser DH, et al. Pancreatitis with arthropathy and subcutaneous fat necrosis. *Arth Rheum* 1983;26:121–126.
209. Sebastiani GD, Passiu G, Galeazzi M, et al. Prevalence and clinical associations of aCL antibodies in systemic lupus erythematosus: a prospective study. *Clin Rheumatol* 1991;10:289–293.
210. Wong K-L, Liu H-W, Ho K, et al. Anticardiolipin antibodies and lupus anticoagulant in Chinese patients with systemic lupus erythematosus. *J Rheumatol* 1991;18:1187–1192.
211. Savi M, Ferraccioli GF, Neri TM, et al. HLA-DR antigens and aCL antibodies in Northern Italian systemic lupus erythematosus patients. *Arthritis Rheum* 1988;31:1568–1570.
212. Faux JA, Byron MA, Chapel HM. Clinical relevance of specific IgG antibodies to cardiolipin. *Lancet* 1989;2:1457–1458.
213. Knight PJ, Peter JB. Occurrence of antibodies to cardiolipin in systemic lupus erythematosus [abstract]. *Arthritis Rheum* 1986; 29:S27.
214. Norberg R, Nived O, Sturfelt G, et al. Anticardiolipin and complement activation: relation to clinical symptoms. *J Rheumatol* 1987;14(suppl 13):149–153.
215. Shergy WJ, Fredich DW, Pisetsky DS. The relationship of aCL antibodies to disease manifestations in pediatric systemic lupus erythematosus. *J Rheumatol* 1988;15:1389–1394.
216. Picillo U, Migliaresi S, Marcialis MR, et al. Longitudinal survey of aCL antibodies in systemic lupus erythematosus. *Scand J Rheumatol* 1992;21:271–276.
217. Ravelli A, Caporali R, Di Fuccia G, et al. Anticardiolipin antibodies in pediatric systemic lupus erythematosus. *Arch Pediatr Adolsc Med* 1994;148:398–402.
218. Kaburati J, Kuwana M, Yamamoto M, et al. Clinical significance of phospholipid-dependent anti-b2-glycoprotein I antibodies in systemic lupus erythematosus. *Lupus* 1995;4:472–476.
219. Romero FI, Amengual O, Atsumi T, et al. Arterial disease in lupus and secondary APL syndrome: association with anti-b2-glycoprotein I antibodies but not with antibodies against oxidized low-density lipoprotein. *Br J Rheumatol* 1998;37:883–888.
220. Derksen RHWH, Biesma D, Bouma BN, et al. Discordant effects of prednisone on aCL antibodies and the lupus anticoagulant (letter). *Arthritis Rheum* 1986;29:1295–1296.
221. Cooper RC, Klemp P, Stipp CJ, et al. The relationship of aCL antibodies to disease activity in systemic lupus erythematosus. *Br J Rheumatol* 1989;28:379–382.
222. Out HJ, DeGroot PH, Hasselaar P, et al. Fluctuations of aCL antibody levels in patients with systemic lupus erythematosus: a prospective study. *Ann Rheum Dis* 1989;48:1023–1028.
223. Hassell KL, Kressin DC, Neumann A, et al. Correlation of APL antibodies and protein S deficiency with thrombosis in HIV-infected men. *Blood Coagul Fibrinolysis* 1994;5:455–462.
224. Rubbert A, Bock E, Schwab J, et al. Anticardiolipin antibodies in HIV infection: association with cerebral perfusion defects as detected by 99mTc-HMPAO SPECT. *Clin Exp Immunol* 1994; 98:361–368.
225. Thirumalai S, Kirshner HS. Anticardiolipin antibody and stroke in an HIV-positive patient [letter]. *AIDS* 1994;8: 1019–1020.

226. Hunt JE, McNeil HP, Morgan GJ, et al. A phospholipid-beta 2-glycoprotein I complex is an antigen for aCL antibodies occurring in autoimmune disease but not with infection. *Lupus* 1992; 1:75–81.
227. Cappell MS, Simon T, Tiku M. Splenic infarction associated with aCL antibodies in a patient with acquired immunodeficiency syndrome. *Dig Dis Sci* 1993;38:1152–1155.
228. Maeshima E, Sakagashira M, Yamada Y, et al. [A case of malignant rheumatoid arthritis with lupus anticoagulant and cerebral infarction]. *No To Shinkei* 1995;47:391–395.
229. Wolf P, Gretler J, Aglas F, et al. Anticardiolipin antibodies in rheumatoid arthritis: their relation to rheumatoid nodules and cutaneous vascular manifestations. *Br J Dermatol* 1994;131: 48–51.
230. Rosler DH, Conway MD, Anaya J-M, et al. Ischemic optic neuropathy and high-level aCL antibodies in primary Sjögren's syndrome. *Lupus* 1995;4:155–157.
231. Castanet J, Lacour JP, Perrin C, et al. Association of eosinophilic fasciitis, multiple morphea and APL antibody. *Dermatology* 1994;189:304–307.
232. Pope JE, Thompson A. The frequency and significance of aCL antibodies in scleroderma. *J Rheumatol* 2000;27:1450–1452.
233. Herrick AL, Heaney M, Hollis S, et al. Anticardiolipin, anticentromere and anti-Scl-70 antibodies in patients with systemic sclerosis and severe digital ischaemia. *Ann Rheum Dis* 1994; 53:540–542.
234. Herrick AL, Oogarah P, Brammah TB, et al. Nervous system involvement in association with vasculitis and aCL antibodies in a patient with systemic sclerosis [letter]. *Ann Rheum Dis* 1994;53:349–350.
235. Stasi R, Stipa E, Masi M, et al. Prevalence and clinical significance of elevated APL antibodies in patients with idiopathic thrombocytopenic purpura. *Blood* 1994;84:4203–4208.
236. Perez de Oteyza C, Lopez Valero I, Romero Barbero JL, et al. [Antiphospholipid antibodies in megakaryocytic thrombopenias]. *An Med Interna* 1994;11:263–267.
237. Font J, Cervera R, Lopez-Soto A, et al. Anticardiolipin antibodies in patients with autoimmune diseases: isotype distribution and clinical associations. *Clin Rheumatol* 1989;8:475–483.
238. Burden AD, Gibson IW, Rodger RS, et al. IgA aCL antibodies associated with Henoch-Schonlein purpura. *J Am Acad Dermatol* 1994;31:857–860.
239. Hergesell O, Egbring R, Andrassy K. Presence of aCL antibodies discriminates between Wegener's granulomatosis and microscopic polyarteritis. *Adv Exp Med Biol* 1993;336:393–396.
240. de la Fuente Fernandez R, Grana Gil J. Anticardiolipin antibodies and polyarteritis nodosa. *Lupus* 1994;3:523–524.
241. Cohney S, Savige J, Stewart MR. Lupus anticoagulant in antineutrophil cytoplasmic antibody-associated polyarteritis. *Am J Nephrol* 1995;15:157–160.
242. McLean RM, Greco TP. Anticardiolipin antibodies in the polymyalgia rheumatica-temporal arteritis syndromes. *Clin Rheumatol* 1995;14:191–196.
243. Kerleau JM, Levesque H, Delpech A, et al. Prevalence and evolution of aCL antibodies in giant cell arteritis during corticosteroid therapy. A prospective study of 20 consecutive cases. *Br J Rheumatol* 1994;33:648–650.
244. Liozon F, Jauberteau-Marchan MO, Liozon E, et al. [Anti-cardiolipin antibodies in Horton's disease]. *Ann Med Interne* (Paris), 1992;143:433–437.
245. Yokoi K, Akaike M, Shigekiyo T, et al. [An elderly patient with Takayasu's arteritis associated with APL antibodies]. *Nippon Ronen Igakkai Zasshi* 1994;31:716–719.
246. Misra R, Aggarwal A, Chag M, et al. Raised aCL antibodies in Takayasu's arteritis [letter]. *Lancet* 1994;343:1644–1645.
247. Espinoza LR, Jara LJ, Silveira LH, et al. Anticardiolipin antibodies in polymyalgia rheumatica-giant cell arteritis: association with severe vascular complications. *Am J Med* 1991;90:474–478.
248. Ina Y, Takada K, Yamamoto M, et al. Antiphospholipid antibodies: a prognostic factor in sarcoidosis? *Chest* 1994;105: 1179–1183.
249. Wang CR, Chuang CY, Chen CY. Anticardiolipin antibodies and interleukin-6 in cerebrospinal fluid and blood of Chinese patients with neuro-Behcet's syndrome. *Clin Exp Rheumatol* 1992;10:599–602.
250. Zouboulis CC, Buttner P, Tebbe B, et al. Anticardiolipin antibodies in Adamantiades-Behcet's disease. *Br J Dermatol* 1993; 128:281–284.
251. al-Dalaan AN, al-Ballaa SR, al-Janadi MA, et al. Association of anti-cardiolipin antibodies with vascular thrombosis and neurological manifestation of Behcets disease. *Clin Rheumatol* 1993; 12:28–30.
252. Papagiannis A, Cooper A, Banks J. Pulmonary embolism and lupus anticoagulant in a woman with renal cell carcinoma. *J Urol* 1994;152:941–942.
253. Malnick S, Sthoeger Z, Attali M, et al. Anticardiolipin antibodies associated with hypernephroma. *Eur J Med* 1993;2:308–309.
254. Zarrabi MH, Zucker S, Miller F, et al. Immunologic and coagulation disorders in chlorpromazine-treated patients. *Ann Intern Med* 1979;91:194–199.
255. Larsson GB, Langer L, Nassberger L. Thiazide-induced kidney damage with circulating antibodies against myeloperoxidase and cardiolipin. *J Intern Med* 1993;233:493-494.
256. Canoso RT, de Oliveira RM. Chloropromazine-induced aCL antibodies and lupus anticoagulant: absence of thrombosis. *Am J Hematol* 1988;27:272–275.
257. Firer M, Sirota P, Schild K, et al. Anticardiolipin antibodies are elevated in drug-free, multiply affected families with schizophrenia. *J Clin Immunol* 1994;14:73–78.
258. Kucuk O, Gilman-Sachs A, Beaman K, et al. Antiphospholipid antibodies in sickle cell disease. *Am J Hematol* 1993;42:380–383.
259. Sallam S, Wafa E, el-Gayar A, et al. Anticardiolipin antibodies in children on chronic haemodialysis. *Nephrol Dial Transplant* 1994;9:1292–1294.
260. Matsuda J, Saitoh N, Gohchi K, et al. b2-Glycoprotein I-dependent and -independent aCL antibody in patients with end-stage renal disease. *Thromb Res* 1993;72:109–117.
261. Sitter T, Spannagl M, Schiffl H. Anticardiolipin antibodies and lupus anticoagulant in patients treated with different methods of renal replacement therapy in comparison to patients with systemic lupus erythematosus. *Ann Hematol* 1992;65:79–82.
262. Phillips AO, Jones HW, Hambley H, et al. Prevalence of lupus anticoagulant and aCL antibodies in haemodialysis patients. *Nephron* 1993;65:350–353.
263. Miyagawa S, Matsuura E, Kitamura W, et al. Systemic lupus erythematosus and aCL antibodies in Klinefelter's syndrome. *Lupus* 1995;4:236–238.
264. Durand JM, Quiles N, Kaplanski G, et al. Lupus anticoagulant and Klinefelter's syndrome [letter]. *J Rheumatol* 1993;20: 920–921.
265. Folomeev M, Kosheleva N, Alekberova Z. Systemic lupus erythematosus with Klinefelter's syndrome. A case report from the USSR [letter]. *J Rheumatol* 1991;18:940.
266. Bajocchi G, Sandri G, Trotta F. Anticardiolipin antibodies in Klinefelter's syndrome [letter]. *J Rheumatol* 1994;21:7.
267. Lousa M, Sastre JL, Cancelas JA, et al. Study of APL antibodies in a patient with Sneddon's syndrome and her family. *Stroke* 1994;25:1071–1074.
268. Rebollo M, Val JF, Garijo F, et al. Livedo reticularis and cerebrovascular lesions (Sneddon's syndrome). *Brain* 1983;106: 965–979.
269. Pettee AD, Wasserman BA, Adams NL, et al. Familial Sneddon's

syndrome: clinical, hematologic, and radiographic findings in two brothers. *Neurology* 1994;44:399–405.

270. Constans J, Le Herissier A, Vergnes C, et al. [Circulating lupus coagulation inhibitor in two sisters, one with disseminated lupus erythematosus and the other with immunologic thrombocytopenic purpura]. *Rev Med Interne* 1992;13:305–306.
271. Olson JC, Konkol RJ, Gill JC, et al. Childhood stroke and lupus anticoagulant. *Pediatr Neurol* 1994;10:54–57.
272. Schoning M, Klein R, Krageloh-Mann I, et al. Antiphospholipid antibodies in cerebrovascular ischemia and stroke in childhood. *Neuropediatrics* 1994;25:8–14.
273. Hellan M, Kuhnel E, Speiser W, et al. Familial lupus anticoagulant: a case report and review of the literature. *Blood Coagul Fibrinolysis* 1998;9:195–200.
274. Molta C, Meyer O, Dosquet C, et al. Childhood-onset systemic lupus erythematosus: APL antibodies in 37 patients and their first-degree relatives. *Pediatrics* 1993;92:849–853.
275. Ida A, Hirose S, Hamano Y, et al. Multigenic control of lupus-associated APL syndrome in a model of (NZW x BXSB) F1 mice. *Eur J Immunol* 1998;28:2694–2703.
276. Asherson RA, Doherty DG, Vergani D, et al. Major histocompatibility complex associations with primary APL antibody syndrome. *Arthritis Rheum* 1992;35:124–125.
277. Arnett FC, Olsen ML, Anderson KL, et al. Molecular analysis of major histocompatibility complex alleles associated with the lupus anticoagulant. *J Clin Invest* 1991;87:1490–1495.
278. McHugh NJ, Maddison RT. HLA-DR antigens and aCL antibodies in patients with systemic lupus erythematosus. *Arthritis Rheum* 1989;32:1623–1624.
279. Baek K, Petri M, Schmeckpeper B. Predictive value of HLA DR and DQ for APL antibodies (aPL) in SLE [abstract]. *Arthritis Rheum* 1994;37:S296.
280. Gulko PS, Reveille JD, Koopman WJ, et al. Anticardiolipin antibodies in systemic lupus erythematosus: clinical correlates, HLA associations, and impact on survival. *J Rheumatol* 1993; 20:1684–1693.
281. Galeazzi M, Sebastiani GD, Tincani A, et al. HLA class II alleles associations of aCL and anti-b2GPI antibodies in a large series of European patients with systemic lupus erythematosus. *Lupus* 2000;9:47–55.
282. Wilson WA, Perez MC, Armatis PE. Partial C4A deficiency is associated with susceptibility to systemic lupus erythematosus in black Americans. *Arthritis Rheum* 1988;31:1171–1175.
283. Wilson WA, Perez MC. Complete C4b deficiency in Black Americans with systemic lupus erythematosus. *J Rheumatol* 1988;15:1855–1858.
284. Petri M, Watson R, Winkelstein JA, et al. Clinical expression of systemic lupus erythematosus in patients with C4A deficiency. *Medicine* 1993;72:236–244.
285. Lockshin MD, Druzin ML, Goei S, et al. Antibody to cardiolipin as a predictor of fetal distress or death in pregnant patients with systemic lupus erythematosus. *N Engl J Med* 1985; 313:152–156.
286. Blank M, Cohen J, Toder V, et al. Induction of anti-phospholipid syndrome in naive mice with mouse lupus monoclonal and human polyclonal anti-cardiolipin antibodies. *Proc Natl Acad Sci USA* 1991;88:3069–3037.
287. Branch DW, Dudley DJ, Mitchell MD, et al. Immunoglobulin G fractions from patients with APL antibodies cause fetal death in BALB/c mice: a model for autoimmune fetal loss. *Am J Obstet Gynecol* 1990;163:210–216.
288. Gharavi AE, Mellors RC, Elkon KB. IgG anti-cardiolipin antibodies in murine lupus. *Clin Exp Immunol* 2989;78:233–238.
289. Hashimoto Y, Kawamura M, Ichikawa K, et al. Anticardiolipin antibodies in NZW x BXSB F1 mice: a model of APL syndrome. *J Immunol* 1992;149:1063–1068.
290. Ginsburg KS, Liang MH, Newcomer L, et al. Anticardiolipin antibodies and the risk for ischemic stroke and venous thrombosis. *Ann Int Med* 1992;117:997–1002.
291. Schulman S, Svenungsson E, Granqvist S, et al. Anticardiolipin antibodies predict early recurrence of thromboembolism and death among patients with venous thromboembolism following anticoagulant therapy. *Am J Med* 1998;104:332–338.
292. Levine SR, Salowich-Palm L, Sawaya KL, et al. IgG aCL antibody titer > 40 GPL and the risk of subsequent thrombo-occlusive events and death. A prospective cohort study. *Stroke* 1997; 28:1660–1665.
293. Finazzi G, Brancaccio V, Moia M, et al. Natural history and risk factors for thrombosis in 360 patients with APL antibodies: a four-year prospective study from the Italian Registry. *Am J Med* 1996;100:530–536.
294. Petri M. Thrombosis and systemic lupus erythematosus: the Hopkins Lupus Cohort perspective. *Scand J Rheumatol* 1996; 25:191–193.
295. Cervera R, Khamashta MA, Font J, et al. Morbidity and mortality in systemic lupus erythematosus during a 5-year period. A multicenter prospective study of 1,000 patients. European Working Party on Systemic Lupus Erythematosus. *Medicine* 1999;78:167–175.
296. Insko EK, Haskal ZJ. Antiphospholipid syndrome: patterns of life-threatening and severe recurrent vascular complications. *Radiology* 1997;202:319–326.
297. Sasso EH, Suzuki LA, Thompson AR, et al. Thromboembolic events in lupus patients with APL Ab (aPL) are not strongly associated with the Factor V mutation of APC resistance [abstract]. *Arthritis Rheum* 1995;38:S314.
298. Pablos JL, Caliz RA, Carreira PE, et al. Risk of thrombosis in patients with APL antibodies and factor V Leiden mutation. *J Rheumatol* 1999;26:588–590.
299. Oger E, Lernyer C, Dueymes M, et al. Association between IgM aCL antibodies and deep venous thrombosis in patients without systemic lupus erythematosus. *Lupus* 1997;6:455–461.
300. Rosove MH, Brewer PMC. Antiphospholipid thrombosis: clinical course after the first thrombotic event in 70 patients. *Ann Intern Med* 1992;117:303–308.
301. Khamashta MA, Cuadrado MJ, Mujic F, et al. The management of thrombosis in the APL antibody syndrome. *N Engl J Med* 1995;332:993–997.
302. Prandoni P, Simoni P, Girolami A. Antiphospholipid antibodies, recurrent thromboembolism and intensity of oral anticoagulation. *Thromb Haemost* 1996;75:859.
303. Krnic-Barrie S, O'Connor CR, Looney SW, et al. A retrospective review of 61 patients with APL syndrome. Analysis of factors influencing recurrent thrombosis. *Arch Intern Med* 1997; 157:2101–2108.
304. Derksen RHWM, de Groot PG, Kater L, et al. Patients with APL antibodies and venous thrombosis should receive long term anticoagulant treatment. *Ann Rheum Dis* 1993;52:689–692.
305. Rance A, Emmerich J, Fiessinger J-N. Anticardiolipin antibodies and recurrent thromboembolism. *Thromb Haemost* 1997;77: 221–222.
306. Levine SR, Brey RL, Kittner SJ. Antiphospholipid antibodies and recurrent thrombo-occlusive events [letter]. *Lancet* 1992; 340:117–118.
307. Levine SR, Brey RL, Salowich-Palm L, et al. Antiphospholipid antibody associated stroke: prospective assessment of recurrent event risk [abstract]. *Stroke* 1993;24:188.
308. Levine SR, Brey RL, Joseph CLM, et al. Risk of recurrent thromboembolic events in patients with focal cerebral ischemia and APL antibodies. *Stroke* 1992;23(suppl I):I29–I32.
309. The Antiphospholipid Antibodies in Stroke Study Group (APASS). Anticardiolipin antibodies and the risk of recurrent

thrombo-occlusive events and death. *Neurology* 1997;48: 91–94.
310. Drenkard C, Villa AR, Alarcón-Segovia D, et al. Influence of the APL syndrome in the survival of patients with systemic lupus erythematosus. *J Rheumatol* 1994;21:1067–1072.
311. Jouhikainen T, Stephansson E, Leirisalo-Repo M. Lupus anticoagulant as a prognostic marker in systemic lupus erythematosus. *Br J Rheumatol* 1993;32:568–573.
312. Wilson WA, Gharavi AE, Koike T, et al. International consensus statement on preliminary classification criteria for definite APL syndrome: report of an international workshop. *Arthritis Rheum* 1999;42:1309–1311.
313. Lockshin MD, Sammaritano LR, Schwartzman S. Validation of the Sapporo criteria for APL syndrome. *Arthritis Rheum* 2000; 43:440–443.
314. Weber M, Hayem G, De Bandt M, et al. Classification of an intermediate group of patients with APL syndrome and lupus-like disease: primary or secondary APL syndrome? *J Rheumatol* 1999;26:2131–2136.
315. Alarcón-Segovia D, Sánchez-Guerrero J. Primary APL syndrome. *J Rheumatol* 1989;16:482–488.
316. Mackworth-Young CG, Loizou S, David J, et al. Primary APL syndrome: features of patients with raised aCL antibodies and no other disorder. *Ann Rheum Dis* 1989;48:362–367.
317. Asherson RA, Khamashta MA, Ordi-Ros J, et al. The primary APL syndrome: major clinical and serological features. *Medicine* 1989;68:366–374.
318. Coull BM, Levine SR, Brey RL. The role of APL antibodies in stroke. *Neurol Clin* 1992;10:125–143.
319. Vianna JL, Khamashta MA, Ordi-Ros J, et al. Comparison of the primary and secondary APL syndrome: a European multicenter study of 114 patients. *Am J Med* 1994;96:3–9.
320. May KP, West SG, Moulds J, et al. Different manifestations of the APL antibody syndrome in a family with systemic lupus erythematosus. *Arthritis Rheum* 1993;36:528–533.
321. Mackworth-Young C, Chan J, Harris N, et al. High incidence of aCL antibodies in relatives of patients with systemic lupus erythematosus. *J Rheumatol* 1987;14:723–726.
322. Asherson RA, Baguley E, Pal C, et al. Antiphospholipid syndrome: five year follow-up. *Ann Rheum Dis* 1991;50:805–810.
323. Mujic F, Cuadrado MJ, Lloyd M, et al. Primary APL syndrome evolving into systemic lupus erythematosus. *J Rheumatol* 1995; 22:1589–1592.
324. Derksen RH, Gmelig-Meijling FH, de Groot PG. Primary APL syndrome evolving into systemic lupus erythematosus. *Lupus* 1996;5:77–80.
325. Andrews PA, Frampton G, Cameron JS. Antiphospholipid syndrome and systemic lupus erythematosus [letter]. *J Rheumatol* 1993;20:988–989.
326. Nachman RL, Silverstein R. Hypercoagulable states. *Ann Intern Med* 1993;119:819–827.
327. Case records of the Massachusetts General Hospital. Weekly clinicopathological exercises. Case 18-1999. A 54-year-old woman with acute renal failure and thrombocytopenia [clinical conference]. *N Engl J Med* 1999;340:1900–1908.
328. Hughes GRV. The APL syndrome: ten years on. *Lancet* 1993; 342:341–344.
329. McNeil HP, Hunt JE, Krilis SA. Antiphospholipid antibodies — new insights into their specificity and clinical importance. *Scand J Immunol* 1992;36:647–652.
330. Love PE, Santoro SA. Antiphospholipid antibodies, aCL and the lupus anticoagulant in systemic lupus erythematosus (SLE) and in non-SLE disorders. *Ann Intern Med* 1990;112:682–689.
331. Bick RL, Jakway J, Baker Jr. WF. Deep vein thrombosis: prevalence of etiologic factors and results of management in 100 consecutive patients. *Sem Thromb Hemostasis* 1992;18:267–274.
332. Eschwege V, Peynaud-Debayle E, Wolf M, et al. Prevalence of APL-related antibodies in unselected patients with history of venous thrombosis. *Blood Coagul Fibrinolysis* 1998;9: 429–434.
333. Zanon E, Prandoni P, Vianello F, et al. Anti-b2-glycoprotein I antibodies in patients with acute venous thromboembolism: prevalence and association with recurrent thromboembolism. *Thromb Res* 1999;96:269–274.
334. Salomon O, Steinberg DM, Zivelin A, et al. Single and combined prothrombotic factors in patients with idiopathic venous thromboembolism: prevalence and risk assessment. Arterioscler. *Thromb Vasc Biol* 1999;19:511–518.
335. Mateo J, Oliver A, Borrell M, et al. Laboratory evaluation and clinical characteristics of 2,132 consecutive unselected patients with venous thromboembolism—results of the Spanish Multicentric Study on Thrombophilia (EMET-Study). *Thromb Haemost* 1997;77:444–451.
336. Heron E, Lozinguez O, Alhenc-Gelas M, et al. Hypercoagulable states in primary upper-extremity deep vein thrombosis. *Arch Intern Med* 2000;160:382–386.
337. Auger WR, Permpikul P, Moser KM. Lupus anticoagulant, heparin use, and thrombocytopenia in patients with chronic thromboembolic pulmonary hypertension: a preliminary report. *Am J Med* 1995;99:392–396.
338. Martinuzzo ME, Pombo G, Forastiero RR, et al. Lupus anticoagulant, high levels of aCL, and anti-b2-glycoprotein I antibodies are associated with chronic thromboembolic pulmonary hypertension. *J Rheumatol* 1998;25:1313–1319.
339. Dahle C, Vrethem M, Olsson J-E, et al. High level of aCL antibodies is an unusual finding in an unselected stroke population. *Eur J Neurol* 1995;2:331–336.
340. Hess DC, Krauss J, Adams RJ, et al. Anticardiolipin antibodies: a study of frequency in TIA and stroke. *Neurology* 1991;41: 525–528.
341. Muir KW, Squire IB, Alwan W. Anticardiolipin antibodies and cerebral infarction [letter]. *J Neurol Neurosurg Psychiatry* 1994; 57:253–254.
342. Trimble M, Bell DA, Brien W, et al. The APL syndrome: prevalence among patients with stroke and transient ischemic attacks. *Am J Med* 1990;88:593–597.
343. The Antiphospholipid Antibodies in Stroke Study Group (APASS). Clinical, radiological, and pathological aspects of cerebrovascular disease associated with APL antibodies. *Stroke* 1993;24:I120–123.
344. Montalban J, Codina A, Ordi J, et al. Antiphospholipid antibodies in cerebral ischemia. *Stroke* 1991;22:750–753.
345. Ferro D, Quintarelli C, Rasura M, et al. Lupus anticoagulant and the fibrinolytic system in young patients with stroke. *Stroke* 1993;24:368–370.
346. Hart RG, Miller VT, Coull BM, et al. Cerebral infarction associated with lupus anticoagulants—preliminary report. *Stroke* 1984;15:114–118.
347. Chancellor AM, Glasgow GL, Ockelford PA, et al. Etiology, prognosis, and hemostatic function after cerebral infarction in young adults. *Stroke* 1989;20:477–482.
348. Brey RL, Hart RG, Sherman DG, et al. Antiphospholipid antibodies and cerebral ischemia in young people. *Neurology* 1990; 40:1190–1196.
349. de Jong AW, Hart W, Terburg M, et al. Cardiolipin antibodies and lupus anticoagulant in young patients with a cerebrovascular accident in the past. *Neth J Med* 1993;42:93–98.
350. Tietjen GE, Levine SR, Brown E, et al. Factors that predict APL immunoreactivity in young people with transient focal neurological events. *Arch Neurol* 1993;50:833–836.
351. Czlonkowska A, Meurer M, Palasik W, et al. Anticardiolipin antibodies, a disease marker for ischemic cerebrovascular events

in a younger patient population? *Acta Neurol Scand* 1992;86: 304–307.

352. Jouhikainen T, Pohjola-Sintonen S, Stephansson E. Lupus anticoagulant and cardiac manifestations in systemic lupus erythematosus. *Lupus* 1994;3:167–172.
353. Christensen K, Herskind AM, Junker P. [Antiphospholipid antibodies and occlusive vascular disease]. *Ugeskr Laeger* 1993;155:2896–2900.
354. Thorp JM, Jr., Chescheir NC, Fann B. Postpartum myocardial infarction in a patient with APL syndrome. *Am J Perinatol* 1994;11:1–3.
355. Ames PR. Antiphospholipid antibodies, thrombosis and atherosclerosis in systemic lupus erythematosus: a unifying 'membrane stress syndrome' hypothesis. *Lupus* 1994;3:371–377.
356. Garrido JA, Peromingo JA, Sesma P, et al. More about the link between thrombosis and atherosclerosis in autoimmune diseases: triglycerides and risk for thrombosis in patients with APL antibodies [letter]. *J Rheumatol* 1994;21:2394.
357. Witzum JL, Steinberg D. Role of oxidized low density lipoprotein in atherogenesis. *J Clin Invest* 1991;88:1785–1792.
358. Vaarala O, Alfthan G, Jauhiainen M, et al. Cross reaction between antibodies to oxidized low-density lipoprotein and to cardiolipin in systemic lupus erythematosus. *Lancet* 1993;341: 923–925.
359. Hamsten A, Norberg R, Björkholm M, et al. Antibodies to cardiolipin in young survivors of myocardial infarction: an association with recurrent cardiovascular events. *Lancet* 1986;1: 113–116.
360. Bick RL. The APL-thrombosis syndromes. Fact, fiction, confusion, and controversy [editorial]. *Am J Clin Pathol* 1993; 100:477–480.
361. Nasonov EL, Noeva EA, Kovalev V, et al. [Cardiolipin antibodies in patients with myocardial infarction and unstable angina pectoris]. *Kardiologiia* 1992;32:32–34.
362. Morton KE, Gavaghan TP, Krilis SA, et al. Coronary artery bypass graft failure — an autoimmune phenomenon? *Lancet* 1986;II:1353–1357.
363. Klemp P, Cooper RC, Strauss FJ, et al. Anti-cardiolipin antibodies in ischaemic heart disease. *Clin Exp Immunol* 1988;74: 254–257.
364. Ferlazzo B, Bonanno D, Quattrocchi P, et al. [Connections between ischemic heart disease and anti-cardiolipin antibody positivity]. *Minerva Cardioangiol* 1993;41:113–117.
365. Cortellaro M, Cofrancesco E, Boschetti C. Cardiolipin antibodies in survivors of myocardial infarction. *Lancet* 1993;342: 192.
366. Sletnes KE, Smith P, Abdelnoor M, et al. Antiphospholipid antibodies after myocardial infarction and their relation to mortality, reinfarction, and non-haemorrhagic stroke. *Lancet* 1992; 339:451–453.
367. Edwards T, Thomas RD, McHugh NJ. Anticardiolipin antibodies in ischaemic heart disease [letter]. *Lancet* 1993;342:989.
368. Phadke KV, Phillips RA, Clarke DT, et al. Anticardiolipin antibodies in ischaemic heart disease: marker or myth? *Br Heart J* 1993;69:391–394.
369. Yilmaz E, Adalet K, Yilmaz G, et al. Importance of serum aCL antibody levels in coronary heart disease. *Clin Cardiol* 1994;17: 117–121.
370. Raghavan C, Ditchfield J, Taylor RJ, et al. Influence of aCL antibodies on immediate patient outcome after myocardial infarction. *J Clin Pathol* 1993;46:1113–1115.
371. Tsakiris DA, Marbet GA, Burkart F, et al. Anticardiolipin antibodies and coronary heart disease. *Eur Heart J* 1992;13: 1645–1648.
372. Derksen RHWM, Hasselaar P, Blokzijl L, et al. Coagulation screen is more specific than the aCL antibody ELISA in defining a thrombotic subset of lupus patients. *Ann Rheum Dis* 1988; 47:364–371.
373. Ferro D, Saliola M, Quintarelli C, et al. Methods for detecting lupus anticoagulants and their relation to thrombosis and miscarriage in patients with systemic lupus erythematosus. *J Clin Pathol* 1992;45:332–338.
374. Jouhikainen T, Julkunen H, Vaarala O, et al. Antiphospholipid antibodies and thrombosis in systemic lupus erythematosus: comparison of three lupus anticoagulant assays and aCL ELISA in 188 patients. *Blood Coagul Fibrinolysis* 1992;3:407–414.
375. Ginsberg JS, Wells PS, Brill-Edwards P, et al. Antiphospholipid antibodies and venous thromboembolism. *Blood* 1995; 86:3685–3691.
376. Simioni P, Prandoni P, Zanon E, et al. Deep venous thrombosis and lupus anticoagulant. A case-control study. *Thromb Haemost* 1996;76:187–189.
377. Metz LM, Edworthy S, Mydlarski R, et al. The frequency of phospholipid antibodies in an unselected stroke population. *Can J Neurol Sci* 1998;25:64–69.
378. Ghirardello A, Doria A, Ruffatti A, et al. Antiphospholipid antibodies (aPL) in systemic lupus erythematosus. Are they specific tools for the diagnosis of aPL syndrome? *Ann Rheum Dis* 1994;53:140–142.
379. Derksen RHWM, Out HJ, Blokzijl L, et al. Detection of the lupus anticoagulant in pregnancy. *Clin Exp Rheumatol* 1992;10: 323–324.
380. Alving BM, Barr CF, Tang DB. Correlation between lupus anticoagulants and aCL antibodies in patients with prolonged activated partial thromboplastin times. *Am J Med* 1990;88:112–116.
381. Nojima J, Suehisa E, Akita N, et al. Risk of arterial thrombosis in patients with aCL antibodies and lupus anticoagulant. *Br J Haematol* 1997;96:447–450.
382. Guglielmone HA, Fernandez EJ. Distribution of lupus anticoagulant and aCL antibody isotypes in a population with APL syndrome. *J Rheumatol* 1999;26:86–90.
383. Long AA, Ginsberg JS, Brill-Edwards P, et al. The relationship of APL antibodies to thromboembolic disease in systemic lupus erythematosus: a cross-sectional study. *Thromb Haemost* 1991; 66:520–524.
384. Ginsberg JS, Brill-Edwards P, Johnston M, et al. Relationship of APL antibodies to pregnancy loss in patients with systemic lupus erythematosus: a cross-sectional study. *Blood* 1992;80: 975–980.
385. Petri M, Roubenoff R, Dallal GE, et al. Plasma homocysteine as a risk factor for atherothrombotic events in systemic lupus erythematosus. *Lancet* 1996;348:1120–1124.
386. Alegre VA, Gastineau DA, Winkelmann RK. Skin lesions associated with circulating lupus anticoagulant. *Br J Derm* 1989; 120:419–429.
387. Alarcón-Segovia D, Pérez-Vázquez ME, Villa AR, et al. Preliminary classification criteria for the APL syndrome within systemic lupus erythematosus. *Sem Arthritis Rheum* 1992;21:275–286.
388. Weinstein C, Miller MH, Axtens R, et al. Livedo reticularis associated with increased titers of aCL antibodies in systemic lupus erythematosus. *Arch Dermatol* 1987;123:596–600.
389. Naldi L, Locati F, Marchesi L, et al. Cutaneous manifestations associated with APL antibodies in patients with suspected primary APL syndrome: a case-control study. *Ann Rheum Dis* 1993;52:219–222.
390. Champion RH, Rook AJ. Livedo reticularis. *Proc R Soc Med* 1960;53:961–962.
391. Sneddon JB. Cardiovascular lesions and livedo reticularis. *Br J Dermatol* 1965;77:180–185.
392. Rumpl E, Neuhofer J, Pallua A, et al. Cerebrovascular lesions and livedo reticularis (Sneddon's syndrome) — a progressive cerebrovascular disorder? *J Neurol* 1985;231:324–330.

393. Burton JL. Livedo reticularis, porcelain-white scars, and cerebral thromboses. *Lancet* 1988;I:1263–1265.
394. Rook A, Wilkinson DS, Ebling FJ. *Textbook of Dermatology 3rd ed.* Oxford, England: Blackwell Scientific Publications, 1979.
395. Yancey Jr. WB, Edwards NL, Williams Jr. RC. Cryoglobulins in a patient with SLE, livedo reticularis, and elevated level of aCL antibodies. *Am J Med* 1990;88:699.
396. Pinol-Aguadi J, Ferrandiz C, Ferrar-Roca O, et al. Livedo reticularis y accidentes carebro-vasculares. *Med Cutan Ibero Lat Am* 1975;3:257–265.
397. Stamm T, Schmidt RC, Lubach D. Livedo racemosa generalisata (Ehrmann). Neurologische, neuroradiologische und histologische Beobachtungen. *Nervenarzt* 1982;53:211–218.
398. Lubach D, Stamm T. Neurologische Veranderungen bei Livedo racemosa generalisata (Ehrmann). Kasuistik und literaturubersicht. *Hautarzt* 1981;31:245–248.
399. Lubach D, Stamm T. Zerebrale gefässerkrankungen bei jüngeren patienten mit livedo rademosa generalisata (Ehrmann). *Fortschr Med* 1982;100:676–680.
400. Jonas J, Kölble K, Völcker HE, et al. Central retinal artery occlusion in Sneddon's disease associated with APL antibodies. *Am J Ophthalmol* 1986;102:37–40.
401. Goldberger E, Elder RC, Schwartz RA, et al. Vasculitis in the APL syndrome. *Arthritis Rheum* 1992;35:569–572.
402. Yasue T. Livedoid vasculitis and central nervous system involvement in systemic lupus erythematosus. *Arch Dermatol* 1986; 122:66–70.
403. Braverman IM. *Skin Signs of Systemic Disease, 2nd ed.* Philadelphia: W.B. Saunders Co., 1981.
404. Acland KM, Darvay A, Wakelin SH, et al. Livedoid vasculitis: a manifestation of the APL syndrome? *Br J Dermatol* 1999;140: 131–135.
405. Johannsson EA, Niemi KM, Mustakillio KK. A peripheral vascular syndrome overlapping with SLE: recurrent venous thrombosis and hemorrhagic capillary proliferation with circulating anticoagulants and false-positive reactions for syphilis. *Dermatologica* 1977;15:257–267.
406. Bazex A, Bazex J, Boneu B, et al. Ulcere de jambe, anticoagulant circulant. Lupus érythémateaux aigu dissémine. *Bull Soc Fr Dermatol Syph* 1976;83:350–352.
407. Cuny JF, Schmutz JL, Jeandel C, et al. Ulcere de jambe et anticoagulants circulants. *Ann Dermatol Venereol* 1986;113:825–826.
408. Selva A, Ordi J, Roca M, et al. Pyoderma-gangraenosum-like ulcers associated with lupus anticoagulant. *Dermatology* 1994; 189:182–184.
409. Barbaud AM, Gobert B, Reichert S, et al. Anticardiolipin antibodies and ulcerations of the leg. *J Am Acad Dermatol* 1994;31: 670–671.
410. Bissonnette R, Tousignant J. Anticardiolipin antibodies and lower leg plaques and ulcers of 45 years duration [letter]. *Int J Dermatol* 1993;32:619.
411. Babe KS, Jr., Gross AS, Leyva WH, et al. Pyoderma gangrenosum associated with APL antibodies. *Int J Dermatol* 1992;31: 588–590.
412. Grob JJ, Bonerandi JJ. Cutaneous manifestations associated with the presence of the lupus anticoagulant. *J Am Acad Dermatol* 1986;15:211–219.
413. Reyes E, Alarcón-Segovia D. Leg ulcers in the primary APL syndrome. Report of a case with a peculiar proliferative small vessel vasculopathy. *Clin Exper Rheumatol* 1991;9:63–66.
414. Alarcón-Segovia D, Osmundson PJ. Peripheral vascular syndromes associated with systemic lupus erythematosus. *Ann Intern Med* 1965;62:907–919.
415. Alegre VA, Winkelman RK. Histopathologic and immunofluorescence study of skin lesions associated with circulating lupus anti-coagulant. *J Am Acad Dermatol* 1988;19:117–124.
416. Dodd HJ, Sarkany I, O'Shaughnessy D. Widespread cutaneous necrosis associated with the lupus anticoagulant. *Clin Exp Dermatol* 1985;10:581–586.
417. Frances C, Boisnic S, LeFebvre CH, et al. Manifestations cutanées rares au cours du lupus: nécrose cutanée étendue superficielle. *Ann Dermatol Venereol* 1986;113:976–977.
418. Frances C, Tribout B, Boisnic S. Cutaneous necrosis associated with the lupus anticoagulant. *Dermatologica* 1989;178:194–201.
419. Wolf P, Soyer HP, Auer-Grumbach P. Widespread cutaneous necrosis in a patient with rheumatoid arthritis associated with aCL antibodies. *Arch Dermatol* 1991;127:1739–1740.
420. O'Neill A, Gatenby PA, McGaw B, et al. Widespread cutaneous necrosis associated with cardiolipin antibodies. *J Am Acad Dermatol* 1990;22:356–359.
421. Del Castillo LF, Soria C, Schoendorff C, et al. Widespread cutaneous necrosis and APL antibodies: two episodes related to surgical manipulation and urinary tract infection. *J Am Acad Dermatol* 1997;36:872–875.
422. Amster MS, Conway J, Zeid M, et al. Cutaneous necrosis resulting from protein S deficiency and increased APL antibody in a patient with systemic lupus erythematosus. *J Am Acad Dermatol* 1993;29:853–857.
423. Gibson GE, Gibson LE, Drage LA, et al. Skin necrosis secondary to low-molecular weight heparin in a patient with APL antibody syndrome. *J Am Acad Dermatol* 1997;37:855–859.
424. Abernethy ML, McGuinn J, Callen JP. Widespread cutaneous necrosis as the initial manifestation of the APL antibody syndrome. *J Rheumatol* 1995;22:1380–1383.
425. Mueh JR, Herbst KD, Rapaport SI. Thrombosis in patients with the lupus anticoagulant. *Ann Intern Med* 1980;92: 156–159.
426. Olive D, Andre E, Brocard O, et al. Lupus erythemateux dissemine revele par des thrombophlebites des membres inferieurs. *Arch Fr Pediatr* 1979;36:807–811.
427. Davies GE, Triplett DA. Corticosteroid-associated blue toe syndrome: role of APL antibodies. *Ann Intern Med* 1990;113: 893–895.
428. Kaufman JL, Karmody AM, Leather RP. Atheroembolism and microthromboembolic syndromes (the blue toe syndrome and disseminated atheroembolism). In: Rutherford RB, ed. *Vascular Surgery, 3rd ed.* Philadelphia: W.B. Saunders, 1989:565–572.
429. Williams H, Laurent R, Gibson T. The lupus coagulation inhibitor and venous thrombosis: a report of four cases. *Clin Lab Haematol* 1980;2:139–144.
430. Digre KB, Durcan FJ, Branch DW, et al. Amaurosis fugax associated with APL antibodies. *Ann Neurol* 1989;25:228–232.
431. Kleiner RC, Najarian LV, Schatten S, et al. Vaso-occlusive retinopathy associated with APL antibodies (lupus anticoagulant retinopathy). *Ophthalmology* 1989;96:896–904.
432. Asherson RA. Subungual splinter haemorrhages: a new sign of the APL coagulopathy? *Ann Rheum Dis* 1990;49:268–271.
433. Sulli A, Pizzorni C, Cutolo M. Nailfold videocapillaroscopy abnormalities in patients with APL antibodies. *J Rheumatol* 2000;27:1574–1576.
434. Blanc P, Barki J, Fabre JM, et al. Superior mesenteric vein thrombosis associated with aCL antibody without autoimmune disease [letter]. *Am J Hematol* 1995;48:137.
435. Liu WH, Lan JL, Chen DY, et al. Renal vein thrombosis in Chinese systemic lupus erythematosus with high titre aCL antibody [letter]. *Br J Rheumatol* 1992;31:787–788.
436. Bregani ER, Corneo G, Pogliani EM. Antiphospholipid antibodies and splenic thrombosis in a patient with idiopathic myelofibrosis (APL antibodies and thrombosis). *Haematologica* 1992;77:516–517.
437. Keegan AD, Brooks LT, Painter DM. Hepatic infarction and nodular regenerative hyperplasia of the liver with associated

aCL antibodies in a young woman. *J Clin Gastroenterol* 1994; 18:309–313.

438. Asherson RA, Chan JKH, Harris EN, et al. Anticardiolipin antibody, recurrent thrombosis and warfarin withdrawal. *Ann Rheum Dis* 1985;44:823–825.
439. Averbuch M, Levo Y. Budd-Chiari syndrome as the major thrombotic complication of systemic lupus erythematosus with the lupus anticoagulant. *Ann Rheum Dis* 1986;45:435–437.
440. Levine SR, Welch KMA. The spectrum of neurologic disease associated with APL antibodies: lupus anticoagulants and aCL antibodies. *Arch Neurol* 1987;44:876–883.
441. Briley DP, Coull BM, Goodnight Jr. SH. Neurological disease associated with APL antibodies. *Ann Neurol* 1989;25:221–227.
442. Levine SR, Deegan MJ, Futrell N, et al. Cerebrovascular and neurologic disease associated with APL antibodies: 48 cases. *Neurology* 1990;40:1181–1189.
443. Munts AG, van Genderen PJ, Dippel DW, et al. Coagulation disorders in young adults with acute cerebral ischaemia. *J Neurol* 1998;245:21–25.
444. Landi G, Calloni MV, Sabbadini MG, et al. Recurrent ischemic attacks in two young adults with lupus anticoagulant. *Stroke* 1983;14:377–379.
445. Levine SR, Welch KMA. Cerebrovascular ischemia associated with lupus anticoagulant. *Stroke* 1987;18:257–263.
446. Frances C, Papo T, Wechsler B, et al. Sneddon syndrome with or without APL antibodies. A comparative study in 46 patients. Medicine (Baltimore), 1999;78:209–219.
447. Harris EN, Gharavi AE, Asherson RA, et al. Cerebral infarction in systemic lupus: association with aCL antibodies. *Clin Exper Rheumatol* 1984;2:47–51.
448. Pope JM, Canny CLB, Bell DA. Cerebral ischemic events associated with endocarditis, retinal vascular disease, and lupus anticoagulant. *Am J Med* 1991;90:299–309.
449. Asherson RA, Khamashta MA, Gil A, et al. Cerebrovascular disease and APL antibodies in systemic lupus erythematosus, lupus-like disease, and the primary APL syndrome. *Am J Med* 1989;86:391–399.
450. Mesa HA, Lang B, Schumacher M, et al. Sneddon's syndrome and phospholipid antibodies. *Clin Rheumatol* 1993;12:253–256.
451. Kurita A, Hasunuma T, Mochio S, et al. A young case with multi-infarct dementia associated with lupus anticoagulant. *Intern Med* 1994;33:373–375.
452. Jura E, Palasik W, Meurer M, et al. Sneddon's syndrome (livedo reticularis and cerebrovascular lesions) with APL antibodies and severe dementia in young man: a case report. *Acta Neurol Scand* 1994;89:143–146.
453. Asherson RA, Mercey D, Phillips G, et al. Recurrent stroke and multi-infarct dementia in systemic lupus erythematosus: association with APL antibodies. *Ann Rheum Dis* 1987;46:605–611.
454. Molad Y, Sidi Y, Gornish M, et al. Lupus anticoagulant: correlation with magnetic resonance imaging of brain lesions. *J Rheumatol* 1992;19:556–561.
455. Levine SR, Kieran S, Puzio K, et al. Cerebral venous thrombosis with lupus anticoagulants: report of two cases. *Stroke* 1987; 18:801–804.
456. Hachulla E, Michon-Pasturel U, Leys D, et al. Cerebral magnetic resonance imaging in patients with or without APL antibodies. *Lupus* 1998;7:124–131.
457. Amoroso A, Del Porto F, Garzia P, et al. Primary APL syndrome and cerebral atrophy: a rare association? *Am J Med Sci* 1999; 317:425–428.
458. Oyama H, Kojima H, Ohta Y, et al. Abnormal cerebral blood flow associated with APL antibody syndrome — four case reports. *Neurol Med Chir* (Tokyo) 1997;37:41–48.
459. Cuadrado MJ, Khamashta MA, Ballesteros A, et al. Can neurologic manifestations of Hughes (APL) syndrome be distinguished from multiple sclerosis? Analysis of 27 patients and review of the literature. *Medicine* (Baltimore) 2000;79:57–68.
460. Fulford KWM, Catterall RD, Delhanty JJ, et al. A collagen disorder of the nervous system presenting as multiple sclerosis. *Brain* 1972;95:373–386.
461. Lavalle C, Pizarro S, Drenkard C, et al. Transverse myelitis: a manifestation of systemic lupus erythematosus strongly associated with APL antibodies. *J Rheumatol* 1990;17:34–37.
462. Hardie RJ, Isenberg DA. Tetraplegia as a presenting feature of systemic lupus erythematosus complicated by pulmonary hypertension. *Ann Rheum Dis* 1985;44:491–493.
463. Oppenheimer S, Hoffbrand BI. Optic neuritis and myelopathy in systemic lupus erythematosus. *Can J Neurol Sci* 1986;13: 129–132.
464. Harris EN, Gharavi AE, Mackworth-Young CG, et al. Lupoid sclerosis: a possible pathogenetic role for APL antibodies. *Ann Rheum Dis* 1985;44:281–283.
465. Marabani M, Zoma A, Hadley D, et al. Transverse myelitis occurring during pregnancy in a patient with systemic lupus erythematosus. *Ann Rheum Dis* 1989;48:160–162.
466. Markusse HM, Haan J, Tan WD, et al. Anterior spinal artery syndrome in systemic lupus erythematosus. *Br J Rheumatol* 1989;28:344–346.
467. Mok CC, Lau CS, Chan EY, et al. Acute transverse myelopathy in systemic lupus erythematosus: clinical presentation, treatment, and outcome. *J Rheumatol* 1998;25:467–473.
468. Watts MT, Greaves M, Clearkin LG, et al. Anti-phospholipid antibodies and ischaemic optic neuropathy [letter]. *Lancet* 1990;335:613.
469. Asherson RA, Merry P, Acheson JF, et al. Antiphospholipid antibodies: a risk factor for occlusive ocular vascular disease in systemic lupus erythematosus and the "primary" APL syndrome. *Ann Rheum Dis* 1989;48:358–361.
470. Tolosa-Vilella C, Ordi-Ros J, Jordana-Comajuncosa R, et al. Occlusive ocular vascular disease and APL antibodies [letter]. *Ann Rheum Dis* 1990;49:203.
471. Heckerling PS, Froelich CJ, Schade SG. Retinal vein thrombosis in a patient with pernicious anemia and aCL antibodies. *J Rheumatol* 1989;16:1144–1146.
472. Wiechens B, Schroder JO, Potzsch B, et al. Primary APL antibody syndrome and retinal occlusive vasculopathy. *Am J Ophthalmol* 1997;123:848–850.
473. Cobo-Soriano R, Sanchez-Ramon S, Aparicio MJ, et al. Antiphospholipid antibodies and retinal thrombosis in patients without risk factors: a prospective case-control study. *Am J Ophthalmol* 1999;128:725–732.
474. Silvestrini M, Cupini LM, Matteis M, et al. Migraine in patients with stroke and APL antibodies. *Headache* 1993;33: 421–426.
475. Silvestrini M, Matteis M, Troisi E, et al. Migrainous stroke and the APL antibodies. *Eur Neurol* 1994;34:316–319.
476. Tsakiris DA, Kappos L, Reber G, et al. Lack of association between APL antibodies and migraine. *Thromb Haemost* 1993;69:415–417.
477. Herkes GK, Cohen MG, Podgorski M, et al. Cerebral systemic lupus erythematosus with apnea in a patient with cardiolipin antibodies and oligoclonal bands. *J Rheumatol* 1988;15:523–524.
478. Khamashta MA, Gil A, Anciones B, et al. Chorea in systemic lupus erythematosus: association with APL antibodies. *Ann Rheum Dis* 1988;47:681–683.
479. Hatron P-Y, Bouchez B, Wattel A, et al. Chorea, systemic lupus erythematosus, circulating lupus anticoagulant. *J Rheumatol* 1986;13:991–993.
480. Hodges JR. Chorea and the lupus anticoagulant. *J Neurol Neurosurg Psychiatry* 1987;50:368–369.

481. Besbas N, Damarguc I, Ozen S, et al. Association of APL antibodies with systemic lupus erythematosus in a child presenting with chorea: a case report. *Eur J Pediatr* 1994;153:891–893.
482. Shimomura T, Takahashi S, Takahashi S. [Chorea associated with APL antibodies]. *Rinsho Shinkeigaku* 1992;32:989–993.
483. Asherson RA, Derksen RHWM, Harris EN, et al. Chorea in systemic lupus erythematosus and "lupus-like" disease: association with APL antibodies. *Sem Arthritis Rheum* 1987;16:253–259.
484. Rose CD, Goldsmith DP. Childhood adrenal insufficiency, chorea, and APL antibodies. *Ann Rheum Dis* 1990;49:421–423.
485. Kirk A, Harding SR. Cardioembolic caudate infarction as a cause of hemichorea in lupus anticoagulant syndrome. *Can J Neurol Sci* 1993;20:162–164.
486. Cervera R, Asherson RA, Font J, et al. Chorea in the APL syndrome. Clinical, radiologic, and immunologic characteristics of 50 patients from our clinics and the recent literature. *Medicine* (Baltimore), 1997;76:203–212.
487. Ziporen L, Shoenfeld Y, Levy Y, et al. Neurological dysfunction and hyperactive behavior associated with APL antibodies. A mouse model. *J Clin Invest* 1997;100:613–619.
488. Menon S, Jameson-Shortall E, Newman SP, et al. A longitudinal study of aCL antibody levels and cognitive functioning in systemic lupus erythematosus. *Arthritis Rheum* 1999;42:735–741.
489. Hanly JG, Hong C, Smith S, et al. A prospective analysis of cognitive function and aCL antibodies in systemic lupus erythematosus. *Arthritis Rheum* 1999;42:728–734.
490. Moder KG, Miller TD, Tazelaar HD. Cardiac involvement in systemic lupus erythematosus. *Mayo Clin Proc* 1999;74:275–284.
491. Asherson RA, Harris N, Gharavi A, et al. Myocardial infarction in systemic lupus erythematosus and "lupus-like" disease. *Arthritis Rheum* 1986;29:1292–1293.
492. Petri M, Perez-Gutthann S, Spence D, et al. Risk factors for coronary artery disease in patients with systemic lupus erythematosus. *Am J Med* 1992;93:513–519.
493. Petri M, Spence D, Bone LR, et al. Coronary artery disease risk factors in the Hopkins Lupus Cohort: prevalence, patient recognition, and preventive practices. *Medicine* 1992;71:291–302.
494. Maaravi Y, Raz E, Gilon D, et al. Cerebrovascular accident and myocardial infarction associated with aCL antibodies in a young woman with systemic lupus erythematosus. *Ann Rheum Dis* 1989;48:853–855.
495. Brown JH, Doherty CC, Allen DC, et al. Fatal cardiac failure due to myocardial microthrombi in systemic lupus erythematosus. *Br Med J* 1988;296:1505.
496. Murphy JJ, Leach IH. Findings at necropsy in the heart of a patient with aCL syndrome. *Br Heart J* 1989;62:61–64.
497. Anderson D, Bell D, Lodge R, et al. Recurrent cerebral ischemia and mitral valve vegetation in a patient with APL antibodies. *J Rheumatol* 1987;14:839–841.
498. Asherson RA, Lubbe WF. Cerebral and valve lesions in systemic lupus erythematosus. Association with APL antibodies? *J Rheumatol* 1988;15:539–543.
499. Galve E, Ordi J, Barquinero J, et al. Valvular heart disease in the primary APL syndrome. *Ann Intern Med* 1992;116:293–298.
500. Leung W-H, Wong K-L, Lau C-P, et al. Association between APL antibodies and cardiac abnormalties in patients with systemic lupus erythematosus. *Am J Med* 1990;89:411–419.
501. Chartash EK, Lans DM, Paget SA, et al. Aortic insufficiency and mitral regurgitation in patients with systemic lupus erythematosus and the APL syndrome. *Am J Med* 1989;86:407–412.
502. Khamashta MA, Harris EN, Gharavi AE, et al. Immune mediated mechanism for thrombosis: APL antibody binding to platelet membranes. *Ann Rheum Dis* 1988;47:849–854.
503. Ford PH, Ford SE, Lillicrap DP. Association of lupus anticoagulant with severe valvular heart disease in SLE. *J Rheumatol* 1988;15:597–600.
504. Asherson RA, Gibson DG, Evans DW, et al. Diagnostic and therapeutic problems in two patients with APL antibodies, heart valve lesions, and transient ischaemic attacks. *Ann Rheum Dis* 1988;47:947–953.
505. Martinez-Lavin M, Fonseca C, Amigo MC, et al. Antiphospholipid syndrome in patients with cyanotic congenital heart disease. *Clin Exper Rheumatol* 1995;13:489–491.
506. Petri M. Pancreatitis: a rare manifestation of systemic lupus erythematosus. *Rheumatology Review* 1992;1:75–79.
507. Lubbe WF, Asherson RA. Intracardiac thrombus in systemic lupus erythematosus associated with lupus anticoagulant. *Arthritis Rheum* 1988;31:1453–1454.
508. Leventhal LJ, Borofsky MA, Bergey PD, et al. Antiphospholipid antibody syndrome with right atrial thrombosis mimicking an atrial myxoma. *Am J Med* 1989;87:111–113.
509. Baum RA, Jundt JW. Intracardiac thrombosis and APL antibodies: a case report and review of the literature. *South Med J* 1994;87:928–932.
510. O'Hickey S, Skinner C, Beattie J. Life-threatening right ventricular thrombosis in association with phospholipid antibodies. *Br Heart J* 1993;70:279–281.
511. Kattwinkel N, Villanueva AG, Labib SB, et al. Myocardial infarction caused by cardiac microvasculopathy in a patient with the primary APL syndrome. *Ann Intern Med* 1992;116:974–976.
512. Ingram SB, Goodnight Jr. SH, Bennett RM. An unusual syndrome of a devastating noninflammatory vasculopathy associated with aCL antibodies: report of two cases. *Arthritis Rheum* 1987;30:1167–1172.
513. Greisman SG, Thayaparan RS, Godwin TA, et al. Occlusive vasculopathy in systemic lupus erythematosus: association with aCL antibody. *Arch Intern Med* 1991;151:389–392.
514. Alarcón-Segovia D, Cardiel MH, Reyes E. Antiphospholipid arterial vasculopathy. *J Rheumatol* 1989;16:762–767.
515. Lecerf V, Alhenc-Gelas M, Laurian C, et al. Antiphospholipid antibodies and atherosclerosis. *Am J Med* 1992;92:575–576.
516. Kupferminc MJ, Eldor A, Steinman N, et al. Increased frequency of genetic thrombophilia in women with complications of pregnancy. *N Engl J Med* 1999;340:9–13.
517. Branch DW, Silver RM, Blackwell JL, et al. Outcome of treated pregnancies in women with APL syndrome: an update of the Utah experience. *Obstet Gynecol* 1992;80:614–620.
518. Laskin CA, Bombardier C, Hannah ME, et al. Prednisone and aspirin in women with autoantibodies and unexplained recurrent fetal loss. *N Engl J Med* 1997;337:148–153.
519. Cowchock S. Autoantibodies and pregnancy loss [editorial]. *N Engl J Med* 1997;337:197–198.
520. Scott JR, Rote NS, Branch DW. Immunologic aspects of recurrent abortion and fetal death. *Obstet Gynecol* 1987;70:645–656.
521. Simpson JL, Carson SA, Chesney C, et al. Lack of association between APL antibodies and first-trimester spontaneous abortion: prospective study of pregnancies detected within 21 days of conception. *Fertil Steril* 1998;69:814–820.
522. Grandone E, Margaglione M, Colaizzo D, et al. Genetic susceptibility to pregnancy-related venous thromboembolism: roles of factor V Leiden, prothrombin G20210A, and methylenetetrahydrofolate reductase C677T mutations. *Am J Obstet Gynecol* 1998;179:1324–1328.
523. Dumenco LL, Blair AJ, Sweeney JD. The results of diagnostic studies for thrombophilia in a large group of patients with a personal or family history of thrombosis. *Am J Clin Pathol* 1998;110:673–682.
524. Kaleli B, Kaleli I, Aktan E, et al. Antiphospholipid antibodies in eclamptic women. *Gynecol Obstet Invest* 1998;45:81–84.
525. Branch DW, Andres R, Digre KB, et al. The association of APL antibodies with severe preeclampsia. *Obstet Gynecol* 1989;73:541–545.

526. van Pampus MG, Dekker GA, Wolf H, et al. High prevalence of hemostatic abnormalities in women with a history of severe preeclampsia. *Am J Obstet Gynecol* 1999;180:1146–1150.
527. Dekker GA, de Vries JI, Doelitzsch PM, et al. Underlying disorders associated with severe early-onset preeclampsia. *Am J Obstet Gynecol* 1995;173:1042–1048.
528. Dekker GA, van Geijn HP. Endothelial dysfunction in preeclampsia. Part II: reducing the adverse consequences of endothelial cell dysfunction in preeclampsia; therapeutic perspectives. *J Perinat Med* 1996;24:119–139.
529. Scott RAH. Anti-cardiolipin antibodies and pre-eclampsia. *Br J Obstet Gynaecol* 1987;94:604–605.
530. D'Anna R, Scilipoti A, Leonardi J, et al. Anticardiolipin antibodies in pre-eclampsia and intrauterine growth retardation. *Clin Exp Obstet Gynecol* 1997;24:135–137.
531. Martinez-Abundis E, Gonzalez-Ortiz M, Cortes-Llamas V, et al. Anticardiolipin antibodies and the severity of preeclampsia-eclampsia. *Gynecol Obstet Invest* 1999;48:168–171.
532. Nagayama K, Izumi N, Miyasaka Y, et al. Hemolysis, elevated liver enzymes, and low platelets syndrome associated with primary anti-phospholipid antibody syndrome. *Intern Med* 1997;36:661–666.
533. McMahon LP, Smith J. The HELLP syndrome at 16 weeks gestation: possible association with the APL syndrome. *Aust N Z J Obstet Gynaecol* 1997;37:313–314.
534. Ornstein MH, Rand JH. An association between refractory HELLP syndrome and APL antibodies during pregnancy; a report of 2 cases. *J Rheumatol* 1994;21:1360–1364.
535. Rix P, Stentoft J, Aunsholt NA, et al. Lupus anticoagulant and aCL antibodies in an obstetric population. *Acta Obstet Gynecol Scand* 1992;71:605–609.
536. Vogt E, Ng AK, Rote NS. A model for the APL antibody syndrome: monoclonal antiphosphatidylserine antibody induces intrauterine growth restriction in mice. *Am J Obstet Gynecol* 1996;174:700–707.
537. Wang Z, Fan Y, Wu G. [Relation between fetal intrauterine growth retardation and aCL antibodies]. *Chung Hua Fu Chan Ko Tsa Chih* 1997;32:623–625.
538. Petri M. Recurrent abortion and APL antibodies: aCL, lupus anticoagulant. In: Schlaff WD, Rock JA, eds. *Decision making in reproductive endocrinology and infertility*, Boston: Blackwell Scientific Publications, 1993:346–348.
539. Gilkeson RC, Patz EF, Jr., Culhane D, et al. Thoracic imaging features of patients with APL antibodies. *J Comput Assist Tomogr* 1998;22:241–244.
540. Asherson RA, Mackworth-Young CG, Boey ML, et al. Pulmonary hypertension in systemic lupus erythematosus. *Br Med J* 1983;287:1024–1025.
541. Chazova IE, Samsonov M, Aleksandrova EN, et al. [Phospholipid antibodies in primary pulmonary hypertension]. *Ter Arkh* 1994;66:20–23.
542. Nakagawa Y, Masuda M, Shiihara H, et al. Successful pulmonary thromboendarterectomy for chronic thromboembolic pulmonary hypertension associated with aCL antibodies: report of a case. *Surg Today* 1992;22:548–552.
543. Anderson NE, Ali MR. The lupus anticoagulant, pulmonary thromboembolism, and fatal pulmonary hypertension. *Ann Rheum Dis* 1984;43:760–763.
544. Luchi ME, Asherson RA, Lahita RG. Primary idiopathic pulmonary hypertension complicated by pulmonary arterial thrombosis. *Arthritis Rheum* 1992;35:700–705.
545. De Clerck LS, Michielsen PP, Ramael MR, et al. Portal and pulmonary vessel thrombosis associated with systemic lupus erythematosus and aCL antibodies. *J Rheumatol* 1991;18:1919–1921.
546. Crausman RS, Achenbach GA, Pluss WT, et al. Pulmonary capillaritis and alveolar hemorrhage associated with the APL antibody syndrome. *J Rheumatol* 1995;22:554–556.
547. Aronoff DM, Callen JP. Necrosing livedo reticularis in a patient with recurrent pulmonary hemorrhage. *J Am Acad Dermatol* 1997;37:300–302.
548. Maggiorini M, Knoblauch A, Schneider J, et al. Diffuse microvascular pulmonary thrombosis associated with primary APL antibody syndrome. *Eur Respir J* 1997;10:727–730.
549. Savin H, Huberman M, Kott E, et al. Fibrosing alveolitis associated with primary APL syndrome. *Brit J Rheumatol* 1994;33:977–980.
550. Kerr JE, Poe R, Kramer Z. Antiphospholipid antibody syndrome presenting as a refractory noninflammatory pulmonary vasculopathy. *Chest* 1997;112:1707–1710.
551. Kochenour NK, Branch DW, Rote NS, et al. A new postpartum syndrome associated with APL antibodies. *Obstet Gynecol* 1987;69:460–468.
552. Argento A, DiBenedetto RJ. ARDS and adrenal insufficiency associated with the APL antibody syndrome. *Chest* 1998;113:1136–1138.
553. Ghosh S, Walters HD, Joist JH, et al. Adult respiratory distress syndrome associated with APL antibody syndrome. *J Rheumatol* 1993;20:1406–1408.
554. Kant KS, Pollak VE, Weiss MA, et al. Glomerular thrombosis in systemic lupus erythematosus: prevalence and significance. *Medicine* 1981;60:71–86.
555. Glueck HI, Kant KS, Weiss MA, et al. Thrombosis in systemic lupus erythematosus. Relation to the presence of circulating anticoagulants. *Arch Intern Med* 1985;145:1389–1395.
556. Nochy D, Daugas E, Droz D, et al. The intrarenal vascular lesions associated with primary APL syndrome. *J Am Soc Nephrol* 1999;10:507–518.
557. Kincaid-Smith P, Fairley KF, Kloss M. Lupus anticoagulant associated with renal thrombotic microangiopathy and pregnancy-related renal failure. *Q J Med* 1988;69:795–815.
558. Leaker B, McGregor A, Griffiths M, et al. Insidious loss of renal function in patients with aCL antibodies and absence of overt nephritis. *Br J Rheumatol* 1991;30:422–425.
559. Spronk PE, Bootsma H, Nikkels PG, et al. A new class of lupus nephropathy associated with APL antibodies [letter]. *Br J Rheumatol* 1994;33:686–687.
560. Jouquan J, Pennec Y, Mottier D, et al. Accelerated hypertension associated with lupus anticoagulant and false-positive VDRL in systemic lupus erythematosus [letter]. *Arthritis Rheum* 1986;29:147.
561. Asherson RA. The catastrophic APL syndrome. *J Rheumatol* 1992;19:508–512.
562. Ostuni PA, Lazzarin P, Pengo V, et al. Renal artery thrombosis and hypertension in a 13 year old girl with APL syndrome. *Ann Rheum Dis* 1990;49:184–187.
563. Pérez-Vázquez ME, Cabiedes J, Cabral AR, et al. Decrease in serum APL antibody levels upon development of nephrotic syndrome in patients with systemic lupus erythematosus: relationship to urinary loss of IgG and other factors. *Am J Med* 1992;92:357–362.
564. Stone JH, Amend WJ, Criswell LA. Outcome of renal transplantation in systemic lupus erythematosus. *Semin Arthritis Rheum* 1997;27:17–26.
565. Stone JH, Amend WJ, Criswell LA. Antiphospholipid antibody syndrome in renal transplantation: occurrence of clinical events in 96 consecutive patients with systemic lupus erythematosus. *Am J Kidney Dis* 1999;34:1040–1047.
566. Asherson RA, Hughes GRV. Hypoadrenalism, Addison's disease and APL antibodies. *J Rheumatol* 1991;18:1–3.
567. Satta MA, Corsello SM, Della Casa S, et al. Adrenal insufficiency as the first clinical manifestation of the primary APL

antibody syndrome. *Clin Endocrinol* (Oxford), 2000;52: 123–126.
568. Yap AS, Powell EE, Yelland CE, et al. Lupus anticoagulant. *Ann Intern Med* 1989;111:262–263.
569. Lenaerts J, Vanneste S, Knockaert D, et al. SLE and acute Addisonian crisis due to bilateral adrenal haemorrhage association with APL antibodies. *Clin Exp Rheumatol* 1991;9:407–409.
570. Rao RH, Vagnucci AH, Amico JA. Bilateral massive adrenal haemorrhage: early recognition and treatment. *Ann Intern Med* 1989;110:227–235.
571. Pelkonen P, Simell O, Rasi V, et al. Venous thrombosis associated with lupus anticoagulant and aCL antibodies. *Acta Paediatr Scand* 1988;77:767–772.
572. Siu SCB, Kitzman DW, Sheedy PF, et al. Adrenal insufficiency from bilateral adrenal hemorrhage. *Mayo Clin Proc* 1990;65: 664–670.
573. Inam S, Sidki K, Al-Marshedy A-R, et al. Addison's disease, hypertension, renal and hepatic microthrombosis in "primary" APL syndrome. *Postgrad Med J* 1991;67:385–388.
574. Ames DE, Asherson RA, Ayres B, et al. Bilateral adrenal infarction, hypoadrenalism and splinter haemorrhages in the 'primary' APL syndrome. *Br J Rheumatol* 1992;31:117–120.
575. Asherson RA, Hughes GRV. Recurrent deep vein thrombosis and Addison's disease in "primary" APL syndrome. *J Rheumatol* 1989;16:378–380.
576. Walz BAE, Silver RD. Addison's disease in "primary" APL syndrome. *J Rheumatol* 1990;17:115.
577. Komesaroff PA, Yung AP, Topliss DJ. Postoperative primary adrenal failure in a patient with aCL antibodies. *J Rheumatol* 1991;18:88–90.
578. Carrette S, Jobin F. Acute adrenal insufficiency as a manifestation of the aCL syndrome? *Ann Rheum Dis* 1989;48:430–431.
579. Carlisle E, Leslie W. Primary hypoadrenalism in a patient with a lupus anticoagulant. *J Rheumatol* 1990;17:1405–1407.
580. Alperin N, Babu S, Weinstein A. Acute adrenal insufficiency and APL syndrome. *Ann Intern Med* 1989;111:950.
581. Denninger MH, Chait Y, Casadevall N, et al. Cause of portal or hepatic venous thrombosis in adults: the role of multiple concurrent factors. *Hepatology* 2000;31:587–591.
582. Egesel T, Buyukasik Y, Dundar SV, et al. The role of natural anticoagulant deficiencies and factor V Leiden in the development of idiopathic portal vein thrombosis. *J Clin Gastroenterol* 2000;30:66–71.
583. Collier JD, Sale J, Friend PJ, et al. Graft loss and the APL syndrome following liver transplantation. *J Hepatol* 1998;29: 999–1003.
584. Asherson RA, Harris EN, Gharavi AE, et al. Aortic arch syndrome associated with aCL antibodies and the lupus anticoagulant: comment on Ferrante paper. *Arthritis Rheum* 1983;26:594–595.
585. Drew P, Asherson RA, Zuk RJ, et al. Aortic occlusion in systemic lupus erythematosus associated with APL antibodies. *Ann Rheum Dis* 1987;46:612–616.
586. Ferrante FM, Myerson GE, Goldman JA. Subclavian artery thrombosis mimicking the aortic arch syndrome in systemic lupus erythematosus. *Arthritis Rheum* 1982;25:1501–1504.
587. Jindal BK, Martin MFR, Gayner A. Gangrene developing after minor surgery in a patient with undiagnosed systemic lupus erythematosus and lupus anticoagulant. *Ann Rheum Dis* 1983; 42:347–349.
588. Bird AG, Lendrum R, Asherson RA, et al. Disseminated intravascular coagulation, APL antibodies, and ischaemic necrosis of extremities. *Ann Rheum Dis* 1987;46:251–255.
589. Collins Jr. RD. Catastrophic arterial thrombosis associated with an unsuspected aCL antibody, following pyelography [letter]. *Arthritis Rheum* 1989;32:1490–1491.
590. Harris EN, Hughes GRV, Gharavi AE. Antiphospholipid antibodies: an elderly statesman dons new garments. *J Rheumatol* 1987;14:208–213.
591. Rauch J, Tannenbaum H, Senécal J-L, et al. Polyfunctional properties of hybridoma lupus anticoagulant antibodies. *J Rheumatol* 1987;14:132–137.
592. Rauch J, Meng Q-H, Tannenbaum H. Lupus anticoagulant and antiplatelet properties of human hybridoma autoantibodies. *J Immunol* 1987;139:2598–2604.
593. Harris EN, Asherson RA, Gharavi AE, et al. Thrombocytopenia in SLE and related autoimmune disorders: association with aCL antibody. *Br J Haematol* 1985;59:227–230.
594. Harris EN, Gharavi AE, Hegde U, et al. Anticardiolipin antibodies in autoimmune thrombocytopenic purpura. *Br J Haematol* 1985;59:231–234.
595. Fabris F, Steffan A, Cordiano I, et al. Specific antiplatelet autoantibodies in patients with APL antibodies and thrombocytopenia. *Eur J Haematol* 1994;53:232–236.
596. Nojima J, Suehisa E, Kuratsune H, et al. High prevalence of thrombocytopenia in SLE patients with a high level of aCL antibodies combined with lupus anticoagulant. *Am J Hematol* 1998;58:55–60.
597. Funauchi M, Hamada K, Enomoto H, et al. Characteristics of the clinical findings in patients with idiopathic thrombocytopenic purpura who are positive for anti-phospholipid antibodies. *Intern Med* 1997;36:882–885.
598. Guzman J, Cabral AR, Cabiedes J, et al. Antiphospholipid antibodies in patients with idiopathic autoimmune haemolytic anemia. *Autoimmunity* 1994;18:51–56.
599. Sthoeger Z, Sthoeger D, Green L, et al. The role of aCL autoantibodies in the pathogenesis of autoimmune hemolytic anemia in systemic lupus erythematosus. *J Rheumatol* 1993; 20:2058–2061.
600. Moore J, Ma DD, Concannon A. Non-malignant bone marrow necrosis: a report of two cases. *Pathology* 1998;30:318–320.
601. Paydas S, Kocak R, Zorludemir S, et al. Bone marrow necrosis in APL syndrome. *J Clin Pathol* 1997;50:261–262.
602. Becton DL, Stine KC. Transient lupus anticoagulants associated with hemorrhage rather than thrombosis: the hemorrhagic lupus anticoagulant syndrome. *J Pediatr* 1997;130:998–1000.
603. Sands JJ, Nudo SA, Ashford RG, et al. Antibodies to topical bovine thrombin correlate with access thrombosis. *Am J Kidney Dis* 2000;35:796–801.
604. Petri M, Baker J, Goldman D. Risk factors for avascular necrosis in SLE [abstract]. *Arthritis Rheum* 1992;35:S110.
605. Mok MY, Farewell VT, Isenberg DA. Risk factors for avascular necrosis of bone in patients with systemic lupus erythematosus: is there a role for APL antibodies? *Ann Rheum Dis* 2000; 59:462–467.
606. Cozen L, Wallace DJ. Avascular necrosis in systemic lupus erythematosus: clinical associations and a 47-year perspective. *Am J Orthop* 2000;27:352–354.
607. Asherson RA, Liote F, Page B, et al. Avascular necrosis of bone and APL antibodies in systemic lupus erythematosus. *J Rheumatol* 1993;20:284–288.
608. Nagasawa K, Ishii Y, Mayumi T, et al. Avascular necrosis of bone in systemic lupus erythematosus: possible role of haemostatic abnormalities. *Ann Rheum Dis* 1989;48:672–676.
609. Mok CC, Lau CS, Wong RW. Risk factors for avascular bone necrosis in systemic lupus erythematosus. *Br J Rheumatol* 1998;37:895–900.
610. Mont MA, Glueck CJ, Pacheco I, et al. Risk factors for osteonecrosis in systemic lupus erythematosus. *J Rheumatol* 1997;24:654–662.
611. Egan RM, Munn RK. Catastrophic APL antibody syndrome presenting with multiple thromboses and sites of avascular necrosis. *J Rheumatol* 1994;21:2376–2379.

612. Mok MY, Isenberg DA. Avascular necrosis of a single vertebral body, an atypical site of disease in a patient with SLE and secondary APLS. *Ann Rheum Dis* 2000;59:494–495.
613. Brewster JA, Quenby SM, Alfirevic Z. Intra-uterine death due to umbilical cord thrombosis secondary to APL syndrome. *Lupus* 1999;8:558–559.
614. Silver RK, MacGregor SN, Pasternak JF, et al. Fetal stroke associated with elevated maternal aCL antibodies. *Obstet Gynecol* 1992;80:497–499.
615. Akanli LF, Trasi SS, Thuraisamy K, et al. Neonatal middle cerebral artery infarction: association with elevated maternal aCL antibodies. *Am J Perinatol* 1998;15:399–402.
616. de Klerk OL, de Vries TW, Sinnige LGF. An unusual cause of neonatal seizures in a newborn infant. *Pediatrics* 1997;100:E8.
617. Tabbutt S, Griswold WR, Ogino MT, et al. Multiple thromboses in a premature infant associated with maternal phospholipid antibody syndrome. *J Perinatol* 1994;14:66–70.
618. Brewster JA, Shaw NJ, Farquharson RG. Neonatal and pediatric outcome of infants born to mothers with APL syndrome. *J Perinat Med* 1999;27:183–187.
619. Milliez J, Lelong F, Bayani N, et al. The prevalence of autoantibodies during third-trimester pregnancy complicated by hypertension or idiopathic fetal growth retardation. *Am J Obstet Gynecol* 1991;165:51–56.
620. Pollard JK, Scott JR, Branch DW. Outcome of children born to women treated during pregnancy for the APL syndrome. *Obstet Gynecol* 1992;80:365–368.
621. Moodley J, Bhoola V, Duursma J, et al. The association of APL antibodies with severe early-onset pre-eclampsia. *S Afr Med J* 1995;85:105–107.
622. Morgan M, Downs K, Chesterman CN, et al. Clinical analysis of 125 patients with the lupus anticoagulant. *Aust N Z J Med* 1993;23:151–156.
623. Lockshin MD. Which patients with APL antibody should be treated and how? *Rheum Dis Clin North Am* 1993;19:235–247.
624. Petri M. Hydroxychloroquine use in the Baltimore Lupus Cohort: effects on lipids, glucose and thrombosis. *Lupus* 1996; 5:S16–S22.
625. Canadian Hydroxychloroquine Study Group. A randomized study of the effect of withdrawing hydroxychloroquine sulfate in systemic lupus erythematosus. *N Engl J Med* 1991;324:150–154.
626. Julkunen H, Hedman C, Kauppi M. Thrombolysis for acute ischemic stroke in the primary APL syndrome. *J Rheumatol* 1997;24:181–183.
627. Takeuchi S, Obayashi T, Toyama J. Primary APL syndrome with acute myocardial infarction recanalised by PTCA. *Heart* 1998;79:96–98.
628. Chambers Jr JD, Haire HD, Deligonul U. Multiple early percutaneous transluminal coronary angioplasty failures related to lupus anticoagulant. *Am Heart J* 1996;132:189–190.
629. Nakajima T, Ando H, Ueno Y, et al. Successful thromboendarterectomy for chronic pulmonary embolism in a patient with systemic lupus erythematosus and APL syndrome. *Jpn Circ J* 1997;61:958–964.
630. Fischer M, McGehee W. Cerebral infarct, TIA and lupus inhibitor. *Neurology* 1986;36:1234–1237.
631. Young SM, Fischer M, Sigsbee A, et al. Cardiogenic brain embolism and lupus anticoagulant. *Ann Neurol* 1989;26:390–392.
632. Bern MM, Lokich JJ, Wallach SR, et al. Very low doses of warfarin can prevent thrombosis in central venous catheters. A randomized prospective trial. *Ann Intern Med* 1990;112:423–428.
633. Levine M, Hirsh J, Gent M, et al. Double-blind randomised trial of a very-low-dose warfarin for prevention of thromboembolism in stage IV breast cancer. *Lancet* 1994;343:886–889.
634. Thrombosis prevention trial: randomised trial of low-intensity oral anticoagulation with warfarin and low-dose aspirin in the primary prevention of ischaemic heart disease in men at increased risk. The Medical Research Council's General Practice Research Framework. *Lancet* 1998;351:233–241.
635. Lockshin MD. Answers to the APL-antibody syndrome? *N Engl J Med* 1995;332:1025–1027.
636. Nasr SZ, Parke AL. Thrombosis in the APL-antibody syndrome [letter]. *N Engl J Med* 1995;333:666.
637. Rapaport SI, Le DT. Thrombosis in the APL-antibody syndrome [letter]. *N Engl J Med* 1995;333:665.
638. Said PB, Martinuzzo ME, Carreras LO. Neutralization of lupus anticoagulant activity by human immunoglobulin in vitro. *Nouv Rev Fr Hematol* 1992;34:37–42.
639. Alarcón-Segovia D, Sánchez-Guerrero J. Correction of thrombocytopenia with small dose aspirin in the primary APL syndrome. *J Rheumatol* 1989;16:1359–1361.
640. Leuzzi RA, Davis GH, Cowchock FS, et al. Management of immune thrombocytopenic purpura associated with the APL antibody syndrome. *Clin Exp Rheumatol* 1997;15:197–200.
641. Espinola-Zavaleta N, Vargas-Barron J, Colmenares-Galvis T, et al. Echocardiographic evaluation of patients with primary APL syndrome. *Am Heart J* 1999;137:973–978.
642. Nesher G, Ilany J, Rosenmann D, et al. Valvular dysfunction in APL syndrome: prevalence, clinical features, and treatment. *Semin Arthritis Rheum* 1997;27:27–35.
643. Aziz A, Conway MD, Robertson HJ, et al. Acute optic neuropathy and transverse myelopathy in patients with APL antibody syndrome: favorable outcome after treatment with anticoagulants and glucocorticoids. *Lupus* 2000;9:307–310.
644. Aringer M, Smolen JS, Graninger WB. Severe infections in plasmapheresis-treated systemic lupus erythematosus. *Arthritis Rheum* 1998;41:414–420.
645. Weisman MH, Bluestein HG, Berner CM, et al. Reduction in circulating dsDNA antibody titer after administration of LJP 394. *J Rheumatol* 1997;24:314–318.
646. Iverson GM, Jones DS, Marquis D, et al. A chemically defined, toleragen-based approach for targeting anti-b2-glycoprotein I antibodies. *Lupus* 1998;7(suppl. 2):S166–S169.
647. Musso M, Porretto F, Crescimanno A, et al. Autologous peripheral blood stem and progenitor (CD34+) cell transplantation for systemic lupus erythematosus complicated by Evans syndrome. *Lupus* 1998;7:492–494.
648. Brodsky RA, Petri M, Smith BD, et al. Immunoblative high-dose cyclophosphamide without stem cell rescue for refractory, severe autoimmune disease. *Ann Int Med* 1998;129:1031–1035.
649. Brodsky RA, Sensenbrenner LL, Jones RJ. Complete remission in severe aplastic anemia after high-dose cyclophosphamide without bone marrow transplantation. *Blood* 1996;87:491–494.
650. Krause I, Blank M, Shoenfeld Y. Anti-DNA and APL antibodies in IVIG preparations: in vivo study in naive mice. *J Clin Immunol* 1998;18:52–60.
651. Shoenfeld Y, Krause I, Blank M. New methods of treatment in an experimental murine model of systemic lupus erythematosus induced by idiotypic manipulation. *Ann Rheum Dis* 1997; 56:5–11.
652. Andersson U, Bojork L, Skanson-Saphir U, et al. Pooled human IgG modulates cytokine production in lymphocytes and monocytes. *Immunol Rev* 1994;139:5–20.
653. Harris EN, Pierangeli SS. Utilization of intravenous immunoglobulin therapy to treat recurrent pregnancy loss in the APL syndrome: a review. *Scand J Rheumatol Suppl* 1998; 107:97–102.
654. Branch DW, Peaceman AM, Druzin M, et al. A multicenter, placebo-controlled pilot study of intravenous immune globulin treatment of APL syndrome during pregnancy. The Pregnancy Loss Study Group. *Am J Obstet Gynecol* 2000;182:122–127.
655. Gordon C, Kilby MD. Use of intravenous immunoglobulin

therapy in pregnancy in systemic lupus erythematosus and APL antibody syndrome. *Lupus* 1998;7:429–433.

656. Birdsall MA, Lockwood GM, Ledger WL, et al. Antiphospholipid antibodies in women having in-vitro fertilization. *Hum Reprod* 1996;11:1185–1189.
657. Sher G, Matzner W, Feinman M, et al. The selective use of heparin/aspirin therapy, alone or in combination with intravenous immunoglobulin G, in the management of APL antibody–positive women undergoing in vitro fertilization. *Am J Reprod Immunol* 1998;40:74–82.
658. Blank M, Shoenfeld Y, Cabilly S, et al. Prevention of experimental APL syndrome and endothelial cell activation by synthetic peptides. *Proc Natl Acad Sci U S A* 1999;96:5164–5168.
659. Blank M, George J, Barak V, et al. Oral tolerance to low dose b2-glycoprotein I: immunomodulation of experimental APL syndrome. *J Immunol* 1998;161:5303–5312.

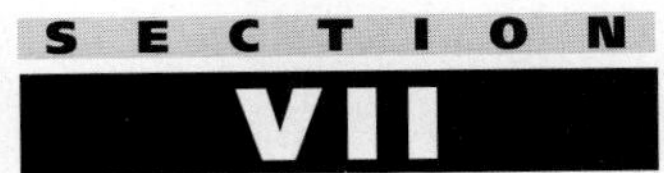

MANAGEMENT AND PROGNOSIS

53

PRINCIPLES OF THERAPY AND LOCAL MEASURES

DANIEL J. WALLACE

> Take pneumonia. It has been treated by bleeding, and got well. It has been treated by brandy and got well. It has been left to itself and got well. And the bleeders, the brandy givers, and the doers of nothing at all, respectively, have had a vast deal to say for themselves and against their rivals. And which of them are to be our guides and masters in the treatment of pneumonia? None of them for a single day, much less for always.
>
> —Latham (1)

FORMULATION OVERVIEW

One of the most difficult and misunderstood aspects of lupus is its management. Before therapy is initiated, the practitioner must determine the type of lupus and, on this basis, formulate a treatment program. Because the prognosis of each clinical subset differs widely, it is essential that the patient database be completed before an educational session is initiated. Have all blood tests, radiographic measures, biopsies, and scans providing information that can affect treatment been performed? Once these prerequisites have been met, the physician should be able to answer the following questions:

1. Does the patient meet the American College of Rheumatology criteria for systemic lupus erythematosus (SLE)?
   a. If not, does the patient meet biopsy criteria for discoid lupus or subacute cutaneous lupus? If not, is the physician satisfied that the patient has SLE, in spite of lacking four criteria? (This distinction is a matter of clinical judgment.)
   b. If not, does the patient have an undifferentiated connective tissue disease (UCTD)? Some patients with clear-cut inflammatory arthritis, a positive antinuclear antibody (ANA), and constitutional symptoms are treated similarly to lupus patients (see Chapter 46, Differential Diagnosis and Disease Associations). About 14% with UCTD evolve to classical SLE.
   c. If so, are related disorders such as mixed connective tissue disease, scleroderma, and dermatopolymyositis excluded?
2. If the patient has SLE, is life-threatening organ involvement present? If not, does the patient have mild SLE?
3. Which subset best describes the disease? Does a particular aspect of the patient's disease require specific considerations, intervention, or counseling (e.g., antiphospholipid syndrome, Ro (SSA) positivity, seizures, inappropriate behavior, concurrent fibromyalgia)?

I occasionally come across patients who have been labeled as having SLE when in fact they do not. The implications of telling a patient that he or she has lupus are tremendous. The emotional and psychologic effects of receiving this diagnosis open up new worlds of powerful and expensive medications, influence career planning and family life, alter one's productivity and lifestyle, and in the United States, makes it difficult to obtain health, life, or disability insurance. If you are not certain of the diagnosis, do not lock yourself in (2).

THE EDUCATIONAL SESSION

All newly diagnosed patients, as well as those who are new to the treating physician, deserve an educational session that includes concerned family members and loved ones. The session is supervised by the physician and may involve other health professionals or use audiovisual aids. Several studies have demonstrated that socioeconomic differences account for the widely divergent outcomes in those with SLE (3,4) (see Chapter 61). It is critical that the patient establish a relationship and a rapport with the physician, speak a common language, keep appointments, take medication as prescribed, have transportation to the medical office, and have access to medical assistance or advice 24 hours a day. Educational and informational literature relating to various aspects of the disease, including therapy, are available from organizations such as the Arthritis Foundation and the Lupus Foundation of America (see Appendix 2 for additional resource information).

TABLE 53.1. ISSUES TO BE COVERED IN THE EDUCATIONAL SESSION

1. What is lupus, and what are its causes?
2. Many types of lupus exist. You have (cutaneous, mild, organ-threatening) lupus erythematosus, which has a (fair, good, excellent) prognosis with treatment.
3. Physical measures include the use of heat, exercise, and diet. Physical, occupational, or vocational therapy may be helpful. Discuss general preventive strategies that relate to osteoporosis, avoiding infections, and immunizations.
4. Psychologic measures include dealing with fatigue, emotional stress (in appropriate cases), physical trauma, family and job problems, and pain. Genetic counseling and a discussion of lupus and pregnancy may be needed.
5. Medication includes salicylates, nonsteroidal antiinflammatory drugs, antimalarials, corticosteroids, cytotoxic drugs, and innovative therapies. Adjunctive measures such as vitamins, birth control, and the prevention of antiphospholipid antibody complications may be helpful.
6. Resource information includes patient education materials, counseling availability, self-help, websites, exercise groups, and useful telephone numbers.

The treatment of lupus erythematosus is divided into three categories: (i) physical and psychologic measures, (ii) drug therapy, and (iii) surgery. The latter is employed occasionally, and the first is infrequently discussed. Table 53.1 summarizes the issues that should be discussed with the patient and family during the educational session.

GENERAL THERAPEUTIC CONSIDERATIONS

Rest And The Treatment Of Fatigue

Fatigue is present in at least one half and up to 87% of all patients with SLE, and it can be their most disabling symptom (5,6). Potentially reversible causes of fatigue should be ruled out first. These include anemia, fever, infection, hypothyroidism, hormonal deficiencies, hyperglycemia, and complications from medication. In SLE, fatigue may be related to cytokine dysfunction as well as to inflammation. The administration of certain cytokines is known to induce fatigue (7), and hypoimmune fatigue syndromes could reflect decreases of the stress response (8) (see Chapters 17, Neuroendocrine Immune Interactions: Principles and Relevance to Systemic Lupus).

Reduced muscle aerobic capacity may play a role (9). The concept of pacing is paramount in managing fatigue. Total bed rest can worsen fatigue as well as promote osteoporosis, muscle disuse, atrophy, and contractures. Overexertion and fatigue denial also are counterproductive. I encourage my patients to pace themselves. An hour or two of morning activity should be followed by a midmorning break. A couple of hours of late-morning activity could be followed by a restful lunch break. Periods of activity followed by periods of rest usually permit most patients with lupus to attain an improved level of functioning and productivity.

Treatment of fatigue requires consideration of the source and contributory factors. Iron deficiency anemia is common because of dietary deficiency, heavy menstrual periods, and/or blood loss resulting from the use of salicylates and nonsteroidal antiinflammatory drugs (NSAIDs). If the fatigue is caused by parenchymal pulmonary disease, oxygen may be helpful; if it is secondary to inflammation, antiinflammatory drugs are used. In addition to corticosteroids, quinacrine and hydroxychloroquine (Plaquenil, Sanofi) are cortical stimulants and may decrease fatigue in patients without organ-threatening involvement (10,11). Dehydroepiandrosterone (DHEA) and selective serotonin reuptake inhibitors [e.g., fluoxetine (Prozac, Dista)] can be useful. Many patients with SLE who have minimal disease activity and normal blood work (other than a positive ANA) complain of profound fatigue. Depression, fibromyalgia, and emotional stress must be excluded as causes. Three surveys have suggested that fibromyalgia or depression are the most common causes of fatigue in SLE (12–14). Secondary fibromyalgia with a concomitant sleep disorder is not uncommon. Some physicians empirically prescribe low doses of thyroid, vitamin B12 injections, or amphetamines for the nonspecific fatigue of SLE; however, the routine use of these agents should be discouraged. Occasionally, I have found methylphenidate hydrochloride (Ritalin, Novartis) to be useful in severe cases. In contrast, the use of agents that promote restorative sleep should be considered.

Exercise, Physical Therapy, and Rehabilitation

A major cause of fatigue in SLE is from deconditioning. Aerobic capacity is 62% of the average expected in healthy, age-matched females (15). Inflamed peripheral muscles in SLE may result in decreased aerobic exercise capacity (9,16). Exercise regimens improved physical functioning and fatigue in two abstracts (17,18). The patient with SLE should remain physically active and avoid excessive bed rest. Exercises that strengthen muscles and improve endurance while avoiding undue stress to inflamed joints are desirable. Activities such as swimming, walking, low-impact aerobics, and bicycling should be encouraged. Recreational activities involving fine-motor movements and placing stress on certain ligamentous and other supporting structures (e.g., bowling, rowing, weight lifting, golf, tennis, jogging) should be considered on an individual basis. Exercises involving sustained isometric contractions increase muscle strength more than isotonic exercises do. Physical measures, such as the use of local moist heat or cold, decrease joint pain and inflammation. Many patients benefit from a whirlpool bath (Jacuzzi), hot tub, or therapy pool, or from merely soaking in a tub of hot water.

Physical therapists instruct patients in strengthening and toning exercises, improved body mechanics, and gait training. No specific measures or treatment approaches are unique for patients with lupus. Joint deformities develop in approximately ten percent of patients; physical and occupational therapies to minimize deformities are desirable in this group. Splints are useful for most patients with carpal-tunnel syndrome related to SLE. Corrective-tendon surgery and joint replacement are helpful in advanced cases.

Occupational therapists instruct patients in the principles of energy conservation and joint protection. They evaluate activities of daily living and advise on the use of devices or aids, such as wrist splints, comb handles, and raised toilet seats, when needed.

Vocational rehabilitation may be important in retraining a patient with SLE who can no longer work in the sun (e.g., farmer, construction worker, fisherman) or perform tasks requiring fine hand-motor function (e.g., typist).

Tobacco Smoke and Alcohol

Smoking impairs oxygenation, raises blood pressure, and worsens Raynaud's among other adverse actions. Two studies have associated smoking with the formation of autoantibodies, including ANA (19,20). A study of 56 patients with SLE failed to show an immunosuppressive effect of tobacco, which has been held to improve ulcerative colitis (21). Brown et al. (22) correlated tobacco use with worse cutaneous-lupus activity than among nonsmokers. Additional comparisons have confirmed that chronic, cutaneous lupus is more common in lupus than in nonsmokers (23), as is SLE (24,25). A Japanese epidemiologic survey (26) associated smoking with a 2.3 odds ratio for developing SLE. Because tobacco smoke contains potentially lupogenic hydrazines (see Chapter 3, The Role of the Environment in Systemic Lupus Erythematosus and Associated Disorders), abstinence and avoiding second-hand smoke are important. The efficacy of antimalarials may be decreased in smokers, perhaps as a result of the effect of tobacco upon the cytochrome P450 enzyme system that metabolizes chloroquines (27).

Although alcohol can worsen reflux esophagitis common in SLE and is not advised in patients taking methotrexate, two studies have concluded that moderate alcohol use was inversely correlated with the presence of SLE (24,25).

Weather and Seasons

Changes in barometric pressure can aggravate stiffness and aching in patients with inflammatory arthritis (28). In other words, whether a climate is hot or cold or wet or dry per se does not influence joint symptoms; barometric alterations do (e.g., hot to cold or wet to dry). I counsel my patients with lupus to expect some increased stiffness and aching in these circumstances and not to feel that they have done anything wrong.

Does increased summer sunlight or seasonal changes affect SLE? In Norway, there are fewer flares in January and more sun sensitive rashes during the summer (29). Sixty-six French lupus patients had significantly more organ-threatening flares during the summer (30). Israeli patients had more phototoxicity in summer months (31), but more joint pains, weakness, fatigue, and Raynaud's during the winter (32).

Pain Management

Patients with lupus have an increased prevalence of pain management problems (33). Patients with inflammatory arthritis respond poorly to analgesics with no antiinflammatory effects. The use of propoxyphene, codeine, or pentazocine in SLE should be limited to postoperative management and other situations. These drugs can induce dependence, have short-lived effects, and do not affect the underlying problem. Antiinflammatory drugs (e.g., salicylates, NSAIDs, corticosteroids) therefore are more effective in treating pain symptoms in SLE. Some patients with chronic pain problems who are unresponsive to simple measures should be referred to pain-management centers, which use measures such as acupuncture, transcutaneous electrical nerve stimulation units, biofeedback, psychologic counseling, and physical therapy to alleviate pain and eliminate narcotic dependence. Other causes of pain in patients with SLE include avascular necrosis, steroid-induced hyperesthesia and fibromyalgia.

Role Of Stress And Trauma

Many studies have shown that certain forms of emotional stress, including depression and bereavement, as well as physical trauma can affect the immune system for example, causing decreased lymphocyte mitogenic responsiveness, lymphocyte cytotoxicity, increased natural killer-cell activity, skin homograft rejection, graft-versus-host response, and delayed hypersensitivity (34–36). Stress, unfortunately, is difficult to quantitate for evaluation of its clinical effects. Could the impairment in T-cell immune functions be responsible for a clinical flare of lupus that is mediated by B-cell hyperreactivity? Have these immune abnormalities been reproduced in patients with lupus? Can the neuroendocrine axis influence immune responses? The results of basic science, animal studies, and psycho-neuro-hormonal-immune links in this area are reviewed in Chapter 17, Neuroendocrine Immune Interactions: Principles and Relevance to Systemic Lupus; this section and Chapter 36 only review human studies.

In 1955, McLeary et al. (37) related the onset of disease to significant crises in interpersonal relationships in 13 of 14 patients with SLE. In 1967, Otto and Mackay (38) compared 20 patients with SLE to 20 controls. The SLE-hospitalized group experienced significantly more stress than other hospitalized, seriously ill controls before the onset of disease. All patients thought that stress provoked their illness. In another study, 18 of 36 patients with SLE (50%)

who were interviewed believed that psychologic factors triggered disease onset, and an additional 25 thought that it was possible (39).

Can stress exacerbate preexisting SLE? Ropes observed 45 serious disease flares in her 160-patient cohort over a 40-year period. Of the 45 patients, 41 believed that emotional stress precipitated their flare (40). Hinrichsen et al. (41) exposed 14 women with SLE, 14 healthy controls, and 12 sarcoidosis patients to acoustic stress. Significant increases in polymorphonuclear leukocyte and lymphocyte counts as well as significant elevations of circulating B and CD8+ T lymphocytes, with a relative reduction in CD4+ T lymphocytes, were noted in the healthy controls but not in the patients with SLE or sarcoidosis. The difference in effects was not steroid related. A follow-up study by this group (42) suggested that patients with SLE have significantly reduced cell mobilization to psychologic stress compared with that of controls.

Recently, Dobkin et al. reviewed various ascertainment methods for evaluating psychosocial distress and were able to correlate it with increased disease activity among 44 lupus patients (43). One study suggested that sexual abuse (a form of chronic stress) raises ANA titers (44).

Most patients with SLE already have abnormal immune function, but it has not been proven that stress further impairs these functions and results in a disease exacerbation (36). Further, patients with lupus vary widely in their responses to stress (45). Nevertheless, I believe that stress reduction is a helpful measure in the overall management of SLE.

No evidence has shown that physical trauma is related to the causation or exacerbation of SLE. I have had many patients, however, whose condition appeared to worsen after major vehicular accidents. Discoid lupus erythematosus (DLE) can develop as a result of physical trauma; King-Smith (46) first observed this in 1926. In 1956, Kern and Schiff (47) reported on five well-documented cases and sent a questionnaire to 400 dermatologists. Of these, 54 reported having treated 78 patients. The most common causes of DLE were blows from various objects, lacerations, and scars. In 1963, Lodin (48) confirmed these findings and noted that ten of 458 Swedish patients (2.2%) with DLE had a documented preceding trauma. These observations were reinforced by Eskreis et al. (49) in 1988 and de Boer et al. in 1997 (50). On the other hand, profound stress or trauma may improve lupus. Ten patients of mine with diffuse, proliferative nephritis living near the epicenter of the 1994 Los Angeles earthquake showed improvements in their sedimentation rates, anti-DNA levels, and 24-hour urine proteins 30 to 45 days after the quake occurred (51). One report of catastrophic antiphospholipid syndrome provoked by trauma has appeared (52). Acute stress may correlate with increased urine neopterin levels, decreased natural killer-cell response, and increased numbers of beta-2 adrenoreceptors on mononuclear cells without a clinical disease flare (53,54).

In summary, several authors have implicated stress as a factor that can induce or exacerbate SLE. However, a definitive study using large numbers of patients and controls with a similar chronic illness is needed before the association can be considered established. Until then, I believe that stress reduction is both prudent and important.

Diet And Vitamins

Patients with SLE should eat three well-balanced, nutritious meals daily. Animal studies suggesting that fish-oil intake might be beneficial in the treatment of autoimmune diseases have led to several human clinical trials based on the findings that eicosapentaenoic acid and docosahexaenoic acid inhibit platelet aggregation, leukotriene B4 production by polymorphs, and 5-lipoxygenase products in polymorphs and monocytes (55–57). Although a small-scale, open-label study suggested immunologic benefits (58) and another an improved sense of well-being (59), in contrast to rheumatoid arthritis, three double-blind, placebo-controlled studies of SLE failed to show any antiinflammatory actions or other clinical benefits, except for a slight lowering in plasma triglyceride and an elevation of high-density lipoprotein levels (60–64). Fish-oil derivatives may prevent miscarriages associated with antiphospholipid antibodies (65). Substituting dietary polyunsaturated fatty acids with saturated fats (which I do not recommend) was suggested in one uncontrolled study (66). A diet high in fatty meats may be associated with more severe disease (67). In some animal studies, caloric restriction was found to suppress autoimmune diseases (55,68), but three clinical reports showed that reduced caloric intake has no effect on parameters such as hemoglobin, serum IgG levels, or antibody titers (69–71).

The ingestion of alfalfa sprouts can induce lupus in primates and might exacerbate human SLE; thus, alfalfa sprouts should be avoided (72–77). The offending agent is probably an amino acid, l-canavanine, which has been shown to alter both T- and B-cell responses (72).

Alcohol and milk may decrease the risk of developing SLE (26). Two controlled studies have found patients with SLE to have increased food allergies (78,79), but the clinical significance of this observation is uncertain (see Chapter 60, Adjunctive Measures and Issues: Allergies, Antibiotics, Vaccines, Osteoporosis, and Disability).

Patients taking large doses of corticosteroids and those who are hypertensive should restrict their salt intake. Some patients with nephritis need to be salt, potassium, and protein restricted. Potassium supplementation may be needed for some patients on diuretics, and patients with anemia often benefit from foods with a high iron content (e.g., red meat). Steroids can increase lipid levels and induce a chemical diabetes, and a low-fat or diabetic diet should be implemented if this occurs.

Almost all of my patients have asked about the efficacy of vitamins in SLE. No controlled studies have been published demonstrating any clear-cut benefits from their use. Low homocysteine levels are more common in SLE, are associated with increased atheroembolic complications, and are treated with the administration of folic acid (see Chapter 44, Serum and Plasma Protein Abnormalities and Other Clinical Laboratory Determinations in Systemic Lupus Erythematosus). Vitamin B_{12} and folic acid can be used to treat specific types of anemias, and vitamin E may improve wound healing. Vitamin B_6 (pyridoxine) is a diuretic and has been used in carpal-tunnel syndrome as an adjunctive agent. In one study, lupus patients had low serum 25-hydroxyvitamin D3 levels (80). Vitamin D, with calcium supplementation, may retard the osteoporosis that is induced by corticosteroids. Other than these nonspecific measures, the judicious use of vitamins by patients with lupus is probably harmless and often has a placebo effect as long as intake is not excessive.

Sun Avoidance, Phototoxicity, and Sunscreens

One study of 125 patients with SLE noted that 73 are sunsensitive (81). In 42 of patients, sun exposure exacerbated systemic symptoms, and in 35, it had a significant effect on lifestyle. The mechanism by which this occurs is controversial, but it is probably related to the action of ultraviolet (UV) light on epidermal DNA, which enhances its antigenicity, allowing anti-Ro to be exposed to the cell surface, which promotes an inflammatory response, and skin production of cytokines, prostaglandins, and oxygen free radicals (see Chapters 28 and 29).

UV light consists of three bands, two of which are important in SLE. UVA light (i.e., 320 to 400 nm) is responsible for drug-induced photosensitivity (i.e., photoallergic reactions) and delayed tanning, and it is constant during the day. It takes approximately 1 hour of UVA exposure to induce sunburn. UVB light (i.e., 290 to 320 nm) is more significant in SLE. It is more pronounced during midday (10 a.m. to 3 p.m.) and causes sunburn readily (i.e., phototoxic reactions).

Hundreds of prescription drugs can cause photoallergic and/or phototoxic reactions. The most common are phenothiazines, tetracyclines, nalidixic acid, sulfa-containing agents, piroxicam, methotrexate, amiodarone, psoralens, phenytoin, and carprofen (82). Photosensitizing chemicals are found in certain perfumes, mercury-vapor lamps, xenon-arc lamps, tungsten iodide light sources, discotheques, color television sets, halogen lamps (83), and photocopier machines (84). The presence of anti-Ro/SSA antibody is associated with photosensitivity in more than 90 of white patients with SLE (85). Fluorescent lights are a source of UVA and UVB, but only rarely might their avoidance be beneficial (86). Clear jacket and bulk covers that control UV emanation without reducing visibility are available and, for all practical purposes, eliminate any risks (87,88).

Although the UV end of the spectrum is the most damaging to lupus skin lesions, heat and infrared exposure also can cause exacerbations. The flares produced by infrared exposure are characterized by a marked increase in erythema of short duration. These are frequently experienced by patients with SLE who work near a hot stove, oven, or furnace for any length of time. One characteristic of DLE and SLE is that skin burns and scalds can produce localized lesions of DLE at the site of trauma (i.e., the Koebner phenomenon) even in apparently normal skin (46–48).

Sunscreens are UV light-absorbing chemical agents in a cream, oil, lotion, alcohol, or gel vehicle. These chemicals can block UVA, UVB, or both. They include aminobenzoic-acid esters (UVB), cinnamates (UVB), salicylates (UVB), benzophenones (UVA, UVB), avobenzone (UVA), anthralites (UVA, UVB), and butylmethoxydibenzomethanes (UVA, UVB). Physical sunblocks containing titanium dioxide and zinc oxide scatter light. A sun protection factor (SPF) value is the ratio of the time that is required to produce erythema through a UVB sunscreen product to the time that is required to produce the same degree of erythema without it. The SPF ranges from 2 (i.e., minimal protection) to 50 (i.e., highest protection). We advise outpatients to use agents with a high SPF (i.e., at least 15). A sunscreen with SPF of 15 will block 93% of UVB, while one with SPF 50 will block only 5% more. Unfortunately, because of irritation, contact dermatitis, and occasional photosensitivity, patient compliance is poor, and it may be necessary to try several compounds before an acceptable block is found. In particular, the alcohol base in p-aminobenzoic acid (PABA) and PABA esters may sting and dry the skin.

Sunscreens should be applied over active and healed lesions and to areas that may burn, including the cheeks, nose, lips, and arms approximately 30 minutes before sun exposure. They can be applied over the scalp hair before going outdoors, and cosmetics may be applied over sunscreens. Two forms of UV light exposure often are overlooked. Skin lesions frequently are more intense on the left cheek and the lateral aspect of the left arm because of UVA exposure while driving a car. If the lesions are primarily distributed in these areas, the physician should inquire whether such exposure might be responsible and advise the patient on avoiding it (89). Merely keeping the window closed or tinting the window may filter the sunlight sufficiently. Automotive glass blocks UVB effectively but not UVA. Another unnoticed source of exposure is UV light that is reflected off the surface of sand, water, cement, or snow, and UV radiation is greater at higher altitudes. For example, the intensity at 5,000 feet is 20 higher than that at sea level. Patients should be cautioned about these sources of danger. A cloudy day only decreases UV exposure by 20 to 40.

Sunscreens block vitamin D activation in the skin, and oral supplementation may be required. An occasional patient develops eye sensitivity to UV light that is not responsive to wearing ordinary sunglasses. Special coated lenses to protect the eyes are available (90). In patients with lupus erythematosus and a definite UV sensitivity, walking a few blocks without any protection usually is permitted. If further exposure is necessary, general measures such as wearing a broad-brimmed hat and long sleeves, as well as using an umbrella can be used; these decrease UV exposure by 30 to 50. When a remission occurs, either spontaneously or induced, greater freedom of sun exposure is permitted. Frequently, otherwise asymptomatic patients have a persistent butterfly erythema that is aggravated by sun exposure, and use of antimalarials and local sunscreens usually controls this if it is severe enough to warrant therapy.

Avoidance of UV exposure has been so overemphasized that many patients are irrational about going out during the day. Unless definite evidence of exacerbations that are provoked by such exposure is noted, normal activities need not be restricted or curtailed. Although it is advisable to caution the patient that sun exposure may cause increased local erythema or development of new skin lesions, the physician should avoid causing a sunlight phobia. The average patient, even one who is photosensitive, usually can walk a few blocks at midday without protection and experience no ill effects. The question of how limited light exposure should be must be determined on an individual basis. The physician must use judgment so that the patient's way of life is interrupted as little as possible. Because sun exposure is greatest midday, outdoor activities should be undertaken in the morning or later in the afternoon.

Antimalarial therapy increases the patient's tolerance to sun exposure even in those who were extremely sensitive to UV light before taking them (91–94). The degree of limitation must be reevaluated frequently, because the tendency to sunlight-induced exacerbation of skin lesions can subside, particularly with disease remission (either spontaneous or drug-induced). Even NSAIDs can be photoprotective (95).

LOCAL THERAPY FOR DISCOID LUPUS ERYTHEMATOSUS AND SYSTEMIC LUPUS ERYTHEMATOSUS

Local treatment is used for isolated lesions of DLE or for refractory skin lesions in patients with DLE or SLE. The most effective, safe, and least scarring type of local therapy is the use of various steroid preparations. These can be fluorinated or nonfluorinated, and they may be of low, intermediate, or high potency (Table 53.2). Most nonfluorinated steroids include hydrocortisone cream or ointment and now are available as over-the-counter preparations in strengths of less than 1%. These agents are less expensive but less potent than the fluorinated preparations, which produce more stinging, dermal atrophy, depigmentation, striae, telangiectasia, acne, folliculitis, and *Candida* superinfection (96). Fluorinated steroids cannot be applied to the face for more than 2 weeks at a time without expecting cutaneous side effects. I have found betamethasone dipropionate 0.05% (Diprolene, Schering) and clobetasol proprionate 0.05% (Temovate, Glaxo Wellcome) creams or ointments to be the most effective dermatologic agents for short-term treatment of discoid lesions, especially in conjunction with antimalarials. Other studies also support this view (97).

These preparations should be used three or four times daily for optimal effectiveness and only applied directly over the lesions. Patients should be warned not to use them on normal skin, because they induce atrophy. Improvement usually is noted within a few days. Unfortunately, recurrences frequently appear within a few days to weeks after the cessation of treatment, but small lesions can be controlled adequately and indefinitely by the intermittent use of this method. Old, indurated, and chronically scaling lesions respond poorly to this form of treatment alone and require occlusive therapy (discussed later), intracutaneous injection, and/or antimalarials. We usually start patients on an intermediate-strength steroid cream or ointment and move up to high-potency agents for resistant lesions. Ointments generally are used for dry skin and creams for oily skin, but the ointment form is more effective than a cream, gel, or lotion. Fluorocarbon-propelled sprays are the least effective. Thin skin is more permeable to topical steroids as well.

The introduction of Actiderm (ConvaTec) patches allows for the improved absorption of high-potency steroids with less irritation. This should replace the use of translucent plastic, steroid-impregnated tape (Cordran Tape, Oclassen), and occlusive dressings such as plastic wrap, which increase percutaneous absorption by a factor of 100 and have been documented to be effective for those with severe DLE (98–102). Airtight occlusion of the skin causes obstruction of the sweat ducts, however, which may exacerbate pruritus and foster bacterial overgrowth on the skin surface. Jansen et al. (103) reported that topical fluocinolone acetonide cream 0.025% (Synalar, Medicis), when applied by massaging into the lesions four or five times daily or by using an occlusive dressing daily, was effective in 43 of 59 patients with DLE. It was necessary to supplement local therapy with antimalarials or corticosteroids in 11 patients. Of these 59 patients, five failed to respond, and 23 who had required antimalarials were able to discontinue them with the consistent use of local medication. All 24 patients who responded well to topical therapy and were followed through two summers did well, except for three who relapsed and required retreatment.

In another study (104), daily application of triamcinolone acetonide 0.5 in a flexible collodion base to recalcitrant DLE lesions was effective in six of seven patients compared with the use of nonmedicated collodion as a control. It may be especially helpful in the external ear, where occlusive dressings are impractical.

Intralesional therapy often is helpful when topical applications fail. Several studies have shown the value of intradermal injections of steroids. Callen as well as other investigators have documented the superiority of this method to

TABLE 53.2. TOPICAL CORTICOSTEROIDS RANKED BY POTENCY (65)*

Group	Generic Name	Brand Name
I. Superpotent		
	Clobetasol propionate cream, ointment, gel, or emollient, 0.05%	Temovate
	Betamethasone dipropionate cream or ointment, 0.05%	Diprolene
	Diflorasone diacetate ointment, 0.05%	Psorcon
	Halobetasol propionate cream of ointment, 0.05%	Ultravate
II. Potent		
	Amcinonide ointment, 0.1%	Cyclocort
	Betamethasone dipropionate cream, 0.05%	Diprolene
	Betamethasone dipropionate ointment, 0.05%	Diprosone
	Desoximetasone cream or ointment, 0.25% and gel, 0.05%	Topicort
	Diflorasone diacetate ointment, 0.05%	Maxiflor
	Fluocinonide cream, gel, or ointment, 0.05%	Lidex
	Halcinonide cream, 0.1%	Halog
	Mometasone furoate ointment, 0.1%	Elocon
III. Midpotent		
	Amcinonide cream or lotion, 0.1%	Cyclocort
	Betamethasone dipropionate cream, 0.05%	Diprosone
	Betamethasone valerate ointment, 0.1%	Valisone
	Diflorasone diacetate cream, 0.05%	Maxiflor
	Fluocinonide cream, 0.05%	Lidex-E
	Fluticasone propionate ointment, 0.005%	Cutivate
	Halcinonide ointment, 0.1%	Halog
	Triamcinolone acetonide ointment, 0.1%	Aristocort A
IV. Midpotent		
	Fluocinolone acetonide ointment, 0.025%	Synalar
	Flurandrenolide ointment, 0.05%	Cordran
	Hydrocortisone valerate ointment, 0.2%	Westcort
	Mometasone furoate cream, 0.1%	Elocon
	Triamcinolone acetonide cream, 0.1%	Kenalog
V. Midpotent		
	Betamethasone dipropionate lotion, 0.05%	Diprosone
	Betamethasone valerate cream, 0.1%	Valisone
	Fluocinolone acetonide cream, 0.025%	Synalar
	Flurandrenolide cream, 0.05%	Cordran
	Fluticasone propionate cream, 0.05%	Cutivate
	Hydrocortisone butyrate cream, 0.1%	Locoid
	Hydrocortisone valerate cream, 0.2%	Westcort
	Triamcinolone acetonide lotion, 0.1%	Kenalog
VI. Mild		
	Alclometasone dipropionate cream or ointment, 0.05%	Alcovate
	Betamethasone valerate lotion, 0.05%	Valisone
	Desonide cream, 0.05%	DesOwen
	Flumethasone pivalate cream, 0.03%	Locorten
	Fluocinolone acetonide cream or solution, 0.01%	Synalar
	Triamcinolone acetonide cream, 0.1%	Aristocort A
VII. Mild		
	Topicals with hydrocortisone, dexamethasone, flumethasone, prednisolone, and methylprednisolone	

*Group I compounds are arranged by potency.

the use of topical or oral steroids in resistant lesions (102,105–107). Triamcinolone suspensions have been the most widely used; these include triamcinolone diacetate 1.25% or 2.5% suspension (Aristocort Diacetate Parenteral), triamcinolone acetonide 10 mg/mL (Kenalog Parenteral, Westwood-Squibb), and 1% or 2.5% aqueous suspension (Meticortelene Acetate Suspension).

Occasionally, acute swelling may occur at the site of injection, but this usually subsides within 24 hours. A local depression also may appear because of tissue reabsorption; this may be noted in five of patients (107) and usually disappears within several months. It is probably a pseudoatrophy resulting from true tissue destruction. James (107) reported nine patients with DLE who were treated in this manner: five had an excellent response, and the benefit was satisfactory in two. Rowell (108) treated 28 patients with multiple intralesional injections of triamcinolone at 3-week intervals. In 13 patients, the injected lesions cleared, and 13 other patients improved. Only two patients did not respond. Smith (109) also described favorable results in 13 patients with DLE. Biopsy studies before and after therapy showed a diminution of follicular plugging and hyperkeratosis in all patients, accompanied by some thinning of the epidermis. Vascular dilatation and cellular infiltration disappeared, and skin atrophy was not observed.

Triamcinolone acetonide in an emollient dental paste (Kenalog in Orabase, Westwood-Squibb), used two or three times daily and at bedtime, is useful for sensitive lupus mucous membrane lesions. A buttermilk or hydrogen peroxide swish or gargle also is effective as an adjunctive agent. Over the long term, systemic antimalarials are more efficacious for lupus mucous membrane involvement.

Joint aches can be managed with topical nonsteroidal gels such as ketoprofen (20%) with or without muscle relaxants (e.g., 1% cyclobenzaprine) if fibromyalgia is also present. These preparations are available from compounding pharmacists.

The transplantation of normal skin to sites of excised quiescent lesions has been successful in a small number of patients (110,111). Transplantation of 4-mm, hair-bearing punch grafts into active plaques of patients with DLE, however, showed recipient dominance, with a decrease in hair survival and the appearance of discoid lesions in the implanted skin (112).

Intralesional administration of *quinacrine* and *chloroquine* was used in the 1950s with good results (91,113, 114), but it was abandoned because of the high incidence of hemorrhagic bullae, local discomfort, erythema, bleeding, and crusting of blood. A newer form of topical chloroquine clearly protects one from UVB (91). Caustic acids, intralesional *gold*, topical *5-fluorouracil*, *nitrogen mustard*, *BCNU* and vitamin D analogs and solid carbon dioxide also have been used (115–118, see Chapter 59, Occasional, Innovative, and Experimental Therapies).

REFERENCES

1. Bean WB, ed. *Aphorisms from Latham*. Iowa City: The Prairie Press, 1962.
2. Wallace DJ, Schwartz E, Chi-Lin H, et al. The rule out lupus' rheumatology consultation: clinical outcomes and perspectives. *J Clin Rheumatol* 1995;1:158–164.
3. Ginzler EM, Diamond HS, Weiner M, et al. A multicenter study of outcome of systemic lupus erythematosus. I. Entry variables as predictors of progress. *Arthritis Rheum* 1982;25: 601–611.
4. Wallace DJ, Podell T, Weiner J, et al. Systemic lupus erythematosus survival patterns. Experience with 609 patients. *JAMA* 1981;245:934–938.
5. Krupp LB, LaRocca NG, Muir J, et al. A study of fatigue in systemic lupus erythematosus. *J Rheumatol* 1990;17:1450–1452.
6. Zonana-Nacach A, Roseman JM, McGwin G Jr, et al. Systemic lupus erythematosus in three ethnic groups. VI. Factors associated with fatigue within 5 years of criteria diagnosis. *Lupus* 2000; 9:101–109.
7. Wallace DJ, Margolin K, Waller P. Fibromyalgia and interleukin-2 therapy for malignancy. *Ann Intern Med* 1988;108:909.
8. Sternberg E. Hypoimmune fatigue syndromes: diseases of the stress response? *J Rheumatol* 1993;20:418–421.
9. Forte S, Carlone S, Vaccaro F, et al. Pulmonary gas exchange and exercise capacity in patients with systemic lupus erythematosus. *J Rheumatol* 1999;26:2591–2594.
10. Wallace DJ. Antimalarial agents and lupus. *Rheum Dis Clin North Am* 1994;20:243–263.
11. Wallace DJ. The use of quinacrine (Atabrine) in rheumatic diseases: a reexamination. *Semin Arthritis Rheum* 1989;18:282–296.
12. Bruce IN, Mak VC, Hallett DC, et al. Factors associated with fatigue in patients with systemic lupus erythematosus. *Ann Rheum Dis* 1999;58:379–381.
13. Tench CM, Mc Curdie I, White PD, et al. The prevalence and associations of fatigue in outpatients with SLE. *Arthritis Rheum* 1998;41:S332.
14. Taylor J, Skan J, Erb N, et al. Lupus patients with fatigue: is there a link with the fibromyalgia syndrome? *Arthritis Rheum* 1998;41:S332.
15. Tench CM, Mc Curdie I, Mc Carthy J, et al. The assessment of aerobic capacity in a group of patients with SLE and its association with fatigue, sleep quality and disease activity. *Arthrtis Rheum* 1998;41:S332.
16. Sakauchi M, Matsumura T, Yamaoka T, et al. Reduced muscle uptake of oxygen during exercise in patients with systemic lupus erythematosus. *J Rheumatol* 1995;22:1483–1487.
17. Ramsey-Goldman R, Chang RW, Dunlop D, et al. Exercise in patients with systemic lupus erythematosus (SLE): pilot study. *Arthritis Rheum* 1995;38:S242.
18. Fitzgerald SG, Manzi S. Physical activity and systemic lupus erythematosus. *Arthritis Rheum* 1997;40:S163.
19. Matthews JD, Whittingham S, Hopper BM, et al. Association of autoantibodies with smoking, cardiovascular morbidity and death in the Busselton population. *Lancet* 1973;ii: 754–758.
20. Regius O, Lengyel E, Borzsonyi L, et al. The effect of smoking on the presence of antinuclear antibodies and on the morphology of lymphocytes in aged subjects. *Z fur Gerontologie* 1988; 21:161–163.
21. Benoni C, Nilsson A, Nived O. Smoking and inflammatory bowel disease: comparison with systemic lupus erythematosus. A case-controlled study. *Scand J Gastroenterol* 1990;25:751–755.
22. Brown K, Petri M, Goldman D. Cutaneous manifestations of SLE associated with other manifestations of SLE and with smoking (abstract). *Arthritis Rheum* 1995;38:R27.
23. Gallego H, Crutchfield CE, Lewis EJ, et al. Report of an association between discoid lupus erythematosus and smoking. *Cutis* 1999;63:231–234.
24. Hardy CJ, Palmer BP, Muir KR, et al. Smoking history, alcohol consumption and systemic lupus erythematosus: a case-control study. *Annals Rheum* 1998;57:451–455.
25. Mc Alindon T, Felson D, Palmer J, et al. Associations of cigarette smoking and alcohol with systemic lupus erythematosus (SLE) among participants in the black women's health study. *Arthritis Rheum* 1997;40:S162.
26. Nagata C, Fujita S, Iwata H, et al. Systemic lupus erythematosus: a case-control epidemiologic study in Japan. *Int J Dermatol* 1995;34:333–337.
27. Rahman P, Gladman DD, Urowitz MB. Smoking interferes with efficacy of antimalarial therapy in cutaneous lupus. *J Rheumatol* 1998;25:1716–1719.

28. Guedj D, Weinberger A. Effect of weather conditions on rheumatic patients. *Ann Rheum Dis* 1990;49:158–159.
29. Haga H-J, Brun J, Mollnes TE, et al. Seasonal variations in activity of systemic lupus erythematosus in a subarctic region. *Annals Rheum Dis* 1998;235.
30. Leone J, Pennaforte JL, Delhinger V, et al. Seasonal influence on risk of systemic lupus aggravation: retrospective study of 66 patients. *Rev Med Interne* 1997;18:286–291.
31. Amit M, Molad Y, Kiss S, et al. Seasonal variations in manifestations and activity of systemic lupus erythematosus. *Brit J Rheumatol* 1997;36:449–452.
32. Krause I, Shraga I, Molad Y, et al. Seasons of the year and activity of SLE and Behcet's disease. *Scand J Rheumatol* 1997;26:435–439.
33. Lindal E, Thorlacius S, Stefansson JG, et al. Pain and pain problems among subjects with systemic lupus erythematosus. *Scand J Rheumatol* 1993;22:10–13.
34. Calabrese JR, Kling MA, Gold PW. Alterations in immunocompetence during stress, bereavement and depression: focus on neuroendocrine regulation. *Am J Psychiatry* 1987;144:1123–1134.
35. Wallace DJ. The role of stress and trauma in rheumatoid arthritis and systemic lupus erythematosus. *Semin Arthritis Rheum* 1987;16:153–157.
36. Wallace DJ. Does stress or trauma aggravate rheumatic disease? *Baillieres Clin Rheumatol* 1994;8:149–159.
37. McLeary AR, Meyer E, Weitzman EL. Observations on the role of depression in some patients with disseminated lupus erythematosus. *Psychosomat Med* 1955;17:311–321.
38. Otto R, Mackay IR. Psycho-social and emotional disturbances to systemic lupus erythematosus. *Med J Aust* 1967;2:488–493.
39. Blumenfield M. Psychological aspects of systemic lupus erythematosus. *Primary Care* 1978;5:159–171.
40. Ropes MW. *Systemic lupus erythematosus*. Cambridge, MA: Harvard University Press, 1976.
41. Hinrichsen H, Barth J, Ferstl R, et al. Changes of immunoregulatory cells induced by acoustic stress in patients with systemic lupus erythematosus, sarcoidosis, and in healthy controls. *Eur J Clin Invest* 1989;19:372–377.
42. Hinrichsen H, Barth J, Ruckemann M, et al. Influence of prolonged neuropsychological testing on immunoregulatory cells and hormonal parameters in patients with systemic lupus erythematosus. *Rheumatol Int* 1992;12:47–51.
43. Dobkin PL, Fortin PR, Joseph L, et al. Psychosocial contributors to mental and physical health in patients with systemic lupus erythematosus. *Arthritis Care Res* 1998;11:23–31.
44. De Bellis MD, Burke L, Trickett PK. Antinuclear antibodies and thyroid function in sexually abused girls. *J Traumatic Stress* 1996;9:369–378.
45. Adams SG Jr, Dammers PM, Sala TL, et al. Stress, depression and anxiety predict average symptom severity and daily symptom fluctuation in systemic lupus erythematosus. *J Behav Med* 1994;17:459–477.
46. King-Smith D. External irritation as a factor in the causation of lupus erythematosus discoides. *Arch Dermatol* 1926;14:547–549.
47. Kern AB, Schiff BL. Discoid lupus erythematosus following trauma: report of cases and analysis of a questionnaire. *Arch Dermatol* 1957;75:685–688.
48. Lodin H. Discoid lupus erythematosus and trauma. *Acta Dermatovener* (Stockh) 1963;43:142–148.
49. Eskreis BD, Eng AM, Furey NL. Surgical excision of trauma-induced verrucous lupus erythematosus. *J Dermatol Surg Oncol* 1988;14:1296–1299.
50. De Boer EM, Nieboer C, Brunyzeel DP. Lupus erythematosus as an occupational disease. *Ann Derm Venerol* 1997;77:492.
51. Wallace DJ, Metzger AL. Can an earthquake cause flares of rheumatoid arthritis or lupus nephritis? *Arthritis Rheum* 1994;37:1826–1828.
52. Barak N, Orion Y, Cordoba M, et al. Catastrophic antiphospholipid syndrome triggered by trauma. *J Rheumatol* 1999;26:1835–1836.
53. Schubert C, Lampe A, Rumpold G, et al. Daily psychosocial stressors interfere with the dynamics of urine neopterin in a patient with systemic lupus erythematosus: an integrative single-case study. *Psychosom Med* 1999;61:876–882.
54. Pawlak CP, Jacobs R, Mikeska E, et al. Patients with systemic lupus erythematosus differ from healthy controls in their immunological response to acute psychological stress. *Brain Behavior Immunity* 1999;13:287–302.
55. Homsy J, Morrow WJ, Levy JA. Nutrition and autoimmunity: a review. *Clin Exp Immunol* 1986;65:473–488.
56. Lee SL, Rivero I, Siegel M. Activation of systemic lupus erythematosus by drugs. *Arch Intern Med* 1966;117:620–626.
57. Robinson DR, Prickett JD, Makoul GT, et al. Dietary fish oil reduces progression of established renal disease in (NZB × NZW)F1 mice and delays renal disease in BXSB and MRL/l strains. *Arthritis Rheum* 1986;29:539–546.
58. Das UN. Beneficial effect of eicosapentaenoic and docosahexaenoic acids in the management of systemic lupus erythematosus and its relationship to the cytokine network: prostaglandins. *Leukotrienes and Essential Fatty Acids* 1994;51:207–213.
59. Walton AJE, Snaith ML, Locknisar M, et al. Dietary fish oil and the severity of symptoms in patients with systemic lupus erythematosus. *Ann Rheum Dis* 1991;50:463–466.
60. Clark WF, Parbtani A, Huff MW, et al. Omega-3 fatty acid dietary supplementation in systemic lupus erythematosus. *Kidney Int* 1989;36:653–660.
61. Kremer JM, Michalek AV, Linninger L, et al. Effects of manipulation of dietary fatty acids on clinical manifestations of rheumatoid arthritis. *Lancet* 1985;i:184–187.
62. Westberg G, Tarkowski A. Effect of Ma-EPA in patients with SLE. A double-blind, crossover study. *Scand J Rheumatol* 1990;19:137–143.
63. Clark WF, Parbtani C, Naylor CD, et al. Fish oil in lupus nephritis: clinical findings and methodological implications. *Kidney Int* 1993;44:75–86.
64. Ilowite NT, Copperman N, Leicht T, et al. Effects of dietary modification and fish oil supplementation on dyslipoproteinemia in pediatric systemic lupus erythematosus. *J Rheumatol* 1995;22:1347–1351.
65. Rossi E, Costa M. Fish oil derivatives as a prophylaxis of recurrent miscarriage associated with antiphospholipid antibodies (APL): a pilot study. *Lupus* 1993;2:319–323.
66. Thorner A, Walldius G, Nillson E, et al. Beneficial effects of reduced intake of polyunsaturated fatty acids in the diet for one year in patients with systemic lupus erythematosus. *Ann Rheum Dis* 1990;49:134.
67. Minami Y, Sasaki T, Komatsu S, et al. Female systemic lupus erythematosus in Miyagi Prefecture: a case-control study of dietary and reproductive features. *Tohoku J Exp Med* 1993;169:245–252.
68. Lom-Orta H, Diaz-Jouanen E, Alarcon-Segovia D. Protein-caloric malnutrition and systemic lupus erythematosus. *J Rheumatol* 1980;7:178–182.
69. Corman LC. The role of diet in animal models of systemic lupus erythematosus: possible implications of human lupus. *Semin Arthritis Rheum* 1985;15:61–69.
70. Fernandes G, Yunis EJ, Good RA. Influence of diet on survival of mice. *Proc Natl Acad Sci USA* 1976;73:1279–1283.
71. Youinou P, Baron A, Garre M, et al. Autoantibodies and protein-calorie malnutrition. *J Rheumatol* 1981;8:174–175.
72. Alcocer-Varela J, Iglesias A, Llorente L, et al. Effects of l-canavanine on T cells may explain the induction of systemic lupus erythematosus by alfalfa. *Arthritis Rheum* 1985;28:52–57.
73. Malinow MR, Bardana EJ Jr, Pirofsky B, et al. Systemic lupus

erythematosus-like syndrome in monkeys fed alfalfa sprouts: role of a nonprotein amino acid. *Science* 1982;216:415–417.
74. Montanaro A, Bardana EJ. Dietary amino acid-induced systemic lupus erythematosus. *Rheum Dis Clin North Am* 1991; 17:323–332.
75. Morimoto I, Shiozawa S, Tanaka Y, et al. l-Canavanine acts on suppressor-inducer T cells to regulate antibody synthesis: lymphocytes of systemic lupus erythematosus are specifically unresponsive to l-canavanine. *Clin Immunol Immunopathol* 1990;55:97–108.
76. Prete PE. The mechanism of action of l-canavanine in inducing autoimmune phenomenon (letter). *Arthritis Rheum* 1985;28: 1198–1200.
77. Roberts JL, Hayashi JA. Exacerbation of SLE associated with alfalfa ingestion (letter). *N Engl J Med* 1983;308:1361.
78. Carr RI, Wold RT, Farr RS. Antibodies to bovine gamma globulin (BGG) and occurrence of a BGG-like substance in systemic lupus erythematosus sera. *J Allergy Clin Immunol* 1972; 50:18–30.
79. Diumenjo MS, Lisanti M, Valles R, et al. Allergic manifestations of systemic lupus erythematosus. *Allergol Immunopathol* (Madrid) 1985;13:32–3326.
80. Muller K, Kriegbaum NJ, Baslund B, et al. Vitamin D3 metabolism in patients with rheumatic diseases: low serum levels of 25-hydroxyvitamin D3 in patients with systemic lupus erythematosus. *Clin Rheumatol* 1995;14:397–400.
81. Wysenbeek AJ, Block DA, Fries JF. Prevalence and expression of photosensitivity in systemic lupus erythematosus. *Ann Rheum Dis* 1989;48:461–463.
82. Anonymous. Drugs that cause photosensitivity. *Med Lett* 1986; 28:50–51.
83. Wildhagen K, Woll R, Deicher H. Case report: systemic lupus erythematosus patients at risk due to unprotected exposure to unsubdued halogen lamps. *Akt Rheumatol* 1993;18:167–169.
84. Klein LR, Elmets CA, Callen JP. Photoexacerbation of cutaneous lupus erythematosus due to ultraviolet A emissions from a photocopier. *Arthritis Rheum* 1995;38:1152–1156.
85. Mond CB, Peterson MG, Rothfield NF. Correlation of anti-Ro antibody with photosensitivity rash in systemic lupus erythematosus patients. *Arthritis Rheum* 1989;32:202–204.
86. Martin L, Chalmers IM. Photosensitivity to fluorescent light in a patient with systemic lupus erythematosus. *J Rheumatol* 1983; 10:811–812.
87. Rihner M, McGrath H Jr. Fluorescent light photosensitivity in patients with systemic lupus erythematosus. *Arthritis Rheum* 1992;35:949–952.
88. Sontheimer RD. Fluorescent light photosensitivity in patients with systemic lupus erythematosus: comment on the article by Rihner and McGrath. *Arthritis Rheum* 1993;36:428–431.
89. Johnson JA, Fusaro RM. Broad-spectrum photoprotection: the roles of tinted auto windows, sunscreens and browning agents in the diagnosis and treatment of photosensitivity. *Dermatology* 1992;185:237–241.
90. Diddie KR. Do sunglasses protect the retina from light damage? *West J Med* 1994;161:594.
91. Langlo L. Efficiency of local application of chloroquine and mepacrine in preventing the effects of ultraviolet rays in human skin. *Acta Dermatolovener* 1957;37:85–87.
92. McChesney EW, Nachod FC, Tainter ML. Rationale for treatment of lupus erythematosus with antimalarials. *J Invest Derm* 1957;29:97–104.
93. Page F. Treatment of lupus erythematosus with mepacrine. *Lancet* 1951;ii:755–758.
94. Sjolin-Forsberg G, Lindstrom B, Berne B. Topical chloroquine applied before irradiation protects against ultraviolet B (UVB)- and UVA-induced erythema but not against immediate pigment darkening. *Photodermatol Photoimmunol Photomed* 1992–1993; 9:220–224.
95. Hughes GS, Francom SF, Means LK, et al. Synergistic effects of oral nonsteroidal drugs and topical corticosteroids in the therapy of sunburn in humans. *Dermatol* 1992;184:54–58.
96. Weston WL. Topical corticosteroids in dermatologic disorders. *Hosp Pract* 1984;19:159–172.
97. Anonymous. Clobetasola potent new topical corticosteroid. *Med Lett* 1986;28:57–59.
98. Garb J. Nevus verrucous unilateris cured with podophyllin ointment. Ointment applied as occlusive dressing; report of a case. *Arch Dermatol* 1960;81:606–609.
99. McKenzie AW, Stoughton RB. Method for comparing percutaneous absorption of steroids. *Arch Dermatol* 1962;86:606–610.
100. Scholtz JR. Topical therapy of psoriasis with fluocinolone acetonide. *Arch Dermatol* 1961;84:1029–1030.
101. Sulzberger MB, Witten VH. Thin pliable plastic films in topical dermatologic therapy. *Arch Dermatol* 1961;84:1027–1028.
102. Witten VH. Newer dermatologic methods for using corticosteroids more efficaciously. *Med Clin North Am* 1961;45:857–868.
103. Jansen GT, Dillaha CJ, Honeycutt WM. Discoid lupus erythematosus. Is systemic treatment necessary? *Arch Dermatol* 1965; 92:283–285.
104. Brock W, Cullen SI. Triamcinolone acetonide in flexible collodion for dermatologic therapy. *Arch Dermatol* 1967;96:193–194.
105. Callen JP. Chronic cutaneous lupus erythematosus. Clinical, laboratory, therapeutic and prognostic examination of 62 patients. *Arch Dermatol* 1982;118:412–416.
106. Callen JP. Intralesional triamcinolone is effective for discoid lupus erythematosus of the palms and soles. *J Rheumatol* 1985; 12:630–633.
107. James AP. Intradermal triamcinolone acetonide in localized lesions. *J Invest Dermatol* 1960;34:175–176.
108. Rowell NR. Treatment of chronic discoid lupus erythematosus with intralesional triamcinolone. *Br J Dermatol* 1962;74: 354–357.
109. Smith JF. Interlesional triamcinolone as an adjunct to antimalarial drugs in the treatment of chronic discoid lupus erythematosus. *Br J Dermatol* 1962;74:350–353.
110. Friederich HC. Skin transplantation and skin grafts in chronic discoid LE. *Hautarzt* 1969;20:119–122.
111. Friederich HC. Results of autotransplantation in chronic discoid lupus erythematosus. *Arch Klin Exp Derm* 1970;237:71–75.
112. Nordstrom RE. Hair transplantation. The use of hair bearing compound grafts for correction of alopecia due to chronic discoid lupus erythematosus, traumatic alopecia, and male pattern baldness. *Scand J Plast Reconstr Surg* 1976;14 (suppl):137.
113. Everett MA, Coffey CM. Intradermal administration of chloroquine for discoid lupus erythematosus and lichen sclerosus et atrophicus. *Arch Dermatol* 1961;83:977–979.
114. Pelzig A, Witten VH, Sulzberger MB. Chloroquine for chronic discoid lupus erythematosus. Intralesional injections. *Arch Dermatol* 1961;83:146–148.
115. Hebra F, Kaposi M. On diseases of the skin, including the exanthemata. Tay W, trans., Hitlon FC, ed. London: The New Sydenham Society 1866–1880, 1874;(4).
116. Sulzberger MB, Wolf J, Witten VH, et al. *Dermatology, diagnosis and treatment. 2nd ed.* Chicago: Year Book Medical Publishers, 1961.
117. Vena GA, Coviello C, Mastrolonardo M, et al. Topical 5-fluoracil in the treatment of discoid lupus erythematosus. Preliminary study over two years. *J Dermatol Treat* 1996;7:167–169.
118. Feliciani C, Amerio S, Mohammad Pour S, et al. IL-1 alpham and TNF alpha in cutaneous lesions of lupus erythematosus are inhibited by topical application of calcipotriol. *Int J Immunopathol Pharm* 1995;8:199–207.

54

SALICYLATE AND NONSTEROIDAL THERAPY

KEYVAN YOUSEFI
MICHAEL H. WEISMAN

The English clergyman Edward Stone first discovered the medical properties of salicylates in 1763 (1). He administered willow bark extract to 50 patients with different illnesses and achieved good results. Specific salicylate use in the treatment of rheumatologic diseases was reported independently by two German physicians; each reported a case series of patients experiencing acute rheumatologic disorders who responded with a significant reduction in joint swelling and tenderness attributed to salicylic acid remedies (1).

Beginning with phenylbutazone in 1953, indomethacin in 1965, and ibuprofen in 1974, enormous quantities of nonsteroidal antiinflammatory drugs (NSAIDs) have been manufactured, tested, and sold worldwide. NSAIDs are among the most commonly prescribed drugs in the world, with estimates as high as nearly $2 billion spent annually in the United States (2). NSAIDs are able to produce analgesia, inhibit platelet aggregation, and reduce fever and inflammation. Their analgesic effects are seen within minutes of intake and become more evident in a few hours. NSAIDs cannot reverse the underlying disease or change the course of the illness responsible for the inflammatory process (3). Despite the fact that the Food and Drug Administration (FDA) has not approved the commercial promotion of NSAIDs in the management of systemic lupus erythematosus (SLE), these agents have been used widely for the treatment of fever, arthritis, pleuritis, and pericarditis in SLE subjects. In a survey done at a medical center population of 925 lupus patients, 84% reported NSAID intake (4).

This chapter discusses the role of these agents in the management of lupus patients, and evaluates some of the major side effects associated with their use. Table 54.1 lists some of the available nonsteroidals and their properties.

MECHANISM OF ACTION

Arachidonic acid is produced in response to chemical or mechanical stimuli by the actions of the enzyme phospholipase A (Fig. 54.1). Arachidonic acid is then catabolized either by cyclooxygenase A to form an unstable endoperoxide called PGH_2, or by 5-lipooxygenase to produce leukotrienes. PGH_2 immediately breaks down to form prostaglandins PGE_2, PGI_2, PGD_2, toxic oxygen radicals, and thromboxane A_2 (5,6). Prostaglandins induce a variety of inflammatory effects such as swelling, erythema, changes in vascular permeability, and neutrophil chemotaxis. They

TABLE 54.1. SOME AVAILABLE SALICYLATES AND NSAIDS

Drug	Dose Range (mg/d)	Half-life	Cost[a]
Salicylates			
Aspirin	1,000–6,000	4–15 hrs	$
Diflunisal	500–1,500	7–15 hrs	$$
Salsalate	1,500–5,000	4–15 hrs	$
Short half-life NSAIDs			
Diclofenac	75–150	1–2 hrs	$$
Etodolac	600–1,200	7 hrs	$$
Fenoprofen	1,200–3,200	2 hrs	$
Ibuprofen	1,200–3,200	2 hrs	$
Indomethacin	50–200	3–11 hrs	$
Ketoprofen	100–400	2 hrs	$$$
Ketorolac[b]	15–150	4–6 hrs	$$
Meclofenamate	200–400	2–3 hrs	$$
Tolmetin	800–1,600	1 hr	$$$
Long half-life NSAIDs			
Nabumetone	1,000–2,000	24 hrs	$$
Naproxen	250–1,500	13 hrs	$
Oxaprozin	600–1,200	49–60 hrs	$$
Piroxicam	20	30–86 hrs	$$
Sulindac	300–400	16 hrs	$$
Meloxicam	7.5–15	15–20 hrs	$$$
COX-2 inhibitors			
Celecoxib	200–400	11 hrs	$$$
Rofecoxib	12.5–50	17 hrs	$$$

[a]Based on Mosby's Gen Rx 10th ed., 2000.
[b]Not recommended for long-term use.
Adapted from Clements P, Paulus H. Salicylate and nonsteroidal therapy. In: Wallace DJ, Hahn B, Dubois EL, eds., *Dubois' Lupus Erythematosus.* Baltimore: Williams & Wilkins, 1997:1109–1116.

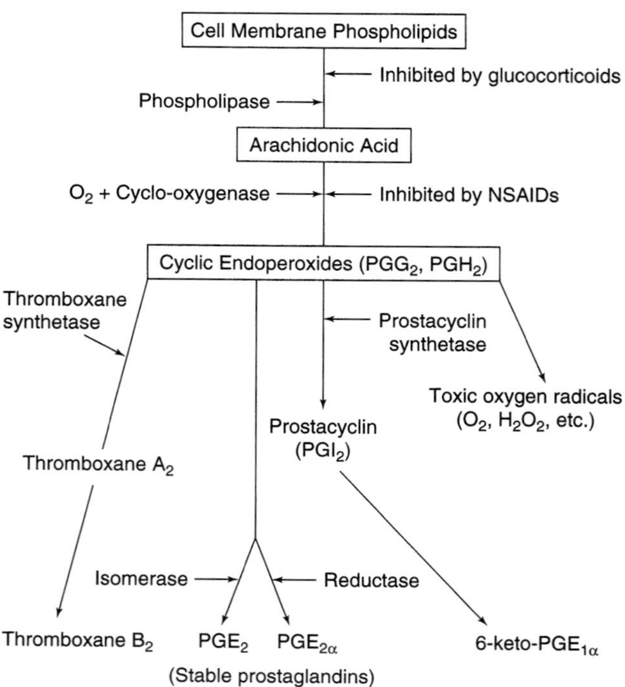

FIGURE 54.1. Cyclooxygenase pathway for arachidonic acid metabolism. (From Clements and Paulus [3], with permission.)

also appear to play a role in several important homeostatic physiologic processes. In the kidneys, they regulate renal perfusion in part by dilating renal vasculture; in the stomach, they protect gastric mucosa from autodigestion by gastric acid. Prostaglandins stimulate bone resorption by their effect on osteoclasts, leading to periarticular bone resorption (7).

By binding to cyclooxygenase A, NSAIDs inhibit the rate-limiting step in the production of prostaglandins. It is now recognized that there are two distinct proteins that possess cyclooxygenase activity, called COX-1 and COX-2. COX-1 is present in many tissues such as renal collecting tubules, platelets, endothelial cells, smooth muscle, and gastric mucosa, whereas the COX-2 gene is expressed in a limited number of cells such as brain neurons, synoviocytes, and smooth muscle cells (8). COX-2 expression has been noted to be intensified in synoviocytes and inflammatory cells of rheumatoid arthritis patients (9). Since COX-1 is a major factor in the normal physiologic processes and functions of organ homeostasis and COX-2 is involved in pathophysiologic events, the concept has evolved that there are "good" and "bad" actions of NSAIDs that can be separated from each other (10). Along this line of reasoning, it is thought that much if not all of the toxicity of NSAIDs is secondary to inhibition of the COX-1 enzyme.

Recently, COX-2 selective inhibitors have been developed and introduced into the market. These agents are highly selective for COX-2 enzymes even at doses significantly higher than the manufacturer's recommended dosage. These drugs have been shown to be as effective as naproxen for pain control in rheumatoid arthritis and osteoarthritis patients. They have been observed to cause serious gastroduodenal injury in large clinical trials at a rate greater than placebo but less than nonselective COX inhibitor (11–14).

COX-2 inhibitors may also have a potential role in the treatment of other diseases because of the discovery that they play a role in a variety of important and sometimes critical biologic processes. A higher level of COX-2 expression is noted in Alzheimer's patients. Epidemiologic studies suggest a delay in progression of the disease in patients taking NSAIDs (15,16). COX-2 agents may also be helpful in retardation of colorectal adenoma growth (17).

Despite a great deal of enthusiasm, there remain to be resolved several safety issues regarding these agents. Cyclooxygenase enzymes seem to play an important role in thrombogenesis. COX-1 enzyme regulates the production of thromboxane A_2, leading to aggregation of platelets and vasoconstriction, whereas COX-2 influences the production of prostacyclin, the enzyme that stimulates vasodilitation. Nonspecific NSAIDs block the production of both COX-1 and COX-2 enzymes, thereby not influencing the thrombogenesis pathway in one direction or another. However, COX-2 inhibitors limit the production of prostacyclin and may favor the aggregation of platelets, ultimately leading to thrombosis and ischemia (10,18). This hypothesis has not yet been evaluated in clinical studies. However, there is a report of four cases of ischemic complications associated with COX-2 inhibitors in patients with connective tissue diseases (mostly SLE) that predispose to thrombosis; the authors state that COX-2 inhibitors could possibly shift the hemostatic balance toward a prothrombotic state in susceptible patients (19).

The COX-2 enzyme is produced in macula densa, medullary interstitial cells, and the cortical ascending limb of the kidney. It appears that COX-2 may play a role in renin synthesis. One may speculate that COX-2 inhibitors could lead to reduced glomerular filtration rate (GFR) and hyperkalemia. In addition, renal blood flow may be affected due to blockage of prostaglandin formation by COX-2 in medullary cells (20,21). In a randomized trial of 75 healthy patients, 60 to 80 years of age, on a sodium-restricted diet, single and multiple doses of rofecoxib decreased the GFR at a rate similar to indomethacin, suggesting that renal toxicity is not spared by drugs specific for COX-2 inhibition (22).

CLINICAL STUDIES

Nonsteroidals were first reported to be clinically useful in the management of lupus by a German group in 1953 (3). Dubois (23,24) reported favorable responses to indomethacin in 18 of 22 lupus patients with arthritis. He also observed improvement in arthralgia in 13 of 17 lupus patients after an average of 16 weeks treatment with ibuprofen. In a Hungarian study, 12 lupus patients with moderately active disease were treated with piroxicam for a mean period of 13 months. Ten patients responded with clinical and immunologic improvements without elevation in serum creatinine and transaminases (25).

Karsh and colleagues (26) undertook the only reported double-blinded, randomized study comparing the clinical effects of aspirin and ibuprofen in lupus patients. They randomized nine patients to receive aspirin and ten to ibuprofen. At the end of a 14-day period, seven of the nine patients in the aspirin group experienced reduction in joint pain and swelling compared to only two in the ibuprofen group. Four in the aspirin group and two in the ibuprofen group developed transaminase elevation. One in the aspirin group and two in the ibuprofen cohort demonstrated an elevation in serum creatinine. In all cases, the hepatic and renal toxicity was reversed upon drug cessation.

Espinoza and colleagues (27) evaluated the effects of indomethacin in six lupus patients with refractory nephrotic syndrome secondary to lupus nephritis. These patients had persistent nephrotic syndrome despite corticosteroid and diuretic management. All six patients had improvement in serum albumin and a reduction in proteinuria. For four patients, these effects persisted for up to several years.

Aspirin has been recommended for the treatment of the antiphospholipid syndrome (28). Patients with this syndrome are at increased risk for recurrent fetal loss as well as arterial and venous thrombosis. There have been several studies measuring the effects of aspirin, alone or in combination with steroids, in fetal and pregnancy outcome in lupus patients.

Gatenby and colleagues (29) reported a reduction rate in pregnancy wastage from 88% to 55% in lupus patients with antiphospholipid antibodies following treatment with low-dose aspirin. Several other studies have confirmed similar findings in lupus pregnancies associated with positive antiphospholipid antibodies (30–32). It appears that low-dose aspirin exerts its antithrombotic effects by blocking the production of thrombaxane A_2, a potent vasoconstrictor and platelet aggregant. Aspirin may also stimulate interleukin-3 production, promoting placental and fetal development (31,32).

DRUG INTERACTIONS

Because lupus patients are often receiving multiple medications, physicians should be aware of potential drug interactions. It is known that NSAIDs blunt the antihypertensive effects of loop and thiazide diuretics (33). These agents also have the potential to increase prothrombin time if taken with Coumadin. Aspirin, in antiinflammatory dosages, was shown to interfere with systemic and renal clearance of methotrexate, leading to higher serum levels (34). There are case reports of renal failure and bone marrow aplasia when methotrexate is taken with aspirin, indomethacin, or naproxen (33,35).

ADVERSE REACTIONS

Adverse reactions are common with NSAIDs. Lupus patients are probably at increased risk for experiencing side effects largely because they often have active multiorgan involvement (36). Other factors such as age and diminished renal function most certainly play a role for toxicity development.

Renal

In the general population, renal adverse reactions associated with NSAID intake are not frequently encountered, but do occur. The most common and worrisome renal side effect is acute reversible renal insufficiency, typically occurring in patients with additional risk factors such as advanced age, plasma volume contraction, or preexisting renal insufficiency (37,38).

It is felt that NSAIDs induce their renal side effects by inhibiting prostaglandin synthesis (3). Prostaglandins most likely play a significant role in maintaining renal hemodynamics in SLE patients. Renal perfusion has been observed to be highly dependent on the vasodilatory effects of prostaglandins (3). Prostaglandins are also observed to play a role in inhibition of T-cell lymphocytes in animal models with lupus nephritis. Administration of prostaglandin analogues improves the renal function in animal models of lupus (39,40).

Kimberly and Plotz (41) reported up to 58% reduction in creatinine clearance as well as increases of serum creatinine to 163% of normal in 13 of 23 lupus patients after a minimum of 7 days of aspirin therapy. These reversible changes were noted to be more prominent in patients with active nephritis and low complement levels.

Ter Borg and colleagues (42) measured the effects of indomethacin after a week of treatment in 13 lupus patients with baseline absence of any significant renal disease. They found an average of 15% reduction in GFR and a normal renal blood flow in the treatment group, with no significant change in the control group.

In two other controlled studies in nonuremic lupus patients, ibuprofen or indomethacin intake led to an average 16% reduction in GFR. Patients with active lupus glomerulonephritis seem to experience larger changes in renal function compared to lupus patients without active nephritis (43–45). There are reports of acute tubular necrosis in lupus patients with ibuprofen, naproxen, and fenoprofen intake (46–48).

There are no long-term observational studies evaluating the effects of NSAIDs in lupus patients. Renal papillary necrosis and chronic renal failure have been associated with prolonged NSAID intake in normal human subjects; however, the actual risks for these complications have not been established (38).

In a case-control study, a twofold increase of chronic renal disease was observed in daily users of NSAIDs. After adjustment for other analgesics, the odds ratio was 10. This increased risk was primarily seen in men older than 65 (49). However, in an occupational risk factor case-control European study evaluating 272 patients with chronic renal failure, an increased risk for nephropathy was not associated with regular nonsteroidal intake (50). Nonetheless, in a Malaysian prospective study of 259 patients with a minimum cumulative total of 1-kg analgesic intake, renal papillary necrosis was confirmed by computed tomography (CT), ultrasound, or intravenous urography in 29 patients who had consumed NSAIDs as the sole or predominant analogue (51). All of these data point to an increased risk for reduction in renal function for lupus patients, especially those with either active renal disease or established renal insufficiency. The potential benefits must be anticipated, with careful monitoring for side effects, when NSAIDs are used in lupus patients with renal compromise or active renal disease.

Gastrointestinal

To the best of our knowledge, there has not been a published study evaluating gastrointestinal (GI) side effects associated with nonsteroidals in lupus patients. In the general population, dyspepsia develops in approximately 10% to 20% of patients who take nonsteroidals on a regular basis. It was 60 years ago that Douthwaite and Lintott (52) found endoscopic evidence of gastric mucosal damage secondary to aspirin intake. Since then, numerous reports have confirmed this finding. Nonsteroidals have direct toxic effects on gastroduodenal mucosa as well as indirect effects caused by the blockade of gastric prostaglandin production (53). The coincident use of corticosteroids and anticoagulants increase the risk of GI bleeding (54,55).

The FDA has approved the commercial promotion of concomitant misoprostol four times daily with nonsteroidals for prevention of NSAID-associated ulcers. Misoprostol, however, is associated with a number of side effects such as abdominal bloating, diarrhea, and increased uterine contractility leading to spontaneous abortion (53). Proton pump inhibitors appear to be effective for prevention of GI mucosal injury caused by nonsteroidals, although more confirmatory studies are needed (56). H2-receptor antagonists were found to be effective in preventing duodenal ulcers but not gastric ulcers in two large randomized studies (57,58).

Nonacetylated salicylates inhibit prostaglandins to a lesser degree and therefore appear to have a lower incidence of GI bleeding. Some of the newer NSAIDs appear to have less gastroduodenal mucosa injury potential. Nabumetone and etodolac have a preferred affinity for COX-2. Recent endoscopic and surveillance studies suggest that these agents have a lower incidence of ulceration (59).

COX-2 inhibitors are the latest addition to the growing number of NSAIDs. In several well-controlled studies, they have been shown to have a significantly reduced incidence of GI toxicity (12–14). They appear to maintain their selectivity even at higher than recommended doses. However, more studies are needed regarding the long-term safety of these agents. COX-2 enzyme may actually play a role in gastroduodenal ulcer healing. In mice, COX-2 protein seems to be involved in the healing of gastric mucosal lesions. COX-2 is also found at the rim of gastrodoudenal ulcers in human models (60,61). These reports suggest that COX-2 inhibitors may retard gastroduodenal ulcer healing induced by other stimuli such as *Helicobacter pylori* or other NSAIDs. Therefore, clinical trials are needed to investigate these preliminary findings.

Hepatic

Mild reversible elevations of serum transaminases with no significant elevation of serum bilirubin or alkaline phosphatase have been reported with salicylate intake in lupus and juvenile arthritis patients (62). In general, administration of salicylates at more than 2 g/d is required to impose a significant risk (63). Aspirin seems to be the most common agent involved in cases of significant hepatic injury, and the mechanism is likely due to a direct toxic effect associated with the orthoacetyl moiety (64). Fries and Holman (65) reported transaminase elevations associated with aspirin intake in 48 of their 192 lupus patients. Travers and Hughes (66) noted transaminase elevations in seven of their 74 lupus patients who were taking aspirin at therapeutic doses. Four of these seven patients were prescribed diflunisal for analgesia in place of aspirin for 2 months without any transaminase elevations. Sulindac has also been observed in a number of cases to lead to transaminitis and even jaundice. In one review it was noted that there are no reports of any significant irreversible chronic hepatic sequelae due to salicylates (36). Wallace recommends aspirin to be continued unless transaminase levels are above 100 IU/dL (3).

Aseptic Meningitis

There are 43 reported cases in the literature of NSAID-induced aseptic meningitis. The majority of these patients present with fever, headache, stiff neck, and a clinical picture similar to infectious meningitis. Analysis of the cerebrospinal fluid (CSF) characteristically demonstrates a high white count, normal glucose, and elevated protein with no bacterial growth (67–71). SLE is the most common underlying disease associated with these reported cases of aseptic meningitis (18 cases). The etiology of this phenomenon is not fully understood. The presence of rash and facial edema, and the disappearance of symptoms after discontinuing the drug suggest a hypersensitivity reaction. A cell-mediated cross-reactivity to a natural constituent similar to ibuprofen has been suggested to occur in SLE patients without prior exposure to the drug (71). In addition, lack of suppressor cells in lupus patients could potentially lead to a more pronounced response (72). Ibuprofen is overwhelmingly the most reported agent associated with aseptic meningitis (>85% of all cases) followed by tolmetin, sulindac, naproxen, and diclofenac (68,73–76).

Dermatologic

Lupus patients are noted to be at a higher risk for developing allergic reactions to all drugs especially antibiotics and, to a lesser extent, NSAIDs (77,78). Nonsteroidals in general are associated with cutaneous reactions, which include angioedema, urticaria, fixed eruptions, exanthema, erythema multiforme, and Stevens-Johnson syndrome. Aspirin, diflunisal, sulindac, and naproxen are associated with approximately a 5% incidence of rash (79,80). A unique photosensitivity reaction has been associated with piroxicam. This reaction usually occurs within 3 days of sun exposure and often presents as a vesiculobullous eruption (81).

Allergic reactions to sulfonamide drugs in particular seem to be more prevalent in lupus patients. Petri and Allbritton (82) demonstrated in a case-control study of 221 lupus patients that 31% exposed to sulfonamide antimicrobials, compared to 12% in the control group, developed allergic reactions such as rash, angioedema, fever, and bronchospasm. Furthermore, six patients developed lupus flare that was confirmed by a physician. In a retrospective study of 340 lupus patients and 306 controls, the prevalence of drug hypersensitivity was 56% compared to 14% in the control group. Again, sulfonamide antibiotics were the most common agents followed by penicillin, cephalosporins, and NSAIDs. Five episodes of lupus flares were noted in the SLE group (83).

Celecoxib, one of the new COX-2 inhibitors, is a derivative of benzenesulfanomide. Due to the concern for cross-reactivity, product labeling for celecoxib advises patients not to use the medication if they have a history of allergic-type reactions to sulfanomides (84). However, case reports of clinical cross-reactivity among sulfanomide antimicrobials and other sulfanomide medications (furosamide, sulfanylureas, and thiazides) are rare (85). Sulfanomide antimicrobials contain an arylamine group at the N4 position that other sulfanomide medications such as celecoxib do not possess. There is also a difference in haptenation, metabolic, and site specificity requirements that very likely result in a low propensity for cross-allergenity (86).

In a small pilot study with 50 lupus patients treated open label for 1 to 9 months with celecoxib for musculoskeletal pain, no differences were noted in the incidence of allergic reactions in the patients with a self-reported history of sulfa allergy compared to those without this history (87).

SUMMARY AND CONCLUSIONS

1. NSAIDs and salicylates can be used with caution in the management of non–organ-threatening SLE inflammation such as arthralgia, serositis, fever, and soft tissue swelling. It has not been established whether any specific agent is superior over any other in the treatment of lupus.
2. Aspirin is recommended for treatment of lupus patients with concomitant antiphospholipid syndrome or other risk factor for thrombosis.
3. Nonacetylated salicylates and COX-2 inhibitors are recommended in patients at risk for gastrointestinal toxicity.
4. SLE patients, especially those with active nephritis, are at increased risk for developing renal toxicity associated with NSAIDs. Nonacetylated salicylates appear to be safer in this situation.
5. Lupus patients on chronic long-term NSAID therapy should be closely monitored, with complete blood counts and chemistry panels, in order to avoid NSAID toxicity. This should occur at a minimum of every 3 months.
6. Drug-drug interactions are a worrisome potential problem in the sicker lupus population.
7. The newer COX-2 inhibitors represent an opportunity to better define risk and benefit in the lupus population. However, there are unsolved problems with the newer agents. More clinical and basic research is required to understand their potential benefits as well as adverse effects with regard to kidney, brain, GI tract, wound healing, and thrombogenic potential.

REFERENCES

1. Hedner T, Everts B. The early clinical history of salicylates in rheumatology and pain. *Clin Rheumatol* 1998;17(1):17–25.
2. Garcia L. Pain-free at last. *Dallas Morning News* Sept 6, 1999;1C.
3. Clements P, Paulus H. Salicylate and nonsteroidal therapy. In: Wallace DJ, Hahn B, Dubois EL, eds. *Dubois' lupus erythematosus*. Baltimore: Williams & Wilkins, 1997:1109–1116.
4. Wallace DJ, Metzger AL, Klinenberg JR. NSAID usage patterns by rheumatologists in the treatment of SLE. *J Rheumatol* 1989; 16(4):557–560.
5. Meade EA, Smith WL, DeWitt DL. Differential inhibition of prostaglandin endoperoxide synthase (cyclooxygenase) isozymes by aspirin and other non-steroidal anti-inflammatory drugs. *J Biol Chem* 1993;268(9):6610–6614.
6. Lee SH, et al. Selective expression of mitogen-inducible cyclooxygenase in macrophages stimulated with lipopolysaccharide. *J Biol Chem* 1992;267(36):25934–25938.
7. Goodwin JS. Are prostaglandins proinflammatory, antiinflammatory, both or neither? *J Rheumatol Suppl* 1991;28:26–29.
8. Hawkey CJ. COX-2 inhibitors (see comments). *Lancet* 1999; 353(9149):307–314.
9. Crofford LJ, et al. Cyclooxygenase-1 and -2 expression in rheumatoid synovial tissues. Effects of interleukin-1 beta, phorbol ester, and corticosteroids. *J Clin Invest* 1994;93(3):1095–1101.

10. Lipsky PE, et al. Unresolved issues in the role of cyclooxygenase-2 in normal physiologic processes and disease. *Arch Intern Med* 2000;160(7):913–920.
11. Lipsky PE, Isakson PC. Outcome of specific COX-2 inhibition in rheumatoid arthritis. *J Rheumatol* 1997;24(suppl 49):9–14.
12. Bjarnason I, et al. A randomized, double-blind, crossover comparative endoscopy study on the gastroduodenal tolerability of a highly specific cyclooxygenase-2 inhibitor, flosulide, and naproxen. *Scand J Gastroenterol* 1997;32(2):126–130.
13. Simon LS, et al. Anti-inflammatory and upper gastrointestinal effects of celecoxib in rheumatoid arthritis: a randomized controlled trial (see comments). *JAMA* 1999;282(20):1921–1928.
14. Langman MJ, et al. Adverse upper gastrointestinal effects of rofecoxib compared with NSAIDs (see comments). *JAMA* 1999; 282(20):1929–1933.
15. Pasinetti GM, Aisen PS. Cyclooxygenase-2 expression is increased in frontal cortex of Alzheimer's disease brain. Neuroscience 1998;87(2):319–324.
16. McGeer PL, Schulzer M, McGeer EG. Arthritis and anti-inflammatory agents as possible protective factors for Alzheimer's disease: a review of 17 epidemiologic studies (see comments). Neurology 1996;47(2):425–432.
17. Eberhart CE, et al. Up-regulation of cyclooxygenase 2 gene expression in human colorectal adenomas and adenocarcinomas. *Gastroenterology* 1994;107(4):1183–1188.
18. McAdam BF, et al. Systemic biosynthesis of prostacyclin by cyclooxygenase (COX)-2: the human pharmacology of a selective inhibitor of COX-2 (published erratum appears in *Proc Natl Acad Sci USA* 1999;96(10):5890). *Proc Natl Acad Sci USA* 1999; 96(1):272–277.
19. Crofford LJ, et al. Thrombosis in patients with connective tissue diseases treated with specific cyclooxygenase 2 inhibitors: a report of four cases. *Arthritis Rheum* 2000;43(8):1891–1896.
20. Harris RC, et al. Cyclooxygenase-2 is associated with the macula densa of rat kidney and increases with salt restriction. *J Clin Invest* 1994;94(6):2504–2510.
21. Harding P, et al. Cyclooxygenase-2 mediates increased renal renin content induced by low-sodium diet. Hypertension 1997;29(1 pt 2):297–302.
22. Swan SK, et al. Effect of cyclooxygenase-2 inhibition on renal function in elderly persons receiving a low-salt diet. A randomized, controlled trial. *Ann Intern Med* 2000;133(1):1–9.
23. Dubois EL. Management of systemic lupus erythematosus. *Modern Treatment* 1966;3(6):1245–1279.
24. Dubois EL. Letter: ibuprofen for systemic lupus erythematosus. *N Engl J Med* 1975;293(15):779.
25. Gergely P. Treatment of systemic lupus erythematosus (SLE) with piroxicam (Hotemin-Egis). *Ther Hung* 1989;37(2):83–85.
26. Karsh J, et al. Comparative effects of aspirin and ibuprofen in the management of systemic lupus erythematosus. *Arthritis Rheum* 1980;23(12):1401–1404.
27. Espinoza LR, et al. Refractory nephrotic syndrome in lupus nephritis: favorable response to indomethacin therapy. *Lupus* 1993;2(1):9–14.
28. Harris EN. Antiphospholipid syndrome. In: Dieppe P, Klippel JH, eds. *Rheumatology*, vol 2. London: CV Mosby, 1998:35.1–35.6.
29. Gatenby PA, Cameron K, Shearman RP. Pregnancy loss with phospholipid antibodies: improved outcome with aspirin containing treatment. *Aust NZ J Obstet Gynaecol* 1989;29(3 pt 2):294–298.
30. Balasch J, et al. Antiphospholipid antibodies in unselected patients with repeated abortion. *Hum Reprod* 1990;5(1):43–46.
31. Kaaja R, et al. Production of prostacyclin and thromboxane in lupus pregnancies: effect of small dose of aspirin. *Obstet Gynecol* 1993;81(3):327–331.
32. Fishman P, et al. Aspirin-interleukin-3 interrelationships in patients with anti-phospholipid syndrome. *Am J Reprod Immunol (Copenhagen)* 1996;35(2):80–84.
33. Nishihara KK, Furst DE. Aspirin and other nonsteroidal anti-inflammatory drugs. In: Koopman WJ, ed. *Arthritis and allied conditions: a textbook of rheumatology*. Baltimore: Williams & Wilkins, 1997:611–654.
34. Stewart CF, et al. Aspirin alters methotrexate disposition in rheumatoid arthritis patients. *Arthritis Rheum* 1991;34(12):1514–1520.
35. Maiche AG. Acute renal failure due to concomitant action of methotrexate and indomethacin (letter). *Lancet* 1986;1(8494): 1390.
36. Kimberly RP. Treatment. Corticosteroids and anti-inflammatory drugs. *Rheum Dis Clin North Am* 1988;14(1):203–221.
37. De Broe ME, Elseviers MM. Analgesic nephropathy (see comments). *N Engl J Med* 1998;338(7):446–452.
38. Buckalew VJ. Nonsteroidal anti-inflammatory drugs and the kidney. In: Greenberg A, and National Kidney Foundation, eds. *Primer on kidney diseases*. San Diego: Academic Press, 1998:291–298.
39. Bennett WM, Henrich WL, Stoff JS. The renal effects of nonsteroidal anti-inflammatory drugs: summary and recommendations. *Am J Kidney Dis* 1996;28(1 suppl 1):S56–62.
40. Kelly CJ, et al. Prostaglandin E1 inhibits effector T cell induction and tissue damage in experimental murine interstitial nephritis. *J Clin Invest* 1987;79(3):782–789.
41. Kimberly RP, Plotz PH. Aspirin-induced depression of renal function. *N Engl J Med* 1977;296(8):418–424.
42. ter Borg EJ, et al. Renal effects of indomethacin in patients with systemic lupus erythematosus. *Nephron* 1989;53(3):238–243.
43. Herrera-Acosta J, et al. La inhibicion de la sintesis de prostaglandinas suprime la reserva funcional renal en pacientes con nefropatia lupica. *Rev Invest Clin* 1987;39(2):107–114.
44. Nagayama Y, et al. Beneficial effect of prostaglandin E1 in three cases of lupus nephritis with nephrotic syndrome. *Ann Allergy* 1988;61(4):289–295.
45. Patrono C, et al. Functional significance of renal prostacyclin and thromboxane A2 production in patients with systemic lupus erythematosus. *J Clin Invest* 1985;76(3):1011–1018.
46. Ling BN, et al. Naproxen-induced nephropathy in systemic lupus erythematosus. *Nephron* 1990;54(3):249–255.
47. Brezin JH, et al. Reversible renal failure and nephrotic syndrome associated with nonsteroidal anti-inflammatory drugs. *N Engl J Med* 1979;301(23):1271–1273.
48. Anonymous. Renal effects of fenoprofen (letter). *Ann Intern Med* 1980;93(3):508–509.
49. Sandler DP, Burr FR, Weinberg CR. Nonsteroidal anti-inflammatory drugs and the risk for chronic renal disease (see comments). *Ann Intern Med* 1991;115(3):165–172.
50. Nuyts GD, et al. New occupational risk factors for chronic renal failure. *Lancet* 1995;346(8966):7–11.
51. Segasothy M, et al. Chronic renal disease and papillary necrosis associated with the long-term use of nonsteroidal anti-inflammatory drugs as the sole or predominant analgesic. *Am J Kidney Dis* 1994;24(1):17–24.
52. Douthwaite A, Lintott G. Gastroscopic observation of effect of aspirin and certain other substances on stomach. *Lancet* 1938;2: 1222–1225.
53. Wolfe MM, Lichtenstein DR, Singh G. Gastrointestinal toxicity of nonsteroidal antiinflammatory drugs (see comments) (published erratum appears in *N Engl J Med* 1999;341(7):548). *N Engl J Med* 1999;340(24):1888–1899.
54. Piper JM, et al. Corticosteroid use and peptic ulcer disease: role of nonsteroidal anti-inflammatory drugs. *Ann Intern Med* 1991; 114(9):735–740.
55. Shorr RI, et al. Concurrent use of nonsteroidal anti-inflammatory drugs and oral anticoagulants places elderly persons at high

risk for hemorrhagic peptic ulcer disease. *Arch Intern Med* 1993; 153(14):1665–1670.

56. Lanza FL. A guideline for the treatment and prevention of NSAID-induced ulcers. Members of the Ad Hoc Committee on Practice Parameters of the American College of Gastroenterology. *Am J Gastroenterol* 1998;93(11):2037–2046.
57. Ehsanullah RS, et al. Prevention of gastroduodenal damage induced by non-steroidal anti-inflammatory drugs: controlled trial of ranitidine. *BMJ* 1988;297(6655):1017–1021.
58. Robinson MG, et al. Effect of ranitidine on gastroduodenal mucosal damage induced by nonsteroidal antiinflammatory drugs. *Dig Dis Sci* 1989;34(3):424–428.
59. Roth SH, et al. A controlled study comparing the effects of nabumetone, ibuprofen, and ibuprofen plus misoprostol on the upper gastrointestinal tract mucosa. *Arch Intern Med* 1993; 153(22):2565–2571.
60. Mizuno H, et al. Induction of cyclooxygenase 2 in gastric mucosal lesions and its inhibition by the specific antagonist delays healing in mice (see comments). *Gastroenterology* 1997; 112(2):387–397.
61. Schmassmann A, et al. Effects of inhibition of prostaglandin endoperoxide synthase-2 in chronic gastro-intestinal ulcer models in rats. *Br J Pharmacol* 1998;123(5):795–804.
62. Carneskog J, Florath-Ahlmen M, Olsson R. Prevalence of liver disease in patients taking salicylates for arthropathy. *Hepatogastroenterology* 1980;27(5):361–364.
63. O'Gorman T, Koff RS. Salicylate hepatitis. *Gastroenterology* 1977;72(4 pt 1):726–728.
64. Seaman WE, Ishak KG, Plotz PH. Aspirin-induced hepatotoxicity in patients with systemic lupus erythematosus. *Ann Intern Med* 1974;80(1):1–8.
65. Fries J, Holman H. *Systematic lupus erythematosus: a clinical analysis*. Philadelphia: WB Saunders, 1975.
66. Travers RL, Hughes GR. Salicylate hepatotoxicity in systemic lupus erythematosus: a common occurrence? *BMJ* 1978;2(6151): 1532–1533.
67. Widener HL, Littman BH. Ibuprofen-induced meningitis in systemic lupus erythematosus. *JAMA* 1978;239(11):1062–1064.
68. Moris G, Garcia-Monco JC. The challenge of drug-induced aseptic meningitis (see comments). *Arch Intern Med* 1999;159(11): 1185–1194.
69. Wasner CK. Ibuprofen, meningitis, and systemic lupus erythematosus. *J Rheumatol* 1978;5(2):162–164.
70. Samuelson CO Jr, Williams HJ. Ibuprofen-associated aseptic meningitis in systemic lupus erythematosus. *West J Med* 1979; 131(1):57–59.
71. Berliner S, et al. Ibuprofen may induce meningitis in (NZB × NZW)F1 mice. *Arthritis Rheum* 1985;28(1):104–107.
72. Fauci AS, et al. Immunoregulatory aberrations in systemic lupus erythematosus. *J Immunol* 1978;121(4):1473–1479.
73. Ruppert GB, Barth WF. Tolmetin-induced aseptic meningitis. *JAMA* 1981;245(1):67–68.
74. Weksler BB, Lehany AM. Naproxen-induced recurrent aseptic meningitis. *DICP* 1991;25(11):1183–1184.
75. Ballas ZK, Donta ST. Sulindac-induced aseptic meningitis. *Arch Intern Med* 1982;142(1):165–166.
76. Shoenfeld Y, et al. Sensitization to ibuprofen in systemic lupus erythematosus (letter). *JAMA* 1980;244(6):547–548.
77. Goldman JA, Klimek GA, Ali R. Allergy in systemic lupus erythematosus. IgE levels and reaginic phenomenon. *Arthritis Rheum* 1976;19(4):669–676.
78. Sequeira JF, et al. Allergic disorders in systemic lupus erythematosus. *Lupus* 1993;2(3):187–191.
79. Anonymous. Cutaneous reactions to analgesic-antipyretics and nonsteroidal anti-inflammatory drugs. Analysis of reports to the spontaneous reporting system of the Gruppo Italiano Studi Epidemiologici in Dermatologia. *Dermatology* 1993;186(3):164–169.
80. Szczeklik A, Gryglewski RJ, Czerniawska-Mysik G. Clinical patterns of hypersensitivity to nonsteroidal anti-inflammatory drugs and their pathogenesis. *J Allergy Clin Immunol* 1977;60(5):276–284.
81. Bigby M, Stern R. Cutaneous reactions to nonsteroidal anti-inflammatory drugs. A review. *J Am Acad Dermatol* 1985;12(5 pt 1): 866–876.
82. Petri M, Allbritton J. Antibiotic allergy in systemic lupus erythematosus: a case-control study (see comments). *J Rheumatol* 1992;19(2):265–269.
83. Wang CR, Chuang CY, Chen CY. Drug allergy in Chinese patients with systemic lupus erythematosus (letter; comment). *J Rheumatol* 1993;20(2):399–400.
84. Co S. Celebrex (celecoxib capsules). In: *Physicians' desk reference*. Montvale, NJ: Medical Economics, 2000:2901–2904.
85. deShazo RD, Kemp SF. Allergic reactions to drugs and biologic agents. *JAMA* 1997;278(22):1895–1906.
86. Patterson R, Bello AE, Lefkowith J. Immunologic tolerability profile of celecoxib. *Clin Ther* 1999;21(12):2065–2079.
87. Lander S, Wallace DJ, Weisman M. Safety and efficacy of celecoxib in SLE patients and SLE patients with a self-reported sulfa drug allergy. *Arthritis Rheum* (abst suppl) 2000;43:S242.

55

ANTIMALARIAL THERAPIES

DANIEL J. WALLACE

Antimalarials are effective nonsteroid drugs for some patients with non–organ-threatening lupus. Unlike other disease-modifying therapeutic agents that are used to treat systemic lupus erythematosus (SLE), antimalarials do not suppress the bone marrow or increase the risk for opportunistic infections.

HISTORICAL PERSPECTIVE

Antimalarials were first used therapeutically in 1630 as an antipyretic (1). They were first employed in the treatment of cutaneous lupus in 1894, when Payne (2) tried quinine. In 1928, Marstenstein (3) reported good results in 22 of 28 patients with discoid and subacute systemic lupus who were treated with pamaquine (Plasmachin), which is similar to quinine in that both are substituted 8-aminoquinolines. In 1938, Davidson and Birt (4) reported excellent results in 19 of 29 patients who were treated with quinine bisulfate. In 1941, Prokoptochouk (5,6) successfully treated 35 patients with discoid lupus erythematosus (LE) by giving daily doses of 300 mg of quinacrine (Atabrine, mepacrine), a compound first synthesized by the Germans during the 1920s but possibly first discovered by Paul Ehrlich a decade earlier (7). During World War II, quinine supplies were cut off by the Japanese, and the U.S. Surgeon General declared Atabrine to be the official drug to treat malaria (8,9). Between 1943 and 1946, 3 million Americans took the drug daily. Anecdotal evidence of its efficacy in treating some skin disorders among British soldiers prompted Page (10) to study the drug for use in the treatment of discoid lupus. Unaware of Prokoptochouk's work, he reported in 1951 its benefits in an uncontrolled study of 18 patients with lupus and two with rheumatoid arthritis (RA), and the report received wide attention. These findings were soon confirmed at the Mayo Clinic by O'Leary et al. (11).

Subsequently, it was shown that other antimalarials also are effective. Chloroquine was patented in 1934 and hydroxychloroquine synthesized by the mid-1940s and shown to be less toxic than quinacrine. In 1953, Goldman et al. (12) reported that chloroquine was helpful in 21 patients, including three with subacute disseminated disease, and in 1954, Pillsbury and Jacobson (13) noted that 15 of 16 patients with SLE taking chloroquine improved. Hydroxychloroquine (Plaquenil) was released in 1955 after it was found to be effective in SLE and RA, with fewer adverse reactions than chloroquine (14–16). Amodiaquin (Camoquin) also was efficacious in SLE, but it was taken off the market in the United States in the early 1970s because of its propensity to induce agranulocytosis (17–19). It is still available in many other countries. Finally, an extremely potent antimalarial, Triquin (which contained chloroquine, hydroxychloroquine, and quinacrine) took advantage of the synergy between quinacrine and the chloroquines. It was released in 1959 after a report claimed that 44 of 45 patients with lupus, mostly antimalarial-resistant, at Boston City Hospital had dramatic responses (20). The preparation sold well until it was withdrawn in 1972 as part of a campaign against the use of combination drugs. Sanofi-Winthrop discontinued the production of Atabrine in 1992, but it is still available from 2,500 compounding pharmacists in the United States who can obtain quinacrine hydrochloride powder from Sigma or ICN chemical suppliers (21).

PHARMACOLOGY OF THE ANTIMALARIALS

Chloroquine

Chloroquine (7-chloro-4-;{4-diethylamino-1-methylbutylamino} (Fig. 55.1). Almost completely absorbed by the gastrointestinal tract, only 10% is fecally excreted. Renal excretion (50%) is increased by acidification and decreased by alkalinization. The drug is bound by plasma proteins and largely deposited into tissues. High concentrations can be found in the liver, spleen, kidney, lung, and all blood elements (2,25–27), as well as in pigmented tissues. Chloroquine is broken down into three *N*-dealkylated metabolites that are of toxologic and pharmacologic importance including desethylchloroquine and bisdesethylchloroquine. Chloroquine and desethylchloroquine competitively inhibit CYP2DI/6-mediated reactions *in vivo* and *in vitro*. The

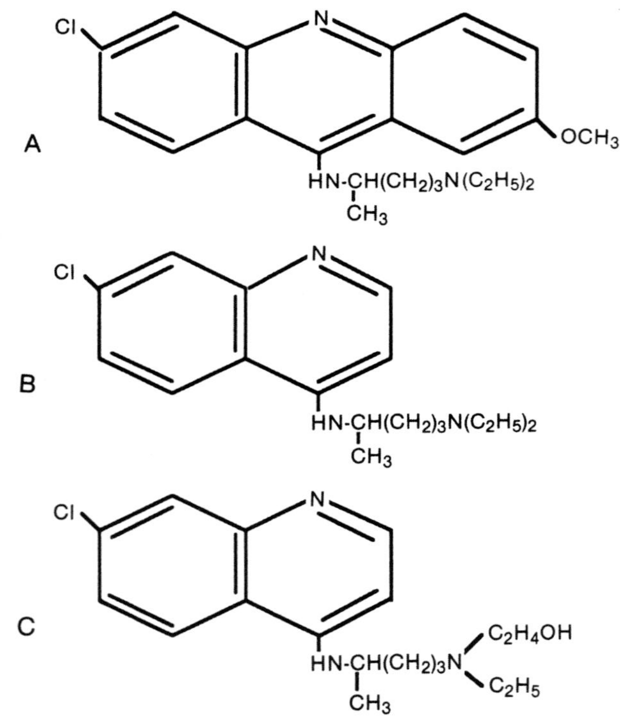

FIGURE 55.1. Structural formulas of commonly used antimalarial drugs. **A:** Quinacrine. **B:** Chloroquine. **C:** Hydroxychloroquine. (From Wallace (311), with permission.)

R (−) chloroquine enantiomer may be more potent, has a longer half-life, and higher unbound plasma concentrations (28–30) The drug readily crosses the placenta and is excreted in small amounts in breast milk. A child receives less than 1% of the maternal dose (31,32).

Chloroquine is slowly excreted with elimination half-lives of 20 to 60 days, but detectable amounts in the urine, red cells, and plasma for as long as 5 years after discontinuation (33). The half-life is governed by dose-dependent kinetics, increasing from 3 hours after a single 250-mg dose to 13 days after 1,000 mg. Chloroquine decreases creatinine clearance by a mean of 10 in 55% of its users, probably by increasing plasma aldosterone levels (34,35). Drug interactions have been reported with ampicillin and methotrexate (chloroquine decreases its bioavailability), but not with aspirin (36–38). It has *in vitro* synergy with cyclosporine and antagonism with d-penicillamine (39).

Hydroxychloroquine

Hydroxychloroquine sulfate (2-[[4-[(7-chloro-4-quinolinyl) amino]pentyl]ethylamin]ethanol sulfate; Plaquenil) is a 4-aminoquinoline that differs from chloroquine by a hydroxyl group at the end of a side chain (Fig. 55.1). The two agents have similar pharmacokinetics. The 200-mg tablets contain 155 mg of hydroxychloroquine base, consisting of equal amounts of (−)-(R) and (+)-(S) enantiomers. The (+)-(S) form has greater bioavailability (40) but a shorter half-life (41). Hydroxychloroquine is broken down into three metabolites: desethylchloroquine, desethylhydroxychloroquine, and bidesethylchloroquine (42). Hydroxychloroquine is 75% to 100% absorbed in the gastrointestinal tract, with 50% in 2 to 10 hours and 50% bound by serum proteins (43–45). Some is conjugated with glucuronide and excreted in the bile, but 30% to 60% is biotransformed in the liver. Excretion occurs in two stages: a rapid one, with a half-life of 3 days; and a slower one, with an overall half-life of 40 days. Forty-five percent is excreted by the kidney, 3% by the skin, and 20% fecally. It takes 6 months to reach a 96% steady state. Much of the drug is deposited into tissues, with the highest concentrations in the adrenal and pituitary glands. Other areas with high concentrations include melanin-containing tissues, liver, spleen, and leukocytes. Inflammatory disease activity does not correlate with drug blood concentrations (46). Hydroxychloroquine is approximately two thirds as effective as chloroquine and half as toxic (47).

The drug may slightly alter kidney function; 15 of 118 patients with RA had a mean 10% decrease in creatinine clearance (34). The dosage must be reduced in patients with renal failure. Dialysis does not help overdosage, because the agent is extensively sequestered (45).

Hydroxychloroquine can interact with digoxin and reduce its levels (a quinidine-like effect) (48). One five-center survey has suggested that hydroxychloroquine administration may decrease the frequency of liver enzyme abnormalities seen in patients with RA who are on methotrexate or salicylate therapy (49), and this has been confirmed by another report (50).

Quinacrine

Quinacrine (6-chloro-9-[-methyl-4-diethylamine]butylamine-2-methoxyacridine; Atabrine, mepacrine, Atebrine, chinacrin, Erion, Acriquine, Acrichine, Palacrin, Metoquine, Italchin) differs from chloroquine only in having an acridine nucleus (i.e., an extra benzene ring) instead of a quinoline (Fig. 55.1). The drug is rapidly absorbed after oral administration. Plasma levels rise in 2 to 4 hours, reaching a peak in 8 to 12 hours (51). Plasma concentration increases rapidly during the first week, and 94% equilibrium is attained by the fourth week. The drug is distributed widely in tissue but is slowly liberated, with the highest concentrations in the liver and spleen and the lowest concentrations in the brain and heart. The liver concentration may be 20,000 times that in plasma. Skin deposits often are clearly visible. Quinacrine crosses the placenta and reaches the fetus. Spinal fluid levels are 1% to 5% of plasma levels. Eighty percent to 90% of the drug is bound to plasma proteins in therapeutic doses, and it has a half-life of 5 to 14 days. It is slowly excreted from the body; less than 11% is eliminated in the urine daily (52).

Quinacrine also can be administered intralesionally (53,54), for discoid lesions, intramuscularly, intravenously, rectally, transcervically, or delivered through a chest tube for malignant pleural effusions (52,55).

MECHANISMS OF ACTION

Light Filtration

One of the major aggravating factors in patients with SLE is ultraviolet (UV) light exposure. More UV radiation is absorbed (Table 55.1) when skin concentrations of antimalarials are higher (44–46). Antimalarials deposited in the skin absorb UV light in a concentration-dependent manner (56–58). Hydroxychloroquine, but not methotrexate, methylprednisolone, or saline, blocked cutaneous reactions induced by UV light (59). Topical chloroquine protects against UVA- or UVB-induced erythema (60). Sontheimer's group (61) has shown that chloroquine modulates UV activation of the c-*jun* proto-oncogene, which protects against UV damage. Ironically, the chloroquines and quinacrine can also induce a photosensitivity reaction (62–64). An antiinflammatory effect or downregulating action on keratinocytic function also might be important (65). Quinacrine can impede photodynamic actions, inhibit laser-induced photosensitivity, and increase UV light tolerance (10), perhaps by scavenging water radicals (66–68).

TABLE 55.1. IMPORTANT MECHANISMS OF ACTION OF ANTIMALARIAL DRUGS

Immunologic actions
Blocks antigen processing by raising intracytoplasmic pH, which depletes cells of their receptor sites with consequent decrease in cytokine production (especially IL-1, IL-6, and TNF-α)
Inhibit natural killer activity, mitogenic stimulation
Impedes formation and helps dissolve immune complexes
Antiinflammatory effects
Inhibits phospholipase A_2 and C
Prostaglandin antagonization
Stabilizes lysosomal membranes
Decreases fibronectin release by macrophages
Blocks superoxide release at multiple sites
UV light absorption
Hormonal actions
Decreased estrogen production
Hypoglycemic, impairs insulin release
Antiproliferative activities
Blocks graft versus host disease
Intercalates with DNA
DNA, RNA polymerase inhibition
Decreased tumor size and chemotherapy resistance
Inhibits platelet aggregation and adhesion
Antimicrobial effects, decrease antibiotic resistance
Anticholinesterase and sympatholytic actions
Quinidinelike cardiac actions, reduction of infarct size
Lowers cholesterol and LDL levels by 15% to 20%

TNF, tumor necrosis factor; IL, interleukin; LDL, low-density lipoprotein.

Immunologic Effects

The principal mechanism of action of hydroxychloroquine and chloroquine relates to their elevation of intracytoplasmic pH. Because antigen processing is an acidic, pH-dependent component, the chloroquines turn off this process by decreasing the number of autoantigenic peptides presenting on the cell surface (69,70). The tendency of chloroquine and hydroxychloroquine to target macrophage-mediated cytokines such as interleukin-1 (IL-1), IL-2, and tumor necrosis factor-α to a greater extent than T-helper cell–mediated cytokines such as IL-2, IL-4, and IL-5 suggests that its sites of action are preferential (71–79). Chloroquine also inhibits interferon-γ production by CD4- and CD8-positive synovial T-cell clones in patients with RA (80), suppresses natural killer cell activity (81,82), and suppresses IL-6 immune activity in a variety of mitogenic stimulation studies (81–90).

Raising the pH of cytoplasm has a profound effect on the lysosomal membranes, which are stabilized (85,91–96). Chloroquine is concentrated in the nuclear and lysosomal fractions of white blood cells (92,97). Chloroquine becomes trapped in lysosomes and alters their pH, which results in an increase in lysosome number and volume. Inclusion bodies (i.e., myelin bodies) containing plasma membrane phospholipid accumulate because of the reversible inhibition of membrane recycling; this remarkable action leads to decreased phagocytosis, chemotaxis, and cell functioning. More specifically, it substantially depletes the cell of its surface receptors (trapping approximately 50% of them), which alters the cell's responsiveness to mitogenic stimuli (44,66,93,94,98). Quinacrine probably has similar actions (66,99–101).

Chloroquine has opposing actions, in that it inhibits the formation of antigen-antibody complexes *in vitro* and enhances the association of such complexes in a dose-dependent fashion (102) or can split them (103). Chloroquine has been used to dissociate antigen-antibody complexes as part of a laboratory technique that is used in typing red blood cells with a positive direct antiglobulin test (104,105). Also, it strips human leukocyte antigens (HLAs) from lymphocyte and platelet membranes (106–108). Clinically, it has been shown to decrease circulating immune complex levels in patients with RA (109).

Chloroquine blocks the DNA–anti-DNA reaction by binding not to the anti-DNA antibody but to the DNA (110). Competition for binding sites on DNA among chloroquine, sodium ions, and anti-DNA antibodies occurs only under nonphysiologic conditions (111). Work from Dubois' and Kunkel's laboratories documented that the binding of quinacrine to nucleoproteins can block the LE cell factor (112–114).

Antiinflammatory Effects

Chloroquine is a strong prostaglandin antagonist (especially against phospholipase A_2) and a weak agonist (115–118). The antagonist effect clearly is demonstrable at concentrations that are reached in human plasma when the drug is used therapeutically (118). Chloroquine reduces prostaglandin synthesis through the inhibition of phospholipases A_2 and C (116,119–121). Antiphospholipase A_2 blockade decreases the actions of bradykinin in synovial fibroblasts, suppresses its algesic effects, and decreases histamine release from basophils (122–126). *In vitro* hexosamine depletion of intact articular cartilage by E prostaglandins is accomplished through the DNA-dependent RNA synthesis of cathepsin-like proteases (127). This can be inhibited by chloroquine through the inhibition of DNA primer.

Chloroquine and hydroxychloroquine also exhibit antiinflammatory actions by decreasing IL-1–induced cartilage degeneration, perhaps through inhibiting elastase (128, 129), fibronectin release by macrophages (130), and reactions that are dependent on sulfhydryl-disulfide interaction (131). Chloroquine inhibits angiogenesis *in vitro*, which results in antiinflammatory effects (132,133).

Quinacrine also is a potent inhibitor of phospholipase A_2, which results in decreased leukotriene and prostaglandin release (117,119,134–143). It is a nonselective antilipolytic agent that decreases prostaglandin E_2 production in a dose-dependent fashion. Thromboxanes B_2 and A_2 are specifically suppressed. Quinacrine also stabilizes cell membranes as a result of its Na-K-adenosine triphosphatase (ATPase) inhibitory effects (141), and it inhibits lysosomal enzymes that are involved in phospholipid catabolism. Strongly concentrated in leukocytes and lysosomes, quinacrine has a stabilizing effect (136). Phagocytosis, chemotaxis, RNA synthesis, and hexose monophosphate shunt burst activity are inhibited by the drug (66,67,144–146).

Chloroquine and quinacrine also are antipyrogens (147–149).

Hormonal Effects

Chloroquine may reduce estrogen production (150) and have an adrenal-stimulating effect (151). In patients with RA and sarcoidosis, it decreases 1,25-hydroxyvitamin D levels (152, 153). A major area of interest concerns its applications in diabetes as a result of the agent's hypoglycemic action. This occurs secondary to chloroquine-induced decreased degradation of insulin (154,155), inhibiting lysosomal proteolysis (156) and, possibly, decreasing insulin-induced loss of receptors (157). Although hydroxychloroquine lowers blood sugars in patients with SLE by a mean 5 mg/dL (158), occasional reports of clinically evident, chloroquine-associated hypoglycemia have been published (159–161).

Quinacrine accumulates in peptide hormone-producing cells (162,163), and it can block prolactin (164,165) and insulin release. Conflicting reports about its effects on 17-ketosteroids have been published (10,125).

Antioxidant Effects

In high doses, chloroquine can inhibit polymorphonuclear oxidative bursts (166). Chloroquine, hydroxychloroquine, and quinacrine block superoxide release by actions at multiple sites on the metabolic pathway (141,145,167–170), which may have a beneficial effect on bronchial asthma (171).

Antiproliferative And Graft Versus Host Effects

Chloroquine interferes with protein synthesis *in vivo* and *in vitro* (172,173). It blocks DNA and RNA biosynthesis and produces rapid degradation of ribosomes and dissimilation of ribosomal RNA. By intercalation, chloroquine inhibits DNA and RNA polymerase reactions *in vitro* and DNA replication and RNA transcription in susceptible cells (174). Chloroquine does not alter the ability to repair damage from UV light–induced DNA excisions (175). It impedes DNA synthesis stimulated by platelet-derived growth factor (176). Interest has focused on its anticarcinogenic properties. Chloroquine can inhibit the replication of Moloney leukemia virus and tumor development in newborn mice (177), be toxic to melanoma cells (178), and inhibit pancreatic adenocarcinoma cell growth (179). Further, it can potentiate hyperthermia therapies with or without radiation (180–182), block Z-DNA formation (183), and enhance chemotherapy cytotoxicity in multiple drug-resistant human leukemic cells (184). Both chloroquine and hydroxychloroquine decreased alloreactivity in three separate studies as part of preventing graft versus host disease among transplant patients (133,185,186).

Quinacrine also binds to DNA by intercalation between adjacent base pairs (187–189). Quinacrine blocks radiation-induced DNA strand breaks and potentiates the antiproliferative effects of radiation (68,189–194). It reduces the incidence of cancer in rats given nitrosourea (195), decreases the number of somatic mutations induced in murine leukemia cells (196), decreases tumor size in mice (182,197), and reverses resistance to vincristine (198). Lymphocytes *in vitro* treated with quinacrine show increased chromosomal aberrations (199).

Antiplatelet Effects

Hydroxychloroquine and chloroquine that accumulate in blood platelets can inhibit platelet aggregation and adhesion in a dose-dependent fashion (200–204). A desludging effect was demonstrated in the retinal veins of 20 patients with RA (205), and additional studies suggested that hydroxychloroquine reduces the size of thrombi and does not prolong bleeding time (202,207,208). As a result, the drug has been used for thromboprophylaxis of postoperative pulmonary emboli in orthopedic patients (209). Quinacrine also can inhibit platelet aggregation, probably because of its antiphospholipase actions or its interaction with 3′,5′-cyclic guanosine monophosphate (cGMP) (210–214).

Antimicrobial Effects

Inhibition of DNA replication may be the mechanism of action for the antimicrobial effects of chloroquine. It does not impede the growth of viruses but does protect the cells against virus-induced cell damage (215). Chloroquine's discontinuation has been associated with flares of viral infections (216). Chloroquine and hydroxychloroquine inhibit replication of the human immunodeficiency virus in T cells and monocytes (217,218), which may account for the negative association between AIDS and SLE (219). Quinacrine has antiparasitic, antiprotozoan, antibacterial, antiviral, and antifungal actions (52). It can prevent resistance to various antibiotics and increase interferon production (220), and perhaps prevent pneumocystis infection (221).

Muscle And Nerve Effects

Chloroquine is a muscarinic receptor antagonist, which results in an atropine-like effect in humans (220,222). The agent also can block dopamine β-hydroxylase (223). Quinacrine is a strong inhibitor of cholinesterase because of its inhibition of cGMP (133,142,224,225). It can block β-agonists, α-adrenergic actions, and norepinephrine (142, 224,226–228). Quinacrine protects mice from lethal amounts of snake venom neurotoxins (229).

Cardiac Effects

Both chloroquine and quinacrine possess quinidine-like actions. Chloroquine increases heart rate, lowers blood pressure, and decreases premature ventricular contractions in humans (230–232). Patients taking chloroquine routinely show electrocardiographic flattening of T waves and a slight prolongation of the QT interval (233). Quinacrine's antiarrhythmic actions occur as a result of slowing inward current and decreasing the automaticity of Purkinje fibers; it can treat atrial fibrillation and prevent ventricular fibrillation (234,235). The antiphospholipase A_2 actions of chloroquine and quinacrine resulted in studies demonstrating that both can decrease acute myocardial ischemic damage in dogs, rats, pigs, and cats (236–245).

Antihyperlipidemic Effects

Animal studies have shown that chloroquine decreases serum bile acid and cholesterol levels by 10% to 20% (246–248). Lysosomotropic agents reduce the proteolysis of many plasma membrane receptors, and chloroquine increases the number of low-density lipoprotein (LDL) receptors (249–252). Alternatively, inhibition of the hydrolysis of internalized cholesterol esters also may lead to increased LDL receptor levels (250,251) (discussed later).

Promotion Of Apoptosis

Defective regulation of apoptosis may be central to the development of autoimmune disease. Meig et al. (206) showed that hydroxychloroquine was able to induce apoptosis in lupus peripheral blood lymphocytes in a dose- and time-dependent manner, and Potvin et al. (253) were able to reproduce this with chloroquine in human endothelial cells. Krieg's group (254) suggested that this could be prevented *in vitro* when CpG dinucleotides activate NF-κB.

CLINICAL STUDIES

Chloroquines: Antilupus Activity

As early as 1956, Ziff et al. (255) noted a favorable response in 11 of 12 patients with SLE who are given antimalarials and commented on the reduction of steroid requirements (Table 55.2). Dubois (256) claimed that 90% to 95% of patients had a favorable response. To evaluate the effectiveness of medication for the treatment of discoid LE, it is essential to know the incidence of spontaneous remissions. In Dubois' (257) studies, 10% of patients had a history of spontaneous

TABLE 55.2. MAJOR CLINICAL TRIALS OF CHLOROQUINES IN SLE

Source	Findings
Ziff et al. (255)	11 of 12 patients had favorable responses; steroid-sparing properties noted
Dubois (256,257)	90% with non–organ-threatening disease improved with hydroxychloroquine; over 300 patients treated
Rothfield et al. (262–264)	27 patients who stopped chloroquine because of macular changes had more flares after 1 year than in either of the prior 2 years while taking it
Callen (261)	33 of 34 given hydroxychloroquine for cutaneous lupus responded (9, excellent; 15, very good; 6, good; 3, fair; 1 poor)
Esdaile et al. (267)	47 patients controlled with hydroxychloroquine were given continued therapy or placebo for 24 weeks; treated group had fewer disease flares and severe disease exacerbations
Williams et al. (269)	71 patients in controlled/placebo trial of articular complaints showed subjective joint pain assessment improvement with hydroxychloroquine
Meinao et al. (271)	24 patient, double-blind study in Brazil; chloroquine was steroid sparing and prevented disease flares

improvement. In the series of Herrman et al. (258), 14% of patients healed spontaneously, compared with 85% or more who improved with antimalarials (259,260). Callen (261) treated 62 patients with discoid lupus at the University of Louisville over a 5-year period, and he reported on 34 who were given hydroxychloroquine. Of these, nine patients were said to have an excellent response, 15 were very good, six good, three fair, and one poor.

Rothfield et al. (262–264) studied the discontinuation of antimalarial therapy on SLE activity in 27 patients who had developed maculoretinopathy. Exacerbations during the 2 years before and 1 year after discontinuation were compared. On this basis, ten patients had more exacerbations during the year after antimalarials were stopped than during either of the 2 previous years while receiving these drugs. Of these, three had no increase in the number of exacerbations, and four had fewer exacerbations after the discontinuation of therapy. The required maintenance dose of prednisone was higher after the discontinuance of antimalarial treatment. The data suggested that chloroquine therapy is a factor in the suppression of disease in ten of 17 patients and is steroid-sparing. Hughes (265) found hydroxychloroquine to be particularly useful for anti-Ro/SSA–positive disease, confirmed its steroid-sparing properties, and advocated combined antimalarial therapy for resistant cases.

The Canadian Hydroxychloroquine Study Group (266,267) studied 47 patients with SLE whose disease was controlled with hydroxychloroquine and randomized them to either continued hydroxychloroquine or placebo for 24 weeks. The hydroxychloroquine group had significantly fewer disease flares and a lower risk of severe disease exacerbation. A 3-year follow-up study by the group confirmed this. Hydroxychloroquine was felt to have a favorable impact on the morbidity and mortality of the Johns Hopkins Lupus Cohort (268).

Nine centers from the Cooperative Systemic Studies of the Rheumatic Diseases studied hydroxychloroquine versus placebo among 71 patients with mild SLE in a 48-week trial. Patient assessment of joint pain significantly improved, and only two patients withdrew because of adverse effects (269). Similarly, Littlejohn's group in Australia noted only 8% of patients with lupus who were given hydroxychloroquine discontinued the drug at 12 months, and only 24% at 24 months (270). A double-blind study of chloroquine in 44 steroid-dependent patients with SLE found it to be steroid-sparing and to prevent disease flares (271). Petri and Yadia (272) negatively associated hydroxychloroquine use with the development of proteinuria. Rothfield's group (273) found hydroxychloroquine to be of value in treating three patients with SLE and hypergammaglobulinemic purpura.

Ruzicka et al. (274) compared acitretin, a retinoid with hydroxychloroquine in 58 patients with cutaneous lupus. Although the drugs were only given for 8 weeks, 50% in both groups cleared; however, the retinoid group had many more side effects.

Antilupus Actions: Quinacrine With Or Without Chloroquines

The results of the last quinacrine-alone clinical trial were published in 1961, but between 1940 and 1961, 20 reports on 771 patients were published (52) (Table 55.3). Remarkable for the similarity of their findings, 27% of patients had an excellent response, 46% improved, and 27% did not respond. Cutaneous and constitutional symptoms improved first, and the chloroquines were superior to quinacrine in treating synovitis.

Combinations of chloroquines with quinacrine have shown favorable results. Ten of 14 patients with chloroquine- or hydroxychloroquine-resistant cutaneous disease cleared their lesions when quinacrine was added in one survey (275), and 13 of 15 cleared their lesions in another (276). Toubi et al. (277) confirmed this in six patients by lowering Systemic Lupus Erythematosus Disease Activity Index (SLEDAI) scores (277).

Adjunctive Useful Actions Of Antimalarials In Patients With Lupus

Antithrombotic Effects

The actions of chloroquines on platelets were reviewed earlier. In 1985, I reported that the antiplatelet effects of hydroxychloroquine were associated with a statistically significant decrease in thromboembolic disease among 92 patients evaluated (278). A follow-up survey suggested that this trend was applicable to patients with anticardiolipin antibody (279). Petri et al.'s (280,281) 393-member lupus cohort has confirmed this in a prospective study, and McCarty and Hellman (282) confirmed it among 121 patients at the University of Indiana.

Antihyperlipidemic Effects

As discussed earlier, antimalarials have an antihyperlipidemic action. In 1990, our group showed that hydroxychloroquine induced a 15% to 20% decrease in serum cholesterol, triglyceride, and LDL levels in 150 patients (283) (Table 55.4). These actions might decrease the hyperlipidemic and atherogenic effects of corticosteroids and suggest a greater adjunctive role for hydroxychloroquine. Hodis et al. (284) confirmed these findings, as did Petri et al.'s (285) longitudinal regression analysis among her 264 patient cohort and the results of other investigators (286–291), including in children (292). Quinacrine also lowered lipid levels in a double-blind, placebo-controlled trial of 16 patients with diabetes (293).

Additional Possible Benefits Of Antimalarials In Patients With Lupus

Fox (294) found that hydroxychloroquine decreased antibody levels in patients with Sjögren's syndrome, most of whom

TABLE 55.3. TWENTY-ONE CLINICAL TRIALS OF ATABRINE IN LUPUS

Investigator	Year	Patients (*n*)	Response (%) Excellent	Improved	None or Doubtful
Prokoptchouk[a]	1940	(35)	?	?	?
Sorinson	1941	51	23	33	43
Page	1951	18	50	33	17
Somerville et al.	1952	23	17	66	17
Cramer and Lewis	1952	6	83	0	17
Wells	1952	12	25	50	25
Sawicky et al.	1952	30	20	50	30
Black	1953	60	17	38	45
O'Leary et al.	1953	40	40	36	25
Courville and Perry	1953	13	38	54	8
Kaminsky and Knallinsky	1953	61	16	62	21
Harvey and Cochrane	1953	62	37	23	40
Kierland et al.	1953	52	33	46	21
Rogers and Finn	1954	45	47	38	15
Helanen	1954	36	28	58	14
Christiansen and Nielson	1956	97	32	40	28
Dubois	1956	61	25	56	20
Nielsen	1956	12	17	75	8
Buchanan	1959	25	28	52	20
Winklemann et al.	1961	67	10	75	15
Lipsker	1995	15	53	27	20
Totals (*n*)		771	209	352	210
Totals (%)		100	27	46	27

[a]Excellent or improved response, 73% (5).
Adapted from Wallace DJ. The use of quinacrine (Atabrine) in rheumatic diseases: a reexamination. *Semin Arthritis Rheum* 1989;18:282–296, with permission.

reported less dryness after 1 to 3 years of therapy. Other studies tend to support this (295,296). Reports also have suggested that hydroxychloroquine or chloroquine ameliorate methotrexate-induced rheumatoid nodulosis or liver function abnormalities (49,50,297) and has analgesic actions (298).

In conclusion, it seems to be generally agreed that antimalarials are effective for cutaneous manifestations, polyarthralgia, pleuritis, and low-grade pericardial inflammation associated with SLE. In addition, some of the associated malaise and lethargy are ameliorated. Antimalarials are of no effect in seriously ill patients with central nervous system involvement, hematologic changes, or renal disease. They help in withdrawing steroid therapy once remission has been induced by steroids and other agents (264,299)

TABLE 55.4. EFFECT OF ANTIMALARIALS ON LIPIDS[a]

Parameter[b]	Group A (*n* = 58)	Group B (*n* = 35)	Group C (*n* = 18)	Group D (*n* = 44)
Cholesterol	180.93 ± 49.44	212.71 ± 36.84	186.22 ± 36.70	204.64 ± 49.44
HDL	59.40 ± 20.30	56.59 ± 14.00	57.41 ± 15.88	53.90 ± 16.95
LDL	101.00 ± 29.62	120.26 ± 32.59	102.41 ± 28.97	127.27 ± 41.10
Triglyceride	106.45 ± 51.41	172.57 ± 99.95	145.05 ± 61.54	128.93 ± 68.48
Medications (ms)				
Mean dose HCQ	386	0	400	0
Mean dose steroids[c]	0	10.83	8	0

[a]All serum levels expressed as mg/dL ± 1 SD. A—HCQ alone; B—steroids alone; C—HCQ and steroids; D—neither HCQ nor steroids.
[b]Important significant comparisons; $p < .05$, group B versus C (cholesterol) and HCQ versus no HCQ (triglyceride): $p < .01$, group A versus D (cholesterol); $p < .001$, HCQ versus no HCQ (cholesterol), HCQ versus no HCQ (LDL), and steroids versus no steroids (triglyceride).
[c]Steroid dose expressed as daily equivalent dose of prednisone.
HCQ, hydroxychloroquine: HPL, high-density lipoprotein.
Adapted from Wallace DJ, Metzger AL, Stecher VJ, et al. Cholesterol-lowering effect of hydroxychloroquine in patients with rheumatic disease: reversal of deleterious effects of steroids on lipids. *Am J Med* 1990;89:322–326, with permission.

and may be useful in diminishing the atheroembolic complications of SLE.

DOSAGE

The dosing schedule used in the treatment of discoid LE varies with extent of the skin lesions and the patient's tolerance of the drugs. Theoretically, it is advisable to begin with a larger initial dosage so that equilibrium can be reached sooner. From a practical standpoint, however, the treatment of discoid LE is not urgent. Although an initial loading dose is advisable for the moderately ill patient with SLE, larger starting doses produce a high incidence of side effects, such as nausea, vomiting, and diarrhea, and therefore discourage the patient from further trials with the drug (300). In our experience, some patients who note gastrointestinal side effects with generic hydroxychloroquine do not have the same problems with brand name Plaquenil.

Hydroxychloroquine usually should be initiated in a dosage of 400 mg daily (given once daily or in 200-mg divided doses). This should approximate 5 to 7 mg/kg/d. Responses usually begin in 2 to 3 months, but the drug does not reach its peak efficacy for 6 to 12 months. In more urgent situations, 600 mg daily may be given for 1 to 2 months. This is associated with a greater incidence of gastrointestinal complications and retinotoxicity if used for more than a few months (301). Smoking may decrease the effectiveness of hydroxychloroquine in cutaneous lupus (302).

Chloroquine usually is given in a dosage of 250 to 500 mg daily; this should approximate 4 mg/kg/d. Chloroquine works within 1 to 2 months but is associated with a 10% incidence of retinotoxicity, compared with 3% for hydroxychloroquine (303). Hence, the eyes should be checked at 3-month intervals for patients on chloroquine and at 6-month intervals for those on hydroxychloroquine. Plasma levels do not correlate with efficacy (304).

As little as 1 g of chloroquine can be fatal to a child, and 3 g can be fatal to an adult. The pills taste bitter, which tends to discourage abuse. Overdoses are managed with mechanical ventilation, epinephrine, activated charcoal, and diazepam (305–308).

If additional therapy is required, quinacrine can be added. It has an established synergy with the chloroquines (20,52,57,275–277,309). Usually, 100 mg are given daily (although up to 200 mg daily can be administered), but as little as 25 mg may be effective. Occasionally, therapy can be initiated with quinacrine as opposed to the chloroquines when ophthalmologic considerations contraindicate the latter's use. Also, quinacrine is a much greater cerebral cortical stimulant than the chloroquines and is used for patients in whom fatigue is overwhelming (310). Quinacrine is not retinotoxic. Its onset of action is 3 to 6 weeks.

In my experience, at least 95% of patients with skin lesions of discoid LE and SLE show moderate to significant benefit from treatment with antimalarials (311). The most common cause of failure is the physician's impatience in giving the drugs adequate time to work. After 1 to 2 years of therapy, antimalarials can be tapered. Hydroxychloroquine is decreased to 200 mg daily for 3 to 6 months, then reduced by eliminating days of the week (e.g., the next decrement from 200 mg daily would be 5 days a week for 3 months, then 3 days a week). One or two tablets per week may be all that is required to suppress skin lesions, and this helps to minimize toxicity. The reader is referred to Bernstein (303) for a more detailed discussion of the issues reviewed in this section.

PREGNANCY

See Chapter 47.

ADVERSE REACTIONS

The adverse reactions to antimalarials are listed in Table 55.5 and discussed here.

TABLE 55.5. TOXIC EFFECTS OF CHLOROQUINE AND HYDROXYCHLOROQUINE[a]

Nervous system[b]	Gastrointestinal system[c]
Peripheral neuropathy	Anorexia
Involuntary movements	Abdominal distention
Difficulty in visual accommodation	Abdominal cramps
Vestibular dysfunction	Heartburn
Nerve deafness	Nausea
Tinnitus	Vomiting
Migrainelike headache	Diarrhea
Lassitude	Weight loss
Nervousness	Eyes
Insomnia	Subjective[c]
Mental confusion	Impaired reading ability
Toxic psychosis	Poor distant vision
Convulsive seizures	Scotomas
Skin and hair	Night blindness
Dryness of skin[c]	Entopic phenomena
Pruritus[c]	Objective
Urticaria[c]	Decreased color vision[c]
Morbilliform rash[c]	Scotoma with or without pigment changes in fundus[c]
Maculopapular rash[c]	Arterial constriction[b]
Desquamating and exfoliating lesions[b]	Retinal edema[b]
Increased pigmentation of skin[c]	Pallor of optic dish[b]
Porphyria cutanea tarda	Pigmentation about macula[c]
Bleaching of hair[b]	Bull's-eye lesion[c]
Hair loss[b]	Loss of corneal reflex[c]
Blood[b]	Deposits in cornea[c]
Leukopenia	Retinopathy[c]
Agranulocytosis	

[a]If given in recommended doses.
[b]Occurs in less than 1%.
[c]Occurs in 1% to 20% given chloroquine and in 1% to 10% given hydroxychloroquine.
Adapted from Kelley WN, Harris ED Jr, Ruddy S, Sledge CB. *Textbook of rheumatology.* Philadelphia: WB Saunders, 1980, with permission.

Generalized And Gastrointestinal Reactions

Considering their remittive potential, antimalarial therapies generally are well tolerated when compared with other disease-modifying drugs. In one study, more than 90% of patients who were prescribed hydroxychloroquine for lupus were still taking the drug a year later (270). Approximately 10% of those receiving hydroxychloroquine and 20% receiving chloroquine complain of anorexia, abdominal distention and cramps, heartburn, nausea, vomiting, diarrhea, and/or weight loss. These symptoms are transient, decrease, or disappear with lower dosing or changing to brand name Plaquenil, and they do not cause long-term sequelae. In Esdaile's group's (300) cohort, 20 of 156 (13%) patients followed for up to 15 years stopped antimalarials due to side effects, half of which were gastrointestinal. Quinacrine may create these symptoms in up to 30% of patients, and diarrhea may be particularly pronounced. It can be alleviated with lower doses or by taking a bismuth suspension (e.g., Pepto-Bismol) with quinacrine. The chloroquines are associated with musculoskeletal, flulike symptoms of aching and fatigue in 5% to 10% of patients, but symptoms resolve within 1 to 2 weeks even if therapy is continued.

Antimalarials rarely are hepatotoxic (52,296). One report of hepatic failure possibly associated with hydroxychloroquine has appeared (312).

Neuromuscular And Cardiac Effects

In 1948, Nelson and Fitzhugh (313) first reported that the chronic administration of chloroquine to rats induces necrosis of cardiac and voluntary muscle. The term *chloroquine neuromyopathy* has evolved over the years; it is clinically evident in fewer than 1% of those taking chloroquine and has been the subject of only about a dozen case reports with hydroxychloroquine (314–329). Patients complain of muscle weakness, numbness, and tingling, and they sometimes have myasthenic symptoms. Active inflammatory myositis, hypokalemia, and steroid myopathy must be considered in the differential diagnosis. A myasthenia gravis–like picture with ptosis occasionally appears, which is reversible with drug discontinuation (330,331). The patient may present with an acute polyneuropathy. Peripheral nerves may demonstrate segmental demyelination and cytoplasmic inclusions in Schwann cells (and in perineural and endothelial cells to a lesser extent). Histopathologic investigation of the muscles reveals a vacuolar myopathy, acid phosphatase–positive vacuoles in type I fibers, and lysosomal hyperreactivity with large secondary lysosomes. Electron microscopy reveals electron-dense curvilinear bodies and concentric and parallel lamellae within the muscle (332). Both skeletal and cardiac muscle can be involved. Muscle enzyme levels only occasionally are elevated. Electromyography reveals fibrillations, positive sharp waves, complex, repetitive discharges, and sometimes a myotonia pattern. Dramatic recovery is associated with discontinuation of the drug. Plasma chloroquine levels do not correlate with the clinical or pathologic picture (333). Muscle enzyme levels only occasionally are elevated. This syndrome does not occur with quinacrine.

Rarely, acute urinary retention, heart block, or a congestive cardiomyopathy has been associated with chloroquine, but not with hydroxychloroquine (334–340).

Cutaneous And Pigmentary Changes

Antimalarials can induce skin dryness, pruritus, pustulosis, porphyria, erythema annulare, urticaria, changes in pigment, rashes, psoriatic flares, and exfoliating lesions (341,342). Approximately 3% of patients have to discontinue the drug secondary to adverse cutaneous reactions (331). Psoriatic flares result from the ability of hydroxychloroquine to interfere with epidermal transglumatase activity, which stimulates epidermal proliferation (343). Quinacrine is associated with a lichen planus or eczema-like eruption that, if ignored, can be the first sign in a chain of events that ultimately leads to aplastic anemia. Any rash resulting from quinacrine requires its immediate cessation (52).

Pigment changes occur in 10% to 25% of those who are receiving long-term chloroquine therapy and in a smaller percentage of those taking hydroxychloroquine (344–347). These adverse effects rarely, if ever, require discontinuing treatment. Gum pigmentation is common (348), and grayness at the roots of scalp hair, eyelashes, eyebrows, and beard may be observed, along with gray streaks in the hair. A blue-black discoloration occasionally is noted on the skin (Fig. 55.2). Chloroquine binds with melanin *in vivo* and *in vitro* by the electrostatic attraction of positively charged drug molecules to negative groups of the melanin polymer; this probably is supplemented by van der Waals forces or charge transfer complexes. These changes are reversible when chloroquine therapy is stopped. Nail beds can be affected and appear to be diffusely pigmented (Fig. 55.3) or to display transverse bands. Chloroquines frequently can cause light sensitivity (349,350) or, rarely, porphyria (351) in patients with SLE.

Quinacrine also binds to melanin. Membrane-bound intracellular quinacrine granules combined with large amounts of iron and sulfur produce asymptomatic black-and-blue marks, especially on the shins and hard palate (Fig. 55.4). Quinacrine also can induce a yellow stain that, like the pigment, is dose related and resolves with cessation of therapy or lowering of the dose. The stain may be evident in up to 30% of patients; it sometimes looks like a suntan and may enhance the patient's appearance (52). All of these changes also are reversible.

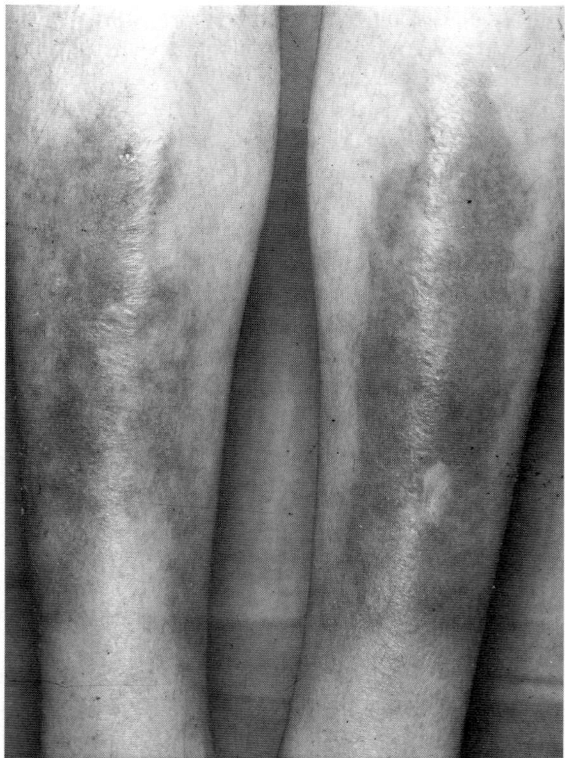

FIGURE 55.2. Blue-black pretibial pigmentation from prolonged antimalarial administration.

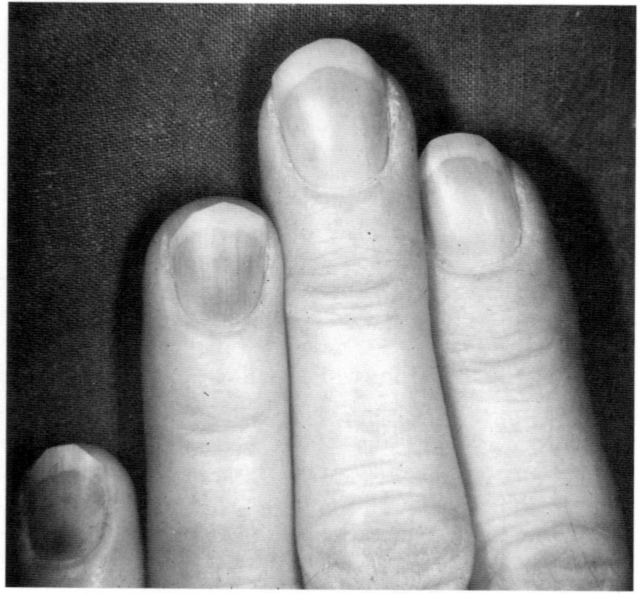

FIGURE 55.3. Nail-bed pigmentation resulting from antimalarial therapy.

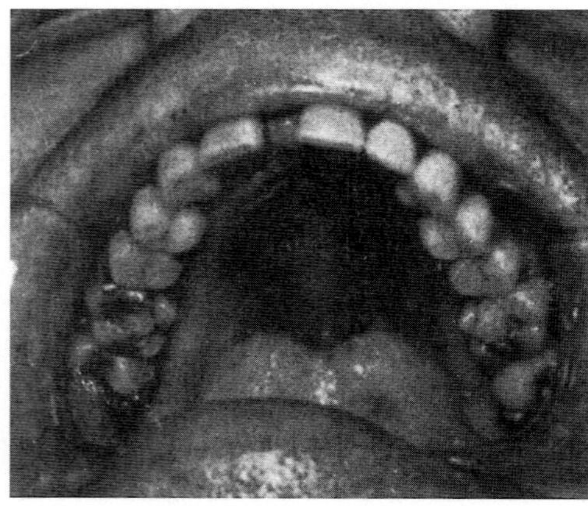

FIGURE 55.4. Blue-black pigmentation on the hard palate caused by antimalarial therapy.

Central Nervous System

Quinacrine and, to a lesser extent, chloroquine, are cerebral cortical stimulants. Engel et al.'s (310) classic study documented electroencephalographic patterns that were compatible with pronounced psychic stimulation in a group of healthy volunteers given 200 to 1,200 mg of quinacrine daily for 10 days. Symptoms of fatigue and mental clouding may be ameliorated. On the other hand, excessive dosing can result in psychosis, seizures, and hyperexcitability (52,256,310,352–354). A 0.4% incidence of reversible, toxic psychosis was reported among 7,604 U.S. soldiers who were given 100 mg of quinacrine daily in World War II and in 28 patients among 30,000 who were treated for malaria (0.1%) (355,356). Central nervous system complications of chloroquine, such as mania or insomnia, have infrequently been noted in SLE (357,358).

Hematologic Toxicity

Hydroxychloroquine has been associated with only one case of agranulocytosis, in a patient who was given 1,200 mg daily (359), which is three to six times the current recommended dose. Chloroquine, but not hydroxychloroquine, has been implicated in some reports with glucose-6-phosphatase deficiency hemolysis (360) and with agranulocytosis (361). Toxic granulation has been observed in the leukocytes of patients receiving long-term chloroquine, which represents large, membrane-bound myelin bodies in mature neutrophils and lymphocyte (362,363).

The prevalence of aplastic anemia among U.S. soldiers in the Pacific during World War II increased from 0.66 to 2.84 per 100,000 after quinacrine's introduction (364). This represented 58 patients, 48 of whom received quinacrine. Of these, 16 were associated with overdoses, and two received other marrow-suppressant drugs concurrently. Wallace's review analyzes these cases, reviews the literature, and suggests ways to prevent this from occurring (52; also see 365,366).

Miscellaneous Effects

Antimalarials may inhibit gastric motility based on their parasympatholytic effects (367), and they may induce hypokalemia (368), and its quinine-like actions are responsible for sensineural hearing loss (369).

Ocular Toxicity

Corneal, Ciliary Body, And Lens Changes

Corneal deposits of chloroquine are observed in 18% to 95% of patients, appear within several weeks, and are symptomatic in 50% of patients (302,370–375). Keratopathy is limited to the corneal epithelium; the pattern can vary from punctate opacities to whirling lines. Visual acuity is not reduced, but patients may complain of halos around light sources and of photophobia. No residual damage occurs, and corneal deposits disappear with drug discontinuation and usually are not a reason to stop therapy. Corneal sensation may be decreased by 50% (376). Because recommended chloroquine doses have decreased over the last 30 years, corneal problems now occur less frequently (377). Two studies were unable to find any corneal changes among 164 patients who were given hydroxychloroquine for 3 to 7 years (378,379). Easterbrook (380,381) reported a 5% to 10% incidence of corneal infiltrates with hydroxychloroquine, but none were symptomatic. A decreased dosage is advised for these patients. Hydroxychloroquine crystals may be seen in the tear film by slit-lamp examination (370). In doses three to six times greater than those currently recommended, quinacrine can induce corneal edema rarely (382,383).

Alterations in accommodation and induction of cataracts rarely occur with long-term chloroquine therapy and have not been reported with hydroxychloroquine or quinacrine (374).

Retinopathy

Since the first report appeared in 1957 (384), approximately 300 cases of chloroquine and hydroxychloroquine retinopathy have been reviewed in the literature. Retinopathy is an often-misunderstood problem that needlessly deters patients from initiating antimalarial therapy. Bernstein's (303) thorough analysis concluded: "I would estimate that the risk of (reversible) retinopathy in patients who are not regularly monitored ophthalmologically is 10% for those receiving chloroquine and 3% to 4% for those receiving hydroxychloroquine at presently recommended dosage levels. With regular and accurate observation and testing, these risks might be reduced substantially."

Clinical Presentation And Pathophysiology

SLE can induce retinal vascular lesions secondary to disease activity that are unrelated to any form of therapy, and macular degeneration is a common feature of the normal aging process. Thus, it is not always easy to implicate antimalarials as the cause of retinal dysfunction. The chloroquines usually take years to induce pathology, and early retinopathy is asymptomatic. Patients with lupus who are aware of the retinotoxicity of antimalarials often complain of visual symptoms weeks after starting therapy; this can be attributed to corticosteroid or nonsteroidal antiinflammatory drug (NSAID) treatment, or to psychopathology.

The most common presenting symptoms are difficulty in reading, photophobia, blurred distance version, visual-field defects, and light flashes. Premaculopathy consists of fine pigmentary stippling of that area. Eventually, it becomes surrounded by a zone of depigmentation encircled by an area of pigment, giving a bull's-eye appearance (Fig. 55.5). Rods and cones (which compose the macula) are particularly sensitive to the chloroquines. With more extensive retinal damage, the arterioles show generalized attenuation and segmental constriction with disk pallor. In the periphery of the fundus, a prominent choroidal pattern and fine granularity of the retina are seen. Many years later, gross pigment changes of hereditary retinal depigmentation may occur, and color vision and the foveolar reflex are lost (374,375,385–388).

Several theories account for chloroquine retinopathy. Retinal pigmented epithelial cells perform as macrophages and digest the discarded outer segments of photoreceptor cells as they are physiologically shed. Lysosomal accumulation (discussed earlier) results in an intracellular buildup of lamellar myelin bodies, which leads to scotoma (389). Alternatively, melanin deposits in the retina produce pigmentation of the rods and cones and of the pigmented cells in the outer nuclear and outer plexiform layers, with result-

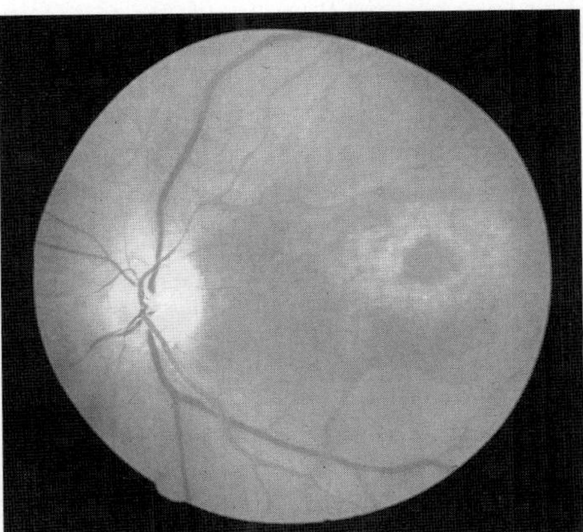

FIGURE 55.5. Bull's-eye macular pigmentation secondary to hydroxychloroquine (1,200 mg/dL for 15 months in a 90-lb woman).

ing pathology (390,391). Platelet-activating factor or chloroquine's effect on inhibiting protein synthesis may play a role (392,393). Cases of retinopathy have been reported, however, in the absence of pigment deposition (394). Chloroquine, but not hydroxychloroquine, breaks down the blood–retina barrier, as documented by vitreous fluorophotometry (394,395).

Important Clinical Studies

The incidence of retinopathy has decreased over the last 30 years, because currently recommended doses of both chloroquine and hydroxychloroquine are approximately 50% of the formerly recommended doses. In 1992, Bernstein (396) reviewed all published cases of hydroxychloroquine retinopathy and those reported by the Food and Drug Administration (FDA) between 1960 and 1990. Only 20 patients fulfilled validated criteria. In 15 of the patients, recommended dosing levels were exceeded, and the remaining five patients took the drug for longer than 10 years.

In 1967, Bernstein (385) first observed that lower chloroquine doses were associated with a lower incidence of retinopathy. In 1966, Voipio (387) believed that patients with lupus are more susceptible to retinopathy than are those with RA. Mackenzie (397) reviewed experiences with over 900 patients with RA. If doses were kept below 5.1 mg/kg/d for chloroquine or 7.8 mg/kg/d for hydroxychloroquine in patients with normal hepatic and renal functions, retinotoxicity did not occur. Marks and Power (398) followed 222 patients who were given a mean of 286 g of chloroquine for a mean of 36 months. Twenty-two developed retinal changes, and only one had decreased visual acuity. These changes were directly related to age, total dose, and duration of treatment. In another study, Marks (399) sent questionnaires to 45 rheumatologists in Great Britain; 23 had never had a patient with antimalarial eye toxicity. Mills et al. (400) reviewed the experience of 347 patients who were treated with hydroxychloroquine. The chief risk factor was a patient age of more than 70 years (in whom preexisting macular degeneration commonly was seen) and a cumulative dose of more than 800 g. Of the patients in this subset, 29 had at least a mild pigmentary maculopathy, but none had decreased visual acuity or altered foveolar light thresholds. Macular changes in patients under the age of 40 years and on doses of less than 600 mg/d of hydroxychloroquine were not seen. Runge (401) reported no cases of retinopathy among 101 patients with RA given hydroxychloroquine for a mean of 20 months. Rynes et al. (378,379,402) also have carried out a number of studies on the effects of antimalarials. In 99 patients (31% of whom had SLE) who were given 400 mg of hydroxychloroquine daily for a mean of 37 months, no retinotoxicity was reported (378), but in a follow-up report 4 years later (403), it was observed in 4% of the patients with RA.

Elman et al. (404) studied 270 patients with RA who were given chloroquine for up to 15 years. They noted that senile macular atrophy is seen in 30% of healthy patients over the age of 65, and that chloroquine toxicity is greater in this group and more difficult to evaluate. Only one patient had clear-cut, drug-induced retinopathy. Two studies from the National Institutes of Health followed over 100 patients (405,406). No differences in retinopathy between the SLE and RA groups were noted, and retinotoxicity from hydroxychloroquine did not occur. Retinotoxicity occurred in 4% of patients with total chloroquine dosages of less than 400 g, in 8% with less than 800 g, but in 50% (two of four patients) with greater than 800 g. Frenkel (407) followed 100 patients for a mean of 3 years on daily dosages of hydroxychloroquine from 200 to 400 mg; no retinopathy was noted. Bell and Boh (408) noted retinopathy in four of 142 patients with RA given hydroxychloroquine but, contrary to previous reports, was unable to relate this to total dose, duration, or age.

Easterbrook (409,410) screened 1,500 patients at the University of Toronto for retinopathy over a 15-year period. Of the 50 cases that were detected, only one patient was on hydroxychloroquine (in a high dosage of 600 mg daily). The chloroquine retinopathy patients were only taking a dose slightly higher than the mean. Chloroquine is associated with progressive visual loss, even after drug discontinuation, because of the long time it is present in tissues (409). One report documented the onset of macular changes in a young man with progressive visual impairment 7 years after stopping the drug (410). A total of seven such cases have appeared, and interpretation is difficult as a result of poor documentation or the likelihood of the macular degeneration of aging being a factor (411–415). The onset of retinotoxicity has never been reported after the cessation of hydroxychloroquine. One large center in Great Britain stopped screening patients taking hydroxychloroquine after failing to find a single case of retinopathy in 73 patients who had taken the drug for more than 18 months (416), and Hughes' London-based group (417) found no cases among 82 patients with rheumatic disease who had taken hydroxychloroquine for at least 1 year.

Three studies conducted in the 1990s found hydroxychloroquine induced "reversible premaculopathy" in 10 of 437 patients (418), retinopathy in one (in whom dosing was excessive) of 1,207 patients (419), and 0 of 758 patients (420). Mavrikakis et al. (421) followed 58 Greek connective tissue disease patients prospectively with eye examinations every 6 months. Two developed new evidence of retinopathy at 6.5 and 8 years, respectively, with appropriate dosing. The lesions were still present 3 years later. In 1998, the Canadian government warned, "Although chloroquine has been used in the treatment of rheumatoid arthritis and discoid lupus erythematosus, it is considered that the potential toxicity of the drug outweighs any anticipated benefits" (422). I agree with the statement, but I find chloroquine useful in patients who live in countries where hydroxychloroquine is not available or prohitively expensive and in patients with severe cutaneous rashes for up to 90 days.

Only one case of questionable retinotoxicity has been reported with quinacrine (423). Zuehlke et al. (424) noted no eye toxicity from quinacrine in 26 patients followed at the University of Iowa over a 30-year period and reviewed the literature. None of the 200 patients treated with quinacrine by Dubois or those that I have treated have evolved retinopathic changes (52).

Once the lesion appears, no specific therapy other than cessation of the antimalarial is required. Although antimalarial excretion can be increased by acidification with ammonium chloride, ascorbic acid, or British antilewisite, nothing indicates that the ocular lesion is improved (385). The best and only treatment is discontinuation of the drug if even equivocal changes of retinopathy occur. Mackenzie and Szilagyi (425) suggested that sunglasses may prevent the retinal lesion. They showed that high-dose chloroquine concentrates in melanin in pigment epithelium, blocking the normal light-absorbing action of melanin and thereby removing its protective mechanism. This has been supported by laboratory studies in rats (426), but it is premature to advocate the use of sunglasses in all patients who are taking antimalarials.

TABLE 55.6. EYE TOXICITY FROM ANTIMALARIAL MEDICATIONS

Cornea	Symptoms of photophobia and halos around light sources, decrease in sensation Usually mild and can come and go; rarely requires drug to be stopped These changes are always reversible with drug cessation; no permanent damage reported Chloroquine: noted in 50% Hydroxychloroquine: found in 5–10% Quinacrine: reported in 5%
Retina	Melanin deposits or lamellar myelin bodies in retinal pigmented epithelial macrophages Clinically presents as scotomas; especially targets rods and cones Must be differentiated from macular degeneration associated with aging Chloroquine: found in 10% after 10 years of continuous use; can be irreversible Hydroxychloroquine: found in 3% after 10 years of continuous use; always reversible if doses of <7 mg/kg/d used and patient not in renal failure Quinacrine: not reported
Monitoring recommendations	Chloroquine: eye examination every 3–4 months Hydroxychloroquine: eye examination every year at doses of 5 mg/kg/d or less; every 6 months at doses up to 7 mg/kg/d; every 3 months at higher doses Quinacrine: no special precautions

Retinal Testing And Clinical Correlates

Ophthalmologists have many techniques that purport to evaluate retinal and macular integrity and function, but most agree to disagree about the optimal sequence of testing. Patients who are taking chloroquine should have an eye examination every 3 months, and every 6 months with hydroxychloroquine. Two helpful reviews of these methods for antimalarial monitoring have been published (374,427).

If color vision is abnormal, testing is inexpensive and reliable; some investigators believe it is the most sensitive method (428). The time it takes to recover macular function after illumination of the retina is known as the macular dazzle test. Although it is thought to be prolonged in patients with early antimalarial maculopathy (429), Easterbrook (430) found that it is abnormal in almost all patients who are on antimalarials and does not distinguish those with retinopathy from those without. Fluorescein angiography shows striking macular uptake. Its sensitivity and specificity ratings are disappointing (374), however, and it was less reliable than color vision testing in a controlled, comparative study (428).

Visual field testing, especially if augmented by Amsler grids, is a simple and inexpensive screen for paracentral scotomas (430). Amsler grids can be self-administered and are easily reproducible in cooperative patients (431). Electrooculography (EOG) reflects the metabolic integrity of the retinal pigment epithelium but correlates poorly with macular changes that are induced by chloroquines. Electroretinography is another technically complex procedure that detects late changes, but it is difficult to interpret in early disease. In addition, many nonspecific abnormal readings are noted in normal patients. Dark adaptation testing probably is of little value. One controlled study found contrast sensitivity testing to be superior to pattern visual-evoked potentials and EOG (432). In a fascinating report, a British survey found that rheumatologists could identify 52 of 65 minor retinal changes in patients on chloroquine and concluded that expensive, frequent eye examinations generally are unnecessary (433). Table 55.6 provides a summary of, and our group's recommendations for, eye toxicity in antimalarials.

When Is Retinal Testing Cost Effective?

Rynes and Alpert et al. (434) estimated that $20 million is spent on retinal testing in the United States for patients taking hydroxychloroquine each year. Two groups have suggested that $126,000 to $200,000 is spent on biannual exams or $74,000 on annual exams to pick up each case of retinopathy (419,435). A recent consensus conference recommended annual eye examinations in low-risk individuals on hydroxychloroquine therapy who have been on the drug for less than 10 years in doses of 6.5 mg/kg/day or less (436).

SUMMARY

1. Three antimalarials that are commercially available in the United States have documented efficacy in the treatment of lupus erythematosus: chloroquine, hydroxychloroquine, and quinacrine.
2. These agents are the safest drugs available and are recommended for patients with non–organ-threatening lupus who require more than sunscreens, steroid salves, or NSAIDs.
3. Chloroquines are most effective for treatment of the following features of LE (in decreasing order): cutaneous lesions, arthritis-arthralgias, fatigue, and serositis. Chloroquine is more powerful than hydroxychloroquine. Quinacrine is most effective for the following (in decreasing order): cutaneous lesions, fatigue, arthritis-arthralgias, and serositis.
4. Chloroquine and quinacrine are effective in 1 to 2 months; hydroxychloroquine often requires a 3- to 6-month wait. Chloroquines and quinacrine are synergistic and can be combined.
5. Antimalarials work by turning off antigen processing by raising intracytoplasmic pH. They also work by blocking damaging UV light, suppressing immune reactivity, promoting apoptosis, inhibiting antibody formation, and blocking prostaglandin and leukotriene synthesis by the inhibition of phospholipase A_2. They also inhibit platelet aggregation and adhesion, decrease membrane receptor sites because of lysosomal membrane accumulation, and are antimicrobial and antiproliferative.
6. Steroid-sparing actions also have been documented.
7. Higher dosing can cause a faster response but also greater toxicity.
8. Generalized gastrointestinal and musculoskeletal complaints are reversible and usually minor. The only serious complication of the chloroquines is retinotoxicity, which is observed in 10% of patients on chloroquine and in 3% of those on hydroxychloroquine. This can be minimized by frequent eye examinations and the use of hydroxychloroquine. Irreversible retinal changes have never been reported in a patient with lupus who was taking hydroxychloroquine in recommended doses for up to 6 years and undergoing eye checks every 6 months (437). Quinacrine is not retinotoxic, but blood counts need to be monitored because it can cause aplastic anemia (rarely).

REFERENCES

1. Leden I. Antimalarial drugs: 350 years. *Scand J Rheumatol* 1981;10:307–312.
2. Payne JF. A postgraduate lecture on lupus erythematosus. *Clin J* 1894;4:223–229.
3. Marstenstein H. Subacute lupus erythematosus and tubercular cervical adenopathy. Treatment with plasmochin. *Z Hart Geschlechskr* 1928;27:248–249.
4. Davidson AM, Birt AR. Quinine bisulfate as a desensitizing agent in the treatment of lupus erythematosus. *Arch Dermatol Syph* 1938;37:247–253.
5. Prokoptchouk AJ. Treatment of lupus erythematosus with acridine. *Z Haut Geschlechtskr* 1940;66:112(abst).
6. Prokoptchouk AJ. Article translated into English. *Arch Dermatol Syph* 1955;71:520.
7. Wallace DJ, Is there a role for quinacrine (Atabrine) in the new millennium? *Lupus* 2000;9:81–82.
8. Office of the Surgeon General. Circular letter no. 153; the drug treatment of malaria, suppressive and clinical. *JAMA* 1943;123: 205–208.
9. Greenwood D, Historical perspective. Conflicts of interest: the genesis of synthetic antimalarial agents in peace and war. *J Antimicrob Chemother* 1995;36:857–872.
10. Page F. Treatment of lupus erythematosus with mepacrine. *Lancet* 1951;2:755–758.
11. O'Leary PA, Brunsting LA, Kierland RR. Quinacrine (atabrine) hydrochloride in treatment of discoid lupus erythematosus. *Arch Dermatol* 1953;67:633–634.
12. Goldman L, Cole DP, Preston RH. Chloroquine diphosphate in treatment of discoid lupus erythematosus. *JAMA* 1953;152: 1428–1429.
13. Pillsbury DM, Jacobson C. Treatment of chronic discoid lupus erythematosus with chloroquine (Aralen). *JAMA* 1954;154: 1330–1333.
14. Cornbleet T. Discoid lupus erythematosus treatment with plaquenil. *Arch Dermatol* 1956;73:572–575.
15. Lewis HM, Frumess GM. Plaquenil in the treatment of discoid lupus erythematosus: preliminary report. *Arch Dermatol* 1956; 73:576–581.
16. Mullins JF, Watts FL, Wilson CJ. Plaquenil in the treatment of lupus erythematosus. *JAMA* 1956;161:879–881.
17. Leeper RW, Allende MF. Antimalarials in the treatment of discoid lupus erythematosus: special reference to amodiaquin (Camoquin). *Arch Dermatol* 1956;73:50–57.
18. Maguire A. Amodiaquine hydrochloride in the treatment of chronic discoid lupus erythematosus. *Lancet* 1962;i:665–667.
19. Pappenfort RB, Lockwood JH. Amodiaquin (Camoquin) in treatment of chronic discoid lupus erythematosus; preliminary report, with special reference to successful response of patients resistant to other antimalarial drugs. *Arch Dermatol* 1956;74:384–386.
20. Tye MJ, White H, Appel B, et al. Lupus erythematosus treated with a combination of quinacrine, hydroxychloroquine and chloroquine. *N Engl J Med* 1959;260:63–66.
21. The quinacrine connection. *Fitzpatrick's J Clin Dermatol* 1994;Jan/Feb.
22. Closson RG. Liquid dosage form of chloroquine. *Drug Intell Clin Pharm* 1988;22:347.
23. Goodman LS, Goodman A. *The pharmacologic basis of therapeutics*, 5th ed. New York: Macmillan, 1975:1045–1069.
24. Okor RS, Nwankwo MU. Chloroquine absorption in children from polyethylene glycol base suppositories. *J Clin Pharmacol Ther* 1988;13:219–223.
25. French JK, Hurst NP, O'Donnell ML, et al. Uptake of chloroquine and hydroxychloroquine by human blood leukocytes in vitro: relation to cellular concentrations during antirheumatic therapy. *Ann Rheum Dis* 1987;46:42–45.
26. Nosal R, Ericsson O, Sjoqvist F, et al. Distribution of chloroquine in human blood fractions. *Methods Find Exp Clin Pharmacol* 1988;10:581–587.
27. Raghoebar M, Peeters PA, van den Berg WB, et al. Mechanisms of cell association of chloroquine to leucocytes. *J Pharmacol Exp Ther* 1986;238:302–306.
28. Berliner RW, Earle DP, Taggert JV, et al. Studies on the

chemotherapy of the human malarials, the physiological disposition, antimalarial activity and toxicity of several derivations of 4-amino-quinidine. *J Clin Invest* 1948;27:98–107.

29. Ette EI, Essien EE, Thomas WO, et al. Pharmacokinetics of chloroquine and some of its metabolites in healthy volunteers:a single dose study. *J Clin Pharmacol* 1989;29:457–462.
30. Ducharme J, Farinotti R, Clinical pharmacokinetics and metabolism of chloroquine. Focus on recent advancements. *Clin Pharmacokinet* 1996;31:257–274.
31. Ette EI, Essien EE, Ogonor JI, et al. Chloroquine in human milk. *J Clin Pharmacol* 1987;27:499–502.
32. Leng JJ, Mbanzulu PN, Akbaraly JP, et al. Transplacental passage of chloroquine sulphate: in vitro study. *Path Biol (Paris)* 1987;35:1051–1054.
33. Rubin M, Bernstein HN, Zvaifler NJ. Studies on the pharmacology of chloroquine. Recommendations for the treatment of chloroquine retinopathy. *Arch Ophthalmol* 1963;70:474–481.
34. Landewe RBM, Vergouwen MSC, Goei The HS, et al. Antimalarial drug induced decrease in creatinine clearance. *J Rheumatol* 1995;22:34–37.
35. Musabayane CT, Ndhlovu CE, Balment RJ. The effects of oral chloroquine administration on kidney function. *Ren Fail* 1994; 16:221–228.
36. Seidman P, Albertioni F, Beck O, et al. Chloroquine reduces the bioavailability of methotrexate in patients with rheumatoid arthritis. *Arthritis Rheum* 1994;37:830–833.
37. Adelusi SA, Salako LA. Protein binding of chloroquine in the presence of aspirin. *Br J Clin Pharmacol* 1982;13:451–452.
38. Ali HM. Reduced ampicillin bioavailability following oral coadministration with chloroquine. *J Antimicrob Chemother* 1985;15:781–784.
39. Dijkmans BA, de Vries E, de Vreede TM. Synergistic and additive effects of disease modifying anti-rheumatic drugs combined with chloroquine on the mitogen-driven stimulation of mononuclear cells. *Clin Exp Rheumatol* 1990;8:455–459.
40. Iredale J, Fieger H, Wainer IW. Determination of the stereoisomers of hydroxychloroquine and its major metabolites in plasma and urine following a single oral administration of racemic hydroxychloroquine. *Semin Arthritis Rheum* 1993;23:74–81.
41. Ducharme J, Fieger H, Ducharme MP, et al. Enantioselective disposition of hydroxychloroquine after a single oral dose of the racemate to healthy subjects. *Br J Clin Pharmacol* 1995;40: 127–133.
42. Iredale J, Wainer IW. Determination of hydroxychloroquine and its major metabolites using sequential achiral-chiral high performance liquid chromatography. *J Chromatogr* 1992;573:253–258.
43. McLachlan AJ, Tett SE, Cutler DJ, et al. Bioavailability of hydroxychloroquine tablets in patients with rheumatoid arthritis. *Br J Rheumatol* 1994;33:235–239.
44. Mackenzie AH. Pharmacologic actions of 4-aminoquinoline compounds. *Am J Med*1983;75(suppl 1A):5–10.
45. Tett SE, Cutler DJ, Day RO, et al. Bioavailability of hydroxychloroquine tablets in healthy volunteers. *Br J Clin Pharmacol* 1989;27:771–779.
46. Tett SE, Day RO, Cutler DJ. Concentration-effect relationship of hydroxychloroquine in rheumatoid arthritis—a cross sectional study. *J Rheumatol* 1993;20:1874–1879.
47. Scherbel AL, Harrison JW, Atdjian M. Further observations on the use of 4-aminoquinolone compounds in patients with rheumatoid arthritis related diseases. *Cleve Clin Q* 1958;25:95.
48. Leden I. Digoxin-hydroxychloroquine interaction? *Acta Med Scand* 1982;211:411–412.
49. Fries JF, Singh G, Lenert L, et al. Aspirin, hydroxychloroquine, and hepatic enzyme abnormalities with methotrexate in rheumatoid arthritis. *Arthritis Rheum* 1990;33:1611–1619.
50. Aponte J, Petrilli M, von Dawson N. Liver enzyme levels in arthritis patients treated with long-term bolus methotrexate. *Arthritis Rheum* 1992;35:126–127.
51. Joint Report of Armored Medical Research Laboratory, Fort Knox, KY, and Commission on Tropical Diseases, Army Epidemiological Board, Preventive Medicine Service, Office of the Surgeon General, United States Army. Plasma quinacrine concentration as a function of dosage and environment. *Arch Intern Med* 1946;78:64–107.
52. Wallace DJ. The use of quinacrine (Atabrine) in rheumatic diseases: a reexamination. *Semin Arthritis Rheum* 1989;18:282–296.
53. Ottolenghi-Lodigiani F. Local intradermal application of acridine preparations for treatment of chronic lupus erythematosus. *Hautarzt* 1955;6:24–27.
54. Thies W. Recent experiences in treatment of chronic discoid lupus erythematosus with atabrine and chloroquine, particularly with local and combined therapy. *Hautarzt* 1955;6:227–232.
55. Wallace DJ. Controversy over sclerotherapy for malignant pleural effusions. *Ann Intern Med*1994;121:150–151.
56. Cahn MM, Levy EJ, Schaffer B, et al. Lupus erythematosus and polymorphous light eruptions; experimental study on their possible relationship. *J Invest Dermatol* 1953;21:375–396.
57. McChesney EW, Nachod FC, Tainter ML. Rationale for treatment of lupus erythematosus with antimalarials. *J Invest Dermatol* 1957;29:97–104.
58. Shaffer B, Cahn MM, Levy EJ. Absorption of antimalarial drugs in human skin: spectroscopic and chemical analysis in the human skin and corium. *J Invest Dermatol* 1951;30:341–345.
59. Lester RS, Burnham TK, Fine A, et al. Immunologic concepts of light reaction in lupus erythematosus and polymorphous light eruption. I. The mechanism of hydroxychloroquine. *Arch Dermatol* 1967;96:1–10.
60. Sjolin-Forsberg G, Lindstrom B, Berne B. Topical chloroquine applied before irradiation protects against ultraviolet B (UVB)- and UVA-induced erythema but not against immediate pigment darkening. *Photodermatol Photoimmunol Photomed* 1992–1993; 9:220–224.
61. Nguyen TQ, Capra JD, Sontheimer RD. 4-Aminoquinoline antimalarials enhance UV-induced c-jun transcriptional activation, *Lupus* 1998;7:148–157.
62. Motten AG, Martinez LJ, Holt N, et al. Photophysical studies on antimalarial drugs. *Photochem Photobiol* 1999;69:282–287.
63. Nord K, Orsteel A-L, Karlsen J, et al. Photoreactivity of biologically active compounds, X: photoreactivity of chloroquine in aqueous solution. *Pharmazie* 1997;52:598–603.
64. Forest SE, Stimson MJ, Simon JD. Mechanism for the photochemical production of superoxide by quinacrine. *J Phys Chem [B]* 1999;103:3963–3964.
65. Sjolin-Forsberg G, Berne B, Eggelte TA, et al. In situ localization of chloroquine and immunological studies in UVB-irradiated skin of photosensitive patients. *Acta Derm Venereol* 1995; 75:228–231.
66. Ferrante A, Rowan-Kelly B, Seow WK, et al. Depression of human polymorphonuclear leucocyte function by anti-malarial drugs. *Immunology* 1986;58:125–130.
67. Rainsford KD. Effects of antimalarial drugs on interleukin-1–induced cartilage proteoglycan degradation in vitro. *J Pharm Pharmacol* 1986;38:829–833.
68. Hissung A, Dertinger H, Heinrich G. The action of ionizing radiation on DNA in the presence of quinacrine. I. UV absorption and fluorescence measurements. *Radiat Environ Biophys* 1975;12:5–12.
69. Fox RI. Mechanism of action of hydroxychloroquine as an antirheumatic drug. *Semin Arthritis Rheum* 1993;23:82–91.
70. Fox RI, Kang H-I. Mechanism of action of antimalarial drugs: inhibition of antigen processing and presentation. *Lupus* 1993;2 (suppl 1):S9–S12.

71. Sperber K, Quraishi H, Kalb TH, et al. Selective regulation of cytokine secretion by hydroxychloroquine: inhibition of interleukin 1 alpha and IL-6 in human monocytes and T cells. *J Rheumatol* 1993;20:803–808.
72. Wallace DJ, Linker-Isareli M, Hyun S, et al. The effect of hydroxychloroquine therapy on serum levels of immunoregulatory molecules in patients with systemic lupus erythematosus. *J Rheumatol* 1994;21:375–376.
73. Picot S, Peyron F, Vuillez J-P, et al. Chloroquine inhibits tumor necrosis factor production by human macrophages in vitro. *J Infect Dis* 1991;164:830.
74. Ertel W, Morrison MH, Ayala A, et al. Chloroquine attenuates hemorrhagic shock-induced immunosuppression and decreases susceptibility to sepsis. *Arch Surg* 1992;127:70–76.
75. Engel W, Morrison MH, Ayala A, et al. Chloroquine attenuates hemorrhagic shock-induced suppression of Kupffer cell antigen presentation and major histocompatability complex class II antigen expression through blockade of tumor necrosis factor and prostaglandin release. *Blood* 1991;78:1781–1788.
76. Zhu X, Ertel W, Ayala A, et al. Chloroquine inhibits macrophage tumour necrosis factor-alpha mRNA transcription. *Immunology* 1993;80:122–126.
77. Picot S, Peyron F, Dondadille A, et al. Chloroquine-induced inhibition of the production of TNF, but not of IL-6 is affected by disruption of iron metabolism. *Immunology* 1993;80:127–133.
78. Bygbjerg IC, Svenson M, Theander TG, et al. Effect of antimalarial drugs of stimulation and interleukin 2 production of human lymphocytes. *Int J Immunopharmacol* 1987;9:513–519.
79. Salmeron S, Lipsky PE. Immunosuppressive potential of antimalarials. *Am J Med*1983;5(suppl):19–24.
80. Landewe RMB, Miltenburg AMM, Breedveld FC, et al. Cyclosporine and chloroquine synergistically inhibit the interferon-gamma production by CD4 positive and CD8 positive synovial T cell clones derived from a patient with rheumatoid arthritis. *J Rheumatol* 1992;19:1353–1357.
81. Ausiello CM, Barbieri P, Spagnoli GC, et al. In vivo effects of chloroquine treatment on spontaneous and interferon-induced natural killer activities of rheumatoid arthritis patients. *Clin Exp Rheumatol* 1986;4:255–259.
82. Pedersen BK, Bygbjerg IC, Theander TG, et al. Effects of chloroquine, mefloquine and quinine on natural killer cell activity in vitro. An analysis of the inhibitory mechanism. *Allergy* 1986;41:537–542.
83. Bygbjerg IC, Flachs H. Effect of chloroquine on human lymphocyte proliferation. *Trans R Soc Trop Med Hyg* 1986;80:231–235.
84. Dijkmans BA, de Vries E, de Vreede TM, et al. Effects of antirheumatic drugs on in vitro mitogenic stimulation of peripheral blood mononuclear cells. *Transplant Proc* 1988;20(suppl 2): 253–258.
85. Hurvitz D, Hirschhorn K. Suppression of in vitro lymphocyte responses by chloroquine. *N Engl J Med* 1965;273:23–26.
86. Hall ND, Goulding NJ, Snaith ML, et al. Antimalarial drugs and the immune system. *Br J Clin Pract* 1987;41(suppl 52): 60–63.
87. van Loenen HJ, Dijkmans BA, de Vries E. Concentration dependency of cyclosporin and chloroquine as inhibitors of cell proliferation and immunoglobulin production upon mitogen stimulation of mononuclear cells. *Clin Exp Rheumatol* 1990;8:59–61.
88. Karres I, Kremer J-P, Dietl I, et al. Chloroquine inhibits proinflammatory cytokine release into human whole blood. *Am J Physiol* 1998;43:R1058–1064.
89. Van den Borne BEEM, Dijkmans BAC, Rooij HH, et al. Chloroquine and hydroxychloroquine equally effect tumor necrosis factor-alpha, interleukin 6 and interferon-gamma production by peripheral blood mononuclear cells. *J Rheumatol* 1997;24:55–60.
90. Bondeson J, Sundler R. Antimalarial drugs inhibit phospholipase A2 activation and induction of interleukin 1 beta and tumor necrosis factor alpha in macrophages: implications for their mode of action in rheumatoid arthritis. *Gen Pharmacol* 1998;30:357–366.
91. Forsdyke DR. Evidence for a relationship between chloroquine and complement from studies with lymphocyte mitogens: possible implications for the mechanism of action of chloroquine in disease. *Can J Microbiol* 1975;21:1581–1586.
92. Zvaifler NJ. The subcellular localization of chloroquine and its effects on lysosomal disruption. *Arthritis Rheum* 1964;7: 760–761(abst).
93. Fontagne J, Roch-Arveiller M, Giroud JP, et al. Effects of some antimalarial drugs on rat inflammatory polymorphonuclear leukocyte function. *Biomed Pharmacother* 1989;43:43–51.
94. Stenseth K, Thyberg J. Monensin and chloroquine inhibit transfer to lysosomes of endocytosed and macromolecules in cultured mouse peritoneal macrophages. *Eur J Cell Biol* 1989; 49:326–333.
95. Fox R. Antimalarial drugs: possible mechanism of action in autoimmune disease and prospects for drug development. *Lupus* 1996;5(suppl 1):S4–S10.
96. Salmeran G, Lupsky PE. Immunosuppressive potentials of antimalarials. *Am J Med*1983;75(suppl 1a):19–24.
97. Jones CJ, Salisbury RS, Jayson MI. The presence of abnormal lysosomes in lymphocytes and neutrophils during chloroquine therapy: a quantitative ultrastructural study. *Ann Rheum Dis* 1984;43:710–715.
98. Labro MT, Babin-Chevaye CB. Effects of amodiaquine, chloroquine and mefloquine on human polymorphonuclear neutrophil function in vitro. *Antimicrob Agents Chemother* 1988;32: 1124–1130.
99. Weismann G. Labilization and stabilization of lysosomes. *Fed Proc* 1964;23:1038–1044.
100. Naimiuchi S, Kumagai S, Imura H, et al. Quinacrine inhibits the primary but not secondary proliferative response of human cytotoxic T cells to allogeneic non-T cell antigens. *J Immunol* 1984;132:1456–1461.
101. Trist DG, Weatherall M. Inhibition of lymphocyte transformation by mepacrine and chloroquine. *J Pharm Pharmacol* 1981;33:434–438.
102. Szilagyi T, Kavai M. The effect of chloroquine on the antigen-antibody reaction. *Acta Physiol Acad Sci Hung* 1970;38:411–417.
103. Wu-Fei C, Nai-Chung K, Ken-Heng T, et al. The inhibition of immunologic response by chloroquine. *Chin Med J* 1964; 83:531–535.
104. Edwards JM, Moulds JJ, Judd WJ. Chloroquine dissociation of antigen-antibody complexes. A new technique for typing red blood cells with a positive direct antiglobulin test. *Transfusion* 1982;22:59–61.
105. Srivastava A, Pearson H, Bryant J, et al. Acidified chloroquine treatment for the removal class I HLA antigens. *Vox Sang* 1993; 65:146–150.
106. Majsky A. The effect of chloroquine on lymphocytic HLA-A and B antigens. *Casopis Lekaru Ceskych (Czech)* 1992;131:560–563.
107. Lombard-Platlet S, Bertolino P, Deng H, et al. Inhibition by chloroquine of the class II major histocompatability complex-restricted presentation of endogenous antigens varies according to the cellular origin of the antigen-presenting cells, the nature of the T-cell epitope, and the responding T cell. *Immunology* 1993;80:566–573.
108. Lucas GF. A survey of platelet serology in UK laboratories (1987): an assessment of the efficacy of using chloroquine-treated platelets to distinguish between platelet-specific and anti-HLA antibodies. The UK Platelet and Granulocyte Serology Workshop Group. *Clin Lab Haematol* 1990;12:185–200.

109. Segal-Eiras A, Segura GM, Babini JC, et al. Effect of antimalarial treatment on circulating immune complexes in rheumatoid arthritis. *J Rheumatol* 1985;12:87–89.
110. Stollar D, Levine L. Antibodies to denatured deoxyribonucleic in lupus erythematosus serum. V. Mechanism of DNA-anti-DNA inhibition by chloroquine. *Arch Biochem* 1963;101:335–341.
111. Reinhard J, Bennett R. Chloroquine inhibition of anti-DNA binding. *Clin Res* 1980;28:77A(abst).
112. Chorzelski T, Blaszczyk M, Langner A. Effect of resochin on the formation of cells in vitro. *Pol Med J* 1966;5:201–205.
113. Dubois EL. Effect of quinacrine (Atabrine) upon lupus erythematosus phenomenon. *Arch Dermatol* 1955;71:570–574.
114. Holman HR, Kunkel HG. Affinity between the lupus erythematosus serum factor and cell nuclei and nucleoprotein. *Science* 1957;126:162–163.
115. Zidovetzki R, Sherman IW, Cardenas M, et al. Chloroquine stabilization of phospholipid membranes against diacetylglycerol-induced perturbation. *Biochemical Pharmacol* 1993;45:183–189.
116. el Tahir KE. Influence of niridazole and chloroquine on arterial and myometrial prostacyclin synthesis. *Br J Pharmacol* 1987;92: 567–572.
117. Horrobin DF, Manku MS, Karmazyn M, et al. Quinacrine is a prostaglandin antagonist. *Biochemical Biophysical Comm* 1977;76:1188–1193.
118. Manku MS, Horrobin DF. Chloroquine, quinine, procaine, quinidine, tricyclic antidepressants, and methylxanthines as prostaglandin agonists and antagonists. *Lancet* 1976;2:1115–1117.
119. Churchill PC, Churchill MC, McDonald FD. Quinacrine antagonizes the effects of Na, K-ATPase inhibitors on renal prostaglandin E_2 release but not their effects on renin secretion. *Life Sci* 1985;36:277–282.
120. Filippov A, Skatova G, Porotikov V, et al. Ca^{2+}-antagonistic properties of phospholipase A_2 inhibitors, mepacrine and chloroquine. *Gen Physiol Biophys* 1989;8:113–118.
121. Matsuzawa Y, Hostetler KY. Inhibition of lysosomal phospholipase A and phospholipase C by chloroquine and 4,4′bis(diethylaminoethoxy) alpha, beta-diethyldiphenylethane. *J Biol Chem* 1980;255:5190–5194.
122. Crouch MF, Roberts ML, Tennes KA. Mepacrine inhibition of bradykinin-induced contractions of the rabbit ear vein. *Agents Actions* 1981;11:330–334.
123. Juan H. Inhibition of the algesic effect of bradykinin and acetylcholine by mepacrine. *Naunyn Schmiedebergs Arch Pharmacol* 1977;301:23–27.
124. Mitchell HW. Pharmacological studies into cyclo-oxygenase, lipoxygenase and phospholipase in smooth muscle contraction in the isolated trachea. *Br J Pharmacol* 1984;82:549–555.
125. Nagy E, Kocsar L. Experiments on the antihistaminic action of Atabrine. *Derm Wschr* 1956;133:265–269.
126. Toll JB, Andersson RG. Effects of mecaprine and p-bromophenacyl bromide on anti-IgE and phospholipase A_2-induced histamine release from human basophils. *Agents Actions* 1986;18:518–523.
127. Fulkerson JP, Ladenbauer-Bellis IM, Chrisman OD. In vitro hexosamine depletion of intact articular cartilage by E-prostaglandins: prevention by chloroquine. *Arthritis Rheum* 1979;22:1117–1121.
128. Kamel M, Bassiouni M. Chloroquine inhibits elastase enzyme activity in vitro. *Clin Exp Rheumatol* 1992;10:99–104.
129. Rainsford KD. Effects of antimalarials drugs on interleukin-1 induced cartilage proteoglycan degradation in vitro. *J Pharm Pharmacol* 1986;38:829–822.
130. Stecher VJ, Connolly KM, Speight PT. Fibronectin and macrophages as parameters of disease-modifying antirheumatic activity. *Br J Clin Pract* 1987;41(suppl):64–71.
131. Gerber DA. Effect of chloroquine on the sulfhydryl group and the denaturation of bovine serum albumin. *Arthritis Rheum* 1964;7:193–200.
132. Inyang AL, Bikfalvi A, Lu H, et al. Chloroquine's modulation of endothelial cell activity induced with basic fibroblast growth factor and human serum: effect on mitogenesis, protease production and cell migration. *Cell Biol Int Rep* 1990;14:35–46.
133. Khoury H, Adkins D, Young S, et al. Hydroxychloroquine for the prevention of acute graft versus host disease (GVHD) in unrelated donor (URD) transplantation:Preliminary results of a Phase II trial. *Blood* 1998;92:1861.
134. Authi KS, Traynor JR. Stimulation of polymorphonuclear leucocyte phospholipase A_2 activity by chloroquine and mepacrine. *J Pharm Pharmacol* 1982;34:736–738.
135. Dise CA, Burch JW, Goodman DB. Direct interaction of mepacrine with erythrocyte and platelet membrane phospholipid. *J Biol Chem* 1982;257:4701–4704.
136. Erman A, Azuri R, Raz A. Prostaglandin biosynthesis in rabbit kidney: mepacrine inhibits renomedullary cyclooxygenase. *Biochem Pharmacol* 1984;33:79–82.
137. Evans PM, Lanham DF. Effects of inhibitors of arachidonic acid metabolism on intercellular adhesion of SV40-3T3 cells. *Cell Biol Int Rep* 1986;10:693–698.
138. Fletcher JE, Kistler P, Rosenberg H, et al. Dantrolene and mepacrine antagonize the hemolysis human red blood cells by halothane and bee venom phospholipase A_2. *Toxicol Appl Pharmacol* 1987;90:410–419.
139. Flynn JT. Inhibition of complement-mediated hepatic thromboxane production by mepacrine, a phospholipase inhibitor. *Prostaglandins* 1987;33:287–299.
140. Hoffman SL, Prescott SM, Majerus PW. The effects of mepacrine and p-bromophenacyl bromide on arachidonic acid release in human platelets. *Arch Biochem Biophys* 1982;215:237–244.
141. Hurst NP, French JK, Bell AL, et al. Differential effects of mepacrine, chloroquine and hydroxychloroquine on superoxide anion generation, phospholipid methylation and arachidonic acid release by human blood monocytes. *Biochem Pharmacol* 1986;35:3083–3089.
142. Lot TY, Bennett T. Comparison of the effects of chloroquine, quinacrine and quinidine on autonomic neuroeffector mechanisms. *Med Biol* 1982;60:307–315.
143. Raz A. Mepacrine blockade of arachidonate-induced washed platelet aggregation: relationship to mecaprine inhibition of platelet cyclooxygenase. *Thromb Haemost* 1983;50:784–786.
144. Baker DJ, Trist DG, Weatherall M. Proceedings: inhibition of phagocytosis by mepacrine. *Br J Pharmacol* 1976;56:346P–347P.
145. Read NG, Trist DG. The uptake of mepacrine horse polymorphonuclear leucocytes in vitro. *J Pharm Pharmacol* 1982;34: 711–714.
146. Tauber AI, Simmons ER. Dissociation of human neutrophil membrane depolarization, respiratory burst stimulation and phospholipid metabolism by quinacrine. *FEBS Lett* 1983;156:161–164.
147. Lot TY. Acute effects of chloroquine on body weight, food and water intake of chicks and rats. *Med Sci Res* 1993;21:3–7.
148. Cranston WI, Hellon RF, Mitchell D, et al. Intraventricular injections of drugs which inhibit phospholipase A_2 suppress fever in rabbits. *J Physiol (Lond)* 1983;339:97–105.
149. Spagnuolo C, Galli C, Omini C, et al. Antipyretic action of mepacrine without blockade of prostaglandin (PG): the kinetics of quinacrine (mepacrine) block. *J Physiol (Lond)* 1980;306: 262–281,283–306.
150. Nicola WG, Chloroquine therapy reduces estrogen production in females. *Boll Chim Farm* 1997;136;447–449.
151. Grundmann M, Bayer A. Effects of chloroquine on adrenocortical function. H. Histological, histochemical and biochemical changes in suprarenal gland of rats on long-term administration of chloroquine. *Arzneim Forsch* 1976;26:2029–2035.

152. O'Leary TJ, Jones G, Yip A, et al. The effects of chloroquine on serum 1,25-dihydroxyvitamin D and calcium metabolism in sarcoidosis. *N Engl J Med* 1986;315:727–730.
153. Palit J, Holt PJL, Still PE, et al. Effect of chloroquine on serum vitamin D in rheumatoid arthritis. *Br J Rheumatol* 1988;27 (suppl):131–132.
154. Quatraro A, Consoli G, Magno M, et al. Hydroxychloroquine in decompensated, treatment-refractory noninsulin-dependent diabetes mellitus. A new job for an old drug? *Ann Intern Med*1990;112:678–681.
155. Smith GD, Amos TA, Mahler R, et al. Effect of chloroquine on insulin and glucose homeostasis in normal subjects and patients with non-insulin dependent diabetes mellitus. *Br Med J* 1987; 294:465–467.
156. de Feo P, Volpi E, Lucidi P, et al. Chloroquine reduces whole body proteolysis in humans. *Am J Physiol* 1994;267: E183–186.
157. Maegawa H, Kobayashi M, Watanabe N, et al. Inhibition of down regulation by chloroquine in cultured lymphocytes (RPMI-1788 line). *Diabetes Res Clin Pract* 1985;1:145–153.
158. Petri M, Ferman D, Goldman D. Hypoglycemic effect of hydroxychloroquine in systemic lupus erythematosus. *Arthritis Rheum* 1994;37(suppl):R24(abst).
159. White NJ, Miller KD, Marsh K, et al. Hypoglycemia in African children with severe malaria. *Lancet* 1987;1:708–711.
160. Abu-Shakra M, Lee P. Hypoglycemia: an unusual adverse reaction to chloroquine. *Clin Exp Rheumatol* 1994;11:95.
161. Shojania K, Koehler BE, Elliott T. Hypoglycemia induced by hydroxychloroquine in a type II diabetic treated for polyarthritis. *J Rheumatol* 1999;26:195–196.
162. Ekelund M, Ahren B, Hakanson R, et al. Quinacrine accumulates in certain peptide hormone-producing cells. *Histochemistry* 1980;66:1–9.
163. Lundquist I, Ahren B, Hakanson R, et al. Quinacrine accumulation in pancreatic islet cells of rat and mouse: relationship to functional activity and effects on basal and stimulated insulin secretion. *Diabetologia* 1985;28:161–166.
164. Rillema JA. Actions of quinacrine on RNA and casein syntheses in mouse mammary gland explants. *Prostaglandins Med* 1979;2:155–160.
165. Rillema JA, Etindi RN, Cameron CM. Prolactin actions on casein and lipid biosynthesis in mouse and rabbit mammary gland explants are abolished by p-bromphenacyl bromide and quinacrine, phospholipase A_2 inhibitors. *Horm Metab Res* 1986;18:672–674.
166. Kharazmi A. Antimalarial drugs and human neutrophil oxidative metabolism. *Trans R Soc Trop Med Hyg* 1986;80:94–97.
167. Hurst NP, French JK, Gorjatschko L, et al. Studies on the mechanism of inhibition of chemotactic tripeptide stimulated human neutrophil polymorphonuclear leucocyte superoxide production by chloroquine and hydroxychloroquine. *Ann Rheum Dis* 1987;46:750–756.
168. Hurst NP, French JK, Gorjatschko L, et al. Chloroquine and hydroxychloroquine inhibit multiple sites in metabolic pathways leading to neutrophil superoxide release. *J Rheumatol* 1988;15:23–27.
169. Miyachi Y, Yoshioka A, Imamura S, et al. Antioxidant action of antimalarials. *Ann Rheum Dis* 1986;45:244– 248.
170. Salmon D, Verdier F, Malhotra K, et al. Absence of effect of chloroquine in vivo on neutrophil oxidative metabolism in human subjects. *J Antimicrob Chemother* 1990;25:367–370.
171. Struhar D, Kivity S, Topilsky M. Quinacrine inhibits oxygen radicals release from human alveolar macrophages. *Int J Immunopharmacol* 1992;14:275–277.
172. Ciak J, Hahn FE. Chloroquine: mode of action. *Science* 1966; 151:347–349.
173. Conklin KA, Chou SC. Antimalarials: effects on in vivo and in vitro protein synthesis. *Science* 1970;170:1213–1214.
174. Bolte J, Demuynck C, Lhomme J. Synthetic models deoxyribonucleic acid complexes with antimalarial compounds. I. Interaction of aminoquinoline with adenine and thymine. *J Am Chem Soc* 1976;98:613–615.
175. Horkay I, Nagy E, Varga L, et al. Effect of chloroquine on DNA synthesis in the skin of DLE patients. *Acta Dermatovener (Stockh)* 1979;59:435–439.
176. Bottger BA, Sjolund M, Thyberg J. Chloroquine and monensin inhibit induction of DNA synthesis in rat arterial smooth muscle cells stimulated with platelet-derived growth factor. *Cell Tissue Res* 1988;252:275–285.
177. Pazmino NH, Yuhas JM, Tennant RW. Inhibition of murine RNA tumor virus replication and oncogenesis of chloroquine. *Int J Cancer* 1974;14:379–385.
178. Inoue S, Hasegawa K, Ito S, et al. Antimelanoma activity of chloroquine, an antimalarial agent with high affinity for melanin. *Pigment Cell Res* 1993;6:354–358.
179. Zeilhofer HU, Mollenhauer J, Brune K. Selective growth inhibition of ductal pancreatic adenocarcinoma cells by the lysosomotropic agent chloroquine. *Cancer Lett* 1989;44:61–66.
180. Djordjevic B, Lange CS, Austin J-P, et al. Potentiation of radiation lethality in HeLa cells by combined mild hyperthermia and chloroquine. *Radiat Res* 1992;130:267–270.
181. Morrow M, Hager C, Berger D, et al. Chloroquine as a hyperthermia potentiator. *J Surg Res* 1989;46:637–639.
182. Thomas R, Vane DW, Grosfeld JL, et al. The effect of chloroquine and hyperthermia on murine neuroblastoma. *J Pediatr Surg* 1990;25:929–932.
183. Kwakye-Berko F, Meshnick S. Sequence preference of chloroquine binding to DNA and prevention of Z-DNA formation. *Mol Biochem Parasitol* 1990;39:275–278.
184. Zamora JM, Beck WT. Chloroquine enhancement of anticancer drug cytotoxicity in multiple drug resistant human leukemic cells. *Biochem Pharmacol* 1986;35:4303–4310.
185. Gilman AL, Beams F, Tefft M, et al. The effect of hydroxychloroquine on alloreactivity and its potential use for graft-versus-host disease. *Bone Marrow Transplant* 1996;17:1069–1075.
186. Schultz KR, Bader S, Paquet J, et al. Chloroquine treatment affects T-cell priming to minor histocompatability antigens and graft-versus-host disease. *Blood* 1995;86:4344–4352.
187. Doglia S, Graslund A, Ehrenberg A. Specific interactions between quinacrine and self-complementary deoxynucleotides. *Anticancer Res* 1986;6:1363–1368.
188. O'Brien RL, Olnenick JG, Hahn FE. Reactions of quinine, chloroquine, and quinacrine with DNA and their effects on the DNA and RNA polymerase reactions. *Proc Natl Acad Sci USA* 1966;55:1511–1517.
189. Voiculetz N, Smith KC, Kaplan HS. Effect of quinacrine on survival and DNA repair in x-irradiated Chinese hamster cells. *Cancer Res* 1974;34:1038–1044.
190. Biller H, Schachtschabel DO, Leising HB, et al. Influence of x-rays and quinacrine (Atebrine) for chloroquine (Resochine)—alone or in combination—on growth and melanin formation of Harding-Passey melanoma cells in monolayer culture. *Strahlentherapie* 1982;158:450–456.
191. Fuks Z, Smith KC. Effect of quinacrine on x-ray sensitivity and the repair of damaged DNA in *Escherichia coli* K-12. *Radiat Res* 1971;48:63–73.
192. Giampietri A, Fioretti MC, Goldin A, et al. Drug-mediated antigenic changes in murine leukemia cells: antagonistic effects of quinacrine, an antimutagenic compound. *J Natl Cancer Inst* 1980;64(2):297–301.
193. Hiller RI. A study of quinacrine dihydrochloride in the human breast in vitro and in vivo. *Am J Surg* 1970;119:317–321.

194. Pfab R, Schachtschabel DO, Kern HF. Ultrastructural studies of the effect of x-rays and quinacrine (Atebrin) or chloroquine (Resochine)—alone or in combination—on Harding-Passey melanoma cells in monolayer culture. *Strahlentherapie* 1985;161:711–718.
195. McCormick DL. Anticarcinogenic activity of quinacrine in the rat mammary gland. *Carcinogenesis* 1988;9:175–178.
196. Bach MK. Reduction in the frequency of mutation to resistance to cytarabine in L1210 murine leukemic cells by treatment with quinacrine hydrochloride. *Cancer Res* 1969;29:1881–1885.
197. Dabancens A, Zipper J, Guererro A. Quinacrine and copper, compounds with anticontraceptive and antineoplastic activity. *Contraception* 1994;50:243–251.
198. Inaba M, Marauyama E. Reversal of resistance to vincristine in P388 leukemia by various polycyclic clinical drugs, with a special emphasis on quinacrine. *Cancer Res* 1988;48:2064–2067.
199. Krishnaja AP, Chauhan PS. Quinacrine dihydrochloride, the non-surgical female sterilant induces dicentrics, rings, and marker chromosomes in human peripheral blood lymphocytes treated in vitro: a preliminary report. *Mutat Res* 2000;466:43–50.
200. Bertrand E, Cloitre B, Ticolat R, et al. Antiaggregation action of chloroquine (English abstract). *Med Trop (Mars)* 1990;50: 143–146.
201. Kinlough-Rathbone RL. *Platelets, drugs and thrombosis. The effects of some other drugs in platelet formation.* Basel: Karger, 1975:124–131.
202. Rosenberg FJ, Phillips PG, Druzba PG. *Platelets and thrombosis. Use of a rabbit extracorporeal shunt in the assay of antithrombotic and thrombotic drugs.* Baltimore: University Park Press, 1974:233–234.
203. Jancinova V, Nosal R, Pterikova M. On the inhibitory effect of chloroquine on blood platelet aggregation. *Thromb Res* 1994; 74:495–504.
204. Ernest E, Rose M, Lee R. Modification of trans-operative changes in blood fluidity by hydroxy-chloroquine. A possible explanation for the drug anti-thrombotic effect. *Pharmaceutica* 1984;4:48–52.
205. Cecchi E, Ferraris E. Desludging action of hydroxychloroquine in rheumatoid arthritis. *Acta Rheum Scand* 1962;8:214–221.
206. Meig XW, Feller JM, Ziegler JB, et al. Induction of apoptosis in peripheral blood lymphocytes following treatment in vitro with hydroxychloroquine. *Arthritis Rheum* 1997;40:927–935.
207. Edwards MH, Pierangeli SS, Liu Z, et al. Hydroxychloroquine reverses thrombogenic properties of antiphospholipid antibodies in mice. *Circulation* 1997;96:4380–4384.
208. Edwards MH, Pierangeli S, Liu XW, et al. Hydroxychloroquine reverses thrombogenic properties of antiphospholipid antibodies in mice. *Circulation* 1997;96:4380–4384.
209. Carter AE, Eban R, Perrett RD. Prevention of post-operative deep venous thrombosis and pulmonary embolism. *Br Med J* 1971;1:312–314.
210. Loudon JR. Hydroxychloroquine and postoperative thromboembolism after total hip replacement. *Am J Med* 1988;85 (suppl 4A):57–61.
211. Matsuoka I, Suzuki T. Mapacrine-induced elevation of cyclic GMP levels and acceleration of reversal of ADP-induced aggregation in washed rabbit platelets. *J Cyclic Nucleotide Protein Phosphor Res* 1983;9:341–353.
212. McCrea JM, Robinson P, Gerrard JM. Mepacrine (quinacrine) inhibition of thrombin-induced platelet responses can be overcome by lysophosphatidic acid. *Biochim Biophys Acta* 1985;842: 189–194.
213. Winocour PD, Kinlough-Rathbone RL, Mustard JF. The effect of phospholipase mepacrine inhibitor on platelet aggregation, the platelet release reaction and fibrinogen binding to the platelet surface. *Thromb Haemost* 1981;45:257–262.
214. Yamakado T, Tanaka F, Hidaka H. Mepacrine-induced inhibition of human platelet cyclic-GMP phosphodiesterase. *Biochim Biophys Acta* 1984;801:111–116.
215. Watson DE. Chloroquine protection against virus induced cell damage without inhibition of virus growth. *J Gen Virol* 1972;14:100–102.
216. Helbling B, Reichen J. Reactivation of hepatitis B following withdrawal of chloroquine. *Schweiz Med Wochenschr* 1994;124:759–762.
217. Sperber K, Kalb TH, Stecher VJ, et al. Inhibition of human immunodeficiency virus type I replication by hydroxychloroquine in T cells and monocytes. *AIDS Res Hum Retrovirus* 1993; 9:91–93.
218. Haartmann M. Resochin bei HIV-Infektion. *Hautarzt* 1992; 43:387.
219. Wallace DJ. Lupus, acquired immunodeficiency syndrome, and antimalarial agents. *Arthritis Rheum* 1991;34:373–374.
220. Ray P, Berman JD. Prevention of muscarinic acetylcholine receptor-down regulation by chloroquine: antilysosomal or antimuscarinic mechanisms. *Neurochem Res* 1989;14:533–535.
221. Podrebarac TA, Jovaisas A, Karsh J. Pneumocystis carinii pneumonia after discontinuation of hydroxychloroquine in 2 patients after systemic lupus erythematosus. *J Rheumatol* 1996; 23:199–200.
222. Muller S, Rother U, Westerhausen M. Complement activation by cryoglobulin. *Clin Exp Immunol* 1976;23:233–241.
223. Sabban EL, Kuhn LJ, Sarmalkar M. Chloroquine and monensin alter the post translational processing and secretion of dopamine beta-hydroxylase and other proteins from PC 12 cells. *Ann NY Acad Sci* 1986;493:399–402.
224. Alund M, Olson L. Release of (14C) quinacrine from peripheral and central nerves. *J Auton Nerv Syst* 1980;2:281–294.
225. Minker E, Kadar T, Matejka Z. Effect of chloroquine and mepacrine on the spontaneous and evoked movements of the rat portal vein. *Acta Physiol Acad Sci Hung* 1980;55:71–80.
226. Lot TY. The in vitro pharmacology of chloroquine and quinacrine. *Med Biol* 1986;64:207–213.
227. Torda T, Yamaguchi I, Hirata F, et al. Quinacrine-blocked desensitization of adrenoceptors after immobilization stress or repeated injection of isoproterenol in rats. *J Pharmacol Exp Ther* 1981;216:334–338.
228. Torda T, Yamaguchi I, Hirata F, et al. Mepacrine treatment prevents immobilization-induced desensitization of beta-adrenergic receptors in rat hypothalamus and brain stem. *Brain Res* 1981;205:441–444.
229. Crossland RD. Effect of chlorpromazine and quinacrine on the lethality in mice of the venoms and neurotoxins from several snakes. *Toxicology* 1989;27:655–663.
230. Harris L, Downar E, Shaikh NA, et al. Antiarrhythmic potential of chloroquine: new use for an old drug. *Can J Cardiol* 1988;4:295–300.
231. Tona L, Ng YC, Akera T, Brody TM. Depressant effects of chloroquine on the isolated guinea-pig heart. *Eur J Pharmacol* 1990;178:293–301.
232. Anigbogu CN, Adigun SA, Inyang I, et al. Chloroquine reduces blood pressure and forearm vascular resistance and increases forearm blood flow in healthy young adults. *Clin Physiol* 1993; 13:209–216.
233. Bustos MDG, Gay F, Diquet B, et al. The pharmacokinetics and electrocardiographic effects of chloroquine in healthy subjects. *Trop Med Parisitol* 1994;45:83–86.
234. Bass SW, Ramirez MA, Avaido DM. Cardiopulmonary effects of antimalarial drugs. VI. Adenosine, quinacrine and primaquine. *Toxicol Appl Pharmacol* 1972;21:464–481.
235. Goodman LS, Gilman A. *The pharmacological basis of therapeutics*, 2nd ed. New York: Macmillan, 1954:1167–1173.
236. Ambrosio G, Bigazzi MC, Tritto I, et al. Limitation of the area

of necrosis induced by quinacrine after coronary occlusion in the dog (English abstract). *G Ital Cardiol* 1985;15:1139–1146.
237. Chiarello M, Ambrosio G, Capelli-Bigazzi A, et al. Inhibition of ischemia-induced phospholipase activation by quinacrine protects jeopardized myocardium in rats with coronary artery occlusion. *J Pharmacol Exp Ther* 1987;241:560–568.
238. Chiariello M, Ambrosio G, Capelli-Bigazzi M, et al. Reduction in infarct size by the phospholipase inhibitor quinacrine in dogs with coronary artery occlusion. *Am Heart J* 1990;120:801–807.
239. Fazekas T, Szekeres L. Effect of chloroquine in experimental myocardial ischemia. *Acta Physiol Hung* 1988;72:191–199.
240. Kimura T, Satoh S. Inhibitory effect of quinacrine on myocardial reactive hyperthermia in the dog. *J Pharmacol Exp Ther* 1985;232:269–274.
241. Moffat MP, Tsushima RG. Functional and electrophysiological effects of quinacrine on the response of ventricular tissues to hypoxia and reoxygenation. *Can J Physiol Pharmacol* 1989;67: 929–935.
242. Otani H, Engleman RM, Breyer RH, et al. Mepacrine, a phospholipase inhibitor. A potential tool for modifying myocardial reperfusion injury. *J Thorac Cardiovasc Surg* 1986;92:247–254.
243. Seguin J, Berta P, Saussine M, et al. Mepacrine, a phospholipase inhibitor (letter). *J Thorac Cardiovasc Surg* 1987;94:312–314.
244. von Bilsen M, van der Vusse GJ, Willemsen PH, et al. Effects of nicotinic acid and mepacrine on fatty acid accumulation and myocardial damage during ischemia and reperfusion. *J Mol Cell Cardiol* 1990;22:155–163.
245. Estevez AY, Phillis JW. The phospholipase A2 inhibitor, quinacrine, reduces infarct size in rats after transient middle cerebral artery occlusion. *Brain Res* 1997;752:203–208.
246. Lafont H, Chanussot F, Dupuy C, et al. Influence of acute injection of chloroquine on the biliary secretion of lipids and lysosomal enzyme in rats. *Lipids* 1984;19:195–201.
247. Matsuzawa Y, Hostetler KY. Studies on drug-induced lipidosis: subcellular localization of phospholipid and cholesterol in the liver of rats treated with chloroquine or 4,4′bis (diethylaminoethoxy)alpha, beta-diethyldiphenylethane. *J Lipid Res* 1980;21:202–214.
248. Sewell KL, Livneh A, Aranow CB, et al. Magnetic resonance imaging versus computed tomographic scanning in neuropsychiatric systemic lupus erythematosus. *Am J Med* 1989;86:625–626.
249. Beynen AC. Could chloroquine be of value in the treatment of hypercholesterolemia? *Artery* 1986;13:340–351.
250. Goldstein JL, Brown MS. The LDL pathway in human fibroblasts. A receptor-mediated mechanism for the regulation of cholesterol metabolism. *Curr Top Cell Regul* 1976;11:147–181.
251. Goldstein JL, Brunschede GY, Brown MS. Inhibition of the proteolytic degradation of low density lipoprotein in human fibroblasts by chloroquine, concanavalin A and Triton WR 1339. *J Biol Chem* 1975;250:7854–7862.
252. Gaafar KM, Abdel-Khalek LR, El-Sayed NK, et al. Lipidemic effect as a manifestation of chloroquine retinotoxicity, *Drug Res* 1995;45:1231–1235.
253. Potvin F, Petitclerc E, Marceau F, et al. Mechanisms of action of antimalarials in inflammation. Induction of apoptosis in human endothelial cells. *J Immunol* 1997;158:1872–1879.
254. Yi AK, Peckham DW, Ashman RF, et al. CpG DNA rescues B cells from apoptosis by activating NfkappaB and preventing mitochondrial membrane potential disruption via a chloroquine sensitive pathway. *Int Immunol* 1999;11:2015–2024.
255. Ziff M, Esserman P, McEwen C. Observations on the course and treatment of SLE. *Arthritis Rheum* 1956;7:332–350.
256. Dubois EL. Antimalarials in the management of discoid and systemic lupus erythematosus. *Semin Arthritis Rheum* 1978;8:33–51.
257. Dubois EL, Martel S. Discoid lupus erythematosus; analysis of its systemic manifestations. *Ann Intern Med* 1956;44:482–496.
258. Herrman WP, Koch H, Hoft G. Catamnestic studies on the course of chronic erythematosus. *Hautarzt (Ger)* 1962;13: 309–315.
259. Merwin CF, Winkelmann RK. Dermatologic clinics. 2. Antimalarial drugs in the therapy of lupus erythematosus. *Proc Mayo Clin* 1962;37:253–268.
260. Winkelmann RK, Merwin CF, Brunsting LA. Antimalarial therapy of lupus erythematosus. *Ann Intern Med*1961;55:772–776.
261. Callen JP. Chronic cutaneous lupus erythematosus. Clinical, laboratory, therapeutic and prognostic examination of 62 patients. *Arch Dermatol* 1982;118:412–416.
262. Rothfield N. Efficacy of antimalarials in systemic lupus erythematosus. *Am J Med*1988;85(suppl 4A):53–56.
263. Rothfield NF. General considerations in the treatment of systemic lupus erythematosus. *Mayo Clin Proc* 1969;44:691–696.
264. Rudnicki RD, Gresham GE, Rothfield NF. The efficacy of antimalarials in systemic lupus erythematosus. *J Rheumatol* 1975;2:323–330.
265. Hughes GR. Antimalarials in SLE. *Br J Clin Pract* 1987;41(suppl 52):10–12.
266. Canadian Hydroxychloroquine Study Group. A randomized study of the effect of withdrawing hydroxychloroquine sulfate in systemic lupus erythematosus. *N Engl J Med* 1991;324:150–154.
267. Canadian Hydroxychloroquine Study Group. A long-term study of hydroxychloroquine withdrawal on exacerbations in systemic lupus erythematosus. *Lupus* 1998;7:80–85.
268. Petri M. Hydroxychloroquine: past, present, future. *Lupus* 1998;7:65–67.
269. Williams HJ, Egger MJ, Singer JZ, et al. Comparison of hydroxychloroquine and placebo in the treatment of the arthropathy of mild systemic lupus erythematosus. *J Rheumatol* 1994;21:1457–1462.
270. Morand EF, McCloud PI, Littlejohn GO. Continuation of long term treatment with hydroxychloroquine in systemic lupus erythematosus and rheumatoid arthritis. *Ann Rheum Dis* 1992;51: 1318–1321.
271. Meinao IM, Sato EI, Andrade LEC, et al. Controlled trial with chloroquine diphosphate in systemic lupus erythematosus. *Lupus* 1996:5:237–241.
272. Petri M, Yadia N. Predictors of new development of proteinuria in SLE. *Arthritis Rheum* 1995;38:S314(abst).
273. Senecal J-L, Chartier S, Rothfield N. Hypergammaglobulinemic purpura in systemic autoimmune rheumatic diseases: predictive value of anti-Ro (SSA) and anti-La (SSB) antibodies and treatment with indomethacin and hydroxychloroquine. *J Rheumatol* 1995;22:868–875.
274. Ruzicka T, Sommerburg C, Goerz G, et al. Treatment of cutaneous lupus erythematosus with acitretin and hydroxychloroquine. *Br J Dermatol* 1992;127:513–518.
275. Feldmann R, Salomon D, Saurat JH. The association of two antimalarials chloroquine and quinacrine for treatment-resistant chronic and subacute cutaneous lupus erythematosus. *Dermatology* 1994;189:425–427.
276. Lipsker D, Piette J-C, Cacoub P, et al. Chloroquine-quinacrine association in resistant cutaneous lupus. *Dermatology* 1995;190: 257–258.
277. Toubi E, Rosner I, Rozenbaum M, et al. The benefit of combining hydroxychloroquine with quinacrine in the treatment of SLE patients. *Lupus* 2000;9:92–95.
278. Wallace DJ. Does hydroxychloroquine sulfate prevent clot formation in systemic lupus erythematosus? (letter). *Arthritis Rheum* 1987;30:1435–1436.
279. Wallace DJ, Linker-Israeli M, Metzger AL, et al. The relevance of antimalarial therapy with regard to thrombosis, hypercholesterolemia and cytokines in SLE. *Lupus* 1993;2(suppl 1):S13–S15.
280. Petri M, Hellmann D, Hochberg M, et al. Arterial thrombotic

events (TE) in SLE: the Baltimore Lupus Cohort Study. *Arthritis Rheum* 1994;37:S297(abst).
281. Petri M, Magder L. Predictors of antiphospholipid antibodies (APL) in SLE: a longitudinal analysis. *Arthritis Rheum* 1995; 38:R24(abst).
282. McCarty GA, Hellman DK. Hydroxychloroquine treatment in 121 patients with antiphospholipid antibody syndrome: clinical and serologic efficacy. *Arthritis Rheum* 1999;42:S368.
283. Wallace DJ, Metzger AL, Stecher VJ, et al. Cholesterol-lowering effect of hydroxychloroquine in patients with rheumatic disease: reversal of deleterious effects of steroids on lipids. *Am J Med* 1990;89:322–326.
284. Hodis HN, Quismorio FP, Wickham E, et al. The lipid, lipoprotein and apolipoprotein effects of hydroxychloroquine in patients with systemic lupus erythematosus. *J Rheumatol* 1993; 20:661–665.
285. Petri M, Lakatta C, Magder L, et al. Effect of prednisone and hydroxychloroquine on coronary artery disease risk factors in systemic lupus erythematosus: a longitudinal data analysis. *Am J Med*1994;96:254–259.
286. Blyth TH, McDonald AG, Capell HA, et al. A comparison of hydroxychloroquine and myocrisin in rheumatoid arthritis; does hydroxychloroquine have a favorable effect on the blood lipid profile? *Br J Rheumatol* 1994;33(suppl 1):149(abst).
287. Powrie JK, Watts GF, Smith GD, et al. Short-term effects of mepacrine on serum lipids, lipoproteins and apolipoproteins in patients with non-insulin dependent diabetes mellitus. *Metabolism* 1994;43:131–134.
288. Podrebarac T, McPherson R, Goldstein R. Lipid profiles and lipoprotein (a) levels in systemic lupus erythematosus and primary antiphospholipid antibody. *Arthritis Rheum* 1995;38: S169(abst).
289. Belmont HM, Kitsis E, McCullagh E, et al. Prospective study of hydroxychloroquine effect on serum lipids in patients with SLE and rheumatoid arthritis. *Arthritis Rheum* 1995;38:S220(abst).
290. Kavanaugh A, Adams-Huet B, Jain R, et al. Hydroxychloroquine: effects on lipoprotein profiles (the HELP trial): a double-bline randomized, placebo-controlled, pilot study in patients with systemic lupus erythematosus. *J Clin Rheumatol* 1997;3:3–8.
291. Rahman P, Gladman DD, Urowitz MB, et al. The cholesterol lowering effect of antimalarial drugs is enhanced in patients with lupus taking corticosteroid drugs. *J Rheumatol* 1999;26: 325–330.
292. Lawrence S, Mc Crindle B, Quinneville J, et al. Dysproteinemia in childhood systemic lupus erythematosus (SLE) and risk factors for premature atherosclerosis and coronary artery disease (CAD). *Arthritis Rheum* 1996;39:S189.
293. Powrie JK, Watts GF, Smith GD, et al. Short-term effects of mepacrine on serum lipids, lipoproteins, and apolipoproteins in patients with non-insulin-dependent diabetes mellitus. *Metab Clin Exp* 1994;43:131–134.
294. Fox RI, Chan E, Benton L, et al. Treatment of primary Sjogren's syndrome with hydroxychloroquine. *Am J Med* 1988;23(suppl 1):82–91.
295. Kruize AA, Hene RJ, Kallenberg CGM, et al. Hydroxychloroquine treatment for primary Sjogren's syndrome:a two year double blind crossover trial. *Ann Rheum Dis* 1993;52:36–364.
296. Fox R, Dixon R, Guarrasi V, et al. Treatment of primary Sjogren's syndrome with hydroxychloroquine: a retrospective, open label study. *Lupus* 1996;5(suppl 1):S31–S36.
297. Combe B, Guttierez M, Anaya J-M, et al. Possible efficacy of hydroxychloroquine on accelerated nodulosis during methotrexate therapy for rheumatoid arthritis. *J Rheumatol* 1993;20:755–756.
298. Middleton GD, McFarlin JE, Lipsky PE. Hydroxychloroquine and pain thresholds. *Arthritis Rheum* 1995;38:445–447.
299. Bell CL. Hydroxychloroquine sulfate in rheumatoid arthritis: long-term response rate and predictive parameters. *Am J Med* 1983;75(suppl 1A):46–51.
300. Wang C, Fortin PR, Li Y, Panaritis T, et al. Discontinuation of antimalarial drugs in systemic lupus erythematosus. *J Rheumatol* 1999;26:808–815.
301. Furst DE, Lindsley H, Baethge B, et al. Dose-loading with hydroxychloroquine improves the rate of response in early, active rheumatoid arthritis. A randomized double-blind six-week trial with eighteen-week extension. *Arthritis Rheum* 1999;42:357–365.
302. Rahman P, Gladman DD, Urowitz MB. Efficacy of antimalarial therapy in cutaneous lupus in smokers versus nonsmokers. *Arthritis Rheum* 1997;40:S58.
303. Bernstein HN. Ophthalmologic considerations and testing in patients receiving long-term antimalarial therapy. *Am J Med* 1983;75(suppl 1A):25–34.
304. Miller DR, Fiechtner JJ, Carpenter JR, et al. Plasma hydroxychloroquine concentrations and efficacy in rheumatoid arthritis. *Arthritis Rheum* 1987;30:567–571.
305. Miller D, Fiechtner J. Hydroxychloroquine overdosage. *J Rheumatol* 1989;16:142–143.
306. Riou B, Barriot P, Riamailho A, et al. Treatment of severe chloroquine poisoning. *N Engl J Med* 1988;318:1–6.
307. Saissy JM, Gohard R, Diatta B, et al. The role of diazepam as monotherapy in the treatment of chloroquine intoxication. *Presse Med* 1989;18:2022–2023.
308. Kivisto KT, Neuvonen PJ. Activated charcoal for chloroquine poisoning. *Br Med J* 1993;307:1068.
309. Rein CR, Fleischmajer R. The treatment of lupus erythematosus and infiltration of the skin with A.P.A. 5533. *Br J Dermatol* 1957;69:174–177.
310. Engel GL, Romano J, Ferris EB. Effect of quinacrine (Atabrine) on the central nervous system; clinical and electroencephalographic studies. *Arch Neurol Psychiatr* 1947;58:337–350.
311. Wallace DJ. Antimalarial agents and lupus. *Rheum Dis Clin North Am* 1994;20:243–263.
312. Makin AJ, Wendon J, Portmann BC, et al. Fulminant hepatic failure secondary to hydroxychloroquine. *Gut* 1994;35:569–570.
313. Nelson AA, Fitzhugh OG. Chloroquine; pathologic changes observed in rats which have been fed various proportions for 2 years. *Arch Pathol* 1948;45:454–462.
314. Avina-Zubleta A, Suarez-Almazor ME, Russell AS. Incidence of myopathy in the use of antimalarials. *Arthritis Rheum* 1993;36: S194(abst).
315. Afifi AK, Bergman RA, Harvey JC. Steroid myopathy. Clinical, histologic and cytologic observations. *Johns Hopkins Med J* 1968;123:157–173.
316. Gerard JM, Stoupel N, Collier A, et al. Morphologic study of neuromyopathy caused by prolong chloroquine treatment. *Eur Neurol* 1973;9:363–379.
317. Hicklin JA. Chloroquine neuromyopathy. *Ann Phys Med* 1968; 9:189–192.
318. Hughes JT, Esiri M, Oxbury JM, et al. Chloroquine myopathy. *Q J Med* 1971;40:85–93.
319. Itabashi HH, Kokmen E. Chloroquine neuromyopathy, a reversible granulovacuolar myopathy. *Arch Pathol* 1972;93:209–218.
320. Leger JM, Puifoulloux H, Dancea S, et al. Chloroquine neuromyopathies: 4 cases during antimalarial prevention. *Rev Neurol* 1986;142:746–752.
321. McAllister HA, Ferrans VJ, Hall RJ, et al. Chloroquine-induced cardiomyopathy. *Arch Pathol Lab Med* 1987;111:953–956.
322. Pearson CM, Yamazaki JN. Vacuolar myopathy is systemic lupus erythematosus. *Am J Clin Pathol* 1958;29:455–463.
323. Ratliff NB, Estes ML, Myles JL, et al. Diagnosis of chloroquine cardiomyopathy by endomyocardial biopsy. *N Engl J Med* 1987; 316:191–193.

324. Robberecht W, Bednarik J, Bourgeois P, et al. Myasthenic syndrome caused by direct effect of chloroquine on neuromuscular junction. *Arch Neurol* 1989;46:464–468.
325. Sewell RB, Barham SS, LaRusso NF. Effect of chloroquine on the form and function of hepatocyte lysosomes. Morphologic modifications and physiologic alterations related to the biliary excretion of lipids and proteins. *Gastroenterology* 1983;85: 1146–1153.
326. Tegner R, Tome FM, Godeau P, et al. Morphological study of peripheral nerve changes induced by chloroquine treatment. *Acta Neuropathol (Berl)* 1988;75:253–260.
327. Whisnant JP, Espinosa RE, Kierland RR, et al. Chloroquine neuromyopathy. *Proc Mayo Clin* 1963;38:501–513.
328. Seguin P, Camus C, Leroy J-P, et al. Respiratory failure associated with hydroxychloroquine neuromyopathy. *Eur Neurol* 1995;35:236–237.
329. Richards AJ. Hydroxychloroquine myopathy. *J Rheumatol* 1998;25:1642–1643.
330. Estes ML, Ewing-Wilson D, Chou SM, et al. Chloroquine neuromyotoxicity. Clinical and pathologic perspective. *Am J Med* 1987;82:447–455.
331. Rynes RI. Side effects of antimalarial therapy. *Br J Clin Pract* 1987;41(suppl 52):42–45.
332. August C, Holzhausen HJ, Schmoldt A, et al. Histological and ultrastructural findings in chloroquine-induced cardiomyopathy. *J Mol Med* 1995;73:73–77.
333. Godeau P, Piette C, Balafrej M. A study of blood chloroquine concentration in patients with retinotoxicity and neuromyopathies. *Semin Hosp Paris* 1979;55:955–957.
334. Verny C, de Gennes C, Sebastien P, et al. Heart conduction disorders in long-term treatment with chloroquine. *Presse Med Paris* 1992;21:800–804.
335. Cubero GI, Reguero JJR, Ortega JMR. Restrictive cardiomyopathy caused by chloroquine. *Br Heart J* 1993;69:451–452.
336. Ihenacho HNC, Magulike E. Chloroquine abuse and heart block in Africans. *Aust NZ J Med* 1989;19:17–21.
337. Guedira N, Hajaj-Hassouni N, Srairi JE, et al. Third-degree atrioventricular block in a patient under chloroquine therapy. *Rev Rhum* (Engl Ed) 1998;65:58–62.
338. Veinot JP, Mai KT, Zarychanski R. Chloroquine related cardiac toxicity, *J Rheumatol* 1998;25:1221–1225.
339. Dhote R, Lestang P, Zuber M, et al. A cause of acute urinary retention: chloroquine induced neuromyopathy. *Rev Rhum* (Engl Ed) 1996;63:69.
340. Reuss-Borst M, Berner B, Wulf G, et al. Complete heart block as a rare complication of treatment with chloroquine, *J Rheumatol* 1999;26:1394–1395.
341. Jimenez-Alonso J, Tercedor J, Jaimez L, et al. Antimalarial drug-induced aquagenic-type pruritus in patients with lupus. *Arthritis Rheum* 1998;41:744–750.
342. Assier-Bonnet H, Saada V, Bernier M, et al. Acute generalized exanthematous pustulosis induced by hydroxychloroquine. *Dermatology* 1996;193:70–71.
343. Wolf R, Lo Schiavo A, Lombardi ML, et al. The in vitro effect of hydroxychloroquine on skin morphology transglumatase. *Int J Dermatol* 1997;36:704–707.
344. Campbell CH. Skin pigmentation with camoquin as a malarial suppressive. *Trans R Soc Trop Med Hyg* 1959;53:215–216.
345. Campbell CH. Pigmentation of the nail-beds, palate, and skin occurring during malarial suppressive therapy with camoquin. *Med J Aust* 1960;47:956–959.
346. Dubois EL. Systemic lupus erythematosus: recent advances in its diagnosis and treatment. *Ann Intern Med* 1956;45:163–184.
347. Kyle RA, Bartholomew LG. Variations in pigmentation from quinacrine. Report of case mimicking chronic hepatic disease. *Arch Intern Med* 1962;109:458–462.
348. Veraldi S, Schianchi-Veraldi R, Scarabelli G. Pigmentation of the gums following hydroxychloroquine therapy. *Cutis* 1992; 49:281–282.
349. Seidman P, Ros AM. Sensitivity to UV light during treatment with chloroquine in rheumatoid arthritis. *Scand J Rheumatol* 1992;21:245–247.
350. Kristensen S, Orsteen A-L, Sande SA, et al. Photoreactivity of biologically active compounds. VII. Interaction of antimalarial drugs with melanin in vitro as part of phototoxicity screening. *J Photochem Photobiol* 1994;B26:87–95.
351. Kutz DC, Bridges AJ. Bullous rash and brown urine in a systemic lupus erythematosus patient treated with hydroxychloroquine. *Arthritis Rheum* 1995;38:440–443.
352. Evans RL, Khalid S, Kinney JL. Antimalarial psychosis revisited. *Arch Dermatol* 1984;120:765–767.
353. Lindeman RD, Pederson JA, Matter BJ, et al. Long term azathioprine-corticosteroid therapy in lupus nephritis and idiopathic nephrotic syndrome. *J Chronic Dis* 1976;29:189–204.
354. Andrews RC. The side effects of antimalarial drugs indicates a polyamine involvement in both schizophrenia and depression. *Med Hypotheses* 1985;18:11–18.
355. Gaskill HS, Fitz-Hugh T Jr. Toxic psychosis following atabrine. *Bull U S Army M Dept* 1945;86:63–69.
356. Lidz J, Kahn RL. Toxicity of quinacrine (Atabrine) for the central nervous system; experimental study on human subjects. *Arch Neurol Psychiatr* 1946;56:284–289.
357. Reis J. Chloroquine induced insomnia in the treatment of systemic lupus erythematosus. *La Presse Med* 1991;20:659.
358. Akhtar S, Mukherjee S. Chloroquine induced mania. *Int J Psychiatr Med*1993;23:349–356.
359. Polano MK, Cats A, van Olden GAJ. Agranulocytosis following treatment with hydroxychloroquine sulphate. *Lancet* 1965;1: 1275.
360. Choudhry V, Madan N, Sood SK, et al. Chloroquine-induced haemolysis and acute renal failure in subjects with G-6-PD deficiency. *Trop Geogr Med* 1978;30:331–335.
361. Kersley GD, Palin AG. Amodiaquine and hydroxychloroquine in rheumatoid arthritis. *Lancet* 1959;ii:886–888.
362. Fedorko M. Effect of chloroquine on morphology of cytoplasmic granules in maturing human leukocytes—an ultrastructural study. *J Clin Invest* 1967;46:1932–1942.
363. Read WK, Bay WW. Basic cellular lesion in chloroquine toxicity. *Lab Invest* 1971;24:246–259.
364. Custer RP. Aplastic anemia in soldiers treated with Atabrine (quinacrine). *Am J Med Sci* 1946;212:211–224.
365. Fishman A, Kinsman JM. Hypoplastic anemia due to atabrine. *Blood* 1949;4:970–976.
366. Schmid I, Anasetti C, Petersen FB, et al. Marrow transplantation for severe aplastic anemia associated with exposure to quinacrine. *Blut* 1990;61:52–54.
367. Minker E, Blazso G, Kadar T. Inhibitory effect on gastric motility of chloroquine and mepacrine. *Acta Physiol Acad Sci Hung* 1978;52:455–458.
368. Jaeger A, Sauder J, Kopferschmitt FF, et al. Hypokalemia as evidence of chloroquine toxicity. *Presse Med* 1987;16:1658–1659.
369. Johansen PB, Gran JT. Ototoxicity due to hydroxychloroquine: report of two cases. *Clin Exp Rheumatol* 1998;16:472–474.
370. Beebe WE, Abbott RL, Fung WE. Hydroxychloroquine crystals in the tear film of a patient with rheumatoid arthritis. *Am J Ophthalmol* 1986;101:377–378.
371. Calkins LL. Corneal epithelial changes occurring during chloroquine (Aralen) therapy. *Arch Ophthalmol* 1958;60:981–988.
372. Cullen AP, Chou BR. Keratopathy with low dose chloroquine therapy. *J Am Optom Assoc* 1986;57:368–377.
373. Hobbs HE, Eadie SP, Somerville F. Ocular lesions after treatment with chloroquine. *Br J Ophthalmol* 1961;45:284–297.

374. Lozier JR, Friedlaender MH. Complications of antimalarial therapy. *Int Ophthalmol Clin* 1989;29:172–178.
375. Maksymowych W, Russell AS. Antimalarials in rheumatology: efficacy and safety. *Semin Arthritis Rheum* 1987;16:206–221.
376. Henkind P, Rothfield NF. Ocular abnormalities in patients treated with antimalarial drugs. *N Engl J Med* 1963;269: 433–439.
377. Kadin M, Dubois EL. Keratoconjunctivitis sicca, corneal and lens changes associated with lupus erythematosus and its treatment. Unpublished observations.
378. Rynes RI, Krohel G, Falbo A, et al. Ophthalmologic safety of long-term hydroxychloroquine treatment. *Arthritis Rheum* 1979;22:832–836.
379. Tobin DR, Krohel GB, Rynes RI. Hydroxychloroquine:seven-year experience. *Arch Ophthalmol* 1982;100:81–83.
380. Easterbrook M. Ocular effects and safety of antimalarial agents. *Am J Med*1988;85(suppl 4A):23–29.
381. Easterbrook M. Is corneal deposition of antimalarial any indication of retinal toxicity? *Can J Ophthalmol* 1991;25:249–251.
382. Ansdell VE, Common JD. Corneal changes induced by mepacrine. *J Trop Med Hyg* 1979;82:206–207.
383. Chamberlain WP Jr, Boles DJ. Edema of cornea precipitated by quinacrine (Atabrine). *Arch Ophthalmol* 1946;35:120–134.
384. Cambiaggi A. Unusual ocular lesions in a case of systemic lupus erythematosus. *Arch Ophthalmol* 1957;57:451–453.
385. Bernstein NH. Chloroquine ocular toxicity. *Surv Ophthalmol* 1967;12:415–447.
386. Krill AE, Potts AM, Johanson CE. Chloroquine retinopathy. Investigation of discrepancy between dark adaptation and electroretinographic findings in advance stages. *Am J Ophthalmol* 1971;71:530–543.
387. Voippio H. Incidence of chloroquine retinopathy. *Ophthalmologica* 1966;148:442–452.
388. Parhami N, Morrell M. Loss of color vision and hydroxychloroquine. *J Clin Rheumatol* 1996;2:117–118.
389. Elner VM, Schaffner T, Taylor K, et al. Immunophagocytic properties of retinal pigment epithelium cells. *Science* 1981; 211:74–76.
390. Lloyd LA, Hiltz JW. Ocular complications of chloroquine therapy. *Can Med Assoc J* 1965;92:508–513.
391. Wetterholm DH, Winter FC. Histopathology of chloroquine retinal toxicity. *Arch Ophthalmol* 1964;71:82–87.
392. Meyniel G, Doly M, Millerin M, et al. Demonstration of the participation of platelet-activating factor (PAF) in chloroquine retinopathy. *CR Acad Sci Paris* 1992;314:61–65.
393. El-Sayed NK, Abdel-Khalek LR, Gaafar KM, et al. Profiles of serum proteins and free amino acids associated with chloroquine retinopathy. *Acta Ophthalmol Scand* 1998;76:422–430.
394. Banks CN. Melanin: blackguard or red herring? Another look at chloroquine retinopathy. *Aust NZ J Ophthalmol* 1987;15: 365–370.
395. Raines MF, Bhargava SK, Rosen ES. The blood-retinal barrier in chloroquine retinopathy. *Invest Ophthalmol Vis Sci* 1989;30: 1726–1731.
396. Bernstein HN. Ocular safety of hydroxychloroquine sulfate (Plaquenil). *South Med J* 1992;85:274–279.
397. Mackenzie AH. Dose refinements in long-term therapy of rheumatoid arthritis with antimalarials. *Am J Med* 1983;75 (suppl 1A):40–45.
398. Marks JS, Power BJ. Is chloroquine obsolete in treatment of rheumatoid disease? *Lancet* 1979;1:371–373.
399. Marks JS. Chloroquine retinopathy: is there a safe daily dose? *Ann Rheum Dis* 1982;41:52–58.
400. Mills PV, Beck M, Power BJ. Assessment of the retinal toxicity of hydroxychloroquine. *Trans Ophthal Soc UK* 1981;101:109–113.
401. Runge LA. Risk/benefit analysis of hydroxychloroquine sulfate treatment of rheumatoid arthritis. *Am J Med* 1983;75(suppl 1A):52–56.
402. Bartholomew LE, Rynes RI. Use of antimalarial drugs in rheumatoid arthritis: guidelines for ocular safety. *Intern Med* 1982;3:66–70.
403. Rynes RI. Ophthalmologic safety of long-term hydroxychloroquine sulfate treatment. *Am J Med* 1983;75(suppl 1A):35–39.
404. Elman A, Gullberg R, Nilsson E, et al. Chloroquine retinopathy in patients with rheumatoid arthritis. *Scand J Rheumatol* 1976;5:161–166.
405. Finbloom DS, Silver K, Newsome DA, et al. Antimalarial use and the development of toxic maculopathy. *Arthritis Rheum* 1981;24(suppl):S82(abst).
406. Finbloom DS, Silver K, Newsome DA, et al. Comparison of hydroxychloroquine and chloroquine use and the development of retinal toxicity. *J Rheumatol* 1985;12:692–694.
407. Frenkel M. Safety of hydroxychloroquine (letter). *Arch Ophthalmol* 1982;100:841.
408. Bell CL, Boh LE. The risk of retinopathy associated with hydroxychloroquine (HCQ) use in patients with rheumatoid arthritis (RA). *Arthritis Rheum* 1989;32(suppl):R32(abst).
409. Easterbrook M. Dose relationships in patients with early chloroquine retinopathy. *J Rheumatol* 1987;14:472–475.
410. Easterbrook M. Useful and diagnostic tests in the detection of early chloroquine retinopathy. *Arthritis Rheum* 1989;32(suppl): R8(abst).
411. Ehrenfeld M, Nesher R, Merin S. Delayed-onset chloroquine retinopathy. *Br J Ophthalmol* 1986;70:281–283.
412. Burns RP. Delayed onset of chloroquine retinopathy. *N Engl J Med* 1966;275:693–696.
413. Martin LJ, Bergan RL, Dobrow HR. Delayed onset chloroquine retinopathy: case report. *Ann Ophthalmol* 1978;10:723–726.
414. Ogawa S, Kurumatani N, Shibaike N, et al. Progression of retinopathy long after cessation of chloroquine therapy (letter). *Lancet* 1979;1:1408.
415. Sassani JW, Brucker AJ, Cobbs W, et al. Progressive chloroquine retinopathy. *Ann Ophthalmol* 1983;15:19–22.
416. Morsman CD, Livesey SJ, Richards IM, et al. Screening for hydroxychloroquine retinal toxicity: is it necessary? *Eye* 1990;4:572–576.
417. Spalton DJ, Verdon Roe GM, Hughes GRV. Hydroxychloroquine, dosage parameters and retinopathy. *Lupus* 1993;2: 355–358.
418. Bray VJ, Enzenauer RJ, Enzenauer RW, et al. Antimalarial ocular toxicity in rheumatic disease. *J Clin Rheumatol* 1998;4: 168–169.
419. Levy GD, Munz SJ, Paschal J, et al. Incidence of hydroxychloroquine retinopathy in 1,207 patients in a large multicenter outpatient practice. *Arthritis Rheum* 1997;40:1482–1486.
420. Grierson DJ. Hydroxychloroquine and visual screening in a rheumatology outpatient clinic. *Ann Rheum Dis* 1997;56: 188–190.
421. Mavrikakis M, Papazoglou S, Sifkakis PP, et al. Retinal toxicity in long term hydroxychloroquine treatment. *Ann Rheum Dis* 1996;55:187–189.
422. Gillis C, ed. *Compendium of pharmaceuticals and specialties*, 33rd ed. Ottawa: Canadian Pharmacists Association, 1998.
423. Carr RE, Henkind P, Rothfield N, et al. Ocular toxicity of antimalarial drugs: long-term follow-up. *Am J Ophthalmol* 1968;66: 738–744.
424. Zuehlke RL, Lillis PJ, Tice A. Antimalarial therapy for lupus erythematosus: an apparent advantage of quinacrine. *Int J Dermatol* 1981;20:57–61.
425. Mackenzie AH, Szilagyi PJ. Light may provide energy for retinal damage during chloroquine treatment. *Arthritis Rheum* 1968;11:496–497.

426. Legros J, Rosher I, Bereger C. Influence of the ambient light level in the ocular modifications induced by hydroxychloroquine in the rat. *Arch Ophthalmol* 1973;33:417– 424.
427. Portnoy JZ, Callen JP. Ophthalmologic aspects of chloroquine and hydroxychloroquine therapy. *Int J Dermatol* 1983;22:273–278.
428. Cruess AF, Schachat AP, Nicholl J, et al. Chloroquine retinopathy. Is fluorescein angiography necessary? *Ophthalmology* 1985; 92:1127–1129.
429. Carr R. Prolonged pharmacotherapy and the eye. A symposium. Chloroquine and organic changes in the eye. *Dis Nerv Syst* 1968;29(suppl 3):36–39.
430. Easterbrook M. Comparison of threshold and standard Amsler grid testing in patients with established antimalarial retinopathy. *Can J Ophthalmol* 1992;27:240–242.
431. Easterbrook M. The use of Amsler grids in early chloroquine retinopathy. *Ophthalmology* 1984;91:1368–1372.
432. Bishara SA, Matamoros N. Evaluation of several tests in screening for chloroquine maculopathy. *Eye* 1989;3:777–782.
433. Fleck BW, Bell AL, Mitchell JD, et al. Screening for antimalarial maculopathy in rheumatology clinics. *Br Med J (Clin Res)* 1985;291:782– 785.
434. Rynes RI, Alpert DA. Antimalarials. Is re-evaluation needed? *J Clin Rheumatol* 1998;4:50–62.
435. MacLean CH, Lee PP, Keeler EB. Cost analysis of routine ophthalmologic screening for hydroxychloroquine retinal toxicity. *Arthritis Rheum* 1999;1996;39:S72.
436. Corzillus CM, Bienfand D, Liang MH. Cost-effectiveness analysis of screening for hydroxychloroquine-induced retinopathy. *Arthritis Rheum* 1997;40:S316.
437. Easterbrook M, Bernstein H. Ophthalmological monitoring of patients taking antimalarials: preferred practice patterns. *J Rheumatol* 1997;24:1390–1392.

56

SYSTEMIC GLUCOCORTICOID THERAPY IN SYSTEMIC LUPUS ERYTHEMATOSUS

KYRIAKOS A. KIROU
DIMITRIOS T. BOUMPAS

Phillip Hench was the first to introduce glucocorticoids (GCs) into clinical medicine when he successfully treated a patient with rheumatoid arthritis (RA) in 1949 (1). The long record of GCs in the management of rheumatic diseases testifies to their clinical usefulness. However, GC benefits occur at a high cost of serious side effects. Therefore, therapeutic strategies aiming to decrease exposure to GC are imperative. The treating physician, optimally a rheumatologist with experience in the management of systemic lupus erythematosus (SLE) (2), should carefully evaluate the patient and attempt to distinguish inflammation due to disease flare from infection, thrombosis, and drug (including GC) adverse effects. Combination therapies of GCs with other immunosuppressive or antiinflammatory agents can help achieve disease control with less exposure to GCs. It is hoped that future research on both SLE pathogenesis and mechanisms of GC action will add safer and more effective therapies to our armamentarium against SLE.

This chapter briefly reviews the basic pharmacology of endogenous and synthetic GCs, the mechanisms of their action at the molecular level, and their antiinflammatory and immunosuppressive effects. Then the pharmacokinetics and drug interactions of GCs are discussed, and the authors' opinions regarding their use in SLE are presented. Lastly, adverse effects of GCs with relevance to SLE is analyzed, and the GC withdrawal syndrome is briefly reviewed.

ENDOGENOUS AND SYNTHETIC GLUCOCORTICOIDS

Steroidogenesis in the adrenal cortex produces endogenous GCs, mineralocorticoids (MCs), and adrenal androgens (3,4). Cortisol (hydrocortisone) is the main human endogenous GC and is secreted primarily in response to adrenocorticotropic hormone (ACTH). Secretion follows a circadian rhythm that achieves maximum plasma concentration at 8 A.M. (16 μg/dL) (3–5). However, in the context of stressful stimuli and hypothalamic-pituitary-adrenal (HPA) axis stimulation, these levels can increase to more than 60 μ/dL, losing their diurnal variation (5,6). The ability of an organism to maintain appropriate GC levels before and during stress is essential for its survival (7,8).

Synthetic GC, more potent and with fewer MC effects than cortisol, have been developed. The biochemical structure of cortisol and synthetic GC is shown in Fig. 56.1 and their pharmacologic properties are compared in Table 56.1. Regulatory mechanisms of synthetic GC with regard to binding to the cortisol-binding globulin (CBG), tissue-specific metabolism, affinity for GC receptors (GRs), and interaction with transcription factors may substantially differ from those of native GC (4,9,10).

The great need for improved synthetic GC with fewer adverse effects and intact antiinflammatory/immunosuppressive action has first generated deflazacort [an oxazoline analogue of prednisolone with a shorter plasma half-life and fewer MC effects (11-13)], then GC with high topical activity but low systemic bioavailability such as budesonide, and lastly the "dissociated" GC (14,15). With regard to deflazacort, it is still controversial whether its adverse effect profile is superior to prednisone (11–13). Studies that used deflazacort doses according to an equipotency ratio to prednisone of 1.2:1 favored deflazacort over prednisone (12), but other studies that used an equipotency ratio of 1.5:1 had discouraging results (13). It is not currently approved for clinical use in the United States. Budesonide is a GC agent structurally related to 16α-hydroxyprednisolone that is characterized by high topical yet low systemic GC activity (and thus fewer adverse effects) due to its rapid first-pass liver metabolism and inactivation. Thus, by design, this agent is suitable only when topical antiinflammatory action is desired such as in asthma (given by inhalation), and in active Crohn's (orally; 16,17). Of special interest and promise to the field of systemic GC therapy appears to be the more recent development of synthetic GC that dissociate their potent activator protein-1 (AP-1) and nuclear factor kappa B (NF-κB) transrepression activities (antiinflam-

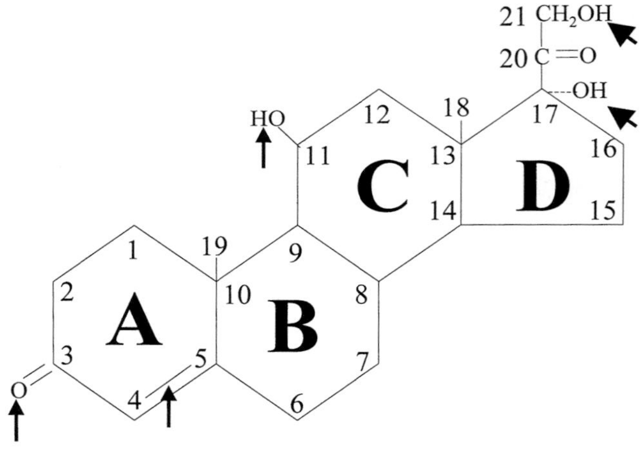

FIGURE 56.1. A: Structure of cortisol (hydrocortisone). All the Δ^4 double bond, 3-keto group, and 11β-OH group are essential for glucocorticoid (GC) function, and the first two are also required for mineralocorticoid activity. The hydroxyl group at C21 is required for mineralocorticoid activity and is present on all natural and synthetic GCs. The 17α-hydroxyl group, present on cortisol and synthetic GCs (but not on corticosterone), enhances GC potency. **B:** Structure of selected common synthetic GCs. The addition of a Δ^1 double bond on cortisol (as in all shown GCs) selectively increases GC activity and delays GC metabolism. The methyl group at position 6α (methylprednisolone) increases GC, over MC, activity even further. Notably, fluorination at the 9α position (fludrocortisone; not shown) greatly enhances GC and MC activity (the latter much more than the former). However, when modified with a Δ^1 double bond and a methyl group substitution at C16α, fludrocortisone loses all MC activity and becomes dexamethasone.

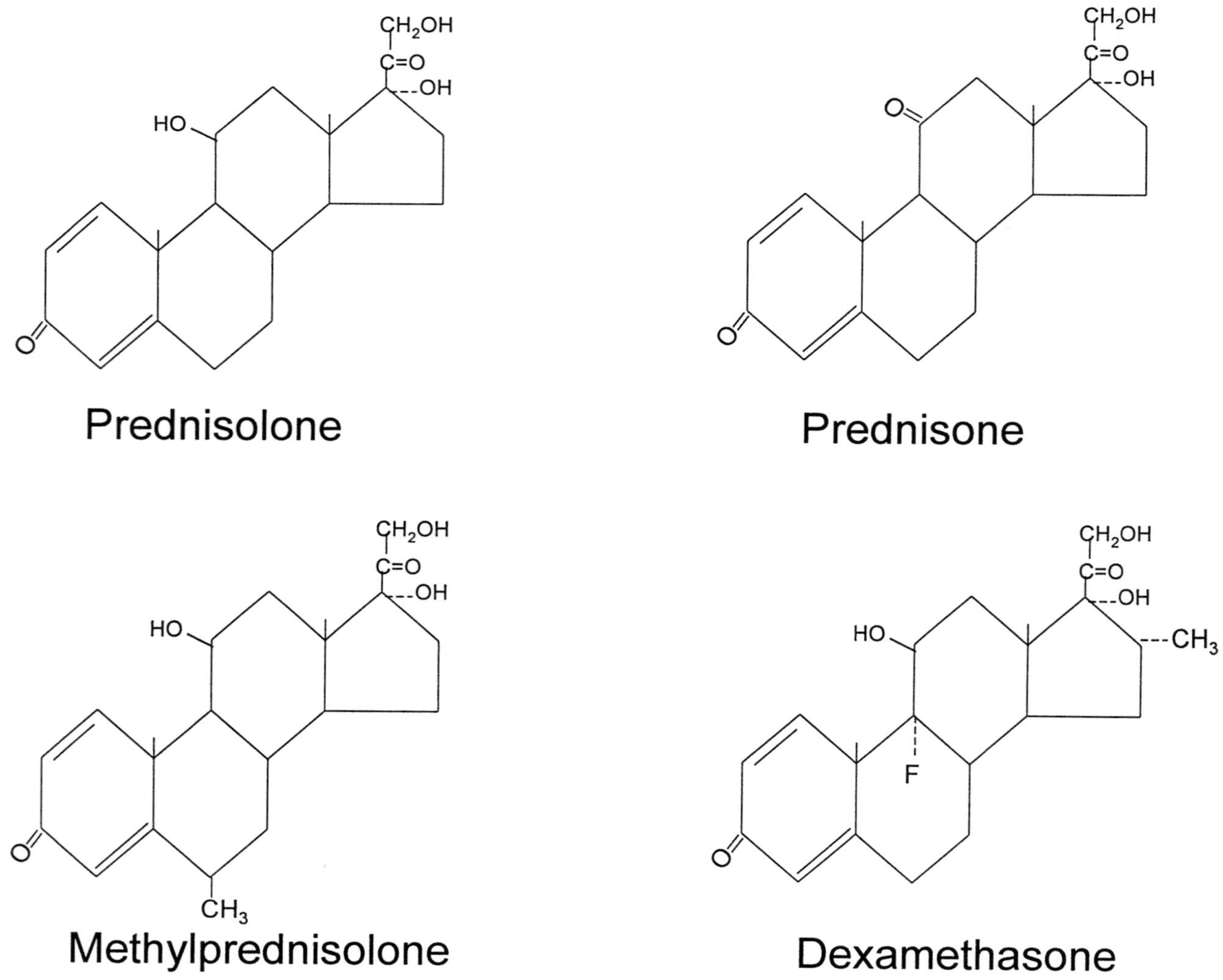

TABLE 56.1. SELECTED ENDOGENOUS AND SYNTHETIC GLUCOCORTICOID (GC) AGENTS

GC Preparation	Equivalent Antiinflammatory Dose (mg)	Mineralocorticoid Activity	Half-life (min)	Biologic Half-life (hours)
Cortisol	20	1	60	8–12
Cortisone	25	0.8	60	8–12
Prednisone	5	0.8	180	12–36
Prednisolone	5	0.8	180	12–36
Methylprednisolone	4	0.5	180	12–36
Triamcinolone	4	0	180	12–36
Dexamethasone	0.75	0	220	36–72

matory) from their weak transactivation ones (see below) that are likely responsible for GC adverse effects (14,15). However, their clinical benefit has yet to be seen. Additionally, it is of some interest that the novel glucocorticoid analogues 21-aminosteroids (or lazaroids), although unable to bind to glucocorticoid receptors, can act as free radical scavengers and membrane stabilizers and share the neuroprotective effect of high-dose methylprednisolone in CNS injury (18).

MOLECULAR MECHANISMS OF GLUCOCORTICOID ACTION

Glucocorticoid effects are mainly mediated via specific GC receptors (GRs). These are conspicuous cytoplasmic proteins and operate as hormone-activated transcriptional regulators (reviewed in refs. 19–22). Hydrocortisone and some other GCs are also capable of binding mineralocorticoid receptors (MRs) with higher affinity than they bind GR and mediating aldosterone-like effects (Table 56.1). GR specificity, at the relatively low baseline body cortisol levels, is maintained because of the action of 11β-hydroxysteroid dehydrogenase-2 (11β-HSD_2), a steroid metabolizing enzyme expressed at MC-sensitive tissues (like the kidney). 11β-HSD_2 metabolizes hydrocortisone to its inactive 11-keto derivative (cortisone) (3,4,7).

Glucocorticoid receptors, when inactive, are bound to certain heat shock proteins (i.e., HSP90, HSP70) and immunophilins (IPs) (19–22). However, upon GC ligation, GRs dissociate from these proteins and translocate to the nucleus, where they bind to glucocorticoid responsive elements (GREs) on DNA with positive [i.e., lipocortin-1 (23)] and negative gene transcription activation effects [i.e., osteocalcin (24)]. Alternatively, GRs through direct protein-protein interactions are able to transrepress function of other transcriptional factors like AP-1 (25–27), NF-κB (15,28), and the signal transducers and activators (STATs) (29). Induction of IκBα transcription by GR and thus indirect inhibition of NF-κB-dependent proinflammatory genes is an example of another sophisticated mechanism of GC action (30,31). Finally, GCs can act postranscriptionally and lead to decreased or increased messenger RNA (mRNA) stability of cytokine genes (32–34).

Besides having GR-mediated transcriptional genomic effects that depend on new protein synthesis and therefore have a delayed onset (at least 30 minutes), GCs may act independently of GRs and thus much more rapidly (within seconds or minutes) (18,35). These GC effects usually occur at relatively large pharmacologic doses and can be either cell surface receptor mediated and therefore specific, or initiated by physicochemical interactions with cellular membranes and nonspecific (18,35). Examples of the former include the negative feedback regulation of ACTH production by hydrocortisone and the behavioral as well as cardiovascular effects of GCs (35,36). On the other hand, inhibition of cation cycling and respiration in concanavalin A–stimulated rat thymocytes constitute nonspecific GC effects (18,35). Interestingly, different GC agents have dissimilar relative potencies when their nonspecific or classic effects are considered (37).

ANTIINFLAMMATORY AND IMMUNOSUPPRESSIVE EFFECTS

The biologic effects of GCs are multiple, affect all tissues, and are essential for body homeostasis during normal or stress conditions. Although in clinical medicine GCs are used to suppress inflammation and pathologic immune responses, a growing number of studies "paradoxically" attribute immune enhancing effects to these agents (7,9,10,38–40). It seems that endogenous GCs have an important overall regulatory role in modulating immune responses that develop to such stressors as infections. For example, GCs act, on the one hand, permissively to help immune responses develop adequately and in a timely fashion to fight the invading organisms, and, on the other hand, suppressively to restrain a potentially deleterious "overshoot" of those same responses (7). Parameters that determine the direction of GC immune effects include primarily the serum levels and timing of GC exposure relative to the initiation of stress. Higher (pharmacologic) levels such as those occurring after the initiation of stress are in general immunosuppressive, whereas lower physiologic levels of GC present before stress initiation may enhance immune responses. Notably, acute stresses (or short exposure to GC) enhance immune responses, while chronic exposure to stress or GC has the opposite effect (38). Endogenous GCs (cortisol) appear to mediate both types of effects. Dexamethasone, however, a synthetic GC, mediates predominantly immunosuppressive effects, a phenomenon that may be explained by dexamethasone's inefficient binding to CBG, its longer half-life, its higher affinity for GRs, and absence of MC effects (Table 56.1) (9,10,38). The immune-enhancing GC effects may be mediated through MR. Augmentation of T-cell proliferation to antigenic stimuli (39), of lymphocyte trafficking to skin and regional lymph nodes [during a delayed type hypersensitivity (DTH) response (38)], of cytokine production [including the macrophage migration inhibitory factor (MIF) (40, 41)], as well as synergy with different cytokines [such as with interleukin-6 (IL-6) in the induction of acute-phase responses] and upregulation of cytokine receptors (7,9,10) are some of these effects.

The antiinflammatory effects of GCs (Table 56.2) are complex, mediated via their GRs, and correlate with dose and duration of GC treatment. At the level of blood vessels, GCs inhibit vasodilatation and vascular permeability, limiting therefore erythema, plasma exudation, and swelling. The inhibitory GC effects on the upregulation of the inducible nitric oxide synthase (iNOS), and therefore NO synthesis, by tumor necrosis factor-α (TNF-α), IL-1β, and interferon-γ (IFN-γ) (42) may contribute to this effect. Neutrophils are affected primarily in their ability to migrate to inflammatory sites. This effect is probably due to inhibition by GC of chemokine synthesis [i.e., IL-8 (43)] and adhesion molecule expression [intercellular adhesion molecule-1 (ICAM-1), E-selectin (44)] and induction of lipocortin-1 [or annexin I (45)]. In patients with RA, inhibition of neutrophil ingress into inflamed joints was seen as early as 90 minutes after pulse GC therapy (46), and was associated with rapid modulation of adhesion molecules and inflammatory mediators in the joints (46,47). Inhibition of synthesis and secretion of inflammatory mediators by the different cells involved in the inflammatory reaction (such as monocytes-macrophages, fibroblasts, and endothelial cells) is central in the action of GC. Eicosanoid generation is inhibited by GC through induction of transcription of lipocortin-1, which is a potent inhibitor of phospholipase A_2 activity (23,48), and inhibition of IL-1β [or lipopolysaccharide (LPS)]-mediated cyclooxygenase-2 (COX-2) induction (49). Additionally, destructive tissue enzymes such as collagenase are downregulated by GC (26,27). Inhibition of cytokine generation constitutes another important antiinflammatory effect. Specifically, synthesis (and sometimes action) of TNF-α, IL-1β, IL-2, IL-3, IL-6, IL-8, granulocyte-macrophage colony-stimulating factor (GM-CSF), and IFN-γ is blocked (15,28,32,43,50,51). On the other hand, synthesis of IL-10 and transforming growth factor-β (TGF-β) cytokines considered to have antiinflammatory properties is either not affected or induced (52–54). The differential effects of various GC therapeutic regimens on cytokine production have been elegantly shown in human arteritis–severe combined immunodeficiency disease (SCID) mice chimeras by Brack et al. (53). SCID mice engrafted with human temporal arteries were studied with regard to the effects of *in vivo* intraperitoneal GC therapy on inflammation of the temporal arteries. Doses of dexamethasone of 0.04 and 0.4 mg/kg for 7 days induced IκBα transcription, inhibited nuclear NF-κB protein expression, and decreased transcription of the NF-κB-regulated genes iNOS, IL-1β, IL-2 and IL-6. Inhibition of IFN-γ could only be achieved by high doses of dexamethasone (4 mg/kg for 4 days) or chronic therapy (0.4

TABLE 56.2. IMPORTANT ANTIINFLAMMATORY AND IMMUNOSUPPRESSIVE EFFECTS OF GLUCOCORTICOIDS

Antiinflammatory effects
- Inhibition of blood vessel dilatation and permeability (i.e., due to downregulation of NO synthesis)
- Inhibition of neutrophil migration to periphery (probably via inhibition of chemokine synthesis and adhesion molecule expression) leading to neutrophilia
- Inhibition of synthesis of inflammatory mediators such as eicosanoids by downregulating phospholipase A_2 (via lipocortin-1 induction) and COX-2
- Downregulation of destructive enzymes (i.e., collagenase)
- Alteration of cytokine balance in favor of antiinflammatory cytokines (i.e., IL-10, TGF-β), while proinflammatory cytokines (i.e., TNF-α, IL-1β, GM-CSF) are suppressed

Immunosuppressive effects[a]
- Lymphopenia[b] (T cells affected more than B cells and CD4 T cells more than CD8 T cells); probably due to lymphocyte redistribution (mainly to bone marrow and spleen) and perhaps apoptosis
- Inhibition of signal transduction events critical for T-cell activation (i.e., early tyrosine phosphorylation, CaM-kinase II activation, calcineurin-dependent transactivating pathways)
- Inhibition of IL-2 synthesis and signaling
- Downregulation of cell surface molecules (i.e., LFA-1, CD2, CD40L) important for full T-cell activation and function
- Inhibition of antigen-presenting cell function (by blocking cell surface expression of MHC class II and CD80 molecules)
- Deviation of immune responses toward a Th2-type cytokine formation (by preferentially inhibiting synthesis of IL-12 over that of IL-4 and IL-10)
- Induction of T-cell apoptosis (of questionable contribution to GC-mediated immunosuppression)

[a]Immunosuppression concerns primarily the cellular and less so the humoral immunity and is more evident with intermediate to high doses of glucocorticoids.
[b]When lymphopenia is associated with lymphocyte migration toward the regional nodes of inflammation, it represents immune enhancement rather than immunosuppression (see text for discussion).
NO, nitric oxide; COX-2, cycloxygenase-2; CaM-kinase II, Ca^{2+} calmodulin–dependent protein kinase II; GM-CSF, granulocyte-macrophage colony-stimulating factor; IL, interleukin; TGF, transforming growth factor.

mg/kg for 28 days). However, TGF-β transcription was not inhibited by any dexamethasone regimen, an effect interpreted by the authors as pathogenetically important for the disease, since TGF-β, depending on the local tissue conditions present, may augment inflammation.

Although GCs induce peripheral neutrophilia, by reducing neutrophil migration to tissues, the peripheral numbers of eosinophils, basophils, monocytes, and lymphocytes decrease upon even a brief exposure to GC (19–22). Lymphopenia has been attributed to redirection of lymphocytes to bone marrow and spleen (55–57), but also to the skin and regional lymph nodes of inflammation sites (38). T-cell numbers decrease more than B cells and CD4 T cells more than CD8 T cells (57). GC immunosuppression is mediated by inhibition of several stages of T-cell activation, including early tyrosine phosphorylation events (58), activation of Ca^{2+}/calmodulin-dependent protein kinase II [CaM-kinase II) (59)], and calcineurin-dependent transactivating pathways (60). As already mentioned, GCs inhibit IL-2 synthesis, which is critical for T-cell proliferative responses (33,61), and additionally inhibit signaling of this cytokine (62). Downregulation of lymphocyte function-associated antigen-1 (LFA-1), CD2, c-*myc*, and CD40 ligand (CD40L), and induction of 3′,5′-cyclic adenosine monophosphate (cAMP) (by inhibiting phosphodiesterase activity) further contribute to T-cell dysfunction (22,63, 64). Glucocorticoids also affect T-cell function indirectly by inhibiting the expression of major histocompatibility complex (MHC) class II and CD80 molecules on antigen-presenting cells (20,22). B-cell function and immunoglobulin synthesis are relatively resistant to the immunosuppressive GC effects. GCs have also important effects in shaping the developing immune responses as they favor deviation to T-helper-2 (Th2)-type cytokine formation by preferentially inhibiting IL-12 synthesis and sparing IL-4 and IL-10 (54,65–67). This effect might suggest that these agents are more potent in the treatment of diseases characterized by Th1-type cytokine predominance, like RA.

The ability of GC to induce apoptosis of double positive thymocytes (65) and activated mature T cells (68) correlates with low cellular levels of bcl-2 and appears to have important implications for maintenance of central and possibly peripheral tolerance as well (65). Interestingly, T-cell receptor (TCR)-mediated activation-induced cell death (AICD) and GC-mediated apoptosis are mutually antagonistic, an effect that may be in part due to downregulation of Fas ligand by GC (65,69). The degree to which GC-mediated apoptosis contributes to immunosuppression is not known, however. Seki et al. (70) correlated clinical resistance to GC in SLE patients with decreased *in vitro* apoptosis of anti-CD3–activated peripheral blood mononuclear cells (PBMCs) (70). In another study, γ/δ T cells, which may be implicated in SLE pathogenesis, showed increased *in vitro* susceptibility to GC-mediated apoptosis (without requiring previous activation), and their *in vivo* downregulation by GC therapy correlated with disease control in SLE patients (71). Both antiinflammatory and immunosuppressive effects of GCs are summarized in Table 56.2.

Glucocorticoid Resistance

Resistance to GC can have many causes. Impaired bioavailability due to decreased GC absorption (i.e., by cholestyramine) or increased GC metabolism (i.e., by hyperthyroidism or drugs such as barbiturates) can occasionally be a cause of GC resistance (72).

Resistance to endogenous GC rarely occurs in the generalized inherited glucocorticoid resistance (GIGR) syndrome characterized by GR abnormalities, high plasma cortisol levels, and the absence of Cushing's syndrome symptoms (73–75). The opposite picture, increased primary GC sensitivity, has also been noted (74). Additionally, an acquired GR abnormality has been observed in a subset of AIDS patients who present with addisonian symptoms and hypercortisolism (76). The acquired, tissue-specific GC resistance, which is clinically more important, has been studied best in steroid-resistant bronchial asthma, where the lack of GC benefit on airway inflammation contrasts with a high incidence of GC adverse effects from other organs (77). Cytokines, secreted in the context of such diseases as bronchial asthma, RA, SLE, and depression, are thought to play an important role in tissue-specific GC resistance, by inhibiting GR function. Proposed mechanisms of such an effect include induction of AP-1 [mutually antagonistic with GR for transactivation effects (26,27)], inhibition of GR translocation, and induction of the beta isoform (GRβ) of GR via alternative splicing of the GR pre-mRNA (77,78). GRβ has been proposed as an important inhibitor of the functionally active GRα (79). In SLE, increased catabolism of hydrocortisone by lymphocytes (80) and resistance to GC-mediated apoptosis of $CD8^+$ T cells have been proposed as mechanisms of GC resistance (70).

PHARMACOKINETICS AND DRUG INTERACTIONS

Oral absorption of GC is excellent. Prednisone is 80% to 90% absorbed when orally administered, whether on an empty or full stomach. Once systemically absorbed, a large fraction of GC (90% for hydrocortisone) binds to serum proteins and only their free fraction is biologically active (3,4). Of the two GC-binding proteins, transcortin, or CBG, binds to GC with high affinity and low capacity, whereas albumin binds with low affinity and high capacity. Since hydrocortisone and prednisolone bind to both CBG and albumin, their protein binding is concentration dependent and varies from 90% at lower doses (i.e., with standard oral doses) to 60% at higher doses. In contrast, methylprednisolone and dexamethasone bind almost exclusively (99%)

to the high capacity albumin and therefore have concentration-independent protein-bound fractions (60% to 70%). The difference in the plasma free concentrations of dexamethasone and prednisolone at standard oral doses may explain the better cerebrospinal fluid (CSF) penetration and better efficacy of the former in the preventive therapy of meningeal leukemia (81). The 11-keto GC derivatives such as prednisone and cortisone are inactive unless reduced by 11β-HSD1 in the liver to their 11-OH analogues prednisolone and hydrocortisone (Fig. 56.1) (3,4). Inactivation of GC occurs predominantly in the liver and involves the sequential reduction of the Δ^4 double bond (the rate-limiting step in cortisol metabolism), and the 3-keto group (Fig. 56.1). Glucuronidation and sulfation follow, which confer water solubility and allow for urine excretion. Additionally, 6β-hydroxylation by the cytochrome P-450 microsomal enzyme CYP3A4 also enhances water solubility and urinary excretion of GC. Serum half-lives of different GC differ and vary from 60 to 300 minutes. However, biologic half-lives of GC are dependent on their tissue levels and are much longer than their serum half-lives (Table 56.1).

Since, in liver failure, decreased conversion of prednisone to its active form (prednisolone) is overcompensated for by reduced clearance of unbound prednisolone (resulting in higher prednisolone concentrations after oral prednisone administration), there is no reason to substitute for prednisone with another inherently active GC agent in these patients. Additionally, low serum albumin does not seem to decrease the unbound concentration of prednisolone, and therefore (mild) dose adjustments of GCs should be based only on the lower clearance of these agents in liver failure and not on the albumin levels per se (reviewed in ref. 82).

In addition to the above-mentioned inhibition of enteric GC absorption by cholestyramine, there are other important drug interactions. Drugs that induce hepatic microsomal enzymes (especially CYP3A4), such as phenobarbital, phenytoin, rifampin, and carbamazepine, increase GC elimination. In contrast, ketokonazole, erythromycin, ethynyl estradiol, and norethindrone inhibit CYP3A4 and can increase GC activity (83). Mifepristone (RU-486), an antiprogestin drug marketed as an abortifacient, has potent antiglucocorticoid properties (at the level of GR) as well (84). Conversely, GC can also reduce the serum level of salicylates (85) and CYP3A4 substrates. Additionally, pulse GCs have been recently shown to significantly increase international normalized ratios (INR), 2 to 6 days after their administration, in patients on oral anticoagulation therapy (86).

GENERAL PRINCIPLES OF GLUCOCORTICOID THERAPY

Uncontrolled disease activity in SLE can be both debilitating and life threatening and thus demands rapid and effective intervention. The value of therapy with high doses of GC (i.e., more than 0.6 to 1 mg/kg/d of prednisone) in dramatically improving SLE survival has been established (already by data from the predialysis era) in patients with diffuse proliferative glomerulonephritis (DPGN) (87,88). Subsequent studies focused on evaluating different strategies of GC use to maintain high effectiveness and yet reduce the risk of the increasingly apparent grave adverse effects. Besides interpersonal variation in GC sensitivity (2,89,90) and risk of adverse effects, it is now clear that long-acting synthetic GCs (i.e., dexamethasone) are the most dangerous agents in the family, and their daily use should be avoided (20,91,92). Ample evidence exists that high GC doses (especially when time intervals between doses are small) for prolonged periods of time are invariably toxic. In fact, Sergent et al. (93) have shown increased infection-related mortality in patients with severe neuropsychiatric SLE (NPSLE) when treated with prednisone doses of more than 100 mg/d for 37 days on average (range 8 to 68 days). On the other hand, low-dose GC (LDGC) therapy (dose equivalent to <7.5 to 10 mg/d of prednisone) appears to be better tolerated but not risk-free, since complications such as growth suppression, osteoporosis, and cataract formation can still occur. Therefore, the ultimate goal of therapy should always be complete cessation of GC, if possible.

Alternate-day GC therapy (ADGC) also has a better safety profile compared to that of daily GC regimens. The incidence of skeletal growth inhibition, HPA-axis suppression, hypertension (HTN), Cushing's syndrome, hypokalemia, overcatabolism, myopathy, and infection has been noted to be reduced (91,92,94,95). However, ADGC effectiveness is less and, excluding perhaps membranous nephritis with nephrotic syndrome (96), its use should be restricted to GC-tapering or maintenance regimens (91,92,94).

Severe or organ/life-threatening lupus manifestations require large doses of GCs. For the purpose of this discussion, doses of 0.6 to 1 mg/kg/d of prednisone [high-dose GC (HDGC)] have been arbitrarily separated from very high doses of GC (VHDGC; 1 to 2 mg/kg/d of prednisone or more), based on two facts. First, HDGC therapy, for up to 6 to 8 weeks, has been considered as one of the standard regimens for the treatment of lupus nephritis (96,97), perhaps the most important and best studied SLE manifestation. Second, for very severe disease manifestations, larger doses (VHDGC) are usually required. Additionally, the latter regimen is probably more toxic, especially if followed for more than a few weeks (93) without appropriate dose tapering. The most effective approach to initiating HDGC or VHDGC for severe SLE disease, and especially when constitutional symptoms (i.e., high fever and prostration) are present, is to administer it in two to four doses per day (20,91,92,94). A notable exception is the management of severe focal or diffuse proliferative glomerulonephritis (FPGN or DPGN) where once-a-day regimens are adequate (96,97). Should the condition prove GC-unresponsive, use of pulse GC and/or additional immunosuppressive agents is necessary. Most disease complications will respond in less than 1 to 2 weeks. However, markers of lupus nephritis (especially proteinuria) may take 2 to 6 weeks to improve (94).

Within 1 to 2 weeks from initiation of therapy, whether a satisfactory response has occurred or a cytotoxic agent has been added to the regimen for refractory disease, tapering of GC therapy should be initiated, according to our opinion (20). The first step is to solidify the GC regimen into a once a day morning GC dose (20,92,94). The daily dose can then be decreased by 5 mg (or 5% to 10%) per week until a dose of 0.25 to 0.5 mg/kg/day is reached and more slowly thereafter, aiming for either a complete withdrawal or, if that is not possible, for LDGC. It may be preferable to follow an ADGC tapering regimen during which the second day's dose is usually first gradually decreased to zero, before decreases of other doses are made (94). Caution should be applied during tapering, as too fast or too slow dose decrements can lead to disease flare/withdrawal symptoms and increased GC toxicity respectively. In the event of a flare during the tapering, the dose is increased to the immediate previous effective level for a few weeks, before the next, perhaps slower, tapering attempt. Less severe SLE manifestations are managed with LDGC or moderate-dose GC (MDGC) accordingly (20,91,92,94,97). Table 56.3 provides an overview of the suggested GC use in SLE.

The importance of other immunosuppressive agents (such as cyclophosphamide, azathioprine, etc.) in helping control the disease while allowing safe tapering of GC (steroid-sparing activity) cannot be overemphasized. DPGN is the best studied SLE complication, and randomized controlled clinical studies have documented the supe-

TABLE 56.3. USUAL REGIMENS OF SYSTEMIC GLUCOCORTICOID THERAPY IN SLE

GC Regimen	Representative Indications	Common Adverse Effects (AE)
Pulse GC (PGC): MP 1 g (15–30 mg/kg)/d or 1 g/m^2 BSA, IV × 1–3 d, monthly as indicated; usually with oral GC (0.5–1 mg/kg/d PDN)	Life or organ-threatening complications (i.e., RPGN, myelopathy, severe acute confusional state, alveolar hemorrhage, vasculitis, optic neuritis)[a] HDGC-refractory disease DPGN or severe FPGN[b]	Same as with HDGC (see below), but overall incidence of AE may be lower, partly because they allow more rapid taper of oral GC doses Special considerations due to large dose and route of administration: fluid overload, hypertension, neuropsychiatric symptoms; *rarely: cardiac arrhythmias—sudden death, seizures, intractable hiccups, GC anaphylaxis*
Very high dose GC (VHDGC): ≥1–2 mg/kg/d PDN IV/PO (start with divided doses)	Life or organ-threatening complications (as for PGC)[a]	Same but more severe than with HDGC Psychosis Risk of severe-fatal infection may be particularly high (avoid use for more than 1–2 weeks)
High-dose GC (HDGC) 0.6–1 mg/kg/d PDN IV/PO Moderate-dose GC (MDGC) 0.125–0.5 mg/kg/d PDN PO	DPGN or severe FPGN (for less than 6–8 weeks)[b] Thrombocytopenia/hemolytic anemia Acute lupus pneumonitis "Lupus crisis"[c] Moderate SLE flares [i.e myositis, severe pleurisy, ophthalmoplegia (except optic neuritis), thrombocytopenia] With PGC, or CY/AZA for severe disease	Same AE for both HDGC and MDGC but incidence and severity are at lower levels with the latter HPA-axis suppression, Cushing's syndrome, hypertension, hypokalemia, hyperglycemia, hyperlipidemia, atherosclerosis, OPN, ON, risk of infection, skeletal growth retardation, glaucoma, cataracts, skin fragility, acne, insomnia, steroid psychosis, mood swings, etc.
Low-dose GC (LDGC) <0.125 mg/kg/d (<7.5 mg/d) PDN PO	Arthritis, mild constitutional symptoms (unresponsive to analgesics/NSAID/AM). Generalized LN Maintenance therapy	Least toxic daily regimen; cataracts, GC-withdrawal symptoms (upon tapering to or below LDGC), skeletal growth retardation can occur; probably minimal OP, ON, HPA-axis suppression
Alternate-Day GC (ADGC)	Membranous nephritis with nephrotic syndrome (2 mg/kg) During tapering GC dose Maintenance therapy (i.e., 0.25 mg/kg for GN)	Decreased adverse effects (i.e., HPA-axis suppression, skeletal growth retardation, infection, Cushing's syndrome) compared to daily regimens OP can occur

[a]Cyclophosphamide therapy, usually IV (IVCY), is often needed as well.
[b]In combination with IVCY.
[c]Lupus crisis refers to the acutely and severely ill patient with high fever, extreme prostration, and other symptoms of active SLE (i.e., pleurisy, arthritis, vasculitic rash), who requires large doses of GC for disease control. Infection has been excluded as the cause of the symptoms.
MP, methylprednisolone; BSA, body surface area; PDN, prednisone; RPGN, rapidly progressive glomerulonephritis; OP, osteoporosis; ON, osteonecrosis; LN, lymphadenopathy; CY, cyclophosphamide; AM, antimalarials; AZA, azathioprone.

riority of intravenous cyclophosphamide (IVCY)-containing regimens over those with GC alone (98–100). Not only is renal scarring prevented with cytotoxic therapy (101), but also a more effective GC tapering scheme can be achieved. Additionally, many observational studies, case series, and case reports favor the use of cyclophosphamide (mainly IV) in other life/organ-threatening SLE complications that may be refractory to GC alone [at appropriately high doses or pulse therapy (102–113)]. Severe NPSLE of nonthrombotic etiology [especially acute confusional state, myelopathy, optic neuritis (102–108)], pulmonary hemorrhage (110), interstitial pneumonitis (111), acute cardiomyopathy (112), and severe vasculitis of other systems such as the gastrointestinal (113) are such examples. In such grave cases, patients might benefit from simultaneous administration of GCs and other immunosuppressives (mainly IVCY) from the outset of the disease. For less severe disease manifestations such as arthritis, serositis, and mild constitutional symptoms, agents such as hydroxychloroquine, nonsteroidal antiinflammatory drugs (NSAIDs, analgesics, and local GCs (i.e., intraarticular) should be given priority, and systemic GCs used only if necessary and at the lowest effective dose (91,92,94). Dehydroepiandrosterone (DHEA), an adrenal androgen with immunomodulatory properties whose serum levels are low in SLE and further decrease with GC therapy, has shown some promise as a steroid-sparing agent for mild-moderate SLE and possibly a small beneficial effect when used in patients with severe SLE (114–117).

The above approach to GC use in SLE is based on the assumption that alternative noninflammatory or nonautoimmune diagnoses have been carefully excluded, before a patient is committed to prolonged immunosuppressive therapy. Infections hold the first priority and they can closely mimic many lupus complications, including acute confusional states, aseptic meningitis, lupus nephritis, lupus pneumonitis, arthritis, and GI vasculitis. Presentations of SLE patients with acute abdomen (AA) are a particularly challenging problem in management. Medina et al. (118) found that although vasculitis correlated with overall SLE disease activity (53% of 36 patients with active versus none of 15 with inactive SLE patients), common surgical diagnoses and primary abscesses (in immunosuppressed patients) were more common. Interestingly, three cases in the active group had abdominal thrombosis and high anticardiolipin titers. Only one patient with hepatic artery thrombosis survived after thrombectomy and 100 mg/d prednisone therapy. In the same study a delay in surgery for more than 48 hours (excluding the cases that had a complete response to HDGC) was associated with much higher mortality, especially in the active group. Once infection was ruled out, however, vasculitis responded to pulse GC (PGC) with or without IVCY (118).

In general, arterial or venous thrombosis without concomitant SLE activity [e.g., cardiovascular accident (CVA) secondary to the antiphospholipid syndrome] requires anticoagulation alone, and increases of GC dosage should be avoided (94,97,103). If thrombotic thrombocytopenic purpura (TTP) is diagnosed, plasma exchanges may be useful (97). Late complications of SLE (119), such as advanced atherosclerosis–coronary artery disease (CAD), scarring nephritis (with high chronicity and low activity indices on kidney biopsy), osteonecrosis, shrinking lung syndrome, and chronic dementia should discourage heroic interventions (93,94,97). Seizures or acute confusional states may not be secondary to SLE and in fact result from hypertension or metabolic/electrolyte abnormalities, whereas psychosis might result from GC therapy itself (93). The probability of these alternative diagnoses substantially increases when SLE activity in other systems is low. In such cases of isolated seizures or psychosis, conservative management (which may include anticonvulsant and psychotropic agents) along with careful monitoring is all that is usually required (93,94).

When managing certain SLE complications with GC, it is often prudent to aim for "reasonable" but not complete resolution of disease activity, since often the latter translates into higher and more toxic GC dosages. For example, asymptomatic hemolytic anemia or idiopathic thrombocytopenic purpura (ITP) with a hematocrit of more than 30% and 20,000 to 50,000 platelets (and no other coagulopathy) does not per se warrant increases of GC therapy (94,97). In more severe cases that invoke long-term HDGC therapy for adequate control, splenectomy or cytotoxic medicines should be considered (94,97).

Pulse Glucocorticoid Therapy

Pulse glucocorticoid (PGC) therapy, usually 1 g (or 1 g/m^2 of body surface area) of methylprednisolone (MP) IV per day for 3 days that may be repeated at monthly intervals, was first used in SLE to treat DPGN (96–98,100,120,121). PGCs are also effective for moderate-severe NPSLE (97, 103,104,106–108,122), pneumonitis (97), serositis (123), vasculitis (124,125), and thrombocytopenia (97,122). One study compared PGC to 100 mg of MP IV and found no difference (126). Another demonstrated an advantage of PGC over oral prednisone at 14 days but not at 28 days (127). It is generally felt that for very severe DPGN (or rapidly progressive glomerulonephritis; RPGN), PGCs work faster than standard oral HDGCs and probably permit both use of MDGCs (0.5 mg/kg/d) at therapy initiation and a faster taper of GC dose (100). However, two randomized controlled trials showed that PGC therapy (monthly for 6 months or for at least 1 year, respectively) was not as effective as an IVCY-containing regimen (monthly for 6 months and then quarterly) for proliferative lupus nephritis (98,100). The second study and especially another more recent National Institutes of Health (NIH) trial (128) that included 5 years of protocol therapy with IVCY, PGC, or both and an extended median follow-up of 124 months, have both suggested that the combination can lead to a better renal outcome than therapy with either agent alone. It appears that concurrent use of both agents offers a therapeutic advantage for severe SLE in general (104,110,129), possibly because of a synergistic effect between the two agents. PGC may have additional nongenomic immediate effects (35) that may allow for a faster and more effective action than conventional HDGC. On the other hand IVCY has better long-term effects on the scarring consequences of inflammation (101) and a very potent ability to suppress humoral immunity (129). Advocates of PGC therapy argue that this therapy may have fewer adverse effects than oral GC alone, partly because it allows a more rapid tapering of the latter. A small case-control study of the authors suggested that use of PGC was not associated with more osteoporosis/osteopenia than use of oral GC alone despite significantly larger cumulative (pulse and oral) GC doses in the first group (130). The cosmetogenic and diabetogenic effects of PGC may be less severe as well (121). However, complications such as glucocorticoid-induced osteonecrosis (GION; 100,131), major infections (100,121), and mood disorders/psychosis (132) can still occur. Seizures (133), dangerous cardiac arrhythmias (134) and anaphylaxis (100) have been rarely reported, as well, with this therapy.

Although MP appears to be the most frequently used GC agent for PGC therapy, megadoses of dexamethasone have also been very effective for the same indications, including severe NPSLE (135). Since there are no head-to-head studies comparing pulse dexamethasone and pulse MP, it is not clear whether there is an advantage to either therapy at equivalent doses. With regard to NPSLE management, both agents appear to be comparable in their capacity to penetrate CSF, based on their protein binding characteristics (see Pharmacokinetics and Drug Interactions, above). In cases of severe brain edema, where agents with low MC activities might be preferable, although both MP and dexamethasone are suitable, the latter might offer a slight advantage (Table 56.1).

Use Of Depot Glucocorticoid Agents

Depot preparations of GC are designed to have long-lasting effects (3 to 4 weeks) after a single intraarticular (IA) or intramuscular (IM) injection. Examples include MP acetate and triamcinolone hexacetonide. IM injections are used for their potent systemic effects and IA injections for their local action in the affected joint. However, even in the latter case, some systemic absorption and GC toxicity can occur (136). Use of IM depot GC can be considered on the rare occasion that parenteral use is desirable but IV access not immediately available. Interestingly, Dasgupta et al. (137), in a controlled trial for polymyalgia rheumatica, used regular 3-weekly (every 3 weeks) IM depot MP acetate injections in comparison with standard oral GC therapy. Adverse effects, especially fractures and weight gain, were less with the depot GC therapy, probably due to the lower cumulative GC dose in that arm of the study (137).

Glucocorticoid Use During Pregnancy And Lactation

Use of GC therapy during pregnancy is indicated primarily to treat active SLE in the mother and probably for incomplete heart block of neonatal lupus in the fetus. Since only fluorinated GCs (e.g., dexamethasone, betamethasone) are able to enter the fetal circulation in significant amounts, as they are only partially metabolized by the placental 11β-HSD_2 (138,139), nonfluorinated GCs (usually prednisone) are used for the first and fluorinated GCs for the latter indication. Saleeb et al. (140), in a recent retrospective study, have found that fluorinated GCs given to mothers with anti-Ro or anti-La antibodies at the time of echocardiographic detection of fetal congenital heart block (CHB), were able to at least prevent progression of second-degree blocks and reverse hydropic fetal changes. However, and of some concern, oligohydramnios was seen more frequently in the treatment than in the placebo group.

When treating the mother for active SLE, the lowest effective GC dose should be employed. Although development of cleft palate has been reported in animal studies with the use of GC (137,138,141), this fact probably carries no clinical significance and should not restrict use of GC when otherwise indicated (138). Other GC adverse effects on pregnancy outcomes include a high incidence of preterm deliveries, which are mainly due to premature ruptured membranes (142–145) and possibly fetal growth restriction (138). Gestational hypertension or diabetes mellitus (DM) (142,144,145) is not uncommon. Additionally, osteoporosis (138,146) and, probably less commonly, maternal cataracts (144), or GION can also occur (138). With regard to osteoporosis, the combination of GC and heparin may be particularly toxic to the bones, and vertebral fractures have been reported (146). Mothers treated with GC during pregnancy may need stress GC doses in the peripartum period, especially when there is prolonged labor/delivery or a C-section is required (138). Careful monitoring of the neonates born to these mothers for development of adrenal insufficiency is also recommended (138). To avoid disease flares that can lead to both disease and treatment complications, patients who are already on hydroxychloroquine should probably be kept on this (relatively safe) therapy during pregnancy (147–149). Additional immunosuppressive medications that may be safe during pregnancy, such as azathioprine, cyclosporin A, and IVIG, should be considered for moderate-severe SLE disease activity (138) and might help decrease GC doses.

Because of their unfavorable adverse effect profile, GCs have lost ground to the combination of heparin and aspirin in treating the pregnancy loss of the antiphospholipid syndrome (APLS) (142,143,145). Additionally, Laskin et al.

(144) found the combination of prednisone and aspirin of no benefit to the treatment of women with autoantibodies (including antiphospholipid antibodies) and recurrent fetal loss (144). However, GC may still have a place in the management of women with APLS secondary to SLE to treat thrombocytopenia or a concomitant SLE flare (145).

The use of prednisone/prednisolone at doses below 20 to 30 mg/day in breast-feeding mothers is probably safe as less than 10% of the active drug enters breast milk (138,139). It is prudent to wait 4 hours after GC intake before breast-feeding, especially when higher doses are necessary (138).

Use Of Glucocorticoids During Stress

Because of the high risk of HPA-axis suppression (see below), patients on chronic GC therapy should be given supplemental GCs during the stress of surgery or moderate-severe illness. Traditional recommendations called for 100 mg of a water-soluble form of hydrocortisone (i.e., sodium succinate) IV every 8 hours, tapered as the patient recovers. However, more recent data have shown that individuals with intact adrenal function rarely generate more than 150 to 200 mg of cortisol even during major surgery (5,150). Based on this information, more recent recommendations argue that 25 mg of hydrocortisone (or its equivalent) should be given daily for 1 to 3 days during minor stress, whereas for moderate and severe stress 50 to 75 mg and 100 to 150 mg, respectively, daily for 1 to 3 days should be given (5,151). Another argument in favor of this approach may be that unnecessarily high GC doses that might interfere with wound healing and increase the risk of infection are avoided (5,151). Glucocorticoid agents with less mineralocorticoid activity than hydrocortisone would be preferable when dealing with fluid-overload states (e.g., in a lupus nephritis patient).

ADVERSE EFFECTS OF GLUCOCORTICOIDS

Both clinicians and patients should be fully aware that adverse effects (AEs) of GC therapy are not uncommon and can in fact be very serious. Although brief courses of high-dose GC therapy (e.g., for bronchial asthma) are probably well tolerated and AEs (e.g., Cushing's syndrome, glucose intolerance HPA-axis suppression), if they occur, are rapidly reversible (72), more prolonged therapy, as is usually the case with SLE patients, invariably leads to complications. Of note, some AEs (e.g., skeletal growth inhibition, HPA-axis suppression, GION, cataracts) occur even with LDGC, and others usually require larger doses of GC before they occur (e.g., infection, psychosis, myopathy, hyperlipidemia). Since susceptibility to GC AEs may vary from person to person, according to individual pharmacokinetic differences, Sarna et al. (90), in order to minimize AEs, have suggested the use of specific GC exposure indices (instead of the absolute or cumulative GC doses) in guiding GC dosing of children with transplants (90). Comorbid conditions and risk factors that may predispose to more severe GC AEs (e.g., hyperlipidemia, hypertension, hyperglycemia-DM, hypokalemia, osteoporosis, personal or family history of cataract or glaucoma, prior exposure to tuberculosis) should be identified prior to institution of GC therapy. Patients and their families should be educated to recognize and promptly report symptoms of such complications as infection (e.g., fever), diabetes, psychosis, and osteonecrosis (joint pain). In parallel, careful clinical and laboratory monitoring for the development of osteoporosis, DM, hyperlipidemia, hypertension, glaucoma, etc., should not be neglected (2). Interventions known to prevent or ameliorate GC AE (summarized in Table 56.4) should be undertaken (2). This is particularly true for GIOP, infection susceptibility, myopathy, and atherosclerosis (see below). Reversal of some AEs (e.g., HPA-axis suppression, Cushing's syndrome, and psychosis) can be achieved with cessation of GC therapy, or at least modification into the safer ADGC or LDGC regimens. Unfortunately, some AEs, like cataract formation, GION, osteoporotic fractures, growth retardation in children, and atherosclerotic vascular events, are irreversible (152).

Iatrogenic Cushing's syndrome (with the typical centripetal body fat redistribution), a characteristic feature of GC excess, can occur in a period of less than 1 month during HDGC therapy (4). It differs from the native Cushing's syndrome in that there is less androgen excess (androgens are suppressed by GC excess) and less hypertension (4). On the other hand, GION, posterior subcapsular cataracts, glaucoma, pseudotumor cerebri, and pancreatitis are more commonly seen.

Chronic Suppression of the Hypothalamic-Pituitary-Adrenal Axis

Suppression of the HPA-axis after chronic exposure to moderate-high doses of GC begins from suppression of corticotropin-releasing hormone (CRH) and ACTH and eventually leads to atrophy of adrenal zones fasciculate and reticularis, the principal cortisol-producing structures (secondary adrenal failure). Exposure to GCs for periods of less than 2 to 3 weeks or for longer periods to low-dose GC (<10 mg/d of prednisone, as long as it is not taken as a single bedtime dose) are considered safe and do not lead to clinically significant adrenal insufficiency (4,72). On the other hand, patients exposed to any doses of >20 mg/d for more than 3 weeks should be considered as having HPA-axis suppression (4,72). These patients need proper GC supplementation during surgical procedures or illnesses. Recovery from suppression varies depending on the intensity of GC exposure but usually lasts from 6 to 9 months and is gradual. CRH secretion recovers first, followed by ACTH, and lastly by cortisol secretion. Additionally, adrenal responsiveness to

TABLE 56.4. SUGGESTED MONITORING AND PREVENTIVE-THERAPEUTIC INTERVENTIONS FOR SELECTED GC ADVERSE EFFECTS[a]

AE	Assess and monitor for	Intervention
HPA-axis suppression	Symptoms of adrenal insufficiency during significant stress (illness or surgery)	Choose low risk GC regimens (LDGC, ADGC) when possible Medical alert bracelet; stress-doses of GC perioperatively or during severe illness
Osteoporosis	BMD at baseline and q12 months thereafter if bisphosphonates are not given (for high risk patients more aggressive monitoring is probably necessary)	Smoking/ETOH cessation; exercise; low salt diet; calcium (1,500 mg/d) and vitamin D (400–800 IU/d); HRT[b]; *bisphosphonates* for high-risk patients (i.e., those starting on >15–20 mg/day of prednisone for more than 2 months, especially if with additional OP risk factors), established OP, or significant bone loss during GC therapy
Osteonecrosis	Unexplained joint/bone pain (perform MRI to detect early GION if plain radiography not revealing)	Avoidance of weight bearing and joint-salvage surgery (core decompression, osteotomy, nonvascularized or vascularized bone grafting) may arrest progression of early ON to bone collapse
Cardiovascular[c] Lipidemia Hypertension Hyperglycemia Obesity	Baseline fasting serum lipid profile (TC, HDL-C, LDL-C, TG) and then yearly TC; symptoms of polyuria, polydipsia; after baseline serum glucose, urinary glucose tests q3–6 months; baseline serum potassium; BP at baseline and every visit; edema, shortness of breath	Diet (to control one or all of hyperlipidemia, hyperglycemia, and hypertension, accordingly) Aerobic exercise Antimalarial therapy (cholesterol-lowering and anticoagulant properties) Lipid-lowering and/or antihypertensive agents, if previous measures not adequate Folate, and vitamins B_6, B_{12}, for elevated homocysteine levels
Infection	Fever; severe lymphopenia[d]; PPD skin test; varicella immune status (before initiation of GC therapy)	Vaccinations for influenza, pneumococcus, tetanus Antituberculosis therapy, if PPD+, or evidence for TB exposure PCP prophylaxis,[e] avoid contact with children vaccinated with OPV[e]
Muscle	Proximal muscle weakness	Muscle strengthening exercises
Psychiatric	Symptoms of depression, psychosis	Antipsychotics as an adjunct therapy to GC dose lowering or cessation
Eye	Visual changes	Decrease/cessation of GC dose (for glaucoma)
PUD	Record other PUD risk factors (NSAIDs, comorbidities)	Gastroprotection (H2-blockers, proton-pump inhibitors, misoprotol)

[a]In general, if GC cessation is not feasible, tapering to LDGC or modification to an ADGC regimen is the safest intervention for most GC adverse effects.
[b]If not contraindicated (i.e., thrombophilia).
[c]APLA, homocysteine, and SLE activity are GC-unrelated but significant cardiovascular risk factors in SLE patients.
[d]Usually when lymphocytes <350/mm^3, but PCP can occur with higher numbers.
[e]For severely immunosuppressed SLE patients (i.e., therapy with GC doses ≥ 20 mg/d of prednisone plus other immunosuppressive agents and/or significant lymphopenia).
BMD, bone mineral density; TC, total cholesterol; HDL-C, high-density lipoprotein cholesterol; TG, triglycerides; BP, blood pressure; PPD, purified protein derivative; TB, tuberculosis; PCP, *Pneumocystis carinii* pneumonia; OPV, oral polio virus; PUD, peptic ulcer disease.

stress normalizes much later than the baseline adrenal cortisol secretion. Patients should be informed about the potential dangers of this important problem, advised not to abruptly discontinue their GCs unless authorized by their physician, and wear medical alert bracelets (4,72). GC withdrawal should start by tapering GC dose to physiologic levels (20 mg of hydrocortisone or 5 mg of prednisone in a single morning dose). Morning serum cortisol levels are measured and only when they are more than 10 μg/dL can the maintenance dose be discontinued. However, these patients may still have abnormal cortisol responses to stress, and coverage should be given when necessary. Next, an acute ACTH test is performed. If 30- or 60-minute cortisol serum levels, after IM, IV, or subcutaneous (SC) injection of 250 μg of cosyntropin (synthetic $ACTH_{1-24}$), are more than 20 μg/dL, adrenal insufficiency is unlikely and stress GC supplementation is no longer necessary. However, exceptions can occur, and if there is any clinical suspicion of adrenal insufficiency (e.g., hypotension after surgery), GC coverage should be given (4,72).

Bone Toxicity

Glucocorticoid-induced osteoporosis (GIOP) and osteonecrosis (GION) are frequent adverse effects of GC and contribute substantially to the morbidity associated with these agents. Recent advances in bone biology have shown that osteoblasts and osteoclasts are both derived from bone marrow precursors and that osteoblastogenesis is a prerequisite for osteoclastogenesis (153). The link is provided by osteoprotegerin ligand (OPGL, also known as ODF, or TRANCE, or RANKL), a member of the TNF-α family of proteins, which is expressed on committed preosteoblastic cells and mediates osteoclast differentiation and activation (153,154). The main histologic findings in GIOP are decreased bone formation rate, decreased wall thickness of trabeculae, a strong indication of decreased osteoblastic work output, and *in situ* death of portions of bone (153). Weinstein et al. (155), by studying a mouse model of GIOP, found that there was an early (7 days after exposure to GC) increase in osteoclast perimeter and bone resorption, an effect that might have been due to OPGL induction by GC (156). On the other hand, chronic GC exposure (27 days) led to decreases in bone turnover and bone formation, probably explained by inhibited osteoclastogenesis and osteoblastogenesis, respectively. Osteoblast function was further compromised as these cells underwent increased GC-induced apoptosis (155). Additionally, the augmented osteocyte apoptosis observed was proposed by the authors as a potential mechanism for GC-induced osteonecrosis as osteocytes are critical in sensing microdamage and regulate bone remodeling accordingly (153). Dysregulation of calcium balance (decreased intestinal absorption and increased urinary excretion), gonadal hormone repression, myopathy, and in SLE downmodulation of DHEA sulfate (DHEAS) are other proposed mechanisms of GIOP (157–160).

Glucocorticoid-induced osteoporosis predominantly affects cancellous bone and the axial skeleton. During the first 3 to 6 months of GC therapy there is a rapid bone loss (up to 12%), which slows down thereafter to 2% to 5% annually (153). SLE patients may have additional risk factors for osteoporosis such as use of sunscreens (inadequate vitamin D formation), inability to exercise due to musculoskeletal inflammation or fatigue, hormonal changes (including premature ovarian failure due to cyclophosphamide therapy), kidney damage, or medications known to induce osteoporosis (heparin, anticonvulsants, cyclosporine) (157). Additionally, the disease itself could theoretically cause bone loss given the recent evidence that activated T cells express functionally active OPGL (161).

Careful evaluation of SLE patients before and after initiation of GC therapy should be performed to identify other potentially modifiable osteoporosis (OP) risk factors and guide further management. Specifically, baseline and every 6 to 12 months thereafter, evaluation of bone mineral density (BMD) is essential to assess bone loss. Markers of bone formation and bone resorption might offer additional help in assessing the effectiveness of current OP-preventive measures. Serum levels of 25-hydroxyvitamin D, luteinizing hormone (LH) (for females), and gonadal hormones can be measured if indicated to help identify potential targets of intervention. General measures for OP prevention including a well-balanced, low-salt diet, and avoidance of alcohol and smoking, and weight-bearing muscle-strengthening exercises should be encouraged. A short-acting GC at the lowest effective dose should be preferentially used, although doses as low as 6 mg of prednisolone per day, on average, may lead to spinal bone loss (162). Unfortunately, alternate-day therapy does not seem to protect from GIOP (157). As a first step to GIOP prevention, calcium and vitamin D intake should be optimized and 1,500 mg/day (by diet or supplements) and 400 to 800 IU/day, respectively, should be taken. Use of pharmacologic doses of vitamin D are discouraged except in the case of documented vitamin D deficiency (163). Active vitamin D metabolites, like calcitriol, have been shown to preserve bone during GC therapy (164), but the relatively high risk for hypercalcemia/hypercalciuria (158) and its potential association with soft tissue calcifications in SLE patients with lupus nephritis (165) make their use less desirable. Thiazide diuretics (with potassium supplementation) might be useful in the case of hypercalciuria (157).

Hormone replacement therapy (HRT) should be instituted in all postmenopausal women, and documented hypogonadism in men and premenopausal women, if there are no contraindications (158,166,167). In SLE patients, estrogen therapy might theoretically induce flares of the disease. However, they appear to be safe, as long as disease (especially nephritis) is not active during initiation of therapy and there is no thrombophilia (168). It is hoped that ongoing studies will answer this question in the near future. Another hormone, DHEA, has recently shown a promising bone sparing effect in SLE patients treated with HDGC (117).

The best evidence regarding effective prevention and treatment of GIOP exists for bisphosphonates, especially during initiation of GC therapy when bone loss is the worse (169–171). While there is some concern with prolonged use of these agents in young individuals, due to their long-term retention in bones (158), this should not discourage physicians from using them when clearly indicated in young SLE patients (e.g., those on HDGC at high risk for, or already with, OP). However, bisphosphonates should not be used in pregnancy or moderate-severe renal failure, and their discontinuation should be considered when GC doses have been substantially tapered with stabilization of BMD. Calcitonin has been recommended for GIOP, but it does not seem as effective (158,163,172). If the above measures fail, bone anabolic agents such as low doses of slow-release sodium fluoride could be cautiously used (159). Other promising therapies for GIOP have, in the meantime, emerged. Specifically, daily SC injections of human parathyroid hormone 1-34 [hPTH (1-34)] in postmenopausal women who also received HRT and calcium supplementation reversed GIOP in the lumbar spine, while control therapy with HRT and calcium alone did not (173). Statins have also shown promise, as they appear to have bone anabolic activity (174), can block GIOP and

GION (175,176), and their use has been associated with lower rates of fractures in preliminary human studies (177,178). Finally, synthetic GCs with dissociated transactivating and transrepressing activities (14,15) have been proposed as potentially bone-sparing GC agents (153).

The pathogenesis of GION remains largely unknown. Proposed mechanisms include blood vessel occlusion by external compression (fat accumulation in the bone marrow), or intravascular flow obstruction by thrombosis or fat embolism (179,180). Apoptotic death of osteocytes, which are considered as mechanosensors and initiators of repair in bone, has been recently proposed as a mechanism of femoral head collapse in the context of GC therapy (153). Pathologically, GION is characterized by empty lacunae in trabeculae and bone marrow necrosis, and later by repair processes such as vascular granulation tissue and appositional (on the dead bone) new bone formation (179). Although pure medullary infarcts are asymptomatic, corticocancellous osteonecrosis can lead to pain and joint destruction depending on the extent and location of lesions (179,180). Symptoms usually take a few months to a few years to develop after GC exposure (179,181,182). Typical sites of involvement include the subchondral regions of convex bone ends such as the proximal and distal femur, and the proximal humerus.

The risk of GION increases with both the dose and duration of GC therapy. However, even GC regimens of short-term high doses (183), adrenal insufficiency replacement doses (184), and intraarticular injections (185) have been implicated. In SLE patients, the reported prevalence of osteonecrosis has varied from 5% to 50% (186–191) with magnitude of GC exposure being the major risk factor (187–191). Interestingly, clinically occult osteonecrosis was noted in 12% of SLE patients, according to one study, and did not progress after 1 year of follow-up (192). Predicting which patients will develop GION is very difficult. Presence of Cushing's syndrome features was shown significant in many studies (188–190), but inconsistent results exist for the presence of antiphospholipid antibodies (186,188,189). Patients should be informed about this potentially very serious GC complication, which often occurs when SLE disease activity is under control, educated how to recognize GION symptoms (e.g., groin pain upon weight bearing), and instructed to avoid high-impact activities (179,180,191). When hip GION is at an early stage, relief of weight bearing is recommended (179,180,191). For this purpose, Simkin and Gardner (180) have suggested the use of crutches with a four-point walking pattern to avoid excessive load on the opposite (at risk) hip. Operative management of precollapse lesions includes core decompression, osteotomy, and nonvascularized and vascularized bone grafts (179,180,191). Advanced disease (stages III to IV by plain radiography according to the Ficat staging system) often requires total joint replacement therapy (179,180,191). Interference with potential key mechanisms of GION such as fat accumulation (i.e., by statins), intraosseous hypertension (i.e., vasodilators), coagulation (i.e., stanozolol), or osteocyte apoptosis (i.e., PTH) may offer additional hope in managing this disease in the near future (153,176,191).

Effects On Intermediary Metabolism: Abnormalities In The Metabolism Of Glucose, Lipids, And Protein

Glucocorticoids induce insulin synthesis but oppose its effects on glucose metabolism predisposing to or aggravating (if already present) diabetes mellitus (DM). These effects of GC are mediated mainly through decreased peripheral utilization of glucose and induction of gluconeogenesis in the liver. The latter is in part due to the increased substrate availability for gluconeogenesis as a result of the GC enhancing effects on lipolysis and protein catabolism (3,4). The hyperglycemic effects of GC may be of particular importance in SLE, a disease with an increased prevalence of DM (6% to 8%) (193–195) and perhaps an increased frequency of the prediabetic insulin resistance syndrome (196).

Dyslipoproteinemias with elevated serum levels of triglycerides (TGs), very low density lipoprotein cholesterol (VLDL-C), and decreased levels of HDL-C and apoprotein A-I can occur in active SLE even before GC treatment (197,198). Nephrosis, when present, is an additional aggravating factor for hyperlipidemia. GCs have an important impact on lipid metabolism themselves as they act permissively to enhance the lipolytic effect of catecholamines and growth hormone (GH) and induce a centripetal body fat redistribution (4). GC can also induce cholesteryl ester synthesis by macrophages *in vitro*, an effect that could be blocked by progesterone (199). Ettinger and Hazzard (200) have shown that administration of 0.35 mg/kg/d of prednisone for 14 days in healthy men increased their levels of VLDL-C, HDL-C, and TGs. In SLE, increases of TC, VLDL-C, LDL-C (197,201), and TGs (197,202) have been noted, and only prednisone doses of >10 mg/d had significant hyperlipidemic effects (195,202). Moreover, Petri et al. (203) have found that an increase in the prednisone dose by 10 mg daily was associated with a 7.5 mg/dL increase in cholesterol levels. Interestingly, antimalarial therapy can counteract this GC effect and decrease cholesterol (203,204).

Despite inducing weight gain as a result of their appetite enhancing effects (203), GCs favor protein breakdown and lead to steroid myopathy and poor wound healing (see below).

Cardiovascular Effects

Hypertension due to GCs occurs at high doses. This is partly due to the permissive effects of GCs on the action of vasoactive substances [angiotensin II (ATII), catecholamines] on the vessel wall and myocardium that result in increased systemic vascular resistance (SVR) and increased cardiac contractility (3,4). Inhibition of prostaglandin E_2 (PGE_2) and kallikrein synthesis by GCs also contributes to their adverse effects on blood pressure (BP). When 11β-HSD_2 functions normally, GC mineralocorticoid effects on BP are unlikely, except perhaps in very high doses of cortisol. In the Hopkins Lupus Cohort, increases of prednisone doses by 10 mg were associated with BP increases of 1.1 mm Hg (203).

Urowitz et al. (205) in 1976 reported the occurrence of accelerated atherosclerosis in premenopausal women with SLE. The prevalence of clinical atherosclerosis manifesting with angina, myocardial infarction, or peripheral vascular disease has been estimated to be 7% to 10% (194, 195,206,207). Subclinical atherosclerosis is even higher (35% to 40%) according to recent studies (208,209). Disease activity of SLE itself is considered at least in part responsible for hyperlipidemia (197,198), and atherosclerosis (208) a process that is now considered inflammatory with evidence of immune activation (210). Experimental evidence that immune complexes (in association with high-cholesterol diet) can induce atherogenesis in rabbits (211) and that lupus sera are capable of accelerating cholesterol uptake by human aortic smooth muscle cells (212) may offer additional support to a pathogenetic association of SLE and atherosclerosis. Along these lines, Rahman et al. (213), in a comparison study of patients with accelerated atherosclerosis with and without SLE, found one less traditional risk factor in patients with SLE, which led the authors to suggest that SLE itself be considered a cardiovascular risk factor, similarly to DM. Importantly, duration of GC therapy was found to be an independent risk factor for development of CAD in SLE (194,195,214), along with older age at diagnosis of SLE, hypercholesterolemia (193–195), and other cardiovascular risk factors including hypertension, obesity (195,208), elevated homocysteine (214), and even antiphospholipid antibodies (198,200,214) and C-reactive protein (CRP) (208). The potential of GCs to aggravate SLE-atherosclerosis, based at least on their adverse effects on serum lipids and BP, cannot be overemphasized, and every attempt should be made to keep their doses at levels below the equivalent of 10 mg of prednisone daily. Moreover, activity of the disease should be adequately controlled, and other cardiovascular risk factors (including homocysteine levels) identified and properly addressed. If dietary measures and antimalarial therapy are not enough to control hyperlipidemia, lipid-lowering agents should be added to the therapeutic regimen.

Neuropsychiatric Adverse Effects

Central nervous system (CNS) GC effects are relatively common. Mood changes are probably the commonest, occurring in half the patients (4). Depression more commonly or euphoria can occur. Additionally, cognitive dysfunction and decreased duration of REM sleep can be seen (4). Rarely and especially with high GC doses, manic behavior, psychosis, or seizures can supervene during therapy, and need differentiation from primary NPSLE (93,132,215). The distinction can be difficult, but the temporal relationship to increases in GC dose, along with lack of focal neurologic signs or CSF abnormalities, suggests the correct diagnosis. Discontinuation or reduction of GC therapy along with phenothiazine suffices to reverse GC-induced psychosis (215). Benign intracranial hypertension (pseudotumor cerebri) occurs only rarely.

Infection

Glucocorticoids predispose to infection and at the same time may mask clinical clues of infection as a result of their immunosuppressive and antiinflammatory effects. On the other hand, reduction of inflammation is probably responsible for the improved outcomes observed when *Pneumocystis carinii* pneumonia (PCP) and *Haemophilus influenzae* meningitis are treated with adjunctive high-dose GC therapy (216,217). The incidence of infection after GC therapy was examined in a meta-analysis by Stuck et al. (218), and was found to be 12.7% (1.6-fold that of the control population). In the same study, patients treated with less than 10 mg of prednisone daily, or a cumulative dose of less than 700 mg, were spared from a higher risk to infection. Besides increasing the incidence of bacterial infections, GC can reactivate latent tuberculosis (TB) or histoplasmosis and predispose to an accelerated form of herpetic keratitis that culminates in blindness (4). Active SLE, by itself, increases the risk of bacterial (219–221), and, more rarely, opportunistic infections (222), probably as a result of several immune system perturbations (reviewed in ref. 223). Therapy with GC further augments the susceptibility of SLE patients to infection (152,219,221,222,224). Interestingly, in one study treatment with GC and cyclophosphamide improved survival but at the same time was associated with sepsis as a cause of death (224). Sepsis has been frequently cited as the first cause of death in SLE patients, being responsible for 19% to 54% of all deaths (152,205,219,221,223,224).

With regard to opportunistic infections, GC at relatively high doses (on average 40 mg or more of prednisone daily) can increase the risk of PCP, especially when combined with other immunosuppressive agents and/or coexistent peripheral lymphopenia (222,225,226). Prophylaxis for PCP should be considered in such patients. Since use of trimethoptim-sulfamethoxazole may be of concern in SLE, alternative prophylaxis regimens should be tried (e.g., dapsone 100 mg/d) (227). Additionally, PPD skin testing will help identify patients exposed to TB who will be candidates for antituberculosis prophylaxis. Notably, for patients on GC doses equivalent to ≥ 15 mg/d of prednisone for 1 month or more, a PPD skin reaction ≥ 5mm of induration is considered positive and warrants preventive therapy (227a). Immunizations with *H. influenzae* type B, tetanus toxoid, and pneumococcal vaccines were found safe and able to induce protective antibody titers in SLE patients (228). However, a trend toward lower protective antibody titers was noted for patients on immunosuppressive agents, perhaps suggesting that immunizations should best be done before initiation of such therapy. Vaccinations for influenza (killed vaccines), pneumococcus, and tetanus (component protein or peptide vaccine) are therefore highly recommended for SLE patients. In contrast, vaccinations with live attenuated viruses such as oral polio, varicella, and measles-mumps-rubella (MMR) should be avoided in immunosuppressed patients as they may lead to disease (227). Notably even contact with children vaccinated with oral polio vaccine (but not MMR) is risky (227).

Steroid Myopathy

Glucocorticoids have permissive actions necessary for normal function of skeletal muscle. However, exposure to fluorinated GC or large daily doses [>30 mg of prednisone (229)] of nonfluorinated GC administered for more than a few weeks [and in one study of cancer patients, within 15 days (230)] can cause a proximal myopathy characterized primarily by atrophy of type IIB muscle fibers (72,91, 229–232). Usually the pelvic girdle muscles (231) are more severely affected, and sometimes respiratory muscle weakness can occur (232). Although muscle enzymes are usually normal, urine creatine (231) and serum lactic dehydrogenase (LDH) (in SLE) might be elevated (232). Exercise (both resistance and endurance) is effective in attenuating GC-induced muscle atrophy (233).

The rare syndrome of acute myopathy of intensive care can occur in critically ill patients treated with high-dose IV GCs and neuromuscular junction–blocking agents (234). These patients develop a severe quadriplegia characterized by impaired muscle membrane excitability and a necrotizing myopathy with loss of thick filaments on muscle histopathology (234–236).

Skeletal Growth Retardation

Children treated with GCs, especially during their prepubertal years, display delayed skeletal maturation and growth (91,237–239). Even regimens considered to be relatively safe, such as LDGC, ADGC, and inhaled or intranasal therapy, have been implicated in growth retardation (239–241), which, of interest, has been observed in one study without concomitant HPA-axis suppression [as assessed by morning serum cortisol levels and standard cosyntropin testing (241)]. Among children treated with ADGC for cystic fibrosis, persistent growth impairment was observed only in boys (but not girls) after cessation of therapy (239). Mechanisms of GC AEs on skeletal growth may include inhibition of chondrocyte insulin-like growth factor-I (IGF-I) production, GH- and IGF-I–receptor expression, GH secretion, collagen type I synthesis, and upregulation of collagenase-3 expression (242,243). GC-treated children respond to GH therapy with increased growth velocity but responsiveness is not optimal and correlates negatively with GC dose (238,242).

Other AEs

Effects of GC on protein catabolism, fibroblast function, and collagen metabolism are probably responsible for suppression of wound healing processes and skin atrophy-purpura. Notably, chronic steroid therapy in SLE patients has been associated with tendon ruptures (244).

Posterior subcapsular cataract formation is not uncommon with systemic, topical, or inhaled GC use, and children may be more susceptible to this complication. Open-angle glaucoma may occur rapidly with topical ocular administration, but may take years before it occurs with systemic GC therapy. Glaucoma, in contrast to cataracts, often resolves with GC discontinuation. Regular ophthalmologic follow-up for both potential AEs is required (245).

There is probably no association between GC use and development of peptic ulcer disease (PUD) or its complications (246). However, concomitant use of NSAIDs confers a higher risk of PUD (247), and the same is probably true when other comorbid conditions [e.g., congestive heart failure (CHF), renal failure, old age] are present (152).

Hypersensitivity reactions and severe anaphylaxis to GC can rarely occur. Intravenous, intraarticular, soft tissue, and intradermal injections have been usually implicated, but association with topical and oral GC use has also been reported (248–250). Asthmatics with atopy may be more susceptible to this complication (248). It has been suggested that injectable epinephrine and diphenhydramine be readily available in rheumatology offices, in case anaphylaxis to GC injections occurs (250).

GLUCOCORTICOID WITHDRAWAL SYNDROME

Symptoms upon withdrawal of GC can be due to either SLE reactivation or adrenal insufficiency. The latter usually occurs with attempts to taper GC below physiologic levels (i.e., 5 to 7.5 mg of prednisone) and consists of anorexia, nausea, weight loss, arthralgias, myalgias, lethargy, weakness, and mild orthostatic hypotension-tachycardia. These symptoms can rarely occur even with normal adrenal function, as defined by normal morning cortisol levels and a normal ACTH stimulation test, and in that case may be due to GC resistance from prolonged LDGC use (4,72).

FUTURE DIRECTIONS

After half a century of continuous GC use in clinical practice, important advances have been made regarding both mechanisms of GC action and the rational usage of these agents for the benefit of our patients. However, much more research and progress is still needed in this field. First, developing new and safer GC agents is of utmost importance. In this direction some progress has already been made with the emergence of the "dissociated" GCs. Yet their alleged improved safety profile over conventional GCs remains to be proven. Second, understanding the pathogenesis of GC-induced adverse effects will help develop more effective interventions for their prevention or treatment. Along these lines, for example, the osteocyte antiapoptotic activity of PTH might explain its promising effects in GIOP (and perhaps GION). Promise with regard to GIOP and GION has been shown recently also for the statins. Blocking OPGL might be another approach to the management of GIOP. Finally, successful research into the mechanisms for GC resistance might help predict effective GC doses before therapy initiation and at the same time allow for design of new therapeutic interventions that will aim to decrease GC resistance. Usage of biologic cytokine inhibitors to downregulate the proinflammatory transcription factors AP-1 or NF-κB that are mutually antagonistic with GR might be one such approach. The design of these therapies for SLE patients should also, however, take into account parallel advances in our understanding of the pathogenesis of this disease.

ACKNOWLEDGMENT

The authors would like to thank Peggy Crow for useful discussion.

REFERENCES

1. Hench PS, Kedall EC, Slocumb CB, et al. Effect of hormone of adrenal cortex (17-hydroxy 11-dehydrocorticosterone: compound E) and of pituitary adrenocorticotrophic hormone on rheumatoid arthritis: preliminary report. *Proc Mayo Clin* 1949; 13:181–187.
2. Anonymous. Guidelines for referral and management of systemic lupus erythematosus in adults. American College of Rheumatology Ad Hoc Committee on Systemic Lupus Erythematosus Guidelines. *Arthritis Rheum* 1999;42:1785–1796.
3. Schimmer BP, Parker KL. Adrenocorticotropic hormone; adrenocortical steroids and their synthetic analogs; inhibitors of the synthesis and actions of adrenocortical hormones. In: Hardman JE, Limbird LE, Molinoff PB, et al., eds. *Goodman and Gilman's the pharmacological basis of therapeutics*, 9th ed. New York: McGraw-Hill, 1996:1459–1485.
4. Orth DN, Kovacs WJ. The adrenal cortex. In: Wilson JD, Foster DW, Kronenberg HM, et al., eds. *Williams' textbook of endocrinology*, 9th ed. Philadelphia: WB Saunders, 1998:517–664.
5. Lamberts SWJ, Bruining HA, de Jong FH. Corticosteroid therapy in severe illness. *N Engl J Med* 1997;337:1285–1292.
6. Jurney TH, Cockrell JL, Lindberg JS, et al. Spectrum of serum cortisol response to ACTH in ICU patients. Correlation with degree of illness and mortality. *Chest* 1987;92:292–295.
7. Sapolsky RM, Romero LM, Munck AU. How do glucocorticoids influence stress responses? Integrating permissive, suppressive, stimulatory, and preparative actions. *Endocr Rev* 2000; 21:55–89.
8. Chrousos GP. The hypothalamic-pituitary-adrenal axis and immune-mediated inflammation. *N Engl J Med* 1995;332: 1351–1362.
9. Wilckens T, Derijk R. Glucocorticoids and immune functions: physiological relevance and potential of hormone dysfunction. *Trends Pharmacol Sci* 1995;16:193–197.
10. Wilckens T, Derijk R. Glucocorticoids and immune functions: unknown dimensions and new frontiers. *Immunol Today* 1997; 18:418–424.
11. Anonymous. Deflazacort—an alternative to prednisolone? *Drug Ther Bull* 1999;37:57–58
12. Lipuner K, Casez JP, Horber FF, et al. Effects of deflazacort versus prednisone on bone mass, body composition, and lipid profile: A randomized, double blind study in kidney transplant patients. *J Clin Endocrinol Metab* 1998;83:3795–3802.
13. Barcelona JAS, Martin MC, Lopez VN, et al. An open comparison of the diabetogenic effect of deflazacort and prednisone at a dosage ratio of 1.5 mg:1 mg. *Eur J Clin Pharmacol* 1999;55: 105–109.
14. Vayssiere BM, Dupont S, Choquart A, et al. Synthetic glucocorticoids that dissociate transactivation and AP-1 transrepression exhibit antiinflammatory activity in vivo. *Mol Endocrinol* 1997;11:1245–1255.
15. Berghe WM, Francesconi E, De Bosscher K, et al. Dissociated glucocorticoids with antiinflammatory potential repress interleukin-6 gene expression by a nuclear factor-κB-dependent mechanism. *Mol Pharmacol* 1999;56:797–806.
16. Greenberg GR, Feagan BG, Martin F, et al. Oral budesonide for active Crohn's disease. *N Engl J Med* 1994;331:836–841.
17. Rutgeerts P, Lofberg R, Malchow H, et al. A comparison of budesonide with prednisolone for active Crohn's disease. *N Engl J Med* 1994;331:842–845.
18. Buttgereit F, Burmester GR, Brand MD. Bioenergetics of immune functions: fundamental and therapeutic actions. *Immunol Today* 2000;21:192–199.
19. Boumpas DT, Paliogianni F, Anastassiou ED, et al. Glucocorticosteroid action on the immune system: molecular and cellular aspects. *Clin Exp Rheumatol* 1991;9:413–423.
20. Boumpas DT, Chrousos GP, Wilder RL, et al. Glucocorticoid therapy for immune-mediated diseases: basic and clinical correlates. *Ann Intern Med* 1993;119:1198–1208.
21. Paliogianni F, Boumpas DT. Molecular and cellular aspects of cytokine regulation by glucocorticoids. In: Goulding NJ, Flower RJ, eds. *Glucocorticoids—milestones in drug therapy*. Basel: Birkhauser, 2001:81–104.
22. Crow MK. Mechanisms of glucocorticoid action on the immune system and in inflammation. In: Andrew L, Paget S, eds. *Principles of corticosteroid therapy*. London: Edward Arnold Limited, 2002:*in press*.
23. Flower RJ, Blackwell GJ. Anti-inflammatory steroids induce biosynthesis of a phospholipase A2 inhibitor which prevents prostaglandin generation. *Nature*, 1979;278:456–459.
24. Stromstedt PE, Poellinger L, Gustafsson JA, et al. The glucocorticoid receptor binds to a sequence overlapping the TATA box of the human osteocalcin promoter: a potential mechanism for negative regulation. *Mol Cell Biol* 1991;11:3379–3383.
25. Paliogianni F, Raptis A, Ahuja SS, et al. Negative transcriptional regulation of human interleukin 2 (1L-2) gene by glucocorticoids through interference with nuclear transcription factors AP-1 and NF-AT. *J Clin Invest* 1991;91:1481–1489.
26. Jonat C, Rahmsdorf HJ, Park KK, et al. Antitumor promotion and antiinflammation: downmodulation of AP-1 (Fos/Jun) activity by glucocorticoid hormone. *Cell* 1990;62:1189–1204.

27. Yang-Yen HF, Chambard JC, Sun YL, et al. Transcriptional interference between c-Jun and the glucocorticoid receptor: mutual inhibition of DNA binding due to direct protein-protein interaction. *Cell* 1990;62:1205–1215.
28. De Bosscher K, Schmitz ML, Vanden Berghe W, et al. Glucocorticoid-mediated repression of nuclear factor-kappaB-dependent transcription involves direct interference with transactivation. *Proc Natl Acad Sci USA* 1997;94:13504–13509.
29. Stocklin E, Wissler M, Gouilleux F, et al. Functional interactions between stat5 and the glucocorticoid receptor. *Nature* 1996;383:726–728.
30. Scheinman RI, Cogswell PC, Lofquist AK, et al. Role of transcriptional activation of IκBα in mediation of immunosuppression by glucocorticoids. *Science* 1995;270:283–286.
31. Auphan N, DiDonato JA, Rosette C, et al. Immunosuppression by glucocorticoids: inhibition of NF-κB activity through induction of IκB synthesis. *Science* 1995;270:286–290.
32. Lee SW, Tsou AP, Chan H, et al. Glucocorticoids selectively inhibit the transcription of the interleukin-1β gene and decrease the stability of interleukin 1β mRNA. *Proc Natl Acad Sci USA* 1988;85:1204–1208.
33. Boumpas DT, Anastassiou ED, Older SA, et al. Dexamethasone inhibits human interleukin 2 but not interleukin 2 receptor gene expression in vitro at the level of nuclear transcription. *J Clin Invest* 1991;87:1739–1747.
34. Paliogianni F, Balow, JE, Boumpas DT. Glucocorticoids modulate the binding of specific proteins to AU-sequences in the 3′-untranslated region (UTR) of interleukin-2 (IL-2) by activating phosphatases 1 and phosphatase 2. *J Allergy Clin Immunol* 1997;99:1954(abst).
35. Buttgereit F, Wehling M, Burmester GR. A new hypothesis of modular glucocorticoid actions: steroid treatment of rheumatic diseases revisited. *Arthritis Rheum* 1998;41:761–767.
36. Orchinik M, Murray TF, Moore FL. A corticosteroid receptor in neuronal membranes. *Science* 1991;252:1828–1851.
37. Buttgereit F, Brand MD, Burmester GR. Equivalent doses and relative drug potencies for non-genomic glucocorticoid effects: a novel glucocorticoid hierarchy. *Biochem Pharmacol* 1999;58: 363–368.
38. Dhabhar FS, McEwen BS. Enhancing versus suppressive effects of stress hormones on skin immune function. *Proc Natl Acad Sci USA* 1999;96:1059–1064.
39. Wiegers GJ, Labeur MS, Stec IE, et al. Glucocorticoids accelerate anti-T cell receptor-induced T cell growth. *J Immunol* 1995; 155:1893–1902.
40. Barber AE, Coyle SM, Marano MA, et al. Glucocorticoid therapy alters hormonal and cytokine responses to endotoxin in man. *J Immunol* 1993;150:1999–2006.
41. Calandra T, Bernhagen J, Metz CN, et al. MIF as a glucocorticoid-induced modulator of cytokine production. *Nature* 1995;377(6544):68–71
42. Geller DA, Nussler AK, DiSilvio M, et al. Cytokines, endotoxin, and glucocorticoids regulate the expression of inducible nitric oxide synthesis in hepatocytes. *Proc Natl Acad Sci USA* 1993;90:522–526.
43. Mukaida N, Morita M, Ishikawa Y, et al. Novel mechanism of glucocorticoid-mediated gene repression. Nuclear factor-kappa B is target for glucocorticoid-mediated interleukin 8 gene repression. *J Biol Chem* 1994;269:13289–13295.
44. Cronstein BN, Kimmel SC, Levin RI, et al. A mechanism for the antiinflammatory effects of corticosteroids: the glucocorticoid receptor regulates leukocyte adhesion to endothelial cells and expression of ELAM-1 and ICAM-1. *Proc Natl Acad Sci USA* 1992;89:9991–9996.
45. Lim LHK, Solito E, Russo-Marie F, et al. Promoting detachment of neutrophils adherent to murine postcapillary venules to control inflammation: effect of lipocortin-1. *Proc Natl Acad Sci USA* 1998;95:14535–14539.
46. Youssef PP, Triantafillou S, Parker A, et al. Effects of pulse methylprednisolone on cell adhesion molecules in the synovial membrane in rheumatoid arthritis. Reduced E-selectin and intercellular adhesion molecule 1 expression. *Arthritis Rheum* 1996;39:1970–1979.
47. Youssef PP, Haynes DR, Triantafillou S, et al. Effects of pulse methylprednisolone on inflammatory mediators in peripheral blood, synovial fluid, and synovial membrane in rheumatoid arthritis. *Arthritis Rheum* 1997;40:1400–1408.
48. Goulding NJ, Godolphin JL, Sharland PR, et al. Anti-inflammatory lipocortin 1 production by peripheral blood leucocytes in response to hydrocortisone. *Lancet* 1990;335:1416–1418.
49. O'Banion MK, Winn VD, Young DA. cDNA cloning and functional activity of a glucocorticoid-regulated inflammatory cyclooxygenase. *Proc Natl Acad Sci USA* 1992;89:4888–4892.
50. Waage A, Bakke O. Glucocorticoids suppress the production of tumor necrosis factor by lipopolysaccharide-stimulated human monocytes. *Immunology* 1988;63:299–302.
51. Beutler B, Krochin N, Milsark IW, et al. Control of cachectin (tumor necrosis factor) synthesis: mechanisms of endotoxin resistance. *Science* 1986;232:977–980.
52. Batuman AO, Ferrero AP, Diaz A, et al. Regulation of transforming factor-β1 gene expression by glucocorticoids in normal human T lymphocytes. *J Clin Invest* 1991;88:1574–1580.
53. Brack A, Rittner HL, Younge BR, et al. Glucocorticoid-mediated repression of cytokine gene transcription in human arteritis-SCID chimeras. *J Clin Invest* 1997;99:2842–2850.
54. Visser J, van Boxel-Dezaire A, Methorst D, at al. Differential regulation of interleukin-10 (IL-10) and IL-12 by glucocorticoids in vitro. *Blood* 1998;91:4255–4264.
55. Fauci AS, Dale DC. The effect of hydrocortisone on the kinetics of normal human lymphocytes. *Blood* 1975;46:235–243.
56. Fauci AS. Mechanisms of corticosteroid action on lymphocyte subpopulations. Redistribution of circulating T and B lymphocytes to the bone marrow. *Immunology* 1975;28:669–680.
57. Ten Berge RJM, Sauerwein HP, Yong SL, et al. Administration of prednisolone in vivo affects the ratio of OKT4/OKT8 and the LDH-isoenzyme pattern of human T lymphocytes. *Clin Immunol Immunopathol* 1984;30:91–103.
58. Paliogianni F, Ahuja SS, Yamada H, et al. Glucocorticoids inhibit T cell proliferation by downregulating proliferative signals mediated through both T cell antigen and interleukin-2 receptors. *Arthritis Rheum* 1992;35:S127.
59. Paliogianni F, Hama N, Balow JE, et al. Glucocorticoid-mediated regulation of protein phosphorylation in primary human T cells: evidence for induction of phosphatase activity. *J Immunol* 1995;1809–1817.AQ16
60. Paliogianni F, Boumpas DT. Glucocorticoids regulate calcineurin-dependent trans-activating pathways for interleukin-2 gene transcription in human T-lymphocytes. *Transplantation* 1995;59:1333–1339.
61. Vacca A, Martinotti S, Screpanti I, et al. Transcriptional regulation of the interleukin 2 gene by glucocorticoid hormones. Role of steroid receptor and antigen-responsive 5′-flanking sequences. *J Biol Chem* 1990;265:8075–8080.
62. Paliogianni F, Ahuja SS, Balow JP, et al. Novel mechanism for inhibition of human T cells by glucocorticoids (GC): GC modulate signal transduction through IL-2 receptor. *J Immunol* 1993;151:4081–4089.
63. Pitzalis C, Pipitone N, Bajocchi G. Corticosteroids inhibit lymphocyte binding to endothelium and intercellular adhesion: an additional mechanism for their anti-inflammatory and immunosuppressive effect. *J Immunol* 1997;158:5007–5016.
64. Bischof F, Melms A. Glucocorticoids inhibit CD40 ligand

expression of peripheral CD4+ lymphocytes. *Cell Immunol* 1998;187:38–44.

65. Ashwell JD, Lu FWM, Vacchio MS. Glucocorticoids in T cell development and function. *Annu Rev Immunol* 2000;18: 309–345.
66. Blotta MH, Dekruyff RH, Umetsu DT. Corticosteroids inhibit IL-12 production in human monocytes and enhance their capacity to induce IL-4 synthesis in CD4+ lymphocytes. *J Immunol* 1997;158:5589–5595
67. Dekruyff RH, Fang Y, Umetsu TD. Corticosteroids enhance the capacity of macrophages to induce Th2 cytokine sythesis in CD4+ lymphocytes by inhibiting IL-12 production. *J Immunol* 1998;160:2231–2237.
68. Tuosto L, Cundari E, Montani MSG, et al. Analysis of susceptibility of mature human T lymphocytes to dexamethasone-induced apoptosis. *Eur J Immunol* 1994;24:1061–1065.
69. Yang Y, Mercep M, Ware CF, et al. Fas and activation-induced Fas ligand mediate apoptosis of T cell hybridomas: inhibition of Fas ligand expression by retinoic acid and glucocorticoids. *J Exp Med* 1995;181:1673–1682.
70. Seki M, Ushiyama C, Seta N, et al. Apoptosis of lymphocytes induced by glucocorticoids and relationship to therapeutic efficacy in patients with systemic lupus erythematosus. *Arthritis Rheum* 1998;41:823–830.
71. Spinozzi F, Agea E, Bistoni O, et al. T lymphocytes bearing the γδ T cell receptor are susceptible to steroid-induced programmed cell death. *Scand J Immunol* 1995;41:504–508.
72. Baxter JD. Advances in glucocorticoid therapy. *Adv Intern Med* 2000;45:317–349.
73. Vingerhoeds AC, Thijssen JH, Schwarz F. Spontaneous hypercortisolism without Cushing's syndrome. *J Clin Endocrinol Metab* 1976;43:1128–1133.
74. Lamberts SW. The glucocorticoid insensitivity syndrome. *Horm Res* 1996;45(suppl 1):2–4
75. Werner S, Bronnegard M. Molecular basis of glucocorticoid-resistant syndromes. *Steroids* 1996;61:216–221.
76. Norbiato G, Bevilacqua M, Vago T, et al. Cortisol resistance in acquired immunodeficiency syndrome. *J Clin Endocrinol Metab* 1992;74:608–613.
77. Leung DY, Spahn JD, Szefler SJ. Immunologic basis and management of steroid-resistant asthma. *Allergy Asthma Proc* 1999; 20:9–14.
78. Pariante CM, Pearce BD, Pisell TL, et al. The proinflammatory cytokine, interleukin-1alpha, reduces glucocorticoid receptor translocation and function. *Endocrinology* 1999;140:4359–4366.
79. Bamberger CM, Bamberger A-M, de Castro M, et al. Glucocorticoid receptor β, a potential endogenous inhibitor of glucocorticoid action in humans. *J Clin Invest* 1995;95:2435–2441.
80. Klein A, Buskila D, Gladman D, et al. Cortisol catabolism by lymphocytes of patients with systemic lupus erythematosus and rheumatoid arthritis. *J Rheumatol* 1990;17:30–33.
81. Balis FM, Lester CM, Chrousos GP, et al. Differences in cerebrospinal fluid penetration of corticosteroids: possible relationship to the prevention of meningeal leukemia. *J Clin Oncol* 1987;5:202–207.
82. Frey BM, Frey FJ. Clinical pharmacokinetics of prednisone and prednisolone. *Clin Pharmacokinet* 1990;19:126–146.
83. Feldweg AM, Leddy JP. Drug interactions affecting the efficacy of corticosteroid therapy. A brief review with an illustrative case. *J Clin Rheumatol* 1999;5:143–150.
84. Spitz IM, Bardin CW. Mifepristone (RU 486)-A modulator of progestin and glucocorticoid action. *N Engl J Med* 1993;329: 404–412.
85. Klinenberg JR, Miller F. Effect of corticosteroids on blood salicylate concentration. *JAMA* 1965;194:601–604.
86. Costedoat-Chalumeau N, Amoura Z, Aymard G, et al. Potentiation of vitamin K antagonists by high-dose intravenous methylprednisolone. *Ann Intern Med* 2000;132:631–635.
87. Pollak VE, Pirani CL, Schwartz FD. The natural history of the renal manifestations of systemic lupus erythematosus. *J Lab Clin Med* 1964;63:537–550.
88. Pollak VE, Dosekun AK. Evaluation of treatment in lupus nephritis: effects of prednisone. *Am J Kidney Dis* 1982;2(suppl 1):170–177.
89. Huizenga NA, Koper JW, De Lange P, et al. A polymorphism in the glucocorticoid receptor gene may be associated with an increased sensitivity to glucocorticoids in vivo. *J Clin Endocrinol Metab* 1998;83:144–151.
90. Sarna S, Hoppu K, Neuvonen PJ, et al. Methylprednisolone exposure, rather than dose, predicts adrenal suppression and growth inhibition in children with liver and renal transplants. *J Clin Endocrinol Metab* 1997;82:75–77.
91. Quismorio FP Jr. Systemic corticosteroid therapy in systemic lupus erythematosus. In: Wallace DJ, Hahn BH, eds. *Dubois' lupus erythematosus*, 5th ed. Baltimore: Williams & Wilkins, 1997:1141–1162.
92. Kimberly RP. Corticosteroid use in systemic lupus erythematosus. In: Lahita RG, ed. *Systemic lupus erythematosus*, 3rd ed. San Diego: Academic Press, 1999:945–966.
93. Sergent JS, Lockshin MD, Klempner MS, et al. Central nervous system disease in systemic lupus erythematosus. Therapy and prognosis. *Am J Med* 1975;58:644–654.
94. Hahn BH. Management of systemic lupus erythematosus. In: Kelley WN, Harris ED, Ruddy S, et al., eds. *Textbook of rheumatology*, 5th ed. Philadelphia: WB Saunders, 1997:1040–1056.
95. Fauci AS. Alternate-day corticosteroid therapy. *Am J Med* 1978;64:729–731.
96. Balow JE, Boumpas DT, Austin HA. Lupus nephritis. In: Brady HR, Wilcox CS, eds. *Therapy in nephrology and hypertension.* Philadelphia: WB Saunders, 1999:130–137.
97. Fessler BJ, Boumpas DT. Severe major organ involvement in systemic lupus erythematosus. Diagnosis and management. *Rheum Dis Clin North Am* 1995;21:81–98.
98. Boumpas DT, Austin HA III, Vaughn EM, et al. Controlled trial of pulse methylprednisolone versus two regimens of pulse cyclophosphamide in severe lupus nephritis. *Lancet* 1992;340: 741–745.
99. Austin HA III, Klippel JH, Balow JE et al. Therapy of lupus nephritis. Controlled trial of prednisone and cytotoxic drugs. *N Engl J Med* 1986;314:614–619.
100. Gourley MF, Austin HA III, Scott D, et al. Methylprednisolone and cyclophosphamide, alone or in combination, in patients with lupus nephritis. *Ann Intern Med* 1996;125:549–557.
101. Balow JE, Austin HA 3rd, Muenz LR, et al. Effect on the evolution of renal abnormalities in lupus nephritis. *N Engl J Med* 1984;311:491–495.
102. Boumpas DT, Yamada H, Patronas NJ, et al. Pulse cyclophosphamide for severe neuropsychiatric lupus. *Q J Med* 1991; 81:975–984.
103. Boumpas DT, Scott DE, Balow JE. Neuropsychiatric lupus: a case for guarded optimism. *J Rheumatol* 1993;20:1641–1643.
104. Baca V, Lavalle C, Garcia R, et al. Favorable response to intravenous methylprednisolone and cyclophosphamide in children with severe neuropsychiatric lupus. *J Rheumatol* 1999;26: 432–439.
105. Boumpas DT, Patronas NJ, Dalakas MR, et al. Acute transverse myelitis in systemic lupus erythematosus. Magnetic resonance imaging and review of the literature. *J Rheumatol* 1990;17: 89–92.
106. Barile L, Lavalle C. Transverse myelitis in systemic lupus erythematosus-the effect of IV pulse methylprednisolone and cyclophosphamide. *J Rheumatol* 1992;19:370–372.

107. Mok CC, Lau CS, Chan EY, et al. Acute transverse myelopathy in systemic lupus erythematosus: clinical presentation, treatment and outcome. *J Rheumatol* 1998;25:467–473.
108. Kovacs B, Lafferty TL, Brent LH, et al. Transverse myelopathy in systemic lupus erythematosus: an analysis of 14 cases and review of the literature. *Ann Rheumatic Dis* 2000;59:120–124.
109. Liu MF, Lee JH, Weng TH, et al. Clinical experience of 13 cases with severe pulmonary hemorrhage in systemic lupus erythematosus with active nephritis. *Scand J Rheumatol* 1998;27:291–295.
110. Fukuda M, Kamiyama Y, Kawahara K, et al. The favourable effect of cyclophosphamide therapy in the treatment of massive pulmonary hemorrhage in systemic lupus erythematosus. *Eur J Pediatr* 1994;153:167–170.
111. Eiser AR, Shanies HM. Treatment of lupus interstitial lung disease with intravenous cyclophosphamide. *Arthritis Rheum* 1994;37:428–431.
112. Naarendorp M, Kerr LD, Khan AS, et al. Dramatic improvement of left ventricular function after cytotoxic therapy in lupus patients with acute cardiomyopathy: report of 6 cases. *J Rheumatol* 1999;26:2257–2260.
113. Grimbacher B, Huber M, von Kempis J, et al. Successful treatment of gastrointestinal vasculitis due to systemic lupus erythematosus with intravenous pulse cyclophosphamide: a clinical case report and review of the literature. *Br J Rheumatol* 1998;37:1023–1028.
114. Van Vollenhoven RF. Dehydroepiandrosterone in systemic lupus erythematosus. *Rheum Dis Clin North Am* 2000;26:349–362.
115. Van Vollenhoven RF, Engleman EG, Mc Guire JL. Dehydroepiandrosterone (DHEA) in systemic lupus erythematosus: results of a double-blinded, placebo-controlled, randomized clinical trial. *Arthritis Rheum* 1995;38:1826–1831.
116. Petri M, Lahita R, McGuire J, et al. Results of GL701 (DHEA) multicenter steroid sparing SLE study. *Arthritis Rheum* 1997;40(suppl):S327.
117. Van Vollenhoven RF, Park JL, Genovese MC, et al. A double-blinded, placebo-controlled, clinical trial of dehydroepiandrosterone in severe systemic lupus erythematosus. *Lupus* 1999;8:181–187.
118. Medina F, Ayala A, Jara LJ, et al. Acute abdomen in systemic lupus erythematosus: the importance of early laparotomy. *Am J Med* 1997;102:100–105.
119. Rubin LA, Urowitz MB, Gladman DD. Mortality in systemic lupus erythematosus-the bimodal pattern revisited. *Q J Med* 1985;55:87–98.
120. Cathcart ES, Idelson BA, Scheinberg MA, et al. Beneficial effects of methylprednisolone "pulse" therapy in diffuse proliferative lupus nephritis. *Lancet* 1976;1:163–166.
121. Kimberly RP, Lockshin MD, Sherman RL, et al. High dose intravenous methylprednisolone pulse therapy in systemic lupus erythematosus. *Am J Med* 1981;70:817–824.
122. Eyanson S, Passo MH, Aldo-Benson MA, et al. Methyprednisolone pulse therapy for nonrenal lupus erythematosus. *Ann Rheum Dis* 1980;39:377–380.
123. Isenberg DA, Morrow WJ, Snaith ML. Methyl prednisolone pulse therapy in the treatment of systemic lupus erythematosus. *Ann Rheum Dis* 1982;41:347–351.
124. Ko SF, Lee TY, Cheng TT, Ng SH, et al. CT findings at lupus mesenteric vasculitis. *Acta Radiol* 1997;38:115–120.
125. Hiraishi H, Konishi T, Ota S, et al. Massive gastrointestinal hemorrhage in systemic lupus erythematosus: successful treatment with corticosteroid pulse therapy. *Am J Gastroenterol* 1999;94:3349–3353.
126. Edwards JC, Snaith ML, Isenberg DA. A double blind controlled trial of methylprednisolone infusions in systemic lupus erythematosus using individualized outcome assessment. *Ann Rheum Dis* 1987;46:773–776.
127. Mackworth-Young CG, David J, Morgan SH, et al. A double blind, placebo controlled trial of intravenous methylprednisolone in systemic lupus erythematosus. *Ann Rheum Dis* 1988;47:496–502.
128. Illei GG, Crane M, Collins L, et al. Long-term follow-up of patients with lupus nephritis (LN) treated with methylprednisolone or cyclophosphamide alone or in combination. *Arthritis Rheum* 1999;42(suppl):S166.
129. Fox DA, McCune WJ. Immunosuppressive drug therapy of systemic lupus erythematosus. *Rheum Dis Clin North Am* 1994;20:265–299.
130. Kirou KA, Yazici Y, Zuniga R, et al. Pulse glucocorticoid therapy is not associated with lower bone mineral density than daily oral glucocorticoids. *Arthritis Rheum* 1998;41(suppl):S302.
131. Massardo L, Jacobelli S, Leissner M, et al. High-dose intravenous methylprednisolone therapy associated with osteonecrosis in patients with systemic lupus erythematosus. *Lupus* 1992;1:401–405.
132. Wada K, Yamada N, Suzuki H, et al. Recurrent cases of corticosteroid-induced mood disorder: clinical characteristics and treatment. *J Clin Psychiatry* 2000;61:261–267.
133. Suchman AL, Condemi JJ, Leddy JP. Seizure after pulse therapy with methylprednisolone. *Arthritis Rheum* 1993;26:117.
134. Moses RE, McCormick A, Nickey W. Fatal arrhythmia after pulse methylprednisolone therapy. *Ann Intern Med* 1981;95:781–782.
135. Fessel WJ. Megadose corticosteroid therapy in systemic lupus erythematosus. *J Rheumatol* 1980;7:486–500.
136. Lazarevic MB, Skosey JL, Djordjevic-Denic G, et al. Reduction of cortisol levels after single intra-articular and intramuscular steroid injection. *Am J Med* 1995;99:370–373.
137. Dasgupta B, Dolan AL, Panayi GS, et al. An initially double-blind controlled 96 week trial of depot methylprednisolone against oral prednisolone in the treatment of polymyalgia rheumatica. *Br J Rheumatol* 1998;37:189–195
138. Bermas BL, Hill JA. Effects of immunosuppressive drugs during pregnancy. *Arthritis Rheum* 1995;38:1722–1732.
139. Kitridou RC. The mother in systemic lupus erythematosus. In: Wallace DJ, Hahn BH, eds. *Dubois' lupus erythematosus*, 5 ed. Baltimore: Williams & Wilkins, 1997:967–1002.
140. Saleeb S, Copel J, Friedman D, et al. Comparison of treatment with fluorinated glucocorticoids to the natural history of autoantibody-associated congenital heart block. Retrospective review of the research registry for neonatal lupus. *Arthritis Rheum* 1999;42:2335–2345.
141. Pinsky L, DiGeorge AM. Cleft palate in the mouse: a teratogenic index of glucocorticoid potency. *Science* 1965;147:402–403.
142. Cowchock FS, Reece EA, et al. Repeated fetal losses associated with antiphospholipid antibodies: A collaborative randomized trial comparing prednisone with low-dose heparin treatment. *Am J Obstet Gynecol* 1992;166:318–323.AQ17
143. Silver RK, MacGregor SN, Sholl JS, et al. Comparative trial of prednisone plus aspirin versus aspirin alone in the treatment of anticardiolipin antibody-positive obstetric patients. *Am J Obstet Gynecol* 1993;169:1411–1417.
144. Laskin CA, Bombardier C, Hannah ME, et al. Prednisone and aspirin in women with autoantibodies and unexplained recurrent fetal loss. *N Engl J Med* 1997;337:148–153.
145. Cowchock S. Treatment of antiphospholipid syndrome in pregnancy. *Lupus* 1998;7(suppl 2):S95–S97.
146. Menashe Y, Ben-Baruch G, Greenspoon JS, et al. Successful pregnancy outcome with combination therapy in women with the antiphospholipid antibody syndrome. *J Reprod Med* 1993;38:625–629.

147. Buchanan NM, Toubi E, Khamashta MA, et al. Hydroxychloroquine and lupus pregnancy: review of a series of 36 cases. *Ann Rheum Dis* 1996;55:486–488.
148. Parke A, West B. Hydroxychloroquine in pregnant patients with systemic lupus erythematosus. *J Rheumatol* 1996;23:1715–1718.
149. Anonymous. A randomized study of the effect of withdrawing hydroxychloroquine sulfate in systemic lupus erythematosus. The Canadian Hydroxychloroquine Study Group. *N Engl J Med* 1991;324:150–154.
150. Kehlet H, Binder C. Adrenocortical function and clinical course during and after surgery in unsupplemented glucocorticoid-treated patients. *Br J Anaesth* 1973;45:1043–1048.
151. Salem M, Tainsh RE Jr, Bromberg J, et al. Perioperative glucocorticoid coverage. A reassessment 42 years after emergence of a problem. *Ann Surg* 1994;219:416–425.
152. Ginzler EM, Aranow C. Prevention and treatment of adverse effects of corticosteroids in systemic lupus erythematosus. *Baillieres Clin Rheumatol* 1998;12:495–510.
153. Manolagas SC, Weinstein RS. New developments in the pathogenesis and treatment of steroid-induced osteoporosis. *J Bone Miner Res* 1999;14:1061–1066.
154. Lacey DL, Timms E, Tan HL, et al. Osteoprotegerin ligand is a cytokine that regulates ostreoclast differentiation and activation. *Cell* 1998;93:165–176.
155. Weinstein RS, Jilka RL, Parfitt AM, et al. Inhibition of osteoblastogenesis and promotion of apoptosis and osteocytes by glucocorticoids. Potential mechanisms of their deleterious effects on bone. *J Clin Invest* 1998;102:274–282.
156. Hofbauer LC, Gori F, Riggs BL, et al. Stimulation of osteoprotegerin ligand and inhibition of osteoprotegerin production by glucocorticoids in human osteoblastic lineage cells: potential paracrine mechanisms of glucocorticoid-induced osteoporosis. *Endocrinology* 1999;140:4382–4389.
157. Cunnane G, Lane NE. Steroid-induced osteoporosis in systemic lupus erythematosus. *Rheum Dis Clin North Am* 2000;26:311–327.
158. Anonymous. Recommendations for the prevention and treatment of glucocorticoid-induced osteoporosis. American College of Rheumatology Task Force on Osteoporosis Guidelines. *Arthritis Rheum* 1996;39:1791–1801.
159. Reid IR. Glucocorticoid osteoporosis-mechanisms and management. *Eur J Endocrinol* 1997;137:209–217.
160. Formiga F, Moga I, Nolla JM, et al. The association of dehydroepiandrosterone sulphate levels with bone mineral density in systemic lupus erythematosus. *Clin Exp Rheumatol* 1997;15:387–392.
161. Kong YY, Feige U, Sarosi I, et al. Activated T cells regulate bone loss and joint destruction in adjuvant arthritis through osteoprotegerin ligand. *Nature* 1999;402:304–309.
162. Hansen M, Podenphant J, Florescu A. et al. A randomized trial of differentiated prednisolone treatment in active rheumatoid arthritis. Clinical benefits and skeletal side effects. *Ann Rheum Dis* 1999;58:713–718.
163. Lukert BP, Kipp D, Broy S. Management of glucocorticoid-induced osteoporosis—first, do no harm: comment on the American College of Rheumatology recommendations for the prevention and treatment of glucocorticoid-induced osteoporosis. *Arthritis Rheum* 1997;40:1548.
164. Sambrook PN, Birmingham J, Kelly PJ, et al. Prevention of corticosteroid osteoporosis: a comparison of calcium, calcitriol and calcitonin. *N Engl J Med* 1993;328:1747–1752.
165. Okada J, Nomura M, Shirataka M, et al. Prevalence of soft tissue calcifications in patients with SLE and effects of alphacalcidol. *Lupus* 1999;8:456–461.
166. Hall GM, Daniels M, Doyle DV, et al. Effect of hormone replacement therapy on bone mass in rheumatoid arthritis patients treated with and without steroids. *Arthritis Rheum* 1994;37:1499–1505.
167. Reid IR, Wattie DJ, Evans MC, et al. Testosterone therapy in glucocorticoid-treated men. *Arch Intern Med* 1996;156:1173–1177.
168. Buyon JP. Hormone replacement therapy in postmenopausal women with systemic lupus erythematosus. *J Am Med Wom Assoc* 1998;53:13–17.
169. Adachi JD, Bensen WG, Brown J, et al. Intermittent etidronate therapy to prevent corticosteroid induced osteoporosis. *N Engl J Med* 1997;337:382–387.
170. Saag KG, Emkey R, Schnitzer TJ, et al. Alendronate for the prevention and treatment of glucocorticoid-induced osteoporosis. Glucocorticoid-Induced Osteoporosis Study Group. *N Engl J Med* 1998;30:292–299.
171. Cohen S, Levy RM, Keller M, et al. Risedronate therapy prevents corticosteroid-induced bone loss. A twelve month, multicenter, randomized, double-blind, placebo-controlled, parallel-group study. *Arthritis Rheum* 1999;42:2309–2318.
172. Healey JH, Paget SA, Williams-Russo P, et al. A randomized controlled trial of salmon calcitonin to prevent bone loss in corticosteroid-treated temporal arteritis and polymyalgia rheumatica. *Calcif Tissue Int* 1996;58:73–80.
173. Lane NE, Sanchez S, Modin GW, et al. Parathyroid hormone treatment can reverse corticosteroid-induced osteoporosis. Results of a randomized controlled clinical trial. *J Clin Invest* 1998;102:1627–1633.
174. Mundy G, Garett R, Harris S, et al. Stimulation of bone formation in vitro and in rodents by statins. *Science* 1999;286:1946–1949.
175. Wang GJ, Chung KC, Shen WJ. Lipid clearing agents in steroid-induced osteoporosis. *J Formos Med Assoc* 1995;94:589–592.
176. Cui Q, Wang GJ, Su CC, et al. The Otto Aufranc Award. Lovastatin prevents steroid induced adipogenesis and osteonecrosis. *Clin Orthop* 1997;344:8–19.
177. Meier CR, Schlienger RG, Kraenzlin ME, et al. HMG-CoA reductase inhibitors and the risk of fractures. *JAMA* 2000;283:3205–3210.
178. Wang PS, Solomon DH, Mogun H, et al. HMG-CoA reductase inhibitors and the risk of hip fractures in elderly patients. *JAMA* 2000;283:3211–3216.
179. Mankin HJ. Nontraumatic necrosis of bone (osteonecrosis). *N Engl J Med* 1992;326:1475–1479.
180. Simkin PA, Gardner GC. Osteonecrosis: pathogenesis and practicalities. *Hosp Pract* 1994;29:51–64.
181. Metselaar HJ, van Steenberge EJP, Bijnen AB, et al. Incidence of osteonecrosis after renal transplantation. *Acta Orthop Scand* 1985;56:413–415.
182. Bradbury G, Benjamin J, Thompson J, et al. Avascular necrosis of bone after cardiac transplantation. Prevalence and relationship to administration and dosage of steroids. *J Bone Joint Surg* 1994;76A:1385–1388.
183. Taylor LJ. Multifocal avascular necrosis after short-term high-dose steroid therapy. A report of three cases. *J Bone Joint Surg* 1984;66B:431–433.
184. Vreden SG, Hermus AR, van Liessum PA, et al. Aseptic bone necrosis in patients on glucocorticoid replacement therapy. *Neth J Med* 1991;39:153–157.
185. Laroche M, Arlet J, Mazieres B. Osteonecrosis of the femoral and humeral heads after intraarticular corticosteroid injections. *J Rheumatol* 1990;17:549–551.
186. Cozen L, Wallace DJ. Avascular necrosis in systemic lupus erythematosus: clinical associations and a 47-year perspective. *Am J Orthop* 1998;27:352–354.
187. Houssiau FA, N'Zeusseu Toukap A, Depresseux G, et al. Magnetic resonance imaging-detected avascular osteonecrosis in sys-

temic lupus erythematosus: lack of correlation with antiphospholipid antibodies. *Br J Rheumatol* 1998;37:448–453.

188. Mont MA, Glueck CJ, Pacheco IH, et al. Risk factors for osteonecrosis in systemic lupus erythematosus. *J Rheumatol* 1997;24:654–662.
189. Mok CC, Lau CS, Wong RW. Risk factors for avascular bone necrosis in systemic lupus erythematosus. *Br J Rheumatol* 1998; 37:895–900.
190. Zizic TM, Marcoux C, Hungerford DS, et al. Corticosteroid therapy associated with ischemic necrosis of bone in systemic lupus erythematosus. *Am J Med* 1985;79:596–604.
191. Mont M, Jones LC. Management of osteonecrosis in systemic lupus erythematosus. *Rheum Dis Clin North Am* 2000;26: 279–309.
192. Aranow C, Zelikof S, Leslie D, et al. Clinically occult avascular necrosis of the hip in systemic lupus erythematosus. *J Rheumatol* 1997;24:2318–2322.
193. Gladman DD, Urowitz MB. Morbidity in systemic lupus erythematosus. *J Rheumatol* 1987;14(suppl 13):223–226.
194. Manzi S, Meilahn EN, Rairie JE, et al. Age-specific incidence rates of myocardial infarction and angina in women with systemic lupus erythematosus: comparison with the Framingham study. *Am J Epidemiol* 1997;145:408–415.
195. Petri M, Perez-Gutthann S, Spence D, et al. Risk factors for coronary artery disease in patients with systemic lupus erythematosus. *Am J Med* 1992;93:513–519.
196. Bruce IN, Gladman DD, Urowitz MB. Premature atherosclerosis in systemic lupus erythematosus. *Rheum Dis Clin North Am* 2000;26:257–277.
197. Ilowite NT, Samuel P, Ginzler E, et al. Dyslipoproteinemia in pediatric systemic lupus erythematosus. *Arthritis Rheum* 1988; 31:859–863.
198. Borba EF, Bonga E. Dyslipoproteinemias in systemic lupus erythematosus: influence of disease, activity and anticardiolipin antibodies. *Lupus* 1997;6:533–539.
199. Cheng W, Lau OD, Abumrad NA. Two antiatherogenic effects of progesterone on human macrophages; inhibition of cholesteryl ester synthesis and block of its enhancement by glucocorticoids. *J Clin Endocrinol Metab* 1999;84:265–271.
200. Ettinger WH, Hazzard WR. Prednisone increases very low density lipoprotein and high density lipoprotein in healthy men. *Metabolism* 1988;37:1055–1058.
201. Ettinger WH, Goldberg AP, Applebaum-Bowden D, et al. Dyslipoproteinemia in systemic lupus erythematosus. Effect of corticosteroids. *Am J Med* 1987;83:503–508.
202. MacGregor AJ, Dhillon VB, Binder A, et al. Fasting lipids and anticardiolipin antibodies as risk factors for vascular disease in systemic lupus erythematosus. *Ann Rheum Dis* 1992;51:152–155.
203. Petri M, Lakatta C, Magder L, et al. Effect of prednisone and hydroxychloroquine on coronary artery disease risk factors in systemic lupus erythematosus: a longitudinal data analysis. *Am J Med* 1994;96:254–259.
204. Rahman P, Gladman DD, Urowitz MB, et al. The cholesterol lowering effect of antimalarial drugs is enhanced in patients with lupus taking corticosteroid drugs. *J Rheumatol* 1999;26: 325–330.
205. Urowitz MB, Bookman AAM, Kehler BE. The bimodal mortality pattern of systemic lupus erythematosus. *Am J Med* 1976; 60:221–225.
206. Abu-Shakra M, Urowitz MB, Gladman DD, et al. Mortality studies in systemic lupus erythematosus: results from a single center: causes of death. *J Rheumatol* 1995;22:1259–1264.
207. Abu-Shakra M, Urowitz MB, Gladman DD, et al. Mortality studies in systemic lupus erythematosus: results from a single center: predictor variables for mortality. *J Rheumatol* 1995;22: 1265–1270.
208. Manzi S, Selzer F, Sutton-Tyrell K, et al. Prevalence and risk factors of carotid plaque in women with systemic lupus erythematosus. *Arthritis Rheum* 1999;42:51–60.
209. Bruce IN, Burns RJ, Gladman DD, et al. A study of myocardial perfusion abnormalities in women with SLE. *J Rheumatol* 1998; 25(suppl 52):72.
210. Ross R. Atherosclerosis—an inflammatory disease. *N Engl J Med* 1999;340:115–126.
211. Minick CR, Murphy GE, Campbell WG. Experimental induction of athero-arteriosclerosis by the synergy of allergic injury to arteries and lipid-rich diet: effect of repeated injection of horse serum in rabbits fed a dietary cholesterol supplement. *J Exp Med* 1966;124:635–652.
212. Kabakov AE, Tertov VV, Saenko VA, et al. The atherogenic effect of lupus sera: systemic lupus erythematosus-derived immune complexes stimulate the accumulation of cholesterol in cultured smooth muscle cell from human aorta. *Clin Immunol Immunopathol* 1992;63:214–220.
213. Rahman P, Urowitz MB, Gladman DD, et al. Contribution of traditional risk factors to coronary artery disease (CAD) in patients with SLE. *J Rheumatol* 1999;26:2363–2368.
214. Petri M. Detection of coronary artery disease and the role of traditional risk factors in the Hopkins Lupus Cohort. *Lupus* 2000; 9:170–175.
215. Ling MHM, Perry PH, Tsuang MT. Psychiatric side effects of corticosteroid therapy. *Arch Gen Psychiatry* 1981;38:471–477.
216. Pareja JG, Garland R, Koziel H. Use of adjunctive corticosteroids in severe adult non-HIV *Pneumocystis carinii* pneumonia. *Chest* 1998;113:1215–1224.
217. McIntyre PB, Berkey CS, King SM, et al. Dexamethasone as adjunctive therapy in bacterial meningitis. A meta-analysis of randomized clinical trials since 1988. *JAMA* 1997;278:925–931.
218. Stuck AE, Minder CE, Frey FJ. Risk of infectious complications in patients taking glucocorticosteroids. *Rev Infect Dis* 1989;11: 954–963.
219. Ginzler E, Diamond H, Kaplan D, et al. Computer analysis of factors influencing frequency of infection in systemic lupus erythematosus. *Arthritis Rheum* 1978;21:37–44.
220. Duffy KN, Duffy CM, Gladman DD. Infection and disease activity in systemic lupus erythematosus: a review of hospitalized patients. *J Rheumatol* 1991;18:1180–1184.
221. Kim WU, Min JK, Lee SH, et al. Causes of death in Korean patients with systemic lupus erythematosus: a single center retrospective study. *Clin Exp Rheumatol* 1999;17:539–545.
222. Liam CK, Wang F. *Pneumocystis carinii* pneumonia in patients with systemic lupus erythematosus. *Lupus* 1992;1:379–385.
223. Iliopoulos AG, Tsokos GC. Immunopathogenesis and spectrum of infections in systemic lupus erythematosus. *Semin Arthritis Rheum* 1996;25:318–336.
224. Bellomio V, Spindler A, Lucero E, et al. Systemic lupus erythematosus: mortality and survival in Argentina. A multicenter study. *Lupus* 2000;9:377–381.
225. Kadoya A, Okada J, Iikuni Y, et al. Risk factors for *Pneumocystis carinii* pneumonia in patients with polymyositis/dermatomyositis or systemic lupus erythematosus. *J Rheumatol* 1996;23: 1186–1188.
226. Porges AJ, Beattie SL, Ritchlin C, et al. Patients with systemic lupus erythematosus at risk for *Pneumocystis carinii* pneumonia. *J Rheumatol* 1992;19:1191–1194.
227. Singer NG, McCune J. Prevention of infectious complications in rheumatic disease patients: immunization, *Pneumocystis carinii* prophylaxis, and screening for latent infections. *Curr Opin Rheumatol* 1999;11:173–178.

227a. Anonymous. Targeted tuberculin testing and treatment of latent tuberculosis infection. American Thoracic Society. *MMWR Morb Mortal Wkly Rep* 2000;49(RR-6):1–51.

228. Battafarano DF, Battafarano NJ, Larsen I, et al. Antigen-specific antibody responses in lupus patients following immunization. *Arthritis Rheum* 1998;41:1828–1834.
229. Bowyer SL, LaMothe MP, Hollister JR. Steroid myopathy: incidence and detection in a population with asthma. *J Allergy Clin Immunol* 1985;76:234–242.
230. Batchelor TT, Taylor LP, Thaler HT. Steroid myopathy in cancer patients. *Neurology* 1997;48:1234–1238.
231. Askari A, Vignos PJ, Moskowitz RW. Steroid myopathy in connective tissue disease. *Am J Med* 1976;61:485–492.
232. Kanayama Y, Shiota K, Horiguchi T, et al. Correlation between steroid myopathy and serum lactic dehydrogenase in systemic lupus erythematosus. *Arch Intern Med* 1981;141:1176–1179.
233. LaPier TK. Glucocorticoid-induced muscle atrophy. The role of exercise in treatment and prevention. *J Cardiopulmon Rehabil* 1997;17:76–84.
234. Lacomis D, Giuliani MJ, Van Cott A, et al. Acute myopathy of intensive care: clinical, electromyographic, and pathological aspects. *Ann Neurol* 1996;40:645–654.
235. Hanson P, Dive A, Brucher JM, et al. Acute corticosteroid myopathy in intensive care patients. *Muscle Nerve* 1997;20: 1371–1380.
236. Larsson I, Li X, Edstrom L, et al. Acute quadriplegia and loss of muscle myosin in patients treated with nondepolarizing neuromuscular blocking agents and corticosteroids: mechanisms at the cellular and molecular levels. *Crit Care Med* 2000; 28:34–45.
237. Allen DB. Growth suppression by glucocorticoid therapy. *Endocrinol Metab Clin North Am* 1996;25:699–717.
238. Allen DB, Julius JR, Breen TJ, et al. Treatment of glucocorticoid-induced growth suppression with growth hormone. National Cooperative Growth Study. *J Clin Endocrinol Metab* 1998;83:2824–2829.
239. Lai HC, FitzSimmons SC, Allen DB, et al. Risk of persistent growth impairment after alternate-day prednisone treatment in children with cystic fibrosis. *N Engl J Med* 2000;342:851–859.
240. Doull IJ, Freezer NJ, Holgate ST. Growth of prepubertal children with mild asthma treated with inhaled beclomethasone dipropionate. *Am J Respir Crit Care Med* 1995;151:1715–1719.
241. Skoner DP, Rachelefsky GS, Meltzer EO, et al. Detection of growth suppression in children during treatment with intranasal beclomethasone dipropionate. *Pediatrics* 2000;105:E23(1–7).
242. Canalis E. Editorial: Inhibitory actions of glucocorticoids on skeletal growth. Is local insulin-like growth factor I to blame? *Endocrinology* 1998;139:3041–3042.
243. Jux C, Leiber K, Hugel U, et al. Dexamethasone impairs growth hormone (GH)-stimulated growth by suppression of local insulin-like growth factor (IGF)-I production and expression of GH- and IGF-I-receptor in cultured rat chondrocytes. *Endocrinology* 1998;139:3296–3305.
244. Furie RA Chartash EK. Tendon rupture in systemic lupus erythematosus. *Semin Arthritis Rheum* 1988;18:127–133.
245. Renfro L, Snow JS. Ocular effects of topical and systemic steroids. *Dermatol Clin* 1992;10:505–512.
246. Conn HO, Poynard T. Corticosteroids and peptic ulcer: meta-analysis of adverse events during steroid therapy. *J Intern Med* 1994;236:619–632.
247. Piper JM, Ray WA, Daugherty JR, et al. Corticosteroid use and peptic ulcer disease: role of nonsteroidal anti-inflammatory drugs. *Ann Intern Med* 1991;114:735–740.
248. Schonwald S. Methylprednisolone anaphylaxis. *Am J Emerg Med* 1999;17:583–585.
249. Lew DB, Higgins GC, Skinner RB, et al. Adverse reaction to prednisone in a patient with systemic lupus erythematosus. *Pediatr Dermatol* 1999;16:146–150.
250. Mace S, Vadas P, Pruzanski W. Anaphylactic shock induced by intraarticular injection of methylprednisolone acetate. *J Rheumatol*1997;24:1191–1194.

57

IMMUNOSUPPRESSIVE DRUG THERAPY

W. JOSEPH MCCUNE
MONA RISKALLA

Immunosuppressive agents are widely used to treat systemic lupus erythematosus (SLE) despite the relative paucity of controlled trials showing their efficacy, especially with regard to prolongation of survival. Most studies have been performed in patients with nephritis. The availability of histology and relatively accurate tests of renal function allow a fairly accurate estimation of the response to therapy; however, the duration of such trials, usually 1 to 5 years, has been much less than the anticipated survival of most patients with lupus. Especially in patients who do not have fulminant disease, long-term trials are required; unless sensitive markers for treatment failure are employed (e.g., doubling of serum creatinine instead of progression to renal failure), prolonged treatment of patients randomized to suboptimal regimens may not be practical.

A meta-analysis that included 440 patients with lupus nephritis in 19 clinical trials concluded that the use of immunosuppressive drugs (azathioprine and/or cyclophosphamide) in addition to prednisone and the use of prednisone alone significantly reduced the risks of end-stage renal disease (ESRD) or death by 12.9% and 13.2%, respectively (1). These findings were consistent with those of Felson and Anderson (2), who in 1984 combined eight clinical trials employing prednisone alone versus prednisone plus azathioprine and/or cyclophosphamide for the treatment of lupus nephritis. They concluded that progression to both renal failure and death was delayed by immunosuppression, particularly in patients with diffuse proliferative nephritis, although statistical significance was lost when the azathioprine- or cyclophosphamide-treated groups were analyzed separately. This chapter focuses on widely used immunosuppressive agents, emphasizing controlled trials, most of which have enrolled patients with lupus nephritis, and reviews the use of the alkylating agents azathioprine, cyclosporine, methotrexate, and mycophenolate mofetil.

ALKYLATING AGENTS

More than a dozen alkylating agents are currently in use. Of these, nitrogen mustard, cyclophosphamide, and chlorambucil have been applied sufficiently widely in the treatment of SLE to warrant discussion. Although there are inherent similarities in mechanisms of action, the clinical effects, both therapeutic and toxic, of the individual alkylating agents differ from each other and may vary depending on the dose, route of administration, duration of administration, and cumulative dose of these agents. Larger cumulative doses of alkylating agents are associated with escalating risk of toxicity, particularly gonadal failure and secondary malignancies. Because alkylating agents are currently essential in the management of some severe forms of lupus, familiarity with strategies to minimize toxicity is important in order to use these drugs with maximal benefit.

The earliest use of alkylating agents, reported by Osborne et al. (3) in 1947, was topical application of nitrogen mustard in cutaneous lupus, followed by the description from Chasis in 1949 of the efficacy of nitrogen mustard in glomerulonephritis (4). Despite the impressive results obtained with nitrogen mustard, however, there is a larger body of knowledge regarding the clinical and immunologic effects of cyclophosphamide, and this agent is reviewed first.

Cyclophosphamide

Cyclophosphamide is a merchlorethamine derivative that is inactive as administered. It is metabolized by mitochondrial cytochrome P-450 enzymes in the liver to a variety of active metabolites, an increasing number of which have been shown to have both therapeutic and toxic actions. These include 4-hydroxycyclophosphamide, phosphoramide mustard, acrolein, and others. Not only the liver but other tissues such as transitional epithelial cells in the bladder and lymphocytes may metabolize the drug, resulting in local toxicity and/or immunosuppression. Cyclophosphamide may have toxic and/or therapeutic effects in cells that are not actively dividing as well as in dividing cells.

Cyclophosphamide is well absorbed orally, and the oral and intravenous (IV) doses are equivalent. Large boluses of cyclophosphamide can be given orally with comparable levels of the parent (i.e., inactive) compound being attained in serum versus those with IV administration. Approximately 20% is excreted by the kidney, and 80% is processed by the liver. Because the effect of organ failure on the half-life of active cyclophosphamide metabolites is poorly understood, no firm guidelines exist for dose adjustment. Patients with creatinine clearances of less than 30 mL/min have increased toxicity from this drug, and doses should be modified accordingly. Cyclophosphamide is incompletely cleared by dialysis; therefore, the dose should be lowered in dialysis patients. The effect of hepatic insufficiency on cyclophosphamide toxicity is poorly understood, in part because the liver is responsible for both the production of active metabolites and their degradation.

The immunologic effects of cyclophosphamide have been described (5,6). Direct effects of cyclophosphamide on DNA resulting in cell death have been identified as the major effect of cyclophosphamide. These effects may occur at any stage during the cell cycle. Direct immunomodulatory effects also may occur and be responsible for the relatively rapid onset of therapeutic efficacy of cyclophosphamide (i.e., within 2 to 4 days) that is seen in some patients at a time when attrition of immunocompetent cells because of the inhibition of cell division would not be expected. Putative mechanisms of action include alteration or macrophage function, increased production of prostaglandin E_2, alteration of gene transcription, and direct functional effects on lymphocytes (5,6). Intravenous cyclophosphamide induces suppression of T-cell activation by a combination of monoclonal antibodies to the CD2 antigen (7,8); however, modulation of T-cell function has not been convincingly shown to play an important role in the treatment of lupus.

Cyclophosphamide produces dose-related lymphopenia. Therapeutic doses of cyclophosphamide produce dose-dependent reduction of both $CD4^+$ and $CD8^+$ T cells (7–9). Intravenous cyclophosphamide reduces the population of $CD4^+$ and $CD8^+$ lymphocytes and B cells, with a more marked reduction of $CD4^+$ lymphocytes and B cells during monthly therapy. Following cessation of monthly therapy, B-cell populations rapidly return to baseline (7), but CD4 populations remain relatively suppressed during less intensive IV cyclophosphamide therapy, resulting in prolonged reduction of the CD4/CD8 ratio (9). Persistent reduction of the percentage of $CD19^+$ lymphocytes and of the CD4/CD8 ratio 6 months after completion of 6 months of therapy has been reported (10). Other studies have suggested specific reduction of B-cell function (11). Reduction of autoantibody production has been demonstrated in patients with SLE who are treated with both oral and IV cyclophosphamide and in patients with rheumatoid arthritis who are treated with oral cyclophosphamide (7,12). Despite reduction of pathogenic autoantibody production, reduction of overall levels of immunoglobulin (Ig) classes IgG, IgA, and IgM, and IgG subclasses has not been observed in our patient population. This suggests that specific suppression of autoantibody production is a function of cyclophosphamide when used in therapeutic doses and may underlie its beneficial action in SLE.

Low doses of cyclophosphamide in both animals and humans can heighten immune responses. This has been noted in both antibody-mediated and cell-mediated immunity, and it has been theorized that low doses of cyclophosphamide could enhance antitumor immunity in humans (13). Low doses of cyclophosphamide accelerate the production of diabetes in the nonobese diabetic (NOD) mouse (14). The mechanism of action of cyclophosphamide in these situations is unclear, but it may represent functional alterations as well as depletion of lymphocyte subsets. These observations suggest that tapering the dose of cyclophosphamide may produce unexpected effects. As a practical matter, however, there are no clinical data to support the hypothesis that during tapering of immunosuppressive drugs, particularly cyclophosphamide, immunosuppression is supplanted by immunostimulation.

Malignancies And Hemorrhagic Cystitis

Development of malignancies following cyclophosphamide administration is well described in patients with rheumatic diseases, particularly rheumatoid arthritis and Wegener's granulomatosis (15). Long-term follow-up studies by Baltus et al. (16) and Baker et al. (17) of rheumatoid arthritis patients treated with oral cyclophosphamide have established an approximately 10% additional incidence of malignancy compared with age-matched controls after a total dose of 30 g. Doses of less than 10 g are almost certainly safer; doses of 100 g or more are even more likely to produce malignancy. The overall incidence of hematologic malignancies in patients receiving more than 30 g of cyclophosphamide may approach 5%. Radis et al. (18) reported a 20-year follow-up of the original study by Baker et al. and showed continued occurrence of cyclophosphamide-induced malignancies, including bladder cancer throughout the 20-year follow-up period. At the completion of this study, only 40% of the original patient population that was treated with cyclophosphamide remained cancer-free.

Myelodysplastic syndromes, specifically monosomy-5 and/or monosomy-7, have been observed in cyclophosphamide-treated patients with rheumatic disease (19). Although there is little data, there is no reason to believe that comparable doses of other alkylating agents such as chlorambucil or nitrogen mustard are safer. An increased incidence of cutaneous malignancies, including melanomas, squamous cell carcinomas, and aggressive basal cell carcinomas, has been observed (20). In addition, there is an increased risk of cervical dysplasia and carcinomas of the cervix and vulva. This risk is also a problem for transplant patients receiving various immunosuppressive drugs (20,21). Intravenous cyclophosphamide (IVC) therapy of patients with lupus has not been associated with a statistically significant increase in the incidence of fully developed cancers, probably because of the lower cumulative doses and the use of IV hydration to protect the urinary tract. This information may be deceptive due to the relative shorter lengths of follow-up obtained thus far.

Hemorrhagic cystitis, presumably induced in part by exposure to the metabolite acrolein, is a premalignant lesion that is identified in 50% of patients who eventually develop transitional cell carcinoma of the urinary tract, particularly the bladder. It is identified in 5% to 17% of oral cyclophosphamide-treated patients (22). Hemorrhagic cystitis is unusual in IV cyclophosphamide-treated patients with lupus, although it has been reported in patients who did not receive IV hydration (23) and in cancer chemotherapy patients receiving high doses. Use of sodium 2-mercaptoethane sulfonate (mesna) has been advocated to reduce the concentration of acrolein and perhaps other toxic metabolites in the bladder. Vigorous hydration and mesna used together may provide the best protection, although there is no established standard of care. Patients with neurogenic bladders may require bladder drainage or irrigation during treatment. In our institution, two patients with decreased urine output who received IVC without bladder irrigation developed severe posttreatment hemorrhagic cystitis.

Hematologic Effects

Compared with other alkylating agents such as nitrogen mustard, the acute effects of cyclophosphamide are relatively benign. Stem cells appear to be quite resistant to cyclophosphamide. After pulse therapy, the nadir of the lymphocyte count occurs on approximately day 7 to 10, and that of the granulocyte count on approximately day 10 to 14 (7). There usually is a prompt recovery from granulocytopenia after 21 to 28 days. In some patients, the recovery period may be prolonged, necessitating longer dose intervals. Prior use of alkylating agents may be associated with delayed recovery. Immunologically mediated cytopenias often improve after treatment with appropriate doses of IV cyclophosphamide, whereas they are more likely to worsen after azathioprine administration. Thrombocytopenia, which rarely occurs as a result of treatment except after prolonged therapy, may signify the onset of a myelodysplastic syndrome.

Other Cyclophosphamide-Induced Toxicity

Cyclophosphamide is toxic to the granulosa cell and, as a consequence, reduces serum estradiol levels and progesterone production, inhibits the maturation of oocytes, and reduces the number of ovarian follicles, ultimately resulting in ovarian failure. Studies in patients with breast cancer receiving cyclophosphamide show increasing toxicity to the ovaries from cyclophosphamide therapy with advancing age. In women with breast cancer in their 40s, 30s, or 20s, the cumulative doses of cyclophosphamide required to produce ovarian failure were 5, 9, or 20 g, respectively (5). Amenorrhea or premature ovarian failure is less likely to occur in patients who receive short-term (approximately 6 months) monthly IV cyclophosphamide.

Patients who are receiving cyclophosphamide may develop transient amenorrhea resulting from their illness (i.e., hypothalamic amenorrhea) or true ovarian failure because of cyclophosphamide. The risk of osteoporosis is increased by amenorrhea regardless of its cause.

Oral contraceptive use was reported to reduce ovarian failure in one uncontrolled series of patients with Hodgkin's disease (24). There is no evidence that administration of progestational agents is protective.

In female animals, administration of a gonadotropin-releasing hormone (GnRH) analogue suppresses the metabolic activity of granulosa cells, reducing the incorporation of tritiated thymidine into ovarian tissues. This treatment protects female rats and primates from cyclophosphamide-induced gonadal damage but not male rats (25,26). Studies of patients with cancer and lupus (27,28) have suggested that administration of depot preparations of GnRH analogue (depot-Lupron) during treatment with cyclophosphamide may be protective. During suppressive treatment patients experience symptoms of estrogen withdrawal, including hot flashes, and have an increased risk of osteoporosis and accelerated vascular disease unless estrogen is added back (29). Studies of women receiving a GnRH analogue for other indications showed endothelial dysfunction as evidenced by reduced dilatation of brachial arteries in response to hypoxic stress that was normalized by adding back estrogen. We have routinely provided estrogen replacement (with progestins, which avoid unopposed estrogen stimulation of the uterus) to women during ovarian suppression except when there is a clear contraindication, utilizing an estrogen in a strength that is intended to restore estrogen levels to slightly less than estimated levels prior to treatment (27).

Cyclophosphamide, a potent teratogen, can cause severe birth defects after administration of as little as 200 mg during early pregnancy (30–34). Reported abnormalities included absent thumbs, absence of the great toes or all toes, palatal abnormalities, and a single coronary artery. Because fertility is preserved in most lupus patients, highly effective contraceptive techniques (e.g., oral contraceptives or injected progestins in appropriately selected patients) should be strongly considered. Use of cyclophosphamide in life-threatening lupus during late pregnancy is controversial, but may be appropriate in special circumstances because fetal loss is extremely likely when severe maternal flares are uncontrolled. Major cyclophosphamide-induced toxicities are felt to occurs during the first half of pregnancy (35,36).

In males, azospermia is expected after extensive treatment and usually is irreversible. Administration of depot preparations of testosterone may be protective. Sperm banking should be considered, although it may be impractical in ill patients.

Infections frequently are observed in immunosuppressed patients with lupus who are receiving prednisone with or without cyclophosphamide or azathioprine. Use of the latter two drugs increases the risk of herpes zoster, and probably also of *Pneumocystis carinii* pneumonia (PCP) (37). Prophylaxis against PCP, now routine in the treatment of Wegener's, has lagged in lupus treatment, perhaps because of reluctance to administer trimethoprim-sulfamethoxazole (TMP-SMX) to lupus patients. We have used TMP-SMX three times weekly in lupus patients known to tolerate this drug, and otherwise have used dapsone (100 mg/day) in patients without glucose-6-phosphate dehydrogenase deficiency. In cyclophosphamide-treated patients with lupus, increased risk of infection has been associated with higher daily doses of prednisone and depression of the CD4/CD8 ratio in circulating lymphocytes (38). Hypogammaglobulinemia should be considered in patients who develop infections (39).

Gastrointestinal toxicity includes nausea and vomiting, constipation, late-onset diarrhea, intestinal dysmotility, and pseudomembranous colitis. Patients occasionally develop significant hepatotoxicity, with elevation of transaminases and jaundice (40,41). Cardiac toxicity may produce cardiac failure and mimic myocardial ischemia. Interstitial pneumonitis and/or fibrosis, proliferation of type II pneumocytes, interstitial inflammation, and interstitial fibrosis characterize pulmonary toxicity (42–44).

Clinical Trials With Cyclophosphamide For Lupus Nephritis

The literature regarding the use of cyclophosphamide in SLE, particularly lupus nephritis and central nervous system lupus, continues to increase at an exponential rate precluding a detailed review of all studies here. Results of controlled trials are summarized in Tables 57.1 and 57.3. In this discussion, trials of monthly bolus cyclophosphamide will be emphasized, but many modified regimens have been proposed, such as weekly or biweekly bolus cyclophosphamide given intravenously and boluses of cyclophosphamide given orally (45,46). These regimens have been reported to be safe and effective in small series. However, long-term data are not available, nor have these regimens been tested in controlled studies. More complicated regimens, including bolus cyclophosphamide synchronized with plasmapheresis and sequential regimens using cyclophosphamide followed by azathioprine have been described.

A 20-year clinical trial comparing most of the regimens that have been widely used to treat lupus nephritis was performed at the National Institutes of Health (NIH) including patients with mostly proliferative nephritis, all of whom were treated with daily oral glucocorticosteroids at the initiation of immunosuppressive therapy (47,49–51). Patients were given (a) no additional therapy, (b) oral azathioprine, (c) oral azathioprine plus oral cyclophosphamide, (d) oral cyclophosphamide, or (e) IV cyclophosphamide. The duration of administration of these agents differed, ranging from approximately 2 to 4 years. The IV cyclophosphamide-treated patients had a variable number of monthly pulses (often three) before being assigned to once-every-3-months cyclophosphamide therapy (Fig. 57.1). There were several key findings: (a) Differences in outcome were not apparent until more than 5 years had elapsed. Until that time, prednisone-treated patients had the same rate of renal failure and death as immunosuppressed patients. This may relate in part to the relatively mild degree of renal compromise in some patients at entry and the use of renal failure or death as end points. After 10 years, however, there were marked differences in renal survival, favoring any regimen that included cyclophosphamide over the administration of prednisone alone. (b) There was a trend for patients treated with either prednisone alone or oral cyclophosphamide to have higher death rates than patients who were treated with

TABLE 57.1. CONTROLLED TRIALS OF CYCLOPHOSPHAMIDE AND/OR AZATHIOPRINE IN THE TREATMENT OF LUPUS NEPHRITIS

Study	Patients (*n*)	Results
Fries et al. (52)	14	P > CTX alone
Garancis and Piering (53)	22	P + CTX > P + AZA
Donadio et al. (54–56)	26	More recurrences with P; P vs. P + CTX = survival, and on dialysis
Ginzler et al. (117)	14	P + AZA = P + CTX
Balow et al. (47)	111	P + IVC > P + AZA + CTX > P + AZA > P
Boumpas et al. (58)	65	IVC for 30 months > IVCX for 6 months > MP
Sesso et al. (60)	29	IVC or MP both unsuccessful
Gourley et al. (59)	80	IVC > MP; trend for IVC + MP > IVC

AZA, azathioprine; POC, oral cyclophosphamide; IVC, intravenous, intermittent cyclophosphamide; MP, bolus methylprednisolone; P, prednisone.

IV cyclophosphamide or azathioprine plus cyclophosphamide. This probably reflects the toxicity of oral cyclophosphamide and ineffectiveness and toxicity of prednisone alone. (c) The combination regimen of oral azathioprine plus cyclophosphamide appeared to work as well as IV cyclophosphamide in terms of progression to renal failure or death. (d) Retrospective analysis suggested that the presence of chronic change on initial biopsy was a poor prognostic factor, predicting a poor outcome unless immunosuppressives were used. (e) In the subset of patients who underwent serial biopsies, progression of chronic change occurred initially in all patients. Immunosuppressive-treated patients appeared to stabilize after an initial period of scarring; prednisone-treated patients had further scarring.

Oral Cyclophosphamide

Most studies of cyclophosphamide have compared cyclophosphamide and prednisone versus prednisone alone. An interesting study by Fries et al. (52) in 1973, however, compared oral cyclophosphamide alone versus prednisone alone for a mean of 9 weeks in 14 patients with lupus, ten of whom had nephritis. Cyclophosphamide failed to control either minor or major manifestations, despite development of leukopenia and significant additional toxicity in many patients. Patients who were changed to prednisone from cyclophosphamide did better. These results suggest that cyclophosphamide and prednisone may act synergistically.

In a randomized trial, Garancis and Piering (53) treated 22 patients with biopsy-proven membranoproliferative glomerulonephritis using low-dose prednisone (approximately 10 mg/d) and 2 mg/kg/d of either cyclophosphamide or azathioprine. After 6 to 36 months, the cyclophosphamide-treated patients had better renal function and fewer deaths (none vs. four).

In another randomized trial, Donadio (54–56) assigned 50 patients with diffuse proliferative glomerulonephritis to treatment either with 6 months of oral cyclophosphamide plus prednisone or with prednisone alone, re-treating patients who subsequently flared with 6 additional months of oral cyclophosphamide. The cyclophosphamide-treated group had fewer flares of renal disease after 2 years and was felt to have a more favorable clinical course. Cyclophosphamide appeared to have a steroid-sparing effect. Patients with advanced renal insufficiency (i.e., creatinine clearance ≤30 mL/min) appeared not to benefit from this regimen. After 4 years, however, there was no difference in progression to death or renal failure between the two groups.

Fu et al. (57) compared daily oral cyclophosphamide with cyclosporine in children with nephritis and found no difference in efficacy. The details of this somewhat atypical protocol are reviewed below (see Cyclosporine).

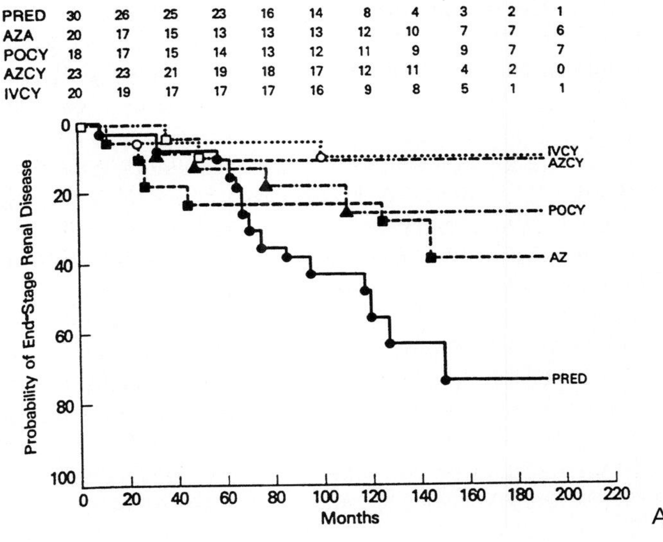

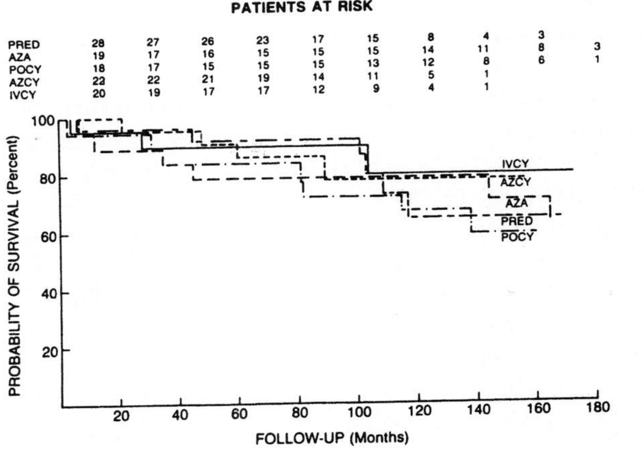

FIGURE 57.1. A: Probability of progression to end-stage renal disease in the study population by treatment group: prednisone only (PRED), azathioprine (AZ), oral cyclophosphamide (POCY), oral azathioprine plus oral cyclophosphamide (AZCY), and intravenous cyclophosphamide (IVCY). Survival curves are shown, with end-stage renal disease as the outcome. The number of patients at risk in each group is shown for each 20-month time point. The curves for the AZCY, IVCY, and POCY groups were significantly different from that of the control (PRED) group (p = .0011, p = .0025, and p = .032, respectively). The AZ group did not differ significantly from the PRED group (p = .09). The Mantel statistic from which the p values (vs. PRED) were obtained was: AZ, 2.872; POCY, 4.619; AZCY, 10.571; and IVCY, 9.169. The 95% confidence intervals at the 120-month (10-year) point were as follows: PRED, 0.67–0.23; AZ, 0.93–0.49; POCY, 0.97–0.53; AZCY, 1.00–0.78; and IVCY, 1.00–0.74. (From Steinberg AD, Steinberg SC. Long-term preservation of renal function in patients with lupus nephritis receiving treatment that includes cyclophosphamide versus those treated with prednisone only. *Arthritis Rheum* 1991;34:945–950, with permission.) **B:** Probability of survival in patients with lupus nephritis by treatment groups: prednisone (PRED), azathioprine (AZA), oral cyclophosphamide (POCY), combined oral azathioprine and cyclophosphamide (AZCY), and intravenous cyclophosphamide (IVCY). (From Balow et al. (47), with permission.)

Bolus Cyclophosphamide In Lupus Nephritis

Monthly bolus cyclophosphamide (IVC), first described as a treatment for lupus in 1984 by Sessoms and Kovarsky (23), is now the best studied immunosuppressive regimen for severe lupus. More than two dozen studies have been published, most of which focus on lupus nephritis. Early experience indicated that 6 months was too short a duration of treatment for patients with lupus nephritis, approximately 50% of whom experienced flares after discontinuation.

These observations were confirmed by Boumpas et al. (58), who compared three regimens in a relatively sick group of patients with lupus nephritis: seven monthly pulses of prednisone, seven monthly pulses of IVC, or seven monthly pulses of IVC followed by maintenance pulses of IVC every 3 months. All groups received oral prednisone. End points, such as doubling of serum creatinine, were relatively sensitive, and differences between the treatment groups were evident after a few years. In this study, seven monthly pulses of IVC followed by an every-3-month maintenance regimen resulted in fewer flares and fewer doublings of serum creatinine compared with seven monthly pulses of cyclophosphamide without maintenance pulses every 3 months or seven monthly pulses of methylprednisolone (Fig. 57.2). The longer IVC regimen resulted in more toxicity, however, particularly ovarian failure. In addition, bolus methylprednisolone was not as effective as long-term cyclophosphamide.

A related study compared bolus IVC vs. bolus methylprednisolone vs. both regimens as treatment for lupus nephritis (59). As in the previously described study, cyclophosphamide was clearly superior to bolus methylprednisolone. Interestingly, although statistical significance was not achieved, there was a strong suggestion that addition of bolus methylprednisolone to bolus cyclophosphamide increased the efficacy of the latter, suggesting that this approach might also be appropriate for "salvage" in patients who do not appear to be responding to bolus cyclophosphamide. Patients who received methylprednisolone pulses had more osteonecrosis than those who did not.

An opposite conclusion was reached by Sesso et al. (60). They compared short-term IVC versus bolus methylprednisolone in 29 patients with severe lupus nephritis. Patients received eight pulses (roughly comparable with the short-term arm on the previously described study by Boumpas et al. (58) in terms of total dose) over a 13-month period without maintenance IVC. This study found no difference in outcome. Survival without renal failure was a disappointing 62% over a mean 15 months of follow-up; 5 of 29 patients (17%) died. The high rate of initial treatment failures in the cyclophosphamide group and shorter-term follow-up could explain the lack of differences in outcome compared with those of other studies.

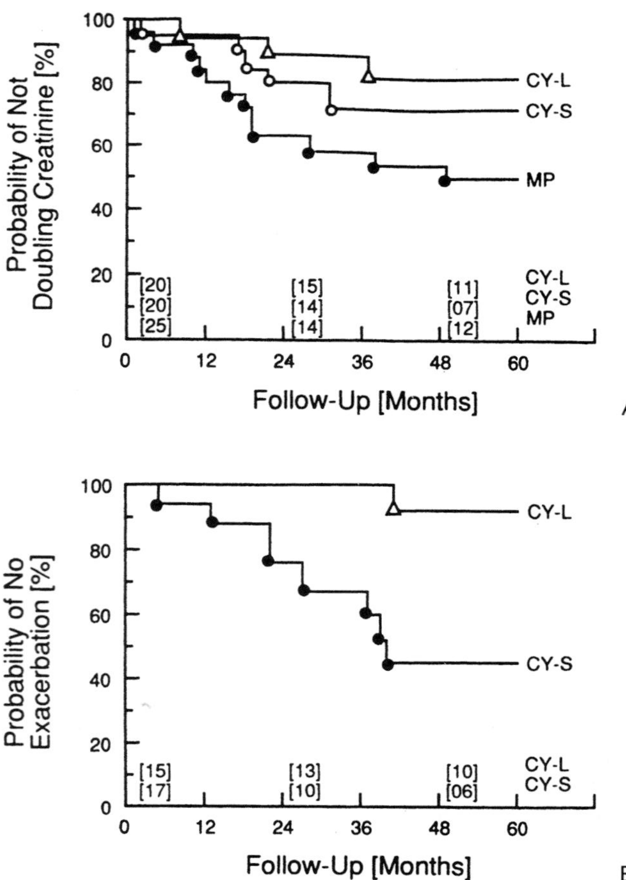

FIGURE 57.2. Treatment of severe lupus nephritis. **A:** Probability of not doubling serum creatinine levels in 65 patients with severe active lupus nephritis randomly assigned to receive: IV methylprednisolone (MP), 1.0 g/m^2 monthly for 6 months; IV cyclophosphamide (CY-S), 0.5 to 1.0 g/m^2 monthly for 6 months; or IV cyclophosphamide (CY-L), 0.5 to 1.0 g/m^2 monthly for 6 months, followed by quarterly infusions for 24 months (Gehan test comparing CY-L with MP, $p = .037$). **B:** Probability of no exacerbation of lupus activity on completion of monthly pulses in groups randomly assigned to receive CY-L and CY-S (Gehan test, $p = .006$). Numbers of patients that remain at risk at various times are shown along the abscissa. (From Boumpas DT, Austin HA, Vaughn EM, et al. Controlled trial of pulse methylprednisolone versus two regimens of pulse cyclophosphamide in severe lupus nephritis. *Lancet* 1992;340:741–745, with permission.)

Boletis et al. (61) compared IVC with ten immunoglobulin infusions and found equivalent results over an 18-month period. Proteinuria actually increased slightly in the IVC group.

A review of these studies, as well as the voluminous literature regarding open trials of cyclophosphamide, and the authors' experience suggests the following:

1. Approximately 80% of patients respond to treatment after 6 monthly pulses, of whom 20% will flare when the frequency of treatment is reduced to every 3 months and continued for an additional 2 years. Gradual reduc-

tion of the frequency of treatment from monthly to every 2 months for 6 months and then to every 3 months may reduce the number of unexpected severe flares. If no immunosuppression is given after the first 6 months, the flare rate approaches 50%. In the event of a partial but unsatisfactory response, continued monthly treatment may be successful.

2. Patients with renal insufficiency average an approximately 30% improvement in creatinine clearance during the first 6 months, but tend to backslide toward baseline values after 1 to 2 years. It is interesting to speculate that this may result from continued glomerular scarring in the apparent absence of inflammation, as described by Chaghac in total lymphoid irradiation-treated lupus nephritis patients (62). However, it is possible that inflammation recurs as immunosuppression is reduced or that other processes such as occult hypertension and hyperfiltration may be important factors.
3. Proteinuria and features of nephrotic syndrome usually improve substantially during the first 6 to 12 months. Patients who are not in complete remission after 6 months (e.g., proteinuria reduced but not yet <1 g) may have continued reduction of proteinuria during less intensive therapy.
4. Treatment of nephrotic syndrome resulting from either class IV or class V nephritis results in reduction of proteinuria, increased serum albumin levels, and improvement of hypercholesterolemia, which otherwise may be severe and relatively refractory to diet or pharmacologic treatment. The substantial reduction of cardiovascular risk that obtains in many cases may outweigh the risk of treatment even in some patients destined ultimately to develop renal failure.
5. Sequential treatment consisting of "induction" of clinical improvement followed by "maintenance" treatment with a less toxic immunosuppressive may reduce toxicity while maintaining disease control. Presently there are published series using azathioprine as a follow-up agent in both adults and children proliferative and membranous nephritis, suggesting that some patients do well with this approach (63–65). In our experience most, but not all, patients remain controlled when this approach is used; some patients flare repeatedly when switched from cyclophosphamide to azathioprine. This approach may be particularly beneficial to individuals who wish to retain fertility. As there is little long-term experience with this approach, further studies are needed. Other potential approaches to sequential therapy include use of cyclosporine or mycophenolate mofetil (or both) after induction of remission with bolus cyclophosphamide.
6. The concept that one should demonstrate that corticosteroids are ineffective in patients with severe nephritis before adding immunosuppressives is clearly obsolete. In some severe cases cyclophosphamide appears to be indispensable, as illustrated in our institution by unsuccessful attempts to avoid using cyclophosphamide in pregnant women by combining multiple less toxic agents, even in the short term. Conversely, in milder cases, prompt treatment with a less toxic immunosuppressive may delay or avoid use of cyclophosphamide.
7. McInnes et al. (66) compared the projected cost of therapy, kidney dialysis, and loss of work of treating 1,130 patients annually with prednisone plus IVC versus that of treating them with prednisone alone. A $50 million savings in patient-care costs and $42 million savings in loss of work costs was projected resulting from the use of IVC.

Intravenous Cyclophosphamide In Nonrenal Lupus

In general, severe nonrenal manifestations of lupus that result from immune complex disease respond more rapidly and completely to IVC plus corticosteroids than to corticosteroids alone. The required treatment duration and size of individual IVC boluses varies with different disease manifestations. For example, severe transverse myelitis may respond to a shorter course of treatment than severe nephritis, and immune-mediated thrombocytopenia may respond to lower than usual doses. During treatment of severe lupus with IVC, improvement of minor manifestations, including constitutional symptoms, fevers, arthralgias, rash, pleurisy, and serologic abnormalities, and reduced prednisone requirements usually occur within 3 months.

Neuropsychiatric Lupus

No clear guidelines exist regarding therapy for neuropsychiatric lupus (NPSLE) with various modalities, including corticosteroids, cyclophosphamide, and/or anticoagulation. Distinction between various primary pathogenic mechanisms, such as immune complex–mediated vasculitis, antibody-mediated cerebral injury, microangiopathy, thrombosis, or secondary causes such as atherosclerosis or infection, is notoriously difficult, and is further complicated by the multifactorial etiology of many events. In many cases, skilled physicians must make a "seat-of-the-pants" decision regarding the use of immunosuppression, anticoagulation, or both, based on clinical, serologic, or magnetic resonance imaging evidence, unless there is biopsy evidence of tissue inflammation or cerebrospinal fluid pleocytosis. In many series, treatment decisions have been made (apparently appropriately) on the basis of clinical judgment, rather than on specific inclusion criteria.

In our hands, active, steroid-refractory cerebral lupus that is adjudged to be secondary to immunologically mediated injury has responded well to IVC with or without bolus methylprednisolone in most cases. Anticoagulation has been used simultaneously when it has been impossible to distinguish thrombotic from inflammatory disease or to rule out the possibility that vascular inflammation is contributing to the development of thrombosis. Neither the presence of antiphospholipid antibodies nor involvement of one or more large vessels rules out use of immunosuppression as opposed to anticoagulation. Boumpas et al. (67) treated nine patients with monthly IVC, three of whom had transverse myelitis and five of whom had focal neurologic findings, seizures, or both. The duration of symptoms ranged from 3 to 45 days. All nine patients had findings suggesting an inflammatory process, including anti-DNA antibodies, and five had cerebrospinal fluid pleocytosis. Five of these patients concomitantly had antiphospholipid antibodies. All patients recovered either partially or completely. These observations suggest that in selected patients who have antiphospholipid antibodies that may not be the major cause of their events, IV cyclophosphamide administration is associated with clinical improvement.

Other series of IVC in NPSLE report favorable results. Neuwelt et al. (68) retrospectively reviewed 31 patients with neuropsychiatric lupus who were treated with IVC and who had failed a variety of prior therapies, including corticosteroids, Coumadin, chlorambucil, and azathioprine. Indications included organic brain syndrome in 55% of patients, strokes in 35%, peripheral mononeuropathies in 32%, seizures in 29%, and transverse myelitis in 16%. Patients with anticardiolipin antibodies were treated with warfarin. Treatment regimens varied from low to high doses of IV cyclophosphamide, and plasmapheresis was added to some patients when they appeared not to improve after IVC. Overall, 61% of patients were reported to improve, of whom 26% were not initially improved after 9 months of therapy and appeared to respond to addition of plasmapheresis. The failure rate for patients with organic brain syndrome was 83%, compared with 37% for other indications. Malaviya et al. (69) treated 14 patients with a variety of focal and diffuse neurologic deficits. All patients except the two with seizures stabilized or improved.

Numerous studies have demonstrated improvement of transverse myelitis with IVC, with or without bolus corticosteroids (70,71). Because of the catastrophic nature of transverse myelitis and the importance of prompt therapeutic intervention, it may be appropriate to have a very low threshold for prompt institution of IVC when this syndrome appears suddenly, with or without concomitant high-dose (e.g., 1 g/m^2) methylprednisolone. In our institution, prompt use of bolus cyclophosphamide for transverse myelitis has been associated with preservation of the ability to ambulate in most patients, although many have continued to have neurogenic bladders.

Ten patients with bilateral corticosteroid-refractory optic neuritis and severe visual compromise were treated with bolus cyclophosphamide for 6 months (72). Ten of 20 eyes recovered completely, six partially, and four did not.

Baca (72a) treated seven children with NPSLE (including seizures, focal neurologic deficits, transverse myelitis, and organic brain syndromes) with monthly bolus cyclophosphamide combined with three initial boluses of 30 mg/kg methylprednisolone. Three patients had anticardiolipin antibodies but were not anticoagulated. Six patients recovered completely and one had a minor residual deficit.

Other Disease Manifestations

Numerous corticosteroid-refractory manifestations of lupus have been reported to benefit from pulse cyclophosphamide in case reports and uncontrolled series, including systemic vasculitis, and gastrointestinal vasculitis and pneumatosis intestinalis (73). Hematologic conditions reported to respond include aplastic anemia (74,75) acquired factor VIII deficiency (76), and acquired von Willebrand disease (77), as well as lupus-induced cytopenias, particularly thrombocytopenia. Thrombocytopenia in active lupus possibly may respond to lower pulses of cyclophosphamide than are necessary to control other disease manifestations. Roach and Hutchinson (78) successfully treated steroid-refractory thrombocytopenia on two occasions in one patient with only 400 mg of IV cyclophosphamide. Boumpas et al. (79) found overall improvement of thrombocytopenia in patients who were treated according to the NIH protocol. Although IV cyclophosphamide should not, in our opinion, be substituted for plasmapheresis and plasma exchange in thrombotic thrombocytopenic purpura (TTP) in patients with lupus, it has been added to plasma exchange for this indication (80,81). Bolus cyclophosphamide alone may be ineffective for lupus-related TTP; two of our patients developed TTP during monthly bolus cyclophosphamide therapy for nephritis, and, despite prompt addition of plasma exchange, one patient died and the other progressed to renal failure.

Several studies suggest that lupus-related interstitial lung disease and bronchiolitis obliterans may respond to monthly cyclophosphamide (82,83). Fukada et al. (84) also noted a response of pulmonary hemorrhage to IVC. In our experience, IVC is associated with control of pulmonary hemorrhage in patients with lupus who appear to be steroid refractory in the majority of cases. Although cases of idiopathic inflammatory myositis have not uniformly responded well to IVC in the published literature, three patients with SLE were reported by Kono et al. (85) to have remission of refractory polymyositis with the addition of IVC.

In summary, these nonrenal manifestations of lupus appear to respond to IVC in most cases when steroid therapy had apparently failed. These results do not establish the superiority of IV over oral cyclophosphamide for these indications, however.

Bolus Cyclophosphamide In Children

IVC has been used successfully in children of all ages, including infants (86). Studies by Lehman and Onel (87) of treatment with IVC for 36 months have shown good disease control and arrest of progression of the chronicity index. This group has also added intravenous methotrexate to IVC in refractory patients with benefit (88). It is our opinion that daily oral cyclophosphamide is clearly less desirable in children with lupus, as it is in adults, because of its toxicity, and that it should not be used as first-line therapy instead of bolus cyclophosphamide.

Combination therapy for severe lupus with synchronized plasmapheresis and cyclophosphamide has been proposed by Euler et al. (89,90). The rationale for this mode of therapy is that the depletion of circulating autoantibodies may stimulate increased activity of lymphocytes and plasma cells that are responsible for immunoglobulin formation, resulting in increased susceptibility to cyclophosphamide. Two regimens have been proposed, one of which involves performing a single pheresis before each of a series of monthly pulses of cyclophosphamide. A controlled trial did not show significant benefit from adding pheresis to IVC. The second, more intensive protocol includes daily plasmapheresis on 3 successive days of 60 mL/kg, followed on days 4, 5, and 6 by three pulses of 12 mg/kg of IV cyclophosphamide. Patients then are treated over a 6-month period with escalating doses of oral cyclophosphamide and 1 mg/kg/d of prednisone that gradually is tapered. This treatment regimen is highly toxic even when granulocyte colony-stimulating factor (GCSF) is employed to treat leukopenia, and deaths have resulted. However, in a patient population with mixed indications for therapy including pneumonitis, nephritis, retinal vasculitis, and pericarditis, there was marked overall reduction of disease activity in 12 of 14 treated patients, and at final assessment eight patients were reported to be clinically well for a mean follow-up time of 6 years. Seven patients developed amenorrhea. This highly complex protocol appears to achieve satisfactory results in most patients when in expert hands, but it has been extremely toxic (90–93). It may represent an intermediate intensity of treatment between conventional and high-dose cyclophosphamide regimens

Aggressive Cyclophosphamide-Containing Regimens

High-dose cyclophosphamide regimens sufficient to arrest production of hematopoietic cells are being tried in lupus. Because stem cells are resistant to cyclophosphamide, the marrow recovers after a period requiring support with cells and colony-stimulating factors. Brodsky and colleagues (94) reported treating patients with severe SLE with 200 mg/kg cyclophosphamide with complete responses in half the patients. There were no deaths.

Autologous stem cell transplantation utilizing high-dose cyclophosphamide with or without additional immunosuppressives is being evaluated in a number of rheumatic diseases. One study reported enrollment of nine patients in a protocol (95), of whom one died during induction and seven ultimately underwent transplantation. Fluid overload occurred in all patients; three required dialysis or hemofiltration and two were intubated. All patients responded clinically and were able to discontinue immunosuppressive medications. The dramatic disease suppression reported appears to exceed that of high-dose cyclophosphamide regimens. However, the short-term toxicity appears to be greater. Across the world the mortality of stem cell transplantation for rheumatic diseases exceeds 10%. This figure may improve with modifications of treatment regimens and criteria for patient selection.

Summary Of IVC Therapy For Lupus

1. There is no evidence that IVC is more effective than oral cyclophosphamide in patients with lupus in the long run, but it is unquestionably less toxic.
2. The dose and duration of IVC required to achieve disease control vary with the disease manifestation. For instance, a subset of patients with lupus nephritis almost certainly requires treatment for at least 2 to 3 years. Many patients with neurologic disease appear to be well controlled after 3 to 6 monthly pulses of IV cyclophosphamide. Relatively low doses that are administered short term may help to achieve control of thrombocytopenia or hemolytic anemia.
3. Prednisone has been employed with oral or IV cyclophosphamide in all studies showing efficacy. Daily oral cyclophosphamide without prednisone was not effective in a single controlled study.
4. High doses of prednisone (≥20 mg/d) administered with IVC increased the risk of infection.
5. The cumulative dose of cyclophosphamide predicts the risk of gonadal injury and risk of secondary malignancies. Intense and prolonged surveillance for malignant and premalignant conditions (especially those resulting from human papillomavirus [HPV]) is indicated in cyclophosphamide-treated patients.
6. Failure of active lupus to respond to IVC does not imply that the disease manifestation is inherently untreatable. Potential interventions include addition of bolus methylprednisolone or another immunosuppressive to IVC, use of nitrogen mustard, high-dose cyclophosphamide or stem cell transplantation, or use of pheresis if a microangiopathy has supervened.
7. The indications for IVC therapy for neurologic disease are poorly characterized. The possibility that an antiphospholipid antibody syndrome exists is not in itself a contraindication to the treatment of apparent inflammatory disease. In catastrophic neurologic disease in which the etiology is unclear, combined anticoagulation and immunosuppression should be considered.

Nitrogen Mustard

Nitrogen mustard (mechlorethamine) is a highly potent alkylating agent with prolonged immunosuppressive and immunomodulatory effects. Although it is infrequently used at the present time, a detailed review is in order, because it appears to be quite efficacious in severe lupus and may have different properties than IV cyclophosphamide. For instance, studies in patients with rheumatoid arthritis show that nitrogen mustard when administered intravenously is effective in suppressing disease activity, whereas IV cyclophosphamide given monthly probably is not.

Nitrogen mustard is administered in its active form and has potent caustic, immunosuppressive, and carcinogenic effects on exposed tissue. These properties are responsible for the high incidence of thrombophlebitis and local irritation at IV infusion sites, as well as for the risk of severe tissue necrosis if the drug is extravasated. These effects also occur during topical application and are responsible for the reports of successful therapy for both cutaneous lupus and other cutaneous diseases, such as mycosis fungoides. Topical application of nitrogen mustard is associated with the induction of primary or secondary malignancies at the application site.

Nitrogen mustard is considered to be a more potent stimulant of nausea and vomiting than cyclophosphamide. Reviews that deal with this side effect generally were written before the introduction of highly effective antiemetic agents or antiemetic combinations, such as the combination of ondansetron, lorazepem, diphenhydramine, and dexamethasone. Judicious use of these agents when coupled with vigorous hydration, both immediately after drug administration to reduce local tissue damage effects and during the period of time that nausea and vomiting may occur, could considerably reduce the immediate toxicity of this drug.

The bone marrow effects of nitrogen mustard differ from those of cyclophosphamide. Hematologic toxicity of nitrogen mustard following the administration of a single course of this drug has been reported to be relatively modest by Dubois (96), who treated patients only after a bone marrow examination to rule out bone marrow hypocellularity. In this setting, the nadir of the leukocyte count is said rarely to fall below 2,500 cells/mL, although the period of leukopenia is far longer than that associated with cyclophosphamide, on the order of 6 weeks. This appears to result in part from the increased toxicity of nitrogen mustard to stem cells. Although reports of secondary hematologic malignancies in nitrogen mustard–treated patients with lupus are rare, patients who were treated with nitrogen mustard for hematologic diseases have an increased incidence of secondary hematologic malignancies, including myelodysplastic syndromes. The rarity of such reports in patients with connective tissue disease may relate in part to the lower cumulative doses that usually are administered in this population, which may relate in turn to the cumbersome nature of this therapy.

Nitrogen mustard is given as a course of approximately 0.3 to 0.4 mg/kg (15 to 20 mg), either as a single IV dose administered in a large amount of fluid over 1 hour and followed by vigorous hydration, or as two divided doses given 12 hours apart. In some patients, courses have been repeated as often as every 6 weeks.

Clinical responses to nitrogen mustard have been observed as rapidly as within several days, and they are more protracted than those to IV cyclophosphamide. During a period when the prognosis of lupus nephritis was poor, outcomes were in general better than those obtained with prednisone alone, although they were worse than those obtained today with improved supportive care and adjunctive agents (Table 57.2). It therefore is difficult to evaluate nitrogen mustard in the context of modern therapeutic adjuncts.

In 1954, Dubois (96) reported the treatment of 33 patients with 20 mg of IV nitrogen mustard. He initially treated most patients with steroids or antimalarials, only adding nitrogen mustard after 2 months of unsuccessful therapy with prednisone. Twenty-six of the 33 patients had renal disease. Interestingly, none of the patients who did not have nephritis benefited from treatment; 13 of 16 nephrotic and seven of ten nonnephrotic patients with renal disease improved. In many cases, he observed diuresis within a few days in patients with nephrotic syndrome. Long-term survival was greater in those patients with nephritis who responded to the treatment. Wallace et al. (97) reviewed the therapy of nephritis in the same practice, including 44 patients receiving 74 courses of nitrogen mustard. After 40 days, improvement of multiple parameters, including urinary sediment, serum cholesterol, steroid dosage, serum creatinine, and urine protein excretion was noted (Table 57.2). The response rate again was noted to be higher in patients with nephrotic syndrome. Favorable responses to one or two courses were said to have lasted for years in some patients.

In 1973, Dillard et al. (98) described the treatment of 17 patients with diffuse proliferative glomerulonephritis using nitrogen mustard. Five patients died of renal failure, four within 6 weeks. The remaining 12 patients improved, seven of whom had no exacerbation of renal disease after a mean follow-up of 33 months. All were reported to have normal renal function and protein excretion at follow-up. Nitrogen mustard was felt to be steroid sparing and to be associated with reduction of the level of activity in serial renal biopsies, although the severity (i.e., chronicity) score was not reduced by therapy. Results were said to be unsatisfactory in patients with high levels of both disease activity and scarring.

Wallace and Metzger (99) reported that administration of one or two courses of nitrogen mustard, 0.4 mg/kg, resulted in improvement of disease activity in two patients with severe nephritis and nephrotic syndrome who failed to respond to monthly IVC, one of whom had failed 32 prior

TABLE 57.2. PARAMETERS 40 DAYS AFTER NITROGEN MUSTARD ADMINISTRATION

	Incidence		Disappeared at 40 Days		
Parameter	*n*	%	*n*	%	Mean Duration of Response (mo)
Hematuria	45/56	80	14/45	31	46
Hyaline casts	28/58	48	11/28	39	33
Granular casts	32/56	57	11/32	34	63
Oval fat bodies	19/56	34	2/19	11	—

	Decreased			
Parameter	*n*	%	Criteria for Decrease	Mean Decrease
Serum creatinine level	13/33	39	≥0.1 mg/dL	0.63 mg/dL
Serum cholesterol level	19/27	70	≥1 mg/dL	99 mg/dL
24-hour urine protein level	31/38	82	100 mg	3,595 mg
Prednisone dosage	26/43	60	≥1 mg	19 mg
Weight	39/57	68	≥0.1 kg	2 kg

From Wallace et al. (97), with permission.

courses of IVC. Topical application of nitrogen mustard has been advocated in severe cutaneous lupus; however, this can result in local induction of malignancy (100). The role of nitrogen mustard in the management of severe lupus is unclear at present. In patients with nephritis, it appears to offer the potential to dramatically reduce severe disease activity for several months after a single intervention, perhaps in patients who have failed cyclophosphamide or pulse steroid therapy.

Chlorambucil

Chlorambucil is an alkylating agent that differs from nitrogen mustard because it does not produce local irritative effects, and from cyclophosphamide because it is not metabolized to acrolein and does not cause hemorrhagic cystitis. In patients with lupus, it is administered orally in daily doses of from 2 to 12 mg. It has been used as an IV bolus in patients with multiple sclerosis (101) or sarcoidosis (102). Chlorambucil is toxic to dividing cells (103), but it also may have immunomodulatory effects. In idiopathic membranous nephritis, reduction of the number of T cells and reduction of the CD4/CD8 ratio resulted from alternating monthly oral prednisone and oral chlorambucil (104). Monthly pulse chlorambucil in multiple sclerosis was reported to disproportionately reduce circulating B cells (101). The dose, rate of administration, and underlying disease probably alter the observed effects of chlorambucil on immune function, as is the case with cyclophosphamide.

Side effects of chlorambucil that may differ from cyclophosphamide include both marrow suppression and malignancy. Recovery of stem cells is less rapid than after cyclophosphamide administration. Published series suggest that substantial difficulty is encountered during treatment resulting from suppression, which may be irreversible, of individual circulating cell lines (red cells, leukocytes, and platelets) (105).

Chlorambucil is a potent oncogen. Its oncogenicity relative to cyclophosphamide is controversial; however, it is in our opinion more dangerous than IVC. Somatic and germ cell mutations (103,105), leukemias, myelodysplastic syndromes, and cutaneous malignancies are increased. Of 144 patients with polycythemia vera who were treated with chlorambucil, 11% developed leukemia after 5.4 years, representing a 13.5-fold increase over patients treated with phlebotomy alone (105a). Patapanian et al. (106) identified significant excess malignancy compared with controls in 39 patients with rheumatoid arthritis after 5 years; three hematologic and eight cutaneous malignancies were identified.

Studies of this potentially useful agent are too limited to permit comparison with other immunosuppressive drugs. However, it almost certainly is effective against lupus when combined with prednisone.

In 1973, Snaith et al. (107) reported improvement of steroid-resistant nephritis in five of five patients and of active lupus in a sixth using chlorambucil, 2 to 5 mg/d. Amenorrhea developed in four patients. In 1974, Epstein and Grausz (108) reported improved survival in 16 of 31 patients with lupus and diffuse proliferative nephritis who received chlorambucil in addition to prednisone, but they also reported serious toxicity, including marrow aplasia in five patients, leading to one death. In Egypt, Sabbour and Osman (109), in a retrospective study of a group of patients with very high mortality (58% over 5 years), found prednisone plus chlorambucil to be associated with better survival than prednisone alone or prednisone plus oral cyclophosphamide. Survival and reduction of proteinuria were markedly better in chlorambucil-treated patients than in other groups; however, the chlorambucil-treated patients were treated much more recently than other groups

There has been little recent work with chlorambucil in lupus; however, it has been extensively studied in idiopathic membranous and proliferative nephritis and nephrotic syndrome. Regimens containing chlorambucil generally have been felt to be effective, and in one study they were found to be superior to monthly pulse cyclophosphamide (110, 111).

Azathioprine

In contrast to cyclophosphamide, azathioprine has not been extensively studied in the past decade as a therapeutic agent in lupus nephritis. The caveats that apply to older studies of nephritis (i.e., potentially confounding effects on renal survival of differences in management of hypertension, use of angiotensin-converting enzyme inhibitors or other measures to prevent progression of renal disease) apply here (Table 57.1). The following controlled studies of azathioprine have yielded disparate results, suggesting that azathioprine is effective in some, but not all, patients.

In the large NIH trial, low-dose azathioprine added to low-dose cyclophosphamide plus prednisone was as effective as IV cyclophosphamide (administered every 3 months) plus prednisone, with comparable mortality and toxicity (50,51,112). Compared with oral cyclophosphamide, renal survival was the same, but there was a trend that failed to reach statistical significance for the combination regimen to be associated with lower mortality. Thus, azathioprine appears to have a cyclophosphamide-sparing effect when used in combination with that drug. Overall outcomes in the NIH study of azathioprine alone plus prednisone (without cyclophosphamide treatment with azathioprine) were intermediate between prednisone and cyclophosphamide-containing regimens and failed to achieve significance, although they were better than prednisone alone.

Donadio et al. (113) randomized 16 patients to azathioprine plus prednisone versus prednisone alone. After 6 months, there was histologic improvement in measures of disease activity (i.e., karyorrhexis, proliferation, fibrinoid deposition, hyaline thrombi, necrosis) in both groups, but there was no difference in outcome after 6 months or after 2 to 3 years (114). Hahn et al. (115) randomized severely ill patients with lupus to prednisone with or without azathioprine over a 2-year period and found no differences in outcome. However, patients with nephritis entered into the azathioprine group were more likely to have severe renal disease with diffuse proliferative glomerulonephritis on biopsy, possibly resulting in underestimation of the efficacy of this drug.

In a study that illustrates the difficulty of distinguishing the toxicity of one drug regimen from the efficacy of alternate therapy, Cade et al. (116) used four different regimens to treat 50 patients with lupus, including prednisone alone, prednisone plus azathioprine, azathioprine alone, and azathioprine plus heparin. Unfortunately, 13 of 15 prednisone-treated patients died, with a mean survival of 19 months, after receiving 60 to 100 mg of prednisone daily for 6 months. In the azathioprine plus prednisone group (which received lower doses of prednisone), nine of 13 patients survived, with a mean survival of 38 months. Compared with the very high-dose prednisone group, azathioprine alone or in combination with either prednisone or heparin produced superior results.

In a double-blind, crossover trial, Ginzler et al. (117) compared azathioprine plus prednisone with prednisone alone and found no benefit.

Recent studies suggest that azathioprine may be most useful either in early stages of nephritis to prevent development of more severe lesions or as maintenance therapy after IVC (as noted earlier). Esdaile (117a) conducted an elegant study in the 1980s at Yale of lupus nephritis patients who received immunosuppression for lupus nephritis. Almost all immunosuppressed patients were treated with azathioprine. When patients who received early biopsies and treatment

TABLE 57.3. CONTROLLED TRIALS INCLUDING BOLUS METHYLPREDNISOLONE, CYCLOSPORIN, OR IV IMMUNOGLOBULIN IN SLE

Author	Therapeutic Arms	Result
Boumpas (58) 1992	IVC short-term IVC long-term Bolus MP	Long-term IVC > short-term Bolus MP < either IVC
Sesso (60) 1994	IVC Bolus MP	Equivalent outcome 38% renal failure/15 months
Gourley (59) 1996	IVC Bolus MP IVC + Bolus MP	IVC > Bolus MP Trend for IVC + Bolus MP > IVC
Fu (57) 1998	CS without P POC + P	Similar renal outcome 38% renal failure/15 months
Boletus (61) 1999	IVC IVIG	Equivalent short-term results

CS, cyclosporine; IVC, intravenous cyclophosphamide; MP, methylprednisolone; POC, oral cyclophosphamide; P, prednisone; IVIG, IV immunoglobulin.

were compared with those who had delayed biopsies and treatment, there was strikingly increased preservation of renal function and reduced mortality in the early treatment group. These patients, who were less sick than those reported in earlier trials described above, appeared to be more responsive to treatment with azathioprine, suggesting that there may be a role for immunosuppressives that are safer than IVC when new-onset, relatively mild nephritis is diagnosed. In our experience, however, some azathioprine-treated patients develop progressive renal disease that responds dramatically to the discontinuance of azathioprine and institution of IVC.

Azathioprine has been used for a variety of nonrenal indications in active SLE. During a controlled trial in patients with active nonrenal lupus, Sztejnbok et al. (118) added azathioprine 2.5 mg/kg/d to prednisone in half the patients. Azathioprine was reported to be unhelpful in controlling acute disease but to be steroid sparing and reduce mortality. A study randomizing patients with well-controlled lupus to continuation or withdrawal of azathioprine has demonstrated more exacerbations in patients who discontinued the drug (119).

Azathioprine has been reported to be effective in severe cutaneous lupus in several series (120–123) and to have a steroid-sparing effect. It has been reported to be useful in treating chronic active hepatitis complicating lupus, as well as nonvirally mediated chronic active hepatitis in nonlupus patients. The relatively slow onset of action as well as the lack of dramatic responses of disease activity to this drug mandate consummate clinical judgment on the part of the treating physician when decisions are made regarding whether use of this agent has been effective.

Summary

Azathioprine appears to be less effective than either cyclophosphamide or nitrogen mustard in arresting active, very progressive nephritis, but it may be effective in both early nephritis and as a maintenance drug after IVC. It appears to be both corticosteroid and cyclophosphamide sparing. Although slow in onset of action, azathioprine is a very useful agent in mild to moderately severe SLE.

Cyclosporine

Cyclosporine (CS) has complex immunologic effects, predominantly inhibition of T-cell gene activation, transcription of cytokine genes, and lymphokine release. In addition, it inhibits the recruitment of antigen-presenting cells and antigen presentation. It is unclear which, if any, of these effects is relevant to the pathogenesis of SLE, except perhaps high-level control of T-cell activation of antibody production (124). It is administered orally or intravenously, with marked variation in bioavailability after oral dosage. Absorption requires formation of an emulsion with bile and can be altered by a variety of gastrointestinal conditions, including diarrhea, malabsorption, and delayed gastric emptying. The drug is highly lipophilic, and levels may be increased in patients with hypocholesterolemia. It is eliminated by cytochrome P-450 with formation of multiple metabolites and excreted in the bile. CS levels are influenced by numerous medications, including rifampin, phenytoin, phenylbutazone, and phenobarbital, which decrease concentrations; and calcium channel blockers, progesterone and macrolide antibodies, and ketaconazole, which increase concentrations. As a consequence, monitoring CS levels is recommended at currently employed doses.

A major adverse effect is nephrotoxicity. Reduction of glomerular filtration may be underestimated because of compensatory hyperfiltration and the increasing contribution of tubular secretion of creatinine to the measured creatinine clearance as renal function declines (125). This side effect appears to be dose related, but it is not completely absent even in studies using doses as low as 2 mg/kg. In a population of 192 adults and children, including 152 with diabetes, who were treated with CS for a mean of 13 months before biopsy, 41 had biopsies that were consistent with CS-induced nephropathy (126). There is an association of nephropathy with maximal dose, mean dose, and cumulative dose before biopsy, but not with blood levels. Deray et al. (127) evaluated 16 patients with autoimmune uveitis who were treated with CS, 5 mg/kg/d initially. CS was adjusted according to the serum creatinine. There was a progressive decline of creatinine clearance throughout the study from the baseline of 120 mL/min to 75 mL/min at 24 months. The glomerular filtration rate (GFR) decreased from 116.8 to 75.3 mL per minute. There was a significant increase in total cholesterol levels. Altman et al. (128) treated patients with rheumatoid arthritis sequentially with the following regimens: first with a nonsteroidal antiinflammatory drug (NSAID), then with CS, 5 mg/kg, then with both. At the end of the study, there was a significant increase in blood urea nitrogen and creatinine levels in nine of 11 patients, and an additive effect of the two drugs was postulated. This side effect, in our opinion, is the major potential limiting factor in its use in SLE.

Compared with alkylating agents, bone marrow suppression is uncommon. Lymphoproliferative syndromes frequently are observed in CS-treated patients with organ transplants, but they are rare in patients with autoimmune disorders. CS appears to have little, if any, ovarian toxicity and has been employed in a limited number of pregnancies without obvious birth defects. Hypertension has been observed in 50% to 80% of transplant recipients. CS impairs the excretion of potassium, uric acid, and magnesium, and it is a notorious cause of refractory gout. It can cause hypomagnesemia and has been implicated in central nervous system toxicity, including headache, tremors, and occasionally, focal neurologic defect. Hirsutism, gingival hyperplasia, and gastrointestinal disturbances may occur.

Application of CS in SLE has been the subject of only a few controlled trials. Balletta et al. (129) randomized ten patients with lupus nephritis to either CS, 3 mg/kg/d, plus prednisone or to prednisone alone. After 12 months, there was no significant change in creatinine or creatinine clearance, but there was a reduction in proteinuria in the CS-treated group. In the treated group, the proteinuria declined from 2.7 to 0.3 g/24 hours, whereas in the prednisone-alone group, proteinuria increased from 2.1 to 2.6 g/24 hours.

In an open randomized trial Fu et al. (57) treated 40 children with World Health Organization (WHO) class III or IV lupus nephritis with either CS (2.5 to 5 mg/kg) alone (without corticosteroids) or prednisolone 2 mg/kg plus cyclophosphamide 2 mg/kg orally (P+C) for 1 year. At entry, all children had growth retardation following >1 year of corticosteroids. Subjects received an intense regimen of corticosteroids just prior to randomization until lupus activity diminished. There was comparable control of disease activity and resolution of proteinuria. Hemolytic complement (CH_{50}) and C3 levels were actually lower at the end of treatment, however. The authors concluded that CS controlled clinical but not serologic activity. The alternate regimen, although quite toxic, was probably effective, suggesting that CS as monotherapy also had some activity in order to achieve comparable results.

A number of open trials have suggested efficacy, using 2.5 to 10 mg/kg CS. Favre et al. (130) treated 26 lupus nephritis patients with CS 5 mg/kg/d, adjusted to achieve through levels of 250 to 350 ng/mL, plus prednisone, reporting a reduction of disease activity and proteinuria compared with baseline after 2 years. They reported an overall reduction of disease activity, stable serum creatinine levels, and slightly improved GFR, with striking reduction of proteinuria. By their estimation, activity was reduced on biopsy, and chronicity was slightly improved. In 1986, Feutren et al. (131) added CS, 5 to 10 mg/kg/d for 9 to 18 months, to prednisone in nine patients with systemic disease, and they reported apparent benefit in six patients and reduction of mean prednisone dose from 0.8 to 0.3 mg/kg/d without changes in DNA antibody titers or complement C4 levels. Proteinuria declined from 1.6 to 0.9 per 24 hours. In another trial, Isenberg et al. (132,133) treated five patients with a relatively large dose, 10 mg/kg/d, of CS, but these patients failed to respond, except for improvement of arthralgias in two. There were complications, including angioedema associated with the decline of Cl esterase inhibitor levels (133), in three patients, increased serum creatinine in three, and a sensation of being unwell in all patients. The study was terminated as a result.

Radhakrishnan et al. (134) treated ten lupus patients with membranous nephropathy, complicated in three cases by mesangial lesions, with CS, 4 to 6 mg/kg/d. Serial biopsies revealed an increase in the chronicity index and an increase in the stage of the membranous nephropathy, which is somewhat analogous to the chronicity index that is applied in proliferative disease. Several patients had reduction of proteinuria.

Tokuda et al. (135) treated 11 women with lupus with initial CS doses of 3 mg/kg/d. Hypertension occurred in 40%, and modest clinical improvement was observed.

Hussein et al. (136) treated five women with lupus nephritis, two of whom were pregnant, using CS plus low-dose prednisone. They noted stable renal function in all but one patient and hypertension in three.

Caccavo et al. (137) in an open trial treated 27 lupus patients who had an unsatisfactory response to either corticosteroids alone or corticosteroids plus an immunosuppressive for 24 months with an initial dose of CS 2.5 to 5 mg/kg. Disease activity, minor manifestations, cytopenias, and neurologic disease improved. Proteinuria was reduced, and the mean serum creatinine increased form 0.89 to 0.96 mg/dL (p = NS)

Dostal et al. (138) treated 11 patients with nephritis with CS, 5 mg/kg/d. After 1 year there was improvement of proteinuria, slight reduction of mean serum creatinine levels, and reduction of the mean Systemic Lupus Erythematosus Disease Activity Index (SLEDAI) from 26 to 4. Hypertension occurred in seven patients. At repeat biopsy, inflammation improved, and "chronic" changes were increased in five patients and reduced in three.

Tam et al. (139) administered CS 5 mg/kg/day to 17 patients with class IV nephritis of whom 12 completed 24 months of treatment. (Three of the remaining patients had azathioprine added.) Reduction of proteinuria was gradual, with only partial resolution at 1 year and further improvement in the subset of patients who reached year 5. Biopsy findings were of interest: no patient had evidence by repeat biopsy of persistence of inflammation at 1 year. There was no increase in chronicity (mean chronicity index 5.1 at baseline vs. 5.7 at 1 year).

Morton and Powell (140) reviewed treatment of mostly nonrenal lupus in 43 patients with CS (mean 4.1 mg/kg/day). Hypertension occurred in 14 patients, and a rise of creatinine >30% in nine. The drug was stopped in 39 of 47 treatment courses because of toxicity or lack of efficacy. Hallegua et al. have suggested that CS is helpful in membranous nephritis (140a).

Cyclosporine has been reported to be well tolerated in pregnancy (136), useful when added to cyclophosphamide for nephritis (141), and has been combined with immunoadsorption in pregnancy (142).

Conclusions

Although the mechanism by which cyclosporine may alter the course of lupus is uncertain, it is likely that it favorably affects some manifestations of lupus, such as proteinuria, over the relatively short period of 1 to 2 years, and may reduce overall disease activity. The outcome of studies in membranous nephropathy will be of great interest. In both controlled and open trials, glomerular filtration has not improved, as would be expected in bolus cyclophosphamide-treated nephritis patients, and some patients have developed hypertension and reduced GFR. Stabilization of GFR might reflect amelioration of nephritis combined with mild toxicity from the drug. Experience with other immunosuppressives (e.g., prednisone, daily cyclophosphamide) emphasizes the importance of long-term follow-up in determining risk vs. benefit. CS still does not have the track record of successful long-term use in lupus shared by cyclophosphamide and azathioprine, and is better suited to empiric use when irreversible injury is not imminent.

Methotrexate

Methotrexate (MTX) is a folate antagonist, which when administered at the doses used in rheumatic diseases has less obvious immunosuppressive effects than alkylating agents or azathioprine. In fact, it may act by other means. There is no convincing association of changes in lymphocyte subsets, surface markers, lymphocyte function, or autoantibody levels with therapeutic effects on rheumatic diseases. It appears to have multiple antiinflammatory effects including increased adenosine levels at sites of inflammation, inhibition of leukotriene B_2 formation, interleukin-1 (IL-1) effects, fibroblast proliferation, and preferential cyclooxygenase-2 inhibition (143,144). Other putative mechanisms of action include inhibition of neutrophil function, interference with the action of IL-1, suppression of lipoxygenase formation, and inhibition of the intracellular enzyme 5-aminoimidazole-4-carboxamide ribonucleotide transformylase (145). It is unclear which mechanisms of action are important in lupus treatment.

Side effects of MTX particularly hepatotoxicity and cytopenias, are well known. Selected aspects will be reviewed. MTX toxicity is increased in patients with depressed renal function, and increases in patients maintained on a stable dose of MTX who sustain a decline in renal function (e.g., from active nephritis) (144,146). Side effects occur less frequently in rheumatoid arthritis patients given 1 mg/day folate, and drug efficacy (against rheumatoid arthritis) appears unaltered. MTX increases homocysteine levels and cardiovascular risk in lupus patients, an effect that is also reduced by simultaneous administration of folate (136–144,146–148).

Pulmonary toxicity, which has been reported in 2% to 7% of patients with rheumatoid arthritis, is characterized by cough, bilateral or unilateral pulmonary infiltrates, and dyspnea (149–153). There is a nonspecific interstitial inflammatory cell infiltrate and an increased number of T cells on bronchoalveolar lavage (151). Reported mortality is 17%, with a 50% recurrence rate on rechallenge and 50% mortality of recurrences. Pneumocystis prophylaxis for patients receiving MTX plus moderate- to high-dose corticosteroids should reduce the number of episodes of PCP pneumonitis requiring distinction from MTX pneumonitis. MTX is teratogenic and an abortifactant (154,155). Rheumatologists have been shown to inadequately identify and address the need for contraception in women taking MTX (156). MTX-induced malignancies appear to be rare. A reversible lymphoproliferative disease can occur, and has been reported to evolve into Hodgkin's disease (157).

Other forms of MTX toxicity, including acute hepatic injury, hepatic fibrosis, stomatitis, and, in high doses, central nervous system toxicity, have been reviewed elsewhere (145).

Methotrexate has gained considerable popularity in the treatment of systemic rheumatic diseases, including rheumatoid and psoriatic arthritis, Wegener's granulomatosis (150,158), and Takayasu's disease (159). In Wegener's the efficacy of MTX appears to be less than that of daily oral cyclophosphamide (as also is the case for IVC).

In SLE, there is a paucity of data. Two early studies, the treatment of seven patients with 7.5 mg/wk for 6 weeks by Dubois (160), and administration of either daily oral MTX, 2.5 mg, or 50 mg of IV MTX weekly by Miescher and Riethmuller (161), produced equivocal results. Rothenberg et al. (162) treated ten patients with MTX, 7.5 to 10.0 mg weekly, of whom seven patients improved. Improvement was noted in myositis, rash, pleurisy, arthritis, and proteinurea, but leukopenia was observed in three patients. Wilke et al. (163) treated 17 patients with lupus using a mean MTX dose of 1 g over 8 months. They reported benefit in 57% of patients and toxicity in 70%, with an increase of toxicity associated with use of diuretics or NSAIDs. They noted elevation of liver function tests and gastrointestinal side effects, but not cytopenia. In an open trial in pediatric patients, Abud-Mendoza et al. (164) treated ten patients with MTX, 5 to 10 mg weekly, in addition to their previous regimens, which in four cases included both prednisone and cyclophosphamide. Of the ten patients, two had a poor outcome, and five had excellent responses with discontinuation of cyclophosphamide and other drugs. Wilson et al. (165) treated 12 SLE patients who lacked renal or central nervous system disease with MTX and noted apparent clinical improvement without change in antibodies to DNA or complement. Corticosteroid dose was reduced in six patients. Hashimoto et al. (166) treated two patients with myositis, fever, and pancytopenia complicating lupus, and they noticed a fall in the number of CD20 positive cells. Walz LeBlanc et al. (167) found MTX to be well tolerated and effective in a review of five patients.

Rahman et al. (168), in a retrospective controlled study, concluded that there was a 60% reduction of the joint count in MTX-treated lupus patients with antimalarial-resistant synovitis vs. 12% in the control group. In this study MTX was not steroid sparing. In a retrospective study Kipen et al. (169) also concluded that MTX had not been steroid sparing. Gansauge et al. (170), in an open trial of

MTX 15 mg/week administered to 22 patients, noted overall improvement.

In a double-blind, randomized, placebo-controlled trial, Carneiro and Sato (170a) treated 41 patients with MTX, 15 to 20 mg/week vs. placebo. After 6 months, compared with the placebo group, MTX-treated patients had significantly more resolution of arthritis, rash, and hypocomplementemia (the most frequent clinical features at entry), and more improvement of the SLEDAI score. Mean prednisone doses at follow-up were increased in the placebo group and significantly decreased in the MTX group.

Conclusion

Methotrexate is relatively safe and well tolerated and helps some lupus patients, particularly those with synovitis. Monitoring of renal function is essential to ensure safety.

Mycophenolate Mofetil

Mycophenolate mofetil (MMF) has established itself as a successful immunosuppressive medication in multiple applications and has a unique mode of action that may be particularly applicable to control of SLE erythematosus. MMF is the morpholinoethyl ester of mycophenolic acid (MPA). MPA was originally isolated from *Penicillium* species in 1896. In the 1960s MPA was found to have antifungal and anticancer activities. In the 1970s, MPA was studied as a treatment for psoriasis. Although it was effective, poor and erratic absorption along with a high incidence of gastrointestinal toxicity limited further study (171).

MPA is a potent, noncompetitive, reversible inhibitor of inosine monophosphate dehydrogenase (IMPDH), a necessary enzyme in the *de novo* pathway of purine synthesis. The *de novo* synthesis pathway is uniquely essential (172) in activated lymphocytes, while most other cells use the salvage pathway of purine synthesis. Not only do lymphocytes primarily depend on the *de novo* synthesis pathway, but activated lymphocytes predominately use the second isoform of IMPDH against which MPA is most specific (172a, 173,174). *In vitro* activities of MPA include inhibition of both T- and B-lymphocyte proliferation in response to mitogenic stimulation (175) and of antibody formation in humans to horse antilymphocyte globulin (172) and tetanus toxoid (176). Suppression of IgG anti–antithymocyte gamma-globulin (ATGAM) antibody production by MMF is greater than that of azathioprine (AZA) (172). MPA also interferes with the production and/or function of adhesion molecules necessary for the migration of lymphocytes to areas of inflammation (177). Studies of various animal models of atherosclerosis and arterial injury demonstrate protective effects of MMF with decreased vessel wall thickening and cellular proliferation (178–180).

MMF is rapidly hydrolyzed to MPA and is 94% bioavailable by the oral route. The drug is reversibly converted to an inactive glucuronide—mycophenolic acid glucuronide (MPAG)—in the liver and excreted into the gastrointestinal tract. Much of MPAG is deglucuronidated by intestinal flora and undergoes enterohepatic recirculation. It is eventually excreted primarily through the kidney (171). Serum drug levels are increased in patients with elevated creatinine. In transplant studies, doses of 2.0 g/d or 3.0 g/d were studied with little gain in efficacy but increased toxicity at the 3.0 g/d dose (181–183). A review of patients at our institution suggests that, in practice, rheumatologists are using dosage ranges between 0.75 and 2.5 g/d for the treatment of SLE, and about 50% of patients cannot tolerate 2 g/day.

MMF has proven to be a potent antirejection agent in experimental animal models (175,184). MMF appears to be effective in experimental autoimmune disease including Heymann nephritis and experimental autoimmune uveitis (185,186). Studies in the Medical Research Laboratory lymphoproliferative (MRL/*lpr*) and New Zealand black (NZB) × New Zealand white (NZW) F1 mouse models of SLE have shown suppression of development of lupus glomerulonephritis, a decrease in glomerular immunoglobulin deposits in MMF-treated mice, and improved survival (187,189–190).

MMF currently has Food and Drug Administration (FDA) approval for prevention of acute allograft rejection in kidney transplantation and for use in cardiac transplantation. MMF has been widely accepted as a more potent agent than AZA in pediatric and adult transplantation. Three large, multicenter, randomized controlled studies of human cadaveric renal transplants have compared MMF with either AZA or placebo. Findings among the studies showed statistically significant decreases in acute rejection and steroid use, suggesting MMF is superior to AZA or placebo (181–183). Studies of lung, liver, and heart transplant elicited similar results (171). A successful trial of renal transplant utilizing MMF without prednisone was reported (190a).

Successful treatments reported in adults with autoimmune diseases include a randomized trial suggesting superiority to or against AZA in Crohn's disease (191). MMF has been explored in the treatment of uveitis, rheumatoid arthritis, Takayasu arteritis, psoriasis, pemphigoid, and pyoderma gangreosum (191a,192–197).

Although extensively studied in transplantation as a replacement for AZA, studies in SLE are limited to a few uncontrolled studies and one recently published trial in lupus nephritis. In 1999, Dooley and Cosio (198) published a report of 12 patients with relapsing or resistant lupus nephritis, most of whom had prior IVC therapy, followed for a mean of 12.9 months. They found significant improvements in proteinuria and improvement or stabilization of serum creatinine in all patients. Although corticosteroid doses in this study were not specifically analyzed, it appears all patients were on significant steroids at the start of therapy, including three patients who received bolus solumedrol and were on less at the end of the study. Briggs et al. (199) reported a series of eight patients with renal disease characterized by proteinuria, two of whom had lupus nephritis. Both had significant improvement in proteinuria on stable prednisone doses, and one improved after being switched from AZA to MMF. Gaubitz et al. (200) studied ten patients with SLE whose systemic and renal manifestations of disease were inadequately controlled on corticosteroids and AZA or cyclophosphamide. All patients had improvement in clinical disease activity measured by the Systemic Lupus Activity Measure (SLAM) with scores decreasing from mean 15.5 ± 5.5 to 8.0 ± 3.3 after 6 months of therapy. The four patients with lupus nephritis on quarterly Cytoxan had modest but not statistically significant improvements in serum creatinine. The mean corticosteroid dose decreased significantly over 6 months. Pashinian et al. (201) reported on eight severe SLE patients who had failed one or two immunosuppressive agents. After 6 months, four of six patients had improvement in SLEDAI scores, and all patients with nephritis had decreased proteinuria. These findings occurred in conjunction with a decrease in mean steroid dose (201). Petri (94) studied 22 SLE patients requiring immunosuppressive therapy placed on MMF. Although eight failed and required cyclophosphamide, most showed sustained improvement in overall disease activity, prednisone, C4, and anti–double-stranded DNA (dsDNA). The ten patients with nephrotic-range proteinuria showed a mild but not significant improvement in proteinuria while on MMF.

In a randomized trial comparing treatment of class IV nephritis with MMF plus prednisone (P) for 1 year vs. oral cyclophosphamide plus P for 6 months followed by azathioprine plus P for 6 months, responses were favorable and equivalent in both groups, with reduction of proteinuria and stabilization of serum creatinine levels (202). Neither regimen resulted in improvement of creatinine levels, which has been seen in some series. This study appears to move MMF into the "big leagues." However, short-term equivalence of outcome needs to be confirmed by long-term clinical follow-up and evidence that renal scarring is prevented by both regimens to the same extent that is accomplished by long-term IVC.

With regard to toxicity, in controlled trials for the prevention of renal transplant rejection, diarrhea was increased in patients receiving MMF, with an incidence of up to 36%, compared to 21% for patients receiving AZA and 14% for patients receiving placebo. Few patients (up to 2%) developed severe neutropenia (absolute neutrophil count $<0.5 \times 10^3$/L). The incidence of malignancies among the patients enrolled who were followed for ≥1 year was similar to the incidence reported in the literature for renal allograft recipients. There was a slight increase in the incidence of lymphoproliferative disease in the MMF treatment groups compared to the placebo and AZA groups. In three controlled studies for prevention of rejection, similar rates of fatal infections or sepsis (<2%) occurred in patients while receiving MMF or control therapy in combination with other immunosuppressive agents (38,203).

Descriptions of toxicity in SLE patients are all anecdotal and in sample sizes far to small to detect significant but rare side effects such as malignancy. The following data are from a compilation of six studies involving MMF and SLE in which adverse events were reported. Out of 81 patients, 21 (26%) had gastrointestinal symptoms—nausea, vomiting, and/or diarrhea. Four patients (5%) had recurrence of herpes stomatitis. Two patients each had vertigo and prurigo. One patient each had severe leukopenia, severe anemia, pancreatitis, and flare of existing vaginal candidosis. Pneumonia and asymptomatic leukopenia each occurred in two patients (197a,198–201).

MMF appears to be a promising agent in the treatment of SLE with a similar and perhaps even less toxic side effect profile than AZA. The recent controlled trial in lupus nephritis will heighten interest in this promising but expensive compound. Because it is substantially more expensive than azathioprine, comparison with this agent is needed. Our impression is that MMF has faster onset of action than azathioprine and may be superior in some cases.

SUMMARY

Immunosuppressive drugs are being applied more widely and more successfully in SLE than previously, with refinement of indications so that treatment in general is becoming more appropriate. The decision to use immunosuppressives should be made with full knowledge that these agents are uniformly toxic, particularly the alkylating agents, in which increasing cumulative dose is unquestionably related to increasing risk of serious consequences, including sterility and malignancy. Although the data most strongly support treatment of severe active lupus nephritis, especially when there is both activity and chronic change and a significant component of proliferation is shown on the renal biopsy, indications are widening. It is reasonable to use IVC for almost any life- or organ-threatening lupus flare that is immune-complex mediated. It is my impression that the vast majority of, if not all, new cases of aggressive nephritis, regardless of histophathology, should be treated if necessary with immunosuppression, particularly cyclophosphamide. Likewise, many hematologic abnormalities, including thrombocytopenia, hemolytic anemia, and some leukopenias, will respond to IVC in much lower doses than those that are required for the treatment of renal disease. IVC alone clearly is inadequate in the treatment of many cases of thrombotic thrombocytopenic purpura. Selected cases of central nervous system disease and additional life-threatening systemic manifestations almost certainly can benefit from cyclophosphamide administration. However, cyclophosphamide is not necessarily the most potent alkylating agent that is available, nor is the IV form of administration preferable in all cases.

Use of azathioprine as an adjunct to prednisone and as a steroid-sparing agent is supported by numerous studies. It is a slow-acting agent that is unlikely to be helpful immediately in fulminant disease. Its major uses appear to be achieving control of minor manifestations and possibly early nephritis, reducing corticosteroid use, and possibly as a maintenance agent in severe lupus after IVC. The role of methotrexate remains unproven, but its lack of a convincing association with induction of malignancies makes it an attractive alternative for the control of some steroid-refractory manifestations of lupus, such as synovitis, provided that renal function is stable. Cyclosporine, on the other hand, remains incompletely tested. Lack of marrow suppression and tolerability in pregnancy are advantages, but its significant nephrotoxicity mandates caution in its use. Ongoing trials in nephritis, particularly membranous nephritis, will yield important results.

Mycophenolate mofetil is a promising but expensive agent that may offer advantages of more rapid onset of action than azathioprine and effectiveness for some disease flares that would otherwise be treated with cyclophosphamide. Its relative potency compared to IVC and azathioprine remains to be clarified. It may be too early to routinely use this expensive drug in place of azathioprine. However, when gonadal toxicity is an issue, substituting MMF for IVC may prove to be reasonable in some patients with nephritis.

It is to be hoped that judicious and early use of more benign therapies, especially antimalarial drugs alone or in combination, antiinflammatory drugs, and low doses of corticosteroids, will reduce or delay the need for more aggressive therapy. Unfortunately, the promise of effective biologic agents in SLE is yet to be fulfilled. In the immediate future, the most promising advances may be drug regimens that take the place of alkylating agents at various stages of disease evolution.

REFERENCES

1. Bansal V, Beto J. Treatment of lupus nephritis: a meta-analysis of clinical trials. *Am J Kidney Dis* 1997;29(2):193–199.
2. Felson DT, Anderson J. Evidence for the superiority of immunosuppressive drugs and prednisone over prednisone alone in lupus nephritis. Results of a pooled analysis. *N Engl J Med* 1984;311:1528–1533.
3. Osborne E, Jordon J, Hoak F, et al. Nitrogen mustard therapy in cutaneous blastomatous disease. *JAMA* 1947;135:1123–1128.
4. Chasis H, Goldring W, Baldwin DS. Effect of febrile plasma, typhoid vaccine, and nitrogen mustard on renal manifestations of human glomerulonephritis. *Proc Soc Exp Biol Med* 1995; 71:565–567.
5. Lynch J, McCune W. Immunosuppressive and cytotoxic pharmacotherapy for pulmonary disorders: state of the art. *Am J Respir Crit Care Med* 1997;155:395–420.
6. McCune W, Fox D. Immunosuppressive agents—biologic effects in vivo and in vitro. In: Kammer GM, Tsokos GC (eds), *Lupus: molecular and cellular pathogenesis.* Totowa, NJ: Humana Press, 1999;37:612–641.
7. McCune WJ, Golbus J, Zeldes W, et al. Clinical and immunologic effects of monthly administration of intravenous cyclophosphamide in severe systemic lupus erythematosus. *N Engl J Med* 1988;318:1423–1431.
8. McCune W. Defective CD2 pathway T cell activation in systemic lupus erythematosus. *Arthritis Rheum* 1991;34:561–571.
9. McCune WJ, Dunne RB, Millard J, et al. Two year follow-up of patients with severe systemic lupus (SLE) treated with pulse cyclophosphamide. *Arthritis Rheum* 1990;33(Suppl):S103.
10. Amano H, Morimoto S, Kaneko H, et al. Effect of intravenous cyclophosphamide in systemic lupus erythematosus: relation to lymphocyte subsets and activation markers. *Lupus* 2000;9(1): 26–32.
11. Takeno M, Suzuki N, Nagafuchi H, et al. Selective suppression of resting B cell function in patients with systemic lupus erythematosus treated with cyclophosphamide. *Clin Exp Rheumatol* 1993;11:263–270.
12. Fox DA, McCune WJ. Immunologic and clinical effects of cytotoxic drugs used in the treatment of rheumatoid arthritis and systemic lupus erythematosus. *Concepts Immunopathol* 1989;7:20–78.
13. Berd D, Mastrangelo MJ. Effect of low dose cyclophosphamide on the immune system of cancer patients: depletion of CD4+, 2H4+ suppressor-inducer T-cells. *Cancer Res* 1988;48:1671–1675.
14. Yasunami R, Bach JF. Anti-suppressor effect of cyclophosphamide on the development of spontaneous diabetes in NOD mice. *Eur J Immunol* 1988;18:481–484.
15. Hoffman GS, Kerr GS, Leavitt RY, et al. Wegener's granulomatosis: an analysis of 158 patients. *Ann Intern Med* 1992;116: 488–498.
16. Baltus JA, Boersma JW, Hartman AP, et al. The occurrence of malignancies in patients with rheumatoid arthritis treated with cyclophosphamide: a controlled retrospective follow-up. *Ann Rheum Dis* 1983;42:368–373.
17. Baker GL, Kahl LE, Zee BC, et al. Malignancy following treatment of rheumatoid arthritis with cyclophosphamide. *Am J Med* 1987;83:1–9.
18. Radis CD, Kahl LE, Baker GL, et al. Effects of cyclophosphamide on the development of malignancy and on long-term survival of patients with rheumatoid arthritis. *Arthritis Rheum* 1995;38:1120–1127.
19. McCarthy CJ, Sheldon S, Ross CW, et al. Cytogenetic abnormalities and hematologic malignancies associated with the use of alkylating agents in rheumatic diseases. *Arthritis Rheum* 1994;37(9):S428.
20. Ginzler E, Feldman D, Giovaniello G, et al. The association of cervical neoplasia (CN) and SLE. *Arthritis Rheum* 1989;32(4 suppl):S30(abst).
21. Nyberg G, Eriksson O, Westberg NG. Increased incidence of cervical atypia in women with systemic lupus erythematosus treated with chemotherapy. *Arthritis Rheum* 1981;24:648–650.
22. Stillwell TJ, Benson RC Jr. Cyclophosphamide-induced hemorrhagic cystitis. A review of 100 patients. *Cancer* 1988;61: 451–457.
23. Sessoms SL, Kovarsky J. Monthly intravenous cyclophosphamide in the treatment of severe systemic lupus erythematosus. *Clin Exp Rheumatol* 1984;2:247–251.
24. Chapman RM, Sutcliffe SB. Protection of ovarian function by oral contraceptives in women receiving chemotherapy for Hodgkin's disease. *Blood* 1981;58:849–851.
25. Ataya KM, Palmer KC, Blacker CM. Inhibition of rat ovarian [3H] thymidine uptake by luteinizing hormone-releasing hor-

mone agonists: a possible mechanism for preventing damage by cytotoxic agents. *Cancer Res* 1988;48:7252–7256.

26. Rivkees SA, Crawford D. The relationship of gonadal activity and chemotherapy-induced gonadal damage. *JAMA* 1988;259: 2123–2125.
27. Slater C, Liang M, McCune W, et al. Preserving ovarian function in patients receiving cyclophosphamide. *Lupus* 1999;6(1): 3–10.
28. Blumenfeld Z, Shapiro D, Shteinberg M, et al. Preservation of fertility and ovarian function and minimizing gonadotxicity in young women with systemic lupus erythematosus treated by chemotherapy. *Lupus* 2000;9:401–405.
29. Blumenfeld Z, Avivi I, Linn S, et al. Prevention of irreversible chemotherapy-induced ovarian damage in young women with lymphoma by a gonadotrophin-releasing hormone agonist in parallel to chemotherapy. *Hum Reprod* 1996;11(8):1620–1626.
30. Gilchrist DM, Friedman JM. Teratogenesis and IV cyclophosphamide (letter). *J Rheumatol* 1989;16:1008–1009.
31. Kirshon B, Wasserstrum N, Willis R. Teratogenic effects of first-trimester cyclophosphamide therapy. *Obstet Gynecol* 1988;72: 462.
32. Enns G, Roeder E, Chan R, et al. Apparent cyclophosphamide (cytoxan) embryopathy: a distinct phenotype? *Am J Med Genet* 1999;86(3):237–241.
33. Greenberg LH, Tanaka KR. Congenital anomalies probably induced by cyclophosphamide. *JAMA* 1964;188:423–426.
34. Toledo TM, Harper RC, Moser RH. Fetal effects during cyclophosphamide and irradiation therapy. *Ann Intern Med* 1971;74:87–91.
35. Ramsey-Goldman R, Mientus JM, Kutzer JE, et al. Pregnancy outcome in women with systemic lupus erythematosus treated with immunosuppressive drugs. *J Rheumatol* 1993;20: 1152–1157.
36. Bermas BL, Hill JA. Effects of immunosuppressive drugs during pregnancy. *Arthritis Rheum* 1995;38:1722–1732.
37. Bradley JD, Brandt KD, Katz BP. Infectious complications of cyclophosphamide treatment for vasculitis (see comments). *Arthritis Rheum* 1989;32:45–53.
38. Morgan MC, Matteson E, Dunne R, et al. Complications of intravenous cyclophosphamide: association of infections with high daily doses of prednisone in lupus patients. *Arthritis Rheum* 1990;33(suppl 5):R27(abst).
39. Tsokos GC, Smith PL, Balow JE. Development of hypogammaglobulinemia in a patient with systemic lupus erythematosus. *Am J Med* 1986;81:1081–1084.
40. Snyder LS, Anderson ML. Cyclophosphamide-induced hepatotoxicity in a patient with Wegener's granulomatosis. *Mayo Clin Proc* 1993;68:1203–1204.
41. Du LT, Rigaud D, Papo T, et al. Cyclophosphamide-induced hepatitis in Wegener's granulomatosis (letter; comment). *Mayo Clin Proc* 1994;69:912–913.
42. Usui Y, Aida H, Kimula Y, et al. A case of cyclophosphamide-induced interstitial pneumonitis diagnosed by bronchoalveolar lavage. *Respiration* 1992;59:125–128.
43. Stentoft J. Progressive pulmonary fibrosis complicating cyclophosphamide therapy. *Acta Med Scand* 1987;221:403–407.
44. Morse CC, Sigler C, Lock S, et al. Pulmonary toxicity of cyclophosphamide: a 1-year study. *Exp Mol Pathol* 1985;42: 251–260.
45. McCune WJ. Oral bolus cyclophosphamide—liberating libation or nauseating nostrum? *J Rheumatol* 1996;23:212–213.
46. Dawisha SM, Yarboro CH, Vaughan EM, et al. Outpatient monthly oral bolus cyclophosphamide therapy in systemic lupus erythematosus. *J Rheumatol* 1996;23:273–278.
47. Balow JE, Austin HA, Tsokos GC, et al. Lupus nephritis. *Ann Intern Med* 1987;106:79–94.
48. Deleted in page proofs.
49. Balow JE, Austin HA, Muenz LR, et al. Effect of treatment on the evolution of renal abnormalities in lupus nephritis. *N Engl J Med* 1984;311:491–495.
50. Austin HA, Muenz LR, Joyce KM, et al. Prognostic factors in lupus nephritis. Contribution of renal histologic data. *Am J Med* 1983;75:382–391.
51. Austin HAI, Klippel JH, Balow JE, et al. Therapy of lupus nephritis: A controlled trial of prednisone and cytotoxic drugs. *N Engl J Med* 1986;314:614–619.
52. Fries JF, Sharp GC, McDevitt HO, et al. Cyclophosphamide therapy in systemic lupus erythematosus and polymyositis. *Arthritis Rheum* 1973;16(2):154–162.
53. Garancis JC, Piering WF. Prolonged cyclophosphamide or azathioprine therapy of lupus nephritis. *Clin Pharmacol Ther* 1973;14:130(abst).
54. Donadio JV, Holley KE, Ferguson RH, et al. Progressive lupus glomerulonephritis. Treatment with prednisone and combined prednisone and cyclophosphamide. *Mayo Clin Proc* 1976;51:484–494.
55. Donadio JVJ, Holley KE, Ferguson RH, et al. Treatment of diffuse proliferative lupus nephritis with prednisone and combined prednisone and cyclophosphamide. *N Engl J Med* 1978;299: 1151–1155.
56. Donadio JVJ, Glassock RJ. Immunosuppressive drug therapy in lupus nephritis: In-depth review. *Am J Kidney Dis* 1993;21 (3):239–250.
57. Fu L-W, Yang L-Y, Chen W-P, et al. Clinical efficacy of cyclosporin A (Neoral) in the treatment of paediatric lupus nephritis with heavy proteinuria. *Br J Rheumatol* 1998;37: 217–221.
58. Boumpas DT, Austin HA, Vaughn EM, et al. Controlled trial of pulse methylprednisolone versus two regimens of pulse cyclophosphamide in severe lupus nephritis. *Lancet* 1992;340: 741–745.
59. Gourley MF, Austin HA III, Scott D, et al. Methylprednisolone and cyclophosphamide, alone or in combination, in patients with lupus nephritis. *Ann Intern Med* 1996;125:549–557.
60. Sesso R, Monteiro M, Sato E, et al. A controlled trial of pulse cyclophosphamide versus pulse methylprednisolone in severe lupus nephritis. *Lupus* 1994;3:107–112.
61. Boletis J, Ioannidis J, Boki K, et al. Intravenous immunoglobulin compared with cyclophosphamide for proliferative lupus nephritis. *Lancet* 1999;354(9178):569–570.
62. Chaghac A, Kiberd B, Farinas MC, et al. Outcome of acute glomerular injury in proliferative lupus nephritis. *J Clin Invest* 1989;84:922–930.
63. Chan T, Li F, Hao W, et al. Treatment of membranous lupus nephritis with nephrotic syndrome by sequential immunosuppression. *Lupus* 1999;8(7):545–551.
64. Chan T, Li F, Wong R, et al. Sequential therapy for diffuse proliferative and membranous lupus nephritis: cyclophosphamide and prednisolone followed by azathioprine and prednisolone. *Nephron* 1995;71(3):321–327.
65. Niaudet P. Treatment of lupus nephritis in children. *Pediatr Nephrol* 2000;14(2):158–166.
66. McInnes PM, Schuttinga J, Sanslone WR, et al. The economic impact of treatment of severe lupus nephritis with prednisone and intravenous cyclophosphamide. *Arthritis Rheum* 1994;37: 1000–1006.
67. Boumpas DT, Yamada H, Patronas NJ, et al. Pulse cyclophosphamide for severe neuropsychiatric lupus. *Q J Med* 1991;296 (new series 81):975–984.
68. Neuwelt CM, Lacks S, Kaye BR, et al. Role of intravenous cyclophosphamide in the treatment of severe neuropsychiatric systemic lupus erythematosus. *Am J Med* 1995;98:32–46.

69. Malaviya AN, Singh RR, Sindhwani R, et al. Intermittent intravenous pulse cyclophosphamide treatment in systemic lupus erythematosus. *Indian J Med Res* 1992;96:101–108.
70. Propper DJ, Bucknall RC. Acute transverse myelopathy complicating systemic lupus erythematosus. *Ann Rheum Dis* 1989; 48:512–515.
71. Barile L, Lavalle C. Transverse myelitis in systemic lupus erythematosus—the effect of IV pulse methylprednisolone and cyclophosphamide. *J Rheumatol* 1992;19:370–372.
72. Galindo-Rodriguez G, Avina-Zubieta J, Pizarro S, et al. Cyclophosphamide pulse therapy in optic neuritis due to systemic lupus erythematosus: an open trial. *Am J Med* 1999;106 (1):65–69.
72a. Baca V, Lavalle C, Garcia R, et al. Favorable response to intravenous methylprednisone and cyclophosphamide in children with severe neuropsychiatric lupus. *J Rheumatol* 1999;26: 432–439.
73. Grimbacher B, Huber M, von Kempis J, et al. Successful treatment of gastrointestinal vasculitis due to SLE with intravenous pulse cyclophosphamide: a clinical case report and view of the literature. *Br J Rheumatol* 1998;37(9):1023–1028.
74. Walport MJ, Hubbard WN, Hughes GRV. Reversal of aplastic anemia secondary to systemic lupus erythematosus by high-dose intravenous cyclophosphamide. *Br Med J* 1982; 285:769.
75. Braun J, Sieper J, Schwarz A, et al. Severe lupus crisis with agranulocytosis and anuric renal failure due to a mesangial lesion (WHO IIB)—successful treatment with cyclophosphamide pulse followed by plasmapheresis (letter). *Br J Rheumatol* 1991;30:312–313.
76. Trotta F, Bajocchi G, La Corte R, et al. Long-lasting remission and successful treatment of acquired factor Vlll inhibitors using cyclophosphamide in a patient with systemic lupus erythematosus. *Rheumatology* 1999;38(10):1007–1009.
77. Viallard J, Pellegrin J, Vergnes C, et al. Three cases of acquired von Willebrand disease associated with systemic lupus erythematosus. *J Haematol* 1999;105(2):532–537.
78. Roach BA, Hutchinson GJ. Treatment of refractory, systemic lupus erythematosus-associated thrombocytopenia with intermittent low-dose intravenous cyclophosphamide. *Arthritis Rheum* 1993;36:682–684.
79. Boumpas DT, Barez S, Klippel JH. Intermittent cyclophosphamide for the treatment of autoimmune thrombocytopenia in systemic lupus erythematosus. *Ann Intern Med* 1990;112:674.
80. Hess DA, Sethi K, Awad E. Thrombotic thrombocytopenic purpura in systemic lupus erythematosus and antiphospholipid antibodies: effective treatment with plasma exchange and immunosuppression. *J Rheumatol* 1992;19:1474–1478.
81. Perez-Sanchez I, Anguita J, Pintado T. Use of cyclophosphamide in the treatment of thrombotic thrombocytopenic purpura complicating systemic lupus erythematosus: two cases reported. *Ann Hematol* 1999;78(6):285–287.
82. Godeau B, Cormier C, Menkes CJ. Bronchiolitis obliterans in systemic lupus erythematosus: beneficial effect of intravenous cyclophosphamide (see comments). *Ann Rheum Dis* 1991;50: 956–958.
83. Schnabel A, Reuter M, Gross W. Intravenous pulse cyclophosphamide in the treatment of interstitial lung disease due to collagen vascular diseases. *Arthritis Rheum* 1998;41(7):215–220.
84. Fukuda M, Kamiyama Y, Kawahara K, et al. The favourable effect of cyclophosphamide pulse therapy in the treatment of massive pulmonary haemorrhage in systemic lupus erythematosus. *J Pediatr* 1994;153:167–170.
85. Kono DH, Klashman DJ, Gilbert RC. Successful IV pulse cyclophosphamide in refractory PM in 3 patients with SLE (letter). *J Rheumatol* 1990;17:982–983.
86. Saberi M, Jones B. Remission of infantile systemic lupus erythematosus with intravenous cyclophosphamide. *Pediatr Neurol* 1998;12(2):136–138.
87. Lehman T, Onel K. Intermittent intravenous cyclophosphamide arrests progression of the renal chronicity index in childhood systemic lupus erythematosus. *J Pediatr* 2000;136 (2):243–247.
88. Edelheit B, Arkachaisri T, Onel K, et al. Combination chemotherapy for refractory lupus nephritis. *Arthritis Rheum* 2000; 43:5321.
89. Euler HH, Guillevin L. Plasmapheresis and subsequent pulse cyclophosphamide in severe systemic lupus erythematosus. An interim report of the Lupus Plasmapheresis Study Group. *Ann Med Interne (Paris)* 1994;145:296–302.
90. Schroeder JO, Euler HH. Treatment combining plasmapheresis and pulse cyclophosphamide in severe systemic lupus erythematosus. *Adv Exp Med Biol* 1989;260:203.
91. Euler HH, Schroeder JO, Harten P, et al. Treatment-free remission in severe systemic lupus erythematosus following synchronization of plasmapheresis with subsequent pulse cyclophosphamide. *Arthritis Rheum* 1994;37:1784–1794.
92. Euler HH, Schroeder JO, Zeuner RA, et al. A randomized trial of plasmapheresis and subsequent pulse cyclophosphamide in severe lupus: design of the LPSG trial. *Int J Artif Organs* 1991;14:639–646.
93. Schroeder JO, Euler HH, Loffler H. Synchronization of plasmapheresis and pulse cyclophosphamide in severe systemic lupus erythematosus. *Ann Intern Med* 1987;107:344.
94. Brodsky RA, Petri M, Jones RJ. Hematopoetic stem cell transplantation for systemic lupus erythematosus. *Rheum Dis Clin North Am* 2000;26:377–387.
95. Traynor A, Burt R. Haematopoietic stem cell transplantation for active systemic lupus erythematosus. *Rheumatology* 1999;38: 767–772.
96. Dubois EL. Nitrogen mustard in treatment of systemic lupus erythematosus. *Arch Intern Med* 1954;93:667–672.
97. Wallace DJ, Podell TE, Weiner JM. Lupus nephritis: Experience with 230 patients in a private practice from 1950 to 1980. *Am J Med* 1982;72:209.
98. Dillard MG, Dujovne I, Pollak VE, et al. The effect of treatment with prednisone and nitrogen mustard on the renal lesions and life span of patients with lupus glomerulonephritis. *Nephron* 1973;10:273–291.
99. Wallace DJ, Metzger AL. Successful use of nitrogen mustard for cyclophosphamide resistant diffuse proliferative lupus glomerulonephritis: report of 2 cases. *J Rheumatol* 1995;22(4):801–802.
100. Vonderheid EC, Tan ET, Kantor AF, et al. Long-term efficacy, curative potential, and carcinogenicity of topical mechlorethamine chemotherapy in cutaneous T cell lymphoma. *J Am Acad Dermatol* 1995;20:416–428.
101. Chiappelli F, Myers LW, Ellison GW, et al. Preferential reductions in lymphocyte sub-populations induced by monthly pulses of chlorambucil: studies in patients with chronic progressive multiple sclerosis. *Int J Immunopharmacol* 1991;13:455–461.
102. Kataria YP. Chlorambucil in sarcoidosis. *Chest* 1980;78:36–43.
103. Steinberg AD. Chlorambucil in the treatment of patients with immune-mediated rheumatic diseases. *Arthritis Rheum* 1993; 36:325–328.
104. Zucchelli P, Ponticelli C, Cagnoli L, et al. Prognostic value of T lymphocyte subset ratio in idiopathic membranous nephropathy. *Am J Nephrol* 1988;8(1):15–20.
105. Cannon GW, Jackson CG, Saumualson CO, et al. Chlorambucil therapy in rheumatoid arthritis: clinical experience in 28 patients and literature review. *Semin Arthritis Rheum* 1985;15:-106–118.
105a. Berk PD, Goldberg JD, Silverstein MN, et al. Increased inci-

dence of acute leukaemia in polycythaemia vera associated with chlorambucil therapy. *N Engl J Med* 1981;204:441–477.

106. Patapanian H, Graham S, Sambrook PN, et al. The oncogenicity of chlorambucil in rheumatoid arthritis. *Br J Rheumatol* 1988;27:44–47.
107. Snaith MI, Holt JM, Oliver DO, et al. Treatment of patients with systemic lupus erythematosus including nephritis with chlorambucil. *Br Med J* 1973;2:197–201.
108. Epstein WV, Grausz H. Favorable outcome in diffuse proliferative glomerulonephritis of systemic lupus erythematosus. *Arthritis Rheum* 1974;17:129–142.
109. Sabbour MS, Osman LM. Comparison of chlorambucil, azathioprine or cyclophosphamide combined with corticosteroids in the treatment of lupus nephritis. *Br J Dermatol* 1979;100(2): 113–125.
110. Reichert LJ, Huysmans FT, Assmann K, et al. Preserving renal function in patients with membranous nephropathy: daily oral chlorambucil compared with intermittent monthly pulses of cyclophosphamide. *Ann Intern Med* 1994;121:328–333.
111. Ponticelli C, Zucchelli P, Passerini P, et al. A randomized trial of methylprednisone and chlorambucil in idiopathic membranous nephropathy. *N Engl J Med* 1989;320:8–13.
112. Steinberg AD, Steinberg SC. Long-term preservation of renal function in patients with lupus nephritis receiving treatment that includes cyclophosphamide versus those treated with prednisone only. *Arthritis Rheum* 1991;34:945–950.
113. Donadio JV, Holley KE, Wagoner RD. Treatment of lupus nephritis with prednisone and combined prednisone and combined prednisone and azathioprine. *Ann Intern Med* 1972;77: 829–835.
114. Donadio JVJ, Holley KE, Wagoner RD, et al. Further observations on the treatment of lupus nephritis with prednisone and combined prednisone and azathioprine. *Arthritis Rheum* 1974; 17:573–582.
115. Hahn BH, Kantor OS, Osterland CK. Azathioprine plus prednisone compared with prednisone alone in the treatment of systemic lupus erythematosus. Report of a prospective controlled trial in 24 patients. *Ann Intern Med* 1975;83:597–605.
116. Cade R, Spooner G, Schlein E, et al. Comparison of azathioprine, prednisone, and heparin alone or combined in treating lupus nephritis. *Nephron* 1973;10:37–56.
117. Ginzler E, Diamond H, Guttadauria M, et al. Prednisone and azathioprine compared to prednisone plus low dose azathioprine and cyclophosphamide plus low dose azathioprine and cyclophosphamide in the treatment of diffuse lupus nephritis. *Arthritis Rheum* 1976;19:693–699.

117a. Esdaile JM, Joseph L, MacKenzie T, et al. The benefit of early treatment with immunosuppresive agents in lupus nephritis. *J Rheumatol* 1994;21:2046–2051.

118. Sztejnbok M, Stewart A, Diamond H. Azathioprine in the treatment of systemic lupus erythematosus: a controlled study. *Arthritis Rheum* 1971;14:639–645.
119. Sharon E, Kaplan D, Diamond H. Exacerbation of systemic lupus erythematosus after withdrawal of azothioprine therapy. *N Engl J Med* 1973;288:122–124.
120. Shehade S. Successful treatment of generalized discoid skin lesions with azathioprine (letter). *Arch Dermatol* 1986;122(4): 376–377.
121. Tsokos GC, Caughman SW, Klippel JH. Successful treatment of generalized discoid skin lesions with azathioprine. Its use in a patient with systemic lupus erythematosus. *Arch Dermatol* 1985;121:1323–1325.
122. Werth V, Franks AJ. Treatment of discoid skin lesions with azathioprine (letter). *Arch Dermatol* 1986;122(7):746–747.
123. Callen JP, Spencer LV, Burruss JB, et al. Azathioprine. An effective, corticosteroid-sparing therapy for patients with recalcitrant cutaneous lupus erythematous or with recalcitrant cutaneous leukocytoclastic vasculitis. *Arch Dermatol* 1991;127:515–522.
124. McCune WJ, Friedman AW. Immunosuppressive drug therapy for rheumatic disease. *Curr Opin Rheumatol* 1993;5:282–292.
125. DeMattos A, Olvaei A, Bennett W. Nephrotoxicity of immunosuppressive: long-term consequences and challenges for the future. *Am J Kidney Dis* 2000;35(2):333–346.
126. Feutren G, Mihatsch MJ. Risk factors for cyclosporine-induced nephropathy in patients with autoimmune diseases. *N Engl J Med* 1992;326:1654–1660.
127. Deray G, Benhmida M, Le Hoang P, et al. Renal function and blood pressure in patients receiving long-term, low-dose cyclosporine therapy for idiopathic autoimmune uveitis. *Ann Intern Med* 1992;117:578–583.
128. Altman RD, Perez GO, Sfakianakis GN. Interaction of cyclosporine A and nonsteroidal anti-inflammatory drugs on renal function in patients with rheumatoid arthritis. *Am J Med* 1992;93:396–402.
129. Balletta M, Sabella D, Magri P, et al. Cyclosporin plus steroids versus steroids alone in the treatment of lupus nephritis. *Contrib Nephrol* 1992;99:129–130.
130. Favre H, Miescher PA, Huang YP, et al. Cyclosporin in the treatment of lupus nephritis. *Am J Nephrol* 1989;9(suppl 1): 57–60.
131. Feutren G, Querin S, Tron F, et al. The effects of cyclosporine in patients with systemic lupus. *Transplant Proc* 1986;18:643–644.
132. Isenberg DA, Snaith ML, Morrow WJ, et al. Cyclosporin A for the treatment of systemic lupus erythematosus. *Int J Immunopharmacol* 1981;3:163–169.
133. Isenberg DA, Snaith ML, Al-Khader AA, et al. Cyclosporin relieves arthralgia, causes angioedema (letter). *N Engl J Med* 1980;303:754.
134. Radhakrishnan J, Valeri A, Kunis C, et al. Use of cyclosporin in lupus nephritis. *Contrib Nephrol* 1995;114:59–72.
135. Tokuda M, Kurata N, Mizoguchi A, et al. Effect of low-dose cyclosporin A on systemic lupus erythematosus disease activity. *Arthritis Rheum* 1994;37:551–558.
136. Hussein MM, Mooij JM, Roujouleh H. Cyclosporine in the treatment of lupus nephritis including two patients treated during pregnancy. *Clin Nephrol* 1993;40:160–163.
137. Caccavo D, Lagana B, Mitterhofer AP, et al. Long-term treatment of systemic lupus erythematosus with cyclosporin A. *Arthritis Rheum* 1997;40(1):27–35.
138. Dostal C, Tesai V, Rychlik I, et al. Effect of 1 year cyclosporine A treatment on the activity and renal involvement of systemic lupus erythematosus: a pilot study. *Lupus* 1998;7:29–36.
139. Tam L, Li E, Leung CB, et al. Long-term treatment of lupus nephritis with cyclosporin A. *Q J Med* 1998;91:573–580.
140. Morton S, Powell R. An audit of cyclosporin for systemic lupus erythematosus and related overlap syndromes: limitations of its use. *Ann Rheum Dis* 2000;59:487–489.
141. Ferrario L, Bellone M, Bozzolo E, et al. Remission from lupus nephritis resistant to cyclophosphamide after additional treatment with cyclosporin A (letter). *Rheumatology (Oxf)* 2000;39: 2180–2000.
142. Maeshima E, Yamada Y, Kodama N, et al. Successful pregnancy and delivery in a case of systemic lupus erythematosus treated with immunoadsorption therapy and cyclosporin A. *Scand J Rheumatol* 1999;28:54–57.
143. Cronstein B. Molecular therapeutics: methotrexate and its mechanism of action. *Arthritis Rheum* 1996;39(12): 1951–1960.
144. Mello S, Barros D, Silva A, et al. Methotrexate as a preferential cyclooxygenase 2 inhibitor in whole blood of patients with rheumatoid arthritis. *Rheumatology (Oxf)* 2000;39(5):533–536.
145. Fox DA, McCune WJ. Immunosuppressive drug therapy of sys-

temic lupus erythematosus. *Rheum Dis Clin North Am* 1994; 20:265–299.
146. Chatham W, Morgan S, Alarcon G. Renal failure: a risk factor for methotrexate toxicity. *Arthritis Rheum* 2000;43(5): 1185–1186.
147. Landewe R, van den Borne B, Breedveld F, et al. Methotrexate effects in patients with rheumatoid arthritis with cardiovascular comorbidity {letter}. *Lancet* 2000;355(9215):1616–1617.
148. Fijnheer R, Roest M, Hass F, et al. Homocysteine, methylenetetrahydrofolate reductase polymorphism, antiphospholipid antibodies and thromboembolic events in systemic lupus erythematosus. *J Rheumatol* 1998;25(9):1737–1742.
149. Cannon GW, Ward JR, Clegg DO, et al. Acute lung disease associated with low-dose pulse methotrexate therapy in patients with rheumatoid arthritis. *Arthritis Rheum* 1983;26:1269–1274.
150. Hoffman GS, Leavitt RY, Kerr GS, et al. The treatment of Wegener's granulomatosis with glucocorticoids and methotrexate. *Arthritis Rheum* 1992;35:1322–1329.
151. Hargreaves MR, Mowat AG, Benson MK. Acute pneumonitis associated with low dose methotrexate treatment for rheumatoid arthritis: report of five cases and review of published reports. *Thorax* 1992;47:628–633.
152. Kremer J, Alarcon G, Weinblatt M, et al. Clinical, laboratory, radiographic, and histopathologic features of methotrexate-associated lung injury in patients with rheumatoid arthritis. *Arthritis Rheum* 1997;40(10):1829–1837.
153. Imokawa S, Colby T, Leslie K, et al. Methotrexate pneumonitis: review of the literature and histopathological findings in nine patients. *Eur Respir J* 2000;15(2):373–381.
154. Janssen N, Genta M. The effects of immunosuppressive and anti-inflammatory medications on fertility, pregnancy, and lactation. *Arch Intern Med* 2000;160(5):610–619.
155. Roubenoff R, Hoyt J, Petri M, et al. Effects of antiinflammatory and immunosuppressive drugs on pregnancy and fertility. *Semin Arthritis Rheum* 1988;18:88–110.
156. Britto M, Rosenthal S, Taylor J, et al. Improving rheumatologists' screening for alcohol use and sexual activity. *Arch Pediatr Adolesc Med* 2000;154(5):478–483.
157. Moseley A, Lindsley H, Skikne B, et al. Reversible methotrexate associated lymphoproliferative disease evolving into Hodgkin's disease. *J Rheumatol* 2000;27(3):810–813.
158. Langford C, Talar-Williams C, Barron K, et al. A staged approach to the treatment of Wegener's granulomatosis. *Arthritis Rheum* 1999;42(12):2666–2673.
159. Hoffman GS, Leavitt RY, Kerr GS, et al. Treatment of glucocorticoid-resistant or relapsing Takayasu arteritis with methotrexate. *Arthritis Rheum* 1994;37:578–582.
160. Dubois E. *Lupus erythematosus. A review of the current status of discoid and systemic lupus erythematosus and their variants*, 2nd ed. Los Angeles: USC Press, 1976.
161. Miescher PA, Riethmuller D. Diagnosis and treatment of systemic lupus erythematosus. *Semin Hematol* 1965;2:338–345.
162. Rothenberg RJ, Graziano FM, Grandone JT, et al. The use of methotrexate in steroid-resistant systemic lupus erythematosus. *Arthritis Rheum* 1988;31(5):612–615.
163. Wilke WS, Krall PL, Scheetz RJ, et al. Methotrexate for systemic lupus erythematosus: a retrospective analysis of 17 unselected cases. *Clin Exp Rheumatol* 1991;9:581–587.
164. Abud-Mendoza C, Sturbaum AK, Vasquez-Compean A, et al. Methotrexate therapy in childhood systemic lupus erythematosus. *J Rheumatol* 1993;20:731–733.
165. Wilson K, Katz J, Abeles M. The use of methotrexate in systemic lupus erythematosus. *Arthritis Rheum* 1991;31(suppl):R39–R30.
166. Hashimoto M, Nonaka S, Furuta E, et al. Methotrexate for steroid-resistant systemic lupus erythematosus. *Clin Rheumatol* 1994;13:280–283.
167. Walz LeBlanc BA, Dagenais P, Urowitz MB, et al. Methotrexate in systemic lupus erythematosus. *J Rheumatol* 1994;21:836–838.
168. Rahman P, Humphrey-Murto S, Gladman D, et al. Efficacy and tolerability of methotrexate in antimalarial resistant lupus arthritis. *J Rheumatol* 1998;25:243–246.
169. Kipen Y, Littlejohn G, Morand E. Methotrexate use in systemic lupus erythematosus. *Lupus* 1997;6:385–389.
170. Gansauge S, Breitbart A, Rinaldi N, et al. Methotrexate in patients with moderate systemic lupus erythematosus (exclusion of renal and central nervous system disease). *Ann Rheum Dis* 1997;56(6):382–385.
170a. Carneiro J, Sato E. Double blind randomized placebo controlled clinical trial of methotrexate in systemic lupus erythematosus. *J Rheumatol* 1999;26:1275–1279.
171. Simmons W, Rayhill S. Preliminary risk-benefit assessment of mycophenolate mofetil in transplant rejection. *Drug Safety* 1997;17(2):75–92.
172. Kimball J, Pescovitz M, Book B, et al. Reduced human IgG anti-ATGAM antibody formation in renal transplant recipients receiving mycophenolate mofetil. *Transplantation* 1995;60: 1379–1383.
173. Ransom J. Mechanism of action of mycophenolate mofetil (review). *Ther Drug Monit* 1995;17(6):681–684.
174. Allison A, Eugui E. The design and development of an immunosuppressive drug, mycophenolate mofetil. *Springer Semin Immunopathol* 1993;14(4):353–80.
175. Eugui E, Mirkovich A. Lymphocyte-selective antiproliferative and immunosuppressive effects of mycophenolic acid in mice. *Scand J Immunol* 1991;33(2):175–83.
176. Burlingham W, Grailer A. Inhibition of both MLC and in vitro IgG memory response to tetanus toxoid by RS-61443. *Transplantation* 1991;51(2):545–547.
177. Allison A, Eugui E. Immunosuppressive and other effects of mycophenolic acid and an ester prodrug mycophenolate mofetil. *Immunol Rev* 1993;136:5–28.
178. Gregory C, Huang X, Pratt R, et al. Treatment with rapamycin and mycophenolic acid reduces arterial intimal thickening produced by mechanical injury and allows endothelial replacement. *Transplantation* 1995;59:655–661.
179. Raisanen-Sokolowski A, Myllarniemi M. Effect of mycophenolate mofetil on allograft arteriosclerosis (chronic rejection). *Transplant Proc* 1994;26(6):3225.
180. Raisanen-Sokolowski A, Vuoristo P, Myllarniemi M, et al. Mycophenolate mofetil (MMF, RS-61443) inhibits inflammation and smooth muscle proliferation in rat aortic allografts. *Transplant Immunol* 1995;3:342–351.
181. European Mycophenolate Mofetil Cooperative Study Group. Placebo controlled study of mycophenolate mofetil combined with cyclosporin and corticosteroids for prevention of acute rejection. *Lancet* 1995;27(345):1321–1325.
182. Tricontinental Mycophenolate Mofetil Renal Transplantation Study Group. A blinded, randomized clinical trial of mycophenolate mofetil for the prevention of acute rejection in cadaveric renal transplantation. *Transplantation* 1996;61(7): 1029–1037.
183. Sollinger H. Mycophenolate mofetil for the prevention of acute rejection in primary cadaveric renal allograft recipients. *Transplantation* 1995;60(3):224–232.
184. Blakely ML, Van der Werf WJ, Dalmasso AP, et al. Anti-B cell agents: suppression of natural antibodies and prolongation of survival in discordant xenografts. *Transplant Proc* 1994;26(3): 1374–1375.
185. Penny M, Boyd R. Mycophenolate mofetil prevents the induction of active Heymann nephritis: association with Th2 cytokine inhibition. *J Am Soc Nephrol* 1998;9(12):2272–2282.
186. Chanaud N, Vistica B. Inhibition of experimental autoimmune

uveoretinitis by mycophenolate mofetil, an inhibitor of purine metabolism. *Exp Eye Res* 1995;61:429–434.

187. Van Bruggen M, Walgreen B. Attenuation of murine lupus nephritis by mycopheolate mofetil. *J Am Soc Nephrol* 1998;9 (8):1407–1415.
188. Deleted in page proofs.
189. Corna D, Morigi M. Mycophenolate mofetil limits renal damage and prolongs life in murine lupus autoimmune disease. *Kidney Int* 1997;51:1583–1589.
190. McMurray R, Elbourne K. Mycophenolate mofetil suppresses autoimmunity and mortality of the female NZB × NZW F1 mouse model of systemic lupus erythematosus. *J Rheumatol* 1998;25(12):2364–2370.

190a. Birkland S. Steroid-free immunosuppression after kidney transplantation with antithymacyte globulin induction and cyclosporine and mycophenolate mofetil maintenance therapy. *Transplantation* 1998;66:1207–1210.

191. Neurath M, Wanitschke R. Randomised trial of mycophenolate mofetil versus azathioprine for treatment of chronic active Crohn's disease. *Gut* 1999;44(5):625–628.

191a. Daina E. Schieppati A. Mycophenolate mofetil for the treatment of Takayasu arteritis: report of three cases. *Ann Intern Med* 1999;130:422–426.

192. Larkin G, Lightman S. Mycophenolate mofetil. A useful immunosuppressive in inflammatory eye disease. *Ophthalmology* 1999;106(2):370–374.
193. Goldblum R. Therapy of rheumatoid arthritis with mycophenolate mofetil. *Clin Exp Rheumatol* 1993;11(8):S117–119.
194. Nousari H, Sragovich A. Mycophenolate mofetil in autoimmune and inflammatory skin disorders. *J Am Acad Dermatol* 1999;40(2):265–268.
195. Haufs M, Beissert S. Psoriasis vulgaris treated successfully with mycophenolate mofetil. *Br J Dermatol* 1998;138(1):179–181.
196. Enk A, Knop J. Mycophenolate is effective in the treatment of pemphigus vulgaris. *Arch Dermatol* 1999;135(1):54–56.
197. Nousari H, Lynch W. The effectiveness of mycophenolate mofetil in refractory pyoderma gangreosum. *Arch Dermatol* 1998;134(12):1509–1511.

197a. Petri M. Mycophenolate mofetil treatment of systemic lupus erythematosus. *Arthritis Rheum* 1999;42:5303.

198. Dooley M, Cosio F. Mycophenolate mofetil therapy in lupus nephritis: clinical. *J Am Soc Nephrol* 1999;10(4):833–839.
199. Briggs W, Choi M, Scheel P. Successful mycophenolate mofetil treatment of glomerular disease. *Am J Kidney Dis* 1998;31(2): 213–217.
200. Gaubitz M, Schorat A, Schotte H, et al. Mycophenolate mofetil for the treatment of systemic lupus erythematosus: an open pilot trial. *Lupus* 1999;8:731–736.
201. Pashinian N, Wallace D, Klinenberg J. Mycophenolate mofetil for systemic lupus erythematosus. *Arthritis Rheum* 1998;41:S110.
202. Chan TM, Li FK, Tang C, et al. Efficacy of mycophenolate mofetil in patients with diffuse proliferative lupus nephritis. *N Engl J Med* 2000;343:1156–1162.
203. *Physicians' desk reference.* Medical Economics, 1999.

58

NONPHARMACOLOGIC THERAPEUTIC MODALITIES

DANIEL J. WALLACE

In addition to medication, physical measures, and psychologic support, the treatment of systemic lupus erythematosus (SLE) may necessitate the use of other nonpharmacologic modalities. These include dialysis and transplantation for end-stage renal disease, lasers for cutaneous lesions and possibly synovitis, apheresis for life-threatening complications of the disease, and lymphocyte depletion through thoracic duct drainage or total lymphoid irradiation for selected patients with refractory disease.

DIALYSIS

Patients with end-stage renal disease from chronic SLE represent 1.5% of all dialysis patients in the United States (1). Two thousand patients with lupus are dialyzed annually; 10% succumb each year.

Uremia

Uremia was the major cause of death in patients with SLE until the 1960s, when dialysis became available. Only a small percentage of dialysis patients have SLE. Between 1977 and 1985, 5,726 persons in Australia and New Zealand were placed on dialysis; only 63 (1.1%) had SLE (2). Despite therapeutic advances, 26 of 128 patients with nephritis who were followed by Wallace between 1980 and 1989 evolved end-stage renal disease that required dialysis (3,4); all but three of the 26 had nephrotic syndrome. Between 1972 and 1993, 104 of 566 patients diagnosed with SLE in Okinawa, Japan, evolved end-stage renal disease (5). The reader is referred to Cheigh and Stenzel's excellent literature review (6).

Uremia and dialysis both are associated with a decrease in the systemic activity of SLE in many, but not all, patients (7,8). Mojcik and Klippel summarized the results in 179 patients in seven studies, and concluded that clinical, serologic, and steroid requirements decreased (9). Szeto noted that most disease flares occur during the first year of dialysis (l0), and a high level of disease activity during this time also was found by Bruce et al. (11). Ziff and Helderman (12) have speculated that the toxic effects of uremia on the immune system are responsible for its ameliorative effects on extrarenal disease. It also is possible that the disease has run its course in some individuals and subsided but, by that time, the chronic renal damage is irreversible.

Reversibility

Some patients who develop renal failure from lupus nephritis can discontinue dialysis. This was true in 41% of Kimberly et al.'s 41 patients; 11 were dialyzed for less than 2 months (13). On the other hand, 37% died. Five were transplanted successfully. Coplon et al. (14) reported on their experience with 28 dialysis patients followed between 1969 and 1980. Of these, eight were dialyzed for a mean of 4.3 months before discontinuation, six deaths occurred in the patients with the highest steroid requirement, seven were transplanted, and only three had extrarenal disease. The first few months on dialysis appear to be critical. A high mortality rate is observed, but many of those who survive can either discontinue dialysis or become candidates for transplantation (15). Acute tubular necrosis superimposed on lupus nephritis can induce transient renal failure (16).

Prognosis

Survival on dialysis is good. Ziff and Helderman's 30 patients had a 67% 5-year survival rate (12), Jarrett et al.'s had 59% (17), and Cheigh et al.'s had 65% in the late 1970s (18). These figures compare favorably with those of non-SLE dialysis patients. Some reports have documented a better survival rate: 71% in Australia and New Zealand at 5 years (2), and 89% in 55% Dutch patients at 5 years (19). Males had a poorer renal survival than females (20), and African American women fare poorly with 58% of 19 dead at 5 years (21). In these studies, nonrenal SLE activity was minimal. Most deaths were related to infection or vascular-access problems.

At the University of California, only three of 12 patients on dialysis for lupus nephritis needed corticosteroids after 31 months' mean observation (22). In 1990, Cheigh et al. (23) presented a follow-up of 59 patients with end-stage renal disease who were seen at New York Hospital between 1970 and 1987. Of these, 86% were female, and mean age was 27.4 years at end-stage renal disease onset. They were followed for a mean of 6.5 years. SLE disease activity at years 1, 5, and 10 was 55%, 6.5%, and 0%, respectively. The 5- and 10-year survival rates were 81.1% and 74.6%, respectively. Erythropoietin decreases the morbidity of patients with SLE on dialysis (24).

Ginzler et al.'s multicenter trial of 1,103 patients with SLE (25) showed that dialysis has little impact in evaluating causes of death in SLE, although dialysis patients have a much higher rate of infection (7,26). Socioeconomic considerations also are important. In the largely indigent group at Los Angeles Harbor-University of California at Los Angeles (UCLA) Medical Center, six of nine dialysis patients died at 1 to 28 months, and five of these six had disease flares (27). The quality of life of patients on dialysis has been reviewed. They tended to have good mental well being but reduced physical function and general health (28).

Hemodialysis Versus Peritoneal Dialysis

The success of hemodialysis in ameliorating disease activity may result from its ability to remove circulating pathogenic immune complexes, complement, and other factors (29). Hemodialysis also has antiinflammatory effects, decreases T-helper lymphocyte levels, and diminishes mitogenic responsiveness (30,31). Three cases of a patient developing SLE while on hemodialysis have appeared (32,32a,33), and while rare, successful pregnancies while on hemodialysis are noted occasionally (34).

In contrast, peritoneal dialysis does not cause these changes. Several studies have documented more reactivation of SLE, higher anti–double-stranded DNA (anti-dsDNA) levels, more thrombocytopenia, and higher steroid requirements with peritoneal dialysis (10,16,30,31). In one center, four of six patients who were started on peritoneal dialysis had to be switched to hemodialysis (35), though this has not been found by others (36). Nossent et al. (19,37) noted among 55 patients that peritoneal dialysis was associated with poorer survival, more serositis, cytopenias, and serologic activity. Switching to it from hemodialysis could reactivate lupus. It is my experience that barring extenuating or unusual circumstances, hemodialysis is preferable to peritoneal dialysis.

TRANSPLANTATION

Patients with lupus account for 3% of all renal transplantations in the United States, or approximately 300 cases per year (38). By 1996, the overall graft survival for all diseases at one year had improved to 93.9% from living donors and 87.7% from cadaveric grafts, compared to 88.8% and 75.7%, respectively, in 1988 (39).

Graft And Patient Survival

By 1975, patients with SLE in the United States were being transplanted, and 150 were transplanted between 1975 and 1980 (40,41). These studies concluded that allografts from a living, related donor have a much better survival rate. Two-year graft survivals averaged 50%. In Australia and New Zealand, 19 transplants performed between 1977 and 1985 were associated with 95% and 83% survival rates at 1 and 5 years, respectively, and with 75% and 70% 1- and 5-year graft survival, respectively (2). In 1987, Roth et al. (42) reported a 93% patient survival and an 84% graft survival at 6 years among 15 patients who were transplanted at their institution. Of 2,510 renal transplants performed at the University of Minnesota between 1969 and 1987, 33 (1%) were for SLE (43), as were 20 of 616 (3%) at Albert Einstein College of Medicine (44). Of Cheigh et al.'s 59 patients with lupus and end-stage renal disease (discussed earlier), 18 were transplanted over a 17-year period (23). Massry's group at Los Angeles County/University of Southern California Medical Center transplanted 64 indigent (60% Hispanic or black) patients with SLE between 1979 and 1992 (45); 80 received cadaveric transplants. Five-year graft and patient survivals were 61 and 86, respectively. Currently, 5-year graft survivals average 70% (19,23,43, 44,46–51). Criswell's group has undertaken three large-scale reviews of transplantation in the cyclosporin era and compared their results with 97 patients to others in a literature review (52–54). Graft survival compared to nonlupus controls was 82 (versus 88%) at 1 year but only 19 (versus 35%) at 10 years. Allograft failure risk was doubled and associated with HLA mismatches, smoking, and delayed allograft functioning (188). An excellent, current review has appeared (55).

Indigent pediatric populations do not do as well. Among 17 children with SLE who were transplanted in Brooklyn (56), 80% and 45% 1- and 4-year graft survivals, respectively, were reported. The availability of cyclosporine has resulted in a decreased use of azathioprine to prevent rejection. One study comparing these drugs in SLE transplants (19 received azathioprine and 17 cyclosporine) documented the statistically significant superiority of cyclosporine in graft survival (57), while another came to opposite conclusions (58).

Antiphospholipid Antibodies

Patients with antiphospholipid antibodies are clearly at an increased risk for thromboembolic events, which can have an adverse effect on graft survival (59–62), the course of dialysis (63) and vascular access viability (64). Stone et al.

identified 25 patients with antiphospholipid antibodies who were transplanted at University of California, San Francisco. Fifteen had thromboembolic events, and ten died (65). Antiplatelet drugs should be employed, and the addition of warfarin may be necessary.

Serologic Features, Disease Recurrence, And Pregnancy

Patients undergoing transplantation may have persistent elevations of antinuclear antibody and anti-DNA antibody titers as well as reduced complement levels. These serologic abnormalities are of little importance and do not affect the outcome of the graft (7,40,42). These abnormalities were present in four of seven patients who were transplanted by our group between 1980 and 1989. Despite this, disease recurrence in the transplanted kidney is rare. Various centers have noted nephritis in zero of 12 patients (66), zero of seven (7), one of 17 (56), two of 15 (42), one of 28 (19), one of 14 (51), and one of 18 patients (40), for a total of six in 111 patients (5). Isolated case reports of disease recurrence suggest that a disproportionate number of these patients had undergone peritoneal dialysis or had active disease at the time of transplantation (67–71). Criswell's group noted nine of 97 cyclosporin treated patients had recurrent lupus nephritis by biopsy (52). Only three had abnormal serologies and one was symptomatic. Their literature review suggested that using serologic parameters or serum-complement levels to evaluate for recurrence was inaccurate (54).

Despite this, most of the allografts were still functioning well (72). Extrarenal lupus activity usually is quiescent after renal transplantation (73). One case of *de novo* SLE in a renal transplant patient has appeared (74).

At Thomas Jefferson University, 35 pregnancies were reported among 24 SLE transplant patients (75). 77% were successful, though many were complicated by preeclampsia and hypertension.

In summary, to achieve the optimal transplant environment, patients should be in remission, be on hemodialysis or no dialysis, and receive an allograft from a living, related donor. Cyclosporine with mycophenolate mofetil and low-dose prednisone now constitutes the immunosuppressive regimen of choice, but this regimen has not been specifically studied in lupus. See Table 58.1.

TABLE 58.1. INDICATIONS FOR APHERESIS IN SYSTEMIC LUPUS ERYTHEMATOSUS

I. Absolute—benefits are clear-cut and often life-saving
   1. Thrombotic thrombocytopenic purpura
   2. Cryoglobulinemia
   3. Hyperviscosity syndrome
II. Relative—acceptable to use when clinically indicated
   1. Severe organ-threatening disease that is underresponsive to steroid and cytotoxic drug therapy.
III. Investigational
   1. Antiphospholipid antibody removal in pregnancy
   2. Anti-Ro/SSA antibody removal in pregnancy
IV. Contraindicated
   1. Mild lupus or nonorgan-threatening lupus

LASER THERAPY

Lasers have been sporadically studied in rheumatoid arthritis since 1980 (76). Evidence has suggested that neodymium:yttrium-aluminum-garnet (Nd:YAG) lasers can decrease synovial proliferation (77), and that gallium-aluminum-arsenide lasers diminish lymphocyte mitogenic responsiveness (78). However, two double-blind, randomized trials in rheumatoid arthritis showed no benefits (79,80).

Carbon-dioxide lasers have been used to treat discoid lupus lesions and telangiectasias. These lesions can be vaporized, but cellular alterations in nonvaporized cells that are several hundred microns away may be responsible for decreased disease activity (81). Argon lasers also have been used (82).

Laser therapy should be regarded as experimental. Preferably, it should be used as part of a well-designed research protocol.

LYMPHOCYTE DEPLETION

Basic Principles

Evidence that the lympholytic actions of alkylating agents, corticosteroids, and radiation were responsible for ameliorating certain disease states has led to investigations of the role of thoracic-duct drainage, total-lymphoid irradiation, and lymphapheresis in rheumatic diseases. Lymphoid tissue occupies up to 3% of the total body weight; this includes 1% lymphocytes, or 10^{12} lymphocytes per 70 kg. Lymphocytes are widely distributed and consist of both long- and short-lived populations. T cells comprise roughly 90% of the lymphocytes in the thoracic duct lymph, 65% in peripheral blood, 75% in the mesentery, and 25% in the spleen; most of these are long-lived. Therefore, thoracic duct drainage and localized radiation remove lymphocyte populations in a different manner than those removed by lymphapheresis (83).

Thoracic Duct Drainage

Pioneered by researchers at UCLA in the early 1970s, cannulation of the thoracic duct followed by removal of billions of lymphocytes clearly improved disease activity in patients with SLE (84). The procedure is not practical for clinical use, however, because it is technically difficult, expensive, frequently complicated by infection, and only can be done once.

Lymphapheresis

On-line lymphocyte depletion has not been studied adequately as a treatment modality for SLE. No commercially available membranes selectively remove lymphocytes without other leukocytes, so only cell separation by centrifugation methods have been used. Because most patients with SLE are lymphopenic, and this is aggravated by the concomitant use of corticosteroids or cytotoxic drugs, it often is difficult to remove the lymphocyte fraction on cell separators. Our studies in patients with rheumatoid arthritis have shown that a 5×10^9 lymphapheresis performed three times a week for 6 weeks can induce a significant lymphopenia that persists for 4 to 6 months (85). Unlike plasma removal, 15% of the body's total blood volume must be extracorporeal to perform a lymphocyte cut on centrifugation devices, and this requires a near-normal cardiovascular and pulmonary status. In addition, blood transfusions may be required. Despite these drawbacks, however, Spiva and Cecere (86) reported that a combination of lymphapheresis and plasmapheresis was clinically beneficial in 16 of 19 patients with SLE on concurrent immunosuppression, and that helper:suppressor T-cell ratios were decreased.

Total Lymphoid Irradiation

Between 1980 and 1997, a total of 17 patients with lupus nephritis and nephrotic syndrome refractory to conventional drug therapy received 2,000 rad of total lymphoid irradiation over a 4- to 6-week period at Stanford University (87–92). Clinical responses were seen within 3 months and sometimes persisted for years. At follow-up ranging from 12 to 79 months, seven patients were off corticosteroids and without nephrosis; however, one patient died, one ultimately required chronic dialysis, and four developed neutropenia, one developed thrombocytopenia, three developed bacterial sepsis, and four developed herpes zoster. T-helper populations (i.e., CD4+ cells) decreased, and selective B-cell deficits documented by diminished pokeweed mitogen-induced immunoglobulin secretion were observed. Both total and serum immunoglobulin-specific IgE levels were not altered. The survival rate at 7.5 years was identical to that of a historical control group treated with steroids and immunosuppressives, with an equal prevalence of serious complications. Genovese et al. published an abstract in 1997 with a long-term follow up on these patients (93). Six of 21 had died, and four developed cancer. 57% were dialyzed.

Trentham et al. (94) at Harvard also used total lymphoid irradiation (for rheumatoid arthritis), but they no longer advocate its use. These authors agree that although short-term benefits are apparent, the high probability of disease recurrence after several months to years limits the physician's options in giving alkylating agents to patients who have already been irradiated (95). Further, a high infection rate is observed, and newer therapeutic strategies (e.g., parenteral cyclophosphamide) probably are superior to total lymphoid irradiation. An Israeli group noted unsatisfactory results in two patients who underwent total lymphoid irradiation (96).

Photopheresis

In extracorporeal photochemotherapy, commonly known as photopheresis, leukocytes obtained at apheresis are treated with ultraviolet A (UVA) irradiation after the patient has received a photoactivatable drug, p-methoxypsoralen (97). Leukocytes reinfused into the patient can function but have diminished responses. Although only 5% of one's total circulating lymphocytes are treated, photopheresis clearly is beneficial for cutaneous T-cell lymphomas. Knobler et al. (98,99) observed modest improvements in eight patients with SLE in an uncontrolled study. The potentially harmful effects of UVA light in SLE, particularly in those with anti-Ro/SSA antibodies, has tempered enthusiasm for this procedure. Photopheresis is being intensively studied for scleroderma and graft-versus-host reactions.

PLASMAPHERESIS

Basic Principles

Apheresis refers to the removal of a blood component (e.g., red-blood cells, lymphocytes, leukocytes, platelets, plasma) by centrifugation or a membrane cell separator, with return of the other components to the patient. Removing 1 L of plasma decreases plasma proteins by 1 g/dL, but because of compartmental equilibration and protein synthesis, 2.5 L of plasma must be exchanged weekly to decrease protein levels. In the intravascular space, 50% of the total IgG and 67% of the total IgM are found. Nine exchanges of 40 mL/kg over 3 weeks leave only 5% native plasma. The removal rate of plasma proteins and components depends on charge, solubility, avidity to other plasma proteins, configuration, synthesis, and uptake rates. In immunologic disorders, the recovery of immunoglobulin levels can be slowed by the concurrent use of immunosuppressive agents. If none are used, then antibody rebound, or the tendency of certain antibody levels to rise rapidly above their prepheresis baseline after initially decreasing, is observed; this often correlates with a disease flare (81). Plasma usually is replaced with a combination of albumin, salt, and water. Certain complications of lupus (e.g., thrombotic thrombocytopenic purpura) necessitate the use of fresh-frozen plasma replacement, because a plasma factor is deficient. When performed by personnel at experienced blood banks or dialysis facilities, plasmapheresis usually is safe; serious complications (e.g., hypotension, arrhythmia, infection) occur less than 3% of the time in this group of sick patients (100). The reader is referred to my detailed reviews of the subject (101,102).

Rationale In Systemic Lupus Erythematosus

Plasmapheresis can remove circulating immune complexes and immune reactants (e.g., free antibody, complement components), alter the equilibrium between free and bound complexes, and restore reticuloendothelial phagocytic function (103). Three different centers have documented reversal of the reticuloendothelial system blockade by plasmapheresis (104–106). In one report (107), plasmapheresis improved suppressor-cell functioning and, in another (108), selectively removed IgG anti-DNA. Steven et al. (109) demonstrated improved bacterial killing by monocytes after plasmapheresis, and in patients with mild disease, Tsokos et al. (110) found no change in proliferative responses to mitogens or lymphocyte subpopulation percentages. In 17 steroid- and immunosuppressive-resistant patients with lupus nephritis, however, Wallace et al. (111) reported normal B- and T-cell counts but diminished mitogenic responsiveness and CD4 levels (compared with pre-plasmapheresis values) after 15 exchanges.

Clinical Studies In Systemic Lupus Erythematosus

The use of plasmapheresis was reported first by Jones et al. in 1976 (112). Follow-up observations brought the conclusion that patients who are the most seriously ill and have the highest levels of circulating immune complexes respond best (113–116). Patients who are treated concomitantly with plasmapheresis, prednisone, and cyclophosphamide do better than those who are treated with prednisone and azathioprine (117), and those who are on prednisone alone may become worse (118). The procedure is well tolerated in children and pregnant women with SLE (119–120).

The most impressive results were reported in patients with lupus nephritis who had active disease and minimal scarring. Of 31 Finnish patients in this subset, 24 responded to treatment (121). Kincaid-Smith's group (122) rebiopsied eight patients with acute crescentic proliferative lupus nephritis several weeks after they received prednisone and cyclophosphamide and underwent plasmapheresis, and they found dramatic improvements in seven. A literature review in 1986 noted that 69% of 42 cases of diffuse proliferative nephritis improved after plasma exchange (123). These and other promising reports (124–126) led to two controlled trials. Lewis' group randomized 86 patients with new-onset proliferative nephritis to oral cyclophosphamide and prednisone, with or without plasmapheresis (127–130). Both groups improved, and no differences in the outcome were noted. Numerous methodologic flaws minimize the value of this study, however (131). Wallace et al. (111,131) restricted their study to 27 patients with nephrotic syndrome who were resistant to a minimum 3-month trial of steroids and cytotoxic drugs. Of these, ten were randomized to continue their therapy, and plasmapheresis was added to 17. After 2 years, seven had a good outcome (i.e., normal serum-creatinine level and resolution of nephrotic syndrome), and seven had a poor outcome (i.e., dialysis or death). All seven who had a good outcome underwent plasmapheresis (p=.026). Of the seven responders, five had undergone pheresis. The poor responders could not be predicted in advance by any of 30 variables used (111,131).

Interest has focused on the removal of anticardiolipin antibody and the lupus anticoagulant by plasmapheresis during pregnancy or in patients who have experienced recurrent thromboembolic episodes (132). Results have been mixed (133–140). Plasmapheresis is safe during pregnancy (141) and can be used weekly for the temporary removal of anticardiolipin (141a,142–144). It is especially helpful if large amounts of the IgM isotype are present (145). The apheretic removal of anti-Ro/SSA in mothers whose fetuses show signs of congenital heart block is currently under study (146–149).

Clark et al. (150) embarked on a study of long-term plasmapheresis in patients with SLE and achieved modest, but not cost-effective, results. Isolated case reports have claimed efficacy for almost every manifestation of SLE. Six French patients with central nervous system lupus had favorable responses (152), and this was confirmed by Neuwelt et al. in a larger study (153). The usefulness of plasmapheresis in cryoglobulinemia, thrombotic thrombocytopenic purpura, and hyperviscosity syndrome is well established (102,154,155), and these complications occasionally occur in patients with SLE. Several reports have suggested that plasmapheresis is useful for pulmonary hemorrhage (156–158).

Euler's group in Germany has devised an innovative approach for the treatment of seriously ill patients with SLE (159). It involves deliberately inducing antibody rebound with plasmapheresis, followed by high-dose intravenous cyclophosphamide to eliminate the increased numbers of malignant clones. Their pulse synchronization technique has resulted in some spectacular successes with long-term, treatment-free remissions (127,159–166). The net result was that pulse/synchronization does not work using conventional cyclophosphamide doses for lupus nephritis (167) or the disease in general (168). Using higher-dose cyclophosphamide can be more effective, though much riskier.

New membrane technologies have enabled selective plasmapheresis to be performed. Membranes that remove cryoproteins (169), anti–single-stranded DNA (170,171), IgG containing circulating immune complexes (172), and anti-dsDNA by immune adsorption (173–181) have been developed. Unfortunately, membranes activate complement and may present additional risks of hemolysis. In my experience, any theoretic cost saving obtained by avoiding albumin replacement is countered by the frequent clogging of expensive membranes, which necessitates termination of the procedure or use of a second membrane. Also, many patients with SLE do not have anti-DNA, and it is only one of many putative autoantibodies that may accelerate the disease process. Flares with treatment also have been reported (182). Further, selective membranes remove fewer plasma proteins than conventional plasmapheresis; this usually is not the practitioner's intent.

Summary

At this time, plasmapheresis should be used only for patients with renal disease who are resistant to corticosteroid and cytotoxic drug therapy, specific disease subsets in which its efficacy is established (e.g., those with hyperviscosity syndrome, cryoglobulinemia, or thrombotic thrombocytopenic purpura), and in those with acute, life-threatening complications of SLE, in each instance in combination with corticosteroids and cytotoxic therapy (Table 58.1).

ULTRAVIOLET A-1 IRRADIATION

McGrath et al. (183–186) have reported modestly beneficial effects of the longer wavelengths of UVA-1 radiation (340 to 400 nm) in open-label, double-blind, placebo-controlled, and long-term follow-up studies. Disease activity indices, cutaneous lesions, and anti-dsDNA levels improved. No side effects were reported. The mechanism by which this might work has been speculated on (187), and these reports await independent confirmation.

SUMMARY: DIALYSIS AND TRANSPLANTATION IN SYSTEMIC LUPUS ERYTHEMATOSUS

Up to 10% of SLE patients evolve end-stage renal disease. Their 5-year survival with optimal care is 80% to 90%.

Hemodialysis has theoretical advantages over peritoneal dialysis, is associated with fewer infections, and perhaps less lupus activity.

The majority of lupus patients have their disease activity improve when uremic.

Graft survival for SLE patients in the United States at 1 year is less than the 93.9% national average, and usually is in the 80% to 90% range.

Transplantation is most successful if lupus is not active at the time of surgery.

Patients with a history of antiphospholipid antibody-related events have a poor outcome.

REFERENCES

1. United States Renal Data System. USRDS 1991. *Am J Kidney Dis* 1991;18(suppl 2):11–27.
2. Pollock CA, Ibels LS. Dialysis and transplantation in patients with renal failure due to systemic lupus erythematosus. The Australian and New Zealand experience. *Aust N Z J Med* 1987; 17:321–325.
3. Pistiner M, Wallace DJ, Nessim S, et al. Lupus erythematosus in the 1980s: a survey of 570 patients. *Semin Arthritis Rheum* 1991;21:55–64.
4. Neumann K, Wallace DJ, Azen C, et al. Lupus in the 1980's: III. Influence of clinical variables, biopsy and treatment on the outcome of 150 patients with lupus nephritis seen at a single center. *Semin Arthritis Rheum* 1995;25:47–55.
5. Iseki K, Miyasato F, Orura T, et al. An epidemiologic analysis of end-stage lupus nephritis. *Am J Kidney Dis* 1994;232:547–554.
6. Cheigh JS, Stenzel KH. End-stage renal disease in systemic lupus erythematosus. *Am J Kidney Dis* 1993;21:28.
7. Brown CD, Rao TKS, Maxey RW, et al. Regression of clinical and immunological expression of systemic lupus erythematosus (SLE) consequent to development of uremia (abstract). *Kidney Int* 1979;16:884.
8. Wallace DJ, Podell TE, Weiner JM, et al. Lupus nephritis. Experience with 230 patients in a private practice from 1950 to 1980. *Am J Med* 1982;72:209–220.
9. Mojcik CF, Klippel JH. End-stage renal disease and systemic lupus erythematosus. *Amer J Med* 1996;101:100–107.
10. Szeto CC, Li PKT, Wong TYH, et al. Factors associated with active systemic lupus erythematosus after endstage renal disease. *J Rheumatol* 1998;25:1520–1525.
11. Bruce IN, Hallett DC, Gladman DD, et al. Extrarenal disease activity in systemic lupus-erythematosus is not suppressed by chronic renal insufficiency or renal replacement therapy. *J Rheumatol* 1999;26:1490–1494.
12. Ziff M, Helderman JH. Dialysis and transplantation in end-stage lupus nephritis (editorial). *N Engl J Med* 1983;308: 218–219.
13. Kimberly RP, Lockshin MD, Sherman RL, et al. Reversible end stage' lupus nephritis. Analysis of patients able to discontinue dialysis. *Am J Med* 1983;74:361–368.
14. Coplon NS, Diskin CJ, Peterson J, et al. The long-term clinical course of systemic lupus erythematosus in end-stage renal disease. *N Engl J Med* 1983;308:186–190.
15. Correia P, Cameron JS, Ogg CS, et al. End-stage renal failure in systemic lupus erythematosus with nephritis. *Clin Nephrol* 1984;22:293–302.
16. Henry R, Williams AV, McFadden NR, et al. Histopathologic evaluation of lupus patients with transient renal failure. *Am J Kidney Dis* 1986;8:417–421.
17. Jarrett MP, Santhanam S, Del Greco F. The clinical course of end-stage renal disease in systemic lupus erythematosus. *Arch Intern Med* 1983;143:1353–1356.
18. Cheigh JS, Stenzel KH, Rubin AL, et al. Systemic lupus erythematosus in patients with chronic renal failure. *Am J Med* 1983; 75:602–606.
19. Nossent HC, Swaak TJ, Berden JH. Systemic lupus erythematosus: analysis of disease activity in 55 patients with end-stage renal failure treated with hemodialysis or continuous ambulatory peritoneal dialysis. Dutch Working Party on SLE. *Am J Med* 1990;89:169–174.
20. Nossent HC, Swaak TJ, Berden JH. Systemic lupus erythematosus after renal transplantation: patient and graft survival and disease activity. *Ann Intern Med* 1991;114:183–188.
21. Krane NK, Burjak K, Archie M, et al. Persistent lupus activity in end-stage renal disease. *Am J Kidney Dis* 1999;33:872–879.
22. Pahl MV, Vaziri ND, Saiki JK, et al. Chronic hemodialysis in end-stage lupus nephritis: changes of clinical and serological activities. *Artif Organs* 1984;8:423–428.
23. Cheigh JS, Kim H, Stenzel KH, et al. Systemic lupus erythe-

matosus in patients with end-stage renal disease: long-term follow-up on the prognosis of patients and the evolution of lupus activity. *Am J Kidney Dis* 1990;16:189–195.

24. Romero R, Novoa D, Perez-Frerria A, et al. Resistance to recombinant human erythropoietin in a hemodialysis patient with lupus reactivation. *Nephron* 1995;69:343–344.
25. Ginzler EM, Diamond HS, Weiner M, et al. A multicenter study of outcome of systemic lupus erythematosus. I. Entry variables as predictors of progress. *Arthritis Rheum* 1982;25: 601–611.
26. Gral T, Schroth P, Sellers A, et al. Terminal lupus nephropathy (TLN) treated with chronic hemodialysis (CHD) (abstract). *Clin Res* 1970;18:150.
27. Sires RL, Adler SG, Louie JS, et al. Poor prognosis in end-stage lupus nephritis due to nonautologous vascular access site associated septicemia and lupus flares. *Am J Nephrol* 1989;9: 279–284.
28. Vu TV, Escalante A. A comparison of the quality of life of patients with systemic lupus erythematosus with and without end stage renal disease. *J Rheumatol* 1999;26:2595–2601.
29. Ng RCK, Craddock PR. End-stage renal disease in systemic lupus erythematosus (letter). *N Engl J Med* 1983;308:15–37.
30. Rodby RA, Korbet SM, Lewis EJ. Persistence of clinical and serologic activity in patients with systemic lupus erythematosus undergoing peritoneal dialysis. *Am J Med* 1987;83:613–618.
31. Wu GG, Gelbart DR, Hasbargen JA, et al. Reactivation of systemic lupus in three patients undergoing CAPD. *Peritoneal Dialysis Bull* 1986;6:6–9.
32. Hernandez-Juras J, Bernis C, Paraiso V, et al. Development of systemic lupus erythematosus in a patient on hemodialysis. *Am J Nephrol* 1992;12:105–107.

32a. Al-Hawas F, Abdalla AH, Al-Sulaiman MH, et al. Development of systemic lupus erythematosus in a male patient after 14 years on hemodialysis. *Am J Kidney Dis* 1997;29:631–632.

33. Kasama RK, Shusterman NH, Rocco MV. The de novo diagnosis of systemic lupus erythematosus in a hemodialysis patient. *J Clin Rheumatol* 1996;2:160–162.
34. Toyota T, Yorioka N, Takahashi N, et al. Successful birth in a hemodialysis patient with SLE. *Nephron* 1993;65:331–332.
35. Kahl LE, Al-Sabbagh R, Greenberg A, et al. Comparison of hemodialysis (HD) and peritoneal dialysis (PD) in systemic lupus erythematosus (SLE) patients with end stage renal failure (ESRF) (abstract). *Arthritis Rheum* 1986;29(suppl):S97.
36. Stock GG, Krane NK. Treatment of end-stage renal disease due to lupus nephritis: comparison of six patients treated with both peritoneal and hemodialysis. *Adv Perit Dial* 1993;9:147–151.
37. Berend K, Nossent H. Reactivation of systemic lupus erythematosus after transfer to peritoneal dialysis. *Nephrol Dial Transplant* 1997;12:2808.
38. Suthanthiran M, Stron TB. Renal transplantation. *N Engl J Med* 1994;331:365–394.
39. Hariharan S, Johnson CP, Bresnahan BA, et al. Improved graft survival after renal transplantation in the United States, 1988-1996. *N Engl J Med* 2000;342:605–612.
40. Amend WJ Jr, Vincenti F, Feduska NJ, et al. Recurrent systemic lupus erythematosus involving renal allografts. *Ann Intern Med* 1981;94:444–448.
41. Cats S, Terasaki PI, Perdue S, et al. Increased vulnerability of the donor organ in related kidney transplants for certain diseases. *Transplantation* 1984;37:575–579.
42. Roth D, Milgrom M, Esquenazi V, et al. Renal transplantation in systemic lupus erythematosus: one center's experience. *Am J Nephrol* 1987;7:367–374.
43. Bumgardner GL, Mauer SM, Ascher NL, et al. Long-term outcome of renal transplantation in patients with systemic lupus erythematosus. *Transplant Proc* 1989;21:2031–2032.
44. Schechner RS, Greenstein SM, Glicklich D, et al. Renal transplantation in the black population with systemic lupus erythematosus: a single center experience. *Transplant Proc* 1989;21: 3937–3938.
45. El-Shahawy MA, Aswad S, Mendez RG, et al. Renal transplantation in systemic lupus erythematosus: a single-center experience with sixty-four cases. *Am J Nephrol* 1995;15:123–128.
46. Kirby JD, Dieppe PA, Huskisson EC, et al. d-penicillamine and immune complex deposition. *Ann Rheum Dis* 1979;38: 344–346.
47. Sokunbi D, Wadhwa NK, Waltzer WC, et al. Renal transplantation in patients with end-stage renal disease secondary to systemic lupus erythematosus. *Transplant Proc* 1993;25:3328–3333.
48. Sumrani N, Miles AM, Delaney V, et al. Renal transplantation in cyclosporine-treated patients with end-stage lupus nephropathy. *Transplant Proc* 1992;24:1785–1787.
49. Arango JL, Henao JE, Mejia G, et al. Renal transplantation in patients with systemic lupus erythematosus. *Nefrologia* 1991; 11:526–530.
50. Contreras-Rodriguez JL, Bordes-Aznar J, Alberu J, et al. Kidney transplantation in systemic lupus erythematosus: experience from a reference center in Mexico. *Transplant Proc* 1992;24: 1798–1799.
51. Goss JA, Cole BR, Jendrisak MD, et al. Renal transplantation for systemic lupus erythematosus and recurrent lupus nephritis. A single-center experience and a review of the literature. *Transplantation* 1991;52:805–810.
52. Stone JH, Millward CL, Olson JL, et al. Frequency of recurrent lupus nephritis among 97 renal transplant patients during the cyclosporin era. *Arthritis Rheum* 1998;41:678–686.
53. Stone JH, Amend WJC, Criswell LA. Outcome of renal transplantation in 97 cyclosporin-era patients with systemic lupus erythematosus and matched controls. *Arthritis Rheum* 1998;41: 1438–1445.
54. Stone JH, Amend WJC, Criswell LA. Outcome of renal transplantation in systemic lupus erythematosus. *Seminars Arthritis Rheum* 1997:27:17–26.
55. Stone JH. End-stage renal disease in lupus: disease activity, dialysis and outcome of transplantation. *Lupus* 1998;7:654–659.
56. Tejani A, Khawar M, Butt KMH. Drug therapy, dialysis and transplantation in children with diffuse proliferative lupus nephritis (abstract). *Pediatr Res* 1987;21:485A.
57. Perri NA, Lipkowitz GS, Honig JH, et al. Cyclosporine markedly improves patient and graft survival in renal transplantation (abstract). *Kidney Int* 1987;31:466.
58. Uchida H, Sugimoto H, Nishimura Y, et al. Renal transplantation for systemic lupus erythematosus and recurrent lupus nephritis. *Transplant Proceedings* 1998;30:3908–3909.
59. Bochicchio T, Garcia-Torres E, Martinez-Lavin M, et al. Adverse outcome after renal transplantation in two patients with primary antiphospholipid syndrome (PAPS) (abstract). *Arthritis Rheum* 1993;36:S117.
60. Lauzurica R, Bonet J, Vaquero M, et al. Recurrence of membranous lupus glomerulonephritis two months after a renal cadaver transplant. *Transplant Proc* 1992;24:108–109.
61. Radhakrishnan J, Williams GS, Appel GB, et al. Renal transplantation in anticardiolipin antibody-positive lupus erythematosus patients. *Am J Kidney Dis* 1994;23:286–289.
62. Jarassa FB, Avdikou K, Pappas P, et al. Late renal transplant arterial thrombosis in a patient with systemic lupus erythematosus and antiphospholipid syndrome. *Nephrol Dial Transplant* 1999;14:472–474.
63. Kaplan B, Cooper J, Lager D, et al. Hepatic infarction in a hemodialysis patient with systemic lupus erythematosus. *Amer J Kid Dis* 1995;26:785–787.

64. Brunet P, Allaud M-F, San Marco M, et al. Antiphospholipids in hemodialysis patients: relationship between lupus anticoagulant and thrombosis. *Kidney Int.* 1995;48:794–800.
65. Stone JH, Amend WJC, Criswell LA. Antiphospholipid antibody syndrome in renal transplantation: occurrence of clinical events in 96 consecutive patients with systemic lupus erythematosus. *Amer J Kid Dis* 1999;34:1040–1047.
66. Mejia G, Zimmerman SW, Glass NR, et al. Renal transplantation in patients with systemic lupus erythematosus. *Arch Intern Med* 1983;143:2089–2092.
67. Cantarovich M, Hiesse C, Lantz O, et al. Renal transplantation and active lupus erythematosus (letter). *Ann Intern Med* 1988; 109:254–255.
68. Kumar V, Kono DH, Urban JL, et al. The T-cell receptor repertoire and autoimmune diseases. *Annu Rev Immunol* 1989;7 657–682.
69. Moorthy AV, Zimmerman S, Mejia G, et al. Recurrence of lupus nephritis after renal transplantation (abstract). *Kidney Int* 1987;31:464.
70. Yakub YN, Freeman RB, Pabico RC. Renal transplantation in systemic lupus erythematosus. *Nephron* 1981;27:197–201.
71. Fernandez JA, Milgrom M, Burke GW, et al. Recurrence of lupus nephritis in a renal allograft with histologic transformation of the lesion. *Transplantation* 1990;50:1056–1058.
72. Nyberg G, Blohme I, Persson H, et al. Recurrence of SLE in transplanted kidneys: a follow-up transplant biopsy study. *Nephrol Dial Transplant* 1992;11:1116–1123.
73. Straka P, Grossman R, Makover D, et al. Disease quiescence following renal transplantation in patients with systemic lupus erythematosus (abstract). *Arthritis Rheum* 1989;32(suppl):S115.
74. Fox L, Zager PG, Harford AM, et al. Lupus nephritis in a pediatric renal transplant recipient. *Pediatr Nephrol* 1992;6: 467–469.
75. McGrory CH, de Horatius DJ, Moritz MJ, et al. Pregnancy after renal transplantation in females with systemic lupus erythematosus (SLE). *Arthritis Rheum* 1996;39:S315.
76. Goldman JA, Chiapella J, Casey H, et al. Laser therapy of rheumatoid arthritis. *Laser Surg Med* 1980;1:93–101.
77. Herman JH, Khosla RC. Nd:YAG laser modulation of synovial tissue metabolism. *Clin Exp Rheumatol* 1989;7:505–512.
78. Inoue K, Nishioka J, Hukuda S. Altered lymphocyte proliferation by low dosage laser irradiation. *Clin Exp Rheumatol* 1989; 7:521–523.
79. Hall J, Clarke AK, Elvins DM, et al. Low level laser therapy is ineffective in the management of rheumatoid arthritic finger joints. *Br J Rheumatol* 1994;33:142–147.
80. Heussler JK, Hinchley G, Margiotta E, et al. A double-blind randomised trial of low power laser treatment in rheumatoid arthritis. *Ann Rheum Dis* 1993;52:703–706.
81. Henderson DL, Odom JC. Laser treatment of discoid lupus (case report). *Laser Surg Med* 1986;6:12–15.
82. Nurnberg W, Algermissen B, Hermes B, et al. Successful treatment of chronic discoid lupus erythematosus with argon laser. *Hautarzt* 1996;47:767–770.
83. Wallace DJ, Klinenberg JR. Apheresis. *Dis Mon* 1984;30:1–45.
84. Nyman KE, Bangert R, Machleder H, et al. Thoracic duct drainage in SLE with cutaneous vasculitis. *Arthritis Rheum* 1979;20:1129–1134.
85. Wallace DJ, Medici MA, Nichols S, et al. Plasmapheresis versus lymphoplasmapheresis in rheumatoid arthritis: immunologic comparisons and literature review. *J Clin Apheresis* 1984;2: 184–189.
86. Spiva DA, Cecere FA. The use of combination plasmapheresis/leukocytapheresis in the treatment of refractory systemic lupus erythematosus. *Plasma Ther Trans Tech* 1983;4:151–164.
87. Chagnac A, Kiberd BA, Farinas MC, et al. Outcome of the acute glomerular injury in proliferative lupus nephritis. *J Clin Invest* 1989;84:922–930.
88. Edworthy SM, Albridge K, Farinas C, et al. Renal outcome and survival of lupus patients treated with total lymphoid irradiation (TLI) compared with two control groups: biologically matched pairs and intention to treat patients (abstract). *Arthritis Rheum* 1989;32(suppl):R20.
89. Solovera JJ, Farinas MC, Strober S. Changes in B lymphocyte function in rheumatoid arthritis and lupus nephritis after total lymphoid irradiation. *Arthritis Rheum* 1988;31:1481–1491.
90. Strober S, Farinas MC, Field EH, et al. Lupus nephritis after total lymphoid irradiation: persistent improvement and reduction of steroid therapy. *Ann Intern Med* 1987;107:689–690.
91. Strober S, Field E, Hoppe RT, et al. Treatment of intractable lupus nephritis with total lymphoid irradiation. *Ann Intern Med* 1985;102:450–458.
92. Terr AI, Moss RB, Strober S. Effect of total lymphoid irradiation on IgE antibody responses in rheumatoid arthritis and systemic lupus erythematosus. *J Allergy Clin Immunol* 1987;80: 798–802.
93. Genovese MC, van Vollenhoven RF, Remey D, et al. Long term follow up in patients treated with total lymphoid irradiation for lupus nephritis. *Arthritis Rheum* 1997;40:S59.
94. Trentham DE, Belli JA, Bloomer WD, et al. 2000-CentiGray total lymphoid irradiation for refractory rheumatoid arthritis. *Arthritis Rheum* 1987;30:980–987.
95. Moskowitz R, Strober S, Trentham D. Total lymphoid irradiation: a viable therapeutic approach for connective tissue disease? *Point/Counterpoint* 1990;7:3–12.
96. Ben-Chetrit E, Gross DJ, Braverman A, et al. Total lymphoid irradiation in refractory systemic lupus erythematosus. *Ann Intern Med* 1986;105:58–60.
97. Mayes MD. Photopheresis and autoimmune diseases. *Rheum Dis Clin NA* 2000;26:75–81.
98. Knobler RM, Graninger W, Graninger W, et al. Extracorporeal photochemotherapy for the treatment of systemic lupus erythematosus. A pilot study. *Arthritis Rheum* 1992;35:319–324.
99. Knobler RM, Graninger W, Lindmaier A, et al. Photopheresis for the treatment of lupus erythematosus. Preliminary observations. *Ann N Y Acad Sci* 1991;636:340–356.
100. Pohl MA, Lan S-P, Berl T. Lupus Nephritis Collaborative Study Group. Plasmapheresis does not increase the risk for infection in immunosuppressed patients with severe lupus nephritis. *Ann Intern Med* 1991;114:924–929.
101. Wallace DJ. Plasmapheresis in lupus. *Lupus* 1993;2:141–143.
102. Wallace DJ. Apheresis for lupus erythematosus. *Lupus* 1999;8: 174–180.
103. Kaplan AA. Therapeutic plasma exchange. *Blackwell Science* (Malden, MA), 1999:159–177.
104. Hamburger MI, Gerardi EN, Fields TR, et al. Reticuloendothelial system Fc receptor function and plasmapheresis in systemic lupus erythematosus. *Artif Organs* 1981;5:264–268.
105. Low A, Hotze A, Krapf F, et al. The nonspecific clearance function of the reticuloendothelial system in patients with immune complex mediated diseases before and after therapeutic plasmapheresis. *Rheumatol Int* 1985;5:69–72.
106. Walport MJ, Peters AM, Elkon KB, et al. The splenic extraction ratio of antibody-coated erythrocytes and its response to plasma exchange and pulse methylprednisolone. *Clin Exp Immunol* 1985;60:465–473.
107. Abdou NI, Lindsley HB, Pollak A, et al. Plasmapheresis in active systemic lupus erythematosus: effects on clinical, serum and cellular abnormalities (case report). *Clin Immunol Immunopathol* 1981;19:44–54.
108. Colburn KK, Gusewitch GA, Statian Pooprasert BS, et al. Apheresis enhances the selective removal of antinuclear anti-

bodies in systemic lupus erythematosus. *Clin Rheumatol* 1990; 9:475–482.

109. Steven MM, Tanner AR, Holdstock GE, et al. The effect of plasma exchange on the in vitro monocyte function of patients with immune complex diseases. *Clin Exp Immunol* 1981; 45:240–245.
110. Tsokos GC, Balow JE, Huston DP, et al. Effect of plasmapheresis on T and B lymphocyte functions in patients with systemic lupus erythematosus: a double blind study. *Clin Exp Immunol* 1982;48:449–457.
111. Wallace DJ, Goldfinger D, Savage G, et al. Predictive value of clinical, laboratory, pathologic and treatment variables in steroid/immunosuppressive resistant lupus nephritis. *J Clin Apheresis* 1988;4:30–34.
112. Jones JV, Cumming RH, Bucknall RC, et al. Plasmapheresis in the management of acute systemic lupus erythematosus? *Lancet* 1976;i:709–711.
113. Jones JV. Plasmapheresis in SLE. *Clin Rheum Dis* 1982; 8:243–260.
114. Jones JV. *The application of plasmapheresis in systemic lupus erythematosus: therapeutic apheresis and plasma perfusion*. New York: Liss, 1982:81–89.
115. Jones JV, Cumming RH, Bacon PA, et al. Evidence for a therapeutic effect of plasmapheresis on patients with systemic lupus erythematosus? *Q J Med* 1979;48:555–576.
116. Jones JV, Robinson MF, Parciany RK, et al. Therapeutic plasmapheresis in systemic lupus erythematosus. Effect on immune complexes and antibodies to DNA. *Arthritis Rheum* 1981;24:1113–1120.
117. Hamburger MI. A long-term study of plasmapheresis (PEX) and cyclophosphamide (C) in systemic lupus erythematosus (SLE) (abstract). *J Clin Apheresis* 1984;2:143.
118. Wei N, Klippel JH, Huston DP, et al. Randomized trial of plasma exchange in mild systemic lupus erythematosus. *Lancet* 1983;i:17–21.
119. Jordan SC, Ho W, Ettenger R, et al. Plasma exchange improves the glomerulonephritis of systemic lupus erythematosus in selected pediatric patients. *Pediatr Nephrol* 1987;1:276–280.
120. Watson WJ, Katz VL, Bowes WA Jr. Plasmapheresis during pregnancy. *Obstet Gynecol* 1990;76:451–457.
121. Von Feldt J, Ostrov BE. The use of cyclophosphamide in the treatment of CNS lupus (abstract). *Arthritis Rheum* 1990;33 (suppl):R21.
122. Kincaid-Smith P, Fairley KF, Kloss M. Lupus anticoagulant associated with renal thrombotic angiopathy and pregnancy-related renal failure. *Q J Med* 1988;68:795–815.
123. Samtleben VW, Gurland HJ. Plasmapheresis in lupus nephritis: rational (sic) and clinical experiences. *Nieren-und Hochdruckkrankheiten* 1986;15:104–108.
124. Lockwood CM, Pussell B, Wilson CB, et al. Plasma exchange in nephritis. *Adv Nephrol* 1979;8:383–418.
125. Sharon Z, Roberts JL, Fennell JS, et al. Plasmapheresis in lupus nephritis. *Plasma Ther* 1982;3:165–169.
126. Wallace DJ, Goldfinger D, Bluestone R, et al. Plasmapheresis in lupus nephritis with nephrotic syndrome. A long-term follow-up. *J Clin Apheresis* 1982;1:42–45.
127. Clough JD, Lewis EJ, Lachin JM. Treatment protocols of the lupus nephritis collaborative study of plasmapheresis in severe lupus nephritis. The Lupus Nephritis Collaborative Study Group. *Prog Clin Biol Res* 1990;337:301–307.
128. Hebert L, Nielsen E, Pohl M, et al. Clinical course of severe lupus nephritis during the controlled trial of plasmapheresis therapy (abstract). *Kidney Int* 1987;31:201.
129. Lewis EJ, Lachin J. Primary outcomes in the controlled trial of plasmapheresis therapy in severe lupus nephritis. *Kidney Int* 1987;31:208–211.
130. Lewis EJ, Hunsicker LG, Lan S-P, et al. A controlled trial of plasmapheresis therapy in severe lupus nephritis. *N Engl J Med* 1992;326:1373–1379.
131. Wallace DJ. Plasmapheresis for lupus nephritis (letter). *N Engl J Med* 1992;327:1029.
132. Neuwelt CM, Daikh DI, Linfoot LA, et al. Catastrophic antiphospholipid syndrome: response to repeated plasmapheresis over three years. *Arthritis Rheum* 1997;40:1534–1539.
133. Kozlowski CL, Johnson MJ, Gorst DW, et al. Lung cancer, immune thrombocytopenia and the lupus inhibitor. *Postgrad Med J* 1987;63:793–795.
134. Derksen RH, Hasselaar P, Blokzijl L, et al. Lack of efficacy of plasma-exchange in removing antiphospholipid antibodies (letter). *Lancet* 1987;ii:222.
135. Fullcher D, Stewart G, Exner T, et al. Plasma exchange and the anticardiolipin syndrome in pregnancy (letter). *Lancet* 1989; ii:171.
136. Passaleva A, Massai G, Emmi L, et al. Plasma exchange in the treatment of acute systemic lupus erythematosus without circulating immune complexes. *Clin Exp Rheumatol* 1985;3: 255–257.
137. Thompson BJ, Watson ML, Liston WA, et al. Plasmapheresis in a pregnancy complicated by acute systemic lupus erythematosus. Case report. *Br J Obstet Gynaecol* 1985;92:532–534.
138. Durand J-M, Lefevre P, Kaplanski G, et al. Antiphospholipid syndrome and plasma exchange (letter). *Nephron* 1994;68:142.
139. Matsuda Y, Tohwo M, Kawanishi T, et al. Therapeutic plasmapheresis for the treatment of pregnant systemic lupus erythematosus patients with antiphospholipid antibodies (abstract). *Arthritis Rheum* 1995;38:S392.
140. Flamholz R, Tran T, Grad GI, et al. Therapeutic plasma exchange for the acute management of the catastrophic antiphospholipid syndrome: beta(2)-glycoprotein I antibodies as a marker of response to therapy. *J Clin Apheresis* 1999;14:171–176.
141. Hubbard HC, Portnoy B. Systemic lupus erythematosus in pregnancy treated with plasmapheresis. *Br J Dermatol* 1979; 101:87–90.
141a. Naesguna E, Yamada Y, Kodama N, et al. Successful pregnancy and delivery in a case of systemic lupus erythematosus treated with immunoadsorption therapy and cyclosporin A. *Scand J Rheumatol* 1999;28:54–57.
142. Kanai Y, Yamazaki Y, Kimura K, et al. Therapeutic plasmapheresis for the treatment of pregnant systemic lupus erythematosus patients with antiphospholipid antibodies. *Lupus* 1998;7(supp 1):114.
143. Nakamura Y, Yoshida K, Itoh S, et al. Immunoadsorption plasmapheresis as a treatment for pregnancy complicated by systemic lupus erythematosus and antiphospholipid antibodies. *Am J Repro Immunol* 1999;41:307–311.
144. Canales MA, Sevilla J, Hernandez D, et al. Efficacy of combined plasmapheresis with immunoglobulin for a gestation with antiphospholipid antibodies and Rh alloimmunization. *Med Clin* (Barcelona) 1999;112:438–439.
145. Kob1ayashi S, Tamura N, Tsuda H, et al. Immunoadsorbent plasmapheresis for a patient with antiphospholipid syndrome during pregnancy. *Ann Rheum Dis* 1992;51:399–401.
146. Epstein AL, Huhta JC, Glickman JD, et al. Transient reversal of congenital complete heart block (CCHB) (abstract). *Arthritis Rheum* 1994;37:S317.
147. Roche B, Lhote F, Chasseray J-E, et al. Fetal congenital heart block and maternal systemic lupus erythematosus: can plasma exchanges play a useful role? *Transfusion Sci* 1992;13:463–466.
148. van der Leij JN, Visser GHA, Bink-Boelkens M, et al. Successful outcome of pregnancy after treatment of maternal anti-Ro (SSA) antibodies with immunosuppressive therapy and plasmapheresis. *Prenat Diagn* 1994;14:1007.

149. Deleted in page proofs.
150. Clark WF, Lindsay RM, Cattran DC, et al. Monthly plasmapheresis for systemic lupus erythematosus with diffuse proliferative glomerulonephritis: a pilot study. *Can Med Assoc J* 1981; 125:171–174.
151. Clark WF, Lindsay RM, Ulan RA, et al. Chronic plasma exchange in SLE nephritis. *Clin Nephrol* 1981;16:20–23.
152. Tanter Y, Rifle G, Chalopin JM, et al. Plasma exchange in central nervous system involvement of systemic lupus erythematosus. *Plasma Ther Transfus Technol* 1987;8:161–168.
153. Neuwelt CM, Al-Baude HA, Webb RL. Role of intravenous cyclophosphamide in the treatment of severe neuropsychiatric systemic lupus. *Amer J Med* 1995;98:32–41.
154. Kambic H, Hyslop L, Nose Y. *Topics in plasmapheresis: a bibliography of therapeutic applications and new techniques.* Cleveland: ISAO Press, 1985.
155. Sinico R, Fornasieri A, Fiorini G, et al. Plasma exchange in glomerulonephritis associated with systemic lupus erythematosus and essential mixed cryoglobulinemia. *Int J Artif Organs* 1983;6(supp 1):21–25.
156. Erickson RW, Franklin WA, Emlen W. Treatment of hemorrhagic lupus pneumonitis with plasmapheresis. *Semin Arthritis Rheum* 1994;24:114–123.
157. Huang D-F, Tsai S-T, Wang SR. Recovery of both acute massive pulmonary hemorrhage and acute renal failure in a systemic lupus erythematosus patient with lupus anticoagulant by the combined therapy of plasmapheresis plus cyclophosphamide. *Transfusion Sci* 1994;15:283–288.
158. Garcia-Consuerga J, Merino R, Alonso A, et al. Systemic lupus erythematosus: a case report with unusual manifestations and favourable outcome after plasmapheresis. *Eur J Pediatr* 1992; 151:581–582.
159. Schroeder JO, Euler HE, Loffler H. Synchronization of plasmapheresis and pulse cyclophosphamide in severe systemic lupus erythematosus. *Ann Intern Med* 1987;107:344–346.
160. Barr WG, Hubbell EA, Robinson JA. Plasmapheresis and pulse cyclophosphamide in systemic lupus erythematosus (letter). *Ann Intern Med* 1988;108:152–153.
161. Clark WF, Dau PC, Euler HH, et al. Plasmapheresis and subsequent pulse cyclophosphamide versus pulse cyclophosphamide alone in severe lupus: design of the LPSG trial. Lupus Plasmapheresis Study Group (LPSG). *J Clin Apheresis* 1991;6: 40–47.
162. Dau PC, Callahan J, Parker R, et al. Immunologic effects of plasmapheresis synchronized with pulse cyclophosphamide in systemic lupus erythematosus (case report). *J Rheumatol* 1991; 18:270–276.
163. Euler HH, Gutschmidt HJ, Schmuecking M, et al. Induction of remission in severe SLE after plasma exchange synchronized with subsequent pulse cyclophosphamide. *Prog Clin Biol Res* 1990;337:319–320.
164. Euler HH, Schroeder JO. Antibody depletion and cytotoxic drug therapy in severe systemic lupus erythematosus. *Transfusion Sci* 1992;13:167–184.
165. Euler HH, Guillevin L. Plasmapheresis and subsequent pulse cyclophosphamide in severe systemic lupus erythematosus. *Ann Med Interne* 1994;145:296–302.
166. Euler HH, Schroeder JO, Harten P, et al. Treatment-free remission in severe systemic lupus erythematosus following synchronization of plasmapheresis with subsequent pulse cyclophosphamide. *Arthritis Rheum* 1994;37:1784–1794.
167. Wallace DJ, Goldfinger D, Pepkowitz SH, et al. Randomized controlled trial of pulse/synchronization cyclophosphamide/ apheresis for proliferative lupus nephritis. *J Clin Apheresis* 1998; 13:163–166.
168. Schroeder JO, Schwab U, Zeuner R, et al. Plasmapheresis and subsequent pulse cyclophosphamide in severe systemic lupus erythematosus. *Arthritis Rheum* 1997;40:S325.
169. Koo AP, Segal AM, Smith JW, et al. Continuous flow cryofiltration in the treatment of systemic vasculitis (abstract). *Arthritis Rheum* 1983;26(suppl):S67.
170. Terman DS, Buffaloe G, Mattioli C, et al. Extracorporeal immunoadsorption: initial experience in human systemic lupus erythematosus. *Lancet* 1979;2:824–827.
171. Traeger J, Laville M, El Habib R, et al. Extracorporeal immunoadsorption of DNA antibodies on DNA-coated collagen films: first results in systemic lupus erythematosus. In: Nose Y, ed. *Plasmapheresis.* Cleveland: ISAO Press 1983:155–166.
172. Snyder HW, Cochran SK, Balint JP Jr, et al. Experience with protein A-immunoadsorption in treatment-resistant adult immune thrombocytopenic purpura. *Blood* 1992;79:2237–2245.
173. el-Habib R, Laville M, Traeger J. Specific adsorption of circulating antibodies by extracorporeal plasma perfusions over antigen coated collagen flat-membranes: application to systemic lupus erythematosus. *J Clin Lab Immunol* 1984;15:111–117.
174. Harata N, Sasaki T, Shibata S, et al. Selective absorption of anti-DNA antibodies and their idiotype positive cells in vitro using an anti-idiotype antibody-affinity column: possible application to plasma exchange. *J Clin Apheresis* 1991;6:34–39.
175. Hashimoto H, Tsuda H, Kanai Y, et al. Selective removal of anti-DNA and anticardiolipin antibodies by adsorbent plasmapheresis using dextran sulfate columns in patients with systemic lupus erythematosus. *J Rheumatol* 1990;18:545–551.
176. Pineda AA. Methods for selective removal of plasma constituents. *Prog Clin Biol Res* 1982;106:361–374.
177. McLeod B, Lewis E, Schnitzer T, et al. Therapeutic immunoadsorption of anti-native DNA antibodies in SLE: clinical studies with a device utilizing monoclonal anti-idiotypic antibody (abstract). *Arthritis Rheum* 1988;31(suppl):S15.
178. Palmer A, Gjorstrup G, Severn A, et al. Treatment of systemic lupus erythematosus by extracorporeal immunoadsorption (letter). *Lancet* 1988;2:272.
179. Schneider M, Berning T, Waldendorf M, et al. Immunoadsorbent plasma perfusion in patients with systemic lupus erythematosus. *J Rheumatol* 1990;17:900–907.
180. Suzuki K, Ishizuka T, Harigai M, et al. Continuous anti-ds DNA antibody apheresis in systemic lupus erythematosus. *Lancet* 1990;336:753–754.
181. Suzuki K, Hara M, Hirigai M, et al. Continuous removal of anti-DNA antibody, using a new extracorporeal immunoadsorption system, in patients with systemic lupus erythematosus. *Arthritis Rheum* 1991;34:1546–1552.
182. Higgins RM, Streather CP, Buhler R, et al. Relapse of systemic lupus erythematosus after extracorporeal immunoadsorption (letter). *Nephron* 1995;69:183.
183. McGrath H Jr. Ultraviolet-A irradiation therapy for patients with systemic lupus erythematosus: a pilot study. *Curr Ther Res* 1994;55:373–381.
184. McGrath H Jr. Ultraviolet-A1 irradiation decreases clinical disease activity and autoantibodies in patients with systemic lupus erythematosus. *Clin Exp Rheumatol* 1994;12:129–135.
185. McGrath H Jr, Martinez-Osuna P, Lee FA. Ultraviolet-A1 (340-400 nm) irradiation therapy in systemic lupus erythematosus. *Lupus* 1996;5:269–274.
186. Molina JF, Mc Grath H Jr. Longterm ultraviolet-A1 irradiation therapy in systemic lupus erythematosus. *J Rheumatol* 1997;24: 1072–1074.
187. Morison ML. UVA-1 phototherapy of lupus erythematosus. *Lupus* 1994;3:139–141.
188. Lockhead KM, Pirsch JD, d'Allessandro AM, et al. Risk factors for renal allograft loss in patients with systemic lupus erythematosus. *Kidney Int* 1996;49:512–517.

59

OCCASIONAL, INNOVATIVE, AND EXPERIMENTAL THERAPIES

DANIEL J. WALLACE

The previous six chapters have discussed conventional therapies for lupus erythematosus (LE). These include general measures, local applications, nonsteroidal antiinflammatory drugs, antimalarials, corticosteroids, and immunosuppressive agents. Occasionally, specific subsets of lupus require additional approaches, and some patients with refractory disease benefit from innovative management. This chapter reviews these management practices and discusses ancillary measures.

MEDICATIONS

Antileprosy Drugs

Dapsone

Dapsone, or 4,4-diaminodiphenylsulphone, interferes with folate metabolism and inhibits para-aminobenzoic acid. It also blocks the alternate pathway of complement activation and neutrophil cytotoxicity (1), and it inhibits superoxide and hydroxyl generation in patients with rheumatoid arthritis (2,3). Its use is limited by its toxicity, which includes sulfhemoglobinemia and methemoglobinemia, a dose-related hemolytic anemia, a "dapsone hypersensitivity syndrome," and aplastic anemia (4,5). In a case reported during 1978, it was said to benefit urticaria associated with systemic lupus erythematosus (SLE) (6). Small series (5,7–16) have reported that dapsone can ameliorate vasculitis, bullae, urticaria, oral ulcerations, thrombocytopenia, lupus panniculitis, and subacute cutaneous lupus. Dapsone may be steroid-sparing, and it can be effective in chloroquine-resistant patients.

Dubois' group found dapsone to be helpful in three of seven patients, but three developed a significant anemia (17). Coburn and Shuster (18) reported that nine of 11 patients with discoid LE improved on 100 mg daily. Lindskov and Reymann (19) gave dapsone to 33 patients with chronic-cutaneous LE — eight had excellent and eight had fair results, but 17 (52%) had no response. Dapsone occasionally can make rashes worse (20,21), perhaps because of its sulfa component.

All patients treated with dapsone should have their baseline glucose-6-phosphate dehydrogenase levels determined; the drug should not be given to individuals with low levels. Complete blood counts should be performed every 2 weeks for the first 3 months and then every 2 months thereafter. Dapsone should be started at a dose of 25 mg twice daily and eventually raised to 100 mg daily. Dapsone also interacts with all oxidant drugs, such as phenacetin and Furadantin (Dura). Concurrent administration of 800 U of vitamin E daily may decrease the degree of dapsone-induced hemolysis (22). Delayed hypersensitivity reactions can occur (23).

I believe that dapsone has a place in the treatment of cutaneous and musculoskeletal lupus, especially when steroids are ineffective or contraindicated. Hematologic toxicity is high, however, and the drug should be used infrequently and cautiously.

Thalidomide

Also known as -N-phythalimidoglutarimide, thalidomide is a highly teratogenic drug with antileprosy and antilupus effects. It has no influence on the complement system, but it can stabilize lysosomal membranes, reduce tumor necrosis factor activity, antagonize prostaglandin, inhibit neutrophil chemotaxis and angiogenesis, and alter cellular and humeral immunity (23–26). Side effects of thalidomide include teratogenicity, fatigue, dizziness, weight gain, constipation, amenorrhea, dry mouth, and a non–dose-related polyneuropathy that is associated with chronic administration (27). Despite these rather significant drawbacks, Barba Rubio et al. (28,29) pioneered its use in discoid LE in Mexico during the mid-1970s. Improvement begins within weeks on doses between 100 and 400 mg daily (30). Knop et al. (31) reported that in 46 patients with antimalarial-resistant discoid LE given 400 mg/day and followed for up to 2 years, 90% had complete or marked regression. Also,

71 relapsed on its discontinuation and improved when it was restarted, and 25 developed a polyneuritis. The drug also can heal antimalarial-resistant lesions (32). 44% of 16 patients at Graham Hughes' London unit had complete cutaneous remissions with thalidomide; another 37% had a partial response (33). Twenty of 23 Brazilians with chloroquine-resistant chronic-cutaneous lupus had clearing of lesions with thalidomide; 52% experienced drowsiness and 22% abdominal distension (24). Other important side effects include amenorrhea and pustuloderma, and possibly thrombosis (34,35,40). Similar favorable responses and toxicity have been noted by others in smaller groups of patients (25,30,36–39). In addition, thalidomide has been used to treat graft-versus-host disease, acquired immunodeficiency syndrome (AIDS), Behcet's syndrome, and rheumatoid arthritis (41,42). It is available in the United States from physicians who have registered with the New Jersey based Celgene Corporation and comply with stringent requirements. Thalidomide should never be used in women who are pregnant or contemplating pregnancy.

Clofazimine

In 1976, Krivanek et al. (43) reported resolution of discoid LE in all of nine patients treated with 100 to 300 mg/day of clofazimine (Lamprene, Novartis) for 3 months, but a follow-up paper (44) found it to be effective only in early, acute-onset lesions. The drug has antileprosy, antibacterial, and antimalarial activity. It is sequestered in macrophages, stabilizes lysosomal enzymes, and stimulates the production of reactive oxidants (45). Two other favorable studies have appeared (46,47), but Dubois' group had no responses among eight patients treated (17). Long-term use of clofazimine in LE can result in cutaneous pigment deposits (48).

Other Novel Immune Suppressives

Most immune-suppressive agents at least occasionally used to manage SLE are reviewed in Chapter 57. A few additional ones deserve mention here.

Cytarabine helped three patients with refractory cutaneous lupus (49), and fludarabine helped one (50). The nucleoside analog, *2-chlordeoxyadenosine (2-CdA)* was given to 12 patients with proliferative nephritis as an infusion. Fifty percent had substantial improvement at the National Institutes of Health (51). Two of three patients who were resistant to cyclosporin or cyclophosphamide improved somewhat with *tacrilimus (Prograf, FK-506)* (52). Several of our renal transplant patients have tolerated *rapamycin (sirolimus, Rapamune, Wyeth Ayerst)*, a recently approved drug similar to tacrolimus that inhibits T-cell activation and proliferation without difficulty (53). The use of novel immune suppressives such as *mizoribine, lobenzarit*, and the 5-lipoxygenase inhibitor *zileuton* (54–56) appear to be safe and have shown antilupus effects in small, open-labeled human trials. Our group has given *leflunomide (Arava, Aventis Pharmaceuticals)* to 18 patients with favorable results (56a).

Gold

In the 1940s and 1950s, gold frequently was used to treat LE. It was thought to be beneficial but toxic (57–60). Reports of this period antedated criteria for defining SLE and rheumatoid arthritis as well as the introduction of lupus serologies. As a result, the *Physicians' Desk Reference* lists SLE as a contraindication for using gold sodium thiomalate (Myochrysine, Merck & Co., Inc.).

In 1983, 16 patients with SLE but without renal involvement were given oral gold at the University of California, San Diego (61). They had fevers, fatigue, arthritis, serositis, vasculitis, rashes, and mouth ulcers. Gold was of modest benefit, with significant improvement noted only in physician assessment and steroid dose reduction. A British group treated 22 patients with biopsy-documented cutaneous lupus with oral gold for up to 1 year (62). Of these, 12 had dramatic clearing of lesions, and five others demonstrated definite improvement. In another report (63), seven of 12 patients who received aurothioglucose (Solganal, Schering) injections had improved arthritis and decreased steroid requirements. Some still are concerned that gold can flare SLE (64), and further studies are needed to define its potential role.

Vitamin A, Beta Carotene, And Retinoids

Beta carotene, vitamin A, and retinoids are related compounds that may have antilupus actions because of their sun-blocking and antioxidant activities. Skin tests with vitamin A have revealed an increased hyperreactivity in patients with SLE and their relatives compared with controls (65), and its oral administration in SLE enhances natural killer-cell activity and mitogenic responsiveness (66).

Beta carotene has been used to treat polymorphous light eruption, erythrohepatic protoporphyria, and discoid LE. Of seven patients with cutaneous lupus, six improved in two reports (67,68), but Dubois and Patterson (69) found beneficial results in only one of 26 patients.

Retinoids inhibit collagenase, prostaglandin E2, and rheumatoid synovial proliferation; interfere with intracellular-binding proteins; and interact with kinases, such as cyclic AMP (70,71). In addition, epidermal antibodies can be altered, and an effect on epidermal cell differentiation may be observed (72). Three retinoids have been evaluated in cutaneous lupus: (i) *isotretinoin (13-cis-retinoic acid; Accutane, Roche Laboratories)*, (ii) *etretinate (Tegison, Roche Laboratories)*, and (iii) the aromatic retinoid *acitretin (Soriatane, Roche Laboratories)*. When given in doses of 40 mg twice daily, isotretinoin induced complete resolution of lesions in eight of ten patients, including several with refractory, subacute-cutaneous lupus (72). In another open trial, it was effective in 20 of 24 patients (30). Other case reports and a literature review have confirmed these findings (73–77).

I have had similar success, but unless the patient is kept on a maintenance dose of 10 to 40 mg daily, recurrences are common. Isotretinoin can cause arthralgias and skeletal hyperostoses (78). Etretinate also may ameliorate cutaneous lesions (79), but extraspinal tendon and ligamentous calcifications have resulted from therapy (80). The drug no longer is available in the United States. A newer aromatic retinoid, acitretin, now is available in the United States. In one paper (81), seven favorable reports were reviewed, and 15 of 20 patients studied had complete clearing of all lesions. This included five of six patients with refractory, subacute-cutaneous lupus. A randomized, double-blind study found that 46 of patients treated with acitretin improved (82). The recommended dose is 20 to 50 mg a day. The teratogenicity of the retinoids is a major concern in treating females of childbearing age. Topical retinoids with sunscreens also may be useful (83).

Danazol

Danazol (Danocrine, Sanofi) is an impeded androgen whose effects in SLE are unclear. It may decrease Fc receptor expression and platelet-associated IgG, can reverse protein S deficiency (84), and also may have a hormonal down-regulating action. Danazol displaces steroids by binding to steroid-binding globulin, which frees the latter compound. Its most promising use so far is for the treatment of idiopathic thrombocytopenia, in which steroid-sparing effects are observed, and after an initial response, low doses can be administered as maintenance therapy (85). Idiopathic thrombocytopenia caused by SLE responds well in some patients to between 400 and 800 mg/day of therapy (86–89). Cervera et al. (90) noted that all of 16 patients given danazol achieved a complete remission when it was started at 200 mg/day and increased stepwise up to 1,200 mg until benefit or toxicity was observed. Several reports also have documented its efficacy in cases of SLE with autoimmune hemolytic anemia (91–94). In addition, danazol has been reported to help patients with persistent, premenstrual LE flares (95). In combination with cyproterone acetate, 11 patients with SLE had fewer exacerbations, and persistent, disabling mouth ulcers disappeared in three (96). Danazol may be effective in discoid LE (97); of 21 patients given danazol in a controlled trial with corticosteroids, all had fewer flares, lower steroid requirements, and higher hemoglobin levels, platelet counts, and C4 complement levels than 20 patients taking steroids alone. Of the 21 patients in the danazol group, however, eight withdrew because of hepatotoxicity, gastric symptoms, or asthenia (98). Occasionally, danazol can worsen SLE (99), and it has been associated with the development of hepatocellular carcinoma in one patient (100) and with hyperglucagonemia in another (101).

Danazol has no role in the management of life-threatening, nonhematologic manifestations of lupus.

Other Hormones

The use of contraceptive and other menses-altering or menses-regulating hormones is discussed in Chapters 16, The Importance of Sex Hormones in Systemic Lupus Erythematosus, and 39, The Use of Exogenous Estrogens, Endocrine System, and Urogenital Tract.

Testosterones

In 1948, Lamb gave androgens to five patients with lupus, but without significant improvement (102). In 1950, Dubois et al. and Fromer (103,104) treated several female patients with massive doses of *testosterone*, both orally and intramuscularly, using as much as 500 to 1,000 mg/day for as long as 5 weeks without benefit.

After a 30-year hiatus, interest in androgen therapy resurfaced. Lahita and Kunkel (105) treated four men and four women with *19-nortestosterone (Nandrolene)* for 2 months to 2 years. The condition of the men grew worse, but some women improved. Minimal masculinization was noted, sedimentation rates and anti-DNA levels decreased slightly, and hemoglobin and white counts both improved. Swaak et al. (106) found that modest improvements were outweighed by hirsutism and voice alterations among 36 patients in a placebo-controlled trial, and Hazelton et al. (107) observed no clinical change in ten patients treated with the drug. A Soviet androgen preparation, Sustanon-250, has been purported to decrease disease activity (108–110).

Dehydroepiandrosterone

Dehydroepiandrosterone (DHEA) is a steroid precursor of androgens, and to a lesser extent estrogens. Produced in the adrenal gland, its levels decline with age. DHEA increases IL-2, soluble-adhesion molecules, and interferon (IFN) while down-regulating interleukin-4 (IL-4), IL-5 and IL-6 (111–113). It increases growth-hormone levels, may improve bone density, fatigue, libido, and cognitive dysfunction (114,115). Although available over the counter as a "dietary supplement", a quality control review of 16 preparations showed that 0 to 150% of what was claimed on the label was actually in the product (116). Van Vollenhove, McGuire and their colleagues at Stanford have studied DHEA for the last decade. In doses of 100–200 mg a day, favorable effects were reported in mild-to-moderate lupus in an open-label study (117), double-blind trial (118), and at long-term follow-up (119,120). In patients with severe SLE, bone density improved but disease activity changes were not statistically significant (121). A multicenter trial showed that DHEA is slightly steroid sparing in a subset of patients with active disease (122). Most of the side effects include acne, facial hair, fluid retention, and headache. There is some concern that DHEA might accelerate a preexisting prostate or gynecologic malignancy. This writer believes that compounded DHEA in doses of 50 to 200 mg a day may be beneficial in lupus patients who have mild fatigue or cognitive impairment after undergoing a gynecologic or prostate evaluation.

Miscellaneous Hormones

A double-blind, crossover trial treating 11 patients with SLE using *tamoxifen*, an antiestrogen, demonstrated no benefits from the drug (123). Prolactin appears to have proinflammatory effects, and interest has centered on the use of prolactin suppression with *bromocriptine* in SLE (see Chapter 44, Serum and Plasma Protein Abnormalities and Other Clinical Laboratory Determinations in Systemic Lupus Erythematosus). In one report, recombinant *growth hormone* reactivated a previously quiescent nephritis (124).

Gamma Globulin

Intravenous gamma globulin delays the clearance of antibody-coated autologous red blood cells, competitively inhibits reticuloendothelial Fc receptor blockade, has anti-idiotypic antibody activity, modulates the release and function of proinflammatory cytokines and adhesion molecule expression, and decreases pokeweed mitogen-induced B-cell differentiation (125–129). Hypogammaglobulinemia with recurrent infections is a rare event in SLE (see Chapter 44), and use of intramuscular gamma globulin to prevent infection in lupus is not uncommon, even though no controlled studies have documented its efficacy (130–132).

Intravenous gamma globulin first was used in a case of lupus nephritis in 1982 (133), and its use has increased since then (134). It may be acutely helpful for autoimmune thrombocytopenia secondary to SLE (135–138) and for the neonatal thrombocytopenia that is seen in children of mothers with SLE (139). Gamma globulin is thought to be useful for serious disease exacerbations (140,141), such as in central nervous system lupus (142,143), pericarditis (145), cardiac dysfunction (146), acquired factor VIII deficiency (147,148), pancytopenia (149,150), refractory cutaneous lupus (151,152), myelofibrosis (153), nephritis (144,154–156), polyneuritis (157), hypoprothrombinemia with the lupus anticoagulant (158), and for preventing recurrent fetal loss in patients with the antiphospholipid syndrome (159–164). Seventeen of 20 Israeli lupus patients with a variety of clinical manifestations responded to therapy (165). In patients with mild disease, little response to gamma globulin has been noted (166).

The use of gamma globulin for the treatment of lupus nephritis is controversial. The drug is expensive and potentially dangerous. The reader should appreciate that it often is ineffective (167) or temporarily effective (168). It can flare disease activity (169), induce acute renal failure (170,171), myocardial infarction (172), aseptic meningitis (173), and vasculitic rashes (174) among other symptoms. Low or absent IgA (seen in 5% with SLE) is a relative contraindication to its administration.

Levamisole

The T-cell immunostimulant drug levamisole, now widely used to manage colon cancer, first was noted to be effective for SLE in 1975, in a case report of an ANA-negative patient (176). The same group subsequently reported that 16 patients treated with levamisole for a minimum of 4 months improved, but no clinical parameters were mentioned (177). Other groups found the drug not only to be ineffective in a total of 17 patients but associated it with serious adverse reactions and no discernible immunologic changes (178–181). Rovensky et al. (182) documented clinical responses in 16 of 20 patients but, in a follow-up report (183), noted that nearly 50% had significant leukopenia or hepatoxicity that required discontinuation of the drug. Ogawa et al. (184) claimed some amelioration of nephritis in 50% of their patients in an uncontrolled study, and Feng et al. (185) treated 17 patients with 150 mg/day for 3 days consecutively every 2 weeks. Of these patients, five had their lupus completely suppressed, and 11 could reduce their steroid doses. Unfortunately, only eight of 17 patients had a positive LE preparation, antinuclear antibodies were not reported, and no statistical analyses were used.

The only controlled trial of levamisole was performed by Hadidi et al. (186). In their study, 26 patients with SLE who had been inadequately controlled by up to 30 mg/day of prednisone were given either 150 mg of levamisole or a placebo weekly for 6 months. Most patients had to have their steroid doses increased, and no improvements were observed.

Antilymphocyte And Antithymocyte Globulin

Because antilymphocyte globulin is immunosuppressive, it has been tried experimentally in a number of patients with SLE. Treatment usually has been combined with steroids and other agents. Fever as well as local and hematologic reactions have been frequent. Results generally are equivocal (187–189). In the largest and only controlled study (190), nine patients given antilymphocyte globulin, azathioprine, and prednisone did no better than those in a prednisone-only treated group. Pancytopenia was reversed in one patient given antithymocyte globulin (191).

Antibiotics

Chloramphenicol and its analogues inhibit antibody production by interfering with nucleic acid synthesis or (192). An analogue of chloramphenicol, thiamphenicol, was given to six patients with lupus nephritis (193). Following a 16-day course of 2 g daily, four patients had increased complement and decreased anti-DNA levels, lower antinuclear antibody titers, and disappearance of glomerular-bound gamma globulin. Sustained remissions function lasted for 9 months to 3 years following a single course of therapy. In 1979, Richmond (194) gave thiamphenicol to 13 patients with lupus nephritis for 2 weeks (195) and then reviewed the drug's record of inhibiting cell-mediated immune reactions and prolonging rat renal allograft survival. Symptomatic improvement was noted in only two patients, but six had serologic improvement. Chloramphenicol (196), *penicillin* (197,198), *sulfonamides* (199–200), *tetracycline* (201), and *streptomycin* (202,203) also have been purported to help in SLE. The usefulness of these approaches is doubtful, however, and no controlled studies are available.

Interferon And Other Antiviral Agents

Interferon (IFN)-alpha induces the formation of anti-DNA and antinuclear antibodies (204). Numerous reports document the induction of SLE in patients who receive the drug for a variety of reasons (205–212) as well as IFN-beta-1a (213). IFN-gamma administered for presumed rheumatoid arthritis induced multisystemic SLE in two patients (214,215). Surprisingly, IFN-alpha (especially intralesional) has been effective in managing patients with refractory discoid and subacute cutaneous lupus (216–219). In one case report (220), *isoprinosine* given to a patient with lupus for a viral infection produced improvement in disease activity.

Thymosin And Thymectomy

Because the thymus gland is an important lymphoid organ in which lymphocytes differentiate, proliferate, and mature, experimental thymectomy has been undertaken to treat SLE, but with uniformly negative results (221–226). The administration of thymosin, or thymic hormone, represents the opposite approach. It increases T-lymphocyte counts, improves lymphocyte responsiveness, and decreases null-cell counts *in vitro* (227–230). Thymulin inhibits cytokine response in SLE (231). Factor V thymosin was given to four patients with SLE, and improvement was claimed in three, with no adverse reactions observed (232). Unfortunately, improvement was not defined or described, nor was the degree of disease activity in these patients stated. Thymus factor X was thought to be useful in a poorly documented report (233).

Vasodilators

Prostaglandin E1 (PGE1) is a vasodilator that can suppress the effector systems of inflammation and both enhance and diminish cellular and immune responses (234). Several case reports have associated PGE1 infusion with improved renal function in lupus nephritis and decreased levels of circulating immune complexes (235–237). PGE1 also ameliorates digital ischemia in SLE (238–240). Renal function also improved in a double-blind, crossover study of ten patients given a thromboxane inhibitor (241) as well as an open-label one (242,243), and the angiotensin-converting enzyme inhibitor *captopril* (244) may be capable of reducing proteinuria.

DRUGS TO AVOID

d-Penicillamine, minocycline, and *sulfasalazine* clearly are effective for rheumatoid arthritis, and d-penicillamine also has antiscleroderma actions. These drugs have been given to patients with SLE who were thought to have rheumatoid arthritis or scleroderma. Because sulfa drugs and tetracyclines may exacerbate lupus (and can be photosensitizing) and d-penicillamine can induce lupus, extreme caution is advised if SLE is suspected (245,246) (see Chapter 42). The issue with sulfasalazine is more problematic because three reports among 15 patients have suggested that the drug is modestly effective for chronic-cutaneous (but not systemic) lupus (247–249). It has been suggested that responders who are less prone to light-sensitive reactions tend to be rapid acetylators (247). I advise against using this drug in view of numerous reports of its exacerbating or inducing SLE (250, see Chapter 60). Certain Chinese and Peruvian *herbs and echinacea* also contain chemicals that are harmful in SLE (251–253).

SHOULD RADIATION THERAPY BE AVOIDED?

Although total lymphoid irradiation has been used to manage SLE (see Chapter 58), anecdotal reports of disease flares in patients undergoing radiation therapy for cancers are widespread. A review of the literature reveals causes of preexisting cutaneous lupus flared by radiation therapy (254–256) and one of widespread pelvic necrosis (257). On the other hand, a definitive 1993 matched-controlled, prospective evaluation of 61 patients with collagen vascular disorders failed to find an increased incidence of reactions compared with the autoimmune group (258). A smaller survey of six lupus patients supports this (259), though scleroderma patients seem to tolerate radiation therapy poorly (260). None of my patients have ever had lupus flares associated with radiation therapy.

MISCELLANEOUS AGENTS AND COMPLEMENTARY THERAPIES

Nearly one half of 707 SLE patients from six centers used some form of complementary therapies (261). In Mexico, patients who used alternative therapies had more disease severity and/or complications (262).

The older literature is replete with references to the successful use of many systemic drugs. *Vitamin B12* and *pantothenic acid* have been reported in controlled studies to be of benefit (263–265). Authorities such as Sulzberger (266) have recommended the use of *vitamin B12, liver extract,* and *bismuth* (267–269) for the treatment of discoid LE. The Russian literature contains numerous reports of the beneficial effects of *methylxanthines, splenin, lysozyme,* and *prospidin* (270–273). Other drugs and modalities that have been tried include *tuberculin* (274); Chinese herbs, especially *T Wilfordii Hook F* (275–283); *arsenic* (284); *heliotherapy* (285); *para-aminobenzoic acid* (286,287); *colchicine* (288); *pentoxifulline (Trental, Hoechst Marion Roussel)* (289) *aminoglutethimide* (290); *sulfasalazine* (291); *hemotherapy* (292); *transfer factor* (293); *auriculo acupuncture* (294); *phenytoin* (295); *hyperbaric oxygen* (296), *sarei-to* (297), *acupuncture* (298), pulsed *magnetic fields* (299), *topical DNCB* (300), the complement inhibitor *nafamostat mesylate* (301); and *sodium diethyldithiocarbamate* (302).

Ayres and Mihan (303,304) reviewed ten papers that evaluated the use of the antioxidant *vitamin E* for discoid lesions. Nine were published prior to 1955, and a recent report suggested no benefits (305). Routine *splenectomy* has been advised in patients without significant hematologic complications (306). *Witchcraft* has even been used successfully (307).

I do not recommend any of these measures.

REFERENCES

1. Reinitz E, Barland P. Adverse reactions to dapsone. *Lancet* 1981;ii:184–185.
2. Christiansen J, Tegner E, Irestedt M. Dapsone hypersensitivity syndrome in a patient with cutaneous lupus erythematosus. *Acta Derm Venereol* 1999;79:482.
3. Chang DJ, Lamothe M, Stevens RM, et al. Dapsone in rheumatoid arthritis. *Semin Arthritis Rheum* 1996;25:390–403.
4. Meyerson MA, Cohen PR. Dapsone-induced aplastic anemia in a woman with bullous systemic lupus erythematosus. *Mayo Clin Proc* 1994;69:1159–1162.
5. Mok CC, Lau CS, Woon Sing Wong R. Toxicities of dapsone in the treatment of cutaneous manifestations of rheumatic diseases. *J Rheumatol* 1998;25:1246–1247.
6. Matthews CNA, Saihan EM, Warin RP. Urticaria-like lesions associated with systemic lupus erythematosus: response to dapsone. *Br J Dermatol* 1978;99:455–457.
7. Fenton DA, Black MM. Low-dose dapsone in the treatment of subacute cutaneous lupus erythematosus. *Clin Exp Dermatol* 1986;11:102–103.
8. Hall RP, Lawley TJ, Smith HR, et al. Bullous eruption of systemic lupus erythematosus. Dramatic response to dapsone therapy. *Ann Intern Med* 1982;97:165–170.
9. Holtman JH, Neustadt DH, Klein J, et al. Dapsone is an effective therapy for the skin lesions of subacute cutaneous lupus erythematosus and urticarial vasculitis in a patient with C2 deficiency (case report). *J Rheumatol* 1990;17:1222–1225.
10. Moss C, Hamilton PJ. Thrombocytopenia in systemic lupus erythematosus responsive to dapsone (abstract). *Br Med J* (Clin Res) 1988;297:266.
11. Ruzicka T, Goerz G. Dapsone in the treatment of lupus erythematosus. *Br J Dermatol* 1981;104:5–356.
12. Yamada Y, Dekio S, Jidol J, et al. Lupus erythematosus profundus report of a case treated with dapsone. *J Dermatol* 1989; 16:379–382.
13. Medina F, Jara LJ, Miranda JM, et al. Diamine-diphenyl-sulfone (DDS) treatment of refractory subacute cutaneous lupus erythematosus (SCLE) (abstract). *Arthritis Rheum* 1993;36: S228.
14. Singh YN, Adya CM, Verma KK, et al. Dapsone in cutaneous lesions of SLE: an open study. *J Assoc Physicians India* 1992; 40:735–736.
15. Park YH, Sunamoto M, Miyoshi T, et al. Effectiveness of dapsone on refractory immune thrombocytopenia in a patient with systemic lupus erythematosus associated with sarcoidosis. *Rinsho Ketsueki* 1993;34:870–875.
16. Cohen J, VanFeldt J, Werth VP. Urticarial vasculitis: a successful treatment with dapsone. *J Clin Rheumatol* 1995;1:249–250.
17. Jakes JT, Dubois EL, Quismorio FP Jr. Antileprosy drugs and lupus erythematosus (letter). *Ann Intern Med* 1982;97:788.
18. Coburn PR, Shuster S. Dapsone and discoid lupus erythematosus. *Br J Dermatol* 1982;106:105–106.
19. Lindskov R, Reymann F. Dapsone in the treatment of cutaneous lupus erythematosus. *Dermatologica* 1986;172:214–217.
20. Alarcon GS, Sams WM Jr, Barton DD, et al. Bullous lupus erythematosus rash worsened by Dapsone. *Arthritis Rheum* 1984;27:1071–1072.
21. Kraus A, Jakez J, Palacios A. Dapsone induced sulfone syndrome and systemic lupus erythematosus. *J Rheumatol* 1992;19: 178–179.
22. Barranco VP. Dapsoneother indications. *Int J Dermatol* 1982; 21:513–514.
23. Barnhill RL, McDougall AC. Thalidomide: use and possible mode of action in reactional lepromatous leprosy and in various other conditions. *J Am Acad Dermatol* 1982;7:317–323.
24. Atra E, Sato EJ. Treatment of the cutaneous lesions of systemic lupus erythematosus with thalidomide. *Clin Exp Rheumatol* 1993;11:487–493.
25. Hasper MF, Klokke AH. Thalidomide in the treatment of chronic discoid lupus erythematosus. *Acta DermVenereol* (Stockh) 1982;62:321–324.
26. Calabrese L, Fleischer AB. Thalidomide: current and potential clinical applications. *Amer J Med* 2000;108:487–495.
27. Ludolph A, Matz DR. Electrophysiologic changes in thalidomide neuropathy under treatment for discoid LE (English abstract). *EEG EMG* 1982;13:167–170.
28. Barba Rubio J, Franco Martinez E. Discoid LE (treatment with thalidomide) (in Spanish). *Med Cut Iber Lat Am* 1977;3: 279–286.
29. Barba Rubio J, Gonzalez FF. Discoid LE and thalidomide. Preliminary results (in Spanish). *Dermatol Rev Mex* 1975;19: 131–139.
30. Lo JS, Berg RE, Tomecki KJ. Treatment of discoid lupus erythematosus. *Int J Dermatol* 1989;28:497–507.
31. Knop J, Bonsmann G, Happle R, et al. Thalidomide in the treatment of sixty cases of chronic discoid lupus erythematosus. *Br J Dermatol* 1983;108:461–466.

32. Hasper MF. Chronic cutaneous lupus erythematosus. Thalidomide treatment of 11 patients. *Arch Dermatol* 1983;119:812–815.
33. Stevens RJ, Andujar C, Edwards CJ, et al. Thalidomide in the treatment of the cutaneous manifestations of lupus erythematosus: experience in sixteen consecutive patients. *Brit J Rheumatol* 1997;36:353–359.
34. Ordi J, Cortes F, Martinez N, et al. Thalidomide induces amenorrhea in patients with lupus disease. *Arthritis Rheum* 1998; 41:2273–2275.
35. Rua-Figueroa I, Erausquin C, Naranjo A, et al. Pustuloderma during cutaneous lupus treatment with thalidomide. *Lupus* 1999;8:248–249.
36. Knop J, Happle R, Bonsmann G, et al. Treatment of chronic discoid lupus erythematosus with thalidomide. *Arch Dermatol Res* 1981;271:165–170.
37. Samsoen M, Grosshaus E, Basset A. Thalidomide in the treatment of chronic lupus erythematosus (English abstract). *Ann Dermatol Venereol* (Paris) 1980;107:515–523.
38. Scolari F, Harms M, Gilardi S. Thalidomide in the treatment of LE (English abstract). *Dermatologica* 1982;165:355–362.
39. Bessis D, Guillot B, Monpoint S, et al. Thalidomide for systemic lupus erythematosus. *Lancet* 1992;339:549–550.
40. Flaguel B, Wallach D, Cavelier-Balloy B, et al. Thalidomide and thrombosis. *Ann Derm Venereol* 2000;127:171–174.
41. Gutierrez-Rodriguez O, Starusta-Bacal P, Gutierrez-Montes O. Treatment of refractory rheumatoid arthritis: the thalidomide experience. *J Rheumatol* 1989;16:158–163.
42. Randall T. Thalidomide's back in the news, but in more favorable circumstances (news). *JAMA* 1990;263:1467–1468.
43. Krivanek J, Paver WK, Kossard S, et al. Clofazimine (Lamprene) in the treatment of discoid lupus erythematosus. *Australasian J Dermatol* 1976;17:108–110.
44. Krivanek JF, Paver WK. Further study of the use of clofazimine in discoid lupus erythematosus (letter). *Australas J Dermatol* 1980;21:169.
45. Zeis BM, Schulz EJ, Anderson R, et al. Mononuclearucocyte function in patients with lichen planus and cutaneous lupus erythematosus during chemotherapy with clofazimine. *S Afr Med J* 1989;75:161–162.
46. Crovato F, Levi L. Clofazimine in the treatment of annular lupus erythematosus (letter). *Arch Dermatol* 1981;117: 249–250.
47. Mackey JP, Barnes T. Clofazimine in the treatment of discoid lupus erythematosus. *Br J Dermatol* 1974;92:93–96.
48. Kossard S, Doherty E, McColl I, et al. Autofluorescence of clofazimine in discoid lupus erythematosus. *J Am Acad Dermatol* 1987;17:86–7871.
49. Yung RL, Richardson BC. Cytarabine for refractory cutaneous lupus. *Arthritis Rheum* 1995;38:1341–1343.
50. Viallard J-F, Mercie P, Faure I, et al. Successful treatment of lupus with fludarabine. *Lupus* 1999;8:767–769.
51. Davis JC Jr, Austin H III, Boumpas D, et al. A pilot study of 2-chloro-2′-deoxyadenosine in the treatment of systemic lupus erythematosus-associated glomerulonephritis. *Arthritis Rheum* 1998;41:335–343.
52. Duddgidge M, Powell RJ. Treatment of severe and difficult cases of systemic lupus with tacrilimus. A report of three cases. *Annals Rheum Dis* 1997;56:690–692.
53. Anon. Sirolimus (Rapamine) for transplant rejection. *Medical Letter* 2000;42:13–14.
54. Hirohata S, Ohnishi K, Sagawa A. Treatment of systemic lupus erythematosus with lobenzarit: an open clinical trial (abstract). *Arthritis Rheum* 1993;36:S228.
55. Hackshaw KV, Shi Y, Brandwein SR, et al. A pilot study of Zileutin, a novel selective 5-lipoxygenase inhibitor, in patients with systemic lupus erythematosus. *J Rheumatol* 1995;22: 462–468.
56. Iwasaki T, Hamano T, Alzawa K, et al. A case of systemic lupus erythematosus (SLE) successfully treated with mizoribine (Bredinin). *Ryumachi* 1994;34:885–889.

56a. Remer CF, Weisman MH, Wallace DJ. Benefits of leflunamide in systemic lupus erythematosus. *Lupus* 2000. In press.

57. Bechet PE. Aurotherapy in lupus erythematosus: study based on further experience of 14 years. *N Y State J Med* 1942;42: 609–614.
58. Crissey JT, Murray PF. Comparison of chloroquine and gold in the treatment of lupus erythematosus. *Arch Dermatol* 1956;74: 69–72.
59. Haxthausen H. Treatment of lupus erythematosus by intravenous injections of gold chloride. *Arch Dermat Syph* 1930;22: 77–90.
60. Pascher F, Silverberg MG, Loewenstein LW, et al. Therapeutic assays of New York Skin and Cancer Unit, Post-Graduate Medical School, New York University-Bellevue Medical Center: aurol-sulfide (Hille). *J Invest Dermat* 1949;13:151–155.
61. Weisman MH, Albert D, Mueller MR, et al. Gold therapy in patients with systemic lupus erythematosus. *Am J Med* 1983;75(suppl 6A):157–164.
62. Dalzier K, Going S, Cartwright PH, et al. Treatment of chronic discoid lupus erythematosus with an oral gold preparation. *Br J Dermatol* 1985;113(suppl):25–26.
63. Singer JZ, Ginzler EM, Kaplan D. Solganol (Aurothioglucose) for treatment of arthritis of systemic lupus erythematosus (SLE) (abstract). *Arthritis Rheum* 1987;30(suppl):S14.
64. Strejcek J. Lecba solemi zlata a systemovy erythematodes (English abstract). *Cas Lek Cesk* 1983;122:469–472.
65. Weissmann G, Rothfield N, Thomas L. Cutaneous hyperreactivity to vitamin A in systemic lupus erythematosus (SLE) (abstract). *Arthritis Rheum* 1962;5:665.
66. Vien CV, Gonzalez-Cabello R, Bado I, et al. Effect of vitamin A treatment on the immune reactivity of patients with systemic lupus erythematosus. *J Clin Lab Immunol* 1988;26:33–35.
67. Haeger-Aronsen B, Krook G, Abdulla M. Oral carotenoids for photosensitivity in patients with erythrohepatic protoporphyria, polymorphous light eruption and lupus erythematodes discoides. *Int J Dermatol* 1979;18:73–82.
68. Newbold PC. Beta-carotene in the treatment of discoid lupus erythematosus. *Br J Dermatol* 1976;95:100–101.
69. Dubois EL, Patterson C. Ineffectiveness of beta-carotene in lupus erythematosus (letter). *JAMA* 1976;236:138–139.
70. Boyd AS. An overview of the retinoids. *Am J Med* 1989; 86:568–574.
71. Harris ED Jr. Retinoid therapy for rheumatoid arthritis. *Ann Intern Med* 1984;100:146–147.
72. Newton RC, Jorizzo JL, Solomon AR, et al. Mechanism-oriented assessment of isotretinoin in chronic or subacute cutaneous lupus erythematosus. *Arch Dermatol* 1986;122:170–176.
73. Formica N, Shornick J, Parke A. Resistant cutaneous lupus responds to isoretinoin (Accutane) (abstract). *Arthritis Rheum* 1989;32(suppl):S75.
74. Green SG, Piette WW. Successful treatment of hypertrophic lupus erythematosus with isotretinoin. *J Am Acad Dermatol* 1987;17:364–368.
75. Rubenstein DJ, Huntley AC. Keratotic lupus erythematosus: treatment with isotretinoin. *J Am Acad Dermatol* 1986;14: 910–914.
76. Shornick JK, Formica N, Parke AL. Isotretoin for refractory lupus erythematosus. *J Am Acad Dermatol* 1991;24:49–52.
77. Dieng MT, Revuz J. Retinoids for cutaneous lupus. *Ann Dermatol Venereol* 1994;121:271–272.
78. Matsuoka LY, Wortsman J, Pepper JJ. Acute arthritis during

isotretinoin treatment for acne. *Arch Intern Med* 1984;144: 1870–1871.
79. Rowell NR. Chilblain lupus erythematosus responding to etretinate. *Br J Dermatol* 1987;117(suppl 32):100–101.
80. DiGiovanna JJ, Helfgott RK, Gerber LH, et al. Extraspinal tendon and ligament calcification associated with long-term therapy with etretinate. *N Engl J Med* 1986;315:1177–1182.
81. Ruzicka T, Meurer M, Bieber T. Efficiency of acitretin in the treatment of cutaneous lupus erythematosus. *Arch Dermatol* 1988;124:897–902.
82. Ruzicka T, Sommerburg C, Goerz G, et al. Treatment of cutaneous lupus erythematosus with acitretin and hydroxychloroquine. *Br J Dermatol* 1992;127:513–518.
83. Seiger E, Roland S, Goldman S. Cutaneous lupus treated with topical Tretinoin: a case report. *Cutis* 1991;47:351–355.
84. Ruiz-Arguelles GJ, Ruiz-Arguelles A, Perez-Romano B, et al. Protein S deficiency associated to anti-protein S antibodies in a patient with mixed connective tissue disease and its reversal by danazol. *Acta Haematol* 1993;89:206–208.
85. Ahn YS, Rocha R, Mylvaganam R, et al. Long-term danazol therapy in autoimmune thrombocytopenia: unmaintained remission and age-dependent response in women. *Ann Intern Med* 1989;111:723–729.
86. Marino C, Cook P. Danazol for lupus thrombocytopenia. *Arch Intern Med* 1985;145:2251–2252.
87. West SG, Johnson SC, Andersen PA, et al. Danazol for the treatment of refractory autoimmune thrombocytopenia in systemic lupus erythematosus (SLE) (abstract). *Arthritis Rheum* 1986;29(suppl):S44.
88. Wong K-L. Danazol in treatment of lupus thrombocytopenia. *Asia Pacific J Allergy Immunol* 1991;9:125–129.
89. Blanco R, Martinez-Taboada VM, Rodriguez-Valverde V, et al. Successful therapy with danazol in refractory autoimmune thrombocytopenia associated with rheumatic diseases. *Brit J Rheum* 1997;36:1095–1099.
90. Cervera H, Jara LJ, Pizarro S, et al. Danazol for systemic lupus erythematosus with refractory autoimmune thrombocytopenia or Evans' syndrome. *J Rheumatol* 1995;22:1867–1871.
91. Cervera H, Jara JL, Pizarro S, et al. Long-term danazol therapy in systemic lupus erythematosus and hematologic onset (abstract). *Arthritis Rheum* 1993;36(suppl):S92.
92. Aranegui P, Giner P, Lopez-Gomez M, et al. Danazol for Evans' syndrome due to SLE (letter). *DICP* 1990;24:641–642.
93. Chan AC, Sack K. Danazol therapy for autoimmune hemolytic anemia associated with systemic lupus erythematosus (case report). *J Rheumatol* 1991;18:280–282.
94. Pizarro S, Medina F, Jara J, et al. Efficacy of danazol therapy vs splenectomy in systemic lupus erythematosus patients with hematologic onset (abstract). *Arthritis Rheum* 1990;33(suppl): S165.
95. Morley KD, Parke A, Hughes GR. Systemic lupus erythematosus: two patients treated with danazol. *Br Med J* (Clin Res) 1982;284:1431–1432.
96. Jungers P, Liote F, Pelissier C, et al. The hormonomodulation in systemic lupus erythematosus: preliminary results with Danazol (D) and cyproterone-acetate (CA) (English abstract). *Ann Med Interne* (Paris) 1986;137:313–319.
97. Torrelo A, Espana A, Medina S, et al. Danazol and discoid lupus erythematosus (letter). *Dermatologica* 1990;181:239.
98. Dougados M, Job-Deslandre C, Amor B, et al. Danazol therapy in systemic lupus erythematosus. A one-year prospective controlled trial on 40 female patients. *Clin Trials J* 1987;24:191–200.
99. Guillet G, Sassolas B, Plantin P, et al. Anti-Ro-positive lupus and hereditary angioneurotic edema. A 7-year follow-up with worsening of lupus under danazol treatment. *Dermatologica* 1988;177:370–375.
100. Weill BJ, Menkes CJ, Cormier C, et al. Hepatocellular carcinoma after danazol therapy. *J Rheumatol* 1988;15:1447–1449.
101. David J. Hyperglucagonaemia and treatment with danazol for systemic lupus erythematosus. *Br Med J* (Clin Res) 1985;291: 1170–1171.
102. Lamb JH, Lain ES, Keaty C, et al. Steroid hormones, metabolic studies in dermatomyositis, lupus erythematosus and polymorphic light-sensitivity eruptions. *Arch Dermat Syph* 1948;57: 785–801.
103. Dubois EL, Commons RR, Starr P, et al. Corticotropin and cortisone treatment for systemic lupus erythematosus. *JAMA* 1952; 149:995–102.
104. Fromer JL. Use of testosterone in chronic lupus erythematosus: preliminary report. *Lahey Clin Bull* 1950;7:13–17.
105. Lahita RG, Kunkel HG. Treatment of systemic lupus erythematosus (SLE) with the androgen 19-nor testosterone (Nandrolene) (abstract). *Arthritis Rheum* 1984;27(suppl):S65.
106. Swaak AJG, Van Vilet Daskalopoulou E, Cutolo M, et al. Effect of nandrolone with decanoate (Deca-Durabolin) on the disease activity of female patients with systemic lupus erythematosus. A double-blind placebo-controlled study. *Rheumatol Int* 1994;13: 237–240.
107. Hazelton RA, McCruden AB, Sturrock RD, et al. Hormonal manipulation of the immune response in systemic lupus erythematosus: a drug trial of an anabolic steroid, 19-nortestosterone. *Ann Rheum Dis* 1983;42:155–157.
108. Folomeev MIu. Use of androgens in the complex treatment of men with systemic lupus erythematosus. *Ter Arkh* 1986;58:57–59.
109. Folomeev MIu, Folomeev IuV. Use of androgens in the complex treatment of men with systemic lupus erythematosus. *Revmatologiia* (Moskva) 1986;4:24–26.
110. Yu MIu, Folomeev IuV. The use of androgens in multiple modality therapy of men with systemic lupus erythematosus. *Ter Arkh* 1986;58:111–114.
111. Suzuki N, Suzuki T, Sakane T. Hormones and lupus: defective dehydroandrosterone activity induces impaired interleukin-2 activity of T lymphocytes in patients with systemic lupus erythematosus. *Ann Med Interne* 1996;147:248–252.
112. Van Vollenhoven RF. Role of sex steroids in the Th1/Th2 cytokine balance: comment on the article by Miossec and van den Berg. *Arthritis Rheum* 1998;41:2105–2115.
113. Straub RH, Zeuner M, Antoniou E, et al. Dehydroepiandrosterone sulfate is positively correlated with soluble interleukin 2 receptor and soluble intercellular adhesion molecule in systemic lupus erythematosus. *J Rheumatol* 1996;23:856–861.
114. Derksen RH. Dehydroandrosterone (DHEA) and systemic lupus erythematosus. *Semin Arthritis Rheum*1998;27:335–347.
115. Himmel PB, Seligman TM. A pilot study employing dehydroepiandrosterone (DHEA) in the treatment of chronic fatigue syndrome. *J Clin Rheumatol.* 1999;5:56–59.
116. Parasrampuria J, Schwartz K, Petasch R. Quality control of dehydroepiandrosterone dietary supplement products. *JAMA* 1998;280:1565.
117. van Vollenhoven RF, Engleman EG, McGuire JL. An open study of dehydroepiandrosterone in systemic lupus erythematosus. *Arthritis Rheum* 1994;37:1305–1310.
118. Van Vollenhoven RF, Engleman EG, Mc Guire JL. Dehydroepiandrosterone in systemic lupus erythematosus. Results of a double-blind, placebo-controlled clinical trial. *Arthritis Rheum* 1995;38:1826–1831.
119. Van Vollenhoven RF, Morabito LM, Engleman EG, et al. Treatment of systemic lupus erythematosus with dehydroepiandrosterone: 50 patients treated up to 12 months. *J Rheumatol* 1998; 25:285–289.
120. Barry NN, McGuire JL, van Vollenhoven RF. Dehydroepiandrosterone in systemic lupus erythematosus: relationship

between dosage, serum levels and clinical response. *J Rheumatol* 1998;25:2352–2356.
121. Van Vollenhoven RF, Park JL, Genovese MC, et al. A double-blind, placebo-controlled, clinical trial of dehydroepiandrosterone in severe systemic lupus erythematosus. *Lupus* 1999;8: 181–187.
122. Petri M, Lahita R, McGuire J, et al. Results of the GL701 (DHEA) multicenter steroid-sparing SLE study. *Arthritis Rheum* 1997;40:S327.
123. Sturgess AD, Evans DT, Mackay IR, et al. Effects of the oestrogen antagonist tamoxifen on disease indices in systemic lupus erythematosus. *J Clin Lab Immunol* 1984;13:11–14.
124. Yap HK, Loke KY, Murugasu B, et al. Subclinical activation of lupus nephritis by recombinant growth hormone. *Pediatr Nephrol* 1998;12:133–135.
125. Stiehm ER, Ashida E, Kim KS, et al. Intravenous immunoglobulins as therapeutic agents (clinical conference). *Ann Intern Med* 1987;107:367–382.
126. Dwyer JM. Manipulating the immune system with immunoglobulin. *N Engl J Med* 1992;326:107–116.
127. Ruiz de Souza V, Kaveri SV, Kazatchkine MD. Intravenous immunoglobulin (IVIg) in the treatment of autoimmune and inflammatory diseases. *Clinical Exp Rheum* 1993;11(suppl 9): S33–S36.
128. Silvestris F, d'Amore O, Cafforio P, et al. Intravenous immune globulin therapy of lupus nephritis: use of pathogenic anti-DNA-reactive IgG. *Clin Exp Immunol* 1996;104(S1):91–97.
129. DeKeyser F, DeKeyser H, Kazatchikine MD, et al. Pooled human immunoglobulins contain anti-idiotypes with reactivity against the SLE-associated 4B4 cross-reactive idiotype. *Clin Exper Rheumatol* 196;14:587–591.
130. Maltaek N, Harreby MS, Thogersen B. Intravenous immunoglobulin administration to a patient with systemic lupus erythematosus and pneumococcal septicemia. *Ugeskr Laeger* 1994; 156:4039–4041.
131. Siber GR. Immune globulin to prevent nosocomial infections. *N Engl J Med* 1992;327:269–271.
132. Swaak AJG, van den Brink HG. Common variable immunodeficiency in a patient with systemic lupus erythematosus. *Lupus* 1996;5:242–246.
133. Sugisaki T, Shiwachi S, Yonekura M, et al. High dose intravenous gamma globulin for membranous nephropathy (MN), membranoproliferative glomerulonephritis (MPGN) and lupus (LN) (abstract). *Fed Proc* 1982;41:692.
134. Gaedicke G, Teller WM, Kohne E, et al. IgG therapy in systemic lupus erythematosus; two case reports. *Blut* 1984;48: 387–390.
135. Howard RF, Maier WP, Gordon DS, et al. Clinical and immunological investigation of intravenous human immunoglobulin (IVIG) therapy in SLE-associated thrombocytopenia (abstract). *Arthritis Rheum* 1989;32(suppl):S75.
136. Maier WP, Gordon DS, Howard RF, et al. Intravenous immunoglobulin therapy in systemic lupus erythematosus-associated thrombocytopenia. *Arthritis Rheum* 1990;33:1233–1239.
137. ter Borg EJ, Kallenberg CGM. Treatment of severe thrombocytopenia in systemic lupus erythematosus. *Ann Rheum Dis* 1992;51:1149–1151.
138. Hanada T, Saito K, Nagasawa T, et al. Intravenous gammaglobulin therapy for thromboneutropenic neonates of mothers with systemic lupus erythematosus. *Eur J Haematol* 1987;38: 400–404.
139. Francioni C, Galeazzi M, Fioravanti A, et al. Long term I.V. Ig treatment in systemic lupus erythematosus. *Clin Exp Rheumatol* 1994;12:163–168.
140. Abdou NI, Yesenosky P, Chou A, et al. Intravenous human immunoglobulin (IVIG) therapy in active SLE: a six month in vivo and in vitro study (abstract). *Arthritis Rheum* 1994;37 (suppl):S406.
141. Corvetta A, Della Bitta R, Gabrielli A, et al. Use of high dose intravenous immunoglobulin in systemic lupus erythematosus: report of three cases. *Clin Exp Rheumatol* 1989;7:295–299.
142. Tomer Y, Shoenfeld Y. Successful treatment of psychosis secondary to SLE with high dose intravenous immunoglobulin. *Clin Exp Rheumatol* 1992;10:391–393.
143. Sherer Y, Levy L, Langevitz P, et al. Successful treatment of systemic lupus erythematosus cerebritis with intravenous immunoglobulin. *Clin Rheumatol* 1999;18:170–173.
144. Lin CY. Improvement in steroid and immunosuppressive drug resistant lupus nephritis by intravenous prostaglandin E1 therapy. *Nephron* 1990;55:258–264.
145. Hjortjoer Petersen H, Nielsen H, Hansen M, et al. High-dose immunoglobulin therapy in pericarditis caused by SLE (letter). *Scand J Rheumatol* 1990;19:91–93.
146. Sherer Y, Levy L, Shoenfeld Y. Marked improvement of severe cardiac dysfunction after one course of intravenous immunoglobulin in a patient with systemic lupus erythematosus. *Clin Rheumatol* 1999;18:238–240.
147. Pirner K, Rosler W, Kalden JR, et al. [Long-term remission after i.v. immunoglobulin therapy in acquired antihemophilic factor hemophilia with systemic lupus erythematosus.] *Z Rheumatol* 1990;49:378–381.
148. Lafferty TE, Smith JB, Schuster SJ, et al. Treatment of acquired factor VIII inhibitor using intravenous immunoglobulin in two patients with systemic lupus erythematosus. *Arthritis Rheum* 1997;40:775–778.
149. Akashi K, Nagasawa K, Mayumi T, et al. Successful treatment of refractory systemic lupus erythematosus with intravenous immunoglobulins. *J Rheumatol* 1990;17:375–379.
150. Ilan Y, Naparstek Y. Pure red cell aplasia associated with systemic lupus erythematosus: remission after a single course of intravenous immunoglobulin. *Acta Haematol* 1993;89: 152–154.
151. Piette J-C, Frances C, Roy S, et al. High-dose immunoglobulins in the treatment of cutaneous lupus erythematosus: open trial in 5 cases (abstract). *Arthritis Rheum* 1995;38:S304.
152. Puddu P, de Pita O, Rufelli M, et al. Intravenous immunoglobulin therapy: modification of the immunofluorescence pattern in the skin of six patients with systemic lupus erythematosus. *Arthritis Rheum* 1996;39:704–708.
153. Aharon A, Levy Y, Bar-Dayan Y, et al. Successful treatment of early secondary myelofibrosis in SLE with IVIG. *Lupus* 1997; 6:408–411.
154. Becker BN, Fuchs H, Hakim R. Intravenous immune globulin in the treatment of patients with systemic lupus erythematosus and end stage renal disease. *J Am Soc Nephrol* 1995;5:1745–1750.
155. Levy Y, Sherer Y, George J, et al. Intravenous immunoglobulin treatment of lupus nephritis. *Semin Arthritis Rheum* 2000;29: 321–327.
156. Buletis JN, Ioannidis PJA, Boki KA, et al. Intravenous immunoglobulin compared with cyclophosphamide for proliferative nephritis. *Lancet* 1999;354:569–570.
157. Lesprit P, Mouloud F, Schaeffer A, et al. Prolonged remission of SLE-associated polyradiculoneuropathy after a single course of intravenous immunoglobulin. *Scand J Rheumatol* 1996;25:177–179.
158. Pernod G, Arvieux J, Carpentier PH, et al. Successful treatment of lupus anticoagulant-hypoprothrombinemia syndrome using intravenous immunoglobulins. *Thromb Haemostasis* 1997;78: 969–970.
159. Carreras LO, Perez G, Vega HR, et al. Lupus anticoagulant and recurrent fetal loss: successful treatment with gammaglobulin (letter). *Lancet* 1988;ii:393–394.

160. Katz VL, Thorp JM Jr, Watson WJ, et al. Human immunoglobulin therapy for preeclampsia associated with lupus anticoagulant and anticardiolipin antibody. *Obstet Gynecol* 1990;76:986–988.
161. Parke AL, Maier D, Wilson D, et al. Intravenous gamma-globulin, antiphospholipid antibodies, and pregnancy. *Ann Intern Med* 1989;110:495–496.
162. Clark AL, Spinnato JA, Pierangeli SS, et al. Intravenous immunoglobulin and the antiphospholipid syndrome in pregnancy (abstract). *Arthritis Rheum* 1993;36(suppl):S276.
163. Kaaja R, Julkunen H, Ammala P, et al. Intravenous immunoglobulin treatment of pregnant patients with recurrent pregnancy losses associated with antiphospholipid antibodies. *Acta Obstet Gynecol Scand* 1993;72:63–66.
164. Gordon C, Raine-Fenning N, Brackley K, et al. Intravenous immunoglobulin (IVIG) therapy to salvage severely compromised pregnancies in SLE and antiphospholipid syndrome. *Lupus* 1998;7:S1–114.
165. Levy Y, Sherer Y, Langevitz P, et al. A study of 20 SLE patients with intravenous immunoglobulin — clinical and serologic response. *Lupus* 1998;8:705–712.
166. Ballow M, Parke A. The uses of intravenous immune globulin in collagen vascular disease. *J Allergy Clin Immunol* 1989;84: 608–612.
167. De Pita O, Bellucci AM, Ruffelli M, et al. Intravenous immunoglobulin therapy is not able to efficiently control cutaneous manifestations in patients with lupus erythematosus. *Lupus* 1997;6:415–417.
168. Schoeder JO, Zeuner RA, Euler HH, et al. High dose intravenous immunoglobulins in systemic lupus erythematosus: clinical and serological results of a pilot study. *J Rheumatol* 1996;23:71–75.
169. Barron KS, Sher MR, Silverman ED. Intravenous immunoglobulin therapy: magic or black magic. *J Rheumatol* 1992;19 (suppl 33):94–97.
170. Pirner K, Rubbert A, Burmester GR, et al. Intravenous immunoglobulin therapy in systemic lupus erythematosus. *Infusionsther Transfusionmed* 1993;20(suppl):131–136.
171. Pasatiempo AMG, Kroser JA, Rudnick M, et al. Acute renal failure after intravenous immunoglobulin therapy. *J Rheumatol* 1994;21:347–349.
172. Elkayam O, Paran D, Milo R, et al. Acute myocardial infarction associated with high dose intravenous immunoglobulin infusion for autoimmune disorders. A study of four cases. *Ann Rheum Dis* 2000;59:77–80.
173. Reed AM, Kredich DW, Schanberg LE, et al. Aseptic meningitis is a common side effect of high dose IVIg in children with autoimmune disease. *Arthritis Rheum* 1997;40:S283.
174. Hashkes PJ, Lovell DJ. Vasculitis in systemic lupus erythematosus following intravenous immunoglobulin therapy. *Clin Exp Rheumatol* 1996;14:673–675.
175. Deleted in page proofs.
176. Gordon BL 2nd, Keenan JP. The treatment of systemic lupus erythematosus (SLE) with the T-cell immunostimulant drug levamisole: a case report. *Ann Allergy* 1975;35:343–355.
177. Gordon BL 2nd, Yanagihara R. Treatment of systemic lupus erythematosus with T-cell immunopotentiator levamisole: a follow-up report of 16 patients under treatment for a minimum period of four months. *Ann Allergy* 1977;39:227–236.
178. Rabson A, Blank S, Lomnitzer R. Effect of levamisole on in vitro suppressor cell function in normal humans and patients with systemic lupus erythematosus. *Immunopharmacology* 1980; 2:103–108.
179. Rosling AE, Rhodes EL, Watson B. Removal of a blocking factor from the sera of patients with systemic lupus erythematosus with Levamisole. *Clin Exp Dermatol* 1978;3:39–42.
180. Scherak O, Smolen JS, Menzel EJ, et al. Effect of levamisole on immunological parameters in patients with systemic lupus erythematosus. *Scand J Rheumatol* 1980;9:106–112.
181. Smolen J, Scherak O, Menzel J, et al. Levamisole in systemic lupus erythematosus (letter). *Arthritis Rheum* 1977;20: 1558–1559.
182. Rovensky J, Cebecauer L, Zitnan D, et al. Levamisole treatment of systemic lupus erythematosus (letter). *Arthritis Rheum* 1982; 25:470–471.
183. Rovensky J, Lukac J, Zitnan D, et al. Results of immunomodulatory therapy in systemic lupus erythematosus. *Int J Immunother* 1986;2:193–198.
184. Ogawa K, Sano T, Hisano G, et al. Levamisole in systemic lupus erythematosus. *Ann Allergy* 1979;43:187–189.
185. Feng PH, Oon CJ, Yo SL, et al. Levamisole in the treatment of systemic lupus erythematosus — preliminary results. *Singapore Med J* 1978;19:120–124.
186. Hadidi T, Decker JL, El-Nagdy L, et al. Ineffectiveness of levamisole in systemic lupus erythematosus: a controlled trial. *Arthritis Rheum* 1981;24:60–63.
187. Brendel W. The clinical use of ALG. *Transplant Proc* 1971;3: 280–286.
188. Morishita Y, Matsukawa Y, Kura Y, et al. Antithymocyte globulin for a patient with systemic lupus erythematosus complicated by severe pancytopenia. *J International Medical Research* 1997; 25:219–223.
189. Herreman G, Broquie G, Metzger JP, et al. Treatment of SLE and other collagenoses with anti-lymphocyte globulin. A propos of 10 cases (in French). *Nouv Presse Med* 1972;1:2035–2039.
190. Pirofsky B, Bardana EJ, Bayracki C, et al. Antilymphocyte antisera in immunologically mediated renal disease. *JAMA* 1969; 210:1059–1064.
191. Hollingworth P, de Vere R, Tyndall ADV, et al. Intensive immunosuppression versus prednisolone in the treatment of connective tissue diseases. *Ann Rheum Dis* 1982;41:557–562.
192. Svec KH, Weisberger AS, Post RS, et al. Immunosuppression by a chloramphenicol analogue in patients with lupus glomerulonephritis (abstract). *J Lab Clin Med* 1968;72:10–23.
193. Weisberger AS, Wessler S, Avioli LV. Mechanisms of action of chloramphenicol. *JAMA* 1969;209:97–103.
194. Richmond DE. Thiamphenicol as an immunosuppressant in active systemic lupus erythematosus with nephritis. *Aust N Z J Med* 1979;9:670–675.
195. Johnson SAM, Meyer O, Brown JW, et al. Failure of chloramphenicol (chloromycetin) in treatment of 3 cases of lupus erythematosus disseminatus. *J Invest Dermatol* 1950;14:305–307.
196. Morris MH. Acute lupus erythematosus disseminate treated with penicillin. *N Y State J Med* 1946;46:917–918.
197. Strakosch EA. Acute lupus erythematosus disseminatus treated with penicillin: report of case. *Arch Dermat Syph* 1946;54: 197–199.
198. Pollak O, Ziskind JM. Death during sulfonamide treatment; finding of liver cells in brain. *J Nerv Ment Dis* 1943;98: 648–655.
199. Weiner AL. Disseminated lupus erythematosus treated by sulfanilamide: report of 4 cases. *Arch Dermat Syph* 1940;441: 534–544.
200. Saha HH, Lumio JT, Mustonen JT, et al. Complete remission of intractable SLE after trimethoprim-sulphamethoxazole therapy for pneumocystis carinii. *Nephrol Dial Transplant* 1995;10: 274–276.
201. Bolgert M, Le Sourd M, Habib G. Subacute lupus erythematosus: exanthematous onset with bullous lesions: treatment with aureomycin (in French). *Bull Soc Franc Dermat et Syph* 1949;56:433–436.
202. Gougerot H, Carteaud A, Desvignes P. Acute eruption in facial lupus erythematosus. Kaposi-Besnier-Libman-Sacks syndrome

apparently healed by streptomycin (in French). *Bull Soc Franc Dermat et Syph* 1949;56:41.
203. Rasponi L. Antibiotics in pemphigus vulgaris and in acute lupus erythematosus. *Postgrad Med J* 1982;58:98–99.
204. Ehrenstein MR, McSweeney E, Swana M, et al. Appearance of anti-DNA antibodies in patients treated with interferon-alpha. *Arthritis Rheum* 1993;36:279–280.
205. Flores A, Olive A, Feliu E, et al. Systemic lupus erythematosus following interferon therapy. *Br J Rheum* 1994;33:787–792.
206. Wandi UB, Nagel-Hiemke M, May D, et al. Lupus-like autoimmune disease induced by interferon therapy for myeloproliferative disorders. *Clin Immunol Immunopathol* 1992;65: 70–74.
207. Ronnblom LE, Alm GV, Oberg KE. Autoimmunity after alpha-interferon therapy for malignant carcinoid tumors. *Ann Intern Med* 1991;115:178–183.
208. Morris LF, Lemak NA, Arnett FC Jr, et al. Systemic lupus erythematosus diagnosed during interferon alfa therapy. *South Med J* 1996;89:810–814.
209. Tolaymat A, Leventhal B, Sakarcan A, et al. Systemic lupus erythematosus in a child receiving long-term interferon therapy. *J Pediatr* 1992;120:429–432.
210. Hory B, Blanc D, Saint-Hiller Y. Systemic lupus erythematosus-like syndrome induced by alpha-interferon (abstract). *Eur J Med* 1992;1:379.
211. Schilling PJ, Kurzrock R, Kantarjian H, et al. Development of systemic lupus erythematosus after interferon therapy for chronic myelogenous leukemia. *Cancer* 1991;68:1536–1537.
212. Machold KP, Smolen JS. Interferon-gamma induced exacerbation of systemic lupus erythematosus. *J Rheumatol* 1990;17: 831–832.
213. Nousari HC, Kimayi-Asadi A, Tausk FA. Subacute cutaneous lupus erythematosus associated with interferon beta-1a. *Lancet* 1998;352:1825–1826.
214. Granninger WB, Hassfeld W, Pesau BB, et al. Induction of systemic lupus erythematosus by interferon-gamma in a patient with rheumatoid arthritis. *J Rheumatol* 1991;18:1621–1622.
215. Garcia-Porrua C, Gonzalez-Gay MA, Fernandex-Lamelo F, et al. Simultaneous development of SLE-like syndrome and autoimmune thyroiditis following alpha interferon treatment. *Clin Exp Rheumatol* 1998;16:107–108.
216. Nicolas JF, Thivolet J, Kanitakis J, et al. Response of discoid and subacute cutaneous lupus erythematosus to recombinant interferon alpha 2a. *J Invest Dermatol* 1990;95(suppl 6):142S–145S.
217. Thivolet J, Nicolas JF, Kanitakis J, et al. Recombinant interferon alpha 2a is effective in the treatment of discoid and subacute cutaneous lupus erythematosus. *Br J Dermatol* 1990;122: 405–409.
218. Nicolas J-F, Thivolet J. Interferon alfa therapy in severe unresponsive subacute cutaneous lupus erythematosus. *N Engl J Med* 1989;321:1550–1551.
219. Martinez J, de Misa RF, Boixeda P, et al. Long term results of intralesional interferon alpha-2B in discoid lupus erythematosus. *J Dermatol* 1993;20:440–446.
220. Haidushka I, Zlatev S. Isoprinosine in patient with systemic lupus erythematosus (letter). *Lancet* 1987;ii:153.
221. Alarcon-Segovia D, Galbraith RF, Maldonado JE, et al. Systemic lupus erythematosus following thymectomy for myasthenia gravis. Report of two cases. *Lancet* 1963;ii:662–665.
222. Chorzelski T, Jablonska S. Coexistence of lupus erythematosus and scleroderma in light of immunopathological investigations. *Acta Derm Venereol* (Stockh) 1970;50:81–85.
223. Dacie JV. Autoimmune haemolytic anaemias. *Br Med J* 1970; 1:381–386.
224. Hutchins GM, Harvey AM. The thymus in systemic lupus erythematosus. *Bull Johns Hopkins Hosp* 1964;115:355–378.
225. Larsson O. Thymoma and systemic lupus erythematosus in the same patient. *Lancet* 1963;ii:665–666.
226. Mackay IR, Goldstein G, McConchie IH. Thymectomy in systemic lupus erythematosus. *Br Med J* 1963;1:792–793.
227. Wilmers MJ, Russell PA. Autoimmune haemolytic anaemia in an infant treated by thymectomy. *Lancet* 1963;ii:915–917.
228. Baxevanis CN, Reclos GJ, Papamichail M, et al. Prothymosin alpha restores the depressed autologous and allogeneic mixed lymphocyte responses in patients with systemic lupus erythematosus. *Immunopharm Immunotoxicol* 1987;9:429–440.
229. Lavalle C, Pizarro S, Drenkard C, et al. Transverse myelitis: manifestation of systemic lupus erythematosus strongly associated with antiphospholipid antibodies. *J Rheumatol* 1990;17:34–37.
230. Scheinberg MA, Cathcart ES, Goldstein AL. Thymosin-induced reduction of null cells in peripheral-blood lymphocytes of patients with systemic lupus erythematosus. *Lancet* 1975;i: 424–446.
231. Safieh-Garabedian B, Ahmed K, Khamashta MA, et al. Thymulin modulates cytokine release by peripheral blood mononuclear cells: a comparison between healthy volunteers and patients with systemic lupus erythematosus. *Int Arch Allergy Immunol* 1993;101:126–131.
232. Goldstein AL, Zatz MM, Low TL, et al. Potential role of thymosin in the treatment of autoimmune diseases. *Ann N Y Acad Sci* 1981;377:486–495.
233. Lasisz B, Zdrojewicz Z, Dul W, et al. Possibility of using TFX (thymus factor X) in the treatment of systemic lupus erythematosus. *Pol Tyg Lek* 1989;44:724–725.
234. Zurier RB. Prostaglandin E1: is it useful? (editorial). *J Rheumatol* 1990;17:1439–1441.
235. Lin CY. Improvement in steroid and immunosuppressive drug resistant lupus nephritis by intravenous prostaglandin E1 therapy. *Nephron* 1990;55:258–264.
236. Nagayama Y, Namura Y, Tamura T, et al. Beneficial effect of prostaglandin E1 in three cases of lupus nephritis with nephrotic syndrome. *Ann Allergy* 1988;61:289–295.
237. Yoshikawa T, Suzuki H, Kato H, et al. Effects of prostaglandin E1 on collagen diseases with high levels of circulating immune complexes. *J Rheumatol* 1990;17:1513–1514.
238. Hauptman HW, Ruddy S, Roberts WN. Reversal of the vasospastic component of lupus vasculopathy by infusion of prostaglandin E1. *J Rheumatol* 1991;18:1747–1752.
239. Constans J, de Precigout V, Combe C, et al. Efficacy of prostacyclin perfusions for the microangiopathy associated with lupus. *Presse Med* 1991;20:3–5.
240. Yoshikawa Y, Mizutani H, Shimizu M. Systemic lupus erythematosus with ischemic peripheral neuropathy and lupus anticoagulant: response to intravenous prostaglandin E1. *Cutis* 1996;58:393–396.
241. Pierucci A, Simonetti BM, Pecci G, et al. Improvement of renal function with selective thromboxane antagonism in lupus nephritis. *N Engl J Med* 1989;320:421–425.
242. Cole EH. Modulation of renal prostaglandin metabolism in therapy of lupus nephritis. *J Rheumatol* 1996;23:1686–1688.
243. Oshida T, Kameda H, Ichikawa Y, et al. Improvement of renal function with a selective thromboxane inhibitor, DP-1904, in lupus nephritis. *J Rheumatol* 1996;23:1719–1724.
244. Shapira Y, Mor F, Friedler A, et al. Antiproteinuric effect of captopril in a patient with lupus nephritis and intractable nephrotic syndrome. *Ann Rheum Dis* 1990;49:723–727.
245. Laversuch CJ, Collins DA, Charles PJ, et al. Sulphasalazine-induced autoimmune abnormalities in patients with rheumatic disease. *Br J Rheum* 1995;34:443–543.
246. Borg AA, Davis MJ, Dawes PT, et al. Combination therapy for rheumatoid arthritis and drug-induced systemic lupus erythematosus. *Clin Rheumatol* 1994;13:522–524.

247. Delaporte E, Catteau B, Sabbagh N, et al. Traitement du lupus erythemateaux chronique par la sulfasalazine: 11 observations. *Ann Dermatol Venereol* 1997;124:151–156.
248. Carmichael AJ, Paul CJ. Discoid lupus erythematosus responsive to sulphasalazine. *Brit J Dermatol* 1991;125:291–294.
249. Artuz F, Lenk N, Deniz N, et al. Efficacy of sulfasalazine in discoid lupus erythematosus. *Int J Dermatol* 1996;35:746–748.
250. Gunnarsson I, Kanerud L, Pettersson E, et al. Predisposing factors in sulphasalazine-induced systemic lupus erythematosus. *Brit J Rheumatol* 1997;36:1089–1094.
251. Hilepo JN, Bellucci AG, Mossey RT. Acute renal failure caused by 'Cat's Claw' herbal remedy in a patient with systemic lupus erythematosus. *Nephron* 1997;77:361.
252. Abt AB, Oh JY, Huntington RA, et al. Chinese herbal medicine induced acute renal failure. *Arch Intern Med* 1995;15:211–212.
253. Gertner E, Marchall PS, Filandrinos D, et al. Complications resulting from the use of Chinese herbal medications containing undeclared prescription drugs. *Arthritis Rheum* 1995;38: 614–617.
254. Balabanova MB, Botev IN, Michailova JI. Subacute cutaneous erythematosus induced by radiation therapy. *Brit J Dermatol* 1997;137:646–663.
255. Eedy DJ, Corbett JR. Discoid lupus erythematosus exacerbated by X-ray irradiation. *Clin Exper Dermatol* 1988;13:202–203.
256. Rathmell AJ, Taylor RE. Enhanced normal tissue response to radiation in a patient with discoid lupus. *Clinical Oncology* 1992;4:331–332.
257. Olivotto IA, Fairey RN, Gillies JH, et al. Fatal outcome of pelvic radiotherapy for carcinoma of the cervix in a patient with systemic lupus erythematous. *Clin Radiology* 1989;40:83–84.
258. Ross JG, Hussey DH, Mayr NA, et al. Acute and late reactions to radiation therapy in patients with collagen vascular diseases. *Cancer* 1993;71:3744–3752.
259. Rafkal SM, Deutsch M. Radiotherapy for malignancies associated with lupus. Case reports of acute and late relations. *Am J Clin Oncol* 1998;21:54–57.
260. Mayr NA, Riggs CE Jr, Saak KG, et al. Mixed connective tissue disease and radiation toxicity. A case report. *Cancer* 1997;79: 612–618.
261. Moore A, Petri MA, Manzi S, et al. The use of alternative medical therapies in patients with systemic lupus erythematosus. *Arthritis Rheum* 1998;41:S133.
262. Ramos-Remus C, Gamez-Nava JI, Gonzalez L, et al. Use of alternative medicine in a consecutive sample of patients with systemic lupus erythematosus. *J Rheumatology* 1997;24: 2490–2491.
263. Goldblatt S. Treatment of lupus erythematosus with vitamin B12: preliminary report of 4 cases. *J Invest DermVenereol* 1951; 17:303–304.
264. Goldblatt S. Cyanocobalamin (vitamin B12) therapy of lupus erythematosus; further observations. *Acta Dermatovener* (Stockh) 1953;33:216–235.
265. Welsh AL. Lupus erythematosus: treatment by combined use of massive amounts of pantothenic acid and vitamin E. *Arch Dermat Syph* 1954;70:181–198.
266. Sulzberger MB, Wolf J, Witten VH, et al. *Dermatology, diagnosis and treatment, 2nd ed.* Chicago: Year Book Medical Publishers, 1961.
267. Berman L, Axelrod AR, Goodman HL, et al. So-called lupus erythematosus inclusion phenomenon of bone marrow and blood: morphologic and serologic studies. *Am J Clin Pathol* 1950;20:403–418.
268. Pascher F, Sawicky HH, Silverberg MG, et al. Therapeutic assays of New York Skin and Cancer Unit, Post-graduate Medical School, New York University-Bellevue Medical Center: aurol sulfide (Hille). *J Invest Dermatol* 1948;10:441–445.
269. Arnold HL. Insoluble bismuth (Subsalicylate) should be revived for treatment of LE in general and SCLE in particular (letter). *Int J Dermatol* 1991;30:377.
270. Benenson EV, Mirrakhimova EM. Clinical effectiveness of prospidin in systemic lupus erythematosus: results of a 6 month follow-up. *Ter Arkh* 1989;61:21–26.
271. Biriukov AV, Stenina MA, Anan'eva LP, et al. Clinical effectiveness of the treatment of systemic lupus erythematosus with preparations of the methylxanthine group and T-activin. *Klin Med* (Mosk) 1987;65:107–111.
272. Glavinskaia TA, Pavlova LT, Dorofeichuk VG. Lysozyme in the combined therapy of erythematosus (English abstract). *Vestn Dermatol Venereol* 1990:21–25.
273. Matveikov GP, Titova IP, Kaliia ES, et al. Immunopathological manifestations of systemic lupus erythematosus and their correction during long-term dispensary observation. *Ter Arkh* 1987;59:27–31.
274. Cannon AB, Orstein GG. Lupus erythematosus: treatment with tuberculin. *Arch Dermatol* 1927;16:8–11.
275. Tu BY. Combined treatment using traditional Chinese medicine and Western medicine of lupus crisis: a report of 10 cases (English abstract). *Chung Hsi I Chieh Ho Tsa Chih* 1986; 6:215–217.
276. Wang BX, Yuan ZZ. A tablet of Tripterygium wilfordii in treating lupus erythematosus. *Chung Hsi I Chieh Ho Tsa Chih* 1989; 9:407–408.
277. Wang ZY. Clinical and laboratory studies of the effect of an antilupus pill on systemic lupus erythematosus (English abstract). *Chung Hsi I Chieh Ho Tsa Chih* 1989;9:452, 465–468.
278. Wanzhane Q, Chenghuane L, Shumei Y, et al. Tripterygium wilfordii hook F in systemic lupus erythematosus. Report of 103 cases. *Chinese Med J* 1981;94:827–834.
279. Yang HT, Zhang JR. Treatment of systemic lupus erythematosus with saponin of ginseng fruit (SPGF): an immunological study (English abstract). *Chung Hsi I Chieh Ho Tsa Chih* 1986; 6:157–159.
280. Yuan ZZ, Feng JC. Observation on the treatment of systemic lupus erythematosus with a Gentiani macrophylla complex tablet and a minimal dose of prednisone (English abstract). *Chung Hsi Chieh I Ho Tsa Chih* 1989;9:133–134, 156–157.
281. Ramgolam V, Ang SG, Lai YH, et al. Traditional Chinese medicines as immunosuppressive agents. *Annals Acad Medicine* (Singapore) 2000;29:11–16.
282. Tao X, Lipsky P. The Chinese antiinflammatory and immunosuppressive herbal remedy *tripterygium wilfordii* hook F. *Rheum Dis Clin NA* 2000;26:29–50.
283. Kao NL, Richmond GW, Moy JN. Resolution of severe lupus nephritis associated with Tripterygium wilfordii hook F ingestion. *Arthritis Rheum* 1993;36:1751–1756.
284. Goldberg LC. Lupus erythematosus: treatment with oxophenarsine hydrochloride. *Arch Dermat Syph* 1945;52:89–90.
285. Ballico I. The cure of lupus erythematosus by means of ultraviolet rays (in Italian). *Raggi Ultraviol* 1930;6:182–187.
286. Zarafonetis CJD. Therapeutic possibilities of para-amino-benzoic acid. *Ann Intern Med* 1949;30:1188–1211.
287. Zarafonetis CJD, Grekin RH, Curtis AC. Further studies on the treatment of lupus erythematosus with sodium para-aminobenzoate. *J Invest Dermatol* 1984;11:359–381.
288. Callen JP. The effectiveness of colchicine for cutaneous vasculitis in lupus erythematosus. *Clin Rheum Pract* 1984;2:176–179.
289. Galindo-Rodriguez G, Esquivel G, Bustamante R. Efficacy of pentoxifylline in the treatment of refractory nephrotic syndrome in lupus nephritis (abstract). *Arthritis Rheum* 1999;42:S214.
290. Etherington J, Haynes P, Buchanan N. Letter to the editor. *Lupus* 1993;2:387.

291. Delaporte E, Piette F, Bourjot D, et al. Treatment of chronic lupus erythematosus with sulfasalazine (abstract). *La Presse Med* 1994;23:95.
292. Kurnick NB. Rational therapy of systemic lupus erythematosus. *Arch Intern Med* 1956;97:562–575.
293. Fundenberg HH, Strelkauskas AJ, Goust J-M, et al. Discoid lupus erythematosus: dramatic clinical and immunological response to dialyzable leukocyte extract (transfer factor). *Trans Assoc Am Phys* 1981;94:279–281.
294. Chen YS, Hu XE. Auricula-acupuncture in 15 cases of discoid lupus erythematosus. *J Tradit Chin Med* 1983;5:261–262.
295. Rodriguez-Castellanos MA, Barba Rubio J, Barba Gomez JF, et al. Phenytoid in the treatment of discoid lupus erythematosus. *Arch Dermatol* 1995;131:620–621.
296. Wallace DJ, Silverman S, Goldstein J, et al. Use of hyperbaric oxygen in rheumatic disease: case report and critical analysis. *Lupus* 1995;4:172–175.
297. Kimura K, Nanba S, Tojo A, et al. Effects of sairei-to on the relapse of steroid-dependent nephrotic syndrome. *Amer J Chinese Medicine* 1990;18:45–50.
298. Lautenschlager J. Acupuncture in treatment of inflammatory rheumatic diseases. *Z Rheumatol* 1997;56:8–20.
299. Khamaganova IV, Berlin IuV, Volkov VE, et al. The use of a pulsed magnetic field in the treatment of lupus erythematosus. *Ter Arkh* 1995;67:84–87.
300. Stricker RB, Goldberg B, Epstein WL. Immunological changes in patient with systemic lupus erythematosus treated with topical dinitrochlorobenzene. *Lancet* 1995;345:1505–1506.
301. Kono K, Tatara I, Takeda S, et al. Nafamostat mesylate therapy for systemic lupus erythematosus with nephrotic syndrome: a case report. *Current Therapeutic Research* 1996;57:438–444.
302. Delepine N, Desbois JC, Taillard F, et al. Sodium diethyldithiocarbamate inducing long-lasting remission in case of juvenile systemic lupus erythematosus (letter). *Lancet* 1985;ii:1246.
303. Ayres S Jr. Discoid lupus erythematosus: thalidomide or vitamin E? (letter). *Int J Dermatol* 1985;24:616.
304. Ayres S Jr, Mihan R. Lupus erythematosus and vitamin E: an effective and nontoxic therapy (letter). *Cutis* 1979;23:4–9.
305. Yell YA, Burge S, Wojnarowska F. Vitamin E and discoid lupus erythematosus. *Lupus* 1992;1:303–305.
306. Johnson HM. Effect of splenectomy in acute systemic lupus erythematosus. *Arch Dermatol Syph* 1953;68:699–713.
307. Kirkpatrick RA. Witchcraft and lupus erythematosus (letter). *JAMA* 1981;245:1937.

60

ADJUNCTIVE MEASURES AND ISSUES: ALLERGIES, ANTIBIOTICS, VACCINES, OSTEOPOROSIS, AND DISABILITY

DANIEL J. WALLACE
BEVRA HANNAHS HAHN

Some of the most common queries that lupologists are asked deal with adjunctive issues. They do not concern treating lupus per se; rather, they relate to handling circumstances that have the potential to impact on the disease. This chapter explores the following five commonly encountered problems: (i) Do patients with lupus have more allergies than others, and in any case, should they receive allergy shots? (ii) Should patients with lupus receive antibiotic prophylaxis before special procedures, and are there any antibiotics that warrant extra caution? (iii) What about immunizations in general? (iv) When and how are lupus patients disabled? And (v) as hormones are used to treat osteoporosis that especially affects patients with lupus because of steroid therapy, what is the optimal treatment for osteoporosis?

LUPUS AND ALLERGIES

Do Patients With Lupus Have More Allergies Than Healthy Individuals?

In 1976, Goldman et al. (1) first documented that patients with lupus had a significantly increased incidence of allergic rhinitis and drug allergy, although IgE levels were not different from those in healthy subjects. In 1985, a Spanish group (2) used Goldman et al.'s methodology and confirmed their data among 63 patients with systemic lupus erythematosus (SLE) compared to 51 autoimmune individuals, and 133 healthy volunteers. Of patients with SLE, 73% had evidence for urticaria, rhinitis, pharyngitis, conjunctivitis, asthma, or allergy to foods, drugs, and insect stings, compared with 37% of others. Sequeira et al. (3) found that 132 patients with SLE had significantly greater drug allergies, skin allergies, and insect allergies than 66 individuals with non-SLE disorders. Interestingly, their family members also had more allergies than the control group. 56% of 44 Israeli patients with lupus had self-reported allergies (4). Elkayam et al. associated SLE flares in atopic patients with higher IgE levels (5), and 36 children of 26 Japanese mothers with SLE had higher IgE levels (6). However, a case-controlled study of 49 lupus patients in England found no increased risk of IgE mediated/associated allergic disorders (7).

If these reports created any doubt concerning antibiotic sensitivity, Petri and Albritton (8) put this to rest in 1992 with an exhaustive case-control study of 221 patients with SLE, their 186 best friends, and 178 relatives from the Johns Hopkins Lupus Cohort. As expected, sulfa antibiotic lupus flares (in 21%) and reactions (defined as rash, hives, fever, asthma, nausea, or lupus flare, and noted in 31%) were the most pronounced. Significantly increased reactions also were found among those given penicillin/cephalosporins, tetracyclines, and erythromycins. A letter to the editor responding to Petri and Albritton's survey confirmed these findings (9). Of 250 drug reactions reported in one center among patients with SLE, 30 were to sulfonamides, 25 to penicillin, 20 to cephalosporin, 19 to tetracyclines, and 18 to erythromycin. This represented 57% of 340 patients with lupus, compared with 14% of their 303 chronic arthritis clinic patients. Forty-seven reactions were to nonsteroidal, antiinflammatory agents. Another survey reported an odds ratio of 2.6 for medication allergies and 1.8 for hives in a case-control study of 195 patients with SLE (10).

An allergic tendency does not appear to be limited to SLE among patients with rheumatic disease. Similar findings, although on a much smaller scale, have been observed in Sjögren's syndrome (11) and systemic vasculitis (12).

Why Do Patients With Lupus Have More Allergies?

The issue of causation has been addressed on several levels. Diumenjo et al. (2) hypothesized three mechanisms: (i) a higher level of hypersensitivity to exogenous antigens, (ii) anaphylactoid products of complement activation, or (iii) cytotropic autoantibodies. Gruber et al. (13) found IgM-anti-IgE (in 27%) and IgG-anti-IgE (in 34%) antibodies among 67 patients with SLE. Significant correlations were observed with articular involvement, with lymphadenopathy, and anti-DNA antibodies as compared to those without the antibodies. IgE levels are increased in SLE, correlate with disease activity and not necessarily allergy (1,14,15). Urticaria and hives are also increased in prevalence and may not represent allergic responses to exogenous antigens.

Should Allergic Patients With Systemic Lupus Erythematosus Receive Allergy Shots (Immunotherapy)?

Immunotherapy (i.e., desensitization protocols) was introduced early in this century to help allergy sufferers, and it became clear that giving immunotherapy to otherwise healthy individuals carried a risk of nonspecific formation of autoantibodies. In a study at Louisiana State University, 40% of patients with allergic rhinitis (one half of whom were receiving immunotherapy) had a positive antinuclear antibody (ANA), compared with 11% who had miscellaneous medical diseases and 10% of healthy controls. This observation did not extend to rheumatoid factor, anticytoplasmic antibodies, or anti-DNA (16). Among asthmatics, seven of 50 (four of whom were receiving immunotherapy) had an ANA of 1:40 or greater, compared with none of 35 patients with miscellaneous medical diseases (17). Phanuphak and Kohler (18) related the onset of polyarteritis nodosa with immunotherapy in six patients. On this basis of studies such as these, as well as of personal anecdotal experiences that autoimmune patients flared their disease after receiving allergy shots, the World Health Organization Working Group of the International Union of Immunological Sciences formally recommended in 1989 that patients with autoimmune disease not receive immunotherapy (19,20). In our own practice, about one half of our lupus-allergy patients have at least a mild flare of symptoms after having allergy shots, and we prefer alternative therapies to desensitization protocols.

LUPUS AND ANTIBIOTICS

Are There Any Antibiotics That Patients With Lupus Should Avoid?

Because patients with SLE tend to develop more infections than healthy people, the choice of optimal antibiotics is a frequently encountered problem. *Sulfonamides* (and, to a lesser extent, *tetracyclines*) are noted for their sun-sensitizing properties, which can flare rashes, occasionally induce fevers, and exacerbate the disease in general (8–10,21–29). *Minocycline* can induce a lupuslike reaction, autoimmune hepatitis and a positive p-ANCA directed against myeloperoxidase (30,31). Among 27,688 acne patients aged 15 to 29, individuals taking minocycline had a 8.5-fold increased risk for developing a lupus reaction (32). Hess recently reviewed some of the speculative mechanisms by which this could occur (33). The above-mentioned antibiotics commonly are prescribed for young women by their dermatologists (for acne) and gynecologists (for urinary-tract infection), who frequently are unaware that treating a patient with lupus warrants special antibiotic considerations. The previous section details the studies that document this (8–10).

On a practical level, we tend to divide antibiotic reactions into those that cause skin rashes or urticaria alone (penicillins/cephalosporins, erythromycins) and those that produce disease flares as well. Sulfa-based antibiotics are well-known provocateurs of disease activity and should be used with extreme caution; preferably, they should be avoided. Although uncommon, *ciprofloxacin* and its relatives can induce a vasculitic reaction (34), arthralgias (35), and flares of SLE (36).

Should Patients With Lupus Receive Antibiotic Prophylaxis?

Although bacterial endocarditis is rare, an established consensus recommends that antibiotic prophylaxis be given to high-risk patients before dental and certain surgical procedures (37). Miller et al. found that 18.5% of 361 lupus outpatients had a heart murmur, but only 13 (3%) had a significant valvular abnormality warranting antibiotic prophylaxis (38). However, patients with SLE, especially those with antiphospholipid antibodies, are at an increased risk for developing cardiac vegetations. These vegetations usually are asymptomatic, and they are noted on two-dimensional echocardiograms approximately 30% of the time (39) (see Chapter 32). Because as many as 40% of patients with lupus have at least one antiphospholipid antibody, and because mitral valve prolapse is more prevalent in patients with SLE we recommend that all of our immune-suppressed patients with lupus receive antibiotic prophylaxis before dental procedures (40). The drug of choice is amoxicillin, although erythromycin, penicillins, and cephalosporins are acceptable alternatives in ampicillin-sensitive patients.

LUPUS AND IMMUNIZATIONS

Should Patients With Lupus Be Immunized?

The issue of immunization is both controversial and misunderstood. This section attempts to clarify the misunderstandings and to summarize the salient points, including the following:

1. Infrequent reports have claimed that immunizations induce systemic lupus (41–50). Older et al. and Shoenfeld et al.'s 1999 and 2000 literature reviews report 24 cases of SLE following vaccination: ten after hepatitis B, three typhoid/paratyphoid, eight "combinations", two anthrax, and one tetanus (51,52).
2. Patients with SLE tolerate most immunizations well, and adverse reactions are uncommon (53). Disease flares, however, may be slightly more frequent than the incidence of spontaneous flares (54).
3. Immunizations are less effective in patients with SLE who are on high doses of corticosteroids. In one survey, protective levels of antibody after immunization were achieved in 90% receiving tetanus toxoid, 88% with *hemophilus influenza* type B, and slightly more than half receiving pneumococcus (54). Antibody responses depend on the concentration of antigen, HLA type, and concurrent medication. Patients with lupus might make more anti-DNA and other autoantibodies after repeated immunizations (56).
4. Immunizations with killed vaccine (e.g., pneumococcus, influenza, tetanus) generally are regarded as safe, but the safety of live vaccines (e.g., polio, mumps, BCG, yellow fever, measles, rubella) has not been established in patients with SLE who are on high doses of steroids or cytotoxics. When somebody living with a severely immune-compromised patient with lupus receives a live vaccine, the patient should avoid secretory contact with them for 2 weeks.

What About Specific Immunizations?

In 1980, Jarrett et al. (57) reported on their experience administering *pneumococcal* vaccine to patients with SLE. Mean antibody levels at both 1 and 12 months following vaccination were significantly lower than those in control patients. However, in follow-up studies (58,59), the persistence of pneumococcal antibodies in immunized patients was found to be protective for a mean of 3 years. In a double-blind, controlled study, Klippel et al. (60) obtained similar results. Concurrent immunosuppression did not affect response (61).

In similar studies of *influenza* vaccination in patients with SLE, Williams et al. (62) noted no disease flares but decreased antibody titers compared with a control group in a double-blind trial. Two other studies have reported similar findings (63). Herron et al. (64) observed that antibody responses are especially decreased in steroid-treated patients; of 20 immunized patients, one experienced a serious flare after injection. Influenza vaccines rarely induce a systemic vasculitis (65). Mitchell et al. (66) attempted to study the kinetics of specific antiinfluenzal antibody production by cultured lymphocytes following immunization, but *in vitro* responses (which have been reported to be decreased) (67,68) did not correlate with *in vivo* changes. Louie et al. reported that four of 11 immunized patients did not develop significant levels of antibodies and one developed new-onset proliferative nephritis (69).

Abe and Homma (70) administered *tetanus toxoid* to 200 subjects with SLE and a similar number of controls. No difference in antibody titer existed between these groups following both primary and secondary immunizations, but a subgroup had lower antibody responses. In one study, the time of appearance of the antibodies and serum titers were normal in patients with SLE (71), but others found lower responses (72) and documented a restricted IgG1 response (73). Nies et al. (74) studied antitetanus toxoid antibody synthesis after booster immunization in SLE and a control group. The patients with SLE had decreased prebooster antibody levels, and one third had a blunted antibody response. It was shown that the blunted response results from poor B-cell responsiveness and is not related to T helper or suppressor function. In an ominous follow-up report (56), this group found increased anti-DNA production *in vitro* following keyhole limpet hemocyanin immunization. This was especially true after secondary immunization and might represent a risk from the repeated immunization of patients with SLE, although there is no evidence that the anti-DNA contains pathogenic subsets.

Severe exacerbations of SLE have been reported after *hepatitis B* vaccines (49,75,76), and the vaccine has been thought to induce lupus (45–48,50). Fifteen lupus patients had a lower antibody index compared with 14 normal controls, and in one unit, all SLE pediatric dialysis patients failed to seroconvert after hepatitis B vaccination (77,78).

Additional reports have examined responses to other microbes. Antibody responses after immunization with flagellin derived from *Salmonella adelaide, Proteus 0X-2*, and *Rickettsia rickettsi* were normal (71,79), decreased with antistreptolysin O, *Escherichia coli*, and *Shigella* sp. (79–82), and both increased and decreased with *Brucella* sp. (81,83).

In summary, we recommend that patients with SLE should receive all necessary immunizations. Children of patients with SLE who are immunocompromised and receive live-virus vaccines should avoid secretory contact with their parent for approximately 1 to 2 weeks, or a rheumatologist should be consulted. They also should be consulted before giving routine, but not necessary, immunizations (e.g., influenza) to patients on steroids or to those with active disease. In 1996, the British Society of Rheumatology Clinical Affairs Committed issued guidelines stating that (i) patients on 40 mg of prednisolone a day should have vaccinations postponed until at least 3 months after immune-suppressive treatment has been stopped, or doses lowered to 20 mg a day, and (ii) though hepatitis B vaccination is usually safe, further study of its role in autoimmunity was recommended (84).

LUPUS AND OSTEOPOROSIS

Prevalence And Risk Factors For Osteoporosis In SLE

The overall prevalence of osteoporosis (defined as atraumatic fractures or bone density more that 2.5 SD below the mean for young, healthy controls) in patients with SLE is 12% to 30%, and the prevalence of fractures is 5% to 8% (85–92). Ramsey-Goldman found fractures in 12.3% of 702 women with SLE, representing a five-fold increased risk (93). High-dose glucocorticoids increased the risk for osteoporosis in some, but not all, studies; older age, postmenopausal state, female sex, and physical inactivity because of severe, active SLE all are important predictors of increased risk (94–97). Studies in children and adolescents suggest that bone mineralization changes occur very slowly (98) and in adult males they barely take place (99). One cross-sectional study (100) showed that among premenopausal women with SLE on glucocorticoid therapy, 23% had osteoporosis. Low bone mass correlated positively with increasing damage from SLE, longer disease duration and cumulative dose of prednisone. In women and men with rheumatic diseases such as SLE requiring glucocorticoid therapy, more than half have osteoporosis (101). Therefore, the physician should employ strategies that prevent osteoporosis, as well as treatment of that condition, in patients with SLE.

Mechanisms Of Osteoporosis In Systemic Lupus Erythematosus

Pathogenic factors that increase risk for osteoporosis in patients not on glucocorticoids include increased disability, physical inactivity, smoking, use of alcohol, genetic predisposition, thinness, femaleness, age over 50 years, menopause, and Caucasian and Asian races (reviewed in references 102–104). In patients with SLE taking glucocorticoids, the risk for osteoporosis and fracture is increased, particularly in patients with other predisposing factors. Glucocorticoids increase risk by reducing absorption of calcium from the gastrointestinal tract, increasing loss of calcium from renal tubules, (these changes in calcium stimulate release of parathyroid hormone), reducing hormone synthesis by pituitary, ovary and testis, and reducing osteoblast formation, proliferation, and adhesion while at the same time activating osteoclasts (102,103). Introduction of prednisone therapy in doses ≥7.5 mg daily (or equivalent) often cause rapid bone loss in the first 6 months of treatment (102).

The Management Of Osteoporosis In Systemic Lupus Erythematosus

As shown in Fig. 60.1, several strategies to prevent or treat osteoporosis are of proven benefit (reviewed in 102–104).

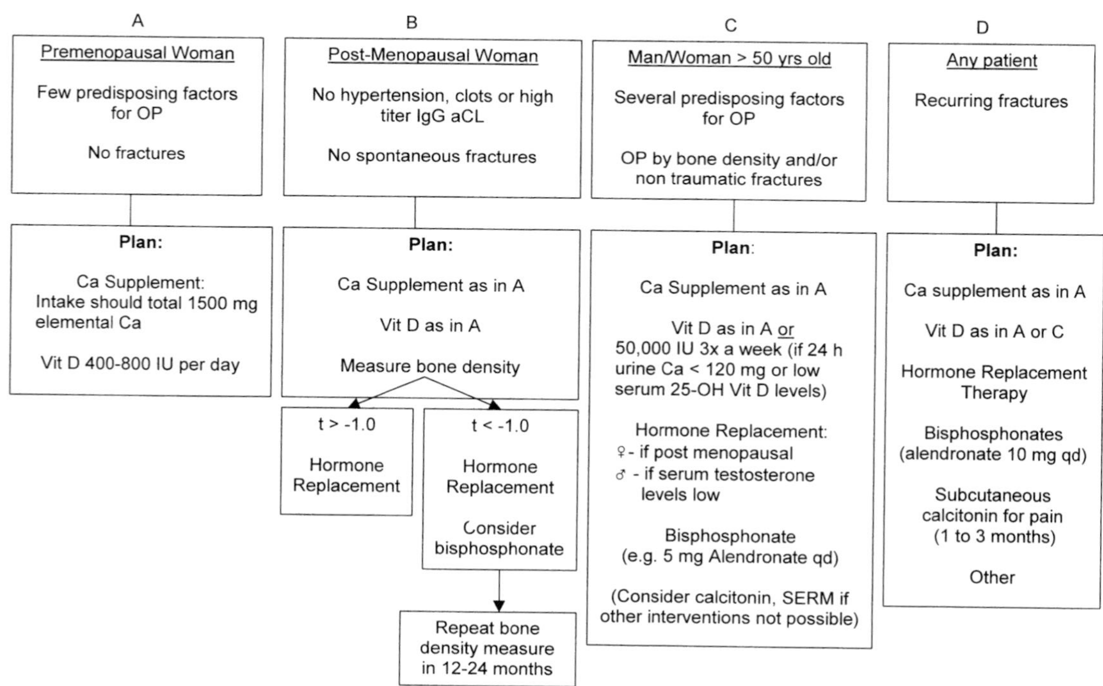

FIGURE 60.1. Algorithm for prevention and treatment of osteoporosis in patients with systemic lupus erythematosus.

These strategies include administration of calcium, vitamin D or metabolites, sex hormones, calcitonin, and bisphosphonates.

Calcium

With regard to administration of supplemental calcium, many studies have suggested measurable benefit, albeit relatively small compared to other strategies. Hahn's group (105) studied patients with SLE and other rheumatic diseases who were treated with glucocorticoids. Administration of supplemental calcium delayed bone loss, although vitamin D (cholecalciferol) and 25-OH vitamin D (calcifidiol) were more effective. Another study (106) showed that calcium supplementation alone decreased bone loss by inhibiting bone resorption in patients taking glucocorticoids. On the other hand, a more recent study (107) comparing calcium alone to other regimens showed that calcium alone did not prevent loss of bone. Calcium plus 1,25-(OH)2 vitamin D (calcitriol) maintained vertebral bone mass in patients (with various diseases) on chronic glucocorticoid therapy better than calcium alone, and calcitonin added to calcitriol and calcium was even more effective in preventing bone loss. Because the average daily intake of calcium in the United States population is only 600 mg — well below the minimal daily requirement — most experts recommend that all patients with SLE on glucocorticoid therapy be supplemented with oral calcium of 500 to 1000 mg elemental calcium content (102,103). Contraindications to this approach include a recent history of renal stones, hypercalciuria, or hypocalcaemia. Calcium supplementation is a good starting point, but additional interventions are desirable for patients with a history of osteoporotic fractures or with low bone density on osteodensitometry or on routine x-rays. In interpreting osteodensitometric data, comparison of a patient's bone mass with the mean for normal young individuals of the same sex and ethnic group, known as a t-score, is as follows: greater than 1 standard deviation below the mean = osteopenia with increased risk for fracture: greater than 2.5 standard deviations below the mean = osteoporosis with greatly increased risk for fracture (108).

Vitamin D

Administration of vitamin D and metabolites to prevent or treat osteoporosis is also controversial. Experts recommend maintenance of minimal daily requirement (400 to 800 IU) to optimize intestinal absorption of calcium (102,103). However, studies in patients receiving chronic glucocorticoid therapy suggest that higher doses of cholecalciferol, or relatively high doses of vitamin D metabolites, are required to demonstrate diminished bone loss. For example, an unrandomized, uncontrolled study (109) administering 50,000 units of cholecalciferol three times a week showed diminution of bone loss in steroid-treated rheumatic disease patients, but a prospective randomized trial of 50,000 units once a week showed no benefit (110). A recent trial (111) of 1,000 units of cholecalciferol plus 500 mg of supplemental calcium daily in glucocorticoid-treated patients with low bone density showed no significant changes in bone density at either lumbar spine or hip over 36 months. In contrast, treatment with an active vitamin D metabolite (1-alpha vitamin D, alfacalcidol), 1 μg plus 500 mg of calcium daily resulted in a 2% increase in vertebral bone mass (no increase in mass in the hip) (111). Doses of calcitriol that prevented bone loss in a prospective randomized trial in patients with asthma on systemic glucocorticoid therapy averaged 0.5 μg per day — a dose at which approximately 25% of patients developed hypocalcaemia (107). In summary, it is sensible to recommend that patients with SLE, especially those on glucocorticoid therapy, take 400 to 800 IU daily of vitamin D to meet minimal daily requirements, but maintenance of bone mass with vitamin D or its metabolites requires large doses (50,000 units of vitamin D cholecalciferol three times a week or 0.5 μg of 1,25 (OH)1 vitamin D calcitriol daily). If the physician elects to use these high doses, it is imperative to monitor calcium levels in urine and serum on a regular basis, since the risks of hypercalciuria and hypocalcaemia are substantial. Therefore, this therapy should probably be reserved for patients with very low 24-hour urine calcium levels (<120 mg) despite oral calcium supplementation, who cannot take hormone replacement therapies, calcitonin, or bisphosphonates, and who are at high risk for osteoporotic fracture.

Sex Hormone Therapy

Sex hormone therapy to prevent osteoporotic fractures in patients with SLE is also somewhat controversial (112). Estrogen administration reduces bone resorption. Because SLE is predominantly a disease of women of child-bearing ages, and because estrogen worsens disease in some mouse strains that develop lupuslike disease spontaneously, there is concern that administration of estrogen or progestogens might worsen SLE. At the time of this writing, a prospective study is underway in the United States to compare flare rates in women with SLE who are randomized to receive 1 year of hormone replacement therapy or placebo. It is the opinion of the authors that administration of hormone replacement therapy to women with clinically stable SLE is usually safe (excluding women with clotting disorders, poorly controlled hypertension, and high titers of IgG antiphospholipid antibodies). Of course, hormone replacement therapy is useful for other purposes, such as reducing hot flashes and maintaining vaginal and bladder mucosal surfaces. Whether the therapy protects against degenerative coronary-artery disease is point of debate, because in a recent study women with myocardial infarctions were not protected from additional cardiac events by institution of hormone replacement therapy (113). With regard to the osteoporosis of SLE, Kung et al. randomized 29 hypogonadal, premenopausal women with SLE to receive either conjugated estrogen/progesterone combination or calcitriol in addition to 1 g of calcium carbonate a day (114). Hormonal replacement therapy, but not calcitriol, prevented bone loss. Two additional studies in women with asthma or rheumatoid arthritis on glucocorticoids showed that hormone replacement therapy in comparison to placebo increased lumbar spine bone density over a period of 1 year (115,116). Therefore, it is likely that estrogen/progestogen therapies help prevent bone loss in menopausal women with SLE. If there are no major contraindications, providing this therapy should reduce osteoporosis and its consequences. In women who cannot take estrogen because of hormone-dependent tumors such as breast cancer, the use of selective estrogen receptor modulators such as tamoxifen or raloxifene to prevent osteoporosis is probably acceptable (117,118): no data are published regarding efficacy or safety in human SLE. With regard to young women with lupus, especially those on glucocorticoid therapy, who develop scanty and infrequent menstrual periods, some experts recommend additional oral contraceptives containing at least 50 μg of estradiol per tablet (102) for the purpose of maintaining bone mass and general health. There are no controlled trials in SLE to support this view, nor to prove that it is safe, but it is logical.

Calcitonin

Calcitonin either subcutaneous or intranasal, may be beneficial in preventing or treating osteoporosis. Calcitonin works primarily by inhibiting osteoclastic function and bone resorption. As noted in the previous section on vitamin D therapies, calcitonin in addition to calcitriol and calcium was more effective at maintaining bone mass than calcitriol plus calcium in patients with asthma on glucocorticoids (107). Other investigators showed patients with chronic lung diseases or sarcoidosis maintained lumbar bone mass when treated with intranasal or subcutaneous calcitonin (119,120). In a 2-year prospective placebo-controlled study in patients with temporal arteritis and polymyalgia, Healey et al. showed stable lumbar spine bone mass in patients on calcitonin (121). Side effects of injectable calcitonin include flushing and nausea. This can be minimized by beginning with low doses such as 50 units a few times a week: the recommended dose effective in the largest number of patients is 100 units daily. Nasal calcitonin is administered as 200 units per day in one spray into one nostril. Local irritation is the main side effect. There may be some analgesic effects of calcitonin: the authors use it primarily in individuals with pain from acute fractures.

Bisphosphonates

Perhaps the most important advance in prevention and treatment of glucocorticoid osteoporosis in the past few years has been the introduction of several generations of bisphosphonates. These drugs work primarily by binding to bone and preventing osteoclastic resorption. In the interval between osteoclastic and later osteoblastic suppression, new bone forms. Several studies have shown efficacy in prevention of bone loss in patients with idiopathic osteoporosis treated with etidronate, pamidronate, alendronate, and residronate (reviewed in 104). Many patients with idiopathic osteoporosis treated with alendronate or residronate show increased density in the lumbar spine over a 2-year period, and some studies have shown small but significant increases in density of the hip. Most importantly, fracture rates are significantly reduced (122,123). Several studies have shown benefits of cyclic etidronate in maintaining bone mass in patients on chronic glucocorticoids (124–127). Palmidronate has also been effective in preventing bone loss in patients treated with glucocorticoids (128). With regard to alendronate, a large randomized prospective study by Saag et al. (129) compared 477 men and women on glucocorticoid therapy treated for 48 weeks with placebo, alendronate 5 mg a day, or alendronate 10 mg a day. The patients on placebo lost bone mass at lumbar spine and femoral neck (mean of −0.4% and −1.2%, respectively). On both doses of alendronate bone density increased in the lumbar spine (mean 2.1 and 2.9% for 5 and 10 mg doses); femoral neck density also increased in the alendronate groups (mean 1.2 and 1.0% for 5 and 10 mg doses). Vertebral fractures occurred in 2.3% of patients receiving alendronate compared to 3.7% in the placebo group; thus, alendronate treatment reduced relative risk for vertebral fracture to 0.6. Patients receiving the 10 mg alendronate dose had a higher incidence of upper gastrointestinal side effects. In a smaller trial (130) in patients with sarcoidosis receiving glucocorticoids, bone density at the distal radius decreased by 4.5% in the placebo group and increased 0.8% in the group receiving alendronate 5 mg a day. Several clinical trials of risedronate have been published. One (124) compared risedronate, 5 mg a day to placebo in women with postmenopausal osteoporosis followed for 3 years; the cumulative incidence of new vertebral fractures was reduced by 41% and nonvertebral fractures by 39%. Bone mineral density increased at the lumbar spine, femoral neck, and midshaft of the radius in the risedronate group. Approximately 17% of patients withdrew from the study because of adverse events — similar in treated and placebo groups. In a similar trial in 1,226 women with postmenopausal osteoporosis and two or more vertebral fractures, 5 mg of risedronate daily reduced vertebral and nonvertebral bone fractures significantly compared to placebo (131). Risedronate also has been studied in glucocorticoid osteoporosis (132). A total of 228 patients with various inflammatory conditions receiving ≥7.5 mg of prednisone a day were randomized to receive placebo or risedronate at 2.5- or 5-mg daily doses and followed for 12 months. The 2.5-mg dose was dropped when other studies showed better efficacy with 5-mg doses. Bone density was lost from the lumbar spine, femoral neck, and femoral trochanter in placebo but not risedronate groups and there was a trend toward decreased vertebral fractures (5.7% in risedronate compared to 17.3% in placebo). The most important side effect of bisphosphonates is gastrointestinal problems, with esophagitis, gastritis, dyspepsia, and abdominal pain. These have occurred in 10% to 15% of study patients — not dramatically higher than in placebo groups. However, in practice, the authors find that gastrointestinal complaints are not unusual in SLE patients receiving bisphosphonate therapies. Each dose of bisphosphonate must be given on an empty stomach, or the drug will not be adequately absorbed. A recent study (133) shows that one weekly dose of alendronate (70 mg) is as effective as daily doses of 10 mg, and this dosing is more convenient and might increase patient compliance. There is some concern about administering bisphosphonates to young individuals, because the effect of decades of storage of these compounds in bone is not known. In summary, there are abundant data proving efficacy of bisphosphonates in osteoporosis, both in terms of maintaining or increasing bone density and reducing new fractures. Similar beneficial effects on bone density have been shown in patients receiving chronic glucocorticoid therapy, and the effects are larger than those seen with supplemental calcium and minimal daily requirement doses of vitamin D. Therefore, the drugs can be recommended for use in patients with SLE, especially those on glucocorticoids, when bone density is low, fractures have occurred, or the patient is at substantial risk for osteoporosis. Whether effects on bone are additive to hormone replacement therapies, and whether such combinations are safe in SLE, remains to be seen.

Other Strategies

Other strategies may be considered for management of patients with SLE who experience repeated bone fractures in spite of the above therapies. Slow release fluoride increases vertebral bone density in individuals with postmenopausal osteoporosis, including those receiving glucocorticoids. One study reported reduction of fractures by this treatment in individuals with postmenopausal osteoporosis (134), although an earlier study with a different fluoride preparation (not slow release) showed an increase in fracture rate (135). The use of fluoride in osteoporosis is controversial, particularly with the demonstrated efficacy of bisphosphonates. It might be used rarely in patients who continue to fracture (particularly vertebrae) in spite of the other therapies we have discussed. Anabolic steroids have been studied in glucocorticoid osteoporosis. Administration of nandrolone decanoate, 50 mg intramuscularly every 3 weeks, resulted in increased density of the radius over 6 months (136). Men with SLE who have low testosterone levels (particularly those on glucocorticoids) might benefit from hormone replacement in terms of bone density and muscle mass. There is some debate as to whether androgens can be administered to men without flaring SLE, but definitive studies are not available. The use of dehydroepiandrosterone (DHEA) may help maintain bone mass in patients with SLE; controlled trials addressing this question have not been published (137). Thiazide therapy lowers renal loss of calcium and has small but measurable benefit on bone density and fracture rates, which disappear shortly after therapy is discontinued (138). This strategy may be useful adjunctive therapy in individuals with high levels of calcium in 24-hour urine collections (>300 mg).

Some evidence suggests that deflazacort is a glucocorticoid that causes less calcium and bone loss than other glucocorticoid preparations (139–141). Several studies have shown less calciuric effects of deflazacort compared with prednisolone, and significantly less loss of vertebral mass, but there is debate about antiinflammatory dose equivalency, and whether at equivalent doses there is relative bone sparing. In general, equivalent antiinflammatory doses are 6 mg of deflazacort to 5 mg of prednisone. The preparation is not available in the United States, but it is approved for use in several European nations and in Mexico (as Calcort, Aventis).

In summary, the optimal strategies for prevention of osteoporosis in patients with SLE include withdrawal of glucocorticoid therapy when possible, control of active disease to maintain physical activity, maintenance of adequate calcium intake, a reasonable exercise regimen, institution of hormone replacement therapies at menopause, and addition of bisphosphonates (or calcitonin) in patients with high risk of osteoporosis or a history of osteoporotic fractures.

DISABILITY

Many lupus patients find it difficult to obtain disability insurance. Historically, Social Security disability with Medicare benefits has been reserved for patients with active, organ-threatening disease even though many of them are working without any obvious impairment.

A handful of studies have addressed the employability of lupus patients. Two early surveys suggested that disability correlated with disease activity, marriage or family responsibilities, and musculoskeletal complaints (142,143). The advent of the Stanford Health Assessment Questionnaire (HAQ), clinical activity, and damage indices resulted in three recent disability surveys with differing results. In Saskatchewan, Canada, only 14% of 160 SLE patients were receiving disability payments, which did not correlate with HAQ scores and suggested only mild functional impairment (144). HAQ scores do not measure psychological impact or deal with concurrent fibromyalgia. Partridge et al.'s university-based group from five centers noted that

40% of 159 newly diagnosed SLE patients had quit work within 3.4 years (145). The predictors of early work disability were not having greater than a high-school education, receiving Medicaid, being without health insurance, having a job requiring physical strength, an income below poverty level, or greater disease activity at diagnosis. Half were African American. Murphy et al. similarly noted that 52% of 46 patients at the University of Pennsylvania (most were African American) had applied for disability as a result of fatigue, musculoskeletal, or neuropsychiatric symptoms (146). The musculoskeletal objective findings were minimal. In our experience, most community-based SLE patients with a high-school diploma are employed. If fibromyalgia is excluded, most disability is found among those with serious organ-threatening disease, neuropsychiatric impairments, and avascular necrosis (147).

REFERENCES

1. Goldman JA, Klimek GA, Ali R. Allergy in systemic lupus erythematosus: IgE levels and reaginic phenomenon. *Arthritis Rheum* 1976;19:669–676.
2. Diumenjo MS, Lisanta M, Valles R, et al. Allergic manifestations of systemic lupus erythematosus. *Allergol Immunol* (Madr) 1985;13:323–326.
3. Sequeira JF, Cesic D, Keser G, et al. Allergic disorders in systemic lupus erythematosus. *Lupus* 1993;2:187–191.
4. Shahar E, Lorber M. Allergy and SLE: common and variable. *Isr J Med Sci* 1997;33:147–149.
5. Elkayam O, Tamir, Pick AI, et al. Serum IgE disorders, disease activity and atopic disorders in systemic lupus erythematosus. *Allergy* 1995;50:94–96.
6. Kasai K, Furukawa S, Hashimoto H, et al. Increased levels of IgE in children of mothers with systemic lupus erythematosus. *Allergy* 1995;50:370–373.
7. Morton S, Palmer B, Muire K, et al. IgE and non-IgE mediated allergic disorders in systemic lupus erythematosus. *Ann Rheum Dis* 1998;57:660–663.
8. Petri M, Albritton J. Antibiotic allergy in systemic lupus erythematosus: a case-control study. *J Rheumatol* 1992;19: 265–269.
9. Wang C-R, Chuang CY, Chen C-Y. Drug allergy in Chinese patients with systemic lupus erythematosus. *J Rheumatol* 1993; 20:399–400.
10. Stron B, Reidenberg MM, West S, et al. Shingles, allergies, family medical history, oral contraceptives, and other potential risk factors for systemic lupus erythematosus. *Am J Epidemiol* 1994; 140:632–642.
11. Katz J, Marmary Y, Liveneh A, et al. Drug allergy in Sjögren's syndrome. *Lancet* 1991;337:329.
12. Cuadrado MJ, d'Cruz D, Lloyd M, et al. Allergic disorders in systemic vasculitis: a case-controlled study. *Br J Rheumatol* 1994;33:749–753.
13. Gruber BL, Kaufman LD, Marcheses MJ, et al. Anti-IgE autoantibodies in systemic lupus erythematosus. Prevalence and biologic activity. *Arthritis Rheum* 1988;31:1000–1006.
14. Elkayam O, Tamir R, Pick AI, et al. Serum IgE concentrations, disease activity, and atopic disorders in systemic lupus erythematosus. *Allergy* 1995;50:94–96.
15. Mikecz K, Sonkoly I, Meszaros C, et al. Serum IgE level in systemic lupus erythematosus. *Acta Med Hung* 1985;42:59–65.
16. Menon P, Menon V, Hilman B, et al. Antinuclear and anticytoplasmic antibodies in allergic rhinitis (abstract). *Clin Res* 1989; 37:40A.
17. Menon P, Menon V, Hilman B, et al. Antinuclear and anticytoplasmic antibodies in bronchial asthma. *J Allergy Clin Immunol* 1989;84:937–943.
18. Phanuphak P, Kohler PF. Onset of polyarteritis nodosa during allergic hyposensitization treatment. *Am J Med* 1980;68: 479–485.
19. World Health Organization/International Union of Immunological Societies Working Group Report. Current status of allergen immunotherapy (shortened version). *Lancet* 1989;i: 259–261.
20. World Health Organization/International Union of Immunological Societies Working Group Report. Current status of allergen immunotherapy (hyposensitization). *Bull WHO* 1989;67: 263–272.
21. Cohen P, Gardner FH. Sulfonamide reactions in systemic lupus erythematosus. *JAMA* 1966;197:817–819.
22. Escalante A, Stimmler MM. Trimethoprim-sulfamethoxasole induced meningitis in systemic lupus erythematosus. *J Rheumatol* 1992;19:800–802.
23. Honey S. Systemic lupus erythematosus presenting with sulfonamide hypersensitivity. *Br Med J* 1956;1:1272–1275.
24. Gordon PM, White MI, Herriot R, et al. Minocycline-associated lupus erythematosus. *Br J Dermatol* 1995;132:120–121.
25. Bulgen DY. Minocycline-related lupus. *Br J Rheumatol* 1995; 34:398.
26. Wiedemann H-R. Minocycline-related lupus in childhood. *Eur J Pediatr* 1994;153:540.
27. Quilty B, McHugh N. Lupus-like syndrome associated with the use of minocycline. *Br J Rheumatol* 1995;33:1198–1199.
28. Gende NST, Bowman SJ, Mowat AG. Lupus-like syndrome in patients treated for acne. *Br J Rheumatol* 1995;34:584–585.
29. Elkayam O, Yaron M, Caspi D. Minocycline-induced autoimmune syndromes: an overview. *Semin Arthritis Rheum* 1999;28: 392–397.
30. Angulo JM, Sigal LH, Espinoza LR. Coexistent minocycline-induced systemic lupus erythematosus and autoimmune hepatitis. *Semin Arthritis Rheum* 1998;28:187–192.
31. Griffiths B, Gough A, Emery P. Minocycline-induced autoimmune disease: comment on the editorial by Breedveld. *Arthritis Rheum* 1998;41:563–570.
32. Starkeboom MCJM, Meier CR, Jick H, et al. Minocycline and lupuslike syndrome in acne patients. *Arch Intern Med* 1999; 159:493–497.
33. Hess EV. Minocycline and autoimmunity. *Clin Exper Rheumatol* 1998;16:519–521.
34. Beuselinck B, Devuyst O. Ciprofloxacin-induced hypersensitivity vasculitis. *Acta Clin Belg* 1994;49:173–176.
35. Terry JB. Norfloxacin-induced arthralgia. *J Rheumatol* 1995;22: 793.
36. Mysler E, Paget SA, Kimberly R. Ciprofloxacin reactions mimicking lupus flares. *Arthritis Rheum* 1994;37:1112–1113.
37. Van der Meer JTM, van Wijk W, Thompson J, et al. Efficacy of antibiotic prophylaxis for prevention of native-valve endocarditis. *Lancet* 1992;339:135–139.
38. Miller CS, Egan RM, Falace DA, et al. Prevalence of infective endocarditis in patients with systemic lupus erythematosus. *J Am Dent Assoc* 1999;130:387–392.
39. Luce EB, Presti CF, Montemayor I, et al. Detecting cardiac valvular pathology in patients with systemic lupus erythematosus. *Spec Care Dentist* 1992;12:193–197.
40. Zysset MK, Montgomery MT, Redding SW, et al. Systemic lupus erythematosus: a consideration for antimicrobial prophylaxis. *Oral Surg Oral Med Oral Pathol* 1987;64:30–34.

41. Ayvazian LF, Badger TL. Disseminated lupus erythematosus occurring among student nurses. *N Engl J Med* 1948;239: 569–570.
42. Mamoux V, Dumont C. Lupus erythematosus disseminatus and vaccination against hepatitis B virus. *Arch Pediatr* 1994;1: 307–308.
43. Brown MA, Bertouch JV. Rheumatic complications of influenza vaccination. *Aust N Z J Med* 1994;24:57–573.
44. Finielz P, Lam-Kim-Sang LF, Guiserix J. Systemic lupus erythematosus and thrombocytopenic pupura in two members of the same family following hepatitis B vaccine. *Nephrol Dial Transplant* 1998;13:2420–2421.
45. Tudela P, Marti S, Bonal J. Systemic lupus erythematosus and vaccination against hepatitis B. *Nephron* 1992;62:236.
46. Guiserix J. Systemic lupus erythematosus following hepatitis B vaccine. *Nephron* 1996;74:441.
47. Mamoux V, Dumont C. Lupus erythemateaux dissemine et vaccination contre l'hepatite B. *Arch Pediatr* 1994;1:307–308.
49. Durand JM, Cretel E, Morange S, et al. Lupus erythematosus triggered by recombinant hepatitis B vaccine. *Clinical Exper Rheumatol* 1996;14:S16.
50. Laoussadi S, Sayag-Boukris V, Menkes C-J, et al. Severe rheumatic disorders associated with hepatitis B virus vaccination. *Arthritis Rheum* 1998;41:S230.
51. Shoenfeld Y, Aharon-Maor A, Sherer Y. Vaccination as an additional player in the mosaic of autoimmunity. *Clin Exper Rheumatol* 2000;18:181–184.
52. Older SA, Battafarano DF, Enzenauer RJ, et al. Can immunization precipitate connective tissue disease? Report of five cases of systemic lupus erythematosus and review of the literature. *Semin Arthritis Rheum* 1999;29:131–139.
53. Turner-Stokes L, Isenberg DA. Immunization of patients with rheumatoid arthritis and systemic lupus erythematosus. *Ann Rheum Dis* 1988;47:529–531.
54. Schattner A, Ben-Chetrit E, Schmilovitz H. Poliovaccines and the course of systemic lupus erythematosus — a retrospective study of 73 patients. *Vaccine* 1992;10:98–100.
55. Battafarano D, Battafarano NJ, Larsen L, et al. Antigen-specific antibody responses in lupus patients following immunization. *Arthritis Rheum* 1998;41:1828–1834.
56. Louie JS, Liebling MR, Nies KM. In vitro anti-DNA production by SLE following KLH immunization (abstract). *Arthritis Rheum* 1984;27:S39.
57. Jarrett MP, Schiffman G, Barland P, et al. Impaired response to pneumococcal vaccine in systemic lupus erythematosus. *Arthritis Rheum* 1980;23:1287–1293.
58. Croft SM, Schiffman G, Snyder E, et al. Specific antibody response after in vivo antigenic stimulation in systemic lupus erythematosus. *J Rheumatol* 1984;11:141–146.
59. McDonald E, Jarrett MP, Schiffman G, et al. Persistence of pneumococcal antibodies after immunization in patients with systemic lupus erythematosus. *J Rheumatol* 1984;11: 306–308.
60. Klippel JH, Karsh J, Stahl NI, et al. A controlled study of pneumococcal polysaccharide vaccine in systemic lupus erythematosus. *Arthritis Rheum* 1979;22:1231–1235.
61. Lipnick RN, Karsh J, Stahl NI, et al. Pneumococcal immunization in patients with systemic lupus erythematosus treated with immunosuppressives. *J Rheumatol* 1985;12:1118–1121.
62. Williams GW, Steinberg AD, Reinersten JL, et al. Influenza immunization in systemic lupus erythematosus. A double-blind trial. *Ann Intern Med* 1978;88:729–741.
63. Brodman R, Gilgillan G, Glass D, et al. Influenzal vaccine response in systemic lupus erythematosus. *Ann Intern Med* 1978;88:735–740.
64. Herron A, Dettleff G, Hixon B, et al. Influenzal vaccination in patients with rheumatic diseases: safety and efficacy. *JAMA* 1979;242:53–56.
65. Mader R, Narendran A, Lewtas J, et al. Systemic vasculitis following influenza vaccination report of 3 cases and literature review. *J Rheumatol* 1993;20:1429–1431.
66. Mitchell DM, Fitzharris P, Knight RA, et al. Kinetics of specific anti-influenza antibody production by cultured lymphocytes from patients with systemic lupus erythematosus following influenza immunization. *Clin Exp Immunol* 1982;49:290–296.
67. Turner-Stokes L, Cambridge G, Snaith ML. In vitro response to influenza immunization by peripheral blood mononuclear cells from patients with systemic lupus erythematosus and other autoimmune disease. *Ann Rheum Dis* 1988;47:532–535.
68. Turner-Stokes L, Cambridge G, Snaith ML. In vitro lymph node and peripheral blood lymphocyte responses to influenza immunization in patients with systemic lupus erythematosus. *Clin Exp Rheumatol* 1989;7:71–74.
69. Louis JS, Nies KM, Shoji KT, et al. Clinical and antibody responses after influenza immunization in systemic lupus erythematosus. *Ann Intern Med* 1978;88:790–792.
70. Abe T, Homma M. Immunological reactivity in patients with systemic lupus erythematosus. Humeral antibody and cellular immune responses. *Acta Rheumatol Scand* 1971;17:35–46.
71. Lee SL, Meiselas LE, Zingale SB, et al. Antibody production in systemic lupus erythematosus (SLE) and rheumatoid arthritis (RA) (abstract). *J Clin Invest* 1960;39:1.
72. Rubin RL, Tang F-L, Lucas AH, et al. IgG subclasses of anti-tetanus toxoid antibodies in adult and newborn normal subjects and in patients with systemic lupus erythematosus, Sjögren's syndrome and drug-induced autoimmunity. *J Immunol* 1986; 137:2522–2527.
73. Devey ME, Bleasdale K, Isenberg DA. Antibody affinity and IgG subclass of responses to tetanus toxoid in patients with rheumatoid arthritis and systemic lupus erythematosus. *Clin Exp Immunol* 1987;68:562–569.
74. Nies K, Boyer R, Stevens R, et al. Anti-tetanus toxoid antibody synthesis after booster immunization in systemic lupus erythematosus: comparison of the in vitro and in vivo responses. *Arthritis Rheum* 1980;23:1343–1350.
75. Senecal J-L, Bertrand C, Coutlee F. Severe exacerbation of systemic lupus erythematosus after hepatitis B vaccination and importance of pneumococcal vaccination in patients with autosplenectomy: comment on the article by Battafarano et al. *Arthritis Rheum* 1999:42;1307–1308.
76. Maillefert JF, Tavernier C, Sibilia J, et al. Exacerbation of systemic lupus erythematosus after hepatitis B vaccination: comment on the article by Battafarano et al. and the letter by Senecal et al. *Arthritis Rheum* 2000:468–469.
77. Gartner S, Emlen W. Hepatitis vaccination of SLE patients. *Arthritis Rheum* 1996;39:R18.
78. Moxey-Mims MM, Preston K, Fivush B, et al. Heptavax-B in pediatric dialysis patients: effect of systemic lupus erythematosus. *Pediatr Nephrol* 1990;4:171–173.
79. Lee AKY, Mackay IR, Rowley MJ, et al. Measurement of antibody-producing capacity to flagellin in man. IV. Studies in autoimmune disease, allergy and after azathioprine treatment. *Clin Exp Immunol* 1971;9:507–518.
80. Cassals CP, Friou GJ, Teague PO. Specific nuclear reaction pattern of antibody to DNA in lupus erythematosus sera. *J Lab Clin Med* 1963;62:625–631.
81. Baum J, Ziff M. Decreased 19S antibody response to bacterial antigens in systemic lupus erythematosus. *J Clin Invest* 1969;48: 758–767.
82. Block SR, Gibbs CB, Stevens MB, et al. Delayed hypersensitivity in systemic lupus erythematosus. *Ann Rheum Dis* 1968; 27:311–318.

83. Meiselas LE, Zingale SB, Lee SL, et al. Antibody production in rheumatic diseases. The effect of brucella antigen. *J Clin Invest* 1961;40:1872–1881.
84. Ioannou Y, Isenberg DA. Immunisation of patients with systemic lupus erythematosus: the current state of play. *Lupus* 1999;8:497–501.
85. Dhillon VB, Davies MC, Hall ML, et al. Assessment of the effect of oral corticosteroids on bone mineral density in systemic lupus erythematosus: a preliminary study with dual energy x-ray absorptiometry. *Ann Rheum Dis* 1990;49:624–626.
86. Kalla AA, Fataar AB, Jessop SJ, et al. Loss of trabecular bone mineral density in systemic lupus erythematosus. *Arthritis Rheum* 1993;36:1726–1734.
87. Kalla AA, Meyers OL, Kotze TJ, et al. Corticosteroid therapy and bone mass comparison of rheumatoid arthritis and systemic lupus erythematosus. *South Afr Med J* 1994;84:404–409.
88. Formiga F, Moga I, Nolla JM, et al. Loss of bone mineral density in premenopausal women with systemic lupus erythematosus. *Ann Rheum Dis* 1995;54:274–276.
89. Hansen M, Halberg P, Kollerup G, et al. Bone metabolism in patients with systemic lupus erythematosus. *Scand J Rheumatol* 1998;27:197–206.
90. Chen CJ, Yen JH, Tsai WC, et al. Decreased bone mineral density in premenopausal patients with systemic lupus erythematosus. *Kao Hsiung I Hsueh Ko Hseuh Tsa Chih* 1996;12:567–572.
91. Kainberger F, Grampp S, Kudlacek S, et al. Bone mineral density and biochemical parameters of bone metabolism in female patients with systemic lupus erythematosus. *Ann Rheum Dis* 2000;59:308–310.
92. Gilboe I-M, Kvien TK, Haugeberg G, et al. Bone mineral density in systemic lupus erythematosus: comparison with rheumatoid arthritis and healthy controls. *Ann Rheum Dis* 2000; 59:110–115.
93. Ramsey-Goldman R, Dunn JE, Huang C-F, et al. Frequency of fractures in women with systemic lupus erythematosus. *Arthritis Rheum* 1999;42:882–890.
94. Li EK, Tam SL, Young RP, et al. Loss of bone mineral density in Chinese patients pre-menopausal women with systemic lupus erythematosus treated with corticosteroids. *Brit J Rheumatol* 1998;37:405–410.
95. Kipen Y, Buchbinder R, Forbes A, et al. Prevalence of reduced bone mineral density in systemic lupus erythematosus and the role of steroids. *J Rheumatol* 1997;24:1922–1929.
96. Houssiau FA, Lefebre C, Depresseux G, et al. Trabecular and cortical bone loss in systemic lupus erythematosus. *Brit J Rheumatol* 1996;35:244–247.
97. Kipen Y, Briganti E, Strauss B, et al. Three year followup of bone mineral density change in premenopausal women with systemic lupus erythematosus. *J Rheumatol* 1999;26:310–317.
98. Trapani S, Civinini R, Ermini M, et al. Osteoporosis in juvenile systemic lupus erythematosus: a longitudinal study on the effects of steroids on bone mineral density. *Rheumatol Int* 1998; 18:45–49.
99. Formiga F, Nolla JM, Mitjavila F, et al. Bone mineral density and hormonal status in men with systemic lupus erythematosus. *Lupus* 1996;5:623–626.
100. Sinigaglia L, Varenna M, Binelli L, et al. Determinants of bone mass in systemic lupus erythematosus: a cross sectional study on premenopausal women. *J Rheumatol* 1999;26:1280–1284.
101. Dykman TR, Gluck OS, Murphy WA, et al. Evaluation of factors associated with glucocorticoid-induced osteopenia in patients with rheumatic diseases. *Arthritis Rheum* 1985;28:361–368.
102. American College of Rheumatology Task Force on Osteoporosis Guidelines. Recommendations for the prevention and treatment of glucocorticoid-induced osteoporosis. *Arthritis Rheum* 1996;39:1791–801.
103. Cunnane G, Lane NE. Steroid-induced osteoporosis in systemic lupus erythematosus. *Rheum Dis Clin N Amer* 2000;26: 311–329.
104. Raisz LG. Osteoporosis: current approaches and future prospects in diagnosis, pathogenesis, and management. *J Bone Min Metab* 1999;17:79–89.
105. Hahn TJ, Halstead LR, Teitelbaum SL, et al. Altered mineral metabolism in glucocorticoid-induced osteopenia. Effect of 25-hyddroxyvitamin D administration. *J Clin Invest* 1979;64: 655–665.
106. Reid IR, Ibbertson HK. Calcium supplements in the prevention of steroid-induced osteoporosis. *Am J Med* 1988;85:887–888.
107. Sambrook PN, Birmingham J, Kelley P, et al. Prevention of corticosteroid osteoporosis: a comparison of calcium, calcitriol and calcitonin. *N Engl J Med* 1993;328:1747–1752.
108. Miller PD, Bonnick SL, Rosen CJ, et al. Clinical utility of bone mass measurement in adults, consensus of an international panel. The Society for Clinical Densitometry. *Semin Arthritis Rheum* 1996;25:361–72.
109. Hahn TJ, Hahn BH. Osteopenia in patients with rheumatic diseases: principles of diagnosis and therapy. *Semin Arthritis Rheum* 1976;6:165–188.
110. Adachi JD, Bensen WG, Bianchi F, et al. Vitamin D and calcium in the prevention of corticosteroid induced osteoporosis: a 3 year followup. *J Rheumatol* 1996;23:995–1000.
111. Ringe JD, Coster A, Meng T, et al. Treatment of glucocorticoid-induced osteoporosis with alfacalciol/calcium versus vitamin D/calcium. *Calcified Tiss Internat* 1999;65:337–340.
112. Buyon JP. Hormone replacement therapy in postmenopausal women with systemic lupus erythematosus. *J Amer Med Wom Assoc* 1998;53:13–17.
113. Hulley S, Grady D, Bush T, et al. Randomized trial of estrogen plus progestin for secondary prevention of coronary heart disease in postmenopausal women. Heat and Estrogen/progestin replacement study (HERS) Research Group. *JAMA* 1998;280: 605–613.
114. Kung AWC, Chan TM, Lau CS, et al. Osteopenia in young hypogonadal women with systemic lupus receiving chronic steroid therapy: a randomized controlled trial comparing calcitriol and hormonal replacement therapy. *Rheumatol* 1999;38: 1239–1244.
115. Lukert BP, Johnson BE, Robinson RG. Estrogen and progesterone replacement therapy reduces glucocorticoid-induced bone loss. *J Bone Miner Res* 1992;7:1063–1069.
116. Hall GM, Daniels M, Doyle DV, et al. Effects of hormone replacement therapy on bone mass in rheumatoid arthritis patients treated with and without steroids. *Arthritis Rheum* 1994;37:1499–1505.
117. Khovidhunkit W, Shoback DM. Clinical effects of raloxifene hydrochloride in women. *Ann Intern Med* 1999;130:431–439.
118. Cummings SR, Palermo L, Browner W, et al. Monitoring osteoporosis therapy with bone densitometry: misleading changes and regression to the mean Fracture Intervention Trial Research Group. *JAMA* 2000;282:1318–1321.
119. Ringe JD, Welzel D. Salmon calcitonin in the therapy of corticoid-induced osteoporosis. *Eur J Clin Pharmacol* 1987;33: 3539–3541.
120. Montemorro L, Schiraldi G, Fraioli P, et al. Prevention of corticosteroid-induced osteoporosis with salmon calcitonin in sarcoid patients. *Calcif Tissue Int* 1991;49:71–76.
121. Healey J, Paget S, Williams-Russo P, et al. Randomized trial of salmon calcitonin to prevent bone loss in corticosteroid-treated temporal arteritis and polymyalgia rheumatica. *Calcif Tissue Int* 1996;58:73–80.
122. Cummings SR, Black DM, Thompson DE, et al. Effect of alendronate on risk of fracture in women with low bone density but

without vertebral fractures: results from the Fracture Intervention Trial. *JAMA* 1998;280:2077–2082.

123. Harris ST, Watts NB, Genant HK, et al. Effects of risedronate treatment on vertebral and nonvertebral fractures in women with postmenopausal osteoporosis. A randomized controlled trail. *JAMA* 1999;282:1344–1352.
124. Diamond T, McGuigan L, Barbagallo S, et al. Cyclical etidronate plus ergocalciferol prevents glucocorticoid-induced bone loss in postmenopausal women. *Am J Med* 1995;98:459–463.
125. Mulder H, Struys A. Intermittent cyclical etidronate in the prevention of corticosteroid-induced bone loss. *Br J Rheumatol* 199433:348–350.
126. Adachi JD, Cranney A, Goldsmith CH, et al. Intermittent cyclic therapy with etidronate in the prevention of corticosteroid induced bone loss. *J Rheumatol* 1994;21:1922–1926.
127. Struys A, Snedler AA, Mulder H. Cyclical etidronate reverses bone loss of the spine and proximal femur in patients with established corticosteroid-induced osteoporosis. *Am J Med* 1995;99:235–242.
128. Reid IR, King AR, Alexander CJ, et al. Prevention of steroid-induced osteoporosis with (3-amino-1-hydroxypropytlident) 1,1 bisphosphonate (APD). *Lancet* 1988;2:1144–1145.
129. Saag KG, Emkey R, Schnitzer TJ, et al. Alendronate for the prevention and treatment of glucocorticoid-induced osteoporosis. Glucocorticoid-Induced Osteoporosis Intervention Study Group. *New Eng J Med* 1998;339:292–299.
130. Gonnelli S, Rottoli P, Cepollaro C, et al. Prevention of corticosteroid-induced osteoporosis with alendronate in sarcoid patients. *Calcif Tiss Internat* 1997;61:382–385.
131. Reginster J-Y, Minne HW, Sorensen OH, et al. On behalf of the Vertebral Efficacy with Risedronate Therapy (VERT) Study Group. Randomized trial of the effects of risedronate on vertebral fractures in women with established postmenopausal osteoporosis. *Osteoporos Int* 2000;11:83–91.
132. Cohen S, Levy RM, Keller M, et al. Risedronate therapy prevents corticosteroid-induced bone loss. A twelve-month, multicenter, randomized, double-bind, placebo-controlled, parallel-group study. *Arthritis Rheum* 1999;42:2309–2318.
133. Schnitzer T, Bone HG, Crepaodi G, et al. Therapeutic equivalence of alendronate 70 mg once-weekly and alendronate 10 mg daily in the treatment of osteoporosis. Alendronate Once-Weekly Study Group. *Aging* 2000;12:1–12.
134. Pak CYC, Sakhaee K, Piziak V, et al. Slow-release sodium fluoride in the management of postmenopausal osteoporosis. A randomized controlled trial. *Ann Inter Med* 1994;120:625–632.
135. Riggs BL, Hodgson SF, O'Fallon MW, et al. Effect of fluoride treatment on the fracture rate in postmenopausal women with osteoporosis. *N Engl J Med* 1990;322:802–809.
136. Adami S, Rlossini M. Anabolic steroid in corticosteroid-induced osteoporosis. *Wien med Wochenschr* 1993;44:395–397.
137. Formiga F, Moga I, Nolla NM, et al. The association of dehydroepiandrosterone sulphate levels with bone mineral density in systemic lupus erythematosus. *Clin Exper Rheumatol* 1997;15: 387–392.
138. Cauley JA, Cummings SR, Seeley DG, et al. Effects of thiazide diuretic therapy on bone mass, fractures and falls: The Study of Osteoporotic Fractures Research Group. 1993;118:666–673.
139. Olgaard K, Storm T, van Wowern N, et al. Glucocorticoid-induced osteoporosis in the lumbar spine, forearm and mandible of nephrotic patients: a double-blind study on the high-dose, long-term effects of prednisone versus deflazacort. *Calcif Tissue Int* 1992;50:490–494.
140. Loftus J, Allen R, Hesp R, et al. Randomized double-blind trial of deflazacort versus prednisone in juvenile chronic (or rheumatoid) arthritis: a relatively bone-sparing effect of deflazacort. *Brit J Rheumatol* 1993;32(suppl 2):39–44.
141. Deflazacort—an alternative to prednisolone? *Drug Ther Bull* 1999;37:57–58.
142. Stein H, Walters K, Dillon A, et al. Systemic lupus erythematosus—a medical and social profile. *J Rheumatol* 1986;570–576.
143. Hochberg MC, Sutton J. Physical disability and psychosocial dysfunction in systemic lupus erythematosus. *J Rheumatol* 1988;15:959–964.
144. Sibley J, Hage M. Disability in a Canadian Lupus Cohort. *Arthritis Rheum* 1998;41:S220.
145. Partridge AJ, Karlson EW, Daltroy LH, et al. Risk factors for early work disability in systemic lupus erythematosus. Results from a multicenter study. *Arthritis Rheum* 1997;40:2199–2206.
146. Murphy NG, Kollvisoot A, Schumacher HR Jr, et al. Musculoskeletal features in systemic lupus and their relationship with disability. *J Clin Rheumatol* 1998;4:238–245.
147. Mikdashi JA, Rus V, Handwerger BS, et al. Risk factors for work disability in acute neuropsychiatric lupus. *Arthritis Rheum* 1999;42:S99.

61

PROGNOSIS, MORTALITY, AND MORBIDITY IN SYSTEMIC LUPUS ERYTHEMATOSUS

DAFNA D. GLADMAN
MURRAY B. UROWITZ

The concept of the clinical spectrum of systemic lupus erythematosus (SLE) has evolved over the last 50 years. Before identification of the LE-cell phenomenon in 1948, the diagnosis of this condition was difficult. In 1971, the preliminary criteria for the classification of SLE, based on knowledge of the disease at the time, were described (1), but they included few laboratory tests. These criteria were revised in 1982 (2) and again in 1997 (3) to include serologic tests that had become more generally available. Many patients who had been labeled as having lupus in earlier studies would not meet the current criteria for diagnosis of the disease; on the other hand, mild cases of SLE in the past would have been overlooked. Therefore, early survival studies included only those patients with severe SLE who could be diagnosed by biopsy or at autopsy; thus, long-term survival was unusual. After the introduction of corticosteroids in 1948, the reported survival times in SLE improved significantly. All of these factors have conspired to produce an improved survival in SLE over time. This chapter examines survival in SLE, predictors for mortality, and causes of death. Other important prognostic outcomes that contribute to morbidity in patients with SLE also are discussed.

SURVIVAL ANALYSIS

Early studies of survival in patients with SLE reported that no more than 50% survived the first 3 years of their illness (4, 5). Merrell and Shulman (6) introduced the life-table method to describe survival in SLE and defined the time of diagnosis of SLE as the start point for calculating disease duration. In their classic 1955 study (6), data extrapolated from 99 cases of SLE predicted that 78% of these patients would be alive 1 year after diagnosis, 67% after 2 years, and 51% after 4 years. Patients who were diagnosed within 2 years of the onset of symptoms had a poorer survival. Subsequent studies demonstrated better survival in the 1960s than in the previous decade (7–10). Dubois' group pioneered large-scale survival studies with reports in 1956 and 1963 (11,12) that included 163 and 520 patients, respectively. In the 1956 survey, the 5-year survival rate was 40%. Of the 60 patients from the presteroid era, or those who were inadequately treated, 50 succumbed within 2 years after diagnosis. The duration of disease from diagnosis to death was divided by Dubois into three periods of observation: (i) 1950 to 1955, (ii) 1956 to 1962, and (iii) 1963 to 1973. This was not an artificial division; 1956 marked the first time that central nervous system (CNS) lupus was treated with high doses of steroids, and 1963 marked the general availability of procedures such as the use of potent nonmercurial diuretics and peritoneal dialysis. The median duration of disease (until death) in the group treated before 1955 was less than 2 years, and by 1973, it had increased to 8.5 years (13).

In 1966, Leonhardt (14) studied 54 Swedish patients with SLE and obtained survival curves from the time of diagnosis of about 90% at 1 year and 70% at 5 years whereas matched normal individuals had 97% and 94% 5-year and 10-year survivals, respectively. Estes and Christian (15) used Merrell and Shulman's methods on 150 patients who were seen between 1962 and 1970, 90 of whom received steroid therapy. The 5-year and 10-year survival rates were 77% and 59%, respectively. Urowitz et al. (16) reported a 5-year survival rate of 75%, while the 10- and 15-year survival rates dropped to 63% and 53%, respectively. In a subsequent evaluation by Lee et al. (17), the first- and second-year survival rates were estimated at 93.1%, and by 5 years, the survival rate decreased only to 91.2%.

Tremendous improvement in survival was evident throughout the 1970s. Urman and Rothfield (18) evaluated the survivorship of 156 patients who were treated at the University of Connecticut between 1968 and 1976, and they compared it with that of 209 of Rothfield's New York

City patients who were treated from 1957 to 1968. Although the validity of comparing two such totally disparate groups has been questioned, the 5-year survival rates were 93% and 70%, respectively. Over 90% received steroids, but less than 1% were treated with immunosuppressive drugs. Improved survival was attributed to better disease understanding, newer antibiotics, use of C3 and anti-DNA to monitor activity, and judicious adjustment of steroid doses. The prevalence of CNS disease decreased significantly between the two groups.

In 1981, Wallace et al. (4,19) evaluated the course of 609 patients who had been followed in Dubois' private practice since 1950. The overall 5-, 10-, and 15-year survival rates were 88%, 79%, and 74%, respectively. Overall survival improved only in those who were diagnosed since 1970. Patients older than 50 years of age had a benign course, and children did well (100% 10-year survival) only if renal disease was not present. At least 100 of the 609 patients were off all medication and in complete remission for at least 5 years. These findings are consistent with those in a report by our group (20) of several patients with severe multisystem disease who were off all medications and were asymptomatic a mean of 75 months later.

Ginzler et al. (21) reported the results of a nine-center study of 1,103 patients in 1982. The 5- and 10-year survival rates were 86% and 76%, respectively. (Note the similarity to the Wallace data.) No improvement in survival was noted in the patients entered between 1965 and 1970 compared with those entered between 1971 and 1976. One-half of the patients received public funding, and they had a significantly lower survival rate. Overall, whites lived longer than African Americans, but this difference was not noted in the privately funded patients.

Other investigators have reported better survival rates in patients with SLE than those found in the Wallace and Ginzler studies. At the Johns Hopkins Hospital, 140 subjects had 94% and 82% 5- and 10-year survivals, respectively (22). A British group (23) observed 98% 5-year survival among 50 patients who were followed for 29 months. Fries and Holman (24) reported that more than 90% of their 193 patients survived for 10 years. Jonsson et al. (25) identified 133 patients with SLE out of 158,572 Swedish individuals. Only nine deaths occurred in these patients, and the 5-year survival rate was 95%. In India, however, patients with SLE have not fared as well, with survival rates of 68% at 5 years and only 50% at 10 years (26). In a large, hospital-based Danish study (27,28), 39 deaths occurred between 1965 and 1983, and an 80% 10-year survival rate was reported, which did not change when patients were divided into those diagnosed before and those diagnosed after 1973. Similarly, a Dutch group (29) that followed 110 patients between 1970 and 1988 noted only 14 deaths, with survival rates of 92% and 87% at 5 and 10 years, respectively. Reveille et al. (30) examined survivorship in 389 patients who were seen at the University of Alabama hospitals between 1975 and 1984. The 89 deaths in this group provided 89% and 84% 5- and 10-year survival rates, respectively. In another southeastern US study of largely publicly funded patients, Studenski et al. (31) reported the outcomes of 411 patients who were observed between 1969 and 1983 at Duke University hospitals in North Carolina. Only patients who were seen within 2 years of diagnosis were considered. The 81 deaths in this group allowed 84% 5-year and 82% 10-year Kaplan-Meier survival curves to be devised. A recent analysis of the Duke University cohort followed between 1969 and 1983 revealed slightly lower survival rates of 82%, 71%, and 63% for 5-, 10-, and 15-year survival (32).

In the nineties, there was continued improvement in the survival rates of patients with SLE in the Western world. In a study of 66 patients from Finland (33), the 10- and 15-year survival rates were 91% and 81%, respectively. Pistiner et al. (34), reviewing data collected in a single practice in Los Angeles, California, reported survival rates of 97% at 5 years, 93% at 10 years, and 83% at 15 years. These authors clearly demonstrate the improved survival in the past decade, because their previous survey (19) demonstrated 88%, 79%, and 74% survival at 5, 10, and 15 years, respectively. Information from the Arthritis, Rheumatism, and Aging Medical Information System (ARAMIS) data bank reveal similar results (35). The most recent data from the University of Toronto Lupus Clinic reveals rates of 93%, 85%, 79%, and 68% for 5-, 10-, 15-, and 20-year survival (36). Almost identical survival rates were reported by Tucker et al. (37) for a cohort of 165 patients followed at Bloomsbury Rheumatology Unit in London, England. A study of 658 patients from Mexico City provides excellent overall survival rates of 96% at 5 years and 92% at 10 years when measured from the time of first symptom. However, the 5-year survival from entry to the cohort was only 91% (38) (Unfortunately, the survival was not calculated from the time of diagnosis and therefore is not comparable to the other reported series). A study of 306 European Spanish patients revealed similar 5-, 10- and 15-year survival rates of 90%, 85% and 80% (39). A multicenter cohort of 513 Danish patients identified survival rates of 91%, 76%, 64%, and 53% for 5-, 10-, 15-, and 20-years, respectively (40). Uramoto et al. (41) compared patients with SLE diagnosed at the Mayo Clinic between 1981 and 1982 to those diagnosed between 1950 and 1979 and found a significant improvement in the survival rates over time. Their patients are older (49 and 46 years at diagnosis) than those included in other cohorts (early thirties). Cervera et al. (42) recently reported a 5-year survival of 95% among a cohort of 1,000 European patients with SLE. However, this was based on duration of follow-up and is not comparable to previous studies, as the patients entered this multicenter study with an average disease duration of 101 months. A recent study from Lund, Sweden demonstrated 93% 5-year survival and 83% 10-year survival (43). The median age at diagnosis for the Swedish cohort was similar to that noted at the Mayo Clinic.

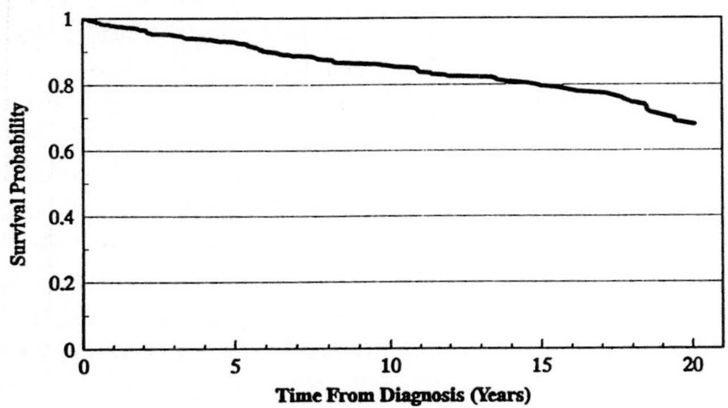

FIGURE 61.1 Survival in systemic lupus erythematosus, University of Toronto Lupus Databank. From Abu-Shakra et al. *J Rheumatol* 1995;22:1259–1264, with permission.

Five-year survival rates were similar to the general population, however, the 10-year survival in the SLE cohort was reduced compared to the rate of 96.3% in the general population.

The improved survival typical of the Western world has not been noted worldwide. It has been suggested that the survival of patients with SLE from India has not improved at all during the 1980s (44). A comparison of patients with SLE who were registered between 1981 and 1985 with those who were registered between 1986 and 1990 revealed that these two groups were similar in demographics and disease characteristics, and in their mortality rates (72% and 78% at 5 years, respectively). Of note, mortality was higher in the first 2 years of disease. Five and 10-year survival rates for SLE patients in Singapore during the period of 1970 to 1980 were 70% and 60%, respectively (45). An additional study from India (46) including patients followed from 1981 to 1993 revealed a cumulative survival of 77% at 5 years and 60% at 10 years. Among black Caribbean patients, poorer survival of only 56% at 5 years has been recorded (47), and a study from Chile (48) shows that 10-year survival of Chilean patients with lupus is somewhat lower than that of patients in several North American centers. In Malaysia, the overall 5- and 10-year survival rates were reported to be 82% and 70%, respectively. The results were lower for Asian Indian patients (70% and 65%, respectively) but were similar in Chinese and Malay patients (83% and 75%, respectively) (49).

In summary, the survival of patients with SLE has improved from 50% at 2 years in 1939 to 5- and 10-year survivals of 70% and 50%, respectively, after the introduction of corticosteroids in the 1950s; to 90% and 80% 5- and 10-year survivals, respectively, in the 1980s; and to almost 70% survival at 20 years in the 1990s (Fig. 61.1 and Table 61.1).

TABLE 61.1. SURVIVAL RATES (%) FOR 5, 10, 15, AND 20 YEARS IN PUBLISHED SERIES OVER THE PAST FIVE DECADES

Author (Ref)	No. of Patients	Outcome Year	Center	5	10	15	20
Merrel & Shulman (6)	99	1953	Baltimore	50	–	–	–
Kellum & Hasericke (7)	299	1964	Cleveland	69	54	–	–
Urman & Rothfield (18)	156	1968	New York	70	63	–	–
Estes & Christian (15)	150	1971	New York	77	60	50	–
Urowitz et al. (16)	81	1974	Toronto	75	63	53	–
Urman & Rothfield (18)	209	1976	Farmington	93	84	–	–
Wallace et al. (19)	609	1979	Los Angeles	88	79	74	–
Boey (45)	183	1980	Singapore	70	60	–	–
Ginzler et al. (21)	1103	1982	Multicenter	86	76	–	–
Jonsson et al. (25)	86	1985	Sweden	97	–	–	–
Malaviya et al. (26)	101	1986	India	68	50	–	–
Gripenberg & Helve (33)	66	1988	Finland	–	91	81	–
Swaak et al. (29)	110	1989	Holland	92	87	–	–
Reveille et al. (30)	389	1990	Alabama	89	83	79	–
Pistiner et al. (34)	570	1990	Los Angeles	97	93	83	–
Seleznick & Fries (35)	310	1990	Stanford	88	64	–	–
Kumar et al. (44)	286	1990	India	78	–	–	–
Wang et al. (49)	539	1990	Malaysia	82	70	–	–
Ward et al. (32)	408	1991	Durham	82	71	63	–
Nossent (47)	68	1993	Curaçao	56	–	–	–
Massardo et al. (48)	218	1993	Chile	92	77	66	–
Abu-Shakra et al. (36)	665	1993	Toronto	93	85	79	68
Tucker et al. (37)	165	1993	London	93	86	78	–
Murali et al. (46)	98	1993	India	77	60	–	–
Blanco et al. (39)	306	1993	Spain	90	85	80	–
Ståhl-Hallengen et al. (43)	162	1994	Sweden	93	83	–	–
Jacobson et al. (40)	513	1999	Denmark	91	76	64	53

REASONS FOR IMPROVED SURVIVAL IN PATIENTS WITH SLE

It may be concluded that the major contributing factors toward improved survival since 1950 are the availability of dialysis, corticosteroids, and improved antibiotic and antihypertensive agents. Further improvement in subsequent decades has resulted from earlier diagnosis and the inclusion of milder cases in the more recent studies. Wallace et al. (19) found a mean interval of 4 years from onset to diagnosis in the 1970s; in 1990, this interval was 2 years (34). This is not supported, however, by the patterns of disease that have been seen over the past two decades (4,41) or by a recent study from Curaçao (47), in which the delay of diagnosis was only 18 months and the patients fared poorly.

The authors of the Dutch study analyzed the pattern of clinical features in patients with SLE over the past two decades (50). They divided their 110 patients, who were followed prospectively in their lupus clinic, into three groups based on their year of diagnosis. Group A included patients who were diagnosed before 1975, group B included patients diagnosed between 1975 and 1979, and group C included patients diagnosed between 1980 and 1985. There were no differences in the age at diagnosis, the age at onset of symptoms that could be related to SLE, or the interval between onset of symptoms and diagnosis in these groups. Moreover, there were no significant differences in the frequency of clinical features at the time of diagnosis. The number and types of exacerbations in these groups were not different after correction for disease duration. Thus, the authors concluded that the use of American College of Rheumatology (ACR) criteria for the classification of SLE, or the availability of laboratory tests for the diagnosis of the disease, have not led to earlier diagnosis of SLE or a change in its clinical pattern during the past two decades.

A recent study from Toronto (51) further investigated the reasons for the improved survival noted among patients with SLE over a 24-year period. These authors had documented the increased survival rates for their patients over that period of time. They divided their patients into three groups, reflecting three periods of admission to their lupus clinic, and compared the survival rates in these groups to those recorded for the general population over the same periods of time. The improved survival in their patients with SLE did not reflect only the general improvement in survival in the population, because the Standardized Mortality Rates decreased over the three periods, from 7.74 in the early 1970s, 3.02 in the late 1980s and early 1990s. Analysis of variance did not reveal significant differences in the age at diagnosis or at enrollment into the clinic, or in disease activity at presentation as measured by the SLE Disease Activity Index (SLEDAI). While there was a reduction in deaths because of infection and other morbidity, there were no differences in deaths related to lupus disease activity. The authors concluded that the improved survival in their patients was not the result of earlier diagnosis and/or a milder form of the disease. Because no new medications for SLE were instituted during the period of study, new treatments could not be considered as the reason for improvement. More appropriate use of conventional therapy was a more likely explanation.

In Chile, Massardo et al. (48) also noted that patients whose disease onset was after 1980 fared better than those who were diagnosed earlier, but they did not compare their patient population with the overall Chilean population. In India, the lack of improvement in survival in their population was thought to result from the general standard of medical care. This lends support to the notion that the improved survival in patients with SLE may have resulted from advances in medical therapy in general, such as improved antibiotics, antihypertensive agents, and the availability of renal dialysis and transplantation, as well as from more judicious use of lupus-specific therapy.

Uramoto et al. (41) recently demonstrated that while the incidence of SLE tripled over four decades between 1950 and 1990, the survival of patients with SLE has improved. They suggested that recognition of mild disease and better approaches to therapy may contribute to the improved survival, but this is not supported by the literature.

MORTALITY RATES

Five major reports have appeared that allow trends in overall mortality rates among patients with SLE to be interpreted. Data from the studies by Cobb (52) and Siegel et al. (53) demonstrate surprisingly low death rates. Between 1968 and 1972 (54) and between 1972 and 1977 (55), improvements in mortality rates were seen in all subsets; both of these studies suggest that mortality in African Americans is accentuated in early adulthood and then declines and that mortality in whites consistently increases with age. Death rates increased earlier in females than in males. These figures cannot be interpreted to imply a greater incidence of SLE in African Americans than in whites, however, because socioeconomic differences between the groups are still large and consequently, influence mortality.

Kaslow (56) also studied mortality patterns in 12 US states that include 88% of all Americans of Asian ancestry. Between 1968 and 1976, the mortality rate for Asian Americans was 6.8 per million person-years, compared with 8.05 for African Americans and 2.8 for whites. Serdula and Rhodes (57) noted the mortality rate in Hawaii (1970–1975) to be 1.89 per million person-years for whites and 14.46 for nonwhites who were almost entirely of Asian ancestry. This finding also implied greater disease severity, increased incidence of SLE, or more socioeconomic hardships among Asian Americans, but these contentions remain to be proven.

Several reports have addressed mortality rates of SLE in Europe. Helve (58) derived a 4.7 per million person-years mortality rate among patients with SLE in Finland, but this study considered only hospitalized patients. Hochberg (59) accessed the Office of Population Censuses and Surveys data from 1974 to 1983 for England and Wales. He concluded that females have a fourfold higher mortality rate than men and that the highest mortality rates were in the 65- to 74-year age group. The annual mortality rate among females fell from 4.47 to 2.99 per million person-years between 1974 and 1983. These mortality patterns are similar to those observed in the United States. In the Danish multicenter cohort (40), the overall mortality rate was 2.9% per year, with a standardized mortality ratio of 4.6. This standardized mortality ratio is identical to that reported for the Toronto cohort (36). A study from Mexico City also identified the mortality rate at 2.4% per year, but does not provide comparative data for the Mexican population (38).

Ward recently demonstrated that in-hospital mortality among patients with SLE admitted through the emergency room is lower at hospitals in which there is more experience caring for patients with SLE (60). Mortality for emergency admissions as a result of SLE was 1.7% for hospitals with high experience compared to 10% for hospital with less experience.

CAUSES OF DEATH

Despite their improved survival, patients with SLE still die at a rate that is three times that of the general population (51). Causes of death may be divided into those related to the SLE disease process itself, those related to therapy, and those from unrelated causes (Table 61.2). Causes related to the SLE include active disease, including nephritis, vasculitis leading to CNS disease or intestinal perforation, intractable bleeding, and end-organ failure (e.g., renal, cardiac, or pulmonary). These certainly have improved with the more appropriate use of steroid therapy, the introduction of antimalarials, and immunosuppressive therapy. Better treatment for hypertension as well as cardiac and pulmonary failure, and the advent of renal dialysis and transplantation, may have averted some of the deaths that otherwise would have resulted from intractable organ failure in these patients.

The primary cause of death may at times be difficult to determine, but early studies followed the detailed protocols that were given in Klemperer's classic paper of 1941 (61). Before 1962, the most common cause of death was progressive renal failure and its associated complications. The incidence of uremia increased from 5% of patients who were treated in the 1930s to as high as 36% in Estes and Christian's report in the 1960s (15), before declining in the 1970s. Since then, uremic demise has occurred much less frequently as a result of better care for patients with end-stage renal disease, including dialysis and the use of cytotoxic therapy for lupus nephritis. Between 1956 and 1973, it decreased from 36% to 14% for all causes of death. The second most common clinical pattern was evidence of active CNS lupus, but with high-dose steroid therapy, CNS lupus became a much less frequent cause of death after 1956 (61). In Dubois' series (62), it decreased from 26% to

TABLE 61.2. PRIMARY CAUSES OF DEATH AND THEIR CONTRIBUTING FACTORS IN SLE

	Primary Cause N (%)	Contributing Factors N (%)
I. Active SLE	20 (16)	38 (30.6)
II. Infections	40 (32)	12 (9.7)
III. Other morbidity related:	38 (31)	2 (1.6)
Acute vascular events	19 (15.4)	
Myocardial infarction	13 (10.5)	
CVA	5 (4)	
Rupture of abdominal aneurysm	1 (0.8)	
Sudden death	10 (8)	
CHF	2 (1.6)	
Pulmonary embolism	2 (1.6)	1 (0.8)
Renal failure	2 (1.6)	3 (2.4)
Pulmonary fibrosis	2 (1.6)	
Others	1 (0.8)	
IV. Unrelated to SLE	13 (10.5)	5 (4)
Malignancy	8 (6.5)	
Suicide/accident	3 (2.4)	
Chronic obstructive lung disease	2 (1.6)	
Aplastic anemia		1 (0.8)
V. Unknown	13 (10.5)	

CHF, congestive heart failure; CVA, cerebrovascular accident; SLE, systemic lupus erythematosus.
From Abu-Shakra M, Urowitz MB, Gladman DD, et al. (36) Mortality studies in systemic lupus erythematosus. Results from a single centre. I. Causes of death. *J Rheumatol* 1995;22:1259–1264, with permission.

8% between 1956 and 1973. The more recent multicenter study (63) revealed mortality because of CNS disease to be reduced to 7%, and in the most recent study from Toronto (36), CNS disease contributed to 5% of deaths.

Most patients in Klemperer's series (61) died from infections because of low resistance and the unavailability of antibiotics. Common bacterial pathogens and tuberculosis accounted for most of these infections (15,64–66); opportunistic organisms were rare in the presteroid era. By 1975, despite the benefits that may follow steroid or cytotoxic therapy, the primary cause of death remained progressive renal damage. The second most common cause was infection, particularly bronchopneumonia caused by opportunistic pathogens. Ropes (67) emphasized that the major causes of death before 1949 were infection, active lupus, and uremia, but that by 1964, they were uremia, infection, and CNS disease.

In 1976, Urowitz et al. (16) demonstrated a bimodal mortality pattern in SLE. Of 81 patients who were studied, 11 died, and six of these died within a year of diagnosis, usually from complications of active lupus or sepsis. All were on high-dose steroids. The remaining five patients died a mean of 8.6 years after diagnosis. None had active nephritis or sepsis. The mean dose of steroids was minimal, and four patients had myocardial infarctions. Their follow-up studies (36,68), as well as the work of others cited in this section, confirmed these findings.

Urman and Rothfield (18) also demonstrated a change in the causes of death as patients with SLE age. Among 209 patients who were studied in New York City from 1957 to 1968, the main cause of 49 deaths was active lupus (excluding uremia; 39%), lupus nephritis (27%), and infection (22%). In 19 deaths among their 156 Connecticut patients who were followed from 1968 to 1976, the causes were lupus nephritis (42%), active lupus (excluding uremia; 21%), and infection (16%).

The multicenter study of 1,103 patients by Rosner et al. (63) reported 222 deaths between 1965 and 1976. As in Urman and Rothfield's report (18), no patient died from a malignancy. The major causes were infection (18%), renal disease (18%), CNS disease (7%), and cardiovascular disease (6%).

Karsh et al. (69) reviewed 94 deaths in 428 patients with lupus nephritis who were seen at the National Institutes of Health between 1954 and 1977. The bimodal pattern first reported by Urowitz et al. (16) was observed. The causes of death were renal complications (40%), vascular disease (25%), and infection (16%). Only one death occurred from cancer, although most of the patients were treated with immunosuppressive drugs.

In a similar study of 138 patients with lupus nephritis who were followed at Guy's Hospital in London between 1964 and 1982 (70), 42 died. Of these, 12 died, usually from active lupus or infection, within a month of starting dialysis. The bimodal curve with late vascular deaths was borne out.

Wallace et al. (19,71) reported their experience with 128 deaths among 609 private patients who were seen between 1950 and 1980. Only 38 of those in the group had kidney disease, but they accounted for 67% of the deaths. The most common causes of death without nephritis were cardiovascular disease (primarily atherosclerotic; 30%), CNS disease (mostly vasculitis; 24%), and sepsis (17%). These authors confirmed Urowitz's finding that most early deaths result from active SLE, and that the preponderance of later deaths result from cardiovascular complications (16).

Information was available on 55 of 67 patients with SLE who died at the University Hospital in Jamaica between 1972 and 1985 (72). Of these, 23 were early demises, and 32 were late. Deaths were caused by infection (37%), renal disease (24%), hemorrhage (17%), and CNS disease (17%). Of 88 deaths observed in a SLE cohort by Studenski et al. (31) at Duke University, 71 resulted from the disease. Reveille et al. (30) reviewed the charts of 389 patients with lupus at the University of Alabama who were seen between 1975 and 1984. Of the 89 patients who died, 74 had a determinable cause of death. The principal causes of death were infection (39%), active SLE (11%), and cardiovascular disease (9%). Pistiner et al. (34) completed a 10-year update of 570 patients with lupus who were seen between 1980 and 1989. None of the patients with discoid or drug-induced lupus died. The most common causes of deaths among patients with SLE were active disease (35%), sepsis (19%), stroke (15%), and cardiovascular disease (15%).

Sepsis, advanced renal failure, left-ventricular failure, and pulmonary embolism were the leading causes of death in the study reported from India (44). Causes of death among 48 Chilean patients with SLE (48) included active SLE in 31 patients, with renal and CNS disease being most prominent. Seventeen patients died with inactive lupus. Four of these 17 deaths resulted from infection, with the others generally resulting from complications of the disease or its therapy. Infection contributed to death in 27 patients. A survey of African blacks who were hospitalized with SLE between 1984 and 1990 in Durban, South Africa, revealed a high mortality rate (73). Causes of death among the 23 patients who died in the hospital included a combination of infection (47%), renal failure (37%), cardiac failure (21%), and neurologic disease (16%). Other causes included pulmonary embolism, diabetic coma, and cardiovascular collapse. Infections and active lupus were the most common causes of death among SLE patients in Singapore (45). These were also the most common causes of death in the European Working Party study (42) and in the Danish study (40). Infection was the most common cause of death in the cohort from London reported by Tucker et al. (37). These authors also reported on four of 16 deaths related to complications of malignancy.

Abu-Shakra et al. (36) reviewed the causes of death in 124 patients with SLE who died during follow-up at the

University of Toronto Lupus Clinic between 1970 and 1994. Active SLE and infection were both primary and contributing factors in a large proportion of the patients (Table 61.2). Patients who died within the first 5 years of diagnosis were more likely to die of active disease, whereas patients who died late in the course of their disease tended to die of atherosclerotic complications, thus demonstrating the bimodal mortality once again. Of the 124 patients who died from 1970 to 1993 in that clinic, 40 have had post-mortem examinations (36). Of these, 21 (40%) had evidence of moderate to severe atherosclerosis at the time of death either as a coexistent finding or as a primary cause of death. This same group of investigators demonstrated that while mortality risks from SLE have decreased over the past 25 years, there was a decrease in mortality related to infection and no decreased mortality because of active SLE. Ståhl-Hallengegre et al. (43) also demonstrated that late deaths among patients with SLE were related to atherosclerosis.

Accelerated atherosclerosis has been identified as a major cause of mortality and morbidity in SLE. Studies at the University of Toronto cohort revealed that at any point in time 10% of the patients will have features of clinical atherosclerosis either manifesting as angina, myocardial cardiac infarction, or peripheral vascular disease alone or in combination. This is comparable to the prevalence of myocardial infarction and angina noted in other, more recently established, lupus cohorts including Pittsburgh (6.7%) and Baltimore (8.3%) (74,75). Ward (76) also has identified atherosclerotic morbidity and mortality among patients with SLE. Bruce et al. (77) further demonstrated that persistent hypercholesterolemia in the first 3 years of SLE was a risk factor for mortality in their inception cohort.

FACTORS ASSOCIATED WITH MORTALITY

Demographic Factors

Several specific factors have been implicated as predisposing factors for mortality in patients with SLE (Table 61.3). These include demographic features, which are unrelated to the disease process itself, such as race, gender, age at onset, and socioeconomic status, including the type of healthcare delivery system that is available.

TABLE 61.3. FACTORS ASSOCIATED WITH MORTALITY

Non-SLE–related factors	SLE-related factors
Demographic	Year at diagnosis
Race	Time of onset to diagnosis
Gender	Disease manifestations
Age at onset	Disease activity at presentation
Socioeconomic status	Treatment
Healthcare delivery system	
Environmental	
Geographic	

SLE, systemic lupus erythematosus.

Race

Race distribution and its influence on SLE prognosis is discussed in Chapter 4, The Epidemiology of Systemic Lupus Erythematosus, and in the previous sections of this chapter. Siegel et al. (78,79) analyzed the relationship between survival and race among a black, Puerto Rican, and white population in a series of 292 cases in the 1960s, and they observed no differences. The 5-year survival rates by group ranged from 62.7% to 65.1%.

In general, whites have a better outcome than nonwhites, with mortality rates being three times higher in nonwhites than in whites (54,56). While race did not appear as an important prognostic factor in a logistic regression analysis of the multicenter study published by Ginzler et al. (21), it was found to be a factor adversely affecting survival of patients with SLE when Cox multivariate analysis was applied to a group of 389 patients by Reveille et al. (30). It has been difficult to separate the effects of race and socioeconomic status, particularly regarding the differences between white and African American patients in the United States. In Reveille et al.'s study (30), white patients with private insurance fared better than African American patients with private insurance; however, there was no difference in outcome when African American patients with and without private insurance were compared. Studenski et al. (31) found that nonwhite race and socioeconomic status contributed independently to mortality. Also, although the overall survival was better for whites than for African Americans in a recent report from Duke University (32), this was related to the socioeconomic status, which was poorer among the African Americans. Abu-Shakra et al. (80) analyzed the factors associated with mortality in patients with SLE who were followed at a single centre. Race was not found to be associated with mortality. Levy et al. (81) identified high unfavorable outcomes among their black and North African patients. This was based on a descriptive analysis, not on a formal statistical evaluation. They suggest that while this may be related to poor socioeconomic status, noncompliance with medical treatment is another factor. Thus, while there may be racial differences in the expression of this disease and its outcome, the effect of race has been confounded by other factors. Wang et al. (49) demonstrated a reduced survival among Asian Indian patients compared to Chinese and Malay patients in Malaysia.

Gender

The relationship between gender and prognosis has been controversial. While Kaslow suggested higher mortality in females than in males with SLE (54), Wallace et al. (19) and

Kaufman et al. (82) demonstrated the opposite: a better prognosis for women than for men. Kellum and Haserick (7) also reported that male SLE was more severe: 34.5% of men were alive at 8 to 10 years, compared with 56.3% of women. Swaak et al. (29), a Soviet group (83), as well as a study by Ward et al. (39), have confirmed these findings. On the other hand, gender did not appear to be a significant predictor in the statistical analysis performed by Ginzler et al. (21). Miller et al. (84), Ward and Studenski (85), and Wang et al. (48) concluded that the spectrum and severity of SLE tended to be the same in males and females. Chang et al. (86) found no statistically significant differences in survival between male and female patients in Taiwan. Abu-Shakra et al. (80) found no effect of gender on prognosis. Thus, the issue of the effect of gender on prognosis in SLE remains unanswered.

Age At Onset

Age at onset of SLE was found to be a significant predictor of survival at both 1 and 5 years in the multicenter study (21), with better survival rates in older patients. Onset of SLE in the pediatric-age group has been associated with a worse prognosis, probably because these patients still may die earlier than their counterparts with older-onset disease (87). Studenski et al. (31) found no significant effect of age on survival (cutoff at 55 years). On the other hand, Reveille et al. (30) found that increasing age of onset adversely affected survival. A comparison with the estimated survival of the age-matched segment of the US population showed that patients with SLE fared worse at all age groups. Abu-Shakra et al. (80) found that older patients (≥50 years) at diagnosis or presentation to the Lupus Clinic were at a slightly higher risk for death than patients who were diagnosed before age 50. Older age also was associated with decreased survival in the study reported by Ward et al. (32). It is of interest that when experimental lupus was induced in young and old BALB/c mice by immunization with 16/6 idiotype in complete Freund's adjuvant, old mice produced fewer antibodies and demonstrated a milder renal lesion than young mice, suggesting that aging modifies development and expression of the autoimmune disease (88). Rood et al. (89) recently observed a significantly higher mortality in patients who developed SLE during reproductive years than in patients who developed lupus in the nonreproductive years. Whether this is an effect of age or hormonal status is unclear.

SLE In Children

Childhood SLE is characterized by more organ-threatening disease than adult-onset SLE (37). In the past childhood SLE was thought to be associated with a poorer prognosis (1). Lupus in children is managed the same way as in adults (90), with particular attention being given to their specific psychosocial needs and special problems (see Chapter 41, Serum and Plasma Protein Abnormalities and Other Clinical Laboratory Determinations in Systemic Lupus Erythematosus). All studies from before 1977 were associated with a less than 50% 10-year survival rate (91–96). Because of the more widespread use of cytotoxic agents, improved antihypertensive agents, dialysis, renal transplantation, cyclosporine, and other diagnostic advances, the 10-year survival now has improved to an average of 85% for children who are treated in optimal settings (97–105). In China, the survival rates are lower, with most recent data revealing a 5-year survival rate of only 76.3% (104). A practice containing largely indigent African American and Hispanic patients in Brooklyn reported a 25% 5-year mortality rate and a 25% 5-year rate of renal failure requiring dialysis (105). Lehman's group in Los Angeles was unable to find any prognostic differences among patients with onset at an age of less than 10 years versus 10 to 20 years (87). Wallace et al. (19) could not find any differences in survival between 55 patients who survived to adulthood and who were diagnosed before 20 years of age versus 409 patients who were diagnosed at a later age. Tucker et al. (37) identified identical 5-year survival rates of 94% among the childhood-onset and adult onset SLE patients.

In summary, the bleak prognosis for childhood SLE that was reported in the 1960s and 1970s has improved substantially. Children now have only a slightly worse outcome than adults.

Older Adults

Idiopathic SLE developing in individuals after the age of 50 years as compared with adults with onset before the age of 50 is characterized by a milder serologic picture, infrequent renal disease, and more serositis and arthritis (106). These patients with older-onset SLE had 92% and 83% 5- and 10-year survival rates, respectively, in Wallace et al.'s 1980 survey (19) and in a study by Baker et al. (107). Fewer elderly patients required corticosteroids, and when they did, lower doses were needed, and for shorter durations (108). Nephritis did not appear to alter overall survival (19). However, Reveille et al. (30) noted that older age of onset was associated with a poorer outcome, and Abu-Shakra et al. (80) noted that patients who were diagnosed or presented at 50 years of age or older had a slightly higher risk for mortality.

Socioeconomic Factors

Dubois et al. (13) concluded that patients who were treated in his private practice did better than those who were treated in publicly funded clinics where he worked. Studenski et al. (31) found that patients with lower socioeconomic background had a worse prognosis; they used Medicaid insurance as a marker of low socioeconomic status, which is not necessarily the case in other practices. The issue of noncompliance with medical therapy was proposed by Levy et al. (81) to be as a factor that must be separated from socioeconomic status. Bruce et al. (109) recently demonstrated that poor compliance was associated with poor outcome with respect to renal disease, but suggested that cultural differences may contribute to noncompliance with medications. Petri et al. (110) demonstrated that both noncompliance and type of medical insurance were important factors in the morbidity of SLE. Karlson et al. (111) studied the relationship between lupus morbidity [defined as disease activity measured by the Systemic Lupus Activity Measure (SLAM)] and socioeconomic predictors in five centers; they found that higher education, private insurance/Medicare, and higher income were associated with less disease activity at diagnosis.

Methods Of Healthcare Delivery

Patients who are treated in different healthcare settings (e.g., private practice, university medical center, prepaid health plan, local clinic, or within a government-controlled system such as the Veterans Administration) probably are different. Therefore, the healthcare setting from which a series of patients with SLE is obtained can influence prognosis. The availability of services and specialists varies widely. Sicker patients often are funnelled into tertiary university centers, thus lowering their reported survival curves for SLE (112). As noted earlier, patients from India, Chile, and the island of Curaçao fared worse in terms of survival than patients from North American centers. Whether this is related to a lack of specialists or to poorer standards of medical care in general is not clear.

In the United States, healthcare is funded by private insurance (e.g., fee for service, managed care, or prepaid health maintenance plan), Medicare, Medicaid (i.e., an extension of the welfare system), cash, or local governments that provide subsidized care to indigent patients. Fessel (113), working with middle-class patients who had at least one family member employed and therefore enrolled in the Kaiser-Permanente prepaid health plan, reported good survivals in patients with SLE. Ginzler et al. (21) studied 1,103 patients with SLE at nine centers and found that privately funded patients had better survival rates than those receiving public funding. Reveille et al. (30) documented that African Americans with private insurance have improved survival compared with those without it.

Reports of patient outcome also probably are influenced by the specialty of the physician who is analyzing the data. For example, Wasner and Fries (114) found that rheumatologists and nephrologists usually agree with each other on general treatment approaches for SLE, but that nephrologists place more emphasis on renal biopsy and use immunosuppressive drugs more frequently. Stewart and Petri (115) recently suggested that patients followed in a health maintenance organization had higher creatinine levels, and less were treated with immunosuppressive agents compared to patients followed by an academic rheumatologist. Ward recently demonstrated that in-hospital mortality among patients with SLE is lower in hospitals that have more experience in looking after patients with SLE (60).

Wallace's group (19,33) has observed higher mortality rates in their clinic patients compared with their private-practice patients. Esdaile et al. (117), on the other hand, found that socioeconomic status had no correlation with health outcomes among Canadian patients with SLE, but all of them had health insurance.

Environment

Environmental considerations, such as climate, occupation, exposure to chemicals, diet, lifestyle, exercise, and drug-induced SLE, are described in Chapters 3, The Role of the Environment in Systemic Lupus Erythematosus and Associated Disorders, 4, The Epidemiology of Systemic Lupus Erythematosus, and 55, Antimalarial Therapies. Whether they influence prognosis is uncertain.

Geography

Geography may be a factor in survival patterns. The incidence and prevalence of SLE in various parts of the world are discussed in Chapter 4. Generally, Canadian, Japanese, and European patients with SLE have outcomes similar to those of patients in the United States. SLE might present differently in certain locales, which may alter prognosis. For example, black patients with SLE in Zimbabwe have an unusually high incidence of renal disease and a low incidence of photosensitivity (118). In India (26), Egypt (119), and Thailand (120), mortality rates are high. However, as noted earlier, the differences in survival that have been noted among patients from India, Chile, or the Caribbean may be related to general medical care and not to certain features related to SLE itself.

Systemic Lupus Erythematosus-Related Factors

SLE factors that may affect prognosis include time between the onset of symptoms and the diagnosis of SLE, change in disease expression over time, presence of specific disease manifestations, overall disease activity, and use of therapeutic modalities.

Year Of Diagnosis

The year of disease onset is a critical factor in the prognostic equation. As noted earlier, the overall survival of patients with SLE has improved dramatically over the last 50 years. Treatment practice has changed and varied depending on the year and location of treatment and the source of healthcare delivery. For example, corticosteroids were used at higher doses and for longer periods in the 1950s; similarly, certain immunosuppressive agents were used more extensively in the late 1960s and early 1970s than they are at present. The advent of steroids, dialysis, newer antihypertensives and antibiotics, and parenteral cyclophosphamide has had an impact on patient survival as well (121).

Time From Onset To Diagnosis

The time difference between onset of symptoms and the diagnosis of SLE has not been formally used as a predictor of survival in SLE. It has, however, been considered as a factor in the calculation of survival rates, because there would be a prolonged survival in those instances where the date of onset of symptoms has been used as the entry point of a survival study. Seleznick and Fries (35) actually demonstrated the point by providing survival rates calculated from first symptom (99%, 96%, and 89% for 1, 5, and 10 years, respectively) and from first visit (96%, 88%, and 64% for 1, 5, and 10 years, respectively). Similar observations were made by Drenkard et al. (38) who showed 96% and 92% 5- and 10-year survival rates calculated from the onset of symptoms as opposed to only 91% 5-year survival calculated from the first visit. Wallace et al. (19) pointed out that the time lag between onset of symptoms and diagnosis in their population did not vary significantly in the three decades of their study and, therefore, might not have influenced the improved survival that was noted over that time period. Their 1990 analysis of 464 patients suggested that the time from onset of symptoms to diagnosis in those older than 60 years is 3.2 years, the longest of any age group (34). Urowitz et al. (51) showed that disease duration to first visit did not vary significantly in the three epochs of their study (i.e., early 1970s, late 1970s to mid 1980s, late 1980s to early 1990s). Most investigators calculate survival rates from the time of diagnosis (6), particularly because not all patients who present with symptoms of SLE go on to develop clear-cut lupus. Only one third of the patients with latent lupus described by Ganczarczyk et al. (122) went on to develop clear-cut SLE. If such patients are included in an analysis of survival, they might yield higher survival rates for the sample population. Of interest in this regard is a paper describing SLE in Iceland (123), which describes a nationwide survey allowing the investigators to include milder cases; the mortality rates in this study are similar to those in other reports.

Change In Disease Expression Over Time

Another important issue is whether the nature of SLE has changed with time. Hashimoto et al. (124) conducted a comparison by decades of 229 Japanese patients who were studied since 1955. They concluded that the incidence of Raynaud's phenomenon, alopecia, oral ulcers, and nephritis has increased in the last decade. In contrast, Wallace's (34) group compared 464 US patients with SLE (diagnosed between 1980 and 1989) with the 520 patients who were seen by Dubois (diagnosed between 1950 and 1963) in the same office. The percentage of patients with organ-threatening disease decreased from 65% to 52%, and acute CNS vasculitis practically disappeared. This might be attributed to earlier recognition and treatment of the symptoms and signs of SLE, an evolutionary change in the disease process, changes in referral patterns, and/or the availability of antinuclear antibody (ANA) testing and other serologic procedures that can help to identify milder cases. Urowitz et al. (51) found that the disease expression did not change in an SLE cohort over a 24-year period; thus, survival could not be attributed to milder disease. Moreover, there was a similar delay from diagnosis to presentation to clinic in patients who were seen in the early 1970s compared with late 1980s.

Effect Of Disease Manifestations

The presence of certain disease manifestations may predispose patients to mortality. Between 1973 and 1985 at the University of Mississippi, 50 deaths occurred in patients with SLE (125). Serositis, nephritis, CNS disease, and leukopenia were associated with a fatal outcome, and the mean interval from diagnosis to death was 4.1 years. Reveille et al. (30) found that thrombocytopenia, nephritis, CNS disease, anemia, and hypertension were associated with a poorer outcome. In the Toronto study (80), renal damage, thrombocytopenia, cardiac complications, hypertension, and lung involvement were associated with mortality by univariate analysis, but the best-fitting multivariate model included renal damage, thrombocytopenia, SLEDAI of 20 or higher at presentation, lung involvement, and age older than 50 years at presentation.

Although CNS disease commonly was found in patients who died with active lupus (36) and has been found to be associated with decreased survival (21), most studies have not confirmed the role of CNS disease as a predictor for mortality. On the other hand, the presence of nephritis carried a poor prognosis for patients with lupus who were followed in hospital centers (19,21,30,113) as well as in outpatient facilities (29). The presence of proliferative and chronic lesions on kidney biopsy specimens was associated with a higher risk of all-cause mortality, particularly in patients with normal serum creatinine (126). Similar results were obtained by Esdaile et al. (127) using the conventional Cox model, although when a time-dependent model was developed, only subendothelial deposits were contributory. Massardo et al. (48) also found that survival curves for World Health Organization types II and III were better than for type IV on univariate analysis. It is of interest that the survival rates calculated for the subgroup of Chilean patients who underwent kidney biopsy was somewhat lower than that of the total population, with rates of 89%, 72%, and 58% for 1, 5, and 10 years, respectively. However, renal disease did not remain significantly associated with prognosis on multivariate analysis once disease activity was in the model. In addition, the Lupus Nephritis Collaborative Group did not find that renal activity or chronicity indices predicted either death or renal failure (128).

Overall Disease Activity At Presentation As A Predictor of Mortality

The assessment of disease activity in SLE has become easier with the development and validation of a number of instruments over the past several years. The most commonly used instruments include: the SLEDAI (129), the SLAM (130), the British Isles Lupus Assessment Group (BILAG) (131), the Lupus Activity Index (LAI) (132), and the European Consensus Lupus Activity Measurement (ECLAM) (133). These indices have been shown to be comparable (134,135). Thus, overall disease activity now can be evaluated as a prognostic factor in SLE.

Indeed, overall disease activity at the time of renal biopsy has been shown to be a prognostic factor for mortality in two cohorts of patients (126,136). It also was demonstrated to be the most important predictor of mortality in other cohorts of patients with SLE (137). Disease activity (as measured by the SLEDAI) at the time of presentation to the Lupus Clinic was a predictor for mortality in a recent study (80). While high SLEDAI (>10) was not a predictor among black Caribbean patients, a high-weighted SLEDAI score, depicting disease activity over the course of disease, was associated with decreased survival in both univariate and multivariate analyses (47). The disease activity index had the strongest association with outcome in Chilean patients with SLE (48). Disease activity, although evaluated by an unvalidated measure, was also associated with mortality in patients from Mexico (38).

The effect of the various factors on survival in SLE is summarized in Table 61.4.

Effect Of Treatment On Mortality

Treatment may be an important factor affecting mortality. Improved therapeutic approaches for SLE may provide better disease control through suppression of the inflammatory process and thus reduce mortality that is related to active disease. There have not been many prospective, randomized, controlled drug trials in SLE. The Canadian Hydroxychloroquine Study Group published its findings of a randomized trial of withdrawal of hydroxychloroquine in patients with stable SLE (138). They found that hydroxychloroquine is effective in controlling disease exacerbations in SLE; patients who continued to take the drug were less likely to have clinical flares than those who were taken off the drug.

That steroids have made a difference in the control of SLE is widely accepted, such that it is considered to be unethical to perform a placebo-controlled trial of steroid therapy in SLE. On the other hand, the contribution of steroid therapy to the changing pattern of mortality and morbidity in SLE has been noted (139). Sturfelt et al. (140) recently noted that prolonged corticosteroid therapy was associated with valvular abnormalities and myocardial infarction in their prospectively studied patient population. Because atherosclerotic complications are a major cause of death, particularly late in the disease, this is an important observation. Petri et al. (141) further demonstrated that an increase in prednisone dose of 10 mg was associated with an increase in cholesterol levels of 7.5, thus predisposing patients to coronary-artery disease, while hydroxychloroquine therapy was associated with a lower serum cholesterol level, possibly protecting patients from coronary-artery disease. Use of medications did not appear as a predictive factor in the analysis performed by Abu-Shakra et al. (80).

TABLE 61.4. RISK FACTORS FOR MORTALITY IN PUBLISHED SERIES

Author (Ref)	Year	Time	Age	Race	Sex	SES	Renal	CNS	BP	Plat	DA
Estes & Christian (15)	1955	A	–	–	–	?	+	+	?	?	?
Wallace et al. (19)	1981	D	+	–	–	?	+	–	–	–	?
Ginzler et al. (21)	1982	E	+	+	–	+	+	–	?	?	?
Studenski et al. (31)	1987	D	–	+	–	+	?	?	?	?	?
Swaak et al. (29)	1989	D	?	?	+	?	+	+	?	?	?
Reveille et al. (30)	1990	D	+	+	–	–	+	?	+	+	?
Pistiner et al. (34)	1991	D	–	–	+	–	+	?	?	+	?
Seleznick & Fries (35)	1991	E	–	–	–	–	+	?	+	?	?
Massardo et al. (48)	1994	A	–	–	–	–	+	–	–	+	+*
Drenkard et al. (38)	1994	A	–	–	–	?	+	–	–	+	+
Abu-Shakra et al. (36)	1995	A	+	–	–	–	+	–	–	+	+*
Ward et al. (3)	1995	A	+	–	–	+	?	?	?	?	?

A, anytime prior to death; D, at diagnosis; E*, at study entry; SES, socioeconomic factors; BP, hypertension; CNS, central nervous system disease; Plat, thrombocytopenia; +, risk factor present; –, risk factor absent; ?, risk factor not assessed or not reported.

The role of treatment as a potential confounder of the relationship between major predictors and mortality was investigated by McLaughlin et al. (126). They found that when the treatment variable was added to the baseline model, the relative risk estimates did not change significantly, suggesting that these estimates were not confounded by the treatment variables that were considered, which included steroid and immunosuppressive drugs.

Spontaneous Remissions

During periods of remission, either no symptoms or minor complaints, such as slight morning stiffness or occasional pleuritic discomfort, may occur. Laboratory abnormalities such as leukopenia, elevated sedimentation rate, and positive ANA may persist or disappear.

SLE can spontaneously improve and remit. Dubois (142) reported that 35 of 520 patients had multiple spontaneous remissions of varying lengths of time not associated with treatment. Some were of 10 to 20 years' duration. Ropes (8,9) noted spontaneous remissions of a few months to several years in 70 of 72 patients. Tumulty (143) in 1954 observed spontaneous remission in 19 of 34 patients who were treated symptomatically. Tozman et al. (20) remarked that four of 160 patients with SLE with a history of severe organ involvement who were followed for a mean of 75 months had no treatment and no disease activity. Gladman et al. (144) described 14 patients who were in clinical remission off steroid therapy, with a follow-up range of 2 to 11 years, despite abnormal serologies. Heller and Schur (145) noted that 13 of their 305 patients (4%) developed clinical and serologic (with ANA becoming negative) remissions between 1967 and 1981 and lasting for at least 18 months; only eight of 13 patients, however, were off all medications. Drenkard et al. (146) defined remission as "at least 1 year during which lack of clinical disease activity permitted withdrawal of all treatment for lupus proper." The period of remission was considered from the time the patient stopped all medications. They did not use a validated disease activity measure to describe disease activity. Of their 667 patients followed for a median of 3.7 years, 156 fulfilled their definition of remission, and 62 went into remission within the first 2 years of disease, and 81 were still in remission at the time of the analysis. The mean duration of first remission was 4.6 years (range 1 to 21 years). Patients who achieved a remission period had increased survival, independently of the effect of other disease manifestations that were associated with increased mortality among their patients. They concluded that lupus was a milder disease than previously considered, and that remission was common. Bruce et al. (147) found that 13% of their 706 patients achieved a 5-year treatment-free period in the course of follow-up. The majority of these still had some evidence of mild disease activity although not requiring therapy. A complete remission (defined as a period of at least 5 years on no medications and with a SLEDAI of 0) was rare, occurring in only 1.6% of the patients. A similar number of patients had serologically active but clinically inactive disease for at least 5 years, requiring no therapy.

Overall, it seems that 2% to 10% of patients who fulfill ACR criteria for SLE can enter true disease remissions that can last for months to years; in other words, they have no symptoms and require no therapy for SLE. This must be remembered when considering therapy for the individual patient or when evaluating the efficacy of treatment.

OTHER OUTCOME MEASURES OF PROGNOSIS IN SYSTEMIC LUPUS ERYTHEMATOSUS

Cumulative Organ Damage

As patients with SLE live longer, their prognosis needs to be assessed by other outcome measures. Individual organ damage, most notably the presence of end-stage renal disease, has been used as an outcome (148). More recently, a global measure of damage namely, the SLICC/ACR Damage Index for SLE has been introduced as a measure of outcome in SLE (149). This measure includes descriptors of nonreversible change that occur after the onset of SLE, whether or not they are related to the disease process or its treatment (Table 61.5). This instrument has been shown to be valid and reproducible (150). Higher damage index scores at presentation were associated with higher mortality in patients with SLE (151). The SLICC/ACR damage index has been found to be a useful measure of morbidity among patients with SLE (152). Stoll et al. (153) identified renal damage at 1 year to be predictive of end-stage renal disease, and pulmonary damage to be predictive of death within 10 years. This study also demonstrated that Afro-Caribbean and Asian patients accumulated more damage than Caucasian patients, suggesting a racial influence on disease expression in this disease. A study of the Montreal cohort, which included only Caucasian patients, revealed that the SLICC/ACR damage index scores predicted poor outcomes defined as either death or hospitalization (154). Nossent (155) found that over an observation period of 71 months the median damage index score was 2.4 in a population of patients from Curaçao. Despite the higher SLICC/ACR damage index scores in this patient population, there was no demonstrable association with poorer survival in that study. The LUMINA study (156) showed that deceased patients experienced more active disease and accrued more damage from the outset of their disease compared to survivors. The Dutch Treatment Study revealed that the SLICC/ACR damage index had the capacity to detect change over time. The SLICC/ACR damage index was found to reflect the impact of cumulative disease activity (particularly with respect to the renal and hematologic systems) and cumulative doses of prednisone. The authors

TABLE 61.5. SLICC/ACR SLE DAMAGE INDEX

Item	Score
Ocular (either eye, by clinical assessment)	
Any cataract ever	1
Retinal change OR optic atrophy	1
Neuropsychiatric	
Cognitive impairment (e.g., memory deficit, difficulty with calculation, poor concentration, difficulty in spoken or written language, impaired performance level)	1
OR major psychosis	1
Seizures requiring therapy for 6 months	1
Cerebral vascular accident ever (score 2 if >1 event)	
OR surgical resection not for malignancy	1,2
Cranial or peripheral neuropathy (excluding optic)	1
Transverse myelitis	1
Renal	
Estimated or measured GFR <50%	1
Proteinuria ≥3.5 g/24 hours	1
OR	
End-stage renal disease (regardless of dialysis or transplantation)	3
Pulmonary	
Pulmonary hypertension (right ventricular prominence, or loud P2)	1
Pulmonary fibrosis (physical and x-ray)	1
Shrinking lung (x-ray)	1
Pleural fibrosis (x-ray)	1
Pulmonary infarction (x-ray)	
OR resection not for malignancy	1
Cardiovascular	
Angina	
OR coronary artery bypass	1
Myocardial infarction ever (score 2 if >1 event)	1,2
Cardiomyopathy (ventricular dysfunction)	1
Valvular disease (diastolic murmur, or a systolic murmur >3/6)	1
Pericarditis x 6 months,	
OR pericardiectomy	1
Peripheral Vascular	
Claudication x 6 months	1
Minor tissue loss (pulp space)	1
Significant tissue loss ever (e.g., loss of digit or limb)	
(Score 2 if >one site)	2
Venous thrombosis with swelling, ulceration, **OR** venous stasis	1
Gastrointestinal	
Infarction or resection of bowel below duodenum, spleen, liver, or gall bladder ever, for whatever cause (score 2 if >one site)	2
Mesenteric insufficiency	1
Chronic peritonitis	1
Stricture	
OR upper gastrointestinal tract surgery ever	1
Pancreatitis	1
Musculoskeletal	
Muscle atrophy or weakness	1
Deforming or erosive arthritis (including reducible deformities, excluding avascular necrosis)	1
Osteoporosis with fracture	
OR vertebral collapse (excluding avascular necrosis)	1
Osteonecrosis (score 2 if >1 event)	2
Osteomyelitis	1
Ruptured tendon	1
Skin	
Scarring chronic alopecia	1
Extensive scarring other than scalp and pulp space or panniculitis	1
Skin ulceration (not resulting from thrombosis) for more than 6 months	1
Premature gonadal failure	1
Diabetes (regardless of treatment)	1
Malignancy (exclude dysplasia) (score 2 if >one site)	2

Note: Damage (nonreversible change, not related to active inflammation) occurring since onset of lupus, ascertained by clinical assessment and present for at least *6 months* unless otherwise stated. Repeat episodes mean at least 6 months apart to score 2. The same lesion cannot be scored twice.
ACR, American College of Rheumatology; GFR, glomerular filtration rate; SLE, systemic lupus erythematosus; SLICC, systemic Lupus International Collaborating Clinics.

concluded that SLICC/ACR damage index is a useful outcome measure (157). Zonana-Nacach et al. (158) used the SLICC/ACR damage index to assess damage among 210 Mexican patients with SLE. They found that damage increased with disease duration so that after 10 years of disease 70% of their patients demonstrated damage recorded by the SLICC/ACR. A Danish study (159) also demonstrated that deceased patients had accrued more damage than patients who remained alive. In a recent multicenter cohort of patients with SLE there was evidence of damage within a mean of 3.8 year after onset. While race and socioeconomic status did not influence early damage, older age at diagnosis of SLE, greater disease activity at diagnosis, and longer disease duration were associated with damage (160).

Non-Caucasian race, longer disease duration, higher disease activity, and lower level of education were associated with more organ damage in SLE in two cohorts of patients from the United Kingdom (161).

Specific Organ Damage In Systemic Lupus Erythematosus

While the overall SLICC/ACR damage index provides a global measure of accumulated damage in SLE, it identifies damage in individual organ systems. Individual organ damage is described elsewhere in this book in the appropriate chapters.

Malignancies In Systemic Lupus Erythematosus

Data concerning the incidence of malignancies in SLE are of great interest, because it is believed that the failure of immune surveillance is a cause of the induction and spread of tumors. In SLE, two reasons for faulty immune mechanisms are known. One involves abnormalities in immune regulation that are associated with the disease process. The second involves long-term treatment with cytotoxic agents, which increases the risk of developing cancer. In fact, cancer is an extremely infrequent cause of death in SLE. Eight large surveys (16,18,19,27,30,31,63,69) were composed of 3,683 patients, and of the 667 who died, 16 had malignancies, representing 2.5% of patients. Approximately 1,000 of the total number of patients had received some type of immunosuppressive treatment; however, these studies did not compare the frequency of malignancy to the general population. In a study of 205 patients with SLE who were followed over 2,340 patient-years, Petterson et al. (162) found a 2.6-fold increased risk for all cancers as compared with that of the total Finnish population. Sweeney et al. (163) did not find an increased frequency of cancers among their cohort of patients with SLE, but follow-up was short. In a more recent study of malignancy in 724 patients with SLE who were followed prospectively for 24 years at a single lupus clinic in Toronto, 24 cancers were identified in 23 patients (3.2%) during 7,233 patient-years of follow-up (164). The most frequent cancer types/sites were hematologic. None of the six patients with hematologic malignancies received cytotoxic drugs before the diagnosis of cancer. Compared with the general population in Toronto, the overall estimated risk for all cancers was not increased in the lupus cohort (SIR, 1.08; 95% CI, 0.70 to 1.62). A 4.1-fold increased risk for hematologic cancers was observed; however, when these malignancies were analyzed separately, only non-Hodgkin's lymphoma was associated with an increased risk (SIR, 5.38; 95% CI, 1.11 to 15.7). Using the cancer rates in patients with rheumatoid arthritis or systemic sclerosis who were in the same geographic area, the risk for cancer was found to be significantly lower in the SLE cohort compared with that of patients with rheumatoid arthritis (SIR, 0.65; 95% CI, 0.41 to 0.96) and patients with systemic sclerosis (SIR, 0.4; 95% CI, 0.26 to 0.60). An increased frequency of non-Hodgkin's lymphoma among patients with SLE also was reported from Denmark (165). Ramsay-Goldman et al. (166) found an increased risk for malignancy in their lupus cohort. Breast, lung, and gynecological malignancies were the most common malignancies observed in the cohort and breast cancer was significantly increased in Caucasian women.

No evidence has shown that antimalarials, nonsteroidal antiinflammatory drugs, salicylates, or corticosteroids increase the incidence of malignancies.

Thus there is no consensus yet on the frequency of cancer among patients with SLE. Use of cytotoxic drugs potentially could increase the risk of cancer, but this association has not been documented in patients with SLE. A large multicenter study is necessary to resolve the issue of malignancy in SLE.

QUALITY OF LIFE IN PATIENTS WITH SYSTEMIC LUPUS ERYTHEMATOSUS

In addition to disease activity and damage, quality of life and disability also are considered important outcomes in patients with SLE (166). These have been measured by the Medical Outcome Study (MOS) Short Form 20 (SF-20) as well as by the SF-36. The quality of life of patients with SLE was found to be reduced compared to healthy controls (167–170). While fibromyalgia has been shown to be a contributor to the reduced quality of life in patients with SLE (169,171), disease activity and damage have been reported to contribute by some investigators (168,172), but not all (169,170,173). It seems that the investigators who used either the SLAM or the BILAG as their disease activity measures were more likely to find a relationship between quality of life and disease activity or damage. This may be related to the fact that these two instruments include items that reflect quality of life as well as damage.

Early work disability was reported in 40% of patients with SLE and was related to low education level, higher physical demands of the job, and higher disease activity at diagnosis (174).

SUMMARY

The information in this chapter can be summarized as follows:

1. Overall survival and duration of disease:
a. More than 90% of patients with SLE survive for at least 2 years after diagnosis, compared with 50% of such patients 30 years ago. More recent surveys reveal an 80% to 90% 10-year survival rate and 70% at 20 years. The mechanism for improved survival over the past five decades is unclear.
b. SLE can become inactive for many years; 15% to 20% of patients at any time have no evidence of clinical activity and are on minimal or no medication.
c. African Americans, males, children, patients who receive care in publicly funded systems, and those with thrombocytopenia have a poorer prognosis, especially if nephritis is present.
2. Mortality rates and causes of death:
a. A bimodal mortality curve in SLE is prevalent. Patients who die within 5 years of disease onset usually have active SLE, high steroid requirements, and infections. Patients who die later usually have evidence of atherosclerotic cardiovascular disease; in contrast, active SLE, infection, and high steroid requirements are uncommon.
b. Most patients with SLE die from active SLE, nephritis, sepsis, and cardiovascular disease. Mortality from CNS disease or malignancies rarely occurs.
3. Other outcome measures in SLE

With improved survival, morbidity and damage related to the disease process or its treatment become important outcomes, as is the quality of life and functional disability of patients with SLE.

REFERENCES

1. Cohen AS, Reynolds WE, Franklin EC, et al. Preliminary criteria for the classification of systemic lupus erythematosus. *Bull Rheum Dis* 1971;21:643–648.
2. Tan EN, Cohen AS, Fries JF, et al. The 1982 revised criteria for the classification of systemic lupus erythematosus. *Arthritis Rheum* 1982;25:1271–1277.
3. Hochberg MC. Updating the American College of Rheumatology revised criteria for the classification of systemic lupus erythematosus. *Arthritis Rheum* 1997;40:1725.
4. Wallace DJ. Prognostic subsets and mortality in SLE. In: Wallace DJ, Hahn BH. *Dubois' lupus erythematosus, 4th ed.* Philadelphia: Lea & Febiger, 1993:606–615.
5. McGehee Harvey A, Shulman LE, Tumulty AP, et al. Systemic lupus erythematosus: review of the literature and clinical analysis of 138 cases. *Medicine* 1954;33:291–437.
6. Merrell M, Shulman LE. Determination of prognosis of chronic disease, illustrated by systemic lupus erythematosus. *J Chron Dis* 1955;1:12–32.
7. Kellum RE, Haserick JR. Systemic lupus erythematosus. A statistical evaluation of mortality based on a consecutive series of 299 patients. *Arch Intern Med* 1964;113:200–207.
8. Ropes MW. Observations on the natural course of disseminated lupus erythematosus. *Medicine* 1964;43:387–391.
9. Silverstein MD, Albert DA, Hadler NM, et al. Prognosis in SLE: comparison of Markov model to life table analysis. *J Clin Epidemiol* 1988;41:623–633.
10. Albert DA, Hadler NH, Ropes MW. Does corticosteroid therapy affect the survival of patients with systemic lupus erythematosus? *Arthritis Rheum* 1979;22:945–953.
11. Dubois EL. Effect of LE cell test on clinical picture of systemic lupus erythematosus. *Ann Intern Med* 1956;38:1265–1294.
12. Dubois EL, Tuffanelli DL. Clinical manifestations of systemic lupus erythematosus. Computer analysis of 520 cases. *JAMA* 1964;190:104–111.
13. Dubois EL, Wierzchowiecki M, Cox MB, et al. Duration and death in systemic lupus erythematosus. An analysis of 249 cases. *JAMA* 1974;227:1399–1402.
14. Leonhardt T. Long-term prognosis of systemic lupus erythematosus. *Acta Med Scand* 1966;445(suppl):440–443.
15. Estes D, Christian CL. The natural history of systemic lupus erythematosus by prospective analysis. *Medicine* 1971;50:85–95.
16. Urowitz MB, Bookman AAM, Koehler BE, et al. The bimodal pattern of systemic lupus erythematosus. *Am J Med* 1976;60:221–225.
17. Lee P, Urowitz MB, Bookman AAM, et al. Systemic lupus erythematosus. A review of 110 cases with reference to nephritis, the nervous system, infections, aseptic necrosis and prognosis. *Q J Med* 1977;46:1–31.
18. Urman JD, Rothfield NF. Corticosteroid treatment in systemic lupus erythematosus: survival studies. *JAMA* 1977;238:2272–2276.
19. Wallace DJ, Podell T, Weiner J, et al. Systemic lupus erythematosus survival patterns. Experience with 609 patients. *JAMA* 1981;245:934–938.
20. Tozman ECS, Urowitz MB, Gladman DD. Prolonged complete remission in previously severe SLE. *Ann Rheum Dis* 1982;41:39–40.
21. Ginzler EM, Diamond HS, Weiner M, et al. A multicenter study of outcome of systemic lupus erythematosus. I. Entry variables as predictors of progress. *Arthritis Rheum* 1982;25:601–611.
22. Fineglass EJ, Arnett FC, Dorsch CA, et al. Neuropsychiatric manifestations of systemic lupus erythematosus: diagnosis, clinical spectrum, and relationship to other features of the disease. *Medicine* 1976;55:323–339.
23. Grigor R, Edmonds J, Lewkonia R, et al. Systemic lupus erythematosus. A prospective analysis. *Ann Rheum Dis* 1978;37:121–128.
24. Fries J, Holman H. *Systemic lupus erythematosus: a clinical analysis.* Philadelphia: WB Saunders, 1975.
25. Jonsson H, Nived O, Sturfelt G. Outcome in systemic lupus erythematosus: a prospective study of patients from a defined population. *Medicine* 1989;68:141–150.
26. Malaviya AN, Misral R, Banerjee S, et al. Systemic lupus erythematosus in North Indian Asians: a prospective analysis of clinical and immunological features. *Rheumatol Int* 1986;6:97–101.
27. Halberg P, Alsbjorn B, Tolle Balslov J, et al. Systemic lupus ery-

thematosus: follow-up study of 148 patients. I. Classification, clinical and laboratory findings, course and outcome. *Clin Rheumatol* 1987;6:13–21.
28. Halberg P, Alsbjorn B, Tolle Balslev J, et al. Systemic lupus erythematosus: follow-up study of 148 patients. II. Predictive factors of importance for course and outcome. *Clin Rheumatol* 1987;6:22–26.
29. Swaak AJG, Nossent JC, Bronsveld W, et al. Systemic lupus erythematosus. I. Outcome and survival: Dutch experience with 110 patients studied prospectively. *Ann Rheum Dis* 1989; 48:447–454.
30. Reveille JD, Bartolucci A, Alarcon GS. Prognosis in systemic lupus erythematosus. Negative impact of increasing age at onset, black race, and thrombocytopenia, as well as causes of death. *Arthritis Rheum* 1990;33:37–48.
31. Studenski S, Allen NB, Caldwell DS, et al. Survival in systemic lupus erythematosus. A multivariate analysis of demographic factors. *Arthritis Rheum* 1987;30:1326–1332.
32. Ward MM, Pyun E, Studenski S. Long-term survival in systemic lupus erythematosus. Patient characteristics associated with poorer outcomes. *Arthritis Rheum* 1995;38:274–283.
33. Gripenberg M, Helve T. Outcome of systemic lupus erythematosus. A study of 66 patients over 7 years with special reference to the predictive value of anti-DNA antibody determination. *Scand J Rheumatol* 1991;20:104–109.
34. Pistiner M, Wallace DJ, Nessim S, et al. Lupus erythematosus in the 1980s: a survey of 570 patients. *Semin Arthritis Rheum* 1991;21:55–64.
35. Seleznick MJ, Fries JF. Variables associated with decreased survival in systemic lupus erythematosus. *Semin Arthritis Rheum* 1991;21:73–80.
36. Abu-Shakra M, Urowitz MB, Gladman DD, et al. Mortality studies in systemic lupus erythematosus. Results from a single centre. I. Causes of death. *J Rheumatol* 1995;22:1259–1264.
37. Tucker LB, Menon S, Schaller JG, et al. Adult and childhood onset systemic lupus erythematosus: a comparison of onset, clinical features, serology and outcome. *Brit J Rheumatol* 1995; 34:866–872.
38. Drenkard C, Vilaa AR, Alarcón-Segovia D, Pérez-Vásquez ME. Influence of the antiphospholipid syndrome in the survival of patients with systemic lupus erythematosus. *J Rheumatol* 1994; 21:1067–1072.
39. Blanco FJ, Gomez-Reino JJ, de la Mata J, et al. Survival analysis of 306 European Spanish patients with systemic lupus erythematosus. *Lupus* 1998;7:159-163.
40. Jacobsen S, Petersen J, Ulman S, et al. Mortality and causes of death of 513 Danish patients with systemic lupus erythematosus. *Scand J Rheumatol* 1999;28:75–80.
41. Uramoto KM, Michet CJ Jr., Thumboo J, et al. Trends in the incidence and mortality of systemic lupus erythematosus. *Arthritis Rheum* 1999;42:46–50.
42. Cervera R, Khamashta MA, Font J, et al. Morbidity and mortality in systemic lupus erythematosus during a 5-year period. A multicenter prospective study of 1000 patients. European Working Party on systemic lupus erythematosus. *Medicine* 1999;78:167–175.
43. Ståhl-Hallengegre C, Jönsen A, Nived O, et al. Incidence studies of systemic lupus erythematosus in southern Sweden: increasing age, decreasing frequency of renal manifestations and good prognosis. *J Rheumatol* 2000;27:685–691.
44. Kumar A, Malaviya AN, Singh RR, et al. Survival in patients with systemic lupus erythematosus in India. *Rheumatol Int* 1992;122:107–109.
45. Boey ML. Systemic lupus erythematosus in Singapore. *Ann Acad Med Singapore* 1998;27:35–41.
46. Murali R, Jeyaseelan L, Rajaratnam S, et al. Systemic lupus erythematosus in Indian patients: prognosis, survival and life expectancy. *National Medical Journal of India* 1997;10: 159–164.
47. Nossent JC. Course and prognosis of systemic lupus erythematosus disease activity index in black Caribbean patients. *Semin Arthritis Rheum* 1992;23:16–21.
48. Massardo L, Martinez ME, Jacobelli S, et al. Survival of Chilean patients with systemic lupus erythematosus. *Semin Arthritis Rheum* 1994;24:1–11.
49. Wang F, Wang CL, Tan CT, et al. Systemic lupus erythematosus in Malaysia: a study of 539 patients and comparison of prevalence and disease expression in different racial and gender groups. *Lupus* 1997;6:248–253.
50. Swaak AJG, Nieuwenhuis EJ, Smeenk RJT. Changes in clinical features of patients with systemic lupus erythematosus followed prospectively over 2 decades. *Rheumatol Int* 1992;12:71–75.
51. Urowitz MB, Abu-Shakra M, Gladman DD, et al. Mortality studies in systemic lupus erythematosus. Results from a single centre. III. Improved survival over 24 years. *J Rheumatol* 1997; 24:1061–1065.
52. Cobb S. *The frequency of the rheumatic diseases*. Cambridge, MA: Harvard University Press, 1971.
53. Siegel M, Holley H, Lee SL. Epidemiologic studies on systemic lupus erythematosus, comparative data for New York City in Jefferson County, AL, 1956–1965. *Arthritis Rheum* 1970;13: 802–811.
54. Kaslow RA, Masi AT. Age, sex, and race effects on mortality from systemic lupus erythematosus on the United States. *Arthritis Rheum* 1978;32:493–497.
55. Gordan MR, Stolley PD, Schinnar R. Trends in recent systemic lupus erythematosus mortality rate. *Arthritis Rheum* 1981;24: 762–769.
56. Kaslow RA. High rate of death caused by systemic lupus erythematosus among US residents of Asian descent. *Arthritis Rheum* 1982;25:414–416.
57. Serdula MD, Rhodes GG. Frequency of systemic lupus erythematosus in different ethnic groups in Hawaii. *Arthritis Rheum* 1979;22:328–333.
58. Helve T. Prevalence and mortality rates of systemic lupus erythematosus and causes of death in SLE patients in Finland. *Scand J Rheumatol* 1985;14:43–46.
59. Hochberg MC. Mortality from systemic lupus erythematosus in England and Wales, 19741983. *Br J Rheumatol* 1987;26: 437–441.
60. Ward M. Hospital experience and mortality in patients with systemic lupus erythematosus. *Arthritis Rheum* 1999,42:891–898.
61. Kelmperer P, Pollack AD, Baehr G. Pathology of disseminated lupus erythematosus. *Arch Pathol* 1941;32:569–631.
62. Dubois EL. Systemic lupus erythematosus: recent advances in its diagnosis and treatment. *Ann Intern Med* 1956;45:163–184.
63. Rosner S, Ginzler EM, Diamond HS, et al. A multicenter study of outcome in systemic lupus erythematosus. II. Causes of death. *Arthritis Rheum* 1982;25:612–619.
64. Davidson AG, Fox L, Gold JJ. Appearance of miliary tuberculosis following therapy with ACTH and cortisone in the case of acute disseminated lupus erythematosus. *Ann Intern Med* 1953; 38:852–862.
65. Harris-Jones JN, Pein NK. Disseminated lupus erythematosus complicated by miliary tuberculosis during cortisone therapy. *Lancet* 1952;ii:115–117.
66. Hill HM, Kirshbaum JD. Miliary tuberculosis developing during prolonged cortisone therapy of systemic lupus erythematosus. *Ann Intern Med* 1956;44:781–790.
67. Ropes MW. *Systemic lupus erythematosus*. Cambridge, MA: Harvard University Press, 1976.
68. Rubin LA, Urowitz MB, Gladman DD. Mortality in systemic

lupus erythematosus: the bimodal pattern revisited. *Q J Med* 1985;55:87–98.
69. Karsh J, Klippel JH, Balow JE, et al. Mortality in lupus nephritis. *Arthritis Rheum* 1979;22:764–769.
70. Correia P, Cameron JS, Lian JD, et al. Why do patients with lupus nephritis die? *Br Med J* 1985;290:126–131.
71. Wallace DJ, Podell TE, Weiner JM, et al. Lupus nephritis. Experience with 230 patients in a private practice from 1950 to 1980. *Am J Med* 1982;72:209–220.
72. Harris EN, Williams E, Shah DJ, et al. Mortality of Jamaican patients with systemic lupus erythematosus. *Br J Rheumatol* 1989;28:113–117.
73. Mody GM, Parag KB, Nathoo BC, et al. High Mortality with systemic lupus erythematosus in hospitalized African blacks. *Brit J Rheumatol* 1994;33:1151–1153.
74. Petri M, Spence D, Bone LR, et al. Coronary artery disease factors in the Johns Hopkins Lupus Cohort: prevalence, recognition by patients and preventive practices. *Medicine* (Baltimore) 1992;71:291–302.
75. Manzi S, Meilahn EN, Rairie JE, et al. Age-specific incidence rates of myocardial infarction and angina in women with systemic lupus erythematosus: comparison with the Framingham study. *Am J Epidemiol* 1997;145:408–415.
76. Ward MM. Premature morbidity from cardiovascular and cerebrovascular diseases in women with systemic lupus erythematosus. *Arthritis Rheum* 1999;42:338–346.
77. Bruce IN, Urowitz MB, Gladman DD, et al. Natural history of hypercholesterolemia in systemic lupus erythematosus. *J Rheumatol* 1999;26:2137–2143.
78. Siegel M, Gwon N, Lee SL, et al. Survivorship in systemic lupus erythematosus: relationship to race and pregnancy. *Arthritis Rheum* 1969;12:117–115.
79. Siegel M, Lee SL. The epidemiology of systemic lupus erythematosus. *Semin Arthritis Rheum* 1973;3:1–54.
80. Abu-Shakra M, Urowitz MB, Gladman DD, et al. Mortality studies in systemic lupus erythematosus. Results from a single center. II. Predictor variables for mortality. *J Rheumatol* 1995; 22:1265–1270.
81. Levy M, Montes de Oca M, Claude-Barron M. Unfavorable outcomes (end-stage renal failure/death) in childhood onset systemic lupus erythematosus. A multicentre study in Paris and its environs. *Clin Exp Rheumatol* 1994;12(suppl 10): S63–S68.
82. Kaufman LD, Gomez-Reino JJ, Heinicke MH, et al. Male lupus: retrospective analysis of the clinical and laboratory features of 52 patients, with a review of the literature. *Semin Arthritis Rheum* 1989;18:189–197.
83. Folomeev M, Alekberova Z. Survival pattern of 120 males with systemic lupus erythematosus. *J Rheumatol* 1990;17: 856–858.
84. Miller MH, Urowitz MB, Gladman DD, et al. Systemic lupus erythematosus in males. *Medicine* 1983;62:327–334.
85. Ward MM, Studenski S. Systemic lupus erythematosus in men: a multivariate analysis of gender differences in clinical manifestations. *J Rheumatol* 1990;17:220–224.
86. Chang DM, Chang CC, Kuo SY, et al. The clinical features and prognosis of male lupus in Taiwan. *Lupus* 1998;7:462–468.
87. Lehman TJA, McCurdy DK, Bernstein BH, et al. Systemic lupus erythematosus in the first decade of life. *Pediatrics* 1989 83:235–239.
88. Segal R, Globerson A, Zinger H, et al. The influence of aging on the induction and manifestations of experimental systemic lupus erythematosus. *J Clin Immunol* 1992;12:341–346.
89. Rood MJ, van der Velde EA, Ten Cate R, et al. Female sex hormones at the onset of systemic lupus erythematosus affect survival. *Brit J Rheumatology* 1998;37:1008–1010.
90. Silverman ED, Lang B. An overview of the treatment of childhood SLE. *Scand J Rheumatol* 1997;26:241–246.
91. Abeles M, Urman JD, Weinstein A, et al. Systemic lupus erythematosus in the younger patient: survival studies. *J Rheumatol* 1980;7:515–522.
92. Coleman WP 3rd, Coleman WP, Derbes VI, et al. Collagen disease in children. A review of 71 cases. *JAMA* 1977;237: 1095–1100.
93. Cook CD, Wedgwood RJP, Craig JM, et al. Systemic lupus erythematosus. Description of 37 cases in children and a discussion of endocrine therapy in 32 of the cases. *Pediatrics* 1960;26: 570–585.
94. Garin EH, Donnelly WJ, Fenell RS, et al. Nephritis in systemic lupus erythematosus in children. *J Pediatr* 1976;89:366–371.
95. Jacobs JC. Childhood-onset systemic lupus erythematosus. Modern management and improved prognosis. *N Y State J Med* 1977;77:22–31.
96. Walravens P, Chase HP. The prognosis in childhood systemic lupus erythematosus. *Am J Dis Child* 1976;130:929–933.
97. Wallace C, Schaller JG, Emergy H, et al. Prospective study of childhood systemic lupus erythematosus. *Arthritis Rheum* 1978;21:599–600.
98. Fish AJ, Blau EB, Westberg NG, et al. Systemic lupus erythematosus within the first two decades of life. *Am J Med* 1977; 62:99–117.
99. Morris MC, Cameron JS, Chantler C, et al. Systemic lupus erythematosus with nephritis. *Arch Dis Child* 1981;56:779–783.
100. Caeiro F, Michielson FMC, Bernstein R, et al. Systemic lupus erythematosus in childhood. *Ann Rheum Dis* 1981;40: 325–331.
101. Platt JL, Burke BA, Fish AJ, et al. Systemic lupus erythematosus in the first two decades of life. *Am J Kidney Dis* 1982;2 (suppl 1):212–222.
102. Glidden RS, Mantzouranis EC, Borel Y. Systemic lupus erythematosus in childhood: clinical manifestations and improved survival in fifty-five patients. *Clin Immunol Immunopathol* 1983;29:196–210.
103. Lacks S, White P. Morbidity associated with childhood systemic lupus erythematosus. *J Rheumatol* 1990;17:941–945.
104. Huang JL, Lin CJ, Hung IJ, et al. The morbidity and mortality associated with childhood onset systemic lupus erythematosus. *Chang Gung Med J* 1994;17:113–120.
105. Tejani A, Nicastri AD, Chen C-K, et al. Lupus nephritis in black and Hispanic children. *Am J Dis Child* 1983;137: 481–483.
106. Wilson HA, Hamilton ME, Spyker DA, et al. Age influences the clinical serologic expression of systemic lupus erythematosus. *Arthritis Rheum* 1981;24:1230–1235.
107. Baker SB, Rovira JR, Campion EW, et al. Late onset systemic lupus erythematosus. *Am J Med* 1979;66:727–732.
108. Dimant J, Ginzler EM, Schlesinger M, et al. Systemic lupus erythematosus in the older age group: computer analysis. *J Am Geriatr Soc* 1979;27:58–61.
109. Bruce IN, Gladman DD, Urowitz MB. Factors associated with refractory renal disease in patients with SLE: the role of patient non-adherence. *Arthritis Care & Res* 2000;13:406–408.
110. Petri M, Perez-Gutthann S, Longenecher JC, et al. Morbidity of systemic lupus erythematosus: role of race and socioeconomic status. *Am J Med* 1991;91:345–353.
111. Karlson EA, Daltroy LH, Lew RA, et al. The independence and stability of socioeconomic predictors of morbidity in systemic lupus erythematosus. *Arthritis Rheum* 1995;38:267–273.
112. Henke CJ, Yelin EJ, Ingbar ML, et al. The university rheumatic disease clinic: provider and patient perceptions of cost. *Arthritis Rheum* 1977;20:751–758.
113. Fessel WJ. Systemic lupus erythematosus in the community.

Incidence, prevalence, outcome, and first symptoms: the high prevalence in black women. *Arch Intern Med* 1974;134: 1027–1035.

114. Wasner CK, Fries JF. Treatment decisions in systemic lupus erythematosus. *Arthritis Rheum* 1980;23:283–286.
115. Stewart M, Petri M. Lupus nephritis outcomes: health maintenance organizations compared to non-health maintenance organizations. *J Rheumatol* 2000;27:900–902.
116. Deleted in page proofs.
117. Esdaile JM, Sampalis JS, Lacaille D, et al. The relationship of socioeconomic status to subsequent health status in systemic lupus erythematosus. *Arthritis Rheum* 1988;31:423–427.
118. Taylor HG, Stein CM. Systemic lupus erythematosus in Zimbabwe. *Ann Rheum Dis* 1986;45:645–648.
119. Sabbour MS, Osman LM. Comparison of chlorambucil, azathioprine or cyclophosphamide combined with corticosteroids in the treatment of lupus nephritis. *Br J Dermatol* 1979; 100:113–125.
120. Chirawong P, Nimmannit S, Vanichayakornkul S, et al. Clinical course of lupus nephritis in Siriraj Hospital. *J Med Assoc Thailand* 1978;61(suppl 1):177–183.
121. Fries JF. The epidemiology of systemic lupus erythematosus, 1950–1990. Conceptual advances and the ARAMIS data banks. *Clin Rheumatol* 1990;9:5–9.
122. Ganczarczyk L, Urowitz MB, Gladman DD. Latent lupus. *J Rheumatol* 1989;16:475–478.
123. Gudmundsson S, Steinsson K. Systemic lupus erythematosus in Iceland 1975 through 1984: a nationwide epidemiological study in an unselected population. *J Rheumatol* 1990;17: 1162–1167.
124. Hashimoto H, Shiokawa Y. Changing patterns in the clinical features and prognosis of systemic lupus erythematosus: a Japanese experience. *J Rheumatol* 1982;9:386–389.
125. Harisdangkul V, Nilganuwonge S, Rockhold L. Cause of death in systemic lupus erythematosus: a pattern based on age at onset. *South Med J* 1987;80:1249–1253.
126. McLaughlin JR, Bombardier C, Farewell VT, et al. Kidney biopsy in systemic lupus erythematosus. III. Survival analysis controlling for clinical and laboratory variables. *Arthritis Rheum* 1994;37:559–567.
127. Esdaile JM, Abrahamowicz M, MacKenzie T, et al. The time-dependence of long-term prediction in lupus nephritis. *Arthritis Rheum* 1994;37:359–368.
128. Schwartz MM, Lan SP, Bernstein J, et al. Role of pathology indices in the management of severe lupus glomerulonephritis. *Kidney Int* 1992;42:743–748.
129. Bombardier C, Gladman DD, Urowitz MB, et al., Derivation of the SLEDAI. A disease activity index for lupus patients. The Committee on Prognosis Studies in SLE. *Arthritis Rheum* 1992;35:630–640.
130. Liang MH, Socher SA, Larsen MG, et al. Reliability and validity of 6 systems for the clinical assessment of disease activity in SLE. *Arthritis Rheum* 1989;32:1107–1118.
131. Hay EM, Bacon PA, Gordon C, et al. The BILAG index: a reliable and valid instrument for measuring disease activity in systemic lupus erythematosus. *Q J Med* 1993;86:447–458.
132. Petri M, Hellmann D, Hochberg M. Validity and reliability of lupus activity measures in the routine clinic setting. *J Rheumatol* 1992;19:53–59.
133. Vitali C, Bencivelli W, Isenberg DA, et al. Disease activity in systemic lupus erythematosus: report of the Consensus Study Group of the European Workshop for Rheumatology Research. II. Identification of the variables indicative of disease activity and their use in the development of an activity score. The European Consensus Study Group for Disease Activity in SLE. *Clin Exp Rheumatol* 1992;10:541–547.
134. Gladman DD, Goldsmith CH, Urowitz MB, et al. Cross-cultural validation of three disease activity indices in systemic lupus erythematosus (SLE). *J Rheumatol* 1992;19:608–611.
135. Gladman D, Goldsmith C, Urowitz M, et al. Sensitivity to change of 3 SLE disease activity indices: international validation. *J Rheumatol* 1994;21:1468–1471.
136. Goulet JR, Mackenzie T, Levinton C, et al. The long-term prognosis of lupus nephritis: the impact of disease activity. *J Rheumatol* 1993:20:59–65.
137. Cohen MG, Li EK. Mortality in systemic lupus erythematosus: active disease in the most important factor. *Aust N Z J Med* 1992;22:5–8.
138. The Canadian Hydroxychloroquine Study Group. A randomized study of the effect of withdrawing hydroxychloroquine sulfate in systemic lupus erythematosus. *N Engl J Med* 1991;324: 150–154.
139. Gladman DD, Urowitz MB. Morbidity in systemic lupus erythematosus. *J Rheumatol* 1987;14(suppl 13):223–226.
140. Sturfelt G, Eskilsson J, Nived O, et al. Cardiovascular disease in systemic lupus erythematosus. A study of 75 patients from a defined population. *Medicine* 1992;71:216–223.
141. Petri M, Lakatta C, Magder L, et al. Effect of prednisone and hydroxychloroquine on coronary artery disease risk factors in systemic lupus erythematosus: a longitudinal data analysis. *Am J Med* 1994;96:254–259.
142. Dubois EL. Systemic lupus erythematosus: recent advances in its diagnosis and treatment. *Ann Intern Med* 1956;45:163–184.
143. Tumulty PA. The clinical course of systemic lupus erythematosus. *JAMA* 1954;156:947–953.
144. Gladman DD, Urowitz MB, Keystone EC. Serologically active clinically quiescent systemic lupus erythematosus: a discordance between clinical and serological features. *Am J Med* 1979;66: 210–215.
145. Heller CA, Schur PH. Serological and clinical remission in systemic lupus erythematosus. *J Rheumatol* 1985;12:916–918.
146. Drenkard C, Villa AR, Garcia-Padilla C, et al. Remission of systematic lupus erythematosus. *Medicine* 1996;75:88–98.
147. Bruce IN, Gladman DD, Urowitz MB. Prolonged treatment free periods in a cohort with SLE. *Arthritis Rheum* 1998;41 (suppl 9):S125.
148. Gladman DD. Prognosis and treatment of systemic lupus erythematosus. *Curr Opin Rheumatol* 1996;8:430–437.
149. Gladman D, Ginzler E, Goldsmith C, et al. The development and initial validation of the SLICC/ACR damage index for SLE. *Arthritis Rheum* 1996:39:363–369.
150. Gladman D, Urowitz MB, Goldsmith C, et al. Assessment of the reliability of the SLICC/ACR damage index for SLE. *Arthritis Rheum* 1997;40:809–813.
151. Gladman DD, Goldsmith C, Urowitz M, et al. The Systemic Lupus International Collaborating Clinics/American College of Rheumatology (SLICC/ACR) Damage Index (DI) for SLE: international comparison. The Systemic Lupus International Collaborating Clinics (SLICC). *J Rheumatol* 2000;27:373–376.
152. Gladman DD, Urowitz MB. The SLICC/ACR damage index: progress report and experience in the field. *Lupus* 1999;8: 632–637.
153. Stoll T, Seifert B, Isenberg DA. SLICC/ACR damage index is valid, and renal and pulmonary organ scores are predictors of severe outcome in patients with systemic lupus erythematosus. *Brit J Rheumatol* 1996;35:248–54.
154. Fortin PR, Abrahamowicz M, Neville C, et al. Impact of disease activity and cumulative damage on the health of lupus patients. *Lupus* 1998;7:101–7.
155. Nossent JC. SLICC/ACR damage index in Afro-Caribbean patients with systemic lupus erythematosus: changes in and

relationship to disease activity, steroid therapy, and prognosis. *J Rheumatol* 1998;25:654–659.

156. Bastian HM, Mickail I, Straaton KV, et al. Factors associated with early death in African-American and Hispanic patients with SLE. *Arthritis Rheum* 1997;40 (suppl 9):S160.
157. Bootsma H, Derksen RHWM, Jaegers SMHJ, et al. Usefulness of the SLICC/ACR damage index in patients with systemic lupus erythematosus. *Arthritis Rheum* 1997;40 (suppl 9):S160.
158. Zonana-Nacach A, Camargo-Coronel A, Yanez P, et al. Measurement of damage in 210 Mexican patients with systemic lupus erythematosus: relationship with disease duration. *Lupus* 1998;7:119–123.
159. Voss A, Green A, Junker P. Systemic lupus erythematosus in Denmark: clinical and epidemiological characterization of a county-based cohort. *Scand J Rheumatol* 1998;27:98–105.
160. Rivest C, Lew RA, Welsing PMJ, et al. Association between clinical factors, socioeconomic status, and organ damage in recent onset systemic lupus erythematosus. *J Rheumatol* 2000; 27:680–684.
161. Sutcliffe N, Clarke AE, Gordon C, et al. The association of socio-economic status, race, psychosocial factors and outcome in patients with systemic lupus erythematosus. *Rheumatology* 1999;38:1130–1137.
162. Petterson T, Pukkala E, Teppo L, et al. Increased risk of cancer in patients with systemic lupus erythematosus. *Ann Rheum Dis* 1992;51:437–439.
163. Sweeney DM, Manzi S, Janosky J, et al. Risk of malignancy in women with systemic lupus erythematosus. *J Rheumatol* 1995; 22:1478–1482.
164. Abu-Shakra M, Gladman DD, Urowitz MB. Malignancy in SLE. *Arthritis Rheum* 1996;39:1050–1054.
165. Mellemkjaer L, Andersen V, Linet MS, et al. Non-Hodgkin's lymphoma and other cancers among a cohort of patients with systemic lupus erythematosus. *Arthritis Rheum* 1997;40: 761–768.
166. Ramsey-Goldman R, Mattai SA, Schilling E, et al. Increased risk of malignancy in patients with systemic lupus erythematosus. *J Invest Med* 1998;46:217–222.
167. Gladman DD, Urowitz M, Fortin P, et al. Workshop Report: Systemic Lupus Erythematosus International Collaborating Clinics (SLICC) Conference on Assessment of Lupus Flare and Quality of Life Measures in SLE. *J Rheumatol* 1996;23:1953–1955.
168. Fortin PR, Abrahamowicz M, Neville C, et al. Impact of disease activity and cumulative damage on the health of lupus patients. *Lupus* 1998;7:101–107.
169. Abu-Shakra M, Mader R, Langevitz P, et al. Quality of life in systemic lupus erythematosus: a controlled study. *J Rheumatol* 1999;26:306–319.
170. Gladman DD, Urowitz MB, Ong A, et al. A comparison of five health status instruments in patients with systemic lupus erythematosus. *Lupus* 1996;5:190–195.
171. Gladman DD, Urowitz MB, Gough J, et al. Fibromyalgia is a major contributor to quality of life in lupus. *J Rheumatol* 1997;24:2145–2148.
172. Stoll T, Gordon C, Seifert B, et al. Consistency and validity of patient administered assessment of quality of life by the MOS SF-36; its association with disease activity and damage in patients with systemic lupus erythematosus. *J Rheumatol* 1997; 24:1608–1614.
173. Hanly JG. Disease activity, cumulative damage and quality of life in systematic lupus erythematosus: results of a cross-sectional study. *Lupus* 1997;6:243–247.
174. Partridge AJ, Karlson EW, Daltroy LH, et al. Risk factors for early work disability in systemic lupus erythematosus: results from a multicenter study. *Arthritis Rheum* 1997;40:2199–2206.

62

EXPERIMENTAL THERAPIES IN SYSTEMIC LUPUS ERYTHEMATOSUS

JOSEF S. SMOLEN

When Moritz Kaposi (1) in 1872 dealt with the therapy of systemic lupus erythematosus (SLE) for the first time in the history of medicine, bed rest, ointments, and plant extracts were the only available remedies for a disease whose cause and pathogenesis were unknown. When Philip Hench et al. (2) introduced glucocorticoids into antirheumatic therapy, it became soon available and was successfully used for SLE (3). However, pathogenetic events were still concealed behind light-microscopic histopathologic descriptions (4), since neither antinuclear antibodies (ANAs), debuting as the lupus erythematosus (LE) cell phenomenon (5), nor indirect immunofluorescence (6) had yet been detected. In contrast, when the epochal National Institutes of Health (NIH) study on pulse cyclophosphamide therapy of lupus nephritis was started a decade before its publication (7), ANAs, most of their subsets relevant for SLE, and the immune complex and complement activating nature of SLE were well established (8,9), but subpopulations of human T cells (10), the first interleukins (11,12), and the genetic associations of SLE with the major histocompatibility complex (13) had been suspected or partly detected but not yet characterized.

Over the past two decades the view on SLE became enlightened by the detection of a plethora of cytokines, chemokines, and similar mediators (14), by the characterization of immunoglobulin and T-cell receptor genes (15,16), by the description of a second cyclooxygenase (17), by the insights into apoptosis and its regulation (18), by the elucidation of a myriad of signal transduction pathways and transcription factors that regulate gene expression (19), and by the imminent description and sequence determination of SLE susceptibility genes (20–22).

Given the fact that SLE in many patients is still incurable and is still associated with significant mortality (23), these advances in basic research will materialize into new therapies. Many approaches are still theoretical and will need subtle realization, but others are already in experimental and even early clinical investigation. In this context it is important to bear in mind that the life-threatening nature of severe SLE may not allow controlled clinical trials early in the development of a new therapeutic regime, but ultimate proof of efficacy must be achieved by adhering to established guidance for clinical trials (24).

The most important therapeutic goal in SLE is the inhibition of the autoantibody-, immune complex-, and complement-mediated inflammation in involved organs and/or destruction of target cells. There are several principal means to achieve such clinical success:

1. Prevention of induction and formation of pathogenic autoantibodies.
2. Prevention of binding or deposition of pathogenic autoantibodies or immune complexes at target cells or tissues.
3. Inhibition of the consequences of immune complex formation in target tissues or cells including inhibition of the inflammatory response.

Some measures may act by more than one of these principal approaches and will be discussed where their higher activity is supposed. On the basis of the recent developments, many pathways can be envisaged to lead to the expected beneficial effects. The principal long-term aim, however, must be cure of the disease, which implies cessation of autoantibody production.

PREVENTION OF INDUCTION OR FORMATION OF PATHOGENIC AUTOANTIBODIES

Autoantibody production to a large number of cell-surface and intracellular antigens, particularly nucleic acids and nucleic acid binding proteins, are a hallmark of SLE. By virtue of the immunoglobulin G (IgG) nature and the hypermutations in V-region genes of most of these autoantibodies (see Chapter 19), it has become evident that they are T-cell driven. The generation of such antibodies usually requires at least interactions of T cells with antigen-presenting cells (APCs) and of B cells with T cells. Such effects are not only mediated by the interaction of antigen/peptide–major histocompatibility complex (MHC) with lymphocyte receptors, but also by a variety of co-stimulatory molecules and cytokines that modulate the T- and B-cell response (see Chapters 9–11). The engagement of the various receptors triggers signal transduction mechanisms that via certain transcription factors lead to the activation of the relevant genes. All these elements can be interfered with.

Peptide Therapy For Tolerance Induction

Tolerization With Antigen-Derived Peptides

As discussed, one of the most important aims in the therapy of SLE is the reduction of pathogenic anti–double-stranded DNA (dsDNA) antibodies. Tolerance induction is one potential approach to achieve this goal. Tolerization is usually achieved by application of antigen (or a mimic) prior to immunization. However, under certain circumstances downregulation of an existing immune response is also achievable.

Since nucleosomes appear to be the major antigenic force driving the SLE immune response (25), nucleosomal antigenic structures may be important candidates for such approach. This is further supported by the fact that antihistone H1 antibodies rather than anti-dsDNA autoantibodies are related to severity of SLE (26), that induction of antibodies to dsDNA is difficult to achieve in experimental animals (27), that human SLE T cells react to nucleosomal antigens by providing B-cell help for anti-dsDNA production (28), and that interaction of autoantibody with nucleosomes rather than DNA may be primarily required for induction of lupus nephritis (29). In fact, in experimental lupus, tolerization to hidden nucleosomal epitopes is effective in inhibiting disease (30). This has not yet been studied in more detail in humans.

Cross-Linking Surface Anti-dsDNA Immunoglobulin

A compound containing four oligonucleotides on a triethylene-glycol backbone (LJP 394) is capable of cross-linking anti-dsDNA on the B cell's surface and to downmodulate anti-dsDNA production *in vitro* and in experimental animals in whom it also improves disease severity and survival (31). Anti-dsDNA was also reduced rapidly in patients with SLE who received LJP 394 (32,32a). Evidence of clinical efficacy has to be shown under controlled clinical settings, and phase II/III randomized controlled trials are currently under way. As a caveat, although there is no evidence that this is the case with LJP 394, DNA surrogates may also activate the immune response (33).

Tolerization With Receptor Peptides

Antibodies can also be downregulated by activating the antiidiotypic network. To this end, a monoclonal anti-dsDNA antibody obtained from Medical Research Laboratory lymphoproliferative (MRL/*lpr*) mice carrying an idiotype, 3E10, which is conserved also in human SLE, and particularly in patients with nephritis, has been recently investigated in a phase I study (34); 3E10 was applied intradermally in a placebo-controlled manner. The data indicate that antiidiotypic antibodies were produced in >50% of patients receiving the vaccine and that this vaccination did not induce flares of the disease over 2 years. Although this approach appears promising, 3E10 is only one of many idiotypes, and it would be surprising if vaccination with one idiotype would lead to downregulation of the total anti-dsDNA response. However, such results were obtained in experimental animals in which it was possible to reduce anti-DNA production (35) or delay epitope-spreading and disease (36) using a number of different peptides derived from anti-dsDNA antibodies. Nevertheless, it should be borne in mind that such peptides could also induce the production of pathogenic autoantibodies (37). Therefore, in patients with SLE, application of this approach may be hampered by the vast heterogeneity of the genetic background and the disease. It is difficult to envisage that a single peptide could become a therapeutic agent for all patients. However, this may be a lesser problem if T-cell determinants responsible for an upregulation of pathogenic autoantibodies generally possess specific qualities (37).

Vaccination with T cells or T-cell receptor (TCR) peptides has not yet been widely employed but has been unsuccessful in an attempt to treat rheumatoid arthritis (38; Breedveld, personal communication).

Inhibition Of T-Cell Activities By Monoclonal Antibodies To T-Cell Differentiation Antigens

Since autoantibodies in SLE are T-cell driven and T cells are pivotal players in the generation of the disease in lupus-prone mice (see Chapter 18), elimination or functional inhibition of T cells constitutes a promising approach. The initial hope for effectiveness of anti-CD4 treatment derived from experimental work (39) does not appear to have materialized in human SLE. Although some reports on improvement of SLE by anti-CD4 (40), and data on analyses of cytokines without further clinical descriptions (41) have been published, such reports of individual cases or small series of patients have not yet been followed by controlled trials, and the apparent mild improvement may not warrant further investigation, provided that the doses employed are viewed sufficiently high. Similarly, anti-CD5 coupled with ricin induced an improvement by 50% of renal manifestations, but only in an open phase I study (42). Although efficient inhibition of T-cell activities could lead to important clinical effects, the targets chosen may not be the optimal ones.

Interference With Co-Stimulatory Molecules

Anti-CD40L (CD154) Monoclonal Antibodies

The generation of an efficient immune response depends on the generation of a second signal by co-stimulatory molecules. Such interactions occur primarily between T cells and APCs, T cells and other T cells, and T cells and B cells (see Chapters 9–11). Co-stimulatory molecules have elicited significant interest in recent years, since inhibition of the interaction of CD40 and its ligand (CD40L or CD154) inhibits T-cell activation, B-cell responses, and autoantibody production. CD40-CD40L interaction between T and B cells is pivotal for antibody production to T-dependent antigens (43). In fact, therapy with anti-CD40L monoclonal antibodies prevents or improves experimental lupus (44). In a preliminary open trial of anti-CD40L (HU5c8) there were signs of significant biologic effects as well as some adverse events (45). Several patients developed thromboembolic complications, which led to a premature halt of the study (A. Vaishnaw, personal communication). Currently, there is considerable interest in attempting to understand the mechanistic basis of this complication following reports of CD40L expression on activated platelets and endothelial cells. In a double-blind, placebo-controlled trial of IDEC 131 anti-CD40L antibody, one similar event (stroke) was reported in the highest dose group, but not otherwise (46).

CTLA-4Ig And Anti-CD80/86 (B7.1/2) Monoclonal Antibodies

Another co-stimulatory pathway is induced by CD80/86 (B7.1/2), which can bind to CD28 and/or cytotoxic T-lymphocyte antigen-4 (CTLA-4) (CD152). CD28 is expressed on T cells, and its interaction with the APC's CD80/86 surface antigens conveys a second signal for cell activation (47). However, CTLA-4 has a higher affinity to CD80/86 than CD28; thus, for example, in the presence of low densities of CD80/86, the interaction is preferentially with CTLA-4 on T cells; engagement of CTLA-4 (without activation of CD28) leads to T-cell tolerance to the presented antigen (47). The fusion protein with an IgG-Fc portion, CTLA-4-Ig, makes use of the high affinity of CTLA-4 to CD80/86. Its application significantly improves murine lupus even if applied late in the disease and reduces autoantibody load (48). Likewise, inhibition of CD86 inhibits humoral immunity (49) and experimental SLE (50). After successful application in psoriasis (51), CTLA-4-Ig is currently undergoing clinical trials in SLE and other autoimmune diseases. Currently, inhibition of co-stimulatory pathways appears to be one of the most promising approaches for treating human SLE.

Interference With The Regulatory Cytokine Network

The available data in experimental animals and human SLE suggest that SLE is a T-helper-1 (Th1)-mediated disease in which a predominant lymphokine is interferon-γ (IFN-γ) (52). Th1 cells are not only involved in cell-mediated immune reactions, but exert B-cell help for the production of IgG2a antibodies (53). On the other hand, Th2 cells that produce interleukin-4 (IL-4) and IL-10 constitute helper cells for the production of other antibody classes and isotypes, and the discussion on the regulatory abnormality in SLE is not yet fully resolved. In fact, it may well be that different cytokines are involved in different types of the spectrum of human SLE. To allow better resolution of this issue, several studies have been performed in experimental animals.

Importantly, IFN-γ knockout mice of both an MRL and New Zealand black (NZB) background do not develop lupus (54). These data as well as the inhibition of glomerulonephritis in lupus-prone animals after application of soluble IFN-γ receptor (55) support the Th1 notion. On the other hand, injection of monoclonal antibody against IL-10 inhibited murine lupus (56), and the authors also discuss involvement of tumor necrosis factor-α (TNF-α) in this context (see below). However, IL-10 in SLE may be primarily produced by monocytes/macrophages in the course of the inflammatory process and may thus contribute to a secondary upregulation of autoantibody production within the background of the disease. Reports on the successful application of anti–IL-4, the prototypical Th2 cytokine, are lacking; in contrast, injection of IL-4 improves murine LE (57). Th1 determination and thus IFN-γ production are mediated by the effects of IL-12, which is also increased in SLE (58), supporting the notion on IFN-γ involvement in the pathogenesis of the disease. Given the current evidence, application of inhibitors of IFN-γ, such as soluble IFN receptors, may be worth studying in SLE.

Stem Cell Transplantation

If one could eradicate the abnormal immune system and replace it with an uncommitted new one, one ought to be able to eliminate all pathogenic cells and their products and in parallel restore the normal immune response. Stem cell transplantation (SCT) is an approach directed at such a goal. SCT is highly effective in patients with hematologic malignancies (59) and some immunodeficiencies. In recent years, relentlessly progressing autoimmune disorders have been a focus for SCT, since the combination of SCT (ideally using autologous stem cells purged from contaminating

T cells) with high-dose, myeloablative cytotoxic therapy allows effective antiinflammatory and immunosuppressive treatment, rescue from the subsequent myeloablation, and reconstitution of the immune system with unprimed cells. The idea behind this procedure is halt of the disease via cytotoxic treatment and prevention of its recurrence via replenishment with a naive immune system. In autoimmune diseases, the use of allogeneic SCT, which has a much higher risk than autologous SCT, appears to be unjustified. Therefore, autologous SCT has been employed in a large number of individual patients or small series of patients, but a multicenter open investigation is ongoing during more recent years with significant success in many patients with SLE who previously had unremitting disease (60). Although controlled trials are still lacking, SCT appears to be a promising approach for the relentlessly progressive patient. Nevertheless, SCT is associated with significant risks that have to be weighed against the risk of the disease; moreover, there are patients who experience recurrence of disease despite SCT (61), and it is unresolved at present if this is due to the nature of the underlying disorder or to technical aspects of the procedure. SCT also constitutes one basis for potential gene therapy (see below).

PREVENTION OF BINDING OR DEPOSITION OF PATHOGENIC AUTOANTIBODIES OR IMMUNE COMPLEXES AT TARGET CELLS OR TISSUES

Elimination Of Autoantibodies And Immune Complexes: Plasmapheresis And Immunoadsorption

The principle of plasma exchange lies in the attempt to eliminate pathogenic autoantibodies and potential circulating immune complexes, preventing their tissue/cell deposition and activation of subsequent events. However, controlled clinical trials have revealed that plasma exchange alone is ineffective in SLE (62) and may even lead to a rebound effect. Combination of plasma exchange with pulse cyclophosphamide therapy (i.e., rapid elimination of existing autoantibodies combined with measures to prevent their reproduction) does not appear to be more successful than pulse cyclophosphamide alone (63,64); moreover, it was associated with higher long-term mortality due to infection, since nonselective elimination of immunoglobulins apparently fostered an immunocompromised state beyond that of the disease and therapy themselves (63). In contrast to plasmapheresis, selective elimination of immunoglobulins (IgG or anti-DNA antibodies) (65,66), in combination with cyclophosphamide therapy, may constitute a promising approach for acute exacerbations of SLE that are difficult to control otherwise, but needs to be proven in controlled trials.

The oligonucleotide LJP 394 (see above) could also, at least in part, act by absorption of anti-dsDNA antibodies (32).

Elimination Of Putative Autoantigens: DNAse

The mechanism of DNA–anti-DNA immune complex formation and deposition is still not fully resolved, and there are several theories supported by experimental evidence (29). Nevertheless, the pathogenicity of anti-dsDNA antibodies and their binding to nucleosomal antigens is undisputed. Elimination of the antigen in an immune complex is a feasible goal to achieve improvement of an immune complex disease. To this end, recombinant human DNAse has been applied in experimental animals and reduced anti-DNA antibodies; however, this did not alter the disease course (67). More recently, recombinant DNAse (rDNAse) was applied to patients with SLE; in this study there were no effects on clinical or laboratory variables of the disease (68).

Competitive Inhibition Of Immune Complex Formation: Heparin And D-Peptides

The detailed mechanisms of immune complex formation and deposition in SLE is still not fully resolved. It has been suggested that, rather than deposition of circulating immune complexes, binding of the circulating, kationic nucleosomal antigens to the glomerular basement membrane may be the important event in lupus nephritis; anti-dsDNA antibodies would subsequently bind to the renally deposited nucleosomal antigens and elicit the inflammatory response (29,69). In experimental animals, the application of heparin, by virtue of its charged nature, could prevent renal disease and improve survival due to competitive inhibition of nucleosomal binding to the glomerular basement membrane (70). Again, clinical trials are missing, but since heparinization is rarely contraindicated in SLE, such therapy might be useful at least as an adjunctive measure to the more conventional strategies.

Immune-complex formation and binding of antigen or cross-reactive substrates to antibody can also be inhibited by application of competing antigens or fragments. In an interesting experiment using D amino acid peptide surrogate, which bound specifically to monoclonal anti-DNA antibodies, renal deposition of these antibodies was inhibited (71). Since D-peptides are not degraded rapidly, such therapeutic approach is of significant interest. However, the generation of autoantibodies probably remains unaffected, and care must be taken not to elicit autoantibody formation with peptide surrogates for dsDNA (33).

INHIBITION OF THE CONSEQUENCES OF IMMUNE COMPLEX FORMATION IN TARGET TISSUES OR CELLS INCLUDING INHIBITION OF THE INFLAMMATORY RESPONSE

Interference With The Activation Of The Complement Cascade

Activation of complement (C′) is of pivotal importance in the generation of most features of SLE. Deficiencies of different components of the early C′ pathway are associated with SLE (see Chapters 6 and 13) and low C′ is associated with active disease, especially active nephritis (9). On the other hand, C′ receptor knockout mice do not develop lupus (72). Monoclonal antibodies to C5, which inhibit the consequences of C5 activation including the late membrane attack complex C5-C9, ameliorate murine lupus even if given after the development of anti-dsDNA antibodies (73,74). A chimeric anti-C5 monoclonal antibody has been developed and is currently studied in patients.

Interference With Fc-Receptor Activation By Immune Complexes

The recent observation of normal renal function despite presence of a full-blown autoantibody repertoire in Fc-receptor knockout (Fcγ-R I/III –/–) lupus-prone mice (75) further emphasizes the dichotomy of the autoimmune and the inflammatory response in SLE. In fact, administration of soluble Fc-receptors also ameliorated murine lupus (76). Further supporting the evidence, the inflammatory changes in SLE are not only complement but also Fcγ-receptor mediated. Thus, blocking interactions of immune complexes with the IgG-Fc receptor appears to constitute another potentially successful modality in human lupus. In this respect it should be borne in mind that high-dose immunoglobulin may also block Fc receptors and that such therapy may improve SLE disease activity by up to 80% (77), but controlled trials have not been performed. An alternative explanation for some efficacy of immunoglobulin preparations could be the presence of anti–anti-DNA idiotypes that could dissolve immune complexes and/or downregulate anti-DNA production (78,79).

Interference With The Proinflammatory Cytokine Network

As already discussed above, although SLE disease is induced by abnormalities of the immune response, the ultimate pathogenic steps are of inflammatory nature, elicited by inflammatory processes. Inhibition of the inflammatory events may not cure SLE, but it may improve or even abrogate the clinical disease manifestations. This is typically exemplified by two models discussed above, the Fcγ-R knockout and the CR knockout mice (72,75). The inflammatory response, even when elicited by immune complexes or complement activation, is mediated at least partly by proinflammatory cytokines. The central proinflammatory cytokine is TNF-α, which mediates all attributes of inflammatory responses and activates IL-1 and IL-6, two additional mediators of inflammation (80). However, the role of TNF-α is currently heavily debated; on the one hand, application of TNF-α can lead to amelioration of murine SLE (81) and the anti–IL-10– induced beneficial effects may be mediated by an increase in TNF-α (56); on the other hand, TNF-α is increased in serum and kidneys of lupus mice (82), TNF-α can induce nephritis (83,84), and TNF-α–deficient mice are resistant to the development of glomerulonephritis (85). Finally, TNF-α levels are high in patients with active SLE and correlate with disease activity and IL-6 levels (86). Thus, interference with TNF-α may ameliorate clinical manifestations in SLE.

The recent availability of TNF-blocking agents has elicited new interest into the effect of TNF-α in SLE, since up to 20% of treated patients may increase their ANA and may develop anti-dsDNA antibodies of low titer (87–89). Moreover, three cases of a mild lupus-like disease have been described that were fully reversible after cessation of the TNF blocker. However, in contrast to other agents used as disease-modifying antirheumatic drugs (DMARDs) in rheumatoid arthritis (RA), no severe manifestations of SLE, such as renal involvement, have been observed, and in patients with RA-LE overlap disease TNF blockade did not lead to exacerbation of disease. Thus, TNF may play a dual role in SLE: it may dysregulate autoantibody production and it appears to be importantly involved in the end stage of the disease process, namely the inflammatory events that ultimately damage the organs. Thus, for inhibition of an acute exacerbation of the disease, TNF blockade may be an effective means, and this is also suggested by data from experimental animals (90,91). Finally, it should be mentioned that other proinflammatory cytokines such as IL-1 also may be involved in the SLE process, and inhibition of IL-1 ameliorates murine lupus (92).

Gene Therapy

Gene therapy could be applied either to correct or replace a defective gene, as has already been successfully attempted in experimental models of SLE (93–95), or to transfer a gene whose product could counteract one of the many important pathogenetic steps in a continuous or an inducible manner. The potential for successful gene therapy will depend on (a) our knowledge of the genetic bases of the disease, (b) our pathogenetic insights, (c) our understanding of the heterogeneity of SLE, and (d) the feasibility and ethics of the chosen approach. In principle, gene therapy even in combination with stem cell therapy is a foreseeable path a few years further into this decade.

Immunomodulating Drugs

These agents are detailed here, since many of them act by antiinflammatory means. However, some inhibit T-cell or B-cell functions, and others may interfere with consequences of several pathways.

The possible involvement of TNF-α in the pathogenesis of SLE, as discussed above, is further suggested by the efficacy of thalidomide in subsets of SLE (96), since thalidomide decreases TNF-α production (97). Thalidomide appears to be particularly effective for treatment-resistant skin lesions, but may also have other effects. It must not be given to women of childbearing potential; neuropathy is a major adverse event induced by thalidomide.

Leflunomide, a new DMARD for rheumatoid arthritis (98), has also been found effective in MRL/*lpr* mice (99). Leflunomide inhibits pyrimidine synthesis and NF-κB production (100). However, in an open study in SLE it had only a mild degree of efficacy (101).

Cladribine (2′-chlorodeoxyadenosine), an effective drug for hairy cell leukemia (102), which by virtue of its nature as a nucleoside analogue leads to specific T- and B-cell depletion, appeared to be efficient in an open trial (103), although it induced severe lymphocytopenia and occasional opportunistic infections.

Mycophenolate mofetil is an inhibitor of purine synthesis and is in use for treatment of transplant rejections. In open trials, disease activity as judged by the Systemic Lupus Activity Measure (SLAM), decreased by about 40% (104,105). However, again, a controlled trial is needed to judge the efficacy of the drug.

Finally, recent advances in our understanding of signal transduction pathways have elicited particular hope for therapeutic usefulness of small molecule inhibitors of various kinases, such as mitogen-activated protein kinases (MAPKs) or Janus kinases (JAKs), or transcription factors, such as NF-κB. Their involvement in the activation of cytokine and many other genes is meanwhile well understood. A number of compounds have been developed (18,106) and some may be useful clinically. Experimental and clinical data of such novel compounds are eagerly awaited.

SUMMARY

There are a number of promising agents, biologics and conventional drugs, awaiting new or further clinical trials in SLE, and new pathways have been entered in recent years (107). Controlled clinical trials in SLE are hampered by the heterogeneity of the disease and the potential acuity and life-threatening nature of its exacerbations. However, only such randomized controlled clinical trials will allow ultimate determination of which of these compounds may be beneficial. Thorough design of study protocols, which may have to include rescue procedures for drug elimination or disease flares, will be necessary. The fact that almost 130 years after Kaposi's initial thoughts on treating SLE this disease still is afflicted with significant morbidity and mortality, and that we still seem far away from curative therapeutic measures, makes further research into new treatment modalities mandatory.

REFERENCES

1. Kaposi (Kohn) M. Neue Beiträge zur Kenntnis des Lupus erythematosus. *Arch Dermatol Syphilol* 1872;4:36–78.
2. Hench PS, Kendall EC, Slocumb CH, et al. The effect of a hormone of the adrenal cortex (17-hydroxy-11-dehydrocorticosterone: compound E) and of pituitary adrenocorticotropic hormone on rheumatoid arthritis: preliminary report. *Proc Staff Meet Mayo Clin* 1949;24:181–197.
3. Grace AW, Combes FC. Remission of disseminated lupus erythematosus induced by adrenocorticotropin. *Proc Soc Exp Biol Med* 1949;72:563–565.

3a. Thorn GW, Boyles TB, Massell BF, et al. Medical progress: the clinical usefulness of ACTH and cortisone. *N Engl J Med* 1950;242:824–834.

4. Klemperer P, Pollack A, Baehr G. Diffuse collagen disease: acute disseminated lupus erythematosus and diffuse scleroderma. *JAMA* 1942;119:331–332.
5. Hargraves MM, Richmond H, Morton R. Presentation of two bone marrow elements: the "tart" cell and the "L.E." cell. *Mayo Clin Proc* 1948;23:25–28.
6. Coons AH, Kaplan MH. Localization of antigen in tissue cells. II. Improvements in a method for the detection of antigen by means of fluorescent antibody. *J Exp Med* 1950;91:1–13.
7. Balow JE, Austin HA, Muenz LR, et al. Effect of treatment on the evolution of renal abnormalities in lupus nephritis. *N Engl J Med* 1984;311:491–495.
8. Koffler D, Agnello V, Kunkel HG. Polynucleotide immune complexes in serum and glomeruli of patients with systemic lupus erythematosus. *Am J Pathol* 1974;74:109–122.
9. Schur PH, Sandson J. Immunologic factors and clinical activity in systemic lupus erythematosus. *N Engl J Med* 1968;278:533–538.
10. Reinherz EL, Schlossman SF. Regulation of the immune response: inducer and suppressor T-lymphocyte subsets in human beings. *N Engl J Med* 1980;303:370–374.
11. Gery I, Gershon DK, Waksman BH. Potentiation of the T-lymphocyte response to mitogens. I. The responding cell. *J Exp Med* 1972;136:128–142.
12. Morgan DA, Ruscetti FW, Gallo RC. Selective in vitro growth of T lymphocytes from normal human bone marrows. *Science* 1976;193:1007–1009.
13. Reinertsen JL, Klippel JH, Johnson AH, et al. B lymphocyte alloantigens associated with systemic lupus erythematosus. *N Engl J Med* 1978;299:515–518.
14. Rossi D, Zlotnik A. The biology of chemokines and their receptors. *Annu Rev Immunol* 2000;18:217–224.
15. Tonegawa S. Somatic generation of antibody diversity. *Nature* 1983;302:573.
16. Davis MM, Bjorkman PJ. T-cell antigen receptor genes and T-cell recognition. *Nature* 1988;332:395–402.
17. Masferrer JL, Zweifel BS, Seibert K, et al. Selective regulation of cellular cyclooxygenase by dexamethasone and endotoxin in mice. *J Clin Invest* 1990;86:1375–1379.
18. Afford S, Randhawa S. Apoptosis. *Mol Pathol* 2000;53:55–63.

19. Firestein GS, Manning AM. Signal transduction and transcription factors in rheumatic disease. *Arthritis Rheum* 1999;42: 609–621.
20. Tsao BP, Cantor RM, Kalunian KC, et al. The genetic basis of systemic lupus erythematosus. *Proc Assoc Am Physicians* 1998; 110:113–117.
21. Wakeland EK, Wandstrat AE, Liu K, et al. Genetic dissection of systemic lupus erythematosus. *Curr Opin Immunol* 1999;11: 701–707.
22. Vyse TJ, Kotzin BL. Genetic susceptibility to systemic lupus erythematosus. *Annu Rev Immunol* 1998;16:261–292.
23. Urowitz MB, Gladman DD. Evolving spectrum of mortality and morbidity in SLE. *Lupus* 1999;8:253–255.
24. Smolen JS, Strand V, Cardiel M, et al. Randomized clinical trials and longitudinal observational studies in systemic lupus erythematosus: consensus on a preliminary core set of outcome domains. *J Rheumatol* 1999;26:504–507.
25. Lu L, Kaliyaperumal A, Boumpas DT, et al. Major peptide autoepitopes for nucleosome-specific T cells of human lupus. *J Clin Invest* 1999;104:345–355.
26. Schett G, Rubin RL, Steiner G, et al. The lupus erythematosus cell phenomenon: comparative analysis of antichromatin antibody specificity in lupus erythematosus cell-positive and -negative sera. *Arthritis Rheum* 2000;43:420–428.
27. Pisetsky DS. The role of bacterial DNA in autoantibody induction. *Curr Top Microbiol Immunol* 2000;247:143–155.
28. Voll RE, Roth EA, Girkotaite I, et al. Histone-specific Th0 and Th1 clones derived from systemic lupus erythematosus patients induce double-stranded DNA antibody production. *Arthritis Rheum* 1997;40:2162–2171.
29. van Bruggen MC, Walgreen B, Rijke TP, et al. Antigen specificity of anti-nuclear antibodies complexed to nucleosomes determines glomerular basement membrane binding in vivo. *Eur J Immunol* 1997;27:1564–1569.
30. Datta SK, Kaliyaperumal A, Desai-Mehta A. T cells of lupus and molecular targets for immunotherapy. *J Clin Immunol* 1997;17:11–20.
31. Jones DS, Barstad PA, Feild MJ, et al. Immunospecific reduction of anti-oligonucleotide antibody forming cells with a tetrakis-oligonucleotide conjugate (LJP 394), a therapeutic candidate for the treatment of lupus nephritis. *J Med Chem* 1995; 38:2138–2144.
32. Weisman MH, Blustein HG, Berner CM. Reduction in circulating dsDNA antibody titer after administration of LJP 394. *J Rheumatol* 1997;24:314–318.
32a. Furie RA, Cash JM, Cronin ME. Treatment of systemic lupus erythematosus with LJP 394. *J Rheumatol* 2001;28:257–267.
33. Putterman C, Diamond B. Immunization with a peptide surrogate for double stranded DNA (dsDNA) induces autoantibody production and renal immunoglobulin deposition. *J Exp Med* 1998;188:29–38.
34. Spertini F, Leimgruber A, Morel B, et al. Idiotypic vaccination with a murine anti-dsDNA antibody: phase I study in patients with nonactive systemic lupus erythematosus with nephritis. *J Rheumatol* 1999;26:2602–2608.
35. Waisman A, Ruiz PJ, Israeli E, et al. Modulation of murine systemic lupus erythematosus with peptides based on complementarity determining regions of a pathogenic anti-DNA monoclonal antibody. *Proc Natl Acad Sci USA* 1997;94:4620–4625.
36. Singh RR, Hahn BH. Reciprocal T-B determinant spreading develops spontaneously in murine lupus: implications for pathogenesis. *Immunol Rev* 1998;164:201–208.
37. Hahn BH, Singh RR, Ebling FM. Self Ig peptides that help anti-DNA antibody production: importance of charged residues. *Lupus* 1998;7:307–313.
38. Breedveld FC, Struyk L, van Laar JM, et al. Therapeutic regulation of T cells in rheumatoid arthritis. *Immunol Rev* 1995; 144:5–16.
39. Wofsy D, Seaman WE. Successful treatment of autoimmunity in NZB/NZW F1 mice with monoclonal antibody to L3T4. *J Exp Med* 1985;161:378–391.
40. Hiepe F, Volk HD, Apostoloff E, et al. Treatment of severe systemic lupus erythematosus with anti-CD4 monoclonal antibody. *Lancet* 1991;338:1529–1530.
41. Brink I, Thiele B, Burmester GR, et al. Effects of anti-CD4 antibodies on the release of IL-6 and TNF-α in whole blood samples from patients with systemic lupus erythematosus. *Lupus* 1999;8:723–730.
42. Stafford FJ, Fleisher TA, Lee G, et al. A pilot study of anti-CD5 ricin A chain immunoconjugate in systemic lupus erythematosus. *J Rheumatol* 1994;21:2068–2070.
43. Grewal IS, Flavell RA. CD40 and CD154 in cell mediated immunity. *Annu Rev Immunol* 1998;16:111–135.
44. Datta SK, Kalled SL. CD40-CD40 ligand interaction in autoimmune disease. *Arthritis Rheum* 1997;40:1735–1745.
45. Davidson A, Lalbachan B, Bhoompally R, et al. The effect of anti-CD40L antibody on B cells in human SLE. *Arthritis Rheum* 2000;43(suppl):S271.
46. Kalunian KC, Davis J, Merrill JT, et al. Treatment of systemic lupus erythematosus by inhibition of T cell costimulation. *Arthritis Rheum* 2000;43(suppl):S271.
47. Bluestone JA. Is CTLA-4 a master switch for peripheral T cell tolerance? *J Immunol* 1997;158:1989–1993.
48. Finck BK, Linsley PS, Wofsy D. Treatment of murine lupus with CTLA4Ig. *Science* 1994;265:1225–1227.
49. Daikh DI, Wofsy D. Effects of anti-B7 monoclonal antibodies on humoral immune responses. *J Autoimmun* 1999;12: 101–108.
50. Nakajima A, Azuma M, Kodera S, et al. Preferential dependence of autoantibody production in murine lupus on CD86 costimulatory molecule. *Eur J Immunol* 1995;25:3060–3069.
51. Abrams JR, Lebwohl MG, Guzzo CA, et al. CTLA4Ig-mediated blockade of T-cell costimulation in patients with psoriasis vulgaris. *J Clin Invest* 1999;103:1243–1252.
52. Seery JP, Carroll JM, Cattell V, et al. IFN-γ paper Antinuclear autoantibodies and lupus nephritis in transgenic mice expressing interferon gamma in the epidermis. *J Exp Med* 1997;186: 1451–1459.
53. Romagnani S. The Th1/Th2 paradigm. *Immunol Today* 1997; 18:263–266.
54. Balomenos D, Rumold R, Theofilopoulos AN. Interferon-gamma is required for lupus-like disease and lymphoaccumulation in MRL-lpr mice. *J Clin Invest* 1998;101:364–371.
55. Ozmen L, Roman D, Fountoulakis M, et al. Experimental therapy of systemic lupus erythematosus: the treatment of NZB/W mice with mouse soluble interferon-gamma receptor inhibits the onset of glomerulonephritis. *Eur J Immunol* 1995;25:6–12.
56. Ishida H, Muchamuel T, Sakaguchi S, et al. Continuous administration of anti-interleukin 10 antibodies delays onset of autoimmunity in NZB/W F1 mice. *J Exp Med* 1994;179:305–10.
57. Santiago ML, Fossati L, Jacquet C, et al. Interleukin-4 protects against a genetically linked lupus-like autoimmune syndrome. *J Exp Med* 1997;185:65–70.
58. Tokano Y, Morimoto S, Kaneko H, et al. Levels of IL-12 in the sera of patients with systemic lupus erythematosus (SLE)—relation to Th1 and Th2-derived cytokines. *Clin Exp Immunol* 1999;116:169–173.
59. Appelbaum FR. Allogeneic stem cell transplantation for the treatment of hematologic malignancies: current indications and challenges. *J Rheumatol* 1997;48(suppl):41–45.
60. Tyndall A, Fassas A, Passweg J, et al. Autologous haematopoietic stem cell transplants for autoimmune disease—feasibility

and transplant-related mortality. Autoimmune disease and lymphoma working parties of the European Group for Blood and Bone Marrow Transplantation, the European League against Rheumatism and the International stem cell project for autoimmune diseases. *Bone Marrow Transplant* 1999;24:729–734.
61. Marmont AM. Stem cell transplantation for severe autoimmune diseases. Progress and problems. *Haematologia* 1998;83: 733–743.
62. Wei N, Klippel JH, Huston DP, et al. Randomized trial of plasma exchange in mild systemic lupus erythematosus. *Lancet* 1983;1:17–22.
63. Aringer M, Smolen JS, Graninger WB. Severe infections in plasmapheresis-treated systemic lupus erythematosus. *Arthritis Rheum* 1998;41:414–420.
64. Wallace DJ, Goldfinger D, Pepkowitz SH, et al. Randomized controlled trial of pulse/synchronization cyclophosphamide/ apheresis for proliferative lupus nephritis. *J Clin Apheresis* 1998; 13:163–166.
65. Gaubitz M, Seidel M, Kummer S, et al. Prospective randomized trial of two different immunoadsorbers in severe systemic lupus erythematosus. *J Autoimmun* 1998;11:495–501.
66. Kutsuki H, Takata S, Yamamoto K, et al. Therapeutic selective adsorption of anti-DNA antibody using dextran sulfate cellulose column (Selesorb) for the treatment of systemic lupus erythematosus. *Ther Apheresis* 1998;2:18–24.
67. Klinman D, Elias K, Shak S, et al. Dnase treatment of DNA-anti-DNA immune complexes in SLE. *Arthritis Rheum* 1996;39 (suppl):S309.
68. Davis JC, Manzi S, Yarboro C, et al. Recombinant human DNaseI (rhDNase) in patients with lupus nephritis. *Lupus* 1999;8:68–76.
69. van Bruggen MCJ, Kramers C, Walgreen B, et al. Nucleosomes and histones are present in glomerular deposits in human lupus nephritis. *Nephrol Dial Transplant* 1997;12:57–66.
70. van Bruggen MCJ, Walgreen B, Rijke RPM, et al. Heparin and heparinoids prevent the binding of immune complexes containing nucleosomal antigens to the GBM and delay nephritis in MRL/lpr mice. *Kidney Int* 1996;50:1555–1564.
71. Gaynor B, Putterman C, Valadon P. Peptide inhibition of glomerular deposition of an anti-DNA antibody. *Proc Natl Acad Sci USA* 1997;94:1955–1960.
72. Monia H, Holers VM, Li B, et al. Markedly impaired humoral immune response in mice deficient in complement receptors 1 and 2. *Proc Natl Acad Sci USA* 1996;93:3357–3361.
73. Matis LA, Rollins SA. Complement-specific antibodies: designing novel anti-inflammatories. *Nature Med* 1995;1:839–842.
74. Wang Y, Hu O, Madre JA. Amelioration of lupus-like autoimmune disease in NZB/W F1 mice after treatment with a blocking monoclonal antibody specific for complement component C5. *Proc Natl Acad Sci USA* 1996;93:8563–8568.
75. Clynes R, Dumitru C, Ravetch JV. Uncoupling of immune complex formation and kidney damage in autoimmune glomerulonephritis. *Science* 1998;279:1052–1054.
76. Watanabe H, Sherris D, Gilkeson GS. Soluble CD16 in the treatment of murine lupus nephritis. *Clin Immunol Immunopathol* 1998;88:91–95.
77. Levy Y, Sherer Y, Ahmed A, et al. A study of 20 SLE patients with intravenous immunoglobulin—clinical and serologic response. *Lupus* 1999;8:705–712.
78. Williams RC, Malone CC, Silvestris F. Eluates from anti-DNA-id affinity columns containing F4+, 3I+, 8.12+ and 16/6+ human IgG myelomas produce specific anti-Id antibodies from intravenous immunoglobulins. *Arthritis Rheum* 1996;39:S307.
79. Hahn BH, Elbling FM. Idiotype restriction in murine lupus: high frequency of three public idiotypes on serum IgG in nephritic NZB/W F1 mice. *J Immunol* 1987;138:2110–2118.
80. Feldmann M, Brennan FM, Maini RN. Role of cytokines in rheumatoid arthritis. *Annu Rev Immunol* 1996;14:397–440.
81. Jacob CO, McDevitt HO. Tumour necrosis factor-alpha in murine autoimmune lupus nephritis. *Nature* 1988;331:356–358.
82. Yokoyama H, Kreft B, Kelley VR. Biphasic increase in circulating and renal TNF-alpha in MRL-lpr mice with differing regulatory mechanisms. *Kidney Int* 1995;47:122–130.
83. Brennan DC, Yui MA, Wuthrich RP, et al. Tumor necrosis factor and IL-1 in New Zealand Black/White mice. Enhanced gene expression and acceleration of renal injury. *J Immunol* 1989;143:3470–3475.
84. Moore KJ, Yeh K, Naito T, et al. TNF-alpha enhances colony-stimulating factor-1-induced macrophage accumulation in autoimmune renal disease. *J Immunol* 1996;157:427–432.
85. Le Hir M, Haas C, Marino M, et al. Prevention of crescentic glomerulonephritis induced by anti-glomerular membrane antibody in tumor necrosis factor-deficient mice. *Lab Invest* 1998; 78:1625–1631.
86. Studnicka-Benke A, Steiner G, Petera P, et al. Tumour necrosis factor alpha and its soluble receptors parallel clinical disease and autoimmune activity in systemic lupus erythematosus. *Br J Rheumatol* 1996;35:1067–1074.
87. Charles PJ, Smeenk RJT, DeJong J, et al. Assessment of antibodies to double-stranded DNA induced in rheumatoid arthritis patients following treatment with infliximab, a monoclonal antibody to tumor necrosis factor alpha: findings in open-label and randomized placebo-controlled trials. *Arthritis Rheum* 2000;43:2383–2390.
88. Smolen JS, Steiner G, Breedveld FC, et al. Anti-TNF alpha therapy and drug-induced lupus-like syndrome. *Ann Rheum Dis* 1999;58(suppl):S217.
89. Enbrel (Etanercept) package insert. Immunex Corporation, Seattle, WA.
90. Su X, Zhou T, Yang P, et al. Reduction of arthritis and pneumonitis in motheaten mice by soluble tumor necrosis factor receptor. *Arthritis Rheum* 1998;41:139–149.
91. Deguchi Y, Kishimoto S. Tumour necrosis factor/cachectin plays a key role in autoimmune pulmonary inflammation in lupus-prone mice. *Clin Exp Immunol* 1991;85:392–395.
92. Schorlemmer HU, Kanzy EJ, Langner KD, et al. Immunoregulation of SLE-like disease by the IL-1 receptor:disease modifying activity on BDF1 hybrid mice and MRL autoimmune mice. *Agents Actions* 1993;39(spec no):C117–120.
93. Hong NM, Masuko-Hongo K, Sasakawa H, et al. Amelioration of lymphoid hyperplasia and hypergammaglobulinemia in lupus-prone mice (gld) by Fas-ligand gene transfer. *J Autoimmun* 1998;11:301–307.
94. Raz E, Dudlet J, Lotz M, et al. Modulation of disease activity in murine systemic lupus erythematosus by cytokine gene delivery. *Lupus* 1995;4:286–292.
95. Khaled AR, Soares LS, Butfiloski EJ, et al. Inhibition of NFκB pathways: p50 antisense reduces anti-dsDNA by 90% in BXSB. *Clin Immunol Immunopathol* 1997;83:254–263.
96. Sato EL, Assis LS, Lourenzi VP, et al. Long-term thalidomide use in refractory cutaneous lesions of systemic lupus erythematosus. *Rev Assoc Med Bras* 1998;44:289–293.
97. Moreira AL, Sampaio EP, Zmuidzinas A. Thalidomide exerts its inhibitory action on TNF-α by enhancing mRNA degradation. *J Exp Med* 1993;177:1675–1680.
98. Smolen JS, Kalden JR, Scott DL, et al. Efficacy and safety of leflunomide compared with placebo and sulphasalazine in active rheumatoid arthritis: a double-blind, randomised, multicentre trial. European Leflunomide Study Group. *Lancet* 1999; 353:259–266.
99. Bartlett RR, Dimitrijevic M, Mattar T, et al. Leflunomide (HWA 486), a novel immunomodulating compound for the

treatment of autoimmune disorders and reactions leading to transplantation rejection. *Agents Actions* 1991;32:10–21.

100. Manna SK, Aggarwal BB. Immunosuppressive leflunomide metabolite (A77 1726) blocks TNF-dependent nuclear factor-kappa B activation and gene expression. *J Immunol* 1999;162: 2095–2102.
101. Petera P, Manger B, Manger K, et al. A pilot study of leflunomide in systemic lupus erythematosus (SLE). *Arthritis Rheum* 2000;43(suppl):S241.
102. Tallman MS, Peterson LC, Hakimian D, et al. Treatment of hairy-cell leukemia: current views. *Semin Hematol* 1999;36:155–163.
103. Davis JC Jr, Austin H 3rd, Boumpas D, et al. A pilot study of 2-chloro-2′-deoxyadenosine in the treatment of systemic lupus erythematosus-associated glomerulonephritis. *Arthritis Rheum* 1998;41:335–343.
104. Gaubitz M, Schorat A, Schotte H, et al. Mycophenolate mofetil for the treatment of systemic lupus erythematosus: an open pilot trial. *Lupus* 1999;8:731–736.
105. Dooley MA, Cosio FG, Nachman PH, et al. Mycophenolate mofetil therapy in lupus nephritis. Clinical observations. *J Am Soc Nephrol* 1999;10:833–839.
106. Lee JC, Kassis S, Kumar S, et al. p38 mitogen-activated protein kinase inhibitors-mechanisms and therapeutic potentials. *Pharmacol Ther*1999;82:389–397.
107. Schwartz RS. The new immunology—the end of immunosuppressive therapy? *N Engl J Med* 1999;340:1754–1756.

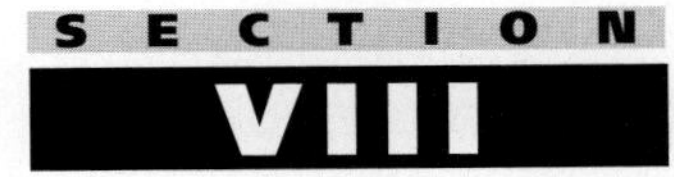

APPENDICES

APPENDIX I

A PATIENT'S GUIDE TO LUPUS ERYTHEMATOSUS[1]

DANIEL J. WALLACE
BEVRA HANNAHS HAHN
FRANCISCO P. QUISMORIO, JR.

PURPOSE OF THIS APPENDIX

When first told they have lupus erythematosus (LE), many patients have never before heard the term. This appendix is intended to help you understand what lupus is, how it may affect your life, and what you can do to help both yourself and your physician in the management of the illness. It will not replace your physician's advice. Because each case of LE is different, only your physician can answer specific questions about your individual situation. It is hoped that by learning facts about LE in nontechnical terms, you may increase your knowledge of the disease. In addition to explaining what lupus is, we have tried to answer other questions that you, your relatives, and your friends may have, such as what causes LE, the difference between cutaneous LE (CLE) and systemic LE (SLE), how the diagnosis is made, and how the illness is treated.

We use easy-to-understand terms throughout this appendix. We also have provided a glossary at the end to explain the more complicated words.

Because many of the most significant studies of LE are fairly recent and are constantly in various stages of exciting change and progress, much of the information that is available is already out of date. If you look up LE in an encyclopedia or medical book, you likely will be confused and maybe even frightened. You do not need to be frightened, and it may interfere with your seeking proper diagnosis and treatment.

A BRIEF HISTORY OF LE

Lupus means wolf in Latin, and *erythematosus* means redness. The name was first given to the disease because it was thought that the skin damage resembled the bite of a wolf.

LE has been known to physicians since 1828, when it was first described by the French dermatologist Biett. Early studies were simply descriptions of the disease, with emphasis on the skin changes. Forty-five years later, a dermatologist named Kaposi noted that some patients with LE skin lesions showed signs that the disease affected internal organs.

In the 1890s, Sir William Osler, a famed U.S. physician, observed that systemic LE (also called SLE) could affect internal organs without the occurrence of skin changes.

In 1948, Dr. Malcolm Hargraves of the Mayo Clinic described the LE cell, which is a particular cell found in the blood of patients with SLE. His discovery enabled physicians to identify many more cases of LE by using a simple blood test. As a result, the number of SLE cases that have been diagnosed during the succeeding years has steadily risen. Since 1954, various unusual proteins (or antibodies) that act against the patient's own tissues have been found to be associated with SLE. Detection of these abnormal proteins has been used to develop more sensitive tests for SLE [i.e., antinuclear antibody (ANA) tests]. The presence of these antibodies may result from factors other than SLE.

WHAT IS LE?

LE usually appears in one of two forms: (1) cutaneous lupus erythematosus (the skin form, CLE); or (2) systemic lupus erythematosus (the internal form, SLE).

Chronic cutaneous lupus (CLE, formerly known as discoid lupus) LE has a particular type of skin rash with raised, red, scaly areas, often with healing in the centers or with scars. These eruptions most commonly are seen on the face and other light-exposed areas. Usually, patients with DLE have normal internal organs. A skin biopsy of the lesion may be helpful in confirming the diagnosis.

Subacute cutaneous lupus erythematosus is a nonscarring subset of lupus that is characterized by distinct immunologic abnormalities and some systemic features.

[1]The material in this appendix has been revised and adapted several times from the original pamphlet by Dubois EL and Cox MB (*Lupus Erythematosus*) in 1976. Copies of this appendix are available from the Lupus Foundation of America and complimentary disks from Dr. Wallace upon request.

SLE is classified as one of the autoimmune rheumatic diseases, in the same family as rheumatoid arthritis, and usually is considered to be a chronic, systemic, inflammatory disease of connective tissue. Chronic means that the condition lasts for a long period of time. Inflammatory describes the body's reaction to irritation with pain and swelling. LE involves changes in the immune system, so that elements of the system attack the body's own tissues. Different organs are affected in each person, and joints usually are inflamed. Inflammation also can involve the skin, kidney, blood cells, brain, heart, lung, and blood vessels. The inflammation can be controlled by medication.

SLE can be a mild condition, but because it can affect joints, skin, kidneys, blood, heart, lungs, and other internal organs, it can appear in different forms and with different intensities at different times in the same person. A large number of people with SLE have few symptoms and can live a nearly normal life. Therefore, while reading about the symptoms, you should not become unnecessarily worried, because all of the symptoms usually do not occur in one person.

How serious lupus is varies greatly from a mild to a life-threatening condition. It depends on which parts of the body are affected. Even a mild case can become more serious if it is not properly treated. (The results usually are good with use of the more recently developed medicines.) The severity of your LE should be discussed with your physician.

In addition to CLE and SLE, there are other variants of lupus. *Drug-induced lupus* afflicts 15,000 Americans each years and results from over 70 different drugs. Fortunately, it goes away when the medicine is discontinued. *Neonatal lupus* reflects the presence of a lupus rash or abnormal heart pacing system in a newborn whose mother has certain lupus autoantibodies. The rash disappears within a few weeks and the children do not have lupus. *Mixed connective tissue disease* or *crossover or overlap* syndromes imply the presence of lupus as well as another autoimmune disorder such as scleroderma (i.e., hardening and thickening of the skin), rheumatoid arthritis or polymyositis (i.e., inflammation of the muscles). Finally, *undifferentiated connective tissue disease* (UCTD) patients often have features of lupus, such as a positive ANA with swollen joints, but do not fulfill the criteria for SLE. Over time, one third evolve lupus or another autoimmune disorder, one third stay as a UCTD, and the process disappears in another third. LE is not infectious or contagious. It is not a type of cancer or malignancy. LE is not related to acquired immunodeficiency syndrome (AIDS).

FREQUENCY OF LE

No one has made an accurate estimate of the number of patients with CLE because many people have mild cases and probably don't know it. There may be as many as 1 million people with SLE in the United States.

The number of new cases of SLE diagnosed by physicians is definitely increasing, for several reasons. After the LE cell test came into use, physicians were able to diagnose the illness correctly in patients who were believed to have other rheumatic diseases, or who were thought to have neurotic complaints. Tests for ANAs and other antibodies, which usually are positive in SLE, have helped physicians to discover even more patients with milder cases, but the tests might be positive in patients without SLE.

Seven of ten patients with CLE and 90% with SLE are women, most of them developing their first symptoms between 15 and 30 years of age. LE is rare in children under the age of 5. It is found throughout the world, however, and affects all ethnic groups and religions.

SLE is more common than rheumatic fever, leukemia, cystic fibrosis, muscular dystrophy, multiple sclerosis, hemophilia, and several other well-known diseases.

WHAT CAUSES LE?

The cause of CLE is unknown. In most cases, the cause of SLE also is unknown, although it is believed that many factors may be involved, including genetic predisposition and environmental factors such as excessive sun exposure, certain medicines, and infections. In families of patients with SLE, it is known that there is an increase in the number of relatives with SLE and rheumatoid arthritis compared with the normal population. Many of the relatives have abnormal proteins, such as ANAs, in their blood, although they may not have any symptoms of the disease.

Some of the genes that increase a person's risk for SLE are known. For example, in the United States, a gene called DR2 increases a person's risk of developing lupus nephritis, although the vast majority of individuals with the gene are healthy.

Many researchers suspect that a special type of immune reaction causes the disease. It is believed that patients develop antibodies against their own tissues, as if they have been vaccinated against themselves. These antibodies are known as autoantibodies ("auto" means self), and the type of allergy is called autoimmunity (or an allergy against oneself). Some of us possess lupus genes. Certain viruses, drugs, chemicals in the environment, or extreme emotional stress might activate the gene. This gene encodes antibodies and/or other products that damage tissue, the net effect of which results in the white blood cells' (i.e., lymphocytes) surveillance system ultimately stimulating the formation of antibodies. Still, the basic question that remains unanswered is what events set off the mechanism that causes antibodies to be produced against one's own tissues. Answering this question may be an important step toward preventing and curing LE.

In perhaps 10% of patients with SLE-type symptoms, the disease may have been caused by medications. The most common of these is procainamide (Pronestyl), which often is used to treat heart irregularities. It is essential that your physician be told of all medications you are taking, including birth control pills and estrogens for menopause, as well as medications purchased over the counter or at health-food stores. Sometimes, medication can flare lupus; for example, sulfa antibiotics can make you more sun sensitive and susceptible to developing rashes.

DIAGNOSIS

The skin rash of CLE may be so typical that an experienced doctor can make the diagnosis by the history and appearance of the rash. If there is any question, a skin biopsy usually helps. It is essential that each patient with CLE have a thorough physical examination, including laboratory tests, to check the possibility of SLE being present.

Diagnosing SLE is more difficult. Finding a definite answer may take months of observation, many laboratory tests, and sometimes a trial of drugs. Because of many different symptoms, some patients are thought to have another disease, rheumatoid arthritis, with swelling of a few or many joints of the hands, feet, ankles, or wrists. If typical skin lesions are present, they are helpful in making the diagnosis. Other findings, such as fever, pleurisy (i.e., painful breathing), or kidney disease, also point to the diagnosis of SLE.

In addition to a complete medical history and physical examination, routine tests are done to learn what internal organs are involved, for example, a blood count to see if there are too few red cells, white cells, or platelets (i.e., cells that are necessary for clotting). A routine analysis of the urine is always done, and a kidney function test using all urine passed in a 24-hour period often is necessary. A chest radiograph and electrocardiogram may be recommended if clinical evidence of problems in the lung or heart is found.

DIAGNOSTIC CRITERIA AND AUTOANTIBODY TESTING

In 1997, the American College of Rheumatology established new diagnostic criteria for SLE. After excluding rheumatoid arthritis, scleroderma, and polymyositis, a diagnosis of SLE can be made if four of the following 11 criteria are met:

1. Butterfly rash on cheeks
2. Cutaneous (discoid) lupus
3. Sensitivity to sunlight
4. Mouth or nose sores
5. Arthritis (i.e., swelling or inflammation of several joints)
6. More than 0.5 g of protein in the urine per day, or cellular casts in a urinalysis
7. Seizures or psychosis
8. Pleuritis or pericarditis
9. Low white blood count, low platelet count, or hemolytic anemia
10. Antibody to DNA or to Sm antigen (i.e., a fairly specific antibody found in about one fourth of patients with lupus), or to antiphospholipid antibody (a false-positive syphilis test, anticardiolipin antibody, or lupus anticoagulant)
11. Positive ANA test

To help confirm the diagnosis, special tests for SLE are performed that measure blood antibodies. These include examinations for ANA, which is the most sensitive test for the disease. Serum complement (i.e., a protein that is decreased during active phases of autoimmune illness) often is measured. Anti-DNA antibody is a specific type of ANA that often is present in the blood of patients with SLE; its presence is helpful in confirming the diagnosis of SLE. Moreover, when the disease is active, especially if the kidneys are affected in SLE, anti-DNA antibodies usually are present in high amounts in the blood. Thus, tests for anti-DNA antibody can be useful in monitoring disease activity in SLE. Again, none of these tests is specific for SLE, and different medical centers may use other diagnostic tests depending on their individual experience tests; consequently, obtaining such a result does not confirm the diagnosis of SLE. All tests must be evaluated by the physician in regard to the signs and symptoms of the patient. Table APPI.1 lists some of the

TABLE APPI.1. PRINCIPAL IMMUNE SEROLOGIES AND THEIR VALUE IN SLE

Autoantibody	% in SLE	% in Normals	Comment
Antinuclear	98	5–10	If absent, it's probably not lupus
Anti-DNA	50	<1	Suggests more serious disease
Anti-Sm	25	<1	The most specific test for lupus
Anti-RNP	25	<1	Many also have MCTD
Antiphospholipid	33	5	1/3 have thromboembolic events
Anti-Ro/SSA	30	<1	Associated with Sjögren's, neonatal lupus, sun sensitivity
Anti-La/SSB	15	<1	Always seen with anti-Ro; may diminish pathogenicity of anti-Ro
Antineuronal	20	<1	Putative marker for CNS vasculitis
Antiribosomal P	20	<1	Seen with psychosis, hepatitis
Low serum complement	50	5	Decreased with inflammation

MCTD, mixed connective tissue disease.

autoantibodies ordered by musculoskeletal specialists concerned about diagnosing or following SLE.

Some patients with a negative ANA may still have SLE. Usually, these patients have anti-Ro/SSA antibody or a positive, nonlesional (i.e., skin that looks normal) skin biopsy using immunofluorescence (i.e., lupus band test). Patients with CLE often have a negative ANA and a positive biopsy from the skin rash.

RESEMBLANCE TO OTHER DISEASES

One problem in diagnosis is that there is no single set of symptoms or pattern of disease. Also, SLE can mimic the symptoms of many other diseases, such as cancers, infections, and hormonal problems, and it can strike many different parts of the body, sometimes confusing even the most experienced physicians. The musculoskeletal pain of SLE often is difficult to differentiate from a syndrome known as fibromyalgia. Formerly termed fibrositis, fibromyalgia is associated with poor sleeping habits, fatigue, tension headaches, numbness and tingling, and irritable bowel symptoms, in addition to spasm and pain in the muscles, especially in the upper neck and back.

SYMPTOMS AND COURSE

The patient with SLE may have periods of severe illness (i.e., flare or exacerbation) with extreme symptoms, intermingled with periods of no illness and complete freedom from symptoms (i.e., remission). The illness comes and goes so unpredictably that no two cases are alike. Even before the discovery of corticosteroids, some patients made a full recovery with treatment by aspirin and rest alone. Although causes for disease flare-ups may be recognized and prevented by the patient, at other times their cause is unknown. Some possibly preventable causes of flare-ups are excessive sun exposure, injuries, insufficient rest, stopping medications that have been controlling the disorder, irregular living habits, and emotional crises. It cannot be emphasized too strongly that abruptly stopping medication, particularly large doses of corticosteroid derivatives such as prednisone, can lead to severe flare of the disease or even a fatal outcome.

SYMPTOMS OF THE DISORDER

The symptoms of SLE are varied, and no two patients have exactly the same ones. Any part of the body can be involved, so symptoms may include one or more of the following in any combination: joint and muscle pain, fever, skin rashes, chest pain, swelling of hands and feet, and hair loss (Fig. APPI.1). Joint involvement in SLE usually is less severe than that occurring in rheumatoid arthritis and usually is nondeforming. You should remember that in most patients, most of the symptoms disappear. This clearing of symptoms is called a remission. Medications usually are necessary to cause remissions, but sometimes they occur spontaneously (i.e., without treatment).

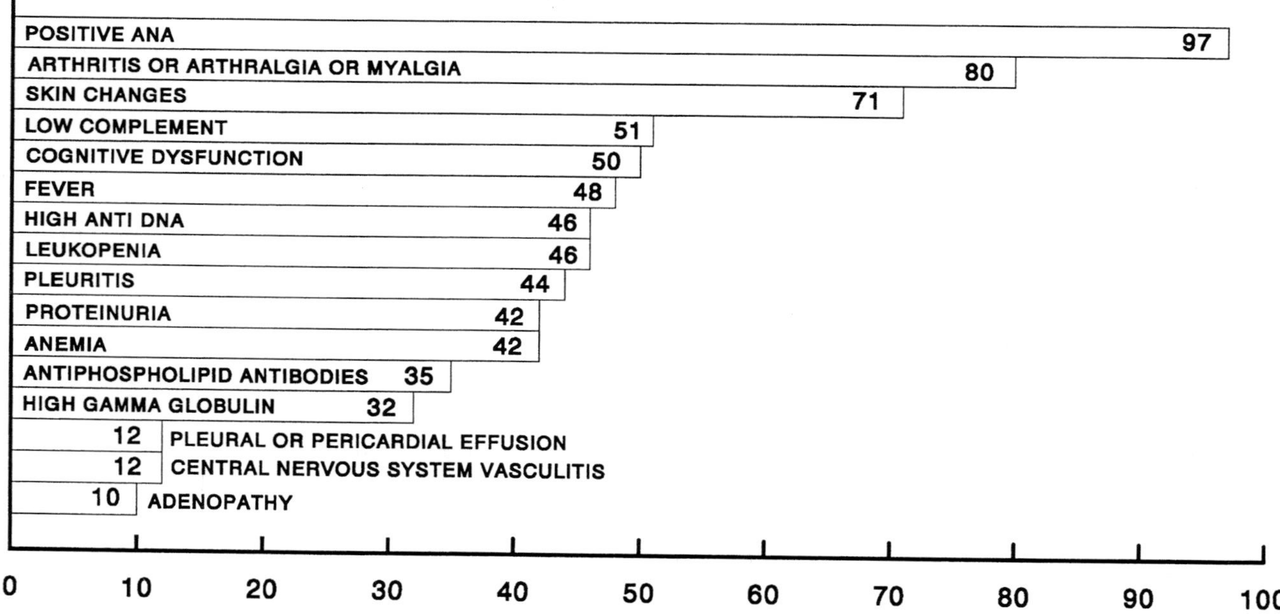

FIGURE APPI.1. Cumulative percentage incidence of 16 clinical and laboratory manifestations of systemic lupus erythematosus (SLE) based on major studies involving nearly 2,000 patients evaluated in seven studies since 1975.

Physicians use the term *remission* or *controlled* rather than *cure* in speaking of the periods when patients are free of symptoms, because both doctors and patients then can be watchful for signs and symptoms, which may be a warning that a flare is beginning. Treatment then can be started before unnecessary damage occurs.

GENERAL SYMPTOMS

Generalized aching, weakness, tiring easily, low-grade fever, and chills commonly are associated with active SLE. Although these symptoms usually are particularly noticeable during flare-ups of the disease, some patients give a lifelong history of low energy, malaise (i.e., generalized discomfort), and inability to keep up an active work schedule. A low-grade rise in temperature (99.5° to 100.5°F), usually in the late afternoon, may be a sign of smoldering LE activity and may appear several days before the patient feels really ill. In the patient with SLE, loss of energy, development of weakness, low-grade fever, or tiring easily is each considered to be a danger sign. It may indicate that new activity of the disease is developing. When any of these early warning signs develop, patients should consult their physician immediately, so that an examination can be made and further treatment prescribed if necessary.

The following symptoms and signs are typically found in SLE:

1. **Skin**: A reddish rash or flush may appear involving the cheeks and nose in a so-called butterfly pattern. Other eruptions resembling CLE may occur in light-exposed areas of the body. Some patients are particularly sensitive to cold. After exposure to cold, the skin of their hands and feet may show several distinctive changes in color. Other patients may notice red, scaling changes on the back of the hands and on the fingers between the knuckles. Small areas of scarring on the scalp may produce baldness, and small red areas on the lips and the lining of the mouth may be related to SLE. Some patients have a definite sensitivity to ultraviolet rays of the sun, and even small amounts of sunlight may make these patients much worse. Easy bruising or pinpoint bleeding into the skin sometimes is related to SLE.
2. **Chest**: Pleurisy, or irritation of the membranes lining the chest, causes painful breathing and is common in patients with SLE. Shortness of breath or rapid heartbeat sometimes is a related symptom. There may be an accumulation of fluid in the chest cavity from inflammatory changes.
3. **Muscular system**: Tiring easily and weakness often are the first symptoms of SLE. Indeed, without these complaints, the diagnosis of systemic involvement in LE is open to doubt. Because they also are common in many other diseases and with plain nervous exhaustion, it is best to let your physician decide on their importance. Weakness occasionally can be caused by corticosteroid drugs. In these cases, a change in medication dose or type often is all that is necessary to return muscle strength.
4. **Bones and joints**: Arthritis, joint swelling, and stiffness are common signs of SLE activity. These may involve only one joint, may move from one region to another, or, rarely, may progress to a deforming arthritis. This, however, rarely is disabling, and it is less frequent than in rheumatoid arthritis. Softening of bone (i.e., osteoporosis) can result from physical inactivity when you are ill and from corticosteroid drugs. Strategies are available to reduce these effects, including calcium, vitamin D, bisphosphonates, and hormonal replacement therapies for menopause.
5. **Blood**: Anemia, or a low red-blood-cell count, is common in patients with LE. There may be a decrease in white blood cells, usually to around 2,500 to 4,000 per mL (normal is 4,500 to 10,000 per mL). The blood platelets, which are necessary for clotting, may become affected. Frequently, abnormalities of proteins in the blood are present as well; sometimes, a false-positive reaction for syphilis occurs when the blood is tested. Of course, this does not mean that the patient has syphilis, because this false reaction is only a manifestation of SLE.
6. **Heart**: In some patients with SLE, swelling of the feet and ankles may occur, as well as shortness of breath or difficulty in breathing after exertion or when lying down. These symptoms may mean that the heart is affected. Fluid may collect in the pericardial sac surrounding the heart; sometimes heart muscle or valves become inflamed. The patient should remember that LE involvement does not always damage the heart permanently, because such changes disappear completely with treatment.
7. **Stomach and intestinal tract**: Pain in the abdomen, nausea, vomiting, diarrhea, or constipation sometimes are associated with SLE. These symptoms may be so severe as to imitate acute appendicitis, a stone in the kidney, or some other condition requiring surgical treatment. If these symptoms appear, it is important for the patient to tell the surgeon that he or she has SLE as well as the type and dosage of medication being taken.
8. **Kidney and bladder**: The kidney serves as the filtering plant of the body, filtering out waste products while preserving the many chemical parts of the blood that are essential for good health. Involvement of the kidney by SLE may cause loss into the urine of some of these essential chemical components, and there may be poor excretion of the waste products that usually are discarded in the urine. Retention and accumulation of the waste products can produce further symptoms that

may require specialized treatment. The development of SLE kidney involvement is painless and should be checked by urinalysis every few months. Kidney biopsy (i.e., removal of a bit of tissue for study under the microscope) may be helpful in confirming the diagnosis or choice of treatment.

9. **Lymph glands, spleen, and liver**: Occasionally, the lymph glands of the neck, under the arms, and in the groin become enlarged. The spleen (an internal organ) also may become enlarged, and SLE hepatitis (i.e., an inflammation of the liver) sometimes develops.
10. **Nervous system** (brain, spinal cord, and nerves): Temporary seizures that resemble epilepsy may be early evidence of SLE, and the diagnosis of SLE is suggested only after other symptoms appear. Mental depression, excitability, unusual worry, headache, mental confusion, forgetfulness, nerves, or even a nervous breakdown can be caused by SLE. Some patients have transient paralysis, stroke, neuritic pains, or poor bladder control related to their disease. Cognitive impairment (difficulty in thinking clearly) is common.
11. **Menstrual periods**: Menstrual periods may become irregular, more or less frequent, or even stop completely for several months. This usually is related to the activity of SLE or to side effects of glucocorticosteroids. When the disease is brought under control, menstrual periods may return to normal.

Thus, a wide range and variety of symptoms may announce the onset of SLE. Some patients, through the entire course of their illness, have symptoms involving only one organ. Others may have symptoms that come and go, and some may begin with one group of symptoms and acquire others as new parts of the body become involved with the SLE process. Remember that before the discovery of cortisone derivatives, 40% of patients improved with rest and aspirin alone.

OTHER CONSIDERATIONS

Early warnings that may indicate a flare-up include chills, fatigue, loss of pep, new symptoms, and fever, such as change from the normal daily temperature to a slight afternoon fever of 99.5° to 100.5°F. If any of these changes occur, the physician should be notified.

The patient with SLE generally can return to his or her regular occupation. Usually, after the illness is well controlled, it does not interfere with full-time work as long as the patient does not become too tired or stressed.

Childbearing

Patients with SLE usually can have successful pregnancies, provided they do not have too much kidney or heart disease. Although many women with SLE feel better during pregnancy, an occasional flare-up can occur. Physicians cannot predict the effect of pregnancy on a particular individual. Whether pregnancy is advisable in your own case should be discussed with your physician before you become pregnant.

Patients with DLE usually have no problems with pregnancy. The safety of many common medications in pregnancy, however, is not well established. Glucocorticoids (i.e., steroids) generally are safe for the fetus and can be continued throughout pregnancy and delivery if needed for disease control. Nonsteroidal antiinflammatory drugs (NSAIDs) and high-dose aspirin should be stopped. Antimalarials are controversial; it may be safest to discontinue them. Active SLE is associated with fetal loss.

A subset of patients with LE and antiphospholipid antibodies (especially those with high levels of anticardiolipin antibody) has been shown to have spontaneous recurrent fetal loss. They also may be at risk for developing blood clots. Children of mothers with SLE who have Ro/SSA antibody are at a slight risk for developing neonatal lupus or congenital heart block.

Contraception

The safest methods of contraception are the use of barrier methods such as diaphragm and jelly, foam, sponges, or condoms. Although birth control pills are safely used by many patients with SLE, the incidence of pill-related complications appears to be higher in these patients than in the normal user, especially in individuals with migraine headaches, high blood pressure, very high cholesterol, and antiphospholipid antibodies. Intrauterine devices are not advisable because of the high incidence of infections connected with their use.

Hormone Replacement Therapy

When women with SLE enter the menopause, either naturally or from the chemotherapy-type medications that sometimes are used to treat SLE, the question of taking estrogen and/or progesterone type hormones arises. Advantages include controlling hot flashes, prevention of dryness and mood swings, and reduced risk of heart attacks, osteoporosis, and fractures. Disadvantages include risking a lupus flare, risks of increased clotting and gallstones, weight gain, fluid retention, and higher blood pressure, as well as a slightly increased risk for breast cancer. Women with lupus and their doctors should weigh the pros and cons before starting this treatment. Treatment always can be stopped if problems do occur.

TREATMENT OF LE

Several effective methods of treatment are available. Unfortunately, all of the medications that are used to treat SLE, including regular aspirin, have some potential dangers, but we must use them, optimally at low levels and for a short time. The one to be used in a particular individual depends entirely on the type of LE that is present. Patients with CLE may be treated with creams or ointments containing corticosteroid medications and sunscreens. With more extensive skin changes, antimalarial drugs often are effective.

Treatment usually is required for months. Stopping medication may produce a flare of skin lesions.

SLE is managed by local treatment for any skin eruptions plus various medications taken by mouth for symptoms such as arthritis, fever, rash, and kidney disease.

Aspirin And NSAIDs (Nonsteroidal Antiinflammatory Drugs)

Aspirin and NSAIDs are not merely pain killers. When taken regularly and as often as prescribed, such as 8 to 16 five-grain tablets daily for adults, aspirin frequently controls fever, pleurisy (i.e., painful breathing), and joint discomfort. Aspirin and NSAIDs should be used with caution in patients who have had stomach ulcers; rarely, internal bleeding may result. When possible, it is advisable to stop these medications 1 week before surgery because of their tendency to slow down blood clotting. Taking the tablets with food often eliminates the stomach upsets that some patients experience. Antacids and a class of drugs known as H2 blockers (Tagamet, Zantac, Pepcid) or prostaglandins (Cytotec) and proton pump inhibitors (Prilosec; Prevacid) frequently help to protect the stomach lining. NSAIDs such as indomethacin (Indocin), naproxen (Naprosyn), or ibuprofen (Motrin) frequently are effective for relieving joint pains as well as pain at other sites of inflammation. Patients with kidney involvement should only take NSAIDs under close medical supervision, and all patients on NSAIDs or aspirin should have blood testing at 3- to 4-month intervals. Newer generation selective COX-2 inhibiting NSAIDs (e.g., Vioxx, Celebrex) may be safer in SLE.

Antimalarial Drugs

This group of medications was first developed during World War II for the treatment of malaria when it became known that quinine, which then was standard treatment for malaria, was in short supply. It was discovered that many patients with LE, especially those who had skin changes of CLE, showed definite improvement after receiving the antimalarial drug quinacrine, although these chemicals also are helpful in systemic types of LE. It should be emphasized that there is no relationship between LE and malaria (which is caused by a small parasite transmitted by mosquitoes).

The exact mechanism of the antimalarial drugs in LE is not known, but by raising the pH of cells (i.e., making them more basic as opposed to acidic), inflammation is decreased. Immune responses also are reduced. In many patients with SLE, the antimalarials appear to make it possible to reduce the total daily dose of cortisone drugs. Another advantage of antimalarials is that they increase resistance to sun exposure and block the appearance of SLE rashes on exposure to ultraviolet light. Antimalarials are not used for the management of patients with organ-threatening involvement (e.g., heart, lungs, kidney, liver), but they are useful in managing skin, joint, and muscle symptoms, as well as fever, fatigue, and pleurisy. These agents often do not take effect for several months. Hydroxychloroquine (Plaquenil) is the only antimalarial approved by the U.S. Food and Drug Administration for lupus and is the safest agent in its class.

Side effects of antimalarials in patients with LE do not often occur, but when they do, they can be important. The most common side effects usually involve the digestive system, with mild nausea, occasional vomiting, and diarrhea. Formerly, certain antimalarials, especially chloroquine (Aralen) and hydroxychloroquine (Plaquenil), were found to affect the eyes when used in doses twice as great as those now prescribed. Therefore, to be certain that no such bad effects occur, patients who are taking these medications must have eye examinations by an ophthalmologist at regular 6- to 12-month intervals. The risk of changes in the retina with Plaquenil is 3 after 10 years of continuous use. These changes are completely reversible with discontinuation of the drug and regular monitoring. Quinacrine (Atabrine) has not been reported to cause eye complications. Any changes in vision should be called to the attention of your physician.

Corticosteroids

The corticosteroid drugs (e.g., prednisone) are used primarily for treating the internal changes that are caused by lupus. However, they also help to heal the skin.

Cortisone and, later, prednisone were the first of the corticosteroid family to be used in medicine, and both they and their successors have been lifesaving in many thousands of patients with many different diseases. They are synthetic forms of hormones that normally are produced by the adrenal glands, which are the small glands above the kidneys. In addition to the beneficial effects of corticosteroids, however, these drugs have unwanted and undesirable side effects that may produce complications when they are taken for long periods.

In some cases of SLE, the physician may choose to prescribe different types of corticosteroid drugs or to prescribe them every other day instead of daily. This method reduces side effects considerably, but it may not be satisfactory for active cases.

The chief action of corticosteroid drugs is to decrease inflammation, so that these drugs control many of the symptoms and signs of SLE that are caused by inflammatory changes (e.g., arthritis and pleurisy). The drugs may be given by mouth in the form of tablets, or by injection into the muscle or joint or directly into the vein.

Another effect of the prednisone-like drugs is their shrinking effect on the adrenal glands. This occurs because the adrenal glands may stop producing the natural hormone, which is of special importance for two reasons. First, the synthetic hormone should not be stopped suddenly, because the adrenal glands may take several months to start production of natural hormone again. A sudden withdrawal of the synthetic hormone leaves the patient without this support and may cause a serious crisis. Therefore, the dosage of corticosteroids should be reduced gradually over several weeks or months, so that the patient's adrenal glands may increase their production of the natural hormone gradually over the same period. Second, any physical or mental stress, surgical procedure, dental extraction, or severe illness may increase the patient's need for large amounts of corticosteroids. When patients have taken corticosteroids for a long time, their own adrenal glands cannot satisfy this increased need, and larger, booster doses of the synthetic drug are required.

Persons who are taking corticosteroid drugs, or those who have taken them during the previous year, should carry with them an identification card or bracelet stating this fact for emergency use (much like the card carried by the diabetic person who must take insulin, or by a person who is extremely sensitive to penicillin).

Two points must be emphasized to every patient with SLE who is taking the corticosteroid groups of drugs. First, the drug should never be stopped suddenly if it has been taken for over 30 days; it should be reduced gradually over a long period (this is best done under the direct supervision of a physician). Second, when any patient is on long-term steroid therapy, he or she may need increased booster doses of the drug before, during, and after any period of general body stresses (e.g., surgery), and he or she should tell the physician or dentist of this possibility.

Because corticosteroids have an appetite-stimulating effect, an effort should be made to avoid excessive weight gain. Damage to weight-bearing joints may occur following long-term steroid treatment and, occasionally, in some patients with untreated SLE. In addition, steroids may induce diabetes, hypertension, cataracts, glaucoma, edema, avascular necrosis, bone demineralization (i.e., osteoporosis), poor wound healing, fragile skin that tears and bruises easily, susceptibility to infections, and ulcers. If the dose of steroids is greater than 15 mg of prednisone each day, people may have increased susceptibility to infections.

Immune Suppressives

Many powerful drugs, such as immune suppressives (e.g., antibody suppressors), are used in the treatment of severe SLE; these immunosuppressive include azathioprine (Imuran), cyclophosphamide (Cytoxan), and methotrexate. These drugs most commonly are used in those with aggressive disease. Indications for these agents are the subject of a great deal of debate, both because they are toxic and their effectiveness has not always been demonstrated, and also because they may decrease steroid requirements. Evidence from the National Institutes of Health suggests that intravenous, intermittent cyclophosphamide in combination with corticosteroids represents the treatment of choice for severe lupus nephritis. Plasma exchange (i.e., plasmapheresis) is a very expensive, blood-filtering procedure whose results are only of uncertain benefit. Its use is reserved for those with life-threatening complications of lupus. Other agents that occasionally are used in LE are nitrogen mustard, retinoid derivatives, leflunomide, gamma globulin, danazol, chlorambucil, dapsone, and cyclosporine.

It is essential that once an effective treatment program has been started, the patient should continue the medication faithfully and not change it without the physician's advice. Severe flare-ups may occur suddenly in patients who stop their treatment abruptly.

COPING WITH LE: HOW CAN YOU HELP YOURSELF?

Physical Measures

1. Be careful in the sun: Two thirds of lupus patients have a problem with ultraviolet A and B (UVA and UVB) radiation from the sun. If you're going to be outside for more than 5 minutes, use a sunscreen. Choose a preparation that has a sun protection factor (SPF) of at least 15 and blocks both UVA and UVB. UVB sun exposure is greatest at midday. Perform your outdoor activities earlier in the morning or later in the afternoon or in the evening. Wear protective clothing. Ultraviolet radiation is greater at higher altitudes. The exposure one gets at sea level in 1 hour is the same that one absorbs in 5 minutes a mile up, as in Denver or Mexico City or on the ski slope.
2. Diet: Lupus patients should eat a nutritious, well-balanced diet. There are some suggestions that fish, or specifically eicosopentaneoic acid in fish oil, might have modest antiinflammatory properties. In double-blind controlled studies, eating the equivalent of two fish meals a week clearly helps rheumatoid arthritis pain. An amino acid, L-canavanine, is found in alfalfa sprouts and can activate the immune system and promote inflammation in lupus patients. Other members of the legume family have only a fraction of the L-canavanine that sprouts do and are safe to use. Lupus patients taking corticosteroids should watch their sugar, fat, and salt intake.
3. When you hurt, apply heat: Moist heat soothes painful joints. Moist heat is superior to dry heat. Hot tubs, saunas, Jacuzzis, or hot showers are useful. We advise ice

or cold applications only for acute strains or injuries for the first 36 hours.

4. General conditioning exercises: Activities such as walking, swimming, low-impact aerobics, and bicycling help prevent muscle atrophy or wasting and decrease your risk for developing thin bones, or osteoporosis. On the other hand, if your joints are swollen or you have fibromyalgia, be careful before doing a lot of weigh lifting, rowing, high-impact aerobics, or engaging in tennis, bowling, or golf. If exercises tire you easily, pace yourself with frequent rest periods.
5. Consult a rehabilitation specialist: Physical therapists assist patients in muscle strengthening programs, exercises, and gait training. Occupational therapists work to minimize stresses to painful areas, evaluate workstations (especially those with computers) to ensure proper body mechanics, and recommend a variety of assistive devices. Vocational rehabilitation counselors may train you for a job that involves less sun exposure or emphasis on repetitive motions involving an inflamed hand or other part of the body.
6. Don't smoke: Tobacco smoke contains an aromatic amine, hydrazine, which can flare cutaneous lupus. Smoking also worsens Raynaud's disease and impairs circulation to a greater extent in lupus patients that in otherwise healthy people.

Develop Preventive Coping Strategies

1. Don't let the weather psych you out: Lupus patients are sensitive to changes in barometric pressure. If the weather goes from hot to cold or wet to dry, one might be a bit achier. This will pass. The best climate for lupus patients is one with the fewest changes in the barometer.
2. Mastering fatigue: Fatigue in lupus is caused by inflammation, anemia, and chemicals known as cytokines, among other sources. Pace yourself. Have periods of activity alternating with periods of rest. Patients who stay in bed all day only become weaker. On the other hand, supermoms who put in a 20-hour day without a break can flare their disease.
3. Have a good doctor-patient relationship: Make sure that your physician is accessible and will assist you when it's important. Work out in advance what to do in case of an emergency. Will your physician advise you if pregnancy is contraindicated, whether or not you can take a birth control pill, know which antibiotics lupus patients need to be careful with, write a jury duty letter, or fill out a disability form if needed? In return, it's vital to keep your appointments, be honest with your physician, take medication as prescribed, and respect the physician's time.
4. Genetic and prognosis counseling: Women with lupus have a 10% chance of having a daughter with lupus and a 2% of having a son with the disease, although there is a 50% chance their offspring will have a positive ANA. Twenty percent of patients with non–organ-threatening SLE will evolve organ-threatening disease, usually within the first 5 years after diagnosis. Patients with non–organ-threatening disease have a near-normal life expectancy if antiphospholipid antibodies are absent. The survival of organ-threatening lupus patients is 75% at 15 years.
5. Pregnancy: 70% of lupus pregnancies are successful. Lupus patients are normally fertile but often don't conceive if they are inflamed. Kidney failure, severe hypertension, and myocarditis are relative contraindications to becoming pregnant. Patients with antiphospholipid antibodies who have miscarried may be given aspirin or heparin during a pregnancy. Mothers with anti-Ro (SSA) antibody should be advised of a 5% to 15% risk of their child being born with a transient lupus rash or a more serious heart problem that can be detected with ultrasounds at weeks 18 and 24. Find out what medicines are safe to take during a pregnancy. Most lupus activity cools down during the second trimester and mild postdelivery flares can occur.
6. Address fevers or infections promptly: Call a doctor if your temperature is over 99.6°F. It could be a lupus flare or an infection. Be careful before taking sulfa-based antibiotics, which are usually prescribed for bladder and female infections. They tend to make lupus patients more sun sensitive and can lower blood counts, and up to 30% of lupus patients are allergic to sulfa drugs.
7. Ask about cognitive therapy: Some lupus patients have difficulty remembering names and dates, balancing their checkbook, and processing thoughts. Termed cognitive dysfunction, cognitive impairment, or "lupus fog," this is a reflection of vascular spasm in that insufficient amounts of oxygen are reaching the brain. These symptoms come and go. Cognitive therapists are psychologists, speech therapists, and physical therapists who can help patients cope with this by initiating biofeedback and specific strategies that improve concentration.
8. Don't be afraid to ask for help: The Lupus Foundation of America (LFA) provides information about doctor referrals, lupus books, patient information brochures, and newsletters. Most local chapters have rap or discussion groups, sponsor guest speakers, and maintain a list of mental health professionals who can assist you. Take the SLESH (systemic lupus erythematosus self-help) course sponsored jointly by the Arthritis Foundation and the LFA.

IS THERE HOPE OF CONQUERING SLE?

There certainly is! A great deal of fast-moving research is going on throughout the world. Medical scientists are interested in SLE not only because they want to help those who suffer from it, but also because they want to find the key to other closely related rheumatic disorders, such as rheumatoid arthritis. We expect laboratory research to improve methods of treatment and, eventually, to provide a means of prevention and cure. Some of the approaches that are being studied include newer antiinflammatory therapies with COX-2 antagonists, chemicals that block or accentuate the effects of "sugar protein" or glycoprotein cytokines, hormones, vaccines with peptides, new forms of immune suppression used in transplant patients, and biologics that block specific parts of the immune system.

GLOSSARY

ACR American College of Rheumatology, a professional association of 5,000 U.S. rheumatologists, of whom 3,800 are board certified; criteria, or definitions for many rheumatic diseases, are called the ACR criteria; Formerly known as the ARA (American Rheumatism Association)

Acute Of short duration

Adrenal glands Small organs located above the kidney that produce many hormones, including corticosteroids and epinephrine

Albumin A protein that circulates in the blood and carries materials to cells

Albuminuria A protein in urine

Analgesic A drug that alleviates pain

Anemia A condition resulting from low red blood cell counts

Antibodies Special protein substances made by the body's white cells for the defense against bacteria and other foreign substances

Anticardiolipin antibody An antiphospholipid antibody

Anticentromere antibody Antibodies to a part of the cell's nucleus; associated with a form of scleroderma called CREST

Anti-DNA Antibodies to DNA; seen in one half of people with SLE and sometimes associated with disease flares and kidney disease

Anti-ENA Extractable nuclear antibodies that largely consist of anti-Sm and anti-RNP antibodies

Antigen Self or foreign substance that stimulates antibody formation

Antiinflammatory An agent that counteracts or suppresses inflammation

Antimalarials Drugs originally used to treat malaria but that are helpful for lupus, such as hydroxychloroquine, chloroquine, and quinacrine

Antinuclear antibodies (ANAs) Proteins in the blood that react with the nuclei of cells; seen in 96% of patients with SLE, 5% of healthy individuals, and in most patients with autoimmune diseases

Antiphospholipid antibody Antibodies to a constituent of cell membranes; seen in one third of patients with SLE; in the presence of a cofactor, these antibodies can alter clotting and lead to strokes, blood clots, miscarriages, and low platelet counts; also detected as the lupus anticoagulant

Anti-RNP Antibody to ribonucleoprotein; seen in SLE and mixed connective tissue disease

Anti-Sm Anti-Smith antibody; is found only in lupus

Anti-SSA Antibody associated with Sjögren's syndrome, sun sensitivity, neonatal lupus, and congenital heart block; also called the Ro antibody

Anti-SSB Antibody almost always seen with anti-SSA; also called the La antibody

Apoptosis Programmed cell death—a normal process for ridding the body of damaged cells

Artery A blood vessel that transports blood from the heart to the tissues

Arthralgia Pain in a joint

Arthritis Inflammation of a joint

Aspirin An antiinflammatory drug with analgesic properties

Autoantibody An antibody to one's own tissues or cells

Autoimmune Allergy to one's own tissues

Autoimmune hemolytic anemia See *hemolytic anemia*

B lymphocyte or B cell A white blood cell that makes antibodies

Biopsy Removal of a bit of tissue for examination under the microscope

Bursa A sac of synovial fluid between tendons, muscles, and bones that promotes easier movement

Butterfly rash Reddish facial eruption over the bridge of the nose and cheeks, resembling a butterfly in flight

Capillaries Small blood vessels connecting between arteries and veins

Cartilage Tissue material covering bone; the nose, outer ears, and trachea primarily consist of cartilage

Chronic Persisting over a long period of time

CNS Central nervous system

Collagen Structural protein found in bone, cartilage, and skin

Collagen vascular disease Antibody-mediated inflammatory process of the connective tissues, especially the joints, skin, and muscle; also called connective tissue disease

Complement A group of proteins that are activated, promote, and are consumed during inflammation

Complete blood count (CBC) A blood test that measures the amount of red blood cells, white blood cells, and platelets in the body

Connective tissue The glue that holds muscles, skin, and joints together

Corticosteroid Any natural antiinflammatory hormone made by the adrenal cortex; also can be made synthetically

Cortisone A synthetic corticosteroid

Creatinine A blood test that measures kidney function

Creatinine clearance A 24-hour urine collection that measures kidney function

CREST syndrome A form of limited scleroderma characterized by C (calcium deposits under the skin), R (Raynaud's phenomenon), E (esophageal dysfunction), S (sclerodactyly or tight skin), and T (a rash called telangiectasia)

Crossover syndrome An autoimmune process that has features of more than one rheumatic disease (e.g., lupus and scleroderma)

Cutaneous Relating to the skin

Cytokine A group of chemicals that signal cells to perform certain actions

Dermatologist A physician specializing in skin diseases

Dermatomyositis An autoimmune process directed against muscles associated with skin rashes

Discoid lupus A thick, plaque-like rash seen in 20% of patients with SLE; if patients have the rash but not SLE, they are said to have cutaneous (discoid) lupus erythematosus

DNA Deoxyribonucleic acid; the body's building blocks; a molecule responsible for the production of all the body's proteins

Enzyme A protein that accelerates chemical reactions

Erythematous Reddish hue

Estrogen Female hormone produced by the ovaries

Exacerbations Symptoms reappear; a flare

False-positive serologic test for syphilis A blood test that reveals an antibody that may be found in syphilis and is falsely positive in 15% of patients with SLE; associated with the lupus anticoagulant and antiphospholipid antibodies

FANA Another term for ANA

Fibrositis or fibromyalgia A pain amplification syndrome characterized by fatigue, a sleep disorder, and tender points in the soft tissues; can be caused by steroids and mistaken for lupus, although 20% of patients with lupus have fibrositis

Flare Symptoms reappear; another word for exacerbation

Gene Consisting of DNA, it is the basic unit of inherited information in our cells

Glomerulonephritis Inflammation of the glomerulus of the kidney; seen in one third of patients with lupus

Hematocrit A measurement of red blood cell levels; low levels produce anemia

Hemoglobin Oxygen-carrying protein of red blood cells; low levels produce anemia

Hemolytic anemia Anemia caused by premature destruction of red blood cells because of antibodies to the red blood cell surface; also called autoimmune hemolytic anemia

Hepatitis Inflammation of the liver

Hormones Chemical messengers made by the body that include thyroid, steroids, insulin, estrogen, progesterone, and testosterone

Human leukocyte antigen (HLA) Molecules inside the macrophage that binds to an antigenic peptide; controlled by genes on the sixth chromosome; they can amplify or perpetuate certain immune and inflammatory responses

Immune complex An antibody and antigen together

Immunity The body's defense against foreign substances

Immunofluorescence A means of detecting immune processes with a fluorescent stain and a special microscope

Immunosuppressive A medication, such as cyclophosphamide or azathioprine, that treats lupus by suppressing the immune system

Inflammation Swelling, heat, and/or redness resulting from the infiltration of white blood cells into tissues

Kidney biopsy Removal of a bit of kidney tissue for microscopic analysis

La antibody A Sjögren's antibody; also called anti-SSB

LE cell Specific cell found in blood specimens of most patients with lupus

Ligament A tether attaching bone to bone and giving them stability

Lupus anticoagulant A means of detecting antiphospholipid antibodies from prolonged clotting times

Lupus vulgaris Tuberculosis of the skin; not related to systemic or discoid lupus

Lymphocyte Type of white blood cell that fights infection and mediates the immune response

Macrophage A cell that kills foreign material and presents information to lymphocytes

Major histocompatibility complex (MHC) In humans, it is the same as HLA

Mixed connective tissue disease When a patient who carries the anti-RNP antibody has features of more than one autoimmune disease

Natural killer cell A white blood cell that kills other cells

Nephritis Inflammation of the kidney

Neutrophil A granulated white blood cell involved in bacterial killing and acute inflammation

NSAIDs Nonsteroidal antiinflammatory drugs, agents that fight inflammation by blocking the actions of prostaglandin; examples include ibuprofen and naproxen

Nucleus The center of a cell that contains DNA

Orthopedic surgeon A doctor who operates on musculoskeletal structures

Pathogenic Causing pathology, or abnormal reactions

Pathology Abnormal cellular or anatomic features

Pericardial effusion Fluid around the sac of the heart

Pericarditis Inflammation of the pericardium

Pericardium A sac lining the heart

Photosensitivity Sensitivity to ultraviolet light

Plasma The fluid portion of blood

Plasmapheresis Filtration of blood plasma through a machine to remove proteins that may aggravate lupus

Platelet A component of blood responsible for clotting
Pleura A sac lining the lung
Pleural effusion Fluid in the sac lining the lung
Pleuritis Irritation or inflammation of the lining of the lung
Polyarteritis A disease closely related to lupus that features inflammation of small- and medium-sized blood vessels
Polymyalgia rheumatica An autoimmune disease of the joints and muscles seen in older patients with high sedimentation rates who have severe aching in their shoulders, upper arms, hips, and upper legs
Polymyositis An autoimmune disease that targets muscles
Prednisone; prednisolone Synthetic steroids
Protein A collection of amino acids; antibodies are proteins
Proteinuria Excess protein levels in the urine; also called albuminuria
Pulse steroids Giving very high doses of corticosteroids intravenously over 1 to 3 days to critically ill patients
Raynaud's disease Isolated Raynaud's phenomenon not part of any other disease
Raynaud's phenomenon Discoloration of the hands or feet (they turn blue, white, or red, especially with cold) as a feature of an autoimmune disease
RBC Red blood cell count
Remission Quiet period, free from symptoms, but not necessarily a cure
Rheumatic disease Any of 150 disorders affecting the immune or musculoskeletal system; approximately 30 of these also are autoimmune
Rheumatoid arthritis Chronic disease of the joints marked by inflammatory changes in the joint-lining membranes, which may have positive rheumatoid factor and ANA tests
Rheumatoid factor Autoantibodies that react with immunoglobulin G (IgG) that are seen in most patients with rheumatoid arthritis and 30% of patients with SLE
Rheumatologist An internal medicine specialist who has completed at least a 2-year fellowship studying rheumatic diseases
Ro antibody See *anti-SSA*
Scleroderma An autoimmune disease featuring rheumatoid-like inflammation, tight skin, and vascular problems (e.g., Raynaud's)
Sedimentation rate Test that measures the precipitation of red cells in a column of blood; high rates usually indicate increased disease activity
Serum Clear liquid portion of the blood after removal of clotting factors
Sjögren's syndrome Dry eyes, dry mouth, and arthritis observed with most autoimmune disorders or by itself (i.e., primary Sjögren's)
Steroids Usually a shortened term for corticosteroids, which are antiinflammatory hormones produced by the adrenal cortex or synthetically
STS False-positive serologic test for syphilis
Synovial fluid Joint fluid
Synovitis Inflammation of the tissues lining a joint
Synovium Tissue that lines the joint
Systemic Pertaining to or affecting the body as a whole
T cell A lymphocyte responsible for immunologic memory
Temporal arteritis Inflammation of the temporal artery associated with high sedimentation rates, systemic symptoms, and occasionally loss of vision
Tendon Structures that attach muscle to bone
Thrombocytopenia Low platelet counts
Thymus A gland in the neck area responsible for immunologic maturity
Titer Amount of a substance, such as ANA
Tolerance The failure to make antibodies to an antigen
Uremia Marked kidney insufficiency frequently necessitating dialysis to stay alive
Urinalysis Analysis of urine
Urine, 24-hour collection All urine passed in a 24-hour period is collected and examined for protein and creatinine to determine how well the kidneys are functioning
UV light Ultraviolet light; its spectrum includes UVA (320–400 nm), UVB (290–320 nm), and UVC (200–290 nm) wavelengths
Vasculitis Inflammation of blood vessels
WBC White blood cell count

APPENDIX II

LUPUS RESOURCES FOR PATIENTS, PHYSICIANS, AND HEALTH PROFESSIONALS

COMPILED BY ELLEN IGNATIUS, JENNY THORN ALLAN, AND KAREN JOHNSON

A wide range of educational and support resources are available to patients with lupus, physicians, and other health professionals. Organizations throughout the country and around the world provide support and hope for patients. Most of these organizations disseminate lupus literature, some promote lupus research, and many provide general educational and support services to patients. A wide range of informative and encouraging literature as well as audiovisual resources that are designed for both patients and physicians are documented at the end of this appendix. They can be obtained singly from the distributors cited. Content varies from personal life-story narratives that captivate the patient to technical treatises of experimental lupus research sure to intrigue the physician. The quality and accuracy of some resource materials are questionable, however; medical information is always in a changing state.

ORGANIZATIONS IN THE UNITED STATES

American College of Rheumatology (ACR), 60 Executive Park S, Suite 150, Atlanta, GA 30329, (404) 633-3777. The ACR, formerly called the American Rheumatism Association, is a professional organization comprised of physicians and scientists (rheumatologists) as well as other health professionals. Health professionals (nurses, physical therapists, occupational therapists, and health educators) make up the Association of Rheumatology Health Professionals Division. The ACR is devoted to the study and treatment of rheumatic diseases, including lupus. The ACR publishes *Arthritis and Rheumatism* (official publication), A & R supplements, special issues, and other professionally oriented publications.

Arthritis Foundation (AF), 1314 Spring Street NW, Atlanta, GA 30309, (404) 872-7100 or 1-800-283-7800. The AF, which has approximately 72 chapters in the United States, works to help patients with rheumatic diseases and their doctors through programs of research, patient services, health information, and professional education and training. The American Juvenile Arthritis Organization (AJAO) is part of the AF. The AF publishes a basic information pamphlet on systemic lupus erythematosus (SLE) as well as pamphlets on topics relating to lupus, such as fibromyalgia, osteonecrosis, osteoporosis, Raynaud's phenomenon, corticosteroid medications, nonsteroidal antiinflammatory drugs (NSAIDs), aspirin, guide to laboratory tests, and others. The AF also publishes *Arthritis Today* (official magazine) and *Bulletin on the Rheumatic Diseases*, which is a professionally oriented newsletter. Individual chapters also publish their own newsletters. The AF also offers an SLE self-help course in selected areas of the country; this 7-week education program includes courses that provide information, skills, and support to persons with lupus and their family to help them cope with the disease.

LE Support Club, 8039 Nova Court, North Charleston, SC 29420, (803) 764-1769. The LE Support Club is a patient-oriented organization that publishes the *LE Beacon* (official newsletter), supplies information on drugs, and maintains and distributes a listing of recommended physicians. All staff members are patients with lupus themselves and will answer questions posed over the phone as best they can. The organization also maintains contact with an advisory board of medical doctors.

Lupus Foundation of America, Inc. (LFA), 1300 Piccard Drive, Suite 200, Rockville, MD 20850-3226, (301) 670-9292. LFA answering services can be reached by calling 1-800-558-0121 (English speaking) or 1-800-558-0231 (Spanish speaking). The LFA, which maintains approximately 100 chapters nationwide, provides patient education services, promotes public awareness of lupus, and funds lupus research. There also are nearly 80 LFA International Associated Groups in over 40 countries. The LFA maintains a newsletter article library containing over 190 current, medically accurate, and appropriately cited and authorized lupus-related articles on a variety of topics. Questions and concerns about lupus can be addressed over the phone by health educators at the LFA national office, and by volunteers at some local chapters. The LFA also publishes *Lupus News* (official newsletter), and local chapters distribute their own newsletters. Local chapters provide support systems for patients with lupus in the form of educational programs, support groups, social activities, and fund-raisers. These types of opportunities for proactive involvement help patients to better cope with their disease. The LFA produces the Facts About Lupus series, a series of brochures on individual topics, as well as various Fact Sheets about lupus and the LFA. Many of the brochures also are available in Spanish. All materials that are available from the LFA have been reviewed and approved by the LFA Patient Education Committee for accuracy. Several pieces of lupus-related literature approved by the Patient Education Committee also are available through the LFA (see Resource Materials section). Lists of additional lupus-related literature and materials will be provided on request.

Lupus Network, Inc. (LN), 230 Ranch Drive, Bridgeport, CT 06606, (203) 372-5795. The LN is an organization that provides information primarily to patients. It supports the sharing of information, whether unorthodox or orthodox in nature. The LN publishes *Heliogram* (official newsletter). It also has a large literature list that covers many lupus topics, such as photosensitivity, cyclophosphamide, and pregnancy.

National Arthritis and Musculoskeletal and Skin Diseases Information Clearinghouse (AMS Information Clearinghouse), 1 AMS Circle, Bethesda, MD 20892-3675, (301) 495-4484. The AMS Information Clearinghouse identifies, collects, processes, and disseminates information about print and audiovisual materials that are concerned with arthritis and musculoskeletal and skin diseases. It is used by physicians, nurses, allied-health professionals, health educators, librarians, mental-health and social workers, and patients as well as their families. The AMS Clearinghouse provides a variety of bibliographies, answers reference questions, and provides information in response to user requests. The AMS Information Clearinghouse also maintains an on-line bibliographic database of information the Combined Health Information Database (CHID) through BRS, an on-line vendor.

National Institute of Arthritis and Musculoskeletal and Skin Diseases (NIAMS), Building 31, Room 4C05, 31 Center Drive, MSC 2350, Bethesda, MD 20892-2350, (301) 496-8188. NIAMS is part of the National Institutes of Health. The NIAMS leads, coordinates, stimulates, conducts, and supports the national biomedical research effort on a broad range of diseases and long-lasting, disabling conditions in the field of rheumatology (e.g., SLE, rheumatoid arthritis), orthopedics, bone and mineral metabolism, muscle biology, and dermatology. NIAMS publishes reprints and brochures, which are available to the general public. An information packet on lupus also is available. *Research Briefings* (official publication) is sent to a select user group. A listing of NIAMS multipurpose arthritis and musculoskeletal diseases centers also is available.

INTERNATIONAL ORGANIZATIONS

There are at least 80 international lupus organizations in 41 countries, including Argentina, Australia, Barbados, Belgium, Brazil, Bulgaria, Canada, Colombia, Czech Republic, Chile, Ecuador, England, France, Germany, Holland, Ireland, Israel, Italy, Jamaica, Japan, Malaysia, Mexico, Morocco, New Zealand, Nigeria, Panama, Paraguay, Puerto Rico, Philippines, Poland, Portugal, Romania, Scotland, Singapore, South Africa, Spain, Sweden, Switzerland, and the West Indies.

Argentina

Asociacián Lupus Argentina (ALUA), Ave. Corrientes 1584 — No. 3, Buenos Aires, 1042, Argentina, +54-11-4371-4444, www.alua.org.ar or www.drwebsa.com.ar/alua

Australia

Arthritis Foundation of Queensland, P.O. Box 807, Spring Hill, Queensland, 4004, Australia

Lupus Support Group Queensland, c/o Jean Barby, Lot 134 Wilkes Rd., Hampton, Queensland 4352 Australia

Lupus Association Tasmania, PO Box 639, Launceston, Tasmania 7250, Australia, 03-6331-9940, www.microtech.com.au/lupustas

Lupus/Scleroderma Group, c/o Arthritis Foundation of South Australia, 1/202 Glen Osmond Rd., Fullarton, 5063 South Australia, 08-8379-5711

Victorian Lupus Association Attn: Enid Elton, 1-154 Balaclava Road, Caulfield, Victoria 3161, Australia, 613-9509-2735, vla@lupusvic.org.au, www.lupusvic.org.au

Lupus Association of NSW, Inc., PO Box 89, North Ryde, New South Wales, 1670, Australia, 02-9878-6055, www.lupusnsw.org.au

Belgium

Association Lupus Erythematosus, Avenue des Jardin, 62/19 B 1030 Brussels, Belgium, +32-2-726-51-52-41

Liga Voor Chronische Inflamitoire Bindweefselziekten (League for Chronic Inflammatory Connective Tissue Disease), Ganzendries 34, B 9420 Erondegem (Erpe-Mere), Belgium, +32-53-80-33-85

Bermuda

The Lupus Association of Bermuda, PO Box HM 1291, Hamilton, HM FX, Bermuda

Brazil

Lupus Society of Brazil, Rua Estela Sezefredo, 59, Sao Paulo, SP 05415, Brazil

Lupus Online, www.lupusonline.com.br.

SOS Lupus Group Rio c/o Maria Buarque, fax 0212-1562-2567 or 0312-1562-2567, *mariaconceicao@hucff.ufrj.br*

Bulgaria

LFA Chapter Phillipopolis, 2 Yosif Shniter Street, Plovdiv, 4000, Bulgaria

Canadian Provinces

Lupus Canada (the umbrella organization), P.O. Box 64034, 5512 4th St. NW, Calgary, Alberta, T2K 6J1, Canada, (800) 661-1468 (toll-free in Canada), (403) 274-5599, (phone/fax), lupuscan@cadvision.com, www.lupuscanada.org

Lupus Society of Alberta, 1301 8th St. SW, Suite 200, Calgary, Alberta, T2R 1B7 Canada, (888) 242-9182 (toll-free in AB) or (403) 228-7956, fax (403) 228-7853, lupuslsa@home.com, *www.lupus.ab.ca*

British Columbia Lupus Society, c/o Shelley Crawford, 895 West 10th Avenue, Vancouver, BC, V5Z 1L7, Canada, (604) 263-4049 or (800) 667-2847 (in British Columbia only), bclupus@telus.net

Lupus Society of Hamilton, 20 Hughson St. Suite 600A, Hamilton, Ontario, L8N 2A1 Canada, (905) 527-2252 (phone/fax), info@lupushamilton.com, www.lupushamilton.com

Lupus Society of Manitoba, Suite 105-386 Broadway Ave., Winnipeg, Manitoba R3C-3R6, Canada, (204) 942-6825

Lupus New Brunswick c/o Nancy Votour, 23-13 Ivan Court, Moncton, New Brunswick E1C 8T3 Canada, (877) 303-8080 (tol-free in NB), (506) 384-6227 (phone/fax), lupus@fundy.net

Lupus Newfoundland and Labrador, PO Box 8121 STN A, Kenmount Road, St. John's NF, A1B 3M9, Canada, (709) 368-8130, lupusnfldlab@nf.aibn.com

Lupus Society of Nova Scotia , PO Box 38038, Dartmouth, Nova Scotia, B3B 1X2, Canada, (902) 425-0358 or (800) 394-0125 (in Nova Scotia only); www.lupusNS.homestead.com

Ontario Lupus Association, 590 Alden Rd. Suite 204, Markham, Ontario L3R 8N2 Canada, (877) 240-1099 (toll-free in ON) or (905) 415-1099, fax (905) 415-9874, ola@lupusontario.org, www.lupusontario.org

Lupus Prince Edward Island, PO Box 23002, Charlottetown PE, C1E 1Z6, Canada, (902) 892-3875

Lupus Québec, 1435 St-Alexandre, Suite 1025, Montréal, Québec, H3A 2G4, Canada, (514) 849-0955

The Lupus Erythematosus Society of Saskatchewan, Box 88, Royal University Hospital, 103 Hospital Drive, Saskatoon, Saskatchewan, S7N 0W8, Canada, (306) 382-7136

China

Zhang Xin, Chief, Department of Rheumatology, Xian Fifth Hospital 710082, Xian City Shaanxi Province, Peoples Republic of China

Czech Republic

Institute of Rheumatology, Na slupi 4 128 50, Praha 2 Czech Republic

Ecuador

Fundación Lupus Eritematoso, Attention Rosario H. Solouzans de Gumsly, Checa 124 y de Agosto, Quito, Ecuador

European Lupus Erythematosus Federation (ELEF)

The members of ELEF are the national organizations of Lupus Groups in Europe. At this time, there are the following 15 countries with 16 organizations: Belgium–FL., Belgium–FR., Finland, France, Germany, Iceland, Ireland, Israel, Italy, The Netherlands, Norway, Portugal, Spain, Sweden, Switzerland, United Kingdom. The website address is www.elef.rheumanet.org.

Finland

Finnish SLE Group, Suomen Reumaliitto, SLE-jaos, Iso-Roobertinkatu 20-22A, 00120, Helsinki, Finland +358-9-476-155, www.reumaliitto.fi

France

Association Française du Lupus et autres Collagenoses (The French Association of Lupus Sufferers & Systemic Rheumatic Diseases), 25 Rue des Charmettes, F 69100 Villeurbanne France +33-04-72 74 10 86

Germany

Deutsche Rheuma-Liga Hessen, L.E. Arbeitskreis, Kohlbrandstrasse 27, D 60385 Frankfurt, Germany

Lupus Erythematodes Selbsthilfegemeinschaft e.V. (Lupus Erythematosus Self Help Association), Ottostrasse 15, D-42289 Wuppertal +49-202-55 92 94

Holland

Lupus Patienten Groep, Postbus 64833, 2506 CE Den Haag, Holland (or the Netherlands)

Nationale Vereniging LE Patienten (National Society LE Patients), Bisonspoor 3004 Holland (or the Netherlands) 3605 LV Maarssen, +31-346-55 24 01

Hungary

Magyar Lupus Egyesület-Hungarian Lupus Society, Adoszam 18157860-1-42 1152 Bpest., Epres sor 4, Hungary, 3060-6433, hsle@freestart.hu

Iceland

The Icelandic League against Rheumatism, Armuli 5, 108 Reykjavik Iceland, +354-553-07 60

Ireland

Cumann Cabhrach Lupus na hEireann (Irish Lupus Support Group Limited), c/o Dominican Day Care Centre, 37 Upper Dominic Street, Dublin 7, Ireland, +353-1-860 10 80

Irish Lupus Support Group Ltd. Cork Branch, 3, Ard Na Greine, Evergreen Rd., Co. Cork, Ireland, 021-496-1375

North Ireland Lupus Group, 10 Downview Rd., Greenisland, Carrickfergus, BT38 8RX Co. Antrim, Northern Ireland, 028-9086-6606, fax 028-9086-0784, *lupus.ni@talk21.com*

Israel

Irgun Ha-Lupus 9e-Yisrael (Israel Lupus Association), Institute of Clinical Immunology, Rambam Medical Center, Rappaport Faculty of Medicine, Haifa, Israel, +972-4-854 28 89

Italy

Gruppo Italiano per la lotta contro il lupus eritematoso sistemico (Italian Group for the Fight Against the Systemic Lupus Erythematosus), Via Arbotori. 14, I 29100 Piacenza, Italy, +39-523-75 36 43

Japan

Susumu Sugai, MD, Kanazawa Medical University, Uchinada-Machi, Kahokugun, Ishikawa-Ken 920-02, Japan

Malyasia

SLE Association of Malaysia, Jabatan Perubatan, UKM Hospital, Bandar Tun Razak, 5600 Cheras, Kuala Lumpur, Malaysia, +603-970-2375, cheng.fan@mailcity.com

Mexico

Lupus Fundacion de Mexico, c/o Dr. J. Humberto Orozco-Medina, Club de Lupus Centro Medico de Occidente, Pedro Buezeta 870-B,Tavascos 3469-306, 44660 Guadalajara, Jalisco, Mexico. +523-813-3001

Morocco

Association of Lupus Victims of Morocco, c/o Akhlij Fatna, 40 Rue des Alpes Maarif, Casablanca, Morocco

Netherlands (See Holland)

New Zealand

Lupus Association of New Zealand c/o Arthritis & Rheumatism Foundation of New Zealand, Inc., PO Box 10-020, Wellington, New Zealand

Nigeria

Lupus Awareness Association of Nigeria, Attention Agu Emmanuel Elochukwu, PO Box 30, Owelli, Awgu Local Government Area, Enugu State, Nigeria

Norway

Lupus Foreningen i NRF, Chr. Skredsviksvei 7, N-1346 Gjettum, Norway, +47-67 14 97 11

Philippines

Arthritis Foundation of the Philippines, Inc. c/o Santo Tomas University Hospital, Room 216-B, España Street, Manila, Philippines

Poland

Instytut Reumatologiczny, Attention Dr. Henryka Maldykowa, ul. spartanska 1, 02-637 Warszawa, Poland

Portugal

Associação de Doentes com Lupus (Association of Patients with Lupus), Praça Francisco, Sá Carneiro No. 11, 2/ Esq., 1000 Lisboa, Portugal, +351-1-846 44 83

Puerto Rico

Apoyo-L c/o Michael Ortiz, Del Carmen No. 7, Juana Diaz, 00795, Puerto Rico, (787) 261-6978

Romania

Clinica Dermatologica, Cluj-Napoca, str. Clinicilor nr. 3, 3400 Cluj-Napoca, Romania

Scotland

Strathclyde Lupus Group Attention Mrs. Jane Ellicott, 6 Hawkhead Road, Paisley, PA1 3NA, Scotland

Singapore

National Arthritis Foundation of Singapore, 336 Smith St. No. 06-302, New Bridge Centre, 0105, Singapore

Lupus Association of Singapore, Balestier Estate, PO Box 460, 9132 Singapore

South Africa

Lupus Support Group Network c/o Arthritis Foundation STVL Branch, PO Box 87360, Houghton, Johannesburg, 2041, South Africa

Lupus Group of South Africa, 11 Firmount St., Somerset West 7129, South Africa, 27-021-852-2992

Spain

Spanish SLE Aid Group, Hospital Clinico, Department Internal Medicina Interno, 170 Villarroel, 08036, Barcelona, Spain

Federación Española de Lupus, Lagunillas 25, locales 3 y 4, 29012, Málaga, Sapin, 952-25-08-26, lupusmalag@arquired.es

Asociation Española de Lupus (Spanish Lupus Association), c/o Martinez de la Rosa, No. 157, 1oB; Esc. Drcha., E-29010, Malaga, Spain, +34-5-261-22-11

Sweden

SLE gruppen (The SLE group), Box 12851, S-112 98 Stockholm, Sweden, +46-8-692-58-33 or -00

Switzerland

Schweizerische Lupus Erythematodes Vereinigung (Swiss Lupus Erythematosus Association), Höhenstrasse 2, CH-8304 Wallisellen, Switzerland, +41-1-830 77 00

United Kingdom

Lupus U.K., St. James House, 27-43 1, Eastern Road, Romford, Essex RM1 3NH United Kingdom +44-1708-73

West Indies

Lupus Society of Trinidad & Tobago c/o Skin Clinic, General Hospital, Charlotte Street, Port of Spain, Trinidad, West Indies

The Hope Foundation of Barbados, 112 First Avenue, Husband Gardens, St. James, Barbados, West Indies

Lupus Foundation of Jamaica, PO Box 560, Kingston 10, Jamaica, West Indies, (876) 803-0082; lupus_foundation@hotmail.com

PATIENT-ORIENTED LUPUS EDUCATIONAL MATERIALS

Informational Brochures, Fact Sheets, And Pamphlets

1. Aranow C, Weinstein A. *Non-steroidal anti-inflammatory drugs*. 2000. Six panels. Discusses the mechanism of action, use, common and uncommon side effects, and brand-name examples. Available from the Lupus Foundation of America, Inc. (301) 670-9292
2. Arthritis Foundation. *Lupus* 20 pp. Informational pamphlet on SLE. Available through the Arthritis Foundation.
3. Wallace D. *Lupus: basics for better living*. 2000. Six panels. Wellness is defined and a wellness lifestyle discussed. Attitude, fitness, nutrition, stress management, and spiritual well-being are addressed. Available from the Lupus Foundation of America, Inc. (301) 670-9292
4. Chartash E. *Cardiopulmonary disease and lupus*. 2000. Six panels. Signs, symptoms, diagnosis, and treatment of inflammation of the heart and lungs are described. Available from the Lupus Foundation of America, Inc.
5. Gluck O. *Anti-malarials in the treatment of lupus*. 2000. Six panels. Describes indications, combination with other medications, dosage, side effects, and considerations in pregnancy. Available from the Lupus Foundation of America, Inc. (301) 670-9292
6. Hahn BH. *Lupus and vasculitis*. 2000. Six panels. Vasculitis is defined, and symptoms, causes, diagnosis, treatment and outcome are addressed. Available from the Lupus Foundation of America, Inc. (301) 670-9292
7. Kassan S. *Sjögren's syndrome and SLE*. 2000. Six panels. Description, laboratory findings, diagnostic tests, associations with lupus, treatment and prognosis. Available from the Lupus Foundation of America, Inc. (301) 670-9292
8. Katz RS. *Immune suppressants and related drugs*. 2001. Six panels. Imuran, cytoxan, and related drugs, how they work, and the beneficial effects as well as the risks. Available from the Lupus Foundation of America, Inc. (301) 670-9292

9. Katz RS. *Steroids in the treatment of lupus*. 2000. Fact Sheet pamphlet. Discusses indications, effects, side effects, dosages, and routes of administration. Available from the Lupus Foundation of America, Inc. (301) 670-9292
10. Klippel JH, Glunz JM. *Kidney disease and lupus*. 2000. Six panels. Incidence, clinical course, diagnostic testing, and treatment of lupus nephritis are explained. Available from the Lupus Foundation of America, Inc. (301) 670-9292
11. Klippel JH. *Medications and systemic lupus erythematosus*. 2000. Six panels. Goals of medical therapy and the principal drugs used in the management of lupus are discussed. Available from the Lupus Foundation of America, Inc. (301) 670-9292
12. Lahita RG. *Lupus in men*. 1996. Six panels. Discusses symptoms, hormonal metabolism, and the psychosocial effects of the diagnosis of lupus on men. Available from the Lupus Foundation of America, Inc. (301) 670-9292
13. Lahita RG. *What is lupus?* 2000. Twelve panels. This comprehensive brochure discusses the types, cause, symptoms, diagnosis, flares, treatment, and prognosis of lupus. Available from the Lupus Foundation of America, Inc. (301) 670-9292
14. Lehman, TA. *Childhood lupus*. 2000. Six panels. Discusses diagnoses, medications, behavior, educating the child and others, anger and depression. Available from the Lupus Foundation of America, Inc. (301) 670-9292
15. Lockshin MD. *Pregnancy and lupus*. 2000. Six panels. Risks and guidelines when planning a pregnancy; Pregnancy outcomes, flares, neonatal lupus, medications, C-sections, and breast-feeding are addressed. Available from the Lupus Foundation of America, Inc. (301) 670-9292
16. Lupus Foundation of America, Inc. Disease fact sheet. 1 p. Defines the disease, dispels common myths, identifies common symptoms, and cites statistics. Available from the Lupus Foundation of America, Inc. (301) 670-9292
17. Lupus Foundation of America, Inc. *Introduction to lupus*. 2000. Six panels. Table of most common symptoms of lupus and the ACR diagnosis list of symptoms; treatment methods, types of lupus; and discussion of cause, prevalence, and prognosis. Available from the Lupus Foundation of America, Inc. (301) 670-9292
18. Lupus Foundation of America, Inc. Late onset lupus fact sheet. 1 p. Describes the statistics of lupus in older populations. Available from the Lupus Foundation of America, Inc. (301) 670-9292
19. Lupus Foundation of America, Inc. Organizational fact sheet. 1 p. Describes the purpose, accreditation, funding, international representation, and public education programs of this nonprofit health agency. Available from the Lupus Foundation of America, Inc. (301) 670-9292
20. Medsger TA. *Lupus in "overlap" with other connective tissue diseases*. 2000. Six panels. Discusses overlap syndromes: rheumatoid arthritis, myositis, scleroderma, mixed connective tissue disease, and Sjögren's syndrome. Chart of frequency of overlap in people with lupus. Discusses heredity and prognosis. Available from the Lupus Foundation of America, Inc. (301) 670-9292
21. Petri M. *Antiphospholipid antibodies in systemic lupus erythematosus*. 2000. Six panels. The effects of antiphospholipid antibodies are described, and the diagnostic tests to determine the presence of anticardiolipin antibodies and the lupus anticoagulant are outlined. Available from the Lupus Foundation of America, Inc. (301) 670-9292
22. Provost T., Sontheimer, RD. *Skin disease in lupus*. 2000. Six panels. Chronic cutaneous lesions, discoid lesions, acute and subacute cutaneous lesions are described. Photosensitivity and treatments are also discussed. Available from the Lupus Foundation of America, Inc. (301) 670-9292
23. Quismorio FP Jr. *Joint and muscle pain in SLE*. 2000. Six panels. Discusses diagnosis and treatment of lupus arthritis, fibromyalgia, avascular necrosis of bone, tendonitis and bursitis, and lupus myositis, as well as drug-induced muscle weakness. Available from the Lupus Foundation of America, Inc. (301) 670-9292
24. Reichlin M. *Laboratory tests used in the diagnosis of lupus*. 2000. Six panels. Outlines the three-prong approach to diagnosing lupus: current symptoms, medical history, and laboratory testing. Available from the Lupus Foundation of America, Inc. (301) 670-9292
25. Rosove M. *Blood disorders in lupus*. 2000. Six panels. Anemia, thrombocytopenia, leukopenia and neutropenia, thrombosis, blood transfusions, and bone-marrow testing are discussed. Available from the Lupus Foundation of America, Inc. (301) 670-9292
26. Rubin RL. *Drug-induced lupus erythematosus*. 2000. Six panels. Medicines that cause this condition are listed in a chart. Also discussed are why this occurs, symptoms, laboratory tests involved in diagnosis, prognosis, and how drug-induced lupus is different from SLE. Available from the Lupus Foundation of America, Inc. (301) 670-9292
27. Shapiro H. *Depression in lupus*. 2000. Six panels. Clinical depression is defined, and frequency, causes, treatment, and prognosis are outlined. Cognitive changes (lupus fog) are discussed. Available from the Lupus Foundation of America, Inc. (301) 670-9292
28. Tuffanelli DL. *Photosensitivity and lupus erythematosus*. 1994. Six panels. The effects of ultraviolet light are discussed. Precautions and ways to provide photoprotection also are described. Available from the Lupus Foundation of America, Inc. (301) 670-9292
29. Wallace DJ, Metzger AL. *Lupus and infections and immunizations*. 2000. Six panels. Reasons for susceptibility to infection are explained, and risks and side effects of various vaccinations are addressed. Available from the Lupus Foundation of America, Inc.

30. Wallace DJ. *Systemic lupus and the nervous system.* 2000. Six panels. How lupus affects the nervous system, symptoms, diagnostic evaluation, and treatment are described. Available from the Lupus Foundation of America, Inc. (301) 670-9292

Books And Booklets Published Since 1985

1. Adams P. *House calls: how we can all heal the world one visit at a time.* San Francisco, CA: Robert D. Reed, 1999. Forward by the comedian and actor Robin Williams and cartoons by nationally syndicated cartoonist Jerry Van Amerongen. This book includes tips on visiting loved ones in the hospital; ways to improve the healing process; how to be a good doctor; and how to be a good hospital patient.
2. Aladjem H. *Understanding lupus.* New York: Charles Scribner's Sons, Revised 1985. 287 pp. Written in conjunction with 30 lupus experts, this book is a comprehensive guide to lupus that is geared toward the patient.
3. Aladjem H. *A patient's story.* Rockville, MD: Lupus Foundation of America, 1986. 15 pp. This booklet presents the fictionalized story of a patient with lupus: her symptoms, diagnosis, treatment, emotional reaction, and acceptance of the disease (extremely easy reading).
4. Aladjem H. *A decade of lupus.* Rockville, MD: Lupus Foundation of America, 1991. 178 pp. This book is a potpourri of articles on various topics that originally were published in *Lupus News* between 1979 and 1989. Topics span psychological, clinical, and research aspects of lupus, including select pieces and interjections about the work of the Lupus Foundation and its key personnel.
5. Aladjem H, Schur PH. *In search of the sun: how to cope with chronic illness and physicians.* New York: Charles Scribner's Sons, 1988. 264 pp. This book chronicles the life story of Aladjem, from her first initial symptoms of lupus to her final triumph of remission. Interspersed among the chapters of her personal story are chapters written by Dr. Peter H. Schur, a lupus expert, who explains the disease and how doctors treat it. The end of the book addresses the importance of good doctor-patient relationships, which contribute to the effective diagnosis and management of the disease. Available from the Lupus Foundation of America, Inc.
6. Blau SP, Schultz D. *Living with Lupus.* Reading, MA: Addison-Wesley, 1993. 264 pp. This comprehensive and informative book is designed for people with lupus, their families, friends, and caregivers. It presents the latest research on possible causes and hopeful treatments, including options other than the standard-drug approach. Available from Addison-Wesley Publishing Company, ATTN: Order Department, 1 Jacob Way, Reading, MA 01867, 1-800-822-6339.
7. Butler B. *The monster under the bed: child rearing when a parent is chronically ill.* St. Louis: LFA, Missouri Chapter, 1990. 30 pp. This booklet is geared toward the parent with a chronic illness, with special insight and examples given by the author, who is a patient with lupus and three children. Available from the LFA, Missouri Chapter, 8420 Delmar Boulevard LL1, St. Louis, MO 63124, (314) 432-0008.
8. Carr RI. *Lupus erythematosus: a handbook for physicians, patients, and their families, 2nd ed.* Rockville, MD: Lupus Foundation of America, 1986. 60 pp. This booklet presents an overview of lupus, with emphasis on SLE. Sections are well delineated and respond to frequently asked questions. Available from the Lupus Foundation of America, Inc. Also available in Spanish.
9. Donoghue PJ, Siegel ME. *Sick and Tired of Feeling Sick and Tired.* New York: WW Norton, 2000. 284 pp. This book offers both understanding and practical guidance for people living with invisible chronic illness, their spouses, families, friends, employers, and physicians. Available from the Lupus Foundation of America, Inc. (301) 670-9292
10. Fransen J, Russell IJ. *The fibromyalgia help book: a practical guide to living better.* Smith House Press, 1996.
11. Heiss G. *Finding the way home: a compassionate approach to illness.* Fort Bragg, CA: QED Press, 1997. 288 pp. This book is based on the author's personal experiences of living with Sjögren's syndrome, and on discussions with hundreds of people who have attended her weekly support groups. It is a book of thoughtful reflections on living with illness.
12. Horowitz M, Brill MA. *Living with lupus.* New York: Penguin Books, 1994. 201 pp. This comprehensive guide provides information explaining the nature of lupus, including causes and diagnosis. The book offers a thorough glossary and resource listing as well. Its easy to understand format answers commonly asked questions and also provides the reader with practical advice about living more comfortably and actively with the disease. Available from Penguin Books USA Inc., 375 Hudson Street, New York, NY 10014.
13. Hughes GRV. *Understanding lupus.* London: Lupus Clinic, Rheumatology Department, St. Thomas Hospital. 1996. 100 pp. This booklet offers a wide range of lupus information, including an explanation of what lupus is, history, clinical features, symptoms, pregnancy, and treatment, all of which is presented in an upbeat manner.
14. Kron A. *Meeting the challenge: living with a chronic illness.* 1998. To order: send $19 (includes S&H) to: Audrey Kron, 7466 Pebble Lane, West Bloomfield, MI 48322.
15. Lahita RG, Phillips RH. *Lupus: everything you need to know.* 1998. Available through the Lupus Foundation of America, Inc. (301) 670-9292

16. Leyden-Rubenstein LA. *The stress management handbook: strategies for health and inner peace.* New Canaan, CT: Keats Publishing. 1999. In her latest book, the author reveals how she helps her clients create their own emotional, physical, and spiritual wellness through the use of guided imagery, inner-voice work, and psychotherapy that is goal-oriented, yet nurturing and humorous.
17. Milstray Wells S. *A delicate balance – living successfully with a chronic illness.* New York: Insight Books/Plenum Publishing Corporation, 1998. 289 pp. A wise, thoughtful approach to helping people with chronic illness understand themselves and find the help they need. Topics include: obtaining the diagnosis, how to be sick in a healthy world, the doctor-patient relationship, disability in the workplace, and treatments.
18. Moore ME, McGrory CH, Rosenthal RS, eds. *Learning about lupus: a user-friendly guide.* 1991. 86 pp. This booklet contains 20 chapters covering various aspects of lupus. It is especially helpful for the newly diagnosed patient who wants to learn the basics. Available from the Lupus Foundation of America, Southeast PA Chapter, (215) 877-9061.
19. Napier K. *Power nutrition for your chronic illness.* New York: MacMillan Publishing. 1998.
20. NIAMS. *Lupus: a patient care guide for nurses and other health professionals.* (revised version of Nass T. *Lupus erythematosus: handbook for nurses, 3rd ed.*). Bethesda, MD: NIAMS, 2001. 130 pp. This spiral-bound book includes chapters on the following: an overview of lupus; advances in lupus research; laboratory tests that are used in the diagnosis and evaluation of SLE; nursing care using a systems approach (e.g., blood, eye, kidney); patient teaching records with worksheets (e.g., salicylates, NSAIDs, antimalarials, steroids, cytotoxic drugs, etc.); psychological implications of lupus; and patient information. Available from NIAMS, through the NIAMS Information Clearinghouse, at no cost. (877) 226-4267
21. Neil AJ. *Meeting the challenge: a young person's guide to living with lupus.* Atlanta: Arthritis Foundation, 1990. 50 pp. This booklet is written in simple terms and is aimed at the adolescent with lupus. Its purpose is to help teenagers or young adults learn about their illness and how to take care of themselves. Interspersed throughout are quotes from youngsters with lupus, making the booklet more personal. Available from the Arthritis Foundation.
22. Phillips RH. *Control your pain!* Hicksville, NY: Balance Enterprises, Inc., 1996. 29 pp. A booklet containing 144 strategies for reducing the pain of lupus. Available from the Lupus Foundation of America, Inc. (301) 670-9292
23. Phillips RH. *Coping with lupus.* Wayne, NJ: Avery Publishing Group, Revised 1991. 256 pp. This book, written by a psychologist, is a guidebook to coping with lupus. The material is comprehensive, ranging from emotional aspects to medications to interacting with people. Many useful and practical solutions to problems are presented. Available from the Lupus Foundation of America, Inc. (301) 670-9292
24. Phillips RH. *Get to sleep! How to sleep well despite lupus.* Hicksville, NY: Balance Enterprises, Inc., 1995. 17 pp. A booklet containing a summary of tips and suggestions on what to do to improve sleep. Available from the Lupus Foundation of America, Inc. (301) 670-9292
25. Phillips RH. *Living well ... despite lupus: 204 surefire techniques for taking charge of your life.* Hicksville, NY: Balance Enterprises, Inc., 1996. Available through the Lupus Foundation of America, Inc. (301) 670-9292
26. Phillips RH. *Successful living with lupus: an action workbook.* Hicksville, NY: Balance Enterprises, Inc., 2000.
27. Pitzele SK. *We are not alone: learning to live with chronic illness.* New York: Workman Publishing, 1987. 335 pp. Available through the Lupus Foundation of America, Inc. (301) 670-9292
28. Rodgers D. *God's plan included lupus.* Baltimore: Noble House, 1998. 137 pp.
29. Samuels R. *When Mom gets sick.* Rockville, MD: Lupus Foundation of America, 1992. 27 pp. Written and illustrated from a 9-year-old's perspective, this is a compelling story based on the experiences of a sensitive and insightful young girl who makes the best from what could be a devastating situation. Available from the Lupus Foundation of America, Inc.
30. Senecal J. *Lupus: the disease with a thousand faces.* Lupus Canada, 1990. 56 pp. This booklet answers some basic questions about SLE, particularly its symptoms, treatments, and effects. The information is easy to find and understand. Available from Lupus Canada. Also available in French.
31. Schned E. *Lupus and you.* Minneapolis, MN: Park Nicollet HealthSource, 1997. To order send $14.95 (includes S&H) to: Catalogue Orders, PNHS, 3800 Park Nicollet Blvd., Minneapolis, MN 55146.
32. Smith *DM. Disability handbook for Social Security applicants.* Arnold, MD: Physicians' Disability Services, Inc., 1995, 1997. 268 pp. This handbook shows patients with lupus how to prove their claims for disability insurance benefits and shows physicians how to evaluate people with SLE and write a report to the Social Security Administration. The handbook includes a Disability Workbook for Social Security Applicants for the patient with lupus (i.e., the claimant) and two copies, one for the patient one for the doctor, of the *Disability Evaluation Guide for People with Systemic Lupus Erythematosus.* Available from the Lupus Foundation of America, Inc. (301) 670-9292

33. Szasz S. *Living with it.* Buffalo, NY: Prometheus Books, 1991. 243 pp. This book is a personal narrative of a woman who was diagnosed with SLE at the age of 13. The story revolves around living with a chronic illness, with emphasis on taking responsibility for the management of that illness. Order from Prometheus Books, 59 John Glenn Drive, Amherst, NY 14228, 1-800-421-0351.
34. The Lupus Foundation of America, San Diego Chapter, Inc. *A rash of creativity.* 1989. 49 pp. This is a booklet of poetry, prose, and drawings by patients with lupus, revealing a wide range of feelings about living with lupus. It is available from the Lupus Foundation of America, San Diego Chapter, PO Box 837, El Cajon, CA 92022.
35. The Lupus Foundation of America, Delaware Chapter. *Learning about lupus: a user-friendly guide, 2nd ed.*. 1997. To order call (610) 649-9202.
36. Wallace DJ, Hahn BH, Quismorio FP Jr. *A patient's guide to lupus erythematosus.* Adapted from the 4th edition of *Dubois' lupus erythematosus.* 1993. Available from the Lupus Foundation of America, Inc. (301) 670-9292
37. Wallace DJ, Quismorio FP Jr, Cox MB. *Lupus erythematosus.* 2001. 18 pp. This booklet covers many aspects of lupus and is presented in a simplified, nontechnical way for the patient with lupus. It provides a good introduction to the disease. Available from the Lupus Foundation of America, Inc. Also available in Spanish.
38. Wallace DJ, Wallace, JB. *Making sense of fibromyalgia.* New York: Oxford University Press, 1999. 242 pp. In the world of confusion about fibromyalgia, among healthcare professionals and patients alike, the authors combine their experience with current research to provide much-needed insight into this syndrome. Complex material is made clear through patient stories, diagrams, and chapter summaries. Also included in information on work issues and innovative remedies.
39. Wallace DJ. *The Lupus book.* New York: Oxford University Press, 2000. 258 pp. This comprehensive book is written for patients, allied health professionals, and others who are interested in understanding this complex illness more fully. Available from the Lupus Foundation of America, Inc. (301) 670-9292
40. Zuckerman E, Ingelfinger E. *Coping with prednisone (and other cortisone-related medicines).* New York: St. Martin's Press, 1999. 208 pp. This is a detailed, practical guide to making treatment with glucocorticoids as effective and trouble-free as possible. It includes exercises, recipes, and tips based on personal experiences.

Audiovisual Resources

1. Gill B, Gill E. *Lupus: an issue for the African-American community.* The Production House, 1993. 28-minute videotape (VHS), color. Any patient with lupus will benefit from the message of this program, but especially those from the African American community, newly diagnosed patients needing reassurance that the future can be both positive and productive, those who have had lupus and are searching for fresh perspectives and encouragement, perplexed friends and family members eager for information and answers on how to comfort their loved ones and receive strength for themselves, and physicians and nurses desiring an enlightened view of the personal struggles of their patients. Available from the LFA, Columbus, Marcy Zitron Chapter, 6161 Busch Boulevard, Suite 76, Columbus, OH 43229, (614) 846-9249.
2. Gill W, Gill E. *Lupus: insights, emotions, encouragement.* The Production House, 1987. This program features discussions with physicians, nurses, patients, and families of patients, and it focuses on strategies for living and building constructive relationships. Its format is four chapters, which can be targeted to specific audiences or used together. The chapters include: (i) insights from a clinical perspective, (ii) insights from a personal perspective, (iii) strategies toward living, and (iv) building constructive relationships. The total video time is 54 minutes. An edited, 14-minute version also is available that is suitable for viewing by general audiences, at health fairs, or clinics. Available from the LFA, Columbus, Marcy Zitron Chapter, 6161 Busch Boulevard, Suite 76, Columbus, OH 43229, (614) 221-0811.
3. Guch J. *Lupus.* 1991. This 30-minute videotape gives an overview of the causes of lupus and an explanation of how this disease affects the people who suffer from it. Available from Films for the Humanities & Science, PO Box 2053, Princeton, NJ 08543, 1-800-257-5126.
4. Horton R, Robbins L. *Voices of lupus.* 1992. 28-minute videotape (VHS), color. This inspiring program uses strong, positive role models to show how women who are afflicted with lupus can help themselves through peer-group support and better communication with their physicians and families. This autoimmune disease affects more than a half-million women from diverse social, cultural, and economic backgrounds. Interviews with patients and physicians demonstrate positive strategies that can help people with lupus, their families, and their physicians to cope better with this painful, unpredictable illness. Available from Films for the Humanities & Science, PO Box 2053, Princeton, NJ 08543, 1-800-257-5126.
5. Lupus Society of Alberta. *Lupus: disease in disguise.* 1990. This program contains two segments: medical information, and patient support. Segment One deals with items such as possible causes, treatment, and the research outlook of lupus. Segment Two contains patient vignettes and information on support groups. The format is 1/2-in. VHS videocassette (23 minutes). Available

from Lupus Society of Alberta, 1301 8th St. SW, Suite 200, Calgary, AB T2R 1B7, Canada, (403) 228-7956.

6. Lupus Foundation of America. *Target awareness*. 1994. This 6-minute video describes what lupus is, who it affects, and the symptoms of the disease. Available from the Lupus Foundation of America, Inc. (301) 670-9292.
7. Maryland Lupus Foundation. *Someone you know has lupus*. This 10-minute video, filmed at Good Samaritan Hospital in Baltimore, details what lupus is and is not, including a discussion of the diagnosis, symptoms, prevalence, occurrence, and treatment. In interviews with Dr. Thomas M. Zizic, Associate Professor of Medicine at the Johns Hopkins University School of Medicine, as well as with several patients, perspectives of both doctors and patients are presented. This videotape is suitable for patients and family members as well as the lay community. Available from the Maryland Lupus Foundation, 7400 York Road, Third Floor, Baltimore, MD 21204, (410) 337-9000 or, within Maryland, 1-800-777-0934.
8. Mellberg K, Urbin Raymond M. *Stories of Lupus*. 1999. This videotape produced by two women with lupus is done in the journalistic style of late CBS newsman Charles Kuralt. Through a series of interviews, this 27-minute documentary reveals the mysterious nature of lupus, and the journey towards wellness and acceptance faced by the diverse group of people who shared their stories. Available from the Lupus Foundation of America, (301) 670-9292.

PROFESSIONAL-ORIENTED LUPUS LITERATURE

Major Lupus Textbooks

1. Lahita RG, ed. *Systemic lupus erythematosus, 34th ed.* San Diego: Academic Press, 1997. 1000 pp.
2. Wallace DJ, Hahn BH. *Dubois' lupus erythematosus, 6th ed.* Baltimore: Williams & Wilkins, 2001. Order from: Lippincott Williams & Wilkins, 530 Walnut St., Philadelphia, PA 19106-3621, or call Customer Service at 1-800-638-0672.

Major Rheumatology Textbooks

1. Kelley WN, Harris ED, Ruddy S, et al., eds. *Textbook of Rheumatology, 4th ed.* Philadelphia: WB Saunders, 1993. Order from WB Saunders, 6277 Sea Harbor Drive, Orlando, FL 32887, or call Customer Service at 1-800-545-2522.
2. Klippel JH, Dieppe PA, eds. *Rheumatology*. Baltimore: Mosby Year Book, 1994. Order from Mosby, Box 1496, Baltimore, MD 21298, or call Customer Service at 1-800-638-0672.
3. Koopman WP, ed. *Arthritis and Allied Diseases, 13th ed.*, 1997. Lippincott Williams & Wilkins, 530 Walnut St., Philadelphia, PA 19106-3621, or call Customer Service at 1-800-638-0672.

SUBJECT INDEX

Note: Page numbers followed by f indicate figures; those followed by t indicate tables.

B

D

G

J

K

L

M

Q

R

S

T

U